KT-472-613

OXFORD MEDICAL PUBLICATIONS

PRICE'S TEXTBOOK OF THE PRACTICE OF MEDICINE

PRICE'S TEXTBOOK OF THE PRACTICE OF MEDICINE

ELEVENTH EDITION

Edited by

SIR RONALD BODLEY SCOTT
K.C.V.O., M.A., D.M., F.R.C.P.

Physician to H.M. The Queen
Consulting Physician, St. Bartholomew's Hospital, and Woolwich Memorial Hospital
Physician, King Edward VII's Hospital for Officers

LONDON
OXFORD UNIVERSITY PRESS
NEW YORK DELHI
1973

Oxford University Press, Ely House, London W.1
GLASGOW NEW YORK TORONTO MELBOURNE WELLINGTON
CAPE TOWN IBADAN NAIROBI DAR ES SALAAM LUSAKA ADDIS ABABA
DELHI BOMBAY CALCUTTA MADRAS KARACHI LAHORE DACCA
KUALA LUMPUR SINGAPORE HONG KONG TOKYO

ISBN 0 19 264155 7
© Oxford University Press 1966, 1973

First Edition 1922
Eleventh Edition 1973

Printed in Great Britain
by Morrison and Gibb Ltd., London and Edinburgh

CONTENTS

SECTION 1
INFECTION AND ANTIBACTERIAL AGENTS

SECTION 2
DISEASES DUE TO INFECTION AND INFESTATION

SECTION 3
DISORDERS DUE TO CHEMICAL AND PHYSICAL AGENTS AND TO CLIMATIC AND ENVIRONMENTAL FACTORS

SECTION 4
GENETIC AND CONSTITUTIONAL FACTORS IN DISEASE

SECTION 5

DISEASES OF THE ENDOCRINE GLANDS

SECTION 6

DISEASES OF THE LIVER, GALL-BLADDER AND PANCREAS

SECTION 7

DISEASES OF THE GASTRO-INTESTINAL TRACT

SECTION 8

DISEASES OF THE HEART AND BLOOD VESSELS

SECTION 9

DISEASES OF THE RESPIRATORY TRACT

SECTION 10

DISEASES OF JOINTS

SECTION 11

GENERAL DISEASES OF THE SKELETON

SECTION 12
DISEASES OF THE URINARY TRACT

SECTION 13
DISEASES OF THE HAEMOPOIETIC ORGANS

SECTION 14
DISEASES OF THE SKIN

SECTION 15
DISEASES OF THE NERVOUS SYSTEM

SECTION 16
DISEASES OF VOLUNTARY MUSCLE

SECTION 17
PSYCHOLOGICAL MEDICINE

PREFACE TO THE ELEVENTH EDITION

With its eleventh edition this textbook completes its half-century and, as a glance will show, departs in some degree from its traditional arrangement. Classifications of disease are notoriously unsatisfactory. The time has passed when a strict anatomico-pathological scheme on the Linnean model would suffice, but it cannot be entirely replaced by one resting on an aetiological basis. Logic has to yield to pragmatism. There are some topics of importance which, although fitting into no pigeon-hole, concern more than one system or group of diseases. We have felt that general articles dealing with such problems avoid tedious repetitions and can provide a wider view of the subject. Thus sections on antibiotics, growth and development, involution and senescence, genetic aspects of medicine, immune mechanisms in disease, the general aspects and chemotherapy of cancer and the therapeutic uses of the corticosteroid hormones appear in the edition.

For the rest, the arrangement of the book remains conventional. Some half-tone plates have been introduced and much new material is included. In addition to the general articles mentioned, the sections on the following subjects have been completely rewritten: the endocrine glands; the liver, gall-bladder and pancreas; the gastro-intestinal tract; the joints; the skeleton; the haemopoietic organs; the voluntary muscles and the skin. All other sections have been carefully revised and brought up to date.

Of our contributors Dr. G. E. Beaumont, Dr. T. C. Hunt, Mr. Ambrose King, Sir Aubrey Lewis, Professor E. F. Scowen and Professor L. J. Witts have retired, having earned our gratitude by their distinguished help and support over so many years. We are deeply indebted to them. It is sad to have to record the deaths since retirement of Dr. W. S. C. Copeman and Sir Alan Moncrieff. The loss of Dr. Dennis Cottom who has written the paediatric articles in the eleventh edition was particularly tragic. His early death has been a serious blow to British Paediatrics. We have been joined by a number of new contributors. They are Professor W. Ferguson Anderson, Dr. John Batten, Professor Cyril A. Clarke, Dr. A. M. Dawson, Professor A. S. Douglas, Mr. T. J. Fairbank, Professor G. Hamilton Fairley, Dr. D. A. G. Galton, Dr. E. J. Holborow, Dr. Michael Mason, Dr. A. Stuart Mason, Dr. C. S. Nicol, Professor A. E. Read, Dr. G. A. Rose, Professor M. Shepherd, Professor J. N. Walton and Professor D. J. Weatherall. Each has an established reputation in the subject on which he writes, and we are delighted to be able to welcome such distinguished reinforcements. It is our hope that with their help *Price's Textbook of the Practice of Medicine* will continue to be a useful work of reference and a guide to current medical practice in Great Britain.

Many have helped in the production of this edition and we must first thank our contributors, upon whose generous labours the success of the book will rest. The publishers, in the person of their representative, Dr. J. C. Gregory, have shown the Editor the courtesy and forbearance which experience leads one to anticipate. Finally, I wish to record my appreciation of the competence and cheerfulness with which my secretary, Miss Marjorie Preston, has borne the heavy burden of her additional duties.

RONALD BODLEY SCOTT

London, N.W.1.
August 1972

CONTRIBUTORS

W. FERGUSON ANDERSON, O.B.E., M.D., F.R.C.P.	*Professor of Geriatric Medicine, University of Glasgow. Physician in Geriatric Medicine, Stobhill Hospital, Glasgow.*
J. C. BATTEN, M.D., F.R.C.P.	*Consultant Physician, St. George's Hospital. Assistant Physician, The Brompton Hospital.*
R. I. S. BAYLISS, M.D., F.R.C.P.	*Physician to H.M. The Queen. Physician and Endocrinologist, Westminster Hospital and King Edward VII's Hospital for Officers, London.*
R. R. BOMFORD, C.B.E., D.M., F.R.C.P.	*Consulting Physician, The London Hospital. Physician, Shahnaz Hospital, University of Meshed, Iran.*
WALLACE BRIGDEN, M.D., F.R.C.P.	*Physician to the Cardiac Department and Physician, The London Hospital. Physician, The National Heart Hospital.*
CYRIL A. CLARKE, C.B.E., Sc.D., M.D., P.R.C.P., F.R.C.O.G., F.R.S.	*Emeritus Professor of Medicine, University of Liverpool. Consulting Physician, Liverpool Royal Infirmary.*
The late DENNIS COTTOM.	*Sometime Physician, Children's Department, St. Thomas' Hospital and Hospital for Sick Children, Great Ormond Street, London.*
A. M. DAWSON, M.D., F.R.C.P.	*Physician, St. Bartholomew's Hospital.*
A. S. DOUGLAS, M.D., F.R.C.P., F.R.C.Path.	*Regius Professor of Medicine, University of Aberdeen. Consultant Physician, Royal Infirmary, Aberdeen.*
T. J. FAIRBANK, M.A., F.R.C.S.	*Senior Surgeon, Orthopaedic and Fracture Departments, United Cambridge Hospitals. Orthopaedic Surgeon, East Anglian Regional Hospital Board.*
G. HAMILTON FAIRLEY, M.A., D.M., F.R.C.P.	*Professor of Medical Oncology, and Director of the Imperial Cancer Research Fund Medical Oncology Research Unit, St. Bartholomew's Hospital. Consultant Physician, Chester Beatty Research Institute, Surrey, and Honorary Consultant Physician, Royal Marsden Hospital, Sutton, Surrey.*
DAVID A. G. GALTON, M.A., M.D., F.R.C.P.	*Honorary Director, Medical Research Council's Leukaemia Unit, Royal Postgraduate Medical School, London. Honorary Senior Lecturer, Department of Haematology, Royal Postgraduate Medical School, London. Consultant Physician, Anaemia Unit, Hammersmith Hospital, London.*
J. D. P. GRAHAM, M.D., F.R.C.P.Ed., F.R.F.P.S., F.R.S.E.	*Reader in Pharmacology and Lecturer in Toxicology, Welsh National School of Medicine. Consultant, United Cardiff Hospitals.*
E. J. HOLBOROW, M.D.	*Consultant Bacteriologist and Member of the Scientific Staff, Medical Research Council Rheumatism Research Unit, Taplow.*
T. A. LLOYD DAVIES, M.D., F.R.C.P.	*Chief Employment Medical Adviser, Department of Employment, London.*

F. O. MacCALLUM, M.D., M.R.C.P., F.R.C.Path.	*Consultant Virologist, The United Oxford Hospitals.*
G. DONALD W. McKENDRICK, M.A., B.M., F.R.C.P.	*Consultant Physician for Infectious Diseases, St. Ann's Hospital, London, and Rush Green Hospital, Essex.* *Consultant Physician, Thurrock Hospital, Essex.* *Lecturer in Infectious Diseases, The Middlesex Hospital, St. Bartholomew's Hospital, and London School of Hygiene and Tropical Medicine.*
R. F. McNAB JONES, M.B., F.R.C.S.	*Senior Surgeon, Ear, Nose and Throat Department, St. Bartholomew's Hospital, London.* *Surgeon, Royal National Throat, Nose and Ear Hospital, London.* *Dean, Institute of Laryngology and Otology, London.*
BRIAN MAEGRAITH, C.M.G., M.A., M.B., B.Sc., D.PHIL., D.Sc., F.R.C.P., F.R.C.P.Ed., F.R.A.C.P.	*Emeritus Professor of Tropical Medicine and Dean, Liverpool School of Tropical Medicine.* *Consulting Physician in Tropical Diseases, Royal Infirmary, Liverpool, and Tropical Diseases Centre, Sefton General Hospital, Liverpool.*
A. STUART MASON, M.D., F.R.C.P.	*Consultant Endocrinologist, The London Hospital.* *Physician in Charge, Diabetic and Endocrine Unit, Oldchurch Hospital, Romford.*
R. M. MASON, D.M., F.R.C.P.	*Physician, Department of Physical Medicine and Rheumatology, The London Hospital.*
C. S. NICOL, T.D., M.D., F.R.C.P.	*Physician in Charge, Venereal Disease Departments, St. Thomas' and St. Bartholomew's Hospitals, London.*
ALAN READ, M.D., F.R.C.P.	*Professor of Medicine, University of Bristol.* *Consultant Physician, United Bristol Hospitals.*
R. W. RIDDELL, M.D., F.R.C.P.Ed., F.R.C.Path.	*Consultant Clinical Bacteriologist, The Brompton Hospital.* *Director of Pathological Services, St. John's Hospital for Diseases of the Skin, London.* *Senior Lecturer in Medical Mycology, Institute of Dermatology, University of London.*
G. A. ROSE, M.R.C.P., M.R.C.Path.	*Consultant Chemical Pathologist, St. Peter's, St. Philip's, and St. Paul's Hospitals, London.*
BRIAN F. RUSSELL, M.D., F.R.C.P., D.P.H.	*Consulting Physician, Skin Department, The London Hospital.* *Consulting Physician, St. John's Hospital for Diseases of the Skin, London.*
SIR RONALD BODLEY SCOTT, K.C.V.O., M.A., D.M., F.R.C.P.	*Physician to H.M. The Queen.* *Consulting Physician, St. Bartholomew's Hospital, and Woolwich Memorial Hospital.* *Physician, King Edward VII's Hospital for Officers.*
MICHAEL SHEPHERD, D.M., F.R.C.P., F.R.C.Psych.	*Professor of Epidemiological Psychiatry, University of London.* *Honorary Physician, Bethlem Royal and Maudsley Hospitals, King's College Hospital and St. Francis Hospital, London.*
R. A. SHOOTER, M.D., F.R.C.P., F.R.C.Path.	*Professor of Bacteriology, University of London.* *Bacteriologist, St. Bartholomew's Hospital, and to the City of London.*
GEORGE A. SMART, B.Sc., M.D., F.R.C.P.	*Director, British Postgraduate Medical Federation.* *Professor of Medicine, University of London.* *Honorary Physician, National Hospital for Nervous Diseases, London.*

JOHN N. WALTON, T.D., M.D., F.R.C.P.
Professor of Neurology, University of Newcastle upon Tyne.
Neurologist, Regional Neurological Centre, General Hospital, Newcastle upon Tyne.
Physician in Neurology, Royal Victoria Infirmary.

D. J. WEATHERALL, M.D., F.R.C.P.
Professor of Haematology, University of Liverpool.
Honorary Consultant Physician (Haematology), United Liverpool Hospitals.

DENIS WILLIAMS, C.B.E., M.D., D.Sc., F.R.C.P.
Senior Physician, National Hospital, Queen Square.
Neurological Physician, St. George's Hospital and King Edward VII's Hospital for Officers, London.

CLIFFORD WILSON, M.A., D.M., F.R.C.P.
Emeritus Professor of Medicine, University of London.
Consulting Physician, The London Hospital.

PLATES

SECTION 1

INFECTION AND ANTIBACTERIAL AGENTS

INFECTION
ANTIBACTERIAL AGENTS

INFECTION

Diseases caused by bacteria and viruses are common and, despite chemotherapy, still kill many patients. They may be naturally serious, or serious because untreated or mistreated, or because they occur in patients who for one reason or another are more susceptible than other people. Until now it has been possible to prevent only a minority by immunization. Some can be prevented by controlling the spread of organisms from patient to patient, but for many diseases this is not yet practicable. It is the intention in this section to review the sources of infection, the routes by which micro-organisms spread, and to note some of the effects of chemotherapy.

Sources of Infection

Sources of infection occur in other people, in animals, or in objects such as soil. Other people may be a source of infection because they are suffering from the disease. Alternatively in some diseases the patient may be infectious during the incubation period, and before the diagnosis is known; or, the infection may be so trivial that no notice is taken of it, although the patient may be as capable of infecting others as those with a florid form of the disease. A patient with this type of infection is referred to as 'a missed case', and is frequently responsible for the introduction or continuation of outbreaks of infection in institutions. The most difficult source to identify and control is the healthy carrier. Carriers may harbour pathogenic bacteria as a late result of suffering from a disease such as typhoid fever or diphtheria, or, as for the staphylococcus, they may carry the organism without a history of disease due to it. In either case they are only likely to be identified by bacteriological examination.

Animals of many kinds are possible sources of infection. In this country in the past milk from tuberculous cows was responsible for an untold number of human cases of tuberculosis. Unpasteurized milk may still contain the causative agent of undulant fever, *Brucella abortus*, or organisms contributed by the milker, such as *Streptococcus pyogenes*. Members of the salmonellae are widespread in the animal kingdom, and are regularly responsible for outbreaks of food poisoning as a result of eating food which has not been satisfactorily preserved, or has been contaminated after preservation or cooking. One of the commoner forms of food poisoning is that caused by animal-derived heat-resistant strains of *Clostridium welchii.* Animal products such as catgut and horse hair may contain organisms originally carried by the animal, and have in the past been responsible for tetanus and anthrax. In other parts of the world, animals may be the reservoir for viral diseases, such as rabies or yellow fever, or for protozoal diseases such as trypanosomiasis.

Pathogenic bacteria found in soil, dust and water have nearly always come from people or animals. Organisms such as the typhoid bacillus readily survive in water. Spore forming organisms, notably the *Clostridia* and *Bacillus anthracis*, can survive for long periods in soil or in dust. Non-spore forming bacteria such as *Streptococcus pyogenes* and *Staphylococcus aureus* can remain alive for weeks or months in dust. Recent work, however, suggests that some dried organisms may be less able to initiate infection than those which have been recently shed by their human host.

Spread of Bacteria and Viruses

People may become infected because they inhale or swallow organisms, or because organisms enter the body through the skin or mucous membranes. Infection with some bacteria and viruses can occur before birth by passage through the placenta.

With such an apparently simple background it has been easy to postulate and to teach general principles of bacterial spread applicable to pathogenic bacteria. Epidemiological studies, greatly aided in recent years by the ability to type organisms within a species, have, however, shown that it may be rash to predict how individual pathogens spread from general principles alone. For some time it will probably be better for the doctor to accept that much more needs to be found out about most viruses and many bacteria before the way in which they spread from patient to patient is known in full detail.

Among the factors that are important before infection occurs are the dose of the organism, the route by which it infects, and the resistance of the individual (a subject discussed on p. 31). For many infections information on some of these heads is missing. Sepsis caused by *Staph. aureus* provides an example. Although the dose needed to start an infection is uncertain, in many patients superficial skin sepsis and wound infections are both autogenous, being derived from the patient's own carrier sites. Of these the nose is the most common, some 30–40 per cent. of normal people being carriers. Transfer of staphylococci from one normal person to another must occur in several different ways, of which one is direct contact. It is also likely that colonization of the nose results from breathing in staphylococci in the air. With the exception, however, of sneezing, respiratory activities do not disseminate staphylococci from the normal respiratory tract, and the sometimes large numbers of staphylococci found in the air are probably dislodged from the skin either by themselves, or more usually, carried on shed skin scales.

Patients with infections of the lung may cough out bacteria. These emerge carried on a spray of particles of different sizes ranging from those large enough to be visible, down to those of a few microns only in diameter. Larger particles fall to the ground within a few feet of the patient. The moisture content of the smaller particles may evaporate and the residual material, perhaps containing micro-organisms, may stay airborne and travel considerable distances. Such particles are known as droplet nuclei.

It has been customary to ascribe the spread of many respiratory infections and some specific fevers to droplet spread. For infections in the lungs this is probably true as the air velocity in the lung at the peak of a cough may approach 300 metres per second at which point large numbers of small particles will be formed. The generalization should not, though, be applied without proof to all infections of the respiratory tract. Although haemolytic streptococci multiply freely in the throat, they are rarely expelled in the sneezes of patients with streptococcal sore throat. As has already been noted, few staphylococci are shed during respiratory activities.

The spread of intestinal organisms has been studied for years, and a great deal is known about it. For some organisms, of which the typhoid bacillus is one, typing methods have more recently provided epidemiologists and public health authorities with the means of tracing routes of spread to a high degree of accuracy.

Advances to come may include the realization that other intestinal organisms as well as the recognized pathogens may pass from person to person. It now appears that organisms in the bowel do not necessarily form a static community. Strains may be changing continually, those being lost being replaced by new strains swallowed in the food. This is probably true, at any rate for hospital patients, for *Escherichia coli* and *Pseudomonas aeruginosa* (*pyocyanea*), organisms that although innocuous in the bowel, can cause infections elsewhere in the body. When more is known about this subject, the treatment of patients with infections of the urinary tract and elsewhere with these organisms may have to include attention to the bacterial content of the bowel, and its origin.

Fortunately intact mucous membrane and skin constitute impassable barriers for most organisms, but lacerations and abrasions are common and organisms may be introduced through insect and animal bites. Deliberate breaks of the skin, by surgical incision or in the course of giving an injection, carry the possibility of introducing infection.

ANTIBACTERIAL AGENTS
THE SULPHONAMIDES AND THE ANTIBIOTICS

Over the last thirty years chemotherapy has entirely altered the picture of infectious disease. Provided that the patient has no complicating condition there are few bacterial diseases which will not respond to proper treatment. So far the only viral infections which can be treated with success are those due to a few of the largest viruses, but for some others, for example influenza, antibiotics have very sharply reduced the mortality by dealing with secondarily invading bacteria.

Although so successful in treatment, antibiotics have only met with modified success in the prevention of infection. On the credit side they can be used for some forms of mass prophylaxis, as in the suppression of dysentery in an institution; or for individual prophylaxis, as in the prevention of recurrences of rheumatic fever by the regular administration of penicillin to prevent haemolytic streptococcal throat infections. Antibiotics have, obviously, also contributed to the prevention of disease by reducing the period of infection, as, for instance in tuberculosis and syphilis. In hospitals they have, however, been responsible for the evolution of strains of bacteria, particularly of *Staph. aureus* and some Gram-negative bacilli, which are not only antibiotic resistant, but which appear to be more virulent than their antecedents. Hospital studies, usually based on typing methods, have shown that cross-infection, defined as the acquisition by a patient of another patient's organisms, occurs far more often than was once thought. Transfer of this sort provides newly evolved bacterial strains with a good chance to survive and spread. It is for this reason that chemotherapy can no longer be considered alone. For good results attention must be paid to the way in which bacteria spread, as well as to how they can be killed in the individual patient.

Unless applied directly to a lesion, antibiotics are not likely to act solely on the organisms causing infection; any other bacteria susceptible to their action will be attacked. This interference with the normal bacterial flora of the patient may produce undesirable results, and even a virtually new disease. Thus the administration of drugs which alter the flora of the alimentary tract may be followed by an overgrowth of yeasts or of staphylococci. In some cases there is erosion of the bowel wall with the production of staphylococcal enterocolitis.

Necessity for Treatment

The majority of infections will resolve in time without specific treatment, but chemotherapy will sometimes save life and can often shorten the illness, prevent complications and save the patient the discomfort incidental to the disease. It is obvious that serious infections should be treated. There is some argument as to whether relatively minor infections should be treated, or whether they should be left to recover unaided. There is, at any rate in theory, complete agreement that in the absence of a clear indication, antibiotics should not be used.

There are several reasons for the reluctance to use antibiotics unless necessary. Treatment may stop development of natural immunity to the infecting organism, although by the time the diagnosis has been made and treatment begun, the immune processes are often under way. Every course of treatment, too, carries with it some risk, either because of the development of hypersensitivity, or because of a toxic effect of the drug itself. Probably the most valid reason for using antibiotics only when necessary is that the proportion of resistant bacteria in a community is directly related to the amount of antibiotic consumed. The mechanism and the rate of development of resistance may be different, but for all antibiotics, the greater the usage, the greater the number of resistant bacterial strains, if resistance is going to develop at all. Once resistance to a drug is acquired, it is usually a permanent property of the organism and the larger the pool of resistant organisms becomes, the less is the value of the antibiotic.

Choice of Drug

Sensitivity tests, correctly performed, and with their limitations understood, are the proper basis for chemotherapy. As normally done they show if an antibiotic can inhibit bacterial growth at a concentration likely to be achieved in the body. Inhibition is all that is needed in the treatment of most infections, as once this is achieved the body's natural defences will remove the cause. Thus a report stating that an organism is sensitive to an antibiotic should normally imply that

TABLE 1

RECOMMENDED DRUGS FOR TREATMENT

	PENICILLIN G	PENICILLINASE-RESISTANT PENICILLINS	AMPICILLIN	CEPHALOSPORINS	STREPTOMYCIN	TETRACYCLINES	ERYTHROMYCIN	CHLORAMPHENICOL	NOVOBIOCIN	NITROFURANTOIN	SULPHONAMIDES	POLYMYXIN	LINCOMYCIN
Actinomycosis	1	—	—	—	—	2	—	4	—	—	—	—	—
Anthrax	1	—	—	—	—	2	—	4	3	—	—	—	—
Brucellosis	—	—	—	—	1+	+1	3	4	—	—	3	—	—
Diphtheria	2	—	—	—	—	2	1	—	—	—	—	—	—
Dysentery—bacillary	—	—	—	—	2	2	—	4	—	—	1	2	—
—infantile	—	—	—	—	—	—	—	—	—	—	—	2	—
Gas gangrene	1	—	—	—	—	2	—	4	—	—	—	—	—
Gonorrhoea	1	—	—	—	2	2	—	4	—	—	—	—	—
Leptospirosis	1	—	—	—	—	2	—	—	—	—	—	—	—
Meningitis *H. influenzae*	—	—	2	—	—	—	—	1	—	—	3	—	—
meningococcal	2	—	2	—	—	—	—	—	—	—	1–5	—	—
pneumococcal	1	—	2	—	3	—	—	—	—	—	3	—	3
Paratyphoid fever	—	—	3	—	—	—	—	1	—	—	—	—	—
Pneumonia *H. influenzae*	3–5	—	2	—	4	1	3–5	4	—	—	—	—	5
Kl. pneumoniae	3–5	—	—	—	4	1	3–5	4	—	—	—	—	—
pneumococcal	1	—	—	2	—	2	2	—	—	—	3	—	3
staphylococcal	1	2	—	2	4	2	2	4	2	—	—	—	3
Strep. pyogenes	1	—	—	2	—	2	2	—	—	—	—	—	3
Psittacosis	—	—	—	—	—	1	—	—	—	—	—	—	—
Staphylococcal infection	1	2	—	2	4	2	2	4	2	—	—	—	3
Strep. pyogenes infections	1	—	—	2	—	2	2	—	—	—	—	—	3
Strep. viridans infections	1	—	—	2	4	—	—	—	—	—	—	—	—
Syphilis	1	—	—	—	5	2	3	4	—	—	—	—	—
Typhoid	—	—	3	—	—	—	—	1	—	—	—	—	—
Urinary infections													
Ps. aeruginosa infections	5	—	—	5	3	3	5	5	—	5	5	1	—
Proteus infections	1–5	—	2	1–5	2	3	5	4	3	2	3	5	—
Esch. coli infections	3–5	—	2	1–5	1	2	5	4	—	1	1	2	—
Strep. faecalis infections	1	—	2	5	3	1	—	4	—	2	5	5	—
Staph. infections	1	2	—	2	2	2	3	4	—	2	3	5	—
Klebsiella infections	5	—	3	1–5	1	2	5	4	—	3	3	2	—

Key to table

1 = drug of choice if infecting strain sensitive.
2 = alternative drug if organisms resistant to first choice, or if patient hypersensitive.
3 = alternative drug usually of lesser activity.
4 = effective drug, but toxicity limits use.
5 = organism resistant to drug, or infection will not respond.

Additional drugs

Fucidin may be used for the treatment of staphylococcal infections, other than those of the urinary tract. Vancomycin and bacitracin may rarely be needed for the treatment of staphylococcal infections or endocarditis, but toxicity severely limits prescription. Cycloserine may be of value in treating tuberculosis and urinary infections, as may kanamycin.

an infection due to that organism will respond to the antibiotic. There are certain recognized exceptions, which come under three rather separate headings.

In a few diseases, notably typhoid fever, demonstration of sensitivity in the laboratory is not a guide to the outcome of treatment. Typhoid bacilli are inhibited by a number of antibiotics, but of those in common use, only chloramphenicol is likely to cure the patient. The reasons for this are not known. Sensitivity tests may also mislead if it is assumed that antibiotics will be effective whatever the condition of the patient. Chronic urinary infections provide a good example. In the presence of obstruction of urinary flow, the chances of curing the infection by chemotherapy are slight, even if the infecting organism is at first sensitive to the drug used. Thirdly, for a very few diseases treatment will only succeed if the antibiotic kills all, or nearly all the bacteria; inhibition of bacterial growth alone is not sufficient. Not all antibiotics are bactericidal. Many are bacteriostatic, and those that are bactericidal will not always kill all organisms exposed to them. Thus in subacute bacterial endocarditis a conventional sensitivity report stating that the streptococcus is sensitive to one or other antibiotic may mislead, if all that has been tested is the ability of the antibiotic to prevent growth. In this disease it is essential to kill bacteria and further tests should be done to choose an antibiotic which will do this. It may be that no single drug can be found that is bactericidal. When this occurs, tests should be done with two, or rarely, more, antibiotics in combination, as together antibiotics may be bactericidal, although not so when used singly. This potentiation of effect is known as synergism. Occasionally the combination of two antibiotics may result in antagonism. In this condition one drug, usually a bacteriostatic one, hampers the action of its bactericidal partner, and the effect is less than that of either drug alone. Antagonism can easily be demonstrated in the laboratory, although the conditions have to be chosen with care. The evidence that it occurs in the treatment of patients is less clear. It has been claimed to occur in the treatment of pneumococcal meningitis, in which the simultaneous administration of penicillin and tetracycline has been said to lead to a higher death rate than if penicillin alone is given, presumably because the tetracycline interferes with the action of penicillin. Antagonism has not been convincingly demonstrated in the treatment of other infections, although this statement would be denied by some authorities, who claim to have seen it, particularly in the treatment of bacterial endocarditis.

It is often necessary to start treatment without laboratory help. The condition may be one which is known to respond regularly to one of the antibiotics; it may be difficult to send specimens to the laboratory, or the patient's condition may be such that treatment has to be started as a matter of urgency before a sensitivity report is available. For many infections this course is not likely to lead to difficulty so long as its empirical nature is recognized and the patient's chemotherapy re-assessed in the light of his clinical progress. It should be avoided if possible in diseases such as endocarditis in which the rational, and possibly life-saving, choice of drug for treatment rests on laboratory findings.

In such infections as meningitis and pneumonia valuable help may be obtained from the laboratory within a few hours from the microscopical examination of a stained film of cerebospinal fluid and sputum.

When the results of treatment conflict with the guidance given by the laboratory, there may be several possible explanations. In time most patients will recover without treatment and the apparently successful treatment of an infection due to an organism said to be resistant to the drug prescribed, does not necessarily mean that the antibiotic has been responsible for the recovery. Discrepancies between the results of sensitivity tests and the outcome of treatment probably occur most often in respiratory infections. As for other infections, the reason may be that the tests have not been well done, but an alternative reason may be that the laboratory has been sent poor material with which to work. The importance of the proper collection of specimens when laboratory guidance in chemotherapy is desired, cannot be over-emphasized.

In deciding which drug to use, the merits of administration by mouth will have to be compared with the advantages of injections. For seriously ill patients and for patients who may fail to take oral preparations there is a certainty about an injection which may recommend it, particularly in the early stages of treatment. Finally the cost should be considered. Many doctors are unaware of the considerable differences in price between the various preparations available.

Duration of Treatment

As a result of experience, supported in many cases by extensive clinical trials, there is general agreement about the length of treatment for many diseases. Tuberculosis, for example, may require months, subacute bacterial endocarditis and actinomycosis weeks, and haemolytic streptococcal infections only days. Difficulties arise when after a reasonable period of treatment the patient has failed to respond and his condition deteriorates. When this occurs the original diagnosis should be carefully reviewed. In some cases, although the original clinical and laboratory decisions were correct, the organisms may be found to have become resistant to the drug used during the course of treatment. Alternatively the original sensitive organism may have been replaced by another and resistant organism which was present only in small numbers at the start of treatment, or the patient may have become infected by entirely new bacteria, derived from himself or by cross-infection from other patients or the staff. For many infections, failure of treatment should be evident within a few days; when it is seen there is usually no benefit to be obtained from persevering with the same drug.

Resistance

Resistant bacteria increase in numbers primarily because antibiotics are used, and the greater the use, the more numerous the resistant strains. There are three main reasons why bacteria are resistant to antibiotics.

Resistance may be a natural property in that the organisms are insusceptible to the action of the antibiotic, or, as in the case of staphylococci and benzylpenicillin, because they produce an enzyme that destroys the antibiotic. They may acquire resistance to an antibiotic during the course of exposure to it, either in the test tube or in the patient during the course of treatment. Thirdly, they may become resistant through the phenomenon of infectious or transferred drug resistance. This recently discovered form by which genetic material conferring resistance can pass from resistant organisms to sensitive ones is of great theoretical and important practical interest. It has been shown to occur in the intestines of animals and man and may occur in the respiratory tract and elsewhere in the body. A disturbing possibility is that resistant non-pathogenic bacteria may be able to transfer resistance to pathogenic bacteria, previously sensitive to antibiotics.

The great frequency of antibiotic-resistant bacteria is, however, the result of their spread from patient to patient, usually in the hospital. In the general population spread occurs less readily. Where it has been studied, for staphylococci, it has been shown that members of the public with resistant strains frequently have had contact with hospitals.

Plainly, in attempting to prevent resistance, antibiotics should only be prescribed when necessary. Hospitals are, however, for the treatment of the sick and the legitimate use of antibiotics in them will almost certainly result in an increasing number of resistant bacteria. Theoretically it should be possible to delay the appearance of resistance by prescribing two antibiotics together. This has been notably successful in the treatment of tuberculosis, but as yet is a policy of only doubtful value for most other infections. The necessity of preventing the emergence and accumulation of resistant bacteria in order that antibiotics may remain effective agents has stimulated research into the routes of hospital cross-infection. This work is beginning to yield valuable results, particularly for staphylococcal infections and infections of the urinary tract, and it is to be hoped that it will also prove of value in other diseases.

THE SULPHONAMIDES

Modern chemotherapy began in 1935 with the description by Domagk of the effectiveness of the first sulphonamide in the treatment of experimental streptococcal infections. There are now many sulphonamides, all of which have the same general structure. Changes in composition are responsible for the varying physical, pharmacological and antibacterial properties.

Sulphonamides are bacteriostatic and owe this action to their ability to compete with para-aminobenzoic acid and so block the enzyme system in the bacterial cells which utilizes para-aminobenzoic acid as a precursor of folic acid. Folic acid is essential for both human and bacterial cells, but they differ in that human cells absorb the vitamin preformed from the diet while bacterial cells are unable to absorb it preformed, and have to make it themselves from para-aminobenzoic acid. The details of this synthesis have become of more importance with the discovery of compounds such as pyrimethamine and trimethoprim that block a later stage of folic acid synthesis in the bacterial cell and that will act synergistically with sulphonamides.

Distribution and Excretion

Although there are individual differences between the sulphonamides, the absorbable compounds are taken up from the bowel and diffuse freely throughout the body, reaching the cerebrospinal fluid in good concentration [Table 3]. An appreciable amount of the dose is usually excreted in the urine in an active form. Non-absorbable sulphonamides are designed to exert their effect within the lumen of the bowel and relatively little is absorbed.

Toxicity and Hypersensitivity

A wide range of toxic reactions may be seen with the sulphonamides, the different compounds varying in the frequency and kind of toxic effect they produce. Gastro-intestinal disturbances and cerebral effects such as depression and confusion are not uncommon. Serious damage has been caused by the precipitation of sulphonamides in the kidney. This hazard may be avoided by keeping the urine alkaline and the patient's water intake adequate. Other toxic reactions include agranulocytosis, aplastic anaemia, thrombocytopenia and hepatitis.

Hypersensitivity to sulphonamides is easily acquired. Hypersensitive patients on re-treatment may show drug reactions and contact dermatitis. Sulphonamides have, rarely, been held responsible for the onset of polyarteritis nodosa. Another rare complication has been the Stevens-Johnson syndrome [see Section 14], particularly following the use of long-acting sulphonamides. Acute haemolytic anaemia is liable to occur when sulphonamides are given to individuals whose red blood cells are deficient in glucose-6-phosphate dehydrogenase [see Section 13].

Preparations

A considerable number of sulphonamides are available, and new preparations are regularly being added to the list. The various preparations may differ in regard to speed of absorption, activity in the body and rate of excretion, but in the final outcome the practical differences between compounds may not be great, as advantages in one direction may be counterbalanced by disadvantages in another. The prescriber's final choice may well depend on experience and local practice. There are three main types. Absorbable sulphonamides are taken up from the bowel and spread rapidly through the tissues. Poorly absorbed sulphonamides are designed to act within the bowel, and relatively little of the drug is absorbed. Lastly there are the long-acting sulphonamides which are absorbed when given by mouth, but which are retained for prolonged periods in the body.

Absorbable Sulphonamides

The choice of absorbable sulphonamides is a wide one. The following are amongst the most used.

Sulphadimidine. This compound is rapidly absorbed. It is one of the most soluble of the sulphonamides and least likely to lead to deposition of crystals in the urine. Since it is not as active as some it should not be used for the treatment of gravely ill patients.

Sulphafurazole. A compound with similar properties to sulphadimidine.

Sulphadiazine. This is one of the more active sulphonamides. It diffuses freely through the tissues, and in particular reaches satisfactory concentrations in the cerebrospinal fluid. Special care must be taken to prevent the deposition of crystals in the urinary tract because it is only sparingly soluble in the urine.

Trisulphonamide Tablets. These tablets are a mixture of sulphathiazole, sulphadiazine and sulphamerazine. The chief virtue of this compound is the lesser risk of crystalluria, due to the fact that the presence of one sulphonamide in the urine does not interfere with the solubility of the others and a lesser amount of each drug can be administered. It can be recommended for use in urinary and other infections.

Poorly Absorbed Sulphonamides

The choice of poorly absorbed sulphonamides is smaller. Among them are:

Succinylsulphathiazole. Since the drug is poorly absorbed, only about 5 per cent. of the dose is available for excretion in the urine, and crystalluria is not a hazard. Sulphathiazole is the active principle, being released by hydrolysis in the bowel.

Phthalylsulphathiazole. This compound differs from the preceding one chiefly in having greater bacteriostatic action in the bowel. The dose is consequently smaller. Poorly absorbed sulphonamides were used originally for the treatment of bacillary dysentery. Results as good or better can be obtained in this disease with absorbable sulphonamides, which many believe should be used in preference.

Long-acting Sulphonamides

New forms of long-acting sulphonamides are still being produced. Time will show which is most useful. Sulphadimethoxine, sulphamethoxypyridazine and sulphormethoxine are among the best known.

Dosage

This is shown in TABLE 2. When using absorbable sulphonamides in the treatment of acute infections it is advisable to give an initial loading dose to procure the necessary blood concentrations as soon as possible. For patients who are unable to take the drug by mouth, treatment should begin with the intravenous injection of a 5 per cent. solution of the sodium salt of the sulphonamide. The injection should be given slowly and care should be taken to avoid extravasation into the tissues. The sodium salt may be given intramuscularly, but the injections are likely to cause pain; they should be spaced out at least three inches apart, and be limited in number. Nerves must be avoided as cases of foot and wrist drop have been reported. Sulphonamides should never be injected intrathecally. This is fortunately not necessary as they diffuse into the cerebrospinal fluid.

To avoid deposition of crystals in the urinary tract the urine should be made alkaline, and the patient's fluid intake should not be below 3 litres in the day.

Antibacterial Activity

Sulphonamides exert a bacteriostatic effect on a considerable number of Gram-positive and Gram-negative organisms. For some species, however, resistant strains are common, and an organism resistant to one sulphonamide can be regarded as resistant to all.

Indications

For most infections sulphonamides have been replaced by more effective and possibly less toxic antibiotics. In a few diseases, for example gonorrhoea, they have in the past been rendered valueless by the predominance of sulphonamide-resistant strains.

Sulphonamides have been the drug of choice for meningitis caused by *Neisseria meningitidis*, but their position is now threatened by the appearance of resistant strains. They are widely used for urinary infections due to the Gram-negative organisms, *Escherichia coli*, *Klebsiella* and *Proteus*, particularly as the drug with which to start treatment before the results of sensitivity tests are known, and for the treatment of the bacillary dysenteries. For both forms of infection, resistant strains are now so common that the value of sulphonamides is less that it was in the past. Sulphonamides may be given together with streptomycin or chloramphenicol for the treatment of pneumococcal meningitis [TABLE 1]. Although the sulphonamides have been superseded for the treatment of gonorrhoea, they are suitable in chancroid and lymphogranuloma venereum. Dermatitis herpetiformis responds well to sulphapyridine. This action appears to be of a different nature from the usual antibacterial activity of a sulphonamide, as many other sulphonamides are without effect.

In surgery the poorly absorbed sulphonamides are used before abdominal operations to reduce the number of bacteria in the bowel.

The long-acting forms of sulphonamides have advantages for the treatment of patients in countries with inadequate medical services and where patients can only be seen at considerable intervals. In countries in which patients can be seen with regularity the short-acting soluble preparations remain the most useful for diseases suggested in this section. The long-acting preparations appear to have no substantial therapeutic advantages.

Sulphonamides should not be used as topical applications because of the significant risk of contact dermatitis.

TRIMETHOPRIM

Sulphonamides act by blocking the enzyme system in the bacterial cell that uses para-aminobenzoic acid as the first stage in the synthesis of folic acid. Other substances have been found that block the next step. Trimethoprim is one of these substances, and when it is used with a sulphonamide the combined effect on a sensitive organism is usually greater than would be produced by either of the drugs acting alone.

The range of activity of trimethoprim closely resembles that of the sulphonamides, and trimethoprim/sulphonamide mixtures are active against the pyogenic cocci, enterobacteria—*Esch. coli*, *Proteus*, *Klebsiella*, *Salmonella*, *Shigella*—gonococci and *H. influenzae*. Tubercle bacilli, *Trep. pallidum* and *Ps. aeruginosa* are resistant.

Resistant strains can develop to sulphonamides and to trimethoprim, although there is hope that development of resistance will be delayed or prevented when both drugs are given together. On the realization of this hope the future value of trimethoprim/sulphonamide compounds depends.

TABLE 2

DOSAGE OF SULPHONAMIDES

ADULTS

ORAL	LOADING DOSE	MAINTENANCE DOSE	INTERVAL
Sulphadimidine, Sulphafurazole, Sulphadiazine, Trisulphonamide (not intravenously)	2–3 G. (1·5 G.–2 G. i.v.)	1–1·5 G.	4–6 hourly
Succinylsulphathiazole	—	2 G.	5 doses in day
Phthalylsulphathiazole	—	1 G.	3 doses in day
Sulphadimethoxine	1 G.	0·5 G.	Daily
Sulphamethoxypyridazine	1 G.	0·5 G.	Daily
Sulphormethoxine	—	1–2 G.	Weekly

Lower doses recommended for urinary infections [TABLE 6].

CHILDREN

ORAL	LOADING DOSE.		MAINTENANCE DOSE		INTERVAL
	0–3 yr.	3–10 yr.	0–3 yr.	3–10 yr.	
Sulphadimidine, Sulphafurazole, Sulphadiazine, Trisulphonamide (not intravenously)	0·5 G. (0·5 G. i.v.)	0·75 G. (1 G. i.v.)	0·5 G.	0·75 G.	4–6 hourly
Succinylsulphathiazole	—	—	0·5 G.	1 G.	5 doses in day
Phthalylsulphathiazole	—	—	0·5 G.	0·75 G.	3 doses in day

So far these compounds have been used with success in the treatment of urinary infections due to Gram-negative bacteria, infections of the air passages, particularly chronic bronchitis, septicaemia and gonorrhoea. Less is known of their value in the treatment of infections caused by the Gram-positive cocci as other antibiotics are available for this purpose.

PENICILLIN

Penicillin was described by Fleming in England in 1929, and was made available for the treatment of patients in 1940–41. Although the first of a long series of antibiotics it remains in many respects the most useful. Penicillin is the product of the moulds *Penicillium notatum* and *Penicillium chrysogenum* and its chemical composition is now known. Early preparations contained several penicillins. The form which, until recently, has been the only one used extensively in medicine is benzylpencillin—penicillin G. It will be described first.

PENICILLIN G (BENZYLPENICILLIN)

Pure benzylpenicillin will retain its potency at room temperature for some years in a dry state. In solution it is much less stable. Solutions at 4° C. deteriorate slowly; at room temperature there is a variable but considerable loss after one day. The activity of other antibiotics is defined in terms of weight, but for penicillin G the Unit is still used although the *British Pharmacopoeia 1968* now gives doses in milligrammes. One Unit is the equivalent of 0·6 microgrammes (μg.) of the International Penicillin Standard, and 150 mg. is approximately equivalent to 250,000 Units of penicillin.

Penicillin is a bactericidal antibiotic, killing bacteria as well as preventing growth. It will, however, act only on bacteria that are growing, and it will not always kill all the organisms in a population exposed to it. This is rarely of clinical significance, but is important in the treatment of a few diseases of which subacute bacterial endocarditis is the outstanding example. Its action is relatively unaffected by minor changes in pH.

Distribution and Excretion

Except perhaps in infants, the gastric juices destroy penicillin G if they are in contact with it for long. If the oral dose is great enough some penicillin will escape destruction and be absorbed lower in the bowel. penicillin is present in the blood. Thus a dose of 500,000 Units will maintain detectable blood levels of penicillin for about 8 hours only. If high continuous blood levels are needed, it may be necessary to give enormous doses of penicillin intravenously or to block renal tubular excretion by the use of probenecid (*Benemid*), 2 G. daily.

The rapid renal excretion of penicillin can be offset to some extent by the use of procaine penicillin, a relatively insoluble compound. Following injection, penicillin is released slowly and continuously from the depot at the injection site giving low, but steady, blood levels for 24 hours or longer. If peaks of penicillin in the blood stream are desired as well, procaine penicillin may be accompanied by crystalline penicillin.

TABLE 3

DISTRIBUTION OF ANTIBACTERIAL DRUGS IN BODY

DRUG	ROUTE ADMINISTERED	URINE	C.S.F.	SEROUS CAVITIES	BILE	PLACENTA
		Proportion of dose	Proportion of blood level			
Sulphonamides	oral	most	high	$\times\frac{1}{2}$	low	$\times\frac{1}{2}$
Penicillin G	intramuscular	60%	low	$\times\frac{1}{4}$	$\times 5$	$\times\frac{1}{2}$
Phenoxymethylpenicillin (Penicillin V)	oral	25%	—	—	—	—
Phenoxyethyl and phenoxypropyl penicillin	oral	60%	—	—	—	—
Methicillin	intramuscular	60%	low	present	present	—
Cloxacillin	oral	35%	low	present	—	—
Ampicillin	oral	30%	—	—	high	—
Cephalosporins	intramuscular	most	—	—	—	—
Tetracyclines	oral	10–30%	low	$\times\frac{1}{3}$	$\times 10$	$\times\frac{1}{4}$
Chloramphenicol	oral	90% most inactive	$\times\frac{1}{2}$	$\times 1$	$\times\frac{1}{2}$	$\times 1$
Erythromycin	oral	3%	0	low	$\times$ 8–64	low
Novobiocin	oral	2%	0	present	conc.	—
Streptomycin	intramuscular	80%	low	$\times\frac{1}{3}$	$\times\frac{1}{3}$	$\times\frac{1}{3}$
Neomycin	intramuscular	approx. 25%	present	present	—	—
Kanamycin	intramuscular	80%	low	low	low	—
Polymyxin	intramuscular	low	0	0	0	0
Vancomycin	intravenous	most	present	present	present	—
Lincomycin	oral	5%	low	—	—	—
Cycloserine	oral	60%	$\times\frac{3}{4}$	present	present	present
Isoniazid	oral	most	diffuses freely in body fluids			
PAS	oral	most	poor	0	0	0
Viomycin	intramuscular	65–100%	$\times\frac{1}{9}$	low	—	—
Fucidin	oral	1%	0	—	conc.	—

In the majority of patients adequate blood concentrations can be produced in this way, but for the systemic treatment of most infections the greater certainty of intramuscular, or occasionally intravenous, injection is preferred. If it is desired to give penicillin by mouth, acid resistant forms of penicillin are available.

Diffusion from the tissues is rapid and following an intramuscular injection the blood concentration of penicillin G rises sharply. The peak, however, is not maintained as the normal kidney removes penicillin from the blood by active tubular secretion. Owing to the rapidity of clearance, increasing the dose will not proportionately extend the period during which

Penicillin diffuses into most parts of the body [TABLE 3]. Approximately 60 per cent. of the injected dose is excreted by the kidney and the resulting concentration in the urine makes possible the treatment of some infections, which elsewhere in the body might be regarded as too resistant (such as those due to *Streptococcus faecalis* and some strains of *Esch. coli* and *Proteus*).

Little penicillin passes through the healthy meninges,

and although the rate of passage is increased with inflammation, massive intramuscular dosage is required for the treatment of meningitis (1 million Units, 2 hourly). Very little penicillin reaches the chambers of the eye.

Toxicity

For practical purposes systemic benzylpenicillin is not toxic. Harmful effects have only been seen in patients with gross renal damage who have received very large doses indeed. In the past penicillin given intrathecally has caused meningeal irritation. This is now thought to have been due to impurities in the penicillin, but a single intrathecal dose should not exceed 20,000 Units.

Hypersensitivity

Reactions to penicillin are probably the commonest form of drug hypersensitivity. Although reactions can occur in patients who have never been given the drug before, the majority are seen in patients who have been sensitized by previous treatment. Generalized reactions usually result from oral, intramuscular or intravenous administrations, but any preparation of penicillin given by any route may cause sensitization and precipitate reactions in sensitive patients. The new semi-synthetic penicillins behave in the same way as penicillin G, in that they sensitize patients, and precipitate reactions in those who are hypersensitive. There is cross-sensitization between penicillin G and the new penicillins.

Generalized reactions are of two types. The first consists of an immediate and acute anaphylactic type of reaction which, unless treated, threatens life. The second form is delayed in appearance, occurring twenty-four hours to four weeks after penicillin has been given. The skin is nearly always involved, and in addition to urticaria and pruritus, there may be fever, eosinophilia, arthralgia and albuminuria. Rarely, exfoliative dermatitis and polyarteritis nodosa have been recorded.

There is, unfortunately, no reliable way by which patients liable to develop generalized reactions can be identified. Skin tests are unsatisfactory, and give misleading results. A negative test does not exclude hypersensitivity and a positive one does not necessarily mean that the patient will have a hypersensitivity reaction when given penicillin. Patients for whom penicillin is prescribed should always be asked if they have received penicillin before, and if there were untoward results. If a negative reply is received, anaphylaxis may still occur. For its immediate treatment adrenaline and sterile syringe and needle should be available.

Reactions to penicillin applied directly to the skin or mucous membrane are of a different nature. In patients who are hypersensitive to topically applied penicillin an eczematous type of change occurs, without disturbances in other parts of the body. This form of hypersensitivity can be detected reliably with patch tests, and is sufficiently common to persuade many dermatologists that penicillin should never be applied directly to the skin.

Procaine penicillin should never be injected intravenously. Inadvertent intravenous injection has been followed by fatal anaphylactic shock. Treatment of generalized hypersensitivity of the delayed type may be particularly troublesome in patients who have been given injections of the longer acting forms of procaine penicillin. To counteract the presence of penicillin in the body, intramuscular injections of penicillinase have been suggested.

Preparations and Dosage

Benzylpenicillin may be given by intramuscular injection as the sodium or potassium salt in aqueous solution. For infections of mild to moderate severity due to sensitive bacteria, a dose of 500,000 Units given twice a day should prove sufficient. For more serious infections, or for infections due to organisms of reduced sensitivity, a larger dose may be needed. As penicillin is virtually free from toxicity, the upper limit is only set by the practical difficulties of injections. Not more than 1 million Units of penicillin can be given in 1 ml. of water, and it is often preferred to use larger volumes for the same dose. For serious infections, a dose of 1 million Units given three to five times in the day is suggested. If a much greater dose is required, as it is on occasion in endocarditis, the possibility should be considered of giving it in continuous intravenous infusion for at least part of the course. TABLES 4, 5 and 6 list other suggested dosage schedules and the dosage for other penicillins.

Antibacterial Activity

Penicillin acts mainly on Gram-positive bacteria. Most of the Gram-negative bacteria are insusceptible, although the *Neisseria* and occasional strains of other species are sensitive.

It is unusual for bacteria to become resistant as a result of contact with the antibiotic, and for at least one organism, *Streptococcus pyogenes*, it is unknown. The all too common penicillin-resistant strains of *Staphylococcus aureus* are only resistant because they produce an enzyme, penicillinase, which destroys benzylpenicillin. Penicillinase-forming strains have apparently not often been produced as a consequence of the use of penicillin in the treatment of patients. The majority of them appear to be the descendants of strains that already possessed the property of forming penicillinase before penicillin was introduced into clinical medicine. Their ubiquity is the result of cross-infection.

Indication for the use of Penicillin G

Because it is a bactericidal antibiotic, and because of its greater efficacy and freedom from toxicity, penicillin G remains the antibiotic of choice for the treatment of infections caused by organisms susceptible to its action. Unless there are substantial reasons to the contrary, it should be considered first for the treatment of all haemolytic streptococcal infections, infections due to penicillin-sensitive strains of *Staph. aureus*, and infections due to the pneumococcus. It is also the drug of choice for the treatment of actinomycosis, anthrax, gas gangrene, erysipeloid, syphilis and gonorrhoea.

Appropriate tests will show the necessity for penicillin G in the treatment of the majority of cases of subacute bacterial endocarditis [TABLE 1].

OTHER PENICILLINS

Phenoxymethylpenicillin (Penicillin V)

This substance has an antibacterial spectrum which is comparable to that of penicillin G, although strains of *Haemophilus influenzae* and *Neisseria gonorrhoeae* are less sensitive to it than to penicillin G. Its chief virtue is that it is resistant to acid and can be given by mouth. In adequate doses, 125–250 mg. 6 hourly, it can safely be used for the treatment of susceptible infections of mild to moderate severity. Like penicillin G it is destroyed by penicillinase.

Phenoxyethylpenicillin and Phenoxypropylpenicillin

These and a number of other penicillins are also acid resistant and can be given by mouth. Among the claims made on behalf of individual members of this group are that they produce higher blood levels and have a slightly increased resistance to penicillinase. So far there is little clinical evidence that they are of greater value in the treatment of infection than is penicillin V.

Methicillin (Dimethoxyphenylpenicillin)

Like the two penicillins in the section above (phenoxyethyl- and phenoxypropyl-penicillin) and those in subsequent sections, methicillin stems from the isolation of the penicillin nucleus, 6-aminopenicillanic acid. This substance is obtained by removing the side chain from penicillin G. Its importance is that a wide variety of new side-chains can be added to it. Some of the resulting compounds have valuable therapeutic properties not possessed by natural penicillins. Methicillin was the first penicillin available which was resistant to the action of staphylococcal penicillinase. It, and cloxacillin, should be considered first for the treatment of infections caused by staphylococci resistant to penicillin G, or for serious staphylococcal infections when treatment has to be started before the sensitivity of the staphylococcus is known.

Methicillin should *not* be used against penicillin-sensitive staphylococci or other penicillin-sensitive bacteria, as weight for weight, it is less active than penicillin G. It is destroyed in the stomach and is of no value if given by mouth. Dosage schedules are suggested in TABLE 4. For intravenous injection 1 G. should be given in 20 ml. of distilled water. The intrapleural and intrathecal dose should be given in 5–10 ml. of water.

Cloxacillin (Isoxazolyl Penicillin)

This penicillin resembles methicillin in its antibacterial activity, but has the advantages that it is active at lower concentrations and, being acid stable, can be given by mouth. Like methicillin the principal indication for cloxacillin is in the treatment of infections caused by penicillin-resistant strains of *Staph. aureus*.

Staph. aureus has unfortunately shown a remarkable ability to develop resistant strains to one antibiotic after another, and strains resistant to methicillin and to cloxacillin (and to the cephalosporins) have been reported and are increasing in numbers. These strains may produce considerable problems in treatment as they commonly also produce large amounts of penicillinase and are often resistant as well to several other antibiotics.

Ampicillin

Ampicillin is another acid-stable penicillin that can be given by mouth. As it retains some activity against Gram-positive organisms while also acting on many Gram-negative bacteria, it has an antibacterial range resembling that of the broad-spectrum antibiotics. It is not resistant to penicillinase and cannot, therefore, be used for resistant staphylococcal infections.

It has been very freely prescribed, particularly for the treatment of urinary tract infections and chronic bronchitis. As with large intravenous doses it diffuses into the cerebrospinal fluid and it may be used for the treatment of meningitis caused by *H. influenzae*, meningococci and the pneumococci. It has not lived up to its early promise in the treatment of enteric fever, but it has been prescribed successfully for the treatment of typhoid carriers. Dosage is given in TABLE 4.

Carbenicillin

Carbenicillin is a penicillin that has lost much of its activity against Gram-positive organisms, but it will act on a variety of intestinal Gram-negative bacteria including *Ps. aeruginosa*. It should be considered along with polymyxin and gentamicin for the treatment of patients infected with this organism. Carbenicillin must be given by injection [see TABLE 4].

CEPHALOSPORINS

These antibiotics stem originally from a mould of the *Cephalosporium* species isolated in 1948 from the sea near a sewage outfall in Sardinia. The original cultures formed several antibiotics: identification and development of commercial methods of manufacture have taken many years. Preparations now available include cephaloridine and cephalothin.

Distribution and Excretion

Both preparations have to be given by intramuscular injection as little is absorbed when they are taken by mouth. They are excreted in the urine [see TABLE 3].

Toxicity and Hypersensitivity

Injections may be painful but serious toxic reactions have not been reported. Patients may develop hypersensitivity reactions, but patients who are hypersensitive to the penicillins do not react to the cephalosporins.

Preparations and Dosage

The properties of cephaloridine and cephalothin are similar. Cephaloridine is more stable in the body than cephalothin, and as the latter is also somewhat less active, it should be injected more frequently. Dosage for cephaloridine is given in TABLE 4.

Antibacterial Activity

The cephalosporins act on organisms sensitive to

penicillin and on some Gram-negative bacteria as well. Their most interesting property is that they are resistant to staphylococcal penicillinase, cephalothin more so than cephaloridine.

Indications

The cephalosporins may be prescribed for the treatment of infections for which penicillin is indicated, but their main use is for the treatment of such infections in patients who have become hypersensitive to penicillin. Streptococcal and staphylococcal infections of the subcutaneous tissues, chest, meninges and blood stream have responded as have infections of the urinary tract. They may not succeed if used alone for the treatment of severe infections such as endocarditis.

TETRACYCLINES

The main members of this group include chlortetracycline, produced by *Streptomyces aureofaciens*, oxytetracycline produced by *Streptomyces rimosus* and tetracycline, which is synthesized from the first two. Chlortetracycline was the first to be discovered in 1948 in the United States. Their properties are so alike that they can be discussed together.

The tetracyclines are of known chemical composition. As powders they are stable at room temperature, but in solution they deteriorate, chlortetracycline more rapidly than its companions. They are bacteriostatic and not bactericidal.

Distribution and Excretion

All three drugs are absorbed from the bowel, and are distributed throughout the body [see TABLE 3], although little passes the intact meninges. Absorption from the bowel is limited, and above a certain point—usually 1·5–2 G. in the day—the blood concentration is not significantly increased by giving a larger dose. They are excreted in the faeces and in the urine.

Toxicity and Hypersensitivity

Drug reactions and contact dermatitis occur very rarely with the tetracyclines. The commonest side-effect in patients given them by mouth is gastro-intestinal irritation. This is rarely sufficient to give rise to concern, but in severe forms, and particularly with larger doses, it may produce nausea, vomiting and diarrhoea. Intravenous administration should not exceed 1 G. in the day, this amount being halved if the drug is also being given by mouth, for with larger doses liver damage has been reported. Tetracyclines are deposited in the teeth during calcification both in the deciduous teeth *in utero* and in the permanent teeth. As varying degrees of pigmentation are produced, unless essential, tetracyclines should not be used for the treatment of women after the fifth month of pregnancy or children in the early years of life.

As they are broad-spectrum antibiotics the tetracyclines alter the bacterial flora of the faeces. In a few patients the alteration permits the overgrowth of yeasts and *Staph. aureus* which are normally present only in small numbers. Occasionally a rapidly progressive staphylococcal enterocolitis may result. The stools become increasingly frequent, are watery in appearance, and consist chiefly of pus cells, red cells, and discarded epithelial cells and enormous numbers of staphylococci. Death may supervene in two or three days, and at post-mortem examination the superficial layers of the intestine will be found to have sloughed, being replaced by sheets of staphylococci. Every attempt should be made to recognize this complication at the onset. The diagnosis is made by the examination of a Gram-stained film of faeces, in which will be seen clusters of staphylococci, usually accompanied by an absence or marked reduction in the normal Gram-negative bacilli. Although cultures may be needed to determine the sensitivity of the responsible staphylococcus, they are not helpful in making the initial diagnosis, as *Staph. aureus* can be isolated from the faeces of 40 per cent. of ordinary hospital patients, and there may not be time to wait for the culture result. Treatment, which is remarkably successful if begun in time, consists of stopping the administration of tetracycline, giving an antibiotic to which the staphylococcus is sensitive—usually erythromycin or neomycin—and correcting the disturbance of blood chemistry which has been produced by the profuse fluid stools.

Overgrowth of yeasts is common. The results may show as soreness in the mouth, or in some patients thrush, which may even extend to the bronchi. Overgrowth in the bowel may cause diarrhoea, and the tetracyclines have become a common cause of pruritus ani. Treatment should include stopping the administration of tetracycline and in severe cases the prescription of nystatin (*Mycostatin*).

In the past renal damage has been caused by epianhydrotetracycline, a toxic epimer formed from tetracycline in the presence of moisture and an acid. The acid was citric acid, included in the drug capsule to increase absorption. Now that this hazard is known, citric acid is no longer used, and toxicity from this cause should not be seen.

Preparations and Dosage

The tetracyclines are available in forms which may be given by mouth, intramuscularly or intravenously. The various routes of administration and dosage are shown in TABLES 4, 5 and 6. They should never be given intrathecally. The intramuscular injection should be made deeply. It is given with procaine hydrochloride. The intravenous injection should be given slowly, or put into a continuous intravenous infusion. As soon as possible intramuscular and intravenous therapy should be stopped, and treatment by mouth begun.

Antibacterial Activity

The tetracyclines are broad-spectrum antibiotics with a bacteriostatic action on many Gram-positive and Gram-negative organisms, rickettsiae and some of the larger viruses of the lymphogranuloma inguinale-psittacosis group. Resistant strains of bacteria are produced by contact with the tetracyclines. This happens infrequently during the treatment of individual patients, but through cross-infection, principally in hospitals, resistant strains of some species are common. Bacteria resistant to one tetracycline are resistant to all.

Almost all the strains of *Staph. aureus* likely to cause epidemic infection in hospital are resistant to the tetracyclines, although it is not known if this is more than an incidental finding. There is also a suggestion that some tetracycline-resistant strains of Gram-negative organisms such as *Proteus* and *Pseudomonas aeruginosa* are more liable to cause disease than their sensitive precursors.

Indications

The tetracyclines are valuable antibiotics when bacteriostatic action is wanted. They should *not* be used when it is vital to kill bacteria, as for example in endocarditis, and probably in osteomyelitis. They should be considered early in the treatment of brucellosis (in combination with streptomycin), rickettsial infections, diseases due to sensitive viruses, and as an alternative to penicillin. They have been extensively used for the suppression of infection in chronic bronchitis, for the treatment of peritonitis, for urinary tract infections and for the treatment of acute amoebiasis, although in this last complaint their action is probably upon the bowel flora rather than on the amoebae. Their wide range of antibacterial activity should not be used by the prescriber as an excuse for failing to make a proper bacteriological diagnosis. Apart from other possible complications of this course of action indiscriminate use of the tetracyclines carries with it the risk of producing resistant strains of bacteria which may be of increased virulence.

CHLORAMPHENICOL

Chloramphenicol was described in 1947 in the United States as the product of *Streptomyces venezuelae*. Preparations now in use are synthesized. It is a bacteriostatic antibiotic of known composition, and is stable. Solutions can be boiled for two hours with no appreciable loss of potency, and at room temperature it keeps indefinitely.

Distribution and Excretion

Chloramphenicol is rapidly absorbed from the bowel and diffuses well throughout the body [TABLE 3], being one of the few antibiotics reaching the cerebrospinal fluid in appreciable concentration. Little chloramphenicol is found in the stools and about nine-tenths of the daily dose is excreted in the urine. Most of the urinary chloramphenicol is present as an inactive nitro-compound, but approximately a tenth of the amount excreted is in an active form.

Toxicity and Hypersensitivity

The most serious effect of chloramphenicol is severe, and sometimes fatal, bone marrow depression. This complication occurs rarely, but is unpredictable, and whilst it probably occurs more often after long and repeated courses of treatment, it has also been reported after short exposure to the drug.

Chloramphenicol is a well recognized cause of drug fever and contact dermatitis.

Preparations and Dosage

It is usually given by mouth and can be given intramuscularly or intravenously. It should not be given intrathecally or intrapleurally [TABLE 4]. Intramuscularly or intravenously the daily dose should be divided into four equal amounts given at 6-hourly intervals. For intravenous administration the dose can be injected as a 10 per cent. solution or added to an infusion; for intramuscular injection a 25–40 per cent. solution is recommended.

Antibacterial Activity

Chloramphenicol is a broad-spectrum antibiotic with a bacteriostatic action on many Gram-positive and Gram-negative bacteria. Contact with it may produce resistant strains, but as in many parts of the world prescription of this drug in hospitals has been restricted on account of the risk of aplastic anaemia, these resistant strains are still uncommon.

Indications

In view of the slight but definite risk of marrow damage, chloramphenicol should only be prescribed when clearly indicated. The indications for it are:

1. *Salmonella* infections. As yet no other drug has been found to be superior to it for the treatment of typhoid fever.
2. Infections in which the causative organism is sensitive to chloramphenicol and resistant to other antibiotics.

ERYTHROMYCIN

Erythromycin is a product of *Streptomyces erythreus*. It was first described in the United States in 1952. It is a stable substance of known composition. In action it is usually bacteriostatic, although it rarely may be bactericidal.

Erythromycin was introduced at a time when antibiotic-resistant strains of staphylococci were becoming dangerously prevalent. As it was recognized that the proportion of bacteria resistant to an antibiotic is directly related to the consumption of the antibiotic, for the first few years of its life the prescription of erythromycin was restricted in many countries. The policy was successful, and for some years erythromycin-resistant strains of *Staph. aureus* were uncommon. As other antibiotics became available for the treatment of penicillin-resistant infections the restrictions on the prescription of erythromycin have been gradually relaxed.

Distribution and Excretion

Erythromycin base is usually well absorbed when given by mouth, although in a few patients absorption may be incomplete. Higher blood levels are produced with erythromycin ester. It is excreted in the bile, in which it is concentrated, and to a variable extent in the urine [TABLE 3].

Toxicity and Hypersensitivity

Erythromycin rarely causes drug reactions and contact dermatitis. Given by mouth it may cause mild gastric irritation, but as the base by mouth or the lactobionate or glucoheptonate given intravenously or intramuscularly, in normal dosage, it is most unlikely to cause toxic effects.

The lauryl sulphate salt of the propionate ester of erythromycin has been accused of producing sensitization. This has resulted in hepatitis in patients given long courses, or in patients receiving two courses of the ester.

Preparations and Dosage

It is prescribed by mouth as the base or as the ester. In view of the possibility of sensitization the former may be preferred. For intravenous or intramuscular use it is given as the lactobionate or the glucoheptonate. The intravenous dose should be dissolved in about 250 ml. of saline and given slowly. It may also be given in a continuous intravenous drip.

Antibacterial Activity

The range of activity of erythromycin closely resembles that of penicillin G, except that it is predominantly bacteriostatic instead of being bactericidal. It therefore inhibits the growth of many Gram-positive organisms, including sensitive strains of staphylococci and a few Gram-negative bacteria including the *Neisseria* and some strains of *H. influenzae*. Unfortunately resistance to erythromycin is acquired easily and it may be seen not uncommonly to develop during the treatment of individual patients.

TABLE 4

SUGGESTED DOSE FOR ADULTS

DRUG	INTRAMUSCULAR	INTRAVENOUS	ORAL	INTRAPLEURAL	INTRATHECAL	OINTMENT	MISCELLANEOUS
Sulphonamides			See	TABLE 2			
Penicillin G	1–5 million Units in 24 hr	Varies	—	20,000 Units	20,000 Units	—	2000 Units/ml. eye drops
Procaine penicillin	600,000–1,200,000 Units in 24 hr	—	—	—	—	—	—
Phenoxymethylpenicillin (Penicillin V)	—	—	125–250 mg. 6 hrly	—	—	—	—
Phenoxyethyl and phenoxypropyl penicillin	—	—	125–250 mg. 4–6 hrly	—	—	—	—
Methicillin	1 G. 4–6 hrly	1 G. 4–6 hrly	—	0·5–1 G.	10–40 mg. daily	—	—
Cloxacillin	250 mg. 4–6 hrly	250 mg. 4–6 hrly	500 mg. 6 hrly	500 mg. daily	10 mg. daily	—	Should not be used in eye
Ampicillin	250–500 mg. 6 hrly	150 mg./kg. daily	250–750 mg. 8 hrly	—	10–40 mg. daily	—	1% eye drops
Carbenicillin	1 G. 4 hrly	1 G. 4 hrly	—	—	—	—	—
Cephaloridine	250 mg.–1·5 G. 6 hrly	—	—	—	—	—	—
Tetracyclines	1 G. in 24 hr	1 G. in 24 hr	0·25–0·5 G. 6 hrly	0·25 G.	Never	0·5–3%	—
Chloramphenicol	2 G. in 24 hr	2 G. in 24 hr	0·25 G. 6 hrly	—	—	1%	0·5% as eye drops
Erythromycin	Not used	1–4 G. in 24 hr	0.25 G.	2–5 mg./ml.	Not used	1%	—
Lincomycin	300–600 mg. 12 hrly	600 mg. 12 hrly	500 mg. 6–8 hrly	—	—	—	—
Novobiocin	500 mg. 12 hrly	500 mg. 12 hrly	0·5 G. 6 hrly	—	—	—	—
Streptomycin (Not Tb)	1 G. 8–12 hrly	1 G. in 24 hr	(not absorbed) 1–2 G. daily	1 G.	25–100 mg. daily	—	—
Neomycin	2–3 G. in 24 hr	—	(not absorbed) 1 G. 4 hrly	0·25%	Never	0·5%	Lotion 0·5%
Kanamycin	0·5 G. 12 hrly	0·5 G. 12 hrly	(not well absorbed) 1 G. 6 hrly	—	100 mg.	5 mg./G.	—
Framycetin (Soframycin)	—	—	(not absorbed) 1–1·5 G. daily	—	—	5 mg./G.	Nasal spray 1·25%
Paromomycin	—	—	(not absorbed) 1–6 G. daily	—	—	—	—
Polymyxin sulphate	25 mg. 6 hrly	0·1 G. in 24 hr	(not absorbed) 0·1 G. 4 hrly	5–10 mg.	5–10 mg. daily	0·1%	—
Polymyxin methane sulphonate	120 mg. 8 hrly	—	0·1 G. 4 hrly	5–10 mg. daily	5–10 mg. daily	—	—
Vancomycin	—	2 G. daily	—	—	—	—	—
Fucidin	—	—	250–500 mg. 6 hrly	—	—	—	—

Indications

Erythromycin may be used instead of penicillin G for the treatment of patients who are hypersensitive to penicillin. It may also be used for the treatment of patients infected by penicillin G-resistant strains of *Staph. aureus* if the organism is sensitive to erythromycin, although for serious infections in patients who are not sensitive to penicillin, methicillin or cloxacillin is likely to be preferred. In view of the occasional poor absorption it is advisable to begin the treatment of gravely ill patients by the intravenous route. To prevent the emergence of resistant strains many authorities advocate the combination of another antibiotic such as novobiocin with erythromycin. In the laboratory combinations of this sort can be shown to delay the production of resistant variants, but in the treatment of patients they have been only partially successful.

In view of its low rate of urinary excretion, erythromycin is unlikely to be of much value in the treatment of infections of the urinary tract. It should be given together with antitoxin for the treatment of diphtheria.

Of the related antibiotics, carbomycin, spiramycin, oleandomycin and erythromycin, erythromycin appears to be the most effective and it should be preferred over other members of this group.

TABLE 5

SUGGESTED DOSES FOR CHILDREN

DRUG	ROUTE	DOSE
Sulphonamides	—	See TABLE 2
Penicillin G	Intramuscular	Only limited by practical difficulties
Penicillin V	Oral	—
Methicillin	Intramuscular	Up to 3 months 500 mg. per day 3 months to 12 years 100 mg./kg. body weight daily
	Intrathecal	Infants 3–5 mg. daily
	Intrapleural	100 mg.
Cloxacillin	Oral and Intramuscular	Up to 2 years ¼ adult dose 3 to 10 years ½ adult dose
	Intrathecal	Infants 3–5 mg. daily
Ampicillin	Oral	Up to 2 years 62·5 mg. 6 hourly 3 to 10 years 125 mg. 6 hourly
	Intrathecal	Infants 5–10 mg. daily
Tetracyclines	Oral	12·5–20 mg./kg. body weight daily
	Intramuscular	50–200 mg. daily
Chloramphenicol	Oral	Newborn not above 50 mg./kg. body weight daily Children 50–100 mg./kg. body weight daily
	Intramuscular	50 mg./kg. body weight daily
Erythromycin	Oral	25 mg./kg. body weight daily
	Intravenous	40–70 mg./kg. body weight daily
Novobiocin	Oral	15 mg./kg. body weight daily
	Intravenous or Intramuscular	15–30 mg./kg. body weight daily
Streptomycin	Oral	0·5–1 G. daily
	Intramuscular	44 mg./kg. body weight daily up to a total of 1 G. daily
Neomycin	Intramuscular	10–15 mg./kg. body weight daily
Kanamycin	Intramuscular	15 mg./kg. body weight daily
Polymyxin	Intramuscular	Up to 2·5 mg./kg. body weight daily
	Intrathecal	Up to 2 years 2 mg. Over 2 years 5 mg.
Vancomycin	Intravenous	44 mg./kg. body weight daily
Fucidin	Oral	22–33 mg./kg. body weight daily as diethanolamine salt
Nitrofurantoin	Oral	5–8 mg./kg. body weight daily
Griseofulvin	Oral	0·25 G. three times a day

LINCOMYCIN

Lincomycin was described in 1963 in the United States as a product of *Streptomyces lincolnensis* var. *lincolnensis*. It is a bacteriostatic antibiotic of known composition and is stable when dry.

Distribution and Excretion

Lincomycin is well absorbed after oral and intramuscular administration and is widely distributed in the body [TABLE 3]. An unusually large concentration is found in bone. When taken by mouth approximately 5 per cent. of the drug appears in the urine, but this figure rises to about half the dose following intramuscular injection.

Toxicity and Hypersensitivity

Few toxic reactions have been reported except that almost half of the patients taking it by mouth may experience loose stools. In some cases treatment may have to be stopped.

Preparation and Dosage

It can be given by mouth, by intramuscular injection or intravenously. Dosages are shown in TABLE 4.

Antibacterial Activity

Lincomycin somewhat resembles erythromycin in that it is active against Gram-positive cocci such as staphylococci, haemolytic streptococci and pneumococci. It differs in that *H. influenzae* and *Neisseria*, that are sensitive to erythromycin, are resistant to lincomycin Lincomycin, however, inhibits Gram-negative anaerobi organisms of faecal origin, *Bacteroides* and *Veilonella*. Resistance to lincomycin appears to be fairly easily acquired.

Indications

Lincomycin could be used for many patients who might otherwise be treated with penicillin or erythromycin and its affinity for bone may lead to it being preferred for the treatment of osteomyelitis. In view of its effect on Gram-negative anaerobes it should be considered for the treatment of faecal peritonitis.

NOVOBIOCIN

Novobiocin is a product of *Streptomyces niveus* and *Streptomyces spheroides* and was first described in the United States in 1955. It is a stable substance of known composition, and is bacteriostatic in action.

Distribution and Excretion

Novobiocin is absorbed from the bowel when given by mouth, and diffuses freely in the tissues, but not into the cerebrospinal fluid [TABLE 3]. It is excreted in the bile, faeces and urine.

Toxicity and Hypersensitivity

Drug reactions and contact dermatitis may occur with novobiocin. In a few patients a yellow pigment may be formed in the plasma. It is apparently a metabolic by-product of the drug, and its presence may interfere with the determination of bilirubin.

Preparations and Dosage

The forms in use are the sodium and the calcium salts. The dosage suggested is shown in TABLE 4. The intramuscular dose may be given in a volume of 5 ml. For intravenous administration the dose should be dissolved in 1000 ml. of saline and given by a continuous drip. Solutions containing dextrose are incompatible with novobiocin, and must not be used. Parenteral administration should only be used for seriously ill patients who are unable to take the drug by mouth: it should be stopped as soon as oral treatment is possible.

Antibacterial Activity

Novobiocin has a range of activity similar to that of penicillin G, including some strains of *Proteus*. Resistance to it is acquired easily.

Indications

Novobiocin has been used for the treatment of infections due to penicillin-resistant organisms, chiefly infections caused by penicillin-resistant strains of staphylococci. It has also been used extensively in combination with another antibiotic in an attempt to prevent or delay the appearance of antibiotic-resistant strains of *Staph. aureus*. Now that penicillinase-resistant forms of penicillin are available it is probable that the usage of novobiocin for both purposes will decline. It should not be used for the treatment of gonorrhoea, but may be of use in the treatment of some *Proteus* urinary infections. The low rate of excretion reduces its value as a urinary disinfectant.

STREPTOMYCIN

The isolation of streptomycin from the mould *Streptomyces griseus* was described in the United States in 1944. It is a stable substance of known composition. Solutions will retain their potency for a month if kept in a refrigerator.

Streptomycin is a bactericidal antibiotic that acts rapidly and is peculiarly sensitive to changes in acidity. The optimum pH for its action is 7·8: at 7 the activity is about one quarter and at pH 6 the activity is only about one twentieth. This characteristic must be borne in mind when using streptomycin for the treatment of urinary infections.

Distribution and Excretion

In patients with normal renal function most of the streptomycin administered is excreted by the kidney. The excretion is glomerular, and is not blocked, as is penicillin, by giving probenecid. Excretion may be impaired in renal failure and toxic serum levels may be unwittingly produced by normal doses. For systemic use it is given intramuscularly. It is not absorbed from the bowel in significant amounts, although it retains its activity in the gut and can be used as an intestinal antiseptic. For distribution in the body see TABLE 3.

Toxicity and Hypersensitivity

Streptomycin may give rise to pain at the site of injection. The most important toxic effect is damage, which may be permanent, to the eighth nerve. With a dosage of 2 G. daily giddiness has occured in between 60–90 per cent. of patients after approximately 4 weeks of treatment. With a dose of 1 G. daily the incidence of giddiness has been reported as dropping to between 10–20 per cent. with the onset delayed until the completion of approximately 6 weeks of treatment. With smaller doses in patients with normal functioning kidneys, the incidence is much reduced. Although not so likely to occur as with dihydrostreptomycin, streptomycin can damage the auditory division of the eighth nerve, and become responsible for lasting deafness. Both forms of eighth nerve damage are seen more often in elderly patients.

Streptomycin is a potent cause of drug reactions and contact dermatitis. Nurses administering the drug are particularly liable to a contact dermatitis of the hands and face. They should protect themselves by wearing gloves.

Dihydrostreptomycin, which is made from streptomycin, is more likely to produce permanent deafness, and may do so with little warning. As organisms resistant to streptomycin are almost certainly also resistant to dihydrostreptomycin, there is little to recommend the latter drug.

Preparations and Dosage

Streptomycin is commonly used as the sulphate. Schedules of dosage for the treatment of infections other than tuberculosis, and of urinary infections, are shown in TABLES 4 and 6. The dosage for tuberculosis is shown in TABLE 7. For this purpose streptomycin should always be given with another drug to prevent the emergence of resistant strains.

Antibacterial Activity

Streptomycin will act on the tubercle bacillus, some Gram-positive cocci and some Gram-negative bacteria, particularly *H. influenzae*, Friedländer's bacillus and *Esch. coli.* Resistance to it develops rapidly and easily and resistant strains are common. If the reaction of the urine is acid the drug will be ineffectual and resistant strains will probably be produced.

NEOMYCIN

Neomycin was first reported in the United States as a product of *Streptomyces fradiae* in 1949. It is a stable antibiotic, containing two active components. It is bactericidal in action, and like streptomycin, becomes more active as the alkalinity of the medium rises.

TABLE 6

SUGGESTED DOSES FOR THE TREATMENT OF URINARY INFECTIONS IN ADULTS

DRUG	OPTIMUM pH OF URINE	DOSE	ROUTE	INTERVAL	LENGTH OF COURSE
Sulphonamides (absorbable)	—	1 G.	oral	6 hourly	7 days, may be extended
Penicillin G	*variable	250,000–500,000 Units	intramuscular	8 hourly	7 days, may be extended
Penicillin V	variable	125–250 mg.	oral	6 hourly	7 days, may be extended
Methicillin	variable	1 G.	intramuscular	6 hourly	7 days, may be extended
Ampicillin	*alkaline	500 mg.	oral	8 hourly	7 days, may be extended
Tetracyclines	acid	0·25 G.	oral	6 hourly	10 days, may be extended
Chloramphenicol	variable	0·25 G.	oral	6 hourly	10 days, should not be extended
Novobiocin	—	0·5 G.	oral	6 hourly	10 days, may be extended
Streptomycin	alkaline	0·5 G.	intramuscular	12 hourly	3 doses
Neomycin	alkaline	0·5 G.	intramuscular	12 hourly	3 doses
Kanamycin	alkaline	0·5 G.	intramuscular	12 hourly	3–5 days
Polymyxin sulphate	no effect	0·1 G.	intravenous		
	no effect	25 mg.	intramuscular	6 hourly	7–10 days
methane sulphonate	no effect	120 mg.	intramuscular	8 hourly	7–10 days
Cycloserine	*variable	250 mg.	oral	12 hourly	14 days
Nitrofurantoin	†variable	100–200 mg.	oral	6 hourly	7 days, may be extended

* = alkaline for *Proteus* † = acid for *Proteus*

Indications

Streptomycin is the sheet anchor of the treatment of tuberculosis. It should always be given in combination with para-aminosalicylic acid or isoniazid, which may potentiate its action and will delay the emergence of resistant strains.

Apart from tuberculosis, the indications are limited. It may be required in combination with tetracycline for the treatment of brucellosis or with sulphonamides for the treatment of plague. Together with penicillin it is usually found to provide a bactericidal combination for the treatment of *Strep. faecalis* endocarditis. Because of the sensitivity to it of *H. influenzae* and Friedländer's bacillus, streptomycin may be used for the treatment of pneumonia due to these organisms, although alternatives are usually available. Urinary infections caused by sensitive organisms are a clear indication. Because of the rapidity of action it is likely that cure will be achieved in a few hours, if at all, and three doses of 1·5 G. in 36 hours should be sufficient. The necessity for an alkaline pH must be remembered.

Distribution and Excretion

Neomycin is not absorbed in appreciable amount from the bowel. When injected it is distributed well throughout the body and slowly excreted in the urine [TABLE 3].

Toxicity and Hypersensitivity

Neomycin given parenterally may cause renal damage, shown by the appearance of albumin, casts, the reduction of renal output and a rising blood urea. These toxic effects are usually reversible. Neomycin is also liable to produce permanent deafness without warning, an accident more likely to happen in patients with pre-existing renal disease and impaired excretion of neomycin. Applied to skin or mucous membrane as an ointment or lotion so little neomycin is absorbed that toxic effects are not produced. Absorption from the pleural cavity and from joints also appears to be too slight to cause toxicity. Intraperitoneal administration of neomycin is not without risk, as it has been thought to be a contributory factor in the production of cardiac arrest. In addition, fatal renal tubular necrosis has followed the intraperitoneal instillation of 3 G. of neomycin.

Drug reactions and contact dermatitis have occurred but are rare.

Antibacterial Activity

Neomycin will act on many bacteria including such Gram-positive organisms as *Staph. aureus*, *Bacillus anthracis* and the tubercle bacillus.

Strains of *Staph. aureus* resistant to it are uncommon but rather surprisingly *Streptococcus viridans*, *Strep. pyogenes* and the pneumococcus are relatively resistant to its action. Strains of a large number of Gram-negative species are sensitive to neomycin. They include the enteric group, *Proteus*, *Pasteurella* and *Brucella*.

Indications

Because of its toxicity neomycin is only given by intramuscular injection as a last resort, as for instance, in the treatment of a subacute bacterial endocarditis, for which no other antibiotic is available. It is given by mouth, either alone or in combination with polymyxin, to reduce the bacterial flora of the bowel in preparation for abdominal operations and in the treatment of hepatic failure, and it has been used for the treatment of bacillary dysentery and staphylococcal enterocolitis. As a topical application it has been used for the treatment of surface infections and it is very widely used as an application to the nostrils to prevent their colonization by *Staph. aureus*. It may be instilled in the pleural space or into a joint cavity, but it should never be injected intrathecally.

KANAMYCIN

Kanamycin is an antibiotic closely resembling neomycin, and was first isolated from *Streptomyces kanamyceticus* in Japan in 1957. It is of known composition, and is stable, withstanding boiling and retaining its potency at room temperature for months. It is bactericidal in action.

Distribution and Excretion

Kanamycin is poorly absorbed from the bowel, but in some circumstances sufficient passes through the bowel wall to produce toxic blood concentrations. After intramuscular injection it diffuses into the tissues, but does not pass in any substantial concentration into the bile, pleural or peritoneal cavities or cerebrospinal fluid [TABLE 3]. It is excreted principally in the urine, 80 per cent. of the injected dose being recoverable.

Toxicity and Hypersensitivity

Kanamycin is a relatively toxic drug which can damage the kidney and the eighth nerve. Toxic effects are more likely to be seen after long courses of treatment, but in patients with impaired renal function blood concentrations may rise rapidly, and permanent deafness may be caused by only short courses. Although normally little kanamycin is absorbed from the bowel, in patients with poor renal function sufficient may be absorbed to produce toxic blood levels. Intraperitoneal administration is not free from risk, as it has been thought to be responsible for cardiac arrest during anaesthesia. It is also possible that it may lead to fatal renal tubular necrosis, as has the intraperitoneal administration of neomycin.

Drug reactions and contact dermatitis have occurred.

Preparations and Dosage

Suggested doses are shown in TABLES 4 and 6. When possible intramuscular injections should be preferred to intravenous, as being less toxic. The intravenous dose should be diluted in glucose saline.

Antibacterial Activity

The antibacterial spectrum of kanamycin resembles that of neomycin, being effective against a variety of Gram-positive and Gram-negative bacteria. Like neomycin it only acts feebly on streptococci. Some degree of cross-resistance exists between kanamycin and streptomycin.

Indications

Kanamycin should be reserved for the treatment of seriously ill patients infected by organisms resistant to other less toxic antibiotics. In the past this has sometimes meant the treatment of severe antibiotic-resistant staphylococcal infections, but for these the new penicillin compounds should be preferred. It may still be needed for the treatment of septicaemia caused by Gram-negative organisms, and perhaps for the treatment of renal tuberculosis due to highly streptomycin-resistant tubercle bacilli. In these cases there is a possibility that the bacilli may also be resistant to kanamycin. For patients known to have normal renal function it may be valuable as a drug for the treatment of urinary infections due to sensitive bacteria, and particularly *Proteus*.

FRAMYCETIN (SOFRAMYCIN)

Framycetin is a product of *Streptomyces decaris*, and was reported in France in 1953. It is a stable substance that is bactericidal in action. It is either the same as one of the components of neomycin or very similar to it.

Distribution and Excretion

When taken by mouth framycetin is not absorbed in significant amounts.

Toxicity and Hypersensitivity

When injected framycetin can cause renal damage and permanent deafness. It is therefore not used systemically. When taken by mouth or applied topically insufficient is absorbed to produce toxic effects. Contact dermatitis is rare.

Preparations and Dosage

Framycetin is prepared for topical use as a cream, lotion, spray or ointment, sometimes in combination with another antibiotic [TABLE 4]. Tablets are available for oral use.

Antibacterial Activity

Framycetin has the same wide range of activity against Gram-positive and Gram-negative organisms as neomycin. Bacteria rarely become resistant to framycetin during the treatment of individual patients but they can be made resistant in the laboratory, and resistant strains are beginning to appear in hospitals as a result of the prophylactic use of the drug.

Indications

Framycetin is a valuable antibiotic for use as a surface disinfectant. It is prescribed for the treatment of superficial infections of the skin and mucous membrane. It has been used successfully as a spray for the treatment of nasal carriers of *Staph. aureus.* As it is not absorbed from the bowel, it has been used for the treatment of diarrhoea of bacterial origin.

GENTAMICIN

Gentamicin is made by *Micromonospora purpurea* and was first described in the United States in 1963. It closely resembles the preceding antibiotics.

Distribution and Excretion

When taken by mouth it is not absorbed in significant amounts.

Toxicity and Hypersensitivity

Giddiness and deafness may occur after parenteral administration particularly in patients with poor renal function.

Preparations and Dosage

Gentamicin is available as the base for injection. If satisfactory levels are to be reached and toxic effects avoided, great care has to be exercised in the size of the dose and the frequency of administration. Calculations should make use of determinations of blood urea and creatinine clearance. Preparations may be available for local application.

Antibacterial Activity

Gentamicin has the same range of activity as the preceding antibiotics, but it is much more active against *Ps. aeruginosa.*

Indications

Gentamicin may become a useful antibiotic for local application, and has been used for burns, bedsores and for nasal carriers of *Staph. aureus.*

Its potential for the treatment of urinary and generalized infections with *Ps. aeruginosa* would seem limited to those centres capable of conducting the exacting control of dosage that is necessary.

PAROMOMYCIN

Paromomycin is a product of *Streptomyces rimosus* forma *paromomycinus.* It was discovered in the United States and first described in 1959. In some of its properties it resembles neomycin and kanamycin, and it has been found to damage animal kidneys and to cause eighth nerve damage in human patients. It is therefore not used for parenteral administration.

Distribution and Excretion

When paromomycin is given by mouth so little is absorbed that generalized toxic effects should not be seen.

Toxicity (by mouth)

Paromomycin given orally may cause loose stools.

Preparation and Dosage

The drug is available as the base. For the treatment of intestinal amoebiasis a five-day course of 1–1·5 G. in divided doses daily is recommended. For bacillary dysentery and for the treatment of hepatic coma the recommended dose is from 2–6 G. daily [TABLE 4].

Antibacterial Activity

Paromomycin resembles neomycin in having a wide spectrum of activity against Gram-positive and Gram-negative organisms. It also has a direct action on *Entamoeba histolytica.*

Indications

Paromomycin appears to be effective against all forms of intestinal amoebiasis. It is also an alternative treatment for bacillary dysentery in the acute and carrier stage. It has been used in the management of hepatic coma.

POLYMYXINS

The polymyxins are products of *Bacillus polymyxa* and were discovered in 1947 by workers in England and the United States. Polymyxins A, B, C, D and E have been described. They are all polypeptides, differing in the number and kind of amino acids they contain. Polymyxins A, C and D are too toxic for use, and only preparations of B and E are available. The closely related antibiotic colistin described in 1953 in Japan as an antibiotic isolated from *Aerobacillus colistinus*, is very similar to, if not identical, with polymyxin E. All the polymyxins are bactericidal.

Distribution and Excretion

Negligible amounts of polymyxin are absorbed when polymyxin is taken by mouth, inhaled as an aerosol or applied to skin, mucous membranes or granulating surfaces. After intramuscular injection it reaches the blood stream and is excreted in the urine [TABLE 3]. It does not pass readily into the cerebrospinal fluid, pleural space or joint spaces.

Toxicity and Hypersensitivity

Polymyxin has the reputation of being a toxic drug. While this is true, it can usually be used with safety if suitable care is taken. Toxicity may show itself in three ways.

There may be local pain at the site of an intramuscular injection. It may occur immediately, and can be prevented by injecting polymyxin in company with a local anaesthetic. A local anaesthetic will not, however, prevent the aching pain which may develop about an hour after the injection. The delayed pain is less likely to be seen with the methane sulphonate preparation, which releases polymyxin at a slower rate and causes less local irritation.

Neurotoxicity is shown by transient flushings and paraesthesiae, the latter frequently being circumoral in distribution. They go when administration is stopped, and leave no permanent damage. They appear to be related to the level of polymyxin in the circulation, and, again, occur less frequently with methane sulphonate preparations.

Not more than 10 mg. daily of the sulphate should ever be injected intrathecally, as serious harm has been reported with amounts greater than this. Intrathecal doses up to 5 mg. daily will rarely produce evidence of meningeal irritation. Doses between 5–10 mg. daily may produce headache and an increase of cells in the cerebrospinal fluid. These effects can be minimized by spacing the intrathecal doses two or three days apart. They disappear on termination of treatment.

Irritation of the kidney, shown by proteinuria and the appearance of red cells and casts, may be seen with normal dosage in patients with adequate renal function. It will go on cessation of treatment and is not an indication for witholding polymyxin. More caution must be exercised in treating patients with poor renal function as increasing nitrogen retention may occur. For these patients the daily intramuscular dose of polymyxin sulphate should not exceed 1–1·5 mg. per kg. body weight and polymyxin should only be given when laboratory facilities are present so that renal function can be checked. The methane sulphonate preparations cause less pain at the site of injection and less irritation of the kidney. In both instances the reduction is presumably due to the slower release of polymyxin from the injection site.

Drug reactions and contact dermatitis are rarely met.

Preparations and Dosage

Polymyxins B and E are usually available as the sulphate or as the methane sulphonate. Dosage is shown in TABLES 4 and 6.

Antibacterial Activity

Polymyxin acts mainly on Gram-negative bacilli. It is notably effective against *Ps. aeruginosa*, an organism frequently resistant to other antibiotics. Cross-resistance is complete between polymyxins B and E and colistin. There is no cross-resistance with other antibiotics. Resistance to polymyxin is acquired only with difficulty.

Indications

Infections with *Ps. aeruginosa* are the prime indication for polymyxin. Urinary infections with this organism will frequently respond to 7–10 days' intramuscular or continuous intravenous administration. Polymyxin may also be valuable for urinary infections caused by Gram-negative bacilli resistant to antibiotics other than polymyxin. It should not be withheld because of unfounded fears of toxicity.

Polymyxin may be the drug of choice for the treatment of meningitis caused by *Ps. aeruginosa* or some other Gram-negative bacteria. It should, of course, only be given after appropriate sensitivity tests. As polymyxin by injection does not reach the cerebrospinal fluid in sufficient concentration it must be given by intrathecal injection.

Polymyxin is less valuable in the treatment of bacteraemia. The blood stream may be cleared, but in parenchymatous organs polymyxin is relatively ineffective, possibly because it combines with constituents of the tissues. It is doubtful if it will ever cure endocarditis, unless surgical removal of the infected tissue or vegetation is possible.

Advantage may be taken of the poor absorbtion of polymyxin to treat respiratory infections with *Ps. aeruginosa* by inhalations as an aerosol, or surface infections of the skin or mucous membrane by topical applications. It may be instilled into the pleural space and into joint cavities. Given by mouth it has been used in the treatment of bacillary dysentery and enteritis caused by enteropathogenic strains of *Esch. coli*.

VANCOMYCIN

Vancomycin is the product of *Streptomyces orientalis* and was described in the United States in 1956. It is a stable substance, solutions retaining their potency for two weeks in the refrigerator. It is bactericidal in action.

Distribution and Excretion

When given by mouth vancomycin is absorbed poorly. Neither is it well absorbed from intramuscular injection, and when given by this route causes pain. It is therefore given intravenously, and following injection diffuses freely in the body [TABLE 3]. It does not normally cross the meninges, but when the meninges are inflamed, vancomycin passes in variable concentrations into the cerebrospinal fluid. A small proportion of the dose is excreted in the bile and faeces, but the majority is excreted in the urine.

Toxicity and Hypersensitivity

Patients may experience hot flushes during the administration of vancomycin. Thrombophlebitis at the injection site is not unusual, and may perhaps be avoided by rotating the veins in use. The most serious toxic complication is damage to the eighth nerve. The likelihood of damage occurring is directly related to the amount of vancomycin in the blood stream. It should not occur in patients with adequate renal function who are receiving normal doses, although it may be seen in these patients with large doses. Impairment of renal function leads to an accumulation of vancomycin in the blood. If vancomycin is given at all to patients with this disability, it must be given with great caution and with daily determinations of the blood vancomycin levels.

Vancomycin can cause drug fever.

Preparation and Dosage

Vancomycin is only given intravenously. The daily dose should not exceed 2 G. [TABLE 4]. It may be given either as 500 mg. every six hours, 1 G. every twelve hours or 2 G. daily in a continuous intravenous infusion. The manufacturer's instructions should be followed in arriving at suitable dilutions for injection.

Antibacterial Activity

Vancomycin has a bactericidal action on Gram-positive organisms including staphylococci, pneumococci, *Strep. faecalis* and *Clostridia*. It has little action on Gram-negative bacteria. Resistance to it is acquired very slowly and it does not show cross-resistance with any other antibiotic in common use.

Indications

There have only been two serious indications for vancomycin, the treatment of resistant staphylococcal infections, and very rarely in the treatment of endocarditis resistant to other antibiotics. The availability of other less toxic drugs for the treatment of resistant staphylococcal infections has greatly reduced the need for its use. If it is prescribed, strict laboratory supervision is essential to ensure that the vancomycin in the blood does not reach toxic levels.

BACITRACIN

Bacitracin was discovered in the United States in 1945. It was given its name because it was obtained from a bacillus resembling *Bacillus subtilis* isolated from a patient called Tracy. Bacitracin is a complex polypeptide. It will retain its potency for months in the dry state and for a week in neutral solutions if kept in a refrigerator. It is prescribed in units and is bactericidal in action.

Bacitracin is so liable to damage the kidney when given by intramuscular injection that it is now used only as a topical application. As it is active almost solely against Gram-positive organisms it is frequently combined with antibiotics such as neomycin and polymyxin for their action against Gram-negative bacteria. It rarely causes drug reactions or contact dermatitis.

FUCIDIN

Fucidin is the sodium salt of fusidic acid, a product of the fungus *Fusidium coccineum*. It was discovered in Denmark and was first described in 1962. Its chemical structure places it in the steroid class.

Distribution and Excretion

Fucidin is absorbed well when given by mouth and diffuses freely in the body. It is excreted, with concentration, in the bile, and the bulk of the drug is excreted in the faeces. Very little is found in the urine [TABLE 3].

Toxicity and Hypersensitivity

Gastric irritation may follow its use.

Preparation and Dosage

Fucidin is given by mouth [TABLE 4].

Antibacterial Activity

Fucidin inhibits the growth of some Gram-positive bacteria, including *Staph. aureus*. Gram-negative organisms, with the exception of *Neisseria*, are mainly insusceptible. There is no cross-resistance with other antibiotics in common use. In the laboratory staphylococci can be made resistant to fucidin fairly rapidly and resistant strains may appear during the treatment of individual patients.

Claims have been made that mixtures of fucidin with penicillin, erythromycin or novobiocin are synergistic.

Indications

It is a valuable antibiotic for the treatment of staphylococcal infection, and particularly, perhaps, for the treatment of bone and joint infections. Its ultimate value will depend on the frequency with which resistant strains emerge.

NITROFURANTOIN (FURADANTIN)

This urinary antiseptic was discovered in the United States in 1952. It is made by chemical synthesis and is slowly bactericidal in action.

Distribution and Excretion

When given by mouth it is well absorbed, but it has no antibacterial action in the serum. About 40 per cent. of the dose is excreted in the urine.

Toxicity and Hypersensitivity

Nitrofurantoin has produced drug reactions in a few patients. It may cause nausea, occasionally with vomiting. This is less likely to happen if the drug is given with a meal rather than afterwards, and, in patients who tolerate it, it may be given for long periods without untoward effects.

Peripheral neuropathy has been described. There is some evidence that this complication occurs when renal function is impaired and there is consequent accumulation of the drug in the blood. Nitrofurantoin should therefore be used with caution, if at all, in the presence of significant renal failure.

Preparations and Dosage

Nitrofurantoin is given by mouth in doses of 100–200 mg. 4 times a day [TABLE 6].

Antibacterial Activity

In the concentration obtained in the urine nitrofurantoin is bacteriostatic and bactericidal for many urinary pathogens. Staphylococci, streptococci, *Esch. coli* and *Proteus* are commonly sensitive to it, strains of *Klebsiella* may be sensitive while almost all strains of *Ps. aeruginosa* are resistant.

Indications

Because of its wide antibacterial action and relative freedom from toxic manifestations, nitrofurantoin should be considered for the treatment of patients with urinary infections when treatment is begun before the sensitivity of the infecting organism is known.

It is valuable as a prophylactic drug, in a dose of 100 mg. 4 times a day, to suppress urinary infection in patients with indwelling catheters or subjected to repeated catheterization provided there is no significant renal failure. It has also been used in long courses to prevent reinfection in children with chronic pyelonephritis and in patients in whom renal stone-formation is feared. It is valueless for the treatment of infections elsewhere than in the urinary tract.

Preparation and Dosage

The drug is usually given by mouth. If this is not practicable, it may be given intramuscularly or intrathecally. Dosage schedules are shown in TABLE 7. It should be given with another agent.

Antibacterial Activity

Isoniazid is bacteriostatic or bactericidal for mycobacteria and particularly for the tubercle bacillus. It has little effect on other bacteria. Large populations of tubercle bacilli may contain strains with increased resistance to isoniazid, and to prevent the emergence of resistant organisms, the drug should always be given in company with another antituberculosis agent, usually streptomycin or PAS.

TABLE 7

DOSAGE OF DRUGS USED IN THE TREATMENT OF PULMONARY TUBERCULOSIS IN ADULTS

SENSITIVE ORGANISMS

DRUG	ROUTE	DOSE
Streptomycin	intramuscular	0·5–1 G. daily, or 1 G. 2 or 3 times weekly
PAS	oral	10 G. daily in 2 equal doses
Isoniazid	oral	200 mg. daily in 2 equal doses

RESISTANT ORGANISMS

DRUG	ROUTE	DOSE
Cycloserine	oral	0·5 G. daily in 2 equal doses
Pyrazinamide	oral	20–35 mg./kg. body weight daily in 3 equal doses
Viomycin	intramuscular	1–2 G. twice weekly
Kanamycin	intramuscular	1 G. daily in 2 equal doses
Tetracyclines	oral	2–4 G. daily in 4 equal doses
Rifampicin	oral	8–12 mg./kg. body weight daily in 3 doses before meals
Ethambutol	oral	25 mg./kg. body weight daily for 60 days; thereafter 15 mg./kg./day

ISONIAZID (INAH)

This synthetic compound is the hydrazide of isonicotinic acid. Its use in the treatment of human tuberculosis was first described in the United States in 1952.

Distribution and Excretion

Taken by mouth, isoniazid is absorbed rapidly, and diffuses freely through the body, reaching concentrations in the cerebrospinal fluid equivalent to those in the blood. It is excreted in the urine [TABLE 3].

Toxicity and Hypersensitivity

Peripheral neuritis is a rare complication of treatment with isoniazid. It is due to a deficiency of pyridoxine, as the urinary excretion of this vitamin is increased during isoniazid therapy. The same mechanism may lead to a sideroblastic anaemia. Both can be prevented by giving pyridoxine, 0·4 G. daily. Drug reactions can occur with isoniazid.

Indications

Isoniazid is one of the most useful drugs for the treatment of all forms of tuberculosis. It is not used in other infections.

PARA-AMINOSALICYLIC ACID (PAS)

The use of PAS for the treatment of tuberculosis arose from the finding that oxygen consumption of the tubercle bacillus was increased in the presence of sodium salicylate. It was therefore thought that related compounds might block oxygen uptake. Of those tested, PAS was found to inhibit the growth of the bacillus best. The first description of its clinical use was in 1946.

PAS is similar in structure to the sulphonamides and to para-aminobenzoic acid. Its action is also probably based on competition with para-aminobenzoic acid.

Distribution and Excretion

Given by mouth PAS is well absorbed. It does not pass into the cerebrospinal fluid. Excretion is in the urine [TABLE 3].

Toxicity and Hypersensitivity

PAS may cause anorexia, nausea, vomiting and diarrhoea. With prolonged treatment hypothyroidism and potassium deficiency may rarely be seen. Patients may become hypersensitive and show drug reactions.

Preparations and Dosage

PAS is given by mouth, usually as the sodium salt. Other salts are also effective and may be used if sodium restriction is important. The dosage is given in TABLE 7.

Antibacterial Activity

PAS is indicated for the treatment of patients with tuberculosis, not for its action alone, but because, when given with another agent such as streptomycin, it will largely prevent the emergence of drug-resistant strains of *Mycobacterium tuberculosis*.

CYCLOSERINE

Cycloserine has been isolated as a product of *Streptomyces orchidaceus* and of *Streptomyces garyphalus*. It was first described in 1955 in the United States and is unusual in that it was introduced for the treatment of urinary infections.

Distribution and Excretion

Taken by mouth, cycloserine is absorbed well and diffuses freely in the body, concentrations in the cerebrospinal fluid being little below those found in the blood. Approximately 60 per cent. of the dose given is excreted in the urine [TABLE 3].

Toxicity and Hypersensitivity

Animal experiments suggested that cycloserine was of low toxicity. In man, however, cycloserine may produce drowsiness, dizziness, mental confusion and convulsions. These side-effects appear to be directly related to the concentration of cycloserine in the blood and are more likely to occur with larger doses. As much of the drug is excreted in the urine, patients with impaired renal function should be watched very closely, as cycloserine may accumulate to toxic levels in the blood. It may also cause drug reactions in hypersensitive patients.

Preparation and Dosage

Cycloserine is given by mouth. The dosages for the treatment of urinary tract infections and tuberculosis are given in TABLES 6 and 7.

Antibacterial Activity

Cycloserine is effective against tubercle bacilli. It also acts on many other bacteria, although the concentrations needed to inhibit growth in the laboratory are usually somewhat high, and not much smaller than those obtainable in the body. Strains resistant to cycloserine may appear during treatment.

Indications

Cycloserine has a part to play in the treatment of patients infected with tubercle bacilli resistant to other agents. To prevent the emergence of resistant strains and because it may be more active in combination, cycloserine should be given with another anti-tuberculosis drug.

Cycloserine has also been used with varying success in the treatment of urinary infections. Because of its potential toxicity it has usually been kept for infections caused by organisms resistant to other antibiotics [TABLE 6].

VIOMYCIN

Viomycin is the product of *Streptomyces floridae* and *Streptomyces puniceus*. It was first described in the United States in 1951. It is used solely for the treatment of tuberculosis, and because of its toxicity is only used for this purpose when the tubercle bacillus is resistant to other agents. In the dry form it is stable: refrigerated solutions retain their potency for a week. In action it is bacteriostatic.

Distribution and Excretion

It is not well absorbed when given by mouth, and must be given by intramuscular injection. It must not be given intravenously on account of possible toxic reactions. There is some diffusion into the cerebrospinal fluid. It is excreted in the urine [TABLE 3].

Toxicity and Hypersensitivity

Viomycin in normal dosage is liable to damage the eighth nerve and the kidney. It should not be given to patients with impaired renal function. All patients receiving the drug should be closely observed for signs of renal damage. Drug reactions occur.

Preparation and Dosage

Viomycin sulphate is given as 2 G. every third day, given in divided doses at a 12 hour interval [TABLE 4].

Antibacterial Activity

For practical purposes the antibacterial activity of viomycin is solely against *Myco. tuberculosis*.

Indications

Viomycin is used only in the treatment of patients with tuberculosis. It is too toxic to be used except as a last resort when the tubercle bacillus is resistant to other antituberculosis drugs. To attempt to delay the appearance of resistant strains another antituberculosis agent should be prescribed with it, even though the organism is resistant.

PYRAZINAMIDE (PYRAZINOIC ACID AMIDE)

Pyrazinamide is a tuberculostatic drug used only for the treatment of tuberculosis. It is liable to cause hepatitis and it should be kept for the treatment of patients infected with tubercle bacilli resistant to at least two of the drugs commonly used. Tubercle bacilli become resistant to it in four to six weeks if it is used alone, and it should therefore always be prescribed with another drug. For infections caused by tubercle bacilli resistant to streptomycin, PAS and INAH, pyrazinamide has been combined with viomycin and with cycloserine.

Patients receiving pyrazinamide should be examined daily for signs of jaundice. Liver function tests should be done at least fortnightly, the most sensitive appears to be the estimation of the serum glutamic oxalacetic transaminase. The drug has also been found to decrease the urinary excretion of uric acid, with an increase of serum uric acid. Regular determinations of blood uric acid are recommended.

Pyrazinamide is given by mouth. Suggested dosage is given in TABLE 7.

RIFAMYCINS

The rifamycins are a new group of antibiotics derived from *Streptomyces mediterranei* isolated in Italy in 1957.

RIFAMIDE

Rifamide is the sodium salt of rifamycin B diethylamide. It is stable at room temperature.

Distribution and Excretion

Rifamide must be given by intramuscular injection. Some 80 per cent. of the dose is excreted in the bile and because of this, bile concentrations may reach very high levels. (In excess of 1000 μg. per ml. as compared with blood levels of 1–2 μg. per ml.)

Toxicity and Hypersensitivity

Pain on injection may occur, but serious side-effects have not yet been reported.

Preparation and Dosage

Rifamide is given by intramuscular injection in a dose of 150 mg. repeated at 6–12 hourly intervals.

Antibacterial Activity

At levels attained in the blood rifamide acts mainly against Gram-positive cocci. It is not affected by staphylococcal penicillinase, and cross-resistance with other antibiotics has not been reported. At the very high concentrations reached in the bile a number of Gram-negative organisms including *Esch. coli*, *Aerobacter aerogenes*, *Proteus*, *Pseudomonas* and *Salmonella* may be sensitive to it.

Indications

Rifamide holds considerable promise as a drug for the treatment of biliary tract infections. It may prove to be a valuable alternative drug for the treatment of infections elsewhere in the body caused by Gram-positive cocci.

RIFAMPICIN

Rifampicin is a semi-synthetic derivative, stable at room temperature and active against mycobacteria.

Distribution and Excretion

When given by mouth and on an empty stomach, rifampicin is absorbed well, and diffuses throughout the body, including into the cerebrospinal fluid. It is excreted in the bile and in the urine.

Toxicity and Hypersensitivity

Rifampicin is well tolerated, but adverse reactions including gastric discomfort, hypersensitivity reactions and perhaps jaundice have been reported. It should not be given during the first three months of pregnancy, and only in cases of necessity during the later months. It is contra-indicated in patients with jaundice or in those hypersensitive to the rifamycins.

Rifampicin may produce a reddish discoloration of the urine, sputum and lacrimal fluid.

Preparation and Dosage

Rifampicin should be taken before meals in a dosage adjusted to the patient's weight on a basis of 8–12 mg. per kg.

Antibacterial Activity

Rifampicin is active against Gram-positive organisms and to a lesser extent against Gram-negative ones, but its chief interest is that it is active at low concentrations against mycobacteria, including *Mycobacterium tuberculosis* and some strains of atypical mycobacteria. Cross-resistance with other groups of antibiotics has not been reported.

Indications

Rifampicin shows the promise of being a valuable drug for the treatment of tuberculosis.

ETHIONAMIDE

This compound is a synthetic derivative from isonicotinic acid, active against tubercle bacilli and, despite its chemical similarity, active against isoniazid-resistant strains. Resistance to it develops rapidly, but given with another antibiotic it has been used successfully by mouth in the treatment of patients with infections due to organisms sensitive to the standard drugs. The usual dose is 125 mg. four times a day.

ETHAMBUTOL

This synthetic antituberculosis drug is absorbed well when given by mouth. It has been recommended with another suitable drug for the treatment of drug-resistant infections. Reversible retrobulbar neuritis has been reported following its use, but if the dosage is restricted to 25 mg. per kg. for 60 days and then reduced to 15 mg. per kg. it is claimed that this complication may be avoided.

NYSTATIN (MYCOSTATIN)

Nystatin is a product of *Streptomyces noursei*, described in the United States in 1951. It is a stable substance that inhibits the growth of yeast-like fungi, but has no appreciable action on bacteria.

Distribution and Excretion

In normal dosage nystatin is not absorbed from the bowel.

Toxicity and Hypersensitivity

Nystatin is most unlikely to cause side-effects due to toxicity or hypersensitivity.

Preparations and Dosage

The usual dose by mouth is 500,000–1,000,000 Units three times a day. For monilial vaginitis it may be used as a tablet containing 100,000 Units or as an ointment containing 100,000 Units per gramme [TABLE 8].

TABLE 8

SUGGESTED DOSES FOR THE TREATMENT OF FUNGUS INFECTIONS IN ADULTS

DRUG	DOSE	ROUTE	INTERVAL	TOPICAL APPLICATION
Mycostatin	500,000–1,000,000 Units	oral	8 hourly	vaginal tablet 100,000 Units ointment 100,000 Units/G. lotion 1%
Amphotericin B	0·25–0·5–1·0 mg. all/kg. body weight	intravenous	dose given over 6 hours once a day	
Griseofulvin	1 G.	oral	daily	—

Antibacterial Activity

Nystatin inhibits the growth of a number of fungi and yeasts, including that of *Candida albicans*. It has no appreciable action on bacteria.

Indications

Nystatin is indicated for treatment of the *Candida albicans* infections of the bowel that occur principally after courses of treatment with broad-spectrum antibiotics. It has also been used prophylactically when tetracycline has been given for long periods, in an attempt to restrain the growth of yeasts in the gut. It is valuable in the treatment of oral and vaginal moniliasis. As nystatin is not absorbed when given by mouth, monilial infections of parts of the body outside the bowel cannot be treated with oral dosage: the drug must be applied directly.

GRISEOFULVIN

Griseofulvin is produced by a number of *Penicillium* species. It was first described in England in 1939, but an account of its remarkable antifungal properties was not published until 1958.

Distribution and Excretion

When given by mouth griseofulvin is well absorbed, and passes to the keratin of the skin, hair and nails in fungistatic concentrations.

Toxicity and Hypersensitivity

Headache and gastric irritation have rarely been reported, as have drug reactions.

Preparation and Dosage

Griseofulvin is given by mouth. The usual daily dose is 1 G. [TABLE 8].

Antifungal Activity

Griseofulvin acts on the fungi responsible for ringworm. It has less action on other pathogenic fungi, and is without action on bacteria. It is ineffective against *Candida albicans*.

Indications

Griseofulvin is indicated for the treatment of ringworms of the skin and nails, including such resistant conditions as *Trichophyton rubrum* infection of the finger nails. As the drug is fungistatic and not fungicidal treatment has to be continued until uninfected new keratin has grown, and administration may have to be continued for months.

AMPHOTERICIN B

Amphotericin B is an antifungal antibiotic isolated from *Streptomyces nodosus*, first described in the United States in 1956. In the dry form it is stable: solutions retain their potency in the refrigerator for 24 hours.

Distribution and Excretion

Oral administration is usually unsatisfactory and the drug is normally given intravenously. Excretion appears to be a slow process, and amphotericin B has been found to be still present in the blood 24 hours after an injection.

Toxicity and Hypersensitivity

Amphotericin B exhibits a range of toxic properties that might preclude its use for systemic treatment if it was not so far the only antibiotic available for a number of deep mycotic infections. Phlebitis has occasionally followed intravenous infusions, and the majority of patients show a febrile response. Headache, nausea and vomiting are not unusual. With long courses and large doses evidence of nitrogen retention in the blood has been seen.

It is claimed that toxic effects have not been seen following the topical application of amphotericin B lotion, and that contact dermatitis is rare.

Preparations and Dosage

Amphotericin B is available as a stable powder, which, for use, is reconstituted in 5 per cent. dextrose solution. The daily intravenous dose should start at 0·25 mg. of amphotericin B activity per kg. body weight and increase to between 0·5 mg.–1 mg. per kg. [TABLE 8]. This amount should be given slowly over 6 hours, the patient being watched for toxic manifestations. Amphotericin has been used intramuscularly with a daily dosage of 20 mg. combined with a local anaesthetic.

It is not yet known how long treatment may have to be continued, but the period will probably be one of weeks. The makers recommend that for patients on prolonged therapy regular liver, kidney and bone marrow studies should be carried out.

Amphotericin B is applied as a lotion at a strength of 1 per cent.

Antifungal Activity

Amphotericin B shows activity against the organisms responsible for cryptococcosis, coccidioidomycosis, histoplasmosis, North American blastomycosis and moniliasis (candidiasis). It has some effect on the ringworm fungi, but apparently not enough to make it of any value as a topical application. It has no significant action on bacteria or viruses.

Indications

Amphotericin B is indicated for the treatment of deep mycotic infections—cryptococcosis, coccidioidomycosis, histoplasmosis, North American blastomycosis, aspergillosis and generalized moniliasis.

NALIDIXIC ACID

Nalidixic acid, a compound of known composition, was synthesized in the United States in 1962. Solutions withstand autoclaving.

Distribution and Excretion

When given by mouth the drug is well absorbed; about 80 per cent. is excreted in the urine.

Toxicity and Hypersensitivity

Nausea and skin rashes have been seen with nalidixic acid, but have not usually been regarded as serious. It should be used with caution in patients with poor renal, hepatic or respiratory function.

Preparation and Dosage

Nalidixic acid is given by mouth. It is available in tablets containing 500 mg. Four grammes should be given in 24 hours in divided doses.

Antibacterial Activity

Nalidixic acid is bacteriostatic and bactericidal for many Gram-negative organisms, but not for *Ps. aeruginosa*. The majority of Gram-positive bacteria are resistant to it. Resistance to it can be produced with ease in the laboratory, and resistant strains have been seen to emerge during the treatment of patients.

Indications

The treatment of infections of the urinary tract has been the chief indication for the use of nalidixic acid.

REFERENCES

GARROD, L. P., and O'GRADY, F. (1971) *Antibiotic and Chemotherapy*, 3rd. ed., Edinburgh.

WILLIAMS, R. E. O., BLOWERS, R., GARROD, L. P., and SHOOTER, R. A. (1966) *Hospital Infection, Causes and Prevention*, London.

R. A. SHOOTER

SECTION 2

DISEASES DUE TO INFECTION AND INFESTATION

DISEASES DUE TO BACTERIAL INFECTION

GENERAL ASPECTS

Infection has been defined as the successful invasion of the tissues of the host by bacteria. Some of its consequences have been described in Section 1. In this section we are concerned with its general clinical aspects.

The normal body possesses defence mechanisms which ensure that such an event is relatively infrequent in spite of the ubiquity of pathogenic bacteria. This natural immunity depends upon mechanical barriers to the entry and spread of micro-organisms, the presence of bactericidal substances in body fluids and secretions and the activity of phagocytic cells. It may be impaired by some general debilitating process or by local tissue injury or it may be overwhelmed by the natural virulence of the organism.

The immediate result is usually to be seen in the invaded tissues where destruction and death of cells become apparent; associated with this local damage are certain general features often attributed to 'toxaemia'. This term has been used in two senses. The first, and more precise, is applicable to infections with bacteria known to produce an exotoxin with specific and clearly defined effects: examples are diphtheria and tetanus. The characteristic features of these two diseases are entirely attributable to exotoxin liberated by the bacteria growing in the local lesion which itself may be trivial and completely overshadowed by the systemic effects of the bacterial toxins.

'Toxaemia' is more often used to describe certain clinical phenomena common to all infective processes. These cannot be confidently ascribed to bacterial toxins alone. Undoubtedly they make a contribution, but the products of the consequent tissue destruction must also be of importance. Significant parts are played, too, by the effects of a raised body temperature; by sweating with resulting loss of water and salts; and by the derangement of function caused by infection of particular organs or tissues. In this sense the term may be convenient, but it is imprecise and does little more than disguise the complexity of the disturbance.

If the local defences prove inadequate to contain the infection, the invading bacteria will enter the circulation. If resistance is low, and the infection overwhelming, the organisms may multiply in the blood stream. This condition of septicaemia is associated with severe general symptoms. Sometimes bacteria escape into the circulation from a focus of infection, but their presence is transient and their numbers few. This is termed 'bacteraemia'; it lacks the serious import of septicaemia. When septicaemia is associated with the formation of abscesses scattered throughout the organs and tissues of the body the condition is called 'pyaemia'. It may result from the lodgement of pyogenic bacteria in capillaries or the dissemination from a local lesion of infective emboli. Systemic pyaemia of the second variety usually reveals itself by multiple lung abscesses. When a tributary of the portal vein is the site of infective phlebitis, portal pyaemia or suppurative pylephlebitis may result with small abscesses studding the liver. The term 'arterial pyaemia' has been used to describe the scattered abscesses seen in acute bacterial endocarditis.

The organisms most likely to lead to septicaemia are *Staphylococcus aureus*, *Streptococcus pyogenes*, pneumococcus, *Neisseria meningitidis*, *Clostridium welchii*, *Pseudomonas aeruginosa*, *Escherichia coli*, and other Gram-negative bacteria. Pyaemia is most often due to *Staph. aureus* but may occur in infections with *Str. pyogenes* and *Esch. coli*. Bacteraemia is common in the early stages of typhoid and paratyphoid fevers and is characteristic of subacute bacterial endocarditis.

The pattern of these general infections has changed in recent years. They are met most frequently as a complication of some chronic debilitating illness such as cirrhosis of the liver or renal failure. They are particularly common in patients with acute leukaemia, rheumatoid arthritis, and systemic lupus erythematosus who have been treated with corticosteroids and other immunosuppressive drugs. They often complicate operations on the urinary and biliary tracts, particularly in the aged. In patients receiving corticosteroids many of the features of infection may be suppressed and multiple pyaemic abscesses are often an unexpected discovery at post-mortem examination.

GENERAL CLINICAL FEATURES

The clinical features of bacterial infection may be divided into those of the local infective lesion, those specific to the particular infecting organism and certain general symptoms and physical signs shared by all such processes. Here only those in the third group are to be considered. The more grave the infection the greater the intensity of these phenomena, although, in all instances, they are similar in kind.

First, there are certain symptoms common to many illnesses: malaise, exhaustion and loss of physical strength. Loss of appetite is usual and, in a seriously ill patient, may be combined with nausea and vomiting. Constipation is the rule, unless the infection is of the alimentary tract when diarrhoea is often a salient symptom; it may occur, too, in septicaemia. Headache is a common symptom of all infections. It is particularly intense when there is some specific local cause such as meningitis or cerebral abscess. It is a feature of the early phase of typhoid and paratyphoid fevers. The mental state in infections is commonly normal. In septicaemia the patient is often unusually alert and unreasonably euphoric. Prolonged infection takes its toll psychologically as well as physically: depression, loss of concentration, and a lowering of morale are common.

With fulminating infection the patient may be stuporose or comatose.

Fever

An elevation of body temperature or fever is an almost invariable accompaniment of bacterial infection. A convenient notion when discussing the temperature of the body is to regard it as consisting of a central core, containing the brain, thoracic and abdominal organs with a variable amount of the deeper parts of the limbs, and a surrounding shell. The temperature of the core is normally maintained at a constant level whatever that of the environment; that of the shell shows wide variations.

Thermometer readings from the closed mouth or the rectum give an indication of the core temperature which in the first normally lies between 96·8°–99·4° F. (36·0°–37·5° C.), being 0·5°–1·0° F. (0·3°–0·6° C.) higher in the second. In a neutral thermal environment axillary and oral temperatures correspond provided the subject is not thin. There is a daily variation of 1·5°–2° F. (0·9°–1·1° C.): the temperature is highest between 5 and 8 p.m., because of heat generated by the day's muscular activity, and lowest in the small hours of the morning. In women the mean body temperature is about 0·3° F. (0·2° C.) higher in the premenstrual phase. Temperature control is often inadequate in infants and in the aged readings are commonly lower than in the young adult.

A constant core temperature is normally preserved by maintenance of the balance between the amount of heat generated by metabolic and muscular activity and the amount lost. In a temperate climate at rest 25 per cent. of the body's heat loss is by vaporization of sweat from its surface, 60 per cent. by radiation to other objects in the vicinity and 15 per cent. by convection currents. The control of body temperature depends on the maintenance of this equilibrium and the details of the mechanism are still uncertain. Receptors are present along the course of the internal carotid arteries which are stimulated by alterations in the temperature of arterial blood, inducing, when it rises, general cutaneous vasodilatation and sweating with consequent loss of heat and vasoconstriction and shivering when it falls. Other thermal receptors are present in the skin, local stimulation of which causes similar general effects as well as purely local dilatation of vessels and sweating. The central mechanism which correlates the information from these receptors and translates it into actions required to maintain a constant core temperature is believed to lie in the hypothalamus.

It is obvious that a rise in the body's temperature must be due to disturbance of this equilibrium, and in bacterial infection this is thought to be due to the liberation of substances known as 'pyrogens'. Lipopolysaccharides have been extracted from a number of bacteria, intravenous injection of which in quantities as small as 0·00001 μg. will cause fever in man. This is not a direct effect of the injected substance but due to its reaction with circulating leucocytes which causes them to liberate 'leucocyte pyrogen'. Pyrogen acts centrally, for it causes no fever in patients with transection of the spinal cord high in the cervical region.

If heat loss from the body were abolished its temperature would rise progressively: this is seen in heat hyperpyrexia and, rarely, as a result of infection. In the majority of infective illnesses, however, the temperature rises to a few degrees above its normal level and there remains constant apart from a variable diurnal oscillation. The thermostatic control has not been destroyed, it has merely been set at a higher level.

Some infections are marked by rigor. This is often the opening event in the fever of pneumococcal pneumonia; it may recur daily in *Esch. coli* infections of the urinary tract or at irregular intervals in the intermittent hepatic fever of Charcot due to cholangitis; it is common in septicaemia and in pyaemia, particularly when an infective embolus breaks loose. It is the characteristic feature of malaria.

At the onset of a rigor the patient complains of feeling chilly; within a few minutes he is shivering; his teeth are chattering and he is demanding to be covered with more and more bed clothes. At this time his skin is dry and cold to the touch. He is pale and the lips a little cyanosed. Although the skin temperature is low, the rectal temperature is rising steadily because the intense cutaneous vasoconstriction reduces the body's heat loss to a minimum while the quantity generated is increased by the involuntary muscular contractions of shivering. This stage lasts for 15–30 minutes. At the end of this period the cutaneous vessels start to dilate, the skin flushes, its temperature rises, the patient begins to feel hot and calls for bed clothes to be removed. Subsequent events take one of two courses. If the rigor initiates a period of sustained fever, the skin remains hot and dry and the temperature elevated. In other instances—of which malaria provides an example—after about an hour sweating starts and rapidly becomes profuse; heat is lost by vaporization of sweat from the body's surface and the temperature falls precipitously until it reaches normal. Most abrupt rises in temperature are brought about by this mechanism. Lesser grades are associated only with chilly sensations.

Hyperpyrexia is defined as a steadily and rapidly mounting body temperature. The skin is hot and dry. There is apathy, followed by stupor, coma and finally by peripheral circulatory failure and death. The rectal temperature may reach 108° F. (42° C.) and even 112° F. (44° C.) has occasionally been recorded. As a result of infection alone, hyperpyrexia is of great rarity in temperate climates. The fundamental fault appears to be abolition of the power to sweat and with it the ability to lose heat by vaporization. It is more likely to occur in the tropics, particularly when humidity is high; in patients who are dehydrated; and in those with some congenital or acquired defect of the sweat glands. Abrupt cessation of sweating may occur with salt depletion complicated by infection. It used to be seen occasionally in acute rheumatic fever with pericarditis.

Certain traditional adjectives are used to describe types of fever or pyrexia. A continuous fever is one in which the temperature is continuously raised above normal and varies less than 1·5° F. (0·9° C.) during the 24 hours. Intermittent describes a fever in which the temperature falls to normal or below at least once in the day, and remittent one in which the diurnal variation exceeds 1·5° F. (0·9° C.) but the temperature does not reach normal.

In most infections the temperature is higher at night than in the morning. Inversion of this pattern is sometimes seen particularly in meningococcal infection, tuberculosis and typhoid fever. Rarely two temperature peaks occur in the 24 hours: this is occasionally a feature of portal pyaemia, of septicaemia with Gram-negative bacilli or *N. gonorrhoeae*, of multiple infections with malaria and of kala-azar.

Periodic fever is a variant less commonly due to bacterial infection. Here periods of pyrexia are separated by afebrile intervals. This pattern is the rule in malaria, relapsing fever, brucellosis and rat-bite fever: the Pel-Ebstein fever seen in some cases of Hodgkin's disease is an example remarkable for its regularity.

The Pulse and Respiration

Fever is accompanied by an increase in the frequency of the heart beat and respiration. With each rise in temperature of 1° F. (0·6° C.) the pulse frequency may be expected to increase by 8 beats per minute in the adult and 12 to 15 in a child. The increase is often greater than expected in scarlet fever, rheumatic fever and pulmonary tuberculosis. A relative bradycardia is one of the classic signs of typhoid and paratyphoid fevers in the early phase of the illness and may also be seen when infection leads to an increase in intracranial pressure, as in meningitis or cerebral abscess.

The respiratory frequency normally increases by 2 or 3 per minute for each rise in temperature of 1° F. (0·6° C.): increase in excess of this usually indicates a respiratory infection.

The Urine

Sweating is usual in the febrile patient and when excessive may lead to sudaminal eruptions. The water lost by this route is one of the factors responsible for the commonly observed reduction in urinary output. The urine is characteristically highly coloured and deposits urates on cooling; a trace of protein is often present while the temperature is elevated.

The Blood

Changes in the circulating blood accompany all bacterial infections. The earliest and most pronounced are in the leucocytes; the typical alteration is an increase in neutrophils which may reach 25,000 per mm^3. or more. Exceptions are typhoid, paratyphoid and undulant fevers in which neutropenia is the rule. The erythrocyte sedimentation rate is invariably increased in acute or chronic infections. Anaemia is unusual in acute infections, unless there is septicaemia; but in many protracted cases it will eventually appear. In form it is normocytic and normochromic.

DIAGNOSIS

Diagnosis of bacterial infection is accomplished in two phases: first the diagnosis of infection, and secondly the identification of the organism responsible. The recognition that infection is present is usually easy when the local and general features of the clinical picture are reviewed. Isolation of the causative bacterium may be less simple, but has an importance which cannot be exaggerated. Precise diagnosis becomes essential now that drugs which are effective, and often specific, exist. This may require bacteriological examination of pus, excreta, or body fluids, depending on the case in question. It may be necessary to start antibiotic treatment before the organism is isolated, but this in no way absolves the physician from taking every step to identify the responsible bacterium by collecting the necessary specimens before specific treatment is instituted.

TREATMENT

Specific antibacterial treatment is reviewed in Section 1 and therapeutic details will be found in the section devoted to individual diseases, but there are certain points reasonably considered here which are relevant to the management of any patient with an infection.

Rest

Rest in bed is essential in the acute febrile stage of any infection, and rest of the affected part, where it is practicable is part of the classic dogma of therapeutics. The bedroom should be at an equable temperature, free from draught and as attractive as circumstances allow. The bed should be placed so that the patient does not face a window or light.

However, prolonged rest carries disadvantages which should not be forgotten in the slavish observation of traditional precepts. Confinement to bed reduces the respiratory excursion, lowers the circulation rate and predisposes to venous thrombosis; it causes wasting of muscle, and leads to mobilization of calcium from the skeleton and thus sometimes to renal calculus. It often results in decubitus ulcer and in postural hypotension. Foot-drop may be caused by the weight of the bed clothes; joints become stiff; contractures occur and constipation and retention of urine are common sequels in the aged. When protracted it wreaks psychological havoc, repressing the aggressive instincts which enable a man to lead a normal competitive life, and fostering a mood of passive compliance in which the outside world loses its meaning and the patient sees himself as the centre of an organization designed solely to administer to his needs and satisfy his whims. As soon therefore as resolution of the infection is established the patient should be encouraged to leave his bed. The resumption of activity must be a gradual process particularly for those who have been ill for a long while.

Nursing Care

Until the introduction of specific antibacterial drugs, the quality of the nursing care often determined the outcome of the illness in patients with severe infections. It retains much importance. It is necessary only to mention a few of the points which demand the nurse's attention. Adequate care of the mouth greatly increases the patient's comfort; frequent changes of clothes will be needed if there is sweating. The care of the skin and treatment of the pressure points by rubbing with alcohol and powdering will prevent bed sores. Regular turning of the patient decreases the chance of pulmonary infection. The encouragement of daily movements of the limbs will help to maintain muscle tone, reduce stiffness of joints, and discourage venous thrombosis.

Diet

Fever is associated with an increase in the metabolism; for each rise in temperature of 1° F. (0·6° C.) the basal metabolism rises by 7 per cent. The caloric requirements in the febrile patient are consequently greater than normal. These considerations are not of moment in short feverish illnesses, but with prolonged infections they assume a great importance. In such patients the daily allowance should be 3000–4000 calories: there is frequently a negative nitrogen balance, thus a liberal allowance of protein is required. The prime considerations are that the diet should be appetizing, that the patient should be able to eat it and that it should not lead to abdominal distension, which is frequently troublesome in the patient with serious prolonged infection. Light meals usually meet these requirements, but there are no other reasons for preferring one article of food to another.

Vitamin requirements and particularly those of the B group are likely to be raised in the febrile patient and a supplement should be prescribed.

Fluid and Electrolyte Requirements

Loss of water is increased in fever by sweating, by increase in the respiration rate and in some instances by diarrhoea. When sweating is profuse, as in the third stage of a rigor, water may be lost at the rate of between 1 and 2 litres per hour. A record of the daily intake and output of fluid is of the greatest help in managing the febrile patient. The minimum quantity of water he requires is that which maintains a urinary output of 1·5 litres daily. When the body temperature is 102° F. (38·9° C.) or above, the daily allowance should be at least 3 litres.

Many ill patients are unwilling to drink, others are too weak to lift a glass. Thus constant supervision and help is required. Iced drinks are inadvisable: it is difficult to drink large quantities and they are taken in sips which favours the swallowing of air, and meteorism.

Electrolyte disturbances are unlikely to occur in short infective illnesses unless some particular feature, such as diarrhoea, which causes loss of potassium is present. Profuse sweating entails loss of sodium. In prolonged infections depletion is common unless circumvented by sodium or potassium supplements.

Water and salts should always be given by mouth when possible. The intravenous route should only be used when the deficit cannot otherwise be made good.

The Bowels

Unless there is some local cause for diarrhoea most infective illnesses are accompanied by constipation, particularly when the patient is elderly, and prolonged rest in bed is necessary. Violent purgatives should be avoided. Liquid paraffin, 15 ml., or Liquid Paraffin and Magnesium Hydroxide Emulsion, B.P.C., 5–15 ml. at night, are usually adequate. If these prove insufficient a glycerin or bisacodyl suppository may be used or a simple enema given.

Impaction of faeces in the rectum is particularly common in the aged. This possibility should not be forgotten. Its relief will usually require digital removal.

Gaseous distension is a common cause of discomfort in the seriously ill patient. It can usually be controlled by attention to the diet and bowels. If these measures are unsuccessful, a rectal flatus tube may be passed or neostigmine methylsulphate given by subcutaneous injection in doses of 0·5–1 mg.

Control of Fever

In most instances no good purpose is served by attempting to lower the body temperature. In particular, antipyretics are inadvisable in all but the most trivial infections: the result is profuse sweating which often makes the patient feel more ill, and this is frequently followed by a rigor which restores the temperature to its previous level. Moreover, antipyretics so pervert the temperature charts that it becomes impossible to judge the effect of antibiotic drugs.

The exceptions to this rule are the trivial short term infective illnesses, hyperpyrexia, and continuous fever of 104° F. (40° C.) or more, causing distress and discomfort. The treatment of hyperpyrexia is a matter of urgency and is fully considered in Section 3. Continuous high fever is best dealt with by sponging with tepid, and later cold, water.

Sleep

A hypnotic will often be required to give the patient with an infective illness adequate sleep. It is important, however, to make sure that sleeplessness is not due to pain or bodily discomfort which requires some different method of relief.

The barbiturate drugs with a medium duration of action are perhaps the most useful: amylobarbitone, 100–200 mg., or butobarbitone, 100–200 mg., are suitable. Chloral Mixture, B.N.F., 15 ml., is also satisfactory. Paraldehyde may also be given rectally (Paraldehyde Enema, B.P.C., 5–6 ml. per kg. body weight, equivalent to 0·5–0·6 ml. of paraldehyde per kg. or by intramuscular injection (Injection of Paraldehyde, B.N.F., 5–10 ml.).

More powerful than these are glutethimide, 250–500 mg., which carries a slight risk of dependence and in large doses depresses respiration, and nitrazepam, 5–10 mg., which is safe and effective.

Other Symptomatic Treatment

The general discomforts of the febrile patient are numerous. Many can be offset by scrupulous attention to nursing and other details already described, but headaches, pains in the limbs, backache and similar symptoms may be sufficiently insistent to demand relief. Undoubtedly the various aspirin and codeine compounds are the most effective agents we possess, but the liability of aspirin to provoke sweating and of codeine to cause constipation must be borne in mind. Suitable preparations are Compound Tablets of Acetylsalicylic acid and Opium, B.P.C., Compound Codeine

Tablets, B.P., Codeine Phosphate Tablets, B.P., 30 mg. and paracetamol, 500 mg. They should be used as sparingly as possible.

REFERENCES

COOPER, K. E. (1969) Regulation of body temperature, *Brit. J. hosp. Med.*, **2**, 1064.
COOPER, K. E. (1969) Fever, *Brit. J. hosp. Med.*, **2**, 1069.
HARDY, J. D. (1961) Physiology of temperature regulation, *Physiol. Rev.*, **41**, 521.

PYREXIA OF UNDETERMINED ORIGIN

A problem which often faces the physician is that of the patient with unexplained fever. In most cases of this kind the temperature falls to normal within 3 or 4 days and uneventful recovery follows. Such short-lived feverish illnesses are commonly attributed to viral infection and this view is probably correct although proof is seldom obtainable. When pyrexia continues without adequate explanation a situation arises which may tax the skill of the most experienced clinician.

CAUSES OF FEVER

A rise in body temperature above normal accompanies a wide range of disorders which may be broadly classified as follows:

Infections. The commonest cause of fever is infection. It may be bacterial, viral, fungal, protozoal or metazoal. It may be generalized in that the process is not confined to one region or system or it may, as in the case of an abscess or bacterial endocarditis, be local.

Some diseases, such as leukaemia, and some drugs, such as the corticosteroids, reduce resistance so that normally harmless bacteria become aggressively pathogenic. These 'opportunist' infections are an increasingly common cause of fever.

Neoplasms. Almost any neoplasm may give rise to fever but it is particularly common when rapid tumour growth leads to necrosis and autolysis. Hypernephroma and metastatic carcinoma of the liver are examples.

Fever is prominent in Hodgkin's disease and occurs, although less frequently, in lymphosarcoma, leukaemia and myelomatosis. In all these it may be difficult to be certain that it is not due to complicating infection.

Tumours may for mechanical reasons be associated with infection which is the cause of fever; lung abscess with bronchial carcinoma and pericolic abscess with carcinoma of the colon illustrate this point.

The Collagen Diseases. Fever is a common feature in many of these. It is often the presenting symptom in systemic lupus erythematosus and polyarteritis nodosa, but occurs at times in all the many members of this group.

Hypersensitivity Reactions. Reactions of this kind are always febrile whether the exciting agent be a drug, foreign protein or unidentified as in the toxic erythemata.

Circulatory Disturbances. Many disturbances of the circulation are associated with pyrexia. Fever accompanies myocardial and pulmonary infarction. It is usual in localized and migratory thrombophlebitis. It follows bleeding into the gastro-intestinal tract, the subarachnoid space, the pleural, pericardial and peritoneal cavities. It accompanies the haemarthrosis of the haemophiliac, the crises of sickle-cell disease and the subperiosteal haemorrhages of scurvy.

Miscellaneous Disorders. Fever is common in a number of disorders which defy precise classification. It is a feature of several metabolic disturbances: acute articular gout, Mediterranean and other periodic fevers, acute intermittent porphyria and thyroid crises. It may occur in cirrhosis of the liver without evidence of complicating infection. It is the rule in profound anaemia of whatever cause and in acute haemolytic states.

High fever accompanies status epilepticus, acute mania and delirium tremens and often occurs during withdrawal of morphine and heroin.

Finally three diseases of uncertain cause are often pyrexial: sarcoidosis, Crohn's disease and acute pancreatitis.

Disturbances of Temperature Regulation. Lesions interfering with the mechanisms controlling the body's temperature lead to pyrexia but are of a different category from the causes already considered. The fault may be central due to a lesion in the hypothalamus or brain stem or it may be peripheral. These last include heat stroke as well as disorders such as anhidrotic ectodermal dysplasia and ichthyosis, where sweating is absent.

Psychogenic Fever. This must be distinguished from factitious fever. Many methods of 'faking a temperature' have been devised sometimes by psychopaths, sometimes by unequivocal malingerers. Their efforts are usually clumsy, and factitious fever can be detected by the bizarre oscillations of the temperature chart and their lack of correlation with the pulse frequency. Suspicion can be confirmed by use of the rectal thermometer.

Many experienced physicians are convinced that fever is at times psychogenic but, as with many physical phenomena thought to be of psychic origin, incontrovertible proof is impossible because all physical causes annot with certainty be excluded.

THE CLINICAL APPROACH

In most patients with pyrexia the cause of fever is immediately obvious, but in a substantial minority it is not. In many of these the illness will be insignificant and of short duration so that lack of precise diagnosis is unimportant. When fever continues for more than 5 days without apparent cause further inquiry is imperative, but if the patient is gravely ill investigation must be put in train without delay.

It is possible here to indicate only one or two points which have particular relevance to this problem. In recording the history, note is taken of recent exposure to infection, both recognized or potential, and to residence abroad. The past history may reveal similar febrile episodes or infections such as enteric fever or brucellosis which may have long delayed febrile complications. Boils or carbuncles may be followed months later by remote staphylococcal infection. The bacteraemia of dental extractions may be the starting point of subacute bacterial endocarditis.

Symptoms referable to anatomical regions or systems may be the clue to localized infection. A history of rheumatic heart disease or of a congenital cardiac defect will raise the question of bacterial endocarditis.

A study of the temperature chart may provide useful evidence. In septicaemia and with active suppuration the fever is usually intermittent, the temperature being high at night and often below normal in the morning. Sometimes in tuberculosis this normal diurnal swing is reversed: in kala-azar two peaks of fever in the day are common. Examples of characteristic temperature patterns are the 'step-ladder' rise of the first week of enteric fever, the tertian or quartan rigors of malaria, the recurrent bouts of relapsing fever and the 'saddle-back' curve of leptospirosis. Pel-Ebstein fever, with alternating 10-day periods of pyrexia and normal temperature, is a rare but diagnostic feature of Hodgkin's disease. Frequently repeated rigors in non-malarious countries are most often due to coliform infection of the urinary tract. Rigors separated by irregular intervals sometimes extending to weeks—the intermittent hepatic fever of Charcot—are characteristic of obstructive cholangitis.

Physical examination may immediately reveal the cause of the fever, but if it does not it is important that it be repeated frequently and meticulously. Often some abnormality appears which resolves the problem. It is perhaps worth noting that physicians sometimes neglect areas such as the testes, the prostate and the uterine adnexa where the explanation of the fever may be found.

Ancillary Methods

In most patients with pyrexia of undetermined cause the eventual explanation is provided by the laboratory. Here it is possible to do no more than indicate the lines investigation should take.

Blood. Anaemia is common with any protracted illness causing fever; it seldom has specific features. However, profound anaemia of any cause may itself be responsible for fever. The white cell picture may indicate leukaemia, glandular fever or some other obvious reason for the patient's illness. Neutrophil leucocytosis favours pyogenic infection; neutropenia is usual in enteric fever and with many viral infections, but may be due to primary bone marrow disease. Eosinophilia occurs in polyarteritis nodosa, sometimes with lymphoreticular neoplasm, with carcinomatous metastases in the liver and with many protozoal and metazoal infestations. Lymphocytosis is found in glandular fever, in toxoplasmosis, in cytomegalovirus infection and in histoplasmosis. Malarial parasites, bartonellae, borelliae, and microfilariae may be seen in blood films.

A rise in the erythrocyte sedimentation rate (E.S.R.) is almost invariable in any feverish illness. Figures in excess of 100 mm. in the first hour by Westergren's method suggest plasma protein changes such as occur in the collagen diseases and myelomatosis. A persistently normal E.S.R. in spite of continued fever suggests that serious physical disease is unlikely.

Bacteriology. Isolation of a pathogenic organism usually establishes the diagnosis beyond doubt and is thus of primary importance. Blood culture is of particular value and gives the essential information in septicaemia, bacterial endocarditis, enteric fever and brucellosis. Cultures of the urine, sputum and faeces, from the throat or paranasal sinuses and from discharges may all provide valuable evidence.

Serology. Serological tests are useful in the diagnosis of enteric fevers and brucellosis, but lack the force of isolation of the bacterium. They are essential in the diagnosis of viral infection; the Paul-Bunnell test is specific for glandular fever and the dye test for toxoplasmosis.

Tests for auto-antibodies, antinuclear factor and rheumatoid factor, and L.E. cell preparations, allow positive diagnosis in some collagen diseases.

Skin Sensitivity Tests. Tests such as the Mantoux and brucellin tests have a limited application in the present context. The same is true of the Kveim test for sarcoidosis.

Biopsy. Needle biopsy of bone marrow, liver, kidney or lymph nodes may provide firm evidence for the diagnosis. Surgical excision of an enlarged lymph node may give essential information. Finally, exploratory laparotomy often provides the only means of certain diagnosis.

Radiology. Radiological examination of the lungs, paranasal sinuses, biliary, urinary and gastro-intestinal tracts, the teeth or the skeleton may yield the clue permitting final diagnosis.

MANAGEMENT

Even when every ancillary aid has been exploited the cause of the fever may still remain undetermined. Such cases can usually be placed in one of two groups. The first contains those patients in whom clinical and laboratory evidence of serious physical disease is lacking. The pyrexia seldom exceeds 99·6° F. (37·5° C.); the patient's appearance is that of health, there is no loss of flesh, the blood count and the E.S.R. are normal. Patients in the second group are undeniably ill; pyrexia is often considerable; there is clinical and laboratory evidence of chronic progressive organic disease in the form of loss of weight, probably anaemia and certainly a raised E.S.R.

Patients of the first group should be advised to increase their physical activities; this step may clarify the situation by rekindling and revealing hitherto occult disease or, if unaccompanied by any deterioration, it will serve to restore confidence which by this time may well be sagging. There are records of patients remaining febrile for many years without cause becoming evident and without deterioration in general health. The question of aetiology has sometimes been begged by the diagnostic label of 'habitual hyperthermia'.

More difficult decisions are required in the second group. The majority of these patients prove to have an infection, malignant disease which is usually generalized, or a collagen disease. Only those with infection are capable of recovery and, with the powerful drugs we now possess, it is unjustifiable to postpone treatment until the academic appetite for precise diagnosis is satisfied. It is logical when faced with this problem to prescribe a 'wide-spectrum' antibiotic in maximum dosage for a week; if fever is not controlled a trial of para-aminosalicylic acid and isoniazid is justifiable, for tuberculosis ranks high among the infections causing pyrexia of undetermined origin. Streptomycin is not sufficiently specific to be of value in a therapeutic test; if any suspicion of subacute bacterial endocarditis exists, penicillin G in a dose of 50 mega Units daily should be given and if the therapeutic response confirms the suspicion it must be continued for 6 weeks. It should be stressed, however, that such therapeutic tests should never be employed until a complete diagnostic impasse is reached.

When these measures prove unavailing, it is reasonable to assume that the patient has an infection resistant to the antibiotics which have been given, some form of cancer, or a collagen disease. Symptomatic relief and temporary control of the last category may be possible and a decision whether to prescribe corticosteroids has to be taken. The dangers and the disadvantages are obvious: in addition to the familiar sequels of prolonged treatment with corticosteroids, undetected infection may advance because of their immunosuppressive action and remain undetected because of their antipyretic effect. Nevertheless, it is usually impossible, probably unjustifiable and certainly inhumane to deny a seriously ill patient the relief which such treatment is likely to give and the risks are much reduced when the potential dangers are appreciated.

If a decision in favour of their prescription is taken, the initial dose should be large—at least 40 mg. of prednisolone daily—and if symptoms are controlled it should be gradually reduced to the lowest amount effective.

If corticosteroid treatment fails to control fever, and indeed even when it succeeds, careful observation and repeated physical examinations must continue until the patient recovers or the diagnosis reveals itself. There are instances in which this revelation is not made until the autopsy.

REFERENCES

GERACI, J. E., WEED, L. E., and NICHOLS, D. R. (1959) Fever of obscure origin—the value of abdominal exploration in diagnosis, *J. Amer. med. Ass.*, **169**, 1306.

GOWER, N. D. (1963) Marrow biopsy in the diagnosis of pyrexia of undetermined origin, *J. clin. Path.*, **16**, 227.

PETERSDORF, R. G., and BEESON, P. (1961) Fever of unexplained origin: Report of 100 cases, *Medicine (Baltimore)*, **40**, 1.

INFECTIONS DUE TO PSEUDOMONADACEAE

GLANDERS

Definition

A disease due to infection with *Loefflerella mallei*, not rare in horses, mules and asses, but only occasionally transmitted to man.

Aetiology

The causative organism, *Loeff. mallei*, is a short non-motile aerobic Gram-negative rod. It elaborates a specific endotoxin, mallein, and can be distinguished antigenically from *Loeff. whitmori*, the cause of melioidosis.

Glanders occurs naturally as an infection of horses, mules and asses and rarely of goats and sheep. Human infection is now of great rarity, but is still seen from time to time in Asia and South America; it usually results from direct contact with an infected animal and is consequently confined mainly to those who work with horses. Laboratory infections have been recorded.

Pathology

Horses are commonly infected from contaminated water troughs or mangers through abrasions of the nasal mucosa. The disease may be acute, with purulent nasal discharge followed by rapidly fatal pulmonary infection, or chronic with granulomatous lymphangitis ('farcy pipes') and lymphadenitis ('farcy buds').

In man the pathological process is marked by cellulitis, necrosis, abscess formation and septic thrombophlebitis.

Symptoms

In man acute and chronic forms both of glanders and of farcy have been described.

In acute glanders the incubation period is about 4 days. An area of cellulitis appears on the nose at the site of infection with a papular eruption rapidly becoming pustular. The inflammatory process spreads centripetally along the lymphatics, forming nodules which ulcerate. Necrosis may affect the nasal bones and cartilages; cervical lymph nodes enlarge and suppurate.

Constitutional symptoms appear early and death, usually with pneumonia, occurs between the tenth and fourteenth days. Enlargement of hilar lymph nodes is common when the lungs are affected. Bacteraemia is not uncommon and may result in multiple abscess formation, suppurative arthritis and meningitis. The leucocyte count is usually not raised.

Chronic glanders resembles the disease seen in the horse. There is a chronic seropurulent nasal discharge associated with scattered subcutaneous and muscular nodules.

Acute farcy results from infection through the skin. Local cellulitis follows with spreading lymphangitis and abscess formation. General symptoms appear and the course resembles that of acute glanders.

Chronic farcy differs from the acute form in the inflammatory reaction being less intense, general symptoms less severe and the course of the disease more protracted. Amyloidosis has been reported as a complication.

Diagnosis

Diagnosis depends upon isolation of the causative organism which is simple when there is suitable material to examine. However, the clinical picture is often misleading and may simulate that of sporotrichosis, cellulitis, typhoid fever or miliary tuberculosis. Suspicion may be aroused by the history of contact with horses and, where infective material is not available for examination, agglutination and complement fixation tests may provide an answer. The skin test with mallein provokes such severe reactions in infected persons that it should not be used.

Treatment

The disease is so rare that the results of chemotherapy are poorly documented. There are reports of successes with streptomycin and with sulphonamides. It is probably advisable to use a combination of these two agents, continuing treatment until all evidence of disease has vanished.

Surgical treatment of suppurating lesions should be as conservative as is safe; manipulation may lead to dissemination of the infection.

Prophylaxis. The destruction of infected animals, identified by skin tests with mallein or by serological methods, has eradicated glanders from most countries.

Every precaution must be taken in nursing to prevent spread of the infection.

Prognosis

If glanders is untreated the mortality exceeds 90 per cent. The effects of chemotherapy on this figure are unknown, but a number of recoveries have been reported.

REFERENCE

MENDELSON, R. W. (1950) Glanders, *U.S. armed Forces med. J.*, **1**, 781.

R. BODLEY SCOTT

MELIOIDOSIS

Definition and Aetiology

A rare disease caused by *Loefflerella whitmori*, an organism related to *Loeff. mallei*, the cause of glanders.

The infection is enzootic in rodents, especially rats, and sometimes other animals including the dog, horse and pig. It has appeared in scattered areas of India, Burma, parts of the Far East, Northern Australia and the United States. It is acquired accidentally by man, probably through contamination of food by urine or faeces of infected animals, usually rats. It does not spread from man to man.

Loefflerella whitmori is a small Gram-negative aerobic organism which can be cultured from the pus of the abscesses that are a common feature of the disease and sometimes from the blood during fever.

Pathology

Lesions resembling those of glanders may develop in any tissue of the body, especially the lungs and the liver.

The lesions are developed about organisms distributed embolically as a pyaemia. They begin as small nodes of cellular reaction the centres of which become necrotic and caseous. The abscesses may become large and confluent in course of time and give rise to signs and symptoms depending on their locality. The organism can usually be cultured from pus obtained from the lesions. Healing may occur in one area and be followed by new abscesses in other parts of the body.

Signs and Symptoms

There are two main clinical forms of the disease, the pyaemic and the septicaemic.

The pyaemic pattern is the more common. Lesions and abscesses form in succession in the organs or connective tissues. Individual lesions commonly occur in the lungs and the liver, causing local signs and symptoms which vary according to the size and severity of the abscesses produced. Local adenitis is common or there may be general glandular enlargement and tenderness. One abscess may follow another in these areas or appear in other parts of the body including the bones, especially the ribs, periosteal tissues and the central nervous system. The physical signs depend on the sites and numbers of the abscesses and the current stage of their development. Constitutional signs are severe. There is emaciation, irregular remittent fever and sweating. There may be anaemia and a moderate leucocytosis.

The development of the disease is slow and progressive. Most cases die. A few, even with numerous abscesses, may survive with treatment.

The septicaemic form of the disease is nearly always fatal. There is a high swinging fever and heavy sweating. The patient is prostrated and frequently shows signs of pulmonary, pleural or gastro-intestinal involvement, including diarrhoea. The liver and spleen enlarge. There is a mild leucocytosis. Some cases may be fulminating with death occurring in a few days. The usual duration is several weeks. Response to treatment is poor.

Diagnosis

This finally depends on the isolation and identification of the organism, either from a focus of pus or from the blood. The organism may be seen in smears made from the pus and recovered by culture or after inoculation of pus into suitable animals.

Agglutinins may be first detected in the serum a fortnight after infection, but are of little diagnostic value.

Treatment

Individual organisms may be shown to be sensitive to certain antibiotics and sulphonamides but the exhibition of these drugs may not affect the course of the disease. In favourable cases sulphadiazine has proved effective in doses of 3 G. daily, continued until the fever has subsided. *Loeff. whitmori* is usually sensitive to chloramphenicol which should be given in the usual doses but in this highly toxaemic disease, the use of this drug has its own dangers, especially in depressing leucopoiesis and the number of circulating thrombocytes. Tetracyclines may also be useful.

Drainage of abscesses is necessary, if possible, and the abscess cavity may be injected with antibiotics.

Nursing is very important and the patient needs good psychological handling as depression is common.

REFERENCE

THIN, R. N. T., BROWN, M., STEWART, J. B., and GARRETT, C. J. (1970) Melioidosis: A report of ten cases, *Quart. J. Med.*, N.S. **39**, 115.

INFECTIONS DUE TO SPIRILLACEAE

CHOLERA

Definition

Cholera is an acute, often fatal, self-limited disease caused by infection with one of the several strains of *Vibrio cholerae*.

Aetiology

The organism multiplies in the gut lumen but does not penetrate beyond the epithelial wall of the gut which remains more or less intact throughout the acute episode. The disease is characterized by very copious, watery diarrhoea, severe watery vomiting, the rapid development of extreme dehydration and muscular cramps, and complications which arise from the physiological effects of the fluid and electrolyte loss, particularly shock and anuria with renal failure.

The disease normally has a limited geographical distribution.

The endemic areas of the three classical strains of cholera are in regions of poverty and poor sanitation and standards of living in India (Bengal and Madras, in particular), East Pakistan and central China. In the last decade a fourth strain of cholera El Tor (see below) which was endemic in Indonesia has appeared in many parts of South-East Asia and the Western Pacific, including Sulawesi (where it was endemic) and other parts of Indonesia, the Philippines, Thailand, Malaysia, Cambodia, Burma and Hong Kong. Small outbreaks or isolated cases have also occurred in places as far west as Iraq and contiguous countries.

Epidemic and pandemic extensions of cholera have happened at irregular intervals along traditional trade routes and other lines of communication between endemic areas and other countries. In the last decade modern air transport has added an important potential factor for spread and there have been several very severe outbreaks in South-East Asia, and recently in Africa south of the Sahara, all caused by the El Tor organism.

The causative organism is *Vibrio cholerae*, a small comma-shaped motile organism which is Gram-negative and grows easily on ordinary media at 99° F. (37° C.). The vibrios are divided into groups depending on their antigenic composition. The three so-called 'classical' cholera vibrios, one or more of which predominated in epidemics and outbreaks before the last decade, were the strains Inaba, Ogawa and Hikojima which have a common H antigen and specific somatic or O antigens. Since 1961, most major appearances of cholera have been caused by a fourth strain, El Tor, which was normally endemic in Sulawesi and possibly elsewhere in Indonesia and which has now largely replaced the classical strains in the traditional endemic cholera areas, except in East Pakistan, and has become established in certain areas of South-East Asia, including the Philippines and Thailand.

The El Tor organism is serologically closely related to the classical strains of cholera vibrios but differs in certain respects. It causes haemolysis *in vitro* in conditions under which the other strains do not and can be identified by specific haemagglutination tests and by its resistance to certain phages which destroy the other vibrios.

The El Tor vibrio was once thought to give rise to only clinically mild disease, but is now recognized as the cause of severe clinical cholera indistinguishable from that induced by the classical strains of the organism. Cholera El Tor is thus accepted as an internationally quarantinable disease.

The cholera organisms appear in nature to be pathogenic only to man. They can be transmitted to animals, but do not produce an equivalent pathological picture.

In man the vibrio remains in the gut contents in which it multiplies in enormous numbers. It is not found in the blood stream.

During the clinical attack the vibrio is found in the faeces and the vomit in astronomical numbers. In infections caused by the classical vibrios the organisms rapidly disappear from the faeces and seldom remain in them for more than 7–10 days after the overt symptoms have subsided.

The vibrio can survive for some days on moist clothing and in slightly dirty water. It does not survive long in clean water and is easily killed by heat and acids.

The infection spreads orally in a community by ingestion of infected water contaminated with excreta from an infected individual, or of other potable fluids including milk, and food such as cold cooked meat, fruit and vegetables which may have been sprinkled with water. Infection also spreads from one person to another by direct contact with the infected stool or vomitus. Occasionally the domestic fly may, under epidemic conditions, act as a mechanical vector.

In endemic areas the disease persists throughout the year, becoming more obvious at certain periods when it is transmitted freely amongst the population. Most cases in endemic areas occur in the hot, moist season, possibly because the rains flush the local filthy water supplies and infect other sources of water. Thus in Bengal the incidence is highest in the early rains, that is to say in May to July and lowest in the dry season.

Outbreaks arise from the introduction of the vibrio by infected persons. Once the disease is introduced into a population it spreads by the same means as above and when sanitation is bad cholera becomes established.

The El Tor organism may often be found in the stool weeks or even months after the clinical attack. One individual in the Philippines (Cholera Dolores) has been passing the same strain at intervals for 8 years. 'Carriers' of this infection therefore exist and are of considerable importance in the maintenance and spread of the disease. In this respect modern fast air travel has also favoured spread to areas in which the requisite bad sanitary standards exist. In the El Tor outbreaks of recent times, the person-to-person mode of spread is regarded as the most important element in transmission. The situation is worsened by the existence of healthy carriers who pass the organism in the faeces but have no obvious clinical effects.

Where sanitary conditions are good, there is little

chance of spread. In non-endemic areas control of cholera will usually follow the ordinary methods of prevention, quarantine, and so forth. Where cholera has developed the local water supplies must be examined and must be protected against infection. Chlorination is successful; failing this, all drinking water should be boiled, and possibly contaminated food avoided.

Some protection may be offered by vaccination with dead vibrios, but there is some doubt about the efficacy of this procedure. The standardized vaccine is given in two doses at an interval of a week for individuals and as a single dose in mass vaccination of populations during an outbreak.

When a population is exposed to infection by no means all become infected and of those infected by no means all show the acute severe effects. The natural barrier to infection is not fully understood, although it is possible that since the organism is so sensitive to acid, an acid gastric secretion may limit the spread of moderate infection by destroying the organism before it can reach the intestine in which it develops.

In a community a cholera outbreak is self-limited and usually dies out soon after reaching its peak. The explanation of this is not clear. There is no evidence that the infected individual develops any immediate immunity against the infection, since he may be re-infected after a short interval. All members of the population appear to be susceptible if exposed, but many may become infected without overt signs. Age and sex have little to do with the spread of infection, except in circumstances where the habits limit the usage of water to a particular group within the community.

Pathology

The pathological changes produced by the organism in the gut itself are minimal. The vibrio develops and multiplies in the lumen along the whole length of the intestine but particularly in the small intestine and does not invade the gut wall. The physiological lesion is the loss of enormous quantities of water and electrolytes from the tissues, via the intestinal lumen. Recent observations on biopsies of the intestinal wall have indicated that even at the height of the infection the epithelium remains essentially intact. It is presumed that the pathogenic activity of the vibrio depends on the production of poisonous substances, probably endotoxins, which are formed during the growth and lysis of the vibrio in the gut lumen content. Experimentally an endotoxin produced from the vibrio has been shown to affect the permeability of physiological membranes to electrolytes and water. This is probably the basic process in the enormous losses of fluid and salt which occur in the disease. It seems possible that in addition to excessive outpouring of fluid and salts into the lumen there is also at some level in the gut a failure of resorption of water and that this in itself may be the major factor in the extreme losses which occur. For such processes to continue an intact epithelium must be postulated so that it can act as an intact organ.

An individual not receiving extraneous fluid may lose 5 or more litres in 24 hours, through diarrhoea and to some lesser extent through vomiting.

The alkaline fluid passed from the intestine contains sodium chloride in isotonic concentration and concentrations of bicarbonate and potassium in excess of those in plasma. The latter may be concentrated as much as five times.

There is a concurrent dramatic removal of extracellular fluid and loss of potassium from the cells. The loss of fluid is reflected in a striking fall of plasma water volume, but the true loss of electrolytes is not reflected in the chemical composition of the plasma. The total chloride concentration may be normal or slightly lowered; the sodium may also be low, but is usually higher in proportion; the potassium concentration is usually little changed, but may be raised, despite the great losses in patients in hypovolaemic shock. The loss of base and bicarbonate leads to varying degrees of acidosis, which can usually be adjusted by therapy.

Other changes in the blood include a rise of blood urea nitrogen which occurs in all cases with haemoconcentration. In anuric cases the non-protein nitrogen of the blood, which includes the urea nitrogen, rises very considerably and may reach several hundred milligrammes per 100 ml.

Parenteral administration of electrolyte solutions will usually rapidly restore the water/electrolyte balance of the body and make up the losses. The evacuation does not, however, as a rule, stop immediately, and may continue for 24 hours or more. In this time the loss of fluid from the intestine may be as much as 15–20 litres, which is replaced volume for volume by the infusion. The evacuation eventually ceases rapidly and the need for intravenous replacement ceases with it.

The initial loss of extracellular fluid and electrolytes shows clinically as sudden and increasing asthenia, rapid loss of weight, visible 'shrinking' of the patient, loss of tone and elasticity of the skin which is stretched over bony prominences, such as the malar bones; the eyes are 'sunken'.

Circulating plasma water is lost and haemoconcentration results with increased viscosity of the plasma with associated rise in concentration of protein. Venous return to the heart and cardiac output are diminished; the blood pressures fall and circulation is maintained by selective reduction of flow through visceral organs, notably the liver and the kidneys. If the situation is allowed to continue (for example, in the absence of fluid replacement) hypovolaemic shock develops, from which the patient may die.

The tissue changes are basically non-specific and are derived from the physiological effects of the loss of water and electrolytes. These include changes in the renal circulation leading, as in other conditions to acute renal failure, with anuria and uraemia. Degenerative changes which occur concurrently in the renal tubules persist for some time after recovery. The circulation through the liver is also restricted and degenerative and necrotic lesions may develop in the centrilobular regions, especially in shocked cases. The gall-bladder and bile-ducts are filled as a rule with dark viscid inspissated bile, following fluid resorption from the ducts. In the shocked case pulmonary oedema may occur as a terminal event.

The stools are watery, of low specific gravity, and

contain flecks of mucus and occasional shreds of epithelium. The so-called 'rice water stool' which is characteristic of the severe case, derives its appearance from the mucus and a background of millions upon millions of vibrios. The stools are always alkaline. Once the severe episode is finished the stools become less frequent and begin to contain more and more faecal matter. Recovery is rapid in this respect.

The urinary output is low during the acute attack, at any time during which anuria may develop. The urine may appear highly concentrated and deeply pigmented but the electrolyte content is low and there is often no sodium or chloride present. In an acute attack the protein present in the urine accounts for the high specific gravity. After recovery the electrolyte concentrations return to normal at a rate dependent on the amount of damage that has occurred in the renal tubules. In anuric cases on recovery there may be a period of several days during which there is diuresis with the passage of large volumes of unconcentrated urine.

Signs and Symptoms

Infection with the cholera vibrio produces a clinical picture which varies from no obvious change to the severe classical watery diarrhoea case. The majority of clinically overt cases conform to the classical picture.

The disease is of short duration, seldom lasting more than five days, and often not more than three. The incubation period is difficult to determine in most cases, but varies anywhere between a few hours to five days.

The classical attack starts with evacuation, which is essentially an uncontrollable diarrhoea which starts mildly, rapidly empties the bowel of faeces and then becomes the urgent passage of voluminous watery stools which appear to contain little more than water and some flecks of mucus, but in fact contain vast numbers of the vibrio which give the fluid an opalescent appearance, readily seen against a dark background by transmitted light.

During evacuation stools are very frequent and are passed effortlessly and completely without control. They are often passed with considerable force as though a tap had been turned on full. There is no pain or colic and the patient is hardly aware that he is evacuating. The same is true of the vomiting, which may come on without nausea as the sudden explosive discharge of volumes of opalescent fluid. Contamination of bedclothing and surroundings is therefore to be expected in cholera and this is particularly important to the doctor or the attendant who gets in the way of either the stool or the vomit; both are highly infective.

Evacuation continues in the untreated case for 3–5 days and is accompanied by a rapid and severe dehydration the progress of which becomes visible, the patient shrinking in front of the observer. Enormous amounts of fluids and electrolytes are lost. The subcutaneous fluid is lost, the skin becomes inelastic and stretched over the underlying tissues, the eyes are shrunken into their sockets, the malar bones prominent. The mouth and tongue are dry; there is extreme thirst and the voice becomes husky.

The patient remains mentally clear, but is usually anxious and restless. As dehydration continues, the blood pressure falls, the pulse quickens and vascular collapse may supervene, the picture closely resembling that of severe heat exhaustion. Once dehydration has become established, muscle cramps may develop. They are frequent, severe, painful, of short duration, and arise particularly in the legs and the back.

During evacuation and dehydration the temperature seldom rises above normal and is frequently subnormal.

From the beginning the urinary volume is reduced and as dehydration proceeds it still further diminishes, even in the milder cases. In severe cases there may be almost complete urinary suppression during the period of the evacuation and the urine passed has a low electrolyte content, and contains albumin and granular casts. When vascular collapse develops there is still further reduction of urine volume, but even without this event, anuria and consequent renal failure and uraemia may develop.

Associated with the dehydration there is rapidly developing haemoconcentration with the usual increase in erythrocyte count and haemoglobin levels and an increase in the viscosity of the blood.

At this stage the combined effects of dehydration and shock will frequently kill the patient. His future in any case is decided by the degree of dehydration and the length of time over which it proceeds before it is corrected, and by the presence or absence of vascular collapse.

The patient may completely recover and from the moment that evacuation ceases is in no further danger. He then passes into the stage of reaction in which there is a rise of blood pressure, an improvement in the volume of the pulse which slows, a return of normal skin colour, a rise of body temperature, sometimes to above normal, and the cessation of evacuation and vomiting. If, however, the vascular collapse continues, changes in the organs may be induced especially in the kidney and acute renal failure or hepatic failure may develop. Such cases usually die and in the late stages have a very high blood urea concentration. Even in these late stages when they are uraemic and oedematous sudden recovery may take place. In some patients the anuria does not develop until two or three days after recovery from the collapse stage and it is therefore necessary to give a guarded prognosis until this period has passed. In some cases after a brief remission circulatory failure may become re-established and the patient may die of shock or cardiac failure.

In the fatal cases, however, the common sequence of events is evacuation followed without remission by vascular collapse.

The progress of the disease is a matter of only a few days and sometimes only a matter of a few hours. Recovery upon restoration of hydration is rapid and remarkable. The shrunken, miserable corpse-like patient rapidly and visibly swells and becomes something approaching normal.

Prognosis depends on the length of time elasping from the onset to the time of replacement of fluid. The governing element is the degree of fluid and electrolyte loss.

The most serious complications are circulatory and renal failure. If anuria develops the outlook is bad.

Cases which develop anuria are usually severely oliguric from the outset. Other complications, such as pneumonia, pulmonary oedema, and gangrene of the extremities in old people in whom the circulation has failed, occur from time to time.

Once the tissue fluid replacement has been achieved, the patient recovers swiftly. The death rate in untreated cases is very high. In properly treated cases it varies from 1–5 per cent.

Diagnosis

The clinical picture of cholera in its worst form is so startling that there is never much doubt about the diagnosis. The condition may occasionally be mistaken for staphylococcal or other food poisoning or choleraic *P. falciparum* infection, in which the syndrome is identical. Malaria may exist concurrently in an individual and in any doubt, a blood film should be examined. Shock and anuria may occur in many other acute conditions, but, with the exception of heat exhaustion, in the absence of severe dehydration.

The diagnosis of an isolated case of cholera may be difficult. Vibrios may be seen in wet specimens of faeces and vomit, but identification of the organism must be carried out bacteriologically. The faeces or material obtained by rectal swabbing should be inoculated direct into alkaline peptone water and incubated at 37° C. for a few hours. The ordinary faecal organisms are controlled by the alkalinity and the vibrio concentrates near the surface of the media. The bacteriological investigation should, however, be left to the bacteriologist. In any case, even when the diagnosis remains in doubt, the treatment of severe dehydration must be undertaken immediately.

Treatment

The vital treatment consists in the replacement of the water and electrolytes. Sodium chloride is probably the most important electrolyte needing immediate replacement but severe losses of potassium also occur and must be corrected.

The replacement of fluid and electrolytes is carried out by intravenous administration of isotonic sodium chloride solution in the first instance.

The amount of rehydration required initially may be estimated from measurement of the specific gravity of whole blood or plasma or from clinical evidence of the patient's condition based on the presence or absence of an easily felt radial pulse, the lowering of pulse pressure as both blood pressures fall, signs of fluid at the pulmonary bases, the facial appearance and condition of the skin. An important factor is the weight. In some clinics a rough estimate of the requirements in a serious case is calculated on the basis of 10 per cent. of the presumed normal body weight expressed as litres; for instance a severely ill man of 50–60 kg. body weight would need up to 5 litres of electrolyte solution for immediate rehydration.

The essential thing is to carry out this replacement as quickly as possible and to judge further treatment by the improvement or otherwise of the patient and the amount of fluid being lost.

It may be necessary, because of the temporary persistence of evacuation, to continue administration of parenteral fluid for 24 hours or longer after initial rehydration. The parenteral fluid requirements at this stage may be considerably reduced by oral administration of diluted isotonic saline containing lactate and potassium chloride.

The intravenous infusion may be given into the jugular vein if the arm veins are collapsed, as they may be in shock, but the latter are usually available after the first litre or two and the needle may be transferred. It is sometimes necessary to cut down on to the arm veins.

The first litre should be run in as quickly as possible, in 5–10 minutes and the second litre in the next 30 minutes. Subsequent infusion may continue at the rate of about 80 drops per minute until the rehydration volume has been given. Thereafter, the amount of infusion depends on the clinical state; it should be continued until the radial pulse becomes full and the pulse pressure is restored to 20–30 mm. Hg.

The fluid is then given at the same rate as the output, which is measured as a routine.

Acidosis is countered by adding lactate, sodium bicarbonate or acetate to the saline solution. A common solution is prepared by mixing 2 volumes of isotonic saline and 1 volume of isotonic sodium lactate (1·75 per cent.). Bicarbonate as an alternative must be added as sterile powder (14–20·5 G. per litre); the solution must not be sterilized by heat. Acidosis, indicated clinically by air hunger and restlessness, is usually controlled during the initial rehydration, i.e. during the administration of the first 3–5 litres in a severe case.

Potassium depletion can be managed by the addition of 5 ml. of a 15 per cent. potassium chloride solution to each litre of infusion. It should not be given until signs of rehydration are evident and the rate of infusion should not exceed 200 ml. per hour.

In rare cases there may be some temporary hyperkalaemia, indicated by electrocardiogram. In these circumstances potassium must not be added to the infusion fluid.

When evacuation ceases, and signs of rehydration are present, intravenous infusion should be stopped and oral fluids substituted.

An input/output fluid balance record should be kept during rehydration.

It is fatal to overload the patient with fluid, particularly if he is in vascular collapse or in anuria.

The first injection of saline brings about almost immediate relief and recovery is usually very rapid. It is rarely necessary to continue intravenous therapy after 24 hours.

If evacuation is continuing during replacement therapy, the fluid input/output record is most important and in these circumstances much larger quantities of intravenous fluid may be given without undue worry.

After recovery a diet rich in potassium and containing such things as fruit juice and coconut milk is advisable.

Acute renal failure and shock in cholera are essentially similar to such emergencies in other acute medical conditions and should be treated accordingly. Infusion of noradrenaline has been found useful by some workers.

The oral administration of tetracycline, 250 mg. 6-

hourly for 48 hours, usually terminates the diarrhoea and removes the vibrios from the stool. The clinical effect is often remarkable and the removal of the infective organism from the intestinal discharge is of considerable public health importance especially in isolated cases. In El Tor infections bacteriological relapse is common; the vibrios sometimes reappear months after clinical cure, especially following purgation. Where evacuation persists beyond 2 days from the beginning of treatment, the drug should be continued until the diarrhoea stops.

In dealing with the immediate attack certain things may require symptomatic treatment and of these, perhaps muscle cramps are the most immediate. Any kind of pain-relieving drug, including anaesthetics, but excepting morphine, may be used. The cramps subside with rehydration.

The patient should be persuaded to take fluid by mouth as soon as the vomiting stops. Careful nursing is essential. In the convalescent state he must be kept quiet in view of the possibility of further vascular collapse.

REFERENCES

LINDENBAUM, J., GREENOUGH, D. B., and ISLAM, M. R. (1967) Antibiotic treatment of cholera, *Bull. Wld Hlth Org.*, **36**, 871.

PHILIPPINES CHOLERA COMMITTEE (1965) A controlled field trial of the effectiveness of cholera and cholera El Tor vaccines in the Philippines: Preliminary report, *Bull. Wld Hlth Org.*, **32**, 603.

PHILLIPS, R. A. (1967) Twenty years of cholera research, *J. Amer. med. Ass.*, **202** (2), 610.

WATTEN, R. H., GUTMAN, R. A., and FRESH, J. W. (1969) Comparison of acetate, lactate and bicarbonate in treating the acidosis of cholera, *Lancet*, ii, 512.

WORLD HEALTH ORGANIZATION (1967) Expert Committee on Cholera, *Spec. Rep. Ser.*, No. 352.

RAT BITE FEVERS

Rat bite fevers, which are world wide in distribution, are due to infection with two distinct organisms, *Spirillum minus* and *Actinobacillus muris*. The organisms occur normally in rats and other small animals and invade man as a result of a bite. Human cases are thus incidental and sporadic. The clinical syndrome is characterized by a relapsing febrile illness of long duration, often with recurring inflammation at the area of the bite wound and involvement of the local lymph nodes. There is also a short-term eruption and muscle and joint pains during the attacks. The mortality is low.

Aetiology

The attack commonly follows a bite but infection may be spread by other means, for example *Actinobacillus muris* may be transmitted in milk, and either infection may be acquired from contaminated food. *Spirillum minus* is a short, rigid body with 2–5 spirals, it stains well with Leishman and readily infects animals. It is found in the tissues, blood, lymph-node juice and peritoneal fluid. *Actinobacillus* can also be recovered from the organs of naturally infected rats especially from the lungs and nasopharynx. It is a Gram-negative pleomorphic micro-organism forming long filaments in culture. It causes the epizootics in mice.

Pathology

The infection may be septicaemic. Spleen, liver and lymph nodes may be enlarged. Arthritis with effusion occurs and renal and hepatic failure may supervene.

Signs and Symptoms

The two infections produce similar clinical pictures which may be difficult to separate. The incubation period in *Spirillum minus* infections is 5–30 days, usually about 2 weeks. In *Actinobacillus* infections it is a little shorter, about 2–10 days. The bite wound often appears to be healing when the illness commences. It then becomes re-inflamed and may develop a chancre-like ulceration with marked regional lymphangitis and adenitis. Onset is marked by a rapid rise in temperature and a remittent fever which may last 2–4 days or as long as a week, followed by a short remission for 3–7 days and further febrile episodes. Relapses occur frequently. An eruption appears as a blue-red or purple mottled erythema on the upper part of the trunk, tending to extend over the trunk and limbs. The spleen is commonly enlarged in *Actinobacillus* infection.

Epidemics, apparently due to contaminated food, have been recorded. The clinical picture differs from that due to rat bite. There is abrupt onset of fever with a maculopapular rash, followed within the first 5 days, by an acute polyarthritis. Bacterial endocarditis has been reported. This form of infection has also been described under the titles of Haverhill fever and erythema arthriticum epidemicum.

Diagnosis

Spirillum minus. The organisms do not occur in great numbers in the blood even at the height of the fever. It is not usually possible to find them in blood films, but they can be found in preparations of oedema fluids from inflamed areas, such as the site of the bite, using dark ground illumination, or in films stained with Leishman or Giemsa. The organisms may be recovered in the blood or tissue fluid of mice inoculated with blood, oedema fluid or lymph-node juice taken from the patient during fever. There is no growth on culture media.

Actinobacillus. Animals are not easily infected with this organism but it can be cultured from blood taken during a period of fever and inoculated into beef infusion broth plus rabbit serum. The presence of infection may also be detected by specific agglutination reactions with the serum from the patient.

Treatment

For infections with *Spirillum minus* organic arsenicals may be used, for example 400–600 mg. neoarsphenamine intravenously at 3-day intervals for 3 doses. Equally successful are penicillin in large doses and streptomycin, 1 G. daily for 10 days.

Actinobacillus infection is best treated with benzylpenicillin, 200 mg. (300,000 Units) six-hourly, or 600 mg. (1 mega Unit) of procaine benzylpenicillin twice a day until the temperature returns to normal, then half the dose for a week. Chlortetracylcine is also effective in the doses given for relapsing fever.

BRIAN MAEGRAITH

INFECTIONS DUE TO ENTEROBACTERIACEAE AND RELATED ORGANISMS

BACTERIOLOGY

The bacteria, the Enterobacteriaceae, to be discussed under this head are *Escherichia coli* and members of the genus *Proteus*. *Pseudomonas pyocyanea* (*Ps. aeruginosa*) is also considered although belonging to the pseudomonadales for it occurs clinically in the same situations as enterobacteriaceae.

All these organisms are Gram-negative. They usually possess flagella and are therefore motile. This property is most evident in some members of the *Proteus* group where it is responsible for the phenomenon of spreading in culture on solid media. They all elaborate endotoxin but it is uncertain whether it is responsible for the clinical features which mark general infection with Enterobacteriaceae. *Ps. pyocyanea* is distinguished by its ability to form a green pigment, pyocyanin, which stains the culture medium surrounding its colonies and may colour discharges from infected patients.

Methods are now becoming available for identifying strains of all three groups of these organisms. When these have been applied to the study of human infection a much clearer pattern should emerge.

EPIDEMIOLOGY

All the bacteria considered here may be inhabitants of the human bowel, *Esch. coli* is constantly present and its discovery elsewhere is taken as an indicator of faecal contamination. The others are less exclusively colonic, and with many related Gram-negative bacilli may be found on grains, plants, in soil and water, and sometimes on the skin.

In the colon these organisms are for the most part harmless residents: some may even have beneficial activities. Outside their normal habitat they are all capable of causing serious infection and invasion is particularly likely to occur when local or general resistance is reduced. A familiar example is to be found in the influence of obstruction on the development of infections of the urinary tract.

HUMAN INFECTION

Local

The Alimentary Tract. Since the alimentary tract is the usual habitat of this group of organisms, invasion of tissues anatomically related is naturally the commonest expression of infection. *Esch. coli* is dominant in these because it enjoys an overwhelming majority in the colon. It is constantly found in cholecystitis, appendicitis, diverticulitis and perforative peritonitis, although in company with other organisms.

It is now accepted that some strains of *Esch. coli* can cause epidemic diarrhoea in infants. Some 20 varieties of these enteropathogenic strains have been recognized: they are distinguished from non-pathogenic organisms by agglutination with specific sera made against their 'O' antigens and are denoted by such symbols as O 55 and O 111.

The Urinary Tract. Acute and chronic pyelitis, pyelonephritis and cystitis are amongst the commonest infections due to this group of bacteria. *Esch. coli* heads the list, but some 13 per cent. are due to strains of *Proteus* and a like proportion to *Ps. pyocyanea.* In many instances some local impediment to urinary flow predisposes to infection. The predominance in women suggests that the invading bacteria usually enter from without, but the precise route they follow has been the subject of unprofitable debate for many years.

Meningitis. Meningitis in the neonate is often due to Enterobacteriaceae and is particularly likely to complicate meningocele. It has also been recorded on a number of occasions as following spinal anaesthesia when the responsible organism has been *Ps. pyocyanea.*

Miscellaneous. These organisms may infect open wounds, areas of chronic infection and devitalized tissues. Metastatic infection is rare. They are often found in the sputa of patients receiving antibiotics, but in these circumstances are of little relevance. They can, however, be a cause of pneumonia in the debilitated.

Ps. pyocyanea is often found in tap water and may resist the conventional antiseptics; it is therefore likely to make an appearance when aseptic technique has been faulty.

General

Septicaemia due to organisms of this group has increased in frequency and importance of recent years. The bacteria most often isolated are *Esch. coli*, *Ps. pyocyanea* and other related Gram-negative bacteria of intestinal origin. About three quarters of these infections appear to be acquired in hospital. They are seen especially in elderly men and middle-aged women, being twice as common in the male as in the female. Infection is almost invariably secondary to some local lesion: in 50 per cent. this is in the urinary tract and in two thirds of these cases the septicaemia follows operation or instrumentation. In a further 20 per cent. the gastro-intestinal tract provides the initial focus. It is a recognized complication of hepatic cirrhosis. In this form of septicaemia the importance of such general factors as prolonged debilitating disease and treatment with corticosteroid drugs is particularly apparent.

The clinical picture may be characteristic. The patient is often an elderly man, weakened by prolonged illness such as malignant disease or chronic urinary retention. The onset is abrupt and may follow operation on the urinary tract. There is often an initial rigor followed by intermittent fever with vomiting and diarrhoea. Serious disturbances in electrolyte metabolism are common and contribute to the gravity of the illness. A rising level of potassium in the serum with falls in those of sodium and chloride is frequently seen. Renal failure is often an additional complication. In some patients profound circulatory failure described as 'bacteraemic shock', is a feature: this is said to be particularly characteristic of *Proteus* septicaemia.

Pseudomonas septicaemia is often accompanied by leucopenia and in the debilitated, in whom it is particularly likely to occur, may give rise to a characteristic ulcerative lesion of the skin, ecthyma gangrenosum. This infection is associated with vasculitis and a generalized Schwartzman reaction with extensive intravascular coagulation has been recorded.

DIAGNOSIS

The diagnosis of infection due to this group of organisms follows the usual principles. There is seldom any difficulty in isolating the bacterium, but it is less easy to be certain that it is responsible for the patient's illness. The Gram-negative bacilli are so commonly secondary invaders of wounds and burns and their constant presence in the bowel makes it hard to know when they should be regarded as pathogenic. There is seldom doubt in a case of septicaemia.

TREATMENT

The details of treatment are discussed fully in the relevant sections and in the chapter on antibiotics. The Gram-negative bacilli have a peculiar facility for developing resistance to antibiotics. This is particularly true of *Esch. coli* and *Proteus* when streptomycin is used in treatment. In the selection of the appropriate drug for the treatment of these infections laboratory tests of sensitivity have abundantly proved their value.

The circulatory failure of 'bacteraemic shock' requires energetic treatment with antibiotics, blood transfusion, intravenous hydrocortisone and possibly vasopressor agents. Electrolyte disturbances require correction.

REFERENCES

DuPont, H. L., and Spink, W. W. (1969) Infections due to Gram-negative organisms: an analysis of 860 patients with bacteremia at the University of Minnesota Medical Center 1958–1966, *Medicine (Baltimore)*, **48**, 307.

Forkner, C. E. Jr., Frei, E. III, Edgcomb, J. H., and Utz, J. P. (1958) Pseudomonas septicaemia. Observations on twenty-three cases, *Amer. J. Med.*, **25**, 877.

Hewitt, C. B., Overholt, E. L., Finder, R. J., and Patton, J. F. (1965) Gram-negative septicaemia in urology, *J. Urol. (Baltimore)*, **93**, 299.

Lewis, J., and Fekety, F. R. Jr. (1969) Proteus bacteraemia, *Johns Hopk. med. J.*, **124**, 151.

McNaught, W., and Stevenson, J. S. (1953) Coliform diarrhoea in adult hospital patients, *Brit. med. J.*, **2**, 182.

Rapaport, S. I., Tatter, D., Coeur-Barron, N., and Hjort, P. F. (1964) Pseudomonas septicaemia with intravascular clotting leading to the generalised Schwartzman reaction, *New-Engl. J. Med.*, **271**, 80.

Tillotson, J. R., and Lerner, A. M. (1966) Pneumonias caused by Gram-negative bacilli, *Medicine (Baltimore)*, **45**, 65.

Weil, M. H., Shubin, H., and Biddle, M. (1964) Shock caused by Gram-negative micro-organisms. Analyses of 169 cases, *Ann. intern. Med.*, **60**, 384.

KLEBSIELLA INFECTIONS

BACTERIOLOGY

Bacteria of the genus *Klebsiella* are Gram-negative capsulate motile bacilli of the family of Enterobacteriaciae. The most important representative is *Kl. pneumoniae* also known as the pneumobacillus, Friedländer's bacillus and *Bacillus mucosus capsulatus*. Other members include *Kl. aerogenes* (formerly *Aerobacter aerogenes*), *Kl. edwardsii*, *Kl. rhinoscleromatis* and *Kl. ozaenae*.

Kl. pneumoniae is found in the upper respiratory passages of some 5 per cent. of healthy individuals and in the stools of a like proportion. Utilizing the capsular antigen some 80 types of Klebsiellae can be recognized. The somatic or 'O' antigens allow further subdivision into groups. *Serratia marcescens*, formerly known as *Bacillus prodigiosus*, is also a member of this group.

HUMAN INFECTIONS

Local

The Respiratory Tract. In man *Kl. pneumoniae* characteristically causes pulmonary infection. Type 1 (A) strains are responsible for about 60 per cent. of cases and most of the remainder are due to Type 2 (B). It is a common secondary invader in patients with bronchiectasis and chronic tuberculosis. It is responsible for about 1 per cent. of cases of acute primary pneumonia. This infection is most frequent between the ages 40 and 60 years and tends to attack debilitated patients. It often gives rise to a serious illness.

In many instances the acute infection becomes chronic with recurrent abscess formation, fibrosis and progressive destruction of pulmonary tissue.

Miscellaneous. *Kl. pneumoniae* is often responsible for infection of the urinary and the genital tracts; it is sometimes recovered from otitis media; occasionally it is the cause of suppurative pylephlebitis and meningitis.

General

Kl. rhinoscleromatis is responsible for rhinoscleroma, a chronic granulomatous disease of the mucosa of the upper respiratory tract seen in South-East Europe. It is uncertain whether *Kl. ozaenae* is the prime cause of ozaena for it is found in patients not suffering from this condition.

General infections with *Kl. pneumoniae* are uncommon but have the same characters as those due to other Gram-negative bacilli. Acute septicaemic, pyaemic and enteric types may be recognized. These forms cause a high mortality. Occasionally a local lesion is associated with transient bacteraemia and this is common in the early phases of an acute pulmonary infection. *S. marcescens* has recently been inculpated as a cause of postoperative septicaemia and of subacute bacterial endocarditis.

DIAGNOSIS

Diagnosis depends on recovery of the organisms from sputum, pus, urine or blood culture. Examination of a Gram-stained film of sputum enables a presumptive diagnosis to be made and effective treatment to be started before the results of culture are known.

TREATMENT

Infections with *Kl. pneumoniae* are always to be regarded as serious and call for energetic and prompt treatment. Details are to be found in the sections on antibiotics and pneumonia.

REFERENCES

ALTEMEIER, W. A., CULBERTSON, W. R., FULLEN, W. D., and McDONOUGH, J. J. (1969) *Serratia marcescens:* a new threat in surgery, *Arch. Surg.*, **99**, 232.

COWAN, S. T., STEEL, K. J., SHAW, C., and DUGUID, J. P. (1960) A classification of the Klebsiella group, *J. gen. Microbiol.*, **23**, 601.

EDMONDSON, E. B., and SANFORD, J. P. (1967) The Klebsiella-Enterobacter (Aerobacter)-Serratia group, *Medicine (Baltimore)*, **46**, 323.

EDWARDS, P. R., and FIFE, M. A. (1955) Studies in the Klebsiella-Aerogenes group of bacteria, *J. Bact.*, **70**, 382.

WEIL, A. J., BEMJAMINSON, M.A., and DE GUZMAN, B. C. (1964) The Klebsiella-Aerobacter-Serratia division: Its role in common infections of man, *Trans. N.Y. Acad. Sci.*, Ser. II, **27**, 65.

R. BODLEY SCOTT

SHIGELLA INFECTIONS

BACILLARY DYSENTERY

Definition and Aetiology

Bacillary dysentery is caused by infection of the wall of the large gut by species of bacteria of the genus Shigella. Such infection on the one hand may lead to acute bacillary dysentery with the passage of blood and mucus and, on the other, to mild diarrhoea or no overt symptoms at all. In between these extremes is a wide range of diarrhoeas with or without blood and mucus which are clinically too numerous and varied to define.

The acute disease is characterized by a severe colitis associated with diarrhoeal faeces containing blood and mucus and at some stage epithelial debris and pus. The course is acute and febrile and may be associated with local or general complications. The disease is serious in its fully developed form and may be fatal. Local epidemics are common.

Infection with Shigella is world wide in distribution and particularly prevalent under insanitary crowded conditions in which food hygiene is neglected, such as obtains in many parts of the tropics.

Infection results from the swallowing of the organism, usually in dirty food or water which has been contaminated with human faeces containing the bacteria. Infected individuals pass enormous numbers of organisms in the stools, particularly in an acute attack, and may continue to pass infective material long after the attack has subsided. Thus, a carrier state not unlike that in typhoid may develop. Four groups of Shigella are recognized: A, *Sh. dysenteriae*; B, *Sh. flexneri*; C, *Sh. boydii*; D, *Sh. sonnei*. Each contains a number of serotypes which do not share antigens. *Sh. sonnei* is an exception, for strains cannot be grouped serologically. The most important clinically are *Sh. flexneri*, *Sh. boydii*, and *Sh. sonnei*. At one time regarded as the most severe form because of its profound toxic effects, but now often considerably milder, is *Sh. dysenteriae*, which is primarily found in hot countries. Infection with *Sh. sonnei*, which causes mild symptoms and sometimes none at all, is widespread and very common in temperate areas.

The organisms are isolated from the faeces or from rectal or sigmoid swabbings and typed by the usual bacteriological methods. Serological investigations in the infected patient are of no diagnostic importance.

Pathology

The organisms multiply in the lumen of the large gut, the wall of which is invaded. An inflammatory reaction ensues which may become very extensive and cause sloughing of the superficial mucosa. Owing to the anatomical distribution of the mucosa, which normally lies in folds transversely across the gut, narrow, shallow, snail-track ulcers develop in serious cases. In very severe infections large areas of the mucosa and submucosa are destroyed and slough. Very acute dysentery with much bleeding results, with excessive secretion of mucus and the discharge of pus. Healing occurs without scarring or with minimal scarring after the subsidence of the infection, but occasionally a postdysenteric colitis may remain after the organisms have gone.

In such circumstances there may be a residual chronic inflammatory reaction in the gut with recurrent superficial ulceration or occasionally abscess formation. Retention cysts produced by blockage of mucus secretion may also develop and from time to time abscess material, mucus and bacilli may be found in the stools.

Inflammatory bacteriologically sterile reactions may occur in tissues remote from the gut, during or subsequent to acute bacillary dysentery, for example in the joints, the eyes (causing iridocyclitis) and the peripheral nerves.

Signs and Symptoms

As stated above, there may be no apparent response to the infection even in cases where the bacilli can be readily recovered from the faeces. This is particularly true in *Sh. sonnei* infections. There may, on the other hand, be sharp diarrhoeic states which are of very short duration and of no particular consequence. These occur commonly in individuals who have recently arrived in an endemic hot area, and are probably caused by ingestion of heavily infected food. Many such bouts of diarrhoea however cannot be bacteriologically identified; some of them are probably not infective, but physiological and result from the effects of ambient high temperature and other physiological factors which may upset the circulation of the gut or the resorption of water from it. In such mild cases of diarrhoea the organisms are seldom recovered.

The acute attack follows an incubation period of variable length which is commonly not more than three days but may be as long as a week or as short as a few hours.

The onset is sudden with gastro-intestinal discomfort, acute diarrhoea, sometimes with nausea and vomiting. The first motions are watery and contain some faecal material but this form of stool is rapidly replaced by the characteristic frequent motions consisting largely of blood and mucus ('red currant jelly') passed in very small amounts at very frequent intervals. The motions consist mostly of mucus and blood with some pus cells and macrophages; there may be some undigested food particles. The passage of the stool is urgent, with tenesmus and severe griping abdominal pain. The abdomen is very tender, especially over the area of the large bowel. The number of motions passed in the day may be as many as 30 to 40 and usually exceeds 20. The patient may have an urgent desire to go to stool which is practically continuous.

An irregular, usually remittent moderate fever accompanies the attack, and persists through the active infection. When treatment is given the fever promptly subsides, the symptoms diminish in intensity and severity and the stools change slowly as their numbers decrease. Blood usually disappears before mucus and the later faeces may become bile stained. The stools become loose and soft and finally of normal consistency. They may continue to contain the bacteria for some time. In the untreated case the acute phase persists for about a week and then gradually subsides. Some cases are very severe and fulminating and death may occur in a few hours or days. The most serious cases may be associated with *Sh. dysenteriae* infection in which, in addition to the dysenteric effects, there is often toxaemia and prostration.

In many cases the characteristic blood and mucus stool may not fully develop and the patient passes frequent wet motions which contain blood and faecal material and are swarming with the organisms. The stools may at times consist of practically nothing but fluid containing mucus, blood and epithelial debris. Occasionally the temperature may reach hyperpyrexic levels or, in patients in whom shock develops, may fall suddenly to subnormal with a corresponding rapid increase in pulse rate.

In severe bacillary dysentery and sometimes in mild cases where there is active and persistent diarrhoea, the loss of fluids and electrolytes from the bowel is considerable and in the more choleraic types may be disastrous, leading to complications such as peripheral vascular failure, very severe salt and water depletion and renal failure. This physiological disturbance is particularly serious in children and needs immediate attention. It adds to the clinical picture the pattern of dehydration, with shrunken eyeballs, tight drawn inelastic skin, and prominent malar prominences.

In the intestine complications may arise from the inflammation. Perforation of the gut, with or without peritonitis, and intestinal haemorrhage following erosion of a large vessel are rare. In the otherwise uncomplicated case as well as in the severer forms, haemorrhoids, polyps and other lesions already present in the gut, such as those caused by bilharziasis, may be exacerbated by the attack.

Diagnosis

Clinical diagnosis in the well-established case is obvious and should be based on the frequent passage of small stools containing macroscopic blood and mucus. The appearance of a sample of stool will help diagnosis. The direct wet preparation reveals an exudate arising from the acute inflammatory process in which will be found erythrocytes, polymorphs, macrophages and mucus.

The stool is usually swarming with bacteria and from it the causative organism can easily be cultivated. Cultivation may also be made from material obtained by rectal swabbing. The faeces should be sent to the bacteriologist as soon as possible. If there is any delay a suitable piece of bloody mucus should be selected from the stool and forwarded in 30 per cent. glycerin in isotonic saline or in other media provided for the purpose. The bacteriologist makes the diagnosis by culture and sugar reactions and other laboratory tests. Serological examination of the patient is not of any great significance.

The diagnosis of the asymptomatic forms of Shigella infection can be made only by isolation of the relevant organisms. It may be suggested by the local existence of an epidemic or of other cases, but bacteriological confirmation is always necessary. Microscopic examination of the stool may indicate the probable diagnosis by disclosure of the inflammatory exudate which also helps to differentiate amoebic dysentery.

Treatment

Treatment of Shigella infection requires the chemotherapy of the organism and the concurrent control of complications, such as dehydration or shock, since these in themselves may kill the patient.

Chemotherapy. Shigella organisms respond to sulphonamides and to many antibiotics. The relatively insoluble sulphonamides, such as sulphaguanidine, succinylsulphathiazole (*Sulfasuxidine*) and phthalylsulphathiazole (*Sulfathalidine*) are usually successful. Phthalylsulphathiazole is the most active and the least likely to be complicated by crystalluria. The dosage in a severe case in an adult is a loading dose of 60 mg. per kg. (usually about 4 G.) followed by half this dosage, 30 mg. per kg. four-hourly until the number of stools is reduced to fewer than 4 in the day. The dosage of 30 mg. per kg. is then continued eight-hourly for a further 3 days. The dosage must not be carried on for more than 10 days.

The soluble sulphonamides are also used but have disadvantages in hot countries and in dehydrated individuals. As chemotherapeutic agents they are, however, extremely successful and may be necessary in cases which do not respond well to the insoluble sulphonamides. Sulphadiazine seems to be the best, given in large doses, up to a maximum of 6 G. in any one day and in divided doses four-hourly, with the usual precaution of providing adequate fluids orally, or keeping the urine alkaline and with a strict fluid input/output account. It is not advisable in cases with extreme dehydration.

Commonly used alternatives are mixtures of sulphonamides, such as *Sulphatriad* in doses of 3 G. initially, then 1 G. four-hourly until the number of stools per day falls to four; thereafter 1 G. six-hourly for 3 days. *Sh. flexneri* and *Sh. sonnei* are readily rendered sulphonamide resistant.

The average severe and mild case of bacillary dysentery responds well to the sulphonamides. Severe cases are more often treated with antibiotics.

Some workers recommend chloramphenicol in doses of 500 mg. six-hourly for 5–7 days.

Tetracyclines in dosages of 2 G. daily in divided doses for up to 5 days are also very successful. Children are given doses in accordance to their body weight.

Streptomycin given orally in doses of 500 mg. twice in the day for 5–7 days regardless of age is also successful.

Combinations of sulphonamides and antibiotics are also commonly used. Examples of these are *Streptotriad* (sulphadimidine, 100 mg., sulphadiazine, 100 mg., sulphathiazole, 100 mg., streptomycin, 65 mg., in each tablet) given in doses of 2 tablets six-hourly for 4 days, and *Guanimycin*, a mixture of streptomycin and sulphaguanidine.

The non-specific effects of dysentery must receive attention concurrently by controlling the dehydration and restoring the fluid and salt balance, and dealing with shock.

Dehydration, when severe, should be countered by intravenous therapy in the usual manner. Where dehydration is excessive the procedure should be the same as in cholera [p. 42]. Milder forms of dehydration can be adjusted by the use of intravenous physiological saline in adults and the use of Darrow's solution diluted 1 in 2 with pyrogen-free water in children. In very severe fluid loss potassium will have to be replaced intravenously or orally. Intravenous administration is given as a solution of not greater than 15 mEq. per litre of saline at about 200 ml. per hour. Oral dosage with potassium chloride, not more than 10 G. per day, is preferable.

Mild cases may be rehydrated by administering water and salt orally. Physiological isotonic saline solution diluted 1 in 4 with water is well tolerated. Potassium chloride, 2 G., may be added six-hourly. In all cases the amount of fluid administered must be limited by the amount of fluid required to restore the physiological balance. This can be estimated in various ways, but for the average patient the clinical estimation is the simplest. In the ordinary course of events not more than 5 litres of fluid will be needed in any one case, and usually less. Overloading with fluid or with potassium may have serious consequences. For this reason all patients should be placed on a strict fluid input/output balance chart.

In infections with *Sh. dysenteriae* a complicating factor may be severe toxaemia which may be relieved by the administration of specific antiserum or concentrated antitoxin. In a suspected case of *Sh. dysenteriae* intoxication specific antitoxin may be given before confirmation of the species is possible, but chemotherapy controls this infection as rapidly and effectively as the others.

REFERENCES

British Medical Journal (1964) Editorial. Drugs for dysentery, **1**, 825.

HUTCHINSON, R. I. (1956) Some observations on the method of spread of Sonne dysentery, *Mth. Bull. Minist. Hlth Lab. Serv.*, **15**, 110.

BRIAN MAEGRAITH

SALMONELLA INFECTIONS

TYPHOID FEVER

Synonyms. Enteric fever; Enterica.

Definition

Typhoid fever is an acute infectious disease characterized by prolonged bacteraemia, continued fever, abdominal symptoms, enlargement of the spleen and, in a proportion of cases, an eruption of rose spots. A relative bradycardia and polymorphonuclear leucopenia are common features.

Aetiology and Epidemiology

Salmonella typhi, the causative organism, is a flagellated Gram-negative rod which is quickly killed by boiling. It is resistant to drying and freezing and may survive for many days in water. It multiplies freely in milk and milk products as well as in shellfish which have lived in sewage-contaminated water. Typing by means of bacteriophages has demonstrated many different strains of typhoid organisms. Over 70 phage-types have been recognized. Phage typing is of great help to the epidemiologist in relating apparently unconnected outbreaks of the disease. Most typhoid strains are Vi-positive (i.e. they contain a Vi antigen) but a few are Vi-negative (see serological diagnosis). Infection takes place through the alimentary tract and is always derived, directly or indirectly, from a human source as man is the only reservoir of the disease. Water, contaminated by sewage, milk or milk products and shellfish such as oysters, mussels and cockles are common vehicles. Outbreaks have also followed consumption of contaminated meats, such as canned corned beef, ice cream, synthetic creams and raw vegetables such as celery or watercress. Laboratory workers have been infected from their cultures and fomites contaminated by excreta may spread the disease. Infected dust does not contribute to spread and typhoid is therefore not a highly infectious disease providing excreta and discharges are disinfected. A strict barrier-nursing technique which includes scrupulous handwashing is necessary to protect attendants.

Typhoid occurs in all parts of the world but is most prevalent in tropical and subtropical countries. Its incidence decreases noticeably with the provision of a pure water supply. Isolated cases or small outbreaks occur in all countries from time to time when food becomes contaminated by a carrier who is usually found to have been associated with some stage of the preparation of the infected food. Similar outbreaks from contamination of a water supply are fortunately much less frequent as they are likely to be devastating. Major epidemics easily develop with the interruption of normal public health services, overcrowding and fall in standards of personal hygiene which occur during wartime. No age is immune but the disease is rare in infants and the elderly. Infection is commonest in those between 5 and 40 years and most statistics show males to be more frequently attacked than females.

Pathology

Typhoid fever is primarily a bacteraemic illness with, as a rule, abdominal symptoms at some stage. After being swallowed, the organisms pass through the mucous membrane of the gut to the mesenteric glands where they multiply. From here they enter the blood stream to invade the liver, spleen and possibly other organs where further multiplication takes place during the remainder of the incubation period. The onset of symptoms is coincident with a further heavier bacteraemia during which organisms reach the Peyer's patches of the small intestine and may lodge in any tissue in the body, thus accounting for the protean manifestations of the disease. This bacteraemia continues for the greater part of the febrile illness and is responsible for the rose spots which are embolic phenomena. The Peyer's patches undergo hyperplasia associated with oedema; this leads to vascular obstruction, necrosis and consequent death of the covering mucous membrane with the formation of ulcers. These ulcers are ovoid in shape with irregular undermined edges; they lie along the long axis of the gut and if extensive may lead to erosion of blood vessels or perforation of the gut wall. Although the characteristic lesions are in the small intestine ulceration may occur in the large gut in severe cases. Inflammation is most severe in the lower ileum which is the commonest site of perforation. Ulcers heal by scarring without causing intestinal obstruction as the scars do not encircle the intestine. The mesenteric lymph nodes are enlarged. Organisms pass from the liver to the gall-bladder and can be cultured from the faeces towards the end of the first week in about 50 per cent. of cases. They appear in greater number in the third week when intestinal ulceration is at its height. Occasionally positive stool cultures have been obtained from contacts a day or two before the development of symptoms.

The acute toxic and degenerative changes found in tissues throughout the body, including the myocardium and kidneys, are those common to severe infections. Zenker's hyaline degeneration of the anterior abdominal muscles, although first described in typhoid, is not specific for enteric fever.

Symptoms

The incubation period averages 10–14 days but may be as short as 3 days or as long as 3 weeks. A long incubation period suggests a waterborne infection. Some patients suffer a brief attack of gastro-enteritis shortly after infection, recovering to remain well throughout the rest of the incubation period.

The severity of an attack of typhoid is related to the virulence of the organism, the size of the infecting dose and the resistance of the patient. Symptomless attacks occur and mild infections are common. Many such transitory illnesses are only recognized when investigations are undertaken because of known contact with the disease.

The first week. The onset is gradual with mild malaise, lethargy, headache and loss of appetite. The patient may complain of sore throat, cough or shivering attacks. Anorexia is usually prominent. It is usual for patients to continue working for the first few days of their illness, this period being known as the *ambulatory phase*. Between the third and the seventh day the symptoms become more severe and the patient usually takes to his bed. Mild upper abdominal discomfort is not infrequent, but constipation is more often present than diarrhoea at this stage. A slight cough is common. The temperature tends to rise in step-ladder fashion with the evening rise being greater by 0·5°–1° F. (0·3°–0·6° C.) than the subsequent morning's fall until it reaches 103° or 104° F. (39·5° or 40° C.). As the week progresses the patient looks and feels more ill, anorexia becomes marked and mild deafness is often present. Vomiting is seldom troublesome and often absent. The tongue is furred and dry, the abdomen is either normal or slightly tender in the hypochondrium and there may be some distension; there are often signs of bronchitis. The pulse rate characteristically remains relatively slow, increasing less than the expected ten beats for each rise in temperature of one degree Fahrenheit. Towards the end of the first week the spleen usually becomes palpable and tender and the rash may appear.

The *rose spots* of enteric fever are characteristic but are only seen in about 10–20 per cent. of cases. They are circular, slightly raised pale pink maculopapules of 2–4 mm. in diameter. They fade on pressure, until they disappear after 3–4 days leaving behind an area of staining. The spots appear in successive crops on the flanks, abdomen and back up to the end of the second week or longer should bacteraemia persist, varying in number from half a dozen to thirty or more; the occasional profuse rash does not necessarily indicate a severe attack. The face and limbs are seldom involved. It should be stressed that rose spots are normally scanty and often a faint pink in colour. They are visible on coloured skin if viewed in a good light.

The second week. The temperature remains raised and may be remittent or continuous in type. The relative bradycardia persists in the early part of the week but this helpful sign is likely to disappear later as tachycardia due to myocarditis develops. The patient is now ill and toxic; sordes appear on the teeth, sticky mucus covers part of the parched mouth and tongue and the lips become dry and cracked. A mental apathy or dullness is common often making it difficult to obtain an accurate history from the patient. Delirium may develop. The abdomen becomes more distended, developing a characteristic doughy, tumid feel on palpation. Diarrhoea may appear, five or six yellow or green stools like pea soup being passed every 24 hours. Colic and tenesmus are not features of the diarrhoea and blood is notable by its absence. The spleen becomes larger; secondary bronchopneumonia is common.

The third week. In favourable cases the temperature starts to fall by lysis about the fifteenth day, toxaemia diminishes, the abdominal symptoms subside and appetite returns, sometimes quite suddenly. Such patients become convalescent in the fourth week.

In unfavourable cases, however, the third week is the danger period, symptoms increase in severity, the patient becomes profoundly toxic passing into the typhoid state of 'coma vigil' in which he lies prostrated and semiconscious, thin, dehydrated, cyanosed and tremulous, unaware of his surroundings yet with eyes open and muttering continuously. Recovery is unusual in such cases but may ensue towards the end of the fourth week. The third week is the period of the two most serious complications of typhoid, perforation of the bowel and intestinal haemorrhage.

The above description is of classical typhoid fever of some severity unmodified by specific therapy. In practice the diagnosis is now seldom delayed beyond the fourteenth day in the severe case and the subsequent course is consequently modified. Coma vigil is seen infrequently.

Even in the untreated case, great variations occur in symptoms and severity. Some attacks are so mild that the patients remain ambulant throughout. Although an insidious onset is usual the illness may begin abruptly with high fever, vomiting and rigors. In the occasional case the onset may be dominated by meningitis or pneumonia due to typhoid bacilli.

Relapses occur in about 10 per cent. of cases, symptoms starting 10 days or so after cessation of specific treatment. The illness is a shorter and milder replica of the first attack, complications being uncommon.

The symptoms in young children show even more variation than in adults. The onset is more likely to be acute with vomiting, convulsions and high fever. Diarrhoea may appear on the first day. In some children cough, fever and raised respiratory rate may simulate lobar pneumonia. Meningism is often present. On the other hand, the symptoms may be vague with sore throat, mild fever, lethargy and loss of appetite. The combination of bronchitis and abdominal tenderness in such a case should suggest typhoid as a possible cause.

Complications

Digestive System. Ulceration of the mouth, gums and throat occurs readily in the absence of careful mouth toilet. A sore red tongue or oral thrush may follow treatment with chloramphenicol.

The most serious complications appear in the third week.

Intestinal perforation occurs in 1–5 per cent. of cases and is responsible for about 25 per cent. of deaths. It mainly affects young adults being rare in the elderly. The first sign may be acute abdominal pain with tenderness and rigidity over the right lower abdominal quadrant. The pulse rises but the temperature drops suddenly. Vomiting appears or increases and bowel sounds diminish. Perforation however may be subacute, slow in onset and with less severe symptoms. It is also likely to appear in the toxic patient who already shows abdominal distension and guarding making diagnosis difficult. In such a case a sudden rise of pulse rate is very suggestive of perforation and if this is accompanied by the disappearance of liver dullness or the appearance of free fluid in the abdomen the suspicion is confirmed. Vomiting is almost always present. Deceptive signs of improvement may appear within an hour or two in typhoid fever as in other forms of perforation and the abdominal signs are of prime importance. Evidence of peritonitis appears within six to eight hours. Although commonest during the third week, perforation may occur later in the illness.

Other complications which may cause abdominal pain include cholecystitis, portal pyaemia, suppurating mesenteric glands, splenic infarction and thrombosis of iliac veins. Slight jaundice is not rare in typhoid. It may be due to hepatitis, cholangitis or haemolysis.

Slight *intestinal haemorrhage* with frank or altered blood in the stools occurs during the third week when sloughs are separating from the Peyer's patches. Severe haemorrhage occurs in about 3 per cent. of cases at this time. Faintness and sweating are associated with a fall in temperature, rising pulse rate and fall in blood pressure. The lack of pain and rigidity and the persistence of liver dullness are the main features which differentiate haemorrhage from perforation until pallor, sweating and air hunger produce evidence of massive blood loss. In the toxic patient sudden alteration of temperature and pulse may be the only signs.

Paralytic ileus is not uncommon in the toxic case. The onset is insidious with vomiting and absent bowel sounds. The distinction between a primary ileus and one secondary to perforation mainly rests on the slower onset in the former.

Respiratory System. Bronchitis is usual and bronchopneumonia or less often lobar pneumonia may appear at any stage. These lung infections are often due to a combination of typhoid bacilli and pneumococci. Pulmonary emboli may complicate deep vein thrombosis during convalescence. Pharyngeal ulceration, due to involvement of the postarytenoid region and resulting in a husky voice, stridor and pain on swallowing is now a rarity.

Blood and Circulatory System. In severe attacks electrocardiographic changes (low voltage tracings with flat or depressed ST segments and inverted T waves) are commonly present when tachycardia and perhaps softening of the first heart sound are the sole clinical signs of involvement of heart muscle. Acute collapse sometimes occurs. Most patients survive such an episode, complete recovery following in due course. Femoral vein thrombosis is a frequent complication in the fourth week. An increase in pulse rate or slight rise of temperature at this stage should lead to examination of the calf for tenderness or swelling. Much less frequent but more serious is arteritis with arterial obstruction leading to pain, numbness and gangrene of extremities. Haemolytic anaemia, probably due to extensive reticulo-endothelial involvement, is not uncommon in toxic cases, but is seldom severe. Haemolysis ceases during convalescence.

Urine. Febrile albuminuria is often present. Typhoid bacilli appear in the urine from the second week onwards in a small proportion of cases. This bacilluria is rarely accompanied by urinary tract infection, such an infection being a necessary precursor to the establishment of pyelonephritis and the development of the chronic urinary carrier state. Retention of urine sometimes occurs in the severely ill.

Locomotor System. One characteristic of periostitis or bone abscess following typhoid is its late appearance either in convalescence or after apparently complete recovery. The tibia is most often affected but no long bone is immune. Pain in the back, 'the typhoid spine', is due to inflammation of ligaments, intervertebral discs or vertebral periosteum, mainly in the lumbar and sacral areas. It usually appears suddenly and may continue for months. 'Cold' abscesses in bone may not give rise to symptoms until years later.

Nervous System. Apathy is part of the disease. Delirium is common but convulsions are unusual in typhoid. Meningitis or encephalitis, with or without paralysis, have been described and a post-typhoid confusional state may persist for weeks or months although ultimate recovery is the rule. Peripheral neuritis with tender, painful toes, mild muscle weakness and depressed reflexes is not infrequent during convalescence after a severe attack.

Other rare complications include vulvovaginitis, orchitis and mastitis. There may be a temporary loss of hair during convalescence.

Carrier State. A patient who continues to excrete typhoid bacilli for some weeks following his attack is known as a convalescent carrier. Providing adequate precautions are taken this condition is not of great significance, the excretor state clearing within a month or two. Should excretion continue for over six months, however, the person has then become a permanent carrier and will remain a potential source of infection to others. Urinary carriers are fortunately much less frequent than intestinal carriers. The organisms multiply in a residual area of chronic typhoid pyelonephritis and appear in the urine fairly constantly while intestinal carriers on the other hand excrete the bacilli intermittently. In these cases the organisms persist in the gall-bladder where they set up a low-grade inflammation often accompanied by gall-stone formation. Viable bacilli can be recovered from different layers of such stones many years after the attack of typhoid. Previous cholecystitis strongly predisposes to the development of the intestinal carrier state, typhoid bacilli passing into the gut from the gall-bladder irregularly. An incidental attack of diarrhoea and the accompanying intestinal hurry may result in typhoid bacilli being easily recovered from the stools. This has been observed in certain known carriers from whom routine cultures have been predominantly unsuccessful.

Diagnosis

Headache and abdominal discomfort associated with fever, cough, lassitude, anorexia and a rising temperature suggest typhoid. Increasing toxaemia, sustained or remittent temperature around 103° F. (39·5° C.) and the onset of diarrhoea with watery green stools in the second week of illness are highly suggestive and the appearance of rose spots in such a case would be diagnostic. The relative bradycardia in the first 10 days or so is a helpful sign in a patient with pyrexia. In most patients, however, typhoid can only be suspected on clinical grounds, confirmation of the diagnosis depending on laboratory investigation. It should be noted that constipation is commoner than diarrhoea in the early stages and that in many patients diarrhoea is absent throughout. Vague upper abdominal discomfort is frequent whilst severe abdominal pain is uncommon in the uncomplicated case.

Special Diagnostic Methods. 1. *Bacteriological.* Culture of organisms from the blood, using both whole blood and blood clot, should be attempted at whatever stage of the disease typhoid is first suspected. This is by far the most important investigation. Positive cultures are most likely in the first 10 days but may be obtained as late as the fourth week. In some cases the organism is recovered from the blood and never from the faeces or urine. Repeated examinations of excreta are often required, negative cultures never excluding the diagnosis. Stools are positive towards the end of the first week in about 50 per cent. of cases and for a variable time thereafter; occasionally organisms have been recovered for a day or two before the onset of symptoms. Typhoid bacilli hardly ever occur in the urine before the tenth day, not often before the fifteenth and in many cases the urine remains sterile throughout.

2. *Serological.* Agglutination tests are of great help in the diagnosis of enteric fevers when cultural methods fail, unequivocal evidence of infection being gained from the Widal reaction in about 90 per cent. of all cases. However, the interpretation of results is not always straightforward. There are three antigens concerned, 'O' (somatic), 'H' (flagella) and Vi. Vi antibodies do not appear with any regularity early in the disease and are therefore of more importance in detecting persistence of infection or a carrier state in a healthy individual than in diagnosis. Antibodies usually begin to appear in the patient's serum between the seventh and tenth days of illness. In the uninoculated and in those who have not previously suffered from typhoid 'O' agglutinins appear first. Although not entirely type specific (*S. typhi* 'O' agglutinins may show a moderate rise in other enteric infections, notably paratyphoid B) most typhoid patients show a fourfold rise of titre within 4 or 5 days of 'O' agglutinins being detected. In patients without previous experience of *S. typhi* antigens a titre of 1:200 'O' agglutinins is highly suggestive of typhoid fever. A fourfold rise of titre is diagnostic. It is quite usual for *S. typhi* 'O' titres to reach 1:1000 or more. In a few patients the level of O antibodies is slow to rise and in others it may never reach a 'diagnostic' level.

'H' agglutinins appear more slowly but tend to persist for longer than 'O' agglutinins both after the disease and after inoculation. Any febrile illness thereafter may cause a sharp rise in 'H' agglutinins. A high 'O' and low 'H' agglutinin titre therefore suggests an active infection whereas a low 'O' and high 'H' titre suggests an anamnestic reaction.

Vi antibodies appear late in the disease. Their main value lies in their persistence in titres greater than 1:10 in the majority of chronic carriers. Up to 10 per cent. of excretors, however, are without Vi antibodies. A steady fall in Vi antibody titre suggests the carrier state has been eradicated. Conversely, the presence of Vi antibodies can be of great use in confirming suspicions about a probable carrier from whom first cultures have been negative.

The level of antibodies in the serum bears no constant relationship to the severity of the illness and relapses are equally common in patients with high or low titres. Intestinal perforations, however, appear to occur more frequently in those with low titres.

3. *Haematological.* The total white cell count is usually normal or depressed to 3000 cells per mm^3. due to a reduction of the polymorphonuclears. Leucopenia is remarkably constant in the acute stage, a total count of over 6000 cells being rare and over 10,000 exceptional.

4. *The Diazo reaction.* When a freshly prepared solution of Diazo reagent is mixed with urine passed between the fifth and fourteenth day of an attack of typhoid a pink froth is formed in about 90 per cent. of cases. False positives are infrequent. This simple test is of some diagnostic help when more elaborate facilities are not available.

Differential Diagnosis

The possibility of typhoid must be considered in any pyrexia of unknown origin and cultures and Widal tests carried out if fever is prolonged. *Any septicaemic illness* may mimic the disease. Paratyphoid, though in general causing a milder illness, can only be differentiated by laboratory methods. The following conditions can cause most difficulty in the early stages.

Bronchitis, tonsillitis, influenza or a simple descending respiratory infection may be suggested by the cough and fever. Lassitude, mental apathy and anorexia are seldom marked in these conditions, however, which usually show a rapid improvement instead of a steady deterioration.

Miliary tuberculosis may show a similar onset with relative bradycardia and a palpable spleen. The temperature is usually more irregular and sweats more profuse than in typhoid. Chest X-ray will eventually confirm the diagnosis in most cases although miliary shadowing may not be evident in the first 10 days.

Tuberculous peritonitis causes a less acute illness but may mimic mild typhoid with fever and abdominal discomfort associated with abdominal distension. The duration of the illness and the appearance of ascitic fluid or palpable masses in the abdomen suggest a tuberculous aetiology.

Suppurative abdominal conditions such as appendicitis and pelvic or perinephric abscess may cause severe constitutional symptoms combined with abdominal pain. Evidence of local infection can usually be found on careful examination and most cases show a polymorphonuclear leucocytosis. The temperature chart is intermittent in character.

Brucellosis commonly causes a relapsing type of fever associated with joint pains and severe sweats. Blood cultures and agglutination tests confirm this diagnosis.

Typhus fever starts more abruptly than typhoid but grave toxaemia is common to both. The rash of typhus, however, is profuse, does not crop and many lesions are petechial. The Weil-Felix reaction and a specific complement fixation test are positive.

In children, the sudden onset with fever, cough and rise in respiratory rate may suggest *pneumonia* or there may be vomiting and neck stiffness necessitating examination of the cerebrospinal fluid to exclude *meningitis*.

Blood cultures taken early in the illness will usually be positive if the patient is suffering from typhoid. Repeatedly negative agglutination tests make enteric fever unlikely though occasionally the appearance of agglutinins is delayed until the fourth week.

Treatment

General. Patients should be nursed in bed in isolation and the Medical Officer of Health notified immediately the diagnosis is made. Concurrent disinfection must be strict. All bed linen should be placed dry in special polythene bags or in disinfectant ('white fluid' or 5 per cent. lysol) on the ward and then disinfected during the laundering process without further handling. Stools and urine should be emptied into 5 per cent. carbolic acid where they should remain for 2–4 hours before being sluiced away. Isolation should be continued until six consecutive negative stool and urine cultures are obtained, specimens being taken on alternate days. Clearance specimens should not be started until at least 48 hours after cessation of specific therapy. Provided nurses observe a strict barrier-nursing technique, including thorough hand-washing after attending the patient, they run very little risk of infection. Skilled nursing attention remains an important part of treatment and a vital one in toxic cases. Such patients must be fed by nurses until the risk of carditis has passed. Mouth toilet should be carried out after each meal; if chewing gum is acceptable, fifteen minutes chewing after feeds helps to keep the mouth clean. Care must be taken to prevent bed-sores developing. The nursing staff must be aware of the need to notify the physicians of any sudden rise or fall in pulse rate or temperature or of the occurrence of abdominal pain. Adequate fluid and calorie intake is essential, the diet in the acute stage being semi-solid with no roughage. Thickened soups, milk, fortified dried milks, eggs, white fish and purée of potatoes will provide the two and a half to three thousand calories required by an adult. Sweetened fruit juices, ice cream and jellies are usually acceptable. If fluids are not taken by mouth or if meteorism is severe they must be administered parenterally. As this seldom needs to be continued for more than 4 days an inadequate calorie intake over the period is less harmful than attempts to give a high calorie intake intravenously. Daily serum electrolyte examinations determine the solutions required which are combined with 5 per cent.

glucose. A small blood transfusion is often helpful in such patients.

Specific. The course and progress of typhoid have been radically changed first by the use of chloramphenicol and more recently by the additional use of corticosteroids. Clinical response in typhoid often does not parallel precisely laboratory sensitivities and chloramphenicol remains the drug of choice. The drug should be given in divided dosage six-hourly up to a maximum of 4 G. per day for an adult for 7 days with 2–3 G. per day for a further 7 days (75 mg. chloramphenicol per kg. per day for the first week, 50 mg. per kg. per day for the second week). The succinate preparation intravenously is valuable in the very ill. A loading dose should not be given at the onset of treatment as this has occasionally been followed by a Herxheimer type of reaction. Relapses are more frequent when treatment is continued for less than two weeks. The response to chloramphenicol is gradual. The patient usually starts to feel better after 48 hours, but the temperature often remains raised for 4–5 days and fresh rose spots may appear during this period in spite of the fact that the organism can rarely be recovered from the blood after starting chloramphenicol. Most typhoid bacilli are sensitive in the laboratory to the tetracyclines but treatment with this group of drugs has proved disappointing.

Ampicillin, in a dosage of up to 1 G. four-hourly (6 G. per day) is a possible alternative to chloramphenicol. When treatment is started on the tenth day or later, however, the response is slow and the temperature may take a week to return to normal. Treatment with ampicillin in the first week is usually followed by a more rapid response. The drug is highly concentrated in the bile and on theoretical grounds should lessen the risk of the development of the carrier state. Combinations of trimethoprim and sulphamethoxazole (*Septrin, Bactrim*) have shown some activity both in the treatment of the acute case and the carrier and are at present under trial.

In the severely ill patient, steroid therapy (combined with chloramphenicol) produces dramatic lessening of toxaemia, fall in temperature and general improvement but with less rapid disappearance of myocarditis. A 5–7-day course in rapidly reducing dosage should start with 40 mg. of prednisolone intramuscularly on the first 2 days. Steroids should never be withheld in the toxic case, but they are not indicated in infections which do not threaten life in view of the theoretically increased risk of perforation. For similar reasons the intramuscular route is recommended.

A 5–7-day course of chloramphenicol or ampicillin is adequate for treating a relapse.

Symptoms and Complications. Diarrhoea requires no specific treatment unless the stools contain an excess of curds when the milk content of the diet must be reduced. Haemorrhage is treated along the usual lines with strict rest, morphine and blood transfusion.

Paralytic ileus requires gastric suction and intravenous fluids with daily electrolyte control. The advisability of surgery for intestinal perforation is debatable; in toxic cases the results of operation are certainly no better than those of medical treatment. This consists of chloramphenicol in doses of 8 G. in the first 24 hours followed by 6 G. daily until the patient improves, combined with gastric aspirations and intravenous electrolytes. Operation is advisable when a sudden perforation occurs in a relatively fit patient.

Anticoagulants should be avoided in deep vein thrombosis so long as intestinal ulceration is still present. They can be considered safe if diarrhoea has ceased and the stools are free from occult blood. Rest and a four-week course of a non-toxic antibiotic such as ampicillin, 3–4 G. per day in divided dosage, are indicated in the later bony complications.

Convalescence has been shortened by the advent of specific therapy, but most patients need a month to recuperate after an attack of moderate severity. As a rule bed rest should be continued until the fourth week and return to activity should be gradual. This is of particular importance if there has been evidence of carditis.

Carriers. Prior to discharge from hospital, following six consecutive negative stool and urine cultures from specimens obtained on alternate days, the Vi antibody should be tested. If this remains raised the carrier state should be suspected and the test repeated in 3 months. Persistence of the agglutinins indicate the carrier state. The Medical Officer of Health must be notified whenever a definite or suspected carrier is discharged from hospital.

In the past, drug treatment of the carrier state has seldom been successful but preliminary results with ampicillin are promising. The drug should be given in divided doses for up to 3 months, starting with 6 G. per day for the first week or two, reducing to 3 G. per day for the remainder of the course. Probenecid, 1 G. twice daily, may be given in addition. Previous gall-bladder disease predisposes to the carrier state and conversely persistance of typhoid bacilli in the biliary tract causes a low grade inflammation and ultimate stone formation. Cholecystectomy should be recommended in the presence of symptoms of gall-bladder disease. It is important to cover the operation with ampicillin and to drain the common bile-duct ensuring that all small stones are removed. About 85 per cent. of excretors will be cured by operation.

The gall-bladder carrier is not a great risk to the community if he is strict in his personal hygiene, thorough washing of hands after visiting the toilet being essential. Carriers must not prepare food for others and in Great Britain are forbidden by law from handling food on sale to the public, whether in shop, restaurant or boarding-house.

Preventive. Active immunization can be achieved with two injections of an acetone- or heat-phenol-killed vaccine usually given as a combination of typhoid with paratyphoids A and B (T.A.B.). A first dose is 0·5 ml. followed by 1·0 ml. four weeks later gives about 80 per cent. protection. These vaccines have been shown to give good protection whereas alcohol-killed alcohol-preserved vaccines have often failed to give any protection. A booster dose is necessary in 2 years if continued protection is required. The vaccine may be used to protect family contacts when a convalescent carrier who will have to prepare the family meals is discharged from hospital. The vaccine causes moderate local and systemic reactions which can be considerably reduced if smaller doses (0·1 ml. for those under 12 years and 0·2 ml. for all others) intradermally replace the normal subcutaneous injection, although protection is probably less certain. Active immunization is not necessary routinely for nurses working in an infectious diseases department.

Prognosis

A fatality rate of 10–25 per cent. has been reduced to less than 5 per cent. with chloramphenicol. The outlook is best in children and worst in the elderly. A delay in appearance of agglutinins may indicate a severe illness but it has been observed in very mild attacks and also in some patients in whom chloramphenicol is started early in the illness. Toxaemic circulatory failure, the commonest cause of death is now usually relieved by steroids leaving perforation as the most serious complication with a fatality rate of about 30 per cent. Periostitis may cause symptoms for months but recovery usually ensues; post-typhoidal mania similarly has a good ultimate prognosis.

Immunity following typhoid is only partial. Second attacks are not rare.

PARATYPHOID FEVER

Aetiology and Pathology

The term enteric fever embraces the typhoid and paratyphoid fevers A, B, and C which in clinical medicine may be indistinguishable. The paratyphoid fevers are ubiquitous but the type differs in different countries. *S. paratyphi B* is the only variety commonly met with in Great Britain and Western Europe while paratyphoid A is prevalent in India and the tropics. Any food or drink may spread paratyphoid but synthetic cream (prepared from processed imported eggs), ice cream, cold meats, shredded coconut and shellfish are common sources in Great Britain of paratyphoid B. Many cases arise in late summer and autumn amongst patients returning from holiday in endemic areas.

Ulceration in paratyphoid B extends throughout the small and large gut but the ulcers are usually shallow.

Symptoms

The incubation period is 7–14 days. The illness is similar to typhoid and in any individual case the distinction between paratyphoid and typhoid must depend on the laboratory. However, certain generalizations are useful. As a rule, paratyphoid is a much milder disease than typhoid although an occasional infection is severe. The onset may be insidious, as in typhoid, or abrupt with diarrhoea and vomiting as in food poisoning. Abdominal pain is more prominent and may be accompanied by vomiting and intestinal guarding suggestive of subacute appendicitis. However, the severity of the constitutional symptoms, particularly the headache, should serve to exclude this possibility. Headache, indeed, is often the main and most striking symptom throughout the illness. Pleural effusion has occurred soon after the onset in some patients.

In spite of high fever, many patients feel surprisingly well while they remain in bed. Abdominal distension is usually mild and in about 50 per cent. of cases constipation persists throughout the illness which, without specific therapy, runs a 3–4 week course. Because toxaemia is less marked myocarditis occurs less often and consequently a relative bradycardia frequently persists throughout. The rash in paratyphoid B is occasionally profuse involving the limbs and even sometimes the face. The patient rarely passes into a state of coma vigil and convalescence tends to be more rapid than in typhoid.

Complications are uncommon although all those occurring in typhoid can arise. Haemorrhage and perforation are rare. Relapses following inadequate therapy however, occur as often as in typhoid and deep vein thrombosis in convalescence is not uncommon. Paratyphoid C is more invasive than the other types giving rise to distant lesions such as arthritis, cholecystitis or abscess formation.

Diagnosis

Diagnostic methods similar to those used in typhoid apply. Blood cultures within the first 10 days are often positive and agglutinins appear in the blood towards the end of the first week. Paratyphoid A and B do not contain Vi antigen and those in paratyphoid C are inconstant. The white cell count shows a leucopenia.

Treatment

The patient should be isolated and treated on identical lines to those suggested for typhoid fever with strict concurrent disinfection. The disease is notifiable in Great Britain. Six negative stool and urine cultures on alternate days are required before declaring a patient free from infection. Convalescent and chronic carriers occur as in typhoid and require similar measures.

REFERENCES

Ashcroft, M. T., Singh, B., Nicholson, C. C., Ritchie, J. M., Sobryan, E., and Williams, F. (1967) A seven-year field trial of two typhoid vaccines in Guyana, *Lancet*, ii, 1056.

Christie, A. B. (1964) Treatment of typhoid carriers with ampicillin, *Brit. med. J.*, **1**, 1609.

Christie, A. B. (1969) Typhoid and paratyphoid fevers, in *Infectious Diseases*, p. 54, Edinburgh.

Huckstep, R. L. (1962) *Typhoid Fever and Other Salmonella Infections*, Edinburgh.

Ministry of Health (1965) *Typhoid and Paratyphoid Fevers*, H.M.S.O., London.

OTHER SALMONELLA INFECTIONS

Synonyms. Salmonellosis; Acute infective food poisoning.

Aetiology

Over a hundred strains of salmonellae have been found to be pathogenic to man. This group of organisms is similar in cultural and fermentation reactions to the paratyphoid bacilli, identification being carried out by agglutination tests. As the organisms may possess up to three O and up to six H antigens, elaborate investigations may be required for specific identification. Many of these antigens are common to different species. Much the commonest of these organisms to cause human disease is *Salmonella typhimurium* (formerly known as *Bacillus aertrycke*); others frequently encountered are *S. enteritidis* (Gaertner's bacillus), *S. montevideo*, *S. newport*, *S. St. Paul*, *S. oranienburg* and *S. thompson*. *S. choleraesuis*, though fortunately uncommon, is highly invasive and the most lethal of the salmonellae.

Sources of Infection

Unlike the organisms of typhoid and paratyphoid, which are confined to man, many salmonellae infect cattle, pigs, rats and mice. The primary source of infection in most outbreaks is a farm animal. Secondary outbreaks arise from human carriers. Any uncooked food liable to contamination by human excreta, as in enteric fever, may act as a source of infection, the food being infected by a carrier or case concerned in its preparation. Processed meats, trifles, custards, cream buns, duck eggs and bulk dried or liquid egg mixtures and dried coconut are the most frequent sources of human infection. Dust-borne infections can occur and have been responsible for repeated outbreaks in a hospital ward.

Pathology

The whole alimentary tract is involved although the changes in the stomach are less marked, a point which distinguishes chemical irritant poisoning. The mucosa is hyperaemic and swollen and Peyer's patches are prominent but ulceration only occurs in severe infections.

Symptoms

The incubation period of infective salmonella gastro-enteritis is commonly 12–24 hours with extremes of 6–48 hours.

The *onset* is abrupt with headache and malaise followed, often in minutes, by nausea, vomiting and diarrhoea. Abdominal pain is frequent, usually central and may be severe. It is often accompanied by guarding and may localize in either iliac fossa. It may be constant or colicky but tends to be relieved when the bowels are opened. Hyperaesthesia of the abdominal skin is a helpful sign which may precede other abdominal symptoms. In some patients diarrhoea and vomiting are delayed for 24 hours, the early symptoms then consisting of headache, malaise and fever. Febrile convulsions are not uncommon at the onset in children and shivering attacks may occur in adults. Meningism may be a prominent sign in toxic cases. It does not necessarily indicate invasion of the blood stream.

Vomiting may continue for days but more often ceases after 48 hours. Diarrhoea is often severe and frequent with the passage of copious watery green offensive stools with mucus and little or no faecal matter, their appearance being highly suggestive of salmonella infection. If ulceration occurs, however, the stools may appear to consist almost entirely of blood. About a third of patients pass blood in their stools at some stage. As fluid is lost in considerable quantities dehydration is common with sweating, hypotension, cramps, oliguria and pre-renal uraemia.

The severity varies from a mild attack of febrile diarrhoea and colic with recovery in 2 days to an illness complicated by severe dehydration and electrolyte disturbance with the blood urea rising to over 300 mg. per 100 ml. In attacks of moderate severity the stools do not return to normal for 7–10 days although the appetite and sense of well-being return much sooner.

In about 8 per cent. of patients the organism is invasive and the illness is *septicaemic*. All salmonella types are capable of producing a septicaemia but *S. choleraesuis* is particularly prone to invade the circulation and is the commonest salmonella cause of bacterial endocarditis. Invasive salmonellosis may present in two ways; in both diarrhoea is insignificant though abnormal stools provide a clue to the diagnosis. There may either be a fulminating onset with high fever, vomiting, peripheral circulatory failure and an occasional loose stool, sometimes followed by evidence of endocarditis or embolic disease in bones, meninges or kidneys. Or, more frequently, patients present with a 'fever of unknown origin' with headache, malaise, cough and bronchitis with an enlarged spleen and occasionally a few rose spots. These patients are constipated but have usually suffered from transient diarrhoea at the onset which may easily be overlooked if not specifically inquired about. They differ from enteric fever in that there is no relative bradycardia and there is usually a leucocytosis. Signs of metastatic infection in bones or elsewhere may appear at any time.

Complications

Dehydration may be obvious within a few hours of the onset or may appear insidiously over some days. The urinary output falls, pre-renal uraemia develops, ketosis leading to further vomiting and fluid loss. Chlorides disappear from the urine. Excessive potassium loss in the stools leads to drowsiness and depressed reflexes. In the septicaemic forms *meningitis* is commonest in infants. *Osteomyelitis* with abscess formation is relatively chronic and a history of diarrhoea within the preceding weeks of a subacute osteomyelitis should suggest the possibility of a salmonella aetiology. *Bacterial endocarditis* and *pneumonia* are likely complications of *S. choleraesuis* infections.

Diagnosis

In most cases this is easy on clinical grounds. An acute febrile gastro-intestinal illness accompanied by the passage of offensive green stools is characteristic. Stool cultures confirm the diagnosis but negative cultures in the acute stage are not uncommon. Negative stool cultures are frequent in the septicaemic forms where blood culture is usually successful. In the invasive type, non-specific salmonella agglutinins develop after the first week. The urinary chloride and blood urea are simple investigations to determine the severity of fluid loss. There is usually a moderate leucocytosis.

The only important differential diagnosis in the gastro-intestinal type is *acute appendicitis*. The presence of headache, the severity of the general symptoms and height of the temperature in salmonellosis all serve to distinguish the two conditions even when the onset of diarrhoea is delayed. *Sonne dysentery* causes a milder illness, vomiting is less prominent, fluid loss is minimal and the stools consist of small quantities of blood and mucus. Invasive salmonellosis is separated from other septicaemic illnesses by blood culture and agglutination tests.

Treatment

The patient should be nursed in isolation and only regarded as non-infectious following three negative stool cultures in convalescence. Food should be withheld until the acute symptoms subside but adequate fluids must be given, starting with Ringer-lactate and glucose solutions flavoured with fruit juices. Dehydration requires parenteral therapy, controlled by electrolyte estimations. Large quantities of glucose saline may be needed. Any potassium deficit must be made good if possible by mouth, 2 G. potassium chloride being given three or four times daily. Tincture of Chloroform and Morphine, B.P.C. (*Chlorodyne*) in 0·6 ml. doses, or chalk and opium mixtures are useful if colic is severe but are not indicated routinely. Diarrhoea continuing after 72 hours can usually be controlled by a diphenoxylate atropine compound (*Lomotil*) which reduces intestinal motility.

Antibiotics are not advised in the treatment of salmonella gastro-enteritis unless septicaemia is suspected. There is no evidence that they shorten the illness in the common type where the infection is limited to the intestine. In addition it is possible that they hinder rather than help the elimination of organisms during convalescence. For *invasive* salmonellosis, on the other hand, full treatment with chloramphenicol as for typhoid fever is mandatory. In the highly febrile toxic intestinal type in which septicaemia is considered unlikely but cannot clinically be excluded, ampicillin, 4 G. per day, should be given until blood culture results are available.

Permanent intestinal carriers are surprisingly rare, probably because invasion of the gall-bladder is exceptional in this condition. The convalescent carrier state, however, may persist for months but clears up spontaneously in under a year in nearly all cases.

Repeated courses of antibiotics are seldom effective in clearing this condition and should be avoided. With strict attention to personal hygiene, including rigid handwashing, a carrier is of little risk to the community.

Prognosis

The over-all mortality is just under 1 per cent. whereas 20 per cent. of *S. choleraesuis* infections are fatal. The infection is serious in neonates. In the elderly diarrhoea may persist for weeks and convalescence is prolonged in any patient who has suffered severe dehydration.

TOXIC SALMONELLA ENTERITIS

If organisms of the salmonella group multiply excessively in food and are subsequently killed by cooking, the relatively heat stable toxin may remain and cause acute food poisoning. The onset is rapid (2–6 hours after ingestion), fever, headache and other infective symptoms are absent and recovery is equally speedy—usually occurring within 12 hours to 3 days. Dehydration may be severe. Confirmation of the diagnosis is difficult unless some of the uncooked, contaminated food is available for examination. If both pre-formed toxin and living organisms are present in food then a biphasic illness may result. Such an attack starting as a toxic enteritis shows evidence of active infection with fever and malaise on the second or third day. There is often a transient improvement between the toxic and infective episodes.

REFERENCES

Black, P. H., Kunz, L. J., and Swartz, M. N. (1960) Salmonellosis. A review of some unusual aspects, *New Engl. J. Med.*, **262**, 811, 864, 921.

Bowmer, E. J. (1964) The challenge of salmonellosis, *Amer. J. med. Sci.*, **247**, 467.

Dixon, J. M. S. (1965) Effect of antibiotic treatment on duration of excretion of *Salmonella typhimurium* in children, *Brit. med. J.*, **2**, 1343.

MacCready, R. A., Reardon, J. P., and Saphra, I. (1957) Salmonellosis in Massachusetts, *New Engl. J. Med.*, **256**, 1122.

Mitchell, R. G. (1965) Urinary tract infections caused by Salmonellae, *Lancet*, i, 1092.

Van Oye, E. (1964) *The World Problem of Salmonellosis*, The Hague.

FOOD POISONING

The term food poisoning is used to describe a number of illnesses in which gastro-intestinal symptoms arise within 24 hours or so of eating food contaminated by bacteria, bacterial toxins or irritant chemicals. The term has disadvantages. For example, the bacillary dysenteries and paratyphoid B are not usually included under this heading although explosive outbreaks of food poisoning can follow contamination of food with these organisms. Conversely, case to case infection is becoming increasingly common in salmonella enteritis which, nevertheless, is an important cause of food poisoning. The diagnosis, however, is worth retaining if these limitations of the term are borne in mind. Prompt notification to the public health authorities of 'food poisoning' without awaiting more accurate bacteriological diagnosis can lead to rapid discovery and suppression of a contaminated source of food. The term is best not applied to allergic skin reactions developing in persons sensitive to certain food-stuffs.

Food poisoning was originally thought to be due to toxic products of protein breakdown formed in the course of bacterial decomposition. Under ordinary circumstances these substances (known as ptomaines) play no part in human illness as they only appear when food is in such an advanced stage of decomposition that it is too repulsive to be eaten.

The causes of food poisoning are:

1. Infective: salmonella enteritis; bacillary dysentery; paratyphoid B.
2. Toxic: salmonellae; staphylococci; *Clostridium welchii* [p. 101]; *Clostridium botulinum* [p. 104].
3. Chemical: accidental contaminants.
4. Mussel poisoning.

In toxic food poisoning organisms multiplying in food produce a relatively heat-stable enterotoxin which gives rise to symptoms within 2–4 hours of ingestion. A combination of toxic and infective episodes can occur if food containing both pre-formed toxin and living organisms is consumed. In 1961 in Great Britain *Salmonella typhimurium* was responsible for 64 per cent. of all incidents of food poisoning, other salmonellae for 32 per cent., staphylococci for 2 per cent. and *C. welchii* for 2 per cent.

TABLE 9

PRINCIPAL FEATURES OF FOOD POISONING

AGENT	INGESTION/ONSET TIME	MAIN SYMPTOMS
Chemical (irritant) . .	Very short, 10 minutes–2 hours	Nausea, abdominal pain, vomiting, sore mouth and diarrhoea
Staphylococcal toxin . .	1–6 hours	Salivation, nausea, vomiting, abdominal pain, collapse and subnormal temperature
Salmonellae	12–48 hours	Abdominal pain, diarrhoea, vomiting, fever
Cl. welchii	8–24 hours	Abdominal pain, diarrhoea and mild vertigo
Cl. botulinum . . .	½–36 hours	Change of voice, diplopia, ptosis, cranial nerve palsies, obstinate constipation
Other 'non-specific' bacteria	3–18 hours	Diarrhoea, abdominal pain, vomiting
Chemical (neurotoxic) .	(i) Early	(i) Early muscular paresis (e.g. organophosphorus compounds such as parathion, 'mussel poisoning')
	(ii) 10–12 days	(ii) Delayed flaccid paralysis (e.g. orthotricresyl phosphate, an oily fluid sometimes mistaken for edible oil)

STAPHYLOCOCCAL FOOD POISONING

Aetiology

Certain strains of staphylococci (*Staphylococcus aureus*) produce an enterotoxin. Food can become contaminated by handlers who have septic skin lesions or who are heavy nasal excretors of staphylococci. Processed meats such as those found in meat pies or shepherd's pie are the commonest sources, but canned meat, milk, cheese and sweetmeats may become infected.

Symptoms

The incubation period is usually 1–2 hours and never more than 6 hours. Nausea and vomiting of dramatic onset are the chief symptoms with upper abdominal pain which may be mild or severe. Diarrhoea follows and prostration with a subnormal temperature and hypotension develop rapidly if a large dose of toxin has been swallowed. In a severe attack the patient's condition deteriorates rapidly for 6 hours or so but recovery is as quick and although transient peripheral circulatory failure is frequent dehydration is rare. Recovery is complete within 48 hours or less.

Diagnosis

The occurrence of severe vomiting in a group of people who have partaken of the same meal a few hours before is strongly suggestive of the diagnosis. Confirmation comes from the recovery of large numbers of staphylococci in the vomit and, if available, in the food. Phage typing will further confirm that the organisms belong to a group known to be capable of forming enterotoxin. If the food was reheated before consumption, however, staphylococci are unlikely to be recovered from either source. It is not uncommon in the case of an elderly person living alone for such a person to be the sole victim. In such a case, the shock, vomiting and abdominal pain may suggest myocardial infarction particularly if no clear history is available and the onset of diarrhoea delayed.

Treatment and Prognosis

No specific treatment is required in the majority of cases and a light diet can be started 24 hours after the onset. In severe attacks intravenous therapy may be necessary. Recovery is rapid even in these severe attacks and death is exceptional. Investigation of an outbreak originating in an institution or bakery entails a clinical examination of the kitchen staff for evidence of septic skin lesions or discharges from the nose or ears.

CHEMICAL FOOD POISONING

The main feature suggestive of food poisoning of chemical origin is the short interval between ingestion and the appearance of symptoms. Patients frequently complain of an abnormal taste, often metallic, within minutes. These symptoms may be accompanied by nausea and abdominal pain, vomiting and diarrhoea following within half an hour.

Chemical food poisoning is usually accidental. It may follow the use of inadequately cleaned containers or the action of acids (for example citric acid in lemonade) on inferior enamel ware. Lead, tin, zinc and antimony poisoning have occurred in these ways.

Neurological symptoms have followed ingestion of food contaminated by pesticides. DDT causes paraesthesiae and limb twitchings. Endrin and similar agricultural sprays cause convulsions. Flaccid paralysis has occurred 2–3 weeks after consumption of ortho-tricresyl phosphate (which has been mistaken for an edible oil). Sodium fluoride when used in error for baking powder has caused diarrhoea and vomiting rapidly followed by paresis.

The possibility of chemical food poisoning should be considered when two or more persons develop abdominal or neurological symptoms shortly after consuming food or drink which will usually have had an abnormal taste. It is important to preserve for the Public Analyst all containers as well as any contents remaining.

MUSSEL POISONING

Illness from eating mussels may be due to typhoid or paratyphoid, enterotoxins, neurotoxins or allergy to shellfish.

Paralytic disease is related to 'red tides', an occasional seasonal discoloration of the sea caused by excessive overgrowth of certain dinoflagellates. These contain a powerful neurotoxin harmless to bivalve molluscs which concentrate the toxin. Circumoral paraesthesiae, weakness, ataxia, headache and vomiting are the predominant symptoms in man.

REFERENCE

MINISTRY OF HEALTH (1965) *Food Poisoning*, London, H.M.S.O.

G. D. W. McKENDRICK

INFECTIONS DUE TO BRUCELLACEAE

PASTEURELLA INFECTIONS

BACTERIOLOGY

The genus *Pasteurella* consists of a number of organisms which are Gram-negative rods showing bipolar staining. From the clinical aspect the two most important members are *P. pestis*, the cause of Oriental plague and *P. tularensis*, the organism of tularaemia. Some bacteriologists would classify the second with the *Brucellae* but majority opinion favours its inclusion in this group.

In addition a number of species exists which are of importance in veterinary medicine, but occasionally cause human infection. These are *P. multocida* (syn. *P. septica*), *P. haemolytica* and *P. pseudotuberculosis*.

HUMAN INFECTIONS

P. multocida causes septicaemia in cattle, pigs, rabbits and poultry. It is apparently carried by normal animals including cats, dogs, foxes and rodents. Human infection usually takes the form of an abscess following a bite from an animal, but an acute respiratory infection may result.

P. haemolytica may cause septicaemia in lambs and pneumonia in cattle and sheep. It has been recovered from human sputum, but its significance is uncertain.

P. pseudotuberculosis causes pseudotuberculosis in guinea-pigs, turkeys, rabbits and other animals. Examples of a typhoid-like illness due to this organism have been recorded in man. It seems probable, however, that it is a relatively common cause of acute mesenteric lymphadenitis in children. It may cause a febrile sore throat with regional lymphadenitis, and both this and mesenteric lymphadenitis have been associated with erythema nodosum.

It is unknown how these infections respond to antibiotic treatment. Plague is remarkably sensitive to the tetracyclines and it is reasonable to suppose that other pasteurella infections would behave similarly.

REFERENCES

ALLOTT, E. N., CRUICKSHANK, R., CYRLAS-WILLIAMS, R., GLASS, V., MEYER, H., STRAKER, E. A., and TEE, G. (1944) Infection of cat-bite and dog-bite wounds with *Pasteurella septica*, *J. Path. Bact.*, **56**, 411.

FREIGANG, B., and ELLIOTT, G. B. (1963) *Pasteurella septica* infections in humans, *Canad. med. Ass. J.*, **89**, 702.

MAIR, N. S., MAIR, H. J., STIRK, E. M., and CORSON, J. G. (1960) Three cases of acute mesenteric lymphadenitis due to *Pasteurella pseudotuberculosis*, *J. clin. Path.*, **13**, 432.

TURNER, T. W., and WILKINSON, D. S. (1969) *Pasteurella pseudotuberculosis* as a cause of erythema nodosum, *Brit. J. Derm.*, **81**, 823.

R. BODLEY SCOTT

PLAGUE

Aetiology

Plague is a bacterial infection caused by *Pasteurella pestis*, a Gram-negative bipolar pleomorphic non-motile aerobic rod, which is encapsulated in the tissues. It is primarily a disease of rodents and is spread accidentally to man by the rat (bubonic plague) or by droplet infection (pneumonic plague).

In all its manifestations plague is a very serious disease with a high mortality in untreated cases.

It is endemic in parts of India and occurs sporadically in many tropical and subtropical countries including Iraq, Iran, Ceylon, Burma, Southern China, Indonesia, and in scattered areas of Africa and Europe. Wild plague occurs, sometimes associated with pneumonic outbreaks, in the Middle East, especially Iran, South-eastern Russia, Mongolia, China, parts of South Africa, South America (including Brazil, Ecuador, Peru and Argentina) and some Western states of North America.

Plague is enzootic in Vietnam and since the development of war in that area has become common in man probably because of war damage to towns and villages with consequent increase of rats and garbage. In 1965–66 over 4500 cases were reported.

P. pestis is very sensitive to heat and sunlight and does not survive outside the body for long, although it will remain for days in sputum or dust in cool moist conditions, and sometimes for weeks in flea faeces. It survives freezing for long periods.

Permanent immunity is usually conferred by an attack. Second attacks are rare.

Plague is naturally an enzootic in rodents, transmitted from animal to animal by fleas.

Man may be infected in two ways: either through the infected flea or occasionally some other arthropod, or through droplet infection from a human case of pneumonic plague.

It has recently been noted in Vietnam that contacts with plague may have the organism growing in the nasopharynx without visible signs of infection. Such individuals are regarded as potential sources of infection to others and require immediate treatment.

Transmission by the Flea. The common vectors are usually rat fleas of which *Xenopsylla cheopsis* is the most efficient and *X. braziliensis* and *X. astia* less so. The human flea and the fleas of cats and dogs or the rodent reservoirs of wild plague only very occasionally act as vectors.

The bacilli are passed in the flea faeces and are rubbed into the tissues through skin abrasions or bites. They are also carried directly on the mouth parts of the flea from previous biting of an infected source.

The commonest mode of infection depends on the blocking of the proventriculus of the infected flea by rapidly multiplying *P. pestis*. The flea is unable to ingest more blood and regurgitation of blood and bacteria occurs when it tries repeatedly to feed. Blocked fleas live for only a day or two but may bite many times in that period and so disseminate the plague organisms more widely than the normal flea.

The rat flea lives for 1–2 years in cool and moist conditions. It lives for a much shorter time in a hot dry climate.

Unblocked fleas infected with plague normally die in about a fortnight but they remain alive in rat nests for months, and so carry the infection over from one season to another.

Epidemiology

Plague exists in two epidemiological forms, urban and wild or sylvatic. The mechanism of transmission differs somewhat, but the basic factors are the same.

The Spread of Urban Plague. Plague exists as an enzootic in wild rodents and is accidently transmitted by fleas to the semi-domestic rat, *Rattus norvegicus*. When the latter dies its infected fleas migrate and infect the domestic rat *Rattus rattus*. When this dies, the infected fleas feed on man and human plague appears. Sporadic cases appear from time to time wherever the disease remains as an enzootic in the reservoir animals. When it becomes epizootic and other conditions are suitable the disease appears in man as an epidemic. The epizootic precedes the epidemic by two or three weeks, and is indicated by a high rat mortality. When the rat population is suitably reduced the epidemic stops.

The pattern of an epidemic of urban plague is thus a slow beginning, a very rapid rise and an equally abrupt fall after some months.

Spread of plague from district to district may result from extension of the enzootic or epizootic or from the carriage of rats from place to place, for instance, on ships or lorries, so that the local population of rodents become infected. Sometimes ambulatory human cases may carry the disease to new areas.

The Spread of Wild or Sylvatic Plague. Plague which exists in certain sparsely populated rural districts as an enzootic of wild rodents, may appear sporadically in man. The infection is kept active by flea transmission from rodent to rodent and man acquires the infection accidentally, for instance when skinning infected wild animals. Epidemics occasionally occur as in urban plague, when semi-domesticated rats become infected after contact with wild rodents. If an epizootic results under these conditions an epidemic may develop.

Wild rodents may migrate considerable distances, and carry plague with them over very wide areas. The domestic rat does not migrate.

Plague spreads rapidly wherever the human population is crowded in insanitary conditions. The disease occurs in temperate climates and in the tropics. It appears most frequently in the cooler weather and during periods of high humidity. The incidence in an endemic area varies greatly from year to year since the spread of the infection to man depends largely on the close association of semi-domesticated and domesticated rats.

Transmission by Droplet Infection. The origin of an outbreak of pneumonic plague is a patient in whom pulmonary complications have developed during bubonic plague. Once established, pneumonic plague spreads from subject to subject by droplet infection. Cold or freezing conditions with relatively high humidity, such as occur when people crowd together in a hard winter, favour droplet spread.

Pathology

The pathological changes seen in plague are caused by a toxic non-specific inflammation with tissue damage, especially affecting the endothelial linings of lymphatics and blood vessels. There is a local lesion at the site of the infection, first appearing as a vesicle and then as a focus of necrosis. The 'bubo' forms in the lymph nodes draining the point of infection. In these nodes acute inflammatory changes occur and commonly lead to extensive suppuration. The blood vessels are congested and there may be haemorrhages into the substance. Small necrotic foci are formed which coalesce to form large abscesses. The tissue of the nodes contains enormous numbers of bacilli. The surrounding connective tissue is oedematous and haemorrhagic and the nodes become matted together. The infection invariably reaches the blood stream and all organs of the body become involved in the inflammatory reaction. The liver and spleen are enlarged, congested and contain characteristic scattered foci of haemorrhagic necrosis. The heart muscle is frequently oedematous, haemorrhagic and contains scattered focal necrotic areas. There may be haemorrhagic pericardial effusion.

The lungs are often seriously involved with acute oedema, congestion and haemorrhage into the alveoli and small bronchioles. Patches of haemorrhagic consolidation may involve most of a lobe. The watery blood-stained sputum partly fills the bronchi and even the trachea. In primary pneumonic plague similar pulmonary lesions develop as a result of inhalation of infected droplets. Bacilli multiply in enormous numbers in the inflamed lung tissue and cause severe toxaemia and bacteraemia. The pulmonary lymph nodes and the contiguous tissues become involved in the same way as superficial buboes within a few hours. Lesions in other organs may appear in primary pneumonic plague but death occurs before these can become extensive.

The early prostration, stupor and delirium of the typical case indicate involvement of the central nervous system, but necropsy does not always show damage to the brain. The cerebrospinal fluid may be turbid with polymorphs and occasionally there may be a frank pasteurella meningitis.

Signs and Symptoms

Plague is commonly classified as bubonic or pneumonic depending respectively on whether the pathological processes develop in the lymph nodes draining the area of the flea bite or primarily in the lungs. There is often no sharp demarcation between the clinical types. In both cases the dominant feature may be active septicaemia with or without localizing signs. In all cases bacteraemia without multiplication of organisms occurs as a transitory phenomenon. It is probable that the 'septicaemic' cases are merely examples of bacterial blood infection in which deep-seated buboes have been formed and perhaps overlooked or in which the node reaction has been inconspicuous.

The clinical picture varies greatly. There may be very little reaction at the point of infection and in some cases the accompanying local adenitis is mild and not progressive. Such cases are called 'pestis minor' or ambulatory plague.

Most cases however become seriously ill after infection and without treatment the mortality is high.

As pointed out above, however, contacts may harbour the organisms in the throat without clinical signs.

Bubonic Plague

The majority of cases develop a bubo in the region of the lymph nodes draining the area infected. There is commonly only one bubo but there may occasionally be several. The incubation period varies from 2–10 days and is usually 3–4 days.

Prodromal symptoms of headache, backache, malaise and apathy may precede the overt attack, but the onset is usually sudden, with rigors and convulsions in children. The temperature rises on the first day up to 104° F. (40° C.) or higher and remains elevated and remittent for the next 2–5 days and then falls slowly or suddenly, depending on the time taken for full development of the bubo. Suppuration and secondary infection of the latter causes a return of fever.

The general appearance of the patient is characteristic. In the early stages he is dull and apathetic, confused, complaining of headache and backache. The stupor and prostration advance, speech becomes slurred, muscular tremors and twitchings develop and the gait becomes unsteady. The tongue is dry and swollen; sordes is common.

The skin is hot and dry, with a blotchy vasodilatation, particularly on the face; the conjunctivae are deeply injected. Petechial haemorrhages appear in the skin and subcutaneous haemorrhages may develop, leading to areas of black discoloration over some of which the skin may become necrotic (the so-called 'black death'). There may also be haemorrhage into the gastro-intestinal tract and from visible mucous membranes.

The pulse during the fever is fast and in severe cases the heart dilates and death may result from cardiac failure. The blood pressure is often low and shock may develop. The respiration rate is fast at the onset and may increase as the disease develops. There is often epigastric pain, nausea and vomiting. The spleen and liver may be moderately enlarged and tender. Moderate leucocytosis is common.

Mental dullness usually increases as the condition progresses, but may give way to restless anxiety and the patient may even become maniacal.

The enlarged node or bubo from the outset causes local pain and tenderness which steadily worsens. It appears within a day of the onset of fever or may be the first sign of the illness.

In 70 per cent. of cases the infective bite occurs on the leg and the groin nodes are involved. The axillary nodes are involved in 20 per cent. The affected node is at first firm and swells rapidly. It is painful and tender; the skin over it is erythematous and hot. The surrounding subcutaneous tissues are oedematous and sometimes haemorrhagic.

A characteristic attitude is adopted in an attempt to gain relief from the pain. Thus, when the bubo is in one groin the patient lies on the other side with his knee flexed and thigh drawn up. When the bubo is in the axilla the arm is held abducted and extended.

The bubo reaches its full size in 2–5 days, by which time the nodes involved are matted together. They may now recede or go on to suppuration, with pointing and discharge of pus to the skin surface. Occasionally large vessels are involved in the necrosis and severe haemorrhage may develop.

Secondary infection is almost inevitable and in cases which recover, chronic indolent ulcers and sinuses may remain.

The course of bubonic plague is short. In outbreaks from 30–90 per cent. of untreated cases may die, most deaths occurring by the fifth day.

The outcome depends to some extent on whether active septicaemia develops.

Septicaemia is always present in pneumonic plague and probably almost always in bubonic, in which it often develops late. Although some patients are septicaemic from the onset the disease is primarily a local one. Once septicaemia has developed death follows rapidly.

Pneumonic Plague

In the terminal stages, pulmonary complications may develop in bubonic plague.

The term 'pneumonic plague' is reserved, however, for those cases in which the lungs are the primary site of infection induced by inhalation of infected material from patients with pneumonic involvement.

Two or three days after exposure, there is an abrupt onset, often without rigor but with chilly feelings and some shivering. The temperature rises rapidly to 104° F. (40° C.) or higher with clinical signs of pulmonary involvement. There is a frequent painless cough. The sputum is mucoid and watery at first, but becomes tinged with blood, and finally red or brown, frothy and bloody. At all stages it is loaded with plague bacilli.

Pain in the chest becomes severe and breathing more and more rapid and difficult, the patient gasping for breath as the pneumonic process develops.

Towards the end there is usually circulatory failure with considerable cyanosis. The physical signs in the chest are equivocal. Signs of heart involvement occur early and are severe. The heart dilates, the blood pressure falls, the pulse quickens and death occurs in 1–3 days, rarely later. Signs of vascular damage are common with haemorrhage from mucous membranes, epistaxis. haematuria and widely scattered petechial or subcutaneous haemorrhages into the skin.

Bacilli are present in large numbers in the blood and sputum from the beginning. There is a polymorphonuclear leucocytosis.

Untreated pneumonic plague is invariably fatal, but modern chemotherapeutic methods have greatly changed the prognosis.

Diagnosis

Clinical diagnosis of plague is of great importance. It is easy in a known outbreak but may be very difficult to make the first diagnosis.

In mild cases, the bubo may be mistaken for other forms of adenitis such as lymphopathia venereum. Bacteriological examination of the node or blood is required.

Tentative diagnosis can be made by the identification of the organisms in dried Gram-stained films of the juice from the early bubo or from the pus. In pus from advanced cases of bubo in which there is secondary infection, it may be difficult to identify *P. pestis*. In septicaemic cases the organisms may be numerous enough to find in a blood film.

Laboratory aids are important so far as the community is concerned, but there is no time to await the results in the individual case and treatment is necessary immediately the disease is suspected. Samples of blood and of node juice or pus should be sent to the nearest bacteriological laboratory.

Examination of dead or trapped rats should be made wherever plague is likely. The characteristic necropsy changes are: diffuse subcutaneous congestion and ecchymosis, enlarged lymph nodes, especially in the neck and the groin, blood-stained fluid in the serous cavities, enlarged pale liver with scattered greyish necrotic areas, enlarged deeply congested spleen sometimes with necrotic foci, congested and oedematous lungs with similar foci. *P. pestis* is present in large numbers in all the organs and tissues.

In rats *P. pestis* must be distinguished from *P. pseudotuberculosis* which produces few effects but may be present in large numbers in the tissues. This can be done by rubbing the suspected material into the shaved belly of a guinea-pig. The animal dies in a few days if plague is present. These methods should be used only by trained personnel.

Treatment

Cases of flea-transmitted plague should be isolated in hospital if possible or in their own homes. Cases of plague pneumonia must be isolated in hospital. Attendants should wear gowns, masks and gloves. In dealing with bubonic plague protective boots are advisable and clothing should be impregnated with DDT.

Nursing is essential, and those concerned in treatment must be properly protected. Incision and drainage of a bubo is not advisable until pointing has occurred. Some relief may be given by fomentation and sedatives, including morphia.

Chemotherapy is effective and has reduced the mortality even in pneumonic cases. In Vietnam the mortality in treated cases varies from 1–5 per cent. The most effective drugs are tetracyclines and streptomycin. Chloramphenicol is also effective. Certain of the sulphonamides are also active, but they have been largely replaced by the antibiotics. Sulphonamide resistance occurs, but antibiotic resistance has not yet become a problem.

In bubonic plague tetracycline is given in doses of 500 mg. 4-hourly until the fever subsides, thereafter 6-hourly for some days. The dose for children is 50 mg. per kg. daily in divided doses.

Streptomycin may be used alone or in combination with sulphonamides. A common regimen is 650 mg. intramuscularly immediately followed by 350 mg. 4-hourly until the temperature has been normal for 2 days. In early bubonic plague it is so effective that some workers claim that a single dose of 1–2 G. is adequate.

In pneumonic plague intramuscular streptomycin should be given in a total dose of 15–20 G. over 10 days. Alternatively, oxytetracycline is given as 500 mg. intravenously followed by 500 mg. orally 3-hourly for three doses, then 6-hourly to a total of 20 G.

Chemoprophylaxis of those exposed to plague, particularly to pneumonic plague, is essential.

Immediate contacts including those in charge of the patient, should be given sulphadiazine, 6 G. daily for 6 days. Other possible contacts should receive half this dose.

Vaccination of those at risk to plague may give some temporary immunity, lasting not more than a few months. Attenuated vaccines are more efficient than killed vaccines in this respect.

TULARAEMIA

Definition

A highly infectious disease, caused by *Pasteurella tularensis* which is normally enzootic in rodents. The clinical picture in man resembles plague and is characterized by an ulcer at the site of infection, enlargement and inflammation of the local lymph nodes and severe constitutional symptoms.

Aetiology

The disease occurs in parts of North America, Scandinavia, Europe, Russia and Japan.

P. tularensis is related to *P. pestis*, the cause of plague, and is a small pleomorphic Gram-negative bipolar coccobacillus which is easily grown on blood agar and egg media.

It occurs in many rodents, including rabbits, hares and squirrels in which it is transmitted by ticks, biting flies, fleas and lice. Man is infected accidentally by the bites of ticks, especially *Dermacentor* spp., *Chrysops* flies or other vectors, or by the bites and scratches of infected animals, and occasionally by insufficiently cooked infected food. Man to man transmission does not occur.

Pathology

The reaction at the site of the infection is basically acute inflammation, with the development of pus and ulceration. The affected tissues contain the organisms. The enlarged local lymph nodes develop like the bubo in plague and undergo acute inflammation, necrosis and pus formation. Necrotic foci surrounded by mononuclear and polymorphonuclear cellular reaction occur in many organs including the liver, spleen and lungs, commonly leading in the latter to bronchopneumonia. In moderately severe cases granulomatous foci of epithelioid cells are found sometimes with giant cells, fibroblasts and peripheral lymphocytic infiltration.

There is a moderate leucocytosis.

Signs and Symptoms

The pattern of the disease in man may be dominated by certain features, such as ulceration, changes in the glands or the eyes and general toxaemia. Nevertheless there is a common background to these syndromes.

The acute case begins suddenly 3–5 days after infection with severe headache, feelings of cold and mild shivers and a rise of temperature to 103° F. (39·5° C.) or higher. The symptoms remain those of any febrile attack for a few days. There follows a short remission, which may last 2–3 days, after which the fever returns and persists for 2–3 weeks, during which the patient suffers severe headache and body pains, heavy sweats and often nausea and vomiting. The fever subsides by lysis.

In most cases the local reaction at the site of infection, which is usually on the fingers or hands, begins a day or two after the fever and general symptoms develop. A papule appears and grows rapidly, usually associated with lymphangitis and enlarging tender regional lymph nodes, commonly in the epitrochlear and axillary groups. Pus formation with ulceration of the local lesion occurs in the majority of cases; in others a papular lesion may persist for months. The ulcers are punched out and heal slowly with scarring. In some cases lymphadenitis may develop without obvious local reaction at the site of infection.

Complications include bronchopneumonia, with *P. tularensis* in the sputum, pleurisy, meningitis, ocular lesions, septicaemia and severe toxaemia, producing the so-called 'typhoid state'.

The mortality rate is usually under 10 per cent.

Diagnosis

There may be a history of contact with the animal reservoirs or of bites by ticks or flies. Local lesions at the site of these bites and the presence of associated lymphangitis and enlargement and inflammation of the local lymph nodes are suggestive. Diagnosis, however, must be confirmed by recovery of the organism from blood cultures or from material obtained from the primary lesions or lymph nodes.

P. tularensis grows readily on blood or egg media but, unlike *P. pestis* will not grow on plain agar. Material from these sources may also be inoculated intraperitoneally into guinea-pigs which are highly susceptible and die within a few days. The organisms can be recovered from their tissues or blood.

Agglutinins against *P. tularensis* develop in the serum during the disease. A rising titre is indicative of the infection. Cross-agglutination with *Brucella* spp. may lead to confusion in the early stages but eventually the specific agglutination can easily be differentiated.

Treatment

Antibiotics are successful in dealing with the infection, particularly streptomycin and dihydrostreptomycin in doses of 500 mg. 8-hourly for 3 days. Chlortetracycline and chloramphenicol will also control the attack, but relapses are said to be more common after their use than with streptomycin.

Patients in a typhoidal state require treatment with the antibiotic until the fever subsides.

A successful vaccine has been prepared for the prophylaxis of those whose occupations expose them to the risk of tularaemia.

BRIAN MAEGRAITH

BORDETELLA INFECTIONS

WHOOPING COUGH

Synonyms. Pertussis; Parapertussis.

Definition

An acute specific infectious disease characterized by paroxysmal attacks of coughing which are commonly followed by an inspiratory 'whoop'.

Aetiology and Epidemiology

The causative organism is a small slender Gram-negative rod discovered by Bordet and Gengou (1906) and named *Bordetella pertussis*. Until recently this species was included in the genus *Haemophilus*. It grows best on media containing blood. An allied organism, *B. parapertussis*, morphologically identical but showing cultural and serological differences has been isolated from a number of outbreaks of mild whooping cough in America but only occasionally in Great Britain. These two organisms are antigenically distinct; infection with parapertussis probably accounts for the occasional rare 'second attack' of whooping cough. An occasional attack, too, may be caused by another related organism, *B. bronchiseptica*. Paroxysmal coughing, rarely accompanied by whooping, sometimes occurs during infection with certain respiratory tract viruses such as adenovirus or para-influenza virus. These illnesses tend to be of much shorter duration than whooping cough.

The disease has a world-wide distribution but is more prevalent and tends to be more severe in colder climates. It is endemic the year round in most urban communities although active immunization has resulted in a great reduction of morbidity. Epidemics in the northern hemisphere usually start in January, reach their height in early spring and tail off in the summer. Ninety per cent. of all cases occur in children under five years, but no age is immune and the disease may affect the newborn or his elderly grandparent. Unlike most other infectious diseases there is little or no passive protection of the new-born child, infection in the first six months of life being particularly serious and by no means uncommon. Most statistics show a slightly greater attack rate in females than males.

Infection is followed by immunity which is usually life long, although illness in the elderly may be due to a waning of this protection which depends on local tissue immunity of the respiratory tract as much as on circulating antibodies. Two attacks in childhood are probably always due to separate infections with *B. pertussis* and *B. parapertussis*.

Whooping cough is highly infectious. Spread takes place through droplets, susceptible contacts in the family circle being unlikely to escape. The disease is unfortunately at its most infectious in the first week or two when diagnosis is difficult or impossible on clinical grounds. Infectivity falls fairly sharply once the paroxysmal phase develops but organisms have been recovered from the severe case as late as eight weeks after the onset. The mild missed case is often responsible for spread of the disease but it is considered unlikely that healthy contacts act as carriers.

Pathology

Inflammation of the respiratory mucous membranes from the trachea to the bronchioles is accompanied by infiltration with polymorphonuclear and mononuclear cells and the production of much mucus. At first, thin, this becomes progressively more viscid until plugs are formed consisting of sticky mucus and cellular debris. This irritant material precipitates coughing, temporary relief following the bringing up of the mucous plugs. Frequently, however, the only result is to move plugs from one bronchiole to another. The whoop is caused by a long drawn inspiration through a larynx narrowed by a combination of spasm and mucus. The primary pathological changes in whooping cough are restricted to the respiratory tract and are not specific. Obstruction of bronchi and bronchioles leads to areas of atelectasis and emphysema and, in severe cases, pneumonia due either to *H. pertussis* or to secondary invaders may ensue. The tracheobronchial glands are usually enlarged. The organisms do not become invasive and have never been isolated from outside the respiratory tract.

Symptoms

The incubation period is commonly 7–10 days. Owing to the insidious nature of the early symptoms it is often impossible to fix the onset accurately, which partly accounts for the more extreme claims of incubation periods ranging from three days to three weeks. In practice a subject who has failed to develop catarrhal symptoms within fourteen days of contact can be presumed to have escaped infection.

Most attacks of whooping cough can be divided into catarrhal and paroxysmal stages.

The *catarrhal stage* starts insidiously with coryza and fever. A dry cough soon develops, the clinical picture at this highly infectious time being indistinguishable from a severe cold. Instead of symptoms lessening after 3–4 days however, the fever remains, the cough increases, occurring in bouts which begin to distress the patient, particularly at night. Vomiting may follow the bouts of coughing. Examination reveals a rise of temperature up to 101° F. (38·3° C.), evidence of mild upper respiratory inflammation and possibly signs of bronchitis, although auscultation of the chest may be quite normal throughout the whole illness.

The *paroxysmal stage* usually develops slowly 4–8 days after the onset of the illness. In some patients no history of catarrhal symptoms is obtainable, the illness starting in such a case with a cough which rapidly becomes paroxysmal. As the character of the cough changes from a simple to a spasmodic one the temperature falls to normal or near normal. It is unlikely to exceed 100° F. (37·8°C.) in the uncomplicated case at any time during the paroxysmal stage and in most instances remains within the normal range.

The fully developed paroxysmal stage in the unimmunized child is unmistakable. The cough occurs in spasms, more frequent at night than during the day, many of them spontaneous but also easily provoked by any outside stimulus such as eating, excitement or clinical examination, especially examination of the throat. A paroxysm consists of a toneless inspiration followed by multiple short sharp coughs with open mouth and protruded tongue. This long expiratory coughing phase is continued until the face becomes congested, the superficial veins engorged and the eyes fill with tears. The eyeballs may protrude and the skin become bathed in sweat, mucus running from the nose and mouth until sometimes a sticky plug of mucus is coughed up. Respiratory distress and cyanosis follow in a severe attack, relief eventually coming from the long drawn inspiration which is accompanied by the whoop so characteristic of the disease. The whoop is often absent throughout attacks in the very young and in the elderly. Vomiting during or after the spasm is usual. Exhaustion readily occurs when several coughing bouts follow one another in rapid succession, as is usual in all but the mildest paroxysms.

In the early paroxysmal stage the cough is only occasional but its frequency soon increases in a case of moderate severity until 15–20 paroxysms occur in the 24 hours. In a severe attack this number may be increased to 40 paroxysms or more and in nearly all patients they are more frequent and severe at night. The course of the illness is very variable. Spasms reach their height as a rule within a week and thereafter may decrease rapidly or may persist for 6 or even 10 weeks. When the spasms have become only occasional and mostly mild the odd severe paroxysm may still occur. The knowledge that severe spasms can occur late in convalescence is of particular importance in infants who need assistance during their coughing bouts. A non-specific respiratory infection in convalescence often leads to a return or worsening of the spasms for a few days.

In between spasms most patients are afebrile and feel well. Examination of the respiratory system is usually unrewarding and often completely negative; signs of atelectasis or areas of rhonchi found on examination will often have disappeared when looked for again a few hours later. The severity of the spasms cause a bloated appearance with puffiness of the eyelids in some patients. A subconjunctival haemorrhage in a child with a history of coughing bouts is almost diagnostic of whooping cough and an ulcer on the fraenum linguae due to the tongue being pushed over the lower incisors is also suggestive.

Complications

These may be mechanical, gastro-intestinal, respiratory or neurological.

Mechanical complications occur solely in the paroxysmal stage as a result of increased pressure in the thorax, abdomen or skull. They appear during or immediately following a severe spasm. Bleeding may occur from any surface or into the brain [see Section 15] but the commonest results of rupture of blood vessels are epistaxis, subconjunctival haemorrhage and petechiae in the skin over the neck and upper chest. Haemoptysis, retinal detachment and bleeding from the ears have all occurred. Herniae or rectal prolapse may appear.

The sole *gastro-intestinal* complication is recurrent vomiting; malnutrition and dehydration may follow. Rarely a problem in older children, this can be severe and dangerous in infants in whom maintenance of an adequate fluid and calorie intake can become difficult if each attempt at feeding stimulates further coughing and vomiting.

As a *respiratory* complication bronchopneumonia may appear at any stage. When it complicates the catarrhal phase response to treatment suggests that it is due to secondary bacterial invaders. Pneumonia at this stage leads to diagnostic difficulties, the nature of the underlying illness becoming apparent as the pneumonia subsides with therapy and the cough starts to become paroxysmal. In the later stages of the disease pneumonia may be due to the *B. pertussis* or to secondary infection, persistence of fever for more than five days after the onset of the paroxysmal stage almost always indicating respiratory complications. Pneumonia at this stage is associated with atelectasis and, although most common at the height of the paroxysmal stage it may occur at any time so long as sticky mucus is being produced. Transient small areas of atelectasis are seen in the majority of cases of whooping cough requiring hospital admission, but are only of consequence if subsequent spasms fail to dislodge the obstructing plug of mucus. Lobar collapse is much less frequent. A combination of unrelieved atelectasis and infection leads ultimately to bronchiectasis.

Apnoeic attacks are extremely dangerous spasms which are limited to infants under a year, most often occurring in those under six months of age. Any such attack may prove fatal and recurrent attacks are common in severe infections. Following a spasm or succession of spasms the infant becomes increasingly distressed, he fails to take a deep post-tussic inspiration, becoming ashen grey or deeply cyanosed. He goes limp, loses consciousness and may be convulsed and die, or, following a few feeble inspiratory efforts, spontaneous respiration may slowly start again and his colour gradually return.

Emphysema is a common finding at autopsy. Spontaneous pneumothorax and subcutaneous emphysema are rare complications the latter being first noticed at the base of the neck from where it spreads to the face and chest wall. Whooping cough may light up a latent primary tuberculous infection and this possibility should always be considered in any child whose recovery is unduly delayed. Paroxysmal sneezing is a rare and uncomfortable form of the disease which is self-explanatory. The repetitive spasmodic sneezing, accompanied by running eyes and nose and puffy face is followed in a few days in most cases by the usual coughing spasms.

Neurological symptoms in whooping cough arise in different ways and although relatively infrequent are always of grave significance. When they follow immediately after a severe paroxysm, anoxia is the commonest cause, as for example convulsions in an apnoeic attack; but petechial or even occasionally massive intracranial haemorrhage may be provoked in similar circumstances and lead to brain damage. Generalized convulsions may prove rapidly fatal or recovery may reveal residual paralysis of which hemiplegia is the commonest. Air embolism has also been postulated as a cause of neurological symptoms. Quite apart from the mechanical effects of severe spasms however, an encephalitic illness with apathy, drowsiness, convulsions or paralyses of upper motor neurone type may complicate a previously mild attack, the neurological symptoms developing in the third or fourth week quite independently of the spasms. The aetiology of this post-whooping cough encephalopathy is uncertain but it is probably a sensitivity type of reaction allied to similar states which may follow other infections such as measles and chickenpox.

Diagnosis

In the early catarrhal stage clinical diagnosis is impossible unless whooping cough can be suspected because of contact with a known case in the preceding fortnight. At the paroxysmal stage the diagnosis is essentially clinical, the history of spasms of coughing, worse at night and accompanied by vomiting being highly suggestive. The appearance of the whoop clinches the diagnosis, but it should be pointed out that typical paroxysms without a whoop are equally diagnostic. The paucity of physical signs in the chest in an illness associated with severe coughing bouts is worth notice.

Two laboratory tests can help in the doubtful case. In the first two weeks culture of the organism should be possible in about 80 per cent. of cases but the method of collection of specimens is important. Cough plates, with a Petri dish containing a modified Bordet-Gengou culture medium may be inoculated by holding them in front of the patient as he coughs. A simpler method is to pass a metal swab pernasally after cleaning the anterior nares. This is highly effective provided the swab is taken immediately after a cough and the culture media inoculated at the bedside. Positive cultures are much less frequent by either method after the third week. As the organism is slow growing, reports are often delayed for 4–5 days by which time the diagnosis is likely to have become clear on clinical grounds. A negative culture never excludes the diagnosis.

The peripheral blood shows an absolute lymphocytosis in the paroxysmal stage with total counts in severe cases of up to 100,000 cells per mm^3. of which perhaps 70 per cent. are lymphocytes. A typical count in an average case would be 15,000–25,000 cells per mm^3. with 50 per cent. or more lymphocytes. (It must be remembered that healthy children of under a year have up to 5000 lymphocytes per mm^3.) The erythrocyte sedimentation rate is normal in uncomplicated whooping cough.

The early differential diagnosis is from acute catarrhal states including the *common cold* and other *viral respiratory infections*. A paroxysmal cough can also be caused by the latter, or by a *foreign body* in the airway, *enlargement of tracheobronchial glands* or a *mediastinal tumour*. In these conditions the cough is harsher, the paroxysms usually briefer and the whoop absent. A low pitched whoop is sometimes heard in laryngitis, including the laryngitis which may appear during the prodromal stage of measles, but this occurs during the inspiration preceding the cough and the croupy cough which follows it is unlike that of pertussis.

Treatment

Patients should be isolated and regarded as infectious for a minimum of three weeks from the onset of the paroxysms. Contacts need not be quarantined or kept away from school. Bed is unnecessary for the older afebrile patient whose spasms are less when up and about in the fresh air. Even quite young children soon learn that excitement or running about provokes spasms and are content to play quietly. They also appreciate having a vomit bowl to hand. Patients sit up during spasms which are eased by supporting the head and body firmly. Small meals given often will help to prevent much weight loss whereas large meals provoke spasms and should be avoided.

Infants present a particular problem as they are unable to sit up unaided. They need to be under constant supervision, the more severe cases requiring hospital admission where oxygen and a suction apparatus must be available at the bedside. Feeding is slow and difficult. When it continually provokes spasms and vomiting frequent small feeds are best given through a nasal tube. The fluid intake must be adequate and weight loss restricted as much as possible, discharge from hospital being delayed until weight gain is satisfactory and the infant has more than regained his admission weight. Routine chest X-ray should be carried out after convalescence is well established in all but the mildest cases of pertussis in order to exclude any areas of residual atelectasis. Mantoux testing is indicated if recovery is slow.

There is no specific therapy for pertussis. Antibiotics have no effect on the uncomplicated case once the paroxysmal stage is established and are not indicated if spasms have been present for 48 hours or more. Tetracycline, however, lessens the duration and the severity of the attack if started early in the catarrhal stage and this is of great value when an infant is a known contact. In such a case the drug should be started at the first signs of upper respiratory symptoms and continued for two weeks in a dosage of 25 mg. per kg. per day. Active immunization is of no help in treatment. Claims have been made for hyperimmune gamma globulin prepared from humans recently vaccinated with *B. pertussis* vaccine but no well-controlled studies have been carried out. Improvement, if any, is certainly not dramatic and as the dose is three injections of 20 ml. intramuscularly on alternate days this method of treatment is not in common use.

Symptomatic therapy is equally disappointing—as indicated by the innumerable drugs recommended. Routine cough mixtures are of unproved value, a warm humid atmosphere being more important for the patient with severe spasms. For the nervous child whose spasms are easily provoked small regular doses of phenobarbitone are helpful but over-sedation should be avoided as it carries with it an increased risk of atelectasis. Atropine Methonitrate Solution, B.N.F., in a dosage of 2 drops four-hourly before feeds, increasing as necessary, is of great help in reducing vomiting in infants.

Haemorrhagic complications call for parental reassurance but no specific therapy. Tetracycline is the best antibiotic for pneumonia unless sensitivity tests on sputum cultures reveal a predominantly insensitive organism. Persistent atelectasis nearly always responds to vigorous physiotherapy, bronchoscopy seldom being necessary. In such cases antibiotic therapy should be prolonged until re-aeration is achieved. An apnoeic attack is treated by inversion of the baby astride the right forearm, secretions being removed from the pharynx with the right index finger while the back is percussed with the left hand. Pharyngeal suction may be required to remove secretions. Once the airway is clear oxygen is administered and artificial respiration continued by rocking until spontaneous respiration is re-established. Convulsions are dangerous if repeated or prolonged and require heavy sedation with intramuscular phenobarbitone, 15 mg. at three months, 30 mg. at three to twelve months increasing to 65 mg. at two years, or intramuscular paraldehyde (0·5 ml. under three months of age, 1 ml. at three to six months, 1·5 ml. six to twelve months). The increased risk of respiratory complications must be accepted.

Prevention

Active immunization is highly effective although constant surveillance of the antigenic structure of the prevalent sero-types is necessary to ensure satisfactory vaccines; 85 per cent. of recent infections in the United Kingdom have been due to the sero-type 1, 3, whereas before 1965 antigen 3 was not included in most vaccines. Three injections of 20,000 million killed organisms are given at 4–6 weekly intervals usually combined with diphtheria and tetanus, the volume of the triple antigen being 1 ml. Inoculation is started at 3–4 months of age with a booster dose given at two years.

Whooping cough in the first few months of life is usually contracted from a brother or sister of school age. As active immunization below three months of age is unreliable, protection for such infants is best achieved by maintaining adequate immunity in older siblings by booster doses.

Pertussis vaccine may cause encephalopathy, drowsiness, fits, meningism or paralysis appearing within 48 hours. It should not be given to any child with a history of previous convulsions nor should further doses be administered if any neurologic symptoms follow the first injection.

Prognosis

Active immunization has greatly reduced the frequency and severity of pertussis. Age is the most important single factor in prognosis, death being rare above five years. In the first year of life whooping cough remains a potentially lethal disease with a mortality now reduced to about 10 per cent. by vigorous antibiotic therapy of the respiratory complications and prompt resuscitation during apnoeic attacks. Five years ago the mortality was around 20 per cent. at this age. Sequelae, all now rare, include bronchiectasis, hemiplegia, convulsions, backwardness and blindness of either cerebral or retinal origin.

REFERENCES

LAPIN, J. H. (1943) *Whooping Cough*, Springfield, Ill.

MEDICAL RESEARCH COUNCIL (1956) Vaccination against whooping cough, *Brit. med. J.*, **2**, 454.

MEDICAL RESEARCH COUNCIL (1959) Vaccination against whooping cough, *Brit. med. J.*, **1**, 994.

PRESTON, N. W. (1963) Type-specific immunity against whooping cough, *Brit. med. J.*, **2**, 724.

PRESTON, N. W. (1965) Effectiveness of pertussis vaccines, *Brit. med. J.*, **2**, 11.

REPORT BY THE PUBLIC HEALTH LABORATORY SERVICE WHOOPING COUGH WORKING PARTY (1969) Efficacy of whooping cough vaccines used in the United Kingdom before 1968, *Brit. med. J.*, **2**, 329.

G. D. W. MCKENDRICK

BRUCELLA INFECTIONS

BRUCELLOSIS

Synonyms. Undulant fever; Malta fever; Abortus fever

Definition and Aetiology

These fevers result from infection with species of bacteria of the genus *Brucella*. These organisms are common infections of domestic animals such as the goat and cow and infection in man is acquired accidentally through consuming infected milk or milk products, handling carcasses or delivering newly-born animals.

The diseases in man are grouped together as the undulant fevers, in which recurring waves of fever appear with intervening apyrexial periods. During the pyrexial episodes there may be considerable illness and toxaemia, the spleen commonly enlarges and there may be changes in other organs. The diseases are debilitating, of long duration and erratic progress. The mortality is low but morbidity is considerable. Undulant fevers were first described in the Mediterranean area where the causative organism is *Brucella melitensis* which occurs in apparently healthy Maltese goats. Transmission occurred in these cases through infected goat milk. Subsequently it was found that the organisms could be transmitted via sheep and cattle, usually again by the consumption of infected milk, or by contact with the uterine discharges. In some hot dry areas there is evidence that the infection may be acquired by the inhalation of dust. *Brucella abortus*, which is a common infection of bovine animals, is also transmitted frequently to man, usually from cattle. A third species *Brucella suis* affects pigs and may produce a similar picture in man. These organisms may infect many domestic animals from any of which man may become infected. It has recently been found that the hare also carries the infection.

Br. melitensis in man is derived usually from the Mediterranean goat, *Br. abortus* most commonly from the cow, and *Br. suis* from swine.

Brucella spp. are small Gram-negative non-motile coccobacilli. The differentiation of the species is made by bacteriological methods; it is often difficult. Infection with *Brucella* spreads from animal to animal by contamination of pasture and through uterine discharges which contain enormous numbers of the organisms. *Brucella* spp. survive for a long time in water or in dust and urine. Although the infections produce abortion in animals this does not seem to be the case in humans. There is an age and sex distribution which depends upon occupation. *Br. abortus* infection is uncommon before the age of 15 and is more common in men than in women. *Br. melitensis* on the other hand occurs commonly in Europe in children under the age of 10, irrespective of sex. This is due to milk drinking.

Pathology

After entry the organisms are carried to the lymph nodes and enter the reticulo-endothelial cells. From these they periodically escape into the blood stream and are carried to all parts of the body. They again enter the histiocytes and multiply and periodically escape into the blood. Inflammatory areas and granulomatous nodules composed of the usual epithelioid and lymphoid cells and sometimes giant cells are developed in the bone marrow, the spleen, which is often enlarged and soft, the liver which is also enlarged, and the kidneys. They also occur at times in bones, joints and tendons and in the nervous tissues. Although the sites of election in cattle are the udders and uterus, mastitis is uncommon and abortion does not take place in these infections in women. In males the seminal vesicles, epididymis and testicles may be involved.

Signs and Symptoms

The incubation period is often difficult to establish, but probably varies from a week to a month. The onset is gradual with the early symptoms of mild fever, malaise, headache, generalized muscular pains and mild gastro-intestinal disturbances. After some weeks or months a pyrexial attack occurs which lasts a few days to some weeks and begins suddenly, sometimes with rigor, and with marked increase in severity of the symptoms, including drenching sweats and severe joint pains. The level of the remittent fever rises steadily for a few days and then settles, finally declining to an afebrile intermission which, after only a few days or some weeks is followed by further pyrexial episodes. It is from this pattern of rise and fall of fever that the disease acquired its name.

With each attack there is enlargement and tenderness of the spleen and to a lesser extent the liver. These organs are usually easily palpable by the time the disease has been established a few weeks. Generalized joint and muscle pains are often severe and so is persistent headache. The gastro-intestinal disturbances range from constipation to distension, discomfort and sometimes diarrhoea. There is usually an accompanying hypochromic anaemia and leucopenia in which the granulocytes are reduced, and the lymphocytes and mononuclear cells increased. Insomnia, depression and considerable debilitation are common. The clinical picture varies widely. In one case gross splenomegaly may be dominant and in another arthritis. Commonly only one joint is involved, but occasionally there may be many and may include the vertebrae. In some, lymph node enlargement is a striking feature. Infection of the liver results in impairment of liver function and may result in cirrhosis. The damage to the pancreas is said to result in diabetes. Lesions of bones cause pain, especially in the vertebral bodies and changes in these may upset the intervertebral discs with characteristic marginal proliferation. The many complications include arthritis, bone abscess, bronchopneumonia, pleural effusion, encephalomyelitis, neuritis, meningitis, endocarditis, myocarditis, osteomyelitis and orchitis. In severe cases during the febrile episodes there may be haemorrhages from the mucous membranes, and a purpuric skin rash. Cases vary tremendously in severity; many are mild and ambulatory with few signs; some are severe and fulminating. The average case lies in between. The patient is ill but usually recovers. *Br. abortus* infections are usually milder than those of *Br. melitensis* and cause an illness which may last for about a year. *Br. melitensis* infection may produce much longer illness.

Diagnosis

The organism can be recovered by culture from the blood especially during a febrile attack, occasionally when the patient is afebrile.. *Br. melitensis* and *Br. suis* are aerobic. *Br. abortus* requires excess carbon dioxide. Organisms may also be recovered from material obtained by spleen, lymph node or bone marrow puncture, and sometimes from the urine and the faeces or from synovial fluid.

Agglutinins appear in the serum within a fortnight of the onset of the primary attack. The two main antigens, A and M, occur in varying amounts in all organisms. Monospecific sera may be prepared but the agglutination test is usually group and not species specific. A titre of 1 in 100 is considered diagnostic of infection and a rising titre is suggestive of the active disease. A complement fixation test has also been elaborated but is group specific.

An intradermal test using an antigen, brucellin, made from brucella culture in broth is of some epidemiological value. After the usual intradermal injection the area is examined 4–36 hours later. In most cases of brucella infection a positive reaction appears as a raised erythematous oedematous plaque; false positives may occur. A negative reaction suggests the absence of the infection. The reaction is group specific and not reliable for diagnosis.

Treatment

Relief from the acute disease may be achieved by the administration of several antibiotics, but eradication of the infection may be very difficult in a given case.

Tetracycline, 2 G. orally in four divided doses daily for 21 days is effective in *Br. melitensis* infection. Where the drug can be tolerated, 3 G. daily gives better results so far as relapse is concerned.

Pyrrolidinomethyltetracycline may be given parenterally in severely ill patients with diarrhoea and vomiting, in doses of 275 mg. intravenously twice daily.

Corticosteroids should be given to severely ill patients over the first few days of antibiotics to avoid the Herxheimer-like reactions which sometimes develop.

A recommended combination which is useful in all infections including *Br. suis* is:

Streptomycin intramuscularly in doses of 1–2 G. daily, tetracycline orally, 2 G. daily, sulphadiazine orally, 4–6 G. daily, all for 3 weeks.

In chronic persistent infections the course of treatment may need repeating several times, or may be combined with the administration of a homologous killed vaccine.

BRIAN MAEGRAITH

HAEMOPHILUS INFECTIONS

BACTERIOLOGY

The bacilli of the genus *Haemophilus* are aerobic, non-motile and Gram-negative. They show considerable variation in morphology. The type species is *Haemophilus influenzae* and the group also includes *H. ducreyi.*

H. influenzae was originally found in the respiratory secretions of patients with influenza in the pandemic of 1890 and the observations were repeated in 1918. It was consequently regarded for a while as the cause of influenza. When swine influenza was shown to be due to a synergism between a virus and *H. suis,* it seemed possible that an analogous process operated in man. This view is no longer held but it remains a possibility that damage to the human lung by the virus of influenza permits *H. influenzae* to display a virulence it does not normally possess.

H. influenzae exists in two forms, encapsulated and non-encapsulated. Encapsulated organisms possess a specific soluble substance concentrated in the capsule which allows them to be separated into six serological types, denoted by the letters a, b, c, d, e and f.

Other members of the haemophilus group, *H. parainfluenzae, H. aegyptius, H. haemolyticus* and *H. parahaemolyticus,* are of little importance as a cause of disease in man.

HUMAN INFECTIONS

There is an interesting change in pathogenicity of *H. influenzae* with increasing years. In the infant and young child it is a virulent organism often causing serious infection. In the adult it is rarely capable of pathogenic activity. This is due to the bactericidal activity of the blood increasing with age, as the individual encounters the organism more and more frequently.

H. influenzae can be recovered from about 30 per cent. of healthy children; only one-fifth of these strains are encapsulated, but of this proportion 80 per cent. are of type b which is the common cause of serious infection. Difficulty arises because the mere presence of capsulated haemophili does not prove their causative role. Sometimes *H. influenzae* is the prime cause of the infection, sometimes it plays a secondary, but none the less significant, part and sometimes it is no more than a harmless bystander.

The initial lesion in children is a nasopharyngitis often associated with fever: from this spread may take place to cause acute sinusitis or otitis media, an acute laryngitis or pneumonia. A particularly dangerous manifestation is acute epiglottitis which rapidly leads to respiratory obstruction and is an urgent indication for tracheostomy. This is usually due to type b strains and is seen in children aged 2–7 years, although occasional instances have been recorded in adults. Further dissemination may result in meningitis or suppurative arthritis. *H. influenzae* is in most countries the commonest cause of suppurative meningitis in early childhood. In one series from Australia it was responsible for 13 of 23 cases below the age of 5 years. Meningitis due to this organism appears to have become more common in the last decade.

In adults infections similar to those described in children may occur, but they are of great rarity. It is possible, too, that in pandemics the influenza virus causes damage to the lungs which permits *H. influenzae* to play an actively pathogenic role.

H. influenzae can be recovered from the purulent sputum of many patients with chronic bronchitis often in relatively pure culture. The part played by the organism is hard to assess but most would agree that it appears to be virulent. Certainly treatment with a tetracycline leads to great clinical improvement; it is probable that *H. influenzae* is pathogenic to respiratory epithelium damaged by chronic bronchitis.

Various members of this group have been recovered from patients with subacute bacterial endocarditis. In this disease their role is little more than saprophytic and it is the only form of human infection recorded as due to *H. parainfluenzae, H. haemolyticus* and *H. parahaemolyticus.*

H. aegyptius (Koch-Weeks bacillus) is a cause of epidemic conjunctivitis.

DIAGNOSIS

Diagnosis depends upon isolation of the responsible organism. In some cases of respiratory infection in adults it remains difficult to assess the part it is playing in the cause of the patient's illness.

TREATMENT

H. influenzae is sensitive to sulphonamides and several antibiotics. For the treatment of meningitis chloramphenicol is the drug of choice. Details are to be found in the section on antibiotics.

An effective type-specific rabbit antiserum was available, but it has been displaced by the antibiotic drugs.

REFERENCE

TURK, D. C., and MAY, J. R. (1967). *Haemophilus Influenzae. Its Clinical Importance*, London.

R. BODLEY SCOTT

CHANCROID

Synonyms. Soft chancre; 'Ulcus molle'; Ducrey's infection.

Definition

An acute localized specific infectious disease due to the entrance of a micro-organism (*Haemophilus ducreyi*) into the tissues of skin or mucous membrane.

Aetiology

The infection is nearly always transmitted during sexual intercourse. Accidental infection is rare. The disease is widespread throughout the world but the incidence is highest in tropical countries. In this country it is not common and is limited, for the most part, to seaports. It is found much more often in men than in women. The figures of incidence for England and Wales in the Report of the Chief Medical Officer of the Ministry of Health for 1970 show 46 new cases in males and 4 in females. It is generally regarded as a disease of the highly promiscuous and the unhygienic. Symptomless carriers are known to exist.

Pathology

The organism, *H. ducreyi* or streptobacillus of Ducrey, is a small, slender, Gram-negative bacillus which is often seen in chain formation but may be found singly or in groups. It may be difficult to find in smears from the open sores because of secondary infection. It is a fastidious organism and usually difficult to grow in culture, although in expert hands media containing defibrinated human or rabbit's blood have given good results. The microscopic picture of chancroid is said to be distinctive and biopsy to be a useful method of diagnosis.

Symptoms and Signs

The incubation period is short, namely 3–5 days in most cases. Occasionally it may be as short as 24 hours. At the site of inoculation, which is nearly always on the genitalia, there first appears a small red papule or pustule which quickly breaks down to form an ulcer. The ulcer is usually very painful and extends quite quickly by local tissue spread. It may also ulcerate deeply and be very destructive. It tends to be irregular in outline, with undermined edges and a narrow zone of bright red erythema at the spreading margin. Surrounding tissue may show an erythematous blush. The floor of the ulcer is uneven and is covered with yellowish slough which exudes pus. The granulations bleed freely on manipulation. The base of the sore is not indurated. Occasionally the granulations become exuberant and elevated above the surrounding surface, so called 'ulcus molle elevatum'. Multiple sores are more common than single ones, in contrast to primary syphilis from which the diagnosis must be made. Auto-inoculation is common. In many cases the regional inguinal lymphatic nodes become involved, after periods varying from 2 days up to 3 weeks from the appearance of the sore. This so-called 'inflammatory bubo' is very painful and develops quickly. The skin over the swelling is reddened: the nodes become matted together and soon suppurate with the formation of a large single abscess. This is likely to break down on the surface of the skin to form a large chancroidal ulcer in the groin. Painful lymphangitis may also occur. Other complications which have been described include haemorrhage from the ulcer, urethral stricture, urethral fistula, phimosis and spreading gangrene.

Diagnosis

The diagnosis is frequently made on clinical grounds, but it is important to try to find the organism by smear or culture. Because of secondary infection, its identification may be impossible unless pus can be obtained by aspiration from an unruptured bubo. An intradermal test, the so-called 'Ito-Reenstierna' test, using a vaccine containing the killed organisms, was employed for a number of years. Opinions of its value still vary but in most centres its use has been discontinued because of the large number of positive tests given by individuals without history or signs of the infection.

Treatment

Local antiseptics are usually ineffective and their use is inadvisable because they may prevent the early diagnosis of syphilis by dark-ground examination. Sulphonamides are effective, but they usually have to be given for periods which entail the risk of sensitization, and are not always successful. Common practice is to give sulphathiazole or sulphadiazine in the dosage of 5 G. daily for 10–14 days. Long-acting sulphonamides, such as sulphadimethoxine may be used instead, in the dosage of 1 G. on the first day and 0·5 G. on succeeding days. By this means the minor toxic effects of sulphonamides are usually lessened. Intramuscular injections of streptomycin are also effective. One or two grammes may be given daily for about 5 days, although in some cases administration has been continued for as long as 2 weeks. Tetracycline, oxytetracycline and chlortetracycline, are all effective and may be given in the dosage of 0·25 G. by mouth every 6 hours until healing is complete. They have the disadvantage that they may mask the early signs of syphilis and that they are expensive. Most of the cases respond to sulphonamides or streptomycin which may be used individually or in conjunction, and these are the remedies of choice. Chloramphenicol by mouth is effective but should not be used because of its potential toxic effects. If any treatment is to be effective, local drainage must be established and this may necessitate dorsal slitting of the prepuce. Suppurating buboes should not be incised, but should be aspirated through healthy skin on one or more occasions.

When treatment is finished and the lesions have healed it is customary to keep the patient under observation for 3 months and to perform serological tests at monthly intervals, because of the possibility that syphilis may have been contracted at the same time and that the primary lesion, with its longer incubation period, may have appeared late and have been obscured.

REFERENCES

GREENBLATT, R. B. (1953) United States Public Health Service, Publication No. 255, p. 1.

KING, A. J., and NICOL, C. S. (1969) *Venereal Diseases*, 2nd ed., London.

CLAUDE NICOL

INFECTIONS DUE TO BACTEROIDACEAE

BACTERIOLOGY

Some thirty species of *Bacteroides* have been characterized. They are Gram-negative, non-sporing and usually non-motile and non-capsulate. Most of them have been found as normal inhabitants of the human mouth, genital tract or alimentary canal.

Those of clinical importance are *Bacteroides fragilis*, *Fusobacterium fusiforme* (*Fusiforme fusiforme*), and *Sphaerophorus necrophorus* (*Fusiformis necrophorus*).

HUMAN INFECTIONS

Fusobacterium fusiforme is associated with *Borrelia vincenti* in Vincent's angina and in fusospirochaetal gingivitis and stomatitis [see Section 7].

Bacteroides fragilis and *Sphaer. necrophorus* can be considered together. They both are found in such lesions as appendix abscess, urinary tract infection, parametritis and endometritis. All strains of *B. fragilis* are resistant to penicillin but sensitive to the tetracyclines.

Infections with *Sphaer. necrophorus* are probably more common than generally appreciated. Those who handle infected animals are liable to localized cutaneous and subcutaneous lesions. Veterinary surgeons, butchers and meat inspectors are particularly at risk. As the organism is often found in the mouth, it may cause ulceration of the tonsillar bed after tonsillectomy or of the gums after dental extraction. It is often isolated from the infected wounds which result from human bites.

Local spread from the alimentary and genital tracts accounts for more severe infections, such as puerperal fever, septic abortion and perforative peritonitis. Suppurative thrombophlebitis may follow with generalized septicopyaemia. Lung abscess, empyema of the pleura, meningitis, suppurative otitis media, suppurative arthritis, bacterial endocarditis and liver abscess are all recorded sequels.

Sphaer. necrophorus is sensitive to penicillin, moderately so to chloramphenicol but resistant to streptomycin.

REFERENCES

BORNSTEIN, D. L., WEINBURG, A. N., SWARTZ, M. N., and KUNZ, L. J. (1964) Anaerobic infections—Review of current experience, *Medicine* (*Baltimore*), **43**, 207.

GILLESPIE, W. A., and GUY, J. (1956) Bacteroides in intra-abdominal sepsis; their sensitivity to antibiotics, *Lancet*, i, 1039.

GUNN, A. A. (1956) Bacteroides septicaemia, *J. roy. Coll. Surg. Edinb.*, **2**, 41.

TYNES, B. S., and FROMMEYER, W. B. Jr. (1962) Bacteroides septicaemia, *Ann. intern. Med.*, **56**, 12.

TYNES, B. S., and UTZ, J. P. (1960) Fusobacterium septicaemia, *Amer. J. Med.*, **29**, 879.

INFECTIONS DUE TO MICROCOCCACEAE

STAPHYLOCOCCAL INFECTIONS

BACTERIOLOGY

Staphylococci are organisms which grow in clusters and stain by Gram's method. Until the introduction of the coagulase test there was no easy way of distinguishing potentially pathogenic strains from those only rarely the cause of disease. Pathogenic staphylococci are now recognized by their ability to form coagulase and are referred to as *Staphylococcus aureus* whether they form golden or white colonies on culture media. Coagulase-negative staphylococci are usually harmless, although they may cause urinary infections and have been responsible for endocarditis after cardiac surgery.

During the process of multiplication, staphylococci elaborate a variety of toxins and enzymes. These include a soluble exotoxin, a number of haemolysins, leucocidin, hyaluronidase and coagulase. This last is an enzyme which reacts with a factor normally present in plasma to cause clotting; several antigenically different coagulases have been isolated, but their practical significance lies in their liberation only by pathogenic staphylococci. Certain strains are capable of producing an enterotoxin which can cause food poisoning and which can be distinguished from the exotoxin. Rarely staphylococci produce an erythrogenic toxin which provokes a scarlatinal rash indistinguishable from that of streptococcal scarlet fever. It is antigenically unrelated to the erythrogenic toxin of *Str. pyogenes*.

Staph. aureus is the one organism above all others liable to develop resistance to antibiotic drugs.

PATHOLOGY

Although the respiratory tract may be invaded initially, the characteristic primary lesion of staphylococcal infection is in the skin or subcutaneous tissues. The organisms gain entry through a breach of surface or by the ducts of sweat glands. They multiply locally; the exotoxin causes necrosis and excites an inflammatory response; the hyaluronidase facilitates their spread; and the coagulase causes thrombosis in the neighbouring vessels. The necrotic area is invaded by neutrophil leucocytes; the inflammatory zone is isolated by a wall of fibrin formed by the activity of the coagulase; and an abscess results.

Infection of unusual virulence or inadequate local defences may allow invasion of the blood stream. A characteristic feature of general staphylococcal infection is the formation of abscesses scattered throughout the body. It is to this process that the name pyaemia is often applied.

EPIDEMIOLOGY

Man is the reservoir of staphylococci. Pathogenic strains can be recovered from the nose in 35–50 per cent. of healthy persons. These carriers are often found to have staphylococci also on their hands, arms, and other parts of their bodies as well as on their clothing. It seems likely that they are the most important source of pathogenic staphylococci, although those with active infection, particularly when it is superficial and open to the air, must make their contribution. The hospital has a particular significance. It is there that strains resistant to antibiotics are bred and hospital workers are likely to become carriers of them. Conditions are unusually favourable to the dissemination of virulent organisms and a fertile soil is provided by the newborn, those recovering from operations, and patients with resistance lowered by prolonged disease.

Phage typing has allowed the paths of infection to be traced with precision and much of our knowledge of staphylococcal infection comes from epidemiological studies in hospital wards. *Staph. aureus* has displaced *Str. pyogenes* from the dominating position it held for so long as a cause of serious infection.

HUMAN INFECTIONS

The common clinical varieties of staphylococcal infection in man divide themselves into local and remote. Local infections are due to the direct invasion of the tissues by staphylococci; remote are the result of infections which the local defences have been unable to contain.

Local Infections

The Skin and Subcutaneous Tissues. These are the commonest sites. The most familiar result of staphylococcal invasion of the skin is the boil or *furuncle* in which infection of a pilosebaceous unit leads to a perifollicular abscess. Finally, a central slough or 'core' separates and healing follows with a variable degree of scarring.

Boils may occur in any area, but are most common on the face, neck, forearms, in the flexures and where tight clothing rubs, as at the waist. Their occurrence indicates some breakdown of the cutaneous defences against infection in the form of excoriation or other minor trauma or some general disease, such as diabetes mellitus, which reduces resistance.

A discharging boil serves as a focus from which staphylococci are disseminated and may infect adjacent areas of skin; consequently recurrent furunculosis is a common problem. It may, too, form the starting point from which infection spreads. Boils around the nares have an evil reputation in this regard for they have been followed by suppurative thrombophlebitis extending to the cavernous sinus.

A *carbuncle* may be regarded as a confluent group of boils. It occurs most frequently on the neck.

The other staphylococcal infections of the skin depend for their characteristics upon the exact site of infection. In *blepharitis* and *sycosis barbae* it is the hair follicles of the eyelashes and the beard which are invaded. In *impetigo contagiosa*, which may also be due to streptococci, it is the ostia of the pilosebaceous follicles and in *Bockhart's impetigo* (folliculitis) those of the sweat glands. *Ecthyma* is due to a staphylococcal infection of the dermis leading to necrosis, ulceration and scarring: it occurs in neglected and undernourished children, usually on the legs, and commonly where trauma or pediculosis has caused a breach of surface. *Staph. aureus* is also the organism usually isolated from infected wounds and abrasions and from abscesses of the breast and other superficial tissues.

Occasional instances of staphylococcal scarlet fever have been reported in which a local staphylococcal infection, such as an axillary abscess, has been accompanied by a scarlatiniform rash indistinguishable from that of streptococcal scarlet fever. In such cases profuse desquamation follows the rash, but the Dick and Schultz-Charlton tests are negative [p. 85].

The Respiratory Tract. Active infection of the upper respiratory tract is rarely due to staphylococci although they so commonly colonize the nasal mucosa. It is possible, however, that nasal carriers are more susceptible than others to staphylococcal pneumonia. This disease may occur as an apparently primary infection, but it is seen more often during epidemics of influenza or as a sequel to measles. It has been suggested that invasion of the lungs by virulent staphylococci is only likely to occur when the respiratory epithelium has been damaged by a preceding infection. Staphylococcal pneumonia is always a serious illness and may be of fulminating onset and great severity [see Section 9].

The Alimentary Tract. *Staph. aureus* may cause an acute enterocolitis of abrupt onset, associated with distension, vomiting and choleraic diarrhoea and resulting in dehydration, electrolyte imbalance and peripheral circulatory failure [see Section 7]. This has been long recognized as an occasional sequel of abdominal surgery. Of recent years the incidence of this grave infection has increased *pari passu* with the increased use of antibiotic and corticosteroid drugs. It is met most often after operations on the stomach, but may complicate such diseases as acute leukaemia when massive doses of corticosteroids are used in treatment. The staphylococcus responsible for this infection is usually of a strain known to form enterotoxin and is almost invariably resistant to two or more antibiotics.

The Genital Tract. *Staph. aureus* is responsible for a few cases of puerperal infection.

Remote Infections

When the local defences are breached by the staphylococcus a general infection of the blood stream may occur or the only evidence of this transgression may be the appearance of an abscess at a site remote from the initial lesion.

In the first instance the severity of the illness is inconstant. There may be profound intoxication with stupor or delirium, remittent fever marked by daily rigors, and rapid deterioration without the appearance of suppurative foci. In patients so ill, death, with signs of peripheral circulatory failure, may occur within a few days. In those who survive longer, metastatic abscesses will begin to form: the most frequent sites are the subcutaneous tissues, the muscles, the joints, and the lungs. Cerebral abscesses, panophthalmitis, multiple abscesses in the renal cortex or the myocardium, and perinephric suppuration are all common. Serous cavities, such as the pleura and the pericardium, may be invaded secondarily, but meningitis is rare. Acute staphylococcal endocarditis occurs in about 10 per cent. of fatal cases.

Sometimes the infection pursues a more leisurely course. There are the usual general features of a chronic septic process: increasing lassitude and weakness, progressive loss of flesh and anaemia. Fever may be trivial or coincide with the eruption of fresh infective foci, episodes which may be separated by intervals of several weeks.

At other times the only sign of remote infection is the appearance of an abscess far removed from the primary lesion. This may take place weeks after the initial infection has resolved, and it is often only when a staphylococcus has been isolated from an abscess that the significance of a furuncle, long since healed, is appreciated. Common sites of such lesions are the perinephric space, the renal cortex (carbuncle of the kidney), the spinal epidural space, and bone. In the last instance the result may be an acute osteomyelitis or a chronic abscess (Brodie's abscess). Acute osteomyelitis may itself form the starting point of a secondary generalized infection.

In many patients with remote staphylococcal infection of the type described, resistance to infection has been lowered by some systemic affection such as rheumatoid arthritis, leukaemia, or systemic lupus erythematosus. Treatment with corticosteroid drugs is often an additional factor. In many with this type of infection its clinical expression is muted and the diagnosis is only reached *post mortem.*

Staphylococcal Food Poisoning

This is discussed in the section on food poisoning [see p. 56].

DIAGNOSIS

There is usually little difficulty in the diagnosis of staphylococcal infection. The organism can readily be isolated from cultures of pus or, in general infections, from the blood itself. In staphylococcal enterocolitis immense numbers of staphylococci are usually visible in direct films made from the stool and they grow rapidly on culture. In staphylococcal food poisoning, organisms can be isolated from the contaminated food, and from the vomitus of the victims; those from both sources can be shown to be of the same phage type and it will be one known to form enterotoxin.

Staphylococci that form coagulase all appear able to cause disease. Fortunately only a few phage types are likely to be responsible for infection which spreads from one patient to another. At present there is no laboratory method by which these epidemic staphylococci can be recognized with certainty. Most, but not all, of them are resistant to the tetracyclines and to mercurial antiseptics, and possession of these qualities does not necessarily imply that a staphylococcus will cause spreading infection.

Staphylococcal infections, like those due to most bacteria, are usually accompanied by neutrophil leucocytosis and by an increase in erthyrocyte sedimentation rate. With abscess formation the leucocytosis often rises as high as 25,000 per mm^3. In some chronic cases of generalized infection there may be leucopenia; where infection is secondary to leukaemia, the blood shows the changes characteristic of the underlying disease.

PROPHYLAXIS

In recent years much attention has been paid to the control of staphylococcal cross-infection in hospital and epidemiological studies have been rewarding. Infection still occurs, but it is now usually possible to trace the source of outbreaks. In open surgical wards with reasonable facilities the wound sepsis rate should not exceed 5 per cent. It is not easy to reduce this figure for a large number of factors are operative. The rate of infection in medical wards is much lower.

TREATMENT

The treatment of the established infection is discussed in the relevant sections and in the article on antibiotics [Section 1].

REFERENCES

Elek, S. D. (1959) *Staphylococcus Pyogenes and its Relation to Disease*, Edinburgh.

Fekety, F. R. (1964) The epidemiology and prevention of staphylococcal infection, *Medicine* (*Baltimore*), **43**, 593.

Williams, R. E. O., Blowers, R., Garrod, L. P., and Shooter, R. A. (1960) *Hospital Infection*, London.

Willis, A. T., and Turner, G. C. (1963) Staphylococci in the hospital environment *J. Path. Bact.*, **85**, 395.

R. Bodley Scott

INFECTIONS DUE TO NEISSERIACEAE

MENINGOCOCCAL INFECTIONS

Harmless infection with meningococci, with the organisms leading a transitory saprophytic existence in the nasopharynx, is common; disease resulting from such infection is relatively infrequent. Three clear-cut syndromes are seen:

1. Meningococcal meningitis, by far the commonest, accounts for over 90 per cent. of clinical illnesses.
2. Acute fulminating septicaemia in which death is likely within a few hours of the onset.
3. Chronic meningococcaemia, a mild low-grade septicaemic illness characterized by fever, rashes and joint pains.

AETIOLOGY AND EPIDEMIOLOGY

The meningococcus (*Neisseria meningitidis*) is a Gram-negative diplococcus often described as intracellular because of the frequency with which it is seen inside polymorphonuclear cells. It is somewhat difficult to grow but culture is usually successful when attempted on chocolate agar under a low oxygen concentration.

Four sero-groups have been differentiated, A, B, C and D. A few meningococci are untypable. In the United Kingdom group A used to be responsible for most epidemics but this group is now becoming rare. In the United States groups B and C predominate. Thirty-seven per cent. of groups B and C meningococci are sulphadiazine resistant.

Meningococci are frequently found in the naso-pharynx where they lead a temporary saprophytic existence with no disturbance of the host. Temporary carriers of this kind play an important role in dissemination of the disease and whereas infectivity is high it is unusual to get two persons in a family ill with meningococcal disease at the same time. Illness results from increased invasiveness, lowered resistance of the patient perhaps playing some part. What is probably more important is the presence of some immunological deficit. In some cases there is a marked deficiency of gamma M immunoglobulin. Such an inherited defect would explain the occasional family outbreak of disease as opposed to symptomless infection.

Under the conditions of overcrowding which prevail in wartime the carrier rate rises, an epidemic starting when this rate exceeds 20 per cent. The disease is world wide. No age is immune but the majority of cases are children. In wartime epidemics occur in crowded barracks among service personnel, particularly after an intake of recruits who are likely to have no immunity to the prevalent strains of meningococci. On the other hand acquired immunity prevents epidemics among seasoned troops under much more crowded conditions (for example on a troop-ship) even though the carrier rate may remain high. The incidence increases when there is a fall in the absolute humidity such as occurs in the winter months in temperate climates and in the dry season in the tropics. Males are more frequently attacked than females.

Transmission of infection is by droplet. Indirect spread is unlikely as the organism is rapidly destroyed by heat and by drying.

PATHOLOGY

Bacteraemia precedes meningitis in all cases and in most persists during the first few days, septicaemic manifestations appearing in many patients. All layers of the meninges are involved in the inflammatory process, an exudate of leucocytes, fibrin and organisms being found in the ventricles, basal cisterns and the subarachnoid space. Though usually thin, this exudate may thicken and become organized in which case the normal cerebrospinal fluid pathways may be blocked. This is particularly likely to occur at the constrictions around the ventricular foramina or at the aqueduct of Sylvius. Internal or external hydrocephalus results from such obstruction with distension of the ventricles and flattening of the cerebral convolutions. Direct spread of purulent inflammation along nerves can cause labyrinthitis or radiculitis. Vessels surrounded by exudate may thrombose, resulting in focal or diffuse encephalitic signs.

Septicaemic lesions may be found in any tissue. Meningococci localize in the vascular endothelium causing vascular damage with a petechial or purpuric rash. Gangrene may follow extensive thrombotic lesions. Massive haemorrhages into the suprarenal cortex occur in fulminating septicaemic cases together with bleeding from mucous and serous surfaces.

The incubation period is thought to be between 3 and 5 days.

FULMINATING MENINGOCOCCAL SEPTICAEMIA

Synonyms. Waterhouse-Friderichsen syndrome; Acute adrenal apoplexy.

Definition

An overwhelming septicaemic illness associated with haemorrhages into the suprarenal cortex and elsewhere, in which death is usual within 4–24 hours of the onset.

Symptoms

The patient is usually a child, often one of under two years of age. The onset is sudden with vomiting and restlessness, frequently waking the child who was quite well on going to bed. There may be abdominal pain. At this stage the patient looks pale, ill and anxious with a tachycardia but usually no fever. The respiratory rate is raised. Within 2–6 hours a petechial rash appears on the face, trunk and limbs, larger purpuric lesions soon following. At times the rash almost seems to appear as one watches the patient, so rapidly may it develop. Toxaemia becomes intense, pallor or cyanosis are striking and the pulse fades into imperceptibility, the blood pressure soon falling to an unrecordable level. Respirations are markedly increased and may be gulping in character. Death usually occurs before the meninges are invaded, signs of meningitis being absent and the cerebrospinal fluid normal. Although delirium may occur, mental clarity to within a few moments of death is often a striking feature. The speed of development of peripheral circulatory failure, toxaemia and death must be stressed. Thrombocytopenia may occur. At autopsy meningococci are present in blood vessels in most tissues throughout the body and haemorrhages are widespread. The essential lesion of the syndrome is the haemorrhagic destruction of the adrenal cortex which is normally visible macroscopically at autopsy. Death, however, is not due to adrenocortical failure as cortisol levels in the peripheral blood remain normal or raised.

Treatment and Prognosis

This is one of the greatest emergencies in medical practice. There is no doubt that if the diagnosis can be made early enough some of these patients can be saved, but delay of half an hour may well prove fatal. Treatment must therefore be begun as soon as the patient is seen with 3 mega Units (1·8 G.) of penicillin intramuscularly and a maximum dose of sulphonamide intravenously if possible or intramuscularly should the veins be collapsed. Prednisolone, 40 mg., or equivalent corticosteroid should also be injected. Treatment in hospital is continued with sulphonamides, penicillin and steroids intravenously while the patient is nursed in an oxygen tent. Success has followed the use of continuous heparin intravenously, 100 Units per kg.

every 6 hours (about 25,000 Units per day), the aim of this treatment being to stop the extensive intravascular coagulation. If the patient can be kept alive for 24 hours there is a good chance of recovery. Steroids are reduced rapidly over the subsequent seven days as improvement is maintained. Blood culture and petechial scrapes will provide bacteriological confirmation of the diagnosis, but laboratory investigation must follow and not precede treatment. A lumbar puncture is time consuming and is only indicated if signs of meningitis develop and meningococci have not been seen in the petechial scrapes.

When recovery takes place permanent replacement therapy with steroids is not required. This suggests that survival is only possible in those in whom cortical damage is minimal at the time treatment is started.

CHRONIC MENINGOCOCCAL SEPTICAEMIA

Synonym. Chronic meningococcaemia.

In certain patients meningococcal infection produces a low-grade septicaemic illness in which there are recurrent attacks of pyrexia with mild shivering attacks. These occur every two or three days and are usually associated with a rash consisting of papules on the trunk and limbs, many of which develop a petechial centre. The rash is sometimes profuse and has been confused with rubella. Some people develop erythema nodosum of the shins and many complain of muscle and joint pains. There is little toxaemia and patients neither look nor feel particularly ill. This illness may persist for weeks or months before burning itself out or ending in meningitis. The diagnosis should be considered in all cases of intermittent fever accompanied by spots. Repeated blood cultures may be required to recover the organism. Immediate recovery follows treatment with penicillin or sulphonamides.

MENINGOCOCCAL MENINGITIS

Synonyms. Cerebrospinal fever; Epidemic cerebrospinal meningitis; Spotted fever.

Definition

Meningococcal meningitis is the commonest type of pyogenic meningitis. It is due to infection with the meningococcus and occurs in sporadic and epidemic forms.

Symptoms

The *onset* is commonly abrupt with fever, headache, malaise and vomiting. In some cases this is preceded by 48 hours of upper respiratory tract symptoms, presumably due to the meningococcal pharyngitis although this has seldom been investigated. With the onset of headache the temperature rises to 102°–103° F. (38·9°–39·5° C.); the pulse may remain relatively slow if there is an appreciable rise of intracranial pressure. The headache is severe, throbbing in character and often most intense over the occiput although it is sometimes confined to the frontal areas. Photophobia is usual and vomiting becomes more frequent and may be projectile. Irritability and delirium are common. Convulsions may occur but deep coma is unusual.

On examination the appearance of the developed untreated case is typical. The patient lies on his side with his back towards the light, resenting any interference though usually remaining fairly quiet while left undisturbed. The apparently semiconscious person may get up to pass urine in a corner of the room. Retention of urine occurs less often than incontinence but is suggested by the appearance of restlessness in a previously quiet patient. Attempts to turn the patient on his back produce clear evidence of cerebral irritation which often makes a satisfactory clinical examination difficult or even impossible. There is marked neck stiffness in such a case due to spasm of the posterior cervical muscles. There may be some head retraction. Back flexion is also severely limited as is straight leg raising due to protective spasm limiting the movement of the inflamed meninges. Kernig's sign is best elicited by flexing the hip to a right angle and observing the degree of limitation of knee extension. Brudzinski's signs (spontaneous flexion of the knees and hips on attempting neck flexion and spontaneous flexion of one leg when passive flexion of the opposite leg is carried out by the examiner) are often positive. There may be a general reduction in superficial and tendon reflexes. External rectus palsy and facial nerve paralysis are the commonest signs of focal neurological involvement. In a patient who has suffered his primary herpetic infection, herpes labialis is almost inevitable and often extensive.

A rash is present in about 40 per cent. of patients. It consists originally of roseolar papules, most of which rapidly become petechial and some purpuric. There is no characteristic distribution, although it is not uncommon for the limbs to be heavily involved with only a few lesions on the trunk. It appears on the second or third day and the mucous membranes may be affected. Meningococci are present in the haemorrhagic lesions.

The clinical picture in infants requires special mention as the younger the child the less typical is the illness. Over twelve months of age there are usually unequivocal signs of meningeal involvement, signs which may be scanty between 6 and 12 months and are often absent before 6 months. The first sign of illness is frequently a convulsion which may be repeated. In between fits the infant is irritable and unwilling to take feeds. Vomiting is usual and often projectile. The infant dislikes being nursed, often crying when picked up and ceasing when returned to the cot. The cry may be high pitched. The temperature may be normal or raised. On examination the infant is seen to lie quietly but usually cries as soon as he is handled. He is pale may be cyanosed and the respiratory rate is frequently high. Neck stiffness is often absent and Kernig's sign negative but the anterior fontanelle is usually tense and may be bulging. Even this sign may be absent however, particularly if vomiting has been severe enough to lead to dehydration.

In the absence of specific treatment some patients start to recover in the third week, some become comatose and die, but the majority enter a chronic phase with progressive emaciation, opisthotonus continued vomiting and the development of hydrocephalus, paralyses and bed-sores. Occasional recovery with severe sequelae may follow this stage but most such patients die. Posterior basic meningitis in infants is a chronic hydrocephalic form of the disease in untreated infants which is now rarely seen.

Following treatment with sulphonamides, vomiting usually ceases within 24–48 hours, the patient also becoming co-operative within this period. Headache in children commonly disappears within a few days but may persist in an adult for up to a fortnight, particularly if he is allowed to sit up or get up too early.

Various forms of the disease have been described in the past but these are mostly only variants in degree from a mild attack in which clinical recovery takes place within 2 or 3 days of starting treatment to a severe illness in which gross evidence of meningitis appears early.

Complications

These are much less numerous since the advent of sulphonamide therapy but are still seen, particularly in patients in whom treatment has been delayed or has been inadequate.

Neurological. Transient palsies of the 6th, 7th or 3rd cranial nerves may appear in the acute stage, normally resolving satisfactorily with the meningitis with ultimate complete recovery. They are due to the involvement of the nerves in their intracranial course through the inflammatory exudate. A mild degree of papilloedema is not uncommon in the acute stage but swelling of the disc of more than moderate degree suggests a focal intracranial collection of pus.

Unexplained fever, intermittent vomiting, drowsiness often of sudden onset or failure to convalesce rapidly in the second week after adequate therapy should make one suspect the onset of hydrocephalus or a subdural effusion, both complications virtually limited nowadays to infancy. The fontanelle, if patent, is found to be tense but the cerebrospinal fluid shows the meningitis to be resolving satisfactorily. The skull may enlarge rapidly. Subdural tapping will confirm the diagnosis of effusion, repeated removal of small quantities of a fluid with a high protein content usually leading to resolution.

If hydrocephalus is the cause of the patient's symptoms the diagnosis will be confirmed by ventriculography.

Encephalitic complications occur. In one type the patient becomes deeply comatose a day or two after the onset, this usually being associated with evidence of diffuse neurological involvement such as bilateral extensor plantar responses and bulbar or other palsies. Over 50 per cent. of these patients die in spite of recovery from the meningitis, respiratory failure or bronchopneumonia being the immediate cause of death. In the second type, focal lesions such as hemiplegia, monoplegia or aphasia appear suddenly. Recovery is the rule with little or no residual disability. Radiculoneuritis causing a flaccid paralysis is now eytremely rare.

Special Senses. Some degree of permanent deafness which may be bilateral occurs in 5 per cent. of cases due to a direct spread of infection to the labyrinth. The deafness may be partial or complete and its presence should always be specifically looked for in convalescence, particularly in the young child. Blindness is now very rare but can arise from an iridochoroiditis, acute optic atrophy from pressure of exudate, or delayed optic atrophy following the development of hydrocephalus.

Urinary Changes. Glycosuria, due to inflammatory changes in the region of the floor of the fourth ventricle, is common. It is associated with a moderate rise of blood sugar and if there has been much vomiting there will be ketosis in addition. The quantity of sugar in the urine seldom exceeds 1·5 g. per cent. and rapidly disappears as the patient improves. Febrile albuminuria is usual.

Other Complications. Arthropathies with turbid effusions into large joints are now infrequent; they resolve with chemotherapy. Heavy purpuric eruptions may become gangrenous, particularly on the buttocks, elbows and lower legs. Gangrene of the digits is also occasionally seen. Pericarditis occurs in about 5 per cent. of cases and may be associated with myocarditis or endocarditis.

Diagnosis

In the ordinary adult case the triad of headache, vomiting and neck stiffness is typical of meningeal irritation and should lead to examination of the cerebrospinal fluid. If photophobia and cerebral irritation are marked and the history short then a diagnosis of pyogenic meningitis is almost certain. In infants the diagnosis is much more difficult and must constantly be borne in mind in any ill baby. Indications for lumbar puncture in any unwell baby are unexplained convulsions, vomiting, fever, dislike of being handled or attacks of pallor or cyanosis.

The essential investigation in the diagnosis of any suspected case of meningitis is examination of the cerebrospinal fluid obtained by lumbar or cisternal puncture. In addition, blood cultures should always be carried out as the organism may not always grow in the cerebrospinal fluid. If a rash is present, scraping of petechiae and immediate Gram staining is a rapid method of confirming a meningococcal infection.

Macroscopically the cerebrospinal fluid varies from slightly turbid to frankly purulent, the number of cells usually lying between 2000 and 10,000 per mm^3. of which over 95 per cent. are polymorphs. In early cases the cell count may number less than 1000 per mm^3. or in some severe cases there may be over 50,000 per mm^3. Following treatment the total count falls rapidly and lymphocytes largely replace the polymorphs. The protein is originally raised to 200–400 mg. per 100 ml. and sugar reduced to 15 mg. per 100 ml. or lower. In acute cases, however, when a lumbar puncture is likely to be carried out within six hours of the onset the sugar level may be within normal limits. In most cases films made from the centrifuged deposit show intracellular and extracellular diplococci. Culture of meningococci is not invariably successful.

Nowadays the cerebrospinal fluid is frequently modified by antibiotics administered prior to the patient's admission to hospital. The total cell count is lower, up to 50 per cent. of the cells may be lymphocytes and organisms may neither be seen nor cultured.

A high protein and a reduced sugar content help to distinguish these 'half treated' cases from aseptic meningitis. Most patients show a leucocytosis in the peripheral blood but this may be absent in the more severe infections.

The differential diagnosis includes:

1. *Other causes of pyogenic meningitis* of which *Haemophilus influenzae* and pneumococci are the commonest. Influenzal meningitis frequently follows an upper respiratory tract infection, otitis media or pneumonia, is usually subacute in onset and is rarely accompanied by a rash. Pneumococcal meningitis, on the other hand, tends to be very acute, coma often appearing within 24 hours. It is frequently secondary to sinusitis, purulent otitis media or pneumonia. The final diagnosis of pyogenic meningitis must rest with the examination of the cerebrospinal fluid.

2. *Tuberculous Meningitis.* Patients suffering from this disease have a longer history, usually of over a week, with an insidious onset. Choroidal tubercles may be present. The cerebrospinal fluid contains under 500 cells per mm^3., most of which are lymphocytes, the protein is high, often over 300 mg. per 100 ml. and the sugar frequently reduced to under 40 mg. per 100 ml. If tubercle bacilli are not seen and if the patient has been treated with antibiotics, the differential diagnosis between a partially treated meningococcal meningitis and tuberculous meningitis may be difficult. Chest radiography, Mantoux testing and daily cerebrospinal fluid examinations combined with close observation without therapy will be necessary to establish the type of meningitis present.

3. *Aseptic Meningitis.* Few patients with aseptic meningitis are toxic and delirium is uncommon. Neck stiffness is also generally less marked. Although in many types, including poliomyelitis, the cerebrospinal fluid examined early in the central nervous system phase shows a predominance of polymorphs this is never above 90 per cent. and the total cell count rarely exceeds 300 per mm^3. The protein is only slightly raised and the sugar level remains within normal limits.

4. *Meningism.* The clinical picture of meningitir, with headache, vomiting and neck stiffness, combined with a *normal* cerebrospinal fluid, is called meningism. Back stiffness and a positive Kernig's sign are present also if the meningism is at all marked. Meningism may appear in any severe infection, including smallpox and typhoid fever but is most often seen in the following common illnesses of childhood: tonsillitis; cervical adenitis; pneumonia, particularly apical; acute pyelitis; salmonella enteritis and certain viral respiratory infections including influenza.

If meningism is at all marked even if one of the above is detected, the cerebrospinal fluid must be examined to exclude a coexistent meningitis. Meningism is commoner in children than in adults.

Subarachnoid haemorrhage is often mistaken for meningitis. The onset in this disease is usually dramatically sudden and the cerebrospinal fluid is evenly blood stained.

Treatment

General. The patient must be nursed in isolation in hospital. There is a real risk of close contacts becoming infected with meningococci although a much smaller one of any such contact becoming ill. Early diagnosis is essential for the best results. On no account should a suspected case of meningitis be treated at home with chemotherapy without confirmation of the diagnosis. Such a procedure is liable to make the causative organism difficult to recover and may seriously jeopardize the patient's chances if he is suffering from one of the less common varieties of meningitis. Exceptions to this rule are only permissible in countries where hospital facilities are lacking. In such a situation under epidemic conditions when the diagnosis of meningococcal meningitis has been confirmed in one or two patients, it is justifiable to treat all cases of meningitis as meningococcal.

The room should be darkened while photophobia is present. Excessive restlessness requires padding of the bed which will need to have cot sides. Paraldehyde, 5–8 ml., intramuscularly for an adult, or 0·2 ml. per kg. for a child is a useful sedative with a wide margin of safety. Soluble phenobarbitone, 15 mg. at 3 months, 60 mg. at 1 year, and 200 mg. in an adult, intramuscularly, may be required to stop convulsions. Fluids will nearly always be retained by mouth within 48 hours of starting specific treatment and parenteral therapy is not usually required in the uncomplicated case. If coma is deep enough to impair the swallowing reflex the airway must be kept clear by nursing the patient semiprone with a slight head down tilt to the bed combined with suction as necessary. Headache requires analgesics. Retention of urine usually responds to carbachol injection, 0·25 mg. in 1 ml. for an adult, but catheterization may be necessary. Neurosurgical investigation becomes necessary if papilloedema is marked or if hydrocephalus is suspected. Subdural effusions require repeated tapping and aspiration of small quantities of fluid.

Following treatment many children are well enough to be discharged from hospital after 2 weeks. They should be kept in bed for at least 5 days following the return of temperature to normal or the disappearance of the headache, whichever is the longer. Adults require a somewhat longer convalescence as too early activity leads to return of headache. They should be mobilized in bed for a week after their symptoms have disappeared before being allowed up. In a straightforward case, a second examination of the cerebrospinal fluid is unnecessary nor is there any need for clearance throat swabs as the organisms are readily eliminated by chemotherapy. Meningococcal infection is notifiable in the United Kingdom. Family contacts should be given a 24-hour course of sulphadiazine and then allowed to return to school or work.

Specific. Sulphonamides have revolutionized the treatment and prognosis of meningococcal infections. Sulphadiazine or sulphadimidine give excellent results when given in full dosage for 2–3 days followed by a smaller dose to complete a seven-day course. Thus the treatment schedule for an adult using sulphadiazine is 2 G. of the soluble sodium salt intramuscularly (or intravenously in the severely ill) followed by 1·5 G. orally four-hourly for 2–3 days; 1·25 G. four-hourly for

3–4 days. A child under three years requires 3 G. per day in divided dosage four-hourly with reduction to 2 G. per day after 2–3 days. On this regime the persistence or return of moderate fever on the fifth or sixth day is not infrequently due to the sulphonamide and subsides once the drug is stopped. Penicillin is instilled intrathecally at the diagnostic lumbar puncture following removal of turbid fluid, 10,000 Units in those under 2 years and 20,000 Units in all other patients. (Intrathecal penicillin is unnecessary in meningococcal meningitis but its use is justified pending confirmation of the meningococcal origin of the infection.) Intramuscular penicillin in large doses is now mandatory in view of increasing illness due to sulphonamide-resistant organisms. Though still rare in the United Kingdom, in the United States over 30 per cent. of cases of meningococcal infection are now due to such strains. Corticosteroids are not required routinely. They are indicated in the presence of peripheral circulatory failure with hypotension and in patients with an excessive purulent exudate in the subarachnoid space as shown by a cell count of over 40,000 per mm^3. or by the appearance of focal neurological signs *after* the onset of treatment.

Prophylactic. Under epidemic conditions in a closed community meningococci can be eliminated by giving 2 G. of sulphadiazine per day for 3 days, or 6 G. for 1 day (adult dose). This is of value in dealing with outbreaks in service populations and is also applicable to treating whole villages under primitive conditions. Family contacts should always be given one day's treatment with sulphonamides. In view of the possibility of the strain being resistant, contacts must also be warned to report to their doctor at the first sign of ill health.

Prognosis

The mortality has been reduced by sulphonamides from 70 per cent. to under 10 per cent. Theoretically no patient should die from meningococcal meningitis as the organism is always sensitive to sulphonamides or penicillin. Many series have produced mortalities of under one per cent. Delay in onset of treatment due to diagnostic errors is the most important factor responsible for the present mortality. The effect of age is significant, the disease having a considerable mortality in the first year of life undoubtedly contributed to by the greater difficulty of diagnosis at this age. The death rate is also higher in the elderly. In the period 1966–68 the annual notifications of meningococcal infection in England and Wales were 407, 293 and 605. The case mortality varied between 26 and 17 per cent.

The severity of symptoms is of little help in assessing prognosis in the acute stage with the exception of the level of consciousness. Deep coma is a grave sign, particularly when this persists or makes its appearance two to three days after starting therapy.

REFERENCES

EICKHOFF, T. C., and FINLAND, M. (1965) Changing susceptibility of meningococci to antimicrobial agents, *New Engl. J. Med.*, **272**, 395.

HOBBS, J. R., MILNER, R. D. G., and WATT, P. J. (1967) Gamma-M deficiency predisposing to meningococcal septicaemia, *Brit. med. J.*, **4**, 583.

MCKENDRICK, G. D. W. (1968) Treatment of pyogenic meningitis, *J. Neurol. Neurosurg. Psychiat.*, **31**, 528.

MCKENDRICK, G. D. W. (1969) Aetiological factors in meningococcal infections, in *Medical Annual*, p. 274, Bristol.

SMITH, M. H. D. (1956) Acute bacterial meningitis, *Pediatrics*, **17**, No. 2, 258.

G. D. W. MCKENDRICK

GONORRHOEA

Definition

An infectious disease due to *Neisseria gonorrhoeae* or the gonococcus.

Aetiology and Epidemiology

The gonococcus is a Gram-negative diplococcus. It is a strict parasite and depends for spread upon direct transference from host to host. It spreads along mucosal surfaces and is also able to penetrate columnar epithelium producing an inflammatory response in the submucosa. It is susceptible to environment and is rapidly killed by drying or by weak antiseptics. It seldom survives for more than a few hours outside the body except under conditions of artificial cultivation.

In 1946 47,343 cases of gonococcal infection were reported in England and Wales, the highest recorded number; the figure fell to 17,526 in 1954, but has since risen to 54,764 in 1970. Factors which have contributed to this recent rise include the symptomlessness of this disease in many women and increasing promiscuity in the general population. Groups with the highest incidence include immigrants of all races, male homosexuals, and adolescents; prostitution also still plays its part. Some irresponsible males attend the clinics with repeated infections.

Modes of Infection

Sexual intercourse is by far the most common and important mode of infection causing involvement of the lower genito-urinary tract in both sexes. Infection may also be transmitted to the rectum in the passive homosexual and to the conjunctival sacs of adolescents or adults, also to those of newly-born infants by contamination with the infected genital secretions of the mother. Occasionally accidental infection occurs in children due to poor standards of hygiene or close contact in bed; little girls are particularly susceptible to infection transmitted from their parents in this way. Spread of infection in schools and hospitals has also been reported in the past.

Diagnosis

The organism is identified by the examination of the infected material by smear and culture, and if necessary by sugar fermentation tests. Staining shows organisms, which appear as Gram-negative diplococci within the cytoplasm of polymorphonuclear leucocytes. Extracellular organisms cannot be accepted as gonococci. Culture on chocolate, haemolysed horse blood, or hydrocele agar takes 24–48 hours: colonies may be more readily identified by the oxidase staining test. Special selective culture medium [Thayer-Martin (TM) VCNT medium] is also of use for testing. Legal proof of gonorrhoea rests upon the demonstration of organisms having all the cultural characteristics of gonococci. Fermentation reactions differentiate the organisms from the other Neisseria. A positive gonococcal complement fixation test in blood serum is only presumptive evidence of gonococcal (or meningococcal) infection past or present, but a positive finding indicates that smears and cultures should be repeated. Recently fluorescent antibody methods have been introduced which can be used on both smears (rapid method) and on 12-hour cultures (delayed method). These tests make possible speedier and more specific positive diagnoses particularly in women.

GONORRHOEA IN THE MALE

This presents as an acute infection of the mucous membrane of the urethra. The disease commonly remains localized to the urethra and its communicating structures, but occasionally it invades the blood stream and affects distant tissues.

Signs and Symptoms

The incubation period is commonly 2–10 days. The clinical onset is variable but at first there is usually a slight tingling discomfort in the urethra, followed by a thin discharge which quickly becomes mucopurulent and then frankly purulent. There is likely to be a variable degree of dysuria and perhaps slight frequency of micturition. The patient usually feels well, but there may be slight constitutional disturbance. On examination the margins of the external urinary meatus are red, oedematous and pouting. There is a yellow or greenish-yellow purulent discharge. It is important to be sure that the discharge comes from within the urethra and not from under the prepuce. The urine is hazy due to pus in the first glass of the two-glass test. If the infection has reached the posterior urethra, a development which takes place in about 10–14 days in the ordinary untreated case but occasionally much more quickly, the patient may complain of increasing dysuria and of frequency of micturition and the second urine glass is also hazy. In severe cases a few drops of blood may appear at the end of micturition, but marked haematuria is rare. Such patients may show evidence of toxic absorption, such as headaches, malaise, increased pulse rate and pyrexia, which is usually of low degree, but may reach 103°–104° F. (39·4°–40° C.) if complications occur. Proctitis may often be symptomless but in some cases there is pain on defaecation with bleeding and a purulent blood-stained discharge.

Treatment

Patients should be advised to assist recovery by refraining from all forms of alcohol and vigorous physical exercise. In most cases these restrictions are only necessary for the first 14 days after treatment is instituted. All patients infected with gonorrhoea should also refrain from sexual intercourse until they have completed a satisfactory period of observation.

Penicillin still remains the antibiotic of choice. Intramuscular injections from 1·2 G. (1,200,000 Units) to 2·4 G. (2,400,000 Units) of procaine penicillin in aqueous suspension are commonly given. The larger dose of penicillin is preferable as an increasing percentage of strains of gonococci are now partially resistant to it. It is also likely to be large enough to cure incubating syphilis. It may be better to use an equivalent unit dose of procaine penicillin fortified with benzylpenicillin combining the advantages of initial high levels with prolongation of effect. If this amount fails, due to infection with the more resistant strains of gonococci, the dosage of penicillin may have to be increased to 4·32 G. (4,800,000 Units).

A single dose of benzylpenicillin, 3 G. (5,000,000 Units) dissolved in 0·5 per cent. lignocaine, has also been used. These various penicillin regimes have been shown to be more effective if supplemented with probenecid, 1 G. by mouth 15–30 minutes before the injection or 0·5 G. six-hourly for 24 hours. By these means excretion from the kidneys is delayed. Oral penicillins have been used in the past. Good results were obtained with phenoxymethylpenicillin (penicillin V) given in doses of 250 mg. three times daily for 3 days or in one or two doses totalling up to 1·8 G. Oral phenoxymethylpenicillin (*Broxil*) in two doses each of 500 mg. with an interval of 4–8 hours was also used. More recently oral ampicillin (*Penbritin*) has been used successfully in single 1 G. or 2 G. dosage either combined with penicillin by injection or with probenecid. With the increase in number of partially resistant strains of gonococci, other drugs than penicillin must be considered as an alternative in the treatment of gonorrhoea.

The sulphonamide drugs were used for the treatment of gonorrhoea in 1937 onwards but by 1947 the cure rate had fallen to 14 per cent. Recently, however, it has been shown that the action of sulphonamides against the gonococcus is appreciably potentiated by the concurrent administration of trimethoprim. A tablet containing trimethoprim, 80 mg. with sulphamethoxazole, 400 mg. (*Bactrim*, *Septrin*) has been shown to be effective in the cure of gonorrhoea using 4 tablets immediately and then 2 twice daily for 4 further days. Streptomycin has given good results in the past when given intramuscularly in single doses of 1 or 2 G. Unfortunately strains of gonococci resistant to streptomycin have now increased in number so that this antibiotic is no longer indicated as resistance to it is usually complete. However, such is not yet the case with kanamycin and a single intramuscular injection of 2 G. or 1 G. daily for 2 or 3 days is effective although expensive and slightly painful. The above mentioned drugs, unlike penicillin, have the advantage of having no effect on treponemes, and, therefore, there is no danger of masking syphilis. Chloramphenicol has given good results but it is potentially dangerous because of its toxic effects; while other and safer remedies are available it should not be used for the treatment of gonorrhoea. The tetracycline drugs are all effective but tetracycline and oxytetracycline are probably a little more so than chlortetracycline: 500 mg. may be given by mouth every 6 hours for 48 hours, but a single dose of 1·5 G. has been claimed to be effective. Intramuscular injections of these preparations have been used but they are apt to cause local pain.

Experience with other antibiotics is small but the following have given good results: demethylchlortetracycline in single doses by mouth of 1·2 G. followed by a further similar dose in 4–6 hours: erythromycin by mouth, 500 mg. every 6 hours for 4 days, totalling 8 G.: spiramycin in single doses by mouth of 2·5 G. or in total dosage of 4–12 G. spread over 1 or 2 days: actinospectacin in single doses of 1·6 G. by intramuscular injection: doxycycline (*Vibramycin*) in a single oral dosage of 900 mg. given on a full stomach.

The effect of successful treatment is diminution of purulent discharge within a matter of hours. A slight mucoid secretion may persist for a few days and then disappear. If there is still discharge a week later without gonococci being found in the tests then this should be considered as a coincidental non-gonococcal urethritis which has not responded to penicillin and should be treated accordingly.

Tests for Cure

It is necessary to ensure that the patient is free from gonococcal infection. The following tests are commonly advocated in the case of men treated for gonorrhoea: clinical observation and testing should occupy 3 months. The patient should be examined at least once in the early morning before passing urine to exclude the presence of urethral discharge and of clinical and microscopic evidence of pus in the urine. The prostatic fluid should be examined microscopically for excess of leucocytes on one or two occasions. Two weeks or more after clinical recovery the walls of the anterior urethra should be inspected with the urethroscope, if the patient has a history of previous urethritis. The blood should be tested for syphilis at the end of 3 months. If the gonococcus reappears in the secretions within 14 days and further sexual intercourse is denied then relapse is probable and the sensitivities of the organisms to antibiotics should be requested and retreatment with either a higher penicillin dosage or another drug given. If, however, the gonococcus reappears more than 14 days after initial treatment and in particular, if further sexual intercourse is admitted then a new infection is indicated and treatment as given on the first occasion will probably be effective.

Local Complications

The following local complications may occur in the male:

1. Infection of the Tyson's (parafrenal) glands and of the para-urethral ducts. Balanitis due to the gonococcus is rare.
2. Infection of Littré's glands and the lacunae of Morgagni.
3. Subepithelial tissue infiltration leading to periurethral abscess, urinary fistula and finally stricture formation.
4. Cowperitis with or without abscess and sinus formation.
5. Prostatitis, with or without abscess formation.
6. Vesiculitis.
7. Vasitis leading to epididymitis often with associated hydrocele.

Evidence of a local complication may be found during the acute, subacute or chronic stages of the disease, but it is probable that in most cases the actual time of invasion is during the acute stage of the infection.

Metastatic Complications

There is no doubt that the gonococcus sometimes invades the blood stream and produces metastatic effects but this is probably a rare happening. The experience of recent years has made it clear that most cases of arthritis and 'rheumatism' occurring in association with genital gonorrhoea, and possibly all cases of metastatic conjunctivitis and iridocyclitis formerly attributed to that cause, are due to an associated 'non-specific' infection which is probably acquired at the same time as the gonorrhoea (see non-gonococcal urethritis and Reiter's disease). However, suppurative arthritis due to the gonococcus occurs occasionally and unless promptly treated may result in destruction of the joint. It seems to be monarticular in most cases and to involve joints such as the knee and wrist. The gonococcus can be found in the joint fluid and the condition responds to penicillin and other antibiotics. Gonococcal septicaemia with endocarditis and pericarditis is a rare complication.

GONORRHOEA IN THE FEMALE

With uncomplicated infections the sites which are likely to be involved are the urethra, cervix uteri, and, sometimes, the vaginal fornices. The urethral symptoms may be similar to those in the male, but urethral discharge is not usually noted by women. Cervicitis may cause backache and vaginal discharge. However, it is most important to note that there is a complete absence of symptoms in up to 50 per cent. of patients. If vaginal discharge is present in considerable amount it is usually due to coexisting infestation with the vaginal parasite, *Trichomonas vaginalis*, which is present in over 50 per cent. of the cases. The patient should be examined and specimens taken in the lithotomy position with a good light. The cervical secretion may be purulent or mucopurulent in appearance. Specimens are taken for smear and culture after careful cleansing with a cotton wool swab. If there is marked frothy vaginitis it is likely to be due to trichomoniasis but slight vaginitis in the fornices may be due to the gonococcus. On applying pressure from behind forwards to the floor of the urethra a bead of pus may appear at the external urinary meatus and should be examined for the gonococcus by smear and culture. The patient should not have passed urine during the 3 hours preceding tests. Investigations will need to be repeated in a few days if negative on the first occasion, and three or four sets of tests may be necessary to confirm the diagnosis. The longer infection has been present the more difficult it becomes to identify the gonococcus.

Proctitis. Proctitis is often symptomless and caused by a direct spread of infection from the genital tract due to contaminated vaginal discharge or menstrual blood flowing over the everted anal mucosa at defaecation. It is a common finding in women with genital gonorrhoea. Inspection by proctoscope and the taking of smears and cultures from the wall of the anorectum should form part of routine investigation.

Treatment

Treatment of uncomplicated infection in the female is the same as in the male with penicillin the drug of choice. Other drugs in similar dosage are also used when indicated as in men.

Tests for Cure

These are most important in women because of the likelihood that the residual infection will be asymptomatic. Smears and cultures from the sites of infection should be taken twice or three times in the first 2 weeks after treatment, then after three consecutive menstrual periods. Serological tests are performed as for men.

Local Complications

The following local and pelvic complications may occur in the female:

1. Skenitis.
2. Bartholinitis and abscess formation.
3. Salpingitis leading to sterility, oöphoritis and pelvic peritonitis.
4. Pyosalpinx, tubo-ovarian abscess and pelvic abscess.

Metastatic Complications

These may occur in the females as a result of trauma to the genital tract. Cases of gonococcal arthritis in which either upper or lower limb joints may be involved have been reported. As in the male, proof of the diagnosis is in the finding of the gonococcus in the joint fluid.

For detailed consideration of the complications of gonorrhoea, local and metastatic, of gonorrhoeal ophthalmia in adults and adolescents, of ophthalmia neonatorum and of gonococcal vulvovaginitis in children and of their treatment, and finally of tests of cure, reference should be made to a textbook of the venereal diseases.

REFERENCES

KING, A. J. (1964) *Recent Advances in Venereology*, London

KING, A. J., and NICOL, C. S. (1969) *Venereal Diseases*, 2nd ed., London.

Lancet (1961) Medical Research Council Working Party, ii, 226.

THAYER, J. D., and MARTIN, J. E. JR (1966) *Publ. Hlth Rep.* (*Wash.*), **81**, 559.

UNITED STATES PUBLIC HEALTH SERVICE (1961) Gonococcus: Procedures for isolation and identification, Publication No. 499.

WORLD HEALTH ORGANIZATION (1961) Gonorrhoea, *Bull. Wld Hlth Org.*, **24**, No. 3.

CLAUDE NICOL

INFECTIONS DUE TO LACTOBACILLACEAE

STREPTOCOCCAL INFECTIONS

BACTERIOLOGY

The streptococci form a large group of micro-organisms distinguished by their spherical or oval shape, their habit of growing in chains and the fact that they are Gram-positive. Classification presents some difficulty. Most species are aerobic, but some are anaerobic or micro-aerophilic. The aerobic streptococci may be subdivided by their behaviour when grown on a blood-agar plate. The colonies of one group are surrounded by a clear zone of complete haemolysis; those of the second by a halo of green discoloration; while those of the third have no effect upon the blood-containing medium. These groups are the β-haemolytic, the α-haemolytic and the non-haemolytic or γ (gamma) type streptococci.

The β-haemolytic streptococci may be further divided into Lancefield's Groups A–Q by means of a precipitin reaction utilizing specific polysaccharide antigens. Over 90 per cent. of human infections are due to streptococci of Group A; they are known as *Streptococcus pyogenes* and are almost always the organisms concerned when the name haemolytic streptococcus is used. Griffiths has subdivided *Str. pyogenes* into a number of serological types designated by Arabic numerals depending upon surface protein antigens (M, T and R). M-antigens are type-specific and are closely related to virulence; 51 antigenically distinct types of M-protein have so far been identified.

Str. pyogenes elaborates a number of extracellular products. Important amongst these are: the erythrogenic toxin, two haemolysins, streptokinase, streptodornase (deoxyribonuclease) and hyaluronidase. Only the first, which is responsible for the rash of scarlet fever, plays a clear cut role in the pathogenesis of human disease. Erythrogenic toxin is antigenic, but although several different varieties probably exist exposure to one produces immunity to all. It is used in the Dick test and its antitoxin in the Schultz-Charlton reaction [see p. 85]. Of the two haemolysins streptolysin O is antigenic and streptolysin S is not; estimation of the antistreptolysin O titre of serum affords some evidence of recent infection with a Group A streptococcus and the same is true of streptokinase and antistreptokinase.

β-Haemolytic streptococci, other than those of Group A, are rarely the cause of disease in man. Strains occasionally incriminated almost invariably belong to Groups B, C, D or G. Those of Group B, commonly cause bovine mastitis and have been isolated from patients with puerperal infection, neonatal sepsis and subacute bacterial endocarditis. Group C streptococci are also animal parasites but have caused cellulitis, tonsillitis, scarlet fever and wound infection in man. Group D strains are closely related to the enterococci and include many which are not β-haemolytic, they are commonly found in infections of the urinary tract. Streptococci of Group G are the cause of epidemic canine tonsillitis and have been responsible for human puerperal infection.

EPIDEMIOLOGY

The only significant sources of haemolytic streptococci are symptomless carriers or sufferers from active streptococcal infection. Infection is only acquired by contact with such persons and consequently the danger is increased by overcrowding and inadequate ventilation. In former times, spread by infected food or milk sometimes took place but this is now virtually unknown.

Group A streptococci can be recovered from the carrier's throat and far less often from his nose, although he may never have been the victim of a recognizable streptococcal infection. Surveys have shown that 5–15 per cent. of normal adults and 10–20 per cent. of normal children may be carriers. It is clear from recent work that nasal carriers are of much greater importance in the spread of disease than those in whom the organism resides in the throat. The rate for nasal carriage in children is between 2 and 5 per cent.

The frequency of clinically evident streptococcal infections of the upper respiratory tract depends upon a number of poorly defined factors. Among these are the virulence of the predominating type of streptococcus, seasonal and climatic conditions and the level of immunity in the population. This last may have considerable importance for infection is not followed by immunity to all types of *Str. pyogenes*, but only to that responsible for the infection in question. Some types, especially Types 12 and 49, are particularly likely to cause nephritis. With this exception specific types of *Str. pyogenes* are not linked with specific clinical syndromes: in any community at one time the same serological types of Group A streptococcus will be responsible for all the varied clinical manifestations of streptococcal infection.

HUMAN INFECTIONS DUE TO HAEMOLYTIC STREPTOCOCCI

General Aspects

The consequences of infection with the haemolytic streptococcus in man can be considered under two heads. There are first the immediate lesions provoked by invasion by the streptococcus and dependent upon its actual presence in diseased tissues; and secondly remote lesions not of this simple causation. These are unique to the haemolytic streptococcus, they follow the height of the infection by two or three weeks and current opinion attributes them to an ill-defined process with an immunological basis.

Immediate Lesions

The Respiratory Tract. The upper respiratory tract, particularly the lymphoid tissue of the nasopharynx, is frequently colonized by the haemolytic streptococcus and in many instances the organism causes inflammatory changes. It is not known what decides whether in any particular patient the streptococcus will behave as an innocuous saprophyte or as an aggressive pathogen. The frequency of streptococcal infection of the upper respiratory tract is greater in cold and damp climates, although the carrier rate may be as high in dry sunny countries, where such infections are of great rarity.

There is a curious variation in clinical patterns which depends upon age. In infants and young children the primary lesion may be a mild nasopharyngeal catarrh, but sequelae such as suppurative lymphadenitis and otitis media often follow; in older children and young adults florid acute follicular tonsillitis is common; in the middle-aged and elderly a catarrhal inflammation is again the usual expression of infection, but suppurative lymphadenitis is rare.

The haemolytic streptococcus may thus be responsible for a wide range of infections of the upper respiratory tract. Pharyngitis, tonsillitis, peritonsillar abscess, otitis media, mastoiditis and sinusitis are all common. Extension of infection may lead to suppurative cervical lymphadenitis, retropharyngeal abscess, Ludwig's angina, thrombophlebitis of intracranial venous sinuses, cerebral abscesses and meningitis. These are all considered in detail in the relevant sections.

Streptococcal pneumonia is now uncommon and usually occurs as a complication of viral pneumonia. It is particularly liable to progress to pyothorax [see Section 9).

Scarlet fever results from local infection, usually of the throat, with a streptococcus producing erythrogenic toxin.

Skin and Subcutaneous Tissue. The haemolytic streptococcus was once a common cause of surgical wound infection and is still frequently responsible for sepsis of cuts and abrasions. It may lead to cellulitis, erysipelas, and streptococcal gangrene. It occurs, usually in association with *Staph. aureus*, in impetigo contagiosa.

Septicaemia. Haemolytic streptococcal septicaemia is now rare. It was once the organism most often responsible for puerperal septicaemia. Invasion of the blood stream was particularly liable to occur with infected wounds. The clinical picture has already been described [p. 31]. Its features are those of severe general infection; in most instances a local lesion affording the streptococcus a mode of entry is evident. Local abscess formation is unusual. At one time almost invariably fatal, streptococcal septicaemia now responds rapidly to antibacterial drugs.

Remote Sequelae

Under this head are grouped a number of diseases which may follow haemolytic streptococcal infection after an interval of 2–3 weeks. None is due to the actual presence of streptococci in the lesion and the mechanisms concerned are not understood. There is a growing body of opinion favouring an immunological explanation for these phenomena.

The diseases which fall into this group are rheumatic fever, acute glomerulonephritis, erythema nodosum, Henoch-Schönlein or anaphylactoid purpura, and possibly some examples of mesenteric lymphadenitis. They are considered in detail in their respective sections. The relationship is most clear cut in the first two. The last three are perhaps best regarded as possible reactions to several different agencies of which streptococcal infection may be one. In rheumatic fever the preceding infection may be with any type of group A streptococcus, but by contrast there are particular types, especially Types 12 and 49, liable to cause acute nephritis.

DIAGNOSIS

The diagnosis of streptococcal infection follows the usual principles. Although some of the clinical pictures such as scarlet fever and erysipelas, are sufficiently characteristic, every effort must be made to isolate the causative organism. In the various upper respiratory tract infections it is even more important. Swabs from the throat or nasopharynx usually provide the material. In other cases swabs from wounds, vaginal discharges, or blood cultures may be required.

It is often valuable, as evidence supporting the diagnosis of rheumatic fever, to be able to prove that a haemolytic streptococcal infection has recently taken place. The organism can seldom be isolated from the nasopharynx and, if it can, there is no proof of it having been the cause of infection. In these circumstances estimation of the antistreptolysin O titre of the serum is often useful. It is above 150 units per ml. in 85 per cent. of patients with active rheumatic fever.

PROPHYLAXIS

It is known that when haemolytic streptococci can be eliminated from the nasopharynx, relapses of rheumatic fever are rare. Isolation is impracticable, for so many carriers exist, but regular administration of an antibiotic or a sulphonamide has proved most effective. There is good evidence, too, that the incidence of rheumatic fever is greatly reduced when acute streptococcal infections are treated promptly and energetically.

Anyone who has had an attack of rheumatic fever should therefore be recommended to take 0·5–1 G. of sulphadiazine daily or 250 mg. of phenoxymethylpenicillin twice daily by mouth for at least five years. Because of the greater risk of infection, prophylaxis is of particular importance for such patients during any period in hospital.

TREATMENT

This is considered in the relevant sections and in the article on the antibiotics.

REFERENCES

DUMA, R. J., WEINBERG, A. N., MEDREK, T. F., and KUNZ, L. J. (1969) Streptococcal infections: a bacteriologic and clinical study of streptococcal bacteremia, *Medicine* (*Baltimore*), **48**, 87.

EICKHOFF, T. C., KLEIN, J. O., DALY, A. K., INGALL, D., and FINLAND, M. (1964) Neonatal sepsis and other infections due to Group B beta-haemolytic streptococci, *New Engl. J. Med.*, **271**, 1221.

MCCARTY, M. (1954) *Streptococcal Infections*, New York.

RAMMELKAMP, C. H., JR (1957) Epidemiology of streptococcal infections, *Harvey Lect.*, **51**, 133.

REINARZ, J. A., and SANFORD, J. P. (1965) Human infections caused by non-group A or D streptococci, *Medicine* (*Baltimore*), **44**, 81.

UHR, J. W. (1964) *The Streptococcus, Rheumatic Form and Glomerulonephritis*, New York.

R. BODLEY SCOTT

SCARLET FEVER

Synonym. Scarlatina.

Definition

Scarlet fever is a specific disease caused by infection with haemolytic streptococci in which a rapid onset with fever, headache, vomiting and sore throat is followed within 24 hours by a punctate erythematous rash.

Aetiology

Two criteria must be satisfied for the rash of scarlet fever to appear, sufficient growth of *Str. haemolyticus* to allow production of a large enough quantity of erythrogenic toxin and a patient who is susceptible to the toxin. If there is insufficient toxin produced the patient suffers either from an inapparent infection or from an infection without a rash (e.g. streptococcal tonsillitis) the severity of the illness in this instance depending on the bacterial protein component, M substance. Thus an attack of tonsillitis without a rash, contracted from a case of scarlet fever does not necessarily imply immunity to scarlet fever. Most strains of haemolytic streptococci produce the same erythrogenic toxin, but three other antigenically distinct toxins are known and infection with a streptococcus elaborating one of these may result in a second attack.

Although scarlet fever is most often due to a throat infection, the illness can complicate streptococcal infection in other sites such as wound or puerperal sepsis, and indeed not all cases of clinical scarlet fever are due to streptococcal infection. Certain strains of haemolytic staphylococci also produce an erythrogenic toxin giving rise to staphylococcal scarlet fever. At the present time severe 'surgical scarlet fever', in which an infected wound is the site of toxin production, is more commonly staphylococcal than streptococcal in origin.

Epidemiology

Scarlet fever mainly affects children between three and ten years of age—an attack often appearing within twelve months of starting school. It is uncommon in adults and rare under a year. Streptococcal infection is endemic throughout the world but scarlet fever is uncommon in the tropics, although the incidence of persons susceptible to erythrogenic toxin is similar to that found in temperate zones. The rarity of the scarlatinal rash appears to be due to a change in skin susceptibility to the toxin in tropical climates. Attacks occur all the year round with an increase in autumn and winter, sometimes reaching epidemic proportions.

Scarlet fever is not highly infectious. The organisms are found in the nose and throat and are spread by droplet, by direct contact or by infected fomites. Septic complications such as purulent rhinitis or a discharging otitis media increase the infectivity. Food-borne outbreaks, most often from contaminated milk, sometimes occur and should be suspected in any explosive outbreak in a closed community. Investigation of the kitchen staff is likely to reveal a heavy streptococcal excretor. Healthy carriers of streptococci are common and may spread the disease but the carrier state is usually intermittent and easily dealt with. It is the unhealthy carrier with an infected discharge who is much more dangerous.

The severity of scarlet fever has waxed and waned over the centuries. The disease was severe at the beginning and the end of the nineteenth century, at one time during this period being the main cause of childhood death in England. It has become progressively milder during the past fifty years, but an increase in virulence may well occur in the future. It has always been more common among the poorer sections of the community where overcrowding contributes to its spread.

Pathology

The rash is caused by damage to the capillary reticulo-endothelial network accompanied by perivascular infiltration with monocytes, changes also seen at autopsy in severe cases in lymph nodes, liver and spleen. Excessive capillary damage leads to a haemorrhagic rash which persists after death while the erythematous rash disappears. The autopsy findings are those common to severe infections with evidence of widespread cellular damage including cloudy swelling and degeneration of heart muscle. They are not specific to scarlet fever.

Symptoms

The incubation period is commonly 2–4 days with extremes of 1–7 days.

The *onset* is sudden, the cardinal symptoms being headache, vomiting and sore throat. In the mild type of case common at the present time, vomiting is seldom prolonged, usually being restricted to one or two episodes at the onset. It is sometimes accompanied by abdominal pain. Convulsions and rigors are uncommon. The temperature rises rapidly but in mild cases may not exceed 100° F. (37·8° C.). In more severe cases with a temperature of 103° F. (39·5° C.) or more there may be an undue degree of tachycardia, the heart rate rising by more than the expected ten beats per minute for each degree Fahrenheit of temperature. Coryza and cough are notable by their absence.

Changes in the mouth are present early in the disease, a generalized redness of the tonsils, palate and uvula increasing in intensity rapidly over the first 24 hours. A patchy white or yellowish mucopurulent exudate appears on the tonsils accompanied by oedema in the more severe case. At first follicular, the patches of exudate often combine to form a continuous membrane on one or both sides. This exudate is confined to the tonsils, only rarely spreading on to the fauces. It is easily removed. In addition to the generalized hyperaemia in the mouth there may be an enanthem on the palate consisting of bright red spots superimposed on the general redness giving rise to a punctate appearance. When this precedes the exanthem it is of considerable help in diagnosis.

The tongue undergoes characteristic changes with remarkable constancy and in these days of mild attacks with fleeting rashes it provides valuable evidence in doubtful cases. In the early stages the whole tongue, with the exception sometimes of the tip, is covered with a white fur through which the papillae project as small red points (*strawberry tongue*). On the second to fourth day the fur starts to peel from before backwards and from the edge inwards until the surface becomes red and raw looking with rather swollen red papillae projecting (*raspberry tongue*). The whole tongue may be slightly swollen but it is rarely sore. This appearance lasts till the seventh day of illness, returning gradually to normal in the second week. These changes are not invariably present in scarlet fever but other signs of the disease would need to be unequivocal for the diagnosis to be made in the presence of a normal tongue.

At the time of the initial faucial inflammation the lymph nodes at the angle of the jaw are swollen and tender. During the eruptive phase there may be a mild generalized non-tender lymphadenopathy. The spleen may be sufficiently enlarged to be just palpable for a few days.

The *rash* normally appears within 24 hours of the onset but may be delayed for two days or occasionally even longer. It commonly appears first on the chest, neck and upper arms, spreading quickly to the rest of the trunk and reaching the legs last. It usually develops within a few hours but is variable in its rate of appearance and also in the areas involved. The trunk is most heavily affected, the rash on the limbs sometimes being indeterminate. The hands and feet normally escape. The face is flushed with, in more severe cases, a striking area of circumoral pallor but this appearance is seen in children febrile from other causes. In the presence of a scarlatiniform rash, however, it can be a striking feature. The rash on the trunk and limbs, and, rarely, on the face, consists of two elements, a diffuse erythema on which are superimposed punctate areas of increased redness (*punctate erythema*) but either of these elements may be absent. The puncta are about the size of goose pimples but in a coarse rash they may be larger and the erythematous element indistinct. The eruption shows a symmetrical intensification on the lower abdomen and groins, the inner aspect of the thighs, the axillae and the back. The rash disappears last from the lower abdomen and upper and inner aspect of the thighs. Miliary sudamina, due to blocking of the sweat glands by the inflammatory process, may be superimposed on the rash, particularly in hot weather. With a heavy erythema linear petechiae appear in the flexures of the elbows (*Pastia's sign*) and in other skin folds. Itching is unusual.

The rash lasts from 6 to 48 hours in most cases but it can remain for a week. It may be followed by peeling of the chest and trunk. Or peeling may start on the tips of the fingers or toes where it tends to be coarser with the skin coming away in large sections. Rarely an incomplete cast of a hand or foot has been shed. Peeling nowadays is an inconstant feature and when it does appear it may be delayed for two or three weeks. Some evidence of it can often be found, however, if a close enough inspection is made of the ears and of the tips of the fingers and toes. In severe cases temporary loss of hair may follow desquamation.

The temperature chart shows no distinctive features, the height of the temperature being closely related to the severity of the infection or the presence of complications. In straightforward cases it is highest at the onset, falling rapidly by lysis as the rash subsides and reaching normal in three to five days.

Varieties

(a) Simple. (c) Toxic.
(b) Septic. (d) Surgical.

Simple Scarlet Fever. Nearly all present-day cases fall into this category—90 per cent. of them being mild while the remainder are moderately severe. In the mild type the patient never appears particularly ill, toxaemia is negligible, the temperature does not exceed 101° F. (38·3° C.) and symptomatic recovery takes place within 3 to 4 days. In the more severe cases the prodromal symptoms are more striking with the temperature reaching perhaps 104° F. (40° C.), the rash heavier and lasting for a few days, while fever and constitutional symptoms may persist for up to a week. Complications are more common in this group.

Septic Scarlet Fever. The characteristics of this type are intense faucial inflammation with exudate and oedema accompanied by widespread local lymphatic spread and later blood stream dissemination of the organisms. Ulceration of the tonsils may spread to the soft palate, the mucous membrane of the mouth being widely excoriated and bleeding at a touch. The profuse seropurulent nasal and oral discharges cause ulceration and sores at the anterior nares, on the lips and at the angle of the mouth. There is considerable painful enlargement of cervical lymph nodes with peri-adenitis and cellulitis. Swallowing is painful and some difficulty in breathing is usual. The temperature is high, the chart being remittent or intermittent in type. Delirium may occur at night but most patients are rational though restless and irritable. The rash may be heavy or scanty. Some patients show septic symptoms of a milder type and recover satisfactorily but in others in whom treatment is withheld death is likely in the second week, following spread of infection to the blood stream. Penicillin therapy has revolutionized the prognosis of septic scarlet fever.

Toxic or Malignant Scarlet Fever. In this rare form of the disease there is profound toxaemia due to rapid dissemination of toxin, but relatively little local spread of infection. An abrupt onset with vomiting, headache, high fever and delirium is rapidly followed by the development of an intense scarlet or purple rash in which there are frequently petechial elements. Bleeding may occur from any mucous membrane. Although there is intense hyperaemia of the throat there is little oedema or exudate and local signs are relatively insignificant. It is the constitutional and cerebral symptoms which dominate the clinical picture. An increasing tachycardia with a gallop rhythm and muffled heart sounds, together with falling blood pressure, signify the onset of circulatory failure. Loss of peripheral vascular tone and toxic myocarditis both contribute to this. Without specific therapy this form of the disease is usually fatal within 48 hours.

Surgical (or Extra-Faucial) Scarlet Fever. Infected burns, scalds, wounds or operation sites or skin lesions such as chickenpox vesicles are the common sources of 'surgical' scarlet fever. The possibility of a staphylococcal aetiology in such cases must be borne in mind.

Complications

There are two distinct groups of complications—those due to spread of the infecting organisms and those due to toxic-allergic reactions.

Septic Complications. Spread of infection may be local by direct extension and through the lymphatics or it may take place via the blood stream. Aspiration pneumonia is rare. Local spread can result in a wide variety of complications such as peritonsillar abscess, purulent rhinitis, sinusitis, purulent conjunctivitis, angular stomatitis, cellulitis, otitis media and cervical adenitis. Septicaemia will rarely be followed by distant metastatic abscesses in bones or joints and occasionally by a purulent pericarditis. Certain of these complications however are much more frequently encountered than others. They may appear at any time but are most frequent in the first few days. When they appear after the twelfth day they may be due to a superimposed infection with a different strain of streptococci. These late septic complications used to be fairly common in the days when scarlet fever cases were nursed in open wards resulting in contact between patients suffering from infections due to antigenically distinct organisms. With the modern practice of isolating scarlet fever patients from each other (unless in a family where one can assume that the same strain is responsible for the different cases) late septic manifestations have become rare.

Otitis Media. The proportionately wider Eustachian tube in young children encourages spread to the middle ear. Infection is often bilateral though earache is usually limited to one side or may be absent. Irritability with increase or return of fever suggests otitis media. The drum is red and tense. The appearance of a serosanguinous discharge from an ear may be the first indication of infection. Frank mastoiditis with pain, swelling and tenderness over the mastoid process may appear early and occasionally there is intracranial spread, leading to meningitis.

Cervical Adenitis. Enlarged and tender lymph nodes in the neck normally become non-tender as the temperature subsides, returning to a normal size more slowly. Fever, malaise and increasing adenitis may appear during the second, third or fourth week unaccompanied by sore throat or pharyngeal signs. The tonsillar and anterior cervical chain are those most frequently involved and suppuration may follow. Although the constitutional symptoms rapidly subside with treatment the glands may be very slow to return to normal, relapse often following too early cessation of treatment. Sometimes secondary tonsillitis precedes the lymphadenopathy.

Purulent Rhinitis. A profuse thin mucopurulent nasal discharge is often associated with sinusitis although the latter may occur without rhinorrhoea. Swelling and redness of the upper and lower eyelids without conjunctivitis suggests infection of the ethmoid.

Toxic-Allergic Reactions. Transient mild albuminuria is common during the febrile stage. Focal nephritis sometimes occurs with red and white cells and protein in the urine but without oliguria, hypertension, oedema or nitrogen retention. Myocarditis is toxic in origin and is the cause of the disproportionate tachycardia sometimes met with.

Rheumatic fever, acute (Type I) nephritis or anaphylactoid (Henoch-Schönlein) purpura may follow one to three weeks after scarlet fever and differ in no way from similar attacks which may follow other streptococcal infections. Nephritis, however, only follows infection with certain nephrotoxic strains, Griffiths Types 12, 4 and 25 being most often incriminated. Gangrene has occurred after severe postscarlatinal purpura—usually anaphylactoid in type though rarely caused by a transient thrombocytopenia.

Diagnosis

The diagnosis of scarlet fever must never be made on the rash alone. Detection of β-haemolytic streptococci in the nose or throat favours scarlet fever but a negative culture does not exclude it even if antibiotics have been withheld prior to the culture being taken. A mild degree of polymorphonuclear leucocytosis is usual but not invariable and a moderate eosinophilia may develop later in the first week.

The *Dick test* determines the state of immunity to erythrogenic toxins; 0·1 ml. of toxin intradermally being followed in 12–24 hours in susceptibles by a circumscribed area of erythema of 1 cm. or more.

A negative reaction should indicate immunity to the toxin. Conversion from a positive test performed on the first three days of a doubtful case of scarlet fever to negative when repeated 7–10 days later is strong confirmation of the diagnosis. In practice, however, the test is seldom used as a diagnostic aid. As not all scarlet fever is due to the same erythrogenic toxin it is not surprising to find about 10 per cent. of persons still Dick-positive immediately following an attack, thereby limiting its value. The test has some application in providing an index of susceptibility to the disease in a community. At the age of two years about 80 per cent. are Dick-positive to standard toxin, the number decreasing to about 30 per cent. at fifteen years and continuing to diminish slowly thereafter. Most infants are Dick-negative at birth, but not those born of Dick-positive mothers from whom there can be no passive transfer of antibodies.

The *Schultz-Charlton reaction* or blanching test depends on the local effect of 0.1 ml. of antitoxin when injected intradermally into an erythematous rash. If the rash is due to scarlet fever it fades within eight hours around the site of the injection. In these days of mild and often short-lived rashes the test is frequently difficult to interpret, and as a negative response does not exclude the diagnosis it is of limited practical value.

The clinical diagnosis is seldom difficult. The symptoms of headache, vomiting and sore throat followed within 24 hours by a punctate erythematous rash are characteristic. The appearance of the tongue is helpful at all stages.

The flushed face with circumoral pallor, common in children with *lobar pneumonia*, together with the abrupt onset, fever and vomiting may suggest scarlet fever. The absence of rash and the appearance of cough with other signs of increasing respiratory distress soon serve to differentiate.

The rash of *rubella* on its second day may be scarlatiniform on the trunk but discrete macular lesions usually persist on the limbs or face. The absence of prodromal symptoms, the minimal throat signs and the enlargement of the posterior cervical lymph nodes are all distinguishing features of rubella. The coarse blotchy rash of *measles*, appearing first on the face after 3–4 days of febrile coryza is unlikely to be confused with scarlet fever.

Scarlatiniform rashes may be caused by many *drugs* including aspirin, quinine, belladonna, phenobarbitone, sulphonamides, arsenical compounds, gold and para-aminosalicylic acid. Malaise and fever are usually absent, as is evidence of local infection. In acute exfoliative dermatitis the rash is more intense but does not show the punctate appearance and the illness runs a more prolonged course. Scarlatiniform rashes may appear in the prodromal period of chickenpox and smallpox and occasionally measles. These are usually short lived and once again the focal signs of streptococcal infection are absent.

Treatment

Patients should be nursed in bed at home until 48 hours after the return of the temperature to normal. They should preferably be in a room of their own and certainly other children should be excluded. Hospital admission is unnecessary for the majority of patients. The disease is notifiable in the United Kingdom. With specific therapy in the uncomplicated case patients can be regarded as non-infectious from the eighth day and provided the respiratory tract is healthy, can return to school fourteen days from the onset. In hospital practice, it is useful to obtain one negative throat culture before discharge. Although this provides no guarantee of detecting all convalescent carriers, the heavy excretor will be revealed and can receive further treatment. Patients remain infectious so long as discharges persist.

Symptomatic drugs are seldom necessary but sore throat can be relieved in the older patient by aspirin gargles. Painful lymph nodes are eased with dry heat, frequently applied. No dietary restriction is necessary but a good fluid intake with sugared drinks should be maintained during the febrile period.

School contacts need not be quarantined but should be kept at home at the first suspicious symptom. Similarly, adult members of the household can continue their normal work unless this entails handling milk or milk products. Rigid quarantine restrictions are clearly illogical while streptococcal tonsillitis without a rash is not a notifiable disease.

Specific. All patients should receive penicillin, the type and route depending on the severity of the attack.

Phenoxymethylpenicillin by mouth for a minimum of 5 days (adult dose 0·25 G. six-hourly) is adequate for most cases of simple scarlet fever but this course should be prolonged to 10 days if clinical recovery is not rapid, discharges persist or any complications appear. In septic cases treatment should start with 0·15 G. (250,000 Units) of penicillin G intramuscularly four-hourly. With satisfactory progress oral penicillin can replace the injections after a few days but the total course should not be less than 10 days. Otitis media and other septic complications are treated similarly and respond rapidly.

Toxic scarlet fever should be treated with penicillin G in larger doses, 0·6 G. (1 mega Unit) intramuscularly immediately followed by 0·3 G. (½ mega Unit) six-hourly. Prednisolone phosphate, 40 mg., should be injected intramuscularly or slowly intravenously if there is marked circulatory failure. It is doubtful if antiscarlatinal serum has any place in modern therapy. Prednisolone is continued in a dosage of 10 mg. six-hourly for the first 24 hours, 40 mg. being given in divided doses during the second 24 hour period, the dose thereafter being reduced by 10 mg. on alternate days.

Abscess formation will necessitate surgical drainage but this must be delayed until the abscess has a well-defined wall and fluctuation is distinct.

Resistant streptococcal carriers nearly always clear with a ten-day course of oral penicillin but tonsillectomy may be required in persons with deeply infected crypts.

Prevention

Passive immunization with antiscarlatinal serum or active immunization with modified toxin are not indicated as these procedures give immunity to the erythrogenic element only and are not without risk. Prolonged prophylaxis with oral penicillin will prevent most re-infections with haemolytic streptococci and is indicated in children who have suffered from rheumatic fever.

Prognosis

Recovery is rapid and complete in nearly all cases. The previously common sequel of chronic otitis media is seldom seen in view of the rapid response of the acute ear infection to treatment. Septicaemia is a dangerous complication of the septic form of the disease, as is pneumonia. Death may occur in toxic cases too rapidly for therapy to be effective. The combination of scarlet fever and diphtheria is always serious but now exceptionally rare in Great Britain. Permanent renal or cardiac damage may follow acute nephritis or rheumatic fever but both these complications are uncommon.

REFERENCE

TOP, F. H. (1960) Scarlet fever, in *Communicable and Infectious Diseases*, 4th ed., St. Louis.

ERYSIPELAS

Synonym. St. Anthony's fire.

Definition

Erysipelas is an acute infectious disease involving the skin, commonly of the face or leg, with resultant erythema and swelling associated with fever and constitutional symptoms.

Aetiology and Pathology

The disease is due to infection with streptococci of Lancefield Group A. No particular strain is responsible for erysipelas so that different manifestations of streptococcal infection, for example, tonsillitis, scarlet fever or erysipelas might result in three individuals infected from a common source. Nevertheless, in the days when cross-infection with haemolytic streptococci was common in institutions the disease tended to spread as erysipelas. The organism enters through a break in the skin but in many cases close examination fails to reveal the site of entry. The frequency of small sores and abrasions in and around the nares is responsible for the face being the site most commonly attacked. Gravitational ulcers, abrasions from ill-fitting shoes or cracks between the toes lead to erysipelas of the lower leg, the second commonest site involved.

The disease is world wide in distribution, most cases being sporadic with a slightly greater incidence in spring and autumn than at other times of the year; the sexes are equally affected. Although no age is immune, erysipelas is mainly a disease of the forty to sixty years age group in whom it appears as a primary infection, the route of entry through the skin being inapparent. In younger patients the disease is more likely to complicate a more obvious lesion such as a burn or a vaccination.

Spread of infection is by direct contact but the infectivity is low as few organisms are shed from the lesion. Pathologically the lesion in uncomplicated cases is confined to the superficial layers of the skin. Streptococci, pus cells and exudate fill the lymphatics, the organisms being most numerous at the spreading margins of the rash.

Symptoms

The incubation period is usually 2–3 days with extremes of 1–7 days.

The onset is abrupt with a sharp rise of temperature to 102° or 103° F. (38·9° or 39·5° C.) accompanied by headache, shivers, malaise and vomiting. Sometimes the illness begins with a true rigor, mental confusion or delirium being not uncommon in older patients. Mild irritation, tightness or discomfort may draw attention to the local lesion but for the first 24–48 hours these symptoms are often overshadowed by the severity of the constitutional upset and consequently overlooked by the patient, particularly when the site of the infection is the leg. By the second day there is clear evidence of local inflammation with redness of the skin which has a distinct raised margin at its junction with the normal skin that can more easily be felt than seen. As the rash spreads peripherally during the subsequent days the erythema in the centre fades and oedema of the skin and surrounding soft tissue increases. Oedema is particularly severe in facial erysipelas with resultant closure of one or both eyes making the patient's features scarcely recognizable. The oedema is worse on the side of the face on which the infection started. Minute vesicles are often present at the onset on the erythematous skin, changing to large vesicles or bullae filled with clear fluid as the lesion progresses. A crust forms after the bullae rupture. In those cases in which the blebs do not appear the skin shows a fine peeling as the rash fades. Some degree of gravitational purpura frequently develops when the lesion involves the calf but this is less common on the face. Without specific therapy the disease lasts from 1–3 weeks.

Complications

Local spread of infection leads to *lymphangitis*—quite common in limb erysipelas—or *cellulitis* with or without abscess formation. Spread of infection to the meninges, cavernous sinus, or blood stream used to occur but is now rarely seen. Albuminuria is usually transient but nephritis occasionally occurs. In an elderly toxic patient *prerenal uraemia* may develop due to an inadequate fluid intake, and *pneumonia* remains a potential hazard in such elderly patients. Recurrent erysipelas may occur in the same situation with intervals of months or years between attacks. A thorough search will sometimes reveal the break in the skin through which the infection enters, but often no such lesion can be found.

Diagnosis

The diagnosis is clinical, laboratory investigation seldom being required. In doubtful or early cases haemolytic streptococci can be recovered from culture of vesicular fluid removed by capillary tube from the small lesions. Some degree of polymorphonuclear leucocytosis is usual. Examination of any patient with severe febrile symptoms must include inspection of the legs otherwise erysipelas of the calf will be missed. In facial erysipelas confusion may arise with ophthalmic herpes zoster. In this condition the rash is originally papular, stopping abruptly at the midline, its distribution being limited to that of the affected nerve. Erysipelas, however, though usually more marked on one side than the other does not confine itself to a nerve distribution and spreads peripherally. Cellulitis causes a much more painful and tender lesion with an ill-defined edge, the distinction from erysipelas being important as incision through the latter must be avoided.

Treatment

The patient should be nursed in bed preferably in isolation; given adequate bed spacing it is quite safe to barrier-nurse patients with erysipelas in an open ward as the infectivity of the disease is low.

Penicillin is the drug of choice, an initial intramuscular dose of 0·6 G. (1 mega Unit) of penicillin G being followed by 0·25 G. of the phenoxymethyl salt four-hourly by mouth for 7 days. This leads to constitutional improvement within 24 hours together with halting of the spread of the rash which dries up within 3–10 days. Local drugs or dressings are unnecessary; dead skin should be removed, bullae opened and the fluid gently mopped away. Scratching must be prevented, by splinting if need be, as must pressure from the weight of the body or bed clothes. Elderly patients suffering from erysipelas involving a leg must be mobilized as soon as the inflammation is subsiding in order to avoid prolonged oedema in convalescence. If oedema persists an elastic stocking should be worn as soon as the skin will tolerate it. Incision of any complicating abscess must be delayed until the erysipelas is under control as too early interference may be followed by septicaemia.

Prognosis

The mortality rate is now very low and complete recovery is the rule. Oedema following erysipelas of the leg in an elderly person may last for months or even permanently.

G. D. W. McKendrick

RHEUMATIC FEVER

Definition

Rheumatic fever is an acute or subacute pyrexial illness with widespread inflammatory lesions in connective tissues, especially those of the joints, the heart, the blood vessels and the hypodermis.

Aetiology

An association between infection with haemolytic streptococci of Lancefield's Group A and rheumatic fever is now universally accepted. The affected tissues are not directly invaded by the organism, but in almost every instance there is preceding streptococcal infection. The evidence for this is clinical and serological. Often there is a clear cut history of an upper respiratory infection 2 or 3 weeks before the onset of rheumatic fever; haemolytic streptococci of Group A may have been isolated at the time of this episode or they may still be recovered from the throat when the patient comes under observation with rheumatic fever. Indirect clinical evidence of the relationship is provided by the infrequent recurrence of rheumatic fever when streptococcal infection is controlled by chemoprophylaxis. Serological examination of patients with rheumatic fever shows an immune response characteristic of recent haemolytic streptococcal infection whatever method of assay is used. Precipitins can be demonstrated; positive complement fixation tests are obtained; there is an increase in the titre of antistreptolysin-O, fibrinolysin and other antibodies [see p. 80]. Observations in epidemics of streptococcal disease show that the immune response in those who subsequently develop rheumatic fever tends to be greater than in those who do not.

Although this association is established it remains uncertain how the lesions are caused. The most widely held view is that the changes are allergic and due to sensitization of the tissues to some product of streptococcal growth. Infection by any strain of Group A haemolytic streptococcus may be followed by rheumatic fever, but only a minority of those acquiring such infections develops this sequel. It has been found that in epidemics of streptococcal disease, rheumatic fever follows in only 3 per cent. Immunity is specific for the serological type of streptococcus and does not extend to others of Group A. There is consequently no protection against repeated infections from different types of streptococci each of which may initiate rheumatic fever in a susceptible individual. It seems probable that a constitutional factor exists and there is good evidence of hereditary predisposition to the disease.

Rheumatic fever is rare before the age of 4 and after that of 30 years; the peak of incidence is about 7. This may well be a reflection of the greater frequency of streptococcal disease at this age. It was noted in the Second World War that when large numbers of young men were brought together in camps under conditions which favoured the spread of streptococcal infection, the incidence of rheumatic fever rose to levels similar to those of childhood. There has been over the last 15 years an undoubted decline in the frequency of the disease and in its severity, although no precise figures are available. This may be due in part to the influence of antibiotics and in part to the improvement in nutrition and general health of the community; it is one aspect of the waning importance of *Streptococcus haemolyticus* as a major pathogen.

Contributory causes are all those influences which favour the incidence or the spread of streptococcal infection. Into this category fall such factors as poverty, overcrowding, malnutrition and damp, together with the greater frequency of the disease in the autumn and winter months. In a negative sense the rarity of rheumatic fever in the tropics is another aspect of this relationship.

Pathology

The hallmark of rheumatic fever is the Aschoff node. It is a fusiform lesion with a central area of necrosis ringed by a fan-like arrangement of epithelioid cells and a perimeter of lymphocytes. As the acute inflammatory changes resolve the nodule is replaced by fibrous tissue.

Rheumatic fever is a generalized affection of connective tissue and Aschoff nodes are scattered throughout the body, being especially common in the heart, the joints, the blood vessels, the subcutaneous tissues and the serous membranes.

In fatal cases the heart will be found to have borne the brunt of the disease. Aschoff bodies abound throughout the myocardium and lesions occur along the lines of closure of the valves, leading to the familiar verrucous vegetations which finally undergo fibrosis and give rise to the valvular defects of chronic rheumatic heart disease.

The Clinical Picture

Onset. The mode of onset is variable. In adults it is frequently abrupt and often follows 10–21 days after an infection of the upper respiratory tract. This may have been an acute tonsillitis, but may be no more than a nasopharyngitis. There is a sudden rise of temperature with chills and, almost at once, complaint of pain in a joint or joints. Epistaxis is a common early symptom. In children the disease often starts insidiously: there may be abdominal pain, vague aches in the limbs—traditionally spoken of as 'growing pains'—skin rashes, lassitude, sweating and sore throats. In this form of 'subacute rheumatism' it is often difficult to fix a date of onset.

General Picture and Course. The patient soon begins to show the usual features of a febrile illness with coated tongue, loss of appetite and constipation. Sweating is often profuse and the sweat is said to have a characteristic 'acid' smell.

Monocyclic, polycyclic and continuous varieties of rheumatic fever have been described, but a classification of more practical utility is into those patients in whom the activity of the disease rapidly subsides and recovery with no or minimal cardiac damage results; those in whom the process remains active for months or years with frequent recrudescences and advancing disability; and those in whom rapidly progressive disease leads to death in a few weeks or months.

Persistent activity is shown by fever, anaemia, leucocytosis and a raised erythrocyte sedimentation rate (E.S.R.) with or without the local manifestations of the rheumatic process discussed in later paragraphs.

The categories of rheumatic fever described above afford but a rough guide to the course of the disease and variations are frequent. Recurrence is common, especially in children, being estimated at 25 per cent. in patients aged 4–13 years. The older the patient the less commonly it occurs. In young adults the disease will often last only 6 weeks, by which time all evidence of activity will have vanished and no sign of heart disease will remain. In younger children, in whom the insidious onset described earlier has been observed, a state of subacute rheumatism with symptoms insufficiently severe to drive the patient to the doctor may persist for months. During this time progressive damage to the heart valves takes place.

Convalescence is often protracted because of the nature of the disease and the frequency of relapses, but this prolonged illness can only too easily come to undermine the morale of the patient and may sometimes foster a pusillanimous attitude in the medical attendant.

Fever. In rheumatic fever the temperature seldom exceeds 102° F. (39° C.). The fever may be remittent or even intermittent and is one of the most sensitive indices of rheumatic activity. Hyperpyrexia was formerly an occasional complication, especially in the presence of pericarditis. It is now of extreme rarity.

Arthritis. Pain, swelling and redness of joints are characteristic features of rheumatic fever. In adults arthritis is the usual initial symptom. The typical picture is of a fugitive polyarthritis, the acute inflammatory changes flitting overnight from one joint to light upon another. Knees, ankles, wrists and shoulders are affected in that order of frequency. The severity of the joint affection varies from a trivial ache to intense pain with swelling, redness and the rapid appearance of effusion. Less commonly several joints show changes simultaneously and, in children, small joints may be affected. Sometimes in adults the arthritis lacks the typical migratory tendency and is strictly monarticular; in such cases the knee joint commonly suffers. In young children arthritis may be absent. It is, perhaps, worth mentioning the fact, that in spite of its name, rheumatic fever may occur without any evidence of articular disease.

When effusion occurs the joint fluid is turbid and contains neutrophil leucocytes, but is sterile on culture.

The Heart. The heart is affected by the disease process in at least 75 per cent. of patients with rheumatic fever. Tachycardia, often disproportionate to the rise in temperature, is the rule, but must not be regarded as unequivocal evidence that the heart has been affected. Convincing clinical proof is provided by the development at the apex of a blowing pansystolic or a short mid-diastolic murmur (Carey Coombs murmur) indicating mitral valvulitis; the development at the base of an early diastolic murmur indicating aortic valvulitis; a pericardial friction rub; or outward displacement of the apex beat due to cardiac dilatation. The electrocardiogram will show pathological changes in the majority of patients if tracings are repeated frequently: prolongation of the PR or QT intervals, abnormal T waves and evidence of intraventricular block are common.

The signs described here are those to be anticipated in an initial attack of rheumatic fever. It is, however, a disease peculiarly liable to recurrence and acute carditis often occurs in patients with well-established chronic rheumatic heart disease. Evidence of activity is then superimposed on pre-existing signs of valvular defect.

Pericarditis occurs in about 10 per cent. of patients and usually in the more severely affected. It commonly develops in the first month. There may be no more than an ephemeral friction rub or it may progress rapidly to massive effusion, although this is now rarely seen.

Cardiac symptoms are much less common than signs in acute rheumatism. Precordial pain is sometimes a complaint, even without signs of pericarditis, and has been attributed to myocarditis. In the rare fulminating cases extreme dyspnoea may result from left ventricular failure or pericardial effusion. Congestive heart failure is rare in the absence of established valvular lesions; when it does occur without these in acute rheumatic fever it is evidence of active myocarditis.

Although chronic rheumatic heart disease is the sequel of acute rheumatic fever, it is not an inevitable one. The younger the patient the more likely is the heart to suffer permanent damage and once established each relapse will add to it. After convalescence there are signs of valvular defect in 60–65 per cent. of patients, but this proves transient in about one-tenth. Follow-up figures also show that between one- and two-fifths of those who appear to have escaped valvular damage show signs of it within 10–20 years. Approximately two-thirds of all patients who have rheumatic fever in childhood eventually develop chronic rheumatic heart disease. All these show lesions of one or more valves: in about 85 per cent. the mitral valve is affected, in 44 per cent. the aortic, in 12 per cent. the tricuspid and in 1–2 per cent. the pulmonary.

The Lungs. Pleurisy is said to occur in 10 per cent. of patients, but is rare in the absence of pericarditis. It may be followed by effusion. Rheumatic pneumonia has frequently been described. It is not seen in more than 1 or 2 per cent. of active cases and these are usually of the severe fulminating variety. The lung shows a mixture of collapse, congestion and oedema with fibrinous exudate and mononuclear infiltration. It appears to be a specific lesion and not, as some have suggested, solely the result of left ventricular failure. Lesser degrees of rheumatic pneumonia are seen which are transient and do not appear greatly to influence the course of the disease.

The Skin and Subcutaneous Tissues. The frequency of sweating disproportionate to the height of the fever has already been noted; it may lead to sudaminal or miliarial eruptions. Various non-specific rashes, such as urticaria or purpura, may be seen. Erythema nodosum and erythema multiforme are occasional accompaniments and probably bear the same relation to preceding streptococcal infection as does rheumatic fever itself.

Erythema marginatum is peculiar to rheumatic fever and thus has a specific significance. It occurs on the trunk and proximal parts of the limbs; lesions may be scanty or numerous, persistent or ephemeral; they consist of circles or irregular areas of apparently normal skin outlined by a thin red erythematous margin. Erythema marginatum occurs in about 8 per cent. of patients with rheumatic fever, particularly in children with the subacute type.

Subcutaneous nodules are found almost exclusively in children and are said to be seen in 20 per cent. of patients with active disease. They vary in diameter from a few millimetres to 2 or 3 centimetres; they arise from tendons and aponeuroses, most frequently on the knees, knuckles, elbows and along the nuchal ridge. Their presence indicates activity of the rheumatic process.

The Nervous System (see Section 15). Sydenham's chorea bears a peculiar relation to rheumatic fever. It usually occurs without other rheumatic phenomena and does not affect the E.S.R. Nevertheless 20 per cent. of patients with chorea later develop rheumatic heart disease and about the same proportion with rheumatic fever later develop chorea.

The Abdomen. Abdominal pain is a common symptom in rheumatic fever in children. The explanation is uncertain; in some instances it has been attributed to rheumatic peritonitis.

Diagnosis

The classical case of rheumatic fever presents no problem, but with the declining incidence of the disease and the frequency of atypical cases diagnostic difficulties do arise.

Acute rheumatic arthritis needs to be distinguished from that due to pyogenic or gonococcal infection, to gout, and from Reiter's syndrome. The articles on these subjects should be consulted. Confusion sometimes arises with rheumatoid arthritis of rapid onset, especially when it is monarticular; the same is true of systemic lupus erythematosus and polyarteritis nodosa. Fever and arthralgia occur also in serum sickness, subacute bacterial endocarditis, brucellosis, acute lymphoblastic leukaemia of childhood—which often offers considerable difficulty—and in the crises of sickle-cell anaemia. In the past distinction from acute osteomyelitis was often a problem and it may be hard to decide whether pericarditis is due to rheumatism or of the acute benign variety.

A therapeutic test with sodium salicylate will often resolve diagnostic difficulties. This drug, given in adequate doses, will always cause the temperature to fall to normal within 48 hours in uncomplicated rheumatic fever.

Clinical Pathology. Anaemia which is normocytic and normochromic rapidly establishes itself; there is some evidence that this is in part a dilution effect and thus more apparent than real. The haemoglobin level is seldom below 9·5 g. per 100 ml. A leucocytosis of 10,000–15,000 per mm^3. is common in the earlier stages, the increase being neutrophil. The E.S.R. is considerably raised throughout the period of active disease and is a useful guide to progress, although, like the blood count it has little diagnostic value.

Indirect support for the diagnosis of rheumatic fever is given by proving that a haemolytic streptococcal infection preceded the onset of symptoms. Laboratory evidence for this is provided by an antistreptolysin-O titre in excess of 200 Todd units per ml. Similar increases can be demonstrated in the antibodies to other streptococcal antigens such as fibrinolysin and streptokinase, but the estimation of antistreptolysin-O is simple and has become the routine test. Transient 'false positive' serological tests for syphilis may occur in the acute stage.

In a proportion of patients with acute rheumatic ever haemolytic streptococci of Group A can be recovered from the nasopharynx. This finding establishes a diagnosis neither of rheumatic fever nor of a preceding streptococcal infection.

The urine usually contains protein during the febrile phase of the disease.

Treatment

The general management of the patient with rheumatic fever does not differ from that of any patient with a prolonged febrile disease.

Rest. Rest should be enforced while there is evidence that the disease process is active and should be absolute when there are signs of active carditis; in these circumstances the patient should be allowed to do nothing for himself; he should be washed and fed and he should make use of a bed-pan and urine bottle. He should be allowed to assume the position he finds most comfortable, although there are theoretical reasons for preferring a sitting posture as demanding least work from the heart. It is wise to regard all children as having active carditis until there is convincing evidence to the contrary, but adults can be allowed more freedom.

There is, in fact, no conclusive evidence that complete rest influences the prognosis and indeed it would be hard to obtain. Nevertheless it is widely believed that those patients who are allowed unrestricted freedom do badly and suffer frequent relapse. This view is not held by all and some even contend that prolonged rest has an adverse effect.

The duration of rest in bed depends upon the persistence of activity of the disease. Only when there is no fever or other clinical sign of activity and when the blood count and the E.S.R. have returned to normal should mobilization be started. Convalescence must be gradual and may need to be prolonged over several months. Relapse is common and enjoins further rest. It is only too easy for morale to suffer during this long period and for the seeds of cardiac neurosis to be implanted. For this reason purposive and positive rehabilitation is important and renewed rest should only be advised when there is no room for doubt that the disease is active once again.

Drug Treatment. The rheumatic process may be suppressed by salicylates or by the corticosteroids. Neither has any great advantage over the other; in some cases toxic symptoms arise from the first, in others the side-effects of the corticosteroid hormones prove troublesome. Corticosteroids bring the symptoms under control more rapidly and some prefer to use them when there is active carditis. There is little support for the view that permanent cardiac damage is less frequent and less severe when these hormones are used. The combination of corticosteroids and salicylates may allow the first to be given in smaller doses and to be withdrawn earlier, while control is maintained with the second. Neither do more than discourage the overt expression of the disease, they do not influence the underlying process. They both appear to prevent the tissue response and reduce the inflammatory reaction without having any effect upon the cause of either.

Salicylates may be given as sodium salicylate, as acetylsalicylic acid or as calcium acetylsalicylate in doses of 1–1·5 G. of the first, or 0·6 G. of the aspirin compounds, every three hours in an adult and proportionately less in a child. The optimum blood level is 30–35 mg. of salicylate per 100 ml. and when this is reached fever abates, joint pain disappears and effusions undergo absorption. The intervals between doses can then be increased to four and later six hours.

Toxic symptoms which may arise from treatment with salicylates are nausea, vomiting, tinnitus, deafness and hyperpnoea. These can often be avoided by starting with a dose smaller than the optimum and gradually increasing it. The addition of sodium bicarbonate increases the excretion of salicylate and only relieves intoxication by reducing the concentration in the blood to ineffective levels. It is not to be recommended.

Corticosteroids may be given as prednisone. It is usual to begin with 10 mg. four times daily; at the end of one week the dose is reduced to 5 mg. four times daily and after a further three weeks it is decreased slowly in the hopes of being able to withdraw the drug after six weeks. Corticotrophin may be used in a dose of 100 Units daily by intramuscular injection for the first week, reducing the daily dose by 20 Units at the end of each week.

It is not always easy to decide how long drug treatment should be continued. Not only are symptoms relieved, but the laboratory indices of activity are also suppressed by treatment with salicylates and corticosteroids. The only course is to reduce the dose slowly, watching for a reappearance of symptoms or a rise in the E.S.R. If these do not take place, further cautious reduction should follow until the drug is withdrawn altogether. Withdrawal is sometimes followed by a 'rebound phenomenon' when activity appears to increase, but dies down after a few days.

Prophylaxis. Tonsillectomy is only indicated when there is unassailable evidence of tonsillar infection or a story of recurrent tonsillitis. It has proved disappointing as a prophylactic measure and should never be undertaken until all sign of rheumatic activity has been absent for two months.

It has been abundantly shown than if infection of the upper respiratory tract can be prevented relapse and recurrence are far less likely. To this end 1 G. of sulphadiazine or 125 mg. of phenoxymethylpenicillin should be taken daily by mouth or 0·9 G. (1·2 mega Units) of benzathine penicillin given by intramuscular injection once a month for a period of at least two years after the initial attack.

Some authorities believe that a course of penicillin at the onset of rheumatic fever is advisable with the aim of purging the nasopharynx of haemolytic streptococci.

Prognosis

The immediate mortality of rheumatic fever is 6·5 per cent. An analysis of published series shows that 10 years after the onset of acute rheumatism 10 per cent. of patients have died, 51 per cent. have chronic rheumatic heart disease and 30 per cent. have recovered completely.

Before antibiotics were used in prophylaxis recurrences and relapses were common. Earlier figures showed that 40 per cent. had a second attack of rheumatic fever within 2 years; 58 per cent. within 5 years and 63 per cent. within 10 years. In one recent series of 101 children receiving a monthly prophylactic injection of penicillin, only one minor relapse had been noted in 5 years.

REFERENCES

CRUICKSHANK, R., and GLYNN, A. A. (1959) *Rheumatic Fever, Epidemiology and Prevention*, Oxford.

HALL, P. (1961) On the prognosis and natural history of acute rheumatic fever and rheumatic heart disease. A study based upon a 25-year material in a Swedish town served by a single hospital, *Acta med. scand.*, **169**, Suppl. 362.

MARKOWITZ, M., and KUTTNER, A. G. (1962) The treatment of acute rheumatic fever, *Amer. J. Dis. Child.*, **104**, 313.

PAUL, J. R. (1957) *The Epidemiology of Rheumatic Fever*, New York.

THE TREATMENT OF ACUTE RHEUMATIC FEVER IN CHILDREN. A Joint Report by the Rheumatic Fever Working Party of the Medical Research Council and the Sub-Committee of the American Council on Rheumatic Fever of the American Heart Association, *Brit. med. J.* (1955), **1**, 555.

INFECTIONS DUE TO OTHER STREPTOCOCCI

α-Haemolytic streptococci include *Streptococcus viridans* and *Streptococcus pneumoniae* (pneumococcus) which is considered later. The first leads a commensal existence in the throat and oral secretions of almost all persons. It is commonly found in carious teeth and is responsible for most periodontal and apical infections. It is the commonest cause of subacute bacterial endocarditis.

The most important non-haemolytic aerobic streptococcus is *Streptococcus faecalis* (enterococcus) a normal inhabitant of the human and animal intestine. It is a common cause of urinary tract infection and a less common one of subacute bacterial endocarditis.

Anaerobic streptococci, of which the best documented is *Peptrostreptocccus putridus*, are probably normal inhabitants of the vagina. They have been incriminated in wound infections, postoperative synergistic bacterial gangrene, anaerobic streptococcal myositis and occasional instances of cerebral abscess.

PNEUMOCOCCAL INFECTION

BACTERIOLOGY

Str. pneumoniae or the pneumococcus is lanceolate in shape, grows usually in pairs or short chains and is Gram-positive. The organism is enclosed within a polysaccharide capsule on the basis of antigenic differences in which more than 80 types of pneumococcus can be recognized. Many of these are of low pathogenicity for man and 80 per cent. of the pneumococci isolated from patients with pneumonia belong to Types I–VIII. Other antigens which are not type specific have been demonstrated, but antibodies against them have little effect upon the invasive capacity of the organism. The pneumococcus produces a hyaluronidase, a haemolysin and autolytic enzymes.

EPIDEMIOLOGY

Forty to seventy per cent. of healthy people carry pneumococci in their upper respiratory tracts: the organisms usually belong to Types with high numbers and are seldom pathogenic. Occasional epidemics of pneumococcal pneumonia have been reported in the past. They have usually occurred in closed communities such as camps and prisons. In such circumstances a high carrier rate of virulent types has been found. The healthy carrier seems to be of greater importance in the spread of infection than the patient with pneumonia.

HUMAN INFECTION

The classic form of pneumococcal infection in man is pneumonia [see SECTION 9]. In the days before antibiotics were available, pneumococcal lobar pneumonia in adults was a common illness with a characteristic and sharp-cut clinical picture. In this form it is now rarely seen, presumably because antibacterial treatment is customarily prescribed before significant invasion of the lower respiratory tract has occurred. In children the usual anatomical pattern of pneumococcal pneumonia has always been lobular. Although lobar pneumonia occurs in healthy adults, it seems probable that the pneumococcus more readily invades a respiratory tract which is not intact. Pneumococcal pneumonia is often obviously secondary, usually to the damage wrought by a virus infection. Bronchopneumonia is often due to the pneumococcus. Reduction in resistance by debilitating illness, surgical operation or treatment with corticosteroids and local changes in the lungs, such as congestion or atelectasis, are all important predisposing causes. A combination of one or more of these factors with the presence in the upper respiratory tract of virulent pneumococci is needed to cause pneumonia. In adults with pneumococcal pneumonia the organisms belong to Types I, II or III in 50 per cent. and to Types I to VIII in 80 per cent. of cases. In children Types I, II and III are important but in a considerable proportion the pneumococcus is of Type XIV.

The respiratory tract is the portal through which most pneumococcal infections enter the body. Some of the most common are due to the direct spread to anatomically related structures: otitis media, mastoiditis and sinusitis are examples in its upper, and empyema of the pleura and pericarditis in its lower reaches. Further extension from the first may give rise to cerebral abscess or meningitis.

In lobar pneumonia, untreated with antibiotics, bacteraemia occurs in 25 per cent. in the first two or three days. From this remote infections may be derived. Suppurative arthritis, usually monarticular, is rare, but well documented. The most serious are peritonitis, meningitis and acute bacterial endocarditis. The third seldom occurs without the second.

Pneumococcal peritonitis may occur as a 'primary' infection. It is typically found in children, especially girls. It was a relatively frequent infection in children with the nephrotic syndrome. There is some reason for thinking that infection is by way of the genital passages for in many pneumococci can be recovered from the uterine cervix. Pneumococcal meningitis may also appear to be 'primary', but a spread from the upper respiratory tract must presumably be responsible. Pneumococci may sometimes give rise to recurrent subacute parotitis.

Acute glomerulonephritis has occasionally been observed to follow pneumococcal pneumonia. There is usually an interval of three or four weeks between the two.

PROPHYLAXIS

Pneumococcal infections are likely to be frequent where there is overcrowding, defective hygiene and inadequate ventilation. The organism is so commonly found in the healthy mouth that isolation is impracticable. It has been shown that inoculation with the capsular polysaccharide of the pneumococcus gives immunity against pneumonia due to types from which the vaccine is prepared. There is seldom justification for such a procedure, but it has proved useful in controlling prolonged epidemics of pneumonia in confined communities.

TREATMENT

The specific treatment is discussed in the section on antibiotics and chemotherapy. The pneumococcus is particularly sensitive to sulphonamide drugs and to various antibiotics and these agents have altered the picture of pneumococcal infection more dramatically perhaps than that due to any other organism. It is, therefore, now only of historical interest that pneumococcal pneumonia was one of the few diseases for which an effective antiserum was evolved.

R. BODLEY SCOTT

INFECTIONS DUE TO CORYNEBACTERIACEAE

DIPHTHERIA

Definition

A disease caused by the Klebs-Loeffler bacillus, *Corynebacterium diphtheriae*, characterized by a membranous exudate at the site of infection which is later followed by distant toxic effects, the chief being circulatory failure and paralyses.

Aetiology

The *C. diphtheriae* is a slender Gram-positive non-motile, non-sporing rod which tends to appear segmented or clubbed. It grows on Loeffler's and tellurite medium and ferments glucose. There are three main strains of bacilli, gravis, intermedius and mitis which show cultural, biochemical and usually toxigenic differences. Gravis and intermedius are the most virulent, growing well on human tissue while mitis strains multiply less readily and remain more superficial. Gravis strains are characteristically fermenters of starch whereas intermedius and mitis are not. All strains produce an exotoxin which is responsible for the majority of the serious complications.

There are virulent and non-virulent forms. Most non-virulent forms belong to the mitis group although occasionally avirulent forms of gravis and intermedius occur. Toxigenic strains may change to become non-toxigenic. Conversely, a non-toxigenic strain can be changed in the laboratory by treatment with bacteriophage into a virulent toxin-producing strain. Although this change has not been shown definitely to occur in the field, it may well do so and it would account for the sudden appearance of diphtheria in a community previously free from the disease. The laboratory distinction between virulent and non-virulent strains depends on culture on Elek plates or by guinea-pig inoculation. The strain can usually be shown to be toxin-producing within 24 hours by the former method. Virulent organisms kill a guinea-pig within 4 days, producing typical changes at autopsy.

Diphtheroids are organisms morphologically similar to diphtheria bacilli which may cause confusion in bacteriological diagnosis. They include Hofmann's bacillus, frequently recovered from the ear and nose but less often from the throat and *Corynebacterium xerosis* obtained from the conjunctiva. These organisms have different sugar reactions from diphtheria bacilli.

Epidemiology

Diphtheria has a world wide distribution with a tendency to occur in epidemic form in autumn and winter. The incidence in Great Britain has been enormously reduced in recent years following the introduction of active immunization. In 1945, 694 persons died of diphtheria in England and Wales, in 1967 none. In the absence of immunization, clinical cases appear to occur more readily in temperate than in tropical zones although there is a high proportion of infection in the tropics as shown by Schick testing. Diphtheria is rare under six months of age and above middle age, being commonest in the 2–10 year olds. Recently the greatest incidence has shifted from the pre-school to the early school group.

The disease is spread by droplet infection from carriers and cases, the latter being the most dangerous source. Anterior nasal diphtheria, which commonly causes only little ill health but copious nasal discharge, is highly infectious. As the organism is resistant to heat, cold and drying, spread by fomites (for example, on clothes, books or toys) is a theoretical possibility but outside hospital this method of spread is of minor importance. In the past, milk has been responsible for an occasional outbreak.

Instead of leading to an increase of the carrier state as was originally feared, active immunization has in fact been followed by the apparent disappearance of carriers. Outbreaks in a community free from the disease for a number of years are due either to the introduction of the organism from outside or possibly to a non-toxic strain mutating to a toxin-producing one.

Pathology

The organisms remain at the site of infection and do not become invasive, constitutional symptoms arising from absorption of the powerful exotoxin. Multiplication of organisms leads to toxin production which causes epithelial necrosis. This is followed by an inflammatory reaction, fibrin and leucocytes entering the necrotic area to form the membrane characteristic of the disease. The membrane is 'false' in that it consists of invaded and necrotic layers of the mucosa and is not an exudate superimposed on an intact surface. The necrotic process is deeper and toxin is absorbed much more readily from the fauces and nasopharynx than from the nose or larynx where there is little soft tissue between mucous membrane and cartilage. Corynebacteria are present at the margin of the membrane, which is adherent and removed only with difficulty and which varies from a thin transparent film to a thick opaque greyish-white plaque. Membrane may extend down the respiratory tract to the trachea and major bronchi where it is less adherent than in the fauces.

When death occurs in the first week the heart is dilated and pale, cloudy swelling and interstitial oedema being seen microscopically. The heart muscle in patients dying later in the disease shows multiple degenerative foci with plasma cells and lymphocytic infiltration together with minute fat granules. These foci may involve the conduction fibres. There are no valvular lesions but intracardiac thrombi sometimes occur. Neurological symptoms are associated with fatty degeneration of the myelin sheaths of peripheral nerves. The kidneys show non-specific inflammatory changes with shedding of tubular epithelium.

Symptoms

The incubation period is commonly between 2 and 5 days with extremes of 1–10 days.

The fauces are most often the site of a diphtheritic infection and as absorption of toxin takes place much more rapidly than from other sites faucial diphtheria is usually associated with most toxaemia. Diphtheritic membrane may be found in the nose, nasopharynx, fauces or larynx. Infection in other sites is rare.

The classification of clinical diphtheria in the first instance is, therefore, an anatomical one. Most cases fall clearly into one of these groups but it must be realized that the membrane is not always limited to one site, for example nasal and faucial or faucial and laryngeal diphtheria not infrequently co-exist.

The acute stage of all types covers the first week where the most prominent symptoms are most likely to be due to the local lesion. Thereafter in the more severe infections the local symptoms fade and the illness is dominated by cardiovascular and later by paralytic symptoms.

Anterior Nasal Diphtheria. This type is of considerable epidemiological importance because of its high infectivity, but it is seldom serious to the patient. The onset is insidious with minimal malaise and fever. The membrane is confined to the front of the nose, usually on the nasal septum. It may be in one or both nostrils. The characteristic signs are a profuse thin blood-stained serous nasal discharge together with small ulcers or crusted sores appearing at the anterior nares, and extending on to the upper lip and cheeks. Little toxin is absorbed and myocarditis and paralysis are accordingly rare. Undiagnosed, the nasal discharge may persist for weeks. It ceases rapidly following treatment.

Posterior Nasal (Nasopharyngeal) Diphtheria. This is a serious and dangerous form similar in all respects to faucial diphtheria with which it is generally associated. The danger lies in the fact that there may be considerable membrane formation in the nasopharynx hidden behind the palate and therefore not easily visible on ordinary throat inspection.

Faucial Diphtheria. The onset is insidious, particularly in children who become quiet and refuse their food. Lassitude, mild headache, malaise and sore throat are associated with a moderate degree of fever though the temperature seldom rises above 101° F. (38·4° C.). Indeed, pyrexia is often absent on the first day or two and may never exceed 100° F. (37·8° C.). It should be noted that sore throat is not a marked symptom and one never complained of by some children.

Membrane is not present at the onset but may be extensive within 24 hours. In the mildest form, it never appears, the fauces being merely injected. Typically, membrane begins on one or both tonsils and may spread on to the pillars of the fauces, the uvula and palate. It may be thin or thick, greyish, yellowish or creamy in colour or, if mixed with blood, a dirty-grey colour. In the early stages it tends to glisten. It can be removed only with difficulty, usually leaving a bleeding surface. The more severe the case, the thinner and less well defined is the membrane. Old membrane, or membrane after treatment with antitoxin is thick and opaque with a sharply defined edge. The extent varies considerably and the possibility of additional membrane on the back of the uvula or palate (posterior nasal diphtheria) must always be considered. In most cases there is an area of inflammation visible as a hyperaemic zone surrounding the membrane separating it from the pale oedematous fauces. With little membrane there is little oedema. Foetor is often striking and characteristic. There is always some degree of cervical adenitis with an element of peri-adenitis but this is not particularly painful and only slightly tender. A serous or blood-stained nasal discharge appears later in many cases. Drowsiness, vomiting, pallor or tachycardia are signs of early toxicity.

The severity of faucial diphtheria is related to the amount of membrane and cases are classified accordingly:

1. *Mild*—tonsillar diphtheria, membrane limited to one or both tonsils.

2. *Moderate*—membrane on the pillars, uvula or pharynx with moderate peri-adenitis.

3. *Severe*—membrane as in moderate but with considerable faucial oedema, gross peri-adenitis, early toxaemia and, in a few cases, skin or mucous membrane haemorrhages.

Severe (Hypertoxic, Malignant, 'Bull-neck') Diphtheria. Severe faucial diphtheria has a high mortality. The patient is usually a child who is restless, irritable and pale. The mouth is open, the face puffy and gross cervical peri-adenitis produces the typical 'bull-neck' appearance. Vomiting is repeated and feeding is difficult. There is a heavy albuminuria. The pulse is rapid and the blood pressure low. Tendon reflexes are often absent. Respiration is rapid and shallow and an ashen cyanosis may replace the pallor. A blood-stained nasal discharge is usual, often accompanied early by sores. Petechial haemorrhages may appear in the skin, particularly in the axillae and over the front of the chest or haemorrhages may be seen in the mouth. These are always a grave sign. The throat shows marked oedema on which is superimposed a thin, filmy, translucent and ill-defined membrane. The foetor on opening the mouth is unmistakable. Death from circulatory failure is likely any time between the fifth and twenty-first day but may occur much later from sudden exertion. Widespread paralyses are to be expected in those who survive long enough.

Antitoxin transforms the filmy membrane after 2–3 days into a thick, opaque separating membrane, the throat returning to normal within a further 7–10 days.

Laryngeal Diphtheria. This is rare over the age of 5 years. The illness is one of progressive laryngeal obstruction with relatively little toxaemia unless associated with faucial diphtheria. The membrane may spread down the trachea into the major bronchi. The symptoms of croup—hoarse voice, inspiratory stridor and croupy cough appear. As these symptoms increase, recession of the chest wall appears with restlessness, pallor and ultimately cyanosis and asphyxia. This development takes from 24 hours to a few days but periodic superimposed attacks of laryngeal spasm may cause acute obstructive episodes early in the illness, any of which may prove fatal. In rare instances, membranous casts are coughed up with relief of symptoms.

Other Sites. Cutaneous diphtheria is rare and usually due to infection of an existing wound, ulcer or skin lesion. Such ulcers have a dark leathery base and tend to be chronic, their diphtheritic nature often remaining unsuspected until peripheral neuritis appears. The conjunctivae, middle ear, umbilicus in the newborn and genital mucous membrane are rare sites of diphtheritic infection. Non-virulent diphtheria organisms are not infrequently cultured from chronic ear discharges.

Complications

The chief are *cardiovascular* and *paralytic*. These two complications are related to the virulence of the infecting strain, the amount of membrane (and hence toxin) formation and the time interval between the onset and the administration of antitoxin. Some degree of myocarditis is present in all cases of faucial diphtheria in which there is membrane formation. The more exotoxin formed the sooner the onset of circulatory and paralytic symptoms. Once toxin is fixed in heart muscle or peripheral nerves it is not affected by antitoxin which can only neutralize circulating toxin.

Acute Circulatory Failure. This is the commonest cause of death. It is due to a combination of peripheral failure and severe myocarditis but it is not always possible to determine clinically which of these elements is of most significance. Cardiovascular symptoms may appear at any time from the third to twenty-first day depending on the severity of the attack. The early signs are tachycardia accompanied by pallor and sometimes vomiting. The blood pressure falls, the heart sounds alter and signs of congestive failure (increase in jugular venous pressure and tender enlargement of the liver) appear. Frank oedema is rare. The common alterations in heart sounds are weakness of the first sound, sometimes softening of the second sound, splitting and the development of presystolic triple rhythm. Slowing of the heart rate in the second week is not necessarily a good sign, as it may be due to heart block. Atrial fibrillation is uncommon. Routine electrocardiograms reveal abnormalities in nearly all cases of faucial diphtheria. Diffuse myocardial damage is indicated by low voltage tracings and by flattened or depressed ST segments with inverted T waves. Damage to the conducting mechanism is present in most fatal cases and all types of heart block from prolongation of the PR interval to complete A-V block are seen. The electrocardiogram is a useful aid in assessing progress but is of little help in prognosis as severe changes with complete block are quite compatible with recovery and conversely sudden death may occur in a patient whose tracings show only moderate changes. Recovery from myocarditis is complete in virtually all patients although in severe cases this may take over three months. Permanent heart block is a great rarity.

Paralytic Stage. The degree of peripheral neuritis, like myocarditis, depends on the amount of toxin fixed in the nerves before the administration of antitoxin. The earlier paralysis appears the more extensive will be the ultimate weakness. Paralyses develop in a remarkably constant order with the *palate* being first affected. In toxic cases a palatal palsy may become evident as early as the seventh day but it most commonly occurs between the third and sixth weeks. Either a change in the character of the voice with the production of a nasal quality or regurgitation of fluids down the nose may be the first indication. On inspection, palatal movement is seen to be diminished or absent. If the palsy is confined to one side this is invariably the side on which membrane has been more extensive, the palsy being due to the local action of toxin on the nerve endings. *Eye palsies* soon follow, blurred vision due to weakness of accommodation being much more common than external ocular palsies although the external recti are sometimes involved.

Peripheral neuritis of the limbs and trunk occurs from the fourth week onwards. This is fairly symmetrical and may be extensive. Sensory symptoms are usually absent although in those who develop peripheral neuritis late it is not uncommon to find a sensory ataxia, perhaps with associated paraesthesiae.

Respiratory failure seldom occurs before the sixth week. It may be due to diaphragmatic and intercostal paralysis, to pharyngeal paralysis with consequent pooling of secretions and airway obstruction, or to a combination of both. If the patient survives this last major hazard, recovery is ultimately complete although it may take six months or more.

A patient who develops palatal weakness in the second week of illness can be expected to suffer extensive paralysis. Conversely, if palatal palsy appears late, in the fifth or sixth week, this is likely to be the sole neurological complication.

Palatal and eye palsies usually recover in 1–3 weeks even in those who ultimately develop extensive peripheral neuritis. There may be a late return of palatal weakness, however, in association with pharyngeal paralysis.

The cerebrospinal fluid shows an increase of protein in severe cases. A rare neurological complication is hemiplegia due to a cerebral embolus from an intracardiac thrombus.

Albuminuria, which is constant and heavy in severe attacks, is present in moderate degree in most faucial cases. At times casts and red cells appear in the urine. Bronchitis, bronchopneumonia and atelectasis (in laryngeal cases) may arise. Otitis media is uncommon. Septic faucial diphtheria due to a mixed infection of diphtheria and haemolytic streptococci is characterized by an atypical membrane, painful lymphadenitis and usually marked toxaemia. The temperature may be higher than is usual in diphtheria.

Diagnosis

Diphtheria is rare in Great Britain at the present time and in recent outbreaks the first cases have been missed. Any serous or bloody nasal discharge or any membranous throat should be regarded with suspicion. Suggestive signs are a membrane spreading on to the fauces which is only removed with difficulty associated with a low-grade fever but a relative tachycardia.

Investigations include nose and throat swabs in all suspected cases, swabs being taken from the edge of any membrane present. It is important to realize that negative swab cultures do *not* exclude diphtheria, especially if an antibiotic has been administered. Nasal swabs are not infrequently positive in faucial diphtheria and swabs from both sites must always be taken. The presence of numerous morphological corynebacteria on direct film is suggestive, but bacteriological confirmation of the presence of virulent diphtheria may take up to 3 or occasionally even 6 days. There is usually a moderate leucocytosis.

Tests of Immunity. The Schick test determines *susceptibility* to diphtheria; 0·1 ml. of toxin is injected intradermally into the forearm and a control solution of heated toxin injected into the other arm. A positive reaction consists of an area of induration and erythema of 10 mm. or more in diameter by the fourth day and indicates susceptibility to the disease. A negative reaction implies immunity to the toxin. Non-specific pseudo-reactions are not uncommon, appear early and disappear within two to three days. Schick tests should be read at four days but if the control is negative a positive result can often be declared with certainty at two days. The test may be useful in diagnosis in a suspected mild case. A Schick test will not be affected by antitoxin if this is withheld for six hours. This can be of help in the differential diagnosis of a carrier from an early case, a negative test excluding toxic diphtheria.

The Moloney test determines *sensitivity* to the products of the diphtheria bacillus and consists of an intradermal injection of 0·1 ml. of toxoid, diluted 1:100. The test is read in 24 hours, a positive indicating that active immunization with toxoid is likely to be followed by a constitutional reaction. Sensitivity to diphtheria toxoid increases with age and the Moloney test should replace the Schick control in those over ten years of age in whom active immunization is contemplated, positive reactors not requiring immunization.

The differential diagnosis varies with each clinical type.

Anterior Nasal Diphtheria. A *foreign body* causes a profuse, often offensive and purulent nasal discharge. Examination with a nasal speculum reveals the cause. Rhinorrhoea from non-diphtheritic infection is seldom blood-stained and there is no membrane. Swabs should always be taken from a persistent nasal discharge.

Faucial Diphtheria. In *streptococcal tonsillitis* the exudate is often more yellow, frequently patchy and always easily removed. It is confined to the tonsil, the rest of the throat showing a generalized bright red erythema. The patient is flushed rather than pale and the temperature is often above 102° F. (38·9° C.). The tonsillar glands are tender.

A *quinsy* causes unilateral faucial oedema, but it is seldom accompanied by membrane formation and the acute pain and tenderness are notable features. There may be a greyish exudate in *Vincent's angina*, but the lesion is ulcerative rather than membranous and the development is insidious. Membranous tonsillitis of non-bacterial origin more closely resembling streptococcal than diphtheritic infections are not uncommon in children.

Infectious mononucleosis may produce a throat lesion with attached greyish membrane and oedema identical to diphtheria. It is the commonest infection to cause real difficulty in diagnosis. Most often such patients, however, show other evidence of glandular fever such as generalized lymphadenopathy, splenomegaly and abnormal mononuclear cells in the peripheral blood. *Acute leukaemia* and *agranulocytosis* may be complicated by oral lesions resembling diphtheria. *Thrush* is usually easily distinguished by the lack of constitutional upset and the presence of multiple small lesions on the buccal mucosa and tongue. *Herpes zoster of the palate* may cause an extensive unilateral lesion but there is little toxaemia, the membrane is strictly limited to one side and discrete herpetic lesions on the buccal mucous membrane or in the external auditory meatus will be found. Hyperacusis, deafness or earache on the affected side are likely to be the first symptoms. The membrane frequently seen following tonsillectomy is confined to the raw area and does not spread. Cursory examination has led to bull-neck diphtheria being mistaken for *mumps*. The pallor, toxaemia, tachycardia and throat lesion of malignant diphtheria should prevent this tragic mistake being made.

Laryngeal Diphtheria. Although diphtheria is now one of the less common causes of croup it must always be considered in the differential diagnosis of this syndrome and antitoxin administered if evidence of a different aetiology is lacking. Infectious croup is usually part of a *laryngotracheobronchitis* of viral aetiology and the acute laryngitis is accompanied by evidence of throat and bronchial infection. *Measles* may present in this way. Occasionally streptococci and *Haemophilus influenzae* cause acute laryngitis with croup. *Catarrhal spasm of the larynx* appears suddenly, usually at night, and clears up in an hour or two though it may recur. This is an allergic phenomenon not uncommonly complicating upper respiratory tract infections in young children.

A low *retropharyngeal abscess* may produce laryngeal obstruction. The abscess can be felt by digital examination of the back of the pharynx and may be visible on throat inspection.

Inhalation of a foreign body may cause difficulty if the history of aspiration is lacking. Sudden choking on change of position or during a coughing bout is suggestive.

Rare causes of laryngeal obstruction include angioneurotic oedema, papillomata and congenital laryngeal stridor. In supraglottic oedema, due to *H. influenzae* epiglottitis, there is severe toxaemia associated with airway obstruction, but no laryngitis. The red swollen epiglottis can be seen.

Treatment

General. All patients must be nursed in bed in isolation, every patient with faucial disease being nursed flat for the first week and kept in bed for a minimum of three weeks. Signs of myocarditis call for a much longer period of recumbency. Mobilization is only begun when clinical and electrocardiographic evidence of myocarditis has subsided. It must be gradual, the well-tried regime of allowing a pillow a week until the patient is propped up in bed forming a satisfactory basis. In the acute stage, all patients must be fed. This programme may be adjusted as required but the importance of rest cannot be overstressed. Should congestive heart failure develop the patient may be more comfortable propped up, but most cases fare better when nursed flat and this position should be maintained if hypotension is marked and dyspnoea minimal. If there is doubt about the wisdom of allowing a certain increase in activity then the proposed increase should be delayed. As complete recovery will ultimately ensue, it is tragic when sudden death occurs because of unwise exertion due to impatience. Peripheral circulatory failure is treated by raising the foot of the bed, administering steroids and nursing in an oxygen tent. Complete rest and quiet are essential. The value of digitalis is doubtful, but if there is clear evidence of venous congestion it should be tried.

Paralytic complications are treated by rest and passive movements followed by active exercises in convalescence. Respiratory difficulties are managed in the same way as those due to poliomyelitis with postural drainage for pharyngeal paralysis and artificial respiration in a cabinet respirator when the diaphragm and intercostals are involved. If both respiratory and pharyngeal muscles are affected, then tracheostomy and intermittent positive pressure respiration are indicated. Convalescence is prolonged following severe paralytic symptoms. Even after muscular power has returned a sensory ataxia of the limbs may limit walking and fine hand movements for weeks.

Three negative nose and throat swabs at weekly intervals should be obtained in all cases of diphtheria before release from isolation.

Specific. Diphtheritic antitoxin must be administered without delay to any patient in whom a clinical diagnosis is made or strongly suspected. Antitoxin therapy must never be withheld while awaiting bacteriological confirmation. Only in a suspected mild case is it ever justifiable to delay six hours after carrying out a Schick test. It is very important that the patient should receive the first dose not later than the third day of the disease. The dose required is dependent on the type of the disease, its duration and the extent of the membrane and is unrelated to the age of the patient. A mild faucial case requires up to 20,000 Units intramuscularly, a moderate one 40,000 to 80,000 Units, half of which should be given intravenously, and a severe case 100,000 to 200,000 Units intravenously. 10,000 Units is usually adequate for anterior nasal disease. The larger doses are indicated when there has been delay in the patient coming under observation. Before giving antidiphtheritic serum (which is a horse serum preparation) a history regarding previous serum injections and possible allergy must be obtained. If this is negative 0·2 ml. of the undiluted serum is injected subcutaneously and if there is no reaction after half an hour then the bulk of the dose can safely be administered intramuscularly. In toxic cases 50,000 Units intramuscularly can serve as the test dose before giving 100,000 Units intravenously, the serum being warmed to blood heat and injected extremely slowly. Risks of severe reactions are greatest following intravenous therapy and must be balanced against the dangers of delay inherent in intramuscular treatment, absorption from this route being slow.

If the patient is shown to be sensitive to horse serum therapy is begun with a small dose subcutaneously which is gradually increased every 20–30 minutes providing there is no reaction. Should a reaction occur, the same or a smaller dose is given depending on its severity. The scheme is as follows:

0·1 ml. of 1 in 20 dilution subcutaneously with 0·05 ml. of 1 in 1000 adrenaline.

0·1 ml. of 1 in 10 dilution subcutaneously with 0·05 ml. of 1 in 1000 adrenaline.

0·1 ml. of undiluted antitoxin subcutaneously.

0·2 ml. of undiluted antitoxin subcutaneously.

0·5 ml. of undiluted antitoxin subcutaneously.

The bulk dose can then be safely given intramuscularly. 1 in 1000 adrenaline solution must be immediately available in a syringe whenever horse serum is administered, as must intravenous hydrocortisone or equivalent prednisolone preparation.

A repeat dose of antitoxin should not be necessary if the correct assessment is originally made. A further dose can, however, safely be given after 2–3 days if the membrane continues to spread. Penicillin should be given to all cases, but in no way replaces the need for antitoxin. It helps to limit spread of infection, but has no effect on any preformed toxin.

Many cases of laryngeal diphtheria respond satisfactorily to prompt antitoxin and penicillin therapy together with nursing in a steam tent. Should respiratory obstruction increase tracheostomy should not be delayed; persistent cyanosis is an absolute indication as is continued restlessness. Membrane is sucked out at operation, patients thereafter being nursed in a steam tent; in infants the tube is removed as soon as possible and certainly not later than the fifth day in order to avoid the risk of a 'retained tube'. Tracheostomy is preferable to intubation or repeated attempts at aspiration of membrane on direct laryngoscopy. Most convalescent and long-term carriers are cleared with a seven-day course of erythromycin. Tonsillectomy is rarely required.

Prophylactic. Passive immunization with 1500 Units of antidiphtheritic serum (A.D.S.) only lasts from two to three weeks and is rarely indicated by itself, but is of use in giving immediate protection to unimmunized close contacts who at the same time receive 0·5 ml. of alum precipitated toxoid (A.P.T.) into the other arm.

Routine active immunization is best carried out with a triple vaccine containing tetanus and pertussis starting at about four months of age. Three injections are necessary at appropriate intervals, booster doses of combined diphtheria and tetanus vaccine being given at school entry and at 8–12 years of age. A.P.T. or purified toxoid aluminium phosphate (P.T.A.P.) are good antigens. Toxoid antitoxin floccules (T.A.F.) is the vaccine recommended for booster doses in older children or for primary immunization from the age of five years. This vaccine contains horse serum proteins and is thus not suitable for those likely to be sensitive to horse serum.

In countries such as Great Britain, where diphtheria is no longer endemic in most areas, elimination of the organism from the affected community should be the aim of the control measures employed. Family and class contacts of the patient form special groups which should be investigated urgently by repeated nose and throat swabbing together with determination of immunization states. Those with positive cultures are isolated and observed daily while virulence tests are proceeding. The treatment of carriers with erythromycin has been mentioned above. If the number of contacts renders close daily observation difficult there is a good case for protecting unimmunized close contacts with a combination of antitoxin (1500 Units) in one arm and 0·5 ml. A.P.T. given into the other arm followed by a further 0·5 ml. A.P.T. 4 weeks later. Those actively immunized within the preceding two years can be regarded as safe while those immunized more than two years previously should receive a booster dose of T.A.F. Carriers discharged from hospital after three negative cultures should be swabbed one to three weeks later as relapse of the carrier state is not rare.

Prognosis

As indicated above, this depends on the infecting organism, gravis strains in general producing more toxin than others, on the position and extent of the membrane, and on the delay in administering antitoxin. Anterior nasal diphtheria is mild while faucial or pharyngeal attacks are likely to be severe. Malignant diphtheria has a mortality approaching 50 per cent. Haemorrhages, 'bull-neck', repeated vomiting and heavy albuminuria are all signs of grave prognosis.

Death in diphtheria in the first week is due either to circulatory failure or to laryngeal obstruction. Myocarditis is particularly likely to prove fatal during the second and third weeks, respiratory failure being responsible for most deaths thereafter. The majority of patients can be considered to be out of danger in seven weeks although in the worst cases death may take place as late as ten weeks from the onset from a combination of respiratory and cardiac failure. The outlook is always grave in infants under a year and the mortality is higher in children under five years than in those over that age. However severe the attack, survival is almost invariably followed by complete recovery without sequelae, although in the severe case this may take up to six months.

Active immunization usually prevents or modifies diphtheria, but severe or fatal attacks may occur.

REFERENCES

Galbraith, N. S., Barnes, J. M., and O'Moore, G. R. (1967) Simultaneous primary immunisation against tetanus and reinforcement of diphtheria immunity in children, *Mth. Bull. Minist. Hlth Lab. Serv.*, **26**, 172.

GROARKE, F. L., ADAMSON, M. I., ELIAS-JONES, T. F., and WHITTAKER, L. (1960) An outbreak of diphtheria: epidemiological aspects, *Brit. med. J.*, **1,** 1607.
KEHR, M. J., TANNAHILL, R. W., ELIAS-JONES, T. F., and WHITTAKER, L. (1960) Observations on a present day outbreak of diphtheria, *Publ. Hlth* (*Lond.*), **74,** 294.

G. D. W. MCKENDRICK

LISTERIA INFECTION

BACTERIOLOGY

Listeria monocytogenes is a Gram-positive non-sporing, motile bacillus which is aerobic or micro-aerophilic. It often occurs in pairs with the two rods disposed end to end at an acute angle. Morphologically it is easily confused with diphtheroids and this mistake, which has frequently been made, suggests that the rarity of human infection is more apparent than real.

EPIDEMIOLOGY

The organism was originally isolated from rabbits and guinea-pigs during a laboratory epizootic in Cambridge. It has since proved to be a common infection in a wide range of animals, including horses foxes, dogs, pigs, mice, rats, birds and recently, chinchillas imported into this country. In farm animals it causes a meningo-encephalitis; intra-uterine foetal infection with abortion occurs in sheep and cattle; in rodents and poultry the usual finding is focal granulomatous necrosis of the liver and myocardium.

The organism has a world-wide distribution, but infection is naturally enough commoner in rural areas than in towns. Outbreaks are uncommon and in animals and man cases are usually sporadic.

HUMAN INFECTION

Listeriosis is commoner in infancy than at other periods, and the only syndrome it causes associated with a characteristic clinical picture is miliary granulomatosis or granulomatosis infantiseptica, which results from intra-uterine infection of the foetus. Often the mother has a mild febrile illness 3 or 4 weeks before confinement; sometimes she has a rigor. Delivery is often premature and about one-third of the infants are stillborn, others die within minutes of birth and a few survive for 2 or 3 weeks. The striking features are dyspnoea with intense cyanosis; diarrhoea is the rule; the spleen and liver are usually enlarged. Small, dark red granulomata are to be found on the posterior pharyngeal wall. Most infants die with circulatory failure, but in some meningitis develops. Post-mortem examination reveals disseminated miliary nodules of necrotic granulomatous tissue.

The other manifestations of *L. monocytogenes* infection are less specific. In children a septicaemic type often terminating in meningitis is common, and indeed, meningitis is the commonest clinical expression of this disease. An oculoglandular form has been described in adults and occasionally an anginose variety associated with lymphadenitis. Pneumonia and empyema of the pleura may result from septicaemia. *L. monocytogenes* has been recovered from the genital tract in women and is said to be a cause of urethritis in men; transmission is assumed to be venereal. Like most micro-organisms it has been the cause of subacute bacterial endocarditis.

Recently it has been recognized that listeriosis is liable to complicate the later stages of malignant disease, and this is particularly true of lymphoreticular neoplasms. In this connexion it ranks as one of the 'opportunist' infections.

Diagnosis

Early diagnosis is essential if any of the infants with miliary granulomatosis are to be rescued. Isolation of the organism is the essential step. Examination of the meconium is the most certain and rapid method, but cultures of blood, urine and where appropriate, of cerebrospinal fluid should be made.

The blood commonly shows a neutrophil leucocytosis and increase in monocytes is exceptional. There is no evidence that this organism can cause glandular fever.

Treatment

L. monocytogenes is susceptible to most antibiotics; penicillin is the drug of choice.

Prognosis

Listeria infection of the newborn is almost inevitably fatal unless treatment is early and energetic. Untreated meningitis is said to carry a mortality of 70 per cent. The oculoglandular and anginose varieties in adults have a favourable outlook, but unless treated, meningitis may supervene.

REFERENCES

DEGEN, R. (1967) Die Neugeborenen-Listerioise und ihr Thoraxröntgen Bild, *Münch. med. Wschr.*, **109,** 79.
GUIN, G. H., GENDELMAN, S., and STEVENS, H. (1965) Listeriosis of the central nervous system: four affected infants, *Clin. Pediat.* (*Phila.*), **4,** 258.
HOEPRICH, P. D. (1958) Infections due to Listeria monocytogenes, *Medicine* (*Baltimore*), **37,** 143.
LOURIA, D. B., HENSLE, T., ARMSTRONG, D., COLLINS, H. S., BLEVINS, A., KRUGMAN, D., and BUSE, M. (1967) Listeriosis complicating malignant disease: a new association, *Ann. intern. Med.*, **67,** 261.
SEELIGER, H. P. R. (1961) *Listeriosis*, New York.

R. BODLEY SCOTT

ERYSIPELOID

Synonym. Erysipeloid of Rosenbach.

Definition

An infection of the cellular tissues of the fingers or hands with the organisms of swine erysipelas, *Erysipelothrix rhusiopathiae*, resulting from injury to the skin arising from the handling of animal or vegetable matter.

Clinical Picture

This is essentially a disease of food handlers and

manipulators. It starts as an erysipelas-like swelling on a finger or the hand. The swelling advances with an easily visible border and may travel up one finger on to the hand and down the adjoining finger. Constitutional disturbance is slight. If untreated, the condition persists for several weeks.

Erysipeloid spreading to a diffuse generalized involvement of the skin is rare. It may be accompanied by fever and arthritis. Still rarer is the septicaemic form in which purpura, joint pains and endocarditis may develop, sometimes with a fatal outcome.

Treatment

It quickly responds to intramuscular injections of penicillin.

REFERENCE

PRICE, J. E. L., and BENNETT, W. E. J. (1951) The erysipeloid of Rosenbach, *Brit. med. J.*, **2**, 1060.

BRIAN F. RUSSELL

INFECTIONS DUE TO BACILLACEAE

ANTHRAX

Synonyms. Wool-sorters' disease; Splenic fever; Siberian plague; Malignant pustule; Charbon.

Definition

Anthrax is an acute infectious disease characterized most commonly by a local skin lesion (malignant pustule). Highly fatal septicaemic, pulmonary and intestinal infections also occur.

Aetiology and Epidemiology

The causative organism, *Bacillus anthracis*, is a large Gram-positive capsulated bacillus which develops a characteristic filamentous appearance when cultured on artificial media. Spores are not found in animal or human tissues, only developing when the organisms come into contact with oxygen. They are extremely resistant to destruction.

Anthrax is primarily a disease of herbivorous animals, particularly sheep, cattle, horses and goats. It is endemic in all parts of the world. Animals become infected from the ingestion or inhalation of spore contaminated food or water. Human infection has almost invariably an animal source although transmission from man to man can take place. In Great Britain most cases still arise from the handling of infected material imported from abroad in spite of the fact that legislation has eliminated the risk from shaving brushes and wool by insisting on sterilization. Pulmonary anthrax used to be a serious hazard among wool workers but this is now prevented by treating the raw wool before processing. Hides cannot be subjected to similar treatment without damage and therefore infection still arises in tanners. Anthrax is an occupational hazard of meat porters, butchers, farmers, veterinary surgeons and workers in the hair and tanning industries. Bone meal (used as a fertilizer) has caused infection. In the United States, imported goat hair, goatskin and carpet wool are the sources of most human infections.

Pathology

The essential local lesion is an acute inflammatory one in which oedema, coagulation-necrosis and haemorrhage are characteristic features. The altered blood is responsible for the black appearance of the local lesion. It is usually possible to isolate the organism from the oedema fluid surrounding the eschar which often has a gelatinous quality.

Symptoms

The incubation period is normally 1–3 days. There are three clinical forms of the disease of which the skin form is the most common.

Malignant Pustule. The site of the infection is an exposed part of the body, commonly the face, neck, forearm or back of the hands. A small red papule forms which rapidly becomes vesicular. This is surrounded by a zone of red non-pitting oedema which develops into a brawny induration by the third day. By this time, a ring of secondary vesicles, sometimes very small, often surrounds the initial lesion which soon becomes covered by a dry almost black scab or eschar. There may be associated lymphangitis with some tender swelling of the appropriate lymph nodes but the lack of pain and tenderness of the primary lesion is often striking. In the early stages, constitutional symptoms are mild and fever slight, but toxaemia appears suddenly as septicaemia develops. A malignant pustule heals with residual scarring in 10 days–4 weeks.

Pulmonary Anthrax (Wool-Sorters' Disease). In this variety of the disease bacilli are inhaled from infected hair or wool. A fulminating pneumonia develops rapidly with cough, dyspnoea and haemoptysis, death occurring within 1–4 days of the onset.

Intestinal Anthrax. This is very rare and is due to eating meat or drinking milk from an infected animal or possibly to eating food contaminated by spores. The symptoms are those of a severe gastro-enteritis. Although serious, it is not, like pulmonary anthrax, invariably fatal.

Diagnosis

In the severe forms the diagnosis is often not suspected until after death. The relative lack of pain in the lesion associated with marked induration and the central black eschar are the characteristics of the malignant pustule. Confirmation comes from culture of the organisms from the haemorrhagic fluid on the edge of the scab but minimal manipulation of the lesion is essential to avoid precipitating a septicaemia. The possibility of anthrax should be considered in the differential diagnosis of any 'blind boil' or in any relatively painless cellulitis occurring on an exposed area of skin, particularly if the patient's occupation leads him into contact with animals or animal products.

Treatment

The patient is nursed in isolation and all attendants should be masked and gloved. In Great Britain the disease is notifiable to the Medical Officer of Health and to the Chief Inspector of Factories. Antibiotics have replaced Sclavo's serum. The treatment of choice is a seven-day course of penicillin and streptomycin although good results have been claimed with the tetracyclines and with chloramphenicol. The malignant pustule is covered with a cold dressing and re-dressed infrequently.

Prophylaxis. Control of the disease in animals by active immunization together with prompt notification and the complete destruction of dead animals by burying them in quick lime will cut down the risk of human infection. Skins, carcasses, wool and similar potentially infected animal products are inspected and where possible disinfected at the port of entry. Increasing use is likely to be made of irradiation for killing anthrax spores in wool and skins. A vaccine has been used successfully in America to protect workers exposed to a definite risk.

Prognosis

Internal anthrax has a mortality of over 90 per cent. Antibiotics have almost eliminated the risk of septicaemia in cutaneous anthrax and death is now exceptional in this form. Recovery takes place in 1–4 weeks from the onset.

REFERENCES

GOLD, H. (1955) Anthrax: report of 117 cases, *Arch. intern. Med.*, **96,** 387.

MINISTRY OF LABOUR (1959) Report of the Committee of Inquiry on Anthrax, Cmd. No. 846, London, H.M.S.O.

TAYLOR, L., and CARSLAW, R. W. (1967) Cutaneous anthrax, *Lancet*, i, 1214.

G. D. W. MCKENDRICK

CLOSTRIDIAL INFECTIONS

Members of the genus *Clostridium* are large Gram-positive rods which are anaerobic or at most micro-aerophilic. All produce endospores; most are flagellated; a few form capsules. In culture they show a remarkable pleomorphism. The majority of the clostridia are soil saprophytes concerned with the active decomposition of organic matter. Those pathogenic to man produce exotoxins which are largely responsible for symptoms of infection. These species are:

1. *Cl. botulinum* is a non-invasive saprophyte which may grow in food-stuffs where it forms a potent exotoxin, responsible for the symptoms of botulism when contaminated food is eaten [p. 104].

2. *Cl. tetani* is only slightly invasive but its exotoxin is so potent that tetanus may result from the most trivial lodgement [p. 102].

3. *The gas-gangrene group* contains a large number of clostridia. The significance of some members as a cause of human gas gangrene is uncertain. The most important in this respect are *Cl. welchii* (*perfringens*), *Cl. oedematiens* and *Cl. septicum*. Less frequently *Cl. histolyticum* and *Cl. bifermentans* are responsible.

In many cases of gas gangrene several species of clostridium are present and it may be difficult to decide which is playing the leading part. The most frequent is undoubtedly *Cl. welchii* of which six types are recognized depending upon the toxins produced. Type A alone gives rise to gas gangrene in man. Type F has been identified as the cause of necrotizing enteritis. Type A forms a number of toxins of which alpha-toxin, a lecithinase, is responsible for many of its effects. *Cl. oedematiens* type A, *Cl. septicum*, *Cl. haemolyticum* and *Cl. bifermentans* also elaborate alpha-toxins which apart from that of the last are immunologically distinct from the alpha-toxin of *Cl. welchii.*

GAS GANGRENE

Clostridial finection is seen most often in wartime when wounds become contaminated with soil. In civilian life perhaps the most common site of infection is the uterus, when it is usually the consequence of criminal abortion. It is seen from time to time after amputation through the upper third of the thigh.

It has been estimated that clostridia can be recovered from some 30 per cent. of war wounds. Usually there is little more than surface contamination and because the organisms are strict anaerobes active multiplication does not occur. In some instances invasion of fascial planes takes place with the appearance of 'anaerobic cellulitis'. This is usually a mild self-limiting infection with moderate toxaemia. Gas gangrene supervenes in less than 5 per cent. of wounds contaminated with clostridia. Gas gangrene is liable to develop in deep, heavily contaminated wounds involving muscle with retained foreign bodies or necrotic tissue. Such conditions reduce the oxygen tension of the tissues and this effect may be heightened by ischaemia until the anaerobic clostridia are able to multiply. Directly this process starts toxins are formed and seep into the surrounding tissues. Alpha-toxin will cause necrosis of muscle by disrupting the lecithin of the cell envelope; collagenases and hyaluronidases facilitate extension by destroying the connective tissue scaffolding: and the invasion spreads with gathering speed through the muscle.

Symptoms

There is an incubation period varying from 9–48 hours with *Cl. welchii* and up to 5 days with *Cl. oedematiens* before the patient begins to complain that the wound is becoming increasingly painful. Within a few hours deterioration in his general condition becomes evident; fever is not a striking feature, but tachycardia and a falling blood pressure give warning of peripheral circulatory failure which may progress rapidly. Anuric renal failure may develop and it has been suggested that the mechanism here is similar to that of 'crush syndrome'. Meanwhile the serous discharge from the wound increases and becomes especially voluminous with *Cl. oedematiens* infection. The foul odour of the discharge is due to other associated anaerobic organisms. The surrounding skin, at first tense and pallid from oedema of the underlying muscle, later becomes dusky and finally covered with bullae containing bloody fluid. Crepitation in the affected muscle is often late and seldom as dramatic as the name, gas gangrene, implies.

General intoxication becomes profound as the necrotizing myositis advances. In fatal cases death occurs after a period of stupor or coma.

Uterine infections show the same sequence of events, but are frequently associated with septicaemia. In many instances, presumably as a result of alpha-toxin activity, this is accompanied by fulminating intravascular haemolysis with haemoglobinuria and anuric renal failure.

Diagnosis

Clostridia may be recovered from wounds without gas gangrene being present and gas formation may occur in some infections with Gram-negative bacilli. The diagnosis is therefore a clinical one based on the characteristic physical signs. Sometimes radiography may help by showing bubbles of gas in the suspected muscle. In the presence of such signs the demonstration in discharges from the wound or uterus of large numbers of Gram-positive bacilli with the morphological characteristics of clostridia, establishes the diagnosis. When doubt exists it is valuable to know the species and type of the clostridia isolated.

Prevention

The prevention of gas gangrene lies in the adequate surgical toilet of wounds likely to be contaminated and the avoidance of measures liable to cause ischaemia. Antitoxin is often given as a prophylactic. The recommended dose is 9000 Units of *Cl. welchii*, 4500 of *Cl. septicum* and 3000 of *Cl. oedematiens* alpha antitoxins; its value is uncertain. There is as yet insufficient information on the benefit of active immunization in man, but in domestic animals it seems established.

Treatment

Treatment of gas gangrene is essentially surgical, consisting of incision, drainage and even amputation, as indicated by the local situation.

Antibiotics are of great value. For an established case penicillin G should be given in massive doses, 1 mega Unit (0·6 G.) 2-hourly. It should also be given prophylactically to patients undergoing high amputation through the thigh because of ischaemia.

Antisera are of dubious value. The doses recommended are 25,000 Units of *Cl. welchii*, 12,500 Units of *Cl. septicum* and 10,000 Units of *Cl. oedematiens* alpha antitoxins every 4–6 hours. Before they are given the not inconsiderable risk of anaphylactic shock should be considered.

Hyperbaric oxygen therapy has been advocated in the treatment of gas gangrene, but its value is not yet established.

REFERENCES

GARROD, L. P. (1958) The chemoprophylaxis of gas gangrene, *J. roy. Army med. Cp.*, **104**, 209.

MACLENNAN, J. D. (1962) The histotoxic clostridial infections of man, *Bact. Rev.*, **26**, 177.

CLOSTRIDIAL ENTERITIS

Cl. welchii can cause an enteritis or gastro-enteritis by multiplying in food which it has contaminated. This is a mild type of food poisoning due to an aberrant Type A, which is markedly resistant to heat and survives boiling for 1–4 hours. The clinical picture is one of abdominal pain and diarrhoea with an onset some 8–24 hours after the offending meal. Vomiting is unusual.

The more severe form known as *enteritis necroticans* came to light during the war years and immediately after the Second World War, when a number of cases were reported from Germany. In this condition there is gangrene of a segment of small bowel, usually in the jejunum.

The cause is food contaminated with *Cl. welchii* Type F which produces little alpha-toxin, but large amounts of beta-toxin, which has lethal and necrotizing activity. It is of interest that Types B and C, although not pathogenic to man, produce much beta-toxin, and cause acute enteritis in various domestic animals.

The clinical picture of enteritis necroticans is not specific. There is an acute onset of central abdominal pain and tenderness with diarrhoea and collapse. Mortality is high and the diagnosis is often made *post mortem*. The value of antiserum is not established. Surgical resection appears to give the best chance of recovery.

REFERENCES

PARRY, W. H. (1963) Outbreak of *Clostridium welchii* food poisoning, *Brit. med. J.*, **2**, 1616.

PARRY, W. H. (1966) The epidemiology of *Clostridium welchii* food poisoning, *Publ. Hlth Rep.* (*Wash.*), **81**, 22.

R. BODLEY SCOTT

TETANUS

Synonym. Lockjaw.

Definition

An infectious disease due to the toxin of *Clostridium tetani* in which paroxysms of muscle spasm are superimposed on a generalized tonic rigidity, the latter most consistently affecting the masseters and trunk musculature.

Aetiology and Epidemiology

The bacillus of tetanus is a slender, spore bearing anaerobic rod, the spores forming at the end of the organism giving it a characteristic drumstick appearance. Spores are highly resistant to destruction by heat or antiseptics and can remain dormant in tissues for months until conditions become suitable for germination. They are present in human and animal faeces and are widely distributed in dust and soil, particularly in highly manured ground. In spite of this the disease is relatively rare in the United Kingdom.

Tetanus follows injury in the great majority of cases.

Puncture wounds, for example, by a nail or rose thorn, are more favourable for the germination of spores than are superficial scratches. Tissue necrosis provides a suitable culture medium for the bacilli so that severe injury, especially one in which clothing or other debris enters the wound increases the risk of tetanus. The disease is thus a particular hazard of wartime and to a lesser extent to farm workers and gardeners. Outbreaks have also occurred in hospitals from contamination of gauze, grey wool, catgut and other surgical materials.

Tetanus is most common in the tropics. Tetanus neonatorum, a highly fatal form of the disease arising from umbilical sepsis, is limited to tropical countries.

Pathology

Although tetanus is almost invariably caused by the introduction of the organism through the skin, the wound may be too small to be detected. Infection through the bronchial or intestinal mucosae has been postulated. The presence of pyogenic cocci in a tetanus contaminated wound increases the risk of clinical tetanus developing by causing increased tissue destruction.

Cl. tetani produces an extremely powerful exotoxin which has an affinity for nerve tissue. A fatal dose is too small to be antigenically active and therefore no immunity follows an attack. The toxin travels along peripheral nerves to the central nervous system and also in the blood stream. Tonic rigidity is thought to be due to the action of the toxin on the neuromuscular end plates, this hypothesis explaining the early rigidity which sometimes develops near a wound. Reflex spasms, on the other hand, are caused by the toxin increasing the excitability of the anterior horn cells in the spinal cord. Once the toxin is fixed in nerve cells it can no longer be neutralized by antitoxin.

There are no specific autopsy changes of tetanus. Secondary effects include pneumonia, myocarditis and vertebral fractures.

Symptoms

The incubation period is commonly 2–21 days. The length of the incubation period is of considerable significance in prognosis and its evaluation, therefore, is important in a particular case. A short incubation period can be accepted as a true one; one can assume in such a case that the organisms started to multiply immediately after entry. In general, the longer the incubation period, the better the prognosis, but severe and fatal attacks may follow an apparent long incubation period—even one up to a hundred days. In such cases, the true incubation period, that is to say, the time from the moment the organisms started to multiply to the onset of symptoms, is probably short although this cannot be determined. This is the likely explanation of fatal cases of tetanus in which the first symptoms appear three weeks or more after the organism has gained entry. In such a case, the spores remain dormant until tissue destruction, sepsis, surgical manipulation or other factors change the environment into one suitable for their germination.

Most cases of tetanus pass through three stages; prodromal stage; stage of tonic rigidity; stage of reflex convulsions.

Prodromal symptoms of fleeting back pain and a general feeling that all is not well often precede muscle spasm by 24 hours. The patient not infrequently has a little difficulty in swallowing at this stage and this may lead him to complain, misleadingly, of sore throat. The difficulty in swallowing increases as the disease progresses.

Trismus (painless spasm of the masseters) is the first indication of *tonic rigidity* and may be the first symptom. Beginning as a slight stiffness in the jaw it may increase until the teeth are firmly clenched and the mouth cannot be opened at all. Measurement of the dental gap (the distance between the incisors) is a useful guide to progress. Involvement of the facial muscles leads to the production of a *risus sardonicus*, the mirthless grin caused by retraction of the angles of the mouth. At the same time the abdominal recti become stiff, the spasm steadily increasing to produce a board-like, but painless rigidity. This increase of tone in the abdominal wall musculature is of great help in differentiating trismus due to tetanus from that due to local causes. As tonic rigidity increases, head retraction and opisthotonus appear, the rigidity reaching its maximum in a severe case in 48 hours. In a mild attack it may take up to seven days to develop. All movements become slow and difficult, including breathing and swallowing. The patient may complain of a tight chest. In a developed case the mirthless grin associated with narrowing of the palpebral fissures and head retraction combine to give a striking and diagnostic appearance. The alteration of the voice due to speaking through clenched teeth with limited palatal movement is also typical.

Tonic rigidity is much less marked in the limbs than in the trunk. In some cases, however, *local rigidity* develops around the site of the wound. This may be severe and may precede trismus by a few days. When this occurs the ultimate attack is usually mild. Local rigidity in a limb can be of help in deciding if a minor wound of doubtful significance is indeed the site of entry.

Reflex spasms (convulsions), due to increased central excitability of nerve cells appear within a few hours of the tonic rigidity in the severe case or may be delayed for up to five days. In mild cases no spasms occur. The time interval between the onset of trismus and the onset of generalized spasms is known as the 'period of onset'. This is of great prognostic importance. Spasms may be spontaneous or precipitated by extraneous stimuli such as noise or nursing attention. At the onset they are usually brief but they increase in severity and duration as well as in frequency as the disease develops. Occasionally the first spasm is severe and may even prove fatal. As a rule convulsions worsen for up to a week and persist for up to 2–3 weeks or occasionally longer. They become intensely painful and are dreaded by the patient. There is a sudden increase of muscle tone with clenching of the jaw, increase in head retraction and opisthotonus combined with extension of the limbs. A severe spasm stops respiration and may cause laryngeal obstruction. The patient becomes deeply cyanosed. Any severe spasm may prove fatal within two to three minutes. In addition to generalized spasms minor twitchings of individual parts are not uncommon. Occasionally laryngeal spasms, severe enough to threaten life, occur without widespread convulsions.

The tendon reflexes in tetanus are usually exaggerated. The disease is essentially afebrile, apart from a terminal hyperpyrexia which is common in fatal cases, although any patient may show a mild rise of temperature of 99° F. (37·3° C.). A more marked degree of fever usually indicates secondary infection such as pneumonia. The mind remains clear. The cerebrospinal fluid is normal.

The course of tetanus is variable. In the most severe cases the first paroxysm may prove fatal, death taking place on the second or third day. Tonic rigidity in severe cases may persist for up to three months. In more moderate attacks reflex spasms persist for 7–10 days, to be followed by a gradual lessening of tonic rigidity until complete recovery some six weeks later.

Complications

The most important are respiratory. The great majority of deaths are due to asphyxia or to collapse-pneumonia secondary to respiratory obstruction, inefficient coughing or dysphagia. Underventilation may be insidious, in which case it is due to tonic chest wall rigidity, or acute either as a result of respiratory arrest or laryngeal spasm during a convulsion. Retention of urine and obstinate constipation are common. Severe spasms may cause laceration of the tongue or compression fractures of vertebrae. Myocarditis may occur.

Diagnosis

The combination of trismus and painless abdominal rigidity in an alert afebrile patient is diagnostic of tetanus. Most local causes of trismus, of which *quinsy* and *dental abscess* are the commonest, are painful and cause fever. Although a proper examination of the mouth may be impossible in such cases there is usually other evidence of local sepsis such as tender and enlarged cervical glands. The neck and back stiffness of tetanus may suggest *meningitis* but headache, vomiting and fever are absent in this disease. Trismus is sometimes seen in *poliomyelitis*. The abnormal cerebrospinal fluid and the later development of facial paralysis serve to differentiate. *Mumps* may cause trismus.

The spasms of *strychnine poisoning* resemble tetanus but there is no tonic rigidity from strychnine, the muscles becoming quite flaccid between the spasms. Board-like abdominal rigidity may suggest peritonitis but this is excluded by the lack of associated symptoms and signs.

Treatment

General. The patient is nursed in a darkened room under conditions of quiet with the minimum of interference. Oral feeding is carried out as long as possible but feeding frequently has to be continued by a nasal gastric tube owing to difficulty in swallowing. A high calorie diet is given. Urinary retention requires catheterization.

Many sedatives have been used in tetanus and in mild cases the choice is of little importance provided that over-sedation is avoided. A satisfactory combination is chlorpromazine, 50 mg., and phenobarbitone, 100 mg., four to eight hourly. Chlorpromazine is particularly valuable as it lessens tonic rigidity in addition to its central sedative action. It is often used in combination with promethazine, 50 mg. of each drug being given four to eight hourly but this combination of drugs should be avoided if there is any tendency to hypotension. When severe spasms are easily provoked, thiopentone, 2–4 ml. intravenously, is given before any major nursing procedure such as catheterization.

Wherever a patient with tetanus is nursed facilities must be immediately available at the bedside for the administration of Suxamethonium Chloride Injection, B.P., 50 mg. intravenously, intubation and artificial respiration during any life-threatening spasm. A gag is necessary to prevent damage to the tongue.

Complete relaxation with tubocurarine combined with tracheostomy and intermittent positive pressure respiration have revolutionized the treatment of severe tetanus. The indications for instituting this regime are:

1. The appearance of major convulsions within 24 hours of the onset of trismus.
2. Spasms severe enough to produce cyanosis.
3. Tonic rigidity of sufficient severity to produce hypercapnoea.
4. Aspiration pneumonia.
5. Inability to swallow.

Tubocurarine is given in 15 mg. doses in hyaluronidase intramuscularly as often as necessary to prevent convulsions and to lessen tonic rigidity sufficiently to allow adequate ventilation. Sedatives are continued in smaller doses. The patient is treated on a similar regime to that used for bulbospinal respiratory poliomyelitis with regular position changes and chest physiotherapy. In the severest cases, complete relaxation may be necessary for over three weeks. On this regime many recoveries have taken place among patients whose prognosis would previously have been regarded as hopeless.

Specific. 50,000 Units of antitetanic serum (A.T.S.) are given intramuscularly half an hour after a test dose. If there is no reaction to this large intramuscular dose within half to one hour, a further 50,000 Units are given slowly, intravenously. Débridement or excision of the wound, if any, is essential. It should be delayed until serum has been given. Penicillin is indicated routinely. As no immunity results from an attack of tetanus, patients should receive active immunization during convalescence.

Prophylaxis

Active immunity with tetanus toxoid requires three doses of toxoid. It is preferably included in immunization schedules of infants as a triple antigen with pertussis and diphtheria. The primary course requires two injections with a one month interval between them, the third following about six months later.

The Tetanus-prone Injury. Any deep or punctured wound, any wound possibly contaminated by soil, any infected wound and any wound associated with devitalization of tissue must be regarded as possibly contaminated with tetanus bacilli. The wound must be excised, penicillin given intramuscularly, and 1 ml. of adsorbed toxoid administered. The use of A.T.S. is no longer regarded as mandatory. If the risk of tetanus is considered great and the patient has never received active immunization in the past, 1500–5000 Units A.T.S. should be used—given in the opposite arm to the toxoid. Arrangements should be made for such persons to complete active immunization later.

Prognosis

The use of relaxants and intermittent positive-pressure respiration has reduced the mortality in neonates from 80 per cent. to about 40 per cent. and in older children and adults from about 50 per cent. to 20 per cent. The outlook in older children and adults is related to the incubation period, the period of onset and the method of treatment. Before the use of relaxants and artificial respiration, death was usual with an incubation period of less than seven days and a period of onset of under 48 hours, but many such patients now survive. A period of onset of over three days carries a good prognosis. The longer the patient survives, the better the outlook. Ultimate recovery is complete.

REFERENCES

Adams, E. B., Holloway, R., Thambiran, A. K., and Desai, S. D. (1966) Usefulness of intermittent positive-pressure respiration in the treatment of tetanus, *Lancet*, ii, 1176.

Adams, E. B., Wright, R., Berman, E., and Laurence, D. R. (1959) Treatment of tetanus with chlorpromazine and barbiturates, *Lancet*, i, 755.

Cox, C. A., Knowelden, J., and Sharrard, W. J. W. (1963) Tetanus prophylaxis, *Brit. med. J.*, **2,** 1360.

Kloetzel, K. (1963) Clinical patterns in severe tetanus, *J. Amer. med. Ass.*, **185,** 559.

Purkis, I. E., and Curtis, J. E. (1965) Severe tetanus: its complications and management, *Canad. med. Ass. J.*, **93,** 1200.

BOTULISM

Definition

Botulism is a rare and frequently fatal form of food poisoning in which a pre-formed bacterial exotoxin causes widespread paralysis.

Aetiology

The causative organism is *Clostridium botulinum*, an anaerobic spore-forming Gram-positive bacillus. Human disease is caused by one of three different types A, B and E which have distinct toxins. The organisms are found in the soil and also occasionally in the faeces of animals, including man. In view of its widespread occurrence in virgin and manured soils the rarity of the disease may appear surprising. However, the clostridia can only multiply under strictly anaerobic conditions and unlike other forms of food poisoning their growth causes a change in the taste of food which develops a characteristic sour odour. Canned and bottled foods, particularly when the processing has been carried out in the home, have been responsible for most outbreaks. The exotoxin of *Cl. botulinum* is the most powerful poison known: it has been estimated that 1 g. would be sufficient to kill many millions of people. The toxin is absorbed from the intestinal tract and acts on the nervous system. Although the clostridial spores may survive boiling for over four hours the toxin is destroyed by heat. Hence, food containing toxin can be rendered safe by re-cooking. In the Loch Maree disaster of 1922 all eight members of a fishing party died after eating sandwiches containing duck paste. Since then there have been only seven cases of botulism recognized in Great Britain.

Symptoms

Symptoms appear 2–36 hours after the ingestion of the toxin, change of voice such as hoarseness often being the first sign. This, however, may be preceded by vomiting. Diarrhoea is unusual. Giddiness, unsteadiness on standing and diplopia are the initial complaints, paralysis of other cranial nerves rapidly following with the development of squints and difficulty in talking and swallowing owing to paralysis of the tongue and pharynx. The abdomen is distended but free from pain. Paralysis spreads to the trunk and limbs and death follows from respiratory failure. There are no sensory changes and consciousness is retained till the end.

The mortality rate has varied from 70 to 100 per cent. in different outbreaks. Death may occur within three hours of ingesting the toxin but is more usually delayed till the third day.

Treatment

Polyvalent (type A and B) antitoxin is available in different centres in Great Britain; 50,000 Units should be given slowly intravenously daily. On theoretical grounds tracheostomy and intermittent positive pressure respiration offer hope of survival. On analogy with tetanus complete recovery would appear to be possible if the patient could be kept alive during the paralytic stage.

REFERENCES

Brocklehurst, J. C. (1957) Fatal outbreak of botulism among Labrador Eskimos, *Brit. med. J.*, **2,** 924.

Koenig, M. G., Spickard, A., Cardella, M. A., and Rogers, D. E. (1964) Clinical and laboratory observations on Type E botulism in man, *Medicine* (*Baltimore*), **43,** 517.

G. D. W. McKendrick

INFECTIONS DUE TO MYCOBACTERIACEAE

The genus *Mycobacterium* contains many organisms pathogenic to man and animals as well as many non-pathogenic species. All those responsible for progressive disease share the quality of staining with difficulty, but of resisting decolorization by strong acids. The human pathogens are *Mycobacterium tuberculosis*, *Mycobacterium leprae*, *Mycobacterium ulcerans*, *Mycobacterium balnei* and a number of strains sometimes described as 'atypical' or 'anonymous'. Those which cause disease in animals include *the murine strain of tuberculosis* (the vole bacillus) and *Mycobacterium paratuberculosis* (Johne's bacillus). Familiar non-pathogenic species are *Mycobacterium smegmatis* (the smega bacillus) and *Mycobacterium phlei* (the Timothy grass bacillus).

TUBERCULOSIS

MYCOBACTERIUM TUBERCULOSIS

In the lesions it causes in the tissues, *M. tuberculosis* appears in the form of straight or curved slender rods with parallel sides: it is often found in groups. It will not stain by Gram's method, but with difficulty takes up carbol fuchsin and other dyes; once stained it resists decolorization by acids and alcohol (Ziehl-Neelsen's stain).

M. tuberculosis is an aerobe, but grows more slowly than most bacteria and demands special media. In culture it shows great variation in morphology and in fluid media virulent strains arrange themselves in microscopic serpentine cords. The organism loses its virulence and its capacity to form cords on repeated subculture.

The tubercle bacillus is susceptible to desiccation, heat and other physical agents, but will resist some of the common antiseptics, possibly because of the hydrophobic characters of the bacterial wall. It can survive for long periods in dust and dried sputum.

Five 'typical' varieties of *M. tuberculosis* exist, the human, the bovine, the piscine, the murine and the avian. The last is pathogenic for man only very rarely, although a few proven cases of human infection have been recorded.

It is usually possible to distinguish the human and bovine types by their cultural characteristics on solid egg media. The first grows luxuriantly in rough colonies and is described as 'eugonic'; the second is 'dysgonic' growing slowly in smooth colonies. These features are not invariable and may be lost on subculture. Virulence tests may be required for certain distinction: the human bacillus is pathogenic for the guinea-pig but virtually non-pathogenic for the rabbit, while the bovine type causes progressive disease in both animals.

The chemical composition of *M. tuberculosis* has been the subject of much inquiry. It varies qualitatively and quantitatively in different cultures depending in part on the media used. Several protein fractions have been extracted and all obtained from any one strain can elicit a positive skin test in animals infected with that strain. Human and bovine strains cannot be distinguished by skin tests. At least two polysaccharides have been isolated which are serologically distinct: they are antigenic, but will not give positive skin tests. Mycobacteria are particularly rich in lipids: these substances resist destruction in the tissues and are thought to be responsible for some of the characteristic reactions evoked by the organism.

ATYPICAL MYCOBACTERIA

In recent years a number of strains spoken of 'atypical' have been isolated from patients with disease clinically indistinguishable from tuberculosis. In many these strains appear to be the undoubted cause of the disease. These organisms are not variants of recognized strains of *Mycobacterium* and thus some prefer to call them 'anonymous' rather than 'atypical'. Classification is still unsatisfactory. Four groups are generally recognized:

Group I. The photochromogens which form pigment in culture only after exposure to visible light.

Group II. The scotochromogens which form pigment on culture in the dark.

Group III. A heterogeneous collection of non-chromogenic strains, sometimes known as the Battey group.

Group IV. The 'rapid growers'.

Mycobacterium kansasii is probably the best known representative of Group I and *Mycobacterium fortuitum* of Group III. Other more elaborate classifications recognize as many as seven groups.

These mycobacteria sometimes appear to be non-pathogenic saprophytes, but are at other times undoubtedly the cause of disease. In one series of 2,916 strains of mycobacteria isolated from sputum 71 (2·5 per cent.) were placed in the anonymous categories. Of these 40 were regarded as associated with active pulmonary disease of which 27 belonged to Group I. Other figures show that anonymous mycobacteria are isolated from between 0·7 and 4·0 per cent. of patients considered clinically to have pulmonary tuberculosis: the vast majority fall into Groups I and III.

Cervical lymphadenitis in children is not infrequently due to Group III strains and occasionally to scotochromogens. Bone lesions have been described and occasional cases of disseminated infection by anonymous mycobacteria are on record. These last are of interest for they have usually been accompanied by blood changes suggesting aplastic anaemia.

There has been some argument over the question of nomenclature. It has been contended that the disease due to infection by anonymous mycobacteria should not be called tuberculosis and that 'mycobacteriosis' would be a more appropriate label. There is some immunological relationship between *M. tuberculosis* and anonymous mycobacteria of Groups I, II and III.

Infection with them may give a positive skin test to tuberculosis. Histologically the lesions in the lungs are indistinguishable from those of tuberculosis although the pattern in lymphadenitis is less specific.

Infectivity seems to be less than that of 'typical' tuberculosis, but the 'anonymous' mycobacteria are far less susceptible to the antibiotics effective against the human and bovine strains. Such infections seem to occur more readily in lungs damaged by silicosis.

HUMAN TUBERCULOSIS

The principal strains responsible for human infections are the human and bovine types of *M. tuberculosis*. Infection with other varieties is rare and, with the exceptions mentioned in earlier paragraphs, unimportant. The human type is commonly found in pulmonary disease and the bovine in tuberculosis of lymph nodes, bones and joints. This difference is not due to any peculiarities of the two strains of mycobacteria, but springs from the fact that the human type is conveyed by inhaled droplets of infected sputum and the bovine by drinking infected milk.

Immunity

The immune mechanisms of tuberculosis differ from those of most bacterial infections. The importance of humoral antibodies is uncertain although their presence can be demonstrated by the usual methods. They exert little bactericidal effect on the bacilli.

The important feature is the alteration in tissue reactivity which occurs as a result of infection. This was established by Koch and the phenomenon bears his name. He showed that if virulent tubercle bacilli were injected subcutaneously into a healthy guinea-pig, the puncture wound healed in a day or two, but fourteen days later a nodule formed at the site of injection which later ulcerated. Subsequently the regional lymph nodes enlarged and caseated. The term 'caseation' is used to describe a form of necrosis characteristic of tuberculosis in which the affected tissue is converted into a homogeneous structureless material with the appearance and consistency of cheese. The process of autolysis is halted before the stage of liquefaction. If the injection was made into a guinea-pig previously infected with tuberculosis the sequence of events would be quite different. Within two days induration would appear at the site of injection to be rapidly followed by ulceration. No enlargement of regional lymph nodes would take place and the ulcer would usually heal rapidly.

The tissues had acquired hypersentitivity, leading to an acute exudative response but localizing the infection. A similar result can be achieved by sensitizing the animal with an injection of killed bacilli. An important difference between the responses is that in the sensitized animal, lymphatic dissemination occurs less readily and the bacilli are fixed locally.

It has been much debated whether the allergic response to a second infection serves any useful purpose. It is naïve to regard it in simple teleological terms as necessarily a mechanism to help preserve the host. There are clearly occasions when it works to his advantage but equally obviously occasions on which it is harmful. There is evidence which suggests that resistance is not dependent on hypersensitivity, for desensitization does not decrease it. Nevertheless it is impossible to induce resistance without at the same time causing hypersensitivity.

Pathogenesis

The interrelations of infecting organism and host are more complex in tuberculosis than in any other infection, largely because the tissue reactions are modified by the development of hypersensitivity to the invading bacilli.

The changes in the tissues are of two kinds, exudative and proliferative. They are best followed in the lung of the experimental animal. In the earliest stage a fluid exudate is seen to surround the infecting organisms; in it are a few neutrophils some of which may contain bacilli. The exudate diminishes, most of the neutrophils perish and phagocytic monocytes appear which engulf the dead leucocytes and the bacilli. This lesion may be microscopic or it may affect an entire lobe depending on the dose of bacilli and the susceptibility of the host. If there has been previous tuberculous infection with resulting hypersensitivity the exudative response is great; if the animal is not hypersensitive it is only moderate. There are three possible sequels. First, there may be complete resolution and restoration of the *status quo ante*: this is likely when the infecting dose is small and resistance is high. Secondly, when the infecting dose is great and hypersensitivity well developed, necrosis and sloughing may result with the formation of a cavity. Thirdly, a proliferative or productive lesion may develop. In this case, the monocytes are followed by epithelioid cells with pale cytoplasm and vesicular nuclei which arrange themselves radially. After two or three weeks fibroblasts, lymphocytes and plasma cells dispose themselves around the circumference of the lesions while in the centre one or more giant cells appear. These may exceed 100 μ in diameter and they contain many dark-staining nuclei ranged round their periphery. This lesion now constitutes the microscopic tubercle, the hallmark of tuberculous infection.

Further growth is by extension or by fusion with neighbouring lesions until a macroscopic tubercle is formed. Its subsequent fate depends on factors not understood. The centre undergoes caseation necrosis when it follows one of three courses. It may rupture into one of the air passages, discharge its contents and leave a cavity; it may become encircled by fibrous tissue and undergo healing with calcification; or it may remain dormant, containing virulent mycobacteria and be stirred to renewed activity years later.

Primary infection in man is commonly pulmonary and the sequence of events has been most fully studied in the lungs. Bacilli, usually contained in droplets of infected sputum, are inhaled and carried to the periphery. A parenchymal lesion develops which may be trivial and cause no symptoms or may be of massive exudative type. Infected material usually passes by the lymphatic vessels to the regional hilar nodes where further lesions appear. In most cases primary tuberculous infection heals rapidly, having passed unrecognized, and leaves a small area of calcification at the periphery of one lung with a similar lesion in the related lymph node. Occasionally it gives rise to progressive exudative disease. The initial parenchymal lesion is called a Ghon's focus and it, together with the infected hilar lymph nodes constitute the primary or Ghon's complex.

Less commonly the primary infection is in the tonsil or the intestine with lymphadenitis in the cervical or mesenteric nodes. This occurs when organisms are swallowed, usually in infected milk.

Once the primary lesion has healed the patient will have acquired hypersensitivity to tuberculoprotein and subsequent infection, which is often termed 'post-primary', will follow a course modified by this fact. Further lesions are due to reinfection from external sources or possibly by the bacilli escaping from lesions within the body. The process tends to be productive, it is usually situated at the apex of a lobe, it shows little tendency to spontaneous healing, and does not spread to the regional lymph nodes. It commonly progresses to cavitation and further spread of the disease takes place by direct extension and by discharge of infective material into the air passages.

Spread of Infection in the Body

M. tuberculosis is an intracellular organism although it is capable of extracellular multiplication in pulmonary cavities and similar situations. Nevertheless its normal habitat limits its methods of spread. The first of these is by simple extension to contiguous structures. The second is by lymphatic dissemination: cells containing bacilli are carried by the lymphatic channels to regional lymph nodes which become the seat of active infection. Chains of lymph nodes may be affected in this fashion and material containing bacilli may enter the thoracic duct and thus the blood stream.

The third route of spread is by the blood stream itself. A caseous lymph node or other lesion ruptures into a vein discharging its content of bacilli into the circulation. This mechanism is responsible for miliary tuberculosis. Finally dissemination may occur by way of the bronchi, alimentary tract or urinary passages. In the first instance, the contents of the cavity may be aspirated into another part of the lung causing tuberculous bronchopneumonia. In the second, infected sputum may lead to laryngeal tuberculosis or be swallowed to cause tuberculous enteritis. In the third, discharges from tuberculosis of the kidney may infect the ureter and the bladder.

Incidence

Attention has already been drawn to the frequency with which primary tuberculosis is clinically silent; it follows from this observation that in tuberculosis the incidence of past infection, of morbidity and of mortality differ widely.

The frequency with which tuberculous infections occur can be judged by the presence of skin hypersensitivity to tuberculoprotein as shown by the Mantoux test [p. 109] and by post-mortem statistics. By both criteria infection becomes more frequent with increasing age. Post-mortem studies indicate that between the ages of 10 and 19 years evidence of past or present tuberculosis is found in 35 per cent. of examinations and over the age of 60 years the figure rises to 85 per cent. In this country a survey some years ago showed that in children aged 15 years, 53 per cent. of country dwellers and 38 per cent. of town dwellers gave positive reactions to tuberculin. The difference was attributed to the higher consumption in the country of unpasteurized milk. 66 per cent. of Army recruits aged 18–20 years were positive reactors. In a random sample of adult non-tuberculous hospital patients 12 per cent. were negative reactors. It seems certain, therefore, that between 80 and 90 per cent. of adults living in the British Isles will have acquired tuberculous infection before they die. These figures may well already require revision and it is clear that the age of primary infection is steadily rising.

The mortality from tuberculosis of all types has shown a tremendous decline which started about 1870, beginning even before the causative organism had been identified. In England and Wales the standardized mortality ratio for this infection for the quinquennium 1851–55 was 1502 and for 1960–64, 21. The fall has been greatly accelerated by the introduction of effective chemotherapy. In England and Wales in 1945, 23,468 persons died of tuberculosis, in 1967 the figure was 2,043. Expressed as deaths per 100,000 living the rates for these two years are 61·5 and 4·2 respectively.

Morbidity has shown a similar trend. The only measure by which this can be gauged is the number of notifications. The number of new cases notified in England and Wales was 52,110 in 1945 and 21,747 in 1962.

The age at which active pulmonary tuberculosis is most frequently recognized is showing a surprising change. For many years it was a disease of young women, but it is now elderly men who are the chief victims. The mortality rate per 100,000 living in England and Wales in 1967 was 0·7 for women aged 25–35 years, but 31 for men of 65–75 years.

Epidemiology

There are two reservoirs from which tuberculous infections spread. The patient with active pulmonary tuberculosis and the tuberculous dairy cow. From the first droplets containing mycobacteria are inhaled and give rise to pulmonary tuberculosis; from the second infection of the cervical or mesenteric nodes, perhaps with later tuberculosis of bones or joints arises. Other modes of transmission are rare. Occasionally a skin abrasion becomes infected and this was once a common occupational risk in butchers. Discharges from sinuses and contaminated excreta may exceptionally be the vehicles of infection and oral transmission has been recorded in infants.

Secondary factors have received much attention. The possibility of some genetic predilection to infection exists. It has been shown, for instance, that when one twin develops tuberculosis, infection of the other occurs in one of three cases when binovular and in three of four when uniovular. Many of the other factors which have been thought to increase the liability to tuberculosis are difficult to analyse. The racial differences may well be due to differences in living conditions, although there is little doubt that American Negroes are more likely to develop a spreading form of the disease. Malnutrition is commonly accompanied by overcrowding which will favour the spread of infection. It seems doubtful whether age has great influence. It was formerly believed that children and infants were more susceptible but it is clear that the age at which primary infection is acquired is steadily rising.

The influence of occupation depends first upon the opportunity it affords the spread of infection and secondly upon the inhalation of the possibly noxious substances. Examples are, the nursing profession where exposure to the risk of infections is frequent and the effects of inhaled siliceous dusts upon the lung.

There are certain diseases in which an undue liability to tuberculosis has long been recognized: chief amongst these are diabetes mellitus, cirrhosis of the liver, chronic alcoholism and the chronic leukaemias. The incidence in these special instances has decreased *pari passu* with the general reduction and with the more effective management of the diseases in question. The high incidence in mental hospitals is presumably due to conditions facilitating the spread of infection.

Prolonged administration of corticosteroid drugs has been shown to reduce resistance to tuberculosis and to reactivate lesions previously considered healed. Because they often suppress the general features of infection, the clinical picture may be unusual and the disease often eludes diagnosis until the process is far advanced.

CLINICAL FORMS OF TUBERCULOSIS IN MAN

LOCAL INFECTIONS

There are few organs or tissues which may not at times be the seat of tuberculous infection. The respiratory, alimentary, urinary and genital tracts, bones, joints, lymph nodes, serous membranes, the meninges, the suprarenal glands, the skin and the liver are commonly affected. The clinical features of tuberculosis of these regions are considered in the relevant sections. The thyroid gland, the salivary glands, the pancreas, the heart and the voluntary muscles are only infected in exceptional circumstances.

GENERALIZED INFECTIONS

Generalized tuberculosis arises through the discharge of infected material from a caseating lesion into the circulation. The lesion in question is often a lymph node which becomes adherent to a vein, finally eroding its wall and pouring its contents into the blood stream. The picture varies with the site of the lesion from which dissemination occurs: when a systemic vein receives the discharge of tuberculous material the lungs may be affected almost exclusively; when a pulmonary vein, the infection is mainly systemic. All intermediate gradations occur.

The acuteness of the process also shows variations. The common form is generalized miliary tuberculosis in which the bacilli disseminated through the blood stream give rise to innumerable discrete tubercles scattered throughout the lungs and other tissues. This type is so called because the tubercles are about the size of a millet seed. There is a fulminating variety which has been named tuberculous septicaemia in which the widespread lesions show a miliary necrosis with little cellular reaction, but with immense numbers of tubercle bacilli. The pathological appearances have been described as non-reactive tuberculosis. Similar lesions have been produced experimentally by the injection of large numbers of virulent bacilli into hypersensitive animals. Finally, a subacute form has been described in which it is believed that intermittent showers of tubercle bacilli enter the blood stream. The different clinical pictures caused by the several processes are not clear cut and it serves no good purpose to try and describe them separately.

Incidence

Generalized tuberculosis may arise in a patient known to have chronic tuberculous infection or in one previously in good health. The classic miliary form is seen most frequently below the age of 10 years. It usually follows within six months of a primary infection. With the age of primary infections becoming progressively later, miliary tuberculosis although far less common than formerly, is now seen relatively more often in the second and third decades of life. It was once a disease of infants and young children and in former times was often noted to follow measles or whooping cough. The acute septicaemic type has been recorded most often in the middle aged and is twice as common in men as in women; the subacute form tends to affect the young adult.

The Clinical Picture

The onset of generalized tuberculosis may be abrupt or gradual, but in all cases the initial symptoms are general. They include vague ill health, fatigue, exhaustion, headache, loss of weight and fever. In the septicaemic form anaemia is often an early feature, and frequently leads to the illness being regarded as a haematological problem.

As the disease establishes itself, the features become more clear cut. The fever is usually intermittent and may reach 103°–104° F. (39·4°–40° C.) in the evening. Occasionally the chart shows an inverted pattern with febrile peaks early in the day. Tachycardia is often disproportionate to the pyrexia, sweats at night may be drenching. Insomnia and headache are troublesome and prostration becomes profound.

After a period of one to two weeks localizing symptoms and signs may appear and it has been customary to recognize two types of generalized tuberculosis; the 'typhoid' and the 'pulmonary'. In the first there is increasing tumidity of the abdomen, and the liver and spleen become palpable. Constipation is the rule. In the second variety there is a cyanotic flush and dyspnoea is out of proportion to the trivial signs of pulmonary disease which amount to no more than scattered crepitations.

In about 90 per cent. of patients with miliary disease tuberculous meningitis develops [see Section 15]. It is the usual conclusion in the classic and subacute forms but less common in the septicaemic group. In the subacute type local lesions such as pleural or pericardial effusion, arthritis or cutaneous tuberculides may appear in successive crops over weeks or months. Finally it terminates in acute miliary tuberculosis and meningitis. In the septicaemic type profound toxaemia with progressive loss of weight, prostration and anaemia usually conclude the illness.

Generalized tuberculosis was probably always fatal before the specific antibacterial agents were available. With adequate treatment 80–90 per cent. of patients now recover. The outlook in the acute septicaemic type remains grave.

Diagnosis

The early diagnosis of generalized tuberculosis was of academic interest before effective chemotherapy existed. It is now a matter of great moment, for the earlier treatment is started the better is the outlook.

Suspicion is naturally aroused when symptoms such as those described appear in the patient known to have or to have had tuberculosis. This type of case is uncommon and the disease more often seems to have arisen *de novo*.

Radiology is often helpful, for the diffuse mottling in radiograms of the lungs is characteristic of miliary pulmonary tuberculosis, but it may only develop after some weeks or, if the disease is mainly extrapulmonary, not at all.

Material obtained by bone marrow aspiration or puncture biopsy of the liver may yield tubercle bacilli or show the characteristic histological lesions.

Even in the absence of clear cut signs of meningitis, examination of the cerebrospinal fluid may show changes indicative of early meningeal invasion.

In the majority, examination of the blood reveals a neutrophil leucocytosis amounting to perhaps 20,000 per mm^3. This serves to exclude enteric fevers. In the septicaemic form profound changes have been described. The commonest is a pancytopenia suggesting aplasia of the bone marrow. Neutropenia is another variation, but a number of cases with a blood picture indistinguishable from that of acute myeloblastic leukaemia have been reported. The erythocyte sedimentation rate is always raised in active tuberculous infection.

M. tuberculosis has only rarely been recovered from the blood in generalized tuberculosis. This method has little practical diagnostic value.

DIAGNOSIS OF TUBERCULOUS INFECTION

This may be said to be at two different levels. The diagnosis of infection, and the diagnosis of disease. Once infection has taken place, the patient will be hypersensitive to tuberculoprotein and will react positively to skin tests with tuberculin. This indicates no more than infection at sometime in the past; it does not mean that the patient has active tuberculosis. Before one can be certain that active tuberculous disease exists, the presence of *M. tuberculosis* should be demonstrated, although its existence frequently has to be inferred from radiological appearances or clinical findings, without awaiting the certainty given by isolation of the organism.

Tuberculin Tests

The demonstration of reactivity to tuberculoprotein is of value in several ways. If there is no reaction a healthy subject must be regarded as never having had a primary infection and as being susceptible. A positive reaction means that at some time or other tuberculous infection has taken place. In an infant it is almost invariably associated with active progressive disease. Conversion from negative to positive indicates a recent primary infection. Negative reactions, which may be misleading, are also seen in the early stages of primary infection and sometimes in overwhelming tuberculous or other infections; in about 60 per cent. of patients with sarcoidosis and about 45 per cent. of those with Hodgkin's disease and similar disorders.

The test is carried out with tuberculoprotein in the form of tuberculin or its purified protein derivative (PPD). Old Tuberculin (OT) is the concentrated filtrate of a steam-killed culture of *M. tuberculosis*. OT.T is derived from human strains and OT.PT from bovine. There is no demonstrable difference between the two, although tuberculin made from the avian type of bacillus can be distinguished antigenically. The purified protein derivative (PPD) is prepared by the precipitation of proteins from OT by trichloracetic acid or a half saturated solution of ammonium sulphate. A special batch of PPD has been adopted by the World Health Organization as a standard and an International Tuberculin Unit is defined as that amount equal in potency to 0·00002 mg. of the standard. PPD has largely superseded OT.

A number of skin tests have been used; the original, long since discarded, was the scratch test of von Pirquet. The routine methods now are the Mantoux intradermal test and the Heaf test. The first is carried out by the injection of 5–10 Tuberculin Units (TU) of PPD, or an equivalent amount of OT, in 0·1 ml. of physiological saline into the skin of the flexor surface of the forearm. A positive reaction is denoted by an area of induration not less than 5 mm. in diameter appearing between 48 and 72 hours after the injection. Oedema and erythema are of no significance. If the reaction to 5 or 10 TU is negative the test is repeated using 100 TU in 0·1 ml. of saline. If this gives a negative result the patient is considered 'Mantoux negative'. With the Heaf test, the tuberculin is applied to the skin and a multiple puncture spring release gun (Heaf gun) makes the intradermal inoculation by pricking through it. A positive reaction varies from four discrete papules to a wide zone of induration. Both these tests are acceptable but the Heaf test is generally to be preferred.

Vollmer's patch test has been used in children. In this a strip of adhesive plaster carrying a piece of gauze soaked in OT and allowed to dry is applied to the skin of the back. A positive result is shown by a red papulo-vesicular eruption 48–96 hours after application. It is said to show good correlation with the results of the Mantoux reaction. A tuberculin jelly test has not proved dependable.

Demonstration of M. Tuberculosis

The most convincing proof that a patient has active tuberculosis is the demonstration of the bacillus in the lesion or in the discharges from it. The material examined may be sputum, fluid from a joint or serous cavity, the contents of a cold abscess or caseating lymph node, the stool, the urine, the cerebrospinal fluid or the aspirate from liver or bone marrow puncture. The discovery of acid alcohol-fast bacilli morphologically resembling *M. tuberculosis* is usually sufficient, but this is only easy when organisms are abundant. Cultures and inoculations into guinea-pigs are both widely used, but have the disadvantage that an answer may not be available for 4–6 weeks with the first method and 4–12 weeks with the second.

Biopsy Methods

Short of demonstrating the *Mycobacterium* the finding of typical tuberculous giant cell systems, especially when there is caseation affords reasonable proof of the diagnosis. Sometimes mycobacteria can be seen in fixed sections. Lymph nodes, ulcers, skin lesions, sinuses and needle biopsy of the pleura, liver and bone marrow provide suitable material.

Serological Methods

Many attempts have been made to devise complement fixation tests and other serological methods as aids to the diagnosis of tuberculosis. All the techniques give a high proportion of 'false positives' and none has yet proved of practical value.

CONTROL AND PROPHYLAXIS OF TUBERCULOSIS

The control of tuberculosis, like the control of most infections, requires the abolition of the reservoirs from which infection spreads. These are patients with active pulmonary tuberculosis, and dairy cattle producing infective milk. In the British Isles, the second has almost disappeared as a significant cause with the pasteurization of milk and the eradication of tuberculosis in dairy cows. As a result bone and joint tuberculosis has become rare and even the formerly common tuberculous lymphadenitis is unusual.

Control of the human carrier is less easy but immense advances have been made. The first step is the segregation and treatment of patients known to have tuberculosis; the second is the routine radiographic examination of contacts, with treatment of any found to be infected; and the third is the nation-wide campaign of case-finding surveys, using mass miniature radiography. The energetic prosecution of these methods together with the discovery of effective chemotherapeutic agents has been responsible for what was once called 'the captain of the men of death' being deposed from its previous eminence.

Experimentally it has been established that the injection of killed tubercle bacilli increases the resistance to tuberculosis, and that attentuated living bacilli are even more effective. There is cross-immunity between human and bovine types. The original attenuated strain of Calmette and Guérin, the Bacille Calmette-Guérin (B.C.G.), has been used extensively in prophylaxis. Considerable differences in invasiveness exist between different strains derived from the original culture, but there is no evidence that the organism can revert to its former pathogenicity. There are, however, at least four examples of B.C.G. giving rise to progressive tuberculosis in man, all in individuals unable to develop resistance to infection. The vaccine prepared from the vole bacillus has been used for the same purpose.

The results of a controlled clinical trial of B.C.G. and vole bacillus vaccine have been published by the Medical Research Council. More than 50,000 children aged 14–15½ years, initially free from active tuberculosis and known contact with the disease, have been followed for an average of 8·8 years. In the control unvaccinated group the annual incidence of tuberculosis was 1·91 per 1000, in the B.C.G. vaccinated group 0·40 per 1000 and in those receiving vole-bacillus vaccine 0·43 per 1000 compared with 2·30 per 1000 in a control group. Thus B.C.G. appeared to reduce infection by 79 per cent. and vole-bacillus vaccine by 81 per cent.

B.C.G. vaccine has been used extensively in the vaccination of various groups, such as nurses and medical students, in whom exposure to infection is likely. The usual method is to vaccinate all those in whom the Mantoux test is negative to 100 TU and who may thus be assumed not to have had a primary tuberculous infection.

TREATMENT

The treatment of active tuberculous infection is considered in detail in the section on antibiotics and in the sections which deal with tuberculosis of the various organs and systems. The basis of specific therapy is a mixture of chemotherapeutic agents, most commonly, streptomycin, isoniazid, and para-aminosalicylic acid. It is becoming clear, however, that sensitivity tests are important in the management of this disease: resistant strains are not rare and amongst them 'anonymous' mycobacteria are gaining in numerical significance.

REFERENCES

FOGAN, L. (1970) Atypical mycobacteria: their clinical laboratory and epidemiologic significance, *Medicine (Baltimore)*, **49**, 243.

GOLDMAN, K. P. (1968) Treatment of unclassified mycobacterial infection of the lungs, *Thorax*, **23**, 94.

KILIGER, I., HAHNE, O. H., and WHITTEN, C. F. (1964) Atypical mycobacteria as a probable cause of chronic bone disease, *J. Pediat.*, **65**, 340.

MARKS, J., and RICHARDS, M. (1962) Classification of the anonymous mycobacteria as a guide to their significance, *Mth. Bull. Minist. Hlth Lab. Serv.*, **21**, 200.

MEDD, W. E., and HAYHOE, F. G. J. (1955) Tuberculous miliary necrosis with pancytopenia, *Quart. J. Med.*, N.S. **24**, 351.

MEDICAL RESEARCH COUNCIL (1963) Third Report of the Tuberculosis Vaccines and Clinical Trials Committee, B.C.G. and vole bacillus vaccines in the prevention of tuberculosis in adolescence and early adult life, *Brit. med. J.*, **1**, 973.

MITCHISON, D. A. (1963) The epidemiology of tubercle bacilli, *Sci. Basis Med.*, 39.

REES, R. J. W. (1959) Experimental approach to the problems of resistance to tuberculosis, in *Lectures on the Scientific Basis of Medicine*, Vol. 7, p. 203, London.

REPORT (1959) A single tuberculin test for epidemiological use: a comparison of the Mantoux and Heaf tests, *Tubercle*, **40**, 317.

RICH, A. R. (1952) *The Pathogenesis of Tuberculosis*, Springfield, Ill.

OTHER HUMAN MYCOBACTERIAL INFECTIONS

M. ulcerans, an organism morphologically identical with *M. tuberculosis*, has been isolated from patients with chronic ulceration of the skin of the extremities in Australia, West Africa, South East Asia and Mexico. In Uganda it has recently been proved the cause of a common and crippling ulcerative disease of the skin, known locally as the Buruli ulcer. This bacillus shows the peculiarity of growing in culture only at temperatures between 25° and 35° C. It can therefore act as a pathogen only in those anatomical areas where the mean temperature is below 37° C.

Another related organism is *M. balnei*. This again cannot multiply at temperatures above 35° C. and has been held responsible for a benign ulcerative lesion usually of the skin of the elbows which often follows abrasions acquired in swimming-pools: for this reason the disorder is sometimes called 'swimming-pool disease'. It was first noted in Sweden.

There is cross-immunity between both these two organisms and B.C.G. gives considerable protection against infection with both species. Vaccines made from them, however, give no protection against virulent bovine bacilli. Surgical excision followed by a course of streptomycin is said to be the most effective method of treatment.

REFERENCES

LINELL, F., and NORDEN, A. (1954) *Mycobacterium balnei*: a new acid fast bacillus occurring in swimming pools and capable of producing skin lesions in humans, *Acta tuberc. scand.*, Suppl. 33, 1.

MACCULLUM, P., TOLHURST, J. C., BUCKLE, G., and SISSONS, H. A. (1948) A new mycobacterial infection in man, *J. Path. Bact.*, **60**, 93.

UGANDA BURULI GROUP (1969) B.C.G. vaccination against *Mycobacterium ulcerans* infection (Buruli ulcer). First results of a trial in Uganda, *Lancet*, i, 111.

R. BODLEY SCOTT

LEPROSY

Leprosy results from infection with *Mycobacterium leprae* or Hansen's bacillus. The disease is characterized by a long incubation period and a chronic course with the development of lesions in the skin and peripheral nerves.

Leprosy has a very wide distribution. It is prevalent in parts of the Middle East, Asia, the Pacific, Africa, Central and South America and occurs in Northern Australia, some of the Pacific Islands and in Southern Europe and the Mediterranean littoral.

It appears particularly in areas where human contact is close and continuous in unhygienic conditions, involving both indigenes and visitors after long exposure.

M. leprae is an acid-fast bacillus morphologically indistinguishable from *M. tuberculosis*. It cannot be grown *in vitro* but can be maintained in the foot pad of mice or in the thymectomized mouse.

Infection probably occurs through the skin and is transmitted via bacteriologically active lesions in the skin or mucous membranes in cases of lepromatous leprosy. The infection seems to be most frequently acquired in childhood, but transmission to adults occurs. There is no congenital transmission.

Little is known of the early stages or mechanics of transmission, although the organism has been found in the skin of apparently healthy individuals.

In the event, the response of the tissues of the infected person determines the ultimate development of the disease.

Where local tissue reaction is vigorous, the multiplication and dissemination of the organism is restricted. Where there is little reaction, the organisms multiply and disseminate freely.

Pathology

In some cases the infection is probably localized and eliminated. In persons in whom leprosy is to develop, the mycobacteria invade the skin, enter the corium and reach the terminal radicals of the peripheral nerves, where they are phagocytosed by Schwann cells. They also enter reticulo-endothelial cells in the dermis. Subsequent events are determined largely by the tissue response of the patient. The organisms may spread locally in the subcutaneous tissue to other areas of the skin via lymphatics and eventually, via the blood, to various organs of the body.

There are two extreme forms of the disease, the *lepromatous* and the *tuberculoid*, with every variety of intermediate development.

Lepromatous leprosy develops in patients with little resistance to the organisms, which are able to multiply and disseminate freely in the tissues. The lepromin reaction is negative. The characteristic skin lesion is the *leproma*, which appears clinically as an indefinitely demarcated macule or area of change in the texture and colour of the skin. Histological section shows some cellular infiltration of the dermis from which the atrophic epithelium is separated by a clear uninfiltrated subepidermal zone. The lesion at first occurs in the terminal nerve twigs which are hyaline and contain many mycobacteria lying with their long axes parallel to the nerve. Fusiform swellings develop in the nerve radicals containing dense masses of organisms, many of which are phagocytosed by histiocytes which degenerate and become the characteristic 'foam cells' of Virchow. There are also additional masses of organisms packed together to form 'globi'. The general cellular reaction is poor and confined largely to the reticular layers of the dermis.

The later stages of lepromatous lesions including nodules are all based on the same pattern of many organisms in the nerve radicals, foam cells and globi and an over-all minimal cellular response.

The eventual involvement of the nerve trunks by large numbers of organisms in lepromatous leprosy causes some swelling of the endoneurium but little cellular response and consequently, except during periods of clinical exacerbation, relatively little neurological damage.

Tuberculoid leprosy occurs in patients with pronounced tissue reaction to the infection. The skin lesions are clearly demarcated and the peripheral nerves are involved. The organism is distributed scantily and the lepromin reaction is positive.

The lesions are divided usually into *major* and *minor tuberculoids* which begin as anaesthetic hypochromic macules and eventually become localized, with raised edges and pebbled surface.

These represent focal granulomata, resembling those seen in tuberculosis, with epithelioid and giant cells and considerable cellular reaction. The dermis and subepidermal zone are involved. Mycobacteria are scanty and are usually found in the cellular reactions involving the nerves.

The granulomatous reactions about the nerve twigs gradually extend centripetally to involve the superficial plexuses and the trunks. The active cellular response results in tumour formation and the resultant pressure eventually destroys the fibrils leading to considerable nerve damage. Cold abscess may develop.

There are two other types of leprous lesions: (1) *Dimorphous*, or intermediate which is unstable both clinically and pathologically and which may develop into either lepromatous or tuberculoid leprosy. Bacilli may be absent or numerous and the lepromin reaction may be positive or negative. (2) *Indeterminate* which may remain static or progress into any of the three other types. This early lesion shows scattered non-specific cellular infiltration which may involve nerve fibres. The lepromin test may be weakly positive.

Other tissues: Tissues other than the skin and nerves may become involved in the development of leprosy, either as a direct result of the infection or indirectly from the effects of nerve damage.

The eyes are frequently involved in both lepromatous and tuberculoid leprosy. The testes are invaded by the organisms in lepromatous leprosy and the parenchyma may be affected leading to physiological effects and the clinical appearance of secondary sexual changes, such as gynaecomastia.

Regional lymph nodes may be involved and if superficial may eventually rupture to the surface producing chronic ulcers with sinuses discharging bacilli. Infiltration and ulceration of the nasal mucosa is common in lepromatous leprosy and may extend to the larynx, trachea and occasionally to the bronchi.

Bone lesions occur in both forms of leprosy but are mostly seen in the tuberculoid form in which non-specific osteitis, osteoporosis and absorption occur as a result of nerve damage and the accompanying vascular and trophic changes. The most severe deformities may result, particularly in association with muscular contractures.

Signs and Symptoms

There is a long incubation period, usually of many years. The onset is nearly always gradual but may be acute with attacks of fever and pain in the peripheral nerves and the appearance of evanescent skin eruptions.

Leprosy in a given patient tends to develop into one of the two extremes, but there may be many intermediate forms. In the majority of cases the appearance of a skin lesion is the first sign of the infection. The earliest lesions may be difficult to differentiate but as they develop slowly over months the differences between lepromatous and tuberculoid usually become more obvious.

Tuberculoid Leprosy. In some cases well-defined local lesions appear and may persist for weeks and months and spontaneously disappear without further development of the disease. In most, however, the initial lesion persists and other lesions develop later. The skin lesions may become minor or major tuberculoids. They occur anywhere on the body and are sharply defined, infiltrated and raised above the surrounding skin. The skin is dry, may be hairless, scaly, pebbled and frequently depigmented; it may be erythematous. The area is analgesic and anaesthetic. Sometimes the lesions appear as large annular areas with a centre of fairly normal skin. Small nerves are thickened and may be palpable in the vicinity of the skin lesions. Larger nerve trunks are often also thickened and palpable. The thickening is due to tissue reaction in the nerve branches and peripheral trunks which may be very greatly thickened. Signs of local neuritis may develop. The thickening is often clearly visible. Destruction of the fibres in an involved nerve trunk leads to corresponding motor and sensory changes in the relevant areas commonly below the knee and the elbow. For instance, damage to the ulnar nerve frequently results in paresis and wasting of the corresponding muscles of the hand and sensory loss in the fingers and palm; wrist-drop commonly develops. Corresponding lesions occur in the legs when the peroneal nerves are damaged; foot-drop is common. The skin over the areas supplied by the damaged nerves becomes cold, shiny and inelastic and sweating stops. The muscles become fibrotic and eventually contract; the bones may become rarefied, decalcified and absorbed. Extreme deformity may finally develop.

The insensitive and atrophic tissues are easily damaged and secondarily infected. Perforating ulcers result at points of pressure, especially over the heads of the metatarsals and the os calcis and on the palms, hands and fingers. The ulcers are often deep and usually secondarily infected. Chronic sinuses form and the underlying bone is often involved. Peripheral nerves other than those of the extremities may be involved, including the great auricular. Damage to the seventh nerve leads to facial palsy. Involvement of the nerves to the eyelids and eyes leads to loss of sensation and interference with eye movements. The blink reflex may be lost and the cornea may become damaged, leading to blindness.

The tuberculoid tumours in the peripheral nerves and trunks may caseate and form cold abscesses. These increase the local pressure on the nerve fibrils and speed up the nerve damage. They cause considerable local pain, tenderness and swelling, and operation is necessary.

Lepromatous Leprosy. The first sign of the infection is commonly the appearance of an indeterminate vague macule in the skin. The affected area is flushed, and slightly shiny, it blends imperceptibly into the surrounding skin without clear demarcation and is not usually anaesthetic. It extends locally to become a lepromatous macule. Other similar lesions may develop around it and coalesce until the areas of skin involved become very extensive. The skin of the face and the lobes of the ears are often affected early by macular lesions and diffuse infiltrations. The skin thickens and becomes oedematous and corrugated, especially in the supra-orbital, frontal and malar prominences and ears, giving rise to the classical leonine features. Hair is lost from the eyebrows and face, but not usually the scalp. Nodular lesions are common. These are painless, intracutaneous or subcutaneous tumours occurring most commonly on the ears, the face and extremities. They vary in number and size. They may become necrotic and ulcerate, discharging enormous numbers of mycobacteria.

Mucous membranes may be involved in the lepromatous processes and may ulcerate and discharge organisms. The nasal and pharyngeal mucosae are frequently involved in this way and considerable damage and deformity may result, especially when secondary infection occurs. The organisms may invade the eyes, causing lesions which include painful iritis and which may lead to blindness.

Dimorphous (Intermediate) Leprosy. The early lesions are slow growing indeterminate partly anaesthetic macules, sometimes with satellite lesions. Later lesions resemble those of tuberculoid or lepromatous leprosy, or both. Annular patches are common, with clear normal-looking central skin and peripheral raised hypopigmented erythematous surrounds, over which there is some sensory loss. Peripheral nerves are involved early and severely, and clinical signs of nerve damage may be present before corresponding skin lesions appear.

Indeterminate Lesions. These are hypopigmented macules which are usually flat, diffuse, with indefinite boundaries and not anaesthetic. Sweating function and hair growth are maintained. Such early lesions are very common in endemic areas.

Reaction States. From time to time exacerbations of lepromatous leprosy occur, usually as a result of over-vigorous drug treatment, in which there is an acute extension of the condition, with rapid expansion of old lesions and appearance of new ones and with notable increase in the numbers of mycobacteria in the lesions. There is usually some fever and the patient is often ill and prostrated with painful swellings of limb joints. This so-called *lepra reaction* may be mild, lasting a few days or severe and continue for many weeks. It may be precipitated by too active treatment.

Other forms of reaction occurring in lepromatous leprosy include the peculiar *erythema necroticans*, described in Central and South America and characterized by lesions on the face and hands which arise from dilatation and thrombosis of capillary vessels, with ulceration and scarring. The picture represents a sudden increase in tissue resistance to the mycobacteria and may be accompanied by the acquisition of a positive lepromin reaction.

Erythema nodosum leprosum may also appear especially during treatment. It is a Herxheimer sensitivity reaction in the form of scattered erythematous cutaneous nodules which develop usually on the extremities and the face but may be generalized. The eruption lasts only a short time and may be accompanied by fever. Unlike the lepra reaction it does not represent an extension of the disease.

Reactions also develop in tuberculoid leprosy. Acute inflammation and ulceration of a single tuberculoid lesion sometimes occurs, without systemic effects, and representing a local 'reaction of recovery'. Occasionally many or all the lesions in a tuberculoid case including those in the nerves may become swollen and tender. The skin lesions may ulcerate.

Diagnosis

The certain diagnosis of leprosy depends on the demonstration of *M. leprae* in the lesions.

The organisms are easily found in lepromatous leprosy, but may be very difficult to discover in other forms of the disease.

A small incision is made through the suspected lesion to uncover the fatty layer beneath the epithelium. This layer is then scraped with the point of the knife and the scrapings are transferred to a slide, dried, fixed by heat and stained for acid-fast bacilli by the Ziehl-Neelsen method. Several lesions should be examined in this way. Smears of scrapings from the mucosa of the nasal septum will usually contain organisms in lepromatous leprosy. Examination of this tissue should not however be substituted for that of suspected lesions elsewhere.

Biopsy samples of the lesions should also be removed for bacteriological and histological examination. Organisms can usually be readily demonstrated in lepromatous and dimorphous lesions. Tuberculoid and lepromatous lesions can be distinguished readily by the histological pattern, but the intermediate stages of dimorphous lesions may be very difficult to define.

Mycobacteria are rarely found in skin or nasal mucosa scrapings in tuberculoid leprosy. Here the diagnosis is often largely clinical, but biopsies of peripheral nerves may be performed and the tissue stained for acid-fast organisms, which are usually present but very scanty.

The Lepromin (Mitsuda) Reaction. The test is carried out by intradermal injection of 0·1 ml. of antigen prepared from bacteriologically strongly positive lepromatous tissue or its extracts. Similar results have been claimed when an antigen prepared from normal skin is used.

The site of injection is examined every 24 hours. The positive reaction appears in two stages. The early reaction develops in 48 hours as oedema and thickening of the inoculated area and local erythema. The late reaction is characterized by considerable local infiltration in the form of a palpable and visible nodule which may undergo central necrosis. It appears after 2–3 weeks and reaches its maximum in 3–4 weeks.

The lepromin reaction is not diagnostic of leprosy as such. It is, however, helpful in assessing the tissue resistance of the individual patient to the mycobacteria.

Where the tissue response is weak, as in lepromatous leprosy, the reaction is negative. In the other forms of the disease the reaction may be weakly positive or negative.

Treatment

Sulphones. The most satisfactory drug is dapsone (diamino-diphenylsulphone or DDS). It has the disadvantage of producing a slow response and may need to be continued over many years, otherwise there may be relapse. Certain toxic effects may occur including gastro-intestinal disturbances and anaemia, the latter largely due to the presence of erythrocyte glucose-6-phosphate dehydrogenase deficiency. Lepra reactions or erythema nodosum leprosum may also be induced if the treatment is pressed too vigorously. DDS should not be given to patients with overt renal disease. DDS is given slowly at first in very small doses which are gradually increased over a period of months to a full dosage.

DDS maintains its effectiveness for years in most patients. In a few, drug resistance develops and other drugs have to be substituted.

DDS is prepared as 100 or 25 mg. tablets.

The following dosage regimen for an adult of 60 kg. (or more) body weight is recommended for any form of leprosy:

First month: 25 mg. once a week
Second month: 25 mg. twice a week
Third month: 25 mg. four times a week

The dose reached in the third month, i.e. 100 mg. weekly may then continue indefinitely, but most workers advise a final dose of 200 mg. weekly in order to minimize the risk of the development of drug resistance.

Doses for children are calculated in proportion to body weight.

Various preparations of DDS are available for intramuscular injection, sometimes used in mass campaigns or where there are difficulties in regular oral administration. The drug is made up in 25 per cent. solution in an oily vehicle and given at weekly or fortnightly intervals, in doses slowly rising from 25 mg. to 1 G.

Other intramuscular agents include solapsone (*Sulphetrone*) given in doses rising slowly from 0·5 ml. to 3·0 ml. (of a 50 per cent. solution) in 3–6 months.

This drug is used in patients recovering from acute reactions in lepromatous leprosy or where DDS is not tolerated.

Other Drugs. These are usually regarded as second-line.

Where there is intolerance or sensitivity to DDS, thiambutosine (*Ciba 1906*; diphenylthiourea, DPT) is commonly used in the following oral doses (for an adult of 60 kg. and upwards):

First month: 250 mg. daily in divided doses
Second month: 500 mg. daily
Third month: 1 G. daily
Thereafter: 2 G. daily

Drug resistance sometimes appears after this drug has been used for more than 2 years. For this reason, DDS is usually introduced in small but increasing dosage in the second year, with equivalent diminution of the thiambutosine, until it is finally replaced.

Thiambutosine is also prepared as a 20 per cent. suspension in arachis oil for intramuscular injection. It is claimed that 1 G. (5 ml. of the suspension) of the drug given intramuscularly once a week is equivalent in activity to 2 G. daily given orally.

Thiacetazone may also be given as an alternative to DDS. The maximum dose of 50 mg. thrice daily should be reached after 3–4 months' increasing dosage. DDS should gradually be substituted over the second and third years, as for thiambutosine.

Clofazimine (*Lamprene*), in doses of 100 mg. (capsule) daily or on alternate days, is sometimes given in long-standing lepromatous leprosy or persistent lepromatous reactions or as a substitute for DDS in drug resistant cases.

Rifampicin (*Rifadin*), a bacterial semi-synthetic antibiotic, also used in tuberculosis, is under trial.

Treatment should be continued in tuberculoid leprosy for at least 2 years. In lepromatous and dimorphous leprosy drug treatment is needed for at least 4 years or for at least 2 years after the disappearance of clinical and bacteriological activity. The latter is estimated by the ratio of uniformly stained and solid forms of *Mycobacterium leprae*, which are regarded as viable, to beaded and disrupted organisms (the morphological index).

Tuberculoid and indeterminate leprosy do not commonly relapse after successful treatment. Lepromatous and dimorphous leprosy may, and some watch should be kept where possible. Some workers recommend a maintenance course of half the normal full dosage indefinitely in such cases.

Treatment of Reactive States. Precipitating causes such as febrile illnesses should be checked.

Minor reactions in tuberculoid leprosy need no treatment as they are usually beneficial. When the lesion is severely affected or in an anatomically important area, the antileprosy drug should be withdrawn and prednisolone, 30 mg. daily for 3 days, should be given and the dosage gradually reduced thereafter. The specific leprosy drug should be reintroduced gradually.

In lepromatous reactions the antileprosy drug should be withdrawn immediately and the patient put to bed. Anti-inflammatory drugs may bring relief. Some authorities advise short courses of sodium antimony tartrate intravenously or stibophen intramuscularly. Most prefer the alternative of chloroquine, 150 mg. (base) twice daily for 2 weeks.

If this is ineffective, corticosteroids are required, for example, prednisolone, 30 mg. daily, the dose gradually reducing to withdrawal in 6–8 weeks. Where there are ocular complications such as iritis, cortisone 1 per cent. solution may be instilled into the eyes during systemic treatment with prednisolone.

DDS is resumed slowly, at low dosage, starting at 5 or 10 mg. weekly and gradually increasing to full therapeutic doses over some months. A low maintenance dose of prednisolone may be needed over the early stages of re-introduction of the DDS.

Management and Prophylaxis. Secondary infection of ulcers, etc. requires treatment by antibacterial agents. Surgical amputation may be necessary and there is a big field for orthopaedic rehabilitation.

The psychological handling of a case of leprosy is of great importance especially when the case is seen in an area in which it is rare or not endemic, such as Europe. For this reason special arrangements are often made for reporting a case to the health authorities. It should be appreciated that tuberculoid leprosy is for practical purposes non-infective and there is no reason why the patient should not be treated accordingly. Both tuberculoid and bacteria-free lepromatous cases should be encouraged to live as normal a life as possible in the community. In many endemic areas isolation has been largely replaced by mass chemotherapy.

Segregation is now seldom practiced.

Recent work has indicated that B.C.G. vaccination may prevent the appearance of lesions in exposed children. This has still to be confirmed statistically, but the evidence is sufficient to warrant B.C.G. vaccination in contacts with lepromatous and dimorphous bacteriologically positive cases.

DDS also appears to offer some protection to child contacts; the dose given is usually half the therapeutic dose.

REFERENCES

British Medical Journal (1968) Leading article. B.C.G. vaccination against leprosy, **1**, 4.

Dharmendra, Nordeen S. K., and Ramannjam, K. (1967) Prophylactic value of DDS against leprosy—a further report, *Leprosy in India*, **39**, 100.

Rees, R. J. W., Waters, M. F. R., Weddell, A. G. M., and Palmer, E. (1967) Experimental lepromatous leprosy, *Nature* (*Lond.*), **215**, 599.

Waters, M. F. R., and Rees, R. J. W. (1962) Changes in the morphology of *Mycobacterium leprae* in patients under treatment, *Int. J. Leprosy*, **30**, 266.

Brian Maegraith

INFECTIONS DUE TO ACTINOMYCETACEAE

ACTINOMYCOSIS

Synonym. Ray-fungus disease.

Definition

A chronic suppurative disease of localized origin, tending to spread into adjacent tissues without being limited by anatomical demarcations. It occasionally becomes disseminated. The causative organism is *Actinomyces israelii* and the clinical types of disease are chiefly cervicofacial, dermal, pulmonary and abdominal.

Aetiology

Actinomyces bovis was first described by Bollinger in 1877 as the micro-organism producing large, hard, sarcomatous-like masses occurring about the jaw bones of cattle, and in the following year Wolff and Israel found a similar organism, now known as *A. israelii*, in human disease. There is reason to believe that *A. israelii*, normally saprophytic in the upper respiratory tract, may become invasive when tissue is injured or otherwise rendered susceptible.

Actinomyces naeslundii may also be an agent of human actinomycosis.

Pathology

The characteristic of the disease is a suppurative lesion often communicating with the surface by a sinus. Pus contains visible granules which, examined microscopically, are seen to have a centre of closely meshed filaments of bacterial dimensions, with a border of radially arranged striations, usually ending in club-shaped bodies. These bodies are regarded as hyaline deposits produced by local tissue reaction.

If granules are not seen in pus from sinuses, sinus walls may be curetted in order to find them. They may become more obvious if pus is vigorously shaken up in sterile water, the deposit then being examined. Alternatively, the pus may be thinly spread in a sterile Petri dish. Microscopical examination is facilitated by crushing the granules between slides. The bacterial filaments are Gram-positive while the clubs are Gram-negative. Culture is difficult, particularly if mixed secondary infection is present, and multiple inocula should be made on various media incubated anaerobically.

Clinical Features

These depend upon the anatomical distribution of the granulomata.

Cervicofacial. When the infection occurs in the jaw and adjacent structures the patient presents a swelling very like a sarcoma, generally about the angle or ramus of the mandible. The swelling may, however, affect the submandibular tissues and lymph nodes rather more than the jaw itself, or even be confined to the glands. The swelling is tender, somewhat painful and not generally so hard as in sarcoma. It may show one or more small zones of softer consistency than the rest of the lump. With progress of the disease, abscesses form and point externally to give rise to multiple sinuses. In most cases there is no obvious source of infection inside the mouth; it is assumed that a carious tooth, or infected gums and periodontal membranes are responsible. The tonsils are sometimes the site of original disease.

Dermal. Granulomata appear in the skin and subcutaneous tissues (1) alone, or (2) complicating the disease in deeper structures.

1. Solitary lesions are rare and have occurred following trauma from an infected tooth, for example on the hands. The initial lesion is a rounded swelling suggestive of tuberculosis rather than pyogenic infection, but it is usually firmer in texture than a tuberculous skin lesion. It also has to be distinguished from a gumma. As the lesion progresses it tends to ulcerate after the appearance of soft dusky-red areas. Pus escaping from the ulcerated parts may contain typical

'sulphur granules'. At this stage, it is not unlike a chronic carbuncle or a suppurating gumma.

2. Similar skin lesions not infrequently occur in association with primary infection of deeper structures. These may have resulted from direct spread of disease or from haematogenous dissemination.

Pulmonary. The possibility of actinomycosis should constantly be borne in mind where indefinite basal physical signs accompany cough, fever and haemoptysis. In some cases a pleural effusion develops early and bacteriological examination of the exudate reveals the nature of the disease. Disease may be unilateral or bilateral. The clinical picture may resemble tuberculosis, but as it progresses the differential diagnosis often lies between actinomycosis, bronchiectasis and necrotizing neoplasm. In the later stages of the disease there is wasting, intermittent fever, purulent expectoration and physical signs of progressive lung infiltration, often involving the pleura. Periostitis of the ribs seen radiologically is strongly suggestive of actinomycosis.

Abdominal. The favourite site of infection is the caecum and appendix region. The disease can manifest itself as an attack of appendicitis, most often acute, in which case the diagnosis is made only at the time of laparotomy. Alternatively, it may present as a slowly growing mass in the right iliac fossa, with some pain, tenderness and constitutional disturbance, in which case suspicion may be aroused as to its nature bearing in mind that this region is a site of election for actinomycosis. Distinction must be made from a swelling due to regional ileitis, to tuberculosis or new growth. There is a tendency for the infection to spread from the ileocaecal region: (1) to the adjacent peritoneum; (2) to the abdominal wall; (3) to the liver; (4) to ovary and Fallopian tubes. For this reason it is rare to find the lesion confined to the appendix by the time operation takes place. Similarly, the first evidence of caecal infection may be the involvement of the parietes in the lower right quadrant of the abdomen, in which case there is always a probability that the infection has spread from the bowel. The liver is sometimes involved alone, that is, without obvious intestinal lesions. The disease can only be distinguished from abscess due to other bacteria by examination of pus obtained by puncture or incision.

Cerebrospinal. The brain, like the skin, may be infected by direct spread from an adjacent lesion, or by way of a general pyaemic process.

Diagnosis

Actinomycosis simulates other chronic inflammatory diseases, for example, pyogenic infection, tuberculoma and gumma. Sarcoma must also be considered in differential diagnosis. The chief reason why actinomycosis goes unrecognized is that the possibility of its existence is so often overlooked. All materials from a suspected case (pus, pleural exudate, sputa, material from liver puncture, excised lymph nodes, etc.) should be carefully examined foı branching bacterial filaments, and the pathologist should have his attention drawn to the possibility of actinomycosis as a diagnosis. Special culture studies can then be instituted in order to identify the causative organism.

Treatment

Penicillin is the drug of choice and must be given in high doses until apparent cure and thereafter in reduced dosage for a further period. Sulphonamides are useful supplements to penicillin. For exceptional cases which prove resistant to penicillin, other antibiotics such as tetracyclines or streptomycin may have to be considered. Surgical procedures require early consideration and any abscess or infected area should be drained, or incised and freely curetted. Pre- and postoperative penicillin therapy is essential and should be maintained for prolonged periods.

Course and Prognosis

These vary greatly and much depends on the degree to which peripheral spread of disease has occurred and whether the infection has become pyaemic. In lesions of the jaw and in skin infections, which are primary and not associated with visceral infection, the prognosis is more favourable than when lungs, liver or intestinal tract are involved. Early diagnosis before secondary infection develops adds greatly to the chance of recovery. Uncertainty as to whether complete extirpation of *A. israelii* has been achieved after apparently successful treatment makes assessment of prognosis difficult. Relapses are common and must be allowed for when planning treatment schedules.

REFERENCES

BATES, M., and CRUICKSHANK, G. (1957) Thoracic actinomycosis, *Thorax*, **12**, 99.

COLEMAN, M. R., GEORG, L. K., and ROZZELL, A. R. (1969) *Actinomyces naeslundii* as an agent of human actinomycosis, *Appl. Microbiol.*, **18**, 420, 427.

COPE, Z. (1938) *Actinomycosis*, London.

GARROD, L. P. (1952) Actinomycosis of the lung: aetiology, diagnosis and chemotherapy, *Tubercle (Lond.)*, **33**, 258.

NOCARDIOSIS

Definition

A chronic suppurative disease of respiratory origin which may undergo haematogenous dissemination. Metastases particularly affect the brain and meninges; the kidney, endocardium, spleen, liver and adrenal gland can be involved. The causative organism is *Nocardia asteroides*. Infection is often 'opportunist' in origin.

Aetiology

The disease is world wide in distribution but is less common than actinomycosis to which it has many resemblances. *Nocardia asteroides* is an aerobic actinomycete which is partially acid-fast and Gram-positive. It has been isolated from the soil and, in contrast to *A. israelii*, is a cause of exogenous infection in man.

Pathology

A pyogenic infection is produced similar to that due to a number of other bacteria. Compared with actinomycosis, there is less sinus formation, extension of disease across fascial planes and fibrosis. It is very uncommon for sulphur granules to develop in the pus. Abscesses in other organs such as the brain often accompany pulmonary disease, but the primary lung lesion sometimes cannot be found. In the lesions Gram-positive branching filaments are found and may reach 50 μ in length. They easily fragment into bacillary forms and since these are partially acid-fast it is possible that occasionally they may be mistaken for *Mycobacterium tuberculosis* or anonymous mycobacteria.

Clinical Features

Disease varies widely in extent from single lesions to widespread consolidation of one or both lungs. Cavitation may develop. Tuberculosis, actinomycosis and histoplasmosis may be simulated. Extension to the pleura is common, but spread to and penetration of the chest wall in advanced cases is less frequent than in actinomycosis. General deterioration of health and appearance of localizing signs elsewhere accompany haematogenous dissemination of disease.

Diagnosis

Nocardiosis has to be differentiated from other pyogenic bacterial infections of the lung and other organs and from tuberculosis, actinomycosis and histoplasmosis. Smears of sputum, pus or gastric lavage concentrates should be stained by Gram's method and for acid-fastness. They should also be cultured aerobically both at 26° C. and 37° C. *Nocardia asteroides* can survive the concentration methods used in tuberculosis diagnostic work and will then grow on Löwenstein-Jensen medium producing colonies which resemble those of certain anonymous mycobacteria. It may be difficult to assess the significance of the isolation of *N. asteroides* from sputum, particularly in subtropical or tropical zones, just as is the case for anonymous mycobacteria. Such isolations may result from pulmonary disease or may merely indicate recently inhaled organisms.

Treatment

A sulphonamide, particularly sulphadiazine, is the drug of choice in contrast to the use of penicillin in actinomycosis. This therapy may be supplemented by trimethoprim on purely empirical grounds; streptomycin has also been used in combination. Fusidic acid may prove a useful treatment. Prolonged therapy is necessary and should accompany and precede surgical treatment. Drainage of abscesses and pleural effusions, and excision of affected lung are sometimes necessary.

Prognosis

This depends on early diagnosis of disease before metastasis has occurred and on efficient chemotherapy. After dissemination infection is difficult to control and may be fatal.

REFERENCES

MURRAY, J. F., FINEGOLD, S. M., FROMAN, S., and WILL, D. W. (1961) The changing spectrum of nocardiosis, *Amer. Rev. resp. Dis.*, **83**, 315.

NEU, H. C., SILVA, M., HAZEN, E., and ROSENHEIM, S. H. (1967) Necrotising nocardial pneumonitis, *Ann. intern. Med.*, **66**, 274.

PEABODY, J. W., and SEABURY, J. H. (1957) Actinomycosis and nocardiosis, *J. chron. Dis.*, **5**, 374.

RICHTER, R. W., SILVA, M., NEU, H. C., and SILVERSTEIN, P. M. (1968) The neurological aspects of *Nocardia asteroides* infection, *Ann. Rev. nerv. ment. Dis.*, **44**, 424.

R. W. RIDDELL

INFECTIONS DUE TO TREPONEMATACEAE

BORRELIA INFECTIONS

THE RELAPSING FEVERS

The relapsing fevers are caused by morphologically indistinguishable spirochaetes belonging to the group of motile treponemata or borrelia. They are characterized by the occurrence of attacks of high remittent fever which appear and subside sharply with intervals of quiescence. There are two clinical forms, which are transmitted by lice and by ticks respectively.

LOUSE-BORNE RELAPSING FEVER

Aetiology

Louse-borne relapsing fever is a serious disease which results from infection with *Borrelia recurrentis* transmitted to man by the human body louse *Pediculus humanus*. The disease is characterized by periods of fever associated with enlargement of the liver and spleen, jaundice and toxaemia. There are seldom more than two febrile relapses. Mortality is high.

It occurs in colder and temperate climates of the world and where lice are common but outbreaks have occurred in cool seasons in Africa, the Middle East, India and South America.

There appear to be many strains of *Borr. recurrentis* with some serological differences. The organism is present in the plasma only during the febrile episodes. It is actively motile in wet preparations and stains readily in dry films; the average length is 15 μ and there are 6–8 spirals. It can be cultured on suitable media or in the chick embryo and can be passaged in monkeys, but does not readily infect other animals until it has been through the monkey. It is therefore only during the febrile period that blood of the patient is infective for the louse, which becomes itself infective 5–15 days later and will remain so for the rest of its life. The infection is not transmitted transovarially, hence individual lice must be infected by a blood meal.

Infection is transmitted not by the bite of the louse, but by the rubbing into abrasions of remnants of damaged lice broken up by scratching. An attack affords immunity to reinfection, which is lost within a year. In endemic areas epidemics are therefore possible every two or three years.

Pathology

Petechial haemorrhages occur under the skin, the

mucosae, pleura, peritoneum and in the brain. The liver is enlarged and hyperaemic; the spleen is considerably enlarged, soft and congested and may be heavily infected. It contains miliary aggregations of mononuclear cells and spirochaetes. The kidneys often show medullary congestion and cortical ischaemia. Spirochaetes are found in intercellular spaces and within the Kupffer cells of the liver and reticulo-endothelial cells of lymph nodes and bone marrow.

Signs and Symptoms

The incubation period varies from 2 to 12 days. There may be prodromal signs for a day or two followed by sudden onset with rigor, prostration, headache, widespread bodily pains, nausea and vomiting. The temperature rises rapidly to 104° F. (40° C.) or higher and continues as a remittent fever. The skin is flushed, the conjunctivae and mucous membranes often injected. Epistaxis is common. The liver and spleen enlarge and are tender. Jaundice is frequent and there may be signs of bronchitis. There may be an erythematous or macular rash which in severe cases is haemorrhagic.

The symptoms and signs develop and continue for about a week. As suddenly as it became elevated, the temperature now falls to normal or subnormal and the patient may temporarily collapse. The symptoms and signs abate and the liver and spleen become smaller. An afebrile period of a few days to 3 weeks follows, to be succeeded by a febrile relapse, similar to the primary attack but usually a little shorter and less severe. It may, however, become more severe than the initial attack and jaundice may appear for the first time. After a few days the fever again abates only to reappear as a second relapse. Sometimes there may be a third or even fourth relapse before the disease finally subsides. In most cases there are not more than two relapses. Thereafter the individual remains immune for months.

The death rate in epidemics may be as high as 30 per cent.

Diagnosis

The disease is often associated with outbreaks of epidemic louse-borne typhus and should always be considered a possibility when such epidemics occur. It may also occur during epidemics of yellow fever which may be very difficult clinically to distinguish from it.

The diagnosis is made by examining the blood during the febrile periods. The spirochaetes are present in the plasma under these conditions but absent in the afebrile intermissions.

The causative organisms are easily found in wet preparations of plasma or blood by dark ground examination, or in thick or thin blood films stained with Leishman or Giemsa. They may be recovered by culture in specific media or by inoculation of monkeys.

Treatment

The louse infestation must be removed. The patient should be treated with DDT and bathed before admission.

Tetracyclines are the drugs of choice, in doses of 500 mg. six-hourly for one day, followed by 250 mg. six-hourly for a week. The course is repeated after one week.

In Ethiopia, success in clinical relief and control of relapse has followed 500 mg. tetracycline intravenously, followed by the same dose next day. To minimize reactions, 300,000 Units of procaine penicillin may be substituted on the first day for the tetracycline.

High dosage with penicillin will also terminate the attack but may not prevent subsequent relapses.

Arsenical drugs were used successfully in the past but are now seldom given.

Severe reactions may develop within an hour of treatment, with rigor, high fever and falling blood pressure. The reactions last 8–12 hours and do not respond to cortisone. They are usually milder after penicillin.

TICK-BORNE RELAPSING FEVER

Non-epidemic or endemic relapsing fever is caused by *Borrelia duttoni*. This is primarily an infection of animals, from which it spreads to ticks and is transmitted from tick to tick transovarially.

The general clinical picture resembles that of louse-borne relapsing fever but the attacks are shorter and more severe and relapses are more frequent.

The disease occurs in the Mediterranean littoral especially North Africa, Eastern Europe, the Middle East, Central Asia, North India, tropical and sub-tropical America, parts of the United States, Central, East and South Africa.

Aetiology

Where rodents are the reservoir, the disease occurs only sporadically in man and depends on man being attacked by ticks infected from the animals. Ticks feed only occasionally on man; usually when he is lying on the ground or working or camping in the bush.

In Central Africa ticks infest human habitations and become infected directly from man. The infection becomes more patchily distributed and often confined to one area or dwelling in a particular village. The African disease differs from the others since man is the only mammalian reservoir. It is transmitted in endemic areas by several species of ticks, such as *Ornithodorus moubata*. The Spanish form of tick-borne relapsing fever can be adapted to transmission by the louse. The tick becomes infected after feeding. Offspring of infected female ticks are infected transovarially; infection may persist through several generations so that only rare contact with a mammalian reservoir may be necessary to maintain the infection in a colony of ticks.

When the tick bites man it pierces the skin and excretes saliva, evacuates faeces and discharges coxal fluid. Spirochaetes are present in all these fluids and may enter the wound made in feeding, or cuts and abrasions, or through unbroken mucous membranes.

The pathology of the disease resembles that of louse-borne relapsing fever.

Signs and Symptoms

The onset and course are much the same as in louse-borne relapsing fever. The intervals between the febrile paroxysms are shorter, being usually less than a fortnight; the febrile periods are slightly shorter and the fever tends to be lower. Spirochaetes are less numerous in the peripheral blood, but again are present only during the febrile episode. The number of relapses is greater; there may be six or more, the complications are more frequent and severe, and include iritis and neurological changes such as seventh nerve paralysis and spastic paraplegia. The febrile episode is often associated with diarrhoea or dysentery. The tendency to haemorrhage is greater than in the louse-borne disease.

Nevertheless, mortality is lower in the latter. Recovery is followed by substantial but temporary immunity to reinfection. Constant exposure in an endemic area results in tolerance.

Diagnosis

Diagnosis is made as in louse-borne relapsing fever except that *Borr. duttoni*, although much less numerous in the blood easily infects other animals in addition to monkeys.

Treatment

Antibiotics have replaced organic arsenicals. One of the tetracyclines given in doses of 500 mg. six-hourly for one day, followed by 250 mg. six-hourly for a week, will produce rapid clinical cure. After an interval of one week, 250 mg. six-hourly is given for a further week, in order to reduce the risk of relapse.

Antibiotics may evoke severe reactions.

Prophylaxis

Louse-borne relapsing fever is gradually disappearing in the world in the face of economic and hygienic advance. The tick-transmitted fevers, however, remain endemic in wide areas owing to the exceptional biological efficiency of the vector.

Tick-infested environments should be controlled with insecticides. The individual should avoid sleeping on floors of infested areas. Bed nets and repellents are advisable.

Brian Maegraith

TREPONEMAL INFECTIONS

SYPHILIS

Definition

A specific infectious disease due to entry of a micro-organism, *Treponema pallidum* into the tissues, either by inoculation into the skin or mucous membrane, or by needle puncture into veins or other deeper tissues (acquired syphilis) or by transmission *in utero* (congenital syphilis).

Acquired syphilis has an early infectious phase covering the first 2 years of the disease and a late non-infectious phase for the remainder of the patient's life. In the early phase, the primary sore or chancre represents the local tissue reaction to the inoculation of treponemes at sexual intercourse. This is followed by a spread of infection via the lymphatics to the regional lymph nodes and the entry of treponemes into the blood stream due to local tissue necrosis of the chancre. This systemic spread of infection results in secondary lesions of skin, mucous membrane and lymph nodes and more rarely of the eyes, viscera, bones and central nervous system. In the late phase inflammatory tertiary lesions, termed gummata, occur in the skin and subcutaneous tissues, bones and viscera, although they are rarely found in the cardiovascular or central nervous systems, which tend to be involved more often in fibrotic and degenerative changes. From the earliest stages formation of circulating antibodies can be detected by serological tests. Any or all of the clinical stages may be omitted and thus the disease in a latent stage often goes unrecognized. With congenital syphilis and blood transfusion syphilis in the adult the systemic signs are the first manifestations of the disease.

Aetiology

T. pallidum is a minute organism which in fresh specimens under dark-ground illumination appears as a white, very delicate corkscrew. Its length varies from 5–24 μ (average 8–10 μ): the distance between individual coils is 1 μ and the width of each coil is 1 μ. It is active on its own ground but slow in moving through the microscopic field. It has been demonstrated in every affected tissue, with the exception of the cornea, the internal ear and the knee joints and possibly the spinal cord in tabetics, as well as in the characteristic lesions of congenital syphilis. It has a life of only a few hours under natural conditions outside the body, but in blood obtained for purposes of transfusion it can remain alive for 72 hours. It is killed at once by drying, by comparatively low degrees of temperature and by much weaker antiseptics than suffice to destroy ordinary pathogenic organisms.

The usual methods of transmission are by sexual intercourse and by way of the placenta to the foetus *in utero*. The person suffering from syphilis is contagious by any form of sex contact during most of the early infectious stage. After the disease has been present for 2 years it is unlikely that he will continue to transmit infection in this way. In the case of the foetus, however, although transmission from the mother is most likely in the first 2 years of her infection, it has occurred much later. Transmission occurs most often in the second half of pregnancy. Accidental infection usually results from contamination of a minute abrasion with secretion from infectious syphilitic lesions, of which the most dangerous are the primary sore, the moist secondary lesions and some of the early lesions of congenital syphilis. The dangers of accidental infections from later lesions are extremely slight but it is possible to infect susceptible animals with biopsy material from them. Even in the earlier stages the risks of accidental infection appear to be slight, presumably because the organism is so susceptible to external agencies. This is shown by the fact that, even when the disease has been highly prevalent, the proportion of extragenital chancres has been low in countries where the standards of personal hygiene are equal to those of Western Europe. A number of instances of infection by transfusion of blood have been recorded, and they have included cases in which the donor was still in the incubation stage of the disease. On the other hand, patients with late syphilis have been used as donors in cases of emergency in a number of instances without harm to the recipients, and it is clear that the older the infection the less likely is the micro-organism to be in the blood stream.

Epidemiology

There has been a steady decline in the morbidity of syphilis. The number of cases at all stages fell from 23,878 in 1946 to 3267 in 1970 in the clinics in England and Wales. The equivalent figures for early infectious syphilis were 17,675 and 1162.

Pathology

It has been shown that after inoculation by scarification, the micro-organism reaches the nearest lymph nodes of a rabbit in half an hour. The syphilitic lesion of every stage is histologically the same—a granuloma composed of a collection of epithelioid cells, plasma cells, numerous small lymphocytes and some giant cells, with obliterative endarteritis of the vessels. The pathology of syphilis as it affects the nervous and cardiovascular systems is discussed in the appropriate sections. Here it may suffice to sketch the main general effects of syphilis on the vessels, since they cause a large proportion of the serious results of syphilitic infection. A common result of syphilitic arteritis of smaller vessels is occlusion with consequent ischaemia of the territory they nourish. In the primary stage the effect is to produce necrosis of the surface tissue of the sore with erosion or ulceration. The epithelium covering the secondary papule is likely to become necrotic and remain adherent as a fine scale, giving the so-called 'papulosquamous' lesion. The vascular supply is most affected in the gumma or tertiary lesion, leading to necrosis and considerable destruction of tissue, but it has been suggested that there is also a tissue hypersensitivity factor at work. Gummata of bones destroy bony tissue but at the same time provoke a reaction by the periosteum whereby new bone is deposited on the surface of the cortex in irregular fashion and destroyed bone is replaced by densely sclerotic new bone. In the long bones, formation of new bone usually keeps pace with destruction but in the flat bones and particularly those of the skull, destruction is likely to predominate, giving, in neglected cases, the appearance of rounded areas of erosion of bone of which the classical example is the 'worm-eaten' skull. At all stages of syphilis healing is by scar tissue. If the inflammatory infiltrate is small, as in some primary and most secondary lesions, the amount of scar tissue is also small. If there is much infiltration, as in some primary lesions and most tertiary lesions, the scarring may be considerable. Scar formation and subsequent contraction occasionally have important effects on viscera, such as the liver, interfering seriously with their functions.

It is well known that syphilis is a milder disease in females than in males, and experimental evidence suggests that the difference is due to some action of female sex hormones.

Symptoms and Signs

For convenience of description, syphilis is divided into primary, secondary and latent stages in the early phase and latent, tertiary and quaternary stages in the late phases. Some prefer to refer to cardiovascular and neurosyphilis separately rather than to a quaternary stage. The diagnosis of the latent stages depends entirely on serodiagnosis. The division at all stages is only empirical, and it is common experience that one stage may merge into or overlap another.

Primary Syphilis. The incubation period varies from a minimum of 9 days to a maximum of about 90 with an average of 28 days. A small papule, the primary chancre, then appears at the site of inoculation: most commonly there is only one lesion, but there may be two or more. The majority occur on the genitals; only 10 per cent. are extragenital. The papule quickly enlarges to a round or oval lesion of varying size: the surface usually becomes eroded, or perhaps more deeply ulcerated: the eroded area is clean and granular and surrounded by a dull-red areola. Beyond the confines of the eroded area the tissues are infiltrated, giving a feeling of thickening or induration when the base of the lesion is palpated between the finger and the thumb. This induration, on account of which the name of 'hard chancre' has been given to the lesion, may become more and more pronounced until in some cases it feels as though there were a button embedded in the tissues. The sore does not bleed easily when scraped but serum oozes freely from it, and this serum usually contains numerous treponemes. It is comparatively painless.

Individual features vary with the site. Thus, the most indurated primary chancres are those on the mucous surface and edge of the prepuce in males, and on the labia, posterior commissure and cervix uteri in females. In the case of a sore at the reflection of the prepuce on the coronal sulcus, when the prepuce is retracted the lesion may flick over like the tarsal plate when the upper eyelid is everted. A sore at the edge of the prepuce may narrow the preputial orifice causing phimosis. Induration may be felt of a sore in the distal urethra, which may not be visible: the patient may complain of haematuria. Sometimes a primary sore occurs at the external urinary meatus and in either case the diagnosis is made by the discovery of *T. pallidum* in the scanty urethral discharge. With primary sores of the glans penis induration is less easy to appreciate but the sore is easy to recognize by its dull-red areola, even contour, eroded centre and indolent progress. Treponemes may be inoculated into the extragenital sites by kissing, licking or biting during love play and have been seen on the lip, tongue, tonsil, eyelid, cheek, neck, shoulder and breast. They have occasionally been inoculated by tattooing or into the finger of a nurse or doctor examining an infected patient. A chancre of a finger nail may be painful, and thus may be mistaken for a whitlow. The commonest site today for an extragenital chancre is the anal canal of a passive male homosexual.

The course of the primary syphilitic sore varies greatly. In some cases the lesion is fleeting, and its apparent triviality may lead to failure to seek advice: the history of a substantial proportion of cases of late syphilis is that the initial lesion was either unnoticed or ignored. Ordinarily, the primary sore which remains untreated lasts 3–10 weeks and after the erosion has healed over, a button of indurated tissue may remain to mark the site. Weeks or months after healing the sore may break down again in the untreated or inadequately treated patient, the so-called 'monorecidive' or chancre redux. When a syphilitic chancre is infected by secondary organisms, ulceration may be more severe, and it may then be painful.

Shortly after the appearance of the primary sore the lymph nodes often become painlessly enlarged: this involvement may be unilateral or bilateral. The affected nodes may reach a large size, bulging under the overlying skin which, however, does not become reddened. The nodes are of firm, rubbery consistency and remain discrete. The character of the swelling and the absence of signs of acute inflammation often give the clue to the nature of the infection. In females the inguinal nodes remain unaffected if the sore is on the cervix as the lymph drainage is to the glands in the pelvis. Syphilitic lymph nodes do not suppurate unless the sore has become contaminated by secondary organisms, so that the presence of suppuration does not necessarily exclude the diagnosis of syphilis. Some time after the local lymph nodes have begun to enlarge and before other signs of secondary syphilis are found, there may be widespread adenitis, which can be appreciated by palpation of the posterior cervical and epitrochlear nodes.

When the sore is from 7 to 10 days old, the serum commonly gives positive serological reactions. The percentage of cases in which positive results to the serological tests are given increases with the duration of the disease until the appearance of lesions of the skin characteristic of the secondary stage. Patients in the secondary stage always have positive serological tests.

Secondary Stage. In general the skin eruptions of secondary syphilis tend to be widespread, non-irritant, discrete, polymorphic, symmetrically distributed, dull-red in colour, rounded in outline and usually infiltrative to touch.

Commonly, a generalized pinkish rash, the *macular or roseolar rash*, appears 6–8 weeks after the sore. It usually appears on the chest, back and abdomen as rose-pink circular spots, varying in size from 5 to 10 mm., which with age may deepen in colour to a dull red. They may be difficult to see, unless the patient is stripped and viewed in a good light. The eruption may also involve the upper part of the limbs but usually misses the face. It fades in a few weeks, leaving little or no staining.

After the fading of the roseola, a patchy loss of pigment may occur, especially in the pigmented zone of the neck of brunettes. It is rarely seen in men. The depigmented areas are circular and of the same size as the original roseolar spots. The condition has been called syphilitic leucoderma of the neck. It is a residual effect which may persist indefinitely, and therefore assist in diagnosis many years later.

The papular eruption follows closely after the roseolar, and takes a number of different forms, the commonest and usually the earliest being dome-shaped, rounded dull-red papules distributed over the trunk, limbs and face. Most are about the size of a pea, but amongst the smaller papules may be larger ones. The papules are discrete and symmetrically distributed. On palpation with the tips of the fingers they feel induraled. The rash is often described as 'polymorphic' which in this instance means there are spots in different stages of development. Thus, among the papules there will be dull-red macules and some papules showing desquamation on their surfaces. This rash can be called maculopapular. Variations of the ordinary, papular eruption are the papulosquamous, squamous, papulopustular and pustular. In the papulosquamous syphilide a large proportion of the papules are covered at their centre by loose scales. The squamous or psoriasiform syphilide is a papular eruption in which scaling is a still more prominent feature. In the papulopustular syphilide the centre of the papule becomes necrotic, and looks rather like an acne spot. When the whole papule breaks down, a pustular syphilide results, resembling a varicellar or a variolar eruption. The term 'pustular' is a misnomer, because the central areas of the spots consist of necrotic tissue and not of polymorphonuclear leucocytes, but it is time-honoured. A more severe form is the type in which the papule breaks down quickly, and the underlying tissue becomes eroded or ulcerated. As the destruction of tissue extends, the secretion dries to a crust. This may become heaped up by a deposit of successive layers with the formation of limpet-like crusts, blackish or greenish in colour due to altered blood, a condition which is called rupia.

Variations of the Papular Syphilide in Different Situations. Round the anus, between the buttocks, on the lateral surfaces of the scrotum, on the labia, on the inner aspects of the upper thighs, and on other warm moist areas of the body, the papular syphilide often becomes large and prominent, forming fleshy-looking masses, rounded in outline, with broad base and flat top. The surface may become greyish-white, due to necrosis, and after separation of the slough, exudes serum packed with *T. pallidum*. These are the broad condylomata or condylomata lata, the most contagious lesions of early syphilis. They tend to become confluent and after the necrotic tissue is shed from the surface, to present a moist, dull-red, eroded surface, fringed with loose epithelium. They are occasionally found between the toes, under pendulous breasts, in the axillae and at the umbilicus.

On the palms and soles the papules appear as flat or slightly raised spots, varying in size from a pea to a sixpence. They scale easily, leaving collars of loosened epithelium surrounding shining papules. The papular syphilide may be well marked on the face with lesions grouped round the mouth and nose and on the forehead following the margin of the hair, the 'corona veneris'; it is also often possible to find many papules in the hairy scalp. On the face, especially above the nasolabial folds and the chin, the papules sometimes form in rings, so called annular syphilides. In some cases the facial lesions may be hypertrophic, especially at mucocutaneous junctions, appearing like condylomata lata: on account of a resemblance to the lesions of yaws, the condition has been called a framboesiform syphilide.

The small follicular syphilide usually appears later than the early papular eruption. Each lesion is related to a hair follicle and they are found in small clusters of minute dusky-red papules on the trunk, particularly the back. Only in pigmented skins are these lesions found in considerable numbers. The lichenoid syphilide, also a later secondary manifestation, occurs as a small, flat, dull-red elevation, a few millimetres wide and often polyhedral.

Recurrent Papular Eruptions. In untreated or inadequately treated patients recurrences of the papular eruption tend to be much more limited in distribution. One form, the corymbose syphilide, appears as one or only a few rather densely packed groups of papules, the diameter of each group being 20–80 mm. or more. In some cases there is a large papule in the centre of the group and around it, separated by a zone of healthy skin, is a group of smaller papules. The chief sites are the extensor surfaces of the arms, the shoulders, back and abdominal wall.

Alopecia. The hair is shed to a varying degree in the secondary stage—syphilitic alopecia. In most cases the thinning is not particularly noticeable unless the hair is cut short: in others there is an obvious patchy loss, giving the sides and back of the head a moth-eaten appearance; exceptionally the patients may become temporarily bald and women may need to wear a wig. The beard and eyebrows and other body hair may be affected.

Lesions of the Mouth and Throat. Before the secondary rash appears on the body the soft palate may become erythematous. Other lesions of the mouth usually make their first appearance with the papular syphilide of the skin. On the mucous surfaces of the lips and the pillars of the fauces the early syphilide is a rounded greyish-white, slightly raised patch—the so-called mucous patch—edged with a dull-red areola, which marks it off from the surrounding mucous surface. The greyish-white appearance is due to necrosis of the superficial tissues. On the pillars of the fauces the lesions may become confluent and, on separation of the slough, form a serpiginous erosion, sometimes known as the 'snail track' ulcer. On the tonsil the lesion tends to ulcerate more deeply. If a mucous patch on the lip crosses the angle of the mouth it becomes fissured and is called a split papule. On the sides of the tongue there may be fissuring and ulcerations and mouth lesions may occasionally become condylomatous. On the dorsum of the tongue the mucosal lesions appear as dull pink, bald spots after the papillae of the tongue have been shed in the necrotic process. The discharge from any of these lesions teems with treponemes and is very infectious. Mucous patches can also be found in the nose, on the septum and the floor. In the larynx, by suitable examination, they can be seen chiefly on the epiglottis and aryepiglottic folds: they are apt to become eroded and ulcerated, causing the husky voice which may occur in patients suffering from secondary syphilis. These lesions of the mouth and throat are more apt to recur than are those of the skin in untreated or inadequately treated patients.

Other Mucous Membranes. Mucous patches also occur on other mucous membranes, such as those of the vulva, at the vaginal outlet, at the posterior commissure, on the cervix, just within the anal canal, and on the glans penis and the mucous surface of the prepuce. Usually these lesions are eroded and appear sharply defined against the background of normal-looking mucous membrane. At these sites they are usually called mucous erosions. On the genitalia, especially on the glans, eroded papules may be mistaken for multiple primary lesions, especially if other signs of secondary syphilis are absent or inconspicuous.

Lymphadenitis. Rubbery, discrete, non-tender enlargement of lymph nodes, especially those of the posterior triangle of the neck, is common in the secondary stages of the disease.

Bones. Aching pains in the long bones—osteocopic pains—may result from mild periostitis at this stage of the disease. X-rays may also show destructive bone lesions, which may occur in the skull.

The Eye. Acute iridocyclitis of one or both eyes occasionally occurs later in the course of secondary syphilis, but is more common in association with recurrent or relapsing lesions. It may be differentiated from iridocyclitis due to other causes by either clinical or serological evidence of early syphilis and by prompt and satisfactory response to antisyphilitic treatment.

Hepatitis, with jaundice and enlargement of the liver, is occasionally found in the secondary stages of syphilis and responds promptly to antisyphilitic treatment. The spleen may also be palpable.

Epididymitis has been reported in a few cases, usually in the form of small nodules, varying in size from a pea to a marble, in the globus major of the epididymis.

Meningitis. From about the sixth month, or even earlier, the patient may develop symptoms and signs pointing to acute syphilitic meningitis [see Section 15]. It is also well to remember that in up to 25 per cent. of cases of secondary syphilis changes have been reported in the cerebrospinal fluid indicating asymptomatic neurosyphilis, although only a small proportion of these patients develop acute meningitis. If untreated most of these patients will ultimately develop clinical neurosyphilis.

Constitutional Symptoms. In some cases, towards the end of the primary stage or on the appearance of the rash, the patient may develop a mild degree of pyrexia, which may be intermittent, continuous or remittent, and accompanied by some constitutional disturbances, such as headache, malaise, and anorexia. Headache is not uncommon and may be severe and persistent if there is acute meningeal involvement. Patients with mucous patches in the larynx develop hoarseness and others may complain of arthralgic pains without clinical joint involvement.

Moderate degrees of anaemia may be found. The red cell count may be slightly reduced, to between 4,000,000 and 5,000,000 with haemoglobin content as low as 10 g. per 100 ml. In early syphilis the total white cells may reach 20,000 per mm.^{3} but levels of 10,000–12,000 are more common. Lymphocytes predominate and may constitute 65 per cent. of the total; this lymphocytosis may persist for months. The erythrocyte sedimentation rate is usually significantly raised.

Tertiary Stage. In general, the first tertiary lesion is likely to appear from 3 to 10 years after infection. Tertiary or gummatous lesions tend to be localized and asymmetrical in distribution and destructive in character.

The gummatous lesions which involve the skin are of three kinds:

1. *The Nodular Cutaneous Syphilide.* This appears as a group of small gummata arising in the skin of one or more isolated areas of the body. The individual nodules vary in size from a pinhead to a pea. They are rounded, dull-red in colour and firm and elastic on palpation. They often become confluent to form a more or less continuous ridge, arranged in roughly concentric circles, or arcs of circles, or as a serpiginous line of varying length. The affected area is often one that is exposed to injury or constant friction, it may be as small as a finger nail or larger than a hand. The individual gummata may degenerate only so slightly as to produce some scaling, or may ulcerate more deeply and become crusted. The lesion extends centrifugally by the development of more gummata, and leaves in its wake an area of skin which may appear normal, be pigmented or, if the nodules originally ulcerated, may now show non-contractile tissue paper-like scars, following the concentric distribution of the lesion. In some cases with ulceration, extension is more rapid than healing, and a large patch of small ulcers of the skin may be left behind the advancing line of involvement. Sometimes the nodules do not resolve as the lesion extends and dull-red rounded or polycyclic plaques of indurated tissue are formed. These become covered with greyish, waxy-looking crusts and the condition has therefore been named:

2. *The Squamous Tertiary Syphilide.* The lesions often resemble those of psoriasis and have been called on that account psoriasiform tertiary syphilides. The commonest tertiary lesion to involve the skin is:

3. *The Subcutaneous Gumma.* This commences deep to the skin in the subcutaneous or other tissue, such as muscle or periosteum, and presents as an isolated rounded subcutaneous swelling of rubbery consistency. The swelling is painless and may be fluctuant as the necrotic centre may be semifluid. At first the skin over it is not discoloured: when first noticed it may be no more than a small nodule but may slowly increase in size to that of an orange. In due course the expanding swelling is likely to become attached to the overlying skin which then shows dull-red discoloration. The central area of skin then becomes involved in the inflammatory process and breaks down with the formation of a sinus which discharges the necrotic centre developing into a gummatous ulcer. This is highly typical in appearance. It is circular in outline following the contour of the original swelling, or polycyclic if confluence of two or more gummata has occurred. The ulcer is sharply punched out with vertical walls leading down to a granular floor covered with clean dull-red granulations. A tough, yellowish-white slough of necrotic tissue, the wash-leather slough, may remain adherent to walls and floor. The skin surrounding the margin of the ulcer shows dull-red discoloration and squamous change. If the gummatous process commences in or subsequently involves periosteum, the floor of the ulcer consists of necrotic bone. The regional lymph nodes are not involved. On healing, the scar indicates the rounded outline of the original lesion.

The mucous membranes of the mouth and throat are often involved in the tertiary stage of syphilis. The process usually starts in submucous tissue or in deeper structures, such as the periosteum of the hard palate or the musculature of the tongue. The soft palate and uvula are particularly common sites and ulceration is likely to cause erosion or perforation, scarring and subsequent deformity. Sometimes the soft palate becomes adherent to the posterior pharyngeal wall. Perforation of the hard palate may result from gummata originating in the roof of the mouth or in the floor of the nose. Ulceration of the tonsil may be deeply destructive. These conditions are remarkable for their chronicity and for the fact that they produce discomfort rather than pain. Similar lesions may affect the submucous tissues of the nasal cavity causing ulceration and extension to bone, and may result in widespread destruction, especially of the nasal septum including the cartilaginous portion. This may collapse with deformity due to a well-marked groove between the nasal bones and cartilage and perhaps to forward tilting of the nares. All these gummata of mucous membrane are more commonly seen in congenital syphilis.

In the tongue discrete gummata may reach the surface and cause punched-out ulcers, but more commonly the process is a diffuse gummatous infiltration of the muscle following the distribution of the vascular supply. In the initial stages the tongue may be swollen, but the condition is painless and seldom attracts attention. The process runs a chronic course and on healing diffuse fibrosis occurs with subsequent contraction and shrinkage. Later, characteristic changes are seen on the surface, giving the appearance known as chronic superficial glossitis. The changes are three in number, and one or any combination of them may be present. First, contraction of fibrous tissue may produce deep irregular fissuring of the surface of the tongue. Secondly, interference with the blood supply of the mucous membrane renders it abnormally vulnerable to minor injury which causes patchy necrosis of superficial epithelium with irregular white areas of leucoplakia, particularly at the margins of the tongue. Similar patches may be found on the mucous surfaces of the cheeks at the angles of the mouth, or of the lips. Thirdly, there is atrophy of the papillae at the sides and tip of the tongue leaving smooth glazed areas. The patient may complain of pain in the tongue and may be sensitive to acids, spices and hot foods. The condition may, however, be symptomless. Discomfort and pain usually subside with healing of the eroded mucous membrane in the course of a few weeks. The changes in the tongue are permanent. Carcinomatous change in a leukoplakic patch is common and is not prevented by antisyphilitic treatment. It is, therefore, most important to take a biopsy from any suspicious infiltrated area.

In the larynx submucous gummata are common and, on laryngoscopy, may be seen as small rounded swellings above the vocal cords. Deeply destructive ulceration may follow and there may be actual sloughing of laryngeal cartilages. In the developing stages there are alterations of voice and later, in untreated cases, laryngeal stenosis may follow.

Tertiary syphilis of bones causes variable symptoms and signs, and may be difficult to diagnose unless the possibility of such involvement is remembered. Those most commonly affected are the tibia, the bones of the skull, the clavicle, sternum and femur, but none is immune and trauma is frequently a predisposing cause. There may be no symptoms or the patient may complain of pain at the affected site—a gnawing, persistent pain of boring character which is worse at night. If the bone is near the surface an irregular hard swelling may be noticed. In long bones the process is likely to involve a limited segment giving rise to an irregular hard swelling as the result of subperiosteal deposits of new bone. Radiologically the new bone formation can be seen on the surface of the original cortex and the cortical bone is seen to be sclerotic, and therefore more radio-opaque than normal, with, perhaps, some invasion of the medullary cavity. In the flat bones, and particularly those of the vault of the skull, the process is destructive, with rounded areas of osteoporosis surrounded by areas of moderate sclerosis—so-called worm-eaten skull. Severe deformities may result when this destructive process involves the nasal bones, the nasal septum and the palate, which are common sites. After a period of ozaena the bridge of the nose may be destroyed or a large perforation suddenly appear in the hard palate. From the nose the process may spread to the skin with disfiguring ulceration of the face. Syphilitic dactylitis is uncommon, but occasionally causes an indolent painless swelling, usually of the proximal phalanx of a finger. Vertebral gummata are rare but have been known to cause retropharyngeal, lumbar or iliac swellings.

Gummata of the liver are now uncommon. The lesions are usually multiple, and grow to a large size and tend to be destructive. On healing, the liver substance may be intersected by sheets of fibrous tissue which reach the surface, dividing the organ into irregular lobes, the hepar lobatum. The condition may cause jaundice and nodular enlargement of the liver may be felt. Portal obstruction may give rise to portal hypertension and splenic enlargement with its customary consequences [see Section 7].

Tertiary syphilis of the testis is now quite rare. It may be a diffuse, slow painless enlargement of the organ, the 'billiard ball' testis. Testicular sensation is lost. Occasionally localized gummata of the testis produce nodules which may ulcerate through the scrotal skin.

The bursae are not often invaded in tertiary syphilis. The parts affected are those most exposed to stress and strain, such as the pre-patellar bursae in women scrubbers. The swelling is of soft rubbery consistency and shows no signs of acute inflammation. It may involve and ulcerate through the skin like a subcutaneous gumma.

Fever occurs in some patients with tertiary syphilis, and the fact that it is due to this disease may be suggested by its response to antisyphilitic treatment. It has been reported particularly in association with gummatous hepatitis. Syphilis should be remembered as a rare cause in cases of persistent pyrexia of unknown origin. Syphilis of the nervous and cardiovascular systems are considered in the relevant sections [see Sections 8 and 15].

Diagnosis

Primary Stage. It is essential that every genital sore and every inflammatory ulcer elsewhere on the body of which the diagnosis is not obvious should be examined for the presence of treponemes. This should be done before any antiseptics have been applied or antibiotics administered. The sore should first be cleaned with a saline swab and its edge scraped with the edge of a scalpel. It should then be squeezed and the serum collected after it has oozed for a few minutes. When the necessary apparatus is at hand it is better to examine the specimen at once by dark-ground illumination: if it has to be sent away, the serum should be allowed to run into a capillary tube, of which both ends may be sealed with candle grease. Spiral organisms other than *T. pallidum* may be seen in specimens obtained from the genitals or the mouth, but they are largely eliminated by taking care to clean the surface of the lesion before collecting the specimen. Organisms should not be accepted as *T. pallidum* unless they are characteristic in appearance and movement. If the lesion is not easily accessible the nearest enlarged lymph node is punctured and a little of the node fluid is aspirated.

Clinically, primary syphilitic sores are distinguished from others by their comparative painlessness, colour, indolence, surrounding infiltration, slighter tendency to bleed, indolent enlargement of neighbouring lymph nodes. The suspicion must always be confirmed by the demonstration of *T. pallidum*. The length of the incubation period is a guide only when the patient has not been exposed to infection within the previous 9 days.

Various conditions which are commonly found on the genitalia may give rise to difficulty in diagnosis. Several of the more important require brief mention. Herpes genitalis, which is commonly seen, appears as grouped vesicles of pinhead size which break down to small circular erosions. They cause slight irritation and are not indurated. Chancroid, which is now rare, has an incubation period of only a few days, the sores are painful and destructive, and the edges are undermined. There may be an accompanying painful bubo which tends to suppurate and to discharge through a sinus.

Scabetic runs on the glans and skin of the penis itch especially at night; they are mound-like, and not eroded or indurated. Other conditions which must be considered in differential diagnosis include lymphogranuloma venereum, granuloma inguinale, squamous-celled carcinoma, herpes zoster, Behçet's syndrome, chemical or physical trauma and circinate balanitis. To exclude the diagnosis of syphilis it is important to repeat the dark-ground test several times until the sore heals and to test the blood serum for syphilis initially at least monthly for 3 months.

Syphilitic chancres in parts of the body other than the genitals are often overlooked, mainly because the possibility of syphilitic infection is not considered. Unilateral tonsillitis should arouse suspicion, especially if associated with painless enlargement of lymph nodes in the upper part of the anterior triangle of the neck on the affected side. Similarly, the clue to the nature of a syphilitic chancre on the lip may be given by enlargement of lymph nodes of the submental or submaxillary groups. A primary sore affecting the terminal phalanx of a thumb or finger often simulates a whitlow; the syphilitic sore is more brawny and more indolent.

Secondary Stage. The macular syphilide is fairly easy to diagnose if the history of a primary sore with indolent enlargement of regional lymph nodes is obtained. The subcuticular, deeply grounded appearance of the spots, which rarely itch and are pink in colour, is supported by the association of positive serological reactions. Other erythemata are brighter red and may be irritable; they often affect the backs of the hands. The ordinary dome-shaped papular syphilide is usually easy to distinguish from a non-syphilitic eruption. The indurated feel of the papule, the tendency to scale, its dull-red copper colour, its distribution on the face, palms, soles and genitals and its association with lesions of the mouth and throat are all valuable diagnostic signs. The different appearances which a papular syphilide presents in different parts of the body such as dry papules on the trunk and limbs and moist papules in the perianal area, on the genitals, and in other moist warm parts, contrast strongly with non-syphilitic dermatoses, which tend to be true to type, wherever situated. The dark-ground test should always be applied to the exudate from the lesions for rapid diagnosis, even with dry papulosquamous syphilides which will first need to be scarified.

Among the eruptions which may be confused with syphilitic rashes is that of urticaria pigmentosa, but with this condition the spots are dark and not raised, and on rubbing the macule a wheal is formed. Seborrhoea is more superficial and is more scaly, the scales being greasy. Pityriasis rosea is often mistaken for syphilis, but the lesions are brighter in colour and more irritable; they tend to become more angular with their centres covered by branny scales. Ringworm is more superficial and irritable, and the fungus may be found in scrapings from its border. Tinea cruris or dhobie itch affects a triangle at the upper and inner part of the thigh; it is brighter red, more irritable and quite superficial. Drug rashes are more inflammatory and irritable: they appear more suddenly, and are usually associated with a history that the patient has taken a drug which is known to cause such an eruption. The eruptions of specific fevers are usually associated with more pronounced constitutional symptoms. The lesions of acne are pustular and show more inflammatory reaction than secondary syphilides: they affect the upper part of the chest and the back between the shoulders, rather than the flanks, loins and limbs. The spots of molluscum contagiosum are white and umbilicated and caseous matter can be squeezed from their centres. Lichen ruber planus is characterized by flatter, smaller, polygonal spots of a violet tinge and waxy appearance: it is more irritable. Psoriasis is usually superficial, bleeds at a number of points when lightly scraped, and affects the extensor rather than the flexor surface of the limbs: the scales are more silvery, and in moist situations the rash remains true to type; contrasting with the syphilide which forms the moist papule or condyloma latum. Lichen planus papules are difficult to distinguish from a lichenoid syphilide on the penis but typically silvery lesions on the mucous membrane of the cheeks may confirm the diagnosis. Varicella is vesicular at one stage and more superficial and irritable. With variola there is a prodromal stage with fever and backache: the spots are of uniform character and appear first on face and wrists. Pemphigus vegetans may bear a superficial resemblance to condylomata lata, but no *T. pallidum* can be found in serum from the lesions, and usually typical bullae can be found elsewhere on the body and limbs.

Syphilitic condylomata have sometimes been diagnosed as haemorrhoids, but they are usually separated from the anal ring by some normal skin. Condylomata acuminata, or genital warts, are granular and pedunculated. The deeper forms are distinguished from ordinary impetigo by the darker colour of the crusts, the circular rather than the linear shape of the lesions, and the greater degree of tissue destruction below the crusts. Scabies is sometimes mistaken for a crusted syphilide, and the reverse is also true. The individual scabetic lesion is often easy to recognize where it has not been scratched, on the wrists and between the fingers, but it is well to remember that scabies and syphilis often co-exist.

Secondary syphilitic lesions of the mouth can usually be diagnosed by the characteristics described. Vincent's angina is a possible source of error, but the condition is painful and the microscopic findings are characteristic. Glandular fever presenting with sore throat, general adenopathy and a skin rash may give rise to confusion, especially as serological tests for syphilis may be positive.

Tertiary Stage. An indolent swelling, or an ulcer preceded by a swelling, should always arouse a suspicion of syphilis. Denial by the patient of a primary sore, or of secondary lesions, is of little importance, for these may never have appeared or have been long since forgotten. The positive serological reactions may mislead, for some swellings and ulcers in syphilitic patients will prove to be malignant. On the other hand, negative serological reactions are strong but not absolute evidence against tertiary syphilis. Biopsy may be of aid in diagnosis. Space does not permit enumeration of the many conditions from which the lesions of tertiary syphilis may have to be diagnosed. An occasional source of error is epithelioma in the mouth, which is more apt to be painful than a gumma and to appear as a lesion with a raised rolled everted edge. The onset of the condition is frequently determined by old syphilitic glossitis and the presence of positive blood serological tests may thus obscure the diagnosis.

Stasis ulceration on the legs may be diagnosed by lesions much less regular in contour, less sharply punched out, and associated with more evidence of acute inflammation and of venous stasis. They tend to occur nearer the ankles.

Treatment

Preventive. The value of any method of prevention of syphilitic infection has always been difficult to determine. Local cleansing and the use of antiseptics have been recommended and practised for many years, but with any such procedure the failures are obvious enough and the successes never known. Clearly no method of disinfection is likely to be successful unless it is promptly applied. The local application of antiseptic may prevent the appearance of the syphilitic chancre without eliminating the disease and if it is used the patient should be followed up with blood tests for at least 3 months.

Prophylaxis by ingestion or injection of antisyphilitic remedies should not be practised, because the effect may be to mask the symptoms for many months without curing the patient. Since the introduction of penicillin for the treatment of syphilis a good deal has been said and written about the desirability of abortive or prophylactic treatment of the patient who has taken a risk of contracting syphilis. To give such treatment is tantamount to accepting the diagnosis, and logically, should be followed by observation and testing for at least 2 years with due restrictions as regards marriage and family life. Quite apart from the prolonged anxiety involved there are obvious disadvantages to the patient, who in most cases can be pronounced free from infection with certainty after 3 months. On the other hand this type of treatment may be necessary in underdeveloped countries where adequate diagnostic tests are not available. Accidental infection of fingers, lips and other extragenital parts is best prevented by avoiding contamination with fresh secretions from patients in the early stages of infection. The patients should be warned of the risks arising from sharing table utensils, crockery and house linen with others. They should not kiss others nor talk directly into people's faces, and articles which they have used should be dipped in very hot water. Doctors and nurses should wear gloves when handling such patients and then wash with soap and water. With modern methods of treatment the exudates cease to be infectious within 24 hours.

Curative. The remedies most commonly employed for the treatment of syphilis have been preparations of (1) arsenic, (2) bismuth, (3) mercury, (4) penicillin, (5) iodine, (6) other antibiotics. The first four and last destroy parasites: iodine promotes the absorption o granulomatous tissue. There is now general agreement that penicillin is the drug of choice and many believe that the use of other remedies in addition is unnecessary and undesirable. The different remedies will be described and their use in the management of syphilis discussed.

Arsenical Preparations. These are organic compounds in which the arsenic is trivalent or pentavalent. At the present time the accepted view in most parts of the world is that their use for the treatment of syphilis is no longer justified.

Mercurial Preparations. Mercury was formerly the main remedy for the treatment of syphilis but in the early 1920s it was almost entirely superseded by bismuth. It was, however, used occasionally when injections were impracticable.

Preparations of Bismuth. Bismuth was applied to the treatment of syphilis in 1921 and it supplanted mercury in all cases for which intramuscular or deep subcutaneous injection of heavy metal was indicated. Before the introduction of penicillin the almost universal practice was to use bismuth, which was more effective and better tolerated than mercury, in conjunction with arsenical preparations for the treatment of syphilis in all stages, except general paralysis.

Bismuth is administered exclusively by the intramuscular route, and many different preparations are available. Insoluble suspensions of bismuth have been those most commonly used for antisyphilitic treatment. Only one of these preparations now remains in the British Pharmaceutical Codex, namely, bismuth oxychloride injection, which is a watery suspension containing 100 mg. per ml.

The toxic effects are few. Care must be taken to avoid injecting preparations of bismuth into veins because they are then highly toxic, and, if an insoluble preparation is used, pulmonary embolism may result.

A slaty-blue line commonly appears at the margin of the gums of patients receiving this treatment, especially adjoining the molar teeth. It is due to the formation and deposition of bismuth sulphide and is only found in association with infection of the gums.

Albuminuria is found occasionally, especially with the soluble preparations. It is an indication to stop bismuth. The urine should be tested before each injection. The place of bismuth in the treatment of syphilis is now restricted to preliminary treatment of some cases of late syphilis before penicillin is given, and its value even in this respect is debatable. For this purpose the insoluble preparations are probably the most satisfactory.

Penicillin. The general properties and the methods of administration of penicillin are described in Section 1. Here it is necessary only to describe: (1) the effect of the drug on the different manifestations of syphilis; (2) the methods of using it for the treatment of syphilis which seem most effective in the light of knowledge available at the time of writing; and (3) the toxic effects which may be encountered in the course of this treatment.

Of the various preparations of penicillin available benzylpenicillin (penicillin G) appears to be the most effective for the treatment of syphilis. Investigative work in the United States indicated that pure crystalline benzylpenicillin gave results which were moderately superior to those obtained with amorphous penicillin.

Penicillin, in appropriate doses, has an effect upon *T. pallidum* which is at least equal to that of the best arsenical compounds, and correspondingly its effects in producing healing of the various manifestations susceptible to the action of the arsenical compounds is at least as satisfactory. Penicillin has, of course, the great advantage over the arsenical compounds that for most patients it is non-toxic, and it is possible to give large doses frequently with impunity. An important therapeutic advantage over the arsenical compounds is that it reaches the foetus *in utero* far more easily. It is effective in preventing infection of the foetus, or in curing the foetus if it is already infected. For the treatment of neurosyphilis, also, the effect of penicillin appears to be superior to older methods of treatment even though the drug appears in the cerebrospinal fluid either in small quantities or not at all after intramuscular administration at ordinary dosage level. Whether penicillin should be used alone or in conjunction with other antisyphilitic remedies will be discussed in the appropriate section.

The effective treatment of syphilis does not require high levels of penicillin in the blood and therefore various preparations have been devised to delay the absorption of penicillin when given by intramuscular injection, suspending it in media which repel body fluids. The effect is to give a prolonged, constant but comparatively low level of the drug in the blood. Effective blood levels of penicillin can be maintained for as long as 24 hours by a single dose of 600 mg. (600,000 Units) of procaine penicillin suspended in 2 ml. of oil or water. This method is therefore applicable to the treatment of out-patients. A further development is the addition of the water-repellent aluminium monostearate in 2 per cent. concentration to an oily suspension of procaine penicillin of fine particle size (PAM). This still further prolongs absorption so that the effect of an average dose may extend over several days. Further prolongation with low levels can be obtained by the use of benzathine penicillin (dibenzylethylenediamine penicillin). A single dose of 2·4 mega Units (1·8 G.) of this preparation is likely to give an effective level of penicillin in the patients blood for about 2 weeks. Unfortunately this preparation is apt to cause local pain at the site of injection but this may be diminished by injecting half of the quantity required into each buttock. By this means the treatment of syphilis with penicillin may be restricted to one or two injections.

Toxic Effects of Penicillin. The general problems of reactions to penicillin and their treatment are considered in Section 1. Here it is necessary only to discuss certain points peculiar to the treatment of syphilis with this drug.

Jarisch-Herxheimer Reaction. This is a focal and general reaction which may follow the use of a rapidly effective drug, such as penicillin or an arsenical, at the commencement of treatment. It occurs in more than 50 per cent. of cases of primary and secondary syphilis in which the first injection may be followed within a few hours by fever, headache, malaise, pain in the joints and limbs and exacerbation of the symptoms and signs of infection. At this stage it is not harmful but the patient should be warned of the possibility that it may occur. Ordinarily the reaction occurs within 12 hours and is over in less than 24 hours from the time of the injection. The cause is unknown and there is little evidence to support the theory that it results from liberation of toxins following the destruction of large numbers of treponemes. In the late stages of syphilis the reaction is less common and usually slight. It occurs in about 25 per cent. of the cases but in most of them there is no more than slight fever of which the patient may be unaware. Occasionally, however, serious results have followed through exacerbation of severe involvement of the central nervous system, thrombosis of a large cerebral vessel or blockage of the ostium of a coronary artery, perforation of the aortic wall or of an aneurysm, or oedema of the glottis in cases of gummatous lesions of the larynx. Such cases are rare and many physicians have used penicillin as the initial remedy in cases of late syphilis without ill effects. Nevertheless, nothing is to be gained by speed and intensity of treatment in these cases and it seems reasonable to adopt some precautionary measures to prevent hazards, however unlikely. It has been suggested that patients with late syphilis should commence treatment with very small doses of penicillin with gradual increase of dosage, but experimental work has shown this to be an ineffective precaution. The reaction appears to be of the 'all or none' type: it does not occur with a minute dose but does occur when the 'trigger' dose is reached and then with full force, irrespective of the size of the dose. The reaction occurs once and is hardly ever repeated. In most cases the reaction can be prevented by a preliminary course of injections of insoluble bismuth which, of course, acts much more slowly and seldom produces this effect. Bismuth, however, will not protect from the Jarisch-Herxheimer reaction in cases of general paralysis. Small doses of steroid hormones, such as prednisone, 5 mg. given before each of the first two injections of penicillin, appear to have been effective in preventing or diminishing the reaction, but higher doses may be needed.

The Effects of Penicillin on the Diagnosis of Syphilis. Penicillin given for other diseases is sometimes a source of confusion in the diagnosis of syphilis. For instance, serious difficulties may arise in the cases of patients treated with penicillin for pneumonia, or for surgical infections, who are later found to have positive serological tests for syphilis. In such cases it is necessary to distinguish between biologically false positive results and true positives which indicate that the patient is suffering from syphilis. The decision requires careful study of the patient, and if necessary, examination and testing of contacts. The treponemal immobilization (TPI) test may help. If the result of careful investigation leaves the diagnosis in doubt and the amount of treatment has been inadequate by accepted standards, then full treatment should be given followed by the necessary observation and tests presently to be discussed.

If the patient has acquired early syphilis and gonorrhoea at the same time, penicillin given for treatment of gonorrhoea may delay or even suppress the lesions of syphilis without curing the patient. On this account it has been customary to observe the following rules when giving penicillin for the treatment of patients with gonorrhoea:

1. All patients with gonorrhoea should have blood taken for routine tests for syphilis before treatment is given.

2. Penicillin should not be used for the treatment of patients with gonorrhoea who also have lesions suggestive of syphilis until those lesions have been fully investigated.

3. All patients treated with penicillin for gonorrhoea should remain under observation with monthly serological tests for at least 3 months.

4. A sharp febrile reaction within the first 24 hours after the use of penicillin for gonorrhoea suggests the possibility of concurrent early syphilitic infection, as it has been shown that the Jarisch-Herxheimer reaction may occur in the incubation period of syphilis.

Iodine Preparations. Iodides promote the absorption of syphilitic granulation tissue and may be useful in the later stages of infection. Potassium iodide is most often given by mouth in doses of 0·3–2 G. thrice daily. It is usually prescribed with alkali to avoid gastro-intestinal disturbances. Most patients tolerate 0·3–0·6 G. three times a day without difficulty, but iodism may result from higher dosage. The benefit to be derived from this remedy is not now sufficient to justify perseverance with it in the face of major discomfort and its use is now usually limited to a therapeutic test to confirm the diagnosis of a gummatous lesion.

Other Antibiotics. No other antibiotic is as effective as penicillin in the treatment of syphilis but some have antitreponemal effect and are useful for the treatment of patients who are sensitized to penicillin. Most experience has been obtained with the tetracyclines. Chlortetracycline, oxytetracycline and tetracycline are all effective. They have the disadvantage that they are best given by mouth and careful supervision is essential to ensure that the drugs are taken.

Good results have also been reported with chloramphenicol but the experimental work suggests that it is less effective than the tetracyclines. Because of its potential toxic effects it should not be used for the treatment of syphilis.

Experimental work suggests that erythromycin may be as effective as tetracycline in the treatment of syphilis but experience with it is less. It is usually given by mouth and because of this and the fact that it is not yet established by experience as a fully satisfactory remedy, close observation and follow-up are essential.

The Treatment of Acquired Syphilis

The main principles to be observed in the treatment of syphilis are as follows: (1) Treatment should begin as soon as possible after a diagnosis has been established. The earlier treatment is begun the better the results. (2) The amount and duration of treatment should be sufficient to ensure the probability of cure but over-treatment should be avoided. (3) Due attention should be given to the general health of the patient. (4) Observation and testing after treatment should be careful and prolonged. There are some failures following all methods of treatment and long observation may be necessary before these can be recognized.

Early Syphilis. It is now generally agreed that penicillin alone is sufficient for the treatment of early syphilis: the addition of other remedies does not increase the efficacy of treatment and adds to the hazards.

The following are accepted methods for the treatment of early syphilis:

1. Ten to twelve daily intramuscular injections, each of 600 mg. (600,000 Units) of procaine penicillin, in watery suspension. This employs relatively few injections which are painless: it avoids admission to hospital.

2. Ten to twelve daily intramuscular injections, each of 600 mg. (600,000 Units) of procaine penicillin in oil with 2 per cent. aluminium monostearate (PAM). These injections can be given every 2 or 3 days with equally good effect. The main advantage of daily administration is that the period of treatment is shortened and the presence of a series of depots in the tissues will prolong treatment for a week or more after the course of injections is finished. Some prefer to commence the course of treatment with a single large injection of 2·4 G. (2·4 mega Units) of the preparation, especially in cases of secondary syphilis. If the patient ceases to attend this dosage is likely to render him non-infectious and gives a possibility of cure.

3. A single dose of 1·8 G. (2·4 mega Units) of benzathine penicillin, of which half is usually injected into each buttock. This has the advantage that only one injection is required and thus may be useful in under-developed countries where follow-up is limited. It has the disadvantage that it gives local pain and may give rise to difficulty if the patient proves to be sensitized to the drug. The percentage cure rate is not quite so high as with multiple injection courses.

4. If the patient is sensitized to penicillin other antibiotics must be used. On the present evidence the remedies of choice are tetracycline, oxytetracycline and erythromycin. Tetracycline is given by mouth in dosage of 30–40 G. over a period of 10–15 days. One method is to give two capsules (0·85 G.) four times daily for 15 days. The recommended dosage of erythromycin is 20–30 G. over a period of 10–15 days, the daily dosage being 500 mg. every 6 hours. If the patient is pregnant it is probably better to use erythromycin because there are some doubts about the possible effects of tetracycline upon the foetus. Experience of these and other substitutes for penicillin in the treatment of syphilis is encouraging but still inadequate and careful follow-up is essential in these cases.

Observation After Treatment. Following treatment with penicillin the patient should remain under close observation with monthly clinical examinations and tests of the blood for the first 6 months, and thereafter examinations and blood tests every 3 months for at least a further 18 months. The cerebrospinal fluid should be obtained by lumbar puncture and tested during the second year of observation. If, however, the blood tests remain positive beyond the expected period, or if a relapse occurs, it is advisable to test the fluid earlier. If the response to penicillin is satisfactory in other respects and tests of cerebrospinal fluid are negative, the fluid need not be tested again.

After two years of observation, cure may be presumed.

Failures of treatment. The critical period for the development of clinical or serological relapse is between the fourth and ninth months after treatment.

The indications for further treatment are three in number:

1. *Clinical Relapse.* When the relapse is of the mucocutaneous or infectious type it may be impossible to be sure that the patient has not been reinfected. Cases of true relapse are partly resistant to treatment and on re-treatment it is advisable to double the original length of the penicillin course and to consider the advisability of giving, in addition, further courses of the drug. The birth of a syphilitic child to a treated syphilitic mother is a form of clinical relapse.

2. *Serological Relapse.* This is said to occur when tests originally negative, as with sero-negative primary syphilis, become positive; tests originally positive become negative and then positive again; tests originally positive show at first no change or decline in the quantitative titre, but subsequently show progressive rise in titre; or when tests of the cerebrospinal fluid, originally negative, become positive. Serological relapse commonly precedes clinical relapse.

3. *Serological Resistance.* This is very rare, if it in fact occurs. The decision as to the period of time after which persistence of positive serological tests is regarded as evidence of failure of treatment of early syphilis is an arbitrary one. In much of the experimental work on the subject the period was fixed at 1 year after treatment. For the routine management, failure may be presumed if the quantitative tests show no fall in titre after 6–9 months of observation, but this may in fact indicate that the patient's original diagnosis was of late and not of early syphilis.

Late Syphilis. After the second year of infection the details of treatment depend largely on the presence or absence of visceral, cardiovascular or neurological involvement, the treatment of which is discussed elsewhere in this book. It is thus important not only to examine carefully the cardiovascular and nervous systems, but also to test the cerebrospinal fluid and X-ray the aorta as part of the routine investigation. If tests of the fluid are negative they are unlikely to become positive later, and the central nervous system is unlikely to be affected.

Latent Syphilis. In these cases the only evidence of the disease is the positive serological tests. In the past it was shown that such patients who received full dosage with arsenicals and bismuth remained in good health after prolonged observation in more than 95 per cent. of the cases, whether or not the serological tests became negative. Penicillin is no more effective than arsenic and bismuth in reversing positive serological tests to negative in these cases. Full assessment of the value of penicillin in these cases will take many years. Its use for the treatment of latent syphilis is based on the reasonable assumption that, being of value for early syphilis, it must also be effective in late syphilis. Penicillin has the advantage of brevity and safety and it is common practice to use it for the latent stages of the disease. Many patients with latent syphilis report improvement in general health after this treatment.

Benign Late Syphilis. The evidence is that prompt healing of cutaneous, mucosal and osseous gummata, and other benign late lesions, follows the administration of 2·4–4·8 mega Units of penicillin. Common practice is to use rather more penicillin, such as from 6 to 9 mega Units spread over 10–15 days. As for early syphilis it is a good practice to give a daily injection of 600 mg. (600,000 Units) of a reliable preparation of procaine penicillin. The results are as good as those obtained with arsenicals and bismuth and the treatment is, of course, much shorter and much safer.

The fact that serological tests remain strongly positive after this treatment in many of the cases is not an indication for further treatment. On the other hand, prolonged observation is important and re-treatment should be undertaken on any evidence of clinical relapse. There is some evidence that steroid drugs may reactivate syphilitic lesions so they are contra-indicated.

Whether it is justifiable to use penicillin in the treatment of these cases of late syphilis without preliminary treatment with injections of bismuth and perhaps iodide by mouth is an open question. The tendency in the United States is to discount the importance of the Jarisch-Herxheimer reaction. There is no doubt that serious effects of this reaction are rare and they present no problem in the majority of cases. There remains the possibility of some serious effect in an occasional case. It is obviously impossible to exclude by clinical examination the contingency of asymptomatic involvement of vital organs, and nothing is to be gained by speed and intensity of treatment in cases of long standing. Some clinicians give preliminary treatment with weekly intramuscular doses of 0·3 G. of an insoluble preparation of bismuth for 3–4 weeks, combining the treatment with 300–600 mg. of potassium iodide by mouth three times a day. Others use prednisone, 5 mg. by mouth before the first two injections of penicillin. If the possibility of a severe Jarisch-Herxheimer reaction is anticipated this dosage may be raised to 5 mg. three times daily for 2 days before the penicillin is started, and continued at the same dose for the first 2 days of the penicillin course.

Asymptomatic Neurosyphilis. In cases of latent syphilis in which positive changes in tests of the cerebrospinal fluid indicate involvement of the central nervous system, it is customary to give a rather longer course of injections of penicillin. Common practice is to give a daily injection of 600 mg. (600,000 Units) of procaine penicillin for 21 days, totalling 12·6 G. In these cases the guide to the efficacy of treatment is the cell count and the protein content of the cerebrospinal fluid. Earliest and most striking is the reduction of the cell count which, in successful cases, returns to normal 10–24 weeks after treatment. The protein content also responds, but rather less promptly. Normal values are usually reached by the sixth month and maintained thereafter. The Wassermann reaction and colloidal tests improve more slowly and may show positive changes for an indefinite period. The response of these tests is more prompt and satisfactory with early than with late asymptomatic neurosyphilis. The usual practice is to give no additional treatment if the patient remains well and the cell count and protein level in the cerebrospinal fluid remain within normal limits. Tests of the cerebrospinal fluid should be repeated at intervals of 6 months for the first year after treatment and thereafter yearly till satisfactory reversal has occurred.

If further treatment is required a second course of penicillin should be given. For the rare failures of treatment with penicillin, pyretotherapy is the best form of supplementary treatment. This may be given by inoculation with the parasite of benign tertian malaria, allowing ten or more paroxysms of fever before suppression with antimalarial therapy. Alternatively, fever may be given by repeated intravenous injections of vaccine such as typhoid-paratyphoid (TAB) vaccine. Pyretotherapy is a highly technical procedure which will be rarely indicated, and should not be undertaken without full knowledge of the technique and of its possible complications.

Syphilis and Marriage. For complete safety the syphilitic patient should be advised not to marry, or if already married not to cohabit with the partner in marriage, until cure may be presumed following 2 years of observation after treatment. This is the kind of advice which is seldom taken and most clinicians are satisfied with lesser standards. If treatment appears to have been successful the risk is probably very slight after a year of observation and, provided that the partner in marriage is made aware of the slight risk, permission to marry or to resume married life may be given at this time.

CONGENITAL SYPHILIS

An infected mother can transmit syphilis to her offspring long after she has ceased to be sexually contagious. In general the more recent her infection the more severe the effects of transmitted infection on the foetus. The theoretical course of the obstetric history of a syphilitic woman is stated in Kassowitz's Law, according to which each pregnancy results in miscarriage progressively later in pregnancy, followed by the delivery of stillborn or macerated foetuses at term, then by living syphilitic infants and finally by healthy infants. This kind of history, which is presumed to be due to gradual attenuation of infection, is seldom obtained. In practice, miscarriages may alternate with stillborn or living syphilitic children and a healthy infant may be born between two who are infected. It has even occurred that only one of twins was syphilitic. It is now generally agreed that infection always occurs from the mother by way of the placenta and that infection is not transmitted in the first 3 months of life. It may be assumed that miscarriage in the first 3 months of pregnancy is not due to syphilis. In the past it has been stated that the syphilitic placenta can be recognized by macroscopic appearances and, with more certainty, by microscopic changes in the chorionic villi. This view is now discredited and it seems clear that examination of the placenta does not help in this diagnosis unless *T. pallidum* can be found, which is seldom possible.

Congenital syphilis is now quite rare. The figures of incidence for England and Wales for 1970 were only 11 cases in infants in the first year of life. Cases diagnosed in older patients amounted to 185. The death rate per 1000 live births of infants under one year was nil.

Symptoms and Signs

The clinical manifestations of congenital syphilis may be divided into three groups: those which appear early, those which appear late, and the stigmata. The early lesions are those which occur in the first 2 years of life. These are, for the most part, infectious and resemble those of secondary syphilis in the adult, the late lesions include gummata indistinguishable from those of tertiary syphilis, and the stigmata are scars of deformities resulting from developing tissues being damaged by the treponemes.

Early. *The Skin and Mucous Membranes.* The syphilitic infant born alive may show an eruption of large, rounded, dusky-red papules surrounded by bullae on the palms or soles containing serum or pus, the so-called bullous eruption of syphilitic pemphigus. The fluid contains *T. pallidum* in large numbers. Some 3–4 weeks after birth or perhaps considerably later, various rashes may appear which are identical in appearance with those found in secondary syphilis. The papular eruption is the commonest. All these eruptions tend to be widespread, involving the whole of the trunk and limbs, but they may be particularly well marked in the napkin area, on the skin round the nose and mouth and on the palms and soles. Annular lesions are particularly common and there may be extensive crusting. In moist areas and where the rash is exposed to friction, the affected areas may become reddened and glazed. Condylomata may be found especially in the anogenital area, and, where the rash is profuse and becomes confluent at the angles of the mouth and nose, ulcerative fissures may form. These sometimes leave radiating linear scars, rhagades, which remain as signs of the disease. Sometimes the skin has a yellowish-brown *café-au-lait* colour, and if as is common, there is much wasting, it may be wrinkled, giving the infant's face the appearance which has been called the 'old man' look. There may be patchy loss of hair, chiefly at the sides and back of the scalp, syphilitic alopecia. Rarely the syphilitic infant may grow an abundant crop of hair, the syphilitic wig. Syphilitic papules may involve the nail beds, causing infiltration and oozing of serum round the nails which may be loosened and shed—syphilitic paronychia. The new nails may be opaque, irregular and narrowed at the base. Mucous patches may be found in the nose, mouth, throat and larynx. The nasal lesions may cause a persistent and blood-stained discharge and nasal obstruction may lead to difficulty in feeding. The nasal discharge is infectious and syphilitic papules may appear at the margins of the nares. Discharge and obstruction give the typical picture of syphilitic snuffles. As the result of laryngeal infection the infants cry may be hoarse and raucous. Anaemia is common in these severely affected infants.

Lymphadenitis. Rubbery discrete non-tender enlargement of the lymph nodes may be noted.

Liver and Spleen. As the result of early syphilitic infection the abdomen may be grossly swollen, due to enlargement of liver and spleen. The enlargement of the liver is due to abnormal persistence of foetal blood-forming islands and to pericellular fibrosis, resulting from the treponemal infection.

The Bones. The long bones may be affected in various ways. In the first six months of life osteochondritis is a common result and may be detected early by radiographic examination. In severe cases the ends of the bones may be very painful and tender, and, because of the pain on movement, the infant may appear to be paralysed, syphilitic pseudoparalysis, or may scream when handled. Swelling of the epiphyseal ends of the bones may be obvious. Pathological fractures and separation of epiphyses are possible sequelae. Radiologically, epiphyses may be enlarged, the epiphyseal line is broad and irregular, and the zone of provisional calcification is sclerotic and shows irregularity like the teeth of a saw. There are irregular patches of osteoporosis in the diaphyses, particularly at the metaphyseal ends, and there is subperiosteal deposition of new bone. In the second 6 months of life the signs of osteochondritis disappear, but the evidence of periostitis persists and becomes more marked. Successive layers of new bone are laid down on the surface of the cortex under the periosteum in regular fashion. Dactylitis may occur in the second year of life. It may cause fusiform swelling of the proximal phalanges of one or more fingers, or, more rarely, toes.

Choroiditis may occur in the early months of life and may be overlooked. Iritis is rare.

Late. Lesions of the tertiary type may appear as early as the third year of life or at any time subsequently. They occur most commonly between the ages of 7 and 14 but may be delayed until adult life. Gummata involving the skin have no features which distinguish them from similar lesions due to acquired syphilis. Gummata of the mouth and throat are particularly common and may result in perforation of the palate and pillars of the fauces. Gummatous destruction of the nasal septum may involve the cartilage and result in collapse of the nasal cartilage which it supports. In consequence the nose may be deformed with a groove at the junction of the nasal bones and cartilage and perhaps upwards tilting of the nares.

The commonest late lesion is interstitial keratitis, which may begin at any age from 4 to 30 years, or even later. Usually it starts in one eye, but in spite of treatment the other is likely to be involved after an interval which may vary from a few weeks to many years. The patient complains of photophobia and pain in the affected eye. At first there is seen to be injection of the sclerotic coat at the margin of the cornea, and from the limbus blood vessels extend into its deep layers, becoming clinically obvious as a pink patch—the salmon patch—or detected only with the aid of the slit lamp and corneal microscope. At the same time there is an exudation of lymphocytes into the deep layers of the cornea, causing haziness or ground-glass appearance of the normally transparent membrane. The condition is frequently associated with iridocyclitis which may be masked by the severity of the process in the cornea. The outcome is variable. The attack may clear in a few weeks without damage to the sight, or it may persist for many months and the patient may be prone to subsequent relapses. Even with severe attacks the damage to sight may be slight, but central opacities of the cornea are a common end result and vision may be grossly impaired in consequence.

Nerve deafness from involvement of the nerve endings of the VIIIth cranial nerve in the internal ear affects some patients who suffer from interstitial keratitis, but occurs rather later. It may occur independently of corneal infection. The result may be bilateral progressive deafness which may become complete. An audiogram shows a typical hearing loss in the high frequency range. Keratitis, nerve deafness and the characteristic deformity of the upper central incisors described below are sometimes called Hutchinson's triad.

Other later effects of congenital syphilis are diffuse interstitial orchitis and effusion into both knee joints without pain or interference with movement, Clutton's joints, which are found at any time from the ages of 5 to 25. Between the ages of 8 and 14, and sometimes earlier, these children may develop gummatous osteoperiostitis of the long bones, particularly the tibiae. The pathology of this condition is the same as that which occurs in adults, but the process is often widespread and may involve the whole length of the bones. Thickening of the tibia is commonly most marked on the anterior surface of the middle third of the bone giving a forward convexity and appearance of curvature, the bowed or sabre-shaped tibia. There is no true curvature of the bone because the periostitis strengthens rather than weakens the cortex. In the early years of life there may be areas of localized thickening of the bones of the vault of the skull—the periosteal or Parrot's nodes.

Congenital syphilis may not only cause anaemia and marasmus in infants and young children, but also delay development and increase the liability to intercurrent infections in infancy and later years. The visceral and central nervous system lesions of congenital syphilis are described in other sections of this book. Aortitis is rarely seen as the result of congenital syphilitic infection.

Stigmata. Scars and deformities result from the lesions which have been described. Facial disfigurement may be due to several causes. Severe and prolonged rhinitis may result in failure of normal development of the bones which surround the nasal cavity. Thus, flattening of the bridge of the nose may give the deformity known as saddle-nose; under-development of the superior maxilla may make it appear that the mandible is overdeveloped—the so-called bulldog jaw, healed periosteal nodes of the frontal bone may give abnormal prominence of the forehead—frontal bossing; and the combination of these deformities is sometimes called the bulldog facies. Corneal scarring with empty blood vessels at the periphery of the cornea, seen on the corneal microscope, rhagades, sabre-shaped tibiae, perforations of the palate and nasal septum, collapse of the nasal cartilage, are all common stigmata. The fundus oculi may show the changes of old healed choroidoretinitis which are usually peripheral and bilateral.

The upper central and other incisors of the permanent dentition may show narrowing at the cutting edge, as compared with the width of the tooth at the gingival margin, together with curving of the margins, antero-posterior thickening and, in some cases, a crescentic notch at the cutting edge—Hutchinson's teeth. Less often the first lower molars show a dome-shaped deformity of the grinding surface to which are attached the undeveloped cusps in the form of four small projections—Moon's molars. The dental dystrophies result from the effect of severe syphilitic infection upon the developing buds of these teeth.

Diagnosis

If there are bullous or other moist lesions *T. pallidum* can usually be found by the dark-ground method without difficulty. Scraping of the dry lesions of the skin may also make it possible to find the organism. The results of serological tests must be interpreted with reserve in the first weeks of life. Infants with negative serological tests may be suffering from incubating syphilis. On the other hand, non-syphilitic infants may give positive serological tests for syphilis if the mothers' tests are positive, due to antibody carry-over across the placental barrier.

In cases of doubt antisyphilitic treatment should be withheld at birth and quantitative tests on the infant should be repeated at weekly intervals. If it is not infected the strength of the test declines progressively to negative, usually within a few weeks. If the titre of the reaction fails to decline or increases over a period of weeks, infection is probable. Confirmatory evidence can usually be obtained from physical examination of the infant and from radiographic changes in the long bones which are present early.

Provided that the possibility of syphilitic infection is remembered the diagnosis should not present great difficulties. The bullous rash may be confused with staphylococcal pemphigus neonatorum, but the former appears earlier and is nearly always found on the palms and soles. Lesions in the napkin area may be mistaken for a napkin rash, but the latter is brighter red in colour and does not extend into the folds of groins and buttocks. The rashes of early congenital syphilis are nearly always associated with other signs.

Treatment

Preventive. The prevention of transmission to offspring is primarily a matter of prevention of infection of mothers. The precautions to be observed in relation to marriage and syphilis and the rules for cohabitation of those who become infected after marriage have been described. Most cases of transmission result, however, from undiagnosed and unsuspected infection, and for this reason all pregnant women should be fully examined and tested serologically during pregnancy. This precaution does not give absolute protection because of the possibility that the mothers may be incubating syphilis when examined or that they may be infected later, but it has certainly prevented many cases of congenital syphilis. Treatment of the syphilitic pregnant woman will almost certainly prevent transmission of infection. In the days of prolonged chemotherapy with arsenicals and bismuth it was the general experience that treatment begun before the end of the fourth month of pregnancy nearly always protected the foetus. Treatment begun later or interrupted for any reason was less certain in its effects but still provided a degree of protection corresponding to the amount and duration of the treatment administered. In this respect penicillin has proved an important advance in efficacy of treatment. Adequate dosage at any stage of pregnancy may be expected to ensure freedom of the offspring from infection in 98 per cent. of the cases. A convenient method is to give the mother a daily intramuscular injection of 600 mg. (600,000 Units) of procaine penicillin in oily or watery suspension for 10–12 days, the total dosage being 6–7·2 G. It is a reasonable precaution to repeat this course of injections of penicillin in the next succeeding pregnancy even though evidence points to the fact that the mother is already cured.

Curative. There is no justification for treating the newly born infant of a syphilitic mother for syphilis as a precautionary measure without first confirming the diagnosis. In cases of difficulty the correct diagnosis can always be made with certainty in due course and the infant is not likely to suffer in consequence. On the other hand to assume the diagnosis and treat before it is confirmed establishes the necessity for prolonged observation, frequent tests of the blood and tests of the cerebrospinal fluid. At the same time a lifelong stigma is attached to the patient which may result in much unhappiness.

When the fact of infection has been established, the infant should be treated with injections of penicillin. Total dosage may be calculated at the rate of 500 mg. (500,000 Units) of penicillin per kg. of body weight. Thus, for an infant weighing 4 kg. the total dosage would be 2 G. (2,000,000 Units). An effective method of giving the treatment would be to give 200 mg. (200,000 Units) of procaine penicillin suspension intramuscularly each day for 10 days.

The result of such treatment in cases of early congenital syphilis are so good that further treatment is usually not required. Treponemes disappear from surface lesions within a matter of hours, lesions heal promptly and serological tests for syphilis usually become negative after periods varying from a few weeks to 4 months and thereafter remain negative. It is rare to find pathological changes in cerebrospinal fluid tested a year after treatment.

If indication for further treatment arises, a further course of injections of penicillin can be given with the likelihood of a good result.

In cases of late congenital syphilis the treatment is similar, with dosage of penicillin based in the same way on body weight. The results are good but it is to be anticipated that in a number of these cases serological tests will remain positive in spite of treatment, and this is not necessarily an indication to continue treatment. On the other hand, evidence of clinical or serological relapse, as already defined, or of continuing activity of infection of the central nervous system, as shown by a persistent high cell count or excess of protein in the cerebrospinal fluid, call for more intensive treatment.

Observation after treatment should be prolonged, and certainly should continue until growth ceases, for, although the results of treatment are excellent, there are likely to be occasional failures. Provided that the patient remains clinically well with, in the case of early infection, negative serological tests, the tests of the cerebrospinal fluid need not be repeated if they are negative at the end of 1 year after treatment.

Certain of the late manifestations appear to run their course irrespective of treatment. Interstitial keratitis is a case in point. Antisyphilitic treatment should certainly be given because the patient is suffering from systemic infection, but additional local treatment is required for the eye to prevent damage to sight. The process is ultimately self-limiting and the administration of steroid hormones holds the inflammatory process in check until spontaneous cure results, reducing residual damage to a minimum. A useful method is to give cortisone acetate suspension in normal saline, 5 ml. per ml., or cortisone ointment 15 mg. per G. base, or both, by local application to the conjunctival sac. The patient is admitted to hospital and the application is made every 2 hours, until the symptoms and signs of the local condition are suppressed, which may take 4 or 5 days. The treatment is then continued at intervals of 4 hours. In severe cases subconjunctival injections of cortisone, 10 mg. in 0·4 ml., may be required in addition. The patient stays in hospital for about 10–14 days and then continues the local applications at home, every 4 hours during the day only, for 4 weeks, then 8-hourly and finally twice daily. After another 4 weeks the treatment can be stopped, although it must be resumed if relapse occurs. The method is likely to give freedom from symptoms, the probability of normal vision, and little or no corneal scarring. Local hydrocortisone, 5 mg. per ml., prednisone acetate, 0·25 per cent., and prednisolone-free alcohol, 0·25 per cent., have also been used successfully. In all these cases the pupil must be kept dilated with 1 per cent. atropine throughout the period of treatment.

Deafness, due to involvement of the VIIIth cranial nerve, and Clutton's joints are other conditions which do not respond to antisyphilitic treatment. There has been some recent evidence which suggests that patients with nerve deafness may benefit from steroid hormones given systemically.

SEROLOGICAL TESTS FOR SYPHILIS

Serological tests for syphilis are of two kinds, the so-called standard tests (STS), and tests for specific antibodies.

The Standard Serological Tests for Syphilis (STS) depend upon the fact that in the course of certain diseases, including syphilis, an antibody-like substance called 'reagin' appears in the serum of the affected patients. Reagin has the property of combining with colloidal suspensions of lipoids extracted from animal tissues which then flocculate. After combining with reagin the lipoidal particles have the power to fix complement. STS are, therefore, of two kinds, complement fixation tests and flocculation tests. Wassermann, who employed the complement fixation technique, was the first to produce such a test for syphilis, in 1906. He employed as his antigen extracts of liver from infants who had died from congenital syphilis and in the belief that it was specific. However, the test also gave satisfactory results with extracts of normal tissues and it soon became evident that neither complement fixation tests nor flocculation tests for syphilis were specific. In the course of years it appeared that reagin was probably present in small quantities in normal human serum but that these quantities were insufficient to give positive STS. In the presence of a number of diseases other than syphilis, however, the quantity of reagin increases and positive tests may be obtained. There have been many modifications of Wassermann's technique and many tests based on the principle of fixation which do not bear his name. It has since been shown that the active principle of extracts of normal animal tissues, such as beef-heart, used for making antigens for the STS is a serologically active phospholipid, called 'cardiolipin'. In the modern standard complement fixation tests for syphilis, cardiolipin, in combination with purified lecithin and cholesterol, is substituted for the crude tissue extracts of the past with considerable increase in sensitivity of the tests, and some think, of their specificity. The purified antigen is considerably easier to standardize than the crude antigens of the past. Among the many flocculation tests employed the Kahn test is probably the best known, but tests such as the Price Precipitation Test, the Kline, Meinicke, Mazzini and V.D.R.L. (Venereal Disease Research Laboratory) tests are all widely used. In cases of early syphilis, reagin can be demonstrated in the blood serum 7–10 days after the appearance of the initial lesion in most cases. It usually disappears 9–16 weeks after successful treatment. In cases of late syphilis it may persist in spite of treatment although the amount may diminish, as shown by fall in the titre of quantitative tests.

Non-syphilitic Reactions to the Standard Tests. These 'false positive' results are of four kinds: (1) Technical false positive reactions which result from errors, such as mistakes in the collection and labelling of specimens, faulty technique in the tests, or mistakes in recording or reporting the final results. Occasional errors of this kind are inevitable and it should be an absolute rule for the clinician that any result which does not accord with the history and physical signs of the patient should be checked by testing another specimen of serum from the same patient. Some laboratories perform several different tests on the same specimen as a routine and this is a good precaution against technical errors. (2) Variations in the normal, giving positive results which are not due to syphilis may also be found occasionally in the cases of some patients who appear to produce an excess of reagin from no detectable cause. In these cases specific tests are negative. (3) Those due to diseases allied to syphilis such as yaws, bejel and pinta, which give positive serological reactions in standard and specific tests, which are identical with those resulting from syphilis. Distinction between these diseases has to be made on clinical grounds. (4) Biological false-positive (BFP) reactions in diseases unrelated to syphilis, such as malaria, vaccinia, virus pneumonia, infectious mononucleosis, typhus, Weil's disease, filariasis and pulmonary tuberculosis which, on occasion, give positive STS. In these cases the amount of reagin is usually small so that quantitative tests are positive at a low titre, and the excess of reagin usually persists for only a few weeks, so that the tests become negative without specific treatment. However, certain chronic diseases, especially leprosy and chronic collagen diseases such as systemic lupus erythematosus may give strongly positive tests and reactivity may continue indefinitely. The fact that such positive reactions are not due to syphilis may be established by applying specific tests for that disease.

The Specific Serological Tests for Syphilis. It has been shown that the serum of syphilitic patients contains an antibody which, in the presence of complement, inhibits the movement of *T. pallidum*, and on this fact is based the test which is now known as Treponema Pallidum Immobilization (TPI) Test. The organisms are extracted from lesions in infected rabbits and suspended in a medium in which they remain motile and virulent for a limited period but do not multiply. On incubation with syphilitic serum and complement derived from guinea-pigs, the organisms lose their motility and cease to be infectious to rabbits. The antibody is distinct from reagin and the test is highly specific, giving positive results only with serum from syphilitic patients and those with yaws and other treponematoses. The test is complicated and can only be done in specially equipped laboratories: the cost is high. The test is not a substitute for the STS. It becomes positive later in the course of early syphilis and, although it becomes negative after successful treatment in cases of early syphilis, once the secondary stage has passed without treatment it is likely to remain positive for the rest of life. Its particular value is in distinguishing between syphilitic and non-syphilitic positive results to STS when other evidence of syphilis is lacking. It is also useful in certain cases of late syphilis, particularly those in which the cardiovascular or nervous system are affected, in which the STS have become negative in the course of time.

Efforts have been made to devise simpler and less costly specific tests which can be used as routine in any laboratory. The test which most nearly fulfils these criteria is the Reiter Protein Complement Fixation (RPCF) Test. This employs as antigen a protein fraction obtained from the non-virulent Reiter strain of *T. pallidum* which can be subcultured on artificial medium. The antigen is prepared from the cultures and is available commercially. The complement fixation technique is used with the Reiter protein antigen substituted for non-specific antigen. The antibody detected by the RPCF test differs from both reagin and 'immobilizing antibody' but the TPI test and the RPCF test agree in about 80 per cent. of the cases. The technique presents no difficulties and the cost of the reagents is not high.

Another specific test is the Fluorescent Treponemal Antibody (FTA) Test. It depends on a technique in which the serum to be tested is applied to a drop of suspension of virulent *T. pallidum* which has been dried on a slide: if specific antibody is present, it adheres to the surface of the treponemes. To this is added serum of rabbits sensitized to human globulin, containing antibodies to human globulin, conjugated with fluorescein isothiocyanate. The specimen is then incubated and observed with the dark-field microscope with a source of ultra-violet light. If the test is positive the anti-human globulin together with the fluorescein adheres to the antibody on the surface of the treponemes and the latter show fluorescence. In a recent modification the group antibody is removed from sera by absorption into ultrasonically disintegrated Reiter treponemes thus enabling detection of the specific antibody alone (FTA–ABS test). In cases of early syphilis both the RPCF and the FTA–ABS test may become positive before the STS. The FTA–ABS test may prove to be particularly useful in the serological diagnosis of early syphilis in the primary stage in cases in which *T. pallidum* cannot be demonstrated because an antibiotic has already been given. After successful treatment of early syphilis, the RPCF and FTA–ABS test may remain positive for longer than the STS and therefore they are not particularly useful in assessing the adequacy of treatment. It must again be emphasized that none of the specific tests is capable of differentiating between syphilis and yaws or the other closely allied treponematoses.

REFERENCES

King, A. J. (1964) *Recent Advances in Venereology*, London.

King, A. J., and Nicol, C. S. (1969) *Venereal Diseases*, 2nd ed., London.

Nabarro, D. (1954) *Congenital Syphilis*, London.

Stokes, J. H., Beerman, H., and Ingraham, N. R. (1945) *Modern Clinical Syphilology*, 3rd ed., Philadelphia.

United States Public Health Service (1968) Syphilis: A synopsis, Publication No. 1660.

United States Public Health Service (1969) Manual of tests for syphilis, Publication No. 411.

Willcox, R. R., and Guthe, T. (1966) Treponema pallidum, *Bull. Wld Hlth Org.*, Suppl. 3.

Claude Nicol

YAWS

Synonyms. Framboesia; Pian.

Aetiology

Yaws is a contagious disease caused by *Treponema pertenue* and characterized by lesions in the skin and bones. The lesions are basically granulomatous and non-destructive in the early stages, but later cause serious tissue damage. The distribution is irregular in the tropics. Yaws is endemic in South America, the West Indies, North and Equatorial Africa, parts of India, Ceylon, Burma, Indonesia, Thailand, Malaysia and the Philippines. It also occurs in Central America and Northern Australia. Under modern conditions as a result of extensive world eradication campaigns using penicillin, the disease is now very restricted in many of its former endemic areas. It cannot yet, however, be regarded as eradicated in these regions and constant supervision is necessary to keep it at its present low level.

T. pertenue is a motile, tightly coiled spirochaete, indistinguishable morphologically from *Treponema pallidum* which causes syphilis. It has not been successfully cultivated *in vitro* but can be transmitted to certain animals, including monkeys and rabbits in which it produces lesions different from those initiated by *T. pallidum.*

The organism is transmitted by direct contact with an infective human case. There are no animal reservoirs. It may survive for a time outside the body in material dropped or scraped from lesions and lying in the soft moist warm earth, for instance on the floor of a native hut. It is not known whether the organism can penetrate the unbroken skin, but it most commonly gains access through abrasions. Flies and cockroaches may occasionally spread the infection. Mechanical transmission from existing lesions is well understood by indigenes in endemic areas, where deliberate infection of infants is sometimes practised.

The disease may remain quiescent for long periods in some areas, especially where control by mass treatment has been carried out, but it is liable to break out if there is any relaxation of this procedure.

Yaws is common in sparsely clothed rural communities living in crowded insanitary conditions where transmission by contact is easy. It is relatively uncommon in towns and cities. Its distribution in the population is thus the reverse of that of syphilis, with which there is a strong cross-resistance; it is possible nevertheless for a patient with active yaws to acquire syphilis and vice versa. The Wassermann and Kahn reactions are positive in the serum, but in contradistinction to syphilis are negative in the cerebrospinal fluid.

The infection is most commonly acquired in early childhood, usually after the age of one. There is no evidence of congenital transmission. The disease may be acquired by non-immune adults, but yaws in adults is usually a manifestation of infection in childhood. Coloured races are much more commonly infected than white.

The lesions and episodes of yaws may be primary, secondary or tertiary depending on the stage of development of the disease in the particular individual. They are alternatively described as early and late yaws.

The primary lesion or 'mother yaw' is self-limited and non-destructive. The subsequent secondary lesions of the skin are basically similar granulomatous formations. Tertiary lesions of the skin on the other hand are destructive. The early lesions of the bone occur during the stage of secondary skin changes and are therefore usually regarded as secondary. They do not cause bone destruction. Tertiary lesions of bone, which develop later, are grossly destructive.

Yaws may not progress beyond the secondary stage. Primary and secondary lesions may overlap but secondary and tertiary do not. The interval between the primary lesion and the development of the tertiary stage may be several years.

Pathology

The basic lesion is a granuloma in many ways resembling that of syphilis. The pathological changes develop on sites in which the treponemata may be found in the primary and secondary skin stages, but not always in the tertiary.

Lesions arise in either the skin and subcutaneous tissue, in the bone or in both. Visceral lesions have not been definitely ascribed to yaws although some authors believe that aortic changes may result from infection. The central nervous system is not affected.

The histological pictures of the primary and secondary skin lesions are identical, although the clinical appearance at a particular anatomical site depends on the local arrangements and structure of epithelium and subcutaneous tissue. In the early stages the epidermis is thickened and the underlying tissue loosely infiltrated with lymphocytes and plasma cells. The infiltration becomes rapidly heavier and a papule develops over which the epithelium is at first thickened with hypertrophic branching epithelial papillae and later thinned.

Eventually the overlying epithelium thins but, unless it is damaged or kept continually moist, does not ulcerate, so that the lesion remains covered by epithelium. When ulceration occurs serous fluid exudes and coagulates over the granulomatous surface which elsewhere remains covered by epithelium.

Treponemata are easily found in scrapings from the upper areas of the granulomatous tissue. Unless there is ulceration and secondary infection the lesion will heal without much scarring, sometimes leaving a thin, tissue-paper scar. Lesions in moist areas, such as the corners of the mouth or the anus and vulva may easily ulcerate and become infected. In other areas, especially in the hands and feet, extensive hypertrophy of the keratinous layers of the epithelium occurs and may lead to remarkable 'horn' formations.

During the secondary stage characteristic changes in the bones commonly appear. They occur in many bones and are represented chiefly by diffuse or local rarefaction of the cortex, especially of long bones and the small bones of the hands and feet, plus periostitis with the deposit of new bone. The periostitis is a cellular, oedematous and painful reaction. Bone lesions are not necessarily associated with skin lesions in the same area and ulceration over them is accidental. The tertiary skin lesions of yaws develop after the secondary stage has subsided. The granulomatous changes are basically the same but ulceration is common and the deeper tissues, including bone, are often involved. The ulceration may be very severe and extensive leading eventually to extreme scarring, and deformity.

Lesions occurring late in the bone or tertiary lesions include foci of rarefaction, necrosis and absorption, particularly of long bones, and localized areas of periostitis with irregular deposit of new bone. The lesions are very destructive and secondary infection is common. Usually few bones are affected.

Signs and Symptoms

The incubation period is 3–6 weeks. The site of the initial lesion varies, but it commonly occurs on the legs or buttocks. The lesion appears first as an erythematous macule then as a nodule which enlarges as the yaw develops, often reaching 2–4 cm. in diameter. The lesion is raised above the surface and the skin over it is usually intact. When the covering epithelium is broken or ulcerated serous fluid exudes from the surface which becomes covered with a yellowish scab. After a few weeks or months it heals, usually without much scarring.

The primary lesion may still be present when the first batch of secondary lesions appears. These are basically similar to the primary lesions, but are multiple and occur in successive crops months or years apart. They may occur anywhere on the skin, but are particularly common on the face, around the mouth and in the vulval cleft, anus and buttocks. They are rare on the scalp. They are uncommon in mucous membranes proper although they occur quite frequently at mucocutaneous junctions. The lesions vary greatly in size, some being inches long and others very small. Each batch of lesions heals spontaneously in a few months, the eruption subsiding completely. Yaws are commonly painless, but they may be itchy and become damaged by scratching. When secondary infection develops local lymph nodes are enlarged. The lesions may become very painful in areas such as the soles and palms where the epithelium is firm. In such areas the granulomatous tissue commonly presents on the medial or lateral aspects of the sole or palm where the epithelium is thinner. In patients with lesions in the soles the attempt to walk on one side or other of the foot has given rise to the term 'crab yaws'.

Ulceration direct through the thick plantar epithelium may occur and is extremely painful and incapacitating. The granulomatous tissue becomes exposed and appears to well up through the thickened hyperkeratotic epithelium which is cracked and turned back. There may be scattered areas of hard keratotic epithelium which eventually fall out leaving punched-out holes; this condition is known as 'clavus'. The plantar skin is often irregularly thickened, dry and peeling and cracked and fissured, which may make walking difficult.

Lesions of the type described above are the commonest in the secondary stage. They may be accompanied by many similar tissue changes which differ considerably in clinical appearance. For example, depigmented macules or papules occur covered with desquamating epithelium. Circinate lesions raised only slightly above the surface and closely resembling fungal infections are common in some endemic areas. Leathery desquamated and papular skin changes occur particularly on the abdomen or the knees and the backs of the hands. Muscle tendons may be involved, especially those of the wrist, producing painless ganglia.

Secondary bone lesions are usually multiple and involve the whole or most of the shaft of the relevant bone. They develop rapidly and resolve spontaneously after a few weeks or months. Relapses are common in the same bone. The bones most commonly affected are the long bones of the legs and forearms and the small bones of the hands and feet. The affected areas are tender and extremely painful. There may be local oedema and aching. Function may be grossly impaired. The prime example is the extensive dactylitis, commonly seen in children and often involving both hands, with swollen, tender, aching and practically unusable fingers. The periosteal deposits of new bone often lead to deformity such as the bending and bowing of the long bones of the limbs.

Late secondary lesions occur in the skull in the maxillary bones, sometimes producing a bar of thickening due to periosteal deposits of new bone across the face on either side of the bridge of the nose known as 'goundou'. The joints are not commonly involved.

The tertiary stage of yaws is commonly seen in persons who have progressed through the primary and secondary stages without adequate treatment but it may appear without any such history. Tertiary lesions may develop years after the secondary lesions have subsided. They may appear in young children but are commonly not observed until after the fifth year.

Tertiary lesions occur again in the skin and subcutaneous tissues and the bones. The basic reaction is a granuloma similar to that of the secondary stage but is more active and destructive, leading to ulceration of the skin which involves the deeper tissue including the bone. A diffuse lesion is produced which may start as a nodule and rapidly become ulcerated. The ulcer is indolent and slowly progressive and resembles that of late syphilis. It usually becomes secondarily infected if unattended and can lead to terrible scarring and deformity, especially when associated with local osteomyelitis.

Certain other tertiary changes occur in the skin, including the so-called 'juxta-articular' nodules, which are firm painless subcutaneous cystic tumours developing near the large joints, especially the knees.

Tertiary palmar and plantar lesions also occur with scarring and considerable contractions.

The tertiary bone lesions are very serious. They develop in few rather than many bones. There is local cortical rarefaction and destruction. Radiology discloses roughly oval areas of rarefaction and necrosis often containing debris and spicules of dead bone which may be discharged to the surface. There is also localized and irregular periostitis, with new bone formation.

Spontaneous fractures sometimes occur, especially of a long bone such as the humerus.

Large nodules on the skull and sternum are common, resulting from irregular thickening and rarefaction of bones, particularly the outer table. Ulceration of the skin over these lesions may occur with sinus formation and secondary infection.

The most destructive lesions occur in the face and involve the hard palate and the nasal processes of the maxillary bone. The whole of these bones may disappear with the tissues over them. The lips and nose are lost and the eyes may be involved and very severe deformity of the face. Healing results in hideous scarring. This condition is known as 'gangosa'.

The course of yaws is normally progressive, moving from primary to secondary and on to tertiary stages, but all variants of this theme occur.

The disease is not congenital and is rare in infants. In the individual case seen in the secondary stage there is no way of telling whether tertiary lesions are likely to develop.

It is therefore essential to treat all cases of yaws especially in the early stages. Treatment is now so effective that the tertiary lesions can be completely avoided.

The prognosis in an untreated case depends on the duration of the disease and the point at which active treatment is given.

Most cases overcome the infection after a few years following the secondary stages. In some, the disease may remain latent. The secondary lesions tend to appear irregularly in overlapping separate crops for a period of two or three years and then subside. Tertiary lesions follow after an irregular interval of years. Spontaneous recovery may occur at any stage.

Diagnosis

The diagnosis is primarily clinical but examination of fluid from skin lesions in the primary and secondary stages will usually disclose the treponemata. Where bacteriological diagnosis is required the surface of the epithelialized lesions or the crust from ulcerated lesions is removed and fluid and scrapings from the granuloma are examined under dark ground illumination for the actively motile organisms.

The Wassermann, Kahn and other similar reactions are positive 3–6 weeks after the appearance of the primary lesions and remain positive throughout the disease until the late healing stage when they may become negative. The titre may also fall or become negative following successful treatment. The reactions are negative in the cerebrospinal fluid. In the latter there may be some increase in protein and lymphocytes.

Differential Diagnosis

Yaws must be distinguished from two very similar diseases *bejel* and *pinta*. *Bejel* occurs mainly amongst Bedouin Arabs in the Middle East and is a form of non-venereal or endemic syphilis usually acquired in young childhood. The early history may offer little help since it corresponds to the development of yaws; moreover, the circinate papules and eruptions and the bone lesions closely resemble those of secondary yaws.

Ulceration of the palate and tonsils and involvement of the nasal bones also occur in the tertiary stages. Spontaneous recovery may take place at any stage.

The differentiation of endemic syphilis from yaws can be made finally only by bacteriological definition of the infecting parasite.

The differentiation of yaws from *pinta* may also be difficult and indeed there is considerable evidence that the conditions may be identical. The granulomatous tissue reaction is less active than in yaws, and the primary lesions progress more slowly. The florid type of lesion seen in yaws does not occur.

Pinta is found in rural areas of Central and South America and in certain Caribbean islands, including Cuba. The causative organism is tentatively called *Treponema carateum* and is morphologically indistinguishable from *T. pertenue*. Transmission occurs in the same way as in yaws. Infection is acquired in childhood or adolescence. It is rare in infants. It is found mostly in dark-skinned populations and rarely in Europeans. There is a much weaker cross-immunity with syphilis than is the case with yaws and coincident infection with syphilis is relatively common.

The basic lesion is a slowly developing subcutaneous granuloma with hypertrophy and later atrophy of the overlying skin in which colour changes occur due to redistribution and loss of local pigment. Mucous membranes are only rarely affected. In the late stages there may be complete depigmentation of both epithelium and corium. Local lymph nodes may be enlarged. Visceral lesions do not occur. The Wassermann reaction is negative in the early stages, becoming positive after some months.

The primary lesion appears at the point of infection as a raised infiltrated plaque which is erythematous or bluish-black and sharply demarcated from the surrounding skin. It spreads slowly with satellite lesions which become absorbed into it. After 6–12 months similar lesions, called *pintids*, appear successively on the limbs and sometimes the trunk. Lesions often coalesce so that large areas of the body become involved. Pintids are painless but may be itchy and become secondarily infected by scratching. They eventually become almost completely depigmented and the skin over them atrophies. The lesions may be arranged symmetrically, for instance on the backs of the wrists. Irregular areas of depigmented or hyperpigmented skin may be scattered over the body including the plantar and palmar surfaces; the latter may become hyperkeratotic and develop contractures similar to those seen in yaws.

Diagnosis is made on geographical and clinical grounds especially when the slowly growing depigmented lesions are arranged symmetrically. Organisms are easily found in early and late lesions. The active disease responds to penicillin but nothing can be done for the changes in pigmentation.

Circinate secondary lesions of yaws often closely resemble clinically those of certain fungus infections such as tinea versicolor in which irregular skin depigmentation may occur. The finding of the treponema in the yaws granuloma or the fungus in skin scrapings determines the diagnosis.

Late tertiary ulceration in yaws in which the treponema may not be found can be differentiated from tropical ulcer, the exudate from which usually shows the characteristic spirochaetes and fusiform bacilli.

Treatment

The only form of treatment now used is penicillin given intramuscularly in a form called PAM, i.e.

procaine penicillin in oil with 2 per cent. aluminium monostearate.

For individual cases treatment usually consists of the following: Adults: 1·2 mega Units given twice with an interval of 3–5 days between the doses (total dose, 2·4 mega Units). Children 5–15 years: half the above dosage. Children under 5 years: a single dose of 0·3 mega Units.

For mass treatment campaigns adults and children over 5 years of age are given 1·2 mega Units as a single dose and children under the age of 5 receive 0·3 mega Units.

The effect of treatment is spectacular in primary and secondary skin and bone lesions. Clinical recovery is extremely rapid and healing may be complete in skin lesions within a fortnight.

In mass treatment single dosage therapy is adequate provided follow-up is carried out. The object is either to treat the individual infective cases, regarded for this purpose as those which have primary or secondary skin lesions, or to treat the total number of people involved with obvious yaws. Mass treatment of yaws with penicillin is most promising so far as eradication of the disease is concerned.

LEPTOSPIRAL INFECTIONS

LEPTOSPIROSIS

Synonyms. Weil's disease or spirochaetal jaundice; Japanese seven-day fever; Swamp fever.

Aetiology

These diseases are caused by species of the spirochaete *Leptospira,* an organism commonly found in rats and other rodents living in or near stagnant water. The distribution of the disease is world wide.

The infection of man is accidental but it may be occupational, associated with contamination of the skin or mucous membranes or of foodstuffs by urine from infected animals. In the British Isles leptospirosis is an occupational hazard in sewer-workers, farmers and fish cleaners.

The clinical conditions which result may vary greatly in severity. In its serious forms the infection carries a high mortality and the characteristic picture is one of fever, jaundice and toxaemia, haemorrhages into the skin and mucous membranes and damage to the kidneys with characteristic changes in the urine including increasing albuminuria. In the milder varieties the features may be those of an influenza-like illness or may resemble benign lymphocytic meningitis.

The species of *Leptospira* concerned are morphologically identical but can be distinguished by bacteriological methods, and the study of their pathogenicity in animals.

Classification is normally made in terms of agglutination reactions and cross-absorption. The type species is *Leptospira icterohaemorrhagiae,* which is commonly associated with the vector rat *Rattus norvegicus.* Increasing numbers of serotypes have been proved to be infective to man.

Leptospirae are slender, actively motile, closely wound spirochaetes of variable length.

They stain well with Romanowsky dyes or silver impregnation methods, and can be cultured on simple bacterial media.

L. icterohaemorrhagiae which causes Weil's disease, a very severe illness in man, infects dogs, cats and occurs as an enzootic in rats, field mice and other small rodents. In these animals, which are the reservoirs of the infection, the organisms invade the blood stream and the kidneys and are passed in the urine to contaminate food, sewers, swamps, paddy fields, ponds and rivers. Man becomes infected by ingesting contaminated food or water, or by the entry of the organisms through damaged skin or mucous membranes.

Leptospira canicola is usually found as an enzootic in dogs in which the urine contains the organism. It is not found in rodents. The infection in man is less severe than that of *L. icterohaemorrhagiae.*

There are many other forms of leptospirosis caused by other species such as *Leptospira bataviae,* and *Leptospira hebdomadis* found in many areas of the world including the Middle East, parts of South-East Asia, including Japan, Indonesia and Thailand, and Eastern Europe.

In the British Isles the infection is most commonly acquired by bathing in canals, the water of which has been contaminated by the urine of rats or dogs.

Pathology

The organisms are usually taken in by man through the mouth or nose and may penetrate the mucosae or the damaged skin. They spread to the blood stream and localize in certain tissues, especially the liver and kidney. They multiply vigorously for two to three weeks and then gradually disappear. Characteristic lesions are focal vascular haemorrhages and degenerative necrotic changes in the liver and kidneys. There may or may not be jaundice. Haemorrhages occur in the muscles, lungs and kidneys. The liver is enlarged and there is centrilobular necrosis. The kidneys show multiple haemorrhages with distal and proximal convoluted tubular necrosis. There is patchy cortical ischaemia and medullary congestion. Death may result, as in so many other acute infections, from acute renal failure with uraemia.

Signs and Symptoms

The incubation period in infections with *L. icterohaemorrhagiae* varies from a few days to 3 weeks but is usually not more than 10 days. There are three stages, the febrile, the jaundiced and the convalescence.

The onset is sudden with a rapid rise of temperature, rigors, severe headache, muscular pains and gastro-intestinal disturbance with nausea and vomiting. The remittent fever lasts about 10 days. Jaundice appears on the fourth or fifth day and deepens rapidly; the stools become clay coloured.

Herpes labialis is common with haemorrhagic vesicles and there may be a petechial macular rash. There is commonly conjunctival congestion, and maybe epistaxis, blood-stained sputum and haematuria.

The urine contains bile pigment and increasing amounts of protein. In cases in which kidney failure appears oliguria develops and may be followed by anuria.

Where haemorrhage is severe there may be some anaemia. There is an early leucopenia which is followed by moderate leucocytosis. Convalescence begins after the second week, and recovery is complete in a further three weeks. Organisms appear in the urine by the third week of the illness. There may be a recrudescence, which may persist for some weeks, but with less severe constitutional damage.

Great variations in severity are noted in leptospirosis, even in the same endemic area. The more severe cases are jaundiced; mild cases are not. Fulminating fatal cases occur with rapidly developing deep jaundice, very severe toxaemia and prostration, delirium and cardiac failure. Death commonly occurs in the second week. The mortality varies from less than 10 per cent. to over 50 per cent.

The number of recognized pathogenic leptospirae is increasing rapidly and now exceeds 30.

The pattern of Weil's disease is followed in varying degrees by most infections, but some, for example *L. canicola* infection, are very mild and are not characterized by jaundice. Renal damage seems to be common to all of them. The clinical picture in a given geographical area is thus essentially local, depending on the infecting organism.

Diagnosis

In the early stages of the disease in known endemic areas a tentative clinical diagnosis is often made in patients with fever, severe conjunctival congestion and pronounced tenderness of the calf muscles.

In the first 10–14 days the organisms may be found in the blood by triple centrifugation. The deposit is examined on dark ground, or by blood culture on broth medium containing inactivated rabbit serum. Guinea-pigs inoculated intraperitoneally with infected blood may develop fever and jaundice within 2 weeks. The animals are infective after two weeks, and the leptospirae will be found in smears of the liver or kidneys or in the blood culture.

Agglutinins appear in the blood of patients by the sixth day and reach a maximum by the third week. Very high titres are developed against stock cultures.

Mass surveys for agglutinins have been successfully carried out using dried blood on filter paper as the source of serum.

In routine agglutination tests a suspension of *L. icterohaemorrhagiae* is used. Agglutination at a dilution of 1 in 20 may with proper controls may be regarded as positive.

The *Escherichia coli* adhesion test is also of value in diagnosis using the patient's serum, a living suspension of leptospira and fresh guinea-pig serum. Where the test is positive *Esch. coli* adhere to the leptospirae.

Treatment

Treatment with antibiotics may be successful if given early, especially in the first 3 days after onset. Benzylpenicillin is recommended in doses of 600 mg. (1 mega Unit) four-hourly for 24 hours and then six-hourly for up to 6 days. Tetracyclines are also active in doses of 30 mg. per kg. orally in divided doses continuously until 48 hours after the temperature becomes normal.

Streptomycin has been used with success combined with penicillin.

The response to antibiotics is much less satisfactory in the later stages of the disease.

Nursing, the correction of water and electrolyte loss, and the management of renal failure are of great importance in the later stages.

BRIAN MAEGRAITH

INFECTIONS DUE TO MYCOPLASMATACEAE

Formerly known as pleuropneumonia-like organisms or PPLO, mycoplasmas are intermediate in size between bacteria and viruses, the smallest reproductive units measuring 100–125 nm. Unlike viruses they can grow in cell-free media providing a protein is present, but they lack a rigid cell wall and thus tend to be highly pleomorphic. All are resistant to penicillin but sensitive to tetracycline.

In nature mycoplasmas are widespread, found in plants and in animals and man as intracellular parasites. Some species are pathogenic. In plants they are thought to cause aster yellows and other diseases, and they are responsible for several infections of economic importance in animals, including bovine pleuropneumonia of cattle.

In man mycoplasmas have been isolated from the mouth and respiratory, genital and urinary tracts. Only two species are known with certainty to cause disease, *M. hominis* type 1 (for which antibodies are present in more than half of adults) produces a febrile sore throat and *M. pneumoniae* which is one of the main causes of the syndrome of primary atypical pneumonia [see Section 9]. From time to time mycoplasmas have been isolated from joints, the pleural cavity and brain abscesses. Although normal inhabitants of the genito-urinary tract they may be found more frequently in the presence of inflammation and it has been claimed that one variety, the T strain, is responsible for some cases of non-specific urethritis.

REFERENCE

TAYLOR-ROBINSON, D. (1971) Mycoplasmas and the evidence for their pathogenicity in Man, *Proc. roy. Soc. Med.*, **64**, 31.

R. A. SHOOTER

INFECTIONS DUE TO RICKETTSIAE

RICKETTSIAL INFECTIONS

TYPHUS FEVERS

Typhus fevers and allied conditions, such as the spotted fevers due to infection with *Rickettsia* spp., are found in many parts of the world.

Typhus fevers are caused by species of *Rickettsia*, which are small pleomorphic organisms intermediate between bacteria and viruses and which occur intracellularly in their hosts, especially in the endothelium of the small blood vessels.

They exist as coccoid or rhomboid forms varying from 1 μ in diameter up to 2·5 μ in length. In any given preparation they vary enormously in form. They are Gram-negative and stain well with Romanowsky dyes. Animals are susceptible to most rickettsiae with exception of the organism responsible for louse-borne epidemic typhus. They can be grown in tissue culture and chick embryo. Most are easily killed by heat. The exception to this is the closely related organism *Coxiella burneti* which causes Q fever. Antiseptics destroy them easily.

The rickettsial infections are usually spread by arthropods especially the louse, the tick, the mite and the flea.

The principal typhus fevers are usually described in terms of their vectors and are divided into louse-borne, flea-borne, mite-borne and tick-borne typhus fevers. Most rickettsial infections occur naturally in small rodents and other mammals, and man is infected accidentally so that the conditions are usually sporadic. They sometimes occur in epidemics, particularly the louse-borne form, which is the only one which can be spread by arthropods from man to man and in which man appears to be the only reservoir.

The specific rickettsiae concerned in these fevers are: *Rickettsia prowazeki*, which causes the louse-borne or epidemic form of typhus and is maintained in man and the louse that feeds on him, *Pediculus humanus*. The only other rickettsial infection in which man is the reservoir is trench fever (*Rickettsia quintana*). *Rickettsia mooseri* causes flea-borne or murine typhus which occurs as a natural infection in rats, mice and other rodents and is transmitted normally by the rat flea *Xenopsylla cheopis* (also the vector of plague). It is occasionally transmitted by the louse. It normally survives by passage from rodent to rodent via the louse or the flea and man is only accidentally infected.

Rickettsia orientalis (or *tsutsugamushi*) causes classical mite-borne typhus. It is found in wild rodents and other animals and is transmitted by mites, the commonest of which is *Trombicula*. Mites also transmit rickettsial pox caused by *Rickettsia akari*. The mite becomes infected in the early stages of its life cycle by taking only one meal of tissue juice. The female transmits the infection transovarially to the offspring, which in turn transmits it to man and normally to other wild animals by the bite. In this way transmission requires at least two generations of mites.

There are several rickettsial infections transmitted by ticks. *Rickettsia rickettsi* causes the spotted fever group of diseases. Normally a parasite of small mammals, it is transmitted accidentally to man by the tick. *Rickettsia conori*, the cause of Mediterranean fever, is transmitted by the dog tick *Rhipicephalus sanguineus*. The dog is the normal reservoir but in South and East Africa wild rodents may act as such and in this case the organism is sometimes referred to as the *Rickettsia conori* var. *pijperi*. Q fever, caused by *C. burneti*, and bullis fever, may also be transmitted by ticks.

Since ticks are regular feeders on animals, infection may be passaged directly through them by biting, or transovarially to the next generation. The usual process is animal to animal via ticks. The biting of man by the tick is accidental and the disease is not transmitted man to man.

The mode of infection of arthropods by rickettsiae is important in relation to the spread of the human disease.

In the louse-borne infection the rickettsiae multiply in the cells of the gut wall of the louse and are eventually passed in its faeces. Man is infected by rubbing the faeces or crushed lice into skin abrasions and not actually by the bite of the louse. Transmission may also occur from the inhalation of dried faeces. There is no known animal reservoir and only the human body louse will transmit the infection. When the louse is destroyed typhus ceases to exist in the endemic area.

In flea-borne typhus the flea is infected when it takes a blood meal from an infected animal and the organisms are eventually passed in the faeces. Man is invaded by the flea and is infected through the faeces in the same way as in the louse-borne infection. The human louse does not appear to take up *R. mooseri* infection but since there is some cross-protection between flea and louse typhus, it has been suggested that from time to time epidemics of the latter may have originated from infection of lice from the flea-borne organism.

Some differentiation of rickettsiae can be achieved

to some extent by the clinical effects of inoculation of infective material into animals. In louse-borne typhus, for instance, blood taken during fever and injected intraperitoneally into guinea-pigs will produce fever in the animals in about 10 days.

Blood from cases of flea-borne typhus injected intraperitoneally into the same animal produces fever in about the same time, accompanied by inflammation of the tunica vaginalis (the so-called 'Neill-Mooser' reaction).

Blood from tick-borne typhus (*R. rickettsi*) injected intraperitoneally into guinea-pigs causes the 'scrotal' reaction of acute inflammation of testes and scrotum.

Blood from cases of mite-borne typhus inoculated in the same way produces no local reaction and no fever, but the animals die and the organisms are found in the peritoneal exudate.

The rickettsiae can be distinguished by bacteriological methods. Cross-antigenicity can be detected in some, but not all, by the Weil-Felix reaction.

Certain strains of *Proteus* agglutinate in the presence of serum from patients suffering from certain rickettsial infections. The agglutinations are associated with the somatic (O) antigen of the *Proteus* some of which, namely *Proteus* OX19, OXK and OX2, are used for the routine identification of rickettsiae by serological examination.

Serum is taken from the patient and set up in serial dilutions against suspensions of the *Proteus* organisms. The test is of value in diagnosis and differentiation. By the tenth day of some rickettsial diseases agglutinins are present in high titre in the serum and the titre thereafter continues to rise for another fortnight and then gradually diminishes. A rising titre after the tenth day is therefore of diagnostic significance. The standard reactions to the Weil-Felix test can be seen in the following table:

Disease	OX19	OX2	OXK
Louse- and flea-borne	+ + + /-	+ + /-	negative
Tick-borne . .	+ + /-	+ + /-	+
Mite-borne . .	negative	negative	+ + +

Other serological tests which are more specific and reliable are agglutination by sera of suspensions of rickettsiae, which can be used with cross-absorption tests.

Complement fixation tests using extracts or suspensions of rickettsiae are also highly specific.

LOUSE-BORNE TYPHUS

Synonyms. Typhus exanthematicus; Epidemic typhus.

Definition

A disease characterized by sudden onset, high remittent fever, severe prostration and toxaemia, a generalized rash appearing on the fifth day and central nervous system symptoms. It is one of the great epidemic diseases of history.

The disease lasts a fortnight to 16 days and in epidemics the mortality is high.

Aetiology

The geographical distribution is determined by the presence of lice amongst the population. Wherever there are lice, there may be epidemic typhus, especially in the colder parts of the world.

The louse transmits the infection when it or its faeces are crushed into abrasions or bites in the skin surface. Lice migrate from person to person and thus help to disseminate the disease. Infection may sometimes occur as a result of inhalation of dried faeces from louse-ridden clothing.

For some reason epidemic typhus may be a relatively mild disease in children. Its severity increases with rising age, until over forty the mortality is very high.

One attack affords considerable and usually life-long immunity. It is not known whether the infection is cured after recovery without treatment or persists for long periods. The so-called Brill's disease is believed to represent a recrudescence occurring long after recovery from the primary attack.

Pathology

The basic lesion in louse-borne typhus is parasitization of the endothelium of the small blood vessels by rickettsiae. This occurs anywhere in the body but particularly in the skin, brain, muscles and heart. The affected cells swell and there is considerable proliferation of vascular endothelium.

Cellular nodules composed of round cells and mononuclear macrophages form around these areas of angiitis, and the vessels, especially in the skin, become cuffed with lymphocytes, plasma cells and sometimes polymorphs.

These changes in the small vessels are followed by irregular thrombosis and haemorrhage. The larger vessels may become involved in the cellular reaction, usually without thrombosis.

These are the characteristic lesions of typhus and are responsible for most of the morbid changes seen at autopsy including the petechial haemorrhages, bronchopneumonia, myocardial damage, the patchy gangrene of the skin and the sloughs in skeletal muscle and subcutaneous tissues. The extensive gangrene of the extremities which may occur is caused sometimes by thrombosis and sometimes by neurological lesions.

Signs and Symptoms

The incubation period ranges from less than a week to three weeks. The onset is abrupt and associated with rigor, headache, muscular pains and fever, which rises rapidly to 103°–104° F. (39·4°–40° C.) and then becomes continuous, with relatively small fluctuations. At this stage the face is flushed and congested, the conjunctivae are injected. The mouth is dry, the tongue is furred and may be trembling. The nose and throat are congested and epistaxis is common. There is abdominal discomfort, with constipation or occasionally diarrhoea, and the spleen becomes palpable within the first few days. By the fourth or fifth day the condition worsens considerably. The patient is prostrated and stuporose, sometimes delirious. He emits a strange unpleasant musty smell which is said to be characteristic. The rash appears on the fifth day, first on the shoulders and in the axillae, then on the abdomen, chest, back and extremities. It rarely develops on the face, the palms or the soles. It consists at first of numerous rose-red macules, which fade on pressure but, after a day or two when the pathological processes in the vessels have sufficiently developed, become dull red and no longer fade. The rash begins to disappear about the tenth day by which time the lesions have become brownish. There is often an additional blotchy mottling of the skin which has the same distribution ('subcuticular mottling'). In severe cases purpuric patches may appear in the skin and bleeding occurs from mucous membranes, leading sometimes to haematemesis, melaena and haematuria.

Nervous system symptoms are always prominent within the first week. The patient sleeps badly and has fearful nightmares. He early develops a tremor of the tongue and often twitchings of limb muscles.

Incontinence of urine and faeces is common and may remain through the illness. Coma may develop in the first week or the patient may become confused and maniacal and need restraining. Some involvement of the respiratory tract is always present, usually bronchitis, which is commonly followed by bronchopneumonia, and sometimes pleurisy and empyema, or terminal gangrene or abscess of the lung.

The lesions which develop in the myocardium may produce clinical effects including tachycardia and myocardial failure. Complications include gangrene of areas of the skin, which is common, and symmetrical gangrene of the extremities. Suppurative parotitis also occurs.

In recovery, the temperature falls by rapid lysis between the twelfth and fourteenth days and is normal by the sixteenth day. In fatal cases, death usually occurs in the second week. Oliguria occurs in most severe cases. Anuria with renal failure and uraemia is a common cause of death.

Treatment

On admission the patient should be given a bath and his clothes disinfested by heat. The patient and his hospital clothes should be deloused once weekly with 10 per cent. DDT powder.

All the usual forms of typhus respond to certain antibiotics, of which chloramphenicol is probably the best. Chlortetracycline and oxytetracycline are also effective.

The results are often dramatic especially in the early stages of the infection. The fever subsides in 2–4 days and convalescence is rapid.

Corticosteroids may be used in the early stages of severe attacks to assist the patient until the specific treatment becomes effective. The use of antisera prepared for certain tick-borne infections is unnecessary.

Chloramphenicol is given in a loading dose of 50 mg. per kg. body weight, followed by 2 G. each day in four divided doses, continued until the temperature has become normal for 48 hours. Relapses may occur in cases treated in the early stages. They may be prevented by repeating the dosage of chloramphenicol for one day a week after the cessation of full therapy.

The tetracyclines are given in similar doses.

Corticosteroids such as prednisolone may be given concurrently with the antibiotics in severe cases.

The prophylaxis of louse-borne typhus depends on louse control on persons and clothing, by cleansing, insecticides such as DDT and repellents. Vaccines of *R. prowazeki* have been used to protect individuals. The most successful is prepared from an avirulent strain maintained in the chick embryo.

Cox vaccine (containing killed *R. prowazeki*) is given in a dose of 1 ml. subcutaneously, repeated in 10–14 days, with a booster dose on exposure.

TRENCH FEVER

Trench fever, due to *R. quintana* and transmitted by lice, is a febrile disease marked by splenomegaly and a maculopapular eruption; bouts of pyrexia may recur over many months. It was of importance in the First World War and in the Second World War outbreaks were reported from the Russian front. Diagnosis is made by recovery of the rickettsia or by specific agglutination or complement-fixation tests; the Weil-Felix reaction is of no value.

MITE-BORNE TYPHUS

Synonyms. Scrub typhus; Japanese river fever; Mite fever.

Aetiology

This form of typhus is caused by *R. orientalis* (or *tsutsugamushi*) which occurs in rural and bush areas throughout the Far East, including Japan, the Philippines, Indonesia and New Guinea.

The reservoirs are small wild animals usually rodents amongst which the infection is transmitted by several species of mites, principally *Trombicula.* During their six-legged larval stage the mites take the only blood or tissue meal of their lives and become infected with the rickettsiae, which the female passes transovarially to the offspring, which infect the mammalian hosts during their single feed. The larval mites attack animals or man with equal freedom, but man is rarely bitten unless exposed for some reason in the geographical area concerned, for example, during war or clearing operations.

R. orientalis is antigenically distinct from other rickettsiae and can be separated from them by the usual methods. The serum from the patient agglutinates only the OXK strain of *Proteus* [p. 141].

The pathology of the disease is similar to that of louse-borne typhus but the vascular damage is less evident. On the other hand general vascular collapse or renal failure frequently occurs.

Rickettsiae have been established as the cause of occasional outbreaks of fever with vesicular eruption. the best documented example is rickettsialpox, first observed in New York City in 1946. The responsible organism, *R. akari*, was shown to be transmitted by a mite, *Allodermanyssus sanguineus*, normally found on mice.

Signs and Symptoms

There is an incubation period of 6–18 days. The onset resembles that of epidemic typhus. An 'eschar' or small necrotic ulcer covered by a black scab develops at the site of the bite of the vector, generally on the trunk. Local lymph nodes are enlarged and there is occasionally general adenitis. The eschar is of diagnostic importance. It persists for about 3 weeks, i.e. usually throughout the disease.

The rash appears between the fifth and eighth days in the form of a macular eruption developing first on the sides of the abdomen and chest and spreading to the extremities. It fades rapidly in a few hours after persisting for some days. The fever is similar to that of louse-borne typhus and lasts for about 2 weeks, falling by lysis over several days. The signs and symptoms are as in epidemic typhus. Death occurs commonly in the second week following general circulatory or renal failure or bronchopneumonia or encephalitis. The mortality varies. It may be as high as 60 per cent. in some outbreaks.

Diagnosis

Diagnosis is made on a knowledge of the locality and circumstances, the discovery of the eschar, a positive Weil-Felix reaction for OXK, with a rising titre reaching its maximum after 3 weeks. The serum of the patient is also taken for tests for specific agglutination of rickettsial suspensions. Blood from the patient may be injected intraperitoneally into guinea-pigs in which death occurs after about a fortnight and the rickettsiae can be identified bacteriologically.

Treatment

Chloramphenicol is specific. See details of treatment of louse-borne typhus.

Vaccines have not been successful in prophylaxis. Protection depends on personal prophylaxis, avoidance of infected areas and animals.

Chloramphenicol and other antibiotics are not successful as suppressives.

TICK-BORNE TYPHUS

Aetiology

There are several forms of tick typhus which are normally enzootic in a wide range of animals, and are conveyed from one animal to another by various species of ticks. Man is infected sporadically and accidentally by ticks seeking a blood meal. Ticks pass the infection transovarially to their offspring which become equally infective to mammals.

The diseases occur in North America (Rocky Mountains), South America, Africa (especially the Mediterranean coastal areas), India and Northern Australia. One form, Q fever, is very widespread [p. 144].

The causative organism of Rocky Mountain spotted fevers and the spotted fevers of South America is *R. rickettsi.* This form of tick typhus affects chiefly rural populations whose work brings them in contact with wild life and tick infested stock, but may be spread through the ticks of domestic animals, including the dog.

Mediterranean fièvre boutonneuse is caused by *R. conori*, which is usually transmitted by the common dog tick *Rhipicephalus*. The dog is the normal reservoir of the infection.

Tick-bite fever in South Africa and East Africa is caused by *R. conori* or *pijperi* which occurs in the veldt. The clinical picture resembles fièvre boutonneuse, easily maintained in experimental animals. Antigenic differences exist between this organism and *R. rickettsi* and *R. conori.*

Pathology

Histopathological changes in the vessels similar to those in endemic typhus, occur in all forms of tick typhus but on the whole the nodular lesions may be less pronounced, except in *R. rickettsi* infections in which thrombi develop in the arterioles and venules and may give rise to thrombonecrotic lesions involving the whole vessel wall. These lesions constitute a destructive angiitis uncommon in other forms of typhus.

In very severe cases of tick typhus there may be extensive gangrene and sloughing of the skin of the scrotum, vulva, fingers and toes.

Signs and Symptoms

Most cases of *R. rickettsi* infection are severe. There are also mild and fulminating fatal cases. The progress of the disease resembles that of louse-borne typhus, except for the duration of the fever and the appearance of the rash.

The incubation period varies from a few days to two weeks. The onset is similar to louse-borne typhus, with the early establishment of remittent fluctuating fever which continues when it declines rapidly by lysis.

A rash resembling that of early measles appears on the third or fourth day. This fades and is succeeded on the fifth to seventh day by a roseolar macular eruption which develops first on wrists and ankles and then rapidly extends over the whole body including the palms, soles and face including the eyelids and the scalp. It sometimes involves the buccal and pharyngeal mucosa. The abdominal wall and the face are least affected. The lesions become progressively more prominent and petechiae develop in them. In severe cases they may become dark red and confluent and some may undergo necrosis. Sloughing, gangrenous and necrotic lesions of the skin, genitalia and extremities occur in late severe cases.

The general course of fièvre boutonneuse is similar to other forms of typhus but is comparatively mild and the mortality is low. The rash is roseolar, unlike that of louse-borne typhus, and commonly spreads to the palms, soles and face. As in mite typhus, there is often a primary lesion (the so-called 'tache noire') at the site of the infecting tick bite.

Diagnosis

The diagnosis of tick typhus is made by the usual techniques, using the Weil-Felix and complement-fixation reactions and agglutination of specific rickettsial suspensions. Blood containing *R. rickettsi* causes a characteristic testicular and scrotal reaction after intraperitoneal injection into guinea-pigs.

Treatment

General prophylaxis consists in burning tick-infected

bush, dipping livestock and eliminating or controlling the reservoir animals. Vaccines have been prepared from attenuated egg-passaged *R. rickettsi* which give some protection. These are most successful when administered subcutaneously at the time of greatest activity of the ticks, i.e. during the spring. The immunity which develops lasts only about a year.

Chloramphenicol and tetracyclines are specific, as for other forms of rickettsial infection [p. 142].

Prednisolone may help modify the severe effects and shorten the disease, in doses of 30 mg. followed in 24 hours by two further doses of 15 mg., and rapidly decreasing doses thereafter.

Formalin-killed vaccines are available against American tick typhus. There is at present no successful vaccine for the African disease.

FLEA-BORNE TYPHUS

Synonym. Murine typhus.

Aetiology

This disease is caused by *R. mooseri*, which normally infects rats. It is transmitted from rat to rat by the rat flea, usually *Xenopsylla cheopis*, which may infest man and transmit infection through its excreta, which may contain masses of the organisms. It is occasionally transmitted in rodents by the rat louse.

Man may be infected occasionally by inhalation of dust containing infected rat, flea or louse faeces. The organism is passed in the urine of infected rats and infection may thus result by contamination of food (sometimes called ship fever).

Flea-borne typhus is world wide in distribution and occurs especially where conditions are unhygienic and conducive to man-rat contact.

R. mooseri has been recovered also from wild rats in many parts of the world.

Only sporadic infections occur in man, whose ectoparasites do not normally transmit the infection. *R. mooseri* is closely related to *R. prowazeki*, and gives a similar Weil-Felix reaction. An attack of one disease immunizes the individual against an attack of the other.

Inoculation of infected blood into the guinea-pig produces fever and the Neill-Mooser tunica reaction [p. 141].

The pathology of flea-borne typhus is basically similar to that of louse-borne. The clinical picture is similar but milder. Complications are infrequent and mortality is low.

Diagnosis

The differentiation from the louse-borne infection may be difficult. Clinically there are no epidemics and the condition is milder.

The Weil-Felix reactions in the two infections are identical. Agglutination by the patient's serum of suspensions of the specific rickettsiae may help to differentiate them. Complement fixation methods may also help, but there is considerable overlap of antigenicity.

Intraperitoneal inoculation of infected blood from the patient into male guinea-pigs produces after 10 days both fever and the Neill-Mooser tunica reaction in *R. mooseri* infection and usually only fever in *R. prowazeki* infection.

Treatment

As with most rickettsial infections, the antibiotics chloramphenicol and the tetracyclines are specific [see p. 142].

There are no successful vaccines. Personal and communal prophylaxis consists essentially in avoidance of rat flea infested areas and the control of the rodent and flea population.

COXIELLA INFECTIONS

Q FEVER

Definition

An acute febrile illness caused by *Coxiella burneti* characterized by sudden onset, general symptoms including headache, and usually the development of interstitial pneumonitis. There is no rash and agglutinins to *Proteus* organisms do not develop.

Aetiology

The causative organism, *C. burneti*, is small and pleomorphic. It is present in the blood during the febrile period. It may also be recovered from sputum, urine or cerebrospinal fluid or from tissues, especially spleen, obtained at necrospsy.

Q fever is an enzootic of many wild and domestic animals transmitted naturally by certain ticks. It is commonly transmitted to domestic stock, including cattle. Ticks infesting livestock easily become infected with *C. burneti* which appears in their faeces. The causal organism is resistant to desiccation and is conveyed to man by inhalation of infected dust, by drinking milk or occasionally by ticks. Infection may also occur through handling infected tissues, secretions, etc. It occurs easily in laboratory workers handling *C. burneti*.

Q fever, with pulmonary involvement, can be reproduced in man by inhalation or intranasal instillation of infective material containing *C. burneti*. Intradermal or intramuscular inoculation of the organism may give rise to fever and rickettsaemia but without pulmonary signs.

Q fever appears sporadically or in explosive outbreaks. It was first described in Australia. It is now known to occur in many parts of the world, including England, Spain, Italy, Greece, the Middle East, tropical and South Africa and the United States of America. During the Second World War localized 'epidemics' occurred amongst troops stationed on the Mediterranean littoral.

Pathology

C. burneti can readily infect many wild and domesticated animals and several species of ticks; transovarial transmission has been described in the latter. Pathological changes in infected animals include moderate enlargement and engorgement of the spleen and small granulomatous lesions in many organs.

In man, post-mortem findings have been described in very few cases. The principal lesions are found in the lungs, especially in the basal zones, in which there are patchy consolidation and thickening of the alveolar walls and perivascular tissues due to accumulations of macrophages and round cells. Polymorphs and red cells occur in minimal numbers. There may be small scattered areas of necrosis and breaking down of alveolar septa. Foci of round cell and macrophage accumulations have been reported in the testes, kidneys and other organs; similar lesions, involving the microglia, occur in the brain. Intracellular and extracellular rickettsiae have been identified in smears of lung, spleen, testes and brain. Vegetative endocarditis has been described in a few cases.

Signs and Symptoms

The incubation period is 2–3 weeks. The onset is usually sudden. There is a wide variation in severity. The clinical picture may show nothing beyond a mild fever lasting only a day or two. In most cases, however, the temperature rises rapidly at first to moderate heights, but may reach 103°–105° F. (39·4°–40·6° C.) after 1 or 2 days. The fever is remittent and swinging. It lasts from a few days to 3 weeks. General symptoms may develop at the onset and persist through the febrile period. Headache and general muscular pains are often severe. Subjective feelings of cold and occasional shivering may occur, but rigor is unusual. Nocturnal sweating and insomnia are common in some outbreaks. Anorexia and nausea are the rule. The upper respiratory tract is not usually involved, but a slight dry cough may develop about the fourth day, accompanied by pain in the chest, which may be localized to one area. The sputum is usually mucoid or mucopurulent and may be blood-streaked; occasional small haemoptyses have been reported. In some patients dyspnoea may be the dominant picture, and there may be cyanosis. Examination of the chest at this stage may reveal localized reduction in air entry, commonly in one or both bases, with occasional crepitations and scattered rales. In seriously ill patients there may be obvious signs of consolidation in one or both bases. The physical signs of lung involvement, however, may vary considerably from day to day and are often evanescent, but evidence of pulmonary changes can usually be demonstrated by radiography which discloses a primary atypical pneumonia involving small areas of one or more lobes. The lesions may progress for a few days and then become stationary, disappearing only slowly. They frequently persist well into convalescence.

Evidence of changes in organs other than the lungs and the spleen is uncommon. In those cases in which the febrile episode continues for weeks, however, signs of liver involvement, including jaundice, may develop and occasionally cardiac valvular defects become apparent.

Relapses occur weeks or months after the initial attack in a small percentage of cases, with recurrence of fever and pulmonary signs and symptoms.

Course

Complications rarely develop. Delirium and signs of acute meningo-encephalitis have been reported. Orchitis has also been described during a severe attack. Some loss of weight occurs during the febrile period and there is considerable weakness, which may persist for weeks after treatment.

Fatal issue is rare. Deaths have been reported in a few natural infections and in a laboratory worker.

Diagnosis

Clinical diagnosis is difficult. A knowledge of the patient's employment especially in regard to contact with livestock is useful. The early stages of Q fever closely resemble those of many other acute febrile illnesses, and in the stage of pulmonary involvement the diagnosis of pneumonia or atypical pneumonia is commonly made. In some areas psittacosis and coccidioidomycosis must be differentiated. Diagnosis depends finally on the recovery of the organism or the results of serological examinations.

C. burneti can be recovered during the febrile stage of the illness by intraperitoneal inoculation of blood or urine into guinea-pigs. The organism is eventually identified in spleen smears from the infected animals. Because of the considerable danger of accidental infection, isolation of the organism should not be attempted except under the proper laboratory conditions.

Diagnosis is usually made by examination of the serum for agglutinins against killed suspensions of *C. burneti* and for complement fixing bodies. Agglutinins appear by the end of the second week and can be identified in most cases by the end of the fourth week. Complement-fixing bodies may be present by the seventh day and are at a high titre by the end of the third or fourth week.

The antibody content of the serum in a given patient should be ascertained early and late in the illness. Diagnosis should be made in the presence of a rising titre of antibodies. Titres of 1 : 8 for agglutination and 1 : 20 for complement fixation are regarded as significant, but considerably higher titres are usually found at a late stage, i.e. weeks and even months after the onset.

No cross-reactions with other members of the rickettsial group occur; serum from a case of Q fever will not agglutinate *Proteus* suspensions and does not contain cold agglutinins.

Treatment

Chloramphenicol and tetracyclines are effective in the doses used for other forms of rickettsial infections.

Treatment results in the fall of temperature to normal in a day or two and rapid resolution of the pulmonary signs. A few cases may relapse shortly after treatment is stopped. These must be immediately re-treated.

Prophylaxis is best achieved by immunization (with formalized vaccine prepared from infected yolk-sac tissue) of individuals likely to be exposed to infection in stock yards, dairies, slaughter-houses, etc. Pasteurization or boiling of milk is necessary in areas known to be infected: the former process may not be efficient. Transmission from patient to patient in a ward is unlikely so long as sterilization of sputum and excreta is carried out. Quarantine and isolation are unnecessary.

BRIAN MAEGRAITH

NEWCASTLE DISEASE VIRUS INFECTION

Newcastle disease virus (NDV) is a member of the myxo group of viruses which affects the respiratory and gastro-intestinal tracts or the central nervous system of fowl. A small number of proven human infections in the form of a mild febrile illness with a unilateral superficial conjunctivitis have been reported in persons closely exposed to infected birds. The incubation period has been only 1–2 days. The illness is of about 7–10 days' duration.

Diagnosis is best made by isolation of the virus from conjunctival exudates by inoculation into embryonated hen eggs or tissue cultures. Tests for rise in antibody may also be made, but the results must be interpreted with caution as no antibodies may be detected even in those in whom the virus has been isolated from the conjunctiva. Cross-reactions with mumps virus antigens may be present.

There is no specific treatment.

FOOT AND MOUTH DISEASE

The virus causing this disease in cattle and occasionally in sheep and swine is one of the smallest known, about 20 millimicrons, and also one of the most stable in ordinary atmospheric conditions. In spite of the widespread nature of the disease in the affected animal, with superficial lesions in the mouth and on the hoofs, the paucity of human cases suggests that man has a relatively low susceptibility. It has been suggested that vesicles on the mouth and lips in humans have been caused by drinking infected milk.

Virus isolation should be attempted from all suspected cases by inoculation of vesicle fluid into guinea-pigs, new-born mice and tissue cultures. Serological tests are also possible in special laboratories.

There is no specific treatment, but 0·5 per cent. sodium hydroxide should be applied to skin lesions.

ORF

Synonym. Contagious pustular dermatitis of sheep.

This is a not uncommon infection of sheep and goats in many countries. It is caused by a virus which is similar in size to the pox viruses, but differs from them in its lack of pathogenicity for embryonated fowl eggs and for laboratory animals, except rabbits to which it may be transmitted by the use of highly concentrated virus. It has been grown in tissue cultures of human amnion. There is no apparent immunological relationship to the pox viruses. The appearance of the virus in the electron microscope is specific, and examination of material from a lesion may confirm a clinical diagnosis.

The disease usually occurs in animals under one year of age. The lesions are present on and around the mouth and hoofs and elsewhere on the skin in areas free of hair. Infection of man occurs most often on the hands and arms, but sometimes on the face and neck. There is usually only a single papule with redness and swelling of the surrounding tissue and no other evidence of disease. A vesicle gradually develops, slowly resolves, and heals without scar.

There is no specific treatment.

MISCELLANEOUS INFECTIONS

The organisms responsible for this group of infections share properties with both bacteria and true viruses. In addition to man they are found in a wide range of birds and animals usually causing mild or inapparent infections, but some members may cause abortion in ewes or dairy cattle and encephalitis. These agents have only been cultivated in living tissues up to the present time, as have the true animal viruses, but in contrast to the latter their growth may be inhibited by sulpha drugs and many antibiotics, the tetracyclines being the most active. Persistent subclinical or low-grade infection may occur in lymphogranuloma venereum and in the lung in psittacosis. Recovery does not appear to be associated with a significant level of neutralizing or protective antibodies. Some members of the group elaborate a toxin, which is demonstrable by its lethal effect on mice when inoculated intravenously. It is not known whether this plays any part in natural infection of man.

REFERENCE

BEDSON, S. P. (1959) The psittacosis-lymphogranuloma group of infective agents, *J. roy. Inst. publ. Hlth*, **22**, 67, 99, 131.

PSITTACOSIS (ORNITHOSIS)

Synonym. Parrot fever.

Definition

A febrile illness in which inflammation of the lung may occur, sometimes a fatal pneumonia and rarely encephalitis, caused by agents whose natural hosts are psittacines of various species (psittacosis) and pigeons, domestic fowl, fulmars, egrets and numerous other avian species (ornithosis).

Aetiology

The disease is caused by agents which occupy a

position midway between the rickettsiae and the true viruses, but will be referred to as viruses. They vary considerably in size depending upon the stage of their development which takes place by binary fission. They possess a deoxyribonucleic acid core but also ribonucleic acid, lipids and carbohydrates. Their natural hosts are various psittacine birds, domestic fowl and wild birds such as pigeons and gulls. In these the virus normally lies dormant, but, if the general health of the bird deteriorates, lethal infection develops. These viruses may be transmitted from avian hosts to man, and person to person communicability is possible though uncommon. Transmission is usually airborne from infected secretions or excreta, but is possible from avian hosts. Other members of this family of viruses, which have domestic animals such as the ewe as their natural host, may also be transmitted to man and produce disease.

Pathology

Infection usually takes place from infected droplets, so maximum damage is found in the lung, but systemic infection also occurs and in fatal cases which will probably have succumbed from pneumonia, pathological changes may be found in other organs, possibly as the result of a toxin produced by the virus. Patchy consolidation of the lung will be present and there may be enlargement of the liver and spleen, haemorrhage into the adrenals and congestion and oedema of the heart, meninges and brain.

Microscopical examination shows proliferation of the lining cells of the alveoli with cellular infiltration of the walls. The alveoli contain an exudate of desquamated cells and phagocytes in which the agent may be found; few polymorphonuclear leucocytes are seen. The bronchi and large bronchioles are comparatively unaffected. Focal necrosis will be present in the hepatic parenchyma and degeneration of the kidney parenchyma may be found. Cytoplasmic inclusions may be found in the cells of the meningeal exudate. Proliferation and degeneration of the lining cells of the capillaries may be seen in the brain. Myocarditis and damage to other parts of the vascular system are not infrequently present.

Symptoms and Signs

The incubation period is about 10 days, with extremes of a few days to two weeks, but in severe cases may appear to have been longer, due to an insidious onset.

Infection most often takes the form of a mild pyrexial or influenza-like illness with abrupt onset and without any localizing signs. In the classical case the onset may be sudden, with severe influenza-like symptoms and a temperature of 100°–102° F. (37·8°–39° C.). The respiration rate may be increased. The pulse may be relatively slow as in typhoid fever. A dry cough may develop and there may be scanty mucopurulent or purulent sputum. Moist rales followed by signs of patchy consolidation appear about the second week. Radiological examination will reveal much more extensive lesions than suspected from the physical signs.

There may be nausea, vomiting, diarrhoea or constipation. In more severe cases albuminuria is not infrequent, hepatomegaly may be present as well as myocardial damage which may be prolonged, and epistaxis and rose spots. The spleen is usually not palpable. Meningitis, encephalopathy and mental depression may all occur. There is usually a leucopenia. Death is from pulmonary insufficiency and toxaemia.

Inadequate treatment favours a relapse.

Diagnosis

In the absence of known contact with sick birds, there is little to differentiate the disease from influenza, Q fever or other virus pneumonia, except possibly the relatively slow pulse and respiratory rate. Mere contact with sick birds is of course not diagnostic and specific diagnosis can only be made by laboratory tests. Complement fixation tests are made with serum collected in the acute stage and again 14–21 days later. If treatment has been begun early the formation of antibody may be suppressed and repeat tests at the fourth or fifth week may be necessary.

If patients are seen in the first day or two of illness, before treatment has been started, the agent may be isolated from the sputum and the blood by inoculation into the yolk sac of embryonated eggs or into mice. The agent may be isolated from the lung and spleen of fatal cases, but only with difficulty in patients who have received antibiotics.

Treatment

Tetracyclines are active against these agents and chlortetracycline is probably the drug of choice. A recommended course is 4 G. daily for two days, then 2 G. daily until recovery. Symptomatic improvement is the rule if large doses are begun early and continued for a week or two. Convalescence should be gradual in those who have had pneumonia or myocardial damage.

Prognosis

This disease carried a considerable mortality rate before the introduction of the antibiotics. Fatalities may still occur in the very young and the elderly, particularly if treatment is not begun early in the disease. Especially virulent strains of virus appear to have been responsible for the high fatality rate in some small outbreaks. General debility may persist for several weeks after the temperature has returned to normal and the disappearance of physical signs in the lungs.

REFERENCE

HARDING, H. B. (1962) The epidemiology of sporadic urban ornithosis, *Amer. J. clin. Path.*, **38**, 230.

F. O. MACCALLUM

LYMPHOGRANULOMA VENEREUM

Synonym. Nicholas-Favre's disease.

Definition

A sexually transmitted infectious disease due to an agent of the species Bedsonia.

Aetiology

It is common in tropical and subtropical climates but relatively uncommon in temperate climates.

The infective agent belongs to a group which includes those of psittacosis, trachoma and inclusion conjunctivitis. The nomenclature is still uncertain. The organisms are in some respects more related to bacteria than viruses. They have been grouped under the heading of Bedsonia or Chlamydia.

The disease is transmitted sexually and usually commences with a transient inconspicuous genital lesion after an incubation period which is rarely less than a week but may be 3–5 weeks.

Signs and Symptoms

Early Lesions. The primary lesion is usually herpetiform but varies in appearance. It is often missed completely and seldom found in women. It may be intra-urethral giving rise to a form of non-gonococcal urethritis. If the lesion is on the external genitalia it may be followed, in a few days to a few weeks, by inflammatory enlargement of the inguinal lymph nodes, the 'inguinal syndrome'. Involvement is usually unilateral but it is sometimes bilateral. The patient experiences pain in the groin and becomes aware of painful tender swellings. The swellings soon become matted together and adherent to skin and deep structures. The iliac nodes at the pelvic brim and the femoral nodes may be involved. Suppuration occurs with multiple small abscesses, bluish-red discoloration of adherent skin, and multiple sinus formation. The sinuses discharge semi-caseous material which may, however, become purulent and blood-stained, due to secondary pyogenic infection. This is the typical clinical picture but there are many variations.

Associated constitutional symptoms are variable but sometimes severe. They include chills, fever, headache, anorexia, nausea, arthralgia and loss of weight. The pulse rate is raised and the temperature may be raised to 103° F. (39·5° C.). In the absence of treatment, clinical recovery may take weeks or months and characteristic scars remain in the groins.

Late Lesions. Late manifestations may appear from a year or two up to many years later. They include the 'anorectal syndrome', commoner in women, with proctitis, rectal ulceration and proctocolitis leading to stricture. Later, anal fistula, perirectal abscess and rectovesical and rectovaginal fistulae may complicate the condition. Malignant changes have followed. There may be chronic lymphatic oedema of the vulva (*esthiomène*) or male genitalia (elephantiasis) sometimes with ulcerative granulomatous and polypoid masses on the surface.

Diagnosis

An intradermal test (Frei's test) was introduced in 1925. As now employed, the antigen is prepared from the infective agent grown in the yolk sacs of developing chick embryos; 0·3 ml. of the preparation is injected into the skin of one forearm and the same amount of control material, made from normal yolk, into the other forearm. The test is read at 48 and 72 hours and, if positive, gives a raised red papule, at least 8 mm. across and surrounded by a variable area of erythema; the control should give no reaction. The test is usually positive within 2–3 weeks of infection but once reactivity is established it may persist for many years and perhaps for life, irrespective of the activity of the infection.

The same specific antigen is used for the complement fixation test and this is more sensitive and reliable than the intradermal test. It usually gives positive results earlier in the course of the disease and a positive result in dilutions of blood serum to 1 in 16 or above is regarded as evidence of active or recent infection with the virus. Persistent lower titres probably indicate past rather than present infection. There is cross-reaction with the infective agent of psittacosis.

In many cases of active disease there is hyperglobulinaemia, and the erythrocyte sedimentation rate is raised.

Treatment

In early cases good results may follow the use of a sulphonamide such as sulphathiazole and sulphadiazine, 5 G. daily in divided doses for 5–10 days. Long-acting sulphonamides, such as sulphadimethoxine may be equally effective in dosage of 1·5 G. on the first day, then 0·5 G. daily. In some cases treatment has to be continued for a longer period.

Tetracycline, chlortetracycline and oxytetracycline have given good results but they are sometimes disappointing. Dosage is 500 mg. every 6 hours for 21 days.

Claims have been made for triacetyloleandomycin in dosage of 1 G. twice daily for 5 days.

In some late cases surgical treatment of the anorectal and colonic complications may be necessary.

REFERENCES

GREENBLATT, R. B. (1953) United States Public Health Service Publication No., 255, p. 38.

KING, A. J., and NICOL, C. S. (1969) *Venereal Diseases*, 2nd ed., London.

CLAUDE NICOL

TRACHOMA—INCLUSION CONJUNCTIVITIS

Synonym. Granular conjunctivitis; Inclusion blenorrhoea of the newborn.

Definition

A specific communicable keratoconjunctivitis caused by an agent or agents belonging to the psittacosis group and characterized by the formation of follicles, papillary hyperplasia and in severe cases pannus and scar formation.

Aetiology

The disease is caused by a specific agent (trachoma-inclusion conjunctivitis = TRIC) which has properties similar to those of the psittacosis-lymphogranuloma venereum group. It may be isolated from infected material by inoculation into the yolk sac of embryonated hen eggs. As a result of extensive investigations in several regions of the world in recent years, ideas about the natural history of the disease and identity of the agents associated with trachoma and inclusion conjunctivitis are changing. Rather than two distinct entities of separate aetiology, it is probable that there is a spectrum of similar organisms, possessing slight antigenic differences which may cause mild or severe infection of the eye, urethritis in the male and cervicitis in the female. Strains of the agent which are indistinguishable by all laboratory tests from some of those associated with so-called inclusion conjunctivitis have been recovered from the eyes of patients with the keratitis, pannus and conjunctival cicatrization characteristic of trachoma. Similarly, agents indistinguishable by laboratory tests have been isolated from the genital tract and eyes of the same patient with clinical trachoma. Infection occurs from contact with other patients with active lesions or from infected fomites. In developed countries in temperate climates, such as Great Britain, it is essentially a sporadic venereal disease. Primary infection of the eyes is usually in infancy or early childhood, but may occur at any age. Recurrent attacks are seen in patients whose lesions have apparently healed. Monkeys and baboons have been infected and showed no immunity to re-infection; the second attack runs a similar course to the original infection, but is often milder.

Pathology

This will vary depending upon the severity of the infection, which in turn may depend upon the mode of infection, the age of the patient, the environment (dirt, secondary bacterial infection) and possibly the strain of infecting organism. In mild infections, usually seen in the newborn and called inclusion conjunctivitis (because inclusions are found), the conjunctivitis is generally most marked in the lower lid. There is infiltration with polymorphonuclear leucocytes, but as lymphoid tissue is absent in this site at birth, follicles will not be seen until the second month. In the adult, follicular hyperplasia with round cell infiltration follows the initial acute polymorphonuclear reaction. In areas where the disease is endemic, generally more serious and called trachoma, the upper half of the conjunctival sac and cornea are said to be more affected than the lower half.

Cytoplasmic inclusions may be seen in the epithelial cells before any other change is visible. The next stage is a subepithelial infiltration of small round cells, particularly plasma cells, with oedema and the formation of minute lymphoid follicles. The exudate is chiefly of polymorphonuclear leucocytes, which are present even when secondary infection is absent. Superficial vascularization of the cornea occurs and finally there is necrosis of the subepithelial tissue of the conjunctiva followed by cicatrization.

Signs and Symptoms

The incubation period varies between 1 and 10 days, but is usually 3–7 days. The onset is usually insidious, but may be acute if the infecting dose is large and by the direct route, as from the genital tract during birth.

In the newborn, infection manifests itself as a mucopurulent conjunctivitis with a swelling of the lids affecting one or both eyes. A discharge has been first seen as early as the first day of life and as late as the fourteenth day. In the early stage the conjunctiva is congested and oedematous. As the disease progresses the conjunctiva becomes thickened with papillary hypertrophy and diffuse infiltration. The acute stage lasts about 10–14 days and the inflammation cannot be distinguished clinically from bacterial or other conjunctivitis. The disease may gradually subside over a period of weeks, but even in mild infections the conjunctiva rarely returns to normal in less than three months. Bacterial infection is more common than in adults. Scarring and pannus, i.e. trachoma, may develop.

In older children and adults, tissues react differently from the newborn. In childhood the disease is frequently mild and unrecognized in the early stages. The pathological changes usually persist longer in adults than in children. When the onset is acute, there may be a very marked papillary hypertrophy of the conjunctiva together with oedema of the upper limbus, subepithelial infiltration and possible pannus and abundant exudate. This stage may persist for several weeks after which, if no secondary infection occurs, the lesion becomes less intense and the exudate decreases. Spontaneous healing may occur in a childhood infection, but in adults the lesion is likely to progress slowly to conjunctival and corneal cicatrization. When this occurs vision eventually becomes distorted as the result of corneal scarring; other complications are ptosis, trichiasis and entropion. Thus the lesion can recover, the end result being inclusion conjunctivitis, punctate keratitis or trachoma.

Diagnosis

In the acute stage and in mild infections a specific diagnosis can only be made on finding cytoplasmic inclusions in epithelial cells. When a purulent discharge is present the lesion in the newborn must be differentiated from gonococcal and staphylococcal ophthalmia. The typical changes described as trachoma are pathognomonic. The introduction of improved laboratory methods of culture, such as tissue culture, for isolation of these agents may help to clarify numerous points.

Treatment

For active trachoma sulphadiazine is given by mouth, 2 G. initially and then 1 G. four times daily for one week. It is advisable to continue with 0·5 G. three times daily for a second week. Simultaneously, chlortetracycline or tetracycline may be given orally, 1 G. daily for two weeks, and drops or ointment may be applied locally. In mass campaigns in some regions it has been convenient, economical and satisfactory to apply chlortetracycline locally as an ointment or oily solution twice daily for 3–6 consecutive days each month over a period of 6 months. Physical signs may persist for several weeks or months after the agent has disappeared as the result of successful treatment or the agent may persist after clinical signs have disappeared. In patients first seen in the later stages of the disease surgical treatment may be necessary because of the entropion and trichiasis resulting from cicatricial changes in the conjunctiva. Improvements in the standard of living aids control of the disease in those countries where it is endemic.

Prognosis

The prognosis is good if treatment is instituted early in the disease, and in children with a mild infection in the primary attack little scarring may occur. However, untreated recurrent infections may result in total blindness in about 1 per cent. and defective vision rendering the patient incapable of independent manual work in another 4 or 5 per cent.

REFERENCE

American Journal of Ophthalmology (1967) Conference on Trachoma and Allied Diseases, **63**, 1041.

F. O. MacCallum

NON-GONOCOCCAL GENITAL INFECTION

Aetiology and Epidemiology

Apart from gonorrhoea, urethritis may result from a number of causes including: infection higher in the urinary tract, pre-existing urethral stricture, the vaginal parasite *Trichomonas vaginalis*, various bacteria, a fungus such as *Candida albicans*, trauma, including the application of antiseptics, neoplasms and viruses such as those of herpes genitalis and the infective agent of lymphogranuloma venereum. An allergic factor may sometimes be involved. In about 90 per cent. of the cases of non-gonococcal urethritis, however, no definite cause has yet been established but the strong presumption is that it is a sexually transmitted infection with either the 'T' strain of mycoplasma or with the TRIC agent of the Chlamydia (Bedsonia).

Signs and Symptoms

In the male the urethral symptoms of discharge and dysuria, which are usually slight, are likely to commence from 10 days to 4 weeks after intercourse. On examination the patient is seen to have mucopurulent urethral discharge, smears from which show pus cells but no organisms; cultures grow no organisms or only a few contaminants. For this reason the condition is sometimes called abacterial or 'non specific' urethritis. One characteristic of the urethritis requires special mention. The urethral secretion is frequently so slight that the patient does not notice it. This may account for the long incubation periods which are sometimes described: for the condition may be present for some time before it attracts attention and may be finally precipitated by a large intake of alcohol. The true incubation period is probably about 10–14 days.

In other cases the patient remains completely unaware of his condition which may come to light in the course of routine examination for some other reason or through the development of a complication. Patients with asymptomatic infection may show no signs of the disease at the time of examination. In order to recognize the signs it may be necessary to examine the patient in the early morning before the first urine has been passed: if the urine has been held for 8 hours or more a urethral smear can be taken and the urine will contain pus threads. Patients with asymptomatic infection are, of course, likely to be infectious to others. In a small number of cases of severe infection the discharge is accompanied by haematuria and symptoms of cystitis, when it is called acute abacterial or haemorrhagic cystitis. In other cases pyuria may be the only evidence of the disease and the condition is then called abacterial pyuria. This urethritis has for some time been a common condition and now seems to be becoming more so. The number of men attending the venereal diseases clinics of England and Wales with evidence of non-gonococcal infection increased from 10,794 in 1951 to 47,292 in 1970. This compares with 37,784 cases of gonorrhoea in men at the clinics in that year.

Female Consorts. The consorts of men with non-gonococcal urethritis nearly always show some signs of inflammation which is presumed to be due to the same cause. Often there are no symptoms but if present they may be due to associated trichomonal vaginitis. The infection causes urethritis, cervicitis and sometimes proctitis. The diagnosis is difficult to make in women because the urethritis is usually slight and the cervicitis has no characteristic features. The new-born infant of such a woman may develop a mild ophthalmia.

Local Complications. The local complications in men and women are similar to those which affect the patients suffering from gonorrhoea [pp. 80, 81] but they tend to be less acute. In particular, ascending infection with inflammation of the uterine adnexa occurs in many cases in females and recrudescence and relapse of tubal inflammation are common. Sterility is a possible sequela.

Systemic Complications. There is some division of opinion as to whether the urethritis associated with Reiter's disease is the same as the uncomplicated condition just described. Up to the point at which the arthritic and ocular lesions occur the urethritis of the so-called 'venereal syndrome' of Reiter's disease appears to take an identical course and, in the absence of absolute evidence, it seems likely that the two conditions are due to the same cause.

Treatment

The same rules as in gonorrhoea about avoiding sexual intercourse and the consumption of alcoholic drinks should be followed. The disease will then respond fairly well to systemic treatment, but in untreated cases signs and symptoms tend to resolve in 6–8 weeks. It is sometimes difficult to distinguish between relapse and reinfection. The penicillins in general are ineffective, but ampicillin, 250 mg. six-hourly for 5 days, is moderately effective. The combination of streptomycin and sulphonamide has given good results in the past although each remedy by itself is ineffective. Streptomycin, 1 G., is injected intramuscularly and this may be followed by sulphathiazole or sulphadiazine, 5–6 G. in divided doses by mouth daily for 5 days. Equally good results are obtained by the combination of streptomycin with a long-acting sulphonamide, such as sulphadimethoxine, in similar dosage, such as 1·5 G. on the first day and 0·5 G. daily for a further 4 days. However, tetracycline and oxytetracycline by mouth seem to be the most effective remedies. Dosage of the tetracyclines ranges between 250 and 500 mg. six-hourly for 5–20 days. Spiramycin (*Rovamycin*) has also given good results, the usual dosage being 500 mg. every 6 hours for 5–10 days. Demethylchlortetracycline, 300–600 mg. twice daily by mouth for 5–20 days, also seems effective, but care should be taken to avoid photosensitivity reactions. The longer course or higher daily dosage of all these antibiotics is particularly indicated when relapse has occurred.

Tests for Cure. These should be no less stringent than those applied after an attack of gonorrhoea. The details of procedure are identical [pp. 80, 81].

REITER'S DISEASE

Synonyms. Brodie's disease; Urethro-conjunctivo-synovial (UCS) syndrome.

Definition

A syndrome of non-gonococcal urethritis, polyarthritis and conjunctivitis or iritis.

Aetiology

In Great Britain and North America it is found in association with sexually transmitted non-gonococcal urethritis. On the continent of Europe, in Asia, and in North Africa, it is more often reported with bacillary or amoebic dysentery or non-specific diarrhoea. In cases following dysentery an early indication of the presence of the syndrome is likely to be a non-gonococcal urethritis and, irrespective of the mode of onset, the subsequent behaviour of the fully developed condition appears to be the same. In some cases of the sexually acquired disease the patient may have active gonorrhoea or the history of recent gonococcal infection. It seems likely that neither gonorrhoea nor the dysenteries are direct causes of Reiter's disease but it has been suggested that damage to the urethral and intestinal mucosae by these infections acts as a predisposing factor. Remedies which are effective for these two conditions neither prevent nor alleviate Reiter's disease. There is some evidence that a familial factor is involved.

Clinical Features

The condition is considerably more common in males than in females. The likely age of onset is between 20 and 40, although younger and older patients are sometimes affected.

The full syndrome consists of non-gonococcal urogenital infection in the form of urethritis, prostatitis and cystitis, in that order of frequency; arthritis which is usually polyarticular; conjunctivitis or iritis and distinctive lesions of mucous membranes and skin, the latter usually termed keratoderma blenorrhagica. In the majority of the cases the full syndrome is not present, a fact which has led to confusion in diagnosis and in nomenclature.

Arthritis. The onset of the arthritis may be acute or subacute and it is likely to be associated with variable pyrexia and tachycardia. In severe cases, particularly those with generalized keratoderma, the patient appears ill and may rapidly become cachectic.

The blood picture shows a moderate normocytic anaemia and slight neutrophil leucocytosis. The erythrocyte sedimentation rate is raised, being more than 100 mm. in the hour in more severe cases; there is elevation of the alpha-2-globulin. Results of the serological tests for the rheumatoid factor are almost invariably negative: lupus erythematosus cells are not found and serum uric acid levels are within normal limits. In less severe cases constitutional changes may be slight and changes in the blood picture and erythrocyte sedimentation rate are proportionately diminished.

The attack of arthritis is usually self-limiting, the course varying from 1 to 18 months. Many patients are prone to recurrent attacks. The joints usually involved are those of the lower limbs, especially the knees, ankles, metatarsophalangeal joints and other small joints of the feet. Sometimes there is widespread involvement of joints which may include those of the hands, elbows, shoulders, sternoclavicular, sacro-iliac and temporomandibular joints. If only one joint is involved it is most likely to be the knee. Suppuration does not occur. Aspirated joint fluid is yellow and turbid containing numerous polymorphonuclear leucocytes with occasional lymphocytes. It is sterile on culture. Synovial biopsies show no characteristic diagnostic features. In the early stages of the disease X-ray changes in the joints are absent or minimal.

Lesions of the Eyes. Conjunctivitis occurs in about half the cases. It is usually bilateral and most marked on the tarsal conjunctiva of the lower lids especially at the lateral angles. Usually it is mild and transient, but occasionally severe and purulent with chemosis. Anterior uveitis sometimes occurs later in the course of a first attack of arthritis and may be preceded by an attack of conjunctivitis. Most commonly it appears months or years after the onset of the disease, by which time the other manifestations may have become symptomless. Some patients suffer as many as 20–30 attacks of uveitis and blindness may eventually result. There is evidence of close correlation between the presence of chronic sacro-iliitis and the development of anterior uveitis. Keratitis and corneal ulceration occur infrequently.

Lesions of Skin and Mucous Membranes. Keratoderma blenorrhagica is found in about 8 per cent. of these patients. It commences on the skin of the soles of the feet in the form of dull-red macules which become vesicular, then pustular and then keratotic. The keratotic patches may be hard and nodular or consist of limpet-like soft masses of scale. The rash is commonly confined to the soles of the feet, but in severe cases it may spread to involve the digits including the nail beds, the limbs, trunk and even the scalp. Lesions of the penis are found in about 25 per cent. of the cases. They are rounded, shallow, red erosions with slightly raised edges and often covered by a thin greyish membrane. Adjacent erosions may coalesce to form larger lesions with a circinate outline. On this account the condition is often called circinate balanitis. In circumcised patients soft keratotic crusts may form on the surface of the lesion. Lesions of the tongue and buccal mucosa occur in about 10 per cent. of cases. They are usually painless superficial erosions, and a particularly common site is the mucosa covering the hard palate. Like those of the penis they are rounded and red and tend to coalesce. Occasionally the surface may be covered by a greyish membrane.

Other Systemic Manifestations. Involvement of the nervous system is rare but peripheral neuropathy has been reported. The cardiovascular system is occasionally affected and aortic incompetence and electrocardiographic changes associated with pericarditis or myocarditis have been described. Lesions of the lungs have also been reported.

The Late Course of the Disease

As stated, acute or subacute attacks of Reiter's disease are usually self-limiting and are likely to subside spontaneously after periods which vary from 1 to 18 months. It seems that few of these patients make a complete and permanent recovery. The late effects fall into five groups:

1. Multiple Attacks without Residual Damage to the Joints. The late episodes of arthritis are sometimes related to sexual intercourse and to fresh attacks, or relapses, of urethritis. The intervals between recurrences vary greatly, from a few weeks or months to a number of years. In recurrent attacks, as with first attacks, the distribution of the arthritis follows no set pattern, for although the knees and feet are usually affected, some patients show more generalized polyarthritis with involvement of the hands and wrists.

2. Painful Deformities of the Feet. The commonest of these is the painful calcaneal spur, related to the posterior attachment of the plantar fascia. Occasionally periostitis of the os calcis may be seen in the X-ray to extend over the entire inferior and posterior surfaces of the bone. A spur may also develop at the site of attachment of the Achilles tendon. Pes planus is sometimes a residual deformity; or in other cases pes cavus occurs and both conditions may be associated with fixed dorsiflexion of all the toes at the metatarsophalangeal joints and hyperflexion at the proximal interphalangeal joints, giving multiple hammer-toe deformities. The hammer-toe deformities and also lateral deviation of the toes at the metatarsophalangeal joints sometimes occur without pes planus or pes cavus.

3. Painful Feet without Deformity. The most usual effects of this kind are tenderness of the heel on walking, localized in the region of the posterior attachment of the plantar fascia to the os calcis, and tendinitis of the Achilles tendon.

4. The Syndrome of Spondylitis. In the course of years a few of these patients develop a condition resembling ankylosing spondylitis. This does not conform to the pattern of classical ankylosing spondylitis, in which progressive spinal stiffness is the predominant symptom. The condition presents with polyarthritis, affecting chiefly the ankles and feet, and spinal stiffness with comparatively little pain follows later. Routine radiographs in relapsing cases of Reiter's disease have shown evidence of chronic sacro-iliitis in 45 per cent. of the cases and in many of them there have been few symptoms of the involvement. Changes in the sacro-iliac joints tend to be progressive and the end result may be their complete obliteration. In a few the process extends to spinal joints and ligaments with the end result of 'poker-back'.

Many patients with classical ankylosing spondylitis have evidence of chronic inflammation of prostate gland and seminal vesicles and some of them suffer from anterior uveitis. Although the significance of this is speculative, it seems likely that there is some relationship between Reiter's disease and ankylosing spondylitis [see Section 10].

5. Recurrent Attacks of Uveitis. As already described, anterior uveitis is usually a late complication of the disease with onset months or years after the initial attack. Patients with chronic sacro-iliitis seem to be particularly prone to recurrent anterior uveitis and a few develop aortic incompetence. Investigation of patients with anterior uveitis of unknown cause has shown that more than 70 per cent. of them have chronic prostatovesiculitis, as compared with 29 per cent. of patients of the same age groups with no history of uveitis or genital infection. Some of the patients with uveitis have been found to be suffering from undiagnosed Reiter's disease and others from ankylosing spondylitis or plantar fasciitis. This association suggests the possibility that the common factor in these conditions is genital infection, in the form of urethritis or chronic prostatovesiculitis.

Differential Diagnosis

In straightforward cases observed in the acute stage this presents no difficulty, but there are many less typical cases in which the diagnosis from other rheumatic diseases presents considerable difficulty. Reiter's disease may have to be distinguished from rheumatoid arthritis, ankylosing spondylitis, gout, psoriatic arthropathy, gonococcal arthritis, acute rheumatic fever and the arthritic manifestation of serum sickness.

Treatment

Bed rest, good nursing and good feeding are essential until the active phase of the attack has passed. The course of the arthritis is not influenced by antibiotics but some of them have a favourable effect on the urogenital infection in many cases. Tetracycline may therefore be given by mouth in doses of 250–500 mg. every 6 hours for 5–20 days. These measures combined with calcium aspirin for the relief of pain, may suffice for mild cases. In more severe cases phenylbutazone (*Butazolidin*), oxyphenbutazone (*Tanderil*), 200 mg. given by mouth twice or three times daily, is usually strikingly effective in relieving pain. The dose should be reduced progressively as the severity of the pain lessens. Steroid hormones may be required in severe cases or in the event of failure to respond to the measures described. In such cases, treatment should commence with 60 mg. daily of prednisone or the equivalent, given in divided doses, slowly reduced to a daily maintenance dose of 15–20 mg.

In a case of severe prolonged painful arthritis the

patient will benefit from the use of light splints at night, but the immobilization must not be constant or prolonged or ankylosis may result. By day the patient should be encouraged to move the affected joints. As soon as the active phase of the arthritis has subsided, the patient should be mobilized and more active physiotherapy should be given.

If keratoderma blenorrhagica and circinate balanitis are present, simple hygienic measures are required to prevent secondary infection in moist areas. If the rash is widespread and severe the patient's general condition is likely to be such that steroid hormones are required and these in sufficient dosage will partially suppress the surface lesions. If not, a 1 per cent. hydrocortisone lotion may be used.

Conjunctivitis is usually mild and requires no treatment; if it is exceptionally severe chloramphenicol eye drops (0·5 per cent.) may be used to control secondary infection. Anterior uveitis, which may recur long after other manifestations of the disease have subsided, requires management by an ophthalmologist. The principles of treatment are dilatation of the pupil with 1 per cent. atropine drops (Atropine Sulphate Eye-Drops, B.P.C.) and the topical use of hydrocortisone (Hydrocortisone Eye-Drops, B.N.F.). In very severe cases it may be necessary to give subconjunctival injections of steroid hormones, or systemic prednisone. This treatment is usually effective in controlling any one attack but even so iridectomy may be required in severe relapsing cases.

It should not be forgotten that Reiter's disease, as seen in Western countries, is commonly associated with communicable non-gonococcal genital infection and the proper management of cases must include investigation of sexual partners.

REFERENCES

CSONKA, G. W. (1965) *Brit. J. vener. Dis.*, **41**, 65.
HANCOCK, J. A. H. (1965) *Practitioner*, **195**, 605.
HARKNESS, A. H. (1950) *Non-gonococcal Urethritis*, Edinburgh.
KING, A. J. (1964) *Recent Advances in Venereology*, London.
KING, A. J., and NICOL, C. S. (1969) *Venereal Diseases*, 2nd ed., London.

CLAUDE NICOL

BARTONELLOSIS

Synonyms. Oroya fever and verruga peruana; Carrión's disease.

Aetiology

Infection with the organism *Bartonella bacilliformis* is transmitted by the bite of female sand flies (*Phlebotomus*). The disease is characterized by two distinct and consecutive clinical patterns, namely, Oroya fever, a severe febrile episode associated with anaemia which may be very severe, and verruga peruana, characterized by the appearance of an eruption consisting of haemangiomata.

In untreated cases especially in epidemics the mortality may be very high because of complicating salmonella septicaemia.

Bartonellosis is limited to the eastern and western slopes of the Andes, in narrow valleys of Peru, Ecuador and Colombia at 2,000–10,000 feet above sea level.

The organism can be recovered from man or the insect vectors. It is a small pleomorphic Gram-negative bacterium-like motile body found in the febrile stage in large numbers inside the erythrocytes and in cells of the reticulo-endothelium throughout the body. It can be cultured in tissue culture or on blood agar. Many species of phlebotomus are vectors; the most widely distributed vector is *P. verrucarum*. The sand flies become infected within a few days of biting an infected host and subsequent transmission takes place through the proboscis during further feeding.

The disease is endemic in well-defined localities. Where non-immunes are collected it may become epidemic. Natives of the endemic areas acquire the disease in childhood and, since some immunity develops, it is seldom seen in adult indigenes.

Pathology

In the first stage there is massive invasion by the organism of the erythrocytes and reticulo-endothelial cells. Extensive haemolysis occurs with resulting anaemia. Diffuse or punctate haemorrhages appear in mucosae and submucous tissues and in serous membranes. There is generalized enlargement of lymph nodes and the liver and spleen are enlarged. The bone marrow is hyperplastic. The organisms are present in great numbers in the cytoplasm of the reticulo-endothelial cells throughout the body. These cells in the spleen and the Kupffer cells of the liver are loaded with yellow-brownish pigment (haemosiderin) which also lies in the tissue spaces. There is marked erythrophagocytosis. Central parenchymal necrosis occurs in the liver.

In the second stage, superficial lesions occur in the skin. They consist of newly formed blood vessels lying in oedematous connective tissue, in which there are haemorrhagic foci and marked proliferating endothelial cells. The endothelium of the blood vessels is hypertrophic and may reduce the effective lumen. Some vessels are compressed by the surrounding proliferating reticulo-endothelial cells. The endothelium of the blood vessels is hypertrophic and may reduce the effective lumen. Some vessels are compressed by the surrounding proliferating reticulo-endothelial cells.

At a later stage fibroblasts invade the tumours, over which the epithelium may be lost. Bleeding may be considerable and secondary infection of individual lesions is common.

There are often deeper subcutaneous nodules which may undergo necrosis. The organisms are found in the cytoplasm of the reticulo-endothelial cells, but in smaller numbers than in the febrile stage.

Signs and Symptoms

Oroya Fever. The incubation period is usually 3 or 4 weeks. The onset is sudden, with fever and rigor. There is increasing malaise and prostration, with headache and severe pains in the long bones and the joints, nausea, vomiting and diarrhoea. Anaemia from haemolysis becomes evident early and progresses steadily; the erythrocyte count may fall to fewer than one million cells per mm^3. There is an appreciable rise in reticulocytes which may present the appearance of macrocytosis. Nucleated erythrocytes also appear in the peripheral blood. The marrow is hyperplastic. There is no haemoglobinuria. The blood pressure falls, the skin becomes wax-like, the mucous membranes blanched. The fever is remittent or intermittent rising to a peak in the evenings and falling in the morning. After 2–6 weeks the signs may gradually subside, or septicaemia commonly due to *Salmonella typhimurium* may cause death, usually between the third to sixth week. In uncomplicated cases or in cases in which the salmonella infection is treated, the prognosis is good.

Verruga Peruana. This syndrome usually follows the febrile illness after some weeks or months but it may begin before the fever is ended. The lesions develop on the skin and mucous membranes, and are particularly prevalent on the face and limbs. The mucous membranes of the mouth, nose and eyes may be affected. They appear as a rule as miliary lesions a few millimetres in diameter, bright or dull red and slightly raised above the surface. They are at first covered with a thin layer of shiny skin but may break down through the skin or even become pedunculated. There are often similar more deeply seated lesions in the subcutaneous tissues which may be some centimetres across and project above the surface. The lesions bleed freely when damaged and easily become secondarily infected. The various types of lesions occur concurrently and appear in successive crops. They persist for some months and occasionally for a year or more. Healing occurs without scar formation unless they have been ulcerated and infected.

Diagnosis

The clinical features of both episodes are characteristic within the endemic areas. Examination of thin blood films stained with Giemsa will reveal the bartonella in the erythrocytes during the febrile illness. The organisms can be seen in the reticulo-endothelial cells in smears from lesions taken in the eruptive stage.

Treatment

There is no specific treatment. The salmonella infection can be controlled with chloramphenicol or tetracyclines in the usual doses.

BRIAN MAEGRAITH

DISEASES DUE TO VIRAL INFECTION

GENERAL ASPECTS

The criteria which lead to the classification of an organism as a virus are smallness of size, obligate intracellular parasitism and resistance to antibiotics. In the true sense a virus is not an organism as it has no independent metabolism, but as we are only interested here in viruses as a cause of infectious disease, they will be considered as such. Although originally described as viruses, the organisms of the psittacosis-lymphogranuloma venereum-trachoma group replicate in a manner resembling bacteria, they are sensitive to sulphonamides and some antibiotics, and are placed in an intermediate position between the rickettsiae and the largest true viruses; they are frequently referred to as the bedsoniae, or more recently as the chlamydia. However, the diseases caused by the psittacosis group and respiratory infection caused by a bacterium, *Mycoplasma pneumoniae*, are included in this section on virus diseases.

Viruses differ from bacteria in their mode of replication. The latter contain within themselves all the necessary apparatus for their reproduction, drawing their nutrients from an artificial culture medium or from the tissues of higher organisms. Viruses are largely nucleoprotein in nature and the nucleic acid fraction is responsible for replication of the whole virus by instructing the synthesizing mechanism of the cell to produce viral rather than cellular components. Thus, for its reproduction the virus uses both cell nutrients and cell machinery.

Studies of bacterial viruses have advanced our understanding of how viral nucleic acids initiate and control the synthesis of specific proteins. Specific bacterial virus material has been produced in the laboratory by mixtures of the specific nucleic acids together with the necessary enzymes under appropriate conditions. The possibility of inducing an animal virus to go through a complete growth cycle in a cell-free system can now be contemplated. Preparations of the nucleic acid from numerous viruses have been shown to be infective when injected into susceptible cells, indeed some viral nucleic acids can, when injected replicate in hosts not susceptible to the whole virus.

It has long been known that most animal viruses grow best in the laboratory in young rapidly dividing cells in embryonated eggs or tissue cultures. Some will grow and cause demonstrable lesions only in cells derived from foetal tissues, in some only human foetal cells will suffice.

Two other, and possibly related, characteristics of viruses have attracted attention recently: first, the ability of some DNA viruses to remain latent or dormant for long periods and, secondly, the capacity of some animal and fowl DNA viruses to produce tumours *in vivo* and alterations in normal cells in tissue culture. Examples of chronic and latent infection in man with possible reactivation on one or more occasions, are cytomegalovirus infection, herpes simplex, serum hepatitis, subacute inclusion encephalitis (measles) and varicella/zoster, and some types of adenovirus lie latent in the tonsils and adenoids of children probably without much injurious effect. For example, herpes simplex in which the primary infection may be symptomless, may as a result of various trigger mechanisms make its reappearance at varying intervals from time to time as 'recurrent herpes'. In the majority of instances this latent herpetic infection lasts a lifetime in spite of the presence of humoral antibodies. Reactivation of these latent viruses may be associated with the use of immunosuppressive drugs in the treatment of various diseases, e.g. leukaemia, and in patients receiving organ transplants.

On the whole, there is little evidence that this persisting infection leads to malignant change; even in human warts, also believed to be due to DNA virus, where there is epithelial hyperplasia for long periods, malignant disease does not develop. Recently, however, several human adenoviruses have been found to cause transmissible sarcomata in day-old hamsters and rats. Specific virus antigens are present although the virus cannot be recovered subsequently from the tumour. A culture of the cells of a lymphosarcoma of the maxilla (Burkitt tumour) in African children may contain an intranuclear herpes-like body (EB virus), but a virus has not yet been isolated. It has been suggested very recently as a result of virological investigations in the United States that there may be an increased risk of cervical cancer in women with a genital infection by a particular type (type 2) of herpes simplex virus. These and many other observations have stimulated a new interest in the possibility that viruses may play a part in the causation of some human cancer.

IMMUNITY

The study of virus infection at the cellular level is a branch of cellular genetics. The interaction between viral and cellular functions shows that infection cannot be dismissed as a disrupting intrusion, it results in an addition of genetic specificity to the cell's endowment. Inevitably the most easily recognized viruses are those that lead to destructive events in their hosts, but in contrast with the situation in bacterial infection even these events occur at the genetic, rather than the metabolic, level. Thus viral activity in animals is directly affected by the genetic make-up of the host. One strain of mice may be resistant to one virus or group of viruses, but susceptible to another; in another strain the position may be reversed; however, resistance is also relative and may vary with the age of the host and the route of infection. Viruses which normally attack the higher mammals can be adapted to small rodents and even cold-blooded vertebrates; it is possible that there are viruses of wild animals with vectors not normally feeding on man, but which might acquire pathogenicity in altered ecological conditions.

The possible association between ABO blood groups and disease in man may extend to viral infections, for instance in one group of young adults infected with influenza A_2 virus when it first appeared, a relative excess of Group O individuals was noted with fewer of group A. All these factors, as well as nutrition, hormone deficiency and environment, are related to susceptibility and resistance, but their roles are more difficult to evaluate than those of the classical immunological processes.

The mechanisms of immunity to viral disease and the processes by which recovery takes place have been receiving increasing attention recently, because of the failure to find potent antiviral agents. Various lines of investigation have indicated that there are cellular factors of importance in addition to the traditional antibodies. Those viruses with a protein coat around their nucleic acid will evoke antibodies in any susceptible host with a functioning antibody-producing system, but there are probably some with a lipoid coat which are not antigenic. Most patients with hypogammaglobulinaemia have long been known not to suffer with undue severity from such viral infections as influenza, poliomyelitis and vaccinia, presumably because some intracellular process brings virus multiplication to a halt. In the case of vaccinia, there are rare patients who can neither form antibody against it nor control virus multiplication; their lymphoid cells appear to be defective and the usual delayed hypersensitivity reaction which occurs with vaccinia does not take place so that progressive, usually fatal, infection occurs.

More than 30 years ago it was shown that certain immunologically unrelated viruses, as well as different strains of the same virus, could interfere with each other's growth in the cell either *in vivo* or *in vitro* when the less pathogenic one was inoculated first. In 1957 Isaacs and Lindenmann found that, in experimental infection with influenza virus, this was due to the formation in the infected cell of a substance they called 'interferon'. Interferons, proteins usually of low molecular weight, can be isolated from the cells, purified and concentrated. When injected in an adequate dose into a cell susceptible to the virus it can interfere with virus replication apparently by preventing synthesis of viral nucleic acid. It seems possible that some such process, sometimes together with delayed hypersensitivity reaction, operates in virus infections to protect the antibody-deficient patients mentioned above, but that one or both of these mechanisms are deficient in patients who develop vaccinia gangrenosum.

Interferon-like substances have been recovered from different kinds of cells infected with many different viruses, but there appears to be some host specificity. An interferon produced in monkey cells is more effective in preventing infection in monkeys and man than is one produced in chicken or rabbit cells. Interferon prepared in cultures of human leucocytes has been used experimentally in the treatment of viral infections of man but the practical value of this use of the material is not yet known. Interferons have also been produced by the injection of non-viral double-stranded RNA.

As in chemotherapy the difficulty may be that many cycles of virus replication have usually occurred before symptoms or signs develop and frequently it may be impossible for sufficient interferon to reach the site of virus activity in time to prevent irreparable tissue damage. Improved methods of early diagnosis together with purified concentrated preparations of interferon for local application, inhalation or even intravenous injection or better still artificial interferon inducers as mentioned above may eventually overcome these drawbacks. Not all viruses produce interferon and there are some between which interference takes place although no interferon-like substance has been isolated. It is obvious that much has still to be learned about the mechanism of viral infection and cellular recovery from it.

Although intracellular mechanisms of defence play a part in the reaction to infection by most viruses, there is no doubt that specific antibodies, either introduced passively or produced actively in response to live or inactivated virus, can prevent or minimize infection if they are present in adequate amount before infection takes place or before the virus has become well-established. This is particularly true of those infections in which viruses are comparatively harmless to the tissue or *target organ* in which *primary multiplication* occurs and from which virus must be carried by the blood stream to other organs before it can cause pathological changes of significance to the patient. An example is the primary multiplication of poliovirus in the intestine. It was long thought that vaccines of inactivated virus would be incapable of producing adequate levels of antibody, but this has proved untrue provided sufficient antigen, in which the protein has not been too severely degraded, is used. Two or three doses may be required.

Attentuated live virus vaccines, of which smallpox and yellow fever are the classical examples, have been favoured by many in recent years on the assumption that they are likely to give protection of long duration, similar to that following natural infection. This would reduce the number of inoculations, for some of the live virus vaccines may be given by their natural routes, for instance intranasally for influenza and orally for poliomyelitis. However all the viruses must be grown in chick embryos or primary cell tissue cultures in many of which there may be latent viruses, thus extensive testing is required to safeguard the individual and progress is slow. Failure to develop attenuated viruses completely devoid of dangerous reactions has retarded their use. On the other hand innocuous strains have frequently been obtained which have lost their antigenic power in the process of attenuation. However, new techniques are making it increasingly possible to develop stable attenuated variants of many viruses, e.g. measles, poliomyelitis and rubella. In a number of regions where the diseases are endemic various combinations of attenuated live virus vaccines against measles, smallpox and yellow fever are being given in a single inoculation by multijet gun.

The addition of adjuvants, such as water in oil emulsion, to inactivated virus vaccines enhances their antigenicity and makes it possible to use smaller quantities, thus more antigens can be included in the usual 0·5–1 ml. dose, but a low rate of slowly developing local reactions reported from these preparations under certain conditions of use has delayed their widespread application. Certain essential bacterial prophylactics for children such as diphtheria and tetanus toxoid, must be inoculated parenterally on several occasions and it is likely that suitable combinations of these with various inactivated virus vaccines, e.g. poliomyelitis and measles, are in use in some countries.

DIAGNOSIS

The clinical diagnosis of some of the classical virus diseases, such as measles, paralytic poliomyelitis, rabies or yellow fever, is relatively easy, but the advent of laboratory techniques has uncovered many mild infections due to these and other viruses. Numerous viruses have been shown to cause illnesses similar to influenza or non-paralytic poliomyelitis, reaffirming the fact that the respiratory tract and central nervous system can react to infection in only a limited number of ways. Early and accurate diagnosis may well become essential for effective treatment because the variation in the structure of nucleic acids of different viruses suggests that the antiviral agents of the future may have a limited range of activity.

Facilities for virological diagnosis, although sometimes limited, are now generally available, but many of the techniques are such that they are not yet as readily accessible as bacteriological methods. Compared with the benefit the patient may anticipate from their results, virological techniques are expensive and it becomes important that they should be applied with propriety.

One of the main features of virus diseases is that clinicians frequently find it difficult to make an aetiological diagnosis due to the general lack of specific diagnostic symptoms or signs except in typical examples of some of the common exanthemata of childhood, acute anterior poliomyelitis and rabies. This is in contrast to the usual confidence in making a provisional diagnosis of a particular bacterial infection. Viruses multiply only inside cells, but if viraemia occurs either in a primary or secondary stage it is possible that one or more different organs may be affected. Practically all the organs can only react in a limited way to such an intracellular infection with the result that a syndrome may be caused by many different viruses and a single virus or type of virus may commonly cause a variety of symptoms and signs or syndromes in different people even within a small community or family during a short space of time. This diagnostic difficulty, in addition to the natural desire for advance in knowledge, has been a stimulus to the development of more rapid methods of diagnosis in order that specific treatment may be applied when it becomes available. As these techniques have improved and been more widely applied numerous unsuspected manifestations of even common virus infections such as rubella and herpes simplex have been revealed.

In any patient with an illness not conforming to one of the standard viral patterns—acute respiratory catarrh, 'influenza', aseptic meningitis or lower motor neurone paralysis—it is advisable to discuss the problem with the virologist.

In general the following types of specimen may be usefully examined if a viral infection is suspected.

Smears for Microscopic Examination

Smears should be made on clean glass slides from scrapings of macules, papules or from the bases of vesicles, conjunctiva, cornea or ulcers or from juice aspirated from lymph nodes and other biopsy material. They should be dried in air and not fixed unless so directed by the laboratory.

Development of the techniques of immunofluorescence and electron microscopy has made it possible to obtain a more rapid specific or provisional diagnosis under certain conditions in a number of virus infections, e.g. herpes simplex, orf, respiratory syncytial virus, smallpox, trachoma and varicella/zoster. These techniques are not available in all laboratories and particular care is necessary in the preparation of specimens from nasopharyngeal exudates, skin lesions, brain biopsy, etc. so it will be necessary to discuss this question beforehand with the laboratory.

Specimens for Isolation of Virus

Isolation and identification of virus or detection of antigen by immunological methods within a day or two of the onset of the illness is the ideal, but, other than in herpes, the pox-group and a few respiratory tract infections there are few virus infections where it is possible.

Vesicle and pustule fluid should be collected in capillary tubing or aspirated and placed in a sterile bottle. The tops of such lesions should also be removed and placed in sterile bottles.

Throat swabs should be collected from all patients with pyrexia of unknown origin and with undiagnosed infections of the respiratory tract and central nervous system of less than 4 days' duration. It is seldom worthwhile attempting to isolate virus from the throat after the fourth day unless vesicles or ulcers are present, even though fever may persist for a week or more. On the other hand some enteroviruses may be present in the throat without local evidence of infection.

Swabs from the nose, throat, conjunctival sac and other suspected sites of virus growth should be broken off into 2 ml. of buffered tissue culture fluid or saline containing a small amount of animal protein, such as bovine serum albumen, in a sterile bottle and stored at 4° C. or lower temperature. If there is going to be a delay in transit to the laboratory the bottles should be packed in ice.

Faecal specimens should be examined from patients with pyrexia of unknown origin, suspected viral infections of the nervous system, the alimentary tract and the respiratory tract of less than 7 days' duration. Isolation of virus from the faeces may be possible for a longer period but excretion may be intermittent and, with rare exceptions, examination of a stool after the tenth day is unrewarding. The recovery of an enterovirus from the faeces is no proof of a causal connexion with the patient's illness; many enteroviruses can cause silent infections and some adenoviruses and polioviruses may be excreted for several months. Faecal specimens may consist of a piece of faeces about a gramme in weight, a rectal swab or 10 ml. of saline enema washings. They may be kept at room temperature for a few hours or at 4° C. for 2 or 3 days but for longer periods should be stored at −20 C. or lower temperature.

Cerebrospinal fluid should be cultured in all instances of suspected virus infection of the nervous system. A positive result will be of more significance than isolation of virus from the throat swab or faeces but the latter must be attempted. Cerebrospinal fluid should be collected in volumes not smaller than 2 ml. and stored and transported at temperatures similar to those recommended for throat swabs.

Urine is not generally suitable for attempts at virus isolation except in certain specific cases such as cytomegalic inclusion disease or suspected congenital rubella although some adenoviruses, measles and mumps have been isolated from the urine.

Brain biopsy and ventricle fluid have yielded virus from cases of suspected cerebral abscess or encephalitis due to herpes simplex virus where culture of the cerebrospinal fluid is usually negative.

Viruses are seldom isolated from the blood in most situations in temperate climates and when this is to be attempted the blood is best anticoagulated with citrate or cresol-free heparin. It is often more convenient to provide the laboratory with one specimen which is allowed to clot; the clot and some serum may then be used for isolation of virus and the serum for antibody tests. Isolation of virus may be attempted within the first 48 hours in all patients with pyrexia of unknown origin with or without a rash or *post mortem* in rapidly fatal illnesses.

In fatal cases of suspected virus infection, heart blood, samples of suspected organs, throat swabs and bowel content should be collected if necropsy is made within 48 hours of death. Specimens should be collected with separate sterile forceps and scissors for each tissue and the latter each placed in a separate sterile bottle. Tissues should be placed at the lowest temperature available, or if no refrigeration is possible, 50 per cent. glycerin in buffered saline should be added.

Serological Studies

Serological tests are the most economical of the laboratory's time and may be positive when attempted virus isolation has failed. Their defect is that with few exceptions these results are of significance only if a rise in antibody titre can be demonstrated in convalescence 2 or 3 weeks after the onset. By this time the patient has usually recovered and the result may no longer be of interest to the physician. However, it remains advisable to provide the laboratory with paired sera when this is possible, particularly from patients with febrile illness of unknown origin and heart disease of uncertain origin. Five to ten ml. of clotted blood in a clean sterile bottle is preferable, though lesser amounts are acceptable from children. Whole blood should not be stored at temperatures below 4° C. Serum from the first specimen is stored at the laboratory and if the possibility of a virus infection still remains after 14–21 days a second specimen is collected and the two specimens are tested together.

Histological Studies

Representative pieces of tissue should be placed in formol saline or other suitable fixative.

ANTI-VIRAL AGENTS

If infection by the psittacosis-LGV-TRIC group of organisms, which respond to tetracyclines, and some members also to sulpha drugs, is excluded, it can be said that until recently no antibiotic or chemotherapeutic agent given in non-toxic doses was known to cut short a virus disease once infection was established. Most of the substances tested had been selected empirically and, although some had interfered with virus growth when given before or at the time of inoculation of the virus in laboratory experiments, all failed when given after infection.

The discovery that the active principle in all viruses is a nucleic acid suggested that, with knowledge of its configuration, an inhibitor might be devised which would interfere with synthesis of the virus. The study of nucleic acid inhibitors had already been pursued in the investigation of normal cell growth and the cause of cancer, thus much basic information was already available. It was soon shown that halogen derivatives of deoxyuridine interfered with the growth of two large DNA viruses, herpes simplex and vaccinia, in tissue culture. From this sprang the observation that 5-iodo-2-deoxyuridine (iodoxuridine) would cure experimental keratitis in rabbits due to herpes or vaccinia and later also experimental herpetic skin infection in guinea-pigs. Controlled trials in man demonstrated the efficacy of the drug in healing dendritic ulcers due to herpes virus in 7–10 days. For the effect of idoxuridine on other forms of herpetic infections see page 205.

The second important group of compounds is the thiosemicarbazones, in particular n-methylisatin-β-thiosemicarbazone (methisazone) which is given orally. This has a prophylactic effect when given in the pre-symptomatic stage of variola and is active against vaccinia. It acts by interfering with protein synthesis in the late stages in the production of infective virus.

Two other recently developed, unrelated compounds, l-adamantanamine hydrochloride and certain iso-quinoline derivatives have been shown in small trials to have a prophylactic effect against influenza A2 and against A2 and B viruses, respectively, if given at the time of exposure.

If animal viruses can be replicated in the test tube without tissue culture, as has recently been reported with some bacterial viruses, it should be possible to study their growth mechanism more fully and we may see the development of rational chemotherapy. However, a complicated intracellular mechanism has to be controlled and progressive cellular damage takes place during the characteristically long incubation period in many virus infections and these effects may prevent the effective chemotherapy of many virus diseases.

Another substance, interferon, has attracted much attention because of its less specific action [see p. 155]. So far it has only been used successfully in man as a prophylactic against vaccinia. There are considerable technical difficulties in the large scale production of interferon from virus infected cultures for clinical use, though in time these may be overcome. Some non-viral synthetic substances induce the formation of interferon in the intact animal, and this is another possible approach to therapy and prophylaxis.

The weight of evidence at present suggests that corticosteroids cause more harm than good in a number of acute virus infections, e.g. acute herpetic keratitis, and their potential dangers should be carefully considered in each case. In patients who have been on corticosteroids for some time when infection takes place, the disease may be more severe than in normal individuals. Results of experimental investigations and some clinical observations suggest that in certain other virus infections involving the central nervous system where an antigen-antibody reaction may be an important part of the pathological process, use of corticosteroids in the early stages to reduce this immunological reaction may hasten recovery.

In most systemic virus infections with an incubation period of 10 days or more, the injection of high titre specific neutralizing antibodies in the form of gamma globulin from pooled plasma obtained from the general population or from recent convalescents during the first week of incubation will probably result in a mild or subclinical infection. If it is given before infection is acquired, it will prevent it. Its effect lasts for about five weeks. The protective action has been clearly demonstrated in infective hepatitis, measles, to a less extent in smallpox, and even to some degree in rabies, when given soon after the bite. The gamma globulin in general use is not effective in chickenpox and in mumps has been shown only to reduce the frequency of complications such as orchitis. It is possible that specific gamma globulin will prove a useful adjunct to treatment with interferon or with the virustatic or virucidal substances which may be developed in the future.

GENERAL CLINICAL FEATURES OF VIRUS DISEASE

Any organ in the body may be attacked by some virus or another so that a wide variety of signs and symptoms may be present in a virus infection, particularly if viraemia occurs and few of these signs or symptoms are associated particularly with virus infections. In addition, some virus infections produce no obvious signs and symptoms, i.e. a silent infection. A number of quite dissimilar viruses produce a similar clinical picture, e.g. virus pneumonia, virus lymphocytic meningitis, and one virus may produce a wide variety of clinical pictures, e.g. coxsackie viruses cause febrile exanthemata, meningitis, myositis. Many virus infections may be accompanied by a rash, but it is its general distribution and progress together with the associated general features of the disease and not the appearance of the rash alone which may cause suspicion of a virus aetiology. Possibly the one general feature which is most suggestive of a virus infection is not a sign or symptom but the type of inflammatory response. This tends to be a leucopenia with a neutropenia in contrast to a leucocytosis with a preponderance of polymorphonuclear leucocytes in bacterial infections. This picture is seen in the blood, cerebrospinal fluid and affected tissues, although if severe necrosis takes place in the latter there may be an infiltration of polymorphonuclear cells. In some diseases such as infectious mononucleosis, hepatitis and cytomegalovirus infection, this mononuclear type of response is much more marked than in others. However, even this type of reaction is not restricted to virus diseases and may be seen in toxoplasmosis. In the upper respiratory tract a large proportion of mild illness is attributed to virus infection, probably rightly so. In the lower respiratory tract there is a tendency to label a particular group of symptoms as a virus pneumonia, but quite frequently this is caused by a bacterium, *Mycoplasma pneumoniae*. Also, when a provisional diagnosis of virus, aseptic or lymphocytic, meningitis is made it is necessary first to eliminate the possibility of tuberculosis and leptospirosis which also produce a lymphocytic response in the cerebrospinal fluid and for which specific therapy is possible.

Virus infections provide certain classical examples of so-called auto-immune disease, e.g. post-infective and post-vaccinal encephalomyelitis and the Guillain-Barré syndrome. Mumps virus is thought to have caused acute thyroiditis followed in some patients by an auto-immune thyroid disorder. Examples among blood diseases which are recognized, although uncommon, are thrombocytopenic purpura following rubella, and haemolytic anaemia which has been associated with a number of virus infections, and mycoplasma pneumonia.

F. O. MacCallum

EXANTHEMATIC VIRUS INFECTIONS

SMALLPOX

Synonym. Variola.

Definition

An acute infectious disease characterized by an unusually constant incubation period, a severe prodromal illness and a peripheral rash which appears on the third day. The rash later becomes vesicular and ultimately leaves permanent pock marks.

Aetiology

There are four viruses in the pox group which may affect man, the viruses of variola major, variola minor, cowpox and vaccinia. These all share a common antigen so that infection with one gives protection, for a time, against all members of the group. These are large viruses which are visible under the high power of the ordinary microscope as intracytoplasmic inclusions (*Guarnieri bodies*) which are aggregates of the actual virus particles—the '*elementary bodies*' *of Paschen*. The viruses are readily visible under the electron microscope which shows them to measure 200–250 micromicrons. Smallpox virus may survive for a year or more in the dry state but is destroyed by moisture.

Epidemiology

Infection is derived directly or indirectly from human sources, no other members of the animal kingdom being affected. The virus enters through the respiratory tract by the inhalation of droplets or dust, only brief and not very close contact being necessary for infection to take place. In this sense the disease is highly infectious and undoubtedly the severity of the ensuing attack is unrelated to the size of the infecting dose, as instances of fulminating fatal cases are known to have followed brief and minimal exposure. Virus may possibly enter through the conjunctivae, but entry through the intact skin without the production of a local lesion is most unlikely. Fomites are important. Intermediaries may carry the virus on their clothes and laundry workers are not infrequently infected by clothes from an undiagnosed patient. Bedding, clothes, rags and bales of imported cotton have all acted as vectors in this way. Flies and other insects occasionally spread the disease. It is debatable whether aerial convection over distances of more than quarter of a mile contributes to the spread. Most workers believe that unexplained cases which appear in many epidemics can be best accounted for by assuming they were infected by a 'missed case' in the epidemiological chain of events. However, there is no doubt that some of these unexplained cases have arisen in persons living within short distances of a smallpox hospital in which one or more patients was being nursed, and as it is known that a very small dose only is necessary to infect, the possibility of aerial spread cannot be dismissed. Nevertheless in the epidemiological investigation of the majority of outbreaks timing is such that a missed case twelve days previously offers the best explanation of what at first may seem to be an unrelated case. Infectivity is not great in the early stages of the disease but it increases rapidly as the rash appears. At the crusting stage the bedding and surrounding atmosphere are heavily contaminated with virus. Fulminating cases have little time to infect others in life especially as they may die before the true rash appears. The severity of the illness inevitably leads to a fair degree of isolation merely by confining patients to bed. Such cases, however, are commonly misdiagnosed and not infrequently spread infection after death, particularly at autopsy.

There is no natural immunity to smallpox, all races and all ages being susceptible if unprotected by previous infection with one of the pox group of viruses. Introduction of the disease into an unprotected community is likely to lead to a widespread epidemic unless stringent isolation and quarantine measures are taken. Smallpox is introduced into Great Britain in winter or spring and only rarely in the summer, December to April being the usual epidemic period in countries where the disease remains endemic.

Dangerous foci of major smallpox, from which most importations arise, exist in India, Pakistan, China and West Africa, but the disease is endemic in most Asian countries and in parts of South America.

Pathology

Following entry of the virus into the respiratory tract, it is believed that it passes to local lymph tissue and later to the liver and spleen through the blood, although no symptoms arise from this presumed viraemia. Certainly there is a heavy viraemia coincident with the onset of symptoms during which the virus reaches the skin, this persisting in diminishing degree for the whole of the first week. The skin lesions of smallpox lie in the deeper layers of the epidermis and may extend into the corium. Oedema and cellular necrosis are followed by vacuolation, the developed vesicles being filled by clear fluid which is often traversed by reticular fibres which divide the vesicle and depress its centre. The fluid becomes turbid when leucocytes infiltrate the lesion, this change developing independently of secondary infection. A crust forms as the pustule dries up. On mucous membranes the lesions are much more superficial and vesicles rupture almost as soon as they are formed. Haemorrhages are widespread in fulminating cases.

It should be stressed that apart from the skin and mucous membranes, there are no autopsy features specific to smallpox. This is particularly important to remember in fulminating cases which may die within 48 hours of the onset of an acute haemorrhagic illness before the appearance of the true rash (*purpura variolosa*). The autopsy findings are those common to acute infectious processes. The liver and spleen, however, are often appreciably enlarged in overwhelming infections. Bronchopneumonia is a common terminal event.

SYMPTOMS

The incubation period is the most constant known among the specific infectious diseases, symptoms appearing in the great majority of cases on the twelfth day from infection. In some instances the incubation period has ranged from 8 to 16 days.

Variola Major

Synonyms. Unmodified major smallpox; Classical epidemic smallpox.

Prodromal Illness. The onset is sudden with chills or rigors, fever, headache and often pain in the back. The temperature rises to 102°–104° F. (38·9°–40° C.). Retching and vomiting are common and prostration may be marked. Abdominal pain is sometimes severe and is likely to be accompanied by muscle guarding. Cough is frequent. The patient is anorexic and thirsty, he may be delirious but in the more severe infections he tends to be rational though slow to respond to questions or commands. In children the illness may start with convulsions. Almost invariably, whether the attack proves to be rapidly fatal or unusually mild, the prodromal symptoms appear suddenly and are severe enough to send the patient forthwith to bed. This is of some epidemiological importance in limiting the number of contacts from the moment the patient has become infective.

The general condition remains much the same for one to two days, but by the third day there may be some improvement accompanied by a fall in temperature, to be followed by return of fever and malaise as the true rash appears. Fleeting erythematous *prodromal rashes* may occur in the groins, axillae or on the trunk during the first two days. They are bright red or dusky red in colour and may resemble scarlet fever or less frequently measles. They disappear within a few hours and are of good prognostic importance. Their main significance lies in the fact that they may lead to diagnostic errors. Petechial rashes appearing in the prodromal period are an integral part of fulminating smallpox, increasing in extent during the brief remainder of the patient's life. When they are confined to the lower abdomen and the upper thighs (the bathing-trunk area) they are pathognomonic of smallpox.

Eruptive Stage. The focal or *true rash of smallpox* appears on the third day, macules being first noted on the forehead, over the malar region, the bridge of the nose and along the sternomastoids with a few on the back, on the forearms and on the backs of the wrists. Within 24 hours many more macules develop and join the original herald spots. The rash starts therefore on the forehead, face, forearms and the back of the chest spreading later to the front of the chest, the upper arms and reaching the legs after 24 hours. Lesions also appear early in the mouth, on the palate, tongue and buccal mucous membrane.

The *distribution* of the smallpox rash is primarily centrifugal both at its onset and at its height. It is markedly symmetrical. Lesions are more numerous on the face, forearms and later on the legs than on the trunk. The rash has a preference for prominences and tends to avoid flexures, although this is a relative matter and in a heavy rash there may be many lesions in, for example, the axilla. Nevertheless, in contrast with surrounding areas the rash here is likely to be less dense. The supraclavicular fossae, the intermammary groove and the antecubital and popliteal fossae similarly show a relative sparing. The rash is heaviest on the supra-orbital, nasal and malar prominences on the face. It is more profuse on extensor than on flexor surfaces and may show patches of confluence over bony prominences such as the elbows. Lesions can be seen on the margins of the pinnae and not uncommonly follow extensor tendons on the backs of the hands and around the ankles. On the limbs, the rash as a rule is more profuse distally than proximally—that is to say, heavier below the elbows and knees than above them. The palms of the hands and the soles of the feet may be heavily involved. On the head and trunk the rash is heavier on parts above than below. Thus there is likely to be more rash on the forehead than the face, on the face than on the chest, on the chest than on the abdomen and on the back of the chest than on the loins. Of all the above points the centrifugal nature of the rash, its symmetry and its predilection for prominences are the most constant. The distribution, however, can be upset by previous skin irritation from tight clothing or preceding skin disease. Over such areas the rash may be confluent.

The characteristic features of the individual lesions and the progress of the disease varies with the different types.

Fulminating Smallpox (Purpura Variolosa)

The onset is sudden, prodromal symptoms are severe and in the exceptional case death occurs within 36 hours with no unequivocal outward or autopsy evidence of the nature of the illness. More usually skin haemorrhages appear on the second day in the groins, flanks and axillae increasing over subsequent days. Haemorrhages are not confined to the skin but are present in the mouth and under the conjunctivae; they may occur from any mucous membrane resulting in haematemesis, haematuria or an intestinal or uterine bleed. In those who survive five days there may be maculopapular elements of true rash on the face or wrists but these are often indistinct and overshadowed by the purpura. At first apprehensive and greatly disturbed by severe headache, backache or abdominal pain, the patient becomes apathetic and hypotonic though usually not delirious. The temperature is not unduly raised. The liver and spleen may be enlarged. There is usually an irritant cough with accompanying signs of bronchitis. Death is inevitable by the fifth day but often takes place earlier.

Malignant Smallpox

Following a severe 48-hour prodromal illness the temperature falls and the patient may even feel well enough for a few hours to sit out of bed. The temperature rises again on the third day and a dusky erythema appears on the face with a macular rash on the upper chest, back and arms. There may be a few petechiae intermingled with the erythema. In malignant smallpox the rash develops slowly and the early stages may be more profuse over the proximal than the distal parts of the limbs. Sometimes the erythema suggests acute sunburn. There may be little change in the rash by the fifth day, general vesiculation being delayed till the tenth day, although many individual lesions, particularly those with a petechial base, will become vesicular earlier. The face shows a confluent, sunburnt appearance and at all stages there is likely to be a bright 'lobster' erythema between individual lesions. The early vesiculation of some lesions and slow maturation of others gives the appearance of cropping. At the papular and vesicular stages the spots are superficial and flat topped with a hot velvety feel. Vesicles may run together with the formation of bullae which collapse as fluid is absorbed, or the skin may be shed leaving a raw painful surface. Pustulation does not occur. In the patient in whom the lesions are confluent on the face and limbs, death usually takes place from toxaemia and fluid loss between the tenth and fourteenth day. If confluence is limited to the face the prognosis is appreciably better. Mucous membrane haemorrhages may occur at any time. Subconjunctival haemorrhages are present in most fatal cases.

The characteristic features of malignant smallpox are the slow evolution of a rather superficial rash with pseudo-cropping—a very different clinical picture from the much better-known classical benign smallpox.

Benign Smallpox

Benign smallpox refers to a common and less fatal type of variola in which the evolution of the rash differs from the malignant variety. The rash may be *confluent* (on face, limbs and part of the trunk), *semi-confluent* (i.e. confluent on the face but not elsewhere) or *discrete*. If there are less than twenty lesions the case is classified as *abortive*. The severity of benign smallpox is closely related to the extent of the rash.

The onset is sudden, as in the other types, and fever is likely to be high. The rash appears on the third day with the distribution already described. The individual lesions appear as macules but in under 24 hours become papules which can be felt when pinched between the finger and thumb. At first 2–3 mm. in diameter they enlarge to 5–6 mm. They are deep set in the skin, remarkably uniform in size and all lesions in any area of skin are more or less at the same stage of development. The lesions on the face scalp, arms and back are usually about 24 hours in advance of those on the legs. On the third day of rash (sixth day of illness) the earliest papules have become vesicles, but close inspection will reveal vesiculation on the summits of some papules at an earlier stage. However, the main rash is never fully vesicular before the fifth day of illness and this is more usually delayed till the sixth or seventh days. Vesicles are circular, raised or pearly in appearance, many being multiloculated and umbilicated. There is often a surrounding erythematous areola, whilst with heavy rashes there is a considerable oedema of the skin between the spots. Pustulation occurs early in the second week but is independent of secondary infection. By the twelfth to thirteenth day the pustules begin to dry up, some from absorption, some from rupture by scratching. Crusts form which separate in a few days, but where the skin is thick—as on the palms and soles—the dried-up unruptured pustules may persist as 'seeds' which may remain for weeks. Variola virus is present in seeds as indeed it is in lesions at all stages from macules to crusts. Small haemorrhages at the base of some lesions or into some vesicles are not uncommon and are not of grave significance, but mucous membrane haemorrhages or heavy bleeding into the rash are always grave signs. The skin eruption may be accompanied by lesions on the conjunctivae, mucous membranes of the mouth and respiratory, genital and intestinal tracts. Vesicles may be seen on the palate while the skin lesions are still indeterminate; they rupture early in the mouth leaving shallow ulcers. Hoarseness or aphonia results from laryngeal lesions and painful swallowing is a troublesome symptom when there are many lesions in the pharynx.

Although the prodromal illness is severe the toxaemia thereafter is less than in the malignant type. The temperature tends to fall during the first three days, rising again with the appearance of the rash. Thereafter it falls by lysis, often reaching normal by the end of the first week. Secondary fever from the eighth to the ninth day onwards is related to the extent of the rash and is accentuated by secondary infection or other septic complication. The fall of temperature during the evolution of the rash is a characteristic of smallpox seldom seen in other exanthemata.

There is usually a generalized mild to moderate degree of lymph node enlargement. The spleen may be palpable. The urine is concentrated and may contain protein. In the uncomplicated case, convalescence starts with the crusting phase and proceeds rapidly. Desquamation, particularly of the feet and hands, may accompany the shedding of the crusts and loss of hair is not unusual.

Modified Smallpox (Varioloid)

Smallpox occurring in a person partially protected by previous vaccination often leads to diagnostic errors. There is no modification of the virulence of the virus which provokes a normal attack in the unprotected. Following vaccination, immunity to the toxaemic element of the virus appears to wane before immunity to the rash-producing element. The prodromal illness is therefore sudden in onset and fairly severe, with the symptoms of an unmodified attack. The rash usually appears on the third day but may do so on the first or second day or may be delayed till the fifth day. It may appear first on the chest or abdomen instead of the face. Individual lesions develop quickly while the appearance of the rash as a whole is extended over a few days. Thus scabs may be present at the same time as papules. The lesions of modified smallpox are small and superficial and may abort. Although the centrifugal distribution may not be so obvious as in unmodified smallpox, counting the lesions will confirm that the peripheral areas are more heavily involved than the central. The predilection of the rash for prominences remains. Frequently the temperature does not rise again with the appearance of the rash—the whole eruptive phase being afebrile.

Variola Sine Eruptione

Smallpox without a rash is not rare in the vaccinated and may also occur in the unvaccinated. A detailed search for lesions to exclude abortive smallpox (less than twenty spots) must be made before this diagnosis is accepted. A 12–48-hour febrile illness occurs 12 days after exposure, followed by a rapid return to health. This form of the disease can only be recognized in persons under surveillance as known contacts.

Variola Minor (Alastrim; Kaffir-pox)

This is a mild form of smallpox due to a less virulent strain of virus. The disease is endemic in parts of Africa and South America. The virus breeds true, an epidemic of minor smallpox never changing to major or vice versa. It differs from major smallpox in its mild course, low mortality and absence of secondary fever and mildness of scarring.

The incubation period is usually 12 days, but may be between 10–15 days. The onset is sudden with similar prodromal symptoms to major smallpox of headache, backache, vomiting, abdominal pain and cough. Some patients have a mild or indefinite prodromal phase. The rash has an identical distribution to the major disease but tends to develop more quickly. Secondary fever is usually absent. The lesions are often more superficial than in variola major but deeper than in chickenpox. Although the mortality is under 2 per cent., fulminating and malignant cases occasionally occur and in a particular patient the distinction between major and minor smallpox is often impossible. In an outbreak of smallpox, however, there is soon no doubt as to whether one is dealing with the major or minor disease.

Complications

Secondary infection of the skin increases the severity and duration of the pustular stage with lymphadenitis and sometimes deeply spreading subcutaneous infection. Staphylococcal *septicaemia*, previously not uncommon, is now a much less frequent cause of late death. Independently of infection of the lesions, staphylococcal sepsis in the form of boils and styes may occur during convalescence. The pock marks or scars on the skin are a normal sequel to smallpox. A temporary *alopecia* is due to destruction of hair follicles by lesions in the scalp.

Eye complications are important though permanent blindness is rare. Lesions frequently arise on the lid margins and are associated with closure of the eye due to oedema. Conjunctivitis is common. Lesions on the scleral conjunctiva normally appear to heal without trouble. A rapidly spreading keratitis, however, may lead to sloughing of the cornea or corneal ulceration may occur and be followed by perforation and panophthalmitis.

With modern therapy *bronchopneumonia* is mostly confined to infants and the aged and otitis media and acute parotitis are similarly uncommon. Laryngitis and tracheitis, however, are frequent and indeed an accepted feature of the malignant disease, the inflammation here being due to the variola lesions.

Albuminuria is usual in severe attacks, but nephritis only occurs when smallpox is complicated by streptococcal infection. As in other exanthemata *post-infective encephalopathy* may arise 5–13 days after the onset but this is a rare complication. Drowsiness, mental changes, signs of meningeal irritation and paraylses of different types have occurred.

Bone and joint complications are of two types—*pyogenic osteomyelitis* and *osteomyelitis variolosa*. In the latter the metaphysis is infected with virus during the viraemia although symptoms do not appear until 2–6 weeks later when the joint becomes involved. The first symptom is swelling of the joint soon associated with pain and tenderness, the elbow being by far the commonest joint to be affected. This complication is confined to children. Detachment and extrusion of the epiphysis may follow but ultimate function is often surprisingly good despite considerable deformity.

DIAGNOSIS

Pre-eruptive Phase. In the absence of known contacts smallpox is unlikely to be considered during the prodromal stage. The combination of severe backache and abdominal pain in a patient taken acutely ill with headache and fever should suggest the possibility but such symptoms may be due to many infections including influenza, pyelitis, meningitis, encephalitis, septicaemia or malaria. These severe prodromal symptoms assume particular diagnostic significance, however, at the stage of the focal rash. The abdominal pain and guarding not infrequently lead to a laparotomy for acute appendicitis but the severe headache should exclude this diagnosis. The appearance of petechiae confined to the bathing-trunk area is pathognomonic of smallpox and a symmetrical spread of haemorrhages from the groins along the flanks to the axillae is characteristic. A more widespread haemorrhagic rash at this stage, however, may be due to smallpox or to any septicaemia, particularly meningococcal, streptococcal or staphylococcal. Acute thrombocytopenic purpura and acute leukaemia are often confused with purpura variolosa. In this form of smallpox the liver and spleen may be enlarged and the white count raised with an increase in the number of primitive cells. The dramatic onset of the illness and the early death in smallpox should exclude blood dyscrasias which seldom kill so quickly. The erythematous prodromal rashes of smallpox are likely to be more confusing than helpful. Their danger lies in the false sense of security engendered by an incorrect diagnosis of, for example, scarlet fever—thereafter scant attention being paid to the focal rash as it develops until it becomes sufficiently pronounced to demand attention and detailed re-examination of the patient.

Eruptive Phase. The focal eruption in its early stages may be confused with measles, severe rubella or a drug (especially a sulphonamide) rash. In malignant smallpox the early rash on the face may be morbilliform but there is no coryza, no Koplik's spots and the development of the rash in these diseases is different, being quick in measles and slow in smallpox. Typhus and the rose spots of typhoid have caused confusion although the distribution of the lesions in these two diseases is central.

Any patient who develops a papular or vesicular rash involving the face on the third day of a febrile illness must be thoroughly examined in a good light even if the lesions are scanty. The particular points in favour of smallpox are a centrifugal distribution, a preponderance of lesions on the extensor surfaces and prominences and evidence of slow progression of the lesions with most spots in any one area at the same stage of development.

The differentiation from chickenpox is important. The disease is not uncommon in adults, particularly immigrants, and the rash may be delayed until the third day of the illness. Chickenpox presents the following distinctive characteristics:

1. The rash appears first on the trunk and is most marked on the chest, trunk, face, scalp, upper arms and thighs. It becomes less dense over the wrists and hands. There are few, if any, lesions on the palms or soles.

2. Successive crops appear for up to five days and the temperature remains raised during this period. Thus it is common to see lesions at all stages from macule to crust in close association.

3. Some lesions always develop quickly so that a few vesicles are present within 24 hours of the appearance of the rash. Vesicles are not seen at this stage in smallpox.

4. The lesions vary in shape and size, many in the flexures being ovoid. They are superficial, on rather than in the skin, unilocular and the majority are not umbilicated.

An extensive rash with little constitutional upset is unlikely to be due to smallpox. A scanty rash, of peripheral distribution, with no constitutional upset at this stage of the rash may well be due to mild or modified smallpox. Proof of successful vaccination within two years makes the diagnosis of smallpox extremely unlikely.

Eczema herpeticum and eczema vaccinatum may produce similar lesions to smallpox but the distribution is usually quite different as the rash is almost confined to the eczematous skin. Generalized vaccinia may prove difficult, especially in a known contact of smallpox, but such a case can safely be admitted to a smallpox hospital if real doubt exists. The rash in erythema multiforme exudativum is normally pleomorphic, may be predominantly vesicular or bullous and often involves the extremities. It may resemble malignant smallpox but the history shows that the rash and constitutional symptoms began together and that vesiculation started early. Acne affects the face, shoulders, back and chest but not the forearms or hands. A papular syphilide shows other evidence of secondary syphilis. A non-specific sensitivity reaction to the protein in calf lymph may cause fever and a papulovesicular rash. This appears ten days to three weeks after vaccination, is heavy on the forearms and hands and variable in extent elsewhere; but the face usually escapes.

Laboratory Diagnosis. The virus laboratory can be of great help in the diagnosis of smallpox and in any doubtful case use must be made of the facilities offered. Provisional results which are available within 2–24 hours have a high degree of accuracy, but are not infallible. Culture of variola virus takes three days or longer. Thus the diagnosis of smallpox must in the first instance always be a clinical one and the action taken must depend on this and can never await the results of virus culture.

The specimens required for investigation depend on the stage of the patient's illness—blood in the prodromal period, smears on slides at the macular stage, lesion tops, vesicle fluid, scrapings from the base of vesicles and crusts from the more fully developed rash. This material is used for:

1. *Gel diffusion test*, the test material being used as antigen. A positive result may be obtained within 2–12 hours. This indicates infection with one of the pox group but does not differentiate variola major, minor or vaccinia. This is a reliable test giving a positive reaction in over 90 per cent. of cases. Pustular material has been known to produce a false positive. A test which becomes rapidly positive indicates smallpox.

2. *Complement fixation test.* The result is available within 24 hours, a positive result having the same reliability and significance as the gel diffusion test.

3. *Virus culture* on the chorio-allantoic membrane of the hen's egg. Confirmation of the presence of variola virus may take from 3–7 days. Vaccinia grows more quickly and is easily differentiated. Variola minor can now be distinguished from variola major by cultural means.

4. *Direct examination* of a stained specimen for elementary bodies. This method has considerable difficulties even for the experienced observer and is therefore seldom relied upon.

5. *Electron microscopy.* Confirmation of a pox group infection is available by this method within 4 hours. It is possible to distinguish between the pox viruses and the herpes viruses (which include the varicella-zoster virus of chickenpox) but not between variola and vaccinia.

Chickenpox virus does not grow on chick embryo. Herpes simplex virus will, but seldom causes difficulty to the virologist.

The blood picture in fulminating smallpox shows a leucocytosis with a lymphocytosis, granulopenia and thrombocytopenia. The total white cell count may exceed 40,000 cells per mm^3., many of which may be primitive cells.

TREATMENT

Procedure and Control. Immediately smallpox is suspected the Medical Officer of Health should be notified and the patient kept where he is. If he is being seen in the surgery, other patients should be sent home after making a note of their names and addresses. In the United Kingdom the Medical Officer of Health can, after seeing the case, get further advice by calling out a member of the panel of smallpox opinion. If the clinical suspicion is upheld the patient is removed to a smallpox hospital. It is of great importance that a patient in whom the possibility of smallpox exists is not admitted to a general or infectious diseases hospital as smallpox is no respecter of routine barrier-nursing techniques. Control of an outbreak in a community with good public health facilities is carried out by the method of ring vaccination. This entails finding the primary contacts (all those persons who have been in contact with the patient from a few hours before the onset of his illness until his removal) and quarantining them in house and garden. The other members of households of the primary contacts make up the secondary contacts; these are allowed to continue their normal activities. Both primary and secondary contacts are vaccinated and the primary contacts surveyed daily till the sixteenth day, their temperatures being recorded daily from the tenth day. Primary contacts with a previously poor vaccination state are given further protection with hyperimmune gamma globulin, 1–1·5 G. being injected intramuscularly 24 hours after vaccination.

General. Patients remain infectious until all the crusts are shed and seeds extruded. Terminal disinfection must be thorough.

Nursing is of extreme importance. The patient should be encouraged to eat whatever he fancies so long as an adequate fluid and calorie intake are maintained. An indwelling polythene gastric tube may be the best way of achieving this. In severe cases intravenous fluids and protein are required but an extensive rash makes parenteral therapy difficult. Tepid sponging to reduce temperature, simple analgesics such as Compound Codeine Tablets, B.P., or Ipecacuanha and Opium Tablets, B.P., 600 mg., and optimistic nursing care form the basis of treatment. Mouth washes are required three times a day and chewing-gum is helpful if it does not cause pain. The eyes are cleaned with normal saline. Should corneal ulceration appear 0·5 per cent. prednisolone and neomycin ointment should be applied twice daily, the pupils being kept dilated with 1 per cent. atropine. Inhalation of Benzoin, B.P.C., may relieve laryngitis.

Skin irritation is not usually severe. Local treatment is of psychological benefit to the patient and the staff, but it is doubtful if it has any effect on the development of the rash. Painting the skin twice a day with a 1 in 5000 solution of potassium permanganate is harmless and comforting. In confluent cases the hair must be cut short and a glycerin mask applied to the face and hands may prove soothing. Olive oil relieves excessive skin tenderness which sometimes follows separation of scabs.

Systemic antibiotics should be started at the vesicular stage to lessen secondary infection. Penicillin or cloxacillin, if penicillin-resistant staphylococci are present in the ward, should be given orally for seven days.

Specific. An antivariola chemotherapeutic agent, N-methylisatin β-thiosemicarbazone, has been developed in the laboratory. This is of no value in treatment. Thiosemicarbazones have been shown to have some protective effect when given in the incubation period. They are toxic drugs, however, and vaccination combined, if necessary, with hyperimmune gamma globulin remains the best method of protection of contacts.

PROGNOSIS

The mortality of unmodified variola major is about 40 per cent. The prognosis in the individual case must be considered under the following headings:

1. *Vaccinal condition of the patient.* Smallpox within ten years of vaccination is rarely fatal and can be expected to show considerable modification; thereafter protection gradually wanes until fatal cases become as frequent as in the unvaccinated. There are, however, many instances of attacks which appear to have been modified by vaccination 30–40 years previously, but it is never possible in any individual case to be certain that its mild nature is in fact related to the earlier vaccination.

2. *Age.* In the unvaccinated the mortality in the first five years of life is over 40 per cent. The mortality falls up to 15–20 years, to rise steadily thereafter until it becomes high once again in the elderly.

3. *The nature of the attack.* Fulminating smallpox is invariably fatal. Malignant confluent smallpox has a 70 per cent. mortality, benign confluent smallpox 20 per cent. and discrete smallpox 2 per cent. Extensive haemorrhages at any stage of the disease carry a grave prognosis. A mild prodromal illness presages a mild attack. The more profuse the pustular rash the worse the prognosis.

4. *The route of entry of the virus.* When infection takes place by inoculation through the skin a mild attack commonly follows (see Vaccinia).

Variola minor has a mortality of 0·5–2 per cent. but the prognostic criteria detailed above for variola major apply equally to this form of the disease. The good outlook is determined by the fact that over 97 per cent. of the cases are discrete.

SMALLPOX HANDLERS' LUNG

A respiratory illness may develop 10–12 days after contact with smallpox in frequently vaccinated highly protected persons. This is seen amongst nurses and doctors. The symptoms are mild dyspnoea, cough, fever and occasionally an erythema multiforme type rash. Chest X-ray shows discoid or reticular lesions. Symptoms improve within a few days but the radiological changes may last for months.

The syndrome is usually considered to be an allergic response to the inhalation of scale dust heavily contaminated by variola. It has never been shown to be infective and is unlikely to be a manifestation of smallpox infection.

REFERENCES

DIXON, C. W. (1962) *Smallpox*, London.

MACRAE, A. D. (1967) Laboratory diagnosis of smallpox, *Mth. Bull. Minist. Hlth Lab. Serv.*, **26**, 189.

MINISTRY OF HEALTH (1964) Memorandum on the Control of Outbreaks of Smallpox, London, H.M.S.O.

RAO, A. R., MCKENDRICK, G. D. W., VELAYUDHAN, L., and KAMALAKSHI, K. (1966) Assessment of an isothiazole thiosemicarbazone in the prophylaxis of contacts of variola major, *Lancet*, i, 1072.

VACCINIA

Definition

Vaccinia is an infectious condition normally produced intentionally by inoculation with vaccinia virus. Accidental infection also occurs. Following the appearance of a vesicular skin lesion antibodies develop which protect against smallpox.

History

Protection against smallpox was achieved for centuries in China and elsewhere by inserting crust material into the nostrils or by skin inoculation of material from a smallpox lesion. The smallpox thus produced by *variolation* was a modified form of the disease with a very low mortality. The skin inoculation method was introduced into England by Lady Mary Wortley Montagu about 1720, but only achieved limited popularity. As inoculated persons are infectious, thus causing the spread of unmodified smallpox, variolation was made illegal in 1840.

By the 18th century it had long been apparent to farmers in England that individuals accidentally inoculated with cowpox were protected against smallpox. In 1796 Jenner made practical use of this fact by inoculating a boy with matter from a cowpox lesion on a milkmaid's hand. Subsequent inoculation of the boy with variolous material failed to produce smallpox.

The source of vaccinia virus in use today is uncertain but it probably originated from cowpox. However, vaccinia and cowpox viruses are now distinct. Vaccinia virus is propagated in healthy calves or sheep, the contents of the vesicles being collected, treated with glycerin and frozen. The glycerinated calf lymph is repeatedly tested for bacteriological contamination. It remains active for at least eight months if stored at low temperature. Vaccine free from bacteria can be prepared by culturing the virus on the chorio-allantoic membrane of chick embryos but the protection afforded seems to be less than that obtained with calf lymph. Because of the slight risk to the vaccinated subject as well as to others inherent in the use of a vaccine containing live virus, search continues for a successful method of preparing a vaccine from killed virus.

Indications

In countries where smallpox is endemic and the risk of contracting smallpox correspondingly high, routine vaccination should be carried out at birth and repeated at one to five-yearly intervals. In non-epidemic countries the wisdom of routine infant vaccination is debated. Those who do not favour routine vaccination argue that the risk of smallpox is so small in such a community that it does not equal the risks of vaccination. Routine vaccination of all infants in Great Britain would lead to approximately 10 per cent. of the population being immune at any one time—too small a figure to prevent spread of the disease; it is postulated that to maintain a completely protected community some six million yearly vaccinations would be necessary and that the death rate from complications would exceed the death rate from smallpox. It is also suggested that smallpox introduced into a totally unprotected community is less likely to lead to modified and hence misdiagnosed cases. The protagonists of these views consider vaccination should be reserved for contacts or likely contacts of known cases and for medical, nursing, hospital and laundry personnel as a routine.

The contrary view is held by the Department of Health which recommends routine infant vaccination. The arguments supporting this view are: (1) complications of primary vaccination in infancy are low; (2) although partial protection cannot be guaranteed after 7–10 years in any particular individual, smallpox attacking a group of persons vaccinated thirty years or more previously will cause fewer deaths than in an unvaccinated group of similar ages (i.e. long-term protection can be expected in a proportion of those vaccinated in infancy); (3) with increasing travel and military service commitments many persons will require vaccination in young adult life and the risks of repeat vaccination are considerably less than those of primary vaccination at this age.

The best age for primary vaccination in infancy is four to five months or between one and two years. Routine re-vaccination at school age is recommended in Great Britain.

Hospital staff should be vaccinated regularly at three-yearly intervals.

Contra-indications

The following are specific contra-indications to routine primary vaccination. They do *not* apply to close contacts of smallpox who must be protected by vaccination.

1. Exposure to infectious diseases.
2. Septic skin conditions.
3. Infantile eczema. An eczematous child must be kept away from a vaccinated person because of the risk of accidental infection.
4. Hypogammaglobulinaemia.
5. Corticosteroid therapy.
6. Pregnancy.
7. Allergic conditions. Sensitivity reactions are more common in such subjects.
8. The presence of intercurrent or chronic illness. Patients suffering from leukaemia are likely to develop generalized vaccinia.

It is preferable not to vaccinate (e.g. the intending traveller) at the same time as carrying out other immunization procedures. If this cannot be avoided then the injection should be given into the arm other than that used for vaccination. Vaccination against yellow fever should precede a smallpox vaccination by at least four days.

Method

An area of skin over the insertion of the deltoid at the junction of the upper and middle thirds of the humerus is cleaned with acetone or ether and allowed to dry. A drop of lymph is placed on the cleaned skin which is then perforated either by scratching or by applying multiple pressure with a sterile needle. In routine primary procedures a 'minimal trauma' technique should be used, either a single scratch $\frac{1}{8}$ in. (3 mm.) long or six to ten pressures over a similar area. The method of multiple pressure involves using a flat sided needle which lies parallel to the skin. With each rapid down movement, the point of the needle is not being driven into the skin but pulls a little epidermis over it with each pressure. The arm should be allowed to dry and no dressing is required until a vesicle appears.

Smallpox contacts should receive three vaccination insertions about 2 in. (5 cm.) apart with $\frac{1}{4}$ in. (6 mm.) scratches. This type of vaccination leads to earlier vesiculation and therefore earlier protection in addition to lessening the chance of failure.

Results of Vaccination

Primary Vaccinia. Irritation begins at the site of inoculation within 48 hours. A papule appears on the third day, vesiculation starting on the fifth day and reaching its maximum by the eighth day. The lesion is surrounded by an area of inflammation and is by now about a centimetre in diameter but its size will depend on the length of the scratch or number of pressures. The contents of the vesicle, which shows umbilication, become turbid and the pustule enlarges slowly till the tenth to twelfth day when it dries up with the formation of a scab. This separates in due course to leave a pitted scar which remains for life. Successful primary vaccination must never be assumed in any patient in whom such a scar cannot be found.

Vaccination is accompanied by viraemia. Headache, fever, malaise and tender axillary lymph nodes commonly occur between the eighth and tenth day. Such constitutional symptoms are slight or absent in babies and in re-vaccinations carried out within ten years.

Accelerated (Vaccinoid) Reaction. This reaction occurs in a partially immune person. The lesion reaches its maximum size within 3–7 days, there is definite vesicle formation and ultimately faint but definite scar formation. There is no constitutional upset.

Local Reaction without Vesiculation. A local reaction reaching its maximum on the second or third day accompanied by elevation, erythema and itching but without vesiculation may be due to immunity but may equally well be a non-specific reaction following a vaccination which has failed to take due to poor technique, faulty lymph or other cause. Immunity is the likely cause of this reaction in the well vaccinated person but this must never be assumed to be the case in the face of a smallpox threat. Re-vaccination should be carried out in such an instance.

No Local Reaction. This may be due to immunity or to failure. A further attempt should be made using fresh lymph.

Immunity to smallpox develops between the eighth and tenth day, antibodies being demonstrable in the blood from the tenth day onwards. Successful vaccination in the first three days following exposure to smallpox will usually protect or modify the disease but protection can never be guaranteed in those vaccinated after contact.

Inspection of Results. The vaccination site should be inspected on or about the seventh day. A 'major reaction' after a primary vaccination consists of a typical vesicle; after re-vaccination a major reaction may either be a vesicle or pustule or an area of palpable induration surrounding a scab or ulcer. Any other local reaction is termed 'equivocal'. Results should therefore be recorded as:

A—major reaction
B—equivocal reaction
C—no reaction.

In the case of B or C at least one further attempt at vaccination or re-vaccination should be made.

The duration of immunity is extremely variable. Complete protection is almost certain for at least two years and often for many more. Fatal smallpox is highly unlikely within ten years and many apparently modified attacks occur twenty years or more after vaccination.

Complications

The commonest complication is *secondary bacterial infection* of the local lesion. This is accompanied by cellulitis, increased lymphadenopathy and fever. Erysipelas or, more rarely tetanus, have occurred.

Vaccinia virus itself may cause complications; an eczematous patient who becomes infected with vaccinia either intentionally or by accident is likely to develop a febrile illness with extensive vaccinal lesions chiefly confined to the eczematous skin (*eczema vaccinatum*). This serious infection, which has a 6 per cent. mortality, may also arise in those whose eczematous condition is virtually quiescent.

Generalized vaccinia in those with normal skin is rare, crops of lesions appearing 7–14 days following vaccination. These are much more superficial than the primary lesion and heal without scarring. The mortality rate is low.

Accidental vaccinal lesions, often around the face and mouth, are due to skin inoculation from the patient's own lesion or from a contact. Keratoconjunctivitis may arise in this way.

Progressive vaccinia (vaccinia necrosum, vaccinia gangrenosum) is a rare but highly lethal complication which is sometimes associated with a quantitative or qualitative defect in gamma globulin but is more likely to be due to a deficient cellular response to the infection. The initial lesion fails to heal, spreading slowly over the weeks with increasing destruction of tissue. Further lesions develop until the infant dies, usually months after the vaccination. Vaccinal osteomyelitis has occurred.

Postvaccinal encephalomyelopathy has varied greatly in its reported incidence, the estimated chance of this complication varying between 1 in 63 to 1 in a million vaccinations, in different countries at different times; all statistics on this subject must clearly be interpreted with caution. Encephalitis less often follows primary vaccination in the first and second year of life than at school age—and is very rarely a result of re-vaccination.

The present evidence in the United Kingdom suggests that the mortality from encephalitis among infants is about 6 per cent. Post-vaccinal neurological illness in infants under two years seems mainly to be an encephalitis associated with viraemia, whereas in older persons central nervous system complications are more likely to be examples of post-infective encephalopathy.

Symptoms of meningo-encephalomyelopathy appear 7–12 days after vaccination. The mortality rate may reach 30 per cent.; of the survivors a few suffer permanent neurological or psychiatric sequelae.

Toxic eruptions of erythema multiforme occasionally appear 7–10 days following vaccination. An irritant papular vesicular rash often most marked on the wrists and hands but usually avoiding the face also occurs—sometimes with a three-week delay. Thrombocytopenic purpura has been recorded.

Treatment

Uncomplicated vaccination requires no treatment other than a loose dry dressing to protect the lesion at the vesicular stage.

The potentially fatal complications of eczema vaccinatum and vaccinia necrosum call for hyperimmune antivariola gamma globulin intramuscularly in a dose of 0·2 ml. per pound body weight.

Interferon applied locally may prove to limit the spread of progressive vaccinia. Preliminary reports of N-methylisatin β-thiosemicarbazone are conflicting.

REFERENCES

DIXON, C. W. (1962) Vaccination against smallpox, *Brit. med. J.*, **1**, 1262.

MINISTRY OF HEALTH (1967) Memorandum on Vaccination Against Smallpox, London, H.M.S.O.

SCIENTIFIC COMMITTEE ON INTERFERON (1962) Effect of interferon on vaccination in volunteers, *Lancet*, i, 873.

CHICKENPOX—HERPES ZOSTER

Aetiology

The relationship between chickenpox and shingles has long been known. Both diseases are due to a virus and the evidence now confirms beyond doubt that the viruses are identical. The varicella-zoster virus is a brick-shaped body measuring approximately 230 micromicrons which can be isolated from chickenpox and zoster lesions. No difference between the viruses isolated from patients suffering from either disease can be detected in the laboratory by electron microscopy, culture or serological means. Inoculation of susceptible children with zoster virus produces clinical chickenpox which spreads to other children as chickenpox.

Herpes zoster does not spread as herpes zoster but may do so as chickenpox; the reverse does not take place. Thus a grandparent with shingles may well cause chickenpox in susceptible grandchildren but the child with chickenpox is no risk to any person who has suffered from the disease and will not give anyone shingles. Following an attack of chickenpox it seems likely that the virus is not completely eliminated from the body but remains dormant—possibly in the posterior root ganglia. This is analogous to the known persistence of herpes simplex virus in cells at mucocutaneous junctions following a primary herpetic infection. Many years later, perhaps as a result of local or general stress, the virus multiplies causing an attack of shingles. If multiplication is considerable there is a spill over of virus in the blood with few or many ‘chickenpox’ lesions in addition. Apart from this association the diseases are quite distinct in clinical practice and affect different age groups. They are consequently considered separately.

CHICKENPOX

Synonym. Varicella.

Definition

An acute and highly infectious disease characterized by a vesicular rash which tends to appear in successive crops.

Epidemiology

The disease is universal although less common in certain areas such as the West Indies. In most urban communities it is endemic the year round with localized epidemics occurring from time to time. It is highly infectious. The majority of patients are children, but it is not uncommon in adults. Due to its high infectivity infection is usually but not invariably acquired at the first contact. The disease is spread mainly by droplet and direct contact but it can also be spread by fomites. Chickenpox is notoriously difficult to contain in hospital where cross-infection follows unless the strictest barrier-nursing technique is observed. There is no doubt that the hands and clothing of the staff can spread the disease. The virus is present in the skin and mucous membrane lesions and has been recovered from the blood. Patients are probably infectious for a period of 24 hours before the appearance of the rash and remain so until the lesions have dried up. Crusts are not infectious.

Pathology

The virus is thought to enter through the nasopharyngeal route, probably multiplying during the incubation period in lymphatic tissue. It reaches the skin during the viraemia which occurs early in the illness. Many other tissues including the lung, liver, spleen, pancreas and suprarenals have been shown to be involved in fatal cases. The skin lesion lies in the cellular epidermis, only rarely invading the corium. The lesion, first macular and then papular, undergoes central liquefaction with resulting vesicle formation. It contains clear fluid which may become turbid from invasion by lymphocytes without secondary infection. Scab formation follows absorption of the fluid or rupture of the vesicle, except on mucous membranes where rupture leaves a shallow ulcer. Multinucleated giant cells containing intranuclear inclusion bodies can be demonstrated at the base of a chickenpox vesicle.

Symptoms

The incubation period is commonly 14–16 days with limits of 11–21 days.

Prodromal symptoms, especially in children, are often insignificant or absent. In adults, however, 48–72 hours of malaise and mild fever may precede the appearance of the rash although these symptoms are seldom severe enough to interfere with the patient's occupation. Headache, shivers and mild backache may occur. Not uncommonly one or two spots appear at the onset but are disregarded until the main crop begins. Occasionally in children the illness starts with vomiting, convulsions and high fever. Fleeting prodromal scarlatiniform rashes may precede the true rash, appearing and fading in a matter of 12 hours or less.

The *eruption* of chickenpox appears first on the trunk but soon spreads to the face, scalp and proximal parts of the limbs. It may be first noticed on the face and sometimes on the mucous membranes of the fauces and palate although lesions here tend to appear after they have been noted on the skin. There is no orderly progression, although the forearms and legs, if involved at all, tend to be affected later. Fresh crops of lesions appear for up to five days while in mild cases there may be no fresh spots after 48 hours. The distribution of the rash is characteristic. There are more lesions on the trunk than on the limbs and more on the proximal than on the distal parts of the limbs. Even in severe attacks lesions are seldom numerous on the back of the wrists, the palms or the soles. There is no predilection for extensor surfaces or prominences, lesions occurring freely in the axillae and other flexures. The normal distribution of the rash may be upset by previous skin irritation. Thus, sunburn may cause a heavy rash on the forearms or a napkin rash an increase of lesions on the buttocks. The face may be heavily involved and there are usually many spots in the scalp.

The individual lesion starts as a macule, rapidly becoming papular, vesicular and then scabbing. Some become pustules. The rapidity of development is characteristic, the lesion taking approximately 24 hours or less to become vesicular. Thus a few vesicles are normally visible on the first day the rash is noted. The lesions are superficial being on, rather than in, the skin, vary in size and shape and are frequently irritant. The vesicles tend to be oval where they lie in line with the natural body creases. The amount of surrounding erythema is variable but not as a rule very striking. Vesicles look like translucent droplets ('dewdrops'), seldom being more than 0·5 cm. in diameter. They are mostly unilocular and umbilication is rare. Confluence of adjacent vesicles is exceptional. Owing to its itchiness the rash is often infected by scratching and then the lesions become enlarged and more inflamed.

The appearance of the eruption in successive crops leads, after a day or two, to the presence at the same time on the same area of skin of lesions at all stages of development, i.e. papules, vesicles, pustules and scabs. On mucous membrane the vesicles rupture early leaving shallow grey ulcers. So long as cropping continues the temperature is likely to remain raised, indeed in more severe cases it rises as the rash develops in contrast to smallpox. Some cases, however, are apyrexial throughout.

Varieties. All severe forms of chickenpox are rare. *Haemorrhagic chickenpox* is characterized by haemorrhages both into the rash and into surrounding skin. There may also be bleeding from mucous membranes. It is usually a fatal disease associated with high fever and severe constitutional symptoms. Predisposing causes are leukaemia or steroid therapy (either current or recent), but haemorrhagic chickenpox may affect a previously healthy individual.

Varicella bullosa is due to a combined chickenpox and haemolytic streptococcal infection. The lesions form large bullae which rupture leaving raw areas. Also due to a combined streptococcal infection, and more serious, is *varicella gangrenosa* in which infection of some lesions is associated with an intense cellulitis and local gangrene. In the past, diphtheria was sometimes responsible for this type.

Most infants are protected by maternal antibody till about six months of age. In the unprotected infant neonatal chickenpox is potentially lethal but may run a mild and uneventful course. The onset is often mild with little constitutional upset but if cropping continues for over three days a severe and possibly fatal attack should be expected. Autopsy in such cases shows extensive visceral involvement.

Complications

Secondary bacterial infection of pocks is usually staphylococcal, localized abscess formation from an infected lesion being the commonest cause of fever after the fifth day. Rarely *septicaemia* and distant staphylococcal infections ensue. Scarlet fever and chickenpox not infrequently occur together due to streptococcal infection of one or more vesicles.

Varicella pneumonia is chiefly seen in adults and is often, though by no means invariably, associated with a severe attack with a heavy rash. Symptoms start on the second to fifth day. Cough, dyspnoea and cyanosis are prominent and haemoptysis is frequent. Examination of the chest may reveal extensive medium crepitations but clear-cut evidence of consolidation is absent and signs are often minimal. Radiography, however, reveals gross nodular opacities throughout both lung fields. It is not uncommon to find marked X-ray changes with minimal cough and shortness of breath. Most patients recover symptomatically in one to three weeks but a few patients succumb in 2–3 days with heart failure and pulmonary oedema. It may be months before complete radiological recovery occurs. There may instead be a permanent fibrosis with ultimately a diffuse 'miliary' calcification first visible 2–10 years after the attack.

Varicella *encephalomyelopathy* starts between the third and tenth days and is unrelated to the severity of the attack. Evidence of neurological involvement is ushered in with headache, stiff neck, vomiting, convulsions, irritability, drowsiness or coma. Peripheral neuropathy or transverse or ascending myelopathy may occur but the commonest central abnormality is a cerebellar ataxia, particularly affecting the arms. The cerebrospinal fluid may be normal or show a rise of cells and protein or protein alone. The prognosis is good, over 80 per cent. recovering completely; about 5 per cent. die, the remainder being left with permanent damage such as personality change or residual paralysis.

Rare complications include *hepatitis, orchitis* and *myocarditis.* Haemorrhagic and fatal chickenpox often occurs in patients undergoing steroid therapy for some other condition.

Diagnosis

Typical cases cause no difficulty, the pleomorphic, vesiculating rash of central distribution being characteristic. Electron microscopy of material from lesions may show herpes virus particles. Culture is slow but is useful in confirmation of atypical cases. A gel diffusion test using vesicle fluid as antigen may give a positive result within six hours but a negative test does not exclude chickenpox. The white cell count is usually normal.

Severe chickenpox may be mistaken for smallpox, although the rapid development and the central distribution of the rash clearly distinguish the two conditions. What is more likely and much more serious is that mild smallpox is mistaken for chickenpox. The differential diagnosis is fully discussed on page 163 but it must be stressed that just as a mild illness does not exclude smallpox, neither does a severe one exclude chickenpox.

Papulovesicular urticaria occasionally causes confusion but the lesions are smaller, seldom involve the face and frequently occur in clusters on the legs. If vesicles are present they are pin-point in size. The lesions of insect bites are similar to those of papular urticaria. Scabies, acne and impetigo all have a different distribution from chickenpox, do not involve the mouth and persist longer. The lesions in eczema herpeticum and eczema vaccinatum are almost confined to the eczematous areas of skin. Pityriasis rosea and a papular secondary syphilide start with discrete lesions but in neither disease does vesiculation follow.

Treatment

The disease is self-limited, the majority of patients requiring no treatment. Patients should be isolated until all the lesions are dry, usually a period of 10–14 days. Mild cases do not need to be kept in bed after the first 48 hours. Skin irritation is helped by the liberal application of calamine lotion, and by oral antihistamines such as promethazine, 25 mg. three times a day for an adult. Prophylactic antibiotics are not required.

Septic complications are treated with the appropriate antibiotics. Varicella pneumonia requires complete rest, oxygen and sedation. Digitalis and diuretics are only indicated if there is evidence of heart failure. It is customary to use penicillin prophylactically in the presence of varicella pneumonia although its value is doubtful. Present evidence suggests that steroids are harmful.

In encephalomyelopathy steroids are indicated (as described for measles) in those patients who develop signs of neurological involvement five days or more after the onset. In the rare case in whom this complication starts earlier than the sixth day the risk of disseminating the virus outweighs any possible advantage. Steroids should thus not be used before the sixth day of illness.

In the patient who develops chickenpox while undergoing steroid treatment the dose must be maintained. It should only be increased if a severe attack appears to be developing.

Prevention

Previous infection confers life-long immunity except for an attack associated with herpes zoster.

No vaccine is available. Gamma globulin is of variable protective value. It is indicated in a dosage of 0·45 ml. per kg. in an attempt to modify a subsequent attack in the following non-immune groups of contacts: (1) infants of under three months of age whose mothers have not had chickenpox; (2) infants born during a maternal attack of chickenpox; (3) those undergoing steroid therapy. Prevention of the above groups from coming into contact with chickenpox, where possible, is a much safer procedure than relying on the use of gamma globulin after exposure.

Prognosis

Death is rare. When it does occur it is due to the haemorrhagic form, to varicella pneumonia or to encephalomyelopathy. The dangerous combination of steroids with chickenpox has been discussed. Chickenpox is often lethal when occurring as a complication of leukaemia.

REFERENCES

BLAIR, A. W., JAMIESON, W. M., and SMITH, G. H. (1965) Complications and deaths in chickenpox, *Brit. med. J.*, **2**, 981.

BOUGHTON, C. R. (1966) Varicella zoster in Sydney, *Med. J. Aust.*, ii, 392.

HAGGERTY, R. J., and ELEY, R. C. (1956) Varicella and cortisone, *Pediatrics*, **18**, 160.

KNYVETT, A. F. (1966) The pulmonary lesions of chickenpox, *Quart. J. Med.*, **35**, 313.

Lancet (1966) Editorial, ii, 431.

G. D. W. McKENDRICK

HERPES ZOSTER

Synonyms. Zoster; Shingles.

Definition

An acute infection of the posterior root ganglion by a neurotropic virus, leading to severe pain in the distribution of the corresponding posterior root, and to the appearance of a crop of vesicles in the cutaneous distribution of the root.

Aetiology

The disease is seen at all ages. In elderly patients it is very often more serious as well as more painful than in the young. The older the subject the more persistent and severe are the painful sequels. It may arise without discoverable cause and with a febrile reaction and considerable malaise. It often happens a few days after exposure to chicken pox. There is little doubt that both are due to the same virus, zoster probably being a manifestation of infection in the partially immune subject. In some instances it follows radiotherapy, the eruption appearing in the segment irradiated.

Pathology

The essential lesion is an acute inflammation of the dorsal root ganglion of the same histological character as the lesion of acute anterior poliomyelitis. Later, degenerative changes occur in the fibres of the dorsal roots and of the peripheral sensory nerves. There is an increased protein and lymphocyte count in the cerebrospinal fluid. There are also widespread changes in the central nervous system sometimes reflected in evidences of acute encephalomyelitis.

Symptoms

There may be an onset with fever which persists for 2, 3 or even 4 days. There is from the first pain at the place at which later the herpetic eruption is to appear. This occurs on the third or fourth day of the illness. At first the rash is a patchy erythema, upon which appear small vesicles filled with clear fluid. From the fifth to the tenth day the vesicles dry up and shrink progressively until a scab is formed. This finally drops off, sometimes leaving considerable scarring. These scars may be anaesthetic to touch, pinprick and temperature sense. The pain before and during the evolution of the cutaneous lesion may be intense. It is of a burning and itching quality, and in frail and elderly persons it may persist as a most intractable post-herpetic neuralgia for months or even years.

Herpes of the ophthalmic division of the fifth nerve is most commonly found in elderly persons. Corneal vesicles may form and burst, causing ulcers, which may spread and end in residual scarring (nebulae), which impairs vision. In addition to the effects upon the eye itself and upon vision there may be reduction in sensation or total anaesthesia in the territory of the fifth nerve, and terrible pain. When sensory loss is slight the small paper-white scars of the herpetic lesions are always anaesthetic, although the surrounding zone may be hyperaesthetic. This is pathognomonic. Instead of anaesthesia in the area there may be distressing hyperaesthesia to light touch or pressure which leads to an almost psychotic state of protective anxiety about, and preoccupation with, the area. Finally, and distinct from the hyperaesthesia, intractable spontaneous pain may present—a pain which dominates the whole of the subject's life. This pain is aggravated by fatigue, worry and physical debility and often induces a neurotic reaction on the part of the patient or a state of depression in which suicide may be contemplated.

Herpes of the geniculate ganglion occasionally occurs. The vesicles are found in the pinna, and there is pain in this region, over the mastoid, and sometimes in the fauces. It causes vertigo and severe facial palsy, which is often irrecoverable (the Ramsay Hunt syndrome). Occasionally a generalized eruption indistinguishable from varicella may follow, or more rarely precede or accompany the zonal lesion. This condition of herpes generalisatus is seen most often in the elderly and particularly when the zoster complicates malignant disease such as leukaemia [see Section 13]. It may be precipitated by corticosteroid therapy.

Localized paralysis may accompany zoster. Thus, in ophthalmic herpes there is occasionally third-nerve palsy, with ptosis and squint. In geniculate herpes, facial palsy with loss of taste over the anterior two-thirds of the tongue is the rule. In herpes of the lower thoracic ganglia there may be paralysis of the oblique abdominal muscles on the affected side. The marked local bulging of the abdominal wall which ensues resembles at first sight the presence of an abdominal tumour. These paralyses do not invariably clear up, though the facial palsy of geniculate herpes does so more frequently than the paralysis of the abdominal muscles. The onset of the illness may reflect the widespread infection of the nervous system, with hemiplegic or paraplegic dysaesthesiae, as well as prostration. The encephalitis and myelitis, which are uncommon, nearly always have a good prognosis. Nevertheless, zoster in the elderly should always be considered a serious disease, because of the possibility of permanent painful disability.

Treatment

Corticosteroids should be used as soon as the diagnosis is made; ACTH gel, 80 I.U. intramuscularly on the first day, 40 I.U. for 3 days and then rapidly tailing off, may cause dramatic resolution and subsequent freedom from pain. There exists the possibility of dissemination as an encephalomyelitis or as diffuse varicella, but in the aged especially the benefits outweigh the risks.

Vesicles should be kept dry and left alone unless there is secondary infection. Analgesics help in the acute phase, but not when post-herpetic pain has developed, when tranquillizers (diazepam, 5 or 10 mg.) and antidepressives (amitriptyline, 25 mg.) may be needed.

A great variety of local applications have been used without avail. Irradiation of the posterior root ganglia is useless. Surgical measures such as division of peripheral nerves, posterior spinal roots or the spinothalamic tract in the cord are equally ineffective. The pain is a central one, not amenable to surgery of peripheral nerve pathways. Frontal leucotomy was advocated, but has fallen into disrepute, being as damaging as it is ineffective. Anterolateral thalamotomy is justified when intractable pain persists. Whether medical or surgical treatment is used it is essential to pay attention to the patient's attitude and life pattern, and to try to divert his preoccupation from the affected area. It is probable that it is in the breaking down the patient's protective attitude to the affected skin that the present vogue of intensive stimulation by massage and by vibrations has its basis.

In this regard it is important to appreciate that the patient's temperament and attitude is intimately bound up with the pain. Granted severe shingles in the elderly, those whose lives are dominated by the local distress have rigid temperaments, and have always been noted for their perfectionist attention to detail, and their inability to 'get their mind' off a problem.

REFERENCES

BIGGART, J. H., and FISHER, J. A. (1938) Meningo-encephalitis complicating herpes zoster, *Lancet*, ii, 944.

DENNY-BROWN, D., ADAMS, R. D., and FITZGERALD, P. J. (1944) Pathologic features of herpes zoster: a note on 'geniculate herpes', *Arch. Neurol. Psychiat.* (*Chic.*), **57**, 216.

RUSSELL, W. R., ESPIR, M. L. E., and MORGANSTERN, F. S. (1957) Treatment of post-herpetic neuralgia, *Lancet*, i, 242.

TAVERNER, D. (1960) Alleviation of post-herpetic neuralgia, *Lancet*, ii, 671.

DENIS WILLIAMS

GERMAN MEASLES

Synonym. Rubella.

Definition

Rubella is a mild, benign infectious disease due to a virus. It is characterized by a long incubation period followed by a short invasive stage with a rash and lymphadenopathy. When a woman is infected in early pregnancy serious foetal damage may occur.

Aetiology

The virus can be grown on a variety of tissue cultures but in only some (for example, primary human amnion) are visible cytopathic effects produced. Growth on vervet monkey kidney (a highly sensitive tissue) must be shown by failure of a challenge inoculation with ECHO Type 11. Virus can be recovered from the nasopharynx from up to 7 days before the rash to 7–14 days thereafter. Culture should be successful in 90 per cent. of patients who show a rash. Viraemia has been detected shortly after virus is first recovered from the throat, reaching its maximum at the time of the rash. Virus is also present in the urine.

The patient is probably infectious from up to 2 days before the rash appears, remaining so for a further 3–4 days. Infectivity is lower than in measles. Spread is by droplet and by close contact. The incidence of the disease is greatest in spring and early summer with epidemics occurring every 4–6 years or so, though with no great regularity. The disease predominantly affects children but many escape and consequently the illness is often seen in adolescents and young adults. Many practitioners believe that second and even third attacks of rubella are common. This should not be accepted on the present evidence in view of the difficulties of diagnosis of the disease. There is no doubt that rubella can be closely mimicked by other virus infections, notably some of the Coxsackie and ECHO groups. It seems more likely that lifelong immunity is usual after rubella, most supposedly recurrent attacks being due to diagnostic error.

Symptoms

The incubation period is normally 16–18 days, with extremes of 14–21 days.

Premonitory symptoms are often absent in children, the rash being the first evidence of the disease. In some children, however, and in most adults a mild prodromal illness from 1 to 3 days precedes the rash. There is a mild fever and a little coryza, sore throat, headache and conjunctivitis. The posterior cervical lymph nodes may be enlarged and tender and this is the commonest, and may be the sole, pre-eruptive symptom. These symptoms commonly subside within 24 hours of the appearance of the rash. The *enanthem* of rubella may appear in the prodromal period or with the rash. It consists of pin-point reddish spots on the palate, some of which may show a very fine vesiculation. As similar changes may be seen in many upper respiratory infections, including measles, scarlatina and infectious mononucleosis, the enanthem is of little help in differential diagnosis. There is usually a mild tonsillar congestion and occasionally a little exudate.

The *lymphadenopathy* is an important and significant feature of the disease. Lymph nodes in any situation may be enlarged and moderately tender but the adenitis is often confined to the posterior cervical glands. The suboccipital and postauricular glands are often enlarged to the size of peas, not infrequently being discovered by the patient. The enlargement starts in the prodromal period but is usually maximal about the time the rash appears. The tenderness subsides within a day or two but palpably enlarged glands may persist for several weeks. Splenomegaly is not uncommon during the acute stage. The conjunctivae characteristically show a mild suffusion coincident with the rash or preceding it in some of those cases who develop prodromal symptoms.

The *rash*, at first discrete and macular, may become slightly papular, morbilliform or scarlatiniform as it develops. It appears first as discrete spots on the face and neck, affecting the circumoral region, the scalp and the skin behind the ears. Sometimes lesions are first seen on the wrists, chest, shoulders or even the legs. They are pale pink macules, smaller than those seen in measles, which tend to appear in clusters. The rash quickly spreads to the trunk and limbs and in most cases it quickly fades. On the second day the face is no longer spotty but appears diffusely erythematous. The rash on the trunk often becomes confluent at this time and may closely resemble scarlet fever although the lesions on the limbs remain discrete. The rash of german measles rarely lasts more than three days. It is not followed by staining of the skin but a minimal fine desquamation is sometimes seen. Although a rash appears in over 90 per cent. of patients over 15 years of age it is frequently absent in younger children. In institutional outbreaks up to 50 per cent. of sero-conversions have occurred in children with no rash and often with no symptoms, although examination has frequently revealed some lymph gland enlargement in these otherwise inapparent infections.

In most patients fever and constitutional upset is mild throughout but temperatures of up to 104° F. (40° C.) occur from time to time in some patients. However, fever subsides with the disappearance of the rash and convalescence is remarkably speedy.

Complications

In childhood complications are distinctly rare. There is so little inflammation of the respiratory mucous membrane that secondary bacterial infection is seldom seen. Post-rubella *encephalomyelopathy* or *polyneuro-*

pathy occasionally occur 5–10 days after the onset. A benign *polyarthritis* affecting young women has been a feature of some epidemics. Joint pain and swelling occurs on the third to eleventh day with a return of fever. Small or large joints may be involved but there is never associated carditis. The condition is benign and subsides spontaneously in 5–10 days. *Purpura*, usually but not invariably associated with a transient thrombocytopenia, has occurred.

Rubella in Pregnancy. Rubella in the first trimester of pregnancy carries a risk to the foetus. The risk is greatest in the first four weeks, becoming progressively less towards the twelfth week. Foetal death and abortion may occur or a damaged infant may survive to be born with some congenital abnormality of which heart disease, deafness, cataract and central nervous system anomalies such as microcephaly, hydrocephalus or mental deficiency are the commonest. Multiple defects may be present. During the first four weeks of pregnancy the risk of foetal damage from the mother developing rubella is approximately 50 per cent., at 5–8 weeks it is 35 per cent., at 9–12 weeks it is 15 per cent. After 16 weeks the risk becomes negligible.

The following recommendations can be made:

1. If a woman in the first 12 weeks of pregnancy comes into contact with rubella, blood should be taken for rubella haemagglutination inhibition antibodies. This test takes under 24 hours to perform. If antibodies are absent, 1·5 G. of hyperimmune gamma globulin should be given. If antibodies are present the patient can be reassured. Should serology not be possible gamma globulin should be administered unless the history of previous rubella is incontrovertible.

2. If a woman contracts rubella in the first 4 weeks of pregnancy there is a strong case for recommending therapeutic abortion providing there are no legal obstacles, unless there are reasons such as age, religion, delayed pregnancy or parental wishes for the pregnancy to continue.

3. When rubella occurs between the fourth and twelfth weeks the risk of an abnormal child being born should be represented to the parents as about 15–25 per cent. and decision with regard to abortion can be taken in the light of all the circumstances.

4. The parents should be reassured and no further action taken when rubella occurs after the first trimester.

It is vital that the diagnosis of german measles should be confirmed beyond reasonable doubt—by no means always an easy task.

Congenital Rubella. Rubella embryopathy is due either to inhibition of cell growth or to cellular necrosis. Defects, which are often multiple, include the following:

- Retardation of growth.
- Eye defects (cataract, glaucoma, retinopathy).
- Heart lesions (patent ductus arteriosus, ventricular septal defect, pulmonary stenosis, interstitial myocarditis).
- Deafness, thrombocytopenic purpura.
- Cerebral defects (mental backwardness, meningo-encephalitis, cerebrospinal fluid pleocytosis).
- Splenomegaly, hepatomegaly, skeletal abnormalities.

Ninety-eight per cent. of infected infants have neutralizing antibody in the IgM series. Virus can readily be isolated from the throat, urine and rectum of infants who have been infected *in utero*, whether or not they show signs of disease. Virus excretion may last up to 12 months.

Diagnosis

Laboratory confirmation of the diagnosis is now possible but takes at least 2 weeks whether from culture of throat washings or examination of paired sera. Neutralizing antibodies appear about the fourth day and reach their peak in 2–3 weeks. The white cell count shows a leucopenia with sometimes an increase in plasma or Türk cells but these changes are not specific. The diagnosis, therefore, remains clinical. The cardinal features are a mild brief illness with a pale pink, discrete rash, enlarged and tender suboccipital or postauricular glands combined with a mild conjunctival suffusion. *Enteroviral infections* (Coxsackie A and some echoviruses) may cause similar illnesses. However, in these infections, the posterior cervical glands are not so likely to be involved, the rash may show a fine petechial element, particularly over the shoulders and the anterior axillary folds and headache with or without aseptic meningitis is likely to be severe.

A mild attack of *measles* may cause difficulty but the more prolonged and pronounced coryza and cough, the presence of Koplik's spots (which do not occur in rubella) a blotchy, dusky rash and the subsequent staining of the skin serve to differentiate. Confusion between rubella and *scarlet fever* is more common. In favour of the latter are the more severe initial symptoms of headache, vomiting (rare in rubella) and sore throat. The circumoral area is usually pale, the tongue changes are characteristic and the eyes are clear and bright. In rubella the rash on the trunk may be indistinguishable from scarlet fever but it remains discrete on the limbs. An eruptive fever which suggests measles on the first day and scarlet fever on the second day is usually rubella.

Many *toxic and drug rashes* may bear a resemblance to rubella but their distribution is more irregular, the lesions are larger and often pleomorphic and the cervical lymphadenopathy is absent. A rubelliform rash may be seen in infectious mononucleosis, but does not appear till the fourth day or later. *Pityriasis rosea* is distinguished by the herald patch, the browny colour of the lesions which are most marked on the trunk, together with the complete well-being of the patient.

Treatment

Patients can be regarded as non-infectious once the rash has faded. No quarantine of contacts is necessary. Treatment is symptomatic with rest in bed during the febrile period.

Prophylaxis

When indicated in pregnancy the dose of gamma globulin required to lessen the risk of foetal damage is 1·5 G.

A living attenuated vaccine is now in widespread use, but there is doubt about the duration of the immunity it produces.

Prognosis

Rapid, uneventful recovery is the rule and immunity is probably long lasting. The possibility of second attacks is discussed above. Complete recovery can be expected in about 80 per cent. of those who develop neurological complications. A few will die, the remainder showing some degree of residual paralysis.

REFERENCES

DUDGEON, J. A. (1967) Clinical aspects of pre-natal and post-natal infection, *Publ. Hlth (Lond.)*, **81,** 268.

FIELD, A. M. (1967) Antibody responses in rubella, *Publ. Hlth (Lond.)*, **81,** 279.

HILL, A. B., DOLL, R., GALLOWAY, T. MCL., and HUGHES, J. P. W. (1958) Virus diseases in pregnancy and congenital defects, *Brit. J. prev. soc. Med.*, **12,** 1.

LÜNDSTRÖM, R. (1962) Rubella during pregnancy, *Acta paediat. (Uppsala)*, **51,** Suppl. 133, 1.

MINISTRY OF HEALTH (1960) Rubella and Other Virus Infections during Pregnancy, No. 101, London, H.M.S.O.

MEASLES

Synonym: Morbilli; Rubeola.

Definition

Measles is a highly infectious disease characterized by respiratory catarrh, Koplik's spots on the buccal mucous membrane and a distinctive maculopapular rash.

Aetiology and Epidemiology

The virus of measles can be cultured on various human and monkey tissues. It is approximately 140 micromicrons in size, is able to survive for long periods at low temperatures but only for a few days at room temperature. Its growth in tissue culture causes the formation of multinucleated giant cells and eosinophilic inclusions both in cytoplasm and nuclei. The virus appears to be identical with the virus which causes giant-cell pneumonia—the latter, therefore, being measles without a rash. The virus of canine distemper is closely allied to that of measles, infection with it in experimental animals giving partial protection against attack by measles virus.

Measles is of world-wide distribution, both sexes being equally susceptible. As it is extremely infectious, few children in an urban community escape attack and thus the disease is relatively infrequent in adults. When introduced into an unprotected community it spreads with great rapidity to persons of all ages, causing many deaths. In Great Britain more than half the cases occur in children under ten. In poor and crowded communities the disease attacks young children, whilst amongst the middle classes the infection is commonly delayed until school age. Nation-wide epidemics occur every two years due to the natural increase by birth of the number of susceptibles. The disease is rare in the first six months of life due to passive protection received from the mother. A diagnosis of measles under this age is always suspect unless the mother has never suffered infection.

Measles in pregnancy tends to cause abortion or premature birth, in the latter case the infant may be born with the disease (*congenital measles*). Measles in early pregnancy, not followed by abortion, carries a slight risk of foetal damage but this is much less than with rubella.

Spread takes place by direct contact or by droplet infection. Fomites are unimportant outside hospital practice. The virus enters through the intact conjunctiva and also through the respiratory tract. Patients are at their most infectious during the prodromal period before the development of the rash.

Pathology

The characteristic lesion of measles is the large multinucleated giant cell which appears in the pharyngeal and bronchial mucosa associated with a general mucosal inflammation. Giant cells are also found in other lymphoid tissue such as the tonsils, lymph nodes, spleen and appendix.

Koplik's spots consist of minute areas of endothelial proliferation which break down into shallow ulcers at the base of which are cells undergoing active mitosis. The rash starts in the superficial vessels of the corium. Plasma and some cells pass through the capillary walls leaving the staining which remains as the erythema subsides. In a heavy rash whole blood contributes to the staining which becomes frankly haemorrhagic.

Fatal cases show bronchiolitis with interstitial infiltration with mononuclear cells. Secondary bacterial bronchopneumonia is almost invariably present.

Symptoms

The incubation period is commonly 10 days to the onset of symptoms—12 days to the appearance of the rash, but varies within 8–12 days.

An illness of infection is occasionally seen, consisting of a transient mild fever sometimes associated with a fleeting rash, the whole episode coinciding with infection and subsiding within a few hours. It is so mild that it is likely to pass unnoticed unless the patient is under medical observation.

The onset is fairly rapid with fever, malaise and irritability. Coryza, sneezing, dry cough and watery eyes rapidly appear. The child suffering from a moderately severe attack presents a typical picture of misery on the second day with running eyes and nose. Croup is not uncommon and diarrhoea also is a frequent symptom in this *catarrhal stage*. On the third day the temperature may fall and the patient improve only to deteriorate again with the appearance of the rash on the fourth day. Transient prodromal rashes—either of morbilliform or scarlatiniform type are not uncommon on the second day in measles and lead to diagnostic and prognostic errors. When such a rash is followed by improvement and fall of temperature on the third day it may be thought, erroneously, that the patient has been fortunate to suffer from a particularly mild attack. Such a belief is confounded when fever returns and the true rash appears a day or two later. Epistaxis is quite common during the catarrhal stage of measles.

Koplik's spots usually appear two days before the rash. They consist of small irregular spots of bright red colour in the centre of which is a minute bluish-white speck. They appear in clusters and are most numerous on the inner aspects of the cheek opposite the molar teeth and near the gum margin. They increase in number until the rash starts, thereafter fading rapidly. Sometimes they are so numerous as to cover nearly the whole buccal mucous membrane. In some cases the red background is insignificant whilst in others it is dominant, the white specks only being visible in a bright light. The spots are always best seen in daylight. Koplik's spots are pathognomonic of measles. As they are frequently present for 48 hours before the rash as well as for a few hours after it begins to appear they are an invaluable diagnostic sign.

The rash appears on the third or fourth day although it is sometimes delayed as long as six days. It is usually accompanied by a sharp rise of temperature and respiratory rate, together with wide-spread medium crepitations audible throughout the lung fields. It is first seen on the forehead, behind the ears and along the hair margin at the back of the neck. It spreads rapidly, sometimes after a day of hesitancy, over the face, neck, trunk and limbs, this period of development lasting from 12 to 48 hours. The individual lesions are at first discrete dusky pink macules but they rapidly enlarge in size to become maculopapular, many cf the lesions running together. This gives the typical blotchy appearance in which large areas of skin are covered by patches of rash with an irregular outline. The confluence is less marked on the limbs. Petechial haemorrhages into the rash are common and are not of grave importance as they merely indicate a heavy rash. Itching is rare.

The eruption fades in the order of its appearance, usually disappearing first from the face after some 2–3 days, sometimes starting to fade from here before it has fully developed on the legs. It leaves behind a brownish staining due to extravasation of plasma. In heavy or haemorrhagic rashes the staining may persist for a fortnight but in general it fades within a few days. With the disappearance of the rash a fine branny desquamation may develop but this is much less constant than staining and is confined to the areas where the rash has been most profuse, usually the face and trunk. With the development of the rash the temperature may continue to rise but it falls by rapid lysis once the rash starts to fade and convalescence thereafter is rapid in the absence of complications. The rapid respiratory rate as the rash appears may suggest pneumonia but the pulse/respiration ratio is little under 4:1 in the absence of this complication. The catarrhal symptoms also reach their maximum at this time, the coryza, cough and generalized wretchedness of the child being striking features in the more severe attacks. The conjunctivitis may cause photophobia which may subside before the rash appears or persist during its development. The tongue is coated, the throat congested and a moderate generalized lymphadenopathy may be present. The spleen may be palpable. In some cases the tongue strips to become similar to the red strawberry tongue of scarlet fever.

Many attacks are milder than the above description, with the rash complicating a 'febrile cold' but with relatively little constitutional disturbance. Abortive attacks in which no rash develops can only be diagnosed with certainty if Koplik's spots are detected (*morbilli sine morbillis*). *Haemorrhagic measles* is fortunately rare. This is a severe and frequently fatal form in which hyperpyrexia and delirium are associated with haemorrhages into the skin and from mucous membranes of the mouth and intestinal tract. It must not be confused with simple measles with a haemorrhagic rash, when the bleeding is confined to the rash, a common manifestation not of serious significance.

Complications

The wide-spread inflammation of the mucosa in the respiratory tract predisposes to secondary bacterial infection and this remains the chief hazard of measles. Otitis media and bronchopneumonia are the commonest complications of the disease.

Otitis media, catarrhal or suppurative, may appear just before, with or following the focal eruption. It most often starts about the fifth day and is a common cause of the temperature failing to settle as the rash subsides. Older children usually complain of earache, but fever or return of temperature may be the only symptoms in the young child. Sometimes a purulent discharge appears without warning. Obvious mastoiditis is now rare.

Bacterial *bronchopneumonia* appears when the rash is at its height or within the next few days. *Haemophilus influenzae*, staphylococci and pneumococci are the commonest bacteria implicated. The dry cough increases, the respiratory rate, pulse and temperature rise, the pulse/respiration ratio falling to less than 4:1, often to about 2:1. The accessory respiratory muscles including the alae nasi are brought into play and the respiratory rhythm becomes inverted with a pause at the end of inspiration. With increasing hypoxia restlessness and cyanosis appear. Postmeasles pneumonia is variable in its course. Whereas the majority of cases clear up with therapy within 7–10 days, some attacks persist for weeks with fluctuation in the temperature chart and physical signs. Permanent lung damage with fibrosis or bronchiectasis may follow recovery in such cases. Death may occur as late as 3–4 weeks after the onset of bronchopneumonia.

Bronchitis can be regarded as an integral part of an attack of measles but *bronchiolitis* is a complication normally due to the virus. This may cause intense respiratory distress in the prodromal stage, possibly progressing to bronchopneumonia which, prior to the development of the rash, is usually due to the measles virus. This is always serious. Mediastinal emphysema leading to subcutaneous emphysema of the neck and anterior chest wall may appear.

In the young child *laryngitis* of sufficient severity to cause croup may dominate the catarrhal stage but usually improves with the development of the eruption. Blepharitis and *suppurative conjunctivitis* can occur but severe corneal ulceration leading ultimately to loss of vision is nowadays very rare. Sinusitis and suppurative cervical adenitis are also uncommon.

The stomatitis of measles sometimes becomes ulcerative towards the end of the first week. In cachectic patients in the past this could be followed by fatal gangrene of the lips and cheeks (*cancrum oris*) but this complication is no longer seen in Great Britain. A purulent *vaginitis* may occur. *Diarrhoea* is common in the catarrhal stage.

Purpura, either thrombocytopenic or non-thrombocytopenic may follow measles. Rapid recovery is usual. The incidence of *acute appendicitis* is higher in measles than can be explained on grounds of chance. Symptoms appear about the time of the rash and are associated with lymphoid hyperplasia in the appendix.

The incidence of postmeasles *encephalomyelopathy* is approximately 0·1 per cent. Symptoms appear 5–10 days after the onset. The usual history is for the temperature and rash to be subsiding with the patient appearing to be well on the way to convalescence when one of the following neurological symptoms appears rather suddenly: retention of urine, drowsiness, irritability, convulsions, vomiting or severe headache. Signs of meningeal irritation may be severe or absent. Any type or mixture of neurological lesion may appear but a transverse or ascending myelopathy, peripheral neuropathy or severe disturbance of consciousness or personality without paralysis are the most common. Fever may recur or the whole episode may be afebrile. The cerebrospinal fluid usually shows a rise of protein but the cells may be within normal limits or show a moderate increase up to 500 per mm^3.

The course is extremely variable. Recovery may follow a brief illness lasting a day or two or a prolonged coma of many weeks' duration. Severe paralyses also frequently disappear completely. On the other hand some sequelae in the form of altered personality, recurrent convulsions or permanent paraparesis or hemiparesis can be expected in about 20 per cent. of survivors. About 10 per cent. of patients with this complication die and between 60 and 70 per cent. recover completely. If there is no improvement in paralytic symptoms four weeks from the onset the chance of complete recovery is considerably diminished, but even with a slow return of function ultimate disability is often surprisingly slight. Routine electroencephalography early in the illness has shown abnormal tracings in all cases of measles, suggesting that brain involvement is part of the disease. Evidence has recently accumulated from electron microscopy and fluorescent antibody studies which indicates that measles virus is the cause of *subacute sclerosing panencephalitis*. This is a rare progressive condition in which behavioural disturbances and fits are followed by the development of involuntary movements, ataxia, mental deterioration and death within a few months. The onset is usually some months or years after the attack of measles [see Section 15].

Measles is a serious disease in the tuberculous. It is particularly liable to cause spread of a latent or a symptomless primary infection. This possibility must always be considered when convalescence is slow and a child fails to thrive. Measles frequently causes reversal of a positive Mantoux test for up to six weeks so a negative test during this period does not exclude tuberculosis. Convalescence should be rapid in measles; persistence of cough may be due to bronchitis, tuberculosis, patchy atelectasis or pneumonia.

Diagnosis

The diagnosis of measles is essentially clinical. The development of a maculopapular rash on the third or fourth day of a coryzal illness with Koplik's spots in the mouth is pathognomonic. Simple laboratory investigations are of little value. Most uncomplicated cases show a leucopenia whilst a polymorphonuclear leucocytosis indicates a suppurative complication. Culture of the virus from nasopharyngeal secretions is too slow for routine use and is only of value in cases with no or indeterminate rashes. Serological tests can also be used in such a case, a fourfold rise of antibody being diagnostic. The characteristic giant cell of measles can often be demonstrated in nasopharyngeal secretions in the catarrhal and eruptive phases.

In the prodromal stage mild measles resembles other upper respiratory infections. The higher temperature, irritability and conjunctivitis, however, in the more severe attacks should make one suspicious. The appearance of Koplik's spots on the second or third day is diagnostic and should always be looked for. Similarly measles must be considered in the differential diagnosis of croup. The higher temperature, coryza and conjunctivitis will differentiate this from diphtheria. Prodromal rashes should not cause confusion as Koplik's spots are usually present at the same time.

In the eruptive stage measles may be confused with rubella, smallpox, typhus, infectious mononucleosis, serum disease and drug eruptions.

The characteristics of *rubella* are its mildness, the absence or brevity of the prodromal symptoms and the presence of enlarged posterior cervical, postauricular and suboccipital glands. The rash is a brighter pink, remains more discrete on the limbs and comes and goes more quickly.

In *smallpox* there may be a morbilliform prodromal rash but confusion with measles occurs more often when the true rash appears on the third day on the face and arms. The more leisurely and regular development of the rash with the appearance of papules is typical of smallpox. In this disease headache, backache, vomiting and abdominal pain are likely to be severe whilst coryzal symptoms are absent.

Typhus may be simulated by measles but again coryzal symptoms are minimal and the rash in typhus rarely invades the face which is always affected in measles. In *infectious mononucleosis* the rash may be morbilliform but otherwise the diseases are dissimilar. *Serum rashes* usually itch and frequently show an urticarial element. Certain drugs, particularly suphonamides, cause a rash indistinguishable from the rash of measles, the diagnosis depending on the history and the lack of confirmatory signs of measles.

Treatment

The disease is self-limiting and in the majority of patients symptomatic therapy is all that is required.

The patient should be nursed in bed until the rash has faded and the temperature has been normal for 48 hours. Isolation within the family is seldom practicable and usually unnecessary as other susceptibles will have been infected before the diagnosis is made.

Limitation of visitors to the household, however, is highly desirable. The patient will probably have some degree of immunity to the prevalent strains of cocci within the family circle but pyogenic organisms introduced by outsiders can easily invade the inflamed and susceptible respiratory mucous membrane. For this reason patients requiring hospital admission should be nursed in separate rooms or in an open ward only if adequate bed spacing (at least twelve feet between the bed centres) is possible.

In a short-lived disease diet is unimportant, an adequate fluid intake being all that is required. There need be no restriction, however, for those who retain their appetites. The mouth and teeth should be cleaned regularly. There is no need to nurse the patient in a darkened room except for the relatively few whose conjunctivitis is severe enough to cause photophobia. An erroneous belief still persists in many quarters that light will permanently damage the eyesight in measles.

Steam inhalation relieves laryngitis and a simple linctus (such as Pholcodine Linctus, B.P.C.) may be required for an irritant cough. If the temperature rises to 104° F. (40° C.) it should be lowered by regular tepid sponging combined with calcium aspirin.

Bacterial complications can largely be prevented by prophylactic antibiotics but these are not required in most cases. They are indicated in the following groups:

1. Those under two years of age.
2. Those already suffering from some other disease.
3. Those with a history of purulent otitis media or frequent catarrhal otitis media.
4. The seriously ill.

The best drug is phenoxymethylpenicillin orally for 5–7 days.

Bacterial complications are treated with antibiotics in the usual way, penicillin being the drug of choice for bronchopneumonia and otitis media. In severe bronchopneumonia in which a multiple bacterial aetiology is suspected combined treatment with ampicillin and cloxacillin is indicated.

Encephalomyelopathy requires lumbar puncture and sedation if there is much irritability. Corticotrophin or prednisolone is worthy of trial and possibly affects the outcome if treatment is started within 12 hours of the onset of neurological symptoms. If delayed for over 48 hours its effect is much more doubtful. The drug chosen should be given in large dosage (100 mg. intramuscularly per day in divided dosage for 2 days) rapidly decreasing, the total course lasting about 10 days. Certain animal experiments suggest that corticotrophin may be of greater value than prednisolone. There is no evidence that convalescent serum or gamma globulin affect this complication.

The uncomplicated case of measles is non-infectious five days after the appearance of the rash and is recovered within a fortnight of the onset. Considerable weight loss may occur in the more severe attack but convalescence is rapid. On the tenth day or so of illness the ears, nose, throat and chest should be examined before declaring recovery to be complete.

Prophylaxis

Isolation and quarantine generally fail to prevent epidemics of measles because of the high infectivity of the disease combined with the difficulty of isolating patients at their most infectious (i.e. during the catarrhal stage). Quarantine of contacts is not recommended. A particularly close watch for early symptoms among contacts, however, can lead to their early isolation.

In ward outbreaks susceptibles should be protected with gamma globulin and separated so that each is surrounded if possible by children who have had the disease. The risk of any second generation cases spreading the disease further is thereby considerably reduced. The ward is quarantined for three weeks during which time non-immunes are not admitted. This long period is necessary as gamma globulin may delay the development of symptoms.

Immunization

Passive immunization can be carried out with a variety of blood products such as plasma, parental or convalescent serum or gamma globulin. The last is the agent of choice. In the first 5 days following exposure a dose of 0·2 ml. per kg. will normally prevent the disease, this temporary immunity lasting 4–6 weeks.

Active immunization is now widely practised. One dose of living attenuated virus subcutaneously (Schwarz strain) gives a solid immunity for some years and the fall in antibody level closely parallels the fall seen after the natural disease. It is therefore likely that immunity will be prolonged.

Prognosis

The mortality rate is closely related to the economic state of the country. In the United Kingdom and America the mortality is approximately one per thousand whereas in some less advanced countries it is over 20 per cent. and measles remains one of the important killers of childhood. Deaths are due either to bronchopneumonia or to encephalomyelopathy. Respiratory complications are more common and consequently the disease more serious in those under two years of age. The disease is likely to be severe in the debilitated child. Permanent pulmonary fibrosis, blindness from corneal scarring and deafness from mastoiditis are all rare sequelae. The prognosis of neurological complications is mentioned above.

REFERENCES

Enders, J. P., McCarthy, K., Mitus, A., and Cheatham, W. J. (1959) Isolation of measles virus at autopsy in cases of giant-cell pneumonia without rash, *New Engl. J. Med.*, **261**, 875.

Lancet (1968) Vaccination against measles, Editorial, ii, 616.

Magnus, H. M. (1967) Measles vaccine—present status, *Med. Clin. N. Amer.*, **51**, 599.

Pampiglione, G. (1964), Prodromal phase of measles: Some neurophysiological studies, *Brit. med. J.*, **2**, 1296.

G. D. W. McKendrick

RESPIRATORY VIRUS INFECTIONS

The viruses which infect particularly the respiratory tract cause a wide spectrum of syndromes which vary from a mild sore throat to fatal pneumonia, but may sometimes cause silent or inapparent infections. In general these viruses are seldom recovered from children or adults in normal health. Some of these syndromes may also be caused by other agents such as psittacosis, *Rickettsia burnetii*, *Mycoplasma pneumoniae*, β haemolytic streptococci and *Coccidioides immitis*. The descriptions of the syndromes, which are set out in TABLE 10 are given in Section 9, but some of the syndromes are discussed briefly here and notes on the various respiratory viruses of the various groups follow. Data on streptococcal infection, psittacosis, Q fever and coccidioidomycosis are found elsewhere.

The main syndromes are influenza; febrile sore throat, pharyngitis and tonsillitis; the common cold; croup or laryngotracheobronchitis in infants; acute bronchitis in children and bronchiolitis in infants; and atypical pneumonia. In most of these syndromes one virus or group of viruses is associated with a preponderance of the cases and will be described with it. However, nearly all of the viruses have been found associated with nearly all the syndromes.

INFLUENZA

Synonym. Grippe.

Definition

An acute febrile illness of short duration with malaise, fever and aches and pains in muscles; signs and symptoms of respiratory tract infection are usually present. In severe cases, tracheitis and pneumonia may occur. Mild and abortive infections are common and subclinical infection is not infrequent.

Aetiology

The disease is usually caused by influenza viruses A or B; influenza virus C tends to cause only sporadic mild illness. A similar type of illness may be caused by a number of other viruses. The influenza viruses occur as filaments and spheres; the latter have a diameter of 80–100 millimicrons. They have an outer layer or envelope of lipoprotein, enclosing a coiled filament of ribonucleoprotein. The three viruses replicate in embryonated hen eggs and influenza A and B in cultures of certain primate tissues.

The human viruses (A and B) may be transmitted to ferrets and mice in which they produce respiratory tract disease. Influenza viruses with similar properties may cause disease of the respiratory tract of horses, swine and domestic fowl, but current strains of these viruses do not appear to affect man. The disease is transmitted by air-borne infected droplets from actively infected persons in the first day or two of illness, from symptomless infections and possibly from infected fomites.

Pathology

The primary lesion is a necrosis of the ciliated respiratory epithelium. Infection starts in the nasal cavity where it may remain or spread down to the lower bronchi and trachea. An acute inflammation of the pharynx with a mononuclear exudate can be found in many patients. In experimental infection in ferrets by the exposure to an aerosol the first lesion seen is necrosis of the nasal respiratory epithelium which is followed rapidly by oedema and leucocytic infiltration of the underlying tissues, but the basal epithelium is left intact. In more severe infections extensive tracheitis and fatal pneumonia may occur. In fatal cases in man one finds patches of lilac-coloured consolidation which are firm with oedema fluid. Microscopically there is destruction of the tracheal and bronchial epithelium and necrotic exudate in the lumen. The bronchioles are distended, their walls hyperaemic and oedematous and there is exudate in the lumen. Alveoli are distended with oedema fluid and haemorrhage and their walls thickened. After recovery from experimental infection in animals epithelial hyperplasia and regeneration may occur quite rapidly in the nasal passages, but much more slowly in the lower part of the respiratory tree. Although fatal influenza virus pneumonia occurs with the above picture, in recent years death has resulted more frequently from secondary infection with *Staphylococcus pyogenes*.

The virus has on rare occasions been isolated from the blood and internal organs and even from the brain; that from the organs was probably derived from the blood. If lesions are present at sites other than the lung, they are typical of toxic changes and the presence of extravasations of blood suggests toxic action causing increased permeability of blood vessel walls.

Signs and Symptoms

The incubation period is 2–3 days. During outbreaks the clinical picture is remarkably uniform. In the majority of patients the illness is only of about three days duration with a sudden onset of headache, malaise, shivering, fever and aches and pains in the limbs. This is followed by a dry non-productive cough in a large proportion of the cases and a sore throat with or without nasal congestion and obstruction in a smaller number. Mild conjunctivitis may be present, but is not characteristic, and virus has not been isolated from the eye.

Encephalomyelitis may follow after an interval of a week or two.

These symptoms and signs disappear in a few days, and the temperature returns to normal, but the patient remains weak for several days more. Patients may tire readily for a further week or two and some are easily depressed. Some patients may have an even milder illness, but a proportion, which varies between outbreaks, may develop pneumonia. This is more likely in the very young and elderly or those with chronic respiratory and heart disease.

Diagnosis

During outbreaks the classical picture is unmistakable, but numerous other viruses can produce a similar syndrome, so that an accurate specific diagnosis cannot be made by clinical means in sporadic cases, and even during an epidemic a varying proportion of illnesses will be due to other viruses. Specific diagnosis can be made in the laboratory by demonstration of the presence of the virus in cultures of throat swabs or garglings and the application of the fluorescent antibody technique to specially collected smears of nasal and pharyngeal mucosa in the first 2 days of illness. The same techniques may be applied to lung and trachea removed *post mortem*, if death has occured within a few days of the onset. If death is from secondary bacterial infection, recovery of the virus may be possible, but will be more difficult. Otherwise diagnosis may be made by the demonstration of a rise in the level of antibodies in convalescence.

Treatment

The prophylactic benefit of inactivated influenza virus vaccines in about 60 per cent. of inoculees when given before the appearance of an outbreak or epidemic has been proved in a number of countries. One of two doses are given depending upon the likelihood of previous exposure of the patient to the expected virus and whether he has received vaccine within the past 18 months. The effect of present vaccines lasts only about 12 months, but the introduction of adjuvant vaccines is likely to give greatly improved results. The general use of attenuated live virus administered intranasally has not been introduced because of technical difficulties in producing material of constant, satisfactory potency which does not cause unacceptable reactions in man. It would obviously have certain practical advantages and also probably give better protection.

The prospects for specific chemotherapy are discussed on page 158.

A biologically active substance, interferon [p. 155], has been shown to be protective in laboratory tests when given before or up to a few hours after the virus, but its activity in man after the onset of symptoms has not been established.

Treatment remains symptomatic and in the majority of cases with self-limiting disease little is needed except analgesics for myalgia and pharyngitis. If pneumonia develops prompt use of large doses of antibiotics, particularly ones known to be active against *Staph. pyogenes*, *Streptococcus pneumoniae* and *H. influenzae* is essential, especially in those with a history of chronic chest disease or heart failure; supportive measures will also be required in the latter.

Corticosteroids should be used in those patients with fulminating pneumonia or encephalopathy or if encephalomyelitis occurs 7–14 days later.

Prognosis

Prognosis is good in the majority of cases, but should be guarded in those with heart disease, the elderly or the very young. Death may occur within 24–48 hours from the effects of the virus alone, either due to the action of the virus on the blood vessel wall or to viral toxin. If secondary bacterial infection is recognized early and treated promptly, bearing in mind the possibility of infection with a resistant *Staph. pyogenes*, the prognosis is reasonably good.

ACUTE FEBRILE SORE THROAT

Synonyms. Unclassified acute respiratory disease; Febrile catarrh.

Definition

An endemic acute febrile respiratory illness usually of short duration, in which nasopharyngitis, tonsillitis and laryngitis may be present, but without signs or symptoms indicative of a specific aetiology.

Aetiology

A large number of viruses have been found in recent years associated with sporadic cases and outbreaks of these relatively minor illnesses [TABLE 10]. All these

TABLE 10

ACUTE RESPIRATORY SYNDROMES AND THEIR CAUSATIVE VIRUSES OR AGENTS

CLINICAL SYNDROMES	VIRUSES
Influenza and febrile influenza-like disease .	Influenza A, B, C, adenoviruses 3, 4, 7, 14 and 21, coxsackie and echoviruses
Febrile sore throat, pharyngitis, tonsillitis .	Adenoviruses 3, 4, 7, 14, 21, influenza A and B, para-influenza, rhinoviruses, enteroviruses, β haemolytic streptococci
Common cold . . .	Rhinoviruses, para-influenza, respiratory syncytial, adenoviruses, influenza A and B, enteroviruses
Croup, laryngotracheobronchitis in infants and young children . .	Para-influenza, respiratory syncytial
Acute bronchitis in children	Respiratory syncytial, rhinoviruses, para-influenza, influenza A and B, *Mycoplasma pneumoniae*
Acute bronchiolitis in infants	Respiratory syncytial, para-influenza, influenza A and B, *M. pneumoniae*
Atypical pneumonia .	*M. pneumoniae*, adenoviruses, psittacosis, *Rickettsia burnetii*

viruses have been isolated in cultures of various mammalian tissues and coxsackie A viruses in newborn mice. Specific antibodies of one type or another may be detected in convalescence. Infection of man takes place by contact with other active cases and probably also with symptomless infections.

Signs and Symptoms

The incubation period is usually 4–5 days.

In the majority of cases there is a gradual onset with minor or catarrhal symptoms and signs, followed by mild fever, sore throat and malaise. In the remainder there is a sudden onset with chills and marked fever with corresponding pulse rate, pharyngitis, cough and myalgia. On examination there will be few abnormal signs except an inflamed pharynx and some cervical adenopathy.

Diagnosis

A specific diagnosis can only be made by isolation of the virus, bacterium or mycoplasma from the respiratory tract and preferably also by the demonstration of a rise in antibodies to the virus or other organism in the blood in convalescence.

Treatment

In older children and adults most of these illnesses are relatively mild and no treatment is necessary other than mild analgesics and gargles to relieve malaise and pharyngitis.

Although there appear to be a large number of viruses concerned, which cause little serious disease in most children, investigation may show that ultimate benefit for adult life may be obtained by a polyvalent vaccine which will reduce the number of virus infections in early childhood, if no other suitable prophylactic or chemotherapeutic agents become available.

Prognosis

Recovery is complete in a relatively short time.

ADENOVIRUSES

This group, which takes its name from the first types isolated, which were found latent in adenoids prepared for tissue culture, include the viruses most commonly associated with this syndrome in childhood. There are at least 31 known serologically distinct types all of which possess one common group antigen, although they may be responsible for a number of quite dissimilar clinical syndromes, in addition to febrile catarrh. Thus types 3, 4, 7, 14 and 21 cause mild respiratory tract disease, occasionally pneumonia and conjunctivitis, type 8 epidemic keratoconjunctivitis and types 1, 2 and 5 mesenteric adenitis in infants and young children. Similar viruses of different serological types have been recovered from other mammals, such as cattle and dogs.

Types 1, 2 and 5 may be recovered from about 25 per cent. of tonsils and 50 per cent. of adenoids, removed from children at operation, by growing the tissue, although no virus may be isolated by inoculation of a suspension of the tissue into cultures of other susceptible cells. These types are seldom associated with respiratory tract disease. They are, however, sometimes found in infants with mesenteric adenitis and may be one of the causes of this condition in which *Pasteurella pseudotuberculosis* has also been incriminated in several countries. Not unexpectedly the same types of adenovirus have been found in the faeces of some infants with intussusception, which in these cases may have been precipitated by enlarged mesenteric glands.

Types 3, 4, 7, 14 and 21 have been commonly associated with outbreaks of febrile catarrh in young servicemen and semi-closed communities of children and adolescents. There is a short period of fever, headache, shivering and sore throat which may be followed by pharyngitis, laryngitis and tracheitis either singly or together. Bronchitis and pneumonia may follow. Types 3 and 4 and 21 occasionally cause severe, even fatal, pneumonia in infants. Illness due to these types of adenovirus is uncommon and usually very mild in the general adult population.

These types, particularly 3, 7 and 14, may also cause pharyngo-conjunctival fever which is most often seen in residential schools and other groups of children. There is fever, acute pharyngitis with or without mucopurulent exudate, cervical gland enlargement and follicular angular conjunctivitis either unilateral or bilateral. There may be little pain in the eye; the lesion is often first noted by friends rather than the patient.

Type 8 has been associated almost entirely with epidemic keratoconjunctivitis particularly in groups whose occupation leads to some conjunctival injury or to some other eye infection, which may provide a suitable site for virus growth. Eight other types were recovered from the eyes of patients with suspected trachoma or conjunctivitis in the Middle East.

Types 26 and 27, which were originally isolated from rectal swabs of symptomless children in a nursery, caused only mild conjunctivitis when swabbed on to the palpebral conjunctiva or mild rhinitis when instilled intranasally in adult volunteers. Virus was recovered from the faeces for 1–2 weeks after the onset of illnesses in which adenoviruses have been thought to be the aetiological agent.

Diagnosis

Adenovirus infection may be suspected in certain diseases such as pharyngo-conjunctival fever, and epidemic keratoconjunctivitis but a specific diagnosis can only be made in the laboratory by isolation of the virus from the throat swabs and faeces and from the results of antibody tests on blood collected in the acute and convalescent stages.

Treatment

Prophylactic vaccines of formolized adenoviruses 3, 4 and 7 have been effective in reducing respiratory tract illness in Service recruits. Live virus vaccine in enteric-coated capsules administered orally has also been effective in similar groups. Because of the relatively mild illness usually produced and the multiplicity of types concerned, it has not been considered worthwhile to develop vaccines for other types or for wider use. There is no specific treatment for the respiratory tract infections, but in epidemics symptomatic treatment and antibiotics will be necessary in severe lower respiratory tract infections in infants. Iodoxuridine may be used in proven type 8 keratoconjunctivitis.

Prognosis

Infections with adenoviruses are usually self-limiting and give rise to little concern except for severe lower respiratory tract illness in infants.

THE COMMON COLD

Definition

An acute illness of a few days' duration, with or without low grade fever, accompanied by inflammation of the mucous membranes of the nasal cavity, and sometimes of the pharynx and larynx.

Aetiology

This disease is caused most frequently by one of a group of more than 80 viruses with special growth requirements and at present known as rhino or coryza viruses, but it may be associated with infection by some other respiratory and enteroviruses. The viruses may be isolated in tissue cultures of human embryo lung or kidney or simian kidney, and may be divided into subgroups according to their tissue preference and the variations in cultural environment required for their growth and their antigenic constitution.

There is now no doubt that rhino viruses by themselves can cause the common cold, but the role played by bacteria is still uncertain. Some organisms may find that the environment created by virus infection provides ideal conditions for their growth and this results in prolongation of the syndrome. It is also possible that in some individuals a mild asymptomatic bacterial infection may provide a more suitable site for virus multiplication.

Infection occurs from contact with other patients with active lesions or with healthy carriers or from infected fomites.

Low temperature (cold weather) does not cause colds, but rapid alterations in the physiological state of the mucous membranes due to changes from warm temperatures indoors to cold outdoors and vice versa may favour growth of the virus; overcrowding in cold weather also favours spread of the virus.

Recent investigations have shown that serological immunity to a particular virus disappears after a number of years, so that second attacks with the same virus may occur, but recurrent colds in a season are most likely due to infection with different viruses (or are possibly allergic phenomena).

The chimpanzee is the only animal which is susceptible to human cold viruses.

Pathology

The main lesion consists of vascular engorgement and oedema of the mucous membranes of the nasopharynx with infiltration of the mucosa and possibly underlying tissues by mononuclear cells. There is little or no necrosis of the mucosal epithelium, but desquamation of superficial epithelial cells occurs. Lymphoid follicles are enlarged. The usually copious exudate is serous or mucous, but later may become purulent; this is not necessarily a sign of bacterial infection.

Signs and Symptoms

The incubation period is 24–72 hours.

The dominant symptoms result from inflammation of the mucous membranes of the nasal passages. The onset is acute with increase in watery nasal discharge, sneezing and possibly slight pyrexia and sore throat. This may disappear in 24 hours or persist for a few days, or rarely a week or two. Congestion of the nasal passages may cause slight malaise for a day or two and, if catarrh continues, the discharge usually becomes thick and purulent. Infection of the sinuses and middle ear may occur and in certain patients subject to chronic chest disease exacerbations of their asthma or bronchitis may occur.

Diagnosis

The clinical syndrome is an obvious one, but its specific aetiology can only be determined by isolation of the virus and antibody tests.

Treatment

There is no specific treatment. Only symptomatic treatment is possible, particularly of secondary bacterial infection by antibiotics in those suffering from complications, e.g. patients with chronic chest disease. Satisfactory vaccines containing one or two types of rhinovirus have been made but general use of rhinovirus vaccines is impractical because of the numerous types of virus which would need to be incorporated. Autogenous vaccines from the patient's nasopharyngeal bacterial flora are thought by some to give benefit to those with frequently recurring colds.

Prognosis

This is always good except in those with chronic chest disease in whom secondary bacterial infection may occur.

CROUP

Croup or obstructive laryngotracheobronchitis in infants and children has been mainly associated with para-influenza viruses. This is an especially serious disease in children under 2 years of age.

PARA-INFLUENZA MYXOVIRUSES

Synonyms. Haemadsorption viruses 1, 2, 3, 4; Croup-associated viruses.

There are four para-influenza viruses affecting man which are so named because they are of similar size and morphology to influenza viruses; like them they contain RNA, possess agglutinins for fowl and guinea-pig erythrocytes and are inactivated by ether. There are group relationships between the various types and with mumps virus, but they are immunologically unrelated to influenza viruses A, B and C. Analogous viruses with similar antigens are found in other mammals, e.g. mice and bovines.

Some strains of type 1 will replicate in fertile hens' eggs, but most strains require cultures of monkey or human tissues. Their growth may not produce visible degeneration of these tissue cultures, but the presence of the virus may be detected by the addition of guinea-pig erythrocytes which are adsorbed to the infected cells (haemadsorption) or are agglutinated by virus in the culture fluid.

For the most part these viruses cause relatively mild respiratory tract disease in adults, but they may cause croup, bronchitis or bronchopneumonia in infants. Illness due to these viruses is thought to be infrequent in adults because of immunity from childhood infection, but an outbreak of mixed infection with influenza A has been described in a home for the aged. In volunteers, inoculated intranasally, infection occurred in the form of a cold or febrile influenza-like illness and took place even in some who had antibodies to the virus. Infection with types 1 and 3 has tended to occur earlier in life than with type 2 in those centres in temperate climates where antibody surveys have been made.

ACUTE BRONCHITIS, BRONCHIOLITIS AND PNEUMONIA IN INFANTS

These diseases may be caused by any of the viruses mentioned above, but the agent most commonly associated is the respiratory syncytial virus (RSV). It tends to appear in localized outbreaks for limited periods infecting a high proportion of children under 5 years of age. Although the clinical picture is often alarming in infants the case fatality rate has been less than 2 per cent. in a number of proven outbreaks. Wheezing is not uncommon with RS virus infection, but asthma tends not to persist when recovery from infection occurs.

RESPIRATORY SYNCYTIAL VIRUS

This RNA virus was first isolated from chimpanzees with a cold in the United States, and called CCA, but not long afterwards it was isolated from sick children in a number of areas. Its name refers to the appearance of infected tissue culture cells, particularly HeLa cells in which giant cells or syncytia are formed. The virus is similar in size to the myxoviruses and resembles them morphologically but does not possess a haemagglutinin. Another differential characteristic is its instability on storage. Because the virus is liable to be killed by freezing and thawing, material from suspected patients should be inoculated directly in tissue cultures or kept at 4° C. until used.

Diagnosis

Diagnosis is made by isolation of the virus from throat swabs in tissue culture and serological tests with blood collected in the acute stage and 14–21 days after the onset of illness. More recently detection of the presence of this virus in cells of aspirated nasopharyngeal washings or tissue culture has been facilitated by the fluorescent antibody technique.

VIRUS PNEUMONIA

Synonym. Atypical pneumonia.

Definition

A diffuse inflammation of the lung in the form of pneumonitis, rather than the pneumonic consolidation seen in bacterial infections, accompanied by general malaise, anorexia, remittent fever and a dry, frequently non-productive, cough. The disease usually lasts 10–14 days and is rarely fatal.

Aetiology

Many rickettsiae, bedsonia and viruses may cause pneumonia, e.g. Q fever, psittacosis, the exanthemata and the numerous respiratory viruses, but these have not been responsible in many patients, in a high proportion of whom cold agglutinins appear in their blood. The aetiological agent in the latter is now known to be not a virus, but an organism of the family mycoplasma which grows on or in an artificial medium, with a very high content of serum. The organism may be recovered from the sputum or possibly from throat washings or swabs and specific antibodies to it appear in convalescence. Infection results from contact with other active cases or symptomless infections.

Pathology

The cold agglutinin-positive case is rarely fatal, so that little information is available. The principal infiltrating cell is mononuclear, which may be found in a few foci in the peribronchial region or in numerous patches throughout a lobe or several lobes. In severe cases oedema of the alveoli and bronchioles will be present. In other types of virus pneumonia there may also be ulcerations and necrosis of the bronchi and various inclusion bodies may be present depending upon the specific virus, e.g. adenovirus, chickenpox, measles, etc.

Signs and Symptoms

The incubation period is 7–14 days.

In a typical case the onset is usually insidious with relatively mild respiratory symptoms; general malaise, fatigue and slight paroxysmal dry cough are followed by a sore throat, possibly mild chest pain and moderately elevated temperature, which is usually biphasic. On examination no abnormal physical signs are found in the lung in many patients; this proportion is as high as 50 per cent. in some outbreaks. However, fine crackling râles which tend to shift to different areas on successive days may be found later in the illness when mucoid or mucopurulent sputum may be produced. An X-ray of the lung will usually show lesions much more extensive and widespread than the patient's illness would lead one to suspect; mottled or ground-glass-like shadows, particularly in the hilar area, or distributed in patches throughout the lung, are characteristic. In an outbreak in a closed community, such as a school or service unit, there are usually a large number of cases of milder illness or colds and even symptomless infections, which may show similar radiological changes, but to a less degree than those seen in typical cases.

Diagnosis

Differential diagnosis from bacterial pneumonia is usually possible from the history, X-ray picture or results of antibiotic treatment. Penicillin will have little or no effect on any virus or mycoplasma pneumonia. A specific diagnosis can only be made in a laboratory where tests for complement-fixing or other antibody on two sera taken in the acute and convalescent stages are possible for a large number of respiratory viruses and for mycoplasma. Isolation of virus or mycoplasma may be attempted in the first day or two of symptoms, but because of the insidious nature of the onset, the patient is usually seen too late unless an outbreak is in progress.

Treatment

Mild cases will recover spontaneously on symptomatic treatment, but in more severe cases due to mycoplasma recovery may be enhanced by chlortetracycline, 4 G. daily for two days, then 2 G. daily until recovery, as used for psittacosis, or demethylchlortetracycline, 300 mg. orally in capsules, three times a day. (For Q fever see p. 194.)

Prognosis

Fatality is rare even from secondary infections or complications. Specific treatment may speed recovery when illness is due to one of the psittacosis group of agents or to mycoplasma.

RESPIRATORY ENTEROVIRUSES

Respiratory Enteric Orphan (REO) Viruses

This group has three serological subtypes, the first of which was found in the stools of healthy children (hence Enteric Orphan), but has since been recovered from the throat and faeces of a few patients with upper respiratory tract disease. The results available at present indicate that this group is relatively unimportant as a cause of illness in man. They are of some general interest, however, as one type was first isolated from an Australian aborigine, all are found in a number of different vertebrates and they produce haemagglutinins.

ECHO Viruses [See p. 195]

Several different members of this heterogeneous group, e.g. types 11, 19, 20 and 28, have been associated with mild upper respiratory tract disease particularly in children. Some of the patients infected with echovirus 11, 19 and 20 also had abdominal pain and diarrhoea and virus was present in the throat and faeces. In echovirus 28 infections, both natural and when induced in volunteers, the illness has been similar to the common cold and this virus is now classed as a rhinovirus. The virus has seldom been recovered from the faeces.

Coxsackie Viruses [See p. 192]

Viruses of both A and B groups have been found associated with mild upper respiratory tract infection. Several types of group A have been recovered from the throats of patients with herpangina and one type from a condition described as acute lymphonodular pharyngitis, but the most important type is A21 (Coe) virus which has been the cause of outbreaks of upper respiratory tract illness in semi-closed communities of young adult males in several countries.

In Group B, types 1, 2, 3, 4 and 5 may all produce mild pharyngitis which is most likely to be seen when these viruses are prevalent in the community and causing lymphocytic meningitis and Bornholm disease.

VIRUS INFECTIONS OF THE NERVOUS SYSTEM

VIRUS MENINGITIS

Synonyms. Lymphocytic meningitis; Benign acute aseptic meningitis.

Pathology

A large number of viruses may occasionally cause a benign meningitis, but it is one of the common syndromes associated with infection by arbo, enterovirus, lymphocytic choriomeningitis, mumps and poliomyelitis viruses, and is seen in glandular fever. In contrast to most bacterial meningitides, mononuclear cells preponderate in the cerebrospinal fluid; one seldom finds more than 1000 per mm^3. of fluid and not infrequently fewer than 100 per mm^3. Protein may be increased in quantity, but the sugar and chloride levels are usually normal, which aids in differentiation from tuberculous infection. Leptospira and toxoplasma may also cause lymphocytic meningitis.

A combination of animal inoculation and tissue culture of blood, throat swab, stool and cerebrospinal fluid collected early in the disease, and serological tests on blood collected in the acute and convalescent stages, should, if most of the available techniques are used, give a positive result in at least 50 per cent. of patients in whom tests for non-viral organisms are negative. A number of the viruses which cause meningitis may be recovered from the throat and faeces of apparently healthy individuals so it is obvious that isolation of a virus from the cerebrospinal fluid will be of much greater aetiological significance. However, polioviruses are practically never isolated from cerebrospinal fluid and the others seldom later than the fifth or sixth day from the onset of meningitis, whereas faeces may be positive for longer periods so the latter specimen must always be cultured.

Antibodies do not as a rule become detectable before the twelfth to fourteenth day from the onset of illness so that the patient has often recovered by the time the second specimen is collected, but paired sera should be obtained whenever possible. Rapid routine complement fixation tests are available for herpes simplex, lymphocytic choriomeningitis, mumps and poliomyelitis viruses and may give a positive result when cultures are negative or confirm the significance of the isolation of a virus. Routine complement fixation tests are not available for the coxsackie and echoviruses, but neutralization tests may be possible in special circumstances in some laboratories.

Some indication of the likely aetiological agent may be obtained from the season and geographical position, but variation in the time of outbreaks other than with arthropod-borne viruses may occur from year to year. There may be diagnostic confusion in patients with bacterial meningitis treated by antibiotics at home before specimens have been collected and who later, when recovery is not immediate, are admitted to hospital. Double infection of the meninges with a bacterium and a virus though probably rare, has been described, as has dual infection with more than one virus.

Prognosis

The prognosis is usually good, but occasional severe cases have been complicated by convulsions, and mental deterioration in late convalescence has been reported. Although a single mild attack of virus meningitis may have little obvious effect, there may also be slight parenchymal damage and the cumulative effect of infection with different viruses at intervals over several years may be great, particularly in those children whc already have some functional impairment.

LYMPHOCYTIC CHORIOMENINGITIS

This is the only virus meningitis for which the term choriomeningitis should be used. It is caused by a virus the natural host of which is the house mouse. For many years it was considered to be the main cause of aseptic meningitis, particularly in the United States, but it is now recognized that only a small proportion of cases of lymphocytic meningitis is due to this virus. Patients are usually found to be residents of mouse-infested premises.

Mild infections, not progressing to meningitis may, occur; otherwise typical cases are indistinguishable from meningitis due to other viruses. In occasional cases virus pneumonia has occurred and even resulted in a fatal outcome. A fatal transplacental infection to a newborn has been described.

Virus may be isolated by inoculation of blood and cerebrospinal fluid collected in the acute stage of the illness, intracerebrally into adult mice known to come from a virus-free stock, or subcutaneously into guinea-pigs. Infected mice, guinea-pigs and monkeys show lymphocytic infiltration of the meninges, particularly the choroid plexus. Complement-fixing antibodies of low titre can usually be detected in convalescence.

There is no specific treatment.

Prognosis is usually good with recovery in a few weeks, but death has occurred as a result of pneumonia, and also possibly from extension of the infection to the brain or cord.

Coxsackie and ECHO Viruses

These two types of virus need special mention for they are isolated from patients with meningitis or acute meningo-encephalitis from time to time in a way which shows they are endemic particularly in the summer months. They both affect the meninges and central nervous system secondarily and frequently cause acute illness with widespread muscle pains as well as giving lymphocytic meningitis (see Coxsackie and Echovirus infections, pp. 192 and 195).

REFERENCES

BOGAERT, L. VAN (1959) Acute encephalitis in childhood, *Brit. med. J.*, **1**, 1201.

CIBA FOUNDATION (1961) *Symposium: Virus Meningo-Encephalitis*, London.

DIMSDALE, H. (1957) Acute encephalomyelitis of virus origin, in *Modern Trends in Neurology*, ed. WILLIAMS, D., London.

MCCONKEY, B., and DAWS, R. A. (1958) Neurological disorders associated with Asian influenza, *Lancet*, ii, 15.

MEYER, H. M. Jr., JOHNSON, R. T., CRANFORD, I. P., DUSCOMB, H. E., and ROGERS, N. G. (1960) Central nervous system syndromes of viral etiology: a study of 731 cases, *Amer. J. Med.*, **29**, 234.

MILLER, H. G., STANTON, J. B., and GIBBONS, J. L. (1956) Para-infectious encephalomyelitis and related syndromes, *Quart. J. Med.*, **25**; 427.

RIVERS, V. M., and HORSFALL, F. L. (1959) *Viral and Rickettsial Infections of Man*, 3rd ed., Philadelphia.

THIRUVENGADAM, L. V. (1959) Disseminated encephalomyelitis after influenza, *Brit. med. J.*, **2**, 1233.

TURNBULL, H. M. (1928) Encephalomyelitis in virus diseases and exanthemata, *Brit. med. J.*, **2**, 331.

F. O. MACCALLUM

ACUTE ANTERIOR POLIOMYELITIS

Synonyms. Infantile paralysis; Heine-Medin disease; 'Polio'.

Definition

An acute infectious disease characterized, in its fully developed form, by local or widespread muscular paralysis due to destruction, by the action of a specific neurotropic virus, of anterior horn cells in the spinal cord or corresponding cells in the medulla.

Aetiology

Before the use of active immunity the disease occurred in both sporadic and epidemic manner. The most severe epidemics have occurred in the countries of northern Europe and North America, but it has appeared with increasing frequency in Australia, New Zealand and South Africa, and such island communities as Malta and Mauritius have not been spared. During the Second World War a particularly virulent form was prevalent in North Africa and the whole Mediterranean littoral.

It showed a marked seasonal variation, being commonest in the hotter months of the year. In northern Europe the incidence usually began to increase towards epidemic proportions in July and slackened off in October or November. Sporadic cases, however, occurred throughout the year. It has been virtually eliminated in the past decade by mass immunization of the child and young adult population with modified virus of types 1, 2 and 3, its eradication in so short a time being one of the greatest triumphs of preventive medicine. Much which follows must seem historical in such fortunate countries.

A conspicuous feature of the disease is its preference for the young, although no age is immune. In the early years of this century its maximal incidence among infants led to its being named 'infantile paralysis' and at that time the greatest number of cases occurred in the second and third years of life.

Over a period of 50 years there has been a steady tendency for the disease to attack older people, and at present the maximal incidence is between the ages of 5 and 10. This curious change in age distribution, taken with the unfortunate fact that the incidence of paralytic poliomyelitis seems to increase rather than to decrease with the improved standards of hygiene in more advanced communities, suggests that whereas in primitive communities children come frequently in contact with the virus in early life and so acquire immunity, those in more advanced communities escaped this early inoculation before the advent of prophylactic vaccination, to fall victims to a virulent attack in later childhood.

The successful transmission of the disease from man to monkeys by Landsteiner and Popper in 1909 and the subsequent researches of Flexner and Lewis and others as to the nature of the infecting agent proved to be landmarks in the development of our knowledge of virus diseases in general and of those of the nervous system in particular. It has culminated in the development of the highly effective oral vaccine which has, of course, contained the distribution of the virus. The pattern of epidemiology remains the same in unprotected communities.

The virus is among the smallest so far identified with a diameter of 27–30 micromicrons. It is distributed widely in the human race and is commonly a harmless inhabitant of the nasopharynx and intestinal canal. It can be recovered from the nasopharyngeal washings and the faeces of both clinical cases and many contacts, as well as from flies and communal sewage in affected areas. It is now recognized that only a minority of the individuals harbouring the virus develop even mild symptoms of disease and that of these not more than a fifth develop paralysis. There is thus a large pool of healthy 'carriers' in any non-immunized community that is affected and these probably play a major role in transmission of the disease. This is in accordance with the known fact that 50 to 80 per cent. of town-dwellers in countries where the incidence of the disease is great have protective antibodies in their sera at a high titre. Three types of the virus have been identified: Type 1 (Brunhilda), which is at present the most virulent and carries the highest incidence of paralysis; Type 2 (Lansing), which can be adapted to be pathogenic to rodents; and Type 3 (Leon). All three have been responsible for paralytic attacks in the human. They are serologically distinct and one type does not confer protection against the natural disease caused by the other types. It has recently become clear that infection with viruses of the Coxsackie and ECHO group is sometimes associated with an illness clinically indistinguishable from paralytic poliomyelitis. It has long been recognized that the aseptic meningitis of non-paralytic poliomyelitis can be mimicked by many other viruses.

A clinically recognizable attack of poliomyelitis, whether paralytic or not, leads to the development of specific antibodies in the blood which with rare exceptions confer lifelong immunity from a further attack. Such antibodies are not present in the sera of individuals from isolated and unaffected communities, or in those of susceptible individuals in affected communities. On the other hand, the high incidence of natural immunity among adults, especially the town-dwellers, in affected populations confirms the belief that subclinical attacks occur during many such persons' lifetimes.

The method of spread of the infection has been a matter of controversy for many years. It has been generally accepted that unaffected carriers play a larger part in the process than do recognizable cases of the disease. Although the participation of flies cannot be excluded, it is clear that the principal agency concerned is human contact. The main matter of dispute has been whether the infection is carried by droplets from the nasopharynx and upper respiratory tract, or by the various methods of faecal contamination from the gastro-intestinal canal. The evidence for droplet spread is strong and epidemiological studies have shown a close association between cases of the disease and human movement in circumstances in which spread by the excreta was unlikely. The undoubted association between tonsillectomy and the development of bulbar poliomyelitis also indicates the nasopharynx as a potential source of infection. On the other hand, the major incidence of the disease in hot weather has always suggested that it was spread by faecal contamination, and there is now convincing evidence that the gastro-intestinal tract acts as a portal of entry for the virus and that in most epidemics it is the principal one. The virus can be recovered from the stools of patients for several weeks after an attack, as well as from those of intimate contacts and from communal sewage. The method of transmission is largely by human contact operating through such agencies as contaminated food, eating utensils and latrines. Although the virus can be recovered from flies in infected areas, the part they play as vectors has not yet been determined. It used to be said that case-to-case infection did not occur, but this is not so. Such occurrences are, however, extremely rare in institutions where cases are treated with careful barrier nursing precautions.

There is still uncertainty as to how the virus, when it reaches a susceptible host in adequate dosage, breaches the defences of the body surface and reaches the nervous system. There is evidence that in so doing it is aided by a lowering of the victim's general resistance, or by local injury, such as tonsillectomy, or by local disturbance such as may cause the diarrhoea which often precedes attacks in which a gastro-intestinal origin of the infection is to be suspected. The virus is capable of transmission along axons, but can only proliferate in the bodies of nerve cells. The axonal route is believed to be important where trauma such as tonsillectomy has directly exposed nerve endings to virus, but it is likely that the infection usually reaches the brain by the blood stream. Virus can be readily recovered from the blood by using tissue culture methods. Examination of the nervous systems of humans, or of experimental animals dying of the disease, shows that the virus is widely distributed in the brain and spinal cord, but reaches its highest concentration in the anterior horn cells of the spinal cord, especially of the lumbar enlargement, the motor nuclei of the brain stem and motor cells of the cerebral cortex. An interesting association has been shown to exist between intramuscular injections such as may be given for purposes of immunization and the development of paralysis in neighbouring muscles during succeeding weeks. This is now believed to be due to the action of poliomyelitis virus determined by the specific local trauma of the injection.

Pathology

The virus of poliomyelitis is an obligatory intracellular parasite, and its action takes place entirely within the nerve cell. The changes seen in the nervous system vary with the virulence of the infection. The virus has a special affinity for the anterior horn cells of the spinal cord and in severe infections these cells in portions of the cord undergo acute necrosis. If the experimentally infected animal is destroyed at this initial stage no lesions other than these cell changes are found, and the rapidly ensuing cellular exudation and meningeal infiltration seen in fatal human cases are not present. The necrosis of nerve cells in the surviving patient is naturally soon followed by phagocytic processes; microglia and polymorphonuclear leucocytes rapidly invade the affected areas and clear away the dead nerve cells. In less severe infections, less acute forms of nerve cell changes are seen, and with these the cellular exudation is almost wholly of amoeboid microglia which fill the perivascular spaces in the affected parts of the cord. Together with leucocytes, they finally overflow into the cerebrospinal fluid. They may appear here even before the development of paralysis, and it was this early indication of meningeal infiltration that led to the view formerly held that a meningitis preceded the involvement of the nervous system. In the affected regions of the grey matter of the ventral horns, some cells always remain unaffected by the virus. Some degree of encephalitis is a constant feature, although it is not usually clinically manifest.

Laboratory Diagnosis

Isolation of Virus. The virus can be isolated from throat and nasopharyngeal washings and from faeces. Material from the throat is most likely to give positive results if collected over the period from 6 days before to 3 days after the onset of symptoms. The best source of virus is probably faeces obtained early in the course of the disease. Specimens may be kept at 4° C. for several days.

Serological tests are unsatisfactory and difficult to interpret because of past infections with other types of poliovirus and cross-reaction with Coxsackie and ECHO antigens. Antibody titre reaches a peak so early—often before the diagnosis is suspected and thus it is seldom possible to demonstrate a significant rise.

Cerebrospinal Fluid. The fluid is clear, colourless or faintly yellow, and under normal or only slightly increased pressure. The levels of chlorides and sugar are normal. The protein content is slightly increased at first and tends to rise during the first 3 weeks after the onset of the disease. The cell content of the fluid is variable. In the majority of cases there is a pleocytosis of 20–100 cells per mm^3. The count is usually a mixed one, with lymphocytes outnumbering the polymorphs in a proportion of two or three to one. In some cases, however, a high proportion of polymorphs may be found at the onset usually giving place to a predominantly lymphocytic increase in subsequent punctures. The fluid may be normal in indubitable cases. The nature and number of the cells seem not to afford any prognostic indications.

Blood. In the early stages of the illness, there is usually a polymorphonuclear leucocytosis, which may reach as high as 30,000. This leucocytosis disappears when the fever abates. Although the clinical picture of the unmodified disease remains unchanged, mass vaccination of the population of the United States of America and of European countries has greatly reduced the incidence of this disastrous infection, has altered the attitude of the community to it, and has increased the native incidence of mild and abortive forms.

Symptoms

Poliomyelitis is now so rare in Europe that a full account of its symptomatology, based upon the experience of the author and others who have witnessed all its ravages, is appropriate.

Infection with poliomyelitis virus in unprotected subjects nevertheless remains a common event and of those so affected only a small proportion develop symptoms of a kind sufficiently definite to permit of a clinical diagnosis. Of these latter probably not more than a fifth are destined to develop paralysis. This has led to the recognition of three degrees of poliomyelitis: (1) 'formes frustes' or abortive cases; (2) pre-paralytic and non-paralytic poliomyelitis; (3) paralytic poliomyelitis. This clinical subdivision is justifiable and useful on practical grounds, but it should be understood that there is no corresponding pathological subdivision and that the three degrees shade off imperceptibly into one another.

'Formes Frustes'. Such cases occur sporadically and are particularly plentiful in times of epidemics. They can rarely be diagnosed with certainty although their nature may be suspected in the presence of an epidemic or retrospectively, when other cases have occurred in the same family or isolated community. The symptoms consist of malaise, headache, mild fever, aching in the back and limbs and sometimes a sore throat, or mild gastro-intestinal upset and are thus common to influenza and other virus infections. The disturbance subsides in 24–48 hours without residual symptoms and the spinal fluid is usually normal.

Non-paralytic and Pre-paralytic Poliomyelitis. The symptoms are similar to those of the abortive case but more intense and prolonged. The onset is often abrupt and fever practically invariable. The temperature is commonly 103° or 104° F. (39·4° or 40° C.) and this pyrexia commonly lasts for 2–4 days and then gradually subsides, sometimes finally and sometimes to rise again a few days later and before the paralysis makes its appearance. Pains in the back and limbs are more severe and flexion of the spine is painful. Vomiting and anorexia are common and in many cases there is diarrhoea. After a day or so the general headache becomes intensified and occipital in position and is associated with the classical symptoms of meningeal irritation, irritability, neck stiffness and photophobia. The muscles of the back and limbs are often tender and may show tremor and depression or loss of their reflexes. There may be retention of urine.

Such a clinical picture in an adolescent, or young adult, in the summer or early autumn is extremely suggestive of poliomyelitis, but to those who have had extensive experience of epidemics the picture seen in young children is highly characteristic. The child is commonly flushed and miserable, and may be drowsy, but presents an appearance of mingled apprehension and restlessness, and may be irritable. In severe infections the child breathes rapidly, appears preoccupied and in a state of tenseness. An ataxic tremor and involuntary muscular jerkings may be present. Extreme fearfulness, and confused and alarming dreams are common. The child is hypersensitive to even the lightest touch and resents being moved. Vomiting, probably of central origin, may also be present. Headache, pain in the neck and back, stiffness of the spine and pain in the back on active or passive flexion, diminution of tendon jerks, and some diffuse weakness all appear in sequence.

During this stage of the illness it is impossible to predict with certainty whether the symptoms will subside, or whether paralysis will suddenly declare itself. If the nature of the disease has been recognized an agonizing period of waiting is inevitable and may be prolonged for 2 or 3 days.

Generally speaking, severe fever and meningeal signs and depression of tendon reflexes are of grave significance, but mild premonitory signs may be followed by severe local or general muscular paralysis. It should be remembered that probably not more than one-fifth of the cases diagnosed, many confirmed by cerebrospinal fluid changes, subsequently develop paralysis.

Paralytic Poliomyelitis. In these cases usually at the height of the constitutional and meningeal disturbance muscular paralysis declares itself. It may be confined to the muscles innervated by the spinal cord—the spinal form—or affect those innervated by the bulbar nuclei either exclusively or in addition to spinal paralysis—the so-called 'bulbar poliomyelitis', or polio-encephalitis.

1. Spinal Form. The onset of paralysis occurs usually between the second and the fifth days of the constitutional disturbance, but may be delayed as long as the tenth day if the fever persists. From the moment of its first appearance it usually reaches its height within 24 hours, but in rare cases it may continue to become more severe for several days, or recrudesce after becoming stationary.

In distribution and severity the paralysis varies over the widest possible extent. At one end of the scale are those cases in which, within a few hours, all four limbs are completely paralysed and the patient is engaged in a life-and-death struggle with respiratory failure. At the other are cases so mild that the paralysis is not recognized till the patient starts to get up. Generally speaking the legs and lower trunk muscles suffer more frequently and severely than the upper parts of the body, especially when diarrhoea has been a feature of the invasive period.

Wherever it occurs, the paralysis is of the flaccid, lower motor neurone type with loss of muscle tone, loss of voluntary power varying from weakness to complete paralysis, and diminution or loss of the corresponding tendon reflexes. This is rapidly followed by wasting, which in severe cases is rapid and intense in degree. Until it has been seen, the rate at which the muscles dissolve under one's eyes can hardly be believed. Such muscles are frequently tender and sometimes show spasm, so that the development of contractures occurs both easily and rapidly. The paralysis is generally much more widespread and severe at its commencement than it is destined to be permanently. At first all four limbs may be completely helpless and later there may be complete recovery in all but one limb. The widely spread temporary paralysis is due to a recoverable affection of nerve cells, whereas the permanent paralysis is the result of actual destruction of nerve cells, by the necrotic lesion. Usually the muscles first affected are the ones that show the greatest permanent damage.

In the rare 'ascending' type the paralysis may gradually ascend from the legs and lower trunk to the upper limbs, and progressive deterioration of the respiratory muscles during the first day or two after the onset of paralysis is relatively common. It is probably due to progressive exhaustion of the nerve cells of the upper thoracic and cervical region, themselves a little damaged, by the failure of the lower thoracic muscles to carry their share of the respiratory burden. In cases where the cervical cord is involved respiratory embarrassment makes its appearance early and in the absence of artificial respiration in some form it may lead to a fatal outcome within a few hours of the onset of paralysis.

In cases which survive, the narrowing down of the initial paralysis begins to show itself after the end of the first week, and any muscle which will recover useful power will have done so before the end of the third month. The paralysed muscles undergo atrophy, which is more rapid and complete in those cases in which there will be no subsequent recovery; they give the reaction of degeneration. They are flaccid from the first, and in the course of time tend to develop a variable degree of contracture, and yet it is common to see a limb which remains permanently flail-like. Any muscle which shows a response to faradism 3 weeks after the onset will usually recover completely. When a limb is paralysed, there is usually marked vasomotor paralysis, and there may be subsequent retardation of growth. Deformities of the body and limbs may arise as the result of the loss of support, which results from the paralysis, from the action of unopposed muscles and from the contractures. Such deformity may involve actual dislocation of joints, as in the shoulder joint, when the deltoid is paralysed and the pectorals escape.

The local lesion of the spinal cord is by no means confined to the grey matter. It may occasionally involve the contiguous white matter of the lateral column sufficiently to give rise to signs of lesion of the pyramidal tract, and in rare cases of other fibres, such as the spinothalamic tract, with a resulting Brown-Séquard syndrome. This is the so-called 'myelitic' form. Paralysis of the cervical sympathetic is occasionally seen when the lower part of the cervical enlargement is involved, with the usual signs of a small pupil and low-lying lid on the affected side. It is, however, generally a transient event.

Disturbances of sensation of an objective kind are rare; they are almost always transient, and amount to blunting of pain and temperature sensibility, from involvement of the spinothalamic tracts which are contiguous to the ventral horns. Subjective disturbances are common, and consist of severe local pains in the limbs, back and neck. Tenderness of the muscles, and pain on moving the joints are sometimes very prominent, and may persist for many weeks. The dominance of the clinical picture by persistent pains in the periphery constitutes the so-called 'neuritic' form of poliomyelitis.

The reflexes, both superficial and deep, are at first lost in the affected region, and indeed are generally absent throughout the body in the early stages of a severe case, from the general effect of the virus upon the nerve elements. In the later stages they return, or remain permanently absent, according as the muscles recover or not. The preservation of a tendon-jerk or any sign of a returning reflex, either deep or superficial, in the early days of the illness is a most useful prognostic indication that the muscles concerned with the reflex will entirely recover.

Retention of urine is common during the first 10 days of the illness, particularly in the case of male subjects where the trunk muscles are involved. It is never permanent.

2. Bulbar Form. Involvement of the muscles innervated by the bulbar nuclei may be present from the onset and may be encountered in the absence of spinal cord symptoms. This is commonly seen in the cases occurring as a complication of tonsillectomy. More often, however, it occurs as an extension of the disease in cases in which the cervical enlargement of the spinal cord is involved and respiratory complications are already present. Its onset is often heralded by mental confusion and drowsiness, acceleration and irregularity of the pulse, irregularity of the respiratory effort and flushing and congestion of the skin and conjunctivae. These symptoms may be confused with those of anoxia. Excessive bronchial secretion occurs and adds to the danger of this grave complication. Paralysis of the pharynx may be unilateral or bilateral, and leads to dysphagia and to the accumulation of secretions in the pharyngeal recesses. Laryngeal paralysis may be partial or complete and may lead to dangerous adductor spasm. Paralysis of the tongue may occur. The palate is commonly involved, giving rise to a nasal speech and regurgitation of fluids down the nose. Unilateral or bilateral facial palsy is common, but similar paralysis of the muscles of mastication is much more rare, but occasionally the patient may be unable to keep the jaw shut. Ocular paralyses are rare and patients showing them are usually moribund. Occasionally, however, spontaneous nystagmus occurring in short bursts and at a rapid rhythm may be seen and is not of particularly sinister significance.

The occurrence of bulbar symptoms is always an event of grave prognostic significance, but if the patient survives the cranial nerve paralyses make a remarkably complete recovery.

Diagnosis

When once paralysis is present the diagnosis of poliomyelitis presents no difficulty. In children a localized paralysis has to be distinguished from such causes of 'pseudoparalysis' as acute rheumatism or osteomyelitis, in which there may be fever and pain with reluctance to move the limb.

In cases of generalized paralysis the group of diseases most likely to be confused with poliomyelitis are the peripheral neuritides, particularly acute infective polyneuritis and acute porphyria. In both of these the paralysis is symmetrical and at first peripheral in distribution and, although slight, some sensory disturbances are usually present. Finding cerebrospinal fluid with a high protein content, but no excess of cells, is a point in favour of polyneuritis. Cases of poliomyelitis affecting both legs and the lower part of the trunk may easily be confused with acute compression of the spinal cord in the dorsal region with a flaccid paraplegia, especially when this is caused by an infective lesion of the spine such as osteomyelitis. Careful attention to the history and the finding of sensory loss with a clear upper level will usually suffice to avoid this mistake.

Isolated bulbar poliomyelitis cannot be confused with focal lesions of the medulla such as syringobulbia, or vascular lesions, but a similar picture may be seen in botulism. It is particularly in abortive cases and in the pre-paralytic stage that difficulty in diagnosis arises. Indeed it is often impossible to diagnose poliomyelitis with certainty, though it may be suspected in the presence of an epidemic or on account of the time of year. In cases showing merely fever, malaise and some generalized muscular pains the differential diagnosis is from influenza, tonsillitis and the exanthems. These are rare in summer and early autumn. More difficult to distinguish are the premonitory phases of other virus diseases, namely infective hepatitis, glandular fever and virus pneumonia.

When signs of meningeal irritation are prominent the diagnosis is from the various forms of meningitis, though it should be borne in mind that all the conditions mentioned above may be associated with 'meningism'.

Pyogenic meningitis usually presents a picture so definite that serious difficulty does not arise, but meningococcal meningitis may start insidiously and tuberculous meningitis relatively acutely. The distinction from these conditions can usually be made with certainty on the cerebrospinal fluid, but this may take a day or two.

Greater difficulty occurs with benign lymphocytic meningitis and with the meningo-encephalitis of mumps which may precede the parotitis as in both cases a pleocytosis similar to that of poliomyelitis occurs with no fall in glucose or chlorides and little increase in protein.

The meningeal reaction to a cerebral or extradural abscess may also give a mixed pleocytosis with a sterile fluid, but here there is usually a considerable increase in the total protein content.

Treatment

The first problem that faces a physician called to see a case of poliomyelitis is disposal. The right policy is to treat poliomyelitis as a directly contagious illness and to refer all patients to a special unit where barrier nursing is possible and full facilities for respiratory management are available. If the case is mild, or the fever already subsiding, absolute bed rest should be enjoined for there is satisfactory evidence that the taking of vigorous physical exercise in the pre-paralytic stage may not only greatly increase the likelihood of paralysis occurring but may also determine its distribution. The patient should remain in bed for 2 weeks after all fever and symptoms have subsided, and get about gradually during the third week. Contact with others should be avoided for 3 weeks after the temperature becomes normal, and for the same time the excreta should be immersed in lysol for 12 hours before disposal. No restrictions need be placed on diet, though at first the appetite may be poor.

In established cases treatment falls into three natural phases:

1. The acute illness lasting from the onset for 2 or at most 3 weeks.
2. The stage of neuronic recovery lasting for 6 months or so from the onset.
3. The stage of adaptation and rehabilitation lasting up to 3 years from the time of the acute illness.

The Acute Illness. Here the primary object of treatment is to ensure the patient's survival. He should be nursed on a soft mattress or ripple bed upon a stiff wire bed or fracture boards. All nasopharyngeal discharge and excreta, linen and feeding utensils should be sterilized and kept separate from those of the other patients and all attendants should wear masks and gowns. The diet should be light but as nutritious as the patient will tolerate.

All muscles showing weakness or paralysis should be put as far as possible in the position of physiological rest. The feet and toes should be supported at right angles to the legs by pillows and a vertical board. The knees should be maintained at 10 degrees flexion by a slender bolster underneath them. If the deltoids are affected the shoulders should be kept abducted by pillows to as near as the patient will tolerate to 90 degrees. The hand should be dorsiflexed at the wrist to 30 degrees with the fingers and thumbs gently flexed round a small woollen cushion. Pain and spasm in muscles may be relieved by hot packs and the discomfort treated with analgesics. From the beginning all joints should be put through their full range of passive movement twice a day. The complete immobility formerly insisted upon is now regarded as harmful and responsible for much of the painful limitation of movements and muscular contractures which were such a tiresome feature of the convalescent phase. Retention of urine is best treated by an indwelling catheter and seldom lasts more than 2 weeks even in severe cases. If cystitis develops it should be treated immediately by the appropriate antibiotic and, if severe, this should be combined with tidal drainage.

The complications of poliomyelitis which threaten life are respiratory failure and bulbar involvement. The patient should always have access to an intensive care unit.

Respiratory failure. Although this commonly develops suddenly during the first 2 or 3 days of paralysis it does not do so without warning. Frequent and careful examination of the chest may reveal the progressive involvement of the intercostal muscles on one or both sides and may be confirmed by asking the patient to count aloud without drawing breath. An initial count of 50 or more may fall to 20 before the patient is conscious of dyspnoea at rest. Spirometer readings should be taken at regular intervals and starting at 3000–4000 ml. may fall on successive measurements to 1200 ml. or so before cyanosis is visible or subjective distress is experienced.

It is often paralysis of the diaphragm which precipitates a respiratory crisis and necessitates the use of a cuirasse respirator. If the emergency develops suddenly, as it often does within 12 hours of the onset of paralysis, the decision to use the respirator presents no difficulty. If it develops gradually over several days from progressive exhaustion of the remaining respiratory muscles a difficult choice has to be made. It is preferable to resort to a respirator too early than too late and a rapidly falling respiratory exchange as indicated by a vital capacity of less than 1500 ml. in an adult is an indication for the use of a respirator.

The effects of respiratory embarrassment are often aggravated by the accumulation of bronchial secretions, frequently excessive in amount, which the patient is unable to cough up. The complication can often be forestalled, especially in children, by postural drainage. The patient is laid face downwards on a thoracic bed with the head and chest sloping downwards at 30 to 45 degrees. In other cases it may be necessary initially to suck out the secretions through a bronchoscope.

When respiratory embarrassment occurs tracheostomy is performed, a well-fitting metal tracheal tube inserted and positive pressure respiration instituted through a humidifier with a respirator of the type designed by Beaver. Later the metal tube is replaced by a plastic or rubber one with an inflatable balloon to secure an efficient closed circuit for the positive pressure in the respirator pump.

Bulbar poliomyelitis. When this occurs in the absence of respiratory involvement or of widespread mesencephalitis it is a relatively benign condition. Dysphagia may necessitate feeding by nasal catheter and the accumulation of secretions in the nasopharynx and upper respiratory passages may require postural drainage or repeated suction. The occurrence of adductor spasm of the vocal cords may require tracheostomy. Recovery is the rule. Bulbar poliomyelitis with mesencephalitis and signs of more generalized polio-encephalitis is usually a terminal event.

It is when it occurs—as it usually does—as a complication on the second or third day of a case of spinal poliomyelitis of the cervical and thoracic cord with respiratory involvement that bulbar poliomyelitis presents a therapeutic problem of the greatest difficulty. It is associated with excessive bronchial secretion and often with laryngeal obstruction which, with a patient already in a respirator, has usually led to rapid death. In an epidemic in Denmark where such cases were common, the mortality was nearly 90 per cent. until the drastic measure of immediate tracheostomy and positive insufflation followed by regular suction was adopted. This procedure reduced the mortality to approximately 25 per cent., and as already outlined is now standard practice. With the modern methods described above it is not uncommon for a patient to survive the immediate emergency only to become permanently dependent upon artificial respiration—a dilemma of a most poignant kind for all concerned.

The Stage of Neuronic Recovery. During this period, which lasts for 3–6 months in severe cases, the objects of treatment are to promote the maximal recovery of nerve cells, and therefore of muscles, to restore function and to prevent contractures and deformities. The patient is best treated in a specialized convalescent unit such as is often associated with orthopaedic centres. Massage and passive movement of limbs should gradually give way to active movements carried out at first with slings or in warm baths and later against progressively increasing resistance. Weight bearing should be assisted by such devices as bannisters, crutches and calipers. Stationary bicycles and boats and the intelligent use of ball games play an important part and progress is more rapid in cheerful and well-run units where group methods are possible and use can be made of the stimulus of competition and emulation.

Care must be taken to prevent the development of deformities and where the trunk mucles are involved the patient should spend several hours a day lying prone on a flat bed to correct the tendency to develop a lower thoracic and lumbar kyphosis. Breathing exercises should be given.

After 6 months it is unlikely that more neurones will recover their function and improvement becomes much slower. It continues, however, for many months or even years by virtue of the increased adaptation of the patient to his disability and by the hypertrophy and taking over of new function by existing muscles.

The Stage of Adaptation and Rehabilitation. This is really a continuation of the above and may last 2–3 years. In it function gradually improves and the patient's range of activity increases. Instrumental devices may be used and in many cases the patient has to be trained for a new occupation, depending upon the nature of the residual paralysis and the natural aptitudes of the individual. After 2 years, operative orthopaedic procedures may be needed to stabilize flail joints or to improve function by tendon transplants.

Specific Measures

Active Immunity. The whole subject of the control of poliomyelitis has been revolutionized by the success of mass active immunization which has superseded all other methods of prophylaxis.

Two forms of vaccine are available. The first, made by the Salk process, is a filtrate of virus-infected tissue cultures inactivated by incubation with formalin. Vaccines against each type of poliovirus are prepared separately and pooled. The final product is tested to exclude live virus and for antigenicity. With early batches the antibody response to type 1 virus was inadequate in about 15 per cent. of those vaccinated, but this defect has now been overcome. Three subcutaneous injections are required: the second a month after the first and the third 8–12 months after the second. Field trials have shown the incidence of paralysis to be reduced in the vaccinated by 75–80 per cent.

The second form, developed by Sabin, consists of attenuated strains of living virus. It is given orally and the immunity which follows is similar to that induced by a natural infection. The theoretical danger is that the attenuated virus might regain its neurotropic character. There is no evidence that this happens and field trials have been carried out in several million subjects. A small proportion of those receiving vaccine do not become infected and show no antibody response.

The method of immunization by live attenuated vaccine could not be simpler. The vaccine contains a mixture of types 1, 2 and 3 poliovirus. 0·1 ml. (3 drops) is given on a lump of sugar, the dose is repeated in 6 weeks and thereafter annually. It is important that the whole family, and if possible the whole immediate population, should be immunized simultaneously.

Course and Prognosis

A good deal has already been said on these aspects of poliomyelitis. In abortive and non-paralytic cases, which represent the majority, recovery is complete, though patients will often notice general lassitude and even a marked loss of weight for some weeks or months after the illness.

Purely local paralysis presents no threat to life and the patient recovers with a varying degree of local disability. It is not uncommon to see cases of complete paralysis of all muscles below one knee or of one shoulder girdle, and spinal deformities may later develop from weakness of the spinal musculature.

The fatality rate cannot be determined with accuracy because of the difficulty of diagnosis in the abortive and non-paralytic varieties. In the past the fatality rate has been 10–15 per 100 paralytic cases, but it has fallen to a much lower figure recently. There is still a higher proportion of deaths in those over 15 years of age.

Cases of generalized paralysis are always in grave danger because of the likelihood of respiratory failure and this complication is the principal cause of death. However, if the emergency is surmounted, remarkable recovery of respiratory function occurs. In part this is due to the development of increased efficiency in the remaining respiratory muscles, including the accessory muscles, but partly to the fact that the initial loss of power in diaphragm and intercostals is often due to exhaustion rather than to irreparable anterior horn cell damage.

In cases surviving the first impact of the disease improvement in muscle tenderness begins after a week or so and recovery of function of muscle begins about the same time. It usually begins first in the muscles last affected, and in cases destined to make a good recovery it continues at a rapid rate for 2–3 months. Recovery of tendon reflexes or the faradic response often precede the return of voluntary power. Muscles which show no sign of recovery then are unlikely to make any useful recovery. After 3 months, recovery continues at a gradually slower rate for another 6 months, but most of the improvement during this period results from the development and adaptation of function in already active muscles rather than from further recovery of nerve cells.

In all but mild generalized cases some degree of permanent wasting and weakness of muscles will remain which may necessitate the use of various appliances to improve function and mobility and various orthopaedic procedures to the same end. In severe cases the patient may be left permanently confined to a spinal chair or wholly dependent for life upon some form of respirator and he is faced with all the problems of psychological readjustment that this implies. Many cases of this sort still exist.

In young children and, to a lesser extent in adolescents, the loss of muscle may lead to serious defects of growth in the limbs and to deformities both of the limbs and the trunk.

The occurrence of bulbar symptoms increases greatly the gravity of the prognosis, but if the patient survives the cranial nerve palsies usually undergo complete recovery.

Second attacks of poliomyelitis have occurred, but are exceedingly rare. They probably result from a susceptible individual encountering at different times strains of the virus which do not confer cross-immunity.

REFERENCES

Affeldt, J. E. (1954) Recent advances in the treatment of poliomyelitis, *J. Amer. med. Ass.*, **156**, 12.

Koprowski, H. (1960) Historical aspects of the development of live virus vaccine in poliomyelitis, *Brit. med. J.*, **2**, 85.

Lacey, B. W. (1949) The natural history of poliomyelitis, *Lancet*, i, 849.

Russell, W. R. (1952) *Poliomyelitis*, London.

RABIES

Synonyms. Hydrophobia; Lyssa.

Definition

This infective disease, rare in Britain, is due to a filtrable virus which is located in the salivary glands and central nervous system. It is transmitted to man and most warm-blooded animals through infective saliva of canines or blood-lapping bats. There is a long and variable incubation period, and a short pyrexial illness of sudden onset characterized by fever, nervous exaltation and violent muscular spasms involving the oesophagus and respiratory system. Once symptoms have supervened, the patient invariably dies.

Aetiology

The disease is generally transmitted either by the licking of a freshly abraded surface of skin or the bite of an infected dog. In Eastern Europe and the Orient, wolves transmit the disease and, owing to extensive laceration of the tissues, a greater proportion of people bitten by them develop the disease than with either dogs or jackals. It has been intimated that wolf bites entail a mortality of 80 per cent. In Trinidad, in 1925 an epidemic of paralytic rabies in man was attributed to the bites of vampire bats, cattle being the original source of infection.

The Virus of Rabies. This belongs to the class of neurotropic viruses that have a special affinity for the grey matter of the nervous system.

Pasteur in 1881 showed that the causal agent of rabies could be transmitted from animal to animal by intracerebral inoculation of infected brain. Serial passage modified the virus. The naturally occurring 'street virus' carries a long incubation period and has the capacity of multiplying in the salivary glands; after some twenty passages the incubation period is reduced to 7 days and the salivary glands are no longer invaded. This modified strain is known as 'fixed virus'.

Some strains of virus when cultivated in the developing chick embryo lose all pathogenic properties although retaining antigenic potency.

Epidemiologically two patterns are recognizable: one which occurs in wild life maintained by many types of mammal such as wolves, mongooses, foxes and jackals and by bats, and an urban type in which the dog alone is responsible, although during an epidemic other domestic animals such as cats and cattle may be infected.

Pathology

Excess of cerebrospinal fluid, petechial haemorrhages of the pia arachnoid and injection of its vessels may be found at autopsy. Histological examination reveals cellular infiltration of the perivascular lymph spaces as well as Negri bodies within the cytoplasm of the nerve cells and their processes. These are globular or ovoid structures, of variable diameter (0·5–25 microns), especially common in the Purkinje cells of the cerebellum and the hippocampus; they are present in the brains of 97 per cent. of dogs infected with street virus.

Symptoms

The period intervening between the bite and the clinical manifestations varies from 1 to 2 months, as a rule, the limits being 11 days to over a year. Face, head and neck bites have a shorter incubation period than those on the arm which have a shorter incubation than those on the leg. The onset is generally sudden, but prodromal symptoms are sometimes noted for a day or two before a hydrophobic syndrome appears. For convenience, three stages are described.

1. The Invasion Stage. This includes prodromal features such as pain in the scar, fever, headache, rapid pulse, anxiety, restlessness, insomnia, irregular and sighing respirations and phases of rushed speaking.

2. The Stage of Excitation. This supervenes in 24–48 hours. There is intense restlessness, mental excitement, hyperaesthesia and hydrophobia which consists of a sudden spasm of the muscles of the mouth, pharynx and larynx and, to a greater or lesser degree, the whole respiratory musculature. An attack may be induced by offering the patient water. As the glass approaches the mouth, the head retracts in a series of spasmodic jerks associated with gasping respirations, while any water reaching the mouth is immediately ejected. The shoulders are elevated, the chest expanded and the sternomastoid and platysma muscles contracted. Later, the synaptic resistance in the reflex arcs become so lowered that a variety of sensory stimuli such as a sudden sound, cold air, strong light, a strange smell and even the suggestion of water may suffice to induce the attack. The voice is altered. Frothy saliva collects in the throat and mouth and is flung off the lips during the attacks which may be characterized by intense fury or the most profound terror. Lastly, opisthotonus and general respiratory spasm are superadded. In the interval the mind is clear, the patient remaining quietly at rest in bed. Examination of the central nervous system reveals, as a rule, nothing more than increased deep reflexes. Glycosuria occurs and vomiting, exhaustion and emaciation characterize the final stage of the illness. During the paroxysm death may occur from dilatation of the right heart, though sometimes near the end the spasms ameliorate or cease altogether.

3. Stage of Paralysis. If the patient survives long enough, paralysis of various types, including ascending spinal paralysis, paraplegia and hemiplegia, may supervene. The patient lies helpless and exhausted, and generally dies in coma. In man this stage is rarely seen in canine-transmitted rabies, but paralytic rabies is commonly encountered in the bat-transmitted variety in Trinidad.

In the Trinidad outbreak all the cases were of this variety, and all proved fatal. The onset is acute, with fever and headache. Numbness and burning sensations in one or both legs, paresis of the legs and retention of urine follow. After 2 or 3 days the paraplegia becomes more complete, and the plantar and tendon reflexes disappear. One limb is commonly affected before the other. In a few days the paralysis begins to ascend, involving the muscles of respiration, articulation and deglutition. There is dyspnoea and restlessness. The sufferer remains conscious, but may be delirious. Sensory changes are of variable intensity. A final brief coma precedes the fatal issue. During this time the temperature swings round 103° F. (39·4° C.), and there is profuse sweating. Hydrophobic symptoms are exceptional, and when present, slight. The cerebrospinal fluid yields an increased globulin content, but is otherwise normal. The duration of the illness is from 4 to 8 days.

Rabies in the Dog. These animals never show the hydrophobic syndrome observed in man. The earliest manifestation appears to be a change in temperament, followed by irritation and exacerbations of vicious fury in which the animal runs amok, biting wildly anything in its path. Later, swallowing becomes difficult, the bark is altered, the jaw drops and general paralysis ensues. Death invariably follows some 2 to 5 days after the first symptoms appear. In dumb rabies the stage of excitation is absent.

Diagnosis

As a rule, little difficulty is experienced in diagnosis, but occasionally tetanus, the cerebral type of typhus fever, bulbar paralysis from any cause, and datura and other poisonings encountered in Oriental countries may need differentiation. The behaviour of the patient at the onset of the disease can easily be mistaken for hysteria or for histrionic behaviour.

Treatment

This is mainly preventive, and in England the muzzling order and the strict quarantine of all imported dogs has led to the virtual eradication of rabies. The author cared for one of the two cases to appear in Britain in the last decade; she was an immigrant, bitten before leaving her home country. In endemic areas canine bites should be promptly treated, and the suspected dog chained up, muzzled and kept under observation. Should the animal be alive at the end of 10 days it is proof that the bitten person has not been infected. This rule, universally followed in Pasteur institutes, is based: (1) on the knowledge that the infected dog never survives longer than 6 days from the onset of its illness; and (2) that the saliva of a rabid dog is never infective for more than 4 days before the onset of symptoms. In suspicious cases, especially the head, face and neck bites, treatment should be commenced without delay and discontinued if the dog survives.

The virus of rabies differs from that of yellow fever in not passing through the intact skin, and where there is a history of being licked by an animal suspected of rabies prophylactic inoculation need not be advised unless fresh skin abrasions were present at the time.

Local Treatment. If seen within 30 minutes, bleeding should be encouraged by the application of a ligature just tight enough to obstruct the venous return and the parts bathed with permanganate solution. All bites and abrasions of the skin should be cleaned immediately with soap or detergent solution. Subsequently, each tooth-mark should be probed separately and cauterized or treated with pure phenol. For 3 days the wound should not be sutured; this particularly applies in the case of face bites.

Specific Measures. Those available are active and passive immunization. For the first a variety of vaccines are available. A subcutaneous injection of virus attenuated on egg white is given on alternate days for 2 weeks, followed by 'booster' doses 1 and 2 weeks afterwards. Passive immunity is provided by the use of hyperimmune antiserum within 2 days of infection but has little value.

Serum reactions occur in more than 10 per cent. of

patients given vaccine. They appear in the form of encephalomyelitis. For this reason antirabic vaccination should not be given unless specific indications exist. The best guide to treatment is the scheme prepared by the Expert Committee on Rabies of the World Health Organization (1954).

Treatment of the Paroxysm. The best thing to do is to keep the patient anaesthetized. In the hands of an experienced anaesthetist with positive pressure respiratory apparatus the curarine analogues may be used to reduce the intense spasms.

Prognosis

By no means all patients bitten by rabid animals die, but once clinical manifestations appear the disease invariably ends fatally. Estimates varying from 5 to 33 per cent. have been made of the death-rate in untreated patients, but of those receiving early antirabic inoculations in Pasteur institutes, not more than 1 per cent. die. The mortality varies with the site of the bite, the interposition of clothing, the number of tooth-marks, the extent of tissue laceration and the rapidity with which efficient local treatment has been instituted. Head, face and neck bites are particularly dangerous, as well as bites from wolves and jackals.

REFERENCE

KENT, J. R., and FINEGOLD, M. (1960) Human rabies transmitted by the bite of a bat, *New Engl. J. Med.*, **263**, 1058.

RIDLEY, A. (1965) A case of rabies, *Brit. med. J.*, **1**, 1596.

DENIS WILLIAMS

COXSACKIEVIRUS INFECTIONS

GENERAL ASPECTS

The Coxsackie viruses received their name from the town where the two patients lived from whom Dalldorf recovered the virus, known as Coxsackie A1, by inoculation of their faeces into new-born mice in 1948. The patients had typical paralytic poliomyelitis and Type 1 poliovirus was also isolated from the stools. The mice which developed paralysis showed inflammatory lesions in the skeletal muscles. Since then about 30 immunological types of virus with similar pathogenicity for new-born mice have been isolated from the throat, faeces and other sites in patients with a variety of illnesses and from some normal persons. The types have been divided into two broad subgroups A (24) and B (6) on the basis of the pathological picture usually found in affected mice. The A group viruses tend to produce diffuse acute inflammation and necrosis of the striated muscles, but two produce anterior horn cell lesions in mice, and laboratory-adapted strains of these cause similar lesions in monkeys. The B group cause focal areas of necrosis of the skeletal muscles and necrotic lesions in the brain, pancreas, liver, embryonic fat pad and myocardium. There are antigenic relationships between some of the A group and all the B group. The present classification is neither rigid nor likely to be permanent; there is already at least one type that is classed by some workers as echovirus type 9 and by others as Coxsackie virus type A23.

As the site of the optimum virus growth in man is the gastro-intestinal tract and the viruses are of the same order and size, and have a similar nucleic acid core and physical and chemical properties to the polioviruses and echoviruses, they are classed with them as enteroviruses. However, as a whole, Coxsackie viruses have much less affinity for motor neurones than the polioviruses and much more for other organs, with the result that they usually produce a viraemia and a broad spectrum of clinical diseases and syndromes of which examples are Bornholm disease, myocarditis and pericarditis, pharyngitis, orchitis, vesicular rashes, and rarely pneumonia, in addition to meningitis, encephalitis and lower motor neurone paralysis. Some examples of the types of Coxsackie A and B viruses which have been found associated with various syndromes are shown in TABLE 11. The division into epidemic and sporadic is meant to be only a rough guide. Those listed as sporadic under some syndromes might cause outbreaks at any time. Some of the B group viruses may interfere with poliovirus infection, but several of the A group might have the opposite effect, converting a mild poliovirus infection into a paralytic one if double infection takes place.

It has not been possible to produce satisfactory complement-fixing antigens from either A or B group viruses which will give specific reactions with human sera in a manner suitable for routine diagnosis. Specific neutralization tests are possible, but are too laborious for use except in special investigations of a small number of patients.

TABLE 11

CLINICAL SYNDROMES ASSOCIATED WITH COXSACKIE VIRUS INFECTIONS

SYNDROMES	VIRUSES	
	Epidemic	*Sporadic*
Aseptic meningitis	A7, A9, B1–6	A1
Paresis, paralysis, encephalitis	A7	A2, A9, B1–5
Pleurodynia, Bornholm disease	B1–5	
Eruptive fever, hand, foot and mouth disease	A4, A5, A9, A16, B1	B3, B5
Herpangina	A2, A4, A5, A6, A8, A10	
Myocarditis or encephalomyocarditis in neonatal period	B1–5	A16, B1–5
Benign pericarditis in adults and children		A1, B1, B3, B5
Upper respiratory tract infection	A6, A10, A21	B1–5
Orchitis		B1–5
'Pyrexia of unknown origin'		A5, B1–5

As these viruses may be present in the throat and faeces of healthy persons, the isolation of virus from them is not of such aetiological significance in relation to the presenting illness as it is from the cerebrospinal fluid, the blood, skin lesions or some affected organ. A rise in antibodies in the blood in convalescence is supportive evidence but not conclusive in a sporadic case.

HAND, FOOT AND MOUTH DISEASE

In the past 10 years many sporadic cases and outbreaks of a syndrome known as hand, foot and mouth disease have been described from different countries. The illness has been caused by infection with coxsackie A group viruses of types 5, 10 and 16. Vesicles which break to form shallow ulcers, are present in the anterior part of the mouth and on the wall of the pharynx. Vesicles may be present only in the mouth but are frequently accompanied by a maculopapular rash which progresses to vesicles on the hands and feet and sometimes elsewhere on the limbs and buttocks. All age groups may be affected and in one case in an elderly female chronic infection with the same type of virus persisted for 2 years.

MENINGITIS, PARALYSIS AND ENCEPHALITIS

Several of the A group and all of the B group have been found associated with disease of the nervous system particularly meningitis, but also with paralysis of limbs and facial muscles similar to that seen in poliovirus infection and occasionally with encephalitis.

Pathology

If meningitis occurs by itself no characteristic lesion will be present. The few recorded fatal cases of central nervous system disease have been infants and young children. In A7 virus infections the pathological lesions have been indistinguishable from those of poliovirus, with perivascular cuffing with lymphocytes in the medulla and degeneration and neuronophagia of motor neurones of the anterior horn cells in the spinal cord. A similar picture is seen in experimentally-infected monkeys although they do not show the extensive involvement of the spinal cord which is commonly seen with poliovirus. In fatal B group infections of the newborn the meninges are oedematous and infiltrated with macrophages. There are areas of focal degeneration scattered throughout the parenchyma of the cerebrum and pons, but widespread in the spinal cord; the cerebellum may also be affected.

Signs and Symptoms

The incubation period is 2–14 days. Onset is sudden with headache, fever and often nausea and vomiting. On examination, stiffness of the neck and possibly the back is found and Kernig's and Brudzinski's signs are positive. If there is only meningitis the patient has usually recovered in a week. There will be moderate pleocytosis of the cerebrospinal fluid, sometimes with polymorphonuclear predominance at the beginning, but always lymphocytic later. Protein may be elevated, but the sugar and chlorides are normal.

If paralysis develops it will be indistinguishable from that caused by polioviruses. It tends to affect the muscles supplied by the facial nerve or those of the limbs and is usually unilateral. Except in coxsackie A7 infections, paralysis has usually been transient. All the paralytic A7 cases in one year in Glasgow were in males.

Encephalitis may occur with or without meningitis. There may be severe headache, confusion, lethargy, paraesthesia, paralysis of cranial nerves, blurring of vision and papilloedema. It is possible that these viruses also attack the cerebellum or vestibular nucleus causing ataxia.

Diagnosis

This can only be made by isolation of the virus from throat swab, faeces and preferably cerebrospinal fluid and from brain and cord *post mortem*. Serum should be collected in the acute stage and about two weeks after onset although serological tests for coxsackie viruses are not routine.

Treatment

There is no specific treatment. The headache may not be relieved by common analgesics including morphine, but may be helped by lumbar puncture. Treatment of paralysed muscles will be the same as in poliomyelitis.

Prognosis

Recovery from meningitis or paralysis is usually rapid and complete, but there may be a long delay, up to a year, in recovery from paralysis, and permanent residual atrophy has been described in a small number of children with A7 virus or with B group infection. The possibility of Parkinsonism occurring rarely cannot be ruled out. Death has resulted from respiratory and circulatory failure in A7 virus infections and fatal encephalitis with or without myocarditis has occurred in B group infections in infants.

PLEURODYNIA

Synonyms. Epidemic myalgia; Bornholm disease; Devil's grip.

Definition

The disease obtained its most common name from the description of cases in outbreaks on the Danish island of Bornholm by Sylvest in 1934. It has been described from many different areas of the world under the various synonyms.

Aetiology

Soon after the first coxsackie virus was described by Dalldorf, in cases of poliomyelitis-like disease, other workers recovered similar viruses from patients with Bornholm disease. All the B group viruses have been incriminated, but not those of the A group. Typical cases have been described where no coxsackie virus has been isolated but an echovirus was present.

Pathology

The symptoms are those of muscle pain and in the mouse focal inflammatory and necrotic lesions are usually produced in the skeletal muscles of the mouse by the B group of viruses. In the very few recorded muscle biopsies from humans, similar changes were seen and isolation of the virus from muscle was also reported.

It is a little surprising that the A group of viruses which produce more generalized myositis in the mouse have not been shown to cause such lesions in man.

Signs and Symptoms

The incubation period is 2–14 days.

The disease is characterized by sudden onset with headache, fever, severe pain in the lower chest and abdomen and sometimes in limbs and lumbar muscles. The pain is usually spasmodic and related to respiratory movement and there may be rapid breathing and suppression of breath sounds. There may be muscle tenderness and cutaneous hyperaesthesia and pleural friction may be heard at some stage but demonstrable pleural fluid is uncommon. The lungs are rarely involved. In an outbreak a small number of patients or other members of the household may have pharyngitis, coryza or meningitis. In widespread outbreaks of the disease, pericarditis and orchitis may also be present in other patients.

The initial acute attack is usually finished in two days but fever and less severe pain may persist for a week. Recurrence of pain and fever at intervals of a few days is not uncommon.

Diagnosis

Differentiation from acute pulmonary and abdominal emergencies is the main concern particularly at the beginning of an outbreak or in sporadic cases. The tendency to have a normal blood leucocyte count or a slight leucopenia is more suggestive of a virus infection. Unfortunately the virus in throat swab or faeces is unlikely to produce disease in new-born mice or tissue culture changes until a minimum of three days have passed, by which time the clinical picture has usually become clearer. However, identification of the virus may be of value if further similar cases are seen in the area.

Treatment

There is no specific treatment so that only symptomatic treatment is required, particularly analgesics. But it is wise to keep in mind the possibility of pericarditis developing later, so convalescence should be gradual.

Prognosis

This is good once the aetiology is recognized.

PERICARDITIS AND MYOCARDITIS

Severe, frequently fatal, myocarditis in the newborn, due to coxsackie B viruses has been reported from several countries and maternal infection with these viruses during pregnancy may be one of the causes of congenital heart disease. In addition, however, it has become evident in recent years that members of the B group, and occasionally some of the A group, may cause pericarditis, with or without myocarditis, in older children and adults. These often occur during a wave of infection when other patients are suffering from Bornholm disease, meningitis or non-specific general malaise and fever.

Pathology

In a single case of A1 infection biopsy was carried out because of the suspicion that the pericarditis was due to tuberculosis. Biopsy revealed a thickened tough pericardial membrane consisting of organized clot and dense fibrous tissue with chronic inflammatory cell infiltration. Valvulitis has also been described in patients with fatal myocarditis.

Signs and Symptoms

The incubation period is a few days to several weeks.

There may be a history of sore throat, fever, headache and pains in the chest, typical of Bornholm disease, or the premonitory symptoms may be very mild and the patient remains ambulant. The signs and symptoms of pericarditis may follow after an interval of a few days or a week or two of improvement with a return of fever. Abnormal electrocardiographic recordings and abnormal levels of serum enzymes indicative of myocardial involvement may be present.

Diagnosis

In the acute stage of the disease virus may be isolated from the throat and faeces and possibly from pericardial fluid, but frequently the possibility of a virus aetiology is not thought of until too late or the pericarditis occurs after the acute stage of illness. It may be possible to demonstrate a rise in antibodies to one of the coxsackie B viruses, but often the diagnosis can only be inferred from a high titre of antibodies to one type of virus which may be known to be present in other members of the family or contacts.

Treatment

There is no specific treatment. For symptomatic treatment see pericarditis.

Prognosis

The prognosis is usually good and recovery commonly takes place in 1–6 weeks, but progression to adhesive pericarditis with a fatal outcome has been described.

ECHOVIRUS INFECTIONS

With the advent of tissue cultures, the scope of the virus laboratory was enlarged so that patients could be studied in larger numbers and surveys for viruses present in the throat and faeces of healthy contacts of patients and of normal (control) individuals became possible. As a result, numerous new viruses were recovered from the faeces of normal persons which produced degeneration of cells in cultures of human and simian tissues, but did not produce clinically recognizable disease in laboratory animals. These were at first called orphan viruses (without a disease), but later the term enteric cytopathogenic human orphan or echoviruses was applied. Subsequently many of these viruses were found to be associated with definite clinical syndromes [TABLE 12], and there are now at least 34 typed viruses in this group.

In addition to the characteristics mentioned above, the echoviruses have properties similar to those of the coxsackie and polioviruses which allows a larger grouping of all three together as enteroviruses. The echoviruses are immunologically distinct from each other and from the coxsackie and polioviruses. They are about 18–25 millimicrons in diameter. They have a central core of ribonucleic acid and a protein coat, and are resistant to diethyl ether. A few have been found more frequently in the throat than in faeces and have been associated with minor respiratory tract disease. At least five types have been recovered from the blood and eleven types from the cerebrospinal fluid, and high titre tissue culture fluids of nine types have produced a febrile illness in inoculated monkeys or chimpanzees. One of the earlier echoviruses, echo 10, was later found to be larger (100 millimicrons in diameter) than the others and it is now classified as one type of another group of Respiratory Enteric Orphan (REO) viruses, some of which are pathogenic for mice. Some strains of echo 9 after passage in tissue culture will produce a myositis similar to that of Coxsackie A group viruses in new-born mice, and this virus is called by some investigators coxsackie A23. Thus it can be seen that no final classification has been achieved, although an attempt has been made to subdivide echoviruses into those which do and those which do not produce a cytopathic effect in cultures of the kidneys of African red grass (*Erythrocebus patas*) monkeys, and also into those which may agglutinate human erythrocytes.

No routine diagnostic complement fixation test is possible with any of these echoviruses because of cross reactions which occur with the antigens available at present. Even in neutralization tests, which are more specific but cumbersome, cross-reactions between types occur.

Signs and Symptoms

The incubation period is usually 5–10 days.

It is not surprising that this large number of immunologically different viruses have been found associated with many different syndromes [see TABLE 12]. Most of these have been associated with several types of virus and many of the viruses with more than one syndrome. The division into 'epidemic' and 'sporadic' is meant to be loose and temporary and merely gives a rough guide to the virus laboratory when arranging for the typing of a virus isolated from an outbreak. Up to the present time more types have been recovered from patients with disease of the central nervous system than with other disorders, but this has possibly been the result of the interest in poliomyelitis and the aetiology of so-called non-paralytic poliomyelitis or aseptic meningitis.

A few types have also been isolated from patients with mild paresis and from the spinal cords of a few cases of fatal bulbospinal paralysis or encephalitis. Cerebellar ataxia has been described in a few patients with echo 9 infection, as have symptoms and signs of ataxia due to damage of the vestibular nuclei and transverse myelitis with echovirus 19.

Skin rashes have been prominent in outbreaks due to echo 9, in some cases rubelliform or morbilliform, and in others petechial. The rashes were often noted in about a quarter of the children of a community, while meningitis occurred in the adults. In echo 16 infection, a maculopapular rash has been the main feature and sometimes with it and with echo 14, the rash has appeared after the fever has subsided, as in roseola infantum.

Although it has been thought for some time that some epidemics of nausea, vomiting and diarrhoea or of diarrhoea alone are due to viruses and two agents transmissible to volunteers were recovered several years ago, attempts to isolate a virus from most outbreaks and to culture the above two agents have been unsuccessful. In two outbreaks of mild disease in premature and new-born infants in a New York hospital, echo 18 was apparently the aetiological agent, and echo 5 in one in England, and in a small outbreak in an infant nursery in France echo 14 was responsible. Echo 11, 19 and 20 have been associated with upper respiratory tract infection combined with vomiting and diarrhoea and in some communities echoviruses have been recovered from stools of a higher proportion of patients with summer diarrhoea than with other complaints. However, if the cause of the common institutional and familial outbreaks of non-bacterial diarrhoea and vomiting is a virus it has not been isolated.

Several echoviruses have been associated with mild influenza or a common cold-like illness. Echo 11 produced the former in children, but diarrhoea in adult volunteers, and echo 28 has been found to produce a disease similar to the common cold in volunteers and is now classed as a rhinovirus. Isolated cases of acute myocarditis in children have been reported associated with echoviruses.

It is possible for overlapping infections of several enteroviruses to occur in a limited area at the same time, making it difficult from a single isolation to determine the aetiological relationship of the agent to the outbreak.

TABLE 12

CLINICAL SYNDROMES ASSOCIATED WITH ECHO VIRUSES

SYNDROME	EPIDEMIC	SPORADIC
Meningitis	4, 6, 9, 16, 30, 31	1, 2, 3, 5, 7, 11, 13, 14, 15, 17, 18, 19, 20, 21, 22, 25
Paralysis and encephalitis	4, 6, 9, 30	1, 2, 11, 16, 19
Eruptive fevers	9, 16	2, 5, 6, 8, 11, 14
Minor respiratory disease with or without enteric disease		7, 8, 11, 20, 22, 25, 28
Pleurodynia		6, 8
Enteritis in infants and children	5, 14, 18	7, 11, 19, 20, 28 (8, 12, 22, 23, 24)

Pathology

With such a variety of clinical pictures the pathological changes will also be heterogeneous and as few fatal cases have been recorded there is little information on the nature of these processes.

Diagnosis

A specific diagnosis can only be made in the laboratory by recovery of the virus from skin lesions, throat swabs, faeces, blood or cerebrospinal fluid and also preferably the demonstration of a rise in neutralizing or other antibody to the virus between a specimen of blood collected in the acute stage and a second collected in convalescence.

Treatment

There is no specific treatment.

Prognosis

Prognosis is almost invariably good except for occasional cases of severe encephalitis. There may be signs of residual parenchymal damage to the brain which may be the cumulative effect of successive infections with a number of echo or other neurotropic viruses.

REFERENCES

ASHKENAZI, A., and MELNICK, J. L. (1962) Enteroviruses, a review of their properties and associated diseases, *Amer. J. clin. Path.*, **38**, 209.

BROWN, G. C. (1968) Coxsackievirus infections and heart disease, *Amer. Heart J.*, **75**, 145.

EVANS, A. D., and WADDINGTON, E. (1967) Outbreak of hand, foot and mouth disease, *Brit. J. Derm.*, **79**, 309.

KIBRICK, S. (1964) Current status of coxsackie and echoviruses in human disease, *Progr. med. Virol.*, **6**, 27.

RAY, G. G., PLEXICO, K. L., WENNER, H. A., and CHIN, T. D. (1967) Acute respiratory illness associated with coxsackie B4 virus, *Pediatrics*, **39**, 220.

SCOTT, T. F. MCNAIR (1962) Clinical syndromes associated with enterovirus and reovirus infections, *Advanc. Virus Res.*, **8**, 165.

ARTHROPOD-BORNE VIRUS INFECTIONS

(ARBOVIRUS INFECTIONS)

GENERAL ASPECTS

The investigations of laboratories which were originally organized to study the epidemiology and control of yellow fever in South America and Africa and subsequently of other laboratories set up in tropical and subtropical areas have led to the discovery in recent years of a large number of viruses from mosquitoes, ticks and mites and a variety of wild and domestic animals, birds and man. There are now more than 200 viruses included under this heading, of which at least 50 have been demonstrated as a cause of human disease.

Nearly all the viruses have been isolated by the inoculation of mice less than 10 days old, usually by the intracerebral route. Most of the viruses are about the same size, 40–50 millimicrons in diameter, a few 60–75 and one or two about 100 millimicrons, are sensitive to ether and sodium desoxycholate and possess haemagglutinins for chick and goose erythrocytes.

Though the viruses which had been associated with encephalitis, e.g. equine encephalitis, Japanese B, Russian spring-summer and St. Louis encephalitis, were formerly thought to be quite different from those causing systemic illnesses, e.g. yellow fever and Rift Valley fever, more recent epidemiological and laboratory studies using new techniques have shown this not to be the case. It is well recognized that the so-called encephalitis viruses may cause systemic illness and belong to different antigenic groups and that viruses causing dengue, Rift Valley fever, yellow fever and similar diseases may be quite unrelated to each other antigenically, but closely related to some of the 'encephalitis-virus' groups. Much of this clarification came as the result of the development by Casals and his colleagues of haemagglutination tests which are used to classify the arboviruses as is seen in TABLE 13. This is of course only a provisional classification of some of the viruses which have been investigated more thoroughly.

Infections with the majority of these viruses occur for the most part in vertebrate hosts other than man and infection is maintained through contact with blood-sucking insects in whom a cycle of virus multiplication usually occurs before transfer to a fresh host. In most instances man becomes infected only by chance interference in the cycle. Some of the infections occur in epidemic waves, others occur yearly with fluctuations in incidence according to rainfall.

Changes in the ecology of mosquitoes, birds and

mammals by the introduction of agriculture or alteration of irrigation systems may precipitate aberrant cycles of virus activity and lead to epidemics of what were previously insignificant arbovirus infections.

Clinical differentiation may be quite difficult when only a febrile illness or encephalitis is present, particularly in some areas where several different groups of viruses may be present at the same time but in some, such as chikungunya, dengue and sandfly fever the presence of joint and bone pains and rashes may be helpful in making a provisional diagnosis.

Vaccines have been developed for the prevention of some of the diseases in man, e.g. yellow fever and Russian spring-summer encephalitis, and for louping ill and Rift Valley fever in sheep, but more widespread control will eventually depend on attempted eradication of the vectors, which in forest areas such as Brazil and Central Africa is likely to be impracticable.

uncommon but there will be stiffness of the neck, weakness of muscles and diminution of the tendon reflexes. A moderate pleocytosis, predominantly mononuclear after the first day or two, is found in the spinal fluid. Most patients make a complete recovery but sequelae such as mental deterioration, epilepsy and spastic palsies may be seen in children. The mortality rate is about 10 per cent.

In E.E.E. there is apparently a smaller proportion of subclinical infections and the disease is more severe. Children have been affected more than adults. The onset is abrupt and patients rapidly pass into a state of lethargy, then stupor or coma. Neck rigidity and Kernig's sign are present. Focal brain damage results in aphasia, diplopia and paralysis. A greater pleocytosis is present in the spinal fluid than in W.E.E.; polymorphonuclear leucocytes predominate early and mononuclears after a few days. Various types of

TABLE 13

GROUP A	GROUP B	GROUP C	BUNYAMWERA GROUP	GUAMA GROUP	MISCELLANEOUS
E.E.E.	Japanese B encephalitis	Apeu	Bunyamwera	Guama	Bwamba
W.E.E.	Murray Valley encephalitis	Marituba	Kairi	Bimiti	California encephalitis complex
Semliki Forest		Oriboca	Cache Valley	Catu	
Chickungunya	St. Louis encephalitis	Caraparu	Germiston		Mengo
O'nyong nyong	West Nile encephalitis				Rift Valley fever
	Dengue 1–4				Sandfly fever
	Yellow fever				Colorado tick fever
	Russian spring-summer encephalitis complex				

GROUP A

The main members of this group are the equine encephalitis viruses (Western, Eastern and Venezuelan), chikungunya and o'nyong nyong.

The former have been found in western and eastern United States, the Caribbean area and South America and can be differentiated by serological tests. Originally the prototype strains of W.E.E., E.E.E. and V.E.E. were recovered in the three areas, western and eastern United States and Venezuela. Later, strains of W.E.E. and E.E.E. were found in the south and V.E.E. further north, which led to the belief that infected birds were transferring the virus during migration south in the winter time or vice versa. However, more recent studies have shown that there are antigenic differences between, for example, the W.E.E. viruses isolated in North and South America.

EQUINE ENCEPHALITIS

Signs and Symptoms

The incubation period in equine encephalitis is 5–20 days. The majority of infections with the arbo viruses are subclinical. When the central nervous system is involved the resulting illness varies little except in its severity and the description given for the western and eastern types of equine encephalomyelitis are representative of this.

In W.E.E. the onset is sudden with generalized headache, nausea, fever and lethargy. Paralysis is

paralysis and mental deterioration occur as sequelae in most patients who survive. The mortality rate is 60–70 per cent.

Pathology

The pathological changes are very much the same in all types, essentially a meningo-encephalitis with only slight infiltration of the meninges. In E.E.E. there is more severe damage to neurones.

Diagnosis

Diagnosis in all cases depends upon isolation of the virus from blood or cerebrospinal fluid if meningitis or encephalitis are present, or from the central nervous system *post mortem* and on the results of antibody tests on sera collected at the onset of illness and about two weeks later.

Treatment

Prophylactic vaccines are available for protection of horses against the equine encephalitides. There is no specific treatment.

Prognosis

The prognosis is not good in equine encephalitis, particularly E.E.E. in man. The fatality rate in those with encephalitis has been as high as 70 per cent. and in those who survive sequelae have been common.

CHIKUNGUNYA

Chikungunya virus was recovered in 1953 from

patients in an epidemic of dengue-like disease in East Africa and has since been found in South India and South-East Asia associated with epidemics of dengue and haemorrhagic fever. Both *Aëdes aegypti* and *A. africanus* are vectors in East Africa.

O'NYONG NYONG

O'nyong nyong is a dengue-like disease which in 1959 swept through Uganda, Kenya, Congo and probably spread into the Sudan. It differed from classical dengue in the sudden onset of high fever and chills followed by joint pains. Many patients found standing difficult and some were so ill that they could not move. It was from the joint weakness that the name was derived. An itchy morbilliform rash appeared about the fourth day. Nearly 90 per cent. of the people in the epidemic area were infected but the oldest age groups were immune. Convalescence was slow, but there were no fatalities.

The virus was isolated from the blood of patients by inoculation of suckling mice. One of the most interesting points about the virus was that the vector was found to be *Anopheles funestus*, a common vector of malaria in East Africa. This was the first time that a carrier of malaria had been shown to transmit a virus disease.

GROUP B

The most important disease-producing members of this antigenically related group produce several types of illness: (1) Japanese B, St. Louis (United States) and Murray Valley (Australia) encephalitis. (2) Dengue and yellow fever. (3) West Nile fever. (4) Russian spring-summer complex.

1. These are all mosquito-borne, particularly by culicines, and small outbreaks tend to occur at intervals of a year or more, probably due to the time and conditions required to build up a number of susceptible animal and avian hosts, e.g. swine and egrets for Japanese B in Japan. Over 90 per cent. of infections in man are asymptomatic or sufficiently mild to be unrecognizable. In the 10 per cent. or less who develop acute encephalitis from Japanese B the mortality rate is 20–50 per cent., being much higher in old people. Twenty per cent. of the survivors have permanent sequelae such as mental defects and physical disorders. St. Louis and Murray Valley infections are milder in every way.

2. Dengue and yellow fever are considered on pages 199, 200.

3. West Nile fever often occurs as an epidemic, sometimes as a serious febrile disease with abdominal pain and vomiting, rash and lymphadenopathy. It occasionally causes fatal encephalitis in the aged.

4. The Russian spring-summer complex are tick-borne, the vector is usually *Ixodes ricinus* or *I. persulcatus*. These usually cause a mild systemic infection in ruminants or small rodents of the forest but occasionally cause death from encephalitis in sheep (louping ill) or generalized disease in monkeys (Kyasanur Forest disease). Until a few years ago this group was only recognized in Russia (Russian spring-summer encephalitis) and Scotland and northern England (louping ill), but a closely related virus is present in Finland and Sweden and much of south eastern Europe (Poland, Czechoslovakia, Jugoslavia, Austria). In 1957 a virus of this group was demonstrated to be responsible for a severe systemic disease involving monkeys and man in the Kyasanur Forest a few miles inland in the State of Mysore in India and another, the Powassan virus, was isolated from the brain of a fatal case of encephalitis in Ontario, Canada.

Signs and Symptoms

RSSE may present in the acute phase as meningitis or meningo-encephalitis, possibly with paralysis; a sub-cortical lesion with extrapyramidal signs; or as the polio-encephalomyelitis type with severe paralysis, usually fatal. In the latter there may be residual paralysis in up to 50 per cent. of survivors. The total mortality rate has been variously reported as 1–20 per cent.

Pathology

RSSE virus attacks particularly the nuclei of the reticular formation, the substantia nigra and the anterior horn of the cervical spinal cord.

Prophylaxis and Treatment

Inactivated virus vaccines are now available for protection against this group, but they are subtype specific; that from RSSE is not protective against Kyasanur Forest disease. There is no specific treatment.

GROUP C AND OTHER GROUPS

In addition to the A and B groups, other smaller divisions have been possible by serological tests, e.g. a C group of viruses from Brazil, a Guama group with several viruses from the Amazon region and one from Trinidad, and a Bunyamwera group including viruses from the United States, Trinidad, South America and southern Africa. Finally there is a large antigenically unrelated miscellaneous group which includes Rift Valley fever, Colorado tick fever, sandfly fever [see p. 203] and numerous others which affect man.

The large majority of these viruses other than groups A and B have been isolated only from mosquitoes or sentinel mice stationed in forest regions and some have been recovered only in a single season in one area where trapping has been continuous over a number of years. In several instances antibody surveys have indicated that these viruses have caused little or no infection in domestic animals or man in the region. Proof of their possible pathogenicity for man depends in some cases on the occurrence of infection in laboratory workers. Although they are of no importance to man at the present time it is possible that, with alterations of the agricultural and economic conditions of some of these areas, an infringement on the rodent or avian-mosquito cycle may result in an alteration or extension of infection to new vectors in closer contact with man and hence to outbreaks of disease.

RIFT VALLEY FEVER

The natural host of this virus is the sheep and it was originally isolated from sick sheep which died with a hepatitis in the Rift Valley in Kenya in 1930. It was recognized that sheep herders and others in areas associated with the diseased animals might develop a febrile illness and infection of laboratory workers handling the virus resulted in a similar illness in a high proportion of them. The virus was of particular interest because it produced necrosis of the liver and, although immunologically unrelated to yellow fever, a reciprocal interference between these two viruses could be shown under the appropriate experimental conditions in mice and monkeys.

Although antibodies to the virus were found in sera of primates from North and West Africa in 1939 and it was isolated from forest mosquitoes in Uganda little attention was paid to it outside virus laboratories. However, in 1950 it suddenly appeared in the Union of South Africa where it caused severe outbreaks of disease with a high mortality in new-born sheep and calves. Infections occurred in farmers and veterinarians, some of whom developed choroidoretinitis with prolonged impairment of vision. The virus was later recovered from species of *Aëdes* and *Culex* mosquitoes.

An attenuated vaccine is now being used to protect non-pregnant sheep and cattle and lambs and calves over 3 months of age in areas where the disease has been present.

COLORADO TICK FEVER

Although this disease was described by the early white settlers in the Rocky Mountains area, a clear clinical description with implication of a tick as the vector was made only in 1930. Until the recent isolation of Powassan virus in Ontario it was the only known tick-borne virus infection in North America. Infection is confined to those in contact with the wood tick *Dermacentor andersoni* in the months of March to June.

The usual clinical picture is that of a sharp onset with fever, malaise, headache and pains of localized and general distribution. A remission for a day or two often occurs after a few days and is followed by a second febrile period. There is no rash or obvious physical signs other than mild inflammation of the throat and conjunctiva. Recovery may be prolonged. Severe meningitis or encephalitis may occur in a small proportion of those infected. Subclinical infections are not uncommon.

Treatment

There is no specific treatment.

REFERENCES

WORK, T. H. (1963) Tick-borne viruses; a review of an arthropod-borne virus problem of growing importance in the tropics, *Bull. Wld Hlth Org.*, **29**, 59.

WORLD HEALTH ORGANIZATION (1967) Arthropod-borne viruses *Wld Hlth Org. tech. Rep. Ser.*, No. 369.

F. O. MACCALLUM

DENGUE FEVER

Synonym. Breakbone fever.

Aetiology

Dengue is caused by a Group B arbovirus. It occurs in most of the tropics and subtropics, especially in coastal areas, from southern North America, South America, West Indies, Mediterranean seaboard, Egypt, Middle East, North, Central and South Africa, Greece, Russia, Turkey, Middle East, India, China, many Pacific islands, Philippines, Thailand, Solomon Islands and Northern Australia.

There are at least four overlapping antigenic strains.

An attack produces immunity against the homologous strain lasting about a year and against other strains for a variable period of months. Epidemics are therefore likely to occur every two or three years in an endemic area.

The vector is the female *Aëdes* mosquito, usually *Aëdes aegypti.*

The virus is present in the blood of human patients for as long as three days after the onset of the illness and possibly for a short time before. The mosquito becomes infective 8–14 days after ingesting blood containing the virus and remains infected for the rest of its life. The virus is injected during the bite of the fly. Transmission depends on the presence of infective vectors and non-immune hosts. Man is the usual reservoir of infection, although some monkeys may carry certain strains of the virus.

Since the vector breeds in hot moist conditions and not in the cold, the disease is often seasonal in its incidence, outbreaks occurring in the wet seasons in the tropics and in the summer and autumn in the subtropics.

When non-immunes are numerous and the local community has been free from disease for more than a year and immunity is low, explosive epidemics may appear which burn themselves out after the majority of the population has been infected.

The pathological changes induced in man are not clearly determined. Classical dengue is not fatal.

The same viruses in certain circumstances cause severe mosquito-borne South-East Asian haemorrhagic fever, which may be fatal [see p. 215].

Signs and Symptoms

The clinical picture varies according to the outbreak or epidemic, the geographical area and the individual. The disease lasts anything from 1–10 days. The incubation period may be only a few days or as long as a fortnight, usually about 5–10 days. There may be some prodromal malaise, headache or shivering. The onset is very abrupt and the patient can often recall the exact time he became ill. The body temperature rises rapidly up to 103°–105° F. (39·4°–40·5° C.), frequently with rigor. The other signs and symptoms begin immediately. The most impressive are severe headache, usually supra-orbital, and associated with tenderness of the orbital muscles, which causes pain on eye movement; intense agonizing pains in the joints, long bones and back, depression and insomnia.

The sharp shooting body pains are accompanied by soreness on pressure over the muscles and tendons and especially at muscle insertions around the joints.

The patient is anorexic and complains of epigastric discomfort. There is nausea and sometimes vomiting may be severe.

Blotchy congestion of the peripheral circulation is common, especially on the face and the hands and is sometimes thought to be a rash. Epistaxis is common.

Photophobia is pronounced and there is puffiness of the eyelids, severe conjunctival injection and sometimes excessive weeping.

The nasopharynx is not affected and unlike influenza, there are no respiratory symptoms.

In general the patient is restless, anxious, depressed. The pulse is at first rapid, but may slow considerably in the first 2–3 days even when the fever is high, thus resembling the pulse in yellow fever. It remains slow until convalescence.

The fever is initially high, it may be remittent or continuous. It falls to normal after 3–4 days usually by crisis, accompanied by sweating and sometimes diarrhoea. The temperature may now remain normal and the patient recovers or there may be a remission, lasting a few hours or one or two days during which the symptoms subside, followed by a second febrile episode in which the temperature rise is only moderate and lasts 2–3 days and ends by lysis.

The two febrile phases separated by a short remission, constitute the classical 'saddle-back' fever which was once considered characteristic of dengue, but which is in fact not always present. A simple remittent fever lasting a few days is probably commoner.

The rash in dengue seldom develops before the fourth or fifth day and may therefore not appear until the second febrile stage. It occurs as a regular feature in some outbreaks and is absent in others. In a given outbreak it may be the characteristic feature of the infection, but some cases will not develop a rash and in others it may be only fleeting and may be missed. It is morbilliform but bright red, and fades easily on pressure. In severe cases some macules become petechial. The eruption, which is itchy, appears first on the dorsum of the hands or feet, and spreads rapidly to the arms and legs and may include the trunk and involve the face. It develops rapidly and begins to fade as the temperature subsides. Fine desquamation follows. Scratching may lead to secondary infection. The pruritus is often the overriding concern of the already depressed sufferer.

Leucopenia with granulocytopenia develops by the third day, the leucocyte count ranging from 2000–4000 cells per mm^3.

In some epidemics there is a general adenitis which is symmetrical or confined to certain groups of glands which are palpable, discrete and only slightly tender. This may or may not be associated with the rash.

Diagnosis

Diagnosis is easy in epidemics and difficult in isolated cases. It is often impossible to separate dengue clinically from phlebotomus fever especially where there is no rash. In the early stages, before the rash develops, dengue may be confused with influenza, but the absence of respiratory involvement is usually indicative.

Certain of the dengue viruses are concerned in the acute haemorrhagic fevers which occur in the East which may be difficult to differentiate in the early stages.

Virological techniques are necessary to identify the organisms.

Treatment

There is no specific treatment but measures are aimed at the control of symptoms such as itching, headache and insomnia.

YELLOW FEVER

Definition and Aetiology

Yellow fever is a febrile illness of short duration resulting from infection with a Group B arbovirus which appears to be the same in all endemic areas, and which is transmitted by certain genera of Culicine mosquitoes, especially *Aëdes aegypti*.

Yellow fever is endemic in many parts of West and Central Africa from Senegal to Angola. Immunity surveys have disclosed that the disease is much more widely spread than was formerly realized, and have shown that it occurs in Kenya, Uganda, Somalia and Zambia. Tanganyika appears to be free. In Uganda the permanent focus of infection is in the forest belt where the disease is enzootic in monkeys. It also occurs in tropical South America in Venezuela, Bolivia, Peru, Colombia and Brazil and is endemic in certain parts of the West Indies, including Trinidad.

Severe cases occurring in non-immunes exhibit fever, slow pulse, progressive albuminuria, vomiting, jaundice and varying degrees of renal, hepatic and circulatory failure. There is a high mortality rate. In indigenes of endemic areas the disease is usually mild.

Yellow fever is much more narrowly distributed than its possible vectors, which abound in many areas, including Asia, in which the disease has never occurred.

The small virus is present in the blood up to the fourth day of disease and occasionally for longer periods. It can be transmitted to rhesus monkeys by blood inoculation or intracerebrally into white mice. After repeated passage it becomes avirulent. This altered virus is the basis of the living attenuated vaccines used for immunization.

A very powerful and long-lasting immunity to subsequent infection is developed by the tenth day of an attack of yellow fever. Successful vaccination also gives rise to very powerful immunity after the same time.

Cross-immunity with certain other viruses occurs and it is believed that some viruses can stimulate and accelerate the production of the immune bodies by the yellow fever virus.

Factors such as these probably protect the children of endemic areas and account for the mildness of the attacks seen in them. The vectors are female mosquitoes, including *Aëdes*. The vector receives the virus by ingesting infected human or animal blood. It becomes infective to man 14–21 days later and remains infective for the rest of its life.

There are three epidemiological forms of yellow fever: the urban, rural and jungle, which differ in regard to vectors and sources of infection.

In urban yellow fever the reservoir is man and the vector exclusively the domestic mosquito *Aëdes aegypti*. In rural yellow fever the reservoir may be man or animals and the vector is again usually *A. aegypti*. In the jungle form of the disease, the reservoir is not man, but certain forest animals and the vectors are various species of *Aëdes* or *Haemogogus*.

Transmission in all areas depends on a supply of vectors, infective reservoirs and suitably non-immune hosts.

Epidemics may develop, where conditions are favourable, but unless the supply of non-immunes is maintained the epidemic will die out as the survivors become immune.

In endemic areas infection is kept going mainly in young children. Infants are not easily infected in the early months because of immunity transmitted from the mother.

Adults native to endemic areas are commonly protected against reinfection as the result of infection in childhood.

Aëdes aegypti breeds in and about human dwellings in small quantities of water lying in artificial containers, tree holes, etc. Breeding may continue through the year, but where rains and dry seasons alternate, transmission is seasonal, and maximal during the rains.

Jungle yellow fever occurs in individuals living or working in forest regions and is transmitted to man by accident.

In Uganda, for instance, it is passed from monkey to monkey by the mosquito *Aëdes africanus*, which normally lives at high levels in the trees and is thus unlikely to transmit the infection to man. Spread to humans probably occurs as a result of accidental infection of some other vector in the forest regions such as *Aëdes simpsoni* which bites an infected monkey descended from the forest. In forest regions of Brazil yellow fever is transmitted from animal to animal by mosquitoes which are found during the day chiefly in the tree tops but which descend at night to ground level and may thus transmit directly to man.

Once the disease is established in humans it may be transmitted from man to man by vectors including *Aëdes aegypti* and may then become epidemic.

Pathology

In the pathology of yellow fever there is little specific. Jaundice is minimal but may be pronounced in fulminating or prolonged cases. There are often petechial haemorrhages beneath the skin and mucous membranes and in the pleura, pericardium and the peritoneum. The lungs may be oedematous and contain moderate haemorrhages. The liver shows characteristic changes and the kidneys are sometimes tense and swollen with scattered medullary congestion and cortical ischaemia.

Altered blood is found in the gastric and intestinal contents and the intestinal mucosa is often covered with petechial haemorrhages most prominent in the upper part of the small intestine and in the stomach.

The degenerative and necrotic changes in the liver tissue occur mostly in polygonal cells of the midzone, but they may spread to the central and peripheral zones and are often associated with widespread fatty degeneration. The cytoplasm of the affected cells undergoes coagulative degeneration and necrosis, breaking up into masses which stain deep pink with eosin (Councilman's bodies). In some cases, but not all, changes also occur in the nucleus, in which the nucleolus disappears, the chromatin is displaced peripherally and the centre is filled with granular acidophilic material (Torres bodies). Neither of these changes is concerned with the actual presence of the virus, which is found in the cytoplasm. This non-specific midzonal necrosis is also found in other conditions than yellow fever, including certain forms of viral encephalitis and severe burns. It is nevertheless sufficiently characteristic to be useful in diagnosis.

Loss of blood by haemorrhage leads to anaemia in severe cases. This may be masked by haemoconcentration if circulatory failure supervenes.

Leucopenia of the order of 3000–4000 cells per mm^3. develops by the third day. There is the unusual feature of granulocytopenia with a 'shift to the left'. Normal leucocyte counts are restored in convalescence.

In severe cases prothrombin is reduced and clotting time increased.

The plasma bilirubin is moderately raised early and increases as clinical jaundice appears. The transaminases are increased but other liver function tests are not always impaired unless there is obvious hepatic failure.

Other changes in the blood depend on the clinical situation and are non-specific. Blood urea nitrogen and non-protein nitrogen rise in the early stages and may reach very high levels in anuric and uraemic cases.

The urinary volume is invariably reduced. In many cases there is oliguria and in severe cases anuria, with accompanying uraemia. The urine has a low chloride content. Albumin escapes in increasing amounts as the disease progresses and may reach levels of several grammes per litre. Tubular casts are present in most cases. In some there may be erythrocytes or frank haematuria. Bile is usually present by the fourth or fifth day.

Signs and Symptoms

The progress of yellow fever depends on whether the patient is partly immune or non-immune.

In endemic areas the disease is usually mild amongst indigenes and especially in children. Non-immunes are highly susceptible in all areas and in them the classical clinical picture develops.

The incubation period is 3–6 days with a maximum of 10 days.

Mild cases may be accompanied by severe headache and some fever, conjunctival injection, nausea and vomiting. Albuminuria occurs early, but is light and rapidly disappears. Recovery occurs in a few days.

In more severe cases the fever starts abruptly, sometimes with rigor, reaches 104° F. (40° C.) or so and then becomes remittent for a few days, subsiding by lysis. The patient complains of headache, backache, bone and joint pains. The skin is congested, the conjunctivae injected and there may be epistaxis. There is usually some epigastric discomfort. The picture may be difficult to distinguish from dengue.

The classical picture, which occurs in previously unexposed subjects, is much more serious and develops in two main phases, separated by an afebrile interval of comparative calm.

The first phase is severe. The onset is abrupt. The temperature rises, frequently with rigor, to 102°–103° F. (38·9°–39·4° C.) and remains at about this level for 3–4 days, subsequently falling to normal. The pulse rate is fast at onset, but drops rapidly in the first 24–48 hours sometimes to as low as 50 beats per minute. The falling pulse rate in relation to the temperature was once regarded as a classical diagnostic sign of yellow fever (Faget's first sign). It presents in two ways, either as a steady pulse with rising temperature or a falling pulse with a steady temperature.

In the early stages peripheral congestion is pronounced, giving the face a blotchy appearance. There is severe conjunctival injection with photophobia and bleeding from the nose and gums. Headache, backache and limb pains are severe. The patient is restless and prostrated, with severe epigastric discomfort, tenderness, anorexia, nausea and vomiting. The vomit contains bile and sometimes also blood swallowed after epistaxis. There is commonly watery diarrhoea and blood may be present in the stool.

Jaundice does not appear as a rule before the fourth or fifth day. It is usually not pronounced and may be no more than an icteric tinge. The yellow colour can sometimes be recognized only by blanching the skin. In some epidemics jaundice may develop rapidly and become intense; the clinical picture then very closely resembles infective hepatitis.

Protein, mostly albumin, appears in the urine on the first day and increases steadily in amount. Tubular casts appear early and the urine volume invariably falls to oliguric levels. Anuria may develop in the later stages.

At the end of the first febrile episode the temperature falls to normal levels, the signs and symptoms subside and the patient feels much better. In severe cases, however, after a few hours the fever returns and the patient passes rapidly into a state of intoxication and prostration. The temperature rises rapidly, but seldom reaches the former levels. The pulse quickens slightly, but remains slow in relation to the fever. The second febrile episode seldom lasts more than eight days. In the late stages of severe cases the pulse rate may suddenly become very fast and there is an equally sharp fall in temperature to normal or below. This phenomenon, which is sometimes called Faget's second or prognostic sign, represents the onset of medical shock, and usually indicates a fatal issue.

In the second febrile phase signs and symptoms present in the first period become exaggerated. Epigastric discomfort, nausea and vomiting are severe. Bleeding from the mucous membranes is general and leads to vomiting of changed blood, the so-called 'black vomit', and to melaena. Petechial haemorrhages occur into the mucous membranes and under the skin and there is persistent bleeding from the nose and lips from which fresh blood may appear in the vomit.

In the classical case, the jaundice increases and bile appears in the urine. The liver is not usually palpable but in some epidemics, fulminating cases may occur in which there is considerable liver enlargement and intense deepening jaundice.

Albuminuria is present throughout the illness. It increases steadily and becomes very pronounced. Oliguria is invariable during the disease and may go on to anuria especially in cases which are markedly oliguric from the start. Acute renal failure with anuria, rising blood urea and acute uraemia, is the commonest cause of death.

The second stage is usually dominated by the signs of renal, hepatic or circulatory failure, singly or together. In fulminating cases there may be no remission, and death occurs in the first few days of the overt illness, usually from acute liver failure.

The patient is usually conscious throughout the illness, but is restless and anxious or deeply prostrated and apathetic. There may be terminal delirium.

The attack lasts as a rule not more than 14 days. In non-immunes the mortality is high, death usually taking place during the second febrile period between the fifth and tenth day. On the other hand, the over-all mortality is low since the vast majority of cases of yellow fever occurring in indigenes of an endemic area are mild and recovery is the rule. Natives of adjacent areas in which the disease is uncommon or absent, however, are liable to develop the full-scale illness during epidemics in which the death rate may be high.

Diagnosis

The clinical diagnosis of the isolated mild case is difficult. In an outbreak it is relatively easy, especially in the non-immune.

The differential diagnosis includes other viral infections such as infective hepatitis, some of which, for example, haemorrhagic fever, may be excluded on geographical grounds. In infective hepatitis a history of exposure to known cases or recent syringe therapy may be helpful; there is a febrile pre-icteric stage, and fever often subsides as the jaundice, which is deeper and more persistent, develops. The liver is usually palpable and may be tender. Fulminating cases of infective hepatitis and yellow fever may be clinically indistinguishable.

The early stages of dengue and allied arbovirus infections may cause some difficulties which may be dispelled by the appearance of the rash or adenitis. Otherwise the clinical progress and serological reactions should make the distinction.

Confusion has often arisen clinically with blackwater fever and falciparum malaria, in both of which jaundice, associated with enlargement and tenderness of the liver, may appear early and deepen rapidly. The discovery of haemoglobinuria or parasites in the blood should settle the issue.

High fever, proteinuria, jaundice and black vomit may occur in both relapsing fever and leptospirosis, both of which may appear in endemic yellow fever areas. Careful parasitological and bacterial examinations are needed to separate these conditions from yellow fever in the early stages.

The specific diagnosis of yellow fever depends on the demonstration of *a rising titre of protective antibody in the serum,* as measured by the mouse protection test. Antibodies are detectable in the serum on the fourth day after the onset and reach their maximum by the tenth day. Thereafter they persist in high titre for many years. Serum samples should therefore be taken from the patient on admission and at intervals subsequently. Assay of antibodies in a single sample of serum may help, for if they are present in high concentration at the onset of a febrile illness or absent late the diagnosis of current yellow fever can be ruled out.

In suitably equipped laboratories the virus may be isolated from blood taken from the patient in the first four days (occasionally up to the tenth day).

At autopsy, the pattern of midzonal liver necrosis described above is a valuable clue to the diagnosis. It can be demonstrated rapidly by frozen section. In endemic areas where autopsies are sometimes difficult to obtain, liver samples are sometimes taken through the abdominal wall with a viscerotome.

Treatment

There is as yet no specific treatment. Sulphonamides and antibiotics are ineffective against the virus.

The patient must be nursed under a mosquito net and kept as quiet as possible. He should be offered soft food containing protein if he will take it, and glucose drinks. Water and electrolyte balance must be adjusted by intravenous infusion of glucose saline in dehydrated patients. Where there is severe diarrhoea, potassium chloride should be given orally if possible or added to the rehydrating fluid. Parenteral plasma or plasma substitutes are needed in shock. Protein hydrolysates may also be given intravenously.

Renal failure must be treated by the standard methods. In all cases each specimen passed should be measured and examined in order to keep check on the development of anuria, which may be sudden.

Parenteral administration of vitamin K may be needed especially in cases in which the vascular and liver damage is considerable.

Prophylaxis

Entomological control of the vector of urban yellow fever, *Aëdes aegypti* is possible in cities and towns. Elsewhere it is not.

Individuals and communities can be protected by vaccination with attentuated virus, prepared from the original 17D strain isolated in Ghana, or from a strain isolated in Dakar, Senegal. Vaccination provides extremely powerful immunity within 10 days of inoculation of the virus. Vaccination should not be carried out in children younger than 9 months and it is usual to allow an interval of 6 weeks between vaccination for smallpox and for yellow fever, although in mass campaigns the vaccines are often given simultaneously. International regulations regard vaccination as providing adequate protection for a period of 10 years.

SANDFLY FEVER

Synonyms. Pappataci fever; Three-day fever.

Definition

An acute non-fatal arbovirus infection which has not yet been grouped and which is transmitted by the sandfly *Phlebotomus* spp.

Aetiology

The distribution depends on the fly which is common in many parts of the tropics and subtropics. The incidence of the disease has been greatly reduced by the use of modern insecticides.

The causal virus is unclassified at present. It is present in the blood of the patient shortly before the onset and for about one day afterwards. The reservoir of infection is man.

The vector is the female *Phlebotomus* or sandfly. These insects are most active and ferocious at night and rest in cool shady places and cracks in stonework during the day. They fly only 100 metres or so from their breeding grounds so that transmission is very local.

The fly becomes infective about a week after ingesting blood in which the virus is circulating; it remains infective for life.

Transmission is seasonal, appearing usually in the late spring or autumn. It is sometimes epidemic in the summer.

All non-immunes are highly susceptible. Some immunity is acquired against the homologous strain, but this is of short duration and in a local epidemic indigenes are usually unaffected. There is some cross-immunity between the various strains of the sandfly virus, but not with dengue.

Signs and Symptoms

The disease is not fatal. It resembles dengue but there is no rash, no adenitis and no saddle-back fever. The whole illness takes only 3–4 days.

The incubation period is 3–7 days.

The onset is very sudden, with a rapid rise of temperature up to 105° F. (40·5° C.), commonly with rigor. The fever is remittent and lasts for 1–4 days resolving by crisis, accompanied by intense sweating and sometimes epistaxis. The signs and symptoms appear as abruptly as the fever. The peripheral circulation is congested; the nasopharynx and conjunctivae are injected. There is photophobia and lacrimation. The main complaints are severe headache, with pain in the back of the orbit, pains and aches in the long bones, joints and back, depression, anorexia, nausea and sometimes vomiting. There may be some bronchitis. The pulse often becomes slow in relation to the fever, but it may be very fast.

There is a leucopenia similar to that in dengue but no rash or adenitis.

Convalescence may be slow because of depression.

Diagnosis

There is as yet no easy laboratory method for making a diagnosis, which depends largely on the clinical picture. The disease is easily recognized during an epidemic, but is often confused with atypical dengue, influenza or the early stages of haemorrhagic fever.

Treatment

Treatment is entirely symptomatic.

BRIAN MAEGRAITH

VARIOUS UNCLASSIFIED VIRUS INFECTIONS

HERPES SIMPLEX

Synonym. Herpes febrilis or labialis.

Definition

An acute infectious disease characterized by superficial vesicles containing clear fluid in the skin and mucous membranes particularly of the buccal area and sometimes on the conjunctiva and cornea and genitalia, but may occur anywhere on the body. Occasionally the primary infection is generalized, affecting many organs, particularly in children or it may cause disease of the central nervous system. The vesicles on the skin usually dry up after 7–10 days and the scabs disappear usually without scarring. Recurrent attacks, usually at the same site, may occur at intervals varying from weeks to years throughout life.

Aetiology

The disease is caused by a medium-sized virus (*Herpesvirus hominis*) about 180 millimicrons in diameter with a deoxyribonucleic acid (DNA) core. There are at least two serological types, I and II. Virus from genital sites is usually type II. Virus from all other sites is usually type I, but may be type II. Primary infection occurs in persons without antibody, usually in children. Recurrent attacks with vesicles occur in persons with antibody who are carriers of the virus and in whom the balance between immunity and virus activity is upset. A closely related virus (B virus), which is normally found in various species of monkeys, may affect man producing encephalomyelitis, usually with fatal consequences.

Pathology

Histologically the lesions in the skin and mucous membranes resemble those seen in chickenpox and zoster. Proliferation of the epithelium is followed by swelling of the cytoplasm and nuclei of basal epithelial cells. As a result of cell necrosis and the production of large amounts of intercellular serous exudate unilocular vesicles are formed beneath the stratum corneum. Multinucleated giant cells with intranuclear inclusions may be found in the base of the vesicles. Necrotic lesions are found in the liver, and adrenals and sometimes in the lung and brain when fatal generalized infection occurs in the newborn or in infants with eczema. In fatal encephalitis, which may occur at any age, there is marked engorgement of the brain and meninges with area of softening, mainly in the cortex, but also in the subcortical white matter. Intranuclear inclusions are found in glial and nerve cells.

Symptoms and Signs

The incubation period in the primary attack is 4–5 days.

The primary attack which usually occurs in childhood is most often subclinical, but may present as a vesicular gingivostomatitis with fever; irritability, malaise and local adenopathy may be present. Mild attacks in children are often misdiagnosed as 'teething'. In adults, there may also be sore throat, adenitis and fever. In a small proportion of patients primary infection may manifest itself as acute meningitis or encephalitis and in others there are vesicles at some area of trauma, such as the eye, where it is a common cause of keratitis with ulceration, the site of a fracture, on the terminal phalanx of fingers where it may simulate a bacterial whitlow, or on the genitalia. Severe widespread infection of the skin may occur in patients with eczema. Rarely, primary infection occurs as a rapidly fatal generalized disease in the neonatal period particularly in premature babies, or in children in the first 2 years of life who are suffering from malnutrition or some other debilitating disease, such as severe measles.

Recurrent attacks may occur at the site of the primary lesion. They are usually precipitated by some febrile illness or metabolic upset, e.g. a common cold, lobar pneumonia, malaria, meningococcal infection or ovulation, psychological disturbance or trauma. After a short period of tingling and itching small painful papules appear which rapidly develop into vesicles containing clear watery fluid. Although usually scattered at primary infection, the distribution of the vesicles, particularly in recurrent attacks on the face, may be similar to those of zoster. The vesicles dry up after 7–10 days leaving a scab which usually drops off without scarring.

Diagnosis

The vesicular eruption on the skin and mucous membranes and the accompanying illness are usually typical, but doubt may arise in impetigo, aphthous ulcers and herpes gestationis, none of which are of virus aetiology. The lesion in herpes simplex infection of eczematous skin may be indistinguishable from that caused by vaccinia. Herpes simplex infections on the face may simulate zoster and herpetic whitlows may be mistaken by the inexperienced for those caused by bacteria. The herpetic whitlow is characterized by excruciating pain, by vesicles which initially contain clear fluid and by extensive transient tissue destruction. The precise aetiology of these lesions, as well as general infection of the newborn, encephalitis and meningitis due to herpes simplex, can only be diagnosed by laboratory methods.

The virus may be isolated from vesicle fluid or scrapings of the base of lesions on skin and mucous membranes, scrapings of conjunctiva or corneal lesions in a primary infection (but less often from a recurrent ulcer of the cornea); from brain biopsy in encephalitis and sometimes from cerebrospinal fluid; rarely from the blood at the onset of a primary infection; from the blood, liver, adrenals, brain and other affected organs in fatal infections. Tissue cultures are the most sensitive medium, but embryonated egg and suckling mice, may be used.

Stained smears of scrapings of the base of ulcers may show giant multinucleated cells but these may also be present in varicella and zoster. Acidophilic intranuclear inclusions may be found in cells of affected tissues.

The immunofluorescence technique may be used on smears from lesions of skin or mucous membranes, biopsy specimens or tissues obtained at autopsy. Electronmicroscopy may be applied to similar specimens.

In a primary infection there is an increase of antibodies in the blood in convalescence which can be measured by various tests. No increase in antibodies can usually be detected after recurrent attacks.

Treatment

In the past a large variety of agents have been used in the treatment of herpes, such as dyes, antiseptics and soothing ointments, but few, if any, have a specific action. Though no infallible treatment for all types of herpes simplex infection has yet been developed, 5-iodo-2′deoxyuridine (idoxuridine) is of benefit in the treatment of herpetic lesions of the skin and eye and probably other sites. The drug is potentially mutagenic and should not be used in pregnant women with the possible exception of a primary infection occurring in the terminal stages of pregnancy. Idoxuridine is insoluble in most common solvents and has no effect when applied as an ointment on the skin. When applied in the form of a solution of 5 per cent. idoxuridine in dimethyl sulphoxide (DMSO), the duration of recurrent lesions is much reduced and the discomfort disappears within hours. Recurrences in the same site are rare after effective treatment. The solution is applied three times a day for 3 days. Herpetic gingivostomatitis can be improved by the use of idoxuridine in orabase which will adhere to the ulcers. Local application of iodine in collodion gives a symptomatic relief. Intensive treatment with continuous application of idoxuridine in DMSO is of value in the treatment of herpetic whitlows. Pain is relieved within hours. The treatment should continue until virus cultures are negative.

Idoxuridine as drops or ointment is of value in the treatment of herpetic keratitis, if used judiciously by an ophthalmologist familiar with the action of the drug. Debridement, carbolization, iodization and the use of antibacterial drugs still have a place in the treatment of this condition and in selected cases of recurrent herpetic corneal ulcers simultaneous use of corticosteroids and idoxuridine have been of value. Corticosteroids should not be used alone.

A small number of cases of herpetic encephalitis have been treated with systemic idoxuridine with variable results, possibly because the diagnosis is usually made too late. Systemic treatment may be attempted in generalized herpetic infection in which the severity of the disease outweighs the risk of possible toxic effect of the drug.

In *eczema herpeticum* it may be necessary to replace loss of fluid and electrolytes and control secondary bacterial infection with antibiotics. Recurrent attacks may be prevented by controlling the trigger mechanism responsible, e.g. use of aspirin when elevation of temperature is expected at the time of ovulation.

Intravenous inoculation of cytosine arabinoside (*Cytarabine*), 2 mg. per kg. per day in a single daily dose for 5 days, may be of value in the treatment of severe infection in patients with leukaemia who are being treated with immunosuppressive drugs.

Prognosis

The ordinary infection is self-limiting unless complicated by secondary bacterial infection, particularly in eczematous infants in whom the disease may be fatal. Corneal lesions are likely to be recurrent and may lead to blindness. Systemic infection of the newborn is usually fatal. Herpes encephalitis may cause permanent damage to the brain with sequelae such as paralysis, mental retardation and behaviour difficulties. This may occur more frequently than is at present realized. All types of infection may be more severe in patients receiving corticosteroids for other purposes.

F. O. MacCallum

MUMPS

Synonyms. Epidemic parotitis; Infective parotitis.

Definition

An acute infectious disease normally characterized by swelling of the parotid or other salivary glands. Although there are a considerable number of complications death is exceedingly rare.

Aetiology and Epidemiology

Mumps is due to infection by a virus which has an affinity for glandular and nervous tissue. It belongs to the group of myxoviruses (which include para-influenza virus 1 and 2). Mumps occurs all over the world being endemic in all large areas of population. Although primarily a disease of childhood no age is exempt; 25 per cent. of cases occur between 0–4 years; 56 per cent. between 5–9 years; 11 per cent. between 10–14 years; and 8 per cent. after puberty. The disease is rare in infants. Localized epidemics are commonest in the spring but may arise at other times of year.

Infection is direct from patient to patient but mild or subclinical infection is not uncommon and is responsible for some spread of the disease. The virus probably enters through the nose or mouth but the site of primary multiplication is uncertain. Some believe it to be in the parotid glands while others consider it takes place in the epithelium of the respiratory tract. A viraemia occurs at the onset of the illness with localization in glandular and nervous tissue.

Pathology

Due to the benign nature of the disease opportunity for pathological study is rare. Inflamed glandular tissue shows oedema and lymphocytic infiltration with debris and leucocytes occupying the lumina of the ducts. Surrounding soft tissue may also become oedematous.

Symptoms

The incubation period is 18–21 days with probable extremes of 14–30 days.

In the majority of cases there is swelling of the parotid glands but it should be realized that mumps without salivary gland involvement is by no means rare. Indeed, in some outbreaks such cases have amounted to approximately 10 per cent. Almost any 'complication' of mumps may appear as the sole manifestation of the disease.

In the common form swelling of one parotid is the first sign of the disease. This may be associated with mild fever and constitutional symptoms which not uncommonly precede the glandular swelling by 1–2 days. Earache or pain in the region of the masseter or shivering with slight sore throat may be premonitory symptoms.

The parotid swelling is at first unilateral; it increases for 2–3 days forming an ill-defined elastic swelling which is frequently much more clearly seen than it is felt. The sulcus between the mandible and the mastoid process is obliterated, the lobe of the ear being pushed upwards and forwards. Only rarely is the skin over the gland reddened or oedematous. The swelling subsides after a few days, sometimes very quickly. Frequently 24–48 hours after the appearance of the first gland the parotid on the other side becomes enlarged. Occasionally the interval between invasion of the two parotid glands is extended up to 7 or even rarely 10 days. The submandibular and sublingual glands may be attacked. Sometimes the former become swollen before a parotid; palpation with one finger in the mouth and another below the jaw will reveal the swelling which lies just anterior to the angle of the jaw. The parotid may escape or may swell in its turn. The lacrimal glands are only rarely involved. The swollen glands are uncomfortable due to tension rather than being acutely painful. The thought or sight of food may cause an increased ache due to salivary secretion. Trismus may occur. The orifices of the ducts, particularly Stensen's ducts, are often swollen and red in the early stages and give useful confirmation that a vague swelling is parotid in origin. A moderate degree of cervical lymph node enlargement may accompany mumps.

Moderate pyrexia, 101°–102° F. (38·3°–38·9° C.) may accompany the onset and persist for a day or two but many attacks remain afebrile throughout especially in young children. A relative bradycardia is sometimes a feature in febrile patients. One attack usually confers life-long immunity.

Complications

The viraemia of mumps may give rise to a wide variety of glandular or neurological manifestations, any one of which may appear in isolation without preceding parotid gland swelling.

Of glandular complications *orchitis* is by far the commonest. This is very rare before puberty but occurs in 20–30 per cent. of postpubertal males. In some outbreaks an incidence of over 50 per cent. has been reported. It appears 7–14 days after the onset although in some instances orchitis precedes the inflammation of the salivary glands. The onset is acute with abdominal or testicular pain, vomiting and considerable fever. The affected testicle rapidly becomes hot, swollen and acutely tender with widespread inflammation affecting the epididymis in addition to the body of the gland. In most instances only one testis is involved, bilateral orchitis arising in about 10 per cent. of those who develop this complication, i.e. an incidence of about 2 per cent. in postpubertal males. The lesion subsides spontaneously within a week, the temperature often falling abruptly on the third or fourth day. Relapse occasionally occurs. In spite of the fact that some degree of testicular atrophy may follow an attack loss of libido or sterility seem to be rare sequelae of bilateral orchitis. Spermatogenesis has been demonstrated even when both testes have appeared to be atrophic.

In the female patient *oophoritis*, with transient pelvic pain and mild fever, is a much less frequent complication.

Pancreatitis is less common than orchitis but leads to diagnostic errors particularly when it precedes the parotitis. Symptoms most often appear on the third to fifth day. Sudden epigastric pain and tenderness is associated with vomiting. The abdominal rigidity normally prevents palpation of the swollen pancreas. The serum amylase is raised and glycosuria may develop in association with a raised blood sugar. Diabetes as a sequel to mumps is very exceptional but undoubtedly may occur even without clinical evidence of pancreatitis. The symptoms of pancreatitis subside rapidly in 3–4 days in most cases.

Other glands which are rarely involved are the thyroid, breast and Bartholin's glands.

The most frequent neurological complication is a benign *aseptic meningitis* which may well be the sole manifestation of the mumps infection, or it may precede or follow the parotitis by a few days. The signs and symptoms are those of a lymphocytic meningitis with headache, vomiting, stiff neck and the development of a positive Kernig's sign. Mental confusion is most uncommon. Focal central nervous system signs are rare, uneventful recovery taking place within 1–7 days in the vast majority of cases. The cerebrospinal fluid shows a raised cell count, commonly between 200–1000 per mm^3., all of which are lymphocytes. It is unusual in mumps for there to be an excess of polymorphonuclear cells in the early stages (as so often occurs in other forms of aseptic meningitis). The protein is raised to between 50 and 100 mg. per 100 ml. Very rarely a severe *meningo-encephalitis* occurs with confusion, paralyses and evidence of widespread brain or cord damage. This syndrome may appear in the second week when it is more likely to be a post-mumps sensitivity reaction (analogous to the encephalopathy of measles and chickenpox). When it appears within the first few days of the attack, however, and is associated with a considerable pleocytosis in the cerebrospinal fluid, a true mumps meningo-encephalitis due to invasion of the central nervous system by the mumps virus is probable. The distinction is of more than academic interest as it affects the decision whether or not to use corticosteroids in treatment.

Nerve deafness is a rare but serious complication because it is usually permanent and complete. It may be accompanied by vertigo, tinnitus and vomiting and is usually ascribed to an auditory neuritis. Fortunately it is normally unilateral. *Facial palsy*, from neuritis of the seventh cranial nerve is rare. Optic neuritis may occur as part of a post-mumps encephalopathy.

Clinical *myocarditis* is infrequent but electrocardiographic evidence of temporary damage to the heart has been demonstrated in 15 per cent. of cases in one study. These changes consist of depression of S-T segments and inversion of T waves in lead V4 or other chest leads. The P-R interval may be prolonged, heart block being the commonest clinical manifestation of heart involvement. Recovery is uneventful.

Acute benign *arthritis* or capsulitis may arise in the second or third week. Usually monarticular and affecting a large joint, the arthritis is accompanied by fever and a raised sedimentation rate. There is little response to salicylates but spontaneous recovery is rapid. Transient *thrombocytopenic purpura* rarely occurs during convalescence from mumps.

The inflammatory oedema of submaxillary mumps has on occasions spread to the glottis and necessitated tracheostomy. Presternal oedema, possibly associated with thyroiditis is sometimes severe and striking. Secondary infection very rarely leads to suppuration of a parotid gland.

Diagnosis

In the straightforward case in which swelling of one parotid is rapidly followed by a swelling on the other side the diagnosis presents no difficulty. In many instances, however, the salivary gland swelling may be unilateral or indistinct or the illness may start with abdominal pain, meningitis or some other 'complication'. A history of contact with mumps approximately three weeks previously is of great help but laboratory confirmation is often necessary in cases without salivary gland involvement. The serum amylase may be raised in mumps irrespective of clinical pancreatitis and is a quick and useful test to employ. The white cell count may show a slight lymphocytosis but this is inconstant, the count often being normal.

Isolation of mumps virus is not as yet a routine diagnostic procedure. Serological testing, however, is simple and reliable although the need to examine paired sera obtained with a week's interval between the specimens means that the diagnosis is restrospective. A fourfold rise in antibody is diagnostic. Antibody to the soluble antigen (mumps S) appears about the third day, increasing rapidly and falling to a low level again in about three months. The virus particle antibody (mumps V) appears later and persists for much longer and is thus often a useful indication of a previous attack.

Unilateral parotitis, especially in an older person, is more likely to be due to a suppurative infection than to mumps. The diagnosis is easily established by watching pus emerge at the duct orifice on massage of the gland. Recurrent parotitis is often of unknown aetiology but its recurrent nature excludes mumps. A duct calculus causes swelling of the gland which is usually intermittent. Sarcoidosis and tumours lead to chronic painless swellings.

Inflammatory swelling of the cervical lymph nodes, especially when accompanied by periadenitis and oedema, may simulate mumps. As a rule, however, a lymph node has a well-defined edge, but this feature may be absent if periadenitis is marked. A dental abscess shows similar features combined with a tooth tender to percussion. The serious error of mistaking bull-necked diphtheria for mumps should not occur if the toxaemia of the patient is taken into account and the fauces thoroughly examined. Septic lymph nodes are generally much more tender than mumps swellings and are usually accompanied by a polymorphonuclear leucocytosis.

Treatment

Mumps is infectious for 2–3 days before the swelling appears, the infectivity thereafter rapidly diminishing. Isolation is recommended for 7 days from the appearance of the last gland to become swollen. Contacts need not be quarantined.

The patient should be nursed in bed until the glands are subsiding. In the case of adult males rest should continue until the twelfth day as early ambulation appears to increase the risk of orchitis developing. There is no specific treatment for mumps and most patients require no symptomatic relief other than a mild sedative or analgesic.

Orchitis is treated by rest, a supportive bandage and analgesics. Two doses of 100 Units of corticotrophin on successive days relieve pain, often dramatically, but the effect on fever and subsidence of the swelling is less clear. There is no evidence that stilboestrol is of any value, nor is incision of the tunica albuginea to be recommended. Patients require reassurance that they will neither be impotent nor sterile as a result of this complication.

Other complications are treated symptomatically. In encephalitic cases steroids should be used as for post-measles encephalopathy only if the onset of neurological symptoms is late and one can be reasonably certain that there is not an active virus encephalitis. Patients with myocarditis should rest until the electrocardiogram has returned to normal.

Prevention

Ordinary gamma globulin is ineffective. The value of gamma globulin prepared from convalescent mumps serum has not been confirmed by controlled study although there is evidence that it lessens the risk of orchitis. There is little application for passive immunity in this disease. A live attenuated vaccine is now licensed for use in the United States. This is given by injection with minimal side-effects, causes no spread of infection to contacts and gives 95 per cent. protection for at least 2 years.

Prognosis

The mortality is very low in spite of the numerous possible complications. Complete recovery from these is the rule apart from the rare neurological deafness and the very rare paralytic meningo-encephalitis which may result in some residual disability. Mumps in pregnancy does not cause congenital malformations.

REFERENCE

HILLEMAN, M. R., BUYNAK, E. B., WEIBEL, R. E., and STOKES, J. (1968) Live attenuated mumps-virus vaccine, *New Engl. J. Med.*, **278,** 227.

CYTOMEGALOVIRUS INFECTIONS

Synonyms. Cytomegalic inclusion disease; Salivary gland virus inclusion disease.

Definition

The cytomegalovirus (CMV) causes widespread infection in man, much of which passes unrecognized. It is responsible for severe infantile infections with resultant death or brain damage. In older children and adults hepatitis or a glandular fever type illness may occur.

Aetiology and Epidemiology

The virus has been classified in the herpes group (with simplex and varicella zoster). Infection is followed by the development of complement fixing antibodies which remain raised for long periods in the same way as occurs after a primary infection with herpes simplex. This indicates a continuing infection with periodic reactivations of virus. About one-third of the population acquire antibody between the ages of 15 and 30 years and it is estimated that some 4 per cent. of adult women excrete CMV at any one time. Although 4 per cent. of pregnant women excrete virus this is usually due to reactivation in the presence of antibody and in such cases the baby is healthy at birth. It often becomes infected however at 3–6 months of age after its passively transferred immunity disappears. When *primary* infection of the mother occurs during pregnancy transplacental infection of the foetus takes place with resultant stillbirth or neonatal illness. The birth of a second infected infant to the same mother has not been known to occur. Spread takes place by droplet infection, but other routes play a part as virus is excreted in the urine and from the cervix as well as in saliva. Young children often excrete virus in the urine for many months but adults, except those on immuno-suppressive drugs (of whom 50 per cent. are excreters), are normally short-term excreters. Fresh blood is another source of infection as 5 per cent. of donors carry CMV on their white blood cells. Stored blood is much less likely to be infectious due to the lability of the virus.

Pathology

The characteristic lesion is the presence of intranuclear and cytoplasmic inclusion bodies in giant cells. Although first recognized in salivary glands in fatal neonatal infections the lesions have now been found in virtually all tissues.

Symptoms

Infection in Infants. As already explained, most infantile infections arise at 3–6 months of age when the maternal transferred immunity is waning. True congenital infection follows a primary maternal illness and results in foetal death or neonatal illness. The classical features of neonatal cytomegalic inclusion disease are jaundice, hepatosplenomegaly, thrombocytopenic purpura and haemolytic anaemia. Extensive neurological involvement with necrotizing haemorrhagic encephalitis causes widespread neurological symptoms and in those who survive cerebral calcification may later be demonstrated on radiology. Severity varies from a combination of most of the above to episodes of transient jaundice, transient purpura or merely failure to thrive. In view of the frequency of neurological involvement mental retardation, often with microcephaly, may follow even mild attacks of CMV infection and it is believed that about 10 per cent. of cases of mental retardation in the United Kingdom are due to this virus.

Infection in the Older Child and Adult. Most infections pass unrecognized and many are probably symptomless. The two commonest syndromes are hepatitis, sometimes with prolonged fever and a glandular fever-like illness with fever, lymphadenopathy and atypical mononucleosis. Sore throat is absent and heterophile antibodies do not appear. Patients suffering from leukaemia and those undergoing open heart surgery, transplant operations or receiving immunosuppressive therapy are particularly liable to be affected by cytomegalic inclusion disease.

Diagnosis

This is dependent on laboratory investigation. The complement fixation test becomes positive in the third to fourth week and a fourfold rise from onset to the fourth week is diagnostic. Virus appears in the urine relatively late, from the fourth week onwards. Urine should be sent to the laboratory in transport medium at 4° C. and not frozen. Liver biopsy may well show the characteristic inclusion bodies and virus can also sometimes be cultured from this material.

In infants the differential diagnosis includes congenital rubella, congenital toxoplasmosis, disseminated herpes simplex, neonatal sepsis, congenital syphilis and erythroblastosis foetalis. In adults CMV infection should be excluded in any case of atypical hepatitis or sero-negative glandular fever. The disease should be considered at all ages in any obscure febrile illness, and particularly in those categories of patients mentioned above as being highly susceptible.

Prognosis and Treatment

About 50 per cent. of infants with generalized cytomegalic inclusion disease die and some 25 per cent. of all cases recognized in infancy suffer permanent mental damage. Complete recovery without sequelae can be expected in the previously healthy older child or adult but the disease may prove fatal in those with underlying illness. The virus is sensitive to idoxuridine but systemic treatment with this toxic drug has not so far resulted in cure. Its use should only be considered in the severe infantile type. There is no other specific treatment.

REFERENCES

CARLSTROM, G., ALDEN, J., BELFRAGE, S., HEDENSTROM, G., HOLMBERG, L., NORDBRING, F., and STERNER, G. (1968) Acquired cytomegalovirus infection, *Brit. med. J.*, **2**, 521.

CONCHIE, A. F., BARTON, B. W., and TOBIN, J. O'H. (1968) Congenital cytomegalovirus infection treated with idoxuridine, *Brit. med. J.*, **4**, 162.

JACK, I., and MCAULIFFE, K. C. (1968) Sero-epidemiological study of cytomegalovirus infections in Melbourne children and some adults, *Med. J. Aust.*, i, 206.

STERN, H. (1968) Isolation of cytomegalovirus and clinical manifestations of infection at different ages, *Brit. med. J.*, **1**, 665.

STERN, H., ELEK, S. D., BOOTH, J. C., and FLECK, D. G. (1969) Microbial causes of mental retardation, *Lancet*, ii, 443.

G. D. W. MCKENDRICK

DISEASES BELIEVED TO BE DUE TO VIRUS INFECTION

ENCEPHALITIS LETHARGICA

Synonym. Epidemic encephalitis.

Definition

An acute febrile disease, formerly occurring sporadically and epidemically, possibly due to the infection of the nervous system by a virus which has not yet been identified. Its principal incidence is upon the upper parts of the nervous system, the cerebrum, basal ganglia and brain stem. Though very definite, it was remarkably polymorphic, and sometimes monosymptomatic, and its type has changed greatly during the passage of an epidemic. The absence of evidence of case-to-case infection necessitated the assumption that infection was transferred by carriers or by those in the presymptomatic stage of infection only.

History

When we read of the influenza epidemic which swept over Europe in 1580 and which was accompanied by a malady so peculiar as to gain the title of 'Schlafkrankheit', and afterwards of the epidemic described by Sydenham in 1675 as 'febris comatosa', the 'sleeping sickness' of Tübingen in 1712 and Dubini's epidemic of the fatal 'electrical chorea' in Northern Italy in 1846, we cannot but agree with von Economo's conclusion that these were epidemics of lethargic encephalitis. The subsequent epidemics of Mauthner's 'nona' in Piedmont in 1891, and also Pfuhl-Leichtenstern's 'haemorrhagic encephalitis' in 1905 have been shown to be similar to lethargic encephalitis, both clinically and pathologically. The malady last became pandemic in Britain and Northern Europe from 1917, reaching a maximum in 1920, and then declined almost to vanishing point over the next 15 years.

In this country sporadic cases of sufficiently definite characteristics to stand up to both clinical and pathological criteria of diagnosis have continued to make their appearance, but they are rare. It should be remembered that many cases thought to be of this nature prove at autopsy to be due to tumours or other causes. On the other hand, the continued appearance of cases of Parkinsonism in young people, sometimes associated with other postencephalitic sequelae, makes it likely that instances of the infection, so mild as not to produce clinically recognizable symptoms, occur. It has been brought to our notice that the history of these epidemics in Europe shows that they occur every half-century or so. The half-century since the last epidemic will immediately follow the publication of the present edition, so, bearing in mind that we are as vulnerable to it as we were in 1580, the reader should be forewarned if not pre-armed.

Aetiology

During the period of its frequent incidence, the disease occurred both sporadically and epidemically, with no centre of spread. It was more prevalent in the cold season of the year. No age was exempt and cases occurred in the seventh decade of life, but it was rare in young children and seemed to be most incident in the first half of adult life. The mode of infection is unknown. According to Von Economo, when once the virus obtains access to the nervous system it spreads, as in other cases of virus diseases of the nervous system, by axonal routes. Its effect remains confined to the nervous system, but the occurrence of progressive nervous sequels long after the acute illness, which is such a feature of the disease, suggests that the virus may survive in the nervous system for long periods of time. This view, expressed a third of a century ago, anticipated the present interest in 'slow viruses' in the central nervous system.

The height of the epidemic incidence of lethargic encephalitis has many times coincided with a severe epidemic of influenza, but no further connexion between the two conditions is known. Von Economo first succeeded in transferring the virus to the monkey by intracerebral inoculation in 1916. Subsequent smaller epidemics in Japan and St. Louis, though conforming in general to the features of the pandemic of 1917–20 have shown sufficiently constant variation in age incidence and death-rate as well as clinical feature to make it seem likely that there exist more than one strain of the virus.

Pathology

The cerebrospinal fluid pressure is raised and in a few of the cases blood or the products of haemorrhage are present. In about one-third of cases the cell count has been normal. In the rest there has been a moderate lymphocytic pleocytosis, with little or no protein increase, sugar and chlorides being normal. No prognostic indications can be derived from the nature of the fluid. The vessels of the brain are markedly congested and full of blood, and the colour shows a characteristic change from the normal throughout the whole of the grey matter, varying from a rosy flush to a deep salmon-pink, giving rise to the term 'the rose-coloured brain'. When hardened in formalin, this colour becomes a heavy purple grey. Both subdural and deeply seated haemorrhages are occasionally found. Von Economo describes the anatomical picture as one of unvarying constancy. It is that of an oedematous and congested brain, with all the grey matter conspicuously reddened in contrast to the white matter, which is of normal colour. There is a non-purulent and, properly speaking, a non-haemorrhagic inflammation of the whole grey matter exclusively, the white matter being uninvolved. There is most conspicuous perivascular lymphocytic cuffing remarkable for the absence of any polymorphs, with an intense cellular infiltration of the grey matter with elements of the microglia, while the neuroglia is unaltered and demyelination does not occur. Accompanying and succeeding these inflammatory changes is a certain measure of neuronophagia, with primary loss of the ganglion cells.

Symptoms

The following account written by James Collier in the first edition is authoritative, and so retained, almost unchanged.

In the acute forms the onset may be with general symptoms, such as shivering, malaise, headache and fever and bodily pains, a thickly coated white tongue and constipation, and sometimes vomiting and persistent hiccough. This train of symptoms usually appears in the story as an attack of 'influenza'. The pyrexia does not usually last longer than a week. Countless such attacks of 'influenza', distinguishable only by the occurrence of transient diplopia, or of slight somnolence, and often even without any such distinguishing features, followed by apparently complete recovery, have been succeeded after long intervals, by the slow onset of the Parkinsonism of lethargic encephalitis. Again, the epoch of infection may apparently give rise to no symptoms at all, and long afterwards an insidious onset of Parkinsonism ensues.

An increasing lethargy is present in many of the cases. In this condition the patient will lie for days without stirring a muscle, taking no heed of his surroundings and passing the dejecta under him unheeding. Yet when roused by command and vigorous bodily stirring, he will wake up and hold an intelligent conversation, lapsing back at once when he is left alone, even though his mouth be half full of unswallowed food. In this condition, flexibilitas cerea may often be demonstrated in the limbs. This state of stupor may last for 3 weeks or longer even in patients who completely recover. It passes away gradually. Unrousable coma is invariably a sign of impending death. Subsequent memory of events during the stuporous state may be remarkably retained. Insomnia may be a troublesome early symptom, and even when the patients are markedly lethargic they will complain that they cannot sleep. Occasionally reversal of sleep rhythm may occur, the patient sleeping soundly all day only to become restless and overactive at night. Lethargy, however, may be absent and the early mental state be that of vivacious excitement, talkativeness and restlessness. In some the first sign may be delirium or mental aberration, which may rapidly develop into acute and violent mania; such cases are rapidly fatal. In those who recover after severe symptoms, considerable mental reduction and self-obvious mental change may persist. Indeed, it has been said that no sufferer from the disease ever regains his original mentality, and it is a common experience to find the personality seriously changed in the way of mental reduction. Complete incapacity for any sustained work, entire change of character, antisocial tendencies, moral perversion and depressed neurasthenic states are not uncommon sequels of the disease, particularly when it occurs in children or adolescents.

Convulsions are rare, but they may undoubtedly occur as in other forms of encephalitis. Indeed, the initial clinical picture may be dominated by convulsion, and closely resemble status epilepticus from other causes.

Ophthalmoplegia and other paralyses in the region of the cranial nerves are most often nuclear in type, but peripheral paralysis of any cranial nerve may be seen, most commonly unilateral paralysis of the facial nerve. The pupils may show every abnormality which a lesion of the nervous system can produce. Inequality, eccentricity and loss of light reflex and ciliary paralysis may occur. The loss of light reflex may be unilateral. The external ophthalmoplegia, being nuclear in origin, involves both eyes in terms of their conjugate movements, and the upward and downward movements are, as a rule, more severely impaired than are the lateral movements. Bilateral ptosis is usual, and is an important and valuable early indication of the disease. The common error is to consider it part of the sleepy state. The nuclear ophthalmoplegia is often irregular, giving rise to strabismus and diplopia. There may be also peripheral paralysis of any of the oculomotor nerve trunks. The degree of the ophthalmoplegia varies in different cases from slight diplopia with hardly noticeable strabismus to complete paralysis of both eyes. It may be rapidly transient or permanently severe. In severe cases which survive there is always some improvement in the degree of paralysis in the course of time.

The diplopia and loss of accommodation cause much defect of vision, but many of the patients complain of a loss of vision in each eye, which is too great for any such explanation, the cause of which is not yet explicable. Papilloedema has been reported in a few cases. It is transient and never reaches a high degree.

Bilateral nuclear facial paralysis and bulbar paralysis are not uncommon. Paralysis of any individual cranial nerve may occur, and also of any individual spinal root, but they always recover.

Symptoms indicative of lesions of the basal ganglia are among the most common features of the disease, and they are often the most persistent. These consist of weakness of movement, rigidity with slowness of movement and spontaneous involuntary movements. The weakness, rigidity and slowness of movement give rise to a peculair immobility of facial and bodily expression and movement. The face is mask-like, the neck stiff and the head moves little and slowly, the trunk bent forward and stiff, the arms held away from the trunk, the whole appearance of the patient closely resembling that of *paralysis agitans*. Rapid fluttering of the eyelids when gently closed is characteristic of this condition. The spontaneous involuntary movements may be of a rhythmic tremulous nature, as in paralysis agitans, or there may be slow rhythmic, choreiform, athetoid, myoclonic, irregular or highly complicated movements: these may be met with at any stage of the malady, but most commonly appear some little time after the acute stage has passed away. Fibrillation and fascicular twitching of the muscles is common in the acute stage. In cases where bulbar symptoms, either of a spastic or flaccid kind, are present, hypersalivation is often troublesome.

In addition to these symptoms and signs, indications of disorder of the cerebral hemispheres may occur. Bilateral spasticity with signs of damage to the pyramidal systems, increased jerks, lost abdominal reflexes and extensor plantar responses are common. Hemiplegia, aphasia and hemianopia may occur. Meningeal symptoms may be marked in the early stages, such as suboccipital headache, painful stiffness of the neck, head retraction, vomiting and Kernig's sign. Indeed, rapidly fatal cases have occurred in which the clinical picture throughout was hardly distinguishable from that of acute meningitis, but without any leucocytosis in the cerebrospinal fluid. A major incidence of the lesions upon the cerebellum gives rise to the picture of acute cerebellar ataxy following a lethargic onset, and the end result may be a condition closely resembling a usual type of disseminate sclerosis. Such cases make a good recovery in the course of time.

Peripheral pains are sometimes severe and are usually quite local. They may be the first signs of the illness, and may persist for months after recovery. They are presumably due to the lesions around the nerve roots which have been already noted.

Since lesions have been found in the spinal cord, it is only to be expected that focal spinal symptoms should be met in rare cases. These are usually acute atrophic paralyses similar to those of poliomyelitis and recover completely. It has been argued, however, that this atrophic palsy is due to a lesion of the spinal roots. More severe lesions may apparently give rise to a condition resembling acute transverse myelitis.

The incontinence which is almost constantly present, even when the lethargy is far from deep, is the result of the lethargy. Transient conscious dysuria may happen in the early stages of the disease. The deep reflexes may be lost in severe cases during the acute stages, and they are usually absent in pre-mortal conditions. Otherwise they tend to be exaggerated, especially if involvement of the pyramidal system is present. The condition of the abdominal and plantar reflexes depends upon the presence of lesions of the pyramidal tracts, when the abdominal reflexes will be absent and the plantar reflexes of the extensor type.

In some cases the initial effects of the disease are so slight as not to call for medical attention, and yet in the course of months, or it may be years, the most serious and completely incapacitating paralysis appears. Such a patient may notice that he sees double, and does not feel well for a few weeks. He recovers, but after a few years begins to manifest the signs of a slowly oncoming Parkinsonism. A similar result in the slow and late development of grievous symptoms may follow any attack of lethargic encephalitis and make the prognosis in this malady difficult.

Diagnosis

A diagnosis of lethargic encephalitis is often made, but must be received with the greatest reserve at the present time. In typical cases the diagnosis presents no difficulty, the rousable stupor, incontinence, ophthalmoplegia and negative, lymphocytic or blood-containing cerebrospinal fluid being so characteristic as to preclude possibility of error. The less usual forms, and especially those with gradual onset and slight symptoms, often present great difficulty and require much care and full knowledge of the possible symptomatology of the disease for their recognition. There is no specific laboratory test for the malady, and the diagnosis must be based upon clinical grounds. Because of this it is impossible, except in retrospect when postencephalitic symptoms develop, to recognize this form of encephalitis from others of similar form due to a different virus. Where meningeal symptoms are prominent, distinction has to be made from other forms of meningitis and from poliomyelitis. Here, the cerebrospinal fluid is of the highest importance, as polymorphonuclear leucocytes occur rarely in lethargic encephalitis. In cases commencing with peripheral pains, excitement, maniacal symptoms or convulsions, careful lookout should be kept for the advent of ptosis, ophthalmoplegia or lethargy, the appearance of which, following such symptoms, should at once suggest the diagnosis. It must be borne in mind that the clinical picture of the disease may be dominated by a hemiplegic condition, and that an apoplexy may occur during the acute stage of the disease. Slight cases of the disease are frequently unrecognized, or are indeed unrecognizable in the early stages, but here the diagnosis can often be made with certainty from the end results; the peculiar ophthalmoplegia, the spontaneous involuntary movements and the paralysis agitans-like syndrome being almost pathognomonic of the malady.

Course

The course of the disease is extremely variable. It may be a slight transient illness lasting a few days, and leaving no sequelae after a few weeks; or a most malignant disease, fatal in a few days. In others, symptoms indicative of fresh lesions may occur repeatedly weeks and even months after the onset.

Sequelae

The disabilities which this malady may leave in its wake are numerous and varied. The mental, paralytic and Parkinsonian end results have already been referred to, but special mention must be made of the so-called oculogyric crises, and of involuntary spontaneous movements, having the general features of habit spasms or tics.

Oculogyric crises. This term is applied to recurring attacks of tonic conjugate deviation of the eyes. This is almost always upwards and is accompanied by wrinkling of the forehead, extension of the neck and in fact all the muscular activity associated with the act of looking upwards. Deviation of the eyes to one side is exceedingly rare. The attacks may occur several times a day or only at an interval of months. They are often specific in their times of occurrence and may be precipitated by a variety of stimuli such as emotion, fatigue or watching a moving picture. The attack may last from a few minutes to many hours and often passes off only after sleep. It is commonly associated with an intense degree of mental depression and while it lasts the patient may experience recurring obsessional thoughts, be impelled to carry out stereotyped movements or develop ideas of reference, particularly feelings of persecution.

Patients suffering from oculogyric crises always show some signs of Parkinsonism. The attacks often grow less frequent over a period of years and may cease completely. Their frequency and duration is in many cases considerably reduced by the regular administration of amphetamine sulphate, 5–10 mg. twice daily.

Postencephalitic tics. A variety of stereotyped involuntary movements are experienced by postencephalitic subjects, usually in association with some degree of Parkinsonism. Rhythmic movements of the jaws, tongue and face are common. Alterations in respiratory rhythm with sighing, gasping inspirations may occur. Torticollis, indistinguishable from the variety found in elderly subjects happens rarely and there may be hideous recurring contortions of the face and trunk and grotesque mannerisms of gait and speech.

Treatment

Nothing being known of the infectivity and mode of spread of the disease, isolation and disinfection are not usually employed. Each case must in England be immediately notified to the public health authorities. No treatment is known which has any specific influence upon the disease. It remains therefore to use those measures which will help to keep the patient alive and those which relieve symptoms. Nasal feeding may be necessary. Relief of the constipation is most important and is often followed by striking improvement in the symptoms. After the acute stage, treatment is concerned with combating the physical and mental listlessness and depression which so often persist and with the restoration of normal mobility and function to the limb. In these, physical and occupational therapy can play a useful part. The treatment of Parkinsonism is considered in Section 15.

Prognosis

A rapid onset and quick development of severe symptoms, marked pyrexia, delirium and maniacal excitement are bad prognostic signs and indicate a rapidly fatal issue. After the third week of the disease, the probabilities are all in favour of survival. The prognosis, however, as to how much permanent damage to the nervous system will eventually remain is hardly possible, since slow improvement may go on for months and even years. Of the acute cases occurring at the height of an epidemic, 40 per cent. are quickly fatal, 30 per cent. are reduced to chronic invalidism and 30 per cent. appear to recover completely (Von Economo). In most of these latter the syndrome of Parkinsonism subsequently appears after an interval which may be a few months or many years, and the weakness, rigidity and tremors, which form this paralysis agitans-like picture persist indefinitely.

REFERENCES

Holt, W. L. Jr. (1957) Epidemic encephalitis: A follow up study of 265 cases, *Arch. Neurol. Psychiat. (Chic.)*, **38**, 1135.

Von Economo, C. (1931) *Encephalitis Lethargica: Its Sequelae and Treatment*, trans. Newman, K. O., London.

Denis Williams

BENIGN MYALGIC ENCEPHALOMYELITIS

Synonyms. Icelandic disease; Royal Free Hospital disease.

Definition

Benign myalgic encephalomyelitis is an acute disease affecting women much more frequently than men, the characteristic features being headache, muscle pains, paralyses, emotional disturbance and sensory symptoms of a bizarre nature. Many institutional outbreaks have been recorded, most involving nursing and ancillary staff in hospitals.

Aetiology and Epidemiology

The causative agent is unknown although the illness is generally believed to be due to a virus infection. Full virological investigations, however, have so far proved negative. A toxic cause, possibly food borne, has been postulated in some outbreaks when the illness has arisen in a close knit community but no support for this thesis has been forthcoming. It becomes less tenable as further investigation during such outbreaks has always revealed scattered sporadic cases occurring in the general community at the time of the institutional epidemic.

The first epidemic to be described occurred in 1948 amongst the general population of Akureyri in Iceland. Since then outbreaks have been reported from many countries. They have mostly arisen among hospital staff where nurses have been affected predominantly, spread to patients only rarely occurring. The disease affects women much more frequently than men and it is rare before puberty. The largest epidemic in Great Britain occurred in the Royal Free Group of hospitals in 1955 when there were nearly 300 cases amongst a hospital staff of 3500. Case to case infection is common although the method of spread is not known.

The pathology is unknown as autopsy material has not become available. Lesions are assumed to be widespread throughout the brain and spinal cord. Attempts have been made recently to dismiss the disorder as a hysterical phenomenon.

Symptoms

The incubation period is uncertain but appears to fall between 5–10 days. The onset is generally insidious with occipital headache, pains in the limbs and giddiness associated with a low pyrexia. Lassitude is often marked and anorexia, nausea or vomiting occur in about 50 per cent. of cases. Mild sore throat is usual. Pain in the neck, shoulders and back is sometimes severe and accompanied by spasm with muscle tenderness. Paralysis of limbs or trunk may arise at any stage and is usually accompanied by pain. Inability to get up from the supine position due to weakness or pain or a combination of both is a frequent complaint. A notable feature is the tendency for the symptoms to fluctuate from day to day.

On examination fever is usually slight (seldom above 100° F. (37·8° C.)) and may be normal throughout most of the illness. There may be evidence of a mild upper respiratory tract infection with throat injection and slight enlargement of the posterior cervical lymph nodes but the main abnormal signs are found in the central nervous system. Neck and back stiffness is usual, nystagmus is frequent and cranial nerve palsies may occur. There are often somewhat bizarre areas of sensory loss which tend to alter from day to day and are usually confined to a paralysed limb. Emotional lability is common, episodes of depression, tearfulness or forgetfulness occurring in the majority of patients. Insomnia with alteration of the sleep rhythm may be troublesome. Hysterical outbursts in a previously normal and well adjusted individual can make interpretation of physical signs difficult. The most characteristic feature is the distinctive type of paresis which tends to have an upper motor neurone distribution, is usually associated with increased muscle tone and reflexes and often with severe pain and spasm. However, the limb may be flaccid in the early stages. Paralysis is never complete, whatever movement remains usually showing a typically jerky quality—'a stuttering paresis'—which becomes most evident during the recovery stage. Plantar reflexes are flexor in spite of increased reflexes in the affected limb. Cranial nerve palsies, bulbar palsy and paresis of respiratory muscles may all occur.

The course is extremely variable. In mild cases with no clear cut evidence of central nervous system involvement complete recovery within 3–4 weeks is the rule. In more severe cases the duration of the illness is closely related to the extent of the paralysis. Periods of improvement may be followed by relapse with a further spread of paresis. Most paralyses recover in 3–4 months although symptoms of debility, both physical and mental, may persist for months or even years. Such patients tire easily and find difficulty in concentrating. Persistent muscle spasms, athetoid movements and Parkinsonian-like symptoms have occurred as permanent sequelae but these are rare.

Diagnosis

The main clinical features are the multiplicity of symptoms including emotional instability associated with low fever, nystagmus and a 'stuttering' hyperreflexic paresis. The disproportion between the severity of muscular weakness and the objective neurological signs is characteristic. The cerebrospinal fluid is nearly always normal but may show a moderate rise of protein. The electromyogram of paretic muscles shows a characteristic reduction of the motor unit potentials on volition with marked grouping which resembles the jerky movements seen clinically. These changes, which are characteristic of the disease, suggest long motor tract involvement. The electroencephalogram may show evidence of diffuse cerebral involvement but the tracings are not specific. The sedimentation rate is normal or raised to 30 mm. in an hour and the white cells show a slight increase of mononuclear cells, some of which are of virus type.

During an outbreak the diagnosis presents no difficulty. The sporadic case, however, may need close observation and investigation. The illness may bear a very close resemblance to *hysteria* and there is little doubt that many cases of this disease are labelled as functional in origin. This is particularly likely to occur when emotional symptoms predominate. In encephalomyelopathy, however, the reflexes are most exaggerated in the affected limb, periodic mild fever occurs, the gag and corneal reflexes are usually present and pain is a prominent symptom. Hysterical paralysis is normally painless.

The resemblance to *poliomyelitis* is only superficial. In that disease the paralysis is flaccid and areflexic, wasting occurs early and the cerebrospinal fluid contains an increase of cells and protein. Sensory symptoms are very rare. *Coxsackie B infection*, however, may cause a similar illness with meningism, muscle pains, tenderness and transient paresis. The illness is acute, fever is prominent and recovery is rapid. Most such paretic cases have an abnormal cerebrospinal fluid.

Treatment

The patient should be nursed on fracture boards in isolation although how long infectivity lasts is unknown. Rest is vital and must be continued well into convalescence as too early return to activity frequently leads to relapse. Analgesics are required to relieve pain. Passive movements of joints affected by paresis should start early but are often difficult to carry out owing to painful spasms. Local (infra-red) heat prior to physiotherapy is helpful in such cases. Calipers may be required in convalescence.

Prognosis

No deaths have been reported. Complete recovery is the rule although convalescence is often slow and it may be months before the patient returns to normal health. Sequelae include athetoid movements, persistent muscle spasms and psychiatric changes.

REFERENCES

ACHESON, E. D. (1959) The clinical syndrome variously called benign myalgic encephalomyelitis, Iceland disease and epidemic neuromyasthemia, *Amer. J. Med.*, **26,** 569.

MCEVEDY, C. P., and BEARD, A. W. (1970) Concept of benign myalgic encephalomyelitis, *Brit. med. J.*, **1,** 11.

PRICE, J. L. (1961) Myalgic encephalomyelitis, *Lancet*, i, 737.

ROYAL FREE HOSPITAL GROUP (1957) an outbreak of encephalomyelitis, *Brit. med. J.*, **2,** 895.

SIGURDSSON, B., and GUDMUNDSSON, K. R. (1956) Clinical findings six years after outbreak of Akureyri disease, *Lancet*, i, 766.

G. D. W. MCKENDRICK

THE HAEMORRHAGIC FEVERS

Aetiology

This group of fevers are probably all of viral origin but some still need differentiation. As in yellow fever, pathological changes occur in the small blood vessels and in the circulation, particularly in the kidneys, sometimes with anuric renal failure, and often associated in the early stages with haematuria. There is usually also some degree of hepatic and pulmonary involvement and sometimes a form of polyarthritis. In severe cases fatal circulatory failure may develop.

The haemorrhagic fevers have been recognized in the East for some time. They first came into global prominence during the Korean war in which seasonal outbreaks of haemorrhagic fevers occurred in troops. Outbreaks have occurred also in Manchuria and South and Central Russia.

Not all these conditions have been associated with recognized viruses, but recent work has considerably helped in defining the situation, especially in South-East Asia (see below).

The vectors in some haemorrhagic fevers have not yet been fully identified. In India (Kyasanur Forest fever) and in the Crimea, ticks transmit the infection. Depending on the viruses and vectors involved the haemorrhagic fevers may occur seasonally, sporadically or as a small localized epidemics. There is a strong possibility that in some areas field rodents may act as reservoirs. In Kyasanur Forest fever epizootics appear in monkeys and transmission is by *Ixodes* ticks.

Mosquito-borne Haemorrhagic Fevers of South-East Asia. In the Philippines, Thailand, Malaysia, Vietnam and eastern India haemorrhagic fevers occur which are commonly referred to as mosquito-borne haemorrhagic fevers of South and South-East Asia.

The disease is seasonal and recurrent. It was first recognized in an epidemic in Manila in 1954, and has since appeared in other towns in the Philippines. It appeared as an epidemic in Bangkok in 1958 and has recurred there regularly since with peaks of incidence every 2 years; since 1964 it has been reported in other towns in Thailand and outbreaks have occurred in Malaysia, including Penang, Singapore, South and North Vietnam and eastern India (Calcutta).

Four types of Dengue virus (of which Type II occurs most commonly) and the Chikungunya virus (originally isolated in East Africa) have been isolated from patients or from the mosquito identified as the vector, *Aëdes aegypti*. On the whole, the disease caused by the latter virus is milder.

The haemorrhagic disease appears in areas in which classical dengue syndromes are occurring simultaneously caused by apparently identical viruses. In most outbreaks children in the age group 3–14 have been affected. This has been particularly notable in Thailand and the Philippines. The original incident in Singapore involved young adults, but in recent outbreaks children have been affected. Except very rarely haemorrhagic fever occurs only in the indigenous population and expatriates are not involved, although both groups suffer from the prevailing dengue.

There is at present no explanation as to why the Dengue and Chikungunya viruses which normally produce relatively mild diseases should sometimes cause such severe and frequently fatal haemorrhagic syndromes. It is thought by some that host factors are involved in the form of a hyperimmune response to sensitization by previous infection with the same viruses. Mutation of the virus may also be concerned.

Pathology

The common cause of death in the Korean outbreaks was circulatory failure associated with acute renal failure with uraemia. Haemorrhages occur in many organs, including the lungs, and pulmonary oedema was sometimes terminal.

There was general capillary dilatation, congestion and haemorrhage, with associated focal necrosis and local cellular reaction. Changes were most often found in the kidneys in which there was pronounced congestion of the medullary vessels with haemorrhages between the tubules. The picture in the cortex was largely that of irregular ischaemia, with which the anuria was associated.

The chief pathological lesions in other organs were associated with capillary damage and with changes in permeability of the endothelium. Fluid may accumulate in endothelial sacs; tissue oedema is common, and there are variable degrees of changes occurring in the organs, depending on the changes in the local circulation. In some forms of haemorrhagic fever tissue damage in the liver may be considerable and associated with overt changes in liver function particularly in circulating transaminases. Haemorrhages may occur in any organ and in some epidemics are particularly notable in the brain and in the heart muscle.

The spleen is commonly enlarged and there may be haemorrhages into the skin, particularly where trauma has occurred. In some cases there is an increase in bleeding time and a reduction in platelets.

In South-East Asian mosquito-borne haemorrhagic fever generalized vascular damage is the most important pathological feature. Necrosis of blood vessels is rarely seen but diapedesis of erythrocytes is common. Focal acidophilic necrosis occurs in the parenchymal cells of the liver and in the Kupffer cells. Frank necrosis of the renal convoluted tubules has not been reported and acute renal shut-down is rare.

Signs and Symptoms

The clinical picture varies with the causal virus and the area in which it is transmitted. The classical picture has been described in haemorrhagic fever in South-East Asia. Most clinical patterns bear some similarity to this since the underlying pathological processes are basically similar.

Mosquito-borne Haemorrhagic Fevers of South-East Asia. The clinical picture has a wide spectrum, varying from severe haemorrhagic fever to a relatively mild dengue-like illness with some haemorrhagic complications. The manifestations vary somewhat from country to country.

There is an acute or gradual onset with fever which is usually mild and lasts for 1–3 days. The patient feels malaise, commonly complains of sore throat, nausea and headache; he sometimes vomits amd may develop an irritating cough. The picture worsens rapidly as the haemorrhagic features develop. Epistaxis is common. There may be haematemesis and melaena. Petechiae and purpuric spots and sometimes frank intracutaneous or subcutaneous haemorrhages appear in the skin of the extremities, the trunk, especially the back and the face.

The fever begins to subside on the third to the fifth day and in severe cases, as the haemorrhagic manifestations develop, the patient goes into medical shock, with cold blotchy skin, falling blood pressures and imperceptible pulse. In this state the fatality rate in outbreaks varies from 15 to 50 per cent. Convalescence rapidly follows recovery from shock and is uncomplicated.

A striking difference between this disease and the haemorrhagic fevers of Korea is the rarity with which renal failure develops, even in affected adults. Death is almost always due to shock.

In the Thai form of haemorrhagic fever the liver is palpable in about half the patients admitted to hospital; in the Philippines it is rarely palpable. Epistaxis is much commoner in the Philippines than elsewhere.

Korean Haemorrhagic Fever. The course of the disease may be divided into three phases.

The first phase begins abruptly with fever which persists for some days. The onset may be associated with rigors, intense muscular and bone pain, nausea and vomiting. The temperature does not usually rise very high, seldom over 104° F. (40° C.). There is early congestion of the skin, nasopharynx and conjunctivae. Epistaxis is common and the vomit may contain blood. Within a day of the onset the pulse often becomes slow, as it does in yellow fever.

About the third day petechiae appear in the skin and the mucous membranes and small subcutaneous haemorrhages may develop. Protein, blood cells and casts appear in the urine. There is usually frank haematuria. From the onset most patients are clearly oliguric. In some, especially during the second phase, this oliguria may develop into anuria with associated uraemia. In this stage there may be either leucopenia or a mild leucocytosis.

In the classical picture the second phase is toxic. The temperature gradually falls but the general condition deteriorates steadily. The haemorrhagic changes are exacerbated, prostration increases, oliguria becomes anuria and the amount of protein passed in the urine steadily rises. The blood pressures during this stage are low in some patients and in some may fall to the point of circulatory failure. Haemorrhages from the nose, stomach, kidneys and lungs increase and bruising of the skin may be pronounced. Associated with the developing medical shock, haemoconcentration appears and masks the anaemia which may result from the bleeding. The rash during this stage may be well advanced and is commonly markedly petechial. It occurs on the chest wall and in the axillae and is associated with haemorrhages in the mucosae, including that of the intestine, so that black blood may appear in the stool.

In certain areas the infection may involve the liver at this stage and some mild degree of jaundice may develop, associated with changes in transaminases and other indications of liver dysfunction. There is sometimes considerable histological hepatic tissue damage.

The second phase of the disease may go on to the characteristic picture of anuria with rapidly developing acute uraemia. Patients who enter this stage have a bad prognosis. In some of them there may develop acute circulatory failure, but in others in association with the uraemia the blood pressure may rise considerably.

In the majority of cases the second phase passes into that of convalescence. This occurs somewhere between the tenth and fourteenth day as a rule and is ushered in by a vigorous diuresis which may persist for some time with the passage of large quantities of dilute urine. In convalescence the blood urea level gradually falls to normal and the leakage of protein from the urine ceases. It is frequently some time before full recovery of renal function occurs.

The other evidence of capillary damage and haemorrhages ceases with the appearance of convalescence.

Complications may occur resulting from capillary haemorrhage and associated tissue reactions, amongst which may be parotitis, orchitis, pancreatitis and in some areas, where the emphasis appears to be in the cerebral or the meningeal vessels, meningo-encephalitis may appear as a clinical syndrome.

The differential diagnosis in many areas includes leptospirosis which can be distinguished by bacteriological diagnostic methods and in which jaundice is much commoner and more severe.

Various forms of typhus may be mistaken for haemorrhagic fevers, but in these haematuria is unusual and diagnosis may be confirmed bacteriologically.

In some areas also relapsing fevers may give rise to some difficulties. But here again the clinical picture is different, the classical relapsing fever pattern of the temperature charts is unique and the organisms should be observable in the blood.

Various forms of purpura may also have to be considered.

The prognosis varies. The death rate is seldom more than about 10 per cent. and the commonest cause of death is renal failure with developing uraemia.

Diagnosis

In outbreaks the clinical diagnosis is sufficient. As the causative agents become known more certain serological and viral methods are being employed, but these are still inadequate to cover the wide range of syndromes.

In South-East Asia immunological evidence of infection with Dengue and Chikungunya viruses can be obtained by serological methods and the viruses have been isolated from the blood in the early days of the syndrome.

Treatment

There is no specific treatment but each clinical feature must be treated on its merits. This particularly includes the management of shock and, in some forms of the syndrome, acute renal failure. Certain antibiotics have been used with success by some workers and in the severe case, particularly in renal failure, the use of corticosteroids in the usual doses is recommended. The administration of vitamin K is also commonly necessary during the haemorrhagic stages.

REFERENCES

American Journal of Tropical Medicine and Hygiene (1965) Symposium on some aspects of hemorrhagic fevers in the Americas, **14,** 789.

BHAMARAPRAVATI, N., PRASONG TUCHINDA, and VIJITR BROONYAPAKNAVIK (1967) Pathology of Thailand haemorrhagic fever, *Ann. trop. Med. Parasit.*, **61,** 500.

Bulletin of the World Health Organization (1966) Summary. Mosquito-borne haemorrhagic fevers in South East Asia and the Western Pacific, **35,** 1.

BRIAN MAEGRAITH

CAT SCRATCH FEVER

This is a systemic illness, the main feature of which is the development of a small pustule usually at the site of a cat scratch, bite or other cutaneous injury most often on the upper limbs, but rarely in the mouth, throat or eye. It is followed 2–6 weeks later by pain, swelling, inflammation and suppuration of the lymph nodes draining the area. This may be accompanied or followed by generalized lymphadenopathy and splenomegaly. Malaise, fever, headache, a macular rash on the extremities, conjunctivitis and meningo-encephalitis may occur. The lymph nodes usually heal after the aspiration of pus or surgical intervention, but occasionally convalescence is protracted.

The aetiology of the condition remains obscure, although an agent of the psittacosis-lymphogranuloma venereum group and atypical acid-fast bacilli have both been suspected. The sera of some patients are positive in the complement fixation test with psittacosis-lymphogranuloma venereum group antigen. This may be merely a manifestation of exposure to a member of the group, feline pneumonitis virus, which is not the cause of cat scratch fever.

The only diagnostic test is the positive skin reaction obtained by intradermal injection of heated pus obtained from another case or from the patient himself. Frei antigen gives a negative reaction.

Histological examination of an affected node in the early stages shows a characteristic granulomatous type of lesion, with small abscesses present in germinal follicles, which progress to areas of necrosis not unlike that seen in tuberculous lesions.

There is no specific treatment. Most cases resolve spontaneously although surgical drainage of suppurating nodes may be necessary.

GASTRO-ENTERITIS

The improved facilities for the diagnosis of bacterial and protozoal gastro-intestinal infections and the introduction of effective therapeutic substances against them in recent years have revealed the presence of various forms of febrile and afebrile gastro-enteritis of unknown aetiology, occurring either in sporadic form or as outbreaks in communities or institutions. These have been assumed by many physicians to be due to viruses and have been called such names as 'epidemic nausea and vomiting', 'winter vomiting disease', 'epidemic diarrhoea' and 'virus gastro-enteritis'.

In the majority of cases no evidence for a viral aetiology has been obtained, even when the latest laboratory techniques for the isolation of viruses have been used.

However, two virus-like agents, 'Marcy' and 'F.S.', transmissible in volunteers were recovered some years ago in the United States from patients with an afebrile and a febrile type of gastro-enteritis respectively, but neither has produced any recognizable changes in any host or tissue culture in the laboratory.

Echovirus 5, 14 and 18 have been found associated on single occasions with small outbreaks of gastro-enteritis in a premature or infant nursery, and echovirus 11 and 20 have been associated with mild gastro-enteritis in older children, but these were apparently unusual occurrences with viruses which usually cause eruptive fevers, meningitis or upper respiratory tract infections. The isolation of some other echoviruses has been reported more frequently from children with summer diarrhoea than from others in the same hospitals, but there has not been any consistent pattern. If a virus or viruses are responsible for epidemics of diarrhoea and vomiting their isolation in the laboratory must await some new technique not available at present.

There is no specific treatment.

REFERENCE

YOW, M. D., MELNICK, J. L., PHILLIPS, C. A., LEE, L. H., SOUTH, M. A., and BLATTNER, R. J. (1966) Enteroviruses in infantile diarrhoea, *Amer. J. Epidem.*, **83,** 255.

MESENTERIC ADENITIS

Cases of mesenteric adenitis and intussusception in infants and young children have on occasion been found to be associated with the excretion of adenoviruses 1, 2 and 5 which are commonly found latent in adenoids and tonsils. A rise in antibodies has been demonstrated in some cases and in these it is conceivable that the primary infection may attack the lymph nodes of the mesentery which, becoming enlarged from inflammation, might form the starting point for intussusception in young infants. These viruses are, of course, only one possible specific cause of these conditions. *Pasteurella pseudotuberculosis* [see Section 7] has also been recovered from enlarged mesenteric glands of children in several countries of Europe and in Great Britain.

F. O. MacCallum

ROSEOLA INFANTUM

Synonym. Exanthem subitum.

Aetiology

Roseola infantum is a disease which mainly attacks infants between the ages of six and twelve months. It is rare over the age of three years. No virus has yet been isolated although its viral aetiology is strongly suggested by its natural history and the apparent subsequent life-long immunity. Case-to-case infection appears to be rare, spread within the family being most unusual. Inapparent infections rather than low infectivity would seem the more likely explanation.

Symptoms

The incubation period probably lies between 9 and 15 days.

The onset is abrupt with high fever and sometimes with a convulsion. The temperature remains raised for from 3 to 4 days during which time there is moderate irritability and the infant is usually off its food but nevertheless looks better than might be expected from the height of the fever. Clinical examination reveals no significant abnormal physical signs. There may be minimal conjunctivitis or pharyngitis. The temperature falls by crisis or rapid lysis on the third or fourth day coincident with the appearance of the rash and symptomatic recovery of the child.

The rash appears when the infant is better or when he is rapidly getting better. It consists of rose-pink discrete macules appearing on the trunk and neck and spreading to the face and limbs. The rash sometimes remains limited to the trunk. It fades in one to two days without sequelae.

Diagnosis

The clinical picture of the rash appearing at or after recovery is quite characteristic. Because of this it is often erroneously ascribed to teething or to sensitivity to some drug given during the febrile period. The absence of coryza, the normal temperature at the time of the rash and the absence of staining distinguish roseola from measles. Before the appearance of the rash the disease should be kept in mind in any infant with a high fever, particularly when this is associated with less constitutional upset than might be expected.

Treatment and Prognosis

No treatment is necessary, recovery being uneventful. Roseola infantum remains a possible cause of death from a febrile convulsion in an infant in whom no explanation is forthcoming at autopsy.

REFERENCE

Krugman, S., and Ward, R. (1968) *Infectious Diseases of Children*, p. 93, St. Louis.

G. D. W. McKendrick

DISEASES DUE TO INFECTION BY PATHOGENIC FUNGI

THE MYCOSES

Numerous fungi are pathogenic to man, and the diseases they cause are conveniently described as the mycoses. Certain infections due to actinomycetes and corynebacteria are not, in fact, fungal in nature although it has become customary to include them in descriptions of this group of diseases. The mycoses may be subdivided as follows:

Epidermal and Mucosal Infections

Ringworm, candidiasis (moniliasis), pityriasis versicolor, erythrasma, trichonocardiosis axillaris, and piedra. Certain infections due to actinomycetes and corynebacteria are not, in fact, fungal in nature although they are often mentioned in connexion with this group of diseases because of their similarity to them.

Ringworm may be acquired, according to the fungus species involved, from contact with infected humans or animals or possibly with soil. It may also be acquired from infected inanimate materials such as floors, clothing and farm apparatus. In contrast, candidiasis develops when excessive proliferation of *Candida albicans*, a normal inhabitant of the human upper respiratory, intestinal or genital tracts, occurs.

Cutaneous and Subcutaneous Infections

Mycetoma (actinomycetoma and maduromycetoma), chromoblastomycosis, sporotrichosis, phycomycosis, rhinosporidiosis, and metastasizing infections of pulmonary and abdominal mycoses (see below).

These infections, apart from metastatic lesions, are acquired as a result of traumatic introduction of the causative fungus into the dermis and deeper tissues.

Pulmonary Infections Sometimes Becoming Disseminated

Cryptococcosis (torulosis), histoplasmosis, coccidioidomycosis, North American blastomycosis, South American blastomycosis, aspergillosis and mucormycosis.

These diseases are not transmitted from person to person but result from the inhalation of air-borne particles containing infective elements, usually spores, of the organism concerned. Some of these diseases, e.g. cryptococcosis and histoplasmosis, may be 'opportunist'.

Treatment

Griseofulvin has a specific action against dermatophytes causing ringworm, and nystatin is used chiefly for local infections due to *Candida albicans*. Amphotericin B has broad-spectrum activity and has proved valuable in treating systemic infections such as cryptococcosis (torulosis). Certain new antifungal agents, amongst which is 5-fluorocytosine, may well prove to be very effective in therapy.

REFERENCES

CLAYTON, Y. M. (1970) Sensitivity of certain ocular fungi to antifungal drugs, *Trans. ophthal. Soc. U.K.*, **89**, 837.

JONES, B. R. (1970) Antifungal drugs for oculomycosis, *Trans. ophthal. Soc. U.K.*, **89**, 819.

RIDDELL, R. W. (1967) Fungal infections, in *Third Symposium on Advanced Medicine*, ed. Dawson, A. M., p. 15, Royal College of Physicians, London.

MYCETOMA

Synonym. Madura foot.

Definition

A chronic granulomatous infection with suppuration simulating actinomycosis. It affects exposed parts of the body, especially the feet. With progress of disease, marked swelling of the part involved may occur and external nodules connected with deeper sinuses appear. From sinuses the purulent and oily fluid exuded contains colonies of the causative organism like the grain in actinomycosis. These may be white or cream-coloured, red, brown or black.

Two types of organisms are concerned in this disease:

1. Actinomycetes giving rise to actinomycetoma. There are a number of causative organisms (*Nocardia asteroides*, *N. brasiliensis*, *Streptomyces madurae*, *S. pelletierii* and *S. somaliensis*). Unlike *Actinomyces israelii*, causing actinomycosis, which is a microaerophilic or an anaerobic organism, these actinomycetes require aerobic conditions for growth.
2. True fungi giving rise to maduromycetoma, including *Madurella mycetomi*, *M. grisea* and *Allescheria boydii* (*Monosporium apiospermum*).

Aetiology

The disease is most common in tropical and subtropical areas where the causative fungi may be found in soil or on plants. The habit of walking barefooted in these areas predisposes to infection. The term 'madura foot' originated from the fact that the disease is endemic in the Madura area of Madras. Males are more commonly affected than females.

Pathology

Numerous small abscesses and sinuses are found in subcutaneous tissues and may communicate with external nodules and lesions of muscle, fascia and bone. In the pus grains may be found, their colour depending on the causative organism. Actinomycetes may be demonstrated by their positive reaction to Gram stain, and true fungi by their broad, ramifying and often irregular mycelium.

Clinical Features

A subcutaneous nodule may develop weeks or months after localized trauma but in many cases there is no such history. The first signs are the presence of one or more hard, painless, subcutaneous nodules on the foot, and more rarely the hands, face and limbs. There is less tendency for lymph nodes and viscera to become involved than is the case in actinomycosis. After several months, swelling increases, the nodules break down and ulcerate, and sinuses are formed which discharge their characteristic exudate. Finally, the parts become riddled with sinuses, exuding foul-smelling, semi-purulent fluid. Even in advanced disease, pain and haemorrhage are conspicuous by their absence. The general health may suffer if secondary bacterial infection becomes predominant resulting in anaemia and toxaemia. Radiographs reveal bone involvement in advanced cases, both destructive and proliferative reactions being present.

Diagnosis

Laboratory identification of the nature of granules occurring in pus establishes the diagnosis. Culture studies are necessary to complete the investigation of the organism concerned.

Treatment

Early surgery is the treatment of choice. In actinomycetoma, sulphonamides are most effective but penicillin or broad-spectrum antibiotics are sometimes indicated. In maduromycetoma there is no effective therapeutic agent.

Prognosis

Lesions usually remain localized with very slow spread into adjacent tissues so that if adequate excision is performed at an early stage recurrence is unlikely. On the other hand, mycetomata rarely heal spontaneously and if neglected may lead to much tissue destruction ultimately necessitating amputation. Failing this, death may occur due to secondary infection.

REFERENCES

ABBOT, P. (1956) Mycetoma in the Sudan, *Trans. roy. Soc. trop. Med. Hyg.*, **50**, 11.

MARIAT, F. (1957) Les principaux actinomycètes aérobies responsables de mycétomes, *Sem. Hôp. Paris*, **5**, 939.

CHROMOBLASTOMYCOSIS

Synonym. Verrucous dermatitis.

Definition

A chronic infection of the skin and subcutaneous tissues caused by one of four closely related pigmented fungi (*Phialophora pedrosoi*, *P. verrucosa*, *P. compactum* and *Cladosporium carrionii*). The disease is characterized by warty lesions which become encrusted and eventually may ulcerate. The lower leg is usually involved, but lesions of elbow, thigh, buttock and other parts occur.

Aetiology

Though the disease has been reported from most parts of the world, it is more common in tropical and subtropical areas. It is thought that the causative fungi contaminate wood and other vegetable matter. Males are affected more frequently than females.

Pathology

Subacute granulomata with giant cells develop at sites of infection and in some zones micro-abscesses are formed. Within these, and within phagocytic cells, the typical brown thick-walled round fungal cells of the causative organism may be found. These cells reproduce by transverse fission and not by budding. They may also be found in skin scrapings of verrucous lesions.

Clinical Features

A papule may form at a known site of injury and gradually extends with the development of satellite lesions. Spread is usually very slow over months or years. Subsequent injury may lead to areas of ulceration. After years of neglect, lymphatic obstruction may give rise to elephantiasis of the extremity.

Diagnosis

The morphology and histology of early lesions may simulate cutaneous tuberculosis; syphilis, leishmaniasis and other fungal infections also require exclusion. The presence of fungal cells in tissue material establishes the nature of the disease which is confirmed by culture studies.

Treatment

Since there are no efficient therapeutic agents for this infection, surgery is at present the only treatment. Therapy with 5-fluorocytosine may prove to be an alternative.

Prognosis

Cure is to be expected if early lesions are widely excised but disease is difficult to eradicate in neglected cases.

REFERENCE

Carrion, A. L. (1950) Chromoblastomycosis, *Ann. N.Y. Acad. Sci.*, **50**, 1255.

SPOROTRICHOSIS

Definition

A chronic subcutaneous infection with little tendency to suppuration. Local dissemination by lymphatics is typical, satellite lesions developing along their course. Rarely widespread dissemination may occur giving rise to visceral and skeletal lesions. The causative fungus is *Sporothrix schenckii* an organism having two distinct growth phases, mycelial and yeast, according to its environment.

Aetiology

The disease is of world-wide distribution. *S. schenckii* has been isolated from timber, soil and plants and it is from such sources that infection is usually acquired. Extensive outbreaks have occurred in mines where pit props were infected with the fungus. Horticultural workers, farmers and labourers are particularly exposed.

Pathology

The histology of the sporotrichotic lesion is usually complex showing areas of chronic granuloma, giant cell reactions and micro-abscesses. Since the fungus cells are very scantily distributed in the lesion, the absence of organisms in the kind of cytological reaction described above should lead to sporotrichosis being suspected. Although the infective phase of *S. schenckii* is filamentous, this structure is no longer maintained when it is introduced into the subcutaneous tissues. Instead, single cells (i.e. yeasts) are formed. Such yeasts as can be found in the tissue lesion are often cigar-shaped, but serial sections may be required to demonstrate them.

Clinical Features

An indolent papule is the commonest mode of presentation, and this may develop two or three weeks after known trauma. It extends slowly and fails to heal in spite of various kinds of local therapy. An ulcer may form with a violaceous border and by this time similar lesions along the lines of draining lymphatics may have become obvious. Sometimes the granuloma commences more deeply in the subcutaneous tissues and though movable at first later becomes attached to the skin. The primary lesion is often referred to as the 'sporotrichotic chancre'. The pus from ulcerated nodules is thin and of small amount unless secondary pyogenic infection becomes predominant.

Rarely extensive lymphatic and haematogenous dissemination may ensue in neglected cases. This may lead to widespread subcutaneous lesions, granulomata of the oral and nasal mucosae, and skeletal metastases; viscera are seldom involved.

Primary pulmonary sporotrichosis has been described associated with lung cavitation.

Diagnosis

The localized subcutaneous lesion with limited lymphatic spread is so typical of sporotrichosis that diagnosis should present no problem. Where disease is more widespread, its persistence despite various forms of treatment should cause one to consider *S. schenckii* infection as a possibility. The most valuable investigation is the culture of biopsy material or pus when the causative fungus can be readily isolated. Inoculation of rodents with homogenates of biopsy material is also a valuable isolation procedure. Sporotrichosis has to be differentiated from syphilis, tuberculosis, leprosy and other fungus infections giving rise to granulomata.

Treatment

Potassium iodide by mouth in ascending dosage up to the limits of tolerance usually brings about a steady resolution. Amphotericin B given intravenously is indicated for those patients who fail to respond to oral iodide therapy and for cases showing widespread dissemination.

Prognosis

Once diagnosis has been established and proper medical treatment instituted prognosis is excellent.

REFERENCES

BROWN, R., WEINTRAUB, D., and SIMPSON, M. W. (1947) Sporotrichosis infection in mines of the Witwatersrand, *Proc. Transv. Mine med. Offrs' Ass.*, Johannesburg.

CRUTHIRDS, T. P., and PATTERSON, D. O. (1967) Primary pulmonary sporotrichosis, *Amer. Rev. resp. Dis.*, **95**, 845.

NORDEN, A. (1951) Sporotrichosis, *Acta path. microbiol. scand.*, Suppl. 19.

PHYCOMYCOSIS

Definition

This is a subcutaneous infection caused by *Basidiobolus meristosporus*, a phycomycete. Features of the disease are the presence of subcutaneous induration of 'rubbery' consistency and the absence of ulceration.

Aetiology

The disease has been reported from Nigeria, Ghana, Uganda and India and probably occurs in other subtropical and tropical zones. The mode of origin of infection is unknown and history of trauma has not been a feature of case reports.

Pathology

A chronic inflammatory reaction is accompanied by the presence of poorly staining broad fungal hyphae with no cross-walls. Eosinophils are numerous and much eosinophilic debris is present around hyphae.

Clinical Features

Indolent and slowly spreading subcutaneous induration occurs in this disease. It may involve a considerable area of a limb or other parts.

Diagnosis

The clinical picture is very characteristic and confirmation of diagnosis is made from the histopathology and culture of biopsy material.

Prognosis and Treatment

It is uncertain whether spontaneous cure occurs or if the disease is self-limiting. Response to oral iodide therapy is good.

REFERENCE

HARMAN, R. R. M., JACKSON, H., and WILLIS, A. J. P. (1964) Subcutaneous phycomycosis in Nigeria, *Brit. J. Derm.*, **76**, 408.

RHINOSPORIDIOSIS

Definition

A chronic infection of the mucous membrane of the nose, eyes, ears and larynx and occasionally of penis, vagina and rectum. The causative organism is *Rhinosporidium seeberi* which is assumed to be a fungus although it has never been cultured.

Aetiology

The disease is world wide and most common in Ceylon and India. It is not known as to how infection is acquired but immersion in stagnant water has been suggested as being responsible in some cases.

Pathology

The lesions usually take the form of polyps which are soft and nodular. Greyish-white areas occur over the pink surface and these consist of large fungal cells (sporangia) containing vast numbers of spores. The surrounding tissues consist of an oedematous, myxomatous stroma infiltrated with chronic inflammatory cells including plasma cells and lymphocytes; esoinophils are scanty. The sporangia are thick-walled and may be as much as 200 μ in diameter.

Clinical Features

Infection at first gives rise to local pruritus and mucoid discharge. After months or years, soft and vascular polyps develop which become pedunculated. As they enlarge they become obvious, for example, at the anterior nares or in the pharynx, and they may give rise to nasal obstruction, dyspnoea and dysphagia. Conjunctival lesions sometimes spread on to the face and into the lacrimal sac. Penile lesions can resemble venereal warts, vaginal granulomata may simulate condylomata, and rectal involvement may be confused with rectal polypi or haemorrhoids.

Diagnosis

This is established by the finding of large numbers of typical sporangia containing innumerable small spores in biopsy material.

Treatment

Adequate surgical excision of early lesions is indicated. Cauterization, in addition, may be necessary where infection is more widespread.

Prognosis

Disease remains localized. Lesions give rise to cosmetic problems, discomfort, later to obstructive effects.

REFERENCE

KARUNARATNE, W. A. E. (1964) *Rhinosporidiosis in Man*, London.

CRYPTOCOCCOSIS (TORULOSIS)

Synonym. European blastomycosis.

Definition

A subacute or chronic infection of the lungs which

frequently disseminates by haematogenous spread particularly to the cerebrospinal system. Metastases may also involve the skeletal system, skin and other organs. The causative organism is *Cryptococcus neoformans*, an encapsulated yeast.

Aetiology

The disease has a world-wide distribution and the causative organism has been isolated from the soil, pigeon droppings, fruit and milk.

Pathology

Where large numbers of encapsulated *C. neoformans* cells are proliferating in the tissues, cysts containing glairy mucoid material are visible on naked-eye examination. In such instances, there may be only slight cellular reaction to the invading fungus seen histologically. On the other hand, where the yeasts are few and the inflammatory reaction considerable, the histology may simulate that of any chronic granuloma. A range of findings between these two extremes are seen both in the primary pulmonary and the disseminated lesions. In cerebral infections, the base of the brain is chiefly involved, the meninges becoming thickened and opaque. Metastases in the brain substance frequently form cyst-like areas and give rise to haemorrhages.

Clinical Features

Primary pulmonary disease may take the form of a minimal lesion, a solitary mass (toruloma), or an area of infiltration, sometimes cavitated. When dissemination occurs, unilateral or bilateral spread of disease gives rise to extensive areas of pneumonitis. Occasionally miliary tuberculosis is mimicked. Meningeal cryptococcosis can have a gradual or sudden onset with headache, vomiting and pain and stiffness in the muscles of the neck. The signs are those of subacute or chronic meningitis, and a diagnosis of tuberculous meningitis has in the past frequently been made. Cerebral infection gives rise to signs of an extending intracranial lesion and to papilloedema. There are often remissions in the course of this infection which may continue for months or for many years.

Bone lesions are osteolytic and unassociated with periosteal proliferation. They occur in approximately 10 per cent. in cases of cryptococcosis. Skin granulomata can take the form of papules, acne-like pustules or subcutaneous abscesses. These may ulcerate and produce glairy pus.

Diagnosis

Cryptococcosis has to be differentiated from neoplastic diseases of the lungs and from other chronic fungal and bacterial infections. Meningeal lesions must be distinguished from those due to *M. tuberculosis*. Skin granulomata may resemble rodent ulcers, gummata or carcinomata.

Cryptococcal infection is known to complicate sarcoidosis, Hodgkin's disease, leukaemia, reticulosis and other conditions in which the immune processes become disturbed. In such instances, the organism proliferates in affected lymph nodes or other tissues.

Diagnosis is confirmed by finding encapsulated budding yeasts in sputum, cerebrospinal fluid, tissue biopsy homogenates or scrapings. They should also be searched for in the glairy pus from ulcerated skin or mucosal lesions. The organisms are best demonstrated by mixing the exudate with nigrosin or India ink. By so doing the capsular material surrounding the yeast cell is clearly demarcated. Cultures should also be made and pathogenicity tests on mice carried out.

No serological or skin tests are of practical value in the diagnosis of this infection.

Treatment

Excision is the treatment of choice for solitary pulmonary lesions or of lesions limited to one or two lobes. An important prerequisite for surgery is the exclusion of metastases in the cerebrospinal and skeletal systems or, as far as possible, elsewhere. Even if no evidence of such spread can be found, cryptococcal meningitis may still develop postoperatively. Isolated dermal lesions should be excised. Amphotericin B has been the chemotherapeutic agent of choice pre- and post-operatively and in meningeal cryptococcosis. More recently, treatment with 5-fluorocytosine has been reported to be effective. In assessing the value of treatment procedures, the known incidence of naturally occurring remissions must be taken into account.

Prognosis

Subclinical infection probably occurs which undergoes spontaneous healing, and it is possible also that disseminated disease is occasionally self-limiting. The development of widespread metastases is of grave prognosis.

REFERENCES

LITTMAN, M. L., and ZIMMERMAN, L. E. (1956) *Cryptococcosis*, New York.

WATKINS, J. S., CAMPBELL, M. J., GARDNER-MEDWIN, D., INGHAM, H. R., and MURRAY, I. G. (1969) Two cases of cryptococcal meningitis, one treated with 5-fluorocytosine, *Brit. med. J.*, **3**, 29.

HISTOPLASMOSIS

Synonyms. Darling's disease; Cave disease; Reticulo-endothelial cytomycosis.

Definition

An inapparent acute, subacute or chronic disease usually of respiratory origin which notably involves reticulo-endothelial cells. Pulmonary infection is most often asymptomatic or benign, but occasionally occurs as a persisting and extending pneumonitis in which cavitation may develop. Widespread reticulo-endothelial dissemination probably follows infection more frequently than is at present recognized and rarely this aspect of the disease becomes the most important clinically. The causative fungus is *Histoplasma capsulatum*, a diphasic organism which grows as mycelium or as yeasts according to its environment. A similar fungus, *H. duboisii*, occurring in parts of Africa is less often responsible.

Aetiology

The disease has a world-wide distribution but is particularly endemic in certain zones, for example, great river basins like the Mississippi valley. *H. capsulatum* has been isolated from soil, dust, air-samples and animal excreta (particularly of chickens). It has been found in old silos and in caves which were visited by subjects who subsequently developed the disease. Infection is acquired through the inhalation of air-borne spores which develop on the mycelium of *H. capsulatum* growing saprophytically in the soil or elsewhere in nature. Laboratory infections may follow the handling of cultures of the organism. The extent to which articles from endemic parts of the world may transmit infection elsewhere is as yet unknown.

Pathology

In the granulomata produced by this fungus, intracellular minute yeast cells, 2–5 μ in diameter, indicate the nature of the disease. The small size may lead to their being overlooked or to confusion with Leishman-Donovan bodies or toxoplasma cells. The yeasts of *H. duboisii* are larger. In the lungs, spleen and notably in the adrenal glands, central necrosis of the granulomata follows and the picture may then simulate tuberculosis. With the process of healing, calcification becomes a particular feature of histoplasmosis.

Clinical Features

Dual infections with *H. capsulatum* and *Myco. tuberculosis* have been known to occur and, because of the similar clinical features of the two diseases, difficulties may arise in differential diagnosis. The similarity of some forms of histoplasmosis to visceral and mucocutaneous leishmaniasis must always be borne in mind. Furthermore, *H. capsulatum* infection may complicate sarcoidosis, Hodgkin's disease, leukaemia and other diseases affecting immune processes.

Certain clinical types of disease are well-recognized:

Solitary Pulmonary Nodule. This is usually situated close to the pleura and simulates lesions of this kind met with in tuberculosis and coccidioidomycosis.

Benign Pulmonary Infection. Disease is usually asymptomatic but may be accompanied by pyrexia and malaise. Zones of pneumonitis seen radiologically may be scattered throughout all lung fields and tend to undergo spontaneous resolution. Healed miliary tuberculosis is mimicked when calcification accompanies this. More severe infections resemble attacks of influenza or atypical pneumonia and are associated with marked fever, lassitude and chest pain. Radiographs show extensive mottling in such cases.

Progressive Pulmonary Histoplasmosis. Subacute and chronic fibrocaseous and cavitated disease is an uncommon sequel of infection by *H. capsulatum.* It has been observed in sanatoria amongst patients assumed to be tuberculous.

Disseminated Histoplasmosis. Haematogenous dissemination giving rise to widespread reticulo-endotheliosis of serious degree may manifest itself at any stage following initial infection. It is rare, however, compared with the very large numbers of cases of benign infection which are known to occur in endemic areas. It should be stressed that this complication can develop many years after original infection, the nature of which may or may not have been recorded. The metastases occur particularly in the liver, spleen, lymph nodes, adrenal glands, bone marrow and in the mucous membranes of the mouth and gastro-intestinal tract. Hepatomegaly, splenomegaly and mucocutaneous ulcerations may be presenting features in disseminated disease. Dissemination has been associated with long-term steroid therapy.

Diagnosis

The development of skin hypersensitivity to *H. capsulatum* antigen (histoplasmin) follows asymptomatic or symptomatic infection. Skin testing is carried out as in the Mantoux test and interpretation of results is the same as for tuberculosis. A positive finding indicates past or present infection. Serological investigations may point to the presence of active disease, precipitins appearing early and complement-fixing antibodies late. A single histoplasmosis skin test may stimulate humoral antibodies to *H. capsulatum* antigen in histoplasmin-hypersensitive subjects. Caution must be exercised when interpreting serological results on blood samples taken more than two days after a histoplasmin skin test.

There is little to distinguish the radiological findings in pneumonitis due to *H. capsulatum* from those due to *Myco. tuberculosis*, other bacteria or viruses, or to *Coccidioides immitis* and other fungi. In healed lesions, a preponderence of discrete and perfectly spherical lesions is suggestive of histoplasmosis.

Search is made for very small yeast cells, often intracellular, in smears of sputum, bronchial aspirates and gastric lavage material stained by Giemsa's method. Marrow and lymph node biopsies should be examined where disseminated disease is considered to be a possibility. Culture studies should also be carried out on the above materials employing both 26° C. and 37° C. for incubation in order to demonstrate the mycelial and yeast phases of *H. capsulatum.* Animal inoculation studies may also prove helpful.

For histological material, detailed study using various staining techniques is required to differentiate the cells of *H. capsulatum* from those of other fungus infections and from leishmaniae and toxoplasma.

Treatment

No specific therapy is needed in the treatment of limited pulmonary infections. Where disease is extending, amphotericin B, administered intravenously, should be considered. Surgery is occasionally indicated particularly for persistent cavitating lesions.

Prognosis

Most pulmonary infections are benign. Disseminated disease does not necessarily carry with it a poor prognosis, but extensive spread left untreated may be fatal. Absence of serum antibodies early in disease, increasing complement-fixing antibody titres during the course of infection, and loss of skin hypersensitivity to histoplasmin are of serious significance.

REFERENCES

CLARKE, B. M., and GREENWOOD, B. M. (1968) Pulmonary lesions in African histoplasmosis, *J. trop. Med. Hyg.*, **71,** 4.

COCKSHOTT, W. P., and LUCAS, A. O. (1964) *Histoplasma duboisii*, *Quart. J. Med.*, N.S., **33,** 223.

COLE, A. C. E., RIDLEY, D. S., and WOLFE, H. R. I. (1965) Bowel infection with *Histoplasma duboisii*, *J. trop. Med. Hyg.*, **68,** 92.

FURCOLOW, M. L., and BRASHER, C. A. (1956) Chronic progressive (cavitary) histoplasmosis as a problem in tuberculosis sanatoriums, *Amer. Rev. Tuberc.*, **73,** 609.

KAUFMAN, L., TERRY, R. T., SCHUBERT, J. H., and MCLAUGHLIN, D. (1967) Effects of a single histoplasmin skin test on the serological diagnosis of histoplasmosis, *J. Bact.*, **94,** 798.

LOOSLI, C. G. (1955) Histoplasmosis, some clinical epidemiological and laboratory aspects, *Med. Clin. N. Amer.*, **39,** 71.

MURRAY, P. J. S., and SLADDEN, R. A. (1965) Disseminated histoplasmosis following long-term steroid therapy for reticulosarcoma, *Brit. med. J.*, **2,** 631.

SWEANY, H. C. (1960) *Histoplasmosis*, Springfield, Ill.

COCCIDIOIDOMYCOSIS

Synonyms. Valley fever; Desert rheumatism; Coccidioidal granuloma.

Definition

An inapparent, acute, subacute or chronic disease of respiratory origin, which closely mimics tuberculosis. Infection is most frequently asymptomatic or benign, but sometimes gives rise to persistent areas of pneumonitis which may caseate and later cavitate. Dissemination is unusual but when it occurs gives rise to cold abscess formation in various viscera, the skeletal system and in the skin and subcutaneous tissues. The causative organism is *Coccidioides immitis*, a diphasic fungus which grows as mycelium or as rounded cells according to its environment.

Aetiology

Endemic zones are limited to the south-western regions of the United States of America and to similar arid zones in Mexico and Venezuela. *C. immitis* has been isolated from the soil of these areas particularly in the regions of excrement-contaminated rodent burrows. Infection results from the inhalation of air-borne spores which are readily and widely disseminated by air currents. Cultures of this fungus very easily give rise to infections in laboratory workers.

Pathology

Epithelioid tubercles and giant cell systems characterize the early lesions produced by *C. immitis*. Infiltrations by neutrophil polymorph cells give rise to so-called 'suppurating pseudo-tubercles' which are less commonly seen in tuberculosis. The granulomata may heal by resolution or fibrosis. Caseation and abscess formation are often present; calcification may occasionally be seen. Within the lesions the causative fungus is easily demonstrated and takes the form of round cells (sporangia) up to 200 μ in diameter. As they mature they form internal spores. These become freed by rupture of the sporangia walls, in this way spreading infection. The lesions may be so similar to those of tuberculosis that it is essential to exclude the presence of acid-fast bacilli before diagnosis is made.

Clinical Features

It is usual for infection to be inapparent or so mild that its nature is overlooked. All degrees of severity of disease can occur depending on the numbers of spores inhaled and the resistance of the subject infected. Coccidioidomycosis may co-exist with tuberculosis. Certain clinical types of disease are well recognized:

Solitary Pulmonary Nodule. This is usually small and can become calcified. It is similar to lesions of this kind met with in tuberculosis and histoplasmosis.

Benign Pulmonary Infection. Symptoms follow exposure to infected dust, the incubation period being one to four weeks. Features of an influenza-like illness first appear, such as malaise and arthralgia. Manifestations of hypersensitivity, such as erythema nodosum, develop one to two weeks after onset of symptoms in about 5 per cent. of infections. Patchy consolidation of the lungs is seen radiologically and a pleural effusion may form. It is usual for resolution to occur after one or two months, but fibrotic or calcified lesions sometimes remain and occasionally thin-walled cavities.

Progressive Pulmonary Coccidioidomycosis. This rarely develops as an immediate continuation of severe primary infection though it may be considerably delayed. General deterioration in health is accompanied by persistent fever. Signs of extending bronchopneumonia become apparent.

Disseminated Coccidioidomycosis. Haematogenous spread of infection may accompany progressive pulmonary coccidioidomycosis. At sites of metastases, granulomata are formed and later give rise to cold abscesses. The meninges and brain, skeletal system, skin and subcutaneous tissues are often involved. An isolated peripheral metastasis is well known. Temporary spontaneous remissions in the course of disseminated infections have been described.

Diagnosis

The development of skin hypersensitivity to *C. immitis* antigen (coccidioidin) follows inapparent or apparent infection. The reading of skin tests is as for the Mantoux test in tuberculosis, and positive results indicate past or present infection. Serological tests are usually negative in mild and early infections, but in more severe cases precipitins appear and, later, complement-fixing antibodies.

Radiologically, coccidioidomycosis simulates tuberculosis and histoplasmosis. In slight infections, the lesions are similar to those met with in various bacterial and viral diseases.

The fungal cells (sporangia) can sometimes be found in smears of sputum, bronchial aspirates and gastric washings. Culture studies must be carried out with caution in view of the infectious nature of the fungus. Both at 26° C. and 37° C. *C. immitis* grows as white filamentous colonies. Specimens of pus and homogenates of biopsy material should be similarly investigated. Animal inoculation is a valuable additional diagnostic procedure.

Treatment

Specific treatment is only indicated in cases of severe and extending pulmonary infection, or when there is evidence of haematogenous dissemination. Administration of amphotericin B intravenously is the treatment of choice but it is not always effective. It should also be used when surgery is contemplated and also postoperatively. Excision of persistent localized lesions, and aspiration or drainage of cold abscesses may be required.

Prognosis

Complete recovery is the usual outcome of even severe primary infections. Progressive disease may undergo spontaneous arrest, but an increasing titre of complement fixing antibody and a loss of skin hypersensitivity are of serious import.

REFERENCES

Ajello, L. (1967) *Coccidioidomycosis*, University of Arizona Press, Tucson.
Fiese, M. J. (1958) *Coccidioidomycosis*, Springfield, Ill.
Forbus, W. D., and Bestebreurtje, A. M. (1946) Coccidioidomycosis, *Milit. Surg.*, **99,** 653.
Johnson, J. E., Perry, J. E., Fekety, F. R., Kadull, P. J., and Cluff, L. E. (1964) Laboratory-acquired coccidioidomycosis. A report of 210 cases. *Ann. intern. Med.*, **60,** 941.

NORTH AMERICAN BLASTOMYCOSIS

Synonym. Gilchrist's disease.

Definition

A chronic granulomatous infection originating as a respiratory disease and readily giving rise to disseminated lesions in skin. The initial pulmonary lesion may be minimal and be associated with extensive dermal manifestations. The causative organism is *Blastomyces dermatitidis*, a diphasic fungus which grows as mycelium or as yeasts according to environmental conditions.

Aetiology

The disease is geographically very limited and is practically restricted to the North American continent. Recent infections have been reported from various parts of Africa. The disease occurs particularly in persons whose occupation involves intimate contact with the soil. Attempts to isolate *B. dermatitidis* from soil and vegetation have been singularly unsuccessful and its distribution in nature remains unknown.

Pathology

Epithelioid cell granulomata together with zones of suppuration characterize this infection. These two types of reaction may vary in degree throughout the lesions. In inflammatory areas the yeasts of *B. dermatitidis*, 10–30 μ in diameter, are found. Considerable epithelial hyperplasia is a feature of skin lesions and micro-abscesses occur in the epidermis and more deeply.

Clinical Features

Pulmonary infection takes the form of subacute suppurative bronchopneumonia. Later the pleura is involved but extension to chest wall is less common than in actinomycosis. With advancing disease the sputum becomes purulent and blood stained. Radiological examination is suggestive of chronic pyogenic bacterial infection or of neoplasm. Untreated disease is usually progressive and gives rise to haematogenous dissemination of infection.

Metastatic lesions occur chiefly in the skin and subcutaneous tissues but are also well known in bones, meninges and brain. Granulomata frequently occur in the spleen and liver, and often also in the urogenital system.

For many years it was thought that the skin became involved by surface inoculation and introduction of *B. dermatitidis* by this route. This was due to the fact that cutaneous and subcutaneous lesions are often the most apparent and presenting signs, the original lung granulomata being minimal or absent. Skin metastases develop as verrucous granulomata having raised serpiginous borders. As these advance to involve new areas of skin, some central healing with scarring takes place. Numerous micro-abscesses cover the extending border and the surface of the granuloma. Centrifugal spread of the lesions continues for months or years and may cause much disfiguration.

Mucous and mucocutaneous lesions involving the oropharynx, larynx or rectum can simulate squamous-cell carcinoma.

Diagnosis

The use of skin tests employing fungus antigen (in this case blastomycin) are less reliable than in histoplasmosis or coccidioidomycosis. Serological tests are also of only limited value.

Radiological findings in early pulmonary infection most commonly show broadening of hilar shadows and limited opacities in the lung fields suggestive of neoplasm or tuberculosis. Later widespread mottling is seen.

The yeast cells of *B. dermatitidis* are present in sputum and bronchial aspirates particularly when these are purulent. The cells may readily be found in the exudate of freshly-opened pustules of skin lesions. Culture studies are performed at 26° C. and 37° C. to isolate the mycelial and yeast forms of the fungus respectively.

Treatment

Therapeutic measures used in the past include oral iodides and intravenous 2-hydroxystilbamidine. Many cases relapsed. Amphotericin B administered intravenously appears to be more effective.

Prognosis

Extending pulmonary disease and the presence of disseminated lesions are of serious import and may prove to be fatal if untreated. Cutaneous blastomycosis with minimal lesions elsewhere is a very slowly progressive but non-fatal condition.

REFERENCES

BUSEY, J. F. (1964) Blastomycosis I. A review of 198 collected cases in Veterans Administration hospitals. Blastomycosis co-operative study of the Veterans Administration, *Amer. Rev. resp. Dis.*, **89**, 659.

EMMONS, C. W., MURRAY, I. G., LURIE, H. I., KING, M. H., TULLOCH, J. A., and CONNOR, D. H. (1964) North American blastomycosis. Two autochthonous cases from Africa, *Sabouraudia*, **3**, 306.

FURCULOW, M. L., BALOWS, A., MENGES, R. W., PICKARD, D., MCCLELLAN, J. T., and SALIBA, A. (1966) Blastomycosis. An important medical problem in the Central United States, *J. Amer. med. Ass.*, **198**, 529.

GATTI, F., DE BROE, M., and AJELLO, L. (1968) *Blastomyces dermatitidis* infection in the Congo. A report of a second autochthonous case, *Amer. J. trop. Med. Hyg.*, **17**, 96.

SCHWARZ, J., and BAUM, G. L. (1951) Blastomycosis, *Amer. J. clin. Path.*, **21**, 999.

SOUTH AMERICAN BLASTOMYCOSIS

Synonym. Paracoccidioidal granuloma.

Definition

A chronic granulomatous disease affecting the mucous membranes of the mouth and nose and contiguous skin areas, and producing lymphadenopathy and systemic spread to various organs. The causative organism is a diphasic fungus. *Paracoccidioides brasiliensis*, which simulates *B. dermatitidis* and which has mycelial and yeast structures depending on conditions of its growth.

Aetiology

The disease is limited to South American countries and to Central America. The causative organism has been isolated from soil but the way in which it produces infection is unknown.

Pathology

The lesions are similar to those of North American blastomycosis except for the fact that the yeast cells of the causative fungus show multiple points of budding. There is a greater tendency for lymphoid tissue to be involved.

Clinical Features

The first lesions usually appear at the mucocutaneous margins of the mouth, nose, conjunctivae or anus. They are proliferative granulomata which eventually ulcerate. Other skin lesions, which are manifestations of disseminated infection. may simulate leishmaniasis or tuberculosis.

It is common for the lymph nodes in the region of initial lesions to become infected and from them sinuses may drain to the overlying skin area. Cervical lymphadenitis may be so extensive as to suggest a neoplastic process.

In systemic infection, splenomegaly is practically always present and, unlike North American blastomycosis, the lymphoid tissues of the intestinal tract are frequently affected. The lungs, bones, adrenal glands and brain are also sites of metastases.

Diagnosis

Skin tests with fungus antigen (paracoccidioidin) are of limited value. In serological tests, the complement fixing antibody titre shows a rise as disease progresses and a fall with improvement.

The causative yeast cells, up to 30 μ in diameter, are very readily found in pus, biopsy scrapings and in encrusted exudate. Around the cells are multiple buds 2–5 μ in size. By culturing at 26° C. and 37° C. the mycelial and yeast phases of *P. brasiliensis* can be grown.

Treatment

Long term amphotericin B therapy is the treatment of choice; sulphonamides are less effective.

Prognosis

If untreated this appears to be invariably fatal. Relapses frequently occur in treated cases.

REFERENCE

FURTADO, T. A., WILSON, J. W., and PLUNKETT, O. A. (1954) South American blastomycosis or paracoccidioidomycosis, *Arch. Derm. Syph. (Chic.)*, **70**, 166.

ASPERGILLOSIS

Definition

A fungus infection which becomes superimposed upon various disease conditions. It is rarely a primary disease in man. It occurs most commonly as a pulmonary infection and gives rise to extensive fungus proliferation (aspergillus mycetoma), necrotizing granulomatous lesions, and Arthus-like eosinophilic infiltrations in allergic subjects. Haematogenous dissemination is an uncommon sequel. The causative organism is almost invariably *Aspergillus fumigatus*, other aspergillus species being rarely involved.

Aetiology

This is a world-wide disease. Though *A. fumigatus* is a frequent contaminant of decomposing vegetation such as composts, mouldy hay and grain, its spores are ubiquitous in urban as well as in rural air. It grows profusely at 37° C. Aspergillosis was once thought to occur mainly in bird fanciers, farm workers and others handling grain, but it is now believed that occupation is not an important aetiological factor. Whereas primary aspergillosis is a well-known disease of birds which simulates tuberculosis, human disease appears to be always associated with pre-existing lung damage.

Pathology

Pulmonary infection develops in areas of infarction,

pneumonitis, tuberculosis, bronchiectasis, carcinoma, leukaemia or lymphoma. *Aspergillus fumigatus* proliferates in closed lesions in the form of branching filaments which may produce mycelial masses. Tissue necrosis and neutrophil polymorph leucocytic infiltration result. Vascular thrombosis is frequently seen in the affected lung areas, and the fungus may penetrate obstructed vessels. Where mycelium proliferates in air spaces, it develops typical greyish-green sporing structures. Growth within old tuberculous, bronchiectatic or other cavities produces fungus masses known as aspergillus mycetomata. The walls of these cavities are usually epithelialized, but where this is not the case fungal invasion may give rise to haemorrhage.

Aspergillus mycelium proliferates in the bronchial exudate of asthmatic subjects and becomes associated with infiltrations of lung parenchyma by eosinophil cells. In this form of aspergillosis the fungus is present in very scanty amount in the bronchi and is not found in the Arthus-like zones of lung infiltration.

Haematogenous dissemination from pulmonary lesions gives rise to metastatic abscesses containing mycelium in skin and subcutaneous tissues, brain, kidney, myocardium and bone.

Clinical Features

Three main types of pulmonary disease occur:

Saprophytic Type. Minor degrees of aspergillus infection are likely to go unnoticed since interest is centred upon the disease condition which led to predisposition to fungus invasion. With the development of more extensive infection, the sputum may become purulent and fever and haemoptysis ensue. Aspergillosis of the pleura occurs in cases of bronchopleural fistula or may follow aspiration of an empyema or intrathoracic surgical procedures. Fungus infection may delay healing of wounds postoperatively.

The aspergillus mycetoma is usually a solitary lesion situated in the upper lobe which develops insidiously over months or years as a spherical mass. It is most commonly discovered accidentally during routine radiography, but haemoptysis may be a presenting symptom. In X-rays it is seen as a rounded tumour-like opacity with a crescentic cap of translucency; movement may be seen on changing the position of the patient. A pulmonary neoplasm may be simulated in radiographs.

Allergic Type. This is a form of pulmonary eosinophilia and occurs in asthmatic subjects. Recurrent attacks of pyrexia, chest discomfort and wheezing are accompanied by expectoration of tenacious sputum and sometimes 'casts'. Serial radiographs show changing areas of shadowing and clearing. After repeated episodes of these hypersensitivity reactions, bronchography has shown the presence of ectasia in bronchi which were previously normal. Bronchograms are typified by the presence of fusiform or saccular dilatations in segmental or subsegmental bronchi with filling distal to dilated zones.

Radiographs in which pulmonary shadowing is visible beyond zones of bronchial obstruction may simulate the appearances associated with neoplastic bronchial obstruction.

Disseminated Type. Haematogenous spread of infection is generally associated with disease conditions in which immunity is reduced. Localizing signs occur at the sites of metastic abscesses in patients suffering from leukaemia, Hodgkin's disease and other malignant conditions, especially in those undergoing long-term treatment with corticosteroids or radiomimetic drugs. The lungs and any other organs may become the sites of aspergillus abscesses.

Diagnosis

Intradermal skin tests of Mantoux type are not used in the diagnosis of aspergillosis. Prick tests with aspergillus antigen are, however, valuable and give immediate reactions in patients with allergic aspergillosis; in saprophytic type aspergillosis there is no response. On the other hand, a positive result is not necessarily indicative of allergic aspergillosis since it may be found in patients with other types of fungal allergy. The serological diagnosis of aspergillosis is of great value since the great majority of patients suffering from aspergillus mycetoma have precipitins in their sera and at least 70 per cent. of those in the allergic aspergillosis group.

Since *A. fumigatus* is ubiquitous and is isolated from the sputum of about 10 per cent. of bronchitic patients and from a higher proportion of asthmatic subjects, its presence in cultures is not conclusive evidence that it is playing a pathogenic role. Most patients suffering from aspergillosis, however, give positive cultures although repeated sputum examinations may be necessary before the fungus is grown. Incubation of cultures is carried out at 37° C. and fungal colonies are always of filamentous type with typical green sporulation.

A sputum eosinophil count should be performed and blood eosinophils estimated if allergic aspergillosis is suspected. Any 'casts' present in the sputum should be sectioned and examined for aspergillus filaments amongst the inspissated mucin and eosinophil cells. A silver impregnation technique should be used.

Treatment and Prognosis

Saprophytic Type. Specific treatment is only indicated when dissemination of infection is likely. Intravenously administered amphotericin B or 2-hydroxystilbamidine may be effective. The appearance of multiple metastases is of serious import. Surgical excision of mycetomata is necessary when recurrent haemoptyses occur or when there is any doubt as to the nature of the lesion. In most instances, they may be left undisturbed without fear of complications.

Allergic Type. The inhalation of antifungal agents such as nystatin or brilliant green solution, and desensitization with aspergillus antigen, have been used in treatment. They are of doubtful value. Corticosteroid therapy may need consideration in certain cases. Recurrent hypersensitivity reactions occurring over the years may lead to much bronchial damage and sometimes death in status asthmaticus.

Disseminated Type. Amphotericin B or 2-hydroxystilbamidine administered intravenously are drugs of choice in this serious complication.

REFERENCES

BRITISH TUBERCULOSIS ASSOCIATION (1968) Aspergillus in persistent lung cavities after tuberculosis, *Tubercle (Lond.)*, **49**, 1.

CAMPBELL, M. J., and CLAYTON, Y. M. (1964) Bronchopulmonary aspergillosis, *Amer. Rev. resp. Dis.*, **89**, 186.

GOWING, N. F. C., and HAMILTON, I. M. E. (1960) Tissue reactions to aspergillus in cases of Hodgkin's disease and leukaemia, *J. clin. Path.*, **13**, 396.

HINSON, K. F. W., MOON, A. J., and PLUMMER, N. S. (1952) Bronchopulmonary aspergillosis, *Thorax*, **7**, 317.

LONGBOTTOM, J. L., and PEPYS, J. (1964) Pulmonary aspergillosis: diagnostic and immunological significance of antigens and C-substance in *Aspergillus fumigatus*, *J. Path. Bact.*, **88**, 141.

SCADDING, J. G. (1967) The bronchi in allergic aspergillosis, *Scand. J. resp. Dis.*, **48**, 372.

MUCORMYCOSIS

Definition

A chronic infection of the respiratory tract disseminating to other organs occurring particularly in patients suffering from diabetes and other debilitating diseases. It is caused by certain species of Mucor, Rhizopus and Absidia (Phycomycetes).

Aetiology

The disease has a world-wide distribution but is uncommon. The causative fungi are frequent saprophytes occurring in nature. They become pathogenic for subjects whose immunity is lowered. The long-term use of corticosteroids and radiomimetic drugs appears to add to predisposition.

Pathology

There are no specific inflammatory reactions. Broad branching fungal filaments showing no transverse walls are present in affected tissues. Thrombosis and infarction are often found when vessels become invaded by the causative fungus.

Clinical Features

Pneumonitis in which phycomycete infection plays a complicating role may be associated with clinical evidence of disseminated disease. The paranasal sinuses, orbit, brain and gastro-intestinal tract may be involved.

Diagnosis

There are no skin or serological tests of value. Exudates should be cultured for the presence of grey-white floccose Phycomycete colonies which may show black sporulation. Caution is required when interpretating culture results since the fungi responsible for this disease are common contaminants.

Treatment and Prognosis

This infection occurs in seriously ill patients and adds to the gravity of prognosis. No specific therapy is known.

REFERENCE

BAKER, R. D. (1957) Mucormycosis. A new disease, *J. Amer. med. Ass.*, **163**, 805.

R. W. RIDDELL

DISEASES DUE TO PROTOZOAL INFECTION

MALARIA

Definition

Malaria is a febrile illness caused by sporozoa of the genus *Plasmodium* of which four species infect man. The parasites are conveyed to man by the female anopheline mosquito. The clinical effects are dependent on the infecting species and the previous exposure of the patient; they include fever which may be periodic, anaemia and enlargement of the liver and spleen.

Aetiology

The species of Plasmodium concerned in human malaria are *Plasmodium falciparum*, *Plasmodium vivax*, *Plasmodium malariae* and *Plasmodium ovale*. These species are distributed within a very wide area stretching from 60° N. to 40° S. latitude.

P. falciparum (malignant tertian) malaria is found in warm, moist climates, most of tropical Africa, parts of India and Pakistan, South-East Asia including Thailand, Vietnam, Indonesia and New Guinea, South and Central America. It occurs irregularly in the Middle East and was formerly present in parts of southern and eastern Europe. It does not occur in West Africa.

P. vivax (benign tertian) malaria is widespread in the tropics and subtropics and in some temperate regions. *P. malariae* (quartan) malaria is much less common; it occurs widely in the tropics especially in East and West Africa, India, Ceylon, South and Central America. *P. ovale* (ovale tertian) malaria is uncommon and is found in irregular areas in East, West and Central Africa and South America. A few cases have been reported in South-East Asia.

All forms of malaria are transmitted in nature by the females of some species of *Anopheles* mosquito. The disease may also be transferred from man to man by the passage of infected blood and is occasionally transmitted across the placenta. It can be induced artificially by infective mosquito bite or intravenous administration of sporozoites.

The life cycle of the parasite begins in the female mosquito when she ingests human blood containing the sexual forms of the parasite (*gametocytes*). In the stomach the male gametocytes liberate flagella which fertilize the female cells. The resultant conjugate pierces the stomach wall and develops beneath the lining membrane to become a cyst in which the infective forms called *sporozoites* appear. These eventually reach the salivary glands and proboscis and are injected into man during the insect bite. The process takes 7–14 days and the mosquito remains infective for the rest of its life. The sporozoites after injection into human tissues pass rapidly into the blood stream and thence to the liver where they enter the parenchymal cells, round off and multiply, producing the first liver cycle of the parasite, the pre-erythrocytic phase (PE), which in the course of 6–8 days matures and divides producing *merozoites*. The liver cell ruptures and the merozoites are expelled either into adjacent liver cells or into the blood stream. In the latter they set up the asexual or erythrocytic (E) cycle which is responsible for the clinical effects.

Up to this point the life cycle is the same for all four species of parasite, but thereafter *P. falciparum* and the other three organisms differ. In *P. falciparum* the parasites in the liver die out after the erythrocytic phase has been initiated. In the others the liver phase persists, forming a succession of parasites which are presumed to pass to development at intervals similar to the pre-erythrocytic period. The persistent liver phase is usually called the exo-erythrocytic or EE cycle.

The life cycles can be summarized thus:

All four parasites:

SP	⟶	PE	⟶	E
(sporozoites)		(primary liver phase: Pre-erythrocytic)		(erythrocytic phase)

This is the only pattern for *P. falciparum*.

In the other species of malaria the persistent liver forms develop and the life cycle may be written.

SP ⟶ PE ⟶ E
PE ↓ EE

In the developed case of clinical malaria, therefore the parasitic patterns are:

P. falciparum .	E form only.
P. vivax .	Both the E and the EE form present.
P. malariae .	
P. ovale .	

As will be seen later, modern chemotherapy and chemoprophylaxis and suppression are based on these life cycle patterns.

The erythrocytic (E) cycle is started by the entry of a merozoite into an erythrocyte. The completion of the cycle takes 48 hours in *P. falciparum*, *P. vivax* and *P. ovale* infections and 72 hours in *P. malariae* infection. In this time the parasite passes through successive stages, beginning with the unpigmented 'ring' consisting of a disc of cytoplasm containing one or more masses of chromatin, corresponding to a nucleus. This becomes actively amoeboid and grows into the *trophozoite*, in which malaria pigment (*haemozoin*) first appears. The chromatin then divides, each portion becoming surrounded by separate collections of cytoplasm to form a *merozoite*.

The mature parasite at this stage is called a *schizont*. The erythrocyte then ruptures and releases the merozoites into the plasma, from which some migrate to further erythrocytes and repeat the cycle or become *gametocytes* which persist in the cells.

Epidemiology

Malaria is transmitted in areas in which there are the necessary *Anopheles* vectors, suitable warm ambient temperature and humidity, a reservoir of infection containing gametocytes (usually the local population) and available suitable new hosts. Malaria seldom occurs at heights above 7000 feet.

Endemicity in a given area depends on local conditions of insect transmission and host reaction. The situation is described as holoendemic where there is heavy continuous transmission, and hyperendemic, mesoendemic and endemic depending on the findings in the population in regard to the incidence of parasitaemia and enlargement of the spleen in relation to age groups.

In the community malaria is classed as stable or unstable. The former occurs in areas in which there is constantly repeated infection, so that the surviving population possesses a notable degree of immunity. Under these circumstances epidemics do not occur. Unstable malaria occurs where transmission is intermittent, for example where it is seasonal or is occurring in populations partly, but inadequately, protected against infection by drugs or entomological control. In such areas, where the population has a variable state of immunity, epidemics may happen.

Individual Resistance to Infection ('Immunity'). The severity and duration of an attack of malaria is modified by the presence in the individual of resistance or 'immunity' to the effects of the infection. Some individuals are naturally more resistant to infection than others. Most are readily susceptible when first exposed, but as a result of long continued or repeated infection some degree of resistance or immunity is gradually acquired to further infection, especially from the same strain of parasite. Subjects who have acquired such resistance or 'immunity' are often referred to as 'immune', but the resistance is not absolute. It shows itself chiefly not so much in prevention of infection as in limiting its extent and clinical effects. It develops specifically against the particular strain of infecting parasite. There may also be some indication of resistance to the homologous species of parasite but not to other species.

The nature of acquired immunity in malaria is still not fully understood. Humoral immune bodies are developed, including highly specific fractions contained within the gamma globulins (which in the case of *P. falciparum* infections in Africa have been shown to have a therapeutic effect in children infected with the homologous strain) but these appear to be maintained for any length of time only in the presence of the E form of the parasite. If the latter is eradicated by treatment or long absence from the endemic area, immunity is lost over a period of months.

Immunity takes time to develop and individuals who eventually acquire it usually suffer severely from malaria in the early years of exposure.

In endemic areas malaria is rare in young indigenous infants, but is increasingly common and severe after the first few months of life. In the first two years the hazards are great, but as the child grows older the attacks of malaria get less frequent and milder. Older children and adults in these areas eventually show well marked resistance to the effects of the infection. If, however, there is some interruption in transmission for any considerable period the acquired resistance is reduced or, in areas where transmission is seasonal, may not fully develop, rendering the individual and the community open to epidemics.

Pathology

In some way not understood the development of the E form of the parasite in the erythrocyte initiates the pathological processes which lead to the tissue changes and clinical patterns of malaria. There is some evidence that the growing parasite may liberate substances into the circulation which affect tissue respiration and it is known that in infections in which periodic fever is established the febrile episodes are related to the late stages of the E cycle, including the rupture of the mature schizonts. The tissue phases of the parasite have no clinical or pathological effect other than locally in the liver tissue.

As in many acute medical conditions, the progress of the disease depends on the balance between the pathological activity of the parasite and the development of resistance by the host. In *P. falciparum* infections the pathological developments usually progress to a fatal issue without treatment. The other infections are usually self-limited.

The invaded erythrocyte is destroyed when the mature schizont ruptures; many unparasitized erythrocytes are also lysed. This leads to anaemia, the degree of which is increased by lysis and phagocytosis of uninfected cells. This is most developed in *P. falciparum* malaria in which the haemolytic processes may become dominant, leading rapidly to severe anaemia, with haemoglobinaemia and haemoglobinuria (blackwater fever). The anaemia leads to anoxaemia which is associated with cellular anoxia of varying degree, a factor of importance in pathological tissue changes.

In severe malaria, particularly in *P. falciparum* infections, circulatory changes are also induced locally in certain organs and generally in the whole cardiovascular system. Local circulatory disturbances lead to physiological and pathological responses of the organs concerned.

Such local circulatory changes account for some of the swelling and enlargement of the spleen and liver seen in the early stages of acute infection before the later cellular processes of hyperplasia have become active. Over-all reduction in renal blood flow results in oliguria and, if persistent, in anuria and acute uraemia. Changes in liver blood flow similarly lead to tissue damage and dysfunction, the latter aggravated by some degree of metabolic respiratory inhibition, as mentioned above. In severe cases centrilobular hepatic degeneration and necrosis results. The normally impermeable endothelium of the brain vessels is affected, causing local leakage of protein and fluid which may result in stasis and clinically in coma. Blood flow changes in endocrine organs such as the adrenal may upset the hormonal balance and lead to profound circulatory and other disturbances. In the later stages of *P. falciparum* infection general circulatory collapse may occur, which in turn may precipitate local effects such as liver or renal dysfunction and failure.

Thus there is much of the pathology of malaria that is essentially non-specific in character. The presence of the parasite in the erythrocyte in some way initiates these processes, which develop and multiply like a chain reaction. At first they are reversible and can be influenced by suitable treatment. Later they may become irreversible and collectively cause the death of the patient in whom the various patterns of fatal malaria will be found, including haemorrhages from the small brain vessels, centrilobular hepatic necrosis and renal anoxia with cortical ischaemia. The development of the final stages is seen in *P. falciparum* malaria. In other forms of the infection the lesions remain largely reversible.

There are in addition specific effects of the infection. For instance, during the development of the erythrocytic phase of the parasite, the haemoglobin of the host cell is broken down by the plasmodium into insoluble and particulate malarial pigment (or *haemozoin*). This escapes from the erythrocyte when the schizont ruptures, and is liberated into the plasma, finally being phagocytosed by circulating or tissue macrophages. Haemozoin appears to have no histotoxic effects in itself, but is found widely distributed in the tissues, either in the macrophage system or interstitially. In large amounts it gives the organs a characteristic grey-black macroscopic appearance.

It was suggested at one time that the loss of haemoglobin which occurs in the synthesis of haemozoin might be associated with some physico-chemical change in the remaining molecules whereby acceptance and discharge of oxygen might be affected adversely. However, all the evidence indicates that there is no change in the dissociation curves of unchanged haemoglobin in malaria and not sufficient disturbance in the chemical environment of the plasma to shift the curves unfavourably to the right. The actual exchange of oxygen in the lungs and at the tissue face thus goes on normally in malaria, until the point is reached at which there is insufficient circulatory pigment available. Anaemia of this degree is only very rarely achieved.

The phagocytic mechanisms of the body become very active in malaria and are specifically active against the particular strain of invading parasites and their products and sometimes the uninfected erythrocytes. These, together with malaria pigment are taken up in great quantity by the Kupffer cells of the liver, the pulp cells of the spleen and the macrophages of the marrow and other tissues. The histiocytes and macrophages become swollen and distended and in some anatomical areas, for instance in the sinusoids of the liver, may cause a degree of mechanical obstruction to the circulation which in turn aggravates such processes as the dynamic alterations in centrilobular hepatic blood flow.

In the acute attack of malaria, E forms of parasites are found in the peripheral blood. Gametocytes may also be present.

The species of plasmodia have differing powers of invasion of erythrocytes. *P. falciparum* invades the erythrocyte at all stages from reticulocyte to mature cell and the erythrocyte infection rate may be very high. *P. vivax* on the other hand, selectively invades young erythrocytes, so that the infection rate is rarely above 2 per cent. partly because in malaria there is some mechanism which, although not acting as an impediment to the production of reticulocytes, inhibits their appearance in the peripheral blood when parasites are present. *P. malariae* invades old erythrocytes so that the infection rate in this disease is normally even lower.

Changes in the size and shape of the invaded erythrocytes occur particularly in *P. vivax* and *P. ovale* infections, in both of which the cells enlarge and become stippled with pigment derived from haemoglobin and staining red with Romanowsky dyes. In the former the erythrocytes retain their normal outlines although their volume is increased. In the latter they become oval. The size and shape of the erythrocytes in *P. falciparum* infections are not affected.

The thin blood film usually shows some anisocytosis and poikilocytosis; in severe anaemia there may be nucleated erythrocytes. The bone marrow response is normoblastic.

In acute malaria there is often a moderate leucopenia, affecting chiefly the granulocytes. The erythrocyte sedimentation rate is raised.

The production of specific immunity to the parasite may effect both the course of the infection and the development of the pathogenic processes involving the host. In acute infections such as *P. knowlesi* malaria in rhesus monkeys or severe *P. falciparum* infections in man, the immediate effects of immune reactions are probably minimal. On the other hand, there is evidence that tissue damage (for example, lysis of unparasitized erythrocytes) may result from auto-immune reactions.

In long-continued or repeated infections the role of immunosensitivity reactions may be much more important. Thus, the so-called 'malarial nephrosis' arising in children infected with *P. malariae* is believed to be due to damage to the glomerular basement membrane by an antibody: antigen complex to which it is sensitized.

The chemical anatomy of the blood depends on factors such as the prevailing state of hepatic and renal function.

There is a rise in plasma bilirubin, which may be considerable in patients with hepatic dysfunction. Liver function tests, particularly the transaminase levels and tests dependent on protein changes, are abnormal in many cases in which no clinical sign of hepatic dysfunction exists.

In oliguric and anuric cases the blood urea is raised; in the latter very high concentrations are rapidly reached.

The electrolyte content of the plasma is determined by the degree of dehydration, vomiting and diarrhoea. In acute lysis the plasma potassium concentration may be an abnormally high.

The plasma protein concentrations vary. In acute malaria there may be little change from normal, or a fall in albumin. At a later stage and particularly in infections which have continued for a long time the albumin is low and the globulin raised, the increase being largely in the gamma globulin fraction. The latter contains a specific antibody.

In blackwater fever haemoglobin is present in the plasma.

The urine should always be examined at all stages in an attack of malaria. The volume is commonly reduced, but anuria may develop suddenly. For this reason each specimen should be measured and examined and reliance must not be placed on the 24-hour collection.

In the acute attack small amounts of protein, usually albumin, escape into the urine, and casts are common. Erythrocytes may be present and in cases with sharp haemolysis, haemoglobin appears macroscopically [see blackwater fever, p. 234].

The electrolyte content of the urine depends on the circumstances; for instance, when there is considerable loss of electrolytes through diarrhoea, sweating or vomiting, there may be no measurable sodium chloride.

The reaction of the urine is not characteristic in malaria. It may be neutral, acid or alkaline, even when haemoglobin is being passed or when the total volume is grossly reduced.

Clinical Patterns of Malaria

The clinical picture of malaria is created by the invasion of the erythrocytes by the parasites. It has been already noted that the latter fall into two main groups so far as the life cycle in man is concerned, namely, *P. falciparum* in which there is no persistent liver infection, and *P. vivax*, *P. malariae* and *P. ovale* in which there is. The same grouping is relevant in the clinical manifestations. *P. falciparum* infection causes malignant malaria, an acute progressive disease beset with complications and often fatal. The other forms of infection which may be considered collectively as the *P. vivax* group of malarias cause more benign illnesses in which complications are uncommon and death rare, and in which the acute attack is self-limited and relapses are common.

The Incubation Period. The time elapsing between the bite of the infected mosquito and the first appearance of fever with parasites in the blood of a non-immune host is roughly the same in all infections, about 10–15 days or longer. In *P. vivax* and *P. malariae* infections acquired in certain geographical areas, for instance, formerly in England, the incubation period may be many weeks or several months. The prepatent period, i.e. the time between sporozoite infection and the first discharge of merozoites into the blood from the PE liver phase is 6–8 days.

Periodicity of Fever. The rupture of the mature schizonts is associated with a febrile paroxysm in many forms of malaria. In infections in which the E phase takes 48 hours to complete, i.e. in *P. falciparum*, *P. vivax* and *P. ovale* infections, the peaks of fever occur every third day when the parasites mature together and every day when they mature in two major batches 24 hours apart. The fevers so produced are called *tertian* and *quotidian* respectively. Some strains of *P. falciparum* mature in less than 48 hours, causing, when all parasites mature together, a periodicity rather shorter than tertian and sometimes known as *subtertian*; this has led to the label ST malaria. *P. malariae* takes 72 hours to complete its E cycle and when all parasites mature simultaneously the febrile episodes occur every fourth day, producing *quartan* fever. Quotidian fever may also occur in this infection.

The febrile response in the *P. vivax* group of malarias differs in some respects in primary attacks and relapses. In the former, some days are needed before the rhythm of parasitic maturation is settled, so that the initial fever exhibits no periodicity; by the end of the first week periodicity is usually established. In relapses the periodicity of the parent attack appears immediately. In *P. falciparum* infections the pattern may be the same, but in many cases no periodic fever appears at any stage. Moreover *relapses* in the sense in which they occur in *P. vivax* infections (i.e. the establishment of the new E cycle by the escape of merozoites from the persistent liver EE phase) do not occur. In *P. falciparum* malaria recrudescences result from an exacerbation of the E phase which has continued from the primary infection.

Reinfection is common in all forms of malaria and may occur in individuals who are currently infected or who have been infected. The clinical picture is dependent on the prevailing acquired resistance.

SIGNS AND SYMPTOMS

THE VIVAX GROUP OF MALARIAS

(Infections with *P. vivax*, *P. ovale* and *P. malariae*.)

Infection with P. vivax and P. ovale (Vivax or benign tertian malaria; ovale tertian malaria).

In the last few days of the incubation period in a primary attack there are often prodromal symptoms of headache, severe backache, limb pains, anorexia, nausea and sometimes vomiting. Mild transient and irregular bouts of shivering and cold feelings are common. In relapses the prodromata are usually absent and the attack develops quickly.

The onset of the primary attack is associated with a rise of temperature to 101° F. (38·3° C.) or higher, which is usually accompanied by shivering and complaints of coldness, but not rigor. Parasites appear in the blood.

Fever: For the first few days or possibly the first week of the primary attack the fever is irregularly remittent or intermittent, with peaks of 103° F.–105° F. (39·4°–40·6° C.) but without clear periodicity. In the vast majority of cases periodic intermittent fever then follows and without treatment continues for 6 weeks to 3 months. The periodicity once established remains the same throughout the attack and subsequent relapses, unless disturbed by other intercurrent febrile infections.

In relapses the fever is periodic from the onset.

The febrile paroxysm: The bursts of fever and the associated signs and symptoms are called paroxysms and are physiologically closely related to similar phenomena which result from other causes, such as the inoculation of T.A.B. vaccine.

Paroxysms are commoner in the day than in the night and for some reason often occur in the afternoons rather than the mornings.

There are typically three stages, the cold, the hot and the sweating.

The cold stage covers the initial sharp rise of temperature to febrile levels. It is usually completed within an hour to an hour and a half. The patient feels increasingly cold and shivery and finally develops rigors. The temperature rises rapidly, but the skin remains pale and may feel cold. The pulse is fast and thready, the blood pressure raised. Nausea and vomiting develop and become worse as the peak of fever is reached. Up to this point external warmth is demanded by the patient and blankets and hot water bottles bring some relief.

Quite suddenly the *hot* stage replaces the cold. The subjective feelings change. The patient now feels hot and feverish, the rigors stop, the pale dry skin flushes, the pulse becomes full and bounding, the blood pressure falls. Nausea and vomiting increase. The patient is restless, excitable and may become incoherent or delirious. The temperature usually remains at about the level reached during the cold stage but may rise still higher. The general picture is that of any other high fever. Blankets and hot bottles are abandoned.

The hot stage commonly lasts longer than the cold and is succeeded by the *sweating* stage.

Sweating usually first appears on the face at the temples and rapidly becomes generalized and heavy. Sweat pours off the patient, soaking pyjamas and bed clothes. The symptoms of fever disappear and the temperature falls within an hour or more to normal or below. The pulse rate slows, vomiting stops and the patient feels a great sensation of relief, and commonly falls into an exhausted sleep from which he wakes refreshed.

The *interval* now follows, in which the temperature remains normal or may show an occasional low peak of fever. The patient feels well until the next paroxysm develops at its due time.

Parasites are present in the peripheral blood throughout the attack. In the vivax malarias all stages of the active E cycle may be seen at some time in the blood, but one particular stage usually predominates at a particular time. Thus, just prior to the development of a paroxysm and in its early stages, schizonts predominate. Late in the paroxysm and early in the interval the commonest parasites are rings and trophozoites predominate later in the interval.

Gametocytes may also be present during an attack and for some months afterwards as the erythrocytes containing them survive for normal periods and are not destroyed by the parasites. They have no significance so far as the clinical attack is concerned.

Anaemia is present in some degree especially in cases which have been active for some time and in individuals who are suffering from chronic or repeated infections.

In the acute case the anaemia is seldom severe. The erythrocyte count is commonly between 3 and 5 million cells per mm^3. In *P. vivax* infections, the mean cell diameter may be raised above normal, due to the increase in size of erythrocytes which contain parasites. In *P. malariae* infections the mean size of the cell is unchanged or slightly reduced.

Reticulocytes are not usually present in increased numbers during the attack. Reticulocytosis is common however in the first 7–10 days after successful treatment.

The *spleen* increases in size but may not become palpable until 10–14 days after the onset of an acute attack. Thereafter the organ size increases slowly. After repeated or continuous infection the spleen may become very large.

In the early stages there is often some pain and tenderness in the splenic area.

There is usually some biochemical, but rarely clinical, evidence of liver dysfunction. In long continued cases the liver is often palpable, especially in children.

In untreated cases paroxysms occur regularly for 6 weeks or longer. Spontaneous clinical cure then ensues and is followed, after a variable interval of clinical quiescence, by a relapse which begins abruptly with paroxysm, rigor and periodicity similar to that of primary attack. The relapse lasts as a rule a rather shorter time than the primary attack and is often less severe. In vivax and ovale tertian malaria relapses cease within three years of leaving an endemic area.

Infection with P. malariae (Quartan malaria; malariae malaria)

Basically the clinical picture is very similar to that of vivax malaria, but there are certain differences.

The incubation period may extend to three or four weeks and sometimes months. The onset may be insidious and the primary attack occasionally starts with a quartan periodic fever. The latter is the commonest periodicity achieved but there may be any variation from this to quotidian, depending on the rhythm of maturation.

The paroxysm often lasts longer than that of vivax malaria with all stages prolonged, and the sweating stage may be followed by some prostration.

Representatives of all stages of the E cycle appear in the peripheral blood, as in vivax malaria, the dominant form at any one time depending on the paroxysm.

Parasites are usually fewer than in vivax malaria. Gametocytes may be present after the first week of the primary attack.

Normocytic anaemia develops which may be milder than that in vivax malaria, but is occasionally severe.

Changes in the spleen and liver are similar to those in vivax malaria.

Untreated the attacks may last for two or more months. Relapses, with febrile periodicity the same as that developed in the original attack, occur at intervals with intervening quiescent periods. Although overt attacks often cease within a few years of infection, the parasite may reappear in the blood from time to time for many years.

After long-continued or recurrent infection, especially in children, a nephrotic syndrome may develop.

FALCIPARUM MALARIA

(Infection with *P. falciparum*: malignant tertian malaria; subtertian malaria.)

Falciparum malaria may be uncomplicated or complicated.

Uncomplicated Falciparum Malaria

The incubation period in a non-immune varies from 8–15 days. Prodromal symptoms, especially severe headache, backache and attacks of shivering occur in the few days immediately prior to the attack.

The onset may be clear cut or insidious.

The overt attack may be introduced by some dominant sign which is particularly common in certain geographical areas, and which may not suggest malaria. Thus diarrhoea resembling dysentery or food poisoning is a not infrequent beginning in parts of the West African coast.

Usually, the onset is brisk and the patient develops moderate fever, with flushed or pale skin which is often damp with sweat. He feels ill and complains of headache, bone and joint pains, particularly backache, which may persist from the prodromal stage. Anxiety and confusion are common and the patient is frequently prostrated. He may appear only moderately ill and the disease is easily mistaken for influenza, especially in non-endemic areas. This appearance is deceptive and dangerous, since at any stage severe and fatal complications may supervene.

In severe cases there may be anxiety, excitement or maniacal outbursts. Light or deep coma may develop as the condition proceeds and may become the dominating clinical picture. In light coma, the patient may be roused and will drowsily attempt to answer questions. When the coma is deep the patient is completely unresponsive and usually incontinent. In such circumstances the condition should be regarded as 'complicated' and treated accordingly [p. 233].

The *fever* is moderate, remittent or intermittent for the first few days and may continue so throughout the illness. In many cases, particularly in some geographical areas, periodic fever may never develop; in others by the end of the first week tertian, subtertian or quotidian periodicity is established with paroxysms resembling those of vivax malaria, but often of shorter duration.

The sweating stage may not be clearly defined. In cases with remittent fever the skin may remain moist throughout. In the intervals between the paroxysms the temperature may remain above normal and the feeling of well-being which accompanies the end of the paroxysms is usually absent.

In some cases there may be only irregular mild remittent fever which declines in intensity in the final stages, even of a fatal attack. Occasionally, heavy infection may exist without any fever.

Parasites are present in large and increasing numbers in the erythrocytes in the peripheral blood. The later stages of schizogony take place in the deep tissue vessels and are thus not normally visible in the peripheral blood except in heavy infections or during complications. Usually, only the rings and early trophozoites are present in blood films. The number of parasites present varies considerably during the day, but steadily increases as the disease progresses. Very high erythrocyte infection rates may occur. Characteristic sickle-shaped gametocytes, which may persist for months, appear after the first week.

Anaemia is often severe, not only because of the destruction of the large numbers of infected erythrocytes, but also because of considerable haemolysis of unparasitized cells. The erythrocyte count in cases of average severity varies from 2·5 to 3·5 million cells per mm^3. In severe cases which have lasted some days there may be fewer than 1 million cells per mm^3. In some cases acute intravascular haemolysis may occur with haemoglobinaemia and haemoglobinuria, giving rise to the syndrome of blackwater fever.

The degree of anaemia may not indicate the degree of haemolysis, since both the erythrocyte count and haemoglobin concentration may be increased by haemoconcentration.

There is usually a moderate leucopenia with granulocytopenia. Malaria pigment may be seen in circulating macrophages and polymorphs.

Nausea and vomiting are common from the onset. Vomiting is sometimes severe and intractable. Epigastric discomfort, anorexia and dyspepsia are usual. Looseness or frank watery diarrhoea is common and may persist from the prodromal stages.

The *spleen* enlarges rapidly and is usually palpable within 10 days of the onset. It continues to enlarge and gives rise to local signs and symptoms including tenderness which may appear before the organ becomes palpable. Acute pain in the splenic region, sometimes referred to the left shoulder, with interference in breathing and some local guarding may occur if infarcts or haemorrhages develop in the substance or subcapsular areas of the organ. Surgical emergencies may develop from accidental or spontaneous splenic rupture or twisting of the pedicle.

After repeated attacks especially in children, the spleen becomes very large; in continually reinfected adults it may eventually become fibrotic and small.

The *liver* is always affected in falciparum malaria. It is usually tender and palpable in the acute attack. In children in endemic areas it is usually enlarged, firm and tender. Liver function is disturbed. Transaminase levels are raised and the thymol turbidity test is positive.

The serum albumin is lowered, at first without much change in globulins, but, with the development of immunity in chronic or repeated infection, the latter, particularly the gamma fraction, are increased.

Serum bilirubin is increased in the majority of cases, with increased output of urobilinogen in the urine. In severe cases clinical jaundice appears.

The urine commonly contains some protein and casts; there may be erythrocytes.

The daily output of urine is low and in cases in which sweating, diarrhoea or vomiting have been severe, dehydration may be considerable, and urinary chloride is low.

Oliguria may develop into anuria in severe cases, with the appearance of the renal anoxia syndrome, including anaemia and rising blood urea.

A syndrome similar to acute nephritis develops sometimes, with oliguria, frank haematuria and high blood urea.

The systolic blood pressure is low and the diastolic may be very low, for example only 40 or 50 mm. Hg. The pulse is full and bounding and usually fast. Vascular failure may develop in severe cases.

The uncomplicated case responds extremely well to specific treatment.

The untreated attack is usually much shorter than that of vivax malaria and often ends fatally. When recovery occurs a temporary resistance has developed which is particularly notable against the same strain of the parasite. While the resistance exists, succeeding infections produce progressively less severe clinical effects.

Recrudescences due to the persistence of the E phase of the parasite usually occur not later than a year from the withdrawal from an endemic area; occasionally they may develop as long as two years later.

Severe anaemia and enlargement of both the spleen and the liver with irregular bouts of 'low' fever occur in individuals suffering from repeated or continuous infection, and the patient may pass into so-called malarial cachexia or gradually recover, with the acquisition of immunity.

The prognosis in a given case depends on the length of time the infection has progressed without treatment, the intensity of the parasitic infection and the clinical state with particular regard to circulatory failure. It must always be guarded since at any time fatal complications may develop.

Complicated Falciparum Malaria (Pernicious Malaria)

Complications may develop without warning at any stage in either a primary attack or a recrudescence of falciparum malaria. They appear most commonly in non-immune patients who have been ill for some time without proper specific treatment and in those who have suffered from repeated attacks or recrudescences which have been inadequately treated.

Complications, or 'pernicious' symptoms should be anticipated in any anaemic patient in whom more than 5 per cent. of the erythrocytes are infected. In such cases multiple infection of single erythrocytes is common and schizonts are sometimes found in the peripheral blood. On the other hand, complications may develop in patients with apparently light infections and little obvious anaemia.

The syndromes of complicated malaria result from the natural progress of the pathological processes concerned, and often appear to involve one or more organ. They are usually classified clinically in this way.

Clinical signs and symptoms related to the central nervous system are collectively classified as *cerebral malaria*. Neurological involvement usually appears during the course of an untreated attack in a non-immune, but may be the first indication of infection. The patient becomes drowsy and passes into coma, from which it may not be possible to rouse him. The physical state depends on the area of the brain principally affected. The pupils are often unequally contracted; the deep reflexes may be abolished or exaggerated. Localized neurological signs may be present. Muscular twitchings, odd movements of the head and neck and convulsions may be prominent, especially in children. Incontinence of urine and faeces may develop.

In some cases consciousness may not be completely lost and the patient will respond to physical stimuli or questioning. In others there may be acute mental disturbances, including mania, sometimes appearing in otherwise apparently normal people.

It is safe to say that almost any nervous symptom or neurological sign may derive from complicated malaria.

Accompanying these syndromes there is usually, but not always, remittent fever and some anaemia. Parasites, mostly rings but sometimes with occasional schizonts, are invariably present in the peripheral blood, often in great numbers.

Some patients may develop hyperpyrexia, the temperature not uncommonly exceeding 106° F. (41·1° C.). The dry skin and central nervous changes, which probably arise from hypothalamic damage, may be easily mistaken for heat hyperpyrexia.

Other complications need no detailed description. Gastro-intestinal syndromes include *dysenteric* malaria, in which the patient passes very frequent stools consisting mainly of blood and mucus in a clinical picture indistinguishable from that of bacillary dysentery, *choleraic* malaria in which there is acute watery diarrhoea and vomiting with dehydration, sometimes indistinguishable from cholera itself, and *bilious remittent fever* in which there is acute hepatic failure with increasing jaundice. Renal syndromes include acute nephritis and anuric uraemia.

One very important complication is the development of acute circulatory failure or shock. Because this picture commonly develops without fever, it is sometimes known as *algid malaria*. The patient passes rapidly into medical shock often associated with coma. He is usually dehydrated, with sunken eyes and pale cold inelastic skin. The pulse is thin and fast; both systolic and diastolic pressures are low, the latter sometimes unmeasurable. The acute reduction of blood volume is associated with some degree of haemoconcentration. Gastro-intestinal discomfort, diarrhoea and severe vomiting with accompanying dehydration often occur. The peripheral blood contains many parasites, some of which may be schizonts.

If this condition is not recognized and treated immediately the patient will die.

Blackwater Fever

In certain cases of *P. falciparum* infection waves of acute haemolysis occur with both haemoglobinaemia and haemoglobinuria. The syndrome is recognized as *blackwater fever*.

The condition occurs most commonly in individuals who have been exposed irregularly in an endemic area of falciparum malaria. Visitors to such an area may develop it after some months or years of chronic or intermittent infection, especially when the infection is inadequately suppressed by chemotherapy or when there is incomplete entomological control. Irregular attacks or recrudescences of falciparum malaria apparently produce some kind of sensitivity reaction in the host tissues which eventually respond vigorously to a further overt infection by acute intravascular haemolysis similar to that seen in favism and associated with fever, often jaundice, and renal insufficiency. This applies to visitors and indigenes alike.

There is some evidence that irregular suppression by quinine is particularly predisposing to an attack of blackwater fever.

The haemolysis leads to severe anaemia which develops suddenly. There may be only one episode of haemolysis or several.

Haemoglobinuria appears suddenly. The urine is dark brown or black if the reaction is acid, red if alkaline or neutral. The concentration of pigment usually lightens and finally clears in 24–36 hours. There may be several waves of haemoglobinuria. The urine during the passage of the pigment contains large amounts of sediment and protein, both of which clear in the non-haemolytic phases. The volume is low and anuria may develop at any time.

Death may follow intractable haemolysis, vascular collapse, or acute hepatic failure, but most commonly results from the development of anuric uraemia. The latter syndrome, which is widely dispersed in acute medical states was first described in blackwater fever.

Clinical diagnosis is made on the history and the presence of haemoglobinuria.

The latter must be distinguished from other causes of haemoglobinuria particularly that arising in glucose-6-phosphate dehydrogenase-deficient individuals in response to drugs such as the 8-aminoquinolines or phenacetin.

P. falciparum parasites may or may not be present in the peripheral blood; they are never more than scanty.

Treatment. Treatment is largely non-specific. Corticosteroids in the early stages are helpful in the usual dosages. Transfusion is usually necessary. Renal failure, dehydration, hepatic failure and shock are treated by standard methods.

Antimalarial therapy is required only when there are substantial numbers of parasites present, which is rare. Chemo-suppression may however be continued during the attack provided quinine is not used.

MALARIA IN IMMUNES

The foregoing descriptions of malaria cover the several forms of the disease as it occurs in the non-immune adult.

As pointed out elsewhere, in individuals who have acquired immunity or resistance to local parasite strains as a result of previous continuous or repeated infection, the effects of further infection are considerably modified. The clinical picture does not usually resemble fully developed malaria. It consists as a rule of malaise, mild fever, headache, backache, anorexia, sweating and feeling unwell and ineffective. More severe attacks develop if immunity is weakened as a result of inadequate dosage of antimalarial drugs or reduction of reinfection by incomplete entomological control. In such circumstances blackwater fever may occasionally develop in indigenes in a *P. falciparum* endemic area.

Immunity capable of such modifications of the clinical attack is acquired by the indigene of an endemic area only after continuous exposure to infection and survival from previous infections. It is a valuable and hard-won possession and should not be taken away lightly, at least until antimalarial measures in the area are assured and permanent. There is now general agreement that the maintenance of immunity is largely dependent on the continued presence of the E phase of the parasite in the blood. This point must be considered in recommending treatment, since eradication of the parasite, for instance in *P. falciparum* infections, will be followed by loss of immunity in a few months and thus to a vicious subsequent attack after infection with the same organism.

Acquired immunity is often limited to the local strain of parasite. Thus immunity to a particular strain does not usually mean that the patient is immune to others of the same species occurring in other geographical areas. Sometimes indigenes of one area, fully equipped to withstand infection with the local strain, will suffer a full-scale attack, as severe as that which might develop in a non-immune, after becoming infected by a strain from another area. The attack in these circumstances must be regarded in the same way as infection in a non-immune.

MALARIA IN PREGNANCY AND IN CHILDREN

Malaria is a common cause of abortion and premature labour. After childbirth the indigene mother often suffers from a relatively acute attack with high fever and other serious symptoms. It is believed that in the final trimester of pregnancy there is a lowering of the acquired resistance to superinfection, i.e. infection with the same strain of parasite.

Labour may be directly complicated by the effects of malarial infection, including severe anaemia (often in this case associated with additional folic acid deficiency) and enlargement of the spleen and liver. In some cases splenomegaly may be a direct obstruction to the expansion of the uterus as the foetus develops, and abortion results.

Malaria in the pregnant woman must be regarded as a potential cause of abortion. Antimalarial drugs are indicated to reduce this risk and to prevent the common post-partum fever due to the disease.

Malaria may occasionally be transmitted across the placenta to the foetus, probably as a result of intra-uterine placental damage.

In children malaria is probably one of the most important causes of morbidity and mortality.

Clinical attacks are rare in the first few months of life for various reasons, including transfer of immune bodies in milk, and the exclusive milk diet.

Thereafter, until the age of two or three years, children become peculiarly susceptible to malaria and prone to complications, so that all forms of the disease may prove fatal.

The clinical picture of malaria in the child depends to some extent on whether the attack is due to a recent acute infection, to frequent reinfection or to long-continued infection.

The acute form, which occurs in the child who has not acquired resistance, especially, for example, in areas in which malaria is seasonal, is often quite different from the disease as seen in the adult.

The child is pale from anaemia, miserable, dull, restless and anorexic. There is moderate fever. The skin is dry and flushed or pale, cool and sweaty. There are frequently severe gastro-intestinal symptoms including vomiting, colicky abdominal pain, wind and diarrhoea. The abdomen is distended and tender. The spleen and liver are palpable and usually tender. Convulsions, meningismus and coma often develop suddenly.

The child, unless treated, will die from the acute attack.

In children in whom the infection has continued for some time, anaemia is severe, the abdomen is distended, the liver enlarged and the spleen steadily increases in size. Weight is lost, and there is puffiness of the face and wasted stick-like limbs. There may be little or no fever. Parasites are present in the blood, but in smaller numbers than in the acute attack.

Without treatment there is a decline, with remissions, which finally leads either to death or the picture of the so-called 'chronic' malaria, in which the child is listless, wasted, with thin limbs, a protuberant abdomen and gross splenomegaly. A spleen of this size is exposed to risk of rupture from external violence, twisting of its extended pedicle, infarct and haemorrhage. Mucous membranes are pale; there may be visible icterus. Secondary vitamin deficiencies are common and lead to changes in the skin and mucous membrane, especially of the mouth and tongue.

DIAGNOSIS OF MALARIA

The diagnosis of active malaria can be made only by the identification of the parasite in its erythrocytic (E) phase.

Discovery of gametocytes is not necessarily evidence of existing active malaria, since these forms of the parasite, although developed during the attack, remain in the relevant erythrocytes for as long as three months and may thus still be present after subsidence or cure of the disease.

Blood Films

Parasites are usually found in stained thick or thin blood films. They are also present in organ or tissue smears, including material from the spleen and bone marrow, but these are rarely examined for diagnostic purposes; there is little evidence that parasites are likely to be discovered in such material when they cannot be found in the blood.

Diagnosis of the presence of the E phase parasites is made by examination of thick films prepared by picking up a drop of blood from a needle prick in the finger or lobe of the ear on to a clean glass slide and spreading it evenly. When thoroughly dry the film is stained in watery solutions of Romanowsky dyes (dilute Giemsa of Field's stain).

On examination under oil with the 2 mm. objective, the cytoplasm of the parasites are stained blue, the chromatin red or reddish blue. The dehaemoglobinized erythrocytes are not stained, but the nuclei of the leucocytes are stained blue and the platelets pink.

Differentiation of the species of parasite may often be made by examination of the thick blood film, but is easier in the thin film. This is prepared by the ordinary haematological methods from a drop of blood picked up on a clean slide and spread evenly along the surface. The film is allowed to dry and is fixed and stained in the usual way with Leishman or Giemsa stain. In this case the erythrocytes remain intact and the parasites, stained as above, can be examined within them.

The finer distinctions of the species of parasite is a technical matter which requires or may require expert help. In the ordinary course of events the physician is concerned only in determining whether the parasites in a particular case are members of the vivax group or are *P. falciparum*, or both.

The erythrocytes containing the parasites are enlarged in *P. vivax* and *P. ovale* infections in both of which fine stippling with Schüffner's dots is also present. In the latter infection the invaded cells are fimbriated. Infected erythrocytes are not enlarged in *P. malariae* infections.

The unpigmented ring forms of *P. falciparum* are usually present in considerable numbers; they may be occasionally few and sometimes very numerous. The rings are usually small and delicate, occasionally heavy. Multiple infection of individual erythrocytes is common. Double chromatin dots may be present in individual parasites. The presence of other forms of the E phase of the parasite is exceptional. There may be characteristic crescent-shaped gametocytes.

In the vivax group of malarias all forms of the E phase, including rings, trophozoites and schizonts appear at some time in the blood. In *P. vivax* and *P. ovale* the rings are usually large and loose, the trophozoites bigger and pigmented. In *P. malariae* these stages are smaller and compact and the so-called 'band form' is common stretching across the erythrocyte. Gametocytes are round and compact.

Relatively few parasites appear in the peripheral blood as compared with the numbers seen in *P. falciparum* infections.

The blood should be examined frequently at intervals in an attack. In *P. falciparum* infections in particular great variations may occur during the day in the numbers of parasites present in the peripheral blood. Hence failure to find parasites on one occasion is not significant. The usual routine is to examine blood films taken in the mornings and in the evenings from the time of admission.

Parasites may be scarce in the blood of patients who have recently taken suppressive antimalarial drugs.

Clinical suspicion of malaria exists wherever the signs and symptoms suggest it in patients who have been exposed in an endemic area. It is essential to obtain a clear geographical history especially in view of modern fast and frequent global movement. Malaria is usually easy to diagnose parasitologically but the blood film may never be examined and the diagnosis may consequently be missed if the physician fails to discover that the patient has been in an endemic area, even for only a few hours, and that malaria must therefore be considered. The combination of periodic or remittent fever, anaemia and splenic enlargement is very suggestive in non-immunes. Anaemia and splenic enlargement are equally suggestive in indigenes in an endemic area.

THE TREATMENT OF MALARIA

The treatment of malaria consists in the administration of the specific antimalarial drug and in dealing with any complicating clinical factors, such as anaemia, dehydration or shock.

Before chemotherapy can be rationally applied in a given case the physician must have assessed the 'immunity' status of the patient and determined the species of the infecting parasites.

For practical purposes patients may be divided into *non-immunes* in whom there is only the recent history of exposure in an endemic area or, in the case of indigenes of one endemic area, exposure in another, and *immunes*, in whom there is a history of continuous exposure in the same endemic area.

The aims of chemotherapy are quite different in the two instances. In non-immunes the object is eradication of all phases of the infection; in immunes it is the control of the infection to the point where the clinical attack can be aborted but without eradication of the E phase of the parasite upon which the integrity of the immunity depends.

The importance of determining the species of parasite is twofold. First, the problems of parasite eradication are different, since in *P. falciparum* only the E phase of the parasite is present, whereas in the other infections both the E and EE phases exist. Second, *P. falciparum* is a dangerous and often fatal infection in non-immunes and the others are usually not.

Drugs which act on the parasite in its E phase are known as *schizonticides*. They are effective against the E forms of all parasites. There are five groups of schizonticide compounds, namely, the 4-aminoquinolines (such as chloroquine), mepacrine, quinine, proguanil and pyrimethamine. These drugs act directly on the E phase of the parasite in the trophozoite or early schizont stage.

The only drugs which act on the EE phase of the vivax group of parasites are the 8-aminoquinolines of which primaquine is the most used.

Drug Resistance

Parasite drug resistance until recently was confined to proguanil and pyrimethamine, to both of which many parasites throughout the world are now fully resistant.

Parasite resistance to chloroquine and other 4-aminoquinolines has now been demonstrated in areas of South-East Asia and South America, but not in Africa. Cross-resistance with mepacrine has also been demonstrated in these parasites.

Where resistance exists it is present at all stages of the parasite life cycle including that in the mosquito. Thus in areas in which resistant parasites occur the relevant drug is useless.

In some of the parts of the world in which chloroquine resistance has been demonstrated, widespread resistance to proguanil and pyrimethamine already exists, and mepacrine resistance is also present. In such areas quinine remains the only effective therapeutic agent until new compounds are discovered.

Toxic Effects of Schizonticides in Therapeutic Dosage

The toxicity of chloroquine is low. There may be some gastro-intestinal discomfort to begin with, usually relieved if the drug is given with adequate fluid. A few patients complain of blurring of vision or patchy scotomata, but these effects are transitory. Occasional skin rashes may occur.

Mepacrine rarely gives rise to toxicity. The only serious complication is an acute psychosis, often maniacal, which appears especially in certain races, such as Malays and Singhalese. The syndrome disappears quickly on cessation of therapy. Intense colouring of the skin occurs but without harmful effect.

Quinine produces nausea, sometimes vomiting, deafness, dizziness and tinnitus. Occasional patients develop an erythematous macular sensitivity rash. In sensitive persons haemoglobinuria occasionally develops. The drug should be avoided in blackwater fever.

The choice of drug depends on many factors, chief of which are the speed and reliability of action, the method of administration required, the toxic effects and the possibility of parasite drug resistance.

Of the schizonticides, the 4-aminoquinolines, mepacrine and quinine are the most active and reliable.

Toxic Effects of the 8-Aminoquinolines

There is little margin between the therapeutic and toxic doses. Mild degrees of cyanosis arising from the production of methaemoglobinaemia are common. Colicky abdominal pain may be present for the first few days of treatment, when the stools are usually loose, and may be bad enough to indicate temporary stoppage of the drug. In glucose-6-phosphate dehydrogenase-deficient subjects haemolysis and haemoglobinuria may arise. Although this haemolysis is self limited, it is usually regarded as an indication to stop therapy.

CHEMOTHERAPY OF MALARIA IN THE NON-IMMUNE

In this section chemotherapy is discussed in the following order: treatment of uncomplicated falciparum malaria; treatment of complicated falciparum malaria; treatment of the vivax group of malarias.

Details of dosage are given for adults only on the basis of 60 kg. body weight. Children accept antimalarial drugs readily in doses corresponding to body weight.

TREATMENT OF P. FALCIPARUM INFECTION

Uncomplicated P. falciparum Malaria

The objective is to eradicate the E phase of *P. falciparum* by using a schizonticide.

In uncomplicated cases the drugs should be given orally, except sometimes in children in whom under special circumstances they may be given intramuscularly.

Recommended schizonticides are the 4-aminoquinolines (in the absence of resistance) and quinine, in that order.

The drugs should be given carefully to make sure they are swallowed and not vomited back. Each tablet should be administered separately with a draught of water.

CHLOROQUINE (*Nivaquine*)
(or any equivalent 4-aminoquinoline.)
600 mg. base (4 tablets) on admission.
300 mg. base (2 tablets) 6 hours later.
300 mg. base (2 tablets) each morning for the next 3 days.

QUININE
650 mg. (2 tablets) twice daily for 7–10 days.
650 mg. (2 tablets) may be given thrice daily for the first 2 days in heavy patients.

NOTE:

In uncomplicated cases of both falciparum and vivax malarias ferrous sulphate in doses of 1 G. per day in divided doses should be given to assist in restoration of haemoglobin levels. The diet should contain adequate protein.

For treatment of drug-resistant infections, see p. 239.

Complicated Falciparum Malaria

Specific drug therapy is essential in complicated malaria and no delay can be tolerated but concurrent immediate treatment of the complications themselves is also vital.

The aim of chemotherapy is again to eradicate the E phase of the parasite by the use of a schizonticide.

The 4-aminoquinolines or quinine may be given intravenously or intramuscularly.

The intravenous route is the most immediately effective.

The drug used intravenously must be given in dilute solution and very slowly. The usual technique is to take up the compound in pyrogen-free water or saline to a total volume of 15–20 ml. and inject slowly through a small needle taking 10 minutes to complete the injection.

Intramuscular administration is made with 5–10 ml. of the solution, injected into the gluteal muscles with aseptic precautions.

DOSAGES RECOMMENDED:

CHLOROQUINE (*Nivaquine*)

Intravenous: 200 mg. (base), repeated in 8–12 hours if necessary, either by syringe or by addition to a saline drip. Not more than 2 doses are likely to be required in the first 24 hours. Oral administration should be given as soon as possible, on the basis of adding to the parenteral dosage to attain the total dosage mentioned above, i.e. in the case of chloroquine 1·5–1·8 G. in 4 days.

In common usage is *Nivaquine Soluble*, a 5 ml. ampoule of which contains 200 mg. (base).

Higher doses are sometimes given but carry some risk of the development of shock.

Intramuscular: Same dosage.

QUININE

Intravenous: 450–650 mg. repeated in 8 hours if necessary, in the same manner as for chloroquine (see above).

Intramuscular: Same dosages.

Treatment of the Complications of Pernicious Falciparum Malaria

It is essential to treat the infection and the complications concurrently. Many of the latter are medical emergencies which will in themselves cause the death of the patient unless controlled.

Acute Anaemia. See section on blackwater fever [p. 234]. Transfusion is necessary when the erythrocyte count falls quickly below 2 million cells per mm^3. even when haemoglobinuria is absent. Where there are signs of circulatory embarrassment the transfusion should be given as packed cells.

The agglutinin pattern is disturbed in malaria and the donor's blood must therefore be cross-matched with that of the patient both in regard to cells and plasma. Blood which should be satisfactory on the basis of blood grouping may be incompatible and should never be used until cross-matched.

The amount of blood administered should be considered as part of the total input of fluid in relation to output, especially in anuric patients. 0·5–1 litre is usually sufficient and there is always risk of circulatory embarrassment which may be fatal if too much is given. In blackwater fever there is often some haemolysis of the introduced cells but this is unavoidable.

In severe anaemia arising in chronic or repeated infection, transfusion is seldom necessary. Recovery usually follows the administration of ferrous iron, treatment of the infection and good diet.

Shock. Shock occurring in algid malaria or as a late event in previously uncomplicated infections requires the usual restoration of blood volume by serum, or protein substitutes. The serum must be matched with the patient's cells.

Dehydration. Dehydration, including that occurring in choleraic malaria, should be dealt with as in other examples of acute water and salt depletion. Potassium losses may also require replacement.

Cerebral Symptoms. These must be treated by ordinary non-specific methods. Recovery will be dependent on concurrent chemotherapy. In coma, corticosteroids in the usual descending doses are often very helpful over the first few hours or days, for example 200–300 mg. of hydrocortisone or the equivalent of prednisolone intramuscularly in the first 24 hours, with half the dose the following day. Dexamethasone has also been used with success.

Hyperpyrexia. The patient must be sponged or sprayed with cold water which is evaporated from the skin with fans. Other methods of cooling may also be used. In most cases the temperature falls in a short time to 101°–102° F. (38·4°–38·8° C.) at which point active treatment should be stopped. The temperature will then usually fall below normal and may subsequently rise, when treatment should be resumed. Too sudden lowering of temperature may lead to the development of shock.

Acute renal failure should be treated on general lines. In grave cases peritoneal dialysis has proved effective.

Other complications are similarly treated by non-specific methods.

TREATMENT OF THE VIVAX GROUP OF MALARIAS

The objective is to eradicate the E phase of the parasite with a schizonticide and the persistent liver EE phase with an 8-aminoquinoline. The drugs may be given together.

The schizonticides in common use are the 4-aminoquinolines and quinine. The 8-aminoquinolines are primaquine or quinocide.

DOSAGES RECOMMENDED:

(1) CHLOROQUINE: 600 mg. (base) immediately.
300 mg. (base) 8 hours later.
300 mg. (base) once on each of the next 3 consecutive days.

PRIMAQUINE: 7·5 mg. (base) twice daily, continued for 10–14 days.

The primaquine may be given at the same time as the chloroquine course or subsequent to it. Quinocide in doses of 7·8 mg. (base) thrice daily may be used instead of primaquine.

(2) QUININE: 650 mg. twice daily for 10 days.
PRIMAQUINE as above (1).

NOTE:

Because of the possible toxic effects of the 8-aminoquinolines patients must be carefully watched or kept in bed. They should be given plenty of fluid. A fluid balance record must be kept; the volume of each specimen of urine should be measured and examined for haemoglobin pigment.

Severe intestinal colic, the appearance of increasing methaemoglobinaemia, visible as 'cyanosis' especially in the finger nails, or of haemoglobinuria indicate cessation of treatment.

THE TREATMENT OF MALARIA IN 'IMMUNES'

In individuals who have been exposed to repeated or continuous infection with malaria parasites the clinical attack becomes much modified and causes relatively little disturbance.

The aim in such cases is to deal with the E phase of the parasite and to contain it at non-clinical levels.

The treatment is the same whatever the infecting *Plasmodium.*

Oral dosages of schizonticides given on one day only are usually adequate, as follows:

CHLOROQUINE (*Nivaquine*): 300 mg. base (2 tablets) or the equivalent dose of AMODIAQUINE (*Camoquin*), i.e. 2 tablets (400 mg. base).

QUININE: 1·5–1·8 G.

MEPACRINE: 300–500 mg. (3–5 tablets).

PROGUANIL: 300–500 mg. (3–5 tablets).

PYRIMETHAMINE: 50 mg. (2 tablets).

TREATMENT OF DRUG-RESISTANT MALARIA

P. falciparum infections

Parasites may be resistant to proguanil (and pyrimethamine) or to the 4-aminoquinolines (and mepacrine) or to both.

(1) Parasites resistant to proguanil and pyrimethamine (provided they are not also resistant to the

4-aminoquinolines) respond to the usual dosage regimen of chloroquine or *Nivaquine* [p. 237].

(2) Parasites resistant to the 4-aminoquinolines usually respond to full doses of quinine, for example, 1·3 G. daily for 10 days. An alternative is the combination of the long-acting sulphonamide sulphormethoxine (*Fanasil*). 1 G., and pyrimethamine, 50 mg., given once, or with the pyrimethamine repeated on the second day. Doses are the same for non-immunes and immunes.

(3) Parasites resistant to all four drugs respond to quinine as in (2) above.

P. vivax group infections

Parasites may become resistant to proguanil and pyrimethamine. Resistance to 4-aminoquinolines and mepacrine has not been reported.

Infections with proguanil (and pyrimethamine) resistant *P. vivax* respond to the usual combination of chloroquine and primaquine [p. 238]. The combination of sulphormethoxine and pyrimethamine has also been shown to eliminate the E parasites and so give clinical cure.

PROPHYLAXIS AND SUPPRESSION OF MALARIA

Prophylaxis implies complete protection from the infection at all stages from the injection of sporozoites.

Suppression implies the control of the E phase of the parasite to subclinical levels, or its eradication.

No drugs can destroy the sporozoites, so that no true prophylaxis exists. However, in *P. falciparum* infections the PE liver phase may be destroyed or aborted by proguanil or pyrimethamine, provided there is no drug resistance. This activity is sometimes referred to as 'causal prophylaxis'.

In all other forms of chemotherapeutic control of malaria the aim is suppression. In *P. falciparum* infections, if the E phase is completely destroyed by the drugs, as it may well be, the result is suppression with radical cure. In the vivax malarias suppression is relatively easy but because of the development of the persistent EE liver phases of the parasites radical cure does not occur.

Individuals who are already infected with malaria should be treated with a full therapeutic course before being placed on a suppressive drug schedule.

The drugs available are the schizonticides, all of which have been used with success.

As a principle it is wise to use as a suppressive some drug other than the one likely to be employed for treatment. Since chloroquine is one of the most powerful and readily available schizonticides, it is commonly reserved for this purpose and either proguanil or pyrimethamine is used for suppression. Nevertheless, chloroquine or some other 4-aminoquinoline is widely taken as a suppressive, despite the generally accepted view that its irregular use may lead to the development of parasite drug resistance. In some areas quinine and mepacrine are also in use.

Suppressive therapy with all drugs except mepacrine should be started just before the individual reaches the endemic area. Mepacrine must be given daily for at least a fortnight before exposure in order to allow the acquisition of adequate blood levels.

Thereafter the drug must be taken *regularly* during the entire stay in the endemic area and for at least a month after leaving it. Regularity is essential.

The suppressive dose is best taken with a meal and with ample fluid.

In suppressive doses these drugs are practically non-toxic. They have no effect on sexual activity or pregnancy.

DOSAGES RECOMMENDED:

CHLOROQUINE (*Nivaquine*): 300 mg. (base), 2 tablets, once weekly,

or

150 mg. (base), 1 tablet, twice weekly.

(Children (in weekly doses) 0–2 years, 37·5 mg.; 3–5 years, 75 mg.; 6–10 years, 150 mg.; over 10 years, 225–300 mg.)

Toxic effects: Minor gastro-intestinal disturbances may occur after first few doses; occasional skin lesions.

PROGUANIL (*Paludrine*): 100 mg., 1 tablet daily.

(Children (in daily doses) 0–1 year, 25–50 mg.; 2–5 years, 50–100 mg.)

Toxic effects: Occasional gastro-intestinal discomfort.

PYRIMETHAMINE (*Daraprim*): 50 mg. (2 tablets) once weekly;

or

25 mg. (1 tablet) twice weekly.

Children (in weekly doses) 0–12 years, 12·5 mg. Thereafter adult dose.

Toxic effects: none.

MEPACRINE: 100 mg. (1 tablet) daily. Adults only.

Toxic effects: Usually very slight. Skin is stained yellow and drug is excreted in the hair. Women often object to the cosmetic effects. Brown-blue irregular skin lesions resembling those of lichen planus may occur if drug is taken over very long periods.

QUININE: 250–325 mg. daily.

(Children in proportion to body weight.)

Toxic effects: Unpleasant effects vary from individual to individual. At worst they include dizziness, tinnitus with some deafness, sometimes nausea and vomiting, occasionally sensitivity skin rashes.

SUPPRESSION OF DRUG RESISTANT MALARIA

P. falciparum infections

Parasite resistance to proguanil and pyrimethamine is now very widespread and resistance to chloroquine and other 4-aminoquinolines has also appeared, with cross-resistance to mepacrine. In the presence of resistance the relevant drug or drugs cannot be successfully used.

The 4-amino quinolines and quinine are active against proguanil or pyrimethamine resistant parasites in the usual doses for non-immunes and immunes. The combination of diaphenylsulphone (DDS), 0·5–1 G. for 1 week, and pyrimethamine has proved successful against pyrimethamine-resistant strains.

Parasites resistant to 4-aminoquinolines respond to proguanil or pyrimethamine and to quinine.

Parasites resistant to all four synthetic drugs usually respond to quinine, but sometimes only to large doses.

Various combinations of drugs have been tried, the most promising of which is sulphormethoxine, 1 G., plus pyrimethamine, 50 mg., given once. Cycloguanil embonate with sulphadiamine (DADDS) has shown some activity against chloroquine and proguanil-resistant *P. falciparum*.

P. vivax and P. malariae infections

Parasites resistant to proguanil and pyrimethamine respond to the 4-aminoquinolines in the usual way. They do not respond to the combination of cycloguanil and sulphadiamine.

No parasites have so far been found resistant to the 4-aminoquinolines or mepacrine.

GLOBAL MALARIA ERADICATION PROGRAMME

Mass control, which it is hoped will lead eventually to eradication, depends on entomological control of the vectors and on chemosuppression aimed at suppressing active malaria in the population and removing the residual reservoirs of gametocyte infections.

Chloroquine, proguanil and pyrimethamine singly or in various combinations have been widely used, either administered as tablets or mixed with household salt. Distribution difficulties and the development of parasite resistance to the drugs have caused retardation of the global programme of eradication which is already suffering from the wide development of insect insensitivity to insecticides.

Repository compounds providing anti-parasitic activity over a long period after a single dose are being tried in eradication programmes. The most widely used is cycloguanil embonate derived from a metabolite of proguanil. A single dose gives protection against *P. falciparum*, *P. vivax* and *P. malariae* for as long as 4 months but, as might be expected, is inactive against strains resistant to proguanil or pyrimethamine. In combination with sulphadiamine it is said to have some action against proguanil-resistant *P. falciparum* [see p.238].

REFERENCES

ADAMS, A. R. D., and MAEGRAITH, B. G. (1971) *Clinical Tropical Diseases*, 5th ed., Oxford.

British Medical Journal (1969) Leading article. Malaria in Britain, **1,** 776.

EDINGTON, G. M., and GILLES, H. M. (1969) *Pathology in the Tropics*, London.

GARNHAM, P. C. C. (1966) *Malaria Parasites and other Haemosporidia*, Oxford.

HARINASUTA, TRANAKCHIT, VIRAVAN, C., and REID, H. A. (1967) Sulphormethoxine in chloroquine-resistant falciparum malaria in Thailand, *Lancet*, i, 1117.

HERRERO, J. (1966) The use of long-acting sulphonamides alone or with pyrimethamine in malaria with special reference to sulformethoxine, *Proc. Third Int. Pharm. Congres.*, Sao Paulo, July 1966, Basel.

Lancet (1969) Leading article. Drug resistant malaria, i, 1245.

MAEGRAITH, B. G. (1967) Biochemical and physiological host:parasite relationships in mammalian malaria, *Protozoology*, **2,** 65.

PETERS, W. (1969) *Chemotheraphy and Drug Resistance in Malaria*, London.

WILCOCKS, C. (1967a, b) Recent developments in tropical medicine, Parts I and II, *Abstr. Wld Med.*, **41,** 241, 325.

WORLD HEALTH ORGANIZATION. SCIENTIFIC GROUP (1967) Chemotherapy of malaria, *Tech. Rep. Ser.*, No. 375.

LEISHMANIASIS

These are diseases caused by infection with protozoa belonging to the genus *Leishmania*. The infection may be general or localized. General infection is caused by *Leishmania donovani* and gives rise to visceral leishmaniasis or kala-azar. Localized infections occur in the skin, producing the oriental sore, caused by *Leishmania tropica* or in the skin and associated mucous membranes producing the clinical picture of mucocutaneous leishmaniasis, caused by *Leishmania brasiliensis*. The parasites are all transmitted to man by species of the sandfly *Phlebotomus* spp.

The relationship between the three species has not yet been fully worked out. *L. donovani* infection produces considerable immunity to further infection with the homologous strain and to *L. tropica*. The latter produces only homologous immunity.

VISCERAL LEISHMANIASIS

Synonyms. Kala-azar; Black sickness; Dumdum fever.

Definition and Aetiology

Visceral leishmaniasis is a disease characterized by a long incubation period and chronic course, remittent fever, leucopenia and enlargement of the spleen and liver. It results from infection with *L. donovani*, acquired via the bite of the sandfly, several species of which transmit the infection.

There are two main types of the disease, the Mediterranean and the Indian. The former occurs in hot moist regions of the Mediterranean littoral including North Africa and in Iran, Iraq, and the Arabian peninsula, Asian Russia and mainland China. The Indian form is found in Assam, and parts of India and Burma bordering the Bay of Bengal.

Visceral leishmaniasis is also found in South and Central America, including northest Brazil, Colombia and Venezuela and in Mexico and Guatemala; it also occurs in West, Central and East Africa, notably in Kenya and Somalia.

The Mediterranean disease is found most commonly in infants and young children and does not occur as epidemics. The Indian form is seen in older children and young adults; it commonly occurred in epidemics, but has practically disappeared as a result of residual insecticide spraying for malaria eradication. The American and African types usually affect young children, adolescents and adults; the former may become epidemic.

The organism is the same for all forms of the disease wherever it occurs. In man it exists in non-flagellate form as very characteristic small oval bodies between 2 and 5 μ in length and containing a large laterally placed nucleus to which the small rod shaped kinetoplast is turned end-on. The parasites, which are known as *Leishman-Donovan bodies*, are found in the cytoplasm of reticulo-endothelial cells or free in the blood plasma. They multiply by fission and the host cell eventually ruptures, liberating the organisms which then infect other cells in which the cycle is repeated. They are carried by blood macrophages to all tissues of the body, where the invasion of the reticulo-endothelial cells is continued.

The vector is the female sandfly, which becomes infected by sucking blood containing parasites from an infected human or animal reservoir. In the insect the parasite rapidly develops into the flagellate leptomonad form which multiplies in great numbers and eventually partially blocks the pharynx and buccal cavity. When the 'blocked' insect attempts to feed the parasites escape into the wound and enter the tissues, where they are taken up by the fixed and mobile macrophages in which they are transformed into leishmania forms and multiply.

Transmission by *Phlebotomus* spp. in this way is probably the only natural method. Occasionally the infection may be transmitted in transfused blood.

In the Indian disease the reservoir is man. In the other forms the infection is a zoonosis. The Mediterranean reservoir is commonly the domestic dog, sometimes the jackal or gerbil. Dogs and foxes are reservoirs in the Americas. In Africa south of the Sahara wild rodents are the main animal hosts.

Pathology

The macrophage system of the host is quickly parasitized by the leptomonads introduced during the bite of the infected sandfly. The parasites are converted into Leishman-Donovan bodies which then multiply and disseminate as described above.

The basic tissue reaction to the infection is a rapid proliferation of reticulo-endothelial tissue throughout the body, particularly in the Kupffer cells of the liver and the macrophage cells of the spleen and bone marrow. The liver and spleen enlarge rapidly as a result of this increase in tissue and associated circulatory changes. The lymph nodes are affected in a similar manner and may be clinically enlarged throughout the body. Other areas commonly involved are the corresponding tissues in the intestinal wall and in the skin. Many of the proliferating cells are heavily infected with parasites. There is little other cellular reaction, beyond irregular lymphocytic infiltration; fibrosis is minimal unless initiated for other reasons, such as the nutritional disturbances which accompany the late stages of the disease. With successful treatment the tissues may return to normal, even though the organs such as the spleen in particular may have been grossly enlarged.

The bone marrow is hyperplastic and characteristic changes occur in the blood cells. A leucopenia resulting from an absolute reduction in granulocytes occurs in uncomplicated cases. There is an absolute reduction in all forms of granulocytes, usually associated with a moderate increase in lymphocytes and mononuclear cells. The total leucocyte count is nearly always considerably reduced, and commonly ranges from 4000 cells per mm^3. to less than 2000; occasionally an intractable agranulocytosis may develop, with corresponding changes in the marrow.

In the majority of severe cases there is also a moderate anaemia arising from hypersplenism, with haemoglobin concentrations of 5–10 g. per 100 ml. The erythrocytes show anisocytosis and poikilocytosis and there may be some nucleated red cells in the peripheral blood.

Erythrocyte osmotic fragility is increased in severe cases, in which the platelet count is often low.

Serum albumin concentration falls, sometimes to very low levels and concentration of globulins concurrently rises; the albumin-globulin ratio is thus reversed. The total protein is usually less than normal. The rise in globulins is mostly in the gamma globulin fraction, which probably indicates the production of antibodies. The erythrocyte sedimentation rate is increased.

The liver function tests are usually deviated; the blood bilirubin is raised and there may be overt jaundice.

Signs and Symptoms

It is believed that infection is always followed by overt disease; inapparent infections do not occur.

The time that elapses between the bite of an infective *Phlebotomus* and the appearance of signs and symptoms varies considerably. The onset may be acute and occur with fever which subsides spontaneously and later reappears irregularly, with few presenting signs until the classical picture emerges several months later.

More frequently, the onset is insidious and the patient may not seek help for several months or longer. A remarkable aspect of the clinical picture is that the really ill patient does not feel prostrated or as ill as he is. He presents emaciated, febrile with gross enlargement of the spleen and liver, but still getting about and often actively resents being put to bed. Commonly the first signs are the progressive enlargement of the spleen and liver, which eventually cause considerable discomfort. The spleen is usually easily palpable by the second month of fever.

In cases with an insidious onset the patient becomes increasingly listless and tired. There are irregular episodes of mild or moderate fever with afebrile remissions and early development of leucopenia. The ill health increases with time and there is progressive wasting which eventually may become extreme despite the common retention of a good appetite. The fever is remittent or intermittent, often with two or three sharp peaks during the day. The pulse rate is fast. The blood pressure is usually low, with a systolic pressure in the region of 100 mm. Hg or lower.

The most striking sign is the enlarging spleen, which grows in size rapidly and over the weeks and months may fill the left side of the abdomen and finally present in the pelvis. The organ is firm and is not tender except when perisplenic or capsular lesions develop. The liver usually enlarges less in proportion but not infrequently its edge is palpable as low as the level of the umbilicus. In some patients the spleen may be grossly enlarged without a corresponding increase in the size of the liver. Occasionally the liver will enlarge more than the spleen.

Jaundice sometimes occurs, but not usually before the third month of the overt disease.

In some patients a generalized lymph node enlargement is a prominent feature; this occurs particularly in certain areas, such as the Sudan.

The skin is usually dry and rough. In dark skinned people patchy hyperpigmentation occurs, particularly on the face, over the malar prominences and temples, sometimes round the mouth. (Hence the early name of 'black sickness' for the disease.)

The hair becomes brittle and falls out, leaving the patient temporarily bald or with patches of alopecia.

The lungs are commonly involved, showing signs of bronchitis or bronchopneumonia.

Diarrhoea is also common, probably arising from infiltration and proliferation of macrophages in the gut walls; there may be frank dysentery, which can be attributed to the disease only when other infections such as *Shigella* have been excluded.

In chronic cases the disease may last 1–2 years or longer.

During the disease there is an evident lack of resistance to other infections. Relapses or recrudescences of malaria are common. Infection of the respiratory tract is frequent and may be fatal. In severely ill children especially when there is bone marrow depression, cancrum oris may develop. Death commonly results from secondary infections of this sort, but in any case the mortality amongst untreated cases is extremely high. The prognosis with treatment is usually good.

Post-kala-azar dermal leishmaniasis occurs especially as a sequel of the Indian form of visceral leishmaniasis. It usually appears about a year after apparently successful treatment for kala-azar, but may develop in individuals with no previous history of the generalized disease. The lesions of the skin, which contain *L. donovani*, occur in several forms, most commonly as scattered hypopigmented macules and irregular patches which are often concentrated over the shoulders and neck but may occur anywhere on the trunk or extremities. Papillomatous nodules which rarely ulcerate and have some resemblance to those seen in leprosy are also common, especially on the face, sometimes in the nasopharynx. These nodular lesions have been reported in the Sudanese infection. The two types of lesion often occur concurrently.

Diagnosis

Diagnosis depends on identification of the parasite, which can usually be found easily in material withdrawn from bone marrow, spleen or liver and in the peripheral blood.

It is common practice to examine smears of bone marrow and of blood in the search for organisms. The marrow is usually taken from the sternum. Splenic puncture is sometimes carried out as an alternative and is said by some to be more reliable in cases in which the parasites are scanty.

Smears of tissue fluid and blood should be dried, fixed and stained by Leishman's or Giemsa's method. The parasites are usually plentiful in the former but may be difficult to find in the blood. They occur mostly within the cytoplasm of the macrophages, but may be found free also, probably following cellular rupture in the preparation of the slide.

In cases where the organisms are not seen in tissue or blood preparations, culture on rabbit blood agar at room temperature may reveal them in the flagellate leptomonad form. Two or three drops of the patient's blood are added to a tube of medium which is incubated at room temperature for up to 3 weeks.

Examination of the blood will show some anaemia and the characteristic leucopenia and granulocytopenia.

Presumptive diagnosis may be made by employing certain tests on serum from the patient, which are dependent on the changes which occur in protein content, especially the increase in gamma globulin. The tests are not specific and may be positive in conditions other than kala-azar. The *formol-gel* test is carried out by adding one drop of undiluted commercial formalin to 1 ml. of serum in a small glass test tube. The mixture is shaken and left at room temperature. In positive cases the fluid becomes opaque and gels within an hour. The test becomes positive within one to two months of the development of kala-azar and becomes negative after restoration of normal serum protein concentrations following treatment. Variations of the reaction are also sometimes used, for instance Chopra's antimony test, in which 4 per cent. urea stibamine is added to a 1 in 10 dilution of serum in distilled water. In positive cases flocculation occurs.

Animals are not easily infected with *L. donovani*, with the exception of the hamster. Inoculation of blood or tissue fluid into animals is rarely used for diagnostic purposes.

Complement fixing bodies can be demonstrated (using an antigen made from Kedrowsky's acid-fast bacillus) early in the disease. It remains positive for some time after treatment and is negative in other forms of leishmaniasis.

A delayed hypersensitivity reaction results from the intradermal injection of 0·2 ml. leishmanin, an antigen made from leptomonad culture. The reaction is read after 48–72 hours; a positive reaction is indicated by local induration of more than 5 mm. diameter. Positive reactions occur 6–8 weeks after recovery from kala-azar and are a sign of immunity to *L. donovani* from any geographical area. In all forms of cutaneous leishmaniasis the reaction becomes positive early and remains so for life.

Leishmanin is sometimes used in epidemiological surveys for the presumptive diagnosis of leishmaniasis. The positive reactions are not species specific.

Treatment

Antimonial drugs are the basis of specific treatment. Sodium or potassium antimony tartrate are the only useful trivalent compounds. They are given intravenously in doses similar to those administered for bilharziasis and, because of their cheapness, are used sometimes in mass campaigns. They are toxic, irritant and have unpleasant side-effects [p. 275]. Pentavalent antimonial drugs, which are not irritant and can be given intramuscularly as well as intravenously, have now largely replaced tartar emetic. Kala-azar acquired in most endemic areas responds readily to such treatment but in the Sudan and East Africa and to a lesser extent in the Mediterranean area the disease may be refractory.

There are many pentavalent antimonial drugs available including stibamine glucoside (*Neostam*), urea stibamine, ethylstibamine (*Neostibosan*) and sodium stibogluconate (*Pentostam*). The dosage regimen of the latter may serve as an example. The drug is supplied in a solution containing 100 mg. pentavalent antimony per millilitre. It is given intravenously or intramuscularly each day for 6–10 days. The maximum daily dose is usually 600 mg. A dose of 200–300 mg. is commonly given as the first injection but side-effects are usually minimal, apart from some nausea and occasional vomiting. Children tolerate the drug well in doses calculated in accordance with body weight.

Urea stibamine is also widely used, especially in India. It is given intravenously daily or on alternate days in rising doses of 50 mg., 150 mg. and 250 mg. The latter dose is continued for 10 days in Indian kala-azar. Two or three courses at intervals of 10 days may be needed in other forms of the disease. This drug produces painful damage to muscle and other tissue and is given only intravenously.

Very rarely, a condition resembling shock may develop after the fifth or sixth injection of antimonials, both trivalent and pentavalent, sometimes accompanied by high fever. General treatment, including adrenaline and blood volume adjustment is needed.

Cases which are refractory to antimony treatment in the usual doses may respond to higher or more prolonged dosages, but as an alternative the diamidine drug, pentamidine, may be used in doses of 3–4 mg. per kg. body weight intramuscularly for 10–12 days. Hydroxystilbamidine isethionate is said to be more effective and less toxic. It is given intravenously in doses of 5 mg. per kg. body weight in adults and 3 mg. per kg. body weight in children, in daily doses for 7–10 days. If necessary the dosage is repeated after 10–14 days.

Indian kala-azar usually responds well to this dosage. Other forms may need more prolonged treatment. After one course, an interval of 10 days without treatment is followed by a further 6-day course; this may be repeated after a further interval of 10 days.

Treatment for other than the Indian form of the disease may be repeated twice, with intervals of 10 days between each course, as for sodium stibogluconate.

The diamidine drugs are toxic. Hypoglycaemia may develop and it is wise, therefore, to give glucose drinks during treatment; glucose may be needed immediately if the blood sugar begins to fall. A few cases of myelitis have been reported following administration of hydroxystilbamidine. Skin rashes may develop in susceptible individuals; such reactions may be minimized by promethazine or other antihistaminics.

Under treatment, *Leishmania* may be expected to be eliminated in about a month.

About 10 per cent. of Mediterranean and African cases relapse in up to 2 years.

Refractory cases may respond to amphotericin B (*Fungizone*). This drug is toxic. The urine should be examined regularly during treatment. If proteinuria develops or if the blood urea nitrogen begins to rise administration should be stopped. The dose is 0·25 mg.–1.0 mg./kg. body weight given slowly intravenously in 5 per cent. dextrose, in a concentration of not more than 0·1 mg. per 1·0 ml. Treatment is given every other day for 3–8 weeks, usually with an antipyretic. Severe reactions respond to prednisolone, 5–10 mg. thrice daily.

Occasionally in very refractory cases excision of the spleen has been effective.

Dermal lesions respond poorly to treatment and may need several courses of antimonials. They are refractory to pentamidine.

CUTANEOUS LEISHMANIASIS

Synonyms. Oriental sore; Delhi or Baghdad boil; Lupoid leishmaniasis.

Aetiology

Lesions of the skin and subcutaneous tissues are caused by infection with *Leishmania tropica*. They occur in a wide area of the world stretching from the Mediterranean littoral to China and South East Russia, including North African countries, the Sudan, Ethiopia, parts of West Africa, most of the Middle East, Iran, Turkistan, Pakistan, India and most of Central and South America. In the latter it is probable that some of the reported cases were caused by *L. brasiliensis*, which is morphologically indistinguishable from *L. tropica*.

Lupoid leishmaniasis occurs in some parts of the Middle East. Considerable areas of skin may be involved. Lesions develop slowly and may heal in the centre, forming irregular annular sores which last for years.

Although kala-azar occurs in many of these countries, the regional distribution of the two conditions does not overlap since infection with *L. donovani* provides considerable immunity to infection with *L. tropica*.

In some areas man is the only significant reservoir of infection, in others, dogs, cats and field rodents, for example the gerbil, are important reservoirs. Thus in northern Iran, the gerbil, which commonly has infective sores on its ears, is the natural reservoir, in Italy the dog acts as such and in Iraq man and not the dog.

The parasites are transmitted in the usual way by the bite of the sandfly *Phlebotomus* spp., the species of vector varying from one locality to another. The lesions are commonly classified as 'wet' and 'dry'. The former occurs most commonly in rural desert areas, the latter in towns and cities. It is believed that the same strain of parasite may give rise to either form of clinical picture.

Cutaneous leishmaniasis is usually endemic, occasionally epidemic. It occurs more in children than adults. One attack confers considerable immunity to superinfection, a fact well known to the local indigenes, who often practice deliberate inoculation in young childhood in order to avoid scarring and deformity at a later age.

Pathology

The leptomonad forms which develop in the vectors are transmitted to man through the skin during the bite of an infective sandfly. The organisms invade the local macrophage cells, are transformed into *Leishmania* forms and multiply vigorously, spreading when the cell ruptures to other cells of the reticulo-endothelium as in the visceral form of the disease. In this case, however, there is no general dissemination and the reaction is purely local. A granulomatous nodule is formed as the corium becomes infiltrated with plasma cells, lymphocytes and proliferating macrophages, many of which are filled with *L. tropica*. The overlying epithelium thins and atrophies and commonly ulcerates. There is extensive peripheral cuffing of the small blood vessels with lymphocytes. Secondary infection via the ulcerated surface is common and complicates the picture by accumulations of polymorphs and pus formation. Scabs of dried secretion and pus may form over the ulcer, which presents with a granulomatous base and infiltrated raised edges and surrounding erythema and oedema, as the inflammatory reaction extends into the subcutaneous tissues. The process seems to be self-limiting. After some weeks or months the parasites disappear and healing gradually takes place, often with considerable scarring.

Signs and Symptoms

The sore appears in experimental circumstances a few weeks or months after the infective inoculation, but in the majority of cases this period is impossible to determine owing to the prevalence of sandfly bites. The lesions may be single or multiple.

The first sign is a small itchy papule which enlarges and becomes more indurated. It may remain as a 'blind boil' and finally subside. More commonly after a few months it ulcerates and a crust of dried serous fluid or pus forms over the ulcer. The crust is repeatedly removed by scratching and the granulomatous bleeding base is exposed and becomes secondarily infected. The lesion remains superficial and rarely involves the deeper tissues. It measures from 1–5 cm. across, but may become larger as tissue destruction results from the secondary bacterial infection. Individual lesions heal in some months with or without treatment. The local lymph nodes are usually enlarged and slightly tender in the acute stages.

The lesions occur commonly on the areas most exposed to the biting sandfly, especially the face, hands, wrists, feet and legs. There is usually only one sore, but there may be several and occasionally many scattered over the body.

The dry form of lesion has a long incubation period and may remain in the papular state for many months without ulceration, or may never ulcerate. There may be no appreciable cross-immunity between this lesion and the 'wet' variety.

There are no general changes, such as leucopenia, in dermal leishmaniasis but occasionally there may be evidence of metastasis in locally enlarged glands.

Diagnosis

Diagnosis is usually obvious clinically in endemic areas. Confirmation is necessary by the demonstration of the parasite. *L. tropica* is not usually found in the exudate from lesions or in material taken from the ulcer itself. It may be found in smears taken by curettage of the base or sides of the cleaned ulcer, but it is better to withdraw material from the indurated margins of the ulcer by inserting a needle or fine drawn glass Pasteur pipette through the normal skin near the edge and directing it towards the lesion. Films made from this material should be dried and stained with Leishman or Giemsa's stain and examined for the parasites which will be found within the macrophage cells or lying free.

The fluid should also be dropped on to rabbit blood agar for culture at room temperature.

In lupoid lesions *Leishmania* are few and often very difficult to demonstrate.

Clinical differentiation from blastomycosis, yaws, syphilis or lupus may be necessary, particularly in lesions in which the parasites are scanty. Parasitological diagnosis clinches the matter. Cutaneous leishmaniasis does not give rise to a positive Wassermann reaction and does not respond to penicillin.

In difficult cases the leishmanin intradermal skin reaction may be very helpful. The antigen is injected into the skin of the forearm in the usual way. A positive reaction is seen after 48–72 hours as a raised erythematous nodule which disappears after a few further days or may occasionally ulcerate.

Treatment

The rural form often subsides spontaneously, with some scarring.

Local treatment with injection of 10–20 per cent. solution of mepacrine hydrochloride or of berberine sulphate into the surroundings of the ulcer is sometimes effective in speeding up the healing. *Pentostam*, 600 mg. in 5 ml. sterile distilled water, is often successful, infiltrated into the surrounds 3–4 times a day, on alternate days. Local applications of carbon dioxide snow, diathermy, X-rays, etc., have been used successfully in refractory cases.

Antibacterial drugs especially antibiotics are needed for dealing with the secondary infection.

General treatment is not indicated, except in cases with multiple lesions or where glandular metastasis is suspected. Pentavalent antimonial compounds are given in the usual doses.

Pentamidine is not effective.

Lupoid lesions heal slowly after systemic treatment. *Pentostam* in the usual doses is indicated.

MUCOCUTANEOUS LEISHMANIASIS

Synonyms. South American leishmaniasis; Espundia; Uta; Chiclero or bay sore.

Aetiology

Mucocutaneous leishmaniasis results from infection with *Leishmania brasiliensis* which is morphologically and culturally indistinguishable from *L. tropica*.

Three main clinical types exist probably caused by variants or nosodemes of the main species *L. brasiliensis*. All are transmitted by the bite of the female sandfly *Phlebotomus* spp.

Classical espundia occurs in Brazil and contiguous

countries in which it is endemic and occasionally epidemic. It affects especially forest workers living in low-lying warm wet and wooded areas, in which the 'wet' form of the disease occurs; in drier arid areas the 'dry' form is common. The infection is a zoonosis, the animal reservoirs being dogs, cats and sylvatic rodents.

Uta occurs in Peru and the north coast of South America. A mild form has been described in Panama and Costa Rica.

Bay sore occurs in Mexico, Guatemala and British Honduras. The causative agent has been labelled *L. mexicana.* In some areas forest rodents act as reservoirs.

Other forms of leishmaniasis exist in South America which are not readily placed in these three main groups, including the chronic pleomorphic variety reported in Venezuela.

Pathology

The basic pathological processes and histological developments are the same as those in cutaneous leishmaniasis. The injection of leptomonads by the infected insect leads to the appearance and multiplication of the *Leishmania* in the cytoplasm of the local cells of the reticulo-endothelial system.

In espundia a primary lesion develops as a nodule in the area of the infective bite and may resolve or go on to ulceration. In a high proportion of cases there is additional invasion of the mucosa of the nose, mouth and pharynx and sometimes of the genitals and the rectum by *Leishmania* which results in a granulomatous reaction followed by secondary infection and gross tissue destruction and finally scarring. The mucosa may be invaded by direct extension of an existing local lesion or by metastasis via the blood stream. This reaction may develop while the primary lesion is still present or after it has healed. In the lesions there is epithelial hyperplasia, and the development of a poor granulomatous tissue consisting of macrophages and chronic inflammatory cells with cellular infiltration of the peripheral sweat glands and hair follicles.

The first lesion appears as a papule which enlarges, ulcerates and may be covered by a crust. The process extends to contiguous tissues and secondary infection is common. Eventually cartilage and bone are destroyed with gross deformity especially in the hard and soft palate, the nose and pharynx.

Parasites are found in the nodules and indurated margins of the ulcers. They are present in the histiocytes and other macrophages and sometimes in polymorphs and fibroblasts and may also be lying free in the tissues.

There is no general dissemination of the parasites. There may be extension to local lymph nodes and metastasis from the initial lesion or the secondary mucosal lesions by a process not clearly understood. The initial lesion or lesions may occur anywhere on the body and there is at present no clear explanation for the appearance of metastatic lesions in the nasal and buccopharyngeal mucous membranes.

Signs and Symptoms

Classical espundia. The first lesions appear at the sites of the sandfly bites, on exposed parts of the body. There may be several initial papules, which develop into nodules and may ulcerate. Alternatively the lesions do not develop beyond the papular or nodular stage and then either remain stationary or retrogress. The ulcerating nodule is the commonest form of initial lesion. The sharply defined ulcers usually become covered with a thin firm crust of dried secretion or seropus with easily bleeding granulomatous tissue beneath. The local lymphatic vessels may become irregularly thickened and new skin lesions may form as a result of ulceration over them.

Metastasis of the infection in the mucous membranes of the face and occasionally the rectum occurs in a high proportion of cases and constitute the outstanding clinical pattern. The development of metastatic lesions seems to have little relation to that of the primary lesions. Metastasis of the *Leishmania* occurs when the latter are still present but may not disclose itself clinically until many years after they have healed. In about 10 per cent. of cases clinical signs of metastasis appear while the primary lesion is still active.

The metastatic lesion commonly becomes first evident clinically on the nasal septum in which an ulcer forms over a rapidly developing leishmanial granuloma. The lesion extends deeply into all surrounding tissue in all directions. Eventually the local tissues, mucous membranes, lips, soft palate and cartilage are all consumed in a destructive process usually associated with secondary infection which may involve the larynx and even the trachea. The bony structures of the nose may become involved in the later stages. Terrible deformity results, and death may occur from respiratory involvement, sepsis and malnutrition from inability to eat.

Lesions of a similar nature may occur on the genitals or in the perianal region, with extensive granulomatous ulceration of the rectum. A papulopustular eruption widely spread over the body sometimes develops in patients with mucocutaneous leishmaniasis.

Uta represents cutaneous development of *L. brasiliensis* infection of the dry type. The lesions are usually confined to the skin and only occasionally occur on mucous membranes. They rarely ulcerate.

Bay sore appears as localized chronic lesions which persist for many years. They are particularly common on the ears, but are found also on other parts of the face and the limbs. The outer ear is slowly eroded by the granulomatous reaction which alternately heals and breaks down over the years. The sore is painless and bleeds easily when ulcerated. Considerable local deformity results.

Many variations in the clinical appearance of *L. brasiliensis* infection have been described, amongst which are the chronic widespread cutaneous changes described in patients in Venezuela. The lesions are pleomorphic and include erythematous macules, papules and nodules, often of considerable size. Diffuse infiltrated areas also occur, with dryness and roughening of the overlying skin. The lesions appear chiefly on the face, ears, arms and legs, especially the hands, elbows and knees. The changes in the face and ears in some cases very closely simulate those of lepromatous leprosy. The course is very chronic and the lesions seldom ulcerate. It is not yet certain whether these variations in the form in which leishmaniasis appears arise from variation in host reaction or in strains of parasite species.

Diagnosis

The demonstration of the parasite in smears taken from lesions or its recovery by culture are needed to confirm the diagnosis. *Leishmania* may be found in material obtained by aspiration or biopsy of lesions in the skin, lymph nodes or by curettage of the ulcerating metastatic lesions. In the latter they are more easily found in the early stages before secondary infection has become extensive.

The organisms like other forms of *Leishmania* can be grown from similar material in blood agar [p. 242].

Where there is difficulty in finding the parasite, the leishmanin skin test performed and described above [p. 242] provides valuable presumptive evidence of *Leishmania* infection. A positive reaction develops early in the disease and continues throughout. The Wassermann reaction is negative.

Clinically, the fully developed case of espundia may be mistaken for yaws, leprosy, syphilis, nasal myiasis or blastomycosis. Differentiation depends on the identification of the parasite.

Treatment

Mucocutaneous leishmaniasis responds less satisfactorily to treatment than other forms of leishmaniasis.

Many workers regard sodium antimony gluconate as the best drug, given intravenously, as for visceral leishmaniasis and repeated if necessary.

Some consider the trivalent antimonial compounds give better results. Antimony sodium tartrate (tartar emetic) in doses of 100 mg. intravenously given every other day for 15 doses is sometimes used. The regimen has to be repeated at intervals. Stibophen (fouadin) has also been used with moderate success.

Pentamidine, in doses similar to those given in kala-azar, has been given with good results in some cases.

Pyrimethamine, 25 mg. twice daily for 2 weeks, plus standard doses of folic acid; half this dose for children of 8–15 and one quarter for younger children, has been used successfully.

Cycloguanil pamoate (*Camolar*) a depot drug derived from pyrimethamine metabolite has been used with effect in a single dose of 5 mg. (base) per kg. body weight, repeated if necessary after some months.

Refractory cases have responded to amphotericin B [see p. 243].

Chloroquine in doses of 600 mg. (base) twice daily for 2 days followed by 300 mg. (base) daily for 2–3 weeks has also been tried with some promising results.

Espundia responds sometimes to arsenical drugs, especially amino-arsenophenol or oxophenarsine given in doses of 5 mg. per kg. body weight on alternate days for 5 doses, repeated after a fortnight.

Antibiotics are indicated for dealing with the secondary infections, but are of no value against the *Leishmania*.

REFERENCE

MANSON-BAHR, C. (1971) Leishmaniasis, in *The Management and Treatment of Tropical Diseases*, ed. Maegraith, B. G., and Gilles, H. M., Oxford.

TRYPANOSOMIASIS

Trypanosomiasis represents the clinical effects of infection with species of the protozoal organism *Trypanosoma*. In African trypanosomiasis the infecting agents are *T. gambiense* and *T. rhodesiense*. In American trypanosomiasis the infecting agent is *T. cruzi*.

AFRICAN TRYPANOSOMIASIS

Synonym. Sleeping sickness.

Aetiology

The two trypanosomes *T. gambiense* and *T. rhodesiense* cause distinct clinical entities, commonly known respectively as gambiense and rhodesiense sleeping sickness.

Gambiense trypanosomiasis develops slowly and may last 3 years or more. It is characterized by infection of the blood stream, involvement and enlargement of the lymph nodes, and eventual infection and involvement of the central nervous system. Rhodesiense infection develops more quickly, glandular involvement is uncommon, infection of the central nervous system is rapid and death often occurs within 12 months.

The trypanosome infections occur within a wide belt of Africa between the latitudes 10° N. and 25° S. Inside this area the distribution is patchy, with regions of high endemicity in West Africa, including Nigeria and the Congo, and in East Africa. Gambiense trypanosomiasis is much the more widely distributed; it occurs mainly in West and Central Africa but also appears in scattered areas of East Africa, particularly Uganda. Rhodesiense infection occurs only in East Africa, particularly in Tanganyika, Uganda and Zambia, Rhodesia and Malawi.

In Africa trypanosomes are transmitted to man by the *Glossina* or tsetse fly. In the vector, which sucks the organisms from the infected host during a blood meal, the parasites develop in 2–3 weeks into so-called *metacyclic* forms which are infective to man. These reach the salivary glands of the insects and are injected at biting.

In the human infection the trypanosomes appear as slender actively motile flagellates of up to 30 μ in length, with finely pointed anterior and blunted posterior ends, an oval centrally placed nucleus and a pin-point sized posteriorly placed kinetoplast, from which the undulating membrane projects, to reach the anterior end of the organism as a free flagellum. With Romanowsky dyes the nucleus stains red and the cytoplasm blue. In wet preparations made from blood or tissue fluid the parasites are seen as actively motile, fast moving bodies lying in the plasma amongst the blood cells which they vigorously disturb.

T. gambiense and *T. rhodesiense* are morphologically identical. They are also indistinguishable from *T. brucei* which infects certain ungulates.

The most important species of *Glossina* (tsetse) flies which transmit the infections are: *G. palpalis*, *G. pallidipes*, *G. tachinoides* and *G. morsitans*. All will transmit *T. gambiense*. The latter is the principal vector of *T. rhodesiense*.

The tsetse flies, both sexes of which carry the infection and which bite by daylight, need shade and moisture for survival and breeding and are consequently found in scrub and shady trees near water. They also need moderate warmth. Dry or hot conditions do not suit them. They do not normally travel far from their breeding grounds but may be carried long distances in motor vehicles or trains. *G. morsitans* is hardy and less dependent on environment than the others. *G. palpalis* and *G. tachinoides*, on the other hand are never found far from shade and moisture. Tsetse flies produce single living larvae. Reproduction is thus very limited. The larvae pupate in the soil and the mature fly is developed in a few weeks. These factors are all significant in the epidemiology of the infection and in its control.

Transmission, which occurs when the tsetse fly inoculates metacyclic forms of the parasite into the tissues at the time of biting, depends basically on man-fly contact. This may occur when both are plentiful but may also occur when the fly is scanty so long as the infection rate is high and there are suitable non-immune human hosts. In most areas man is the reservoir of the infection, but certain wild or domestic animals, notably the large antelope, may sometimes act as such.

Infection occurs without regard to age and sex when exposure is comparable, but in many areas it depends on occupation, since one particular group, for instance, the men or the women, may be more exposed, e.g. during fishing, than the other.

In endemic areas, populations which have been exposed for long periods to repeated infection often develop some kind of resistance which modifies the clinical attack. In these areas the average case is often mild or apparently so, although at any stage it may become acute and even fatal. The classical picture is most commonly seen in epidemics, but is not rare in endemic areas.

Pathology

The metacyclic organisms injected at the site of the bite are quickly transformed into trypanosomes which invade the blood stream and lymphatics, the lymph nodes (mostly in the case of *T. gambiense* infection) and later the central nervous system. Other organs, including the heart and the spleen, may be involved.

Lymphocyte and plasma cell infiltration occurs at the site of the bite in both types of infection. Metacyclic trypanosomes may be present initially but within 48 hours transformation to the rapidly-multiplying, fully-developed trypanosomes has taken place.

In both types the lymph nodes draining the bite area become infected, enlarged and undergo similar cellular changes, with oedema and vascular congestion. The blood now becomes infected. Glandular involvement, most obvious in gambiense infection, may remain localized or may become generalized. In an erratic manner the gland tissue becomes invaded by fibroblasts and finally by fibrosis. The glands may be unaffected in rhodesiense infections. In both infections trypanosomes surrounded by cellular reactions are sometimes present in the interstitial tissues, especially of the heart, and are ultimately replaced by fibrous tissue with consequent disturbance of function.

In a few weeks in rhodesiense infections, and in a few months in gambiense infections, the central nervous system becomes invaded by the trypanosomes. A leptomeningitis results at first to be followed by the development of a meningo-encephalitis, with perivascular cuffing with lymphocytes and occasional Mott cells, which are modified macrophages with lobulated eosinophilic cytoplasm and eccentric nuclei. There may be some endothelial proliferation of the vascular walls, leading to endarteritis and even obliteration. The lesions are seen best in the pia in which there may also be small haemorrhages and scattered Mott cells. Trypanosomes, often in groups or nests, are scattered about the brain substance, sometimes with and sometimes without microglial proliferation and local 'softening'. Neuronal changes are late and rarely pronounced. The brain is often oedematous, evidenced at autopsy by a 'wet' brain with markedly flattened convolutions.

The choroid plexus is often severely congested and infiltrated with lymphocytes; and sometimes with large numbers of parasites.

The upper region of the cord may show similar changes.

The cerebrospinal fluid is affected soon after the central nervous system is invaded. The pressure is moderately raised and the cellular content rises to 10–50 cells or more per mm^3. mostly due to lymphocytes and occasional Mott or plasma cells. The fluid rarely contains sufficient cells to produce turbidity. The protein content is moderately increased and rises as the disease progresses. It is seldom much in excess of 100–150 mg. per 100 ml. The globulin content usually gives rise to a tabetic type of colloidal gold curve. Trypanosomes are frequently present in the early stages of nervous system involvement but are invariably found in the late stages.

Signs and Symptoms of Gambiense Trypanosomiasis

In populations in an endemic area, gambiense sleeping sickness is frequently clinically mild. In a given individual, however, it may either continue to run a mild course or may suddenly become exacerbated and end fatally. Fulminating cases appear from time to time in all areas, in which the central nervous system is involved early, with rapidly advancing meningo-encephalitis or in which acute severe septicaemia develops, again leading to a fatal issue.

The classical picture of the disease, known as sleeping sickness, occurs commonly in non-immune visitors infected in an endemic area, but also appears in indigenes, especially during epidemics.

The disease begins with a tumour at the site of the fly bite, followed after a short interval by the stage of invasion in which first the blood then the lymph nodes become involved. Finally, this is followed by invasion of the central nervous system and meningo-encephalitis.

The full progress of the disease normally takes 2–3 years but may exceptionally be completed in less than a year.

A red swelling and sometimes a wheal occurs at the site of the bite within a few minutes. This quickly subsides and is replaced in about a week by a firm tender reddish violet nodule which may be 2·5 cm. or more in length and surrounded by a diffuse erythematous and sometimes slightly oedematous plaque-like area. The nodule is itchy and scratching may lead to secondary infection and ulceration. Fluid withdrawn from the tumour after the first 24 hours usually contains trypanosomes. Earlier there may be some metacyclic forms. The lesion lasts 1–2 weeks and subsides without scarring unless ulceration has occurred.

The stage of invasion begins 10 days to 3 weeks after the bite (the incubation period) in many cases but may be delayed months or even years in some individuals.

The onset, which is very difficult to determine in indigenes of an endemic area because of other causes of similar symptoms, is accompanied by fever, tachycardia, malaise, headache and sometimes insomnia. Trypanosomes appear in the peripheral blood but, at this early stage, are relatively few, only one or two being present per oil immersion field. Later they become more numerous but are plentiful only in rare cases.

In some individuals a characteristic rash develops as large irregular or roughly annular patches of transient erythema sometimes with a clear centre, usually on the trunk, especially the back, and occasionally on the face and limbs. The rash fades in a few hours and tends to reappear at intervals thereafter. It is difficult to detect in a coloured skin.

Involvement of the lymph nodes occurs soon after the onset, or may be the first overt sign of infection. The affected glands, of which the first may be those draining the bite area, are moderately enlarged, firm and discrete, with the skin freely movable over them. They usually appear in batches, particularly in the posterior cervical region (Winterbottom's sign) but there may be generalized adenitis.

A gland takes several months to reach its maximum size and may remain enlarged for years. Eventually it becomes replaced by fibrous tissue, diminishing in size to a mere fibrous nodule. In any one anatomical group of glands it is common to find some enlarged, some fibrosed. Glands do not suppurate unless secondarily infected.

Glandular enlargement is the common finding but in individual cases and occasionally in localized epidemics, it may not be prominent or may be absent, even when the blood is heavily infected.

Active trypanosomes can usually be found in the fluid withdrawn from an enlarged gland.

The spleen and liver may both be moderately enlarged. Serous effusions have occasionally been reported in joint cavities and the pleural and pericardial spaces. These are commoner in rhodesiense infections.

The disease reaches this stage of development in some months. Thereafter the dominating factor is the invasion of the central nervous system and the resultant meningo-encephalitis, which causes the classical 'sleeping sickness'.

The patient becomes progressively apathetic and confused. He is irritable when roused, sometimes emotional or depressed. His memory fades and his personality disintegrates. He sleeps more and more and may have to be aroused to eat. Finally, he fails even to feed himself or falls asleep during a meal and lies curled up on the ground, saliva and bits of the meal dribbling from his mouth. Coma eventually develops.

In this stage various signs of malnutrition develop and complicate the picture. The patient is thin and asthenic, vitamin deficiencies are prominent. The face, in contrast to the miserable wasted body is puffy especially round the eyelids and the malar region, producing a rather surly moon-shaped look which is highly characteristic.

Neurological signs may appear at any stage in this period. They vary considerably from patient to patient.

Muscular cramps and deep seated sharp pains are common over the long bones, deep pressure, especially over tendons, eliciting severe pain. Spatial sensation may be lost with corresponding slow shuffling unsteady gait. Inco-ordination of movements is common, especially in the hands and legs. The knee-jerks are present until late in the disease.

The early motor signs usually occur on the face, and fingers. Fine tremor of the lips and tongue develop; speech becomes slow and slurred and later incoherent. Paresis of the facial muscles is common, leading to protrusion of the lower lip, with dribbling of saliva, and changes round the orbit which are accompanied by excessive lacrimation. Tremor of the hands becomes severe and interferes with ordinary movements. Muscle twitching in the face, forearms and calves are common.

Progress of the central nervous lesions is usually continuous but may be slow and subject to intermittent remissions and exacerbations.

The patchy glandular enlargements may be present throughout. Trypanosomes are usually still present in the gland fluid, and often in the blood. They are usually found in the spinal fluid.

The final stages are accompanied by the effects of malnutrition, dehydration and sometimes anuria and uraemia. There may be cardiac dilatation and failure, with associated oedema. Incontinence of faeces and urine is common.

Trophic sores frequently appear in patients who have had no one to care for them, and, with secondary infection may be a cause of death. Other intercurrent infections, especially pneumonia and dysenteries may prove fatal, and occasionally there may be an acute extension of the encephalitis, with an accompanying trypanosome septicaemia.

In untreated cases the outlook is very bad. Modern drugs have considerably improved the prognosis even of late cases and treatment is usually successful in the early stages.

Mild or apparently mild clinical pictures are the

usual pattern in endemic areas, but the classical case is seen in these areas during epidemics.

The patient sometimes complains of headache, and there is usually lymph node enlargement especially in the posterior triangle of the neck but occasionally this may be absent although the blood is infected. In later stages there may be some disturbance of sleep rhythm, personality changes, muscular tremors, slurring speech, with the typical 'swollen' facies.

Trypanosomes are present in the blood and gland juice and in the later stages in the cerebrospinal fluid.

Although in many cases the disease is apparently mild, it is not easy to indicate the prognosis with certainty, since some may progress slowly to give the classical picture and others may develop sudden and fatal exacerbations. The form the disease takes may be a matter of local strains or of the development of acquired resistance.

In epidemics the earlier cases are usually mild, but an increasing proportion develop classical symptoms as the epidemic progresses.

Diagnosis

Diagnosis depends on the discovery of the parasite in the blood, lymph node juice (or other tissue fluid) or the cerebrospinal fluid.

Blood. Wet preparations are made by placing a drop of blood on a coverslip face downwards on a microscope slide. The preparation may be ringed with petroleum jelly. Examination under the 16 mm. objective will disclose the trypanosomes wriggling actively in the plasma between the cells.

Thick or thin films prepared and stained as for malaria enable the final identification to be made. *T. gambiense* and *T. rhodesiense* cannot be differentiated.

Where infection is suspected and parasites cannot be found in smears of blood, lymph node or tissue fluid, 5 ml. of blood is withdrawn into citrate and centrifuged at 1000 r.p.m. for 10 minutes. The supernatant is removed and centrifuged in the same way. The supernatant is then spun at 2500–3000 r.p.m. for 10 minutes and the whole of the deposit examined for trypanosomes.

Tissue Fluid from Lymph Nodes. An enlarged soft gland is chosen and lifted between the finger and thumb until the skin over it is fixed and tight. After sterilizing the skin with alcohol and allowing to dry, a medium-sized thoroughly dry, sterile hypodermic needle is inserted into the gland substance. The gland is then gently massaged. A syringe is attached to the needle and the fluid withdrawn. The volume of material obtained in this way is very small but should be sufficient for several wet preparations and smears which should be examined as for blood. The smears should be allowed to dry and are then fixed and stained by the Giemsa or Leishman technique. *T. gambiense* can usually be detected by this method, but *T. rhodesiense* may not. The latter is best sought in the blood.

Cerebrospinal Fluid. The pressure is measured, and the deposit obtained after centrifuging the fluid is examined as above for cells and trypanosomes.

The cellular content and protein concentration of separate samples of the fluid are determined by the usual methods.

Cells seldom rise above 50–100 per mm^3. Protein is only moderately increased over normal, ranging from 40 to 150 mg. per 100 ml. in overt cases.

Mass diagnosis is made by examination of blood or gland tissue or both. Lumbar puncture is not usually performed except when indicated.

Signs and Symptoms of Rhodesiense Trypanosomiasis

The pathological processes and clinical course are basically the same as in gambiense trypanosomiasis but are usually accelerated so that death occurs in 9–12 months from the onset.

The distribution of the disease which occurs only in East Africa in Zambia, Southern Rhodesia, Malawi, Mozambique, Tanganyika, Uganda corresponds to that of the main vector *Glossina morsitans*.

The incubation period is about the same or shorter. The onset is associated with fever and sometimes rigor. Lymph nodes are usually little involved. Trypanosomes appear early in the blood, often in relatively large numbers. In the early stages scattered fleeting subcutaneous areas of oedema are not uncommon. Serous effusions occur more frequently than in *T. gambiense* infection and myocardial damage is more prominent and severe, both early and late. The myocardial effects lead to a rapid pulse rate which persists.

The central nervous system is involved early, usually within 4–6 weeks of the onset. Mental symptoms are often prominent but the full picture of sleeping sickness rarely develops, probably because of the short duration of the illness.

Diagnosis is made as above.

Prognosis in the untreated case is generally bad, although in certain geographical areas mild forms of the disease exist.

TREATMENT

Chemotherapy. The object of chemotherapy is to remove the parasites from the blood, tissues and cerebrospinal spaces.

Drugs

FOR TRYPANOSOMES IN BLOOD AND TISSUE: NOT FOR PARASITES IN THE CENTRAL NERVOUS SYSTEM.

Suramin (*Antrypol*): An organic substituted urea. Provided as powder. Usually made up in 10 per cent. solution in sterile pyrogen-free distilled water.

Dosage: 20 mg. per kg. body weight. Maximum single dose 1 G. Intravenous.

Pentamidine isethionate: A diamidine compound provided as powder. Usually made up in 10 per cent. solution in sterile pyrogen-free distilled water.

Pentamidine methanesulphonate (*Lamidine*) may be used as an alternative.

Dosage: 3–4 mg. (base) per kg. body weight. Maximum single dose 300 mg. Intramuscular.

FOR TRYPANOSOMES IN THE CENTRAL NERVOUS SYSTEM.

(Note: Melarsoprol and melarsonyl potassium also act on blood and tissue parasites.)

Melarsoprol (Mel B): Organic pentavalent arsenical with dimercaprol (British Anti-Lewisite: BAL). Provided in ampoules of 3·6 per cent. solution in propylene glycol for intravenous injection. Fluid is viscous; administered in dry syringe through large bore dry needle.

Dosage: 3·6 mg. per kg. body weight. Maximum single dose 5 ml. (180 mg.).

Melarsonyl potassium (Mel W, *Trimelarsan*): on trial as an alternative for melarsoprol in gambiense infections only.

Tryparsamide: Organic pentavalent arsenical. Once the main line of attack on trypanosomes in the central nervous system. To some extent superseded by melarsoprol, but still of potential value for mass treatment of large numbers of cases of gambiense infections. Powder made up as 20 per cent. solution in sterile pyrogen-free distilled water.

Dosage: 30 mg. per kg. body weight. Maximum single does 2 G.

Nitrofurazone (*Furacin*): Used in cases, usually of rhodesiense infestation which have proved resistant to melarsoprol. Supplied in tablets of 100 mg.

Dosage: 10 mg. per kg. body weight. Maximum single dose 500 mg. Oral.

Very toxic. May produce severe polyneuropathy (and haemolytic anaemia in glucose-6-phosphate dehydrogenase deficient individuals); heart may be involved as in beriberi. Thiamine should be administered concurrently.

Dimercaprol. British Anti-Lewisite (BAL). Used to counter toxic effects of arsenicals.

Dosage: 3 mg. per kg. body weight. Intramuscular.

Treatment Regimens

GAMBIENSE INFECTIONS:

1. *Very early cases*, a few weeks from onset, may respond to treatment aimed at trypanosomes in the blood and tissues. All other cases require treatment for infection of the central nervous system.

Blood and tissue infection only.

(i) Suramin. Since the drug sometimes causes renal damage it should not be given to patients with any form of kidney disease or dysfunction. In treatment of trypanosomiasis, a test dose of 0·2 G. is given intravenously and specimens of urine are examined. If proteinuria, casts and/or erythrocytes appear the drug is discarded and pentamidine substituted. If there is no renal reaction, 1 G. is given intravenously on days 1, 3, 7, 14 and 21, making a total of 5 G. in 3 weeks. If the patient is acutely ill with fever, smaller doses are given in the early stages of treatment, as follows: Day 1: 0·25 G.; day 3: 0·5 G.; day 7: 0·75 or 1 G.; days 14, 21: 1 G.

(ii) Pentamidine is used as an alternative to suramin. The drug is given in doses of 250–300 mg. intramuscularly for 10 consecutive days, or every other day for 10 doses.

2. *Cases with central nervous system involvement.* These require removal of trypanosomes from the blood and tissues and from the central nervous system.

Melarsoprol may be used by itself or, where the patient is febrile, in combination with suramin.

Dosage Regimens

(i) Melarsoprol only.

Day 1	Melarsoprol	5 ml. (180 mg.)
Day 2		5 ml. (180 mg.)
Day 3		5 ml. (180 mg.)
Interval of 7–10 days.		
Day 11 or 14		5 ml. (180 mg.)
Day 12 or 15		5 ml. (180 mg.)
Day 13 or 16		5 ml. (180 mg.)

(ii) Suramin in combination with melarsoprol.

Day 1	Suramin	0·2 G. Test dose
If no renal toxicity:		
Day 3	Suramin	0·25 G.
Day 6		0·5 G.
Day 10		0·75 G.
Day 17		1 G.

Then follow with melarsoprol as in (i) above.

(iii) Suramin in combination with tryparsamide.

Given only in special circumstances, for instance where there is an outbreak and many cases need treatment or if mass therapy is intended.

Day 1	Suramin	0·2 G. Test dose
If no toxicity proceed as follows:		
Day 3	Suramin	1 G.
Day 6		1 G.
Day 10		1 G.
Day 17		1 G.
Day 24		1 G.
Follow after 5–7 days by:		
Day 29 or 31	Tryparsamide	1 G.
Day 34 or 36		2 G.
Day 39 or 41		2 G.
Day 44 or 46		2 G.
Day 49 or 51		2 G.

RHODESIENSE INFECTIONS

The trypanosomes should be considered in all cases to have involved blood, tissues and the central nervous system.

(i) Melarsoprol. The regimen used for gambiense infections is usually regarded as too vigorous for rhodesiense trypanosomiasis. The following is recommended for adults of 50 kg. or more. Note that the *total* dosage is higher than that for gambiense.

Day 1	0·5 ml. (18 mg.)
Day 3	1 ml. (36 mg.)
Day 5	1·5 ml. (54 mg.)
7 day interval.	
Day 13	2·5 ml. (90 mg.)
Day 14	2·5 ml. (90 mg.)
Day 15	2·5 ml. (90 mg.)
7 day interval.	
Day 23	5 ml. (180 mg.)
Day 24	5 ml. (180 mg.)
Day 25	5 ml. (180 mg.)

(ii) Suramin in combination with melarsoprol. This combined course is needed if the patient is febrile and seriously ill.

Suramin: as for gambiense (ii, above).
Melarsoprol: as in (i).

(iii) Nitrofurazone. In cases resistant to melarsoprol. For an adult of 50 kg or more:

Days 1, 2	500 mg. daily.
Days 3–7	500 mg. thrice daily for 5 days.
Interval of 7 days	
Days 15–20, or 22	Repeat 500 mg. thrice daily for 5–7 days.

Note: Give thiamine, 25–50 mg. daily intravenously, or other vitamin B compound, say, *Becosym*, 1–3 ampoules daily intramuscularly.

The patient should be kept at rest on a high protein diet. If febrile, the short course of suramin recommended above (1, (i)) should be given before the nitrofurazone is started.

Toxicity of Arsenicals

All these compounds are toxic, especially in the presence of vitamin deficiencies or febrile illness. Melarsoprol should be avoided, for instance, in patients with influenza or during an influenza epidemic.

Melarsoprol, melarsonyl potassium and tryparsamide have the usual toxic disadvantages of arsenical compounds. They may cause gastro-intestinal disturbances with diarrhoea and/or vomiting. Dermatitis, sometimes exfoliative, may occur after prolonged treatment.

There are two common toxic developments with the Mel compounds. Reactive encephalopathy appears as muscle twitching and some somnolence in about 10 per cent. of treated individuals. The drug should be withheld and recovery is usually rapid. After an interval the dosage may be cautiously renewed. Haemorrhagic encephalopathy develops in a few cases and is fatal. The patient rapidly becomes comatose with stertorous breathing and succumbs in a few hours or days.

Tryparsamide sometimes causes optic nerve damage which may lead to permanent atrophy and blindness; the onset is indicated by increasing dimness of vision, photophobia, lacrimation and ocular pain.

Dimercaprol may relieve acute arsenical toxicity in doses of: 3 mg. per kg. intramuscularly four-hourly for 2 days, six-hourly for 1 day and twelve-hourly for 10 days.

Chemoprophylaxis

Pentamine given intramuscularly as a single dose of 200–250 mg. will protect against *T. gambiense* infection for 3–6 months, and has been widely used for this purpose in endemic areas.

Intravenous injection of a single dose of 1 G. suramin also gives some more limited protection lasting 6 weeks to 3 months.

Chemoprophylaxis is not successful in *T. rhodesiense* infections.

AMERICAN TRYPANOSOMIASIS

Synonym. Chagas' disease.

Aetiology

This disease occurs irregularly in Central and South America from Mexico to the Argentine, and in certain islands of the West Indies. The distribution of the vector is much wider and includes some of the southern North American states. The disease does not occur outside of the Americas.

The causative organism is the pleomorphic *Trypanosoma cruzi* which closely resembles the trypanosomes of the African disease, except that it has a large oval posteriorly placed kinetoplast. It exists in two forms in the host, i.e. as the trypanosomes in the blood stream and tissue fluids and as the leishmanioid form in the tissue cells.

The infection in most areas may be regarded as an enzootic in a variety of animals including rats, the armadillo, pigs, cats and dogs, and is acquired accidentally by man. In some districts, however, it is transmitted from man to man via the vector and man may be the only reservoir.

The disease is transmitted by large biting reduviid bugs belonging to the family *Triatomidae*, of which *Panstrongylus megistus* and *Triatoma infestans* are the commonest. All stages of the bugs may transmit the infection, the adult being the most important.

The bugs thrive in dirty unhygienic environments associated with man or animals and the disease is consequently seen most frequently in the lowest economic groups of a community. They are active mainly at night when transmission most commonly occurs. The bug is infected by sucking blood containing trypanosomes from either the human or the animal reservoir. The parasites eventually become converted into the infective metacyclic forms in the mid- and hindgut in 2–3 weeks.

The bug is now infective to the mammal and remains so for the duration of its life.

Transmission occurs by the introduction into human tissues of the metacyclic parasite in the faeces of the bug passed during feeding. The usual sequence of events is that in response to the bite the victim fingers or scratches the area and accidentally rubs the faeces into the bite wound or cuts or abrasions, mucous membranes such as the conjunctiva and sometimes the intact skin.

Infection occurs most commonly in children who are bitten as the bug crawls over the face during the night.

Transmission across the placenta has been reported. Occasionally infection may result from accidentally swallowing live or dead bugs. Other insects including the bed bug can be infected artificially but are of no importance in natural transmission.

Pathology

The metacyclic forms cause a brisk tissue response at the point of entry into the host. A small subcutaneous swelling appears consisting of localized oedema, cellular infiltration and the parasites. The infection spreads via the lymphatics to the local lymph nodes which become enlarged, oedematous and infiltrated with lymphocytes and plasma cells. The trypanosomes reach the blood stream within a few days. The parasites distributed in this way enter local tissue cells and undergo multiplication in leishmanioid form; the invaded cells finally rupture, liberating large numbers of trypanosomes into the tissue spaces and the blood stream. These later invade fresh tissue cells and the leishmanioid cycle is repeated. In this way the cells of many tissues become destroyed. The process occurs particularly in the Kupffer cells of the liver, the macrophages of the spleen and in striated muscle, especially the cardiac muscle. The lesions developed in the latter are responsible for much of the more serious clinical effects.

In the acute form of the disease which occurs particularly in infants and young children, extensive and progressive myocardial damage develops within a few weeks. In less severe cases, which may survive, fibrosis gradually replaces the destroyed tissue and chronic myocardial disturbances may appear in later life.

Other organs may be seriously involved, including the thyroid; goitre is associated with the infection in some regions. Meningo-encephalitis may develop and cause early death; there is some perivascular cuffing and granulomata consisting largely of microglial cells may be scattered through the brain substance around trypanosomes or leishmanioid forms of the parasite. In such cases the changes in the spinal fluid include an increase in mononuclear cells and protein; trypanosomes may be present.

The nerve plexus of the oesophagus and colon are sometimes damaged by the tissue reaction to the infection. The hollow organs dilate and may become enormous, giving rise in subacute and chronic cases to characteristic mega-oesophagus and megacolon.

The trypanosomes may be found in the blood, by direct examination or biological methods, over many years in chronic cases. They are present in largest numbers in the initial acute attack and relapses.

Signs and Symptoms

The disease appears in acute, subacute and chronic forms.

The acute disease is commonest and most severe in infants and young children usually between the ages of 1 and 6 years. It may occur, however, in any non-immune individual who becomes infected.

The incubation period is difficult to determine in some cases but usually ranges from a few days to 3 weeks.

The onset of the clinical disease is usually sudden, but is commonly preceded by local reactions to the inoculation of infective material, especially on the face.

The first sign of infection is a swelling which appears within a few hours at the site of inoculation. This develops most frequently on the forehead, eyelids, conjunctiva, cheek or lips, but may be found anywhere on the exposed body. The lesion presents as a small firm raised infiltrated erythematous plaque surrounded by an area of loose oedema (the so-called *chagoma*) which may become extremely painful. It reaches maximum size in 3–4 days and gradually subsides over the next few weeks. The skin over the area may desquamate; suppuration may develop only if scratching leads to secondary infection.

The local lymph nodes are involved in the first few days. They enlarge and become firm and slightly tender; they remain discrete. There may be loca oedema and erythema. Occasionally there is no chagoma and the enlarged glands may be the first sign of infection.

Apart from the chagoma, patches of local hard oedema may develop particularly in the face, and commonly involving the eyelids and cheek on one side (*Romana's sign*). The oedema may remain localized or spread over the cheek into the neck or to the other side of the face. Sometimes it appears bilaterally from the beginning. It may disappear in a few days or persist for weeks.

The skin over the oedematous area is erythematous and blotchy, producing the effect of bruising. The lacrimal glands are commonly swollen and there is often excessive lacrimation; the conjunctiva is intensely congested and the eyelids are often glued together with dried secretion.

Similar patches of hard oedema may occur from time to time elsewhere on the body, including the legs, scrotum and abdominal wall. General anasarca may occasionally be seen in infants.

The general reactions start with a moderate remittent fever which persists for some weeks. It may become very high and continuous especially in infants.

The pulse rate is very fast and there are often mitral bruits. Where the myocardial damage is especially severe, acute fatal cardiac failure develops within a week of the onset. In most cases, however, the condition steadily worsens with increasing signs of heart involvement over the course of several weeks.

The cardiac muscular damage may cause sudden dilatation and failure, the usual terminal event, but this may be preceded by changes in rhythm, such as atrial fibrillation or heart block.

Pulmonary involvement is frequent with fast respiration, bronchitis or bronchopneumonia.

The spleen becomes palpable in the first fortnight but is seldom prominent. In addition to the local glands involved in the originally infected area, there is often a generalized mild glandular enlargement.

In some cases there may be a transient morbilliform or urticarial rash. There is usually little indication of involvement of the central nervous system; occasionally, especially in infants, severe meningo-encephalitis develops with the usual changes in the cerebrospinal fluid and the patient dies in coma or convulsions, with or without concurrent cardiac signs.

The acute stage lasts a variable time. Cases with acute severe cardiac involvement may die in a few days. In those with less severe cardiac damage recovery may occur after a few weeks, sometimes with residual signs, sometimes with apparent remission which may be followed in adolescence or adult life by signs of fibrotic myocardial damage.

There may be occasional return of acute symptoms with fever and signs of myocardial involvement in older children who usually give a history of previous acute attacks (the so-called subacute form of the disease). In such cases a series of mild recrudescences may occur over some years, with eventual recovery, permanent cardiac signs or death during an exacerbation.

Many individuals may escape the early severe attacks

and present in adolescence or adult life with signs of myocardial damage. These may represent the first signs of infection or there may be a long history of subacute attacks and remissions. Mega-oesophagus and/or mega-colon are sometimes present in the later stages of chronic infections.

These so-called chronic forms of the disease may have parasites present in the blood and detectable by direct examination. More often the diagnosis depends on biological or serological investigations [see below].

Sudden death from cardiac causes is common in chronic cases.

In endemic areas the number of chronic cases is always considerably greater than that of acute attacks.

Diagnosis

Clinical diagnosis of acute infection in children in endemic areas is usually obvious where there is a unilateral or bilateral facial oedema, a chagoma with local enlargement of lymph nodes and later signs of myocardial damage.

Confirmation depends on the demonstration of trypanosomes in the blood or lymph node tissue fluid and occasionally in the cerebrospinal fluid.

Thick and thin blood films prepared and examined as for African trypanosomiasis will usually contain *Trypanosoma cruzi* in the early stages of acute infections in children and sometimes in exacerbations of subacute infections. In chronic cases they are present in the blood from time to time in very small numbers and are easily missed.

Where the infection is suspected and trypanosomes are not found by direct blood examination, indirect methods are needed. The parasites can be cultured from the blood on special (NNN) medium, in which they take about 3 weeks to develop. The commonest indirect method is, however, xenodiagnosis, in which laboratory raised triatome bugs free from infection with *T. cruzi* or other trypanosomes are allowed to suck blood from the patient and are subsequently kept for 1–3 months and examined for metacyclic parasites.

Mice and puppies are easily infected with citrated or fresh unclotted blood from the patient injected subcutaneously or intraperitoneally. Trypanosomes appear in the animal blood in 1–3 weeks and leishmanioid forms can be found in the tissues, especially the cardiac muscle.

T. cruzi must be distinguished from other trypanosomes, particularly *T. rangeli*, which appears in many of the same parts of the world and can be sometimes found in human blood and reduviid bugs caught wild. *T. rangeli* has a very small rounded kinetoplast, easily distinguished from the large oval body in *T. cruzi*. It does not cause symptoms in man.

Very specific antigens have been prepared from *T. cruzi* especially in Venezuela for complement-fixation reactions with the patient's serum. Positive results are obtained in most cases of the chronic myocardial disease and appear at the usual time in acute infections. They represent presumptive evidence of infection. Some slight cross-reactions occur in sera from cases of cutaneous leishmaniasis.

The complement fixation test should be associated with other diagnostic methods wherever possible.

Treatment

Treatment is at present unsatisfactory. The drugs which are effective in the African disease are not active in *T. cruzi* infections.

The major difficulty is to find a drug or combination of drugs which will deal with both blood trypanosomes and tissue leishmanioid parasites. Many compounds will remove the trypanosomes, including Bayer 7602, Cruzon M.3024, primaquine, pentaquine, but these are ineffective against the tissue forms. Recent studies of nitrofurazone, furazolidone and furaltodone which are toxic drugs have failed to produce better results. Attempts to eliminate the trypanosomes for long enough to minimize or prevent leishmanioid formation have also failed.

Control depends on elimination of the vectors which can be locally achieved with insecticides such as DDT. Some control of infection of the bugs may result from the use of trypanocidal drugs in active cases, but in the long run success will depend on improvement in housing and living standards.

REFERENCES

Transactions of the Royal Society of Tropical Medicine and Hygiene (1968) Seminar. Trypanosomiasis, **62**, 120.

WORLD HEALTH ORGANIZATION (1969) Comparative studies of American and African trypanosomiasis, *Tech. Rep. Ser.*, No. 411.

AMOEBIASIS

Definition and Aetiology

Amoebiasis is the condition of harbouring the protozoon *Entamoeba histolytica*. The organism may live for long periods in the lumen of the large intestine as a commensal, without invading the intestinal wall. When invasion occurs lesions are developed in the mucosa which may give rise to clinical amoebic colitis or to extra-intestinal lesions. Invasion may sometimes occur with only localized lesions which do not cause overt signs or symptoms (inapparent amoebiasis).

The infection is world wide, occurring especially unhygienic conditions in warm climates.

E. histolytica is a parasite of man but is occasionally found in other animals. Infection is normally acquired by swallowing the cysts of the organism passed in the faeces of an infected patient and contaminating food-stuffs or water. Cysts survive for some days in faeces but do not withstand drying or disinfectants, including chlorine.

Excystation occurs in the lower part of the small intestine and the upper part of the large intestine. Each viable cyst liberates a 4-nucleated amoeba which subsequently splits into single nucleated entamoebae which may survive and multiply in the lumen or invade the intestinal wall.

Under conditions still not fully understood but which involve a relatively slow movement through the intestinal lumen, some trophozoites of *E. histolytica* form cysts which are eventually excreted in the faeces.

In acute diarrhoea, cysts are not formed and the trophozoites as such are passed. In general, the diarrhoeic soft stool contains the entamoeba and the formed stool contains the cysts. Once the cyst is formed it does not excyst in the lumen but must be ingested before liberating the trophozoite.

Pathology

Infection with *E. histolytica* produces effects which vary considerably from patient to patient in the same endemic area and also vary from one endemic area to another. Infections acquired in the tropics as a rule have more pathogenic effect than those in temperate countries.

The pathogenicity of the organism is not understood, and it is often difficult to determine whether a particular strain of parasite is pathogenic or not. Most contain trypsin which is capable of digesting the epithelium of the gut wall but some strains will produce lesions in humans and animals and some will not. Some live in the intestinal lumen and never penetrate the epithelium; many others will remain for long periods as commensals surviving solely in the gut lumen, and then suddenly invade the wall. Strains of *E. histolytica* which give rise to small cysts less than 10 μ in diameter seldom produce lesions. Those which produce larger cysts may or may not be invasive. Swellengrebel believed that the parasite is normally a commensal, living in the lumen or on the epithelial surface but not penetrating until special circumstances exist which are suitable to invasion. Clinical evidence suggests that in a given host a strain of parasite may, over long periods, alternate between pathogenicity and existence as a commensal. This view is widely accepted. It is therefore important to distinguish carefully between infection, i.e. the survival and multiplication of the parasite in the gut, and invasion, which implies the penetration of the epithelium. Factors which may affect the activity of *E. histolytica* in the gut, apart from the inherent properties of the strain itself, are believed to include the environment, i.e. the lumen contents including the bacteria, mucous secretion and possibly injury to the epithelium.

The primary infection with *E. histolytica* always occurs in the large intestine. The amoeba may penetrate the gut wall forming specific abscesses and ulcers and may involve adjacent structures. It may spread extra-intestinally via the local blood flow to the liver and other organs.

The lesions may occur anywhere in the wall of the large gut but are found most commonly in the caecum, sigmoid colon and rectum. In very severe acute cases there may be extensive multiple lesions in all areas of the large intestine, including the rectum; the terminal ileum may also be involved.

The basic lesion follows amoebic invasion through the intestinal epithelial wall. The process results largely from digestion of the tissues by the amoebae, so that in the early stages there is liquefaction of the tissues beneath the broken mucosa, penetrating in the first instance as far as the muscularis mucosae. At the periphery of the lesion there are groups of amoebae, but relatively little inflammatory cellular response, unless there is secondary infection. Deep to the muscularis mucosae, however, cells begin to accumulate as the muscle layer 'bulges' downwards and finally ruptures, liberating *E. histolytica* trophozoites into the submucosa in which they spread laterally, giving rise to the characteristic 'flask-shaped' lesions. On the surface of the gut the lesion presents as an ulcer with undermined edges and an irregular base made up of lysed debris; pus is present only when there is secondary infection. Trophozoites of *E. histolytica* are found in the tissues at the advancing boundaries of the lesions in which there is very little inflammatory vascular reaction and a limited round cell response. When secondarily infected, the margins are infiltrated with polymorphs and amoebae may be difficult to find.

In some cases the deeper layers of the gut wall may be invaded by the parasite which may induce a lytic and mildly cellular response in the muscle layers and connective tissues.

The granulomatous mass so produced in which secondary infection is common is known as an *amoeboma* and may reach considerable size and come to involve the surrounding tissues. Occasionally the invasion by *E. histolytica* extends right through the gut wall and causes perforation and leakage into the peritoneum, giving rise to amoebic peritonitis.

Extra-intestinal spread of amoebic infection, in addition to contiguous local developments such as described above, arises from embolic distribution of parasites in the blood and lymph vessels. This process is probably repeated frequently in the natural evolution of the disease, since it is usually easy to find vessels in the vicinity of an intestinal lesion containing active trophozoites of *E. histolytica* and the parasite may also be found in serial section in local lymph vessels and nodes in areas of the intestinal wall near the amoebic lesion. In most cases, however, it seems that the tissues in which the amoebae finally become held, are able to destroy them. Sometimes the parasites survive and multiply, invading the tissue and producing extra-intestinal lesions which are pathologically the same as those in the gut, the basic process being lysis of the tissue cells with minimal inflammatory response.

The commonest extra-intestinal lesions occur in the liver, eventually producing large abscesses containing the so-called 'anchovy sauce' pus, which consists of lysed necrotic liver tissue and which is normally bacteriologically sterile. The edges of the abscess consist of changed liver tissue infiltrated with *E. histolytica*, but without inflammatory cellular infiltration. Beyond is the normal liver tissue. Unless secondary infection has occurred there is no fibrotic reaction, but infected abscesses may eventually be walled off by a fibrous capsule. Healing takes place by regeneration of the hepatic tissue.

An amoebic liver abscess spreads without pressure signs in the liver tissue and may rupture eventually into the abdominal cavity or through the diaphragm into the pleural cavity where it may extend into the lungs. It may also penetrate into the pericardium. Further embolic spread may occur and in this way new lesions may be set up in any part of the body, including the lungs and the brain.

Contiguous tissues may become involved by direct extension where abscesses, for instance, have burst through the skin or where surgical wounds have been made. Amoebic infection of the skin occurs in this way. Again the basic lesion is lytic disintegration of the tissue cells, usually with the addition of the effects of secondary infection. *E. histolytica* trophozoites are usually found in great numbers in the discharge from such lesions, which may be very extensive.

The development of the amoebic liver abscess represents the final stage in a process which is still not understood. It is not clear why embolic lesions may develop in one case and not in another, or why in the same individual seeding of the liver with amoebae from the gut results at one time in the local destruction of the parasite and on another occasion in its survival and the initiation of an abscess. Sensitivity reactions may play a part in such acceptance of the parasite by the host tissues, or mechanical factors may be involved, such as the development of infarcts arising from portal venous obstruction by amoebic emboli. There are probably many intermediate stages between the embolic distribution of the parasite and the appearance of the abscess. Wide seeding of amoebae in the liver tissue may occur in the small portal venous radicals, with some local cellular response or even local abscess when severe intestinal lesions are induced in animals. Individual reactions of this sort resolve and do not normally go on to gross abscess formation. The process is sometimes regarded as amoebic hepatitis. Biopsy has never clearly revealed such lesions in man, but controversy still exists regarding the frequency with which such episodes may occur, and their relation to abscess formation.

Signs and Symptoms

Many individuals who become infected with pathogenic strains of *E. histolytica* never show clinical signs of the infection although the parasite may exist in the lumen contents for many years. In such persons the parasite either behaves as a commensal and does not invade the mucosal wall or gives rise to minimal localized invasion which produces no clinical effects. The commensal organism may remain permanently inactive or may suddenly penetrate the epithelial wall and set up lesions which eventually may lead to clinical effects.

In other individuals infection with the same parasite leads not only to survival of the organism in the gut but to immediate invasion with the production of lesions and clinical signs and symptoms.

The onset may be fairly clearly defined and appear within a week or two of a known infection, but it is usually more insidious. There may be some looseness of stools and mild diarrhoea which eventually subsides, but tends to recur at intervals (*amoebic colitis*). Some cases begin with looseness and pass on to *amoebic dysentery*, with the passage of six to ten blood-stained mucous motions in the day. There is usually no pain, colic or tenesmus as there is in bacillary dysentery and the patient may at first show few general reactions. There is seldom fever or toxaemia and the patient can usually continue with his work. The passage of loose stools continues for a few days or weeks and then ceases. Remission follows, usually of weeks or months, sometimes years, during which there may be occasional loose motions and periods of constipation. Eventually a new attack of loose diarrhoea or dysentery follows and is itself succeeded by another remission. The sequence of repeated attacks of dysentery interspersed with remissions is the common pattern of the disease, which may continue in this way for many years. Complications may develop at any stage.

More severe and sometimes fulminating and complicated cases of amoebic dysentery occur, especially in association with malnutrition, debilitation and concurrent infections. Severe cases are sometimes common in certain geographical areas, amongst particular racial groups. They are usually associated with extremely poor standards of living and nutrition, but may occasionally occur in otherwise apparently well nourished healthy people.

The complications of intestinal amoebiasis are essentially local, and include occasional erosion of large blood vessels, with severe haemorrhage or perforation of the gut with peritonitis. Peritonitis in acute dysentery may be generalized and indicated by increasing abdominal distension, hiccoughs and vomiting. Localized perforation with local peritonitis occurs in milder cases and especially a severe ulcerating colitis. Extension of infection in the gut wall and contiguous tissues to form an amoeboma is not uncommon. The firm inflammatory mass can be felt through the abdominal wall, usually in the region of the caecum or sigmoid colon, and has to be differentiated from carcinoma and other tumours. It is usually tender, particularly when examined *per rectum*, fixed, and may cause radiological signs of irregular constrictions of the gut lumen. It does not always respond well to specific treatment, probably because of the secondary infection which is almost invariably present. There may be several tumours of this sort along the wall of the large intestine.

The commonest and most important remote complication of intestinal amoebiasis is liver abscess.

The abscess usually shows itself during a remission and not often in an acute attack, but takes a long time to develop so that the timing of its presentation in relation to the intestinal infection may be fortuitous. There may be amoebic cysts in the stool, but in many cases these cannot be found and there may be no evidence of intestinal lesions.

There is often but not always a history of previous attacks of dysentery and remissions or of amoebic hepatitis. Liver abscess may appear in a person with no recognizable history of dysentery. It does not appear in the initial acute attack.

The majority of liver abscesses occur in the right lobe. They are usually large and single but occasionally there may be several small abscesses. The lesions arise from coalescence of embolic foci in which parasites have become caught in the smaller portal venous radicals and multiply with cellular reactions; the process is quickened by the development of infarcts.

The patient feels discomfort and fullness in the liver region, and later pain and tenderness, which become increasingly severe. The liver is enlarged, particularly in the affected lobe and there is restriction of movement in the corresponding region of the diaphragm and sometimes referred shoulder pain. This stage in which the abscess is growing may take some weeks and may be accompanied by irregular bouts of remittent fever and marked sweating. There is a moderate leucocytosis. There may be short remissions in which the local signs subside but as the abscess grows the signs and symptoms return and become worse. The patient may present looking desperately ill but often without feeling as prostrated as would be expected. The skin is sallow and moist with sweat; there is seldom jaundice. There is a high swinging remittent or intermittent fever and a leucocytosis of 15,000–20,000 cells per mm^3. Peaks of fever are common at night and may be followed by drenching sweats. The patient complains of severe local tenderness and pain, often referred to the right or left shoulder depending on the location of the abscess. The liver is palpable and tender, especially over the affected lobe. When the abscess is in the right lobe there is frequently bulging of the chest wall in the area, with widening of the intercostal spaces and intense localized tenderness over the lesion. The affected lobe is enlarged upwards as well as downwards so that radiologically the diaphragm is raised and irregular and may be fixed, or show practically no movement.

If the diagnosis is not made at this stage the abscess progresses to involve very considerable areas of the liver and may rupture through the abdominal wall or the diaphragm, into the peritoneal cavity or sometimes into the pericardium.

There are commonly signs of involvement of the lungs, in the right base in particular, and in cases in which there has been extension into the pleural cavity and lungs from the liver abscess, cough with expectoration of anchovy sauce pus containing amoebae. When the lesion has resulted from direct embolism of organisms and not from extension of a liver lesion, the sputum contains whitish pus in which the active trophozoites can be found.

Other extra-intestinal lesions produce localizing signs depending on their anatomical situation, and may or may not be accompanied by general reactions.

In an attack of intestinal amoebiasis, and sometimes in active recrudescences, the patient may complain of pain in the liver region and the liver is moderately enlarged and tender. In acute cases there is irregular remittent fever and profuse sweating. There is usually a moderate leucocytosis. In acute attacks associated with dysentery *E. histolytica* trophozoites are commonly found in the stools. In attacks occurring in remissions, there may or may not be cysts. The symptoms subside with treatment and abscess does not form. To some physicians this picture represents amoebic hepatitis: others hold that hepatitis as such does not occur. The issue has not yet been settled.

Diagnosis

Diagnosis of intestinal amoebiasis depends on identification of *E. histolytica* or its cysts in the stool or in swabbings or scrapings of the intestinal wall made during sigmoidoscopy or proctoscopy.

During acute dysenteric attacks the active amoeboid trophozoites are present in the loose mucus and bloody faeces, sometimes in great numbers, sometimes relatively scanty. Repeated examination of warm freshly passed stools should be carried out, since the number of organisms passed in an individual case varies very considerably from motion to motion and from day to day. Examination of stale cold stools is unsatisfactory, since the amoebae present will be dead and 'rounded up'. Faecal smears stained to show the nuclei of the parasites may be useful in these circumstances, but diagnosis should be made only on identifying the actively motile entamoeba containing ingested erythrocytes and protruding large clear pseudopodia. There is no accompanying cellular exudate, such as is seen in bacillary dysentery.

In remissions the formed stools will usually contain the cysts. Trophozoites are not found. Various methods of faecal concentration may help when cysts are scanty. It is also useful sometimes to give the patient a saline purge and to examine the result for cysts, and possibly at a later stage for amoebae.

E. histolytica must be differentiated from other amoebae which occur in human faeces, only one of which is known to cause pathological lesions in man, *Iodamoeba bütschlii.*

Some cases give no clinical history but pass cysts freely in the stools. These may be infected without invasion or have small lesions which do not present clinically. Others have a suggestive history of intermittent diarrhoea or dysentery and remission, but no parasites can be found. The latter present considerable difficulty for the physician. On theoretical grounds the diagnosis should not be made until parasitological evidence is available, but this attitude is often disregarded. No doubt in this way some genuine infections are included and possible extra-intestinal lesions may be prevented by treatment, but there must be many incorrect diagnoses made. So long as there are no serious psychological effects and so long as other possibilities, especially carcinoma, are excluded, this probably does not matter.

The diagnosis of amoebiasis finally depends on the demonstration of the trophozoite or the cyst, except in amoebic liver abscess where clinical diagnosis may be sufficient to warrant treatment. Certain immunological reactions may be helpful in deciding the diagnosis of syndromes such as amoeboma or post-dysenteric amoebic colitis in which the parasite may be extremely hard to find. The complement fixation test, using extracts of *E. histolytica* (in culture) as an antigen, the gel diffusion, latex agglutination haemagglutination and fluorescent antibody tests are being studied. These tests when positive indicate that tissue infection has occurred but since they remain positive for long periods, do not distinguish between present and past. The fluorescent antibody test is considered by some to be the most sensitive, and might well be the most useful in routine laboratories, using either serum or faecal smears and slide smears of cultures of *E. histolytica* as antigen.

The tests may be used to distinguish the commensal infection (the true carrier state) from one in which invasion has occurred without clinical signs (inapparent or symptomless amoebiasis).

The diagnosis of extra-intestinal amoebiasis depends on the location of the parasite and on the search for evidence of intestinal infections.

Some physicians claim that there is no such entity as hepatitis in amoebic infection, but this presupposes that once the *E. histolytica* becomes established in the liver tissue, abscess is inevitable. This may not always be the case. Severe signs referable to the liver occurring in a remission should be regarded as indicating an abscess, and the full-blown picture of swinging fever, leucocytosis, acute hepatic pain, bulging chest wall and local tenderness and the raised and fixed diaphragm should make the clinical diagnosis straight forward. In such cases failure to find cysts in the stool should not affect the specific treatment. Where there is reasonable certainty of liver abscess, removal of the contents by aspiration needle must be considered. Attempts at aspiration of the pus for diagnostic purposes are unjustified unless anti-amoebic therapy is begun immediately and facilities for therapeutic aspiration are at hand. Trophozoites of *E. histolytica* can be found in 80 per cent. of cases if the material is examined immediately after aspiration.

In pulmonary involvement, the diagnosis may sometimes be confirmed by finding the active amoeboid trophozoite in the sputum. Trophozoites may also be present in the pleural fluid or in the pericardial fluid in cases in which the liver abscess has extended in these regions.

TREATMENT

The basis of treatment is the destruction and elimination of *E. histolytica* in the intestine and in the tissues.

There are many drugs which will act directly or indirectly on the amoebae in the gut, some that will act on the parasites in the tissues and some which will do both.

Drugs chosen for treatment are determined by the type of amoebiasis. The effectiveness of a given drug depends on its limiting toxicity, its mode of action and the site of the infection.

Of the existing drugs, the one with the widest range of activity against both gut and tissue infection and the least toxicity is metronidazole (*Flagyl*).

Drugs with powerful activity on the parasite in the tissues are emetine, dehydroemetine and to a lesser degree chloroquine.

A wide variety of agents act directly on the amoebae in the gut. These include diloxanide furoate and di-iodohydroxyquinoline, and arsenical compounds or mixtures including *Milibis* and carbarsone.

The following details of treatment are recommended by the Durban authorities, who are commonly regarded as the most experienced.

Severe Amoebic Dysentery. Ulcerative Post-dysenteric Amoebic Colitis

(i) If the patient is able to take drugs orally, metronidazole, 800 mg. thrice daily for 5–10 days.

(ii) An alternative is the following combined treatment, which may be preferable in extremely severe cases in which early oral treatment is difficult.

Emetine, 1 mg. per kg. body weight, maximum daily dose of 65 mg. usually given in 2 doses, 8 hours apart, intramuscularly. Alternatively dehydroemetine, 90 mg. daily intramuscularly. Both drugs are given for 10 consecutive days.

Emetine and dehydroemetine have certain toxic effects (less pronounced in the latter) and are contra-indicated in patients with cardiac lesions. The patient should be immobilized during treatment and the effect on the heart monitored by repeated ECG. If signs of cardiac involvement develop the drugs must be stopped.

Tetracycline, 500 mg. six-hourly. Begin intravenously and switch to same dosage orally. Given concurrently with the emetine.

Diloxanide furoate, 500 mg. thrice daily for 10 days orally.

Note: Dehydration can often be dealt with orally and will help control diarrhoea. Severe dehydration must be adjusted by intravenous infusion of isotonic saline, as required.

Moderate Dysentery. Amoebic Colitis

(i) Metronidazole as above.

(ii) Emetine or dehydroemetine for 3–5 days as above, with tetracycline and diloxanide as above:

or tetracycline (oxytetracycline or chlortetracycline), 250 mg. six-hourly for 10 days, with diloxanide furoate, 500 mg. thrice daily for 10 days. Chloroquine, 600 mg. at once, 300 mg. after 6–8 hours, then 300 mg. twice daily for 10 days. (The chloroquine is given to minimize the development of liver complications.)

Complications of Intestinal Amoebiasis

Peritonitis developing in acute severe dysentery is treated with gastric suction and parenteral replacement of fluid and electrolytes. Haemorrhage with falling blood haemoglobin may need immediate transfusion. In the rare event of intussusception surgical action may be necessary.

No surgical procedures should be undertaken until anti-amoebic treatment has commenced.

Infection with no Apparent Clinical Signs

Individuals infected in Europe and passing cysts do not require treatment.

People infected in the tropics or in whom there is a clear history of previous clinical incidents should be treated, especially if serological tests are positive, indicating that invasion has taken place.

Food handlers passing cysts should also be treated where practicable, bearing in mind the likelihood of reinfection in highly endemic areas.

A wide choice of drugs is available for those without previous history. For example:

Metronidazole, 400–800 mg. thrice daily for 5 days.

Diloxanide furoate, 500 mg. thrice daily for 10 days.

Di-iodohydroxyquinoline, 600 mg. thrice daily for 21 days.

Tetracycline, 250 mg. six-hourly for 7 days.

Where there is a previous history, amoebic colitis may be taken to exist. Treat as for moderate amoebic dysentery (above).

Other Drugs

Antibiotics with direct action on amoebae are sometimes used in moderately severe cases of amoebic colitis or for clearing infections in inapparent amoebiasis:

Paromomycin, 500 mg. six-hourly orally for 7 days.

Fumagillin, 20 mg. thrice daily for 10 days.

Aminosidine sulphate, 1 G. daily intramuscularly for 5 days (also successful in dysentery and extra-intestinal lesions).

Niridazole, is an extremely powerful amoebicide and has been used in amoebic dysentery and amoebic liver abscess in doses of 25 mg. per kg. body weight daily for 7–10 days. There is general agreement, however, that the side-effects are too severe for general use.

Arsenicals are successful in clearing moderate dysentery and colitis but the relapse rate is high if they are used alone. They are often used in combination with other drugs. Carbarsone in doses of 250 mg. twice daily orally for 10 days is still used extensively in areas where the cost of other treatment is uneconomic. *Milibis*, a pentavalent arsenical containing bismuth is sometimes used successfully in chronic amoebic colitis in doses of 250 mg. thrice daily for 7 days. Again, relapse rate is high.

Extra-intestinal Infections

Acute extra-intestinal amoebiasis will usually respond to metronidazole in the doses quoted above, for 5–10 days. Emetine and dehydroemetine are also successful and preferred by some physicians; they are given in the usual doses and with the usual precautions for 10 days. Aminosidine (see above) has also been used.

Once the extra-intestinal infection has been controlled, possible residual infection in the intestine is treated with metronidazole (if necessary, as the original treatment may have cleared the intestinal amoebiasis) or with a combination of tetracycline, diloxanide and chloroquine (as detailed above).

Amoebic Liver Abscess

Small abscesses may regress with drug regimens only and without aspiration. Well advanced abscesses require aspiration, which should be performed with a wide-bore needle attached to a syringe. Aspiration is indicated where there is a palpable mass and persistent local tenderness, where the diaphragm is raised and fixed or when there is no response to drug treatment.

The patient is given morphine or pethidine, the local skin is infiltrated with local anaesthetic and the needle inserted with full aseptic precautions. The pus withdrawn is examined immediately; amoebae are usually present but will not be easily identifiable if the pus is allowed to stand for more than an hour before examination. As much pus as possible is removed by gentle suction. Syringe aspiration may be repeated daily if large quantities of pus are present. It is seldom necessary to use continuous drainage and surgical interference should be avoided except in cases where no pus can be found by needle in a patient with persistent signs and no response to drugs.

Anti-amoebic therapy should be instituted immediately the diagnosis has been made and confirmed. Metronidazole alone, in the usual doses, is often all that is needed. Alternatively emetine or dehydroemetine may be given for 10 days. Chloroquine is usually given in addition in doses of 600 mg. (base) immediately followed in 8 hours by 300 mg. daily for 12–28 days.

For the residual intestinal infection give diloxanide furoate, 500 mg. thrice daily for 10 days; if dysenteric signs are present, add tetracycline in the usual doses.

Amoebic liver abscess usually responds rapidly to treatment with regression of symptoms and general improvement which is maintained. The abscess cavity shrinks rapidly and is ultimately replaced by regenerated liver tissue without scarring.

Test of Cure

In intestinal infections relapses or recrudescences may occur weeks or months after treatment.

As a routine consecutive stools should be examined for several days for cysts not earlier than 1 month after the completion of treatment. Ideally, this examination should be repeated at 3-monthly intervals for a year. The latter is seldom possible especially in individuals treated as outpatients, and the result of the examination after a month have commonly to be accepted.

In the follow-up of severe dysenteric cases or cases of ulcerative amoebic colitis, cure is measured in terms of absence of infection and the retreat of rectal ulceration.

The progress of a liver abscess may be followed by injection of X-ray opaque iodide solution into the abscess cavity but this is seldom necessary. Radioactive scanning has also been employed for this purpose and for diagnosis of lesions not identified by aspiration.

REFERENCES

Elsdon-Dew, R. (1969) Amoebiasis: Its meaning and diagnosis, *S. Afr. med. J.*, **43**, 483.

Powell, S. J., MacLeod, I., Wilmot, A. J., and Elsdon-Dew, R. (1966) Metronidazole in amoebic dysentery and amoebic liver abscess, *Lancet*, ii, 1329.

Stamm, W. P. (1970) Amoebic aphorisms, *Lancet*, ii, 1355.

World Health Organization (1969) Expert Committee on Amoebiasis, *Tech. Rep. Ser.*, No. 421.

COCCIDIOSIS

The intracellular sporozoa *Isopora hominis* and *I. belli*, which some authorities consider is identical to and others separate from *I. hominis* sometimes occur in man. (See also Toxoplasmosis.)

The sporocysts or oocysts which are passed in the faeces (and have been observed in duodenal aspirates) are the only forms of the parasite so far observed in human infections. It is believed that the full cycle resembles that of *Isospora felis* which infects cats. The parasite is thus presumed to invade and develop in the epithelium of the small intestine. The mature oocyst contains four sporozoites which are probably liberated in the intestinal lumen and penetrate the epithelial cells. Schizogony (and eventually sporogony) take place therein and merozoites penetrate other contiguous cells. In this way shallow lesions are found which heal easily but may initiate the diarrhoea which is the major clinical feature.

The infection is commoner in warm environments including parts of India, the Middle East, South-East Asia and the South Pacific than in temperate. It follows ingestion of food or drink contaminated with ripe oocysts (i.e. containing sporozoites). Clinical signs may appear in about a month. The patient develops diarrhoea which is usually mild although the stool may contain blood, pus cells and mucus. There may be intestinal colic. Eosinophilia is usual. The episode usually lasts about a week. Oocysts which are elongated and tapering, 20–30 μ in length, contain within the clear thin wall the segmenting sporoblast or the four fully developed sporozoites. They appear in the faeces a day or two after the onset and may persist. They are sometimes accompanied by Charcot-Leyden crystals. They may be found in the faeces of apparently healthy individuals. Cysts of *Eimeria* sp. have also been found in human faeces. The clinical picture is self limited. There is no specific treatment.

BALANTIDIASIS

Aetiology

Balantidiasis, balantidiosis or ciliate dysentery, is a form of dysentery resulting from infection with a large ciliate protozoan parasite *Balantidium coli.* The condition is widely distributed but not very common.

The parasite occurs as a trophozoite, an active oval ciliate organism up to 200 μ in length and 80 μ in width, or as cysts, which are smaller and rounded. *Bal. coli* is a parasite of pigs and occasionally other animals, including the monkey and guinea-pig. Man acquires the disease from the pig by swallowing cysts passed in formed stools.

Bal. coli may act as a commensal in man, living in the lumen of the large intestine. It may at times invade the mucosa and submucosa of the gut, leaving irregularly circular surface ulcers, with undermined edges and necrotic base. The lesions closely resemble those of amoebiasis.

The infection may remain entirely asymptomatic and is discovered by finding the parasite in the stools. In most cases there is an insidious onset with loose stools, followed by frank dysentery with bloody mucoid stools resembling those of acute severe amoebiasis. The course becomes chronic with remissions and exacerbations. Extra-intestinal lesions, such as liver abscess do not occur. Death may result in untreated acute cases.

Diagnosis

Diagnosis in the acute phase is made by discovering trophozoites in the stools or sigmoidoscope scrapings and in the quiescent stage by finding the cysts.

Treatment

Oxytetracycline and chlortetracycline have proved the most effective therapeutic agents, in doses of 500 mg. thrice daily for 10 days. Alternatively, arsenical drugs such as acetarsol (*Stovarsol*) may be given orally, 250 mg. thrice daily for a week.

GIARDIASIS

Aetiology

Giardiasis or flagellate diarrhoea results from infection with the flagellate *Giardia lamblia*, a pear-shaped organism 10–18 μ long and possessing a ventral sucker.

Infection follows swallowing the cysts which are passed in the stool. In a given infection cysts may continue to be passed at irregular intervals over many years. The trophozoite inhabits the jejunum and duodenum. It may reach the bile-ducts.

In light infections there are usually no clinical results, but in heavy infections, the large numbers of organisms sticking to the mucosa with suckers cause diarrhoea and discomfort, with the passage of yellowish greasy stools in which there may be excess fat. A common picture is one of insidious onset of persistent looseness and mild steatorrhoea, the latter presumably due to malabsorption from the mucosa covered with parasites which may be present in large numbers in the stool.

There may be demonstrable malabsorption of fat, vitamin A and xylose.

Treatment

Mepacrine given in the form of tablets of hydrochloride is effective in doses of 100 mg. thrice daily for 5–7 days. Relapses may occur.

Chloroquine is also active, in doses of 300 mg. base once daily for 5 days.

Metronidazole is very successful in doses of 400 mg. thrice daily for 5 days.

BRIAN MAEGRAITH

TRICHOMONIASIS

Definition

An infective disorder of the genital tract due to *Trichomonas vaginalis*, and usually transmitted by sexual intercourse.

Aetiology

T. vaginalis is oval or pear-shaped, measuring 15–25 μ in its long axis and provided with four flagella and an undulating membrane which give it a characteristic jerky motility in fresh secretions.

T. vaginalis can usually be identified by direct microscopic examination of freshly obtained secretion in a wet film or hanging drop preparation. It grows well on various media and a combination of smear examination and culture provides the most effective diagnostic method.

Trichomoniasis in Males

This usually presents as low-grade, non-gonococcal urethritis, commoner in coloured than in white patients. The incubation period is from 1 to 3 weeks. The diagnosis is made by finding the organism in smear, or culture. In some cases, however, there are no symptoms and the signs may be slight. but 'comma like' threads may be seen in the first urine specimen. As far as the evidence goes it seems that about 15 per cent.

of all cases of non-gonococcal urethritis in males are due to this cause. The organism has also been found in the preputial sac, in prostatic secretion, seminal fluid and urine. In some cases the condition may be self-limiting in men, and in general the longer the infestation has been present the more difficult it is to identify the organism. However, the organism tends to persist in patients having pre-existing urethral stricture or stenosis of the external urinary meatus. Complications are not known to occur.

Trichomoniasis in Females

Infestations in females are commonest during the years of greatest sexual activity but also occur after the menopause and occasionally seen in female infants shortly after birth. Transmission usually occurs during sexual intercourse but may occasionally result from accidental contamination from a lavatory, from towels or clothing or from improperly sterilized gloves and instruments used for examination. Infestation may occur with an intact hymen when transmission has taken place by close genital contact without penetration. In other patients there has been no recent sexual contact and the condition has been long-standing when the diagnosis is made. Trichomoniasis is frequently associated with other sexually transmitted infections in women: approximately 50 per cent. of women with gonorrhoea have been found to have trichomoniasis in addition.

The incubation period, as in the male, is from 1 to 3 weeks. In many cases the patient complains of vaginal discharge which is thin, yellow and offensive. If it is profuse it may cause vulvitis and intertrigo. The patient may complain of dyspareunia and the passing of a vaginal speculum may be painful. Sometimes, however, symptoms are minimal or absent. In typical cases the vaginal wall is reddened and the vaginal secretion is thin, yellow, offensive and perhaps frothy. There may be red, punctate spots on the vaginal surface of the cervix, the so-called 'strawberry cervix'. The pH of the vaginal secretion varies from 6 to 8, as compared with the normal reading of 4 to 5. Infection of the lower urinary tract due to the same cause is present in at least a quarter of the cases. This may cause dysuria and frequency. Skenitis and Bartholinitis are occasionally associated. Endocervicitis is probably due to associated non-gonococcal infection and it is controversial whether *T. vaginalis* ever penetrates into the upper genital tract.

Diagnosis

Diagnosis depends on finding the organism in smear or culture or both. It is essential to exclude gonorrhoea and other venereal infections which may be present coincidentally. Non-gonococcal genital infection is also frequently present in addition but may only be evident after the trichomoniasis has been successfully treated. Vaginal thrush due to *Candida albicans* is often associated. *T. vaginalis* has not been found in the mouth, conjunctival sac or rectum of either sex.

Treatment

The treatment of choice is metronidazole (*Flagyl*) by mouth. Dosage may be 200 mg. three times daily after meals for 7 days but 400 mg. twice daily for 5 days is equally effective. The toxic effects have been slight but occasionally the drug causes slight gastric and intestinal irritation or a skin rash. There has been no evidence of damage to the foetus *in utero* but as a precaution the manufacturers have advised that it should not be given till after the third month of pregnancy. One course of treatment is likely to be effective in over 80 per cent. of cases. Some of the remainder who do not absorb the drug well will respond to a second course at double the routine daily dosage; others appear to harbour bacteria in the vagina capable of breaking down metronidazole and may need additional local treatment. The possibility of re-infection by further sexual intercourse should always be considered, however, in treatment failures. Sexual partners should therefore be examined and treated as indicated. If for any reason metronidazole by mouth is contra-indicated, local treatment will have to be given with vaginal pessaries of a mercurial or pentavalent arsenical preparation (*Penotrane*, SVC). The patient should insert one or two pessaries at night for 2 weeks. Treatment usually gives effective symptomatic relief but recurrence is commonly due to spread from other sites of involvement in the genito-urinary tract. Cases of skin sensitivity reactions to the arsenical preparation have been reported.

Alcohol should be avoided during treatment.

REFERENCES

Dunlop, E. M. C., and Wisdom, A. R. (1963) *Brit. J. vener. Dis.*, **41**, 85.

King, A. J., and Nicol, C. S. (1969) *Venereal Diseases*, 2nd ed., London.

Trussell, R. E. (1947) *Trichomonas Vaginalis and Trichomoniasis*, Springfield, Ill.

Claude Nicol

TOXOPLASMOSIS

Definition

A disease of man and animals, of world-wide distribution, caused by a small protozoon, *Toxoplasma gondii*, which may be transmitted to the foetus *in utero* by an infected mother or acquired by some means as yet unknown in childhood or in adult life. The majority of acquired infections probably pass unnoticed but the parasite may give rise to a wide variety of symptoms and signs of differing severity and variable duration. Depending partly upon the age of the person when infected, they tend to be so grouped that four main clinical types of illness may be recognized.

1. *CONGENITAL:*

This form is characterized by encephalomyelitis, cerebral calcification, hydrocephalus and choroidoretinitis; with symptoms either apparent at birth, or appearing soon afterwards.

2. *ACQUIRED:*

(i) *Cerebrospinal:* most frequent in children in whom the most typical manifestations are those of an acute meningo-encephalitis.

(ii) *Lymphatic:* characterized by the enlargement of one of more groups of lymph nodes, with at times fever of several weeks' duration and marked constitutional disturbance.

(iii) *Exanthematous:* the form most frequently found in adults, presenting as an acute febrile illness with a widespread maculopapular rash, a diffuse interstitial pneumonitis, myocarditis and at times meningo-encephalitis.

(iv) *Latent:* where infection by *T. gondii* gives rise to no symptoms or signs of the disease, and diagnosis can only be made by means of laboratory tests. Latent infections are found only in adults, and are probably always acquired after the age of childhood.

Aetiology

The causal organism was first discovered in 1908, in a small North African rodent, the gondi (*Ctenodactylus gundi*), and it was named *Toxoplasma gondii* (Nicolle and Manceaux). It is a protozoan which has very recently (1970) been shown to be a coccidian parasite closely related to *Isospora*. It is probable that infection may be normally acquired by ingestion of oocysts passed in the faeces of infected animals, including the cat. The parasite invades the superficial epithelial cells of the intestinal wall where it undergoes schizogony and eventually sporogony, with development of oocysts which are passed in the faeces and infect further hosts after ingestion. Experimentally, toxoplasmosis may be transmitted to mice and other suitable animals by ingestion of infected brain tissue containing cysts.

T. gondii is an intracellular parasite found usually in the endothelial cells, the mononuclear leucocytes or the tissue cells. Free living forms may also be found in the tissue fluids of the host. In this free extracellular form, the parasite is a slender crescent-shaped organism, with one end rounded and the other pointed, measuring from 4 μ to 6 μ in length, its breadth being around 2 μ. Intracellular forms often lose the crescent shape, becoming pear-shaped, oval or rounded when they may readily be confused with *Leishmania*. In dry films stained by Wright's or Giemsa's methods, the cytoplasm is blue, the granular nucleus, which is single and fills about one-quarter of the cell, stains a reddish-purple and will be seen near the rounded extremity, whilst towards the pointed end there is a small deeply staining red granule, the paranuclear body. The parasite multiplies by longitudinal fission within the endothelial and tissue cells of its host. With virulent strains these cells rupture early, releasing the parasites which then invade fresh cells, thus enabling the parasite to multiply extremely rapidly; though, in the light of present knowledge, with doubtful benefit to itself, since it may result in an overwhelming and rapidly fatal infection of its host. With less virulent strains the cells often remain intact, allowing reproduction to continue until they become greatly distended by 80 or more parasites; their nuclei are then extruded, and the hypertrophied, cyst-like structures that remain, packed with parasites, are known as pseudocysts. Within them the parasites seem to be in a resting or inactive stage, causing little tissue damage or cellular reaction, the cyst wall probably affording protection from any circulating antibodies, thereby enabling a chronic infection to become established.

T. gondii can be cultivated in the laboratory if living tissue cells are used. It propagates most readily on the chorio-allantoic membrane of the developing chick embryo at 95°–99° F. (35°–37° C.) if protected from bacterial contamination and dehydration. The embryo usually dies between the seventh and tenth days.

Epidemiology

Toxoplasma gondii has been found in many species of mammals and birds, and also in certain reptiles. The first authenticated report of human infection was made in 1923, since when human infections have been recorded in many European countries, including Great Britain; in the Middle East; Ceylon; North, Central and South America; Australia and Hawaii. Infection has recently been recorded in some areas of Japan and in West Africa. The incidence of toxoplasmosis in man is not known yet, but subclinical infections are probably much more frequent than it is generally realized. Recent surveys using serological tests have shown that positive reactions, suggesting a past infection, may be given by 10–50 per cent. of the adult population in many areas. Such figures should, however, be treated with caution, since doubt has been cast on the validity of some of the tests used, it having been found that they are not specific for *T. gondii*.

Although little is known as yet about the transmission of the parasite to humans it is probable that many patients have been infected by swallowing oocysts discharged in the faeces of infected reservoir animals. Rodents, cats and dogs in particular are thought to be a possible source of infection. Recent evidence from Japan indicates that toxoplasmosis in swine may be an important source of human infection. Cattle, sheep and goats are also frequently infected with *Toxoplasma*.

Neonatal infections appear to be conveyed transplacentally to the foetus from an infected mother, who almost invariably remains free from any symptoms of the disease herself. If the infection is acquired early in pregnancy by the mother, abortion will probably result, or if the pregnancy continues the foetus will be so extensively damaged that it will be stillborn. Infection late in pregnancy may result in the infant being free from any signs of the disease at birth, and several weeks or even 2 or 3 months may elapse before signs and symptoms appear. Later offspring from such mothers, with one possible exception, have never yet been born with toxoplasmosis. It seems probable that if the mother became infected during the puerperium the disease could be transmitted to the infant if it was breast-fed, as lactating laboratory mice have conveyed the parasite to their offspring in the milk.

Laboratory workers handling *Toxoplasma* have several times acquired very severe or fatal infections, though by what means remains unknown.

Of the many prevailing surmises on the mode of entry of the parasite into the human body, the majority of those who have studied the disease consider there are at least three possible routes:

1. The commonest via the gastro-intestinal tract,

following the ingestion of infected food presumably containing oocysts from the faeces of reservoir animals.

2. The respiratory tract, by inhalation of droplets containing cysts of the parasite.

3. Contact with infected tissue.

It is not yet known whether the vegetative forms of *Toxoplasma* are as vulnerable to human gastric juice as they are to that of experimental animals; nor is it known how resistant the pseudocysts are to storage, desiccation, cold or heat. Since they occur quite frequently in the muscles of animals used as food, the eating of raw or insufficiently cooked meat would seem a likely source of infection. The pseudocysts have also been found in the ovaries of hens; it is therefore possible that eggs could convey the infection. Recently toxoplasmosis has been recognized in cattle and the disease has been transmitted to calves, both congenitally and in the milk. In some rural areas in Great Britain unpasteurized milk is still the only form available, and this could well provide another source of infection should the disease become common in cattle.

It has already been mentioned that *Toxoplasma* are present in the bronchioles and probably in the sputum of human cases of toxoplasmosis with pneumonitis, and this is true of domestic animals with clinical evidence of the disease. Moreover, respiratory symptoms are a much more prominent feature of the disease in most animals than they are in man, and thus those looking after such sick animals might well become infected by the inhalation of infected droplets, and also possibly through the conjunctiva, since animals have been infected by this route.

Infection via the skin is also possible through the handling of infected tissues as it is known that *Toxoplasma* can penetrate closely shaved skin and it is therefore not improbable that some human infections may be caused by the parasite entering through cracks and small abrasions in the skin. This would certainly explain the increased proportion of positive serological reactions that has already been observed, in veterinary surgeons, slaughterhouse workers and in particular in those handling rabbits.

Komiya and colleagues in Japan have recently demonstrated both vegetative and cyst forms of *Toxoplasma* in the diaphragmatic muscle of pigs, and a corresponding high presumptive infection rate (dye test and toxoplasmin skin reaction) in swine slaughterers. They consider that infection is acquired from cysts conveyed by hand to mouth and also by direct invasion of vegetative forms through small abrasions and other lesions on the skin.

Pathology

The lesions in the intestinal epithelium are very superficial and may show no reaction beyond immediate damage to the invaded cells. In the artificially infected cat they appear most frequently in the ileum, in the epithelium of the lower third of the villi and to a lesser degree in the macrophages of the intestinal tissue. In the infected cells Zaman and Colley (1970) have recently described endogenous parasites including mature schizonts, merozoites, microgametocytes and microgametes.

Following infection of the gut or after feeding with infected brain tissue, some parasites may be distributed throughout the body by the blood stream and become established in the cells of the reticulo-endothelial system, and also in the parenchymal cells. Localization occurs in many organs, more often in the brain, lung, liver or spleen, parasites often being found also in the kidney, suprarenal glands, bone marrow and lymph nodes. Muscle fibres are also invaded, in particular those of the heart, as well as the skeletal muscles. They may also be found within phagocytic cells and living free in the intracellular fluids of the affected organs.

The typical lesions are small focal areas of necrosis surrounded by a zone of inflammation containing lymphocytes, mononuclear and plasma cells. Hypertrophied cells distended with parasites, the so-called pseudocysts, are often seen. Serous exudates are commonly found in the various body cavities.

In congenital cases lesions predominate in the brain, spinal cord, retina and choroid. Inflammation often extends to the ependyma, causing ventricular block and hydrocephalus. As well as the typical necrotic foci, minute granulomata are also found in the brain, which calcify if the affected infant survives long enough. The lesions in the central nervous system are not very marked, and often sections must be searched with the greatest diligence before they are seen.

In the acquired adult infections, which usually pass unnoticed, the lesions are often found accidentally. Rarely there is a widespread dissemination of the parasite with lesions throughout the body, though more often the predominant feature is an interstitial pneumonitis with thickening of the alveolar walls and infiltrations of giant and plasma cells. There may also be scattered areas of purulent bronchiolitis. Inflammatory and necrotic areas are also quite frequently found in the liver, spleen and heart muscle, and encephalitis has occurred in several adult cases, though it is seldom as predominant a feature as in congenital infections, or in the acquired infections of children.

CLINICAL FEATURES

As knowledge of toxoplasmosis increases, and as more clinical reports become available, so does it appear that the sharply demarcated clinical syndromes that were described in the earlier accounts of the disease are not clear entities, apart from the fairly clear-cut distinction between congenital and acquired infections.

Whilst it is still true that there is a preponderance of certain clinical features in children, and others which appear with greater frequency in adults, the clinical manifestations of acquired toxoplasmosis seem to be no longer sufficiently exclusive to one or other age group to justify the old subdivision into the acquired infection of childhood and the acquired infection of the adult.

Congenital Toxoplasmosis

Acute infections with widespread dissemination of the parasites and necrotic lesions in many organs, in particular the lungs, the heart, liver, spleen, kidney, suprarenal glands and lymph nodes have been described, but occur very infrequently in congenital toxoplasmosis. Subacute infection is the common form, with predominating neurological symptoms which may be noted at birth or shortly afterwards. If the foetus is infected very early in pregnancy, the disease will reach an advanced stage *in utero*, and cases have been recorded where the pregnancy having continued to term was followed by an obstructed labour owing to the development of hydrocephalus in the foetus.

In the typical subacute congenital infection, the symptoms and signs may be subdivided into:

1. Those due to the presence of parasites within the body; these may be called primary symptoms and signs.
2. Those secondary to the principal lesions caused by the parasite, namely encephalomyelitis and choroidoretinitis. The common primary signs are fever, with a fluctuating temperature which may at times be subnormal; jaundice, which has been described in about one-third of all congenital cases; purpura, which occurs infrequently, and a maculopapular rash, which is extremely rare. Anaemia and leucocytosis, with an absolute increase in monocytes and lymphocytes, are found in about one half of all cases, and the liver and spleen are not infrequently enlarged.

The signs secondary to encephalomyelitis most frequently found are muscular twitchings and convulsions; stiffness of the neck, paraplegia, respiratory weakness and cyanosis, which at times may be due to an interstitial pneumonitis; vomiting and diarrhoea. Hydrocephalus develops in the majority of infected infants and rapid enlargement of the head may occur. At times when there is early and extensive cerebral damage microcephaly may be found. The cerebral lesions become calcified if the infant survives long enough and may later give rise to Jacksonian convulsions, and the majority of infants who survive for a number of years are mentally deficient.

The ocular findings most frequently include microphthalmia, the small eyes being in striking contrast to the enlarged head; nystagmus, which may result either from poor fixation due to choroidoretinitis or from the lesions in the central nervous system; vitreous opacities and choroidoretinitis. The lesions are nearly always bilateral and cause blindness or very severe impairment of vision in those infants who survive. The majority of infants, however, die within the first few weeks of life.

Acquired Toxoplasmosis

Cerebrospinal. In the earlier accounts of toxoplasmosis this form of the disease was usually considered to be not only the invariable manifestation of infection in children, but also confined solely to them. Meningoencephalitis has, in recent years, been reported many times in adults with the disease, but it is seldom the initial feature of the attack, usually occurring as a complication of the exanthematous form towards the end of the first or second week of the illness, not infrequently after the acute stage has subsided and recovery appears to have commenced.

The cerebrospinal form is probably still found more frequently in children, in whom it tends to be the predominant feature of the illness. The onset is marked by fever, very severe headache, vomiting and delirium. Convulsions often occur a day or two later and the picture presented may suggest a brain tumour. Deafness is often found, and very occasionally choroidoretinitis has been recorded, but it is not a constant feature as in the congenital infections. The attacks are frequently severe and often rapidly fatal, with death following within a few days of the onset. Some infections run a more chronic course, but not necessarily with a more favourable outcome, since death may occur several weeks after the commencement of the illness. Complete recovery is, however, by no means uncommon, without the development of any sequelae, even when the attack has been exceedingly severe.

Lymphatic. Some of the earlier accounts of toxoplasmosis mentioned that a generalized enlargement of lymph nodes was occasionally observed, but it is only in recent years that the lymphatic form has been recognized as a clinical type that occurs without any of the other manifestations of the disease. It has been stated quite recently that probably the commonest manifestation of acquired toxoplasmosis in man yet known is a lymphadenitis resembling glandular fever. The total number of cases of this form of infection reported to date does not yet seem large enough to confirm the above statement. Although the lymphatic form is not usually described as occurring predominantly in children, nearly all the recorded cases have been found between the ages of 5 and 15 years.

As with most infectious illnesses, there is a fairly wide range in the severity of the attack and there seems to be no practical advantage in adopting the classification which divides this form into three main clinical groups since they do not appear to differ except in severity.

A proportion of these cases have a sudden febrile onset, often with a rigor, and fatigue is a common premonitory symptom which precedes the onset by several days. The fever usually rises rapidly to about 104° F. (40° C.) and is frequently accompanied by catarrhal symptoms, cough, headache and pain in the back. At times the throat is sore and there may be abdominal discomfort and diarrhoea. These symptoms and the fever nearly always precede the glandular enlargement and it may be a week or more before the enlarged glands are first observed. The fever usually lasts for 2–3 weeks but occasionally may be present a few days only. At times, in adult infections, the fever may continue for 6–7 weeks, with a high initial temperature of about 105° F. (40·5° C.) slowly subsiding to about 102° F. (38·9° C.) some ten days after the onset, subsequently it may fluctuate between 100° F. (37·8° C.) and 101° F. (38·3° C.) for 2–3 weeks before slowly returning to normal. Although there are no complications, and recovery invariably follows, the febrile cases often require a prolonged convalescence, fatigue being a very prominent feature for 3 or 4 months following an attack.

A large number of cases are afebrile and free from any symptoms apart from, at times, some initial tenderness in the region of the enlarged glands; the general health remains unaffected by the infection. Others remain unaware even of the enlarged glands which are found during some routine examination.

The characteristic feature of this form of toxoplasmosis whatever degree of severity it may assume, is enlargement of one or more groups of lymph nodes. Those most frequently affected are the cervical, suboccipital, axillary and inguinal groups. A radiograph of the chest may also reveal enlargement of the hilar glands. Enlargement of the cervical glands is fairly constant and they are nearly always the first glands to become affected, other groups becoming enlarged after an interval of several days or even 1–2 weeks. The glands are usually firm, discrete and vary in size from that of a hazel-nut to that of a walnut. They are usually painless, though there may be some initial tenderness during the first week or two of the illness. There is no inflammation of the skin overlying the glands and suppuration does not occur.

Another very characteristic feature of all cases whether febrile or afebrile is the persistence of the glandular enlargement; enlarged lymph nodes usually can be found 6–9 months after the onset of the attack.

Exanthematous. Although many clinical forms have been described in adults, the most typical is an acute febrile illness of sudden onset, sometimes marked by rigors, soon followed by the appearance of a generalized maculopapular rash which is absent from the palms of the hands and the soles of the feet, and which closely resembles the rash of typhus or Rocky Mountain spotted fever. There may be a disseminated myositis giving rise to severe aching pain in the muscles, or at times to myocarditis when the heart muscle is involved. The outstanding feature, however, is a diffuse, interstitial pneumonitis resembling an atypical virus pneumonia, which frequently runs a rapid course with severe dyspnoea, cyanosis and respiratory failure. Enlargement of the liver and spleen will be found in a few cases and encephalitis has been a feature of several acute cases in adults.

DIAGNOSIS

Clinical Diagnosis

Even presumptive evidence of *Toxoplasma* infection is rarely obtainable on clinical findings alone, except in infants. A combination of convulsions, hydrocephalus or microcephaly, choroidoretinitis and calcified areas in the brain, seen in a radiograph, strongly suggests toxoplasmosis when found in infancy, and in older children a similar picture, together with blindness or serious impairment of vision and mental deficiency makes a similar diagnosis equally probable. In adults clinical diagnosis is extremely difficult and it is more likely to be considered under the differential diagnosis of an unidentified infection than as a probable diagnosis by itself.

Laboratory Findings

The usual routine laboratory investigations give little help in toxoplasmosis.

Blood. Anaemia of moderate degree is usual, particularly in infants, though the haemoglobin is seldom less than 12·3 g. per 100 ml. or the red cell count below 4 million. The leucocytes are usually slightly increased in numbers, from 9000 to 12,000 being a common finding with a considerable increase in lymphocytes and monocytes in many cases, the increase in monocytes being of lesser degree but much more constant. In several proved cases eosinophils have been raised, reaching 14–20 per cent. of the differential count.

Cerebrospinal Fluid. This is often xanthochromic in cases with encephalomyelitis. Protein: usually considerably increased, the increase being relatively greater than that of the cells. Sugar: normal in amount or slightly decreased. Cells: leucocytes are often present in large numbers, with a very considerable range, an average or usual figure being around 500 per mm^3., though counts of 60 and 1600 are often recorded; erythrocytes are usually present but in lesser numbers.

Definitive Diagnosis

The definitive diagnosis of toxoplasmosis by the direct isolation of *T. gondii* from the patient is frequently not possible and therefore indirect methods are also employed, and provided that a full range of investigations is carried out, with consistent findings, a diagnosis of toxoplasmosis may still be established with reasonable certainty.

Morphological Identification of Toxoplasma. During the acute stage of the infection the parasite may sometimes be found in stained smears of bone marrow, in material obtained by splenic puncture or in the centrifuged deposits of exudates, cerebrospinal and ventricular fluids. Fresh cover-slip preparations should also be examined. Smears should likewise be made from a portion of any tissues removed at biopsy or autopsy, and these should be stained with Giemsa; the other portions should be fixed, and thin sections made, which should be stained with haematoxylin and eosin, and then very carefully examined with an oil immersion lens. The parasites in the pseudocyst form are those most easily recognized after a little experience.

Biological Identification of Toxoplasma. Material obtained from a suspected case of toxoplasmosis should be inoculated into laboratory animals, which must be free from naturally occurring infection in themselves. Mice, hamsters and guinea-pigs are the most satisfactory animals, and at least six mice and two guinea-pigs must be used before any reliance can be placed on the test. Similar material to that used for making stained smears should be injected intracerebrally into the mice and intraperitoneally into the guinea-pigs. The animals should be watched for signs of illness; if after a month all have remained well, passage to another group of animals should be undertaken by the inoculation of tissues from one half of the first group. Where illness develops, exudates should be carefully examined, and if *Toxoplasma* are not found, part of these fluids should be inoculated into other animals. Smears should be made, and carefully examined, from the brain, lung, liver, spleen and the peritoneal lining of any animals that die. The parasite may be found after the primary inoculation and it is frequently isolated after the first passage. For practical purposes not more than three passages should be performed since it is quite exceptional for the parasite to be recovered if the first three passages have proved to be fruitless.

Direct demonstration of the parasites has only been

possible in about one half of the total number of human cases so far described.

Indirect Methods of Diagnosis

Complement Fixation Test. An antigen derived from chick-embryo cultures should be employed and the test serum should be examined within 24 hours of taking the blood, as complement-fixing activity may develop spontaneously after a longer period. Complement-fixing antibodies develop 3–4 weeks after infection occurs and may persist for several years in fairly high titre, although they often disappear during convalescence. Some 10 per cent. of healthy adults give a positive result with this test but a titre of over 1: 8 suggests a recent infection.

Neutralizing-Antibody Test. Infection with *T. gondii* leads to the formation of antibodies in the blood which may persist for many years after recovery. They may be demonstrated by their ability to prevent infection of the chick embryo with *Toxoplasma*, or the development of skin reactions in the rabbit. Although all human sera produce an erythema with oedema of the rabbit's skin within 24 hours of injection this usually fades after 4 days. If, however, any *Toxoplasma* are present and are not neutralized by antibody, a typical lesion will develop around the site of the injection after 3 or 4 days, becoming fully developed about the eighth day. The test is performed by injecting intracutaneously mixtures of the patient's serum with living *Toxoplasma*, obtained from cultures, in a shaved area on the back of a rabbit. Several dilutions of the *Toxoplasma* suspension are made in order to obtain the neutralizing titre of the serum. This test is not very reliable and it should not be used unless other tests are also performed.

Toxoplasmin Skin Test. The toxoplasmin is prepared from a special strain of *Toxoplasma* which are killed by irradiation from a germicidal electric lamp. Intradermal injections of suitable dilutions of toxoplasmin and a control antigen are made in the skin of the patient, and the area is observed after 48 and 72 hours. A positive reaction, indicating infection by *Toxoplasma*, consists of an area of erythema and induration exceeding 10 mm., present after 48 hours, with an absence of reaction in the area of the control. The test is more reliable than the neutralizing-antibody test, but, like the former, it does not indicate the state of activity of the disease, positive reactions being given by from 10 to 20 per cent. of apparently healthy people.

Methylene Blue Dye Test. If films, made from a suspension of parasites and normal serum, are stained with alkaline methylene blue, the parasites will appear as rounded, deeply stained bodies; if, however, the serum contains specific antibodies together with an 'accessory factor', some modification takes place in the cytoplasm of the parasite so that they no longer accept the stain. Until quite recently great reliance was placed on this test, but it is now known that it is by no means specific for *Toxoplasma*, a positive result being obtained also with *Sarcocystis*, *Trichomonas vaginalis* and *Trypanosoma lewisi* and probably other parasites. These findings do not necessarily invalidate the dye test, though the interpretation of the test when low titres are obtained is not easy. It is probably wise to insist that for a diagnosis of active toxoplasmosis to be justifiable, not only must the dye test and the complement fixation test be positive, but their respective titres should be not less than 1: 128 and 1: 8. In practice it will be found that the complement fixation test is nearly always positive with a dye test titre of 1: 128.

Differential Diagnosis

1. In infants when jaundice is present and the liver and spleen are enlarged, it must be distinguished from erythroblastosis foetalis. Birth injury, bacterial meningitis, foetal infection with many viral diseases may also present somewhat similar features.

2. In older children, with neurological abnormalities, it must be distinguished from tuberculous meningitis, disseminated sclerosis, cerebral angiomatosis and also from brain tumours.

3. In adults with acute infections, typhus, Rocky Mountain spotted fever and atypical pneumonia are the most likely causes of confusion. Toxoplasmosis should also be considered when evidence of past or existing encephalitis or myocardial disease is found where the cause remains unexplained. Pseudocysts occur frequently in the skeletal muscles and have at times been mistaken for sarcosporidia.

4. The lymphatic form will almost certainly be mistaken for glandular fever in the majority of cases, and it seems highly probable that if this form of toxoplasmosis is much more common than is generally realized, many of the 'clinical diagnoses' of glandular fever where the blood picture is atypical and the Paul-Bunnell test negative, may in fact be toxoplasmosis, since of the total number of such cases in any year, a very small proportion indeed will even arouse a suspicion of toxoplasmosis. It is certainly true that in many an outbreak of fever accompanied by glandular enlargement, giving a clinical picture that suggests glandular fever, laboratory confirmation may be obtained for only some 10–20 per cent. Enlarged glands may frequently be present in such cases 5–6 months later.

The persistence of the glandular enlargement may also at times arouse suspicion of Hodgkin's disease.

TREATMENT

Animal experiments have been made in which a very wide range of drugs have been tested, and whilst a number have had some effect, very few have encouraged clinical trials in human infections.

Pyrimethamine (*Daraprim*) appears to be the most successful drug in the treatment of toxoplasmosis when given concurrently with sulphadiazine. Both drugs need to be given in heavy doses. A useful regimen is as follows. On the first day, pyrimethamine orally, 50 mg., followed in 6–8 hours with 25 mg.; on the following 13 days, 25 mg. daily. Sulphadiazine: A single dose of 2 G., immediately followed by 1 G. six-hourly, continued for 14 days. Alternatively, *Sulphatriad* in doses of 3 G. immediately, and 1 G. four- to six-hourly may be used.

Folic acid and vitamin B complex should be given in the usual doses concurrently.

In animals other sulphonamides may cure early and light infections. The most active is sulphapyrazine. Broad-spectrum antibiotics including tetracycline and chlortetracycline are also active in large doses in heavy infections.

Cortisone or prednisolone has been used in ocular toxoplasmosis.

PROGNOSIS

The lymphatic form of toxoplasmosis runs a benign course, recovery being apparently invariable, and the prognosis is therefore excellent. Of the other forms of toxoplasmosis the great majority of recorded cases have ended fatally to date, but until the true incidence of the disease is known with accuracy, the case mortality will probably continue to be disproportionately high, since the majority of diagnoses will be amongst the most severe infections, with a large number obtained after post-mortem examination. Until a few years ago, recovery was the exception, but an increasing proportion of recoveries from the clinical forms of toxoplasmosis have more recently been recorded.

The congenitally acquired infections usually have a fatal termination either within the first few months of life, or in early childhood with a few years of survival marred by greatly impaired vision or blindness, and retarded mental development. Acute toxoplasmosis in children, marked by involvement of the central nervous system, have usually had a fatal termination, though there have been several reports of complete recovery, no sequelae being apparent. In adults a greater number of recoveries have been recorded, the outlook being more favourable when the respiratory symptoms predominate, even though the mortality with this form remains high. Encephalitis was considered unusual in adults a few years ago; during the last 5 years it has been a feature of a considerable proportion of the diagnosed infection in adults, with a fatal termination in about one half. Laboratory infections have not been numerous but they have been exceptionally severe, nearly all of them being fatal.

In recent years evidence based on serological tests has been accumulating, though the findings cannot be accepted without reserve, since, apart from many technical difficulties making the tests often unreliable, the dye test, which was considered the most satisfactory, has recently been shown to give positive reactions with a number of other protozoa. Despite these objections, it appears that the latent or subclinical form of toxoplasmosis is common, and that the clinically recognizable infections are extremely rare. Thus it is probably true to say that whilst the case mortality from the disease toxoplasmosis remains very high, the mortality following infection by *Toxoplasma* is extremely low.

REFERENCES

ADAMS, A. R. D., and MAEGRAITH, B. G. (1971) *Clinical Tropical Diseases*, 5th ed., Oxford.

British Encyclopaedia of Medical Practice (Medical Progress) (1960–69) Annual reviews of progress in tropical medicine, London.

HUTCHISON, W. M., DUNACHIE, J. F., SIIM, J. C., and WORK, K. (1970) Coccidian-like nature of *Toxoplasma gondii*, *Brit. med. J.*, **1**, 142.

TROWELL, H. C., and JELLIFFE, D. B. (1958) *Diseases of Children in the Subtropics and Tropics*, London.

ZAMAN, V., and COLLEY, F. C. (1970) Observations on the endogenous stages of *Toxoplasma gondii* in the cat ileum, *Southeast Asian J. trop. Med. Publ. Hlth*, **1**, 457.

BRIAN MAEGRAITH

PNEUMOCYSTIS PNEUMONIA

Synonym. Interstitial plasma cell pneumonia.

Incidence

Pneumocystis pneumonia has been recognized in Europe for 30 years as a frequent and sometimes epidemic disease of premature and debilitated infants between the ages of 4 weeks and 4 months. The disease is uncommon in Britain and the United States. Pneumocystis pneumonia has been reported in adults usually as a complication of leukaemia or lymphoma, but one or two instances in previously healthy persons have been recorded. Small epidemics affecting three or four members of one family have been observed.

Aetiology

The disease is associated with the presence of the organism *Pneumocystis carinii* in the lungs. However, *Pneumocystis carinii* has not yet been successfully cultured and Koch's postulates have not been fulfilled. It is probably protozoal but this has not been finally determined. It exists widely in laboratory and wild animals but the disease has not been transmitted experimentally. The organism is presumably a pathogen of low virulence which causes disease only when antibody formation is defective or resistance is otherwise impaired.

Pathology

At autopsy the lungs are airless, dry and of a tan colour. The alveolar walls and interstitial tissues are thickened and usually heavily infiltrated by mononuclear or plasma cells. However, this is not a feature in those patients with virtual absence of the plasma cell-lymphocyte series as is the case in congenital agammaglobulinaemia. For this reason the condition is better known as pneumocystis pneumonia rather than interstitial plasma cell pneumonia. The alveoli are packed with an amorphous eosinophilic foamy exudate containing occasional cysts, 3·5 μ in diameter and numerous basophilic round bodies 0·5 μ in diameter, both of which are thought to be alternative forms of the parasite. The bodies are best demonstrated by the periodic acid-Schiff, Giemsa or Gomori methenamine silver methods of staining.

Clinical Features

The onset is insidious and the course subacute. The incubation period is considered to be approximately 1–2 months and the duration of the disease, from the onset of symptoms, some 4 weeks. The disease is characterized by fever and progressive pulmonary failure, the severity of which is out of proportion to the physical signs in the chest. Some degree of eosinophilia is common in the peripheral blood.

Radiographs show a characteristic symmetrical ground-glass cloudiness, spreading outwards from the hila of the lungs, of increasing intensity and extent. Areas of lobular collapse and emphysema may produce a finely mottled or honeycomb effect. Interstitial or mediastinal emphysema and pneumothorax may occur.

There is a clear association between congenital and acquired hypogammaglobulinaemia and pneumocystis pneumonia. The infection may also complicate an exaggeration of the physiological fall in gamma globulin which occurs in early infancy. Various malignant diseases of the reticulo-endothelial system, treatment with corticosteroids, irradiation, chemotherapy and antibiotics predispose either by interfering with immune processes, by inhibiting the growth of other organisms in the respiratory tract or by damaging lung tissue. In a few adult cases normal gamma globulin levels have been present. In 10–25 per cent. of all affected infants pneumocystis pneumonia is associated with cytomegalovirus infection, and cases in adults have also been associated with cytomegalic inclusion disease or cryptococcosis.

Diagnosis

The diagnosis is usually made at autopsy, but the subacute course, the type of patient and the discrepancy between the severity of the illness and the radiograph on the one hand and the paucity of physical signs in the chest on the other may lead to a presumptive diagnosis which can only be confirmed in life by lung biopsy.

Treatment

No specific treatment is available. Antibiotics fail to cause definite improvement and antiprotozoal drugs are also of doubtful value.

Prognosis

The course is that of progressive pulmonary failure and death occurs by asphyxia. The mortality has been estimated by various authors at anywhere between 10 and 100 per cent.

REFERENCES

British Medical Journal (1962) Pneumocystis pneumonia, Leading article, i, 625.

Burke, B. A., Krovetz, L. J., and Good, R. A. (1961) Occurrence of *Pneumocystis carinii* pneumonia in children with agammaglobulinemia, *Pediatrics*, **28**, 196.

Hennigar, G. R. *et al.* (1961) *Pneumocystis carinii* pneumonia in an adult, *Amer. J. clin. Path.*, **35**, 353.

McKay, E., and Richardson, J. (1952) *Pneumocystis carinii* pneumonia associated with hypogammaglobulinaemia, *Lancet*, ii, 713.

McNeal, J. E., and Yaeger, R. G. (1960) Observations on a case of pneumocystis pneumonia, *Arch. Path.*, **70**, 397.

Rubin, E., and Zak, F. G. (1960) *Pneumocystis carinii* pneumonia in the adult, *New Engl. J. Med.*, **262**, 1315.

R. Bodley Scott

TROPICAL EOSINOPHILIA

Synonyms. Tropical pulmonary eosinophilia; Eosinophilic lung; Tropical eosinophilic asthma; Weingarten's syndrome.

Definition

An allergic condition characterized by persistent high eosinophilia associated with varying degrees of pulmonary signs and symptoms.

Aetiology

The majority of cases result from infection with nematodes, usually filarial worms, not adapted to man. In some cases the cause is not known.

The condition occurs widely throughout the world especially in Africa, India and the Far East.

Pathology

The syndrome is not fatal. The characteristic feature is high persistent absolute eosinophilia associated with leucocytosis which may reach very high figures.

The pulmonary changes are often minimal but may resemble viral pneumonitis radiologically. The mucoid sputum may contain epithelial cells and clumps of eosinophils.

Signs and Symptoms

The clinical pattern varies considerably.

The patient may present with indefinite symptoms of cough and chest pain without pulmonary or radiographic signs. There may be some irregular history of asthmatic attacks and sometimes episodes of urticaria.

In the classical case there is paroxysmal coughing which is worse at night. Paroxysms may be violent and repeated several times during the night. In many patients the attacks resemble asthma. There is a feeling of chest constriction and often dull aching pain over the front of the chest. Sweating may be profuse after a paroxysm.

Physical signs in the chest are equivocal. In the well developed case there are sibilant or sonorous rhonchi. heard over both lungs and sometimes coarse basal crepitations.

Radiological examination usually reveals that the hilar shadows are enlarged and blurred. Transverse branching striations may cross the lung fields and in some cases there is discrete rounded soft mottling especially prominent in the bases. These signs disappear quickly after treatment.

The Blood. The leucocyte count is raised and ranges from extremes of 10,000–100,000 cells per mm^3. with a common range of 15,000–40,000 cells per mm^3. Normal eosinophils constitute from 25 to over 80 per cent. of the total cells. The other cells are unchanged.

The leucocyte count and numbers of eosinophils vary in the patient from time to time.

Diagnosis

The total number of eosinophils per mm^3. should

exceed 3000. The leucocyte count should not be below 10,000 cells per mm³. It is usually higher and may be very high; the bone marrow, however, shows normal leucopoiesis except for a predominance of eosinophils.

The radiographic picture and lung signs may be mistaken for tuberculosis, but the changes occur in the bases and not the apices of the lungs and acid-fast bacilli are absent.

In the majority of cases the syndrome represents an allergic response to infection with a filarial worm, usually one not adapted to man but sometimes one, such as *W. bancrofti*, which normally infects man. Evidence of this infection should be sought in the history, for example, the area of exposure, and by the use of skin sensitivity and complement fixation reactions. For the allergic skin reaction 0·1 ml. of a suitable antigen (made from adult worms, for example, the dog heart worm *Dirofilaria*) is injected intradermally in the forearm. A positive reaction is indicated by a large wheal with pseudopodia developing 20–30 minutes later. Serum should be taken for complement fixation tests using the same antigen.

Response to treatment with diethylcarbamazine may offer confirmatory evidence of filarial infection.

Treatment

Cases due to filarial worm infections respond dramatically to large doses of diethylcarbamazine as follows: 6 mg. per kg. body weight thrice daily for 5 days, given as tablets in adults or syrup in children.

In a few cases complete cure is not effected by this treatment. A second course of diethylcarbamazine should then be given not earlier than 4 weeks from the first.

Late relapses are treated in the same way.

In the first few days of treatment there is often remittent fever, oedema of the face and skin reaction, including urticaria. These allergic responses can be regarded as diagnostic. They may be relieved by giving antihistamine drugs for the first five days of treatment. Bronchial spasm may be relieved by adrenaline or aminophylline.

It is noteworthy that before the filarial origin of the majority of cases was realized, arsenicals were regarded almost as specific drugs for the treatment of the syndrome. They are now seldom used.

Corticosteroids have been used successfully in refractory cases.

BRIAN MAEGRAITH

DISEASES DUE TO METAZOAL INFECTION

TREMATODES

INTESTINAL FLUKES

In most of these trematode infections man is infected only accidentally and the organisms live in wild or domestic animals.

The life cycles have much in common.

The adults are leaf-shaped hermaphrodite motile worms which may be minute or several inches in length.

They are attached to the intestinal wall by muscular suckers, and operculate eggs with undeveloped ova are passed in the faeces. Hatching takes place either in water or in a fresh-water mollusc intermediate host, from which cercariae are eventually discharged. The cercariae encyst to form metacercariae either on various forms of vegetation or in intermediate hosts including reptiles, fish or molluscs.

Human infection occurs as a result of ingesting metacercariae from which the larva is released in the small intestine to mature into the adult.

There are two sub-orders of intestinal flukes which occur in man, the most important of which are the Distomata. Of the Amphistomata the only common infection is due to *Gastrodiscoides hominis* a natural infection of pigs which occurs in man in India and is found in the colon, particularly in the caecum, and may in heavy infection give rise to diarrhoea or mucous colitis.

FASCIOLOPSIASIS

Aetiology and Pathology

The most important of the Distomata is *Fasciolopsis buskii*, a common infection of pigs and dogs which frequently infects man in South-East Asia and in other parts of the Far East. The operculated eggs are passed in the faeces and hatch in fresh water. The miracidia develop in certain snails, including *Segmentina*; eventually cercariae are produced which encyst on water plants.

Man is infected by ingesting metacercariae encysted on various water plants, especially the water chestnut, water caltrop, the water bamboo and water hyacinth. In South-East Asia where these roots are eaten raw, the infection commonly occurs in children. After ingestion, adults mature in the small intestine. The adults are large, measuring as much as two inches long, and are attached to the duodenal and jejunal mucosa. In heavy infections the stomach and large intestine may be involved. Eggs first appear in the faeces in about three months. The large flukes may directly damage the intestinal wall with associated local inflammatory and cellular reactions, including concentrations of eosinophils. Ulceration or abscess may occur at the points of attachment of the flukes. Rarely there may be frank haemorrhage resulting from erosion of vessels. There is commonly an excessive secretion of mucus leading to mucous diarrhoea.

Apart from the local effects there may be severe toxic reaction. There may be allergic oedema of the face and legs and, not uncommonly, ascites. Anorexia, diarrhoea, nausea and vomiting may persist and in severe cases death may result.

The infection is associated with a moderate eosinophilia and there may be a leucopenia.

The ordinary infection is not of very serious consequence, but heavy infections may cause considerable prostration and illness and even death in young children. The infection must therefore be regarded as serious.

Diagnosis

Diagnosis is made by the discovery of the eggs and on occasions the adults in the stool.

Treatment

Treatment consists of the administration of tetrachloroethylene in the usual doses [p. 296].

INFECTION WITH OTHER INTESTINAL FLUKES

Infection with *Heterophyes heterophyes* is common in parts of the Middle East.

Man is infected by eating raw fish containing metacercariae.

The adult is small, and is attached to the wall of the small intestine by its suckers. The eggs are passed in the faeces. They contain a fully developed miracidium which initiates the usual life cycle.

At the point of attachment of the adults in the intestine there may be mild inflammatory cellular reaction, sometimes with superficial necrosis and excess mucous secretion; diarrhoea results.

In some cases the adult penetrates the mucosa and may reach the mesenteric vessels and so pass to the brain and other organs, including the heart. In the heart myocardial damage may result from mild cellular reaction to the parasites and sometimes changes may be evoked on the cardiac valves.

Diagnosis is made by the discovery of eggs or adults in the faeces.

Treatment is unsatisfactory but claims have been made for piperazine adipate which is said to deal with up to 50 per cent. of infections in the usual dosages.

In the Far East infection with *Metagonimus yokogawai* may occur. Man is infected accidentally by eating raw or inadequately cooked fish or shrimps, containing the infective metacercariae.

The very small adults are attached to the duodenum. They may penetrate the mucosa and deposit their eggs in the submucosal tissue. Mature eggs are passed in the faeces.

The pathological lesions are similar to those caused by *Heterophyes*, but the adults commonly invade the deeper layer of the mucosa with infiltration into the intestinal wall, ulceration or erosion of the mucosa and excessive secretion of mucus. As a result of the deep invasion of the mucosa, eggs may reach the blood vessels or lymphatics of the intestine and get carried to various organs, including the heart, brain and the spinal cord. In these sites granulomatous reactions occur giving rise to local damage and associated functional disturbance. The invasion of the intestinal submucosal tissues by the adults is usually associated with little damage.

The condition is diagnosed by the discovery of the eggs and adults in the stool.

There is no specific treatment although chloroquine has been successful in some cases.

THE LUNG FLUKE

The trematode parasite *Paragonimus westermani* is found in man in many parts of the Far East, in South America and in localized areas of West Africa and the Congo.

The adult flukes are about half an inch in length, are hermaphrodite and produce brown operculated eggs which may reach 120 μ in length.

The eggs are coughed up in the sputum or swallowed and passed in the faeces. After their escape they mature in water. A miracidium emerges and invades snails of the genus *Semisulcospira* within the liver of which development takes place. The cercariae liberated from the snail enter crayfish and crabs and encyst in the muscles and other tissues to become metacercariae.

Pathology

Man becomes infected by swallowing raw or inadequately cooked secondary host tissues. In the small intestine the metacercariae excyst, penetrate the intestinal walls and pass through the abdominal cavity, the diaphragm and the pleura into the lungs, where they tend to lodge peripherally. A capsule of inflammatory and fibrous tissue forms round each developing parasite, which starts producing eggs within 6 weeks.

The capsule may enlarge and eventually rupture into a bronchiole so that the contents, including the eggs, are coughed up as sputum. There are usually only a few parasites present in any one human infection. Many intermediate hosts other than man exist. Aberrant flukes may lodge in organs other than the lungs, including the liver, the peritoneum, skeletal muscle and the brain or the cord. The presence of the worms in these areas may lead to localizing signs and symptoms.

Signs and Symptoms

The patient is usually seen at the stage where the cysts have developed in the lungs and the eggs and other cyst contents are being coughed up by the patient.

The migration of the metacercariae does not normally give rise to signs and symptoms. These occur as a result of the reaction of the host tissues to the presence of the parasites and their eggs. There may however be some fever and when the parasite reaches the lungs there is often cough with increased sputum, commonly streaked with blood.

In the classical case there may be some degree of haemoptysis or the sputum is flecked with blood and bright yellow spots which on examination will be found to contain the eggs. Where there is full pulmonary development the patient complains of shortness of breath, chronic cough and chest pains. There is evidence of persistent bronchitis or bronchiectasis and sometimes pleural effusion. At this stage, where the cyst has formed in the lungs, radiology may be helpful in the diagnosis; the site and extent of the lesion which is usually singular may be determined by serial tomography.

In other areas of the body the presence of the parasites produces symptoms depending on the location. They may be in the walls of the intestine producing enteritis or in the liver, producing hepatitis and so forth. In the brain they commonly give rise to attacks of Jacksonian epilepsy.

The symptoms are most severe in the first 5 or 6 years of the infection. They persist for very long periods since the worm survives for as long as 20 years.

Diagnosis

Diagnosis depends on the recovery of the characteristic eggs from the sputum or faeces. In the sputum the eggs commonly occur as masses of golden-brown material in which they are tightly packed together. Parasites may occasionally be removed by biopsy from areas other than the lungs. Eggs may also be found in the stools in patients who have swallowed their sputum or occasionally where there have been intra-abdominal lesions.

Complement fixation tests are sometimes useful and reactions to the injection of antigen into the skin are now commonly used to map areas of endemicity of the infecting parasite.

Treatment

Chloroquine has been fairly successful when given in large doses. Emetine has also been claimed to be successful.

The best drug is bithionol (*Actamer*) given as 30–50 mg. per kg. every other day in divided doses over a period of 20–30 days. The patients are rapidly freed from eggs and improve clinically even after the first few days of treatment. The side-effects are mild; there may be some abdominal pain and diarrhoea and a little nausea and vomiting.

LIVER FLUKES

The common infections with liver flukes are those caused by *Clonorchis sinensis* and *Opisthorchis viverrini* or *O. felineus* in South East Asia and the Far East and by *Fasciola hepatica* which occurs in many parts of the world.

Clonorchiasis and opisthorchiasis constitute a serious menace to the health of the communities in which they occur.

CLONORCHIASIS

Aetiology

This infection is found in the Far East, including China, Indonesia, Korea, Japan, North Vietnam and Formosa.

It may occur in man, cats and other animals.

The hermaphrodite fluke measures about an inch in length. The eggs are small and operculated, each containing a miracidium. They are ingested by *Bulimus* (*Bithynia*) snails and in due course cercariae emerge from the snail and penetrate fresh water fish in which they encyst in the muscles, becoming metacercariae.

Pathology

The definitive hosts, including man, become infected by eating flesh containing metacercariae. These excyst in the duodenum, ascend the common bile-duct and enter the bile capillaries, where they mature. The cycle takes about 4 months, when eggs appear in the faeces. The number of adults in a given infection may be very large. In the bile capillaries there is local inflammatory reaction with dilatation of the biliary canals containing the worms. There is localized hyperplasia of the epithelium and pericholangitic fibrosis.

New bile capillaries are formed in these areas.

Masses of eggs may escape from the damaged canals and bile-ducts into the parenchyma. Around these, granulomatous reactions are set up which are later walled off by fibrous tissue, with consequent interference with the lobular pattern of the liver and considerable fibrosis. The ultimate damage to the liver depends largely on the numbers of worms and the degree to which the worms and eggs escape into the liver tissue. With light infections the effects are minimal. With heavy infections there may be considerable enlargement and extensive fibrosis of the liver.

Liver cirrhosis accompanied by portal hypertension appears on occasion in areas where the liver fluke infection is associated with alcoholism or with some other toxic factor.

In some areas carcinoma of the liver and even carcinoma of the pancreas have been reported in association with the liver fluke infection.

The interference with the circulation and flow of the bile following the obstruction and fibrosis of the bile-ducts may give rise to mild jaundice, but this is seldom severe.

In children especially the effects of the infection are associated with a general toxic reaction not unlike that seen in fasciolopsiasis, with emaciation, cachexia and even death.

Signs and Symptoms

The clinical picture is dependent on the degree of infection. In heavy infections there is a chronic relapsing cholangitis and enlargement of the liver, which may present two or three fingers' breadth below the costal margin with a firm and often slightly tender edge. There is some increase in bilirubin in the blood and sometimes clinical jaundice. Changes develop in liver function, indicated especially in the transaminases. Systemic manifestations include tachycardia, giddiness, tremors, muscular cramps, depression and varying degrees of toxaemia. The spleen is rarely enlarged. A mild remittent fever is common.

Diagnosis

Diagnosis depends on the discovery of the eggs in the faeces or of eggs and adults in fluid aspirated from the duodenum.

In some geographical areas the endemicity has been mapped out by the use of antigens made from adult worms and injected intradermally.

Less severe infections may cause few symptoms or signs and there may be no measurable liver dysfunction although the organ is moderately enlarged and firm.

Treatment

There is no really satisfactory treatment. Large

doses of chloroquine have been given with some success. Good results have been claimed with hexachloroparaxylol (*Metol*), 100–200 mg. per kg. body weight, given in three divided doses after meals for 5 days. Bithionol is not effective. Secondary infection in the bile-ducts is dealt with by giving tetracycline, 500 mg. 6-hourly for up to 10 days.

Control of the infection depends on the control of the snails, improvement in hygienic habits and adequate cooking of food before consumption. Since raw fish is the mainstay of the national diet in the endemic areas, changes in eating habits are extremely difficult to bring about.

OPISTHORCHIASIS

Aetiology

This infection occurs in North Eastern Europe, Russia, India, Japan and particularly in north eastern Thailand and surrounding territories.

Man and other animals, including the cat and dog, become infected by eating raw fish containing metacercariae. The life cycle of the parasite is very similar to that of *Clonorchis*.

Pathology, Signs and Symptoms

The clinical picture and the patterns of parasitological and pathological changes are the same as in clonorchiasis. Although the liver is often considerably enlarged there is rarely any evidence of portal hypertension and associated enlargement of the spleen. The picture thus contrasts with that of late bilharziasis. Liver function changes are as in clonorchiasis.

Diagnosis

Diagnosis is made by the discovery of eggs in the faeces or eggs and adults in the duodenal juice.

Treatment

Treatment is unsatisfactory. Some success is claimed for chloroquine, 300 mg. of the base twice daily for 2 weeks, followed by the same dose 3 days in the week for a total of 5 weeks. This often limits the egg output and improves the clinical condition. The drug acts on adults in the bile-ducts and also probably on the eggs. The dosage of chloroquine is heavy and side-effects are common. These can be relieved by oral glucose and administration of vitamin B complex. They include nausea, vomiting, anorexia, dimness of vision and sometimes scotomata, dizziness, vertigo, headache and skin rashes.

In cases with obvious biliary obstruction the chloroquine should be accompanied by vitamin K given as menaphthone sodium bisulphite injection, 5–10 mg. intramuscularly, daily.

Bithionol is not successful. Hexachloroparaxylol is sometimes effective (see Clonorchiasis). Tetracycline should be given for the secondary biliary tract infection.

FASCIOLIASIS

Aetiology

Fascioliasis is widely distributed but is much less common than other liver fluke infections. It results from eating metacercariae of the sheep liver fluke *Fasciola hepatica* which encyst on vegetation, including grass and watercress. The adults are an inch or more in length. They mature in the biliary tract about 4 months after infection.

Pathology and Signs and Symptoms

Pathological changes occur in the walls of the invaded bile-ducts, with epithelial hypertrophy, desquamation, dilatation, fibrosis and cystic dilatation of the lumen. The adults may erode the duct lining, and masses of eggs and sometimes adults may escape into the parenchyma causing local granulomatous reactions which are later replaced by fibrosis or occasionally become abscesses. There is at first general enlargement of the liver, but in severe cases with massive fibrosis the organ may be ultimately reduced in size. Portal hypertension rarely develops except in the presence of other liver insults.

Ectopic larvae may be distributed to any tissue. Adults may be found in the blood vessels, the brain, the orbit and the subcutaneous tissues. These ectopic parasites are usually surrounded by granulomatous reactions in which the worm may live for months and is eventually replaced by giant cell tissue and fibrosis. Large numbers of larvae may become caught up in the liver in this way [see visceral larva migrans, p. 299]. A form of pharyngeal fascioliasis called *Halzoun* occurs in the Middle East, resulting from the lodging of adults in the submucosa after ingestion of infected mutton. This may give rise to serious obstruction to the air passages.

In the severe case the picture is one of chronic or recurrent cholangitis with moderate jaundice and irregular remittent fever. There is heavy sweating, abdominal pain, right hypochondrial tenderness and pain over the gall-bladder region, persistent diarrhoea and vomiting of bile-stained fluid. There is usually high eosinophilia, anaemia and moderate leucocytosis.

Diagnosis

Diagnosis is confirmed by finding the eggs in the faeces. Some help may be obtained by serological tests, including complement fixation, using an antigen made from adult worms.

In the visceral larva migrans syndrome the granulomata containing larvae may sometimes be found in liver biopsy.

Treatment

Treatment is unsatisfactory. Chloroquine has been tried with equivocal results in doses of 300 mg. daily for 30 days. This regimen produces unpleasant side-effects. It relieves the clinical picture temporarily, but relapse is common. Bithionol (*Actamer*) has been successful in some cases, in doses of 30–50 mg. per kg. body weight every other day for 10–15 doses. Some success was claimed with hexachloroparaxylol, as in other liver fluke infections. In the state of larva migrans some success has been claimed with large doses of diethylcarbamazine (*Banocide, Hetrazan*).

REFERENCE

HARINASUTA, C., and HARINASUTA, T. (1971) Fluke infections, in *Management and Treatment of Tropical Diseases*, ed. Maegraith, B. G., and Gilles, M. M., Oxford,

SCHISTOSOMIASIS

Synonym. Bilharziasis.

Definition and Aetiology

Schistosomiasis is caused by infection with the blood fluke *Schistosoma.* Three major species of this trematode infect man, i.e. *S. japonicum* (causing Asian schistosomiasis), *S. mansoni* (causing intestinal schistosomiasis or bilharziasis) and *S. haematobium* (causing genito-urinary schistosomiasis or bilharziasis). The clinical pictures presented depend upon the infecting species and may be basically intestinal or genito-urinary, although more general complications are common. The lesions are primarily associated with the dissemination of the eggs of the worm in the relevant tissues.

The geographical distribution of the infections will be discussed below in the accounts of the diseases caused by the three species.

The life cycle of all three species of *Schistosoma* is essentially the same.

The adults exist as males and females which vary in length from 7 to 25 millimetres. The female is long and slender and is commonly found wrapped in and protruding from the gynaecophoric canal of the male. The paired worms live in the venous vessels about the gut and pelvis, where the female lays her eggs in the terminal radicles of the portal venules often temporarily migrating from the male to do so. The eggs are laid separately in rows and the vessels then contract upon them.

Local necrosis of the vessel wall occurs as the embryo within the egg develops and the egg escapes into the tissues and, if near the surface epithelium, passes out of the body into some hollow viscus such as the intestine or urinary bladder. Eggs containing fully developed embryos are passed in the faeces or urine and many eventually reach water, in which they hatch, liberating the ciliated larva or miracidium which swims freely and must penetrate the intermediate host snail within a few hours.

Within the snail, the species of which are specific for the species of *Schistosoma* concerned, further development takes place in the liver tissue and eventually in 4–8 weeks the next stage larvae or cercariae escape into the water. These are fork-tailed and swim freely for some hours fork first, until they penetrate the skin of the definitive host, in this case man.

Man is usually infected in this way when working, wading or swimming in infected water, but he may also become infected by drinking water containing cercariae. In endemic areas children are infected at an early age and the infection rate increases rapidly to high figures during adolescence and adult life. In some areas where endemicity is particularly high, practically the whole young child, adolescent and adult population exposed is infected. There is sexual or social variation in incidence only when habit and occupation affect the frequency of exposure.

In man, within 24 hours the cercariae reach the peripheral venules and are carried via the heart to the pulmonary circulation in which some may become caught and eventually destroyed. Other larvae escape into the systemic circulation and are carried through the hepatic artery to the portal circulation in which they mature. Eventually paired adults reach the mesenteric and pelvic venules, eggs are laid and the cycle is repeated.

In most endemic areas, *S. japonicum* exists in both man and animals, including the water buffalo, cattle, sheep, dogs, pigs and rats. These animals constitute an important reservoir of infection and pose a serious problem in control. In Formosa, the infection occurs in animals not in man. In Thailand, a small focus of infection exists in which no animal reservoirs have been found.

In both *S. mansoni* and *S. haematobium* infections man is the only important reservoir, although baboons, monkeys and rodents have been found naturally infected with the former.

Basic Pathology

The clinical and pathological patterns which result from the infection depend on the species of *Schistosoma* involved and on the reaction of the host tissues to the worm and its products, particularly the egg. As in all helminth infections the complicated tissue response to the presence of the worm includes the development of sensitivity: immunity processes which influence both the cellular and clinical pictures. The tissue response depends in the first instance on the presence of eggs containing the living miracidium. Eggs which escape to the surface usually cause little damage during their passage through the tissues, but those which remain commonly stimulate the production of cellular granulomata, which develop more vigorously in some tissues, such as the liver, than in others, such as the stomach wall. Some granulomatous reactions also occur round dying or dead worms, but the live worm at any stage seldom invokes much local response, although it is often responsible for the more general allergic reactions. In the later stages of the disease complications arise largely as the result of fibrous replacement and extension of granulomatous lesions, especially in the liver, the intestines, the urinary bladder, ureters and kidneys and in the lungs. These lesions will be discussed in the sections dealing with specific infections.

The initial clinical developments are to a considerable extent determined in the first instance by the anatomical distribution of the adult worms. Thus in *S. japonicum* infections, the adults find their way to venules of both the superior and inferior mesenteric veins and so affect both the small and large intestinal tissues; *S. mansoni* adults invade mainly the inferior mesenteric veins, and so the large gut. In *S. haematobium* infections most adults are found in the vesical and other pelvic venous plexuses and some occur in the inferior mesenteric veins. The pathological effects are thus found in the urinary bladder and other parts of the genito-urinary tract.

The first evidence of infection often develops at the site of the penetration of the cercariae, where a slight itchy papular eruption may develop. The tissue reaction is mild and reflected in some vasodilatation and round cell infiltration. The larva penetrates the skin by cellular lysis initiated by enzymes which presumably assist its movements in the deeper tissues to the point where it enters the blood stream via a venous capillary. Migration to and through the lungs is accompanied by little local or general reaction in the early stages, although some small vessels may be injured and cause minute haemorrhages in the alveoli. As the worms mature in the portal vessels in the liver and later in the mesenteric and pelvic veins, their tissues provide an antigenic stimulus to the production of antibodies and after some weeks an allergic general reaction commonly develops, indicated clinically by fever, malaise, epigastric discomfort, cough and bronchitis and sometimes an urticarial rash. These manifestations begin before the worms are completely mature and egg laying has started. They are common in *S. japonicum* and *S. mansoni* infections. From this stage onwards, allergic antibody-antigen reactions of one grade or another influence the clinical and pathological progress of the infections.

The eggs containing living miracidia are the chief pathogenic agents and are responsible for initiating most of the local tissue changes. Subsequent developments depend on the extension of these lesions and on their physiological and pathological effects on the body of the host. The anatomical distribution of the adult worms in the mesenteric and pelvic veins determines to some extent the initial distribution of the eggs in the tissues, and so the clinical picture.

Many eggs which have passed from the venules in which they were laid, escape through the tissues to the urine and faeces. These cause little tissue damage. Others pass into the blood stream and are seeded to the liver or via the systemic circulation to all tissues of the body, where they are eventually arrested in small vessels and set up ectopic cellular reactions, the effects of which vary with the location.

Most of the eggs remain in the tissues into which they originally escaped. In the course of 2–3 weeks, while the contained miracidia are still living, these eggs set up the characteristic granulomatous response which is the basis of all subsequent developments. It is believed that the miracidium secretes some toxic substance which stimulates the cellular response. The cellular response consists largely of lymphocytes, plasma cells, macrophages and eosinophils. Later, epithelioid cells appear and a granuloma is formed similar to that seen in tuberculosis. After some weeks the larva dies and the egg shell may calcify. Under these circumstances giant cells may be formed; there is a lymphocytic and fibroblastic infiltration at the periphery of the lesion and eventually the granuloma may be replaced by fibrous tissue.

The local effects of such cellular and granulomatous reactions to the eggs depends on the relevant tissue. For example, in the liver fibrosis may eventually result in portal hypertension, ascites, enlargement of the spleen and gastric and oesophageal venous varices.

Regression of granulomatous lesions without fibrosis may occur without treatment, especially when superinfection is restricted or absent. Such regression is commonly seen in adults who were heavily exposed as children and subsequently were less exposed or unexposed.

Immunity reactions, as mentioned above, are set up in schistosomiasis. Little is known about the importance of these reactions but evidence is accumulating to show that a fair degree of resistance to superinfection may be acquired in circumstances in which there is frequent or continuous exposure, as in individuals working in irrigated rice fields. Certain humoral antibodies can easily be demonstrated in the blood, but it is not certain whether these are relevant to resistance to infection. The allergic manifestations of the disease are undoubtedly important in deciding its development and the general body responses.

The clinical picture varies widely in infections caused by the same species of parasites, not only from host to host, but from one geographical area to another. It is probable that the intensity of the infection may be a major factor in determining the ultimate response to a given host, but this is a very difficult point to determine except in terms of the clinical severity of the case and the history of exposure. In Egypt, for example, infection with *S. mansoni* and *S. haematobium* produce very severe clinical patterns quite unlike those seen in many parts of Africa further south, especially in areas where exposure is relatively light as compared with that in Egypt. Repeated reinfection is obviously part of this process but it is again difficult to assess its relevance, especially with the development of acquired resistance to superinfection. Other factors are also probably concerned, including the nutritional status of the individual, and regional variation in the prevalent strains of the parasite. Anaemia from blood loss and sometimes from hypersplenism may occur.

Other Forms of Schistosomiasis in Man

In parts of tropical Africa human intestinal schistosomiasis is sometimes caused by *S. intercalatum*, the terminal-spined eggs of which closely resemble those of *S. haematobium*. This worm is normally a parasite of cattle and sheep. Rare infections of man with *S. matthei*, also a parasite of animals, have been reported. *S. bovis* infection has occurred, involving the urinary tract.

Schistosomal dermatitis, or swimmer's itch, is locally recognized in many parts of the world and arises as a reaction to invasion by cercariae of schistosomes of birds and mammals. The diseases do not progress beyond this stage. On mild exposure, prickling and itching sensations occur at the site of entry within an hour and persist. Later there is a macular or urticarial eruption. Papules form in 18–24 hours and are intensely itchy; some lesions vesiculate and as a result of scratching become secondarily infected. The reaction subsides in about a week. The first exposure may not produce a very vigorous response but the reaction often, but not always, becomes more pronounced with subsequent exposure, due to the development of some kind of sensitivity. Heavy exposure in a sensitized subject may cause general allergic reactions.

In sensitized subjects the penetration of the cercariae of human schistosome infections, especially *S. japonicum* may occasionally produce similar dermatitis.

About twenty species of animal schistosomes are known to cause dermatitis.

Helminthological Diagnosis of Infection

The diagnosis depends finally on the demonstration of the worm or its eggs in the tissues or excretions, usually the faeces and urine. Discovery of adults is accidental during life, when they may be discovered in biopsy material, but at autopsy they may readily be found in the various plexuses of the intestinal or genito-urinary tracts or in the liver substance.

Clinical diagnosis depends on the discovery of the eggs of the particular species infecting the host.

The eggs can be readily distinguished by their size and shape [see section on specific infections below]. In freshly passed eggs in active untreated cases the living ciliated miracidium can be seen moving within the confines of the shell and may be hatched out by exposure to large volumes of water.

In *S. haematobium* infections the eggs are usually easily found in the deposit from centrifuged urine, especially when there is obvious haematuria. Miracidia can readily be hatched from urine sediments. It is rarely necessary to use concentration methods on the urine. Eggs may also be present in material obtained from rectal biopsy.

In *S. japonicum* infection eggs may be discovered in the faeces by direct examination of faecal smears, but in many cases concentration methods are required [see below]. Sometimes rectal biopsy may be necessary. Some authors recommend combining these methods of examination, including hatching.

In dysenteric heavy infections the eggs of *S. mansoni* are usually easy to find by direct faecal examination, but in lighter infections they may be very difficult to discover and routine diagnosis usually demands some concentration technique [see below]. Eggs are often easily found in rectal biopsy material when they are difficult to find in the faeces, and, in suitable circumstances it is probably advisable to check the diagnosis in this way, and also by hatching.

In both *S. japonicum* and *S. mansoni* infections eggs and associated granulomas may also sometimes be found in liver biopsy material and in the sputum.

Differentiation of Eggs

Eggs can easily be identified under the low power of the microscope.

SPECIES	SIZE OF EGG	SHAPE
S. haematobium	120–170 × 70 μ	well developed terminal spine
S. mansoni	120–170 × 70 μ	well developed single lateral spine
S. japonicum	100 × 65 μ smallest and most variable	no spine, but a small tubercle or hook laterally

Quantitative Estimation of Egg Output

Urine or faecal suspension is passed through hardened filter paper by vacuum, schistosome eggs being retained by the paper. The paper is then placed on a few drops of saturated aqueous ninhydrin solution in a flat dish and the colour reaction developed by incubating at 60° C. for 1 hour. The stained paper is examined by transmitted light, after mounting in a drop of water. Eggs which contain a miracidium stain deep purple, and are easily recognizable and countable. The total number of eggs passed daily can be calculated in this way (Bell's technique). A simpler quantitative technique has recently been designed by Kato; 50 mg. of stool is sieved through fine wire mesh, spread on a microscope slide and covered with a strip of glycerin-soaked celluloid. By this method schistosome eggs can be easily counted and the eggs of other helminths are equally distinguishable.

Faeces. Eggs may often be found in faecal smears prepared in water or saline on a microscope slide and covered with a coverslip. It is usual, however, to employ some method of concentration either in glycerol, in which the eggs are undamaged and hatchable, or in formol ether, in which the miracidia are killed.

Urine. The deposit from a specimen of urine which has been allowed to stand or has been centrifuged is examined on a slide under a coverslip. Eggs are usually present in such preparations in cases with haematuria and often when pus is being passed.

The chances of finding eggs are best during activity, usually in specimens passed over the period 10.00 to 14.00 hours. This specimen is to be preferred to the terminal specimen passed at the end of micturition, which was formerly advised.

Hatching. When eggs containing viable miracidia are exposed to large volumes of water the larvae escape and swim freely in the fluid near the surface.

Urine: S. haematobium. The urine is gently centrifuged and the supernatant poured away. The sediment is covered with the same volume of tap water and left for several hours at room temperature in the tropics or at about 25°–30° C. in temperate areas. Miracidia will be seen with a hand lens swimming near the surface.

Faeces. 15–20 g. of faeces is emulsified in about a litre of water and the emulsion is poured into a flask with a narrow neck so that the fluid level rises into the neck. Hatching takes place at room temperature in hot countries in the course of 3–5 hours or sooner. The miracidia can be detected as minute bodies swimming about in an inch of water below the meniscus. They should be examined by hand lens in transversely directed bright light.

Rectal Biopsy. This is useful in all infections. It is performed through a proctoscope. The rectal wall is swabbed and the material examined. Eggs may often be present. Biopsy is then carried out with fine forceps not more than 6 cm. above the anal mucocutaneous junction. The tissue is removed from the superficial layers of the mucosa and bleeding is controlled by gentle swabbing, and in rare instances where bleeding is severe, by rectal packing.

The tissue is divided into two portions. One piece is crushed between two slides and examined for eggs under the low power of the microscope. The other is fixed in 1 per cent. formalin for histological examination.

Diagnosis by the Detection of Immune Bodies, and Sensitivity

Antibodies can be found in the blood of persons infected with schistosomes from about the fourth week, i.e. before the eggs begin to appear in the excreta; of these, the most powerful are the complement fixing bodies. Using antigens made from adult worms the detection of these antibodies can be a very useful diagnostic technique; only 2–3 per cent. of false positives appear in populations in non-endemic areas. The reaction is group- rather than species-specific. A positive complement fixation test is rendered negative some months after successful treatment.

The detection of serum antibodies by other methods, such as precipitation and cercarial Hüllen reaction (C.H.R.) is possible in a high proportion of cases but is not usually regarded as a safe diagnostic procedure.

In screening populations during surveys of endemicity the intradermal skin test can be useful, using antigen prepared from adult worms, of species of *Schistosoma* infecting man or animals (usually *S. spindale*). A volume of 0·1 ml. antigen is injected intradermally and the result read 20 minutes later. A positive reaction is shown by the development of a wheal with pseudopodia which has a diameter of 2–3 times that of the wheal caused by the injection. In non-immune areas false positives are found in 2–5 per cent. of the population. Over 90 per cent. of individuals infected for more than 6 weeks give positive reactions.

Except for specific purposes, such as surveys, serological or skin sensitivity techniques cannot replace the search for eggs.

Treatment

The treatment of all forms of human infection is basically the same but the response differs according to the species. Unless contra-indicated, treatment is usually given in all grades of infection however low the output of eggs. It has not yet been determined whether very light infections cause serious or permanent lesions or whether the effects of such infections may regress without treatment.The decision as to whether such infections should be treated (in view of the possible risks of therapy) consequently varies from worker to worker.

The results of treatment vary according to the infecting parasite, the worm load, and the pathological effects already induced in the host.

Trivalent Antimonials. The most commonly used drugs are the trivalent antimonials. Probably the most successful is the sodium or potassium salt of antimony tartrate (tartar emetic). Ammonium antimony tartrate is sometimes used as an alternative.

Other trivalent antimonials are also widely used, including stibophen or fouadin, which can be given intramuscularly, and antimony lithium thiomalate (*Anthiomaline*) given intramuscularly. They all have fewer side-effects than tartar emetic but are less effective against the schistosome infection.

Sodium or Potassium Antimony Tartrate. The drug must be prepared to B.P. standards, i.e. contain less than 5 parts of lead per million. It is made up as a 6 per cent. solution in 5 per cent. glucose and administered slowly intravenously, well diluted with pyrogen-free water or saline. The greatest care must be exercised during the injection to avoid leakage into the tissues, which causes inflammation, necrosis and sloughing. A common dosage regimen is as follows: For each 15 kg. body weight 0·5 ml. of a 6 per cent. solution is given for each dose, to a maximum of 2 ml. per dose, for individuals weighing 60 kg. or more. Children below 15 kg. in weight are not given the drug. This dose is given on alternate days on 12–16 occasions.

BODY WEIGHT KG.	VOLUME OF 6 PER CENT. SOLUTION OF TARTAR EMETIC	DRUG PER DOSE	TOTAL DOSE
15+	0·5 ml.	30 mg.	360–480 mg.
30+	1 ml.	60 mg.	720–960 mg.
45+	1·5 ml.	90 mg.	1080–1440 mg.
60+	2 ml.	120 mg.	1440–1920 mg.

S. haematobium infections respond very well to 10–12 doses and it is not usually necessary to continue beyond this point. Unfortunately both *S. mansoni* and *S. japonicum* respond less favourably and the regimen in these infections is usually extended to the full 16 injections.

In all three infections it may be necessary to repeat the schedule after the test of cure has been applied [see below].

The side-effects of the administration of sodium or potassium antimony tartrate are unpleasant and include cough, a feeling of chest constriction and dyspnoea during and immediately after the injection. Nausea is common and vomiting may follow the injection especially if it is given too soon after a meal. The pulse is quickened after injection as a rule but with reasonable precautions serious consequences can be avoided by having the patient recumbent during the injection and at rest for some hours afterwards. Toxic effects on the heart, shown by the electrocardiogram, include changes in the T wave and the isoelectric levels. These become more notable as the course of treatment continues. Other toxic effects developing during a course of antimonial therapy include severe vomiting, diarrhoea and jaundice. These are indications for stopping therapy. Death may follow an injection but only rarely. Tartar emetic and other drugs containing antimony are contra-indicated in cases with heart disorders and renal or hepatic disease.

It is usually held that side-effects are minimized by diluting the drug solution and injecting it slowly.

Thus, it is the practice in Europe to make the solution up to 10–15 ml. with pyrogen-free water or saline and inject over a period of about 10 minutes. In Egypt, during mass treatment campaigns, however, the drug is regularly injected rapidly and directly as the 6 per cent. solution, without serious side-effects.

The oral administration of tartar emetic is being tried in China in mass campaigns with good results but severe side-effects.

Other Antimony Compounds. Stibophen (fouadin) may be used where intravenous therapy presents difficulty. The drug is presented as a 6·4 per cent. solution. It is given intramuscularly with the usual aseptic precautions, in successive doses on alternate days as follows: 1·5 ml.; 3·5 ml., then 5 ml. on each occasion for a total of 10–15 doses.

Side-effects are mild, but in mass campaigns in Egypt it has been found that there is a higher mortality rate than with tartar emetic, largely due to shock, which may develop after the fourth or fifth dose.

Rapid elimination of eggs from the excreta occurs after a course of treatment but relapses are commoner than with tartar emetic. The drug works best in *S. haematobium* infections and is used as routine treatment of *S. japonicum* infections with some success in the Philippines.

Antimony lithium thiomalate (*Anthiomaline*) may also be given intramuscularly in doses equivalent to 20 mg. metallic antimony daily or every other day for 15–20 doses.

Antimony dimercaptosuccinate (*Astiban*, TWSb) is widely used and has had success in all forms of schistosome infections. It has the advantages over tartar emetic of being administered either intramuscularly or intravenously with relatively few side-effects. A few deaths have been reported during therapy with the drug. In *S. haematobium* infections it acts very quickly on the eggs and the egg-laying capacity of the female worms. It is less successful in the other infections. It is given in 10 per cent. solution in doses of up to 8 mg. per kg. (maximum single dose, 500 mg.) every other day for 5 doses. The maximum total dosage for adults is 2·5 G. Results with equivalent doses are very good in children.

Non-antimonial Compounds. Niridazole (*Ambilhar*) is a very effective antischistosomal drug recently introduced by Ciba. It is considered to be the drug of choice for treatment of *S. haematobium* infections in doses of 25 mg. per kg. body weight for 7 days.

It has been used extensively for treatment of *S. mansoni* infections and appears to be as good an antiparasitic drug as the antimonials. Similar satisfactory antiparasitic results have been reported in a limited number of *S. japonicum* infections.

Side-effects are common and usually mild. Anorexia, nausea, abdominal pain and occasionally vomiting have been recorded, but these are not more severe than with other antischistosomal drugs. They are reversible on withdrawal of the drug, but except in the circumstances noted below, this is seldom necessary.

In some patients reversible electrocardiographic changes occur on the 3rd–5th day of treatment and may persist for several days after treatment. Most workers regard these as not clinically significant.

In the treatment of *S. haematobium* infections the side-effects have been negligible and the drug can be given safely and effectively to outpatients. It is particularly well tolerated by children.

This is not always the case with other infections. Neuropsychiatric effects and changes in the electrocardiogram have been recorded in both *S. mansoni* and *S. japonicum* infections. These have included hallucinations, delirium, confusion and occasionally loss of consciousness and convulsions. There have been a few deaths but the effects are usually reversible on withdrawal of the drug; concurrent administration of barbiturates may reduce the severity of the neuropsychiatric side-effects.

It is generally agreed that these severe toxic effects occur most commonly in individuals with severe liver damage and fibrosis in whom collateral circulation has been established, allowing a higher systemic concentration of the drug to develop and possibly some concomitant failure of its metabolism in the liver. For this reason, the drug is regarded by some as having limited value in well developed or heavy *S. mansoni* or *S. japonicum* infections although it works well in light infections.

Thioxanthones have also been found to be effective against schistosomiasis, particularly *S. haematobium* infection.

Lucanthone (*Miracil D; Nilodin*) may be given in a total dosage of 60 mg. per kg. body weight over 3 days, in twice-daily doses of 10 mg. per kg. This regimen often causes side-effects and a lower daily dose given for a longer period is often substituted, such as 10 mg. per kg. for 10 days.

The drug has unpleasant side-effects including nausea, vomiting, epigastric pain, diarrhoea, giddiness, muscular twitchings, insomnia and depression. The skin may stain yellow. These effects make it very difficult to tolerate. Recently lucanthone has been combined with a resin to produce a compound which disintegrates slowly in the intestine, lowers the rate of absorption but not the ultimate effective level in the blood, and so reduces the side-effects very considerably.

Hycanthone, a hydroxymethyl perivative obtained from lucanthone by the action of *Aspergillus sclerotiorum* and said to be the active metabolite of lucanthone, is under trial in *S. haematobium* and *S. mansoni* infections. The drug is given in doses of 3 mg. per kg. body weight orally for 3 days or as a single injection of 3 mg. per kg. intramuscularly. Some side-effects including headache, giddiness and nausea have been noted after oral dosage but are less intense after intramuscular injection. Parasitological results are promising in both infections. Some deaths have been recorded.

Some success has been obtained in *S. haematobium* infections with the lucanthones, but the responses of the other infections have been poor. Relapse after treatment is common.

Mass Therapy. Mass therapy of schistosomiasis is used on a large scale to control the disease in endemic areas, especially in China and Egypt. In the latter tartar emetic is administered in the dosage regimen given above, for 12–16 doses. The results vary widely through the country and are best with *S. haematobium* infections.

The drug is injected as a 6 per cent. solution, often undiluted and quickly, with relatively few side-effects. As alternatives, *Astiban* and stibophen have been tried, also with good results.

Test of Cure

The definition of cure in an individual case depends on the effect of the treatment in removing eggs from the excreta. A most important factor is, of course, the possibility of reinfection.

In individuals who are not likely to be infected after treatment, the disappearance of eggs and their continued absence after three months (i.e. long enough to cover the first probable relapses) can usually be regarded as 'cure'. In those who become exposed again following treatment, eggs from new infections can appear at any time after about 6 weeks–2 months. To test the value of a drug, therefore, selected patients should be kept from infection for at least 3 months.

The results of treatment may be expressed as 'cure' (i.e. the absence of eggs in the excreta as determined by the usual techniques) or as 'reduction in egg output'. The latter, based on the quantitative examination of big samples, is the more reliable, and is independent of the initial egg output.

A few relapses, due to the survival of worms which were probably not fully developed at the time of treatment, may occur after 3 months.

Prevention and control of schistosomiasis depends on dealing with the human infection and controlling the vector snails. In the former, mass therapy with tartar emetic is the commonest procedure. This has had little effect on the incidence of the disease in the endemic areas concerned but has had a definite impression on the clinical patterns which have become milder. Snails are controlled by many methods, including the use of copper sulphate and organic compounds in the water in which they live and breed. The prospects of advance by means of medical and social education are slow, but in the long run, success could be achieved by change of human habits so that the infective faeces or urine were not allowed to reach water in which the eggs could hatch and the miracidia infect the snails.

SCHISTOSOMIASIS HAEMATOBIA

Synonyms. Urinary schistosomiasis or bilharziasis; Vesical schistosomiasis.

Aetiology

The disease arises from the presence of adults of *S. haematobium* in the vesical and pelvic venous plexuses.

Schistosomiasis haematobia is found only in Africa and the Middle East, except for a small focus near Bombay in India. The chief endemic area is the Nile Valley. The infection extends across the North African coastal areas to Morocco, through the Sudan and Ethiopia to large areas of East Africa, South Africa and Madagascar and Mauritius, across equatorial Africa to the west coast countries from Senegal to South West Africa. It is endemic in parts of Israel, parts of Saudi Arabia and the Yemen, Syria, Iraq and Iran. There are small endemic foci in Portugal and Cyprus.

Man is the main reservoir and in many areas the only reservoir; baboons and monkeys have been found naturally infected.

The principal intermediate host is the snail *Bulinus* spp. In some areas, for example in Portugal, *Planorbarius* sp. act as hosts.

Pathology

The development of the pathological changes following the laying of eggs and their escape into the tissues is described above. Because of the distribution of the egg-laying females, the lesions develop in the early stages primarily in the urinary bladder and ureters, later in the kidneys and the seminal vesicles and prostate or vagina, cervix and uterus. Eggs may be seeded to any part of the body and set up granulomatous reactions followed by fibrosis which may give rise to local clinical signs.

The characteristic changes are seen in the bladder. Eggs are deposited in venules in the walls, and penetrate into the tissues. Many pass through the mucosa into the urine, but many also remain in the local tissues and set up granulomatous reactions some of which break down and others are replaced by fibrous tissues. Eggs in the bladder wall commonly calcify after the death of the miracidia. In this way the bladder wall becomes irregularly granulomatous and fibrous, with loss of elasticity and considerable calcification contracture and limitation of volume. Granulomatous papules, polyps and inflammatory papillomata form on the surface, which may ulcerate, with considerable bleeding. Secondary infection is common and aggravates the condition by setting up chronic cystitis and by causing abscess formation in the bladder wall.

Lesions develop peripherally and the ureters, urethra and contiguous organs become involved in similar pathological processes. In the ureters there is frequently irregular dilatation and constriction in the lower third with scattered granulomata, eggs, calcification and fibrosis. Secondary infection may spread to these regions and ascend to the pelvis of the kidney. Hydronephrosis and pyonephrosis are not uncommon late sequels. It is generally agreed that there is some relationship between late schistosomal infection and the appearance of carcinoma of the bladder in some areas, notably Egypt.

Similar lesions develop in the pelvic organs and lead eventually to chronic fibrosis, with secondary infection, abscess and sinus formation; changes in the skin of the perineal region may occur and occasionally localized elephantiasis develops, for example in the penis.

Eggs are distributed widely in *S. haematobium* infections, but gross changes in organs other than those mentioned are unusual. Eggs are commonly found in granulomata in the rectal mucosa.

Signs and Symptoms

There may be some mild dermatitis at the site of entry of the cercariae, lasting a few days. Thereafter no further signs appear for about 3–6 weeks, when the allergic general reaction to the nearly mature worms becomes manifest, with fever (often daily peaks), malaise, cough and sometimes a papular or urticarial rash. There is an accompanying moderate eosinophilia. This syndrome is not usually severe and subsides in a few weeks; it may often be so mild as to be unnoticed.

Eggs may appear in the urine from 6 weeks onwards after infection. At first they are unaccompanied by local signs or symptoms, but in the course of a few more weeks or months these begin to develop. The first signs are often frequency with some urgency and tenderness over the bladder. Blood appears in the urine at the end of micturition and later may be present in the whole specimen passed. Clots are common and may cause considerable discomfort when passed. Pus is usually present by the time the haematuria is well established and may precede it. At this stage there are often episodes of acute cystitis with the usual symptoms.

As the bladder lesions develop, frequency increases, micturition may become precipitate and there is incontinence with persistent dribbling, as the volume of the bladder is reduced by contraction and ultimately by calcification of the wall, which can readily be seen radiologically. Signs of involvement of other organs gradually develop. The ureters become tortuous and irregularly dilated and constricted, pyelitis may succeed the chronic cystitis and eventually signs of pyelonephrosis may appear and be followed by anaemia. Inflammatory granulomatous masses may form almost anywhere in the pelvic tissues.

The progress of the clinical picture depends on many factors, some of which appear to be governed by the geographical locality in which the infection occurs. Thus the pattern in Egypt is usually much more advanced than elsewhere in Africa, probably because of the intensity of infection and reinfection. In many parts of East and West Africa only minimal effects are suffered by infected individuals. Infection is seen most commonly in children, who seem little affected even when haematuria is present and pathological changes in the bladder and uterus advanced. On the other hand, single fresh infections in completely non-immune Europeans often produce severe early signs and urinary and vesical symptoms which demand urgent treatment.

Carcinoma of the bladder is common in some *S. haematobium* endemic areas, and many authorities consider there is a causal relationship.

Diagnosis

For identification of eggs in urine and rectal biopsy, see above.

The maximum output of eggs in the urine occurs during activity. The most satisfactory specimens for finding eggs are therefore urine samples collected between 10.00 and 14.00 hours. Such samples are more reliable than those taken at the end of micturition, as formerly advised.

Cystoscopy is commonly employed to examine the lesions in the bladder and is a useful method of checking progress. Lesions in the bladder are most conspicuous in the trigone, where whitish bilharzial tubercles may be seen in early cases. These ulcerate and extend to form papillomata, which may become extensive, with bleeding ulcerated surfaces. In these regions and sometimes scattered irregularly over the surface there occur the characteristic 'sandy patches', or areas of roughened hard mucosa filled with calcified eggs. Biopsy of the bladder wall will reveal typical granuloma formation, fibrosis and necrosis, with eggs containing living miracidia or eggs which are calcified.

Radiological methods will reveal the changes in the bladder and ureters. Marked calcification of the bladder wall, with considerable reduction in volume, motility and contractility, is a common finding in severe late cases.

Carcinoma cells may sometimes be found in the urine.

Treatment

This infection responds better than the others to chemotherapy [see above for details]. Regression of lesions may occur in the absence of treatment.

The anatomical local damage to the bladder, ureters and pelvic organs only occasionaly require surgical operation. Control of secondary infection is essential, and should be obtained by the administration of wide-spectrum or specific antibiotics. The cystitis responds to the usual methods of therapy; considerable relief is obtained by controlling this infection and keeping the urine alkaline with citrates.

SCHISTOSOMIASIS MANSONI

Synonyms. Intestinal schistosomiasis; Intestinal bilharziasis; Bilharziasis mansoni.

Aetiology

The disease results from infection with *Schistosoma mansoni*, the adults of which live principally in the inferior mesenteric veins of the large intestine.

Schistosomiasis mansoni occurs in Africa and in parts of the West Indies and South America to which it was imported by the slave trade. It is present in Africa in many of the areas in which *S. haematobium* occurs, but is more localized. Foci have been found in a few parts of the Middle East, for example in Saudi Arabia and the Yemen, but it is much less common there than *S. haematobium* infection. There are endemic areas in Brazil, Venezuela and Surinam and in certain West Indian islands, including Puerto Rico, Dominica, St. Lucia and Martinique.

As a result of migration from Puerto Rico to North America, the disease is commonly met in certain big cities in the latter, notably New York.

Man is the main reservoir, but in some areas it is possible that the infection may be a zoonosis, with baboons, monkeys or rodents as animal hosts.

The principal intermediate hosts are the snails *Biomphalaria* spp. in Africa and *Australorbis* spp. in the Western hemisphere.

Pathology

The basic pathological changes have been described above. The distribution of the oviparous females leads to initial concentration of the lesions in the intestinal walls and contiguous structures. In the walls of the large intestine and lower small intestine characteristic granulomata form with mucosal changes not unlike those in the bladder, leading to irregular thickening, ulceration and haemorrhage, the formation of granulomatous papillomata, and extensive fibrosis, sometimes with narrowing of the lumen. Secondary bacterial infection is common.

Eggs are carried freely to the liver and become caught up in the finer lateral branches of the portal veins and venules. The usual cellular granulomata are developed around them and after the death of the embryo, fibrotic replacement commonly occurs. The result, over a long period and when the seeding of eggs has been heavy, is the development of an extensive characteristic periportal fibrosis which leads in severe cases to steadily rising portal venous pressure and the picture of portal hypertension. In this syndrome one of the earliest signs is increase in the size of the spleen. This organ enlarges progressively and may eventually occupy most of the left half of the abdominal cavity. The combination of the enlarged irregularly fibrosed liver and the enlarged spleen is commonly called 'Egyptian hepatosplenomegaly'.

Eggs commonly escape into the lungs, often during the early stages of the disease, and evoke granulomatous reactions which cause the prolongation of the early clinical signs of infection. Later they may cause arteriolar fibrosis and pulmonary circulatory obstruction, leading to the picture of pulmonary hypertension and cor pulmonale. Severe lung damage in the late stages is usually associated with hepatic fibrosis and portal hypertension and there is evidence that when the latter has developed, the collateral circulations allow the easier access of eggs to the lungs.

Eggs may form ectopic lesions in any part of the body. They may be found for instance in the brain or cord, kidneys and myocardium. The skin may be involved.

Signs and Symptoms

Penetration of cercariae may produce a temporary dermatitis. The allergic reaction which occurs 3–6 weeks later, is often severe, with onset of fever, sometimes with rigors and heavy sweating, nausea, vomiting, abdominal discomfort with fullness over the liver, which may be tender and slightly enlarged, diarrhoea and a dry unproductive cough with dyspnoea. An urticarial or papular rash may develop. The patient feels ill and prostrated. This stage may continue for some weeks.

Eggs are excreted 6 weeks–2 months from the time of infection and may be found in smears of the diarrhoeic stool. The development from this stage depends on egg deposition in the tissues and the reaction to them.

In the early stages the clinical pictures are sometimes divided clinically into the dysenteric and the hepatosplenic, with all variations between. In the former there is diarrhoea with blood and mucus, abdominal pain and discomfort, loss of weight and anaemia. Eggs are easily found in the dysenteric stool. In the hepatosplenic variant, there is more abdominal discomfort and progressive enlargement of the liver and the spleen. Eosinophilia is moderate. Another common form which is seen in Egypt is one in which the pulmonary signs are prominent, and eggs may be found in the sputum. Patients with pulmonary involvement commonly cough up sputum streaked with blood, and may do so at irregular intervals through the course of the illness, even when it is moderate rather than severe.

The acute picture usually settles in a few weeks and there may be periods of recrudescence and remission for some time until the clinical results of the intestinal damage and complications such as portal hypertension become manifest.

The colon becomes thickened, tender and spastic, especially in the sigmoidal and caecal regions, and can often be easily palpated. The liver is usually palpable and tender.

The affected gut mucosa ulcerates and secondary infection occurs and the patient suffers from periodic bouts of dysentery in which, in addition to mucus and blood, there may be notable amounts of pus and epithelial debris. In some areas of the large intestine the granulomatous and inflammatory reactions may cause the production of polyps which may be visible on sigmoidoscopy and which may prolapse when in the lower rectum. Tumours which can be palpated as tender masses are particularly common in the caecal and sigmoidal areas. These may cause the patient considerable discomfort and present radiological pictures which may be easily mistaken for other inflammatory masses such as amoeboma or even for carcinoma. Patients with long-standing pericolic lesions often develop pronounced clubbing of the fingers, even in the absence of pulmonary complications.

In the late stages fibrosis of the gut wall may lead to considerable constriction of the lumen and obstruction to faecal passage, the picture closely resembling that of carcinoma.

Periportal fibrosis in the liver leads to the syndrome of portal hypertension in many advanced cases, with great splenic enlargement, ascites, the establishment of superficial and deep collateral circulation, visible on the abdominal and chest walls and presenting as dilatations and varices of the veins of the lower oesophagus and the stomach. These varices may give rise to serious haemorrhages which may be fatal.

Pulmonary arterial hypertension not infrequently accompanies the syndrome of portal hypertension. It may develop independently. Eggs are found in the bloody sputum.

In highly endemic areas the disease takes on a serious form in individuals constantly exposed to infection and reinfection. In other regions it may produce comparatively few clinical effects. Again, it would seem that the intensity of the infection is the governing factor in the development of the clinical picture.

Diagnosis

Methods of identifying the characteristic lateral-spined eggs in the faeces and in intestinal biopsies are described above.

The examination of the patient by sigmoidoscopy or proctoscopy is indicated. Eggs are commonly found in rectal snips.

In the differential diagnosis, other causes of pericolic tumour, distortion and constriction must be eliminated, especially carcinoma.

Treatment

S. mansoni infection responds less favourably than *S. haematobium* infection to treatment with antimonials, of which sodium antimony tartrate and *Astiban* are the most satisfactory. Niridazole is effective but toxic effects may be serious in cases with hepatic fibrosis.

Lucanthone (*Miracil D*) is not a satisfactory alternative.

Treatment of complications is very important. Splenectomy relieves some cases of portal hypertension in the early or middle stages and some success has been obtained by tying the hepatic artery in advanced cases.

The treatment of the syndrome of portal hypertension as a whole is carried out on the usual lines. Antischistosomal treatment in a patient with severe hepatic fibrosis and collateral circulation may seed the systemic blood with dead or dying worms which may also reach the liver. A decision on whether to treat the infection or not will have to be reached in each individual case on its merits. Most cases benefit by treatment.

SCHISTOSOMIASIS JAPONICA

Synonyms. Asiatic schistosomiasis; Katayama disease; Yangtze River fever.

Aetiology

The disease is caused by *S. japonicum* the adults of which inhabit the small branches of the superior and inferior mesenteric veins.

It is limited to the Far East in parts of China (especially the Yangtze basin), Japan, the Philippines and Celebes. In these areas it is endemic and enzootic. In Formosa it occurs only as an enzootic. In a small focus in southern Thailand a few human cases have been found but transmission has stopped. An active focus has been found recently in Khong Island in South Laos; this may be a menace in the proposed local irrigation programmes which are part of the larger Mekong River development scheme.

S. japonicum infects many animals readily and in most of the endemic areas these creatures act as important reservoirs of infection. Animals of particular importance in this respect are the domestic water buffalo and cattle, dogs, cats, pigs and rodents.

The intermediate snail host is the amphibious *Oncomelania* spp. which inhabits irrigation canals, slow-flowing streams, and ditches, and contiguous fresh-water swamps and pools.

Pathology

S. japonicum produces the most severe form of schistosomiasis in man. The female lays many more eggs than that of the other species. The general reactions are the same as in the other infections. The pathological lesions are primarily developed in the intestinal walls but are widespread. The general development is similar to that in *S. mansoni* infection. The liver is involved early and severely as in *S. mansoni* infection and the picture of enlarged liver and spleen, with portal hypertension, ascites and the development of collateral circulation with gastro-oesophageal varices is common. Pulmonary hypertension and fibrosis is less common and ectopic lesions in the central nervous system much more common than in *S. mansoni* infections.

Signs and Symptoms

There may be some dermatitis at the point of entry of the cercariae. The general allergic reaction occurs early, sometimes within a fortnight of infection and is severe with swinging fever, often urticaria and subcutaneous oedema, nausea, vomiting, diarrhoea, liver tenderness and enlargement. There is often tenderness along the region of the large intestine and the colon may be palpable, especially in the sigmoidal region. Signs of bronchitis or scattered bronchopneumonia are common with a dry cough and dyspnoea. Radiologically this stage appears as scattered mottling of variable size.

The reaction lasts for some weeks and is associated with a high eosinophilia.

This toxaemic picture is sometimes called Yangtze River fever or Katayama fever.

As the disease progresses the changes in the intestines lead to dysenteric signs and symptoms which are severe but intermittent. Eggs are commonly present in the bloody mucoid stool. There are bouts of remittent or intermittent fever. The colon becomes palpable and tender. The liver and spleen are enlarged and tender and in the later stages the picture of hepatosplenomegaly with portal hypertension commonly develops. The high eosinophilia which develops in the early febrile stage is considerably reduced as the disease progresses.

Haematemesis, melaena and hepatic intoxication and coma are common in advanced cases.

At all levels of infection, the disease caused by *S. japonicum* is more severe and progressive than the other forms of human schistosomiasis. Complications due to ectopic distribution of eggs are common, especially in the brain, where space-occupying tumours result from ectopic eggs and sometimes adults. The neurological accompanying signs depend on the locality of the lesion.

Diagnosis

Eggs are usually easier to find in the stools than in *S. mansoni* infections but concentration methods rather than direct examination of faecal smears are usually necessary. Rectal snips are useful.

Treatment

This is the most difficult infection to treat. So far, tartar emetic either parenterally or orally has given the best results. The long course of 16 doses or its equivalent in antimony content, is needed. Good results have been obtained with *Astiban* and with stibophen.

The allergic febrile syndromes which occur during the maturation of worms are sometimes relieved by cortisone or prednisolone in corresponding doses.

Treatment of complications is non-specific.

REFERENCES

Cowper, S. G. (1971) *A Synopsis of African Bilharziasis*, London.

Jordan, P., and Webbe, G. (1969) *Human Schistosomiasis* London.

CESTODES

THE CYCLOPHYLLIDIAN TAPE WORMS

The commonest cestode worms which infect man in the tropics and subtropics are the Cyclophyllidian tape worms *Taenia saginata* and *Taenia solium*, the dwarf tape worms *Hymenolepis nana* and *H. diminuta*, and the dog tape worms *Echinococcus granulosus* and *E. multilocularis*. With the exception of *Echinococcus* spp. which occurs solely in the larval form in man and the adult form in animals, all these worms develop as adults in man. *T. solium* also occurs in the larval form in man.

The presence of the adult worm in the gut seldom causes serious consequences, although there may occasionally be some ill health and possibly loss of weight.

Most of the large tape worms occur as single infections but multiple infections are possible. In the case of the dwarf tape worms *Hymenolepis* multiple infections are usual.

In all adult infections the worms attach themselves by the head to the small intestinal mucosa. They have no buccal cavity or alimentary tract and absorb their nutriment through the integument. The body of the worm, which is composed of large numbers of segments or strobila, hangs down along the lumen of the intestine. The presence of the adult worm is usually discovered accidentally by the passage of segments in the faeces. Allergic manifestations may occur occasionally in the host but are unusual.

INFECTION WITH TAENIA SAGINATA

The common beef tape worm is a human parasite and is found in wide areas of the world. The large, white and ribbon-like regularly segmented worm may measure more than 20 feet in length, the broadest segments being three-quarters of an inch across. The head is minute and provided with four sucking discs without hooks. With these it attaches itself to the mucosa of the small intestine. From the neck immature segments develop continuously and are pushed down by the formation of further segments which may eventually number a thousand. The mature segments are hermaphrodite. Fertilization occurs and the uterus of the fertilized segments become loaded with eggs. The gravid segments break off from the lower end of the worm as active and contractile units which escape separately through the anus or are passed in the stool.

The patient usually becomes aware of the infection by discovering the escaping segment.

The diagnosis of the species of tape worm is made by examining the segment after immersion in water and compression between glass plates. The uterus has a central stem with up to 20 lateral branches, mostly containing eggs. The genital pore is lateral.

It is important to differentiate *T. saginata* from *T. solium* infection in which the larval forms may exist in man. The larval forms of *T. saginata* are not found in man. In the ordinary course of events the segments do not discharge eggs until after passage to the surface. The eggs so passed or liberated by the disintegration of gravid segments are swallowed by cattle in the intestine of which the larvae are liberated and pass to the tissues, where cysts (cysticerci) are formed containing the head of the future adult. Beef containing these organisms is called 'measly'. On the consumption of such beef the intestinal infection with the adult *T. saginata* develops in man.

Diagnosis

Diagnosis is made by examining the gravid segments. Eggs are found in the faeces in relatively few cases, since they are liberated only after the segment has been damaged or has escaped from the body.

Treatment

Formerly, male fern extract was used with a good deal of success. Modern treatment is more effective and less toxic.

Mepacrine is commonly used. The patient is starved for 24 hours and given a barbiturate. A tube is passed and left overnight so that the end reaches the duodenum. On the following morning 1 G. of mepacrine hydrochloride in 100 ml. of warm water is introduced through the tube by means of a syringe and half an hour later 2 oz. of magnesium sulphate in warm water is introduced in the same way. The tube is then withdrawn and a warm drink is given.

Within one to two hours the deeply stained and contracted intact worm is commonly passed.

The same dose of mepacrine may be given by mouth but usually causes vomiting.

Dichlorophen (*Antiphen*) has been used successfully. An effective dose is 6 G. orally as a single dose, or the same dose on each of two successive days. No previous preparation of the patient is necessary; the drug sometimes causes colic and transient mild diarrhoea. This drug breaks up the segments of the worm so that the gravid segments alone are passed immediately after treatment. The head is not passed and is destroyed *in situ*. It is therefore difficult to determine immediately whether the parasite has been eradicated for at least 3 months after treatment.

The synthetic drug niclosamide (*Yomesan*) is successful in doses of 2 tablets, each containing 500 mg. given orally and repeated after an hour. A purge is given the following day when large portions of the worm (but not the scolex) are usually passed. The action on the worm is similar to that of dichlorophen.

INFECTION WITH TAENIA SOLIUM

In its developmental stages this worm follows much the same course as *T. saginata*. The infection is acquired by eating 'measly' pork containing cysticercal larvae

(*Cysticercus cellulosae*) developed in the animal tissues following the ingestion of eggs.

The development of the adult in man is similar to that of *T. saginata*.

CYSTICERCOSIS

Unfortunately when man swallows eggs of *T. solium*, cysticerci develop in his tissues in the same way as in the pig. The larvae liberated after ingestion of the eggs penetrate the intestinal mucosa and are carried by the circulation to all parts of the body. They are eventually caught somewhere and encyst. When cysts develop in sensitive physiological centres such as the brain localizing signs and symptoms may develop. For example, cysts in the brain may lead to attacks of Jacksonian epilepsy or other neurological signs.

Cysticerci also develop in connective tissue and voluntary muscles. Damage is seldom caused until the worm has died and tissue reaction has taken place around it. After death the cysticerci commonly become calcified. Lesions which result from cysticerci may produce symptoms many years after the infection. The possibility of cysticercosis must always be considered in individuals who have lived in areas in which the tape worm is common. The prognosis in cerebral cases is bad so far as cure is concerned, but a fatal issue is uncommon.

In some patients cysticercosis complicates intestinal infestation. The disintegration or damage to gravid segments, forced by reverse peristalsis into the stomach, is sometimes thought to account for such auto-infection, but it is probable that the patient reinfects himself with eggs liberated from damaged segments in the lower bowel.

Diagnosis

Diagnosis is made by the discovery and examination of the gravid segments of the worm after passage via the anus or in the stool, or by the identification of adult worms discharged after treatment. In gravid segments, the uterus has a central stem with 8–10 lateral branches. The head of the worm is about 1 mm. in diameter and is armed with two rows of hooks.

Diagnosis of cysticercosis depends on palpation of cysticerci under the skin or their discovery by biopsy or X-ray of the limbs for the detection of calcified cysts. X-rays of the skull do not usually reveal cysts which may be present in the brain.

Treatment

The treatment recommended for *T. saginata* is effective with *T. solium*. Although dichlorophen and *Yomesan* cause disintegration of segments which may lead to the escape of large numbers of eggs in the stool, and could thus lead to the development of cysticercosis following ingestion, there seems to be no contra-indication for their use.

Treatment of cysticercosis is palliative. The drugs used for the treatment of the adult worms have no obvious effect. This is particularly true in the case of epileptic effects.

INFECTION WITH HYMENOLEPIS NANA AND HYMENOLEPIS DIMINUTA

The dwarf tape worms are cosmopolitan in distribution.

Infections occur largely in dirty environments.

H. nana is a small worm measuring less than 5 cm. in length and about 1 mm. in breadth. The head is provided with 4 suckers and a ring of hooks, with which the adult attaches itself to the intestinal wall. The gravid segments liberate eggs which are passed in the faeces.

Infection results from swallowing the embryonated eggs and there is thus no larval cycle in an intermediate host. Other animals besides man are infected, including rats and mice, but normally the infection is passed from man to man. Auto-infection is common.

Infection is usually multiple and occasionally very heavy.

Heavy infections give rise to severe diarrhoea and toxaemia with nervous symptoms particularly in children, in whom convulsions are common.

H. diminuta is a common parasite of small rodents and is rarely found in man. It is larger than *H. nana* and requires an intermediate arthropod host in which it occurs as a cysticercus. The rat flea *Xenopsylla cheopis*, the common vector of plague, is one of the hosts of this tape worm. Man becomes infected by accidentally swallowing the flea. Multiple infections are common and the diagnosis is made by finding the eggs in the stools.

Treatment of hymenolepis infections is as for other tape worms.

HYDATID INFECTION

Aetiology and Pathology

Infection with the unilocular cyst of *Echinococcus granulosus* is widespread in an irregular way throughout the world and is particularly common in cattle- or sheep-rearing countries, such as Argentina, South Africa and Australia. It occurs in many parts of Europe and the Middle East.

Infection with the multilocular cysts of *Echinococcus multilocularis* (*E. alveolaris*) is much more restricted and is largely confined to Middle and Eastern Europe. Infections have been reported from South America, Australia and England (one case).

The adult worm lives in the small intestine of the definitive host, usually the dog, the fox, the wolf or the cat. The animals become infected by ingesting viscera of the intermediate hosts, including cattle and sheep, which are infected with the larvae of the worm. Eggs are discharged in the faeces of the definitive hosts and are swallowed by man following direct contamination especially from dogs.

After the egg is swallowed the larva escapes into the duodenum and migrates through the intestinal wall. It is carried away in the mesenteric vessels and becomes lodged in tissue capillaries particularly in the liver and the lungs. Larvae may survive and develop slowly in the tissues over many years as 'hydatid' cysts.

The cyst of *E. granulosus* is unilocular. It has a double wall composed of an outer laminated layer and an inner nucleated so-called 'germinal' layer. From this latter are budded off rounded cellular masses which eventually themselves become cystic. These are the so-called 'brood capsules' from the inner walls of which the heads of the worm (scolices with rostellar hooklets) bud and invaginate. The capsules may remain attached to the parent cyst or float free in the milky fluid contents forming the so-called 'hydatid sand'. If the wall of the original cyst or 'mother cyst' is ruptured, the brood capsules or daughter cysts escape and may become seeded in contiguous tissue or elsewhere where they develop into further hydatid cysts. There is usually a vigorous fibrotic reaction around the cyst, which becomes encapsulated; in the late stages the capsule may become calcified, providing a highly characteristic X-ray picture.

In some areas of the world the cysts are multilocular. Infection with such cysts produces slightly different clinical effects and it is usual to regard the worm which gives rise to them as a separate subspecies *E. multilocularis* which infects carnivores including the fox, and rodents. In multilocular cyst infections the reaction of the host is more vigorous but with less fibrosis. The cysts contain many small cavities filled with fluid containing broken membrane and occasionally scolices. Central necrosis of such lesions is common, but fibrous capsulation is incomplete.

Signs and Symptoms

The clinical effects of the presence of a hydatid cyst are commonly the results of local pressure or immunosensitivity reactions arising from the host reaction to antigens in the worm or its products.

When the larva becomes established in the tissues it is surrounded by cellular infiltration, largely lymphocytes, plasma cells and eosinophils. A granulomatous mass is formed and later a cellular fibrous tissue develops and encapsulates the cyst, the walls of which may eventually calcify.

Pus appears only if the dead larva becomes secondarily infected. Where the cyst is developing local tissue damage may occur with associated functional disturbances, but large cysts may develop in the liver or the lungs without causing prominent physical signs and may be discovered by accident. In some regions of the body, however, growing cysts may give rise to clinical signs at an early stage. This is particularly true in bone, in which both kinds of cysts become cellular, syncytial and may invade the bone structure leading to erosion and sometimes spontaneous fracture.

Hydatid cyst is one of the classical causes of hepatomegaly which may be symptomless and which must be differentiated from amoebic liver involvement or hepatic tumour.

Large cysts give rise to signs resulting from compression which are seen most commonly in the liver or the lungs. In the latter they may be associated with pleural effusion or with rupture of the cyst into a bronchus, which leads to the sudden coughing up of quantities of saline fluid containing cyst debris and not infrequently to an acute and sometimes very severe anaphylactic reaction. After rupture of such a cyst the daughter cysts may spread ectopically.

Alveolar hydatid may develop in the lungs and other organs, sometimes in bones. The common site is the liver in which it forms a spongy very slow-growing tumour which becomes necrotic centrally and spreads peripherally. Metastatic parasitic lesions are common and the general picture resembles a slowly developing carcinoma. It is believed that many infections recorded at autopsy in adults were probably acquired in childhood. The prognosis is very bad.

Echinococcal infection produces immunosensitivity in the host in which violent anaphylactic reactions may develop following leakage of cyst fluid into the tissues.

There is eosinophilia which may rise sharply during anaphylactic crises.

Diagnosis

Diagnosis is often made by physical signs plus the Casoni skin reaction in which 0·1 ml. of an antigen prepared from sterile hydatid fluid is injected intradermally into the arm of the suspected individual. A positive reaction develops within 15–20 minutes forming a large wheal with many pseudopodia and several centimetres in diameter, surrounded by a brilliant red arteriolar flare.

The complement fixation reaction may also help, using the same antigen; the test is highly specific.

The examination of suspected tissues by X-ray may be helpful in cases where the cyst walls become calcified or in cases involving bone.

Treatment

Most cases of well developed hydatid cyst require surgical treatment but explorations should never be carried out until precautions have been taken to prevent the fluid from escaping into the tissues. It is wise, for instance, when dealing with a cyst in the liver to aspirate first and fill the cavity with a weak solution of formalin. Tissue contamination at subsequent operation can be prevented by various surgical techniques including marsupialization. This is particularly important when operating on cysts of the liver through the thoracic wall. The escape of any quantity of fluid from the cyst in a highly sensitized person may lead to very grave anaphylaxis. Facilities for dealing with such emergencies should therefore always be available and aspiration, etc., should not be performed except where surgical help is immediately available.

No drugs have any specific effect on this infection.

THE PSEUDOPHYLLIDIAN TAPE WORMS

These constitute the other great group of tape worms which infect man. The most important is the fish tape worm *Diphyllobothrium latum* which occurs around the Finnish lakes and the Caspian Sea.

INFECTION WITH DIPHYLLOBOTHRIUM LATUM

Aetiology

Man becomes infected by ingesting uncooked fish flesh containing the larval stage of the parasite, the so-called *sparganum*. The adult worm is sometimes over 30 feet in length and takes three months to mature. It lives, like the other tape worms, in the small intestine attached to the mucosa by a small head which contains suckers but no hooks. Infection with more than one adult at a time is not uncommon.

Other hosts carrying the adult are the dog, the pig and the cat and allied species. The definitive host passes faeces containing eggs which mature in water and eventually hatch producing a larva which is taken up by a copepod, usually *Cyclops* species. In these copepods the so-called procercoid stage develops. When the copepod is ingested by fresh water fish the procercoid larva escapes and encysts in muscle tissue as the plerocercoid phase or sparganum.

Signs and Symptoms

The clinical picture in man is gastro-intestinal and may include acute abdominal pain and discomfort with diarrhoea. There may be emaciation and convulsions in children, a high degree of eosinophilia, localized oedema and other manifestations of allergy. In a few cases megaloblastic anaemia resembling pernicious anaemia may develop, resulting from competition between the worm and the host for vitamin B_{12}.

Diagnosis

Diagnosis is made by the identification of the operculated thick-shelled yellow eggs in the faeces or of the adult worm after treatment.

Treatment

Treatment is the same as for other tape worms. The anaemia responds to administration of vitamin B_{12} or the removal of the worm.

INFECTION WITH DIPHYLLOBOTHRIUM MANSONI

Man may also become infected with *Diphyllobothrium mansoni* as a result of ingestion of the larvae in raw fish, frogs, fowls or snakes.

Infection of the tissues sometimes results from direct contact with flesh containing spargana; for example, when raw meat is used as a poultice. The sparganum may develop in practically any tissue of the body except bone. There is some cellular reaction around the larva which may move from place to place. When the larva dies the cellular reaction increases and it may be replaced by pus. In this way large abscesses may form particularly in loose tissue such as the orbit. The affected region is inflamed, swollen and intensely painful. It is said that elephantiasis may occasionally result from subsequent lymphatic obstruction.

In such forms of sparganosis treatment is local. Ethyl alcohol is sometimes injected together with local anaesthetic and the subcutaneous lesions are excised. One form of sparganum proliferates by branching and may result in very extensive lesions in which local treatment is valueless.

Under such conditions some success has been obtained by the use of arsenicals. The results of using more modern drugs are not presently available.

NEMATODES

FILARIASIS

Definition

Filariasis occurs in man as a result of infection with certain filarial worms including *Wuchereria bancrofti*, *Brugia malayi*, *Loa loa* and *Onchocerca volvulus*. Infections with *Wuchereria bancrofti* and *Brugia malayi* are commonly called bancroftian and Malayan filariasis respectively. *Loa loa* produces a clinical condition called loiasis, and *Onchocerca volvulus*, onchocerciasis.

A general reaction commonly called tropical eosinophilia consisting of pulmonary symptoms and high eosinophilia often results from the presence in the human tissues of unadapted filarial larvae. This syndrome, which may arise from other causes, is described elsewhere [see p. 267].

BANCROFTIAN AND MALAYAN FILARIASIS

Aetiology and Pathology

Bancroftian filariasis is spread widely in the tropics and subtropics, from the West Indies, South America as far south as the Argentine, southern Spain, the African Mediterranean seaboard, West, Central and East Africa, the islands adjacent to Africa, including Madagascar, the Middle East, India, South East Asia, Southern China, Korea, Indonesia, Northern Australia and certain Pacific islands including Samoa and Fiji. Until recently it existed in the southern and south-western United States.

The distribution of Malayan filariasis is more restricted. In some areas it occurs alone, in others it overlaps the bancroftian infection, for example, in Indonesia. It is found in India, Ceylon, South East Asia, and New Guinea, either widespread or in relatively circumscribed areas.

The development of the worms in man in the two infections is the same. It takes six months or longer for the larva to develop to the adult stage. The adults survive in the human for years. They are fine, filiform worms up to 10 cm. long, lying coiled in lymphatics and lymph nodes especially in the region of the pelvis and the genitalia. Females produce sheathed embryos in large numbers which eventually reach the blood stream and appear in the peripheral blood.

Periodicity of Microfilariae

In many endemic areas the microfilariae of *W. bancrofti* appear in the peripheral blood in greatest numbers at night, between 10 p.m. and 2 a.m. and are scarce or absent during the day.

The explanation of this nocturnal periodicity is not known but it is extremely useful from the point of view of diagnosis and is probably important in relation to the infection of vectors. In some areas in the Pacific the microfilariae of *W. bancrofti* do not have a nocturnal periodicity and may be found during the day.

Transmission of bancroftian filariasis is carried on by mosquitoes, the most widely distributed vectors being species of *Culex*, *Aëdes* and *Anopheles*. The common vector in many areas is *Culex fatigans*.

The periodicity of the microfilariae in Malayan filariasis is similar in some respects to that of bancroftian filariasis but recently two forms of periodicity have been recognized, representing epidemiologically distinct microfilariae.

The 'periodic' form of Malayan filariasis which has the usual nocturnal periodicity is transmitted by certain species of *Mansonia* breeding in water containing the water-lettuce *Pistia* or other plants, and by species of *Anopheles* breeding in pools and ditches. This form of filariasis is found in deforested and swampy areas, such as rice fields, suitable for the breeding of the vectors. Man is infected easily but animals only with difficulty. Man is therefore regarded as the only significant reservoir.

The 'semiperiodic' or 'subperiodic' form of microfilaria of *Brugia malayi* reaches maximum numbers in the peripheral blood during the day or early evening and may be present throughout the day. It is transmitted almost exclusively by certain species of *Mansonia* which breed in forest swamps. It can be transmitted to wild animals including monkeys and to domestic animals, including dogs and cats. These animals thus constitute important reservoirs of infection and have to be considered in planning measures to control transmission.

Transmission

The vector becomes infected by ingesting blood containing infective microfilariae. These escape from their sheathes, penetrate the wall of the insect's gut and are eventually transformed to the infective larvae which reach the proboscis in 2–3 weeks. The flies are then infective and transmit infection by passing the larvae to man during the bite.

In a given area transmission depends on the presence of a sufficient number of suitable vectors, an adequate reservoir of infection (usually human), and an adequate infection rate in the vectors.

The human reservoir is infective to mosquitoes during only part of the clinical disease, since infective microfilariae appear in the blood during the inflammatory and early obstructive stages and not usually in the later stages. In the advanced stages of elephantiasis microfilariae are rarely present and the patients are non-infective.

In some areas the human reservoirs may consist principally of individuals with little or no clinical reaction but with large numbers of microfilariae circulating in the blood.

Pathogenesis of Filarial Infections

It is generally agreed that continued reinfection over a long period is necessary for the full development of the clinical picture, which occurs much more commonly in indigenes than in visitors. There is no racial immunity but some acquired resistance is developed and the consequent immunosensitivity reactions play an important part in the pathogenesis of certain features of the disease.

Differences in age and sex incidence in endemic areas depend largely on differences in opportunities of infection.

The clinical consequences of infection and the presence of microfilariae in the blood are seldom recorded in very young children under the age of two years, although they may occasionally occur earlier.

The full manifestations of the disease develop in youth or early adult life. Certain features such as hydrocele or elephantiasis persist throughout life.

In all filarial infections the background of the pathogenesis is the infection with the adult worm and subsequently with the microfilariae. In some infections, for example in bancroftian and Malayan filariasis, the adult is the major pathogenic agent. In other forms of filariasis the main factor may be the microfilariae. Sometimes both are involved; this is to a varying degree true of all infections.

In addition to the mechanical and structural tissue changes caused by the adult worms or microfilariae, an immunosensitivity state is induced in the host by the infection which explains many of the clinical and pathological manifestations. The manifestations of the immunosensitivity state vary from one infection to another and from one case to another, but in all infections allergic phenomena occur, which may vary from localized oedema to severe anaphylaxis and appear histologically as tissue reactions dominated by eosinophils associated with a high eosinophil count in the peripheral blood. The effects of some infections may also be influenced locally by secondary bacterial infection.

In one way or another these processes play a part in the development of all filarial infections, although the resultant clinical pictures differ considerably and must therefore be examined separately.

Pathology

In the pathology of bancroftian and Malayan filariasis the basic phenomena are similar. The adults inhabit lymphatic vessels and nodes. The microfilariae are first expelled into these areas and later into the blood stream. The most marked reactions occur in the lymphatics and nodes and are believed to be brought about more by the presence of the adults than the microfilariae. The local tissue responses probably occur in areas where the passage of the worm is obstructed or where the worm has been injured or has died and begun to degenerate. Local reactions often occur, however, in areas in which no current trace of the worm can be found.

The development of the disease falls naturally into three phases, the inflammatory, the obstructive and elephantiasis.

In the *inflammatory stage* the characteristic lesion is an acute granulomatous lymphangitis which progresses slowly but is subject to exacerbations, causing very acute lymphangitis characterized by perivascular infiltration with lymphocytes and eosinophils. At this stage the vessels are palpable and may be exquisitely tender.

A non-specific reticulo-endothelial reaction occurs around dead worms with the formation of epithelioid cells and giant cells. Local abscesses may form in vessels or glands if secondary infection ensues and may discharge through the skin.

In the ordinary course of events cellular granulomatous tissue accumulates and gives rise to nodules which press on the lumen of the lymphatics and may obstruct them. The endothelium may also become hypertrophic, leading to lymphothrombosis and endovascular occlusion. Eventually the granulomatous tissue and the occluded vessels are replaced by fibrous tissue.

Associated with the acute exacerbations are some local soft or hard oedema and erythema of the skin, which is usually linear when lymphatics are involved.

The *obstructive phase* develops gradually. Affected lymphatics become dilated, tense with lymph and distorted, producing varices, associated with nodules of granulomatous tissue, so that the area appears as a lobulated, irregular, subcutaneous mass.

Obstruction arises from interference with the flow of lymph from the area which the affected vessels drain. Sometimes dilated lymph vessels may rupture into the surrounding tissues or into a hollow viscus, producing local signs such as ascites.

Lesions similar to those in the vessels develop in the lymph nodes and further obstruction to local lymph flow is created in this way. The obstruction leads to localized oedema which is at first soft but later becomes firm and persistent. Gradually the tissues involved take on the appearance of elephantiasis.

Elephantiasis is primarily due to obstruction of the lymph flow and may be associated with some concurrent obstruction of the venous circulation. The changes in the tissues are not specific to filariasis since they will result equally well from lymphatic obstruction due to other causes such as carcinomatous glands.

There is gradual thickening of the skin and subcutaneous tissues. The epithelium thickens irregularly and warty excrescences appear as the result of local hypertrophy and hyperkeratosis.

The connective and fatty tissues become oedematous and subsequently myxomatous and are irregularly infiltrated with round cells and eosinophils. The subcutaneous lymphatics and lymphatic spaces multiply. They may become distended and lobulated and rupture on to the surface.

In the limbs the muscles are first hypertrophic and later atrophic.

Eventually the thickened heavy tissue begins to hang in folds, causing local inflammation and finally fibrosis. In bancroftian filariasis any area of the body may be affected but certain anatomical regions, particularly the legs, are very commonly involved. In Malayan infections the lower limbs are commonly involved, but genital involvement is very rare. The development of elephantiasis varies amongst individuals and in geographical regions. In some areas with high infection rates the incidence of elephantiasis is low, in others it is very high. In a given region one patient may develop elephantiasis, another not.

In an individual case the development may stop at any stage, but usually not before some clinical signs of obstruction have appeared. In some regions, infection may continue for years without clinical evidence other than microfilariae in the blood. Such 'silent' cases are important reservoirs of the infection.

Worms are rarely found in the tissues involved in elephantiasis, but they may sometimes be discovered in the obstructed vessels, or in lymph nodes, and calcified dead worms can be detected by X-ray.

Signs and Symptoms

The 'incubation' period depends upon the length of time necessary for the worm to reach maturity, which is between 8 and 12 months. It is thus rare for very young children to show any signs of infection.

The clinical features in the early stages may be separated roughly into inflammatory and obstructive. This division is artificial and all stages may overlap. Thus, acute inflammatory episodes may occur from time to time in cases in which obstructive changes are well developed, or even in those with some degree of elephantiasis. In those with well-established elephantiasis, however, they are usually absent.

Most cases of advanced filariasis give a history extending over 2 or 3 years of previous repetitive involvement of lymphatics or glands in anatomical areas related to those in which elephantiasis has developed. This history may be absent and varices, hydrocele or elephantiasis may be the only evidence of the infection.

The onset occurs commonly in children and young adults after frequent exposure. It is usually slow and insidious but there may be an early short febrile episode preceding the inflammatory stage. It is always difficult to distinguish this so-called 'elephantoid' fever from others which are endemic to the area. It may be accompanied by the first attack of local lymphangitis. Subsequent febrile attacks are associated with exacerbations of local inflammatory lesions.

The *inflammatory phases* are varied in distribution and intensity. They consist essentially of recurring intermittent episodes of acute lymphangitis and lymphadenitis, confined to certain anatomical areas in which obstructive lesions may later develop. They are sometimes accompanied by general febrile reactions, and are usually severe and intensely painful.

Lymphangitis. Attacks of lymphangitis usually last only a few days. Lymphatics anywhere in the body may be involved. The commonest sites are superficial vessels in the extremities, particularly in the legs, testes and cord in bancroftian infections and the legs or arms (not the genitalia) in Malayan infections. Attacks tend to recur at intervals in the same anatomical areas.

The affected vessels are easily palpable and acutely tender. The overlying skin is turgid or oedematous and there are streaks of erythema running along the course of the vessels. The area is painful, tender and often itchy; scratching may lead to secondary infection. The lymphangitis is centrifugal in its distribution, commonly starting in lymphatic vessels near glands and proceeding peripherally. In the legs, the femoral and malleolar vessels are most frequently affected, more often unilaterally than bilaterally.

The lymphatics of the spermatic cord and testes are commonly involved in bancroftian filariasis and funiculitis and orchitis are frequent and severe manifestations of the early disease. Inflammation of these areas is very rare in Malayan filariasis.

Vessels anywhere in the body may be involved, and cause local effects. For instance, inflammation of the abdominal lymphatics may present a clinical picture resembling an acute abdomen.

Occasionally abscesses may form about disintegrating worms and pus may be discharged and persistent sinuses formed.

Lymphadenitis. Associated with such bursts of lymphangitis is some degree of local lymphadenitis. The glands become swollen, firm and tender with oedema and erythema of the overlying skin. Adenitis usually accompanies local lymphangitis but may occur independently. Glands in the femoral, inguinal and epitrochlear regions are commonly involved.

The obstructive lesions in these areas may go on in bancroftian infections to hydrocele which is probably most commonly caused by filariasis in endemic regions.

The pattern of acute inflammatory episodes repeated at intervals of weeks or months may last some years but gradually subsides as the obstructive phase develops. The two phases thus frequently overlap.

Obstructive changes develop in parts of the body in which inflammatory reactions have occurred. They may appear without any previous history of inflammatory reactions.

Obstruction is usually progressive and may be associated with irregular outbreaks of local inflammatory reactions.

The signs of obstruction include oedema, varices of local lymph vessels, accumulations of fluid in body cavities and eventually elephantiasis.

Varicose lymphatic vessels are distended with lymph. In superficial areas they are particularly common in the femoral, inguinal and testicular region. Deeper lymphatics may be involved including those of the abdomen.

The vessels may rupture and discharge their contents either on to the surface or into a body cavity or a viscus.

Lymph scrotum occurs when the lymph drainage to the scrotum is obstructed and the swollen tense varicose vessels rupture on to the skin surface. Such a picture usually occurs in the process of development of local elephantiasis.

The skin becomes scattered with small vesicles which burst and liberate lymph. The surface then becomes wet and secondary infection is common. The whole scrotal skin may be involved.

Hydrocele. Effusion into the cavity of the tunica vaginalis commonly results from early obstruction and inflammation of the lymphatics draining the testicular region. The hydrocele so developed may be unilateral or bilateral. It contains clear or milky fluid in which microfilariae may be present. Hydrocele is very common in bancroftian infection and very rare in Malayan. It has recently been reported in infection with *Onchocerca volvulus*. There is commonly a history of previous attacks of orchitis, and funiculitis and the cord is almost invariably irregularly thickened due to changes in the lymphatics and accumulations of nodules of lymphocytic tissue.

The regional inguinal glands are involved.

Lymphatic obstruction gives rise to other accumulations of fluid including ascites, pleural effusion and synovitis. Lymph or chyle ascites may arise from rupture of vessels into the peritoneal cavity.

Sometimes vessels containing chyle burst directly into the genito-urinary tract, causing chyluria, in which the patient passes a mixture of chyle and urine usually mixed with blood.

If the milky urine is allowed to stand it settles into three layers, an upper thin layer of fat, a deep middle layer of lymph and urine containing microfilariae and a deposit of debris, erythrocytes and other cells.

Elephantiasis. It is usually accepted that in geographical regions in which filarial infection occurs most cases of elephantiasis arise from the infection, but it is not always possible to confirm this in any particular case because elephantiasis may be the end result of any chronic obstruction to lymph flow. In many cases there is a history of repeated local lymphangitis or adenitis with remissions of variable length and a gradual increase of tissue damage over some years. However, there may be no such history and the patient may first be seen with fully developed elephantiasis.

The distribution of elephantiasis in the body is dependent to some extent on the infecting worm and the endemic area. In bancroftian infections the lower extremities with or without the scrotum are most commonly involved especially the leg below the knee; the upper extremities, breasts and labia may also be affected.

The distribution of Malayan elephantiasis is somewhat similar except that although the legs are often affected, genital involvement is very unusual.

Episodes of secondary infection are common in elephantiasis particularly where the skin is lying in folds. These are probably basically of minor importance, but may lead to local scar tissue and abscesses.

In elephantiasis of the leg the oedema appears slowly in the lower half of the limb, gradually spreading from the ankle to the knee and in some cases to the thigh. The lesion commonly stops at the knee. In the early stages the oedema is soft but in the course of months or years it becomes hard and myxomatous. The epithelium hypertrophies and becomes irregular and the subcutaneous tissue thickens, becomes fibrotic and myxomatous. Enormous and grotesque enlargements of limbs result. Changes in other parts of the body progress in essentially the same way.

In the scrotum tumours of immense proportions may develop. In such cases the penis is not commonly involved in the elephantiasis, but is retracted within the tumour so that the patient may have great difficulty in micturition.

The testes are dragged down but not functionally damaged, although the cords may be greatly lengthened. This is an important point to remember in surgical removal of the elephantoid mass.

The progress of filariasis is slow and it usually takes many years for elephantiasis to develop.

The clinical effects may stop at any stage. Elephantiasis is more common in natives of any endemic area who suffer repeated infection over long periods than in the visitor.

Once elephantiasis starts it may be difficult to stop, since chemotherapy of the infection may not affect the degree of lymph obstruction already attained.

Diagnosis

The acute stages of filariasis must be distinguished from other causes of lymphangitis, lymphadenitis, funiculitis and orchitis.

The obstructive stages and elephantiasis may be difficult to differentiate, except by the exclusion of other causes of obstruction of lymph flow, such as metastatic carcinoma.

Calcified worms may occasionally be seen in radiographs of glands or elephantoid tissue. Occasionally, lymph nodes have been removed in the search for adults but this is unwise in a condition in which lymphatic obstruction is likely to develop.

In the intermediate stages of the disease microfilariae may be found in the blood if it is examined at the appropriate time. The blood should be examined by wet preparations, in which the microfilariae may be seen moving amongst the erythrocytes, or by stained thick films as for malaria.

It is important to take the blood at the right time in order to pick up microfilariae with nocturnal or diurnal periodicity.

If microfilariae are not found on first examination venous blood may be added to formalin solution in the proportions of 1:8 and the mixture centrifuged and the deposit examined for the dead microfilariae. Alternatively, a few millilitres of blood haemolysed in dilute tepol is passed through a millipore filter which collects the microfilariae (Bell).

Microfilariae may be observed in wet preparations or stained smears of body fluids taken from a hydrocele sac for instance or the abdominal cavity. They are present in the urine in chyluria.

Complement fixation, using an antigen made from the dog heart worm or from the adult worm of human infections, is a valuable diagnostic method. A positive reaction, however, indicates past or present infection.

Skin sensitivity tests, using similar antigens, have been used with equivocal results. A volume of 0·1 ml. antigen is injected intradermally and the reactions, in the form of a wheal with pseudopodia, occurs within 15–20 minutes.

Treatment

Diethylcarbamazine (*Banocide, Hetrazan*) is the only effective drug. It is made up in tablets containing 50 mg. diethylcarbamazine citrate (25 mg. base).

It is employed as follows: 2 mg. (citrate) per kg. 3 times a day for up to 21 days, starting with 2 mg. per kg. once the first day, twice the second and three times on the third day.

Treatment in cases of relapse should be repeated after 6 months.

Mass treatment is commonly given as a single dose of 6 mg. (citrate) per kg. once weekly for 12–24 doses for *W. bancrofti* infections and for 6–8 doses for *B. malayi* infection.

With the exception of hydrocele and elephantiasis of the scrotum, labia or breast, surgical procedures are unsuccessful. The scrotal mass may be removed with safety as long as the surgeon remembers that the testes are intact and should be separated out at the beginning of the operation and eventually transplanted to the thighs. Surgical treatment for elephantiasis of the legs is not successful.

In the relatively early stages where the oedema of the legs is still soft the swelling of the limbs can be substantially relieved by swathing the limb in sorbo rubber and then bandaging it tightly. In this way, especially with temporary elevation of the limb, the oedema can be very greatly reduced.

The psychological handling of patients with filariasis or suspected of it is important, particularly in visitors to endemic areas who have been exposed for only short periods. Exposures of between 3 months and a year do not usually give rise to any serious consequences and although some inflammatory changes may occur, elephantiasis is extremely unlikely.

Diethylcarbamazine gives rise to acute allergic reactions in the first few days of treatment, since it rapidly kills off the microfilariae. These reactions include acute oedema, often involving the face and neck, short term remittent fever, local oedema and sometimes urticaria. They can be avoided or modified by the routine use of antihistamine drugs such as promethazine (*Phenergan*) during the first 4 or 5 days of treatment.

Allergic responses to treatment can also be controlled by corticosteroids in the usual doses.

The long term results of treatment with diethylcarbamazine are sometimes satisfactory but in a heavily infected case repeated courses may be necessary, since adult worms frequently survive.

LOIASIS

Definition and Aetiology

Infection with the filarial worm *Loa loa* is confined to certain regions of tropical Africa, particularly the equatorial rain forests and forest fringes in a narrow band of territory, stretching roughly from west to east between latitudes 10° N. and 5° S. In this area the distribution of the infection is irregular. Areas of intense infection occur in Eastern Nigeria, Camerouns, Congo and in some parts of East Africa.

The adult worms are shorter and thicker than those of *W. bancrofti* and have certain additional distinguishing features. They exhibit rounded bosses on an otherwise smooth cuticle. Both sexes may appear in the human connective tissues but worms are usually found singly. Maturation takes from 6 to 12 months. The life history in the human host is not fully known.

The adults wander about the body in the tissue planes and from time to time may appear beneath the skin.

Man is the only important reservoir of the infection although there is some evidence that monkeys may also carry the infection. Many patients infected with *Loa loa* may show microfilariae in the blood, but this is by no means always the case and it may be very difficult to find microfilariae in a given individual.

The actively motile sheathed microfilariae which closely resemble those of *Brugia malayi* are found in the blood in greater numbers during the day than during the night, although this diurnal periodicity varies considerably from patient to patient.

The vectors are species of the fly *Chrysops*, only the females of which are concerned in transmission.

The fly ingests infective microfilariae when feeding on the human host, and becomes infective to man 10–12 days later when the infective larvae reach the proboscis. In a given fly these larvae usually escape within the next few weeks.

The fly breeds in densely shaded, slowly running streams or stagnant pools, with a sandy, muddy bottom containing decaying vegetation. The adults live high in the canopy of the forests, but are attracted by movement in open spaces and may come down to ground level, for example in rubber plantations where the cover has been removed.

They bite chiefly in the shade during the day, but not at night or in direct sunlight.

The bite may produce a severe local reaction, especially in those sensitized by previous bites.

Clinical Signs and Symptoms

The effects of infection with *Loa loa* may be so trivial as to escape notice, or may be severe, painful and temporarily incapacitating. The severity of the reaction is believed to be related to the intensity of the infection. The usual clinical signs are largely due to the presence of the adult worm, which wanders freely in the superficial connective tissue planes of the host. Local clinical signs arise either from the current presence of the worm, for instance, when it moves across the conjunctiva, or from the effects of its recent passage, as in calabar swellings. The microfilariae in the blood are not important pathogenic agents.

As in all filarial infections, general and local allergic phenomena are pronounced. There is a very high eosinophilia, which may reach 80 per cent. of the total leucocyte count, and sometimes macular, erythematous or urticarial skin rashes.

Calabar Swellings. These tumours are rapidly developing localized masses of intense oedema which occur particularly in areas of the body exposed to trauma, such as the wrists and ankles and the orbit. They may occur before the full maturation of the worm, i.e. within a few months of infection, but they more commonly appear a year or more after infection. There is usually only one swelling at a time, but there may be several. Localized subcutaneous oedema is preceded by sharp pain and itching. A swelling develops in a few hours, becoming several inches across. It remains this size for some days and then subsides slowly. It may last as long as 1–2 weeks, especially in areas which are constantly being injured.

Tumours in an individual patient tend to arise at irregular intervals of weeks or months in the same anatomical areas. They usually remain stationary but may migrate slowly. Occasionally several calabar swellings in succession may occur in the same or in different areas but there are usually long intervals between their appearance.

The tumour causes pain and discomfort especially where the subcutaneous tissue is firm; where the latter is loose, for example in the orbit, there may be no discomfort but the swelling is often very extensive. Most serious effects occur in the region of large joints, for example, the ankles, knees and wrists where the swellings may persist for some time. Irritating pruritus over the affected area is common and scratching may give rise to secondary infection.

In some cases there may be irregular erythematous or oedematous areas scattered over the body and sometimes a macular rash may develop particularly in the region in which a calabar swelling has occurred. Occasionally a whole limb may be oedematous and in a few instances some degree of elephantiasis may develop.

Migrating Adults. Adult worms are seen from time to time moving rapidly with an undulant movement in the subcutaneous tissues, especially where these are loose. The worm can often be distinguished clearly beneath the skin. Local reactions are minimal except in some regions, particularly the eye, where there may be pruritus, severe pain and rapid development of intense oedema. The movement of the worm across the conjunctiva which takes a few minutes is a characteristic feature of the infection. One patient described the symptoms under these circumstances as feeling as though the eye 'had been kicked by a horse'.

Diagnosis

Diagnosis is usually made on the grounds of the history of exposure and of calabar swellings, a very high eosinophilia, the identification of an adult worm removed from the tissues or the discovery of the microfilariae in the peripheral blood.

When the worm is seen crossing loose connective tissue, one end should be fixed by forceps and the creature extracted through a nick in the skin. Care should be taken not to damage the worm, as this may give rise to very severe local allergic reactions. The operation must be performed as aseptically as possible.

Microfilariae are searched for in thick stained blood films or in wet preparations taken during the day. They are not easily found in many cases, and diagnosis is frequently made in their absence.

Antigens made from adults or from dog filarial worms are used for intradermal sensitivity and for complement fixation tests. These are largely group specific and only of general use in assessing the diagnosis.

Treatment

Diethylcarbamazine citrate in the dosage used for *W. bancrofti* infections is the most effective drug. Several courses of treatment are needed to eradicate the infection.

The allergic reactions to treatment are often very severe and include fever, oedema and urticaria. They can usually be controlled by antihistamine drugs, which should be given as a routine over the first five days of treatment. Corticosteroids are rarely required.

ONCHOCERCIASIS

Onchocerciasis results from infection with the so-called 'blinding' filarial worm *Onchocerca volvulus*, which is transmitted by species of *Simu.ium*, commonly known as 'buffalo flies' or 'black flies'.

The clinical picture is characterized by the appearance of subcutaneous nodules, changes in the skin and ocular lesions. There is usually a very high eosinophilia.

Aetiology

Onchocerciasis occurs in many localized areas in East, West, Central, North and North East Africa and in areas of South and Central America. It is present in pockets in the Yemen.

Onchocerca volvulus is responsible for all human onchocerciasis. Man is the definitive host and reservoir of the infection.

The infective larvae are introduced at the time of biting by the vector. Maturation of the worm takes several months. The adult worms are white and filiform and the females are much longer than the males. They mate and become established in an intimate tangle, usually in the subcutaneous lymphatic spaces, where they lead to the formation of characteristic nodules. Occasionally adults are found free in the tissue spaces. They survive for long periods.

In the gravid female, which is ovoviviparous, the uterus is filled with eggs containing larvae in all developmental stages. The unsheathed larvae, or microfilariae, migrate into the tissue spaces and sometimes lymph vessels and nodes. They exist as free moving parasites most commonly found in the tissues lying beneath the skin epithelium. The presence of the microfilariae in these areas leads to the development of the characteristic skin lesions.

Active microfilariae may appear in the scleral conjunctiva, the cornea, the anterior chamber, and the uveal tract. They may also occur in the vitreous and have recently been reported in the lens. Reports of their presence in the posterior segment of the eye have been challenged.

When biting, the *Simulium* fly ingests microfilariae which penetrate through the stomach wall and develop in the thoracic muscles. Larvae infective to man reach the proboscis in about a fortnight. Only female flies transmit the infection.

Simulium introduces its proboscis at an angle into the tissues and consequently becomes infected only by the more superficially placed microfilariae. For this reason early and active lesions are important in transmission, whereas the late burnt-out lesions, in which the few microfilariae lie in the deeper tissues only, are not.

Transmission occurs where vectors and infective human hosts are present together. In most endemic areas the infectivity rate of the fly is high. The transmission is determined mainly by the ecology of the *Simulium* which requires hot moist and shady conditions for breeding. Larvae are attached to stones, vegetation or crustaceae and require fast running well oxygenated water. The flies are thus limited to the vicinity of rapid streams, usually in high or undulating rocky country. These streams are often dry in the summer months, during which the fly disappears. The onset of rains is marked by a sudden return of *Simulium* in large numbers.

The adults rest under leaves or grass and seldom fly far from the parent water. They may be found occasionally many miles from the breeding grounds. They bite at any time during the day. In Africa the bites are most frequent on the legs; in America, where the *Simulium* is commonly found resting in the shelter of the leaves in coffee plantations, bites are commoner on the head and neck.

In endemic areas infection of man occurs at any age. Infection is to some extent an occupational risk, fishermen and plantation workers being particularly exposed. Visitors to an endemic area may also become infected.

The development of the clinical picture is dependent on the intensity and repetition of infection. Signs of infection seldom appear before the second or third year of life.

Pathology

The lesions are derived from the presence of adults and/or microfilariae and from the general tissue reactions, such as immunosensitivity, resulting from the infection. Secondary bacterial infection may complicate the skin lesions, particularly as a result of scratching.

Nodules, which may be single or multiple, contain numbers of intertwined adults of both sexes. They consist of a fibrous mass in the centre of which the coiled worms lie in what appear to be endothelial-lined spaces. There is a variable degree of scattered lymphocytic infiltration of the fibrous tissue in which there may be some microfilariae. The latter are also present in considerable numbers in the subepithelial tissues above the tumour, in which the adults may survive for years.

The fibrous mass is often lightly attached to underlying bone, but the overlying skin is free. On section the tumour appears as a circumscribed concentric mass of fibrous tissue with a honeycombed central area containing the worms. The latter may become calcified after death and initiate a giant-cell foreign body reaction.

Skin Lesions. Actively motile microfilariae are found in the subepithelial and deeper subcutaneous tissues in many areas of the body. Early in an infection there are very few changes in the dermis. There is no cellular reaction about the microfilariae unless they are dead, in which case there is some round cell infiltration. Later lesions show irregular thickening of the epithelium, reduction in sweat and sebaceous glands and some disruption of the superficial elastic layers in which there may be microfilariae. There may be some subdermal cellular infiltration and dilatation of lymphatics. Oedema resulting from sensitivity reactions may be present with or without eosinophils and there may be an irregular inflammatory reaction from secondary infection. In the late lesions the epithelium is atrophic and often depigmented, all layers of the elastic tissue are fragmented, cellular and irregular fibrous reactions are common and microfilariae are absent or found only in the deeper tissues.

Ocular lesions result from the presence of microfilariae. Changes similar to those in the skin develop in the conjunctivae. Living microfilariae may be seen moving about in the substantia propria of the cornea. Cellular infiltrations consisting of plasma and lymphatic cells occur round dead microfilariae and when confluent give rise to visible nummular 'opacities'. The corneal membranes remain intact, and the lens is rarely involved.

Microfilariae are often present in the anterior chamber. So long as they are alive they promote little or no reaction, but when dead they fall to the bottom and become involved in a mild cellular reaction which may lead to fibrosis with involvement of the iris and later glaucoma. The ciliary body may be affected in a similar manner with secondary glaucoma and cataract. The iris pigment clumps. Fundal changes, including clumping of the pigment, atrophic choroiditis and optic atrophy have been reported in infected individuals in some endemic areas, but it is not yet certain whether these are caused by the infection.

Signs and Symptoms

Signs of onchocerciasis are seldom seen in indigenes less than one year old. They usually appear after the age of 3 years. Because of the slow progress of the physical signs and the symptoms, early lesions are seldom seen unless looked for and the patient eventually presents with a well-developed picture. The first indication may be the appearance of a nodule or skin lesions, or both. Eye lesions develop late and are uncommon in children.

Nodules develop as small subcutaneous tumours which take several years to reach their full size. They vary from a few millimetres to several centimetres in maximum length. Some occur occasionally in deeper tissues and may be impalpable.

They are usually obvious, raised above the general skin surfaces and are found most commonly over bony surfaces such as the skull, ribs and trochanters and other areas where the tissues are exposed to pressure. Unless there is secondary infection, they seldom cause symptoms, although occasionally the overlying skin undergoes episodic hyperaemia and oedema from local allergic reactions.

The number of nodules varies from individual to individual and from geographical area to area. There may be few or hundreds. When they are multiple they may appear in a series of disconnected groups. There is also an uneven distribution on the body. In Africa nodules are usually found more on the trunk and limbs than on the head. In America, they are commonest on the head.

The explanation of the appearance and distribution of nodules is not clear. They are said to occur at some confluence of lymphatic channels or where there is traumatic lymphatic obstruction, as in carrying strapped head loads or lying on the hips. It has been suggested also that the relative infrequency of nodules on the head in Africa and their frequency in America may be associated with the limited migration and slow maturation of the larvae acquired during the *Simulium* bite, which occurs most commonly on the lower legs in the former case and on the head and neck in the latter.

Skin lesions develop insidiously. When fully active they cause considerable itching and discomfort and scratching may be followed by complications due to secondary infection. Where large areas of the skin are involved there may be temporary but serious interference with working capacity. The signs vary from time to time in a given patient, with episodes of intense exacerbation interspersed with periods of relative quiescence, but the general progress is continuous. The final state is the so-called 'burnt-out' lesion which gives rise to no symptoms.

The early pruriginous stages often involve wide areas of skin. In Africa the lesions are found on the legs, thighs, buttocks and lower trunk, less commonly on the shoulders, arms and face. The skin is slightly thickened, raised above the surroundings and sometimes hyperpigmented. There may be some desquamation of the keratinous layers. Over-all thickening and wrinkling of the skin may give rise to so-called 'lizard' or 'elephant skin'. These are often local episodes of oedema and erythema. At irregular intervals or continuously the affected skin is intensely itchy. Scratching commonly causes secondary infection which may appear as scattered lesions resembling scabies or occasionally as inflammation of the whole area, especially on the face giving the appearance of erysipelas. In American infections the lesions are commonest on the face, head and neck and may be accompanied by irregularly developing hard oedema of parts of the face and ears.

Late lesions, which are often seen on the legs in Africans, present without symptoms. The skin is thin, atrophic, inelastic and irregularly depigmented.

Ocular Lesions

The incidence of eye lesions varies with the endemic area. In America they are common; in some regions the incidence exceeds 20 per cent. of infected individuals. Similar high figures have been recorded in some parts of Africa, for example in Northern Ghana, but in other areas the incidence is low.

Ocular lesions with clinical features are most commonly seen in patients with nodules or skin lesions on the head or face.

Eye lesions develop late in patients in whom nodules and/or skin lesions are already obvious and well developed. They are commoner in individuals with nodules or skin lesions on the face, head and neck. The most advanced lesions are usually found in adults.

Ocular lesions often follow a progressive development which tends to be slow and painless in the African form of the disease and in the American form more rapid and painful, especially in daylight.

The first sign of involvement is mild episodic conjunctivitis. Later, small round opacities may develop in the cornea, usually in the inferior medial quadrant and sometimes accompanied by some vascular engorgement and occasionally eyelid oedema and photophobia.

Pannus may appear on the inferior segment. Corneal ulceration occurs only after secondary infection or injury.

Microfilariae may be distinguished in the cornea or aqueous with a slit lamp; they commonly occur in groups attached tail to tail. Dead microfilariae and the associated inflammatory cellular response appear as a grey or brown mass usually in the inferior medial aspect of the anterior chamber. The reactions at thi stage may involve the iris, with generalized loss of pigment producing a grey spongy background with scattered clumps of pigment. This change is very striking in the normally brown-eyed African. The iris is eventually distorted, producing a pear-shaped pupil with the apex pointing downwards and medially.

The iridocyclitis which develops is slowly progressive and painless in the African but may be rapid and painful in the American form of the disease. Eventual complications include glaucoma and secondary cataract.

Microfilariae may be seen in the vitreous, which, however, usually remains clear.

In some endemic areas fundal lesions occur which are believed by some workers, but not all, to be onchocercal in origin. The characteristic picture, which resembles atrophic choroiditis, is accompanied by some degree of optic nerve atrophy and eventually blindness. Retinal changes may be present with or without anterior eye lesions.

Blindness in onchocerciasis results occasionally from complicated corneal opacities, associated with trachoma or injury, and more often from iridocyclitis complicated by cataract and secondary glaucoma. Patients with retinal lesions are usually blind or nearly so, but, as pointed out, this has not yet been proved to be due to the onchocercal infection.

Other Complications

Mild elephantiasis and hydrocele or even lymph scrotum occasionally occur in patients infected with onchocerciasis. In hydrocele, microfilariae of *Onchocerca* have been recovered from the fluid.

Very high eosinophilia is common in established onchocerciasis.

Unless the eye is involved, the infection causes little harm to the individual. The skin lesions usually progress for some years and then slowly recede to the 'burnt-out' stage. Nodules remain unchanged for years and may contain living adult worms even after several courses of treatment.

Diagnosis

Nodules must be distinguished from other subcutaneous tumours. In case of doubt it is probably better to excise and examine a nodule histologically than to probe it with a needle in order to examine the fluid for eggs or larvae. Needling may evoke a local allergic reaction. A snip taken from the overlying skin usually contains actively motile microfilariae.

Diagnosis of onchocerciasis is usually made by removing a fragment of skin and examining it after teasing out in saline.

The affected skin is lifted by inserting the tip of a hypodermic needle bevel upwards. After cleaning with alcohol and allowing to dry, a fine shaving is removed with a sterile razor blade, cutting parallel to the bevel of the needle. The object is to remove a sample of epithelium and immediate subepithelial tissue without bleeding. (Blood may contain other microfilariae.) The specimen is teased out in a drop of saline on a microscope slide, covered with a coverslip and examined under the low power of the microscope. Free-swimming larvae will be seen in the fluid near the edges of the preparation. No anaesthetic is needed for the skin, but cocaine should be instilled in the eye before removing a similar fragment of the conjunctiva with a pair of fine scissors. No stitching is necessary.

With the slit lamp, microfilariae may be found in the cornea or anterior chamber (usually the inferior nasal angle).

Differentiation of microfilariae depends on the absence of a sheath and the distribution of the nuclei. In most cases the discovery of numbers of microfilariae in the skin or conjunctival snips or in the eye is sufficient.

Treatment

Surgical removal of nodules and the contained adult worms is commonly practised especially when the tumours are on the head or are causing discomfort.

Chemotherapy depends on the use of diethylcarbamazine citrate, which destroys the microfilariae and eventually most of the adults, or on suramin (*Antrypol*) which kills the adults but has no direct effect on the microfilariae. The drugs are sometimes used in combination.

The usual treatment consists in a course of diethylcarbamazine which may be repeated at intervals if cure is not immediately obtained.

Where there is no or minimal ocular involvement, a total daily dose of 3 mg. per kg. body weight is given in 3 divided doses for 2 days; this is doubled over the next 2 days, trebled over the following 2 days and finally quadrupled and continued for 15 days. The final dose achieved is 12 mg. per kg. body weight per day.

If ocular lesions are present, the initial dose is reduced to 1 or 0·5 mg. per kg. Allergic eye reactions can be prevented or relieved by instillation of 5 per cent. cortisone acetate or by administration of 25 mg. cortisone four times a day for the 2 days prior to giving the diethylcarbamazine and for the first 4 days of treatment.

Since diethylcarbamazine rapidly destroys the microfilariae, allergic reactions are common in the first few days of treatment, including congestion and oedema of the conjunctivae, generalized pruritus, often most severe over skin lesions, and oedema, especially of the face. There may also be an urticarial rash.

These reactions are relieved or prevented by antihistamine drugs in the usual doses, given over the first 5 days of treatment.

Suramin is given intravenously in the same dosage schedule as for trypanosomiasis. An initial small dose of 100 mg. is usually given and the urine is examined for erythrocytes, protein and casts. If there is any renal reaction the drug is contra-indicated. Many workers have reported severe toxic reactions to the use of suramin in onchocercal infections.

On the other hand, since the drug acts on the adults and has little effect on the microfilariae the immediate allergic signs which follow the administration of diethylcarbamazine are usually absent with suramin.

Various regimes in which both drugs are employed in rotation have been designed, for instance, diethylcarbamazine followed by suramin, followed by diethylcarbamazine.

REFEERNCE

WORLD HEALTH ORGANIZATION (1966) Expert Committee on Onchocerciasis, *Spec. Rep. Ser.*, 335.

OTHER FILARIAL INFECTIONS

DIPETALONEMA PERSTANS

Infection occurs in West, Central and East Africa northern South America, Brazil, northern Argentina and Trinidad.

The adults live in the body cavities. The unsheathed microfilariae are found in the blood; there is no periodicity.

The infection is usually without clinical effects, but eosinophilia, subcutaneous swellings resembling calabar swellings, skin oedema and pruritus, sometimes fever, lymphadenopathy and joint and bone pains have been attributed to it. These manifestations respond to diethylcarbamazine.

From time to time, neurological and psychological disturbances have been blamed on perstans infection. Two cases have been recorded recently of microfilariae resembling those of *A. perstans* being found in the cerebrospinal fluid. In one case there were headache, dizziness, vomiting and other cerebral signs before the patient was admitted to hospital in a stuporose state. The cerebrospinal fluid was under pressure and contained 80 cells per mm^3. and numerous microfilariae. The evidence is not altogether convincing in view of the possibility of co-existing occult infections with other filarial worms.

DIPETALONEMA STREPTOCERCA

Infection with *Dipetalonema streptocerca* occurs in West Africa. It is transmitted by *Culicoides* sp. Adults may be found in subcutaneous tissue, usually in the shoulder girdle and upper arms. The small unsheathed larvae occur in the skin immediately below the epithelium on the upper trunk and arms; they can be identified in skin snips, as in onchocerciasis. The infection rarely causes clinical signs. An acute, intensely itchy erythematous eruption of the arms and trunk has been recorded and there is a suspicion that the worm may occasionally be involved in the production of elephantiasis. The rash responds well to diethylcarbamazine.

MANSONELLA OZZARDI

This infection is found in parts of South America and the Caribbean Islands. The vector is *Culicoides* sp. The adults are present in fatty tissue, usually beneath the peritoneum and in other body cavities. The unsheathed larvae are present in the peripheral blood. Inguinal adenitis, erythematous skin rashes, sometimes with oedema, joint pains and severe headache and eosinophilia have been attributed to the infection. Conflicting reports have been given of the action of diethylcarbamazine.

DRACONTIASIS

Synonym. Guinea worm infection.

Definition

Infection with the nematode *Dracunculus medinensis*.

Aetiology

The guinea worm is found scattered over Africa, including West Africa, Central and East Sudan, Egypt, the Middle East, Turkey, Southern Russia, India, South East Asia, the Caribbean and North and South America. The distribution is patchy depending on the presence of vectors and suitable environmental conditions.

The clinical effects are produced solely by female worms. The male has not been found in the human host. The female may measure up to 3 feet in length most of which contains uterus.

The gravid female eventually reaches the surface of the body of the host. A vesicle forms near the head. Ulceration follows and the anterior end of the worm is exposed. Enormous numbers of free-swimming larvae are then ejected through prolapsed portions of the uterus whenever the lesion comes into contact with water.

The larvae which escape from the female eventually enter the crustacian *Cyclops*. They will survive for some days in clean water and for several weeks in dirty water or liquid mud. The intermediate host becomes infective to man in about a week to a fortnight. Man becomes infected by swallowing water containing infective *Cyclops*. The larvae escape into the duodenum and penetrate the wall of the small intestine. The development thereafter goes on in the connective tissue and full maturity is reached in about a year.

Cyclops is found in abundance in standing dirty water or puddles, in ponds, in wells, pits and in the village water supplies.

Infection is common in conditions in which the same supply of water is used for drinking and for washing.

Infection is rare under the age of 4 years, but thereafter steadily increases to become maximal in the young adult.

In some areas it is seasonal; in others it is continuous throughout the year. Infection with a single worm is common, but multiple infections may occur.

Signs and Symptoms

No clinical signs or symptoms occur until the female reaches the stage where larvae are on the point of discharge. A few hours before this the worm reaches the surface of the skin and some local erythema and tenderness develops over the head. There may be at this stage some general severe allergic reactions including generalized pruritus, urticaria, nausea, vomiting and diarrhoea. The local changes are, however, usually the important ones and the general reactions subside as the local lesion develops.

The female appears in the legs and the feet in about 90 per cent. of cases, but may present anywhere, including the scrotum, the back and even the eyeball. It is often visible or palpable under the skin for the greater part of its length.

The patient complains of sharp pain at a site corresponding to the head of the worm, where a papule develops. In the course of one or two days the area becomes indurated, the central region is raised and a vesicle forms and ruptures. In the superficial ulcer so formed the head of the worm is usually visible. On contact of the lesion with water milky fluid escapes. This contains enormous numbers of active larvae which have been ejected from the uterus. Ejection of larvae thereafter continues intermittently when the affected part is exposed to water.

The tissues about the presenting head become indurated, oedematous, reddened and very tender. Where the lesion develops near a joint there may be considerable interference with activity. The local lesion heals in about 6 weeks, provided there is no secondary infection, but the latter is common and serious complications involving joints, especially the ankles and knees, may develop.

Worms may come to lie under the surface but fail to mature and die before they reach the surface. Under such circumstances they remain as cord-like masses, palpable below the skin and these may either become secondarily infected and produce abscesses or become calcified and visible on X-ray.

Aseptic abscesses may be produced by the rupture of immature females. Such accidents may be accompanied by severe general allergic reactions.

There is a high eosinophilia during the active stages.

In the absence of secondary infection the worm will continue to discharge larvae until the uterus is empty, which may take several weeks. Rapid healing then occurs if the worm is artificially removed without damage, but serious effects may result if it becomes broken, since rupture and retraction lead commonly to secondary infection and abscess formation.

Diagnosis

The development of the local lesion is characteristic. The head of the worm can be identified in the uncomplicated ulcer and larvae can be found in the fluid extruded when the lesion is immersed in water. The body of the worm under the skin is also usually clearly visible and palpable for its whole length.

Treatment

Treatment depends on the area involved. The local lesion must be kept clean and secondary infection avoided. In the absence of available chemotherapy the worm is best extracted by the ancient method of winding it up. The local lesion is treated with wet compresses until discharge of embryos stops in one or two days. The head of the worm is identified and grasped by forceps or thread and coaxed out with one hand, with the other massaging the skin and underlying worm in the direction of its head. The worm is tense and surprisingly resistant. When a sufficient length has been exposed, the worm is tied to a match stick which is slowly wound at intervals over the period of treatment. In this way the worm can be removed *in toto* a few inches at a time, provided it is not broken. If it breaks it should be left *in situ* and not removed surgically. A wide-spectrum antibiotic or sulphonamide may be given during removal of the worm, and the stick and rolled worm should be covered with a sterile dressing and the area kept as clean as possible.

Involvement of joints involves special care, especially when there is pus formation, when it may be necessary to aspirate the abscess and immobilize the limb.

Niridazole, 25 mg. per kg. body weight in two divided doses daily for 5–7 days, kills the worms *in situ*. Local pain, tenderness and swelling are relieved in 24–48 hours. This drug seems to be the most efficient agent yet discovered. Thiabendazole in doses of 25 mg. per kg. body weight daily for 3 days is also claimed to be successful. With drug therapy physical removal of the worm is usually not required.

The best way to deal with guinea worm is to control the infection at source. This can be done in water not used for drinking by destroying *Cyclops* with DDT. Adequately protected wells and water supplies, built so as to avoid splashing and puddles of water, are effective in preventing the spread of the infection.

TRICHURIASIS

The whipworm, *Trichuris trichiura*, is a very common parasite of world-wide distribution, especially found in the tropics. There are two sexes which measure up to 5 cm. (2 in.) in length. The female is larger than the male. The anterior part of the worm is slender and threadlike; the posterior portion is thicker and cylindrical. The worms are attached to the intestinal wall by the heads which may be inserted deep into the mucosa. They are commonly found in the caecum and upper large intestine. The females discharge characteristic barrel-shaped eggs which are operculated at both ends and are commonly stained by bile.

Infection arises from swallowing eggs which become infective about 2 weeks after being passed in the faeces. The embryos escape in the small intestine and eventually migrate to the large bowel wall where they become adult. Light infections produce no signs or symptoms, but heavy loads of worms may cause serious consequences in children, including volvulus and even prolapse of the rectum.

Diagnosis

Diagnosis is made by recognizing the eggs in the stool and by finding the occasional adult in the anal region.

Treatment

Chemotherapy is unsatisfactory. Infection is cleared in about half the cases by thiabendazole, given in doses of 25 mg. per kg. body weight twice daily for 3 days. Controlled trials in hospital of dichlorvos, an organophosphorus anticholinesterase compound, have shown that it is very active against *Trichuris*. Further trials are in progress, but there is some doubt over the safety of the drug in areas where there is widespread use of dichlorvos in insect control.

STRONGYLOIDIASIS

Aetiology and Pathology

Infection with *Strongyloides stercoralis* occurs in many parts of the world particularly in the East, South America and Africa. The completion of the life cycle of the worm is complicated and very dependent on environmental conditions. The eggs hatch in the human host and larvae are passed in the faeces. These usually develop into free living adults and this cycle may be repeated for some time. Eventually, however, filiform larvae are formed, which pierce the human skin, reach the heart and escape from the pulmonary vessels into the alveoli and so into the intestine.

The males are passed in the faeces, but the fertilized females penetrate the mucosa where they lay eggs which hatch. The larva escapes into the lumen, thence to the stool, and the cycle is repeated. Sometimes filiform larvae develop during the passage of the recently hatched larvae down the intestine. These may pierce the mucosa or the skin near the anus and repeat the tissue life cycle within the body, thus giving rise to auto-infection.

In a given individual infection may persist in this way for years.

In very heavy infections the damage to the mucosa is severe and even death may result.

Signs and Symptoms

The ordinary degree of infection produces no clinical signs, except some gastro-intestinal discomfort, epigastric pain, and diarrhoea.

In some individuals, usually many years after the initial infection, and in chronic infections, the most pronounced lesions occur in the skin as sensitivity reactions to wandering larva.

A blotchy urticaria develops with an arteriolar flare, and a rapidly moving erythematous serpiginous lesion appears, which moves visibly under the skin and is particularly evident on the upper parts of the limbs and the trunk. These lesions appear suddenly and are transitory. Individual lesions subside in a few hours but the manifestations as a whole may go on for some days with quiescent intervals. Sometimes oedema of a limb has been recorded.

Areas of very itchy oedema, erythema and urticaria, especially around the anus may also occur during strongyloid infection, possibly caused by penetration of filiform larvae passed in the faeces and the local sensitivity reactions resulting therefrom.

Lesions of deep tissue arising in the mucosa and in the viscera in auto-infections in particular, give rise to disseminated visceral larva migrans which may be fatal.

Diagnosis

The diagnosis is made by finding the motile larva in the stool. This must be distinguished from the hookworm larva, but under normal conditions the latter does not appear in the faeces until some days after it has been passed. It is difficult to define the larva in the skin eruptions.

Treatment

The best drug for therapy is thiabendazole, 25 mg. per kg. body weight, given daily for 3 days.

No preparatory purgation or starvation is necessary.

ANCYLOSTOMIASIS

Synonym. Hookworm infection.

Definition

Infection with the nematodes *Ancylostoma duodenale* or *Necator americanus*.

Aetiology

The distribution of hookworm covers most of the world. *A. duodenale* occurs in temperate climates in Europe, in the Middle East, North Africa and in certain areas of the Far East. It may occasionally occur under special conditions (for example in the moist warm environment of mines) in the colder parts of Europe.

N. americanus is much more widely spread in the tropics including Africa, South Africa, the Middle East, India, the Far East, Central and South America, the southern and western United States, and the Caribbean. It also occurs in Indonesia, Thailand and New Guinea. The worms occur concurrently in many areas.

Man is the natural host and harbours the adults in the small intestine. Embryonated eggs are passed in the faeces.

The adults of *A. duodenale* measure up to half an inch (1 cm.) in length; the female is just larger than the male, the body slightly curved and tapered at both ends.

Adults of *N. americanus* are smaller, finer and tapered. The head in both sexes is bent back.

Eggs passed in the faeces develop in warm moist soil and hatch in about 5 days. The active larva migrates to the soil and feeds on organic matter. After some development the infective filiform larva reaches the ground surface and eventually penetrates the human skin. By the third day after penetration it reaches the lungs and, in the same manner as ascaris, the bronchi, trachea and intestine. Adults mature in the upper parts of the small intestine in 3–5 weeks after infection, and attach themselves to the mucosa. Eggs are laid in the lumen and pass out in the faeces. The freshly passed egg is non-infective and there will be no further development of the larva if the faeces is allowed to dry. Development and hatching of the larva occurs only when the faeces are permitted to remain in contact with damp, preferably light or sandy soil at a suitable temperature.

The larva can penetrate any exposed area, including the buttocks, but entry commonly occurs through the legs and feet.

The infection is primarily associated with filthy living conditions, the indiscriminate shedding of faeces and the habit of going bare-foot.

Pathology

The pathological processes initiated by the infection in a given case depend primarily on the number of worms present. An adult attached to the mucosa causes the loss of 0·03 to 0·1 ml. of blood per day. Since infection with a 1000 worms or more is not unusual, the amount of blood lost in this way may be considerable, despite the fact that some 40 per cent. of the iron lost may be resorbed from the gut.

In some hosts but not in others a heavy load of worms thus causes anaemia. It is now believed that anaemia results only in those in whom the over-all iron reserves are deficient. Another important factor involved in the production of anaemia in hookworm infection may be lack of protein in the diet, particularly protein which contains the amino acids necessary for the synthesis of the globin fraction of haemoglobin.

The clinical patterns produced by the hookworm thus arise essentially from the failure of haemopoiesis to replace the blood loss in individuals in whom the iron reserves are deficient.

As in ascaris, however, changes in the lungs during the passage of the larvae may be sufficiently frequent and numerous to produce local pulmonary effects.

The anaemia is essentially hypochromic and microcytic or normocytic. The bone marrow response is mostly normoblastic but in a proportion of cases where some folic acid deficiency co-exists there may be a megaloblastic element. It is probably for this latter reason that replacement of the iron stores alone will not always fully restore the normal haemoglobin level.

Signs and Symptoms

Mild infections produce no obvious signs. Heavy infections in those deficient in iron reserves produce the characteristic anaemia. The low iron reserve may result from long continued bleeding, incomplete haemoglobin synthesis or reduced iron intake. The situation is exacerbated in the later stages of pregnancy. In many cases the explanation for the low iron reserve is not readily available. Unless the worm load is dangerously high it seems that anaemia will not develop if the iron stores are adequate and sufficient iron is being supplied in the diet.

In the average anaemic case the haemoglobin concentration is of the order of 6–8 g. per 100 ml. The erythrocytes are hypochromic and commonly microcytic. In children there is a characteristic picture of a pale individual with an oedematous puffy face, protuberant abdomen, and sometimes ascites and oedema of the legs. The patient complains of epigastric discomfort and shortness of breath. Various signs of malnutrition are also commonly present. The patient is mentally dull and retarded.

When the infection is heavy and the iron reserves are low or absent, the anaemia becomes excessive, and the haemoglobin concentration may fall as low as 2–1·5 g. per 100 ml. Some patients continue working even with this degree of anaemia.

Under these extreme circumstances, death may occur from anaemia. Otherwise, in most infections some balance is established between the patient and his infection and few serious effects result until some extra demand for iron occurs, as in pregnancy, or circumstances develop in which the iron intake is reduced. Some authorities hold that certain vegetables taken normally in the diet may interfere with the absorption of iron by forming insoluble phytates. In estimating intake it should be reckoned that only about 10 per cent. of the iron in the diet is available. Since the synthesis of haemoglobin requires not only iron but also the synthesis of the protein fraction, the protein intake in the diet probably constitutes an important factor in determining the level of anaemia induced by a given worm load. Certain amino acids which are essential in globin synthesis must apparently be supplied in the diet. These are more plentiful in animal protein but may be supplied by the right kind of vegetable protein.

Diagnosis

The diagnosis depends on the discovery of the eggs of the worm in the faeces. An estimate of the total number of eggs per gramme of faeces will give some indication of the worm load but it is notoriously difficult to determine in this way the number of worms involved. The only reliable method is to count the worms passed after treatment.

The presence of eggs in the stools merely confirms the presence of worms in the intestine. It does not mean that the patient is suffering from hookworm disease.

In the East, hookworm eggs must be distinguished from the longer, narrower, but otherwise very similar eggs of *Trichostrongylus* spp.

Treatment

Bephenium naphthoate (*Alcopar*) is the best drug both for individual and for mass therapy. A single dose of 2·5 G. of the base is usually effective for *Ancylostoma*, but 2·5 G. of the base should be given daily for three days for *Necator* infections. Children may be given half the above dosage, at any age.

A satisfactory alternative is a combination of tetrachloroethylene and bephenium naphthoate. A dose of 4–6 ml. of tetrachloroethylene is given in the morning on an empty stomach, followed by bephenium, 2·5 G. (base).

Normally only one course of treatment is necessary since the number of worms which survive is usually too few to cause clinical effects. There is no point in attempting total eradication in individuals who may subsequently become reinfected.

Bephenium has a low toxicity and is extremely effective. It is particularly useful in cases with very severe anaemias and in children. It may be given in the presence of ascaris infection.

Since it is bitter and causes nausea it should be given on an empty stomach or mixed with sugar. Bephenium is expensive; where economic considerations are paramount tetrachloroethylene may be subsituted.

Tetrachloroethylene is given in capsules containing 1 ml. or on a spoon mixed with sugar and water.

Purgation beforehand is unnecessary but is useful

afterwards. The drug should not be used in alcoholics and is potentially dangerous in constipated ill children.

It should never be given alone in the presence of ascaris infection.

The dose of tetrachloroethylene for adults, depending on size and weight, is between 2 and 4 ml. given once and followed two hours later by an efficient saline purgation. In children the dose in 0·1 ml. per kg., up to the adult dose.

For the treatment of mixed hookworm and ascaris infection, the best treatment is undoubtedly bephenium.

Failing this, the ascaris infection can be removed by piperazines and tetrachloroethylene given 3 days later.

Biscomate (*Jonit*) has recently been found equally effective against *A. duodenale* and *N. americanus*. It is given orally at 12-hourly intervals after a meal. The adult dose is 100 mg. after breakfast, 100 mg. after supper on the first day, followed by 100 mg. after breakfast the next day. The total dose is thus 300 mg. Side-effects are mild and transient. They include nausea, vomiting and abdominal pain, and occasionally dizziness.

Worming will eventually be followed by restoration of the haemoglobin concentration, but the process is slow unless iron is added to the diet. The best combination for the treatment of hookworm anaemia is therefore worming followed by the administration of ferrous iron salts, usually as ferrous sulphate in doses of 1 G. daily in three divided doses and continued for up to 3 months.

If the patient presents with a haemoglobin concentration of under 2 g. per 100 ml. the initial doses of iron may be given parenterally. Transfusion even at this stage is usually unnecessary and is undesirable.

The haemoglobin concentration after iron therapy and worming may not always reach normal levels. In some cases this is due to folic acid deficiency (which may be corrected by 5 mg. three times daily for some weeks); in others it may be due to protein deficiency, and must be corrected by diet. In any case, the treatment of hookworm anaemia should always include a well balanced high protein diet.

REFERENCES

British Medical Journal (1968) Hookworm infection. Leading article, **2**, 788.

GILLES, H. M., WATSON WILLIAMS, E. J., and BALL, P. A. J. (1964) Hookworm infection and anaemia, *Quart. J. Med.*, **33**, 1.

ENTEROBIASIS

Definition

Infection with *Enterobius vermicularis*, the thread worm or pin worm, is one of the commonest and most widespread gastro-intestinal worm infections.

Aetiology

The geographical distribution is uninfluenced by climate; it is very largely dependent on dirty living conditions and self infection.

The worm is a human parasite, small, white and threadlike. The males have coiled tails and are about half the size of the females which may reach about a half an inch (1 cm.) in length. The females only are usually found in the active case since most males are destroyed in the intestine. The adults live free in the lumen of the small and large intestines. They have an alimentary tract and feed from the intestinal contents. The females emerge from the anus on to the perineal and perianal skin. Here they die and disintegrate, liberating large numbers of characteristic eggs, which adhere to the skin or the clothing and are transferred thence to towels and fingers. The embryonated eggs rapidly develop and become infective. When swallowed, larvae escape in the intestine and male and female worms develop.

Signs and Symptoms

Infection rarely gives rise to symptoms, unless very heavy. However, the migration of the female worms through the anus to the surrounding skin which occurs most commonly at night may cause local symptoms including severe itching, which may interfere with sleep. Scratching may result in secondary infection of the skin. The fingers and nails become infected with eggs and the patient is thus continually reinfected. This occurs especially in children. Infection may also occur via linen and towels contaminated with eggs. Cross-infection of members of a family is thus extremely common and where one member is found infected, the remainder of the family should be examined for infection.

Diagnosis

In heavy infection the patient may discover the female worms by finding them on his fingers after scratching. Sometimes the worms may be seen in the stool, but the eggs are rarely found in the faeces since they adhere firmly to the perianal skin. The latter is scraped with a blunt blade or rubbed with a suitable swab immediately on awakening in the morning. The usual practice is to employ a swab consisting of a piece of cellophane fastened sticky side out on the end of a wooden stick. This is gently rubbed over the perianal surface. The eggs adhere to the cellophane which can then be opened out sticky side down on a microscope slide and examined under low power for the characteristic unilaterally flattened eggs. Eggs may sometimes be found contaminating the urine in females.

Treatment

Self infection must be stopped by treatment of the infection and cleansing the skin areas concerned. The child's hands may be temporarily protected by gloves, etc. Palliative or antihistamine ointments may be rubbed on the perianal skin to relieve the itching but these are not very successful. The best chemotherapy is the administration of piperazine salts, as for ascaris.

ASCARIASIS

Synonym. Round worm infection.

Definition

Infection with *Ascaris lumbricoides*, the largest of the round worms which infect man. It occurs in all parts of the world where living conditions are dirty. Clinical signs appear only in heavy multiple infections and are largely due to the mechanical effects of the worms in the intestinal lumen.

Aetiology and Pathology

The adult worms are large, white and cylindrical with pointed ends. The males have curled tails. The females measure up to 25 cm. (10 in.) and are 5–7·5 cm. (2–3 in.) larger than the fully developed male. The adults live freely in the lumen of the small intestine. They have an alimentary tract and derive their nourishment from the intestinal contents. In children with very heavy infections the amount of food lost in this way may be sufficient to disturb the nutritional balance.

Whether they are fertilized or not the females pass eggs which escape into the faeces. An infective larva is eventually developed in the fertilized eggs. The eggs are very resistant to antiseptics, heat and dryness. They are frequently blown about in the dust. Man is infected by swallowing the embryonated eggs. Heavy infections indicate gross faecal contamination of the environment. Ascariasis thus represents a classical 'dirt infection'.

The fertilized infective eggs hatch in the small intestine and produce larvae which penetrate the wall of the intestine and are carried in the circulation to the lungs where they lodge for a short time, then penetrate the alveoli and are eventually expelled via bronchioles, bronchi and the trachea. They are swallowed, pass through the stomach, and reach the small intestine, where they develop into adults. The development of large numbers of larvae in the lungs may cause a pneumonitis, with signs and symptoms, including cough and blood-stained sputum in which larvae may sometimes be found. There are often in addition allergic manifestations including a high eosinophilia. The combination of pneumonitis, allergic signs including high eosinophilia and associated generalized adenitis is sometimes called Loeffler's syndrome.

Signs and Symptoms

Infection with a few worms is not usually accompanied in the early stages by overt clinical effects, except occasional gastro-intestinal discomfort and mild diarrhoea, but the adults may suddenly appear in the stool or wander into the stomach whence they may be vomited or ascend the oesophagus and escape via the nasopharynx. Sometimes worms ascend the common bile-duct and cause obstruction associated with severe cholangitis and jaundice. The pancreatic duct may be invaded in the same way. The clinical picture of the heavily infected child in whom there may be hundreds of worms is the undernourished, underweight child with a protuberant belly, with constant intestinal discomfort, frequent diarrhoea, often visible peristalsis and complications which include intestinal obstruction, perforation or volvulus.

Diagnosis

Diagnosis is made either by the discovery of the adult worm or of the eggs in the stools.

Treatment

For ascaris infection the best form of treatment is undoubtedly the piperazine compounds which may be given as the citrate, the adipate or phosphate. In moderate infections the drug is successful in a single dose of 4 G. for the adult followed 24 hours later by a saline purge to ensure the passage of the worms. Children are given single doses as follows: weight less than 20 kg.: 3 G.; weight over 20 kg.: 4 G.

Bephenium hydroxynaphthoate (*Alcopar*) is also satisfactory. The adult dose is 2·5 G. of the base (5 G. of the hydroxynaphthoate) as a single dose given orally without previous preparation of the patient. Children and infants can be given half this dose quite safely.

In cases with diarrhoea the treatment may need to be repeated on two or three successive days. Treatment with bephenium is of particular value since it is also successful for the treatment of hookworm and can thus be safely administered in the patient with both infections. Treatment of hookworm by drugs which do not eliminate ascaris may be dangerous in heavy multiple infections since the ascaris worms may become disturbed and over-active leading to severe complications, including volvulus.

LARVA MIGRANS

Synonym. Creeping eruptions.

Aetiology

Ancylostoma and *Necator* are the only hookworms which normally reach full development in man.

Certain other related but unadapted round worms may infect man without full completion of the life cycle. Under such conditions so-called 'creeping eruptions' may develop. These may appear in the early stages of infection with human hookworm at the site of the penetration of the larva, as an itching irritating rash.

Signs and Symptoms

Some time after infection, unadapted larvae wander under the skin and the characteristic creeping eruption of larva migrans develops. The commonest parasite responsible for such lesions is the hookworm of the dog and the cat, *Ancylostoma brasiliensis* or *Ancylostoma caninum*.

A small papule appears at the site of entry of the larva which subsequently moves about irregularly in a serpiginous tunnel in the corium beneath the epithelium. The larva wanders very slowly and does not develop further. The lesion is at first erythematous, then becomes raised above the skin surface; finally vesicles develop with some local infiltration with eosinophils and lymphocytes. The lesion is commonly surrounded by an arteriolar flare.

It occurs commonly in the feet, hands and buttocks and is associated with intense local pruritus which leads to scratching and secondary reinfection. The lesion behind the advancing larva becomes dry and scaly.

More transient and rapidly moving lesions sometimes with pronounced arteriolar flare occur in infections with *Strongyloides stercoralis*. Somewhat similar lesions may result from aberrant larvae of flies, for instance the larvae of the horse bot fly, *Gasterophilus*. In these, each lesion contains a single minute larva hatched from eggs deposited originally on the hairs. The cattle warble fly *Hypoderma* produces a much larger larva which gives rise to similar lesions.

Treatment

The treatment of creeping eruption is local. Cauterization or cooling agents such as spraying with ethyl chloride or exposure to carbon dioxide snow, usually kill the larvae.

In some cases the infection may be stopped by antihelminthic drugs the best of which is probably thiabendazole, 25 mg. per kg. body weight twice daily for 2 days.

VISCERAL LARVA MIGRANS

Aetiology and Pathology

Lesions produced by nematode larva under the skin are paralleled by similar reactions to unadapted larvae in the viscera of the host. This may occasionally occur in unsuitable conditions in nematode infections in the natural hosts, for example, in heavy *Strongyloides stercoralis* infections.

In man the commonest lesions due to larva migrans in the viscera are those caused by the dog and cat ascarids, *Toxocara canis* or *Toxocara cati*.

Children are most commonly infected. Infective eggs are ingested; the larvae escape, invade the mucosa and reach the mesenteric venules and lymphatics and eventually the viscera. Here they are caught up, commonly in the liver or lungs. No further development of the larva occurs, but it may remain alive for many months and single, multiple or miliary granulomatous lesions may develop, the number depending on the number of larvae.

The lesions may be found at autopsy or biopsy of the appropriate tissue. They are small and in the liver are usually situated in the tissue beneath the capsule. They may also be found in the heart, the kidneys, lungs, striped muscle, the brain, the eyeball and elsewhere.

Histologically they resemble an early tubercule with an outer ring of lymphocytes and polymorphs or eosinophils and an inner layer of histiocytes and epithelioid cells and sometimes giant cells. In early newly formed lesions the living larva lies in the centre of the granuloma and can sometimes be mechanically expressed. It later becomes necrotic and calcified. When secondary infection occurs the lesion becomes purulent. The granuloma eventually becomes walled off by concentric fibrous tissue.

Signs and Symptoms

Clinical signs depend on the number of lesions and their situation. There is nearly always a marked eosinophilia and where the lesions appear in the lungs the picture may closely resemble that of tropical eosinophilia, sometimes with severe respiratory distress.

There is often some degree of splenomegaly. When the liver is invaded it may be enlarged and palpable. Urticarial rashes may occur.

Diagnosis and Treatment

This is based on a history of possible infection (for instance, association with kennels), clinical and laboratory findings which usually include a considerably raised white cell count with high eosinophilia (up to 80 per cent.).

Intradermal injection of antigen made from adult *Toxocara* will, in suitable cases, result in the appearance in 15–30 minutes of a large wheal with pseudopodia and peripheral arteriolar flare. Complement-fixation reactions with the same antigen and the patient's serum are often positive. Haemagglutination tests have also been used successfully. Lesions may sometimes be discovered by liver biopsy.

Treatment is unsatisfactory. Diethylcarbamazine given in high doses may be useful. Thiabendazole in the usual dosage has also been tried successfully.

WANDERING SWELLINGS

Larval lesions may occur in deeper tissue than those in larva migrans. These are solid small oedematous tumours which may move slowly from one area to another, in the course of days or weeks.

The commonest cause of such lesions is the developing round worm *Gnathostoma spinigerum*.

Infection with this nematode occurs in many parts of the East including India, Thailand and China.

The reservoir animals are dogs and cats in which adults are found in the stomach. Eggs are passed in the faeces, hatch in the water and larvae are ingested by *Cyclops*. Fish eat the *Cyclops* and the larvae encyst in the muscles. The ingestion of the larvae thus occurs only in those areas of the world such as Thailand in which raw fish is regularly consumed.

The usual sign is a single migratory subcutaneous swelling which may occur anywhere, but is particularly common on the face and the hands and feet. The swellings vary in size and may reappear intermittently in one place or wander from one area to another.

They are usually itchy and painless, but are occasionally accompanied by a deep boring pain. The swellings are firm and do not pit or suppurate.

Histologically there is intense oedema of the tissue and an inflammatory eosinophilic infiltration. The worm may be visible in some swellings through the skin or in a mucous membrane as in the vagina or cervix uteri.

In *Gnathostoma* infection the lesions are caused not by the larva but by the immature adult. Systemic reactions may occur concurrently, including paroxysmal coughing, and, where the worm involves the kidney tissue, haematuria. Cases of spontaneous haemo- or pneumothorax have been described.

Diagnosis

Diagnosis is often made in relevant geographic areas by removal of the lesion containing the worm.

It is usually curative as there is rarely more than one parasite involved.

Treatment

The best treatment is incision of the lesion and removal of the worm.

EOSINOPHILIC MENINGO-ENCEPHALITIS

This occurs sporadically and occasionally in small outbreaks in certain Pacific Islands, notably Tahiti and Hawaii and in South-East Asia, including Vietnam, Thailand and Malaysia.

The disease is caused by the invasion with mechanical damage of the central nervous system, brain and sometimes cord, by developing adults of nematodes, most commonly *Angiostrongylus cantonensis*, the rat lungworm, and sometimes *Gnathostoma spinigerum*. Secondary inflammatory reactions of an allergic nature occur and give rise to eosinophilic infiltrations of tissue and cerebrospinal fluid. The cerebrospinal fluid is at high pressure and cloudy with cells which are mostly eosinophils; rarely the larva may be found in the fluid.

The clinical picture develops within a few weeks of eating raw or inadequately cooked snails, fresh water shrimps, slugs (*Angiostrongylus*) or fish or other flesh (*Gnathostoma*) harbouring the larvae of the worms. It varies according to the area affected. Commonly the patient shows signs of meningeal involvement with stiffening of neck and paresis of eye muscles. There is fever and prostration. Recovery is spontaneous in most cases without sequelae.

Diagnosis is difficult. It is presumptive in endemic areas where the intermediate hosts are known to have been eaten. Various immunological techniques are being studied.

Anthelmintic drugs are not successful in treatment. Corticosteroids may prove valuable during the acute illness.

BRIAN MAEGRAITH

TRICHINIASIS

Definition.

A disease caused by the adult and embryo forms of the nematode worm *Trichinella spiralis*.

Aetiology

Infection is acquired by eating raw or underdone pork in which the larvae have encysted. After being liberated by the digestion of the cyst walls by gastric juice, the larvae attach themselves to the mucosa of the duodenum and jejunum. Within two days they develop into mature adults; the male measures $1 \cdot 5 \times 0 \cdot 04$ mm. and the female $3–4 \times 0 \cdot 6$ mm. Following copulation the male may die, and the gravid female bores into the mucosa and begins to deposit viviparous larvae ($100 \times 6\ \mu$). Each female may deposit some fifteen hundred larvae in the lymphatics and lacteals of the host's small intestine between the seventh and fortieth day at a rate of one each half hour. The female then dies. The larvae reach the blood stream and become widely distributed to all tissues. They leave the capillaries and settle between muscle fibres, enter serous cavities and even the cerebrospinal fluid. The invasion of striated muscle causes necrosis, hyaline degeneration and a cellular response consisting of neutrophils, eosinophils and lymphocytes. The reaction about the coiled trichina produces the cyst which begins to calcify in 6–18 months, and in which the larvae may survive for 25 years, although they often die within 6 months. The heaviest infestation occurs in the diaphragm, gluteus, pectoral, deltoid, gastrocnemius and intercostal mucles. The extra-ocular and laryngeal muscles, the masseters and tongue may also be involved. In some cases there may be as many as a thousand trichinae per gramme of muscle. The embryos are unable to establish themselves in cardiac or smooth muscle.

Epidemiology

The parasite can infect a wide variety of carnivorous and omnivorous animals. The chief reservoir for human infection is the pig, particularly swine fed on uncooked garbage, but rats, foxes, dogs, cats and bears are often infected. The cysts do not calcify in pork and may easily be missed unless meat inspection is meticulous. Epidemics, which are usually small, are often confined to a family and follow the ingestion of under-done pork, sausages or other products containing pork.

The geographical distribution of trichiniasis depends upon a number of variables. Consumption of undercooked pork is, of course, the primary factor. In some countries little pork is eaten; in others it is under a religious ban; in China traditional methods of cooking the meat ensure that all the larvae are killed.

Trichiniasis was formerly a common infestation in the United States, but its incidence has been greatly reduced by public health measures.

Clinical Features

The symptoms are extremely variable and depend largely upon the degree of infection. The ingestion of heavily infected meat may cause gastro-intestinal symptoms during the first 1–4 days. Nausea, vomiting, colic and diarrhoea may occur. Following the seventh day the migration of the larvae usually causes muscular stiffness, pain, tenderness and weakness, fever which may reach 104° F. (40° C.), oedema, especially of the face, urticaria, neutrophilia and eosinophilia. The fever is often remittent and may continue for several weeks. Backache is a common symptom, and swallowing, speech and respiration may cause difficulty. Headache, delirium and psychic or visual disturbances may suggest encephalitis; hemiplegic or localized paralysis occasionally occurs. Splinter haemorrhages may be seen under the nails or in the conjunctivae, and although the parasite does not settle in cardiac muscle, T wave inversion may be seen in severe infestation.

Diagnosis

In light infection the diagnosis may be extremely difficult. Laboratory methods are helpful in retrospect. If a portion of the suspected meat can be obtained, it should be ground up, digested with hydrochloric acid and pepsin for an hour and examined by means of a dissecting microscope. Examination of the stools for the adult worms is useless, but on occasion the larvae can be found in the blood during the migrating phase. Whole blood is laked by adding ten volumes of 3 per cent. acetic acid and the centrifuged deposit is examined. From ten days after infection the larvae may be found in muscle. Suitable sites for biopsy are the tendinous insertions of the deltoid or gastrocnemius muscles. Portions of the muscle are compressed between plate glass and examined under the low-power microscope. Early on, the larvae lie parallel to the muscle fibres and may be difficult to recognize; they do not begin to coil until the seventeenth day of infection. After encystment the spiral appearance is characteristic. Routine histological methods rarely reveal the parasites but show only a myositis. In acute infection the peripheral blood eosinophils may reach 70 per cent. of a total of 10–20,000 leucocytes per mm^3. and an eosinophilia may persist for 5–7 years. The intradermal skin test (0·1 ml. of 1 in 10,000 dilution of dried powdered trichinae dissolved in saline) is usually not positive before the end of the third week. The local reaction may be immediate or delayed; false positives are common and cross-reactions occur (e.g. with *Trichuris*). The skin test remains positive for about seven years. Precipitin and complement fixing antibodies are more specific but may not be positive in very severe infection. The serum immunological tests revert to negative after a year.

Treatment

No specific treatment is known. Should the condition be suspected in the intestinal phase, an anthelmintic such as piperazine citrate should be given in doses of 1–1·5 G. twice daily for 7 days. An anthelmintic should also be given if corticosteroids are used because the adult worm persists longer in these circumstances. Adrenal corticosteroids or corticotrophin will reduce the acute manifestations of the disease and are of particular value when the central nervous system is invaded. Analgesics should be prescribed and possibly antihistamine drugs may reduce the allergic manifestations. Thiabendazole has been reported as an effective helminthicide in trichiniasis. It is still in the stage of therapeutic trial and is commonly prescribed in doses of 25 mg. per kg. body weight twice daily for 5–7 days.

Trichinellae can be killed by cooking, freezing or irradiation. Smoking, salting or pickling alone does not kill the parasite, for which cooking at a minimum oven temperature of 350° F. (175° C.) for 40–50 minutes per pound, freezing at 0° F. (−18° C.) for at least 24 hours or a temperature of 5° F. (−15° C.) for 20 days is required.

Prognosis

This largely depends on the severity of the infection. In epidemics the mortality rate may vary from 1–30 per cent. but over-all it must be extremely low.

REFERENCES

Gould, S. E. (1945) *Trichinosis*, Springfield, Ill.
Most, H. (1965) Trichinellosis in the United States, *J. Amer. med. Ass.*, **193**, 871.

R. Bodley Scott

ARTHROPODS

MYIASIS

Myiasis occurs when fly larvae invade animal tissues. The larvae, which are obligatory tissue parasites, may be introduced directly by the fly, or indirectly, in foodstuffs. The larva of one fly, the Congo maggot, acts as an ectoparasite of man.

Myiasis is usually cutaneous or involves the mucous membranes, especially those of the nasopharyngeal cavities.

Lesions in the skin may be shallow and migratory, resembling larva migrans resulting from invasion by the larva of *Ancylostoma braziliense*, or deep, leading to the production of single 'boils' containing the larva. In some infestations the larvae burrow deep or otherwise reach the mucous membranes or cavities of the nasopharynx and other areas, including the ear, eye and vagina causing very extensive damage.

Gastro-intestinal myiasis arises from accidental swallowing of larvae in stale foodstuffs. Occasionally this may lead to invasion of the intestinal wall.

A short account of the more important human fly infestations follows:

Shallow Larva Migrans Type of Lesion

Gastrophilus spp. (the Horse Bot or Warble Fly). The larva, which hatches from eggs deposited on the hairs of the host, penetrates the skin and then burrows a serpiginous tunnel parallel to the surface, producing a lesion very similar to the 'larva migrans' produced by nematode larvae. The leading end of the lesion moves a few millimetres a day and the infestation may last for months.

A squirt of ethyl chloride or the local application of ice will kill the larva which can be removed by incision.

Hypoderma spp. (the Cattle Bot or Warble Fly). The larva, which is much larger than that of *Gastrophilus*, burrows deeper but migrates slowly and may cause lesions some distance from the point of entry. There is usually swelling and tissue inflammation as the larva reaches the surface and surgical removal may be necessary.

Deep Boil-like Lesions

Dermatobia Hominis (the Human Bot or Warble Fly). The fly deposits eggs on another arthropod, usually a mosquito, which carries them to the warm-blooded host. Larvae are produced rapidly and penetrate vertically to the surface. They do not migrate, but give rise to an inflammatory swelling which grows as the larva develops. By the third or fourth week a tender intensely itching 'boil' has developed which may be extremely painful especially during the active movements of the larva within the cavity, through the open mouth of which the posterior end of the larva protrudes from time to time. After about 6 weeks the mature larva escapes and drops to pupate in the soil. Secondary infection is usual and there is often accompanying lymphangitis and local adenitis.

The larva may occasionally be squeezed out (an extremely painful performance) but is better extracted under anaesthesia by aseptic incision. Antibiotics should be given to deal with the secondary infection.

Cordylobia Anthropophaga (Tumbu Fly or Blowfly). Eggs are deposited on clothing especially when laid out on the ground or polluted dry sand for laundering. The larvae hatch and penetrate the skin vertically, producing lesions very similar to those of *Dermatobia*, but developing in the course of 2–3 weeks.

The larva can usually be expressed readily by covering the opening in the 'boil' with a drop of liquid paraffin. The posterior end of the larva extrudes and is covered with another drop of oil. The larva withdraws and re-emerges to continue the struggle to breathe. More oil is applied and eventually the whole larva can be expressed from the lubricated cavity. A dressing is applied and wide-spectrum antibiotics are given to deal with the secondary infection.

Tissue Invasion

Callitroga or Cochliomyia spp. (the Screw Worm Flies). These are found in the southern United States and in South America. The fly deposits its eggs in open wounds or damaged tissue or wet discharging surfaces. The larvae burrow deep and invade tissues extensively including even cartilage and bone. Secondary infection is the rule and deep filthy stinking lesions result. When the nasal cavities or middle ear become involved extension to the meninges and brain may occur. The larvae develop in about 3 weeks to 2 months, escape and pupate in the soil. The lesions are most commonly seen in the nasal mucosa and cause painful local swelling. Larvae may be sneezed or coughed out, they are pink and about 2 cm. in length and shaped roughly like a screw.

Treatment consists of removing larvae after swabbing or spraying the area with ether or chloroform in oil. Secondary infection requires treatment with antibiotics. Prevention is a matter of screening the individual especially when there are discharging wounds or sinuses.

Chrysomyia spp. This fly, which occurs in the East and North East Africa, lays its eggs in cuts and wounds or on wet mucous membranes such as the nose, lips and conjunctivae. The progress after the larva burrows into the tissues is much the same as in *Callitroga* infections but the larva develops by the end of a week to the stage at which pupation can occur. Lesions may be very severe and extensive and commonly involve the eye and the orbit.

Somewhat similar lesions are produced by tissue invasion by the larvae of many other flies, including the sheep botfly *Oestrus* spp. and the 'flesh' flies *Sarcophaga* spp. and *Wohlfahrtia* spp. In most instances the larvae are laid on existing stinking wounds or orifices with smelly discharges. In the case of *Wohlfahrtia*, the larvae are believed to be able to pierce the unbroken skin.

Treatment consists, as above, in removal of the larvae and dealing with the local secondary infection.

Ectoparasitic Larva

Auchmeromyia Luteola (the Congo Maggot Fly). This lays eggs in dry sandy soil, for example, on the floor of huts. The small elongate larvae which hatch within 2 days, attach themselves by spines and hooks to the skin of the human host at night and suck blood. When replete, in about 20 minutes, they fall back to the soil. The process may be repeated nightly until the development of the larva is completed. This may take some weeks. Pupation takes place on the ground. Most infestations result from sleeping on bare floors. Proper bedding and repellants are the only satisfactory preventive measures until housing can be improved.

Intestinal Myiasis

Fly larvae are sometimes found in freshly passed human faeces or even in vomit. The larvae, which may be those of many flies, including *Musca*, *Fannia* and *Sarcophaga*, indicate accidental infection from swallowing eggs or larvae in infested food. Sometimes, especially in *Sarcophaga* infection, invasion of the intestinal mucosa occurs with symptoms resembling those of colitis which may persist for months. The larvae passed may be at all stages; even pupae have been recorded. Purgation and enemas usually relieve the condition. Larvae have also been observed in urine, but the source of these has not always been clear. In most cases there is probably contamination from faeces.

LICE

Lice which infest man are: *Pediculus humanus corporis* (the body louse), *P. hum. capitis* (the head louse) and *Phthirus pubis* (the crab louse). These arthropods are obligatory parasites of man.

The louse has a flat body and an indistinctly segmented thorax. It has no wings. There are six legs modified for grasping. The female lays up to five eggs (also called 'nits') in the day. These adhere to the hairs and hatch in about 8 days; the nymphs undergo three moults and mature in 14 days. The life span is 4–6 weeks.

Lice take two blood meals daily. The bite causes considerable local irritation and leaves small haemorrhagic lesions which, in the case of the body louse, are often found concentrated in the waist line.

P. hum. corporis attaches itself to body hair and commonly migrates, especially to coarse clothing, where it will survive for a day or longer; in cold conditions it may survive for a week on clothing. *P. hum. capitis* attaches itself to the scalp hair. Both avoid light.

These lice are spread during close contact with an infested person. They migrate from the host during exercise or during fever.

Relapsing fever (*Borrelia recurrentis*) is transmitted by crushing infected lice and introducing infective material through skin lesions, usually the result of scratching. An infected louse may remain infective for a month.

The *Rickettsia* of exanthematic (louse-borne) typhus are conveyed via the faeces of infected body lice in the same way. Trench fever (*R. quintana*) may be similarly transmitted.

The cysticeroid stage of the dog tapeworm *Dipyllidum canis* may develop in the body louse and is occasionally transmitted to man (usually to children) when the louse is swallowed.

The crab louse *Phthirus pubis* is broader and flatter than the other lice. It has six abdominal segments and has powerful claws on the second and third legs. It clings to hairs in the pubis and groin but may occasionally wander to other hairy skin. The bite is similar to that of the body louse. It does not normally transmit infections to man.

Infestation with lice can be eliminated by dusting with DDT powder (10 per cent.). Three dustings at weekly intervals will remove adults and nits completely. As an alternative for head lice, liquids containing DDT (1 per cent.) and various solvents and emulsifiers, including benzyl benzoate and *Tween* 80 (NBIN is an example). The crab louse may be dealt with similarly or by using emulsions containing lauryl thiocyanate.

Resistance to DDT has developed in some strains of *Pediculus hum. corporis* but not in *P. hum. capitis* or *Phthirus pubis*. Gamma BHC or pyrethrum powders are alternatives to DDT; some resistance to the former is suspected.

In the treatment of head lice the DDT powder can be applied to the head and neck directly. The hair should be cut short.

Some preparations of DDT especially oil suspensions and wall sprays may cause toxic effects in man.

Cleanliness, frequent thorough washing and avoidance of contact with other infested individuals are necessary to prevent further infection.

Louse infested clothing is best dealt with by heat. A hot iron is useful for getting into the folds where the lice tend to congregate.

FLEAS

Fleas are small laterally compressed wingless ectoparasitic arthropods with mouth parts adapted to piercing and sucking. Some have combs on the head or thorax or both. Others are combless. They are moderately species specific for a given host but will migrate to other hosts in suitable circumstances.

Eggs are dropped haphazard and hatch in 3–4 days into active larvae which are commonly found in dust. In the resting stage the larva or the adult may remain dormant for months.

The two major families are both important to man.

The *Pulicidae* include *Pulex irritans* the human flea, *Xenopsylla* sp. commonly found on the rat and vector of bubonic plague and various fleas of rats, mice, dogs and cats. The *Tungidae* include *T. penetrans* (the Chigoe of Jigger Flea) the female of which burrows beneath the human skin and causes serious incapacity especially when secondarily infected.

Flea bites appear as small discrete erythematous sometimes petechial spots, which are usually very irritating, especially in individuals already sensitized to them.

Medically, the most important flea is *Xenopsylla cheopis* which is the major vector of bubonic plague in man. Other species of *Xenopsylla* may also transmit human plague and other genera and species of fleas may be concerned with transmission of *Pasteurella pestis* as a zoonosis.

Murine typhus (*Rickettsia mooseri*) is spread from rats to man by the bite of *Xenopsylla* sp., and maintained as an infection in rats via the rat louse.

The cysticercoid stage of the rat tapeworm *Hymenolepis diminuta* may develop in the body cavity of human, rat and mouse fleas. Swallowing these arthropods leads to human infection with the adult worm.

The dog tapeworm *Diphylidium caninum* may, on rare occasions, be similarly transmitted to man.

Dog and cat fleas can be controlled in the animals by frequent washing. DDT is used for dusting dogs or their kennels with heavy infections. Toxic effects may result.

Houses may be cleared by spraying with 5 per cent. DDT, rat runs by dusting DDT powder (8–10 per cent.).

Protection against biting from xenopsylla suspected of being infected with plague may be achieved by dusting the environment with DDT or using DDT impregnated clothing.

Resistance has developed in many fleas against DDT and its analogues. Gamma BHC and organophosphorus compounds are alternatives but resistance may also be developed against them.

OTHER ARTHROPODS

MILLIPEDES AND CENTIPEDES

Millipedes (*Diplopoda*) have no venom fangs and in any case cannot bite man. Some, however, secrete highly irritant fluid from the segments, which can produce a severe local dermatitis. They may act as intermediate hosts for *Hymenolepis diminuta* if accidentally swallowed.

Centipedes (*Chilopoda*) are provided with poison glands at the base of the first pair of mandibular legs. A duct leads to the claws on these appendages which serve as fangs. Large centipedes, such as *Scolopendra* spp. secrete sufficient venom to cause severe local and even general reactions.

At the site of the bite there is immediate burning pain, which subsides in about half an hour. There is some transient erythema and a little oedema in most cases but in some there may be considerable swelling and pain, which subside only slowly and may leave some residual tenderness for days. Occasionally the local lymph nodes become enlarged and tender and there may be mild fever, headache and some prostration.

A single death has been reported.

Treatment consists in injection of local anaesthetic in the bitten area, as in scorpion sting, and codeine or other palliative general therapy. The application of cold or of mild alkaline solutions or ammonia may relieve the immediate local effects.

TICKS

Ticks as intermediate hosts and vectors of disease are discussed in the relevant accounts of rickettsial infections, relapsing fever and virus infections.

Tick paralysis may result from the injection of toxins especially by the wood tick *Dermacentor andersoni*, which is found in the United States and Canada. It occurs in both man and animals. There is mild fever, ascending symmetrical flaccid paralysis and may be death from respiratory failure. In the early stages there may be only mild constitutional symptoms; later there is sometimes severe toxaemia. The syndrome appears in 1–5 days after implantation of the tick, especially the female, in the tissues, usually in the neck region. It occurs most frequently in the spring and early summer.

Tick paralysis has also been reported after invasion by *Ixodes* spp. and the nymphs of *Amblyomma* spp.

It must be distinguished from viral infections, especially poliomyelitis.

In early cases dramatic improvement may follow the removal of the ticks.

MITES

The relevant sections on mites as vectors of disease, including rickettsial and viral infections should be referred to. Scabies is discussed elsewhere. Certain species cause dermatitis in man. For instance, the bite of the tropical rodent mite *Ornithonyssus* is responsible for irritating and itchy dermatitis in individuals living in rat infested areas. The so-called 'straw itch' or 'grain itch' results from infestation with *Pediculoides* spp. which burrow into the epidermis and produce red and sometimes petechial and very itchy spots upon which vesicles and pustules may develop. *Tyroglyphidae*, which infest cereals, flour, etc., also cause mild skin reactions. Dust from stored cereals or straw infested with mites may act similarly.

Harvest mites (*Trombiculidae*) are notorious in producing severe itchy dermatitis which may be haemorrhagic. Allergic reactions are common. Only the 6-legged larvae attack man.

LINGUATULIDS (PENTASTOMATA: TONGUE WORMS)

The adults of these primitive segmented arachnids *Armillifer* spp. live in the nasal and body cavities of reptiles, birds and some mammals. They are found in various parts of Africa and the Far East. Eggs are swallowed by man, larvae hatch in the intestine and migrate into various organs, especially the liver, spleen, lungs and the intestinal wall. Here nymphs become developed and encyst, producing local clinical effects, or calcifying and remaining inert, often first noticed on X-ray. Multiple infection in the liver may give rise to enlargement of the organ and jaundice. Intestinal obstruction has been reported.

SPIDER BITES

The bites of certain genera of spiders are accompanied by the injection of powerful toxins which can cause serious poisoning and even death in man.

The Black Widow spider *Latrodectus* spp. is probably the best known of the dangerous arachnids. Species are found in many parts of the world including the United States, South America and Europe. Man is bitten usually by the female, which has a round body about a centimetre (half an inch) long, with a shiny black abdomen marked ventrally with a characteristic red hour-glass pattern.

The spider lives in a tube of coarse web which is built in sheds and outbuildings including lavatories. Bites often occur in the latter.

The bite may cause little disturbance except for some local stinging pain, oedema and erythema. In more serious cases the local effects are followed by a general reaction which includes pain spreading from the bite wound to surrounding areas and eventually to the chest and abdomen; severe muscle pains and spasms occurring mostly in flexor muscles and causing the patient to double up. Sweating and excessive salivation are common, as are severe epigastric pain, abdominal rigidity, fever and tachycardia. Circulatory collapse is likely to occur in children.

Arachnid poisoning has been reported in South American states including Chile, in Assam and in Australia. The spider in South America is *Loxosceles laeta*. The bite causes a painful local reaction sometimes with widespread oedema which may involve a limb. In the course of a week blisters appear at the bite and are followed by a gangrenous patch which sloughs off leaving a large ulcer. Healing occurs with scarring.

In Assam spider bites said to be due to *Chilobrachys* are acquired by tea pickers, usually involving the backs of the hands or fingers in which extensive coagulation and consequent blocking of circulation occur, resulting eventually in the loss of the affected digit.

In Australia bites caused by the notorious funnel-web spider, *Atrax robustus* have caused serious reactions and even death.

Treatment

Intravenous administration of calcium gluconate relieves the muscle spasms. Successful antivenines have been prepared.

SCORPION STING

Many of the genera and species of scorpions found in the subtropics and tropics are sufficiently poisonous to cause serious intoxication and occasionally death. It is wise therefore to regard all scorpion stings seriously. The prognosis in a given case depends on the scorpion concerned and the age and health of the subject stung. Children are more seriously affected than adults, presumably because of the relative size of the dose received.

Scorpions shelter during the day in cracks and under stones, in wood piles and shoes. They are more active at night. Stings are the reward of the unwary. The venom is injected by a sting situated in the posterior abdominal segment. The attack comes with the tail bent forward over the body.

The effects of the sting vary. There is always an

extremely painful and sometimes agonizing local reaction. A red wheal appears at the site of the sting puncture; the surrounding tissue becomes oedematous and may ooze blood. There is a pronounced arteriolar flare.

General reactions may be immediate or delayed for some hours.

The patient in the severe case is in agony. Because of the action of the venom on the autonomic nervous system, he is usually also sweating, salivating and weeping; there is often violent sneezing. Nausea and vomiting are common. The patient complains of headache, and dizziness. There may be muscle tremors. He is restless and in severe cases may become comatose and die of respiratory failure or vascular collapse.

In most cases the whole syndrome subsides in a few hours.

Treatment

As in snake bite, the offending creature should be secured and identified, since in some areas specific antitoxins are available.

Relief of the local pain is best secured rapidly by injection of 1 or 2 per cent. procaine (*Novocain*) or the equivalent into and around the area stung. In difficult cases the injection may be repeated. Alternatively, emetine hydrochloride, 60 mg., may be injected into the sting.

General treatment consists of dealing with complications such as shock and administering antivenine, when available. Sympatholytic drugs such as *Rogitine* help to control the autonomic effects.

SNAKE AND SEA SNAKE BITES

SNAKE BITE

Aetiology

Poisonous snakes occur in many parts of the world and are especially prevalent in the tropics. It is extremely difficult to assess the importance of snake bite in a community, but in some agricultural areas, for example in India and South East Asia, it is considerable.

It is important whenever possible to identify the snake which has bitten the patient, since the administration of specific antivenine is much more successful than the polyvalent type.

For this purpose the snake should be preserved whole or at least the head and a few inches of the body and tail provided.

It is necessary first to decide whether the snake is really poisonous. This can be done by examining the teeth and identifying the fangs which are prominent and sharp and set in the upper jaw or maxilla. The examination should be made carefully with forceps since active venom may be present on the fangs or in the poison glands after death.

Classification

The main groups of snakes can be separated thus:

(1) ELAPIDAE (COBRAS, MAMBAS, ETC.).

Fangs fixed in the upper jaw, below or in front of eyes, with few or no other teeth in the maxilla.

Head covered with large scales, lateral nostrils.

Very poisonous.

(2) COLUBRIDAE (BOOMSLANGS, TREE SNAKES, ETC.).

Fangs fixed and at rear of rows of maxillary teeth.

Large head scales. Nostrils lateral.

Not usually dangerous to man.

(3) VIPERIDAE (VIPERS AND PIT VIPERS).

Fangs erectile, lying posteriorly against the palate in a retracted sheath of mucous membrane when relaxed; upright or slightly forward when erected. Often two or more *in tandem* on either side, but no other teeth in maxilla.

Head usually covered with small scales, occasionally with large scales. Nostrils placed vertically.

(i) NO 'PIT' OR DEPRESSION IN THE HEAD BETWEEN THE EYE AND THE NOSTRIL.

Viperidae (Vipers, adders, etc.).

Some mildly, some deadly poisonous.

(ii) 'PIT' PRESENT BETWEEN EYE AND NOSTRIL.

Crotalinae (Pit vipers, rattle snakes, etc.).

Very poisonous.

(4) HYDROPHIDAE (SEA SNAKES).

Found in Eastern sea waters.

Fangs below eyes; most anterior teeth in maxilla.

Long thin body, small head no appreciable neck, large head scales. Wide flanged tail.

Several genera, including *Lapemis*, *Enhydrina* and *Hydropis*.

Very poisonous.

Clinical Features

As most snakes are of nocturnal habit, bites occur most commonly at night.

The physical effects of the bite are determined primarily by the amount and toxicity of the venom injected, but in some areas it is thought that the nutritional status of the victim may play a part in the reaction, since the mortality and morbidity associated with the bites of the same snake vary, sometimes seasonally, amongst communities.

There is great fear of snake bite and a wide tendency to regard any unidentified injury, particularly of the feet, as due to a snake. Patients may arrive at a clinic shaking with fear over a scratch or thorn prick. It is therefore necessary first to decide whether a bite has been inflicted or not.

In many cases there is no question. The patient knows he has been bitten and usually brings the dead snake with him or knows enough about the local hazards to describe it.

Unobstructed bites show two clean puncture wounds set up an inch apart. Most bites are not fully effective and the local skin may be lacerated or scratched because of deviation of the fang by clothing or movement of the victim. In poisonous snake bite there are rarely any other teeth marks. A row of punctures indicates a bite by a non-poisonous snake, which may nevertheless be dangerous because of the introduction of anaerobic bacteria.

Even when there is no doubt about the patient having been bitten by a poisonous snake, the syndromes of 'envenomation' may not develop since venom is not invariably injected during even obvious and successful bites. In most cases oedema develops round the area of the envenomated bite. Absence of local oedema after some hours probably means that venom has not been injected.

Venoms

Most snakes secrete venom in which there are both neurotoxic and haemotoxic factors. Some secrete venom in which one or other factor predominates. Thus, the venom of Elapids is largely neurotoxic and that of vipers commonly, but not always, haemotoxic.

In dealing with snake bite therefore some knowledge of local snakes and their venoms is essential.

Neurotoxic effects develop rapidly, involving the respiratory centre early and sometimes fatally. Death occurs in a few hours or days. Haemotoxic effects take longer to develop. They include shock, capillary bleeding, haemolysis and coagulation or anticoagulation; bleeding from the bite wound may be severe. Death often occurs later than with neurotoxic poisoning, for example, after a week or more.

Local tissue damage in the region of the bite may occur in both elapid and viperid envenomation but is commoner and usually more severe in the latter.

The venoms of sea snakes contain neurotoxic and haemotoxic elements, including a powerful anticoagulant. They are unique in producing severe local damage to skeletal muscle, causing necrosis and liberating myoglobin which may escape in the urine and be mistaken for haemoglobin.

Antivenines

Antitoxins can be made for individual snake venoms (monovalent or specific) or for mixtures (polyvalent), by injection of the relevant venoms into horses. The antitoxin develops in the serum and is usually freed from albumin before being issued.

In any given case the specific antitoxin is more effective in controlling the effects of envenomation than the polyvalent. The identification of the serpent responsible for the bite is therefore of cardinal importance when specific antivenines are available.

Antivenines are available for the treatment of many envenomations including various species of cobra, vipers and sea snakes.

Treatment

The management of snake bite naturally falls into the categories of immediate or first-aid treatment and subsequent treatment.

Immediate Treatment. The bitten area should be immobilized if possible. This may delay the absorption of some venom from the site.

There is some doubt concerning the value of applying a tourniquet, but it is probably wise for psychological reasons alone and might also impede further absorption of the venom. The tourniquet should be applied in the area most suitable for controlling the circulation, for example, above the elbow when the forearm or hand is bitten, sufficiently tight to interrupt the venous return but not to cut off the arterial supply. It must be loosened for a minute or so every 10–15 minutes and should be taken off altogether as soon as the patient can be given further treatment.

Incisions are not advisable. They often cause more serious and permanent injury than the bite. Suction is also of doubtful value.

The local application of potassium permanganate is valueless, but on the other hand, the injection of soap solution into the region of the bite is advised in some parts of India for viper bite. Analgesics may be given, but morphine should be avoided.

The main thing is to reassure the patient, relieve pain and get him to hospital as quickly as possible.

Subsequent Treatment. This consists in dealing with the complication of envenomation and giving antivenine if necessary. If signs of systemic poisoning are apparent and the snake has been identified, the specific antivenine should be given immediately if it is available. Otherwise, a polyvalent antivenine should be used.

If there are no signs of systemic poisoning the decision depends on the appearances of the bite wound and a knowledge of the snake concerned.

In Europe, where the viper rarely causes a fatal accident, antivenine is usually unnecessary but in areas where the snakes may be deadly it is probably advisable to give it even hours after the bite.

Anaphylactic reactions to serum injection are the greatest hazard of antivenine administration. Where possible the patient should be tested for sensitivity but even this may not be adequate as a negative skin reaction may occasionally be found in a susceptible individual.

Intravenous injection is commonly preferred to intramuscular.

Seriously poisoned patients should also be given corticosteroids.

Complications including bleeding or oozing from the bite wound must be dealt with promptly. Serious and rapidly developing anaemia may result from neglecting such bleeding in viperine bites. Respiratory failure occurs in severe neurotoxic poisoning and may call for continuous artificial respiration.

Anuric uræmia is the common cause of death after viper bite. The results of peritoneal dialysis appear to be promising.

A broad-spectrum antibiotic should be given, since the snake bite is often dirty and local damage may be exacerbated by infection. Where there is severe laceration even in non-venomous bites tetanus antitoxin may be advisable or a 'booster' dose of toxoid given in those already protected.

The application of ice to the affected area is said to reduce the risk of local necrosis and to delay the spread of the venom.

Venom sprayed or 'spat' into the eyes by certain

cobras in Asia and Africa causes a painful conjunctivitis and palpebral oedema. In the absence of cuts or abrasions the situation is not dangerous. It is relieved by washing with milk or other bland fluids or by the instillation of diluted antivenine.

REFERENCES

ADAMS, A. R. D., and MAEGRAITH, B. G. (1966) *Clinical Tropical Diseases*, 4th ed., Oxford.

BRITISH ENCYCLOPAEDIA OF MEDICAL PRACTICE (MEDICAL PROGRESS) (1960–9) Annual reviews of progress in tropical medicine, London.

DAVEY, T. H., and LIGHTBODY, W. P. H. (1961) *Control of Disease in the Tropics*, 2nd ed., London.

FAIRLEY, N. W., WOODRUFF, A. W., and WALTERS, J. (1961) *Recent Advances in Tropical Medicine*, London.

MAEGRAITH, B. G. (1965) *Exotic Disease in Practice*, London.

MANSON-BAHR, P. H., ed. (1960) *Manson's Tropical Diseases*, 15th ed., London.

NATIONAL ACADEMY OF SCIENCE (1962) Tropical health, *National Research Council, U.S.A.*, Publication 996.

BRIAN MAEGRAITH

SECTION 3

DISORDERS DUE TO CHEMICAL AND PHYSICAL AGENTS

AND TO CLIMATIC AND ENVIRONMENTAL CAUSES

ACUTE POISONING

INDUSTRIAL TOXICOLOGY

DISORDERS DUE TO CLIMATIC, ENVIRONMENTAL AND OTHER PHYSICAL FACTORS

ACUTE POISONING

INTRODUCTION

THE INCIDENCE AND EPIDEMIOLOGY OF POISONING

In many countries the number of patients who suffer from some form of acute poisoning is increasing. This phenomenon is marked in Britain. Between the years 1957 and 1969 the estimated number of discharges from hospitals in England and Wales of patients suffering from poisoning increased many fold whereas the home population increased by a few per cent. Similarly the number of persons who died from all forms of poisoning in England and Wales rose from 4277 in 1955 to 6398 in 1963 but subsequently declined to 4855 in 1969, an approximate incidence of 1 in 10,000 population annually. The crude death rate per million for England and Wales was 99·4 in 1969.

To a large extent this is related to the increased consumption of drugs taken to allay anxiety, induce sleep or relieve pain. These substances have a steeply additive effect when taken together or in conjunction with alcohol and the combination has probably given rise to fatal accidents. Drugs are often the chosen means of attempted suicide. There has been an absolute increase in the last 10 years in the incidence of suicidal attempts among women.

The means employed has changed for both sexes from violence to poison. Carbon monoxide (utility gas) is no longer the most common lethal agent, accounting for approximately 36 per cent. of deaths in 1969, a marked decline. This trend may be due to an improvement in therapy, particularly first aid, a decrease in the carbon monoxide content of domestic gas and a swing by the section of the public which attempts self-poisoning towards pills and tablets and away from the sordid image of the 'gas oven'. Sedatives come first at 41 per cent., and aspirin at 6 per cent. An increasing number of poisoning episodes are due to self-poisoning with the newer depressants—hypnotics, sedatives and tranquillizers, frequently ingested as a mixture of pills. The relative incidence of poisoning due to pure barbiturate has, therefore, fallen but the incidence due to all forms of cerebral depressants has risen. This is reflected in mortality and morbidity. Availability plays a large part in the cause of an accident or the choice of a means of suicide. The usual place in which acute poisoning takes place is at home, where coal-gas poisoning is of great importance. Death from this agent frequently occurs before treatment can be begun, whereas it is otherwise with barbiturates.

Chronic poisoning of any kind is likely to be due to exposure at work. Contemporary engineering practice, hygiene regulations and educative effort have reduced the incidence despite a great increase in the handling of toxic materials. An individual has less chance of surviving acute poisoning than a traffic accident (although much less likely to be involved) but this is largely due to the lethality of carbon monoxide. Once admitted to hospital less than 2 per cent. die. There are always more deaths from self-poisoning than from accident, except during the first 15 years of life; in England and Wales during 1969 there were 917 deaths from accidental poisoning and 3938 from deliberate self-poisoning. Nevertheless, distressingly large numbers of young children suffer from acute poisoning. In 1969 there were 146 deaths compared to 4709 in adults. Carbon monoxide accounted for 109. In the year 1967 20,670 children were admitted to hospital suffering from poisoning. Obviously few of them die, nevertheless, poisoning is an important cause of death in hospital at ages 0–5 years and 25 per cent. of all admissions for poisoning are of children. The vast majority of them are between the ages of 2 and 5 years. The agents involved are similar to those affecting adults, with, additionally, medicines (ferrous sulphate, sympathomimetics), cleanser-disinfectants (turpentine, detergents) and fuel (paraffin, oil, petrol). The period of life for peak incidence of poisoning is from 35 to 50 years of age, for deaths from 40 to 60 years, but the rate is disproportionately high in old persons, though falling. One-third of the latter cases are accidents, frequently caused by carbon monoxide and due to inability to smell domestic gas or failure to handle apparatus correctly, but the number of suicides among old people is large. Women are more inclined to resolve a marital or emotional crisis by resort to poison than are men, so that a high percentage of hospital patients suffering from overdosage with cerebral depressants or aspirin are females and they have probably attempted suicide during the course of a reactive depression.

The incidence of poisoning varies with the season, summer being the busier time for numbers, but winter the more anxious time because of complications such as bronchopneumonia. About 15 persons each year die of non-accidental poisoning inflicted by others (various degrees of culpability are included) in this country and less than 60 die from therapeutic misadventure, i.e. a fatal outcome directly attributable to treatment with drugs. This is usually due to hypersensitivity on the part of the patient, often with an element of allergic reaction in it, but may be due to gross overdosage from careless prescribing or dispensing. If the toxic reaction or 'side-effect' is a part of the known pharmacological activity of the drug, it should be predictable although not in degree. If it is an allergic reaction it is not predictable in relation to time or dosage, but to elicit a history of allergy should make the physician cautious when prescribing.

THE DIAGNOSIS OF POISONING

In acute poisoning diagnostic aids are at a disadvantage because of the urgency for treatment, the frequently collapsed state of the patient and the tendency for special skills to be less readily available at the time when cases commonly present. It may be that the promptness or otherwise of applying remedial measures is the determining factor for survival. If the degree of poisoning is mild, delay is permissible but the severity of an apparently mild poisoning may advance quickly. Diagnosis has, therefore, to be made without the benefit of procedures which are too time-consuming, although these should be initiated and the results considered when available. There may be nothing characteristic about the case as it presents and an empirical approach will then be inevitable. Nevertheless, the number and efficacy of specific antidotes has increased and it is highly desirable not to misuse them. Non-specific measures such as tracheobronchial suction, gastric suction and lavage, and intravenous infusion are not without hazard if a mis-diagnosis has been made. Personal history may be unobtainable due to disorientation, anxiety, fantasy, fear or restlessness on the part of the patient, or to loss of consciousness. It may be deliberately misleading. Detail obtained from relatives or friends may be much distorted by grief, anger and dismay. The opportunities for the doctor in charge to be cognizant of the patient's life-history are less than heretofore. The essential information required is the patient's age, the presence of constitutional or chronic disability (as diabetes mellitus or phthisis) or recent severe illness, the nature of his employment, and more specifically, the nature, amount and time of taking, the poison, if known. An official information service on poisons was established in Britain in 1963. It consists of an index of brief data on approximately 10,000 products —medicinal, cosmetic, horticultural and domestic— which is available to professional inquirers by telephone at all times. The aim is to provide information on the content of a wide range of products, not by any means all toxic, and an outline of suggested first-aid treatment if this is requested. Case handling remains the responsibility of the doctor in charge of the patient but further consultation is available by telephone. The relevant telephone numbers are: London 01–407–7600; Edinburgh 031–308–2477; Cardiff 02–22–33101; Belfast 02–32–30503. Information must be recorded at all stages of case-handling. Physical examination of patients suffering from acute poisoning should be conducted with especial thoroughness, a balance being struck between urgency and deliberation.

Identification of Poisons in Body Fluids

Despite the earlier statement to the effect that treatment should be initiated without benefit of laboratory identification of poisons it is becoming easier to obtain this information. This benefit has largely resulted from the current tendency to admit cases of poisoning to designated hospitals which are specially equipped to handle them. Preparedness for this task should include the capacity to detect and measure carbon monoxide, alcohol, salicylate, iron and barbiturate in blood, and phenothiazines in urine in addition to the general clinical aids of blood counts, pH, Pco_2, electrolytes and other tests.

The presenting features of poisoning are numerous and often little that is pathognomonic can be obtained from them. Pain results from irritation but many poisons obtund it. The main sites of injury are at the points of absorption—alimentary canal, skin or lungs; the points of excretion—kidneys, skin, lungs, colon; and at the places which are most sensitive or where poison is concentrated—stomach, liver, kidneys, central nervous system. External signs of locally-acting poisons are apparent and may be diagnostic. The odour of the breath may be helpful (vinous, utility gas). Vomiting and diarrhoea are the most common signs of poisoning, but there are many other causes for them. The most difficult distinction to make is that between food poisoning (bacterial or toxic) and poisoning due to noxious food (metals, plants, domestic poisons in children). The liver, as the chief site of detoxification, is affected by most poisons, sometimes severely, e.g. by phosphorus, but there are no signs which distinguish hepatic failure due to endogenous and exogenous toxins. Fever is not usually a sign of poisoning, but febrile illness may complicate it. Depression of respiration with hypoxia and hypercapnia is a common occurrence. Measurements of Po_2, Pco_2 and pH of blood, or a simple measure of arterial oxygen saturation may be of value. Any patient who is unconscious for a number of hours may accumulate fluid in the lungs and develop rhonchi. Soft rales at the bases of the lung with tachypnoea, quick pulse, leucocytosis and fever suggest bronchopneumonia. All patients who have been unconscious for more than 4 hours should have an X-ray of the chest done in order to detect patchy collapse of the lungs. Occasionally there is froth at the mouth and dullness of percussion at the bases with poor oxygenation, which is indicative of acute pulmonary oedema.

Circulatory failure with hypotension is a feature of severe poisoning by depressant drugs. High blood pressure due to stimulant drugs is a transient phenomenon and seldom of importance. Abnormal behaviour may be due to mild poisoning and it is sometimes difficult to distinguish the effects of psychosis from those due to drugs. Sudden illness characterized by partial or complete loss of consciousness are often due to poison. Examination of the nervous system is of particular importance in toxicology, especially in unconscious patients in whom signs of intracranial disturbance should be sought with care. Neurological signs occur commonly, e.g. those of peripheral neuropathy in poisoning with metals. The corneal reflex is easily lost, or nystagmus detected and this is of little significance, but loss of the pharyngeal or 'gagging' reflex or the presence of Babinski's sign is a serious matter. Depressants may cause ataxia, slurred speech and confusion, progressing to stupor, coma and death. Nausea and weakness are common. Certain postural defects, e.g. wryneck after phenothiazines may be met with. Sensation is seldom lost after poisoning except with loss of consciousness or from chronic neuropathy, but quinine causes blindness.

If the bladder is palpable it should be drained by firm pressure or, if unavoidable, by catheter, and urine sent for analysis (aspirin, barbiturate); incontinence is a sign of deep depression. A fluid balance chart is an essential part of management, as renal function may be temporarily depressed, or diuretic therapy embarked upon. Two samples of blood should be withdrawn initially, 10 ml. with sodium edetate and 15 ml. which is allowed to clot. These are used to determine electrolytes, haematocrit value, specific poisons, or urea and sugar levels.

The formed elements of the blood and the marrow cells are sensitive to repeated exposure to poisons, e.g. anaemic and leucopenic reactions to benzene (benzole), punctate basophilia in lead poisoning, purpura due to phenacetin. Changes in blood pigment occur, e.g. carboxyhaemoglobin (CO), methaemoglobin (aniline) and cyanhaemoglobin (HCN). Eczematous skin lesions may be caused by repeated use of drugs including aspirin, sulphonamide, antibiotic or more exotic medicaments such as gold. Pruritus is often due to drugs. Much attention has recently been concentrated on the ability of certain drugs to induce abnormalities in the foetus. Clearly, the effect of poisons may present in a bewildering variety of ways.

PRINCIPLES OF TREATMENT OF POISONING

Certain principles are applicable to most cases of acute poisoning.

Initial Assessment

The first step is to classify the severity of the individual case by an assessment of the nature and amount of the poison taken, the time since exposure to it, the level of consciousness and the existence of complications of age, shock, respiratory inadequacy and complicating disease. The absence of bowel sounds and failure to respond to painful stimuli with other evidences of coma are indicative of severe depressant poisoning. The state of the reflexes and the pupils is not very helpful.

Safeguarding Respiration

If the patient's breathing is obstructed, it is essential to clear the airway at once. This may be done by direct inspection and digital exploration, by employing a laryngoscope and using a mechanical sucker with the patient in the dorsal decubitus position with the head well extended, or by using a bronchoscope and sucker and inserting a Magill tube with or without a cuff. The services of an anaesthetist are often employed for the latter procedure. After clearing the airway and allowing a brief period for adjustment the ventilatory state may be assessed by means of a Wright's spirometer and inflation of the lungs with air, oxygen or a mixture, undertaken if the minute volume is inadequate. Precise figures in litres/min. which are acceptable vary with the rate and depth of respiration and the size of the patient but 6 litres/min. may serve as a guiding line for an adult. Oxygen may be administered in a variety of ways, depending on the adequacy or otherwise of spontaneous breathing: (1) By mouth-to-mouth breathing as an emergency method of resuscitation. It is necessary to compress the upper abdomen and to pinch the victim's nostrils (in an adult) while exhaling repeatedly into the mouth for 10 minutes. Over-inflation must be avoided in children. This process delivers an intermittent current of mixed 'dead-space' and alveolar air to the lungs which is efficacious in resuscitating apparently drowned persons, children in particular. It is of less value in poisoning where the respiratory mechanisms may be severely depressed. (2) By use of an Ambu bag which provides air or oxygen by manual compression of a reservoir connected to a face-piece and one-way valve. (3) By classical artificial respiration, of which the Holger Nielsen method is often preferred. In this the victim is laid prone and the operator kneels facing the patient and compresses the chest by leaning on outstretched hands placed on the scapulae. Inspiration is caused by lifting the victim's arms up and forwards, and the cycle repeated. (4a) As a continuous flow of 6 litres of oxygen per minute delivered through warm water to a non-cuffed tube in the trachea; or (4b) in an oxygen tent. (5a) As an intermittent flow from a valved bag to a cuffed endotracheal tube; (5b) a close-fitting mask with a non-return valve; or (5c) a plastic face-mask. Methods (4b) and (5c) though commonly used give the poorest oxygenation and may contribute to CO_2 retention. If spontaneous respiration is inadequate, it may be supplemented by a mechanical respirator. These machines are either driven by oxygen pressure or electrically and may be set to deliver a preset time-cycled tidal rhythm or to be triggered by the patient's breathing and reinforce it. The former type of machine will not fail if depression deepens, but accurate adjustment of the tidal volume to a physiological level is not easy. On occasions of prolonged respiratory inadequacy with evidence of retention of carbon dioxide, tracheostomy may be performed. All this should be done in close collaboration with an anaesthetist.

During the period of diminished consciousness it is essential that the patient be nursed on his side to reduce the risk of inhaling secretions. He should be turned over regularly, e.g. 2-hourly, and a power-driven tilting bed may be a great help to the nursing staff in carrying out this part of the patient care.

Administration of 2 ml. nikethamide injection intramuscularly may be helpful while control of respiratory function is being organized but there is no place for repeated administration of analeptic drugs in the treatment of acute poisoning. The need to give antibiotics, e.g. 150 mg. (250,000 Units) of benzylpenicillin by injection twice daily and 250 mg. of ampicillin thrice daily by mouth to patients who are febrile, show a leucocytosis or have evident signs of infection or oedema in the lungs, must be seriously considered. A broad-spectrum antibiotic may be preferred. This may be supplemented or replaced by an antibiotic precisely suited to the bacteriology determined if there is evidence of bronchopneumonia, but antibiotics, particularly broad-spectrum antibiotics should not be given as a prophylactic routine. Collapse of the lung is often relieved by vigorous physiotherapy but if it persists for a day, as revealed by radiography, bronchoscopy and direct inflation should be employed. Acute pulmonary oedema should be treated vigorously by bronchial suction, injection of frusemide, 10 mg., and digoxin, 0·5 mg. Assisted respiration by a time-cycled respirator with oxygen delivered with sufficient force to inflate the lungs may be needed. Vigorous prosecution of a diuretic technique or the use of the haemodialyser may reverse the tendency to form fluid in the lungs. If the oedema is the result of inhalation of an irritant, an injection of mepyramine maleate, 25 mg., may be given. Sometimes the obstruction is not due to pulmonary fluid but to outpouring of saliva and mucus; this can be stopped by injection of 1 mg. of atropine sulphate. If foaming in the trachea is particularly troublesome inhalation of an aerosol of 50 per cent. solution of ethanol in water, with intermittent tracheal suction, may clear it. Other measures include venesection in acute heart failure, and aminophylline injection, 0·25 g., if there is bronchoconstriction. It is important not to repeat the administration of aminophylline routinely or there is some danger of poisoning—drowsiness and convulsions.

Removal of the Poison

This may be simply a matter of washing a contaminant from the skin, e.g. acid, or conjunctival sac, e.g. lime, or of rescuing a patient from a poisonous atmosphere, e.g. coal-gas, but removal of swallowed poisons is more difficult. If the patient has an active pharyngeal reflex, digital stimulation of the fauces should be tried and the stomach emptied by drinking a solution of brine, and vomiting. Care should be taken to place children 'head down' while emesis is induced and performed. Injection of apomorphine hydrochloride is not recommended as it is slow to act and toxic. Other emetics, such as salts of copper and syrup of ipecacuanha are likewise not recommended on the grounds that giving one poison is no way to treat another. If the primary poison is a depressant ipecacuanha may fail or inhalation of vomitus take place. Gastric and tracheal suction will then have to be performed and a relatively simple procedure has been unnecessarily complicated. Gastric suction and lavage is too frequently carried out. Most often it is of no value and may do harm if applied without critical appraisal. Extra care must be taken with the young or old, with frail persons, with those who show evidence of previous abdominal surgery, or with those who have swallowed a corrosive. Strong acid or alkali is generally considered to be a contra-indication to gastric intubation for fear of rupture of the viscus, but after lysol or oxalic acid poisoning lavage has been carried out with benefit. If the poison has been swallowed more than 4 hours previously, suction-lavage should be omitted, except in the case of poisoning by aspirin, and mixtures containing aspirin, paracetamol and phenacetin when large accretions of the drug may be recovered after many hours.

During the performance of lavage the patient should be kept head down and semi-prone on a table tilted to 15 degrees. This manoeuvre reduces the probability of inhalation of fluid. The trachea should be closed with a cuffed tube if the patient has no pharyngeal and coughing reflexes, an anaesthetist being asked to attend to the respiratory function meanwhile. In all cases a soft rubber tube should be used, the tip dipped in liquid paraffin and suction applied before lavage. After insertion of the tube to the mark, 250 ml. of warm water at a time is poured into a funnel on the end of the tube and later siphoned out into a bucket. Special washing fluids are seldom indicated. After aspirin or iron pill poisoning a 1 per cent. sodium bicarbonate solution may be used, and milk or calcium lactate will detoxify oxalic acid. The sucker can be used between washes. A total of 1·5 litres is generally enough for an adult and the volume is reduced for smaller patients. The first wash should be kept apart, all being bottled, sealed, labelled and transmitted directly to the analyst so that a chain of factual evidence is available on demand for medico-legal purposes. If thought fit a demulcent (50 ml. of liquid paraffin shaken up with 100 ml. of warm water) may be poured in. When the tube is withdrawn it should be nipped firmly; the throat and mouth should then be cleared by suction or swabs.

In all cases a fluid balance sheet should be maintained and a regime of mild diuresis instituted if there is no evidence of renal failure. A variable degree of dehydration is commonly encountered. If the patient is conscious ample fluid may be given by mouth under supervision. If the patient is not capable of swallowing, two 500 ml. volumes of 5 per cent. dextrose may be infused with one such of normal saline separating them. On no account should forced diuresis be instituted routinely. If oliguria persists it is wise to have the blood urea level measured. If the rate of clearance of the poison by urinary excretion is not likely to be satisfactory due to ingestion of a large dose, a known high blood level of the poison, or an expected slow rate of excretion, this may be hastened by instituting a diuretic regime or by some form of dialysis. In the case of salicylate poisoning, the kidneys are likely to be able to function well and the diuresis can be achieved by administering 10 g. of sodium bicarbonate by stomach tube, intravenous infusion of 5 per cent. dextrose-water and M/5 sodium lactate in excess of the estimated fluid deficit, and intravenous injection of an osmotic diuretic. For this purpose 500 ml. of a 10 per cent. solution of mannitol may be injected in divided doses. Fluid loss must be replaced as a brisk diuresis may occur. Frusemide injection, 10 mg., may be included in the regime. Phenobarbitone being largely excreted by the kidney is also susceptible to diuretic therapy but the lactate solution should be omitted and saline substituted. Drugs such as amylobarbitone which are largely detoxified in the liver are not cleared in active form in the urine. Diuresis is not applicable, but dialysis may succeed. There is always a danger of precipitating pulmonary oedema if forced diuresis is practised routinely.

Dialysis may be applied in cases where the method can clear the poison more rapidly than the kidney or where there is renal failure as a complication of the poison, whether or not the latter is excreted in the urine. Two types of dialysis are available. In intermittent peritoneal lavage a specially balanced solution is run into the pelvic peritoneum via a sterile plastic tube inserted through the abdominal wall, and siphoned out after a time. Haemodialysis is practised with a 'blood-washing' machine. When prognosticating in the case of sedative poisoning it is important to know if the substance is dialysable, as are glutethimide and phenobarbitone, how much of it is firmly bound to protein, whether it is concentrated in body fat (short-acting barbiturates), and how long it is likely to take to disappear unaided. If there is a high blood level of a long-acting barbiturate and the patient is in coma dialysis should not be withheld. It is particularly successful with the alcohols, barbiturates and related hypnotics (in particular with glutethimide), salts such as bromide, all salicylates and the amphetamines but it is not applicable to most other poisonings. It has been found that not more than 1 per cent. of patients admitted to hospital with poisoning need be considered for this therapy.

Maintaining the Circulation

A decline in the efficient action of the cardiovascular system is common in acute poisoning but not immediately alarming except in asphyxial poisoning due to carbon monoxide or cyanide, or following inhalation of gases such as methane, carbon dioxide and hydrogen sulphide, or obstruction of breathing. Patients who have lain in a stupor for many hours may merely be cold, in which case they may be stripped of clothing and wrapped in warm blankets, but they should not be artificially warmed. They will be dehydrated and they may be in a state of shock with low blood pressure (under 80 mm. Hg in an adult). Infusion of 5 per cent. dextrose in water is the usual treatment of dehydration and makes a convenient vehicle for intravenous injection of drugs in solution. A sample of blood should be withdrawn for estimation of electrolytes. If the electrolyte balances are upset as a result of sweating, vomiting, diarrhoea, chemical acidaemia or altered respiration, appropriate infusions may be used to correct the disturbance. Plasma expander may be helpful when there is hypovolaemia, as in severe and prolonged depressant poisoning, but care must be taken to avoid plethora on recovery. Full oxygenation is essential. These measures, preceded by raising the foot of the bed by 5–10 cm., usually restore the circulation. They may be supplemented by one initial intramuscular injection of methylamphetamine hydrochloride, 10 mg. External cardiac massage and electrical defibrillation have restored life to an apparently dead patient. Cardiac arrest is usually associated with respiratory failure and the chance of success is not necessarily prejudiced by the poison.

Use of Stimulants and Antidotes

Steroids have not proved to be of obvious value in acute poisoning unless there is a powerful element of local irritation. The analeptic drugs are not specific in action. They are ineffective in all severe depression. They do not shorten the period of unconsciousness. On occasion a general stimulant such as injection of nikethamide may rouse a young alcoholic, or temporarily improve vital functions in a patient suffering from an overdose of barbiturate. Selected patients may thus be improved to a degree which makes it easier to supervise them while organizing measures for recovery. On occasion it is necessary to use a sedative when the poison is a central stimulant, e.g. intramuscular injection of 4 ml. of paraldehyde in an adult, but this should be avoided if at all possible. No attention is now paid to antidotes such as charcoal or permanganate which were formerly left in the stomach after lavage, but there is an increasing number of specific, and therefore highly effective, antidotes available when the precise cause of the poisoning is known, e.g. nalorphine for morphine, pralidoxime for anticholinesterase poisoning.

POISONING DUE TO ASPHYXIANT GASES AND FUMES

Introduction

Gases and fumes are extremely poisonous and are the cause of some thousands of deaths in Britain each year. This result may be brought about in a number of ways: (1) The gas may not support life, e.g. methane, and may be present in a concentration high enough to exclude air. (2) The fume may be an irritant, e.g. chlorine, and induce asphyxia from bronchospasm and acute pulmonary oedema. (3) The gas may have a toxic action on the central respiratory mechanisms, e.g. carbon dioxide. (4) The gas may inhibit the carriage of oxygen by haemoglobin, e.g. carbon monoxide. (5) It may inhibit its acceptance by the tissues, e.g. cyanide. The most important of the asphyxiant gases, because it is the most commonly met with, is carbon monoxide.

CARBON MONOXIDE POISONING

Synonyms. Utility gas poisoning; Coal-gas poisoning.

Definition

The toxic effects of inhalation of carbon monoxide.

Aetiology

Carbon monoxide (CO) was for long the most common of all causes of death by poisoning. It is produced when carbon is incompletely oxidized and is a colourless, odourless gas which readily mixes with air to produce an asphyxiant, inflammable explosive mixture. It is widely used as a source of heat and to a small extent for illumination; great quantities are produced and used industrially.

Domestic Poisoning. In 1963 deaths from carbon monoxide poisoning in England and Wales numbered 3300 but fell to about 1760 in 1969, a decrease of 47 per cent. and are declining further. This satisfactory trend may reflect improvements in techniques of rescue and first-aid without, and of treatment within, the hospital but it must also reflect the decrease in lethality which has resulted from the reduction in the carbon monoxide content of utility gas as a consequence of the widespread use of natural gas. By far the most important source in connexion with poisoning is the domestic supply, utility gas being a mixture of washed coal-gas and water-gas, the latter formed when steam is passed over red hot coke. The final mixture contains 5–15 per cent. of carbon monoxide to which an unpleasant odoriferous substance is added as a means of detection. In suicide or accident the escape of utility gas is almost invariably complicated by inadequacy of ventilation and the elaborate measures frequently taken by suicidal persons to ensure this are diagnostic. In accidents the source of gas may be a leak from faulty apparatus—old pipes, connexions, taps, cookers, pokers, rings, fires, geysers, refrigerators—or due to incomplete burning of a fuel such as coke, coal, oil, or butane in an ill-designed or ill-ventilated burner, or a 'blow-back' due to a draught. If the gas escapes through a layer of earth, it may well be odourless and is the more dangerous. The exhaust fumes of internal combustion engines contain 10 per cent. or more of carbon monoxide, especially if the carburettor is faultily adjusted, and a small car may produce lethal quantities in 10 minutes if the engine is left running in a closed garage. The smoke of open fires contains carbon monoxide which may accumulate if ventilation is poor and this gas is responsible for death in many victims of conflagration. Persons at the extremes of life are peculiarly susceptible to this poison. In children it is usually an accident, in people over 60 years of age it may equally be suicide or accident. A disproportionately high percentage of persons dying from this poison are old and the peak incidence occurs in winter when ventilation is frequently restricted.

Industrial Poisoning. This is much less common than domestic poisoning because carbon monoxide is used frequently in attempts at suicide, which largely take place in the home which is also the site of most accidents. Repeated exposure to small concentrations, with minimal ill effects, occurs in garages, tunnelling, mining and metal working and at times in busy city streets.

Properties and Actions of Carbon Monoxide. This substance exerts its effect as a result of its affinity for haemoglobin which is 200 times that of oxygen. The pigment formed, carboxyhaemoglobin, is pink in colour. An estimate of the percentage of it may be made by comparing a dilution of the affected blood, if not anaemic, with standard solutions. Spectroscopic examination will display the absorption bands characteristic of the pigment and may be used as a confirmatory test. Patients exposed to an atmosphere which contains carbon monoxide readily accumulate abnormal haemoglobin and suffer from deprivation of oxygen to the tissues. Neurones are peculiarly susceptible to oxygen lack and all persons suffering from hypoxia due to carbon monoxide exhibit mental changes which vary from 'intoxication' to coma. The maximum allowable concentration in air is 100 parts per million for long exposure and 400 parts per million for a brief exposure. Anything in excess of this will give a rise to symptoms of poisoning and 0·2 per cent. in air can prove fatal.

Post-mortem Appearances. Characteristic appearances are of cherry pink lividity (not always present) and a similar colour in the blood, muscles and internal organs. Carboxyhaemoglobin may be detected in the blood. The other appearances are those of asphyxia—oedema and punctate haemorrhages in the cortex, basal ganglia, beneath the pericardium and in the lungs, which may show patchy consolidation. If the patient has survived some days in coma the basal ganglia may show softening and staining. Patches of blistering may be present at pressure points. Putrefaction is alleged to be delayed.

Pathology

The toxic effect of carbon monoxide is essentially due to anoxia as a result of the blockage of oxygen transport. The lesions found in the central nervous system may result from any anoxic episode and are not characteristic of carbon monoxide. The prime neurological manifestation is coma and focal neurological damage with resulting monoplegia may occur. A common central lesion found *post mortem* is anoxic damage to the globus pallidus which may be detected by serial section of the basal ganglia. Equally frequent are necrotic lesions of the grey and white matter of the hemispheres of varying extent and pattern. Lesions of Ammon's horn are seen, but less frequently. Attempts have been made to correlate these appearances with the pattern of the illness. The clinical type in which fatal neurological complications set in some 2–3 weeks after apparent initial recovery has been associated with the occurrence of scattered focal demyelination in white matter.

Symptoms

No ill effects are felt if the level of saturation in the blood is less than 10–15 per cent. of the haemoglobin; at 20–30 per cent. there is a complaint of throbbing frontal headache, dyspnoea, muscular weakness, tinnitus and giddiness. In fit persons nausea, dimness of sight, double vision and marked weakening of will-power and of strength occur at about 40 per cent. Extreme restlessness and hysterical unco-operativeness is common. Anything beyond this level is dangerous, the pulse and respiratory rates increase and sudden collapse may occur if the patient exerts himself to escape his danger. Above 50 per cent. stupor may occur, asphyxial convulsions have been recorded and death is known. Usually 60–80 per cent. saturation is recorded in fatal cases. Patients who have disabilities of the oxygen-carrying mechanism (emphysema, phthisis, myocardial infarct, anaemia) are thereby made more susceptible and may die with much lower saturation levels in blood. The simultaneous presence of cerebral depressants such a alcohol or barbiturate militates against recovery. Primary anoxic anoxia is followed by local anoxia consequent upon cerebral oedema.

Diagnosis

This can be established beyond doubt by spectroscopy and an unsuspected degree of poisoning by this agent has been found at post-mortem examination. The smell of utility gas on the victim's clothing implies that there has been a recent exposure to it and may help to confirm such a history, which is usually unequivocal. The clinical aspect is very variable. Carboxyhaemoglobin may give rise to a pink colour in the skin if the blood is sufficiently highly saturated, if there is no anaemia, and if the exposure has been fairly sudden. It is more often seen in cases of industrial accident than exposure to utility gas. In the latter, the facies is more often grey and sweating or livid, the lips blue or flecked with foam. The respiratory rate is usually increased, and the excursions shallow, but may be apparently normal. Cheyne-Stokes respiration may occur in comatose patients. Carbon monoxide is not an irritant but fumes associated with exposure to it may well be, in which case hyperpnoea will be disproportionately severe. In many mild cases there is little serious involvement of the cardiovascular system. The pulse rate and the blood pressure may be raised; in severe poisoning the blood pressure falls and the pulse is thready and irregular with many extrasystoles. The heart dilates rapidly after exposure to gas, and death, if it occurs, is usually due to acute circulatory failure. The pupils dilate, but the light reflex is only lost late and limb reflexes remain brisk. In deep coma an extensor plantar response may be elicited, with exaggerated limb reflexes, increased muscle tone and trismus. Coma with a flaccid musculature is a bad sign. The body temperature may be low if the patient has lain neglected for long, and vomiting and incontinence may occur. Hyperpyrexia may occur later, with neurological involvement. Glycosuria and albuminuria are commonly noted; hypoglycaemia is described. As the circulation is restored by treatment, patches of erythema may appear on the skin and progress to blisters. They are found on the areas subjected to pressure as the patient lay unconscious, or on the areas of naturally poor circulation and should not be confused with thermal burns.

Treatment

Prophylactic. It is essential that preventive measures be applied rigorously in industry and that domestic plant be properly installed and well maintained. Adequate ventilation of premises is a safeguard of prime importance.

Therapeutic. Having removed the patient from further exposure to the gas, a check should be made that the airway is not obstructed. If necessary, a swab or sucker should be employed to clear it. Artificial respiration (mouth-to-mouth and Holger Nielsen methods) may be needed and should be supplemented as soon as possible with oxygen given from a manually controlled bag by a tight-fitting mask with a one-way valve. This may be sufficient to restore adequate breathing and is the preferred method of first-aid. As soon as the patient has moved to an ambulance, efforts at resuscitation should be continued by wrapping up warmly and giving oxygen or 5 per cent. carbogen. If spontaneous breathing is re-established but inadequate, the latter mixture will usually stimulate ventilation and speed the excretion of carbon monoxide. On reaching hospital the patient's condition should be assessed and blood taken for estimation of carboxyhaemoglobin saturation, haemoglobin and electrolytes. Carbogen therapy may be carried out for 15 minutes by which time the saturation should be lowered to a safe level and it may be replaced by oxygen for as long as thought necessary. Prophylactic use of antibiotics is justifiable if it seems probable that vomit has been inhaled. Dehydration should be corrected by infusion of dextrose-water if necessary and blistering treated as for burns. Transfusion of blood is scarcely profitable. Intravenous injection of digoxin may be called for if acute heart failure is slow to respond to the relief of hypoxia. When impaired consciousness persists after carboxyhaemoglobin in the blood has been lowered to a negligible level a lumbar puncture may be performed and the pressure of the cerebrospinal fluid measured. Should this prove to be grossly elevated, as is probably the case, an intravenous infusion of 500 ml. of 10 per cent. solution of mannitol may be given, or an injection of frusemide, in the expectation of relieving cerebral oedema. In a few hospital centres facilities have been created for patients to be placed in a chamber as soon as possible after admission to hospital and while receiving oxygen by portable apparatus. The chamber is then filled with hyperbaric oxygen. At 2 atmospheres pressure there is no discomfort to attendants, the oxygen dissolved in plasma is raised from 0·25 to 3·8 vols per cent. and the rate of dissociation of CO from haemoglobin is greatly increased. Despite the unavoidable delay in submitting a gassed patient to this therapy, and the elaborate nature of the device, the results claimed from its use, in particular the absence of late neurological sequelae of severe poisoning, are encouraging.

Prognosis

A close watch must be kept for complications due to a prolonged hypoxia, such as renal failure, gangrene, breakdown of wounds and ulcers, or pulmonary oedema, and for progressive paralysis of limbs due to hypoxia and local pressure. Neurological sequelae are well known; they may pass off after a few days or leave residual disability, but they may only appear after 20–30 days. A period of disorientation and restlessness is usual and strict rest in bed is necessary for a number of days even after slight degrees of poisoning. In older persons this may be extended to 2–3 weeks with advantage. There is little apparent correlation between the depth of unconsciousness present when a patient is first seen and the ultimate outcome. If the degree and duration of severe hypoxia has damaged vital centres, the period of coma may be prolonged but can be followed by partial or complete recovery; impairment of memory and of mental powers is usual. Rigidity of muscles and increased tone of the limbs is a sign of severe poisoning. Persons over 60 years of age who are unconscious for 24 hours are in danger of losing life. Repeated exposure may lead to a detectable polycythaemia; continuous exposure leads to cumulation and severe poisoning; chronic poisoning is scarcely possible.

OTHER ASPHYXIANT GASES

METHANE

Methane is present in natural gas, mines (fire-damp) and areas of still air where vegetation decays. It is inflammable. It is not irritant nor does it combine with haemoglobin, but in high concentration will exclude air and fail to support life. Exposure to a pocket of this gas may cause sudden loss of consciousness with the appearances of asphyxia—stupor, cyanosis, stertor, convulsions, rapid pulse and raised blood pressure.

Treatment

Treatment is by rescue and oxygenation.

CARBON DIOXIDE

Carbon dioxide is a heavy, colourless, odourless gas which collects in undisturbed atmospheres, e.g. 'choke damp' and 'black damp' in mines, or over fermenting grain. Great quantities are used in industry. Five per cent. carbon dioxide in inspired air is a powerful stimulant to respiration and cardiovascular action, but higher concentrations overstimulate and 30 per cent. rapidly causes failure of the vital centres. Early symptoms due to moderate concentrations are dyspnoea, dizziness, ataxia and vomiting. They are relieved by return to normal atmosphere. High concentrations may rapidly induce coma and prove fatal.

Treatment

Treatment consists of rescue, clearing the airway and oxygenating fully.

CYANIDE

Cyanide (CN) causes the death of some 40 persons each year, few of them by accident. It is used extensively in industry as a salt and in the form of the gas as a fumigant in ships and warehouses; 100 p.p.m. is lethal to vermin, and dangerous. Accordingly, the latter use is controlled by the Hydrogen Cyanide (Fumigation) Act of 1937. Prussic acid is a 4 per cent. solution and this liquid may be absorbed through skin. Various nitriles used industrially release CN. Acrylonitrile exerts an additional toxic effect on the central nervous system. Cyanide action is the result of inhibition of cytochrome and other enzymes which transport oxygen in the tissues. Asphyxial death may, therefore, occur in the presence of oxygen, and the blood is bright red in colour, partly from cyanhaemoglobin and partly from oxyhaemoglobin. If the gas is inhaled, consciousness may be lost suddenly and convulsions and death follow in a few minutes, but if a solution of a salt or of methyl cyanide is taken on a full stomach, absorption may be delayed and detoxification keep pace with it. The patient may feel dizzy, dyspnoeic and vomit or even survive a period of stupor. Post-mortem appearances are similar to those of carbon monoxide poisoning. On first opening the body an odour of bitter almonds may often be detected.

Treatment

Treatment is directed to detoxifying the cyanide. Mouth-to-mouth breathing should not be practised without a valved airway and artificial respiration is only meaningful if it is used to drive into the lungs the vapour of amyl nitrite from vitrellae which have been crushed into a swab placed over the nose and mouth. As soon as practicable 10 ml. of a 3 per cent. solution of sodium nitrite should be injected intravenously, followed by slow injection of 25 ml. of a 50 per cent. solution of sodium thiosulphate. It is desirable that these materials be available at designated points in workshops where cyanide is a hazard and that personnel be trained to use them at once in an emergency. At this stage oxygen may be administered, respiration supported and gastric lavage considered. As the cyanide radicle exerts its inhibitory influence on oxygen transport by chelating with the iron atom in cytochrome B its effect might be reversible if a more powerful and inessential chelating agent could be provided at the site of action before irreversible anoxic damage has been done. Treatment has been attempted with hydroxycobalamin and with cobalt edetate (*Kelocyanor*). The latter substance may be injected intravenously in a dose of 0·3–0·6 G., followed by 50 ml. of hypertonic dextrose.

POISONING DUE TO DEPRESSANTS OF THE CENTRAL NERVOUS SYSTEM

The greater number of chemical agents involved in acute poisoning are depressants of the central nervous system. The most important are ethyl alcohol and barbiturate. In combination these have a steeply additive effect and may cause accidental death. This may come about because the drinker is seeking oblivion by reinforcing his drink with a sedative or because he mistakenly thinks that the hypnotic will prevent his 'hangover'. Of recent years a variety of synthetic non-barbiturate sedatives, hypnotics and tranquillizers has been introduced into medical practice in an attempt to retain and extend the useful qualities of barbiturate while reducing the risks from overdosage and the likelihood of drug dependence. The most important of these drugs in our present context are the tranquillizers because so much is prescribed (15·4 million N.H.S. prescriptions during 1969 in England, plus 13·1 million for barbiturates) for such a variety of reasons. Inevitably such drugs are involved increasingly in self-poisoning. Another disturbing feature is the frequency with which mixtures of these and other drugs are taken in the course of one episode. Of the more commonly prescribed drugs chlorpromazine (*Largactil*); chlordiazepoxide (*Librium*); diazepam (*Valium*); methaqualone and diphenhydramine (*Mandrax*) and nitrazepam (*Mogadon*) may be encountered.

ETHYL ALCOHOL POISONING

Alcoholic intoxication is dealt with in this section mainly on its acute toxic action and its physical effects. Section 17 should also be consulted for a consideration of alcoholism from the viewpoint of the psychiatrist.

ACUTE ALCOHOL POISONING

Synonyms. Drunk; Drunkenness.

Aetiology

More than £1000 million is spent on alcoholic beverages each year in Britain. These drinks contain varying percentages of ethanol—say 5 per cent. in beer, 10 per cent. in wine, 20 per cent. in reinforced wines, 40 per cent. in spirits. Custom has decreed that approximately the same amount of alcohol (10 ml.) is provided in the measure which is usually employed for each. Excessive consumption within a short period of time may produce a state of general anaesthesia which is characterized by slow induction, a poor therapeutic index and a prolonged effect. Any stage of this condition may be termed drunkenness, but the medical man is usually involved only when innocence or misjudgement leads to severe overdosage, or again, when the dulling of mental acuity leads to antisocial behaviour, or to involvement in accidents. The effect of any given concentration will vary in different individuals according to their physical and mental state at the time of onsumption. Alcoholism *per se* is not a crime except ı relation to being in charge of a road vehicle, where 0 mg./100 ml. has been designated in The Road 'raffic Act of 1967 as the upper permissible limit.

Ethyl alcohol is a colourless, inflammable liquid with fiery taste and a characteristic odour which is very ifferent when fresh and when stale as on the breath of n alcoholic. Dangerous amounts may be absorbed by ıhalation, but usually it is swallowed. Undiluted pirits irritate the mucosae and produce an acute astritis. Alcohol is rapidly absorbed from the small ıtestine and to a degree from the stomach. The rate of bsorption is greater if the stomach is empty and after concentrated drink; it is delayed if fatty food is resent. Alcohol is distributed throughout the body 'ater, and obese persons, unless dropsical, are at a disdvantage compared with lean people of the same 'eight. Peak blood levels are reached in about an hour fter a single dose, maintained for 2 hours when quilibrium is reached, and then decline in a linear ıshion. Urine usually contains some 25 per cent. more lcohol than does an equal volume of blood taken at ıe same time. More than 90 per cent. of absorbed lcohol is broken down in the liver to acetaldehyde, nd in the tissues to acetate. This step is catalysed by n enzyme system which may become deficient from ıck of vitamins or be inhibited by prior administration f the drug disulfiram (*Antabuse*). The consequent ccumulation of aldehyde is toxic. The rate of disposal f alcohol remains very constant over a wide range of ›ncentrations (about 10 g. per hour) so that if a large ›se has been absorbed recovery is delayed. The ıtabolism of ethanol bears a relation to that of carboydrate. If the latter is stimulated, the rate of disposal ıay increase in some patients. A small amount, roportional to the level in the blood, is excreted in the rine and breath. The latter forms the physical basis of ıe 'breathalyser' test applied by the police to persons ıspected of driving while unduly under the influence f alcohol.

athology

In cases of fatal coma there is usually a high blood vel and alcohol is present in the alimentary canal and the urine. The stomach may show evidence of acute ıtarrh, and oedema of the cerebral cortex is often seen. atty infiltration of the liver [see Section 7] is met with ter long-continued alcoholic excess. Portal cirrhosis only met with in a small proportion of chronic coholics who may be under care for acute intoxication though alcoholism looms large in hospital practice relation to hepatic failure. Dietary deficiency of tamins and protein possibly plays a more fundaental role in the aetiology of cirrhosis than ethanol such, but alcoholics frequently suffer from malıtrition.

ymptoms

The blood supply to the brain being copious the epressant effects of alcohol may be felt within a few inutes of taking a drink on an empty stomach. They e a little dizziness accompanied by release of psychic hibitions leading to euphoria. It is largely for this effect that alcohol is consumed, but the speed and degree to which euphoria is attained will depend on a balance of absorption, distribution to the brain and to the rest of the body, metabolic degradation, the mental state of the drinker, and to some extent habituation. If the blood level rises above approximately 50 mg. per 100 ml. slight impairment of visual acuity, slurring of speech, and loss of refined physical and mental capacities occur, and lateral nystagmus can usually be elicited. Often there is evident reddening of the conjunctivae. Up to 150 mg. per cent. the pattern of symptoms is similar, with steady progress towards impairment of physical attainments, and half of a group of normal people might be said to show evidence of intoxication. At 300 mg. per cent. most people are grossly affected, with ataxia, double vision, tremor, incoherent speech, flushed skin, sweating and increased heat loss, marked loss of mental capacity and perhaps nausea or emesis. Higher concentrations produce motor paralysis and loss of consciousness and the fatal concentration is from 0·5 to 0·8 g. per 100 ml. Coma may supervene with surprising speed in susceptible persons, who pass quickly through the stages of anaesthesia. The victim is pale, collapsed, flaccid and sweating. The pupils dilate, breathing is stertorous, the pulse bounding, but blood pressure is not often raised. At the dangerous stage coma deepens, the pulse becomes thready, pressure low and respiration shallow. The body temperature falls. Death from respiratory and circulatory failure may occur or recovery take place slowly. Inhalation of vomit is always a danger and many of the unexpected deaths are due to obstruction of the airway.

Diagnosis

Diagnosis is not always easy, for persons suffering from effects of injury (in particular injury to the head) may have been given alcohol and smell of it. Injury frequently complicates drunkenness and the effects of hypnotic drugs closely resemble those due to alcohol. The combination is highly dangerous and not recognizable by clinical examination. An estimate of urinary or blood alcohol level may be helpful, but does not exclude other causes of stupor. Where there is any doubt, the patient should be kept under observation, a lumbar puncture performed and the skull examined by radiography. The urine should always be examined for sugar, albumin, barbiturate and salicylate. It is highly desirable only to make a diagnosis of alcoholic coma when other causes, particularly injury to the head, cerebrovascular disasters and diabetes, have been excluded by general and specific examinations.

Treatment

The condition of 'hangover' may be treated by bed rest, a sedative such as chlorpromazine, 50 mg., phenobarbitone sodium, 200 mg., or soluble aspirin, 650 mg., and an antacid mixture, with bland diet and ample fluids. A state of stupor demands immediate attention to the airway and to oxygenation; gastric suction may well be of value as recent drinking may have taken place. Correction of dehydration with 5 per cent. dextrose in water intravenously may be needed if the patient has been in a stupor for some hours. Conservation of warmth is desirable, but not heating. Some physicians administer 50 ml. of Strong Injection of Dextrose, B.P.C., and 20 Units of insulin. Massive doses of vitamins (C and B complex) have been given, but unless the patient clearly suffers from malnutrition there is not likely to be any evident benefit. The performance of tracheobronchial toilet and full oxygenation may lighten coma dramatically, or allay restlessness during recovery.

Prognosis

Recovery usually takes place within 24 hours, leaving nervous irritability, headache, fatigue, acute gastritis, and evidence of any injury sustained during the period of amnesia and analgesia. Coma is, of course, more serious. Any patient in this state may die of the effects of exposure and of dehydration, but usually there is a complication such as obstruction of breathing, bronchopneumonia or other disease. Acute over-indulgence is more serious when it complicates chronic alcoholism in the older patient.

ACUTE COMPLICATIONS OF CHRONIC ALCOHOLISM

Definition

The chronic alcoholic has been defined as a person who is not able to control his consumption of alcohol although he knows its disastrous results. This is drug dependence.

Pathology

Primarily, this is a mental disorder and is in the province of the psychiatrist [see Section 17] but there are in relation to this state a number of acute manifestations of toxicity which may properly be considered here. Some persons drink to excess in a regular rhythm and are only encountered by a doctor when acutely intoxicated; some persons have a compulsion to drink to excess on the irregular occasions when they indulge. A few have, on these occasions, an attack of amnesia which may be a prodromal symptom of dependence. Once established, chronic indulgence may be associated with undernourishment and be complicated by peripheral neuropathy, cerebral degeneration (Korsakoff's syndrome) [see Section 15] or impairment of hepatic function [see Section 7]. Episodes of acute intoxication in such persons do not differ from those considered above, but the immediate condition is often serious because the amount of alcohol consumed in a bout of drinking by such patients tends to be large and because of the disabilities and diseases associated with the chronic alcoholism.

Symptoms

The alcoholic often has a high colour, with coarsened features and dilated venules in the nose and cheeks and is cyanosed when cold. The conjunctivae are red and the eyes watery or 'glassy'. There is a noticeable tremor of the hands and perhaps of the lips and he or she is restless in demeanour, may show compulsive movements of a bizarre type, is garrulous but irascible and has a notably poor memory. The chest may be wheezy and there is usually a complaint of morning catarrh which is complicated by vomiting. Constipation interrupted by diarrhoea is often a feature of the condition. On examination there may be evidence of peripheral neuropathy, of enlargement of the liver or of impaired hepatic function, of renal failure, of serious lung disease, or delirium tremens or other psychosis.

Treatment

Alcohol dependence has a poor prognosis. As a preliminary treatment and usually as a consequence of an acute episode, the patient may be put to bed. All alcohol should be withdrawn. If the symptoms of physical dependence are no worse than tremor, weakness, cold sweats, absence of appetite and insomnia they will pass off in 48 hours (the 'drying-out' period). Injection of a sedative, paraldehyde, 4 ml., or phenobarbitone sodium, 200 mg., or chlorpromazine hydrochloride (*Largactil*), 50 mg., will allay restlessness. A gastric antacid relieves dyspepsia and permits of the intake of frequent drinks or small nourishing feeds. Multiple vitamins, C and B complex, e.g. *High Potency Injection Parentrovite* or *Vitavel Syrup* by mouth, may be given as a supplement. If vomiting and diarrhoea persist, tremor and nightmares may herald the onset of acute abstinence syndrome characterized by hallucinosis with agitation (delirium tremens, 'D.T.'s'). This is a grave condition if not relieved, as the patient may die of exhaustion. Drug therapy is directed towards sedation which may be achieved by giving increasing doses and combinations of paraldehyde, 4–12 ml., phenobarbitone sodium, 200 mg., chlorpromazine, or hyoscine hydrobromide and other sedatives, but not morphine. Bronchopneumonia has to be treated energetically. Relief of dehydration and correction of electrolyte imbalance as determined by examination of blood, feeding by gastric tube if possible, and massive doses of vitamins are all needed. Convalescence is apt to be prolonged and continued sedation will be needed; the regimen should be planned between the psychiatrist and physician. If neuropathy is evident, aneurin hydrochloride, 10 mg., may be given by intramuscular injection on alternate days for 2 weeks and then by mouth.

METHYL ALCOHOL POISONING

Methanol is a clear, colourless, inflammable liquid with a fiery taste.

Aetiology

Some 12 million gallons of methanol are issued each year. This alcohol is widely used as an industrial solvent, as a fuel and in 'anti-freeze'. Ethylene glycol mixtures have similar toxic effects. While it is possible to become intoxicated by inhalation of the vapour of methanol, it is most usual to take it in drink. Frequently this is in the form of methylated spirits or denatured alcohol, one of a variety of mixtures of 5–10 per cent methanol in ethyl alcohol to which various distinguishing colours or flavours have been added. This fluid has the attraction of cheapness and may be mixed with more customary beverages. The acute intoxication which results from over-indulgence differs in no way from that due to ethanol, but it is alleged that the type of person who indulges this vice may be more often excited or violent when drunk. Group outbreaks of serious poisoning occur when drink is heavily contaminated in ignorance.

Pathology

The products of catabolism of methanol (formaldehyde and formic acid) are much more toxic than the products of ethanol, and the concentration of formates in the urine may indicate the severity of poisoning. A feature of the poisoning is, therefore, a metabolic acidosis with a fall in plasma bicarbonate (possibly below 20 mEq. per litre) and a fixed acid acidaemia. Methanol is also partially and slowly excreted in urine and exhaled unchanged. It is less readily catabolized in the presence of ethanol. The relation between the dose taken and the toxic effect is variable; 15 ml. may be fatal. The retina is peculiarly susceptible to methyl alcohol or its first product, formaldehyde.

Symptoms

After a delay of 12–24 hours during which the victim may have sobered, there is a return of nausea, vomiting and dizziness, with pain in the eyes, photophobia and flashing lights. The illness progresses rapidly and dilated and sluggish or fixed pupils may be accompanied by loss of vision, dyspnoea, excitement or stupor and collapse. The patient is pale, apprehensive and sweating, the urine scanty and acid. Cardiac irregularity is a feature of severe poisoning.

Treatment

All who may have ingested methyl alcohol should be admitted to hospital so that gastric suction may be performed. If signs of toxicity develop, regular estimations of electrolyte and urea levels, plasma bicarbonate and the blood and urinary pH should be made. An ophthalmologist should be consulted. Intravenous infusion of 5 per cent. dextrose-water or half mixture with saline is advisable after vomiting and should be continued until the estimated deficit has been replaced and a flow of urine is obtained. It may need to be supplemented by 100 ml. of an 8 per cent. solution of potassium citrate by gastric tube in each 24 hours. If oral fluids are not retained and hypopotassaemia requires correction, 1 litre of isotonic solution (1·14 per cent.) of potassium chloride should be infused very slowly in 24 hours into the tubing of the dextrose-saline drip. It may be necessary to replace the estimated base deficit by means of a 5 per cent. solution of sodium bicarbonate if the fall in pH of the blood becomes alarming, but 2 G. 3-hourly by stomach tube is safer. Many physicians advocate the administration of 35 ml. of ethanol by mouth, as a 20 per cent. solution followed by half quantities 4-hourly for 5 days. The urine should be examined regularly. Oliguria due to renal damage produces a scanty urine of high specific gravity with casts, albumin and red cells. This complication is well known. It calls for immediate cessation of potassium supplementation. Renal failure may be suspected and intermittent haemodialysis must be considered seriously. Cerebral depressants should be avoided. It is important to ensure that the patient is fully oxygenated. Haemodialysis may also be considered in order to correct the formic acidaemia.

BARBITURATE POISONING

Aetiology

Barbiturates are formed by structural variations in the side-chain of malonyl urea. Soluble sodium derivatives of the common barbiturates exist. The pharmacological action of all of them is the same—depression of the nervous system—but structural variations result in differences in the rate of absorption and in distribution. These factors permit of the classical arrangement of barbiturates into long-acting—phenobarbitone (*Gardenal*, *Luminal*) and barbitone (*Veronal*); medium duration—pentobarbitone (*Nembutal*), amylobarbitone (*Amytal*), butobarbitone (*Soneryl*); short-acting—quinalbarbitone (*Seconal*) and cyclobarbitone (*Phanodorm*); and the ultra-short-acting barbiturate—thiopentone sodium (*Pentothal*). Peak concentrations of medium or short duration barbiturates in blood and brain may occur 1–2 hours after oral ingestion; barbitone and phenobarbitone require 4–8 hours.

The ultra-short-acting barbiturates are largely bound to plasma protein or stored in body fat from which they are subsequently cleared and degraded in the liver; the long-acting drugs such as phenobarbitone are little bound to plasma protein and mainly cleared by urinary excretion. The medium duration drugs are bound to a greater degree than is phenobarbitone, detoxified in the liver and tissues and excreted; the short duration ones are also excreted quickly. The other major factors in determining the degree and duration of depression are the dose absorbed and the extent to which the patient is habituated. Undoubtedly the 'short' and 'medium' duration barbiturates are the more dangerous as they cause a speedy and profound depression and are not readily dialysable as is phenobarbitone. The duration of the coma is less but the severity is greater.

A knowledge of these facts helps to determine the most suitable treatment for severe intoxications with individual barbiturates. In addition to pure barbiturates, there are mixtures with synergists, e.g. amylobarbitone sodium and quinalbarbitone sodium (*Tuinal*), pentobarbitone sodium and carbromal (*Carbrital*); and with antagonists, e.g. amylobarbitone and dexamphetamine sulphate (*Drinamyl*). Of the dangerous drug combinations, by far the most important is alcohol and barbiturate because of the frequency with which it occurs. The severity of the resulting depression and the ease with which a lethal dose may be unwittingly consumed should be appreciated. About one-third of all cases of acute poisoning admitted to hospital are due to barbiturate. Fortunately, the majority of these are mild. In Britain about 2000 persons die of it each year. In addition, this group of drugs is responsible for a great amount of drug dependence and chronic poisoning. Recently there has arisen a dangerous habit among addicts of self abuse by intravenous injection of a 'solution' of the contents of a capsule of barbiturate.

Symptoms

All stages of depression from mild confusion and sleepiness to coma may be encountered. Therapeutic doses of hypnotic barbiturates will induce natural sleep in suitable circumstances. All of them have an anticonvulsant action, phenobarbitone in particular. If the patient is roused, diplopia, nystagmus and some ataxia may be noted. The subjective reaction to pain in conscious patients is less intense, but barbiturates are not analgesics in therapeutic doses. Larger amounts cause stupor with diminution or absence of some reflexes. The pupils vary in size and are not a reliable guide to depth of depression. The limb reflexes may be diminished, but plantar responses are usually normal. Respiration is always impaired; the rate may be increased and breathing shallow, or slow and stertorous. Ventilatory turnover may with advantage be assessed with a Wright's spirometer. In all cases ventilation is diminished and hypoxia and hypercapnia result. This leads to peripheral vasodilatation, tachycardia, weakening of the cardiac muscle, and ultimately hypovolaemic and respiratory failure.

Retention of urine is common; it may contain sugar as well as barbiturate. If the poisoning is severe, profound coma ensues, body temperature falls and reflexes are lost. Marked hypothermia has been recorded. If this state persists death will take place; if recovery is delayed, pulmonary oedema, bronchopneumonia or renal failure may occur. Localized bullous erythema, not necessarily at pressure points is quite common; porphyrinuria or hyperthermia are unusual complications. The stage of recovery is occasionally characterized by acute excitement, especially if stimulant treatment has been used or if the patient is addicted to barbiturate.

Diagnosis

Diagnosis may be made on a clear history and the findings of general anaesthesia with depressed respiratory and circulatory functions, but the history is often obscure and loss of consciousness may be due to injury, disease, other drugs, or a combination of these. The urine or first stomach washing may be tested for barbiturate, but this drug is taken by so many persons that a positive cobaltous chloride test in urine is not diagnostic of an overdose. Of more value is an estimate of barbiturate in blood. The test takes about 2 hours to perform. Experienced biochemists may state the kind of barbiturate present with some confidence from the peak absorption band detected from the sample or by chromatographic analysis. Values of more than 10 mg. per 100 ml. for phenobarbitone or barbitone, 5–10 mg. per 100 ml. for amylobarbitone, and 3–5 mg. per 100 ml. for pentobarbitone and quinalbarbitone denote high levels of absorption, but the relation between blood level and clinical condition is variable and not to be relied upon for purposes of prognosis since so many patients have acquired tolerance to this drug.

Treatment

Mild degrees of intoxication need no treatment, but patients should be admitted to hospital for fear of adverse developments. In all comatose patients it is necessary to exclude other causes of unconsciousness and to take samples of blood, urine and perhaps of cerebrospinal fluid, for examination. Treatment then consists of the application of general principles [p. 313] with additional methods in selected cases. The first part consists of ensuring a clear airway by vigorous exploration. In all deeply unconscious patients or in case of doubt a cuffed endotracheal tube should be inserted. Only then should the state of oxygenation be estimated whether by clinical observation or refined techniques such as serial measurement of Po_2 and Pco_2 and direct measurement of ventilatory turnover, and measures instituted to correct defects—consultation with an anaesthetist; tracheobronchial suction; inflation of the lungs; administration of oxygen; physiotherapy to the thorax and X-ray of the lung fields. Patchy collapse must be relieved, if necessary by bronchoscopy. Prophylactic antibiotic treatment should not be given as a routine. When it seems probable from the history and findings (e.g. the presence of vomitus in the mouth; the practice of gastric washing without an endotracheal tube; fever and abnormal signs on examination of the lung fields) that infection is to be feared appropriate treatment should be instituted. The second part of treatment, which does not wait on completion of the measures outlined, consists of gastric suction and lavage. This should not be done as a routine and requires careful technique. The third stage consists of a regular check on blood pressure and pulse rate and the correction of dehydration. Mild hypotension may be relieved by tilting the foot of the bed upwards. A single intramuscular injection of 5 mg. of metaraminol may hasten restoration of normal pressure in many cases, but if systolic pressure is consistently below 80 mm.Hg in a young person and 90 mm.Hg in a patient over 50 years of age a degree of hypovolaemic shock may be suspected. Intravenous infusion is required. The choice and volume of fluid is determined by whether or not there has been much vomiting (unlikely in barbiturate poisoning), if there is any sign of pulmonary oedema, if forced osmotic diuresis by mannitol infusion (more successful in phenobarbitone poisoning than overdosage with amylobarbitone) is to be undertaken, or if the therapy is designed solely to increase circulatory blood volume, when plasma or plasma expander will be the better choice. If the bladder is easily palpable it may be catheterized aseptically after a preliminary attempt to empty it by firm pressure has failed. The fluid balance should be recorded. On recovery, all patients should be referred to a psychiatrist.

Special measures applicable to selected patients are as follows:

1. In prolonged coma with retention of carbon dioxide consideration of the use of mechanical respirators and the necessity for tracheostomy.

2. Treatment of pulmonary oedema by relief of heart failure and reduction of extracellular fluid volume. Controlled dehydration may be achieved by giving injection of frusemide or 500 ml. of 10 per cent. mannitol, and these measures supplemented by digoxin, aminophylline, bronchial suction and positive pressure oxygenation with a time-cycled respirator.

3. Analeptics sometimes increase respiratory and reflex activity for a time but do not shorten the duration of coma or increase the rate of excretion of barbiturate. They can only be of slight value, and that where respiration is depressed and skilled attention in short supply. They should not be used routinely and there is no discernible advantage in any particular one.

4. When blood levels are high and the patient in coma, and positive evidence of adequate renal function has been obtained, diuresis may be induced by injection of 500 ml. of 10 per cent. solution of mannitol, urinary volume measured at regular intervals by release of an indwelling catheter, and an equal volume of dextrose in water infused during the succeeding period. There is a danger of pulmonary oedema, and of hypopotassaemia. This technique should not be applied routinely to cases of self-poisoning.

5. Haemodialysis. This is successful in patients with phenobarbitone, barbitone or glutethimide poisoning in whom prolonged coma endangers life. It is less successful with the shorter-acting barbiturates, but the dialysis may be improved by adding plasma protein to the washing fluid. It is very successful in severe aspirin poisoning. It is of obvious value when renal failure complicates the poisoning, e.g. mercury, and is the only hope when lethally high blood concentrations of a dialysable poison have been demonstrated. If haemodialysing apparatus is not readily available, or in small children, peritoneal dialysis may be practised as a less effective alternative. Warmed dialysing fluid (commercially available as *Impersol*) may be modified with advantage by the addition of 5 per cent. by volume of reconstituted plasma and 5 per cent. by volume of sterile 0·5 per cent. solution of sodium bicarbonate. An alkaline fluid increases the transfer of barbituric acid across the peritoneal membrane and protein binds the drug so that it is not reabsorbed.

Prognosis

The longer the patient remains in a stupor without attention the poorer is the prognosis. Extremes of age, the presence of concomitant disease (particularly of the respiratory or circulatory systems), and the simultaneous use of alcohol or other depressant drug militate against recovery. The short-acting barbiturates are apt to cause profound depression, but the duration of the crisis is brief; with phenobarbitone there is more likelihood of complications such as bronchopneumonia or renal failure, since the coma is prolonged.

OTHER SEDATIVES, HYPNOTICS AND TRANQUILLIZERS

The traditional sedatives have been supplemented by a great number of new compounds, all of them with undesirable side-effects. Distribution to the public of such drugs is restricted as they are included in Schedule IV of The Pharmacy and Poisons Act, 1933, but depressed patients obtain them on prescription and may attempt self-poisoning with them. The general principles of treatment apply to these patients with certain specific additions.

GLUTETHIMIDE

This drug (*Doriden*) is a powerful hypnotic which in overdosage may cause profound coma. The drug is soluble in alcohol which, therefore, increases the speed of absorption, is distributed preferentially in body fat and is metabolized in the liver.

Symptoms

Fluctuations in the depth of unconsciousness are particularly marked with glutethimide and death from sudden apnoea may occur unexpectedly. The pulse rate is high and the pupils dilated and fixed, partly as a result of an atropine-like action of the drug. The heart muscle is weakened and severe hypotension often occurs. Acidaemia is also common, partly respiratory in origin but also metabolic.

Diagnosis

This is made on the history and findings, confirmed by estimation of blood level of the drug. The method is as for barbiturate and a level of more than 3 mg. per 100 ml. is likely to be serious, unless the patient is tolerant to the drug.

Treatment

Treatment is as for barbiturate poisoning but there are one or two special points. As this drug is fat-soluble it may be worthwhile to use an emulsion of castor oil and water for gastric lavage if that is to be performed, and/or to deliver a dose of 50 ml. of the oil into the stomach. Forced diuresis is of little value as a means of increasing clearance of the drug but intermittent haemodialysis is very effective. The risk of sudden failure of respiration may be related to increased intracranial tension which will be indicated by deepening coma, the development of papilloedema and a high pressure of cerebrospinal fluid. Intravenous frusemide, 20 mg., or mannitol, 500 ml. of 10 per cent. solution, may relieve this condition.

METHAQUALONE

This drug is of recent origin and has become very popular. It is available by itself (*Melsedin*) or compounded with the depressant antihistamine diphenhydramine as *Mandrax*. The latter is a powerful hypnotic, readily absorbed and acts quickly. The level of methaqualone in blood may be measured, and anything above 3 mg. per 100 ml. is likely to produce significant depression.

Symptoms

These are essentially similar to barbiturate but there are certain additional features. Exaggerated limb reflexes, increased tone in the limbs often with an extensor plantar reflex and minor jactitations in an unconscious patient make one suspect a heavy overdose of methaqualone. Tachycardia, electrocardiographic abnormalities, hypotension, and respiratory inadequacy are common. Bleeding has been noted, e.g. in gastric aspirate, but is uncommon. Pulmonary oedema is liable to occur and other tissues, e.g. the tongue and pharynx, may be affected.

Treatment

There are no differences from the treatment of barbiturate poisoning but forced diuresis is best avoided because of the risk of pulmonary oedema. There is doubt as to the value of haemodialysis, which may act primarily by relief of oedema. Intravenous frusemide, 20 mg., might well be tried as a first measure, then 500 ml. of 10 per cent. solution of mannitol. This drug is excreted as inactive metabolites; the primary line of therapy, therefore, is to promote detoxification by attention to respiration, circulation, hydration, electrolyte balance, warmth and general nursing principles.

SEDATIVES AND TRANQUILLIZERS

The number of such substances in frequent use is increasing and 15·4 million prescriptions for such drugs were issued during 1969 in England alone. Three which are of significance from the frequency with which they are taken in attempts at self-poisoning are chlordiazepoxide (*Librium*), diazepam (*Valium*) and more recently nitrazepam (*Mogadon*). Many patients take these drugs daily for long periods of time and may thus become tolerant of them. They are only dangerous when combined with alcohol or other and more powerful sedatives, or ingested in large amounts.

Symptoms and Treatment

Patients suffering from poisoning of sufficient severity to warrant admission to hospital are not deeply unconscious. Some depression of respiration may be noted, and low blood pressure and a slow pulse. No special measures such as forced diuresis need be undertaken. There is, as yet, limited experience of self-poisoning with nitrazepam.

BROMIDES

Bromide poisoning is still encountered although to a much less extent than formerly, most often in elderly patients with diminished renal function. Stupor seldom occurs but states of confusion are met with such as an acute toxic psychosis with hallucinations, or a milder degree of confusion with slurred speech and ataxia. These may be superimposed on chronic poisoning which is characterized by dulling of the faculties, constipation, anorexia, acneiform rashes and a purplish colour of the facial skin. In younger persons the cause may be consumption of a ureide containing bromide, e.g. carbromal or bromvaletone (e.g. *Persomnia*) and stupor may then be attained. Mild states of dependence occur and acute overdose may complicate this.

Diagnosis

Diagnosis of bromide poisoning may be most surely made by the finding of more than 50 mg. of bromide per 100 ml. in blood.

Treatment

Only rarely will it be necessary to take active steps to safeguard respiration. More often hypotension may call for simple measures such as tilting of the bed or the injection of 10 mg. of methylamphetamine hydrochloride. Natural replacement of bromide by chloride can be hastened if the patient is given an intravenous infusion of equal parts of dextrose-water and saline and a diet containing ample fluid and salt. This may be supplemented with ammonium chloride, 3 G. per day for a week, by mouth.

CHLORAL HYDRATE

The consumption of drugs which act by release of trichlorethanol has increased with the introduction of dichloralphenazone (*Welldorm*) and triclofos (*Tricloryl*). Poisoning occurs in old people and in children. The effects of acute overdosage are often mitigated by vomiting, but chloral is more toxic than alcohol and taken in gross overdoses has caused death from depression of respiration and failure of the circulation.

Treatment

In addition to applying general measures it may be desirable to perform gastric suction-lavage with one-half per cent. solution of sodium bicarbonate in order to counter local irritation.

PARALDEHYDE

Paraldehyde poisoning is rare, but this sedative is much more toxic than ethanol in equal volume. It has been given inadvertently in overdose by mouth and injected parenterally in an attempt at suicide. A twelve hour period of coma with low blood pressure and hyperventilation may result, but seldom does death occur. Acidaemia and haematemesis are complications which may arise.

ANTICONVULSANTS

Anticonvulsant poisoning is most often due to phenytoin sodium (*Epanutin*). The effect of this drug is rather prolonged. Gross overdosage causes a stuporous condition which is treated as for barbiturate poisoning. Lesser amounts of phenytoin, e.g. 0·5 G. per day, may cause drowsiness, ataxia and confusion. Depression of the blood-forming organs has occurred and also cases of megaloblastic anaemia. Toxic nephrosis has been recorded. Many drugs of this type are available and produce similar effects. Patients take a notably long time to recover after acute primidone (*Mysoline*) poisoning, and methoin (*Mesontoin*) is more potent than hydantoin and should be treated with great respect. Succinimides exert little acute toxicity.

ANTIHISTAMINES

Most, but not all, of the antihistamines are depressants of the central nervous system in adults, but in children may produce similar effects to those seen in small animals—excitement, tremor and convulsions. Chlorpheniramine (*Piriton*) is a stimulant; cyclizine, diphenhydramine, mepyramine and promethazine are sedatives. All of these drugs are readily absorbed and rapidly detoxified. They can not readily be detected in the urine.

Symptoms

The effects vary considerably. In self-poisoning in adults stupor with mydriasis, hypotension with tachycardia and abnormal rhythm, and depression of respiration indicate a relatively severe poisoning. In children the dosage is usually less and ataxia, excitement or drowsiness and hyperreflexia leading to convulsions are more usual. The latter condition is dangerous as apnoea may occur.

Treatment

There is no specific treatment and diuresis is not necessary as these compounds are rapidly detoxified. The main difficulty concerns the child with minor convulsions. If a sedative is called for, intramuscular paraldehyde is perhaps the safest but half the normal dosage (calculated by weight) should be given at first and close attention paid to continuing adequacy of respiration.

DERIVATIVES OF PHENOTHIAZINE

Tranquillizers derived from phenothiazine—trifluoperazine (*Stelazine*), chlorpromazine (*Largactil*)—may produce drowsiness and slurring of speech or, in higher doses, stupor characterized by depression of the circulation and flaccidity of muscle disproportionate to the depth of anaesthesia. Arrhythmia is common. Amnesia for the episode of overdosage is usually complete although the patient was conscious. Many untoward side-effects from continued use in recommended dosage have been noted—fever, granulocytopenia, anaemia, rash, cholestatic jaundice, bizarre dyskinesia and rigidity of the muscle groups. Any of these may follow acute self-poisoning.

Treatment

Hypotension in adults who have ingested phenothiazine derivatives may require intravenous infusion; at all times oxygenation has to be attended to. Benzhexol hydrochloride (*Artane*), 5 mg., may be given by mouth for spasmodic dystonia such as torticollis, and repeated 8-hourly for 2 days.

ASPIRIN AND SALICYLATE

Under this heading are included accidental poisoning in children with aspirin, methyl salicylate (oil of wintergreen) or sodium salicylate, and self-poisoning in adults with aspirin.

Aetiology

In children, poisoning may arise by over-enthusiastic dosing for therapeutic purposes or in a toddler who gains access to a bottle of liniment or of aspirin tablets; salicylate is the third most frequent cause of acute poisoning in this age group. Some 4–18 per cent. of admissions of poisoned children to hospital are due to it, but scarcely any of them die. The number of such hospital admissions in England and Wales for salicylate poisoning rose from 1440 to 4710 from 1960 to 1964 but deaths fell from 14 to 3, whereas in adults admissions rose from 2340 to 7140 and deaths from 216 to 252. In adults, aspirin is a common means of self-poisoning, particularly in young women, the peak incidence being at about 20 years of age. The drug can be obtained readily; the amount consumed is frequently very great (30 G. or more) and is in multiples of the customary 300 mg. tablets.

Pathology

Deaths are infrequent in young persons but over 40 years of age it more readily proves fatal. In approximately 3 per cent. of adult patients, especially if there is a complicating prior metabolic or pulmonary abnormality, this outcome may be expected.

At post-mortem examination the stomach may contain white gritty residues which give a blue colour with a hot solution of ferric chloride. The mucosa is reddened and there are eroded and haemorrhagic patches. Aspirin has an antiprothrombin effect and frank purpura may be seen on the skin or the parietal pleura. Pulmonary oedema may be present. The urine contains salicylate as does the blood.

Symptoms

In a child being treated with sodium salicylate the first evidence of poisoning may be drowsiness, pallor, heavy breathing and twitching, followed by demonstrable ketonuria. After swallowing methyl salicylate there is a delay before the onset of these symptoms. The child's breath or vomitus smells of oil of wintergreen and convulsions are particularly likely to complicate matters. In adults who have taken aspirin, salicylism occurs—dizziness, pallor, sweating, noises in the ears, blurred vision and a feeling of alarm, thirst, and possibly of epigastric pain. Vomiting is common, but does not invariably take place. A variable amount of haematemesis may be present. On absorption aspirin causes a respiratory alkalaemia consequent upon overbreathing, complicated by dehydration and loss of electrolytes, due to hyperpnoea, sweating and vomiting. The scanty urine is alkaline at this stage. After a variable period of time buffering mechanisms may fail when acidaemia, scanty acid urine and ketonuria will be present in spite of continued hyperpnoea. Absorption of the drug leads to hyperpnoea, stupor accompanied by twitching, a rising pulse rate and an elevated temperature and blood pressure. If neglected this condition will progress, and death may occur suddenly from respiratory failure or more slowly from circulatory failure and pulmonary oedema. Reflexes remain brisk until near the end. If a diuresis is induced the level of salicylate falls and recovery takes place, but renal function may be impaired by the drug and care must be taken to ensure that the kidneys are working. Oliguria is usually a consequence of dehydration, but sugar, protein and casts may be found in the urine.

Diagnosis

The history is usually quite clear. Powdered aspirin is often seen in the mouth or in vomitus. The urine contains salicylate as does the product of gastric suction and the blood. Pallor, sweating, hyperpnoea and acid urine are indices of severity. Unlike children the majority of adults remain more or less conscious and can, therefore, co-operate in stating the nature of the poisoning. This relative freedom from central depression does not mean that they do not need treatment; unconsciousness is a sign of severe poisoning as is a plasma salicylate level of 50 mg. per 100 ml. and more. Respiratory alkalaemia in adults persists for several hours; hypopotassaemia is frequently present.

In children marked toxicity may be present at a plasma level of 30–35 mg. per 100 ml., acidaemia occurs more readily and with it, coma.

Treatment

Treatment is directed towards removal of the poison and minimizing its effects. In less severe cases (generally those adults with a serum total salicylate level under 50 mg. per 100 ml.) it may be sufficient to perform bronchial toilet and wash out the concretions of aspirin from the stomach with warm tap water or a solution of 0·5 per cent. sodium bicarbonate. Methyl salicylate is relatively insoluble and if less than 4 hours have passed since it was swallowed a purge of 10 G. sodium sulphate in 100 ml. water may be of value to a child, despite the consequent loss of water and salts. In severe aspirin poisoning in adults, a tube should be left in the stomach and 100 ml. water and 2 G. bicarbonate given hourly. To this may be added 0·5 G. of potassium chloride. Dehydration should be speedily reversed by intravenous infusion of 5 per cent. dextrose in water after estimation of the probable deficit, and progress be checked hourly. If there has been much vomiting, it is better to use normal saline and 5 per cent. dextrose in equal proportions. This regime usually leads to an alkaline diuresis and excretion of large amounts of salicylate, with recovery.

If, however, the patient is dangerously intoxicated, with altered blood pH, is grossly hyperpnoeic, or is producing a scanty acid urine, more heroic measures are called for. If necessary the blood pressure should be raised by infusion, and injection of vitamin K given (10 mg. phytomenadione) and one of several measures tried in order to eliminate salicylate or prevent its worst effects: (1) Forced alkaline diuresis which, if successful, should be continued until the plasma salicylate level has fallen below 40 mg. per 100 ml. Intravenous infusion is given at a rate of 2 litres in each of the first 2 hours and 1 litre per hour thereafter. Sodium bicarbonate solution (2 per cent. w/v), 5 per cent. dextrose or laevulose and normal saline, are given in rotation in that order in aliquots of 500 ml. One gramme of potassium chloride may be added to each of these bottles should the serum potassium level fall to 3·5 mEq. per litre or below. The infusion must be discontinued if there is no diuresis or if there are signs of pulmonary oedema. (2) Infusion of 100–200 ml. of 10 per cent. solution of mannitol (injection of mannitol). This treatment works well, but a necessary preliminary is to make sure that the kidney is functioning by obtaining a specimen of urine which should have a specific gravity greater than 1·020 if there is oliguria, or by giving an infusion of 1 litre of M/5 lactate and recording a rise in output from a catheter. Fluid lost by diuresis is replaced in the form of injection of dextrose, of lactate, of saline, or of appropriate mixtures of them. Serum potassium levels should be checked. Bicarbonate may be included in the cycle of infusions. (3) A period of 6–8 hours of intermittent haemodialysis. (4) Partial exchange transfusion of blood in a child. (5) Intermittent peritoneal dialysis with 2 litres of a suitable solution every hour. (6) Intravenous injection of a relaxant and mechanically controlled respiration. The simplest and possibly most effective is the first of all these. Water and electrolyte balance must be watched during diuresis. Mannitol may be included in measure 1 (above) if the diuresis is not satisfactory.

Prognosis

Prognosis is usually good unless 8–12 hours have elapsed since the drug was taken and hyperpnoea is well established. The later stages of severe poisoning are difficult to reverse. A weakness in current therapy would seem to be failure to realize the possible severity of this poisoning so that active treatment may be instituted in the early stages.

ACETANILIDE, PHENACETIN, AMIDOPYRINE, PHENYLBUTAZONE AND PARACETAMOL

Aetiology

These, the lesser analgesics used in proprietary mixtures for the relief of headache, are depressants of the central nervous system but have other and more serious effects if used continuously over a long period of time. Acetanilide may liberate aniline which gives rise to methaemoglobin. Phenacetin may also give rise to altered blood pigment and is recognized as a cause of nephropathy [see Section 12]. Amidopyrine (*Aminopyrine*) may cause agranulocytosis in sensitized persons, as may phenazone and its derivatives (*Saridone*). The mechanism of this abnormality due to amidopyrine is not fully explained but it is akin to that of apronal (*Sedormid*), thrombocytopenia—the development of a specific antibody to the white blood cells of allergic patients. Skin eruptions due to these drugs occur in large numbers of persons [see Section 14]. Paracetamol is toxic to the liver and heart.

Symptoms

Acute overdosage may cause delirium followed by stupor. Altered blood pigments may cause cyanosis (methaemoglobin) and the symptoms of acute anaemia. Agranulocytosis may precede acute pharyngitis, fever, weakness and toxaemia. Blood dyscrasia can only be diagnosed by haematological examination. Renal failure secondary to acute intravascular haemolysis has been encountered.

Treatment

Usually no treatment is needed for altered blood pigment other than rest in bed and full oxygenation if there is dyspnoea. In extreme cases infusion of 25 ml. of a 1 per cent. solution of methylene blue or fresh blood may be given. Depression of bone marrow or hepatic functions are grave condtions which deserve most serious consideration; nephropathy is most often discovered at post-mortem examination.

ACUTE MORPHINE AND HEROIN POISONING

Under this heading are included poisoning due to the naturally occurring alkaloids of opium—morphine and codeine, the semi-synthetic derivative diamorphine (heroin) and the purely synthetic substances pethidine, methadone, phenadoxone and pholcodine.

Aetiology

Poisoning occurs by accident in children, by accident or self-administration in adults and from therapeutic misadventure in either. Children are unusually susceptible to the acute effects of drugs of this class. Tolerance and addiction to these drugs are easily and quickly developed. Such occurrences are rare in Britain with the exception of intravenous self-administration of heroin (frequently combined with cocaine) by heroin-dependent patients. The number of persons who indulge this vice is not known with accuracy but approximately 2500 heroin addicts are registered under the provisions of the Dangerous Drugs Act of 1967. Gross overdosage may occur at any time despite the development of tolerance, as a result of anxiety on the part of the addict to increase the effect of the drug or more usually to exploit a success in penetrating a vein. Repeated and extensive thrombophlebitis makes this manoeuvre increasingly difficult.

Pathology

Death is due to respiratory failure and the classical signs of asphyxia will be present. A quantity of alkaloid may be demonstrable in the urine, stomach, liver and other organs. Heroin is converted to morphine *in vivo*.

Symptoms

In moderate doses all of these drugs have a dual effect in non-habituated persons. Postural hypotension is a feature of mild overdosage in ambulant cases and intravenous injection of pethidine has caused circulatory collapse. Depression of the central nervous system is manifested by analgesia, suppression of cough and slowing of the rate of breathing. Stimulation manifests itself as euphoria, restlessness (pethidine may be convulsant), nausea (especially after codeine), bradycardia due to vagal stimulation, and pin-point pupils. After pethidine the pupils may be dilated. As absorption progresses the patient becomes drowsy and sinks into a stupor which, after morphine, is characterized by stertorous or irregular breathing with a slow pulse rate and profuse sweating. Diminished breathing causes retention of carbon dioxide with consequent respiratory acidaemia and excretion of a scanty acid urine. Pethidine causes a dry skin and fast pulse. The cerebrospinal fluid pressure is raised. Codeine is a wealing agent and puffiness of the face or eyelids is a feature of poisoning with this drug in children. Generalized urticaria may be seen. The limbs are flaccid but reflexes present until near the end. Heroin misuse does not usually give rise to these symptoms because of tolerance. Gross intravenous overdosage causes collapse and sudden death. The precise role of cocaine (a drug which may cause convulsions, followed by apnoea or cardiac arrest) and of heroin (a respiratory depressant which also causes pulmonary oedema) in this is not clear. The use of unclean hypodermic syringes which may be shared leads to outbreaks of viral hepatitis [see Section 6] which is apt to be severe in these undernourished and self-neglecting patients, and to infective cellulitis or septicaemia. These factors complicate the drug toxicity.

Additionally there is the problem of an acute withdrawal syndrome which may be considered to be a form of acute toxicity, albeit a negative aspect of it. In a heroin-dependent person some 24–48 hours after the drug was last administered, or within one hour of being given either of the morphine antagonists (nalorphine and levallorphan) there ensues malaise, sneezing, rhinorrhoea and watering of the eyes, abdominal cramp and deep anxiety and depression. Disturbances of the autonomic nervous system include labile pulse rate and blood pressure, vomiting and diarrhoea, cold sweats and goose flesh. If the condition is severe, as it might well be if nalorphine is given to an addict, hallucinosis, excitement and even convulsions may ensue with danger to life.

Diagnosis

The history is, as always in acute poisoning, of extreme value. Coma with marked respiratory depression (especially slowing of the rate) and consequent hypoxaemia and hypercapnia may arouse suspicion of the cause. After morphine, miosis, bradycardia and sweating are notable; after pethidine these signs are absent. Toxicological examination of urine, blood or gastric contents may take too long to be of value in managing acute cases. The heroin addict can usually be detected by inspection of the limbs for evidence of repeated injections, combined with his state of self-neglect. He is severely constipated. Shortly after taking the drug he feels well and is not likely to seek advice. The state of withdrawal is described above. Heroin is excreted in the urine in the form of morphine which can be detected by gas-liquid chromatography.

Treatment

The primary defect being depression of respiration, this should be controlled by bronchoscopy, suction, intubation and assisted respiration with oxygen. Meanwhile, 15 mg. of injection of the specific antagonist, nalorphine, may be given intravenously and repeated. Gastric suction-lavage may then be performed if desirable and the usual attentions necessary to a patient in coma paid to the state of the circulation, water and electrolyte balance, renal function, and prevention of spread of pulmonary infection.

Acute withdrawal symptoms will be precipitated in heroin or morphine-dependent persons and convulsions may ensue. The treatment of the withdrawal syndrome is a matter for the physician and the psychiatrist working conjointly. Opiates should not be given except when nalorphine has precipitated severe symptoms. It is only lawful for a limited number of designated physicians who staff the drug-dependence clinics to prescribe heroin for the state of heroin dependence (Misuse of Drugs Act, 1971) but every doctor must judge for himself of the best treatment in emergency. Morphine sulphate intravenously should suffice to counteract the most violent effects of nalorphine in an addict. Heavy sedation with chlorpromazine or barbiturate is usually necessary. Attention to the fluid and electrolyte balance and nutrition, and vigorous treatment of infection is also important. Most physicians endeavour to replace heroin-dependence with a less severe dependence on methadone taken orally, others attempt a total withdrawal. Some success has been achieved in shifting addicts from heroin (intravenous) to methadone (oral).

Prognosis

Children and old persons are peculiarly susceptible to these drugs and some persons display hypersensitivity to them. Codeine and pethidine are less likely to produce dangerous poisoning than is morphine or heroin. Neglect of the patient during the first 8–12 hours is very harmful as depression is most severe at that time. The prognosis of heroin-dependence is poor.

POISONING BY CEREBRAL STIMULANTS

The majority of the drugs which poison the nervous system are depressants, but a few stimulants are of importance. These are the plant alkaloids cocaine and strychnine and the synthetic amines related to amphetamine. The latter have become familiar of recent years as habit-forming drugs. Another group of drugs which have a similar action and may be very toxic are the amine oxidase inhibitors. These are prescribed for depression of mood but less frequently than a few years ago, largely because of the introduction of the tricyclic psychostimulant drugs, of which imipramine and amitriptyline are favoured.

STRYCHNINE

The alkaloid of *Strychnos nux-vomica* is prescribed as a 'tonic', frequently in pill form with iron. Such medicines may attract children and the majority of cases of poisoning occur thus.

Aetiology

Strychnine facilitates the spread of impulses through the reflex arcs of the spinal cord and to a lesser extent the brain. All external stimuli may, therefore, give rise to widespread motor discharges which cause tonic convulsions.

Symptoms

After a delay pending absorption, the patient may suddenly cry out, grimace and convulse. Opisthotonos is a common feature. Convulsions recur with increasing frequency and are initiated by any disturbance. Consciousness is retained unless clouded by hypoxia. Death may result from asphyxia.

Treatment

A sedative should be administered as soon as possible, e.g. 2–4 ml. of paraldehyde or 300 mg. of pentobarbitone sodium intramuscularly. Efforts should be made to keep the airway clear by inserting a short curved tube. The patient should be conveyed at once to hospital, oxygen being administered en route if needful. On arrival a state of anaesthesia should be instituted at once, possibly with intravenous thiopentone sodium and a short-acting relaxant, e.g. suxamethonium. Gastric suction and bronchial toilet may then be performed if needful. If convulsions occur on lightening the anaesthesia, a regime of controlled respiration under relaxants should be maintained. Strychnine is detoxicated in a few hours and it is desirable that the patient be kept in a darkened quiet room under observation by a silently efficient nurse during that time.

COCAINE

Cocaine occurs naturally in the leaf of *Erythroxylum coca*; there are a number of related synthetic compounds such as amethocaine and butacaine.

Aetiology

Cocaine hydrochloride is a central stimulant, a powerful euphoriant, a drug of dependence, and a local anaesthetic. It potentiates the effects of adrenaline. As an addictive substance, its distribution is controlled by the regulations of the Dangerous Drugs Act (now replaced by the Misuse of Drugs Act, 1971). On occasion when it or a congener is used in excessive amount to produce anaesthesia of a mucosal surface, e.g. before bronchoscopy, dangerous quantities may be absorbed. For this reason it is usual to apply such drugs in the form of an aerosol of an accurately measured volume of solution. Idiosyncrasy may be met with or excessively rapid absorption from a raw surface may defeat this precaution.

Symptoms

In small amounts cocaine enhances mental activity and causes excitement. The skin is pale and the pupils dilated. In dangerous doses convulsions occur and death from asphyxia may follow obstruction to breathing or prolonged fits. Ventricular fibrillation is another lethal complication to be feared since cocaine and adrenaline increase cardiac irritability and give rise to extrasystoles. This may well be the cause of sudden death in addicts who take intravenous heroin and cocaine.

Treatment

Prevention is much better than cure in this case but, if the situation permits, the convulsing patient should be given intravenous thiopentone sodium immediately, followed by a muscle relaxant, and tracheal intubation should be performed. Respiration may then be controlled. If cardiac arrhythmia becomes troublesome injection of propranolol may prevent the development of ventricular fibrillation. If the cause of collapse is ventricular fibrillation, external cardiac massage and the use of an Ambu bag or other form of controlled respiration may be instituted while an electrical defibrillator is obtained and applied. Cocaine is rapidly detoxicated, so that these measures may save life.

AMPHETAMINE AND ITS CONGENERS

A large number of synthetic amines related to ephedrine have been used for their euphoric and arousing effect, as vascoconstrictors of the nasal mucosa or as bronchodilators. Prescribing these drugs, many of which, such as dexamphetamine and phenmetrazine, are addictive, requires the most careful consideration and their distribution is controlled by inclusion in Schedule IV of the Poisons Rules and the new Misuse of Drugs legislation. Abuse from self-medication occurs, and a form of psychosis has resulted from it. Recently an epidemic occurred of self-administration of methylamphetamine intravenously. This dangerous habit produces immense stimulation and rapid and severe drug dependence of the amphetamine type. In addition to the danger of psychotic or convulsive episodes there is the special liability to cardiovascular disaster. The hazards of group-sharing of contaminated syringes are the same as those found in heroin addicts and indeed it is in part the same patients who indulged in this habit since the prescribing of heroin has been rigidly controlled.

Aetiology

Sympathomimetic amines stimulate the cardiovascular system by releasing catecholamines and acute poisoning may take the form of an excessive effect of this kind. Many of them are inhibitors of the enzyme amine oxidase which catalyses the destruction of the important amines adrenaline, noradrenaline and 5-hydroxytryptamine, and most MAO inhibitors in overdosage cause restlessness and twitching. The amphetamines are convulsants, particularly in children. When taken orally as tablets they are not severely toxic, however, and seldom prove fatal. Frequently they are taken by adults in conjunction with a barbiturate and this complicates the picture.

Symptoms

The euphoria, excitement, tremor, dilated pupils, dry mouth and aggressive talkativeness which characterize moderate dosage increase to anxiety, disorientation, hallucinosis and jactitation after large doses or intravenous administration. The patient may pass into restless stupor. The pulse rate is fast, blood pressure elevated and the face red. An erythematous or macular rash commonly appears and reflexes are brisk. The condition may persist for 12 hours. Drug-dependence of the amphetamine type is usually met with as a group activity amongst irresponsible young people who misuse the drug by oral consumption of tablets of such preparations as dexamphetamine sulphate, or combinations with barbiturate, e.g. *Drinamyl.* Bouts of amphetamine-taking may be alternated with the taking of barbiturate in an attempt to gain sleep. Continued or frequent usage leads to tolerance which may progress to a remarkable degree. The severity of symptoms is not therefore readily correlated with the level in blood. The drug is excreted in the urine, largely unchanged. Being a base it is more readily excreted in acid than in alkaline urine and this fact can be made to play a part in therapy.

Diagnosis

It may be important to distinguish between a toxic episode of this nature in a neurotic patient and a paranoid episode in a psychotic. Mental depression rather than stimulation may be the main feature, if the patient has been used to taking the drug. Convulsions and little evidence of stimulation may be detected, and coma occur with gross overdosage.

Treatment

The only treatment usually required is sedation with 4 ml. of paraldehyde or 300 mg. of phenobarbitone sodium given intramuscularly, and rest in a quiet place. If convulsions occur a period of full control by the anaesthetist as described for strychnine poisoning may be necessary. The acute psychosis met with after repeated massive dosage usually resolves in 7–30 days. Since this drug is excreted by the kidney diuretic treatment may logically be considered but if it is undertaken an attempt should be made to render the urine acid by adding 1 G. of ammonium chloride to each of two 500 ml. bottles of infusion of 5 per cent. dextrose given with 200 ml. of 10 per cent. mannitol in the first hour. Serum electrolytes and urinary pH should be monitored regularly.

AMINE OXIDASE INHIBITORS

These drugs were used freely for the treatment of psychotic depression and, more recently, for hypertensive disease. The former class of patient is particularly liable to self-poisoning. There are two main groups of compounds—hydrazines, of which phenelzine (*Nardil*) and isocarboxazid (*Marplan*) are widely prescribed, and non-hydrazines, of which tranylcypromine (*Parnate*) and nialamide are popular. These drugs are particularly liable to increase the potency of other drugs which may be taken at the same time and thus induce toxic effects from ordinary doses. The effect may be a result of inhibition of hepatic enzymal systems which play a part in detoxifying these drugs. Of the substances so affected alcohol, pethidine, morphine, imipramine and barbiturate are noteworthy. It is only to be expected that an MAO inhibitor will potentiate the action of any amine which is normally detoxified by this enzyme system. Noteworthy are catecholamines (adrenaline-noradrenaline) and serotonin (5-hydroxytryptamine). An unexpected hazard has been revealed. Patients who are under treatment with MAO inhibitors should not eat certain foods, e.g. cheese and banana which have a high content of vaso-active amines detoxified normally by MAO, or they may suffer a cardiovascular disaster.

Symptoms

Elevation of mood may progress to dizziness, tremor, excitement and restlessness but these drugs are not convulsants. Insomnia is likely to be notable. It is difficult to give a logical explanation why a compound which inhibits an enzyme system which catalyses destruction of noradrenaline in the tissues should cause hypotension, but this apparently paradoxical result is the main systemic effect of overdosage with many of these substances, e.g. pargyline (*Eutonyl*). Combination with a sedative of the promazine group may prove lethal. Profound hypotension occurs and may persist for 1–2 days. With it hyperpnoea, hyperpyrexia and hyperreflexia may be observed. The limbs may be quite rigid or opisthotonos occur. The differential diagnosis from strychnine poisoning may not be easy.

Treatment

There is no specific treatment but infusion of plasma will counter hypotension. Sympathomimetics, e.g. metaraminol or methylamphetamine, should be avoided. In no circumstances should sedative treatment be given for hypomania.

PSYCHOSTIMULANT DRUGS

The introduction of reasonably effective drugs which relieve depression of mood has inevitably led to copious consumption. These drugs take some days or weeks to exert a beneficial action and patients are particularly exposed to the hazard of self-poisoning during this period. The most widely prescribed compounds are imipramine (*Tofranil*) and the closely related substance amitriptyline. Both drugs are rapidly absorbed, detoxified in the liver and metabolites excreted in the urine within 24 hours. In additon to their complex actions in modifying the distribution, interaction and metabolism of bioactive amines they exert some atropine-like effect.

Symptoms

Imipramine in overdosage has profound effects on the cardiovascular system which are particularly notable in children—hypotension, complicated by oliguria or apnoea, and arrhythmia leading to cardiac arrest. In adults the cardiovascular system is less severely affected and amitriptyline may cause hypertension and tachycardia. The central nervous system is always excited despite loss of consciousness and reflexes are exaggerated, convulsions occur (especially with amitriptyline in children) and body temperature is grossly abnormal.

Treatment

The prognosis is hazardous but the duration of severe poisoning is relatively short. Propranolol may be tried for cardiac arrhythmia and an anticholinesterase such a pyridostigmine or neostigmine has been advocated. Diuresis is not likely to be helpful as active drug is not cleared by the kidney. Other severe symptoms must be treated symptomatically and full oxygenation and proper circulation maintained while detoxification takes place.

POISONING BY IRRITANTS AND CORROSIVES

LIQUIDS

Aetiology

There is a range of substances which cause intense irritation and possible destruction of tissue at the site of contact. The severity of the resulting chemical burn is related to the agent involved, its concentration, the duration of exposure and the efforts made to remove it. Substances such as mineral acids (hydrochloric, sulphuric and nitric acids) or strong alkalis (sodium and potassium hydroxides and ammonia) may cause loss of tissue. They are infrequently used by suicidal persons, occasionally swallowed in error, and also give rise to minor accidents at work. Should the eyes be affected, the effect may be serious. Certain irritants (hydrochloric acid, phosgene, ammonia, nitrous fumes) are more or less gaseous and may affect severely the eyes, nose, upper respiratory tract and lungs, but any corrosive which has been swallowed may also be inhaled with froth and mucus. All irritant corrosives have systemic effects when absorbed. Acid and alkali cause violent disturbances of the acid-base equilibrium. Oxalic acid, oxalates and phenolic products have a profound effect on the central nervous system which may outweigh the irritant action. Should the patient survive there may be serious late sequelae due to stricture of the oesophagus or pylorus or renal failure.

Symptoms

Burns of the skin due to splashing of concentrated sulphuric acid or phenol may be painless but pain in the mouth, chest or abdomen occur immediately after ingestion of most corrosives. External burns of the chin due to dribbling from the mouth usually occur. Retching, vomiting and the passage of altered blood or mucosal shreds is accompanied by coughing, spasm of the glottis, cyanosis and collapse. The patient may die quickly from perforation of the alimentary canal, acidosis or asphyxia. If the occasion is less dramatic consciousness is not lost; there will be thirst and repeated vomiting, made worse by attempts to drink, and peripheral circulatory failure is likely to develop.

Treatment

Treatment may be considered under three headings. (1) Contaminated clothing should be removed and external burns washed with soap and water. Pethidine hydrochloride, 50–100 mg., should be given, the areas lightly dressed and the patient transferred to a centre which specializes in treating burns. If this is not possible, an anaesthetic may be given, neutralization at the surface attempted with sterile solution of sodium bicarbonate and débridement carried out while plasma or plasma expander is infused and the patient treated as for a thermal burn. (2) External burns to the eye should be treated at once with copious washing. In the case of lime (which is markedly adherent) a fresh 10 per cent. solution of ammonium tartrate is effective. (3) Internal burns from strong caustic may be so severe that no local treatment is possible. If the patient can swallow, a pint of milk, followed by soap solution and then 15 g. of magnesia will effect some neutralization and cause emesis. In a few cases it may be possible to give an anaesthetic, clean the mouth and throat, intubate the trachea and control respiration and then gently pass a soft small bore tube into the stomach. Suction and lavage with warm saline (not bicarbonate) may then be practised, but there is always the fear of tearing the corroded oesophagus and stomach. Gastric and intravenous drip therapy, oxygen, and probably whole blood or plasma and antibiotics will be needed. Careful checks must be made to determine the degree of damage to renal function, whereat phenol is particularly active.

OXALIC ACID AND OXALATES

Not more than 14·2 g. of potassium oxalate may be freely purchased at one time, but this is enough to cause severe poisoning if ingested by a compulsive suicide or taken in error for Epsom salts, which it resembles. A strong solution will produce the caustic effects of an acid, but additionally there is depression of the central nervous system, the muscles and the heart. This is probably due to an acute deprivation of ionized calcium as a result of the formation of insoluble oxalate. Consciousness is lost soon after ingestion and death from cardiac and respiratory failure during or after convulsions is to be feared.

Treatment

Treatment may be begun by giving a pint of milk and inducing emesis if the patient is capable of responding, and should include gastric lavage with diluted lime water as a chemical antidote. 10 g. of calcium lactate may be left in the stomach. Respiration must be fully safe-guarded at all stages. Intravenous calcium gluconate may be tried if tetany supervenes but has little effect in lightening coma.

PHENOLIC SUBSTANCES

A variety of creosotes and cresols exist; in most cases of poisoning these agents are swallowed compulsively by depressed women at home. The cresols are less irritant, depressant to the nervous system and lethal than the creosotes. On swallowing a cresol mixture there is some pain and vomiting, but phenolic substances are local anaesthetics and vomiting is not a marked feature of the episode. The patient feels dizzy, becomes ataxic and rapidly loses consciousness, and may be found in coma, cold, cyanosed and with slow stertorous breathing. Recovery of consciousness takes many hours. Oliguria is a common complication.

Detergents are less toxic than creosote or cresol. The incidence of severe poisoning has declined since these substances largely replaced cresols, creosotes and oxalate as domestic cleansers.

Treatment

Gastric suction and lavage, using a soft tube, is possible and of value. It should be continued until the returns are relatively free of phenolic odour. Respiration should be safeguarded, stimulants avoided and subsequently a close check kept on renal function. Ingestion of detergent needs little treatment—emesis if practicable and milk as a demulcent.

IRRITANT GASES

Chlorine, hydrochloric acid fume, carbon disulphide, ammonia, phosgene and nitrous fumes are irrespirable. They are most frequently met with in industrial plants and affect the victims of accident. Chlorine and ammonia may cause accidents in the home. The former will be released when disinfectant containing bisulphate (acidic) is mixed with bleaching powder, e.g. in cleaning a lavatory pan, and has thus affected a large number of housewives. Solutions of hypochlorite, e.g. parazone, are irritant but not caustic if ingested. Nitrous fumes may gather over stores of dressed silage on farms. In low concentrations they cause irritation of the eyes, nose and throat; in higher concentration the patient may be congested, coughing severely and show evidence of acute tracheobronchitis and hypoxia. Pulmonary oedema consequent upon damage to the alveoli is the danger. It may follow after an initial period of improvement, particularly after phosgene poisoning. Carbon disulphide, additionally, causes much excitement and restlessness which may be followed by collapse. Hydrogen sulphide has a characteristic odour of rotten eggs but the intensity of the smell gives no indication of the concentration of this most toxic gas. In low concentrations it produces a severe conjunctivitis and irritates the mucosae. In higher concentrations, 300–500 p.p.m., it causes loss of consciousness. CS (Riot Control) gas is an intensely irritant lacrimator which may be inadvertently encountered in situations of civil disturbance.

Treatment

Treatment of an irritant gas poisoning is essentially symptomatic. After rescue, first-aid consists of washing affected parts, especially the conjunctivae, treating burns and safeguarding respiration. Injection of atropine sulphate, 1 mg., or of mepyramine maleate, 50 mg., may limit the outpouring of fluid in the upper respiratory tract. It will be necessary to supplement this treatment with tracheobronchial suction, aeration of the lungs, oxygen and possibly antibiotics. Acute heart failure has to be guarded against.

POISONING BY AGENTS COMMONLY FOUND IN THE HOME

Aetiology

The majority of acute poisoning takes place in or near dwelling places. Much of it is deliberate and suicidal in intent. Serious attempts at self-poisoning usually involve utility gas, barbiturate or aspirin, but less deliberate attempts may involve any substance which is to hand and thought to be toxic. In addition there are accidents. Frequently these concern young children who ingest poison in play; or accidental consumption by adults due to toxic substances being stored in unlabelled containers or in an unsuitable place.

NON-BACTERIAL FOOD POISONING

Aetiology

Acute gastro-intestinal upset due to ingestion of infected food is referred to in Section 2. It is a common disease. Much more rarely the cause is ingestion of food contaminated with a chemical. Frequently this is a metal dissolved by preparation of an acidic food in an unsuitable container. The number of persons involved may be relatively high if communal feeding is involved.

Symptoms

The heavy metals are astringent, taste metallic and act as emetics. Generally within an hour of ingestion of the meal persons are affected by nausea, vomiting, pallor with sweating, colic and diarrhoea. Systemic effects of heavy metal poisoning are seldom in evidence. Heavy contamination with bacterial toxin may also act quickly but there is usually a delay of 8–24 hours after ingestion of infected foodstuffs.

Diagnosis

The nature of the episode may arouse suspicion whereupon any possible food source, e.g. sour fruit cooked in a copper pot, should be submitted to analysis.

Treatment

No treatment may be needed if brisk evacuation has occurred and has ceased; otherwise a saline purge may be indicated, followed by a gastro-intestinal sedative such as Chalk and Opium Mixture, B.P.C. If the gastro-enteritis is severe enough to cause dehydration and collapse, the patient is better in hospital where readings of electrolyte values should be made and appropriate infusions given. Desferrioxamine by mouth might be tried experimentally, or edetate by injection.

BLEACHES AND CHLORINATED GERMICIDES

Aetiology

Chlorine-releasing antiseptics may be swallowed compulsively by women or accidentally by children.

The accidental or unexpected release of chlorine from bleaching powder by mixture with acidic solutions of bisulphate has been referred to (see Irritant Gases). Several cleansers designed for use on vitreous enamel and chinaware release chlorine.

Symptoms

These substances cause irritation of the gastro-intestinal tract with cramp, vomiting, diarrhoea and coughing, gasping and irritation of the eyes and nose.

Treatment

Emesis, or lavage with fresh 0·1 per cent. solution of sodium thiosulphate ('hypo') will remove chlorine from the stomach. If the lungs are gravely irritated, pulmonary oedema is to be feared and it is always wise to admit the patient to hospital, to give a prophylactic antibiotic, and to have oxygen available. Injection of 1 mg. of atropine sulphate may dry excessive secretion of the mucosa, but will not modify oedema due to alveolar damage.

OTHER ANTISEPTICS

Aetiology

Iodine solution is less often used than formerly, but occasionally is the cause of acute irritation by ingestion in a child. Potassium permanganate in strong solution is also an irritant. A tablet inserted in the hope of causing abortion has been known to cause corrosion of the vault of the vagina. When ingested, boric acid ('boracic') and borates cause an acute gastro-enteritis after a delay of several hours; if absorbed thus, or as a result of application to a raw surface as an antiseptic, it is a convulsant in infants. The occurrence of a generalized bright erythema a few days later is characteristic. This substance is now excluded from proprietary toilet powders for infants.

Treatment

In all cases of ingestion of irritants, it is important to attempt emesis as soon as possible. After iodine one may give bread and milk, starch or 0·1 per cent. solution of thiosulphate by mouth.

PARAFFIN (KEROSENE)

Aetiology

This agent is responsible for some 10 per cent. of admissions to hospital in acutely poisoned young children. The substance is ingested in error for 'lemonade' having been stored in a 'soft drink' bottle and forgotten. The colour (pink or blue) is bleached out after a time.

Symptoms

Kerosene causes nausea, pallor, vomiting and diarrhoea if ingested. Frequently there is pulmonary irritation due to inhalation of fumes or liquid which spreads rapidly to the alveoli. The resulting pneumonitis may be serious. Paraffin is not readily absorbed from the intestine.

Diagnosis

Diagnosis is made on the history, the odour of paraffin and the symptomatology.

Treatment

Emesis should not be induced, nor gastric suction performed unless prior cuffed intubation of the trachea has been accomplished. The greatest danger from paraffin is a chemical pneumonitis following upon inhalation, otherwise the substance is not very toxic. 200 ml. of medicinal liquid paraffin, in which kerosene is soluble, may be given. Oxygen and antibiotics will probably be needed. Hydrocortisone should be given intramuscularly 6-hourly for 2 days if there is pneumonitis.

METALDEHYDE

Aetiology

Compressed tablets of meta fuel (a polymer of acetaldehyde which is used as a fuel by campers, and by gardeners to kill slugs) may be ingested by young children.

Symptoms

After some delay repeated vomiting and diarrhoea occur. Effects on the central nervous system include increased reflex tone leading to convulsions, respiratory and circulatory collapse with loss of consciousness. They have proved fatal.

Diagnosis

Diagnosis is almost entirely by the history and inspection of residues, which, if dry, are inflammable. Gastric contents contain aldehyde.

Treatment

To attempt emesis at once is important. Every child suspected of having ingested metaldehyde should be given gastric toilet. If consciousness is lost, preparation should be made for control of respiration and sedative treatment as for strychnine poisoning.

NAPHTHALENE

Aetiology

Children may consume portions of certain air-freshener cubes which contain naphthalene; mothball contains paradichlorbenzene which is less toxic. Absorption occurs with ease and less than 1 g. of naphthalene may prove lethal to a small child.

Diagnosis

Excitement leading to convulsions and loss of consciousness is the feature of immediate concern. Vomiting and diarrhoea follow closely. Sequelae of gravity are hepatitis, nephropathy and haemolytic anaemia.

Treatment

If the poisoning is severe it may be necessary to induce anaesthesia in order to control convulsions. Gastric toilet may be performed with advantage, using a solution of sodium bicarbonate, and 100 ml. of it being left in the stomach. Infusion of lactate or of dextrose-saline solution, or of blood if severe haemolysis has taken place, and intramuscular injection of hydrocortisone may all help but the most dangerous complication is renal failure. Intermittent haemodialysis may be the only way to relieve it.

HALOGENATED HYDROCARBON SOLVENTS

Wide use is made of this group of chemicals as solvents in industry and at home because they are non-inflammable, non-combustible and do not make explosive mixtures with air.

Aetiology

Some, e.g. methyl chloride and bromide, are used as fire extinguishers and refrigerants and the fumes when liberated in an enclosed space may prove toxic. Men working in chemical plants, or children who may play with such things have been affected. Carbon tetrachloride is used as a solvent for grease, oil and rubber, as a fire extinguisher and for dry cleaning on a domestic scale. If it is used to extinguish a fire in enclosed premises it may be decomposed and release the colourless toxic gas phosgene. This substance releases hydrochloric acid in the alveoli and may cause fatal pulmonary oedema after a delay of 6–12 hours. Tetrachloroethane is more potent than carbon tetrachloride. It is a solvent for cellulose acetate, a constituent of varnishes and of film base. Trichloroethylene and perchloroethylene are extensively used in the dry cleaning of clothes, the former as a 'spotting fluid' domestically, the latter on a commercial scale. Accidents occur by inhalation of heavy vaporous residues in dry-cleaning vats and by ingestion of fluids from unlabelled bottles. Mild addiction by inhalation of fumes has been described in work people and in young persons who sniff 'glue', i.e. adhesives with this type of solvent in them.

Symptoms

All of these substances affect the central nervous system. They cause giddiness, intoxication, weakness, nausea or vomiting, and loss of consciousness. In addition, individual substances produce particular effects. Methyl chloride may cause a prolonged diminution of visual acuity, anaemia or oliguria after the initial episode. Methyl bromide is a deadly poison with a characteristic delay of 12–48 hours before symptoms appear. Pruritus is often noted at this time; contamination of the skin causes blistering. The patient becomes giddy and is pale, sweating, with dilated pupils. Delirium may develop and become severe. Mild cases recover but pulmonary oedema, renal failure or convulsions may prove fatal. The vapours of trichloroethylene or of carbon tetrachloride may result in a clinical picture like that of halothane anaesthesia. Repeated exposure to small amounts or to tetrachloroethane may give rise to toxic hepatitis, nephropathy or neuropathy. At the onset, this illness is difficult to diagnose as the symptoms are not characteristic of the cause. 'Sniffing' causes drunkenness.

Treatment

Consciousness when lost may usually be restored by removal from the fumes, which often lie at floor level, and adequate oxygenation. Parenchymatous damage is more difficult to deal with and treatment is directed towards the relief of the affected organ.

POISONING BY METALS

ARSENIC

ACUTE POISONING

Aetiology

Arsenic is a severe irritant poison. No industrial accidents involving its use have been notified for several years and it is no longer used as a spray to destroy potato tops or in sheep dip or rat poison. The use of penicillin in the treatment of syphilis has removed organic arsenicals from the causes of therapeutic misadventure. White arsenic (arsenious oxide) is a white, gritty powder, poorly soluble but tasteless. It was available in the form of weed-killer and as such has been used for homicide. Arsenic may, rarely, contaminate foodstuffs. Arsine is a gaseous by-product of certain industrial processes. Poisoning by ingestion of arsenic is now rare.

Pathology

Post-mortem examination of fatal cases reveals that the rugae of the stomach are inflamed, and acute irritation of the intestine is also present. There is much mucus and flakes of white material may be attached to the gastric mucosa. Arsenic in the lumen of the alimentary canal, or in the organs, may be recovered and estimated.

Symptoms

White arsenic has no taste, and intense thirst, epigastric pain and vomiting may be delayed for an hour after ingestion. Severe gastro-enteritis, however, inevitably follows and leads to collapse, with pallor, sweating and low blood pressure. Mucosal shreds may be passed in a watery stool.

Treatment

In acute arsenical poisoning, gastric lavage with

1 per cent. solution of sodium thiosulphate may be practised and the presence of arsenic confirmed. A course of dimercaprol, 4 mg. per kg. every four hours for 2 days intramuscularly followed by 2 mg. per kg. twice daily for 7 days may then be given, but in chronic poisoning BAL is of no value. Dehydration and loss of electrolytes must be checked and transfusion of whole blood will be of value if there is severe haemolysis. Pethidine hydrochloride may be given to relieve colic, or morphine used to check diarrhoea. A careful check on the urinary output is essential, and suppression of urine may require treatment by peritoneal or haemodialysis.

CHRONIC POISONING

Symptoms

Chronic poisoning manifests as anorexia, excess salivation, malaise, weakness and wasting of muscles, anaemia and similar disturbances of vague aetiology. These symptoms may follow an acute attack. The weakness may progress to a severe neuropathy. The skin is usually affected. Erythema, a mottled brown pigmentation (raindrop pigmentation), keratinization of the palms and soles and ridging of the nails have been described [see Section 14]. Rarely cirrhosis of the liver may be encountered.

Treatment

BAL has been used successfully in the treatment of toxic reactions arising during therapy with arsenic, in particular exfoliative dermatitis and agranulocytosis but the place of this drug in the treatment of a long-established poisoning is very doubtful.

ARSENIURETTED HYDROGEN (ARSINE)

Aetiology

This poisonous gas may be evolved when ores containing arsenic are processed or tanks which have contained pickling fluids or acids with arsenical contaminant are cleaned.

Pathology

On inhalation an acute intravascular haemolysis takes place which produces symptoms of anaemia, haemoglobinuria and jaundice. This is an uncommon cause of purpura. Oliguria, liver failure and death may occur.

Symptoms

Malaise, headache, shivering and passage of urine with altered blood pigments in it may take place within a few hours of exposure. It is deeply stained as with bile. Jaundice and severe anaemia follow within a day or two and in fatal cases lead to stupor.

Treatment

Arsine poisoning is a case where prevention is better than cure. There is no specific treatment for the condition but intensive care may well save life. The most serious complication is renal failure with tubular necrosis consequent upon hypovolaemia, reduction in renal circulation and the effect of the poison. An appropriate course of intermittent haemodialysis may save life. Early treatment of pulmonary oedema may be called for.

GOLD

Aetiology

This is usually a form of iatrogenic disease, the poisoning resulting from injection of gold salts for the treatment of rheumatic disease. Susceptibility varies widely.

Symptoms

Any of the toxic effects of a heavy metal may result, but the majority of patients (40 per cent. in one series) suffer from dermatosis, a lesser number from nephrosis, hepatic involvement or depression of marrow function.

Treatment

Therapy with gold should cease at the first evidence of toxic reaction and a course of dimercaprol be given.

IRON

Aetiology

The victims of this poison are commonly young children who are attracted by colourful sugar-coated pills containing a salt of iron, perhaps with strychnine in addition, purchased as a tonic or prescribed for the treatment of hypochromic anaemia. The pills tend to adhere to the gastric mucosa and a high concentration of ionized metallic salt is achieved locally. This acts as a corrosive.

Symptoms

At a variable time after ingestion the child is seen to be pale and thereafter vomits. The vomitus may be blood stained. Respiration is hurried, the pulse fast and the child may complain of backache or pass a loose, dark and offensive stool. Circulatory failure after gastro-enteritis may cause death but if immediate danger passes there may be delayed effects. After an interval of apparent recovery, colic and melaena may return and the child become drowsy and lapse into a stupor interrupted by irritable crying, twitching and restless convulsive movement. If this dangerous phase is safely passed hepatitis or nephropathy may be noted after 1–2 weeks. Some months afterwards symptoms of pyloric stenosis may require attention. Serum iron levels should be recorded throughout the first week of the illness as a guide to the likelihood of an attack of encephalopathy. The urine should be examined for bile salts, bilirubin and urobilin throughout a 3-week period and liver function tests performed before the patient is discharged from hospital.

Treatment

It is important that attempts to produce emesis be advised as soon as possible and that thorough gastric lavage be performed in hospital, preferably with 1 per cent. of solution of bicarbonate. A solution of 0·2 per cent. desferrioxamine should then be used and a portion left in the stomach. This compound is a peptide iron-acceptor related to apoferritin. It should also be injected intramuscularly (2 G. 12-hourly for 2 days) and infused intravenously (not more than 80 mg. per kg. in 24 hours).

MERCURY

Aetiology

Due to increased care in handling this metal and its salts very few cases of poisoning now arise from industrial sources. Quicksilver is volatile and creates a hazard by inhalation, but there is no danger to children who break a clinical thermometer in the mouth, other than the chance of a cut tongue. The salts are poisonous, mercuric chloride (corrosive sublimate) especially so, whereas mercurous chloride (calomel) is merely a purgative. If, however, catharsis fails it may be absorbed. Teething powders containing calomel have been implicated in the cause of acrodynia (pink disease) in infants and are no longer in use. The majority of cases of acute mercurial poisoning are due to the ingestion of a fluid made by dissolving a solution tablet (0·5 g.) of corrosive sublimate. This is a lethal dose. Mercurial diuretics, e.g. mersalyl, may cause stomatitis, gastritis or skin eruptions in susceptible persons or those in whom the renal condition is such that delay in excretion of the mercury occurs. Intravenous injection has caused fatal ventricular arrhythmia. Mercurial salts are used as dressings to protect seed from attacks by insects and have caused the death of countless birds but little human intoxication. Alkyl mercurials are used as fungicides and are frequently applied as an aerosol or smoke in enclosed premises.

Symptoms

Ingestion of the corrosive salt is followed at once by burning pain, blood-stained vomiting and diarrhoea. The mouth becomes red and sore and the mucosa ulcerates. There is a continuous flux and much pain from the bowels for several days. Oliguria is inevitable and the chief danger to life lies in renal or hepatic failure, but complete recovery is very possible. Subacute or chronic poisoning may affect the central nervous system, giving rise to erethism, tremors and degenerative lesions. Excessive salivation, foetor and a blue line on the gums occur. The alkyl mercurials in particular cause nervous symptoms. Rare forms of mercurialism include dermatosis in adults, acrodynia in infants, granulocytopenia and opacity of the optic lens.

Treatment

First-aid by administration of white of egg followed by repeated emesis is important and gastric lavage should be carried out. A course of dimercaprol treatment should be started without waiting to see if oliguria is severe. It can always be cut short if troublesome and penicillamine tried instead. Renal failure must be treated symptomatically, and haemodialysis may be needed. The illness is likely to be a prolonged one and strict attention to the hygiene of the mouth and the skin is important.

ACUTE LEAD POISONING

Aetiology

Acute poisoning occurs much less frequently than chronic poisoning [see p. 343] but it will follow the ingestion of soluble salts of the metal, or it may occur as an acute episode in the course of the treatment of chronic poisoning. To some workmen acute poisoning is an industrial hazard, most frequently following accidental inhalation or contamination of the skin with tetramethyl and tetraethyl lead. In children the condition follows ingestion of lead paint. Most of the paints used by amateurs do not contain lead and are harmless when ingested.

Symptoms

The initial symptoms are metallic taste in the mouth, severe vomiting (the presence of lead chloride may give the vomitus a white appearance), colic and passage of black stools. Circulatory collapse may occur and encephalopathy is a well known complication. Cramps in the muscles are less serious. Complicating sequelae include hepatitis, renal failure and anaemia.

Diagnosis

Acute lead poisoning may be diagnosed with confidence if the serum lead level is in excess of 0·07 mg. per 100 ml. or if a 24-hour specimen of urine contains 0·15–0·30 mg. of lead per litre. Porphyrinuria is usually found at the same time.

Treatment

Gastric lavage should be performed and 500 mg. of D-pencillamine left in the stomach. This dosage should be repeated orally three times per day for several days, and is especially useful in treating children. Adults may be treated with the chelating agent calcium disodium edetate (*Versene*), 30 mg. per kg. intravenously per day for a few days, in divided doses well diluted in dextrose injection. If the most alarming feature of the attack is encephalopathy this infusion should be replaced with diuretic treatment with intravenous injection of frusemide (*Lasix*), 20 mg., or of 100 ml. of 10 per cent. solution of mannitol to relieve intracranial oedema, and the edetate given intramuscularly during the diuresis, reverting to the intravenous route as soon as possible.

INACTIVATION OF METALS BY CHELATION

Dimercaprol (BAL). This may be given in suitable cases (acute poisoning by arsenic or mercury salts) by deep intramuscular injection of a 5 per cent. solution in oil (Dimercaprol Injection, B.P.) in a dose of 0·04–0·06 ml. per kg. body weight, repeated 4-hourly for 2 days, 4 injections on the third day, then twice daily for 5 days. This course should be modified for individual patients. It may be repeated after an interval of a few days. This drug is a local irritant and a generalized poison but it is important to push it to tolerable limits.

Sodium Calciumedetate (Calcium EDTA, Calcium Disodium Edetate). This is a salt of the cyclic organic ethylenediamine tetra-acetic acid. If injected intravenously it will combine with any available metal to form a firmly bound inactive complex which is readily excreted, or itself excreted in 6 hours. It is available as a 20 per cent. solution in 5 ml. ampoules (1 G.) which is best given diluted to 50 ml. with dextrose-water (2 per cent. final concentration). This may be infused slowly, twice daily for 5 days, and repeated after a week. In an emergency 100 ml. may be given to an adult twice during the first day. Calcium trisodium pentetate (Chel 330) is a similar substance given in a dose of 1 G. at a time.

Desferrioxamine Mesylate. When given orally this renders iron inabsorbable and inactive but in acute poisoning has to be administered early to be of much value in this respect. Given parenterally it greatly increases the rate of excretion of the absorbed metal. Intramuscular injections are painful and rapid infusion may cause an anaphylactic reaction. Initial dosage is 1–2 G. intramuscularly, dissolved in water for injection of 5–10 ml. and intravenous infusion of not more than 15 mg. per kg. in 24 hours. One may then carry on with intramuscular treatment for a further day or two.

D-Penicillamine. This is a degradation product of penicillin and acts as a powerful chelating agent for certain metals, notably copper. It is prepared in the form of a white powder, which forms an acid solution. Acetyl-D-penicillamine is less toxic and possibly more effective in sequestering mercury and lead. A dosage of 250 mg. four times a day for 10 days may be tried in acute poisoning with these metals.

POISONING DUE TO PLANTS AND ALKALOIDS

Aetiology

Poisonous plants may be classified into three groups—irritants, centrally acting poisons, and a miscellaneous group. They are most often ingested by children at play, but the number of such episodes is declining. Atropine and its congeners are the most important poisonous alkaloids because the most frequently occurring, but medicinal sources by far outstrip natural ones.

IRRITANT PLANTS

These may contain resins (e.g. cathartics), essential oils (e.g. apiol which is an ingredient of 'female pills'), alkaloids (e.g. colchicine) or saponins (e.g. spurge). The red berries of *Arum maculatum* (Cuckoo Pint or Lords and Ladies) is rather a favourite. It contains an irritant.

Symptoms

Burning pain with excoriation of the lips, vomiting, diarrhoea, colic or collapse follow shortly after ingestion, but severe episodes are uncommon.

Treatment

Emesis may be initiated with brine if it has not already occurred. Gastric lavage is often rewarding. If colic is severe pethidine may be injected. In the rare event of diarrhoea and vomiting resulting in dehydration and collapse the child should be admitted to hospital and appropriate infusions given.

NEUROTOXIC PLANTS

Aetiology

The seeds of the laburnum tree, *Cytisus laburnum L.*, are probably the most common source of this type of poisoning in children. They contain an alkaloid cytisine which is also found in broom and lupin seed. Nicotine, the alkaloid of tobacco, is used as an insecticide in the form of dust or spray. Liquid forms readily penetrate unbroken skin and by this means or by inhalation may prove very toxic, especially to non-smokers. The harmful effects of tobacco smoking, especially the relation as an aetiological factor to the increased incidence of cancer of the lung is almost certainly not due to the content of nicotine, but the toxic effect on the heart probably is. It has been referred to elsewhere, also the relation to peptic ulceration and chronic respiratory disease. Coniine is found in the hemlock plant, *Conium maculatum*, which may be chewed by children who fashion from it a hollow blow-pipe. Other poisonous plants of a similar structure are the Water Hemlock or Cowbane (*Cicuta virosa*) which has a rootstock which resembles a parsnip. It may be eaten by children at play; it contains a virulent poison, cicutoxin. The Water Dropwort (*Oenanthe crocata*) contains a similar toxin. Aconite is found in monkshood, *Aconitum napellus*, which is alleged to have been mistaken for horseradish. Serious poisoning from plants is not common.

Symptoms

About an hour or less after ingestion of a plant source, the victim becomes pale, dizzy and ataxic, probably vomits (cytisine and nicotine) or has diarrhoea and becomes anxious and restless. Bradycardia may be notable and there is twitching, weakness of the muscles and hypotension. Smoking tobacco causes peripheral vasoconstriction, tachycardia and bronchoconstriction. The interval is much less and the effect more severe with a contamination by liquid nicotine. Consciousness is not lost, unless terminally when the patient convulses. Aconite gives rise to a characteristic tingling in the mouth and throat before emesis occurs. Bradycardia and peripheral circulatory failure are marked features of the illness with nicotine and aconite. The others are dangerous convulsants.

Treatment

This is purely symptomatic—oxygenation, support for the circulation, gastric lavage where appropriate followed by control of dehydration. Convulsions may have to be controlled as for poisoning by strychnine [p. 328] which is an alkaloid in the same class.

ATROPINE AND HYOSCINE

Aetiology

Solanaceous alkaloids occur in a number of plants which include Deadly Nightshade, *Atropa belladonna* (patchy in its distribution) Henbane, *Hyoscyamus niger L.* and Woody Nightshade or Bittersweet *Solanum dulcamara* (widely disseminated). The berries are attractive to children, but are not commonly a source of poisoning today. Atropine and hyoscine are widely used medicinally for their property of blocking parasympathetic nerve action, e.g. as a pre-anaesthetic medication, but it is other applications which make them the cause of accidents to children and adults. Typical uses are in eyedrops which may be given too frequently to young children and track into the throat, in antacid and spasmolytic mixtures, in an old-fashioned liniment which may be swallowed by error or in plaster form applied in error to a raw surface. Hyoscine is a sedative and is used in tablet form to prevent motion sickness, morning sickness and in conditions characterized by anxiety and tremor. Children may ingest the tablets.

Symptoms

Atropine causes dryness of the mouth with thirst, flushed skin with fever, dilated pupils, tachycardia, irregular breathing, and excitement which may be maniacal in children, but in adults usually takes the form of visual hallucinosis. Hyoscine has similar peripheral effects, but may produce stupor. Solanine which is present in Bittersweet causes vomiting and diarrhoea.

Diagnosis

The diagnosis may be confirmed by injecting 0·1 mg. of carbachol subcutaneously. Normally this causes bradycardia, a fall in blood pressure and sweating. If the patient is atropinized, no such action is observed. A few drops of urine instilled into the conjunctival sac of a cat will produce dilatation of the pupil after half an hour. This test is more sensitive than any chemical one.

Treatment

Treatment is largely symptomatic but neostigmine, 0·5 mg., may help. It is more important to ensure proper oxygenation, to control fever by sponging and to give ample fluids than it is to apply stimulant or depressant drugs. Photophobia may require that nursing be carried out in a darkened room.

FUNGI

Aetiology

In Britain there are some 20 poisonous fungi but only the bulb agarics are important. The Fly Agaric, *Amanita muscaria*, a handsome scarlet and white-spotted fungus is unmistakable. It contains muscarine among other toxic principles. Much more important, because it is more easily mistaken for an edible fungus, is *Amanita phalloides*, the Death Cap, which contains five toxic peptides. Fortunately it is limited in distribution. As this poison withstands cooking and a portion of one or two grammes of fungus may prove fatal, it is wise not to eat mushrooms from a doubtful source.

Symptoms

After a delay of 24 hours (with *A. phalloides*) a violent attack of nausea, colic, pallor, vomiting and diarrhoea heralds disaster. It is then usually too late to prevent absorption of the poison and the prognosis is related to the amount ingested. Colic, dehydration and peripheral circulatory failure is usual. Renal and hepatic failure may follow after some days of apparent recovery. If serum transaminase levels are measured repeatedly the parenchymal damage may be expected but not prevented. Death may occur after 5–10 days. *A. muscaria* causes a state of excitement, with hallucinations, miosis, gastro-intestinal upset and (rarely) convulsions.

Treatment

Treatment can only be symptomatic and may not be of avail after ingesting *A. phalloides*. Infusions of blood and of solutions of electrolytes may be necessary. Injection of atropine sulphate, 1 mg., repeated hourly will control the worst effects of parasympathetic stimulation from muscarine. Repeated measurement of levels of blood constituents and corrective therapy is necessary. Renal failure may require treatment by dialysis.

POISONING WITH PESTICIDES

Aetiology

The increasing use of insecticides and weed-killers, both in the suburban garden and in the field, has lead to an increase in cases of acute poisoning by these substances.

Rodenticides. The commonly available rat-killer contains warfarin in concentrations which are not likely to affect human beings adversely. There are several extremely toxic substances available but they are used only by the professional pest control officer who is responsible for safe handling. They include thallium and fluoroacetate.

Insecticides. There are two main types of insecticides easily available to the general public: (1) halogenated hydrocarbons such as DDT and gammexane; and (2) organophosphorus compounds such as malathion.

Symptoms

Those of the first group are readily absorbed if ingested, inhaled, or if a solution is allowed in contact with the skin. They are cerebral stimulants and may cause headache, dizziness and disorientation. With active compounds such as dieldrin or after oral ingestion of gammexane by a child, convulsions, coma and death have been recorded. Treatment is purely symptomatic but these compounds are detoxified rapidly so that every effort should be made to maintain respiration and circulation for a day or two. The organophosphorus compounds are anticholinesterases and accordingly give rise to symptoms of overactivity of the cholinergic functions—bronchospasm and outpouring of mucus, or pulmonary oedema with anoxaemia; salivation, diarrhoea, vomiting, sweating, mydriasis (a deceptive symptom as it may merely imply droplets of spray in the conjunctival sac); tachycardia, hypotension, muscular twitching and spasms; dizziness, headache, convulsions and coma.

Diagnosis (Group 2)

Serum and red cell cholinesterase levels are markedly reduced in all cases of poisoning by anticholinesterase but initially diagnosis has to be made on the history and findings.

Treatment (Group 2)

Initial treatment is to wash contaminated skin with soap and water, which may suffice in a mild case. This may be supplemented, if symptoms increase, by repeated injection of atropine sulphate (say 1 mg. intravenously every 15 min.) until some evidence of the relief of the worst symptoms of parasympathetic overactivity is obtained. This treatment does not affect the neuromuscular or the central actions of the poison which are the source of danger to life. Adequate oxygenation is a primary necessity and should take precedence of drug therapy in all cases. Thereafter atropinization is kept up if necessary for many hours and coincidentally therapy with pralidoxime begun. The latter drug is a specific reactivator of cholinesterase. It may be given initially intravenously in a dose of 0·5 G. and repeated.

WEED-KILLERS

Aetiology

These have given rise to less trouble than have insecticides but poisoning can occur by absorption from the skin or by inhalation of dinitro-orthocresol (DNOC) or by inhalation or ingestion of paraquat. DNOC is a hazard to the man spraying crops who may spill a concentrate, be careless about personal hygiene, or suffer unexpected exposure to a spray.

Symptoms

DNOC is a powerful stimulant to catabolic activity and it causes an increase in oxygen consumption, rise in body temperature and loss of weight which may go unperceived until a crisis occurs which resembles acute thyrotoxicosis. Anxiety, restlessness, and insomnia may progress to convulsions. There is marked sweating, raised temperature and tachycardia.

Diagnosis

The skin in a person exposed to DNOC is stained yellow. The substance may be measured in blood and 5 mg. per 100 ml. is a toxic level.

Treatment

The skin should be washed thoroughly and the patient kept cool by external means. Chlorpromazine, 50 mg., or paraldehyde, 4 ml., may be injected intramuscularly as a sedative. Body temperature and fluid and electrolyte balance must be attended to. Cardiac arrhythmia may first be treated by injection of propranolol. If this fails procainamide may be tried.

PARAQUAT

This substance, a derivative of dipyridilium, is a universal weed-killer which acts by destroying chlorophyl. It is relatively harmless when applied to the skin, or if a little of the spray is inhaled, but ingestion of anything other than a trivial quantity may prove fatal. This is usually an accidental occurrence.

Symptoms

Some days after the initial gastro-intestinal upset the victim becomes progressively breathless and ill. The lesion is a progressive cellular proliferation of the lungs (alveolitis) which leads to dyspnoea, anoxaemia which may cause death or prolonged illness.

Treatment

Immediate emesis and gastric lavage may limit absorption. Forced diuresis and haemodialysis may remove it. Little is known of other therapy but hydrocortisone might well be tried.

POISONING BY ADDER BITE

Aetiology

The adder (*Viper berus*) is common in hilly or rocky districts of England, Wales and Scotland but is absent from urban areas and from Ireland. It is a thickset short snake with bold V-shaped marks on its back, shy in habit but armed with twin fangs and venom. Most bites are found on the hands or bare feet and ankles, usually in children and always take place during the summer months.

Symptoms

After the initial shock and pain of the bite, which leaves a twin puncture, there may be local swelling and discoloration, colic, pallor and vomiting. This may be all that happens in an adult or strong child, but if the viper was highly venomous or the child weak, there may ensue restlessness, collapse, spreading oedema, ecchymosis or gangrene. Death is unlikely.

Treatment

Application of a light tourniquet which should be released intermittently after one hour may limit absorption of venom, but cutting at the site to induce haemorrhage is merely mutilating. Symptomatic first-aid by 'mouth to mouth' breathing and by head-down posture may be applied to correct the initial collapse which is largely due to fear; alcohol should not be given. The affected part should be put at rest and breathing safeguarded during removal to hospital. Systemic injection of 100 mg. of hydrocortisone has been suggested and may be tried. Commercially-available polyvalent antivenom, derived from different species of viper, is of little value in England. It is notoriously an allergen and should, therefore, be omitted. It may, of course, be lifesaving in tropical countries. Antibiotics and tetanus antitoxin should be considered.

POISONING BY INSECT STING

Aetiology

Bees and wasps carry a hollow sting by which they can inject a mixture of active polypeptides and amines which causes pain, itch and vascular and tissue damage, which is usually confined to the affected area. On occasion the venom is absorbed into the blood stream and may cause anaphylactic shock which has proved fatal. On rare occasions the site of the sting is itself dangerous due to the effects of acute oedema, e.g. in the tongue or throat.

Symptoms

There may be a syncopal attack from pain and fear, an acute bronchoconstriction and hypotension from allergy, or asphyxial symptoms from choking.

Treatment

Bee stings should be wiped away with the edge of a blunt knife. Wasps do not leave their sting behind. If anaphylactic symptoms appear, injection of adrenaline, 0·25 ml., and an intramuscular or oral antihistamine, e.g. injection of promethazine hydrochloride, 10 mg., may be administered and the patient admitted to hospital for observation. Acute respiratory obstruction may call for speedy tracheal intubation or for tracheostomy.

REFERENCES

British Medical Association (1958) *Recognition of Intoxication*, London.

British Medical Association (1960) *Alcoholism and Road Safety*, London.

Clemmesen, C. (1959) The treatment of poisoning during the past 25 years: a retrospective review, *Dan. med. Bull.*, **6**, 209.

Dukes, D. C., Blainey, J. D., Cumming, G., and Widdowson, G. (1963) The treatment of severe aspirin poisoning, *Lancet*, i, 329.

Edson, E. F. (1960) Applied toxicology of pesticides, *Pharm. J.*, **185**, 361.

Graham, J. D. P., and Parker, W. A. (1948) The toxic manifestations of sodium salicylate therapy, *Quart. J. Med.*, **17**, 152.

Haldane, J. (1895) The action of carbonic oxide on man, *J. Physiol.(Lond.)*, **18**, 430.

Heasman, M. A. (1961) Accidental poisoning in children, *Arch. Dis. Childh.*, **36**, 390.

Matthew, H., ed. (1970) *Acute Barbiturate Poisoning*, Amsterdam.

Meyler, L. (1966) *Side Effects of Drugs*, Vol. V, London.

Norman, J. N., and Ledingham, I. McA. (1967) Carbon monoxide poisoning: investigations and treatment, in *Carbon Monoxide Poisoning*, Progress in Brain Research, Vol. 24, ed. Bour, H., and Ledingham, I. McA., Amsterdam.

J. D. P. Graham

EPIDEMIC DROPSY

Synonym. Argemone poisoning.

Definition

A condition characterized by oedema, vascular changes and cardiac insufficiency, resulting from the ingestion of the seeds of the Mexican poppy (*Argemone mexicana*) or their products.

Aetiology

Epidemic dropsy is most commonly seen in India, especially in Bengal, Bihar, Orissa, Madhya Pradesh and Uttar Pradesh. It has been recorded in Mauritius, Fiji and South Africa.

The toxic agent is an alkaloid sanguinarine which inhibits the end stages of carbohydrate metabolism. The effects thus resemble those of vitamin B_1 deficiency both clinically and physiologically. It is contained in the seeds of the Mexican poppy (*Argemone mexicana*) which sometimes grows as a weed amongst the mustard or wheat crops. The seed is very similar to the mustard seed, and may be mixed with the latter accidentally or deliberately as an adulterant in the manufacture of mustard oil, which is widely used for cooking in many parts of India.

The incidence of epidemic dropsy in India depends to some extent on the issue of the first season's oil; there is some evidence that the toxicity of the oil may be reduced during storage. It is highest during the rains or soon after, i.e. in July and August, and lowest in April.

Breast-fed infants and children under 4 years of age are not often affected, presumably because they do not have access to the oil. All other age groups may be affected. The racial distribution of the condition depends on dietetic habits. Wherever mustard oil is eaten and there is a possibility of contamination, epidemic dropsy may appear. The appearance of the syndrome is independent of the presence of rice in the diet. It appeared in South Africa in individuals after eating flour made from badly sieved wheat.

Pathology

The basic physiological changes and their consequences closely parallel those in acute wet beriberi. Early oedema is associated with increased capillary permeability; late oedema and the rapid serous effusion into the pericardium, lungs, pleural cavity and peritoneal cavity are associated with cardiac failure. There is a generalized acute vasodilatation, affecting the capillaries and small vessels, especially of the skin, heart muscle and uveal tract. Irregular formation of new blood vessels takes place, particularly in the subcutaneous tissues. In some cases haemangiomata (so-called 'sarcoids') develop and may become small pedunculated tumours which bleed readily. Haemorrhage may also occur from mucous membranes. There may be some secondary normocytic orthochromic anaemia.

Vascular dilatation in the iris and ciliary body commonly leads to raised intra-ocular pressure. Glaucoma and blindness from optic atrophy may result.

Vascular engorgement of the skin, liver and other organs is seen at necropsy. The heart muscle is often intensely congested and oedematous. Where cardiac insufficiency is evident the characteristic engorged and enlarged liver is present.

Symptoms and Signs

The clinical picture varies widely. Many cases are mild and except in 'epidemics' may be overlooked. Some outbreaks are notable for the severity, others for the mildness of the syndrome.

The onset is insidious in most cases. There is usually a history of a few days of loss of appetite, nausea and diarrhoea, followed by the appearance of oedema. The severe case may, however, begin suddenly and end fatally in a few days.

Oedema is present in all cases. Other signs vary in

intensity from one case to another and from one outbreak to another.

The oedema appears rapidly. It is soft and easily pitted and mostly confined to the legs. It becomes worse if the patient is allowed to walk about. Occasionally, there may be general anasarca, with effusion into the pleural and pericardial cavities. Terminal lung oedema may occur.

The patient is chiefly concerned with the severe dyspnoea which is constant and worsened by exertion. The blood pressure is low, especially the diastolic, and the pulse is fast and thready. In severe cases the heart is dilated, the apex beat displaced to the left and the base extended to the right. Apical systolic murmurs are common. The electrocardiogram may show evidence of myocardial damage, with sinus tachycardia and extrasystoles. Acute heart failure may develop with atrial fibrillation and enlarging tender liver. Fatal heart insufficiency may develop steadily or appear suddenly.

Peripheral vascular changes are present in most cases. Dilated vessels give the skin an irregular bluish mottled appearance, which may be present from the onset in severe cases, or develop after the oedema in moderate cases. Subcutaneous telangiectases or haemangiomata become visible in some patients. The latter may develop into small tumours or 'sarcoids' up to half an inch across and raised above the surrounding skin, or sometimes sessile. Sarcoids bleed freely if injured; they gradually reduce during convalescence. Hyperaesthesia, tingling of the skin and tenderness of the calf muscles are prominent signs in some cases. The knee-jerks may be absent. General effects vary. There may be mild fever. Nausea is the rule and there is often vomiting. Watery diarrhoea is common.

Glaucoma is one of the most serious complications. In some outbreaks up to 10 per cent. of those affected may exhibit raised intra-ocular tension, with or without local pain and associated with dimness of vision and contracted visual fields.

Diagnosis

Diagnosis is easy in a recognized outbreak but may be difficult in isolated cases. A knowledge of the patient's diet is essential.

Acute oedema appearing in several members of a family or of a community known to use mustard oil is highly suggestive. Wet beriberi, and famine oedema may cause confusion. Information about the diet, or lack of it, is important in differentiating epidemic dropsy from these conditions, which usually develop more slowly. In the former there may be prominent associated nervous signs and a vigorous response with diuresis to thiamine therapy. Both may occur concurrently with epidemic dropsy.

Treatment

Rest in bed is essential. Mustard oil or other possible sources of the toxic agent should be excluded from the diet.

In diarrhoeic cases an initial saline purge may be given. The cardiac insufficiency may or may not respond to digitalis. Thiazide or other diuretics may help.

Dietary deficiencies should be adjusted. Vitamins A, B, C and D may be required, and can be supplied most easily in the form of vegetable extracts, cod-liver oil and fruit juices. Epidemic dropsy, unlike beriberi, does not respond to vitamin B_1. The salt intake should be limited in the acute stages.

Bleeding from haemangiomata can be controlled by pressure. Glaucoma requires operative treatment. It does not usually respond to eserine. Convalescence is slow.

Course and Prognosis

In the average case the signs, especially those related to the cardiovascular system, subside upon rest in bed and are exacerbated on exertion. In some cases the cardiac signs are progressively severe and fail entirely to respond to treatment, the patient dying from cardiac failure in a few days.

The death-rate is usually about 5 per cent., but varies from outbreak to outbreak, reaching as high as 50 per cent.

Prognosis in the individual case should be guarded. It depends chiefly on the cardiac state. It is bad where there is decompensation. Serious cardiac failure may develop at any stage.

HEPATIC VENO-OCCLUSIVE DISEASE

Definition and Aetiology

A disease of children arising from occlusion of the sublobular and central hepatic veins by swelling and intimal proliferation, associated in its late stages with centrolobular cirrhosis and portal hypertension [see Section 6].

It occurs in the Caribbean area, Israel and India and is believed to be caused by ingestion of toxic alkaloids in various kinds of 'bush tea', probably brewed from *Senecio* (ragwort) or *Crotalaria.*

Signs and Symptoms

Children are affected between the ages of 1 and 5. They are usually of the poorest class and undernourished but are not commonly suffering from clinical evidence of protein-calorie malnutrition.

The disease has been described in three stages. The acute stage, which often follows an illness such as pneumonia, presents with loss of weight and rapid enlargement of the liver and development of ascites. In the second phase the enlargement of the liver remains but is asymptomatic. In the third or chronic stage liver cirrhosis is present, with increasing portal hypertension. The child is thin, with stick arms and legs and a protuberant belly. The liver is enlarged and there is ascites and oedema of the legs. Complications of the portal hypertension occur and the prognosis is grave.

Treatment

Treatment is symptomatic. Paracentesis may be necessary and diuretics improve the patient's comfort and reduce the frequency of tapping. Antibiotics are given to deal with intercurrent infections. Recovery is commonly rapid, but in some cases progressive hepatic fibrosis may develop.

VOMITING SICKNESS OF JAMAICA

Definition

A disease due to vegetable poisoning, probably by the unripe Ackee fruit, seen occasionally in Jamaica, predominantly in young children in poor economic circumstances, and characterized by coma and sometimes death. A somewhat similar syndrome has been described in America following ingestion of white snake root.

Aetiology and Signs and Symptoms

There is very good evidence that the syndrome is caused by a poison which temporarily blocks gluconeogenesis in undernourished individuals with low reserves. The most probable source of the toxin is the unripe fruit or the seeds of the Ackee plant (*Blighia sapida*), which contains polypeptides which have this physiological effect and produce in animals a profound fall of blood glucose and depletion of hepatic glycogen.

The clinical picture begins suddenly in apparently well children. There is nausea and severe and repeated vomiting, sweating, convulsions and rapidly deepening coma ending in death. Less seriously affected patients undergo a period of violent vomiting and then recover. Occasionally a child may pass directly into coma.

The most striking laboratory finding is a dramatic drop of glucose concentration in the peripheral blood, which may fall below 10 mg. per 100 ml. A corresponding depletion of glycogen has been shown by biopsy or at necropsy.

Treatment

Treatment consists in intravenous injection of 50 ml. of a 50 per cent. glucose solution. The child may become conscious during the injection, which can then be stopped. Glucose drinks are then given by mouth and the patient is watched for a further 24 hours. If recovery is not immediate, 10 per cent. glucose solution is continued by intravenous drip and followed by nasogastric feeding, as required.

LATHYRISM

Definition

An acute spastic paralysis, with sudden onset, associated with muscular pains and incontinence of urine.

Aetiology and Signs and Symptoms

The syndrome has been reported from many parts of the world including the Mediterranean littoral, Africa, Iran and India.

It appears in those who eat the lathyrus pea, usually late in the season after the crop has been stored. In times of drought and famine the incidence in the relevant areas is often higher because more people eat the pea in lieu of other crops which have failed to survive the calamity.

The clinical effects are possibly caused by a poison in the Akta weed which commonly contaminates the lathyrus crop.

Treatment

There is no specific treatment, but some relief is obtained in malnourished cases by the administration of vitamins, including vitamin A.

BRIAN MAEGRAITH

INDUSTRIAL TOXICOLOGY

GENERAL

Poison may enter the body in three ways. First, fat-soluble substances may be absorbed through the skin. Secondly, dusts and sprays may settle on the lips and be involuntarily swallowed. Thirdly, entry may be gained through the respiratory tract. Absorption of toxic dusts, sprays, vapours and gases through the lungs is the commonest mode of poisoning in industry.

NOTIFIABLE INDUSTRIAL DISEASES

Under the Factories Act, 1961 (and Regulations) any medical practitioner called in to attend a patient whom he believes may be suffering from one of the following diseases contracted in a factory is statutorily required to send notice (in any convenient form) to H.M. Chief Inspector of Factories, Ministry of Labour, London, S.W.1:

- Aniline poisoning
- Anthrax
- Arsenical poisoning
- Cadmium poisoning
- Carbon bisulphide poisoning
- Chrome ulceration
- Chronic benzene poisoning
- Compressed air illness
- Epitheliomatous ulceration due to tar, pitch, bitumen, mineral oil or paraffin
- Lead poisoning
- Manganese poisoning
- Mercurial poisoning
- Phosphorus poisoning
- Toxic anaemia
- Toxic jaundice
- Tricresyl phosphate poisoning
- Triphenyl phosphate poisoning

For arsenic, beryllium, cadmium, lead and mercury, manganese, poisoning is defined as acute, subacute or chronic disease of any organ due to the substance, compound or any alloy. Aniline poisoning is held to include poisoning by a nitro or amide derivative of benzene or chlorobenzene or a homologue of benzene or chlorobenzene. Benzene poisoning includes abnormality of the blood or present exposure to benzene. The requirement to notify poisoning by triphenyl phosphate or tricresyl phosphate is confined to the anticholinesterase action of these substances.

Certain diseases, known as the Prescribed Diseases, are assumed, for the purpose of payment of Industrial Injuries Benefit, in the absence of proof to the contrary, to arise from the conditions and circumstances of work. Though the prescribed diseases include notifiable disease, the requirement resting on medical practitioners to give notice of notifiable disease remains.

Historically, four stages in the medical supervision of workmen exposed to toxic hazards can be distinguished. First, the counting of symptomatic cases of poisoning, secondly, the counting of cases in which physical signs may be detected before symptoms, even if the interval between the occurrence of symptoms and signs is short, thirdly, the introduction of preclinical test to identify deviations from accepted physiological norms, and fourthly, the detection of abnormal substances and/or normal substances in body tissues, particularly in blood or urine, in amounts which exceed the body's power of excretion, storage detoxication and compensatory processes. To take lead as an example, the four stages are represented first by poisoning with symptoms noticeable to the workman, secondly by weakness of muscle groups (usually the wrist) detectable on medical examination, thirdly by a falling or low haemoglobin, and fourthly by estimation of the lead burden of whole blood for which the upper accepted limit is 80 μg. per 100 ml. Whilst rapid progress is being made in defining preclinical tests and vital criteria for many substances and their metabolic effects (e.g. mercury, organo-phosphorus compounds, benzene, arsenic, carbon monoxide), the supervision of workmen exposed to fibrogenic dusts is only just beginning to advance beyond the stage of diagnosis of overt disease or detection of preclinical signs.

MAXIMUM ALLOWABLE CONCENTRATIONS (M.A.C.)

For many poisons which are absorbed through the respiratory system, it is possible to fix with reasonable certainty a level of atmospheric pollution which if exceeded is likely to result in disease or abnormalities, defined at any of the above four stages. The body's response to toxic substances is to the total dose on a continuous scale with imperceptible intervals. The four historical stages described above are arbitrarily chosen on points on the scale. The maximum allowable concentration (M.A.C.) or threshold limit value (T.L.V.) are time-weighted means, applicable to an 8-hour day and 40-hour week, of atmospheric pollution which, however long-continued or however often repeated do not result in demonstrable injury. In fact, of course, a response by the body is occurring and M.A.C.s are not levels of nil effect. A list of M.A.C.s (Dust and Fumes in Factory Atmospheres, 1968) is published by the Department of Employment. During the course of a working day, considerable variations in the level of pollution above and below the M.A.C. occur, hence the importance of a time-weighted mean. In estimating atmospheric pollution, air samples should be taken (either by samplers in appropriate places in the factory or by samplers worn by the workman) in the breathing zone over a sufficiently long period to nullify variations in the level of pollution. In practice, this latter requirement makes representative sampling very difficult as the length of time over which an air sample is taken depends on the half-life of the pollutant (or its metabolites) in the body or target organ. For example, if benzene is the pollutant, sampling is required for 20–30 minutes, if lead, for 3–6 months, if a fibrogenic dust, for infinity (or a life time). In spite of these difficulties, estimation of airborne pollutants is a valuable way of ensuring the best engineering practice is adopted. Once this is done, further inquiries into the safety of the factory or plant can only be by application of refined medical techniques in the study of persons working in the plant. Life time follow-up of individuals, determination of age at and cause of death, is becoming increasingly important as long-term effects (e.g. cancer of the bladder) of industrial chemicals are being recognized.

For some substances having an acute effect (e.g. hydrogen cyanide, hydrogen sulphide) the M.A.C. may be very close to the level (ceiling level) which must not at any time be exceeded: for these substances the M.A.C. becomes a ceiling level.

PRINCIPLES OF PREVENTION

The substitution of a non-toxic substance for a toxic substance eliminates hazard. If this is not possible, total enclosure of processes involving the use of toxic substances should be attempted. Dusts may in some processes be suppressed by spraying with water. Usually, total enclosure is difficult and recourse must be had to local exhaust ventilation to draw dusts, sprays and gases away from the workman. This may be supplemented by blowing clean air at the workman. Low volume, high velocity exhaust draughts applied close to the point of origin of dusts, sprays and gases are more effective than low velocity exhaust ventilation. General ventilation which may be required for other reasons will not prevent toxic hazards. The use of respirators is not to be recommended for routine and planned use. Quite apart from doubt about their efficiency for long use, including liability to leak (up to 10 per cent. of inspired air) between the face and the face-piece, they are uncomfortable and the eye-pieces steam up. Workmen are unable to tolerate them for long periods. For special circumstances, positive pressure airline respirators may be necessary. The importance of clean working, and the wearing of clean working clothing, cannot be over-emphasized. Desirably, workmen employed on hazardous processes should bath and change their clothing before going home. Impervious gloves, aprons, goggles play a part in protection against acids and alkalis and against substances absorbed through the skin but may increase the chance of dermatitis developing. Respirators, if used, should be of a pattern approved by H.M. Chief Inspector of Factories; some approved respirators with low resistance to breathing, have filters which will trap 97 per cent. of dust particles down to 0·25 μ in size. Working for prolonged periods wearing respirators is too uncomfortable to be practicable. Great care must be taken to ensure that the proper and appropriate filter is used in respirators worn to protect against gases, vapours and sprays. Sufficient and appropriate respirators and, if necessary, self-contained oxygen breathing apparatus, together with life lines, must be kept for emergency rescue operations.

Factories, docks, railway premises, warehouses, etc., are subject to the Factories Act, 1961. Many industrial processes are the subject of statutory regulations aimed at controlling and preventing poisoning.

METALLIC POISONS

CHRONIC LEAD POISONING

Synonyms. Plumbism; Saturnism.

Aetiology

Apart from a few cases arising from contamination of food or water with lead and the deliberate use of lead compounds as abortifacients, poisoning is due to the absorption of lead or its compounds during the course of work. Organic compounds of lead are discussed on page 347.

1. Industrial poisoning. Lead and lead compounds are used very widely in industry. The compounds of lead commonly occurring in industry are litharge (PbO), red lead (Pb_3O_4), white lead or lead carbonate ($PbCO_3$), basic lead carbonate ($PbCO_3$:PbO:H_2O) and the oxides of lead PbO_2 and Pb_2O_3, and alloys of lead (e.g. solder). Most industrial cases of lead poisoning arise from absorption of lead through the respiratory system following work in an atmosphere contaminated with dust of lead compounds or with lead fumes produced when lead and lead compounds are heated to about 400° C. or higher (as in shipbreaking when steel plates covered with lead paint or backed with putty are cut with an oxyacetylene flame). Metallic lead is said to be not poisonous, possibly because it is poorly absorbed from the gut, but lead poisoning occurs in motor car discers who grind lead solder fillings of car bodies giving off fine particles of lead solder into the air. Employment in domestic forms of plumbing does not give rise to lead poisoning.

In Britain, certain industries are subject to regulations made under the Factories Act, 1961. These industries are: manufacture of accumulators, rubber industry, manufacture of lead compounds, lead smelting, heading of yarn, vitreous enamelling of glass or metal, tinning of hollow ware, certain processes in the manufacture of pottery (including frit and glaze mixing, colour grinding and blowing, lithographic transfer), painting of vehicles and the use of lead paint. With the exception of the two last mentioned occupations, the 15,000 workers in the scheduled processes are subject to statutory regulations including periodic medical examination. About a further 15,000 persons are employed in lead processes not subject to regulations. Shipbreaking (especially of warships where lead putty is used as well as lead paint), motor ear discing (i.e. polishing the surface of body panels and wings made good by filling with lead solder) are major sources of lead poisoning not subject to special regulations (though the factory occupier is subject to the general provision of the Factories Act applying to all factories, to prevent the emission of a noxious fume or dust into the respirable atmosphere).

Lead poisoning is a reportable industrial disease. In 1970, 70 cases of lead poisoning were notified; about half were in scheduled processes. Evidence exists which suggests that industrial lead poisoning is much commoner than these figures suggest, possibly by as much as five times.

2. Contamination of food and water. Beer and cider drawn through lead pipes, the solution of lead by vinegar, lemon juice, cider, home-made wine from lead glaze on old-fashioned earthenware pots, water (especially if soft or acid) allowed to stand in contact with lead pipes or cisterns have all been reported as causing lead poisoning. Owing to the Public Health Act, 1936, and regulations, the chances of lead poisoning from a public supply of water or from commercially prepared food or drink are remote. Even so, small quantities of lead are present in many waters and also in sophisticated diets. The maximum limit for lead in drinking water is 0·1 parts per million and in beverages 0·2 parts per million. In the past, some cosmetics, especially face powder, contained lead carbonate and still do in the Far East where cosmetics are a common cause of lead poisoning. In the late 1920's, an outbreak of lead poisoning occurred in Australia among children who after a period of drought, ingested flakes of white lead paint by licking raindrops off railings. Subsequent deaths from chronic nephritis were reported. Lead paint should never be used indoors; in particular, lead paint is dangerous to children if used on toys, cots, bedrails, etc., as these may be bitten or licked by children. For paint to be used on children's furniture or toys, the Home Office has fixed an upper limit of 0·5 parts per million (0·5 μg. per g.).

3. Traditionally lead in the form of lead oleate was used to procure abortion, but cannot now be widely used, as lead oleate is in Part I of the Poisons Schedule. Historically, women lead workers were said to abort. Cases of poisoning have been reported following very prolonged use of lead lotions as dressings for ulcers.

Pathology

Lead is deposited in bone in a similar manner to calcium. Conditions which favour the deposition of calcium favour the deposition of lead. During acidosis, lead is removed from the bone and excreted in the faeces and urine. Normal faeces may contain up to 0·28 mg. of lead per 24-hour sample and normal urine up to 0.027 mg. per litre. Lead is transported by being absorbed (in the form of fine particles which can be seen on electron microscopy) on the envelope of red cells. Only about 3 per cent. of lead in the blood is in solution in the serum in the form of lead phosphate or lead lactate. The combustion of petrol to which organic lead compounds are added pollutes the air with lead oxide, some of which is absorbed through the respiratory tract and some deposited on vegetation. Whilst no harmful effects have been demonstrated from this pollution, the blood of an adult not occupationally exposed to lead, may contain up to 0.04 mg. of lead per 100 ml.

The symptoms and biochemical changes in lead poisoning are similar to those of porphyria. Strong evidence exists to suggest that lead affects the co-enzyme A cycle interfering with the metabolism of glycine (which presumably takes place in the liver). In particular, the acetyl CoA pathway is blocked causing deviation to the succinic acid pathway. An excess production of δ-aminolaevulic acid and porphobilinogen results with consequent increased excretion of δ-aminolaevulic acid, porphobilinogen and coproporphyrin III in the urine. The symptoms and signs of lead poisoning and porphyria show a remarkable degree of similarity both in type and incidence. In porphyria, an unknown factor (Goldberg's factor X) is postulated to explain neuropathy; if a similar factor operates in lead poisoning (and there is no evidence that it does), gastro-intestinal symptoms, paresis and paralysis, demyelination of peripheral nerves, encephalopathy, psychoses, common to both lead poisoning and porphyria can be explained in this way. The percentage incidence of symptoms in both conditions is almost identical. In addition, lead interferes with the formation of haemoglobin, almost certainly in the bone marrow, after the stage of protoporphyrin. The combination of iron with haem is inhibited. Occasionally a sideroblastic anaemia may be present and in children a fast moving haemoglobin similar to HbA_2. An action on the maturation of the red cell series cannot be excluded. The life of the red cell is shortened (in severe cases to about 40 days) and this, combined with interference with the synthesis of haemoglobin, results in anaemia. Degraded ribonucleic acid is deposited around the mitochondria of the red cell stem cells in the bone marrow. Basophilic punctuate (stippled) cells appear in the blood, and though not pathognomonic of lead absorption, are present in larger numbers than with other poisons. Nucleated red cell precursors in the bone marrow are stippled. The precise composition of the basophilic substance is not known with certainty but it is probably degraded ribonucleic acid. The kidney tubules show eosinophilic intracellular inclusions.

Symptoms

The earlier symptoms of lead poisoning are vague and only elicited in reply to questions. The commonest are indigestion, vague abdominal discomfort and aches and pains in the limbs often described as 'rheumatism' or 'fibrositis'. Lassitude, fatigue and headaches are frequent. Though constipation is a classical symptom of lead poisoning, nowadays it appears to be infrequent. About half the cases complain of diarrhoea. Each of these symptoms may occur alone or in any combination.

Abdominal colic. Abdominal colic is now an infrequent complaint. When it occurs, it is usually of sudden onset, centralized around the umbilicus and of a tearing nature. Vomiting may occur. Occasionally constipation, which may precede the onset of colic by about one week, may be sufficiently severe to cause stercoral ulcer of the rectum. Lead colic may be mistaken for an acute surgical emergency and instances of laparotomy and other surgical interventions are constantly recurring. The small gut is in spasm and colic is due to spasm of the gut above rings of tonically contracted intestine. The lesser degrees of colic are not infrequently treated as 'indigestion' or duodenal ulceration, a diagnosis which is supported by radiographic reports of a spastic duodenum.

Muscular paralysis. Muscular paralysis and paresis are classical signs of lead poisoning but in Britain, because of improved industrial conditions, they are rarely seen nowadays. The signs are of a lower motor neurone lesion but whether the damage is to the nerve fibres or myoneural junction, or how the damage is produced, has not been unequivocably established. Recent experimental work suggests that nerve conduction is delayed. Muscular wasting may be present, but fasciculation and sensory changes are absent. Some cases may mimic progressive muscular atrophy (due to the toxic action of lead on the anterior horn cells) and in these fasciculation is usually present. Signs of degeneration of the pyramidal tracts may be present very occasionally. Paresis and paralysis affect the muscle group most used; in industrial workers these are the extensor muscles of the wrist and fingers. Loss of synergic extension of the wrist causes weakness in the flexor muscles. The brachioradialis and the abductor pollicis longus usually escape, the former more often than the latter. In men using the upper arms, the adductor and external muscles of the shoulder (spinati, deltoid, biceps, brachialis and brachioradialis) are affected. In the lower limbs, the muscles supplied by the common peroneal nerve are most often affected though the tibialis anterior commonly escapes. In considering what muscles are most used, recreations (e.g. bicycling) must be taken into account. Abductor paralysis of the larynx reported at the beginning of the century no longer occurs, but occasionally facial palsy may be seen.

Cerebral effects. Though occurring but rarely, epileptiform fits, followed by unconsciousness due to encephalopathy, may be the first signs of lead poisoning. Many such cases may be mistaken for space-occupying lesions of the brain. Primary optic atrophy occurs occasionally. Headache, insomnia, irritability, apprehension, pathological fear, and confusion are frequent: occasionally acute toxic dementia and delirium may occur. Some of these changes may persist. Permanent damage to the cerebrum may ensue especially in children in whom lead intoxication is a cause of mental retardation which may be more frequent than hitherto thought.

Tremor may be due to weakness of the muscles or it may be an early sign of encephalopathy.

Physical Signs

Patients with lead poisoning usually have a pallid appearance, but this pallor is not due to overt anaemia. The pallor has a yellow tinge and not infrequently the question arises whether the patient is jaundiced. A malar flush may be present, but this is more apparent than real because of the contrast with the pallid skin.

In the presence of lead colic, the abdomen is soft

and scaphoid. The distinction between lead colic and abdominal catastrophies may be very difficult. A blue line (Burtonian line) around the gingival margins is due to the deposition at the end of the capillary loops of lead sulphides formed by lead absorbed into the circulation and sulphur compounds present in the mouth where dental hygiene is poor. In the presence of other symptoms, a blue line is highly suggestive, but it may occur in the absence of symptoms. It is indicative of lead absorption rather than lead poisoning. A blue line may also occur around the anus.

Blood changes. The earliest changes in the blood are anisocytosis and poikilocytosis shortly followed by a fall in haemoglobin (which may, however, remain within accepted range of normality). The red cells are normocytic or slightly microcytic, but occasionally the blood picture may be mistaken for pernicious anaemia. Punctate basophilia is usually, but not always, found. The relation between the level of punctate basophilia and the degree of symptoms shows much variation. A level of 5000 punctate cells per million red cells (counting coarse punctate cells using dark ground illumination) is suggestive of poisoning or incipient poisoning. Fine punctate cells are of little significance. A mild reticulocytosis is common and the reticulocyte count may rise to a high level simulating the reticulocyte crisis of pernicious anaemia, when lead absorption is stopped and the patient treated with chelating agents. A mild secondary sideroblastic anaemia may occur very occasionally. A few normoblasts may appear in the peripheral blood.

The changes in the bone marrow are not specific but stippled erythroblasts may be found. Changes in the red cells precede a fall in haemoglobin by an interval depending on the balance between lead absorption and excretion and storage. Quite suddenly haemoglobin falls but the fall seldom proceeds below about 11·0–11·5 g. per 100 ml. blood. This is an important differentiation from other anaemias. At this level, symptoms begin to appear.

Renal changes. The passage of large quantities of lead through the kidney, as may occur when a patient is treated without removal from exposure to lead, may give rise to gross albuminuria apparently associated with a nephrosis. The excretion of δ-aminolaevulic acid is increased and coproporphyrin III is excreted in large amounts. Like punctate basophilia the presence of large quantities of coproporphyrin III in the urine is not pathognomonic. Symptoms may occur in the presence of comparatively small quantities of coproporphyrin III and be absent when large quantities are present in the urine. Normal urine may contain up to 100 μg. of coproporphyrin III per litre. The presence of 1500–2000 μg. of coproporphyrin III per litre of urine (calculated to a specific gravity of 1·016) in men and 500–1000 μg. per litre of urine in women is very suggestive of excessive lead absorption. Authors writing at the beginning of the century were convinced that lead caused interstitial nephritis. Today, lead nephropathy is rare but there is little doubt that it does occur from time to time. Glucose and amino acids may appear in the urine especially in children. Albuminuria may occur occasionally (usually being preceded by excretion of amino acids) even before chelating agents are given.

Cardiovascular system. Lead has the historical reputation of causing arteriosclerosis. One recent study of lead workers (and retired lead workers) showed that they suffer an increased mortality due to all causes and relatively large numbers of deaths are due to cerebral haemorrhage, cerebral thrombosis and cerebral arteriosclerosis.

Gout. The association between lead poisoning and gout seems to be fortuitous.

Differential Diagnosis

The diagnosis is not difficult providing the possibility of lead poisoning is kept constantly in mind. In workmen, a precise occupational history, listing the substances handled by the workman or to which he may be exposed, should raise suspicions. Workmen often give general descriptions for their work such as vehicle builder or chemical process worker, and it may be found on inquiry that they are engaged in discing of motor car bodies or grinding lead chromate. A low haemoglobin or raised punctate basophilia should raise suspicions, but neither is specific to lead. Occasionally, confusion may arise with pernicious anaemia, but in the latter disease the coproporphyrin excretion is raised only slightly; other causes of anaemia, such as piles or a bleeding peptic ulcer, need exclusion. Lead poisoning should be considered in the diagnosis of fits, especially if followed by unconsciousness. Unexplained abdominal symptoms, both acute and chronic, may be due to lead poisoning. Unnecessary surgery has been carried out but on the other hand it is essential to remember that acute appendicitis, perforated peptic ulcer, intestinal obstruction, gall-stone colic, renal colic, may, and do, occur in cases of persons occupationally exposed. Sometimes more than one person has been affected by a common cause but isolated cases may occur. Occasionally, hysterical paralysis may occur in a lead worker, but it is usually spastic and may be associated with stocking and glove anaesthesia, or hemi-anaesthesia or hysterical aphonia.

Treatment

The first and most important step in treatment is to prevent further absorption of lead, which in industrial cases means suspending the patient from work.

The older methods of therapy, potassium iodide, sodium citrate, the induction of acidosis by the administration of ammonium chloride, have been superseded by chelating agents. Of the versenate type of compounds, sodium calciumedetate (*Calcium Disodium Versenate*) is usually chosen because its calcium content prevents removal of calcium from the bone. In severe cases, *Calcium Disodium Versenate*, 3 G. in 600 ml. of 5 per cent. glucose in distilled water, is best administered by intravenous infusion over a period of two hours. From 4 to 8 such infusions may be given in 24 hours, but excessive dosage should be avoided because versenate compounds may give rise to a renal tubular failure and necrosis. The urinary output of lead should be observed and may rise as high as 13 mg. per 24 hours. More recently penicillamine has become available as an agent which binds metals. D-penicillamine given orally in doses of 600–1500 mg. per day causes a marked rise in the urinary excretion of lead and a fall in the excretion of δ-aminolaevulic acid and coproporphyrin. The use of calcium versenate and D-penicillamine in an attempt to increase the lead excretion of workmen or other persons still exposed to lead is dangerous, as renal damage may result.

Cortisone should not be given as severe symptoms may be precipitated. A high calcium diet is beneficial.

The administration of calcium by mouth usually relieves colic in about 2 days, or if preferred 15 ml. of a 20 per cent. solution of calcium gluconate or 10 ml. of a 10 per cent. solution of calcium chloride may be given cautiously by slow intravenous injection. Intravenous administration should be reserved for severe cases as the patient feels hot and may vomit after the injection. The action of calcium is to relax the spastic contraction of the gut above a tonic ring. Atropine sulphate, 1 mg. may be given subcutaneously.

Lead encephalopathy should be treated by lumbar puncture. When fits are relieved, chelating agents should be administered. Palsy and paresis should be treated by support applied according to the usual surgical principles and by physiotherapy.

Prognosis

Chronic lead poisoning is not a direct cause of death except when encephalopathy is present.

Prevention

Lead poisoning has been eliminated from the pottery industry (with the exception of lithographic transfers) by the substitution for lead of a low solubility or leadless glaze.

If a non-toxic substance cannot be substituted for lead or lead compounds (e.g. plastic instead of lead paints for outdoor use), the prevention of industrial lead poisoning depends on environmental control associated with strict personal hygiene of exposed workers. Processes should be enclosed to prevent the escape of dust and fumes. A good example of this is the modern method of manufacturing lead carbonate (white lead), in which lead acetate is treated with carbon dioxide to form lead carbonate which drops directly into linseed oil (in which it is preferentially absorbed). If enclosure is not practicable, local exhaust ventilation should be installed to exhaust dust and fumes. The dry rubbing down of lead paint and the spraying of lead paint is prohibited. Where lead compounds are liable to be spilled on the floor, the floor should be impervious and kept wet. The wearing of respirators should not be relied on in routine preventive measures.

Personal cleanliness is important. Careful and thorough scrubbing of the hands and nails with ample soap and running water before eating or drinking is essential. Protective clothing should be provided for work, and preferably, workmen should have a separate set of clothing and bathe completely (using shower baths) before dressing to go home. No food should be eaten in workplaces and smoking should be prohibited. This means that a high standard of washing, sanitary and cloakroom accommodation is required. Nail biters should not be employed on lead processes.

The amount of dust and fumes present in the atmosphere should be monitored periodically especially in places where pollution is especially likely to occur. The maximum allowable concentration of lead in the air is 0·2 mg. per m³. for an 8-hour day, 40 hours a week.

Hours of work should be strictly limited; many persons affected by lead are found to be working long hours and hence increasing their absorption. Young persons and women are prohibited from working in some lead trades. Pregnant women should not be employed but this may be a counsel of perfection, as the women may not know they are pregnant when abortion is most likely to occur. Drinking milk has no preventive effect.

In the past, a distinction has been made between lead absorption and lead poisoning. This distinction is becoming less clear. Whilst it is true that lead, in small quantities, may be absorbed without causing symptoms or signs, it is now appreciated that lead absorption and lead poisoning must be thought of as two ends of a spectrum.

In between, there is a wide area in which the metabolism of the body is altered—and if this alteration is allowed to proceed, deviations from physiological norms will precede the occurrence of symptoms and signs of lead poisoning. Whilst the boundaries between 'normality', acceptable lead absorption, asymptomatic poisoning and symptomatic poisoning are arbitrary, it is inexcusable to allow a workman to proceed to asymptomatic poisoning or to symptomatic poisoning. The following standards are accepted by most authorities.

	NOT OCCUPATIONALLY EXPOSED ADULT	ACCEPTABLE LEAD ABSORPTION	ASYMPTOMATIC POISONING: EXCESSIVE LEAD ABSORPTION	POISONING
Blood lead μg. per 100 ml. whole blood	up to 40	40–75	75–100	above 110
Urinary coproporphyrin μg. per L.	less than 80	80–400	400–1500	above 1500
Urinary aminolaevulic acid mg. per L.	0·6	0·6–2	2–4	above 4
Haemoglobin g. per 100 ml. blood	men 14·6	men 14·6	men 14·6–13·6	men less than 13·6
	women 13·6	women 13·6	women 13·6–12·6	women less than 12·6

The above indices frequently do not run parallel: the significance of a single abnormal index must be assessed clinically. However, the continued presence of an abnormality suggests that investigation is needed.

Near catastrophies have resulted from estimating lead in serum. Lead should be estimated on whole blood (collected in sesquestrinated tubes) the result adjusted for P.V.C. (or if this is not available, for haemoglobin). Blood lead is a good index of hazard to the workman; 80 μg. per 100 ml. whole blood correspond to an air pollution of 0·2 mg. lead per m^3. However, repeated venepuncture required for the estimation of blood lead is not acceptable in Britain; the best way of supervising workmen is to undertake serial (usually monthly) estimations of coproporphyrin and to calculate individual and group moving averages. Semi-quantitative estimation of coproporphyrin based on the Donath method is adequate for this purpose. Persons in whom coproporphyrin excretion is raised should be submitted to investigation (including estimation of blood lead). This view may be modified when the application of micro-methods for the estimation of blood lead which allow lead to be estimated in 0.01 ml. blood obtained by skin puncture are perfected. The estimation of the excretion of lead in the urine is an unreliable index quite apart from the risk of contamination. Estimation of urinary lead is mostly used as an aid to retrospective diagnosis as it rises steeply after chelating with E.D.T.A. in a person with a lead body burden. The urine of non-occupationally exposed persons may contain up to 80 μg. lead per litre urine and a lead worker may excrete up to 200 μg. per litre urine without apparent harm. The administration of chelating agents as a prophylactic for lead workers has been suggested but is to be strongly deprecated because the consequent passage of large quantities of lead through the kidneys and may induce nephrosis. A falling haemoglobin must be regarded as ominous. A haemoglobin of 13 g. per 100 ml. of blood in men (or 12 g. in women) or below is a sign that investigation is required to determine the cause of the anaemia, and in particular whether this is due to lead. A haemoglobin of 12 g. per 100 ml. of blood or below in men (11 g. in women) is a strong indication for the suspension from lead processes, at least until the cause of anaemia is determined. The use of appropriate copper sulphate solutions (Van Slyke's method) to determine specific gravity of blood is a convenient screening method of estimating the haemoglobin, applicable in industrial conditions to large numbers of workers.

Provision exists under the Factories Act for examinations of persons employed in scheduled occupations (see above, but there are many other industries where the risk of lead poisoning is present) to be examined periodically at intervals varying from 7 days to 3 months, but usually 1 month, by the Appointed Factory Doctor (a medical practitioner appointed by H.M. Chief Inspector of Factories for this purpose) who has statutory powers of suspension. Normally, suspension is required for about 3 months and if alternative work cannot be arranged, the workmen necessarily incurs financial loss. Such considerations must not influence the decision whether a workman is fit or not fit to continue work.

Sufficient emphasis cannot be given to the fact that valuable as haemoglobin estimations, coproporphyrin III excretion and punctate counts are, they remain screening methods, indicating to the physician where special attention is needed, both in the care of individual workers and in the investigation of the failure of environmental control.

LEAD TETRAETHYL, LEAD TETRAMETHYL

Aetiology and Pathology

Lead tetraethyl and lead tetramethyl, often referred to as organic lead compounds, are used as anti-knock agents in petrol, in the proportions varying between 0·08 and 0·12 per cent. Both may be absorbed through the lungs (but the methyl compound has a lower vapour pressure than the ethyl). Lead tetraethyl is fat-soluble and rapidly absorbed through the skin; lead tetramethyl is only slowly absorbed. For these reasons lead tetramethyl is safer. In addition, the conversion of lead tetramethyl to lead trimethyl in the liver seems to proceed more slowly than the corresponding conversion of lead tetraethyl to triethyl lead so that excretion, mainly in the urine, can keep pace. The conversion to the tri-compound is thought to be necessary before toxic effects are caused.

Symptoms

Lead tetraethyl has a specific and selective action on nervous tissues. Psychic and neurological lesions of any severity may be produced, but the mental changes usually predominate.

Mental disturbances include sleeplessness, headache, bad dreams, mental excitement, hallucinations and delusions. Early symptoms may be mistaken for an anxiety state. Later, anxiety may be extreme. Sleep is difficult and broken. Restlessness may assume violent proportions. Mania, confusion and dementia may follow and schizophrenia may be simulated. Paranoid ideas may occur. Severe exposure may be followed by convulsions. Suicidal tendencies may be present.

Signs

The blood pressure, particularly the diastolic pressure, falls and this sign may develop before the onset of symptoms. Other early signs are weakness and tremor, and muscular pain may be present. The tremor of lips, tongue and the limbs is usually coarse and jerky and made worse by attempts at control. Blurred vision and diplopia due to weakness of the extrinsic muscles of the eye may be present and vertigo is not infrequent.

Blood lead levels are raised and the total excretion of lead is increased though the faecal/urinary proportion is normal. Urinary coproporphyrin excretion may be slightly, though not invariably, increased. The classical signs of inorganic lead poisoning are absent though occasionally the punctate red cell count is increased.

Lead tetramethyl, for the reasons given above, is likely to produce less severe symptoms and signs than lead tetraethyl.

Treatment

Contaminated skin should be thoroughly washed with kerosene and, if splashed, the eyes irrigated with copious quantities of a bland lotion. All contaminated clothing should be removed and disposed of with care.

Calcium Disodium Versenate and penicillamine increase the excretion of lead and should be given [see p. 345] and it is desirable to give two or three repeated 7 day courses (interrupted by suitable intervals) after acute symptoms have subsided. Psychological disturbances should be treated symptomatically with barbiturates, but morphine should not be given. In suitable cases, with acute psychotic symptoms, electroconvulsive therapy may be beneficial, simplifying the management and treatment of severely disturbed cases.

Prevention

Strict environmental control, including the provision of positive pressure airline respirators, thorough and complete washing with an entire change of clothes after work, the provision of protective clothing, gloves and goggles is essential. Exposed workers should have their urinary excretion of lead estimated periodically and if this rises above 120 μg. per litre they are at hazard. Cleaning sludge from tanks which have contained petrol is dangerous. Besides the danger of absorption through the skin, atmospheric concentrations up to 60 mg. per m^3. of air inside the tank may be found. In cases of difficulty H.M. District Inspector of Factories should be consulted before the tank is entered. The maximum allowable concentration cannot be fixed with certainty but it is *below* 0·15 mg. per m^3. of air.

Carburettors should not be tested (especially in confined spaces) with petrol containing lead, nor should such petrol be burnt in blowlamps.

CHRONIC MERCURY POISONING

Synonyms. Hatter's shakes; Danbury shakes.

Aetiology

Any person who is exposed to mercury and its salts for more than a short period may suffer from mercury poisoning. Some organic mercury compounds (e.g. methyl mercury iodide) are so toxic that poisoning may occur after minimal exposure.

Mercury is mined in the form of sulphide in Spain, Yugoslavia, Italy, China, Mexico, California and Russia and the ore is subject to refining. Such workers are at considerable risk. In this country, thermometer makers, scientific instrument makers, laboratory workers, hatters (who paint or 'carrott' mercury nitrate on to felt), surgical dressing makers, direct current electric meter repairers, makers of electrical apparatus, pharmaceutical workers, finger-print experts, paint makers and photo-engravers are potential victims. The 'silvering' of mirrors and the manufacture of chlorine (by the electrolysis of brine) may cause mercury poisoning. Sailors in submarines may be affected. Inunction of mercury ointment or the continued taking of blue pill and calomel may cause poisoning. In children, the continued administration of teething powders has been blamed as one cause of pink disease.

Organic mercury salts (phenyl mercury acetate, ethyl mercury phosphate, methyl mercury guanidine) are used as fungicides and the makers of these substances and seed dressers may suffer from poisoning. Methyl mercury iodide is so toxic that it should not be made.

Pathology

The vapour pressure of mercury is high, much higher than would be expected for a metal. Comparatively small quantities of mercury (such as may be found in mercury gas seals in scientific apparatus) may cause poisoning. The major portion of entry of vapour is through the respiratory system, but mercury is also absorbed through the skin and gut. The normal average daily intake in food is up to 0·005 mg. but substantial quantities can be leached from amalgam stoppings (especially if new) in teeth. Mercury is excreted in faeces and urine, a fact which may explain the non-correlation between urinary excretion and atmospheric concentration of vapour to which workers are exposed. Mercury has a selective action in the nervous system and kidneys but may be found in all organs. Inorganic salts are concentrated mainly in kidney and organic salts mainly in the nervous system.

INORGANIC MERCURY POISONING (INCLUDING ELEMENTAL MERCURY)

Symptoms

Erethism. Erethism is a peculiar psychological disorder in which timidity, anxiety, lack of decision, failure of concentration, depression, over-reaction to criticism are prominent. Erethism is important as it is an early sign, but one which is often ascribed to 'nervous debility', a diagnosis which appears to be substantiated if recovery (as it nearly always does) follows a holiday. If exposure is not stopped, headache, fatigue, drowsiness or insomnia are frequent and in severe cases hallucinations and dementia may supervene.

Vasomotor disturbances. Blushing, excessive sweating, nearly always accompany erethism. Dermatographia may be present.

Physical Signs

Tremor. Early in the disease, tremor develops. The synonyms hatter's shakes and Danbury shakes arose from the painting or carrotting of mercury nitrate on to felt for hats. Hatters used to live in Danbury, a suburb of New York. The process is no longer employed. It starts as a fine tremor but later may be coarse and convulsive. Tremor of the corners of the mouth often appear before other tremors. Tremor affects the hands, arms, feet, legs and may also affect the tongue and face. It is best demonstrated by serial specimens of handwriting or the square drawing test.

Speech. Scanning speech, with slurring and hesitancy (in addition to that which may result from erethism) is not uncommon.

Motor and sensory disturbances. Ataxia, spasticity, loss of postural sense, loss of sensation to pinprick and light touch may be present in severe poisoning.

These lesions, which may be of any severity and distribution, are due to the diffuse effect of mercury on the nervous system. Cases of mercury poisoning have been mistaken for disseminated sclerosis.

Mercuria lentis. Nearly all workers who have been exposed to elemental mercury for a year or more show a brownish golden staining of the anterior capsule of the lens visible with a slit lamp. Though a sign of absorption of mercury, its occurrence is not related to the onset of poisoning. Opinions differ whether it is due to local rather than general absorption of mercury, probably either may cause it.

Kidney. The effects of mercury on the kidney are not fully understood. Many workers exposed to mercury excrete glucose and amino acids for short periods. Transient albuminuria is not uncommon and occasionally this may become persistent. Occasionally albuminuria may be massive and deaths from nephrosis (tubular damage) have been reported. The daily normal excretion of mercury in the urine is 5–10 μg. Though mercury excretion does not appear to bear any relation to the onset of symptoms of poisoning, workers excreting more than 450 μg. a day (or 300 μg. per litre, specific gravity 1·016) should be considered at hazard (and removed from exposure), though it must be admitted, excretion levels 2 or 3 times greater may occur without discernible harm. An unexplained observation is that the onset of nephrosis is often preceded by a fall in urinary excretion of mercury from previously high levels.

Mouth, gums, teeth. Excessive salivation, loosening of teeth, are signs of advanced poisoning and are unlikely to be seen in industrial practice. As recently as 1950, however, it was noticed that many workers 'carrotting' felt had lost molar teeth in their upper and lower jaws. Teeth may be black and a blue line, similar to that in lead absorption, may be present at the gum margins.

Blood. A mild hypochromic anaemia may be present.

Skin. Mercury fulminate is especially liable to cause dermatitis and small indolent ulcers, known as powder holes. Mercury sulphide may have similar effects.

Treatment

Exposure to mercury or its salts should be stopped and the fluid intake increased. Dispute exists as to the value of dimercaprol (BAL) and chelating agents; some authors do not consider that the excretion of mercury in the urine is increased and others believe that they may increase the albuminuria.

Prevention

Mercury poisoning is undoubtedly much more common than previously thought. Usually exposure to the salts of mercury can be controlled by substitution, total enclosure or exhaust ventilation. In the circumstances in which it is used the control of elemental mercury may be difficult. The amount used should be kept to the minimum and, wherever possible, all mercury should be in closed vessels. All spilled mercury should be recovered immediately but in some operations where spillage is to be expected, arrangements should be made for this to be into water. Benches and floors should be impervious. A common and dangerous fault is the collection of mercury in the cracks of floors. Benches should be decontaminated by washing with a slurry of equal parts of sublimed sulphur and slaked lime.

Medical examination of workers exposed to mercury to detect erethism, changes in writing, alterations in the square drawing test or albuminuria is of little value. Such signs are too late to be of assistance in prevention. Recently developed semi-automated techniques for estimation of mercury in urine allow large numbers of such estimations to be performed whereas previously the labour involved was prohibitive. Estimation of mercury in urine should be compulsory for all workers exposed to mercury for more than a few days. Besides being of value in assessing hazards to individual workers (see above), moving group averages are a good index of environmental control. Probably because of absorption through other routes, the urinary excretion of mercury can only seldom be correlated with the maximum allowable concentration in the air (which is 0·1 mg. per m^3.).

ORGANIC MERCURY POISONING

All the symptoms and signs ascribed to inorganic mercury poisoning may, and do occur, in poisoning by organic mercury compounds. The distinction made between the two forms of poisoning is unreal except that many organic mercury compounds have a highly selective action on the nervous system causing degeneration of the cerebral hemispheres, cerebellum and spinal roots, posterior columns and peripheral nerves. Psychological disturbances varying from mild erethism to gross disturbance of memory and intelligence occur. Hallucinations are common. Methyl mercury iodide causes optic atrophy (with concentric constriction of vision) and focal degeneration of the cerebrum, especially of the occipital cortex. Aryl compounds (i.e. compounds in which the hydrocarbon radical contains a benzene ring, e.g. phenyl mercury acetate) appear to be less toxic than alkyl compounds. Even so, erethism is common among workers exposed to them. In the manufacture of organic mercury compounds the strictest precautions are necessary. Seed dressing is undertaken seasonally and there seems little doubt that the intermittent exposure resulting therefrom saves seed dressers and agricultural workers from severe poisoning. Even so, mild symptoms are common. The daily urinary excretion of more than 30 μg. of mercury should be regarded as a warning sign. The maximum allowable atmospheric concentration for organic mercury is 0·01 mg. of mercury per m^3.

ARSENICAL POISONING

Aetiology

Arsenic forms three oxides, trioxide As_2O_3 (commonly used in industry), pentoxide As_2O_5 (used in insecticides) and tetraoxide As_2O_4. Metallic arsenic is reputed, probably inaccurately, not to be poisonous. Arsenic salts are used in insecticides, weed killers (now prohibited in Britain and many other countries), fungicides, and in the manufacture of glass, enamels and pharmaceutical preparations. Arsenic may be added to alloys to increase hardening and heat resistance. Arsenic compounds are usually absorbed by inhalation of dust but some dust may settle on the lips and be swallowed. Arsine (AsH_3, arseniuretted hydrogen) is a gas which may be evolved accidentally if nascent hydrogen is liberated in the proximity of arsenic salts.

Pathology

Arsenic combines with the —SH radicle and in this way inhibits many enzyme systems including the pyruvate oxidase system (which accounts for the similarity between the polyneuritis of vitamin B_1 deficiency and arsenic poisoning). Normal viscera may contain up to 5 parts per million of arsenic. Arsenic is stored in all the viscera and tissues but selectively in the nails, hair and skin. The elimination of arsenic, through the faeces, urine and secretions (including milk) takes place over a very long period. Arsenic acts as a protoplasmic poison. Lead arsenate is broken down in the body to arsenic and lead. Arsine causes acute haemolysis of red cells.

Chronic Arsenical Poisoning

In industry, apart from the deliberate or accidental swallowing of arsenic compounds, arsenical poisoning is chronic. The main lesions affect the skin and mucous membranes, which undergo dark pigmentation (melanosis). In addition a number of arsenic compounds (e.g. sodium arsenate) are primary irritants producing acute and subacute dermatitis. Hyperkeratosis is a common result. The nails may show broad white bands. Occasionally, peripheral neuritis may result from industrial arsenical absorption. Perforation of the nasal septum may occur. Very rarely a toxic hepatitis, with jaundice, may occur.

Cancer of the skin and lungs (occurring in sheepdip makers) are causally related to exposure to arsenic.

Arsine (Arseniuretted Hydrogen) Poisoning

Two classical accidents occurring in industry may cause arsine poisoning. First, if acid comes in contact with a chipped enamelled iron pan and the acid is contaminated with arsenic, nascent hydrogen is evolved, leading to the formation of arsine. Secondly, dross from alloys, particularly from aluminium alloys, selectively absorbs arsenic. If this dross comes in contact with acid or is washed with an acid water or, with some drosses, exposed to moist air, arsine is evolved. Naturally-occurring peat water is sufficiently acid to give rise to this effect.

Arsine causes acute intravascular haemolysis. Haemoglobinuria (port wine urine) is noted early. Renal failure may ensue. Chronic exposure to arsine gives rise to jaundice, which may be mistaken for infective hepatitis, until several fellow workers have been similarly affected.

Organic Arsines

Chlorvinyldichlorarsine (Lewisite), phenyldichlorarsine and phenarsasine chloride (Adamsite) are acute skin vesicants and pulmonary irritants.

Treatment

Further absorption of arsenic should be prevented by removal from exposure. No specific treatment is known and the administration of dimercaprol (BAL) is usually without effect in inorganic arsenic poisoning. Unless exposure to arsine has been gross, recovery usually occurs within a few days, but blood transfusion may be required. Workmen or soldiers splashed with organic arsines, should have their clothes removed (with suitable precautions adopted by attendants), be washed, put to bed and kept warm. An ointment containing 5 per cent. dimercaprol may be applied to the affected skin. The maintenance of asepsis is important if blisters appear.

Prevention

Prevention consists of: (1) substitution, if possible, by a non-toxic substance; (2) enclosure of processes and exhaust ventilation; (3) the wearing of protective clothing, including gloves, aprons, respirators, as may be appropriate; (4) provision of shower baths and changing facilities; and (5) periodic medical examination. Provided that the circumstances in which arsine is liable to be produced are recognized no difficulty should occur in adopting the necessary measure to avoid its evolution.

CADMIUM POISONING

Cadmium compounds may give rise to acute or chronic illness depending on the dose, route of absorption and exposure. In the acute form, ingested cadmium salts give rise to gastro-intestinal irritation. Inhaled, cadmium fume causes painful cough and dyspnoea which may be followed by pulmonary oedema, bronchopneumonia and proliferating pneumonitis. Chronic cadmium poisoning may follow prolonged exposure to concentrations of cadmium fume too low to cause acute symptoms and also exposure to cadmium oxides and other dust. The condition is insidious in onset and may supervene after a latent period after cessation of exposure. Loss of smell is a prominent symptom of continued exposure to cadmium-containing dusts. Rhinitis, ulceration or perforation of the nasal septum and a yellow discoloration of the teeth may occur. Anaemia has been reported. Renal calculi are not uncommon. The predominant features are, however, pulmonary emphysema and proteinuria, occurring separately or together. The emphysema is atrophic in nature and results in severe decline in pulmonary function. Cadmium is excreted through the renal glomeruli but it is unlikely that damage to the glomeruli accounts for the albuminuria. Damage to the renal tubules can be demonstrated both histologically and biochemically but this damage is unlikely to be of sufficient degree to account for the whole of the proteinuria.

When the proteinuria first appears, traces of α- and β-globulins can be found, but soon low molecular weight albumin (5000–20,000) appears. Partly from the study of human subjects exposed to cadmium and partly as the result of experimental animals, cadmium has been shown to upset the early metabolism, presumably in the liver, of normal serum albumin, in a way which is consistent with fission of the albumin molecule along its length. One or more fragments containing lysine and cystine are metabolically removed. The albuminuria characteristic of cadmium poisoning arises from the excretion of these residues. In poisoned animals up to 40 per cent. of circulating serum albumin may be in this form. Men with chronic cadmium poisoning excreted from 1 to 3·2 g. of protein per litre of urine but the amount excreted is not correlated with the 'dose' of cadmium. It should be noted that boiling only partially precipitates the protein/albumin in the urine: a further precipitation is obtained following the addition of salicylsulphonic acid. Whether the lesions described above are reversible seems doubtful. Hypercalciuria, glycosuria (of the renal type), amino-aciduria, impaired re-absorption of water, impaired acid excretion and hyperchloraemic acidosis are found. Death may follow from right heart failure or renal failure. Cadmium inhibits the enzymatic oxidation of ketoglutamate. In a small group of male workers inhaling cadmium dusts, an excess incidence of cancer of the prostate has been observed, but further investigations are needed to confirm the existence of an industrial hazard.

CHROMIUM

Chromium is prepared from chrome-iron ore. Refinery workers, being exposed to the inhalation of dust of hexavalent chrome compounds, suffer a significant increase in the incidence of cancer of the lung. Chrome plating, in which chromic acid is decomposed electrically, results in bubbles of hydrogen, coated with chromic acid (a trivalent compound), being liberated. Chrome plating operatives suffer from ulceration of the nasal septum which proceeds within a few weeks to perforation of the cartilagenous septum. Apart from the trick that some operatives learn of whistling through the hole, it is asymptomatic. Contact between the skin and chromic acid results in small indolent ulcers (at flexures and minor abrasions) known as chrome holes. Ointments containing E.D.T.A. have been advocated for the palliation and treatment of chrome ulcers but they possess no advantage over bland preparations.

MANGANESE

Manganese salts, particularly the dioxide, are widely used in industry. Manganese dioxide is a major constituent of electric dry batteries. Manganese causes progressive degeneration of the basal ganglia especially the globus pallidus and substantia nigra resulting in symptoms and signs similar to Parkinsonism. A mask-like face, monotonous voice, rigidity and tremor result. Cramp-like pains in the legs and thighs at night are early symptoms. Compulsive crying and laughing occur and in severe cases a peculiar gait known as the 'cock walk of von Jaksch' may be present. Retropulsion and propulsion are marked. Severe manganese poisoning such as occurs in manganese ore miners in Morocco has not been reported from this country but mild cases have been reported. Very rarely hypothyroidism (presumably due to lesions of the infundibulum) may occur [see also Section 5].

BERYLLIUM POISONING

This is described in Section 9.

ZINC

Zinc fume is very irritating to the nose and upper respiratory passage. Probably zinc is the active constituent in brass which causes metal fever or brass-founders' ague, a condition characterized by transient fever and muscular pains occurring on Monday after returning to work following the week-end. The cause is the deposition of a zinc protein complex on the epithelium of the bronchial tree.

NICKEL

Nickel salts are irritating to the skin. Nickel carbonyl, which is a gas, is highly toxic causing immediate headache and dizziness and after a latent period of a few hours, acute respiratory distress. Atelectasis, haemorrhage and necrosis of the lung are found at autopsy. Chronic exposure to nickel carbonyl is causally related to cancer of the ethmoid sinuses. No cases have occurred in Britain from occupational exposure after 1924 when the process of refining was modified.

PHOSPHORUS

Subacute and chronic phosphorus poisoning occurs in three forms: (1) chronic phosphorus poisoning; (2) triorthocresyl phosphate poisoning; (3) poisoning due to organo-phosphorus compounds. Though not a metal from the chemical point of view, phosphorus acts as one.

CHRONIC PHOSPHORUS POISONING

Synonym. Phossy jaw.

Aetiology

Inhalation of the fumes of white (or yellow) phosphorus especially in the presence of dental infection or caries may be associated with the formation of small sequestra in the lower jaw. Red phosphorus does not cause phossy jaw. Massive necrosis of the mandible or superior maxilla no longer occurs in Britain.

Pathology and Symptoms

In growing bone, a characteristic phosphorus band occurs under the epiphyseal cartilage, especially in long bones. In adult bone, the Haversian canals are obliterated by dense bone. Ill-defined hyperaemia of the gum margins occurs and this may be accompanied by an underlying alveolar irregularity which, in time, may release spicules of bone. These gingival and alveolar changes are infrequently seen in ordinary dental practice, but are common among persons exposed to the inhalation of phosphorus fumes. In edentulous persons, inflammation of the crest of the alveolus may occur with fragmentary necrosis of bone. A few exposed persons may develop small sequestra of the lower jaw, and these are usually associated with dental sepsis. Suppurative osteomyelitis may occur. No clear evidence of disturbance of the calcium and phosphorus balance in exposed persons has been demonstrated.

Treatment

Immediate surgical and antibiotic therapy with removal of sequestra results in rapid recovery. Not infrequently sequestra may separate without intervention.

Prevention

Fumes should be controlled by enclosing the process as much as possible and by exhaust ventilation. All persons exposed to the inhalation of phosphorus should maintain a high degree of oral and dental hygiene. Periodic dental examinations are essential and desirably a pre-employment examination should be performed. The Berne Convention, 1906, which prohibited the use of white or yellow phosphorus in the manufacture of lucifer matches, eliminated phossy jaw from among match makers. Phosphorus sesquisulphide is now employed, a perfect example of the elimination of a toxic hazard by the substitution of a non-toxic alternative.

White phosphorus ignites spontaneously in moist air. If splashed on the skin, the part should be immersed in water. Temporary removal from water allows the phosphorus particles to burn and show their position. Under water, they can be removed with forceps. A dressing of 1 per cent. copper sulphate watery solution should be applied.

TRICRESYL PHOSPHATE

Tricresyl phosphates are used as plasticizers in the manufacture of plastics and added to oil have valuable lubricating and anti-corrosive properties. Tricresyl phosphates may be accidental contaminants of adhesives and oils. Extensive outbreaks of poisoning have occurred when contaminated oils and fats have been used for cooking.

Tricresyl phosphates, being easily soluble in fat, are absorbed through the skin which is the main portal of entry in industry, but they may be ingested accidentally as in mass outbreaks of poisoning due to the use of contaminated oil or by failure to wash fingers and hands properly. The destruction or safe disposal of containers which have held tricresyl phosphate is important.

Triorthocresyl phosphate is neurotoxic for man and hens. The *para* and *meta* isomers are not neurotoxic but commercial preparations of these contain 3 per cent. or more of triorthocresyl phosphate.

Triorthocresyl phosphate causes a chromatolysis of the cells of the anterior horn of the spinal cord and motor nuclei of the medulla and pons, degeneration of the posterior columns and pyramidal tract and destruction of the myelin sheaths and of peripheral nerves. These changes are probably secondary to a perivascular infiltration and hyperplastic fibrosis of the small arteries. Cholinesterase is inhibited irreversably.

Paresis is worse in the muscles most used with wasting of the muscles served by the affected nerves. Usually, dorsiflexors of the foot and extensors of the wrist are affected. Retrobulbar neuritis and failure of the respiratory muscles may occur. Pain in the affected limbs is constant but sensory loss is inconstant. Paralysis may be permanent.

ORGANO-PHOSPHORUS COMPOUNDS

Aetiology

Organic phosphorus compounds are widely used in horticulture and agriculture as pesticides, being sold in preparations of varying strength, under a large number of proprietary names, usually intended for use as sprays. Organic phosphorus compounds are absorbed through the lungs, gut and skin. The effect of repeated doses is additive.

Pathology

Organic phosphorus compounds combine with the – SH radicle and act by causing inhibition of cholinesterase. This leads to hypersecretion of the glands, contraction of smooth muscle, slowing of the heart, fasciculation of muscles and central depression of respiration and coma. In addition, some compounds have a narcotic effect and some cause damage to the nerve tracts of the brain and spinal cord. Some compounds inhibit other enzymes, and synergistic effect may occur if pairs of compounds are absorbed. Any simple list of organo-phosphorus compounds is necessarily incomplete but among the more important are parathion, schradan, T.E.P.P. (H.E.T.P.), azinphos-methyl, demeton, demeton-methyl, dimefox, ethion, mercarbam, mevinphos, oxydemeton methyl, plenkapton, phosphamidon and sulfotep. Various proprietary names are used for preparations containing these compounds. The L.D.50's vary from 0·5–2000 mg. per kg. of body weight. Di-isopropylfluorophosphonate (D.P.F.) has similar effects to organo-phosphorus compounds and is used in the treatment of myasthenia gravis, paralytic ileus and glaucoma. Carbamates are used as insecticides but depression of cholinesterase produced by carbamates is much more shortlived than that produced by organo-phosphorus compounds.

Symptoms

Early symptoms are anorexia and nausea, often with mental confusion and a sense of unreality. These symptoms may occur during exposure. Vomiting, abdominal cramp, sensation of cold, sweating and salivation soon follow. Giddiness, apprehension and restlessness may be noticeable. Later, muscular twitchings, especially of the eyelids and tongue, and diplopia may be noticed. Generalized twitching, proceeding to convulsions, occur as poisoning progresses. Diarrhoea, tenesmus, loss of sphincter control, ataxia and mental confusion are usual in severe poisoning. Difficulty in breathing, either from bronchospasm, pulmonary oedema or from depression of respiratory muscles, or a combination of these effects, is an advanced and serious symptom. Death may ensue from coma (with convulsions) or from respiratory failure.

Signs

The patient is pale, collapsed and the pulse is slow. The pupils are constricted. Respiration is weak and laboured and frothy sputum may be present in large quantities, sufficient in some cases to cause severe respiratory embarrassment.

Cholinesterase occurs in red cells and pseudo-cholinesterase in the plasma. For the control of exposed workers or in the course of treatment of a patient, serial estimation of plasma pseudo-cholinesterase or total blood cholinesterase activity is sufficient. Pseudo-cholinesterase falls before cholinesterase: pseudo-cholinesterase activity recovers quickly but cholinesterase is only restored when red cells are renewed. Cholinesterase activity is estimated by enzymic hydrolysis either by measuring the pH change in the substrate (which is the basis of a field method) or by manometric measurement of CO_2 evolved in a Warburg apparatus. The latter method is to be preferred. The results are expressed in Warburg units (μl. of CO_2 formed per minute by 1 ml. of blood or plasma at 37° C.) Normal values are pseudo-cholinesterase 80–150, average 100, cholinesterase 80–150, average 100. The activity of whole blood is in proportion to the red cell/plasma ratio depending on whether cholinesterase or pseudo-cholinesterase is estimated. Desirably, the normal for each worker should be established before exposure starts. Reduction to 75 per cent. of normal indicates excessive absorption. A hazard to the patient arises if levels are reduced to 50 per cent. of normal and serious hazard arises if the reduction is to 30 per cent. of normal.

Treatment

All contaminated clothing should be removed and the skin washed with soap and water. If possible a blood sample should be taken before starting treatment for the estimation of cholinesterase. Five ml. of venous blood should be drawn into a dry syringe and expelled carefully (to avoid haemolysis) into a dry tube containing an anticoagulant. Laboratories undertaking the estimation of cholinesterase activity have been designated by the Ministry of Agriculture from whom a list is obtainable.

P2S (pyridine-2-aldoxime methanesulphonate) and P2AM (PAM) (pyridine-2-aldoxime methiodide) are specific cholinesterase reactivators. (The abbreviation PAM is unfortunate as confusion with PAM, penicillin aluminium monosterate, may occur.) P2S is more soluble in water than P2AM and is recommended in doses of 1 G. dissolved in 6 ml. of water by intravenous injection. Stocks are kept in designated hospitals and laboratories throughout Britain. Repeated doses may be necessary at intervals of 3–4 hours especially as some organo-phosphorus compounds (e.g. parathion) are metabolized in the liver to more toxic forms. P2AM may be harmful in the treatment of carbamate-induced cholinesterase activity.

In the absence of specific cholinesterase reactivators, atropine sulphate in doses of 1–2 mg. should be given. In mild cases this may be sufficient to relieve symptoms, but if symptoms are not relieved or progress, further doses should be given at intervals of 10–30 minutes. Failure to respond, or incipient convulsions, makes the use of specific therapy urgent.

Careful watch should be kept on respiration. Respiratory failure is very liable to occur suddenly and fatally without warning. This watch should be maintained continuously for at least 48 hours even if symptoms have been mild. If failure occurs, respiration should be maintained artificially, preferably by mechanical means. Care should be taken to keep the airway clear. Excessive production of sputum, still more the onset of pulmonary oedema, may call for the passage of an intratracheal tube or a tracheostomy. No hesitation should be felt in performing either of these two procedures if there is any interference with the airway which cannot be quickly controlled. Morphine, theophylline, aminophylline should not be given.

Prevention

All persons manufacturing, packing or using organo-phosphorus compounds should observe strict precautions to avoid absorption. Protective clothing, goggles, face-masks, gloves, boots, should be worn as necessary. It should be remembered the skin is an important portal of entry and all splashes should be immediately washed off. No eating, drinking or smoking should be allowed in the presence of organo-phosphorus. Care is needed in the transport by car, rail and ship of organo-phosphorus compounds and, in particular, special care is needed to see that food (e.g. wheat) is not accidentally contaminated (e.g. from a broken package). Containers should be carefully collected and washed or buried. Under no circumstances should they be used for the transport of any other substance or returned to scrap unless special arrangements are made. Organo-phosphorus compounds may be sprayed from aeroplanes, and a serious risk of crashes, due to diplopia in the pilot, exists if strict precautions are not taken.

All plant should be enclosed, but in agricultural use this may not be possible so it may be necessary to insulate the operative, e.g. a tractor driver should work inside a totally enclosed cabin.

All persons regularly exposed to organo-phosphorus compounds should have their circulating cholinesterase levels estimated regularly though no statutory requirement for this exists. The Agriculture (Poisonous Substances) Act, 1962 applies to the agricultural use of organo-phosphorus compounds.

BENZENE AND ANILINE AND NITRO AND AMIDO DERIVATIVES

Benzene may be distilled from coal-tar, but it is usually fractionated during the distillation of crude oil. Phenol has an OH group attached to the benzene ring.

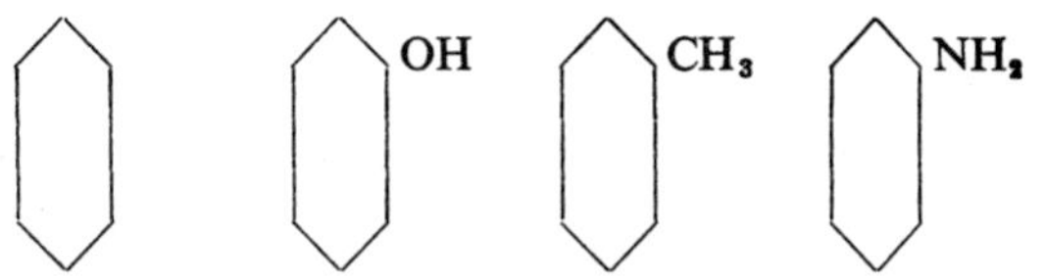

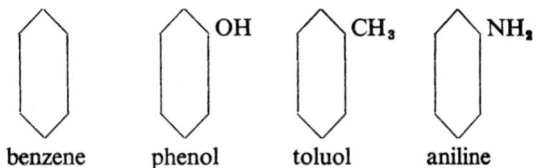

benzene phenol toluol aniline

Nitro derivatives of benzene and phenol (i.e. attachment of one or more NO_2 groups to the ring) include nitrobenzene, trinitrotoluene and dinitrophenol. Amido derivatives (i.e. the attachment of an NH_2 group to the ring) include aniline. There are, of course, a very large number of other derivatives, most of which are toxic, not described here. Remote derivatives of aniline, β-naphthylamine, benzidine, auramine and magenta are implicated as causative agents in cancer of the renal tract and bladder.

BENZENE

Aetiology

Benzene should not be confused with benzine. The latter is a straight chained hydrocarbon; petrol (or gasoline) and naphtha are mixtures of these hydrocarbons. The term benzol has no precise meaning.

Nearly all cases of benzene poisoning arise from industrial exposure to vapour which is absorbed through the lungs. Occasionally, the continued use of preparations containing benzene (especially if in ill-ventilated places) for removing grease from clothes may cause poisoning. Benzene is highly inflammable and may create explosive mixtures with air.

In industry, benzene is widely used as a solvent but its use in this respect is diminishing. Even so, benzene may be used in practically any form of industry; industries in which benzene is a known hazard are the chemical and pharmaceutical industries, rubber industry, blending of motor fuels, linoleum and celluloid industries, manufacture of glues and artificial manure, electrical appliances, photogravure and printing and in industries where adhesives are used, for example, in the manufacture and repair of boots and shoes, cameras, motor car manufacture and repair, sealing of cans and the making of cardboard boxes. In the manufacture of rainproof coats, rubber dissolved in solvents containing benzene is spread over the garment. The same occurs in the manufacture of artificial leather except that nitrocellulose is used instead of rubber.

Benzene appears as a contaminant of other solvents, for example, toluene and xylene. Commercial toluene may contain as much as 11 per cent. of benzene. Descriptions such as toluene 90 refer to the distillation point and bear no direct relationship to the purity. Paints and paint thinners may contain benzene and, at one time, paint strippers commonly contained up to 50 per cent. of benzene.

In Britain there has recently been a marked reduction of the use of benzene, and when the Benzene (Limitation of Use) Regulations come into force, the use of benzene (or a liquid containing more than 1 per cent. of benzene) as a solvent except in a closed system (subject to some minor exceptions) will be prohibited.

Pathology

Up to 40 per cent. of absorbed benzene is metabolized to phenol, which is further metabolized to phenylsulphuric acid and phenylglucuronic acid. Oxidation of phenol to orthodihydroxybenzene (catechol), paradihydroxybenzene (hydroquinol) and 1,2,4, trihydroxybenzene (hydroxyhydroquinol) may occur. Phenylsulphuric ('free phenol') and phenylglucuronic acids ('conjugated phenol') are excreted in the urine. If exposure has been heavy, phenol appears in the urine in addition. The amount of phenol, combined and free, in the urine, bears a linear relationship to the immediately preceding absorption of benzene. After the lapse of a 12–24 hours, the total phenols in the urine return to normal or near normal (less than 30 mg. per litre of urine (specific gravity 1·016)). The rise in phenol excretion during each day and the slower rise in resting or morning levels of phenol over the working week is a useful index of benzene absorption by industrial workers. Benzene is excreted unchanged through the lungs and may be recovered from breath, but in industrial practice this is complicated by the fact that it is nearly always absorbed through the lungs.

The most important effect of benzene is on the bone marrow, where, after a short period of stimulation, continued absorption of benzene causes aplastic anaemia, agranulocytosis, thrombocytopenia, leukaemia or erythromyelosis. How these effects are produced is not known but it seems possible that some of the metabolic products of benzene, including phenol and unknown intermediates, may be mitotic poisons. Some of the other changes occurring in chronic benzene poisoning, such as purpura or gastro-intestinal haemorrhage, can be explained as the result of the depression of the bone marrow but if the theory of mitotic poisoning is accepted, they may be due to the direct effect of the metabolites of benzene on proliferating cells.

Symptoms

Benzene poisoning occurs in two forms (1) acute, (2) chronic.

Acute Poisoning. Inhalation of high concentrations of benzene (from 3000 to 20,000 parts per million of air) causes euphoria, giddiness, excitement and loss of consciousness. Recovery is usual on removal to clean air, but very occasionally artificial respiration may be needed. Sequelae are most unlikely but if exposure has been very severe, signs of degeneration of the central nervous system and psychological disturbances may follow.

Chronic Poisoning. The maximum allowable concentration of benzene for an eight-hour working day is 25 parts per million of air, but evidence exists to suggest that this should be reduced to 10 parts per million. Inhalation of benzene in quantities in excess of 10–25 parts per million for more than 2–3 days, is followed by a transient leucocytosis. Very soon this is followed by a reduction in the number of granular cells in the peripheral blood. An inversion of the polymorph/lymphocyte ratio occurs (though to calculate this the absolute number of cells should be used). Depression of all cellular elements of the bone marrow ensues, and may lead to aplastic anaemia, agranulocytosis and thrombocytopenic purpura. Myeloid and erythro-leukaemia occur more frequently than has hitherto been suspected; occasionally, leukaemia may follow aplasia of the bone marrow. A mixed type of leukaemia (Di Guglielmo syndrome) is a common manifestation of these leukaemic changes. An aleukaemic phase is common. Rather than attempt the categorization of haematological changes, largely on a semantic basis, the term chemical-induced dysplasia of the bone marrow may be preferred. The characteristic change is active but ineffective cell formation in the bone marrow, so that whilst the bone marrow is infiltrated with cells of the erythroblastic or lymphocytic series, the peripheral blood shows depression of the cellular elements with only the occasional presence of abnormal cells. Lymph nodes may be infiltrated with lymphocytic cells and enlarged so that the aleukaemic lymphocytic leukaemia may need to be distinguished from lymphosarcoma. Serum B_{12} is normal.

Studies of groups of workers exposed for some months to high atmospheric pollution with benzene (at present thought to be 100 parts per million or more) show a significant excess of chromosome aberrations. This excess seems to be age related and also influenced by age of starting exposure. In the groups of workers showing this excess, severe haematological effects have occurred in some individuals; whether chromosome aberrations occur in the absence of haemotological effects is not known.

Differential Diagnosis

Usually no difficulty is experienced in identifying the cause of the blood changes, but in any unusual or unexplained blood dyscrasia it is worth remembering benzene as a possible cause. Occasionally, prolonged anaemia may cause cases to present in an unusual manner, for example, as dementia, optic neuritis or cardiac failure.

Treatment

Exposure to benzene should be stopped immediately. Mild cases recover without further action. More serious cases require rest in bed, barrier nursing to avoid infection and a good diet. Blood transfusion may be required to support the bone marrow in aplastic anaemia. The administration of ascorbic acid is thought to be beneficial. Any effect on the blood which proceeds beyond the earliest changes is an absolute bar to further exposure to benzene.

Prognosis

Removal from exposure at the stage of inversion of the polymorph/lymphocyte ratio and of mild depression of the bone marrow, results in recovery. Established cases of blood dyscrasia carry a grave prognosis.

Prevention

In spite of objections on technical grounds, a non-toxic or less toxic solvent can nearly always be substituted for benzene. If this cannot be effected, enclosure of the processes to prevent escape of vapour is usually impossible and reliance has to be placed on local exhaust ventilation to remove fumes from the workroom combined with adequate general ventilation. In arranging for ventilation systems it should be remembered that benzene is highly inflammable and flame proof electrical apparatus and motors may be essential. Periodic red cell and white cell counts and haemoglobin estimation are seldom practicable. Determination of the urinary excretion of phenol is a valuable screening test and a rise of 120 mg. of phenol per 1 litre of urine (specific gravity 1·016) over the course of a working day (i.e. difference between morning and evening excretion) or the excretion of 150 mg. per litre of urine at the end of the day corresponds to an atmospheric concentration of 25 parts per million of benzene breathed for 8 hours. Any preparation containing $2\frac{1}{2}$ per cent. or more of benzene is potentially harmful, but whether a lower percentage is safe cannot be said with certainty.

TOLUENE (TOLUOL), XYLENE

Toluene is metabolized to benzoic and hippuric acid. Xylene is metabolized to toluenic acid and methyl hippuric acid. Possibly because of different metabolites, toluene and xylene are much less toxic than benzene. Report of blood dyscrasias due to toluene and xylene are rare and before accepting these reports the presence of benzene as a contaminant must be excluded. Acute effects, dizziness and loss of consciousness may occur from exposure to toluene and xylene but again, are far less likely than with benzene. Toluene and xylene, but particularly xylene, irritate the nasopharynx. Both toluene and xylene are highly inflammable.

VINYL CHLORIDE

Men emptying stills used to polymerize vinyl chloride to make polyvinyl chloride may suffer asymptomatic absorption of the terminal phalanges. The reason is not known.

ANILINE

Anilism is the term given to poisoning by aniline and by nitro and amido derivatives of benzene. Though substances such as nitrobenzene may have additional specific effects, there are common symptoms and signs, particularly cyanosis, to justify the use of a convenient generic term.

Aetiology

Aniline is a colourless oily liquid which darkens on exposure to light. It is used in the manufacture of dyes, in chemical industry, in cloth pressing and cloth dyeing, in the rubber industry and in the extraction of resins. Aniline is absorbed through the skin but most industrial poisoning results from the inhalation of vapour. Occasionally, dust of aniline compounds may be inhaled or swallowed after settling on the lips. Freshly dyed shoes and laundry marks in marking ink on diapers and dyed blankets may cause anilism.

Aniline reduces haemoglobin to methaemoglobin. Cyanosis is not seen if the patient is anaemic (haemoglobin less than 6 g. per 100 ml.).

Acute Poisoning

Headache, weakness, shortness of breath, giddiness followed by convulsions and unconsciousness may supervene sufficiently quickly to constitute a danger of death from collapse. The patient is cold, the pulse rapid and cyanosis is intense.

Chronic Poisoning

Similar symptoms may develop slowly and less severely; often the exposed person makes no complaint but is noticed to be blue by his fellows. Fatigue, nausea, unsteady gait and peripheral neuritis may be observed. Cardiac arrhythmias (including atrial fibrillation) and anginal symptoms may follow either immediately or after an interval of several days. The red cells show intracellular inclusions (Heinz bodies) and punctate basophilia. With continued exposure anaemia develops.

Treatment

Severe cases require supportive treatment and inhalation of oxygen. An intravenous injection of methylene blue, 1–4 mg. per kg. body weight in 1 per cent. solution, usually relieves cyanosis. Though methylene blue will form methaemoglobin, the reaction is reversible and because of the electrical potentials involved (redox system) causes methaemoglobin to revert to haemoglobin. Methylene blue given in tablets of 60–300 mg. daily by mouth may be preferred. Mild cases of cyanosis recover without treatment.

Prevention

Poisoning by aniline is most common in hot weather when multiple cases may occur. Respirators should be worn if it is necessary to bend over vats containing aniline (or amido or nitro derivatives) and positive pressure air respirators may be required if tanks have to be entered. All contaminated clothing should be removed immediately and skin washed with warm (not hot) water. Baths should be taken at the end of each day's work and working clothes changed for clean clothes.

TRINITROTOLUENE

Synonym. T.N.T.

Aetiology

Trinitrotoluene is a high explosive and naturally is used more in wartime than in peace. In handling trinitrotoluene, regulations relating to explosives must be observed. Trinitrotoluene is a pale crystalline solid, with a faint pinky-yellow colour and is handled in four forms, a flake, prepared by cooling molten trinitrotoluene on a revolving drum, crushed flake passed through rollers, crystalline powder made by cooling molten trinitrotoluene in pans, slab or biscuit made by allowing trinitrotoluene to solidify in shallow pans. Trinitrotoluene may be used as an explosive either alone or mixed with ammonium nitrate (amatol) or barium nitrate (barytol), aluminium powder and other materials (amatax, ammonal, minol, pentolite, burrowite).

Trinitrotoluene may be absorbed through the skin, respiratory system or by swallowing. In industrial practice, inhalation is the most important portal of entry but skin absorption and ingestion cannot be ignored. Trinitrotoluene is metabolized in the liver to 2:6 dinitro-4-hydroxylaminotoluene, 2:6 dinitro-4-aminotoluene and possibly 2:4 dinitro-6-aminotoluene. These substances appear to be conjugated withg lycuronic acid and further detoxication takes place resulting in the excretion of trinitro-benzyl alcohol and dinitroaminobenzyl alcohol. Ingham's improvement of the Webster test (due to the presence of 2:6 dinitro-4-hydroxylaminotoluene) may be applied to the urine to indicate exposure.

Trinitrotoluene causes liver damage which may vary from fatty degeneration to hepatic necrosis. Though the liver damage is toxic in origin, animal experiments suggest that it is influenced by diet. Protein, especially sulphur-containing amino acids, are protective. Depression of the bone marrow occurs and aplastic anaemia may result. Urinary coproporphyrins are increased and the rise is proportional to the severity of poisoning.

Symptoms and Signs

For convenience the effects of trinitrotoluene are divided into (1) absorption, (2) poisoning. It must be understood, however, that there is no clear line of demarcation and every gradation between absorption and fulminating poisoning may occur.

Absorption. Trinitrotoluene adsorbed locally will colour the clothing and skin a yellow-orange. Excretion of metabolites in the sweat will also cause staining. After laundering with alkaline soaps, the areas of clothing where sweating is profuse (e.g. axillae and groin) will be fixed a bright pink colour.

Cyanosis. A mild degree of absorption of trinitrotoluene may produce a lilac colour in the ears, lips and tongue. In part, this is thought to be due to vasoconstriction (and diminishes when the worker becomes animated) and in part, it may be due to methaemoglobinaemia. A more serious form of cyanosis is described below.

Blood Changes. A mild degree of anaemia is common but if the haemoglobin falls more than 1 g. per 100 ml. of blood, the condition must be regarded as serious. Depression of the bone marrow occurs. Persons exposed for several months appear to develop a tolerance and establish an equilibrium with a rise in haemoglobin. Reticulocytosis, punctate basophilia and Heinz bodies appear. A moderate leucocytosis and monocytosis is common. Aplastic anaemia may occur.

Poisoning. The patient complains of considerable fatigue and that he is not refreshed by sleep. Nausea and vomiting, with sickly feelings in the abdomen and occasional hunger pains, may occur. The tongue is usually clean. Substernal pains of the anginal type are common.

The facies is pinched, with white and pink tints, superimposed on a pale muddy complexion. Sallowness is present when there is incipient jaundice. Loss of weight is an early sign and continued loss is ominous.

Anilism of a severe degree may be present, the lips, tongue and gums being of an ashen slaty-blue colour. Methaemoglobin is found in the blood, but in about 2 per cent. of cases sulphaemoglobin occurs. The occurrence of sulphaemoglobin is serious as, unlike methaemoglobin, the body has no means of recovering the fixed haemoglobin.

Abdominal symptoms are due either to gastritis or to liver damage. The stomach empties quickly, gastric rugae are hypertrophied and the pylorus is irritable. Liver damage may be slight, giving rise to no more than incipient jaundice, but the danger of progressive damage ending in acute necrosis is considerable. In patients subject to intermittent exposure, regeneration of the liver lobules may occur. Toxic jaundice due to trinitrotoluene (or to any other cause) is notifiable to H.M. Chief Inspector of Factories. The bone marrow depression may result in a toxic anaemia (also notifiable to H.M. Chief Inspector of Factories). Usually the anaemia is normocytic and accompanied by agranulocytosis and a low platelet count. Purpura may occur.

Dermatitis. Trinitrotoluene is a sensitizing agent to the skin and may cause dermatitis. Personal susceptibility may play a part, but even more important are clean methods of working.

Treatment

Immediate removal from contact with trinitrotoluene is essential. The finger nails should be scrubbed with ether until no pink coloration is obtained with alkaline alcohol. So far as is possible a high protein diet should be given and fats reduced to a minimum.

Prognosis

If liver damage is detected in the early stages recovery occurs, but otherwise the prognosis is grave. The prognosis of toxic anaemia is good with repeated blood transfusions.

Prevention

Strict environmental control is required including good general and local exhaust ventilation to remove dust and fume. Respirators of an approved pattern should be worn for dusty jobs such as the breaking of biscuits. Periodic estimation of atmospheric contamination with trinitrotoluene should be undertaken. The plant should be kept scrupulously clean. Prevention of absorption through the skin is difficult to control, but rests on two pillars, clean working and the use of barrier creams. Dirty workers should not be employed, nail-biters excluded and long nails discouraged. Complete change of working clothes and full bathing before changing into ordinary clothes is desirable. A bath register should be kept. As many of the workers exposed to trinitrotoluene are women, the provision of boudoirs for the application of barrier creams to the face, hands and arms encourages their use. Supervision of the application of barrier creams is desirable. Barrier creams should not contain oil or fat. The use of gloves may increase the risk of absorption as powder gets inside the gloves. No food or drink should be taken in workplaces and, similarly, the use of lipsticks should be prohibited. Smoking is, in any case, prohibited owing to the explosive risk.

Medical supervision and selection of workers is essential. Attention should be paid to cleanliness and a history of jaundice, gastro-intestinal disturbance and dermatitis. All workers should be subject to periodic medical examination (in daylight) at least once a month, preferably once a week, for cyanosis. An incidence of 10 per cent. of cyanosis suggests that conditions are unsatisfactory and in these circumstances one in 500 workers will suffer from toxic jaundice. Statutory provision exists for the keeping of a health register (Factory Form 605). No worker should start the day's work on an empty stomach; so far as possible steps should be taken to ensure that all workers have a good diet, high in protein and ascorbic acid, and avoid alcoholic spirits, confining drinking to reasonable quantities of beer (which may be assumed to have a flushing effect). Fats (e.g. fried fish) should be avoided. The Chemical Works Regulations, 1922, apply to the manufacture of trinitrotoluene.

NITROBENZENE

Synonym. Oil of mirbane.

Nitrobenzene is an oily liquid smelling of bitter almonds; it is used in the manufacture of aniline, quinoline and in perfume, paints and shoe and floor polishes. Occasionally it is used as an abortifacient. Alcohol favours absorption. Nitrobenzene may be absorbed through the skin, by swallowing and by inhalation. Vomiting, drowsiness, which may proceed to synope and death may follow absorption. Absorption of large doses may cause death within 20 minutes. Anilism with intense cyanosis follows less acute exposure. The urine is dark mahogany colour due to the presence of para-aminophenol. Contaminated clothes should be removed immediately and contaminated skin washed either with water or preferably with vinegar or weak acetic acid.

DINITROBENZENE

Dinitrobenzene is used in the manufacture of aniline dyes and is itself an explosive. Probably because it is a solid it appears, in practice, to be less harmful than nitrobenzene. The effect of dinitrobenzene is similar to that of nitrobenzene.

DINITRO-ORTHO-CRESOL (DNOC)

4:6 Dinitro-*ortho*-cresol is a yellow solid which is used widely in agriculture and horticulture to kill weeds, ova, insects and fungi. It is usually applied as a spray in a watery solution of sodium salt. For the control of locusts, it may be applied as a dust or in oil. DNOC may be absorbed through the skin or lungs and by swallowing. DNOC increases the metabolic rate. Early symptoms are a feeling of well-being, followed by thirst, sensations of heat and exhaustion. The pulse rate is increased and fever may be high. Loss of weight may be considerable, up to 10 kg. in a few weeks. The basal metabolic rate is increased, perhaps as much as 400 per cent.

DNOC stains the skin yellow and may cause dermatitis. Anything more than pale yellow staining of the skin suggests that DNOC is not being handled safely.

Besides the skin staining, similar staining may be found *post mortem* in the brain and other tissues. The tissues are dehydrated, petechial haemorrhages present in the brain, lungs, kidneys and liver. The liver shows signs of degeneration. DNOC is a cumulative poison and is excreted slowly. It is absorbed through the skin, alimentary and respiratory tracts.

Treatment

Immediate removal from exposure, thorough washing of the skin and change of clothing is essential. Absolute rest should be enforced. No specific antidote exists and the patient should be kept cool by removing clothing, tepid sponging, air movement, etc. The electrolyte balance should be carefully watched. Atropine should not be given. Barbiturates may be administered to relieve anxiety.

Prevention

Agricultural workers are most liable to be at risk and poisoning is most likely to occur in the summer (partly because of the seasonal use of DNOC and the vaporization of sprays). Chemical process workers may also be exposed. Workers should wear masks, protective clothing, helmets, respirators and gloves. Thorough washing with a change of clothes is desirable at the end of each day's work. In factories, exhaust ventilation should be applied.

Because spraying with DNOC for agricultural and horticultural purposes is usually done in hot weather, operatives may be thirsty (quite apart from the thirst arising from DNOC absorption). Fresh drinking water should be provided as considerable danger of drinking contaminated water arises. A weekly record of the weight of all exposed persons should be kept and, if possible, all persons exposed to DNOC should have the level of DNOC in the blood estimated at least once a week. Intravenous blood samples should be taken 8 hours after last exposure to avoid false peaks. If the blood level of DNOC rises to 20 μg. per ml. of whole blood or above, the workman should be immediately removed from work and rested. If the level of DNOC is between 10–20 μg. per ml. of whole blood, the estimation should be repeated in 48 hours and if there has been a rise, the workman should be removed from contact until the level has fallen to 5 μg. per ml. At least 6 weeks should elapse before the patient returns to exposure. The urinary excretion of DNOC is an unreliable guide to absorption.

DINITROPHENOL

Only 2:4 dinitrophenol (*alpha*-dinitrophenol) is toxic. It is a yellow crystal used in the dye industry, for the preservation of wood and as an explosive. It is absorbed in the same way as DNOC and has a similar effect in raising the basal metabolic rate. The skin may be stained yellow but the urine is a deep orange colour owing to the presence of 2-amino-4-nitrophenol.

At one time dinitrophenol was used to treat obesity but its use has been abandoned as it caused bilateral cataract. Cataract started to appear from between 3–18 months after taking the first dose. When used in this way, other toxic symptoms included urticaria, exfoliative dermatitis, jaundice, peripheral neuritis, loss of discrimination between sweet and salt taste, and a fullness in the ears.

HYDROCARBONS AND HALOGENATED HYDROCARBONS

PETROL, NAPHTHA, BENZINE

These are widely used as solvents. All are highly inflammable. Inhaled in sufficient concentrations, all are narcotics producing giddiness, intoxication and unconsciousness. Reports of chronic toxic effects on the bone marrow must be treated with reserve unless it can be proved that contamination by benzene was absent. Prolonged exposure may cause headache, drowsiness, conjunctivitis and vague digestive symptoms. Being fat solvents, they may potentiate the action of skin irritants leading to dermatitis.

METHYLENE CHLORIDE (METHYLENE DICHLORIDE)

Methylene chloride is used as a paint remover and, in the artificial silk industry. At one time it was proposed as an anaesthetic. Methylene dichloride is very irritant to the skin and if used in the presence of a fire may degenerate to form phosgene.

CARBON TETRACHLORIDE

Carbon tetrachloride is widely used as a solvent, for example, as a vehicle for rubber, the extraction of fats and in the chemical and paint industries. Some domestic grease-removing preparations contain substantial proportions. It is not inflammable and is employed in some forms of fire extinguishers. In contact with hot metal, however, carbon tetrachloride decomposes to form phosgene, so if used in this way, the room must be vacated immediately after the fire is out.

Acute Effects

In high concentrations, the inhalation of carbon tetrachloride produces narcosis but in practice this is a rare occurrence. The characteristic of acute poisoning is the period of delay, about 2–3 days, following exposure which precedes the onset of nausea, vomiting (thought to be of central origin), psychic and motor disturbances of the nervous system which may end in epileptiform fits, unconsciousness and death. Gastro-intestinal haemorrhage, haemoptysis, pulmonary oedema, optic neuritis and paresis of the limbs may all occur.

Chronic Effects

The acute disease may progress to renal and liver damage, but these usually follow prolonged exposure to relatively low concentrations. Though liver damage and portal necrosis has attracted much attention, the action of carbon tetrachloride is first shown by its effect on the kidneys.

Oedema and gross albuminuria due to tubular necrosis develops but in non-fatal cases may subside without having apparent after-effects.

The premonitory symptoms of carbon tetrachloride poisoning have been neglected. Vague nausea and digestive disturbances, vomiting and diarrhoea, inertia and mental hebetude, occurring first in bouts, but later more continuously, should be regarded as warning symptoms. Workers exposed to carbon tetrachloride develop an excessive dislike for its smell and premonitory symptoms may be induced by smelling it.

METHYL CHLORIDE

This is used in the chemical industry and was, at one time, used as the cooling fluid in refrigeration. For the latter use, it has been replaced by the Freons which are virtually non-toxic. Symptoms of poisoning include nausea, vomiting and restlessness followed by somnolence. Dimness of vision may occur. Later the temperature, pulse and respiration may rise temporarily. Oliguria and evidence of acute nephritis occur in about half the cases.

METHYL BROMIDE

Methyl bromide is used in fire extinguishers, and as a refrigerant, fumigant, insecticide and in the chemical industry. Few substances have higher powers of penetration and methyl bromide will quickly penetrate leather and concrete. Except when high concentrations are inhaled its action is delayed for 4–48 hours, causing abrupt nausea, vomiting, headache, giddiness and collapse, sweating with a normal temperature, dimness of vision and diplopia. Psychotic changes, euphoria, confusion and delirium may be prominent. Trismus and opisthotonos may be seen. The pupils are dilated. Convulsions and anuria may occur in severe cases. Tracheobronchial irritation and pulmonary oedema are common. The outcome is usually fatal in the presence of pulmonary oedema, convulsions, anuria and extensive burns but otherwise recovery is complete. Treatment is supportive. Methyl bromide appears to be metabolized to methylmercapturic acid which is excreted in the urine. Methyl bromide is irritant to the skin, producing burns with marked blistering surrounded by erythema and oedema but which rarely penetrate the whole dermis.

TETRACHLORETHANE

This is highly toxic but it has now been replaced by less toxic solvents. Being a good solvent for cellulose acetate, it was a major constituent of 'dope' used for coating aeroplane wings in the First World War and in the cellulose film industry. Inhalation of high concentrations cause narcosis and death. Chronic poisoning occurs in two forms (which may be concurrent), gastrohepatic which may proceed to acute necrosis of the liver and polyneuritic affecting particularly the small muscles of the hands and feet.

TRICHLOROETHYLENE (TRICHLORETHYLENE, TRILENE)

Trichlorethylene is used in many industries including the engineering industry as a degreasing agent and fat solvent. Though trichlorethylene has replaced more toxic solvents, such as carbon tetrachloride, it is not without danger. It is absorbed in the form of vapour through the lungs, part is excreted unchanged through the lungs, but the remainder is metabolized to trichloroethanol and trichloroacetic acid which are excreted in the urine. Trichloroacetic acid can be recovered from the blood. The maximum allowable concentration of trichlorethylene is 100 parts per m^3. of air and concentrations of trichloroacetic acid in excess of 5 mg. per 100 ml. blood and 100 mg. per litre of urine (specific gravity 1·016) indicate excessive absorption.

Trichlorethylene is a narcotic and anaesthetic. Sleepiness, weariness and mild drunkenness are common in exposed workers. Prolonged exposure may be associated with optic neuritis, and neuritis of the other cranial nerves (especially the trigeminal nerve which results in insensibility of the cornea). Vague nausea is common. Toxic jaundice and nephrosis occur rarely. Workers heavily exposed to trichlorethylene for more than a short period show considerable personality changes including diminution in memory and comprehension. Addiction to trichlorethylene is almost certainly much more common than recognized. A number of sudden deaths of workmen undertaking exercise (e.g. running up stairs or bicycling) after exposure to trichlorethylene have been reported. Specific pathology is absent.

Prevention

Good general ventilation is essential in establishments using trichlorethylene but it is usually impossible totally to enclose degreasing processes. Degreasing baths of trichlorethylene should be properly designed to prevent carry over of liquid and vapour when the article is removed and the top of the bath should be refrigerated to condense vapour. For dry cleaning clothes, trichlorethylene has generally been replaced by perchlorethylene which is safer. On heating, trichlorethylene (which is not inflammable) decomposes to hydrochloric acid and in the presence of naked flame to phosgene. Smoking should be prohibited in the presence of trichlorethylene vapour.

ORGANO-CHLORINE COMPOUNDS

Aetiology

Organo-chlorine compounds are used as insecticides and pesticides. Aldrin and dieldrin are used as house sprays in mosquito control and endrin and endosulphan as horticultural sprays for pears, apples, cherry trees and blackcurrant bushes. Dieldrin is more toxic than aldrin which is changed into dieldrin in the body. Organo-chlorine compounds are absorbed through the skin, gut and respiratory system.

Pathology

Organo-chlorine compounds act as central nervous system poisons though the mechanism of this action is not known. Organo-chlorine compounds are deposited in fat and once deposited are virtually not excreted even over the subject's lifetime. The fat of sheep and cattle grazing on grass dressed with dieldrin contains appreciable quantities of this compound. For man, oral doses of dieldrin in excess of 10 mg. per kg. produce acute illness, symptoms occurring within 20 minutes and, in no instance, has a latent period of more than 12 hours been substantiated.

Symptoms and Signs

Three syndromes may be distinguished depending on the dose and toxicity of the organo-chlorine compound absorbed: (1) A few large doses stimulate the central nervous system culminating in one or more convulsions; if death does not occur, recovery is prompt and no significant residual changes follow. (2) A larger number of moderate doses may produce, without warning, loss of appetite, loss of weight and convulsions. (3) Many relatively small doses may cause one or more convulsions without other symptoms.

Hyperexcitability and hyperirritability are common. Coma may follow convulsions. In persons exposed over a period, a condition indistinguishable from idiopathic epilepsy may be presented. Even before the development of fits, the E.E.G. shows epileptiform changes. Myoclonic jerks may be noted by exposed persons, and may be the precursor of convulsions.

Treatment

Immediate removal from contact is essential. Clothes should be removed and the skin thoroughly washed. No specific treatment exists.

Prevention

Absorption of organo-chlorine compounds should be controlled as described under organo-phosphorus compounds. A history of excitability, irritability or jerks of the muscles or limbs should be regarded seriously. Changes in serial electroencephalograms of the spike and wave type seen in petit mal may be used to indicate that the exposed person is at hazard. Estimation of dieldrin in the blood may similarly be used. Symptoms are rare if the blood level of dieldrin is below 50 μg. per 100 ml.

OTHER SUBSTANCES

CARBON BISULPHIDE

The main use of carbon bisulphide is in the artificial silk industry but it is also widely used in other industries as a solvent. It is employed in chemical and pharmaceutical manufacture, the rubber industry, the making of waterproof cements and transparent paper, as a solvent in matches and in rat poison containing phosphorus [p. 352]. Besides being highly toxic, it is also extremely inflammable so much so that the heat from an ordinary electric light bulb may cause an explosion. Special recommendations about the handling and storage of carbon bisulphide exist (Factory Form 83B).

Possibly because of the restrictions necessary for the safe-handling of carbon bisulphide, cases of poisoning are rare in this country. Symptoms and signs of poisoning are of three types: (1) mental disturbance, at first characterized by extreme weariness, apprehension, loss of memory, accompanied by irritability progressing to a manic psychosis and dementia (indeed, in the last century, many artificial silk workers were admitted to asylums and the occupational origin of their illness not diagnosed); (2) striatopallidal degeneration with tremor and stiffness, optic atrophy and peripheral neuritis affecting the motor sensory nerves, especially of the face and forearms may occur; (3) nausea, vomiting and epigastric pain, which though suggesting an abdominal lesion, are possibly of central origin. Exposure to hydrogen sulphide formed when carbon bisulphide decomposes causes chronic conjunctivitis. The presence of carbon bisulphide in the urine is shown by the formation of a black precipitate when Fehling's solution is added.

Recovery is usual following removal from exposure but if exposure has been severe, residual dementia and neurological degeneration may persist. All persons exposed to carbon bisulphide should be carefully observed for personality changes, which may be cyclical.

Evidence is accumulating that groups of workers exposed to air concentrations of carbon bisulphide above the M.A.C. (20 parts per million) suffer an excess of death ascribed to coronary diseases. In Britain, it may be that exposure at this level was associated with war-time conditions.

NITROGLYCERINE

Synonyms. NG; glycerine trinitrate.

When absorbed into a kieselguhr, nitroglycerine is known as dynamite. Nitroglycerine causes vasodilatation consequent upon which headaches, often severe, may be suffered by persons unused to exposure. It is readily absorbed through the skin and also as a vapour through the lungs.

ETHYLENE GLYCOL DINITRATE

Synonyms. E.G.D.N.; Nitroglycol.

Ethylene glycol dinitrate is added to dynamite in proportion up to 40 per cent. as an antifreeze agent and to improve explosive power. The vapour pressure of E.G.D.N. is about 80 times greater than that of T.N.T. so that workers exposed to the mixture inhale (and absorb) a much higher quantity of total nitrates than if exposed to T.N.T. alone. Like T.N.T., E.G.D.N. is also absorbed through the skin. In rats an injection of E.G.D.N. causes a fall in blood pressure thought to be brought about by its metabolic products, ethylene glycol mononitrate, inorganic nitrites and by unconverted E.G.D.N. This mechanism is thought to account for cases of sudden cardiac deaths, unaccompanied by significant pathology, which has been reported among workers, who exert themselves after a few days' interval during which they have not been exposed. Typically, such deaths occur on Monday or Tuesday after a week-end not at work. Since improvement (including the introduction of mechanized processes) in environmental conditions, these deaths no longer occur in Britain.

QUINONE AND HYDROQUINONE (OCULAR OCHRONOSIS)

After being converted to hydroxyphenylpyruvate and homogentisate, tyrosine is further metabolized by the enzyme homogentisic oxidase. Homogentisic acid is hydroquinone acetic acid. Failure of this mechanism: (1) through the congenital absence of homogentisic oxidase as in alcaptonuria; or (2) by overloading the mechanism by excessive absorption of benzene ring-containing substances such as carbolic acid (which used to occur when carbolic dressings were used for long periods), results in deposition of hydroquinone acetic acid in avascular tissues and its excretion in the urine (which darkens on standing). Ochronosis is the term given to the accompanying thickening and staining of cartilage, the conjunctiva and cornea. Ocular ochronosis results from exposure to the vapours of quinone or hydroquinone in the photographic processing industry. The cornea develops a sepia-like stain, traversing the whole of its substance, across the area exposed. The conjunctivae are affected, particularly in the interpalpebral area. Vision is seriously affected, objects being surrounded by a coloured haze and sight may be reduced to finger counting only. Corneal grafting may be necessary. In industry, enclosed processes, preventing the escape of vapour, should be used.

OCCUPATIONAL CANCER

Persons engaged in some trades may be exposed to known carcinogens. Occupations with an accepted excess incidence of cancer are:

Asbestos: Bronchial carcinoma; mesothelioma [see Section 9].

Nickel carbonyl: Cancer of the ethmoid; since the process of refining nickel was improved in 1924, no case has been attributable to nickel carbonyl.

Hexavalent chromates: Bronchial carcinoma; in smelting of chrome ores to produce bichromates. Trivalent salts of chrome used in chrome plating are not carcinogenic.

Isopropyl oil: Nose, exposure to oily residues left behind after distilling isopropyl alcohol (which itself is not carcinogenic).

Wood dust, especially hard woods: Adenocarcinoma of mucous membrane covering middle ethmoid; first noticed in the High Wycombe furniture manufacturers who are exposed to dust of hard woods, especially beech, oak and mahogany, may also (but to less extent) be associated with exposure to dust of soft wood.

Polycyclic hydrocarbons: Bronchial carcinoma; polycyclic hydrocarbons of the benzpyrene and benzanthracene type may occur in the air of vertical retort houses gas works.

Benzene: Leukaemia [see Section 13].

Arsenic: Skin, bronchial cancer in manufacturers of sheep dips.

Ionizing radiations: Blood, bone, lung, skin [see p. 364].

β-Naphthylamine, α-naphthylamine, benzidine, orthotolidine, 4-aminodiphenyl, 4-nitrodiphenyl: Cancer of bladder and renal tract. The latent period varies considerably but the peak incidence is from 11 to 18 years.

Tar, pitch, bitumen: Cancer of skin, polycyclic hydrocarbons.

Mineral oil: Cancer of skin, especially of scrotum; polycyclic hydrocarbons in mineral oil.

Cadmium: Cancer of prostate. Makers of nickel-cadmium batteries.

In preventing occupational cancer the first step should be to substitute a non-carcinogenic or less carcinogenic substance. This has been done in the case of mule spinning for which regulations were made permitting only the use of non-mineral oil or acid treated oil. In the engineering industry, the use of solvent-washed mineral oil (or the dilution of oil with 'suds' to form cutting oils) reduces the carcinogenic potency. Solvent-washed oils contain about a third of the carcinogenic fractions of unwashed oil. Avoidance of contact and personal cleanliness is another principle but is very difficult to apply: there is no excuse for wearing oil-stained underclothes and though bathing after work is desirable, it is seldom possible to remove all the oil ingrained into the skin.

Early diagnosis is essential, if hope of cure is to be held out. Engineering operatives exposed to contact with oil, workers with tar, pitch and bitumen, should be warned and told to report any skin lesion to their medical adviser. The number of persons involved make the organization of periodic medical examination impracticable in the engineering industry; further a workman should be able to notice early changes in his skin better than a physician who sees him (say) every 6 months. Deaths from skin cancer should be avoidable: if they do occur, it is often because a lesion has not been reported by an elderly man who, through lack of a bathroom, is unused to examining his skin. Persons who leave the industry by retirement or for other reasons should be instructed to continue self inspection of the skin. This was arranged for mule spinners by the issue through the Union of a special warning card.

β-Naphthylamine and benzidine are intermediates in the manufacture of synthetic dyes, α-naphthylamine and benzidine are used as mordants in dyeing textiles; all three substances have been incorporated into anti-oxidants employed in the rubber industry, including the manufacture of tyres, boots and shoes and industrial belting. Workers exposed to β-naphthylamine, α-naphthylamine and benzidine or substances contaminated with even small amounts of them, suffer an excess incidence of cancer of the bladder. Though other parts of the epithelium of the renal tract may undergo malignant change, it is the bladder which is especially affected. The distinction between non-malignant papilloma of the bladder and cancer of the bladder can no longer be maintained. Carcinogenesis results from the urine-borne metabolic products not clearly identified but possibly similar to conjugates of anthranilic acid produced in the metabolism of tryptophan. Auramine and magenta are not themselves liable to produce cancer though they may be made from carcinogenic intermediates. Rat poison containing α-naphtholthiourea has now been discontinued. The use of benzidine as a laboratory reagent is highly undesirable.

Persons who have been exposed should be submitted to exfoliative cytology of the urine every 6 months. The appearance of malignant cells frequently precedes symptoms by a long time, and not infrequently precedes the discovery of tumours on cystoscopic examination.

The manufacture and use of the major bladder carcinogens is now strictly controlled by the Carcinogenic Substances Regulations, 1967: indeed some can only be made or used after permission is granted by the Chief Inspector of Factories.

PNEUMOCONIOSIS

Pneumoconiosis means dust on the lungs. Logically, all pulmonary lesions arising from the inhalation of dust should be called pneumoconiosis. Except in the most unusual circumstances, pneumoconioses arise from the inhalation of dust during the course of work, Pneumoconioses may be described as:

1. BENIGN: iron, tin, barium, antimony.
2. FIBROTIC: (i) silica, silicates (including asbestos).
   (ii) mixed dust, including coal, iron ore.
3. INFLAMMATORY: vanadium, manganese, beryllium, hard metal, cadmium, aluminium.
4. ALLERGIC: cotton dust (byssinosis), mouldy hay (farmer's lung), osmium, platinum salts.

The inhalation of some dusts (e.g. hexavalent chrome compounds, arsenic, asbestos, polycyclic hydrocarbons evolved in the manufacture of coal-gas) is causally related to an excess of respiratory cancer among exposed occupational groups, but this is not usually classified as a pneumoconiosis. (Smoking habits must be taken into account when individual cases of bronchogenic cancer may be due to occupation causes.) Toxic gases (e.g. hydrogen cyanide, hydrogen sulphide, phosphine, arsine) may enter the body through the lungs and exert a systemic effect without specific damage to the pulmonary system.

Pneumoconioses are identified either by indicating the causal agent, e.g. silicosis, talcosis, stannosis, or by the nature of the work involved, e.g. coal miners' pneumoconiosis, knife grinders' phthisis. Because of the legal considerations involved, pneumoconiosis has been defined by the National Insurance (Industrial Injuries) Regulations, 1959, SI. 467 as 'fibrosis of the lungs due to silica dust, asbestos dust or other dust, and includes the condition of the lungs known as dust reticulation but does not include byssinosis'. Reticulation is neither a clinical nor a pathological entity but a descriptive term used to describe X-ray appearances of the lung. The result of this definition is that the legal and medical views on pneumoconiosis differ and that the former give undue emphasis to the fibrotic form of lesion. On the other hand, the social consequences of fibrotic lesions greatly outweigh those arising from other forms of pneumoconiosis.

In certain occupations, known as scheduled occupations, the occurrence of pneumoconiosis is presumed (without the onus of proof resting on the workman) to be the result of occupational exposure. Workers in scheduled occupations should be examined periodically by the Pneumoconiosis Panels of the Ministry of Pensions and National Insurance. Any person employed in any occupation (whether scheduled or not) may apply to the Pneumoconiosis Panels for certification as suffering from pneumoconiosis, and if certified, is entitled to assessment for industrial injury benefits. In Great Britain, coalmining contributes two-thirds of the approximately 1600 new cases of pneumoconiosis (excluding byssinosis) certified by the Pneumoconiosis Panels each year. Other major industries involved are pottery, quarrying and dressing of rock (including sandstone and granite), slate mining and quarrying, the manufacture of refractory bricks (heat-resisting silica bricks for the lining of furnaces), furnace dismantling, foundry work especially fettling (the removal of silica particles from iron and steel castings), iron mining, calcining and grinding of sand or flint, china clay getting, manufacture of scouring powders, boiler scaling, metal grinding and exposure to asbestos (weavers of asbestos, insulating materials, pipe laggers).

The clinical aspects of pneumoconiosis are considered in detail in Section 9.

ELECTRICITY

ELECTRICAL INJURIES AND ELECTROCUTION

Aetiology

In Britain, the potential of the domestic electric supply is almost always 230–250 volts alternating current of 50 cycles per second. Generally, industrial lighting supplies are the same. The majority of electric motors are run at 400 volts or more. The conductor rail potential of underground and suburban electric railways is 660 volts. Overhead conductor wire on electric railways may be at up to 25,000 volts. Overhead transmission cables of the National Grid Electricity System vary from 11,000–400,000 volts. Lightning flashes involve potentials of 100–1000 million volts, with a current of some 20,000 amperes for less than one millisecond.

Deaths from electrocution average about 145 a year; about half of these occur from electrical accidents in the home. Deaths from lightning stroke number about 10 a year. In judicial electrocution in U.S.A., an alternating current of 500–2000 volts, 100 milliamperes, is applied for two minutes.

Pathology

From experiments on sheep, it appears that the body resistance varies inversely with the voltage, so that the strict application of Ohm's law (Voltage = Impedance or resistance × Amperes) is not possible. In the circumstances of nearly all electrical accidents, the degree of contact of the body with the electrical conductor affects the total resistance very considerably. The degree of contact depends on the surface area of the body in contact with the live conductor at the point of entry, the degree of insulation of the body from the negative conductor, which, very often, may be the earth, the moisture on the skin, and the pressure of the body against the conductor (e.g. clasping by the hand).

The internal impedance of the body to the passage of electricity is about 500 ohms but skin impedance varies by several orders of magnitude so that the total body resistance varies considerably.

Passage of electricity through the body causes heating and skin burns (often with marked underlying necrosis) and internal injury may result. The degree of heating is determined by the product of the voltage and current. Arcing-over from a high potential conductor to the body reduces the voltage passing through the body and may account for some recoveries by shock from high tensions. Apart from heating, the effects of the passage of electricity through the body occur instantaneously as the electricity enters the body.

In only about 3 per cent. of fatalities has it appeared that the current passed through the respiratory centre. By far the commonest path through the body is from an upper limb to either the opposite upper limb or to the feet. In these circumstances (applicable to about 97 per cent. of fatalities) death results either from: (1) hypoxia due to tetanic contraction of the chest muscles: cyanosis may be severe even though the airway is patent; (2) ventricular fibrillation.

In order to cause ventricular fibrillation, the passage of current through the cardiac muscle must fall either within the refractory period preceding the T wave or in the period between the fall of the R wave and the S wave and lasts for 5–8 milliseconds. Currents greater than a few amperes do not cause fibrillation (which, if burns do not cause death, is another reason for recovery from shock sustained from high tension overhead cables). The frequency of alternating current influences the chance of fibrillation. This is greatest at 50 cycles per second (half cycle = 10 milliseconds) diminishing as the number of cycles per second is diminished or raised above this level. Unfortunately, 50 cycles per second has been chosen as the standard for Britain. The number of amperes passing through the body determine the effects of electricity. At 50 cycles per minute these are:

	MEN *Milliamps*	WOMEN *Milliamps*
No sensation	0·4	0·3
Slight tingling	1·1	0·7
Painful shock but muscular control retained	9	6
Painful shock, 'let-go threshold', mild muscular contractions	16	10
Severe muscular contractions, breathing difficult	23	15
Possible ventricular fibrillation or asystole		
shock of 0·3 seconds	1000	1000
shock of 3·0 seconds	100	100

Muscular contractions may be sufficiently severe to throw the patient to the ground; whether the patient falls backwards or forwards depends on the strength of contraction of the extensor or flexor muscles. Usually the extensor muscles are strongest.

In terms of volts, practical experience shows that the threshold of sensation is about 12 volts, the threshold of pain is below 20 volts and the 'hold on' voltage is about 25 volts. In Britain, the lowest recorded fatal shock voltage is 60 volts. Few fatalities occur below 100 volts and these in unusual circumstances.

Shocks from direct current are rarely fatal unless death results from burns. In death from lightning (or other very high voltages) gross tissue disruption may be found and a common site for this is the scalp and brain. The victims' clothes may have been torn off. These effects are due to the intense electrostatic changes generated and these, according to normal electrical laws, repel each other.

Symptoms

A patient recovering from an electric shock may be severely collapsed. Severe pain may be experienced from skin burns or from muscular and ligamentous injuries or dislocations of joints (due to severe muscular contractions). Less severe shocks may be followed by faintness. Anxiety states are common sequelae and coronary occlusion may occur as a late complication. Retrograde amnesia is common. Neurological sequelae, including Parkinsonism, have been reported but they are rare.

Treatment

A man in contact with an electrical conductor must be removed by a safe method, i.e. by switching off the current, the use of insulated gloves or an insulated pole, or, if no other means is available, by standing on a dry rubber mat or wearing dry rubber boots. The clothes rather than the body should be held. Not only may the rescuer be killed if safe means of rescue are not employed, but the injured person is not saved; this cannot be stressed sufficiently.

Most cases of electric shock recover spontaneously though burns may need treating. For an unconscious patient, immediate resuscitation is required. A safe procedure is to start artificial respiration and if the pulse cannot be felt to give a sharp blow on the precordium. If the pulse still cannot be felt external cardiac massage should be continued until a defibrillator is available. (In the presence of contraction of the chest muscles, mouth to mouth artificial respiration may not be effective.) The whole of the body should be examined for burns as the point of entry of electricity may be shown by no more than a small puncture but considerable underlying tissue damage may be present. Surgical treatment may be needed. Fractures of bone (including skull and spine) may be found. Attention should be paid to the electrolyte balance.

Prevention

The need for the safe design and installation of electrical circuits and apparatus is obvious but the necessity of proper maintenance is often forgotten. All portable electrical appliances should be tested periodically and under no circumstances should frayed flexes be permitted. A number of fatalities have occurred because domestic sockets have not been properly guarded; children being at particular risk because they are likely to poke their fingers or metal needles into the contact holes. Proper earthing of apparatus should be provided but whether, in certain circumstances, earthing is safer than double insulation is a matter for expert electrical advice. Water is a good conductor of electricity and electric apparatus should not be employed in bathrooms and damp places unless properly designed and insulated for this purpose. All electricians should be trained in artificial respiration and external cardiac massage. Unfortunately, many electrical accidents occur in small factories and other places where the standard of discipline and maintenance is poor.

IONIZING RADIATIONS

Aetiology

During the First World War, some 800 girls were employed in U.S.A. painting instruments and watch dials with luminous paint containing radium and mesothorium. In doing this, they developed the habit of pointing their brushes with their lips. Many of the girls developed anaemia, agranulocytosis and some developed osteitis and sarcoma of bone. During the Second World War, an enormous and rapid increase in the use of radium in luminizing instrument dials took place. As the result of the rigid enforcement of preventive practices, no ill effects ensued in Britain. In 1962, one woman employed on luminizing during the war died of myeloid leukaemia but whether this was a coincidental occurrence of leukaemia or due to occupational exposure cannot be answered. X-rays, including fluoroscopic techniques and gamma rays, are being increasingly used for the non-destructive examination of metal articles. Radio-isotopes are now in daily use in research and development laboratories. X-rays, other ionizing radiations and radio-isotopes are widely used for diagnosis and therapy in medical practice. Nuclear fission is now being employed as a source of power for the generation of electricity as well as for 'atomic' bombs. Thallium 204 is widely used in industry where limited powers of penetration are required as in thickness gauges: the use of radium has proved too hazardous (except for some military equipment) and has been very largely replaced by tritium.

Nature of Ionizing Radiations

Ionizing radiations are capable of splitting off orbital electrons from normal electrically neutral atoms, leaving behind positively charged ions. Ionizing radiations may be either electromagnetic waves or corpuscular in nature.

X-rays are electromagnetic radiations, travelling at the speed of light, usually produced by directing a high velocity stream of electrons at a metal surface in a vacuum. It should be noted that the wavelength of X-rays in Ångström units (1A° = 10^{-8} cm.) is $\frac{24000}{\text{voltage.}}$

Gamma radiations are similar to X-rays but have a shorter wavelength. The most important sources of gamma rays are cobalt^{60}, iridium^{192}, caesium^{137}, thulium^{171} and radium.

Beta radiations are particulate and are negatively charged electrons originating from the nuclei of radio nuclides. They leave their parent nuclei at speeds approaching that of light but slow down quickly. For this reason they have low powers of penetration, in air a few metres and in human tissue about a centimetre. Beta particles may be emitted either alone or with gamma rays. When beta particles are stopped in matter, secondary gamma radiation (*Bremsstrahlung*) may be produced and this may be significant as a cause of damage to the tissues.

Alpha particles are helium nuclei (two protons and two neutrons). Alpha particles are relatively heavy (atomic weight 4 or some 7000 times the mass of the beta particle), carry a double positive charge, have low powers of penetration (about 50 μ in tissue) and travel at 12,000–18,000 miles per second. Alpha particles are produced by the decay of naturally occurring radioactive substances such as radium and uranium and by the artificial element plutonium (which is also a strong alpha particle emitter). Because of their large mass and double charge of electricity, alpha particles produce dense ionization along their paths.

Protons are positively charged nuclei, have no or little industrial application.

Neutrons are particles of nearly the same mass as protons, but carrying no electrical charge, have great powers of penetration. In collisions with the atomic nuclei of the substance they are traversing, secondary emission of ionizing radiations occurs. The main use of neutrons is in the generation of atomic power by the fission of uranium^{235} and in the production of radio-isotopes.

Units of Measurement

The unit of activity of radioactive materials is the curie. One curie is the quantity of any radioactive material in which $3{\cdot}7 \times 10^{10}$ atomic disintegrations occur per second. The energy of radioactive emissions is measured in electron volts. One electron volt (eV) equals $1{\cdot}6 \times 10^{-12}$ ergs. One thousand electron volts equal 1 KeV and 1 million electron volts equal 1MeV. Of special importance is measurement of absorbed dose of ionizing radiation for which the rad is the unit. One rad equals 100 ergs per gramme of absorbing medium (e.g. human tissue). One thousandth part of a rad is called a millirad or m.rad. The rem is a unit of radiation dose in tissue which takes into account the biological effectiveness (R.B.E.) (see below) of equal absorbed doses of different kinds of ionizing radiations, rads × R.B.E. = rems. In the last few years, the term quality factor (Q.F.) has been preferred to R.B.E.

The biological effects of ionizing radiations are the

result of the transfer of energy to the tissues along their path. The relatively heavy alpha particle transfers more energy per linear unit than X-rays. One rem is equal to 1 rad of ionizing radiation (produced by 200 KV X-rays) absorbed into tissue. For practical purposes the Q.F. of X-rays, gamma rays, beta particles is 1 and for alpha particles, fast neutrons and protons is 10, i.e. similar biological effects will arise from one-tenth of the absorbed dose.

Measurement

Ionizing radiations may be measured in terms of: (1) total dose, measured by a photographic film suitably developed or a moving quartz fibre; (2) rate at which the dose is received, measured by a Geiger counter or scintillation counter.

Natural Radiation and Artificial Radiation

Man is exposed to ionizing radiations from various natural sources. Cosmic radiations are about twice as great near the poles of the earth as at the equator and terrestrial radiations vary according to the geophysical formation of any particular locality. In Britain the natural background radiations deliver a dose of 2 m.rem per week.

Very little information exists on the dose to the bone marrow from radioactivity ingested in foodstuffs but over the two-year period 1958–59 this was of the order of 20–30 m.rem; the dose from the natural sources to the bone marrow was 160–200 rem.

Buildings protect their inhabitants from cosmic radiations but the materials used in building, especially granite, may have slight radioactivity; chalk and limestone have a low natural radioactivity. Internal exposure due to K^{40} and C^{14} accounts for one-fifth of the total soft tissue dose. K^{40} is present as a constant fraction (10^{-9} curies per g.) of the natural potassium content of the body. About 2 m.rem per year are contributed by C^{14} formed in the atmosphere as the result of cosmic radiation. Internal exposure from naturally occurring radium (R^{226}) and mesothorium is of especial interest because these substances are metabolized like calcium and preferentially deposited in bone, hence subject the bone marrow to alpha, beta and gamma radiation. Strontium (Sr^{90}) is preferentially deposited in bone where it decays into its daughter nuclide yttrium (Y^{90}).

The individual dosage from man-made sources of irradiation may vary widely from the average for the whole population. Individual dosage depends on the use of diagnostic radiology, radiotherapy and possibly on occupational exposure. In England and Wales the average *per capita* dose has been estimated to be 25 m.rem per year but for individual persons the dose, for example from diagnostic X-ray of the lumbar spine, may be 1·5 to 100 m.rem to the bone marrow and up to 400 m.rem to the female gonads. In X-ray of the chest, considerable variation in dosage occurs according to the technique employed but in miniature mass X-rays of the chest, gonad doses of the order of 0·1–0·2 m.rem in women and 0·01–0·7 m.rem in men have been observed.

TABLE 14

THE 30-YEAR INTEGRATED DOSE FROM VARIOUS SOURCES IN UNITED KINGDOM

(Medical Research Council, 1960)

SOURCE OF RADIATION	ANNUAL DOSE RATE M.RAD PER YEAR
Natural background . . .	Range 85–106
Medical radiology: 1957 level* .	19
Miscellaneous sources . . .	Less than 0·5
Fall out:	
Maximum value for mean dose rate in any 30-year period from nuclear explosions up to November 1958	1·2

*If the diagnostic technique of 10 per cent. of hospitals showing highest doses was improved to average standard of other hospitals studied by M.R.C. Committee, this would be reduced to 10 m.rad.

It is not possible to say categorically that any dose of radiation will be without effect. The acceptable limit for the whole body dose is 200 rem (Medical Research Council, 1956) over a lifetime.

Action of Ionizing Radiations

Transfer of energy from ionizing radiations results in the production of ions. In the body the primary effect is the production of ions followed by alteration in the chemical structure of enzyme systems. As much of the body consists of water, H^+ and OH^- ions are produced, and possibly other highly reactive radicles, and presumably these ions influence enzyme systems. Depending on the intensity of effect, cellular death may ensue or there may be gross disturbance of metabolism. Cells undergoing mitosis are most sensitive to ionizing radiation, and chromosome damage may induce malignant changes and genetic abnormalities. It must be emphasized that induced mutations do not differ in quality from those which occur 'naturally'. Further, a malignant change in one cell does not necessarily mean tumour formation. Body tissues vary in their sensitivity to ionizing radiation and broadly this sensitivity depends on the frequency of mitosis. Considerable repair process in tissues and metabolic process occurs, providing the dose and dose rate allow of this.

Effects of Ionizing Radiations

The effects of ionizing radiations depend on:

1. Dose: In adults, the effects of whole body ionizing radiations (excluding the long-term possibility of malignant disease and genetic consequences) are:
   - 50 rem—possible blood changes but no overt illness.
   - 50–100 rem—blood changes likely, some minor injury but no disability.
   - 100–200 rem—mild illness in some individuals.
   - 200–500 rem—illness with rising mortality.
   - 500 rem—case mortality up to 50 per cent.
   - over 500 rem—rapidly rising mortality.
   - over 1000 rem—fatal.

2. The nature of the radiation: Alpha particles are of little significance when received from an external source (mainly because of low powers of penetration) but when originating from deposits in bone may cause aplastic anaemia and osteosarcoma.
3. The tissue or organ subject to radiation. The lymphatic tissues, bone marrow, germinal epithelium of the testes and the cornea are especially sensitive. Brain and muscle are the least sensitive.
4. The manner of administration. The dose may be received almost instantly or over a period, either fractionally at intervals or continuously. There is some evidence to suggest that doses over a period, need to be slightly bigger to produce the same effect. A dose received over a brief period is generally more damaging.
5. In the case of radio-nuclides, absorbed into the body (radium, Na^{24}, C^{14}, I^{131}, Sr^{90}) the half-life of the radio-nuclide and its rate of excretion. Further, the distribution of radio-nuclides is important. For example, Na^{24} is distributed generally and I^{131} is concentrated in the thyroid.

Radiation Syndromes

With extremely high doses, 2000 rem and over, death may occur in a few minutes to a few hours, apparently due to damage to the brain and nervous system. With less severe, but still lethal dose, the order of events depends on the dose and whether a particular organ has been the target for most of the dose. Nausea and vomiting appear almost at once, to be succeeded by diarrhoea. A temporary phase of improvement may occur after 48 hours to be followed about the fifth day by vomiting, diarrhoea (which becomes bloody), dehydration, haemoconcentration, profound disturbance of the electrolyte balance, circulatory collapse and death. If the patient lives sufficiently long, all cellular constituents of the blood will be severely depressed. Epilation and erythema of the skin are likely after the first week.

With lower (though potentially fatal) doses, initial symptoms of nausea, vomiting and diarrhoea occur and are followed by temporary amelioriation. After about 3 weeks, loss of appetite, extreme fatigue, breathlessness and fever appear. Infection is a serious risk. A severe leucopenia is present and immature and abnormal white cells are found in the blood. At about the sixth week agranulocytosis, aplastic anaemia, thrombocytopenia, purpura and intestinal ulceration may cause deterioration. Where death does not occur, recovery is likely to be very prolonged. Signs of target damage may appear, e.g. an acute myocarditis if the heart has been grossly radiated. As the radiation must have passed through the skin, erythema of the exposed area starts about the end of the first week to be followed by blistering and exfoliation. Small bleeding areas appear. A panarteritis is nearly always present and this may cause gangrene, e.g. of fingers and toes. If the patient does not die, contractures are usual. The regenerated skin is atrophic and telangiectases are common. Hairs are absent or sparse.

With smaller (and sublethal) doses, acute symptoms are mild or absent but after an interval leucopenia and depression of all the cellular elements of the blood, diarrhoea and epilation may be observed.

Internal radiation does not produce radiation syndromes but acts on the tissue in which radioactivity is concentrated (e.g. bone).

Effect on Specific Tissues

Lymphatic system. Leucopenia is an early sign of over-exposure. Exposure to ionizing radiations appears to be related to the occurrence of leukaemia, for example in persons treated by X-rays for spondylitis.

Gonads. The germinal epithelium of the testes is more sensitive than that of the ovaries.

Bone marrow. All elements of the bone marrow are severely depressed, leading to agranulocytosis, aplastic anaemia and thrombocytopenia. Abnormal and immature cells are found in the blood. Myeloid leukaemia is a late complication.

Blood Vessels. Increased permeability, oedema of the vessel wall and surrounding tissues and haemorrhage occur.

Gastro-intestinal system. The epithelium ulcerates and haemorrhage is made worse by the vascular changes.

Eyes. A postcortical cataract is very likely to develop.

Skin. The skin effects of large acute doses are described above. Early effects are best demonstrated by serial photographs of the finger nails and serial examination of the fingerprints. Healed skin is atrophic and sensitive to damage. The chronic radio-dermatitis affecting early radiologists was typified by atrophy, hyperkeratosis, ulceration together with underlying panarteritis. Malignant changes were frequent. The condition was very painful.

Bone. Radium selectively deposited in bone may cause an osteosarcoma (as well as depression of the bone marrow). Areas of necrosis may develop.

Genetically Permissible Dose

Because ionizing radiations may accelerate mutations, they are of considerable genetic importance. In this respect, the population dose (i.e. the dose received by all individuals averaged over the population) is significant. The genetic dose to a population is the dose which if it was received by each person from conception to the mean age of childbearing (assumed for purposes of calculation to be 30 years) would result in the same burden to the population as do the actual doses received by the individuals. Over and above the dose from natural radiation, the average genetic dose should not exceed 5 rem.

Much confusion has been occasioned by the use of the term threshold dose, implying that effects do not occur until a limit has been exceeded. Certainly, effects are more likely with big doses, and if the dose is small enough the chances of effects occurring may be negligible. Such a concept, however, fails to take into account the large number of persons exposed to medical use of radiations (about 1 in 10 persons are subject annually to diagnostic procedures). In the long run, the number of cases of disease will be the product of the size of the population at risk, the years of exposure and the probability in each year of development of the disease.

In Britain, the genetic dose averaged over the population from natural background can be assumed to be 3 rem before 30 years of age. The International Commission on Radiological Protection (1958) has recommended that any additional genetic dose should be reduced to 5 rem over 30 years and 'apportioned' as follows:

Occupational exposure 1·0 rem	5 rem
Exposure of special groups 0·5 rem	
Exposure of population at large 2·0 rem	
Reserve 1·5 rem	

For persons over 18 years of age and for critical organs (gonads, bone marrow, lens), the cumulative occupational exposure from external and internal radiations should not exceed $D=5(N-18)$ where D=dose in rem, N=age in years, which means the maximum weekly occupational exposure to the gonads is 0·1 rem.

Prevention

Protection against external radiations is based on: (1) distance from the primary source and any secondary source (gamma and X-rays diminish in proportion to the square of the distance and beta radiations slow down rapidly); (2) provision of absorbing barriers (e.g. lead, barium, concrete); (3) limitation of the period of exposure; (4) the use of unidirectional beams by fitting suitable collimators to the source; (5) avoidance of scatter and reflection of radiations; (6) wearing of protective clothing; (7) personal monitoring (wearing of photographic badges or dosimeters) to determine the dose received; (8) environmental monitoring. For monitoring purposes, the exposure is expressed in rads, as the air dose rather than the body dose is measured and also because physical instruments of measurement cannot take into account the variable factor of biological effectiveness. For practical purposes, however, the Q.F. is unity for the commonly met radiations. The definition of safe procedures and monitoring requires expert physical knowledge, and the advice of a health physicist is essential.

The basic principle of industrial protection embodied in the Ionizing Radiation (Sealed Sources) Regulations, 1969 and Ionizing Radiation (Unsealed Radioactive Substances) Regulations, 1968, is that of adequate shielding of source and/or distance from the source as the inverse square law applies for which a barrier (or other suitable demarcation) is created beyond which the dose rate to which an occupationally exposed person (classified worker) can be exposed does not exceed 2·5 m.rem per hour and for other workers 0·75 m.rem per hour. Exposure at these levels for a 40-hour week would correspond to 5 rem per year and 1·5 rem per year respectively (as recommended by the International Commission on Radiological Protection). Only classified workers are required to submit to medical examination.

All persons about to take up work necessitating exposure to ionizing radiations should be subject to medical examination but periodic medical examination has little part to play in control. The pre-employment examination should be in great detail to provide basic records in the event of a catastrophe. Special attention should be paid to the blood, the presence of sepsis, enlargement of lymph nodes and to the skin. Blood films should be examined for atypical cells. Particular attention should be paid to a history of previous occupational or medical exposure. Pregnant women should not be employed in occupations involving exposure to ionizing radiations, or otherwise exposed if at all avoidable. This, however, is a concept of perfection as women may not know they are pregnant when the foetus is most at hazard.

The handling of unsealed sources such as radium, thorium and caesium should follow the usual principles of enclosure, exhaust ventilation of operating booths and boxes. All operating surfaces should be impervious, monitored for contamination and washed thoroughly at frequent intervals.

Radioactive wastes must be disposed of safely. This may involve dilution so that radioactivity is below an acceptable level, concentration into a small bulk for dumping in disused mines or at sea, or other chemical treatment.

REFERENCES

Very few substances used in industry can be said to be harmless; many are toxic and some very toxic. References to the substances described in this Section and to the many other substances not included will be found in the following publications.

BARNES, J. (1967) *Pesticides*, 3rd Symposium on Advanced Medicine, Royal College of Physicians, London.

BROWNING, ETHEL (1953) *Toxicity of Inorganic Solvents*, M.R.C. Industrial Health Research Board Report No. 80, London, H.M.S.O.

BROWNING, ETHEL (1961) *Toxicity of Industrial Metals*, London.

HUNTER, D. (1969) *The Diseases of Occupations*, 4th ed., London.

KING, E. J., and FLETCHER, C. M., eds (1960) *Industrial Pulmonary Diseases*, London.

LLOYD DAVIES, T. A. (1957) *The Practice of Industrial Medicine*, 2nd ed., London.

MEREWETHER, E. R. A., ed. (1954) *Industrial Medicine and Hygiene*, London.

SCHILLING, R. S. F., ed. (1960) *Modern Trends in Occupational Health*, London.

T. A. LLOYD DAVIES

DISORDERS DUE TO CLIMATIC, ENVIRONMENTAL AND OTHER PHYSICAL FACTORS

EXPOSURE TO HEAT

INTRODUCTION

The clinical effects of exposure to high ambient temperatures result from: (1) interference with the mechanisms regulating heat production and loss and the body temperature; (2) cardiovascular disturbances, usually associated with the processes of acclimatization; and (3) disturbances in the water-electrolyte balance in the tissues. The clinical pictures associated with the first are heat pyrexia and hyperpyrexia and thermogenic anhidrosis. Those determined by changes in water and salt balance are the syndromes of heat exhaustion, i.e. predominant salt depletion and predominant water depletion.

The syndromes may appear as entities or may be associated.

HEAT HYPERPYREXIA

Synonyms. Heat stroke; Hyperthermia.

Definition and Aetiology

Heat pyrexia is a rise of body temperature following exposure to intense heat as in the desert or in an engine room. In mild forms of the syndrome the patient is conscious and sweating. When the oral temperature rises to 106° F. (41·1° C.), with central nervous signs and absence of sweating, the condition is regarded as hyperpyrexia; it should be noted, however, that the syndrome may develop at body temperatures below this. When the onset is very rapid and the picture is accompanied by coma and generalized anhidrosis it is commonly called heat stroke.

The pyrexia arises as a result of exposure to heat and not to light. Exposure must be continuous, usually for hours. Short exposures to very high temperatures seldom precipitate the hyperpyrexic syndrome.

Hyperpyrexia occurs most commonly in subjects who are unacclimatized to very high ambient temperatures or to heavy work at more moderate temperatures (as in mines). It may appear in any race (although less commonly in pigmented individuals), either sex and at any age. It appears more commonly in obese persons. Predisposing factors are usually associated with interference with evaporation of sweat or its production. These include excessive or ill-ventilated clothing, lack of air movement especially in enclosed spaces, and existing febrile illness. Over-production of body metabolic heat as in hyperthyroidism or from excessive muscular activity may also serve as an initiating factor. Excessive intake of alcohol may in itself predispose to heat stroke by increasing the metabolic production of heat, by peripheral vasodilatation and by causing dehydration.

The syndrome may be precipitated by the administration of sweat-inhibiting drugs such as atropine. It is a foreseeable risk in individuals with congenital defect of sweating.

Pathology

The primary pathogenic process in the development and progress of hyperpyrexia is usually considered to be a central failure of sweating, resulting in serious interference with loss of body heat. This view has recently been challenged by some workers who have described cases with very high fever and sweating.

The pathological lesions seen at autopsy in hyperpyrexic patients depend on whether the cause of death was predominantly the very high body temperature or the development of medical shock. In the former case the lesions are primarily neuronal, with degeneration and sometimes necrosis of the nerve cells especially in the cerebellum (where the Purkinje cells are chiefly involved) and the cerebral cortex; in cases which have survived for some days the damaged areas may be infiltrated with glial cells. In shocked cases there may be brain oedema, vascular congestion and scattered small haemorrhages in the brain substance. The lesions are commonest in the deep layers of the cerebral cortex and in the region of the basal nuclei; the cerebellum may be unaffected.

Pathological lesions in other parts of the body result largely from the current vascular failure. They include centrilobular necrosis in the liver and the usual picture of renal anoxia with ischaemic glomeruli and tubular degeneration. In shocked cases there are often petechial haemorrhages into endothelial and mucous membranes particularly in the upper small intestine, peritoneum and pleura.

Clinical Picture

Moderate rise in the body temperature occurs commonly on exposure to heat especially during exercise. In most instances the body is able to adjust the situation readily and the resulting pyrexia, which is neither serious nor of long duration, is accompanied by sweating and minimal signs of central nervous involvement, including restlessness and anxiety.

If the temperature continues to rise, hyperpyrexia may supervene. This usually develops quickly, sometimes dramatically. The onset of clinical signs is abrupt and often without prodromal symptoms, although some patients may complain for a few hours before the onset of intense thirst, headache, dizziness, restlessness and may become progressively confused; some may observe an increasing failure of sweating after exercise.

When the syndrome has developed, the patient exhibits three cardinal features. There are cerebral signs and symptoms, a hot dry skin and very high oral and rectal temperatures.

In most cases the patient is restless, disorientated,

delirious or comatose when he is first seen. When the onset is very rapid, coma develops quickly and deepens. Convulsions and muscular twitching in the limbs may be present. The signs of cerebral involvement vary in form and in intensity in individual patients, and their severity usually depends on the degree and duration of the high fever.

The skin is usually flushed, occasionally pale. It is dry over the whole body, due to absence of sweating; cyanosis of the face and lips is common.

The oral temperature is 106° F. (41·1° C.) or higher, sometimes over 110° F. (43·5° C.); the rectal temperature is about 1° F. (0·6° C.) higher. The pulse is fast, 130 beats or more per minute. There may be soft systolic murmurs and transient changes in the electrocardiogram, with diphasic and inverted T waves indicating myocardial dysfunction, and occasionally disturbances of rhythm. The blood pressure is normal unless shock has appeared. In the latter event the temperature falls rapidly, sometimes to below normal.

The respiratory rate is high. Breathing is shallow at first, becoming stertorous and later intermittent or with Cheyne-Stokes rhythm. There is sometimes extreme hyperpnoea, which may lead to alkalotic tetany. In the late stages accompanying shock, there may be progressive evidence of pulmonary oedema. Watery diarrhoea, sometimes with dark blood, is common and may lead to dehydration; there is often incontinence.

If there is concurrent salt depletion, the volume of urine will be low and there is little excretion of salt. Where there has been prodromal thirst, heavy consumption of fluid may cause temporary polyuria. In shock, anuria and uraemia may develop.

The serum non-protein nitrogen is usually raised and there is commonly a decrease in numbers of thrombocytes.

Diagnosis

The triad of high fever, dry skin and cerebral signs, associated with the history of continued exposure to high environmental temperatures usually makes the tentative diagnosis obvious.

Definite diagnosis must distinguish hyperpyrexias from other causes of which by far the most important is falciparum malaria. The blood must always be examined for parasites. Other conditions in which hyperpyrexia may occur include typhus fevers, tetanus, meningococcal or pneumococcal meningitis and cerebral accidents especially when involving the pons.

Treatment

Effective cooling is required in order to reduce the rectal temperature to about 102° F. (38·9° C.) within one hour.

A slatted table similar to that devised by Guthrie is advisable in geographical or occupational areas where heat hyperpyrexia is a possibility. This provides cooling by convection and evaporation by spraying as much as possible of the body with cold water, combined with active air movement. Alternatively the naked patient may be placed in a tub containing water and ice chips. The body and limbs should be massaged during cooling to promote the peripheral circulation. Consciousness often returns by the end of cooling, with improvement in breathing and pulse rate.

The rectal temperature is checked every 3 minutes. When it has fallen to 102° F. (38·9° C.) the patient is transferred to bed in a cool room. As a rule the temperature continues to fall, reaching about 100° F. (37·8° C.). If the body temperature is allowed to fall much lower than 102° F. (38·9° C.) during active cooling it may subsequently fall rapidly to subnormal and shock may develop.

In many cases there may be further rises of temperature occurring 12–24 hours after the initial cooling. These can usually be controlled by tepid sponging. The temperature regulation may continue unstable for up to a week; the ability to sweat returns in favourable cases within a few hours to several days after cooling.

Unfavourable responses may occur in cases in which the hyperpyrexia has persisted for some hours or longer before treatment, or in which the initial cooling has been too slow, or allowed to continue until the temperature is too low. Acute renal failure occurs in some cases, with progressive uraemia. Jaundice, sometimes associated with centrilobular hepatic degeneration, appears in some patients, usually in those in whom peripheral vascular collapse has occurred.

Chlorpromazine may be given in doses of 25–50 mg. intravenously, in conjunction with physical cooling. It is especially useful in cases in which restlessness or convulsions are prominent.

Antimalarial drugs should be given parenterally if there is any reason at all to suspect falciparum malaria whether or not facilities for immediate diagnosis of parasites in the blood are available.

Shock should be dealt with by the administration of oxygen and intravenous infusion of 5 per cent. glucose in isotonic saline with the usual precautions. Cardiac stimulants such as amphetamine, strophanthus and digitalis have been recommended but are of unproven value. Metaraminol is useful in hypotensive patients in doses of 5–10 mg. intravenously or 200 mg. added to 500 ml. saline dextrose, given by intravenous drip. Corticosteroids have been advised by some authors in view of the occasional occurrence of adrenal haemorrhages.

Sequelae are predominantly neurological. The commonest are persistent or recurrent headache, attacks of dizziness, insomnia, varying degrees of amnesia and personality changes. There may be signs of cerebellar and occasionally pyramidal dysfunction. Most sequelae clear with time; ataxia is said to be the most persistent.

Prognosis

The untreated case of hyperpyrexia will die, death resulting from the high temperature, or from medical shock. In the latter case the pulse rate rises and the temperature rapidly falls. The skin becomes pale, slightly cyanosed and sometimes moist. The blood pressures fall catastrophically and the circulating blood volume is reduced, associated with a rise in apparent haemoglobin concentration.

With adequate treatment the mortality is low in cases caught in time. Over-all mortality varies from 20 to 30 per cent. Death occurs within two days in hyperpyrexia in most cases; some cases survive with high fever for over a week. Death in later cases usually occurs from shock.

Prognosis is dependent on the height and duration of fever before treatment is commenced, and on the development of shock. It is worse in cases with very acute onset, with a very high fever or early development of shock.

ANHIDROTIC HEAT EXHAUSTION

Synonyms. Thermogenic anhidrosis; Tropical anhidrotic asthenia; Heat exhaustion type II.

Definition and Aetiology

A syndrome which develops after months of continuous exposure to a hot environment (usually humid), characterized by exhaustion, partial and irregularly disposed loss of sweating and the appearance on the trunk and upper limbs of vesicular skin lesions (mammillaria or milaria profunda). The syndrome may or may not be associated with disturbance of water-electrolyte balance or of the cardiovascular system. There is no generally accepted explanation of the anhidrosis. The chloride content of the sweat is usually high, suggesting some 'exhaustion' of the glands. In the anhidrotic areas where the mammillaria occur, changes are found in a proportion but not all of the sweat glands; hypertrophied keratotic tissue appears to obstruct the gland ducts, leading to retention of secretion and rupture into the contiguous epithelium which becomes disorganized and forms the characteristic vesicle. The failure of sweating is regarded by some authors as central, by others as peripheral; some suggest it results from hormonal imbalance.

Clinical Picture

The syndrome develops in persons who have been exposed for at least several months to high ambient temperatures, usually in moist conditions. When developed it may prevent the patient from doing active work, but it is usually swiftly amenable to treatment. Occasionally the anhidrosis may become complete and in these circumstances heat hyperpyrexia may occur. Most patients give a history of recent prickly heat which improved shortly before the anhidrotic heat exhaustion began to develop.

During the hot period of the day the patient complains of fatigue even at rest. During and after physical work he becomes increasingly asthenic and disinterested. He suffers in addition frontal headache, some giddiness and tachycardia, with palpitations. Subjective feelings of uncomfortable warmth may be experienced, with 'tightness' of the skin areas in which the mammillaria begin to appear. At this stage the breathing is often fast and exaggerated. Most patients note an increasing reduction in sweating on the body but not on the face or in the axillae. The symptoms ease with rest. Gradually over some weeks they become more severe and periods of rest become longer, until the patient is practically unable to work.

When seen in the exhausted state the patient is often restless and apprehensive.

The pulse rate is fast and respiration deep and fast. Blood pressures are usually normal.

The oral temperature is commonly between 99° and 102° F. (37·2° and 38·9° C.).

The skin is dry over large areas of the trunk and limbs. Sweating is free on the face and neck and the groin, axillae, palms and soles are usually moist.

Mammillaria are scattered in the dry areas of the skin, especially on the trunk and the proximal parts of the limbs. The area involved is covered with myriads of discrete papules, most of which are capped with a minute vesicle containing clear fluid. There is no erythema about the lesions, which distinguishes them from those of prickly heat, and the skin hairs are not involved, as they are in so-called 'goose flesh'. There is usually no pruritus. The mammillaria commonly develop first on the arms and may spread to the trunk, or appear in unassociated areas.

Lesions are not found where sweating is active and are thus seldom present on the head and neck.

Diagnosis

In mild cases it is difficult to distinguish this syndrome from malingering. Localized absence of sweating after exercise (or administration of pilocarpine) is the important point in such cases, which may present before the skin lesions have developed. When facilities are available the chloride content of the sweat may be measured; it is usually high in the genuine case.

The presence of febrile illnesses must be excluded, particularly malaria.

Identification of mammillaria on patches of anhidrotic skin and their differentiation from the lesions of prickly heat usually establishes the diagnosis in the febrile exhausted patient.

In the absence of concurrent salt depletion the chloride content of the urine is normal.

Treatment

In the absence of salt or water depletion or both, the only treatment required is rest in a cool room. The fever, fast pulse and dyspnoea rapidly subside. The mammillaria disappear slowly and are usually succeeded by some desquamation. Ability to exercise begins to return in a few days. Sweating becomes normal in about 2 weeks.

Relapse is common. The patient should therefore be removed from the hot environment.

HEAT SYNCOPE

Synonyms. Exercise-induced heat exhaustion; Heat collapse.

Definition and Aetiology

Syncope, giddiness or fatigue arising during exposure, resulting from pooling peripheral venous blood with failure to maintain the cerebral flow, in the absence of demonstrable salt or water depletion.

The condition is seen in unacclimatized individuals very soon after exposure to heat. Residents in hot climates are usually affected only when performing excessive exercise or when there is a sudden rise of environmental temperature or humidity.

Clinical Picture

In mild cases the patient feels increasingly dizzy and nauseated. He complains of epigastric discomfort and blurred vision; he often yawns repeatedly and may have an urgent desire to defaecate. The attack usually comes on after prolonged standing or sudden change of posture, for example, standing after sitting or lying down. He is intensely pale; the skin is cold and clammy and there is often excessive sweating on the forehead and palms.

Relief may be obtained by sitting or lying down but the patient may faint, as the systolic blood pressure falls rapidly.

At first the pulse is fast, but it is often slow after the faint.

More serious patterns with raised rectal temperature (up to 102° F. (38·9° C.)) occur in individuals who have been over-exercising.

Recovery is rapid in cool surroundings. However, if the patient has to remain in the heat, he may not recover completely for some hours. After a few days of exposure acclimatization is effected in most individuals and heat syncope will occur only after violent exercise.

Some individuals appear more susceptible than others.

Diagnosis

The circumstances in which the episode takes place and the rapid recovery of the patient are diagnostic.

Alternative causes of loss of consciousness must be excluded. Syncope may occur in moderate salt or water depletion, and loss of consciousness may induce heat stroke.

Treatment

In the patient suffering from heat syncope some degree of salt depletion may have already become established. In such cases salted drinks should be given. Otherwise rest in the recumbent position in cool surroundings, with fluids by mouth is all that is immediately required. The salt/water balance in each case must be determined and the patient should be kept from unnecessary exertion until acclimatization can be established.

WATER DEPLETION HEAT EXHAUSTION

Synonym. Water deficiency exhaustion or dehydration.

Definition

Water depletion resulting from inadequate replacement of water losses arising from prolonged sweating. The picture is characterized by pronounced thirst, with fatigue, giddiness, and developing oliguria and fever. In advanced cases delirium may be followed by coma and death.

Aetiology

The severest form of the syndrome develops in individuals entirely deprived of fresh-water intake, as when stranded in a desert or adrift at sea. During working hours in the tropics, water intake usually fails to keep pace with losses in sweat, in insensible perspiration and in respired air. The deficit which results (voluntary dehydration) is usually made good in leisure hours, if water is available. When water is limited, however, the deficit remains and may build up. Even in these circumstances, however, no clinical effects may become evident unless there are sudden further demands due to increased activity or intercurrent diarrhoea and vomiting.

The clinical features of water depletion are presumed to be dependent on the following changes in water-electrolyte balance in the body.

As water depletion develops there is eventually a reduction in volume and increase in osmolarity of the extracellular fluid. Water then moves from the cells to the latter, the reverse of the situation in salt depletion. Despite the rising plasma sodium concentration, resorption of this ion via the renal tubules increases and potassium excretion continues unchecked. The osmolarity of the extracellular fluid thus rises out of proportion to that of the diminished intracellular fluid. Some reduction in plasma volume occurs and the concentrations of sodium chloride, urea and protein rise; since fluid loss is shared by the erythrocytes, there is, however, no corresponding rise in haematocrit.

Clinical Picture

The earliest and most impressive symptom of water depletion is thirst, with dry tongue and mouth, difficulty in eating and swallowing, and anorexia. Fatigue is progressive. Weight is rapidly lost. The patient feels weak and becomes apprehensive and panicky. He is restless and may become hysterical and unco-ordinated. The situation is often worsened by excessive and incautious activity. The lips, mouth and throat are dry and the voice hoarse. Delirium develops, then coma and finally death. Survival time ranges from hours up to 10 days, depending on the ambient temperature and the patient's muscular activities (for example walking in the heat).

The urinary output per day is low in individuals in any state of water depletion. When the syndrome has developed it is low from the beginning and falls to 300–500 ml. Oliguria may give place to anuria especially after the advent of shock in the late stages.

In the early stages the skin is unchanged but as the syndrome develops it becomes 'dehydrated', inelastic and stretched over the bony prominences, especially of the face.

The pulse rate quickens, the pulse pressure falls and the effects of standing after lying recumbent become exaggerated. Finally the pulse rate becomes very fast and vascular failure may develop. The body temperature rises and in some cases hyperpyrexia may supervene.

The breathing rate increases and cyanosis may appear. In the late stages tetany may follow hyperventilation.

Recent work has shown that in voluntary water

depletion the sweat rate falls with the body weight (used as a measure of water loss), indicating that even at this early stage depletion is potentially dangerous, especially if extra work is suddenly demanded.

Diagnosis

Water depletion may sometimes be difficult to distinguish from salt depletion, and the two conditions may occur concurrently, although one or other predominates.

The circumstances in which the syndrome develops are usually diagnostic. Since relatively more water than salt is lost in heavy sweating, the appearance of water depletion in those already in voluntary depletion is more rapid than that of salt depletion. The extreme thirst and the absence of adequate available water supply are important diagnostic points. In water depletion, muscle cramps do not occur, vomiting is uncommon, sweating is diminished, the concentrated urine contains appreciable amounts of chloride, the plasma sodium concentration is raised above normal.

In endemic areas the possibility of falciparum malaria must be excluded by examination of the blood.

Treatment

The patient should rest in bed in a cooled room. He should be given a high fluid intake, orally if possible, otherwise parenterally. The temperature may be reduced by sponging. Body weight should be measured daily and a fluid intake/output record must be kept.

If the patient can take fluid orally, he should be given up to 8 litres in the first day as cool flavoured drinks containing, with the food, a normal amount of salt. The volume of each specimen of urine passed should be measured.

Fluid replacement by the intravenous route is needed in serious dehydration and unconscious patients. If the case is one of obvious water depletion, 5 per cent. glucose may be administered. If there is any possibility that salt depletion exists, isotonic saline should be given, as below [p. 373]. The total fluid needed in 24 hours is rarely more than 4–5 litres.

Clinical recovery is prompt, with rapidly increasing urinary output and return to normal weight.

Complications such as anuria require standard treatment. Coexistent falciparum malaria may require parenteral therapy.

SALT DEPLETION HEAT EXHAUSTION

Synonyms. Heat exhaustion type I; Salt-deficiency heat exhaustion.

Definition

A syndrome brought about by loss of salt and its inadequate replacement following prolonged sweating. It is characterized by fatigue, nausea, vomiting, giddiness, muscular cramps and varying degrees of dehydration and cardiovascular disturbances, including circulatory failure in severe cases. The body temperature is seldom raised much above normal.

Aetiology

The condition is seen most frequently in individuals who have been carrying out hard work in hot conditions, with salt intake inadequate to replace the losses of sodium and chloride during heavy sweating. The deficit of sodium is believed to be the factor of primary significance in the development of this form of heat exhaustion.

It occurs particularly in individuals unacclimatized to working in a hot environment. It may appear in either sex at any age. Predisposing factors include co-existent febrile illnesses, especially malaria, and gastro-intestinal disturbances involving diarrhoea and vomiting.

When an individual in favourable salt balance is exposed to heat, physiological salt-saving adaptations occur in a few days, involving reduction of sweat salt content and maximal resorption of sodium and chloride by the renal tubules. When first exposed to hot working conditions, he may lose well over a litre of sweat per hour containing as much as 4 g. salt per litre. In this way he may become salt-depleted before acclimatization can occur unless he compensates for the excessive losses by increasing salt intake. When he has become acclimatized, as is the case in permanent residents in the tropics or in adapted workers in hot environments such as mines, he is able to remain in salt balance with relatively small increase in intake. A minimal intake is undesirable, however, since it makes the individual vulnerable to abnormal losses of electrolytes arising from vomiting or diarrhoea or the reduction in intake during anorexia.

Clinical Picture

Salt depletion heat exhaustion presents in a wide range of severity. Mild cases are of little clinical consequence and are easily combated. Severe cases are dehydrated and shocked.

There is usually a prodromal stage lasting several days from the first feeling of fatigue, with headache, anorexia, mild nausea, fleeting muscle cramps, giddiness and sometimes unsteadiness of gait and sometimes 'spots in front of the eyes' and tinnitus. The patient sweats freely and the urinary output is low.

The onset in the moderate and severe case is usually accompanied by nausea and some vomiting, especially following the ingestion of large volumes of water. The vomiting is frequently succeeded by muscular cramps.

The patient is exhausted and asthenic; there is almost always some recent loss of weight. In the more severe case he may be restless and anxious or lightly comatose. Otherwise, central nervous signs are not obvious.

The oral temperature is seldom raised above normal. In severe cases it is subnormal. The skin is cold, pale, moist and inelastic; when dehydration is severe, it is stretched over the bony prominences such as the malar bones and the facies is pinched and the eyes look sunken. There may be profuse sweating.

The pulse rate is fast in most cases; the volume is small. In the mild and moderate case the systolic blood pressure commonly ranges from 100 to 110 mm.Hg. The vascular system is, however, unstable and a considerable increase in heart rate and fall of blood pressure occurs when the patient suddenly stands after being in the recumbent position. Under these circumstances he feels very dizzy and may faint.

In severe cases oligaemic vascular failure develops. The shocked patient is usually comatose. He has a pale clammy skin, very fast shallow pulse and a low systolic blood pressure. At first the diastolic pressure may be maintained but it falls as the shock progresses and may become unmeasurable. The circulating blood volume is diminished. The breathing is fast and shallow, deep, stertorous or intermittent. Pulmonary oedema may occur in the late stages.

There is usually persistent nausea and most patients vomit. In many cases vomiting is followed by muscular cramps, fleeting or severe, occurring especially in the legs, arms and abdominal muscles. Muscle cramps occur in two cases in three. They are often precipitated by a large intake of unsalted water. They may last several minutes and are agonizing and dreaded by the conscious patient; they occur in the comatose patient, causing stirring and restlessness. Tetanic carpopedal spasm has been reported.

Renal Function. In mild forms of the syndrome there may be some reduction in urinary output. The urine is moderately concentrated and contains negligible amounts of sodium chloride. In severe cases the urinary output is considerably reduced and may be of the order of only 300–500 ml. per day. Sodium chloride is usually absent. In shocked patients there may be anuria with developing uraemia.

The Blood. Plasma and whole blood sodium and chloride concentrations are reduced in severe cases; changes in potassium concentrations are not consistent. Due to haemoconcentration arising from loss of circulatory plasma volume, the haemoglobin concentration, erythrocyte count and haematocrit are raised, plasma protein is raised and blood urea N is always high. The latter continues to rise in shocked cases in which anuric uraemia has developed.

Diagnosis

The history of exposure to hot ambient temperatures or hot working conditions, the appearance of the patient, vomiting, muscle cramps, oliguria and the absence of sodium chloride in the urine are diagnostic. In severe cases other causes of shock must be excluded. Falciparum malaria must always be excluded by examination of the blood for parasites.

The chloride content of the urine should be measured if facilities exist. In salt depletion the output may be 1–3 g. per litre of urine, or less.

Distinguishing salt depletion from predominant water exhaustion may occasionally be difficult in circumstances where the urinary chloride cannot be estimated; in water exhaustion the chloride content is normal.

Treatment

The object is to restore the electrolyte-water balance and the blood volume. This is done by administration of salt solution (never water only).

The patients should be put to bed in a cooled ventilated room.

Mild cases can be treated orally with 5 or more litres of water in the first 24 hours containing a total of about 25 g. salt, given in fluids and foods such as soups and fruit drinks; salt tablets should be avoided as they are not always absorbed.

Severe and shocked cases need parenteral fluid. 500 ml. of isotonic saline is given quickly, in 15–20 minutes. An initial 500 ml. plasma may be given in shock. Thereafter the infusion may be given more slowly, up to 5 litres in the first 24 hours. As soon as the patient can retain oral fluids parenteral treatment should be stopped. It is seldom necessary to continue it beyond the first day.

Throughout treatment the volume of each specimen of urine passed should be measured in order to watch for the development of anuria.

The urinary chloride concentration should also be estimated from time to time during parenteral therapy. When it begins to rise, saline glucose solution (1 part isotonic saline: 2 parts isotonic glucose) should be substituted for isotonic saline.

Response to treatment is rapid unless renal complications have developed. There is no reason why the patient should not return to work after undergoing a period of acclimatization.

HEAT CRAMPS

Painful cramps similar to those described in salt depletion heat exhaustion may occur in voluntary muscles in individuals working in the heat, such as miners, sugar-cane cutters and firemen.

They occur after heavy sweating and concurrent drinking of large quantities of unsalted fluid. This suggests that the muscle spasms may be due to extracellular salt dilution rather than to salt depletion as such. As in the latter, however, water apparently moves into the cells causing over-dilution or so-called 'water intoxication'.

The cramps appear late in the working day, after some hours of hard work. They are intensely painful and commonly involve the legs and the arms. They last a minute or so, and recur at intervals for hours. Occasionally they are very severe and incapacitate the patient. Involuntary muscles usually escape. The chloride concentration in urine passed during the cramps is considerably reduced.

Most severe attacks respond to the single intravenous administration of 300–500 ml. isotonic saline in 5–10 minutes. Salt balance is later adjusted orally while the patient rests in a cool room. Mild attacks respond to salt given orally.

REFERENCES

LEITHEAD, C. S., and LIND, A. R. (1964) *Heat Stress and Heat Disorders*, London.

WORLD HEALTH ORGANIZATION (1969) Health factors involved in working under conditions of heat stress, *Tech. Rep. Ser.*, No. 412.

BRIAN MAEGRAITH

EXPOSURE TO COLD

INTRODUCTION

The adverse effects of cold upon the human body are of two kinds. In the first, which may be called 'cold injury', exposure of one anatomical region, usually one foot or both feet, to intense cold causes local tissue damage. In the second, hypothermia, a low circumambient temperature leads to a fall in that of the body, sufficient to cause serious constitutional disturbance.

COLD INJURY

Cold injury is for obvious reasons virtually limited to the extremities, although it has occurred elsewhere with surface cooling for induction of hypothermia for surgical purposes. Two main varieties can be recognized.

IMMERSION FOOT

This has been common in survivors of shipwreck and in those whose feet have been immersed for long periods in water which is cold, but not freezing. It was a familiar problem in soldiers serving in the trenches during the First World War and was then called 'trench foot'.

The underlying disturbance is an intense arterial spasm without irreversible damage to vessels or skin. Clinically in the initial ischaemic phase the foot is cold and white, this is followed by hyperaemia when it becomes red, hot and throbbing. Ischaemia may be sufficiently prolonged to cause a neuropathy with burning paraesthesia, often lasting for months.

Treatment is to warm the foot gently in the first phase and to cool it equally gently in the second.

FROST BITE

The distinction from immersion foot is largely one of degree. The exposure to cold is more prolonged and the temperature lower. In frost bite there is occlusion of small vessels due to thrombosis, endothelial damage and aggregations of erythrocytes. The skin is affected by the consequent ischaemia as well as by the direct action of low temperature. The ischaemia is not succeeded by hyperaemia, for it depends on vascular occlusion and not on vasospasm.

Treatment consists of allowing the foot to regain normal temperature by careful insulation at bed rest in a warm room. Active warming is to be avoided. Smoking must be prohibited. The foot must be carefully protected from injury and here this term includes tight bandaging, physiotherapy and drainage of blisters. Vasodilator drugs, especially nicotinamide and hexamethonium, appear to have some value.

American experience in the Korean war proved that nearly 50 per cent. of survivors of frost bite were left with permanent disability, including pain, cold feet, stiff joints, numbness and hyperidrosis.

HYPOTHERMIA

Hypothermia may be induced or accidental. The first is extensively used in 'open heart' surgery to reduce the metabolic needs of the body, and is not considered here. Accidental hypothermia is now recognized as a common and serious event, particularly in the elderly. Its importance was first fully appreciated in the United Kingdom during the unusually cold winter of 1963. In 1957, 7 persons were certified in England and Wales as dying from excessive cold; in 1963 the figure rose abruptly to 148. It is likely that this represents only a trivial proportion of the total victims of hypothermia.

Aetiology

Observations on Channel swimmers have shown that trained athletes can maintain a normal internal body temperature for as long as 15 hours when the skin temperature and that of the sea in which they are swimming is only 59° F. (15° C.), or 39° F. (21·74° C.) below the normal central body temperature. This illustrates the importance of the 'core' and 'shell' concept of temperature regulation [see Section 2]. In others exposed to extreme cold, the core temperature eventually begins to fall: this is particularly true of the elderly who are more sensitive to cold, but it is a hazard, too, in mountain climbers immobilized by accident or fog.

In old people both exogenous and endogenous factors conspire to make accidental hypothermia common. Those living alone in poor circumstances, occupying inadequate and underheated houses, often underclad and underfed, are especially vulnerable. The crisis is often precipitated by a fall, an accident, a stroke or a myocardial infarction, which leaves the victim immobile on the floor. In other instances a respiratory infection, a confusional state or senile dementia prevents him from summoning help. Unconsciousness from alcohol or other addictive drugs and the increased heat loss due to medication with the phenothiazine and barbiturate drugs are additional factors. Myxoedema has long been recognized as having particular importance in this respect, but is found in not more than 10 per cent. of patients with hypothermia. In climbers and walkers, cold, wet clothes and exertion to the point of collapse are important causes.

Pathology

It is difficult to distinguish *post mortem* between changes due to hypothermia and those of coexisting disease. They are seldom striking: a fatty metamorphosis is common in the myocardium, the liver and the kidneys. Acute gastric erosions and submucous haemorrhages occur in about 50 per cent.; pancreatitis is frequent and multiple visceral infarcts are the rule.

Clinical Picture

Three grades of hypothermia are usually described: (1) The rectal temperature lies between 98·4° and 90·0° F (36·9° and 32·2° C.). In this stage the body shows a physiological reaction to cold by cutaneous vasoconstriction, shivering, a rise in blood pressure and pulse rate and diuresis. All these responses are most marked at 95° F. (35° C.). In the elderly, shivering is often slight and both it and vasoconstriction are abolished by chlorpromazine.

(2) The rectal temperature is between 90° and 75° F. (32·2° and 23·9° C.). The muscles become rigid and shivering ceases, although a fine tremor is evident in electrocardiograms. The skin is pale, cold and dry. Pupillary reactions are sluggish, tendon reflexes depressed and the blood pressure and respiratory rate fall. Stupor passes into coma and consciousness is lost at about 80° F. (26·7° C.). Spontaneous respiration ceases about 77° F. (25° C.).

(3) With rectal temperatures below 75° F. (23·9° C.) life is impossible for more than a short time; indeed, death usually occurs at 77° F. (25° C.). There is a case on record of a young Negress who survived a rectal temperature of 64° C. (17·8° C.).

The first grade is common enough in the elderly and usually reversible without medical aid. It frequently escapes recognition because a low reading thermometer, the indispensable diagnostic instrument, is still possessed by few.

The second grade is our chief concern here and it too will often evade diagnosis, because the standard clinical thermometer only records temperatures between 95° and 110° F. (35° and 43·3° C.). The patient is stuporose or comatose. There is extreme pallor with a puffiness of the face which mimics myxoedema. The respiratory rate, the pulse frequency and the blood pressure fall progressively. Atrial fibrillation with a slow ventricular rate is common. A pathognomonic change appears in the electrocardiogram in the form of the J-wave (junctional deflection), an extra deflection at the junction of the QRS complex and the ST segment, usually best seen in lead V4.

Haemoconcentration shown by a raised haematocrit reading is a feature in some cases. The blood urea level is often raised and the plasma bicarbonate level falls. Myocardial and skeletal muscle damage is suggested by increased serum levels of creatinine kinase and α-hydroxybutyrate dehydrogenase.

Treatment

Prevention of accidental hypothermia is theoretically simple, but hard to translate into practical terms. Regular visiting of the elderly and the provision of satisfactory, well-heated housing, adequate clothing and enough food would virtually abolish the problem, but economic and other reasons make the early implementation of any such programme unlikely. For climbers, an easily portable double polythene sleeping bag with an air space between the two layers, has proved an efficient method of conserving heat.

Experience has shown that rapid warming is dangerous in accidental hypothermia. The intense peripheral vasoconstriction is suddenly replaced by a generalized dilatation of skin vessels, which precipitates hypovolaemic circulatory failure. The patient should be wrapped in a blanket in a normally warm room, and the body temperature allowed to rise at a rate of 1° F. (0·55° C.) an hour. If this is not achieved, the room temperature should be raised to 80°–90° F. (26·7°–32·2° C.).

Almost all these patients are dehydrated and a solution of 5 per cent. dextrose or a low molecular weight dextran should be given intravenously. Salt is not usually needed and care must be taken not to overload the circulation. Respiratory infection is constantly present and an antibiotic should always be prescribed: one of the tetracyclines is appropriate. Hydrocortisone in doses of 100 mg. should be given intravenously 6–8 hourly. Thyroxine should be avoided unless there is good reason for suspecting hypothyroidism. This decision is often difficult; the facies may resemble that of myxoedema and the serum cholesterol level is elevated in only about 35 per cent. of patients with hypothyroidism.

Prognosis

The death rate of patients admitted to hospital with accidental hypothermia is probably in excess of 60 per cent. Many have some grave underlying disease such as a cerebral or a myocardial infarction, which contributes to this high figure, but it remains a serious and frequently lethal disorder. There is some evidence that in survivors, temperature regulation is impaired.

REFERENCES

B.M.A. Memorandum (1964) Accidental hypothermia in the elderly, *Brit. med. J.*, **2,** 1255.

Duguid, H., Simpson, R. G., and Stowers, J. M. (1961) Accidental hypothermia, *Lancet*, ii, 1213.

Emslie-Smith, D. (1958) Accidental hypothermia. A common condition with a pathognomonic electrocardiogram, *Lancet*, ii, 492.

Pugh, L. G. C. E. (1966) Accidental hypothermia in walkers, climbers and campers: Report to the Medical Commission on Accident Prevention, *Brit. med. J.*, **1,** 123.

Read, A. E., Emslie-Smith, D., Gough, K. R., and Holmes, R. (1961) Pancreatitis and accidental hypothermia, *Lancet*, ii, 1219.

R. Bodley Scott

SECTION 4

GENETIC AND CONSTITUTIONAL FACTORS IN DISEASE

GROWTH, DEVELOPMENT, INVOLUTION AND SENESCENCE
GENETIC FACTORS IN DISEASE
IMMUNE MECHANISMS IN DISEASE
DISEASES OF CONNECTIVE TISSUE
GENERAL ASPECTS OF NEOPLASTIC DISEASE
DISORDERS OF METABOLISM
DISORDERS OF NUTRITION

GROWTH, DEVELOPMENT, INVOLUTION AND SENESCENCE

GROWTH

Growth is a highly complex process which is ill understood. Not only does it involve over-all increases in height and weight but also growth in various organs and their ability to function optimally at different times throughout the life span. In a child failure to gain weight is as indicative of ill health as is weight loss in an adult. Tissues may evolve either by an increase in the number of cells present or by growth in size of the individual cell. This is a dynamic process in which new cells are laid down and old cells are removed, the rate of production exceeding that of disintegration during the period of childhood. It is interesting that the fraction of the life-span occupied by growth is considerably greater than in other mammals.

Rates of growth vary at different times so that it is useful to have percentile charts reflecting the average height and weight at different stages of maturity for the population under consideration. They are essential not only for determining individual status but are also needed to follow the longitudinal pattern of growth. For example, a child with coeliac disease may be on the 50th percentile channel for height until 6 months old, then falling to below the 3rd percentile until a gluten-free diet is instituted when normal growth potential is regained [FIG. 1].

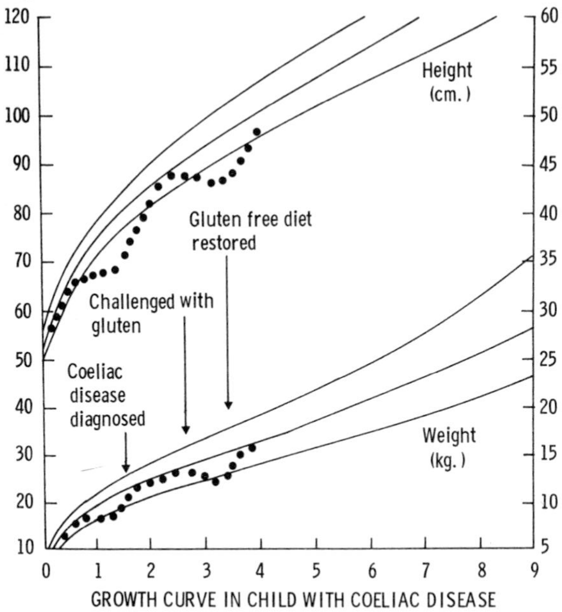

FIG. 1.

Growth and development of the human organism proceed together from conception to maturity. By convention growth implies an increase in size coupled typically with cell division whereas development refers to increasing maturation and functional complexity. Often the more mature organ is the larger but as with the thymus and with lymphoid tissue this is actually smaller in the mature adult than in the child. The brain achieves its adult weight of 1400 g. at the age of 6 years and although it no longer increases in bulk it is certainly not fully developed from a functional standpoint.

Growth is a well co-ordinated harmonious process which follows a sigmoid curve. Although growth is continuous the rate at which it progresses is far from constant. Essentially there are two cycles of rapid growth separated by a period of relatively slower uniform increase. The first period extends from intra-uterine life to the pre-school era gradually decelerating to the age of four. A typical full-term baby weighing 7 lb. (3180 g.) might gain 15 lb. in the first year, 7 lb. in the second and 4–5 lb. in the third year. The second major increase in the velocity of growth takes place around puberty starting at about 10 years in girls and being over by 13 years when menarche occurs. Commonly this is about one year later in boys. Growth in height is more noticeable than weight in this phase and much of an individual's ultimate height is achieved at this time, it is in fact unusual for girls to grow more than 2 or 3 inches after the end of the puberty growth spurt.

It is important to appreciate the changing rates of growth throughout infancy and childhood since factors affecting growth have a much greater impact when they are applied at a time of maximal increase. This is well illustrated by 9-year-old identical twins one of whom is 3 inches shorter than her sister. She suffered a period of severe malnutrition associated with gastro-enteritis from the age of 2–5 months. Had this illness occurred at a later age it is unlikely that she would have sustained this degree of growth retardation. Again a cerebro-vascular catastrophe in childhood results in an infantile type of hemiparesis with characteristic shortening of the affected limbs.

PATTERNS OF GROWTH

Scammon (1930) showed that although most organs follow a general growth curve, various tissues have a characteristic growth pattern. He computed the percentage increment occurring in each year of life from birth to maturity for different organs. He found that the general type of sigmoid curve applied to most external dimensions, to the muscles, the respiratory, and gastro-intestinal systems and to the spleen, kidneys and cardiovascular system. There were in addition three other types of growth curve. The genital type with minimal increment until the onset of puberty. The neural type representing the brain, eyes, meninges and the head dimensions where growth is rapid in early childhood so that 60 per cent. of the total is achieved by age two. Finally the lymphoid type where tissues reach a size considerably in excess of their ultimate size by the age of 10 and then regress to adult dimensions by 18 [FIG. 2]. Although these figures were achieved by careful measurement, clinical observation suggests that the tonsils and adenoids are largest around the

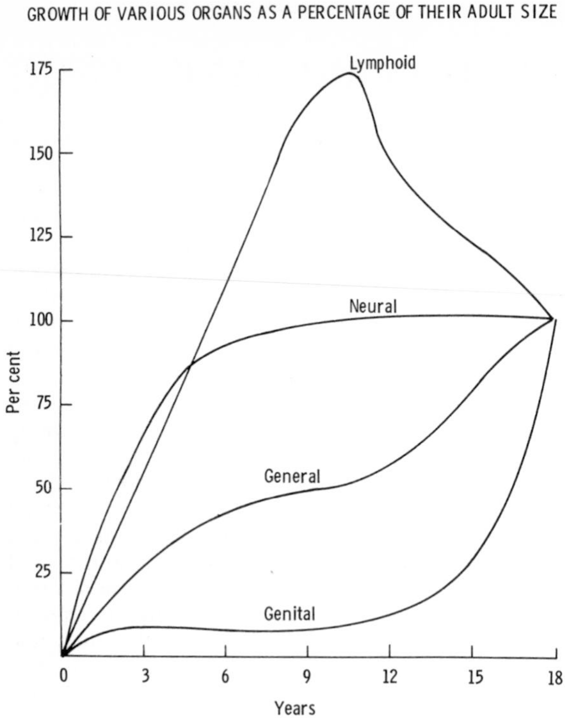

FIG. 2.

fifth birthday and tend to diminish in size thereafter. Other tissues may have their own growth characteristics, the adrenal grows rapidly in the last trimester of pregnancy so that at birth it is proportionally nine times as large as it is in adult life. After birth, like the uterus, it diminishes in size and thereafter follows a genital type pattern.

Growth in Height

For the clinician growth in stature is of particular concern. This is mediated by the creation of new cartilage cells at the ends of bones, the process of chondroplasia. These cells become calcified and incorporated in bone, the process of osteogenesis. Normally these two activities take place synchronously but if the production of new cartilage cells is halted by infection or undernutrition osteogenesis may continue, so that a zone of increased density results and is visible on an X-ray (Harris' lines). Both activities require thyroxine and growth hormone, and although these are complementary thyroxine is predominantly concerned with osteogenesis and growth hormone with chondroplasia. At puberty, androgens and to a lesser extent oestrogens promote skeletal maturation (osteogenesis) more than linear growth. It is well known that androgens given to achieve a growth spurt may result in greater skeletal maturation but cause closure of epiphyses and ultimate dwarfism.

The changing body proportions are interesting. At birth the head occupies one quarter of the total body length and the ratio of the crown to pubis, pubis to ground is 1·8:1 due to the long body and comparatively short limbs; this changes gradually so that as the legs grow more than the body the proportion becomes 1:1 at adolescence, the head now taking up only 1/7th of the total height [FIG. 3].

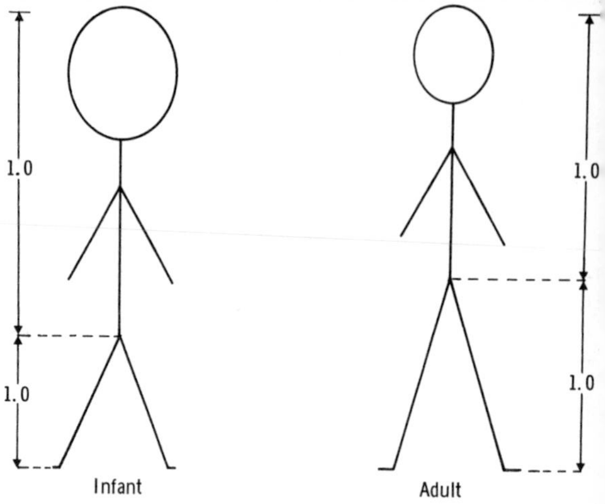

DIAGRAM TO ILLUSTRATE CHANGING BODY PROPORTIONS

FIG. 3.

Failure to achieve the transition to adult proportions will occur if skeletal maturation occurs without linear growth. This is the position in achondroplasia when cartilage production is deficient so that the patient has characteristically infantile proportions with short limbs and a relatively large head.

Developmental and Chronological Age

The life-span is conveniently divided into a number of stages based on age.

AGES OF MAN

PERIOD	AGE
Neonatal period	First month
Infancy	First year
Pre-school	1–5
School	5–11
Pubescence	11–14
Adolescence	14–18
Maturity	18+

Age is used to determine the time at which an individual attends school, when he can undertake employment, or assume civil responsibility, but if one considers a class of 13-year-olds it is clear that there are wide differences both in size and maturity. Although these features are exaggerated at puberty they are present in all age groups and attempts have been made to define developmental or physiological age as distinct from chronological age.

Physical landmarks such as the time at which primary and secondary dentition appear or the onset of menstruation are useful in assessing developmental age. Recently the use of radiographs to establish skeletal maturity has become popular. Here the centres of ossification present and the extent of epiphyseal fusion are compared against standards. A number of atlases are available to make this comparison, and Tanner and

Whitehouse have suggested a system whereby a number of bones are scored in relation to their time to reach maturity so that when an X-ray is compared with their atlas a skeletal index is obtained. It is found that skeletal age or dental age are a better indication of maturity than are height and weight. Skeletal maturation in girls is in advance of boys and maturity is reached some 2 years earlier although they tend to be shorter than boys of comparable age. Equally there is good correlation between skeletal age and the age of onset of menstruation, an early menarche can be predicted in girls with an advanced bone age.

During infancy thyroxine plays a dominant role in determining the rate of skeletal maturation. In the foetus without a thyroid maternal thyroxine is insufficient for normal bone development and retardation of osteogenesis may be noted before other overt signs of cretinism are apparent. Hypothyroidism at any age in childhood is associated not only with delay in the time at which epiphyseal centres arrive but also with disorganized fragmented osteogenesis giving a diagnostic picture of epiphyseal dysgenesis. At puberty the role of thyroxine is taken over by the sex hormones and androgens in particular potentiate skeletal maturation.

FACTORS AFFECTING STATURE

1. Genetic influences
   (a) Familial
   (b) Chromosomal, e.g. Turner's syndrome
2. Prenatal damage
   (a) Intra-uterine infection, e.g. rubella
   (b) Placental insufficiency
3. Malnutrition
   (a) Generalized, e.g. coeliac syndrome
   (b) Cellular, e.g. Fallot's tetralogy
4. Hormonal causes
   (a) Lack of growth hormone
   (b) Excess corticosteroids
   (c) Lack of thyroxine
   (d) Premature androgen secretion
5. Bone disorders
   (a) Chondrodystrophies, e.g. Morquio's disease
   (b) Metaphyseal dysostoses
6. Others

Intra-uterine Malnutrition

A small or abnormal placenta may result in the birth of a baby of low weight at full term. Such babies continue to grow at a suboptimal rate and are sometimes termed primordial dwarfs. A number of types of intra-uterine dwarfs are recognized, the bird-headed type described by Seckel in which there is a small skull with a beaked nose and receding chin, the Russell-Silver type which is thought to be due to placental insufficiency in early pregnancy. These children are of normal intelligence and have a relatively large head with micrognathos; hemihypertrophy, syndactyly, hypospadias and sexual precocity may also be found. Bone age is retarded but they may exhibit different degrees of skeletal maturation depending on which wrist is used to estimate it. The third type of intra-uterine growth failure is sometimes seen in twin pregnancies when one twin is much smaller than the other, again the shorter stature continues into postnatal life. The muscle cells were examined in one child with primordial dwarfism and found to be larger than normal but grossly reduced in number. Like dwarfism due to chromosomal anomalies there is no response to treatment with growth hormone.

Growth and Postnatal Nutrition

In this country failure to grow in length is more likely to be due to malabsorption than to malnutrition. In coeliac disease retardation of linear growth is not only an important diagnostic sign but restoration of normal stature is the best index of adequate treatment. Although the child with an untreated coeliac syndrome will be short it is usual for him to make good the retardation when on a gluten-free diet. In Sheldon's follow-up of 57 cases of coeliac disease there were only 6 who were stunted in adult life and all these had had a long delay of 7 years or more between the onset of the condition and the start of a gluten-free diet.

It is useful to differentiate between short stature in childhood and permanent stunting in adult life. Although malnutrition or malabsorption cause a slowing down in linear growth this is usually made good later so that the ultimate height is normal. Accelerated growth at 3–4 times the normal rate may take place when a hypothyroid child is given thyroxine. Recovery from periods of undernutrition may be slower but eventually the original percentile channel is resumed. From animal work it seems that the ability to catch up depends on the stage at which the malnutrition occurs. If they are malnourished when cell division is complete there is no difficulty in attaining a normal weight for the species. When the malnutrition occurs *in utero* or at an early age when cells are still dividing they may never catch up and these animals are shown to have fewer cells in various organs.

Short Stature

Dwarfism is an unfortunate term applied to persons who are conspicuously smaller than others of their kind. Stature depends not only on the rate at which a person grows but for the length of time growth continues. Delayed puberty may cause concern in a child who is apparently dwarfed at age 14 but whose skeletal age is perhaps 12 and who will continue growing until he has a puberty growth spurt at 16. This pattern tends to occur in families and is sometimes called constitutional delayed growth. It serves to emphasize that height and the rate at which it is achieved may vary widely.

Genetic Factors. Growth is influenced by racial characteristics and by familial patterns within a particular ethnic group. As growth progresses familial resemblances become more noticeable. Facial appearance, dental and skeletal maturation as well as ultimate height follow a genetically predetermined pattern.

Major disruption of genetic influences may occur with chromosomal anomalies. Turner's syndrome of ovarian dysgenesis has 45 chromosomes with an XO or XO/XY pattern. The clinical picture of dwarfism, webbed neck, low hair line, cubitus valgus and associated renal or cardiovascular anomalies is well known. Here the short stature is further accentuated by the failure to have a pubertal growth spurt. Down's syndrome (mongolism) with an extra small chromosome 21 or 22 tends to be below the 3rd percentile for height, but it is in the other trisomic conditions that growth retardation is most marked. In Patau's 13–15 trisomy or Edwards' syndrome 17–19 trisomy gross mental and physical retardation are present.

Intra-uterine Infection

Foetal growth is remarkably rapid due to an innate capacity for cellular division so that normal growth-promoting factors such as thyroxine or pituitary growth hormone are little involved. On the other hand noxious influences such as drugs, radiation or viral infections which inhibit cell division will have a profound effect. Either growth and normal development of particular structures may be prevented or the whole foetus may be stunted. The thalidomide tragedy was a vivid example of a drug inhibiting the growth of limb buds. The rubella virus may cross the placenta during the first trimester of pregnancy and initially it was thought to cause mainly deafness, cataracts or cardiovascular anomalies but it is now clear that microcephaly and dwarfism together with hepatomegaly, thrombocytopenia, bone lesions and other defects are common. Infants in whom there is transplacental infection with cytomegalovirus, or with toxoplasmosis, or syphilis all are small at birth. Most of these infants are also mentally retarded since brain development is proceeding fast and is easily halted by any toxic influence.

Cellular Malnutrition

Studies have shown that in protein deprivation as in kwashiorkor the cell size is grossly reduced whilst the rate of cell multiplication is little affected. This is shown both by histological techniques and by measuring the ratio of total protein to DNA. Cheek and others have shown that in calorie malnutrition or hypoxia, cell division is diminished although protein synthesis continues so that larger cells with abundant cytoplasm are produced. This occurred in patients with cyanotic congenital heart disease and in infants with gross anaemia. Inadequate oxygen supply at a cellular level can result in growth retardation and although Mehrizi and Drash showed this to be most marked in the cyanotic group there is a significant inhibition of growth when the effective cardiac output is reduced. In a series of children with a patent ductus arteriosus there were more than three times the average whose height fell below the 10th percentile. Again there was a marked acceleration of linear growth after the ductus was closed surgically.

Other alterations of the cellular milieu may also inhibit growth. An inability to excrete hydrogen ions in renal failure or in renal tubular disorders causes acidosis with resulting growth failure. In glycogen storage disease there may be an acidosis but it is suggested that lack of available carbohydrate leads to excess utilization of protein for metabolic needs so that less is available for incorporation into the cells.

Hormonal Causes

Hypopituitarism. This arises from a lack of secretions by the pituitary gland and usually presents as dwarfism. Although all the tropic hormones may not be deficient there is commonly a deficiency of growth hormone either alone or associated with or lack of TSH, ACTH or gonadotrophins. The majority of patients have no anatomical cause for the condition although it may be due to a craniopharyngioma or can follow a fractured base of skull or an encephalitis. Rarely it has been described in other conditions affecting the hypothalamic region such as neurofibromatosis, Hand-Schüller-Christian disease or tuberose sclerosis.

Growth failure in idiopathic hypopituitarism may be noted by the age of one year in about 30 per cent. but typically the child is three to four at the time of diagnosis although he appears younger and may have truncal obesity with flabby musculature and thin limbs. Bone age and dentition are markedly delayed although the ratio of upper to lower segment is normal. Sexual infantilism usually persists into adult life although gonadotrophins may be produced in late adolescence. The diagnosis is confirmed by finding a lack of growth hormone following insulin hypoglycaemia and is often associated with a low serum protein-bound iodine (P.B.I.) and diminished I^{132} uptake. A metyrapone test may be positive and there is an increased sensitivity to insulin. Treatment with human growth hormone results in the restoration of normal growth rates in the majority of patients.

The commonest hormonal cause of dwarfism today follows the use of high-dose corticosteroids in the treatment of asthma, collagen diseases or the nephrotic syndrome. Kerrelyn and de Kroon found that growth retardation was minimal with doses of prednisolone, 3 mg. per $m.^2$ body surface (average body surface aged nine is $1m.^2$). Above this level skeletal maturation and growth in height were impaired whilst catch-up growth tended to be slow and variable. It is interesting that despite the retardation of bone age puberty occurred normally in these children.

Maternal deprivation is an accepted cause of growth retardation and recently Powell, Brasel, Raiti and Blizzard have proved that psychologically disturbed children in abnormal home environments have deficiencies of growth hormone and ACTH secretion. Removal of the child to a more normal situation was accompanied by improved levels of growth hormone production.

Lack of Thyroxine. Lack of thyroid in infancy results in the typical appearance of cretinism with associated mental retardation. If it occurs later (after the age of three) linear growth is impaired but permanent cerebral damage is unlikely. The term juvenile myxoedema is used to describe this condition whilst infantile hypothyroidism is preferable to cretinism. Maternal thyroxine crosses the placenta and although linear growth can be normal at birth in totally athyreotic infants there may be evidence of delay in skeletal and cerebral development. Often the diagnosis is not achieved before 2 months when the classical features of lethargy, constipation, pallor, hoarse cry and rough skin together with bradycardia and abnormal reflexes become apparent. Investigations reveal a low P.B.I. with an absent or diminished uptake of I^{132} by the thyroid.

There is epiphyseal dysgenesis together with low values of alkaline phosphatase. Treatment with increasing doses of thyroxine results in a rapid increase in growth velocity.

Premature Secretion of Androgens. Sexual precocity in children results initially in a growth spurt but skeletal maturation advances more rapidly than growth in height so that early closure of the epiphyses means that the ultimate height will be reduced.

Dwarfism due to Bone Disorders

In achondroplasia there is a genetically determined abnormality of the epiphyses of long bones which results in dwarfism with a comparatively long body and short proximal limb bones. Other storage diseases such as Hurler's syndrome (gargoylism), Morquio's disease or Scheie's syndrome in which mucopolysaccharides are laid down in these epiphyses all result in short stature. Dwarfism is often the result of multiple fractures in osteogenesis imperfecta and may also be present in the various types of metaphyseal dysostosis.

REFERENCE

RUBIN, P. (1964) *Dynamic Classification of Bone Dysplasias*, Chicago.

GROWTH CHANGES AT PUBERTY

Pubescence is the era of accelerated growth which takes place together with the development of the secondary sex characteristics. In girls it begins at about 10–11 years and is complete by thirteen, while in boys it tends to be about one year later. There may be individual variation, but events follow a definite time-table.

In females the beginning of the growth spurt is associated with thelarche, the development of the breast tissue. Initially small breast buds appear behind the nipple and may cause concern if they are unilateral or if they precede other signs of puberty by some months. In a recent series inequality of breast growth was noteworthy in 7 per cent. Tanner describes stages of breast development from the pre-adolescent phase in which there is solely elevation of the papilla. Stage II with elevation of the breast as a small mound. This breast bud gives rise to Stage III with enlargement of the breast and areola with no separation of the contours. Stage IV occurs in about 75 per cent. when there is projection of the papilla and areola as a secondary mound beyond the breast. In the mature Stage V there is recession of the areola to the general contour of the breast.

Shortly after the appearance of breast buds there is the development of pubic hair which in both sexes goes through stages of maturation eventually spreading to the inner surface of the thighs.

The growth of axillary hair takes place much later and is not apparent until after the onset of menstruation in about one third. Although menarche is regarded as the end point of pubescence full reproductive maturity may not be reached for some months since the early cycles are frequently anovular [FIG. 4].

Pubertal development in boys begins with enlargement of the testes and with changes in the skin of the scrotum. Not until almost a year later is there enlargement of the penis which at first is mainly in length. This is followed by further growth of the testes and darkening of the scrotal skin. These changes are associated with the appearance of pubic hair and the enlargement of the larynx. This part of the process occupies about 2 years and occurs at the time of the maximum growth spurt; however, a further 2 years are required before the genitalia reach adult size and shape. It is during this period that the growth of axillary and facial hair occur, but it is frequently only poorly developed at the time of the first ejaculation. During puberty changes occur in the male breast with enlargement and pigmentation of

SEQUENCE OF CHANGES AT PUBERTY IN GIRLS

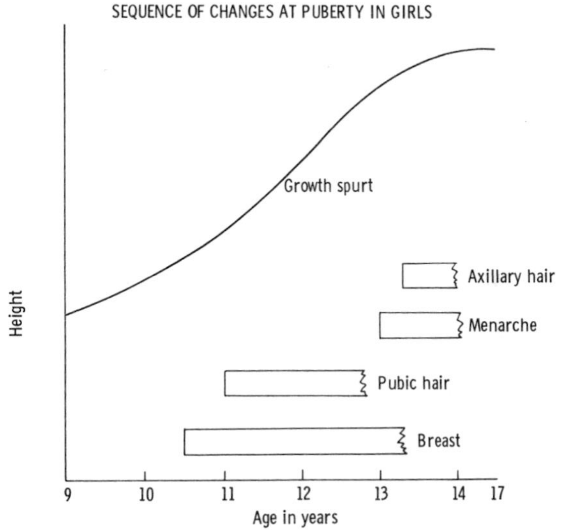

FIG. 4.

the areola, in about 30 per cent. there is gynaecomastia of puberty which may be a response to the presence of circulating oestrogens. In both sexes there is hypertrophy of the apocrine sweat glands and increased sweat production with its characteristic odour. This occurs synchronously with the appearance of axillary hair.

Hormonal Control of Puberty

Production of gonadotrophins by the pituitary is under control of the hypothalamus which in turn is subject to impulses from other parts of the central nervous system. Small quantities of gonadotrophins may be detected in the urine from prepubertal children but it begins to be readily apparent $2\frac{1}{2}$–3 years before menarche. The release of gonadotrophins stimulates the gonads to produce oestrogens and androgens which in turn are responsible for the physical changes of puberty. The gonadal secretions themselves operate a feed-back mechanism so that high oestrogen levels will inhibit the pituitary secretion of the gonadotrophins and so cause gonadal atrophy. If on the other hand there is no oestrogen production as in the gonadal dysgenesis of Turner's syndrome then very high gonadotrophin levels are found.

In addition the adrenal cortex enlarges in size and is responsible for the formation of two-thirds of the urinary neutral 17-ketosteroids with one-third coming from the testes. Adrenal androgens are involved in stimulating the development of pubic and axillary hair since again this occurs in patients with Turner's syndrome who have no gonadal secretion. There is evidence that the follicle stimulating hormone (FSH) and the interstitial cell stimulating hormone (ICSH) which is identical with the luteinizing hormone (LH) are primarily concerned with maturation of the testes. FSH stimulates spermatogenesis while ICSH causes the Leydig cells to produce androgens. These together with adrenal androgens cause the development of the scrotum, prostate, and seminal vesicles. At the same time they provoke the increase in muscle development and the change in laryngeal characteristics.

In girls, oestrogen output rises sharply between 8 and 11 years and a cyclical pattern is noted at an early stage some 2–3 years prior to menarche. Only very small quantities of androgens are detectable in normal females and although progesterone affects all the secondary sex organs it is only after they have developed under oestrogenic influences.

Deviations in Pubertal Development

Either single facets of puberty may occur before their anticipated time or the entire process of pubertal development may occur precociously.

Premature Thelarche. The premature development of breast tissue is not uncommon in girls. It occurs around the second year of life and may persist for months or years and occasionally only one side is affected. Although there may be considerable hyperplasia of the breast the nipples and areola do not increase in size and remain unpigmented. Likewise there are no other signs of oestrogen activity such as changes in the epithelium of the vagina and no increase in height. It is thought to be due to local sensitivity to a normal level of circulating oestrogens.

Premature Adrenarche. This is the name given to the precocious appearance of sexual hair without any other signs of puberty. It is commoner in girls and may occur in the pre-school era. There may be profuse growth of pubic hair and after it has been present for some years sparse axillary hair may be found although there is no generalized hirsutism. There may be a slight increase in the rate of linear growth but no breast changes or enlargement of the clitoris. The condition has also been called premature pubarche but there is evidence that it is due to small quantities of adrenal androgens, so the name precocious adrenarche is to be preferred. When it occurs in boys it may be differentiated from full sexual precocity in that there is no enlargement of the penis, testes or prostate. The condition is benign and is followed in due time by a normal puberty.

Precocious Puberty. The early secretion of gonadotrophins is the basis of a true precocious puberty which follows the normal developmental stages to completion. It may be due to the presence of gonadotrophin-secreting tumours or to intracranial lesions but is more often idiopathic and sometimes has a familial incidence. It should be distinguished from sexual precocity in which some features of puberty are lacking and in which early secretion of gonadotrophins is absent. This may result from interstitial tumours of the testes, from the ingestion of oestrogens or from ovarian neoplasms.

Idiopathic precocious puberty can occur at a very early age and Wilkins states that in a series of 310 girls there were 70 pregnancies before the age of 14, 18 having occurred under 10. Precocious puberty may be due to an intracranial tumour, or it may follow meningitis or encephalitis and is sometimes seen in association with hydrocephalus. Although cerebral causes were found in only 14 per cent. of cases it is interesting that it was six times commoner to find an intracranial cause in boys than in girls. Other uncommon causes of precocious puberty include polyostotic fibrous dysplasia, Silver's syndrome of intra-uterine dwarfism and rarely it may occur together with hypothyroidism.

REFERENCE

Marshall, W. A., and Tanner, J. M. (1969) Variations in the pattern of pubertal changes in girls, *Arch. Dis. Childh.*, **44**, 291.

DEVELOPMENT

Growth is concerned primarily with the acquisition of size, whereas development is concerned with maturation and the acquisition of skills which will enable the child to react purposefully within his environment. All children are different but each follows a sequence of development which is continuous from conception to maturity. The rate of progress varies with the individual and newly acquired skills may be lost or reinforced. For example, the child who is just learning to walk may be unable to do so after being kept in bed for a week with an intercurrent illness.

Development does not necessarily follow an uninterrupted course, but basically it is dependent upon the maturation of the nervous system which follows a fairly circumscribed time-table. This predominates at first, so that there is less variation in achieving earlier landmarks, but later intrinsic capacity is increasingly modified by the child's environment. As with growth, maximal changes take place in the first 3 years and experiences during this period may have a greater impact than physical or psychological events later in childhood.

All the sensory modalities are present in a full-term baby and during the first 6 months they become integrated so that the infant may react to sensory stimuli with motor activity. Initially tactile, thermal and pain receptors are most important and although vision and hearing are present in the neonatal period the baby is little influenced by what he hears and sees. By 4 months of age binocular vision is developing and infants come to recognize familiar patterns of movement, touch and sound so that the basis of memory is established.

It is convenient to discuss this under three headings: (1) motor development; (2) the development of language; and (3) social development, since if development does not follow its expected course it is usually lack of achievement in one or more of these fields that gives rise to concern. Development in all fields is a function of intelligence but some features are more closely dependent than others on this. For example, the child who speaks early is likely to be of superior intelligence whilst early sitting and walking can sometimes be achieved by a mentally subnormal child.

MOTOR DEVELOPMENT

The early neonatal reflexes disappear during the first 3 months of life and are replaced by voluntary movements. Motor development is, more than other skills, dependent on myelinization of the nervous system and therefore in the premature baby an appropriate time allowance must be made for this. TABLE 15 illustrates the orderly sequence of events in the motor development of an average child. There is variation in that some infants may be walking by 9 months, others may never make any attempt to crawl but generally the time-table is observed.

TABLE 15

6 weeks	Moves head from side to side when supine.
3 months	Lifts head and shoulders when prone.
6 months	Sits with minimal support. Pulls himself into sitting position. Rolls from supine to prone.
9 months	Sits without support. Can stand holding on to support, beginning to crawl.
12 months	Pulls to standing position and lets himself down again.
15 months	Walks without help. Crawls upstairs.
18 months	Runs with a stiff gait.
2 years	Walks up and down stairs alone. Jumps from a low object.
2½ years	Walks on tip-toe.
3 years	Stands on one foot.

In addition to the motor activities involved in locomotion and the control of posture, co-ordination of eye and hand movements are associated with the acquisition of motor skills. In assessing the integrity of motor development these also should be considered. In TABLE 16 is a series of achievements which are commonly present at each age and which are easy to test. They can of course be amplified and extended in the older child until they become part of a formal intelligence test.

TABLE 16

Birth	Responds to stimulation of palm with a reflex grasp.
4 months	Reaches for objects.
6 months	Picks up cube from table. Simple purposive manipulations, e.g. banging, shaking rattle, etc.
8 months	Transfers toy from hand to hand.
10 months	Pincer grip with finger and thumb.
1 year	Claps hands.
14 months	Places one object on another.
8 months	Builds tower of three bricks.
2 years	Copies horizontal line.

Delay in Walking

Retarded motor progress in an otherwise normal child may be in keeping with a particular family pattern. Equally the deprived child may be late to walk but learns rapidly when appropriate encouragement is provided. Most, but not all, mentally retarded children are late to sit and walk and this is particularly apparent when it is accompanied by hypotonia as in mongolism or the Prader-Willi syndrome. Other causes of reduced muscle tone such as benign hypotonia or idiopathic hypercalcaemia are responsible for motor delay. In children with cerebral palsy gross hypertonia may make walking impossible, and even in mildly affected infants the increased tone with or without proprioceptive impairment may impede walking and make the child appear unduly clumsy.

Providing the nervous system is intact orthopaedic abnormalities less commonly prevent attempts at walking although in the child with congenital dislocation of the hip the gait will be abnormal. Rickets probably causes motor delay as much because of the accompanying hypotonia as from bony damage. Obese infants are sometimes slow to walk and other who are less venturesome may be late to walk without assistance.

The Development of Language

Learning to talk is a highly complex activity which involves co-ordination of many systems. The child learns by mimicry. On the input side he must be exposed to meaningful sounds which he can hear and learn to discriminate one from another. He must then comprehend the content of the sounds and initiate an appropriate verbal response. Children carry out simple commands such as waving goodbye long before they can vocalize, so it is likely that hearing and understanding precede the ability to communicate by words.

Speech sounds (phonemes) are characterized by their acoustic frequency. Low frequency vowel sounds ranging from 250 c.p.s. 'a' to 2000 c.p.s. 'ee' give power and force to articulation while the higher frequency consonants from 500 c.p.s. 'mm' to 8000 c.p.s. 'ss' are more concerned with intelligibility. The simpler vowel sounds develop first and vocalization in the early months consists mainly of sounds resembling 'a', 'o', 'e'. High frequency consonants are the last sounds to be acquired, and infantile speech with the omission of 'sh' and 'th' is common in children starting school. Lisping in which 'r' is replaced by the lower frequency 'w' is often regarded as an attractive feature of verbalization in infancy.

If the child is not able to hear sounds above a certain frequency then the noises he hears are meaningless and he will not learn to speak. He is not deaf in that he reacts to sounds but fails to make an accepted response and is thought to be 'dumb' or stupid. If in a simple sentence the consonants are not heard, e.g. --ea-e -o -o-e, it is not recognizable although with the same number of vowels omitted it becomes pl--s- g- h-m- (please go home). High-tone deafness may be a sequel to neonatal hyperbilirubinaemia and is important to recognize as it can be helped by the provision of a hearing aid.

Babies vocalize from birth, usually the stimulus is discomfort and the response is crying, but by one month they are making throaty noises which over the next few weeks give way to conventional cooing sounds. By about 4 months they will turn towards a sound and shortly afterwards there is the babbling, razzing phase in which the baby delights in making repetitive chains of sound. Gradually, by about 9 months, the infant is beginning to imitate the intonations and rhythm of the speech he heard but no words can be discerned and it remains jargon. At the age of a year two or three sound sequences may be repeated and he is eagerly accredited with having uttered his first word.

The rate at which a child's vocabulary increases is highly variable. On an average, by 18 months he has slowly increased to about 20 words but this rises to almost 250 by the age of 2 years. More important, he is now using sentences although at first they tend to be short imperatives such as 'give me', 'dat mine'. Nouns and verbs predominate in 2-year-old speech and it is not until three that he may achieve mastery of personal pronouns. Gradually adjectives and adverbs are introduced but frequently the flight of ideas appears to exceed the verbal code available for their expression. By 4 years prepositions and conjunctions are in use although the word 'and' is frequently used as the sole means of stringing together involved clauses. As learning develops at the perceptual level the ability to discriminate sounds is allied with the power to retain and recall auditory images and to integrate them with impressions gained from visual and tactile stimuli. The feed-back of hearing his own voice enables the child to modify his speech so that he learns the sounds which will provoke the intended response in his listener. By this servo mechanism patterns of language are corrected and simple mimicry gives way to an expanding system for the verbal exchange of ideas.

Delayed Speech. Delay in speaking up to the age of two or two-and-a-half is not uncommon, and often it may be found that parents or siblings were equally late. Speech when it arrives in these children is clear and progresses rapidly. The term developmental mutism is used for a group in which speech is delayed until after 3 years in children who are seemingly normal in other respects. They appear to comprehend and develop normally in motor and social fields. When speech does occur it is confused and indistinct although eventually by the age of eight normal language is acquired. This is three times more common in boys and may be associated with left-handedness.

In any child who is late to speak it is essential that hearing is investigated. Losses greater than 30 decibels may slow the development of speech or even make it impossible. A high-tone loss severely impairs speech. The term dysacusis (sensory auditory aphasia) is sometimes used to describe the condition in which there is lack of auditory perception although auditory acuity is intact. Although hearing is possible comprehension of the spoken word is impaired.

Mental retardation is the commonest cause of failure to talk by the age of two and is associated with delay in all other spheres. In the child with cerebral palsy late speech may be due both to intellectual impairment or even when this is absent, to dysarthria. Other disorders of sound production with anatomical or functional abnormalities of the tongue, lips, teeth and palate tend to render speech unintelligible. Infantile autism often presents with failure to talk but in addition there is an over-all inability to relate normally to persons or circumstances. The autistic child appears to be in a world of his own and may carry out complicated repeated manoeuvres or show illogical anxiety especially to any changes in routine. Commonly speech is delayed until six or later although in moments of stress occasional words may be forthcoming. Less commonly an autistic child who has previously spoken normally may discard speech. If and when vocalization occurs, it is not used for communication but may remain a parrot-like repetition of the same words endlessly reiterated, a condition referred to as echolalia.

The deprived child is also late to talk and may initially be thought to be autistic since they also have difficulty in relating to people. On the other hand they do not show bizarre behaviour and when they are encouraged to speak, words are used normally to convey information. Elective mutism rarely causes diagnostic difficulty since speech development has been normal up to the time at which the child elects to stop talking. It is commoner in shy, timid, negativistic children and may be selective so that the child is mute only at school or may talk to only one parent at home. Language is sometimes delayed in twins although this is said to improve if they are separated.

REFERENCES

Ingram, T. T. S. (1968) Speech disorders in childhood, *Pediat. Clin. N. Amer.*, **15**, 611.

Morley, M. E. (1957) *The Development and Disorders of Speech in Childhood*, Edinburgh.

SOCIAL DEVELOPMENT

Social development is concerned with the exciting transition from complete dependence on the mother to adolescent self-sufficiency. It is determined both by the individual's personality and the environment in which he 'grows-up', but despite external factors certain patterns of social behaviour appropriate to age can be distinguished. The infant's earliest social activity is smiling which is present by about 6 weeks of age. Usually it is in response to another face although Spitz and Wolf have shown that a mask with only the eyes present is an acceptable stimulus at 3 months. The baby becomes increasingly discriminating and by 6 months will only smile and turn towards a familiar face. By 9 months he will give and take toys, will attempt to hold a cup and enjoys playing simple games. Towards his first birthday there is the casting stage in which objects are persistently thrown on the ground. Over the next 6 months the ability to speak and walk greatly increases his capacity for social exchanges. He helps to undress himself, learns to turn door knobs and by 18 months has some measure of bowel control.

Gradually from 18 months to 2 years he insists on imitating adults and enters into a play relationship with other members of the family, becoming more conscious of his own rights as a member of the family. The 2-year-old enjoys exploring and testing his own environment, he dislikes being restrained and this can result in temper-tantrums. His desire for self-assertion prevents him obeying commands and often this negativistic phase is one of stubborn opposition. During the period between two and three he will play with other children although he tends to be self-centred and possessive, finding it very difficult to share toys. There are rapid changes of mood, when in only minutes he will revert from clinging affection to violent kicking and screaming. It is important to recognize that this is a normal developmental pattern on which more flexible human relationships are built.

The pre-school child spends much time in imaginative play in which reality and fantasy are closely mingled. It is at this time that he becomes interested in his body and is constantly asking questions about this and every other topic. He may desire independence but needs to be frequently reassured that the warmth of maternal protection and interest is not far away.

Basic personality patterns are established during the pre-school years. The child's idea of himself is derived from his parents, if he feels that he fulfils their expectations and that he is a source of pleasure and pride he comes to look upon himself as a person of importance. Equally, if he is made to feel that he is an unwanted burden to his parents he sees himself as unworthy and inadequate. Most children experience both extremes and learn to form a composite picture of themselves, which is gradually translated into patterns of behaviour whereby they come to know what is allowed and what they may expect of others.

The sequence of social development through school years involves the association in gangs, the interest in organized sports, the preference for members of the same sex with provocative disparagement of the opposite sex. Later there is criticism of adults and an insistence on fairness and the rights of each individual group. As the child gets older the customs and mores of the culture play a more dominant role, but as with growth or motor development, it is fascinating how similar is the pattern.

DENNIS COTTOM

INVOLUTION AND SENESCENCE

In developed countries throughout the world there is an increasing number of elderly people and in the United Kingdom trends indicate that there will, in the next 25 years, be even more individuals over 75 years of whom the majority will be women. The classical survey by Chebotaryov and Sachuk of 27,181 people of 80 years and over has demonstrated clearly that women outlive men, as of the females examined 94 per cent. were widowed and in individuals of 100 years and over there were 52 men and 363 women. In the last 30 years the expectation of life for men of 65 years has increased by little more than 6 months while women have now an extended span of more than 2 years. The old require much more attention from both doctors in general practice and hospital than the younger age groups; there is an increasing number of older men who have been worried about physical illness committing suicide, and of first admissions of the elderly to mental hospital.

Ageing is a process of unfavourable progressive change associated with decline in vigour and ending in death. It is theoretically possible to envisage an individual who grows old but who is free from disease, and indeed an élite of the elderly has been described who become old but in whom the accepted stigmata of ageing are absent. In the practice of clinical medicine two distinct processes are intertwined—ageing and ageing with pathological changes. Thus knowledge is required about gerontology, which is the study of ageing, and geriatric medicine, which is the medical care of the elderly person. Chronological age does not necessarily reflect true or biological age and the various organs of the body do not age at the same rate in any individual.

Gerontology in its scientific approach to ageing is a new study, but for centuries physicians, and before that magicians and alchemists, have endeavoured to prolong life. In spite of the great advances in scientific knowledge the cause of ageing remains obscure and complex.

In the attempt to understand ageing at cellular level it is convenient to consider two types of cells.

1. The fixed post-mitotics. These are specialized cells which do not undergo division and in which the age of the individual cell therefore corresponds with the age of the organism. An example is the neurone.

2. The inter-mitotic cells. These may be undifferentiated, such as the basal cells of the epidermis, or differentiated as in the case of hepatic cells. In both cases the life of such a cell ends with its division, and in studying tissues (compounds of inter-mitotic cells) the age of individual cells cannot be determined.

Great difficulty arises in determining which structural alterations in cells result from age alone since hypoxia produces gross microscopic change. Four changes in the ageing cell have been described: change in nucleo-cytoplasmic ratio with progressive increase in the size of the nucleus, decrease in the quantity of active protoplasm, decrease in water content and physical alteration in the nature of colloid. Doubt has been cast on these classically described changes since in inter-mitotic tissues such as the spleen, smooth muscle, sex glands, adrenal, liver, kidney and thyroid these findings probably represent vascular degeneration rather than primary ageing change.

Theories of ageing include variation in dividing cell quality ('faulty copying'), loss or damage among fixed post-mitotic cells and colloidal changes in molecules.

Deterioration of the Copying Mechanism. Ageing could result from alteration in the structure of the deoxyribonucleic acid (DNA) molecule which would introduce errors into the coded information needed for protein synthesis. This is thought to be unlikely. However, mistakes could occur in the transmission of information from the molecule to the cell where proteins are constituted. This transfer of information is carried out by messenger ribonucleic acid (RNA). Liver cells in old rats produce more RNA than comparable cells from young animals, and it has been suggested that some of the RNA molecules of the old rats contain errors and thus appropriate information is not given for the creation of a specific enzyme. The deficiency stimulates the formation of additional RNA molecules as a compensatory mechanism; when this compensation fails and the cell can no longer produce an excess of RNA death follows.

Falling Cell Turnover. It has been suggested that 'exhaustion' of cells occurs and that something is used up in a cell or that some noxious substance enters the cell. With ageing there is an accumulation of pigmented bodies, the age pigments (lipofuscin). As age advances, these substances occur in increasing amounts in the cells of the heart, brain and adrenals. It has not been shown conclusively that the age pigments interfere with cell function.

Replacement of Cells with those of Inferior Quality. Cells which have undergone genetic, mutational or immunological change might cause senescence. Studies of human lymphocytes using tissue cultures provoked by artificial means into cell division showed an increasing variation with age in chromosomal constitution. Auto-immunity has been suggested as a cause of ageing. In sera of old normal humans there is a striking increase in the incidence of positive reaction for each of the four auto-immune factors for which specific tests are readily available (rheumatoid factor, antinuclear, antithyroid and antigastric parietal cells). While the well-recognized auto-immune diseases are not commoner in old age, three diseases of an immune or probably immune nature do seem chronologically related to ageing: cold-antibody-type auto-immune haemolytic anaemia, amyloidosis, and maturity-onset diabetes. The immunological theory postulates that ageing is a consequence of increasing immunogenetic diversification of the dividing cell populations of the body. The diversifying cells lose the ability to recognize 'self' and a low-grade prolonged histo-incompatibility reaction sets in analogous to a chronic auto-immune state and manifested as ageing.

Cell Death. Szilard's theory of ageing is based on the assumption that individual cells in essential tissues die on a random basis from chance hits by some harmful environmental factor. When a certain critical number of cells is lost in this tissue death of the individual occurs. Subsequent authors have suggested cosmic radiation as one factor.

Failure of Enzymes. The activities of a number of intracellular enzymes are reduced in senescent animals; those tissues whose cells retain regenerative capacity exhibit little change in enzyme activity with senescence whereas those which contain fixed post-mitotic cells show alteration with age. Age-associated impairment in enzymatic activity is most likely to be found in those cells which regulate specialized physiological functions.

Molecular Ageing. Most work on molecular ageing has been done on collagen which forms the main fibrillary structure of connective tissue and accounts for approximately one-third of the total body protein. There is assumed to be no turnover of collagen in the body and the collagen with which an individual is born persists throughout life, although new collagen may form in response to trauma. Collagen is a trihelical polypeptide with plastic qualities and the collagen molecule ages by the increase in production of intermolecular bridges and in association with this the fibres lose their elasticity.

Ageing is a complex phenomenon with many processes involved, but to relate deterioration in function with structural changes in cells seems in the present state of knowledge impossible.

'NORMAL' OLD AGE

Measurements made on older people in whom there was no clinical evidence of disease are recorded; an attempt is thus made to describe a physiology of the elderly. There is difficulty in this as average values of most physiological functions show a linear decline over the entire span of adult existence. Under resting conditions most of the physiological characteristics important in regulating the internal environment are maintained even in advanced age; for example, there is no change in the pH of arterial blood or the levels of arterial blood sugar, although the rate of readjustment of these values to basal levels following displacement is slower in the old than in the young. No significant variation with age occurs in either plasma or blood volumes per kilogram body weight. Hence any reduction in plasma volume in elderly people is the result of disease rather than of age alone. The total body weight increases slowly up to about the age of 60 years and then declines. From studies of body water content which is distributed mainly in muscle and very little in fat and bone there appears to be a systematic fall in lean body mass with advancing age and an increase in total body fat. A decrease in intracellular water in the ageing human has also been shown and is a reflection of the reduction of metabolizing cells in the elderly. This conclusion is confirmed by the determination of the potassium content of the body which falls with age; basal metabolism is reduced with age due to a loss of functioning tissues.

In considering the cardiovascular system of older people the cardiac output falls gradually with age and both systolic and diastolic levels of blood pressure increase with advancing years. American figures compare closely with a much smaller series reported from Rutherglen [TABLE 17].

More important than the mean blood pressure is the upper limit which can be regarded as normal and figures obtained from the Rutherglen Consultative Health Centre are given below [TABLE 18].

Simultaneous determinations of arterial blood pressure and cardiac output have shown that the calculated work of the left ventricle diminished with age. The increasing duration of systole with advancing age suggests that myocardial function is reduced and it seems correct to conclude that myocardial reserve is diminished and excess demands may induce cardiac failure more readily in the old than in the young.

The specific gravity of morning urine does not change significantly with age but if the intake of water is restricted for at least 12 hours prior to the collection of the specimen, concentration is impaired compared with the young. The resting renal blood flow and glomerular filtration rate diminish with age and both the excretory and reabsorption capacities of the renal tubules decrease with increasing age. Thus as people grow older renal function gradually deteriorates and as all functions of the kidney decrease at about the same rate it can be concluded that nephrons are lost in their entirety; although the remaining units are adequate to maintain renal function under resting conditions, reserve capacities are substantially reduced in the ageing individual.

Vital capacity diminishes as people grow older. This may be partly explained by diminution in muscle strength. Gas exchange is relatively little affected in ageing. It is possible that the excessive dyspnoea on

TABLE 17

MEAN BLOOD PRESSURE

Age	UNITED STATES* Men Systolic	Diastolic	Women Systolic	Diastolic	RUTHERGLEN Men Systolic	Diastolic	Women Systolic	Diastolic
65–74	148	81	160·2	83·7	159	86	167	86
75–79	154·3	79·4	156·6	79·3	167	86	172	87
80–84	—	—	—	—	170	88	183	89
85–89	—	—	—	—	166	87	179	94

* (Vital and Health Statistics, Ser. 11. No. 4, 1–40, 1964)

TABLE 18

USEFUL UPPER LIMITS

Age	*Men* Systolic	Diastolic	*Women* Systolic	Diastolic
60–69	195	100	200	102
70–79	204	104	215	106
80–89	215	108	230	110

exertion in old people is attributable to a reduction in the vital capacity of the lungs brought about by increasing rigidity of the thoracic cage.

When thyroid function is examined no change is found in the level of protein bound iodine with increasing age. Total uptake of radioactive I^{131} over 24 hours is the same at all ages although initial uptake is slow in the elderly. The response of the thyroid to a maximal physiological stimulus is not changed significantly with age. Recent experiments utilizing thyroxine labelled with radioactive iodine have shown that ageing in man is accompanied by decrease in the secretion rate of thyroxine.

When adrenal cortical function is considered the capacity of the adrenal cortex to produce adrenal cortical hormones is not diminished during senescence when stimulation is adequate.

The physiological mechanisms of thirst, temperature regulation, posture and pain may be altered in old age. The majority of elderly people admitted to geriatric units are dehydrated and many are suffering from faecal impaction. Temperature elevation may not be found in acute infections associated with fever in younger people. Survivors of accidental hypothermia have been shown to have a resting central temperature which is low, and on exposure to cold falls progressively and abnormally due to impairment of the increase in heat production and decrease in heat loss normally evoked by exposure to cold. This abnormality of body temperature regulation is probably a major aetiological factor in accidental hypothermia of the elderly. In some patients hypothermia can occur two or even three times in the same or successive seasons and postural hypotension due to impaired baroreceptor reflexes is a common finding in patients who have survived accidental hypothermia. Thus these patients may have had a central lesion in the brain which causes disturbance of both temperature regulation and vasomotor control. An elderly person who has sustained fracture of the femur may not complain of pain but may only state that he or she cannot move the leg, and in a recent clinical study of myocardial infarction in patients aged 65 years and over only 19 per cent. of the total had a classical onset with substernal or epigastric pain. The diagnosis of acute abdominal emergencies in the elderly is also made difficult by the relative absence of pain.

Diagnosis is not easy in the elderly patient as there is the need to find enough time to elicit an accurate history; older people are often deaf or may not understand the questions and when previous history is discussed may have forgotten past illnesses including the operative procedure that was carried out many years ago. Inattention, deafness, confusion and the joy of reminiscing make for a long and tedious history taking. It is often essential to have assistance from a relative. Diagnosis in older people is usually multiple and no longer can the physician cling to the single diagnosis theory of his student days. The fascination of geriatric medicine to the clinician lies in the difference in the symptomatology of disease between the elderly and the young. The insidious onset of illness is characteristic and the tendency of the elderly patient to attribute symptoms to ageing and fail to report them to the doctor frequently results in the illness being diagnosed at a late stage. The patient with Addisonian anaemia may present with oedema of ankles, severe breathlessness or fainting attacks. Breathlessness may be the initial complaint in coronary thrombosis or where a change of cardiac rhythm has occurred and the onset of atrial fibrillation has developed.

There is no greater diagnostic problem than the fall in an old person. Apart from being a common cause of death a fall is usually precipitated by some underlying illness. Myocardial infarction, anaemia, heart block, chest infection and neoplasm are some examples and on occasion the fall may be caused by therapy as, for example, a hypotensive agent being prescribed with excessive zeal. The patient with a history of falls presents a problem in diagnosis which demands investigation; not only must any injury which has occurred as a result of the incident be treated but search must be made to find out why the patient fell.

Clinical Findings

Certain facts about the normal changes of ageing are known and the following results were obtained from healthy older people.

Hair Growth. Complete baldness in men showed no trend with ageing, while partial baldness revealed a significant increase with age.

Vision. The ability of the eye to accommodate decreases throughout life due to changes in the substance of the lens and more than 90 per cent. of older people require glasses for near vision.

Deafness. The incidence of deafness due to causes other than wax in ears increases with age. In women it changed from 2·8 per cent. at 60–64 years to 8·3 per cent. at 85–89 years, and in men from 3·0 per cent. at 70–74 years to 9·1 per cent. at 85–89 years.

Reflexes. Abdominal reflexes in healthy older people (60–89 years) were absent in 21 per cent. of men and 58 per cent. of non-adipose women and in 68 per cent. of adipose healthy women. Absence of tendon reflexes in healthy older people is a rare phenomenon apart from the ankle-jerk in men (5 per cent.). Hand-grip decreases with age in men and women, reflecting the lessening muscle power.

Vibration Sense. In men and non-adipose women vibration sense was found to be absent at ankle and patella in 8–10 per cent. in 60–69 age range, in 16–25 per cent. in 70–79 age group, and in 30–40 per cent. in 80–89 age range.

In both sexes height decreases with age more so in women than men and kyphosis is more common in women and, when measurements of the kyphotic angle are taken, increases with age in both sexes. The chest expansion of men and women decreases with age and the decrease is particularly significant for men.

The mean haemoglobin level of healthy elderly people does not differ from that found in younger people, being in a recent series 13·6 g. per 100 ml. in men and 13·1 g. per 100 ml. in women.

Studies of heart size with increasing age are complex but it would appear that the significant increase in the cardiothoracic ratio with age is probably due to actual increase in heart size in men and to a decrease in the transverse chest diameter with the heart size remaining unchanged in women. Further work on the cardiac silhouette with the influence of kyphosis eliminated statistically confirms a significant positive association between cardiac silhouette and age for men but not for women.

In older subjects there is a deterioration in the quality of sleep with a high incidence of nocturnal awakenings but the total amount of sleep seems much the same as for younger age groups, largely due to falling asleep earlier, finally awakening later or taking mid-day naps.

NUTRITION OF THE ELDERLY

Many people eat less as they grow older, and it has been shown that the total calorie requirements fall with age. Symptoms of sufficient severity to induce an old person to consult his doctor are not often due to malnutrition but present indications are that there may be a phase of clinical malnutrition which may lead to poor health, apathy and disinterest. A person may be in a satisfactory state of nutrition but have no adequate nutritional reserves, so that an illness such as pneumonia may precipitate a stage of nutritional deficiency. Physical or mental incapacity may lead to deficient intake of necessary food substances, and a frequent cause of failure to feed properly is depression due to bereavement. Old people do not always buy wisely, so that income may be sufficient but spent on inappropriate food, and it is extremely difficult to change the food habits of elderly people. Though there is little protein deficiency among the elderly in Britain, a study of 60 women over the age of 70 years living alone showed that some diets were ill-balanced and also provided too little protein, vitamin C, vitamin D, calcium and iron, and a striking deterioration in health and nutrition was found in the late 70's in this series.

Low levels of vitamin C, vitamin B_{12}, folic acid and thiamine may be found in elderly people but it would seem from reported surveys that clinical malnutrition may not be evident. Riboflavine deficiency creates a problem in diagnosis because blood levels of this nutriment cannot be correlated with the patient's clinical state, and further investigation will be required to find out if riboflavine deficiency in the elderly exists as a separate entity.

Accurate biochemical assessment of nicotinamide and pyridoxine is also difficult.

Potassium deficiency in man can be induced in the normal person by giving a potassium-deficient diet for 4–8 weeks and this condition has been described with increasing frequency due to dietary deficiency in the elderly. Osteomalacia due to lack of vitamin D as a result of defective dietary intake and lack of exposure to sunshine may be commoner than has been reported, particularly in elderly women. Nutritional osteomalacia has occurred in adults due to dietary lack of vitamin D, when the diet contained less than about 70 Units of vitamin D per day. The usual history is of avoidance of fatty foods or to being a strict vegetarian. In osteomalacia, as in iron deficiency anaemia, it is difficult to assess the part played by malabsorption. It has been suggested that osteomalacia might contribute to the skeletal rarefaction found in old age; that meals designed for the elderly should contain a high proportion of protein with an adequate supply of calcium, iron and vitamin D and be prepared in such a way that the whole meal is eaten. Vitamin C may require to be provided separately, as food planned for older people may have to be kept hot for long periods as, for example, in a meals-on-wheels service. The problem of food supplementation is extremely complex, as flour with added iron does not appear to improve haemoglobin levels in anaemic individuals. Much work has been done recently in sideropenia (serum iron below 50 μg. per 100 ml.) and in one study this condition was found in approximately 40 per cent. of patients admitted to an acute geriatric ward, and in the present state of knowledge these low serum iron levels associated with raised total iron binding capacity and lowered iron saturation suggest widespread iron deficiency.

Evaluation of subclinical malnutrition presents great difficulty, and one possible sign of this condition, namely, sublingual lesions, could not be improved by supplementing the diet with vitamin C. Subclinical scurvy may be an additional factor in maintaining haemorrhage from the gastro-intestinal tract, initially precipitated by aspirin or alcohol, and in such cases poor dietary intake of vitamin C seems the most probable explanation for the low leucocyte ascorbic acid levels observed. The leucocyte ascorbic acid levels have been shown to fall steadily with advancing age in patients with gastro-intestinal haemorrhage and in those with uncomplicated peptic ulcer. This might indicate the need to give supplementary vitamin C to elderly patients with peptic ulceration.

Patients who have had a partial gastrectomy must be followed up carefully and for a long time, as following this operation loss of weight, anaemia, steatorrhoea and bone changes have been described. Atrophic gastritis is common in the elderly, even in the absence of gastro-intestinal symptoms. The consequent reduction in secretion of acid and intrinsic factor results sometimes in impaired absorption of vitamin B_{12} and in such cases additional factors, such as chronic infection which increases requirements for vitamin B_{12} or dietary deficiency, may produce pathological reduction of vitamin B_{12} in the serum. Borderline levels of serum B_{12} and folate are not uncommon in the elderly but the significance of such findings is not clear. Older people who are depressed (perhaps recently bereaved), with a fear of ultimate poverty, the mildly confused, and those with odd food habits, must be supervised, as must the group who are immobile because of physical disease and who depend on others for their food. Those who require prolonged analgesic therapy, especially with aspirin, should be watched for dietetic deficiency. Older people who come to the doctor complaining of lassitude, apathy and weakness, call for further investigation. Apart from obvious anaemia such a syndrome may indicate sideropenia, potassium deficiency and perhaps deficiency of vitamin C, vitamin B_{12} or folate. Such symptoms in the elderly are non-specific and may unfortunately also be a manifestation of incipient cerebrovascular disease, intercurrent acute infection or depression. There are clear indications for giving dietary advice and vitamin supplements to any old person who has recently had a febrile illness, undergone a surgical operation, or sustained injury.

Certain diseases are discussed as their management is specialized and differs from that described for younger people.

NEUROLOGICAL DISEASES

STROKE

The commonest neurological disorder in elderly people is a stroke and at present this is most often due to an infarction of the brain. It is not proposed to deal with the aetiology here nor to enter into the routine treatment which is described in Section 15. The special problems of the elderly, however, merit attention. In the treatment of a cerebral catastrophe, once the diagnosis has been established every effort must be made to save life in the initial phase. In many cases the patient will be unconscious and the aim will be to prevent death from asphyxia, from dehydration or from toxaemia. Routine measures are employed to this end but certain important points must be stressed. If the patient is semiconscious then efforts should be made to communicate with him, as from the beginning explanation, encouragement and instructions must be given. If the patient responds, a drink of water should be administered by the physician to find out if the patient can swallow. This particular observation is most important and is one which should be undertaken by a doctor. In the elderly, if the patient cannot swallow, it is the usual practice to administer normal saline by subcutaneous drip with hyaluronidase. This solution is given alternating with 5 per cent. dextrose in sterile water and 2500 ml. are advised in the 24 hours. If subcutaneous fluids are being used for more than 24 hours then biochemical control is essential and the serum urea and electrolytes must be watched. The use of a subcutaneous drip in this initial phase avoids the dangers associated with either intragastric or intravenous medication in older people.

The immobile patient is always at risk but especially in the period immediately following admission to hospital; this is the time when bedsores are most likely to develop and an alternating pressure mattress is useful at this stage, bearing in mind that nothing will take the place of highly skilled nursing and regular changing of position of the patient in bed. The paralysed limb may feel cold to the touch and relatives or nurses may desire to warm the limb so that an unguarded hot-water bottle may be placed against a paralysed limb and, as the patient cannot move the leg away and may have no sensation in the leg, a burn may result. Watch must be kept for the possibility of overflow urinary incontinence and faecal impaction.

Once the initial phase of resuscitation is concluded the general positioning of the subject in bed is important so that permanent deformities do not occur. Care must be taken to treat foot-drop by a pillow or covered board at the end of the bed and to avoid making the foot-drop worse by having the bedclothes too firmly stretched across the lower part of the bed. At this stage, if the patient cannot swallow, then intragastric feeding may be required and special watch must be kept for the development of parotitis or submandibular gland infection. Passive movements of both arms and both legs and all joints should now be commenced with as much active movement as the patient can undertake.

Rehabilitation in a more positive way will now be starting and the patient is allowed out of bed when he is conscious, afebrile, has no tachycardia and looks as if he could get up. This feeling of well-being is rather indefinite but is sensed both by the patient and by those who are constantly with him.

The surgical treatment of cerebrovascular disease and the use of anticoagulants are dealt with elsewhere [Section 15].

Incontinence of urine is common following a stroke in the elderly and if the brain damage is severe or if mental impairment was present before the stroke the incontinence is likely to be persistent; the patient may have no knowledge of his bladder function. With lesser degrees of brain injury and if the patient is mentally alert, control is likely to be quickly regained.

It is worth recording the frequency of incontinence on a special chart and differentiating between incontinence during the day and at night as patients who are only incontinent at night usually have less severe mental damage and a better prognosis. Such a chart encourages interest in the condition and helps to promote progress.

Other factors which adversely influence the cure of the incontinence are poor general health of the patient and local abnormalities of the urinary tract, such as obstruction to the outflow of urine, muscular weakness, or bacterial infection.

Following a stroke, the patient may only have one good hand and movements may be clumsy causing difficulty for the male in handling the urinal, and incontinence may be accidental in nature. The usual investigation of incontinence is required and the treatment consists in a number of procedures which must be integrated and, among these, simple nursing procedures are of the greatest importance. The patient should be encouraged to get out of bed as soon as his progress will allow and the time up should be gradually increased; this in itself will often cure mild degrees of incontinence. If the patient is out of bed he should be taken to the lavatory every 2 hours and if bedfast there should be hourly attention to his toilet needs. Fluids should be restricted in the evenings and constipation, as it aggravates the tendency to urinary incontinence, should be corrected. A rectal examination is therefore necessary in these cases.

Drug therapy may be of help in three ways: a tranquillizing drug such as thioridazine may improve the patient's mental state if he or she is restless or aggressive and on occasion anticholinergic drugs may be useful when the bladder is small. Examples of these are atropine, propantheline bromide and emepronium bromide, and lastly, if infection is present the appropriate antibiotic should be used.

Commodes of modern type are of value and incontinence pads are useful for the bed case. Day and night urinal appliances are available for male patients but the patient must be able to co-operate in their use. In bedfast male patients the most successful method has been to keep the urinal in position between the legs, associated with the use of incontinence pads. Following a stroke the usual cause of faecal incontinence is faecal impaction of the rectum.

The rehabilitation of the hemiplegic is a team effort, involving physical rehabilitation where the elderly person is taught to use to the maximum the amount of functioning brain tissue which has been left to him. Mental rehabilitation also is necessary where every effort to overcome emotional disturbance is made; the patient may be depressed and this will be a common occurrence rather than a rarity; separate and distinct therapy may be necessary to overcome this condition. Lastly, social rehabilitation is important as while the hemiplegic is undergoing treatment in the hospital, every endeavour must be made to fit his social background to suit his residual disability. This may mean alteration to the house or a new house or a completely different way of life from that to which the patient has been accustomed, and all this can be planned while the patient is undergoing therapy.

The hospital rehabilitation team is composed of the doctor in charge of the case, the nursing staff, the physiotherapist, the occupational therapist, the medico-social worker, the speech therapist and, not infrequently the chiropodist.

Principles of Rehabilitation in the Hemiplegic

Whenever the patient can sit in a chair bed-end exercises are commenced. The patient uses the end of the bed in order to raise himself from his chair and attempts to grasp the end of the bed. Initially both hands—the palsied and the good—may require to be placed on the end of the bed and the patient shown what to do. If the end of the bed is used, a bed-end board (a piece of wood between the uprights at the end of the bed to prevent the patient's feet from slipping under the bed) is placed in position. The patient pulls himself up from a sitting position to a standing position and initially the help of a physiotherapist will be required. The patient should wear outdoor shoes; a patient who cannot stand should not be attempting to walk. Many modifications of these bed-end exercises are used; once the patient is standing he endeavours to raise his palsied leg up on top of the bed-end board or, if the exercise is being performed in a physiotherapy department, on top of a piece of wood about 2 inches high. He will then practise raising the good leg which means standing on the palsied leg and is much more difficult. A further useful exercise is that the patient is asked to take side steps along the bar moving the feet laterally to one side and then the other. By these exercises the patient's sense of balance and posture is restored.

After bed-end exercises the next step is walking with a fixed support, e.g., a wall-bar or parallel bars. A full length mirror is useful at this stage and practice in standing up and sitting down should be encouraged. Walking on the level with a mobile support such as a 'Zimmer' walk-aid is now encouraged and eventually the patient will progress to walk with a 'Warral' tripod stick, then a walking stick and finally with no support. Stair-work is necessary and a staircase with two stout banisters should be used. During this phase of rehabilitation speech therapy may be indicated.

In the hemiplegic patient inability to abduct the arm and reach above the head is a serious handicap in dressing and one of the reasons for putting both arms through a full range of movement from the commencement of the illness is to prevent a 'frozen' shoulder. Full scapulohumeral movement is obtained by the use of a pulley and a rope, the patient exercising the affected shoulder by using his good arm. For the more specialized techniques books on geriatric medicine should be consulted.

In the lower limbs a common deformity is plantar flexion and inversion and this requires correction which can be achieved by a well-fitted boot with an inside iron and outside T-strap. Inversion is corrected by the iron and the foot-drop is controlled by a back stop incorporated in the iron. Sometimes a toe-spring is necessary to prevent foot-drop.

The occupational therapist will co-operate with the physiotherapist in the rehabilitation programme with the final aim of helping the patient to regain independence in the general activities of daily living and to retain the ability to enjoy the social aspect of community life which combats the effects of loneliness in old age.

Complications

Oedema of the affected limb may occur and this may be improved by insisting that the patient when sitting up should place the affected leg on a pouffe or stool, while diuretics of the thiadiazine group or frusemide may help to alleviate the condition if swelling persists, and a crepe bandage applied from the foot upwards may also be of use.

On occasion bullae will appear on a hemiplegic hand or arm which resemble a burn. There is usually no inflammation about the edge of the bullae and they are very similar to those seen in phenobarbitone poisoning. The bullae are usually treated by careful aspiration of fluid leaving the skin intact and applying an acriflavine dye. These bullae have considerable medicolegal implications as the relatives may assume that the patient has been burned when this is not so.

Persistent pain in an arm or leg following a hemiplegia is not uncommon and diagnosis is frequently rendered difficult by the inability of the patient to give an accurate account of the pain. Pain and stiffness of the shoulder joint, 'the frozen shoulder', is frequently seen and every endeavour must be made to avoid this complication by the use of passive movements of the joints on both sides from the beginning of treatment. It is essential to X-ray the shoulder and the cervical spine before treatment is commenced. Short-wave diathermy and pulley exercises may help, while infiltration of the affected shoulder joint with 5 ml. of a 2 per cent. procaine solution may render movement possible.

A painful shoulder joint may be associated with problems of posture. The shoulder capsule is stretched due to the muscular weakness associated with the weight of the paralysed arm. The use of an appropriate arm rest to raise the height of the arm of the chair on the affected side may relieve the pain.

Pain in the paralysed leg may also occur and careful examination including a radiograph should be made to exclude fracture or osteo-arthritis.

The difficulties which sometimes present in the rehabilitation of the hemiplegic have been called mental barriers to recovery and the clinical picture presented by the patient varies from day to day; it is the relative, nurse or physiotherapist who directs attention to the patient's difficulties and not the patient himself. Some of these barriers to recovery are a defect in comprehension where a patient may respond correctly to a simple request but fail completely with a more elaborate instruction. There may be neglect of the hemiplegic limbs despite good recovery of motor power and sensation. Denial of disease where the patient states that his limb is normal when it is obviously paralysed or when he rejects ownership of a limb. Other difficulties encountered include disturbance of body image, space blindness, where the patient cannot appreciate the layout of a ward although he can see clearly, apraxia, where there is loss of ability to initiate purposeful movements in limbs not paralysed, perseveration, memory loss, synkinesia, loss of confidence, depression, sustained inattention, emotional lability and a catastrophic reaction following attempts at physiotherapy. It is essential to make a diagnosis of these difficulties and some, especially depression, are amenable to treatment while others may well improve spontaneously.

The phenomenon of mouthing in the elderly, in which the patient while awake chews and licks her lips although her mouth is empty and she may be edentulous, has recently been described. This mouthing appears to be related to tension and stops momentarily if the subject closes her eyes or if a physician touches an area around the mouth. Most of the patients are unaware that they are mouthing and the condition seems to be caused by lesions in the mouth area of the vermis of the cerebellum.

The emotional lability of the hemiplegic who readily changes from laughter to crying without any reason will improve if it is ignored and reassurance and encouragement to the patient and relatives are of great value in treating this condition.

Particular attention must be paid to the care of the eyes in patients who have had a hemiplegia. On occasion the eye will be vulnerable and it is recommended that an eye-pad be worn if there is any evidence of damage to the 5th or 7th cranial nerves. Watch must be kept for any inflammation which may develop and this must be treated immediately.

PARKINSONISM

The treatment is as for younger people, see Section 15]; if L-dopa is used the initial dosage must be small, e.g. 125 mg. twice a day with gradual increase at longer intervals than for younger people to a lower maintenance level, e.g. 1·5 G. per day.

In the older patient it is important to remember the use of psychotherapy, and here the doctor must stimulate the patient's desire for recovery and may help by equipping his patient better for the acts of daily living. Suits with zip fasteners instead of fly-buttons should be obtained, shirts with collars attached should be used, and a special watch should be kept for the onset of mental depression. In the physiotherapeutic treatment of such cases it is important to remember that on occasion the use of raised heels, adjusted to the height to suit the individual patient by a Roehampton sabot, will tend to put the patient off balance anteriorly and will thus help him walking and especially improve his ability to turn round. Concentration of effort on individuals with this illness will often produce surprisingly good results.

Older people with Parkinsonism can suddenly become much worse and this can occur on transfer from their own home to hospital or after stopping drugs, e.g., benzhexol hydrochloride, abruptly and also with an acute infection. The patient becomes more rigid and does not speak, the skin feels warm, there is usually a history of decreasing mobility and intake of food and fluid, and there may be a rise in temperature especially at the beginning of the illness, but no leucocytosis unless infection is the precipitating factor. Such patients require fluids either subcutaneously with hyaluronidase or by intragastric drip, and a concentrated preparation of vitamin B complex with ascorbic acid (*Parentrovite*) intravenously has been recommended with benzhexol hydrochloride in small doses, e.g., 2 mg. three times a day if this substance has been discontinued abruptly.

INCONTINENCE IN THE ELDERLY

Incontinence of urine and faeces is present when such excreta are passed repeatedly otherwise than into suitable containers, and when this occurs outwith the patient's control. Incontinence is a symptom and not a disease and accordingly the causes will be numerous. Treatment will depend on aetiology and has to be flexible and purposeful to obtain results.

INCONTINENCE OF URINE

General Causes. Organic cerebral disease is the most important cause of incontinence of urine in old age and here the primary lesion is disease of the blood vessels of the brain, atherosclerosis, thrombosis, embolism or haemorrhage, resulting in dementia or hemiplegia, or Parkinsonism. Senile and arteriosclerotic dementia are associated with a progressive deterioration of habits and personality resulting in incontinence of urine. In these conditions the voluntary control of micturition is abolished and the reflex character of the act becomes more pronounced. When the central controlling mechanism is upset, the bladder becomes more active and of smaller capacity with the resultant clinical symptoms of frequency and urgency. There is loss of the normal warning period between the first desire to micturate and micturition itself and spontaneous contractions of the bladder occur early in filling. When this loss of control is associated with mental confusion, the patients are often unaware of being incontinent. In such cases palliative and nursing measures become extremely important. The patient should be kept out of bed as much as his general condition will allow and regular supervised visits to the lavatory, or bedpan or urinal rounds, should be a routine of geriatric wards and also when old people are nursed at home. Restriction of fluid after 6 p.m. reduces the amount of urine secreted during the night and rectal examination is necessary regularly to detect faecal impaction. Tranquillizers are sometimes of value in the management of the case where agitation is a feature, and the antidepressants may help where depression is a cause of mental disturbance. The anticholinergic drugs are useful in mild incontinence when the patient is sensible and synthetic oestrogen preparations by mouth may be of value in women. Appliances in the form of rubber urinals for men for day and night wear are available and plastic pants used with incontinence pads for women.

Local Causes affecting the Urinary Tract. Block to outflow of urine. In elderly men this occurs most commonly because of prostatic hypertrophy and the incontinence is of the overflow variety. The advice of the urologist should be sought immediately and catheterization postponed if possible until he has examined the patient. Other forms of obstruction are those due to stricture, carcinoma of the prostate, bladder neck hypertrophy and stones, while phimosis and balanitis may be the cause of difficulty in micturition and may also cause incontinence.

Gynaecological conditions. Urethral carbuncle, vaginitis and uterine prolapse are causes of this type of incontinence, while stress incontinence brought on by laughing or coughing is often due to weakness of the bladder sphincter and the pelvic wall. This type of incontinence is often amenable to surgical care and the advice of the gynaecologist should be obtained.

Urinary infection. With the possible exception of an acute urinary infection it is unlikely that infection by itself is an important cause of incontinence. It will, however, tend to perpetuate incontinence and attempts to cure it should be made. When the infection persists a block to the urinary flow should be looked for and the presence of renal or bladder stone excluded.

Other Causes. Urinary incontinence may be due to acute illness where consciousness is clouded, and treatment should be directed to the primary disease, the incontinence usually being of a temporary nature. Retention of urine with overflow incontinence should always be excluded in the elderly.

In terminal illness incontinence may be a manifestation of the failing powers of the body. It should be noted that physical handicaps such as hemiplegia may give rise to accidents with the urinal and here accurate observation of the patient is essential. In some instances the practical measure of providing a commode may be rewarded by success.

BONE DISEASE IN THE ELDERLY

Osteoporosis is fully described in Section 11, but there is still doubt about the aetiology and it has been suggested that this process is simply one of senescence.

Osteomalacia from a simple lack of vitamin D is not rare and while intestinal malabsorption and renal tubular defects are other causes, in recent years this disease has occurred especially in elderly women living alone. In older individuals this illness may coexist with osteoporosis and must be considered when there is a raised serum alkaline phosphatase, but this is not always present. The diagnosis is difficult in the elderly patient and is made on the history of muscular aches and weakness often so vague that the patient has been dismissed as neurotic. The main radiological abnormality is bone rarefaction and occasionally the diagnostic features of pseudofracture (Looser's zone) are noted. Biochemical tests on venous blood should show a normal or low serum calcium and a low serum phosphorus or a low serum calcium and a normal serum phosphorus, increased alkaline phosphatase and normal serum creatinine, protein, electrolytes and blood urea. Urine tests should reveal a low calcium:creatinine ratio, a high phosphate clearance, a low percentage tubular reabsorption of phosphate and a high phosphate excretion index. Unfortunately in older patients with osteomalacia the urinary indices are not infrequently of little diagnostic help and the induced hypercalcaemia test of Nordin and Fraser and iliac crest biopsy will be necessary to confirm the diagnosis. Faecal fat and nitrogen excretion tests will exclude steatorrhoea as a cause of the osteomalacia.

Treatment

This will depend on the cause of the osteomalacia but if it is nutritional then small daily doses of 1000 to 5000 I.U. of vitamin D should suffice. If the bone disease has been due to other causes, for example, previous partial gastrectomy or malabsorption then much larger doses will be required.

MENTAL DISORDERS

The importance of diagnosis in mental disease of the elderly cannot be over-emphasized as treatment cannot be successful unless a clear understanding of the patient's illness and difficulties is reached. It is worth stressing the importance of the acute confusional states as this group comprises almost 8 per cent. of mental disorders seen among the over 60's in mental hospitals.

Mental confusion in the elderly resembles the fit or convulsion of the infant; both are symptoms and not diagnoses; both require investigation. Confusion is characterized by disordered awareness of the environment, which may be revealed by disorientation for time, place or persons. Some common causes are infection, drugs (especially barbiturates, benzhexol and digoxin), cerebral infarction, cardiac failure, severe anaemia, uraemia and metabolic disorders such as diabetes or potassium depletion.

The temporary mental confusion so commonly seen following removal from home and associated with change of environment may indicate the presence of a slowly progressive mild deteriorating process. With reassurance and patience the old person will recover from the confusion but will show signs, even when better, of her mental deficit.

A broad spectrum of persistent or relapsing mental abnormality due to vitamin B_{12} deficiency has been described in the absence not only of anaemia but also of megaloblastic erythropoiesis or any clinical evidence of subacute combined degeneration of the cord; folate deficiency may also be a cause of dementia. Further collaboration between the biochemist and the psychiatrist is indicated to clarify the significance of altered calcium metabolism in the mental disorders of the elderly.

An endeavour in the geriatric assessment unit should be made to help the patient with confusion by reassurance and by informing the patient constantly where she is. The patient's name should be in large print on her bed so that she should be called by her own name, and once admitted, the bed should not be changed in position so as to give the patient an opportunity to relate herself to her surroundings. Thioridazine in liquid form (*Melleril Syrup*) in a dose of 12·5–25 mg. two or three times a day is of use in calming such patients. While the diagnosis and treatment of the mental state is proceeding, a plan of physical rehabilitation should be commenced. The patient, if bedridden, should where possible, be mobilized, and providing the physical condition permits, gradual and increasing active exercises encouraged. The advice of the physician trained in geriatric medicine should be available in the mental hospital and a scheme of rehabilitation should be organized just as in the geriatric unit with nurses, physiotherapists, occupational therapists and where necessary chiropodists and speech therapists, all playing a part.

DRUG THERAPY IN THE ELDERLY

In the drug therapy of the elderly, owing to the frequent occurrence of multiple diagnoses, it is essential to deal with the most urgent condition first as it is seldom possible to treat simultaneously all the symptoms of which an elderly person may complain. The elderly patient seldom mentions a purgative or a sleeping tablet if asked about previous drug therapy so that leading questions must be employed. In giving directions to older people about the use of drugs, the greatest care should be taken to explain exactly what is meant and to try to make the medicine-taking as simple as possible. Complicated drug schedules should be avoided and the instructions should be written down so that the relatives, if any, or the district nurse, may see clearly what has been ordered.

The absorption of drugs given orally will not be changed by age alone and will be unimpaired unless the patient has had a previous gastro-intestinal operation. The elimination of drugs in the elderly may be delayed due to impairment of renal function, previous damage to the liver, or by decrease in metabolism, or by an increase in the proportion of body weight represented by fat; decline in the efficiency of the cardiovascular system may result in delayed distribution and elimination of drugs.

Iatrogenic disease is common in older people due to drug therapy. Potassium deficiency can occur if thiadiazine diuretics, frusemide or ethacrynic acid are used daily or on alternate days. Mental confusion is readily precipitated in older people by drug administration and attacks of transient cerebral ischaemia are not infrequently produced by hypotensive agents especially if combined with thiadiazine diuretics. Care must be exercised in using hypotensive agents in older people and before prescribing such drugs the blood pressure should be taken lying and standing. The phenothiazine derivatives, for example, chlorpromazine, promazine and thioridazine, have varying degrees of toxic action. Chlorpromazine can cause cholestatic jaundice, postural hypotension, interference with temperature regulation, Parkinsonism or dyskinesia—a hypokinetic syndrome with spasms of muscles of head and neck. Benzhexol does cause mental confusion on occasion when used in Parkinsonism. Nitrofurantoin and phenylbutazone have also been followed by intrahepatic jaundice.

The dangers of digitalis therapy in the elderly have been described and such toxicity may be the reason for refractory cardiac failure. Elderly patients require smaller maintenance doses often of the order of 0·25 mg. 3–5 days a week. Digitalis toxicity is more likely to occur when the level of potassium is decreased by diuresis or diarrhoea or when blood calcium levels are increased.

Barbiturates are usually contra-indicated in the elderly and giddiness, persistent drowsiness and skin rashes can follow the administration of such substances. If an hypnotic is indicated, chloral hydrate in the form of dichloralphenazone, 1·3–2 G., or triclofos, 1–2 G. as tablets, or triclofos syrup, 1 G. in 10 ml., are useful preparations, while glutethimide, 0·25–0·5 G., is a useful alternative drug.

The use of soap and water enemas are now only of historical interest as a large enema can produce a shock-like reaction in old people and more elegant preparations, such as Fletcher's enema, are now available.

The sensitization of skin following even the use of the most innocuous bland preparation in the treatment of a leg ulcer is not uncommon. The substance is harmless at first but the skin becomes sensitive, and irritation is produced. The elderly diabetic who seems well controlled on an oral antidiabetic substance must be followed up as the diabetic condition may improve so that hypoglycaemia may eventually be produced. Recently an interaction between bishydroxycoumarin and chlorpropamide was described whereby serum concentration of chlorpropamide was increased.

If an antibiotic is indicated in an old person it is always worth inquiring if this substance has been previously administered as even a drug as free of side-effects as penicillin can produce an untoward or allergic reaction, and this inquiry should be made before the antibiotic is given. Streptomycin is especially dangerous because of its ototoxicity if it is given to elderly people with impaired renal function, and nitrofurantoin and phenylbutazone can cause neuropathy.

The rules should be to avoid polypharmacy as much as possible, to give simple instructions to the patient and the patient's attendants, and to use fluid preparations where available.

THE PREVENTIVE APPROACH

Future work with elderly people will involve members of the health team, based on the general practitioner health centre, in the routine visiting of certain groups of 'at risk' individuals. Those over 70 years living alone, those recently bereaved, those compulsorily retired, may be cited as examples, and the iceberg of unreported illness in older people could thus be detected at a much earlier stage. In most countries the failure of self-reporting of illness in older people has been discovered. Chiropody, adequate nutrition, interests and activity, pre-retirement training, and re-employment after retirement, combined with an active health education programme should decrease morbidity in the elderly. Another useful service is a follow-up visit by the social worker, district nurse or health visitor, to each patient discharged from a geriatric unit. The endeavour to keep older people fit is a wise policy for any country with an increasing number of elderly citizens.

REFERENCES

ADAMS, G. F., and HURWITZ, L. J. (1963) Mental barriers to recovery from strokes, *Lancet*, ii, 533.

ANDERSON, W. F. (1971) *Practical Management of the Elderly*, 2nd ed., Oxford.

CHEBOTARYOV, D. F., and SACHUK, N. N. (1964) Sociomedical examination of longevous people in the U.S.S.R., *J. Geront.*, **19**, 435.

EXTON-SMITH, A. N., and STANTON, B. R. (1965) *Report of an Investigation into the Dietary of Elderly Women Living Alone*, London.

MACMILLAN, A. L., CORBETT, J. L., JOHNSON, R. H., CRAMPTON SMITH, A., SPALDING, J. M. K., and WOLLNER, L. (1967) Temperature regulation in survivors of accidental hypothermia of the elderly, *Lancet*, ii, 165.

NORDIN, B. E. C., and FRASER, R. (1956) A calcium-infusion test: urinary excretion data for recognition of osteomalacia, *Lancet*, i, 823.

PATHY, M. S. (1967) Clinical presentation of myocardial infarction in the elderly, *Brit. Heart J.*, **29**, 190.

POWELL, D. E. B., THOMAS, J. H., and MILLS, P. (1968) Serum iron in elderly patients, *Geront. clin.* (*Basel*), **10**, 21.

RUSSELL, R. I., WILLIAMSON, J. M., GOLDBERG, A., and WARES, E. (1968) Ascorbic acid levels in leucocytes of patients with gastrointestinal haemorrhage, *Lancet*, ii, 603.

SHOCK, N. W. (1968) The physiology of ageing, in *Surgery of the Aged and Debilitated Patient*, ed. Powers, J. H., Philadelphia.

STRACHAN, R. W., and HENDERSON, J. G. (1965) Psychiatric syndromes due to avitaminosis B_{12} with normal blood and marrow, *Quart. J. Med.*, **34**, 303.

STRACHAN, R. W., and HENDERSON, J. G. (1967) Dementia and folate deficiency, *Quart. J. Med.*, **36**, 189.

WOLLNER, L. (1967) Accidental hypothermia and temperature regulation in the elderly, *Geront. clin.* (*Basel*), **9**, 347.

WOOLHOUSE, H. W. (1967) *Aspects of the Biology of Ageing*, London.

W. FERGUSON ANDERSON

GENETIC FACTORS IN DISEASE

The science of genetics is of increasing importance in medicine partly because more is now known about the basic facts of inheritance and partly because, with the control of infections, genetic disorders are relatively more frequent than they were.

Before proceeding further it may be useful to define the main genetic terms used in this Section.

Definition of Terms

Allelomorph (Allele). One of two or more contrasted

genetic characters situated at the same locus on the chromosome.

Autosome. Any chromosome other than the sex chromosomes. In man there are 22 pairs of autosomes.

Centromere. The point at which the two chromatids of a chromosome are joined, and the region of the chromosome which becomes attached to the spindle during cell division.

Concordance. When both members of a pair of twins exhibit the same trait they are said to be concordant.

Cross-over (Syn. Recombination). The exchange of genes between homologous chromosomes which takes place at meiosis.

Discordance. When only one twin has the trait they are said to be discordant.

Dominant Inheritance. A character is said to be dominant if the gene controlling it produces the same effect in the heterozygous as in the homozygous state.

Expressivity. The degree to which the effect of a gene is expressed. If the gene is controlling a disease some of those inheriting it will be more severely affected than others, e.g. in neurofibromatosis some individuals will have skin tumours, pigmentation and bone changes, whereas others will have pigmentation only.

Genotype. Strictly, the total genetic make-up of an individual. The term, however, is often used to denote the make-up of an individual with regard to a given pair of alleles, e.g. a blood group A individual may be of genotype AA or AO.

Heterozygous. Possessing two different genes (alleles) at the two corresponding loci of a pair of chromosomes.

Homozygous. Possessing similar genes (alleles) at the two corresponding loci of a pair of chromosomes.

Isochromosome. A type of chromosomal aberration in which one of the arms of a particular chromosome is duplicated because the centromere divides transversely and not longitudinally during cell division. The two arms of an isochromosome are therefore of equal length and contain the same genes [FIG. 5].

Meiosis. The type of cell division which occurs during gametogenesis and results in the halving of the somatic number of chromosomes so that each gamete is haploid.

Mitosis. The type of cell division which occurs in somatic cells.

Monosomy. Lack of one chromosome of an homologous pair, hence the individual only has 45 chromosomes.

Non-disjunction. The failure of two homologous chromosomes to pass into separate gametes either at meiosis or mitosis.

Penetrance. A dominant gene is said to have full penetrance when the character it controls is always evident in an individual possessing the gene. A gene controlling a recessive character is said to be fully penetrant if the character is invariably manifest when the genes are present in double dose.

Phenocopy. A condition which is due to environmental factors but resembles one which is genetic.

Phenotype. The manifest genetic make-up of an individual, e.g. the information available from examination of a single individual, without reference to any family (breeding) data.

Polyploidy. Duplication of the entire basic set of chromosomes more than the normal twice. Hence every chromosome is represented three or more times. (e.g. triploidy with three basic sets; tetraploidy with four basic sets, etc.).

Satellite. A short segment constricted from the rest of a chromosome.

Sex-linkage. A gene is said to be sex-linked when it is on either the X or the Y chromosome. If it is situated on the non-pairing part of the Y it can never cross on to the X and will therefore always be handed from father to son. If a gene is on the X a man will pass it on to his daughters and a woman to either son or daughter.

Translocation. This happens when two pieces of chromosome (not of the same size) are broken off from two non-homologous chromosomes and their positions exchanged (reciprocal translocation). The result is then that one chromosome will have too little chromatin and the other too much.

Trisomy. Where one chromosome is represented by three homologues as opposed to the normal two. Hence the individual has 47 chromosomes.

Tylosis. One of many forms of dyskeratosis. The most conspicuous feature is great thickening of the skin of the palms and soles, and hyperidrosis is also commonly present. Rarely tylosis is confined to the soles. It is inherited as a dominant trait.

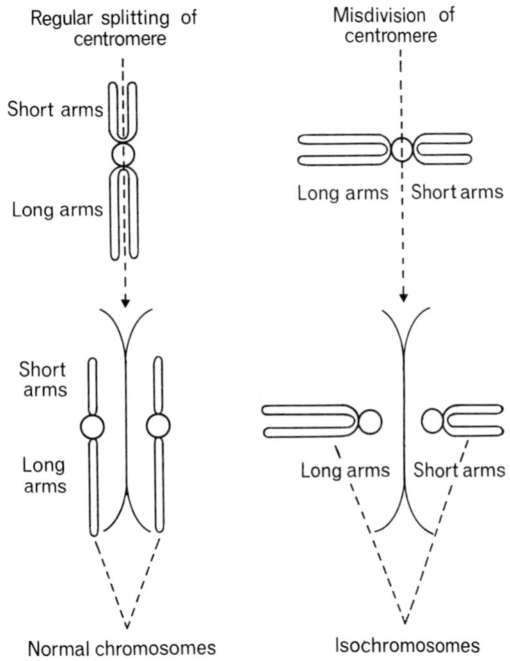

FIG. 5. Isochromosomes. [From Harden, D. G. (1965) in *Chromosomes in Medicine*, ed. Hamerton, J. L., Heinemann, London.]

X-chromosome (Fragmentation of). Some patients with Turner's syndrome have one normal X chromosome and a fragment only of the other X.

PATTERNS OF PEDIGREES

The behaviour of genes in families will next be discussed and methods described of how the various types of inheritance are recognized.

The single gene Mendelian type of pedigree in which affected and unaffected individuals segregate in well-defined ratios is the corner-stone of classical medical genetics. Much more often, however, illness is caused by a subtle interaction between genetic and environmental factors. When this is so it is usually not one gene but many, each with a small and additive effect, which are responsible for the inherited component.

Autosomal Dominant Inheritance

FIGURES 6 and 7 show two situations. In FIGURE 6 we are dealing with a rare gene, e.g. that responsible for

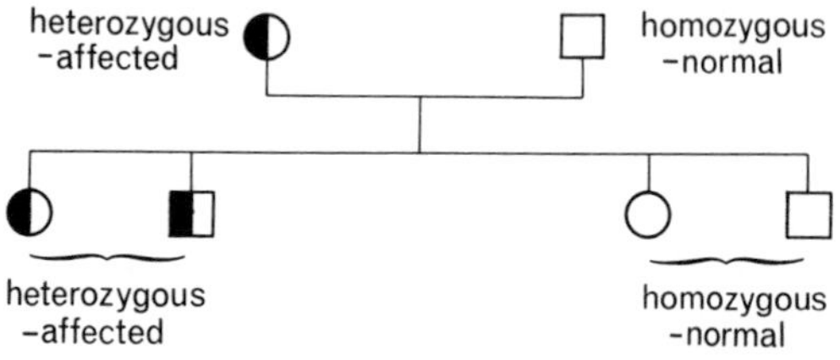

FIG. 6. A dominant trait occurring only in the heterozygous state, e.g. Huntington's chorea.

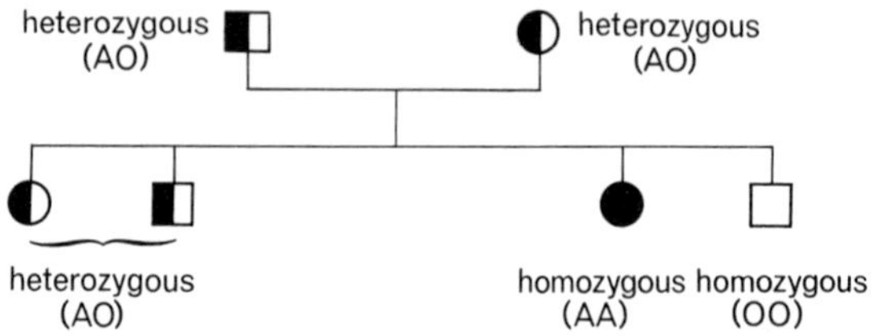

FIG. 7. Mating between two individuals heterozygous for a common dominant trait, e.g. blood group AO (typing as group A because A is dominant to O).

Huntington's chorea. This will originally have arisen as a mutation, and being dominant, will have manifested itself from the beginning. If the heterozygote does not often reproduce (and the fitness of patients with Huntington's chorea is much lower than that of controls), homozygotes are not likely to occur, and if they did, would certainly not be viable. Therefore, the chance of any given offspring having the disease if one parent be affected and the other normal is one in two and the risk is similar for subsequent siblings (chance has no memory). In FIGURE 7 is shown a common and innocuous trait in which an individual heterozygous for blood group A (and therefore genotypically AO) has married someone of the same blood type. Because A is dominant to O, the offspring are, on average, three group A to one group O, but the A's are of two genotypes, AO and AA.

In general, diseases controlled by dominant genes and therefore manifesting in the heterozygotes are less damaging than recessives. This may be partly due to the fact that the abnormal gene is only present in single dose, but additionally, if a dominant gene is disadvantageous enough in the heterozygous condition to prevent reproduction it will be selected against and rapidly disappear. A recessive, on the other hand, however lethal it may be in the homozygote, will (since the carriers are normal) have ample opportunity to spread through the population. This is even more likely to happen than might be expected since carriers of some deleterious recessives probably have increased fertility.

Another peculiarity of dominant inheritance is that characters inherited in this manner are of varying seriousness in different individuals, the degree of severity being known as the expressivity of the gene. When the effect is so reduced that the individual carrying the gene appears quite normal, the trait is said to be 'non-penetrant'. This can cause a good deal of uncertainty when families are being studied, as the gene seems to 'skip' a generation (which in fact it does not do). Part of this variability in expression is dependent on the normal allele which has been received from the unaffected parent and which accompanies the abnormal gene in the heterozygotes. That this is so can be proved because it can be demonstrated that sib-sib correlations for the expressivity of a given disease are stronger than the parent-sibling ones. This is because the affected sibs will all have the same normal allele (from their unaffected parent) and this will be a different one from that possessed by their affected parent.

Autosomal Recessive Inheritance

These characters also usually occur equally often in males and females, and the parents of patients are as a general rule normal, though both must be heterozygous carriers of the gene concerned. Since related individuals are more likely to be carrying the same gene, affected children are not infrequently the offspring of cousin marriages, and it is also a fact that the rarer the recessive trait, the higher the proportion of consanguineous parental matings in the families of affected individuals.

FIGURE 8 shows the general situation. If a child is

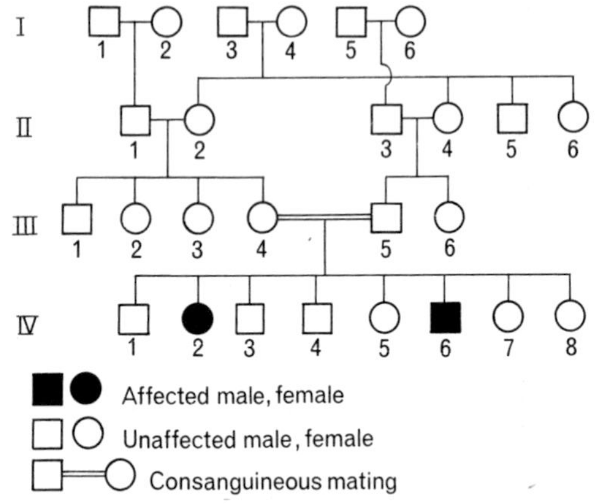

FIG. 8. Pedigree pattern of an autosomal recessive trait. [McKusick, V. A. (1962) in *Principles of Internal Medicine*, ed. Harrison, T. A. *et al.*, 4th ed., McGraw-Hill, New York.]

born with an autosomal recessive trait (e.g. albinism, fibrocystic disease, phenylketonuria) the risk of subsequent offspring being affected is one in four. Phenylketonuria, however, requires further comment. With treatment, affected girls may survive, marry genotypically normal men and produce children who, though heterozygous, would all be expected to be phenotypically normal. However, phenylalanine from the affected mother (who often relaxes the strictness of her diet in pregnancy) can cross the placental barrier and render *all* the children mentally defective. This is a loose example of a 'phenocopy' (see below).

If an affected individual marries a homozygous normal person, none of the children will be affected but all will be carriers. It is unlikely that an affected individual will marry a heterozygote unless there is inbreeding or the gene is common, but when they do, half the children will be affected, just as they would if the trait were controlled by a dominant gene. If two affected (and therefore homozygous) people marry, one would expect all their children to be affected, but this is not invariably so because, though the phenotypes of the two parents are the same, the genes controlling them can be at different loci. The same phenotype can therefore be produced by different genotypes, and furthermore an environmental cause can produce the same phenotype as a genetic one, e.g. the congenital deafness caused by rubella is indistinguishable from the purely inherited type [see phenocopy, p. 397].

Intermediate Inheritance

The terms 'dominant' and 'recessive' are often incorrectly used, and indeed are sometimes almost interchangeable. For instance, if the heterozygote in a 'recessive' condition can be detected by a sensitive test, it is not completely recessive. Also, if a 'dominant' condition is clearly recognizable in the heterozygote and yet the homozygote for this gene is affected in a different way, it is inaccurate to call the character a dominant one, and it would be better to refer to such genes as being 'intermediate' in effect. FIGURE 9 demonstrates this.

The term 'co-dominant' is used to describe allelic characters which are both expressed when they come together in the heterozygote—such as the blood group antigens A and B; in an individual of blood group AB both manifest equally.

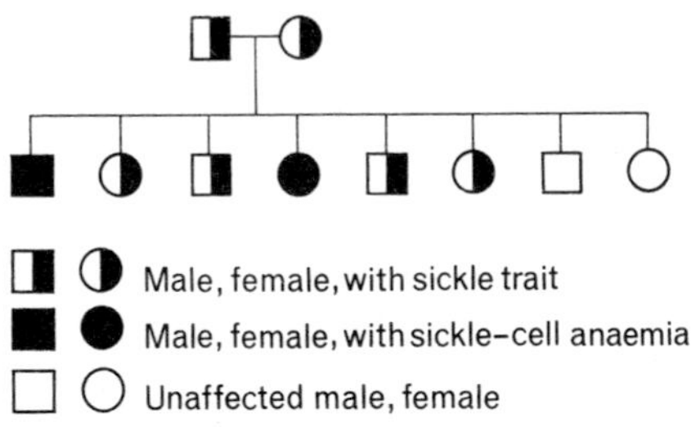

FIG. 9. Pedigree pattern of an autosomal intermediate trait as illustrated by sickle state. The anomaly in the heterozygote can be revealed if the oxygen tension of a drop of blood is lowered. [McKusick, V. A. (1962) in *Principles of Internal Medicine*, ed. Harrison, T. A. *et al.*, 4th ed., McGraw-Hill, New York.]

Sex (X)-linked Recessive Inheritance

X-linked genes can be dominant or recessive in just the same way as autosomal ones, but since a man has only one X chromosome, if he is carrying an X-linked gene it will always manifest, whether it is dominant or recessive in the female. Also, he will always hand on the gene to all his daughters and to none of his sons. FIGURE 10 illustrates the pattern of sex-linkage with the recessive X-linked gene responsible for haemophilia. It will be seen that the daughters of a carrier female are half carriers and half normal, and that the same pattern (though not the same result) applies to her sons—they are half *affected* and half normal. A haemophilic man cannot transmit the disease to any of his sons so that provided his spouse is not a carrier the sons can be sure of being normal. Women are hardly ever affected because the gene is rare and they would have to be homozygous for it [FIG. 10].

Sex (X)-linked Dominant Inheritance

Dominant sex-linked genes are rare, vitamin D-resistant rickets being the best example of a disease and the Xg blood group of a trait inherited in this way. Half the daughters of an affected woman will have the condition, and all the daughters (but none of the sons) of an affected man. It will be appreciated that in a large series of cases, females with the trait (because of their two X chromosomes) will occur twice as often as males. In the case of vitamin D-resistant rickets the hemizygous affected males tend to have the disease more severely than do the heterozygous affected females [FIG. 11].

Y-linkage

Y-linkage has not been definitively proved in Man though possibly hairy ears are an example. It has, however, been shown by unusual inheritance of the Xg blood groups in some families that occasionally genes can cross over from the X to the Y. Furthermore, if the male-determining genes, which are on the short arm of the Y chromosome, cross over to the X, a sperm carrying this abnormal X (known as X^y), if it fertilized an egg, would produce an XX^y zygote, which would explain some abnormal types of sex differentiation.

Sex-limited Inheritance

Some characters are influenced by sex without being sex-linked—the gene being carried on an autosome but only manifesting in one sex. Frontal baldness appears to be an autosomal dominant in men, but in women it behaves like a recessive, a woman needing to have the gene in double dose. Haemochromatosis in the reproductive period is sex-limited to the male because menstruation and parturition are safety valves in the female.

The inheritance of testicular feminization is an interesting genetic problem for the affected male does not reproduce, the normal females are carriers and therefore the pattern of inheritance could be that of a sex-linked recessive. However, it could equally well be a sex-limited autosomal dominant, but since the males are sterile, there is no easy means of testing which theory is correct.

Multifactorial Inheritance

This type of inheritance is, as the name implies, not dependent on one single gene (or pair of alleles) for which the individual is homozygous or heterozygous. It is not even dependent on genes only, but on the

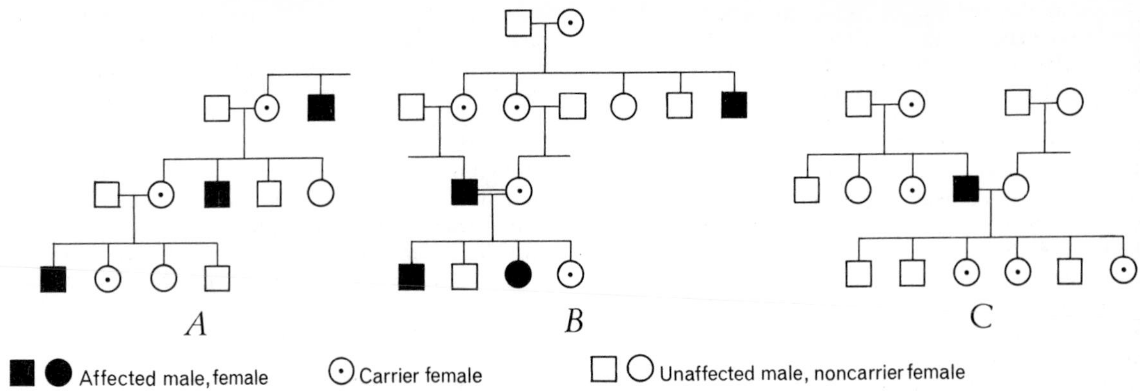

FIG. 10. Pedigree patterns of a sex-linked recessive trait, e.g. haemophilia. A. Note the 'oblique' pattern. B. An affected female can result from the mating of an affected male and a carrier female, as in the case of a consanguineous marriage shown here. C. An affected male mating with a normal, non-carrier female has all normal sons, all carrier daughters. [McKusick, V. A. (1962) in *Principles of Internal Medicine*, ed. Harrison, T. A. *et al.*, 4th ed., McGraw-Hill, New York.]

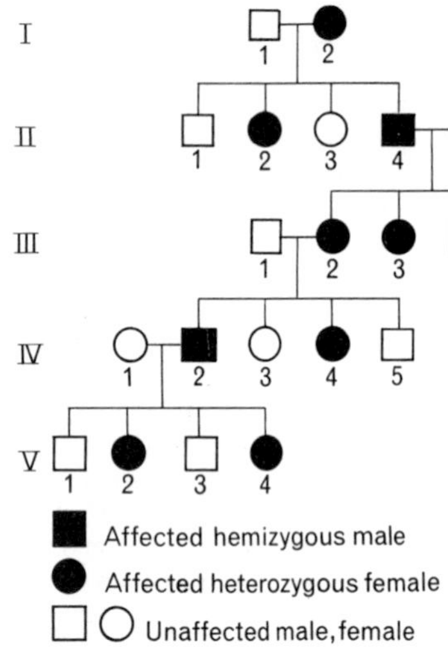

FIG. 11. Pedigree pattern of a sex-linked dominant trait. [McKusick, V. A. (1962) in *Principles of Internal Medicine*, ed. Harrison, T. A. *et al.*, 4th ed., McGraw-Hill, New York.]

environment as well, and many factors, genetic and other, are at work. The genes responsible will all have varying but small effect, and have varying dominance, and it is not easy to differentiate between the inherited and the environmental components. Characters dependent entirely on inheritance and controlled by many genes are known as 'polygenic', but the term multifactorial is loosely used for these as well.

A great many diseases where there clearly is an inherited component and yet no definite pattern of inheritance—such as duodenal ulcer—fall probably into the multifactorial group, there being all degrees of susceptibility just as there are all degrees of tallness or shortness. In duodenal ulcer there are racial and sex differences, and environmental ones such as cigarette smoking, but the genes responsible are additive. This is easy to visualize, but it is still unexplained what actually switches from 'no disease' to 'disease'. However, there is probably a threshold beyond which, if an individual has enough genes predisposing to the disease, and also the environmental factors favour its expression, he will develop the illness.

In connexion with sex difference and disease, Carter (1965) has done some very interesting work showing, for example, that in congenital hypertrophic pyloric stenosis (much commoner in boys than in girls) when a *girl* (i.e. the 'wrong' sex) has the disease she has more affected relatives than does a boy. The female baby is evidently usually more resistant than the male, but when she does develop the disorder, it is because she has a high concentration of predisposing genes, and this is why more of her relatives will also have a positive family history.

Fraser Roberts (1970) gives a very simple introduction to the principles of quantitative variation, which are based on the resemblances between relatives. For each step further away in relationship, the number of genes in common with one's relatives is halved. A parent passes on to a child half his or her chromosomes; a parent and his child therefore have half their genes in common. Clearly, the child will pass on half the genes derived from that particular parent, so a grandparent and a grandchild will have a quarter of their genes in common, and so on. With a rare dominant autosomal gene, it will be clear that half the children of a person in whom it appears will receive it, a quarter of his grandchildren and an eighth of his great-grandchildren. Half the parents and sibs of an affected person therefore resemble the patient, and half do not, and the likelihood of the other types of relative being affected can be calculated in a similar way. With multifactorial inheritance, however, many genes are combining together to produce the end result. On the *average*, half of the genes are making the sib or parent just like the subject, while half of them are making them no more like him than would be an unrelated subject. The difference is that, because there are many genes, occurring in different combinations, instead of half the sibs or parents being totally like and half totally unlike, all the parents and all the sibs are tending to be half-like. All the uncles and aunts are tending to be one-quarter like; all the cousins one-eighth like. These measures of resemblance are termed regressions, and multifactorial inheritance would

TABLE 19

EMPIRIC RISKS FOR SOME COMMON DISORDERS (IN PERCENTAGES)

[From Emery, A. E. H. (1971) *Elements of Medical Genetics*, by courtesy of the author and E. & S. Livingstone, Edinburgh.]

Disorder	*Incidence*	*Sex Ratio M: F*	*Normal Parents Having a Second Affected Child*	*Affected Parent Having an Affected Child*	*Affected Parent Having a Second Affected Child*
Anencephaly	0·20	1:2	2	—	—
Cleft palate only	0·04	2:3	2	7	15
Cleft lip ± cleft palate	0·10	3:2	4	4	12
Club foot	0·10	2:1	3	3	10
Cong. heart disease (all types)	0·60	—	1–4	1–4	—
Diabetes mellitus (early onset)	0·10	1:1	3	3	10
Dislocation of hip	0·07	1:6	4	4	10
Epilepsy ('idiopathic')	0·50	1:1	5	5	10
Hirschsprung's disease	0·02	4:1			
male index			2	—	—
female index			8	—	—
Manic-depressive psychoses	0·40	2:3	10–15	10–15	—
Mental retardation ('idiopathic')	0·30 –0·50	1:1	3–5	—	—
Pyloric stenosis	0·30	5:1			
male index			2	4	13
female index			10	17	38
Schizophrenia	1.00	1:1	14	16	—
Scoliosis (idiopathic, adolescent)	0·22	1:6	7	5	—
Spina bifida	0·30	2:3	4	—	—

follow the pattern indicated if there were no dominance and all the genes were intermediate in effect. Even though this is not so it can still be shown that the incidence of a disease such as duodenal ulcer falls off in the relatives of patients in the proportions that would be expected on the above hypothesis.

GENETIC ADVICE

The commonest request is for information about risks to subsequent children when one has already been born with an abnormality. Advice should always be given in terms of probability, never certainty, and a helpful yardstick is that about one pregnancy in 30 (that is of all pregnancies) will produce a serious developmental abnormality which appears early in life (Fraser Roberts, 1970).

Precise information can only be given in the minority of cases which show clear-cut Mendelian inheritance and these have already been mentioned. More often, particularly in common conditions, the genetic component can only be assessed empirically and TABLE 19 gives some examples.

Detection of Carriers

This necessarily only concerns recessive or 'intermediate' inheritance and TABLE 20 lists some of the more important conditions where heterozygotes can often be recognized. The technique of amniocentesis can sometimes be of use here.

TWINNING

A study of twins is a commonly used technique in genetic research but there has recently been a growing awareness of its limitations. Some of these are as follows:

1. Bias in the collection of twin data. Concordance is much more likely to be reported in monozygotic twins than discordance (an editor is unlikely, for instance, to accept a report of appendicitis occurring in only one of a pair of monozygotic twins).
2. There is a multiplicity of twin types. The monozygous and dizygous forms are well known, but in addition two sperm may fertilize an ovum at the same time so that although the maternal genes are similar the paternal ones differ. Furthermore, monozygous twins are not always both of the same sex and 'identical' twins have even been reported in which one of the pair was normal and the other a mongol.
3. Twinning may affect pathology. For example, cerebral palsy is more frequent in twins than in single births and there is possibly an increase in cancer in twins compared with the single born.

TABLE 20

DETECTION OF THE CARRIER STATE IN SOME AUTOSOMAL AND SEX(X)-LINKED DISORDERS

AUTOSOMAL

Trait	*Abnormalities in the Heterozygotes*	*Remarks*
Amaurotic family idiocy	Coarse abnormal granules in leucocytes present	50 per cent. of granulocytes and 5 per cent. of mononuclear cells affected in homozygotes and heterozygotes.
Hurler's syndrome	Metachromasia, i.e. fibroblasts stain red with toluidine blue O	For Hunter's syndrome (sex-linked) see below. In Morquio's syndrome, where the mucopolysaccharidose storage is limited to the skeletal system, the heterozygotes are not detectable by this method.
Fibrocystic disease of the pancreas	1. Cytoplasmic metachromasia demonstrable (readily distinguishable from that seen in the mucopolysaccharidoses)	
	2. Spock test positive	The Spock test depends on a globulin fraction found in the serum of patients and their parents which causes a disorganized movement of respiratory tract cells in rabbits.
	3. Sodium content of sweat	The sodium content of sweat rises with age and there is little difference between known heterozygotes and normal controls of the same age group. However, in affected cases the sodium content is higher than in controls.

X-LINKED

[From Emery, A. E. H. (1971) *Elements of Medical Genetics*, by courtesy of the author and E. & S. Livingstone, Edinburgh.]

Disorder	*Abnormality*
Haemophilia A	Factor VIII reduced.
Haemophilia B	Factor IX reduced.
G-6-PD deficiency	Erythrocyte G-6-PD reduced.
Congenital agammaglobulinaemia	*In vitro* immunoglobulin synthesis by lymphocytes reduced.
Lesch-Nyhan syndrome	Hypoxanthine-guanine phosphoribosyl transferase in skin fibroblasts reduced. Two populations of cells.
Hunter's syndrome	Granules in skin fibroblasts.
Ocular albinism	Patchy depigmentation of retina and iris.
Vitamin D-resistant rickets (hypophosphataemia)	Serum phosphorus reduced.
Duchenne muscular dystrophy	Serum creatine kinase raised.
Becker muscular dystrophy	Serum creatine kinase raised.
Diabetes insipidus (nephrogenic)	Urine concentration diminished.
Fabry's disease (angiokeratoma)	Urine glycolipids (ceramide hexosides) increased.

Nevertheless it may be very rewarding to study discordant monozygotic twins for this may point to the environmental factor in the disease. Another aspect of twin research which may be useful is the study of the frequency of a condition in twins compared with that in the single born, such as in cancer mentioned above.

LINKAGE AND ASSOCIATION

Genes are said to be linked when they, or more accurately the loci (positions) which they occupy, are situated on the same chromosome. The reason for saying 'locus' rather than 'gene' is that at any given locus the gene may be one or other of a series of allelomorphs, e.g. either the blood group gene for A, *or* B, *or* O. It will consequently be realized that a gene linked to the ABO blood group locus will sometimes be inherited with one allele and sometimes with another.

Furthermore, the possibility of crossing-over must be considered because occasionally genes will change places and two characters will appear together in several members of a family and may become separated in others.

There are only a few firm autosomal linkages in Man and these are listed in TABLE 21. Sex linkage, which is much commoner, is a different problem and dealt with separately.

One of the autosomal linkages will now be discussed to show some of the problems encountered.

The Nail-patella Syndrome and the ABO Blood Group Locus

The nail-patella syndrome, inherited as an autosoma dominant with full penetrance, is characterized by absent or hypoplastic patellae, nail dystrophy, abnormalities of the elbow joints and the presence of iliac horns, and FIGURE 12 illustrates part of a family with the condition.

At first sight there might not appear to be linkage at all as in generation I the nail-patella syndrome appears in an A individual (I.1), in the next in two O people (II.1, the proposita, indicated by an arrow, and II.3), in the next in an A and an O (III.2 and 4), and in the next in an O (IV.1). In fact, however, the linkage is only masked by the dominance of group A. The proposita (II.1) has received the nail-patella gene with her group O, and she has handed them on together to her son, III.2. As, however, the mother of III.2 was group O he must have received O from her and A

TABLE 21

KNOWN AUTOSOMAL LINKAGES

[Adapted from Renwick, J. H. (1969) *Brit. med. Bull.*, **25,** No. 1, by courtesy of the author and Editor.]

References marked * are in Renwick, 1969.

LINKAGES	SOURCE	REMARKS
Lutheran blood group and secretor loci.	Mohr, 1951*	Not assigned to a particular chromosome.
Elliptocytosis and the Rhesus blood group locus.	Chalmers and Lawler, 1953*	Elliptocytosis is controlled by genes at one of two loci, only one of which is linked to Rh. The linked form of the disease tends to be a less severe than the unlinked one. Neither gene is assigned to a particular chromosome.
Nail-patella syndrome and ABO blood group locus.	Renwick and Lawler, 1955*	Not assigned to a particular chromosome.
Haemoglobin-β and haemoglobin-δ loci.	Ceppellini, 1959*	Not assigned to a particular chromosome and of little clinical importance, but there is a form of thalassaemia in which both genes are deleted.
Pulverulent cataract and the Duffy blood group locus.	Renwick and Lawler, 1962*	Assigned to chromosome 1.
The transferrin locus (Tf) and the serum cholinesterase locus (El).	Robson, Sutherland and Harris, 1966*	Not assigned to a particular chromosome.
Albumin (Al) and group specific component (Gc) loci.	Weitkamp, Rucknagel and Gerschowitz, 1966*	Not assigned to a particular chromosome.
ABO blood group and adenylate kinase (Ak) loci.	Rapley, Robson, Harris and Smith, 1968*	Not assigned to a particular chromosome.
Sclerotylosis and the MNS blood group locus.	Mennecier, 1968*	Not assigned to a particular chromosome. Sclerotylosis is distinct from tylosis and characterized by atrophy of the skin as well as hyperkeratosis.
The alpha locus of haptoglobin and chromosome 16.	Robson *et al.*, 1969	Probably chromosome 16.
Myotonic dystrophy, the ABH secretor locus and the Lutheran locus.	Renwick *et al.*, 1971	The amniotic fluid is foetal in origin, at least from the 12th week of gestation.

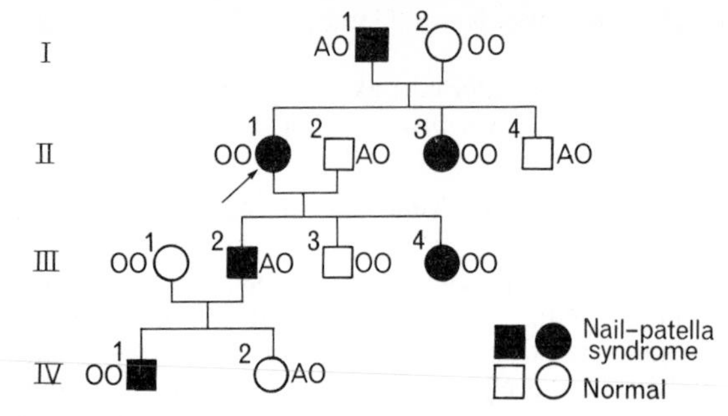

FIG. 12. Nail-patella syndrome. [Clarke, C. A. (1964) *Genetics for the Clinician*, 2nd ed., Blackwell, Oxford.]

from his father. He types as an A individual because A is dominant to O and the linkage of the syndrome with O is masked by this dominance of A. In generation IV it will be seen that III.2 has handed on the condition with O again. The situation is not due to crossing-over —if it were, IV.1 would have received the nail-patella deformity with A.

FIGURE 13 shows what happens when crossing-over does take place. Here the nail-patella syndrome is linked with group A_1, as in I.1, II.1, II.5 and III.2. Crossing-over has occurred at gamete formation in I.1, after the birth of II.5 and before the birth of II.7, who is, as will be seen, blood group A_1 and yet is *not* affected. It will be noticed that the other A individuals in this family

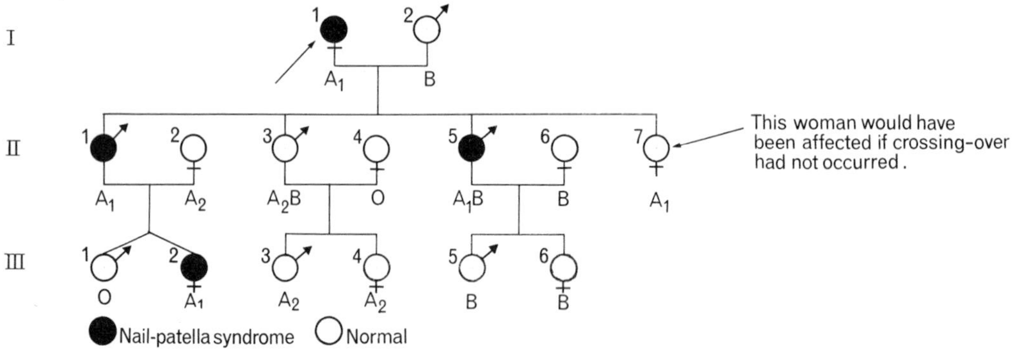

FIG. 13. Nail-patella syndrome. [Clarke, C. A. (1964) *Genetics for the Clinician*, 2nd ed., Blackwell, Oxford.]

who are unaffected are A_2 and not A_1. (A_1 and A_2 are alleles and are distinguishable.)

The cross-over value of about 12 per cent. agrees with that found in many other families. It is calculated by looking at those individuals where the linkage can clearly be seen, i.e. II.1, II.3, II.5, II.7, III.1, III.2, III.5 and III.6. In one case out of the 8 (12 per cent.) where the linkage could be detected a *new* combination is seen instead of the previous one, and this is quite close linkage. If the cross-over value reaches 50 per cent. it will be clear that there is an equal likelihood of the characters occurring separately as there is of them occurring together, and therefore there is no linkage at all, but 'free recombination'.

It is of great interest that Renwick on analysing the linkage data from 27 pedigrees of the nail-patella syndrome found that crossing-over occurred twice as often in women as in men, and in men less frequently as they grew older. If this is characteristic of many loci, it would mean that there would be less recombination, i.e. shuffling, of the paternal than the maternal genes.

Association is a basically different problem from linkage, characters appearing together in the population more frequently than would be expected by chance, e.g. the association between blood group O and duodenal ulcer. Nevertheless, where only a limited number of individuals is available it may be difficult or impossible to distinguish between the two. For example, tylosis and carcinoma of the oesophagus sometimes occur together in families. This could be due either to an association or to two linked genes, one for the tylosis and the other for the carcinoma, but with linkage crossing-over would sometimes occur, and then in a particular family some members would have the cancer without the tylosis.

Sex (X)-linkage and the Mapping of Chromosomes

Numerous genes, for example those controlling the Xg blood group system, glucose-6-phosphate dehydrogenase production, colour vision, haemophilia, the Duchenne type of muscular dystrophy, agammaglobulinaemia and the Xm serum protein group are X-linked —that is, they are known from a consideration of pedigrees to be situated on the X chromosome. By studying families in which *two* X-linked characters segregate (the Xg blood group system is often used as one) it is possible to infer from the frequency of crossing-over how closely the various genes are linked on the X chromosome (the method of calculating the cross-over value has already been given and one 'map unit' is equal to 1 per cent. of crossing-over). Using this method a map has been constructed [FIG. 14] and this shows that there are two clusters of genes on the X which have been reliably mapped in relation to one another, but there is an unmapped section of unknown length between them. Search is continuously being made for an X-linked trait which is at a measurable distance from *both* clusters and can therefore bridge this gap. New genes (not referred to here) are constantly being located but all so far have belonged to one of the two clusters.

Mapping the autosomes is much more difficult [see TABLE 21] but there are situations which clinicians should

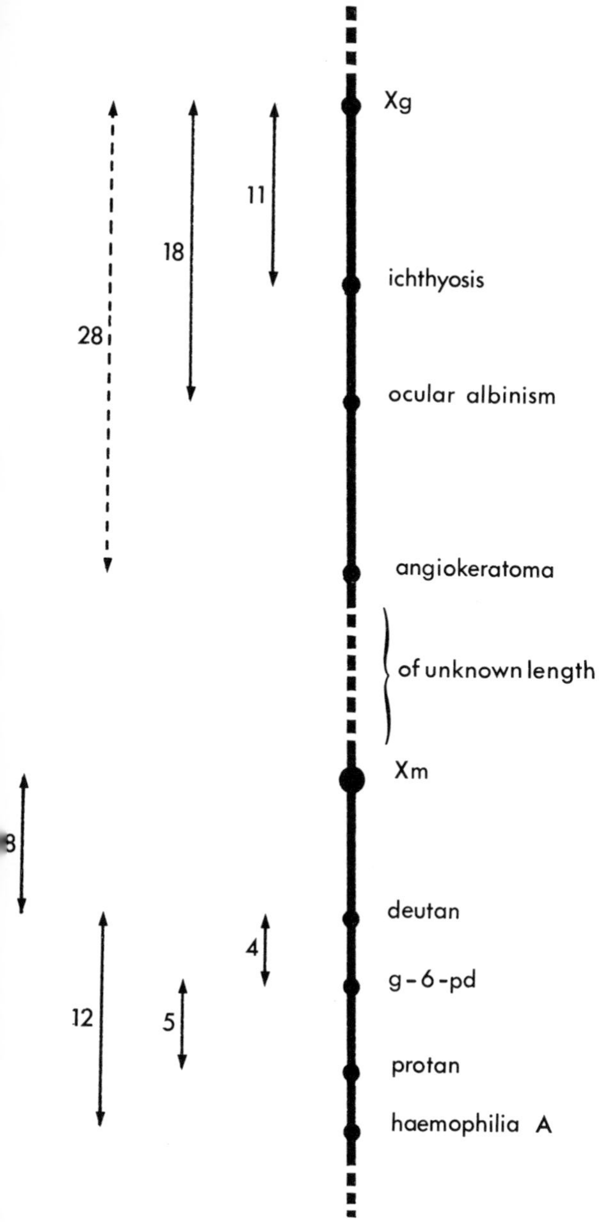

FIG. 14. Tentative map of the human X chromosome with the best guess at present of the location of the Xm locus in relation to previously known loci. Distances are in map units. [Berg, K. (1967) *Bull. European Soc. hum. Genet.*, **1**, 46.]

be on the look-out for. Thus, if a mongol (trisomic for chromosome 21) were found to be of blood group AB and to have one group AB and one group O parent, the clinician would know that the ABO blood group locus was situated on chromosome 21. Alternatively a patient with combined lesions may be informative, for example the baby who suffered from fibrocystic disease (a recessive) and the *cri du chat* syndrome. The latter is characterized by mental deficiency and a curious mewing cry due to weakness and underdevelopment of the upper part of the larynx and is caused by a deletion of the short arm of chromosome 5. It was found, using the Spock test,* that only the mother was a carrier for fibrocystic disease whereas both parents should have been. The deduction was that because of the deletion the child had not received the normal allele from her father and therefore that the gene controlling fibrocystic disease might be on the short arm of chromosome 5 (both parents were chromosomally normal). The hypothesis rests entirely on the reliability of the Spock test for heterozygosity for fibrocystic disease, and more work is needed before the theory could be upheld. It remains, however, a useful example of one way to tackle a genetic problem.

An entirely new way of mapping chromosomes is by means of mixed cell cultures. The procedure is to mix animal cells from two species, each set of cells having particular genetic markers, and to grow them for many generations in culture. When this is done with cells from mice and men, many of the human chromosomes are lost, and with them some of the markers, and so it is probably justifiable to assign these markers to the lost chromosomes. Another application is in the investigation of cancer, since in the mouse normal cells are 'dominant' to malignant ones but malignancy returns when certain chromosomes are lost in the hybrids (Harris, 1971).

GENETIC POLYMORPHISM

Genetic polymorphism is a type of variation in which individuals with clearly distinct qualities exist together in a freely interbreeding single population. Ford (1940) defined the condition as 'the occurrence together in the same habitat of two or more discontinuous forms or "phases" of a species in such proportions that the rarest of them cannot be maintained merely by recurrent mutation'. This definition excludes several very familiar types of variation. For example, the white, Mongolian and Negroid races of Man do not constitute a polymorphism since when interbreeding occurs the hybrid populations are intermediate and variable. Again, continuous variation, as in human height or blood pressure, is not an example of polymorphism. In these examples many genes are at work and the variation is brought about by the cumulative effects of segregation taking place at many loci, and not by 'switch' genes giving rise to distinct alternative forms.

Furthermore, segregation in human populations into normals and phenylketonurics or normals and achondroplasics are not examples of polymorphism.

What do fall into the definition are many enzyme and blood group systems, certain of the haemoglobinopathies and, perhaps most important from the practical point of view, polymorphisms of drug metabolism and pharmacological responses. In each case the problem is to find out the selective advantages and disadvantages which keep the various 'morphs' in balance. In non-human work it can often be demonstrated that heterozygous advantage is the mechanism, but in Man there is only one certain example of this, that of the individual

* Spock and his colleagues found that affected individuals and carriers contain an abnormal globulin which interferes with the normal rhythm of the cilia on the respiratory tract tissue of rabbits.

TABLE 22

RESULTS OF INTERMITTENT DOSAGE REGIMENS IN TUBERCULOSIS PATIENTS OF BOTH ACETYLATOR PHENOTYPES

REGIMEN	FREQUENCY OF DRUG ADMINISTRATION	ACETYLATOR PHENOTYPE	NUMBERS OF PATIENTS	
			FAVOURABLE RESPONSE	POOR RESPONSE
Streptomycin, 1 G. plus.	Twice weekly	slow	75	7
isoniazid, 14 mg. per kg.		rapid	33	3
ditto	Once weekly	slow	49	11
		rapid	33	22
ditto	Daily for first month then once weekly	slow	61	3
		rapid	28	9
ditto plus Pyrazinamide,	Once weekly	slow	58	9
90 mg. per kg.		rapid	18	16

Data from the Madras Tuberculosis Chemotherapy Centre by the kind permission of Dr. D. A. Mitchison.
Favourable response = sputum conversion, i.e. disappearance of tubercle bacilli. *Brit. med. J.* (1967) **4**, 230, and *Lancet* (1967) Annotation, ii, 977.

who, heterozygous for normal and sickle-cell haemoglobin (HbA/Hbs), is at an advantage over the normal because he is protected against malaria and clearly better off than the homozygous sickler who dies young. Malaria is also probably responsible for the high incidence of G6PD deficiency in some areas, and here again we have what appears to be a wholly deleterious trait, liable to cause haemolytic anaemia when pamaquine or fava beans are taken, yet with a frequency of 10 per cent. or more in some malarious areas. More often we simply do not know whether or not heterozygous advantage exists and in one troublesome polymorphism, that of the Rhesus blood group system, the baby who develops Rh haemolytic disease is always a heterozygote.

What can be said with a fair degree of certainty is that people with certain blood group phenotypes are more liable to have a particular disease than are others, e.g. duodenal ulcer is common in patients who are group O, and cancer of the stomach, pernicious anaemia, and (possibly) smallpox are associated with group A. However, it must be remembered that gene frequencies will not alter in subsequent generations unless the disorders operate before reproduction is over.

As was mentioned above, the pharmacogenetic polymorphisms are important. For example, the metabolism of isoniazid (dependent on acetyl coenzyme A) is under simple genetic control, rapid acetylation of the drug (present in about 50 per cent. of Caucasians) being dominant to slow, and TABLE 22 shows that the rapid acetylator is at a very significant disadvantage in the bacteriological response of tuberculosis to treatment when the drug (with streptomycin) is given rather infrequently. Conversely, the slow inactivators are much more liable to develop polyneuritis as a result of the treatment [TABLE 23].

Another example is that of the hypotensive drug hydrallazine, which again is polymorphically acetylated in the liver, and it has been shown that the acetylator phenotype is of importance clinically because the finding

TABLE 23

THE DEVELOPMENT OF POLYNEURITIS IN PATIENTS ON ISONIAZID THERAPY

INACTIVATOR PHENOTYPE	NO POLYNEURITIS	POLYNEURITIS	TOTALS
Rapid	58	2	60
Slow	66	17	83
TOTALS	124	19	143

$\chi^2 = 8{\cdot}87 \quad P < 0{\cdot}01$

Based on Devadatta, Gangadharam, Andrews, Fox, Ramakrishnan, Selkon, and Velu (1960). *Bull. Wld Hlth Org.* **23**, 587.

of antinuclear antibodies is more frequent in slow than in rapid acetylators, and of 12 patients who developed the systemic lupus erythematosus syndrome which this drug sometimes causes, all were slow acetylators and possessed antinuclear antibodies.

Another drug implicated in the acetylator polymorphism is phenelzine, and it has been shown that severe side-effects are far more common in those patients who are slow acetylators of isoniazid.

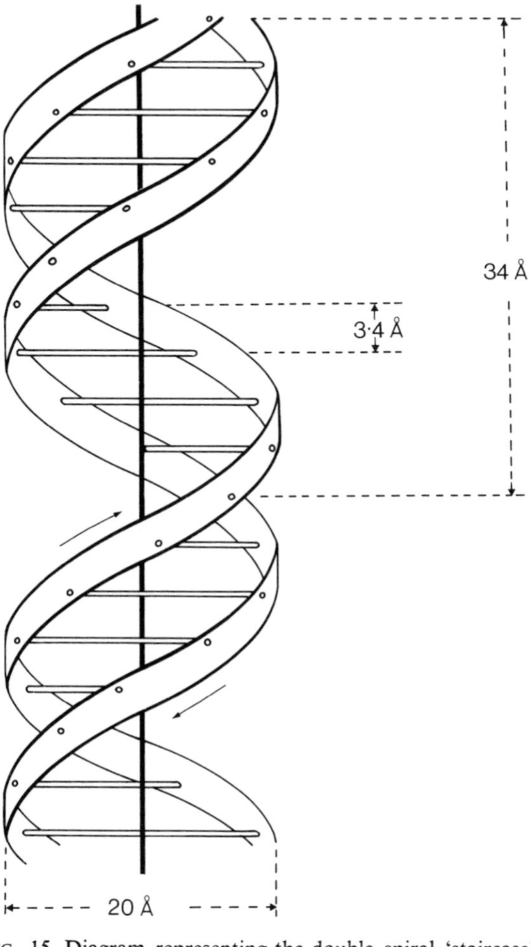

FIG. 15. Diagram representing the double spiral 'staircase' of the DNA molecule, giving dimensions in Ångstrom (one hundred millionth of a centimetre) units. The outer bands represent the phosphate-sugar chains and the horizontal rods the paths of the bases holding the chains together. The arrows indicate that the sequence of bases goes one way in one chain and the opposite way in the other. The vertical line represents the axis of the molecule. [Clarke, C. A. (1964) *Genetics for the Clinician*, 2nd ed., Blackwell, Oxford.]

Two examples of a 'drug response' polymorphism where one phenotype is rare are now mentioned. The first concerns diphenylhydantoin, which occasionally, in the usual clinical doses, causes ataxia and nystagmus, and this has been shown to be due to an inability to hydroxylate the drug, and the same defect has been disclosed in siblings of the affected person. The second relates to methaemoglobinaemia caused by phenacetin because of the patient's relative inability to de-ethylate the drug to paracetamol. In these circumstances, phenacetin is metabolized to a much greater extent than usual along minor pathways to hydroxyphenetidin and to hydroxyphenacetin, both of these being potent causes of methaemoglobinaemia. The same defect was shown to be present in a sister of the patient.

These examples show that a knowledge of genetic polymorphism is of considerable importance in clinical medicine and likely to become more so.

CHROMOSOMES

DNA

Chromosomes are composed of desoxyribonucleic acid (DNA) and a molecule of this consists of two chains, each made up of a desoxyribose phosphate backbone and a series of purine and pyrimidine bases which pair with those on the opposite chain (Watson and Crick, 1953). The molecule is constructed like a double spiral staircase of which the phosphate backbones form the 'banisters' and the nitrogenous bases the 'steps'. The pyrimidine bases are thymidine and

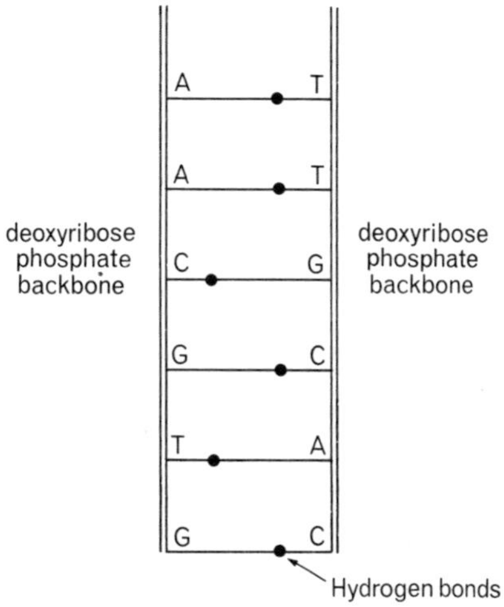

FIG. 16. Diagram showing the way in which the nitrogenous bases of DNA are paired, facing inwards from the phosphate-sugar chain and joined together by hydrogen bonds. [Clarke, C. A. (1964) *Genetics for the Clinician*, 2nd ed., Blackwell, Oxford.]

cytosine and the purines adenine and guanine. Thymine normally always pairs with adenine (mnemonic ts and as) and guanine with cytosine (mnemonic Gc) [see FIGS. 15 and 16]. A single molecule of DNA may have as many as 10,000 purine-pyrimidine pairs and its molecular weight is about 6,000,000.

The two chains reproduce themselves by unwinding and separating and the bases then pick up new partners —guanine plus its sugar and phosphate if cytosine is needing one, and adenine plus its sugar and phosphate if thymine is, and so on. Each new double chain consists therefore of one old and one fresh chain (the 'semi-conservative' mode of replication).

Goulian, Kornberger and Sinsheimer have recently (1967) made the great advance of synthesizing DNA *in vitro*. They put the tritium-labelled DNA of a virus in a test tube with the bases adenine, guanine and (instead of thymine), bromouracil, and added the enzyme polymerase. This caused artificial DNA to be formed round the natural one and the two could be separated because bromouracil is heavier than thymine. This artificial DNA was found to be capable of reproducing itself, and if this were the case in Man it might be possible in the future to attach a needed gene to harmless viral DNA and use this as a vehicle for delivering it to the cells of a patient with a hereditary defect.

The vital importance of DNA is that it can initiate the transmission of information to the amino acids in the cytoplasm so that they can form correct polypeptide sequences and hence the right proteins. For example,

G—C
C—G
A—T

would carry a different message from that of

A—T
G—C
T—A

A gene is therefore that portion of DNA responsible for coding a single polypeptide sequence, and this functional unit is also known as a cistron. It is, of course, vastly smaller than a DNA molecule.

Although the genetic information arises in the DNA of the nucleus, yet the proteins are manufactured in the cytoplasm in small particles called ribosomes. 'Messenger' ribonucleic acid (m RNA) (similar to DNA but with only one strand and with one different base) transmits the correct order of the bases, and 'transfer' RNA (t RNA) picks up the necessary amino acids from the nucleotide pool and assembles them.

It has been shown by Crick *et al.* (1961) in the bacteriophage T 4 that:

1. Three of the four bases form a 'word' which codes for an amino acid. If all four bases formed the 'word' this would only produce sixteen combinations—4 × 4—and there are twenty amino acids, so this was unlikely. Three bases will make 64 combinations (4 × 4 × 4), i.e. too many, but there are several 'words' which code for the same amino acid.
2. The code is 'read' in one direction. If a mutation consisting of the addition of a purine or pyrimidine base takes place, the coding is altered after the addition. If, however, a base is shortly afterwards deleted in the DNA of the phage, the order goes back after it to the original correct sequence, and the same result is obtained if, after the first addition, two further bases are added. It will be seen that either of these procedures will restore the DNA sequence to its original form.

Another way in which the DNA can be altered is by the substitution of one base for another. If this occurs within one triplet, it only alters one amino acid—the one coded for by that triplet. It does not alter the amino acids controlled by the 'words' on either side of the mutated 'word'.

In Man, in sickle-cell haemoglobin the single substitution of the amino acid valine for glutamic acid is enough to change HbA to HbS, this being a mutation in the sense of alteration. Another type of mutation in the base sequence of the DNA can result in no corresponding amino acid being formed, and therefore none of a given protein (for instance an enzyme), and this may account for many of the biochemical blocks in the inherited metabolic disorders.

By a new technique, Gurdon and his colleagues (1971) have shown that oocytes taken from the frog *Xenopus laevis* synthesize haemoglobin when they are injected with rabbit haemoglobin messenger RNA and haemin.

It will be appreciated that what has been discussed is at the molecular level, whereas what follows concerns whole chromosomes—that is, structures which can be studied under the microscope.

Techniques and Chromosome Identification

Chromosomes can only be seen in actively dividing cells, and it is therefore usually bone marrow, peripheral blood and skin which are investigated.

Bone marrow cells are most often looked at in leukaemia and they are therefore examined without culture in order to obviate the normal leucocytes overgrowing the leukaemic ones. For most other investigations peripheral blood (where it is the lymphocytes which are studied) is taken and incubated in a medium containing amino acids and vitamins and there is a 2–3 day interval before preparations can be made. With skin it is at least one and sometimes several weeks before results are obtainable.

In cultures, colchicine is added after the requisite incubation time, and this halts the process of cell division so that the chromatids remain attached by the centromere. The cells are next caused to swell by exposure to a hypotonic solution, and this enables the chromosomes to spread out so that they are more readily analysable. They are then fixed and stained. A chromosome is described and classified according to three criteria: (1) its length; (2) the position of the centromere; and (3) distinguishing features such as the presence of satellites. By the techniques of fluorescence and of Giemsa staining it is now possible to identify individual chromosomes.

In FIGURE 17 is shown how, by convention, the 22 pairs of autosomes are arranged and numbered in decreasing order of size. The X and Y are not numbered. Any chromosome pair can be allotted to one of seven groups and sometimes, but not always, it is possible to differentiate the chromosomes within these groups. The groups are 1–3, 4–5, 6–12 including X, 13–15, 16–18, 19–20 and 21–22 including Y. In the Patau classification the seven groups are labelled with the letters A to G.

By means of labelling the chromosomes with tritiated thymidine it is possible to observe the rate of synthesis of DNA and this is mentioned again when discussing the Lyon hypothesis.

CHROMOSOMAL ABNORMALITIES

Non-disjunction

At cell division homologous chromosomes may fail to separate and pass one into each gamete; instead *both*

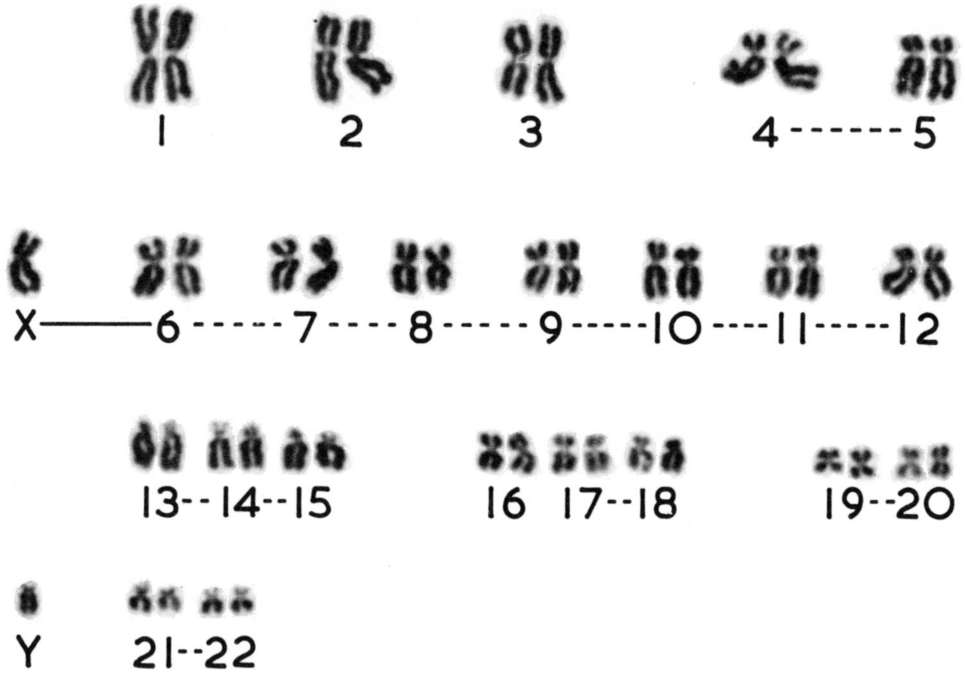

FIG. 17. A normal male karyotype. Magnification × 1,350. Agreed description of the human mitotic chromosomes.

Group A (1–3) Large chromosomes with approximately median centromeres. The three chromosomes are readily distinguished from each other by size and centromere position.
Group B (4–5) Large chromosomes with submedian centromeres. The two chromosomes are difficult to distinguish, but chromosome 4 is slightly longer.
Group C (X and 6–12) Medium-sized chromosomes with submedian centromeres. The X chromosome resembles the longer autosomes in this group, from which it cannot be distinguished. This large group is the one which presents major difficulty in identification of individual chromosomes.
Group D (13–15) Medium sized chromosomes with nearly terminal centromeres ('acrocentric' chromosomes).
Group E (16–18) Rather short chromosomes with approximately median (in chromosome 16) or submedian centromeres.
Group F (19–20) Short chromosomes with approximately median centromeres.
Group G (Y and 21–22) Very short, acrocentric chromosomes. The Y chromosome is usually distinguishable from the autosomes of this group.

[Roberts, J. A. Fraser (1970) *An Introduction to Medical Genetics*, 5th ed.]

members of a pair pass into the same gamete and the other is left without a chromosome of that pair. This is known as non-disjunction and can happen either with the autosomes or with the X and Y, and in the case of the autosomes the individual who received the extra chromosome is known as trisomic for that pair.

Non-disjunction in the Autosomes

Mongolism (Down's syndrome) is caused by trisomy 21, and the much rarer Edwards and Patau syndromes (both characterized by mental retardation and various physical congenital defects) by trisomy of the 16–18 and of the 13–15 groups respectively. It is probable that the mental deficiency of these three disorders is due to the increase in chromatin and that it is not specific for trisomy of any particular chromosome.

Translocation in the Autosomes

Although the majority of cases of mongolism are due to non-disjunction, in about 5 per cent. of cases, and especially in younger mothers, no additional chromosome is present but simply extra chromatin resulting from an exchange of parts from one chromosome (14 or 15) to another non-homologous one (No. 21)—that is a translocation has occurred. FIGURE 18 shows diagrammatically the various types of gamete which a translocation carrier can make, some of which for various reasons are more likely to be formed than others.

It must be emphasized that FIGURE 18 demonstrates gametes and that they will be joined in the zygote by normal gametes from the normal parent. Those gametes therefore which contain the translocated chromosome *and* a chromosome 15 or a chromosome 21, or both [FIG. 18, c, f or g] will, when the normal parent's chromosomes 15 and 21 are added to them at fertilization, give rise to an individual with too much chromatin; furthermore, those individuals who are effectively trisomic for chromosome 21 will be mongols. The offspring arising from a gamete containing the translocated chromosome only [FIG. 18, b] will have almost exactly

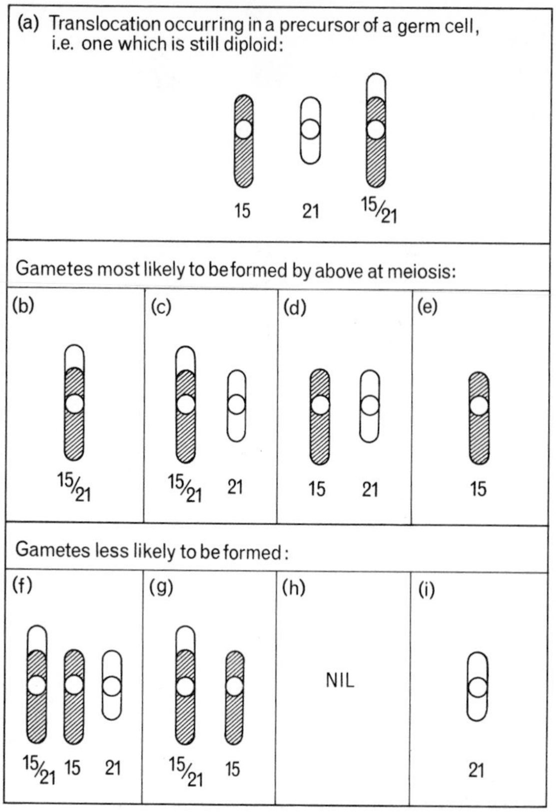

FIG. 18. Mongolism. Translocation involving 15 and 21. From (b) to (i) are gametes which will be joined at fertilization by a normal 15 and a normal 21 chromosome from the other parent. [Adapted from Carter *et al.* (1960) *Lancet*, ii, 678.]

the normal amount of chromatin and will therefore be normal, though a carrier. An individual arising from the normal gamete [FIG. 18, d], and paired with a normal one from the other parent, will be normal and have normal offspring. The combination with (e), (h) and (i) would be lethal.

From the point of view of genetic advice it is very important to know whether mongolism is caused by a translocation or by non-disjunction in a parent. In the former, one parent (probably the mother) will be a carrier, and about one in four of her subsequent children are likely to be mongols, as are about one in four of the children of any member of a family who is carrying the translocation. The risks for non-disjunction cases (by far the commonest) are shown in TABLE 24.

TABLE 24

RELATIONSHIP OF MATERNAL AGE TO TRISOMY 21

MATERNAL AGE	RISK OF OCCURRENCE	RISK OF RECURRENCE
20–30	1:1500	1:500
30–35	1:750	1:250
35–40	1:600	1:200
40–45	1:300	1:100
45-up	1:60	1:20

[From Redding and Hirschhorn (1968) March of Dimes Original Article Series, Vol. iv, No. 4, by courtesy of the authors and of The National Foundation, New York.]

The Patau syndrome can similarly be caused by a 13 to 15 translocation but here it is much commoner to

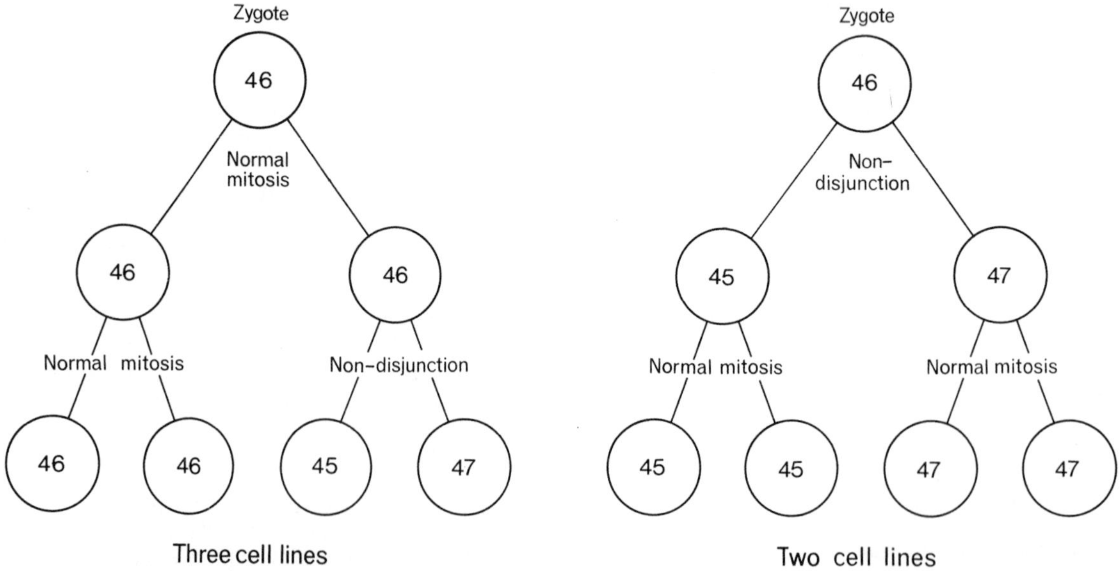

FIG. 19. The production of chromosome mosaics by mitotic non-disjunction after the formation of a normal zygote. [Harnden, D. G. (1965) in *Chromosomes in Medicine*, ed. Hamerton, J. L., Heinemann, London.]

find carriers than affected infants. The reason for this is probably that 13 to 15 trisomy receives a bigger quantity of extra chromatin, chromosomes 13 and 15 being bigger than 21, and the effective trisomy would be lethal.

Mongol Mosaicism

The non-disjunction described above is meiotic and so *all* the cells are abnormal and the zygote will have a uniformly abnormal number of chromosomes. Sometimes, however, non-disjunction occurs after the zygote has been formed, and it is then mitotic, so that two or more cell lines may be established and it is this which is known as chromosomal mosaicism [see FIG. 19]. Mongol mosaics may be normal mentally but have some of the physical stigmata of mongolism such as the facies or the abnormal palm print patterns, and the latter are, in fact, a sensitive index to the presence of trisomy although they do not correlate well with the mental condition of the patient.

Mosaicism may also explain the occurrence of more than one mongol in a family when this is not due to a translocation. It is then assumed that some of the gametes, either maternal or paternal, have 24 chromosomes, the extra one being a second chromosome 21.

Deletion

A disorder due to deletion of the short arm of chromosome 5 is the *cri du chat* syndrome. Deletions are referred to in the section on the mapping of chromosomes and in that on leukaemia.

Non-disjunction in the Sex Chromosomes

Because men and women are respectively XY and XX with regard to sex chromosomes, the consequences of non-disjunction are different in the two sexes and TABLE 25 shows the simplest possibilities.

TABLE 25

SHOWING THE EFFECTS OF NON-DISJUNCTION IN THE SEX CHROMOSOMES

		Normal male gametes	
		X	Y
Abnormal female gametes	O	XO	YO
	XX	XXX	XXY

XO Abnormal female (Turner's syndrome)
YO Almost certainly inviable
XXX Abnormal female (triple X)
XXY Abnormal male (Klinefelter's syndrome)

		Abnormal male gametes	
		XY	O
Normal female gametes	X	XXY	O
	X	XXY	XO

XXY Klinefelter's syndrome
XO Turner's syndrome

Note: These abnormal gametes are produced if the non-disjunction occurs at the *first* meiotic division. If it occurs at the second meiotic division (which is effectively mitotic), XX and YY sperm could also be produced, and four different types of abnormal offspring could result, XXY, XO and XXX as above and also XYY. Males with this last chromosome constitution, XYY (produced by non-disjunction in a Y-bearing sperm) are described below.

Though clinically immaterial which partner is responsible, it is interesting to know that this point can sometimes be decided, either by colour vision studies, or more efficiently, by means of the sex-linked blood group system Xg. Because it is X-linked, males can only be either Xg^a or Xg, whereas in women there are three possibilities—Xg^aXg^a (homozygous positive), XgXg (homozygous negative) and Xg^aXg (the heterozygote). Since the frequency of the heterozygote is as high as 36 per cent. in Europe, many families will segregate for Xg^a and Xg. Using this blood group it has been shown that in Turner's syndrome the non-disjunction is more usually paternal (74 per cent. of cases) whereas in Klinefelter's syndrome it is more usually maternal (60 per cent. of cases).

The clinical features of Turner's syndrome are well known and most cases have 45 chromosomes (particularly those with webbing of the neck), the missing chromosome being an X, and the patients therefore usually chromatin negative. However, about one-fifth of patients are chromatin positive and the explanation for this may be: (1) that they are mosaics, e.g. XO/XX; (2) possessors of a normal X and an isochromosome of the long arm of the X [see p. 397 and FIG. 1]; or (3) carriers of a normal X and part of the second one ('fragmented X').

The shortness of stature and the other somatic abnormalities frequently associated with an XO sex chromosome complement are not present in females who have a normal X and an isochromosome of the short arm of the X; they *are* present, however, when the isochromosome is formed of the two long arms. It appears, therefore, that the genes influencing height and the other somatic characters which are abnormal in XO females are situated on the short arm of the X chromosome, and that for normal development of these characters in the female the short arms of two X chromosomes should be present. It would seem that genes present on the long *and* short arms of *both* X chromosomes are necessary for the development of a functioning ovary.

It is important to recognize Turner's syndrome since after the age of 12, oestrogens can be administered to bring about spurious menstruation which is helpful for psychological reasons. Furthermore, a definite diagnosis also enables a prognosis of permanent infertility to be given with almost complete certainty.

In Klinefelter's syndrome the clinical features are well known and most males with the syndrome have 47 chromosomes and are chromosomally XXY, and they are therefore chromatin positive on nuclear sexing. As to be expected, because of the two XXs there is a low incidence of colour blindness comparable to that found in normal women. Some cases are mosaics, e.g. XY/XXY, but those of this karyotype who have been described do not appear to be less affected than those in whom all the cells are XXY. A few patients, for unknown reasons, are chromatin negative and have the normal complement of 46 chromosomes with an XY sex pair.

In the XYY syndrome the males are usually very tall and it was originally thought from a study of patients in maximum security hospitals that the behavioural disturbances of the men were primarily determined by their abnormal genotype. However, this is now less certain as the results of population surveys suggest that the original finding may have been due to bias in ascertainment.

In the 'triple-X' female (XXX) with 47 chromosomes, the surprising thing is that the women show very little physical abnormality and are sometimes fertile. It may be that as only one X chromosome per cell needs to be working (see the Lyon hypothesis, below) an extra non-working X does not much interfere with normal function. It would be expected that these women would produce some chromosomally abnormal offspring—on average half their sons should be XXY and half their daughters XXX—but so far those children who have been investigated have been normal.

The Lyon Hypothesis

Mosaicism was referred to on page 411 and in the examples given the individuals were always abnormal, but the Lyon hypothesis suggests that *all* women are mosaics with regard to their two X chromosomes. This is an important concept and well worth serious study.

Lyon (1961) postulates that at about the twelfth day after fertilization one of the X chromosomes in every cell of the female foetus becomes inactive. *Which* of the two Xs does so is decided at random for every cell, but once it is decided, all the descendants of that cell follow the same pattern. The result is that about half the somatic cells of the female will have an inactive maternal X chromosome and the paternal one will be 'working', whereas the opposite will be the case in the remaining half. In men the single X will always be working in all the cells. Lyon showed that this was certainly the case in mice, as female animals which were carrying a dominant gene for coat colour on their maternal X and a recessive allele on their paternal one did show patchiness of coat colour—just what would be expected if sometimes the dominant gene was in action and sometimes the recessive one.

The hypothesis explains why too much or too little chromatin does not greatly upset the mental or physical development of individuals where an X chromosome is concerned, but trisomy or monosomy for any of the autosomes is highly damaging. The hypothesis also explains why women are in many ways so little different from men—if both their X chromosomes were active they would have twice as many X-linked genes as males, which they do not. This can actually be tested when a dosage effect might be expected, for example in glucose-6-phosphate dehydrogenase production it is found that normal women do *not* make twice as much of the enzyme as do normal men.

Barr Body

In the somatic cells of the normal female, lying closely adjacent to the nuclear membrane, can be seen a small stainable body which is present in only a very small proportion of cells from males. Sexing therefore from the buccal membrane or the skin has become a routine procedure. The absence of a Barr body (syn. chromatin negative), however, does not necessarily mean that the individual is a male, but merely that there are not two X chromosomes. This is of some importance when a patient presents with some male and some female sex characters.

It is thought that the Barr body is the inactive X and tritium labelling shows that it synthesizes DNA very late. The fact that it is tightly coiled (hence the deep staining) may prevent the production and release of messenger DNA which transmits the chemical instructions from the genes.

CHROMOSOMES AND ABORTIONS

In about a quarter of spontaneous abortions the chromosomes are abnormal whereas in legalized abortuses the figure is around 2 per cent.

TABLE 26 gives the type of distribution of chromosomal abnormality in 120 karyotypes from spontaneous abortions.

The very high incidence of autosomal trisomy (53·3 per cent.) represents about 13 per cent. of all recognized spontaneous abortions and probably about 1·3 per cent. of all conceptions and this contrasts markedly with the figure of 0·2 per cent. for autosomal trisomy in live births, suggesting that such trisomy usually ends in abortion. On the other hand, trisomy of the sex chromosomes (XXX, XXY, XYY), well known in the general population, has not as yet been seen in abortuses.

Monosomy, mainly XO, also has a high incidence but surprisingly few abortuses are recognized with autosomal deficiencies, probably because they are lethal at such an early age that they have not been investigated. The high frequency of XO abortions is somewhat unexpected since individuals with Turner's syndrome can lead a reasonably normal though sterile life. The data in fact suggest that the XO condition at conception may be as high as 0·7 per cent. and that approximately 98 per cent. of the resulting foetuses are aborted (Polani, 1966).

CHROMOSOMES AND LEUKAEMIA

The Ph_1 Chromosome and Chronic Myeloid Leukaemia

The Philadelphia (Ph_1) chromosome is the typical

karyotype abnormality found in the majority of cases of chronic granulocytic leukaemia and results from the partial deletion of the long arm of one of the G group of chromosomes (number 22). It can be found both in the marrow cells and in peripheral blood cultures in the acute phases, but during haematological remissions, either natural or following chemotherapy or radiotherapy, the Ph_1 cell line disappears from the blood though it persists in the marrow. It has been detected only in the immature granulocytes, erythroblasts and megakaryocytes suggesting a possible common stem cell origin for these, since other tissues do not show the abnormality.

In children under 15 years of age, chronic myeloid leukaemia appears in two forms, a juvenile and an 'adult' type, and the presence or absence of the Ph_1 chromosome provides the most certain method of distinguishing them though they also differ in their haematological and clinical features. The juvenile form is Ph_1 negative, with thrombocytopenia usually present and the total white cell count not as high (rarely over 100,000/per mm.^{3}) as in the 'adult' form which is Ph_1 positive. Another striking difference is the increased level of Hb-F (from 15 to 55 per cent.) in the juvenile form whereas this is not the case of Ph_1 positive cases even when the disease occurs in infancy. The juvenile type has a poorer response to chemotherapy than the adult form, and the mean survival time after diagnosis is much reduced.

It is uncertain whether the Ph_1 finding is a sequel to the disease or precedes it but studies on two cases of identical twins, one with chronic granulocytic leukaemia and Ph_1 positive and the other normal and lacking the Ph_1 chromosome, suggest that it may be acquired rather than inherited. On the other hand it has been demonstrated in the blood and marrow of two patients before clinical symptoms developed.

TABLE 26

DISTRIBUTION OF CHROMOSOME ABNORMALITIES IN SPONTANEOUS ABORTIONS

[From Walker, S. (1969) in *Selected Topics in Medical Genetics*, edited by Clarke, C. A., by courtesy of the author.]

	ABNORMALITY	NO. OF ABORTUSES	TOTAL	PERCENTAGE
Monosomy	XO	24	26	21·7
	Double monosomy* (XO+autosome)	2		
Trisomy	A (1–3 group)	5	64	53·3
	B (4–5 group)	2		
	C (6–12 group)	7		
	D (13–15 group)	9		
	E (16–18 group)	21		
	F (19–20 group)	2		
	G (21–22 group)	15		
	Double trisomy†	3		
Triploidy††	XXY	15	23	19·2
	XXX	6		
	XYY	2		
Tetraploidy§		3	3	2·5
Mosaicism and others		4	4	3·3
TOTAL		120	120	

* 44 chromosomes in all
†† 3 sets of autosomes and 3 sex chromosomes
† 48 chromosomes in all
§ 4 sets of autosomes and 4 sex chromosomes

Chromosomes and Acute Leukaemia

1. General. There is good correlation between the cytogenetic data and the state of remission or relapse but the abnormal findings are almost certainly secondary to the disease. Aneuploidy is usually demonstrable in the marrow of untreated leukaemia and in relapse, whereas in remission the normal diploid mode is restored, in contrast to the marrow findings of the Ph_1 chromosome in chronic granulocytic leukaemia.

2. In mongolism (Down's syndrome). Mongols are particularly liable to acute leukaemia, the incidence being about 15 times as high as in the general population, and their susceptibility may be related to the primitive lobulation in their polymorphonuclear leucocytes, which could be the result of trisomy 21. An abnormality in the opposite direction, however, makes the matter puzzling, for in acute myeloblastic leukaemia

cell lines have been observed which are monosomic for chromosome 21.

There may also be an increased risk of acute leukaemia in patients with Klinefelter's syndrome and other congenital aneuploid anomalies, but the evidence is still slight.

3. In other diseases. Patients with Fanconi's aplastic anaemia are prone to leukaemia and this may be due to the high frequency of minor chromosome abnormalities observed in cultured lymphocytes, though they are not so readily seen in marrow cells. Similar chromosome damage has been reported in Bloom's syndrome (characterized by dwarfism and light sensitivity) inherited as an autosomal recessive.

Irradiation and Leukaemia

As is well known there is an increased risk of leukaemia in the Hiroshima and Nagasaki survivors, in patients after radiotherapy for ankylosing spondylitis, and after radioactive phosphorus therapy for polycythaemia vera. Of particular interest is the report in which three apparently normal patients, previously exposed (by accident) to whole body radiation, showed an abnormally small chromosome, indistinguishable from a Ph_1, in both marrow and peripheral blood cells (Goh, 1966).

Drugs and Leukaemia

Benzene is leukaemogenic and, correspondingly, chromosome aberrations have been described in persons previously exposed to the drug. Recent investigations on users of lysergic acid diethylamine (L.S.D.) suggest that this drug may have severe cytogenetic effects, causing chromosome damage not only in the users themselves but also in children born to mothers who took L.S.D. while pregnant.

REFERENCES

Carter, C. O. (1965) The inheritance of common congenital malformations, in *Progress in Medical Genetics*, Vol. 4, ed. Steinberg, A. G., and Bearn, A. G., New York.

Crick, F. H. C., Barnett, L., Brenner, S., and Watts-Tobin, R. J. (1961) General nature of the genetic code for proteins, *Nature* (*Lond.*), **192**, 1227.

Ford, E. B. (1940) in *The New Systematics*, ed. Huxley, J., Oxford.

Goh, K. (1966) Smaller G chromosome in irradiated man, *Lancet*, i, 659.

Gurdon, J. B., Lane, C. D., Woodland, H. R., and Marbaix, G. (1971) Use of frog eggs and oocytes for the study of messenger RNA and its translation in living cells, *Nature* (*Lond.*), **23**, 177.

Goulian, M., Kornberg, A., and Sinsheimer, R. L. (1967) Enzymatic synthesis of DNA, *Proc. nat. Acad. Sci.* (*Wash.*), **58**, 2321.

Harris, Henry (1971) Cell fusion and the analysis of malignancy, *Proc. roy. Soc. B*, **179**, 1.

Lyon, Mary F. (1961) Gene action in the X-chromosome of the mouse (*Mus musculus* L.), *Nature* (*Lond.*), **190**, 372.

Polani, P. E. (1966) Chromosome anomalies and abortions, *Develop. Med. Child Neurol.*, **8**, 67.

Renwick, J. H., Bundey, Sarah E., Ferguson-Smith, M. A., and Izatt, Marian M. (1971) Confirmation of the linkage of the loci for myotonic dystrophy and ABH secretion, *J. med. Genet.*, **8**, 407.

Roberts, J. A. Fraser (1970) *An Introduction to Medical Genetics*, 5th ed., London.

Robson, E. B., Polani, P. E., Dart, S. J., Jacobs, P. A., and Renwick, J. H. (1969) Probable assignment of the alpha locus of haptoglobin to chromosome 16 in man, *Nature* (*Lond.*), **223**, 163.

Watson, J. D., and Crick, F. H. C. (1953) The structure of DNA, *Cold Spr. Harb. Symp. quant. Biol.*, **18**, 123.

Cyril A. Clarke

IMMUNE MECHANISMS IN DISEASE

GENERAL ASPECTS

INTRODUCTION

The immune character of specific hypersensitivity was demonstrated when Richet in 1902 elicited anaphylactic shock in dogs with the second of two spaced injections of sea-anemone extract. In the investigation of immune phenomena in general much confusion at first arose from the puzzling contrast between, on the one hand, the beneficial immunity—that is, enhanced specific resistance to infection—conferred by, say, antitoxic antibodies against tetanus or diphtheria, and, on the other, the deleterious effects such as anaphylaxis that were equally clearly attributable to antibody. The explanation of this paradox began to appear when von Pirquet a few years later pointed out that, looked at from the biological rather than the clinical point of view, both effects evidently reflect aspects of the same *altered reactivity* that develops in the individual as a result of initial exposure to antigen. This altered reactivity, however mediated and expressed, von Pirquet called 'allergy'. It subsequently became increasingly clear that hypersensitivity is a more characteristic accompaniment of allergy than immunity. Initial lodgement of alien biological material in the tissues of the normal subject may stimulate various non-specific mechanisms of inflammation to the extent that the foreign material itself is irritant. In the subject rendered hypersensitive by previous contact, a subsequent encounter activates tissue mechanisms of inflammation through recognition of a different property of such biological material—its foreignness, more particularly its *specific* foreignness. In this way, through specific antigen-antibody interaction, or through the interaction of antigen with specifically sensitized immune cells, mechanisms of tissue defence are brought to bear on a much wider range of alien substances, irrespective of their intrinsic irritant properties.

The biological function of allergic hypersensitivity may indeed be wider than used to be thought. The development of the immune system was for long attributed chiefly to the advantage of being able to muster, on challenge, specific immune mechanisms to augment tissue defence against microbial invasion. In the last decade, however, the idea of 'immunological surveillance' has gained acceptance. This postulates that the ability of the immune system to recognize foreignness, and to activate destructive inflammatory responses as a result, provides a weapon not only against invading micro-organisms, but in Burnet's words 'against cells which by mutation, damage or viral action have developed aberrant antigenic determinants'. According to recent studies in comparative immunology, adaptive immunity has in fact evolved exclusively within the vertebrate subphylum. This, with the now universally accepted fact that the finely discriminant barrier to homograft acceptance—again exclusive to vertebrates—is immunological in nature, lends weight to the argument that an immune function of primary evolutionary importance is policing new antigens that may arise at cell surfaces within the vertebrate body, and producing immune contrivances for destroying the aberrant cells that carry them.

The notion of immunological surveillance recognizes, perhaps more clearly than the concept of immunity, that hypersensitivity is a normal sequel to contact with antigen, not a disease *per se*. To overcome the challenge presented by micro-organisms seeking lodgement in the tissues, or check the proliferation of a clone of mutant cells, the destructive manifestations of specific hypersensitivity need not necessarily exceed the microscopical level—the level at which clinically we recognize immunity. But there are circumstances where the degree, extent, nature or effect of the tissue response to an immune reaction may be such as to constitute a disability in itself. This may happen when, for example, antigen is presented to the tissues of the hypersensitive individual in large doses, or repeatedly, or when hereditary or other factors unduly influence selection of the immune mechanism of hypersensitivity, as in atopic individuals. It may also happen in the context of immunological surveillance when the antigen involved is not an abnormal component of mutant cells, but a constituent of the normal cells of a particular organ or tissue—that is, when the reaction is an autoimmune one.

Miescher and Muller-Eberhard (1969) describe immunopathology as 'a term intended to cover all immune phenomena and immune reactions which are associated with disease, regardless of whether they are helpful, inconsequential or harmful to the host'. This chapter deals with the last of these situations, where immune mechanisms produce disease; excluded from discussion here are aspects of immunopathology related to immunity deficiency syndromes, paraproteinaemias and myelomatosis, and lymphoid neoplasia.

IMMUNE EFFECTOR MECHANISMS

The immune functions of the body have two aspects, afferent and efferent. The afferent side deals with recognition of antigen, its processing, and other events leading up to induction of the immune response, while on the efferent side are the specific effector mechanisms, cellular or humoral, activated by renewed contact with antigen to put immune responses into practical effect. These dual functions are performed by macrophages, lymphocytes and plasma cells originating in the lymphoid tissues of the bone marrow, thymus, lymph nodes and spleen, and in the gut (tonsils, adenoids, Peyer's patches and appendix). Between them, these organs maintain a continual supply of cells that are immunologically competent—that is to say, cells of the lymphoid series qualified to respond to antigenic stimuli reaching them through the afferent side of the immune system, and to undertake effector roles on the efferent side, whether by direct specific interaction with antigen or by production of antibody capable of such specific interaction.

A major part of the cell population of the lymphoid tissues is small lymphocytes, most of them sessile; but a proportion of the lymphocyte population is mobile in the blood and lymph. These mobile lymphocytes recirculate from the lymph nodes via the lymphatics and thoracic duct to the blood, through the white pulp of the spleen, and, leaving the blood stream again through the post-capillary venules in the lymph nodes, rejoin the lymphatic flow into the thoracic duct. The cells of this recirculating pool Gowans identified as immunologically competent in the sense defined above. Originating in the thymus, they constitute a majority of the small lymphocytes in the blood, and the principal cell type in thoracic duct lymph. They are antigen-sensitive cells, responding to antigenic stimuli by transforming into large pyroninophilic 'blast' cells and undergoing mitosis. *In vivo* proliferation of pyroninophilic cells can be seen following antigenic stimulation in the paracortical region in lymph nodes and in the periarteriolar lymphocytic sheaths in the white pulp of the spleen, both traffic areas of the recirculating lymphocyte pool. When white cells from the blood are cultured *in vitro*, addition of antigen causes a similar transformation of a proportion of lymphocytes, provided they come from an individual previously immunized to the same antigen. Antigen-induced proliferation of cells competent to respond to a given antigenic stimulus thus implants an 'immunological memory' of the same antigen that is the basis of allergy, and hence of the hypersensitive response.

It is from this population of long-lived 'memory cells', morphologically indistinguishable from the general run of small lymphocytes, that effector cells of immune responsiveness are drawn. It is thought that each of these cells carries receptor sites specific for only one (or a few related) antigenic determinants, the whole population representing the range of specific immune responsiveness of the individual concerned, as determined by his genetic endowment with regard to protein synthetic mechanisms. Interaction of these effector cells with antigen may have more than one outcome. First, activated cells become capable of producing destructive changes through direct cytotoxic effects. Secondly, stimulation of these cells may result in antibody production. Proliferation of antigen-sensitive lymphocytes of thymic origin does not itself appear to produce direct descendants that are specific antibody-formers. It seems rather that in response to some antigenic stimuli at least these cells co-operate with other lymphocytes (possibly sessile in the lymphoid tissues and originating from the bone marrow) and facilitate both mitosis and maturation of the latter to antibody-forming plasma cells in response to the specific stimulus of antigen.

The two main effectors of immune responses are antibody and activated lymphocytes produced this way.

TISSUE REACTIONS MEDIATED BY ANTIBODIES

Immunoglobulin Classes

Antibodies belong to the immunoglobulin fraction of the serum proteins and are synthesized and secreted by plasma cells maturing from lymphocyte precursors present in all lymphoid tissue except the thymus. Although conforming to a common molecular structure in which two pairs of polypeptide chains (light (L) and heavy (H)) are covalently linked by disulphide bonds to form the single or repeating unit of the finished molecule [FIG. 20], immunoglobulin molecules display a remarkable inner heterogeneity that reflects the highly complex genetic patterns directing synthesis of their constituent peptide chains.

Analysis by electrophoresis and ultracentrifugation shows the wide range of molecular size and charge that exists among immunoglobulin molecules. Immunological analysis shows their heterogeneity in much greater detail. Here separated immunoglobulins, or their constituent fragments or polypeptides are treated as antigenic proteins and antisera raised against them in a different species. The ability of such antiglobulin antisera to discriminate different types and classes of immunoglobulins is based on their specific reactivity with different antigenic determinants on the L or H chains, which in turn represent different amino acid sequences, with their conformational implications for the molecule as a whole. It is now thought, moreover, that this specific reactivity of antibody—the ultimate expression of immunoglobulin heterogeneity—is itself determined by amino acid sequences at the antigen-combining site on the antibody molecule, and that these sequences are unique for each antigenic determinant involved in the elicited immune response. In addition, heterogeneity of structure is at least as important in the remaining parts of the immunoglobulin molecule since it is these that determine the range of the biological activity that antibody molecules can display as immune effectors of tissue reactions.

TABLE 27 shows some of the physical and immunological features of the five classes of immunoglobulins so far distinguished. As free proteins in the body these show very wide differences in distribution and behaviour. In healthy adults the total free IgG (about 80 g.) is distributed equally between the blood and the interstitial tissues, about a quarter passing across capillary walls each day and the same amount returning via the thoracic duct. The macromolecular IgM, on the other hand, is mostly intravascular. In man only IgG among the immunoglobulin classes passes the placenta and reaches the foetal circulation, and this is due not to simple filtration, but to active transport across the trophoblastic cells of the placenta. In the major immunoglobulin class, IgG, four subclasses differing in biological behaviour are distinguished on physico-chemical and immunological grounds. Different forms of IgA also normally coexist; these are monomeric

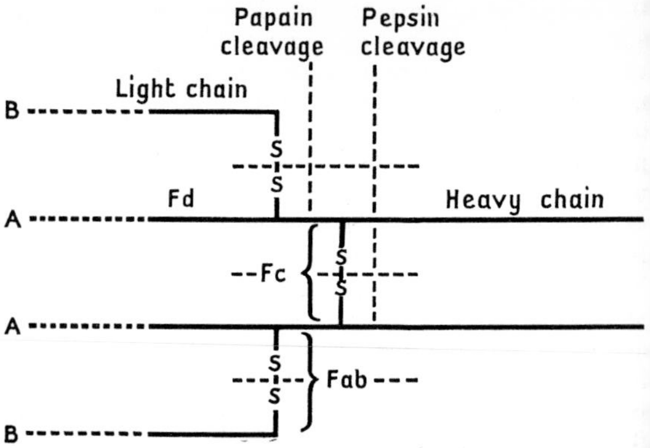

FIG. 20a. Immunoglobulin structure; diagram of proposed 4-chain structure (after Porter). Dotted lines show sites of: papain cleavage, producing two Fab portions and one Fc portion; pepsin cleavage producing F $(ab')_2$; and disulphide-bond reduction producing two light and two heavy chains. The amino acid sequences at the N-terminal (dotted) ends of the chains are variable and form the regions carrying specific combining sites. [Holborow, E. J. (1968) *An ABC of Modern Immunology*, The Lancet Ltd, London.]

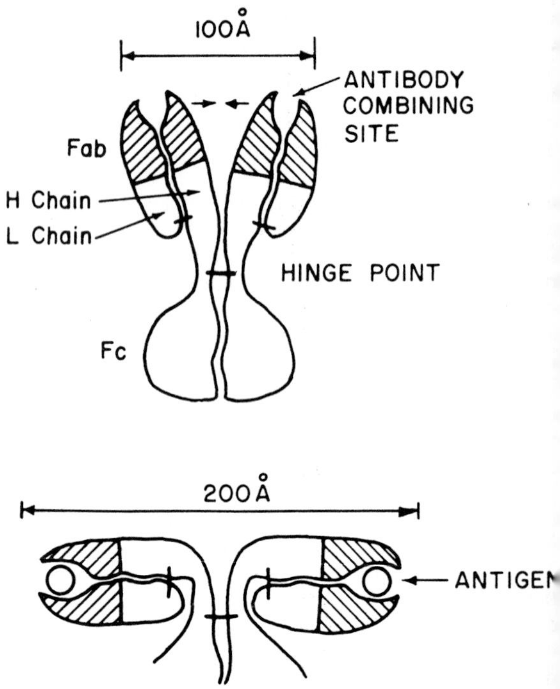

FIG. 20b. Model of IgG structure. On combination with antigen (lower figure) the length of the molecule approximately doubles. The curved interfaces between chains represent stretches of affinity resulting from non-covalent interchain forces. [Rose, B., Richter, M., Sehon, A., and Frankland, A. W., eds. (1968) *Allergology*, p. 101, Excerpta Medica Foundation, Amsterdam.]

serum IgA, and the IgA which is the predominant immunoglobulin in the external secretions (saliva, tears, gastro-intestinal juices). This is a dimer, and carries an additional 'secretory piece' on the molecule. As yet, no antibody activity has been identified in IgD, and little is known of its behaviour. IgE has a very marked affinity for cell surfaces, which presumably accounts for the very low level of this protein in the serum.

Thus, although antibodies in the shape of immunoglobulin molecules are initially secreted into the lymph, blood or tissue fluids in the immediate environment of the plasma cells that produce them, their subsequent distribution in the body is largely determined by the properties of the immunoglobulin class to which they belong. (It may be mentioned here also that a given plasma cell synthesizes only one class of immunoglobulin, as the striking homogeneity of individual myeloma paraproteins would suggest.) Furthermore, since the biological effects of antigen-antibody interaction are also to a great extent dependent upon the class of antibody involved, the site at which antigen-antibody encounter takes place has an important bearing on its outcome, as the next section will show.

action takes place not systemically, but locally. At a mucosal surface for example, such as the eye, nose or bronchus, local activation and release of these same agents produces immediate conjunctivitis, rhinorrhoea or bronchospasm.

The immediate anaphylactic tissue response is directly brought about by antibody possessing an uniquely developed property of fixing firmly to tissues. This property is demonstrated in the classical Prausnitz-Kustner (P-K) test which makes use of another manifestation of local anaphylaxis, the weal response to a skin prick with test antigen. When a small quantity of serum from an individual who shows such a skin response to a given antigen is injected into the skin of a normal unsensitized person, a reaction at the injection site can, after a necessary interval, be elicited by a subsequent challenge with the same antigen. What is relevant here is that the challenge may be withheld for

TABLE 27

PROPERTIES OF HUMAN IMMUNOGLOBULINS

	IgG	*IgA*	*IgM*	*IgD*	*IgE*
Molecular weight	150,000	180,000[1] 390,000[2]	900,000	150,000	200,000
Serum level mg./ml.	5–16	1·25–4·25	4·7–17	about 0·3	about 0·003
Valency (no. of antigen-combining sites)	2	2	5	—[3]	—[3]
Half-life (days)	25	6	5	—	—
Light chain types	κ, λ	κ, λ	κ, λ	κ, λ	κ, λ
Heavy chain class	γ	α	μ	δ	ϵ

[1] Serum IgA (monomer). [2] Secreted IgA (dimer + secretory piece). [3] Not yet known.

TYPES OF ALLERGIC DAMAGE DUE TO ANTIBODY

The most useful classification of tissue-damaging hypersensitivity reactions at present available is that devised by Gell and Coombs on the basis of initiating mechanisms—that is, the circumstances of the initial reaction between antigen and antibody. They distinguish three types of initiating mechanism involving humoral antibody.

Type I Reaction (Anaphylactic)

The signs and symptoms of generalized anaphylaxis that may follow within minutes the parenteral injection of foreign serum, protein or drugs, or sometimes even insect bites or stings in a sensitized individual include a marked fall in blood pressure with profound and possibly fatal shock, intense dyspnoea and urticaria. They occur because combination of antigen with antibody activates enzymes in the tissues and causes the release of vaso-active agents—histamine, serotonin, slow-reacting substance and kinins—which increase capillary permeability, alter vascular tone and stimulate contraction of smooth muscle. General anaphylaxis is rare in man, however; far more commonly, with antigens like pollen or house dust, the antigen-antibody inter-

several days after the initial passive sensitization; yet when the challenge is eventually made, it elicits an immediate unequivocal specific reaction. The essential feature of such tissue-sensitizing antibodies (cytotropic antibodies, or reagins) is this ability to become adsorbed to and persist on cell surfaces, more especially the surfaces of basophil (mast) cells and other mesenchymal cells that produce histamine and other pharmacologically active agents. In effect, such cells become 'allergized' with respect to antigen; and it is only when cell-bound in this way that reaginic antibody is able to produce an anaphylactic response as a result of its specific interaction with antigen.

In man, reaginic antibodies belong to immunoglobulin class IgE, and so far as present knowledge goes, are the chief if not the only direct mediators of human anaphylactic hypersensitivity of immediate type. In the commonest clinical manifestations of the latter, such as allergic asthma, hay fever and eczema, serum IgE levels are often significantly raised, sometimes to several times normal values. IgE is a normal human immunoglobulin, and most normal people produce some reaginic antibodies, but a familial incidence of reaginic hypersensitivity (atopy) is generally held to exist, and doubtless reflects an increased tendency, for reasons perhaps partly genetic and partly environmental, to respond to certain foreign antigenic stimuli by making antibodies in the IgE class, perhaps abetted by an undue sensitivity of the 'allergized' cells themselves.

Type II Reaction (Cytotoxic)

Type I reactions follow from free antigen reacting in the tissues with cell-bound antibody. We have next to consider tissue damage arising from the interaction of free circulating antibody with antigen already forming part of a cell surface or a tissue membrane. Such antigen may be a normal integral component, or may have been initially separate and have become bound by surface adsorption. In either case one result of an encounter with specific antibody is damage to the membrane carrying the antigen, and if this is a cell membrane, lysis and death of the cell.

A familiar illustration of the cytotoxic action of antibody through cell membrane damage is immune haemolysis following incompatible blood transfusion. To reproduce such haemolysis in the test-tube complement must be added to the mixture of incompatible red cells and serum, and it is characteristic of most cytotoxic antibodies that they achieve their effect by directing the cytotoxic action of serum complement toward a specific target cell in this way. Complement was the name given by Bordet to this cytotoxic principle in serum. It is now known that eleven distinct complement components (C1, which has 3 sub-components, and C2–9) interact in sequence to produce membrane damage finally by enzymic action. The process is initiated by the combination of the first component of complement with an immune complex of antigen and antibody. In such complexes the conformation of the immunoglobulin molecules is altered in such a way as to expose certain sites on the Fc portion of the H chain which can then interact with C1 and activate its enzyme component; this in turn mediates the participation of C2 and C4. These jointly catalyse attachment to the cell surface of C3, which generates a new enzymic activity enabling C5, C6 and C7 to interact with the cell surface. At the altered site thus produced C8 and C9 now react sequentially further to modify the cell membrane, and finally to produce a lesion and cell lysis. This complex sequence (much over-simplified in this brief account) is activated and carried through to lysis most efficiently by antigen-antibody complexes at the cell surface in which the immunoglobulin component is IgM, and the haemolytic efficiency of such 19S antibody has long been recognized. However, immune complexes in which the immunoglobulin is IgG may also have considerable complement-fixing properties, although molecule for molecule IgG antibody is less efficiently lytic. IgA and IgE complexes on the other hand have little or no power to fix complement.

Each step in the complement fixation sequence is subject *in vivo* to the action of numerous activators and inhibitors; and at several points short of final lytic activity intermediate compounds are produced which themselves have important biological effects. These are: (1) anaphylotoxins, which are histamine releasers and hence the means by which formation of complement-fixing IgM and IgG immune complexes can lead to altered vascular permeability and smooth muscle contraction; (2) leucocyte chemotactic factors; and (3) opsonizing factors which promote phagocytosis locally by causing immune complexes to adhere to the surfaces of red cells, leucocytes or platelets (immune adherence) and indeed to the surfaces of phagocytic cells themselves, in this way considerably enhancing the function of the latter.

Cytotoxic antibodies are not invariably complement-fixing. In haemolytic disease of the newborn where placental bleeds of Rhesus-positive red cells have provided an antigenic stimulus for production of anti-Rh isoantibodies by a Rhesus-negative mother, the destruction of foetal red cells is due to IgG 'incomplete' antibody passively acquired across the placenta. Complement is not involved here, for it cannot be demonstrated on the antibody-coated cells, and there is little intravascular haemolysis. It appears that the cytotoxic action of the anti-red cell antibody is due rather to its opsonizing effect, the red cells being cleared from the circulation and destroyed later by the phagocytic cells of the spleen. In auto-immune haemolytic anaemia, where the body is actively producing auto-antibodies directed at antigens present as normal surface components of its own red cells, examples occur of antibodies that are complement fixing, and of antibodies that are not, although both are able to bring about eventual destruction of the red cells they combine with. The adsorption of foreign substances on the surfaces of blood cells acting as 'innocent bystanders' can also lead to immune cytolysis and it is thought that this mechanism underlies some drug hypersensitivities manifested as thrombocytopenic purpura or haemolytic anaemia. *Sedormid* purpura, for example, was shown to be associated with the appearance in patients taking this drug of antibodies that react with platelets in the presence of the drug, but with neither drug nor platelets separately. The drug thus appears in such cases to act as a hapten made antigenic by binding to platelets as carrier, and the resulting immune response produces antibody with specificity for the *Sedormid*-platelet complex as a whole. A similar mechanism probably operates in the haemolytic anaemia seen occasionally during treatment with stibophen, quinidine, and more rarely still, penicillin. The comparative rarity of these drug-induced immune blood dyscrasias presumably reflects the instability of most drug-cell complexes and their resulting very poor antigenicity.

It is not surprising that examples of Type II antibody-mediated cell damage are most easily found among blood dyscrasias, where cells can readily be tested for antibody and complement. Damage brought about essentially in the same way by the action of specific antibody and complement is seen also in the kidney, where it affects not individual cell surfaces but the integrity of the glomerular basement membrane itself. Animal experiments clearly show the nephritogenic properties of complement-binding antibodies directed at glomerular basement membrane antigens, and that appropriate immunization with the latter can induce an auto-immune glomerulonephritis on the same basis. In man evidence from immunofluorescent studies is now beginning to come forward that in at least some cases of chronic glomerulonephritis immunoglobulin is bound in linear fashion to the injured basement membrane together with complement. Furthermore, when carefully eluted from the damaged kidney tissue, this immunoglobulin (usually IgG) has proved to be not only specifically reactive with antigens present in normal basement membrane (as shown, again, by immunofluorescence) but also on injection into monkeys, to localize selectively in the renal glomeruli, and to produce an acute glomerulonephritis.

Type III Reaction (Damage by Immune Complexes)

So far, we have considered the effects of immune reactions on local tissues when the participating antibody (Type I reaction) or antigen (Type II reaction) is already bound, for one reason or another, at the surfaces of cells or membranes. When both participants in the antigen-antibody encounter are freely circulating and soluble the immune complexes that result are no less able to provoke tissue responses, especially when complement is activated in the reaction; but the distribution of tissue damage is now independent of localizing effects due to antigen or antibody separately, and is determined instead by the site of deposition of the immune complexes formed. This in turn is greatly influenced by their solubility.

The classical instances of tissue responses mediated in this way by immune complexes are the Arthus reaction and serum sickness, representing respectively effects due to insoluble and soluble complexes. In the experimental animal, the Arthus reaction is a localized acute necrotizing vasculitis, initially appearing about 4 hours after injecting soluble antigen locally in the presence of circulating precipitating IgG antibody. Essential to its development is the coexistence of a high serum concentration of antibody and a high extravascular concentration of soluble antigen; the resulting contrary diffusion gradients lead to antigen-antibody interactions under conditions favouring formation of precipitates, which are deposited in considerable amounts in the local vessel walls. Fixation of complement follows, with production of the biologically active intermediates already noted, increased vascular permeability, and—characteristic of the Arthus reaction—attraction of leucocytes, especially polymorphs, which engulf and digest the immune precipitates. In doing so they contribute significantly to local tissue damage through the high concentration of acid hydrolytic enzymes released from their activated lysosomes.

In man Arthus reactions of this type occur in comparable situations when antigen is introduced extravascularly in the presence of high titre intravascular precipitins. These conditions used to occur in patients receiving repeated therapeutic serum injections, and may become commoner again with increasing use of heterologous antilymphocyte serum as an immunosuppressant. In pulmonary disease due to certain inhaled organic antigens, such as thermophilic actinomyces (farmer's lung) and *Aspergillus fumigatus* (bronchopulmonary aspergillosis), serum precipitins against these fungal antigens commonly develop and an Arthus type of reaction can often be elicited by skin-testing these patients with the appropriate antigen. Cellular infiltrates in the lung lesions of some patients, moreover, resemble those seen in Arthus reactions.

The serum sickness that in man and animals follows a single large injected dose of foreign serum, is, in contrast, a generalized condition, with onset after about 10 days. The signs and symptoms arise when antibodies to the foreign protein begin to appear at a time when the latter is still present in the body in considerable amount. Some of them—bronchospasm, vomiting, diarrhoea, urticaria and shock—are immediate anaphylactic responses due to IgE antibody binding to and involving mucous membrane, skin and smooth muscle in its interaction with antigen. More prolonged effects on the joints, heart and especially the kidneys are brought about by immune complexes formed in the circulation by combination of IgG antibody with persisting antigen. FIGURE 21 shows the temporal relationship between the latter events. After an initial drop due to equilibration between intra- and extravascular fluids serum levels of antigen fall slowly; but

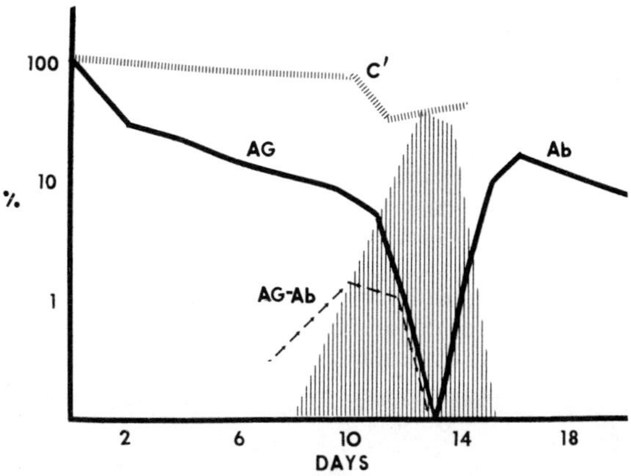

FIG. 21. 'One shot' serum sickness in the rabbit. 250 mg./kg. isotope-labelled bovine serum albumin injected intravenously at day O. With the appearance of antigen-antibody complexes (AG–Ab) there is a fall in serum complement (C′) and the appearance of lesions in heart, blood vessels, joints and kidneys (shaded area). With elimination of complexes free antibody (Ab) appears in the serum, and the inflammatory lesions subside. [Redrawn from Cochrane, C. G., and Dixon, F. J. (1969) in *Immunopathology*, ed. Miescher, P., and Muller-Eberhard, H. J., Vol. 1, Grune and Stratton Inc., New York, by permission.]

after a week or so the rate of loss from the serum increases sharply, and soon free antigen is replaced by free antibody. The phase of rapid antigen loss represents elimination due to interaction with newly-formed antibody. Antigen-antibody complexes begin to form in a milieu at first of gross, and later of moderate antigen excess. As in the classical quantitative precipitin curve, immune complexes formed in antigen excess are soluble. It is during this phase, when soluble complexes are circulating in the blood, that acute inflammatory lesions begin to occur in the joints, heart and kidney. When formed under appropriate conditions of moderate antigen excess complexes attain a critical macromolecular size which favours their trapping by basement membranes or by the internal elastic laminae of blood vessels. Once trapped on membranes, their complement-fixing property is enhanced, and the inflammatory changes ensue. Immunofluorescence shows that in the kidney of experimental serum sickness immune complexes are deposited on the glomerular basement membrane in a pattern that is characteristically granular and irregular, and contrasts with the smoothly linear attachment of specific antibasement membrane antibody described above. Electron microscopy of affected glomeruli shows electron-dense aggregates deposited on the epithelial side of the basement membrane.

In 'one-shot' serum sickness the scattered lesions are transient, since with increasing antibody production soluble complexes are no longer formed, and recovery occurs. Acute post-streptococcal glomerulonephritis is probably a parallel condition, for here too, although renal biopsies taken during the attack have shown immunoglobulin, complement and streptococcal antigen bound to the glomerulus, complete recovery is the rule. Chronic progressive disease can develop, however, when conditions are such that new soluble complexes are forming constantly in the blood. Experimentally, daily injections of small amounts of soluble antigen produce this effect, and thus it might be expected to occur clinically when this situation is reproduced by disease. A striking example recently discovered is malarial nephrosis in African children. Here the parasite (*P. malariae*) has been constantly present in the blood from infancy, and when, for reasons as yet unexplained, tolerance towards it is lost and antibody begins to be formed during early childhood, the conditions favour the formation of soluble complexes with malarial antigen [FIG. 22], nephrosis develops, and renal biopsy

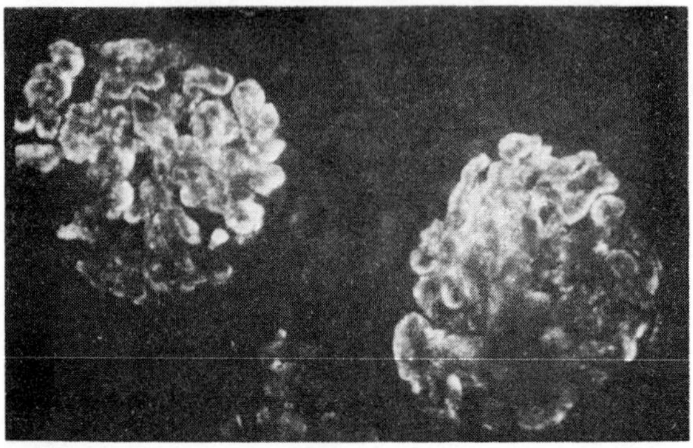

FIG. 22. Cryostat section of renal biopsy from an African child with malarial nephrosis, treated with fluorescein-labelled antihuman IgG antibody and viewed on a fluorescence microscope. Staining of the IgG component shows the immune complexes deposited in granular fashion on the glomerular basement membrane. [Courtesy of Dr. V. Houba.]

shows the characteristic deposits of immunoglobulin, complement, and in this case, *P. malariae* antigen. Another well-authenticated clinical example of soluble complex disease is seen in the nephritis of systemic lupus erythematosus. In this condition serum antinuclear autoantibodies are present, including antibodies against deoxyribonucleic acid (DNA) and in some cases it has been possible to show that in the serum free anti-DNA may alternate with free DNA. In the lupus kidney, membranous glomerular lesions are prominent, and immunofluorescence, again, shows that immunoglobulin is bound, with complement, to the glomerular basement and that this immunoglobulin has antinuclear (including anti-DNA) activity. Furthermore, DNA itself is present at the affected membrane sites.

ALLERGIC TISSUE DAMAGE DUE TO SENSITIZED CELLS

In individuals sensitized by previous exposure, application of certain chemicals to the skin produces a local dermatitis that takes 24 hours or so to develop. The substances that produce this contact hypersensitivity have in common the property of reacting with skin proteins to form hapten-protein conjugates of potent antigenicity in the individual concerned. Skin hypersensitivity arising in this way is a common cause of acute or chronic allergic contact dermatitis associated with exposure of the skin to metals, solvents, resins, some simple reactive chemicals like picryl chloride or dinitrochlorobenzine, cosmetics, antibiotics and other drugs.

Contact hypersensitivity resembles in kind delayed hypersensitivity—formerly known as bacterial allergy, and represented by the tuberculin reaction; this is another relatively slowly developing hypersensitivity reaction elicited by injecting a protein or hapten-protein conjugate into the skin of an appropriately sensitized subject. Contact hypersensitivity and delayed hypersensitivity reactions are highly specific and share the characteristic feature that for the eliciting antigen specificity resides as much in the protein-carrier as in the hapten carried. This is unlike antibody-mediated (immediate or anaphylactic) hypersensitivity, where the response is hapten-specific and independent of the protein used as hapten-carrier in eliciting it. Landsteiner and Chase in 1942 showed that contact hypersensitivity induced in guinea-pigs to the simple chemical picryl chloride could be transmitted to normal guinea-pigs by injecting them with living peritoneal exudate cells from hypersensitive animals, but not by antiserum, however potent, and this introduced the notion that lymphoid cells themselves can effect immune responses directly, without antibody as intermediary.

The essential histological change in delayed hypersensitivity reactions in the skin is local tissue damage in the neighbourhood of an infiltrate of mononuclear cells, made up of lymphocytes and monocytes, and it is now thought that both of these cell types contribute to producing the lesion. The lymphocytes are drawn from the recirculating pool of immunologically competent, and in this case, immunologically active cells, already sensitized and thus arrested at the site of local concentration of antigen by specific interaction with it. This interaction liberates chemotactic factors which cause infiltration of blood monocytes, cells that have originated from rapidly proliferating precursors in the bone marrow, and eventually contribute 80–90 per cent. of the inflammatory cells in the delayed hypersensitivity lesion. It is these monocytes which are evidently the non-specific (in the immunological sense) effectors of actual tissue damage, for in the Chase type of transfer experiment recipients deprived by irradiation of these bone marrow precursors cannot mount delayed reactions. That the interaction of sensitized lymphocytes with antigen produces a biological effect on monocytes is demonstrated *in vitro* by the inhibition of macrophage migratory activity brought about by adding antigen to tissue cultures containing both normal macrophages and lymphocytes from specifically sensitized donors. This promises to be a useful method of studying delayed hypersensitivity *in vitro*.

A similar histological picture of lymphocyte and macrophage infiltration is seen in homografts, e.g. skin, undergoing rejection. Failure to establish skin transplants between genetically dissimilar individuals is due to immunological sensitization, as Medawar showed, and his classical experiments on induction of acquired immunological tolerance of skin homografts in mice, and more particularly his demonstration that tolerance could be terminated by adoptive immunization using transferred lymphoid cells, though not immune serum alone, established clearly that cell-mediated rather than humoral immunity provides the major effector mechanism of homograft rejection. Furthermore, guinea-pigs that had rejected skin homografts gave delayed hypersensitivity reactions to intradermal injection of killed cells, or cell-free extracts, from the same skin donor; while their own lymphocytes excited a typical delayed hypersensitivity when injected intradermally into the same donor. To elicit the latter, however, the lymphocytes had to be living, thus reproducing essentially the conditions of the Chase passive transfer system, except that now sensitized lymphocytes were being injected locally into skin in which transplantation antigens were naturally present.

Thus contact hypersensitivity, delayed hypersensitivity and the homograft reaction are examples of tissue damage brought about by cell-mediated immunity. As well as producing inflammatory changes through the agency of macrophages and monocytes, sensitized lymphocytes are apparently capable of direct cytotoxic effects on cells carrying the antigens in question. *In vitro* models suggest that such target cells can be killed either by specifically sensitized lymphocytes, or by normal lymphocytes in the presence of very small amounts of antibody (possibly antibody of a special class). If these models represent *in vivo* events, they will provide new insight into mechanisms of immunological surveillance and tumour immunity.

From the point of view of immunity, the most direct immune effector mechanism is neutralizing antibody, exemplified by antitoxins against diphtheria or tetanus, and by some viral antibodies, which achieve their main biological purpose merely by combining with antigen. But neutralization of micro-organisms is seldom simply a matter of antitoxin production, and the evolution of immune responsiveness has produced in addition the versatile range of more complex effector mechanisms described above which use specific antigen-antibody interaction as a means of recruiting and intensifying phagocytosis, microbial lysis and the accompanying manifestations of inflammation. A direct role for antigen-sensitive lymphocytes in immunity is less clearly defined, although their ability to mobilize macrophages on activation, and to co-operate in antibody production are clearly of importance. The direct cytotoxic potential of immunologically competent lymphocytes may prove to have more biological significance, as suggested earlier, in tissue surveillance, controlling the emergence of aberrant cell clones within the body.

Thus both humoral and cellular immune effector mechanisms normally act largely through invoking tissue-damaging responses. The examples given here show that the same mechanisms are at work whether the antigens they are directed against are foreign to the body, or whether, as happens in a variety of circumstances, they are self-antigens and the subject of autoimmune responses. Whichever the case, it is when immune effector mechanisms operate above the physiological level, or are directed at tissue components essential to normal function, that the responses they evoke take on the character of disease. Some of the clinical consequences that may then ensue are described in Section 2.

REFERENCES

BURNET, SIR MACFARLANE (1969) *Cellular Immunology*, Cambridge.

GELL, P. G. H., and COOMBS, R. R. A., eds (1968) *Clinical Aspects of Immunology*, 2nd ed., Oxford.

MIESCHER, P. A., and MULLER-EBERHARD, H. J., eds (1969) *Textbook of Immunopathology*, New York.

E. J. HOLBOROW

DISEASES OF CONNECTIVE TISSUE

ANATOMICAL AND PHYSIOLOGICAL CONSIDERATIONS

The connective tissue forms the scaffolding of the body. In different regions and organs it has undergone modifications which enable it to meet specific local requirements, but its basic design remains constant throughout. In essence, it is made up of cells and fibres set in an amorphous matrix or ground substance. Under this general head must be included ligaments, tendons, fascia, joint capsules, the corium, the loose connective tissue, parts of the vascular tree and finally cartilage and bone. The specialized functions served by the last two have been associated with such structural modifications that their consideration is more conveniently relegated to a separate section. Here the term 'connective tissue' is used to describe all the other components listed.

The connective tissue is of mesenchymal origin and its basic cellular element is the fibroblast: in bone and cartilage the analogous cells have acquired additional functions and are known as the osteoblast and the chondroblast. Other cells constantly present include the tissue mast cell and the macrophage; the first is concerned with the production of heparin and hyaluronic acid and the main activity of the second is to act as a scavenger. The fibroblast is the pivotal unit of connective tissue for it is responsible for elaboration of the fibrillary elements and of the ground substance.

The fibrous components of connective tissue are of three kinds: collagen, reticulin and elastic fibres. It seems likely that reticulin is closely related to collagen, indeed it may well be its precursor. Collagen is a protein containing about 25 per cent. of glycine and two unique amino acids, hydroxyproline and hydroxyglycine. It takes the form of wide straight unbranching white bundles and is of high tensile strength, but of low elasticity. Collagen is believed to be formed by the fibroblast; it is metabolically almost inert; and it makes up 30 per cent. of the body's total protein.

Reticulin fibres are found in the parenchymatous organs and in the lymph nodes and spleen. They possess most of the properties of collagen, but the fibrils are smaller and stain readily with silver. Most workers believe that reticulin is immature collagen.

Elastic fibres are highly refractile and of yellow colour: they are larger than those of collagen and show branching. They are readily extensible and resist destruction by such agencies as heat, enzymic digestion and changes in pH. They contain much glycine, but no hydroxyproline nor other amino acid with reactive side chains. Their formation is ill-understood, but they are probably closely related to collagen.

Collagen fibres predominate in such structures as ligaments, tendons and joint capsules where strength and pliability are required. Elastic fibres are found where the property of elasticity is important; they abound, for instance, in the media of the aorta and the ligaments of the foot.

The amorphous ground substance of connective tissue is normally in the form of a gel filling the interstices between cells and fibres. It has a complex composition of mucoproteins and mucopolysaccharides derived from fibroblasts, and water, ions, glucose, cell metabolites and proteins resulting from the constant interchanges between cells and plasma. At least seven acid mucopolysaccharides have been identified, including hyaluronic acid, chondroitin and various chondroitin sulphates. Several are apparently specific for certain tissues: thus chondroitin is only found in the cornea. The mucopolysaccharides are metabolically active and show a rapid turnover. The ground substance is the medium through which pass all materials entering or leaving the cells, and it has been suggested that the mucopolysaccharides act like ion-exchange resins. Hyaluronic acid is responsible for the gelatinous character of the ground substance and for some of its water-binding capacity. The enzyme hyaluronidase removes hyaluronic acid from the connective tissue meshwork, greatly increasing its permeability.

Connective tissue is ubiquitous and it cannot escape playing some part whenever any organ or tissue suffers structural damage or change. There are, however, a number of disorders in which it appears to be primarily affected and these are conveniently considered together. Tissues of mesenchymal origin show a tendency to react to disease in a systematized fashion. This propensity is best developed in the haemopoietic system, but it is shared, too, by the connective tissue and it is in particular these generalized disorders which concern us in this chapter. In some of these the basis appears to be a genetic one and the defect is limited to one component: examples are the abnormality of elastic fibres characteristic of Marfan's syndrome and of collagen in the Grönblad-Strandberg syndrome. In others one specialized form of connective tissue is affected and these include the generalized diseases of bone and cartilage. They possess features which make their discussion in a separate section desirable.

Finally, there is a group in which the connective tissue shows systematized pathological changes of an inflammatory type. Their cause is unknown and they are sometimes spoken of as the 'collagen' or 'collagen vascular' diseases. They are included in this chapter because the generalized connective tissue change does afford some connecting link between them, but their inclusion does not infer aetiological unity. At the present time they still offer a challenge to the nosologist.

HEREDITARY, FAMILIAL AND CONGENITAL DISEASES OF CONNECTIVE TISSUE

MARFAN'S SYNDROME

Synonyms. Dolichostenomelia; Arachnodactyly.

Definition

Marfan's syndrome is an inherited disorder of the mesenchyme manifest by abnormalities of the skeleton, the eyes and the cardiovascular system and probably due to a defect in elastic fibres.

Aetiology

The disorder is inherited as a simple Mendelian autosomal dominant. The sexes are equally affected and there is no specific racial predisposition. Sporadic cases do not exceed 15 per cent. of the total. It has some features of an abiotrophy.

Pathology

The only characteristic changes are to be found in the media of the great vessels. They are degeneration of elastic fibres and the appearance of cystic areas filled with metachromatic material; later the elastic fibres fragment and decrease in number, while the proportion of collagen and smooth muscle increases. This process, which is not specific for Marfan's syndrome, is known as cystic medial necrosis.

Clinical Features

The main abnormalities are found in the skeleton, the eyes and the cardiovascular system.

The patients are often tall, but the abnormal bodily proportions are more significant than the increase in stature. The extremities are disproportionately long and their distal bones even longer. This results in the characteristically elongated fingers and toes which has given it the name of arachnodactyly. The abnormal proportions may be evident at birth, but become more obvious after puberty. Longitudinal growth is everywhere excessive, resulting in dolichocephaly, a high palatal arch, a long narrow face and prognathism. The patients are said to resemble portraits painted by El Greco. Common deformities are funnel or pigeon breast, pes planus, recurrent dislocations and kyphoscoliosis. They usually appear between the ages of 11 and 15 years. The musculature is often underdeveloped and hypotonic; postural defects and pain due to them are common sequels. Bone age judged radiologically is normal.

In the eye ectopia of the lens is to be found in 50–70 per cent. of patients; its presence may be shown by tremor of the iris (iridodonesis) or it may only be detected with a slit lamp. Other ocular abnormalities sometimes associated are heterochromia of the iris, blue sclerotics, myopia and undue liability to retinal detachment.

The cardiovascular component of the syndrome suggests an abiotrophy, for it makes its appearance some years after birth and is progressive. It is the consequence of cystic necrosis of the aortic media. The onset has been noted as early as the fifth year and as late as the sixtieth. There is steadily progressive dilatation of the aorta, usually leading to incompetence of the aortic valve and sometimes associated with dissecting aneurysm. The changes are more striking in males, possibly because they are more likely to be engaged in hard physical work.

Occasionally other abnormalities both of the cardiovascular system and elsewhere have been noted, but it seems likely that they are only coincidental. They include atrial septal defect and various disorders of conduction. The exception is the lesion known as Miescher's elastoma, marked by the appearance of small nodules or papules in the skin of the neck.

Formes frustes of Marfan's syndrome have frequently been reported. Such a diagnosis must be accepted with reserve: aortic medionecrosis is not specific and the skeletal features may not be conclusive. Ectopia lentis is generally held to be the hallmark of the disease although some observers claim that the cardiovascular and skeletal abnormalities 'breed true' in the absence of ocular abnormalities.

Treatment

No definitive treatment exists, but surgical repair of the dilated aorta and operation for the relief of pectus excavatum have been undertaken with success in several patients.

Prognosis

Most patients die from the cardiovascular component of the syndrome. The average age of death for males is 43 years and for females 46 years: in one large series the range was from 9 to 73 years.

REFERENCES

KEECH, M. K., WENDT, V. E., READ, R. C., BISTUE, A. R., and BIANCHI, F. A. (1966) Family studies of the Marfan syndrome, *J. chron. Dis.*, **19**, 57.

SINCLAIR, R. J. G., KITCHIN, A. H., and TURNER, R. W. D. (1960) The Marfan syndrome, *Quart. J. Med.*, **29**, 19.

EHLERS-DANLOS SYNDROME

Synonyms. Cutis hyperelastica; Dermatorrhexis; Cutis laxa.

Definition

A congenital hereditary disorder of connective tissue leading to hyperelasticity of the skin and hypermotility of the joints and possibly due to a defect in the arrangement of collagen fibres.

Aetiology

The Ehlers-Danlos syndrome is probably inherited as a simple autosomal dominant of low penetrance. Most of the cases have been reported in Europeans and the incidence in the male is about twice that in the female.

Pathology

Information is scanty, but the available reports suggest that the normal orderly meshwork of collagen fibres in the skin is lacking and adhesion between bundles is absent. Small cysts containing fat are found in the subcutis.

Clinical Features

Changes are usually evident at birth, but become more obvious with increasing years. They are found mainly in the skin and joints.

The skin has a velvety feel and is strikingly hyperextensible, recalling that of the india rubber man of the circus, in addition it is unduly fragile: wounds gape and heal poorly, leaving a 'tissue paper' scar. These are particularly common on the knees. Sutures tear through the skin readily and dehiscence of wounds is common. Although wounds bleed little, bruising is often excessive and a general haemorrhagic state is sometimes associated. At pressure points, subcutaneous 'spherules' the size of peas are often found.

Hyperextensibility of joints is the second characteristic, resulting in 'double jointedness'. The articulations are often unstable and recurrent dislocations and effusions are common. The underdeveloped and hypotonic muscles often lead to kyphoscoliosis.

Numerous associated anomalies have been reported including diaphragmatic hernia, diverticula of the gastro-intestinal tract, dissecting aneurysm of the aorta and sundry congenital cardiac and renal defects. Some regard blue sclerotics, epicanthic folds and 'lop' ears as integral components of the syndrome.

Treatment

No curative treatment exists. It should be noted that surgery is hazardous in these patients, because of the friability of the skin and the poor healing of wounds.

Prognosis

The disease does not shorten life unless there is some associated anomaly which proves lethal.

REFERENCE

SAEMUNDSSON, J. (1956) Ehlers-Danlos syndrome; a congenital mesenchymal disorder, *Acta med. scand.*, **154**, Suppl. 312, 399.

GRÖNBLAD-STRANDBERG SYNDROME

Synonym. Pseudoxanthoma elasticum.

Definition

An inherited disorder of connective tissue characterized by changes in the skin, the retinae and the arteries.

Aetiology

About 65 per cent. of the recorded cases are in women. There is no racial predisposition. The syndrome is probably inherited as a partially sex-limited autosomal recessive, but its behaviour suggests an abiotrophy.

Pathology

Aggregates resembling fragmented bundles of collagen, but with the staining properties of elastic fibres, are found in the deeper layers of the corium. In the eye, tears occur in Bruch's membrane and in the arterial walls elastic elements undergo degeneration. It is uncertain whether the primary change is in elastic fibres or whether some degenerative process affecting the collagen gives it the property of staining like them.

Clinical Features

The characteristic lesions appear during the second decade in the skin of the face and folds of the neck which becomes thickened and grained with intervening elevated yellow polygonal patches. These constitute pseudoxanthoma elasticum. The changes may be minimal. Subcutaneous calcification is common.

In the eye the lesions consist of 'angioid streaks' which are ruptures in Bruch's membrane. They are seen as brown-grey linear streaks in the retina, four or five times as wide as the veins. They may form the starting point of haemorrhages or proliferative changes. Partial loss of vision is usual. The retinal lesions appear in the second decade.

Arterial changes are common and appear in the third decade. Obliterative disease and intermittent claudication are common, but haemorrhage is more important. This is most often gastric, but may be subarachnoid, renal, uterine or intra-articular. It is presumed to be of arterial origin, but its exact cause is unknown. This syndrome must be remembered as a cause of haematemesis [see Section 7].

Treatment

No definitive treatment exists, although cosmetic surgery may be helpful on occasion.

Prognosis

This depends upon the liability to haemorrhage. Haematemesis and subarachnoid haemorrhage have both proved fatal.

REFERENCE

GOODMAN, R. M., SMITH, E. W., PATON, D., BERGMAN, R. A., SIEGEL, C. L., OTTESEN, O. E., SHELLEY, W. M., PUSCH, A. L., and MCKUSICK, V. A. (1963) Pseudoxanthoma elasticum: a clinical and histopathological study, *Medicine (Baltimore)*, **42**, 297.

HURLER'S SYNDROME AND RELATED DISORDERS

Definition

A group of inherited disorders of mesenchymal tissues characterized by skeletal deformity, enlargement of the liver and spleen, corneal opacity, deafness, mental defect and heart disease.

Aetiology

This group of diseases is due to a genetic disorder of mucopolysaccharide metabolism the exact nature of which is still unknown. The urine contains an excess of these substances. The first described and best known member is Hurler's syndrome or gargoylism. Four other types are now recognized which show minor clinical differences as well as biochemical ones. All are inherited as autosomal recessives except type II (Hurler's syndrome) which is an X-linked recessive.

Pathology

The mucopolysaccharidoses are 'storage diseases'. The affected cells contain what are thought to be products of perverted fibroblastic activity and accumulations occur within fibroblasts in fasciae, tendons, blood vessels, heart valves and the meninges. In other tissues different cells are affected; thus chondroblasts and osteoblasts, neurones, ganglion cells and reticulo-endothelial elements may all be laden with these products of disturbed fibroblastic metabolism. Two more polysaccharides, chondroitin sulphate B and heparitin sulphate, have been found in the urine in Hurler's syndrome.

The mucopolysaccharides which show a metabolic disturbance in this group are chondroitin sulphate B, heparitin sulphate and keratosulphate. They are excreted in excess in the urine. In types I and II both the first two mucopolysaccharides are present in the urine, in type III the excess excretion is of heparitin S, in type IV of keratosulphate and in type V of chondroitin sulphate B.

Clinical Features

In Hurler's syndrome (type I) the patients are normal at birth, but evidence of disease appears in the second year. When fully developed the appearance is characteristic. There is dwarfism with a large head and saddle nose, its tip being splayed and nostrils gaping. The skull often shows scaphocephaly and hypertelorism. The lips are large and the teeth small and malformed. Upper respiratory infections are the rule. The neck is short; kyphosis is usual; the hands are broad and the fingers clawed and spatulate. The movement of joints is often restricted.

The abdomen is usually protuberant, partly due to enlargement of the liver and spleen which may be extreme. Umbilical hernia is almost constant.

Corneal opacity occurs in 70 per cent., but appears to be lacking in those with the sex-linked type of disease. Deafness is unusual. Mental retardation may only be mild; in other cases there is steady deterioration and eventual idiocy. Heart disease usually makes its appearance and is often the cause of death: both valvular defects and cardiomyopathy have been reported.

Radiological changes are often striking. The sella turcica has been described as 'shoe shaped', being long, attenuated and with an anterior projection. The vertebrae are often wedged and show a beak-like projection anteriorly. The medullary cavities of the long bones are enlarged.

In some cases the circulating neutrophils have contained large granules staining lilac with toluidine blue. These are thought to be mucopolysaccharide in nature.

The other varieties are clinically similar; the difference lies in one or other feature of the syndrome being accented. In type II (Hurler's syndrome) corneal opacity does not occur and the general disturbance is milder; in type III (Sanfillipo syndrome) the neurological defect is greater; in type IV (Morquio-Brailsford syndrome) bone changes are severe and characteristic, corneal opacity is usual and aortic incompetence common; in type V (Scheie syndrome) stiff joints, corneal opacity, aortic incompetence and a striking coarseness of the features are found.

Treatment

There is no treatment for this syndrome.

Prognosis

Those with type I usually die before the age of 20 years, commonly from heart disease. In the other types adult life is often reached but a full span seldom achieved.

REFERENCES

BRANTE, G. (1952) Gargoylism: a mucopolysaccharidosis, *Scand. J. clin. Lab. Invest.*, **4**, 43.

McKUSICK, V. A., KAPLAN, D., WISE, D., HANLEY, W. B., and MAUMENEE, A. E. (1965) The genetic mucopolysaccharidoses, *Medicine* (*Baltimore*), **44**, 445.

FIBRODYSPLASIA OSSIFICANS PROGRESSIVA

Synonym. Myositis ossificans progressiva.

Definition

A disease of great rarity and unknown cause characterized by progressive ossification in tendons, ligaments and aponeuroses.

Aetiology

Familial incidence is rare, possibly because sufferers from this disease rarely have children. The unaffected parent of a patient has been noted to show the characteristic microdactyly (see below) in several instances. The disease has been recorded in identical twins. Males are more often affected than females in the proportion of 3 to 2.

It has been suggested, on somewhat flimsy evidence, that the disease is inherited as a Mendelian dominant with irregular penetrance.

Pathology

The early changes are unknown and it is more than likely that the young osteoid tissue with numerous osteoblasts which is seen in established lesions is only a reaction to some preceding damage. The earlier title of 'myositis' has been replaced by 'fibrodysplasia' for the disease is now recognized as one of fibrous tissue structures and not of muscle.

Clinical Features

The onset is sometimes in foetal life, but usually in childhood before the age of 10 years. Transient swellings, which may be painful, appear in connexion with the ligaments, fasciae and tendons of the neck, back and later of the limbs. Their development and resolution, often lasting only a few days, may be accompanied by fever. Ossification in the sites of the swellings follows and gradually the affected structures are replaced by sheets or bars of bone until the patient is rigid and immobilized. The muscles of the tongue, heart, larynx, diaphragm, perineum, eye and anterior abdominal wall usually escape.

The only other abnormality, and it is almost constant, is microdactyly of the great toe which usually possesses only one phalanx. Similar changes are found in the thumbs in about half the patients.

Treatment

It is doubtful whether any treatment is effective, although some reports suggest that corticosteroids, if given sufficiently early, may arrest the progress of the disease.

Prognosis

These patients may survive until old age although they are commonly much disabled.

REFERENCE

McKUSICK, V. A. (1960) *Heritable Disorders of Connective Tissue*, 2nd ed., St. Louis.

THE COLLAGEN DISEASES

SYSTEMIC LUPUS ERYTHEMATOSUS

Synonyms. Disseminated lupus erythematosus; Libman-Sacks disease.

Definition

A chronic progressive inflammatory disease of undetermined cause affecting loose connective tissue. The lesions are scattered in time and space involving organs in an apparently random fashion and giving rise to variable and bizarre patterns of disease.

Aetiology

Females are much more frequently affected than males: earlier reports suggested a preponderance as high as 95 per cent. in women, but this has fallen with wider recognition of the disease to about 85 per cent.

The median age of onset is 25 years and in 80 per cent. of cases it lies between 10 and 40 years, but extremes of 5 and 67 years are recorded.

The annual incidence of newly diagnosed cases in New York and in Sweden is about 10 per million.

It is doubtful whether any racial predilection exists although in the United States the incidence in Negroes is higher than that in the population at large.

There have been several reports of siblings being affected by systemic lupus erythematosus. In addition, such abnormalities as hypergammaglobulinaemia or a biological false positive Wassermann reaction have been noted in close relatives of sufferers from the disease.

The pathogenesis of systemic lupus erythematosus remains uncertain. There is no evidence that bacterial or viral infection plays a part. Endocrine influences may be of importance in view of the female predominance, and there is evidence to suggest that a high mortality runs parallel with a high urinary level of oestrogens. Genetic factors are clearly of significance as shown by the familial incidence of the disease and of abnormalities of the plasma proteins.

There are several drugs capable of provoking a reaction which closely simulates systemic lupus erythematosus. Chronologically the first of these is hydrallazine, a hydrazine formerly used as a hypotensive agent. Eight to thirteen per cent. of patients receiving this drug develop a syndrome clinically, serologically and pathologically indistinguishable from systemic lupus erythematosus. Seventy-four per cent. of those affected have a past history of 'rheumatic disorder'. Withdrawal of the drug is usually followed by improvement, but in two-thirds some symptoms persist, often for years, and may recur long after it has been discontinued. Hydrallazine is spoken of as 'uncovering the lupus diathesis', but what this means and how it is brought about remain obscure.

The second drug to have this effect is procainamide and, as hydrallazine is now seldom prescribed, it occupies pride of place. In this syndrome fever and skin rashes are less common than in systemic lupus erythematosus and lymphadenopathy and renal disease have not been observed. A past history of rheumatic disease is rare. Fifty per cent. recover within 2 weeks of withdrawing the drug and most of the remainder after treatment with corticosteroids. Symptoms persist in 1 in 7. The L.E. cell test becomes negative in about 20 weeks. It is uncertain how this disorder is related to the hydrallazine syndrome, but it appears to be more benign and more frequently reversible.

A similar syndrome has been recorded after isoniazid which is chemically related to hydrallazine. Other drugs reported as producing this syndrome are the anticonvulsants (phenytoin, methoin, troxidone, primidone and ethosuximide) and occasionally penicillin, tetracycline, streptomycin, griseofulvin, the sulphonamides, aminosalicylic acid, phenylbutazone, thiouracil, reserpine, methyldopa, guanoxan and the oral contraceptives.

Exposure to sunlight may provoke a violent cutaneous reaction and be followed by systemic spread in a patient previously believed to have simple discoid lupus erythematosus. Infection, emotional stress and physical hardship have all been blamed for exacerbation or precipitation of the disease.

Perhaps the most generally accepted hypothesis is that systemic lupus erythematosus is an 'auto-immune disease'. Undoubtedly it is possible to demonstrate the presence in the patient's serum of antibodies directed against many of his own tissues. The L.E. cell test which is discussed later is undeniably an immunological phenomenon and proves the presence of antinuclear antibodies. The protagonists of this view claim that the production of these auto-antibodies can hardly be fortuitous and must be causally related to the tissue damage; their opponents maintain that there is no proof that their formation is the cause of the disease and it may well be the result. Certainly the auto-immune hypothesis is the only constructive aetiological explanation so far devised.

Further elaboration of this view necessitates a plunge into the turbid waters of current immunological theory. Those who support it usually accept the clonal selection doctrine of Burnet and suggest that the fundamental fault is a profound weakness, possibly genetic in origin, of the normal mechanisms of immunological homeostasis. This, they maintain, allows the establishment of 'forbidden clones' capable of reacting with 'self' antigens. As the disease progresses there is a gradual increase in the number of these forbidden immunologically competent cells and a corresponding increase in the number and diversity of the auto-antibodies they elaborate.

Pathology

Macroscopically the changes in systemic lupus erythematosus are often unimpressive. They consist of a mixture of serositis, pneumonitis, contracted kidneys, verrucous endocarditis and enlargement of the spleen, liver and lymph nodes. The picture is often complicated by infection.

Microscopically there are four main features. The first is fibrinoid degeneration of collagen and intercellular connective tissue. This consists of the deposition of dense refractile homogeneous acidophil material having the staining reactions of fibrin. It is not specific for this disease. It is probably derived from plasma proteins or from degraded nucleoprotein. It does not originate, as was once thought, from collagen.

The second histological feature is vasculitis which some consider the fundamental lesion. There is damage to the endothelium of small vessels with necrosis, thrombosis and ischaemic change distal to the obstruction. In particular organs modifications of this pattern give rise to characteristic appearances such as the 'onion skin lesions' in the spleen and the 'wire-loop' lesions in the kidneys.

The third change consists of nuclear degradation and haematoxylin body formation: it is the tissue equivalent of the L.E. cell phenomenon (see below). Haematoxylin bodies, so described because they stain purple with this stain, are about the size of cell nuclei and may occur in clumps. They are commonly seen in the lymph nodes, kidneys, spleen, lungs and heart. They are of nuclear origin and probably due to the action of L.E. factor upon mesenchymal cell nuclei.

Finally, in all the affected tissues, as well as in lymph nodes and spleen, aggregates of lymphocytes and plasma cells abound. The supporters of the autoimmunity hypothesis believe these to be 'immunologically competent cells' active against the tissues which show evidence of damage.

Clinical Features

The clinical picture of systemic lupus erythematosus defies succinct description. It is one of great complexity, because the course of the disease is so variable and because almost any organ or combination of organs or tissues may be implicated.

Course and Onset. The course of systemic lupus erythematosus varies from one of fulminant rapidity which may prove fatal in 6 weeks to one of extreme chronicity extending over 20 years or more. It is usually episodic, in that one manifestation will bring the patient under observation and this will be followed after an interval by another and then another. In rapidly progressive cases one incident follows another without the first resolving; when the course is more protracted some degree of remission separates them.

At the onset, episodes of fever and some loss of weight are usual. The commonest initial complaint is of pain and swelling of joints and this may precede other evidence of systemic lupus erythematosus by many years. Other causes for the patient first seeking advice are unexplained fever, skin eruptions and symptoms due to pleurisy, pericarditis, anaemia or kidney disease. The diagnosis may be made in this early stage when the subsequent course will be modified by treatment. If the disorder is not recognized, symptoms wax and wane, being due now to affection of one organ and now of another; irregular periodic fever is usual and there is gradual deterioration in general health with loss of weight and anaemia. Finally, disease of the kidneys with renal failure and hypertension, congestive heart failure or intercurrent infection brings the illness to a close after a course ranging from a few weeks to many years.

Fever is present at some time in 80–90 per cent. of patients. It is a common early symptom and frequently episodic, related to the appearance of disease in a fresh anatomical site. It may, of course, also be due to secondary infection.

The Joints and Muscles. Between 80 and 90 per cent. of patients have at some time symptoms referable to the joints. In about 50 per cent. they constitute the initial complaint. There may be no more than fleeting or recurrent arthralgia or the changes may be indistinguishable from those of rheumatoid arthritis, although rarely so destructive and often asymmetrical or otherwise 'atypical'. Arthritis may precede other clinical or laboratory evidence of systemic lupus erythematosus by as long as 20 years. Synovial biopsy often shows surprisingly little change. Radiological evidence of erosions is rare.

The picture of polymyositis may dominate the scene with electromyographic and characteristic histological changes. Extreme weakness and muscular atrophy may occur.

The Skin. *Discoid lupus erythematosus* may perhaps be regarded as a benign variant of the systemic disorder in which lesions are limited to the skin. Occurring commonly in adults, the 'butterfly area' of the face, the forehead, chin, lower lip and ears are usually affected. The lesions are well-defined circular, oval or irregular patches with thickened red periphery and pale atrophic centre. The surface is covered with white or grey scales and horny follicular plugs may be seen. The patches may remain unchanged for long periods or extend slowly in one area while resolving to leave an atrophic scar in another, sometimes after a preliminary reticulate telangiectasia.

Other sites affected are the vertex with scarring, baldness, erythema and follicular plugging; the buccal mucosa with leukoplakia and eroded areas; the hands where there may be red infiltrative patches on the volar aspect of the phalanges, perniosis around the nail folds, subungual splinter haemorrhages and telangiectasia of the finger tips.

In perhaps 50 per cent. of patients with discoid lupus erythematosus the disease later becomes systematized. The distinction is not always easy and depends upon clinical evidence of affection of other systems and positive serological tests.

In *systemic lupus erythematosus* any of the cutaneous lesions described as features of the discoid variety may occur. In addition others are frequent and some kind of eruption is noted at some time in 65–80 per cent. of patients: in some 25 per cent. it is the presenting symptom. The rashes are often non-specific and may be due to infection or allergy. Urticaria is common. Diffuse erythema especially on areas exposed to light is frequent and undue photosensitivity is often found. Indeed, prolonged exposure to sunlight, as in sunbathing, appears to cause systematization of the discoid type.

Raynaud's phenomena occur in 10–20 per cent. and vasculitis may cause purpura, infarcts of the finger tips and even digital gangrene. Subcutaneous nodules resembling those of rheumatoid arthritis are found in 5 per cent. Occasionally, chronic ulceration of the legs is associated with cryoglobulinaemia. Thrombocytopenia may be responsible for purpura.

The Respiratory System. About 50 per cent. of patients develop pleurisy at some time during the disease and in half these it is associated with a pleural effusion. It is a not uncommon opening event and may be bilateral.

Pulmonary infiltrations occur in about 30 per cent. they are often due to secondary infection, but may be of specific cause. Radiologically they appear as ill-defined shadows or linear areas of atelectasis usually in the lower lobes.

The Cardiovascular System. Some affection of the heart is almost constant on post-mortem examination. In 40–50 per cent. there is the typical verrucous endocarditis of Libman and Sacks. Murmurs are commonly heard: they are usually functional, but mitral stenosis and incompetence, and aortic incompetence have all been observed. Pericarditis occurs in about half the patients and is not rare as a cause of the presenting symptoms. Disturbances of conduction and rhythm are uncommon and although myocarditis is usually slight it is occasionally severe. Hypertension is a common complication and subacute bacterial endocarditis a rare one.

The Alimentary System. Symptoms referable to the gastro-intestinal tract are common, but usually of non-specific origin. They may be attributable to such causes as corticosteroids or aspirin, but they can be due to affection of the bowel or peritoneum by systemic lupus erythematosus. It is of interest that ulcerative colitis has been reported in this disease. Pancreatitis has occasionally been associated and Sjøgren's syndrome is recognized as closely related.

The connexion between disease of the liver and systemic lupus erythematosus is complex. The organ is often found to be enlarged and tests of liver function may be abnormal. Liver damage may, of course, sometimes be due to complicating disease. There is a group of cases starting like viral hepatitis, but usually in young women with amenorrhoea, striae and genital hypoplasia, and progressing to a condition of chronic jaundice with relapsing fever. In many of these there is a positive L.E. cell test and in a few other signs of systemic lupus erythematosus. This disorder has been called 'lupoid hepatitis' [see Section 7]. Occasionally, too, acute hepatitis is associated with a positive L.E. cell test and this has been described as 'hepatic lupus'. The relationship between these two conditions and true systemic lupus erythematosus is uncertain.

The Kidneys. Renal disease develops in 50–75 per cent. of patients with this disease. In some it is non-specific and due to pyelonephritis or hypertension. Specific damage may take place at any time, but generally speaking it appears early and the longer it is deferred the less likely it is to occur. It is the main factor in determining the outcome of this disease.

The urine usually contains protein, but this may be due to fever. There is no doubt that the specific lesions may be present without albuminuria. Renal biopsy is often of great value in establishing the diagnosis when there are no other signs of systemic lupus erythematosus or of assessing the prognosis when there is no albuminuria.

The clinical form of kidney disease varies. The nephrotic syndrome is not rare and may antedate the evidence of the disease by many years. When there is only albuminuria with the presence of cells and casts, about one-third show little change over several years while in the remainder hypertension and renal failure develop rapidly. Uraemia is the cause of death in about 20 per cent.

The Nervous System. In about one-third of patients nervous symptoms occur at some time. They may be secondary to such factors as corticosteroid treatment, hypertension, infection or uraemia.

Psychosis is not rare: it is usually intermittent and coincides with activation of the underlying disease, but is occasionally chronic and progressive. Pathological anxiety, emotional lability, mental deterioration, depression, obsessional trends, paranoia and hallucinations may all occur.

Convulsions are common and may antedate other signs of the disease by years. Cranial nerve palsies and lesions of the cord have been recorded: peripheral neuropathy is rare, but may take either the symmetrical or mononeuritic form. Cerebral haemorrhage may complicate hypertension or thrombocytopenic purpura.

In about one patient in ten there is papilloedema which is not necessarily associated with hypertension. Retinal haemorrhages are common and fluffy exudates along the line of the vessels, known as 'cytoid bodies', may be seen. Episcleritis and iridocyclitis may be additional complications, but all these changes are non-specific.

The Haemopoietic System. The lymph nodes are palpably enlarged in about half the patients at some time. There is no specific pattern and the enlargement is often secondary to infection. Splenomegaly has been recorded in between 8 and 40 per cent. of cases in different series. It is variable, often associated with enlargement of the liver and unrelated to changes in the blood.

Anaemia is the rule. It is often due to secondary causes such as uraemia or haemorrhage. At times it is frankly haemolytic and of the auto-immune type with a positive Coombs antiglobulin test. Cold agglutinins are often present. It is not rare for the Coombs test to be positive without evidence of excessive haemolysis. In some instances patients present with auto-immune haemolytic anaemia, a positive Coombs test and no evidence of systemic lupus erythematosus except a positive L.E. cell test. The position of these cases is not clear but many develop systemic symptons later.

Leucopenia is common in this disease and white cell antibodies have been demonstrated. There is no specific change in the differential leucocyte count and eosinophilia is rare.

Thrombocytopenic purpura may be the opening event in this disease and may remit after splenectomy.

Further evidence of the underlying disease may be delayed for some years. About 30 per cent. of patients show a reduced platelet count at some time. The Evans syndrome of thrombocytopenia and haemolytic anaemia is not rare. Circulating anticoagulants have been reported in a number.

There is an increase in the serum gamma globulin in about 85 per cent. of cases and this change may long precede evidence of systemic lupus erythematosus. It is usually diffuse and not of the monoclonal type. In a small number, probably about 1 per cent., cryoglobulinaemia is present and may be associated with Raynaud's phenomena or ulcers on the legs. The changes in the plasma proteins are responsible for the greatly increased erythrocyte sedimentation rate.

Diagnosis

The diagnosis of systematized lupus erythematosus requires both clinical and laboratory data. It is necessary to show that more than one organ or tissue is affected by the disease process and to establish the presence of circulating auto-antibodies. Before discussing this problem in greater detail it will be wise to consider briefly the tests which indicate the existence of auto-antibodies.

The Lupus Erythematosus (L.E.) Cell Test. This is the most important of the laboratory tests used in the diagnosis of systemic lupus erythematosus. The L.E. cell is a neutrophil containing a homogeneous mass of basophilic material in its cytoplasm. Its formation is essentially an *in vitro* phenomenon, but it is analogous to the haematoxylin body seen in the tissues. When an injured neutrophil is exposed to the serum of a patient with this disease, the nucleus degenerates into a homogeneous mass which is extruded and phagocyted by a healthy neutrophil. Three components are required: a factor which is found in the serum of patients with systemic lupus erythematosus (L.E. factor), nuclear material and actively phagocytic neutrophil leucocytes.

The L.E. factor cannot be distinguished from normal gamma globulin, but it appears to be an antibody directed against nucleoprotein. It is believed to displace histones from their normal combination with desoxyribonucleic acid with which it then combines. It seems likely that complement is not needed for this test.

A number of techniques for carrying out the L.E. cell test have been devised and their sensitivity varies considerably. It is usually carried out by examining films made from the buffy coat of incubated defibrinated blood. The L.E. factor can also be detected by agglutination of polystyrene particles coated with nucleoprotein. This method shows good correlation with the L.E. cell test.

The L.E. cell test is not entirely specific. It is positive at some time in 80–85 per cent. of patients with systemic lupus erythematosus. Positive tests are found also in 10–15 per cent. of patients who would be regarded from the clinical point of view as having rheumatoid arthritis. They occur also in some patients with haemolytic anaemia, hepatitis, nephritis and discoid lupus as well as in occasional instances of other collagen diseases. The only inference to be drawn is that a fundamental relationship must exist between these diverse diseases.

Antinuclear Factor (ANF). The sera of patients with systemic lupus erythematosus contain antibodies other than L.E. factor which bind specifically with somatic cell nuclei. An immunofluorescent method is commonly used for their demonstration. Antinuclear antibodies fixed to cell nuclei can be detected by antihuman-globulin, conjugated with a marker of fluorescein. Sections of rat's liver are heated with the test serum, washed, heated with antihuman globulin-fluorescein, washed again and examined under ultra-violet light. Fluorescent staining of the nuclei indicates a positive result. This staining may assume different patterns which are believed to indicate specific antibodies. Homogeneous staining is given by antibody to deoxyribonucleoprotein (L.E. factor); speckled by antibody to a saline-soluble to nuclear protein; a nucleolar pattern by antibody to nucleolar RNA; and peripheral staining by antibody to free DNA.

Wassermann Reaction. A 'biological false positive' Wassermann reaction has been reported in 10–20 per cent. of patients with systemic lupus erythematosus. This means a positive immunological reaction to the lipoid antigens commonly used, but a negative *Treponema pallidum* immobilization test which is regarded as completely specific for syphilis. The antigen here is cardiolipin. This curious anomaly has been noted years before the development of other signs of the disease; it is also common in auto-immune haemolytic anaemia.

Rheumatoid Factor. The serum of some 75 per cent. of patients with rheumatoid arthritis contains a factor which reacts with gamma globulin. Its presence can be demonstrated by the Rose-Waaler test or by the use of polystyrene latex particles coated with gamma globulin. A positive test is found in 30–40 per cent. of patients with systemic lupus erythematosus.

Coombs' Antiglobulin Test. This test which demonstrates the presence of incomplete auto-antibodies against erythrocytes [see Section 13] is characteristic of auto-immune haemolytic anaemia. It is usually positive when anaemia of this type occurs in systemic lupus erythematosus, but often, too, when the disease is unassociated with anaemia.

Antinuclear antibody tests are extremely sensitive and may give weakly positive results in many disorders and sometimes in normal persons. A strongly positive test is that suggestive of systemic lupus erythematosus and a high titre is of greater significance than the pattern of fluorescence. The test is positive in 95–100 per cent. of patients with this disease. The L.E. cell test is positive in 80–85 per cent. It is quite exceptional to find the second positive when the first is negative.

The peripheral pattern of immunofluorescence is unusual in diseases other than systemic lupus erythematosus and occurs particularly in the seriously ill. It disappears during spontaneous or steroid-induced remission. The behaviour of the other antibodies is inconstant.

In systemic lupus erythematosus most antinuclear antibodies belong to the IgG class of immunoglobulins.

Differential Diagnosis

The differential diagnosis of systemic lupus erythematosus cannot be discussed at length, because it is clear from the previous paragraphs that almost any disease may be mimicked.

Difficulty arises most frequently, perhaps, when the onset is acute with fever and the general features of an infective illness. The diagnosis can, often, only be settled by failure to isolate an organism and the finding of a positive L.E. cell test. Problems arise, too, when only one system is involved at the onset of the illness; examples often encountered are auto-immune haemolytic anaemia, thrombocytopenic purpura, the nephrotic syndrome, or rheumatoid arthritis. Even when a positive L.E. cell test is found the diagnosis should seldom be made until evidence of more diffuse disease appears. In the case of rheumatoid arthritis the differential diagnosis often becomes a semantic dispute.

Treatment

Controlled therapeutic trials in systemic lupus erythematosus are clearly impossible and, because the disease shows such immense variations, it is impossible to be certain of the long-term effects of treatment.

Corticosteroid drugs have been constantly shown to control the inflammatory features of the disease. It is uncertain how greatly they affect its subsequent course. A few prolonged remissions have been noted in the presence of advanced renal disease if high enough doses are used, but although the progress of the lesion in the kidney is slowed, the *status quo* is not restored. Nevertheless, these drugs are the only certain means we have of controlling symptoms and it is almost always necessary to make use of them, although side-effects are common.

Laboratory evidence of favourable response is usually seen. The false positive Wassermann reaction becomes negative in 20–30 per cent.; the L.E. cell test becomes less strongly positive; the serum gamma globulin level falls; the erythrocyte sedimentation rate becomes normal in 50 per cent.; excessive haemolysis ceases; and in 60 per cent. the platelet count rises to normal figures.

In the acute stage, doses of prednisolone of 40–100 mg. daily will be required. Once symptoms are under control the dose is reduced slowly until the lowest level at which they are suppressed is found. In an occasional case more satisfactory results are obtained with ACTH, 40 Units daily. Treatment with corticosteroids can seldom be discontinued once it has been started.

It has been suggested that the effect of the corticosteroids is to interfere with the auto-antigen-antibody reactions which are believed by many to be the cause of the disease. Other methods aimed at reducing antibody formation have been advocated and these include radiotherapy and the use of cytotoxic drugs. The first is rarely applicable, but the second has been exploited recently. The earlier drugs used included the nitrogen mustards, the ethylenimines and the folic acid antagonists. More recently the purine antagonists have been favoured, particularly 6-mercaptopurine and azathioprine (*Imuran*). The results so far have been disappointing and they should only be used when the corticosteroids have failed or when some absolute bar to their employment exists.

Aspirin has been used extensively for the joint pains as it has in rheumatoid arthritis.

Exposure to sunlight should be avoided and drugs, such as sulphonamides, which may cause photosensitization should not be prescribed. Skin lesions often respond well to powerful topical corticosteroids under an occlusive dressing or to injections of 1 per cent. triamcinolone, 0·1–1·0 ml. into the lesion. The cutaneous lesions will also respond to hydroxychloroquine (*Plaquenil*), 400–1200 mg. daily by mouth, but as this causes some risk of ocular complications local treatment is preferable.

Where necessary local applications such as mexenone, 4 per cent. (*Uvistat*), may be used as a screen against ultra-violet light.

Prognosis

The prognosis of systemic lupus erythematosus is difficult to assess. It is bad in children and in women during the reproductive period of life. Four large series from New York show 75 per cent. survival after 3 years and 50–60 per cent. after 10 years. In a recent prospective study one-third of the patients died over an 8-year period of observation: the estimated 5-year survival for the series was 77 per cent., and for 10 years 59 per cent.

The effect of pregnancy seems slight. An occasional woman deteriorates and improves when pregnancy is terminated, but natural variations in the disease could well explain these few cases. Fertility is unimpaired and the babies are healthy, although L.E. factor may be transmitted across the placenta. The frequency of abortion and stillbirth are somewhat increased.

It is not always easy to determine the cause of death even on post-mortem examination. Renal disease is often the deciding factor and tends to occur early or not at all. Involvement of the central nervous system and severe vasculitis are unfavourable features. In round figures 20 per cent. die from uraemia, 20 per cent. from heart failure, 15 per cent. from infection and the remainder of miscellaneous, and sometimes ill-understood, causes.

REFERENCES

Dubois, E. L., and Tuffanelli, D. L. (1964) Clinical manifestations of systemic lupus erythematosus: computer analysis of 520 cases, *J. Amer. med. Ass.*, **190**, 104.

Estes, D., and Christian, C. L. (1971) The natural history of systemic lupus erythematosus by prospective analysis, *Medicine* (*Baltimore*), **50**, 85.

Harvey, A. M., Shulman, L. E., Tumulty, P. A., Conley, C. L., and Schoenrich, E. H. (1954) Systemic lupus erythematosus: review of the literature and clinical analysis of 138 cases, *Medicine* (*Baltimore*), **33**, 291.

Hill, L. C. (1957) Systemic lupus erythematosus, *Brit. med. J.*, **2**, 655, 726.

Larson, D. L. (1961) *Systemic Lupus Erythematosus*, London.

Richardson, J. (1963) *Connective Tissue Disorders*, Oxford.

Talbott, J. H., and Moleres Ferrandis, R. (1956) *Collagen Diseases*, New York.

Taylor, R. T. (1970) Systemic lupus erythematosus, *Brit. J. hosp. Med.*, **4**, 653.

NECROTIZING ANGIITIS

A number of syndromes are recognized in which widespread but patchy inflammatory lesions in the arterial system appear as the fundamental morbid change. These are clearly not of direct bacterial cause and their characters suggest an abnormal immune response. The classification of these disorders is still undecided and the relationship between different syndromes uncertain. Some authorities believe they should be classified according to the size of the artery affected, others prefer the anatomical distribution of the lesions as a basis. It has recently been claimed that these arterial diseases can reasonably be grouped under one head as 'necrotizing angiitis'. The lesions, which are mainly due to ischaemia, may be visceral, cutaneous or affect both areas. The following classification is purely descriptive:

I Mainly affecting muscular arteries:
- Polyarteritis nodosa
- Malignant granuloma
- Giant-cell arteritis

II Mainly affecting small arteries:
- Cutaneous vasculitis
- Anaphylactoid purpura

POLYARTERITIS NODOSA

Synonyms. Periarteritis nodosa; Kussmaul's disease.

Definition

Polyarteritis nodosa is a disease of unknown cause marked by focal inflammatory lesions in small and medium-sized arteries. The changes are usually widespread, but are sometimes limited to one organ or tissue.

Aetiology

Polyarteritis nodosa is an uncommon disease. Its incidence is not known and it is uncertain whether it is becoming more common, as is often claimed, or whether it is detected more frequently. It may occur at any age; it has been reported in an infant of 10 days and in a man of 78 years, but most cases are seen between the ages of 20 and 50 years. Males are affected three times more often than females; no race is immune.

The cause of the disease is unknown. A suggestion that it represented a hypersensitivity reaction was made many years ago and this hypothesis is dutifully repeated in every review. The evidence in its favour is twofold: similar arterial lesions can be found, first in hypersensitivity induced experimentally in rabbits, and secondly in patients dying from serum sickness. Indeed polyarteritis has been reported as following serum sickness. There is a personal or family history of allergic disease in 15 per cent. of patients. This view leaves unexplained the progressive nature of the disease.

Many observers have been struck by the frequency with which there is a preceding history of infection, and particularly of haemolytic streptococcal infection. A considerable proportion of these patients show an increase in antistreptolysin O titre and the association of polyarteritis and rheumatic fever is more frequent than can be explained by chance. A bacterial cause in the more exact sense can be regarded as excluded, but a bacterial allergy of the type postulated as the cause of rheumatic fever remains a possibility.

It has been suggested that polyarteritis might be a manifestation of drug allergy. It has been recorded as following the sulphonamides, penicillin, mercurials, organic arsenicals and thiouracil.

Finally, an auto-immune origin has had its supporters. Some of the 'markers', such as hypergammaglobulinaemia and a response to corticosteroids, are present. Other disorders of this type are rarely associated, although concurrent auto-immune haemolytic anaemia and systemic lupus erythematosus have been noted. Auto-antibodies can only rarely be demonstrated. The evidence is, therefore, far from convincing.

Pathology

The basic lesion in this disease is a focal panarteritis. The inflammatory process starts in the media with neutrophil infiltration and fibrinoid necrosis; it spreads to the adventitia and the intima and the cellular infiltrate becomes eosinophilic. Thrombosis may follow in the affected vessels with ischaemic damage in the territory nourished by them. Aneurysm formation is rare. Occasionally granulomatous lesions with striking eosinophilic infiltration are seen, particularly in the respiratory tract.

In the more chronic cases the larger vessels bear the brunt of the disease; in the rapidly progressive type the small vessels are mainly affected and the condition is one of acute necrotizing angiitis. The lesions of polyarteritis are usually widespread, but are sometimes localized to one organ; typical changes may be limited, for instance, to the appendix, the uterus or the gall-bladder.

Clinical Picture

Onset and Course. In about 50 per cent. of patients the onset of the disease is acute with fever, disproportionate tachycardia, aching in the limbs and abdominal pain. In the remainder it is more insidious and there may be a longer or shorter period during which symptoms are referable to one organ or system. The most striking examples are those with pulmonary localization of the disease; they differ in many respects from other cases, and it has been suggested that a reasonable clinical subdivision would be into pulmonary and extrapulmonary types. Even when there is no pulmonary localization, a history of preceding respiratory infection can be obtained in 45 per cent.

In about 9 per cent. of cases polyarteritis supervenes upon polyarthritis of rheumatoid type. Occasionally the initial features are limited to the skin.

The onset, therefore, may suggest a disease process limited to one organ or system or a generalized disorder, and a disturbance of the first type may pass rapidly into one of the second. When the symptoms are generalized and of acute evolution, the clinical picture is often not specific and the label of 'pyrexia of uncertain origin' may be applied until characteristic features appear.

The course of polyarteritis nodosa is variable. At one end of the scale is a fulminating disease with prostration, fever, tachycardia and wasting which proves fatal in a few weeks, at the other one in which symptoms remain localized and activity subsides after a few months with complete recovery. All gradations between these two occur.

The Respiratory System. About 30 per cent. of patients with polyarteritis nodosa have respiratory symptoms. These give a history of pulmonary disease preceding, sometimes by years, the development of systematized polyarteritis. There may have been chronic bronchitis, pneumonia or asthma. The pneumonia often fails to resolve normally and seldom responds to antibiotics. Asthma, which may antedate generalization by as long as 7 years, is usually accompanied by a striking eosinophilia.

Respiratory symptoms, if they are not the prelude or opening event, rarely develop later; when present they tend to dominate the clinical picture throughout the course of the disease. They may be associated with granulomatous lesions in the upper respiratory tract or in the lungs themselves, lesions which are quite exceptional with extrapulmonary types of polyarteritis. The matter is discussed in the section on Wegener's granuloma [p. 433].

Radiology of the chest may show various appearances. Most commonly there is diffuse irregular mottling; sometimes massive localized shadows indicate pulmonary granulomata and these may cavitate; sometimes there are small fugitive infiltrations.

In general, the outlook for the patient with the pulmonary form of polyarteritis is poor.

The Alimentary System. Abdominal pain occurs at some time during the course of the disease in about 70 per cent. of patients. Infarction of the bowel, the liver and the spleen are common; gangrene and perforation of the bowel may occur; acute pancreatitis, melaena and retroperitoneal haemorrhage are all recorded. In spite of these manifold lesions, abdominal pain may be difficult to explain: it is frequently localized in the right upper quadrant and suspicion is often drawn to the gall-bladder.

The Cardiovascular System. Polyarteritis nodosa is, of course, essentially a vascular disease and its effects are mainly due to ischaemia or haemorrhage.

Occasionally palpable nodules form on superficial arteries. Although it is these which give the disease its name, they are rare. They often appear in crops and may be accompanied by an increase in fever and in general symptoms. They may be so small as to be just palpable or measure 1 cm. or more across.

Raynaud's phenomena are common, especially as an early symptom. They may progress to peripheral gangrene.

The coronary arteries are affected in about 60 per cent. of patients. It is particularly common in children. Ischaemic pain is rare and infarction exceptional. In spite of the lack of symptoms, electrocardiographic changes are frequently noted. Transient dry pericarditis may occur at any stage of the disease.

Hypertension is common in polyarteritis. In different series it has been observed in 45–60 per cent. of patients. It is usually associated with polyarteritic lesions in the kidneys.

The Genito-urinary System. The kidneys are found to be affected in 90 per cent. of cases at autopsy. The renal changes have been divided into two groups: first, a widespread necrotizing glomerulitis and, secondly, a collection of assorted lesions including glomerulonephritis and polyarteritis of larger vessels. The first is associated with rapidly progressive renal failure without hypertension; in the second group hypertension is the rule and often progresses to a malignant stage. It is variously estimated that 25–65 per cent. of deaths in polyarteritis nodosa are due to renal failure. Polyarteritis is one cause of the nephrotic syndrome.

The urine shows abnormalities in 90 per cent. of cases. Proteinuria is almost constant and haematuria common.

Orchitis has been reported on a number of occasions.

The Nervous System. The central nervous system suffers in about 20 per cent. of patients with polyarteritis. Encephalopathy is common. Meningeal symptoms and fits are frequently seen in the younger patients. Intracerebral and subarachnoid haemorrhage may occur.

In another 20 per cent. the peripheral nerves are affected. This may take the form of a peripheral neuropathy of the ascending type. There is often an associated myopathy and limb pain is common. In the majority, however, the disability is due to mononeuritis multiplex. This syndrome is characteristic of polyarteritis; it is due to ischaemic damage to peripheral nerve trunks caused by obliteration of their nutrient arteries. First one peripheral nerve is picked out, then another; the onset in each case is sudden and the distribution of the lesions asymmetrical. There is little or no recovery of function.

The Eyes. The frequency with which the eyes are affected has been variously estimated as 20–75 per cent. The lesions are varied: iridocyclitis, ophthalmoplegias, pupillary abnormalities, arterial occlusions, toxic retinopathy and focal vascular damage to the choroid are all described. In addition the changes of hypertensive disease are common.

The Skin. Rashes occur in 25 per cent. of patients. The pathognomonic nodules have been described in an earlier paragraph. Other specific changes are livedo reticularis and patchy cutaneous gangrene. In addition, non-specific eruptions such as urticaria, purpura and erythema nodosum are seen.

The Locomotor System. Arthralgia is common and in 35 per cent. there is transient or persistent arthritis. In some 9 per cent. of patients polyarteritis develops against a background of what appears to be chronic rheumatoid arthritis. It may be difficult to distinguish between rheumatoid arthritis, complicated by rheumatoid neuropathy, and polyarteritis nodosa.

Diagnosis

The clinical picture is often not characteristic in the early stages. Fever, undue tachycardia, mild anaemia and leucocytosis for which there is no obvious explanation should always arouse suspicion of this disease. Support is given by demonstrating affection of more than one system. The discovery of nodules is diagnostic. Ultimate proof depends upon finding the typical histological changes of the disease: a node, if one can be found, is most likely to give a positive result; muscle and nerve biopsy is less dependable.

The Blood. A moderate orthochromic anaemia is the rule. Rarely there is an associated auto-immune haemolytic anaemia with a positive antiglobulin test. Leucocytosis is usual, but seldom in excess of 15,000–20,000 per mm^3. Eosinophilia is common in pulmonary cases and may be intense; in one instance eosinophils amounted to 75 per cent. of a leucocytosis of 25,000 per mm^3. The E.S.R. is constantly raised, usually to a considerable degree. This presumably depends upon the hypergammaglobulinaemia which is commonly present.

Occasionally a positive L.E. cell test is obtained and rather more frequently antinuclear factor can be demonstrated. In patients starting with rheumatoid arthritis there may be a positive test for rheumatoid factor.

Treatment

There is no specific treatment for this disease. If it appears to have arisen as a result of hypersensitivity, it is logical to remove the agent which is under suspicion. Since many believe streptococcal infection to play a part, a preliminary course of penicillin has been advocated. Little obvious benefit follows such treatment.

Corticosteroids undoubtedly bring about temporary improvement and control acute symptoms. It is doubtful whether they influence greatly the final result. In addition to their usual disadvantages they are thought to carry other dangers in polyarteritis. It has been suggested that the frequency of thrombosis is increased, that the onset of malignant hypertension is accelerated and that neuropathy is aggravated. In spite of these dangers, some of which are hypothetical and others imponderable, it is difficult to deny a seriously ill patient the one drug which will certainly relieve his present distress. If the decision to use corticosteroids is taken, it is essential to give sufficient completely to suppress symptoms. In terms of prednisolone, a daily dose of 60 mg. will probably be required and the dose should be slowly reduced until the lowest level at which there is complete suppression is found.

Prognosis

Polyarteritis nodosa varies from a fulminating disease fatal in three months to an indolent complaint with full recovery after a year or less. It has been estimated that over-all mortality is less than 50 per cent. The average duration of activity is between 6 and 12 months, by the end of this time most patients will either be well or dead. Residual disability, apart from that due to nerve lesions, is unusual.

Kidney disease carries a bad prognosis and accounts, in different series, for 25–65 per cent. of the deaths. Pulmonary lesions also have a grave outlook.

In one small controlled trial, 13 of 21 patients treated with corticosteroids were living after 3 years and 10 after 5 years. There was no conclusive evidence that the treatment had prolonged life when comparison was made with a control series.

REFERENCES

Bleehen, S. S., Lovelace, R. E., and Cotton, R. E. (1963) Mononeuritis multiplex in polyarteritis nodosa, *Quart. J. Med.*, **32**, 193.

Davson, J., Ball, J., and Platt, R. (1948) The kidney in polyarteritis nodosa, *Quart. J. Med.*, **17**, 175.

Miller, H. G., and Daley, R. (1946) Clinical aspects of polyarteritis nodosa, *Quart. J. Med.*, **15**, 255.

Report to Medical Research Council by the Collagen Diseases and Hypersensitivity Panel (1960) Treatment of polyarteritis with cortisone: results after 3 years, *Brit. med. J.*, **1**, 1399.

Rose, G. A. (1957) The natural history of polyarteritis, *Brit. med. J.*, **2**, 1148.

Rose, G. A., and Spencer, H. (1957) Polyarteritis nodosa, *Quart. J. Med.*, **26**, 43.

MALIGNANT GRANULOMA

Synonyms. Giant-cell granuloma of respiratory tract; Lethal midline granuloma; Wegener's granuloma; Granuloma gangraenescens; Non-healing granuloma.

Definition

A rare disease of unknown cause in which progressive granulomatous ulceration of the respiratory tract may later be followed by systemic arterial lesions indistinguishable from those of polyarteritis nodosa. The term Wegener's granuloma is usually reserved for cases in which systemic spread has taken place.

Aetiology

The cause of this disorder is unknown. It may well be that two distinct diseases are being considered under this head; the problem is discussed in the section on pathology.

The age incidence is between 12 and 75 years with most patients being between 35 and 55. Wegener's granuloma is believed by many to be a variant of polyarteritis nodosa.

Pathology

Two histological types of granuloma of the upper respiratory tract can be recognized. In the first, or Stewart, type the cellular infiltrate consists of lymphocytes, plasma cells and atypical histiocytes; there is much necrosis, many small haemorrhages and considerable destruction of bone and cartilage. A proportion of this type eventually proves to have been wrongly classified and declare themselves as frankly reticulosarcomatous. Most of the remainder continue localized to the nose and adjacent tissues, but a few develop systemic vascular lesions and it is for this reason that the two forms of nasal granuloma are considered together.

In the second, or Wegener, type the necrotizing granulation tissue contains giant cells reminiscent of those of tuberculosis, but with densely staining nuclei and a more eosinophilic cytoplasm. Vasculitis may be evident in the granuloma and in the majority of instances systemic arterial lesions eventually develop;

the final result is not to be distinguished from polyarteritis nodosa of the acute type.

Clinical Picture

The Stewart type of granuloma starts in the nose or, less commonly, in the maxillary sinus or the mouth. The earliest symptom is nasal discharge. It leads to local destruction of tissue, including bone and cartilage. Systemic symptoms are usually attributable to secondary infection and haemorrhage; aspiration pneumonia is common.

The Wegener type also presents with nasal symptoms such as obstruction and discharge. Less frequently it starts in the ear, orbital region or skin. An exactly similar granuloma may develop in the lung when it is usually regarded as the pulmonary form of polyarteritis nodosa. In the nose, local destruction is relatively slight; but after a period, which may be only a few months or may extend to several years, systemic symptoms appear and the features become those of fulminating polyarteritis. Death is usual in 4 or 5 months from the onset of the generalized stage.

It is likely that further experience of malignant granuloma will establish the separate identity of the Stewart and Wegener types. At present it seems justifiable to describe them together for their distinction is not absolute.

Diagnosis

The task of initial diagnosis usually falls to the otorhinolaryngologist. Distinction has to be made from other nasal tumours and granulomata. Reticulosarcoma offers the greatest difficulty. Biopsy is essential and should allow the two types to be distinguished.

In the systemic stage anaemia, leucocytosis, eosinophilia and a raised E.S.R. are the rule. There is often hypergammaglobulinaemia.

Treatment

There is general agreement that radiotherapy is the most effective treatment in the Stewart type of granuloma. Only low doses are required. If the disease can be arrested reparative surgery will probably be needed.

In the Wegener type radiotherapy is usually applied when the disease is localized; it may be questioned whether much benefit results. Once the process has become systematized the treatment is that of polyarteritis nodosa.

Prognosis

In the Stewart type of granuloma the disease may be arrested and, in one series, 40 per cent. survived between 6 and 8 years. Wegener's granuloma is probably always fatal, although the length of time before the disease enters its terminal generalized phase is variable and may extend to 5 years or more. Once this stage is established the average survival is about 5 months.

REFERENCES

FRIEDMANN, I. (1964) The pathology of midline granuloma, *Proc. roy. Soc. Med.*, **57**, 289.

WALTON, E. W. (1958) Giant-cell granuloma of the respiratory tract (Wegener's granulomatosis), *Brit. med. J.*, **2**, 265.

GIANT CELL ARTERITIS

Synonyms. Cranial arteritis; Temporal arteritis; Polymyalgia rheumatica; Anarthritic rheumatoid disease.

Definition

A subacute inflammatory disorder of unknown cause affecting larger arteries, particularly the temporal and occipital vessels and less often the aorta and its branches.

Aetiology

The cause of giant cell arteritis is unknown. It is regarded by some as a variant of polyarteritis nodosa and it has sometimes been observed in like manner to follow an acute infection. It is a disease of the elderly; the mean age of onset being 70 years. In one series the range was from 60 to 85 years. Women are affected twice as frequently as men.

Pathology

This disease is a generalized, or potentially generalized, granulomatous panarteritis. Symptoms arise almost exclusively from cranial arteries, but post-mortem examinations invariably reveal diffuse arterial disease. The media bears the brunt of the damage, showing a mixture of necrosis and granulomatous inflammation with the presence of giant-cells. The intima shows diffuse fibrous thickening. Thrombosis is common.

Clinical Picture

There is often a preliminary period of illness of insidious onset with malaise, loss of weight, muscular pains, arthralgia, depression and fever, reaching perhaps 100° F. (38° C.) at night. These symptoms last on an average for 5 months before the diagnosis is established. The nature of the malady is often not appreciated until some striking symptom or group of symptoms points to the diagnosis. Perhaps the most common of these is headache which often lacks specific features, but in a proportion has those which led to the term 'temporal arteritis'. In these the onset is often abrupt; pain is usually of great intensity and may be accompanied by such tenderness of the scalp that to brush the hair or rest the head on the pillow is agonizing. The headache is usually temporal and when this is so the temporal arteries may be thickened, tender and non-pulsatile with reddening of the overlying skin. At other times the occipital arteries are affected and tender nodules may be felt in the scalp. Diffuse arterial occlusions may lead to actual necrosis of the skin. Occasionally there are no local signs of arteritis and the symptoms are those of intermittent claudication of the jaws with pain on biting or chewing.

Ocular disturbances occur in at least 50 per cent. of patients and usually follow the onset of headache, although they may be the presenting feature. Sometimes the interval is as short as 2 days and it has been as long as 6 months: the average is about 4 weeks. Ophthalmoplegia and loss of vision may occur. The first is less common; it is probably due to arterial occlusion, occurs early and usually recovers in 6–8 weeks. The second is the more frequent and by far the more serious. Partial or complete loss of vision may occur in one or both eyes. Visual impairment of some degree is observed in about 50 per cent. of patients. The onset is usually abrupt, involving the whole or part of the field and becoming complete in the area affected within 24 hours. The visual loss is often segmental at first, spreading within a few days to affect the whole field. The ophthalmoscopic appearances are usually less striking than the degree of impairment of vision would suggest. The arteries are thin and empty; there is often oedema of the disc and of the retina itself; in severe cases a cherry-red spot is to be found at the macula. The abnormal signs disappear within days and rarely leave more than ischaemic optic atrophy. In about half the patients both eyes are affected, usually consecutively. If the second eye has not suffered within two months of the first, it is likely to escape.

Once affected there is little chance of improvement and the usual result is complete blindness.

Other cranial arteries are more rarely affected by giant cell arteritis, but evidence of diffuse or localized cerebral ischaemia, including dementia, convulsions, cranial nerve palsies and hemiplegia, has often been recorded. Peripheral neuropathy is even more rare, but mononeuritis multiplex is reported.

Diffuse myalgia is almost invariable in the opening stages and may become sufficiently intense to dominate the clinical picture. Such patients were formerly regarded as suffering from a separate disorder to which the name 'polymyalgia rheumatica' was given; it is now accepted as one expression of giant-cell arteritis.

Myalgia with morning stiffness is the characteristic feature and the muscles of the shoulder girdle, neck, pelvic girdle, lumbar spine and thighs are affected in this order of frequency. They are often painful and tender, but weakness is not striking.

Arthralgia is common but synovitis is unusual and seldom more than transient.

Symptoms arising from disease of the aorta and its branches are unusual. Giant-cell arteritis is one of the causes of the aortic arch syndrome and appears to have been the basic pathological change in some examples of 'pulseless disease' [see Section 8]. It may cause aneurysm or lead to occlusion of mesenteric or limb arteries. Intermittent claudication is not rare. It is quite exceptional for the renal arteries to be affected.

Diagnosis

Diagnosis is easy when the temporal arteries are affected. The severity of the headache should at once arouse suspicion of temporal arteritis, expecially in a patient over the age of 60 years. Biopsy of the inflamed artery will establish the diagnosis, but is seldom required, for if an artery is obviously inflamed there can be little doubt of the diagnosis. The picture of 'polymyalgia rheumatica' is characteristic, but in those without these distinguishing features it may be difficult.

Examination of the blood usually shows a mild orthochromic anaemia with a haemoglobin level around 11 g. per 100 ml. There may be moderate leucocytosis, but this is inconstant. The E.S.R. is greatly raised, often exceeding 100 mm. in the first hour by the Westergren method. There is often some increase in the α_2-globulin fraction of the serum proteins.

Treatment

Early treatment with corticosteroids is of the greatest importance. They will control the headache, the fever and the myalgia, but, far more important, there is good evidence that they will prevent ocular complications if given early enough. If visual impairment has already occurred improvement is most unlikely. Treatment should be continued for at least 6 months from the onset of headache.

Prednisolone or its equivalent may be used. The initial dose in terms of the first should be 10 mg. four times daily and once suppression is achieved, it should be gradually reduced to the lowest quantity which will control symptoms.

Some recommend the simultaneous use of anticoagulant drugs.

Prognosis

The mortality of giant-cell arteritis is between 10 and 15 per cent. Some 75 per cent. of patients recover within 30 months of the onset of the disease. In occasional instances signs of systemic affection persist, sometimes for years. In untreated cases blindness results in 20–25 per cent., but in those who receive full doses of corticosteroids before the onset of visual impairment the incidence is reduced to 9 per cent.

REFERENCES

HAMILTON, C. R. JR., SHELLEY, W. M., and TUMULTY, P. A. (1971) Giant-cell arteritis: including temporal arteritis and polymyalgia rheumatica, *Medicine* (*Baltimore*), **50**, 1.

HART, F. D. (1969) Polymyalgia rheumatica, *Brit. med. J.*, **1**, 99.

MEADOWS, S. P. (1966) Temporal or giant-cell arteritis, *Proc. roy. Soc. Med.*, **59**, 329.

PAULLEY, J. W., and HUGHES, J. P. (1960) Giant-cell arteritis or arteritis of the aged, *Brit. med. J.*, **2**, 1562.

RUSSELL, R. W. R. (1959) Giant-cell arteritis, *Quart. J. Med.*, **28**, 471.

CUTANEOUS VASCULITIS

This term covers a number of conditions in which primary vascular disease, thought to be of allergic origin, is responsible. The clinical pictures include purpura, with or without necrosis; haemorrhagic or necrotizing papules; vesicles or bullae, proceeding to ulceration; foci of panniculitis also proceeding to ulceration and destruction of fat cells with fatty discharge and subsequent healing with a dispersed scar. The type of lesion depends on the size of the vessel involved.

Erythema nodosum is a tender nodular erythematous eruption on the fronts of the legs, sometimes on the extensor aspects of the forearms and thighs, and elsewhere. After passing through the colour changes of bruising, the lesions resolve within a few weeks without ulceration, scarring or atrophy. Recurrences are rare.

It represents a reaction of vascular hypersensitivity;

the sensitizing agents include tubercle bacilli, streptococci, meningococci and other bacteria and viruses. In the United States a common cause is coccidioidomycosis. The lesions may also develop when chemotherapeutic or antibiotic drugs release bacterial products to which the patient is sensitized. It is one of the ways in which sarcoidosis [see Section 9] may present.

Erythema nodosum leprosum is an exacerbation reaction of lepromatous leprosy during treatment, mimicking erythema nodosum clinically but differing histologically. The scars may ulcerate.

Its course may follow an upper respiratory infection. The patient is usually a child or young adult and the initial complaint is of tender swellings in the fronts of the legs and sometimes in the forearms. The lesions are obtuse nodules with ill-defined margins: there may be more than a dozen on the two limbs. After passing through the colour changes described above, slow resolution occurs over 3–6 weeks and no trace is left. Malaise is usual and arthralgia, especially of the knees, is common. Recurrences may occur in cases of streptococcal origin.

Rest in bed until the nodules have subsided is advisable. The treatment is purely symptomatic.

If the tuberculin reaction is undergoing or has recently undergone conversion it is particularly important to avoid contact with open tuberculosis. Every patient requires full investigation to determine the cause.

Erythema induratum (*Bazin*). This is a tuberculide localized to the calves by the inadequate circulation of young women with perniosis.

Darier-Roussy sarcoid. Resembles Bazin's disease but does not ulcerate. The histology is that of sarcoidosis.

Erythema induratum (*Whitfield*). This is also known as nodular vasculitis and presents as recurring tender subcutaneous nodules in the legs, usually in women aged 30–45 years. The cause is uncertain but in some hypersensitivity to a distant tuberculous focus appears responsible.

REFERENCE

Winkelmann, R. K., and Ditto, W. B. (1964) Cutaneous and visceral syndromes of necrotising or 'allergic' angiitis: a study of 38 cases, *Medicine* (*Baltimore*), **43**, 59.

ANAPHYLACTOID PURPURA

Synonyms. Schönlein-Henoch syndrome; Rheumatic purpura; Peliosis rheumatica; Purpura abdominalis; Haemorrhagic capillary toxicosis.

Definition

A syndrome of which the major components are purpura and various exudative skin lesions; pain and swelling of joints; intestinal colic often with melaena or blood-stained mucus in the motions; and haematuria.

Aetiology

Anaphylactoid purpura is predominantly a disease of children. The mean age of onset is 5–7 years and not more than 10 per cent. of cases occur over the age of 12. It is generally held to show a male predominance, but recent series have recorded the two sexes as equally affected. In Great Britain there is a seasonal peak of incidence in February with a lesser one in October.

The basic morbid change is a wide-spread, but focal, inflammation of small arterioles and capillaries. The lesions have the histological features of a hypersensitivity reaction, but the allergen or allergens remain uncertain. The majority of patients are taken ill 2–3 weeks after an upper respiratory tract infection and thus present a parallel with the victims of acute rheumatic fever and acute nephritis. From some 30 per cent. a Group A β-haemolytic streptococcus can be recovered and there is some rise in the antistreptolysin and other antibody titres, but analysis shows that these findings do not differ significantly from those in a control group of non-rheumatic children. Other suspected allergens include many different foods, but in every instance the evidence is as unconvincing as it is for the haemolytic streptococcus. The cause of this disease thus remains unknown.

Pathology

The essential change, as explained earlier, is widespread focal vasculitis. In the skin, nodular perivascular infiltrations consisting of neutrophils and eosinophils, are seen in the dermis. Necrotizing inflammatory foci with thrombosis in small arterioles are common, and the lesions are surrounded by haemorrhage. In the kidneys there is a patchy affection of the glomeruli which show fibrinoid deposition and endothelial proliferations. Renal vein thrombosis is recorded.

Clinical Picture

Onset. In most patients a history of upper respiratory tract infection some two or three weeks previously can be obtained. The onset is usually subacute with headache, anorexia and fever which seldom exceeds 102° F. (38·9° C.). In about 60 per cent. a rash, accompanied by articular or abdominal pain, is the presenting symptom; in 20 per cent. joint pains alone bring the patient under observation and in the remaining 20 per cent. the cause is abdominal pain. In every instance other features of the syndrome appear later.

The Skin. The skin rash must be regarded as a *sine qua non* of this syndrome. It has been said that exceptionally it may be absent, but in such cases diagnosis is virtually impossible. The characteristic eruption of anaphylactoid purpura is seen on the buttocks, the backs of the elbows, the extensor surfaces of the arms and legs and on the ankle and foot. The face is occasionally affected, but the trunk is usually spared. The rash starts as pink, non-irritating papules, within a few hours becoming haemorrhagic and flattening although still remaining palpable. In 35 per cent. the lesion is primarily urticarial, resolving to be replaced by purpura. The red purpuric rash fades through purple to brown and disappears in about 3 weeks. Repeated crops are common.

Local oedema, affecting the periorbital tissues, the dorsum of the hand or the feet is sometimes an opening event. Oedema of the glottis has proved fatal. The eruption may take almost any form—vesicular, bullous or pemphigoid. Rarely necrosis of the skin ensues.

The Joints. Articular symptoms occur in 70 per cent.

of patients. They are present early in the course of the disease and seldom last more than a week. The knees and ankles are most commonly affected, less often the hips, wrists and elbows, and only exceptionally the small joints of the hands and feet. Pain is often more impressive than objective evidence of joint disease. Swelling is commonly periarticular and effusion into the joints uncommon. One or more joints may be affected and the migratory pattern, so characteristic of acute rheumatic fever, is not seen.

The Alimentary Tract. Abdominal symptoms are a feature in one-third of the patients. They may be the initial complaint and cause the patient to seek surgical advice. Pain is variable in intensity, usually colicky and central, but sometimes located in the right iliac fossa. Vomiting is common and there may be haematemesis. Diarrhoea is unusual, but melaena, or stools containing blood-stained mucus, may occur. Tests of the faeces for occult blood are usually positive. Enough protein may be lost in the stool to reduce significantly the serum level.

The symptoms may suggest intestinal obstruction and intussusception is a well-recognized complication. Perforation is also recorded, but is fortunately rare. Surgical exploration may become necessary and carries no undue risk. At operation the terminal ileum is usually affected, but the disease may be much more extensive. The common finding is a haemorrhagic oedema of the intestinal wall and subperitoneal ecchymosis with the thickened segment of bowel forming the intussusceptum.

The Kidneys. In 20–50 per cent. of patients with anaphylactoid purpura there are urinary abnormalities which indicate kidney disease. Their appearance is often late; in 25 per cent. it is more than a month after the onset of the disease. Haematuria, gross or microscopic, is the commonest and often out of proportion to the albuminuria. The majority recover completely and not more than 5–10 per cent. of patients are left with evidence of chronic renal disease. Urinary abnormalities may last for 6 months and still disappear, but if still present after 2 years there is almost certainly irreversible kidney disease. An occasional patient dies with renal failure early in the course of the illness; in some a nephrotic syndrome ensues, but the usual outcome is the picture of chronic nephritis with a mounting blood pressure.

Other Systems. Damage to the nervous system with transient paresis or convulsions is a rare symptom. Intra-ocular haemorrhage is recorded, and perichondritis of the pinna was a feature of one series.

Related Syndromes. Many authorities believe all types of necrotizing angiitis to be variants of the same disease process. Polyarteritis nodosa and anaphylactoid purpura can usually be distinguished from one another, but rarely intermediate forms are encountered which defy classification. There are in addition two uncommon syndromes which are best considered with anaphylactoid purpura.

Purpura fulminans is essentially a disease of children: not more than 10 per cent. of patients are adults. There is a sudden onset a few days after an infection with extensive ecchymoses on the extensor surfaces of the limbs; fever, vomiting and peripheral circulatory failure rapidly supervene and death occurs on the 3rd or 4th day.

An exactly similar clinical picture may result from septicaemia, especially meningococcal (Friderichsen-Waterhouse syndrome) or due to Gram-negative organisms, but it is well established that a non-infective form exists which can be regarded as a fulminating variety of anaphylactoid purpura.

Purpura necrotica is again a disease of children. The onset is usually abrupt with fever, diarrhoea and vomiting, cramps and collapse; in others general symptoms are less dramatic. In all, however, haemorrhages, varying in diameter from 2 mm. to 4 cm., appear in the skin of the face and limbs, often with urticaria and painful swollen joints. Intestinal and renal symptoms are rare. A striking feature of the skin lesions is the way in which one part may show resolution while another is clearly advancing. Later, necrosis occurs in the centres of the haemorrhagic areas and extends sometimes as far as underlying soft tissues. Healing eventually takes place, but recovery is protracted. Purpura necrotica has been regarded as a clinical counterpart of the Schwartzmann phenomenon.

Diagnosis

It is seldom difficult to distinguish anaphylactoid from other forms of purpura (see Section 13) and from other types of necrotizing angiitis. There are examples which are difficult to classify, and the possibility of an infective cause for the more acute forms, such as purpura fulminans, must not be forgotten.

The laboratory affords little help unless biopsy of a skin lesion is undertaken, and this is seldom necessary or justifiable.

The blood shows no diagnostic changes in the typical case. There is no anaemia; moderate neutrophilia often with some eosinophilia is usual; the platelet count is normal and the erythrocyte sedimentation rate raised. The tourniquet test is mildly positive in 25 per cent. The level of serum albumin may be reduced by loss into the alimentary tract.

In purpura fulminans changes in the coagulation process occur secondary to the vasculitis. There is extensive intravascular clotting with a fall in the platelet count and fibrinogen level, and increase in fibrinolytic activity.

Treatment

Treatment is largely symptomatic. Rest is advisable in the early stages of the disease, for increased activity will often cause a fresh outcrop of purpura. The corticosteroids have proved disappointing. Corticotrophin is more effective than the cortisone derivatives given by mouth. It has little effect on the purpura, but will control joint pain, localized oedema and the abdominal symptoms. Indeed, if abdominal pain is not relieved by this means, it is evidence that there is an irreversible lesion, such as an intussusception, requiring laparotomy. Relapse is likely directly the corticotrophin is withdrawn. Surgery should not be delayed when intussusception, obstruction or perforation is suspected.

In purpura fulminans, energetic treatment with corticosteroids, blood transfusion, oxygen and intravenous heparin has proved successful.

Course and Prognosis

Anaphylactoid purpura is usually a benign disorder, ending spontaneously in 6–8 weeks. In 10 per cent. there is a relapsing course, sometimes over years, with recurrences of purpura, oedema and haematuria.

The most serious sequel is renal disease. Not more than 5–10 per cent. develop chronic nephritis. Eighty to ninety per cent. show urinary abnormalities at some time; 50 per cent. of these are clear after 3 months and 80–90 per cent. after 2 years.

Rarely abdominal complications, acute renal failure or oedema of the glottis are responsible for death early in the course of the disease.

REFERENCES

ALLEN, D. M., DIAMOND, L. K., and HOWELL, A. (1960) Anaphylactoid purpura in children (Schönlein-Henoch syndrome). Review with a follow-up of the renal complications, *Amer. J. Dis. Child.*, **99**, 833.

BYWATERS, E. G. L., ISDALE, I., and KEMPTON, J. J. (1957) Schönlein-Henoch purpura, *Quart. J. Med.*, N.S.**26**, 161.

GAIRDNER, D. (1948) The Schönlein-Henoch syndrome (Anaphylactoid purpura), *Quart. J. Med.*, N.S.**17**, 95.

HJORT, P. F., RAPAPORT, S. I., and JØRGENSEN, L. (1964) Purpura fulminans: Report of a case successfully treated with heparin and hydrocortisone. Review of 50 cases from the literature, *Scand. J. Haemat.*, **1**, 169.

PROGRESSIVE SYSTEMIC SCLEROSIS

Synonym. Scleroderma.

Definition

Systemic sclerosis is a disease of unknown cause in which the main features are a diffuse indurative change throughout the connective tissues, due to increased deposition of collagen, and obliterative lesions of small arteries. The process usually declares itself first in the skin and subcutaneous tissues; visceral lesions appear at a later date, particularly in the digestive tract, the lungs, the kidneys and the heart.

Aetiology

Systemic sclerosis affects females three times more frequently than males. It may occur at any age, but in most instances the onset is between 20 and 50 years. It has been described in most races. Familial cases have occasionally been reported.

The cause of systemic sclerosis is unknown. It has been noted, like other diseases of this group, sometimes to follow infection. In conformity with current popular doctrine attempts have been made to establish it as an 'auto-immune' disease. It has been reported in association with haemolytic anaemia, Sjøgren's syndrome and rheumatoid arthritis. There is seldom a positive L.E. cell test, but circulating antinuclear factor can often be demonstrated by special techniques and the Rose-Waaler test is positive in about 30 per cent. of cases. The histological changes, especially in the kidney, may be difficult to distinguish from those of systemic lupus erythematosus and the dividing line between this disease and systemic sclerosis and between systemic sclerosis and dermatomyositis may be hard to draw with confidence. There is some association between scleroderma and malignant disease, although it is far less definite than in the case of dermatomyositis.

Pathology

Histological study of the skin shows oedema in the early stages which is followed by fibroblastic proliferation and deposition of collagen. Later the collagen fibres may undergo hyaline change and calcium may be deposited. In the smaller arteries obliterative thickening of the intima is common with occasional fibrinoid degeneration.

A patchy irregular fibrosis is common in the lungs and in the myocardium. In the kidneys the changes are likewise patchy; the affected glomeruli show thickening of the basement membrane with subsequent obliterative changes. The end result is often an irregularly scarred and contracted kidney.

Clinical Picture

Onset and Course. Systemic sclerosis is usually a chronic disease of insidious onset. Many patients have survived more than 30 years. Occasionally, however, it runs an acute course with death in a few months; when this occurs renal failure is usually the cause.

It is a generalized disorder and the initial symptoms may indicate affection of any one of several systems. In at least 75 per cent. of patients the onset is with Raynaud phenomena and skin changes in the hands. In others gastro-intestinal disturbances, cardiac, pulmonary or even renal symptoms may occupy the centre of the stage. Malaise, loss of weight, low fever and myalgic pains are common whatever the type of onset.

The Skin. Vascular disturbances of the Raynaud type are common and provide the opening symptoms in about 80 per cent. of patients. They may precede by many months the appearance of more definite cutaneous changes.

The types of skin lesion are three:

1. *Circumscribed scleroderma or morphoea.* This usually appears on the trunk and in young adults. It starts as an erythematous patch which rapidly becomes a hard waxy plaque with a violaceous halo. Its relationship to systemic sclerosis is unknown. It usually resolves in about 5 years and no visceral lesions occur. In the early stages distinction from systemic sclerosis may be impossible.

2. *Acrosclerosis of Sellei or sclerodactyly.* Here the sclerodermatous process affects mainly the skin of the hands, feet and face. It is not to be distinguished from other types of systemic sclerosis except that it tends to progress slowly and visceral lesions are often late in appearing.

3. *Diffuse progressive type.* Sclerodermatous lesions appear mainly on the trunk; the extremities and face are often spared and visceral lesions are early and severe.

In the second and third types the changes follow the

same sequence: first, the skin is oedematous, the folds are obliterated and it has a glossy waxy appearance; in the next stage, the indurative process starts and the skin cannot be lifted from the subcutaneous tissues; the final stage is one of atrophy with firm attachment of skin to underlying structures. In this phase subcutaneous calcification (calcinosis), both circumscribed or diffuse, may take place; ulceration of the skin is frequent; branched hair-like telangiectases appear and patches of pigmentation and depigmentation occur. The densely adherent skin may immobilize the fingers and convert the hands into rigid useless claws; it may hamper respiratory movements or prevent the jaws from being opened.

The combination of sclerodactyly, subcutaneous calcinosis and telangiectasia is sometimes known as the Thibierge-Weissenbach syndrome.

The Gastro-intestinal Tract. The whole length of the alimentary tract may be affected in systemic sclerosis. Atrophy and fibrosis of the tongue is common. Most frequently, however, symptoms arise from disease of the oesophagus: dysphagia, belching, regurgitation of food and epigastric discomfort all occur. The lower third of the oesophagus shows striking radiological abnormalities, dilatation and loss of peristalsis being the most common. These changes often occur early and may antedate the skin lesions. They are said to be present in 65 per cent. of patients with systemic sclerosis.

Comparable changes have been recorded in the small bowel and even in the rectum. They may lead to a malabsorption syndrome.

The Heart. The heart is seldom affected early and symptoms of heart disease are relatively uncommon, appearing in only some 10 per cent. of patients. The features are those of cardiomyopathy with congestive heart failure and conduction defects. Occasionally pericarditis occurs. Chronic cor pulmonale may develop secondary to diffuse pulmonary fibrosis.

The Lungs. Fibrotic changes in the lungs are common, but usually develop late. Increasing dyspnoea and unproductive cough are the usual symptoms.

The changes are often patchy and radiologically many different patterns may be seen. A diffuse mottling is common in the early stages and this is often replaced by a 'honeycomb' appearance. Irregular fibrosis may give rise to focal emphysema and recurrent spontaneous pneumothorax be a complication. Pulmonary hypertension occasionally develops.

Respiratory movements are often restricted by adhesion of the thickened skin to the chest wall.

The Kidneys. Albuminuria is common in systemic sclerosis and post-mortem figures show the kidneys to be affected in 75 per cent. of patients. Clinical evidence of significant renal disease is rare. It may occur early or late in the course of the illness and is rapidly progressive, terminating in renal failure. Hypertension is unusual.

The Locomotor System. Gross disease of joints is rare, although the deformity of the hands is often mistaken for that of rheumatoid arthritis. Arthralgia is a common complaint and the immobility produced by the scleroderma leads to osteoporosis. Myalgia is frequent in the early stages and myositis is a constant finding *post mortem.* Occasionally tenosynovitis with a persistent and striking crepitus is a feature of the disease.

Diagnosis

Diagnosis offers little difficulty when the disease is established. It is less easy when Raynaud phenomena are the only symptoms. Occasionally it is hard to decide whether a sclerodermatous lesion is of the benign circumscribed type or whether it is the harbinger of systemic sclerosis. The presence of general symptoms, perhaps with dysphagia, will point the diagnosis. There is usually little difficulty in distinguishing systemic sclerosis from dermatomyositis, but scleroedema adultorum [see Section 14] may present a problem. The possibility of confusion with rheumatoid arthritis has already been mentioned.

There are two uncommon conditions which can be mistaken for systemic sclerosis. *Werner's syndrome* is a disease of early adult life characterized by loss of subcutaneous fat, baldness and cataracts; the skin is drawn tight over the underlying bones, but there is no true sclerodermatous change. It is probably inherited as an autosomal recessive. In *Rothmund's syndrome* there is circumscribed atrophy of the skin over the face and the buttocks, rapidly progressive cataracts and telangiectasia; it usually occurs in childhood.

The Blood. There are no specific changes. A mild orthochromic anaemia may be present; the white blood cell count is usually normal; the E.S.R. is raised. There is often an increase in the γ-globulin fraction of the serum proteins.

The Urine. Albuminuria is the rule and when there is 'true scleroderma kidney' casts and red blood cells are found in the deposit.

Radiology. An opaque meal will demonstrate the changes already described in the lower part of the oesophagus. In early cases they are best shown by ciné-radiography. Such a finding will confirm the diagnosis in a doubtful case. Dilatation and sluggish peristalsis often with changes in mucosal pattern may be found in the small intestine. Films of the chest may show cardiac enlargement, diffuse interstitial pulmonary fibrosis or 'honeycomb lung'. Subcutaneous calcinosis is commonly demonstrable in the fingers and in some of the more chronic cases calcinosis universalis is sometimes found.

Biopsy. The histological changes in the skin are not sufficiently specific for dogmatic diagnosis, particularly in the early case where the clinical features are not characteristic. At this stage there is often little more than an increase in collagen fibres.

Treatment

There is no specific treatment for systemic sclerosis. Many drugs have been recommended, but none has stood the test of time. It has been stated that benefit results from potassium para-aminobenzoate in divided doses of 12 G. daily continued for many years, but the original claims have little support. The corticosteroid hormones may give some transient euphoria, but have no other beneficial action; indeed it has been said that the condition of the skin and the kidneys is made worse by their use.

Surgery may sometimes be inevitable. Gangrenous fingers may need amputation; ulcers may not heal until a plaque of calcium has been evacuated. Sympathectomy will relieve Raynaud phenomena in about 30 per cent. of patients.

Judicious physiotherapy can do much to lessen the patient's discomforts.

Prognosis

Systemic sclerosis is a disease of great chronicity; 70 per cent. survive more than 5 years and 60 per cent. more than 10. Rarely it runs an acute course when death from renal failure may occur in less than 6 months.

REFERENCES

CULLINAN, E. R. (1953) Scleroderma (diffuse systemic sclerosis), *Proc. roy. Soc. Med.*, **46**, 507.

FARMER, R. G., GIFFORD, R. W. Jr., and HINES, E. A. Jr. (1960) Prognostic significance of Raynaud's phenomena and other clinical characteristics of systemic scleroderma. A study of 271 cases, *Circulation*, **21**, 1088.

ORABONA, M. L., and ALBANO, O. (1958) Progressive systemic sclerosis (or visceral scleroderma), *Acta med. scand.*, **160**, Suppl., 333.

THANNHAUSER, S. J. (1945) Werner's syndrome (progeria of the adult) and Rothmund's syndrome: two types of closely related heredo-familial atrophic dermatosis with juvenile cataracts and endocrine features. A critical study with five new cases, *Ann. intern. Med.*, **23**, 559.

DERMATOMYOSITIS

Definition

A disease of unknown cause in which diffuse inflammatory changes occur in skin and muscle. It is probable that no distinction should be drawn between dermatomyositis and some forms of polymyositis in which the skin is more or less completely spared.

Aetiology

Dermatomyositis affects females twice as frequently as males and most cases occur between the ages of 30 and 50 years. It is, however, not rare in children and in one large series the ages of the patients ranged from 2 to 76 years. It has been recorded in identical twins. There is no racial predilection.

The cause of dermatomyositis is unknown. Like many other collagen diseases it has been noted to follow infection, but there is no evidence that it has an infective basis. It shows some association with other diseases of this group and may occur in subjects of rheumatic fever. There is a suggestion that it may fall into the category of auto-immune disease, but there is yet little support for this view.

There is an association in adults with malignant disease and in 15–18 per cent. there is an underlying neoplasm. It may be epithelial or mesenchymal in origin, but carcinoma of the breast and of the ovary are probably the most common. The skin eruption usually appears before the tumour is recognized and it has been suggested that antibodies, evoked in some way by the tumour, cross-react with other tissue antigens. Remission in the dermatomyositis has been claimed after extirpation of the growth.

Pathology

The muscle fibres show degenerative changes with fragmentation, vacuolation and loss of striation; in the early stages the fibrils are separated by oedema fluid and there are occasional collections of lymphocytes, plasma cells and histiocytes. Eventually the damaged fibres are replaced by dense collagenous fibrous tissue. The intramuscular arteries show intimal thickening and sometimes thrombosis.

The changes in the skin are similar to those of scleroderma with thinning of its layers and a diffuse increase in collagen. Calcinosis may be evident in the late stages.

Systemic lesions may be found *post mortem*, particularly in the gastro-intestinal tract, the heart and the kidneys.

Clinical Picture

The onset of dermatomyositis is usually insidious and preceded by some weeks of malaise with muscular aching, weakness and fatigue. In about 25 per cent., however, it appears abruptly.

The commonest initial complaint, occurring in one-third of patients, is swelling of, or an eruption on, the face. The other areas in which the rash occurs most frequently are the V of the neck, the extensor surfaces of the limbs, the trunk and, characteristically, the extensor aspects of the knuckles, elbows and knees. The buccal mucosa may be affected with ulceration, oedema, redness and crusted erosions.

In the early stages the eruption is an erythema often associated with telangiectasis which gives it a peculiar heliotrope colour. When it affects the face and is accompanied by periorbital oedema, the appearance is diagnostic. The oedema may be brawny, pitting, or merely an increase in the turgor of the skin. As the acute stage recedes the lesions become more scaly with pigmentation, atrophy and telangiectasia. In the later phases alopecia and diffuse calcinosis may occur and the appearances closely resemble those of scleroderma.

Muscular weakness is a constant feature and in the acute stage stiffness and pain are common. These two symptoms depend upon the degree of oedema; it may be sufficiently intense to give the muscles a doughy feel. In some patients pain is agonizing. The muscles most affected are those of the pelvic and shoulder girdles and the neck, but none is constantly spared. With resolution of the acute stage the inflamed muscles waste.

The skin and muscles are independently affected: in some cases the cutaneous manifestations completely overshadow the muscular. When the reverse occurs, the label of polymyositis is more appropriate, but it is doubtful whether any real distinction should be made between dermatomyositis and polymyositis without skin lesions, see Section 16].

Visceral symptoms are uncommon. In a few patients

dysphagia occurs and the oesophagus shows abnormalities similar to those of systemic sclerosis. Electrocardiographic abnormalities may prove the presence of myocarditis. Pulmonary fibrosis is a rare sequel and splenomegaly and lymph node enlargement are occasional findings.

It is justifiable to distinguish between the disease in childhood and that in adults which is described in the preceding paragraphs. In children the typical skin changes are accompanied by anorexia, fatigue and rapidly followed by weakness of the shoulder girdle and pelvic muscles with pain and dysphagia. Widespread ulceration of the alimentary tract is common and haemorrhage from these ulcers a common terminal event. In the chronic stage widespread subcutaneous calcinosis is the rule.

Diagnosis

The picture in the usual case is characteristic, but the distinction has to be made from systemic sclerosis and sometimes from scleroedema adultorum [see Section 14]. In a few cases myasthenia gravis, motor neurone disease, trichiniasis and pellagra require consideration.

The Blood. There is often a mild orthochromic anaemia with a slight neutrophilia. A few instances of marked eosinophilia have been reported. The E.S.R. is much raised in the acute stage. There is usually an increase in the levels of C-reactive protein and α_2-globulin in the serum; a significant rise in the γ-globulin is rare. The serum transaminase figures are raised and give a good indication of the extent and activity of the myositis. The L.E. cell test is rarely positive, but rheumatoid factor can often be demonstrated.

The Urine. Albuminuria is usual in the acute stages. While muscle wasting is in progress there is creatinuria.

Electromyography. The electromyogram shows characteristic alterations with a pseudomyotonic reaction, occasional high frequency discharges and waves of low amplitude and duration on voluntary contraction.

Biopsy. Muscle biopsy may provide conclusive evidence of the diagnosis, but the changes are not entirely specific and may even be absent in the early stages.

Treatment

The first task is to determine whether there is an underlying malignant tumour and to treat it appropriately. Its presence is more likely when the patient is of middle age or over.

In the acute stage the symptoms can be controlled with corticosteroids and their use is almost obligatory although it is uncertain whether they influence the final outcome. They should be given in doses sufficient to suppress the activity of the disease: in an adult 60–80 mg. of prednisolone daily or an equivalent amount of any other corticosteroid preparation will probably be required. When the symptoms are under control the dose should be gradually reduced until the lowest quantity effective is determined. Steroid treatment should be continued until the disease is apparently inactive; transaminase estimations are useful in determining progress. During the phase of acute myositis the use of anabolic agents has been advocated. Their value is uncertain. Methandienone (*Dianabol*), 5–10 mg. daily by mouth, or nandrolone (*Durabolin*), 25 mg. by intramuscular injection weekly, may be given.

Physiotherapy is of great importance. Splintage to rest acutely inflamed muscles and to prevent deformity is invaluable. Directly the acute stage is over more active treatment should be instituted.

Prognosis

Dermatomyositis is a serious disease. At least 50 per cent. of patients die, usually within three years of the onset; 25 per cent. die within one year. The cause of death may be intercurrent infection and the impeded respiratory movement makes the lungs particularly vulnerable. A few die from myocardial disease or renal failure. In children perforation of or haemorrhage from gastro-intestinal ulceration is common.

Removal of an associated neoplasm may be followed by some improvement in the dermatomyositis, but complete recovery does not appear to have been recorded. These patients more often die of their dermatomyositis than of their tumours.

In those who survive considerable disability and muscular wasting, often with diffuse calcinosis, is common.

REFERENCES

BANKER, B. Q., and VICTOR, M. (1966) Dermatomyositis of childhood, *Medicine (Baltimore)*, **45**, 261.

DOWLING, G. B. (1955) Scleroderma and dermatomyositis, *Brit. J. Derm.*, **67**, 275.

EVERETT, M. A., and CURTIS, A. C. (1957) Dermatomyositis. A review of 19 cases in adolescents and children, *Arch. intern. Med.*, **100**, 70.

WILLIAMS, R. C. (1959) Dermatomyositis and malignancy: a review of the literature, *Ann. intern. Med.*, **50**, 1174.

SJØGREN'S SYNDROME

Definition

A disease of unknown cause characterized by keratoconjunctivitis sicca, xerostomia and often associated with rheumatoid arthritis.

Aetiology

Ninety per cent. of the patients are women and the onset is usually at the time of the menopause. There is a close association between this disorder and other collagen diseases. Originally rheumatoid arthritis was regarded as an integral part of the syndrome, but xerostomia and keratoconjunctivitis sicca may occur alone or in association with systemic lupus erythematosus, polyarteritis nodosa, systemic sclerosis or Felty's syndrome.

Auto-antibodies can often be demonstrated. The L.E. cell test is frequently positive; antinuclear and rheumatoid factors may be present in the serum. It has been suggested that the causative mechanism is similar to that of Hashimoto's disease [see Section 5], but this has not yet been established.

Pathology

The lacrimal and salivary glands show a dense

lymphocytic infiltration which in the early stages leads to their enlargement. As the disease progresses the glandular elements atrophy, degenerate and are replaced by fibrous tissue. Gastric mucosal atrophy is common.

Clinical Picture

The complaint is of dryness of the mouth and eyes and sometimes also of the nose, pharynx and vulva. In the early stages the lacrimal and salivary glands may be increased in size, but later they shrink. Alopecia is not unusual.

Associated diseases are common and their symptoms may dominate the picture.

Diagnosis

The diagnosis is from other causes of salivary and lacrimal gland enlargement (Mikulicz's syndrome) of which sarcoidosis, lymphatic leukaemia and lymphosarcoma are the most common. It usually offers little difficulty, but can be established when necessary by biopsy. The association with rheumatoid arthritis often provides the clue.

Treatment

No treatment affects the process significantly. The corticosteroid hormones will sometimes give temporary relief and their use is followed by disappearance of the glandular enlargements.

Closure of the lacrimal punctum and 'artificial tears' of 1 per cent. methyl cellulose help to relieve the ocular symptoms.

Prognosis

Sjørgren's syndrome does not threaten life, although once symptoms appear they persist. The prognosis is that of the associated disease.

REFERENCES

Bunim, J. J. (1961) A broader spectrum of Sjøgren's syndrome and its pathogenetic implications, *Ann. rheum. Dis.*, **20,** 1.

Denko, C. W., and Bergenstal, D. M. (1960) The sicca syndrome (Sjøgren's syndrome), *Arch. intern. Med.*, **105,** 849.

WEBER-CHRISTIAN DISEASE

Synonym. Relapsing febrile nodular non-suppurative panniculitis.

Definition

A disease of unknown cause in which focal inflammatory lesions appear in the panniculus adiposus associated with fever and rarely with evidence of visceral disease.

Aetiology

This is a disease of adults, seen more often in women than in men. There is some doubt whether it should be regarded as a collagen disease, but current opinion favours its inclusion in this group. It has been attributed in the past to hypersensitivity to drugs and to bacterial allergy. It is rarely, if ever, associated with other collagen diseases and there are none of the 'markers' of an auto-immune process.

Pathology

The lesions in the panniculus pass through three stages. First there is focal degeneration and necrosis of the fatty tissue with an aggregation of inflammatory cells; these are replaced by macrophages and at this stage the lesion contains many foam cells; finally the cellular infiltrate disappears and fibrosis follows.

Clinical Picture

The disease is marked by the appearance of nodules, 2 cm. or more in diameter, in the subcutaneous fat, particularly of the arms, thighs, chest wall and buttocks. At first they are rounded and tender, later the skin becomes adherent, reddened and often oedematous. Finally the nodule resolves to leave a saucer-like depression of fat atrophy, often with a faint brown staining of the skin. Nodules may coalesce to form sizable plaques. They tend to occur in crops and in the early stages are accompanied by fever and malaise.

Systemic disease is unusual. Sometimes there is enlargement of the liver and spleen. Occasional cases are recorded in which the heart and abdominal organs have been affected. The lesions have usually been situated in the fatty tissues within the body cavities.

Diagnosis

This disease has to be distinguished from others which lead to the formation of nodules in the panniculus. Thrombophlebitis, sarcoidosis and erythema nodosum may all give rise to confusion.

There are no characteristic changes in the cytology or the chemistry of the blood. Biopsy will usually clinch the diagnosis.

Treatment

There is no specific treatment. Corticosteroids will usually control the acute symptoms, but appear to have no sustained beneficial effect.

Prognosis

Only rarely has this disease proved fatal and then in cases with visceral lesions. Although long remissions occur, relapses are frequent.

REFERENCES

Lever, W. F. (1949) Nodular non-suppurative panniculitis (Weber-Christian disease), *Arch. Derm. Syph.* (*Chic.*), **59,** 31.

Oram, S., and Cochrane, G. M. (1958) Weber-Christian disease with visceral involvement: an example with hepatic enlargement, *Brit. med. J.*, **2,** 281.

BEHÇET'S SYNDROME

Definition

A chronic relapsing disease of unknown cause affecting many systems, but having as its most frequent symptoms recurrent aphthous ulceration of the mouth and genitalia, and uveitis.

Aetiology

Behçet's disease has been reported most frequently in young men from countries bordering on the Eastern Mediterranean, but increasing numbers of cases are being recognized in Japan as well as in the temperate Western countries.

Its cause remains unknown and it is included in this section for convenience and not because it is generally accepted as qualifying as a collagen disease. It was first regarded as an infective process and Behçet believed it to be due to a virus; no supporting evidence for this view exists. More recently the belief that it is an auto-immune disorder has gained ground. Antibodies against oral mucosa were found in 17 of one series of 40 patients, and the response to chlorambucil and steroids might be taken as pointers in this direction. Vasculitis is a basic feature of the lesions, and this is often acknowledged to be of auto-immune origin. A raised serum fibrinogen level has been noted in some patients, together with reduced fibrinolytic activity. These two have been recorded in some 40 per cent. of patients with cutaneous vasculitis.

Pathology

Biopsy studies have been made on numerous occasions. The basic lesion appears to be similar in all tissues and to consist of perivascular cellular collections, consisting principally of lymphocytes and histiocytes. These infiltrates are related particularly to small venules which may show swelling of the endothelium and even thrombosis.

Clinical Picture

The clinical picture is one of great complexity, which does not lend itself to succinct description. It is a disease of great chronicity in which febrile episodes occur at irregular intervals, the course sometimes extending over 15–20 years. During these episodes one or more of the focal features of the disease appear and later resolve. The incidence of the various lesions is difficult to assess because they attract the attention of different specialists.

Buccal Cavity. Recurrent aphthous ulceration of the mouth probably occurs in every case and most authors agree that the diagnosis cannot be upheld in its absence. The lesions start as small nodules—periadenitis mucosa necrotica—and progress to the familiar aphthous type.

Eyes. The ocular lesions are common and serious. Uveitis with hypopyon is said to be the commonest but conjunctivitis, iridocyclitis, choroiditis, optic neuritis and retinal vein thrombosis are all described. They are usually progressive and blindness is the almost inevitable result.

Skin. The classical skin lesion of Behçet's disease is the aphthous type of ulcer on the scrotum or labia. Almost as frequent is a nodular infiltration closely resembling erythema nodosum. It is said to occur in 30 per cent. of cases. Pustules, impetigo, folliculitis, pyoderma and erythema multiforme are all frequent accompaniments.

Joints. An inflammatory type of arthritis, affecting particularly the knees and less often the ankles, hands and wrists, is recognized with increasing frequency as part of the syndrome.

Cardiovascular System. Thrombosis of larger veins occurs commonly. It is usually superficial and focal: it is recorded in more than 25 per cent. of cases. Pericarditis has been noted in a few patients.

Epididymitis. Recurrent epididymitis is a recognized feature. It resolves spontaneously after a few days.

Central Nervous System. Affection of the nervous system occurs in between 10 and 25 per cent. of cases. It has been suggested that it is in some way different from other manifestations of the disease, but this seems unlikely. It is usually episodically progressive and carries a serious prognosis. Some authors recognize three types: a brain stem syndrome progressing to bulbar palsy, a meningomyelitis and an organic confusional state leading to dementia. Almost any region of the central nervous system may be attacked.

Diagnosis

Diagnosis is often difficult and depends upon the presence of the classic triad of iritis with recurrent buccal and genital ulcers. The last two must be regarded as the diagnostic *sine qua non*.

The laboratory is of little help. A neutrophil leucocytosis and a raised erythrocyte sedimentation rate are the rule in the febrile episodes. With neurological lesions a pleocytosis of the cerebrospinal fluid occurs; granular cells and lymphocytes are usually present in equal numbers. The protein content is raised.

A peculiar reactivity of the skin has been reported. An intradermal injection of saline is followed by formation of a papule which progresses to a pustule.

Treatment

In most instances corticosteroids will suppress the acute inflammatory episodes, and prolonged continuous treatment will keep the disease under control. Recent reports have suggested that increasing the fibrinolytic activity of the blood with phenformin and ethyloestranol may lead to improvement. These drugs are prescribed as phenformin hydrochloride (long-acting), 50 mg. twice daily with ethyloestranol, 2 mg. four times daily, both by mouth. Treatment needs to be continued for at least 6 months.

The immunosuppressive cytotoxic drugs have been used widely. Optimistic claims have been made of late for chlorambucil, 0·1–0·2 mg. per kg. body weight by mouth.

Prognosis

Behçet's syndrome runs a prolonged course and may eventually burn itself out after 15–20 years. When the eye is affected, the outlook is poor in respect of sight and most patients eventually become blind. Neurological lesions must be regarded as extremely serious; they usually progress and in a high proportion prove fatal.

REFERENCES

BERLIN, C. (1960) Behçet's disease as a multiple symptom complex, *Arch. Dermatol.*, **82**, 73.

FRANCE, R., BUCHANAN, R. N., WILSON, M. W., and

SHELDON, M. B. Jr. (1951) Relapsing iritis with recurrent ulcers of the mouth and genitalia (Behçet's syndrome), *Medicine* (*Baltimore*), **30,** 335.
MASON, R. M., and BARNES, C. G. (1969) Behçet's syndrome with arthritis, *Ann. rheum. Dis.*, **28,** 95.
PALLIS, C. A., and FUDGE, B. J. (1956) The neurological complications of Behçet's syndrome, *Arch. Neurol.*, **75, 1.**
WOLF, S. M., SCHOTLAND, D. L., and PHILLIPS, L. L. (1965) Involvement of nervous system in Behçet's syndrome, *A.M.A. Arch. Neurol.*, **12,** 315.

OTHER COLLAGEN DISEASES

A number of other diseases which are generally regarded as falling into the group of collagen disorders are considered elsewhere in this book. They are thrombotic thrombocytopenic purpura [see Section 13]; scleroedema adultorum [see Section 14]; and pulseless disease (Takayasu's arteriopathy) [see Section 8].

R. BODLEY SCOTT

GENERAL ASPECTS OF NEOPLASTIC DISEASE

THE NATURE OF NEOPLASIA

Neoplasia is a disorder of growing cells, usually irreversible and progressive, that does not arise in response to a functional need, and proceeds from its inception independently of the physiological mechanisms that regulate the growth and function of the tissue in which it arises.

Features of Neoplastic Growth

The property of neoplastic growth resides in the affected cells, as can be shown by the experimental transmission of malignant tumours by the transference of single cells to other animals, and by the phenomenon of metastasis whereby identical colonies of tumours are established in distant organs and tissues by the detachment of single cells or clumps of cells from the primary tumour. The property of neoplastic growth is thus heritable, and it is also stable, since it is perpetuated in the descendants of the primary tumour as long as the host survives, and in the case of successive transplants or tissue cultures of experimental tumours, for long after the death of the original host.

Benign and Malignant Neoplasms

Neoplastic growth differs from normal growth in respect of many structural and functional deviations, but it is not possible to select any one feature that is peculiar to all forms of neoplastic growth and is never associated with normal growth. Neoplasms show a wide range of structural and behavioural diversity, and structural disorderliness is often but not necessarily accompanied by disorderly behaviour. The least disorderly neoplasms, exemplified by the simple lipoma, and mammary fibro-adenoma are usually *benign* in their effects on the host. Structurally they are tumours composed of uniform cells more or less closely resembling the cells of their tissue of origin, and often organized into structural assemblies such as bundles, sheets, acini, tubules, or papillary formations more or less characteristic of those tissues. Such tumours usually grow slowly, acquire a vascular supporting stroma from the neighbouring tissue, they push aside and may compress the surrounding structures but do not damage them, and they remain confined to the site of origin.

In contrast, the most disorderly neoplasms are usually *malignant* in their effects on the host. They are composed of cells that vary greatly in size and shape and in their cytological details, and their histological organization is so imperfect as to be scarcely recognizable. Nevertheless, many malignant neoplasms have a highly organized structure closely resembling that of their tissue of origin and the behaviour of a tumour cannot always be predicted from its histological features. Unlike benign neoplasms, the capacity of malignant growths to organize a vascular stroma is often poorly developed and large parts of the tumours become necrotic.

The special feature of malignant tumours that dominates their behaviour and leads to the death of the host, is their relationship with the neighbouring tissues. The cells invade, infiltrate and destroy neighbouring tissues, disrupt the walls of lymphatics and veins, enter these vessels, and are carried to lymph nodes, and in the blood stream to distant tissues where secondary deposits grow.

Characteristics of Neoplastic Tissues

The basic defect in neoplastic growth remains unknown, if indeed there is a single defect common to all neoplasms. The older hypotheses on the nature of neoplastic change were based on observations on the most extreme examples of malignant growth. Thus excessive growth rate was thought to be a special characteristic of malignant growth. But the growth rate of malignant tissues is now known to be as variable as that of normal tissues, and is often lower than that of the tissue of origin.

Neoplasia is often associated with disturbed differentiation, but malignant growth is compatible with a high degree of differentiation and structural and functional maturation. Well-differentiated but metastasizing thyroid carcinoma may resemble normal thyroid tissue, and it manufactures normal thyroglobulin. Complex proteins such as haemoglobin, the immunoglobulins, insulin, and keratin are produced by the tumour cells in erythraemic myelosis, myelomatosis, pancreatic islet-cell tumours, and keratinizing squamous-cell carcinomas. Thus disturbances of differentiation and maturation alone cannot account for the phenomena of neoplasia.

The breakdown of homeostatic regulation has also been invoked to explain the disorderly character of neoplastic growth. In a sense this view is tautologous, being implied in the definition of neoplasia. However, cell and tissue growth are regulated by numerous extrinsic mechanisms many, perhaps most of which, are likely to be implicated in both neoplastic and normal growth. *Conditional neoplasms* are characterized by exacting environmental requirements without which they cannot grow at all. Nevertheless, in the absence of the necessary conditions, the neoplastic cells survive in a dormant state until these conditions are restored, when active growth is resumed. In man the best examples of conditional neoplasms are the hormone-dependent carcinomata of mammary, prostatic and endometrial origin, the growth of which is heavily influenced by changes in the hormonal environment (see below). Thus the basic defect of neoplasia, though expressed by the manner in which neoplastic cells grow, does not reside either in the phenomenon of growth itself, in the capacity for structural and functional differentiation and maturation, or in many of the regulating mechanisms that control growth.

Changes in the hormonal environment represent a class of growth-regulating mechanisms acting at long range, but cell growth is also under the control of locally operating mechanisms disturbances of which may prove to be more important as factors in neoplastic growth. Thus, in the case of skin, the growth rate, thickness, degree of keratinization, pigmentation and development of the appendages, though site specific and genetically determined, are under the long-range control of hormonal influences that become operative at puberty, and differ in the sexes. But the operation of local factors is shown by the formation of callus at sites subjected to unaccustomed wear and tear. The regulating factor is thought to be a feed-back control of the rate of mitosis in the basal layer of the epidermis determined by the rate of loss of surface squames, and a humoral factor, the epidermal chalone, is thought to mediate the transfer of information from the squamous layer to the basal layer. The role of chalones in the local growth regulation of skin and other tissues is the subject of much investigation and it is perhaps premature to speculate on their importance in neoplastic growth.

In the case of some benign tumours it is possible that the local growth-regulating mechanisms are normal. For example, the lipoma is a benign tumour the tissue of which is structurally indistinguishable from adipose tissue, but it often increases in size in wasting subjects. The local control of fat-cell proliferation appears to be determined by fat storage. This control might be retained in the lipoma, and the disturbance might reside primarily in lipid metabolism which is directed towards storage, and not to breakdown as in the normal depot fat in a wasting subject. Minimal disturbances in the enzyme system regulating the synthesis of neutral fat have been found in lipomata and could alone account for their growth. Similar minor abnormalities in enzyme systems are the only defects known in some well-differentiated benign experimental hepatomas, aptly named 'minimal-deviation' tumours.

Characteristics of Neoplastic Cells

Like neoplastic tissues, the cells composing them may be characterized by many abnormal features, but a neoplastic cell cannot be defined by any constant feature not present in at least some normal cells. Neoplastic cells have been examined by physical, chemical, histological, cytological, cytochemical, biochemical, cytogenetic and immunological methods. They have been examined in the living state by light microscopy, phase contrast and interference microscopy, by their growth characteristics in tissue culture, and after transplantation into other tissue and organs of the host animal, and those of syngeneic, allogeneic, and xenogeneic hosts. They have been studied by electron microscopy in ultrathin sections, and by surface scanning. The surface membranes of malignant cells have been much studied by a variety of methods in the hope that light would be thrown on the nature of metastasis.

A largely unresolved requirement in the examination of malignant cells by any method is the selection of suitable normal cells for comparison. Thus, in myeloblastic leukaemia, whatever the nature of the investigation, leukaemic blast cells should be compared with normal myeloblasts, but methods for separating these in sufficient numbers from normal bone marrow are only now being developed. In lymphoblastic leukaemia, the normal counterpart of the undifferentiated blast cell is unknown, and the customary use of normal marrow or normal small lymphocytes for comparison is not valid. The same objection applies to much quantitative work on neoplasms arising in other tissues.

A common feature of neoplastic cells examined by every known method is their tendency to acquire increasingly abnormal characteristics as the disease advances. These abnormalities appear to reflect the progressive disorganization of growth during the life history of the tumour, and none can be cited as a constant feature of neoplastic cells.

Cytogenetic studies in particular have been valuable in defining the mechanism underlying the tendency to increasing disorganization in the life history of malignant tumours. Recognizable chromosomal abnormalities are found in only a minority of human and experimental tumours, but when present they often provide information on the behaviour of the cells as members of the tumour population. Thus an abnormal chromosome may serve as a *marker*. It may be present in all the cells examined or in only a few. In the former case, serial examinations during the life of the tumour may show an unchanging pattern, indicating that all the cells in the tumour population are genetically similar and constitute a stable *clone*. In the latter case serial examinations may show an increase in the proportion of cells bearing the marker chromosome suggesting that these cells were the descendants of a single cell that had undergone a genetic change that was stable, and conferred a growth advantage on the cell line bearing it, and would eventually lead to the replacement of the remaining cells by the new clone. Some tumours show multiple karyotypic abnormalities; serial examinations show many of them to be inconstant and variable, and the emergence of stable dominant clones is not a regular finding. Nevertheless, cytogenetic studies indicate that tumour cells tend to be genetically unstable and that within the tumour-cell population there is constant competition for survival with selection favouring the perpetuation of stable clones which confer some property enabling them to survive at the expense of their competitors.

In man, karyotypic variability with the emergence of more or less stable clones, themselves subject to further variation and selection, has been demonstrated in mammary and uterine cervical carcinoma, and in testicular neoplasms, but only one human neoplasm, chronic myeloid leukaemia, is known to be constantly associated with a highly characteristic and perhaps specific marker chromosome. In the course of this disease also, the progressive enhancement of its malignant character is sometimes associated with the appearance of cell lines bearing additional chromosomal abnormalities, some of which are sufficiently stable to be perpetuated as clones. These additional abnormalities are not entirely random deviations. Certain configurations have been observed in many patients, suggesting that some parts of the genetic material are inherently unstable. The significance of genetic change in carcinogenesis is discussed further below.

Immunological Properties of Tumours

There is much current interest in the immunological properties of tumour cells. Several experimental tumours and a few human tumours possess antigenic determinants that are specific for the tumours and distinct from any of the known antigens of the adult host tissues. Before the recognition of tumour-specific antigens, the immunological aspects of tumour growth had been neglected for many years. The discovery of the histocompatibility antigens showed that most of the earlier studies purporting to have demonstrated immunological reactivity against tumours had in fact demonstrated only reactivity against foreign tissue. As in the case of cytogenetic abnormalities, it is not yet clear whether the presence of tumour specific antigens is a basic property of all neoplasms or a secondary phenomenon prominent in a few. There is evidence that some tumour-specific antigens cross-react with, and are perhaps identical with, antigens present in foetal tissues, and their presence in tumours may result from the reactivation of parts of the total genome that normally function only in the embryo and foetus. According to one view, an immunological defect is fundamental to the nature of neoplastic growth. During embryological development and throughout life every cell in the body is, according to this view, under immunological 'surveillance', perhaps by repeated physical contact with lymphocytes which recognize cells bearing an abnormal antigenic structure and destroy them. If an antigenically abnormal cell escapes surveillance, it may proliferate as a 'forbidden' clone and initiate a neoplasm.

Whether or not tumour-specific neoantigens confer the property of neoplastic growth on cells bearing them, it seems probable that immunological surveillance plays a part in controlling the growth of tumours once initiated. Patients bearing transplanted kidneys have a higher than expected risk of developing malignant lymphomas, and malignant neoplasms transferred from kidney grafts taken from affected donors. The increased risk is thought to be due to the continuous immunosuppressive therapy administered to the recipients to weaken or abolish the immunological reaction against the foreign kidney. A higher than expected incidence of spontaneous neoplasms has not, however, been reported in mice receiving repeated injections of antilymphocytic serum from the time of birth.

Current investigations of the immunological reactivity of patients suffering from many forms of malignant disease have not shown a consistent immunological defect.

THE CAUSATION OF NEOPLASTIC DISEASE

Knowledge of the factors that predispose to neoplastic growth has been won from clinical, pathological, epidemiological and experimental observations, but it is not known whether all the known predisposing factors convert normal cells to malignant cells through a single common mechanism. Of practical importance is the recognition that exposure to specific carcinogens is responsible for several forms of occupational and industrial cancer, and evidence is accumulating suggesting that many forms of cancer in man result from exposure to carcinogenic influences in the environment. Ionizing radiations, including ultra-violet light, and many naturally occurring and synthetic chemicals are carcinogenic for man. In animals, many forms of malignant disease are caused by viruses; so far no form of human malignant disease is yet known to be caused by a virus, but circumstantial evidence suggests that some may be.

Industrial cancer may be regarded as a special case of environmental cancer in which a defined population is exposed to identifiable carcinogenic factors in special circumstances over ascertainable periods of time. Industrial carcinogens are chemical or radioactive substances, and in a few cases, the conditions of exposure to non-industrial environmental carcinogens in closely studied populations have left no doubt of a direct relation between the supposed carcinogens and the malignant diseases recorded.

Well-known occupational and industrial carcinogens and the diseases caused by them are the following:

1. Scrotal cancer of chimney sweeps exposed to soot: the first occupational cancer, recognized and described by Percivall Pott in 1774; scrotal cancer of workers exposed to shale oils containing carcinogenic hydrocarbons; pitch warts and epidermoid cancers of the skin of workers handling pitch.
2. Lung cancer from exposure to radioactive minerals in the mines of Joachimstal, Schneeberg and others; asbestos-workers' lung cancer.
3. Epidermoid cancers of the skin of the hands in pioneer radiologists and surgeons unaware of the danger of uncontrolled exposure to ionizing radiation; epidermoid cancer of the skin of the face and hands of fisherman exposed to sunlight.
4. Bone sarcomata in watch-dial painters who pointed their brushes charged with radioactive luminous paint by licking them.
5. Transitional-cell carcinoma of the urothelial tract (renal pelvis, ureter, bladder, and urethra) in workers in the aniline-dye, chemical, rubber, cable, and other industries and occupations involving exposure to α- and β-naphthylamine.

6. Malignant mesothelioma of the pleura in miners exposed to asbestos-rich minerals.

7. Erythroleukaemia and other myeloproliferative diseases in workers exposed to benzene fumes.

8. Epidermoid cancer of the skin in workers exposed to arsenic.

The intensity of exposure to carcinogens in the occupational circumstances mentioned leads to an incidence of cancer so high that the relationship between the exposure and the ensuing disease is accepted as causal. In other circumstances in which the incidence of a particular neoplasm is only slightly higher than is found in the general population, the operation of a carcinogen of low potency may be suspected but is difficult to establish. Thus, the incidence of nasopharyngeal cancer and of Hodgkin's disease has been reported to be increasing in indoor woodworkers exposed to sawdust.

Environmental Carcinogens

It is more difficult still to detect carcinogens in the general environment where the level of exposure and therefore the incidence of malignant disease suspected to be caused by them are likely to be extremely low, while the number of potential agents is very large indeed. Statistical analysis was required to establish a raised incidence of leukaemia in patients suffering from ankylosing spondylitis who received therapeutic irradiation to the spine, and in the populations of Nagasaki and Hiroshima who were exposed to the radioactive fall-out following the detonation of atomic bombs in 1945. In both circumstances the maximal incidence of leukaemia was recorded between 5 and 10 years of the exposure, and in both the incidence could be related to the intensity of exposure. In the populations exposed to the atomic bombs the incidence of mammary cancer was increasing between 20 and 25 years after exposure. Detailed statistical analysis was also required to show that about 5 per cent. of all cases of malignant disease, including leukaemia, in children below age 10 is attributable to radiation received *in utero* in connexion with diagnostic radiological procedures.

In the situations quoted there was good reason for suspecting radiation as a carcinogen, and the investigations were deliberately planned to test the hypothesis. It is much more difficult to detect an environmental carcinogen when its presence is suspected because of a rising incidence of one form of cancer in a population, or a notably high incidence in a geographical region, in a racial, ethnic, social or other definable group. In some cases certain associations are well established but the nature of the carcinogenic factor remains elusive. Thus oat-cell, undifferentiated, and squamous-cell carcinoma of the lung but not adenocarcinoma, are strongly associated with cigarette smoking, and there is evidently a weaker association between cigarette smoking and carcinoma of the larynx and carcinoma of the bladder; the incidence of breast cancer is higher in nulliparae than in multiparae, and lower in mothers who breast-feed their babies; the highest incidence of cancer of the uterine cervix is found in prostitutes, and the lowest incidence in nuns; the association in this disease is with an early age of first sexual intercourse, and with promiscuity; carcinoma of the penis is excessively rare in males circumcised in early infancy, and more common in the uncircumcised than in males circumcised in late childhood; epidermoid cancer of the buccal cavity is associated with betel-nut chewing, and cancer of the lip was formerly associated with the smoking of short clay pipes. A specific carcinogen has not been identified in any of the cases cited.

Tests of Carcinogenicity

Ionizing radiation, the carcinogenic hydrocarbons, and the naphthylamines are carcinogenic for small laboratory animals, as well as for man, and it would appear logical to use these animals to test suspected substances for carcinogenicity. The use of Butter Yellow, at one time added to margarine as a colouring agent was prohibited when it was found to cause liver cancer in laboratory rodents. Since then many governments have introduced legislation whereby all types of food additives, whether intended as colouring agents, flavouring agents, or preservatives, must be submitted to tests of carcinogenicity, and some governments require similar tests for pharmaceutical products, cosmetics, and chemicals used in industry and agriculture.

The interpretation of the results of carcinogenicity tests is fraught with difficulty. Different animal species vary greatly in their susceptibility to carcinogens, and in any one species the effect of a given agent varies according to the dose, frequency, and route of administration, and the sex and age of the animals. A compound may be carcinogenic for one species only because it is metabolized in a unique manner, one of the products being the active carcinogen. Arsenic is an established carcinogen for man but not for any laboratory animal. Negative results are sometimes obtained when known carcinogens are administered to specific-pathogen-free animals. In some cases supposed 'carcinogens' are thought to activate latent oncogenic viruses. In others carcinogenicity can be demonstrated only when the test substance is administered by a non-physiological route in massive doses for long periods. The significance of such results is very uncertain in assessing the possible hazards to man.

Known and Suspected Environmental Carcinogens

Chemical Carcinogens. In spite of the difficulties, several groups of substances likely to be widespread in the environment, if only sporadically and in minute amounts, are accepted as powerful carcinogens likely to be responsible for much human malignant disease. Sporadic cancer of the bladder is as likely as industrial bladder cancer to be caused by carcinogens in the urine, and trace amounts of aromatic amines are being sought in cigarette smoke, pharmaceutical dyes, drinking water derived from polluted rivers, food additives and plastic food containers. Carcinogens might also arise from the metabolic breakdown of tryptophan.

Cancer of the oesophagus and gastro-intestinal tract may be produced in laboratory animals by the continuous feeding of a diet contaminated with trace amounts of aflatoxins, which are substances liberated by several species of saprophytic Aspergillus. Aflatoxins are amongst the most powerful carcinogens known, and they can occur whenever the appropriate moulds grow on many foodstuffs during harvesting, storage or transport. They have not yet been proved to cause oesophageal or gastro-intestinal cancer in man but are under suspicion.

The nitrosamines are causing increasing concern as potential carcinogens. In experimental conditions they are the most potent of all carcinogens and are active at high dilution and with very short periods of exposure. Some nitrosamines are produced by fungi, others have been found in edible fruits in the Transkei where there is a high incidence of oesophageal and liver cancer.

Nitrosamines are produced when amines react with nitrites and with nitrates under reducing conditions, and are synthesized by many bacteria. It is possible that they might be formed in the stomach from nitrogen in food, or in the bowel by bacterial synthesis.

Arsenic has been mentioned as a known carcinogen for man, and chromium and nickel have been under suspicion. Several metallic compounds are carcinogenic in animals. An iron-dextran complex commonly used for the treatment of iron deficiency by intramuscular injection was withdrawn for some years because it was found to induce sarcomata in rats and later in several other species of laboratory animals, when injected in massive doses.

The carcinogenic status of natural hormones and of synthetic compounds with hormonal activity is uncertain. In some circumstances carcinogenesis is strongly influenced by the hormonal environment, and the administration of hormones for long periods may increase the likelihood of malignant disease by disturbing the endocrine balance without being primary carcinogens. Hormones are used medicinally, as contraceptives, in cosmetics, and in food derived from animals that have received them as growth promoters.

The incidence of thyroid carcinoma is increased five-fold in goitrous populations, and goitrogenic agents must therefore be considered as potential if indirect carcinogens. Some have induced thyroid tumours in animals. Many commonly used nuts and vegetables are thought to decrease the absorption of iodide, and certain pesticides and the antithyroid drugs block the uptake of iodide by the thyroid, or its incorporation into organic iodine-containing compounds.

The prevailing opinion is that most of the common malignant neoplasms in man are induced by chemical carcinogens in the environment, or produced within the body by bacterial or cellular metabolism. If this opinion is confirmed, much cancer may prove to be preventable.

Oncogenic Viruses

Many neoplasms in laboratory animals and wild animals are of viral origin, and an increasing number of animal neoplasms are suspected to be of viral origin. No human neoplasm is yet known to be caused by a virus, but there is circumstantial evidence that some tumours will prove so to be. Even in the animal tumours of viral origin, the relationship between the presence of an oncogenic virus and the initiation and subsequent growth of the neoplasm is highly complex, and much influenced by endocrine and immunological factors. Wild mice carrying the polyoma virus are tolerant to it and do not develop tumours. In laboratory conditions the polyoma virus will induce multiple neoplasms in different tissues. The leukaemogenic properties of the Gross leukaemia virus could be demonstrated only when inoculated into newborn mice belonging to a strain not carrying it. Gross leukaemia also illustrates the importance of the target organ; mice heavily infected with the virus do not develop leukaemia if the thymus is removed soon after birth, but leukaemia develops if the animals are provided with a thymus from a normal animal. Some radiation-induced murine leukaemias are now known to be of viral origin. The virus is tolerated in the intact animal, but when the thymic lymphoid tissue regenerates rapidly after having been depleted by radiation, the thymic cells become susceptible to infection and become leukaemic. Similarly, the mouse mammary carcinoma virus is not oncogenic unless the mammary gland is activated by the appropriate hormonal environment.

Oncogenic viruses are not a specific taxonomic group. Some, like the leukaemogenic viruses, are RNA viruses, others like the polyoma virus are DNA viruses composed of a central core of DNA, a protein coat, and some have also outer envelopes of host-cell membrane ('complex viruses').

The latter include the herpes viruses that are becoming increasingly suspect as potential oncogenic agents. They are known to be causal agents in several naturally occurring animal tumours including the Lucké renal carcinoma of the leopard frog, Marek's disease of chickens, as well as in the malignant lymphomas in owl monkeys and marmosets experimentally induced by the Saimiri herpes virus of squirrel monkeys.

A herpes-like virus (EBV) was isolated from cultures of Burkitt's lymphoma by Epstein and Barr, but has not been isolated from tumours obtained directly from the patients. However, all patients have been found to contain antibodies against EBV in their sera. Antibodies are present in the sera of a high proportion of normal adults, and the proportion of positive reactors increases during childhood and adolescence, but the antibody titres are not as high as those of 'Burkitt' sera except in persons who have recently had infectious mononucleosis (IM), a disease known to occur only in persons whose sera do not contain anti-EBV antibodies. The highest titres are found in the sera of patients whose Burkitt lymphoma has been successfully treated by chemotherapy. The sera of patients with Burkitt's lymphoma also react with suspensions of Burkitt's lymphoma cells, and the reaction is thought to indicate the presence of specific neoantigens on the cell surface. Apparently identical neoantigens are present in cultured lymphocytes from patients suffering from IM.

The relationship between EBV, Burkitt's lymphoma and IM is unknown, but it is suggested that infection with EBV is common in man and usually tolerated, that a minority who escape infection and reach adolescence without acquiring antibodies are likely to succumb to IM when they are infected, and that a much smaller minority, predisposed by unknown factors, possibly holoendemic malaria in tropical Africa and New Guinea, react by developing Burkitt's lymphoma.

Though speculative, this hypothesis is consistent with what is known of the circumstances in which viruses induce neoplasms in animals. The only other condition in which the serum consistently contains high-titre anti-EBV antibodies is the nasopharyngeal carcinoma found in East Africa and China. Here again, the possibility of a single virus causing more than one type of neoplasm is consistent with the facts of animal oncology.

Carcinoma of the uterine cervix has a greatly differing incidence in different social groups. The strong association with sexual activity and with promiscuity have raised the suspicion of a transmissible aetiology. Herpes virus hominis type II has been removed from the genital tract of a higher proportion of patients than control subjects, but the significance of the finding is not yet clear.

Action of Carcinogenic Agents

Somatic Mutation Hypothesis. The mechanism or mechanisms underlying the change from normal to neoplastic growth brought about by ionizing radiation, chemical carcinogens and oncogenic viruses are unknown, but the change affecting the normal cell, once established, is transmitted through successive generations as long as the tumour survives, and it remains stable even though it renders the economy of the cell unstable and susceptible to profound disturbances affecting its growth and function. Evidence already discussed suggests that some neoplasms behave as a clone and are descended from a single transformed cell. The transformation of a single cell leading to a stable heritable change has been attributed to a mutation affecting the genetic material. In support of this somatic mutation hypothesis was the fact that most of the chemical carcinogens and ionizing radiations are mutagenic. However, genetic 'point' mutations in the classical sense, affecting the DNA of the germ cells at a single gene locus, are excessively rare events and can be demonstrated only in organisms that reproduce rapidly and can be bred in enormous numbers. Most tests for mutagenicity are performed in bacteria, fungi, or species of fruit fly (*Drosophila*) whereas tests for carcinogenicity are performed in mammals. Somatic mutation in its original sense of minimal random change in the DNA may account for some clonal neoplasms but there are too many inconsistencies for it to be accepted as a general hypothesis of neoplastic change. It cannot account for the many neoplasms that develop at multiple sites in a tissue that is already abnormal. Examples are the epidermoid carcinomas arising in skin damaged by long exposure to sunlight, or to contact with carcinogenic hydrocarbons, the neoplastic lesions of mycosis fungoides developing after many years in abnormal skin, the multiple adenocarcinomata arising in the lesions of polyposis coli and adenomatous polyps, several types of carcinoma-in-situ arising in the mammary ducts, the uterine cervix, the skin, the urothelium, the multifocal lymphomas and plasmacytomas arising in the epithelium of the upper respiratory tract, and Burkitt's lymphoma.

In most of the examples cited the neoplastic change appears to be the last of several steps in the progressive alterations taking place over an extensive area of tissue.

The somatic mutation hypothesis was valuable as long as it was thought that stable and heritable alterations in cells could be transmitted only through alterations in the DNA itself. However, all the phenomena of embryonic development, tissue differentiation, cell differentiation and maturation involve the transmission of stable heritage changes without any genetic change in the DNA.

Normal growth, from the first division of the zygote, is a precisely regulated process, subject to locally and distantly operating controlling influences. Each tissue passes through four critical stages in its life history, undifferentiated growth, differentiation, maturation, and functional activity. Some adult tissues, especially nervous tissue and muscle, lose their capacity to replace dead cells by cell division; others, like skin and mucous membranes, the gastro-intestinal tract, the bone marrow, and the lymphoreticular system, retain throughout life, a flexible mechanism for continuous cell renewal from a pool of non-functional stem cells. The parenchymal cells of the kidney and the salivary glands have a limited capacity for cell renewal to replace loss, and those of the liver have a considerable regenerative capacity. None of these tissues is replenished from a pool of non-functional stem cells.

The coding device for all the developmental steps and functional activities described in every tissue resides ultimately in the deoxyribonucleic acid (DNA) code which is represented in its entirety in the nucleus of every cell of the body, and is called the *total genome*. However, only a small fraction of the total genome is utilized in adult cells. Thus the erythroblast nucleus contains the codes for synthesizing mucin, keratin, and pepsin, but erythroblasts synthesize haemoglobin but not the other proteins. That part of the total genome utilized in the life of a functional cell is called the *effective genome*, and the adult cells of each specific tissue utilize effective genomes specific for that tissue. Proliferating tissues with the stem-cell type of renewal mechanism possess a greater range of developmental possibilities than those of parenchymal tissues. Thus a haemopoietic stem cell may develop into a megakaryoblast, or a myeloblast, and in some species into a lymphoblast, but not into a mucin-secreting cell. It is a differentiated cell in so far as its developmental potentiality is restricted to three or four lines of blood cells; the restriction arises in embryonic development, and once established is stable, permanent and heritable. The haemopoietic stem cell has a choice of utilizing one of four effective genomes which results in its further development exclusively on one of four lines. The choice appears to be determined by outside influences, of which the hormone erythropoietin is the best characterized and channels development to erythropoiesis. The haemopoietic stem cell thus has a *facultative genome* from which one of four effective genomes may be selected. Tissue metaplasia results from the selection of part of the facultative genome not ordinarily utilized. In tissue culture, basal epidermal cells that normally give rise by division to cells that synthesize keratin will give rise to mucin-secreting cells when exposed to high concentrations of vitamin A, but again produce keratinizing cells when the medium is replaced by the original culture medium. In this case an environmental factor determines the selection of one of two alternative effective genomes.

Thus the phenomena of cell growth, differentiation, and maturation may be described in terms of an orderly sequence of differential utilization of the total genome. At each step the selected portion of the genome that will be actively or potentially utilized is stabilized and transmitted to successive generations. The epigenetic mechanisms responsible for this sequence are unknown, but their elucidation is the crucial problem of developmental biology. The two main hypotheses are, first, that the genome is inert until activated by an epigenetic influence, and second, that the genome is actively masked and that the selection of a portion of it for activity depends on a process of unmasking.

Functional cells utilize their effective genome by transcribing the information coded in its DNA on to messenger ribonucleic acid (mRNA) which is the template on which the translation of the code into protein takes place on the ribosomes in the cytoplasm. The process of translation involves the assembly of amino acids into polypeptide chains in the order determined by the sequence of base triplets on the RNA template; each triplet codes for one amino acid which is transported to the appropriate site and placed in position by a specific transfer RNA. Whether a particular polypeptide is synthesized at all, and if so, the rate of synthesis and the cessation of synthesis, are regulated in bacteria by a system of feedback control involving some end product related to the activity of the protein concerned, and a system of regulating genes in close proximity to the DNA responsible for the synthesis of the protein. A similar control mechanism is postulated, though not established, for mammalian cells.

The replacement of cells in self-renewing systems is precisely adjusted to physiological need, and the capacity for renewal is flexible. In response to massive haemorrhage, or haemolysis, erythropoiesis proceeds six times faster than normal, and at high altitudes erythropoiesis is permanently, though reversibly, adjusted to maintain a high red cell count. When the subject returns to low altitudes the red cell count reverts to normal. All proliferating tissues are subject to similar control and it is possible that normal cells divide only in response to a specific stimulus.

The processes described suggest that the initiation of neoplastic change could arise by a mechanism not directly involving the DNA, but nevertheless conferring the required properties of stability and heritability on the cells. Such a mechanism would account for several phenomena not explained by the classical hypothesis of somatic mutation, particularly the multiple neoplasms and carcinoma-in-situ arising in a large field of tissue, and the multiple neoplasms in different tissues that can be induced by some chemical carcinogens and some oncogenic viruses. One basic difference between chemical and viral carcinogenesis supports the view that the neoplastic change may be initiated at different sites within the cells. This is the finding that the neoantigens in chemically induced tumours differ from one another even when several tumours of the same histological type are induced in the same animal by a single carcinogen, whereas, in viral carcinogenesis, the same neoantigen appears in all the tumours induced by a particular virus in more than one species of animal. This finding is in accord with evidence from other sources that parts of the viral genome become incorporated in the genome of the host cell and take over part of the direction of its activities. The transformation effected would appear to be specific, and far removed from the random event required by the somatic mutation hypothesis.

The increased incidence of neoplastic disease in many inherited disorders does not necessarily implicate an abnormality of the DNA as the final cause of the neoplastic change, and several different mechanisms seem to be involved in different diseases. Examples are as follows:

1. Xeroderma pigmentosum is a hereditary disorder, transmitted as an autosomal recessive, in which the skin is one of several tissues affected. The skin is abnormally sensitive to light, and progressive hyperplastic changes with multicentric basal-cell and squamous-cell carcinomata and less often malignant melanoma occur. The malignant change is clearly a secondary phenomenon and identical to that found in normal skin exposed to a more intense carcinogenic stimulus. The same applies to another multisystem hereditary disorder inherited as an autosomal recessive, epidermodysplasia verruciformis. Warty lesions appear in childhood, become increasingly numerous and several types of epidermoid carcinoma develop, including intra-epidermal carcinoma-in-situ (Bowen's disease), basal-cell and squamous-cell carcinoma. Wart virus, though widespread in the warty skin lesions cannot be demonstrated in the cells of the malignant lesions. This is reminiscent of the Shope papilloma-virus lesions in rabbits in which the virus can be recovered from the warty lesions but not from the malignant epidermoid carcinomata that develop from them.

2. Polyposis coli is inherited as an autosomal dominant, and there is a high risk of malignant change developing in affected persons, though the malignant change occurs in only a small proportion of the numerous polyps. Chromosomal abnormalities that vary from case to case have been described and are considered to be secondary. The nature of the risk is unknown.

3. Several hereditary conditions with cytogenetic abnormalities carry an increased risk of leukaemia, but the risk is far less than in the diseases just described. In Down's syndrome and D-trisomy one member of a particular pair of chromosomes is duplicated, but in Fanconi's syndrome the chromosome abnormalities are inconstant and variable.

4. Several hereditary immunological deficiency syndromes carry a high risk of malignant lymphoma. The Wiskott-Aldrich syndrome is inherited as an X-linked recessive, and is characterized by thrombocytopenia and eczema as well as by gross immunological deficiency. The ataxia-telangiectasia syndrome (Louis-Bar) is inherited as an autosomal recessive, and other similarly inherited cases, less well characterized, are associated with amyloidosis. It is not known whether the increased risk of neoplasia in these conditions is related to the genetic disturbance, or to the immunological defects

caused by them. The incidence of malignant disease is higher than in the inherited conditions not associated with immunological deficiency.

5. Nephroblastoma (Wilms' tumour). This is an embryonal tumour with a high incidence in children with multiple congenital anomalies, including cases of hemihypertrophy, aniridia, and hypospadias. Chromosomal defects have been described.

6. Retinoblastoma is an embryonal tumour with a high risk of developing in both eyes. There is a strong familial tendency, with a high incidence in the sibs of affected children.

We may summarize by saying that the aetiology of neoplastic growth remains unknown, that a single final cause is unlikely, that known carcinogenic factors include ionizing radiations, chemical carcinogens, and viruses (not yet established for man) and that predisposing factors include immunological, genetic, developmental and endocrine disturbances. It is probable that chemical carcinogens are responsible for the majority of the common malignant diseases of the respiratory, gastro-intestinal and urinary tracts.

METABOLIC EFFECTS OF NEOPLASMS

Most of the harmful effects of malignant tumours are caused by their local effects on neighbouring structures. They are locally destructive to the tissues they invade, and although they advance along paths offering the least resistance, they infiltrate and destroy the walls of lymphatics, capillaries, venules, veins, arterioles or larger arteries, nerve sheaths, and bone; they invade, encircle, and obstruct the tubular structures of the respiratory, gastro-intestinal, and genito-urinary tracts and their associated glands and ducts, and they ulcerate mucous membranes and skin, while their plaque-like deposits on serous membranes exude fluid, often in large quantities.

The clinical consequences of these local effects are essentially fortuitous and depend on the anatomical position of the tumour. At certain sites, tumours or their metastases may produce profound systemic disturbances as a result of the damage they cause to vital tissues or organs. The symptoms resulting from this damage may be the first of which the patient has complained, and may not at first raise a suspicion of underlying malignant disease. In some instances the diagnosis is easily made from the history and physical examination, while in others sophisticated investigations may fail to reveal the underlying cause. Examples are the following:

1. *Uraemia* resulting from bilateral ureteric obstruction due to a pelvic tumour. Pelvic examination will usually suffice to detect its presence.

2. *Partial or complete bone marrow failure* resulting from widespread skeletal deposits of metastatic carcinoma (usually secondary to mammary, prostatic bronchial, renal, or thyroid carcinoma, malignant melanoma, or neuroblastoma). The patients may have had a primary tumour excised years before, or the primary tumour may remain small and undetected at the time of presentation. The presentation is with anaemia, neutropenia or thrombocytopenia in varying combinations. Myelomatosis may also present in this way, the patient having at no time experienced bone pain. The finding of leucoerythroblastic anaemia suggests a diagnosis of secondary carcinoma, melanoma, or neuroblastoma, and rouleaux formation and background protein in the blood films suggest a diagnosis of myelomatosis, in which leucoerythroblastic anaemia is less common. Occasionally the earliest abnormal finding in the peripheral blood in carcinomatosis is eosinophilia with as many as 150,000 eosinophils per mm.[3]. Bone marrow examination permits the recognition of myelomatosis, secondary melanoma and neuroblastoma, and when carcinoma cells are found, a positive L-tartrate-sensitive acid-phosphatase reaction suggests a prostatic origin. The radiological appearance of the bones may give some indication of the nature of the disease. Metastases from prostatic carcinoma are usually osteoplastic, those from mammary carcinoma only occasionally are.

3. *Acute hypercalcaemia* resulting from widespread skeletal deposits of metastatic carcinoma (see 2. for the common primary sites) or from myelomatosis. In this type of hypercalcaemia, the loss of bone calcium is due to a local effect of the malignant cells on the surrounding bone, mediated in some cases by the action of osteoclasts, and the severity of the condition is related to the surface area of bone tissue in contact with tumour cells. Hypercalcaemia may also result from the release of hormone-like substances from extraskeletal tumours in the absence of skeletal metastases, but skeletal metastases must be carefully sought before concluding that they are not present. Widespread but diffuse infiltration of bone may not give rise to pain and may not be detected radiologically until considerable demineralization has occurred. Recent active discrete deposits may cause pain but may not be visible on plain X-rays. However, they are sometimes surrounded by a hyperaemic zone in which reactive new-bone formation is taking place. Tracer doses of radiofluoride are concentrated in these areas, and permit their early detection. The presence of leucoerythroblastic anaemia provides supporting evidence of skeletal involvement and the presumptive diagnosis is clinched by finding malignant cells in a bone marrow aspirate or trephine specimen preferably taken from a site of suspected involvement. In rare cases, usually of metastatic disease from a primary mammary cancer, the spleen and liver are enlarged as a result of myeloid metaplasia, but these patients are usually thrombocytopenic, and it is not safe to attempt a needle biopsy of the liver. Skeletal X-rays may show at least some demineralization even though discrete metastases or irregularities in the bone pattern are not visible.

4. *Diabetes insipidus* resulting from deposits of tumours (other than those arising primarily in the hypophysis) in the neighbourhood of the hypothalamus and hypophysis. The nature of the tumours may be suggested by their radiological appearances, and a full skeletal survey is desirable to reveal other deposits. Eosinophilic granuloma and Hand-Schüller-Christian disease may present in this way.

5. *Hypoadrenalism* resulting from replacement of

both adrenals by metastatic carcinoma. Bronchial carcinoma is the commonest source of this.

6. *Hepatorenal encephalopathy* resulting from extensive replacement of the liver or kidneys by secondary carcinoma. This is a terminal condition usually readily recognized by physical examination, and the search for a primary tumour is academic and rarely undertaken.

The above examples refer to the distant effects of tumours growing in specific organs or tissues. Certain profound general effects associated with tumours, usually but not necessarily disseminated, may cause clinical disability before the onset of any symptoms resulting from the local effects of the tumour, but cannot be related to the involvement of any particular organs or tissues. Neuromuscular disorders and disturbances of coagulation are discussed below.

7. *Neuromuscular disorders* of several types are associated with carcinoma arising from the bronchus, breast, stomach, rectum, ovary, and other organs, and with malignant lymphoma. Minor degrees of proximal muscle weakness and wasting associated with diminution or loss of tendon reflexes are found in a small proportion of cases of carcinoma on routine examination. These changes rarely cause symptoms but occasionally give rise to severe disability in patients not known to be suffering from a malignant disease, and the neuromyopathy may antedate the discovery of the neoplasm by months or years. The neurological disturbances are occasionally associated with small localized tumours and disappear when the tumour is excised.

The commonest disorder is of the neuromyopathic type described above, but predominantly sensory neuropathies occur, as well as mixed types. In some cases the disorder is essentially myopathic with myasthenic features, while in others the findings simulate those of motor neurone disease. Cerebellar dysfunction has been associated with ovarian adenocarcinoma, and occasionally with carcinoma of the breast and lung, but carcinoma of the lung accounts for the majority of cases of all types of neurological disturbances. The cause of the carcinomatous neuromyopathies remains unknown, but they are not due to the physical presence in or near nervous tissue of the tumours or their metastases. In all suspected cases it is essential to exclude the local infiltration of nervous structures by appropriate investigation. A rapidly progressive and lethal leucoencephalopathy due to widespread multifocal demyelinating lesions throughout the white matter of the central nervous system occurs rarely in cases of disseminated malignant disease, most often of malignant lymphoma and Hodgkin's disease. It is thought to be of viral origin, and the victims are patients with a profound defect in their immunological reactivity.

8. *Disturbances of blood coagulation* may cause the presenting symptoms in cases of unsuspected though often widely disseminated malignant disease, almost always of mucin-secreting adenocarcinoma arising in pancreas, stomach, bronchus, prostate, or colon. Migratory thrombophlebitis has been associated with cancer for a century, but the existence of disseminated intravascular coagulation and microangiopathic haemolytic anaemia has been recognized only recently; malignant disease is one of the causes of microangiopathic haemolytic anaemia [see Section 13].

Successive thrombotic episodes in superficial veins or in the veins draining muscles and viscera, result from a hypercoagulable state of the blood believed to be initiated by the thromboplastic activity of substances released from mucin-secreting carcinoma cells. In some cases, sometimes associated with eosinophilia, non-bacterial thrombotic endocarditis is found, usually involving the mitral valve; secondary arterial embolic disease affecting arteries in the brain, limbs, heart, kidneys or other viscera may supervene.

In microangiopathic haemolytic anaemia a high proportion of the red cells in stained blood films show characteristic abnormalities in size and shape (small irregular fragments, triangular cells, helmet cells, and burr cells) believed to result from mechanical damage caused by the passage of the cells under pressure through arterioles of fine calibre across which fibrin strands are enmeshed. The fibrin strands are laid down in vessels passing through and in intimate contact with deposits of tumour which damage their endothelium and liberate thromboplastic substances. The extensive deposition of fibrin consumes the plasma fibrinogen, leading to a fall in its concentration, while the activation of the fibrinolytic system results in the release into the blood of the breakdown products of fibrin and fibrinogen. The widespread intravascular coagulation consumes platelets and results in thrombocytopenia. Thus a patient with severe microangiopathic haemolytic anaemia presents with a low haemoglobin concentration, a high reticulocyte count, thrombocytopenia, a blood film showing the distorted red cells already described, and polychromatic cells and macrocytes indicating increased red cell production. The plasma fibrinogen concentration is low and fibrin degradation products may be identified in the serum. In less severe disease the red cell abnormalities may not be apparent. The condition may appear in many forms of disseminated malignant disease including the malignant lymphomas and leukaemias as well as carcinoma. In extensive reticulum-cell sarcoma confined to the skin, the red cell abnormalities may be striking even though haemolysis does not occur.

Malignant Cachexia and the Metabolism of Bulky Tumours

Tumours also affect the host by their own metabolic activities. When the total mass of tumour tissue is very large in relation to the body weight, some effect on the general metabolism would be expected either as a result of the diversion of essential nutrients from the tissues of the host to the tumour, or as a result of intoxication by metabolites liberated by the tumour. 'Malignant cachexia' has often been attributed to these effects without definite evidence. It is surprising that patients with widespread deposits of metastatic malignant disease often remain well nourished until the onset of one or more secondary phenomena resulting from local effects leads to cachexia. Such secondary phenomena include extensive ulceration of skin and other epithelial surfaces with supervening infection, or compression of tubular structures with subsequent infection resulting from poor drainage, and anorexia resulting from obstructive dysphagia, from persistent vomiting, or from the prolonged use of opiates administered to relieve pain. Some authorities have attributed malignant cachexia entirely to such secondary effects. However, cachexia not secondary to local effects has been associated with small tumours, and has disappeared following their excision. Malignant cachexia in man requires detailed metabolic investigation, for its explanation remains unknown.

There are indeed few instances of gross interference with metabolism resulting from the activities of massive tumours. Patients suffering from *chronic myeloid leukaemia* lose weight because their basal metabolic rate is greatly raised, and this is attributed to the metabolic activity of the total mass of granulocytic tissue which may be 100 times larger than the normal total granulocyte mass. *Raised serum urate levels* are associated with extensive deposits of cellular tumours whose nuclei account for a substantial fraction of the total nucleic acid content of the body. The raised serum urate levels reflect the enlarged total body pool of nucleic acids. Clinical gout occurs in *myeloproliferative disorders* associated with raised serum urate levels, but not in *lymphoproliferative disorders* and *myelomatosis* in which equally high levels are found. In rare cases of *lymphosarcomatosis* and *lymphoblastic leukaemia* in which cell turnover is excessively rapid, the metabolic breakdown of the purines of the nucleic acids leads to the production of urate at a rate beyond the excretory capacity of the kidneys. The urate concentration exceeds the maximum solubility and microcrystals of urate precipitate in the renal tubules, pelves and ureters. The microcrystals confer a consistency of mud on the urine, and obstructive oliguric nephropathy results. This syndrome, though rare in untreated disease, is not uncommon when massive breakdown of tumour cells occurs rapidly during cytotoxic therapy. In this situation the administration of the xanthine oxidase inhibitor, allopurinol, reduces the concentration of urate by causing part of the total metabolites of the purines to be excreted as xanthine and hypoxanthine; the solubility of the three metabolites is independent, the concentration of any one of them does not reach saturation, and crystallization does not take place.

Anaemia is rarely attributable to a specific metabolic effect of tumours. When iron deficiency resulting from chronic blood loss or malabsorption are excluded, there remain cases in which defective iron transport results from hypotransferrinaemia; this is found in many wasting diseases and chronic infections and is not specific for malignant disease. Rarely, patients later found to have acute leukaemia or malignant lymphoma present with megaloblastic anaemia resulting from folate deficiency. The malignant disease becomes overt only when folate therapy is begun, and it is inferred that the malignant tissue functions as a folate trap.

A characteristic form of anaemia resulting from a selective aplasia of the erythropoietic cells in the bone marrow is sometimes associated with the presence of a thymic tumour, usually of benign encapsulated spindle-cell or lymphocytic type though occasionally infiltrating or metastasizing to the pleura. In some cases the anaemia remits after the tumour has been removed, but the precise relationship is obscure, and the same type of anaemia has occurred following the removal of similar tumours when the patients were not anaemic. The patients are usually elderly women, and some have myasthenia gravis.

Fever in malignant disease is usually accounted for by infection, haemorrhage, or necrosis, but these do not explain the fever of Hodgkin's disease, chronic myeloid leukaemia or renal cortical carcinoma. Dying neutrophil leucocytes release pyrogen that is believed to cause the fever accompanying infections; in chronic myeloid leukaemia, the fever subsides when the leucocyte count is lowered by treatment, and is likely to be due to leucocyte pyrogen. The cause of the fever of Hodgkin's disease and renal cortical carcinoma is not known.

Pruritus is a common symptom of Hodgkin's disease, and may precede the appearance of any lesions detectable by physical examination by many months. Hilar and mediastinal-node involvement may be revealed in chest tomograms, deposits in the spleen and liver in technetium-99m scintiscans, and involvement of the pelvic and para-aortic nodes in lymphadenograms. Hepatic involvement may be suggested by abnormalities in the liver function tests, especially an increase in the serum concentration of alkaline phosphatase. Negative results of these investigations do not exclude active disease, and laparotomy should be undertaken when persistent unexplained pruritus is accompanied by fever, sweats, weight loss, a raised erythrocyte sedimentation rate, and a raised alkaline phosphatase content of the neutrophil leucocytes. The spleen may contain deposits of Hodgkin's disease even when not enlarged, and should be removed.

The hyperviscosity syndrome is a feature of those cases of Waldenström's macroglobulinaemia and myelomatosis in which the concentration of paraprotein in the serum is high enough to increase its viscosity sufficiently to impede the microcirculation in the tissues. The effect of immunoglobulin molecules on the viscosity of the serum depends on their size, shape, and extent of polymerization as well as on their concentration. IgM increases viscosity at lower serum concentration than IgG, and within a narrow range, small increases in the concentration lead to great increase in the viscosity. The effect of IgA is similar when it is polymerized, but the relationship between the concentration of unpolymerized IgG and the serum viscosity is linear except in the subclass IgG_3 which behaves more like IgM.

Increased serum viscosity causes weakness and exhaustion, headache, drowsiness, haemorrhages from the nose, gums, gastro-intestinal or genital tract, visual disturbance, isolated neuropathies, congestive cardiac failure, and coma. The sequence of symptoms varies from patient to patient, but in any one case the sequence is usually the same whenever the serum concentration of the paraprotein reaches the critical level for that patient. The symptoms are often preceded by a regular sequence of changes in the fundi that provide a warning of their impending onset. The fundal veins become first dilated, then tortuous, and later their calibre becomes irregular; finally constrictions alternate with dilated segments, give a beaded or 'string of sausages' appearance, and papilloedema, exudates and haemorrhages appear. The symptoms and signs may be rapidly relieved by removing blood, separating and discarding the plasma, and returning the red cells to the patient. The removal of as little as one litre of blood may suffice in some cases. Plasmapheresis is most easily performed with a continuous flow cell separator.

Cryoglobulins are immunoglobulins that precipitate when cooled. They occur in some cases of myelomatosis and Waldenström's macroglobulinaemia as well as in non-malignant conditions. They precipitate in the superficial capillaries and subpapillary venules or outside the vessels in the coldest parts of the skin where they produce microinfarcts. The affected areas are painful, and at first show livid purplish discoloration within which dark brown or blackish necrotic patches appear. The lesions occur on the coldest parts of the skin, usually on the extensor aspects of the limbs and are more numerous distally. Perforation of the anterior part of the nasal septum is often found.

Amyloidosis is found in some 3 per cent. of cases of myelomatosis and Waldenström's macroglobulinaemia and in some cases of long-standing Hodgkin's disease. The main clinical consequences result from involvement of ligaments, fasciae, tendons, synovial membranes, nerves, the liver, the tongue, the larynx, and the myocardium. The carpal tunnel syndrome, focal amyloid deposits in joints and overlying the limb and trunk musculature, macroglossia, hoarseness due to laryngeal involvement, firm enlargement of the liver, and cardiomyopathy are the commoner manifestations. In rare cases coarse purpuric spots appear in clusters over the cheeks, neck, and upper chest. Biopsy of the rectal mucosa offers the best chance of establishing the diagnosis.

Nicotinamide deficiency and *hypoproteinaemia* occur in a small proportion of patients with the carcinoid syndrome who have massive tumour deposits in the liver. The tumour acts as a tryptophan trap, diverting its metabolism to the synthesis of 5-hydroxytryptamine, and away from its major pathways to protein synthesis and the synthesis of nicotinamide. Affected patients develop pellagra-like skin lesions, and become hypoproteinaemic.

Metabolic Effects of Small Tumours

The effects described above are brought about by the metabolic activities of large masses of tumour tissue and are not usually a feature of the early stages of the same diseases, although they may be responsible for the first symptoms.

Profound metabolic disturbances, however, are associated with the activities of quite small tumours which would otherwise remain undetected until they are large enough to cause local manifestations. The association in some instances is so frequent that the appearance of the characteristic syndrome should immediately arouse the suspicion of the presence of a neoplasm, whereas in others, the systemic disturbance, though characteristic, is only rarely associated with a particular neoplasm and is more commonly due to other causes. An example of the former type is phaeochromocytoma, the functional tumour of chromaffin tissue, which releases catecholamines, especially noradrenaline. These cause attacks of paroxysmal hypertension and a variety of vasomotor phenomena. All the functional tumours of the endocrine organs are of this type. An example of the latter type is the association of *acute haemolytic anaemia* with *ovarian tumours* usually *teratomas*, including *dermoid cysts*, occasionally *pseudomucinous cystadenocarcinoma*. Marked spherocytosis is usually present, and splenectomy, if performed, fails to relieve the anaemia. Subsequently, removal of the ovarian tumour is followed by relief of the anaemia. The pathogenesis of the anaemia remains unknown, but is thought to involve autoimmunization. Between these two extremes are a wide variety of manifestations, most of which are poorly understood. Attempts to classify them are necessarily arbitrary and provisional, and the basis of the attempts depends on the standpoint adopted.

From the medical standpoint, metabolic disturbances caused by small tumours are important because they are clinically harmful, and because they provide information that prompts the search for a tumour the presence of which would otherwise remain unsuspected; in some cases the symptoms may be relieved by removing the tumour. In an increasing number of cases, some at least of the metabolic disturbances can now be attributed to the production by the tumour of substances with powerful hormonal or pharmacological activity often closely resembling or even identical with normally occurring substances. In many cases, however, including the ovarian tumours causing haemolytic anaemia, the relation between the tumour and the metabolic disturbance remains obscure.

From the biological standpoint, the release by tumours of substances with powerful hormonal or pharmacological activity should be regarded as a special case of the disturbed metabolism of the tumour cells. Some identifiable products of tumour cells cause no metabolic disturbances but are clinically useful indicators of the presence of a tumour, especially when almost every tumour of a specific type releases the substance: in some instances changes in the serum concentrations of the substances reflect the activity of the tumour. Examples of such substances are α-fetoprotein associated with hepatocellular carcinoma, L-tartrate-sensitive acid-phosphatase with prostatic adenocarcinoma, leucine-aminopeptidase with pancreatic carcinoma, chorionic gonadotrophin with trophoblastic tumours, and lysozyme with monocytic leukaemia. Some of the substances produced by the tumour cells are also produced by their normal counterparts, but others are not normally associated with the tissues of origin. An isoenzyme of alkaline phosphatase resembling placental alkaline phosphatase biochemically and immunologically has been found in the serum and in the tumour in some cases of carcinoma of the lung, breast, uterus, ovary, colon, and of malignant lymphoma and myelomatosis. Other isoenzymes of alkaline phosphatase have been found in association with malignant tumours arising in the lung, gastro-intestinal tract, pancreas, and liver. The clinical importance of these isoenzymes is that the raised serum levels do not indicate the presence of metastases in the bones or the liver. The anomalous synthesis of alkaline phosphatase by tumours is unexplained, but presumably involves the utilization of part of the facultative genome that is normally inactive, and it has been suggested that this synthesis is mediated by the activity of a virus incorporated into the genome.

Metabolically active products that have been identified in tumours and sometimes in the serum are also of two main types, namely those characteristically produced by the tissue from which the tumour arose, and those not known to be produced by the tissue of origin. The former type includes all the hormones and substances with hormonal activity produced by the classical functional endocrine tumours and by those more recently described, which arise in normal anatomical structures appropriate to the endocrine tissue concerned, or in ectopic sites often associated with that tissue in embryological development. Characteristically, the production of the hormones is unphysiological and not subject to the homeostatic control that regulates their secretion by the normal endocrine glands. To a large extent the resulting syndromes are explicable in terms of the overproduction of hormones of known activity, and when two or more hormones are produced by the same tumour, the variations in the clinical manifestations may be explained by the differing proportions in which the several hormones are represented. However, persistent and striking symptoms that disappear when the tumour is removed often remain unaccounted for by any known hormone or pharmacologically active agent. From the biological standpoint, the production of specific hormones by the functional endocrine tumours is analogous to the production of the identifiable but apparently functionally inert substances by specific tumours.

The functional endocrine tumours are considered elsewhere in this volume, as are the *carcinoid tumours* [see Section 7] that release several pharmacologically active substances including 5-hydroxytryptamine and other tryptophan metabolites, histamine, and the proteolytic enzyme kallikrein, as well as unidentified substances the presence of which is inferred from the pharmacological effects not accounted for by the substances already known. It should be noted that, in contrast to the functional endocrine tumours, only a minority of carcinoid tumours produce pharmacologically active substances, and of those that do, only a small proportion cause the carcinoid syndrome, because the active products of those tumours whose venous blood drains into the tributaries of the portal vein are inactivated in the liver. When metastases of those tumours grow in the liver, however, the active products are released into the systemic circulation.

The carcinoid tumours illustrate the difficulty in deciding whether the metabolic products of tumours are appropriate to the presumptive tissue of origin. Most carcinoid tumours arise from the epithelium of those parts of the gastro-intestinal tract and its derivatives that contain argentaffin cells and the tumour cells are thought to arise from these cells. Similar argentaffin-cell tumours, occasionally responsible for the carcinoid syndrome, arise from ectopic gastro-intestinal epithelium within ovarian or testicular teratomas. However, some tumours responsible for the carcinoid syndrome do not resemble the classical argentaffin-cell tumours in any respect and arise from bronchial epithelium, the pancreas, the thyroid and elsewhere. Some apparently monomorphic pancreatic islet-cell tumours have been responsible for the carcinoid syndrome, and have also released gastrin, with the production of peptic ulceration (Zollinger-Ellison syndrome), and insulin. Whatever the embryological derivation of the tumour cells they appear to be capable of synthesizing and releasing a greater variety of specific products than is the case with any normal cell, but their activities, unlike those of normal cells, are not integrated with the physiological requirements of the host.

Aberrant Hormone Production by Non-Endocrine Tumours

Hormonally active substances are produced by tumours arising from many tissues that do not secrete them. The synthesis of these substances by the tumour cells is thought to require the utilization of parts of the facultative genome that is inactive in the cells of the normal tissue, and whatever causes the activation is independent of the physiological requirements of the body. Substances so far identified in association with non-endocrine tumours include those with the activity of vasopressin, antidiuretic-hormone, renin, adrenocorticotrophic hormone, melanophore-stimulating hormone, follicle-stimulating hormone, thyroid-stimulating hormone, parathormone, calcitonin, prostaglandins, glucagon, and insulin. As in the case of carcinoid tumours, the hormone-like substances are produced by only a minority of the tumours of each type, although the incidence of clinical syndromes resulting from their activity is higher than was formerly believed. The metabolic disturbance may precede the onset of any symptoms caused by the local effects of the tumour, while in other cases in which the primary tumour has been treated, it results from the development of recurrence or of metastases. The commoner syndromes are now summarized:

The adrenocorticotrophin syndrome (*ectopic-ACTH syndrome*) is especially associated with oat-cell and undifferentiated carcinoma of the lung, but has also been described in association with thymoma and with carcinoma of the stomach, pancreas (islet-cell), neuroblastoma, thyroid, including medullary carcinoma, parotid, ovary, testis, breast, colon, stomach, and with thymic tumours. It may also be associated with carcinoid tumours, including bronchial carcinoids. The clinical features resemble those following the administration of ACTH and are attributable to a substance having adrenocorticotrophic properties. This has been found in large amounts in the tumours. The adrenocorticotrophic activity of the serum is greatly elevated but in contrast to the findings in Cushing's syndrome due to other causes is not suppressed by the administration of adrenal corticosteroids, indicating that the pituitary is not the source. When the secretory activity of the tumour is relatively low and the tumour only slowly progressive, the symptoms closely resemble those of Cushing's syndrome, but they are often atypical. More rapidly growing tumours may secrete large amounts of ACTH-like substance over a short period, and the adrenal cortex is under maximal stimulation. The patients complain of severe muscle weakness, they have a cushingoid facies and may become diabetic. The adrenal output of cortisol is very high and this leads to excessive loss of potassium in the urine. The administration of ACTH does not lead to any increase in the serum cortisol level, or in the urinary excretion of its metabolites.

The patients sometimes become deeply pigmented, and this results either from the similarity of structure of the peptide produced by the tumour to adrenocorticotrophin which has melanocyte-stimulating activity, or from the production of another slightly different peptide resembling the melanocyte-stimulating hormone more closely.

Hypercalcaemia has been described already as resulting from massive skeletal involvement by malignant tumours. It may also result from the secretion by small tumours of a substance having parathormone activity, and may subside when the tumour is resected only to reappear with the growth of metastases. The parathyroid glands are not involved. A parathormone-like substance has been isolated from the tumours. It occurs most commonly in association with carcinoma of the bronchus, breast, renal cortex, and ovary, and the clinical manifestations depend partly on the duration of the exposure to the parathormone-like substance, and partly on the intensity of the stimulation. In the slowly developing syndrome, calcific corneal deposits and metastatic calcification with nephrocalcinosis may occur, but more commonly the syndrome appears too rapidly for their development. In breast cancers a substance resembling 7-dehydrocholesterol has been demonstrated, but it is not known whether it is released or whether it affects calcium metabolism.

The hyponatraemic syndrome may result from hypocorticism due to adrenal replacement by metastatic tumour. Bronchial carcinoma is a more common source of bilateral adrenal metastases than other primary tumours. The symptoms are those of hypocorticism with extreme lethargy, mental confusion and drowsiness. In these cases the serum potassium concentration is normal. In rare cases of oat-cell carcinoma of the bronchus hyponatraemia may occur in association with a raised plasma volume. The haemoglobin concentration, the packed-cell volume, and the blood urea concentration are low, while the osmolality of the urine is high. In these cases the adrenals are not infiltrated by growth and the hyponatraemic state is thought to arise from the effects of a vasopressin-like peptide with antidiuretic activity that has been identified in the tumours. The urinary sodium loss is increased by the reduced secretion of aldosterone which follows the haemodilution.

The carcinoid syndrome has been mentioned in connexion with bronchial adenoma and other non-argentaffin-cell tumours. It also occurs rarely in association with oat-cell and undifferentiated bronchial carcinoma.

Hypertrophic pulmonary osteoarthropathy (*HPOA*) is especially associated with peripheral lung carcinoma and pleural mesothelioma, but, like all the other conditions discussed, it occurs in only a minority of patients. The patients complain of severe pain in the wrists, ankles, and sometimes knees, and the joints are hot and swollen. There is almost always marked clubbing of the fingers and toes, though this sign is much more common in the absence of HPOA, and some patients have gynaecomastia, which may also occur in the absence of HPOA. HPOA is much more specifically associated with lung cancer than is clubbing, and may precede the onset of chest symptoms by several years. The pain may disappear instantly when the lung is resected, though the physical signs and radiological changes resolve only slowly. The cause of HPOA remains unknown. In some cases with gynaecomastia, high levels of urinary oestrogens are found. In some of these, the high levels persist after the tumour has been resected, but in one case, the levels of serum follicle-stimulating hormone activity were higher in the venous effluent from the tumour than in the arterial blood, and the resected tumour contained large amounts of both follicle-stimulating and luteinizing hormone.

Hypoglycaemia, though usually associated with insulin-secreting β-cell islet tumours of the pancreas also occurs occasionally in association with other tumours, especially retroperitoneal fibrosarcoma, spindle-cell sarcoma, pseudomyxoma, haemangiopericytoma, and even less commonly with bronchial and gastric carcinoma. Histochemical examination of all tumours is essential to make sure that they do not contain the granules characteristic of pancreatic islet β-cells, indicating an origin in ectopic islet tissue. The symptoms occur especially in the early mornings, when fasting, or after exercise, and are relieved by food. During attacks the blood sugar level may fall to 50 mg. per 100 ml. In some cases substances with insulin-like activity have been isolated from the tumours, but the plasma insulin levels have not been raised. Tolbutamide administered intravenously does not raise the plasma-insulin concentration as it does in insulin-secreting islet-cell tumours.

Hyperthyroidism, usually not clinically significant, is commoner in association with some tumours than would be expected by chance, notably in gastro-intestinal and ovarian tumours. In some trophoblastic tumours the symptoms disappear after successful cytotoxic therapy, and in some cases there is evidence of the production by the tumour of a substance with thyroid-stimulating properties.

CHEMOTHERAPY OF MALIGNANT DISEASE

Chemotherapy specific for malignant disease would exploit some property of malignant cells not shared with normal cells. No such property is yet known and chemotherapy still involves the use of agents known as cytotoxic drugs that damage growing cells. The great majority of these drugs interfere with one or more of the cellular processes concerned in the preparation for cell division, or with the mechanical process of mitosis when the newly formed chromosomes of the two daughter cells move apart. Because the process of cell division is common to normal and malignant growing cells, cytotoxic drugs are entirely non-specific in their effect on malignant disease, and cannot destroy malignant cells without also destroying normal growing cells. However, normal growing cells from different tissues vary in their susceptibility to cytotoxic drugs, though the reasons for this variation are largely unknown, and malignant growths also vary in their sensitivity to these drugs. In a few instances the malignant cells are just sensitive enough in relation to the sensitivity of the most vulnerable normal growing cells for worthwhile effects to be obtained by treatment. In this respect only, some selectivity of action is possible. Indeed without it, chemotherapy would not be possible at all. Practical chemotherapy is a compromise in which the attempt to destroy the greatest possible number of tumour cells has to be balanced against the inevitability of causing damage to the normal proliferating cells that are essential to life.

So far, only two forms of malignant disease, both excessively rare, can be eradicated by treatment with cytotoxic drugs, but the explanation for the marginally increased susceptibility of the tumour cells in relation to that of the most vulnerable normal proliferating cells is not known. The two diseases are choriocarcinoma in women, of which over 70 per cent. of patients are curable by chemotherapy, and Burkitt's lymphoma, of which over 70 per cent. of the patients with early disease are curable. In Burkitt's lymphoma, the margin of safety is so small that when the total bulk of the tumour is large, the total dose of cytotoxic drug required to destroy all the tumour cells is higher than the largest dose compatible with the survival of normal proliferating cells. Advanced tumours therefore cannot be eradicated by chemotherapy but by reducing the size of the tumour masses, useful though temporary palliation can often be achieved. The great majority of human neoplasms are far less responsive to chemotherapy than Burkitt's lymphoma, and good palliation rather than cure is all that can be attempted.

The Actions of Cytotoxic Drugs

The mitotic cycle includes the following phases after the preceding cell division: (1) the 'first gap' (G_1) of variable duration in which active synthetic processes have not been shown to occur; (2) the phase of deoxyribonucleic-acid (DNA) synthesis (S) in which the cell synthesizes from simple organic molecules the purine and pyrimidine bases adenine, guanine, cytosine and thymine, combines them with deoxyribose to form the corresponding deoxyribosides, and with phosphate to form the deoxyribotides adenylic acid, guanylic acid, cytidylic acid and thymidylic acid which are assembled in an order determined by that present in the parent chain into the double helix of the new DNA chain. At the end of the S phase the total amount of DNA in the cell is exactly double the amount present at the beginning. The whole process requires not only a rapid uptake of the simple molecules from which the DNA is synthesized but an assembly of enzymes that control each step in the process, and a source of energy. (3) The 'second gap' (G_2) of variable duration before the final phase (4) of mitosis itself in which the DNA threads shorten by spiralization and become condensed into the two sets of compact daughter chromosomes that move apart along the mitotic spindle to form the nuclei of the two daughter cells, each of which receives an identical set of chromosomes. A population of cells continuously engaged in the process of division is said to be 'in cycle'.

Most cytotoxic drugs are thought to act on the S phase or on the process of mitosis, but the damage expressed during the vulnerable phase may have been inflicted before the cell enters it. Cytotoxic drugs are grouped for convenience as shown in Table 28 but the classification gives no information on the precise mode or site of action of the drugs or on their chemical structure.

CLASSES OF CYTOTOXIC DRUGS

THE BIOLOGICAL ALKYLATING AGENTS

These are synthetic compounds of great chemical diversity that have in common the ability to add alkyl groups to a wide range of electronegative groups under the mild aqueous conditions that prevail in the living cell. The cytotoxic alkylating agents have two or more active groups, and it is thought that they destroy growing cells by causing damage to the DNA chain by cross-linking the adjacent guanine molecules on a strand of DNA or the molecules on adjacent strands, thus mechanically preventing the uncoiling of the strands and so halting the replication of the DNA. Although the alkylation of DNA may be the basic mechanism by which the cells are killed there are many differences in the pharmacological properties of the alkylating agents in different chemical classes and in those of the members of each class. Some alkylating agents cause conspicuous breaks in chromosomes, while others at lower equivalent doses cause no visible chromosome damage but prevent cell division and lead to the production of polyploid giant cells.

In any one alkylating agent the alkylating groups become active as a result of hydrolysis, and the rate of hydrolysis which depends on the structure of the whole molecule determines a large part of the biological reactivity. In some, such as chlorambucil and melphalan, the rate of hydrolysis is entirely dependent on the properties of the molecule itself, while in others, such as busulphan, the rate is dependent on the availability of suitable groups that can be alkylated. Cyclophosphamide is an inactive compound from which alkylating compounds are liberated only by enzymic breakdown mainly in the liver.

Alkylating agents differ greatly in their physicochemical properties, and consequently in their biological effects. Highly reactive compounds like mustine hydrochloride are vesicants and can be administered only intravenously, intra-arterially, or into serous cavities. Because of its high reactivity, mustine is particularly valuable clinically when it is important to obtain a rapid response, for example to relieve toxaemia in generalized Hodgkin's disease, or superior vena caval obstruction from bronchial carcinoma. It is less useful for maintenance therapy. Milder agents like cyclophosphamide may also be administered intramuscularly or orally, while highly insoluble compounds like busulphan are suitable only for oral administration. They may be

TABLE 28

CONDITION	BIOLOGICAL ALKYLATING AGENTS	FOLIC ACID ANTAGONISTS	ANTIMETABOLITES		CYTOTOXIC ANTIBIOTICS	PLANT ALKALOIDS	MISCELLANEOUS
			ANTIPURINES	ANTIPYRIMIDINES			
Choriocarcinoma (A)	HN2^{2}, Ml^{2}, Cy^{2}	MTX^{1}	MP^{2}		DAC^{2}	VCR^{2}	
Burkitt's lymphoma (A)	Ml^{1}, Cy^{1}	MTX^{1}					
Lymphoblastic leukaemia (B_1)	Cy (M^{3})	MTX (M^{1}) MTX (i.θ)	MP (M^{2})	Ara-C (IND^{3}) Ara-C (i.θ)	DR (IND^{2})	VCR (IND^{1})	Pred (IND^{1},^{2}) L'ase (IND^{3})
Generalized Hodgkin's disease (B_1)	HN2 (Comb^{1}) Cy (Comb^{2}) Chl (Comb^{3})					VLB (Comb^{2} and ^{3}) VCR (Comb^{1})	Pred (Comb^{1,2} ^{3} PCZ (Comb^{1,2} and ^{3})
Chronic myeloid leukaemia (B_1)	B^{1} Bu^{1}		MP^{2}				DBM^{2} HU^{2}
Chronic lymphocytic leukaemia (B_1)	Chl Cy						Pred^{s}
Disseminated plasmacytoma (B_1)	Cy Ml						U^{2}
Myelomatosis (B_2)	Ml, Cy						Pred^{s}
Waldenstörm's macroglobulinaemia (B_2)	Cy, Ml, Chl						Pred^{s}
Ovarian adenocarcinoma (B_2)	Cy, Ml, Chl, Th, HN2 (i.s.) Th (i.s.)			FU			
Acute myeloid leukaemia (B_2)	Cy (Comb^{2})	MTX(Comb^{2})	MP (Comb^{1}) THG (Comb^{1})	Ara-C (Comb^{1})	DR (Comb^{1})	VCR (Comb^{2})	Pred (Comb^{1}) ? L'ase (Comb^{1})
Nephroblastoma (Wilms' tumour) (B_2)					DAC	VCR	
Reticulum-cell sarcoma (B_2)	Cy (Comb^{1})		MP (Comb^{2})	Ara-C (Comb^{2})	DR (Comb^{2})	VCR (Comb^{1})	PCZ (Comb^{1})
Neuroblastoma (C_1)	Cy (Comb)					VCR (Comb)	
Seminoma (C_1)	Cy, Ml, Chl						
Testicular teratoma (C_2)	Chl (Comb)	MTX (Comb)			DAC (Comb) DAC		
Mammary carcinoma (C_2)	Cy (Comb) HN2 (i.s.)	MTX (Comb)		FU (Comb)			
Gastro-intestinal carcinoma (C_3)				FU			
Soft-tissue sarcomas (C_3)	Chl (Comb)	MTX (Comb)		FU (Comb)	DAC (Comb)		
Epidermoid carcinoma (C_3)	Cy, HN2 (i.art.)	MTX MTX (i.art.)			Bleo		
Malignant melanoma (C_3)	Ml						L'ase
Lymphosarcoma (B_2)	Cy (Comb)	MTX MTX (i.θ)		Ara-C (i.θ)		VCR (Comb)	Pred Comb)

KEY TO TABLE

A = tumours curable by chemotherapy alone.
B_1 = conditions in which chemotherapy is the treatment of choice, and is highly effective in more than 50 per cent. of the cases, but is essentially palliative.
B_2 = as B, but chemotherapy effective in less than 50 per cent. of the cases, and usually less successful than in B_1.
C_1 = conditions in which good palliation is obtained occasionally.
C_2 = conditions in which some benefit is occasionally conferred.
C_3 = conditions in which temporary regression usually of doubtful benefit is observed.

Superscripts
^{1} = treatment of choice.
^{2,3} = second-, third-line drugs.
s = useful in special circumstances.

Parentheses

comb[1,2] = drug best administered in combination with other named drugs carrying same superscript number.
IND[1,2] = drug used to induce remission, in combination with other drug carrying same superscript number.
M[1,2] = drug best administered for maintenance therapy. Superscript indicates suggested order of administration.
i.θ = suitable for intrathecal administration.
i.art. = suitable for intra-arterial administration.
i.s. = suitable for intrapleural or intraperitoneal administration.

Drugs

HN2 = mustine hydrochloride	MTX = methotrexate	DR = daunorubicin	L'ase = L-asparaginase
Ml = melphalan	MP = mercaptopurine	Bleo = bleomycin	PCZ = procarbazine
Cy = cyclophosphamide	Ara-C = cytosine arabinoside	VCR = vincristine sulphate	DBM = dibromomannitol
Chl = chlorambucil	FU = fluorouracil	VLB = vinblastine sulphate	HU = hydroxyurea
Th = triethylenethiophosphoramide	DAC = dactinomycin	Pred = prednisolone	U = urethane
Bu = busulphan	THG = thioguanine		

used in maintenance therapy for months or years and their dosage adjusted in relation to the response and to the side-effects.

The clinical usefulness of the alkylating agents is determined by their efficacy, their convenience in administration, their immediate and delayed toxicity, and by their side-effects. All are mutagenic in experimental animals but the risks in man are not well understood; they are also teratogenic and are to be avoided during the first 16 weeks of pregnancy. All are myelosuppressive, and in practice this property is the chief limiting factor in treatment because bone marrow aplasia resulting from overdosage is often irreversible. The effect on haemopoietic cells relative to that on other growing cells whether normal or malignant varies; it is so great in the case of busulphan, that the usefulness of this drug is practically limited to haemopoietic neoplasms; cyclophosphamide has relatively less effect on the platelet counts than other alkylating agents.

Because the antitumour effect of the alkylating agents is in most diseases small in relation to their myelosuppressive effect, it is usually necessary in order to obtain worthwhile benefit, to administer these drugs at an order of dosage close to the limits of bone marrow tolerance. Meticulous and continuous supervision is therefore essential if these drugs are to be used to the greatest advantage and with safety.

Alkylating agents damage lymphocytes, and unlike other cells, non-dividing small lymphocytes as well as those in the mitotic cycle are vulnerable. Alkylating agents are therefore immunosuppressive, especially when administered continuously for long periods.

Anorexia, nausea and vomiting are common side-effects of alkylating agents that limit their acceptability to some patients. Most patients vomit within 2 hours of receiving mustine hydrochloride, but not before 5 hours of receiving cyclophosphamide or melphalan intravenously. Orally administered cyclophosphamide often causes anorexia, sometimes nausea and less often vomiting. These effects are less often caused by melphalan and chlorambucil, but a patient intolerant to one of these three drugs may accept one of the other two without difficulty. At high dosage, melphalan and cyclophosphamide administered intravenously, and cyclophosphamide but not melphalan, administered orally at low daily dosage for several months cause alopecia in women and sometimes in men. All alkylating agents administered for long periods cause amenorrhoea and hot flushes in women of child-bearing age. Busulphan often causes skin pigmentation not usually in the distribution characteristic of Addison's disease, but a minority of patients, treated continuously for several years, rarely for less than one year, develop a wasting syndrome resembling Addison's disease but lacking evidence of adrenal cortical hypofunction. There is evidence, however, of defective but reversible pituitary responsiveness as shown by the metyrapone test. Busulphan also causes the appearance of giant hyperchromatic polyploid cells in many tissues, and very rarely damages the pulmonary alveolar cells with consequent exudation of fibrin and subsequent intra-alveolar fibrosis. Cyclophosphamide has also caused the wasting syndrome and pulmonary fibrosis. Cyclophosphamide is activated in the liver, and some of its metabolites are excreted in the urine. They often cause hyperaemia of the urothelium and microscopic haematuria and occasionally dysuria and gross haematuria.

After varying periods of time, malignant cells, but not normal cells become resistant to alkylating agents. Further treatment with the same or with any other alkylating agent, still causes bone marrow depression and other toxic effects but no longer influences the tumour. It is believed that resistant cells acquire the property of excising cross-linked parts of the DNA chain and restoring functional continuity. Some tumours such as ovarian adenocarcinoma, Hodgkin's disease, lymphosarcoma and lymphoblastic leukaemia remain sensitive to other types of cytotoxic drugs when they have become resistant to alkylating agents, but when chronic myeloid leukaemia becomes resistant to busulphan, the most commonly used alkylating agent, treatment with other drugs of any class is only partially effective.

Occasional patients develop allergic reactions to alkylating agents, usually in the form of irritating generalized blotchy maculopapular rashes that become confluent and later desquamate. These reactions are specific for the drug concerned and the treatment may be safely continued with another alkylating agent.

Highly reactive alkylating agents like mustine are taken out of the circulation within a few minutes of injection and are fixed by alkylation to the tissues. More slowly reacting compounds and those with a slower spontaneous hydrolysis rate are eliminated through the kidneys before they have exerted their maximum possible effect. Thus in uraemia, the toxic effect of agents like chlorambucil, cyclophosphamide or melphalan is greatly increased.

Clinical Uses

Alkylating agents, alone or in combination with other drugs or radiotherapy are now indispensable in the treatment of Hodgkin's disease, lymphocytic lymphoma (including Burkitt's lymphoma, lymphosarcoma, chronic lymphocytic leukaemia, follicular lymphoma, Waldenström's macroglobulinaemia), plasma-cell tumours (myelomatosis and extramedullary plasmacytoma), chronic myeloid leukaemia, lymphoblastic leukaemia. They are less useful but have a place in the management of histiocytic lymphoma (reticulum-cell sarcoma), testicular seminoma, ovarian adenocarcinoma, mammary carcinoma, neuroblastoma, nephroblastoma, and embryonal sarcoma. Their value in bronchial carcinoma and gastro-intestinal carcinoma is doubtful. However, with the exception of Burkitt's lymphoma, in the early stage of which alkylating agents may effect a cure, and perhaps chronic myeloid leukaemia, in the treatment-responsive stage of which alkylating agents alone, especially busulphan, provide the best method of controlling the disease, the other conditions are best treated by a carefully prepared programme of management in which alkylating agents have a place alongside other methods of treatment. Examples illustrating the circumstances in which they are used are Hodgkin's disease and chronic lymphocytic leukaemia [see Section 13].

In patients with mammary carcinoma alkylating agents should not be considered until the possibilities of surgery, radiotherapy, endocrine ablative surgery, and hormone therapy have been exhausted. They have a place alone or in combination with other drugs, especially vincristine and fluorouracil, only in the presence of disseminated disease refractory to other methods of treatment. Nevertheless, worthwhile regressions are observed often enough to merit trial. Cyclophosphamide is the most convenient drug.

THE ANTIMETABOLITES

The antimetabolites are synthetically prepared structural analogues of naturally occurring substances that play essential parts in the metabolism of proliferating cells. The antimetabolites differ structurally from their normal counterparts only very slightly and compete with them by a variety of mechanisms, to interfere with their specific functions in the synthesis of the pyrimidine and purine bases, their assembly into nucleotides, or their incorporation into the DNA chain. These processes are blocked at different stages in the S phase of the cell cycle by different antimetabolites, and the affected cells fail to divide and often die, though it is not understood how this happens.

Antimetabolites like all other cytotoxic drugs affect normal as well as malignant proliferating cells, and the margin of safety is therefore narrow. This greatly limits their usefulness in practice. The three main types of antimetabolite are analogues of folic acid, of the purines, and of the pyrimidines. Tumour cells, but not normal proliferating cells eventually become resistant to antimetabolites, but because the several types of agent act by different mechanisms there is no cross-resistance between them. A tumour that has become resistant to a folic acid antagonist may still respond to a purine antagonist, or to a pyrimidine antagonist.

Folic-Acid Antagonists. Folic acid, which cannot be synthesized by mammalian cells, plays an essential part in the biosynthesis of the nucleic acids, and of several amino acids, and in amino acid metabolism. To become metabolically active it has to be reduced in two steps to tetrahydrofolic acid (FH_4) by a specific enzyme, folate reductase (DFR). FH_4 transfers single carbon groups from suitable donors such as serine to the precursor molecules for the purine skeleton. Two transfers for the carbon atoms at positions 2 and 8 are required. FH_4 also donates a methyl group to deoxyuridylic acid (UMP, the deoxyribotide of uracil) thus converting it to deoxythymidilic acid (TMP, the deoxyribotide of thymine), while itself becoming oxidized to dihydrofolate (FH_2). To continue its metabolic activity FH_4 must be regenerated from FH_2 by the action of DFR. The conversion of UMP to TMP is the rate-determining step in DNA synthesis, and if it is blocked DNA synthesis cannot proceed.

Methotrexate (MTX) the folic acid antagonist in current clinical use, is the 4-amino-N^{10} methyl-substituted analogue of folic acid. It blocks the conversion of folic acid to FH_4 because it binds DFR irreversibly; its affinity for DFR is much greater than that of folic acid itself so that the blocking action of MTX cannot be reversed by treatment with folic acid at high dosage. It can, however, be bypassed by folinic acid (CF) which is 5-formyl FH_4, already fully reduced.

Experimental and human tumours originally sensitive to MTX may acquire resistance rapidly, but the normal proliferating tissues retain their original sensitivity. In some laboratory situations resistance to MTX has been shown to be due to the increased capacity of the tumour cells to synthesize DFR, while in others resistance has been shown to be due to reduction in the permeability of the cells to MTX. Thus tumour cells become resistant in different ways and attempts to overcome resistance would require knowledge of the underlying mechanism in each case.

Methotrexate is readily absorbed from the gut, and may be administered intravenously, intramuscularly and intra-arterially. It does not pass the blood-brain barrier, and must be administered intrathecally in the treatment of meningeal leukaemia or lymphosarcoma. Although it enters cells readily, it is also rapidly excreted unchanged by the kidneys, so that the effect of a given dose administered by intravenous injection is much less than that of the same dose administered by prolonged intravenous infusion. In uraemic subjects, however, an intravenous dose is cleared slowly from the blood stream and the toxicity greatly increased. The killing power of a single dose administered by injection against proliferating normal or malignant cells is limited not only by the excretion rate but also by the proportion of cells in the S phase in the population at risk. The enhancement of activity by prolonging the duration of an infusion is due to the trapping of an increasing number of cells in the population at risk, as they enter the sensitive phase of the cell cycle.

The major immediate toxic effects of methotrexate are seen in the buccal mucosa, the gastro-intestinal tract, and the bone marrow. Buccal ulceration is an early sign, and if administration is continued after the appearance of an ulcer, extensive confluent and extremely painful ulceration ensues. If the platelet count is falling rapidly the ulcers may be haemorrhagic. Intestinal ulceration may cause abdominal pain and diarrhoea. Methotrexate causes megaloblastic change in the bone marrow, neutropenia and thrombocytopenia, and the blood films show macrocytosis and hypersegmentation of the neutrophils. These changes are seen also in the films of patients on long-term methotrexate therapy whose blood counts are substantially normal. Severe toxic effects include transient alopecia and confluent maculo-erythematous rashes mainly on the face and neck, and in the flexures, and the perineum; the rashes become purpuric before the adjacent normal skin if the platelet count falls.

Patients receiving continuous methotrexate therapy either on a daily or twice-weekly basis succumb more often than normal subjects to upper respiratory and pulmonary infections which tend to run a prolonged course; herpetic lesions on the lips may not heal until the methotrexate is withheld. Increase in the serum levels of alkaline phosphatase and transaminases sometimes occurs during prolonged intra-arterial infusions of methotrexate. Rarely, hepatic fibrosis has been recorded during long-term oral or intramuscular methotrexate therapy, and more rarely still fibrinous exudation into the pulmonary alveoli which has resolved when the administration was stopped. Foetal abnormalities and abortion were recorded when aminopterin, an analogue of methotrexate, was administered during early pregnancy, and are likely to be caused by methotrexate also.

Clinical Uses

Methotrexate, alone or in combination with other drugs is now indispensable in the treatment of lymphoblastic leukaemia, choriocarcinoma in women, Burkitt's lymphoma, and lymphosarcoma. It is sometimes effective when administered by prolonged intra-arterial infusion in the treatment of epidermoid carcinoma of the skin and mucosae of the head and neck. Its value is more difficult to assess in the treatment of mammary cancer and of soft tissue sarcomata because there is no way of predicting the small proportion of patients likely to respond well. An even smaller proportion of patients suffering from other forms of malignant disease have responded to methotrexate, and no general recommendations of practical value can be made. The use of methotrexate is illustrated in the treatment of lymphoblastic leukaemia [see Section 13] and choriocarcinoma.

Choriocarcinoma is so rare and its manifestations, complications, and response to treatment are so varied that useful experience in its management can be accumulated only in special centres, where cure rates exceeding 70 per cent. are obtained. The two features that contribute to this high rate are first, the relative sensitivity of the tumour cells to methotrexate and other cytotoxic drugs in relation to that of the normal proliferating cells, and second, the fact that during apparent remission, early relapse can be detected by recording an increase in the amount of human chorionic gonadotrophin in the urine; intensive therapy must be resumed and continued until the concentration remains repeatedly below the background level of luteinizing hormone from which it cannot be distinguished by current assay methods. A test of comparable sensitivity for determining the end point of therapy is not available in any other human malignant disease; in myelomatosis, for example, paraprotein, at the lowest detectable concentration in the serum represents approximately 50 g. of tumour.

Several regimes of intensive chemotherapy involving the use of methotrexate alone or in combination with other drugs have proved effective in the treatment of choriocarcinoma; the methotrexate may be administered by intravenous infusion continued for several days, or by injections repeated 8 to 12-hourly for 48–72 hours, or by daily injections repeated several times. In each of these regimes it is necessary to counteract the toxicity by injections of folinic acid at suitable intervals.

PURINE ANALOGUES

6-Mercaptopurine (MP), and 2-amino-6-mercaptopurine (thioguanine) are the best known purine analogues. MP is inactive until it has been converted within the cell to its ribonucleotide. This competes with the normal ribonucleotide, inosinic acid, by blocking its conversion to adenylosuccinic acid and to xanthylic acid which are precursors of adenine and guanine deoxyribotides. The excess inosinic acid, and perhaps MP itself, suppress the *de novo* synthesis of inosinic acid at any early stage by feed-back inhibition. MP also interferes with the synthesis of the hydrogen acceptor nicotine-adenine dinucleotide (NAD). The final effect of MP is to suppress DNA synthesis. *In vivo* MP is powerfully myelosuppressive, and clinically this is its main toxic property. Damage to the gastro-intestinal epithelium usually occurs only at higher dosage and hepatotoxicity is very rare. Like the alkylating agents and methotrexate, mercaptopurine is teratogenic and immunosuppressive.

MP is usually administered orally and is well tolerated, only occasionally causing nausea and diarrhoea, and hardly ever mouth ulcers. It is metabolized to thiouric acid by the enzyme xanthine oxidase, and its activity is therefore prolonged if it is administered in combination with the xanthine-oxidase inhibitor allopurinol. Allowance should be made for this effect when allopurinol is administered to reduce the load of purine metabolites derived from breaking down tumour cells excreted as uric acid. MP occasionally causes jaundice with evidence of liver cell damage.

MP is an indispensable drug in the treatment of lymphoblastic leukaemia and the acute myeloid leukaemias, and it is also of some value in busulphan-resistant chronic myeloid leukaemia.

PYRIMIDINE ANALOGUES

5-Fluorouracil (FU) and cytosine arabinoside (Ara-C) are the best known pyrimidine analogues. FU is uracil in which the hydrogen atom at position 5 has been replaced by a fluorine atom. Like uracil it is converted within the cell to its deoxyribotide. The false deoxyribotide competes with the naturally occurring deoxyribotide for the enzyme thymidylate synthetase which converts the normal substrate to deoxythymidylic acid by transferring a methyl group from methylenetetrahydrofolate to position 5 of the uracil moiety. Methylation of the fluoro-substituted deoxyribotide does not occur. The inhibition of deoxythymidilic acid synthesis results in the failure of DNA synthesis and so in the death of proliferating cells. FU is thus specially toxic to the mucosa of the buccal cavity and of the gastro-intestinal tract, to the bone marrow, to embryonic tissues, and it is also immunosuppressive. In clinical practice the pattern of toxicity differs from that resulting from methotrexate administration. Diarrhoea is usually the first sign of toxicity, followed by evidence of bone marrow depression with megaloblastosis, and by ulceration of the tongue more often than of the mucosa of the lips, palate, and cheeks characteristic of methotrexate toxicity.

FU is administered intravenously by injection or infusion, the latter being less toxic but also less effective. It is well tolerated. The margin between toxic damage and therapeutic efficacy is too narrow for FU, used alone, to be a useful drug in practice, but it is occasionally effective in mammary, urothelial, gastric and colorectal carcinoma and ovarian adenocarcinoma. It is probable that it will prove more useful when administered in combination with drugs of other classes.

Cytosine arabinoside (Ara-C) is an analogue of cytidine in which the ribose moiety is replaced by its stereoisomer D-arabinose. It is phosphorylated within the cell by the enzyme deoxycytidine kinase, and is thought to inhibit the reduction of cytidilic acid to deoxycytidilic acid, thus blocking DNA synthesis. *In vivo* it is powerfully myelosuppressive, causing severe megaloblastosis and marrow hypoplasia.

Ara-C may be administered intravenously by injection or by infusion, intramuscularly, subcutaneously, and intrathecally. It is apt to cause nausea and vomiting but is otherwise well tolerated. In experimental leukaemic animals the leukaemia can be eradicated if the size and frequency of doses are adjusted to obtain the correct balance between the tumouricidal effect and bone marrow destruction on the one hand, and bone marrow regeneration on the other. The commonly used clinical schedule of daily intravenous injection for 3–10 days may not be the most effective.

Ara-C is one of several drugs used, usually in combination, in the treatment of acute myeloid leukaemia, lymphoblastic leukaemia, and lymphosarcoma.

CYTOTOXIC ANTIBIOTICS

In the course of testing bacterial filtrates for antibiotic activity, several were found to be powerfully cytotoxic and therefore unsuitable as antibiotics. However, some were found to cause the regression of transplanted tumours in laboratory animals, and the less toxic agents were submitted to clinical trial. The clinically useful antibiotics dactinomycin, mitomycin C, mithramycin, and daunorubicin were isolated from filtrates of bacteria in the genus *Streptomyces*. These antibiotics are structurally varied and they differ in the mechanism whereby they influence division, though the effect of all is to inhibit the synthesis of ribonucleic acid, and hence to block protein synthesis. In Great Britain mitomycin C and mithramycin have been little used. Both dactinomycin and daunorubicin are myelosuppressive and immunosuppressive.

Dactinomycin is the most active of a large group of actinomycins. It combines with DNA and blocks its template activity in directing the synthesis of messenger RNA. As with the alkylating agents, guanine moieties are favoured binding sites, and the cross-linking of adjacent strands of DNA interferes with their separation.

Dactinomycin is active when administered intravenously, but not when administered by mouth. Extravasation causes severe necrotizing effects. At therapeutic doses of 10 μg. per kg. of body weight administered daily for 5 days it is usually well tolerated, but may cause anorexia, nausea and vomiting, and diarrhoea. Overdosage causes profound bone marrow damage, destruction of mature lymphocytes, erythema, thinning and ulceration of the buccal mucosa and gastro-intestinal tract, and intense erythema of the skin with exfoliation, thinning and ulceration. Even at therapeutic dosage, previously irradiated areas of skin become erythematous. In experimental systems dactinomycin is immunosuppressive, damages germinal epithelium, and is teratogenic and carcinogenic.

It is now an essential drug in the treatment of nephroblastoma (Wilms' tumour) in children, it is occasionally effective in other embryonal tumours and in testicular teratoma. Dactinomycin causes regression of metastatic deposits in recurrent nephroblastoma, but it is used to greatest advantage in conjunction with surgery and radiotherapy in the management of the localized primary diseases. Injections are given before the affected kidney is excised, and several further courses are administered after the completion of a radical course of postoperative radiotherapy. The recurrence rate is much lower in patients so treated than when chemotherapy is omitted, and it is possible that the results might be even better if dactinomycin were administered in combination with or alternating with vincristine.

The value of dactinomycin alone or in combination with other drugs is less certain in the treatment of embryonal sarcomas and teratoma but its use should always be considered because of the occasional dramatic response. Drugs that have been combined with dactinomycin are methotrexate and chlorambucil, but the superior efficacy of multiple-drug regimes has not been established.

Daunorubicin, like dactinomycin, blocks the transcription of the genetic code from DNA to messenger RNA, and it damages the DNA by becoming bound to the bases, thus preventing cell division. Its chief immediate toxicity at a single therapeutic dose of 1 mg. per kg. of body weight is to the bone marrow, but higher doses damage the gastro-intestinal mucosa, cause lymphoid atrophy and alopecia. Long-term administration damages the conducting system in the heart, and this effect has led to sudden death from cardiorespiratory collapse. Daunorubicin is irritant to the tissues and must be administered intravenously through a fast-running saline drip. Extravasation is painful and causes severe tissue necrosis.

Daunorubicin at moderate dosage is useful in combination with other drugs in the treatment of acute myeloid leukaemia and lymphoblastic leukaemia, but because of its powerful myelotoxicity it is not suitable at higher dosage for use as the sole agent. There is no cross-resistance between daunorubicin and any of the other antileukaemic agents, and its inclusion with other agents in treatment programmes would be expected to reduce further the likelihood of resistance emerging. Regimes of treatment suitable for routine use are still being developed [see Section 13].

THE PLANT ALKALOIDS

Colchicine and deacetylmethylcolchicine. Colchicine, extracted from *Colchicum autumnale*, and long used in the treatment of gout, is a powerful cytotoxic agent at higher dosage. It arrests cell division at metaphase by damaging the mitotic spindle. It is too toxic for clinical use, but the deacetylmethyl-analogue has been used in the treatment of chronic myeloid leukaemia.

The *vinca alkaloids* have a variety of toxic effects other than those on dividing cells. In spite of their close structural similarity VLB and VCR differ strikingly in their toxic properties. The most serious property of VCR is to cause damage to the axons of peripheral nerves, first manifest in the longest fibres. The first clinically observed effects therefore are depression and loss of the ankle reflexes; paraesthesiae in the toes, and later weakness of the dorsiflexors and evertors of the foot appear. These effects occur only rarely with VLB, after prolonged treatment or when high doses sufficient to cause marked bone marrow depression are used. VCR, however, almost always causes some degree of neuropathy at commonly used doses that do not depress the bone marrow. VCR frequently causes severe constipation and occasionally prolonged ileus, thought to result from an effect on the autonomic plexuses; VLB does not have this effect. VCR, but not VLB, occasionally causes pain in the jaw, teeth and gums, which begins 1–2 days after an injection and passes off within 3 days. Some patients who have received weekly injections of VLB for several months develop persistent pain in one of the large joints, usually the shoulder, which abates when the injections are discontinued. Both VLB and VCR cause tissue necrosis if leakage outside a vein occurs. Both drugs are immunosuppressive.

Vinblastine is an indispensable drug in the management of generalized Hodgkin's disease. VLB is often administered in combination with an alkylating agent because the remission rate is higher than when either drug is used alone and because the onset of resistance is less likely. VLB administered intra-arterially has occasionally been effective in causing sufficient regression in extensive epidermoid carcinomas arising in the facial region to permit radical radiotherapy. It has also been reported as useful in the treatment of gliomata when administered intra-arterially.

Vincristine is an indispensable drug in the treatment of lymphoblastic leukaemia, lymphosarcoma (poorly differentiated lymphocytic lymphoma), and histiocytic lymphoma (reticulum-cell sarcoma), and is sometimes effective in the treatment of Hodgkin's disease, neuroblastoma, and nephroblastoma. Because of its neurotoxic effects it is rarely possible to administer it alone sufficiently frequently at a dosage high enough to be effective in any of these conditions, and it is used to greatest advantage in combination with other drugs.

There is some evidence that when VLB and VCR are administered together their antineoplastic effect is additive. Thus a response equivalent to that given by a full dose of either drug administered alone would be obtained by using half doses of both drugs with a corresponding reduction in the neurotoxic effect of the VCR and of the myelosuppressive effect of VLB.

MISCELLANEOUS DRUGS

Dibromomannitol (*DBM*) is one of a series of halogenated sugars with cytotoxic properties. It is thought to acts as an alkylating agent. It is well tolerated when administered orally at a daily dosage of 200 mg. per m^2. but often causes anorexia, nausea, and vomiting at higher dosage. It is a powerful myelotoxic agent, and is effective in the treatment of chronic myeloid leukaemia. Stabilization of the leucocyte count is more difficult to achieve than is the case with busulphan, but DBM is sometimes effective in busulphan-resistant patients, and its chief value lies in this. Treatment is begun with a 5-day course at a daily dose of 500 mg. per $m.^2$, and after an interval up to 8 weeks to permit observation of the trend in the leucocyte count, an attempt is made to stabilize the leucocyte count by using continuous therapy at a daily dose between 100 and 200 mg. per m^2.

Hydroxyurea, structurally the simplest cytotoxic drug, inhibits the reduction of the ribonucleotides to the corresponding deoxyribonucleotides and so interferes with DNA synthesis. Its effect, though powerful, is short-lived. It is myelotoxic and useful in the management of chronic myeloid leukaemia, particularly in busulphan-resistant cases. It is more difficult to stabilize the leucocyte count with hydroxyurea than with busulphan, and the count often rises steeply when administration is stopped.

Urethane, whose mode of action is unknown, was one of the first cytotoxic drugs submitted for clinical trial. It is myelotoxic and was formerly used in the treatment of chronic myeloid leukaemia. Its disadvantage is that, at therapeutic doses it causes flatulence, anorexia, nausea and vomiting, and nowadays its use is confined to the treatment of patients suffering from myelomatosis that has become resistant to melphalan or cyclophosphamide.

Procarbazine, a methylhydrazine derivative, whose mode of action is unknown, is an indispensable drug in the management of generalized Hodgkin's disease. It is effective in patients who have become resistant to alkylating agents and the vinca alkaloids. It is, however, a powerful myelotoxic drug, and also frequently causes anorexia, nausea and vomiting. When used alone, resistance develops more rapidly than is usually the case when drugs of other classes are used alone. Procarbazine is therefore almost always administered in short courses in combination with vincristine or vinblastine, cyclophosphamide or mustine, and prednisolone; it is usually administered orally at a daily dose of 100 mg. per $m.^2$ for 14 days. Procarbazine may also be administered intravenously. It is sometimes effective in the treatment of lymphosarcoma and reticulum-cell sarcoma.

L-*Asparaginase* represents an entirely different class of chemotherapeutic agent from all others. The L-asparaginases are proteins with enzyme activity, splitting an amino group from the amino acid L-asparagine which becomes converted to aspartic acid. The enzymes are produced by several birds, one order of mammals (Caviidae), and by several genera of bacteria. The detailed structures of the enzymes vary according to their source, and those of bacterial origin have glutaminase activity, believed to reside in the asparaginase molecule itself. The preparations in clinical use, or under trial in Great Britain are derived from bacteria, two from strains of *Escherichia coli*, and one from a strain of *Erwinia caratovora*, a plant pathogen.

The antitumour activity of L-asparaginase was first demonstrated in several strains of murine leukaemia, which could be cured if sufficiently high doses were administered. The antitumour effect was attributed to the action of asparaginase in destroying the body pool of asparagine which was required by the tumour cells and which they were unable to synthesize. The lack of toxicity of the asparaginase for the mice was explained by the capacity of all the normal cells to synthesize asparagine: thus they were independent of an external supply of asparagine.

L-Asparaginase therapy was found to be effective in inducing remissions in children suffering from lymphoblastic leukaemia who had become resistant to all other forms of treatment. About 30 per cent. of patients respond. L-Asparaginase has been administered at doses comparable to those that have cured murine leukaemia, but in the human disease, the remissions are always temporary, they cannot be prolonged indefinitely by maintenance therapy, and if the treatment is administered in courses, the disease usually becomes resistant after the second course. Further remissions may sometimes be obtained if asparaginase from another source is used.

Asparaginase therapy is usually deferred until the patient has become resistant to other methods of treatment. It is not used early in the disease, because the remission rate is lower than with other drugs, especially prednisolone and vincristine in combination. However, asparaginase therapy is undergoing trials as one of a group of drugs used in programmes of intensive therapy aiming at eradicating the disease. Asparaginase is administered intravenously; 28 daily injections are given.

Asparaginase preparations, being proteins, are antigenic, and allergic reactions can be troublesome. They commonly take the form of shivering attacks, chills, urticarial reactions, or respiratory difficulty resulting from bronchospasm, and usually appear after the 10th day of treatment. Some patients can be desensitized by administering a series of doses throughout the day, starting at very low dosage, and increasing the dose with successive injections. The administration of diphenhydramine also helps to minimize allergic reactions in some cases.

Other side-effects of currently available asparaginase preparations are fever, anorexia and nausea, which affect about one in four patients. The enzyme is less innocuous than was formerly supposed, and the synthesis of at least two serum proteins, fibrinogen and albumin is impaired during therapy. Serum fibrinogen levels may fall by 90 per cent. during the first week of treatment, but the level subsequently returns to normal although the treatment is continued; this suggests that the liver cells normally obtain part of their asparagine from an external source and require time to replace the loss by increasing their own synthetic activity. The serum albumin levels usually fall by less than 50 per cent. The haemoglobin concentration of anaemic patients who remit during asparaginase therapy often rises less rapidly than would be expected, and this may indicate that erythroblasts depend in part on externally derived asparagine for haemoglobin synthesis. Finally there is evidence that asparaginase depresses immunological capacity.

Apart from lymphoblastic leukaemia, other malignant diseases have not been found to be regularly sensitive to asparaginase. In myeloblastic leukaemia, the myeloblast count, when raised, frequently falls during the first week of treatment and subsequently rises. This effect may be analogous to that described for serum fibrinogen levels. The leukaemic blasts depend in part on an external source of asparagine, and require time to increase their own synthetic capacity. It is not known whether the effect is of therapeutic value.

PRINCIPLES OF CHEMOTHERAPY

From the previous section, it will be appreciated that the majority of cytotoxic drugs are effective only in a limited range of conditions, that their antitumour activity depends on the same properties that render them harmful to normal growing cells, and that any selectivity they possess against malignant tissues depends on the same type of variation in growth characteristics that is found in normal growing tissues. Therapeutic efficacy is almost always obtained only at the cost of considerable toxicity, and because of this it is never justified to begin chemotherapy without careful consideration of the maximum benefit likely to be obtained in relation to the toxic effects certain to be produced. The aims of treatment, and therefore its strategy, vary according to the disease. In choriocarcinoma and early Burkitt lymphoma, the aim is to eradicate the tumour, and the prospects of doing so are sufficiently good to justify the production of toxic effects, in the expectation that no further treatment will be required, and that the toxic effects will not be permanent. In Hodgkin's disease, the aim is good palliation, and therefore chemotherapy in one form or another will be necessary for the rest of the patient's life. A policy of treatment must be planned in the expectation that the patient will live for many years; in this circumstance it is not justified to incur a burden of toxic effects out of proportion to the benefits conferred. On the other hand chemotherapy must be administered at doses likely to be effective. There is no justification for using cytotoxic drugs at low doses as placebos as is done all too frequently. This type of treatment may cause cumulative toxicity and yet be totally ineffective in its antitumour activity.

The strategy of clinical chemotherapy is based on the necessity for achieving a balance between maximal destruction of the tumour cells and an acceptable burden of toxic effects. Two assumptions, based on experimental work and not fully established in human malignant disease, underlie the practice of chemotherapy. The first is that tumour-cell growth, being largely independent of the homeostatic control that regulates the growth of normal cells, proceeds exponentially, and the second is that at a given dose, some chemotherapeutic agents destroy the same proportion of cells whatever the size of the population at risk. Thus the same dose that reduces a population of 10 million cells to 1 million cells would be required to reduce a population of 10 cells to 1 cell.

In some circumstances tumour cells almost certainly do grow exponentially, and are more likely to do so when they grow in a free-living state in optimal conditions for the inflow of oxygen and nutrients and the removal of metabolites. Such conditions apply more closely to undifferentiated leukaemic cells growing in the bone marrow than to a 'solid' tumour, where the vascularization is precarious, and overcrowding leads to massive necrosis. Even in undifferentiated leukaemic-cell populations, however, there is evidence that only a proportion of the cells are 'in cycle' and growing exponentially. Even if the exponentially growing cells are considered as a separate sub-population, the total increase in that sub-population will proceed exponentially only if all the daughter cells in each generation live to divide again. There is evidence that a variable proportion of the actively proliferating cells in each generation die, so that the doubling time of the sub-population is longer than the generation time of its cells. The doubling time of the whole population (that is the sum of the exponentially dividing sub-population and the resting cells) is longer still. In undifferentiated free-living tumour-cell populations therefore, the doubling time is determined by the relative proportions of resting cells and dividing cells, the death rate in the dividing-cell population, by the generation time of the dividing cells, and by the survival curve of the resting-cell population. In solid tumours with differentiation the relatively simple condition just described is complicated by the following features: first, the stromal and vascular components account for a variable and often substantial proportion of the tumour mass; secondly, some of the component cells differentiate and the mature cells may have a long life span during which they may elaborate a specific product, for example keratin or mucin, that adds materially to the bulk of the tumour. Regional necrosis resulting from vascular insufficiency adds to the non-proliferating part of the tumour. Thus a large tumour may increase in size from factors other than cell division, and the proportion of undifferentiated cells proliferating exponentially may be relatively small. The doubling time of the tumour mass will be very long in relation to the generation time of the proliferating tumour cells. Nevertheless the whole tumour may increase in size exponentially, as shown for example in serial radiological measurements of discrete cannon-ball metastases in lung parenchyma.

The hypothesis of the exponential cell-killing effect of cytotoxic drugs is important because, in theory, it points to the possibility of killing every cell in a given population. Thus, if a course of treatment destroys 90 per cent. of tumour cells, then with an initial population of 10^9 cells, a series of nine similar courses would reduce the population to a single cell, and there would be a 90 per cent. chance that a tenth course would destroy that cell. The hypothesis has been successfully applied to several experimental tumours, and its success led to attempts to eradicate human lymphoblastic leukaemia by repeated courses of intensive chemotherapy. It seems likely, however, that for some drugs, the survival curves for tumour-cell population are hyperbolic rather than exponential; the percentage of cells killed by a given dose of drug falls increasingly rapidly as the cell population declines.

In spite of the qualifications just summarized, the exponential growth of tumours and the exponential cell-killing effect of cytotoxic drugs are probably the most accurate available descriptions on which to plan clinical chemotherapy, and are accepted in the following account.

EXTENT OF CONTROL OF TUMOUR GROWTH ACHIEVED BY DIFFERENT METHODS OF USING CYTOTOXIC DRUGS

FIGURES 23 and 24 illustrate the effect on the growth of a population of tumour cells under the influence of chemotherapy administered by two methods in different clinical circumstances, at different time intervals. The two methods are as follows: the first [FIG. 23, curves 2 and 4; FIG. 24, curves 1, 2 and 3] represents a course of treatment with one drug, or several drugs in combination, at sufficiently high dosage to destroy a substantial fraction of the tumour, assumed to be the same fraction in every course of treatment; the second [FIG. 23, curves 1a and 1b] represents continuous chemotherapy with one drug or several drugs in combination, at low dosage designed for maintenance therapy. In FIGURE 23, curves 1 and 1a, the dosage is such that the number of tumour cells destroyed is exactly balanced by the number of new cells produced, resulting in a steady state, whereas in curve 1b, the dosage is the same, but some of the tumour cells have become resistant to the treatment and are increasing in number more rapidly than the sensitive cells which are still being destroyed at the same rate as they are produced; thus the continuous treatment previously effective in maintaining a steady state is no longer effective.

Both FIGURES 23 and 24 are divided into 4 sections, A, B, C, and D, which relate the clinical effects of the tumour to the total number of cells. Thus in section A the number of tumour cells is too small to be detected by any known means; in section B their presence can be detected by laboratory methods (for example, human chorionic gonadotrophin assay in choriocarcinoma, serum acid phosphatase assay in prostatic carcinoma, paraprotein assay in myelomatosis) but not by clinical or radiological means; in section C, the tumour is large enough to give rise to physical signs or radiological abnormalities, but the patient has no symptoms; in section D, the patient has symptoms.

This subdivision is admittedly artificial and the extent to which it can be applied to different forms of malignant disease varies greatly, but it is useful to illustrate the principles of chemotherapy.

Maintenance Therapy

FIGURE 23 (curve 1a) shows that continuous therapy at low dosage, that prevents the tumour from growing but does not reduce its size, provides excellent symptomatic control when applied to a tumour that has been already reduced by more aggressive treatment (curve 2) below the size at which it causes symptoms. However, the same treatment is useless if administered when the tumour has advanced into section D and is giving rise to symptoms. No matter how long the treatment is continued, the total number of tumour cells will not decrease and the symptoms will persist. At best, the treatment will prevent the situation deteriorating. The use of busulphan at low daily dosage for maintenance in chronic myeloid leukaemia after an initial course at higher dosage illustrates the practical application of curves 2 and 1a, while the onset of busulphan-resistance is illustrated by curve 1b.

Maintenance therapy is only practicable in conditions that respond to drugs which can be safely administered for long periods without incurring insupportable side-effects, and which do not rapidly engender resistance.

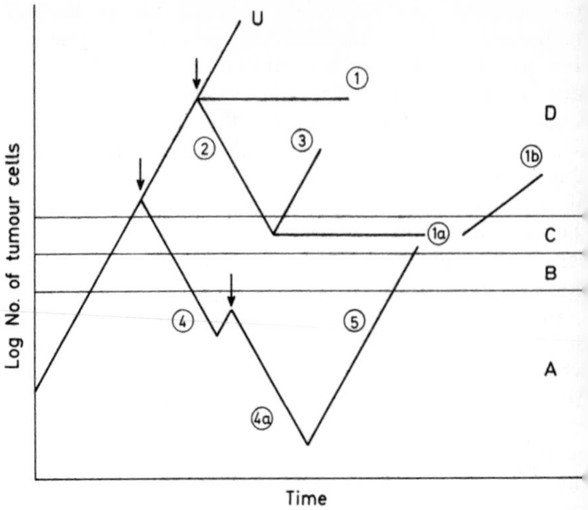

FIG. 23. The effect of chemotherapy on the size of a tumour-cell population. The clinical condition is shown in relation to the number of tumour cells.

Sections A, B, and C: the patient has no symptoms; A, no evidence of the presence of tumour; B, the presence of tumour is shown by special laboratory tests only; C, there is radiological or clinical evidence of disease. *Section D:* the patient has symptoms. The tumour growth is assumed to be exponential (U). Three courses of chemotherapy (2, 4, 4a) at the same dosage destroy the same proportion of tumour cells whatever the total number of cells when the treatment is begun (indicated by arrows). In 2, the symptoms are relieved, but clinical or radiological evidence of disease persists; in 4, symptoms are relieved, all clinical and laboratory evidence of the presence of tumour disappears; in 4a, the treatment is given to an apparently healthy patient. After the effect of the treatment has worn off, the tumour grows at the same rate as before; in 3, symptoms return rapidly; after 4, the further growth is arrested by course 4a; and in 5, the return of symptoms is delayed. Maintenance therapy at low dosage that sustains a steady state does not relieve symptoms in 1, and does not cause any tumour regression in 1a; maintenance therapy is continued in 1b, but the tumour has become resistant to the treatment.

Single-course Therapy

A single course of treatment at high dosage given to a patient in an advanced state of relapse with symptoms may completely relieve the symptoms [FIG. 23, curve 2] but at the end of the course, if maintenance therapy is not given, the tumour will resume its growth at the same rate (U) as before, and in a short time the symptoms will return (curve 3). The same course of treatment administered at an earlier stage of relapse will produce a better effect in that all evidence of active disease will disappear (curve 4) and the time before symptoms return will be much longer than in situation 2. The length of remission will be still further increased if a second similar course is administered as soon as possible after the first (curve 4a), but the possibility of doing so will depend on the toxic effects brought about and the speed of recovery. It will be noted that treatment 4a is given to a patient who has no evidence of active disease and who considers himself to be well. Until recently physicians have been reluctant to administer further treatment in these circumstances, because they were unwilling to inflict distressing and potentially dangerous toxic injury to fit patients whom they knew they could not cure, or were most unlikely to cure. However, attitudes have changed since it has been demonstrated beyond doubt that carefully planned intensive therapy was to the patients' long-term advantage in particular forms of malignant disease, especially choriocarcinoma, Burkitt's lymphoma, Hodgkin's disease, histiocytic lymphoma (reticulum-cell sarcoma), poorly-differentiated lymphocytic lymphoma (lymphosarcoma), lymphoblastic leukaemia, perhaps acute myeloid leukaemia, nephroblastoma, neuroblastoma, embryonal sarcoma, disseminated testicular seminoma, teratoma, and ovarian adenocarcinoma.

Once the desirability of attempting more than relief of symptoms is accepted, the logical inference is to continue treatment as far beyond the limit shown in FIGURE 1, curve 4a, as the patient will tolerate. In correct practice the possibility of doing so is severely limited by the toxicity of the available drugs, which limits the amounts that can be administered and determines the intervals at which courses of treatment can be repeated. FIGURE 24 illustrates the consequences of varying the interval between courses of treatment.

Curve 1 illustrates the outcome when four courses of treatment are administered, each course being started when the patient complained of symptoms. The symptoms are successfully relieved by each course, but clinical or radiological evidence of disease persists throughout, and the condition of the patient at the end of the period is substantially the same as at the beginning. If the same series of four courses were begun when the disease was at a less advanced stage (for example, in section C of FIG. 24), and the intervals between the courses were the same, the disease would be controlled to the extent that the patient would be free of symptoms throughout the period, but as before his over-all condition would not have improved.

If a series of courses designed to relieve symptoms on the lines of curve 1 is planned, but symptoms recur

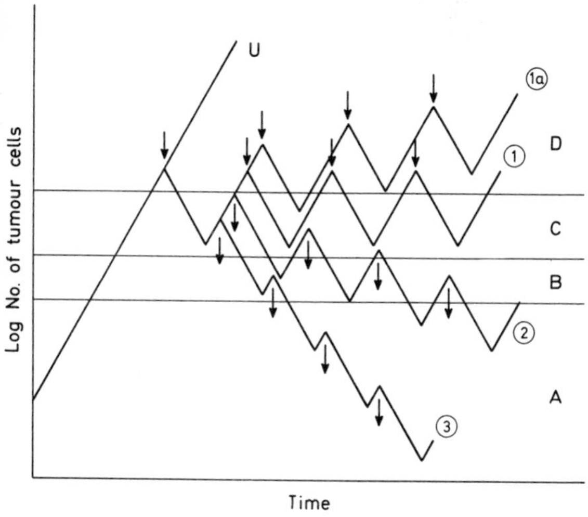

FIG. 24. The effect of varying the interval between courses of treatment at the same dosage on the size of a tumour-cell population. Letter symbols as in FIG 23. In 1, the interval between courses does not prevent the return of symptoms, but is short enough to maintain an essentially steady state. In 1a, the intervals are rather longer, and after the second course the treatment fails to relieve symptoms. In 2, the second course is begun before the return of symptoms, and the third is begun when there are no clinical or radiological signs of the disease, although the presence of tumour is revealed by special tests. In 3, the intervals between courses are short enough to permit considerable reduction in the size of the tumour-cell population.

before the patient has fully recovered from the toxic effects of the first course there will be no possibility of controlling the disease with this form of treatment, because only two alternatives are available. Either treatment must be deferred until the patient has recovered from the toxic effects (curve 1a), or the dosage used in each course must be reduced. The effect will be the same, in that the disease will continue to advance and the treatment will no longer relieve the symptoms. On the other hand, courses of treatment that can be repeated at frequent intervals without incurring insupportable toxicity will lead to progressive reduction in the total number of tumour cells [FIG. 24, curves 2 and 3] and so will lengthen the duration of remission. Curve 3 shows that the most satisfactory result follows when successive courses are administered at very short intervals. The symptoms are relieved after the first course, all clinical and radiological evidence of disease disappears after the second, while after the third evidence of activity is not obtainable at all. In choriocarcinoma, the line dividing section A from section B could be drawn lower in the figure, because the assay of HCG in the urine permits the recognition of a smaller number of tumour cells in the body (about 10^6) than can yet be achieved with any other tumour, and this assay is used to determine the end-point of treatment. No comparable assay of minimal tumour activity is available for any other human malignant disease.

Advantages of Multiple-Drug Therapy

The use of several drugs in sequence or in various combinations is now common practice and is justified by the following considerations: first, the need to reduce the likelihood of the development of resistance; second, the need to reduce the severity of toxic effects; third, the hope of increasing the therapeutic effect by synergism, or by the use of drugs acting independently by different mechanisms and affecting tumour cells at different stages in the cell cycle.

Sequential therapy was an inevitable result of the introduction of new drugs. For ethical reasons, new drugs were first given only to patients who had become resistant to the drugs already available, and as more new drugs were found to be effective, patients were treated by using each drug in turn, usually in the order in which they were introduced, the change from one to another being determined by the onset of resistance, or poor tolerance.

The acquisition of *resistance*, though highly characteristic of malignant cells is not confined to them. Thus patients with idiopathic cold haemagglutinin disease become resistant to chlorambucil, those with systemic lupus erythematosus become resistant to immunosuppressive drugs, while under experimental conditions, resistance to busulphan can be induced in normal lens epithelial cells. The nature of resistance to cytotoxic drugs by cells that were formerly sensitive is unknown and is unlikely to be the same in all cases. There are experimental systems in which resistance may be shown to arise by a genetic change akin to mutation in a very small number of tumour cells in a large population. The change is stable, heritable, and confers a selective advantage on the cells bearing it, enabling them to replace the original population. The initial change is considered to arise by chance and to be a rare event. If the population were exposed to two drugs simultaneously, a mutant cell resistant to one drug would be as likely to be killed by the other as sensitive cells, and the same reasoning would apply to a mutant cell resistant to the second drug. Since mutation is always a rare event the chance of a single cell bearing two independent mutations conferring resistance to both drugs would be infinitesimally small: it would be the reciprocal of the product of the frequency of each mutation. The frequency of resistant mutants arising would be correspondingly lower if more than two drugs were administered simultaneously.

The toxic effects that accompany an effective course of treatment with any particular drug may be insupportable. If two drugs of equal efficacy but acting independently and having different limiting toxic effects are each administered at one half of the dosage necessary to obtain the desired effect, their therapeutic actions will summate, but their specific toxic effects will be one half of those resulting from the full dose, if the ratio of the toxic effects and the therapeutic action is the same at all dose levels. A further reduction in toxicity would result if more drugs were added. Several examples of the exploitation of this phenomenon were given in the section on individual cytotoxic drugs.

Synergism would be expected if two drugs having a comparable antitumour effect acted by unrelated mechanisms. Thus a drug acting only on cells actively synthesizing DNA (S-phase cells) would affect the proliferating cells in a tumour only if its administration were continued long enough to permit all those cells to enter the S phase, but those tumour cells that were out of cycle during the period of exposure would not be affected at all. If a second drug, active also against resting cells, were administered simultaneously, the proportion of susceptible cells in the tumour would be correspondingly greater than if an equivalent dose of the S-phase active drug had been administered instead. Unfortunately, little is known about the basic mechanisms of action of most of the available drugs, and the combinations that have proved useful in practice have largely been chosen empirically and the basis of selection has depended more on the desire to minimize toxicity than on an established rationale of differential mechanism of action.

The possibility must be considered also that certain drug combinations deemed suitable from the standpoint of tolerance, might be antagonistic. Thus a drug that reduced the proportion of cells entering the S phase would limit the efficacy of a drug that acts only on cells in the S phase. Without doubt, improvements in multiple drug therapy will depend on a better understanding of the mechanisms of action of the drugs. The number of drugs available and the numerous variations in dose schedules that are possible with each one makes it increasingly unlikely that effective schedules will be devised empirically. It is indeed possible to show by means of mathematical models which define the growth characteristics of tumour-cell populations and of regenerating normal cell populations, that the chance of devising schedules of treatment that will cause irreversible damage to normal proliferating cells and yet fail to destroy the tumour cells is higher than the chance of devising a safe schedule that will prove effective in eliminating all the tumour cells.

Chemotherapy Records

The expectation of life in several forms of advanced malignant disease has been increased by cytotoxic chemotherapy. On the other hand chemotherapy is inevitably hazardous and potentially lethal because of the toxic effects of the drugs, and thus imposes a grave responsibility on the clinician. A patient may receive repeated courses of treatment with ten or more different cytotoxic drugs during as many years, and it is clearly essential that the records of the treatment, of the response to it, and of the toxic effects produced, be kept in such a way that at all stages it must be possible to survey every detail of the previous course of the disease, to discover exactly which drugs had been administered, by which routes, and in which doses and combinations, and to review the indications for which each course of treatment had been administered, and the criteria by which its efficacy had been assessed. It is important to be able to find out rapidly whether the response to recent courses of treatment was as satisfactory and as long lasting as the response to earlier courses, and whether the severity of the toxic effects was greater than before. This information makes it possible to plan the future treatment rationally. Hospital records are not adapted for retrieving the information in a form that permits the exacting assessment essential for the most efficient management of patients receiving chemotherapy with cytotoxic drugs. Long experience has shown that the simplest way of recording the essential information is by the use of a chart with a linear time scale on which the details of all drugs administered are entered by a system of bars indicating the doses and the dates on which the treatment was begun and ended. Most cytotoxic drugs are myelotoxic, and the trends in the haemoglobin concentration, platelet, total leucocyte and neutrophil counts provide the best index of bone marrow depression. The chart should include a section with a logarithmic scale for plotting the platelet and leucocyte counts. The details of treatment and the blood counts are entered at every visit and other clinical, radiological or biochemical details relevant to the particular case are entered also. Potentially dangerous trends resulting from the treatment are much more easily appreciated by the inspection of the chart than is possible from hospital records or from numerical data in tabular form. The intervals between courses of treatment indicate the duration of remissions, and the extent to which control of the disease is being maintained or lost can be appreciated at a glance. The charts are as indispensable in the practice of chemotherapy as are conventional ward temperature charts in the management of febrile illnesses.

ENDOCRINE THERAPY

Prostatic, mammary, and endometrial carcinoma have some of the characteristics of the *conditional neoplasms* (Foulds) of experimental oncology. Conditional neoplasms grow in certain specific environmental conditions; when the conditions are altered the neoplasms regress but do not die. They persist in a non-proliferating state of *residual neoplasia* and resume active growth when their specific requirements are restored. At any time some or all of the cells in a conditional neoplasm change their character by acquiring the capacity to grow in the absence of the specific conditions that were previously essential. Alteration of the specific conditions will now lead to regression of that part of the neoplasm that has retained its conditional character, but not of the part that has lost its former dependence on those conditions. Conditional neoplasia in hormone-dependent tissues may be regarded as an expression of differentiation. The growth of these tissues is determined by their hormonal environment, and in the absence of the appropriate stimuli the tissues remain dormant. When such a tissue becomes neoplastic its capacity for growth may remain wholly or partly dependent on hormonal stimuli for some time. Thus prostatic carcinoma and its metastases, like normal prostatic epithelium may regress and remain dormant following orchidectomy, but unlike the normal epithelium, some or all of the deposits of the carcinoma will at some stage acquire the capacity to grow in the absence of testicular control. Treatment with oestrogens is as effective as orchidectomy, and is thought to suppress testicular activity by inhibiting the production of pituitary gonadotrophins. However, oestrogens may have a direct inhibitory effect on the carcinoma, because regression may be occasionally observed in orchidectomized patients in relapse.

Normal adult prostatic epithelial cells secrete acid phosphatase, but lose their capacity for doing so after orchidectomy. Prostatic carcinoma cells often secrete acid phosphatase, and the trend in the serum concentration provides an index of the activity of the disease. Following orchidectomy or oestrogen treatment, the serum acid-phosphatase level falls to the normal range. In relapse, however, the tumour cells may secrete acid phosphatase although they are no longer under the influence of androgens, and no longer respond to oestrogen therapy. On the other hand, the tumour cells responsible for the relapse may no longer secrete the enzyme, and in this circumstance serial estimations of the serum acid phosphatase do not provide a warning of impending relapse.

Mammary carcinoma is less often hormone dependent than prostatic carcinoma. Pre-menopausal women may respond to oophorectomy and the response is usually attributed to oestrogen deprivation. Patients who relapse after oophorectomy may respond to bilateral adrenalectomy or to hypophysectomy, and the response is attributed to the removal of oestrogens of adrenal origin. Androgen therapy also induces remission in 25 per cent. of pre-menopausal patients, and a proportion of these patients who relapse while receiving androgens will respond again to oophorectomy. At the time of the menopause, and for the 5 years before and after, patients rarely respond to endocrine ablation therapy or to hormone therapy. Elderly women are more likely to respond to oestrogens than to androgens and this effect is difficult to explain, particularly as adrenalectomy or hypophysectomy are sometimes effective when these patients relapse.

About one third of patients suffering from disseminated endometrial carcinoma respond to treatment with progestational agents, administered continuously for months or years until one or more of the metastases lose their sensitivity. Patients whose disease has recurred following a previous hysterectomy respond as well and as frequently as those who present with disseminated disease. Even numerous large pulmonary deposits may regress during progestogen therapy. Regression is usually evident within 3 months of starting the treatment, and when no significant change has occurred after 3 months, the patient is unlikely to benefit by continuing the treatment.

FURTHER READING

ANDERSON, E. G. (1966) Non-metastatic syndromes associated with carcinoma of the bronchus. 1. The endocrine syndromes, *Hosp. Med.*, **1**, 11.

BARTTER, F. C. (1970) The syndrome of inappropriate secretion of antidiuretic hormone, *J. roy. Coll. Phyns Lond.*, **4**, 264.

BOESEN, E., and DAVIS, W. (1970) *Cytotoxic Drugs in the Treatment of Cancer*, London.

BRAIN, LORD, and MORRIS, F. H., eds (1965) *The Remote Effects of Cancer on the Nervous System. Contemporary Neurology Symposia*, Vol. 1, New York.

CLINE, M. J. (1971) *Cancer Chemotherapy. Major Problems in Internal Medicine*, Vol. 1, Philadelphia.

COLE, W. H., ed. (1970) *Chemotherapy of Cancer*, Philadelphia.

FAIRLEY, G. H. (1969) Immunity to malignant disease in man, Goulstonian Lecture, *Brit. med. J.*, **2**, 467.

FORREST, A. P. M. (1971) Hormonal influences in breast cancer, *Proc. roy. Soc. Med.*, **64**, 509.

FOULDS, L. (1969) *Neoplastic Development*, Vol. 1, New York.

HERON, J. R. (1966) Non-metastatic syndromes associated with carcinoma of the bronchus. 2. The neuromuscular syndromes, *Hosp. Med.*, **1**, 106.

LAURENT, J., DEBRY, G., and FLOQUET, J. (1971) *Hypoglycaemic Tumours*, Amsterdam.

STOKER, M. G. P. (1971) Oncogenic viruses, Leeuwenhoek Lecture, *Proc. roy. Soc. Med.* (in press).

STOLL, B. A. (1969) *Hormonal Management in Breast Cancer* London.

D. A. G. GALTON

DISORDERS OF METABOLISM

INTRODUCTION

Every disease process is associated with quantitative or qualitative changes in some aspects of metabolism. Often these are of minor importance; often their correction is crucial to recovery; sometimes they may themselves endanger life though they are not the initial cause of the illness; and at times the biochemical disturbance may play an over-all part in the production of the clinical syndrome.

A metabolic disorder may arise in the purest form as a result of some genetic abnormality, for genes control metabolism via specific enzymes; chemical poisons may also induce changes which are quite obviously and directly metabolic. A genetic 'abnormality' may exist without producing symptoms or ill health. Under certain conditions, however, for example when specific drugs are given, an illness may be precipitated; some patients with hepatic porphyria behave in this way. Again, detoxication of drugs may be inefficient as a result of a genetically determined defect in the required metabolic pathway. Subjects with such a make-up have a high incidence of toxic reactions to the drug concerned. Probably the best example of such an effect is to be found in the case of isonicotinic acid hydrazide, where persons with a defective acetylation mechanism are very prone to suffer from toxic neurological abnormalities when they receive the drug in normal therapeutic doses.

In general, patients suffer from symptoms and these may be produced by functional abnormalities which may arise long before any structural changes can be detected. Thus more and more, with the advance of medicine and with the desire for earlier diagnosis, it becomes necessary to search for the metabolic derangements which so frequently account for the patient's discomfort and which may so often be improved even when the underlying cause is not curable.

It will be obvious, therefore, that the subjects included under this section are often of general importance and are not necessarily related only to one specific disease.

BASAL METABOLIC RATE

By basal metabolism is meant the metabolism of an individual when he is lying down, completely relaxed, and in the postabsorptive state, i.e. about twelve hours after the last meal.

During sleep metabolic processes take place even more slowly than in the so-called basal state described above. On the other hand food, particularly protein, will increase the metabolic rate, this increased metabolism being largely due to increased hepatic activity. The metabolic rate (the rate of heat production) of an individual is usually measured indirectly by measuring the rate of oxygen consumption (or CO_2 production, or both) and by calculating from this the rate of heat production. In practice the rate of oxygen consumption is the usual measurement which is made and a respiratory quotient of 0·85 is assumed. The individual is made to breathe from and into a closed system containing oxygen and also soda-lime to absorb the exhaled carbon dioxide. The rate of oxygen consumption, corrected to standard temperature and pressure, and the amount of heat produced when this enters into the combustion of foodstuffs, is calculated on the assumption that one litre of oxygen at Standard Temperature and Pressure (S.T.P.) corresponds to the release of 4·83 kilocalories. This is then, conventionally, divided by the surface area of the individual, expressed in square metres, and itself calculated indirectly from the height and weight of the person concerned. A 'normal' average value is obtained from tables and this is subtracted from the found value. This difference is then divided by the 'normal' average value and multiplied by one hundred, the figure being expressed as a percentage above or below normal.

It can be seen that there are several assumptions in the derivation of this figure which are of questionable accuracy. It is also out of keeping with modern practice to express a result as 'plus' or 'minus' a percentage of an arbitrary normal and this method of expressing a result may effectively disguise the real state of affairs, for the actual rate of heat production is not indicated. To say that the B.M.R. of an obese person is 'normal' only means that the basal metabolism of that individual has increased in proportion to his increase in calculated surface area; it gives no indication of the actual rate of heat production, a figure which is of much greater interest when considering metabolic balance. Furthermore, even in the normal, metabolic rate is not strictly related to surface area and in abnormal states there may be great differences in the ratio of metabolically active tissue to surface area. This is well illustrated by subjects who are severely undernourished, for their basal metabolic rate, expressed conventionally in terms of surface area is very low, whereas in terms of metabolically active tissue the reduction is much less. In such subjects, the discrepancy seems mainly to be caused by a greatly increased extracellular fluid volume (shown, when extreme, as famine oedema) which increases the calculated surface area without contributing anything to the metabolic rate.

Determination of metabolically active tissue is difficult and is in itself somewhat arbitrary. It is unlikely to be used in routine clinical practice with existing methods of estimation. The B.M.R. itself is rapidly being discarded by many clinics. Its chief use has been the determination of thyroid function, but on account of its many inherent fallacies, its non-specific nature (it is increased in patients with, e.g. pyrexia, anaemia, certain cardiovascular diseases, leukaemia and certain other malignant diseases and in patients with a phaeochromocytoma as well as in hyperthyroidism) and because there are now many other effective ways of measuring thyroid activity, it has lost its previous importance to the discerning physician.

SALT AND WATER METABOLISM

General Considerations

Water contributes 50–70 per cent. to the total body weight. This body water can be divided into extracellular and intracellular compartments. The extracellular water is distributed in a multiplicity of 'spaces', the chief being the interstitial fluid and the plasma. Extracellular water is also present, however, in the gut, in the secretions of exocrine glands and such places as joint cavities and subarachnoid spaces. Urine in the bladder is not included in estimation of extracellular water.

There is less water in fat cells than in others and thus the proportion of the body weight which is due to water is an inverse function of the degree of obesity. In the obese the total body water may be less than 50 per cent. of the body weight, whereas in lean subjects it may be about 70 per cent.

'Extracellular water' and 'total body water' can each be estimated in a variety of ways; total body water by measuring the dilution of deuterium or of tritiated water, and extracellular volume by measuring the dilution of substances such as insulin, bromide, chloride or thiocyanate which are supposed not to enter cells to any significant extent. Intracellular water cannot be measured directly, but an estimate can be obtained by subtracting the ascertained volume of extracellular water from that found for total body water. TABLE 29 gives the volumes of the various spaces in an average man weighing 11 st. (70 kg.).

TABLE 29

Total body water	42 litres
Extracellular water	14 litres
Composed of:	
Plasma water	3·0 litres
Interstitial fluid	10·5 litres
Other extracellular compartments.	0·52 litres

Cell membranes are freely permeable to water and it can thus be assumed that for all practical purposes the osmolarity of the various body compartments is of the same order, minor differences occurring as a result of differences in hydrostatic pressure. Most of the osmotic pressure of extracellular fluid results from the presence of electrolytes, the main cations being

Na^+ and the main anions being Cl^-, HCO_3^- and in plasma, protein. In intracellular fluid the most abundant cations are K^+ and Mg^{++} and the main anions are organic phosphates, sulphate, bicarbonate and protein.

Although the capillary wall is freely permeable to ions and molecules of small size, there are nevertheless differences in ionic concentration in plasma compared with interstitial fluid. This is partly because the proteins in plasma are acting as anions and this affects the over-all distribution of ions in accordance with the Donnan equilibrium—the concentration of diffusible anions in interstitial water is 1·05 of that in the plasma whereas for diffusible cations the factor is 0·95. The other reason for small differences in plasma and interstitial fluid electrolyte concentration is that equilibrium concentrations are attained with respect to water. Plasma may contain significant amounts of lipids (especially great in such conditions as the nephrotic syndrome) which will result in significantly lower whole-plasma electrolyte levels although the concentration in plasma water will be the same as in interstitial water, except for the Donnan correcting factors. It will be noted that the concentrations are expressed as milli-equivalents per litre (mEq. per litre). In any solution, the total concentration of anions must equal that of cations when they are both expressed as mEq.

Both sodium and potassium ions are diffusible across cell membranes and the high intracellular potassium concentration and high extracellular sodium concentration is maintained by active cellular energy requiring metabolic extrusion of sodium ion—the so-called 'sodium pump'.

It is obvious, therefore, that a number of mechanisms must exist to control not only the concentration and distribution of the various ions in the different body compartments, but to regulate the total quantities of these substances and of water in the body.

Changes in extracellular osmolarity result in appropriate shifts in the partition of water between the extra- and intracellular compartments. At the same time there are changes in the sensation of thirst and in the concentration of the urine which is being secreted. Thus, if there is an increase in extracellular osmolarity there will be a shift of water from the cells and at the same time, owing to stimulation of Verney's osmoreceptors, a greater quantity of antidiuretic hormone will be released from the posterior pituitary, resulting in the secretion of only small volumes of concentrated urine. Furthermore, a sensation of thirst will be induced, which in normal circumstances will cause water drinking. All of these effects will tend to restore the extracellular osmolarity to normal.

Substances such as urea, and to a lesser extent glucose have similar concentrations on either side of cell membranes whereas Na^+ and Cl^- have not. Changes in Cl^- or other anions can easily be accommodated by inverse changes in the ever available and readily disposable HCO_3^-, whereas there is no immediate way of compensating for changes in the concentration for Na^+. This last ion thus becomes the major unit which controls extracellular osmolarity and, since changes in concentration are much more precisely regulated than changes in total quantity, gains or losses in extracellular sodium tend to be associated with similar gains or losses in extracellular water or volume.

The volume of extracellular fluid tends to be kept constant: (1) by the equilibrium established by the differences in capillary and interstitial hydrostatic pressure and the osmotic pressure of plasma proteins, coupled with (2) control of plasma volume, aldosterone secretion evidently being of great importance in this.

The precise ways in which the rate of aldosterone secretion is regulated are still being worked out, but almost certainly baroreceptors in the carotid arteries and in the right atrium are concerned. In addition angiotensin II from the kidney and a stimulatory substance from the central nervous system (perhaps from the pineal) are probably concerned. Conditions which result in diminution of blood volume or in sequestration of blood into the systemic venous system cause a marked increase in aldosterone secretion with a consequent retention of sodium and loss of potassium. When hyperaldosteronism is stimulated in this way, the sodium retention is accompanied by water retention (presumably via ADH secretion) so that there is an increase in extracellular fluid volume to the extent that gross oedema may occur. By contrast, conditions resulting in an increase in plasma volume produce a fall in aldosterone output. Aldosterone secretion also appears to be stimulated by a raised concentration of potassium and depressed when the concentration is low. It should be noted that primary hyperaldosteronism (Conn's syndrome) is not usually accompanied by oedema [see Section 5].

DEHYDRATION

Dehydration is the body state which results from an abnormally low water content. This lack of water may affect both intracellular and extracellular compartments, or the major deficiency may occur in only one of them.

In the last resort, too little body water must occur as a result of a negative body water balance, hence it arises from any condition which results in the loss of water being greater than the intake plus the metabolic production of water. Water intake is controlled largely by thirst and loss occurs in urine, faeces, in any pathological loss of body fluids such as from intestinal fistulae, vomitus or burns, and as evaporation from the skin and lungs. When active sweating is not occurring, this loss by evaporation is called 'insensible loss' and most of it occurs in the lungs. Its precise measurement is very difficult and to some extent it depends upon the metabolic rate. In the adult it may amount to between 600 and 1000 ml. per day and this loss is obligatory, resulting largely from the saturation by water vapour at body temperature of the air which ventilates the lungs.

Water Dehydration

Water dehydration thus occurs whenever the sum of the water intake plus the water derived from metabolism is insufficient to cover insensible loss plus the 500 ml. or so, which is the minimum content of urine and faeces compatible with the full secretion of waste products. Typically this situation arises when a patient is too ill or too weak to obtain or to ask for water to drink and in special conditions such as on rafts after shipwreck. Intense thirst is a prominent feature of this form of dehydration, but the total loss of intracellular fluid is greater than that of extracellular fluid, and, until the dehydration is severe, there is only a relatively slight increase in the haematocrit and haemoglobin values. There is, however, a considerable diminution in the volume of urine which is highly concentrated. The mouth becomes dry and thirst intense. When the water deficiency becomes severe, the face becomes pinched and 'grey' and there is a diminution in muscular power. There may also be emotional lability and, when the dehydration is very severe, confusion and hallucinations.

Water taken by mouth is rapidly absorbed and produces improvement in the general condition in a matter of minutes.

'Sodium' Dehydration

Whenever the loss of sodium from the body is greater than the intake, there is, as a result of the ADH mechanism, a corresponding net loss in body water. The situation arises in conditions such as vomiting or diarrhoea or in profuse sweating.

Thirst is not a feature of this form of dehydration, the patients suffering more characteristically from languor, apathy, muscular cramps, weakness and fatigue. Headache may be present and also a tendency to syncope on standing. Nausea and vomiting which accentuates the dehydration may occur; the skin lacks its normal elasticity and may become wrinkled. Reasonable volumes of urine are passed until the dehydration becomes very great. There is marked diminution in extracellular fluid and plasma volume so that hypovolaemia and hypotension may ensue. At this stage the haemoglobin concentration and the haematocrit may be markedly raised and the patients may enter a state of oligaemic shock, with cold, clammy skin and peripheral cyanosis. Stupor and even sudden death may then occur. At first the concentration of sodium in the plasma remains in the normal range, but in the severe stages it falls. Gastric emptying is delayed when salt depletion occurs and considerable periods may consequently elapse before adequate quantities of saline can be absorbed from the alimentary tract. It is thus usually advisable to give salt solution intravenously.

Combined Sodium and Water Deprivation

It is of course exceptional for patients to become initially deficient either purely of water or of sodium. For example in profuse sweating water and sodium are lost—water relatively more than sodium. But thirst results in the drinking of large quantities of fluid usually containing little or no sodium. Any excess may be passed in the urine and the patient may thus be dehydrated even though large volumes of urine may be passed. If very large volumes are ingested the sodium concentration may fall so low that early symptoms of water intoxication may occur, though this is rarely severe in the absence of renal disease.

Over-hydration Due Mainly to Excess Water—Water Intoxication

This occurs as the result of an excessive quantity of body water relative to sodium. It usually arises only in the presence of deficient renal function, whether this be due to renal disease or is occurring in association with some general metabolic disturbance such as is found in Addison's disease.

It has been noted to follow the administration of large watery enemas to children with megacolon and to follow the over-enthusiastic efforts to produce sodium depletion in patients with cardiac failure. Rarely, in patients with bronchogenic carcinoma, in attacks of acute porphyria or in a variety of other uncommon conditions low concentrations of serum sodium are found and it is supposed that in some at least there is an inappropriately great secretion of antidiuretic hormone. Sometimes, however, this low [Na^+] may be due to decreased 'sodium pump' activity with resultant entry of Na^+ into cells.

Restlessness, muscle twitching, confusion and, later, convulsions and coma are the main clinical features. It seems probable that these effects are due to excessive intracellular water, since treatment by the intravenous administration of hypertonic saline (e.g. 50–100 ml. of 5 per cent. solution) causes a rapid improvement. This form of therapy should not be undertaken as a routine merely because an asymptomatic low concentration of serum sodium happens to be found.

Over-hydration Due to Combined Water and Sodium Retention

If the combined retention is great enough it leads to oedema formation, the excessive fluid being retained in the interstitial spaces. It occurs in conditions leading to secondary hyperaldosteronism such as congestive heart failure, cirrhosis of the liver and the nephrotic syndrome. It is treated by measures which result in sodium and hence water depletion, such as the restriction of sodium intake to less than 20 mEq. (0·5 g. NaCl) per day, and the use of organic mercurial, or thiazide diuretics. Spironolactone (*Aldactone A*), an aldosterone antagonist, may also be used in conjunction with these measures.

POTASSIUM

As previously pointed out, body potassium is largely situated inside cells. The total body content of potassium is about 3700 mEq. (148 g.) in an adult man and of this only about 80 mEq. (3·2 g.) is extracellular. The normal concentration of potassium inside cells is about 150 mEq. per litre (14–20 mg. per 100 ml.). It is to be emphasized that a low extracellular (and therefore plasma) potassium concentration does not inevitably accompany low intracellular potassium concentrations. Indeed, as in some cases of untreated diabetic coma, the plasma potassium concentration may be higher than normal in spite of a cellular depletion of potassium; under these circumstances a certain amount of sodium may have entered cells. On the other hand low concentrations of plasma potassium are usually associated with some cellular depletion of potassium. Since it is not practicable to estimate intracellular potassium in clinical practice, as with all other clinical problems involving water and electrolytes, a general clinical appraisal of the situation is just as important as a determination of the plasma concentration in deciding on the likelihood of potassium depletion.

Hypopotassaemia

In equilibrium the intake and loss of potassium is equal. With a normal diet this is in the order of 65 mEq. (2·5 g.) per day. The kidney in general does not secrete urine containing potassium at a lower concentration than the plasma. With a urinary volume of, say, 1000 ml. per day at least 4–5 mEq. (160–200 mg.) of potassium must be lost each day in the urine even if there is no intake, and additional potassium is lost in the faeces. Urinary losses may be much bigger than the normal intake in such conditions as diabetic acidosis, so-called base-losing nephritis, the post-operative state, Cushing's syndrome, Conn's syndrome, overdosage with steroid compounds such as cortisone, and as a result of the long term use of diuretics, particularly of the thiazide group, and in association with alkalaemia.

A frequent cause of potassium depletion is excessive loss from the alimentary tract and this may, or may not, be associated with deficient intake. Thus pyloric stenosis, gastro-enteritis, ulcerative colitis, steatorrhoea and continuous aspiration of intestinal contents as carried out after operations on the alimentary tract and in paralytic ileus, may all lead to potassium depletion. It has also been reported as resulting from the misuse of purgatives.

Excess body potassium occurs in Addison's disease and in renal deficiency, otherwise it is almost always the result of therapy when more potassium has been given than can be excreted.

A lowered potassium concentration can occur either in extracellular fluid or in cells or in both. It is by no means clear precisely what part extracellular and what part intracellular potassium defect plays in the over-all potassium deficiency syndrome. The most striking clinical manifestations are changes in the electrocardiogram [FIG. 25], paralysis of voluntary muscle and cardiac arrest.

The plasma concentrations at which these manifestations occur are by no means constant and depend to some extent upon other ionic concentrations; they are, for example, more marked at a given potassium level in the presence of a high sodium or calcium level and in the presence of an acidosis. Lowered potassium concentrations increase the excitability of cardiac muscle and enhance this same effect of digitalis. Paroxysmal tachycardia, whether 'spontaneous', or associated with digitalis therapy may be precipitated by hypopotassaemia. No serious cardiac changes should occur with concentrations above about 2·5 mEq. per litre (10 mg. per 100 ml.) and such changes are preceded by electrocardiographic changes which, though not specific for hypopotassaemia, serve as a good clinical index of the situation. Death may occur at a concentration of about 1·5 mEq. per litre (6 mg. per 100 ml.) or lower.

Other changes, perhaps not so striking and not carrying the same urgent danger, are intestinal ileus and changes in the renal tubules. The latter is associated with deficient concentrating power and deficient ability to secrete hydrogen ions and to form ammonia. Polydipsia may be a prominent symptom. The renal lesions consist of cloudy swelling and increased granularity of the cells of the collecting tubules and papillae and it has been suggested that such kidneys are more susceptible to pyelonephritis.

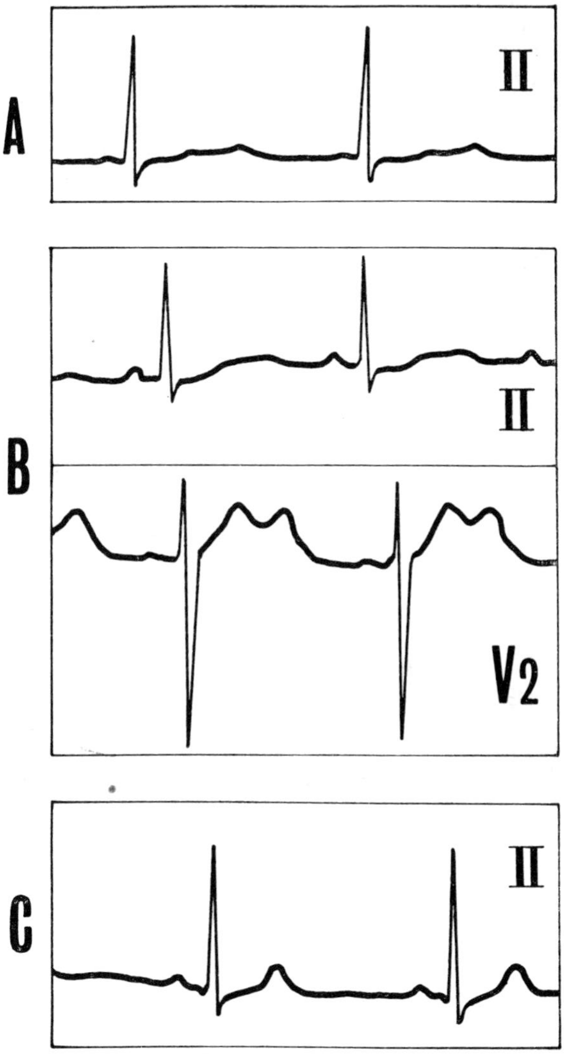

FIG. 25. Electrocardiographic record, showing the effects of potassium depletion in a patient with muscular paralysis following transplantation of the ureters.

A. On admission. Serum K 1·5 mEq. per litre.

B. After potassium therapy. Serum K 2·5 mEq. per litre.

C. After recovery. Serum K 4·5 mEq. per litre.

Hyperpotassaemia

High extracellular potassium concentration may also be associated with voluntary muscle paralysis and in both cases the deep reflexes may be preserved in the early stages. It is not always possible on clinical examination to distinguish between the two forms of paralysis, but a consideration of the clinical history, an examination of the electrocardiogram or, of course, an estimation of the plasma potassium concentration will give quite unequivocal information. High plasma potassium concentrations are associated with electrocardiographic changes quite different from those of hypopotassaemia [FIG. 26]. Again, the levels at which these changes occur are not constant and depend on other ionic concentrations, but no serious complications should take place unless the plasma concentration is over 7·5–8 mEq. per litre (30–32 mg. per 100 ml.). Death from cardiac arrest is liable to occur in the region of 10 mEq. per litre (40 mg. per 100 ml.) and it may not be preceded by muscle paralysis. Marked bradycardia resulting from heart block may occur and give clinical warning of the situation. For a discussion of the role of potassium metabolism in the 'periodic paralysis' syndromes the reader should see the section on that subject.

In summary, a careful clinical appraisal and immediate past history is indispensable to use in conjunction with biochemical analysis of the serum in order to assess the state of a patient with regard to sodium, potassium and water balance. During the management of a patient who has or who may develop changes in the balance of these substances, accurate measurement of the intake and of the losses is of vital importance. Fluids lost should be kept, measured and analysed. Rapid changes in body weight can be regarded as being due to equivalent fluctuations in total body water. For guidance the daily volume and crude approximate composition of a number of body secretions is given in TABLE 16.

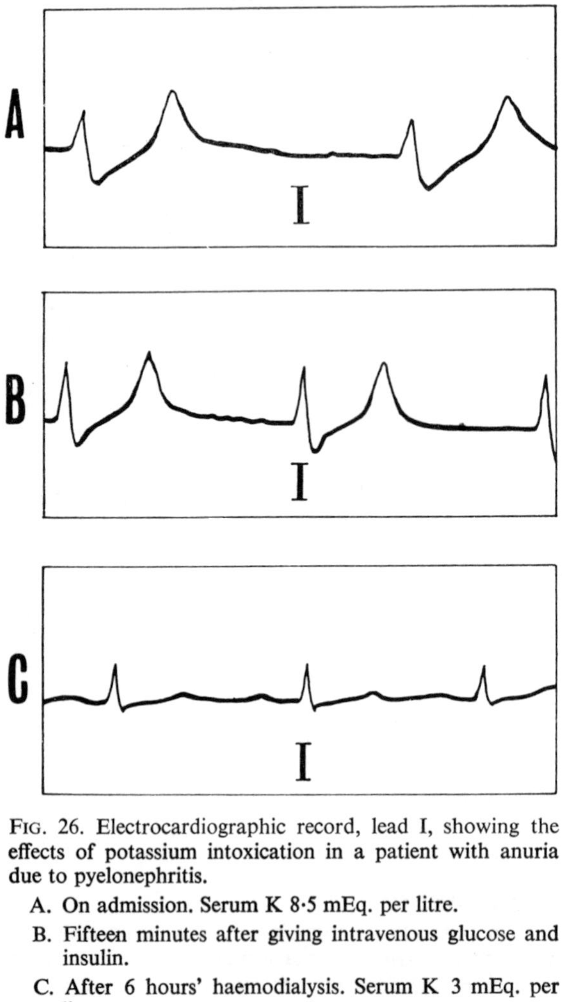

FIG. 26. Electrocardiographic record, lead I, showing the effects of potassium intoxication in a patient with anuria due to pyelonephritis.

A. On admission. Serum K 8·5 mEq. per litre.

B. Fifteen minutes after giving intravenous glucose and insulin.

C. After 6 hours' haemodialysis. Serum K 3 mEq. per litre.

TABLE 16

		mEq. per litre		
SECRETION	DAILY VOLUME	*Na*	*K*	*Cl*
Saliva . . .	1500	10	25	10
Stomach . .	2500	40	8	140
Pancreas . .	700	136	4	50
Bile . . .	500	136	4	105
Small intestine	3000	136	4	120

REFERENCES

BLACK, D. A. K. (1957) *Essentials of Fluid Balance*, Oxford.

ELKINTON, J. R., and DANOWSKI, T. S. (1955) *The Body Fluids: Basic Physiology and Practical Therapeutics*, Baltimore.

GAMBLE, J. L. (1954) *Chemical Anatomy, Physiology and Pathology of Extracellular Fluid*, 6th ed., Cambridge, Mass.

MARRIOTT, H. L. (1950) *Water and Salt Depletion*, Springfield, Ill.

MAXWELL, M. H., and KLEEMAN, C. R. (1962) *Clinical Disorders of Fluid and Electrolyte Metabolism*, New York.

ROSS, E. J. (1959) *Clinical Effects of Electrolyte Disturbances*. Proceedings of a Conference at the Royal College of Physicians, London.

WELT, L. G. (1959) *Clinical Disorders of Hydration and Acid-Base Equilibrium*, 2nd ed., Boston.

WOLF, A. V., and CROWDER, N. A. (1964) *An Introduction to Body Fluid Metabolism*, Baltimore.

REGULATION OF HYDROGEN ION CONCENTRATION

General Considerations

In this section the Brønsted-Lowry terminology, where appropriate, will be used and no reference will be made to some of the older, confusing and often illogical or inaccurate concepts.

The reader will more easily obtain a clear picture of the complicated interaction concerned in what is often referred to as 'acid-base' regulation if he thinks of it in terms of hydrogen ion regulation in the first place and regards all associated phenomena from that point of view.

Free hydrogen ion, H^+, in excess of free hydroxyl ion, OH^-, is what confers acidic properties upon a solution. Water partially dissociates into H^+ and OH^-

$$H_2O \rightleftharpoons H^+ + OH^-$$

the equilibrium being such that the concentrations of H^+ and OH^- ($[H^+]$ and $[OH^-]$) are each about $10^{-6\cdot8}$ gEq. per litre or $10^{-3\cdot8}$ mEq. per litre at 98·6° F. (37° C.). The *product* of the concentrations of these two ions $10^{-13\cdot6}$ remains constant regardless of what other substances may be dissolved in the water. Some substances may cause an increase in $[H^+]$ with a proportionate decrease in $[OH^-]$ (acids) and others a decrease in $[H^+]$ with a corresponding increase in $[OH^-]$ (bases). Acids are substances which increase the hydrogen ion concentration of a solution—substances which donate hydrogen ions or protons; bases are substances which decrease hydrogen ion concentration —substances which accept hydrogen ions or protons.

The pH of a solution is the logarithm (to the base 10) of the reciprocal of the hydrogen ion concentration, i.e. for neutral solutions at 98·6° F. (37° C.) pH = 6·8. Since the product $[H^+] \times [OH^-]$ remains constant, it is obvious that increasing $[H^+]$ of a solution—making it more acid or decreasing its pH—will automatically result in a corresponding decrease in $[OH^-]$, and vice versa.

The normal pH of the plasma of arterial blood is 7·4 (corresponding to $[H^+]$ of ·00004 mEq. per litre) with a range of + or − 0·05. When the $[H^+]$ is higher than this (pH lower) a state of acidaemia exists; conversely alkalaemia is present when the pH is higher than the above level. A state of acidosis can be said to exist when changes occur which would have resulted in a rise in $[H^+]$ above normal, were it not that compensating mechanisms had in fact successfully contained the rise to within the normal range; alkalosis bears a similar relationship to alkalaemia.

The $[H^+]$ of the plasma and extracellular fluid is not necessarily the same as that in cells, indeed intracellular $[H^+]$ may differ in different organs. This problem is being investigated by various means, one of them using the weak acid dimethadione (HDMO) the dissociated anion of which (DMO^-) probably does not pass across cell membranes; at the moment no method of estimating intracellular $[H^+]$ is easily applied to man, particularly in acute clinical situations. It is not proposed to discuss the problems concerned with intracellular hydrogen ion regulation, since knowledge of the subject is as yet too limited to have substantial clinical applications.

On the other hand $[H^+]$ in extracellular fluid is readily determined and a good deal is known of its regulation and of the clinical changes which occur when this regulation is insufficient. The rest of this section therefore will consider only changes in extracellular $[H^+]$ with the exception of the buffering action of the haemoglobin in red blood cells.

The Buffer Systems

The body fluids contain very efficient buffer systems so that the addition or removal of large quantities of H^+ results in comparatively small changes in $[H^+]$ or pH, though it must be remembered that, because pH is a logarithm_{10} expression, a change of 0·3 represents a twofold change in $[H^+]$. These buffer systems are so efficient that only about 5 out of every 10^6 hydrogen ions which may be added to the blood will remain as undissociated H^+ and cause a change in pH; the action is, of course, immediate and automatic. Quantitatively the most important buffer is haemoglobin the total effect of which is some six times greater than that of the plasma proteins, though both contribute an important part to the buffer system. Theoretically the system $H^+ + HPO_4^{--} \rightleftharpoons H_2PO_4^-$ should also be an effective buffer system at plasma pH, but the phosphate concentrations are too small for this system to make any substantial contribution.

However efficient a buffer system may be, there is, of course, always *some* change in $[H^+]$ when H^+ is added or removed. In average normal arterial blood the pH change, because of the buffering action of the above system, would be about −0·3 for every 7·2 mEq. H^+ added.

Respiratory Regulation

The system $H^+ + HCO_3^- \rightleftharpoons H_2CO_3$ acts as a buffer, but at pH 7·4 it is not very efficient, for $[HCO_3^-]$ is about 20 times $[H_2CO_3]$ and a buffering agent is most effective when the two forms are present in about equal concentration. Nevertheless, this system is of very great importance in H^+ regulation, not because of its chemical buffering action, but because H_2CO_3 is in equilibrium with dissolved CO_2, the over-all situation being represented thus:

$$H^+ + HCO_3^- \rightleftharpoons H_2CO_3 \rightleftharpoons CO_2 + H_2O$$

If one applies the Law of Mass Action to this system $K \times [H^+] \times [HCO_3^-] = [H_2CO_3]$ where K is a constant

$$\therefore \frac{1}{[H^+]} = K\frac{[HCO_3^-]}{[H_2CO_3]} = K^1\frac{[HCO_3^-]}{pCO_2}$$

where K^1 is a different constant to K because of the substitution of pCO_2 for $[H_2CO_3]$. pCO_2 is the partial pressure of CO_2 in solution and is, of course, at constant temperature (37° C.) and in a given solution (plasma) strictly proportional to $[H_2CO_3]$

$$\therefore \text{Log}_{10}\frac{1}{[H^+]} = pH = \text{Log}_{10} K^1 + \text{Log}_{10}\frac{[HCO_3^-]}{pCO_2}$$

It can thus be seen that the *ratio* of $[HCO_3^-]$ to Pco_2 is related to pH and that at any given pH the concentration of bicarbonate is automatically determined by the partial pressure of CO_2 in the solution.

Now CO_2 is a substance with a very rapid turnover, for it is constantly being produced by catabolic processes and excreted via the lungs at a rate varying from about 15,000 to over 30,000 mEq. per day. Thus, a slight difference between CO_2 production and its removal by the lungs will result in a change in its concentration in solution and hence in $[H^+]$ *and* $[HCO_3^-]$. In this way, if respiratory ventilation is somewhat less than that which is necessary to keep the alveolar partial pressure of CO_2 to the normal level of 40 mm. Hg, this value will rise.

The CO_2 in arterial blood is in equilibrium with, and at about the same pressure as, that in the alveoli; hence when underventilation occurs the amount of dissolved CO_2 will rise. This in turn will increase $[H_2CO_3]$ and this, as pointed out above will cause an increase in $[H^+]$ or a fall in pH. Conversely, overventilation will produce a rise in pH. It is obvious from these considerations that poor respiratory regulation will in itself be reflected in poor pH regulation.

The respiratory regulation described above is normally mainly determined by the Pco_2 of arterial blood, but the hydrogen ion concentration of arterial blood also plays a part. Increased arterial Pco_2 or increased $[H^+]$ (decreased pH) results in increased pulmonary ventilation so that a reduction in arterial Pco_2 and hence $[H^+]$, towards normal will follow. The control is rapid in its action and follows closely on the heels of the buffering action of haemoglobin and plasma proteins.

Renal Regulation

A slower and more prolonged regulatory effect is produced by the kidneys which exert their control by regulating the secretion of hydrogen ion and of bicarbonate ion. Just as the excretion of a molecule of CO_2 by the lungs effectively rids the body of one H^+, so the excretion of one HCO_3^- by the kidney results in one H^+ becoming available to the body. With the usual European diet and with normal metabolism some 40–60 mEq. of hydrogen ions are produced each day and these must ultimately be eliminated by the kidney if long-term equilibrium is to be maintained.

Bicarbonate is present in glomerular filtrate in much the same concentration as in the plasma. Most of it is reabsorbed in the proximal tubule however, the rate and extent depending largely on CO_2 tension. Hydrogen ions are secreted into the lumen and these combine with bicarbonate to form carbonic acid which either diffuses back into tubular cells or dissociates into CO_2 and H_2O, the former diffusing back into the tissues.

In the distal tubule this secretion of hydrogen ions is not related to plasma CO_2 tension but depends upon the presence of the enzyme carbonic acid anhydrase in the tubular cells. This enzyme accelerates the formation of H_2CO_3 from CO_2 and H_2O and, owing to the dissociation of H_2CO_3 into H^+ and HCO_3^-, there is always a plentiful supply of these ions. H^+, or alternatively K^+, may be switched through the cell membrane into the lumen of the tubule in exchange for Na^+. The maximum difference in $[H^+]$ which the tubular cells can thus produce is about 1:800—which corresponds to a urinary pH of about 4·7. The total amount of hydrogen ion which can be secreted in this way is, however, very small and two other mechanisms exist whereby much larger quantities can be eliminated without lowering the urinary pH to this extreme limit.

1. HPO_4^{--} ions are present in the tubular fluid and these form a buffer system with $H_2PO_4^-$ and H^+ thus:

$$H^+ + HPO_4^{--} \rightleftharpoons H_2PO_4^-$$

Phosphate is normally present in sufficient quantities in the urine for this buffer system to have a significant regulatory effect. It ceases to be very efficient below about pH 5·5 and above about pH 8.

2. NH_3 can be formed from amino acids by the tubular cells. H^+ can then unite with this to form NH_4^+ which is excreted as one of the urinary cations.

When an acidaemia exists this process of H^+ secretion occurs rapidly, but when there is an alkalaemia, H^+ secretion is much diminished and there is a tendency for increased amounts of K^+ to be exchanged for tubular Na^+.

It has already been mentioned that CO_2 is so readily diffusible that the CO_2 in most body fluids approximates to that in the alveoli. It is a curious fact, therefore, that when proper technical precautions are taken, the urinary CO_2 is usually found to be higher than that of the arterial blood. A possible explanation is that a CO_2 gradient is maintained from the renal cortex to the medulla, so that the Pco_2 at the papillae may be kept high by the counter-current mechanism of the loop of Henle. Alternatively, it has been suggested that urine of different pH may be produced by different tubules and that CO_2 is not diffusible across the renal pelvis or bladder. As a further possibility it has been suggested that carbonic anhydrase is deficient in the renal tubular urine and that the dissociation of H_2CO_3 into H_2O and CO_2 occurs so slowly that by the time this has happened the urine has reached a part of the collecting system through which CO_2 cannot diffuse. Whatever the explanation, it has been found that when the urine is about pH 5·5 or less the urinary Pco_2 is only 2 or 3 mm. Hg greater than that of the arterial blood, at urine pH 6·5 the urinary Pco_2 may be about 60 mm. Hg and at urine pH 8 the Pco_2 may be well over 100 mm. Hg.

It must be realized that, with slight modifications because of the slightly different constants for urine, the relationships between $[H^+]$ or pH, Pco_2 and $[HCO_3^-]$ must remain those which have been discussed above. Thus, if the concentration of any two of these constituents in the urine is fixed by renal regulatory mechanisms, the concentration of the third will be automatically determined. Whether renal regulation occurs in fact on two of the constituents only, or whether all three are actively involved, is not yet clear.

Whatever the intimate mechanism, the over-all urinary secretion of H^+ and $^-HCO_3$ is affected by plasma Pco_2, [Cl] and $[Ca^{++}]$, by the intracellular concentration of K^+, and by aldosterone secretion.

Causes of Inefficient Regulation of $[H^+]$

It can be seen from the above that acidaemia or alkalaemia may occur either when the rate of addition or removal of H^+ from body fluids is so great that the control systems are overwhelmed or when some abnormality exists which makes the system of control inefficient. Ventilation which is inadequate (as, for example in chronic bronchitis and emphysema) to allow escape of CO_2 to occur at its rate of production unless alveolar Pco_2 rises to abnormally high levels, will result in a high arterial Pco_2 and hence a high $[HCO_3^-]$ and a high $[H^+]$ (a low pH) or acidaemia. Conversely, over-ventilation, as in hysterical over-breathing, will be followed by a decrease in arterial Pco_2 and hence in a decrease in $[H^+]$ (raised pH or alkalaemia) and a low $[HCO_3^-]$. By contrast, if the failure to maintain a normal pH arises because of too great a change in the rate at which hydrogen ions are introduced or removed from the blood and extra-cellular fluid, the respiratory control being normal, an accumulation of H^+ or acidaemia will result in increased ventilation so that Pco_2 will fall and consequently $[HCO_3^-]$ will *decrease*. Conversely, an alkalaemia or abnormally low $[H^+]$ will depress ventilation so that arterial Pco_2 will rise and hence $[HCO_3]$ will *increase*.

Various biochemical indices are used to help in the delineation of hydrogen ion status, but it can be seen that a true picture can only be obtained if *two* of the three variables pH or $[H^+]$, $[HCO_3^-]$ and Pco_2 are determined. Since, however, many laboratories use only one measurement, such as serum CO_2 content or combining power, which usually gives an approximate idea of [HCO_3^-], it is convenient to classify acidaemia and alkalaemia into *respiratory* and *non-respiratory* depending upon the initial site of the abnormality. The term 'non-respiratory' is preferred to 'metabolic', for acidaemia resulting from the ingestion of large quantities of acid, or from failure of the kidney to secrete H^+, is not strictly metabolic, though the changes are similar.

It will be apparent that wherever the initial abnormality has arisen the control of [H^+] is continued in the other parts of the system. Thus, the acidaemia of diabetic ketosis arises as a result of the metabolic production of abnormally large quantities of H^+ together, of course, with the corresponding anions of beta-hydroxybutyrate⁻ and acetoacetate⁻. The change in plasma pH will be limited by the buffer systems, but it will nevertheless fall. As a result of this, the ratio $\frac{[HCO_3^-]}{P_{CO_2}}$ must correspondingly fall and this must mean a fall in [HCO_3^-], even if there were to be no change in CO_2. However, ventilation is markedly stimulated and this produces a fall in P_{CO_2} from which it follows that [HCO_3^-], must fall even further. At the same time, H^+ is excreted by the renal tubules in large quantities, and in addition, the kidney passes large quantities of the organic anions acetoacetate⁻ and beta-hydroxybutyrate⁻ which must be accompanied by equivalent amounts of cations. Owing to the limited [H^+] which can be achieved by the tubular cells, H^+ can only form a fraction of the cation requirement. A large part of the deficiency is made up by the NH_4^+ which is produced by tubular cells, and the rest mainly by Na^+ and K^+, which depletes the body of these two cations.

Method of Identifying the Type of Abnormality of [H^+]

The whole process can be represented graphically as shown in FIGURE 27. The line AB represents the

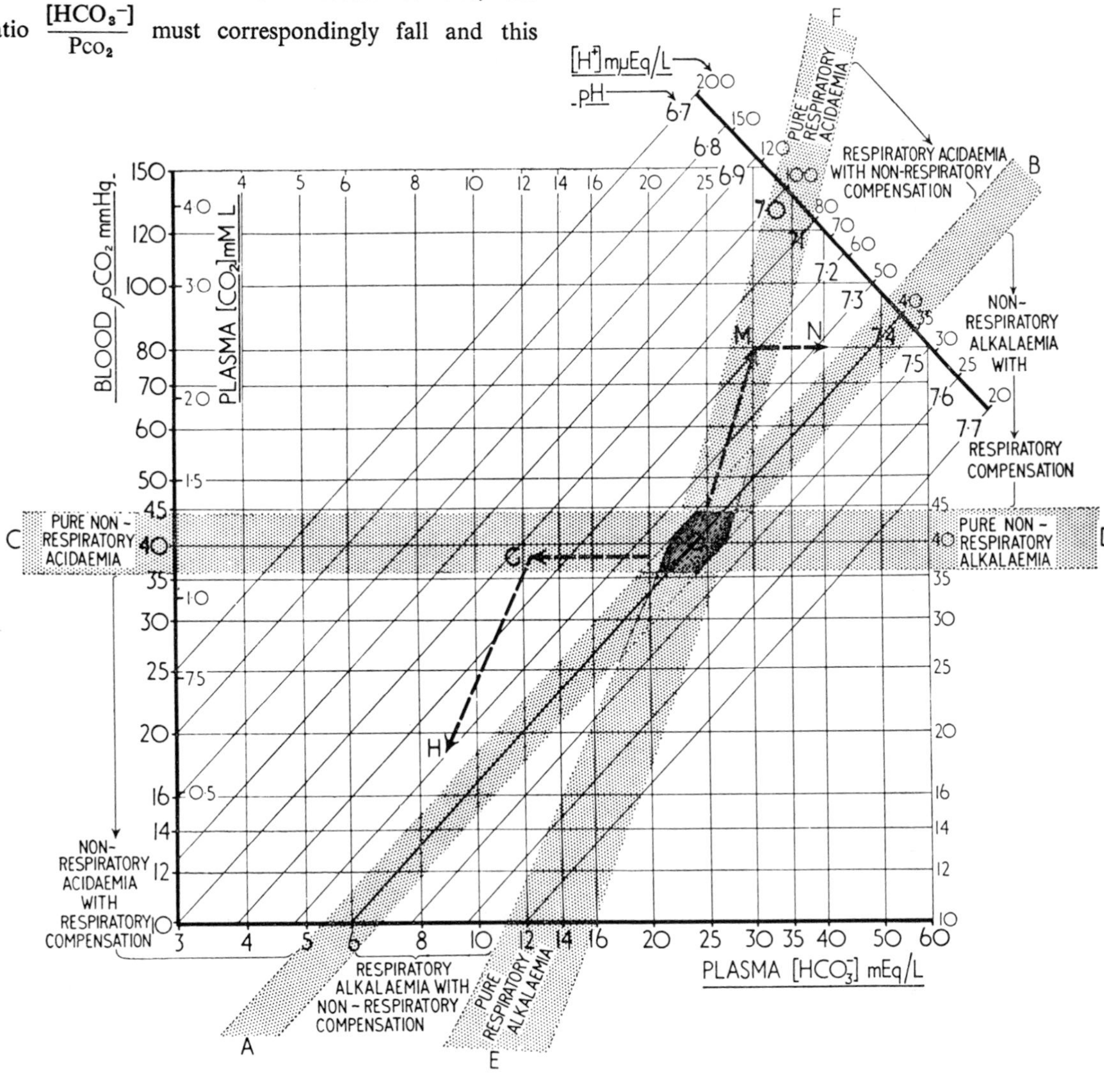

FIG. 27

[Modified by kind permission of Dr. E. J. M. Campbell from a diagram in *Clinical Physiology.*]

normal pH value of 7·4 and the shaded area shows the normal variation of ±0·05. Lines parallel to this give the various pH (or corresponding [H^+] values) within the extremes compatible with life. The horizontal shaded band CD represents the normal range of Pco_2 and the scale on the ordinate represents Pco_2 and the corresponding values of dissolved CO_2 in mm.Hg per litre. The sloping shaded band EF represents the relationship between Pco_2 and [HCO_3^-] in normal blood when no form of compensation for the pH change (such as renal excretion of H^+) can occur except for the buffering action of haemoglobin, plasma proteins, etc. This can obviously be determined experimentally *in vitro*. The area at the intersection of the shaded bands shows the normal arterial range.

In order to delineate the true position of a patient with regard to H^+ regulation, a laboratory determination of any *two* of the three variables Pco_2, pH and [HCO_3^-] is required. If Pco_2 and *total* plasma CO_2 content are determined the [HCO_3^-] value can be calculated by deducting the value for dissolved plasma CO_2 in mm.Hg per litre, corresponding to the estimated Pco_2, from the found value for total plasma CO_2 content. When a point corresponding to the analysis of a patient's blood is plotted, an indication of the type and degree of abnormality and of the amount of compensation can be obtained. The reason for this may be seen if one considers the sequence of events in, say, diabetic acidaemia as it might occur on the chart, and also what might happen in chronic bronchitis.

Parameters used in the Astrup Technique

It can be recalled from the above discussion that blood contains buffers (largely haemoglobin, plasma proteins, and bicarbonate). The normal amount of these buffer bases (BB)—for they are hydrogen acceptors—in blood of pH 7·38 at a Pco_2 of 40 mm. Hg is BB = (40·8 + 0·36 × Hb in g. per 100 ml.) mEq. per litre. Naturally, if hydrogen ions are added to or removed from blood the amount of available BB will be decreased or increased. The difference between the *actual* buffer base which is formed in a specimen of blood and the *normal* buffer base for that specimen is called the base excess (BE) by Astrup. In normal conditions this will have the value 0; it will be positive under conditions of alkalaemia and negative in acidaemia. The other parameter defined by him is the *Standard Bicarbonate*, which is the concentration of bicarbonate in mEq. per litre found in the plasma derived from whole blood in which the haemoglobin has been fully oxygenated and which has been equilibrated to a Pco_2 of 40 mm. Hg. It is thus a bicarbonate concentration which would be maintained if the respiration remained adjusted to keep the Pco_2 at 40 mm. Hg.

If a specimen of blood is equilibrated with CO_2 at various partial pressures and the resultant values of pH are recorded, the plot of log Pco_2 against pH will be, to all intents and purposes, linear. The *slope* of the line will depend upon the buffering action of the blood and can be formed by making pH measurements when the blood has been equilibrated at two different partial pressures of CO_2. The *position* of the line will depend upon the base excess, BE.

Nomograms have been prepared from experimental data on which the curves for BB and BE are plotted on a graph where the ordinate is log Pco_2 and the abscissa is pH. Because the Standard Bicarbonate is always measured at 40 mm. Hg Pco_2, it bears a strict relationship to pH and is also plotted on the abscissa [FIG. 28].

The Astrup apparatus has been designed so that a specimen of blood can easily be equilibrated at different levels of Pco_2 and the consequent pH measured with great accuracy. From these figures a line can be drawn on the nomogram and BB, BE and Standard Bicarbonate can be read. The value of BE × 0·3 × body weight in kg. will give the number of milliequivalents of acid if the value is positive, or of base if the value is negative, which would have to be given to bring the pH of the extracellular fluid back to normal. Owing to the buffering action of intracellular anions the value for the whole body would probably be considerably greater, but in clinical practice it is safer to act on the amounts determined for extracellular fluid and then make further blood measurements. The Standard Bicarbonate is a value obtained regardless of respiratory regulation and hence is a measure of the non-respiratory component of the situation. BE is a measure of the resultant of respiratory and non-respiratory effects.

Clinical Examples

Diabetic Acidaemia. When, owing to the deranged metabolism, an excess of H^+ is produced the pH will fall, and until a respiratory change occurs there will be little or no change in Pco_2. At this stage the point relating CO_2 and [HCO_3^-] will move in the horizontal shaded band to the left of the normal area as shown by the line OG. When the respiratory mechanism is stimulated by the increased [H^+], however, causing increased ventilation, this will lower Pco_2 and the value will fall *parallel* to the almost vertical sloping band and towards—but usually not reaching—the normal pH band as shown by the line GH.

Chronic Bronchitis. In this condition pulmonary ventilation may become seriously deficient in spite of increased respiratory effort. The Pco_2 rises, the blood parameters travelling up the sloping shaded band so that the pH falls (line OM). The kidney then starts to secrete H^+ so that the situation will move to the right towards, but not reaching, the normal pH region (line MN). (If anoxia becomes significant, the resultant increased metabolic production of H^+ will offset to some extent the renal compensation.)

Acidaemia

It will be apparent from the above discussion that the causes of acidaemia can be divided into respiratory and non-respiratory. The respiratory causes are all conditions which result in inadequate ventilation, conditions resulting in weakness of the respiratory muscles—such as myasthenia gravis, in mechanical inadequacy of the thoracic cage—such as advanced ankylosing spondylitis, or in greater stiffness of the thoracic contents—such as obesity, can all result in CO_2 retention. Diseases of the respiratory tract itself such as chronic bronchitis and emphysema or obstruction of the air passages will obviously result in deficient

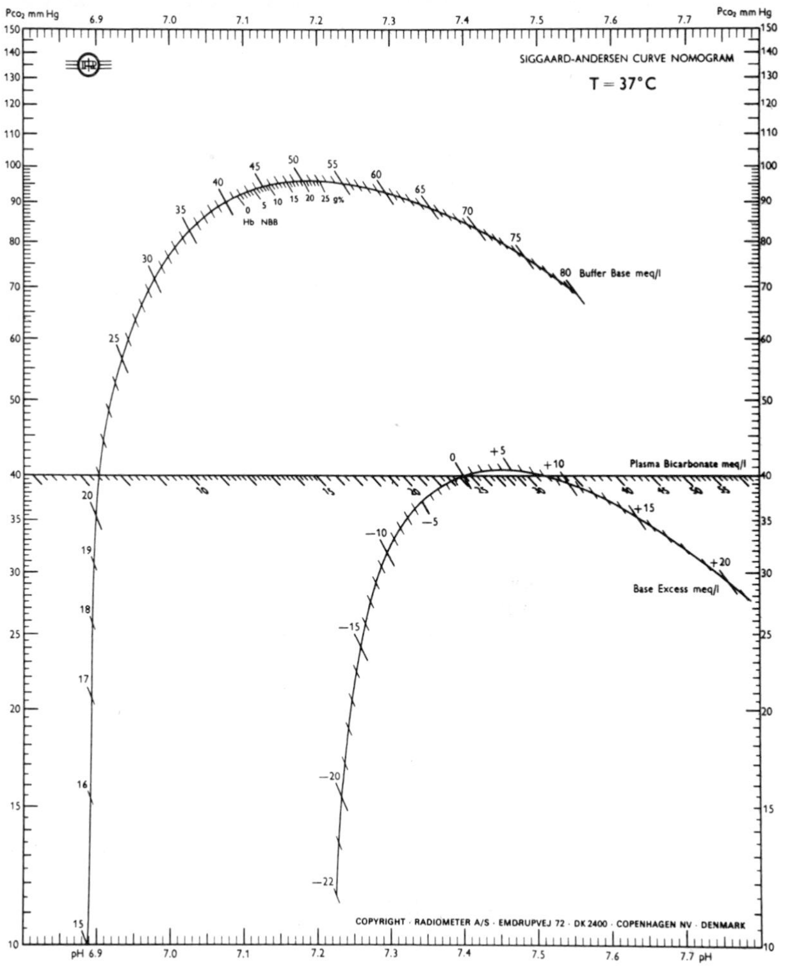

FIG. 28. The Siggaard-Andersen nomogram used in conjunction with the Astrup apparatus. Since haemoglobin is the major buffer base component, values are given along the buffer base line. By means of this the accuracy of the pH and Pco_2 measurements can be checked if the haemoglobin content of the blood sample is known.

ventilation. Finally, depression of the centres controlling respiration, either by disease processes, or by drugs, will cause ventilation to become deficient and hence produce a respiratory acidaemia.

Non-respiratory acidaemia is perhaps of commoner occurrence than the respiratory forms; the causes can conveniently be grouped into alimentary, metabolic and renal.

The alimentary causes result either from the ingestion of acids or of substances which when metabolized give rise to large quantities of H^+ (such as NH_4^+ in ammonium chloride $\rightarrow NH_3 + H^+$, or methyl alcohol which is broken down to formic acid), or from the loss of fluid (as in diarrhoea or a biliary fistula) which has a lower $[H^+]$ than plasma.

Any metabolic process which results in a greatly increased rate of H^+ production may result in acidaemia. Such a situation occurs under conditions of hypoxia or where cellular oxidation processes cannot be continued at the normal rate, so that 'anaerobic' metabolism occurs; the acidaemia occurring after cardiac arrest is a striking example. Whenever energy production by the normal carbohydrate pathways is impaired as in severe diabetes mellitus with deficient insulin activity, keto-acids are produced very rapidly. These, being strong acids, are almost completely dissociated so that there is a very rapid production of H^+, and thus a very marked acidaemia.

Simple renal failure will result in acidaemia if the patient continues to take an average European diet the metabolism of which results in the production of greater amounts of H^+ than of OH^-. There are, however, various diseases affecting the renal tubules in which the urinary pH is rarely lower than about 6. The production of NH_4^+ may also be impaired so that marked acidaemia may occur as a result of the H^+ retention. Acidaemia is also particularly prone to occur in patients whose ureters have been transplanted into the bowel. Here, the acidaemia probably results partly because the bowel re-absorbs more H^+ than OH^- and partly because infection, ascending up the transplanted ureters, damages the distal tubules and impairs their power to secrete H^+ efficiently.

In any solution the total concentration of cations, expressed as equivalent weights (or mEq.) is always equal to the similarly expressed concentration of anions. It follows, therefore, that quantities of H^+ entering the blood stream will always be accompanied by corresponding amounts of anion. Such anions are divisible into two categories: (1) those which can give rise to CO_2 and water, H^+ being incorporated in the process; (2) those which cannot give rise to CO_2 and water.

The importance of this is that anions in the first category can in effect be excreted as CO_2 through the lungs so that no cation other than H^+ need be lost with them. On the other hand anions of the second category must be excreted in the urine accompanied by equivalent amounts of cation. Naturally, where the rate of production of CO_2-producing anions is great enough they, too, may be secreted in the urine accompanied by cation. As has been shown, there is a limitation to the rate at which H^+ can be secreted and this, together with NH^+ is often insufficient to reach the equivalent of the amount of anion which is excreted. Thus large amounts of other cations, most notably Na^+ and K^+ and to some extent Ca^{++} are excreted, so depleting the body of these substances. The sodium depletion entails a corresponding depletion of extracellular water [q.v.] so that this form of dehydration is often present in association with acidaemia. The potassium deficiency, if great enough, can of itself result in impairment of renal tubular function so that even greater deficiency in renal regulation may occur. If the condition is very longstanding osteomalacia may result from calcium deficiency.

The main symptom of acidaemia as such is an increase in the depth and rate of respiration, though this only becomes apparent when the degree of acidaemia is quite severe. The breathing is deep and relatively quiet, though owing to the rapid air flow there may be a hissing sound. This type of breathing is known as acidotic breathing or Kussmaul's respiration. As described above sodium loss and dehydration, potassium and calcium loss may also occur: these may produce their characteristic symptoms which are described elsewhere.

Alkalaemia

The causes of alkalaemia can usefully be placed into the same categories as the causes of acidaemia. Respiratory alkalaemia is not common, but it is usually due to overbreathing on the part of hysterical individuals. The most common cause of alkalaemia used probably to be the ingestion of large quantities of alkaline mixtures by patients suffering from peptic ulcer, but this cause has become unusual since reversible adsorbents such as aluminium hydroxide have become more fashionable. Alkalaemia may also be found in patients with pyloric stenosis who vomit large quantities of acid, i.e. H^+. It should be noted, however, that balance studies have suggested that some of these patients have an alkalaemia affecting the extracellular fluid, but that the hydrogen ion concentration of intracellular fluid is abnormally high. Alkalaemia, when found in association with renal failure, has usually resulted from the treatment of the latter with excessive quantities of alkali. In alkalaemia K^+ instead of H^+ tends to be exchanged for tubular Na^+ so that alkalaemia is usually associated with K^+ deficiency. Conversely potassium depletion is usually accompanied by a mild degree of alkalaemia, a combination seen, for example, in Cushing's syndrome and in Conn's syndrome.

There may be no symptoms even in the presence of quite a severe alkalaemia. However, loss of appetite, nausea and vomiting may occur and may be accompanied by headache and mental abnormalities. Many of these symptoms might, however, arise from the other abnormalities accompanying the alkalaemia, and slow shallow respirations and tetany are the only clinical symptoms which can definitely be ascribed to alkalaemia *per se*. The kidneys may become damaged, the urine containing blood and casts. If the alkalaemia is severe enough and is not treated, death in coma may occur.

Treatment of Altered [H^+]

The treatment of acidaemia or alkalaemia must obviously depend ultimately upon treating the cause, if this is reversible. It may, however, be urgently necessary to deal directly with a severe disturbance of hydrogen ion concentration. If the kidneys are undamaged they will rapidly rectify any H^+ abnormality provided the renal blood flow and glomerular filtration rate are adequate. This, particularly in acidosis of non-respiratory origin, usually requires intravenous administration of adequate quantities of fluid containing a physiological concentration of sodium ion. In non-respiratory acidosis a considerable proportion of the anion can with advantage be HCO_3^- or lactate, both of which are CO_2-producing and so effectively assist in the elimination of H^+. Potassium and calcium deficiencies if present will also have to receive specific attention. Severe alkalaemia is unusual unless there is renal damage and in this case the kidney is frequently unable to excrete large quantities of anion. Adequate quantities of strong acids cannot therefore readily be given unless the anionic component can be readily metabolized. Ammonium chloride may be used effectively (but not in patients with liver disease, because of the toxic action of the ammonium ion, which is normally removed by the liver). The ammonium ion is metabolized in a way not yet fully understood and H^+ is liberated, thus increasing hydrogen ion concentration and combating the alkalaemia.

Alkali Reserve

In the above discussion this term has been carefully avoided, since it has no really precise meaning and it may actually be misleading. Originally applied to the plasma bicarbonate concentration, and implying that the concentration of cations (largely Na^+, which were erroneously conceived of as alkaline) corresponding to this was available 'in reserve' to deal with any increase in non-metabolizable anions (erroneously called acid radicles) which might occur, the term is now sometimes referred to the plasma total CO_2 content ($HCO_3^- + CO_2$).

REFERENCES

ASTRUP, P., JORGENSEN, K., ANDERSEN, O. S., and ENGEL, K. (1960) The acid-base metabolism—a new approach, *Lancet*, i, 1035.

BRØNSTED, J. N. (1923) Einige Bemerkungen über den Begriff der Saüren und Basen, *Rec. Trav. chim. Pays-Bas*, **42**, 718.

CAMPBELL, E. M. J. (1963) Hydrogen ion (acid: base) regulation, in *Clinical Physiology*, 2nd ed., ed., CAMPBELL, E. M. J., DICKINSON, C. J., and SLATER, J. D. H., p. 202, Oxford.

CHRISTENSEN, H. N. (1963) *pH and Dissociation. A Learning Program for Students of the Biological and Medical Sciences*, Philadelphia.

DAVENPORT, H. W. (1958) *The ABC of Acid-Base Chemistry*, 4th ed., Chicago.

KAUFMAN, H. E., and ROSEN, S. W. (1956) Clinical acid-base regulation—the Brønsted schema, *Surg. Gynec. Obstet.*, **103**, 101.

WARDENER, H. E. DE (1967) *The Kidney*, 3rd ed., London.

IRON METABOLISM

The body contains a total of somewhere between 2 and 6 g. of iron. Of this total a few hundred mg. are found as an essential part of various oxidative enzymes and of myoglobin. About 3 g. is present in haemoglobin and the rest, amounting to between 0·5 and 2·5 g. with a great individual variation, is situated in organs such as the liver, spleen and bone marrow, which contain large numbers of reticulo-endothelial cells. Owing to the normal breakdown of red blood cells, some 20–25 mg. of iron are liberated from haemoglobin each day and this quantity is liberated into the plasma. The same quantity is of course removed from the plasma and since the total quantity of plasma iron is only 3–4 mg., it can be seen that the turnover is very rapid indeed. In plasma, iron is transported bound to a β_1-globulin, transferrin, some eight genetic varieties of which have been identified. Plasma transferrin is normally only about one third saturated with iron, the normal concentraton of which is 90–150 μg. per 100 ml. although the total iron binding capacity of normal plasma is 270–400 μg. per 100 ml.

Iron is stored in combination with the protein apoferritin as ferritin, a compound which is readily demonstrated on electron microscopy and which has magnetic properties. Although normally in cells most iron is stored in the form of ferritin, as iron overloading occurs a greater proportion is found in the protein complex haemosiderin, which is probably composed of increasing aggregations of denatured ferritin.

The daily loss of iron from the body is only of the order of about 1 mg. in the male and an average of 2 mg. in women with normal menstruation. During pregnancy the requirement increases to 2·5–3 mg. because the iron requirements of the foetus and placenta are slightly greater than that saved by the cessation of menstrual losses. In childhood, iron requirements are somewhere between those for adult men and women. The daily loss must of course be made good by absorption of iron from the gut; since in the absence of bleeding the daily loss of iron remains very constant, the regulation of the iron content of the body must be achieved by control of this alimentary absorption. In normal man only a very small proportion of food iron is absorbed and this renders precision in studies of the over-all process technically very difficult to achieve—even when radioactive isotopes are employed. It may be stated, however, that of the 15–20 mg. of iron in the daily food intake something less than a tenth, probably only 3–4 per cent. is absorbed. This absorption occurs mainly in the duodenum and is more readily effected when the iron is in the ferrous state, which probably accounts for the observed absorption-enhancing effect of ascorbic acid. It would seem certain that iron can be absorbed elsewhere in the small intestine, but that conditions such as the redox potential and the pH are optimum in the duodenum. Absorption can still occur in the absence of free hydrochloric acid in the gastric secretion, but it tends to be diminished after partial gastrectomy. In states of iron deficiency and whenever erythropoiesis is stimulated (even though there may be a normal amount of iron in the body) there is an increased iron absorption, whereas in states of iron overload, iron absorption is usually depressed. However, the long continued ingestion of abnormally large quantities of iron, as may occur in patients who are unnecessarily given medicinal iron, or in the Bantu whose diet contains large quantities of iron derived from cooking vessels, may overwhelm this regulatory effect and result over the years in the accumulation of abnormal quantities of iron in the tissues. In addition, presumably as a result of an inherited defect, patients who ultimately develop haemochromatosis must absorb more than the required quantity of iron from a normal food intake. The condition does not usually become evident until about the age of 40 years in males and this would only entail the absorption of about 2–4 mg. iron per day. In this condition most of the iron is situated in parenchymatous cells, and fibrosis with destruction of the organ concerned takes place, whereas in patients in whom excess of iron has been brought about by multiple transfusions (e.g. in aplastic anaemia) most of the iron seems to be in the reticulo-endothelial system where it is relatively harmless. Sometimes, however, such patients do develop hepatic cirrhosis, diabetes mellitus and other features of haemochromatosis. These facts have been variously interpreted, some believing that so far as tissue destruction is concerned it is simply a matter of the amount of iron which determines its deposition in parenchymal cells, whereas others think that for some metabolic reason, it is deposited from the start in the parenchyma in patients with haemochromatosis. In all these conditions of iron overload the plasma transferrin tends to be nearly saturated so that the plasma iron concentration is some 2–2·5 times normal and approaches the total plasma iron binding capacity.

An iron-binding protein (gastroferrin) has recently been demonstrated in normal human gastric juice. The protein was shown to be absent in patients with haemochromatosis and to be reduced in iron deficiency anaemia caused by blood loss. Gastroferrin may regulate iron absorption—normal levels inhibit the absorption of the excessive amounts of iron present in a normal diet, reduced levels allowing enhanced absorption in iron deficiency anaemia and absence of the protein allowing the increased iron absorption of haemochromatosis.

Owing to the high iron content of haemoglobin (about 0·47 mg. iron per ml. of blood when the haemoglobin concentration is 14 g. per 100 ml.) it will be obvious that long continued blood loss may easily result in iron deficiency. What measurements have been made would suggest that rarely more than 20–30 per cent. of the total daily food intake of iron (i.e. about 4–6 mg.) can be absorbed even under conditions of maximum requirements; there is thus little margin to allow for excessive iron loss. Stored iron can readily be mobilized and this occurs after phlebotomy, even in patients with haemochromatosis. Thus a patient who is losing iron by bleeding at a rate slightly in excess of its absorption will require a considerable time before all the stores are depleted and hence before an iron-deficiency anaemia becomes manifest.

The term sideropenia has been used to describe the condition of iron deficiency, recognized by a low serum iron concentration and less than 16 per cent. saturation of the total iron binding capacity of the serum, with a normal haemoglobin. Careful double blind studies have shown that any symptoms present in such patients can be as well relieved by placebo as by iron administration but of course treatment may prevent the subsequent development of iron deficiency anaemia.

GEORGE A. SMART

CALCIUM METABOLISM

The adult human body contains 1 kg. of calcium of which 99 per cent. is located in bone. The plasma calcium concentration is normally about 8·8 to 10·3 mg. per 100 ml., although the exact range depends upon the method used. Of the total calcium in the plasma about one-third is protein-bound, mainly by albumin, and of the remaining two-thirds about 0·5 mg. per 100 ml. is complexed by organic acids of low molecular weight such as citrate, leaving an ionized fraction of about 5–6 mg. per 100 ml., again the exact value depending upon the method of analysis used. There are no known functions in the human subject for either the protein-bound or complexed fractions of calcium. The ionized calcium appears to be the important fraction both with regard to the deposition of calcium salts and the excitability of nervous tissues. It follows that when total plasma calcium is measured, it is important also to measure plasma total proteins and to make allowances for any deviation from the normal in the latter. This can be done by adjusting the calcium by 0·75 mg. per 100 ml. for every 1 g. per 100 ml. deviation in the proteins from the arbitrary value of 7·0 g. per 100 ml.

Plasma calcium is regulated by at least two hormones and possibly more. Of these, by far the most important in the adult human subject is that secreted by the parathyroid glands and known as parathyroid hormone. This hormone is a polypeptide of molecular weight approximately 10,000 and it is known to have several independent physiological actions. Firstly, it causes a release of calcium from bone by stimulating the osteoclasts. Secondly, it reduces urinary calcium, possibly by increasing renal tubular reabsorption of calcium, although this point has still to be proved. These two effects are synergistic in leading to a rise in the plasma calcium. Normally, sufficient parathyroid hormone is secreted to maintain the plasma calcium level in the normal range and without this secretion the level falls to 6–7 mg. per 100 ml. A third and entirely independent effect of parathyroid hormone is to decrease the renal tubular reabsorption of phosphate thereby causing a fall in plasma phosphate.

Parathyroid hormone is slow in action and takes some hours to cease acting and the remarkable constancy of the plasma ionized calcium leads one to suppose that there must be a second mechanism for maintaining this constant level. During the last ten years it has been shown that there is indeed a second hormone, namely calcitonin, which is relatively rapid in its effects and which lowers plasma calcium. Calcitonin is also a polypeptide of about 10,000 molecular weight and in man is secreted mainly by the 'C' cells of the thyroid. Calcitonin acts by inhibiting bone reabsorption and this causes a fall in plasma calcium and phosphate. There are some suggestions in the literature that hypocalcaemic factors may be secreted by the adrenals, the anterior pituitary and the parotid glands. However, the evidence has all been from animal studies and there is none as yet that applies to man.

Vitamin D, in physiological doses (up to 400 International Units per day) seems to play a permissive role, allowing the parathyroids to maintain the plasma calcium at a normal level. Thus, in vitamin D-deficiency rickets the plasma calcium may be low, although on the other hand it is sometimes normal. Vitamin D, in very large doses (1–5 mg. per day or 40,000–200,000 I.U. per day), is also able to raise the plasma calcium independently of the parathyroids. This is accomplished in two ways. First, it promotes calcium reabsorption from bone and may thus cause hypercalcaemia even on a calcium-free diet. Secondly, it promotes the absorption of dietary calcium in the intestinal tract. The normal dietary intake of calcium is about 1 gramme per day, of which there is a net absorption of some 250–350 mg. per day which of course is excreted into the urine in the case of a normal adult in calcium balance. In vitamin D deficiency this absorption from the intestinal tract is blocked, and on the other hand large doses of vitamin D can increase the absorption very greatly.

The diffusible plasma calcium is completely filtrable by the renal glomeruli so that about 8,400 mg. per day are presented to the renal tubules, and a very large proportion of this calcium must be reabsorbed in the renal tubules. The normal urinary calcium in Great Britain is 120–350 mg. per day in adult males and 100–300 mg. per day in adult females. It should be noted, however, that the upper limits quoted are not rigid since there are undoubtedly normal individuals in this country with urinary calcium values considerably higher. It must also be noted that the normal range is apparently lower in the United States and in some other countries, and is lower in children. Hypercalciuria is common in cases of renal calculi, and the most common causes of such hypercalciuria are idiopathic hypercalciuria and primary hyperparathyroidism. In idiopathic hypercalciuria it is now possible to lower the urinary calcium not only by restricting dietary intake, but also by administration of thiazide diuretics and/or cellulose phosphate. Whilst thiazides act directly on the renal tubules, cellulose phosphate reduces the intestinal absorption of calcium.

HYPOCALCAEMIA

A low plasma calcium may be due to vitamin D deficiency, steatorrhoea, chronic renal failure, or the various types of hypoparathyroidism. The characteristic symptom is tetany which affects all muscle whether smooth, skeletal, or cardiac. Carpopedal spasm and laryngeal stridor are manifestations of skeletal tetany. The effect on cardiac muscle can be revealed by the E.C.G. which shows a prolonged QT interval. These motor symptoms, however, are part of an even wider nervous disorder which affects the sensory system leading to paraesthesiae, affecting especially the hands and the circumoral region, and the brain, causing depression, psychotic behaviour, convulsions and epilepsy. Prolonged hypocalcaemia leads to calcification of the basal ganglia and also to various ectodermal disorders, with loss of hair, atrophy of the nails with fungal infections, and cataracts. The occurrence of epilepsy or cataracts in unusual clinical circumstances is an indication for the measurement of plasma calcium.

There are two useful signs of pre-tetany when the plasma calcium is low but not sufficiently low to cause overt tetany. Firstly, Trousseau's sign, carpal spasm which is elicited by applying a sphygmomanometer cuff to the arm and inflating above systolic pressure for three minutes. Secondly, Chvostek's sign, the ability to induce twitching of the facial muscles around the mouth, nose and eyes by tapping over the various branches of the facial nerve as they emerge from under the parotid gland.

HYPERCALCAEMIA

Hypercalcaemia of any cause may give rise to a variety of symptoms as follows:

1. Gastro-intestinal disturbances are common with anorexia, nausea, vomiting and constipation.
2. Mental symptoms include fatigue, depression, psychosis and even dementia.
3. Thirst and polyuria result from an impairment in the ability of the renal tubules to attain a high urinary osmolarity.

Nephrocalcinosis may occur at a remarkably early stage, although overt renal damage, as shown by raised blood urea, takes a long time to develop. Hypercalcaemia may eventually lead to renal failure.

Whenever hypercalcaemia of long standing is suspected, corneal calcification should be sought. To observe this sign, a slit lamp is not necessary, a simple torch and small magnifying glass being adequate. The calcification is seen as a linear and granular deposit just inside the junction of the cornea and sclerotic and generally at the medial and lateral borders (3 o'clock and 9 o'clock). It should be noted, however, first, that corneal calcification is probably a sign of raised calcium × phosphate product rather than of hypercalcaemia itself, and secondly that calcification may persist for some time after the cause has ceased to operate, although it does gradually disappear.

The main causes of hypercalcaemia are listed in TABLE 30. Since the cortisone test plays such an important role in the differential diagnosis of hypercalcaemia, the usual response to this test is also shown in the table. The test is performed by administering either cortisone, 50 mg., or hydrocortisone, 40 mg., 8-hourly for ten days and then gradually tailing off the dose and measuring the plasma calcium on days 0, 5, 7 and 10 or more often. It should be noted that the characteristic response to the test is subject to exceptions just as are all general rules in medicine. Thus there are undoubtedly cases of primary hyperparathyroidism with osteitis fibrosa cystica which have shown a fall in plasma calcium with a cortisone test. This hardly effects the value of the test however, since the diagnosis is generally not in doubt when osteitis fibrosa cystica is present.

TABLE 30

THE CAUSES OF HYPERCALCAEMIA AND RESPONSE TO THE CORTISONE TEST

CAUSE	CHANGE IN PLASMA CALCIUM
1. Primary hyperparathyroidism	No change
2. Vitamin D-overdose . .	Falls to normal
3. Vitamin D-sensitive states:	
(a) Hypercalcaemia of infancy . . .	Falls to normal
(b) Sarcoidosis . .	Falls to normal
4. Carcinoma of any type, or myelomatosis; with or without bone secondaries . .	May fall to normal
5. Immobilization . . .	Insufficient data
6. Thyrotoxicosis . . .	Insufficient data
7. Addisonian crisis .	Falls to normal

REFERENCES

ALBRIGHT, F., and REIFENSTEIN, E. C. (1948) *The Parathyroid Glands and Metabolic Bone Disease*, Baltimore.

FOURMAN, P., and ROYER, P. (1968) *Calcium Metabolism and the Bone*, Oxford.

G. A. ROSE

Footnote

In this section the term 'phosphate' is used as an abbreviation for 'inorganic phosphate'.

COPPER METABOLISM

The body of a normal adult contains 100–150 mg. of copper, the highest concentrations being found in liver, kidney, heart, brain and pancreas. About 98 per cent. of the copper in plasma is associated with the α_2-globulin, caeruloplasmin, so called because of its blue colour. This protein, which contains eight atoms of copper per molecule, has a molecular weight of approximately 160,000. Its concentration can be measured in various ways, usually by determining the oxidase activity of serum which correlates with its copper content. Non-caeruloplasmin copper is bound to serum albumin and it is in this active form that copper is transported from the intestine to the tissues. Copper is also a normal component of red blood cells, where at least 80 per cent. is present in the form of erythrocuprein, a colourless protein with a molecular weight in the region of 33,000. The daily adult requirement of copper is about 2 mg., an amount contained in even moderately poor diets. Although copper deficiency gives rise to anaemia, and demyelinating disease of the nervous system in animals, no disorder resulting from copper deficiency alone has yet been reported in man.

Albinism, an inherited disorder characterized by failure in the pigmentation of skin, hair and eyes, results from a deficiency in the cupro-enzyme tyrosinase. Hepatolenticular degeneration (Wilson's disease) is usually associated with lowering of the serum copper and decreased caeruloplasmin levels. It is probably due to a genetically determined impairment in the synthesis of caeruloplasmin. Copper deposited in the cornea, liver, brain and kidney may be responsible for some of the manifestations of this disease. It has been suggested that copper accumulation causes the release of enzymes from lysosomes which results in cell damage. The level of serum caeruloplasmin has been reported to be depressed in multiple sclerosis.

A rare disorder of infants has been described in which there is oedema, hypoproteinaemia, anaemia, hypoferraemia and hypocupraemia with lowering of caeruloplasmin. Kwashiorkor, various malabsorption syndromes and the nephrotic syndrome may lead to hypocupraemia.

Hypercupraemia, asymptomatic as far as is known, is seen in hepatic cirrhosis (particularly in primary biliary cirrhosis), hyperthyroidism, after oestrogen and androgen administration, in most acute and chronic infections, in the collagen disorders, in various malignant diseases and in a number of anaemias.

REFERENCES

Adelstein, S. J., and Vallee, B. L. (1961) Copper metabolism in man, *New Engl. J. Med.*, **265**, 892–897 and 941–946.

Scheinberg, I. H., and Sternliet, I. (1960) Copper metabolism, *Pharmacol. Rev.*, **12**, 355.

MAGNESIUM METABOLISM

The body content of magnesium is about 2000 mEq., it is the second most plentiful intracellular cation. About half the body's magnesium is in bone and the rest is equally distributed between muscle and other soft tissues, liver and striated muscle having high concentrations (15–20 mEq. per kg.). Measurements of serum magnesium by atomic absorption techniques indicate values ranging from 1·6–2·1 mEq. per litre. In adults the average daily magnesium intake is of the order of 25 mEq., mostly derived from green vegetables. Absorption is normally from the small intestine though colonic absorption can also occur. Calcium appears to influence magnesium absorption possibly by competition in a common absorptive process. Usually about a third of the magnesium intake is excreted in the urine, though under conditions of deprivation renal excretion is markedly reduced (to less than 1 mEq. per day).

Magnesium is a cofactor in many key enzyme systems, particularly those that hydrolyse and transfer phosphate groups, including the phosphatases and those concerned in the reactions of adenosine triphosphate. It is essential for the stabilization of DNA, RNA and ribosomes and in the binding of messenger RNA to ribosomes.

Magnesium or calcium depletion causes increased neuronal excitability and neuromuscular transmission whereas magnesium excess has a curare-like action on the neuromuscular junction and may cause general anaesthesia.

Magnesium Deficiency

It has not been possible to cause symptomatic magnesium depletion by dietary restriction alone; probably because marked renal conservation of magnesium occurs. To produce clinical effects it is necessary for an inadequate intake to be aggravated by loss of gastro-intestinal fluids or malabsorption.

Magnesium depletion can exist without reduction in serum magnesium levels, conversely hypomagnesaemia may be present when the cellular magnesium content is normal. However, a lowered serum level is usually indicative of magnesium depletion in the appropriate clinical context. Estimations of erythrocyte magnesium or urinary excretion are also useful in detecting depletion of the element.

Magnesium deficiency causes neuromuscular dysfunction indicated by hyperexcitability and sometimes behaviour disorders. Tetany, major or minor epilepsy, ataxia, vertigo, tremor, muscle weakness, depression, irritability and psychosis may be associated with magnesium deficiency and are reversed by repletion. There is no clinical difference between the tetany of calcium and that of magnesium depletion. The electrocardiogram can be helpful in distinguishing hypocalcaemia from magnesium deficiency, in the former there is prolongation of the QT interval whereas in the latter there is depression of ST segments and inversion of T waves in the precordial leads. Manifestations of magnesium deficiency rarely occur unless the serum magnesium level is less than 1 mEq. per litre.

The main causes of symptomatic hypomagnesaemia are indicated in Table 31.

TABLE 31

CAUSES OF SYMPTOMATIC HYPOMAGNESAEMIA

Gastro-intestinal disorders
- Malabsorption syndromes, including non-tropical sprue
- Malabsorption due to extensive bowel resection
- Bowel and biliary fistulas
- Prolonged nasogastric suction with administration of magnesium-free parenteral fluids
- Prolonged diarrhoea

Protein-calorie malnutrition
Alcoholic cirrhosis
Pancreatitis
Endocrine disorders
Hyperparathyroidism and hypoparathyroidism
Hyperaldosteronism
Diabetic coma
Renal diseases
Glomerulonephritis, pyelonephritis, hydronephrosis, nephrosclerosis and renal tubular acidosis
Alcoholism
Diuretic therapy (mercurials, ammonium chloride and thiazides)
Malignant osteolytic disease
Porphyria with inappropriate secretion of antidiuretic hormone
Excessive lactation
'Idiopathic'

[Reproduced from *The New England Journal of Medicine*, (1968) **278**, No. 13, p. 713, by permission of the Editor and Dr. Walker and Dr. Parisi.]

Magnesium Excess

Magnesium excess occurs most frequently in renal failure and it is dangerous to give magnesium salts to such patients. Cardiac conduction defects develop at serum levels of 5–10 mEq. per litre with an increase in the PR interval and QRS duration and an increased amplitude of the T wave. Tendon reflexes are reduced as the concentration reaches 10 mEq. per litre and respiratory paralysis and general anaesthesia occurs at about 15 mEq. per litre. Still higher concentrations cause cardiac arrest in diastole.

Magnesium Therapy

Magnesium therapy is indicated when the clinical features of magnesium depletion occur and when this is confirmed by low serum, erythrocyte, urinary or tissue magnesium levels. The sulphate salt is available in 10, 25 or 50 per cent. concentrations, the rate of intravenous infusion should not exceed 1·5 ml. of a 10 per cent. solution per minute. Magnesium sulphate has also been used as a sedative in the treatment of pre-eclampsia and eclampsia. Oral magnesium supplements are preferable to intravenous injections when there is no urgency and up to 10 mEq. of magnesium hydroxide can be given daily by mouth without causing alteration of bowel habit in many instances.

REFERENCES

HANNA, S., MACINTYRE, I., HARRISON, M., and FRASER, R. (1960) The syndrome of magnesium deficiency in man, *Lancet*, ii, 172.

WALKER, W. E. C., and PARISI, A. F. (1968) Medical progress: Magnesium metabolism, *New Engl. J. Med.*, **278**, 658, 712, 772.

THE PLASMA PROTEINS

Recently techniques such as electrophoresis, immuno-electrophoresis, chromatography and ultracentrifugation have been developed by which the various plasma proteins can be separated and identified with a refinement which was not previously possible. As a result certain specific changes in plasma proteins have been shown to be related to particular disease entities, other plasma proteins have been found to exist in different forms according to the genetic character of the individual, the functions of many of the protein fractions have been defined and by the use of isotopic techniques knowledge is being accumulated concerning the turnover of proteins in health and disease. A brief review of the subject is presented here.

Plasma proteins consist of albumins and globulins and these components can be fractionated by a number of methods:

Paper electrophoresis which separates groups of proteins with different electrical charges has replaced the use of concentrated salt solution, e.g. ammonium sulphate, where fractionation was incomplete. The following groups are found normally in order of decreasing mobility: albumin, α_1-globulin, α_2-globulin, β-globulin and γ-globulin. When plasma rather than serum is electrophoresed a sixth fraction containing fibrinogen appears between the β- and γ-globulins.

Immuno-electrophoresis by which technique at least 23 distinct serum proteins can be recognized. Unfortunately quantitative assessment of these proteins is difficult to obtain as yet.

Ultracentrifugation which separates proteins of different molecular size reveals 4 main components in normal serum, a high molecular weight 20-S* fraction of macroglobulin, a 7-S fraction containing γ-globulin, a 4·6-S fraction containing albumin and other proteins, and a 3·3-S fraction containing various lipoproteins.

Albumin makes up 55–65 per cent. of the total serum proteins, the normal range of concentration being 4–5·5 g. per 100 ml. The molecular weight of albumin is approximately 69,000 and this, combined with its high concentration in plasma and its higher net electrical charge results in albumin contributing a major portion (about 75 per cent.) of the colloid osmotic pressure (oncotic pressure) of the plasma. Thus, in conditions associated with lowered plasma albumin concentration (less than 2 g. per 100 ml.) oedema occurs. For such oedema fluid to accumulate an increase of aldosterone secretion must occur so that the total body content of sodium, and then that of water mediated by increased antidiuretic hormone, increase sufficiently. Hypoalbuminaemia may result from decreased protein intake as occurs in malnutrition, from impaired absorption in the malabsorption syndromes, from decreased synthesis in liver diseases or debilitating conditions (for the liver is the site of albumin synthesis), from increased loss of albumin from the body via the kidney in the nephrotic syndrome, from the skin in certain exudative conditions, e.g. burns, pemphigus and from the gastro-intestinal tract in various gastric and intestinal lesions—the protein-losing gastro-enteropathies, and finally from an extremely rare genetically determined deficiency in albumin synthesis which, surprisingly, causes only a slight tendency to dependent oedema.

Considerable interest has developed in the so-called protein-losing gastro-enteropathies which were demon-

* S (Svedberg unit) is a unit indicating the rate of sedimentation under standard conditions.

strated to be due to abnormal protein loss into the digestive tract by using a synthetic isotope-labelled polymer of similar molecular size to albumin. This abnormal leakage may occur in many diseases of the stomach or intestine, e.g. gastric carcinoma, hypertrophic gastritis, regional ileitis, various types of steatorrhoea and ulcerative colitis.

In some patients no underlying gastro-intestinal disorder can be detected and the term 'idiopathic hypoproteinaemia' is used to describe this condition. Hypogammaglobulinaemia as well as hypo-albuminaemia probably explains the frequency of infections, while eosinophilia, lymphopenia and chylous ascites may occur less often than the cardinal sign of oedema.

A second genetic abnormality, not associated with any disease process, has been described in which a double albumin peak is found on electrophoresis.

Serum proteins may act as vehicles for the transport of sparingly soluble substances and by absorbing water-soluble substances of small molecular size, may prevent the loss of these from the blood stream. In this respect albumin is important in the transport of free fatty acids and probably also of certain trace metals.

The γ-globulins are electrophoretically least mobile on conventional paper electrophoresis with buffer at pH 8·6. Most antibodies are γ-globulins, however by the technique of immuno-electrophoresis it has been found that antibodies also move to the α- and β-globulin positions on conventional electrophoresis. Plasma proteins with antibody activity are now referred to as immunoglobulins and five classes are recognized at present, IgG (previously termed γ-globulin), IgA, IgM (macroglobulin), IgD and IgE. The basic unit of an immunoglobulin consists of 4 polypeptide chains, 2 of these are heavy chains (MW 50,000–70,000) and 2 are light chains (MW about 20,000). There are two types of light chain, κ and λ which can be combined with four types of heavy chain termed γ in IgG, α in IgA, μ in IgM, σ in IgD and ε in IgE. All but the IgM molecule remain as single units with a MW of about 140,000, whereas the IgM molecule consists of 5 units linked by-S-S- bridges, hence the term macroglobulin.

Usually little synthesis of γ-globulins occurs in the foetus but placental transfer of IgG results in a cord blood level equal to or even higher than that in maternal serum. This level falls after birth until the child's γ-globulin producing cells take over at about 2–3 months. IgM and IgA production begins at about the same time but neither of these immunoglobulins pass across the placenta.

IgA is found particularly in saliva and intestinal secretions and colostrum where it has a higher MW than IgG, though serum IgA has a similar MW to IgG. The difference is due to the addition of a β-globulin, MW about 50,000, termed 'transport' or secretory piece and a structure linking three molecules of IgA to one transport piece has been considered.

The average concentration of IgA in normal serum is about 200 mg. per 100 ml. The IgA globulins contain isohaemagglutinins and antibodies against insulin and thyroglobulin. It is possible that IgA has some function in protecting mucosal surfaces. IgA deficiency sometimes occurs in patients with coeliac disease, with ataxia telangiectasia, the nephrotic syndrome and certain leukaemias.

The *IgM* globulin makes up 5–8 per cent. of the normal serum immunoglobulins; in adults its mean serum concentration is about 100 mg. per 100 ml. The isohaemagglutinins, cold agglutinins, rheumatoid factor and antibody to somatic antigens of Gram-negative bacteria are usually IgM globulins.

IgM levels are lowered in most patients with untreated coeliac disease but can be raised by a gluten-free diet. The lowered levels are probably due to decreased synthesis which may be a reflection of the generalized lymphoreticular dysfunction of coeliac disease. It is not known whether the increased incidence of gastro-intestinal neoplasia and reticulosis is related to the deficient immunoglobulin synthesis.

IgD levels in normal serum range from 0·3 to 40 mg. per 100 ml., the mean level being 3 mg. per 100 ml. The role of IgD is not as yet understood.

IgE is a newly isolated immunoglobulin which appears to have reaginic activity—levels are raised in asthma, hay fever and eczema and there are many other similarities between IgE and reagin. High levels of IgE are found in patients with parasitic infections. IgE sensitizes the surfaces of mast cells causing histamine and slow-acting substances to be released in response to allergen without the intervention of complement.

As would be expected the plasma concentration of γ-globulin tends to be higher than normal in patients who are producing increased amounts of antibody—those with 'auto-immune diseases', e.g. Hashimoto's disease. A non-specific increase in γ-globulin is found in many chronic inflammatory diseases and other disorders of unknown aetiology, e.g. sarcoidosis, the collagenoses, malignant disorders and chronic liver disease. Hypogammaglobulinaemia is normally found in the first few months of life and is more marked in premature infants. It may also result from loss of γ-globulin in the urine in the nephrotic syndrome or into the gut in the protein-losing gastro-enteropathies.

Congenital agammaglobulinaemia may occur in one of two forms—a rare familial alymphocytic form affecting the sexes equally, associated with thymic aplasia and usually fatal before the age of 2, and a milder sex-linked recessive type predominantly affecting boys. In both forms frequent bacterial infections are not followed by antibody formation though viral infections tend to be resisted in the normal way. As might be expected when the marrow or lymphoid tissue is examined plasma cells are reduced or absent. Traces of γ-globulin can still be detected (less than 100 mg. per 100 ml.) in these patients by the more refined techniques mentioned previously. Acquired agammaglobulinaemia is usually not familial and may be associated with thymomas, chronic lymphatic leukaemia, myelomatosis, and other reticulo-endothelial disorders.

There appears to be a high incidence of allergic reactions in patients with congenital and acquired agammaglobulinaemia and a rheumatoid-like syndrome is common. Close relatives of the patients may also exhibit these abnormalities along with hyper- or hypogammaglobulinaemia. Treatment of infections with antibiotics and prophylaxis by administration of gamma globulin may prove life-saving.

The α-globulin fraction represents a heterogeneous group of proteins which have only their electric charge in common. Both lipoproteins and glycoproteins with a high carbohydrate content are present. The carrier proteins for thyroxine and cortisol, thyroxine-binding globulin (TBG) and transcortin are both α-globulins and these proteins also serve as a transport medium for fat-soluble vitamins and copper. An increase in α-globulins is seen in acute inflammatory conditions, various neoplasms, leukaemias, etc. Very high levels of α_2-globulin occur in the nephrotic syndrome. Increased amounts of TBG and transcortin resulting from oestrogen excess in pregnancy or following drug therapy are responsible for the high total serum content of the hormones in these conditions. This is, however, not associated with hormonal over-activity since the level of physiologically effective free hormone is not increased. Familial increases and decreases of TBG have been reported. Lowered α-globulin levels are uncommon and not usually of clinical significance.

The β-globulins are also heterogeneous and have a high lipoprotein content. Transport of iron is mediated by a specific β-globulin termed transferrin, of which there are eight known different genetic types. It has been shown that the tolerance to intravenous iron depends on the amount of transferrin in the plasma. Such symptoms as sneezing, flushing, nausea and vomiting may occur if transferrin is low, e.g. in pernicious anaemia, whereas there is high tolerance in chronic iron deficiency anaemia. Caeruloplasmin, a copper-carrying protein may be lowered in amount in some cases of Wilson's disease. Another group of β-globulins, the haptoglobins are also genetically determined. These proteins which are not present at birth combine with liberated haemoglobin which does not 'spill over' into the urine to cause haemoglobinuria till the haptoglobins are saturated. A homogeneous increase in β-globulin may sometimes occur in myelomatosis.

The paraproteins are atypical proteins which do not normally occur in the blood, e.g. myeloma globulins, pathological macroglobulins, Bence-Jones proteins, the C-reactive protein and cryoproteins.

The myeloma globulins may have the electrophoretic mobility of γ-, β- or rarely α_2-globulins, producing homogeneous peaks on the paper strip. On immuno-electrophoresis they can be shown to belong to the immunoglobulin classes IgG, IgA, IgD or IgE with either κ or λ light chains. Malignant proliferation of a single group or clone of plasma cells causes production of this homogeneous immunoglobulin fraction: a monoclonal gammopathy. These abnormal proteins do not have antibody activity. Sometimes the level of paraprotein remains low and there is no depression of normal immunoglobulin synthesis—such patients have a better prognosis.

The *Bence-Jones proteins* are found in the urine of about 50 per cent. of patients with myelomatosis, and have been shown to represent one or other of the light chains of the immunoglobulins. Sometimes only light chains are produced by the malignant plasma cells but on other occasions complete immunoglobulins are produced as well as the light chains. They can be recognized in urine by their precipitation on heating to 45–55° C. but immunological methods are much more sensitive.

Heavy chain disease (Franklin's disease) has recently been described where the neoplastic cells make an excess of the Fc fragment of the heavy chains of the IgG molecule. This protein gives a narrow peak between the β- and γ-globulin regions on paper electrophoresis and also appears in the urine. The disease usually affects middle-aged men who present with either painful tender enlarged lymph glands or with weakness and weight loss. In some instances there is an unusual redness and oedema of the soft palate. The prognosis is poor and death follows within a few months.

Macroglobulins (IgM immunoglobulins) are present in small amounts in normal sera but pathological macroglobulins usually differ in molecular size from the normal proteins and are present in much greater amounts. They run largely with the β- and γ-globulins on paper electrophoresis and are best recognized by ultracentrifugal studies. Certain antibodies are macroglobulins, e.g. some thyroid antibodies, the cold agglutinins of acquired haemolytic anaemia and the rheumatoid factor. *Waldenström's macroglobulinaemia*, a chronic condition associated with generalized lymphadenopathy, hepatosplenomegaly and a haemorrhagic diathesis is characterized by high levels of macroglobulin probably produced by the abnormal lymphoid type cells. A similar increase in macroglobulins is found in *purpura hyperglobulinaemica*, commonly presenting as chronic purpura, especially of the legs, in older women.

C-reactive protein which is not present in healthy people is recognized by the formation of a precipitate with pneumococcus-C-polysaccharide. In numerous bacterial infections, rheumatic fever, myocardial infarction and carcinomata it appears in the serum during the acute phase and disappears usually when the acute symptoms and fever abate.

Cryoproteins will precipitate in the cold and redissolve on warming. Both cryoglobulins and cryofibrinogens may be found due to some unknown abnormality or as a result of a known disease process, e.g. myelomatosis, leukaemias, lymphomas, collagenoses, chronic infections and the nephroses. Patients usually manifest some type of cold sensitivity such as atypical Raynaud's phenomenon, urticaria, cyanosis and ulceration of extremities. Vascular occlusions or bleeding disorders may be prominent features. Sera and plasma stored at 4° C. and observed at 24 and 48 hours reveal a precipitate of cryoprotein which clears on warming. More than 16 mg. per cent. of cryoglobulin and over 100 mg. per cent. of cryofibrinogen are usually accepted as abnormal values. Other abnormalities of plasma proteins, e.g. macroglobulinaemia may also be present. Treatment is directed to the underlying disease and obviously the patient should avoid exposure to cold.

REFERENCES

Jarnum, S. (1963) *Protein-losing Gastroenteropathy*, Oxford.
Schoen, R., and Sudhof, H., eds (1963) *Biochemical*

Findings in the Differential Diagnosis of Internal Diseases, Amsterdam.

AMYLOIDOSIS

Definition

Amyloidosis is the term applied to a group of syndromes which have in common the deposition in the tissues of an apparently amorphous metachromatically staining material.

Aetiology and Pathology

Classification of the amyloidoses is still tentative but two main types can be recognized: a 'primary' group in which no other pathological process responsible for the lesions can be found, and a 'secondary' group with which some underlying cause such as chronic suppurative conditions (e.g. osteomyelitis, tuberculosis, lung abscess, bronchiectasis), malignant tumours, reticuloses, rheumatoid arthritis, regional ileitis, ulcerative colitis, chronic pyelonephritis and myelomatosis is associated. Primary amyloidosis may occur in familial or sporadic forms; it may affect many tissues or it may be localized, either confined to a particular system or organ, or very rarely as an isolated tumour of amyloid tissue. It was previously thought that the distribution of the deposits could be used to differentiate primary and secondary amyloidosis, the 'typical' amyloid deposits in liver, spleen, intestine and adrenals occurring in the secondary variety and the 'atypical' distribution in tongue, heart, skin and nerves occurring in the primary form. This distinction has not withstood critical examination and all forms of amyloid are now separated into two histological patterns according to the site of initial deposition. In perireticulin amyloidosis, amyloid is first deposited along reticular fibres particularly in the intima and inner portion of the media of blood vessels. In contrast, in pericollagen amyloidosis, amyloid is deposited along collagen fibres in the adventitia, outer media and intervascular connective tissue. Only one fibre system is affected in a given case of amyloid. When the distribution of amyloid is 'typical', intimal deposition is always present, whether the amyloidosis is of primary or secondary type. The 'atypical' distribution of amyloid invariably shows the adventitial type of distribution whether of primary or secondary origin.

Nature and Pathogenesis of Amyloid

Amyloid is a form of connective tissue which can be shown by electron microscopy to consist of fibrils measuring 80–100 A° in diameter and several thousand A° in length. Coating the fibrils are small amounts of most of the connective tissue acid mucopolysaccharides (particularly heparin sulphate) and plasma proteins. One of these proteins which is invariably present in human amyloid substance is a glycoprotein designated amyloid 'P' protein. This has not been detected in normal tissues but traces of it are present in adult plasma.

It is now generally agreed that amyloid fibrils are produced within the cytoplasm of reticulo-endothelial cells, either those which normally form reticulin or those which synthesize collagen, and subsequently extruded from the cells. The nature of the stimulus causing these cells to produce amyloid is uncertain but in secondary amyloidosis the major factor appears to be over-exposure to antigens or toxins.

Incidence

While amyloidosis is a rare cause of death, it occurs more frequently than is generally realized. Significant amyloid deposits are found in 0·5–1·0 per cent. of routine hospital autopsies. In certain ethnic groups amyloidosis is not uncommon, e.g. the dominantly-inherited, atypical neuropathic amyloidosis in part of Portugal and the recessively-inherited, typical nephropathic amyloidosis which accompanies familial Mediterranean fever. The major form of sporadic primary amyloid disease occurs in the fifth and sixth decades, whereas secondary amyloidosis can occur at any age.

Classification of the Amyloidoses

This is shown in TABLE 32.

Clinical Manifestations

The clinical manifestations of secondary amyloidosis may be masked by the underlying disease process and depend on the organs affected by the deposits. *Renal* involvement leads characteristically to a nephrotic syndrome and later to chronic renal failure. When the rate of deposition of amyloid is slower and less extensive, blood vessels tend to be involved causing nephrosclerosis and hypertension and protein loss may be less marked. Renal vein thrombosis can complicate amyloidosis affecting the kidneys and lead to a rapid exacerbation of the nephrotic syndrome.

Hepatomegaly is common but evidence of liver failure, e.g. jaundice and hepatic coma is rare. A specific defect of plasma coagulation factor X has been described in some cases of severe hepatic amyloidosis. *Splenomegaly* is seldom more than of moderate degree. *Gastro-intestinal* involvement leads to chronic diarrhoea and a malabsorption syndrome. In secondary amyloidosis extensive deposition in the *adrenals* may cause adrenocortical failure. Amyloid *neuropathy* may be the result of vascular lesions or compression atrophy. *Myopathy* affects principally the tongue and heart. In *cardiomyopathy* lesions are frequent in the bundle of His and heart failure is accompanied by a low ECG voltage, arrhythmias and digitalis sensitivity. *Skin* involvement may present with purpura, or with flat brownish papules and the elements of the triple response may be impaired.

The inherited amyloidoses present in diverse manners and although amyloid is widely deposited, the kidneys, peripheral nerves and ganglia and the heart bear the brunt of the disease. Familial Mediterranean fever is a genetic disorder, particularly affecting peoples of Mediterranean stock. It presents with recurrent attacks of fever accompanied by pain in the abdomen, chest, skin or joints or with amyloidosis leading to renal failure. It belongs to the perireticulin histological type. The other syndromes seen are familial febrile urticaria, deafness and amyloidosis, familial cardiomyopathy and peripheral neuropathy affecting either the arms or the legs.

Sporadic primary amyloidosis may be diagnosed in

some patients who later are found to have myelomatosis but even in the absence of this complication excessive plasma cells of normal appearance may be found in the marrow.

Diagnosis

Amyloidosis may be suspected clinically but like sarcoidosis the diagnosis rests on the histological appearance of biopsy material. The Congo red test is unreliable. Gum biopsy is painful and may give negative results even in advanced disease.

Prognosis and Treatment

In primary familial amyloidosis the prognosis varies in the different syndromes. In familial Mediterranean fever death occurs at an early age from renal failure; the course is more benign in the syndromes of febrile urticaria and the neuropathies. Patients with cardio-

TABLE 32

CLASSIFICATION OF THE AMYLOIDOSES
(after Muckle, 1969)

DISTRIBUTION	FIBRE ASSOCIATION	HEREDITARY	SPORADIC
Generalized	Pericollagen	1. Neuropathy, legs (Portugal) 2. Neuropathy, arms (N. America) 3. Neuropathy plus carpal tunnel syndrome (N. America) 4. Cardiomyopathy (Denmark)	Secondary: with myelomatosis Idiopathic: classical 'primary'
Generalized	Perireticulin	1. Nephropathic (familial Mediterranean fever, Israel) 2. Nephropathic (similar syndrome, Derbyshire in United Kingdom)	Secondary: 1. chronic infection 2. malignancy Idiopathic: nephropathic
Localized	Pericollagen	—	Dermal
Localized	Mostly pericollagen, others not known	1. Senile cerebral 2. Dermal 3. Corneal	1. Senile (cerebral, pancreatic, pulmonary, cardiac, seminal) 2. Diabetic (pancreatic islets) 3. Tracheobronchial diffuse 4. Focal, nodular (pulmonary, ureteric) 5. In or with neoplasms (carcinoma of skin, medullary carcinoma of thyroid)
Tumoral	Mostly pericollagen, others not known	—	Hepatic, dermal, pulmonary

unreliable and not without risk, it should not now be used. There is a high incidence of rectal infiltration in most varieties of amyloidosis and rectal biopsy is now the diagnostic procedure of choice. It is essential that the biopsy includes a substantial portion of submucosa with its vasculature and it is usually possible to distinguish between perireticulin and pericollagen deposits. Renal biopsy is also a valuable method of diagnosis, though because of its risks and because the kidney may be little affected in primary amyloidosis, it is best to reserve this procedure for patients who show evidence of renal involvement, e.g. albuminuria, hypertension, haematuria or uraemia. Liver biopsy is not often indicated because of the risk of haemorrhage. Hepatic deposits are frequently uneven so the procedure is

myopathy present later in life and die in a few years from heart failure. The average survival from onset of symptoms in the sporadic primary amyloid syndromes is usually about 3 years. In secondary amyloidosis treatment of the underlying disease may slow the progress of the disorder. Unfortunately no specific treatment is available which will cure any form of amyloidosis.

REFERENCES

DAHLIN, D. C. (1949) Secondary amyloidosis, *Ann. intern. Med.*, **31**, 105.

MELLINKOFF, S. M., SNODGRASS, R. W., SCHWABE, A. D., MEAD, J. F., WEIMER, H. E., and FRANKLAND, M. (1962) Familial Mediterranean fever, *Ann. intern. Med.*, **56**, 171.

MISSMAHL, H. P. (1969) Amyloidosis, in *Textbook of*

Immunopathology, ed. MIESCHER, P. A., and MULLER-EBERHARD, H. J., Vol. II, p. 421, New York.

MUCKLE, T. J. (1969) Association of Clinical Pathologists, trainee pathologists teaching tape. A short account of human amyloidosis.

RUKAVINA, J. G., BLOCK, W. D., JACKSON, C. E., FALLS, H. F., CAREY, J. H., and CURTIS, A. C. (1956) Primary systemic amyloidosis: a review and an experimental, genetic and clinical study of 29 cases with particular emphasis on the familial form, *Medicine* (*Baltimore*), **35**, 239.

GEORGE A. SMART

PHENYLKETONURIA

Synonyms. Phenylpyruvic oligophrenia; P.K.U.

The association of mental retardation with the excretion of phenylpyruvic acid in the urine was noted by Folling in 1934 but it was Bickel and Woolf's (1953) suggestion that the retardation might be avoided by a diet low in phenylalanine that led to present day interest in the condition.

Phenylketonuria is a genetically determined disease transmitted as an autosomal recessive. The incidence in the population is about 1 in 15,000, boys and girls being equally affected. Characteristically these patients have blonde hair with blue eyes and fair skin. Eczema occurs in 25 per cent. and non-specific skin rashes are common. Such children may present in the early weeks of life with vomiting, undue irritability and convulsions but more often diagnosis is delayed until slow developmental progress causes concern, usually around 6–9 months.

The untreated patient is likely to be seriously retarded with an I.Q. below 50, many are microcephalic and show a variety of purposeless tic-like movements. Widely spaced incisor teeth, partial syndactyly together with increased muscle tone occurs in a proportion of cases.

Pathology

The essential amino acid, phenylalanine, is normally oxidized to tyrosine under the influence of the enzyme phenylalanine hydroxylase. Lack of the enzyme causes phenylalanine to accumulate in the blood and spinal fluid, this in turn is converted to phenylpyruvic acid which is excreted in the urine. The excess of phenylalanine also prevents the normal formation of melanin from tyrosine which is responsible for the lack of pigment in these patients. Other pathways of tyrosine metabolism are affected so that the reaction tyrosine to adrenaline is inhibited and patients with phenylketonuria have low levels of adrenaline in plasma. More important, the excess phenylalanine or its by-products cause damage to the developing brain and there is evidence to suggest that the delayed myelinization may be related to the low levels of 5-hydroxytryptamine (serotonin) found in these children. Other workers (Perry *et al.*, 1970) suggest that the deficiency of glutamine found in mentally retarded phenlyketonuric patients plays a dominant role in preventing normal cerebral maturation.

Diagnosis

The diagnosis may be suspected by the child's appearance or if there is a family history of retardation. It is confirmed by finding a raised phenylalanine level in the blood or phenylpyruvic acid in the urine, when it gives a green coloration with ferric chloride. If treatment is to prevent mental defect it must be instituted early and screening programmes have been devised to detect it in all newborn infants. Since in Britain only 50–70 children each year are born with this condition it is a major undertaking for relatively small return.

Urine tests dependent on the detection of phenylpyruvic acid have been in use for some years and a ferric chloride impregnated stick (*Phenistix*) has been widely advocated. This proved to be only partly effective and about 50 per cent. of children with phenylketonuria escaped diagnosis in the neonatal period. If this method is to be effective the baby must have been having a normal milk intake for some days so that blood levels of phenylalanine in excess of 15 mg. per 100 ml. are present, only then will its metabolites be detectable in urine.

The Guthrie test is now preferred. This has the advantage that it measures phenylalanine itself and is likely to be positive at an earlier stage. The test is carried out on blood, a drop being collected on to filter paper between the 6th–14th day of life. It depends on the competitive inhibition of growth of *Bacillus subtilis* by the phenylalanine analogue B-2-thienylalanine. Samples containing more than a certain concentration of phenylalanine overcome the inhibition and the bacteria flourish. Positive tests with more than 6 mg. phenylalanine per 100 ml. are selected for further study. Values in the 10–20 mg. range are very likely to have phenylketonuria, particularly if the values are rising rapidly and if there are phenylalanine metabolites detectable in the urine. Values up to 10 mg. per 100 ml. may be found in some heterozygotes and in some patients in which there is delay in developing the enzyme, phenylalanine hydroxylase.

Patients with values of over 20 mg. per 100 ml. of phenylalanine with low tyrosine, should be treated although about 20 per cent. of this group will be of normal intelligence with or without treatment. There remains a group usually with values in the 10–20 mg. range with hyperphenylalaninaemia. These infants have normal tyrosine levels and do not excrete phenylpyruvic acid in the urine. They escape mental retardation and both they and their parents have a normal response if given a phenylalanine load.

Treatment

These children are treated with a synthetic diet low in phenylalanine but complete in other nutrients. Such milks are commercially available as *Cymogram* or *Lofenalac* and should be started as soon as the diagnosis is confirmed. Progress is controlled by keeping the blood phenylalanine level in the 2–4 mg. range. Complete exclusion of phenylalanine may cause growth failure and too rigid dietary control can be associated with rashes, intestinal bleeding and megaloblastic anaemia. The diet is unpalatable and may be rejected by children in the 2–3 year age group but there is solid evidence that adequate dietary control can prevent the gross mental defect, fits and eczema seen in untreated patients. It is not as yet known for how long the diet must continue. Hsia (1969) suggests that all infants with a phenylalanine level of over 20 mg. per 100 ml. should be treated for 5 years and that they should be challenged once or twice during the first 2 years to ensure that the enzyme is still deficient. Other workers are less ready to stop the diet in children who are progressing well.

REFERENCES

Hudson, F. P., Mordaunt, V. L., and Leahy, I. (1970) Evaluation of treatment begun in first three months of life in 184 cases of phenylketonuria, *Arch. Dis. Childh.*, **45,** 5.

Perry, T. L., Hansen, S., Tischler, B., Bunting, R., and Diamond, S. (1970) Glutamine depletion in phenylketonuria, *New Engl. J. Med.*, **282,** 761.

GALACTOSAEMIA

Galactosaemia is a rare inborn error of metabolism which is inherited as an autosomal recessive. Absence of the enzyme galactose-l-phosphate uridyl transferase prevents the normal conversion of galactose to glucose, so that galactose-l-phosphate accumulates in various tissues, and is thought to be responsible for the clinical manifestations of the disease.

Symptoms commonly present in infancy when following milk feeds, vomiting and jaundice associated with hepatomegaly occur. Weight gain is poor and there may be diarrhoea and an increased tendency to bleed. If the condition is not recognized cataracts and mental retardation result. The diagnosis is suggested by finding a reducing substance in the urine and this may be identified as galactose by chromatography. There may also be proteinuria and a generalized amino-aciduria. Lack of the enzyme in red blood cells may be demonstrated and serves to establish the diagnosis. In addition to the classical disease a less severe form may occur with short stature, a tendency to hypoglycaemia and later cirrhosis.

Treatment

Early recognition is important if a lactose-free diet is to prevent mental deterioration. Sometimes the disease remains unsuspected since in an ill, vomiting infant the intake of lactose may be insufficient for reducing substances to appear in the urine. Lactose-free milks, such as soya bean substitutes (e.g. *Galactomin*) are well tolerated and a low lactose intake is necessary throughout childhood. Mental retardation is unlikely if the diet is relaxed after the age of 5 years but the translucency of the lens may be impaired. The carrier state may be detected by finding lower levels of the enzyme uridyl transferase in the red cells or by an abnormal response to a galactose tolerance test.

REFERENCES

Hsia, D. Y. Y. (1967) Clinical variants of galactosaemia, *Metabolism*, **16,** 419.

Komrower, G. M., and Lee, D. H. (1970) Long-term follow-up of galactosaemia, *Arch. Dis. Childh.*, **45,** 367.

FRUCTOSAEMIA

Synonym. Hereditary fructose intolerance.

Like galactosaemia, this is an inborn error of metabolism which is inherited as an autosomal recessive. Unlike galactosaemia, symptoms are delayed until breast-feeding is replaced by bottle feeds with added sucrose. Normally this is hydrolysed to glucose and fructose but lack of fructose-l-phosphate aldolase prevents further breakdown of fructose-l-phosphate which then accumulates. If an affected infant is given a feed containing sucrose he may vomit and have symptoms of hypoglycaemia. As feeding continues there is failure to gain weight, anorexia and hepatomegaly. Fructose is detectable in the urine and later there is renal tubular damage so that a Fanconi syndrome develops with amino-aciduria, renal acidosis and phosphaturia.

The diagnosis is confirmed by giving a fructose load (3 g. per m.^{2} or 0·25 g. per kg.) given intravenously as a 25 per cent. solution) which results in a marked fall of blood glucose and phosphate. It is probable that the accumulation of fructose-l-phosphate inhibits phosphorylase activity and impedes the breakdown of glycogen to glucose. A partial form of late onset has been described in children who voluntarily learn to avoid sugars. They develop cirrhosis and tend to be retarded although, unlike galactosaemia, cataracts have not been described. Interestingly they have noticeably good caries-free teeth. The condition should be differentiated from galactosaemia and from tyrosinosis when it occurs with hepatomegaly, a multifactorial tubular leak and renal rickets. Treatment consists of the exclusion of cane sugar and fruits from the diet. Sorbital in fruit squashes which is converted to fructose should also be avoided. The prognosis is good with proper dietary supervision.

REFERENCES

Cornblath, M., *et al.* (1963) Hereditary fructose intolerance, *New Engl. J. Med.*, **269,** 1271.

Levin, B., Oberholzer, V. G., Snodgrass, G. S. A. I., Stimmler, L., and Wilmers, Mary J. (1963) Fructosaemia—an inborn error of fructose metabolism, *Arch. Dis. Childh.*, **38,** 220.

Dennis Cottom

THE FREE AMINO ACIDS IN THE PLASMA AND URINE

For many years free amino acids have been known to occur in blood and urine. With the advent of the sensitive techniques of paper and ion-exchange column chromatography studies of normal and abnormal amino acid metabolism have advanced rapidly. The amino acid pattern of plasma has a fairly constant composition which roughly simulates the amino acid content of the tissue proteins. Alanine and glutamine are present in the highest concentration in the plasma, whereas in the urine glycine and histidine are most abundant. Amino acid excretion is surprisingly constant in an individual over many years, and there is little difference in the pattern in the two sexes except for an increased histidine excretion in pregnancy. In the cerebrospinal fluid the amino acid content is lower than in plasma and the pattern somewhat different.

An ever increasing number of diseases has been described in which the urinary content of free amino acids is altered in some way either by a general increase in amino acids or by an increase in a limited number of amino acids. A generalized amino-aciduria usually starts with hypersecretion of amino acids which are normally less well reabsorbed by the renal tubules. Later all amino acids are affected. Three sets of circumstances may lead to such an excretion pattern. First, an increased plasma amino acid content may cause an 'overflow' amino-aciduria. Secondly, a normal or low plasma content may be associated with an amino-aciduria due to overloading of an intact reabsorption mechanism by an increased glomerular filtration. This occurs in normal pregnancy. Thirdly, impaired tubular reabsorption amino acids may occur.

Specific types of amino-aciduria may be congenital or acquired. If a particular enzyme is missing, the precursor of the reaction accumulates and if no alternative metabolic pathway is available, this substance and its products may have harmful effects on tissues and be excreted in excess in the urine. In acquired disorders, where there is usually tissue breakdown, taurine and β-amino-iso-butyric acid are excreted in excess.

At least five group-specific mechanisms in the proximal tubule are involved in the active reabsorption of amino acids, each under separate genetic control:

1. For the dibasic amino acids lysine, arginine and ornithine, which is shared with cystine and is common also to the gut mucosa.
2. For a large group of aliphatic and aromatic amino acids (the 'Hartnup' group), also common to the gut.
3. For the dicarboxylic acids glutamic and aspartic acids.
4. For glycine and the imino acids proline and hydroxyproline.
5. For the β-amino acids and taurine.

Recessively inherited defects of processes (1), (2) and (4) are responsible for the abnormalities of cystinuria, Hartnup disease and glycine-imino-aciduria respectively.

Numerous classifications of the amino-acidurias have been proposed. The one shown in TABLE 33 was suggested by Soupart in 1962 and is both rational and comprehensive.

REFERENCES

HARRIS, H., and MILNE, M. D. (1964) Section XVIII, in *Biochemical Disorders in Human Disease*, ed. THOMPSON, R. H. S., and KING, E. J., London.

SOUPART, P. (1962) in *Amino Acid Pools*, ed. HOLDEN, J. T., p. 220, Amsterdam.

OBESITY

Obesity is a state in which there is an abnormally great amount of neutral fat in the storage depots of the body.

The tendency to become obese affects members of certain races more than others, and a tendency to obesity is found to run in families; it is difficult, however, to determine the relative importance of heredity and of feeding habits in these instances. Obesity tends to develop in both men and women in middle age, and in women it frequently begins after childbirth.

The 'Caloric Balance'

The fact that fat is being deposited without a corresponding decrease in other tissues indicates that more calories are being ingested than are converted to heat, and lost as organic compounds in the urine, faeces and breath. The opinion is often given that some people get fat though they eat very little whereas others, who are enormous eaters, remain thin. This may be true, for in normal people there are wide variations, not only in basal metabolism, but in the amount of energy needed to carry out a given task. More important still is the likelihood that those with a tendency to become obese are on the whole much more physically inactive than those who remain lean.

It is certainly true that no differences have been found between the percentage absorption of food in fat and lean people and no evidence has been found that the body will automatically 'burn off' energy-supplying nutrients which are taken in excess of requirements.

A person, when obese, requires much more energy than when thin not only for basal requirements but to accomplish similar physical activities. This acts to some extent as a regulator of body weight, for if a normal person, hitherto in caloric balance, increases his energy intake he will gain weight until the extra energy required to live his normal daily life is equal to the extra energy intake. In actual practice it is probable that such a person will cease to be quite as active as he was previously, so that he will gain somewhat more weight than might be expected from simple calculation. However, once the new equilibrium is reached he will cease to gain further weight.

It would seem to be reasonably clear that appetite and activity are the two main factors which ultimately regulate body weight. There is no evidence that increased activity follows increased intake of food, indeed, the reverse is probably more frequent. Thus, appetite regulation would seem to be the most important single control factor in weight regulation. What controls appetite is still not fully known. There are hypothalamic centres, stimulation of which produces satiation and others whose destruction results in the complete removal of any inclination to take food; the factors which stimulate or inhibit these centres are not known although it has been suggested that increased glucose utilization or increased heat production might result in decreased appetite. Other chemical factors may be important, for example, substances concerned in fat metabolism.

Causes

Presumably, in a few patients who, for example, become obese after encephalitis, there may have been damage to the hypothalamic centres. In most, however,

TABLE 33

CLASSIFICATION OF AMINO-ACIDURIAS

TYPE OF DISORDER	DISEASE	AMINO ACIDS IN URINE	CLINICAL FEATURES
Congenital metabolic block involving one or more amino acids.	(1) Phenylpyruvic oligophrenia.	Phenylalanine and derivatives, indole-acetic acid and derivatives.	Mental defect, deficient pigmentation, eczema, muscular hypertonicity.
	(2) Alkaptonuria.	Homogentisic acid, tyrosine and phenylalanine.	Urine dark on standing, pigmentation of cartilage, arthritis.
	(3) Maple-syrup-urine disease.	Valine, leucine and isoleucine and their α-keto acids.	Mental defect, vomiting, muscular hypertonicity, characteristic smell of urine.
	(4) Hyperphosphatasia.	Phospho-ethanolamine.	Widespread new bone formation.
	(5) Arginine - succinic aciduria.	Arginosuccinic acid.	Mental defect.
	(6) Idiopathic hyperglycinaemia.	Glycine.	Poor growth, mental defect, epilepsy, vomiting.
	(7) Histidinaemia.	Histidine.	Slight mental and physical defects.
	(8) Hyperprolinaemia.	Glycine, proline and hydroxyproline.	Sometimes associated with hereditary nephritis and deafness.
Congenital or acquired defect of convoluted tubule.	(1) Essential cystinuria.	Cystine, lysine, arginine, ornithine.	Cystine calculi, may have similar defect in bowel. Short stature.
	(2) Hartnup disease.	General increase in neutral amino acids, indican and indole-acetic acid.	Pellagra-like rash, mental defect, attacks of cerebellar ataxia associated with infections.
	(3) De Toni-Debré-Fanconi syndrome.	General increase.	Rickets or osteomalacia, glycosuria, hyperphosphaturia.
	(4) Cystinosis.	Cystine.	Cystine deposits in liver, spleen, marrow, renal tubules.
	(5) Heavy metal intoxication.	General increase.	—
	(6) Oxalic lithiasis.	Glycine.	Oxalic acid calculi.
	(7) Glycine-imino-aciduria.	Glycine and the imino acids proline and hydroxyproline.	Harmless.
	(8) Lipoidic nephrosis.	General increase.	Nephrotic syndrome.
Secondary to some other congenital metabolic upset.	(1) Wilson's disease.	Proline, citrulline, cystine, etc.	Cirrhosis, extrapyramidal syndrome, Kayser-Fleischer ring.
	(2) Galactosaemia.	General increase.	Nutritional failure, hepatosplenomegaly, cataracts, mental defect.
	(3) Laevulosaemia.	General increase.	Similar to galactosaemia.
	(4) Lowe's syndrome.	General increase.	Glaucoma, cataracts, mental defect, poor temperature control, acidosis.
	(5) Miscellaneous, e.g. gargoylism, etc.	—	—
Secondary to some acquired metabolic upset.	(1) General systemic disturbances, e.g. kwashiorkor, fasting, radiation, hepatic coma, pernicious anaemia, etc.	Taurine, β-amino-iso-butyric acid.	—
	(2) Liver disorders, e.g. viral hepatitis, cirrhosis, hepatic coma.	General increase.	—
	(3) Vitamin D deficiency, rickets and osteomalacia.	General increase.	—
	(4) Vitamin C deficiency.	Proline, hydroxyproline, later general increase.	—
	(5) Toxic compounds, e.g. mercury, lead, etc.	General increase.	—
	(6) Hypokalaemia.	General increase.	—
	(7) Hyperparathyroidism (primary or secondary).	General increase.	—

a variety of social and psychological factors seem to be the most important stimuli to increased food intake. Eating habits developed in youth may be carried into middle age when energy expenditure has become diminished; psychological disturbances may produce either diminished or increased food intake; in the latter case the gratification derived from the food takes the place of other unsatisfied emotions.

Endocrine abnormalities are sometimes associated with increased weight. Hypothyroidism, for example, usually lowers the energy requirements (by lowering both B.M.R. and physical activity) more than any concomittant decrease in appetite. Hypogonadism also is very prone to be associated with extra fat deposits, particularly in the breasts, abdomen, hips and thighs and it seems possible that the obesity associated with mild degrees of hypopituitarism may well be accounted for by the resulting combination of hypothyroidism and hypogonadism. Increased activity of the adrenal cortex, frequently results in obesity. In Cushing's syndrome, where the main excess secretion consists of cortisol, the fat is deposited on the face, neck and trunk, the limbs being relatively spared—though these look thinner than they really are, because of the diminution in musculature.

In patients with attacks of hypoglycaemia, whether spontaneous or induced in diabetics by too much insulin, the appetite is unduly stimulated and there is a tendency to develop obesity. Finally, the onset of obesity is particularly common at puberty, at the menopause and in women after childbirth. In cases such as these there is presumably some underlying endocrine abnormality which ultimately results in a greater calorie intake than expenditure. Recently, a 'fat mobilizing factor' has been found in the urine of patients and animals who are losing weight and this may well be of endocrine origin, indeed, a substance with fat mobilizing properties has been isolated from the anterior pituitary. Although this may well turn out to be of considerable importance, the precise role of such factors in the mechanism of obesity has yet to be determined.

It is also possible that in some obese patients there may exist an abnormality of fat metabolism (perhaps connected with the above substances), whereby the rate of fatty acid synthesis exceeds the rate of its utilization unless an abnormally high proportion of the body weight is composed of adipose tissue. The fat in adipose tissue is normally in a rapid state of turnover. The outflow of calories from the blood stream, in the form of free fatty acids, is about three times that due to glucose. There is probably a turnover of 1000 to 2000 kilocalories per day in normal adipose tissue, about this energy value of glucose being converted into fat, and the same value of free fatty acid being liberated into the plasma. It is clear that under conditions of over-all calorie balance this synthesis and release of free fatty acid must proceed at the same rate. If for any reason the rate of synthesis should exceed the rate of breakdown, energy utilization in the rest of the body remaining the same, there must be an increase in food intake if other tissues are not to be used for energy purposes. Thus, if in some way such a metabolic change were to be associated with a stimulation of appetite, it could be a cause of obesity. Such a situation probably exists as a genetic abnormality in mice, but, if it exists as a fundamental defect rather than an adaptive mechanism in man, it is likely to be fairly rare.

Effects of Obesity

Obesity is one of the main causes of ill health in countries with a high standard of living. The expectation of life is much shorter than for individuals of normal weight and the incidence of most diseases is greater in the obese than in the normal. Very roughly, the expectation of life decreases by 1 per cent. below the normal for every one pound weight above normal. Obesity appears to be a particularly striking predisposing factor in diabetes mellitus and in cardiovascular disorders; moreover the death rate from diabetes mellitus is about 250 per cent. greater in obese than in normal people and death from cardiovascular diseases is some 60–70 per cent. greater in the obese than in the normal.

Symptoms

General lassitude and weariness, dyspnoea on exertion, aches and pains, particularly in the knees and lumbar spine, maceration and infection of the skin, and sometimes varicose veins and oedema of the ankles, are the main complaints of the obese. In addition, however, there may be symptoms associated with hypertension or diabetes mellitus, conditions closely associated with the obesity itself.

The pain in the knees and back is not surprising when one considers the extra weight which has to be carried, 50–100 lb. (23–45 kg.) being not at all uncommon. This alone will tend to produce dyspnoea, but the position is aggravated by the extra stiffness of the thoracic cage and its contents which greatly increases the work required for respiration. Sometimes in extreme obesity this is so great that under-ventilation occurs with resultant oxygen deprivation and carbon dioxide retention. The oxygen deprivation may ultimately result in secondary polycythaemia. Such individuals may suffer from an irresistible urge to fall asleep and this has been thought to be due to carbon dioxide retention with consequent narcosis; the Pickwickian syndrome is the name which has been given to the condition.

Treatment

There are three main factors to be considered: (1) to correct any obvious underlying cause; (2) to restrict the daily calorie intake below the daily calorie requirements; and (3) to increase, if possible, the general activity of the patient.

When there is any obvious endocrine or metabolic disturbance the main line of treatment must be to correct it. Psychological disturbances may exist, but they do not usually require prolonged psychiatric treatment although sometimes this is essential. In the vast majority of cases, however, the main line of treatment will consist in considerable restriction of the calorie intake. Many diets have been devised for this, but it is often very difficult to ensure that the patient will adhere to them satisfactorily—mainly because of the rigidity or, failing this the complicated nature of the instructions. For this reason a considerable contribution was made by Marriott when he introduced the diet shown below. This is suitable both for simple obesity and for obese patients with diabetes mellitus who do not require insulin. A patient will generally lose at least 2 lb. weight per week when on this diet.

REDUCING DIET

(Devised by H. L. Marriott (1949) *Brit. med. J.*, **2**, 18.)

1. Eat or drink as much as you like (or can get) of: Lean meat, poultry, game, rabbit, hare, liver, kidney, heart, sweetbread—cooked in any way, but *without addition of flour, breadcrumbs or thick sauces.*

Fish (not tinned) boiled or steamed only; no thick sauce.

Eggs, boiled or poached *only.*

Potatoes, boiled, steamed, or baked in skins, but not *fried, roast, sauté or 'chips'*; not potato powder.

Other vegetables of all kinds (fresh, tinned or dried) cooked in any way *not involving the use of fat.*

Salad and tomatoes *without oil or mayonnaise.*

Beetroot, radishes, watercress, parsley.

Fresh fruit of any kind, including bananas. Also bottled fruit if bottled without sugar. *Not tinned or dried fruits (including dates, figs and raisins).*

Sour pickles, *not sweet pickles or chutneys.*

Clear soup, broth, Bovril, Oxo, Marmite.

Salt, pepper, mustard, vinegar, Worcester sauce (no other sauces).

Saccharin for sweetening.

Water, soda-water and non-sweetened mineral waters.

Tea and coffee (milk only as allowed below).

2. You may have milk (not condensed) up to half a pint daily. *No cream.*

3. You may have three very small pieces of bread per day, and take them either one at each main meal or all three at one meal as desired (*'very small'* means *not exceeding* 1 *oz.* (28·5 g.)).

4. You may have *nothing else whatever*: particularly note that this means:

No butter, margarine, fat or oil (except for cooking meat, *not fish*).

No sugar, jam, marmalade, honey, sweets, chocolate, cocoa.

No puddings, ices, dried or tinned fruits, nuts.

No bread (except as above), cake, biscuits, toast, patent reducing breads, cereals, oatmeal, Allbran, Ryvita, Vitawheat.

No barley, rice, macaroni, spaghetti, semolina, sausages, cheese.

No cocktail savouries, alcohol (beer, cider, wines and spirits).

Weigh before you begin, and thereafter weekly, on the *same* scales in the same clothes and at the same time of day.

Total starvation for prolonged periods has been put forward as a satisfactory form of treatment because, surprising as it may seem, patients treated in this way do not feel particularly hungry after the first 12–24 hours. This regime, however, must be carried out in hospital and even under carefully controlled conditions is not without danger for sudden death from cardiac causes have been reported to occur. It has been shown, as one might expect, that such treatment results in a substantial loss in lean body mass as well as in adipose tissue. When one considers these disadvantages along with the inconvenience and expense of prolonged hospitalization, and when one discovers that a high proportion of those who have successfully lost weight in this way rapidly relapse shortly after they return home, complete starvation appears to be a form of therapy which should not be lightly advocated.

Diets with an abnormally high fat content have been advocated as producing weight loss without a prescribed restriction of food intake. In so far as these work they do so largely by producing an automatic reduction in the total daily intake of calories. Until the long-term effect of such diets, e.g. on atherosclerosis is known, it is doubtful if they should be prescribed.

Restriction of fluids is sometimes advocated, but there is little point in this. Fluid retention does *not* cause obesity. The main virtue of restricting fluids with meals is that dry food, which cannot be washed down, is not so attractive and thus less will probably be eaten. It is quite often observed that an obese person will maintain weight for anything up to two weeks even though the calorie intake is considerably less than the energy expended. This is due to fluid retention, and if the patient is followed for long enough it will be found that the retained fluid is always ultimately eliminated.

Appetite depressants are frequently advertised and at one time dextro-amphetamine was widely used for this purpose. In view of the habituation which may occur with compounds of this type, and in view of their widespread misuse, they should no longer be prescribed, nor should any preparation containing them. Other drugs are marketed which are claimed to suppress appetite without producing the psychological side-effects of the amphetamines but none of them is strikingly efficacious.

Controlled trials in which the effect of fenfluramine was compared with other compounds suggested that this substance did in fact have some weight-losing effect and the biguanides phenformin and metformin have also been reported to induce weight loss in non-diabetic obese subjects without inducing hypoglycaemia. It should be emphasized, however, that any effect which these drugs may have is relatively slight, and it remains essential to impress upon the patient, who usually wants an easy way to slim, that drugs are no substitute for cutting down the food intake.

To instil a real desire to lose weight is an absolutely essential beginning to successful treatment.

Results of Treatment

Some obese patients feel light-headed at times while they are losing weight and most of them feel the cold. At first it requires much effort of will to restrict the food intake, but the ability to do this improves with training and all this should be explained to the patient.

The improvement in general well-being is often quite remarkable and quite enough to illustrate to the patient how important it is to be rid of the excessive weight. When diabetes mellitus is present the symptoms usually recede and sometimes even the glucose tolerance test will become normal. Where a patient is hypertensive the measured blood pressure nearly always falls and symptoms such as headache frequently disappear. The fall in measured blood pressure is partly brought about by the decrease in the size of the patient's arm relative to the sphygmomanometer cuff, but there is probably also a decrease in the true blood pressure. It has been shown that the over-all prognosis as to life improves markedly in those patients who successfully slim and remain slim. In spite of this, the over-all long-term results in most published series are very dismal. The majority of obese patients will lose weight for the first six or twelve months of treatment, but there is a great tendency for them to return to their old habits.

LIPODYSTROPHIA PROGRESSIVA (BARRAQUER-SIMONS DISEASE)

Definition

This is a condition in which there is loss of subcutaneous fat, the loss usually being confined to the upper part of the body.

Aetiology

About 80 per cent. of the reported cases are females. The onset tends to occur in early life, in about half of all cases being before the age of 10 years, and in about three-quarters before the age of 20 years. In the relatively few males who have been reported with the condition, the onset was before the age of 10 years in nearly 90 per cent.

A history of infection preceding the onset has been frequently noted, but in view of the frequency of infections in childhood there seems to be no convincing evidence that these infections were causal.

Two endocrine abnormalities have been noted to occur in a significant proportion of cases, namely, hyperthyroidism and either frank diabetes mellitus or a high blood sugar curve, which is sometimes of the 'lag' type. Insulin resistance is sometimes found in those cases which have diabetes mellitus.

Symptoms and Signs

Apart from the psychological disturbances resulting from the abnormal appearance, there are no real symptoms associated with the disease, the patients being in good health; patients in whom there is either associated hyperthyroidism or diabetes mellitus may of course have symptoms and signs associated with those conditions.

Characteristically, there is a great loss of subcutaneous fat from the face, neck, upper limbs and trunk, whereas the buttocks and legs may be normal or even have some excess of fat. The loss of fat gives a superficial appearance of emaciation, but closer inspection reveals the muscles to be normal in size and the outlines of the more superficial ones can readily be seen through the skin.

Occasionally cases are seen where the fat has left the lower limbs and is normal on the upper part of the body. It has also been suggested that the relatively common condition in females of obesity of the lower limbs associated with a normal amount of fat on the upper part of the body may be an allied condition.

Treatment

There is no treatment, the condition, once established, remains more or less stationary, and the expectation of life is unaffected by the lipodystrophy.

REFERENCES

DAVIDSON, S., MEIKLEJOHN, A. P., and PASSMORE, R. (1959) *Human Nutrition and Dietetics*, Edinburgh.

KEKWICK, A., and PAWAN, G. L. S. (1960) *Lancet*, **i**, 1190.

KEYS, A., and BROZEK, J. (1953) Body fat in adult man, *Physiol. Rev.*, **33**, 245.

MAYER, J. (1953) Genetic, traumatic and environmental factors in the etiology of obesity, *Physiol. Rev.*, **33**, 472.

SOCIETY OF ACTUARIES (1959) *Build and Blood Pressure Study*, London.

STRANG, J. M. (1959) in *Diseases of Metabolism*, 4th ed., ed. DUNCAN, GARFIELD G., Philadelphia.

THE AMERICAN JOURNAL OF CLINICAL NUTRITION (1960) *Symposium on Energy Balance*, **8**, 527.

VAN ITALIE, T. B. (1959) Physiologic aspects of hunger and satiety, *Diabetes*, **8**, 226.

WERTHEIMER, E., and SHAPIRO, B. (1948) *Physiol. Rev.*, **28**, 451.

WOHL, M. G., and GOODHART, R. S., eds (1960) *Modern Nutrition in Health and Disease*, 2nd ed., London.

GEORGE A. SMART

DIABETES MELLITUS

Definition

Diabetes mellitus is not a disease, but includes a variety of related disorders of metabolism, having in common an increase in blood sugar, usually accompanied by glycosuria. In many of these there is also a greater or lesser tendency to ketosis, which is the most important immediate danger; and an increased liability to various forms of vascular degeneration, which are the most serious long-term risks.

Prevalence

The prevalence of diabetes in a community depends on how diabetes is defined for this purpose. Studies of glucose tolerance curves in populations (as in the Guy's—Bedford survey of 1962) show a gradual rise in continuous sequence from the normal to the undoubted diabetic. The prevalence of diabetes, as measured by this criterion, thus depends on what degree of abnormality of sugar tolerance is held to constitute diabetes.

Briefly, the position in Western European and American countries appears to be as follows. Using the ordinarily accepted criteria for diagnosis to be mentioned later, detection drives have shown an over-all incidence of the order of 13 per 1000, half of whom are known diabetics and half undetected. The latter are mostly over the age of 40 and are usually obese. They frequently remain undetected till they present with an established complication. If lesser degrees of abnormality in the glucose tolerance test or abnormalities in the cortisone-loaded glucose tolerance test are accepted as evidence of diabetes then the incidence of subclinical diabetes is very much higher. In the survey mentioned, for instance, 130 per 1000 of a supposedly normal adult population showed a blood sugar of more than 120 mg. per 100 ml. two hours after taking 50 g. of glucose by mouth. In any population studied there are also a large number of other glycosurics with normal or near-normal blood sugars, some of whom are potential diabetics and some have low renal thresholds.

It seems likely that there are in the British Isles some 340,000 known diabetics and about an equal number undetected, together with an unknown number of potential ones. Since diabetes is mainly a disease of the older age groups and the population is ageing, the prevalence is likely to rise.

Though insulin has revolutionized the outlook for the diabetic in certain respects—the expectation of life of a 10 year old diabetic child is now 45 years instead of 1·3 years in the pre-insulin era—it has not prevented an alarming incidence of complications, particularly retinopathy, nephropathy and arteriopathy in those who have had the disease for some years. How far these complications are due to factors which cannot be controlled by treatment and how far to avoidable poor control of the diabetic state is a major problem.

Aetiology

Knowledge is quite incomplete, but two factors of importance have been recognized, an inherited tendency and over-nutrition.

There are two kinds of evidence for an hereditary tendency. First, a history of diabetes in one or more blood relatives is much commoner in diabetics than in non-diabetics; and secondly, concordance (i.e. both twins developing diabetes) is several times as common in identical twins as in fraternal twins. Identical twins indeed often develop diabetes of about the same severity, within a short time of each other. How far diabetes mellitus is genetically homogeneous and how the tendency is inherited is uncertain. It has been suggested that it is homogeneous, that the tendency is inherited in a simple recessive manner and that if all potential diabetics lived to the age of 90, the numbers actually developing the disease would be in accordance with this hypothesis.

The importance of over-nutrition is shown by the fact that over the age of 40 some 80 per cent. of patients developing diabetes are, or have been, considerably overweight. Broadly speaking, both the incidence and mortality of diabetes after middle age vary directly with the degree of obesity; and in both World Wars the incidence and mortality fell with rationing.

It appears likely that when the inherited tendency is strong enough, the subject develops diabetes in childhood or youth without becoming fat. If the inherited tendency is less strong, the disease becomes manifest only when precipitating factors 'bring out' the inherited predisposition. The most important of these are obesity and pregnancy, though infection may act temporarily in the same way, and so possibly may trauma and nervous shock. Recent studies have implicated Coxsackie B4 virus infection as a possible aetiological factor.

The disease is apparently commoner in urban than in rural communities, and in Jews than in Gentiles. These differences may well be due to habits as regards diet and physical exercise. It is possible that trauma, like any other form of shock, may hasten the time at which a person with latent diabetes manifests symptoms. The absence of increased prevalence of the disease in the battle casualties of the World Wars indicates that trauma can play no more important part than this.

Pathology

In 1889 Minkowski produced diabetes experimentally by removing the pancreas from a dog. Langerhans had described his islets in 1869, and the hypothetical internal secretion of the pancreas was named 'insuline' long before it was isolated. The final extraction in 1921 after only a few months' work by Banting, then a young orthopaedic surgeon, and Best, a junior graduate assistant, was one of the great medical events of the century.

The pathogenesis at that time appeared deceptively simple. Lack of insulin due to a defect of the islets reduced the ability of the tissues to utilize glucose, which therefore accumulated in the blood, and was excreted in the urine. Impaired oxidation of glucose led to a hold-up in the metabolism of fat, so that intermediary products accumulated in the blood and led to ketosis. It soon became apparent, however, that this was an over-simplification. Histological studies on the pancreas showed that whereas in some human cases various changes are found in the islets, in at least 25 per cent. these appear normal, at least to light microscopy. Further, a number of patients have now survived total pancreatectomy and presumably have no insulin secretion of their own. They have been found to develop a moderate degree of diabetes easily controlled by 40 Units of insulin a day. A similar type of diabetes is seen with some cases of haemochromatosis and chronic pancreatitis. Since many 'idiopathic' diabetics require well over 100 Units a day, their diabetes cannot be due to a simple lack of insulin secretion.

A great deal of experimental evidence has implicated other endocrine glands, particularly the anterior pituitary and adrenals. Indeed, the condition has been produced in suitable animals by injections of anterior pituitary extracts, and more recently of purified growth hormone. This fits in with the clinical observation that mild diabetes is seen in some cases of hyperpituitarism, and often arises during steroid therapy.

Survival in the animal organism depends, amongst other things, on an homeostatic mechanism which maintains the blood sugar in a fairly narrow range between 70 and 160 mg. per 100 ml. This depends on an interaction between a number of substances known directly or indirectly to raise the blood glucose (including pituitary and adrenocortical hormones, adrenaline, glucagon, insulinase, insulin antagonists) and insulin which alone lowers it. An animal would not survive long if lack of food led to hypoglycaemia and unconsciousness. Hence mechanisms for raising the blood sugar and preventing hypoglycaemia in starvation are of more immediate importance than is insulin. Broadly, a diabetic may be regarded as behaving as if in a state of starvation—making inappropriate use of mechanisms for raising the blood glucose; and some features of uncontrolled diabetes, such as the production of glucose from protein and fat sources and the resulting ketosis are the same as those found in starvation.

There have been three main theories of the action of insulin: (1) That it is necessary for the adequate utilization of glucose within the cells. This is the peripheral 'under-utilization' of glucose theory. (2) That it prevents the over-production of glucose in the liver. This is the central 'over-production' of glucose theory. (3) That it facilitates the transport of glucose and other substances across the cell membrane. This is the impaired 'cell permeability' theory.

All recent evidence suggests the third is the most important function of insulin. Having facilitated transport across the cell membranes it may also take part in enzymatic reactions within the cells of muscle and adipose tissue, which lead to the utilization of glucose, and to its storage as glycogen and fatty acid. Whether insulin directly controls gluconeogenesis in the liver or whether the latter is a secondary effect of the failure of glucose to gain access to the cells is uncertain.

Insulin is formed in the β cells of the islets of Langerhans and released from those cells when the glucose concentration in the pancreatic artery rises. One theory of diabetes suggests that an excessive secretion of a diabetogenic factor by the anterior pituitary—either growth hormone or something very like it—leads to exhaustion of the β cells.

Insulin then passes from the pancreas to the portal vein and so to the liver, where some is split by an insulinase into the A and B chains of insulin and some is conjugated with protein. From the liver it passes to the general circulation, where it is exposed to various anti-insulin factors or antagonists. These include pituitary and adrenal cortical hormones and other antagonists. Although the nature of insulin antagonists in idiopathic diabetes remains in doubt, there appears to be some factor in maturity onset diabetes that impairs the action of insulin on muscle but not on fat. The so-called synalbumin antagonist, much studied by Vallance-Owen, may be derived from the B chain of insulin and may constitute an inborn error of metabolism, forcing the pancreas to secrete more insulin in a continuous effort to overcome the inhibitory effect of the antagonist; frank diabetes would occur when the pancreas could no longer fulfil these excess demands. However, there are other theories concerning insulin antagonists and the fact remains that immuno-reactive insulin is present in the plasma of diabetics but its biological potency is obviously poor.

From the general circulation insulin has to reach the cells. Butterfield, by studying arterial and venous insulin differences in the human forearm, claims to have demonstrated diminished insulin clearance from the blood vessels in diabetes. He suggests that the deposition of mucopolysaccharides in the basement membrane of the capillaries, which is certainly the basis of some of the complications of diabetes, may indeed be a factor in the causation of the disease by hindering the clearance of insulin from the circulation.

Just as there appears to be a continuous gradation in sugar tolerance from the normal to the fully diabetic, so it is unlikely that there is a single 'cause' for diabetes. Its causation is likely to be multifactorial and any or all of the mechanisms mentioned may prove to be important.

Clinical Picture

The classical onset with severe thirst, polyuria and loss of weight is seen in a minority, perhaps one-third of cases. Lack of energy, muscular weakness, mild thirst and some loss of weight are found in perhaps another third, if inquiry is made about them. Constipation from dehydration is occasionally the presenting symptom. Definite increase in appetite is unusual, though it is a safe generalization in this country that real loss of weight with an increased appetite means either thyrotoxicosis or diabetes mellitus. Pruritus vulvae and varying degrees of vulvitis are common in women, but generalized pruritus due to diabetes must be excessively rare, if it ever occurs. Men occasionally notice that spots of urine on their trousers dry leaving a white deposit, balanitis is not uncommon, and some complain of impotence.

A few patients are virtually symptomless, the glycosuria being discovered when the urine is examined as a routine for life insurance or other purposes. Almost one-fifth present with symptoms of complications. Of these a very few patients are first seen in diabetic coma, or with severe neuropathy. Others are detected by ophthalmologists who see micro-aneurysms or other evidence of diabetic retinopathy, in antenatal clinics and by gynaecologists among women referred for vulvitis. A few are discovered by testing the urine of patients with boils and other staphylococcal skin infections.

It may be said that a majority of diabetics fall into one of two groups. The older and fatter tend to have mild symptoms with an insidious onset, more often present with a complication, have little tendency to ketosis and are relatively insensitive to insulin. They are often called the 'maturity onset' type. The younger and thinner more often have severe and classical symptoms, with a definite onset, are very liable to ketosis and are sensitive to insulin. They are called the 'juvenile onset' type. Though this division into types is useful, it is by no means absolute. In particular, older diabetics sometimes develop a 'juvenile onset' type and easily go into ketosis.

Physical examination shows nothing in mild uncomplicated diabetes. In severe cases there may be weakness and wasting with some degree of dehydration. In more severe cases a dry brownish tongue, the odour of acetone in the breath and an enlarged tender liver may indicate that the patient is in impending coma. As many patients have complications by the time they consult a doctor, no initial examination of a diabetic is complete without examination of the eyes for lenticular opacities and retinopathy; of the skin for septic infections; of the legs for loss of knee- and ankle-jerks and other signs of diabetic neuropathy, and of the feet for loss of pulsation in the dorsalis pedis and posterior tibial arteries or other signs of impaired blood supply. The urine should be tested for protein and an X-ray of the chest should be taken.

Diagnosis

Urine Testing. The importance of routine urine testing for sugar will be evident from what has already been said. 'Clinitest' is a satisfactory and trouble-saving substitute for Benedict's test, provided the makers' instructions are followed exactly. A positive result indicates that a reducing substance is present in the urine, but not that the substance is glucose. 'False positives' may be due to drugs such as aspirin, salicylates, chloral hydrate and ascorbic acid, or to the presence of other sugars, of which lactose in pregnant and lactating women is the only one of clinical importance. 'Clinistix' is a simple and valuable means of distinguishing glucose from other reducing substances, but gives no indication of the amount of glucose in the urine.

In practice slight colour changes (i.e. a green colour) should be ignored, or left for elucidation by a biochemist. A definite reduction (i.e. yellow or red) in an untreated patient with definite thirst and polyuria, is for practical purposes diagnostic of diabetes, and further investigations are unnecessary. If a definite reduction is found in a patient with no symptoms or with doubtful symptoms, it is best to proceed to a glucose tolerance test.

The urine should also be tested in every case of suspected diabetes by Rothera's sodium nitroprusside test or 'Acetest' and Gerhardt's ferric chloride test for the presence of ketone bodies. The clinical significance of these two tests is often not understood. The nitroprusside test is specific for ketone bodies, but is extremely sensitive so that it may be positive in the presence of a clinically very mild ketosis. A red or purple colour with the ferric chloride test may be produced by ketone bodies or by drugs, notably aspirin and salicylates and sodium aminosalicylate. In the former case the test will be negative if performed on boiled urine, since ketone bodies are volatile. The ferric chloride test, however, is relatively insensitive, and therefore if both tests are positive a ketosis of some severity is present. The practical significance of different findings with these tests is summarized in TABLE 34. 'Acetest' is a convenient portable form of the sodium nitroprusside test.

Blood Sugars and the Glucose Tolerance Test. In each case the patient should have been eating a normal amount of carbohydrate for at least a week before the test, since a normal person after a few days on a reduced carbohydrate diet may show an abnormal blood sugar curve. For this reason patients found to have glycosuria, without definite diabetic symptoms and without ketosis, should never be put on a diet until the diagnosis has been confirmed by further investigations.

A clinically probable diagnosis of diabetes mellitus can be confirmed by estimating a single blood sugar 1–1½ hours after a meal containing at least 50 g. of carbohydrate. If this is over 180 mg. per 100 ml., the diagnosis is confirmed.

In symptomless glycosuria and in any case in which the diagnosis is really in doubt, it is wise to perform a glucose tolerance test. A normal blood sugar curve (i.e. a fasting blood sugar of under 110 mg. per 100 ml., rising to less than 180 mg. per 100 ml. in half an hour and returning to the fasting level within 2–2½ hours) with sugar in one or more corresponding specimens of urine indicates a lowered renal threshold or renal glycosuria. This is a harmless anomaly and requires no treatment. The so-called 'lag storage' or 'steeple' curve in which the blood sugar at half an hour rises to above 180 mg. per 100 ml. but returns to the fasting level within the usual time is also usually regarded as a harmless anomaly. In frank diabetes the fasting blood sugar is above 110 mg. per 100 ml., rises above 180 mg. per 100 ml. and either continues to rise or fails to return to the fasting level in 2–2½ hours. Provided the carbohydrate intake over the previous week has been adequate, and provided other causes of abnormal sugar tolerance, i.e. sepsis, thyrotoxicosis, severe liver disease,

TABLE 34

SUGAR	NITROPRUSSIDE TEST	FERRIC CHLORIDE TEST	SIGNIFICANCE
+++ i.e. 2 per cent. or more	–	–	Probably diabetes mellitus but no immediate danger or urgency.
+++	+	–	Diabetes mellitus with mild ketosis (or biguanide therapy).
+++	++	++	Diabetes mellitus with severe ketosis requiring urgent investigation and treatment.
+++	–	+	Probably a diabetic who has taken aspirin or salicylates.
–	+	–	Mild ketosis due to other causes, e.g. vomiting in children or starvation.

hyperpituitarism and hypercortico-adrenalism can be excluded, a curve in which the blood sugar rises above 180 mg. per 100 ml. at half an hour and does not return to the fasting level at 2–2½ hours should be regarded as indicating diabetes mellitus. It may be added that the chief value of the glucose tolerance test is in excluding diabetes mellitus, and there is never any indication to perform it on a known diabetic under treatment with insulin.

TREATMENT

The decision whether to treat a patient by diet alone or with hypoglycaemic drugs or with insulin depends on the severity of the symptoms, the presence or absence of complications and the patient's age and weight, and not on the results of special investigations such as the glucose tolerance test. Obese adult patients with mild diabetes and no ketosis nearly always can and should be treated with a diet which will reduce their weight. Underweight patients with severe symptoms and especially with ketosis should always be treated with insulin, and so should children. In the case of adult patients whose weight is in the normal range and who have no ketosis and no complications, it is justifiable to try the effects of a moderate reduction of the carbohydrate in the diet, with or without hypoglycaemic drugs.

Treatment will therefore be described under the following headings:

1. Treatment by diet alone.
2. Oral hypoglycaemic drugs.
3. Use of insulin.
4. Treatment of ketosis.

Treatment of Obese Patients by Diet Alone

Such patients are usually over middle age and have mild diabetic symptoms or no symptoms. They quite frequently, however, have some complication, such as retinopathy, by the time they come for treatment. The treatment is that of obesity [p. 494]. If such patients adhere to a diet of 1200–1400 calories, diabetic symptoms, such as thirst and polyuria, disappear, and the hyperglycaemia and glycosuria are usually rapidly controlled. If the weight is substantially reduced or reduced to normal, such patients are often able to eat a more liberal diet without a return of the diabetic state. But if the weight is allowed to increase again, the diabetic state returns. Appetite suppressants are of little avail, except that biguanides act as mild appetite suppressants and are thus the best hypoglycaemic drugs for obese patients.

Difficulty arises with overweight patients who fail to lose weight, especially if they have complications such as retinopathy or obliterative arterial disease. Insulin should be avoided if possible, since such patients are usually insulin-resistant, and if treated with large doses of insulin, their weight only increases further.

Oral Hypoglycaemic Drugs

Two types are available—sulphonylureas and biguanides.

Sulphonylureas. Credit is usually given to Janbon and his colleagues of Montpellier who noted the hypoglycaemic action of a thiazole compound which they were trying out in typhoid fever in 1942. This was studied further by Loubatières. The introduction for clinical purposes of carbutamide, now abandoned on account of its toxic effects, followed on the work of Franke and Fuchs in Germany in 1955.

The compounds most used are tolbutamide, which is short-acting and should be given in doses of 500 mg., 2–4 times a day; and chlorpropamide which is long-acting and should be given in doses of from 100 to 500 mg. first thing in the morning. Both drugs occasionally cause skin rashes, mild gastro-intestinal disturbance and rarely a cholestatic jaundice. Chlorpropamide may also produce an intolerance to alcohol. Both can produce hypoglycaemia, particularly if the patient eats irregularly, but this is never serious with therapeutic doses. Other sulphonylureas are acetohexamide, 250-1500 mg. daily in a single morning dose, and glibenclamide, 2·5–20 mg. daily—usually 10–15 mg. in the morning with or immediately after breakfast. The latter drug is weight for weight 50 times as potent as chlorpropamide, but appears to have little therapeutic advantage, except that it is said to have less side-effects and rarely causes flushing with alcohol.

Sulphonylurea drugs act by promoting the release of insulin from the β cells of the islets of Langerhans. Thus they are effective only in diabetics who have some islet tissue and produce some insulin of their own; and have no effect in pancreatic diabetes. In the United Kingdom it is generally held that they should not be used for obese diabetics who should be controlled by diet alone. They are most successful in middle-aged and elderly diabetics who are of about normal weight, who are not liable to ketosis, but whose hypoglycaemia is not controlled by dietary restriction alone. As mentioned below, they should never be used in children, the young, nor in severe diabetics of any age who are liable to ketosis. It is useless to prescribe them along with insulin. In the United States their use is now discouraged on the grounds that they may increase the risk of cardiovascular complications. This view is not shared by most European authorities.

Biguanides. The hypoglycaemic action of synthalin was known in the 1920's but toxic effects contra-indicated its clinical application.

The compounds most frequently used are phenformin, of which the normal dose is 25 mg. three or four times a day, and metformin of which the dose is 500 mg. three or four times a day. Phenformin is also available as slow release capsules of 50 mg. to be taken once or twice a day. Both may produce nausea, vomiting and sometimes diarrhoea. Some patients can tolerate half the dose stated above (i.e. half one tablet three or four times a day). These drugs do not depend on the presence of insulin and the pancreas. In animals they appear to inhibit the oxidation of glucose, to promote anaerobic glycolysis and also to enhance the passage of insulin into the cells. How they act in man is uncertain, but they are known sometimes to produce a mild ketosis or keto-acidosis, which is not in itself serious, but may cause confusion in diagnosis.

Since these drugs act in a different manner from the

sulphonylureas the effects are additive and patients who fail to achieve control in the first instance with sulphonylureas, or who subsequently lose it, may be controlled on a sulphonylurea plus a biguanide (e.g. tolbutamide, 500 mg., plus phenformin, 12·5 or 25 mg., three or four times daily). Biguanides can be given along with insulin and it has been claimed that some 'brittle' diabetics are better controlled in this way than on insulin alone.

Most experts think it unwise to attempt to treat any young diabetic with these drugs or any combination of them, since apart from the fact that the attempts are usually unsuccessful the long-term results are unknown. Older patients on doses of up to 40 Units of insulin daily may sometimes be successfully changed on to drugs. The trial is best made in hospital since occasionally a rapid deterioration of the diabetic state ensues. If the change is made outside hospital half the usual dose of insulin should be given on the first two days of drug treatment, and the patient should be instructed to test his urine regularly with 'Acetest' tablets until satisfactory control with drugs has been achieved. Accurately measured diets are not necessary with these drugs. Patients of normal weight can eat their usual diet. Patients who are overweight should have their carbohydrate restricted as for obesity [p. 494].

The Use of Insulin

Underweight patients must be treated with insulin since a diet of low calorie value would only lead to further loss of weight. It is important that the objectives of treatment with insulin should be understood. These are:

1. To enable the patient to live as normal a life as possible, earn a living and take part in ordinary activities. To achieve this it is necessary for him to learn more about the management of his own illness than is considered wise in any other condition. The main part of the work of a physician treating diabetics is to teach them how to look after themselves.
2. To keep the patient free from any symptoms of diabetes and from anything more than minor and occasional symptoms of hypoglycaemia throughout the 24 hours; and free from ketosis at any time.
3. To keep the urine as free from sugar as possible and the blood sugar as near normal as possible, provided the attainment of this does not interfere with (1) and (2). It is, for instance, misguided to achieve a sugar-free urine for most of the day, if this means that the patient has hypoglycaemic attacks so frequently that he is unable to earn his living, or that he has to spend most of his spare time testing his own urine and weighing out his food. There is, however, considerable room for skill in attaining (3) within the limits set by (1) and (2).

Insulin is destroyed by the gastric secretion, and therefore cannot be given by mouth. It is usually injected subcutaneously, though it can also be given intramuscularly and intravenously.

It is biologically standardized and is supplied in strengths of 20 Units per ml., 40 Units per ml. and 80 Units per ml. British Standard insulin syringes (B.S.I. 1619) available in 1 ml. and 2 ml. sizes with Luer mounts have a number of advantages and should always be prescribed. Since on these 1 ml. is divided into twenty divisions, each division corresponds to 1, 2 or 4 Units. Insulin should, therefore, be prescribed in multiples of 2 or 4, and not of 5 and 10.

There are unfortunately nine different preparations available in different strengths in Great Britain at the present time. The important ones are:

Insulin Injection, B.P., Soluble Insulin. 'Regular' or 'clear' insulin. Available in strengths of 20, 40 and 80 Units per ml. Acts quickly and strongly. Action starts within half an hour and lasts 6–8 hours with doses up to 40 Units, but up to 12 hours with very large doses. Hypoglycaemic symptoms most commonly occur 2–4 hours after injection, but may be delayed up to 8 hours or more with very large doses.

Soluble insulin is used:

1. In diabetic coma and severe ketosis [q.v.].
2. Three doses of soluble insulin a day, i.e. one dose before each main meal is often employed temporarily when specially strict control is necessary, e.g. at the beginning of treatment, during infections, before and after operations, in the latter months of pregnancy and in patients with active pulmonary tuberculosis.
3. Two doses of soluble insulin a day, i.e. before breakfast and before the evening meal, was for many years the standard treatment for all diabetics on insulin. It is still a useful method for those who are used to it and prefer not to change, for diabetics who are difficult to control on a single dose of any insulin and for those requiring very large doses. More than 60 Units of any insulin in one dose should be avoided if possible, on account of the danger of severe hypoglycaemia and many diabetics who have been on a large single dose of a long-acting insulin feel much better when transferred to two doses of soluble. On this regime one-third of the carbohydrate should be taken at breakfast and one-third in the evening meal, with a small lunch and tea and a snack at mid-morning and last thing at night.

Protamine Zinc Insulin Injection, B.P., 'Cloudy' Insulin. Available in strengths of 40 and 80 Units per ml. Though few if any new diabetics are now started on this type of insulin, there are many long-standing diabetics who still take it.

It is prepared as a suspension which must be shaken before use, consisting of insulin hydrochloride combined with protamine and zinc. It is slowly liberated and absorbed from the site of injection and is thus 'long-acting'. Its action does not begin for 3 or 4 hours but lasts from 12 to 24 or more, according to the dose. When it is given before breakfast, hypoglycaemic attacks occur in the second half of the day or during the following night. It is, therefore, generally considered wise that the dose of P.Z.I. should be adjusted so that the specimen of urine passed on rising should contain a small amount of sugar. Some diabetics are satisfactorily controlled on a single dose of P.Z.I. given before breakfast. In these cases the action of the insulin must presumably be lasting for more than 24 hours. Others require a mixture of P.Z.I. and soluble insulin. The carbohydrate in the diet should be distributed in the proportion of approximately one-fifth at breakfast, at lunch, at tea and at supper, with a snack during the morning and last thing at night.

The usual method is to start with P.Z.I. and increase the dose until the urine passed on rising contains a small amount of sugar. If, when this is achieved, urine passed in the morning or early afternoon contains large amounts of sugar, soluble insulin is added to the morning injection. Theoretically the P.Z.I. and soluble insulin should be given in separate injections since P.Z.I. contains an excess of protamine, and mixed with the soluble this converts an unknown amount of soluble insulin to protamine insulin. In practice, satisfactory results are often obtained by mixing the two in the same syringe according to the following technique:

1. Inject air equivalent to dose of P.Z.I. into P.Z.I. bottle; withdraw needle.
2. Inject air equivalent to dose of soluble into soluble bottle and draw required amount of soluble into syringe.
3. Transfer needle to previously prepared P.Z.I. bottle and draw into syringe the amount of P.Z.I. required.
4. Withdraw needle from P.Z.I. bottle and give injection immediately.

The object of this routine is to avoid transferring P.Z.I. to the bottle of soluble insulin.

By varying the proportions of P.Z.I. and soluble insulin, it is possible to control many diabetics on a single morning dose, the main disadvantage of the regime being the danger of hypoglycaemic reactions at night.

Insulin Zinc Suspensions (I.Z.S., Danish 'Semilente', 'Lente' and 'Ultralente'). It was found that the phosphate previously used as a buffer inhibited the delaying action of the zinc. The Danish preparations consist of insulin precipitated with very small quantities of zinc and resuspended in an acetate buffer without the addition of any protein or protamine. The length of action was found to vary with the size and form of the insulin particles. Insulin Zinc Suspension (Amorphous), B.P. (Danish Semilente, available in strength of 40 Units per ml.), has an action lasting up to about 16 hours. Insulin Zinc Suspension (Crystalline), B.P. (Danish Ultralente, available in strength of 40 Units per ml.), has an action lasting up to 30 hours or more. A mixture of the two, consisting of 3 parts of amorphous to 7 of crystalline, Insulin Zinc Suspension, B.P. (Danish Lente, available in strengths of 40 and 80 Units per ml.) has an action of approximately 24 hours, and has been introduced as the preparation likely to control most diabetics when used in a single dose.

It is the variety most used in this country. The effect is much like that of a mixture of P.Z.I. and soluble, except that hypoglycaemic reactions appear to be less common. With a single morning dose, these may occur during the morning or afternoon but rarely, if ever, at night. Local reactions to the injection are much rarer than with the older insulins. The carbohydrate in the diet should be distributed in three main meals, a quarter each at breakfast, lunch and tea, with a snack during the morning and a small supper in the evening.

Mixtures in any proportions desired can, however, be made up from the amorphous and crystalline preparations, and will remain stable at ordinary temperatures. The action of I.Z.S. (Lente) can be lengthened by adding I.Z.S. crystalline (Ultralente) or shortened by adding I.Z.S. amorphous (Semilente); or a mixture of any proportions of I.Z.S. crystalline and I.Z.S. amorphous can be made up to suit an individual patient. Insulin zinc suspensions cannot be mixed with P.Z.I. or soluble insulin.

Isophane Insulin Injection, B.P. (NPH Insulin). Isophane insulin is slightly longer acting than soluble but can be mixed with it in the same syringe. Some diabetics requiring a small dose of insulin can be controlled on a single morning dose of isophane. Two doses of isophane a day, or two doses of isophane mixed with soluble insulin twice a day are often successful in the control of difficult or 'brittle' diabetics.

Control of Insulin Dosage. Good control means first a state in which the patient feels well, leads a normal life and is free from symptoms, and this is more important than normal biochemical findings. Further, the correct dose of insulin can only be determined when the patient is at home and leading a normal life, though the myth of 'stabilization' in hospital still persists. Patients with a normal renal threshold can usually be controlled satisfactorily by urine tests. Few, if any, such patients can maintain a sugar-free urine throughout the day without periods of hypoglycaemia. One should, however, aim to get the urine sugar-free at some time during the day, even if temporary glycosuria occurs after the main meals. In determining how far this has been achieved, a record of a patient's own urine testing over a day or two of normal activities is of more value than is a single urine test or even a blood sugar under the abnormal circumstances of a visit to the doctor or the diabetic clinic. Reasonably intelligent and co-operative patients can all be taught to use the 'Clinitest' apparatus.

If a patient, particularly an elderly one, is too easily controlled and shows constantly sugar-free urine without hypoglycaemia, one should suspect a high renal threshold. If a patient has frequent hypoglycaemic attacks, but is rarely or never sugar-free, one should suspect a low renal threshold. In such cases the approximate level of the threshold can be determined by performing a series of simultaneous blood and urinary sugar estimations. Patients with low and high renal thresholds should have this information clearly marked on their records. The main indications for blood sugars in the control of treatment occur in dealing with such patients.

Some patients remain well controlled on a given dose of insulin for long periods. Others need more or less frequent adjustment of their doses. Sudden loss of control with heavy glycosuria or ketosis may be due to:

1. Infections such as colds, influenza, urinary

infections, boils, injection abscesses or pulmonary tuberculosis.

2. Mistakes in measuring insulin, a leaking syringe or failure to take insulin.
3. Worry or 'aggravation'.
4. Serious dietary indiscretions.

Hypoglycaemia may be due to:

1. Too large a prescribed dose or a mistake in measuring the dose of insulin.
2. Missing a meal.
3. Unusual exertion.
4. A combination of 2 and 3.
5. There is some doubt how important are hypoglycaemic reactions due to change from beef to pork insulin, but they can occur.

Diabetes mellitus arises in a minority of patients treated with steroids, presumably in patients who are already potential diabetics. The diabetes is usually not severe. If the steroid treatment is necessary, it should be continued, and the diabetes should be treated with hypoglycaemic drugs or with insulin in the same way as any other type. Similarly, diabetes may be precipitated or aggravated by thiazide diuretics. Ideally they should be avoided. If they are essential, their use may increase the insulin requirements.

'Brittle' Diabetics. When the causes of loss of control mentioned have been eliminated, a few diabetics still seem to vary from day to day or hour to hour, so that they are particularly difficult to control. Such patients are all best treated on two injections a day.

Several regimes may be tried:

1. Two doses a day of a long-acting insulin such as isophane, Semilente or Lente.
2. Two doses a day of soluble may be tried with a small quantity of P.Z.I. added to the second injection, which is given before tea instead of before supper.
3. It has been claimed that the addition of a biguanide (e.g. phenformin, 12·5 or 25 mg. three times a day) will lower the insulin requirements and produce better control in such patients.

Insulin Resistance. Occasionally, the amount of insulin needed to control a diabetic rises steeply to 1000 or more Units a day. This appears to be due to the development of insulin antibodies and the passive cutaneous anaphylaxis test is positive. In this condition alone steroids have the effect of lowering the insulin dosage.

Hypoglycaemia. The usual symptoms are a sense of apprehension, hunger, sweating, trembling, palpitation and unsteadiness, which may progress to stupor, coma and convulsions. Some patients become emotionally unstable, or aggressive or behave as if they were drunk. With protamine zinc insulin headaches and lassitude may be complained of, particularly in the early morning; and nocturnal reactions may occur in which the patient may have night sweats or may pass into a convulsion without waking up. A few patients become unconscious almost without warning and old people may develop prolonged confusion. It is wise to think of hypoglycaemia whenever a patient receiving insulin complains of an unusual sensation or behaves in an unusual manner.

All diabetics on insulin should carry sugar (or glucose tablets) and take 2–4 lumps (10–20 g.) as soon as they recognize the symptoms. Many semi-comatose and unco-operative patients can be brought around if their heads are held firmly under the arm and spoonfuls of syrupy sugar solution are forced into their mouths. If the patient is comatose, glucose should be given intravenously in doses of 10–20 G. This is most conveniently administered as 33⅓ per cent. or even 50 per cent. glucose in a 20 ml. syringe. As an alternative glucagon, 1 mg., may be given intramuscularly. This should be followed by sugar orally as soon as the patient is conscious.

Local Reactions to Insulin. A few patients suffer from painful, red, itching bumps which appear at the site of each insulin injection, and last about 36 hours. They appear to be due to a form of sensitization. Sometimes they can be avoided by changing to a different brand of the same type or to a different type of insulin. In rare intractable cases desensitization may be attempted.

Insulin Fat Atrophy. Curious hollows at the sites of injection due to disappearance of subcutaneous fat are sometimes seen in children and adult females, rarely in adult males. They can occasionally be disfiguring. No treatment is constantly effective, though it has been claimed that persistence in injecting the insulin into the tissue at the base of the hollow will cause it to fill up. The simplest course is to advise the patient to use 80 strength insulin and to make injections into the lower abdomen, the buttocks and the tops of the thighs, where loss of subcutaneous fat is unlikely to be noticed and may be welcome.

Management of Intercurrent Illness. Many cases of ketosis and coma would be prevented if it were generally realized by both patients and doctors that diabetics with intercurrent illnesses, particularly infections, often need an increase in their insulin dosage. On no account should insulin be discontinued or the dose reduced because the patient is unable to eat his ordinary diet, as this leads to ketosis and coma. If a patient is unable to eat his usual diet on account of an intercurrent illness, he should take his usual dose of insulin (or a larger one) and take the carbohydrate of the diet either in the form of sugar in water or lemonade, or as some kind of carbohydrate in fluid form. This can easily be arranged if it is remembered that 10 g. of carbohydrate can be taken as:

Sugar . .	2 large lumps or 2 teaspoonfuls
Glucose. .	⅓ oz. or 2 teaspoonfuls
Orange juice .	4 oz.
Milk . .	7 oz.
Horlicks .	2 heaped teaspoonfuls
Ovaltine .	2 heaped teaspoonfuls

Diets for Patients on Insulin. The argument between the protagonists of 'fixed' and 'free' diets is to some extent a matter of words. No one seriously suggests that a diabetic on insulin should be free to gorge on sweets one day and eat almost nothing the next; and no one now attempts to make patients weigh all food eaten. Both accept the need for some degree of control, but differ as to how the control should be exercised. A reasonable compromise is to ask patients to learn to measure their carbohydrate foods by weighing them until they can guess standard 10 g. (⅓ oz.) carbohydrate portions of different foods fairly accurately, and thereafter to weigh them occasionally as a check on their ability to guess. They can thus limit themselves to a prescribed amount of carbohydrate and a prescribed distribution of carbohydrate among the meals for the day without undue hardship. Protein foods and fat are allowed in 'average' amounts, though patients should be warned to avoid an excess of fat in view of the probable association between a high fat intake and atherosclerosis.

The distribution of carbohydrate foods in the day varies with different insulin regimes, and may have to be adjusted by a process of trial and error for individual patients. TABLE 35 shows some of the properties of different insulins and the kind of distribution of carbohydrate generally found most suitable for the commonly used regimes:

Patients with severe diabetes are best admitted to hospital for rapid control. Others can start treatment successfully at home, preferably with the help of a district nurse.

TABLE 35

Type of insulin	*Strengths available in Units per ml.*	*Length of action*	*Time of maximum effect (when hypoglycaemic attacks are most likely)*	*When given*	*Suggested distribution of carbohydrate in diet (for total of 200 g. per day)*					
					Breakfast	Mid-morning	Lunch	Tea	Evening meal	Last thing
SOLUBLE OR ISOPHANE	20, 40, 80	Small doses ½–6 hours Large doses ½–10 or 12 hours	2–5 hours after injection 2–8 hours after injection	About 20 minutes before breakfast and evening meal	60	10	40	20	60	10
P.Z.I. AND SOLUBLE	40, 80	4–24 hours or more	Afternoon, evening, night or early morning	About 20 minutes before breakfast	50	10	40	40	50	10
I.Z.S. LENTE	40, 80	2–24 hours	Morning or afternoon	About 20 minutes before breakfast	50	10	50	50	30	10
							or			
					50	20	60	30	30	10

In arranging a diet for an intelligent and knowledgeable patient, it is usually enough, therefore, to prescribe the total amount of carbohydrate and how it should be distributed throughout the three or four main meals of the day. Such patients can then select such portions of whatever carbohydrate foods they prefer. Less intelligent patients may need to have the exact foods they should take written out for them.

No exact rules can be laid down for the total amount of carbohydrate. This will depend on the age, weight, appetite and habits of the particular patient, and may vary for an adult by anything from 120–350 g. or more, which with average amounts of protein and fat will correspond roughly to 1200–3500 calories. Growing children and adolescents should be given larger amounts of carbohydrate in proportion to their weights than adults. The aim should be to provide a diet which satisfies patients' appetites but keeps them from getting fat.

In either case, a patient who is not in ketosis can be placed immediately on the diet considered likely to be suitable for his age and occupation. In hospital rapid control of more severe cases can usually be obtained by starting soluble insulin in doses of from 16 to 24 Units three times a day, 20 minutes before the three main meals; and by increasing or decreasing the dose according to the results of urine tests. When satisfactory control has been attained, two doses of soluble insulin or an equivalent single dose of a long-acting insulin may be substituted for three doses of soluble.

In milder cases starting treatment at home, it is usually satisfactory to begin with a single small dose of a long-acting insulin, and to increase this gradually according to the results of urine tests. It will usually be found satisfactory to start with a dose of 12 or 20 Units and to increase this by 4 or 8 Units at each visit.

Treatment of Patients with Ketosis

The treatment of coma is considered under complications. Patients with mild ketosis (positive nitroprusside test, negative ferric chloride test) should have their dose of insulin increased by one-quarter or one-third, and should be seen again within a few days. Patients with severe ketosis (positive nitroprusside and ferric chloride tests), whether new or known diabetics, should be treated vigorously, preferably in hospital.

The ketosis is abolished most rapidly by giving soluble insulin and either glucose or carbohydrate feeds at frequent intervals. In some cases it may be enough to continue with the patient's usual diet and give a dose of soluble insulin before each of the three main meals. In more severe cases the following regime will be found useful:

STAGE I (4-hourly insulin and glucose)

Forty grammes of glucose in water or lemonade, with 20 Units of soluble insulin subcutaneously every 4 hours. The urine is tested 4-hourly and the insulin dosage increased or decreased as necessary. This is continued until the urine is free from ketone bodies. If the patient is vomiting the glucose must be given by intravenous drip.

STAGE II (thrice daily insulin and fluid or semi-solid carbohydrate feeds)

		Carbohydrate in grammes
Insulin—7.30 a.m.		
8 a.m.	Tea made with milk from allowance.	
	Porridge made from 1 oz. (30 g.) oats *or* breakfast cereal, 1 oz. (30 g.) .	20
	Glucose *or* sugar, 20 g. .	20
	Milk from allowance.	
	Orange juice, 4 oz. (120 ml.), with glucose, 10 g. . .	20
		60
10 a.m.	Lemonade (fresh lemon juice and water), glucose, 10 g.	10
	2 plain biscuits . . .	10
		20
12 noon	Clear soup, meat *or* yeast extract.	
Insulin—1.30 p.m.		
2 p.m.	Milk pudding made from:	
	Semolina, rice, sago, tapioca, ½ oz. (15 g.) .	10
	Milk from allowance.	
	Glucose *or* sugar, 20 g. .	20
	Orange juice, 4 oz. (120 ml.), with glucose, 10 g. . .	20
		50
6 p.m.	Tea, with milk from allowance.	
	4 Cream crackers *or* water biscuits	20
	Butter from allowance.	
		20
8 p.m.	Clear soup, meat *or* yeast extract.	
Insulin—9.30 p.m.		
10 p.m.	Remainder of milk from allowance.	
	Horlicks *or* Ovaltine, ½ oz. (15 g.)	10
	4 Cream crackers . .	20
	Orange juice, 4 oz. (120 ml.), with glucose, 20 g. . .	30
		60
	Daily allowance of milk, 1 pint (600 ml.). . . .	30
	Daily allowance of butter *or* margarine ½ oz. (15 g.)	
	Total carbohydrates .	240

STAGE III (thrice daily insulin and light diet)

		Carbohydrate in grammes
Insulin—7.30 p.m.		
Breakfast—8 a.m.	Tea *or* coffee, with milk from allowance.	
	Boiled *or* poached egg.	
	Bread *or* toast, 2 oz. (60 g.) .	30
	Butter from allowance.	
	Marmalade *or* jam, 1 oz. (30 g.)	20
	Orange juice, 4 oz. (120 ml.)	10
		60
Mid-morning	Meat *or* yeast extract.	
	2 Water biscuits . .	10
		10
Insulin—11.30 a.m.		
Lunch—12 noon	Steamed fish *or* rabbit *or* chicken, a small portion.	
	4 Boiled potatoes, 3 oz. (120 g.)	20
	Cabbage, spinach, cauliflower, as desired.	
	Ice Cream, 2 oz., Grapes, 2 oz. (60 g.), *or* bananas, 2 oz. (60 g.) . . .	10
	Orange juice, 4 oz. (120 ml.), with glucose, 10 g. . .	20
		50
Tea	Tea, with milk from allowance.	
	Digestive biscuits, 1 oz. (30 g.)	20
		20

		Carbohydrate in grammes
Insulin—6 p.m.		
Supper—6.30 p.m.	Clear soup *or* meat *or* yeast extract.	
	4 Cream crackers . .	20
	Rice, semolina, sago, ½ oz. (15 g.)	
	Milk from allowance . .	20
	Glucose *or* sugar, 10 g. (as milk pudding) .	
	¼ pint jelly *or* stewed apple, 5 oz. (150 g.) . .	10
	Glucose *or* sugar, 10 g. .	10
		60
Bedtime.	Remainder of milk from allowance.	
	Ovaltine or Horlicks, ½ oz. (15 g.) . . . . . *or* 2 plain biscuits	10
		10
	Daily allowance of milk, 1 pint (600 ml.). . .	30
	Daily allowance of butter or margarine, 1 oz. (30 g.)	
	Total carbohydrates .	240

From Stage III the patient can be changed back to his usual diet and insulin regime.

Surgical Operations on Diabetics

Emergency Operations. In an emergency a diabetic patient with glycosuria, but without ketosis, can safely be operated on without preliminary treatment. If the patient is found to have a ketosis of any severity (nitroprusside and ferric chloride tests positive), the operation should, if at all possible, be postponed for a few hours while the ketosis is treated vigorously with frequent doses of soluble insulin. The dose must depend on the patient's previous dose, the severity of the ketosis, the degree of urgency and the experience of the physician, but 20–40 Units of soluble insulin hourly would be safe and suitable for most patients. As such a patient is likely to be dehydrated, he should also be given one or two litres of normal saline intravenously. The drip should be continued through the operation period and changed to 5 per cent. glucose as soon as blood sugar figures approach normal. One of the main difficulties is the diabetic patient who presents in ketosis with symptoms suggesting an abdominal emergency. Patients with ketosis alone may have vomiting, abdominal pain, tenderness, rigidity and a leucocytosis, which improve rapidly when the ketosis is corrected. In doubtful cases the history is of more value than the physical signs. If thirst and polyuria preceded the abdominal symptoms, it is likely that the whole picture is due to diabetic ketosis. If the abdominal symptoms preceded the thirst and polyuria, it is more likely that the ketosis is the result of acute abdominal disease.

Planned Operations. Diabetic patients should be in hospital for a few days before operation for regulation of the diabetes. Those on a small dose (i.e. under 20 Units) of a long-acting insulin can remain on this regime. Those on a larger dose should be changed temporarily on to two or three doses of soluble insulin.

A patient on insulin should preferably be the first on the operating list in the morning. Supper and a late evening snack should be given as usual the night before, but nothing by mouth after midnight. In the morning, the patient should be given ½ to ⅔ the usual morning dose of insulin, followed by 50 ml. of 50 per cent. glucose intravenously. For operations of any length or severity a 5 per cent. glucose drip should then be set up and kept going till the patient can take carbohydrate feeds again by mouth. If the operation takes place in the afternoon, nothing should be given by mouth for the previous six hours.

In the case of patients who are well controlled on hypoglycaemic drugs these are best omitted on the day of operation.

It is necessary to emphasize that hypoglycaemia is the main danger, and temporary hyperglycaemia in the operative and immediate postoperative period is of no importance. It is wise to take a blood sugar at the end of the operation to serve as a guide to post-operative treatment.

The object in the postoperative period is to give carbohydrate either as intravenous 5 per cent. glucose or as fluid carbohydrate feeds, covered by adequate amounts of soluble insulin, until the patient can return to his normal diet or regime. A ratio of 1 Unit of insulin to 2 G. of glucose will usually be found satisfactory. A minimum of 160 G. of glucose a day, i.e. 40 G. and 20 Units soluble insulin 6-hourly should be maintained, the amount of insulin being varied according to the results of urine tests. The stage I, II and III diets for treatment of severe ketosis [p. 505] can be used satisfactorily with or without minor modifications for most such patients.

Pregnancy in Diabetics

Insulin therapy has made pregnancy practically as safe for the diabetic as for the non-diabetic mother, provided she has the benefit of strict and skilled diabetic supervision. It has not, however, done the same for the foetus. Up till 1950 the foetal loss rate from intra-uterine death, obstetric complications and neonatal death was about 40 per cent. In the last decade better care of the diabetic mother, better anaesthesia and the practice of early delivery has reduced this rate in some centres to about 10–14 per cent.

It is known that women who subsequently develop diabetes, as well as diabetic women, tend to have large babies; and also that the high foetal loss rate is evident before the onset of the diabetes, particularly in the previous 2 years. It is also known that diabetic women show an undue incidence of hydramnios and toxaemia of pregnancy. Diabetic babies, apart from their size, usually have a tough leathery skin with coarse features. There is oedema of the skin and subcutaneous tissues. The heart, liver and spleen may be pathologically enlarged, and there is a high incidence of congenital abnormalities. The babies are usually slow and lethargic and subject to cyanotic attacks in the first few days of life. It seems likely that such babies may be hypoglycaemic shortly after birth, but it is unlikely that this accounts for the high early neonatal death rate. In practice, oxygen seems more important than glucose. Babies that survive this period are often difficult to feed and rear at first, but then develop normally.

There is no doubt that strict control of the diabetes is essential. The insulin requirements of pregnant diabetic women undergo variations, and usually increase considerably as the pregnancy proceeds. Further, the renal threshold commonly falls between the third and fifth month, which makes good control more difficult. Such women should be under close supervision and should be seen at short intervals. Those on large single doses of a long-acting insulin should be changed to two or three doses of soluble insulin a day. When control is difficult, such patients may have to be admitted to hospital once or twice during the pregnancy, and all should be admitted by the thirty-second or thirty-third week. Many authorities now favour Caesarean section between the thirty-sixth and thirty-eighth weeks. This reduces the incidence of toxaemias and foetal deaths, which are commonest in the last week or two of pregnancy, and avoids prolonged labour and obstetrical difficulties, but is open to the objection that it may increase the neonatal death rate by adding prematurity to the babies' difficulties. There is often a rapid fall in the mother's insulin requirements early in the puerperium.

PROGNOSIS

TABLE 36 (prepared from the experience of the Joslin Clinic, Boston, Mass., by the Statistical Department of the Metropolitan Life Insurance Co.) shows the average expectation of life of American diabetics at different ages compared with that of the general population.

TABLE 36

EXPECTATION OF LIFE IN YEARS

AGE	MALE		FEMALE	
	Diabetics	*Population*	*Diabetics*	*Population*
10	43·6	59·0	45·0	64·3
15	39·3	54·2	40·7	59·4
20	35·4	49·5	36·8	54·6
25	32·1	44·9	33·6	49·8
30	29·3	40·3	30·9	45·0
35	26·3	35·7	28·0	40·3
40	22·8	31·2	24·6	35·6
45	19·3	26·9	21·2	31·1
50	16·1	22·8	17·7	26·7
55	13·1	19·1	14·6	22·6
60	10·6	15·8	11·9	18·6
65	8·8	12·8	9·6	15·0
70	7·1	10·1	7·4	11·7

While such figures provide a general guide, the prognosis for an individual diabetic depends on many factors. Diabetics now die of the complications of the disease, particularly arteriopathy in all forms, and nephropathy, rather than of diabetes. Bad prognostic signs are the presence of an established complication, lack of intelligence, unwillingness or inability to co-operate, persisting obesity and a severe diabetes, particularly if of an unstable type. Good prognostic signs are the absence of any sign of complications, good intelligence and co-operation, normal weight and height and a mild easily controllable type of diabetes. It is wise to observe a diabetic patient for some time before hazarding any kind of prognosis.

Advice is often asked about the possibility of children of diabetic parents developing the disease. Briefly, if two diabetics marry, all the children will be potential diabetics, but it seems that only about half will develop the disease. If a diabetic marries a non-diabetic in whose family there is no history of diabetes, the chances of the children developing diabetes are small.

COMPLICATIONS

Diabetics appear more liable than normal persons to suffer from infections, particularly staphylococcal skin infections, pulmonary tuberculosis and urinary infections (commoner in women), from cataracts and from various forms of arterial degeneration. Diabetic ketosis and coma, nephropathy, neuropathy, retinopathy and a rare form of 'true diabetic cataract' may be regarded as true complications of diabetes.

Diabetes and Pulmonary Tuberculosis

Diabetics should have their chests radiographed as a yearly routine, and pulmonary tuberculosis should always be remembered as a possible cause of unexplained loss of weight or deterioration in diabetic control, though it is now a rare one. Patients with diabetes and active pulmonary tuberculosis should be treated with a liberal high carbohydrate diet and enough insulin to ensure good control. It is often necessary to give such patients two or three injections of soluble insulin a day, and to vary the dose frequently to obtain good control. It has been claimed also that isoniazid impairs carbohydrate tolerance and may increase insulin requirements.

Arteriosclerosis and Obliterative Arterial Disease in the Legs

It is probable that diabetics are more liable than non-diabetics to all forms of arterial degeneration, including coronary and cerebral artery disease and obliterative arterial disease in the legs. The reason is unknown, as is the pathogenesis of arteriosclerosis in general. It has been suggested that arteriosclerosis is an inevitable part of certain forms of diabetes, but some physicians with great experience believe that its onset is delayed by strict treatment. Obesity appears to be a factor, and this is an additional reason for encouraging obese diabetics to reduce their weight.

Obliterative arterial disease in the legs presents in diabetics more often as gangrene than as intermittent claudication. The reverse is the case in non-diabetics. Arteriography shows that this is due to the fact that the obstruction in the arteries of diabetics is more in peripheral vessels than in the femorals and popliteals. The incidence is related to age rather than to the severity or duration of the diabetes. The treatment of intermittent claudication does not differ from that in non-diabetics, and drugs are equally ineffective.

Foot Complications

Diabetic feet are affected by: (1) sepsis; (2) ischaemia; and (3) neuropathy.

Sepsis usually complicates one of the other processes, but is sometimes seen alone as a web space abscess, which started as a result of infection in the toe cleft. Such abscesses usually have to be incised.

A typical acutely ischaemic foot is very painful, pale and cyanosed and cold to the touch. More chronic ischaemia can be recognized by the absence of hairs, blanching on elevation, lowered temperature and the absence of pulsation in the posterior tibial and dorsalis pedis arteries, though the last is the least reliable sign.

The typical neuropathic lesion is the perforating ulcer over pressure points and very occasionally a neuropathic (Charcot) joint, but areas of gangrene may also occur.

It is important to realize that the incidence of foot complications can be reduced by regular foot precautions and chiropody. Older diabetics should be taught to wash, dry and powder their feet daily. Drying and powdering between the toes is particularly important to prevent fungus infestations which may be the start of septic infections and gangrene. Toe-nails should be cut straight across by someone with good eyesight, and corns should be treated cautiously by experienced chiropodists.

When foot complications do occur, rational treatment depends on an assessment of how far the lesions are due to sepsis, ischaemia or neuropathy. Any sepsis present should be treated first. Ideally the responsible organism should be cultured, but it is often difficult to obtain a pure culture, and hence a broad-spectrum antibiotic such as ampicillin has to be used.

Apart from the points mentioned above the greatest help in diagnosis is that, whereas neuropathic lesions are painless, ischaemic lesions are usually extremely painful, at least in the early stages.

Neuropathic ulcers, provided an X-ray of the foot shows no involvement of bone, heal rapidly if sepsis is controlled and all pressure is removed. The problem then is to prevent further pressure by the use of surgical shoes or occasionally by orthopaedic procedures. Areas of neuropathic gangrene can be treated by local conservative measures—mere nibbling away of the affected tissue.

Ischaemic lesions, other than very small ones in old and enfeebled subjects, require surgery. Aortography followed by vascular surgery is practicable in a small minority of diabetic patients. The majority of those with ischaemic gangrene will require an amputation through healthy tissue. The sooner this is done, once the diagnosis has been made, the more likely will it be that the patient will obtain a satisfactory prosthesis and walk again. Sympathectomy is occasionally of value in superficial ischaemic skin lesions. It is useless in more extensive lesions and in intermittent claudication.

Diabetic Coma

Diabetic coma is one of the most serious of medical emergencies and one with a considerable mortality, unless it receives skilled and speedy treatment and constant attention. It cannot be emphasized too often, therefore, that most cases of diabetic coma are preventable. The exceptions are occasional patients with undiagnosed diabetes, who present in coma without ever having consulted a doctor, and a few patients who are either too stupid, too unco-operative or too ill-disciplined to learn to avoid it, however much effort is expended on their education. Coma can occur if a patient has an infection or if he stops taking insulin, but it occurs most commonly from a combination of these causes. A patient with an infection cannot eat his normal diet, and therefore stops taking his insulin. Many cases of coma would be prevented if both doctors and patients understood how to deal with infections and intercurrent illnesses as outlined on page 503. The usual cause of diabetic coma is increasing ketonaemia, which induces a metabolic acidosis and loss of intracellular fluid and electrolytes, often exaggerated by vomiting. Insulin action is much impaired by ketosis. In rare cases coma is due to a hyperosmolar state associated with very high blood sugars, extreme dehydration and no significant ketosis.

The main clinical features of diabetic coma are listed in TABLE 37 and contrasted with those of hypoglycaemic coma, though the big difficulty in practice is usually not in diagnosing between these conditions, but between diabetic coma and other varieties of coma occurring in a diabetic.

TABLE 37

	Diabetic	*Hypoglycaemic*
History.	Missed insulin. Infection, etc.	Missed meal. Unusual exertion, etc.
Onset.	Slow.	Rapid.
Skin.	Dry.	Sweating.
Tongue.	Dry.	Moist.
Pulse.	Small volume.	Bounding.
B.P.	Reduced.	Normal or raised.
Breath.	May be acetone.	No acetone.
Eyeball tension.	Reduced.	Normal.
Respiration.	Deep and slow 'air hunger'.	Rapid and shallow.
Urine.	Sugar. Ketones + +.	May be sugar. No ketones.
Blood sugar.	Usually 400 mg. per cent. or over.	Less than 60 mg. per cent.
Plasma CO_2.	Diminished.	Normal.
Dextrostix.	High B.S.	Low B.S.

Diabetic coma is a major emergency and should, if at all possible, be treated in a hospital with facilities for urgent biochemical investigations, but treatment should be begun without waiting for the results of such investigations. If the practitioner is certain of the diagnosis of severe diabetic coma, he should give 100 Units of soluble insulin before sending the patient to hospital.

Wherever the patient is to be treated, he should be placed in a warmed bed and nursed on his side. A specimen of urine should be obtained immediately by catheter. If blood sugar estimations are not available, the catheter should be left in position, so that regular specimens can be obtained.

Treatment consists in:

1. Adequate doses of insulin. Give 100 Units (80 intramuscularly and 20 intravenously) as soon as diagnosis is made. Take blood for blood sugar. If this is over 600 mg. per 100 ml., give further 100 Units by same routes. Repeat blood sugar at 1½-hour intervals and adjust further insulin dosage accordingly. If the blood sugar has fallen significantly, the dose of insulin should be halved; if it is the same, the dose should be increased by 50 per cent.; and if it has risen the dose should be doubled. If no facilities for blood sugars, give 100 Units and then 40 Units hourly. Amount of sugar in urine gives no indication of blood sugar until this falls below 300 mg. per 100 ml.

2. Replace water and salt deficiency. Set up intravenous drip and give normal saline, 1 litre in 15 minutes, a second in the first hour and then continue more slowly; 6 or 8 litres of parenteral fluid in the first 12 hours or so is not an excessive amount. The blood pressure should be taken half-hourly, and if this falls or if other signs of circulatory collapse appear, blood (or dextran or plasma) should be given in place of the saline solution. In hyperosmolar coma half normal saline in large quantities is required.

In severe cases of coma there is often a metabolic acidosis with deep, sighing (Kussmaul) respiration and a plasma bicarbonate of less than 12 mEq. per litre. In this event give 1 litre of normal saline, followed by 500 ml. of isotonic (⅙ molar) sodium bicarbonate solution. Follow this by 1 litre of normal saline and a further 500 ml. of isotonic sodium bicarbonate, and thereafter normal saline. It is rarely necessary to give more than 1 litre in all of the bicarbonate solution.

3. Empty the stomach.

Patients in diabetic coma often have dilated stomachs containing quantities of fluid, which may be regurgitated and inhaled. The stomach should therefore be evacuated by means of a small stomach tube, and the tube may be left in position to allow of repeated gastric suction. Patients are also sometimes extremely constipated with palpable scybala in the colon. As soon as the patient is out of danger from ketosis and dehydration, olive oil should be given per rectum and followed by plain water enemas.

4. Look for and treat any infections (boils, injection abscesses, pulmonary tuberculosis, etc.) which may be present. Benzylpenicillin, 300 mg. (500,000 Units) twice daily, should be given prophylactically even if no infection is found.

5. When the blood sugar has fallen to 300 mg. per 100 ml., or if blood sugars are not available, when the sugar in the urine diminishes, substitute 5 per cent. glucose for the saline solution, and give at the rate of 1 litre every 4–6 hours. Once the patient is conscious and the blood sugar is normal, give sips of water, followed by milk and fluid carbohydrate feeds. Transition to a normal diet can be conveniently planned by using the diets provided for the treatment severe of ketosis [p. 505].

Once ketosis is controlled, the greatest danger is hypokalaemia. 10 ml. of Potassium Chloride Injection, B.P. (contains 1·5 g. or 20 mEq. of potassium) should therefore be added to each litre of 5 per cent. glucose. The total potassium deficit may be in the order of 200 mEq., but the rate of replacement by the intravenous route should not exceed 20 mEq. per hour, unless there is close biochemical or electrocardiographic control. Once the patient can swallow it is better to give the potassium by mouth as *Slow K* or *Kloref*, tablets of which contain 8·0 or 6·5 mEq. of potassium respectively. These tablets should be prescribed for 2 or 3 days, or until the patient is taking a full diet. Patients who have been in deep coma should not be allowed to sit up or otherwise exert themselves for several days.

Occasional patients with excessive hyperglycaemia develop coma without ketosis—so called hyperosmolar coma; they should be treated with smaller doses of insulin than those mentioned above and with half normal rather than normal saline.

Eye Complications

Impairment of vision in diabetics may be due to temporary changes in refraction, associated with change in water balance; to lenticular opacities or to retinopathy. Slowly progressive impairment of vision is more often due to cataracts than to retinopathy. Rapid loss of vision, fortunately rare but sometimes leading to complete blindness, is usually due to advanced retinal disease.

Transient Changes in Refraction. Blurring of distant vision from myopia may occur in untreated diabetics, and the sudden onset of myopia in any patient should raise a suspicion of diabetes and lead to testing of the urine. But visual symptoms of this kind are commonly encountered shortly after starting treatment with insulin due to changes in hydration of the lens. The patient should be dissuaded from seeking glasses or new glasses until it is seen whether the blurring disappears after the diabetes has been satisfactorily controlled for 4 weeks.

Lenticular Opacities. Two kinds of cataract occur in diabetics. It is usually stated that ordinary senile cataract is commoner in diabetics than in the general population, though this has been denied by one or two observers of large series, who claim that if sufficiently careful examination is made, the incidence is about equal. The treatment is the same as in non-diabetics. 'True diabetic' cataract or 'snow-flake' cataract is very much rarer, and occurs in adolescence or early adult life. It is said that it is reversible and may improve or even disappear with strict treatment of the diabetes.

Retinophathy. The prevalence of retinal changes increases with the duration of the diabetes; few patients who have had the disease for more than 15 years will have normal retinae. In older patients there is often a mixture of diabetic and hypertensive changes.

The earliest change is the appearance of capillary micro-aneurysms, tiny sharply defined rounded spots, venous in colour and much smaller than most haemorrhages. These are aneurysms of communicating branches between the capillaries of different layers of the retina. If carefully looked for, they can sometimes be seen as the only change in the retinae of quite young patients who have had diabetes for a number of years. The later changes are round 'deep' haemorrhages and small, irregularly shaped, yellowish-white, 'hard' or 'waxy' exudates. 'Fluffy' or 'cotton wool' exudates are occasionally also seen, even in the absence of hypertension.

Some diabetics also show changes in the veins which may be proliferative or non-proliferative. In the latter, the veins in some areas may be 'beaded', or overfilled and tortuous, or may be thrown into loops and coils. In the proliferative form, 'retinitis proliferans', new vessels are formed, which may in time grow into the vitreous. If vitreous haemorrhages then occur, organization of the clot may lead to retinal detachment; retinitis proliferans with haemorrhages and retinal detachment being the usual cause of sudden and rapid deterioration of vision in diabetics. Such patients are also liable to glaucoma.

In older patients, the picture of diabetic retinopathy is often complicated by the addition of hypertensive changes narrowing of the arterioles, superficial flame-shaped haemorrhages and 'cotton wool' exudates. It is likely that good control of diabetes delays the onset of retinopathy, and it has been claimed that the earliest changes in young diabetics are reversible by strict treatment. Once retinopathy has become established, stricter treatment of the diabetes makes disappointingly little difference.

Retinopathy is probably part of a generalized vascular process, since capillary fragility as measured in the arms is increased in diabetics with retinopathy. There is no evidence that drugs have any effect on the course of diabetic retinopathy, except that clofibrate given over long periods may reduce exudates and in a few cases may improve the prognosis.

In 1952 significant improvement was noticed in the retinopathy of a diabetic who had developed spontaneous hypopituitarism. Since then a number of patients have been treated either by surgical hypophysectomy or by the implantation of radioactive yttrium. There is no doubt that improvement has followed these procedures in some cases. A main difficulty is that if one waits till retinitis proliferans is established, the operation is usually too late to do good; while it is unjustifiable to operate on patients without retinitis proliferans, for in some of them the prognosis as regards vision is quite good. These must still be regarded as experimental procedures; and some may consider them rather mutilating for use in the treatment of a condition which does not threaten life.

Recently photocoagulation has been used in the treatment of retinopathy. A multicentre trial is in progress, and it is too early yet to say whether this measure will improve the long-term prognosis.

Nephropathy

If the urine of diabetics is tested for protein as a routine at every visit, a surprising number are found to have intermittent or continuous proteinuria. This may be due to acute cystitis or chronic pyelonephritis, nephritis, arteriosclerotic kidney, heart failure and so on. Symptomless urinary infections are common, particularly in females.

In 1934 Kimmelstiel and Wilson described a histological picture in the kidneys of diabetics characterized by the presence of discrete islands or nodules of hyaline material in the glomeruli. This intercapillary glomerulosclerosis came to be regarded as the pathological basis of the diabetic nephropathy which is one of the diabetic's most serious long-term risks. But the matter is not so simple. It appears that the Kimmelstiel-Wilson lesion may be associated with clinical nephropathy, but each may occur without the other. Further, the electron microscope has revealed changes in the basement membrane of the glomeruli in young patients with diabetes of short duration, long before proteinuria or any clinical sign of nephropathy appears. Patients with nephropathy are usually middle-aged or over, more often female than male, with a history of diabetes for many years. In a classical case, intermittent or continuous proteinuria which may last several years without other signs, is followed by slight or massive oedema of the dependent parts, severe hypertension and retinopathy, which may lead to failing vision; but many cases do not follow the classical course. Characteristically, the insulin requirements fall as the renal disease advances. When the oedema is gross, it is associated with low plasma protein, and can sometimes be controlled to some extent by a high protein, low sodium diet. Otherwise treatment has no effect, and death from renal failure, cardiac failure or cerebral haemorrhage occurs up to about 10 years from the first manifestation of a renal complication. It seems likely that intercapillary glomerulosclerosis and retinopathy are both manifestations of a single vascular degenerative process. It is probable that really good control of the diabetes delays or prevents the onset of these complications, but once they are established, control of the diabetes does not prevent their progressive course.

Neuropathy

This differs from all the other complications in that most of its manifestations are reversible; and when reversed rarely, if ever, recur. Moreover, those that are not reversed reach a certain level and do not progress. The onset of neuropathy often precedes the diagnosis of diabetes; may occur shortly after the initiation of treatment or later in the course of the diabetes, but probably always follows a long period of poor control, even though good control may have been established shortly before the onset of neuropathic manifestations. It is thus unlikely that it is caused by atheroma or other angiopathy since these are progressive and irreversible; and likely that it is caused by some kind of metabolic disturbance associated with long-standing poor control. The diabetes may be very mild in patients presenting with neuropathy.

Diabetic neuropathy can, for convenience, be divided into a few different clinical pictures, but all combinations of these are seen and there is no justification for subdivision into many different syndromes.

Subacute Neuropathy. There is usually a definite onset of pain and weakness in the legs, together with various combinations of weakness, loss of tendon reflexes, hyperalgesia and autonomic denervation. Sensory loss is inconspicuous or absent. The pain is of a peculiar character, often described in bizarre terms. All the manifestations may be asymmetrical. There is often a long preceding history of muscle cramps in the legs. Characteristically, the illness progresses for weeks or months and then recovers partially or completely and does not relapse.

Insidious Neuropathy. Pain and muscle weakness are absent and sensory loss and loss of reflexes are the main features. Tendon reflexes may return but less often than in the subacute neuropathy.

Autonomic Neuropathy. Various forms have been described. Diabetic diarrhoea is characteristically worse by night than by day and may be associated with considerable urgency. Other causes of diarrhoea must be excluded. Impotence occurring early in the disease may be due to anxiety, but later on it is usually neuropathic and rarely reversible. Male hormones are useless and should not be prescribed.

Paralysis of the bladder, pupillary abnormalities, disturbances of sweating, disturbances of blood pressure regulation leading to postural hypotension and syncope, and 'hypoglycaemic unresponsiveness', have all been attributed to autonomic neuropathy. The theory of the latter is that the warning symptoms of hypoglycaemia are a sympathetic response. In the presence of a sympathetic neuropathy the patient may become unconscious without warning symptoms.

Trophic Ulcers. The neuropathic nature of these ulcers is demonstrated by the fact that unlike ischaemic lesions they are painless. A patient walks about on a corn or callus over a pressure point without discomfort. Necrosis of the underlying tissues and a perforating ulcer results. The ulcers heal rapidly, if all pressure is removed (usually by rest in bed) and infection is controlled, but often recur. Regular chiropody for the removal of corns and hard skin prevents many of them.

Treatment. The subacute neuropathy may be a very severe illness confining the patient to bed for weeks or even months. Powerful analgesics may be needed and may fail to control the pain adequately. The condition always improves and may recover completely after a time.

In general terms, the occurence of neuropathy in any form demands close control of the diabetes; though the immediate results of initiating good control are often very disappointing and may even be followed by a temporary progression of the disability.

SPONTANEOUS HYPOGLYCAEMIA

Functional or reactive hypoglycaemia occurring 2–4 hours after meals is fairly common in psychologically unstable individuals and is much the commonest form of spontaneous hypoglycaemia. The main complaints are faintness, weakness, tremulousness, hunger and feelings of nervousness. In contrast to cases of organic hyperinsulinism the condition is not progressive, neurological disturbances and true coma do not occur, the fasting blood sugar is normal and the attacks are not brought on by fasting for 24–48 hours. Similar attacks of alimentary reactive hypoglycaemia occur some hours after meals in patients whose pyloric sphincters have been removed. This should not be confused with 'dumping attacks' [see Section 7] which come on soon after meals.

In reactive hypoglycaemia a glucose tolerance test shows a lag curve with a high peak of blood sugar eventually falling to hypoglycaemic levels 3–4 hours after glucose. Plasma insulin levels rise more slowly than normal to a late, often exaggerated, peak. It is important to establish that the symptoms are accompanied by hypoglycaemia and cured by glucose; the symptoms themselves are common to many anxiety states or may be due to such drugs as the monoamine oxidase inhibitors.

The treatment for this condition is a low carbohydrate diet, avoiding particularly sugar and the more easily assimilable forms of carbohydrate. Sedation may be helpful in anxious patients and abstinence from tobacco is occasionally curative

By comparison, other causes of spontaneous hypoglycaemia are very rare. It is found occasionally in hypopituitarism and hypocortico-adrenalism (glucocorticoid deficiency), in advanced liver disease (failure to store glycogen) and in hypothyroidism. It has been seen in chronic barbiturate addiction and in response to alcohol, and is occasionally self-induced with the aid of either insulin or excessive doses of one of the sulphonylurea drugs. It is seen in children, occurring idiopathically or as a manifestation of sensitivity to the amino acid, leucine. It has been described as a curiosity in large non-pancreatic fibromas and sarcomas. Finally, it occurs in organic hyperinsulinism and it is important that cases due to this cause should be diagnosed, since though they are very rare, surgery may provide a complete cure.

HYPERINSULINISM

Pathology

Hyperinsulinism is usually due to a small islet-celled adenoma (1–2 cm. in diameter) which probably has no predilection for any part of the pancreas, but is more likely to be found when it is in the body or tail. In 10 per cent. of cases two or more adenomata are present. More rarely the tumour is a carcinoma and metastasizes to the adjacent lymph nodes and the liver. Occasional cases have been attributed to generalized hyperplasia of islet-cell tissue.

Symptoms

The main difficulty in diagnosis is that patients with attacks of the kind of symptoms usually associated with hypoglycaemia (apprehension, tachycardia, shakiness, sweating; weakness and 'fainting', directly due to glucose deficiency within the nerve cells) usually turn out to have the functional hypoglycaemia mentioned above, whereas patients with islet-cell tumours are apt to present with bizarre attacks or peculiar neuropsychiatric manifestations, which are easily misdiagnosed as hysteria, epilepsy, alcoholism, cerebral tumour (particularly hypothalamic tumour) or psychosis. It is, therefore, in neurological, neurosurgical and psychiatric departments and in the observation wards of mental hospitals that such patients are most likely to be found. This diagnosis should be considered in any peculiar neuropsychiatric illness, particularly if associated in the earlier stages with episodes of change of mood or loss of consciousness, in which sweating is noticed. Attacks are most common on waking in the morning and the frequency and severity of attacks are progressive. Later, convulsions and irreversible neurological changes or psychosis may be added. In the middle-aged and elderly transient hemiparesis is not uncommon.

Diagnosis

The method used to determine the blood sugar is important in this diagnosis. Methods which measure blood glucose, such as those employing glucose oxidase, give figures 10 (or occasionally more) mg. per 100 ml. lower than those in common use. The difference is relatively unimportant in the diagnosis of diabetes, but most important in the diagnosis of hypoglycaemia. In this section, therefore, but not in that on diabetes mellitus, the figures quoted are those for blood glucose, as determined by a glucose oxidase method. In attacks of hyperinsulinism the blood glucose is usually 40 mg. per 100 ml. or less. Since the diagnosis often has to be made between the attacks the following tests may be employed.

Prolonged Fast. The patient should be admitted to hospital and given nothing but unsweetened fluids for 48 hours. In the presence of an insulinoma the blood glucose usually falls to 30 mg. per 100 ml. If hypoglycaemic symptoms occur 25 G. of glucose intravenously (50 ml. of 50 per cent. glucose) produces a dramatic improvement.

Glucagon Test. Glucagon, 1 mg., is given intramuscularly. In normal persons and in those with insulinomas there is a short, sharp rise in blood glucose within 30 minutes. This is followed in patients with insulinomas by a fall to hypoglycaemic levels (below 40 mg. per 100 ml.) the same fall does not occur in normals nor in most other forms of hypoglycaemia.

Tolbutamide Test. Sodium tolbutamide, 1000 mg. in 20 ml. of distilled water, is given intravenously to a patient in the fasting state. The blood glucose is measured at 30-minute intervals for 3 hours. All patients show a fall in blood glucose in the first and second hour. By 120–180 minutes, however, that of normals has returned to at least 70 per cent. of the initial level, while that of patients with insulinomas either shows no rise or remains below 70 per cent.

It is not usually necessary to terminate any of these tests on account of hypoglycaemia, but intravenous glucose should be at hand, and the patient observed throughout the test. If a diagnosis of insulinoma is strongly suspected the glucagon test is preferred because there is less danger of hypoglycaemia.

Treatment

The immediate treatment in an attack is the administration of intravenous glucose as for insulin hypoglycaemia [p. 503]. Many insulin-secreting adenomata have now been successfully removed, with complete relief of symptoms. A second operation has occasionally been necessary when more than one adenoma was present. When the diagnosis of spontaneous hypoglycaemia is certain and no tumour can be found in the pancreas, it is usual to perform a subtotal pancreatectomy. No treatment is possible for malignant tumours with metastases, for alloxan which destroys normal islet cells, does not appear to affect neoplastic ones. However, diazoxide, a non-diuretic thiadiazine, is often effective in controlling the hypoglycaemia.

REFERENCES

MALINS, J. (1968) *Clinical Diabetes Mellitus*, London.

WRIGHT, P. H., ASHMORE, J., and MALAISSE, W. J. (1970) Diabetes mellitus and hypoglycaemia, in *Biochemical Disorders in Human Disease*, ed. THOMPSON, R. H. S., and WOOTTON, I. D. P., 3rd ed., London.

RICHARD R. BOMFORD
A. STUART MASON

GLYCOGEN STORAGE DISEASE

Synonym. Von Gierke's disease.

Glycogen storage disease results from an inability to convert glycogen to glucose so that glycogen accumulates in the liver and the child develops symptoms of hypoglycaemia. The condition is inherited as an autosomal recessive and commonly causes impaired growth so that most children with glycogen storage disease are below the third percentile for height. Despite this they are usually intellectually normal.

In infancy it may present with vomiting, difficulty in feeding, irritability or even with convulsions due to the low blood sugar. Marked hepatomegaly is found but the spleen is not palpable. A number of enzymes are involved in this metabolic pathway and the clinical severity varies with the enzyme affected. In milder cases the diagnosis may be made only when liver enlargement is found on routine examination.

An increasing number of enzyme defects are being described. Those due to absence of glucose-6-phosphatase (Type I), lack of the debranching enzyme (Type III) or diminished phosphorylases (Types V and VI) account for 80 per cent. of the total.

Type II differs from the other defects in that the glycogen is normal and the glycolytic pathway is intact. The abnormality is due to the lack of lysozymal maltase so that glycogen accumulates within the cell and is not available for normal degradation. Clinically it presents with cardiac failure due to massive left ventricular hypertrophy as the glycogen builds up within the muscle cells of the myocardium.

Type IV is rare, only four cases having been described. The abnormal glycogen, amylopectinose, sets up a fibrotic reaction leading to cirrhosis and death in infancy.

Glucose-6-Phosphate Deficiency (Type I)

This is commonly diagnosed in the first year of life when infants with hepatomegaly are found to have a low blood glucose often with ketosis. These infants are liable to become hypoglycaemic after a four-hour fast and do not respond to injections of adrenaline or glucagon. The level of lactate is raised and impairs the excretion of uric acid so that limited periods of fasting may result in marked acidosis with tachypnoea and collapse. In this type there is an inability to convert fructose or galactose to glucose so that following an oral or intravenous load there is no rise in glucose but lactate is increased. Liver biopsy confirms the excess of glycogen together with complete absence of the enzyme, glucose-6-phosphatase.

Amylo-1, 6-Glucosidase Deficiency (Type III)

Like Type I this accounts for approximately 30 per cent. of the patients with glycogen storage disease. The symptoms tend to be milder and hypoglycaemia may not develop unless fasting is continued for 10–12 hours.

TABLE 38

GLYCOGEN STORAGE DISEASE

CLASSIFICATION			
DEFICIENT ENZYME	TYPE	EPONYM	OTHER NAME
Glucose-6-phosphatase	I	Von Gierke's	Hepatorenal glycogenosis
Lysozymal-1, 4-glucosidase (acid maltase)	II	Pompes'	Generalized glycogenosis
Amylo-1, 6-glucosidase (debranching enzyme)	III	Cori's	Limit dextrinosis
Amylo-1, 4→1, 6-transglucosidase	IV	Andersen's	Amylopectinosis
Muscle phosphorylase	V	McArdle's	—
Liver phosphorylase	VI	Hers'	—

In this type there is a poor response to glucagon after an overnight fast but a normal rise in blood sugar after adequate feeding. This is due to the fact that after starvation the glycogen molecules will have the structure of limit dextrins since the outer branches which are accessible to phosphorylase have already been degraded. Following a meal newly synthesized normal glycogen can be exposed to phosphorylase and the blood glucose rises. The rate of glycogenolysis is slowed so that glycogen accumulates in both erythrocytes and leucocytes. The diagnosis is substantiated by finding diminished enzyme activity either in a liver biopsy or in the leucocytes.

Phosphorylase Deficiency (Types V and VI)

Absence of muscle phosphorylase results in an inability to carry out vigorous exercise, although quiet muscular activity is possible. Intravenous provision of glucose, fructose or lactate restores normal activity. Since there was no rise in lactate levels it was suggested by McArdle (1951) that this was a myopathy due to a failure in muscle glycogen breakdown. Muscle from these patients shows a considerable excess of glycogen associated with absent phosphorylase activity. In this type the diagnosis is usually made in adult life since the disease is confined to muscle. Low levels of phosphorylase in liver results in a mild form of glycogen storage disease in which the hypoglycaemic response to adrenaline or glucogen is almost normal and in which there is lack of phosphorylase in white cells. Phosphorylase deficiency may be found in association with other enzyme defects.

Prognosis and Treatment

In the severe form of glucose-6-phosphatase deficiency (Type I) stunting and death in early childhood may occur. Mild intercurrent illnesses may cause diarrhoea with severe dehydration and acidosis which requires intravenous therapy with glucose and sodium bicarbonate. In the milder form attempts to diminish glycogen deposition with a high protein intake are unimpressive. On the other hand, frequent feeds including a night feed are useful in preventing hypoglycaemic attacks. Enteric-coated carbohydrate and diazoxide may both have a place in preventing symptoms due to a low blood sugar. Surgery in which the portal vein is brought into the systemic circulation so by-passing the liver may offer some hope in the future.

Where more than one member of a family is affected, the second sibling has the same type of disease as the first affected child, although the severity may vary. Enzyme studies may detect the heterozygote and examination of amniotic fluid can sometimes be used to diagnose the condition *in utero*.

REFERENCE

Whelan, W. J., and Cameron, M. P., eds (1965) *Control of Glycogen Metabolism*, Boston.

Dennis Cottom

DISTURBANCES OF PORPHYRIN

The porphyrins are substances which are related to the synthetic pathways used in the production of

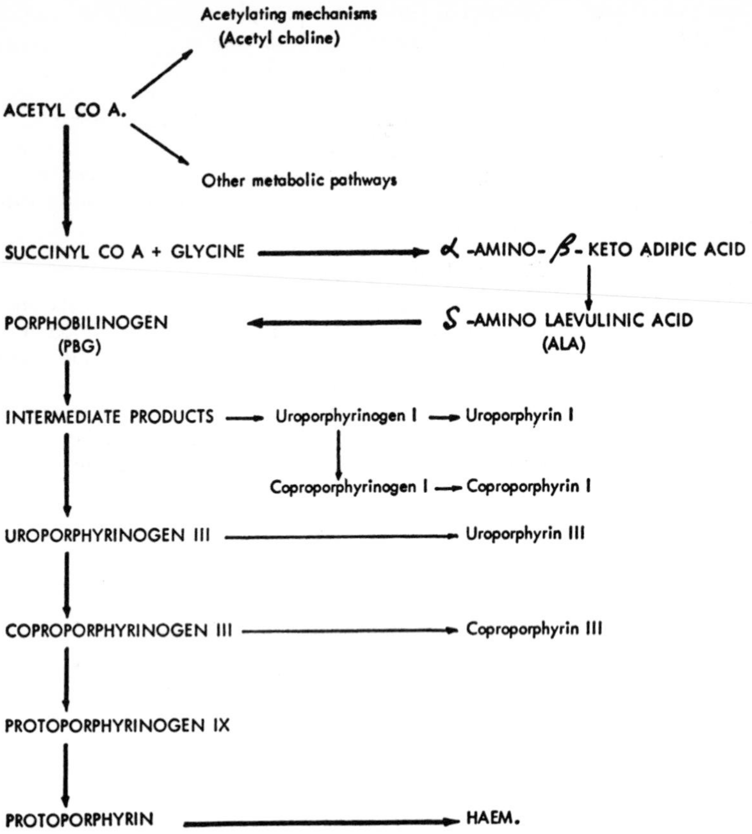

FIG. 29. An outline of the steps involved in the synthesis of haem.

haem and hence of haemoglobin, myoglobin and the cytochromes. The steps in this pathway are shown in FIGURE 29 and some of the structural formulae which explain the anabolic stages and the nomenclature are given in FIGURES 30 and 31.

It will be seen that synthesis of haem takes place by

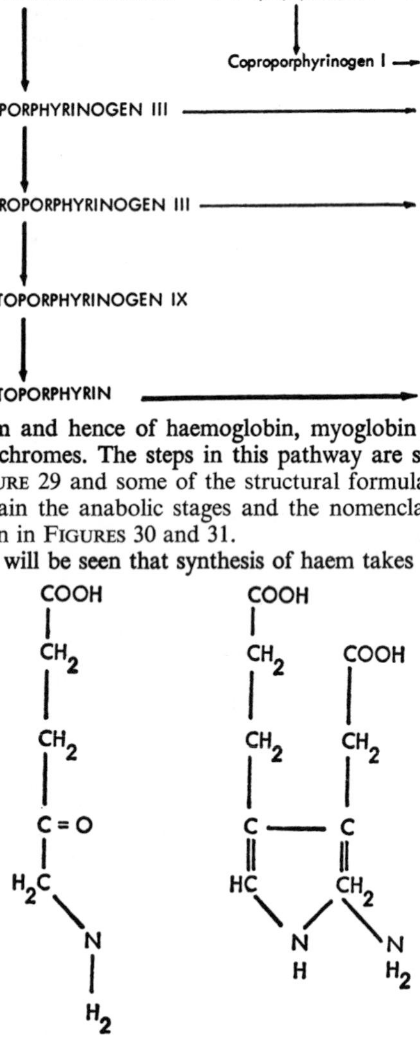

ALA PBG

FIG. 30. Structural formulae of ALA and PBG to show how one molecule of PBG can be formed from two molecules of ALA.

the series III isomers and that series I isomers are, if anything, by-products. This synthesis can probably occur in cells generally, but the most important organs in which it takes place are the bone marrow and the liver.

The condensation of glycine with succinyl CoA by δ-aminolaevulinic acid synthetase requires pyridoxal phosphate as a co-factor and this synthesis of δ-aminolaevulinic acid (ALA) seems to be the rate-limiting reaction in the whole chain leading to haem formation. The reaction occurs within the mitochondria, ALA diffusing through the mitochondrial membrane into the cell sap where the synthesis is carried as far as coproporphyrin III. Coproporphyrin III diffuses into the mitochondria, where it is converted to protoporphyrin IX which is then chelated with iron to form haem. Haem acts as an inhibitor to the synthesis of δ-ALA synthetase so completing the feed-back control loop.

There are a number of inherited conditions and a number resulting from various toxins which are associated with the excretion in the urine of large amounts of ALA and porphobilinogen (PBG), of various porphyrins in the urine and/or faeces, or of a combination of excess ALA+PBG and porphyrin excretion.

Those associated with excessive production of ALA and PBG have been shown to be associated with greatly increased δ-ALA synthetase activity in the liver. Many of the drugs which are known to increase the hepatic activity of δ-ALA synthetase are also liable to precipitate an acute illness in those patients carrying the abnormal porphyric gene and it would seem that they probably act either by inhibiting that part of the gene which *suppresses* δ-ALA synthetase production or by interfering with the feedback suppression of δ-ALA synthetase production by haem.

Since the inherited abnormalities are also associated with *increased* liver δ-ALA synthetase activity and the patients seem to be unduly sensitive to the action of porphyrinogenic drugs, it would seem likely that it is that part of the gene which controls the *suppression* of δ-ALA synthetase production which is involved.

Many patients with such an inherited abnormality may never have any manifestations of the disease. They may, however, be precipitated by appropriate drugs or they may occur spontaneously. In relation to such spontaneous attacks excessive quantities of steroids such as dehydroepiandrosterone have been found in the urine of some patients and these substances were shown to increase ALA synthesis.

THE PORPHYRINURIAS

This term is used, as recommended by Rimington, 'for minor disorders of porphyrin metabolism caused by another disease, or certain drugs or chemicals, in which the clinical features are not directly attributable to the porphyrin abnormality'.

Lead intoxication is perhaps the most important state resulting in porphyrinuria, for it has been advocated that the detection of increased quantities of urinary porphyrins in lead workers should be used to screen them for lead intoxication. Certain anaemias, other toxic chemicals such as aniline, sulphonamides and arsenicals may also be associated with porphyrinuria.

THE PORPHYRIAS

The porphyrias are a series of conditions associated with abnormal porphyrin metabolism in which this metabolic disorder most probably plays a significant part in the symptomatology.

They can be broadly divided into the erythropoietic and the hepatic porphyrias according to the anatomical source of the products of porphyrin metabolism. The classification adopted, certainly somewhat oversimplified, is illustrated in FIGURE 32.

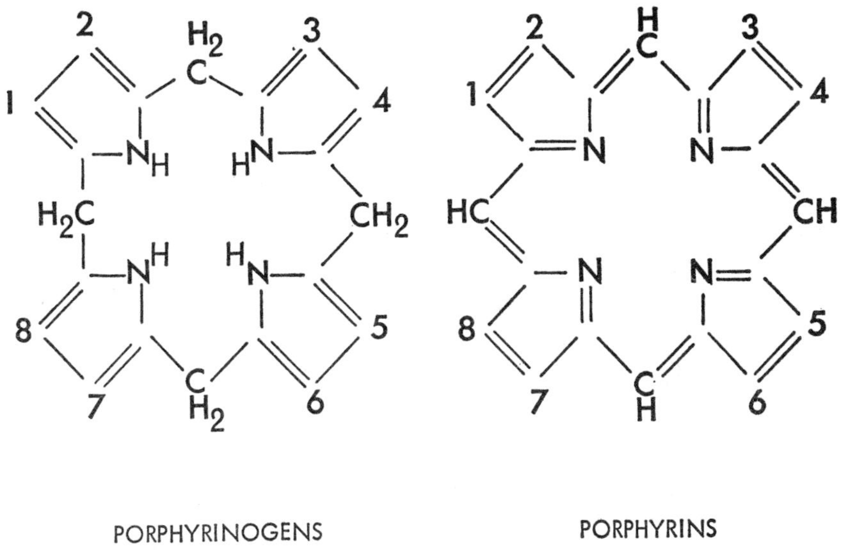

FIG. 31. The essential differences between the porphyrinogens and the porphyrins (whether Series I or III) are shown in the upper part of the figure. In the lower, tabular part are shown the differences in side chains between the *uro- copro-* and *proto-* compounds. It can be seen that in the Series III compounds, one of the four PBG molecules has been rotated through 180 degrees during the condensation, whereas this has not occurred in Series I.

Compound	Side Chains							
	1	2	3	4	5	6	7	8
Uros I	Ac	P	Ac	P	Ac	P	Ac	P
Copros I	M	P	M	P	M	P	M	P
Uros III	Ac	P	Ac	P	Ac	P	P	Ac
Copros III	M	P	M	P	M	P	P	M
Proto IX	M	V	M	V	M	P	P	M

M = $(-CH_3)$ Ac = $(-CH_2COOH)$ P = $(-CH_2-CH_2-COOH)$ V = $(-CH=CH_2)$

ERYTHROPOIETIC PORPHYRIAS

Two conditions can be included under this heading: (1) congenital porphyria; and (2) erythropoietic protoporphyria.

Congenital Porphyria

This condition is very rare, the symptoms are apparent from a very early age and it is probably inherited as a Mendelian recessive characteristic.

The clinical abnormalities are pinkish staining of the napkin, severe photosensitivity resulting in vesicle formation and often in subsequent scarring of the skin and deformity of the fingers, sometimes hypertrichosis, a pinkish discoloration of the teeth, anaemia —usually haemolytic, and splenomegaly.

Examination of the blood by fluorescence microscopy shows that about 5 per cent. of the red cells exhibit a red fluorescence and this has been shown to be due to the abnormal presence of uroporphyrin I. In the bone marrow some 50 per cent. of the normoblasts show this fluorescence and it is confined to the nucleus.

The urine contains excessive quantities of uroporphyrin and coproporphyrin mainly of series I— i.e. not compounds in the normal chain of haem synthesis. The faeces contain excessive quantities of coproporphyrin I.

In order that uroporphyrin I should be produced from PBG the enzyme PBG deaminase is necessary, whereas for the production of uroporphyrin III both PBG deaminase and another enzyme, uroporphyrinogen isomerase, must be present. It would seem likely therefore that owing to a genetic abnormality, some at least of the red cell series are deficient in uroporphyrinogen isomerase with the result that excessive quantities of the series I isomers are produced. These porphyrins are liberated into the plasma and accumulate in the tissues causing the pink staining and the cutaneous photosensitivity.

When the haemolytic anaemia is severe, splenectomy often has a beneficial effect on the blood picture and in a number of cases there has been reported to be a reduction in photosensitivity. This improvement is presumably because the splenectomy and resultant decrease in haemolysis causes a diminution in erythropoietic activity and hence a decrease in the production and release of the abnormal erythropoietic porphyrins.

Erythropoietic Protoporphyrin

This condition was at one time thought to be very rare—probably because the urine does not contain any excess of ALA, PBG or of porphyrin. Faecal porphyrins, however, may be increased. Affected individuals develop intense pruritus and burning of the skin followed by urticaria and weal formation. Chronic eczematous changes may occur but there is no blistering, scar formation or hypertrichosis.

The erythrocytes contain large amounts of protoporphyrin IX and coproporphyrin and fluoresce red under ultra-violet light. Fluorescent normoblasts can be found in the bone marrow.

In one family the disease can be traced through three generations and it would seem that it is transmitted as a Mendelian dominant.

Biochemical changes very similar to those found in erythropoietic protoporphyria may be induced by griseofulvin.

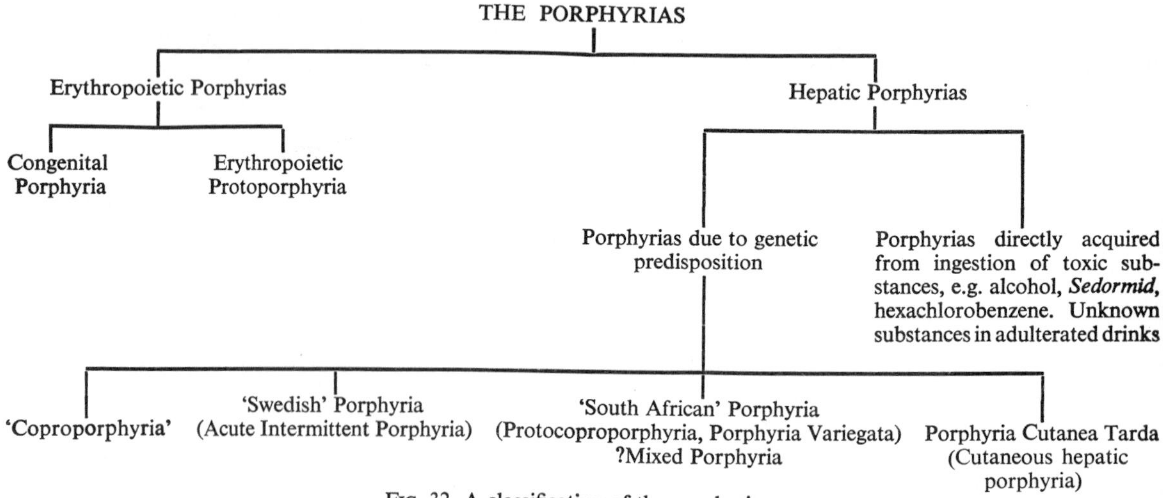

FIG. 32. A classification of the porphyrias.

HEPATIC PORPHYRIAS

Some of the hepatic porphyrias are due to genetic abnormalities and in some there is no evidence of such a constitutional cause, various toxins being the sole responsible factors. However, patients who carry a genetic trait may exhibit no clinical abnormalities but these may be induced by various chemical agents. For this reason it is always important to investigate families of porphyric patients, even if some chemical agent appears to be the aetiological factor. The compounds present in excess tend largely to be those found in or derived from the normal pathways of haem synthesis.

General Symptomatology

There are two groups of symptoms which may occur in the hepatic porphyrias. Those referable to the alimentary tract, cardiovascular system, and nervous system form one group, and the other is confined to photosensitivity and skin lesions. The biochemical cause of the first group is unknown, but the symptoms tend to occur when large quantities of ALA and PBG are excreted (though neither compound can be incriminated). By contrast photosensitivity and susceptibility to minor trauma are associated with the production of large quantities of porphyrins. These are photosensitizing agents and presumably are responsible for the clinical manifestations.

Only the first group of symptoms occur in Swedish or acute intermittent porphyria and light sensitivity is never found. In porphyria cutanea tarda only skin lesions occur, manifestations of the other group being very rare, and then mild, and in such patients liver damage is frequent. This may result in a diminished excretion of porphyrins into the alimentary tract producing an increased concentration in the tissues resulting in enhanced skin sensitivity to light. In South African porphyria both types of symptoms may occur and when those of the first group are present the patients secrete large quantities of ALA and PBG in the urine.

Symptoms Referable to the Alimentary Tract, Cardiovascular System and Nervous System. Abdominal pain is of fairly acute onset and is characteristically very severe. It may be colicky or continuous and may be associated with vomiting and with constipation or sometimes with diarrhoea. The pain may be generalized, but often is mainly experienced in the right iliac fossa or in the epigastrium. Many patients with abdominal pain as a presenting symptom are admitted to surgical wards as emergencies.

The commonest neurological disturbance is motor weakness or paralysis. This may affect the upper or lower limbs only, or it may be much more profound, most of the body musculature being affected, so that respiratory failure or the inhalation of food or saliva may constitute a grave danger and require tracheostomy. The paralysis is usually of the lower motor neurone type, but sometimes evidence of lack of upper motor neurone function can be obtained. Incontinence, or retention of urine is sometimes encountered.

Sensory disturbances are less common, but areas of sensory loss, of diminution or of hyperaesthesia or paraesthesia may sometimes be found.

Epilepsy, generalized or Jacksonian in type may occur and this may be particularly dangerous, for it may lead to the therapeutic use of barbiturates with a possibly fatal consequence.

Many patients exhibit mental disturbances, the pattern of which, from patient to patient, may cover the whole spectrum of mental abnormalities, some having been legally certified as insane. It has been suggested that George III of Great Britain suffered from porphyria and that this was the cause of his mental illness.

Many patients have sinus tachycardia and some develop transient hypertension. Occasionally a variety of minor E.C.G. changes may be found. The sinus tachycardia may be an important sign for, whilst it is still present, it indicates that the patient has not yet emerged from the acute attack of the disease.

Pathologically the lesions in the peripheral nerves resemble those produced by isonicotinic acid hydrazide, motor nerves being more affected than sensory and long fibres more than short. It has been suggested that in AIP (q.v.), as in isonicotinic acid hydrazide intoxication, the lesions may be produced by a pyridoxal phosphate deficiency. In the case of AIP this would result from an increased consumption of pyridoxal phosphate which is necessary in the condensation of glycine and succinyl CO-A by δ-ALA synthetase to form δ-ALA. (See section on porphyrin metabolism.)

Cutaneous Manifestations. In these patients with cutaneous manifestations the lesions are seen in areas exposed to light and it may well be that considerably more exposure is necessary in some types of disease than in others to produce the cutaneous lesions. Increased pigmentation of the hair and skin is common. The skin may develop vesicles and bullae which burst, become infected and cause resultant scarring and sometimes marked deformity. The skin is also particularly susceptible to trauma, vesicles occurring after minor blows on it; there is a decreased reaction to histamine.

Hepatomegaly and jaundice are sometimes seen in those patients exhibiting mainly cutaneous lesions and are often associated with alcoholism or the ingestion of other toxins, as will be discussed later.

Hepatic Porphyrias of Genetic Origin:

'Swedish' Porphyria—Acute Intermittent Porphyria (AIP). The genetic trait which gives rise to this condition has been shown by Waldenström to be quite common in Sweden although, of course, the gene is also present in the population of other countries and it appears to be a dominant.

Except for the occasional presence of increased skin pigmentation, skin manifestations have never been seen in the condition. The predominant characteristic is the acute onset of attacks of abdominal pain, often accompanied by the neurological and cardiovascular abnormalities described above. The attacks may vary from mild intermittent bouts of abdominal discomfort to a fulminating fatal illness. There may be mild fever and a leucocytosis which make the differentiation from an acute abdominal emergency more difficult. Many carriers of the gene never have any symptoms. Attacks may be initiated by a variety of drugs and barbiturates; those with an allyl group are very often the offenders; it would seem likely that barbiturates given after the onset of an attack may precipitate dangerous neurological symptoms in a high proportion of cases. Sulphonamides and alcohol have also been incriminated, and more recently certain steroids including those contained in some oral contraceptives.

The attacks may clear up completely and rapidly or it may be many years before the patient fully recovers. Some patients have evidently developed irreversible damage to the brain, for they have remained permanently insane. The mortality rate of acute attacks is about 25 per cent.

The characteristic biochemical finding is the urinary excretion of greatly abnormal amounts of PBG and of ALA. Freshly passed urine is of normal colour and does not fluoresce but it darkens and gives a red fluorescence after standing, for the PBG condenses *in vitro* to form uroporphyrin. Between attacks abnormal amounts of PBG and ALA continue to be excreted in the urine and by urinary examination for these substances the asymptomatic carriers of the gene can be detected.

'South African' Porphyria—Protocoproporphyria, Porphyria Variegata, also Mixed Porphyria. The recognition of this condition, also associated with a dominant gene but distinct from that concerned in Swedish porphyria, was made clear by Dean and Barnes who traced all of their many cases to a pair of Dutch settlers who came to South Africa in 1688. It seems possible that a similar entity encountered in other countries is due to the same genetic abnormality.

In this condition abdominal and neurological symptoms are more frequently found in females and cutaneous manifestations in males. This is possibly due to the greater exposure to sunlight and ingestion of alcohol and hence liver failure among the men. It would seen that considerable exposure to light is necessary to produce the skin lesions, hence patients with the trait living in temperate climates may not develop skin lesions and so they may symptomatically simulate Swedish porphyria.

Biochemically the urine content has a high level of ALA and PBG during the acute phases of the disease, whereas during remissions the faecal content of protoporphyrin and coproporphyrin is high.

Porphyria Cutanea Tarda (PCT). In these patients skin lesions are manifested, but usually after childhood. Abdominal and neurological lesions are unusual. It is generally recognized that a large consumption of alcohol is frequently associated with the disease, but because very few chronic alcoholics get porphyria, Waldenström investigated the families of some of his cases and found several 'latent' subjects. Some degree of liver damage is almost invariably found in the patients with skin lesions. It would seem that during the latent period an abnormal amount of protoporphyrin and coproporphyrin is found in the faeces and that the urinary secretion of porphyrins increases markedly during the attacks.

It has been shown by Ippen and confirmed by others that multiple venesections will produce marked clinical improvement in most patients with porphyria cutanea tarda. Mild to moderate hepatic siderosis is usually found in patients with PCT but this need not be completely eliminated before the improvement occurs.

Alcoholics with PCT may show considerable improvement if they stop drinking, but even those who continue to drink may be improved by repeated venesection.

Coproporphyria. A few individuals have been found who characteristically secrete large amounts of coproporphyrin III in the faeces, and relatives have been found with the same anomaly. This condition has been alleged to be benign, but at least three cases are known where severe abdominal pain and neurological lesions were precipitated by barbiturates, PBG being found in the urine during the attacks.

Porphyrias Directly Acquired from the Ingestion of Toxic Substances:

Alcoholic Cutaneous Porphyria. It has been shown that the consumption of large quantities of alcohol will, after a variable delay, increase the urinary output of coproporphyrin III. Most chronic alcoholics do not develop porphyrin sensitivity but again in most of the cases, the largest group being found among the Bantu alcoholics, there is no evidence of a hereditary factor. Faecal porphyrins are not increased but excessive porphyrins are found in the urine. It would seem that such cases are different from Waldenström's porphyria cutanea tarda.

Porphyria Due to Other Toxic Substances. An outbreak of porphyria due to the ingestion of the seed-dressing hexachlorobenzene has been reported from Turkey. Skin sensitivity was the main manifestation and large quantities of uro- and coproporphyrins were found in the urine and faeces. Urinary PBG was only found in severe cases.

Sulphonal has been reported as giving rise to porphyria and experimental porphyria can be produced by *Sedormid* and by a number of other compounds.

Treatment

Treatment must in the first place be preventive by withholding known precipitating agents. Secondly, during an acute attack symptomatic treatment is essential and no sedative containing barbiturate should be given. Serum electrolyte concentrations should be watched, for a few patients have been found with very low osmolarity due, it would seem, to an inappropriate oversecretion of antidiuretic hormone. Some of the severe cerebral symptoms might result from this and dramatic response to water restriction can occur. So far as any specific treatment is concerned, it has been claimed that improvement occurs with adenosine-5-monophosphate, but this requires further evaluation.

Experimentally, a reduction in δ-ALA synthetase activity can be achieved by increasing available glucose and an abnormally low protein and carbohydrate intake has been shown to increase the urinary output of ALA in a patient with AIP. It is thus encouraging to know that the abdominal symptoms of AIP have been thought to have been alleviated by a diet high in carbohydrate together with insulin injections.

Intermittent haemodialysis has also been claimed to produce an improvement in symptoms, but the author has seen one patient in whom it was entirely without effect. It is very difficult to assess the effect of any remedy in a condition with such an unpredictable course, but it would seem rational and harmless to give supplements of pyridoxine or its derivatives.

Until the relatives of patients with porphyria have been examined, to determine whether or not they carry the trait, they should under no circumstances be given any substance likely to provoke an acute attack.

It is not easy to determine precisely whether such a

relative is a carrier of the abnormal gene or not. A loading dose of 50 g. of glycine followed by hourly collections of urine in which the ALA output is measured may enable a diagnosis of AIP to be made during periods of remission, but the over-all efficiency of this test is still to be proved.

REFERENCES

DEAN, G., and BARNES, H. D. (1955) The inheritance of porphyria, *Brit. med. J.*, **2**, 89.

DE MATTEIS, F. (1967) Disturbance of liver porphyrin caused by drugs, *Pharmacol. Rev.*, **19**, 523.

GOLDBERG, A., and RIMINGTON, C. (1962) *The Diseases of Porphyrin Metabolism*, Springfield, Ill.

GRANICK, S. (1966) The induction *in vitro* of the synthesis of δ-aminolaevulinic acid synthetase in chemical porphyria: a response to certain drugs, sex hormones and foreign chemicals, *J. biol. Chem.*, **241**, 1359.

IPPEN, VON H. (1961) Allgemein Symptome der späten Hautporphyrie (Porphyria cutanea tarda) als Hinweise für deren Behandlung, *Dtsch. med. Wschr.*, **86**, 127.

RIDLEY, A. (1969) The neuropathy of acute intermittent porphyria, *Quart. J. Med.*, n. s. **38**, 307.

WALDENSTRÖM, J., and HAEGER-ARONSEN, B. (1963) Different patterns of human porphyria, *Brit. med. J.*, **2**, 272.

GEORGE A. SMART

DISORDERS OF NUTRITION

THE VITAMINS

Definition

Vitamins are organic substances, distinct from proteins and carbohydrates, which are present in small quantities in food and which are necessary for the normal nutrition of the body. A substance which by this definition is a vitamin for one species of animal is not necessarily so for another, depending on the ability of the animal to synthesize the substance. For example, ascorbic acid or vitamin C is a vitamin for man and for guinea-pigs, but not for dogs or cats.

The vitamins can be divided into those which are water-soluble and those which are fat-soluble. Since their nature was at first quite unknown, they were labelled with the letters of the alphabet—A, B, C, D, more or less in the order of their discovery. It was soon clear, however, that these were not all pure substances, and with further discovery and labelling in different centres, the nomenclature became chaotic. It is therefore preferable to refer, where possible, to the established chemical name of the vitamin. This is especially important for members of the B complex, but not for the fat-soluble vitamins, since here the various members of a given group have a qualitatively similar physiological action. The daily requirements of the vitamins are measured in milligrammes or microgrammes and this implies that they are not necessarily destroyed in the reactions in which they participate and that their actions may in part be catalytic.

To many of the vitamins a particular role has been ascribed—they act as coenzymes or form part of the structure of a coenzyme involved in vital metabolic processes. Deficiency of the vitamin and hence of the coenzyme interferes with the enzymatic process involved, leading to impaired synthesis of some metabolite or to the accumulation of excessive amounts of the precursors of the reaction which themselves may be toxic.

Vitamin Deficiency Diseases

If the diet contains less than the requisite minimum of a vitamin for long enough, symptoms and signs develop. Although disease entities are ascribed to various vitamin deficiencies, such pure deficiencies rarely occur except under experimental conditions.

Such dietetic deficiencies are rare in the British Isles where vitamin deficiencies are most commonly associated with conditions interfering with absorption, such as steatorrhoea. Where dietetic deficiencies do exist they are usually associated with some social or psychological abnormality, such as chronic alcoholism or dietary faddism. This inability to synthesize the vitamin may not be absolute, e.g. intestinal bacteria can synthesize vitamin K, solar radiation converts 7-dehydrocholesterol into vitamin D_3 and renders the animal independent of vitamin D in the diet.

THE FAT-SOLUBLE VITAMINS

Vitamin A

This substance is contained in liver (the richest source in the normal diet), butter, cheese, eggs and fish-liver oils. It can be formed in the body, however, from the carotenes, and good sources of these are green vegetables, apricots and red palm oil. The International Unit of vitamin A is the equivalent of 0·6 μg. of β-carotene. There are two very similar compounds, both having a similar physiological action. One vitamin, A_1, is found in mammals and salt-water fish, whereas the other, vitamin A_2, is found in fresh-water fish.

Vitamin A can be estimated in the plasma, and the curve obtained by frequent plasma estimations after an oral dose has been used as an index of the efficiency of fat absorption. The minimal daily dose required to protect against deficiency has been shown by human experiments to be about 20 I.U. per kg., or 1300 I.U. for an adult man. In order to allow for storage and to supply a safe margin, however, about 2500–5000 I.U. per day of vitamin A should be ingested. If the carotenes are the sole dietary source then the intake should be about 7500–10,000 I.U.

Vitamin A forms part of the molecule of rhodopsin or visual purple, and hence one of the first signs of deficiency is a high dark-adapted rod threshold. This is not the same as poor night vision, although naturally night vision is inevitably poor when the dark-adapted rod threshold is very high. When light strikes the rod rhodopsin breaks down to retinine and a protein opsin, but the manner in which this reaction yields nervous excitation leading to vision is unknown. Rhodopsin is then reformed from retinine by a series of reactions occurring during dark-adaptation. The cones also require vitamin A for regeneration of the pigment for colour vision (visual violet). Psychological factors are also very important in determining how well a person can manage in the dark, and may well result in complaints of defective night vision in the absence of vitamin A deficiency.

Other manifestations in man of vitamin A deficiency are: xerophthalmia, follicular hyperkeratosis of the skin and keratinizing metaplasia, particularly of the respiratory epithelium, the urinary tract and the pancreas. Xerophthalmia is the most serious of these lesions. Keratinization of the cornea and conjunctivae occurs, and also Bitot's spots, which are thickened, opaque, triangular lesions of the conjunctiva. Infection may supervene to cause a panophthalmitis and resultant total destruction of the eye.

Hyperkeratosis of the hair follicles, particularly on the extensor surface of the limbs, producing the so-called goose skin or phrynoderma also occurs, but it is not absolutely certain that this is entirely due to vitamin A deficiency. It was not produced in experimental vitamin A deficiency when this was studied at Sheffield.

Changes in the respiratory epithelium have been described in children, and it has been suggested that vitamin A deficiency, resulting from malabsorption of fat, may be a factor in producing the lung infections associated with congenital cystic disease of the pancreas.

Vitamin A deficiency resulting from faulty diet is practically never seen in European communities. It is, however, prevalent in parts of Asia, notably in China and India, and in Africa.

Hypervitaminosis A may lead to loss of hair, generalized desquamation and pigmentation. Hepatomegaly and raised intracranial pressure may be present. An acute vitamin A intoxication may follow the ingestion of polar bear liver which has a very high content of the vitamin.

Vitamin D

Vitamin D is the generic term applied to a group of sterols with antirachitic activity. Vitamin D_2 (calciferol) is produced by the irradiation of ergosterol, while vitamin D_3 is formed by irradiating 7-dehydrocholesterol and occurs naturally in butter, egg yolk and fish liver oils. Dihydrotachysterol is a synthetic sterol with low antirachitic activity at a level of intake at which vitamins D_2 and D_3 are effective, though in high doses it has a vitamin D-like action.

The vitamin D compounds are soluble in fat or organic solvents but insoluble in water. In man the antirachitic activity of vitamins D_2 and D_3 are equivalent although patients may become resistant to D_2 but not to D_3. The International Unit (I.U.) of vitamin D is 0·025 mg. of calciferol, i.e. one gramme of calciferol = 40,000 I.U.

Vitamin D can be absorbed from the gut or through the skin, absorption from the gut being aided by bile and therefore being diminished in obstructive jaundice. Steatorrhoea also decreases absorption of the vitamin. Vitamin D_3 is formed in the skin by exposure to radiation in the wavelength 230–313 mμ. In the serum vitamin D is transported with the α-1 and α-2 globulins and after a single large dose of the vitamin can be detected in the serum for several months.

Vitamin D has important actions on calcium and phosphate metabolism. Its main action is to enhance the absorption of calcium from the gut by acting directly on the calcium transport mechanism; a secondary increase in phosphate absorption may also occur. In physiological doses vitamin D increases phosphate absorption by the renal tubules but at higher dose levels renal phosphate excretion is increased.

Vitamin D deficiency results in rickets in the child and osteomalacia in adults [see Section 11] but evidence for a direct action of the hormone on bone is incomplete. Increased bone resorption has been reported after infusion of large amounts of vitamin D_3; this action is dependent on the presence of parathyroid hormone and is depressed by calcitonin. A minimal amount of the vitamin is also required for the normal action of parathyroid hormone on bone. There is a time lag of about 12 hours after administration of vitamin D before its metabolic effects are apparent—its effects are mediated through new protein synthesis and can be blocked by inhibitors of this process.

The daily requirements of the vitamin are not known with certainty, the amount required varying with age and is affected by pregnancy and lactation. A mean daily intake of 10 μg (400 Units) will prevent rickets in childhood and this amount may be sufficient during pregnancy. Smaller amounts will suffice in adults.

Deficiency of vitamin D is accompanied by hypophosphataemia and less frequently hypocalcaemia; the alkaline phosphatase is usually raised.

Intravenous vitamin D_3 causes a significant increase in the fasting serum phosphate in patients with vitamin D deficiency. Treatment with vitamin D is indicated in rickets, osteomalacia and hypoparathyroidism. Rickets and osteomalacia may arise because of nutritional deficiency of vitamin D, malabsorption syndromes, liver disease and certain renal disorders. Patients with renal failure are relatively resistant to vitamin D and large doses may be required, sometimes by the parenteral route. Hypoparathyroidism is associated with hypocalcaemia and hyperphosphataemia. Treatment is aimed at restoring a normal level of serum calcium; vitamin D_2 is the drug of choice, starting with 1·25–5 mg. for the first few days and then reducing to a maintenance dose of 1–2 mg. daily, calcium supplements may be needed initially but if the diet is adequate can be omitted when the serum calcium is normal. Repeated checks of serum calcium are required and even after stabilization the serum calcium should be checked every few months to avoid hypercalcaemia.

Vitamin D intoxication causes nausea, vomiting, muscular weakness, anorexia, thirst, polyuria, convulsions and coma. Hypercalcaemia may also cause renal failure and metastatic calcification. Treatment comprises withdrawal of the vitamin, a high fluid intake, corrections of water and electrolyte imbalance and hydrocortisone administration. Phosphate or sulphate infusions may be needed to correct severe hypercalcaemia. The idiopathic hypercalcaemia of infancy is due to excessive vitamin D intake but in some cases excessive sensitivity to the vitamin may be responsible.

Vitamin E

Vitamin E is found in the germ of cereals, and in green vegetables. There are several compounds which have vitamin E activity. They are all tocopherols, and of these, alpha-tocopherol is probably the most potent.

Vitamin E acts as an anti-oxidant, preserving vitamin A and delaying the onset of rancidity in fats. As might be expected, the vitamin is itself rapidly destroyed by rancid fats.

Recently a syndrome of anaemia, reticulocytosis, thrombocytosis and oedema has been described in low birth-weight newborn infants fed on artificial milk formulae containing relatively large amounts of poly-unsaturated fatty acids. Vitamin E levels were low in these infants, the mean being 0·18 mg. per 100 ml. (normal in breast fed infants or adults being 0·4 mg. or more). Treatment with vitamin E as α-tocopherol (75–100 mg. daily) caused a rise in serum levels and clinical improvement. The mechanism of haemolysis is uncertain but it may be related to the anti-oxidant action of tocopherol. In vitamin E deficiency lipid peroxides accumulate in the erythrocyte membrane and may bind free-SH groups, thereby damaging the membrane and reducing the life span of the cell. Oedema may result from increased capillary permeability from a similar type of damage.

Vitamin K

Vitamin K is present in a large variety of foods and notably in green vegetables. In addition, however, bacteria normally present in the intestine can synthesize the vitamin, and for this reason the daily requirement is unknown.

Two naturally occurring compounds with vitamin K activity are known, K_1, or 2-methyl-3-phytyl-1, 4-naphthoquinone, and K_2, or 2-methyl-3-difarneryl-1, 4-naphthoquinone. The former is the compound present in green plants and the latter is produced by bacteria. It has been found that the removal of the side chains does not result in a loss of vitamin activity, and the simple synthetic compound 2-methyl-1,4-naphth quinone, menaphthone (menadione), is frequently used therapeutically. Many other compounds now are known which possess vitamin K activity, some of them being water soluble.

Vitamin K is necessary for the liver to form prothrombin and deficiency results in a fall in the prothrombin content of the blood. When the level is less than about 15 per cent. of normal, spontaneous haemorrhage occurs. The first manifestation of this is usually haematuria, but spontaneous haemorrhage, which may prove fatal, may occur in any organ of the body.

Bile must be present in the alimentary tract for vitamin K to be absorbed, and deficiency is therefore almost inevitable in any long-standing jaundice of the hepatic or obstructive type. To give the compound by mouth is quite useless in these circumstances, but intramuscular injection is fully effective if liver function is not unduly diminished.

The levels of prothrombin, and factors VII, IX and X may be low even in the normal full term infant but in premature infants levels of the factors may be even lower causing haemorrhagic disease of the newborn. Routine prophylaxis with administration of 0·5–1 mg. of vitamin K_1 or K_3 parenterally to the newborn infant is to be recommended. The benefit of prophylactic administration to the mother is less certain. In established haemorrhagic disease 0·5–1 mg. of vitamin K_1 or K_3 should be given intravenously to avoid haematoma formation. Large doses of vitamin K can produce a Heinz-body anaemia with hyperbilirubinaemia and kernicterus but small doses in the region of 1 mg. are safe. This toxic effect is only seen with the synthetic and water-soluble analogues and does not arise with the naturally occurring vitamin K_1.

Steatorrhoea, whether idiopathic or resulting from pancreatic or other disease, is also at times associated with vitamin K deficiency, and this can be corrected by giving large doses such as 3–5 mg. daily by mouth, though injections may have to be given in severe cases. It is possible that the water-soluble compounds may be the most effective when steatorrhoea is present.

The plasma prothrombin level is used as an index of vitamin K nutrition. It is only valid, however, when there is no liver disease (since liver cells produce prothrombin, vitamin K being necessary in the process) and when no drugs of the dicoumarin group have been given. This group of drugs, which are used as anti-coagulants in conditions such as coronary occlusion, antagonize the action of vitamin K. Overdosage, resulting in very low prothrombin levels and spontaneous haemorrhage, is not rapidly counteracted by vitamin K compounds; the most effective, vitamin K_1, takes 4–12 hours to raise the prothrombin level. Ten to twenty milligrammes by mouth is effective and not much slower in action than parenteral treatment. In an emergency vitamin K_1 can be given intravenously (20–50 mg.) slowly at a rate not exceeding 5 mg. per minute. More rapid administration may cause facial flushing, sweating, chest pain, cyanosis and hypotension. Vitamin K_3 is far less effective in the treatment of drug-induced hypoprothrombinaemia. The patient may be refractory to further anticoagulants for several weeks after administration of vitamin K_1.

Doses of vitamin K far in excess of the therapeutic amounts do not produce any toxic symptoms.

THE WATER-SOLUBLE VITAMINS

Vitamin B_1—Aneurine or Thiamine

Foods rich in aneurine are cereals (where it is mainly found in the germ and the pericarp), legumes, pulses and nuts, pork, ham and bacon, liver, kidney and eggs. It occurs in animal tissues mainly in the pyrophosphate form.

The vitamin has been isolated, identified chemically and synthesized. It is usually measured in milligrammes but 1 International Unit is defined as 3 μg. of aneurine hydrochloride.

Like all vitamins, aneurine was originally estimated biologically, but it is now usual to convert it to thiochrome and to estimate this substance fluorimetrically.

The requirements of aneurine vary with the energy value and carbohydrate content of the diet, but approximately 0·3 mg. per 1000 calories is the minimum intake. Thus, an adult will require something like 1 mg. per day.

Aneurine forms an essential part of two coenzymes which are important in the decarboxylation of the alpha-ketoacids. In aneurine deficiency, pyruvic acid accumulates in the blood and this finding can be used as an estimate of the deficiency, particularly if the production of pyruvic acid in response to a test dose of glucose is measured. It is probably the toxic effects of the accumulating alpha-ketoacids which play a large part in the production of beriberi, the condition resulting from aneurine deficiency.

In addition, thiamine is a co-factor for transketolase involved in the metabolism of pentose via the hexose monophosphate pathway. Evidence of a defect in this pathway has been found in alcoholics with Wernicke's syndrome. Estimations of aneurine deficiency can also be made by measuring the output of the vitamin in the urine by the thiochrome method.

Deficiency of aneurine gives rise to beriberi [p. 529], and to pathological changes in the brain which have been described by Wernicke and which are associated with the clinical manifestations of clouded consciousness, ophthalmoplegias of various types, and nystagmus. Treatment is with large doses of thiamine by the intramuscular or intravenous routes usually combined with other B group vitamins.

In western countries deficiency is usually associated with chronic alcoholism where a high carbohydrate intake is associated with a low intake of vitamin B_1. Under these circumstances the manifestations are usually those of peripheral neuritis or of mental changes rather than that of wet beriberi. Wet beriberi is characterized by the high output type of cardiac failure with warm extremities and a bounding pulse, the condition resembling heart failure due to hyperthyroidism, anaemia, cor pulmonale, or Paget's disease. The condition is cured by treatment with aneurine hydrochloride, 20 mg. thrice daily for 2 weeks.

In the world as a whole aneurine deficiency is most frequently seen among populations whose main cereal is rice. When the pericarp is removed from this cereal, practically no aneurine is left unless the rice has first been partly cooked.

Reactions to large doses of aneurine have occurred which have occasionally been fatal. These have probably been hypersensitivity reactions, however, since they followed injections of the vitamin. Two types of reaction have been described, one resembles anaphylactic shock and occurs after numerous previous injections, and the other presents symptoms like hyperthyroidism with tremors, palpitation, excitement, giddiness and insomnia.

Riboflavin

Riboflavin is a bright yellow substance with a yellow-green fluorescence. It is widely distributed in natural food-stuffs but milk, cheese, eggs, liver, green vegetables and yeast are particularly good sources. It is rapidly destroyed when exposed to light, so that considerable loss occurs in substances like milk. Riboflavin is also synthesized by intestinal bacteria, and some of this is absorbed and utilized—a process known as refection, which is common to most of the vitamin B complex. Riboflavin has been isolated and is synthesized on a large scale. It is measured in milligrammes of pure substance. The quantity present in natural products can be determined biologically by its effect on the growth of rats or chicks, or microbiologically by its stimulating effect on *Lactobacillus casei* (the usual method).

The minimal requirement of riboflavin is about 0·6–0·7 mg. per day, but, since animal experiments indicate that the optimum is about twice this, a daily intake of 1·5–1·8 mg. for an adult woman or man, has been recommended.

This vitamin forms part of the coenzyme flavin mononucleotide, concerned in the oxidation of carbohydrate, and the coenzyme adenine dinucleotide, which forms part of xanthine oxidase. They act as coenzymes in many oxidation-reduction reactions. It is also associated with the retinal pigments.

Riboflavin deficiency in man manifests itself by a dermatitis of seborrhoeic type affecting the skin of the nose and round the mouth and of the scrotum or vulva, and by a superficial glossitis which starts with loss of 'fur' in patches from the dorsum and later the tongue is smooth and occasionally fissured and painful; some observers describe the colour as magenta. It is possible that corneal vascularization and degeneration of the corneal epithelium also occurs. Riboflavin deficiency often occurs in pellagra and signs of the deficiency have been observed to be precipitated when nicotinic acid has been given. During the Second World War neurological abnormalities, particularly optic atrophy with blindness and also deafness, were observed in prisoners of war, and it has been suggested that riboflavin deficiency played a part in these conditions.

None of the signs described above occurs specifically as a result of ariboflavinosis. Thus, although the presence of any of them might suggest that the patient is deficient in riboflavin, the proof must lie in recovery when the pure vitamin is given. The excretion of riboflavin in the urine can be measured, but it is not a reliable index of the nutritional state. The riboflavin content of the plasma or of white blood corpuscles can also be measured microbiologically, and these probably are reasonable indices of possible deficiency. In well-nourished individuals the mean plasma level is 0·8 μg. per 100 ml. for free and 3·2 μg. per 100 ml. for total riboflavin. In white blood corpuscles the mean total riboflavin content is 252 μg. per 100 ml.

Manifestations of riboflavin deficiency tend to occur in communities who develop pellagra and where milk is not consumed; it is seen most commonly in Africa, China and India. It is sometimes seen in patients with steatorrhoea, and riboflavin should always be given with aneurine and nicotinamide to patients who have long periods of intravenous glucose as their sole source of nourishment, or who have to receive long courses of wide-spectrum antibiotics which prevent the occurrence of refection.

Nicotinamide (Vitamin B_7)

Nicotinamide and nicotinic acid are equally effective as vitamin B_7, but in bodily tissues the vitamin is present practically exclusively as nicotinamide. Moreover, whereas nicotinamide produces no untoward reactions, even when taken in large quantities, nicotinic acid in amounts of 25 mg. or more causes intense flushing of the skin, and headaches. In vegetable tissues, however, the vitamin is nearly all present as nicotinic acid. The amino acid tryptophan can be converted by the tissues to nicotinamide and thus can also fulfil the role of vitamin B_7. The vitamin is present in cereals, though in maize it is probably present in a bound form, from which it does not become available for human nutrition. The vitamin is also present in good quantities in meat, liver and yeast. It is synthesized by bacterial flora and part of this is available to the body.

The vitamin B_7 content of foodstuffs is usually estimated by a chick-growth method, but for samples of biological fluids it is more usual to measure the growth stimulation of *Lactobacillus arabinosus*.

The requirements of nicotinamide are not easy to estimate, partly because of the role of tryptophan, partly because of the process of refection, and partly because of the occurrence of the vitamin in forms unavailable to the body. It is probable that 10–20 mg. per day are entirely adequate.

The vitamin forms part of the pyridine nucleotide coenzymes known as nicotinamide-adenine dinucleotide (NAD^+) previously known as coenzyme I or DPN^+ and as nicotinamide-adenine dinucleotide phosphate ($NADP^+$) formerly known as coenzyme II or TPN^+. The pyridine nucleotides are coenzymes for a number of transhydrogenases which catalyse oxidation-reduction reactions, e.g. of lactate to pyruvate.

Nicotinamide is excreted in the urine partly as N^1-methyl nicotinamide, a substance which has a blue fluorescence. This substance can readily be measured and it falls to very low levels in patients suffering from nicotinamide deficiency.

Deficiency of vitamin B_7 is the major factor in the production of pellagra [see p. 530]. It seems to be most common in maize-eating communities. In European communities, apart from the poor of maize-eating areas, it is seen mostly in conjunction with chronic alcoholism, in steatorrhoea and in mental hospitals. Deficiency can also occur after prolonged treatment with wide-spectrum antibiotics.

The dermatitis of this condition particularly affects exposed areas and is associated with skin pigmentation. Recently a pellagrous dermatitis has been described in patients with the carcinoid syndrome. Here the pellagra is probably due to both inadequate intake and absorption of nicotinic acid and to decreased endogenous formation of nicotinic acid from tryptophan. It has also been described in Hartnup disease, an inborn error of metabolism, and during isoniazid therapy. Whatever the cause pellagra should be treated with nicotinic acid, 100 mg. thrice daily or preferably with a similar dose of nicotinamide.

Pyridoxine (Vitamin B_6)

Three compounds occurring in foodstuffs have vitamin B_6 activity, pyridoxine, pyridoxal and pyridoxamine. Although the last two compounds are the ones found in the tissues as part of decarboxylating and transaminating enzymes, the first is the more effective when given by mouth. This is probably because it is not so readily utilized by intestinal organisms as the others, so that a greater proportion is absorbed. Pyridoxine is also concerned in the oxidation of unsaturated fatty acids and seems to be necessary for normal adrenal cortical function. Further, it appears to be necessary for the normal metabolism of tryptophan and when supplies are deficient, an abnormal tryptophan derivative, xanthurenic acid, appears in the urine. This forms the basis of suggested tests for vitamin B_6 deficiency. Vitamin B_6 is widely distributed in foodstuffs, the richest sources being yeast, wheat germ, liver, pulses and cereals. The exact daily requirement is not known, but on the basis of animal experiments it is probably about 1·5 mg. per day.

Experiments on man have shown that B_6 is essential for human nutrition. The symptoms which arise are many and varied; mental depression and confusion, seborrhoeic skin lesions round the nose, eyes and mouth, cheilosis and glossitis, albuminuria, hypochromic anaemia and granulopenia have all been induced by deficiency and have been subsequently cured by giving pyridoxine. Some cases of pellagra appear to require pyridoxine in addition to nicotinamide and riboflavin.

Pyridoxine-responsive hypochromic anaemia is associated with a normal or raised body store of iron and excessive amounts of iron in the marrow. The defect may be due to deficient assimilation of iron into the mature erythrocytes. Because the marrow contains sideroblasts this condition is included in the group of 'sideroblastic anaemias'. Pyridoxine therapy, 150 mg. per day, should be given to patients with sideroblastic anaemia and to those with hypochromic anaemias which have not responded to iron when other causes of anaemia have been excluded.

There are several compounds similar to pyridoxine, which antagonize its action and act as anti-vitamin B_6 substances. The most potent of these is desoxypyridoxine. The substance is useful experimentally, but so far does not seem to have therapeutic applications.

Pantothenic Acid

Pantothenic acid is very widely distributed and this may account for the fact that certain evidence of deficiency in man has not yet been produced. It forms part of the prosthetic group of coenzyme A, an important enzyme concerned in acetylation. It seems also to be concerned with the function of the adrenal cortex, since animals deficient in the substance show evidence of cortical deficiency together with definite histological lesions in the adrenal cortex. Also pantothenic acid-deficient pregnant rats give rise to young with no eyes and abnormalities of the central nervous system. It has been suggested that deficiency of this nutrient was responsible for a syndrome characterized by a subjective feeling of burning in the feet and legs and seen in prisoners of war in the Far East in the Second World War.

Biotin

This substance is excreted in the faeces and urine in greater quantities than it is ingested; it is probably synthesized in very adequate quantities by intestinal organisms. Avidin, a protein in egg-white, combines with biotin and renders it unavailable. In man, deficiency of biotin has been produced by feeding large quantities of egg-white, and the chief manifestations were a scaly dermatitis, anaemia and muscle pains.

It is very unlikely that spontaneous biotin deficiency occurs in man.

Choline

Choline is probably necessary in human nutrition in amounts of about 500 mg. per day. The requirement, however, is almost certainly related to the intake of other substances such as methionine. Animals deficient in choline develop fatty livers and haemorrhagic lesions in the kidney.

Choline is one source of labile methyl groups, it is also concerned as a lipotrophic factor in preventing the undue deposition of fat in the liver, it is concerned in the formation of phospholipids and it is necessary for the formation of acetylcholine.

Choline is frequently used in the therapy of liver disease, but it seems possible that a large part of choline given by mouth is broken down in the intestine to trimethylamine, so that it is more likely to be effective when given parenterally than by mouth.

Inositol

The function of inositol in nutrition is not known and there is no evidence to suggest that deficiency of this substance occurs in man.

Para-aminobenzoic Acid

There is no evidence that this substance must be present in the human diet; it is part of the molecule of folic acid. It is necessary for the metabolism of many pathogenic organisms and metabolic pathways involving this substance are blocked when sulphonamides are present in sufficient quantities. The molecules are very similar and this was the first known example of the antimetabolic action of compounds structurally related to substances occupying key places in metabolic processes.

Folic Acid and Citrovorum Factor or Folinic Acid

Folic acid (pteroylglutamic acid) occurs widely in foodstuffs, mostly in the form of the conjugates, pteroyltriglutamic acid and pteroylheptaglutamic acid. It is converted in the body in the presence of vitamin C to folinic acid (citrovorum factor) which is active and which is itself effective when given in appropriate cases of anaemia. Folic acid is also synthesized by the intestinal flora and this probably forms an important part of the total intake.

Folic acid in the form of tetrahydrofolic acid is involved in the transfer of the formate unit in the biosynthesis of purines, serine and glycine. Interference with its function in purine biosynthesis explains the effect of folic acid antagonists in leukaemic processes.

Megaloblastic anaemias of various types respond to folic acid. This includes true pernicious anaemia, but here such treatment is dangerous, since subacute combined degeneration of the cord may be precipitated; it seems probable that what little vitamin B_{12} there may be available is utilized for haemopoiesis when folic acid is given, thus precipitating evidence of B_{12} deficiency in the central nervous system. Some cases of macrocytic anaemia, usually associated with steatorrhoea or pregnancy, do not respond to vitamin B_{12} but are responsive to folic acid or citrovorum factor. When folic acid is given to patients with steatorrhoea the megaloblastic anaemia usually responds, the stools become less watery and the glossitis may heal.

Nutritional folate deficiency is uncommon except in pregnancy in the United Kingdom though it is sometimes seen in old people or in patients with psychiatric disease or in patients on restricted diets.

Milder degrees of folate deficiency are commoner particularly in conditions associated with cellular proliferation, e.g. pregnancy, lactation, prematurity and infancy. Certain diseases may be complicated by folate deficiency, e.g. leukaemia and the myeloproliferative disorders, haemolytic anaemias, sideroblastic anaemias, Crohn's disease, rheumatoid arthritis and tuberculosis. It is assumed that the dietary intake is insufficient to meet the increased tissue needs.

Certain drugs may induce a megaloblastic anaemia responsive to folic acid though the mechanism of action of the drugs is uncertain. They include barbiturates and other anticonvulsants and alcohol. Trimethoprim may inhibit folate reductase and thus cause megaloblastic anaemia responsive only to folinic acid.

Diagnosis of folate deficiency is easy in the appropriate clinical context if the marrow is megaloblastic. However in minor degrees of folate deficiency the haematological features may not be diagnostic. The blood film may show only increased anisocytosis with occasional macrocytes or hypersegmented neutrophils and in the marrow some of the developing polychromatic erythroblasts may show only early megaloblastic changes.

Laboratory evidence of folate deficiency is obtained by a microbiological assay of the serum or red cell content of the vitamin using *Lactobacillus casei*. The normal serum folate concentration is between 3 and 25 ng. per ml. and that of the red cells 100–800. The urinary excretion of formiminoglutamic acid (Figlu) can also be increased after a loading dose of histidine.

The normal daily adult requirement of folate is about 100–200 μg. of folic acid, the average diet in the United Kingdom contains some 150–200 μg. per day after cooking though the readily available folate may be less than this amount. During pregnancy folate requirements are increased three-fold.

The only need for folic acid is in the treatment of folate deficiency. Folic acid is available as 5 mg. tablets or as a 15 mg. per ml. solution for parenteral use. Usually 5–15 mg. daily are given orally in patients with folate deficiency and this dose is adequate in most patients with malabsorption syndrome, though sometimes injections are required. If folic acid is being given as a therapeutic trial in a patient with megaloblastic anaemia the physiological dose level, 100 μg. per day, is used since this will not cause a haematological response in a patient with vitamin B_{12} deficiency. Folic acid is now given along with iron as a routine during pregnancy. One hundred to 300 μg. daily of folic acid is probably sufficient, administration usually being restricted to the second half of the pregnancy. Masking of vitamin B_{12} deficiency by treatment with folic acid is a possible danger.

Vitamin B_{12} (Cyanocobalamin or Hydroxocobalamin)

This vitamin, which contains cobalt, is Castle's extrinsic factor. Liver extracts also contain hydroxycobalamin, and there are several other derivatives; the active form of these may be coenzyme B_{12} in which the vitamin is linked with the nucleoside adenosine. Its biochemical actions are only partly understood but it has been shown to participate in the isomerization of certain dicarboxylic acids and it may be involved in the conversion of ribonucleotides to deoxyribonucleotides. Deficiency leads to megaloblastic anaemia, to superficial glossitis, to the neurological lesions of subacute combined degeneration of the spinal cord and to a general lack of well-being and a defect in memory is common.

Vitamin B_{12} deficiency rarely arises from deficient intake except in the case of strict vegetarians such as Vegans. Failure of B_{12} absorption may be due to gastric or intestinal causes. In pernicious anaemia intrinsic factor production is defective usually because of an auto-immune gastritis where antibodies to components of the parietal cells and intrinsic factor are formed. Intrinsic factor normally binds to vitamin B_{12} and enhances its absorption in the ileum. Total gastrectomy always causes failure of B_{12} absorption and this is also defective in about one third of patients after partial gastrectomy. Gastric carcinoma is sometimes associated with vitamin B_{12} deficiency. Intestinal causes of impaired B_{12} absorption include disease or resection of the ileum, and conditions with abnormal intestinal flora, e.g. jejunal diverticulosis, regional ileitis, strictures and blind loops.

Deficiency of vitamin B_{12} can be inferred from the clinical picture and the finding of a megaloblastic anaemia associated with a histamine-fast achlorhydria. A reticulocyte response occurring on the fifth, sixth or seventh day after injection of 100 μg. of the vitamin is also good evidence of deficiency. A microbiological assay of the vitamin shows serum values between 100–1000 $\mu\mu$g. per ml. in normal patients. In patients who have received treatment with B_{12} after inadequate investigation it is sometimes necessary to confirm malabsorption of the vitamin. This can be done by the Schilling test where the patient is given an oral test dose of radioactive B_{12} followed by an injection of non-radioactive B_{12} to ensure maximum urinary excretion of the labelled vitamin over the next 24 hours when the urine is collected. Results vary in different laboratories but most normal subjects excrete 10 per cent. or more of the label in 24 hours whereas those with pernicious anaemia excrete less than 5 per cent. To distinguish impaired absorption due to lack of intrinsic factor from that due to intestinal disease the test can be repeated with intrinsic factor which allows separation of the two conditions.

Vitamin B_{12} is available in three forms, cyanocobalamin, hydroxocobalamin and in combination with other substances. Hydroxocobalamin is retained in the body to a greater extent due to its ability to bind with proteins. A maintenance dose of 200 μg. of hydroxocobalamin monthly by injection suffices in the long term maintenance of a patient with pernicious anaemia. The vitamin is very free of side-effects though occasional hypersensitivity reactions have occurred.

Vitamin C

The role of ascorbic acid as a vitamin in primates and in the guinea-pig results from the absence of the enzyme converting L-gluconolactone to ascorbic acid in these species. Ascorbic acid is an essential cofactor in the formation of collagen which has a high content of hydroxyproline, being necessary for the addition of a hydroxyl group to the C-4 position of proline in the presence of collagen proline hydroxylase. The vitamin is also considered to be necessary for the conversion of folic to folinic acid. During infections the urinary excretion of ascorbic acid is reduced even with a normal intake presumably due to increased tissue requirements. Delayed wound healing after surgery has been attributed to vitamin C deficiency. Low levels of the vitamin are seen in some patients with hyperthyroidism and in neoplastic diseases, pregnancy and lactation and in patients suffering from peptic ulceration probably due to the low vitamin C content of certain gastric diets.

Vitamin C is widely distributed, green vegetables, citrus fruits and potatoes being particularly good sources of the substance. It is, however, easily destroyed in cooking, because it is rapidly oxidized when heated in air, and because in many foodstuffs in which it occurs, ascorbic acid oxidase is also present. This rapidly destroys the vitamin whilst the foodstuff is being warmed up in the initial stages of cooking. In general, vegetables cooked for large numbers of people contain very small amounts of ascorbic acid, whereas home-prepared vegetables are much more satisfactory. This is because it is not easy, on a large scale, to raise the temperature of vegetables rapidly to boiling point and so destroy the ascorbic acid oxidase before it has oxidized much of the ascorbic acid. In the home, vegetables can be 'blanched' in boiling water, and this rapidly destroys the ascorbic acid oxidase.

Ascorbic acid can readily be estimated chemically, since it will reduce methylene blue or the dye, 2, 6-dichlorophenolindophenol.

The requirements of ascorbic acid are not exactly known, but human experiments have shown that a daily dose of 10 mg. will cure clinical scurvy and is sufficient to prevent the onset of scurvy at least for over a year. Ascorbic acid is utilized, however, more rapidly than usual during stress and when infections are present, so that the League of Nations Technical Commission's recommendation of 30 mg. per day is probably about right. The National Research Council (U.S.A.) recommends 75 mg. per day, and this would seem to allow a considerable margin of safety.

Ascorbic acid deficiency can be estimated by a saturation test devised by Harris, in which the vitamin is given in a dose of 5 mg. per 1 lb. body weight each morning. The ascorbic acid content of the urine secreted between 4 and 7 hours after the test dose is estimated each day, and this shows a sharp rise after the procedure has been repeated a sufficient number of days to saturate the subject. Normally only 1 or 2 days are required for saturation.

Deficiency can also be estimated by a determination of the ascorbic acid content of leucocytes and platelets. A concentration below 2 mg. per 100 g. indicates severe depletion. Estimation of the ascorbic acid concentration in plasma is not so useful.

SCURVY

Scurvy is a disease characterized by subcutaneous ecchymoses, ulceration and haemorrhage of the gums, anaemia, debility and failure of wounds to heal.

Aetiology

Until about 150 years ago scurvy was the scourge of sea voyages and was a factor of paramount importance in naval warfare. Owing to this disease, sea-going fleets had to be relieved every 10 weeks so that the men could be rehabilitated ashore. It was asserted that, when Lind's recommendation of a daily ration of 1 oz. of lemon juice was implemented, it was equivalent to doubling the fighting strength of the British Navy. A further example of the effects of the disease on sea voyages is furnished by Anson's journey round the world; during 3 months of the voyage more than half the men on two of the ships died from scurvy.

Scurvy also was seen until comparatively recently in infants fed on dried milk powders (see infantile scurvy) but, owing to prophylactic measures, this, too, is rarely seen among European communities.

At the present time in western society, scurvy is most usually seen among old people (particularly men) of meagre means, who are living by themselves —so-called 'bachelor's scurvy'. In them it appears because of a deficient intake of foods containing vitamin C and tends to occur in the late spring.

Pathology

It is generally agreed that the fundamental defect in scurvy is a failure to deposit adequate amounts of intercellular material, of collagen, osteoid material or of dentine. Haemorrhages occur into the skin, subcutaneous tissues, under the periosteum and into the joints, pleura and pericardium. Furthermore, bones are not adequately calcified, the structure of growing bone is disorganized and wounds do not heal properly. Ascorbic acid is also necessary for the proper maturation of erythrocytes and anaemia of variable type also occurs in scurvy.

Symptoms and Signs

Scurvy usually has an insidious onset and it is difficult in patients who present all features to assess the earliest manifestations. However, in experiments on human volunteers who had been saturated with the vitamin it was noted that after some 17–20 weeks of ascorbic acid deprivation hyperkeratosis of the hair follicles began to appear. This was usually first seen on the outer aspect of the upper arms and was also seen on the back, buttocks, backs of the thighs, calves and shins. Affected follicles became plugged with keratinous material and the hair became coiled up inside. Following this, the capillaries round the follicle became dilated and filled with blood and, finally, haemorrhage occurred. After about 30 weeks, haemorrhages occurred in the tips of the interdental papillae of the gums and later swelling and more gross degrees of haemorrhage appeared. Bacterial examination of the gums of patients with scurvy reveals that they are infected with large numbers of Vincent's spirochaetes and anaerobic fusiform organisms. Also, after about 30 weeks, scars which had been made before deprivation of ascorbic acid became livid and red, and at about this time freshly made wounds failed to heal properly. Subcutaneous ecchymoses also occurred at about this time in one subject, but in the experimental disease large subcutaneous ecchymoses did not appear to feature so prominently as they do in the spontaneously occurring condition. Two experimental subjects experienced sudden cardiac pain, electrocardiographic changes being found. It seems probable that these symptoms might have resulted from haemorrhage into the heart muscle and a similar occurrence or haemorrhage into the pericardium might well account for the sudden deaths which were a feature of florid scurvy before measures of preventing and curing the disease were known. During the experiments carried out at Sheffield, it was also noted that subjects, who already had acne before ascorbic acid deprivation, experienced an exacerbation of this condition at a time when manifestations of scurvy were developing.

Although anaemia is a feature of naturally occurring scurvy it did not occur in the experimental subjects. This may well underline the fact that under natural conditions man rarely suffers from deficiency of one nutrient, and scurvy, as seen in clinical practice, is almost certainly associated with deficiencies of other nutrients as well as of ascorbic acid.

Diagnosis

The concurrence of subcutaneous ecchymoses, hyperkeratosis of the hair follicles with perifollicular haemorrhages, and swollen haemorrhagic gums, should suggest the diagnosis at once, and a total and differential white blood count should exclude leukaemia, a condition which can resemble scurvy very closely. In mild cases, however, where the skin lesions are the only clinical manifestation, it is not possible to make a diagnosis without laboratory aids, the lesions themselves not being pathognomonic of scurvy. Either the saturation test or the level of ascorbic acid in the white cell and platelet layer (see vitamin C) should help to establish the diagnosis. The diagnosis can also be established by the response to ascorbic acid, since healing and retrogression of the lesions occur rapidly when adequate treatment is given.

Treatment

Prophylaxis. The diet should contain at least 10 mg. of ascorbic acid per day and preferably more than 30 mg. (see vitamin C).

The established disease is best treated: (1) by giving 1 G. of ascorbic acid daily for 5–10 days followed by a daily intake of 30 mg. or more, (2) by accompanying this by a good nutritious diet of high vitamin content (since other nutrients than vitamin C will almost certainly have been in poor supply).

It should be noted that healing occurred in subjects with experimentally produced scurvy when they were given as little as 10 mg. of ascorbic acid per day. It would seem, however, that, since it is quite harmless to give saturating doses of ascorbic acid, it would be better to do this and thus ensure that a maximum therapeutic effect is obtained.

Prognosis

Untreated, and with a continuation of a scorbutic diet, death will occur. With all but the most serious cases in which sudden death can occur, however, the response to treatment is entirely satisfactory.

GEORGE A. SMART

RICKETS

Definition

Rickets is a systemic disease of early childhood resulting from lack of vitamin D. Although it is now uncommon in Western Europe, it remains a world-wide nutritional problem and is being seen with increasing frequency in immigrant children in Britain.

Aetiology

Human skin contains a substance 7-dehydrocholesterol which is activated by ultra-violet light and converted to vitamin D, which is then absorbed into the circulation. In temperate zones lack of sunshine together with its filtration through glass or smoke render it an inadequate stimulus to vitamin D formation and rickets is likely to appear unless protective supplements are provided in the diet. An infant requires 400 I.U. vitamin D each day and since breast milk and cow's milk contain only 10–20 I.U. per pint some additional provision is necessary.

Nutritional rickets is particularly common in premature babies and is liable to occur at any time when growth is rapid. Well nourished infants on a high carbohydrate intake may show early signs of rickets in the first 6 months, but it is seen in a florid form around 2 years of age. There is an increased tendency for it to occur in coloured children.

Pathology

Rickets is primarily a disorder of bone in which osteoblastic activity and matrix formation of bone proceeds normally but in which there is a lag in the rate of mineralization. Osteomalacia is the corresponding condition in adults. The physiological basis of either condition is a lack of inorganic phosphate in the extracellular fluid with or without a lowered calcium.

Vitamin D is a generic term given to a group of steroids including vitamin D_2, calciferol, or more accurately, ergocalciferol and vitamin D_3, cholecalciferol. It is required for normal absorption of calcium and phosphate from the intestine and for control of phosphate excretion by the renal tubules. If it is deficient the ionic levels of phosphate and calcium in the extracellular fluid are insufficient to allow the precipitation of bone salts on the protein matrix. The phosphate concentration is of prime importance so that if it is severely reduced little calcium is taken up by bone and its serum level may be within the normal range. Due perhaps to the stresses acting on the structurally weakened bone, there is an increased activity of osteoblasts and the consequent release of the enzyme alkaline phosphatase into the blood.

Typical values in a child with longstanding rickets might be: calcium 8·8 mg. per 100 ml., phosphate 2·1 mg. per 100 ml., alkaline phosphatase 86 K.A. units. In a febrile illness or in starvation, tissue breakdown may provide a rise in phosphate so that more calcium is taken up by bone. The serum calcium may then fall to a level at which tetany can occur, presenting in the young infant either as laryngeal stridor or simulating a convulsion.

In rickets the orderly process of ossification at the ends of long bones is greatly disorganized. Section through the epiphyseal region shows a broad zone in which there is deficient mineralization of cartilage cells. Capillaries invade the degenerating cartilage and osteoblasts proliferate so that osteoid is laid down in an irregular manner. The highly vascular, poorly calcified zone does not possess the normal rigidity of ossifying cartilage and is liable to be compressed and deformed by external forces. This results in epiphyses being compressed laterally to give the typical widened, knobbly deformity of rickets. At the same time angulation of long bones may follow displacement of the yielding rachitic metaphysis. Later, as poorly mineralized osteoid is laid down under the periosteum the bone takes on a thickened, bulky appearance without its normal rigidity, so that it may bend under the stress of weight bearing.

Clinical Features

Early Rickets. Infants who were born prematurely and who have been breast fed without supplements of vitamin D are at risk and may have signs of rickets before the age of 3 months. Defective mineralization also affects membrane bones so that the infant may be noted to have a softened skull which can be indented by pressure like a table-tennis ball, the so-called craniotabes. Thickening of the wrists or costochondral junctions may be apparent. More often early rickets is an incidental finding in a child with an infection, sometimes diagnosed when the bones on the chest X-ray are noted to be abnormal.

Fully Developed Rickets. As the disease progresses the infant appears hypotonic and ligaments are weakened, the abdomen becomes distended and the liver is easily palpable at a lower level than normal. These infants are unduly irritable, often look pale and are said to sweat excessively.

Although rickets is a generalized disease it is the bones which are mainly affected. The inadequate mineralization of the membrane bones of the skull result in the anterior fontanelle remaining open until age two or later. The sutures are widely separated and thickening of the parietal and frontal bones gives the appearance of a 'hot-cross bun' head. The excess of osteoid laid down in the frontal bones produces typical bossing. Dentition is often delayed and not only may the teeth erupt out of order but the enamel is hypoplastic and extensive caries is common.

The enlargement of the costochondral junctions of the ribs becomes visible as well as palpable forming a rickety rosary. At the same time the pull of the diaphragm on the softened lower ribs causes a horizontal depression called Harrison's sulcus. If there is respiratory obstruction the upper ribs may also be pulled in leaving the sternum unduly prominent and results in the classical pigeon chest appearance.

The enlarged epiphyses at the wrists and ankles are often the major presenting sign. At the ankles the wide band of proliferating cartilage separating the shaft from the centre of ossification in the epiphysis may give the impression of a double epiphysis. As the child supports himself on his arms the humerus and bones of the forearm become bent outwards and the clavicles may have a sharp upward kink. With weight-bearing the lateral bending of the femora and tibiae may result in a bow-leg or knock-knee deformity. In addition bowing and medial torsion of the tibia causes the femur to be externally rotated to prevent toeing-in so that the hip joint is unstable and a waddling gait is the result.

X-ray Appearances

Radiological changes provide not only diagnostic confirmation but the best way of assessing healing. A film of the wrists will show irregularity of the epiphyseal plate and its distortion by pressure in the centre so that it is widened, concave (cupped) and frayed. The distance between the radius and ulna and the carpal bones is increased as the wide rachitic metaphysis is not radio-opaque. The bone shaft shows a coarse trabecular pattern due to the increase of non-calcified matrix. For the same reason the periosteum may have a double contour and appears to be widely separated from the underlying cortex. Within two weeks of starting treatment a zone of preparatory calcification is laid down in the distal end of the metaphysis and is separated from the shaft by osteoid tissue which gradually becomes mineralized. The bone is laid down in a more compact organized manner and calcification extends from the shaft until it unites with the line of preparatory calcification as healing proceeds.

Diagnosis

The clinical picture of rickets is characteristic and when associated with typical X-rays and biochemical changes the diagnosis is rarely in doubt. In chondrodystrophies, such as Hurler's syndrome, there may be a scoliosis, swollen costochondral junctions together with hepatomegaly and abnormal epiphyses on X-ray, but there is no biochemical disturbance. Craniotabes and bowing of the legs may occur in osteogenesis imperfecta but commonly this is associated with blue sclera and evidence of multiple fractures.

Two other conditions may mimic rickets both clinically and radiologically. Hypophosphatasia is a disease in which there is marked disorganization of mineralization at the ends of long bones. It is inherited as an autosomal recessive and is characterized by very low values of alkaline phosphatase often with normal serum levels of calcium and phosphorus. Again dentition is disturbed but unlike rickets there tends to be premature fusion of skull sutures, sometimes resulting in raised intracranial pressure. There are many variants of metaphyseal dysostosis, most are familial and due to an excess of non-mineralized osteoid, the epiphyses may appear radiologically very similar to rickets. Although of short stature, these children are biochemically normal and may be harmed if given high doses of vitamin D in an effort to correct the bony abnormality.

Rarely, rickets can be associated with neurological symptoms, either with convulsions and behaviour disorders primarily associated with hypocalcaemia, or it may mimic a myopathy. Gross hypotonia, lordosis with a waddling gait and diminished reflexes may precede overt radiological changes. If this occurs with a greenstick fracture a temporary 'pseudo-paralysis' may add to the diagnostic confusion, although by this stage hypophosphataemia is well established.

Treatment

The dosage of vitamin D was originally quoted in International Units based on a standard assay in rachitic rats. One microgramme (μg.) of calciferol is equivalent to 40 I.U. Rickets may be prevented by providing a daily intake of 400 I.U. vitamin D (10 μg.) during the first 2 years of life. It is particularly important when growth is at its maximum and during winter months when the natural supply of vitamin D is limited. Most artificial milks contain 400 I.U. vitamin D added to each quart (1200 ml.) and for breast-fed infants cod-liver oil or preferably a preparation such as *Adexolin* containing 400 I.U. in five drops is given daily as a supplement.

In established rickets moderately large doses of calciferol, 4000 I.U. (100 μg.), may be given for 1–2 months. The higher dose reduces the likelihood of hypocalcaemic tetany and is not likely to cause toxic symptoms if given for a limited period. Some workers advocate a single massive injection of vitamin D of 600,000 I.U. (1·50 G.) but there is then the danger of overdosage with lassitude, anorexia, polyuria and nephrocalcinosis. Active rickets is uncommon over 3 years of age but despite adequate dietary vitamin D the bony deformities resulting from earlier deficiency may persist and require orthopaedic correction.

Other Forms of Rickets

Coeliac Rickets. Rickets can occur in malabsorption syndromes when absorption of fat-soluble vitamins is inadequate. In children with coeliac disease treatment with a gluten-free diet may allow growth to be resumed and if added vitamin D is not provided rachitic changes may appear.

Renal Rickets. When tubular reabsorption of phosphate is impaired the resulting hypophosphataemia leads to rachitic changes in bone. This may be associated with other tubular defects such as renal tubular acidosis when there is an inability to excrete hydrogen ions or it can be part of a multifactorial tubular defect in which there is also glycosuria, proteinuria and amino-aciduria (Fanconi syndrome). This occurs in cystinosis when there is deposition of the sulphur-containing amino acid in the cornea and throughout the reticulo-endothelial system. In Lowe's syndrome it is associated with mental retardation, cataracts and other ocular defects.

Familial Vitamin D Resistant Rickets. This condition is characterized by an inability to reabsorb phosphate in the renal tubules so that hypophosphataemia and rickets result. It is inherited mainly as a dominant and causes short stature with badly deformed bone structure. As in all patients with a renal tubular leak large doses of vitamin D are required. Unlike nutritional rickets milligrammes rather than microgrammes are needed. Doses of 40,000–80,000 I.U. (100–200 mg.) or more are commonly used.

Refractory Rickets with Hypocalcaemia. Rarely rickets is seen in children who do not have an excessive phosphate leak but who require larger doses of vitamin D than normal to prevent rickets. 2000–4000 I.U. (50–100 μg.) a day are necessary. Unlike those with familial resistant rickets hypocalcaemic symptoms may occur.

REFERENCES

EVANS, R., and CAFFEY, J. (1958) Metaphyseal dysostosis resembling vitamin D refractory rickets, *Amer. J. Dis. Child.*, **95**, 640.

HARRISON, H. E. (1961) Vitamin D and calcium phosphate transport, *Pediatrics*, **25**, 231.

STOOP, J. W., SCHRAAGEN, M. J. C., and TIDDENS, H. A. W. M. (1967) Pseudo-vitamin D deficiency rickets, *Acta paediat. (Uppsala)*, **56**, 607.

DENNIS COTTOM

BERIBERI

Definition

Beriberi is a nutritional disorder appearing in several clinical forms in areas of the world where people exist for long periods on a staple diet deficient in vitamin B_1 (thiamine).

Aetiology

It is prevalent in parts of the East and Far East, where milled polished rice is the staple diet and also occurs from time to time in Europe, the Americas and Africa. The development of the syndrome may be precipitated in individuals living on a marginal diet, by diarrhoeal diseases, by pregnancy and lactation and by hard manual work.

A syndrome very similar to dry beriberi may develop in chronic alcoholics who deny themselves food over long periods.

Pathology

The main lesions occur in the cardiovascular system and the nervous system. In acute wet beriberi the heart is hypertrophied and dilated, the right side being predominantly affected; there is evidence of congestive cardiac failure, including peripheral oedema, especially in the legs but sometimes general, and sometimes pulmonary oedema. There are commonly effusions of fluid into the pleural, pericardial and peritoneal cavities. Various degrees of these changes may be found in the intermediate syndromes. In the polyneuritic or dry form of beriberi degenerative changes are found in the nervous system, especially in the peripheral nerves, the spinal cord and pons and medulla. In the spinal cord the posterior columns and both nerve roots may be involved. Demyelination of the peripheral nerves occurs and, in long-standing cases, fragmentation of the nerve fibrils. Any peripheral nerves may be involved with corresponding changes in the relevant muscle and skin areas—most often the sciatic, ulnar and median. The vagi, phrenic nerves and autonomics may also be affected.

Signs and Symptoms

The clinical picture usually develops in individuals who have subsisted at least for months on a deficient diet. Although the two main syndromes of beriberi are traditionally described as 'dry' and 'wet' most clinical pictures are mixed and contain elements of both.

Dry beriberi presents a predominantly neurological picture and appears only after long periods of deficiency.

Early signs include easy development of fatigue, 'heaviness' and stiffness of the legs, and irregular areas of changed or heightened sensations in the limbs.

The muscles of the limbs, particularly those of the calves, become painful and tender on pressure. General symptoms include insomnia, dyspnoea and palpitations.

An ascending symmetrical peripheral neuropathy gradually develops, with increasing muscular weakness and wasting particularly notable in the legs. Foot-drop and, later, wrist-drop develop. The gait becomes ataxic and the finer movements of the fingers and wrists are impeded. Eventually the picture becomes one of flaccid paresis or paralysis, with absent reflexes and muscular wasting. Sensory changes are less pronounced; there is often loss of sensation over the tibial regions and uncomfortable and irritating hyperaesthesia of the soles of the feet. This latter resembles the so-called 'burning feet' syndrome which is believed to be associated with pyridoxine deficiency.

The polyneuritic pattern dominates the clinical picture but is often associated with other evidence of thiamine deficiency or other vitamin deficiency.

Where the syndrome is well advanced and chronic, the effect of therapeutic thiamine administration is limited, and permanent neurological damage may result. In earlier cases the prognosis is better.

A somewhat similar clinical state may be induced by chronic alcoholism and occasionally from ingestion of poisons including arsenicals and fats. Neuropathies occurring in areas and circumstances in which neural beriberi occurs may also be caused by arboviruses.

Wet beriberi may occur in either chronic or acute forms.

In the chronic form there is often considerable neurological damage, but in addition there are cardiac changes and prominent oedema, most marked in the lower limbs but sometimes general and accompanied by serous effusions. The muscular wasting caused by the nerve damage may be marked by local oedema, but there is usually considerable muscular tenderness, most easily elicited in the calf muscles.

Cardiac disturbances become evident as dyspnoea and palpitations with tachycardia. The heart is usually enlarged to the right and systolic murmurs are frequent. The liver is enlarged and tender.

Sudden death from cardiac failure may occur.

Cardiac beriberi may be the terminal stage in either of the above forms. The acute syndrome may also appear without warning in an apparently well person who has been subsisting on a deficient diet. The picture is one of rapidly developing congestive cardiac failure coming on in the course of a few days with gross generalized tissue oedema and effusions into the pleural, pericardial and peritoneal cavities. The pulse is fast, thin and irregular and there are well marked electrocardiographic changes which occur in the T waves and isoelectric levels.

The patient is extremely distressed and sudden death is common in the absence of treatment.

Wernicke's encephalopathy results from acute deprivation of thiamine and sometimes from chronic alcoholism. It begins with anorexia and vomiting, usually without nausea, followed by diplopia, nystagmus and ptosis. The patient becomes apathetic, his intelligence and personality deteriorate, coma ensues and ends in death.

At necropsy vascular lesions are found in the brain in the region of the third ventricle. Except in the very late stages, the syndrome may be reversed by administration of thiamine.

Infantile beriberi develops suddenly in the early months of life in breast fed infants of mothers living on deficient diets but often themselves exhibiting no clinical signs of deficiency. It is characterized by anorexia, vomiting and generalized oedema accompanied or preceded by oliguria. The child cries constantly and may go into meningismus or convulsions and may die suddenly from heart failure unless treated with thiamine.

Neurological signs are uncommon, but the very characteristic 'pathognomonic plaintive whine' is sometimes ascribed to aphonia.

Diagnosis

Dry beriberi must be distinguished clinically from other examples of polyneuritis and muscle weakness. The social and dietary history often point to the diagnosis and confirmation can be obtained by measuring thiamine excretion in the urine.

Wet beriberi must be distinguished in the same way from other causes of congestive heart failure. In the typical acute form the only other syndrome likely to cause confusion is epidemic dropsy and the astonishing response to parenteral thiamine is itself diagnostic.

Sudden heart failure and oedema in a breast fed infant should lead to the suspicion of infantile beriberi wherever the socio-economic background exists.

Treatment

Thiamine hydrochloride (aneurine) should be administered parenterally at first and continued orally as required.

Severely affected cases with cardiac disturbances and oedema must be treated at rest in bed and should be given 50 mg. intravenously, very slowly, taking 10–15 minutes over the injection. A further dose of 50 mg. may be needed intramuscularly for the next 2–3 days after which 10 mg. is given thrice daily by mouth until recovery.

The response is remarkable. The cardiac condition steadily improves and the oedema subsides. Diuresis comes on very rapidly and is a good indication of successful treatment, and indeed, of diagnosis.

Less acutely ill cases can be treated orally with doses of 20–30 mg. daily until convalescence.

The response of neurological beriberi to thiamine is much less satisfactory. Daily doses of 15–30 mg. may be given orally to begin with and B complex vitamins added to the diet.

Severe cardiac failure in infantile beriberi requires the usual general treatment and slow intravenous injection of 25 mg. This dose may be repeated intramuscularly for a further 1–2 days, followed by oral doses of 5–10 mg. daily for some weeks. Less severe cases should receive the same dosage intramuscularly for the first 3 days, followed by the oral dosage. The mother should be given 10 mg. thiamine orally twice daily and placed on a good diet.

General treatment includes adjustment of the dietary content of vitamins and protein.

PELLAGRA

Definition

Pellagra is caused by deficiency of the vitamin niacin or nicotinic acid, often in association with protein deficiency.

Aetiology

Pellagra is characterized by glossitis, gastro-intestinal disturbances, symmetrically disposed dermatitis and changes in the central nervous system.

It appears in many parts of the world, especially where the populations survive on a diet of maize without adequate meat, milk or other protein sources. A similar protein-deficient diet with wheat as the staple food-stuff is not pellagragenic. This seems to be because the nicotinic acid content of maize is unavailable, although adequate in amount and similar to that in wheat. Shortage of protein intake leads to deficiency of tryptophan, an amino acid which is essential for the synthesis of nicotinic acid in the body.

Pathology

Deficiency of nicotinic acid interferes with the synthesis of certain nucleotides which are essential for tissue respiration; the effects are therefore widely distributed in the body. The pathological processes are non-specific and include varying degrees of inflammation of the skin and mucosal surfaces and later atrophy and pigmentation.

Signs and Symptoms

All grades exist between acute and chronic pellagra. The onset is gradual with slowly developing skin and mucosal lesions, asthenia and mental depression and psychosis. Signs of other deficiencies, for instance cheilosis, are almost always present.

The dermatitis is symmetrically disposed on the parts

of the body commonly exposed to sunlight, particularly the hands and wrists, the legs and the dorsum of the feet, the face (with 'butterfly' distribution of the lesions) and the front and back of the neck. The skin which becomes involved first develops intense erythema resembling sunburn, then becomes vesicular and scaly. It thickens, with a rough irregular desquamating surface which changes slowly from red to brownish. Eventually the epithelium may atrophy. In the fully developed stages remarkable increases in pigmentation occur especially in normally dark-skinned people, in whom the whole affected area, especially the hands and the feet become very heavily pigmented and may crack and desquamate, resembling the 'black enamel crazy pavement' skin of kwashiorkor.

The tongue becomes acutely swollen, inflamed and irregularly denuded of papillae; the tip is reddened and sore. The over-all colour changes from red to a very characteristic magenta. Later there may be fissuring and ulceration. Spiced or hot food and drinks are intensely irritating and the patient may become anorexic as a consequence.

Changes also occur on the mucosa of the mouth and lips. The stomatitis may be as severe as the glossitis, and fissuring at the angles of the mouth is usual.

Dyspepsia is usual and there is sometimes severe diarrhoea. Some cases remain constipated. The stools are light coloured and contain little free fat.

Nervous signs and symptoms are invariable and range from severe headache and neurasthenia to various psychotic states including depression and dementia. There may be signs of peripheral neuritis and paraesthesia such as burning feet resulting from deficiencies of other essential substances.

The personality changes which occur are sometimes so pronounced that the patient is unjustifiably placed in a mental hospital.

Pellagra may last for years untreated. Death occurs from intercurrent infection.

Diagnosis

The features of fully developed pellagra are the symmetrical dermatitis, the glossitis, the gastro-intestinal disturbances and the mental changes. In the relevant socio-economic environment these cases should present no difficulty. Diagnosis may be difficult in early cases, but may be established by measuring the output of N-methyl-nicotinamide in the urine. If this is less than 1 mg. in the day, pellagra is probably present.

Treatment

The severely ill patient should be placed on a well balanced protein diet with adequate riboflavin, thiamine and vitamin B complex and given nicotinamide, 100 mg. 6-hourly orally daily for 3–4 days, followed by 200 mg. daily for a fortnight or longer, as required. The vitamin is absorbed rapidly after oral administration. There is no need to give it parenterally. Nicotinic acid should be avoided because of possible acute vasodilator effects.

The response is prompt with rapid improvement in the physical and mental condition. The patient should be maintained on a diet adequate in calories and proteins and with added yeast extract.

Brian Maegraith

PROTEIN DEFICIENCY

Since most cereal foods contain enough protein to supply most of the bodily needs when sufficient calories are ingested, protein deficiency rarely results from dietetic insufficiency without an accompanying deficit of calories. Some of these proteins are deficient in some of the essential amino acids and have been called second-class proteins, but it has been shown that a small addition of first-class protein supplies adequate amounts of these missing amino acids, so that the biological value of the mixture is high. In certain areas, where roots such as tapioca supply an appreciable portion of the total calorie intake, protein deficiency without calorie deficiency may occur.

Aetiology and Pathogenesis

In those parts of the world where food is generally available in adequate quantities, protein deficiency occurs mainly as a result of conditions which prevent adequate food intake, such as anorexia nervosa or obstructions of the oesophagus, or which interfere with absorption. In some areas, however, social customs and dietary habits may result in protein deficiency, particularly in children at the time of weaning.

Abnormalities of the digestive organs, such as idiopathic steatorrhoea, chronic pancreatitis and the results of a variety of surgical mutilations may all result in protein deficiency either from malabsorption or from loss of protein into the lumen of the bowel, and may produce a similar picture to that found resulting from a dietetic deficiency. Liver disease may interfere with protein synthesis, and conditions with massive proteinuria such as the nephrotic syndrome may result in protein abnormalities, but produce a different picture from that of true deficiency. During infections and after any form of trauma in well-fed subjects, there is a considerable breakdown of protein and resultant loss of nitrogen; this is very difficult to prevent and may occur even when the protein intake is much above normal. It seems to be part of the bodily reaction which occurs as a result of trauma and is probably mediated by overaction of the adrenal cortex. In extensive burns the situation is greatly intensified, since, in addition to the loss just described, there is a considerable direct loss of protein in seepage from the burned area.

Symptoms and Signs

It is difficult to separate the symptoms and signs of deficient protein intake from that of semi-starvation, although in children the striking signs of kwashiorkor (q.v.) may occur. Unlike acute starvation, where ketosis is prominent and hunger after a day or two is absent, long-standing undernutrition is not associated with ketosis (provided about 150 g. of carbohydrate per day are ingested), and hunger and thoughts of food are a dominant feature of the mental make-up; for all else there is apathy and depression. Muscle wasting is very evident and this is associated with weakness and, most strikingly, with great lack of endurance.

Bradycardia, hypotension, a small heart and slight anaemia also occur and examination of the serum proteins may reveal them to be low, a finding, however, which is not always present, even in the presence of famine oedema. The basal metabolic rate is also lowered but this is more apparent than real, because in undernutrition there is a high extracellular fluid volume relative to total body weight; nevertheless it does seem that there is a slight reduction in the metabolic rate of the tissues themselves. More striking, however, is the decrease in the over-all daily expenditure of energy which may be only about half that of the normally fed individual. A loss of about 30 per cent. of the lean body weight is the maximum which can occur without loss of life.

Treatment

Where the deficiency is the result of some pathological condition this must, of course, be corrected. Where the deficiency has resulted simply from lack of adequate food it is advisable to increase the amount of food gradually, since cases of congestive heart failure have occurred when large amounts of food have been given to semi-starved individuals. The main necessity is to supply adequate calories, about 3000–3500 being the level ultimately to be achieved, with at least 300 of them in the form of protein. There is a rapid return to normal weight, but it may take as long as a year before full functional normality is attained.

GEORGE A. SMART

PROTEIN CALORIE MALNUTRITION

This label covers a wide group of very important diseases which together constitute the most important paediatric public health problem in emergent tropical countries.

The syndromes range from *kwashiorkor* resulting from protein deficiency in the presence of adequate calorie intake (usually largely in the form of carbohydrate) to *marasmus* arising from over-all gross reduction of protein and calories. Kwashiorkor and marasmic kwashiorkor, in which the calorie intake is relatively low, occur subsequent to weaning. Marasmus is commonly seen in a younger age group, amongst infants.

KWASHIORKOR

Definition

Kwashiorkor is the local name (meaning 'the deposed one') given to a malnutrition syndrome first described in indigenous African children. A similar clinical pattern is now known to occur in many parts of the world, especially in the tropics.

The syndrome appears most commonly in children between the ages of 6 months and 4 years. It is particularly common in late breast fed, weaning or recently weaned children. It may occur in other age groups, and even in adults.

Distinguishing features are apathy and peevishness, retardation of growth, changes in the pigmentation of the skin and in the pigmentation and texture of the hair, muscular wasting, oedema, anaemia and fatty, necrotic or fibrotic changes in the liver.

Nutritional dermatoses are commonly but not invariably present.

Aetiology

Kwashiorkor is generally considered to be the result of severe protein deficiency arising from the intake of a diet low in protein and relatively high in calories, usually supplied as carbohydrates. Secondary deficiencies of individual vitamins may develop. Many cases are complicated by the effects of malaria, helminth infections (especially hookworm) and bacterial infections. These complications are not direct aetiological factors, although they may considerably modify the clinical picture. The syndrome occurs in their absence.

Pathology

The oedema is sometimes said to be associated with the low serum albumin content, but there is no obvious direct relationship. There is some evidence of salt retention.

Changes in the skin vary from patient to patient. Patchy change in pigmentation commonly occurs, which is often indistinguishable from those arising from genetic factors. There may be scattered areas of both hyper- and hypo-pigmentation. Where dermatoses are present the histological changes resemble those described in deficiencies of the particular vitamins concerned.

Changes occur in the texture and pigmentation of the hair. In the latter case, the custom has been to refer to 'depigmentation' but since there appears to be qualitative as well as quantitative change, the term 'dyspigmentation' is better.

The Liver. Post-mortem examination and biopsy commonly reveal fatty degeneration and infiltration, first seen in the periphery of the lobules. The cells of the whole lobule may be involved. During successful treatment the fatty changes regress. Various degrees of fibrosis, sometimes gross, may be seen, especially in patients who have had the syndrome for some time. These changes are believed to be late developments of the same process which results in the earlier fatty changes, i.e. the essential protein deficiency, associated with relative excess of carbohydrate.

The Pancreas. Degenerative changes have been described, varying from atrophy of the acinar cells with diminution in content of granules to hyaline changes, dilated tubules and periacinar, perilobular and sometimes periductal fibrosis. In advanced cases large areas of acinar tissue may be replaced by fibrous tissue. The islets may be affected.

Examination of the duodenal contents in severe cases has revealed reduction in amounts of amylase, trypsin and lipase, normal quantities being restored after successful treatment.

Other Tissues. Atrophic changes in the salivary glands have been described. Muscular atrophy is often considerable, although it may be masked clinically by oedema. Some workers have reported atrophic changes in the intestinal wall. Lesions of the kidneys occur in some cases, the most striking features of which are glomerular hyalinization and pericapsular fibrosis.

Symptoms and Signs

The syndrome comprises some combination of the following features: (1) retarded growth, especially evident during late breast feeding and weaning; (2) muscular wasting and oedema; (3) alterations in skin and hair pigmentation and texture. Various forms of nutritional dermatoses are common but are not invariably present. Biopsy or necropsy reveals the liver changes described above; these are presumed to be present in some form in all cases. Mortality is high in untreated cases.

The syndrome is most easily described as it occurs in the infant. Trowell draws a striking picture of the mother 'unwrapping a miserable imp who immediately grizzles and cries and avoids the light'. The child is apathetic, rarely resists examination and tends to stay where he is put instead of wandering off like a healthy child. The state of the child is one of 'peevish mental apathy'.

The child is retarded for its age in both weight and stature. It may not, however, look emaciated since the subcutaneous fat and prevailing oedema may give a superficial appearance of good nutrition. The essential muscular wasting may become obvious only as the oedema subsides during treatment. It is prominent in the occasional case in which the oedema is minimal.

Changes in the texture and colour of the hair occur in all races, but are probably best seen in the African, in whom the black curly coarse wool may be replaced by reddish, grey or white straighter silky hair, sometimes over the whole head, sometimes only over the temples and vertex. Dyspigmentation may occur without change in texture.

In the original description of kwashiorkor, dermatosis was present. It is now generally agreed that dermatoses, although extremely common, are not an essential part of the clinical pattern. The commonest skin change is one of pigmentation, which may occur without apparent change in skin texture. In many cases the development of hypo- or hyper-pigmentation probably represents the initial change in the development of more serious skin lesions. The commonest form of the latter appears on areas exposed to irritation, such as the napkin area, the back, the buttocks and thighs. The areas usually affected in pellagra, such as the hands and face, escape.

Early lesions are described by Trowell as 'sharply defined black varnished patches . . . which rapidly enlarge'. The affected hyperpigmented skin becomes dry, cracks, scales and peels off, sometimes in 'large enamel-paint' plaques, half an inch or more across. The area beneath is depigmented, and is easily damaged and infected, especially in the napkin area. The general picture has been called 'crackled' or 'crazy pavement' skin. Many cases show an almost universal dry scaling dermatosis which is often particularly prominent in the lower legs. Other forms of skin change include the so-called elephant skin, the skin being thickened, fissured and either hyperpigmented or often unchanged in pigmentation. Bullous changes associated with secondary infection and ulceration in the pelvic region have also been described. The black scaling peeling dermatosis is easily recognized and its association with the kwashiorkor syndrome is generally accepted. On the other hand, the origin of some of the other skin changes mentioned is often difficult to decide, and factors such as exposure, and particularly onchocercal and other skin infections must be carefully excluded as far as possible before accepting such lesions as related to the malnutrition syndrome. The skin lesions respond well to treatment.

Most patients are patently oedematous. The oedema is characteristically soft and easily pitted. It is most obvious in the legs and extends into the genitals and thighs and sometimes the buttocks. The arms, especially the forearms and hands are involved. Oedema of the face especially around the eyes and nose is common.

Most infants with kwashiorkor are notably pot-bellied, a feature which is often exaggerated by the way they sit upright, with their legs out in front of them. There may be some oedema of the belly wall but there is rarely free fluid in the peritoneal cavity. The liver is nearly always palpable. The firm edge may be felt an inch or more below the costal margin; there is usually no tenderness.

Gastro-intestinal disorders are common. Most patients suffer from indigestion and diarrhoea is very common, the infant passing numerous semi-liquid or yellowish stools containing undigested food. There may be some steatorrhoea, with the passage of bulky soft offensive stools, also containing undigested food.

Various signs of vitamin deficiencies are common. Cheilosis, angular or general stomatitis, changes in the eyes, including Bitot's spots and xerophthalmia may be present. Photophobia is common.

Anaemia is present in some degree. Where there are no parasitic infections, it is mild and orthochromic. Ancylostomiasis, malaria and schistosomiasis all affect the final blood picture. The red cell count commonly lies between 2·5 and 3·5 million cells per mm^3. Where there is iron deficiency, for example, in the presence of heavy hookworm infection, the anaemia may be hypochromic. In severe cases there may be some macrocytosis, probably due to the presence of reticulocytes. Megaloblasts are not present. The bone marrow response is normoblastic.

Serum albumin is low. This is regarded as a reflection of liver dysfunction. The globulins may or may not be increased.

The blood chemistry varies with the condition of the patient. Both chloride and fixed bases may be reduced.

Liver biopsy reveals fatty or fibrotic changes depending on the stage of the syndrome and the length of its duration.

Course

The development of the untreated case is steadily retrograde. The child becomes increasingly dull and apathetic; the retardation of growth continues; the gastro-intestinal symptoms, oedema and skin and hair changes progress, and various signs of vitamin and other deficiencies develop. There is a very high mortality in untreated cases. Nevertheless, the response to treatment is good in the vast majority unless the syndrome has progressed too far before treatment is commenced.

Diagnosis

The combination of retarded growth, especially in infants during weaning or postweaning, alterations in skin and hair pigmentation and oedema, usually with some grade of dermatosis establishes the clinical diagnosis. Biopsy of the liver revealing fatty or fibrotic changes confirms it.

The diagnosis of kwashiorkor is usually made in the oedematous stage. Dermatosis and vitamin deficiency signs are not essential for the diagnosis. Signs of deficiency of a particular vitamin are very common complicating factors of the syndrome in a particular area and account for some of the wide variation of clinical patterns described.

Kwashiorkor must be distinguished from marasmus. The relation between kwashiorkor on the one hand and marasmus on the other seems to depend largely on the adequate calorie intake and excess carbohydrate in the diet in the former. In both cases there is an acute deficiency of protein.

Other causes of oedema must be considered. Nephrotic syndrome resulting from *P. malariae* infection may produce a similar degree of generalized oedema and discomfort, but occurs as a whole in an older age group. The liver changes in Indian infantile cirrhosis and hepatic veno-occlusive disease must also be considered in the differential diagnosis.

Treatment

Seriously ill cases are dehydrated and are deficient in electrolytes including potassium.

Replacement should be by mouth except in the most advanced cases, in which diarrhoea is severe and fluid loss is rapid. Intravenous infusion of Ringer's lactate and glucose solution or of half-strength Darrow solution plus 2·5 per cent. glucose is indicated. Lactate is omitted if vomiting is severe. The infusion is at first given rapidly, up to 40–50 ml. per kg. body weight. If the subcutaneous method is used, glucose is omitted. Intraperitoneal and also bone-marrow infusion has been used successfully. Infection is controlled with broad-spectrum antibiotics.

Children in shock may be given an initial intravenous injection of plasma; this is seldom needed. Intravenous protein hydrolysates have been given to extremely advanced cases.

The potassium contained in these fluids is usually adequate to adjust for loss of the electrolyte. When diarrhoea is very severe the potassium levels in the plasma should be checked and more given if required.

Most children can be treated orally or by gastric tube (which should not be left in position). Various fluids have been recommended containing sodium, potassium and calcium, and chloride and bicarbonate (to counteract acidosis; omitted when there is severe vomiting). These are given over the first 24 hours after admission in volumes of 120–200 ml. per kg. body weight per day. Magnesium salts (usually the hydroxide) are usually added as most cases have some deficiency of this electrolyte and early restoration improves the chance and speed of recovery.

Blood transfusion is seldom required, but in cases with severe anaemia slow infusion may be essential.

Food should be given orally in frequent small amounts.

Most children with kwashiorkor have no appetite and it is often necessary to feed them by intragastric tube. Milk or milk products form the most satisfactory basis. Intestinal enzymes are depressed, lactase most of all; lactose should therefore be avoided, since in excess it leads to exacerbation of diarrhoea.

Sucrose is often used, but some children may be intolerant to most sugars. In such circumstances fructose is indicated, but is unfortunately too expensive for general use.

Many mixtures have been recommended. Sai, in West Africa, reports excellent results with skimmed milk, casein, vegetable fat and sucrose. The mixture is prepared and made up as required in water. The volume of fluid is calculated after taking into account other fluids administered; a total of about 150 ml. per kg. body weight is usually adequate.

The dietary intake in the sick child should be 30–60 calories and 1–1·5 G. protein per kg. body weight per day. This is increased gradually to 100–120 calories and 3–4 G. protein per kg. per day as the patient improves.

In cases with persistent watery diarrhoea electrolyte therapy should be followed by milk diluted 1:1 with water and the mixture of skimmed milk, sugar, etc. substituted slowly as the diarrhoea lessens.

After a few days some solid food may be added and the child is offered re-constituted milk as it wishes.

Nutritional Rehabilitation and Convalescence. The most important factor is the training of the mother or the family who have the care of the child. The mother should, if possible, stay with the child through the early days of treatment and be taught preparation and provision of the foods required.

Prevention of kwashiorkor in the long run depends on proper feeding over the weaning period and local foods should be assessed for this purpose and the preparation taught. Various formulations have been devised, for example Incaparina in Latin America and certain foods based on soya bean, which has a relatively high and well balanced protein content.

The long-term attack on kwashiorkor and marasmus depends on improvement of feeding, training in feeding techniques, improved food habits and, in some areas, population control. This involves extensive health education and ultimately improved national economy and agriculture, and is thus a long, slow haul.

A good mixed diet is gradually substituted for milk as the patient improves, and may replace the milk after several weeks. The proportions of protein to carbohydrate in the convalescent diet must be kept within normal limits.

Vitamins, if introduced, should be given in the form of cod-liver oil or vegetable extracts. Purified vitamins are seldom necessary and may be harmful.

It may be necessary to give iron. Very anaemic cases require immediate transfusion. A small transfusion often helps the progress of even moderately anaemic patients.

Parasitic infections should be diligently sought out and treated. Bacterial infections, even when they appear trivial, should be treated, if possible, with antibiotics. Malaria should be treated immediately with synthetic antimalarials.

The usual lipotrophic factors such as methionine are not in themselves of any appreciable benefit in dealing with the fatty liver lesion.

Prognosis

Mortality in the untreated cases ranges from 30–40 per cent. and occasionally even higher. Many children will die within a day or two of being first examined and placed on treatment. Once treatment has been successfully started, however, the prognosis rapidly improves. Mortality in properly treated cases should be less than 10 per cent.

Treatment must be continued over a long period and be carefully supervised, otherwise relapses are common.

Milder untreated syndromes in children may progress into adult life as a stage of subnutrition in which one or more of the essential features of kwashiorkor may be emphasized.

MARASMUS

Marasmus arises from subsistence on a diet which is deficient over-all and in which there is no excess of carbohydrate. The marasmic child is much under weight. The muscles are grossly wasted. The skin is thin to the pinch, since the subcutaneous fat is lost, and is tightly stretched over the bony prominences and the protuberant belly. Oedema may occur in the extremities but is not pronounced. Changes do not occur in the hair and skin texture unless there are concurrent specific deficiencies. The liver and pancreas are usually normal.

Treatment requires replacement of fluid and electrolytes and adjustment of diet as in kwashiorkor.

Marasmic children usually retain their appetites and are consequently easy to feed. They can usually move rapidly from a diet of about 50 calories and 1·5 G. protein to 120–150 calories and 3–5 G. of protein per kg. body weight per day.

Intercurrent infections, especially pneumonia, are dangerous and require prompt and effective treatment. Malaria must be diagnosed and treated immediately; worm infections can usually be left until the patient has recovered.

Anaemia should be dealt with as in kwashiorkor.

REFERENCES

Bowie, M. D., Barbizat, G. O., and Hansen, J. D. L. (1967) Carbohydrate absorption in malnourished children, *Amer. J. clin. Nutr.*, **20**, 89.

Chaudra, R. K., Pawa, R. R., and Ghai, O. P. (1968) Sugar intolerance in malnourished infants and children, *Brit. med. J.*, **2**, 611.

Jelliffe, D. B., ed. (1970) *Diseases of Children in the Subtropics and Tropics*, 2nd ed., pp. 161–214, London.

World Health Organization (1967) Requirements of vitamin A, thiamine, riboflavine and niacin, *Spec. Rep. Ser.*, No. 362.

World Health Organization (1968) Joint FAO/WHO Expert Committee on Nutrition, *Techn. Rep. Ser.*, No. 377.

Brian Maegraith

SECTION 5

DISEASES OF THE ENDOCRINE GLANDS

DISEASES OF THE ENDOCRINE GLANDS

INTRODUCTION

Endocrinology is based as much as any other branch of medicine on scientific principles derived from experimental biology, applied physiology and biochemistry. Clinical suspicion of the presence of an endocrine disorder will always depend upon the physician's assessment of the patient's symptoms and upon the physical findings, but the existence of most endocrine disorders can and must be confirmed by objective tests. In many instances these involve direct measurement of the amount of hormone secreted by the gland in question. Because physical, environmental, psychological and many other factors may influence the concentration of a hormone in blood or urine, it is essential that these assays are carried out under standardized conditions, particularly when the degree of hyper- or hypo-secretion is marginal, and dynamic stimulation or suppression of the gland may be required if the results are to be interpretable. In other instances more indirect, and therefore less precise, parameters of glandular function have to be used. Despite the development of methods for the direct measurement of certain hormones, there is still a tendency to continue to use these indirect tests, an undesirable, time-consuming and uneconomical practice for the patient, the physician and the laboratory. Thus such non-specific tests as the response to a water-load in the diagnosis of adrenal insufficiency must be abandoned as outmoded and replaced by direct hormone assay.

It is essential that scientific confirmation of the clinical diagnosis is obtained before treatment is begun. Failure to observe this golden rule makes subsequent confirmation of the diagnosis difficult or temporarily impossible as, for example, when a patient suspected of hypothyroidism is treated with thyroxine and only later investigations of thyroid function are instituted.

The effect produced by an endocrine gland depends not only upon the amount of hormone it secretes but also upon the responsiveness of the target organ or tissue, and racial and genetic factors. Thus certain diseases of apparent endocrine origin are due to failure of responsiveness of the end organ (e.g. pseudohypoparathyroidism and nephrogenic diabetes insipidus) or to genetic or racial factors (e.g. some instances of excess or sparse facial hair). Only in so far as these conditions mimic endocrine disorders should they be considered part of endocrinology, which is not the proper repository for any ill-understood syndrome of uncertain aetiology. Obesity, for example, is often erroneously attributed to endocrine disturbances, just as anorexia nervosa was in the past. There is increasing evidence that these two conditions are the opposite sides of the same coin and that both may be the expression of a psychological disorder. There is, however, no doubt that psychological factors and generalized organic disease profoundly affect endocrine function as exemplified by the amenorrhoea associated with grief, fear or anxiety, and the retarded growth and sexual development seen in patients with steatorrhoea, congenital cyanotic heart disease or chronic renal dysfunction.

THE HYPOTHALAMUS AND PITUITARY GLAND

PHYSIOLOGICAL CONSIDERATIONS

The Hypothalamus

The hypothalamus is a centre that regulates many diverse functions such as the circulatory, respiratory, autonomic nervous and emotional systems. It also contains nuclei that regulate body temperature, sleep rhythm, appetite and sexual maturation. In the context of endocrinology it serves as an essential link between the cerebrum and adenohypophysis over which it exerts control by the secretion of chemotransmitters which appear to be peptides similar in structure to vasopressin and oxytocin. These chemotransmitters are carried to the pituitary by the portal capillary network of blood vessels. Some have a stimulating action and promote the release of such pituitary hormones as adrenocorticotrophin (ACTH), thyroid-stimulating hormone (TSH), growth hormone (HGH) and the gondadotrophic hormones (FSH and LH). Others have an inhibitory action and suppress the release of prolactin and also possibly of gonadotrophins. In childhood both follicle-stimulating hormone (FSH) and luteinizing hormone (LH) are present in the adenohypophysis but their release until the onset of puberty is either not promoted by release factors or is inhibited by chemotransmitters of hypothalamic origin. A disturbance of this hypothalamic control is the probable cause for 'idiopathic' precocious puberty [p. 606], and in adult life for secondary amenorrhoea induced by emotional disturbances. Various neuropsychotropic drugs influence hypothalamic function. Reserpine, for example, may depress the secretion of the prolactin-inhibiting chemotransmitter so that prolactin is released and gynaecomastia or galactorrhoea occur [p. 595].

The Pituitary Gland

From the anterior lobe of the pituitary gland (the adenohypophysis), which is developed from Rathke's pouch as an outgrowth of the primitive buccal cavity, six polypeptide hormones are secreted. These are growth hormone, adrenocorticotrophin, thyroid-stimulating hormone (TSH), follicle-stimulating hormone, luteinizing hormone or testicular interstitial-cell stimulating hormone (ICSH) as it is called in the male, and prolactin. From the posterior lobe (the neurohypophysis), an outgrowth from the floor of the third ventricle, two short-chain polypeptides, the antidiuretic hormone (vasopressin; ADH) and oxytocin, are released. These are synthesized in the hypothalamus and pass down the axons of the hypothalamo-hypophyseal tract to be stored in the neurohypophysis whence they are secreted into the blood stream.

The physiological actions of these hormones are discussed elsewhere in this section in relationship to the diseases caused by their disordered secretion. By the use of immunoassay techniques the plasma and urinary concentrations of these polypeptide hormones can be measured in certain research centres although in some instances the sensitivity of the method allows only measurement of increased and not normal or subnormal levels.

Control of Anterior Pituitary Function

The secretory activity of the adenohypophysis is regulated by at least two separate mechanisms. One is the feed-back mechanism whereby the hormone secreted by a target gland influences the release of its trophic hormone from the pituitary. Thus, for example, a fall in the plasma cortisol level will stimulate increased ACTH secretion and enhance adrenocortical activity, whereas a rise in plasma cortisol level or exogenous administration of cortisol or its synthetic analogues will suppress ACTH secretion and reduce adrenocortical activity. In many instances it seems that this feed-back mechanism influences both the hypothalamus and the adenohypophysis so that a rise in the plasma cortisol level suppresses the secretion of the corticotrophin-release factor from the hypothalamus and also reduces the secretory activity of the pituitary ACTH-forming basophil cells.

The second mechanism controlling pituitary secretory activity is neural and operates via the hypothalamus and its chemotransmitters. This system overrides the feed-back mechanism and is activated by many non-specific factors and stresses including psychological ones.

Growth Hormone

Human growth hormone (HGH) is a polypeptide containing 187 amino acids of known sequence and is secreted by the acidophilic cells of the adenohypophysis. It is prepared from human pituitary glands obtained at autopsy. Only human and monkey GH are effective in man. The biological actions of HGH are diverse and potentiated by the presence of insulin and thyroxine. Promotion of growth with widening of the cartilaginous epiphyseal disc and increased lengthening of the bones is associated with retention of nitrogen, potassium and phosphate. It seems that HGH and insulin act synergistically to convert amino acids to protein in this anabolic action. HGH promotes the breakdown of fat, causing a rise in the plasma free fatty acid level and a tendency to ketonuria. Glucose utilization is inhibited, probably at the peripheral cellular level, and thus glucose tolerance is impaired. Prolonged administration or over-secretion of HGH causes hyperglycaemia, glycosuria and insulin resistance.

Although HGH is essential for normal growth of children, a no less important role at this age and in adults is its regulation of metabolic homeostasis. A rise in blood sugar after a meal induces increased secretion of insulin and a reduction in the HGH plasma level. Glucose transport, uptake and conversion to glycogen and fat is promoted by the insulin. As the blood sugar level falls, more HGH is secreted with the result that glucose oxidation is inhibited and mobilization of fat raises the plasma free fatty acid (FFA) level. By these mechanisms energy supplies are assured and the blood sugar level is maintained despite an irregular intake of food. The action of HGH seems particularly important in maintaining energy supplies during prolonged fasting and during exercise which itself stimulates secretion of growth hormone.

The secretion of growth hormone is irregular and appears to occur in intermittent bursts. The plasma level varies considerably from time to time during the day and often the night values are higher than during the day. In adults the normal basal fasting level is 0–5 ng. per ml., but higher levels up to 20 ng. per ml. are found in children. Several different mechanisms regulate the secretion of HGH. There is a negative feed-back control between the plasma glucose level and HGH secretion, mediated via the hypothalamus which controls the output of growth hormone from the adenohypophysis by a growth hormone-releasing chemotransmitter. A second mechanism, also mediated via the hypothalamus, is of neural origin, and trauma, exercise and other forms of stress stimulate HGH secretion irrespective of the blood glucose level. A possible third controlling mechanism is the plasma amino-nitrogen level; infusion of arginine or ingestion of *Bovril*, for example, stimulate the release of growth hormone.

TESTS OF HYPOTHALAMIC-PITUITARY FUNCTION

Function of the hypothalamic-pituitary system can often be assessed indirectly by measuring the secretory activity of the target glands. When hypofunction of the target gland is found, the distinction between a primary disorder of that gland and failure of the hypothalamic-pituitary system to secrete adequate amounts of the related trophic hormone is made by studying the response of the target organ to stimulation with exogenously administered trophic hormone. Conversely the distinction between hypersecretion as a result of primary target gland disease and increased secretion of trophic hormone may be made by administration of the hormone produced by the target gland which will suppress the excessive activity of the hypothalamic-pituitary axis. In many clinical circumstances, such as chronic adrenal insufficiency [p. 581] on the one hand and Cushing's syndrome on the other [p. 582], these manoeuvres, despite being indirect, have proved practical and usually reliable.

With the advent of radio-immunoassay techniques the plasma level of many trophic hormones can now be measured directly. The sensitivity of the method may be such that increased secretion is easier to detect than hyposecretion, it being difficult to distinguish between a low normal and a pathologically subnormal value. Often the assay must be carried out under carefully defined circumstances. For example, although the plasma level of FSH and LH are relatively constant in the male, in women important variations occur in relationship to the menstrual cycle [p. 604] and hence blood samples must be taken at a specific time to obtain interpretable results. The recent administration of a naturally occurring hormone (or one of its synthetic analogues) by suppressing the hypothalamic-pituitary axis, may make the measurement of the plasma level of the corresponding trophic hormone meaningless. In patients suspected of hypothalamic-pituitary hypofunction the distinction between low normal and pathologically subnormal plasma trophic hormone levels can often be made by procedures that stimulate the secretion of the particular trophic hormone in question.

Adrenocorticotrophin

Methods for assessment of ACTH secretion by the pituitary gland are discussed in the section on page 579. The finding of increased adrenocortical activity does not of itself indicate whether there is increased pituitary ACTH production or some primary disease of the adrenal glands, but the distinction can often be made, albeit indirectly, by the dexamethasone suppression test [p. 579]. Hypersecretion of ACTH can be measured directly by radio-immunoassay of the plasma ACTH level. Diminished secretion of ACTH is less readily assessed by direct measurement of the plasma ACTH concentration under basal conditions because the difference between normal and subnormal levels is so small. Thus a number of procedures have been evolved which test the cerebro-hypothalamic-pituitary-adrenal system, directly or indirectly, and which will in a normal subject increase the secretion of ACTH and hence adrenocortical activity. Of the several methods that have been used, the response to insulin-induced hypoglycaemia (insulin tolerance test) is in practice the most useful and can in addition be used to provide information about growth hormone secretion (see below). Brief mention will also be made of the other tests sometimes used.

Lysine-8-Vasopressin Test. Synthetic vasopressin acts in a manner similar to the corticotrophin-release factor secreted by the hypothalamus. Its administration stimulates the adenohypophysis to liberate ACTH. Ten pressor units are injected intramuscularly, and blood is taken before the injection and 30 and 60 minutes afterwards for measurement of the plasma 11-hydroxycorticosteroid level [p. 578]. In patients with normal pituitary function, and also with normal adrenocortical responsiveness as determined by prior administration of exogenous ACTH [p. 579], the initial plasma 'cortisol' level is 5 μg. or more per 100 ml. This should rise 30 or 60 minutes after the injection of lysine-8-vasopressin to 15 μg. or more per 100 ml. and the incremental increase above the pre-injection concentration should exceed 5 μg. per 100 ml. An absent or subnormal response indicates impaired anterior pituitary secretory function in respect of ACTH. Vasopressin may cause intestinal cramps and constriction of the coronary arteries. This test should not therefore be carried out in patients with coronary artery disease, hypertension, angina or an abnormal ECG.

Metyrapone Test. This test provides information concerning the ability of the hypothalamus to secrete the corticotrophin-release factor, the pituitary to respond by increased secretion of ACTH and the adrenal cortex to respond in turn to stimulation by the ACTH. The biosynthesis of the adrenal glucocorticoid hormone, cortisol, involves the addition of an hydroxyl group (=OH) at the C-11 position in the molecule of the immediate precursor substance 11-deoxycortisol (Compound S). This is achieved by an 11-beta-hydroxylase enzyme [see FIG. 34, p. 555]. To a degree which may vary from one person to another, metyrapone (*Metopirone*) inhibits this enzyme and 750 mg. four-hourly for six doses suppresses cortisol biosynthesis. The normal hypothalamus responds by increased secretion of the corticotrophin-release factor and the normal pituitary by increased secretion of ACTH which stimulates the adrenal cortex to form 11-deoxycortisol rather than cortisol. The increased secretion of 11-deoxycortisol is reflected in a rise in the urinary excretion of 17-oxogenic steroids but the extent of this rise varies according to the degree of inhibition exerted by metyrapone on the 11-hydroxylating enzyme. An increase of 10 mg. or more in the 24-hour excretion of 17-oxogenic steroids, either on the day of metyrapone administration or on the following day, indicates the ability of the hypothalamic-pituitary system to secrete ACTH in response to the lowered plasma cortisol level and the ability of the adrenal cortex to respond in turn to the ACTH. A negative response may be due to the enzymic inhibition being incomplete so that the resultant of the decreased cortisol production and the increased 11-deoxycortisol synthesis causes no significant change in 17-oxogenic steroid excretion; or it may be due to diminished pituitary ACTH secretion or to primary adrenal unresponsiveness although the last can readily be excluded by showing a normal adrenocortical response to stimulation with exogenous ACTH [p. 579].

Thus an increase in 17-oxogenic steroid excretion after metyrapone indicates a normal hypothalamic-pituitary-adrenal feed-back mechanism. Failure of urinary 17-oxogenic steroid excretion to increase is less informative as this may occur in some normal subjects, because of incomplete inhibition of 11-hydroxylase, as well as in patients with panhypopituitarism and after hypophysectomy. Failure of the test to promote increased secretion of ACTH does not necessarily mean that other stimuli, such as stress or hypoglycaemia, will also fail to activate the hypothalamic-pituitary system to secrete ACTH.

Before the metyrapone test is performed all corticosteroid compounds and exogenously administered ACTH must be withheld for at least 3 days. During the test the patient must be observed carefully because of the possibility of precipitating acute adrenal failure characterized by a fall in blood pressure, vomiting, headache or drowsiness.

Insulin Tolerance Test. This test has particular advantages over the lysine-8-vasopressin and metyrapone tests because it assesses the function of the whole cerebro-hypothalamic-pituitary-adrenal system. In determining the responsiveness of this axis, particularly in patients who have had prolonged treatment with glucocorticoid hormones in pharmacological dosage [p. 577], it provides more reliable information, and it is a more informative test when there is partial or complete hypofunction of the adenohypophysis. Carried out under constant medical supervision, with 40 per cent. glucose solution in readiness for intravenous injection if symptoms of hypoglycaemia become severe, the test is not dangerous, and it has the additional advantage of stimulating in normal subjects the secretion of growth hormone. Thus in the investigation of hypopituitarism it provides information about the secretion of both ACTH and HGH [p. 544].

An intravenous cannula is inserted and control samples of blood are taken 30 and 45 minutes later. Insulin (glucagon-free) is then injected through the needle in an amount that will reduce the blood glucose level to 40 mg. per 100 ml. and induce symptoms of neuroglycopenia. In patients with hypopituitarism, who are insulin sensitive, the test should initially be carried out with 0·1 Units per kg. body weight, but if an adequate degree of hypoglycaemia is not induced 0·15 or 0·2 Units per kg. body weight is used. In patients with acromegaly who are insulin-resistant, 0·2 or 0·3 Units insulin per kg. body weight may be required. After the insulin has been injected blood samples for plasma 11-hydroxycorticosteroids are taken every 10 minutes for one hour, and every 15 minutes for a second hour. Larger samples of blood are taken 30 and 60 minutes after the insulin injection for estimation of HGH.

A normal cerebro-hypothalamic-pituitary-adrenal response is shown by a control 'cortisol' level of at least 5–6 μg. per 100 ml.; an increase to 18 μg. or more after the induction of hypoglycaemia; and by an incremental rise above the control level of at least 7 μg. per 100 ml. This test is of value in detecting diminished secretion of ACTH, in which plasma 11-hydroxycorticosteroid levels will not reach normal levels. It is, of course, necessary to check that the adrenal glands are responsive to ACTH by doing an ACTH stimulation test [p. 579] if a subnormal response to insulin-induced hypoglycaemia is obtained.

Human Growth Hormone

The secretion of growth hormone is often irregular, occuring in bursts, so that the measurement of the fasting basal HGH plasma level may be misleading unless it is grossly raised as may be the case in patients with acromegaly [p. 543]. In the investigation of suspected hypopituitarism or in determining the cause of dwarfism, basal HGH plasma levels are of no value because the sensitivity of radio-immunoassay methods cannot distinguish between low normal and abnormally low values. Much more useful information is obtained by using techniques, appropriate to the condition under investigation, that either suppress or stimulate the secretion of HGH.

Glucose Tolerance Test. In gigantism or acromegaly the normal feed-back mechanism regulated by the blood glucose level becomes abnormal. Instead of the plasma HGH level falling when the blood glucose level rises, the HGH remains high and unchanged. Conversely in HGH deficiency the rise in the plasma growth hormone level, that normally occurs 3–4 hours after glucose administration when the blood sugar level is low or falling, may not take place. This may be used as a screening test in the investigation of children with dwarfism, but a more reliable indication of growth hormone deficiency is obtained from the response to insulin-induced hypoglycaemia.

Insulin Tolerance Test. This test is carried out as described above [p. 541]. In normal subjects the plasma HGH level rises to 50–70 ng. per ml. 30–60 minutes after the insulin has been injected and a satisfactory degree of hypoglycaemia has been induced (40 mg. glucose per 100 ml.). Subnormal responses are found in most patients with diminished HGH secretion.

Pyrogens, Arginine, 'Bovril'. A number of other tests have been used to stimulate HGH secretion in patients suspected of isolated growth hormone deficiency or panhypopituitarism. The production of pyrexia by injection of a bacterial pyrogen stimulates the same pathways as the insulin-tolerance test but it is more unpleasant for the patient. The response to raising the plasma amino-nitrogen by infusion of arginine is unpredictable as a stimulus to HGH secretion in some instances and appears more effective in women than men. More consistent and reliable results are obtained by the insulin-tolerance test provided that a hypoglycaemia of 40 mg. per 100 ml. is induced. Recently *Bovril* has been proposed as a simple and reliable test of HGH secretion in children. The response to 20 g. *Bovril* per 1·5 $m.^2$ body-surface in about 160 ml. hot water, with blood samples (capillary or venous) taken before and at 30-minute intervals thereafter for 2½ hours, appears to give results as reliable as those obtained with the insulin tolerance test; the maximum response is of the order of 20–30 ng. per ml. HGH and abnormally low levels with little or no increase in plasma growth hormone levels occur in HGH deficient children [p. 547].

Other Trophic Hormones

Consideration of the hypothalamic-pituitary secretion of other trophic hormones is considered elsewhere in this chapter; thyroid-stimulating hormone on page 552, FSH and LH on page 604 and ADH on page 548.

HYPERPITUITARISM

Excessive secretion of one or more of the pituitary hormones may result from a primary pituitary or a primary hypothalamic disorder. The endocrine manifestations depend upon which particular hormone is secreted in excess and when as sometimes happens more than one hormone is involved a mixed picture is produced. In addition to the endocrine features there may, when a tumour is present, be neurological symptoms and signs due to pressure on surrounding structures.

Increased secretion of ACTH causes Cushing's syndrome which is discussed in the section on the adrenal cortex [p. 582]. Premature secretion of gonadotrophins causes precocious puberty [p. 606], and during the reproductive years in the female an imbalance in the liberation of FSH and LH will cause menstrual disorders. Inappropriate secretion of prolactin causes gynaecomastia, sometimes associated with galactorrhoea [pp. 594 and 595]. Hypersecretion of TSH might be expected to cause hyperthyroidism but perhaps surprisingly there is no experimental or pathological support for this, and the pathogenesis of Graves' disease is discussed on page 558. Increased secretion of TSH is, however, thought to be responsible for goitre formation in conditions of the thyroid gland associated with reduced biosynthesis of thyroxine and tri-iodothyronine [p. 552]. Increased secretion of ADH is discussed on page 550. Increased secretion of growth hormone causes gigantism before and acromegaly after puberty.

Sometimes tumours, usually malignant, of non-endocrine tissue secrete substances which appear identical, biologically and immunologically, to certain pituitary hormones. The endocrinopathies caused by tumours of non-endocrine origin are discussed on page 550.

Increased secretion of a pituitary trophic hormone also occurs when primary hypofunction of its corresponding target gland fails to operate the normal feedback mechanism. In myxoedema due to primary thyroidal failure, for example, high TSH levels are found in the plasma, and similarly high ACTH plasma levels occur in patients with Addison's disease of the adrenal glands. This increase in trophic hormone secretion in the face of target gland failure makes it possible to distinguish between a primary disorder of the target gland and failure of that gland secondarily to pituitary hypofunction.

Clinical manifestations due specifically to increased pituitary trophic hormone secretion in response to target gland failure are uncommon. In Addison's disease, however, the pigmentation is directly related to the increased secretion of ACTH before adrenocortical substitution therapy is instituted. Many of the clinical symptoms associated with the menopause have been attributed to increased secretion of gonadotrophins in the presence of ovarian failure, but hypothalamic dysfunction also is involved [p. 613].

GIGANTISM AND ACROMEGALY

Definition

Gigantism and acromegaly are both the result of excessive secretion of growth hormone. If the onset occurs before fusion of the epiphyses, gigantism develops with rapid and excessive skeletal growth. Acromegaly develops when the onset of excess growth hormone secretion occurs after fusion of the epiphyses, and is characterized by overgrowth of many tissues, particularly bones which increase in thickness but not in length. There is also a striking enlargement of the acral or terminal parts of the body, particularly the hands, feet and certain elements of the head and face.

Aetiology

Gigantism starts in childhood and is usually obvious by the age of 10. Acromegaly develops in adult life, most commonly in the third decade; the condition is slightly more common in women than men.

Pathology

Gigantism is usually associated with diffuse hyperplasia of the acidophilic cells in the adenohypophysis; less commonly there is an adenoma. Acromegaly is usually associated with an acidophilic adenoma which may show certain histological features suggestive of a carcinoma but the tumour does not metastasize and grows very slowly, often remaining stationary in size for many years. Enlargement of the sella turcica is common, but not invariable, and the clinoid processes may be eroded. Often the tumour expands upwards, pressing on the optic chiasma. Later in the course of the disease the tumour may destroy other functioning pituitary tissue and the picture of panhypopituitarism develops. The prolonged secretion of excess HGH causes enlargement of skeletal muscles and the viscera.

Symptoms

Hypersecretion of growth hormone in the prepubertal period causes an increase in stature relative to the patient's chronological age. The excess growth is most marked in the long bones; the span exceeds the height, and the lower measurement from the symphysis pubis to the soles is greater than the distance from the crown to the symphysis pubis (upper measurement). A parallel increase in muscular development makes the patient strong and well-proportioned. There may at this stage be sexual precocity suggesting that the primary disorder resides in the hypothalamus. Later, features of acromegaly may be added, and symptoms and signs of neurological involvement may develop if an expanding tumour is present.

The onset of acromegaly is often so insidious that neither the patient nor his close relatives may be aware of the striking changes that produce the characteristic acromegalic appearance. The face is elongated and enlarged with coarse features, thickened skin and subcutaneous tissue; the lips, tongue and nose are enlarged. The mandible is prominent (prognathism) and the lower teeth often separated by growth of the jaw. The frontal sinuses enlarge causing beetling of the brow. Enlargement of the hands may necessitate repeated alterations in the size of a wedding ring, and of the feet a larger size in shoes. Hypertrophy of the larynx makes the voice deep and husky. Excessive sweating is common and this hyperhidrosis is a rough clinical guide to the activity of the disease process. The thorax is enlarged and the spine kyphotic, stiff and often painful. Tingling and numbness of the extremities may occur; in some instances one of the earliest manifestations of acromegaly is the carpal tunnel syndrome [Section 15]. The thyroid gland is often enlarged in response to excess secretion of HGH rather than TSH because the PBI level and radio-iodine kinetics do not indicate hyperthyroidism. Thyrotoxicosis is uncommon although it may be suspected because the nervousness, anxiety, impaired concentration and raised basal metabolic rate are all direct consequences of increased HGH secretion. Because of the fat mobilizing action of growth hormone, acromegalic patients are seldom obese. About 30 per cent. develop overt diabetes mellitus, particularly those with a family history of diabetes, and thirst and polyuria may be the presenting symptoms. All the viscera are enlarged; the heart may be 2–3 times its normal weight and intractable cardiac failure is not uncommon in the later stages of the untreated patient.

Amenorrhoea in the female, and loss of libido and potency in the male, may occur. Some patients exhibit gynaecomastia and galactorrhoea [pp. 594, 595]. A high normal or raised serum calcium level is found in about 16 per cent. of patients. This returns to normal in about half after successful treatment of the acromegaly. Persistence of hypercalcaemia should suggest primary hyperparathyroidism which is a well recognized association of acromegaly [p. 571]. About 20 per cent. of acromegalic patients have a raised serum phosphate level. Contrary to previous belief this is a poor index of increased growth hormone because satisfactory treatment, as judged by a reduction in the plasma level of HGH, is not necessarily associated with a fall in the phosphate concentration.

Many patients complain of headache as their presenting symptom, and an expanding acidophilic adenoma may cause visual field defects. Destruction of other pituitary cells may result in panhypopituitarism with loss of muscular strength, hypogonadism and secondary myxoedema.

Diagnosis

The patient's appearance is usually pathognomonic and old photographs will show progressive changes in the facial appearance. X-rays may show hypertrophy of the frontal sinuses, prognathism of the mandible, tufting of the terminal phalanges and in some cases enlargement of the pituitary fossa with erosion of the clinoid processes. Exostoses may develop at the sites of muscle origins and insertions. Periosteal new bone formation on the anterior surfaces of the vertebrae and on the long bones is common. The anteroposterior dimensions of vertebrae in lateral X-rays is increased. The presence or absence of osteoporosis is controversial, but pathological fractures are very uncommon.

Thickening of the lips and the husky voice may suggest myxoedema at first glance but in acromegaly there is hyperhidrosis and the skin is greasy rather than dry and scaly. Hyperthyroidism may also be suggested by the thyroid enlargement, the sweating and glycosuria, and must be excluded by appropriate tests.

Specific confirmation of the diagnosis can usually be obtained by radio-immunoassay of plasma HGH. The serum basal level invariably exceeds 10 ng. per ml. and usually 20 ng. per ml. In marginal cases the response of growth hormone to glucose should be studied [p. 542]. The normal fall in HGH associated with a rise in blood sugar does not occur and the growth hormone titre remains persistently high.

Persistence of hypercalcaemia after treatment should suggest the presence of associated primary hyperparathyroidism. HGH causes phosphate retention by reducing renal phosphate excretion and may mask the usually increased phosphaturia found in hyperparathyroidism [p. 572].

Treatment

The urgency for treatment will depend upon the severity of the patient's headaches, the rate of progression of the disease in respect of its endocrine manifestations and, most important of all, the extent of damage to the visual pathways. Hence the need for regular assessment of the patient's visual fields by perimetry. Increased experience with the natural history of acromegaly and improved therapeutic techniques have rightly influenced medical opinion in favour of early treatment in order to prevent the development of diabetes mellitus, acromegalic cardiomyopathy and neurological complications.

Present experience suggests that implantation of the pituitary with radioactive gold, which emits γ-particles, or yttrium (β-particles) are less effective in reducing hypersecretion of HGH than α-irradiation. The best results, as judged by the reduction in the plasma HGH level, are achieved by hypophysectomy. The transorbital or transnasal route is less disturbing to the patient than a craniotomy and is preferred in cases without enlargement of the sella turcica. Complications of surgery by the transethmoidal or trans-sphenoidal route include hypopituitarism, diabetes insipidus which may be temporary or permanent, nasal rhinorrhoea of cerebrospinal fluid and recurrent meningitis. Complete reversal of the endocrine manifestations cannot be expected but progression of the disease can be arrested and if undertaken early enough may induce some remission of the physical acromegalic features. Treatment of diabetes mellitus may be needed, and in the later stages substitution therapy for panhypopituitarism is necessary.

Prognosis

Acromegaly is a deceptively slowly progressive disease. Although without treatment many patients live until they are aged 50 or 60, they die of potentially preventable cerebral complications, diabetes mellitus, acromegalic cardiomyopathy which is singularly unresponsive to treatment, or panhypopituitarism. With early and effective treatment the disease can be arrested.

HYPOPITUITARISM

Deficiency of only one of the pituitary trophic hormones can occur, and this monotrophic deficit may be confined to growth hormone, thyrotrophin, adrenocorticotrophin or gonadotrophin resulting in dwarfism, secondary hypothyroidism, adrenocortical insufficiency or secondary hypogonadism respectively. Such isolated and selective deficiencies are relatively uncommon. In the case of growth hormone, dwarfism without any other endocrine abnormality will develop [p. 547]; similarly a selective deficiency of gonadotrophins will cause primary or secondary amenorrhoea in women without stigmata of any other endocrine disease [p. 607]. More often, despite the clinical picture being dominated by the apparent hyposecretion of only one trophic hormone, careful investigation will reveal a combined deficiency of one or more of the other trophic hormones. The clinical syndromes that result depend upon the age of the patient.

ADULT PANHYPOPITUITARISM

Synonyms. Simmonds' disease; Sheehan's syndrome.

Definition

A condition caused by partial or complete destruction of the adenohypophysis leading to deficient secretion of trophic hormones with failure of gonadal, thyroidal and adrenocortical function.

Aetiology

Panhypopituitarism occurs twice as commonly in women as men. The usual age incidence is 20–60 years. The commonest cause is infarction of the adenohypophysis as a result of severe obstetrical haemorrhage and shock (Sheehan's syndrome); hence, the higher incidence in women. Pituitary destruction may also result from a suprasellar tumour or cyst (craniopharyngioma) or an intrasellar neoplasm (chromophobe adenoma, carcinoma, or as a late result from an eosinophilic tumour causing gigantism or acromegaly). Less commonly the pituitary is destroyed by a chronic granulomatous lesion (tuberculoma, syphilitic gumma or Hand-Schüller-Christian disease). Ablation of the pituitary by hypophysectomy or implantation of yttrium or radio-gold seeds may be performed in the treatment of Cushing's syndrome or acromegaly, and to control a metastasizing carcinoma of the breast or the retinal complications of diabetes mellitus when vision is threatened.

Pathology

The adenohypophysis is shrunken and fibrosed in Sheehan's syndrome. When replaced by new growth, the sella turcica may be expanded by an intrasellar tumour or flattened from above by a suprasellar cyst; the clinoid processes may be eroded, and the optic chiasma compressed. Craniopharyngiomas often contain areas of calcification that give a characteristic radiological appearance. The target glands are atrophic and weigh less than normal.

Symptoms

The target glands usually manifest their failure in a definite sequence; growth hormone deficiency occurs first, usually without any clinical symptoms. Gonadal failure then develops and amenorrhoea is the first clinical disturbance, to be followed by hypothyroidism and finally adrenocortical insufficiency. In Sheehan's syndrome there is a characteristic initial failure to establish lactation although the patients have done so after previous pregnancies.

Usually the onset of the disease is insidious with weakness and an apathy which often precludes the patient seeking medical advice until the condition is far advanced. Amenorrhoea is the rule and occurs early; impotence in the male and loss of libido in both sexes are the result of diminished androgen secretion but are seldom the subject of complaint. Pubic, axillary and body hair become sparse, and in men the frequency of shaving is reduced. The genitalia and breasts atrophy. The skin of the face becomes soft, wrinkled and pale with a yellow tint; the pallor (alabaster skin with loss of areolar pigmentation in the female) is in part due to lack of melanophore-stimulating hormone and in part due to an anaemia, which may be the presenting symptom and only responds to hormonal substitution therapy.

The onset of thyroid failure is characterized by puffiness of the face and eyelids, dryness of the skin, bradycardia, constipation, slurred croaky speech and the mental changes associated with myxoedema [p. 567]. The patient becomes more apathetic, complains of the cold and may lapse into hypothermic coma. Clinical evidence of adrenal insufficiency is usually not marked. The characteristic pigmentation of Addison's disease does not develop, and sodium depletion and hypotension are seldom pronounced because aldosterone secretion continues in the absence of ACTH. There is a tendency to hypoglycaemia, and an increased liability to infection and inability to withstand physical and psychological stress. Coma may occur late in the course of the disease and is due to hypothermia, hypoglycaemia or pressure on the midbrain or hypothalamus.

Cortisol deficiency aggravated by lack of thyroid secretion may promote water retention, often associated with low plasma sodium and chloride levels but normal blood urea, serum potassium and haematocrit values. This water intoxication may constitute another cause of coma.

In patients with a pituitary tumour, neurological manifestations may dominate the clinical picture. Headaches are common and may be bitemporal or referred to the frontal area in the midline above the nasion. Pressure on the optic nerves causes a variety of visual defects depending on the position of the optic chiasma in relation to the tumour. The blind spot may be enlarged; colour vision, especially for red, may be impaired. Visual field defects range from an upper temporal quadrantic defect to a bitemporal or homonymous hemianopia or unilateral blindness with optic atrophy. The tumour may involve the oculomotor nerves or cause pyramidal signs, uncinate epilepsy or mental deterioration by invasion of the frontal lobes.

Diagnosis

Clinical evidence of deficient function of two or more target glands should always suggest a pituitary cause rather than primary disease of the target glands, and laboratory confirmation of gonadal [p. 605], thyroidal [p. 553] and adrenocortical [p. 578] failure is obtained by appropriate tests. In hypopituitarism the urinary excretion of gonadotrophins is low or absent, whereas in primary gonadal failure it is normal or high. In hypothyroidism secondary to pituitary failure the serum cholesterol level is seldom as raised as it is in primary myxoedema, and thyroidal activity, as judged by the gland's uptake of radio-iodine or the serum protein-bound iodine, can be increased by injections of thyroid-stimulating hormone. Administration of ACTH will, in hypopituitarism, enhance adrenocortical activity as shown by a gradual stepwise increase in the plasma level of 11-hydroxycorticosteroids or the urinary excretion of 17-oxogenic steroids or 11-hydroxycorticosteroids.

Severe weight loss seldom occurs in panhypopituitarism and there should be no confusion between this condition and anorexia nervosa, a disease practically confined to women aged 15–35 and characterized by amenorrhoea, emaciation, downy hair on the face and back, cold purple-blue extremities and bright bird-like activity.

Treatment

Surgical treatment is essential when the cause of the hypopituitarism is a supra- or intra-sellar tumour that by pressure on the optic chiasm threatens vision, produces incapacitating headaches or involves adjacent intracranial structures.

Substitution therapy for the endocrine deficiencies should start with cortisone, 25 mg. in the morning and 12·5 mg. in the afternoon. Thyroxine, 0·1 mg. each morning, is then added and it is important not to start treatment for hypothyroidism, which is often the most obvious clinical abnormality, without first giving cortisone because of the risk of thyroxine accentuating the adrenocortical deficiency. The thyroxine is increased at fortnightly intervals until the patient is taking 0·2–0·4 mg. each morning. Later substitution therapy for gonadal deficiency is added. Androgenic hormones (fluoxymesterone, 2·5 mg. daily or on alternate days by mouth, or methyltestosterone sublingually, 5 mg. daily, for women; and in men fluoxymesterone, 5–20 mg., or methyltestosterone, 25–50 mg. daily) will increase the sense of well-being, the growth of pubic and axillary hair, and libido in both sexes. In women secondary sexual characteristics can be restored and cyclical uterine bleeding induced with ethinyloestradiol, 0·02–0·06 mg. thrice daily, or alternatively a 'contraceptive pill' of high oestrogen content such as *Conovid-E* daily, either being given for the first 21 days of each calendar month.

During an intercurrent illness or a surgical operation the dosage of cortisone must be increased [p. 590] and administered intramuscularly, or as hydrocortisone hemisuccinate or 21-phosphate intravenously if there is impaired absorption because of vomiting or diarrhoea.

Selected patients, both male and female, with primary gonadotrophin deficiency may now be treated for infertility with human FSH and chorionic gonadotrophin (LH) for a limited period of time to induce conception [p. 610].

The treatment of hypopituitary coma depends upon its cause but often several factors, such as hypothermia and hypoglycaemia, contribute to its development. The patient should be nursed in a warm room between blankets with only gentle additional heat given from warm bottles. Hydrocortisone hemisuccinate, 100 mg., should be injected intravenously every 8 hours. Hypoglycaemia is combated with an intravenous injection of 40 ml. of 20 per cent. glucose and hydration maintained thereafter by infusing 1–1·5 litres glucose saline per 24 hours, taking care to avoid overloading the circulation and raising the central venous pressure.

Prognosis

With proper substitution therapy the prognosis is usually good, provided the primary cause, if it is a tumour, can be controlled. Left untreated the patient will eventually die of bronchopneumonia or in coma.

PREPUBERTAL PANHYPOPITUITARISM

Definition

Prepubertal panhypopituitarism results from partial, seldom complete, destruction of the adenohypophysis or dysfunction of the hypothalamo-pituitary system. Although there is a deficiency of all the trophic hormones in varying degree, in the prepubertal child the clinical picture is usually dominated by lack of HGH with resultant dwarfism. Evidence of gonadotrophin deficiency appears later. Puberty fails to occur and the picture is a combination of dwarfism and sexual infantilism (hypogonadism).

Aetiology

The commonest cause of prepubertal panhypopituitarism is a craniopharyngioma. Other causes include an intrasellar tumour, chronic granulomatous lesions (tuberculous meningitis, Hand-Schüller-Christian disease) and perinatal brain trauma. In many instances the cause of the hypothalamo-pituitary dysfunction is never determined.

Symptoms

The clinical picture is usually dominated by dwarfism [p. 547). Rarely, severe and repeated episodes of hypoglycaemia occur due to HGH deficiency or lack of cortisol secretion secondary to ACTH deficiency. At this age hypothyroidism, sufficiently severe to be clinically diagnosable, is usually due to primary thyroidal disease and seldom caused by lack of TSH.

Rarely pituitary and hypothalamic dysfunction lead to obesity, disturbance of skeletal growth, diabetes insipidus and hypogonadism—a syndrome first described by Fröhlich and also called dystrophia adiposogenitalis. The usual cause is a craniopharyngioma or chromophobe adenoma. Dwarfism usually occurs but sometimes growth hormone is secreted in normal amounts, and in the absence of gonadotrophin secretion eunuchoid skeletal proportions [p. 598] develop in the late teens. Fröhlich's syndrome sometimes develops in middle age when in addition to obesity, somnolence and diabetes insipidus, there is secondary hypogonadism characterized by impotence and infertility in the male and amenorrhoea and infertility in the female.

In addition to the endocrine disorders, neurological features may develop [Section 15], and even dominate the clinical picture.

Diagnosis

Confirmation of the deficiency of the pituitary trophic hormones is obtained by appropriate tests. The visual fields must be carefully plotted at regular intervals as a tumour may be slow to reach sufficient size to press on the optic chiasma. X-rays of the skull may confirm the presence of the typical suprasellar calcification often seen in a craniopharyngioma. Air encephalography may be required to determine the size of the tumour and its degree of extension.

Fröhlich's syndrome is often erroneously diagnosed in obese children who have associated delayed puberty and whose external genitalia are partially concealed in a pad of suprapubic fat. The syndrome should not be considered unless there is good evidence of an intracranial lesion. It must also be distinguished from the Laurence-Moon-Biedl syndrome, a rare congenital familial disorder characterized by obesity, hypogonadism, dwarfism, mental deficiency, polydactyly and retinitis pigmentosa.

Treatment

Neurological complications may call for surgical treatment followed by X-ray therapy, especially if vision is threatened. Substitution hormone treatment is given to correct hypothyroidism [p. 566], hypoadrenalism [p. 581], hypogonadism [pp. 598 and 607] or lack of the antidiuretic hormone [p. 549].

Prognosis

If the primary intracranial cause can be controlled or is not progressive, the prognosis is good in terms of life-span provided adequate substitution therapy is given. Cortisone or cortisol (hydrocortisone) is given to correct the secondary hypoadrenocorticism; thyroxine to make good the secondary thyroidal failure; and at the appropriate age androgens are given to boys and oestrogen and progestogen to girls. Satisfactory sexual maturation can be achieved but infertility persists although in selected cases later in life spermatogenesis or ovulation can be induced temporarily to allow conception to occur. The prognosis in terms of dwarfism is less satisfactory and is discussed on page 548.

DWARFISM

Definition

Dwarfism is defined as shortness of stature that is below the third percentile for children of the same age and racial origin.

Aetiology

The causes of dwarfism are many, and in clinical practice lack of growth hormone is less often the aetiological factor than other conditions. Shortness of stature is a common accompaniment and consequence of many systemic disorders such as malnutrition, malabsorption due to coeliac disease or mucoviscidosis, chronic hypoxia due to cyanotic congenital heart disease, chronic renal disease associated with acidosis or azotaemia, asthma, and prolonged administration of corticosteroids for the treatment of such conditions as asthma or Still's disease. Present evidence suggests that corticosteroid therapy suppresses the pituitary secretion of growth hormone and also antagonizes its peripheral action. Dwarfism also occurs in untreated primary hypothyroidism (cretinism and juvenile myxoedema), idiopathic hypoparathyroidism, gonadal dysgenesis (Turner's syndrome) and hypoprolinaemia. Premature secretion of androgenic hormones, as occurs in the adrenogenital syndrome [p. 587] and other causes of precocious sexual development [pp. 602 and 606] promote epiphyseal fusion in advance of the normal age and hence induce dwarfism. The shorter stature of women as compared with men is largely the result of the menarche occurring some 2 years earlier in girls than pubescence in boys.

Genetic factors are important in determining skeletal growth, and shortness of stature, which may or may not be of sufficient degree to be defined as dwarfism, is commonly due to familial influences. Members of such families, in addition to shortness of height, may have some retardation of skeletal maturation and in some adolescence is also delayed. Unresponsiveness of the peripheral tissues to normal growth hormone levels is the cause of dwarfism in African pigmies.

Growth Hormone Deficiency. Deficiency of HGH secretion is seldom manifest to a marked degree during the first 12–18 months of life because during this time the increase in body length is largely independent of growth hormone secretion. In some instances, however, failure of growth occurs antenatally so that the baby, who is not born prematurely, has a low birth weight and fails to grow normally during the postnatal period.

In the majority of cases the aetiology of HGH deficiency is unknown. In others there is a history of brain damage during or after delivery. Some children have a suprasellar cyst (craniopharyngioma) but an intrasellar tumour is rarely present, nor are the other conditions that cause prepubertal hypopituitarism [p. 546]. Under these circumstances lack of growth hormone is usually associated with deficiency of other trophic hormones although this may not be clinically apparent and is only revealed by laboratory investigations.

Selective absence of growth hormone alone may occur as an idiopathic or inherited familial disorder. The deficiency is seldom clinically manifest until the child is aged 2 years or more. Dwarfism may also occur as a result of maternal deprivation. Seemingly this is an emotionally induced disorder, unassociated with malnutrition, and characterized by low plasma growth hormone levels which do not rise in response to stimuli such as hypoglycaemia that normally enhance HGH secretion [p. 540]. Correction of the maternal deprivation results in a resumption of a normal growth rate and normal plasma HGH levels.

Symptoms

Dwarfism may be a relatively minor feature in a child suffering from a systemic disorder such as gluten-sensitive enteropathy, asthma or cyanotic congenital heart disease. But in other systemic disorders, such as renal acidosis, it may be the presenting manifestation.

Dwarfism due to HGH deficiency is usually manifest after the age of 2 years. By this time the rate of growth has already begun to diminish and thereafter the flattened growth curve deviates progressively from the third percentile. This is in contradistinction to small but otherwise normal children with a family history of short stature in whom the height is only just below the third percentile. In these children the growth curve tends, with increasing age, to approach or run parallel with the third percentile. Some children with an isolated deficiency of HGH may present with severe and recurrent episodes of hypoglycaemia.

Many dwarfed children, whether due to endocrine or general systemic disease, do not come under medical supervision until puberty fails to develop; this hypogonadism is the reason for the parents seeking advice. These children have infantile skeletal proportions, the upper measurement from the crown to the symphysis pubis exceeding the distance from the symphysis pubis to the soles. They are in no way grotesque in appearance; usually they have a normal intellect and may be likened to 'Tom Thumb'. In boys the testes may be undescended and in neither sex does puberty occur except in those with monotrophic growth hormone deficiency. Sometimes neurological complications dominate the clinical picture in those with panhypopituitarism; thyroidal or adrenal insufficiency is seldom clinically striking. In all cases, except those caused by premature androgen secretion, skeletal maturation is delayed. The plasma phosphate and alkaline phosphatase levels tend to be low.

Diagnosis

A diagnosis of dwarfism may be immediately obvious if the child's height is grossly abnormal. Often however the diagnosis can only be made in young children by repeated measurements of height over a period of time and comparison of the growth curve with that of normal children. Additional evidence in favour of the diagnosis may be obtained by assessment of skeletal maturation and dental development. X-rays of the skull may show evidence of a craniopharyngioma, and the visual fields must be carefully plotted at regular intervals.

Dwarfism must be distinguished from other skeletal abnormalities such as achondroplasia, osteogenesis imperfecta, rickets and kyphoscoliosis due to spinal caries, poliomyelitis, syringomyelia or vertebral hemiatrophy.

Once a diagnosis of dwarfism has been made, its cause must be established by consideration of the various aetiological factors enumerated above. Often the systemic diseases that give rise to dwarfism are diagnostically obvious but sometimes they are occult and investigatory procedures may be required to exclude such conditions as steatorrhoea or chronic renal disease.

Only after exclusion of systemic diseases, panhypopituitarism and racial or familial influences should serious consideration be given to the possibility of a selective deficiency of HGH. A useful initial screening test for this is to study the plasma growth hormone level during a glucose tolerance test. Normally the plasma HGH level rises 3–4 hours after the glucose has been given at a time when the blood sugar is low [p. 540]. Failure of the HGH level to rise makes further more searching investigations justifiable. An insulin tolerance test [p. 541] and an arginine or *Bovril* test should be done [p. 542]. If these are abnormal, the response of the patient in terms of nitrogen retention should be studied during a short period of HGH administration. Children deficient in growth hormone secretion show a greater degree of nitrogen retention and fall in blood urea than those who are not HGH deficient.

Treatment

The treatment of dwarfism depends upon its cause. Control or cure of a generalized systemic disease is usually followed by a rapid growth spurt and the patient eventually achieves a normal height. Treatment of precocious puberty [p. 587] or congenital adrenal hyperplasia (adrenogenital syndrome) enhances the growth rate provided therapy is initiated before epiphyseal fusion has occurred; even then some degree of stunting is common in patients with the adrenogenital syndrome. The retardation of growth due to prolonged corticosteroid therapy may be mitigated by giving the medication on alternate days or changing to ACTH. Synthetic anabolic hormones, related to testosterone, have been used to promote growth in children with familial shortness of stature not due to HGH deficiency. A growth spurt may be induced initially but the long-term benefit is seldom rewarding because premature epiphyseal fusion and skeletal maturation result.

In patients with growth hormone deficiency due to panhypopituitarism or a monotrophic HGH defect, treatment with growth hormone is available in certain centres but limited by the availability of the hormone which has to be extracted from pituitary glands removed at autopsy. Injections are given twice weekly. After an initial satisfactory response, some 25 per cent. of patients fail to continue to grow in height and this unresponsiveness is due to the development of antibodies to HGH. The antigenicity of the growth hormone is probably the result of some alteration in its molecular structure during extraction or purification. In cases of panhypopituitarism concurrent substitution therapy for adrenocortical and thyroid deficiency must also be given.

Prognosis

The prognosis in terms of stature is good when the cause of the dwarfism is a systemic disease that can be cured or adequately controlled. The outlook for patients with growth hormone deficiency is less certain, partly because treatment with HGH has not been available for a sufficient length of time to assess its value and partly because 25 per cent. of patients develop antibodies to the material currently available.

DIABETES INSIPIDUS

Definition

Diabetes insipidus is a condition caused by deficient secretion of the antidiuretic hormone (ADH). This deficiency may vary in degree, even in the same patient from time to time, and is characterized by the excretion of large volumes of dilute but otherwise normal urine. The resulting dehydration induces the dominant symptoms of thirst and polydipsia, the severity of which is related to the degree of ADH deficiency and the magnitude of the polyuria.

Nephrogenic diabetes insipidus is a rare congenital and hereditary sex-linked disorder which affects male children. In this condition there is no deficiency of ADH but an anatomical and physiological anomaly of the distal tubules and collecting ducts of the kidneys makes them unresponsive to the antidiuretic hormone.

Aetiology

Deficient secretion of ADH may occur at any age and in either sex when there is damage to the hypothalamus, where the octapeptide hormone is synthesized; to the hypothalamo-hypophyseal tract which carries the hormone to the posterior lobe of the pituitary; or to the posterior lobe of the pituitary where the hormone is stored before release into the blood stream. Most commonly the cause is idiopathic but damage to these structures may be produced by a craniopharyngioma or some other pituitary or parapituitary tumour, benign or malignant. Metastases from a mammary or bronchial carcinoma or a melanoma may be responsible. Diabetes insipidus may follow head injuries, intracranial operations or hypophysectomy. Other causes include chronic granulomatous lesions such as sarcoidosis, syphilitic gumma, tuberculoma, eosinophilic granuloma, Hand-Schüller-Christian disease and basal meningitis. Rarely it is a congenital hereditary disease distinct from the nephrogenic form mentioned above.

Symptoms

Often the onset of the condition is sudden or becomes manifest over a period of only a few days. Intense thirst is usually the first symptom noted by an adult, and is made intolerable by any attempt at fluid restriction. In previously non-enuretic children, bed-wetting is often the presenting symptom.

Polyuria occurs by day and by night, with considerable disturbance of sleep. The urine output varies from 4 to 20 litres a day depending upon the patient's body weight, the solute load provided by salt and protein metabolites being excreted in the urine and the degree of ADH deficiency. Fluid loss causes dehydration with weight loss, constipation and sometimes a low-grade pyrexia.

Depending on the cause there may be neurological signs of an expanding pituitary tumour, or symptoms or signs of deficient secretion of trophic hormones from the adenohypophysis. Concurrent deficiency of ACTH secretion may to some extent mitigate the severity of diabetes insipidus because the volume of urinary water excreted is related to the solute load provided by salt and protein metabolites; anterior pituitary failure, hypothyroidism, diminished adrenocortical activity and anorexia diminish this solute load.

Diagnosis

A careful search must be made for the primary cause of the diabetes insipidus, and also for evidence of other endocrine or intracranial abnormalities. A number of indirect tests have been advocated for establishing deficient ADH secretion, such as the infusion of hypertonic saline which by increasing the plasma osmolality would in a normal person stimulate ADH secretion and induce an antidiuresis (Hickey-Hare test). Another indirect test involves the injection of nicotine or the smoking of a cigarette which normally stimulates the hypothalamus to secrete ADH and induce an antidiuresis.

In practice there are two relatively simple steps that will establish a diagnosis of diabetes insipidus. The first is to show that, after the patient has been totally deprived of fluid over several hours so that his body weight has fallen by 5 per cent., the specific gravity of the urine does not rise above 1·010. As it is difficult by ordinary techniques to measure the specific gravity of small urine volumes, more reliable results can be obtained by measuring the osmolality of the urine by the freezing-point depression method. A normal person subjected to this degree of dehydration will attain a urinary osmolality of 800 mOsm. or more, whereas a patient with diabetes insipidus or hysterical polydipsia will fail to achieve this degree of urinary concentration.

Having established that the kidneys cannot conserve water in the face of severe dehydration, the second essential step is to show that the renal tubules are responsive to exogenously administered ADH. A diuresis is established by infusing 5 per cent. glucose intravenously and the bladder emptied every 15 minutes. When the urine volume exceeds 5 ml. per minute, 100 m-Units of aqueous vasopressin is injected intravenously followed by an infusion of 5 m-Units per minute for one hour. In normal subjects and in patients with true diabetes insipidus a marked antidiuresis will occur, the urine volume falling to less than 1 ml. per minute and the urinary osmolality rising to 600–800 mOsm. per kg.

Diabetes insipidus must be differentiated from other causes of polyuria such as diabetes mellitus, chronic renal disease, conditions associated with hypercalcaemia [p. 483], aldosteronism [p. 585] and other prolonged potassium-depletion states, and hysterical or compulsive polydipsia. In diabetes mellitus the hyperglycaemia induces an osmotic diuresis and the glycosuria imparts a high specific gravity to the urine. In the polyuria and low urinary specific gravity (hyposthenuria) of such renal diseases as chronic glomerulonephritis, pyelonephritis, hydronephrosis, polyarteritis nodosa and myelomatous involvement of the renal tubules, there is usually evidence of intrinsic renal disease and failure of the polyuria to be checked by administration of ADH. In aldosteronism and other conditions associated with hypokalaemia and depletion of body potassium, the renal tubular cells show vacuolation and respond poorly, if at all, to ADH. In hyperparathyroidism [p. 571] and other hypercalcaemic conditions, polyuria unchecked by ADH may occur and is attributable to renal damage induced by deposition of calcium in the tubular cells. In nephrogenic diabetes insipidus the abnormal distal convoluted tubules and collecting ducts are unresponsive to ADH.

Often the most difficult distinction is between diabetes insipidus and hysterical polydipsia, although the latter is confined to women with other evidence of psychological disturbance. Whereas patients with diabetes insipidus produce a urine of higher osmolality after vasopressin than after dehydration, the reverse is the case in compulsive water drinkers irrespective of how low the urinary osmolality is. Furthermore the response to a therapeutic trial of vasopressin is different in the two groups. In patients with diabetes insipidus 5 Units vasopressin tannate in oil injected intramuscularly checks the polyuria and stops the polydipsia; the patient feels much better as normal hydration is achieved. In hysterical polydipsia the vasopressin tannate in oil checks the polyuria but the patient continues to drink excessively and develops headaches and malaise from over-hydration.

Treatment

Whenever possible, treatment should be directed to correcting the underlying cause of the diabetes insipidus. Control of the polyuria is essential but must be looked upon as symptomatic treatment. Substitution therapy with ADH is the logical form of treatment, but as will be mentioned later, other forms of treatment are often as effective and more acceptable to the patient. ADH may be given as pituitary snuff administered several times daily by nasal insufflation; this may be effective in mild cases but is liable to induce sensitization characterized by asthmatic attacks. Many patients can be controlled better with a nasal spray containing synthetic lysine-vasopressin (as opposed to normal human arginine-vasopressin) in a concentration of 50 Units per ml. One or two applications of the spray to each nostril are given 3–7 times daily as required. More severe cases may require intramuscular injections of vasopressin tannate in oil in a dose of 0·3–1 ml. (3–5 Units) daily, on alternate days or bi-weekly depending upon the individual's response. It is important to warm the ampoule in hot water and to shake it well before drawing up the solution. Some patients find the injections painful and occasionally an unsatisfactory response is achieved because of poor absorption of the vasopressin from the site of injection.

By mechanisms that are not yet fully understood members and derivatives of the thiazide diuretic group of compounds and also chlorpropamide (*Diabinese*), a sulphonylurea hypoglycaemic agent, often prove effective in controlling the polyuria of diabetes insipidus, increasing the urinary specific gravity and allaying the thirst. Patients may respond better to one diuretic compound than another, and sometimes become resistant to the action of one but responsive to that of another. The greater the polyuria, the larger is the reduction in urine volume. Most patients respond best to a long-acting compound, such as 10–25 mg. clorexolone (*Nefrolan*). Asymptomatic hypokalaemia may develop but potassium balance can be maintained by giving 3–4 tablets *Slow-K* daily. Such treatment is often preferred by the patient to lysine-vasopressin spray or pitressin tannate injections as being less erratic in its control of the symptoms. It is also effective in nephrogenic diabetes insipidus.

The place of chlorpropamide in the treatment of diabetes insipidus is still uncertain. Its action is to decrease the renal free-water clearance, and hence it is ineffective in nephrogenic diabetes insipidus. The smallest effective dose, usually 100–150 mg., should be used and the maximum dose should seldom exceed 250–300 mg. This form of treatment has to be abandoned if symptoms of hypoglycaemia develop.

Prognosis

After head injuries, intracranial operations or hypophysectomy diabetes insipidus may be only a temporary event. Due to other causes, it is usually permanent but is well controlled by treatment and the patient lives a normal life-span provided the cause is not a malignant condition.

ENDOCRINOPATHIES ASSOCIATED WITH NON-ENDOCRINE TUMOURS

A number of different endocrine syndromes may develop in association with tumours, nearly always malignant, that are not of endocrine origin. These neoplasms may arise in a wide variety of organs including the bronchi, thymus, breast, thyroid, pancreas, kidney, trachea, ovary and uterus as well as in mesenchymal tissue. Although a particular endocrinopathy is commonly associated with a tumour of a particular organ, such a relationship is not invariable. Indeed some neoplasms elaborate more than one hormonal substance at the same time and so produce a mixed endocrine picture. The precise chemical structure of the hormones produced by tumours of non-endocrine origin has not been established but in many instances these substances have a biological and immunological action identical with the comparable naturally occurring hormone.

The ability of 'non-endocrine' neoplasms to elaborate hormones is somewhat surprising but the explanation probably lies in the fact that all cells inherit an identical complement of DNA. Fundamentally all cells are totipotential and have all the coded information required for the synthesis of all proteins including protein hormones or part of their constituent amino-acid sequences. The normal failure of non-endocrine tissue to synthesize hormones is ascribed to 'repressors' which mask specific segments of the DNA molecule. It seems possible that when a cell becomes malignant this normal repression is withdrawn allowing the unmasked DNA to promote protein synthesis foreign to the tissue concerned.

Ectopic ACTH Secretion. Secretion of a hormone biologically and immunologically identical with ACTH is most commonly associated with an oat-cell carcinoma of the bronchus. Other sites of the primary tumour include the thymus, thyroid, pancreas, breast, trachea and oesophagus. In some instances a benign bronchial adenoma or carcinoid tumour has been the source. The consequences of the excess ACTH secretion are more often biochemical than clinical, probably because the patient does not often survive long enough to develop the familiar picture of Cushing's syndrome [p. 582]. There are, however, exceptions in which Cushing's syndrome has antedated by months or even years the discovery of a tumour of non-endocrine origin. Greatly enhanced adrenocortical activity associated with very high plasma and urinary cortisol levels and often excessive corticosterone secretion are found in these patients and leads to marked but not invariable hypokalaemic alkalosis. Diabetes mellitus is often more severe than in Cushing's syndrome of primary endocrine origin and oedema is often an early manifestation. As in other endocrinopathies due to tumours of non-endocrine origin, the manifestations of hormone production are relieved by surgical removal of the primary growth or ameliorated with deep X-ray therapy or cytotoxic drugs. A relapse usually occurs if metastases develop because these too secrete ACTH.

Ectopic ADH Secretion. Secretion of antidiuretic hormone may occur from an oat-cell bronchial carcinoma or from malignant or benign tumours of other organs. In some patients a symptomless dilutional hyponatraemia due to water retention may be a chance finding. In others there are manifestations of water intoxication with nausea, vomiting, irritability and mental confusion but without oedema. Characteristic features of inappropriate secretion of ADH are continued urinary excretion of sodium despite hyponatraemia which may be as low as 105 mEq. per litre, and a urinary osmolality greater than that of the serum. Restriction of water intake may improve the patient's symptoms but often better results are obtained symptomatically by giving a salt-retaining hormone such as 9-alpha-fluorohydrocortisone (fludrocortisone) in a large dose of 4 mg. daily. Dilutional hyponatraemia may also occur after head injuries and in patients with benign or malignant cerebral tumours or non-malignant pulmonary diseases.

Ectopic Parathormone Secretion. Hypercalcaemia due to secretion of a substance seemingly identical with parathormone may occur in association with neoplasms without radiological or post-mortem evidence of skeletal metastases. The clinical picture may be dominated by the primary disease such as oat-cell bronchial carcinoma, lymphadenoma or an ovarian or uterine carcinoma; alternatively the presenting features may be those of hypercalcaemia [p. 483], namely constipation, thirst, anorexia, nausea, polyuria and mental confusion which may suggest cerebral metastases. The serum calcium level is raised and the serum phosphate level low; usually the concentration of alkaline phosphatase is normal unless there are hepatic metastases. Administration of cortisol [p. 589] often but not invariably fails to lower the serum calcium level, and when some reduction is obtained a normal level is seldom achieved or sustained.

Hypoglycaemia. Maligant tumours not derived from the pancreatic islet cells may induce hypoglycaemia, and this is particularly associated with large neoplasia of mesenchymal origin such as mesotheliomata or fibrosarcomata. In some instances the primary tumour has been a bronchial carcinoma from which insulin and glucagon could be extracted. In the great majority of cases, however, radio-immunoassay has failed to show high plasma levels of insulin and the hypoglycaemia has been attributed to an unknown humoral substance that inhibits the release of glucose from the liver.

Ectopic Secretion of 5-Hydroxyindoles. Secretion of 5-hydroxytryptamine (serotonin; 5-HT) and 5-hydroxytryptophan (5-HTP) may occur from malignant tumours originating in the bronchus, stomach, pancreas and parafollicular 'C' cells of the thyroid gland [p. 565] as well as from carcinoid tumours. The predominant clinical symptoms ascribable to the excess 5-hydroxyindole secretion are diarrhoea with hyperperistalsis and oedema. Some patients also exhibit flushing of the face probably more related to associated secretion of kinins than 5-hydroxyindoles.

Ectopic Gonadotrophin Secretion. Gynaecomastia, usually but not invariably accompanied by pulmonary osteoarthropathy, may occur in association with tumours of various non-endocrine tissues, particularly oat-cell bronchial carcinomas. Increased levels of oestradiol have been found in the plasma and urine of such cases. This excessive production of oestrogens is related to the secretion of gonadotrophins by the malignant cells. The development of precocious puberty in children with a malignant hepatoblastoma may be due to the same mechanism.

Ectopic Growth Hormone Secretion. The cause of pulmonary osteoarthropathy with its marked increase in subperiosteal new bone formation is uncertain. Often the condition is caused by a bronchial carcinoma or Hodgkin's disease, and may be associated with gynaecomastia. Some patients, if they survive long enough, develop acromegalic-like features. Very high levels of growth hormone have been found in the plasma of these patients. In the absence of increased plasma levels of FSH and LH in one such case, it is possible that the gynaecomastia was caused by ectopic HGH or prolactin secretion.

Ectopic TSH Secretion. Thyroidal overactivity associated with a malignant tumour that secretes thyrotrophin is the least common and least well substantiated of the endocrinopathies of non-endocrine origin. Thyroidal overactivity has been observed particularly in patients with choriocarcinomata and also in those with malignant tumours of the bronchus, gastro-intestinal tract, prostate and reticulo-endothelial system. In at least one instance the thyroid-stimulating substance has had the biological and immunological characteristics of TSH of pituitary origin.

Erythrocytosis. Although strictly speaking not an endocrinopathy, humoral substances (erythropoietin or a related compound) secreted by various tissues may cause an increased red blood cell count and haemoglobin concentration without a concomitant increase in white corpuscles or platelets, thus serving to distinguish erythrocytosis (erythraemia) from polycythaemia rubra vera but not from 'stress' polycythaemia in which the high red cell count is raised due to a chronically reduced plasma volume of unknown cause. Erythrocytosis has been described in association with renal tumours and cysts including hydronephrosis, haemangioblastoma of the cerebellum, uterine fibroids, hepatomas and tumours of the ovary or adrenals usually of a virilizing nature.

THE THYROID GLAND

PHYSIOLOGICAL CONSIDERATIONS

The thyroid gland develops from a median outgrowth from the floor of the pharynx, descends into the neck where it bifurcates, and together with two branchial bodies forms the thyroid lobes. Vestiges of the descending stalk may persist as the foramen caecum at the back of the tongue, the thyroglossal duct and the pyramidal lobe, and may give rise to cysts. Failure of descent may in some instances be a cause of congenital hypothyroidism. The normal adult gland, consisting of two lateral lobes joined at their lower poles by an isthmus, weighs 20–30 g. Usually it is situated in the neck, but sometimes is partially or wholely retrosternal.

The function of the thyroid gland is to synthesize, store and secrete the two thyroid hormones, thyroxine and tri-iodothyronine, of which iodine is an essential constituent [FIG. 33]. The amount of iodine ingested daily is normally 100–200 μg., and this is derived from marine fish, vegetables grown in iodine-containing soil, meat, cow's milk, water and table-salt to which iodide or iodate has been added. Iodine is absorbed from the gastro-intestinal tract as iodide and is concentrated from the serum by the thyroid gland. This trapping of iodide is enhanced by thyroid-stimulating hormone (TSH) and inhibited by thiocyanates and perchlorates, substances long known to be goitrogenic. The trapped iodide is oxidized to iodine, and mono- and di-iodotyrosine formed by iodination of tyrosine. The organification of iodine is inhibited by thiouracil and carbimazole compounds. Coupling of two iodotyrosine molecules leads to the formation of tri-iodothyronine and thyroxine which are stored in combination with a glycoprotein as thyroglobulin. The two hormones, tri-iodothyronine and thyroxine, are released from thyroid colloid by proteolytic enzymes which are activated by TSH, and pass through the walls of the acini into the blood stream. At the same time mono- and di-iodo-tyrosine are released from linkage with thyroglobulin and broken down by dehalogenases so that iodine is conserved within the gland for further use.

In the blood stream about 80 per cent. of the hormonal iodine is thyroxine and the remainder tri-iodothyronine. About three-quarters of the thyroxine is bound to a specific thyroxine-binding globulin (TBG), 15 per cent. to a prealbumin and 10 per cent. to albumin. Only about 0·05 per cent. of the thyroxine is non-protein bound or 'free'. This free thyroxine is *in vitro* in equilibrium with the protein-bound thyroxine and the unoccupied binding sites, which explains why free thyroxine is a better indication of thyroidal function than the total serum thyroxine or the protein-bound iodine which are influenced so much by the concentration of the carrier proteins.

The synthesis of thyroidal hormones is normally regulated by TSH through a reciprocal 'feed-back' mechanism dependent upon the levels of these hormones in the blood stream. A fall in the blood level increases the output of the thyrotrophin release factor from the hypothalamus into the portal veins which run to the adenohypophysis. This factor stimulates the secretion of TSH from the pituitary; more iodide is trapped by the thyroid gland and more thyroxine and tri-iodothyronine are released from thyroglobulin stored as colloid. The formation of thyroid hormones also requires adequate amounts of dietary iodine. When the daily intake falls below about 100 μg., the hormonal output is reduced. This stimulates TSH secretion and the gland enlarges in an attempt to 'make bricks without straw'. Thus iodine deficiency is a potential cause of goitre formation.

The physiological effects of thyroid hormones are widespread, being mediated through influences on cellular metabolism in all tissues. Skeletal growth, sexual maturation and mental development all require normal thyroid function. The calorigenic action induced by increased oxidation and oxygen consumption is reflected in the metabolic rate. The cardiac output and rate are influenced by thyroid hormones, which also

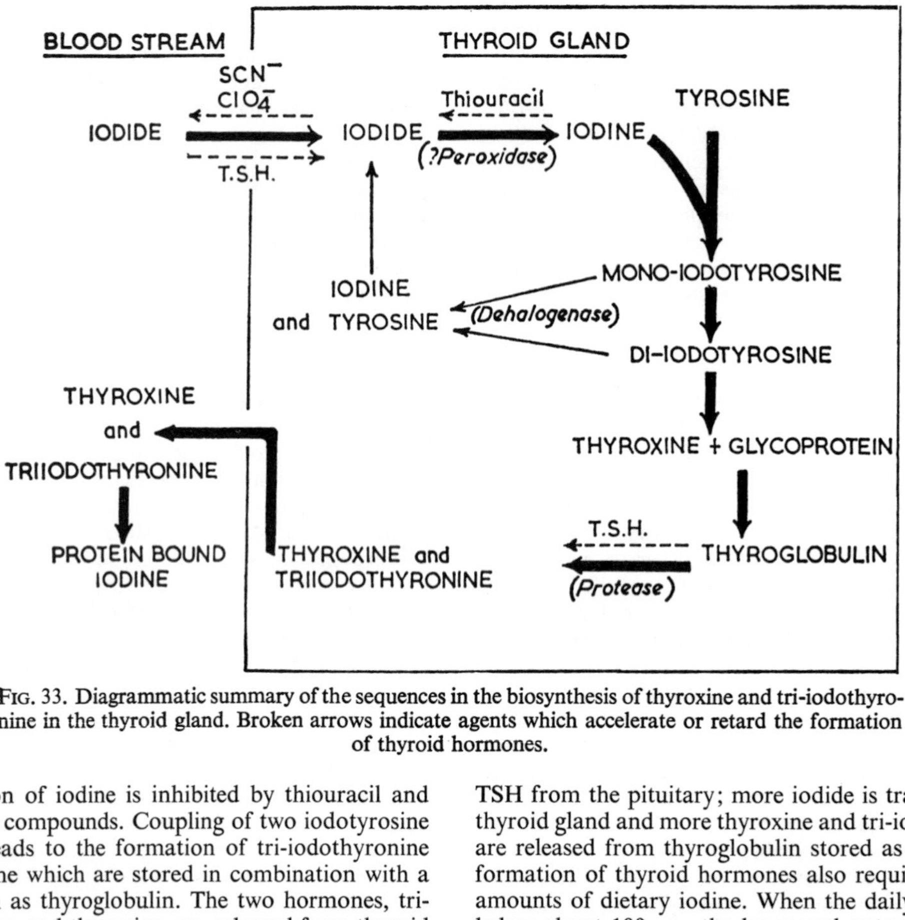

FIG. 33. Diagrammatic summary of the sequences in the biosynthesis of thyroxine and tri-iodothyronine in the thyroid gland. Broken arrows indicate agents which accelerate or retard the formation of thyroid hormones.

increase peripheral utilization of glucose and the conversion of liver glycogen to glucose. Protein catabolism is enhanced in hyperthyroidism and this finds clinical expression in muscle wasting and weakness with increased excretion of nitrogen, phosphorus and potassium. The serum level of cholesterol is in part controlled by thyroid hormones, being raised in thyroid deficiency.

TESTS OF THYROID FUNCTION

The size of the thyroid gland is no indication of its secretory function. Whether or not a goitre is present, tests of thyroid function are used to establish whether the patient is hyperthyroid, euthyroid or hypothyroid. If the patient proves to be thyrotoxic, further clinical and laboratory tests may be necessary to determine whether this thyroidal hyperfunction is due to Graves' disease or to an autonomous toxic 'adenoma'. If the patient is hypothyroid, further tests must be carried out to determine the cause of the hypofunction, and particularly to decide whether the hypothyroidism is primarily due to thyroidal disease or secondary to a pituitary disorder. A wide variety of tests each measuring different facets of thyroid function and iodine metabolism are available. Which one is most likely to prove helpful in establishing the diagnosis depends on the clinical problem presented.

Basal Metabolic Rate. Properly performed this is a helpful, albeit indirect, test of thyroid function. It is particularly useful in confirming a diagnosis of hypothyroidism which, apart from severe malnutrition and the nephrotic syndrome, is the only condition associated with a low B.M.R. This test is less helpful in patients with hyperthyroidism because the B.M.R. is also raised in patients with an anxiety state. Other conditions that elevate the basal metabolic rate are cardiac failure, anaemia, pyrexia, phaeochromocytoma and certain blood dyscrasias and reticuloses.

Protein-Bound Iodine. The amount of iodine that can be precipitated with the plasma proteins is a widely used measure of the amount of circulating thyroid hormones in the plasma. Technically the method is difficult and the results are influenced by the concentration of thyroxine-binding proteins present in the plasma. The normal range is 3·5–8·0 μg. per 100 ml. Values in excess of 8·0 μg. are found in most patients with hyperthyroidism, but, because the thyroxine-binding proteins may be reduced in thyrotoxicosis owing to hepatic dysfunction, some 15 per cent. of hyperthyroid patients have PBI values in the upper normal range. High values are also found in patients who take iodides, usually in the form of cough mixtures or asthma cures, and in those who over the previous 6–12 months or even longer have taken clioquinol (*Entero-Vioform*) or have had X-ray investigations involving the administration of contrast material for cholecystography, pyelography or myelography. High values also occur in pregnancy and in patients taking oestrogens or oestrogen-containing contraceptive pills because under these circumstances the plasma concentration of thyroxine-binding proteins is often increased. A raised PBI level may temporarily be further elevated after treatment of hyperthyroidism with ^{131}I, and also occurs in some patients with virus or auto-immunizing thyroiditis, in whom the protein-bound iodine is composed of abnormal iodoproteins which differ from thyroxine (T-4) and tri-iodothyronine (T-3) in not being extractable from the plasma with acid-butanol.

PBI levels below 4 μg. per 100 ml. are found in hypothyroidism but, because in some cases of myxoedema the plasma level of thyroxine-binding protein is raised, some 25 per cent. of patients may have a PBI level within the lower normal range. Low concentrations of these proteins and hence of PBI also occur in patients with the nephrotic syndrome, during corticosteroid administration and in some patients with Cushing's syndrome or acromegaly. A congenital absence of thyroxine-binding globulin occurs as an inherited dominant X-chromosome linked trait; despite a very low PBI these males are euthyroid and have a normal plasma free thyroxine concentration. An injection of a mercurial diuretic may for 48 hours interfere with the chemical estimation of PBI and give a falsely low result.

Tri-iodothyronine Resin Uptake. The uptake of radioactive tri-iodothyronine (T-3) by a resin is a procedure for measuring the amount of free thyroxine binding protein (mainly TBG) in the plasma that is not bound with thyroidal hormones. Radioactive T-3 is added *in vitro* to the patient's serum. Those binding sites on the plasma proteins not already saturated take up the T-3. The remaining unabsorbed radioactive T-3 is then absorbed on to a resin, and the radioactivity of the resin measured. In hyperthyroidism a large proportion of the TBG binding sites are occupied by thyroxine so that the proportion of the radioactive T-3 absorbed on the resin is greater than normal.

Conversely in hypothyroidism a smaller number of sites on the carrier proteins are occupied. More of the radioactive T-3 is therefore taken up by the thyroxine-binding proteins and less is absorbed on the resin which has a radioactivity of less than normal. The advantages of this test is that it is technically more easy to perform than the estimation of PBI and the result is not influenced by previous administration of iodine-containing compounds. On the other hand, alterations in thyroxine-binding protein capacity, as in pregnancy, nephrosis and oestrogen administration for example, influence the result, but do so in an opposite direction from that found in the estimation of the PBI. Thus an increase in TBG will increase the PBI but reduce the T-3 resin uptake. Abnormal results also occur in patients taking phenytoin or salicylates, substances that interfere with the protein-binding of thyroidal hormones.

Serum Total Thyroxine and Thyroxine Resin Uptake. ^{125}I- labelled thyroxine can be used to measure the resin uptake of thyroxine, as an alternative to measuring the resin uptake of tri-iodothyronine, and also for determining the serum total thyroxine, as an alternative to measuring the PBI. The normal ranges have to be determined by each laboratory using the technique because the results are influenced by technical variations and the reference serum used as a normal control. The serum total thyroxine has a range in the order of 4–11 μg. per 100 ml. and the resin uptake ratio a range of 0·92–1·20.

Free Thyroxine Index. By multiplying the serum total throxine by the thyroxine resin uptake (or the PBI by the T-3 resin uptake) the 'free thyroxine index' can be derived. This correlates well with the free thyroxine concentration measured directly by physicochemical methods. The free T-4 index compensates for changes in thyroxine-binding protein capacity and is one of the most accurate indications of thyroidal secretory function. Using the ^{125}I-labelled thyroxine technique the normal range for the free thyroxine index is of the order of 4·5–11·5.

Radio-iodine Uptake. Two isotopes, ^{131}I with a half-life of 8 days and ^{132}I with a half-life of 2·4 hours, are used to measure the uptake of iodine. Essentially the test is a measure of the trapping function of the gland and is an indirect and sometimes misleading index of thyroidal hormone synthesis. Ideally the uptake should be measured at a time when no appreciable discharge from the gland has occurred, but for a variety of reasons ^{131}I is usually counted 24 hours after administration and ^{132}I after 4 hours. The amount of radio-iodine trapped in the gland is expressed as a percentage of the total dose given. Two factors, other than thyroid trapping, influence the result. One is the elimination of the radio-iodine by the kidney; renal clearance of iodide is variable but if high, less iodine is available for concentration by the thyroid gland. The second is the size of the stable iodide pool with which the radio-active tracer is mixed. If this is large, less radio-iodine will enter the thyroid; whereas if there is iodine deficiency more of the tracer will be taken up by the gland.

High uptakes of radio-iodine occur in hyperthyroidism because the gland is being stimulated by LATS [p. 558]; and also in iodine deficiency when the gland is being stimulated by TSH; in dyshormonogenesis; in patients who have recently stopped taking an anti-thyroid drug and in some cases of auto-immunizing thyroiditis depending on the degree of thyroidal fibrosis.

A reduced uptake of radio-iodine occurs in primary or secondary hypothyroidism; in patients whose secretion of TSH is suppressed by administration of thyroxine or tri-iodothyronine and in those with a large stable iodine pool as a result of ingestion of iodide or injection of radio-opaque contrast media.

TSH Stimulation Test. The intramuscular injection of 5–10 Units of thyrotrophic hormone daily for 3 days will increase the low uptake of radio-iodine in patients with hypothyroidism secondary to pituitary disease but will have no such influence when there is primary thyroidal hypofunction. This test can also be used to confirm whether or not a patient, who has already been started on thyroxine therapy because of a supposed diagnosis of hypothyroidism, really has primary thyroidal hypofunction. The exogenously administered T-4 will suppress the uptake of radio-iodine by suppressing TSH secretion and must be continued during the test. Injections of exogenous TSH will increase the uptake of radio-iodine as compared with the pre-injection control value in patients with responsive thyroid glands but not in those who have primary thyroidal hypofunction.

Tri-iodothyronine Suppression Test. Whereas administration of T-3 will suppress the secretion of TSH and reduce the thyroidal uptake of radio-iodine in normal subjects and also in those with increased TSH secretion such as occurs in iodine deficiency, it has no such effect in patients with Graves' disease in whom the thyroidal overactivity is due to increased LATS production [p. 557]. Equally in hyperthyroidism due to an autonomous toxic 'adenoma' no significant suppression of radio-iodine uptake will occur in response to T-3. Tri-iodothyronine, 40 μg. eight-hourly is given for 6 days, and the uptake of radio-iodine measured before and afterwards. This test is particularly valuable in differentiating a high radio-iodine uptake in hyperthyroidism from that due to iodine deficiency. In the former there is no marked reduction in radio-iodine uptake whereas in iodine deficiency and other conditions with increased TSH secretion the uptake is suppressed to 50 per cent. of the value obtained before T-3 was given. This test is also helpful in determining the causation of bi- or uni-lateral exophthalmos. Failure of suppression is common but not invariable in patients with the ophthalmic form of Graves' disease before there is clinical evidence of hyperthyroidism.

Thyroid Scan. A scintiscan (or gammascan) with ^{131}I is useful in differentiating between a toxic nodular goitre showing a 'hot' nodule and Graves' disease with over-all increased radioactivity. It is also of some limited value in the diagnosis of thyroid cancer when the finding of a 'cold' nodule poorly demarcated from the surrounding tissue suggests a malignant growth, but cysts and benign adenomas may give a similar appearance and the precise diagnosis can only be established by biopsy and histological examination. The finding of ectopic thyroidal tissue that takes up ^{131}I is also suspicious of a thyroid carcinoma, particularly the follicular differentiated type [p. 564] but is also observed in potentially hypothyroidal or overtly cretinous children with an undescended thyroid gland lying in the line of the thyroglossal duct [p. 566].

Thyroidal Antibodies. Although not a test of thyroid function, the presence of circulating thyroidal antibodies can be helpful in determining the causation of a goitre. Two different types of antibody may develop. One is directed against thyroglobulin and is revealed by the precipitin test, which is positive in 70 per cent. of patients with Hashimoto's thyroiditis but negative in simple goitre, drug-induced goitre and in dyshormonogenesis, or the more sensitive tanned red cell haemagglutination test (TRC) which is positive in high titre (dilutions of 1:25,000–1:2,500,000) in patients with Hashimoto's thyroiditis but may also be positive in high or medium titre (1:2,500–1:25,000) in other thyroid diseases. The second type of antibody is complement fixing (CFT) and directed against a microsomal fraction of the thyroid cell. This is positive in medium or high titre (a dilution of 1:20 or more) in 98 per cent. of patients with Hashimoto's thyroiditis and in 83 per cent. of patients with primary myxoedema. The CFT is also positive but usually in lower titres in 60–70 per cent. of patients with thyrotoxicosis, in a third of patients with a non-toxic nodular goitre and a slightly lesser proportion of patients with thyroidal carcinoma.

Long-acting Thyroid Stimulator. LATS is a third and special type of thyroid antibody found in many patients with Graves' disease. This is discussed on page 558.

SIMPLE NON-TOXIC GOITRE

Synonyms. Simple goitre, non-toxic, colloid goitre and non-toxic nodular goitre are synonyms that indicate that the thyroidal enlargement is unassociated with hyperthyroidism or with malignant changes in the gland. The terms endemic goitre and sporadic goitre derive from epidemiological surveys and indicate, albeit superficially, an aetiological reason for the thyroidal enlargement.

Definition

Any non-malignant enlargement of the thyroid gland unassociated with hypersecretion of thyroid hormones constitutes a simple non-toxic goitre. By convention the term is further restricted to the absence of any auto-immune disorder involving the thyroid gland and is confined to those instances in which the thyroidal enlargement is caused by some disturbance in iodine metabolism which leads, because of a tendency to reduced secretion of thyroidal hormones, to increased secretion of the thyroid-stimulating hormone (TSH). It is this increased secretion of TSH that is thought responsible for the enlargement of the thyroid gland.

Aetiology

Iodine Deficiency. Deficiency of iodine limits the biosynthesis of thyroid hormones, and this stimulates the hypothalamus to secrete increased amounts of the thyrotrophin-releasing factor and this in turn promotes the adenohypophysis to secrete more TSH. The thyroid gland hypertrophies and, judging by the infrequency of clinical hypothyroidism, this compensates satisfactorily for the iodine lack.

There are many causes of iodine deficiency. The commonest is dietary, which occurs in certain parts of the world, particularly areas remote from the sea such as the Alps, Pyrenees, Himalayas, Andes, Congo and around the Great Lakes of North America, where the soil and water contain so little iodine that goitre is *endemic*, affecting more than 10 per cent. of the population. It has been estimated that 200 million people in the world today have a simple goitre as a result of absolute iodine deficiency.

Simple goitre also occurs *sporadically* particularly if areas where there is a relative iodine deficiency or the patients' eating habits result in a low dietary intake. In these circumstances goitre is much more common in females than males, and often first appears at the time of puberty when the demand for thyroidal hormones is increased. During pregnancy further enlargement of the thyroid, or the development of a goitre for the first time, is common because partial iodine deficiency is intensified by the increased excretion of iodide by the mother's kidneys and by the iodine requirements of the developing foetus. Some women experience thyroid enlargement in association with menstruation, and also at the time of the menopause.

Dyshormonogenesis. Another cause of simple goitre is an inborn error of iodine metabolism that results from a partial deficiency of one of the several enzymes concerned in the biosynthesis of the thyroidal hormones. These enzymatic defects may involve [FIG. 34] the ability

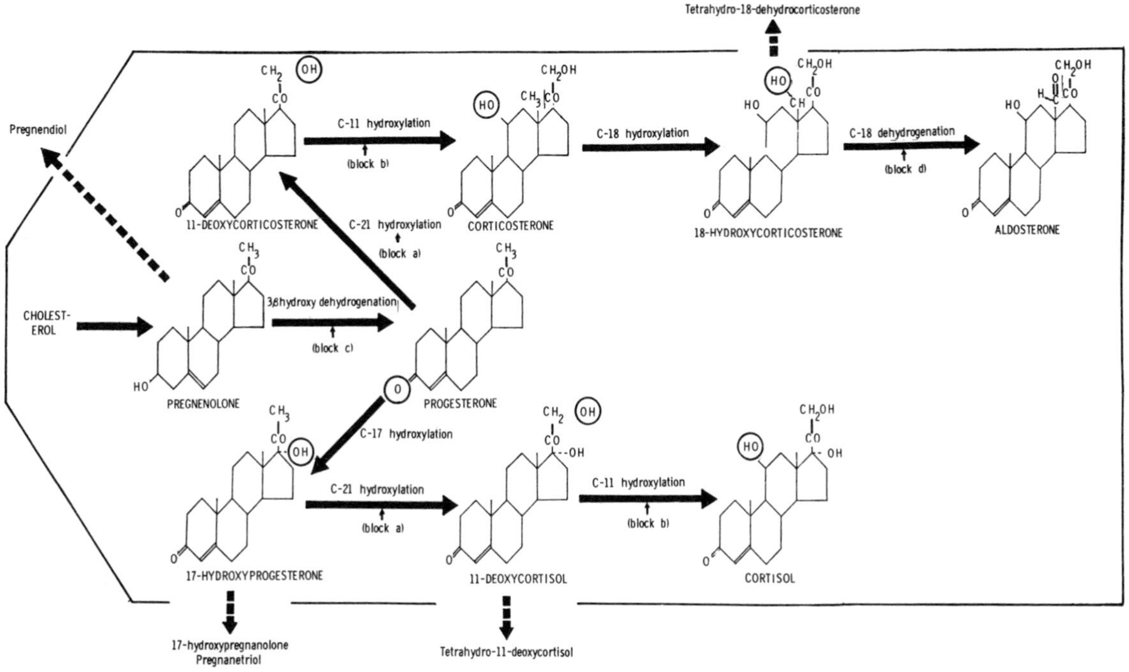

34. The principal steps in the biosynthesis of aldosterone and cortisol in the adrenal cortex. A deficiency of one of the enzymes, C-21-hydroxylase (block a), C-11-hydroxylase (block b), 3-β-hydroxy-dehydrogenase (block c) or C-18-dehydrogenase (block d) results in the urinary excretion of the precursor metabolites indicated by the broken arrows.

of the gland to accumulate (trap) iodide from the serum; the ability of the gland to organify iodine with tyrosine; impairment of the dehalogenation of iodotyrosines with the result that excessive loss of iodine-containing compounds occurs in the urine; the inability to couple iodotyrosines; and the synthesis of abnormal iodoproteins. In some instances these enzymatic defects are hereditary and linked with other congenital defects, e.g. deafness. Depending on the hypothalamic-pituitary response and the degree of enzymatic defect the patient may be euthyroid or become hypothyroid; many remain euthyroid because of the increased TSH secretion and the responsiveness of the thyroid gland.

Goitrogens. An indirect deficiency of iodine may be induced by substances which interfere with the trapping of iodide by the thyroid gland or with its subsequent synthesis to thyroxine or tri-iodothyronine. In addition to thiouracil, carbimazole and perchlorate which are used in hyperthyroidism to restrain thyroid hormone synthesis, other goitrogenic compounds include cyanates, cobalt, para-aminosalicylic acid (PAS), resorcinol and possibly sulphonylurea compounds used for the treatment of diabetes mellitus. 'Cabbage goitre' is attributable to organic cyanides in vegetables of the Brassica group; in Tasmania it has been shown that goitre in schoolchildren is due to feeding them milk from cows fed on a particular species of kale.

Iodide Excess. A special and relatively uncommon form of goitrogen is the prolonged ingestion of excessive amounts of iodide that may be contained in cough medicines and asthma cures (e.g. *Felsol*). It is well recognized that high intrathyroid concentrations of iodide inhibit the organification of iodine with tyrosine and hence reduce the biosynthesis of thyroidal hormones. In most patients, for reasons unknown, a high iodine intake is associated with reduced trapping of iodide by the thyroid gland. In others, because of enhanced TSH secretion and failure to adapt to the high iodine intake, excessive amounts of iodide enter the gland; the production of hormone diminishes and the patient develops an 'iodide goitre' and may become myxoedematous.

Pathology

Under the stimulus of TSH, there is uniform hyperplasia of the thyroid which becomes firm, smooth and uniformly enlarged. The epithelium lining the acini becomes columnar and projects in plicated folds into the centre of the vesicles. At a later stage the degree of hyperplasia becomes less marked in some areas of the gland, and colloid fills the acini with flattening of the lining cells. The gland is now asymmetrical and lobulated. Still later, usually after the age of 30, nodules begin to develop. These are not adenomas but functionally inert areas between which foci of hyperplastic thyroid tissue supply the hormonal needs of the body. The nodules may be single or multiple, and generalized or confined to one part of the gland.

Symptoms

Simple goitre is much more common in women than men and usually first develops at the time of puberty. Initially the gland is only slightly enlarged and, depending on the cause of the iodine deficiency, it may remain so or gradually increase in size, progressing through the asymmetrical lobulated colloid goitre stage to the final nodular stage after the age of 30.

Usually the patient's only complaint is of a swelling in the neck, but if the thyroid gland grows in size and particularly if it is retrosternal, pressure symptoms develop. Displacement and distortion of the trachea causes cough, stridor and dyspnoea, especially at night when the patient lies in a particular position. Compression of the jugular veins causes venous engorgement and facial congestion. Less commonly there is dysphagia and rarely hoarseness of the voice due to compression of a recurrent laryngeal nerve, but this development should always suggest the possibility of malignant change. A sudden increase in the size of the gland or in the severity of pressure symptoms is usually caused by haemorrhage into a cyst or malignant degeneration.

Thyroid function is usually normal and there are seldom signs or symptoms of hypothyroidism. In areas of endemic goitre, however, where the degree of iodine deficiency is marked, hypothyroidism may occur, and the greater the severity of iodine lack, the earlier will thyroid enlargement develop and the more likely are males to be affected as well as women. In cases of sporadic goitre which progress to the nodular stage hyperthyroidism may develop in the sixth or seventh decade (see nodular toxic goitre). Malignant changes are rare and least common when there are multiple nodules.

Diagnosis

In every case of simple goitre, a direct or indirect cause of iodine deficiency or dyshormonogenesis should be sought but often the exact aetiology remains uncertain. The condition must be distinguished from Hashimoto's thyroiditis by the history, absence of thyroidal antibodies and if necessary by drill biopsy. Malignant change is suggested if one area of the gland is hard or adherent to surrounding structures or if there is recurrent laryngeal palsy. Some of the differentiating features are set out in TABLE 39 [p. 564].

Hyperthyroidism must always be excluded by clinical assessment and laboratory investigation. In simple non-toxic goitre the PBI and plasma thyroxine levels are normal. Because of iodine deficiency the uptake of radio-iodine may be increased, but the isotope is retained in the gland for longer than in hyperthyroid patients who quickly discharge the labelled thyroid hormones into the blood stream.

Prophylaxis

Absolute or relative deficiency of iodine must be prevented by prophylactic administration of sodium iodide, or the more stable sodium iodate, in a proportion of 1 part to 40,000–100,000 parts of sodium chloride. This use of iodized salt has proved strikingly effective in reducing the incidence of goitre in such endemic areas as Switzerland and around the Great Lakes of North America, and should be universally adopted as the most satisfactory method of ensuring an adequate dietary intake of iodine. In situations where iodized salt proves impracticable, intramuscular injection of 4 ml. iodized oil (*Neo-Hydriol*), providing 1·6 G. iodine, may prove effective in supplying sufficient iodine to prevent the development of goitre or reduce the degree of enlargement. Such prophylaxis may prove effective for as long as 3 years.

Treatment

Once a goitre has developed, the treatment will depend on its cause, on the patient's age and on the duration of the disease. When a goitrogen is responsible, withdrawal of this will usually be followed by regression of the thyroid enlargement. When absolute or relative iodine deficiency is the cause, regression and prevention of further enlargement may be achieved in infancy and childhood by administration of potassium iodide, 60 mg. daily. After puberty these measures are seldom effective except in thyroid enlargement associated with menstruation or pregnancy. In adolescents and young adults simple goitre is best treated with thyroxine, 0·1–0·3 mg. given daily for several years. By suppressing the pituitary secretion of TSH, enlargement of the thyroid may be prevented and some regression in size is achieved in more than 50 per cent. of cases, particularly if the goitre is of recent origin.

Once the goitre is of long-standing and nodular changes have developed, medical treatment is seldom effective. Often no treatment is required for patients with multinodular goitres but thyroidectomy is indicated if the gland is cosmetically unsightly, if there are pressure symptoms, if hyperthyroidism develops, or if sudden focal enlargement, hoarseness of the voice or adherence to surrounding structures suggest that malignant degeneration has occurred. After thyroidectomy, replacement therapy with thyroxine, 0·1–0·3 mg. daily, should be given for the rest of the patient's life to prevent the remaining thyroid tissue from hypertrophying and to prevent the development of hypothyroidism as a result of exhaustion atrophy of the glandular remnant.

Prognosis

Successful control of simple goitre depends upon prophylaxis. Once established, administration of iodides is only effective in early or mild cases. Thyroxine will control puberty goitres and those due to an inborn error of iodine metabolism. Once nodular changes have occurred no treatment short of thyroidectomy is effective and this must be followed by replacement therapy with thyroxine. In older people with nodular goitres the onset of hyperthyroidism may be insidious, and only manifest by atrial fibrillation and cardiac failure. Malignant degeneration is sufficiently rare as not to constitute a serious hazard.

HYPERTHYROIDISM

Hyperthyroidism or thyrotoxicosis is a clinical state resulting from the oversecretion of thyroidal hormones. It can be caused by diffuse overactivity of the gland as occurs in Graves' disease or as the result of localized overactivity due to a single hyperplastic nodule ('toxic adenoma') or to several less well-defined overactive foci in a nodular goitre of long-standing. Because of certain fundamental differences in aetiology, age-incidence, clinical manifestations and treatment, the two conditions of Graves' disease and toxic nodular goitre will be considered separately.

GRAVES' DISEASE

Synonyms. Thyrotoxicosis; Exophthalmic goitre; Toxic goitre; Basedow's disease; and Primary hyperthyroidism because the condition may arise in a previously normal thyroid gland.

Definition

Graves' disease is characterized by diffuse, usually uniform, enlargement of the thyroid gland accompanied by symptoms and signs caused by excessive secretion of thyroid hormones. Often in addition there are characteristic ocular abnormalities, and less commonly skin lesions (pretibial myxoedema) or changes in the fingers (acropachy).

Aetiology

Graves' disease is much more common in females than males, and usually occurs between the ages of puberty and the menopause, although children are not exempt. A genetic or constitutional predisposition is strongly suggested by a familial incidence, particularly in the mother or the sisters of the proband, of Graves' disease or other thyroidal disorders such as myxoedema or Hashimoto's thyroiditis. Since Graves' disease is now recognized as the probable consequence of a special type of thyroidal antibody, LATS (see below), it is likely that the condition is related to an inherited instability of immunological tolerance; this view is supported by finding evidence of auto-immune dysfunction or overt auto-immune diseases, such as pernicious anaemia associated with gastric parietal-cell antibodies, Addison's disease of the adrenals associated with adrenal antibodies, disseminated lupus erythematosus, antinuclear factor and thyroidal antibodies, in the female relatives of the thyrotoxic proband. Although difficult to obtain convincing scientific support, there is a clinical suspicion that in predisposed subjects Graves' disease may develop as the result of an emotional disturbance. The mechanism by which this is effected is not yet understood.

Although it might be supposed that Graves' disease was the consequence of excessive secretion of TSH, in a manner analogous to Cushing's syndrome due to bilateral adrenal hyperplasia being the consequence of excessive secretion of ACTH, there is now convincing evidence to the contrary. First, the plasma level of TSH is not raised but is abnormally low in patients with Graves' disease. Secondly, Graves' disease has on rare occasions occurred in patients with panhypopituitarism and also in those who have had a total hypophysectomy. Thirdly, the activity of the thyroid gland in Graves' disease is not suppressed by administration of T-4 or T-3, as are the adrenal glands when dexamethasone is given to patients with Cushing's syndrome due to excess ACTH secretion.

There is, moreover, convincing evidence of a humoral substance, other than TSH, that is responsible for stimulating the thyroid gland in Graves' disease. Because in bioassay methods this substance has a thyroid-stimulating effect that occurs later and is more prolonged than TSH, it is known as the long-acting thyroid stimulator (LATS). Present evidence indicates that LATS is not a modified form of TSH but is chemically and immunologically distinct, although the two substances presumably share a common thyroid-stimulating molecular grouping. LATS is a gamma-globulin with all the characteristics of an IgG antibody produced by lymphocytes. What stimulates the production of this immunoglobulin is unknown, but possibly the complementary antigen arises from the thyroid gland itself. With improving bioassay techniques and by concentrating the gamma-globulin fraction, high titres of LATS are found in many patients with Graves' disease. Although the serum level of LATS does not correlate well with the severity of the patient's hyperthyroidism, there is a close relationship between the LATS titre and thyroidal activity as judged by the rate of ^{131}I turnover. High LATS titres are usually found in patients with pretibial myxoedema but there is a poor relationship between the ocular manifestations of Graves' disease and the plasma LATS level. Thus the exophthalmos has been attributed to another humoral agent, the exophthalmos producing substance, for which bioassay methods are as yet unsatisfactory and its site of origin unknown.

In patients with Graves' disease the LATS titre may or may not diminish spontaneously in response to treatment with antithyroid drugs. In those patients in whom it does diminish, a remission persists when the antithyroid medication is stopped; persistence of LATS is likely to be associated with a relapse. High LATS titres may persist in patients with Graves' disease whose hyperthyroidism has been 'cured' by thyroidectomy or radioiodine. In such instances the patient is euthyroid because not enough functioning thyroidal tissue remains to secrete an excess of thyroidal hormones. On rare occasions the persistence of high LATS titres is revealed by a euthyroid woman, previously thyrotoxic, giving birth to a baby with congenital thyrotoxicosis. This situation is attributable to LATS crossing the placenta and stimulating the foetal thyroid gland.

Pathology

The thyroid gland is uniformly enlarged with a marked increase in vascularity. Colloid is scanty and the acini vary in size. The epithelial cells are cubical or columnar and project into the vesicles as plicated folds. Infiltration of the gland with foci of lymphocytes (lymphorrhages), plasma cells and areas of fibrosis indicating focal thyroiditis is common and related to the presence of thyroglobulin and microsomal antibodies in the patient's serum. The histological appearance is modified by treatment. Antithyroid drugs accentuate the hyperplasia which is suppressed by iodide administration with increased formation and storage of colloid and a reduction in vascularity.

In patients with exophthalmos the orbital tissues are infiltrated with lymphocytes, plasma cells, macrophages, mast cells and an increase in metachromatic mucopolysaccharide ground substance. The extra-ocular muscles are hypertrophied and later may become infiltrated and fibrosed. In pretibial myxoedema the dermal tissues contain increased amounts of mucopolysaccharides consisting mainly of hyaluronic acid.

Symptoms

The onset is usually insidious but may be quite rapid. The patient complains of tiredness, palpitations and consciousness of the heart's action, shortness of breath on exertion, nervousness and anxiety, muscular weakness, tremor of the hands or diarrhoea. Relatives may draw attention to the thyroid enlargement or stariness of the eyes. Direct inquiry may elicit a preference for cool weather and intolerance of heat, a good or increased appetite despite weight loss, generalized excessive sweating not confined to the axillae, and oligomenorrhoea. There may be oedema of the ankles.

The patient is tense, talkative and restless. The thyroid, unless retrosternal, shows slight or moderate generalized enlargement, sometimes more marked in one lobe than the other. The gland feels smooth, is firmer than normal, not tender nor fixed to surrounding structures. Pressure symptoms or signs are uncommon. A systolic, or systolic and diastolic, bruit may indicate the increased vascularity of the gland. The skin is warm and pink; cold clammy palms are a sign of anxiety, not of hyperthyroidism. The outstretched hands and fingers have a fine tremor. The pulse is rapid and does not slow to normal levels during sleep. The rhythm is usually regular in patients under 40, but in older or long-standing cases atrial fibrillation may develop. As a consequence of peripheral vasodilatation the pulse is full and bounding with a collapsing quality. When the raised forearm is grasped in the examiner's palm, the hyperdynamic circulation can be clearly felt. A tapping right ventricular impulse is felt to the left of the sternum, and a systolic murmur caused by the high cardiac output is often audible over the pulmonary area. Rarely there is generalized lymphadenopathy and slight enlargement of the spleen.

Ocular manifestations may be slight or dominate the clinical picture. Widening of the palpebral fissures due to retraction of the upper lids is common, and often associated with lid-lag. Some degree of exophthalmos is common, and this may be symmetrical and bilateral or unilateral, in some instances preceding any evidence of thyroid overactivity.

Uncommon clinical features of Graves' disease are acropachy (clubbing) of the fingers, and pretibial myxoedema which more often occurs late in the course of the disease usually when the patient has been rendered euthyroid but continues to have a high plasma LATS titre. Often the skin lesions on the lower legs are symmetrical with a well-defined raised serpiginous margin, itching and tenderness of the thickened infiltrated area.

Congenital Thyrotoxicosis. Before birth, hyperthyroidism in the foetus may be suspected if the foetal heart rate is unduly rapid, and if the mother has been treated in the past for thyrotoxicosis, and persists in having pretibial myxoedema or marked exophthalmos. At birth the baby is emaciated and hyperkinetic; it may have a goitre and diarrhoea. The diagnosis, once suspicion is aroused, is usually clear on clinical grounds alone. The disease is self-limiting because of the half-life of the maternal LATS transferred across the placenta. Unless the thyroidal overactivity is controlled within the first 2 months of life that the condition occurs, the infant may die. Carbimazole, 2·5 mg. once or twice daily, will control the disorder and can gradually be withdrawn during the second month of life.

Complications

Cardiac Failure. Dyspnoea on exertion is a common complaint in patients with hyperthyroidism, who have no evidence of cardiac failure. The shortness of breath is ascribed to the increased oxygen demands due to the increased metabolic rate and in part to weakness of the respiratory muscles. In long-standing neglected cases, in older patients and those who develop atrial fibrillation, frank right-sided cardiac failure may develop with a raised jugular venous pressure, tender hepatomegaly and sacral or ankle oedema. By contrast patients with a toxic nodular goitre more commonly present with atrial fibrillation and cardiac failure because they usually belong to an older age group and may have pre-existing hypertensive or ischaemic heart disease.

Ocular Manifestations. Ocular manifestations of Graves' disease may be divided into the non-infiltrative and the infiltrative types. The characteristics of the *non-infiltrative ophthalmopathy* have been described above, but both forms may occur not only in patients with obvious Graves' disease but also in those with no present evidence and no past history of hyperthyroidism. Ocular features in the absence of thyroidal hyperfunction may pose diagnostic problems suggesting, because often the disorder is confined to only one eye, a retro-orbital disorder, an orbital tumour or a new-growth arising in the paranasal sinuses. Despite the absence of clinical evidence of hyperthyroidism and a normal uptake of radio-iodine and a normal PBI or free thyroxine index, a proportion of these patients, particularly in the later stages, have an abnormal T-3 suppression test [p. 554] which is helpful in establishing the diagnosis. More than half these patients also have TRC or CFT antibodies [p. 554].

In *infiltrative exophthalmos* the patient often complains of a feeling of grittiness in the eyes, lacrimation and diplopia. Oedema and injection of the conjunctivae is associated with swelling of the eyelids and periorbital oedema. Oculomotor paresis most commonly involves the superior and lateral rectus muscles. Progressive exophthalmos, sometimes more marked in one eye than the other, may lead to corneal ulceration, papilloedema, optic atrophy and finally panophthalmitis (*malignant exophthalmos*). Fortunately this grave complication, more common in men than women, usually runs a self-limiting course over a number of months or years.

Pretibial Myxoedema. This is an uncommon complication characterized by circumscribed areas of raised, thickened and indurated skin over the shins. Like exophthalmic ophthalmoplegia, these changes often become more conspicuous after the hyperthyroidism has been treated.

Thyrotoxic Myopathy. Many patients with Graves' disease complain of, or on clinical examination are found to have, muscular weakness and wasting involving the proximal muscles of the shoulder girdle or pelvis. Electromyographic abnormalities are found in about 80 per cent. of cases. This thyrotoxic myopathy is associated with fasciculation and diminished or absent tendon reflexes. Improvement occurs when the hyperthyroidism is controlled as also is the rare condition of thyrotoxic periodic paralysis which is manifest by episodic weakness of the trunk and limb muscles. Rarely myasthenia gravis develops as a coincident disease with thyrotoxicosis; the myasthenia is not cured by rendering the patient euthyroid, and it seems probable that both conditions are the consequence of an autoimmune disturbance.

Thyroid Crisis. Very rarely a thyroid crisis or storm may develop, usually as a complication of thyroidectomy in an inadequately prepared patient or as a sequel to an acute infection. The clinical features, attributed to the sudden flooding of the circulation with thyroidal hormones, sympathetic nervous overactivity and eventual adrenocortical failure, are irritability, confusion, delirium, hyperpyrexia, extreme tachycardia and diarrhoea. Untreated the condition may lead to stupor and finally coma (apathetic crisis).

Carbohydrate and Calcium Metabolism. Glycosuria and a diabetic glucose tolerance curve may be observed, but usually revert to normal when the hyperthyroidism is corrected. Radiological evidence of osteoporosis is not uncommon in older patients with Graves' disease but is seldom associated with symptoms. A proportion of patients, usually those who are severely hyperthyroid, have a raised serum calcium and a low serum phosphorus level with symptoms sometimes of acute hypercalcaemia [p. 483]. A hydrocortisone test [p. 570] usually, but not always, lowers the hypercalcaemia to within the normal range. Control of the hyperthyroidism restores the calcium level to normal and thus excludes the possibility of associated hyperparathyroidism.

Diagnosis

The clinical diagnosis of Graves' disease is often obvious but should always be confirmed by at least one test of thyroid function before treatment is instituted. The total serum thyroxine level and the thyroxine index require only a sample of blood and are more reliable than the PBI which because of changes in the thyroxine-binding protein level may sometimes give misleading results [p. 553].

In the early phases the condition may be confused with an anxiety state in which the tremor is usually coarse, the skin cool, the palms moist and the sleeping pulse not accelerated. The distinction is often difficult because many patients with Graves' disease have a coincident anxiety state. At this early stage tests of thyroid function may be equivocal but harm seldom results if the patient is kept under observation and time is used as a diagnostic ally to clarify the diagnosis. Alternatively a tri-iodothyronine suppression test [p. 554] can be done. This procedure is particularly helpful in mild cases of hyperthyroidism and also in elucidating the cause of unilateral exophthalmos in a patient who has no signs of thyroid overactivity and in whom other causes of unilateral proptosis, such as orbital and retro-orbital tumours or an aneurysm of the internal carotid artery, have to be considered in the differential diagnosis.

Hyperthyroidism should be considered in the differential diagnosis of weight-loss, diarrhoea, atrial fibrillation or cardiac failure without evident cause.

Treatment

Graves' disease is treated with antithyroid drugs, radio-iodine or thyroidectomy. Which of these methods is used depends upon the patient's age, the size of the goitre, the response to treatment in the past, the wishes of the patient and the preferences and experiences of the physician and surgeon.

Propranolol. This is a β-adrenergic blocking agent of great value in the symptomatic control of certain thyrotoxic features. It reduces the heart rate whether the patient is in sinus rhythm or has atrial fibrillation being treated with digoxin. Thus it reduces the patient's cardiac consciousness and palpitations. Excessive sweating, nervousness and tremor are less. It may also increase muscle power in thyrotoxic myopathy. The initial dose for 48 hours should be 10 mg. four times a day and thereafter 40 mg. four times a day. The particular uses of this drug as an adjunct to the management of hyperthyroidism are discussed below. Occasional patients complain of indigestion from its use but this can usually be overcome by reducing the dosage. Propranolol should not be given to patients with bronchial asthma nor to those in cardiac failure.

Radio-Iodine. ^{131}I is usually restricted to the treatment of patients aged 40 or over. It is the method of first choice in patients in the older age groups and constitutes an absolute indication for the treatment of recurrent hyperthyroidism after thyroidectomy irrespective of the patient's age. This is because of the high incidence of complications, such as recurrent laryngeal nerve palsy or hypoparathyroidism, after a second or third thyroidectomy. Although many attempts have been made to determine scientifically the optimal dose of ^{131}I required to render a particular patient euthyroid, none has proved reliable. Thus the dosage is largely empirical depending on the severity of the symptoms and is usually in the range of 4–10 millicuries. Maximum improvement from a given dose is not achieved for 3 months. During this time the patient's thyrotoxic symptoms can be controlled with propranolol, 40 mg. four times a day, which does not interfere with subsequent tests of thyroid function. Three months after ^{131}I treatment thyroid function is re-assessed. About 60 per cent. of patients are euthyroid after a single dose, and the remainder require a smaller second or rarely even a third dose. The important complication of radio-iodine treatment is hypothyroidism which may develop soon after the treatment or more insidiously with the result that within 10 years about 40 per cent. of patients become hypothyroid. For this reason radio-iodine treated patients must be kept under surveillance and replacement therapy with thyroxine, 0·2–0·3 mg. daily, given if hypothyroidism occurs.

Antithyroid Drugs. The use of antithyroid drugs such as carbimazole or propylthiouracil is the treatment of choice in children and adults under the age of 25 years with Graves' disease, provided that the patient does not have a large unsightly or retrosternal goitre. The usual dose of carbimazole is 10 mg. 8-hourly or 100 mg. propylthiouracil 8-hourly. The side-effects of carbimazole are probably slightly less than those with thiouracil and include rashes, gastro-intestinal intolerance, drug fever, an arthritis resembling acute rheumatic fever, generalized lymphadenopathy and, most important of all, agranulocytosis which usually presents with a sore throat. Every patient taking antithyroid drugs must be told to stop treatment at once if a sore throat develops and report for a leucocyte count. Rarely carbimazole causes thinning of the scalp hair.

This treatment is given for 18–24 months, but about 40 per cent. of patients relapse when therapy is stopped. It is common practice to start treatment with the dosage given above and, after about 6 weeks, when the hyperthyroidism is controlled, to reduce the dose to an amount that keeps the patient euthyroid. It is often difficult to find the correct maintenance dose, the patient tends to swing between hypothyroidism and hyperthyroidism, and the goitre usually increases in size. An alternative and easier scheme is to give, throughout the 2 years of treatment, the antithyroid drug in full dosage and to prevent the development of hypothyroidism by adding after the first month of treatment 0·1 mg. thyroxine daily and after the second month 0·2 mg. daily. This combination of an antithyroid drug and thyroxine keeps the patient euthyroid throughout and prevents further enlargement of the gland.

If an adult patient relapses after stopping treatment with antithyroid drugs, thyroidectomy or alternatively but less commonly radio-iodine treatment should be used to render the patient euthyroid. In children it is often preferable to continue antithyroid drug therapy often for many years and perform thyroidectomy when the patient is aged about 18 years.

Antithyroid drugs can also be used to control hyperthyroidism in pregnant women. When the diagnosis is made during the first trimester of pregnancy, thyroidectomy is probably the treatment of choice. When the condition develops later in pregnancy antithyroid drugs are used in the minimum effective dosage and stopped 3–4 weeks before delivery. Antithyroid drugs are secreted in the mother's milk so breast feeding cannot be allowed if the mother has to resume antithyroid medication after delivery.

Subtotal Thyroidectomy. Surgical treatment of Graves' disease is indicated when there are symptoms or signs of pressure from the goitre; when the gland is retrosternal or so large as to be cosmetically unsightly; when there is a relapse after medical treatment; when the gland is nodular; in patients who dislike the prolonged surveillance required for medical treatment, particularly those in the age range 25–40 years; and in women who develop Graves' disease during the first trimester of pregnancy. The patient is prepared for operation with carbimazole, 10 mg. 8-hourly, and propranolol, 40 mg. four times a day for 3–6 weeks. During the 10 days before operation tablets of potassium iodide, 60 mg. thrice dialy, are given to reduce the vascularity of the gland. With modern surgical technique haemorrhage or sepsis is uncommon and the important postoperative complications are damage to a recurrent laryngeal nerve, tetany due to parathyroid deficiency [p. 574] and hypothyroidism, the incidence of which increases gradually over a period of 6 years to 6–10 per cent. A recurrence of hyperthyroidism develops in a similar proportion of cases and is best treated with radio-iodine.

Treatment of Complications

Cardiac Failure. The patient should be confined to bed or an arm-chair. Digoxin should be given in full dosage, 0·75–1·0 mg. intravenously, followed by 0·25 mg. orally twice daily. Diuretics should be given to relieve peripheral oedema and pulmonary congestion. Carbimazole, 10 mg. 8-hourly, is given, and when the patient is clinically euthyroid the carbimazole is stopped and definitive treatment with radio-iodine given 4–7 days later. Carbimazole is then resumed for a further 3 months, and thyroid function assessed a month later. If the patient is euthyroid but still fibrillating, digoxin is stopped and 3 days later the patient's heart converted to sinus rhythm by D.C. counter-current shock.

Ocular Manifestations. There is no certainly effective treatment of the ocular manifestations that occur in Graves' disease and often all that can be done is to protect the eyes and conserve vision until the condition has run its course. In many instances progression of the ocular symptoms is arrested and some remission of the eye signs occurs when the hyperthyroidism is controlled and the patient becomes euthyroid, irrespective of the treatment used to achieve this. Hypothyroidism, as a result of treatment, must be avoided because this appears to aggravate the exophthalmos, and whenever appropriate, sodium thyroxine, 0·2–0·3 mg., should be given daily. To reduce the periorbital oedema, the patient should be given diuretics and sleep propped up in bed. Instillation of drops of methyl-cellulose or liquid paraffin at night may prevent dryness or abrasion of the cornea. Protection from wind or dust is achieved by a carefully applied eye patch or windshields attached to the side-arms of spectacles. Local instillation of guanethidine sulphate 5 per cent. eye-drops twice daily may relieve the feeling of grittiness and reduce the lid retraction by blocking adrenergic nervous impulses. Benefit is usually evident within a week but if ineffective this treatment should not be prolonged further. Guanethidine locally may improve the conjunctival injection and the periorbital oedema but has no influence on the degree of exophthalmos or the ophthalmoplegia. Tarsorrhaphy may be necessary to prevent or control corneal ulceration and is also useful later in restoring symmetry of the palpebral fissures when one eye is more effected than the other. In some patients with progressive malignant exophthalmos and a degree of oedema that makes tarsorrhaphy impracticable, heroic doses of prednisone, 120–140 mg. daily, may under careful hospital supervision have a dramatic effect; if improvement occurs, it is usually possible to reduce the dosage gradually after a month or 6 weeks. Failure of response to corticosteroids, relentless protrusion of the orbital contents and progressive reduction in visual acuity call for surgical decompression which may be accomplished by removal of the supra-orbital plate (Nafziger's operation), removal of the zygoma to allow lateral decompression or removal of the floor of the orbit. X-ray therapy to the orbit or pituitary fossa, hypophysectomy or total ablation of the thyroid gland have not been of proven value in this dangerous situation.

Pretibial Myxoedema. Fluocinolone or betamethasone cream should be applied nightly and covered with an occlusive plastic film such as *Saranwrap*. The amount of ointment should be kept to a minimum and rubbed well into the affected areas. Later the frequency of treatment can be reduced to 2–3 times weekly or monthly depending on the patient's response.

Thyroid Crisis. This is a grave emergency. Propranolol, 5–15 mg., is given by slow intravenous injection to reduce the peripheral manifestations of the extreme hyperthyroidism, to slow the tachycardia and to improve the mental state. Thereafter the drug can be given orally in a dose of 40–80 mg. four times a day. An intravenous infusion of glucose saline is started and 100 mg. hydrocortisone hemisuccinate or 21-phosphate given to counter any adrenocortical insufficiency. The hyperpyrexia, if it persists, is treated with ice-packs and sponging with cold water and alcohol.

Prognosis

Before drugs or thyroidectomy were available for the treatment of Graves' disease, a number of patients after a period of hyperthyroidism became spontaneously euthyroid and several years later developed myxoedema. In retrospect it seems likely that destruction of the thyroid gland was produced by auto-antibodies, and it is now recognized that some 10 per cent. of patients with Hashimoto's thyroiditis give a history of previous thyrotoxicosis. The incidence of hypothyroidism after thyroidectomy is higher in patients who have circulating thyroidal antibodies, particularly of the complement-fixing type, before operation but the incidence of hypothyroidism after radio-iodine treatment cannot be correlated with the pre-treatment level of thyroid antibodies.

It is not known why some patients treated with antithyroid drugs may have a permanent remission when therapy is stopped whereas others relapse. The explanation may lie in the disappearance of LATS.

NODULAR TOXIC GOITRE

Synonyms. Secondary hyperthyroidism, because the overactivity develops in a patient with a pre-existing goitre; Toxic adenoma; Toxic nodular goitre.

Aetiology

Although absolute or relative iodine deficiency is responsible for the simple colloid goitre and the subsequent nodular goitre [p. 555], the cause of the supervening hyperthyroidism is unknown. Patients with a nodular toxic goitre are usually aged 50 or more, and although women predominate, the increased female sex incidence is not as marked as in Graves' disease.

Pathology

The changes in the gland are a combination of those

seen in nodular goitre and in hyperthyroidism. The acini vary in size and in the amount of colloid they contain. Fibrosis is widespread. The excessive secretion of thyroid hormones usually arises in hyperplastic epithelium lying between the nodules and much less commonly from a single overactive nodule, the so-called 'hot nodule' because of its avid uptake of radio-iodine.

Symptoms

The brunt of the disease falls upon the cardiovascular system and the metabolic disturbances, so prominent in Graves' disease, are less evident, because the patient is older and the tissues less responsive to thyroid hormones. The patient may present with high output cardiac failure, and few symptoms and signs to implicate the thyroid gland (*masked hyperthyroidism*). Increased fatigue, palpitations, shortness of breath, swelling of the ankles and an initial loss of weight followed by a gain when oedema fluid accumulates are the usual symptoms. The thyroid is asymmetrically enlarged and may contain a single 'hot' nodule or more often multiple nodular areas of hyperplasia. Atrial fibrillation and right-sided cardiac failure are common. Displacement and compression of the trachea cause stridor and cough. Ocular manifestations are much less striking than in Graves' disease. Stariness of the eyes, due to lid retraction, and lid-lag reflect the increased sympathetic tone, but exophthalmos and diplopia are rare.

Diagnosis

The diagnosis is best confirmed by the free thyroxine index or the PBI. A scintiscan may be helpful in showing that the uptake of radio-iodine is confined to a single nodule or is more widespread in several areas of the gland. A toxic nodular goitre must be considered in the differential diagnosis of cardiac failure, particularly in older patients even with coexisting hypertension or myocardial ischaemia. The stariness of the eyes is often the clue to the correct diagnosis.

Treatment

After pre-operative preparation as described on page 560, subtotal thyroidectomy is the treatment of choice. Radio-iodine may be used and is particularly suitable for the elderly and those who have heart failure. Recurrences are common after ^{131}I treatment and larger doses are required than for the treatment of Graves' disease. When the patient is euthyroid, atrial fibrillation should be converted to sinus rhythm by D.C. countercurrent shock. Permanent medication with thyroxine, 0·2 mg. daily, should be given to prevent hypothyroidism or the development of further nodular hyperplasia.

THYROIDITIS

Very rarely the thyroid gland is infected with pyogenic organisms (acute suppurative thyroiditis) or becomes involved by sarcoidosis, tuberculosis or syphilis. Much more commonly inflammatory changes develop in three distinct conditions. The first is probably caused by a number of different viral agents; the second is the expression of an autoimmune disorder of uncertain primary aetiology; and the third, of unknown aetiology, is best known by the eponymous name of Riedel's thyroiditis until more is known of its causation.

NON-SUPPURATIVE THYROIDITIS

Synonyms. Viral thyroiditis; Acute or subacute (non-suppurative) thyroiditis; de Quervain's thyroiditis.

Definition

An acute non-suppurative inflammation of the thyroid gland, usually of relatively sudden onset and associated with constitutional disturbances and sometimes transient hyperthyroidism in the initial stages.

Aetiology

The disease occurs more commonly in women than men, and perhaps particularly in those who have pre-existing thyroid enlargement. The cause is uncertain but there is increasing evidence from rises in antibody titres that a number of different viruses may be implicated. The most commonly encountered is the Coxsackie virus but the influenza, adenoviruses, ECHO and mumps organisms have appeared in some instances to be responsible. Aetiological proof is hard to establish and it is possible that the rise in viral antibody titre may be an anamnestic response.

Pathology

Usually there is a generalized swelling of the epithelial cells of the thyroid gland and widespread infiltration with plasma cells and lymphocytes. Sometimes these changes are more focal.

Symptoms

The onset may be sudden with pain and tenderness in the front of the neck, which may radiate upwards to the ears. Sometimes the thyroidal involvement is preceded by an upper respiratory infection or by a few days of general malaise with tiredness, low-grade fever and headache. The patient complains of a 'sore throat' and pain on swallowing. The unwary doctor may consider this in reference to the oropharynx and failing to find any infection of the tonsils or faucial area may not appreciate that the patient has a 'sore throat', i.e. a thyroid gland which in fact is tender to the touch and uniformly enlarged. During the first few days of the thyroiditis the patient feels generally ill and has a raised temperature. During this time there may be symptoms and signs of hyperthyroidism attributable to the sudden release of thyroidal hormones from the inflamed gland. The total white cell count is usually normal but there may be a relative lymphocytosis and the sedimentation rate is raised. Characteristically the PBI and plasma thyroxine levels are raised but the acutely inflamed gland takes up little or no radio-iodine. The disease runs a variable course in degree of severity and duration, lasting a few days to several weeks. Relapses are common but usually each recurrence is progressively less severe.

Viral thyroiditis is a more common disease than is generally recognized, largely because the complaint of sore throat with dysphagia attracts the doctor's attention to the oropharynx rather than the enlarged tender thyroid gland.

Treatment

Mild attacks subside spontaneously or in response to simple analgesics. More severe cases respond with symptomatic relief of the thyroidal swelling and tenderness, the fever and the constitutional disturbance to prednisone, 5–20 mg. daily. Such treatment should be continued for 3 weeks and then withdrawn gradually. Relapses are common and may require treatment with another course of prednisone.

Prognosis

In most instances there are no sequelae, and the condition is readily distinguishable from Hashimoto's thyroiditis (see below) by the low titre or absence of thyroidal antibodies and the low uptake of radio-iodine. Thyroidal antibodies rarely persist in viral thyroiditis and hypothyroidism is an uncommon sequela.

HASHIMOTO'S THYROIDITIS

Synonyms. Lymphadenoid goitre; Struma lymphomatosa.

Definition

A chronic inflammatory disease of the thyroid gland produced by thyroid antibodies and characterized by a goitre. In the later stages hypothyroidism is common. There appears to be a continuous spectrum with Hashimoto's thyroiditis in a euthyroid goitrous patient at one end and myxoedema in a patient with no palpable thyroid tissue at the other.

Aetiology

Hashimoto's thyroiditis is much more common in women than men, and usually develops between the ages of 30 and 50. The histological changes and the presence in the patient's serum of antibodies in high titre to thyroglobulin and to thyroid cells indicate an autoimmune disturbance, but what initiates the production of thyroid antigens or disturbs immunological tolerance to promote antibody formation is unknown.

Pathology

The thyroid gland is moderately enlarged, smooth and rubbery firm. There is diffuse lymphocytic infiltration and the parenchyma is replaced in some areas by deposits of lymphoid tissue and in others by fibrous tissue. In the later phases of the condition, the thyroid gland is represented by a fibrotic remnant.

Symptoms

The patient may present with a moderate-sized goitre which is smooth and painless and usually not sufficiently large to cause pressure symptoms. The gland is not attached to skin or surrounding structures. As the condition progresses, the gland enlarges and symptoms of hypothyroidism develop. Finally the gland may become progressively fibrotic and impalpable, the patient presenting with myxoedema. The uptake of radio-iodine varies according to the stage of the disease. Late in the course of the disease it may be low, but more often in goitrous patients it is normal or high, despite evident hypothyroidism, because of the small iodine pool consequent on destruction of functioning thyroidal tissue. The free thyroxine index is normal or low. T.R.C. and C.F.T. antibodies are usually present in high titre. The increase in circulating antibodies is often associated with a rise in the concentration of serum gamma-globulins and positive flocculation tests.

Diagnosis

Hashimoto's thyroiditis may be confused with a simple non-toxic goitre [p. 555] but the late onset of thyroidal enlargement and the high antibody titres serve to make the distinction. The differentiation from viral thyroiditis is made on clinical grounds by the absence of tenderness of the gland.

Treatment

Administration of thyroxine, 0·2–0·3 mg. daily for the rest of the patient's life, will reduce the size of the goitre and correct any coincident hypothyroidism. Rarely thyroidectomy is required for cosmetic reasons, to establish a histological diagnosis or to relieve pressure symptoms.

RIEDEL'S THYROIDITIS

Synonyms. Riedel's struma; Ligneous thyroiditis; Woody thyroiditis.

Aetiology

This is a very rare condition of unknown aetiology. It has been suggested that the pathology is analagous to retroperitoneal fibrosis. Usually older patients are affected, and there is no preference for females.

Pathology

The whole gland is replaced by dense avascular fibrous tissue which first involves one lobe and then spreads throughout the thyroid and to surrounding structures in the neck.

Symptoms

The patient may present with a goitre or with symptoms and signs due to involvement of the structures in the neck. The thyroid is woody hard and fixed to the skin and surrounding structures. Hoarseness due to laryngeal nerve involvement is common and there may be stridor from tracheal compression. Hypothyroidism is a late complication.

Diagnosis

Riedel's thyroiditis is clinically indistinguishable from thyroid carcinoma, and the diagnosis can only be established by biopsy.

Treatment

Ideally total thyroidectomy should be carried out but often this is not possible because of the adherence of the gland to surrounding structures. The most that may be achieved by surgery is relief of the tracheal constriction. Thyroxine, 0·2–0·3 mg. daily, should be given for the rest of the patient's life.

TABLE 39

DIFFERENTIAL DIAGNOSIS OF A NON-TOXIC GOITRE

	SIMPLE COLLOID GOITRE	HASHIMOTO'S THYROIDITIS	THYROID CARCINOMA
Consistency of goitre	Soft or firm	Firm	Firm or hard
Type of goitre	Diffuse or nodular	Diffuse or nodular	Diffuse or nodular
Recent increase in size	May occur	May occur	Common
Discomfort and pressure symptoms	Occasional; mild	Occasional; mild	Frequent; may be severe
Fixation	Never	Very rare	Common
Laryngeal palsy	Very rare	Very rare	Common
Cervical lymph node involvement	Never	Very rare	Common
Hypothyroidism	Rare	Common	Rare
T.R.C. test positive*	Rare	Nearly always	Rare
C.F.T. test positive*	Rare	Nearly always	Frequent
Hypergammaglobulinaemia and flocculation tests positive	No	Usual	No
Sedimentation rate	Normal	Often raised	Often raised
Radio-iodine uptake	Normal or high	Normal, high or low depending on stage of disease	Normal
Free thyroxine index or PBI	Usually normal	Low or normal	Normal

* T.R.C. = tanned red cell agglutination test; C.F.T. = complement fixation test (p. 554).

CARCINOMA OF THE THYROID

Thyroid carcinoma is rare, constituting only about 0·5 per cent. of deaths from malignancy.

Aetiology

When the condition occurs in children, there is often a previous history of X-ray therapy to the head, neck or anterior mediastinum, as for the treatment of a thymic tumour in infancy. Even quite small doses of irradiation in children seem to precipitate thyroid carcinoma.

Pathology

Malignant growths of the thyroid can be divided into the rapidly lethal undifferentiated anaplastic type and the much more benign slowly-growing differentiated papillary and follicular types. The solid carcinoma composed of spheroidal or spindle cells arising from the parafollicular cells of the gland is considered under the separate section on medullary-cell carcinoma (see below).

Papillary tumours are for the most part unencapsulated. Follicular tumours are also slow growing but encapsulated. Anaplastic tumours are composed of variously shaped cells and are rapidly invasive.

Symptoms

Most patients with carcinoma of the thyroid present with a nodule or more diffuse enlargement of the gland which feels firm or frankly hard. A history of sudden increase in size is common and often there are complaints of discomfort such as choking or tightness. Severe pressure symptoms, such as stridor, dyspnoea or dysphagia, may occur, and laryngeal palsy with hoarseness of the voice is not uncommon.

A *papillary carcinoma* is the commonest form of thyroid neoplasm and occurs in all age groups but is the type most commonly found in children and young adults. It usually presents as a single hard nodule in a previously normal thyroid gland and spreads to adjacent lymph nodes and occasionally to the lungs and bones. The course even with lymph node involvement or more distant metastases is usually very protracted with survival in excess of 10 years in more than half the patients.

The *follicular carcinoma* occurs most commonly in middle-aged patients with a previous goitre. The presenting symptom may be a solitary nodule or hoarseness of the voice due to involvement of a recurrent laryngeal nerve. Because of blood-borne dissemination to the skeleton or lungs, the patient may present with a pathological fracture, backache, a leuco-erythroblastic anaemia, or dyspnoea from pulmonary metastases. Lymph node metastases occur less frequently than in papillary carcinomas but bony and pulmonary metastases are more common. About half the patients survive 10 years.

Anaplastic carcinomas occur in older patients. They grow extremely rapidly to involve the skin and surrounding structures in the neck causing hoarseness, stridor and dysphagia. The pain, redness and swelling in the neck may even suggest an acute inflammatory lesion. Most cases are inoperable by the time of diagnosis and lethal within a few months.

The functional ability of thyroid cancers to take up iodine is related histologically with colloid formation and is confined to the papillary and follicular types.

Many of these tumours are TSH-dependent, the uptake of radio-iodine being enhanced by thyroid ablation and pretreatment with carbimazole and suppressed by administration of thyroxine.

Diagnosis

Although a rare condition, the possibility of thyroid cancer should always be considered in a child who presents with a solitary nodule in the thyroid; in an adult who has discrete, firm, enlarged lymph nodes in the neck particularly if there is an associated goitre; and in older patients who have noticed a sudden increase in the size of the thyroid gland particularly if this is associated with hoarseness of the voice, dysphagia, stridor or dyspnoea.

Malignant change very seldom arises in a gland which contains multiple nodules and less than 5 per cent. of solitary nodules prove neoplastic on histological examination. Often what feels clinically like a solitary nodule proves to be a benign 'adenoma' composed of several small nodules made up of small and large follicles containing colloid, cysts and areas of hyperplastic epithelial cells. Nevertheless, because it is impossible from clinical examination to judge its nature, the policy rightly continues to be removal of solitary nodules especially if these fail to take up radio-iodine. The differentiation of thyroidal carcinoma from a simple goitre and Hashimoto's thyroiditis is summarized in TABLE 39.

Treatment

Whenever possible in differentiated carcinomas of the papillary or follicular type, total thyroidectomy and removal of invaded lymph nodes is carried out. In some instances partial thyroidectomy is possible with a reduced liability to postoperative hypoparathyroidism or laryngeal palsy. Replacement therapy with sodium thyroxine, 0·3 mg. daily, is given thereafter to suppress TSH secretion as well as to prevent the development of hypothyroidism. If metastases, other than in local lymph nodes that can be removed surgically, develop deep X-ray therapy is given or radio-iodine can be used if the metastasis is TSH-dependent and concentrates the isotope. Sometimes the metastases can be made more avid for iodine by pre-treatment with carbimazole and withdrawal of thyroxine substitution therapy. An anaplastic carcinoma has usually advanced too far for surgical removal and is best treated with radiotherapy.

Prognosis

The prognosis in the papillary and follicular types of thyroid cancer is extremely good and progression of the disease, even without treatment, is usually slow over many years. Anaplastic tumours advance rapidly usually ending fatally with tracheal involvement in a few months.

MEDULLARY-CELL CARCINOMA OF THE THYROID

Definition

A rare variety of thyroid carcinoma, which arises from the parafollicular cells, is the so-called medullary-cell carcinoma. This is often associated with phaeochromocytoma and also with diarrhoea induced by the secretion from the malignant cells of a humoral substance.

Aetiology

In many instances there is a strong family history of goitre, diarrhoea over many years of death from hypertension secondary to a phaeochromocytoma. The inheritance, the multifocal origins of the parafollicular-cell tumours within the thyroid gland, the association with phaeochromocytomata which are often bilateral, and the wide variety of other autonomic abnormalities that may be present suggest that some single unknown factor may govern the growth of all these different tissues.

Pathology

The thyroid tumour may be single or multiple. It is a solid not anaplastic growth with neither papillary nor follicular differentiation. The stroma contains varying amounts of amyloid and may show some calcification. Spread occurs locally to neighbouring lymph nodes and may extend to the mediastinum or more distant sites. Benign or malignant, functioning or non-functioning, phaeochromocytomata, often bilateral, may be present as well as intestinal ganglioneuromatosis and mucosal neuromas of the lips, tongue and eyelids.

Symptoms

The condition may present as a single nodule in the thyroid gland. Progress of the growth may be very slow over many years. Diarrhoea due to intestinal hurry and unassociated with mucus or blood may be a presenting symptom or develop during the course of the illness. The severity of the diarrhoea is related to the size of the tumour and the degree of its extension beyond the neck. Removal of the tumour stops the diarrhoea which returns if metastases develop. Thus there is good reason for supposing that the intestinal hurry is due to a humoral substance liberated by the malignant parafollicular cells. Present research suggests that prostaglandins (fatty acid derivatives that stimulate plain muscle) may be the responsible factor rather than kinins or 5-hydroxytryptamine for the flushing attacks experienced by some patients with this syndrome. Some patients present a rather characteristic appearance with thickened lips, small mucosal neuromas on the tongue, lips and eyelids, pes cavus and a high arched palate. Other patients have symptoms caused by a phaeochromocytoma without any apparent tumour of the thyroid gland. Often the adrenal tumours are bilateral and may be malignant.

In these patients high urinary or plasma levels may be found of catecholamines and their metabolites, of 5-hydroxytryptamine or its excretory product 5-hydroxyindole acetic acid, of prostaglandins or of calcitonin.

Diagnosis

The tumour in the thyroid may be thought to be a simple non-toxic nodule, and the differentiation can only be made histologically although associated diarrhoea will suggest strongly a medullary cell carcinoma. The differential diagnosis of the diarrhoea may present considerable difficulty unless the primary cause in the neck is recognized.

Treatment

The thyroid tumour should be removed surgically, and a total thyroidectomy done because of the likelihood of other impalpable multifocal centres of new-growth being present. In patients with familial phaeochromocytoma the adrenal tumour(s) should be removed surgically and a gamma-scan of the thyroid made with ^{131}I. Any suggestion of a non-functioning thyroid nodule should lead to thyroidectomy.

Prognosis

The prognosis is variable from 1 to 30 years depending on the rate of progression of the medullary carcinoma. Failure to recognize the patient's hypertension as due to a phaeochromocytoma leads to cardiac failure or a cerebrovascular accident. The prognosis is poor when the phaeochromocytoma is malignant.

HYPOTHYROIDISM

The clinical picture produced by insufficient secretion of thyroid hormones depends upon the age of the patient at which the deficiency occurs, upon the duration of the deficiency and upon its degree. Congenital deficiency of thyroid hormones causes cretinism in infancy. In older children the lack is manifest as juvenile myxoedema, in which dwarfism is the prominent feature, and in adults the clinical picture is known as adult hypothyroidism or myxoedema depending upon the severity of the disease. In addition to deficiency of thyroid hormones caused by some primary abnormality affecting the thyroid gland, secondary hypothyroidism may occur as a consequence of diminished or absent secretion of thyroid-stimulating hormone in hypopituitarism [p. 543].

CRETINISM

Synonym. Infantile hypothyroidism.

Definition

A condition resulting from varying degrees of thyroid deficiency in foetal or early neonatal life and characterized by retarded development, particularly marked in the skeletal and central nervous systems.

Aetiology

Cretinism may occur in endemic or sporadic forms. *Endemic cretinism* is found in areas of severe iodine deficiency where endemic goitre is prevalent, and in most instances the mother of the affected child has a goitre.

Sporadic cretinism is rare. Usually it is due to congenital absence of thyroid tissue (*athyreosis*) or failure of the embryonic gland to descend into the neck. Thyroid deficiency may also arise from partial or complete absence of one of the several enzymes required for the biosynthesis of thyroidal hormones. In the rare cases of dyshormonogenesis [p. 555] cretinism is associated with a goitre (*goitrous cretinism*) and is often an hereditary familial disorder, sometimes associated with other congenital defects such as deafness (Pendred's syndrome). Sporadic cretinism may also occur in an infant born of a hyperthyroid mother who has been treated during pregnancy with too large doses of an antithyroid drug which crosses the placenta and depresses thyroidal activity in the foetus.

Pathology

The changes depend upon the cause of the hypothyroidism. In developmental abnormalities of the gland no thyroid tissue or only a small nodule of ectopic tissue in the line of the thyroglossal duct may be found. In endemic cretinism a goitre may be palpable and the gland is usually atrophic and fibrosed. When an enzymic defect is the cause, the gland is hyperplastic.

Symptoms

The infant is lethargic, falls asleep during feeding, fails to thrive and is constipated. Physical signs may not be discernible until the second month. The abdomen is prominent and an umbilical hernia often present. The face is broad and puffy; the nose is flat, and the lips and nostrils thickened. The tongue is enlarged and protrudes from the mouth. The skin is dry, thickened and sallow. Supraclavicular pads of fat make the neck appear short. The fontanelles are slow to close and skeletal development, as judged by the radiological appearance of ossification centres, is delayed. The infant's temperature may be subnormal. The hair is often dark, the eyes wide set and the infant's cry is hoarse. Dentition is delayed. Mentally the infant is stolid and retarded.

Diagnosis

Cretinism should be suspected in any infant with an umbilical hernia or a neonatal goitre. The single most helpful step in diagnosis is a radiological skeletal survey which will show delayed development and pathognomonic dysgenesis of the ossification centres. The plasma thyroxine level is low as is the PBI in most cases except some with dyshormonogenesis and abnormal iodoproteins in the blood. In athyreosis the uptake of radio-iodine is absent, and in maldescent of the thyroid gland a small area of activity in the line of the thyroglossal duct may be found. In endemic cretinism the uptake of radio-iodine may be normal or increased; and an increased, normal or decreased uptake may occur in dyshormonogenesis depending upon the particular enzyme that is deficient. The ECG usually shows flat T-waves and low voltage QRS complexes.

Rarely cretinism is confused with mongolism, a condition that can be recognized at birth from the characteristic mongoloid eyes, the short little finger, the abnormal palmar and plantar creases and the fine silky hair. Macroglossia may also occur in babies born with exomphalos.

Treatment

In endemic goitrous areas the occurrence of cretinism can be prevented by prophylactic administration of iodide to the mother during pregnancy. To avoid permanent mental deficiency cretinism must be recognized and treated early but unfortunately, when thyroid deficiency has been marked in foetal life, the changes may be irreversible. The appropriate dose of sodium thyroxine ranges from 0·025 mg. daily or on alternate days in a neonate to 0·2 mg. daily later in childhood. The exact amount required is judged by the state of the bowels, skeletal development, the ECG, the serum cholesterol level and the child's physical and mental progress. Overdosage is manifest by diarrhoea, and by accelerated growth and skeletal development as judged by the time of the appearance of the ossification centres; it also makes the child over-excitable.

Prognosis

The outlook depends upon the severity and duration of thyroid deficiency before treatment is started, and no intellectual improvement can be expected in the older child with established cretinism. Foetal deficiency may induce irreversible changes in skeletal and mental development no matter how soon treatment is begun in the neonatal period.

JUVENILE MYXOEDEMA

Definition

Hypothyroidism, which is not present in the neonatal period or in infancy, but first develops in children aged 4–12 and in whom dwarfism is usually the presenting feature.

Aetiology

The cause of the hypothyroidism is not always clear but in some cases the thyroid gland has not developed properly and ectopic thyroid tissue, which produces sufficient thyroid hormones to meet the needs in infancy, fails to do so as the child grows.

Symptoms

In most instances the presenting symptom is shortness of stature. The child may be rather plump with supraclavicular pads of fat but more obvious evidence of thyroid deficiency is lacking and intellect is usually unimpaired. The skeletal proportions are infantile with the upper measurement, from the crown to the symphysis pubis, exceeding the lower measurement from the symphysis to the ground. X-rays show retarded skeletal development and characteristic epiphyseal dysgenesis. Instead of a single focus of ossification in an epiphysis, multiple stippled foci appear. This pathognomonic change is often best seen in the head of the femur but other epiphyses may be involved depending upon the age of onset of thyroid failure.

Diagnosis

The diagnosis is readily confirmed by finding epiphyseal dysgenesis. The PBI is low, but the uptake of radio-iodine in a small area of aberrant thyroid tissue may be increased in an attempt to synthesize sufficient amounts of thyroid hormone. The ECG shows low voltage QRS complexes and flat T-waves. The serum cholesterol level is raised. Hypothyroidism must be considered in the differential diagnosis of any patient with dwarfism.

Treatment

The response to thyroxine, starting with 0·1 mg. daily and increasing after a month to 0·2 mg. and then 0·3 mg. depending on the child's age, is dramatic. This treatment must be continued for the rest of the patient's life.

Prognosis

The prognosis is excellent. Even when the condition has been overlooked and the patient presents in the late teens with dwarfism and primary amenorrhoea in the female or infantile genitalia in the male, normal growth and sexual maturation can be achieved with treatment.

MYXOEDEMA

Synonym. Adult hypothyroidism.

Aetiology

Thyroid deficiency in the adult is much more common in women than men, and usually occurs between the ages of 30 and 50 years with a particular prevalence at the time of the menopause. The cause of the hypothyroidism is often not clear and has in the past been attributed to idiopathic atrophy. Because circulating thyroid antibodies are found in over 80 per cent. of patients with primary myxoedema, it seems probable that auto-immune processes are responsible in most cases; whether these patients represent the ultimate stages of Hashimoto's thyroiditis, in which goitre formation has escaped recognition or never occurred, is as yet uncertain. Myxoedema due to thyroidal atrophy is three times more common than that due to typical lymphadenoid goitre but antibodies to thyroglobulin and thyroid microsomes occur in both as do antibodies to other tissues such as gastric parietal cells and intrinsic factor. Less common causes of myxoedema than atrophic fibrosis or Hashimoto's thyroiditis are radio-iodine used for the treatment of hyperthyroidism [p. 557], virus thyroiditis [p. 562] and too extensive a thyroidectomy. Myxoedema may also be induced by prolonged exposure to goitrogens, such as resorcinol-containing ointment applied to varicose ulcers and the ingestion of iodine-containing cough and asthma cures [p. 556].

Hypothyroidism may also develop secondarily to failure of TSH secretion which is usually an integral part of the syndrome associated with panhypopituitarism [p. 545] but occasionally occurs as a monotrophic pituitary deficiency.

Pathology

The changes in the thyroid gland depend upon the cause. In idiopathic atrophy, in panhypopituitarism and after radio-iodine, little or no thyroid tissue is palpable in the neck. At autopsy the thyroid remnant is fibrosed and shrunken, weighing 3–5 g. instead of the normal 30 g. In Hashimoto's thyroiditis the gland is enlarged; the epithelium is hypertrophied and infiltrated with plasma cells and lymphocytes. Goitrogens also cause thyroidal enlargement and epithelial hyperplasia.

In long-standing cases mucinous material is widely

distributed throughout the extracellular spaces. Atherosclerosis is advanced, and sometimes there is cardiac enlargement and a pericardial effusion.

Symptoms

The severity of the condition varies considerably, epending on the duration and degree of thyroid deficiency. The onset is so insidious that the changes so striking to the alert physician may be completely unnoticed by the patient and the patient's immediate relatives. Complaints are few and often vague. Tiredness, lethargy, constipation, intolerance of cold, stiffness, and aching of muscles attributed to 'rheumatism', or weakness with tingling in the hands (carpal tunnel syndrome) may be presenting symptoms. Deafness may take the patient to the otologist, or menorrhagia to the gynaecological department. Occasionally mental disturbances with hallucinations and paranoia (myxoedema mania) may lead to admission to a psychiatric ward. Neurological symptoms such as epileptiform seizures, drop attacks and ataxia are not uncommon. Atherosclerosis may cause angina pectoris or intermittent claudication.

The appearance of the patient is usually pathognomonic. The face is expressionless, broad and bloated. The eyelids are puffy. The lips and nostrils are thickened. There is a malar flush with a surrounding yellow tinge to the skin caused by carotenaemia. The skin feels dry and coarse; it is thickened by mucinous infiltration but does not pit on pressure. Sweating is absent. Body hair is sparse and short. The voice is croaky and speech is slurred due to mucinous infiltration of the tongue and vocal cords. Cerebration is slowed and memory poor. The tendon reflexes are 'suspended', a normal contraction is followed by a delay before the muscle relaxes. The heart rate is often slow unless anaemia or cardiac failure is present. Three types of anaemia may occur in association with hypothyroidism—iron deficiency with hypochromia often secondary to menorrhagia, a normochromic normocytic anaemia which responds to thyroxine, and a macrocytic anaemia due to vitamin B_{12} deficiency associated with parietal-cell and intrinsic factor antibodies.

About 75 per cent. of myxoedematous patients have hypertension attributable, in the presence of a reduced cardiac output, to increased peripheral vascular resistance which involves also the cerebrovascular circulation. In about one quarter of such cases adequate therapy reduces the blood pressure to normal.

Hypothyroid Coma. In neglected cases the patient may lapse into coma, particularly during spells of cold weather. Usually hypothermia is an important feature. Bleeding from the gastro-intestinal tract, increased bruisibility and cerebrovascular accidents are common in this situation. Myxoedema is but one of several causes of hypothermic coma. Profound damage to skeletal and cardiac muscle is associated with a raised plasma SGOT level, increased creatine kinase and alpha-hydroxybutyrate dehydrogenase. The ECG may become grossly abnormal with prolongation of the P-R interval, widening of the QRS complexes, flattening or inversion of the T-waves, and the development of a J-wave immediately after the R-wave and preceding the ST segment.

Diagnosis

The PBI and plasma thyroxine levels are abnormally low, and the uptake of radio-iodine is greatly reduced. The serum cholesterol is usually raised above 350 mg. per 100 ml. but this change is less common when the thyroid deficiency is secondary to pituitary failure. The history and evidence of gonadal failure supported by laboratory evidence of adrenocortical hypofunction will usually indicate a pituitary deficiency, but long-standing thyroidal failure may induce myxoedematous hypofunction of the adenohypophysis. The distinction between primary and secondary thyroidal failure can be made by radio-iodine studies before and after administration of TSH which will activate the thyroid gland in hypopituitarism but not in primary thyroidal failure [p. 539].

At first sight hypothyroidism may be confused with the nephrotic syndrome, and myxoedema must be considered in elucidating the cause of anaemia or menorrhagia. Although some weight gain occurs, marked obesity is seldom if ever the presenting feature of thyroid deficiency. The sedimentation rate is often increased, probably as a result of increased circulating immunoglobulins. The protein content of the cerebrospinal fluid may also be raised.

Treatment

Substitution therapy with sodium thyroxine should be started cautiously because any sudden increase in metabolism may precipitate angina pectoris, myocardial infarction or cardiac failure. Thyroid extract should not be used, being an impure substance of uncertain biological activity that deteriorates on storage. The initial dose of thyroxine should be 0·05–0·1 mg. daily depending on the patient's age and the duration of the hypothyroidism. In younger patients with a short history the larger dose can safely be used. After a month the dosage is increased by 0·05 mg. and thereafter at 2-weekly intervals by 0·05 mg. until the patient is taking 0·2–0·3 mg. each morning. The biological half-life of sodium thyroxine is such that a single daily dose, rather than divided doses, should be used. The optimal dose, which never exceeds 0·4 mg. daily, is best judged by the patient's appearance, sense of well-being and the plasma thyroxine level. The requirements of thyroxine may be 0·1 mg. higher during the cold winter months than in the summer. Similar increased demands should be met during puberty, pregnancy or lactation. Older patients usually require a somewhat smaller dosage of thyroxine than younger ones. Hypercholesterolaemia, when due to thyroid deficiency, is rapidly corrected by substitution therapy, and the cholesterol level and the tendo Achillis relaxation time are guides to the correct dosage. The ECG usually reverts to normal. Iron or vitamin B_{12} may be required to correct any concurrent anaemia depending on its cause.

Patients with myxoedema secondary to pituitary failure must be treated cautiously because thyroxine may accentuate adrenocortical deficiency. Cortisone should always be given concurrently with the thyroid hormone.

Myxoedema coma is treated by warming the patient gently between blankets, infusing hydrocortisone hemi-succinate or 21-phosphate intravenously providing a clear airway, correcting carbon dioxide retention and giving tri-iodothyronine, 10 μg. thrice daily by gastric tube or intramuscularly. Although the blood sugar level may be raised, intravenous glucose may promote intracellar transfer of carbohydrate.

Prognosis

In most cases the response to treatment is excellent although it may be several months before the patient is completely well. The patient must understand clearly that treatment will have to be continued for the rest of her life. All the symptoms and signs of myxoedema, including the mental changes, are usually reversible provided substitution therapy is not too long delayed. Many patients complain of muscular aches and pain ('rheumatism') as they become euthyroid, but this discomfort soon passes. Manifestations of atherosclerosis, such as angina, are sometimes improved by thyroxine and sometimes aggravated.

Myxoedema coma carries a grave prognosis.

THE PARATHYROID GLANDS

PHYSIOLOGICAL CONSIDERATIONS

The parathyroid glands are concerned with the endocrine control of calcium homeostasis. They are small lenticular bodies, 6 mm. long by 2 mm. wide, and yellow-brown in colour. Usually there are four glands arranged in pairs along the posterior inner border of the lobes of the thyroid but there may be only one or as many as eight. The glands may be embedded within the substance of the thyroid gland or displaced to lie along the course of the trachea or in the anterior mediastinum. The parathyroid glands secrete parathormone, and also, to a much lesser extent, calcitonin which is formed by cells derived from the embryological ultimobranchial glands which become embedded partly in the parathyroid glands and to a greater degree in the thyroid gland where they are represented by the non-colloid containing parafollicular or 'C' cells.

Parathormone

Parathormone is a straight-chain peptide. No trophic hormone of pituitary origin that regulates the rate of parathormone secretion has been detected, and the secretion of the hormone is directly controlled by the serum ionic calcium level, a fall in serum calcium stimulating parathormone secretion and vice versa.

Parathormone has two separate and distinct actions. It mobilizes calcium from the bones, an action similar to and synergistic with vitamin D, and like vitamin D it also enhances intestinal calcium absorption. The resulting hypercalcaemia usually leads to increased urinary calcium excretion. The second action of parathormone is on the renal tubules where it increases phosphate excretion by reducing tubular reabsorption of phosphorus filtered by the glomeruli. Thus in hyperparathyroidism the serum concentration of calcium is raised by increased bone reabsorption and that of phosphorus is lowered by enhanced renal excretion. In parathyroid deficiency the converse occurs.

Calcitonin

Calcitonin, secreted by the parafollicular 'C' cells of the thyroid gland and also by the parathyroid glands, is a peptide containing 32 amino acids. Its action, which is rapid and more evident under experimental conditions in young growing animals, is to lower the serum concentrations of both calcium and phosphorus. The lowering of the serum calcium level is responsible for a reduction in urinary calcium excretion. Its action seems to be related to the inhibition of bone resorption. Its role in calcium homeostasis in man is still uncertain. High levels of the hormone are present in the serum of patients with a medullary carcinoma of the thyroid gland [p. 564] but no changes in the serum calcium level or in bone structure have been observed. Clinical experiments show that exogenous calcitonin in man lowers the hypercalcaemia caused by osteolytic metastases and may relieve the bone pain in Paget's disease. Its future clinical value may lie in the treatment of Paget's disease, of osteoporosis or in retarding the bone wastage found in advancing age, chronic corticosteroid therapy or prolonged immobilization. At the present time these uses are experimental and material is only available for research purposes.

Calcium Balance

The external balance of calcium depends upon the intake and absorption of calcium from the intestinal tract, and its loss in the urine and faeces. The amount taken in depends on the dietary supply, and absorption is modified by the phosphate content of the diet, large amounts tending to increase faecal loss. The absorption of calcium is also facilitated by vitamin D and other unknown, but possibly related, substances which may be elaborated in some patients with sarcoidosis. The action of vitamin D and these related compounds is inhibited by corticosteroids (see below). The plasma calcium level is regulated by intestinal absorption, urinary loss and by the amount of calcium being mobilized from the skeleton by resorption and the amount being deposited in new or maturing bone.

TESTS OF PARATHYROID FUNCTION AND METABOLIC BONE DISEASE

Parathormone Assay

The availability of increased amounts of pure human parathormone has made possible immunoassay of parathyroid hormone in plasma. This technique is as yet not widely practised but may in the future prove decisive in the diagnosis of parathyroid dysfunction.

Serum Calcium Level

The serum calcium level depends to some extent on the analytic method used and with improved techniques the normal range has become narrower. The exact normal values must be determined by each laboratory, but is in order of 9–10·5 mg. per 100 ml. in adults, 9–11·5 mg. in infants and 8–12 mg. in premature infants. The total serum calcium is comprised of free ionized calcium, calcium which is chelated mainly with citrate, and calcium bound to carrier-protein. To avoid fluctuations due to circadian variation, the blood should be taken before breakfast. Venous occlusion must be avoided because the total serum calcium value is related to the serum albumin concentration which is increased by venous stasis. Because a large proportion of the total serum calcium is carried by albumin, the plasma protein level must be estimated in parallel with the calcium, and correction made to the calcium values depending on the serum albumin levels on the basis that each gramme of protein absorbs about 0·8 mg. calcium.

Many factors influence the serum calcium level. Low values occur in hypoparathyroidism; when there is reduced absorption of calcium from the intestine due to dietary deficiency, malabsorption or vitamin D deficiency; in chronic renal disease (renal osteodystrophy); and when the serum albumin level is depressed.

Hypercalcaemia occurs in hyperparathyroidism; when there is excessive intestinal absorption of calcium due to overdosage with vitamin D; in the milk-alkali syndrome which used to develop in patients with peptic ulceration who drank large volumes of milk and took absorbable alkalis such as sodium bicarbonate for the relief of pain; and in a small proportion of patients with sarcoidosis. A high serum calcium level may occur when there is excessive destruction of bone due to myelomatosis, Paget's disease and osteolytic metastases. Rarely hypercalcaemia occurs in association with certain reticuloses and other malignant diseases in which there are no bone metastases, and the increased resorption of bone calcium is attributable to the secretion by the malignant tissue of a parathormone-like substance [Section 4]. Hypercalcaemia may occur also in hyperthyroidism.

Serum Phosphate Level

The serum inorganic phosphate level in normal adults is 3–5 mg. per 100 ml., but may be slightly higher during an active growth phase in children. A high serum phosphate level occurs in chronic renal disease of sufficient severity to cause azotaemia and diminished phosphate excretion. It is a characteristic finding in hypoparathyroidism of any cause, and occurs in some cases of acromegaly but not sufficiently often to be of diagnostic value.

A low serum phosphate level is found in hyperparathyroidism, particularly the primary idiopathic form, but later in the course of the untreated disease the level may rise to normal when impairment of renal function occurs from nephrocalcinosis or renal lithiasis. Hypophosphataemia also occurs in vitamin D deficiency and in the Fanconi syndrome [Section 12] and other renal tubular defects that impair phosphate reabsorption.

Alkaline Phosphatase

The enzyme alkaline phosphatase is produced by many tissues, notably bone, the liver and the intestines. The normal serum concentration of the total amount of the enzyme derived from all sources ranges from 3 to 13 King-Armstrong units per 100 ml. Increased levels occur when there is increased osteoblastic activity such as occurs in hyperparathyroidism, particularly when there is clinical or radiological evidence of bone disease, in Paget's disease (osteitis deformans), in osteomalacia from any cause [Section 11], and to a lesser degree in patients with healing fractures or widespread bone metastases. The alkaline phosphatase level is also raised to about 20 K-A units in growing children.

An increase in alkaline phosphatase activity is commonly found in the serum of patients with liver disease, and particularly high values are found in obstructive jaundice, hepatic metastases causing destruction of liver tissue and in ascending cholangitis. In these conditions the serum level of the enzyme 5-nucleotidase is increased and this makes it possible to distinguish an increase in serum alkaline phosphatase of liver origin from that due to bone disease in which the 5-nucleotidase is normal.

Hydrocortisone Suppression Test of Hypercalcaemia

The hypercalcaemia of hyperparathyroidism has to be distinguished from other causes of a raised serum calcium level. This can usually be done by observing the effect on the serum calcium level of hydrocortisone (cortisol) given for 10 days in a dose of 40 mg. eight-hourly. In hyperparathyroidism the serum calcium level does not change significantly but almost always in other causes of hypercalcaemia the serum calcium level falls significantly, usually into the normal range.

Tubular Reabsorption of Phosphate

In hyperparathyroidism less of the phosphate filtered by the glomeruli is reabsorbed by the renal tubules, so that the percentage tubular reabsorption of phosphate (TRP) is decreased. The test involves measuring the clearance of phosphate and also of creatinine (as an index of glomerular filtration rate) so that the amount of phosphate filtered by the glomeruli can be calculated and the amount finally excreted in the urine measured. This test may be of value in equivocal cases of hyperparathyroidism and the best discrimination between the normal and the abnormal is achieved if the patient has for 3 days before the test a high phosphate intake. This is obtained by a diet containing 1550 mg. phosphorus and 600 mg. calcium, and in addition giving an extra 1550 mg. phosphorus in the form of Na_2HPO_4 and NaH_2PO_4 in separate gelatin capsules three times daily before meals. The test is only valid when there is no azotaemia. Under these conditions of a high phosphate intake the normal percentage tubular reabsorption of phosphorus is 65–77, and lower values are obtained in patients with hyperparathyroidism.

Bone Biopsy

Biopsy of bone, usually of the iliac crest, is a special test that can be of considerable clinical and research value in difficult cases of metabolic bone disease. It will distinguish between osteoporosis and osteomalacia because the latter condition shows the osteoid seams to be widened and uncalcified [see Section 11].

In most cases of parathyroid or metabolic bone disease only a few of these tests are necessary to establish an accurate diagnosis. The clinical and radiological findings, the serum calcium, phosphorus and alkaline phosphatase levels, and in cases of established hypercalcaemia the hydrocortisone suppression test, usually provide sufficient information to reach the correct diagnosis.

HYPERPARATHYROIDISM

Overactivity of the parathyroid glands may occur under three distinct circumstances. In *primary* hyperparathyroidism the excess secretion of parathormone is due to an idiopathic primary disorder of the glands and is unassociated with any recognized previous disturbance of calcium metabolism. *Secondary* hyperparathyroidism may develop secondarily to any condition that lowers, or tends to lower, the serum calcium level and which therefore acts as a stimulus to parathormone secretion. The *tertiary* form is an extension of secondary hyperparathyroidism in which the prolonged hypocalcaemic stimulus to the parathyroid glands results in the eventual development of autonomous parathormone-secreting parathyroid adenomata.

TABLE 40

TYPES AND DIFFERENTIAL DIAGNOSIS OF HYPERPARATHYROIDISM

TYPE OF HYPERPARATHYROIDISM	CAUSE	PARATHYROID PATHOLOGY	SERUM CALCIUM	SERUM PHOSPHORUS	SERUM ALKALINE PHOSPHATE	BONE CHANGES
Primary	Idiopathic	Adenoma, hyperplasia or carcinoma	Raised	Low	Normal or raised if bone disease is present	None, or osteitis fibrosa generalisata or cystica
Secondary	Malabsorption syndromes	Hyperplasia	Low or normal	Normal	Raised	Osteomalacia ± osteitis fibrosa
	Chronic renal disease	Hyperplasia	Low or normal	High	Raised	
Tertiary	Malabsorption syndromes	Adenomata	High	Low	Raised	Osteomalacia ± osteitis fibrosa
	Chronic renal disease	Adenomata	High	Normal or high	Raised	

PRIMARY HYPERPARATHYROIDISM

Synonyms. When clinical or radiological evidence of metabolic bone disease is the presenting or dominant feature of primary hyperparathyroidism the terms osteitis fibrosa generalisata or, if cysts are present in the bones, osteitis fibrosa cystica generalisata, are used to describe the skeletal changes.

Definition

Primary hyperparathyroidism is a condition in which for reasons unknown the parathyroid glands secrete excess parathormone. The clinical manifestations are symptoms due to renal calculi, hypercalcaemia or metabolic bone disease.

Aetiology

Primary hyperparathyroidism is a rare condition of unknown cause. The disease occurs more commonly in women than men, usually at the age of 30–60 years. Sometimes multiple adenomata of the parathyroid glands are associated with tumours of the adenohypophysis (eosinophilic causing acromegaly, or chromophobe adenomata causing pressure effects or hypopituitarism) and also with adenomata of the islet cells of the pancreas, a combination known as *endocrine adenomatosis* (Schmid's syndrome). The finding of multiple adenomata in either the parathyroid glands or the pancreatic islets should stimulate investigation for the other.

Pathology

The commonest cause of primary hyperparathyroidism is a single adenoma in one parathyroid gland which may vary in diameter from a few millimetres to 3 cm. Sometimes multiple adenomata are present. Less commonly there is hyperplasia of one or all parathyroid glands which may have a combined weight of 2–70 g. or more compared with a normal of about 120 mg. In less than 4 per cent. of cases the cause of primary hyperparathyroidism is a carcinoma.

Increased urinary excretion of calcium and phosphorus may lead to the formation of renal calculi composed of calcium phosphate or oxalate, and these may develop without evidence of increased urinary calcium excretion. Calcium is also deposited in the renal parenchyma but only rarely is this sufficient to be detectable by X-rays (nephrocalcinosis). Associated pyelonephritis is common.

Increased resorption of calcium from the bones causes generalized skeletal rarefaction with the development in some cases of cysts, particularly in the femora, humeri, mandible, clavicles or ribs. The bones are thinned and the marrow replaced by yellow-red osteoclastic giant-cell tumours which may deform the bone and predispose to pathological fractures. Why some patients but not others develop clinical or radiological evidence of bone disease in hyperparathyroidism is not known, but it is possible that bone changes are more evident in long-standing cases in which the dietary intake of calcium has been low.

Symptoms

Hyperparathyroidism is usually of many years' standing before clinical manifestations develop. Nowadays patients with this condition are often first diagnosed by the chance finding of a high serum calcium and a low serum phosphate level without any volunteered symptoms to suggest hyperparathyroidism. These cases, diagnosed 'by mistake', merit treatment if the later complications and clinical manifestations of the disease are to be avoided.

Clinical hyperparathyroidism usually presents in one of three different ways. The commonest presentation is a renal disorder due to a calculus causing colic, haematuria or renal infection. About 5 per cent. of patients with renal lithiasis prove to have primary hyperparathyroidism, and the incidence rises to about 15 per cent. in those with recurrent renal calculi. Nephrocalcinosis causes considerable disturbance of renal tubular function leading to polyuria, thirst and polydipsia. Left untreated primary hyperparathyroidism may terminate in renal failure.

The second mode of presentation is related to the hypercalcaemia. The onset of symptoms is usually gradual, the patient complaining of weight loss, anorexia, nausea, weakness, drowsiness, thirst and polyuria. Often mental changes are prominent, and features of anxiety or agitated depression may confuse the diagnostician. About 15 per cent. of such patients have a peptic ulcer and a higher proportion complain of dyspepsia. Hence in patients with unexplained 'indigestion' or with peptic ulceration, the serum calcium level should always be measured. A number of instances of acute or chronic pancreatitis have been observed in patients with primary hyperparathyroidism. Sometimes the onset of hypercalcaemia is sudden and associated with an acute and marked rise in serum calcium to 14–20 mg. per 100 ml. This results in a shock-like state with vomiting, pyrexia and coma. Unless recognized and treated promptly death may occur from anuria or cardiac arrest.

The third and least common method of presentation is metabolic bone disease. A pathological fracture may occur or the patient may complain of backache, pain in the bones on jolting or walking downstairs, or simply of 'rheumatism'. A cyst in the jaw (epulis) may take the patient to a dentist or deformity of a bone to an orthopaedic surgeon. Bowing of a long bone or kyphosis may develop.

Physical signs which specifically suggest primary hyperparathyroidism are uncommon except those related to skeletal changes. Rarely a tumour is palpable in the neck or displaces the trachea or oesophagus on radiological examination. Metastatic calcium deposits under the conjunctiva or at the lateral corneal edge, crescentic in shape and quite unlike the circular ring of arcus senilis, may cause a pathognomonic keratopathy, sometimes better seen by slit-lamp examination. Muscular weakness and hypotonicity due to hypercalcaemia may be marked and sometimes in the later stages the patient has a curious waddling gait.

Diagnosis

The clinical diagnosis of primary hyperparathyroidism can usually be confirmed by the cardinal biochemical abnormalities of an increased serum calcium level and a lowered serum phosphate level. These are the *sine qua non* of the condition, but in mild cases repeated serum calcium determinations may be necessary, and due allowance must always be made for the serum albumin level in interpreting the serum calcium value [Section 4]. A low phosphate dietary intake (430 mg. daily) for 3 days tends to increase the serum calcium level and may raise it from the upper range of normal to the unequivocally abnormal. In obscure cases measurement of the serum ionized calcium level as determined by dialysis, the percentage of tubular reabsorption of phosphate [Section 12], the urinary calcium excretion whilst the patient is on a low calcium diet providing 400 mg. daily, and increased urinary excretion of hydroxyproline (normal adult range 15–55 mg. per 24 hours) may help in establishing the diagnosis.

X-rays may show characteristic subperiosteal erosions of the phalanges, and loss of the lamina dura round the teeth. In osteitis fibrosa cystica the radiological changes are usually characteristic and the serum alkaline phosphatase is raised.

In long-standing cases of primary hyperparathyroidism biochemical confirmation often becomes difficult because renal damage leads to an increase in the serum phosphorus level and a reduction in the serum calcium level to normal. In these circumstances the distinction between primary hyperparathyroidism and the secondary or tertiary forms becomes difficult (see below) although in the last two types there is usually a long history of renal disease, ectopic calcification is more common and bone biopsy may show evidence of osteomalacia as well as osteitis fibrosa.

Primary hyperparathyroidism must be differentiated from other conditions that cause hypercalcaemia [p. 570], but in most of these the serum phosphorus level is not so characteristically low as it is in parathyroid overactivity. The distinction can usually be made by the hydrocortisone suppression test [p. 570] which will usually decrease the hypercalcaemia found in myelomatosis, sarcoidosis, reticuloses and malignant diseases.

The bone changes in hyperparathyroidism must be distinguished from the localized but sometimes multiple lesions caused by osteoclastoma (focal osteitis fibrosa or circumscripta) which usually affects young adults. Paget's disease (osteitis deformans) with an enlarged head, bowing of the legs, and a very high serum alkaline phosphatase level and radiologically a 'moth-eaten' skull seldom presents diagnostic difficulties. In myelomatosis the E.S.R. is markedly raised and a characteristic abnormal protein is usually present in the plasma; Bence-Jones proteinuria may occur and the radiological appearances should not cause confusion. In sarcoidosis skeletal changes are rare and usually confined to the feet or hands; the radiological appearances should cause no confusion and a chest X-ray may show hilar lymphadenopathy. Polyostotic fibrous dysplasia is a unilateral skeletal disorder associated with areas of brown pigmentation in the skin and precocious puberty in girls; the serum calcium and phosphorus levels are normal.

Treatment

Symptoms due to acute hypercalcaemia must be treated by lowering the serum calcium level. This may be achieved by infusing dilute phosphate solution, each litre containing 11·5 g. Na_2HPO_4 and 2·58 g KH_2PO_4. Initially 500 ml. of this solution is infused over 4 hours and the serum calcium level measured again. If necessary a further 300 ml. can be infused. Alternatively the hypercalcaemia can be reduced by chelation with sodium EDTA, 200 mg. per kg. body weight being infused intravenously over $\frac{1}{2}$–1 hour. Calcitonin is also of value in this situation.

Primary hyperparathyroidism is treated surgically. Difficulty may be experienced in locating an adenoma particularly if it occupies an ectopic site. All four glands should, if possible, be identified because a relapse will occur if there are multiple adenomata and only one is removed. When hyperplasia is present, three of the enlarged glands should be removed and sub-total removal of the fourth carried out. The chief postoperative complication is hypocalcaemic tetany, the treatment of which is described on page 575.

Prognosis

To some extent the prognosis of the skeletal changes depends upon how long the disease has been present before treatment is instituted. As a rule there is striking improvement in the bone disease but usually little improvement in the renal damage. Pyelonephritis may be difficult to control; hypertension may develop and become progressive, and renal function deteriorate further. Hence the necessity for early treatment before renal involvement is advanced.

SECONDARY AND TERTIARY HYPERPARATHYROIDISM

Synonyms. Renal or uraemic osteodystrophy and, particularly in children, renal rickets are terms used to describe the bone changes that may occur in association with chronic renal disease.

Definitions

Secondary and tertiary hyperparathyroidism are conditions that may develop in response to any primary disease that lowers or tends to lower the serum calcium level. In a sense *secondary hyperparathyroidism* is a physiological response to a low serum calcium level, and is characterized by compensatory hyperplasia of the parathyroid glands with increased secretion of parathormone in an attempt to maintain a normal serum calcium level. *Tertiary hyperparathyroidism* is a pathological extension of the secondary form; autonomous single or multiple adenoma develop in the previously hyperplastic glands and the serum calcium level is raised above normal.

Aetiology

Secondary or tertiary hyperparathyroidism may develop in steatorrhoea due to such malabsorption syndromes as coeliac disease, gluten-sensitive enteropathy and after gastrectomy. The other important aetiological factor is long-standing renal disease of any cause, usually associated with azotaemia and particularly marked in growing children. Under these circumstances, for reasons unknown, resistance to vitamin D develops or there is failure to convert calciferol to biologically active metabolites, with the result that calcium absorption from the intenstine is reduced.

Pathology

The bones may show the changes of osteomalacia attributable to the underlying primary disease or generalized osteitis fibrosa produced by the parathyroid overactivity, or a combination of both. Some degree of osteosclerosis is also common. In tertiary hyperparathyroidism the bone changes may be indistinguishable from those found in the primary form, but because of associated hyperphosphataemia, induced by renal failure, ectopic calcification is more common.

Symptoms

The clinical picture may be dominated by manifestations of the predisposing disorder. In other instances metabolic bone disease is the presenting feature with skeletal pain and deformity, rickets in children, or a waddling gait. In almost all cases osteomalacia is the most striking radiological and histological finding attributable to the poor intestinal absorption of calcium induced by the primary disease. To this is added osteitis fibrosa generalisata in varying degree but particularly so in tertiary hyperparathyroidism in which it may be more prominent than osteomalacia.

In secondary hyperparathyroidism the serum calcium level is low or normal (never supranormal) and the serum phosphate level is normal or elevated. In tertiary hyperparathyroidism, hypercalcaemia is found but this may only become persistently apparent after calciferol has been given for the control of secondary hyperparathyroidism and stopped because of the development of a raised serum calcium level. The serum phosphate level is depressed in malabsorption syndromes, and normal or more often raised when the underlying cause is renal disease. In both secondary and tertiary forms the alkaline phosphatase is usually raised, in general depending on the degree of osteomalacia. Radiological evidence of ectopic calcification in the arteries or subcutaneous tissues is much more common in tertiary than primary hyperparathyroidism.

Treatment

In secondary hyperparathyroidism due to malabsorption, correction of the underlying disorder and treatment with calciferol will suppress the stimulus to parathyroid overactivity. In cases due to renal disorders treatment with large doses of vitamin D, 1·25–12·5 mg. per day, may be required depending upon the individual response, and there is a liability to acceleration of ectopic calcification unless the hyperphosphataemia is corrected by regular oral administration of 50–100 ml. aluminium hydroxide in divided doses to impede intestinal phosphorus absorption.

In tertiary hyperparathyroidism, partial parathyroidectomy is indicated as the only means to reduce the autonomous parathyroid overactivity, the hypercalcaemia and control the metabolic bone disease.

Prognosis

In malabsorption syndromes the prognosis is good but in chronic renal disease the prognosis is grave both in terms of the skeletal changes and the underlying kidney disorder.

HYPOPARATHYROIDISM

Definition

Hypoparathyroidism is a condition in which biochemical changes and symptoms result from insufficient secretion of parathormone.

Aetiology

The commonest cause of hypoparathyroidism is the inadvertent removal of or damage to the parathyroid glands during thyroidectomy. It may also occur after surgical treatment of primary or tertiary hyperparathyroidism. In these circumstances the deficiency of parathormone secretion may be temporary, due to trauma, oedema or interference with the blood supply to the remaining parathyroid tissue, or it may be permanent.

Much less commonly hypoparathyroidism may be an hereditary or sporadic idiopathic disease attributable, when hereditary, to the inheritance of a sex-linked or autosomal genetic defect. An hereditary, sometimes familial, sex-linked form may occur in boys and is usually manifest early in life. Often there are no other congenital defects and the prognosis is good if the diagnosis is made early. A non-sex-linked form may occur in association with embryological failure of development of the third and fourth branchial clefts. In this condition the thymus also fails to develop and the resultant immunological deficit usually results in early death from infection or diarrhoea. In about 10 per cent. of sporadic or hereditary cases there is associated adrenal insufficiency, associated with auto-antibodies to parathyroid and adrenocortical tissue.

Pathology

The decrease in parathormone secretion causes increased tubular reabsorption of phosphorus, decreased resorption of skeletal calcium and reduced intestinal absorption of calcium. The serum level of phosphorus rises and that of calcium falls. The urinary excretion of calcium is reduced. The lowered serum calcium level is responsible for the increased excitability of nervous tissue, the cataracts that may develop and the other clinical manifestations noted below.

Symptoms

Manifestations of hypoparathyroidism may develop within 48 hours of thyroidectomy or parathyroidectomy. The nursing staff may be the first to notice that the patient is unexpectedly anxious or irritable. In severe cases hallucinations, delusions or dementia may occur. Often the patient's first complaint is of tingling or numbness round the mouth or in the fingers or toes. At this point latent tetany may be revealed by tapping over the facial nerve and inducing contraction of the lips and facial muscles (Chvostek's sign)—a phenomenon sometimes found in perfectly normal people—or by inflating a sphygmomanometer cuff to a little above the systolic blood pressure for 3 minutes and inducing a *main d'accoucheur* (Trousseau's sign). As the serum calcium falls further, overt tetany may be manifest by carpopedal spasms. Painful cramps cause flexion at the elbows and wrists, and the hollowed hands are flexed at the metacarpophalangeal joints with extension of the thumb and fingers (*main d'accoucheur*). There may be plantar flexion of the feet and adduction of the toes. Spasm of the facial and masseter muscles causes risus sardonicus. The laryngeal muscles may be implicated causing hoarseness and stridor (laryngismus stridulus) and lead to a mistaken diagnosis of recurrent laryngeal nerve palsy. Generalized epileptiform convulsions may occur.

In idiopathic hypoparathyroidism or in long-standing untreated cases of the acquired disease changes in ectodermal tissue are common. Cataracts develop; the skin is coarse and dry; the scalp hair falls out and the nails are brittle and deformed; there may be infection with moniliasis. Papilloedema and raised intracranial pressure may occur with radiological evidence of calcification in the basal ganglia of the brain. When the onset of hypoparathyroidism occurs before the permanent teeth are mature, they become ridged and malformed.

Diagnosis

The recognition of postoperative hypoparathyroidism as the cause of tetany is seldom a problem. The serum phosphorus is raised above 4·5 mg. per 100 ml. and the serum calcium lowered to 8·5 mg. or less per 100 ml. The ECG shows prolongation of the Q-T interval in hypocalcaemia. Lesser degrees of acquired hypoparathyroidism may be manifest by symptoms of depression or an anxiety state. Such symptoms are however, particularly in patients who previously had hyperthyroidism, often psychogenic and not due to a minor degree of hypoparathyroidism. Patients who have undergone thyroidectomy should routinely have their serum calcium and phosphorus levels measured before leaving hospital. If the serum calcium level is marginally low or there is doubt as to the cause of the patient's psychological state, an EDTA infusion test should be done. Sodium EDTA in a dose of 70 mg. per kg. body weight is infused in isotonic saline intravenously together with 2 per cent. procaine over a period of 2 hours. In patients with normal parathyroid function, the serum calcium level falls, because of chelation of calcium with EDTA, to about 7 mg. per 100 ml. at the end of the infusion. Thereafter the level rises gradually to reach its previous original value in 12 hours. When there is parathyroid deficiency, the rise in the serum calcium level is delayed.

Idiopathic hypoparathyroidism and long-standing untreated cases of the acquired form of the disease present a considerable problem in differential diagnosis. Tetany may not be manifested in these cases despite a surprisingly low serum calcium level when this is eventually measured. The differential diagnoses involve epilepsy, cataracts, emotional disturbances which in a child may be misinterpreted as mental deficiency, and papilloedema and raised intracranial pressure suggesting a cerebral tumour. The hair, skin and nail abnormalities may take the patient to the dermatologist.

Tetany occurs in a number of other conditions that cause hypocalcaemia or alkalosis which reduces the serum level of ionized calcium. The differentiation of these conditions is seldom difficult [TABLE 41, p. 576].

Treatment

The acute symptoms of hypocalcaemia are promptly relieved by raising the serum calcium level by the slow intravenous injection of 20 ml. of a 10 per cent. solution of calcium gluconate. Vitamin D_2 (calciferol), 1·25 mg. thrice daily, is started and the serum calcium level measured daily. As soon as the level begins to rise maintenance therapy, which, depending on the cause of the hypoparathyroidism may be either temporary or permanent, is given with calciferol or pure dihydrotachysterol in amounts that maintain the serum calcium level at 9·5 mg. per 100 ml. The dose of vitamin D_2 required varies between 0·25 and 1·25 mg. once or twice daily, and of dihydrotachysterol between 0·25 and 1·0 daily. Patients' requirements vary from time to time and continued biochemical supervision is necessary. In most instances the serum phosphorus level takes longer to fall to normal than the calcium level to rise. The response to calciferol and dihydrotachysterol is delayed so the dosage should seldom be increased more frequently than every 4–6 weeks. Particularly careful supervision is required in the late stages of pregnancy and after delivery because at this time there may be enhanced sensitivity to calciferol and hypercalcaemia may develop. All patients should be told the symptoms of hypercalcaemia (thirst, polyuria, headaches, vomiting, diarrhoea and lethargy) and must report to hospital if these develop.

Oral supplements of calcium may be required (calcium lactate, 2 G. thrice daily, equivalent to 0·78 G. calcium daily; calcium gluconate tablets of which 18 provide 1 G. calcium daily; or the more palatable *Sandocal* effervescent tablets each of which provides 0·4 G. calcium).

Prognosis

Many cases of acquired postoperative hypoparathyroidism improve spontaneously after some weeks because the remaining parathyroid tissue hypertrophies or recovers from the operative trauma. Recovery from symptoms of tetany should not induce a false sense of security as many patients adapt to a low serum calcium level only to develop the other manifestations of chronic hypocalcaemia later. Hence the necessity for estimating the serum calcium level. In some instances of acquired hypoparathyroidism and in all idiopathic cases lifelong treatment is required. The prognosis is good in most idiopathic cases provided the diagnosis is made early before cataracts or brain damage have developed.

PSEUDOHYPOPARATHYROIDISM

Pseudohypoparathyroidism is a very rare condition of unknown aetiology which is genetically transmitted as a dominant trait with incomplete penetration depending on sex as females are affected twice as frequently as males. The condition is characterized by parathyroid glands which are normal or hyperplastic but there is apparent failure of the tissues to respond to parathormone.

Symptoms

Clinical manifestations are usually declared in early life with mental deficiency, epilepsy or tetany. The patient is usually short in stature, has a rounded face with frontal bossing of the skull. Characteristically the hands are stubby with shortness of the metacarpal and phalangeal bones of the first, fourth and fifth digits. Ectopic deposits of bone may develop in muscles, tendons, connective tissue and skin. All the other features of hypoparathyroidism (see above) may be present.

Diagnosis

This is suggested by the characteristic clinical appearance and features, by the hyperphosphataemia, the hypocalcaemia and by the absence of proteinuria, azotaemia or other evidence of renal disease.

The condition is distinguished from idiopathic or acquired hypoparathyroidism by the Ellsworth-Howard test, in which the urinary excretion of phosphate is measured for 5 hours after an intravenous injection of 40 B.P. Units (200 U.S.P. Units) of parathormone of biological potency proven in a normal control subject. The degree of increase in phosphaturia is compared with that during a control period of similar duration on the previous day after an injection of saline. In idiopathic or acquired hypoparathyroidism the increase in phosphate excretion is of the order of ten-fold, whereas in pseudohypoparathyroidism the increase is less than three-fold.

Occasionally pseudohypoparathyroidism is confused

with ankylosing spondylitis because of calcification of the vertebral ligaments. The age of onset, the normality of the sacro-iliac joints and the characteristic appearances of the hands and face make a clear distinction.

Treatment

This is the same as for hypoparathyroidism but usually higher doses of vitamin D or dihydrotachysterol are required to control the serum calcium level and to prevent epilepsy. Often treatment is not begun early enough to prevent mental subnormality.

PSEUDO-PSEUDOHYPOPARATHYROIDISM

Pseudo-pseudohypoparathyroidism probably represents an incomplete form of pseudohypoparathyroidism without the metabolic abnormalities of raised phosphate and lower calcium levels. In such cases the characteristic features of the hands, the facies and calcification exist.

TABLE 41

CAUSES AND DIFFERENTIAL DIAGNOSIS OF TETANY

CAUSE	SERUM			REMARKS
	CALCIUM (9–11 mg./100 ml.)	PHOSPHORUS (3–5 mg./100 ml.)	BICARBONATE (24–31 mEq./litre)	
Low calcium intake, vitamin D deficiency, malabsorption of calcium (e.g. steatorrhoea)	Normal or Low	Low	Normal	Serum calcium and phosphorus levels depend on degree of secondary hyperparathyroidism
Hypoparathyroidism	Low	High	Normal	
Respiratory alkalosis due to hyperventilation	Normal	Normal	Low or Normal	Blood pH high
Metabolic alkalosis due to persistent vomiting or excessive intake of alkalis	Normal	Normal	High	Hypochloraemia
Renal failure with azotaemia	Normal or Low	High	Low	Usually proteinuria and raised blood urea. Calcium level depends on the degree of secondary hyperparathyroidism. Liability to tetany offset by acidosis. Hypertension.
Renal tubular acidosis	Low	Low	Low	Liability to tetany offset by acidosis.

THE ADRENAL GLANDS

PHYSIOLOGICAL CONSIDERATIONS

The two adrenal glands, each of which normally weighs 4–7 g., are composed of an outer cortex and an inner medulla which are developmentally, histologically and physiologically distinct. The cells in the yellow-brown cortex are arranged in three layers—an outer zona glomerulosa, a middle zona fasciculata of lipid-containing storage cells, and an inner zona reticularis. A large number of steroidal hormones are secreted by the adrenal cortex and, depending on their main physiological action, these are classified as mineralocorticoids, glucocorticoids, androgens and, of lesser clinical importance, progesterone and oestrone.

Aldosterone

The chief mineralocorticoid is aldosterone, which is secreted by the cells of the zona glomerulosa, and acts on the distal renal convoluted tubules where it enhances the reabsorption of sodium in exchange for potassium and hydrogen ions. It also increases the reabsorption of sodium in exchange for potassium in the glands responsible for the secretion of sweat, saliva, tears and gastric juice. Aldosterone plays an important role in the regulation of the body's sodium balance. The mechanism by which aldosterone secretion is controlled is still not wholly understood. Pituitary control via ACTH is slight and probably unimportant both physiologically and clinically. The most important regulatory system is the renin-angiotensin mechanism.

Renin is a proteolytic enzyme which is liberated from the juxtaglomerular apparatus composed of the juxtaglomerular cells, located in the media of the afferent glomerular arterioles, and the macula densa, a plaque of specialized cells situated in the nephron at the junction between the ascending limb of Henle's loop and the distal tubule. This segment of the nephron lies in contact with the glomerulus from which it originates and its cells are contiguous with the juxtaglomerular cells. Renin acts on an α-2-globulin in the plasma to form a decapeptide angiotensin I which in turn is converted by a circulating enzyme to form the octapeptide angiotensin II. This substance is the primary stimulator of the adrenocortical zona glomerulosa to secrete aldosterone.

The plasma volume, the extracellular concentrations of sodium and potassium and the over-all balances of these ions influence the secretion of renin and aldosterone. If the total exchangeable body sodium is high, the plasma levels of renin and aldosterone are low so that sodium is eliminated in the urine, and conversely when there is sodium depletion the plasma levels of these compounds are raised so that sodium is conserved by the distal renal tubules. Thus aldosterone secretion is enhanced by a low sodium intake, haemorrhage and dehydration. It is also increased by a high potassium intake. Aldosterone secretion is depressed by a high salt intake, expansion of the extracellular fluid volume and by potassium depletion.

Desoxycorticosterone (DOC) and the synthetic compound 9-alpha-flurohydrocortisone (fludrocortisol, *Florinef*) are two substances with strong mineralcorticoid activity and are used for the correction of aldosterone deficiency in Addison's disease and after total adrenalectomy. The latter compound is usually preferred because it can be given by mouth whereas DOC has to be administered by intramuscular injection.

Glucocorticoids

The chief glucocorticoids secreted by the human adrenal cortex are cortisol (hydrocortisone) and to a lesser extent corticosterone. The secretion of glucocorticoids is regulated by the release of ACTH from the basophil cells of the adenohypophysis. The release of ACTH is mediated by a corticotrophin-release factor, a polypeptide related to oxytocin and vasopressin, which is released from the median eminence of the hypothalamus and passes in the portal venous system to the anterior pituitary gland. This hypothalamic control of the secretion of ACTH and hence of glucocorticoids is provoked by 'stress' due to such factors as surgery, infections, noxious chemical agents, environmental factors and emotional disturbances. This mechanism provides a means for the temporary elevation of the plasma cortisol level, and takes precedence over a second method of control whereby the secretion of ACTH is regulated by the plasma level of cortisol. When the plasma cortisol level rises the release of ACTH is suppressed, and when the level falls more ACTH is liberated. This feed-back mechanism is of importance in maintaining the plasma level of cortisol within physiological limits throughout the day.

Glucocorticoids have a wide range of physiological actions. They promote the formation of glucose from protein. An excess of cortisol leads to hyperglycaemia, and a deficiency to hypoglycaemia particularly after fasting. The catabolism of protein is enhanced and hypersecretion of cortisol induces a negative nitrogen balance, muscle wasting, cessation of growth, thinning of the skin and osteoporosis. Glucocorticoids influence the renal blood flow and a deficiency is associated with an inability to eliminate a water load. Cortisol has an effect on sodium and potassium metabolism similar to that of more powerful mineralocorticoids, such as aldosterone, but is much less potent in this action. Excess may cause sodium retention and a rise in blood pressure, whereas a deficiency results in renal loss of sodium, potassium retention and hypotension. Glucocorticoids play an important role in modifying the responses of the organism to infections, trauma and all types of physical and psychological stress. A deficiency lowers the ability to withstand any stress and death may occur suddenly from hypoglycaemia and hypotension. Excess cortisol, on the other hand, reduces the normal defensive responses to inflammation, and this effect, mediated through depression of immunological response, is used to suppress the rejection of an organ-transplant and also to control the manifestations of auto-immune diseases.

Glucocorticoids influence the central nervous system. Psychological disturbances and EEG abnormalities are common in both hypo- and hyper-secretion. Some patients develop an addiction to glucocorticoids which is unrelated to physiological requirements.

Synthetic Glucocorticoids

A large number of compounds have been synthesized with an action similar to cortisol. Cortisone is converted in the liver to cortisol. Others, such as prednisone and prednisolone, have a less potent effect on sodium metabolism and clinically less often induce oedema or hypertension. For this reason they are preferred for the treatment of conditions in which the therapeutic objective is to suppress inflammation or hypersensitivity reactions.

Androgens

A number of hormones with varying degrees of androgenic activity are secreted by the adrenal cortex. Normally these compounds are not secreted until puberty, after which their secretory rate is at least in part under the control of ACTH secretion. Together with other androgenic hormones elaborated by the interstitial cells of the testes and to a lesser extent by the ovaries, these compounds enhance protein anabolism and promote the development of male secondary sexual characteristics. Their anabolic action is shown by an acceleration of skeletal growth which is eventually limited by fusion of the epiphyses, and by an increase in muscular development and strength. Maturation of the scrotum, penis, prostate and larynx in the male, and of the clitoris in the female depend upon androgen secretion. These hormones promote the growth of facial and body hair, increase the greasiness of the skin and enhance the liability to acne. In both sexes androgens increase sexual libido.

TESTS OF ADRENOCORTICAL FUNCTION

Techniques are available for measuring the concentration in the plasma and urine, and also the secretory or production rates, of individual adrenocortical hormones but these methods are too complex for routine use although they may be essential under especially difficult diagnostic situations. For clinical purposes procedures which measure groups of hormones or their metabolites in plasma or urine are usually sufficiently informative.

Plasma 11-Hydroxycorticosteroids. A rapid and simple method is available for measuring compounds in plasma with a Δ^4-3-ketone structure associated with an hydroxyl (-OH) group at the C-11 position in the steroidal molecule. These 11-hydroxycorticosteroid compounds comprise in man cortisol and corticosterone, hence the colloquial but incorrect term the plasma 'cortisol' level. The chemical reaction is dependent on fluorescence which is not produced by synthetic compounds such as prednisone, dexamethasone or fludrocortisone. The great merit of this technique is that samples of plasma can be rapidly assayed. The normal range of 11-hydroxycorticosteroids in a blood sample taken between 9 and 10 a.m. is 5·7–23·7 μg. per 100 ml. with a mean of 14·7 μg. per 100 ml. The level changes during the day and this is discussed on page 579 under circadian rhythm. Because of a rise in the particular protein (transcortin) that carries cortisol in the blood stream, high 'cortisol' values are found in pregnancy and when oestrogens (including oral contraceptive pills) are being taken. Mepacrine and spironolactone interfere with the chemical analysis.

The measurement of *urinary steroids* and their metaboliets usually requires the collection of a complete 24-hour sample. Preferably the urine should be collected under refrigerated conditions but if this is not possible 5 ml. chloroform should be added to the bottle which should be well shaken after the addition of each urine specimen.

Urinary 11-Hydroxycorticosteroids. This rapid screening method is similar to that used for measuring 11-hydroxycorticosteroids in plasma. It estimates mainly free unconjugated cortisol and its metabolite 20-hydroxycortisol. The results of this procedure are more closely related to the true production rate of cortisol from the adrenal glands than, for example, the urinary excretion of 17-oxogenic steroids (see below). In adults the normal upper limit is 350 μg. per 24 hours. Glucose does not interfere with the estimation but mepacrine may produce fluorescence for as long as 5 weeks after stopping its administration.

Increased excretion of 11-hydroxycorticoids occurs in Cushing's syndrome and is of particular value in distinguishing this condition from obesity of non-endocrine origin. The value rises when the adrenal glands are stimulated with ACTH or as a result of indirect stimulation of the pituitary gland to secrete ACTH. Decreased 11-hydroxycorticosteroid excretion occurs in adrenal insufficiency, panhypopituitarism, myxoedema and during administration of synthetic corticosteroid compounds which suppress ACTH secretion.

Total 17-Oxogenic Steroids (and 17-Hydroxycorticosteroids). The 17-oxogenic steroids are derived from C-21 compounds which, when the side-chain at the C-17 position is cleaved by oxidation during analysis, yield 17-oxosteroids. These compounds are largely derived from metabolites of cortisol and its inactive precursors. The normal range in adult females is 5–18 mg. per 24 hours and in adult males 6–22 mg. per 24 hours. Before puberty and in the elderly lower values are found. The presence of glucose in the urine will give falsely low values unless special measures are adopted.

Decreased excretion of 17-oxogenic steroids occurs usually in Addison's disease, panhypopituitarism, myxoedema, during administration of synthetic glucocorticosteroids such as dexamethasone which depress ACTH secretion, and in conditions associated with a reduction in glomerular filtration rate. Increased secretion is found in many but not all cases of Cushing's syndrome, in some patients with obesity, during administration of ACTH and as a result of indirect stimulation of the pituitary to excrete ACTH by administration of metyrapone [p. 541] and other stimuli such as insulin-induced hypoglycaemia or vasopressin.

Neutral 17-Oxosteroids. Urinary neutral 17-oxosteroids are compounds derived from both androgenic and glucocorticoid hormones, and are therefore an imperfect index of the amount secreted of either. In the male about two-thirds of the total represents metabolites of androgens and glucocorticoids of adrenal origin, and one-third arises from androgens of testicular origin. In the female almost all the 17-oxosteroids are normally metabolites of adrenocortical hormones. The normal range of 17-oxosteroids in adult males aged 15–45 years is 5–25 mg. per 24 hours and in adult females of the same age range it is 3–20 mg. per 24 hours. Before puberty and later in life lesser amounts are excreted.

Low levels are found in primary adrenal insufficiency, although significant amounts may be derived from the testes in the male, and in adrenal insufficiency secondary to panhypopituitarism and in myxoedema. The excretion is depressed by administration of synthetic glucocorticoids, and also in malnutrition, any chronic wasting condition and in liver diseases with impaired hepatic metabolism of steroidal hormones. High levels are found in the adrenogenital syndrome [p. 587] and in virilizing tumours of the adrenals or gonads, in some cases of Cushing's syndrome [p. 582] and during administration of ACTH.

Response to ACTH. The response of the adrenal cortex to stimulation with exogenous ACTH is essential in confirming the diagnosis of Addison's disease, and helpful in differentiating primary adrenal failure from that secondary to pituitary failure or suppression.

A plasma sample for 11-hydroxycorticosteroids is taken between 9 and 10 a.m. and a 24-hour urinary collection made for estimation of 11-hydroxycorticosteroids or 17-oxogenic steroids. ACTH-gel is then injected intramuscularly in a dose of 40 mg. twice daily for 3 days. A second plasma sample is taken 5 hours after the ACTH injection on the morning of the third day and urine is collected on the last day also. In normal subjects the plasma 'cortisol' level on the third day rises to over 60 μg. per 100 ml. and there is a parallel increase in urinary steroid excretion, the output of 17-oxogenic steroids exceeding 40 mg. per 24 hours.

In patients with Addison's disease no significant increase in plasma or urinary steroid levels occurs, and usually but not always the pre-ACTH plasma 'cortisol' level is low. In secondary adrenal atrophy due to pituitary failure or suppression, the ACTH causes a step-wise increase in the plasma and urinary steroid levels although these seldom reach in 3 days the same degree of elevation found in normal subjects.

A rapid screening test for hypoadrenocorticism can be carried out with a synthetic polypeptide comprising the first 24 amino acids of ACTH. A sample of blood is taken between 9 and 10 a.m. for the estimation of 11-hydroxycorticosteroids. An injection of 250 μg. *Synacthen* dissolved in 0·5–1·0 ml. saline is injected intramuscularly and a second blood sample is taken 30 minutes later. The criteria of a normal response are a pre-injection value of 5 μg. or more per 100 ml., an increment greater than 7 μg. and a level after 30 minutes in excess of 18 μg. per 100 ml. irrespective of the initial control value. A normal response excludes Addison's disease but no patient on the basis of a subnormal response should be committed to life-long substitution therapy until the more exacting ACTH-gel test described above has confirmed adrenocortical unresponsiveness.

Plasma 'Cortisol' Circadian Rhythm. In normal unstressed subjects at rest the plasma 11-hydroxycorticosteroid values vary during the day, being higher in the early morning than late at night. Blood samples are taken at 6 a.m., 12 noon, 6 p.m. and at midnight. The highest levels are normally found between 6 and 10 a.m. and the lowest between midnight and 4 a.m. This circadian rhythm is almost always disturbed in patients with Cushing's syndrome and the midnight plasma 'cortisol' level, provided the sample is taken without disturbing the patient, is not as low as normal and exceeds 5–8 μg. per 100 ml. The circadian rhythm may also be lost in patients with a head injury or any chronic debilitating illness.

Response to Dexamethasone. The suppressive action of dexamethasone on ACTH secretion as reflected by a lowering of the plasma 'cortisol' level or the urinary excretion of 17-oxogenic steroids is of particular value in establishing the diagnosis of Cushing's syndrome and also in deciding whether the Cushing's syndrome is caused by adrenal hyperplasia, an adrenal adenoma or carcinoma, or an ACTH-producing 'non-endocrine' tumour.

A plasma sample and 24-hour urine collection are obtained before dexamethasone is given for 3 days in a dose of 0·5 mg. six-hourly. On the third day another blood sample is taken and a 24-hour urine collection made. On the fourth day the dose of dexamethasone is increased to 2 mg. six-hourly. This is continued for 3 more days when a third blood sample and 24-hour urine collection are obtained on the last day.

In normal subjects the plasma 'cortisol' level will suppress below 6 μg. per 100 ml. on a dose of 0·5 mg. dexamethasone six-hourly in contrast to patients with Cushing's syndrome who will not show this degree of suppression. The higher dosage of dexamethasone may help to establish the pathological cause of the Cushing's syndrome. Patients with bilateral adrenal hyperplasia usually show significant depression in contrast to those with an autonomous tumour (benign or malignant) of the adrenal gland or an ectopic ACTH-producing tumour who usually do not suppress.

Similarly the smaller 0·5 mg. dose of dexamethasone will usually reduce the urinary excretion of 17-oxogenic steroids to 2 mg. or less per 24 hours in patients who do not have Cushing's syndrome but this distinction may not be absolute in patients with 'simple' obesity. The larger dose of 2 mg. dexamethasone six-hourly will reduce the urinary excretion of 17-oxogenic steroids to 2 mg. or less per 24 hours in normal subjects and those with 'simple' obesity, whereas patients with Cushing's syndrome due to bilateral hyperplasia will not suppress to this degree and usually excrete 3 mg. or more 17-oxogenic steroids per 24 hours. Although exceptions occur little or no suppression is usually achieved when the cause of the Cushing's syndrome is an adrenal tumour or an ACTH-producing 'non-endocrine' carcinoma.

11-Oxygenation Index. This test is of particular value in establishing the diagnosis of congenital adrenal hyperplasia in infants [p. 587], because a complete 24-hour urine specimen, so difficult to obtain accurately in a baby, is not required and the estimations can be made on a casual urine specimen of 75–100 ml. The 11-oxygenation index is the ratio of those 17-oxogenic steroids that do not have an oxygen function at the C-11 position (the 11-desoxy group) to those that do (the 11-oxygenated group). Thus the 11-desoxy group [Fig. 34], which includes such substances as pregnanetriol, 11-deoxycortisol and its metabolite tetrahydro-11-deoxycortisol, are excreted in excess when there is an enzymatic defect in the biosynthesis of the normal 11-oxygenated group of compounds comprising cortisol and its metabolites tetrahydrocortisol and tetrahydrocortisone. The ratio of 11-desoxy to 11-oxygenated compounds is normally less than 0·7. The index is raised above this level in infants and adults when there is deficiency of 21-hydroxylase or 11-hydroxylase enzyme systems. With this technique reliable diagnostic results are obtained in 95 per cent. of cases. A falsely high index may occur during the first week of life when the mechanism for the biosynthesis of cortisol is late to mature but does so during the second week, and also in infants with severe malnutrition associated with malabsorption, hyponatraemia and diarrhoea.

ACUTE ADRENAL INSUFFICIENCY

Synonyms. Adrenal crisis; Adrenal apoplexy.

Definition

A relatively uncommon condition caused by acute deficiency of normal adrenocortical secretion, and characterized by hypotension, mental changes, hypovolaemic shock, hypoglycaemia, stupor and coma terminating in death unless recognized and treated promptly.

Aetiology

As a result of the severe dyshormonogenesis in the adrenal biosynthesis of cortisol, acute adrenal deficiency may occur in the postnatal period of infants with the syndrome of congenital adrenal hyperplasia [p. 587].

In adults acute adrenal insufficiency may be the presenting manifestation of untreated chronic Addison's disease [p. 581]. Either atrophy or tuberculosis of the adrenal glands may be the cause in these patients who, usually for social or psychiatric reasons, have failed to seek adequate medical advice.

More commonly acute adrenal deficiency occurs in adrenalectomized or Addisonian patients who fail to increase their maintenance dose of cortisone and/or fludrocortisone in the face of vomiting and diarrhoea which impede absorption of the orally administered corticosteroids and promote loss of sodium and water. Such circumstances may arise from an intercurrent infection, minor trauma, a surgical operation, the vomiting of pregnancy, parturition or psychological stress—conditions that normally all call for increased secretion of cortisol or aldosterone.

Similarly an acute adrenal crisis may develop in a patient whose hypothalamic-pituitary-adrenal system has been in the recent past or is currently being suppressed by administration of therapeutic doses of glucocorticoids, and who fails to increase the dosage in the event of some stressful situation [p. 590].

Much less commonly an acute virulent infection may involve the adrenal glands and cause haemorrhagic necrosis. When this occurs in infants or young children with meningococcal septicaemia, it is called the Waterhouse-Friderichsen syndrome. Acute infarction of idiopathic origin has also been described in new-born infants and in pregnancy. It may rarely occur as a complication of retrograde venography of the adrenal glands, a procedure sometimes used for determining on which side an adrenal tumour is situated.

Pathology

The clinical picture is due to a deficiency of aldosterone or cortisol or both. Lack of aldosterone causes a reduction in plasma volume due to urinary loss of sodium and water, hypotension and circulatory collapse. Glucocorticoid deficiency is responsible for hypoglycaemia, profound weakness and stupor. The changes found in the adrenal cortex depend upon the aetiology.

Symptoms

The onset of acute adrenal insufficiency is usually sudden and its progression rapid. The patient becomes profoundly weak, apathetic and mentally disturbed, cold, peripherally cyanosed and pale due to vasoconstriction. The blood pressure falls and the pulse pressure is reduced. Nausea, vomiting, abdominal pain and diarrhoea add to the dehydration and weight-loss. A rise in temperature to 101° F. (38° C.) or more is common, associated with a rapid pulse of poor volume. A branny desquamation of the skin may develop in 36–48 hours. Oliguria and death may follow a short period of coma.

Diagnosis

The recognition of acute adrenal failure depends largely upon the clinical picture and the patient's previous history. A sample of blood should be taken at once for measurement of the plasma 11-hydroxycorticosteroid level, the blood glucose concentration (*Dextrostix* may qualitatively confirm the presence of hypoglycaemia), and other indirect parameters of adrenal insufficiency such as hyponatraemia, hypochloraemia and a raised serum potassium level. The ECG may show tall Gothic T-waves indicative of hyperkalaemia. The results of none of these investigations should be awaited before instituting treatment on the basis of a clinical diagnosis. A plasma 'cortisol' level of 5 μg. or less per 100 ml. will strongly support the diagnosis retrospectively, whereas in patients with hypotension due to non-adrenal medical or surgical conditions the plasma 'cortisol' level is usually 20 μg. or more per 100 ml.

Prophylaxis

Adrenalectomized and Addisonian patients must know that increased amounts of glucocorticoids and of mineralocorticoids (usually 9-alpha-fludrocortisol) must be taken if they are subjected to any increased stress. They should always carry a card or bracelet stating their current therapy. So also must patients who have received in the recent past or are currently receiving glucocorticoid therapy; they must be familiar with their treatment and its possible consequences [p. 589]. As a routine all patients must be asked before any surgical procedure whether they have had 'steroid' or 'cortisone' treatment.

Treatment

Hydrocortisone hemisuccinate or 21-phosphate, 100–300 mg., should be given intravenously at once, the dose depending on the gravity of the clinical state. An intravenous infusion of glucose saline is started and after an initial 500 ml., given quickly, 1·5 litres daily is infused with 100 mg. hydrocortisone intravenously every 8 hours. Fludrocortisone, 1–4 mg., is given by mouth but if the patient is vomiting deoxycortone acetate, 5–10 mg. in sesame oil (DOCA) is injected intramuscularly. If the blood glucose is low, additional glucose, 40–60 ml. of a 40 per cent. solution, is injected intravenously. In cases where an acute infection is the cause, penicillin is given parenterally.

Prognosis

Unless the condition is recognized and treated promptly the outlook is grave and death may occur in less than 24 hours. Once the patient has been successfully rescued, the prognosis is excellent provided proper supervision is maintained in the future.

CHRONIC ADRENAL INSUFFICIENCY

Synonym. Addison's disease.

Definition

A disease with an incidence of about 4 per 100,000 people in London characterized by malaise, progressive weakness, weight-loss, pigmentation and in some instances gastro-intestinal symptoms. Untreated the condition is slowly progressive usually but may proceed rapidly to acute adrenal insufficiency (see above) and present as an adrenal crisis often precipitated by physical or emotional stress.

Aetiology

Chronic adrenal insufficiency usually manifests itself in adult life but may occur at any age. In two-thirds of cases the cause is atrophy of the adrenal glands and this occurs more often in women than men. In these cases adrenal antibodies may be demonstrated in the serum, and there may be associated endocrine or other diseases attributable to auto-immune mechanisms, e.g. hypoparathyroidism, pernicious anaemia, diabetes, cirrhosis, alopecia or thyroid disorders. Some cases are associated with amenorrhoea in the female or infertility in the male; in these, antibodies to the theca interna cells of the ovaries and the interstitial cells of the testes are often demonstrable.

Addison's disease may also be due to destruction of the adrenal cortex by tuberculosis, often secondary to previous and forgotten infection of the lungs, or of the peritoneum, endometrium or urinary tract. Tuberculous infection is the cause in about one-third of the cases of Addison's disease and affects men and women equally. Rarely chronic adrenal insufficiency is caused by other chronic granulomatous conditions, amyloidosis, haemochromatosis or metastases, particularly from a bronchial carcinoma.

Adrenal insufficiency is an inevitable consequence of total adrenalectomy for Cushing's syndrome or for control of a metastasizing carcinoma of the breast. Some of the features, such as pigmentation, may sometimes occur in the dyshormonogenesis that causes congenital adrenal hyperplasia [p. 587] but in this the picture is more often that of acute adrenal insufficiency.

Chronic adrenal deficiency of glucocorticoid and androgenic secretions, but not of aldosterone, occurs secondarily to panhypopituitarism [p. 544] and occasionally to an isolated deficiency of ACTH production.

Pathology

Depending on the cause, the adrenal glands are atrophic, fibrosed, infiltrated or calcified. The patient is wasted and pigmented. The heart is small. The clinical and biochemical features are due to deficient secretion of both aldosterone and glucocorticoids. Lack of cortisol is responsible for the malaise and weakness, inability to withstand stress, hypoglycaemia after fasting and a reduction in renal blood flow which may induce a moderate rise in blood urea. In response to the low plasma cortisol level increased amounts of ACTH are secreted, and the skin pigmentation is attributable either to this or to a concurrent increase in the secretion of the melanophore-stimulating hormone (MSH). Both these trophic hormones share similar amino-acid sequences.

Lack of aldosterone causes increased urinary loss of sodium, dehydration, hypovolaemia, hypotension, hyperkalaemia and a modest rise in blood urea.

Symptoms

In most instances the onset is insidious and the course slowly progressive. The initial symptoms are malaise, tiredness and loss of weight. Occasionally amenorrhoea or infertility in the male may be the presenting symptom. Pigmentation may be the first manifestation and antedate any other symptoms by many years. Later anorexia and nausea, attributable to sodium depletion, develop. Vague abdominal discomfort may occur sometimes associated with diarrhoea which on analysis of the faeces is found to be associated with steatorrhoea. Symptoms due to hypoglycaemia are not common. Untreated the patient may become progressively weaker, bedridden and develop contractures of the legs, or may present in a terminal state of acute adrenal insufficiency [p. 580].

On examination there is evidence of dehydration and weight-loss. The patient may be so weak that any muscular effort is impossible, and male patients may be compelled to shave sitting on a chair. The most characteristic and striking finding is a light brown or brownish-black pigmentation. Patients of Afro-Asian origin may notice an increase in their normal pigmentation. The pigment is often seen on the buccal mucosa inside the cheeks or on the gums around the incisor teeth. Externally it is often most marked in the creases of the palms, on the elbows and knees, in old scars and on pressure areas such as round the waist, over the shoulders when shoulder straps rub and round the thorax from tight brassière straps. Axillary and pubic hair is sparse. Postural hypotension is common but a low supine blood pressure is a late sign, and in older patients the blood pressure may be normal but rise to mildly hypertensive levels with treatment. Leucoderma occurs in some patients, and is a non-specific accompaniment of other auto-immune diseases.

Because of haemoconcentration the serum levels of sodium and chloride are usually normal except in the later stages when an adrenal crisis is imminent or has already developed. The blood sugar is usually normal except after prolonged fasting. The serum potassium and the blood urea levels are raised slightly above normal.

In many instances the plasma 'cortisol' level between 9 and 10 a.m. is within the normal range, and such patients, although able to produce sufficient glucocorticoids to meet basal requirements, develop adrenal insufficiency when subjected to stressful situations that increase steroidal demands. Similarly the urinary excretion of 11-hydroxycorticoids and of 17-oxogenic steroids is in the low normal range or subnormal. The essential step in confirming the diagnosis is to show that the plasma 'cortisol' level or the urinary excretion of cortisol and its metabolites do not rise on administration of exogenous ACTH [p. 579]. Very rarely the 'stress' of this investigation may provoke acute adrenal insufficiency; the patient must therefore be hospitalized and hydrocortisone hemisuccinate or 21-phosphate be in readiness if any untoward symptoms suggesting acute insufficiency arise. Adrenal antibodies should be sought for and X-rays of the chest and renal areas taken to show whether there is evidence of pulmonary tuberculosis, quiescent or active, or of adrenal calcification.

Diagnosis

Chronic adrenal insufficiency should be suspected in any patient with weakness, weight-loss and pigmentation although a careful search may have to be made for the last. In addition to the more obvious flagrant cases of Addison's disease, lesser degrees of adrenal insufficiency may occur and these can only be diagnosed by determining whether or not the response to ACTH stimulation [p. 579] is normal. When pigmentation is not pronounced, the condition must be distinguished from an anxiety state or depression, a distinction which may not be easy despite a careful psychiatric appraisal because mental and EEG changes are common in Addisonian patients and improve with treatment.

The pigmentation must be distinguished from that due to racial factors, haemochromatosis which is slatey-blue in colour, hepatic cirrhosis, Crohn's disease, malignant diseases, untreated hyperthyroidism, steatorrhoea, chronic renal disease, long-standing skin irritation due to dermatitis or lice and dirt (vagabond's disease) and that due to certain drugs, namely the blue-grey argyria produced by silver nitrate and the rain-drop pigmentation caused by arsenic.

Salt-losing nephritis may induce a clinical and biochemical picture similar to Addison's disease but proteinuria, casts and often evidence of renal infection are usually present in the former.

The distinction between adrenal insufficiency due to Addison's disease and secondary to pituitary failure is seldom difficult on clinical grounds alone. In the latter pigmentation does not occur and by contrast the skin is often abnormally pale; the clinical picture is usually dominated by hypothyroidism or hypogonadism; and ACTH induces a step-wise increase in plasma 'cortisol' and in urinary 11-hydroxycorticoid and 17-oxogenic steroid excretion.

Treatment

Oral administration of cortisone or cortisol causes a striking improvement in the patient's sense of well-being. The dosage depends upon the patient's age, whether his occupation is sedentary or manual and to a lesser extent on the degree of adrenocortical insufficiency. The usual dosage range is 25–75 mg. cortisone or 20–70 mg. cortisol daily in divided doses. The patient must learn about his disease and how the dosage of glucocorticoid may have to be increased temporarily by 25–100 mg. cortisone or 20–80 mg. cortisol in the event of an intercurrent infection, trauma or a psychological disturbance.

Although many Addisonian patients feel well on cortisone or cortisol alone, they may continue to have a slightly raised blood urea level and further improvement in well-being can be achieved by giving 9-alpha-flurohydrocortisone as a replacement for the aldosterone deficiency. Thus in all but the mildest case fludrocortisone should be given in a dose which ranges from 0·1 mg. on alternate days to 0·2 mg. and seldom more daily. The precise amount is judged by the patient's weight, blood pressure, sense of well-being and the serum levels of urea, potassium and sodium. Overdosage of fludrocortisone causes an excessive increase in weight and sodium retention leading to a raised jugular venous pressure, oedema, headaches and hypertension. When glucocorticoid and fludrocortisone are given in combination, the patient can eat a normal diet and there is no need for additional salt.

The patient should always carry a card or bracelet bearing the diagnosis of his disease and his current therapy.

Prognosis

With modern treatment and proper supervision, the outlook for a patient with chronic adrenal insufficiency is excellent. The pigmentation fades, pregnancy can be safely undertaken and the life-span is normal.

ADRENOCORTICAL HYPERFUNCTION

Overactivity of the adrenal cortex may be due to hyperplasia or a benign or malignant tumour. Depending upon the particular hormone or group of hormones secreted in excess, a number of different syndromes may develop. Hypersecretion of glucocorticoids gives rise to Cushing's syndrome: of androgens to precocious puberty in boys and to virilization in females; and of aldosterone to hypertension, hypokalaemia and a low plasma renin concentration. Rarely an adrenal tumour may secrete excessive amounts of oestrogens and cause feminization in the male. Some adrenocortical carcinomas have little endocrine activity and others may present a mixed endocrinopathy.

CUSHING'S SYNDROME

Synonyms. Adrenocortical hyperfunction; Hyperadrenocorticism.

Definition

A syndrome produced by the excessive secretion of glucocorticoids from the adrenal cortex, and characterized by obesity of particular distribution, hypertension, diminished glucose tolerance, increased protein catabolism, amenorrhoea in the female, and an increased liability to infection.

Aetiology

Cushing's syndrome may occur at any age but is usually seen in the third or fourth decade. The incidence is much higher in women than men. About 75 per cent.

of cases have bilateral adrenal hyperplasia induced by hypersecretion of ACTH and this is due in some 25 per cent. of such cases to a chromophobe or basophil adenoma of the pituitary which eventually becomes clinically or radiologically detectable. In other instances an abnormality of the hypothalamus or even higher centres leading to increased production of the corticotrophin release factor may be the basic disturbance rather than a primary pituitary disorder as originally postulated by Cushing. In the remaining 20 per cent. of Cushing's syndrome the cause is an adrenal tumour, the incidence of an adenoma or a carcinoma being about equal. (About 8–10 per cent. of cases are caused by an ectopic ACTH-secreting 'non-endocrine' tumour [p. 550].)

These ectopic foci of ACTH-secreting tissue are usually tumours arising in organs derived from the embryological foregut, most commonly an oat-cell carcinoma of the bronchus, a bronchial adenoma, carcinoma of the pancreas, a carcinoid tumour usually of the bronchus and non-teratomatous ovarian tumours. In these circumstances the features of Cushing's syndrome are often atypical and may be more biochemical than clinical because the degree of adrenocortical hypersecretion is intense and the patient may not live long enough to develop the usual clinical picture of Cushing's syndrome. However, in some instances, particularly when the ectopic ACTH-producing tumour is benign, the clinical features of apparently typical Cushing's syndrome may antedate by several years the recognition of the primary 'non-endocrine' tumour.

The clinical and biochemical features of Cushing's syndrome are directly attributable to the excess secretion of glucocorticoid hormones and can be reproduced by the prolonged administration of large doses of cortisone, cortisol, corticosterone, synthetic glucocorticoid analogues or of ACTH. Inhibition of protein anabolism is responsible for the thinning of the skin, muscle wasting, osteoporosis and cutaneous striae which develop in areas where the deposition of fat on the trunk is most marked. Muscular weakness is due to the wasting and also to potassium depletion. Diminished glucose tolerance and in some cases frank diabetes mellitus are due to increased gluconeogenesis.

Pathology

The adrenal glands may be hypertrophied, the hyperplasia being most marked in the zonae reticularis and fasciculata, but the size of the glands is a poor index of their secretory function. In some cases of adrenal hyperplasia there may be a small pituitary chromophobe or basophil adenoma or there may be an ectopic ACTH-secreting tumour of non-endocrine origin. Alternatively an adenoma, in one or both adrenals, or a carcinoma is present in one adrenal gland. When the tumour is unilateral, there is usually some degree of atrophy of the contralateral gland due to suppression of ACTH secretion. Hyalinization of the pituitary basophil cells (Crooke's changes) occurs in Cushing's syndrome and also in patients given large doses of corticosteroids.

The bones are osteoporotic and this may lead to pathological fractures or the collapse of vertebrae. Hypertension may cause left ventricular hypertrophy and nephrosclerotic changes in the kidneys.

Symptoms

The onset of the disease is usually gradual over several months and in some instances starts after pregnancy. The patient may complain of obesity; menstrual irregularity; acne and hirsutism in the female; impotence in the male; generalized weakness; bruising; backache or symptoms related to hypertension or diabetes mellitus. Amenorrhoea is common in the female. Psychiatric disturbances, usually depression, may be the presenting abnormality.

The patient's appearance is often characteristic and the time of onset of the disease may be judged by comparison with old photographs. The face is rounded and the complexion a purple plum colour; an excess of hair is common on the upper lip and jaw in women. Acne may be present on the face, chest and shoulders. In contrast to the slender arms and legs, the trunk is obese. The skin is thin and wrinkles when picked up between the thumb and index finger. Purple striae develop round the hips, abdomen, flanks and anterior axillary folds. Bruises and ecchymoses are common. The blood pressure is usually raised and there may be left ventricular hypertrophy. This pathognomonic clinical picture may be much less marked in the early stages of the syndrome. The typical truncal obesity may be absent and the diagnosis may be suggested only by amenorrhoea, acne and hirsutism.

The fasting blood glucose level is often normal but the glucose tolerance curve is usually diabetic and there may be glycosuria. In a quarter of patients some slight degree of polycythaemia is present. A low serum potassium and a high serum bicarbonate level may occur and the extent of these changes depends upon the degree of adrenocortical overactivity. Thus marked hypokalaemic alkalosis is particularly common in patients with an ectopic ACTH-secreting tumour of non-endocrine origin. Pathological fractures of the ribs or wedging of the vertebrae may be seen radiologically. Seldom is there clinical or radiological evidence of a pituitary tumour.

Diagnosis

Two problems surround the diagnosis of Cushing's syndrome. The first is to confirm that adrenocortical hypersecretion is present and the second, and more difficult, is to determine the underlying pathological cause of the increased glucocorticoid secretion because this influences treatment.

The most accurate method for confirming increased glucocorticoid secretion is to measure the cortisol production rate by an isotope dilution technique. Unfortunately this method is only available in special centres, but in most instances the diagnosis can be confirmed by more simple chemical methods. Although the plasma 11-hydroxycorticosteroid level may be in the normal range between 9 and 10 a.m., it is almost invariably raised above the upper normal limit of 5–8 μg. per 100 ml. at midnight provided the patient is undisturbed, physically and emotionally, when the blood sample is taken. Thus the normal cortisol circadian rhythm [p. 579] is blunted and the usual fall in the plasma 11-hydroxycorticoid level does not occur at night. The 24-hour urinary excretion of 11-hydroxycorticosteroids [p. 578] is usually raised above the upper normal limit of 350 μg. per 24 hours, and values of 400–7000 μg. or more may be found. Because of variations in day to day adrenocortical activity in some patients, several 24-hour urine collections may have to be analysed. The urinary excretion of 17-oxogenic steroids may be normal or raised, and this determination is less helpful in establishing the diagnosis than the plasma 'cortisol' level at midnight and the urinary excretion of 11-hydroxycorticosteroids. Particular diagnostic difficulties may arise in 'simple' obesity of non-endocrine origin when there may be increased urinary excretion of 17-oxogenic steroids but excretion of 11-hydroxycorticosteroids per 24 hours is usually normal. Also helpful in confirming adrenocortical overactivity is the dexamethasone suppression test using 0·5 mg. six-hourly as described on page 579.

Once evidence of excess adrenocortical activity has been established, the underlying pathological cause must be defined. In infants bilateral hyperplasia, and in prepubertal children an adrenal carcinoma is the usual cause. In adults a tumour of non-endocrine origin secreting ACTH should be suspected if there is profound muscular weakness associated with a marked lowering of the serum potassium level and an elevation of the serum bicarbonate concentration. Careful physical examination, and radiological studies may reveal an ectopic ACTH-producing tumour.

The main problem, after excluding a tumour of non-endocrine origin, is to distinguish between adrenal hyperplasia, an adrenal adenoma or an adrenal carcinoma. If facilities are available the distinction may be made by measuring the plasma ACTH level. Between 8 and 10 a.m. the normal ACTH concentration is 12–60 pg. per ml; in cases of bilateral hyperplasia the ACTH level is raised (40–200 pg. per ml.) and when an autonomous adrenal tumour is present the plasma level of ACTH is undetectable. Until this assay procedure is more widely available, more indirect methods of differentiation must be used.

The most helpful test is the response to dexamethasone using a daily dose of 8 mg. [p. 579] but exceptions occur in which the activity of an adrenal adenoma is suppressed. The response to ACTH is not reliable. A marked rise in the urinary excretion of 11-hydroxycorticoids or 17-oxogenic steroids will suggest adrenal hyperplasia whereas a lesser response would be expected if an adenoma or carcinoma were present. Only if there is no response to ACTH is the test strongly suggestive of an autonomous adrenal tumour. In most cases of adrenal carcinoma the urinary excretion of 17-oxosteroids is high, often exceeding 30 mg. per 24 hours. In some cases of adrenal adenoma the 17-oxosteroid excretion is low and in cases of hyperplasia it is usually normal or slightly raised.

Unless the pathological diagnosis seems clear from biochemical tests, particularly the degree of suppression obtained with dexamethasone, physical methods may be required to distinguish between hyperplasia and a tumour. An intravenous pyelogram may show downward displacement of one kidney by a suprarenal tumour. X-rays and tomograms after presacral insufflation of oxygen may show bilateral adrenal hyperplasia or a unilateral tumour but often the radiological appearances are difficult to interpret and deposits of fat may be misleading. By passing a catheter via the femoral vein into the inferior vena cava, retrograde venography may delineate a tumour in one or other gland but this is a procedure not without risk.

Treatment

An adrenal adenoma or carcinoma must be removed, and because the contralateral gland is likely to be atrophic, cortisone must be given over the operative period [p. 590] and ACTH may be required post-operatively to activate the remaining gland.

The choice of treatment for bilateral hyperplasia is more controversial. If there is doubt as to the underlying pathology, adrenal exploration should be carried out. If hyperplasia is found, bilateral total adrenalectomy is performed, as this avoids the possibility of subsequent hyperplasia and hypertrophy of the adrenal remnant if partial adrenalectomy is done. When the response to dexamethasone strongly suggests bilateral hyperplasia, the choice lies between adrenalectomy or pituitary X-irradiation. In children deep X-ray therapy may be tried first, followed if unsuccessful by adrenalectomy. In adults conventional X-ray therapy induces a remission in less than 50 per cent. of cases. The intrasellar implantation of radioactive gold or yttrium seeds induces a satisfactory remission in 50 per cent. of cases also, and a partial remission in the remainder, but this procedure is not without complications such as meningitis, diabetes insipidus (temporary or permanent), CSF rhinorrhoea of cerebrospinal fluid and hypopituitarism. For these reasons total adrenalectomy is still in most instances the treatment of choice, particularly in women who later may wish to have children.

When the cause of the Cushing's syndrome is an ACTH-secreting tumour of non-endocrine origin, remission may be achieved by removal or irradiation of the primary tumour. Adrenal hypersecretion is likely to recur if metastases develop. Control of the endocrinopathy may then be achieved by the use of aminoglutethimide [Section 4].

Prognosis

Untreated Cushing's syndrome usually ends fatally within 5 years, death being due to the cardiovascular complications, diabetes or an intercurrent infection. In a number of patients, however, the course of the disease is punctuated by periods of spontaneous remission. The prognosis in an adrenal carcinoma is bad because metastases develop early. The outlook in patients with bilateral hyperplasia or an adenoma is good. Rarely after total adrenalectomy for bilateral hyperplasia and despite adequate substitution therapy with cortisone and fludrocortisone, the patient becomes deeply pigmented due to hypersecretion of ACTH or melanophore-stimulating hormone from a pituitary tumour that may have to be removed surgically if local pressure symptoms or signs develop.

PRIMARY ALDOSTERONISM

Synonyms. Hyperaldosteronism; Conn's syndrome.

Definition

A condition caused by the autonomous hypersecretion of aldosterone (and possibly also in some instances of other mineralocorticoids) and characterized by hypertension and renal wasting of potassium sometimes of sufficient degree to cause hypokalaemic alkalosis, and occasionally muscular weakness or periodic paralysis.

Aetiology

The excess aldosterone secretion usually arises from one or more cortical adenomas, a condition that is more common in women than men and occurs in the age range 30–60. Much less commonly there is bilateral adrenal hyperplasia and this tends to occur in a younger age group (10–20 years) with an equal sex incidence. Very rarely a carcinoma is the cause.

Pathology

In 75 per cent. of cases there is an adrenal adenoma, 1–4 cm. in diameter, with a characteristic orange-yellow colour on section. The excess potassium loss in the urine, induced by exchange of potassium for sodium in the distal convoluted renal tubules, produces a nephropathy characterized by vacuolation of the tubular cells with isosthenuria, polyuria unresponsive to antidiuretic hormone, and a liability to chronic pyelonephritis. The muscular weakness and episodic paralysis are attributable to potassium depletion. Sodium retention occurs and may be reflected by an increase in total body exchangeable sodium and a serum concentration in the high normal range or above. Oedema does not develop; the explanation for this is not entirely clear but may be related to a rise in the glomerular filtration rate or to a compensatory decrease in the reabsorption of sodium by the proximal convoluted renal tubules.

Symptoms

Patients with aldosteronism usually present in one of two ways; either with manifestations of hypertension or, in women more often than in men, with muscular weakness, sometimes sufficiently severe to cause episodic paralysis, hyporeflexia and rarely paraesthesia or tetany. The blood pressure is usually moderately elevated, retinopathy mild and cardiac hypertrophy slight or absent. However, in younger patients the hypertention may be more marked but malignant hypertention is rare. Less commonly polyuria and polydipsia are prominent features, suggesting diabetes insipidus; recurrent pyelonephritis may occur.

In any patient with hypertension of unexplained cause, primary aldosteronism should be considered in the differential diagnosis. Attention to the diagnosis may be drawn by an ECG showing evidence of hypokalaemia (flattening or inversion of the T-waves with apparent prolongation of Q–T interval due to the development of U-waves). Characteristically the serum potassium level is low, often being less than 3·5 mEq. per litre; the serum bicarbonate 30 mEq. per litre or more; and the serum magnesium level may be low. In very rare instances the serum potassium level may be persistently normal. The serum sodium level is normal or slightly elevated, and there may be proteinuria, casts and bacteriological proof of secondary renal infection.

Diagnosis

Careful estimation of the serum potassium, bicarbonate and sodium concentrations on a number of occasions is often the basis for diagnosing primary aldosteronism. Proof of a pathological loss of potassium is obtained by measuring the 24-hour urinary potassium excretion which may be 25 mEq. or more despite a serum potassium level of 3·5 mEq. or less per litre. The urinary pH is usually neutral or alkaline, and the specific gravity or osmolality is only slightly raised by dehydration [Section 4] or administration of ADH.

Measurement of the total exchangeable sodium, which is usually increased, and of the total exchangeable potassium, which is usually low, also provide indirect support for the diagnosis. A simple balance study measuring the urinary excretion of sodium and potassium may be helpful. On a high sodium dietary intake (150–200 mEq. daily), more potassium will be excreted in the urine than is ingested in the diet (a negative potassium balance) and at the end of a week the serum potassium level is likely to be unequivocally subnormal. When the dietary sodium intake is then reduced to low levels (22 mEq. daily), less potassium is excreted and the patient shows a positive balance with a return of the serum potassium level to near normal. Spironolactone given for 4 weeks in a dose of 100 mg. four times a day will provoke a natriuresis and potassium retention but, more significantly, will usually reduce the blood pressure to normal limits in those patients with primary aldosteronism who will benefit from surgery.

When the diagnosis is in doubt recourse must be made to more sophisticated investigations. In primary aldosteronism the normal renin-angiotensin control of aldosterone secretion is suppressed so that the plasma levels of renin and angiotensin II are in the low normal or undetectable range, and in special centres these substances can be measured by immunoassay methods. It is important that the blood sample for the assay of its renin content is taken when the patient is on a low sodium intake and has been standing for some hours. Excess aldosterone or aldosterone metabolites may be present in the urine and the aldosterone production rate, measured by an isotopic dilution technique, is increased, but this also occurs in secondary aldosteronism. The aldosterone secretion rate may be influenced by the serum potassium level and the state of the potassium balance. When potassium depletion is marked, the expected increase in aldosterone secretion may not be prominent. Under these circumstances a diagnostic procedure that may be helpful is to give 10 mg. desoxycortisone acetate (DOCA) intramuscularly every 12 hours for 3 days. In normal subjects and those with hypertension due to causes other than aldosteronism, there is a depression in the aldosterone secretion rate which is little influenced in patients with Conn's syndrome.

Intravenous pyelography, adrenal venography and aortography may all be helpful in determining whether the adenoma is in the left or right adrenal gland. The left gland is twice as commonly the site than the right side, but often the adenoma is too small to be detected radiologically and multiple adenomas may be present in both glands.

Differential Diagnosis

Primary aldosteronism must be distinguished from other causes of hypertension associated with hypokalaemia.

Thiazide Diuretics. These, when given for the treatment of hypertension, before adequate investigation of the cause, may add to the diagnostic confusion by inducing a low serum potassium level.

Cushing's Syndrome. Excess cortisol or corticosterone secretion in Cushing's syndrome or adrenocortical overactivity produced by an ectopic ACTH-secreting tumour may induce hypokalaemic hypertension but the clinical features seldom cause diagnostic difficulties and in Conn's syndrome the urinary excretion of glucocorticoids is normal.

Essential or Renal Hypertension. Hypertension associated with secondary hyperaldosteronism may occur in patients with rapidly progressive or malignant hypertension; in such cases the plasma sodium concentration is usually low and the plasma volume reduced. In addition to excessive potassium excretion, the urinary loss of sodium is usually high in relation to the degree of hyponatraemia; azotaemia and acidosis, rather than alkalosis, are present and the total exchangeable sodium is decreased in contrast to the increase found in primary aldosteronism. Administration of 250 mEq. potassium daily usually restores the serum potassium level to normal in these cases of secondary hyperaldosteronism in contrast to Conn's syndrome in which potassium loading, despite considerable potassium retention, fails to restore a normal potassium level unless the dietary sodium intake is restricted, a procedure that limits the exchange of sodium for potassium in the distal renal tubule. Nor should it be forgotten that hypertensive patients may have coincidental reasons for hypokalaemia such as the excessive use of *purgatives*, of *liquorice products* or *chronic diarrhoea*.

Juxtaglomerular Hyperplasia. Hypokalaemic alkalosis may also be found in a rare ill-understood syndrome unassociated with either hypertension or oedema. In this condition there is hypertrophy of the juxtaglomerular apparatus and increased amounts of renin, angiotensin II and aldosterone in the plasma and urine. The clinical features of this syndrome, named after Bartter who first described it, include failure to thrive, growth retardation, hypogonadism and hypokalaemic tetany. These patients are normotensive and for reasons unknown are resistant to the pressor action of angiotensin.

Periodic Familial Paralysis. This should not give diagnostic difficulties when there is a family history, no biochemical abnormality other than hypokalaemia and no hypertension.

Congenital Adrenal Hyperplasia. In one rare adrenal enzymatic defect, 17-β-hydroxylase deficiency, the affected female develops hypertension, hypokalaemia and has primary amenorrhoea [p. 607].

Treatment

Before surgical exploration of the adrenal glands, the patient should be repleted with potassium by giving a high-potassium low-sodium diet. The administration of spironolactone (*Aldactone-A*), 200–400 mg. daily in divided doses, will speed the repletion and control the hypertension. If at operation a tumour is found, this is removed, but the other gland must also be carefully palpated. If no tumour can be found, the left adrenal gland should be removed, and sectioned for evidence of a tumour. If none is found, half the right adrenal should be removed and sectioned similarly. If no adenoma is found, the remainder of the right gland (total adrenalectomy) is removed if the evidence for aldosteronism is strong; when the evidence is less certain, the remaining half of the right adrenal is left and the patient watched for 6 months. If the clinical and laboratory features of aldosteronism persist at the end of this time, the remaining adrenal tissue should be removed or the patient treated with spironolactone. Cortisone substitution therapy [p. 590] should be given over the period of the operation, and may be required later (in conjunction with fludrocortisone) depending on the extent of the adrenalectomy.

Prognosis

Without treatment aldosteronism is fatal, the patient usually dying of hypertensive vascular complications. The response to surgery depends upon the duration of the disease and the reversibility of any secondary renal damage, but often is very satisfactory.

EXCESSIVE SECRETION OF ANDROGENS

The effect of hypersecretion of androgenic hormones depends upon the age and sex of the patient. Females of any age exhibit virilization as shown by increased muscular development, hirsutism and enlargement of the clitoris. In males the condition often passes unnoticed when the onset is in adult life but produces precocious puberty in the pre-adolescent boy [p 586]. The androgenic compounds concerned are testosterone, dehydroepiandrostenedione and Δ^4-androstenedione which is converted to testosterone in the peripheral tissues. These hormones may be elaborated in the adrenal glands, by an interstitial-cell tumour of the testis [p. 603], by the ovaries in some cases of the Stein-Leventhal syndrome [p. 611] or by an ovarian tumour [p. 613].

Excessive androgen production of adrenal origin occurs in the dyshormonogenesis that causes congenital adrenal hyperplasia (see below) or when there is an androgen-secreting adrenal adenoma or carcinoma. When a tumour is present, the onset and progression of the disease are usually rapid; the patient may complain of discomfort in the area of the neoplasm, and, as the tumour is autonomous, the urinary 17-oxosteroid excretion is not suppressed by dexamethasone [p. 579].

ADRENOGENITAL SYNDROME

Synonym. Congenital adrenal hyperplasia (CAH).

Definition

A rare condition caused by partial or complete deficiency of certain adrenocortical enzymes essential to the biosynthesis of cortisol, and characterized by virilization in the female and precocious puberty in the male. Depending upon the particular enzyme and the degree of its deficiency, there may be associated features of glucocorticoid deficiency, hypertension or increased sodium loss in the urine.

Aetiology

The particular enzyme defect and its degree are genetically determined, usually being inherited as an autosomal recessive trait with clinical expression in the homozygous state. Females are more often affected than males, and the age at which the disorder is first manifest depends upon the completeness and nature of the enzyme defect. At least six different enzymes may be deficient, and the four most common are shown in FIGURE 34.

C-21 Hydroxylase Defect. The most frequent abnormality, occurring in 90 per cent. of cases, is deficiency of the C-21 hydroxylating enzyme, which results in failure to insert an hydroxyl group in the C-21 position of the corticosteroid side chain. This impairs the biosynthesis of both cortisol and aldosterone [block *a* in FIG. 34]. Deficient cortisol production enhances ACTH secretion with compensatory adrenocortical hyperplasia. Increased amounts of 17-hydroxyprogesterone are formed with increased urinary excretion of its three main metabolites, 17-hydroxypregnanolone, pregnanetriol and 11-oxopregnanetriol. Two separate forms of C-21 hydroxylase deficiency occur. In the milder form the chief clinical manifestation is virilization in the female and pseudo-precocious puberty in the male. The more severe form occurs in about one third of cases and is associated with excessive loss of sodium in the urine leading to hyponatraemia, hyperkalaemia and metabolic acidosis. In such cases aldosterone production is markedly deficient and the increased biosynthesis of progesterone and 17-hydroxyprogesterone, which antagonizes the renal tubular action of aldosterone, contribute to the excessive natriuresis.

C-11 Hydroxylase Defect. The next most common abnormality is a deficiency of the C-11 hydroxylating enzyme [block *b* in FIG. 34]. This also impairs the biosynthesis of cortisol and corticosterone. Increased amounts of 11-deoxycortisol and 11-deoxycorticosterone are formed which induce hypertension in addition to virilization as a feature in patients with this particular defect.

3-β Hydroxydehydrogenase Defect. This rare defect [block *c* in FIG. 34], early in the biosynthesis of adrenocortical hormones, leads to decreased production of progesterone and hence of cortisol, aldosterone and androgen also. Thus the clinical features in the new-born infant may be different from those normally encountered; males may show pseudohermaphroditism and females normal genital development. Such infants seldom survive unless diagnosed early and treatment of the acute adrenal insufficiency [p. 580] is corrected.

C-18 Dehydrogenase Defect. This rare abnormality [block *d* in FIG. 34] causes aldosterone but not cortisol deficiency and hence the adrenal glands are not hypertrophied. There is accumulation of 18-hydroxycorticosterone and increased urinary excretion of this compound's tetrahydro derivative which is not suppressed by administration of dexamethasone. The patient suffers the consequences of excessive urinary sodium loss but is not virilized or pigmented. The condition is treated by deoxycortisone by injection or fludrocortisone by mouth which suppresses the excess urinary excretion of tetrahydro-18-hydroxycorticosterone by reducing the enhanced renin-angiotensin stimulus attempting to increase aldosterone production.

Other even rarer enzymatic abnormalities may occur. Absence of the enzyme that converts cholesterol to pregnenolone results in deficient production of cortisol, aldosterone and androgens. The adrenal gland is filled with lipid and the patient usually dies soon after birth of acute adrenocortical insufficiency. The same enzyme deficiency is present in the ovaries and testes with the result that all patients with this defect appear as phenotypic females. Another rare abnormality is the 17-β-hydroxylase defect. This impedes the biosynthesis of 17-hydroxyprogesterone from progesterone [FIG. 34] and the resultant cortisol lack enhances ACTH production with increased formation of 11-deoxycorticosterone and corticosterone. The patient is hypertensive and hypokalaemic. This defect has so far been described only in females and also involves their ovaries. Thus in addition to symptoms of potassium depletion and hypertension, they also suffer primary amenorrhoea and lack of secondary sexual characteristics.

Pathology

The adrenal glands are enlarged and the hypertrophy is most marked in the zonae reticularis and fasciculata. The changes in the genital tract depend upon the severity of the enzyme deficiency and the degree of excess of androgen production.

Symptoms

If the enzyme deficiency is severe, excess androgen secretion will occur *in utero*, and a female child may be born with an enlarged clitoris, variable fusion of the labia and a rudimentary vagina that may not open to the exterior. In some instances a complete penile urethra is found. The baby is therefore a female pseudohermaphrodite having ovaries but no testicular tissue, and may be thought to be a boy with bilateral cryptorchidism. Indeed it may, on examination of the external genitalia alone, be impossible to distinguish between a female pseudohermaphrodite and a bilaterally cryptorchid male child particularly if there is associated hypospadias. Hence the need to establish the genetic sex by examination of a buccal smear or of polymorphs [Section 4]. Male infants with congenital adrenal hyperplasia may show precocious development of the external genitalia at or soon after birth.

In cases with marked enzyme deficiency vomiting,

dehydration and failure to thrive may result from cortisol deficiency, and unless this acute adrenal insufficiency of glucocorticoid secretion is recognized and treated promptly the prognosis is grave.

With lesser degrees of enzyme deficiency clinical manifestations may not appear until later. Male children may show precocious puberty [p. 602] and girls have an enlarged clitoris, hirsutism and acne. In both sexes there is increased skeletal growth and muscular development, but the androgens accelerate epiphyseal closure and thus induce skeletal maturation and thickset dwarfism. Girls with this condition may present with primary amenorrhoea and lack of secondary sexual characteristics. Boys have testicular atrophy because gonadotrophin secretion is suppressed by the high level of adrenal androgens in the plasma, and hence are said to have pseudo-precocious puberty.

The least severe forms of enzyme deficiency may not be apparent until after puberty. In males the testicular atrophy causes infertility but the secondary sexual characteristics are within the normal range or exaggerated by the increased androgen secretion. In females there is secondary amenorrhoea, infertility, hirsutism, acne, laryngeal development, increased musculature and poor secondary sexual characteristics.

Diagnosis

When the phenotypic sex is in doubt at birth, the genetic sex must be established by examination of a buccal smear for Barr bodies [p. 412]. Except in severe cases with a critical degree of glucocorticoid deficiency, the serum sodium and potassium levels are normal. The plasma level of 11-hydroxycorticosteroids is usually within the normal range because excess ACTH may partially overcome the block in cortisol biosynthesis although there is little adrenocortical reserve in the face of stress. Indeed, sometimes the plasma 11-hydroxycorticoid level is raised probably due to the formation of excess amounts of 21-desoxycortisol which will flouresce in the analytic method used. Thus it is important to emphasize that the plasma 11-hydroxycorticoid ('cortisol') level is useless in establishing the diagnosis and may be positively misleading. Similarly the urinary excretion of 17-oxogenic steroids is normal or increased because abnormal precursor metabolites will be estimated by the method used.

The essential findings in establishing the diagnosis are an increase in 17-oxosteroid excretion relative to the patient's age and the presence in the urine of abnormal metabolites such as pregnanetriol (upper normal limit in adults 2·5 mg. per 24 hours and usually less than 0·1 mg. before puberty), 17-hydroxypregnanolone, 11-oxopregnanetriol and tetrahydro-11-deoxycortisol.

Because of the difficulty in collecting accurately a complete 24-hour urine specimen in an infant, the most useful method for establishing the diagnosis in most instances is the 11-oxygenation index [p. 579].

Premature virilization in the male may be due to an adrenal tumour which produces increased urinary excretion of 17-oxosteroids and pregnanetriol. A testicular tumour, usually palpable, may produce increased amounts of urinary 17-oxosteroids but not of pregnanetriol. Congenital adrenal hyperplasia can be distinguished from an adrenal tumour by showing suppression of 17-oxosteroid excretion on administration of dexamethasone in a dose of 8 mg. daily [p. 579]. Other causes of precocious puberty are discussed on page 602.

In the female the differential diagnosis may be more difficult on clinical grounds, particularly in older patients, but the presence of increased amounts of 17-oxosteroids with abnormal metabolites in the urine, and the suppressive effect of dexamethasone are characteristic. Precocious puberty gives rise to premature but normal sexual hair, not to hirsutism. An androgen-secreting adrenal tumour is usually not suppressed by dexamethasone nor is an arrhenoblastoma which may be felt on bimanual palpation. The most difficult distinction is from the Stein-Leventhal syndrome [p. 611] and idiopathic hirsutism. In neonatal female infants the clinical picture of pseudohermaphroditism may be due to the administration of testosterone, methyltestosterone or progestogens to the mother during the early months of pregnancy, but in these cases the urinary excretion of 17-oxosteroids is normal.

Treatment

The essential step is to provide adequate substitution therapy for the defective biosynthesis of glucocorticoids. Cortisone, 25–37·5 mg., or prednisone, 5–7·5 mg., daily is usually sufficient, but the exact dosage is that which reduces the urinary excretion of 17-oxosteroids to the level normal for the patient's age or alternatively renders the 11-oxygenation index [p. 579] normal. Occasionally better control is achieved by the depot intramuscular injection of prednisolone trimethylacetate (100 mg. every 3–4 weeks). In patients with sodium loss, flurohydrocortisone may be necessary in a dose of 0·1 mg. daily. The patient or parents must be warned of the necessity to increase the dose of glucocorticoid in the face of any physical or severe psychological stress.

In a female pseudohermaphrodite plastic surgery may be required to correct the genital abnormalities when the condition is diagnosed in childhood. If the diagnosis is not made until after puberty and the patient has been brought up as a boy, it is often wiser to support the male role and use plastic surgery to make the external genitalia more masculine.

Prognosis

With adequate substitution therapy the prognosis is good particularly in the milder cases unassociated with hypertension or sodium loss. Females treated from early childhood have successfully borne children. In severe cases plastic surgery may be required to correct the genital anomalies, and there is always the danger of an acute adrenal crisis due to glucocorticoid deficiency unless the amount of substitution therapy is increased in situations of stress.

CARCINOMA OF THE ADRENAL CORTEX

Clinical Features

A malignant tumour of the adrenal cortex may

develop at any age, but this is a rare condition. Rapid invasion of surrounding tissues and metastases in the liver usually occur early so that the prognosis is poor. Sometimes the tumour may induce no significant endocrine manifestations. The patient complains of discomfort in the renal area and weight-loss; usually a mass is palpable which can only be differentiated from a renal lesion by an intravenous pyelogram. At laparotomy the tumour may prove irremovable because of local invasion or widespread hepatic involvement.

In other instances the carcinoma secretes one or more of the different groups of hormones normally synthesized in the adrenal cortex. If only one group is produced a relatively 'pure' endocrine picture, e.g. Cushing's syndrome in the case of glucocorticosteroids [p. 582], is produced; if several different groups are secreted a 'mixed' endocrine picture is seen.

Feminization in the male may be produced by an adrenal tumour, which is a carcinoma in 80 per cent. of cases and a benign adenoma in the remainder. The age incidence is 20–60 years. The clinical features are gynaecomastia in almost every case, with obesity and a palpable tumour in more than half the patients. There may be pain in the area of the tumour. Libido is reduced and testicular atrophy is common. In some cases Cushingoid features are also present. The urinary excretion of oestrogens is increased and the output of 17-oxosteroids is normal or raised.

Treatment

Whenever possible the tumour should be removed. If this proves impossible, and endocrine features are prominent, some suppression of hormonal biosynthesis may be achieved with aminoglutethimide in a dose of 0·75–2 G. daily in divided oral doses. This substance interferes with steroidal biosynthesis by blocking the conversion of cholesterol to pregnenolone [FIG. 34] and thus depresses the synthesis of aldosterone, cortisol and other hormones which have in common this early synthetic step. This drug can also prove helpful in control of the Cushingoid features induced by an ACTH-secreting tumour of 'non-endocrine' origin [p. 550]. Its main side-effects are anorexia, vomiting, somnolence, ataxia, fever and an erythematous macular rash. Another compound used for the control of an adrenocortical carcinoma is *o,p*^{1}-DDD which induces atrophy or necrosis of the adrenal cortex. Side-effects are common, involving the gastro-intestinal and central nervous systems. Life may be prolonged for a few months but the discomfort to the patient seldom justifies this form of treatment.

SYSTEMIC CORTICOSTEROIDS IN NON-ENDOCRINE DISEASES

Apart from their value as replacement therapy in acute and chronic adrenal insufficiency, panhypopituitarism and congenital adrenal hyperplasia (the adrenogenital syndrome), corticosteroids are used systemically in the treatment of a wide variety of non-endocrine conditions. In these the therapeutic rationale depends upon the non-specific suppression by corticosteroids of the inflammatory response and of the manifestations produced by a hypersensitivity or antibody-antigen reaction. The steroid dosage usually exceeds normal physiological requirements and is therefore termed pharmacological. Diseases which may respond to corticosteroid therapy include rheumatoid arthritis, ankylosing spondylitis, Reiter's syndrome and acute rheumatic fever; pemphigus, exfoliative dermatitis and other skin diseases; asthma, sarcoidosis and some cases of chronic bronchitis; the nephrotic syndrome, disseminated lupus erythematosus, cranial arteritis, polyarteritis nodosa and Wegener's granulomatosis; thrombocytopenic purpura, haemolytic anaemia and chronic lymphatic leukaemia; ulcerative colitis and some cases of Crohn's disease; sympathetic ophthalmia, non-bacterial iridocyclitis or keratitis and some cases of malignant exophthalmic ophthalmoplegia. Corticosteroids play an important role in the prevention of the rejection phenomenon after organ transplantation. The indications for corticosteroid treatment are discussed elsewhere but except in those conditions where it is life-saving, steroid therapy is seldom the treatment of first choice because of undesirable and potentially dangerous side-effects.

Cortisone is marketed in 25 mg. tablets and the many synthetic analogues (prednisone, prednisolone, methylprednisolone, triamcinolone, paramethasone, betamethasone and dexamethasone) are available in tablets which contain an amount of steroid with an anti-inflammatory action approximately equivalent to that of 25 mg. cortisone. In general the side-effects of all these compounds are similar with the notable difference that the synthetic analogues cause less sodium retention than cortisone and so are less likely to induce hypertension, oedema and urinary potassium loss. For this reason the synthetic analogues are used in preference to cortisone. No one analogue is strikingly superior in therapeutic action to another, and although one preparation may suit a particular patient better than another, in most instances prednisone is the steroid of first choice. The incidence of side-effects depends upon the dosage used, the duration of treatment and the individual response of the patient.

Mooning of the face and obesity of the trunk and neck with sparing of the limbs are common. Other Cushingoid features—acne, hirsuties and purple striae on the flanks and upper part of the thighs—may develop if the dose is large enough. These changes occur less often with triamcinolone which may cause anorexia and weight-loss. Some patients develop amenorrhoea.

Gastro-intestinal complications are common. About 25 per cent. of patients complain of dyspepsia and of those 5 per cent. have radiologically proven peptic ulcers. Haemorrhage or perforation may occur and the latter may be difficult to diagnose because the steroid treatment tends to mask the usual symptoms and physical signs. Similarly the manifestations of an acute infection are obscured, and a staphylococcal or pneumococcal septicaemia may develop with minimal constitutional disturbance, rise in temperature or increase in leucocyte count. Uncontrolled unrecognized infection is the most common complication to cause death, and about 25 per cent. of patients who die while having corticosteroid therapy do so from infection.

There is an increased liability to venous, coronary and cerebral thrombosis. The calf and pelvic veins are most commonly affected, particularly in patients confined to bed and may give rise to pulmonary emboli. Diabetes mellitus develops in some 5 per cent. of patients particularly when the steroid dosage is high and in those with latent glucose intolerance who might be expected to develop diabetes later in life. The frequency of osteoporosis is difficult to determine because lesser degrees may not be radiologically detectable. This is a complication of prolonged treatment and may be manifested by a crush-fracture of a vertebra particularly in patients with rheumatoid arthritis. Aseptic bone necrosis, most often of the femoral head, may occur and has been attributed to fat emboli. This complication has proved very disabling in patients receiving corticosteroid therapy after renal transplantation. Nitrogen loss from protein catabolism may also be the cause of a myopathy characterized by muscular weakness and wasting which occurs most often in patients treated with large doses of triamcinolone. Prolonged treatment may cause cataracts.

Additional side-effects may develop in children treated with corticosteroids. Acute pancreatitis may occur, and a number of cases of pseudotumour cerebri have been described. This syndrome, also called inappropriately benign intracranial hypertension, is characterized by headache, vomiting, a raised intracranial pressure and papilloedema which may lead to blindness. Usually the condition seems to develop when the dose of glucocorticoid is reduced and can be relieved by increasing the dosage again, to be followed by a very gradual weaning process.

The most important and common side-effect, specific of children having prolonged steroid treatment for the control of such conditions as asthma or the nephrotic syndrome, is retardation of growth, which can result in permanent dwarfism. When retardation does occur, as judged by slowing of the growth rate and delay in skeletal maturation, the dosage of corticosteroids must be kept to the absolute minimum that controls the manifestations of the primary disease. Some evidence suggests that corticosteroids on alternate days or treatment with ACTH is less likely to inhibit growth.

Many patients taking corticosteroids experience an increased sense of well-being and even euphoria which makes them reluctant to stop treatment and induces a state of steroid addiction. About 5 per cent. of patients have mental disturbances which range from increased mental activity and insomnia to a frank psychosis, and are particularly common in those with a history of previous mental instability.

Contra-indications

Unless necessary to save life, corticosteroids in pharmacological dosage should be avoided in patients with a peptic ulcer or a previous history of peptic ulcer, haematemesis or melaena; in those with past or present mental instability and when an acute or chronic bacterial infection, including tuberculosis, is present unless antibacterial treatment is given concurrently.

Adrenal Suppression

Corticosteroids inhibit the secretion of ACTH probably by depressing the secretion of the corticotrophin release factor from the hypothalamus. As a consequence with prolonged treatment a degree of anatomical atrophy of the adrenal cortex occurs as shown by a reduction in the weight of the adrenal glands. On stopping corticosteroid treatment there may be a delay before the atrophic adrenal glands respond to ACTH or before the pituitary secretes ACTH, and it may be several months before the hypothalamic-pituitary-adrenal axis functions normally. Initially both the ACTH and cortisol plasma levels are abnormally low. After a month or two the plasma ACTH level rises to normal or above normal if the adrenal glands remain unresponsive. Thus patients who are currently having corticosteroid therapy or have been treated with these compounds in the past may develop adrenocortical insufficiency if exposed to any stress normally associated with increased cortisol secretion.

Reactivation of the adrenal responsiveness to ACTH can be achieved during the gradual withdrawal of corticosteroid therapy by giving injections of corticotrophin-gel, 40 mg. twice daily for 3–4 days. At the end of this time the plasma 11-hydroxycorticosteroid level 5 hours after the last ACTH injection should be greater than 40 μg. per 100 ml. Failure to maintain a normal plasma 'cortisol' level [p. 579] between 9 and 10 a.m. during the 3 days after stopping the ACTH injections implies deficient secretion of corticotrophin from the adenohypophysis and this is usually found only in patients who have had high corticosteroid therapy continuously for a number of years. In most patients the pituitary-adrenal axis will appear to function normally but this does not necessarily mean that increased secretion of ACTH will occur in the face of stress, i.e. the hypothalamic-pituitary axis is not working normally. This suppression of the hypothalamic-pituitary axis may also occur in patients receiving prolonged ACTH therapy. To test this an insulin tolerance test [p. 542] may be done but this is quite impracticable if the patient needs urgent surgical treatment. For this reason the measures outlined below should be adopted.

Prophylaxis

Any patient currently receiving corticosteroids will require increased amounts during a surgical operation, labour or any other severe stress. Cortisone cover is also necessary for any patient who has had a prolonged course of steroids during the previous 18 months. A similar regime is used when surgery is necessary in an adrenalectomized or Addisonian patient, in congenital adrenal hyperplasia [p. 587] and when adrenal exploration is undertaken in a patient with Cushing's syndrome. Twenty-four hours and again 6 hours pre-operatively the patient is given 100 mg. cortisone acetate intramuscularly in addition, if currently taking steroids, to his usual dose. On completion of the operation another 100–200 mg. cortisone acetate is injected intramuscularly. Subsequent treatment depends upon whether the patient vomits. If possible, 50 mg. cortisone is given by mouth four times on the first postoperative day and the dosage is thereafter gradually reduced stepwise. If the patient vomits, 200–400 mg. hydrocortisone hemisuccinate intramuscularly or intravenously is given in divided doses on the first two postoperative days and then oral treatment continued. A major surgical operation normally stimulates the adrenal cortex to secrete 200–400 mg. cortisol, and it is safer to give too much cortisol rather than too little. The blood pressure and pulse rate must be carefully watched, and more steroid given if hypotension develops or the tachycardia is disproportionate to the severity of the operation.

Patients, who have stopped their steroid therapy for more than 18 months, do not necessarily require cortisone cover, but should be watched carefully during the operation period. If either they or the type of patient described in the preceding paragraph develop hypotension during the operation, 200 mg. hydrocortisone, 21-phosphate or hemisuccinate should be injected intravenously and cortisone given intramuscularly or by mouth, as outlined above, in the postoperative period.

THE ADRENAL MEDULLA

PHYSIOLOGICAL CONSIDERATIONS

The cells of the adrenal medulla and other parts of the sympathetic nervous system are of ectodermal origin, being derived from the primitive neural ridge. Two types of tissue are present—neuroblasts or mature ganglion cells and chromaffin cells, so-called because their intracellular granules stain brown with chromic acid. Accessory medullary tissue may be present as pea-sized chromaffin bodies which lie along the line of the carotid arteries and aorta, particularly near the kidneys at the origin of the superior and inferior mesenteric arteries (organs of Zuckerkandl).

Two hormones, adrenaline (epinephrine) and noradrenaline (norepinephrine) are secreted by the adrenal medulla. Noradrenaline is concerned with control of the circulation. A fall in blood pressure causes increased noradrenaline secretion which results in peripheral vasoconstriction and a rise in both systolic and diastolic blood pressure; reflex slowing of the heart rate occurs and there is little change in cardiac output. Adrenaline also influences the circulatory system but is more concerned in combating the metabolic consequences of stress. It raises the blood sugar level by mobilizing glucose from hepatic glycogen, increases oxygen consumption and causes bronchiolar dilatation. Adrenaline causes over-all vasodilatation of the blood vessels, a marked increase in heart rate and cardiac output, and a rise in systolic blood pressure but the diastolic level falls or remains unchanged because of the decreased peripheral vascular resistance.

Adrenaline and noradrenaline are metabolized to metanephrine and normetanephrine and then to 3-methoxy-4-hydroxymandelic acid (vanilmandelic acid, VMA) [FIG. 35]. Only small amounts of adrenaline and noradrenaline are excreted in the urine. Normally the urinary excretion of metanephrine and normetanephrine is less than 1 mg. a day and of 3-methoxy-4-hydroxymandelic acid 2–6 mg. a day.

PHAEOCHROMOCYTOMA

Synonym. Chromaffinoma.

Definition

A benign or malignant tumour of chromaffin tissue causing excessive secretion of adrenaline or noradrenaline which leads to hypertension and peculiar symptoms which often draw attention to the diagnosis.

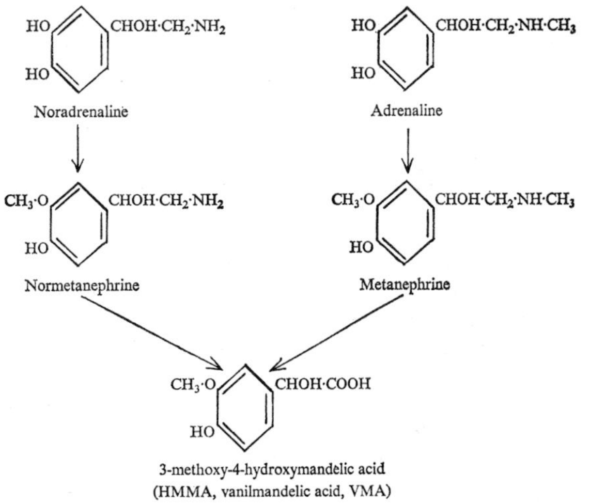

FIG. 35. The degradation of adrenaline and noradrenaline to 3-methoxy-4-hydroxymandelic acid.

Aetiology

The clinical features are directly related to the hypersecretion of adrenaline and noradrenaline. No age group is immune but the condition is diagnosed most often between the ages of 20 and 40. In some instances there is a familial incidence. Phaeochromocytomata may occur in association with neurofibromatosis, familial hyperparathyroidism or von Hippel-Lindau disease. A strong familial incidence is also found in patients with a medullary carcinoma of the thyroidal parafollicular 'C'-cells [p. 569].

Pathology

The tumour is usually benign but may be malignant and produce catecholamine-secreting metastases. The great majority of tumours are located in the abdomen and 90 per cent. are found in the adrenal glands, the right side more commonly than the left. Only rarely is the tumour situated in the thorax or neck.

In 10 per cent. of cases the tumours occur bilaterally in the adrenal glands and this incidence is even higher in children, of whom 24 per cent. have bilateral adrenal tumours and 40 per cent. have multiple tumours. The tumours vary in size, are very vascular and well encapsulated. Secretory potential is not related to size. On section the tumour is yellow-brown in colour and composed of characteristic polygonal cells with a granular cytoplasm; often there is evidence of haemorrhage or necrosis.

Symptoms

Phaeochromocytoma can mimic many other conditions. Most patients complain of attacks, usually lasting 10–15 minutes and sometimes much longer, characterized by profuse sweating, palpitations sometimes associated with cardiac irregularity, nervousness and apprehension, coldness and pallor, angina, dyspnoea, pounding in the head, nausea, vomiting and abdominal pain. These episodic features may occur spontaneously or be induced by physical exertion, emotional disturbances, minor operative procedures or palpation of the abdomen, and are associated with high blood pressure levels. In most cases hypertension is the cardinal finding. The blood pressure, although it fluctuates, may be persistently elevated or alternatively the hypertension may be paroxysmal. About one-third of all patients have glycosuria often only in association with an attack and a diabetic glucose tolerance curve is found in a quarter.

In some cases abdominal pain, hypotension and circulatory collapse may develop from necrosis of or haemorrhage into the tumour. Similar hypotensive episodes have been observed in patients with a phaeochromocytoma that secretes predominantly adrenaline rather than noradrenaline. These hypotensive episodes associated with abdominal pain and fever with a leucocytosis may suggest some intra-abdominal catastrophy such as a ruptured viscus or septicaemia.

Diagnosis

Pyrexia, a raised metabolic rate, a leucocytosis, hyperglycaemia, glycosuria, apprehension, sweating and cardiac irregularity may suggest a variety of diagnoses ranging from hyperthyroidism, coronary insufficiency, diabetes mellitus, menopausal symptoms or an anxiety state to some intra-abdominal surgical emergency. The clinical diagnosis may be particularly difficult if an episode of hypertension, unrecorded by the doctor, is followed by hypotension and circulatory collapse. The diagnosis is more likely to be made when hypertension is present, and although the incidence of the disease is only about 1 in every 1000 hypertensive patients, the possibility of phaeochromocytoma should be kept in mind, particularly if the patient sweats excessively or gives a history of paroxysmal symptoms. Rarely the combination of hypertension, fever, proteinuria and urinary casts suggests pyelonephritis.

The essential step in confirming the diagnosis is to demonstrate an excess of adrenaline, noradrenaline or their metabolites in the urine [FIG. 35]. A useful screening test is the measurement of 4-hydroxy-3-methoxymandelic acid (HMMA; VMA) in the urine, but in paroxysmal cases this may not be increased except during an attack. Patients with phaeochromocytoma usually have a greater than normal increase in the urinary excretion of noradrenaline when they are tipped from the supine to the horizontal position.

A number of pharmacological but indirect tests have been used to establish the diagnosis. When the hypertension is persistent, the intravenous infusion of 5 mg. phentolamine causes a fall in blood pressure but to be of diagnostic significance this reduction of systolic pressure should be at least 50 mm. Hg. In normotensive patients a variety of provocative tests have been used to induce a hypertensive attack. Histamine and tyramine have been used for this purpose but false positive and false negative responses have been obtained; these tests have a certain morbidity and cannot be recommended as reliable. At the present time the glucagon provocative test is under investigation. After a stable pressure has been recorded over several minutes, 1 mg. glucagon is injected into the tubing of an intravenous infusion of 5 per cent. glucose. Thereafter the blood pressure is recorded every 30 seconds for 5 minutes. A positive response is shown by a rise of 20–30 mm. Hg in both diastolic and systolic pressures. If the patient experiences any untoward symptoms the blood pressure can be reduced by the intravenous injection of 5 mg. phentolamine.

Having established that a phaeochromocytoma is present, the next step is to determine its location if possible. A palpable mass may be present in the abdomen or the position of the tumour may be inferred by a rise of blood pressure after deep palpation of one particular area. Chest X-rays should be done to exclude an intrathoracic tumour. The differential assay of the amounts of adrenaline and noradrenaline in the urine may be helpful in predicting the site of the phaeochromocytoma. When an excess of both adrenaline and noradrenaline is present, the tumour is usually located in the adrenal medulla or in the organ of Zuckerkandl. When only noradrenaline is present, the tumour may be anywhere in the abdomen, neck or thorax. Being highly vascular, these tumours can often be located by aortography and this investigation is particularly indicated in children who have a high incidence of multiple tumours.

In malignant tumours that produce catecholamines, dopamine and its metabolite homovanillic acid may be excreted in the urine, whereas these compounds are not secreted by benign phaeochromocytomata.

The accurate determination of urinary catecholamines and their metabolites depends on the absence of interfering substances in the urine which include metabolic excretory products of bananas, mono-amine oxidase inhibitors, methyldopa (*Aldomet*), phenothiazines, tetracycline and vitamins.

Treatment

The hypertension and other manifestations of excess catecholamine secretion can largely be prevented by such alpha-adrenergic blocking agents as phentolamine and phenoxybenzamine, and also by alpha-methyl-*p*-tyrosine (α-MT) which inhibits the hydroxylation of tyrosine to dopa, an essential step in the biosynthesis of adrenaline and noradrenaline. Phentolamine, 5 mg. intravenously, has a relatively short duration of action and is best used for the control of paroxysmal attacks and during handling of the tumour at surgical removal. Phenoxybenzamine has a longer duration of action and may be given orally or intravenously. An effective dose is usually 1 mg. per kg. bodyweight per day but in some cases as much as 200 mg. daily is required to control the blood pressure. Because of α-adrenergic blockade, the excess catecholamines act unopposed upon the β-receptors and induce a potentially dangerous tachycardia which can be controlled by propranolol in a dose up to 40 mg. three times a day or 1–5 mg. given by slow intravenous injection. The precise amount required can only be judged by the response of the heart rate. The advantage of α-MT in a dose up to 2 G. daily is that it controls symptoms, including the tachycardia, by decreasing the synthesis of catecholamines. In patients with phaeochromocytoma the blood volume is often reduced by long-standing vasoconstriction, and there is a marked tendency to dangerous hypotension postoperatively because of vasodilatation and hypovolaemia. This must be avoided by pre-operative preparation of the patient with phenoxybenzamine, usually with propranolol in addition, or preferably with α-MT for a period of at least 5 days. If the patient has cardiac failure due to catecholamine cardiomyopathy a longer period of pre-operative preparation will be required.

The most satisfactory treatment is surgical removal of the tumour. Premedication with hyoscine is preferred to atropine which causes a greater degree of tachycardia. Cyclopropane and trichlorethylene should be avoided as anaesthetic agents because they increase the release of catecholamines and may induce a ventricular tachycardia or arrhythmia. Control of the blood pressure during handling of the tumour at operation is best achieved by intravenous phentolamine. Postoperative hypotension is prophylactically avoided by proper pre-operative preparation and by blood transfusion to replace any operation loss and to maintain a normal central venous pressure when vasoconstriction is relaxed. Rarely is it necessary to infuse noradrenaline (12 mg. per litre of glucose-saline).

After removal of the tumour and recovery from the operation, the urinary excretion of HMMA (VMA) should be measured to ensure that all tumour tissue has been removed. The estimation should thereafter be repeated annually to detect a recurrence, and this is particularly indicated in cases with a familial incidence.

When the tumour is malignant and inoperable long-term treatment with α-MT will control the patient's symptoms.

Prognosis

Unless treated promptly phaeochromocytoma is a potentially fatal condition, death usually being due to ventricular arrhythmia, acute left ventricular failure with pulmonary oedema or a cerebral haemorrhage. Occasionally the patient dies of hypotension after a hypertensive paroxysm, haemorrhage into or necrosis of the tumour, or postoperatively. Surgical treatment usually induces a complete remission of the clinical manifestations and the hypertension, except when multiple tumours are present or renal damage causes persistent hypertension.

NEUROBLASTOMA

Synonym. Sympathoblastoma.

Definition

A highly malignant tumour of sympathetic nerve-cell tissue which occurs in infancy or childhood and produces clinical manifestations locally or as a result of metastases.

Aetiology

The tumour usually arises from the adrenal medulla but may occur elsewhere in the retroperitoneal or retropleural spaces.

Pathology

The tumour grows rapidly and is very cellular; it is composed of round cells often arranged in rosettes. Widespread metastases occur early.

Symptoms

The disease may present as abdominal enlargement due to a retroperitoneal mass or as a result of metastases. Pepper's syndrome occurs during the neonatal period and is characterized by hepatomegaly due to metastoses a retroperitoneal mass, absence of jaundice or ascites and progressive weakness and emaciation. Hutchison's syndrome occurs in childhood and is characterized by proptosis and a raised intracranial pressure due to metastases in the skull, a retroperitoneal mass and a rapidly downhill course. In many of these cases increased amounts of 3-methoxy-4-hydroxymandelic acid, dopamine and homovanillic acid may be excreted in the urine, and help to distinguish the condition from a retroperitoneal sarcoma, a Wilms' tumour or a benign phaeochromocytoma.

Treatment

Radical surgery followed by radiotherapy may cure the condition when the tumour is confined to the abdominal cavity. The prognosis is grave when metastases have developed.

ENDOCRINE DISORDERS OF THE BREAST

PHYSIOLOGICAL CONSIDERATIONS

The breasts are composed of exocrine glandular tissue, comprising the acini and the duct system running from the terminal acinar buds to the nipple, and supporting connective tissue and fat. At birth there may be some mammary enlargement with secretion of 'witch's' milk due to the influence of maternal oestrogens. This quickly subsides, and the breasts remain rudimentary until puberty, of which mammary development is one of the earliest signs. Under the influence of oestrogens the ducts grow and branch, and considerable amounts of fat are deposited around the ductal tissue. Under the influence of progesterone the rudimentary acini develop into swollen buds. It is not uncommon for the breasts to become enlarged and somewhat tender during the week before menstruation, an effect ascribed to increased progesterone secretion during the luteal phase of the menstrual cycle. It is also not uncommon for one breast to be somewhat smaller than the other, and sometimes unilateral hypoplasia is marked and permanent. This emphasizes how much the ultimate size of the breasts depends upon the responsiveness of the mammary tissue to hormonal stimulation as well as the actual plasma level of the hormones concerned. During *pregnancy* there is a marked increase in the branching of the terminal ducts and in the number and size of the acini. These changes are attributable to the high plasma levels of oestrogens and progesterone and also possibly to increased secretion of growth hormone, prolactin and placental lactogen. At term *lactation* is initiated by the secretion of prolactin from the eosinophilic cells of the adenohypophysis which has previously been held in check by a prolactin-inhibitory factor of hypothalamic origin. The ejection of milk is dependent on a neurohumoral reflex initiated by stimulation of the nipple by suckling and the subsequent release from the hypothalamus of oxytocin which stimulates the myoepithelial cells surrounding the terminal ducts and acini. Regression of mammary development occurs with cessation of breast feeding and is even more marked, amounting to atrophy, after the *menopause* when ovarian failure leads to diminished secretion of oestrogens and progesterone.

In the male, breast development does not normally occur but some enlargement of the acinar tissue immediately behind the nipple and not just the deposition of fat, i.e. true gynaecomastia, is commonly found in adolescent boys. In about a quarter the gynaecomastia is unilateral and in most instances resolves spontaneously over a period of 2–3 years. Breast enlargement may also occur at the other end of the life-span in males. At this age gynaecomastia usually has a sinister significance (see below) but in a number of instances no pathological cause is found.

ATROPHY OF THE BREASTS

Oestrogen Deficiency. Atrophy of the breasts or failure of mammary development occurs in conditions of secondary gonadal failure due to failure of secretion of gonadotrophins from the pituitary gland as occurs in panhypopituitarism or isolated deficiency of FSH or LH secretion. Infarction of the pituitary as a consequence of severe post-partum haemorrhage (Sheehan's syndrome) invariably leads to failure of lactation and mammary atrophy. Primary ovarian failure as in Turner's syndrome [p. 608] and other forms of ovarian dysgenesis is associated with poor mammary development. Virilizing tumours of the adrenals or ovaries and the syndrome of congenital adrenal hyperplasia [p. 587] are associated with poor breast development but in these patients hirsutism is a more prominent primary complaint. Malnutrition from any cause, but particularly anorexia nervosa [Section 17], is associated with atrophy of the breasts. In all these conditions treatment must be directed at curing the underlying cause. In some, substitution therapy is required, and cyclical treatment with oestrogens and a progestational agent in the doses recommended on page 608 will correct the hypogonadism and promote breast development.

End-Organ Failure. Young women are often concerned at what they consider to be inadequate breast development. In some instances these patients are underweight but their other secondary sexual characteristics and functions are normal. Often the size of the breasts is not below the normal range but the patients are obsessed by their smallness. Reassurance as to normal sexual function and normal sexuality and, an explanation that the ability to feed a baby is unrelated to breast size may relieve their anxiety to some extent. In some patients administration of a contraceptive pill with a relative high oestrogen content (e.g. *Conovid-E*) may improve breast development and the situation may be further helped by the inunction nightly of 25 mg. stilboestrol in 1 g. lanoline for a period of about 2 months. Just as it is the physician's duty to use psychotherapy to assuage the patient's sense of inadequacy, equally he must warn against the dangers of many of the surgical procedures advocated to increase breast size. Injections of paraffin wax or silicone is to be condemned because of the subsequent development of chronic suppurating inflammatory sinuses. Probably the most 'physiological' surgical procedure is the transplantation of gluteal fat to the retromammary area, but the surgical complexity of this procedure has tended to be replaced by the use of prostheses, usually siliconized bags filled with silicone or dextran solutions. Although often initially pleasing to the patient, the ultimate results with the development of sinuses, herniation of the prosthesis and distortion of the normal breast contour are frequently unsatisfactory. The patient's interests are usually better served by psychotherapy, an explanation as to the current 'mammary cult' and the wearing of a padded brassiere.

HYPERTROPHY OF THE BREASTS

Premature development of the breasts occurs in precocious puberty [p. 606] and may arise as an isolated abnormality, sometimes unilateral, in prepubertal girls as young as 3-years old without other evidence of precocious puberty.

Rarely excessive mammary development starts at puberty and progresses so that the breasts become enormous and grotesque. The cause of this condition is unknown but histologically there is hyperplasia of the periductal fibrous tissue. Judging by the skin temperature, the rubor and the dilated veins, the blood flow to the breasts is enormous. The condition may advance to such a degree that the weight of the breasts makes it impossible for the patient to stand upright. At present the only satisfactory treatment is plastic surgery which may also be indicated in obese patients with pendulous breasts who have succeeded in losing weight.

'Chronic Mastitis'. Recurrent fibro-adenomatosis of the breasts is thought to be due to an imbalance between oestrogen and progesterone secretion. Once it is established that the condition is not malignant, the recurrence of tender nodules can often be prevented or mitigated by giving norethisterone, 15 mg. daily from days 15 to 25 of each menstrual cycle.

GYNAECOMASTIA

Definition

Gynaecomastia is characterized by enlargement and often tenderness of the mammary tissue in the male breast. It may be bilateral or unilateral, first on one side and then on the other.

Aetiology

Gynaecomastia occurs in a large number of seemingly unrelated conditions. In adolescent males some degree of temporary gynaecomastia lasting 1–3 years is sufficiently common to be considered physiologically normal. Its main significance is the embarrassment the patient suffers and the teasing he receives from his school-mates. Although formerly attributed to excess oestrogen secretion or to an imbalance between oestrogens and androgens, there is no laboratory support for this belief. It seems more likely that this transient gynaecomastia is related to growth hormone secretion, and the breast enlargement usually diminishes concurrently with the cessation of growth.

Gynaecomastia is uncommon in patients with hypogonadism secondary to hypothalamo-pituitary dysfunction and is much more common when there is hypogonadism due to primary testicular failure as occurs, for example, in Klinefelter's syndrome [p. 599]. It occurs commonly in men who are given oestrogens for the control of prostatic carcinoma; in those (usually transvestists) who deliberately take oestrogens to attain mammary development; and in those who unwittingly do so by massaging their scalp with oestrogen-containing hair creams to prevent baldness.

It also occurs in patients with hepatic cirrhosis, and may develop in patients recovering from severe malnutrition as a result of re-feeding. Gynaecomastia not infrequently occurs in patients with chronic renal failure when they are treated by long-term haemodialysis.

The gynaecomastia sometimes found in patients with oat-cell bronchial carcinoma, usually but not invariably associated with pulmonary osteoarthropathy, has been ascribed to the ectopic secretion of gonadotrophins, growth hormone and/or prolactin. Gynaecomastia occurs rarely with other pulmonary lesions of a chronic infective nature. The condition has also been observed in association with hypothyroidism, thyrotoxicosis, acromegaly, paraplegia, and feminizing tumours of the adrenal cortex or testis.

A number of drugs may induce gynaecomastia. Spironolactone is a common offender when used as a diuretic in the treatment of patients with ascites of cirrhotic origin or for the control of hypertension caused by aldosteronism. Other drugs, probably by an action on the hypothalamus, may induce gynaecomastia, and these include amphetamine, reserpine, chlorpromazine and methyldopa.

Symptoms

The enlargement of the mammary tissue is seldom marked but often the breast is tender to the touch. The condition must be distinguished from adiposity of the breast. In true gynaecomastia the hypertrophied breast tissue is felt immediately behind the nipple as thickened and tender, whereas in obesity the whole structure is flabby and uniformly enlarged.

Treatment

Treatment depends on the cause. Removal of an oestrogen-secreting tumour will cure the condition as will resection of or X-ray therapy to a bronchial carcinoma. Withdrawal of a precipitating drug will be followed by a remission of symptoms. In adolescent gynaecomastia mastectomy is seldom indicated because of the spontaneous remission that occurs in due course, but surgical intervention may be required in patients with Klinefelter's syndrome to relieve embarrassment.

Prognosis

The prognosis depends upon the cause. Mammary carcinoma may develop in male transvestists who take an excess dosage of oestrogens over a prolonged period of time.

GALACTORRHOEA

Definition

Galactorrhoea is the inappropriate secretion of milk.

Aetiology

The factors responsible for galactorrhoea are ill-understood. It is nearly always associated with amenorrhoea and related to some pituitary or hypothalamic abnormality. Pending better understanding of the mechanisms involved, a number of eponyms are used to describe the syndromes in which galactorrhoea occurs. The Chiari-Frommel syndrome occurs in the post-partum woman who has ceased to feed her baby. It may persist indefinitely but is usually transient. There is no X-ray evidence of a pituitary tumour. The del Castillo syndrome occurs spontaneously in women who have not been pregnant. The sella turcica is of normal size and the galactorrhoea tends to be persistent. In the Forbes-Albright syndrome the galactorrhoea occurs spontaneously or *post partum*. The sella turcica is enlarged radiologically and the condition is permanent. In some instances galactorrhoea may occur in association with Cushing's syndrome [p. 582] due to bilateral adrenal hyperplasia attributable to excess ACTH secretion from the adenohyphosis. It has also been observed in hypothyroidism associated with amenorrhoea.

Symptoms

The amount of milk produced is usually small but sufficient to be an embarrassment and annoyance to the patient. The lactation may be spontaneous or only occur on pressing the breasts.

Treatment

When galactorrhoea is associated with Cushing's syndrome or evidence of a pituitary tumour, hypophysectomy or the implantation of yttrium seeds is the treatment of choice. In the Chiari-Frommel and del Castillo syndromes the galactorrhoea usually ceases when clomiphene, 50 mg. once or twice daily, is given for 7–10 days. This treatment may also correct the amenorrhoea. When the galactorrhoea and amenorrhoea are associated with hypothyroidism, treatment with thyroxine quickly corrects the situation.

DISEASES OF THE GONADS

DISEASES OF THE TESTIS

PHYSIOLOGICAL CONSIDERATIONS

The early embryonic development of the testes is from the medulla of the primitive genital ridge. During the later part of foetal life the testes descend from the posterior abdominal wall through the iliac fossae and inguinal canals to reach the scrotum at or shortly after birth. Normal adult testes are located in the scrotum, measure 4 by 2·5 cm. and have a firm consistency. They are composed of two distinct elements, the seminiferous tubules and the interstitial or Leydig cells.

The *seminiferous tubules* are separated into lobules by septa of connective tissue. The cells lining the tubules are undifferentiated until puberty, when under the influence of the follicle stimulating hormone (FSH), spermatogenic and Sertoli cells develop. Spermatozoa are formed from the germ cells and as they develop and pass towards the lumen of the tubule adhere to the Sertoli cells which are attached to the basement membrane and project perpendicularly into the lumen. Mature spermatozoa pass into the epididymis on the posterior aspect of the testis and thence via the vas deferens to the posterior urethra. Normal spermatogenesis requires secretion of testosterone by the interstitial cells and also of an oestrogenic hormone, which probably originates from the Sertoli cells or possibly the Leydig cells or both. Thus spermatogenesis is defective when Leydig cell function is deficient and androgen secretion is reduced. The cells of the seminiferous tubules are also sensitive to temperature and unless this is lower than the rest of the body temperature, differentiation and maturation are arrested. The germinal epithelium may be irreparably damaged if the testis is not within the scrotum at the time when FSH is secreted at puberty.

The *interstitial cells* secrete testosterone. They are arranged in clumps surrounded by a stroma of connective tissue. These cells are prominent at birth but involute during childhood to become prominent again at puberty as a result of stimulation by the interstitial-cell-stimulating hormone (luteinizing hormone). The Leydig cells are less sensitive to temperature than the seminiferous tubules and will secrete testosterone if the testis is retained within the abdominal cavity. Testosterone is the most potent naturally-occurring androgen, and the androgenic steroids secreted by the adrenal cortex are not sufficient to prevent the development of hypogonadism (eunuchoidism) in a castrated male or in patients with Leydig cell deficiency. During foetal life the secretion of testosterone is responsible for the development of the male genital tract; during and after puberty it is essential for normal spermatogenesis, the growth of the accessory sexual organs, the development of male secondary sexual characteristics, skeletal maturation and muscular growth.

Gonadotrophin Control. FSH is responsible for spermatogenesis, and LH (or the interstitial-cell-stimulating hormone) for Leydig cell activity with consequent secretion of testosterone. Total castration leads to increased plasma levels of both FSH and LH as measured by radio-immunoassay techniques. Administration of testosterone or other potent androgens depresses the pituitary secretion of LH but has little influence on FSH production unless given in large dosage when, in addition to the anticipated atrophy of the Leydig cells, the seminiferous tubules also become atrophic. Conversely failure of Leydig cell function is associated with an increase in the plasma LH titre. Selective failure of spermatogenic tissue increases the plasma FSH level, and administration of oestrogen suppresses the secretion of both FSH and LH. Clomiphene [p. 610] increases the secretion of both gonadotrophic hormones and its uses in the treatment of secondary hypogonadism or seminiferous tubular failure is still under investigation.

TESTS OF TESTICULAR FUNCTION

Although failure of the hormonogenic function of the Leydig cells almost invariably leads to impaired spermatogenesis, the converse is not the case. Tests of testicular function must therefore assess androgen secretion by the interstitial cells and the production of spermatozoa by the seminiferous tubules.

Spermatogenic Function. The assessment of seminiferous tubular function is best determined by a history of the previous ability to procreate and by examination of at least two specimens of semen obtained after 3, and preferably 5, days of sexual abstinence. The specimen should be collected direct into a warmed polystyrene container, and this should be kept in the patient's trouser pocket until delivered to the laboratory within 2 hours. A normal ejaculate has a volume of 2 ml. or more, and less than 1·5 ml. may signify abnormality. The fluid normally contains not less than 20 million sperms per ml. Fertility may occur with a lower count than this provided that the motility of the sperms is particularly marked. Indeed the motility and morphology of the spermatozoa is probably more significant than the total number per ml. Motility declines rapidly after the specimen has been obtained, but within 3 hours at least 40 per cent. of the sperms should be motile. The morphology should be normal in 40–60 per cent. of the sperms. The ejaculate should be tested for the presence of fructose in patients with azoospermia because its absence indicates maldevelopment or occlusion of the vasa deferentia or seminal vesicles.

Androgenic Function. The adequacy of androgenic secretion by the Leydig cells can be assessed only after puberty. Normal secretion is indicated, at clinical examination, by the accessory sexual organs and the secondary sexual characteristics, particularly the size of the penis and scrotum, the development of the prostate and larynx, and the growth of pubic, axillary, peri-anal, facial and body hair. Changes in these parameters are often less striking when Leydig cell function is lost after full sexual maturation has been achieved. Skeletal development is a good index of androgen secretion, particularly in the immediate postpubertal period. Precocious puberty increases bone growth and epiphyseal development, but the epiphyses close early and growth is stunted. Androgen deficiency delays epiphyseal closure; growth continues for an abnormally long time and eunuchoid skeletal proportions are obtained in which the span is greater than the height, and the lower measurement from the symphysis pubis to the ground is much greater than the upper measurement from the crown to the symphysis pubis.

Although testosterone is metabolized and excreted as a 17-oxosteroid, it constitutes so small a proportion of the total 17-oxosteroid urinary output that diminished Leydig cell function is not detectable by ordinary chemical methods. More information is obtained by measurement of the plasma testosterone concentration or by the testosterone production rate, but these are procedures still confined to research laboratories.

Gonadotrophin Secretion. The distinction between primary testicular failure and that secondary to a disorder of hypothalamo-pituitary function can be made by measurement of the plasma or urinary levels of gonadotrophins. Primary testicular failure after puberty is associated with increased gonadotrophin levels, and the more specific separate failure of tubular or Leydig cell function may be reflected by increased plasma levels of FSH in the former and of LH in the latter. Total gonadotrophin urinary excretion, which measures by bioassay both FSH and LH, is a poor index of Leydig-cell failure and is more strikingly increased in defective spermatogenesis. Testicular failure as a consequence of diminished gonadotrophin secretion, which may occur in panhypopituitarism [p. 544] or as an isolated monotrophic deficiency, is characterized by abnormally low levels of FSH.

Testicular Biopsy. In many patients with spermatogenic or androgenic deficiency, testicular biopsy is an essential step in establishing an accurate diagnosis and determining the prognosis. The procedure is simple to perform and best carried out under a short-acting general anaesthetic. The biopsied tissue should be preserved in Bouin's fluid and not in formalin or formol-saline which makes histological interpretation of tubular function difficult. Testicular biopsy is indicated in an infertile couple when the man on two separate occasions shows azoospermia or a sperm count of less than 20 million per ml., particularly if the mobility of the spermatozoa is poor. In seeking the cause of infertility, investigation of the male is often deferred until the wife has been subjected to examination under anaesthesia and salpingography. Because about one-third of all cases of infertility are due to a defect in the male, this is illogical [p. 600].

Testicular biopsy is also indicated in some patients with hypogonadism [p. 598] particularly when high gonadotrophin levels imply primary testicular disease. The nuclear sex, assessed by examination of buccal squames or leucocytes, and determination of the patient's sex chromosomal complement in the karyotype may be necessary to define testicular deficiency of genetic origin [p. 598].

CRYPTORCHIDISM

Synonyms. Undescended testis; Testicular maldescent.

Definition

Cryptorchidism is defined as the absence of one or both testes from the scrotum. It is essential to decide whether the condition is unilateral or bilateral, and also to define the exact position of the gonad. The gland may be *intra-abdominal* and in this condition no gonadal tissue is palpable. The testis may be located in the *inguinal canal.* It may occupy an *ectopic* site lying outside the inguinal canal in the perineum, anterior to the symphysis pubis, between the layers of the anterior abdominal wall or in the femoral canal. It is most important to distinguish true cryptorchidism from the much commoner condition of pseudocryptorchidism (see diagnosis).

Aetiology

The causes of cryptorchidism are many but in most instances no anatomical or endocrine abnormality is detectable. Sometimes the condition is clearly related to an anatomical abnormality such as a congenital inguinal hernia. Rare causes of bilateral cryptorchidism include ill-understood endocrine deficiences in foetal development, abnormal sex chromosome constitution such as Klinefelter's syndrome [p. 599], testicular agenesis or anorchism of unknown causation, aplasia of the tubular germinal epithelium, and pituitary hypofunction which may be generalized or confined to selective gonadotrophin deficiency. Rarely the condition may be confused with female pseudohermaphroditism in which a female child becomes virilized by excess androgenic secretion because of congenital adrenal hyperplasia [p. 587]. Cryptorchidism also occurs in male pseudohermaphroditism [p. 618]. These endocrine abnormalities are uncommon and do not apply when the cryptorchidism is unilateral.

The incidence of *unilaterally* undescended testis is some four times more common at birth than the bilateral form, and far less often corrects itself spontaneously. The incidence of bilaterally undescended testes is 3 per cent. in full-term infants but may be as high as 20 per cent. in those born prematurely but corrects itself in the majority by the age of 3 months. After the age of one year the incidence of bilateral cryptorchidism is only 0·2 per cent.

Pathology

Maldescended testes are liable to torsion, trauma, irreversible degeneration of the seminiferous tubules and malignant change after puberty, particularly when the gonad is retained in the abdomen or associated with an intersex abnormality. Tubular development becomes histologically abnormal in the undescended testis from the age of 5 onwards, and progressively so thereafter; hence the necessity for early treatment.

Symptoms

Testicular maldescent may be first noticed at routine postnatal examination, or the diagnosis may be delayed until the first school examination when the finding of true cryptorchidism is even more significant. Only rarely does maldescent of the testes continue unnoticed into adult life and then presents as infertility or malignant degeneration.

Diagnosis

It is most important that unilateral or bilateral maldescent of the testes is distinguished from the clinically unimportant condition of pseudocryptorchidism in which one or both gonads, retracted by the cremasteric muscle, lie high in the scrotum or in the inguinal canal. Some 80 per cent. of patients referred with cryptorchidism prove to have pseudocryptorchidism, and sometimes the distinction can only be made by repeated examination in warm surroundings with warm hands. In patients with pseudocryptorchidism the testes descend into the scrotum at puberty and no treatment is required. Cryptorchidism must also be differentiated from concealment of the testes in obese boys with a large pad of suprapubic fat often associated with some delay in the onset of puberty.

Treatment

An intra-abdominal testis will never descend spontaneously into the scrotum and because of the possible risk of malignant change later in life and certain failure of spermatogenesis, orchidectomy is recommended. Equally an ectopically located testis will never descend spontaneously and orchidopexy to place the gonad in the scrotum is indicated during the first few years of life. Early operation is also indicated when maldescent is associated with a hernia. Persistent non-descent, unilateral or bilateral, at the age of 5 is an indication for surgical treatment, and because of the degeneration that starts to develop in the seminiferous tubules at this time, the modern practice is to operate sooner rather than later. A short course of 4000 Units of chorionic gonadotrophin may be given intramuscularly thrice weekly for 3–6 weeks at this age, but if unsuccessful orchidopexy should not be delayed later than the age of 8 years.

MALE HYPOGONADISM

Synonyms. Eunuchoidism; Eunuchism.

Definition

Strictly speaking the term hypogonadism could be used to describe deficiency of either one or both of the two functions of the testes, namely the secretion of testosterone by the interstitial cells and the production of spermatozoa. In clinical practice hypogonadism is restricted to describing the clinical state resulting from deficient androgen secretion, and infertility or sterility to describe failure of spermatogenesis. The term eunuch is applied to an anatomically castrated male and eunuchoid to a patient with the clinical features of hypogonadism who is not devoid of his gonads. Hypogonadism usually causes infertility [p. 600] but failure of spermatogenic function may occur without hypogonadism.

Aetiology

Hypogonadism may be due to a congenital or acquired primary disorder of the testes or secondary to failure of the hypothalamo-pituitary system to secrete gonadotrophins.

Primary Hypogonadism. *Congenital causes* of primary testicular interstitial cell failure include developmental defects such as anorchia, genetic defects such as occur in Klinefelter's syndrome [p. 599], dystrophia myotonica, the Laurence-Moon-Biedl syndrome [p. 546] and male pseudohermaphroditism [p. 618]. *Acquired causes* of primary testicular failure of testosterone secretion result from torsion or surgical damage to the blood supply during correction of bilateral herniae during childhood, X-irradiation, surgical removal of the testes, and infections such as bilateral mumps orchitis in the postpubertal phase, tuberculosis, leprosy or syphilis. Testicular atrophy may also occur in haemochromatosis due to the deposition of iron in the gonad, and in patients with hepatic cirrhosis.

Secondary Hypogonadism. Failure of gonadotrophin secretion may be an expression of panhypopituitarism [p. 544] and is then associated with deficient secretion of other trophic hormones. Rarely it occurs as an isolated monotrophic deficiency of unknown aetiology. In these cases there is no evidence of spermatogenesis and Leydig cells may be totally absent on histological examination of testicular tissue obtained by biopsy. In some patients hypogonadism due to an isolated deficiency of gonadotrophin secretion is associated with anosmia due to atrophy of the olfactory lobes (Kallmann's syndrome). Functional secondary hypogonadism may be due to malnutrition or metabolic disorders such as steatorrhoea, chronic renal disease or any other severe debilitating condition. Depression of gonadotrophin secretion may also be induced by a feminizing adrenal tumour that secretes oestrogens or administration of oestrogens for the control of a metastasizing prostatic carcinoma. Hypogonadism may also be self-induced by male transvestists who take large doses of oestrogen to achieve mammary development.

Symptoms

The clinical manifestations of hypogonadism depend upon the age of onset and the degree of androgen deficiency. Unless there is some obvious testicular abnormality, the condition is seldom recognized until after the time of normal puberty, when the parents first become concerned about their son's small genitalia and failure to mature. The penis and scrotum are small; the prostate rudimentary, the larynx underdeveloped and the voice unbroken. Pubic hair is absent or sparse. Facial and axillary hair is usually absent. The skin is soft and hairless. The patient is often slender and has poor muscular development. There is a lack of drive and aggressiveness. Gynaecomastia is common. The bone age at adolescence is less than the chronological age, and failure of the epiphyses to close may result in increased growth of the long bones, so that the patient later in life may be tall with the span greater than the height, and the lower measurement from the symphysis pubis to ground greater than that from the crown to the symphysis pubis (eunuchoid habitus). Libido and erections are much diminished or absent.

Partial loss of androgenic function, or its onset after

maturation has been achieved, causes less striking sexual and somatic effects. Facial and body hair is sparse and pubic hair has a female distribution with a horizontal upper border. The skin is delicate and fine wrinkles appear around the mouth and eyes. The complexion is sallow and there may be a mild degree of anaemia. Androgen deficiency reduces libido and the patient may therefore not complain of impotence and lack of erections.

Diagnosis

The degree of hypogonadism is best assessed by clinical examination to determine the extent of androgenization. This clinical assessment must of course be correlated with the degree of virilization that would be anticipated at the particular age of the patient. Precise quantitation of androgen secretion can be made from the urinary excretion of testosterone or measurement of the testosterone production rate, both involving technically difficult procedures not widely available. The urinary excretion of 17-oxosteroids is not a sensitive measure of androgen production. In an adult the time of onset of hypogonadism may be known from the patient's history and confirmed from the skeletal proportions and the radiological bone age.

The distinction between primary and secondary hypogonadism may be possible on clinical findings if there is clear evidence of other trophic hormone deficiencies or of intracranial disease. Gynaecomastia is more common in primary hypogonadism. The urinary excretion of total gonadotrophins may be helpful in making the distinction. High levels are found in post-adolescent patients with primary testicular disease but the bioassay method usually used largely reflects FSH excretion and this is more increased when there is both Leydig cell and seminiferous tubular disease than when there is only Leydig-cell failure. High plasma levels of LH are found in interstitial-cell deficiency and of FSH in spermatogenic failure of primary testicular origin. Testicular biopsy [p. 597] and determination of the nuclear sex or karyotype analysis may be necessary to establish the diagnosis, particularly in Klinefelter's syndrome.

Often the main problem is determining the cause of hypogonadism in a boy aged 14–18. In addition to the endocrine and genetic causes discussed above and undetected or inadequately treated juvenile myxoedema [p. 567] which is associated with shortness of stature, asymptomatic generalized metabolic disease may be present such as renal acidosis or other forms of chronic renal disease, or steatorrhoea. After exclusion of these causes, the main problem is the recognition of 'idiopathic delayed puberty'. This, like general metabolic causes of hypogonadism, is usually associated with shortness of stature, attributable to a delayed pubescent growth spurt, rather than the normal or increased height found in primary hypogonadism. Unless there is a history of late onset of puberty in other members of the family, idiopathic delayed puberty is a diagnosis that can only be made by exclusion, but most boys with this condition are fat; their small genitalia are concealed by a suprapubic pad of fat and appear relatively even smaller because of the size of their trunk. These children are gluttonous, often keen swimmers and have over-protective mothers. Their condition is often misdiagnosed as Fröhlich's syndrome [p. 546].

Treatment

The underlying cause of the hypogonadism should be corrected but this is seldom possible unless the condition is due to hypothyroidism or is secondary to a pituitary tumour amenable to treatment, or to some non-endocrine disorder such as steatorrhoea or chronic renal disease. Stimulation of the gonads with gonadotrophins is the logical treatment for secondary hypogonadism but injections over a prolonged period are seldom practicable and treatment with chorionic gonadotrophin, 1000 Units thrice weekly for three months, is largely reserved for patients whose puberty is delayed until the age of 17, although the value of any treatment in idiopathic delayed puberty is difficult to assess because normal maturation occurs in the fullness of time.

For most cases of established hypogonadism, replacement therapy with androgens is the treatment of choice. Initially long-acting esters of testosterone are given by intramuscular injection, such as testosterone enanthate, 250 mg., or a combination of esters in the form of *Sustanon 250* at monthly intervals. This should be continued until an adequate degree of virilization has been achieved. Thereafter maintenance therapy can be provided by sublinguinal adsorption of methyltestosterone, 25–50 mg. daily, or oral administration of the synthetic more potent androgen fluoxymesterone, 5–10 mg. daily. Androgen therapy sometimes causes sodium and water retention, acne or gynaecomastia. Rarely orally administered androgens cause cholestatic jaundice.

Prognosis

The prognosis depends upon the cause. Androgen therapy causes a striking improvement in physical, sexual and mental development but permanent infertility must be expected.

KLINEFELTER'S SYNDROME

Synonym. Seminiferous tubule dysgenesis.

Definition

A particular variety of male hypogonadism characterized by one or more extra X chromosomes and manifest by partial or complete hyalinization of the seminiferous tubules, small testes, azoospermia and varying degrees of androgen deficiency. Common clinical associations are gynaecomastia and intellectual subnormality. The secretion of gonadotrophins is increased and there may be a moderate reduction in urinary 17-oxosteroid excretion.

Aetiology

By the definition used here all patients with Klinefelter's syndrome have a chromatin-positive nuclear sex [p. 616] due to one or more extra X chromosomes. Instead of the normal 46 karyotype, the total number of chromosomes ranges from 47 to 49 because the sex chromosome complement is XXY, XXYY, XXXY or

XXXXY. When more than two X chromosomes are present, the cell nuclei may show more than one chromatin dot. This chromosomal abnormality is probably due to non-disjunction of the sex chromosomes during gametogenesis in one of the parents, probably the mother, and the extra X chromosome is responsible for the maldevelopment of the testicular germinal epithelium in the patient. Occasionally sex chromosome mosaicism is found and two cell populations, one XY and the other XXY, are found.

Patients with clinical features similar to those found in Klinefelter's syndrome have been described who have a chromatin-negative nuclear sex and 46 chromosomes with an apparently normal XY complement. In such cases the testicular histological appearances are often atypical. In the past these patients have been termed 'chromatin-negative Klinefelter's syndrome' and the aetiology attributed to some unidentified chromosomal structure anomaly. It is more likely that these cases represent a heterogeneous group arising from a number of different causes and, despite similar but non-specific clinical features, should not be related to Klinefelter's syndrome.

Pathology

A testicular biopsy shows degeneration of the seminiferous tubules which are shrunken and hyalinized. Less obvious changes are present in the interstitial cells which are present in large clumps.

Symptoms

Clinically the condition does not declare itself until after puberty. Gynaecomastia [p. 594] may be the presenting feature. Secondary sexual characteristics are often poorly developed but the degree of lack of androgenization is very variable. Later in life infertility is the main complaint. The testes are small. Depending on the degree of hypogonadism, the habitus is eunuchoid and the legs abnormally long compared with the length of the trunk. An inconstant but unusual feature is that the span and the height are sometimes about equal, whereas in most cases of severe hypogonadism from other causes the span exceeds the height. Intellectual impairment of varying degree may occur, being least marked in those with a chromosomal pattern of 47/XXY, and more marked in those with more than two X chromosomes. Patients with an XXXXY constitution are not only mentally retarded but have an almost pathognomonic facies with epicanthic folds and slanting palpebral fissures; the testes are usually impalpable and the scrotum very rudimentary. Kyphoscoliosis may be present and the little finger curves inwards.

Diagnosis

Determination of the nuclear chromatin sex and preferably also karyotype analysis are essential to the diagnosis of Klinefelter's syndrome. Although testicular biopsy is helpful, the findings are not pathognomonic and may also occur in Reifenstein's syndrome [p. 600] and in mumps orchitis. The urinary and plasma levels of gonadotrophins are high-normal or pathologically increased, a finding which serves to distinguish this type of hypogonadism from that secondary to hypothalamo-pituitary dysfunction. Further aspects of the differential diagnosis are discussed on page 599.

Treatment

Androgen therapy will correct the manifestations of hypogonadism but will have no effect on the azoospermia. Such treatment should, however, be used cautiously in patients with subnormal intellect because enhanced libido may lead to socio-sexual misdemeanour. If gynaecomastia is cosmetically embarrassing plastic surgery is indicated.

MALE INFERTILITY

Definition

An inability to induce conception due to a defect in spermatic function constitutes male infertility.

Aetiology

The causes of male infertility are many. Sterility or subfertility occurs in most cases of hypogonadism [p. 598] when androgen secretion by the Leydig cells is subnormal. Infertility also occurs despite normal androgen production if there is some primary defect in spermatogenesis or an anatomical abnormality of the spermatic tract. Since about one-third of infertile marriages are due to some defect in the male, attention should be paid to the quality of the husband's semen [p. 596] before prolonged investigations of the wife are instituted.

Anatomical Causes. *Bilateral cryptorchidism* is a common cause of male infertility, particularly if steps are not taken until puberty to bring the testes into the scrotum. Hence the necessity for early treatment of this condition [p. 597]. *Trauma* to the testes, particularly during herniotomy in childhood, or as a result of torsion, is another common cause of impaired spermatogenesis later in life. *Varicocele* has an adverse effect on fertility even when the varicocele is unilateral, usually being confined to the left side. Ligation of the spermatic vein may in such cases restore the sperm count and morphology to normal. *Retrograde ejaculation* of semen into the urinary bladder may be a cause of infertility after prostatectomy. Azoospermia may be due to congenital or post-inflammatory *atresia of the vasa deferentia*, a situation suggested by finding aspermia associated with a normal histological appearance on testicular biopsy. *Irradiation* of one testis for the treatment of a seminoma without adequate protection of the other gonad will cause infertility.

Infections. Any infection involving the testes or epididymides, such as mumps in the postpubertal period, tuberculosis, gonorrhoea, leprosy, syphilis and *Esch. coli* infections, may cause testicular atrophy and infertility. Repeated attacks of epididymo-orchitis may be associated with an anatomical abnormality such as hypospadias and lead to postpubertal atrophy of the testes, azoospermia and a variable degree of deficient androgen secretion with or without gynaecomastia (Reifenstein's syndrome). Spermatogenesis may be temporarily depressed in any acute illness, and sterility may be the consequence of any chronic generalized debilitating condition.

Chromosomal Abnormalities. In *Klinefelter's syndrome* [p. 599] infertility is the rule. It also occurs in patients with sex chromosome mosaicism giving an XO/XY or XO/XY/XYYY constitution. These cases have testes which show complete germinal aplasia; their stature is usually short and they have webbing of the neck and other somatic abnormalities similar to those found in Turner's syndrome in the female [p. 608]. In these patients with *male Turner's syndrome* the XY cell-line is doubtless responsible for the presence of testes, and the XO cells are influential in causing defective masculine sexual development.

Gonadotrophin Deficiency. Infertility may result from panhypopituitarism [p. 544] or an isolated deficiency of gonadotrophin secretion. Arrest of spermatogenesis due to failure of maturation of spermatogonia may be recognized by testicular biopsy and is usually the consequence of deficient FSH secretion. Deficient secretion of both FSH and LH gonadotrophins is manifest by absence of both Leydig's cells and tubular atrophy. Sometimes such monotrophic gonadotrophin deficiency is associated with anosmia (Kallmann's syndrome). Such patients are best recognized by the absence or low level of 'total gonadotrophins' in the urine, by additional evidence of hypothalamo-pituitary deficiency (insulin tolerance test, p. 541) except in those cases in which the gonadotrophin deficiency is an isolated defect, and by the findings on testicular biopsy.

Autoimmune Disease. In rare instances infertility has been found to be due to autoantibodies that agglutinate the spermatozoa. Infertility due to autoantibodies to interstitial cell tissue has also been found in patients with Addisonian adrenal insufficiency due to adrenocortical autoantibodies.

Idiopathic Causes. Aplasia of the germinal cells may occur for unknown reasons. In these patients the testes are small and there is complete azoospermia. The patient is normally virilized and has normal skeletal proportions. Testicular biopsy shows absence of germinal epithelium and the tubules show only Sertoli cells (del Castillo syndrome). As in other conditions with primary testicular failure, gonadotrophin secretion is increased; in these cases the plasma FSH level rather than the LH titre is high.

Symptoms

A careful history and complete physical examination are essential in elucidating the cause of male infertility. A seminal specimen should be examined on at least two occasions and often a testicular biopsy is necessary to establish the underlying reason for the defective spermatogenesis. Estimation of the urinary excretion of total gonadotrophins or of the plasma levels of FSH and LH may be required to determine whether the disorder is of primary testicular origin or secondary to a hypothalamo-pituitary disorder.

Treatment

The treatment of infertility depends upon its cause. Surgical correction of anatomical abnormalities is of prophylactic importance in cryptorchidism [p. 597] and is successful in some cases of obstructive azoospermia and varicocele. When infertility is secondary to generalized pituitary failure or monotrophic deficiency of gonadotrophic secretion, fertility may temporarily be induced by the administration of human FSH and human chorionic gonadotrophin to provide LH. Such treatment is still in an experimental stage of development. FSH from human pituitary extracts is scarce but that extracted from human menopausal urine is more widely available and given in conjunction with human chorionic gonadotrophin may improve seminiferous tubular function sufficiently for pregnancy to be induced. Such treatment is only indicated when the plasma or urinary levels of gonadotrophins are abnormally low and testicular biopsy shows maturation failure of spermatogenesis.

Treatment with testosterone has been claimed of value in patients with oligospermia, the rationale being that the testosterone initially induces azoospermia and on stopping treatment there is a rebound with an increase in the sperm count. In practice it seems that testosterone treatment is mainly successful by improving epididymal and vasal function, ejaculation and spermatogenic motility. Sublingual methyltestosterone, 10 mg. daily, or fluoxymesterone, 5 mg. daily, may be used for this purpose.

Unless some detectable and remediable cause for infertility is found, treatment is usually unsatisfactory, as for example in complete germinal aplasia. More important than the total count in oligospermia is the motility of the sperms and this may be improved by the measures outlined above, by attention to the patient's general health, the avoidance of suspensory bandages or tight underwear which may raise the scrotal temperature, and by restricting intercourse to every second or third day. In some instances improvement has followed injections of vitamin B_{12}, a response which should not yet be dismissed as a placebo effect.

IMPOTENCE

Definition

Inability to achieve normal sexual intercourse due to persistent inability to have or sustain an erection constitutes impotency.

Aetiology

Penile erection and ejaculation depend upon a spinal reflex at the sacral (parasympathetic nerves derived from S.2, 3 and 4 through the nervi erigentes) and the lumbar levels (sympathetic nerves derived from L.2 and 3). No less important are psychological stimuli from the higher cerebral centres which together with androgen secretion govern libido. Temporary impotence is common in any generalized organic illness, and also at times of psychological stress.

Local causes of impotence include hypo- and epispadias, Peyronie's disease and Leriche's syndrome (atherosclerosis of the iliac arteries or aorta leading to intermittent claudication in the thighs and impotence). Prostatectomy may also be followed by impotence. *Neurological disorders* that may cause impotence include diabetic neuropathy, in which impotence may be a very early complaint, other causes of peripheral neuritis, tumours or injuries to the cauda equina, spina bifida, disseminated sclerosis, tabes dorsalis and syringomyelia. Lesions of the cerebral temporal lobes are also sometimes associated with impotence. Sympathetic ganglionic blocking drugs, used for the reduction of hypertension, may cause impotence, or more often failure of ejaculation. Most patients with *hypogonadism* [p. 598] experience impotence.

In practice the commonest cause of impotence is a *psychological* disturbance. Sometimes this is an expression of a depressive illness but more often it is of a complex psychoneurotic nature particularly when the onset of the impotence occurs early in life.

Symptoms

In hypogonadism, particularly if present since puberty, the patient seldom complains of impotence because he has little or no libido and may never have experienced normal sexual intercourse. Patients with an acquired organic neurological cause for impotence often complain bitterly because they have a normal libido but fail to achieve an erection under any circumstances. This is particularly the case in patients with mild diabetic neuropathy who may be unaware that they are diabetic. Patients with a depressive illness may present with impotence, often at the instigation of their wives, but a careful history soon shows the true nature of their illness.

Functional or psychoneurotic impotence can often be diagnosed from the history. Early morning erections associated with a full urinary bladder are good evidence of normal physiological and anatomical function. So also is a history that the patient is potent with a partner other than his wife or vice versa, or that he achieves a sustained erection only under certain circumstances. Psychological factors are always responsible for premature ejaculation. Impotence early in the sexual life of a man usually indicates inhibitions, social or moral, but may be an expression of un-self-recognized homosexuality, fetishism or transvestism. When impotence develops later in life, physical illness, business anxieties, pressure of work, marital disharmony or frigidity in the female may be causative factors. It is important to recognize 'relative impotence' in men whose racial proclivity demands frequent intercourse and whose sexual prowess diminishes with increasing years.

Treatment

In hypogonadism, whether primary or secondary [p. 598], potency can be restored or initiated by administration of androgens [p. 599] although this will not usually influence the associated infertility. Neurological causes can seldom be treated effectively and certainly this is the case in most patients with diabetes mellitus however well their blood sugar level is controlled.

Theoretically psychological impotence should be treated by psychotherapy or psychoanalysis but often this is a prolonged, unrewarding, expensive and depressing experience for the patient. It is only indicated when more simple superficial methods fail. In most instances counselling of one or both partners is the corner-stone of treatment. A frank discussion of the problem, an explanation of the frequency of the condition, encouragement, a dissolution of parental censures and heightening of libido by injections of testosterone [p. 599] often effect a cure.

MALE SEXUAL PRECOCITY

Definition

Sexual precocity is defined as the onset of puberty at an age of less than 10 years. It occurs less commonly in boys than girls [p. 606].

Aetiology

Premature sexual development may be due to the inappropriately early secretion of gonadotrophins (true precocity) or to congenital adrenal hyperplasia, or to an androgen-secreting tumour (pseudo-precocity).

True Precocity. This is so called because full sexual maturity is achieved and may occur as a result of a tumour or inflammatory lesion involving the hypothalamus or pituitary gland. Such conditions may cause intracranial symptoms or signs. Sometimes increased gonadotrophin secretion occurs as an idiopathic 'constitutional' anomaly without evidence of any other abnormality. In cases where the precocious sexual development is caused by inappropriately early secretion of gonadotrophins, the size of the testes is proportionate to the development of the other sexual organs; and the excretion of 17-oxosteroids is in the normal range for adolescence at about 4 mg. or less per day. Testicular biopsy shows maturation of both the seminiferous and Leydig cells, and gonadotrophins are present in the plasma or urine in amounts commensurate with adolescent levels.

Pseudo-precocity. In pseudo-precocity there is precocious development of secondary sexual characteristics but sexual maturity does not occur. Pseudo-precocity is more common in the male than the true form caused by premature gonadotrophin secretion. It occurs as a dominant feature in congenital adrenal hyperplasia [p. 587]. Due to an enzymatic defect in the biosynthesis of cortisol with a reduction in the plasma cortisol level, excess ACTH is secreted and the adrenal output of androgens is increased. Increased androgen secretion may also arise from an adrenal tumour, usually malignant at this age, and less commonly from an interstitial-cell tumour of the testis which can usually be detected by palpation. In all these conditions the urinary excretion of 17-oxosteroids is much increased relative to the patient's chronological age. As a result of suppression of gonadotrophin secretion from the adenohypophysis, the testes are small in comparison to the development of the penis and scrotum, and spermatogenesis does not occur.

Symptoms

In addition to premature development of the external genitalia, there is rapid skeletal growth and muscular development. The larynx develops and the voice 'breaks' prematurely. Facial and body hair appears. Libido is enhanced and may cause considerable psycho-social sexual difficulties. Under the stimulus of early androgen production, the epiphyses tend to fuse early so that the ultimate stature in the untreated patient is short.

Other symptoms depend on the cause. Patients with a hypothalamic or parapituitary tumour may have a visual field defect due to pressure on the optic chiasm, headaches, diabetes insipidus or somnolence, features that are conspicuously absent in constitutional precocious puberty.

Diagnosis

Diagnosis depends upon the physical findings, the size of the testes, the urinary excretion of 17-oxosteroids, and sometimes upon testicular biopsy. In premature virilization caused by a malignant adrenal tumour, dexamethasone does not reduce the urinary excretion of 17-oxosteroids as it does in patients with congenital adrenal hyperplasia [p. 587]. The distinction between a cerebral tumour and constitutional factors as a cause of increased gonadotrophin secretion is largely based on the absence of any other symptoms or signs in the latter. In doubtful cases air encephalography may be required to exclude a tumour.

Treatment

Treatment depends upon the cause. Precocious sexual development is readily controlled in congenital adrenal hyperplasia by substitution therapy with cortisone or prednisone [p. 588]. Adrenal and testicular tumours must be removed surgically but the prognosis is usually poor in the former because of the development of hepatic metastases. Hypothalamic or parapituitary tumours threatening vision or causing raised intracranial pressure require surgical treatment or radiotherapy.

In constitutional precocity suppression of gonadotrophin secretion and a reduction in the plasma testosterone level may be achieved with medroxyprogesterone acetate which has to be continued for several years until the boy reaches the normal age of puberty. Treatment is started with the long-acting intramuscular preparation (*Depo-Provera*) in a dose of 100 mg. every 2 weeks. Later the dosage may be increased to 300 mg. every 2 weeks. When progression has been arrested, it may be possible to continue to control the situation with oral administration of medroxyprogesterone acetate but the precise dose and route of administration can only be determined by the patient's response. Although this is at present the only effective treatment known, it must still be considered experimental because its influence on skeletal development is undetermined; the side-effects of a steroidal compound that has to be given in high dosage for several years are undefined; the compound may possibly accelerate osseous development; and it is not known whether hypothalamic-pituitary function will function normally when the suppressive action of medroxyprogesterone is withdrawn on stopping treatment.

TESTICULAR TUMOURS

Aetiology

Benign or malignant tumours of the testis are uncommon and the incidence is highest in cryptorchidism or when there is some sex chromosome abnormality. These neoplasms usually occur between the ages of 10 and 30 years.

Pathology

Germinal-cell Tumours. Tumours arising from the seminiferous tubular cells are usually malignant. *Seminomas* grow relatively slowly, metastasize to the para-aortic glands and are radio-sensitive. *Teratomas* also arise from germinal cells and may contain many different tissues; when chorionic cells predominate, the tumour is classified as a *choriocarcinoma.* Teratomas metastasize early to the abdominal lymphnodes or via the blood stream to produce cannon-ball secondaries in the lungs. More than half the cases have metastases when first seen and even at this stage the primary may be very small or undetectable clinically.

Interstitial-cell Tumours. These arise from the Leydig cells and are very rare. They are usually benign, particularly during the first decade of life, when they are a cause of precocious puberty [p. 602]. In the prepubertal child gynaecomastia is seldom present but this is common in adults and may be the only apparent endocrine abnormality in the older age group.

Symptoms

Testicular tumours usually cause painless enlargement of the testis, and attention may be drawn to the swelling by trauma of no aetiological relationship or by a dull dragging discomfort in the groin. The tumour is usually diffuse, firm and smooth, and seldom attached to the skin. A very malignant choriocarcinoma may induce pain and swelling to a degree that mimics acute epididymo-orchitis. Sometimes the primary tumour is silent and the condition first presents as the result of abdominal or pulmonary metastases.

Interstitial-cell tumours may present as precocious puberty in childhood and rarely occur in adult life.

Diagnosis

Increased amounts of gonadotrophins may be excreted in the urine or found in the plasma of patients with a seminoma or teratoma, particularly a choriocarcinoma. The gonadotrophin increase is helpful in diagnosis and in following the course of the disease and the response to treatment. The distinction from other local testicular swellings such as gummata, chronic inflammatory conditions, particularly tuberculous epididymitis, or a hydrocele is seldom difficult on clinical findings alone.

In interstitial-cell tumours the urinary excretion of 17-oxosteroids is abnormally high for the child's chronological age and very high values are common in adults. Usually the tumour is palpable and the site of the increased 17-oxosteroid production not in doubt. When there is no palpable tumour in the scrotum, the distinction between a testicular or adrenal origin for the 17-oxosteroids can usually be made by measuring the amount of dehydro-iso-androsterone (DHA) in the urine as this constitutes the major proportion of 17-oxosteroids derived from an adrenal but not from a testicular tumour.

Treatment

The tumour should be removed surgically and depending on its nature, block dissection of the regiona lymph nodes and radiotherapy may be necessary

Teratomas, particularly choriocarcinoma, are difficult to control but may respond, when metastases are present, to methotrexate, chlorambucil and actinomycin D, usually in combination.

Prognosis

The outlook after early treatment of a seminoma is good with a 5-year survival rate better than 80 per cent. The prognosis in a teratoma is variable depending on the degree of malignancy. Choriocarcinoma carries a very poor outlook. The prognosis for a benign interstitial-cell tumour is excellent.

DISEASES OF THE OVARY

PHYSIOLOGICAL CONSIDERATIONS

The early embryonic development of the ovary is from the cortex of the primitive genital ridge. Until the onset of puberty the ovaries remain inactive, but then are stimulated by gonadotrophins which are secreted in increased amounts for about 2 years before the menarche. Normal adult ovaries during the reproductive phase of life measure about 3 cm. in length and 1–1·5 cm. in width and thickness. They are composed of an outer layer of cubical germinal epithelium surrounding the cortex and an inner medulla composed of connective tissue containing blood vessels and lymphatic spaces. In the cortex are many thousands of Graafian follicles, each formed from a group of cells derived from the germinal epithelium. One cell in each group develops into an ovum; the remainder proliferate to form a mass of cells (the discus proligerus) around the ovum and an outer layer of the cells which constitute the membrana granulosa. Enveloping each follicle is an outer theca externa composed of fibrous tissue and an inner theca interna which is more vascular and cellular.

Ovulation

Only very few of the Graafian follicles ever mature. Each month, during reproductive life, the granulosa cells in a follicle proliferate in response to follicle-stimulating hormone (FSH), and secrete follicular fluid which surrounds the ovum. The follicle migrates to the surface of the ovary, ruptures and liberates its ovum into the peritoneal cavity, whence it usually passes down the Fallopian tube to the uterine cavity.

The ruptured follicle is filled with blood clot, and, under the influence of FSH and the luteinizing hormone (LH) cells from the theca interna and the granulosa layer, differentiate to form the corpus luteum. If the ovum is not fertilized, the corpus luteum atrophies after ten days leaving a fibrous scar, the corpus albicans. If pregnancy occurs, the corpus luteum persists for about seven months.

Gonadotrophins

Follicle-stimulating hormone (FSH) is secreted by the adenohypophysis in response to a releasing factor produced in the hypothalamus. Judging by immunoassay estimations of plasma FSH levels, two peaks of secretion superimposed on a basal secretory level occur during each menstrual cycle, a small inconstant rise during the last day or two of menstruation and a much more marked and constant peak around the time of ovulation. FSH is primarily responsible for the development of the Graafian follicle. In combination with the luteinizing hormone, it promotes the secretion of oestrogens, and a surge in the secretion of both gonadotrophins is necessary to induce ovulation.

FSH for therapeutic purposes can be extracted from human pituitary glands obtained at autopsy, or from human menopausal urine. From the first source supplies are limited and from the second expensive. Such FSH is mainly used in the treatment of women with infertility due to gonadotrophin deficiency which may be an expression of over-all pituitary failure or a monotrophic defect of primary pituitary origin or secondary to hypothalamic dysfunction. Overdosage may induce multiple ovulation and hence multiple foetuses.

Luteinizing hormone (LH) is also secreted by the adenohypophysis in response to a releasing factor liberated by the hypothalamus. The plasma level of LH as measured by radio-immunoassay reaches a single peak, superimposed on a basal secretory level, at the time of ovulation being associated with a rise in body temperature, an increase in pregnanediol excretion as a metabolite of progesterone, and in some patients by *mittelschmerz*. In conjunction with FSH, LH is responsible for ovulation and the development of the corpus luteum. In the ovary previously stimulated by FSH, LH promotes the secretion of oestrogen and progesterone. Luteinizing hormone is biologically very similar to human chorionic gonadotrophin (HCG) extracted from the urine of pregnant women. Thus HCG is usually used as a source of LH and finds its place in conjunction with FSH in the treatment of infertility of pituitary or hypothalamic origin.

Although both FSH and LH can now be measured in plasma by radio-immunoassay methods which are not yet widely available, gonadotrophin secretion has for many years been assessed by a bioassay procedure using an extract of a 24-hour urine sample. This method measures 'total' urinary gonadotrophins (FSH and LH). Its meaningfulness has been increased by expressing the results obtained in relationship to an international reference preparation (IRP) made from human menopausal urine, but it is often difficult to interpret the significance of an isolated value because of the fluctuations that occur during a menstrual cycle. In women during the reproducing phase of life the normal range lies between 0·15 and 0·5 mg. per 24 hours in terms of the second. IRP–HMG. Zero or low levels are less than 0·15 mg. per 24 hours, and in menopausal women high total gonadotrophin levels of 2·0–8·0 mg. or more are found.

Control of Gonadotrophin Secretion

During reproductive life the secretion of gonadotrophins is regulated by a number of control mechanisms. Release factors liberated by the hypothalamus stimulate the secretion of FSH and LH from the adenohypophysis, and the output is sustained at a relatively uniform basal level. Surges of FSH secretion towards the end of menstruation and of both FSH and LH at the middle of the cycle are responsible for ovulation, and these temporary increases in gonadotrophin output probably originate in higher centres outside the hypothalamus but operating through it. It is these higher centres, perhaps located in the pre-optic centres and influenced by cortical function, which are apparently disturbed in patients who experience anovulatory menstruation and probably also in those with psychogenic or so-called hypothalamic amenorrhoea [p. 610].

In addition to the influence of neurogenic and hypothalamic activity, the secretion of gonadotrophins is regulated by feed-back mechanisms effected by ovarian hormones. Oestrogens suppress FSH secretion probably by depressing hypothalamic function and also LH secretion. LH secretion is also suppressed by androgens and probably also by progesterone.

Ovarian Hormones

Oestrogens and progesterone are secreted in a cyclical manner as each Graafian follicle matures and its corpus luteum is formed.

Oestrogens are synthesized by the cells of the theca interna and corpus luteum in response to both FSH and LH. Oestrone and oestradiol are the primary ovarian oestrogens and are freely interconvertible. Oestriol is a metabolite of oestradiol and has its main effect on the cervical and vaginal epithelium, whereas oestrone and oestradiol chiefly influence the uterine endometrium. In pregnancy the feto-placental unit produces large quantities of oestriol, the urinary excretion of which can be used as an index of placental efficiency. During the menstrual cycle oestrogens reach their highest peak of urinary excretion at the time of ovulation, and are responsible for proliferation of the uterine endometrium. They are also responsible for the development and maintenance of secondary sexual characteristics and accessory sexual organs. At puberty they stimulate epiphyseal growth and may play a part in the eventual fusion of the epiphyses. Because the menarche occurs some two years earlier than testicular maturation, the pubertal growth spurt and cessation of further skeletal development takes place earlier in girls than in boys.

Naturally occurring, semi-synthetic and synthetic oestrogens are available for therapy. The natural compounds have the advantage of not causing nausea or vomiting but are relatively inactive by mouth. The synthetic compounds are cheap and effective by mouth but more liable to cause side-effects.

Progesterone is secreted by the corpus luteum in response to stimulation by LH. Small amounts appear in the urine as the inactive metabolites pregnanediol and pregnanetriol during the luteal phase of the menstrual cycle. Increased secretion of progesterone after ovulation induces secretory and predecidual changes in an endometrium which has already proliferated in response to oestrogen. The rising plasma level of progesterone eventually suppresses the release of pituitary gonadotrophins; the corpus luteum regresses and the reduced secretion of oestrogen and progesterone causes the uterine mucosa to be shed and menstruation to occur. Progesterone has a depressive action on the central nervous system which may in part be the cause of the psychological changes experienced by some women during the premenstrual phase, a time when there is an increased liability to irritability, epilepsy in predisposed subjects, kleptomania and suicide.

Progesterone is not effective by mouth and is now seldom used therapeutically. It has been replaced by synthetic compounds (progestogens) which have a similar action and may be given orally or parenterally.

TESTS OF OVARIAN FUNCTION

Assessment of ovarian function after puberty is largely the concern of the gynaecologist but collaboration with a physician is often helpful when ovarian dysfunction is secondary to some generalized disorder or to an endocrine disease not primarily ovarian in origin. Although after adolescence the adequacy of oestrogen secretion can often be inferred from the degree of development of the secondary sexual organs and the secondary sexual characteristics as judged by simple clinical examination, more sophisticated investigations may be necessary to establish that the production of oestrogen and progesterone is normal and that ovulation is occurring.

Oestrogen Secretion

Vaginal Smear. Serial examination of the superficial epithelial cells obtained by swabbing the lateral wall of the upper third of the vagina provides useful information concerning oestrogen secretion. The degree of cornification of these cells increases during the follicular phase, reaching its maximum at the time of ovulation. A low cornification index indicates deficient oestrogen production. During the luteal phase, with adequate progesterone secretion, the cells have up-curled edges and assume the appearance of a child's paper boat.

Urinary Oestrogen Excretion. The urinary excretion of oestradiol, oestrone and oestriol can be measured chemically but there is such individual variation from person to person, and in the same woman during different menstrual cycles, that isolated measurements may provide little information of clinical value.

Examination of Cervical Mucus. A dried smear of cervical mucus taken during a normal follicular phase shows, under the microscope, crystals with the appearance of a fern. This 'ferning' is good evidence of adequate oestrogen secretion. During the luteal phase 'ferning' is not normally seen, and its occurrence at this time in the menstrual cycle is evidence of progesterone deficiency.

Progesterone Secretion

As mentioned above, the absence of adequate progesterone secretion is reflected by persistence of 'ferning' of cervical mucus during the luteal phase. Progesterone has a slight calorigenic action that influences the basal body temperature, and its secretion provides positive rather than negative evidence as judged by this criterion.

Basal Body Temperature. The patient's temperature is recorded each morning on waking and the result charted. Normally a biphasic response is observed with a pre-ovulatory fall followed by a thermal rise of 0·6–1·0° F. at the time of ovulation. Often the records are difficult to interpret and the temperature may have to be recorded over a period of several months before conclusions can be drawn as to whether or not ovulation is occurring.

Pregnanediol Excretion. Ovulation associated with increased secretion of progesterone leads to increased urinary excretion of pregnanediol, a metabolite of progesterone. In a normal luteal phase following ovulation, pregnanediol excretion usually exceeds 2 mg. per 24 hours.

Endometrial Biopsy. Histological examination of the endometrium provides valuable information as to oestrogen secretion in the follicular phase, and as to progesterone secretion when carried out just before menstruation is due.

Ovarian Anatomy

The size of the ovaries is difficult to determine by bimanual palpation unless gross enlargement is present. Gynaecography, a procedure involving the injection of air into the peritoneal cavity and then X-raying the pelvis in the Trendelenburg position, has been used to determine ovarian size. This is more satisfactorily achieved by laparoscopy which permits direct visualization and biopsy of the gonads.

Gonadotrophin Versus Ovarian Failure

The distinction between primary ovarian failure and that secondary to deficient gonadotrophin secretion can often be made from collateral evidence of other trophic hormone deficiencies [p. 604]; in some instances gonadotrophic deficiency occurs as a monotrophic abnormality. Measurement of 'total gonadotrophin' in a 24-hour urine sample may be helpful in making the distinction [p. 604] but the procedure is not entirely satisfactory, partly because of the basic imprecision of the method and partly because both FSH and LH are measured. More meaningful information will be obtained when the radio-immunoassay of FSH and of LH in plasma is more widely available.

A more dynamic test of ovarian responsiveness to stimulation is to measure the 24-hour urinary oestrone excretion 7 days after a single intramuscular injection of 18,000 Units of pregnant mare's serum which has FSH activity. A normal response is shown by urinary excretion of 15–80μg. oestrone per 24 hours. Because the material contains foreign protein, an intradermal sensitivity test should be done before the serum is injected intramuscularly. A subnormal output, indicating ovarian unresponsiveness, is associated with less than 15 μg. oestrone per 24 hours. A supramaximal response, greater than 100 μg., may occur in the polycystic ovary syndrome [p. 611] and may induce acute ovarian enlargement and abdominal pain. When this condition seems likely from the history and physical examination, laparoscopy is preferred to aid diagnosis.

FEMALE SEXUAL PRECOCITY

Definition

Female sexual precocity is defined as the onset of puberty, and in particular of menstruation, before the age of 10 years. This precociousness is more common in females than males [p. 602].

Aetiology

Precocious puberty in the female may be due to an oestrogen-secreting tumour of the ovary or adrenal cortex, or much more commonly to the premature secretion of gonadotrophins. In 90 per cent. of cases precocious puberty is due to inappropriately early secretion of gonadotrophins and in most instances no abnormality can be found to explain this. Such idiopathic or 'constitutional' precocious sexual development may occur at an age as early as 18 months with development of mammary tissue and associated with maturation of the vulva. Further progression, resembling in every way normal puberty, leads to cyclical ovulation and menstrual loss. The secondary sexual characteristics, the breasts and other accessory sexual organs develop normally. There is rapid skeletal growth, but usually the epiphyses fuse early so that the ultimate stature is short. In all other respects girls with constitutional sexual precocity develop into normal women.

Premature secretion of gonadotrophins may less commonly occur in association with a tumour or inflammatory lesion involving the hypothalamus or pituitary gland. Such conditions may cause intracranial symptoms or signs. Premature gonadotrophin secretion may also occur in some cases of polyostotic fibrous dysplasia (Albright's syndrome, Section 11).

Excessive oestrogen secretion as a cause of precocious puberty is usually due to a malignant tumour of the adrenal cortex or a benign granulosa-cell tumour of the ovary. A mass may be palpable and the urinary or plasma levels of gonadotrophins are low or absent because of hypothalamo-pituitary suppression.

Symptoms

Precocious sexual development may be manifest at an early age, particularly in those cases due to constitutional premature secretion of gonadotrophins. The sexual development resembles in all its stages the changes that occur in a normal menarche. The condition must be distinguished from gynaecomastia which may occur at any early age in some girls but is unassociated with further sexual development until the age of 10–12 years. When excess gonadotrophin is due to an intracranial tumour or inflammatory lesion there may be local manifestations such as headaches, visual disturbances, diabetes insipidus, somnolence or evidence of raised intracranial pressure. Oestrogen-secreting tumours of the ovary or adrenal cortex may give rise to local symptoms.

In girls with constitutional precocious puberty the major problem is in socio-sexual behaviour, and pregnancy may occur as in the celebrated Peruvian girl who at the age of 5 years was delivered of a normal child by Caesarean section.

Diagnosis

The differential diagnosis between premature gonadotrophin and oestrogen secretion can be made by estimation of FSH and/or LH in the plasma or urine. Constitutional precocious puberty is chiefly diagnosed by exclusion of the less common causes of the condition. In Albright's syndrome the precocious sexual development is associated with fibrous cysts in scattered areas of the skeleton, sometimes causing deformity of the affected bone, and by characteristic irregular patches of brown pigmentation of the skin.

Premature menstruation due to an oestrogen-secreting tumour is usually not cyclical nor is it associated with ovulation. The plasma and urinary levels of FSH and/or LH are low, and lack of ovulation is shown by the absence of pregnanediol in the premenstrual urine on repeated occasions. The distinction between precocious sexual development induced by oestrogens or gonadotrophins is often best made by examination of the ovaries at laparoscopy.

Treatment

Treatment depends upon the cause. Oestrogen-secreting tumours must be removed surgically but the prognosis is not good in patients with a malignant adrenocortical carcinoma which usually metastasizes early. Premature gonadotrophin secretion due to a detectable symptom-producing intracranial lesion may require intracranial surgery or radiotherapy. The majority of cases are due to constitutional factors and suppression of gonadotrophin secretion is best attempted with medroxyprogesterone acetate as described on page 603.

FEMALE HYPOGONADISM

The term female hypogonadism implies total or partial failure of both the ovulatory and the hormonal secretory functions of the ovaries. After adolescence the interrelationship of these two activities is in the female much more obviously expressed by menstruation than is spermatogenesis in the adult male. Thus, often the most striking clinical manifestation of female hypogonadism is amenorrhoea. The second most common mode of presentation is failure of development of secondary sexual characteristics or disorders of skeletal growth. Only rarely is infertility the chief complaint and this topic is not considered further, being largely a problem for the gynaecologist.

Amenorrhoea is traditionally divided into primary and secondary types depending upon whether or not menstruation has ever occurred. The use of these terms is here different from the meaning implied in other endocrine disorders in which 'primary' signifies failure of the target gland itself due to some primary disorder, whereas 'secondary' indicates failure of the target gland as a consequence of hypothalamo-pituitary dysfunction.

PRIMARY AMENORRHOEA

Definition

Failure of menstruation to occur at or after the normal age of puberty constitutes primary amenorrhoea.

Aetiology

The age of the menarche varies considerably and may be delayed until 16 or even later. A delayed onset of menstruation sometimes runs in families.

Non-Endocrine Diseases. Local or general non-endocrine disorders may cause primary amenorrhoea. Local causes include imperforate hymen, in which secondary sexual characteristics are usually well developed, and acute or chronic pelvic inflammation. Any serious generalized disorder, inflammatory, metabolic or psychiatric, may delay the menarche by inhibiting the release of gonadotrophins. Particular offenders are renal acidosis or unrecognized chronic renal disease, malabsorption syndromes and anorexia nervosa starting at the time of puberty.

Endocrine Diseases. Amenorrhoea occurs as an expression of panhypopituitarism; it is usually associated with dwarfism which tends to be the presenting symptom at an earlier age. However, in patients with only partial pituitary failure, as may occur with a craniopharyngioma [p. 545], failure of secondary sexual characteristics to develop or primary amenorrhoea may be the presenting complaint. Gonadotrophin deficiency may occur as an isolated monotrophic disorder but this is rare. A not uncommon cause of delayed puberty is juvenile myxoedema [p. 567]; the features of hypothyroidism may be minimal and difficult to recognize, whereas the major manifestations are those of hypogonadism. Congenital adrenal hyperplasia [p. 587] if unrecognized and untreated is a cause of primary amenorrhoea because the excessive secretion of adrenal androgens inhibits the release of pituitary gonadotrophins. Such cases are seldom difficult to recognize because of the evidence of virilization.

Genetic Chromosomal Abnormalities. Some of 25 per cent. of patients with primary amenorrhoea prove to have chromosomal abnormalities such as Turner's syndrome [p. 608], mosaicism with an XO cell-line, or an extra X-chromosome. Some triple-X ('super') females may have a normal mentrual history while others have primary or early secondary amenorrhoea. Although now recognized as not being due to a chromosomal abnormality but to failure of the peripheral tissues to respond to androgens, patients with the testicular feminizing syndrome usually present with primary amenorrhoea or infertility.

Idiopathic Ovarian Dysgenesis. In a proportion of cases of primary amenorrhoea no explanation for the failure of ovarian development is found. Such cases exhibit failure of secondary sexual characteristics and often have a eunuchoid habitus with disproportionately long arms and legs as compared with the trunk. Determination of the nuclear sex, karyotyping and laparoscopic examination with biopsy of the gonads is essential to distinguish these patients from those with simple delayed puberty or the testicular feminizing syndrome. Further chromosomal studies may well show that patients currently diagnosed as idiopathic ovarian dysgenesis are mosaics with an XY cell-line.

Symptoms

With the exception of Turner's syndrome and congenital adrenal hyperplasia, ovarian hypofunction can seldom be predicted until after the time of normal puberty. In addition to amenorrhoea, secondary sexual characteristics fail to develop and the accessory sexual organs remain rudimentary and infantile. Pubic and axillary hair is sparse. The breasts are prepubertal. The hips are narrow, muscular development is poor and often there is little subcutaneous fat. The mental outlook is often immature.

The effect of hypogonadism on skeletal development depends upon the cause. Stunting of growth, due to genetic influences, is the rule in Turner's syndrome which may be recognized by other congenital abnormalities [p. 609]. Dwarfism and infantilism occur in panhypopituitarism, and growth is retarded in juvenile myxoedema, and stunted by early epiphyseal fusion in congenital adrenal hyperplasia. In ideopathic delayed puberty, in selective failure of gonadotrophin secretion and in primary ovarian failure, the lack of oestrogens delays fusion of the epiphyses and, in the presence of normal growth hormone secretion, skeletal development continues for an abnormally long time. The patient is tall and has a eunuchoid habitus, the span exceeding the height, and the distance from the symphysis pubis to the ground being several inches more than that from the crown to the symphysis pubis.

Diagnosis

It is essential to exclude by clinical examination and appropriate investigations, such disorders as steatorrhoea, chronic renal disease, tuberculosis, diabetes, thyroid deficiency, Turner's syndrome or some other chromosomal anomaly, and adrenal or pituitary disorders. If nothing abnormal is found on rectal examination and inspection of the vaginal orifice, further investigation should be deferred until the patient is 16 or 17 depending on her mental maturity. The patient's mother, who often is the person most concerned, should be reassured that nothing will be lost by deferring treatment. If menstruation has not occurred by the age of 16 or 17, pelvic examination and laparoscopy under general anaesthesia is carried out. The urinary excretion of total gonadotrophins, and the oestrone excretion after administration of FSH extracted from human pituitary glands, or from menopausal urine or in the form of pregnant mare's serum [p. 604] are used to distinguish primary ovarian failure from that secondary to hypothalamo-pituitary disease.

Treatment

Although the logical treatment of primary amenorrhoea due to hypothalamo-pituitary dysfunction is to give gonadotrophins, such treatment is seldom in the long term practical. In most cases of primary amenorrhoea in which there is no correctable underlying cause, substitution therapy with oestrogens and progestogens is the treatment of choice. Although ovulation will not be induced nor the patient's infertility influenced, a striking change in the patient's physical and mental development is achieved. Ethinyloestradiol, 0·02–0·05 mg. twice daily, is given for the first 21 days of each calendar month, together with a progestogen, such as norethisterone acetate, 5 mg. daily, for the last 10 days of the 21-day course of oestrogens. When regular menstruation has been established and satisfactory development of secondary sexual characteristics attained, cyclical treatment with a 'contraceptive pill' of high oestrogen content, such as *Conovid-E*, will sustain the feminity of the patient.

Prognosis

This depends upon the cause of the primary amenorrhoea. When there is a correctable underlying disorder, such as thyroid deficiency or gluten-sensitive enteropathy, the outlook is good in terms of both menstruation and fertility. In patients with delayed puberty the prognosis is also good and after a few months of cyclical bleeding induced by oestrogen and progestogen therapy, spontaneous menstruation may occur. In other cases of primary amenorrhoea, particularly those with a chromosomal anomaly, infertility is of course permanent and substitution therapy will have to be continued until the patient reaches the age of the normal climacteric [p. 612].

TURNER'S SYNDROME

Synonyms. Ovarian (or gonadal) dysgenesis, agenesis or aplasia; Bonnevie–Ullrich syndrome.

Definition and Aetiology

Turner's syndrome is a rare congenital abnormality in a phenotypic female and caused by an abnormality in the sex (XX) chromosomal complement. The cardinal manifestation is a menstrual disorder, usually primary amenorrhoea, associated with dwarfism.

In its classical and commonest form, Turner's syndrome is due to absence of an X chromosome so that the patient has a chromatin-negative nuclear sex and an XO chromosomal complement with only 45 chromosomes. The clinical manifestations comprise primary amenorrhoea associated with a wide but variable variety of somatic abnormalities.

In other cases the nuclear sex may be either chromatin positive or negative. In the chromatin positive patients there is not a total loss of the second X chromosome but it is abnormal. In others, chromatin negative, the second X chromosome is represented by an abnormal small chromosome which in some instances represents a deleted Y chromosome. In all these patients there is ovarian agenesis or dysgenesis because of the absence of a normal fully functional second X chromosome.

Some patients with features of Turner's syndrome have mosaicism such as XO/XX, XO/XXX, XO/XY or XO/XYY, and depending on the chromosomal complement the chromatin nuclear sex is positive or negative. In mosaicism the clinical state of the patient depends upon the relative proportions of the two distinct cell-lines, and may range from the classical picture of Turner's syndrome when the XO line predominates to a relatively normal woman when the other XX or XXX line predominates. In patients with XO/XY or XO/XYY mosaicism partial masculinization may be present manifest by phallic enlargement with an imperfect testis on one side and a streak ovary on the other.

Pathology

In classical XO Turner's syndrome the ovaries at laparotomy or laparoscopy are represented by white fibrous streaks on the broad ligament. In mosaicism some active ovarian tissue may be found, and some testicular tissue may be present in mosaics with a complement of Y chromosome. Other pathological findings largely depend on the associated somatic abnormalities. Aortic coarctation may be the cause of death from hypertension, cerebral haemorrhage from a berry aneurysm or rupture of the aorta. A proportion of cases have renal abnormalities, such as a horse-shoe kidney.

Symptoms

Classical XO Turner's Syndrome. Classical XO Turner's syndrome is seldom recognized until the age of puberty when the patient fails to mature sexually and presents either with primary amenorrhoea or shortness of stature. A prepubertal diagnosis may be made if webbing of the neck is marked, hypertension in the arms due to coarctation of the aorta is discovered, or there is congenital lymphoedema. The last, affecting the feet, legs or hands, may be present soon after birth and subside a few months or years later. Sometimes the lymphoedema persists and lymphangiography shows hypo- or aplasia of the lymphatics. Congenital lymphoedema is not pathognomonic of a chromosomal abnormality and may occur without evident cause and unassociated with later ovarian dysfunction.

After the expected age of puberty the clinical features of classical XO Turner's syndrome are usually characteristic. The patient has primary amenorrhoea and is dwarfed, seldom attaining a height in excess of 5 ft. Secondary sexual characteristics are poorly developed. The breasts are rudimentary and the wide spread nipples give the chest a shield-like appearance. The external genitalia are poorly developed, and pubic and axillary hair is present but scanty. Webbing of the neck is usually pronounced; the elbow shows a wide carrying angle (cubitus valgus); the epicanthic folds may be exaggerated and the posterior hairline is low. The nasal bridge may be flattened and the ears low-set with auricular malformation. Mental intelligence may be subnormal and there is an increased incidence of colour blindness because the gene for colour vision is carried on an X chromosome. The plasma and urinary gonadotrophin levels are usually high. Growth hormone secretion is normal. Up to the age of 10 years, bone age, as judged radiologically, is normal but skeletal maturation ceases at the expected time of puberty and the epiphyses fail to fuse. Failure of the patient, in the face of normal growth hormone secretion, to develop the expected eunuchoid skeletal proportions [p. 598] is presumably due to some unexplained end-organ unresponsiveness of the cartilagenous cells and related to the chromosomal abnormality; alternatively it may be due to absence of gonadal hormones which, synergistically with growth hormone, stimulate skeletal development. In early adult life osteoporosis may become apparent, and is probably related to deficient oestrogen secretion.

Turner's Syndrome due to an Abnormal X Chromosome or Mosaicism. In patients with ovarian agenesis or dysgenesis caused by an abnormality in the second X chromosome, deletion of a Y chromosome or mosaicism, the clinical picture is more variable. Somatic abnormalities tend to be less prominent but are more likely to be present when webbing of the neck is marked. Patients with loss of the short arm of the second X chromosome are usually indistinguishable from those with classical XO Turner's syndrome. Those with loss of the long arm of the second X chromosome may have a normal stature and absence of other somatic stigmata. Some patients with mosaicism may have sufficient ovarian tissue to experience occasional or even normal menstruation for a few years after adolescence, and such patients therefore present with secondary amenorrhoea. Those with a deleted Y chromosome or XO/XY mosaicism may have phallic enlargement with otherwise normal if immature female external genitalia. Such cases may be confused with 'true' hermaphroditism [p. 616] particularly if an imperfect testis is found on one side and a streak ovary on the other.

Diagnosis

In classical XO Turner's syndrome the diagnosis is often obvious to the practised eye. The shortness of stature may have to be distinguished from other causes of dwarfism [p. 547], and other causes of primary amenorrhoea and female hypogonadism [p. 607] may also have to be excluded. Webbing of the neck is not pathognomonic: it may occur in women or men who have normal or near-normal sexual function and development, and also in the Klippel-Feil syndrome in which there is synostosis of the cervical vertebrae.

Confirmation of the clinical diagnosis is made by karyotype analysis with careful investigation for mosaicism in atypical cases, and laparoscopic examination for the presence of streak ovaries.

Treatment

Coarctation of the aorta should be corrected surgically and webbing of the neck, if cosmetically unacceptable, can be improved by plastic surgery. After the normal time of puberty the development of menstruation and enhancement of the secondary sexual characteristics should be initiated by cyclical substitution therapy with oestrogens and progestogens [p. 605].

Prognosis

Patients with ovarian dysgenesis remain permanently infertile and many never exceed 5 ft. in height. Adequate secondary sexual characteristics can be developed with appropriate hormonal therapy. A proportion of these patients develop hirsutism due to a hilus-cell tumour in one of the dysgenetic streak ovaries, and unexplained hirsuties merits laparotomy.

SECONDARY AMENORRHOEA

Definition

Cessation of menstruation in a woman who has previously experienced normal regular periods constitutes secondary amenorrhoea.

Aetiology

The commonest causes, depending on age, of secondary amenorrhoea and pregnancy and the menopause [p. 612]. The latter may be difficult to recognize when it occurs at an unusually early age, and may have to be differentiated from the other causes of secondary amenorrhoea mentioned below.

Non-endocrine Diseases. The menstrual cycle is readily disturbed by any non-endocrine systemic disease of an acute or chronic nature. In such cases the amenorrhoea is usually transient and constitutes an unimportant feature in the patient's over-all clinical illness.

Psychogenic or Hypothalamic Amenorrhoea. Inhibition of menstruation without detectable structural abnormality may occur in response to psychological disturbances which appear to influence the hypothalamus with a consequent failure of gonadotrophin secretion affecting particularly the release of LH. Fear of, or a great desire for, pregnancy; bereavement; change of surroundings or occupation or shift work may all be associated with amenorrhoea usually lasting only a few months. More severe psychological disturbances may lead to more prolonged amenorrhoea. This was common in women taken prisoners of war before malnutrition or maltreatment occurred. This syndrome is particularly common in patients with anorexia nervosa, menstruation ceasing concurrently with the weight loss or even preceding it.

Endocrine Diseases. Amenorrhoea or oligomenorrhoea is common in patients with Cushing's syndrome, in hyperthyroidism and in those with a pituitary or parapituitary tumour or infarction of the adenohypophysis (Sheehan's syndrome). Inhibition of gonadotrophin secretion may be induced by oestrogens, progestogens or androgens of either endogenous or exogenous origin. Thus, amenorrhoea occurs in association with androgen secreting tumours of the adrenal glands or ovaries [p. 582] and in congenital adrenal hyperplasia of late onset. In such cases there is usually associated evidence of virilization [p. 583]. Similar manifestations occur in the polycystic ovary syndrome [p. 611]. A number of women fail to resume menstrual periods after stopping the contraceptive pill [p. 615].

Monotrophic failure of FSH, LH or both may occur without apparent cause. Such patients may be difficult to distinguish clinically from those with 'psychogenic hypothalamic' amenorrhoea, and may in fact represent part of a continuous spectrum. Infertility is often a pressing complaint in addition to the amenorrhoea.

Amenorrhoea also occurs in a proportion of patients with adrenal insufficiency caused by adrenal antibodies [p. 581].

Symptoms

The amenorrhoea may come on suddenly or be preceded by a phase of oligomenorrhoea. The occurrence of hot flushes and other menopausal symptoms indicates that ovarian failure is the primary cause. In patients with panhypopituitarism there is concomitant evidence of other trophic hormone deficiencies. In those with excess androgen secretion, evidence of hirsutism or virilization [p. 619].

Diagnosis

The cause of secondary amenorrhoea can usually be determined from the patient's history and the clinical examination. Additional tests of ovarian function and other investigations may be required in certain cases; the distinction between ovarian and pituitary deficiency may require estimation of the urinary total gonadotrophin excretion.

Treatment

The treatment of secondary amenorrhoea depends upon its cause. When there is evidence of adequate oestrogen secretion, as judged by examination of the secondary sexual characteristics, the cytology of the vaginal epithelium and the fern test [p. 605], a 'medical D. and C.' can be induced by giving a potent progestogen such as 17-hydroxyprogesterone caproate in a single intramuscular injection of 375 mg. which under these circumstances will precipitate a menstrual period 2–3 weeks later. Such a test shows that the ovarian secretion of oestrogens is adequate and that the genital tract is capable of a normal response. Cyclical withdrawal bleeding can be induced with the 'contraceptive pill' or serial administration of oestrogens and progestogens, but such treatment seldom re-establishes normal spontaneous menstruation.

Clomiphene citrate is of particular value in the treatment of secondary amenorrhoea due to psychogenic disorders or apparent monotrophic gonadotrophin secretory failure due to hypothalamic dysfunction. In psychogenic cases, particularly those associated with marked weight loss, this treatment should be deferred until the patient's weight has been restored to normal and the psychological conflict resolved. Clomiphene is mainly effective when there is evidence of some oestrogen secretion and total gonadotrophin secretion is not so abnormally high as to indicate unresponsive primary ovarian failure. Its action appears to be that of an anti-oestrogen judging by the fact that it temporarily reduces cornification of the vaginal epithelial cells and may induce hot flushes. By blocking the oestrogen feed-back control of the hypothalamus, it promotes the secretion of gonadotrophic release-factors from the hypothalamus and thereby stimulates the secretion of both FSH and LH from the pituitary gland. Clomiphene treatment is therefore useless in patients with total ovarian failure and in those with a pituitary disease causing deficient synthesis of gonadotrophins. The initial dose should be 50 mg. daily for 5–10 days. If no response occurs, the course should be repeated 6 weeks later. Further unresponsiveness should be followed by 100 mg. daily for 5–10 days, and in some instances as many as 5–10 courses are required at six-weekly intervals to effect a response. Side-effects include a brisk ovarian reaction characterized by gonadal enlargement, abdominal bloatedness or frank abdominal pain, hot flushes, and visual blurring—symptoms that call for cessation or a reduction in dosage. In many patients with secondary anovulatory amenorrhoea a normal menstrual pattern occurs spontaneously after one or more courses of clomiphene.

FSH of human pituitary origin, or extracted from female menopausal urine, followed by LH in the form of human chorionic gonadotrophin may be used to stimulate ovarian function in appropriate cases, but the expense of such treatment limits its use to the correction of infertility rather than just secondary amenorrhoea.

POLYCYSTIC OVARY SYNDROME

Synonyms. Sclerocystic ovary syndrome; Stein-Leventhal syndrome.

Definition

This is a poorly defined clinical syndrome which probably does not represent a single disease entity. In its fully developed classical form it is characterized by the triad of infertility due to failure of ovulation, secondary amenorrhoea and enlarged pearly white ovaries with a thickened capsule and containing multiple small cysts. More than half the patients have hirsutism, and a much smaller proportion may show slight clitoral enlargement. There is a tendency for the patient to be obese. In less classical cases oligomenorrhoea rather than amenorrhoea is present; ovulation may occur infrequently and hirsutism may not be marked.

Aetiology

This clinical syndrome occurs most commonly between the ages of 16 and 30 years. Often the production rates of testosterone and of androstenedione, a weakly androgenic compound that is converted to testosterone in the peripheral tissues, are increased; and this is held responsible for the hirsutism. Although each individual follicle produces an abnormally small amount of oestrogen, the total production rate of oestrogens is usually normal, probably because of the large number of follicles present. This finding is compatible with the small amount of oestrogenic material present in the follicular fluid (see below) and the abnormally great increase in oestrogen secretion that occurs when the ovaries are stimulated with exogenously administered FSH. The urinary excretion of total gonadotrophins is usually normal but may be increased. Such findings are of little help in indicating whether the primary disorder resides in the ovaries or the adrenal cortex. Alternatively an imbalance in the secretion of FSH and LH due to a disturbance in the hypothalamo-pituitary area could be the primary abnormality or secondary to defective steroidogenesis in the adrenal cortex or the ovaries. If the syndrome is not a single entity, as the clinical findings and response to various therapeutic regimes suggest, the primary cause may vary from one patient to another, and explain why conflicting results have been obtained by different methods of treatment.

Ovarian Dysfunction. Analysis of the fluid removed from follicular cysts suggests an abnormality in ovarian steroidogenesis. In some cases there is evidence of lack of activity of the enzyme that forms androstenedione from its precursors. In other cases a high androstenedione and a low oestrogen concentration in the fluid suggests reduced activity of the enzyme that converts androstenedione to oestradiol and oestrone; in such patients the ovaries both *in vivo* and *in vitro* show an abnormally great androstenedione production rate.

Adrenocortical Dysfunction. That a primary adrenocortical disorder can cause polycystic ovaries is suggested by their occurrence in some women with congenital adrenal hyperplasia [p. 587] or a benign virilizing adrenocortical adenoma. The development of polycystic ovaries is presumably attributable to changes in FSH and/or LH secretion. About half the patients with the idiopathic polycystic ovary syndrome, and particularly those with marked hirsuitism, show a suppression in the production rate of C-19 steroids, which include androstenedione, when given dexamethasone. Fractionation of the 17-oxosteroids excreted in the urine from such patients may show an increase in compounds synthesized only in the adrenal cortex and not in the ovary. In these cases the response to dexamethasone, with suppression of ACTH secretion, suggests that the adrenal cortex is the primary site of the syndrome. In other patients suppression of C-19 steroid production is only achieved by giving dexamethasone and oestrogens in combination, suggesting that the ovaries play an important part in the increased biosynthesis of androstenedione and other C-19 steroids.

Gonadotrophin Dysfunction. Conflicting results have been obtained by radio-immunoassay of FSH and LH in patients with the polycystic ovary syndrome. Even if a consistently abnormal secretory pattern were found, it would be difficult to decide whether this was the primary cause or secondary to ovarian and/or adrenocortical dysfunction.

Endocrine Interrelationships. The interrelationships between the ovaries, the adrenal cortex and the hypothalamo-pituitary area make it difficult to determine the primary disorder in a syndrome which is likely to prove heterogeneous in origin. Nor does the therapeutic response, in terms of resumption of ovulatory menstruation, to wedge-resection of the ovaries, adrenocortical suppression with dexamethasone or administration of clomiphene citrate help to define the primary site of the disorder.

Pathology

In the classical Stein-Leventhal syndrome the ovaries are large although this may not be detectable by bimanual palpation. The capsule is thickened and glistening white. The cut surface shows multiple small persistent follicular cysts with hyperplasia of the theca interna. Corpora lutea or corpus luteum cysts are absent. The uterine endometrium usually shows early proliferative changes. The degree of cornification of the vaginal epithelial cells is low but this is probably an expression of increased androgen rather than diminished oestrogen secretion.

In less classical cases the histology of the ovaries is more variable, and there is poor correlation between the ovarian pathology and the clinical manifestations. Corpora lutea may be present, evidence of ovulation may be found and the endometrium may show hyperplasia with cystic glandular changes.

Symptoms

The clinical picture is variable, but classically the patient has oligomenorrhoea which becomes increasingly severe and finally gives place to amenorrhoea. Infertility, as a result of non-ovulation, is a common presenting feature. Hirsutism may be marked and be the main reason for the patient seeking medical advice. Evidence of more marked virilization, apart from slight enlargement of the clitoris, is uncommon. A proportion of patients are obese. Essential to the diagnosis is the presence of polycystic enlarged ovaries, but this may not be detectable by physical examination.

In less classical cases the amenorrhoea may be primary but this is rare. More often oligomenorrhoea occurs and ovulation may take place during some cycles so that infertility is relative rather than absolute.

Diagnosis

The triad of oligomenorrhoea or amenorrhoea, infertility and hirsutism will suggest the polycystic ovary syndrome, and ovarian enlargement may be confirmed by pelvic examination. If no enlargement of the ovaries can be felt, hormonal investigations are unlikely to be helpful. The excretion of urinary 17-oxosteroids is likely to be normal or slightly increased, so also is the total urinary gonadotrophin excretion. Confirmation of the diagnosis depends upon assessment of the size and the macroscopic and microscopic appearances of the ovaries. This can most satisfactorily be achieved by laparoscopy which gives more reliable information than gynaecography or culdoscopy. When hirsutism is marked and oligomenorrhoea or amenorrhoea is present, other causes must be excluded, such as mild cases of congenital adrenal hyperplasia [p. 587] in which virilization may be delayed until after puberty; an androgen-secreting adrenal tumour which may or may not induce some manifestations of Cushing's syndrome by an associated increased secretion of glucocorticoids; or an ovarian tumour [p. 613]. The 11-oxygenation index [p. 579] and the suppression of increased 17-oxosteroid excretion by dexamethasone are helpful in detecting congenital adrenal hyperplasia; the response to dexamethasone and ACTH as well as fractionation of 17-oxosteroids may help to define an adrenocortical tumour; and laparotomy is usually necessary to diagnose an ovarian tumour unless a mass can be felt. The more difficult differentiation is from idiopathic hirsutism [p. 619] in which menstruation is usually normal but the diagnosis is particularly hard to make when there is associated oligomenorrhoea.

Treatment

In view of the uncertain aetiology of the polycystic ovary syndrome, treatment is controversial. Wedge-resection of the ovaries provides the most effective treatment in terms of restoration of ovulatory menstruation and fertility. It also has the advantage of allowing exclusion of an ovarian tumour. Clomiphene citrate is effective in restoring menstruation and fertility in about 80 per cent. of patients, but on withdrawal of treatment amenorrhoea may return and often clomiphene has to be given cyclically over a prolonged period of time. The response may be marked and, to avoid further ovarian enlargement and pain, the dosage should be kept to the minimum that is effective. In a proportion of cases, particularly those with a slightly raised urinary excretion of 17-oxosteroids and hirsutism prednisone, 2·5 mg. thrice daily, may restore normal menstruation, but does not consistently induce ovulation.

Prognosis

The most satisfactory form of treatment, particularly when bilateral ovarian enlargement is marked, is wedge-resection. In some cases this has improved the symptoms only temporarily and hence has been restricted to those patients who wish to become pregnant. In others wedge-resection has provided a more permanent cure. No form of treatment appears to reduce the hirsutism once it has become established. Treatment at an early stage with small doses of prednisone together with the sequential or combined contraceptive pill may, however, prevent or reduce progressive hypertrichosis [p. 619].

FUNCTIONAL UTERINE BLEEDING

Menorrhagia (heavy or prolonged menstrual loss) and metrorrhagia (increased frequency of menstruation) may be caused by local structural disease of the genital organs, systemic disorders particularly of the blood with a reduction in platelets, myxoedema and disturbances involving the secretion of gonadotrophins or ovarian hormones. When no organic cause can be found on gynaecological examination and curettage, the condition is attributed to a primary or secondary disturbance of ovarian endocrine function.

This functional bleeding is not uncommon at the extremes of reproductive life, but is most common at the time of the menopause when it corrects itself spontaneously with the establishment of amenorrhoea. In some instances functional uterine haemorrhage in middle-life can also be shown to be due to failure of ovulation, attributed to some disturbance in the secretion of gonadotrophins. Under the prolonged stimulus of oestrogen from a Graafian follicle, the endometrium becomes hyperplastic and cystic (Swiss cheese). The lack of progesterone, as a consequence of failure of ovulation and of a corpus luteum to form, may result, when the oestrogen level falls, in a seemingly normal period (anovulatory menstruation) or more often in menorrhagia or metrorrhagia preceded by one or two missed periods. An endometrial biopsy will show a proliferative endometrium without any of the secretory changes induced by progesterone, and should be carried out to exclude genital carcinoma before hormone therapy is started.

The bleeding can usually be stopped with a progestogen such as norethisterone acetate, 5–10 mg., or norethisterone or norethynodrel, 10–20 mg. daily for a few days. On stopping treatment withdrawal bleeding occurs. Thereafter a 'contraceptive pill' with a high progestogen content (*Gynovlar*, *Anovlar*) can be used to regulate the menstrual loss. After several months it may be possible to stop this treatment; regular spontaneous menstruation or menopausal amenorrhoea may ensue.

THE MENOPAUSE

Synonym. The climacteric.

Definition

A syndrome characterized by amenorrhoea, vasomotor disturbances and often a wide variety of other symptoms which occurs when ovarian activity ceases physiologically or after oophorectomy or irradiation of the ovaries.

Aetiology

The menopause normally occurs between the ages of 40 and 55. The cause of menopausal symptoms is not known, but there is good reason for believing they are not all due to the same factor. The amenorrhoea is clearly a consequence of failure of ovarian endocrine function. The hot flushes have been attributed on scant evidence to the increased secretion of gonadotrophins. Many of the other manifestations seem to be expressions of anxiety, depression, or a hypothalamic functional disturbance.

Pathology

The ovaries become fibrosed and no longer contain ova. All the accessory sexual organs atrophy and the secondary sexual characteristics regress. Senile vaginitis, kraurosis vulvae and leucoplakia may occur.

Symptoms

Menstruation may cease abruptly, or the periods may become progressively more scanty or occur less frequently. The incidence, frequency and intensity of hot flushes vary considerably. They may occur at times of anxiety or without any apparent precipitating cause. Only the upper part of the body is affected; the feeling of intense heat may or may not be associated with flushing of the skin. Increased perspiration may wet the hair and be particularly troublesome at night. Other more variable symptoms include palpitations, dizziness, shortness of breath, headaches, fatigue, anxiety, irritability, weepiness and sleep disturbances. Depression leads to overeating and an increase in weight which may aggravate degenerative arthritis. Later complications include pruritus vulvae, senile vaginitis, leucoplakia and postmenopausal osteoporosis.

Diagnosis

The diagnosis is usually clear but menopausal amenorrhoea without other symptoms must be differentiated from other conditions which cause cessation of menstruation. Irregular or prolonged bleeding may suggest uterine carcinoma which must be excluded by endometrial biopsy.

Treatment

Many patients are improved by being allowed to discuss their symptoms and express their fears about waning attractiveness and sexuality. This and a mild sedative by day, such as amylobarbitone, 30–50 mg. thrice daily, and a non-barbiturate hypnotic at night are all that is required in the majority of cases. Oestrogen therapy is mainly of value in controlling the hot flushes. The minimal effective dose should be used and given cyclically for the first 21 days of each calendar month for 3 months. The dosage ranges from 0·01 mg. daily to 0·05 mg. thrice daily of ethinyloestradiol, and this should be reduced gradually over the next 6 months. Some patients experience nausea and vomiting with any synthetic or semi-synthetic oestrogen, but are able to tolerate conjugated equine oestrogens in the form of *Premarin*, 0·625 mg. once or twice daily. Withdrawal bleeding may occur, but ceases when the dosage of oestrogen is reduced. Its continuation necessitates a diagnostic curettage. Persistence of hot flushes and other symptoms is usually the result of psychological disturbances. Many patients have early morning waking as an expression of their depression which may become so severe that they develop involutional melancholia. In these cases a striking improvement is achieved with antidepressive drugs with or without the use of oestrogens.

OVARIAN TUMOURS WITH ENDOCRINE ACTIVITY

Ovarian tumours which have endocrine activity are rare but are important in the differential diagnosis of other conditions. Although several different histological types have been described, from the practical endocrine point of view these tumours can be divided into two distinct groups—those that secrete oestrogens and those that produce androgens.

Symptoms

Oestrogen-secreting tumours, composed of granulosa or of theca cells, cause precocious puberty [p. 606] if they develop in childhood. More commonly they arise later in life and cause postmenopausal bleeding, a proliferative endometrium and a resurgence of female secondary sexual characteristics.

Androgen-secreting tumours are less common. They may be composed of cells resembling interstitial testicular tissue (arrhenoblastoma and hilus tumours). Hilus-cell tumours, although rare, appear to occur with increased incidence in patients with Turner's syndrome. The clinical picture is of amenorrhoea, due to suppression of pituitary gonadotrophin secretion, hirsutism and evidence of virilization [p. 582]. In about two-thirds of cases a unilateral ovarian tumour can be palpated bimanually, and such a finding is most helpful in suggesting the diagnosis. Other causes of hirsutism and virilization enter the differential diagnosis and these are discussed on page 620.

MEDICAL ASPECTS OF THE CONTRACEPTIVE PILL

The contraceptive pill can modify or induce a wide variety of metabolic processes and changes which may cause clinical manifestations that come within the sphere of the physician. This section is concerned with these disorders rather than the use of oestrogenic and progestogenic compounds as antifertility agents.

Pharmacology

Contraceptive pills are composed of a progestogenic compound to which is usually added an oestrogenic substance. At the present time six different progestogens are used. Of these, five (norethisterone and its acetate, norethynodrel, lynoestrenol and ethynodiol acetate) are derivatives of 19-nortestosterone, whereas one (megestrol) is derived from 17-hydroxyprogesterone and has less oestrogenic and potentially androgenizing properties. The two oestrogenic substances used are ethinyloestradiol and mestranol, its 3-methyl ether derivative.

Therapeutics

There are three main types of contraceptive pill. The *combined pill* contains an oestrogenic and progestogenic compound in varying proportions and is taken from the 5th day after the onset of menstruation until the 20–22nd day. The *sequential pill* comprises an oestrogenic compound taken from the 5th day until the 14–16th day, followed by a combined oestrogenic and progestogenic tablet for the next 5–7 days. The *progestogenic* pill, currently under further scrutiny, is composed of chlormadinone acetate and is taken continuously. Of these the combined pill is the most effective as a contraceptive agent; present evidence suggests that chlormadinone is the least effective and may possibly become increasingly less effective with continued use; the sequential pill occupies an intermediate place in effectiveness. Nevertheless, as an antifertility measure, the least effective of these agents is equal to all mechanical contraceptive devices.

Mode of Action. The contraceptive pill exerts its antifertility action by a number of different mechanisms. The combined and probably the sequential pills suppress the surges that normally occur in FSH and LH secretion as evidenced by suppression of the normally increased plasma level of FSH early in the follicular phase and the normally increased levels of both FSH and LH at the time of ovulation. Thus ovulation is suppressed. In addition progestogens increase the viscosity of cervical mucus, thereby preventing the entrance of spermatozoa into the uterus; this action is pronounced with chlormadinone which does not suppress ovulation. A third site of action is on the uterine endometrium where a situation unfavourable for nidation of the fertilized ovum is created.

Side-effects

A large number of side-effects may be induced by the contraceptive pill but these must be considered in relationship to the number of women using this method to prevent pregnancy. It is estimated that more than 1 million women in the United Kingdom take the contraceptive pill which has a world-wide usage in excess of 18 million women. Some of the side-effects are attributable to the oestrogenic component and some to the progestogen used in the pill. Thus the incidence and type of side-effect depend to some extent upon the particular tablet used, and the ratio of oestrogen to progestogen. Some side-effects tend to be more pronounced during the first few cycles during which the pill is taken, and may diminish with continued use. Such common side-effects as *nausea* and *vomiting*, *abdominal bloatedness*, *tenderness of the breasts* and *weight gain*, which occur in about one-third of women due to fluid retention, are attributable to the oestrogenic moiety. Weight gain may also occur as a result of the anabolic action of the progestogen. In some patients *headaches*, during the week before menstruation, and *pre-menstrual tension* with enhanced *irritability* occur, and are seemingly related to the progestogenic component. On the other hand some women experience a reduction in pre-menstrual tension. In most cases no change in *libido* is noted but some women experience increased sexual desire in the absence of fear of pregnancy; others have a reduced libido and this is likely to occur in association with *depression*, or rarely with a psychotic disorder, which is more prominent when the progestogenic to oestrogenic ratio is high.

Vascular Disorders. Cramps in the legs and pain in varicose veins are not uncommon in women using an oestrogen-containing contraceptive pill. The incidence of deep vein thrombosis with subsequent pulmonary embolism is increased 10-fold, rising from 1 case per 20,000 in control subjects to 1 case per 2,000 in those using the 'pill'. The incidence of cerebral arterial thrombosis is also increased 8-fold, most commonly the middle cerebral artery being involved and the vertebrobasilar system in 25 per cent. of cases. As yet there is no unequivocal evidence of an enhanced liability to coronary thrombosis. These thrombotic disorders are more liable to occur in women aged 35 or over, and are probably related to the observed increase in platelet adhesiveness and the increased plasma levels of clotting factors VII and X. Such changes are induced by synthetic and not naturally-occurring oestrogens, and are most marked when the oestrogenic to progestogenic ratio is high, as in the sequential regime. Progestogens alone do not seemingly induce such changes. The incidence of thrombotic disorders is higher in women of blood groups A, B and AB than those of group O but this predisposition is not sufficiently great to be of practical clinical significance.

In a small proportion of patients hypertension is aggravated or induced by the use of the contraceptive pill, and cases of malignant hypertension have been observed in which discontinuation of the regime has restored the blood pressure to normal. There is evidence that aldosterone secretion may be enhanced by the contraceptive pill, or that by this mechanism fluid retention and an increase in plasma volume and cardiac output are induced.

Jaundice of the cholestatic type may in rare instances be induced by the contraceptive pill, in some cases being attributable to the oestrogenic and in others to the progestogenic component. Such cases are more common in women who have had cholestatic jaundice as a complication of earlier pregnancies.

Metabolic Changes. Administration of the 'combined' contraceptive pill, which has been most studied, induces a number of metabolic changes. The oral glucose tolerance test is mildly impaired and some 10 per cent. of women develop evidence of biochemical but not of clinical diabetes. There is also an increase in the serum levels of cholesterol, triglycerides and lipoproteins but seldom beyond the upper normal range. Such changes may conceivably predispose to atherogenesis but such an effect will not become clinically discernible for many years.

Oestrogens in the contraceptive pill increase the plasma levels of transcortin, the carrier protein of cortisol, and of thyroxine-binding globulin. As a consequence the plasma *cortisol* and *protein-bound idoine* values may be raised above the upper normal limits and give misleading information unless the physician is aware that the patient is taking the contraceptive pill.

Rheumatic Manifestations. A small proportion of patients taking the contraceptive pill develop arthralgia, morning stiffness of joints or muscles and may show objective evidence of synovitis. This clinical picture simulates rheumatoid arthritis and in some patients the diagnosis is further confused by the development of L.E. cells and an increase in antinuclear antibodies. In some instances Raynaud's phenomenon develops. At present it is uncertain whether these rheumatic manifestations are connected with contraceptive therapy or represent the development of unrelated rheumatoid arthritis which goes into a spontaneous remission when the contraceptive pill is discontinued. There is some evidence that contraceptive medication may aggravate the symptoms and manifestations of pre-existing disseminated lupus erythematosus.

Amenorrhoea. For at least two cycles after stopping the 'combined' contraceptive pill, the urinary excretion of oestrogens, pregnanediol and total gonadotrophins is reduced. This effect is most marked during the first cycle, but the majority of women rapidly re-establish spontaneous ovulation and menstruation. A very few have persistent amenorrhoea which usually responds to administration of clomiphene citrate [p. 610].

Acne. In some women acne is much improved by administration of the contraceptive pill; in others it is made worse. The response obtained probably depends on several factors, the most important of which is the oestrogenic to progestogenic ratio.

Contra-indications

The contraceptive pill should not be used, according to present evidence, in women who have bad varicose veins; in those with a previous history of venous thrombosis or cerebral thrombosis; in patients with active liver disease or a history of pregnancy jaundice; in women with chronic renal disease and those with hypertension from any cause; in patients who suffer severe attacks of migraine, particularly if these are focal; and in women who have any form of blood disease. Oral contraceptives should not be used by women who have had a carcinoma of the breast or cervix.

Non-contraceptive Uses

The contraceptive hormonal pill can be used to establish regular menstruation in women whose periods are erratic; to control menopausal menorrhagia not due to structural organic causes such as fibroids [p. 613]; to prevent dysmenorrhoea; and to relieve premenstrual tension or control acne although in these two conditions the most effective preparation may be found only by trial and error. The sequential regime may be used to induce 'menstruation' in patients with primary or secondary amenorrhoea [pp. 607 and 609] where more radical treatment is inappropriate or ineffective in promoting normal ovarian function. Suppression of ovarian activity is also of value in the control of hirsutism in some patients [p. 619].

INTERSEX

Definition

To the practising clinician the term intersex is most usefully restricted to describe a patient who as a result of some congenital abnormality has accessory sexual organs showing a combination of both male and female characteristics. There is therefore doubt on examination of the external genitalia as to whether the patient is a phenotypic male or female. The term has also been used in a much wider sense to include, at one end of the spectrum, homosexuals and transvestists but in such cases there is no ambiguity as to the patient's phenotypic sex. If the definition of intersex is restricted to those with ambiguous external genitalia, a case of Klinefelter's syndrome [p. 599] would not be considered an intersex because, irrespective of the precise sex chromosomal complement, the patient is a phenotypic male with testes. Similarly, a woman with classical XO Turner's syndrome [p. 608] is not an intersex because, despite the shortcomings of her secondary sexual characteristics after adolescence, she is anatomically female as judged by her external genitalia.

PHYSIOLOGICAL CONSIDERATIONS

Sexual Development

The development of the sexual organs takes place *in utero* in three main stages.

Determination of Genetic Sex. The genetic sex of an individual is determined at the time of fertilization of the ovum. Normally the ovum carries one X chromosome and the spermatozoa either an X or a Y chromosome. Fertilization of an ovum by a Y-carrying sperm results in a male XY zygote, whereas fertilization by an X-carrying sperm produces a female XX zygote. By their action on specific chemical processes, these sex-determining genes control the subsequent differentiation and development of male or female gonads.

Differentiation of the Gonads. During the fifth week of embryonic development an undifferentiated or neutral gonad develops from the urogenital ridge. This primitive bipotential gonad is composed of a cortex and a medulla. At this phase there is no evidence from the appearance of the gonads or from the primitive urogenital area whether the embryo will develop into a male or a female. Later an XX genotypic foetus develops ovarian tissue from the cortex of the primitive bipotential gonad and the medulla involutes. In a foetus of XY constitution the medulla develops into a testis and the cortex involutes.

Development of the Genital Tract. The development of a normal female or male genital tract depends in part upon hormonal influences exerted by the differential gonad and in part upon unknown controlling factors during and after the 10th week of foetal development. The female sexual apparatus is derived from the Müllerian system, and the male apparatus from the Wolffian system. The ovary itself plays little or no part in the organization of the female sexual apparatus, so that even in the absence of an ovary (or a testis) there is a fundamental basic tendency to the development of an internal and external female sexual tract with regression of the Wolffian system.

The testis exerts its effect in two ways. First it suppresses the Müllerian system. This action is confined to the side on which each testicle is situated and is mediated locally by an unknown mechanism seemingly unrelated to androgen secretion. A disorder at this stage, associated with subsequent development of the testis, leads to an apparently normal male child who will have a uterus. The second stage of male sexual development, notably penile growth, is dependent upon testosterone secretion. Delayed or inadequate hormonal secretion at this time will lead to a hypertrophied clitoris rather than a normal prepubertal penis. Thus an imperfectly developed male gonad may fail to exert sufficient influence to overcome the inherent basic tendency to female genital development with the consequence that the external genitalia and adnexa may be wholly or partially female.

Assessment of Sex

The 'sex' of an individual may be judged from several different standpoints.

Chromosomal or Genetic Sex. The chromosomal or genotypic sex is determined by the X and Y chromosomes. By special techniques the two normal X chromosomes can be identified in the dividing cells of a normal genetic female, and two normal X and Y chromosomes in the dividing cells of a normal genetic male. The technique for identifying these chromosomes is difficult and time consuming. Many dividing cells, preferably from different tissues, may have to be examined. Often it is difficult to detect mosaicism when there is more than the normal single cell-line. Furthermore, the proportions of two or more different cell-lines may vary from one tissue to another.

Nuclear or Chromatin Sex. In a normal XX genotype female microscopical examination of buccal squames or polymorphonuclear leucocytes will show that more than 50 per cent. of the cells have a chromatin dot (Barr body) in their nucleus. This represents the second of two X chromosomes and thus implies that the sex chromosomal complement is XX. In contrast 90 per cent. of the cells of a normal XY genotypic male do not show this chromatin dot. The determination of the nuclear sex involves a much simpler procedure than identifying the X and Y chromosomes in dividing cells but it has serious limitations because a chromatin-positive cell may have more than the normal complement of two X chromosomes and have an XXX, XXY or XXXY composition. In these cases in which more than two X chromosomes are present, a proportion of the cells may show more than one Barr body but no information as to the presence of a Y chromosome will be obtained. Conversely a chromatin-negative cell, suggesting an XY chromosomal complement, may have an XO or XYY chromosomal composition.

Gonadal Sex. The gonadal sex depends upon whether testicular or ovarian tissue is present. In early embryonic development this is largely determined by the patient's genotypic sex.

Phenotypic Sex. The phenotypic sex is judged from the anatomy of the external genitalia, associated to some extent after adolescence by the assessment of the degree of development of male or female secondary sexual characteristics.

Psychosexual Orientation. The psychosexual orientation or 'gender role' of an individual usually follows the sex in which the child is brought up, and this in turn usually depends upon whether the infant at birth or in the neonatal period is considered by the mother, the doctor who delivers her, or the midwife as male or female. Exceptions to this rule may occur for physiological or psychological reasons. For example, a male pseudohermaphrodite [p. 618], with testicular tissue but brought up as a girl, may later in life exhibit masculine interests and pursuits. Homosexuals and particularly transvestists may for psychological reasons wish to adopt a psychosexual role opposite to their phenotypic and genotypic sex and in direct variance to the sex in which they have been reared.

Aetiology of Intersex

Most cases of intersex are caused by some detectable or as yet undetectable chromosomal abnormality, or by some abnormal hormonal influence. Sometimes the cause remains unknown although, with improved methods of karyotyping, unexplained cases in the past may now be shown to have mosaicism. Chromosomal abnormalities may result from non-disjunction, deletion of an X or Y chromosome, isochromosomal formation of either the long or short arm of an X chromosome, or the development of mosaicism due to non-disjunction or anaphase lagging. Chromosomal abnormalities tend to disorganize sexual development at an early embryonic stage whereas chemical or hormonal abnormalities tend to do so at a later stage.

Not all sex chromosomal abnormalities cause ambiguity of phenotypic sex. Mention has already been made of anatomical males who in Klinefelter's syndrome have karyotypes 47/XXY, 48/XXXY, 49/XXXXY or mosaicism 46/47 XY/XXY. Some phenotypic males have a 47/XYY karyotype. These individuals are usually excessively tall and well built. They may have mild mental deficiency and exhibit violent and aggressive antisocial behaviour which lands them in prison. Preliminary reports indicate these XYY males secrete excess testosterone and have unexpectedly high urinary levels of luteinizing hormone. Similarly some women with sex chromosome abnormalities show little or no ambiguity of their external genitalia. For example, those with extra X chromosomes, e.g. 47/XXX or 48/XXXX, may appear perfectly normal, although their secondary sexual characteristics are often poorly developed, and give birth to healthy children. These women may have primary amenorrhoea, however, or develop secondary amenorrhoea at an early age. As in many patients with sex chromosomal abnormalities, mental retardation is not uncommon.

TRUE HERMAPHRODITISM

Definition

A very rare condition characterized by the presence of ovarian and testicular tissue in the same individual.

Aetiology

The cause of true hermaphroditism is often obscure. Most cases appear to have a normal 46/XX karyotype; much less commonly an apparently normal male

46/XY chromosomal constitution has been found. In recent years with improved methods of chromosomal analysis an increasing number of hermaphrodites have been shown to be mosaics such as XX/XXX, XX/XY, XX/XXYY and XX/XXY/XXYY. It has been suggested that in some instances of XX/XY mosaicism, double fertilization of an ovum by two sperms, one carrying an X and the other a Y chromosome, may have occurred. In those cases with a 46/XX composition, and no evidence of mosaicism after a careful search, it is possible that there has been translocation of the short arm of a Y chromosome with the short arm of an X chromosome.

Pathology

The gonadal composition is variable. A testis may be present on one side with an ovary on the other, an ovary or testis on one side and an ovotestis on the other, or ovotestes on both sides. The anatomy of the adnexa usually corresponds to the sex of the gonad on that particular side. The external genitalia show varying degrees of ambiguity.

Symptoms

The degree of ambiguity in the appearance of the external genital apparatus is very variable as would be expected from the different aetiological factors and from the proportions of the two different cell-lines in mosaics. Hypospadias with a perineal urethal opening is the most obvious and common finding. Sometimes a gonad may be palpable in an inguinal canal or in one of the genital clefts. More often no gonadal tissue is palpable but a gonad is found at operation for repair of an associated hernia. The scrotum may be bifid and the vagina rudimentary. After puberty male or female secondary sexual characteristics may appear but are seldom well developed. Some patients may appear as normal females and hermaphroditism unsuspected until a laparotomy is carried out for the investigation of primary amenorrhoea.

Diagnosis

Hermaphroditism or pseudohermaphroditism should be suspected in any child born with ambiguous external genitalia. Radiological studies may be required to determine the urogenital anatomy. Karyotype analysis may be helpful particularly to establish mosaicism, but confirmation of the diagnosis requires laparotomy and histological examination of the gonads and adnexa.

Treatment

Treatment depends upon the age at which the diagnosis is made and the anatomy of the external genitalia. In infants and young children an intra-abdominal testis or an ovotestis or ovotestes should be removed and the child reared as a female. If the diagnosis is only made later in life, the sex in which the child has been brought up should largely govern treatment but much will depend on the external genitalia, the psychosexual orientation and wishes of the patient, and the histology of the gonads at laparotomy. Intra-abdominal testes or ovotestes should be removed. Plastic surgery and oestrogens or androgens, as appropriate, are then used to make the external genitalia and the psychosexual orientation more compatible with the sex chosen. Such hormonal treatment will develop the appropriate secondary sexual characteristics and plastic surgery may allow heterosexual intercourse. The patients must be apprised of their infertility if they contemplate marriage.

FEMALE PSEUDOHERMAPHRODITISM

Definition

A rare condition in which a genetically XX female with ovaries has varying degrees of masculinization of the external genitalia. Later in life the untreated condition is usually associated with primary amenorrhoea, hirsutism and lack of secondary sexual characteristics.

Aetiology

The commonest cause of female pseudohermaphroditism is congenital adrenal hyperplasia [p. 587] due to 21-hydroxylase deficiency. As a result of deficient biosynthesis of cortisol, excessive ACTH secretion occurs and the adrenal glands are stimulated to secrete increased amounts of androgens. Much less commonly virilization of a female foetus may occur when such compounds as androgens, norethisterone, ethisterone and related substances are given to the mother at a critical stage of pregnancy. Even less commonly an androgen-secreting tumour in the mother, such as an arrhenoblastoma, may virilize a female foetus. Rarely the condition is unassociated with any evident source of androgens and can then only be differentiated from true hermaphroditism by laparoscopy and biopsy of the gonads.

Pathology

Masculinization occurs after the Müllerian-duct system has differentiated into a normal uterus, Fallopian tubes and upper part of the vagina. Differentiation of the urogenital sinus is, however, incomplete, and presents a more or less male configuration. There is usually marked hypospadias with the lower part of the vagina leading into the urethra just before it opens on to the surface at the base of the phallus. The labial folds are fused and resemble a scrotum devoid of testes; the clitoris may be so enlarged as to resemble a penis. In the adrenogenital syndrome there is marked adrenocortical hyperplasia.

Symptoms

At birth the clitoral enlargement or hypospadias, the partial or complete fusion of the labia and the rudimentary vagina without an obvious opening to the exterior may suggest that the infant is a boy. Later in childhood the absence of testes may provoke the parents to seek medical advice. Later still excess androgen secretion in congenital adrenal hyperplasia promotes muscular development, rapid skeletal growth that terminates with premature fusion of the epiphyses, stunted stature and infantile or prepubertal skeletal proportions. At the expected time of puberty menstruation does not occur and female secondary sexual characteristics fail to develop. Hirsutism may become marked and be accompanied by other features of virilization. In less severely affected cases menstruation and some mammary development may occur.

Diagnosis

It is most important that any dubiety as to the infant's true phenotypic sex is resolved as soon as possible after birth. In the adrenogenital syndrome proper early treatment and the minimum of plastic surgery can convert a female pseudohermaphrodite into a normal female child who later will become a normal woman in every respect. Indecision as to the infant's sex may result in the child being considered a male with hypospadias and undescended testes, and reared as a boy. The diagnosis can usually be established early by showing a chromatin-positive nuclear sex, and an abnormal 11-oxygenation index in the urine [p. 579]. The urinary excretion of pregnanetriol and 17-oxo-steroids, relative to the child's age, are increased but such investigations are seldom necessary in the presence of an increased 11-oxygenation index. If there is marked deficiency of cortisol biosynthesis, the infant may vomit, become dehydrated and fail to thrive [p. 580].

Treatment

When the diagnosis is made, as it should be, early in infancy, the child is treated with cortisone or hydro-cortisone in a dose sufficient to suppress excessive ACTH secretion and to reduce the increased androgen production by the hyperplastic adrenal cortices [p. 582]. Plastic surgery may be required to correct the external genital abnormalities. In those rare instances when the diagnosis has been missed in infancy and the child has been reared as a boy, it is often best in adolescence, particularly if breast development or menstruation occurs, to perpetuate the male psychosocial role to which the patient is accustomed. The ovaries should be removed; the breasts reduced in size by plastic surgery and phallic development further enhanced by administration of testosterone [p. 599].

Prognosis

Provided treatment is started early in patients with congenital adrenal hyperplasia, the prognosis in regard to life and normal femininity with the capacity to pro-create is good. Unrecognized insufficiency of cortisol secretion may cause death in an Addisonian crisis. Congenital adrenal hyperplasia is often genetically determined and the parents must be warned of the likelihood that subsequent children may be similarly affected. The patient must be advised that she may procreate children with an adrenocortical enzymatic defect, but this should not constitute a bar to marriage and pregnancy in the face of modern effective methods of treatment.

MALE PSEUDOHERMAPHRODITISM

Definition

A rare condition in which a genetically XY male with testes has varying degrees of feminization of the external genitalia.

Aetiology

Despite wide variations in the feminization of the internal or external genitalia, patients with male pseudohermaphroditism have a 46/XY karyotype. It appears that either the primitive male gonads fail to suppress the Müllerian system or the later embryonic testes fail to secrete adequate amounts of androgen, or there is a congenital failure of the peri-pheral tissues to respond to testosterone. Thus the genital tract fails to evolve along masculine lines, and after puberty there is failure of the secondary sexual characteristics to develop masculine features.

Pathology

The testes show in adult life apparently normal interstitial cells, but spermatogenesis is absent and this is attributable to failure of the spermatogenic tissue to respond to testosterone or to the abnormal location of the gonads. Rudimentary female adnexa may be present.

Symptoms

The clinical picture is very variable, and predomi-nantly masculine, indifferent and feminine types are distinguished.

In the *masculine type* hypospadias commonly occurs, and the testes may be undescended, lying in the abdomen, inguinal canal or hernial sacs, or located in the labio-scrotal folds. Laparotomy may show un-expectedly some poorly developed evidence of a female genital tract such as a rudimentary uterus and Fallopian tubes.

In the *indifferent type* the external genitalia may be so ambiguous that without further study it is impossible to decide whether the child is male or female. Hypo-spadias with a perineal urethral opening, a bifid scrotum and a rudimentary vagina may be present. Such cases tend to be reared as girls. In both the mascu-line and indifferent types, some degree of androgeniza-tion and development of secondary male sexual characteristics is common at adolescence. Muscular development occurs with some growth of facial and sometimes body hair. Failure of breast development and primary amenorrhoea may be the first suggestion that the affected child, brought up as a girl, is in fact not a genetic female.

In the *feminine type* the degree of femaleness may be so marked that no suspicion as to the true genetic or phenotypic sex of the child is raised until in late adolescence she presents with primary amenorrhoea or infertility. This extreme form of male pseudoherma-phroditism has been termed the *testicular feminization syndrome*. These patients have a normal female appear-ance, a tendency to eunuchoidal skeletal proportions, good breast development and are often attractive. Axillary hair is absent and pubic hair scanty. The labia are small and the vagina ends blindly. The testes, which produce both testosterone and oestrogens may be intra-abdominal or lie in the inguinal canal, in hernial sacs or even in the labia. The condition is often in-herited, occurring in siblings and in the descendants of female carriers who show such traits as scanty sexual hair or a delayed menarche. Biochemical studies have shown that in the testicular feminization syndrome testosterone secretion is normal, and the female secondary sexual characteristics are attributable to the action of oestrogens, the effect of which is unopposed because the peripheral tissues fail to respond to testosterone.

Diagnosis

In infancy and early childhood it is important that male pseudohermaphroditism is distinguished from female pseudohermaphroditism by determining the nuclear and chromosomal sex and, in the case of female pseudohermaphroditism due to congenital adrenal hyperplasia, by the urinary 11-oxygenation index [p. 579] and excretion of 17-oxosteroids. The condition must also be distinguished from true hermaphroditism and atypical cases of Turner's syndrome with XO/XY mosaicism [p. 609]. In most cases radiological examination of the urogenital sinus and laparotomy are required to establish the precise diagnosis.

Treatment

In the masculine and indifferent types of male pseudohermaphroditism the testes should be removed because of the high incidence of malignant change which may reach 20 per cent. after the age of 30. In the masculine type the child is often best reared as a boy, and plastic surgery and later testosterone used to reinforce the male external genitalia and the male psychosexual orientation. The same treatment is usually best in those with more marked ambiguity of the external sexual apparatus.

In the testicular feminization syndrome a different approach is indicated because of the strongly female attributes of the patient, 'her' female psychosexual orientation, the late age at which the patient presents, and the fact that 'she' may already be married to a man and having satisfactory sexual intercourse. No hint of the patient's genetic sex should be given, and the testes should be removed because of their liability to malignant change. Before gonadectomy, oestrogens should be prescribed to prevent hot flushes developing because the testes are the source of the patient's endogenous oestrogen secretion. The patient must be warned that she will always be infertile and menstruation will not occur.

HIRSUTISM

PHYSIOLOGICAL CONSIDERATIONS

The growth of terminal hair, which is coarse and relatively long, is little influenced by gonadal hormones in such areas as the scalp, eyebrows and also the forearms and legs, sometimes being marked on the limbs long before the advent of puberty. Pubic, axillary and to some extent hair on the extremities is dependent upon gonadal hormone secretion, and appears first at the time of puberty, pubic preceding axillary hair by about 2 years. In the male facial and chest hair-growth is promoted by testosterone secretion from the testes. The difference between hair-growth in males and females is quantitative rather than qualitative, and so also is the degree of hairiness in normal women and those suffering from hirsutism. It is usual for the pubic hair in the male to extend upwards to the umbilicus in an inverted V, whereas characteristically the female escutcheon has a horizontal upper border although in many women upward extension along the linea alba is common.

A number of factors effect the growth of terminal hair in post-pubertal life. *Racial origin* has a profound influence, those of dark complexion and Mediterranean or Celtic stock being more hairy than those of blond Scandinavian origin. Conversely the American Red Indian is relatively hairless and so also are those of Oriental stock. The *sex* of the subject has a well recognized influence on the growth of body hair, and this is related to the greater circulating level of testosterone in men. Despite this the extent of body hair at the lower end of the normal male biological distribution curve overlaps with that at the upper end of the normal female curve. *Sensitivity* of hair follicles to androgenic hormones varies considerably from one individual to another and also in different members of the same family. The responsiveness of hair follicles in different areas is also variable. Thus some women show a much greater growth of terminal hair on the lower abdomen and thighs than on the face or chest, whereas others show the converse. The *age* of the subject also affects hair-growth which does not develop on the face or body until puberty is established. After the menopause, pubic and axillary hair regresses although often at this time there is an increase in facial hair. *Hormones* play a prominent role in promoting normal pubic and axillary hair-growth in both sexes and facial hair in the normal male. The most potent are testosterone and androstenedione which is converted to testosterone. These compounds are secreted by the mature gonads and by the adrenal cortex in both sexes. Androgenic hormones also have the effect of causing recession of scalp hair over the temples. Thyroxine influences hair growth in all areas, not only those normally stimulated by androgenic hormones, and hence has a direct action on hair follicle activity.

Definition

Hirsutism is defined in the female as an excess of body or facial hair. There is, however, no sharp dividing line between a normal and pathological degree of hairness because of the wide variation dependent upon racial and genetic influences.

Aetiology

Idiopathic Hirsutism. In the great majority of women no endocrine pathology can be found to explain the excessive growth of hair. This idiopathic type of hirsutism is attributable to increased responsiveness of the hair follicles or to an increase in androgen secretion of adrenocortical or ovarian origin. In about one-third of patients the plasma testosterone level is within the normal range but in others the production rate of testosterone is increased. Idiopathic hirsutism commonly starts soon after puberty but may not be sufficiently marked to present as a clinical problem until the age of 20. Its rate of progress is slow.

Endocrinopathies. Other causes of hypertrichosis are

the polycystic ovary syndrome [p. 611]; tumours of the ovaries [p. 613] such as arrhenoblastoma, and hilus-cell or granulosa-cell tumours; androgen-secreting tumours of the adrenal cortex; Cushing's syndrome; and congenital adrenal hyperplasia due to an enzymatic defect in the biosynthesis of cortisol [p. 587]. In Cushing's syndrome [p. 582], irrespective of its cause, hirsutism is seldom the presenting complaint. Congenital adrenal hyperplasia is an uncommon cause of late onset hirsutism except when the enzymic defect is mild, and hypertrichosis and amenorrhoea are the presenting features occurring after the expected time of puberty.

Iatrogenic. Hirsutism may occur as a consequence of the administration of androgens, synthetic anabolic hormones, cortisone or ACTH. Phenytoin, used in the treatment of epilepsy, and diazoxide, used in the control of hypoglycaemia or hypertension, may both induce generalized hypertrichosis without significant increase in axillary or pubic hair, and without virilization.

Symptoms

The distinction between pathological hirsutism and a normal degree of hirsuties is often difficult to make, and due allowance must be made for the patient's colouring and racial origin. Although the patient may not present until she is 20–25 years old, idiopathic hirsutism is usually slowly progressive from puberty onwards, and is unassociated with menstrual disorders or evidence of virilization. A more substantial increase in androgen secretion and a greater likelihood of a discernible endocrine abnormality are probable when the degree of hypertrichosis is marked; when its onset is later and its progression more rapid; when recession of frontal scalp hair is present; when stigmata of virilization such as clitoral enlargement, hypertrophy of the larynx with deepening of the voice, and a reduction in mammary development occur; and when menstrual disorders such as oligo- or amenorrhoea are present.

Diagnosis

More than 98 per cent. of patients complaining of increased hairiness have idiopathic hirsutism. In the absence of menstrual dysfunction, evidence of virilization, and late onset in life further investigation is seldom justified. When such additional features are present, however, the exclusion or identification of an ovarian or adrenal lesion is necessary. Estimation of the 17-oxosteroids is seldom informative except when there is an androgen-secreting tumour of the adrenal cortex; normal values are often found in patients with masculinizing ovarian tumours. The 11-oxygenation index, and the response to ACTH and dexamethasone may be helpful in defining an adrenocortical lesion [p. 579]. Ovarian tumours are notoriously difficult to detect clinically or biochemically; laparoscopy to establish the polycystic ovary syndrome, or laparotomy with bisection of the ovaries to exclude a neoplasm may be necessary.

Treatment

In the absence of a discernible cause for hirsutism the treatment is essentially symptomatic. Contrary to popular belief shaving does not make the hair growth more vigorous or coarse. An electric razor is the best form of treatment for severe cases, but there is considerable variation in the most satisfactory type and make of razor for each individual. For emotional reasons many women refuse to use a razor on certain, particularly facial, areas although they do so readily on their legs or axillae. In less severe cases bleaching of the hair and chemical or wax depilation, particularly the latter is adequate. Electrolysis is favoured by some but often leads to a morocco-leather appearance of the skin in addition to being expensive, time-consuming and liable to induce acne.

In certain selected cases, where the degree of hirsutism is particularly marked and the presence of polycystic ovaries is suspected, suppression of hair growth may be achieved by prolonged treatment with small doses of prednisone, 2·5 mg. two or three times daily to reduce adrenocortical activity, combined with cyclical administration of a 'contraceptive pill' to suppress ovarian function.

REFERENCES

Alexander, W. D., and Harden, R. McG. (1967) The assessment of thyroid function, *Hosp. Med.*, **1**, 669.

Bartter, F. C., Pronove, P., Gill, J. R., and MacCardle, R. C. (1962) Hyperplasia of the juxtaglomerular complex with hyperaldosteronism and hypokalaemic alkalosis, *Amer. J. Med.*, **33**, 811.

Besser, G. M., and Landon, J. (1968) Plasma levels of immunoreactive corticotrophin in patients with Cushing's syndrome, *Brit. med. J.*, **2**, 552.

Bishop, P. M. F. (1966) Intersexual states and allied conditions, *Brit. med. J.*, **1**, 1255.

Doniach, D., Hudson, R. V., and Roitt, I. M. (1960) Human auto-immune thyroiditis: Clinical studies, *Brit. med. J.*, **1**, 365.

Ferriman, D. (1969) *Anovulatory Infertility*, London.

Fourman, P., and Royer, P. (1968) *Calcium Metabolism and the Bone*, 2nd ed., Oxford.

Gabrilove, S. L., Sharma, D. C., Wotiz, H. H., and Dorfman, R. I. (1965) Feminizing adrenocortical tumours in the male, *Medicine (Baltimore)*, **44**, 37.

Goolden, A. W. G. (1967) Diagnostic uses of radioisotopes; the investigation of thyroid disorders, *Hosp. Med.*, **1**, 927.

Greenwood, F. C., Landon, J., and Stamp, T. C. B. (1966) The plasma sugar, free fatty acid, cortisol and growth hormone response to insulin, *J. clin. Invest.*, **45**, 429.

Harrison, T. S., Bartlett, J. D., and Seaton, J. F. (1967) Exaggerated urinary norepinephrine response to tilt in phaeochromocytoma, *New Engl. J. Med.*, **277**, 725.

Hobbs, J. R., Bayliss, R. I. S., and MacLagan, N. F. (1963) The routine use of ^{132}I in the diagnosis of thyroid disease, *Lancet*, i, 8.

Howorth, P. J. N., and MacLagan, N. F. (1969) Clinical application of serum-total-thyroxine estimation, resin uptake and free-thyroxine index, *Lancet*, i, 224.

Irvine, W. J., ed. (1967) *Thyrotoxicosis*, Edinburgh.

Jackson, D., Grant, D. B., and Clayton, B. E. (1968) A simple oral test of growth hormone secretion in children, *Lancet*, ii, 373.

Loraine, J. A., and Bell, E. T. (1966) *Hormone Assays and their Clinical Application*, Edinburgh.

Loraine, J. A., and Bell, E. T. (1968) *Fertility and Contraception in the Human Female*, Edinburgh.

Mattingly, D., and Tyler, C. (1967) Simple screening test for Cushing's syndrome, *Brit. med. J.*, **2**, 394.

Muller, S. A. (1969) Hirsutism, *Amer. J. Med.*, **46**, 803.

Nieman, E. A., Landon, J., and Wynn, V. (1967) Endocrine

function in patients with untreated chromophobe adenomas, *Quart. J. Med.*, **36,** 357.

OLIVER, D. O. (1968) The diagnosis and management of phaeochromocytoma, *Hosp. Med.*, **2,** 1279.

PECILE, A., and MULLER, E. E, eds (1968) *Growth Hormone*, Amsterdam.

PRUNTY, F. T. G. (1967) Hirsutism, virilism and apparent virilism and their gonadal relationship, *J. Endocr.*, **38,** 85 and 203.

RIMOIN, D. L., BORGAONKAR, D. S., ASPER, S. P., and BLIZZARD, R. M. (1968) Chromatin-negative hypogonadism in phenotypic men, *Amer. J. Med.*, **44,** 225.

ROSS, E. J., MARSHALL-JONES, P., and FRIEDMAN, M. (1966) Cushing's syndrome: diagnostic criteria, *Quart. J. Med.*, **35,** 149.

ROSS, E. J., PRICHARD, B. N. C., KAUFMAN, L., ROBERTSON, A. I. G., and HARRIES, B. J. (1967) Preoperative and operative management of patients with phaeochromocytoma, *Brit. med. J.*, **1,** 191.

R. I. S. BAYLISS

SECTION 6

DISEASES OF THE LIVER, GALL-BLADDER AND PANCREAS

THE LIVER

GENERAL CONSIDERATIONS

The liver in the normal adult weighs approximately 1500 grams. It is situated in the right upper abdomen largely under the right lower ribs. It consists of a mass of parenchymal cells which are traversed by systems of blood vessels, lymphatics, nerves and bile-ducts. The organ has a double blood supply and in the normal subject the portal vein supplies almost two-thirds of the hepatic circulation, the remainder being provided by the hepatic artery. Total liver blood flow in normal subjects is about 1·5 litres per minute. The liver is divided into lobules and these lobules possess a central hepatic vein, and at the periphery there are several portal 'triads', that is collections of supporting stroma containing a branch of the portal vein, the hepatic artery and a bile ductule. Blood flows from these blood vessels via the sinusoids and between the parenchymal cells, leaving via the central hepatic vein. An important cell found in the liver is the Kupffer cell which is particularly prominent in the hepatic sinusoids. This cell is a part of the reticulo-endothelial system and undertakes important storage and immune processes.

The liver has the following important functions:

1. It produces bile and through the bile salts contained in this digestive secretion it facilitates the absorption of fat and fat-soluble vitamins. Bile salts form micelles and solubilize small particles of lipid. The bile salts found in human bile are conjugates of cholic, chenodeoxycholic and deoxycholic acids. These acids are conjugated with taurine or glycine. Bilirubin in the bile is produced largely from the breakdown of senescent red blood cells, though recently evidence has been produced to show that there is some bilirubin formed from haem compounds produced in sites such as the kidney and bone marrow and liver. In haemolytic states the amount of bile pigment transported to the liver is excessive and the serum bilirubin rises [see Section 13].

2. The liver produces a large number of proteins and is the site of synthesis of all the plasma proteins except the immunoglobulins. Of the hepatic proteins albumin is the most important; 10–15 g. of albumin are synthesized in the liver per day and the liver is also the site of production of important binding globulins such as that which binds iron (transferrin), copper (caeruloplasmin) and various combinations of globulin and lipid called lipoproteins. The liver is also the site of production of the proteins concerned in blood coagulation and of amino-acid degradation to alphaketo-acids and ammonia. Ammonia is then converted in the liver to urea by a series of enzymes acting in the Krebs urea cycle.

3. Carbohydrates in the form of glucose and galactose are metabolized in the liver and the end result of this process is the synthesis of glycogen. Glucose undergoes phosphorylation to glucose-6-phosphate prior to its conversion to glycogen. The polymer, glycogen, is stored in the liver and breakdown of this substance (glycogenolysis) is facilitated by several series of enzymes.

4. The liver plays an essential part in fat metabolism. It is able to utilize free fatty acids released from fat depots in order to provide energy. It also converts free fatty acids to triglyceride and other lipids. Neutral fat can be split by the liver to glycerol and free fatty acid. Free fatty acid is in turn oxidized to acetyl Co A units which either undergo complete oxidation or recombine to form aceto-acetic acid. This latter compound is important because it is one of the ketone bodies appearing in the blood and urine in severe diabetes and because it is unable to be further metabolized in the body. The normal liver contains fat—usually about 5 per cent. of its weight. In certain circumstances such as diabetes, starvation, and alcoholic liver disease this amount is much increased.

5. The liver also plays a central role in the breakdown of steroid hormones such as cortisol, testosterone and oestrogens. These hormones undergo degradation, conjugation and excretion in the bile. Antidiuretic hormone is also removed from the circulation by the liver. Many drugs are also altered by the liver so that they become more water soluble and can hence be excreted in the urine. An important system of enzymes exists in the smooth endoplasmic reticulum which is responsible for much of this function. It has been recently demonstrated that this drug metabolizing system can be altered by drugs so that an increased or decreased concentration of enzyme may result. This in turn will alter the speed at which drugs are metabolized. It has been shown, for example, that barbiturates are very potent inducers of the enzymes responsible for the conjugation of bilirubin.

6. The liver also has important storage functions and amongst the substances stored are iron, vitamin B_{12} and folic acid. The amount of B_{12} stored in the liver is sufficient for some two to three years use even if B_{12} absorption fails completely.

LIVER FUNCTION TESTS

There are a certain number of biochemical investigations which can be performed on patients with suspected liver disease. These are collectively known as the liver function tests and although they have proved to be extremely useful in clinical practice it must be remembered that they are in no way specific for the presence of liver disease and many of them are abnormal in conditions which do not primarily affect the liver. Recently these tests have been added to by the incorporation of further immunological tests which can be performed on blood and by the application of techniques of hepatic scintiscanning and ultrasonic scanning.

BLOOD TESTS

The Serum Bilirubin

The normal serum bilirubin is from 0·2 to 0·8 mg. per 100 ml. The amount of pigment which is conjugated is normally small and the van den Bergh reaction is therefore negative. In patients who are jaundiced the serum bilirubin rises and in the range of 2–3 mg. per 100 ml. the degree of pigment retention is sufficient to cause the patient to become visibly icteric. In severe jaundice the serum bilirubin reaches 20–30 mg. per 100 ml. or more. Elevation of the serum bilirubin of this order should lead to a determination of the amount of conjugated and free pigment present. Although no precise delineation of cases into obstructive or liver cell jaundice can be obtained in this way, the fact that there is a large percentage of conjugated pigment, i.e. 90 per cent. or more, is rather suggestive of obstructive jaundice and more equal concentrations of conjugated bilirubin are more suggestive of a liver cell lesion.

In patients with haemolytic jaundice even where there is severe haemolytic anaemia the serum bilirubin rarely reaches more than 5 or 6 mg. per 100 ml. unless there is liver cell damage as well. In this type of jaundice the retained pigment is all of the unconjugated variety—van den Bergh negative.

The Serum Alkaline Phosphatase

This is a most useful test of liver cell function. The normal serum enzyme level is 3–13 King-Armstrong units per 100 ml. (or 1·5–4 Bodansky units per 100 ml.), though in adolescents it is higher. The enzyme has several origins. Much is produced from bone, some is produced in the liver and a further part is produced in the intestinal mucosa. In pregnancy a further contribution to the maternal serum level is from the placenta.

In patients with liver cell disease or in patients with obstructive jaundice the serum alkaline phosphatase may be raised. Although levels over 30 K-A units are suggestive of obstructive jaundice this can readily occur in patients with liver cell disease and it is wrong to assume that such levels are always indicative of obstruction. Further, the height of the alkaline phosphatase does nothing to indicate the level of obstruction when this type of jaundice occurs. A recent method of differentiating between bone disease and liver disease has been the introduction of the estimation of the enzyme 5′ nucleotidase. The serum level of this enzyme is only raised in liver disease and therefore is able to differentiate between liver disease and bone disease when the alkaline phosphatase is raised. There are also techniques for isolating the various types of alkaline phosphatase and thus detecting their origins.

The Serum Proteins and Flocculation Tests

The flocculation tests have largely disappeared from clinical practice. They are in any case non-specific tests of liver function and really depend on the fact that certain heavy metals produce precipitation of abnormal globulins in serum. Much more value can be obtained from estimating the total serum proteins and that fraction made up by the albumin and globulin. In health the serum proteins have a normal total level of 6–8 g. per 100 ml. of which the albumin accounts for 3·5–4·5 g. and the globulins for the rest. In chronic liver cell disease there is diminished production of albumin and altered distribution so that the serum level falls often to below 3 g. per 100 ml. and there is a risk of oedema formation. Conversely the serum globulin levels rise as these proteins are not all produced by the parenchymal cells in the liver and there is often hyperplasia of the reticulo-endothelial structures such as the spleen where they are produced. More value can be obtained by estimating the separate globulin fractions and electrophoresis allows these to be divided into alpha-1, alpha-2, beta and gamma globulins [see Section 4]. It is characteristic of chronic liver cell disease that there is a rise in beta and particularly gamma globulins. It is also characteristic of obstructive jaundice that the alpha-2 and beta globulins are raised and this knowledge is sometimes helpful in making a diagnosis. The serum cholesterol is often elevated in obstructive jaundice. Further analysis of the various immunoglobulin fractions using immuno-electrophoresis has not been of great diagnostic help in liver disease for it is quite common for one or all of the several fractions making up the immunoglobulins to be increased. In acute liver cell disease such as is seen in infective hepatitis the serum albumin is maintained as long as the disease does not become chronic and there is an associated increase in beta and gamma globulins.

Enzyme Levels

Of the various enzymes liberated from the damaged liver cell most value is obtained from estimating the serum levels of the serum glutamic oxaloacetic transaminase (S.G.O.T., aspartate transaminase) of which the normal level is less than 40 units per ml., and of serum glutamic pyruvic transaminase (S.G.P.T., alanine transaminase). Both of these enzymes are elevated in patients with liver cell damage and in those with severe liver cell injury the elevation may be to 1000–2000 units per ml. In patients with obstructive jaundice the elevation of these enzymes is much less and usually below 200–300 units per ml. Of the other enzymes which may be released into the serum the so-called 'liver specific' enzymes such as sorbitol dehydrogenase, fructose-1-phosphate aldolase, and ornithine carbamyl transferase have all proved to be rather insensitive. However, lactic dehydrogenase remains a good, but non-specific, test of liver damage. When separated into its isoenzymes its diagnostic usefulness is increased. Isocitric dehydrogenase levels can also be helpful and as they are likely to be elevated only in patients with liver disease they are a more specific but not particularly sensitive measure of liver cell damage.

Bromsulphthalein (B.S.P.) Excretion

This is probably the most sensitive test of liver function that is available. It cannot be carried out in the presence of jaundice. It depends on the fact that the dye bromsulphthalein is largely removed from the circulation by the liver. B.S.P. traverses the liver cell where it is conjugated with glutathione prior to excretion in the bile. An abnormal retention of B.S.P. in the serum following a loading dose is, therefore, evidence of impaired removal. This usually means that there is liver cell damage and/or abnormal communication between the portal and systemic circulations. The test can be done in two ways.

Simple. In order to do this a 5 per cent. concentration of the dye (5 mg. per kg.) is given intravenously; 45 minutes later a blood sample is removed from the opposite arm and the amount of dye retained is estimated. If there is more than 5 per cent. retention at 45 minutes this is abnormal and, therefore, synonymous with impaired hepatic function.

Complex. It is possible by using continuous infusion of B.S.P. at two known concentrations to determine two liver factors called S (storage), and Tm (transport maximum) for this dye. These are extremely sensitive measures of liver function. Both are usually impaired in liver disease, but in certain conditions one may be more impaired than another. The details of the method used are beyond the scope of this book.

It should be remembered that B.S.P. can cause unpleasant reactions in patients, particularly on second and subsequent administration. It is also highly irritant and must be completely injected intravenously. It is wise to have intravenous hydrocortisone available when any tests of B.S.P. excretion are being performed. Because of the fact that B.S.P. has some drawbacks and because it is not completely removed by the liver and it is metabolized to some extent by other organs there has been a tendency to look for other suitable dyes which can be used. The most satisfactory, though it is expensive, is indocyanine green (I.C.G.), which is also used as a test of liver cell function and can, in a similar way to B.S.P., be used for estimating total hepatic blood flow.

URINE AND STOOL TESTS OF VALUE IN LIVER DISEASE

The identification of bile pigments in the urine by means of the *Ictotest* tablet test, which is based on the purple colour produced by the bile pigment with a diazo dye is a valuable and sensitive test for bile pigment. The estimation of urobilinogen and urobilin can also be of value, though the tests are a little more complex. Using Ehrlich's aldehyde reagent a positive test for urobilinogen at a dilution of 1 in 20 of fresh urine shows the presence of excess of this pigment. This is found in the presence of liver cell disease and in haemolysis. It also occurs, of course, when both these abnormalities are present together. The determination of faecal stercobilin (normal 100–200 mg. per 24 hours) is occasionally of value in the patient with haemolysis when values are elevated.

SCANNING OF THE LIVER

A recent useful technique which has been introduced in the field of hepatic investigation has been hepatic scintiscanning. For this a radioactive substance which is taken up by the liver, is injected intravenously, and by using a scanning device an isotopic 'map' of the liver can be obtained. This gives details of the liver size and homogeneity, as well as some idea of its function. Two types of compound have been used; a group of substances taken up by the reticulo-endothelial system, the best examples of this being colloidal gold or 99 Tc (technetium). A further group of compounds taken up by the liver cell itself include ^{131}I Rose Bengal. The type of scan is similar in each instance. In patients with filling defects in the liver due to tumours, abscesses or cysts the scan has the appropriate defect(s) in it. In patients with chronic liver cell disease there may be diminished total uptake of the isotope together with an alteration in hepatic size and configuration. Most important of all, there is an increased uptake of the radioactive scanning material by the spleen. Scanning techniques have been extremely valuable, particularly so in the detection of cysts, tumours and abscesses within the liver and to a lesser extent in the diagnosis of cirrhosis [PLATE 1].

RADIOLOGY OF LIVER DISEASE

The most important radiological techniques used in the investigation of patients with liver disease are the following:

The Detection of Oesophageal Varices by Barium Swallow [PLATE 1]. This is valuable evidence of portal hypertension and it is of some importance to recognize that varices may be found not only in the oesophagus, but in the stomach, and duodenum. Filling defects in the fundus of the stomach may cause some diagnostic confusion.

Portal Venography [PLATES 1 and 2]. This is an important technique particularly in patients who are being considered for portacaval anastomosis. It consists of the injection of radio-opaque contrast medium into the spleen of the patient and the identification of opacification of the portal vein and any tributaries, and the liver by using multiple films. It is also useful in identifying a collateral circulation in patients with, for example, abnormal neurological disorders which could be part of the syndrome of hepatic encephalopathy. The other technique of use is the identification of the hepatic artery and its branches by coeliac axis angiography.

Coeliac Axis Angiography. This is useful in the detection of hepatic tumours, and in patients with cirrhosis changes in the intrahepatic arteries are also seen. Coeliac angiography can also be used in patients who have undergone splenectomy for identifying the patency or otherwise of the portal vein. Films are made of the contrast medium returning in the portal vein after prior coeliac axis injection.

NEEDLE BIOPSY OF THE LIVER

Though there is a range of biochemical and scanning tests that will give some indication of liver function, the only way of detecting changes in liver structure is by biopsy. This may conveniently be done with a needle technique. The usual apparatus is the Menghini needle. This is a cutting needle which is quickly inserted and withdrawn from the liver whilst suction is maintained to keep the severed biopsy within the barrel of the needle. A 'nail' prevents the biopsy being sucked into the aspirating syringe, and being fragmented. The following are the indications for liver biopsy, providing that other simpler tests have been used. It is helpful in the diagnosis of:

1. Jaundice, where it can confirm a diagnosis of liver

cell or obstructive jaundice, but is unable to deliniate the cause of the liver cell disease or the site of the obstruction.

2. It is of value in the diagnosis of neoplastic disease of the liver, particularly if a nodule can be biopsied directly.

3. It is of value in the diagnosis of various disorders such as the reticuloses, lipoidoses, and amyloidosis, which infiltrate the liver.

4. It is of value in the diagnosis of hepatic cirrhosis, though occasionally the toughness of the liver and fragmentation may make histological interpretation difficult.

5. It is of use in the identification of the cause of hepatomegaly where this is uncertain.

Contra-indications

No patient should be subjected to needle biopsy of the liver unless this is absolutely indicated. Certain precautions are necessary and these are as follows:

1. Ascites, if it is present, must be tapped.

2. Examination of the blood to exclude a haemorrhagic state is essential, and if deficiencies are found either in the prothrombin concentration or in other tests these must be corrected.

3. Blood must be cross-matched in case of haemorrhage after the biopsy.

4. The technique is best avoided in the presence of deep jaundice due either to obstruction or more particularly where this is due to liver cell disease.

The biopsy, when obtained, should be stained with haematoxylin and eosin, as well as by a technique which shows reticulin. In certain cases it may be necessary to stain for iron or amyloid or copper with appropriate techniques.

REFERENCES

Hepatic Structure

RAPPAPORT, A. M. (1963) Acinar units and the pathology of the liver, in *The Liver. Morphology, Biochemistry, Physiology*, ed. Rouiller, C., Vol. 1, p. 265, New York.

Liver Function Tests

LEEVY, C. M. (1961) Dye extraction by the liver, in *Progress in Liver Disease*, ed. Popper, H., and Schaffner, F., Vol. 1, p. 174, New York.

MCAFEE, J. G., ANSE, R. G., and WAGNER, H. N., Jr. (1965) Diagnostic value of scintillation scanning of the liver, *Arch. intern. Med.*, **116**, 95.

MCCARTHY, C. F., READ, A. E. A., ROSS, F. G. M., and WELLS, P. N. T. (1967) Ultrasonic scanning of the liver, *Quart. J. Med.*, **36**, 517.

WILLIAMS, R., KREEL, L., and BLENDIS, L. M. (1967) Coeliac axis catheterization: uses and value in portal hypertension, in *The Liver*, Vol. 19 of the Colston Papers, p. 125, ed. Read, A. E., London.

Liver Biopsy

SHERLOCK, S. (1962) Needle biopsy of the liver: a review, *J. clin. Path.*, **15**, 291.

THE LIVER IN GENERAL DISORDERS

The liver is involved in a large number of generalized diseases. A brief account will be given of some of these disorders in this section.

Diseases of Carbohydrate Metabolism

Diabetes. Both patients with the juvenile (insulin sensitive type) or the maturity onset (insulin insensitive type) of diabetes may exhibit hepatic enlargement. In the juvenile type this is seen in about 10 per cent. of patients and is particularly common where diabetes is difficult to control. The hepatomegaly is usually associated with increased glycogen deposition in the liver. In the maturity onset type when patients are often obese there is a considerable incidence of hepatomegaly which in this type of disease is due to fatty infiltration of the liver.

It should be remembered, too, that the patient with acute diabetic ketosis will occasionally complain of severe abdominal pain which is likely to be due to stretching of the capsule of the liver by glycogen deposition. This is an important symptom and may be wrongly attributed to the presence of intra-abdominal disease. Patients with diabetes also have a higher than normal incidence of hepatic cirrhosis amounting to about twice the incidence in a normal population. It is also recognized that patients with cirrhosis have a high incidence of complicating diabetes and about 30 per cent. of cirrhotic patients have been shown to have abnormal glucose tolerance. The resulting diabetes is usually mild and responds to treatment with oral hypoglycaemic agents or small doses of insulin. The basis for this association is unknown but at least it has been demonstrated that in the cirrhotic patient with abnormal glucose tolerance there is an abnormal resistance to insulin activity. Following a portacaval anastomosis diabetes may be exacerbated and this is then of some clinical importance as diabetic coma may then be confused with hepatic coma complicating the postoperative state.

The Glycogenoses. This is a group of disorders of glycogen metabolism. There is resultant retention of glycogen in the tissues, including the liver, and because of the failure of glycogen breakdown, hypoglycaemia results. There are six main varieties of the disease, the commonest type of which is von Gierke's disease in which glucose-6-phosphatase is deficient in the liver and the kidney. The other types where there is liver involvement and glycogen infiltration is type 3 or Cori's disease where deficiency of a debranching enzyme leads to infiltration of the liver and heart muscle with glycogen, and type 6 (Hers' disease) where the liver is involved due to deficiency of a liver phosphorylase. The clinical picture is similar in these disorders. The liver is enlarged, the patient who is a young child, shows failure of physical and sexual development and there are episodes of severe hypoglycaemia. There is no splenomegaly and this is a point of some clinical importance. The diagnosis rests on the demonstration of an impaired response of the serum glucose level to the effects of glucagon which normally stimulates hepatic glycogenolysis and produces a rise of the blood glucose. In patients with a negative response to this test liver biopsy tissue will demonstrate deficiency of the appropriate enzyme and abnormal concentration and structure of hepatic glycogen. These diseases are difficult to treat. The patients often die in childhood and the only treatment has consisted of frequent glucose feeds to overcome hypoglycaemia and resulting chronic brain damage. The operation of portacaval transposition has been used in those cases where the defect is confined to the liver. The operation consists of dividing the inferior vena cava and the portal vein and re-anastomosing these vessels so that glucose absorbed from the digestive tract is diverted via the inferior vena cava into the peripheral circulation where the glucose is required and blood from the lower half of the body is used to perfuse the portal vein and to maintain hepatic blood flow. A few patients only have been treated in this way, but considerable improvement has been noted in one or two of them.

Amyloid Disease. Amyloid may be deposited in the liver producing hepatomegaly. Chemically amyloid consists of protein with a small amount of carbohydrate. The material is deposited as fine fibrils. The older classification of amyloidosis into primary and secondary is no longer used. Depending on the histological site of deposition amyloid disease is now classified as perireticular amyloidosis, where there is a deposition in and around small blood vessels, and pericollagen amyloidosis, where there is involvement of organ connective tissue. Perireticular amyloidosis is the form commonly seen. It involves the spleen, the kidneys and the liver. It complicates chronic diseases such as tuberculosis, rheumatoid arthritis, some reticuloses and ulcerative colitis. Prolonged suppuration in bone or lung is another rare cause. The patient shows an enlarged, smooth, nontender liver and there may be evidence of proteinuria or oedema. Diagnosis depends on aspiration liver biopsy and staining with appropriate dyes such as Congo red. Material for biopsy may also be obtained by hepatic, renal or rectal biopsy. The latter avoids the risk of haemorrhage from the liver and kidney which may be increased in patients with amyloid disease. The older dye absorption test which depended on the fact that amyloid material took up certain basic dyes such as Evans blue and Congo red have largely been replaced by the biopsy procedures. Perireticular amyloid of atypical distribution is also found in familial Mediterranean fever. This is an inherited disorder characterized by attacks of fever and features of renal failure due to deposition amyloid tissue in the kidneys. The liver is not usually involved. Pericollagen amyloidosis is a rare condition. It may complicate myeloma.

The Liver in the Porphyrias

There are two types of porphyria which involve the liver:

1. Acute intermittent porphyria is a disorder in which the liver synthesizes excess porphyrin precursors, namely delta amino laevulinic acid and prophobilinogen. Clinically it is associated with attacks of severe abdominal pain and vomiting together with peripheral neuritis and mental disturbance. The patient passes dark urine during the attacks which contains excess copro- and uroporphyrin, together with porphobilinogen. Attacks may be precipitated by the administration of drugs, particularly barbiturates, and by alcohol. These precipitate attacks by increasing the synthesis of delta amino laevulinic acid by producing enzyme induction in the liver. The disease may be fatal, due to respiratory failure consequent upon ascending peripheral neuritis.

2. Porphyria cutanea tarda is often associated with alcoholism so that the patient may have a history of heavy drinking and may present with hepatomegaly. This is due to hepatitis or cirrhosis. Excerabations of the porphyria are associated with bouts of deterioration in liver function perhaps related to alcoholism. Another important cause of excerabation is the administration of oestrogens, as for example in patients with carcinoma of prostate. The symptoms of this type of porphyria are due only to the presence of a rash. This is present on exposed surfaces and shows blistering and chronic scarring.

Lipoid Storage Diseases

This group of diseases is associated with the deposition in the cells of the reticulo-endothelial system of abnormal deposits of lipid material. The important diseases which affect the liver and spleen are:

Gaucher's Disease. This is a disease which affects principally Jews and in which deposits of cerebroside are found in the reticulo-endothelial system. This material is not abnormal but cannot be metabolically degraded. The characteristic physical signs are of hepatomegaly, massive enlargement of the spleen and generalized pigmentation of the skin. Pingueculae (yellow wedge-shaped fatty thickenings) may also be found in the sclera. The long bones are also involved so that the lower ends of the femora are classically expanded (hock bottle femora). Diagnosis depends on the demonstration of abnormal Gaucher cells, that is reticulo-endothelial cells containing a fibrillary cytoplasm packed with cerebroside. There is no specific treatment for this disease, though splenectomy may be required for abdominal discomfort, and radiotherapy may be useful if there is severe bone pain [Section 11].

Niemann-Pick Disease. This disease is also found in Jews and produces hepatosplenomegaly. The characteristic cell is different from that in Gaucher's disease and the material deposited is a phospholipid (sphingomyelin). The disease is, unlike Gaucher's disease, almost confined to infancy and patients die before the age of 2 years with an enlarged liver and spleen, mental deficiency, blindness and deafness. Diagnosis is suggested by the history, the physical signs and confirmed by the finding of typical ovoid foamy cells 20–40μ in diameter which contain the abnormal lipid [Section 13].

Hepatic Granulomata

Hepatic granulomatous lesions have a common histological structure consisting of an area of central necrosis and giant-cell formation surrounded by epithelioid cells, lymphocytes and a reticulin capsule. The granulomata are found in a wide variety of diseases so that their identification on a liver biopsy examination suggests the following possible diagnoses—sarcoidosis, tuberculosis, brucellosis, syphilis, ascariasis and infective mononucleosis.

With the exception of sarcoidosis, the lesions, although numerous, do not interfere with hepatic function. Widespread granulomata formation in sarcoidosis is, however, occasionally associated with pre-sinusoidal portal hypertension and even cirrhosis.

Ulcerative Colitis

The following hepatic abnormalities occur in ulcerative colitis. The commonest lesion is fatty infiltration, particularly in the ill patient. Hepatic cirrhosis is a further complication and this may be accompanied by bleeding oesophageal varices. The cause of the cirrhosis is unknown. Obviously syringe hepatitis is a possible cause in those who have had blood transfusions, whilst the fact that ulcerative colitis sometimes accompanies chronic active hepatitis [see p. 639] suggests the importance of autoimmune processes.

Portal bacteraemia has been demonstrated in patients with ulcerative colitis and this could be a factor in the production of pericholangitis (which may produce cholestasis), sclerosing cholangitis—an obliterative fibrosis of intra- and extrahepatic ducts—and occasional cases of hepatic duct cancer. Another possibility is that these lesions could be produced by irritant bile salts such as lithocholic acid—produced from normal bile salts by bacterial action in the abnormal gut and re-secreted in bile. Certainly in the experimental animal lithocholic acid produces bile-duct damage and stone formation.

Fatty Liver

Fatty change in the liver is found in a wide variety of diseases such as diabetes, obesity, ulcerative colitis, malnutrition and as the result of certain liver cell poisons such as alcohol.

The liver is enlarged and smooth and is not tender. In extreme cases the patient may be icteric either due to accompanying liver cell dysfunction or as a result of compression of biliary canaliculi. Fat occupies each liver cell and in cases due to alcoholism there may be areas of focal hepatic necrosis, and condensation of perinuclear cytoplasm—Mallory's alcoholic hyalin. Hepatic fat is derived from many sources. There may be increased hepatic deposition associated with a local failure of lipoprotein synthesis consequent on damage to the endoplasmic reticulum. Increased depot and dietary fatty acid mobilization are further factors. Failure of lipoprotein lipase to hydrolyse triglyceride in the serum may also lead to increased hepatic retention of fat. The mechanism probably varies with the cause. Despite support from animal work it is now thought that fatty infiltration of the liver does not cause cirrhosis. In the alcoholic, fatty degeneration may be followed by cirrhosis, but this is variable and depends on some continuing action of alcohol rather than the fatty change itself.

The Liver in Pregnancy

Of the identifiable hepatic disorders occurring in pregnancy the following are the most important:

Recurrent Cholestatic Jaundice. This is an obstructive type of jaundice which is seen in the last trimester of pregnancy. In some patients the jaundice may be mild and the only prominent symptom is pruritus. In others the jaundice may be deeper and the condition recurs with subsequent pregnancies. The disorder is a benign one, though there is an accepted risk of premature delivery of the foetus. The cause of the disorder is unknown, but it is likely that a steroid produced in pregnancy interferes with bilirubin excretion. Some support for this is suggested by the fact that those mothers who develop recurrent cholestasis of pregnancy are the same patients who show jaundice of an obstructive type following the use of the contraceptive pill. The disorder is variable in distribution and seems commonest in the Scandinavian countries and in certain parts of South America. Apart from the slight risk to the foetus and the prominent pruritus the prognosis of this disorder as regards hepatic function is excellent. It should be noted that even in the normal pregnant subject abnormalities of bromsulphthalein excretion are seen during pregnancy, so that presumably an identical though subclinical type of lesion due to steroid secretion is present during normal pregnancy.

Viral Hepatitis. This is a common disorder in the pregnant patient. Serum hepatitis may result from blood transfusion or venepuncture and close contact with a young family who may be excreting the virus of infective hepatitis increases the risk of this type of viral hepatitis as well. Usually the disease runs a classical course, but there seems, too, to be a risk of increased severity of hepatitis in pregnancy and a tendency for lethal hepatic necrosis. This is certainly so in tropical countries where there is a high mortality both to the mother and foetus. The foetus, however, is not usually born with evidence of viral hepatitis transmitted from the mother.

Drug Lesions in Pregnancy. Many drugs may be given in pregnancy and may injure the liver or produce other biochemical disorders of importance to the foetus. Chlorpromazine and other phenothiazines may cause obstructive jaundice, and the pregnant patient is extremely susceptible to certain antibiotics, in particular tetracycline, which may produce a severe and fatal fatty infiltration of the liver in the last trimester of pregnancy. Jaundice, nausea, vomiting and haematemesis are the usual symptoms and death is from progressive hepatic failure. Drugs given to the pregnant woman or neonate may on occasions potentiate jaundice and kernicterus. These drugs include the sulphonamides which displace bilirubin from its albumin binding site, the antibiotic novobiocin which prevents conjugation of bilirubin in the liver, and vitamin K which increases the production of bilirubin from red blood cells.

Another lesion to be remembered which may be connected to the abnormal metabolism of cholesterol with succeeding pregnancies is the possibility of jaundice due to gall-stone formation.

REFERENCES

Diabetes Mellitus

MEGYESI, C., SAMOLS, E., and MARKS, V. (1967) Glucose tolerance and diabetes in chronic liver disease, *Lancet*, ii, 1051.

Glycogen Storage Disease (*Surgical Treatment*)

RIDDELL, A. G., DAVIES, R. P., and APLEY, J. (1967) Portacaval transposition in the treatment of glycogen storage disease, in *The Liver*, Vol. 19 of the Colston Papers, ed. Read, A. E., London.

Hepatic Granuloma

Sarcoidosis
PORTER, G. H. (1961) Hepatic sarcoidosis. A cause of portal hypertension and liver failure, *Arch. intern. Med.*, **108,** 483.

Amyloid
COHEN, A. S. (1967) Amyloidosis, *New Engl. J. Med.*, **277,** 574, 628.

Ulcerative Colitis
VINNICK, I. E., and KERN, F. (1963) Liver disease in ulcerative colitis, *Arch. intern. Med.*, **112**, 41.

Pregnancy (Recurrent Idiopathic Jaundice)
SVANBORG, A., and OHLSSON, S. (1959) Recurrent jaundice of pregnancy, *Amer. J. Med.*, **27,** 40.

JAUNDICE

The accumulation of bile pigment in the serum is associated with a yellow discoloration of the skin, conjunctivae and mucous membranes called jaundice. The level of serum bilirubin has to reach approximately 3 mg. per 100 ml. before such a change is noted clinically.

There are classically three types of jaundice. These are:

1. *Obstructive jaundice*. In this situation there is obstruction either in the common bile-duct, both hepatic ducts or in the biliary ductules or canaliculi inside the liver. It can therefore be classified as either intra- or extrahepatic.
2. *Liver cell jaundice*. In this condition there is a failure of the liver cell to take up and conjugate bilirubin and to deliver it to the biliary canaliculi for excretion.
3. *Haemolytic jaundice*. In this situation which is accompanied by haemolytic anaemia the amount of bilirubin delivered to the liver is in excess of its excretory capacity. It therefore collects in the serum in the unconjugated form.

OBSTRUCTIVE JAUNDICE

Clinical Picture

Patients with obstructive jaundice have usually experienced a gradual onset of the condition, as serum bilirubin levels take some days, or longer, to reach a maximum. The jaundice is of variable intensity, but with complete obstruction serum bilirubin levels may be 30 mg. per 100 ml. or more. The jaundice is usually accompanied by persistent itching, though this is not invariable, and this phenomenon is thought to be due to the deposition of irritant bile salts in the skin. The patient may complain of pain, particularly if the cause lies in the obstruction of the common bile-duct by gall-stones or by a growth at the head of the pancreas. In a similar way there may be gross weight loss in patients with neoplastic disease. Pale stools and dark urine are universal accompaniments of this form of jaundice. The intrahepatic causes of obstructive jaundice include various drugs, one form of viral hepatitis (obstructive hepatitis) and wide intrahepatic spread of malignant tissue as is sometimes seen in patients with carcinomatosis or Hodgkin's disease. The *physical signs* of obstructive jaundice include icterus and hepatomegaly. In chronic cases the spleen may become enlarged and in patients with neoplastic disease enlargement of supraclavicular glands on either side of the neck may be a feature. Rectal examination may reveal secondary deposits in the pouch of Douglas, and this is an important part of the physical examination of the jaundiced patient. It is also important in patients with chronic obstruction to look for deposits of cholesterol, particularly around the eyelids (xanthelasma) and on bony points or sites of pressure. An important physical sign is occasionally seen in patients with neoplastic obstruction of the common bile-duct below the cystic duct and this is the presence of a spherical tumour felt under the hepatic free margin, which is an enlarged gall-bladder. This is called Courvoisier's sign and is not seen in patients with obstructive jaundice due to biliary calculi. Masses may be found in the abdomen suggesting a primary neoplasm in the stomach, colon or elsewhere, and in such patients examination of the stools for occult blood and precise localization by radiology are important.

Diagnosis

Characteristically, in obstructive jaundice the liver function tests show a raised serum bilirubin of variable extent, a high percentage of conjugated bilirubin in the serum, negative flocculation tests, raised alpha-2 and beta globulins, and moderately raised transaminases, though this may be more elevated in patients with chronic obstruction due to accompanying liver cell dysfunction. Most important of all, there is a raised serum alkaline phosphatase usually in excess of 30 K-A units. The urine contains bile and in cases of complete obstruction is free of urobilinogen. The stools are pale because of lack of biliary pigment and accompanying steatorrhoea.

It is, of course, most important in all patients with obstructive jaundice to inquire about the taking of drugs. Drugs which cause obstructive jaundice include the phenothiazines. Rare examples are due to the contraceptive pill, anticoagulant drugs, butazolidine, chlorpropamide and amitriptyline. Treatment is related to the cause and in the case of extrahepatic obstruction requires surgical intervention.

LIVER CELL JAUNDICE

Aetiology

The usual causes of liver cell jaundice are two, namely hepatitis usually due to the virus of infective or syringe hepatitis and the action of certain poisons and drugs. A classical example of this latter is carbon tetrachloride, used in fire extinguishers and dry cleaning, which causes severe fatty infiltration of the liver and other organs. Other examples of drugs causing liver cell injury include the monoamine oxidase inhibitors used in the treatment of depression and the anaesthetic agent halothane.

Clinical Picture

The onset of liver cell jaundice is usually rapid, the patient's degree of jaundice increasing to a maximum within a day or two of the onset of the disorder. The patient often feels unwell, there is not usually persistent itching and on examination the liver may be enlarged or decreased in size and there may be splenomegaly. It is important to look for evidence of chronic liver cell disease as a basis for acute liver cell dysfunction so that signs like spider naevi, palmar erythema, gynaecomastia, and clubbing are important. If liver cell jaundice is severe then the patient may show evidence of a bleeding tendency and there may be evidence of hepatic encephalopathy and oedema formation, the latter due to a fall in the serum albumin levels.

Diagnosis

The liver function tests apart from showing a high serum bilirubin show abnormal flocculation tests, a rise in the beta and gamma globulins, a normal or raised alkaline phosphatase, and most important of all, considerable elevation of the transaminases. In patients with acute liver cell disease associated with necrosis of the liver there may be a polymorphonuclear leucocytosis in the peripheral blood. The urine of patients with liver cell jaundice contains bile pigment and an excess of urobilin or urobilinogen may be demonstrated.

Treatment

Treatment depends on the cause, but surgery must be avoided.

HAEMOLYTIC JAUNDICE

Clinical Picture

The patient with haemolytic jaundice shows only mild icterus and the urine does not contain bile pigment. It does, however, contain excessive urobilinogen, and may be darker than normal, as may the stools. The liver function tests are normal unless the patient has developed biliary calculi associated with chronic haemolysis and these may then cause a picture of biliary obstruction with raised alkaline phosphatase. The patient with haemolytic jaundice may show splenomegaly and there may, on occasions, be hepatomegaly [see Section 13].

Diagnosis

Examination of the blood will show other features suggestive of haemolysis, such as macrocytes and reticulocytes in the peripheral film. Examination of the bone marrow in patients with haemolysis shows evidence of erythroid hyperplasia. Important tests to determine the nature of the haemolytic process include a history of taking of drugs, examination of the red cells for the detection of antibody coating (Coombs test), an L.E. cell preparation, an electrophoresis of the haemoglobin and a blood culture.

Treatment

This depends on the cause and may include corticosteroids and splenectomy. Surgery may be needed for complicating gall-stones.

REFERENCES

Billing, G. H., and Lathe, G. H. (1958) Bilirubin metabolism in iaundice, *Amer. J. Med.*, **24**, 111.

Sherlock, S. (1962) Jaundice, *Brit. med. J.*, **1**, 1359.

Sherlock, S. (1968) Chronic cholanditides: Aetiology, diagnosis and treatment, *Brit. med. J.*, **3**, 515.

THE CONGENITAL HYPERBILIRUBINAEMIAS

Aetiology

These diseases are inherited disorders of bilirubin metabolism, the abnormality consisting of elevation of the serum bilirubin usually intermittent and without other signs of liver disease or significant haemolysis.

Clinical Picture

The disorder is usually found in children or young adults and is noticed first as the appearance of icterus. The icterus may be intermittent, tends to be found when the patient has some intercurrent illness such as influenza or gastro-enteritis and may be familial. At these times the patient may complain of tiredness and fatigability. The urine may or may not contain bile as the type of bilirubin found in the serum can either be of the unconjugated or conjugated variety.

UNCONJUGATED HYPERBILIRUBINAEMIA

This is Gilbert's disease and probably consists of several conditions of varying biochemical aetiology. The patient is icteric but there is no bile in the urine and there is no evidence of severe haemolysis. Certain drugs can produce a lesion of this type and examples of these are male fern extract used in the treatment of tape worm infestation, cholecystographic contrast media and novobiocin. The defect in the Gilbert type of congenital hyperbilirubinaemia seems to be one of a low bilirubin uptake into the liver though glucuronyl transferase levels in the liver are also dimished. The rest of the liver function tests and biliary excretion pattern are normal. Although the unconjugated hyperbilirubinaemia of Gilbert's disease is benign, one type, the so-called Najjar-Crigler lesion is much more severe, usually dates from birth and is associated with very intense jaundice. The lesion here is a complete lack of glucuronyl transferase in the liver so that bilirubin cannot be conjugated. The very high unconjugated bilirubin levels cause kernicterus and the patient usually dies with severe brain damage. One type of rat has been described with a similar type of inherited lesion, that is a lack of hepatic transferase. This is the so-called Gunn rat. Recently severe unconjugated hyperbilirubinaemia has been successfully treated with phenobarbitone which improves bilirubin conjugation. A rare type of unconjugated hyperbilirubinaemia in the absence of haemolysis has been described by Israels as 'shunt' hyperbilirubinaemia. The cause for this is apparently increased bone marrow turnover of bilirubin.

CONJUGATED HYPERBILIRUBINAEMIA

In this type of hyperbilirubinaemia the patient excretes bile in the urine and it is likely that the defect here is one of transfer of bile from the liver cell to the biliary apparatus. The lesion is of two types depending on whether there is or is not an abnormal pigment found in the liver cells. The abnormal pigment is probably a melanin and gives its name to the Dubin-Johnson syndrome where the presence of the pigment can be recognized by the black colour of the liver (black liver jaundice) on needle biopsy or on inspection of the liver surface. The other type of conjugated hyperbilirubinaemia is the so-called Rotor syndrome. In the conjugated hyperbilirubinaemias there may be abnormalities of the other liver function tests, particularly the alkaline phosphatase and also the B.S.P. excretion, if the excretion pattern is followed longer than the usual 45 minutes. These both suggest that the lesion is one of a defect of transport of bilirubin into the biliary apparatus.

Diagnosis

The importance of the congenital hyperbilirubinaemias is that they are, with the exception of the Najjar-Crigler syndrome, benign. They should not be mistaken for hepatic or biliary disease and operations or long periods of hospital observation, supposing that the patient has such a disorder, are obviously to be avoided. These patients live a normal span of life providing they are not the victims of unnecessary operations or investigations.

REFERENCES

Billing, B. H., Williams, R., and Richards, T. G. (1964) Defects in hepatic transport of bilirubin in congenital hyperbilirubinaemia: An analysis of plasma bilirubin disappearance curves, *Clin. Sci.*, **27**, 245.

Dubin, I. N., and Johnson, F. B. (1954) Chronic idiopathic jaundice: A review of 50 cases, *Amer. J. Med.*, **24**, 268.

Israels, L. G., Suderman, H. J., and Ritzmann, S. E. (1959) Hyperbilirubinaemia due to an alternate path of bilirubin production, *Amer. J. Med.*, **27**, 693.

Powell, L. W., Hemingway, E., Billing, B. H., and Sherlock, S. (1967) Idiopathic unconjugated hyperbilirubinaemia (Gilbert's syndrome): A study of 42 families, *New Engl. J. Med.*, **277**, 1108.

HEPATITIS

INTRODUCTION

Hepatitis—an acute inflammatory disorder of the liver can be due to a variety of pathogenic agents. These include the virus of yellow fever and the virus (or viruses) of infective hepatitis and serum or syringe hepatitis. The virus causing infective mononucleosis is a further cause of hepatitis as are certain of the enteroviruses and herpes group. Neonatal or giant-cell hepatitis may sometimes be due to herpes simplex infection and a more recently recognized cause of this disease is rubella virus. The agent causing Q fever is occasionally associated with hepatitis and a virus is presumably responsible for the hepatitis transmitted from certain green monkeys (Marburg agent). Recently interest has been centred on the isolation of cytomegalovirus (CMV) from some patients with hepatitis. This has largely occurred in patients with debilitating diseases and particularly where immunosuppressive drugs have been used. The disorder seems to be particularly likely to be associated with obstructive (cholestatic) features.

The most important spirochaetal causes of jaundice are those associated with leptospirosis (Weil's disease) and canicola fever, whilst the spirochaetes of the genus *Borrelia recurrentis* which cause relapsing fever are also associated in severe cases with a hepatitis. The jaundice associated with secondary syphilis is not due to the spirochaete causing this disease but to complicating syringe hepatitis which was extremely common complication of its treatment a few years ago.

The number of agents causing hepatitis is large and distinction of one from the other may be difficult. This is because there is difficulty in recognizing with any certainty the causative agent—particularly when this is likely to be infective or syringe hepatitis—and because the histological pattern in the injured liver is similar in most instances whatever the cause. Further, drug lesions may be indistinguishable and the whole pattern of diffuse hepatic injury from spotty areas of micronecrosis through to massive necrosis of the liver is a theme resulting from a host of infective and toxic agents. This can make diagnosis difficult.

VIRAL HEPATITIS

INFECTIVE HEPATITIS

Definition

An acute inflammation of the liver due to an unknown virus or viruses.

Aetiology

This disease is almost certainly caused by a virus but at the time of writing none has been consistently isolated from patients with the disease. A large number, some of them almost certainly associated viruses, have been isolated from suspected cases. The disease is transmitted principally by the oral-faecal route. Chimpanzees may act as occasional carriers. The disease is common, particularly in young people, 20,000 cases occurring annually in this country where it is notifiable. It is common within the family group and particularly so where conditions of hygiene are poor and for this reason epidemics are not unknown in wartime, and are liable to occur where there is faecal pollution of, for example, drinking water or food such as shell-fish. Though causing severe systemic upset in many patients the disease has, on the whole, a good prognosis.

The Australia antigen (now known as hepatitis associated antigen—HAA) is identifiable in the blood of a considerable percentage of patients with viral hepatitis and is thought to be particularly associated with serum hepatitis. Studies at the Willowbank Centre in the United States have in any case shown that two clear-cut and clinically definable syndromes may be produced by inoculation into humans of the same infective material so that the association of HAA with infective hepatitis may mean that we are in fact dealing with SH virus in many cases of so-called infective hepatitis. The antigen is important, as although it does not represent the hepatitis virus itself it can be looked for in, e.g. blood donors and workers in dialysis units and appropriate precautions such as exclusion from a donor programme made. Rarely, in this country, it is possible that chronic liver disease may be associated with its continuing presence in the blood stream. This, it seems, is more common in America and Africa.

Pathology

The liver is usually enlarged and the principal changes are shown on histology. Here there is scattered damage to the hepatic lobule, changes being particularly marked around the centrilobular veins. There is also a marked inflammatory exudate in the portal zones consisting largely of lymphocytes and mononuclear cells. With severe infective hepatitis fibrosis may commence in the expanded portal zones but progression to cirrhosis is most unusual. Other changes are found in the alimentary tract and in the kidney, where there may be minor catarrhal changes in the villi and in the glomerular apparatus. In the patient with acute necrosis of the liver complicating acute infective hepatitis the liver is small and shrunken and on cutting shows a very characteristic picture of small isolated areas of liver cell tissue between which the liver cells are completely lost and the tissue consists of blood cells and some connective tissue. Repair of the liver from this stage usually involves the formation of a true hepatic cirrhosis.

Clinical Picture

Following an incubation period of 2–6 weeks the patient presents with a sudden onset of profound anorexia, nausea and vomiting with abdominal distention and some pain or tenderness under the right costal margin. The patient is pyrexial at this stage, which usually lasts from 3 to 7 days. Less common manifestations in this pre-icteric stage include skin rashes, arthralgia and the symptoms of meningism. Physical signs at this stage are minimal, but may include hepatomegaly and there is often hepatic tenderness. The urine may show the presence of bilirubin before the patient is icteric and certainly sensitive tests of liver function, particularly the serum transaminases are raised at this stage. In many patients the disease may remain anicteric but in the classical case the icteric phase of the disease begins after a few days. The jaundice develops rapidly, the temperature returns to normal and the patient feels much better. Usually at this stage the appetite improves and the abdominal symptoms disappear. Physical signs now include hepatomegaly, and the spleen is enlarged in about 30 per cent. of cases. Together with the splenomegaly, there may be enlargement of some of the lymph nodes in the root of the neck on the right-hand side. The jaundice is of variable duration usually lasting 2 weeks or so and during this phase, though the icterus is of varying depth, the patient is improving.

Diagnosis

The diagnosis of the disease is easy when there is an epidemic in progress, or when there have been similar cases within the family unit. Isolated cases may be difficult to diagnose in the pre-icteric phase, but usually the diagnosis is obvious when the person is young and when the signs are those of acute liver cell jaundice. Confusion may also occur in the elderly where mental symptoms may be more common. Help may be obtained from the liver function tests which show a raised serum bilirubin, transaminase values usually greater than 600 units per ml., positive flocculation tests and a raised beta and gamma globulin in the protein strip. The serum albumin is normal in all except severe cases. The stools are pale and the urine shows the presence of bile pigment and decreased urobilinogen. Urobilinogen reappears with the clearing of the jaundice. The urine may occasionally contain protein, due to minimal renal involvement. A liver biopsy done at this stage would show generalized changes throughout the hepatic lobule, but usually such procedures are not necessary unless there is diagnostic difficulty. The prothrombin time may be lengthened and there may be a poor response to the injection of vitamin K, suggesting a liver cell lesion. The differential diagnosis of the classical case includes hepatitis due to drugs and poisons, viral hepatitis associated with glandular fever, acute alcoholic hepatitis and the virus hepatitis associated with cytomegalic virus disease and Coxsackie virus infection. The most important differential diagnosis is between this disease and drug jaundice.

Treatment

The patient is confined to bed while he is feeling unwell and certainly if there is fever and icterus is present. No specific treatment is required in the average case apart from bed rest, which should be continued until the patient's jaundice has faded and the biochemical tests are approaching normal. The diet should be low in fat, not because this has any remarkable medicinal properties, but simply because the patient feels nauseated by fatty foods and an attempt to maintain nutrition is most important at this stage. Plenty of glucose drinks and a high protein diet are also useful ways of ensuring the rapid return of liver function to normal. Serious signs and symptoms include jaundice which lasts for more than a month, persistent vomiting and the appearance of the signs of chronic liver disease including persistent splenomegaly, ascites and the cutaneous signs of liver disease such as spider naevi. In patients with prolonged jaundice there is certainly a place for corticosteroid therapy. This produces a reduction in the serum bilirubin and an improvement in some of the other liver function tests, notably the transaminases and B.S.P. excretion. The patient begins to feel better and the appetite improves. Prednisone, 40 mg. a day, should be employed for 7–10 days and, providing the icterus has started to fade, the dose may then be cut down slowly to a maintenance one of 5 mg. three times a day. This should usually be kept on for a month or so after the jaundice has disappeared. It should be noted, however, that corticosteroid therapy is not indicated in the average case. The disease is only infectious in the pre-icteric and early icteric phase, therefore it is unlikely that the icteric patient is infectious to those who are involved in his nursing care. A point of some importance is that the disease can be transmitted from blood taken for biochemical investigation if the needle used happens to prick the skin of persons taking blood samples. In such cases prophylaxis with gamma globulin should be employed and this is also wise in those at risk with chronic intercurrent disease and perhaps in young children and pregnant women. A dose of gamma globulin of 0·1 ml. per kg. body weight will give protection against viral hepatitis for about 4 months providing that the patient is not already incubating the disease. It is of no use in the treatment of the established disease and will in many cases only modify hepatitis rather than prevent its appearance. It could, too, be a double edged weapon; the patient with mild hepatitis without jaundice or symptoms may in fact be rather more of a risk to his colleagues than the classical case. However, those at risk need gamma globulin. There should be no difficulty in differentiating acute infective hepatitis of the classical type from obstructive jaundice, providing that a complete history, physical examination and all the special investigations are considered carefully.

Complications

The complications of this disorder are shown in the accompanying figure [FIG. 36]. These will be briefly described.

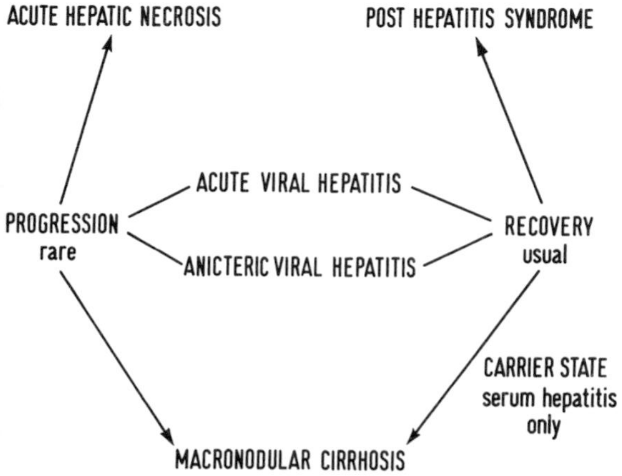

FIG. 36. The course of viral hepatitis.

Obstructive Hepatitis. This used to be called 'cholangiolitic hepatitis' and its precise anatomical cause is unknown. Suffice it to say that in some patients viral hepatitis produces a predominantly obstructive picture with prolonged jaundice, itching and liver function tests showing an obstructive profile. Further, on liver biopsy the signs of liver cell damage may be minimal and there may instead be marked cholestasis. These cases, in particular, are liable to be confused with surgical obstructive jaundice. For this reason it is well worthwhile considering the use of a corticosteroid test; this involves the oral administration of prednisone or some other corticosteroid for 4–5 days and noting the amount by which the serum bilirubin falls. A significant fall, that is greater than about 8 per cent. per day, signifies that obstruction is not likely to be due to a surgical, i.e. extrahepatic lesion. There are, however, exceptions to this. The treatment of obstructive hepatitis is with corticosteroid drugs usually continued for 4–8 weeks. The long-term prognosis is good.

Acute Hepatic Necrosis. This is a very serious complication of acute infective hepatitis and carries a mortality of 80 per cent. or more. In this process the liver is completely destroyed and the patient passes rapidly into hepatic failure. Symptoms suggestive of this complication include persisting deep jaundice, vomiting, and anorexia. The onset may be catastrophic at the beginning of acute infective hepatitis or it may occur after the patient has apparently started to recover. If the patient leaves his bed too early in an ordinary attack of hepatitis it is possible that this complication can be precipitated. He lapses into coma with bleeding from the gums and into the skin, ascites and deepening jaundice. The liver size diminishes. The white blood count may show a polymorphonuclear leucocytosis instead of the classical leucopenia seen in the classical form of the disease. Treatment is unsatisfactory and usually consists of giving neomycin by mouth, administration of large amounts of glucose and potassium orally, and the use, at least in some centres, of massive doses of corticosteroids. Recently trials have been made of exchange blood transfusion and hepatic perfusion through the liver of a donor animal such as a pig. The results on the whole have been disappointing and though some startling recoveries have occurred these have usually turned out to be temporary.

Hepatic Cirrhosis. The persistence of viral hepatitis into a chronic phase is rare, although it is likely that a certain percentage of patients who have had hepatitis may develop a macronodular cirrhosis. The numbers are few, but well documented cases of this progression are present in the literature. The transformation is suggested when the patient develops continuing jaundice, fever, splenomegaly and cutaneous signs of chronic liver disease. However, the change is usually a very insidious one and the patient seems to be free of signs and symptoms often for many years following the viral infection. The precise way in which cirrhosis develops is unknown. Recently agreement has been reached concerning the terminology of the disorders associated with either clinical or biochemical progression following infective hepatitis. Chronic active (aggressive) hepatitis [see p. 639] is synonymous with progression to multilobular cirrhosis, whilst a further type of progressive lesion, chronic persistent hepatitis, is not a forerunner of cirrhosis, and although patients may complain of ill health and the serum biochemistry may be abnormal, histological changes are limited to the portal tracts and basic hepatic architecture is not disrupted.

Aplastic Anaemia. There have been recorded recently several cases of acute aplastic anaemia occurring after acute viral hepatitis. The cause for this is unknown, but presumably the virus damages the bone marrow and this complication, though rare, is often fatal [see Section 13]. Some observers have also suggested that there is a relationship between Down's syndrome and infective hepatitis and there may be an increased incidence of foetal abnormalities in patients who are pregnant when they sustain infection with this virus. Certainly, in pregnant women the disease is often very severe, particularly is this so in tropical countries.

Post-hepatitis Syndrome. Patients who have had infective hepatitis are often unwell for some weeks after the disease has apparently disappeared, at least as judged by the liver function tests. The precise cause of the symptoms is unknown, but there is no doubt that many patients complain of severe degrees of tiredness, nausea and dyspepsia which they did not have before the illness. Many of these symptoms may be psychogenic, but it would be unwise to label them all as such and wiser to appreciate that many patients with this disease need a long period of convalescence before they are entirely fit to return to their work. It is also conventional to suggest that the patient abstains from alcohol for some months. This is based on the fact that some degree of relapse can occur if alcohol is taken. It is likely that the risk is very much over-emphasized but this seems reasonable advice, at least for the first 3 months of the convalescent period.

SERUM HEPATITIS

This disease is also an acute viral infection of the liver and it is believed by most people that the virus is different from that which causes infective hepatitis. The differences between the diseases are best summarized in the following way:

1. The incubation period of serum hepatitis is much longer than that of infective hepatitis. It is of the order of 6 weeks to 6 months.

2. The disease is *not transmitted* by the faecal-oral route (though this view has been challenged in the Willowbank study) and contaminated blood or blood products carry the infective agent. It is, therefore, a risk for any patient in the 'hospital environment', i.e. who is receiving blood or certain blood products or who has had injections with contaminated needles or who has undergone procedures such as tattooing or dental extraction.

3. The disease sometimes has a different *clinical picture* but this is difficult to differentiate clearly from infective hepatitis. Certainly the mortality is much higher and figures of the order of 12–20 per cent. have been quoted, which is in striking contrast to the very low mortality of infective hepatitis. The prognosis is bad, particularly when there is severe intercurrent illness, such as cancer.

4. *Protection* from the disease with gamma globulin is probably not as effectively obtained as in infective hepatitis.

5. The virus of serum hepatitis may remain in the blood stream of some patients for many years, and therefore they may be *potential carriers* of the disease. Blood and blood products from such people would therefore be likely to produce the disease in those patients who were treated with them. In contrast the virus is not present in the faeces of patients with serum hepatitis as it is in infective hepatitis. In recent years, it has been suggested that the difference between infective hepatitis and serum hepatitis is due to the differences in the route of inoculation of the same virus, and they are not different diseases due to different viruses. The answer to this important problem will only be solved when the virus can be isolated and viral antibody neutralization tests performed.

Serum hepatitis is becoming a more important disease as larger volumes of blood are being used for techniques such as open heart surgery and renal dialysis, and blood products such as fibrinogen are employed. In countries where financial reward is offered to blood donors there is a fairly high risk of contaminated blood being given to patients. In this country the risk is negligible but a recent survey in the United States estimated that one patient in 100 undergoing an average transfusion of 3 units of blood would develop serum hepatitis, and figures from Japan are even higher than this. The risks from fibrinogen, antihaemophilic globulin and pooled plasma are of particular importance, the only fractions of blood which are safe are albumin, plasminogen and gamma globulin. The detection of HAA is of great importance, and blood for transfusion is now examined in this way.

REFERENCES

Viral Hepatitis

GRADY, G. F., CHALMERS, T. C., and the BOSTON INTER-HOSPITAL LIVER GROUP (1965) Viral hepatitis in a group of Boston hospitals, *New Engl. J. Med.*, **272,** 657.

HAVENS, W. P. (1962) Viral hepatitis. Clinical patterns and diagnosis, *Amer. J. Med.*, **32,** 665.

Obstructive Hepatitis

DUBIN, I. N., SULLIVAN, B. H., LE GOLVAN, P. C., and MURPHY, L. C. (1960) The cholestatic form of viral hepatitis, *Amer. J. Med.*, **29,** 55.

Serum Hepatitis

MOSLEY, J. W. (1966) Transfusion-associated viral hepatitis, *Anaesthesia*, **27,** 409.

Australia Antigen and Hepatitis

SHULMAN, N. R. (1970) Hepatitis associated antigen, *Amer. J. Med.*, **49,** 669.

DRUG HEPATITIS

Aetiology

Various drugs and poisons attack the liver and produce varying degrees of damage. The important types of reaction that are seen are classified as follows:

1. Damage mainly confined to the intrahepatic biliary apparatus.
   (i) Cholestasis.
   (ii) Cholangiolitis.

2. Damage to the liver cell, either necrosis or fatty change.
   (i) Part of a general hypersensitivity reaction.
   (ii) Confined to the liver.

3. Damage to the centrilobular hepatic veins with venous obstruction.

Pathology and Clinical Picture

Drugs Causing Biliary Obstruction. The groups of drugs which cause biliary obstruction are easily divisible into two because of the different types of reaction that these two main groups produce. Both will produce the clinical picture of obstructive jaundice. The histological features of the two lesions, however, are different. *Cholestasis* is associated with simple bile plugging, that is deposits of bile are seen in the centrilobular area and it is thought that this type of reaction involves a lesion in and around the biliary canaliculi. There is no inflammatory damage and thus no infiltrate in the portal zones. The liver returns to normal if the causative drug is withdrawn. The drugs producing this type of lesion include methyltestosterone and other similar testosterones and nortestosterones, particularly where there is substitution in the 17-alkyl position in the steroid ring. The lesion is produced in a high percentage of patients on these drugs, the severity being proportional to the duration and dose used, so that some may develop icterus and other patients will show abnormalities suggesting obstruction with a raised serum alkaline phosphatase and abnormalities of B.S.P. excretion. The jaundice produced by the contraceptive pill is an example of this type of reaction, at least in most of the cases that have been described. The lesion due to these latter agents is selective in its frequency, being rare in this country and commonest in Scandinavia and South America.

In *cholangiolitis* the hepatic lesion is different. There is a portal cell infiltrate, cholestasis, and evidence of scattered liver cell destruction. The type of drug which produces this reaction is variable. The phenothiazines, particularly chlorpromazine, certain antidiabetic drugs such as chlorpropamide, anticoagulant drugs such as phenindione and antidepressive drugs such as amitriptyline are examples of this group. The picture is one of obstructive jaundice but with the exception that the serum transaminases may be more raised than with cholestasis. The patient usually develops symptoms 10 days to 3 weeks after taking the drug and the illness gradually disappears after the drug is withdrawn. Occasionally the patient may be jaundiced for many months and develops a syndrome very similar to that of primary biliary cirrhosis. There is thought to be a hypersensitivity factor in the production of this type of lesion for only a small percentage of patients treated with these drugs in fact sustain liver damage and in some the blood may show an eosinophilia and eosiniphils may be prominent in the portal cell infiltrate. This type of drug lesion does not respond to corticosteroids and there is little that can be done except to make sure that the offending drug is withdrawn, though recovery has been noted even when it is continued.

Liver Cell Damage. Drugs causing liver cell damage are some ten times as frequent as those that cause damage to the biliary system. Two types of pattern are seen:

Part of a General Hypersensitivity Reaction. This type of lesion is fortunately rare. It is seen with a wide variety of commonly used drugs such as sulphonamides, butazolidine, anti-epileptic drugs, and gold. The reaction is a total hypersensitivity one and the liver damage produced is a mere incident in the picture. Evidence of pulmonary damage with asthma and pulmonary infiltration, alimentary damage with stomatitis, intestinal ulceration, renal damage with oliguric renal failure, albuminuria and skin damage with various types of dermatitis are seen with accompanying jaundice due to liver cell involvement. The mortality from this type of reaction is high.

Hepatitis-like Injury. The important drugs which cause this type of lesion are the monoamine oxidase inhibitors (hydrazine type), the drugs used for the treatment of tuberculosis, i.e. para-aminosalicylic acid and isonicotinic acid, and the anaesthetic agent halothane. The clinical picture is of jaundice with the symptoms of hepatitis following 1–3 weeks after the use of these agents. There are no differences between the clinical picture and that of acute infective hepatitis though the disease is usually much more severe and the mortality is higher. The patients with this type of lesion are thought to have some abnormal susceptibility to the drug and the lesion is rare. In a recent survey of halothane jaundice only a small percentage of patients were thought to have had jaundice as a result of exposure to this anaesthetic. Halothane does not usually cause liver damage on its first administration, but patients who have multiple operations with several exposures to this agent are particularly at risk. The initial sign is pyrexia and abnormalities of liver function tests after an operation for which halothane has been used. This is a warning that if the agent is used again severe hepatic damage with acute hepatic necrosis may occur.

Hepatic Poisons. Exposure is rare, but known poisons are carbon tetrachloride, the toxins of various mushrooms such as *Amanita phalloides* and various hydrocarbons which are used in industry. These drugs are general cell poisons and apart from producing liver damage they usually produce renal and brain damage as well. The characteristic histological finding is an acute fatty infiltration of the organs. Tetracycline may act as a cellular poison in some patients, and an acute fatal fatty infiltration of the liver due to high dosage of this drug in pregnancy is recorded. Damage in the liver in these circumstances seems to be due to an action of the poison on the endoplasmic reticulum. Carbon tetrachloride poisoning is usually seen in patients who have been dry-cleaning clothes in improperly ventilated rooms; it occasionally results from the letting off of fire extinguishers or from oral consumption of the material usually in someone with acute alcoholic intoxication. The mortality in these cases is high.

Hepatic Venous Obstruction. There are certain substances, e.g. urethane, which are known to cause an endophlebitis of the radicles of the hepatic vein and hence produce hepatomegaly and changes similar to those of the Budd-Chiari syndrome.

REFERENCES

Cook, G. C., and Sherlock, S. (1965) Jaundice and its relation to the therapeutic agents, *Lancet*, i, 175.

National Halothane Study. Summary (1966) *J. Amer. med. Ass.*, **197**, 775.

Popper, H., Rubin, E., Gardiol, D., Schaffner, F., and Paranetto, F. (1965) Drug induced liver disease, *Arch. intern. Med.*, **115**, 128.

Sherlock, S. (1966) Prediction of hepatotoxicity due to therapeutic agents in man, *Medicine* (*Baltimore*), **45**, 453.

CIRRHOSIS OF THE LIVER

Definition

Cirrhosis of the liver is a chronic disorder of varying aetiology where the liver shows cellular damage, fibrosis and the formation of regeneration nodules. The disease has been variously classified, but an acceptable up-to-date classification is as follows:

Hepatic cirrhosis may be micronodular, macronodular, or mixed.

Pathology

Micronodular Cirrhosis. In this type of cirrhosis the regeneration nodules formed following hepatic injury are small. They are 3–4 mm. in diameter and the liver is often large and uniformly granular. This type of cirrhosis was previously called portal, septal or Laennec's cirrhosis. It is often associated with alcoholism.

Macronodular Cirrhosis. Macronodular cirrhosis is associated with large regeneration nodules one to several cm. in diameter. In general the cause is unknown, though some cases may follow hepatitis. The liver is coarsely nodular and may be larger or, more characteristically, smaller than usual.

Mixed Cirrhosis. The regeneration nodules are of varying size.

The Complications of Cirrhosis

The following complications may result from the cirrhotic process in the liver:

Portal Hypertension. This results from a blockage of hepatic venous outflow from the hepatic lobules due to the pressure of enlarging regeneration nodules. To some degree the portal hypertension is also explained by the increased 'arterialization' of the hepatic sinusoids due to the increased proportion of blood that the hepatic artery provides for the cirrhotic liver. The results of portal hypertension are the opening up of communications between the portal and systemic circulation and particularly the enlargement of peri-umbilical veins and veins in the mucosa of the lower oesophagus and in the fundus of the stomach, *which can rupture and produce severe bleeding*. The other complication of portal hypertension is that it tends to localize fluid retention so that ascites is a feature of cirrhosis rather than ankle oedema.

Liver Cell Failure. Failure of liver cell function due to the liver cell disease results in hypoalbuminaemia and fluid retention. It is also associated with icterus in many patients.

Portosystemic Encephalopathy. Shunting of some of the breakdown products of protein digestion from the portal circulation to the systemic, results in an intoxication of the brain with the presence of confusion and drowsiness leading to coma. Certain other neurological syndromes may also result from this intoxication.

Metabolic Consequences. The breakdown of certain hormones including hydrocortisone and oestrogens may be delayed in patients with liver cell disease. In the case of the latter this may result in the appearance of changes in the skin which are thought to depend on the vasodilator properties of excess circulating oestrogens and possibly other substances. These changes include spider naevi, which are vascular abnormalities produced by arteriolar dilatation [FIG. 37]. These are usually seen on the skin of the neck, arms and trunk, the lesion consists of a central raised red spot, the dilated arteriole, and a leash of vessels running from it. Though a few spiders may be found in normal subjects the presence of large numbers, particularly with changing distribution of the lesions, is suggestive of hepatic disease. Other abnormalities include an erythema of the palms and soles of the feet, due to a dilatation of skin blood vessels. Clubbing may also be found and, in the male subject with cirrhosis, gynaecomastia and atrophy of the testes may also result from this abnormality of metabolism. Certain changes in the nails, which probably do not depend on oestrogen levels, include opacification of the nail bed, giving rise to 'white' nails or leuconychia; in patients with con-

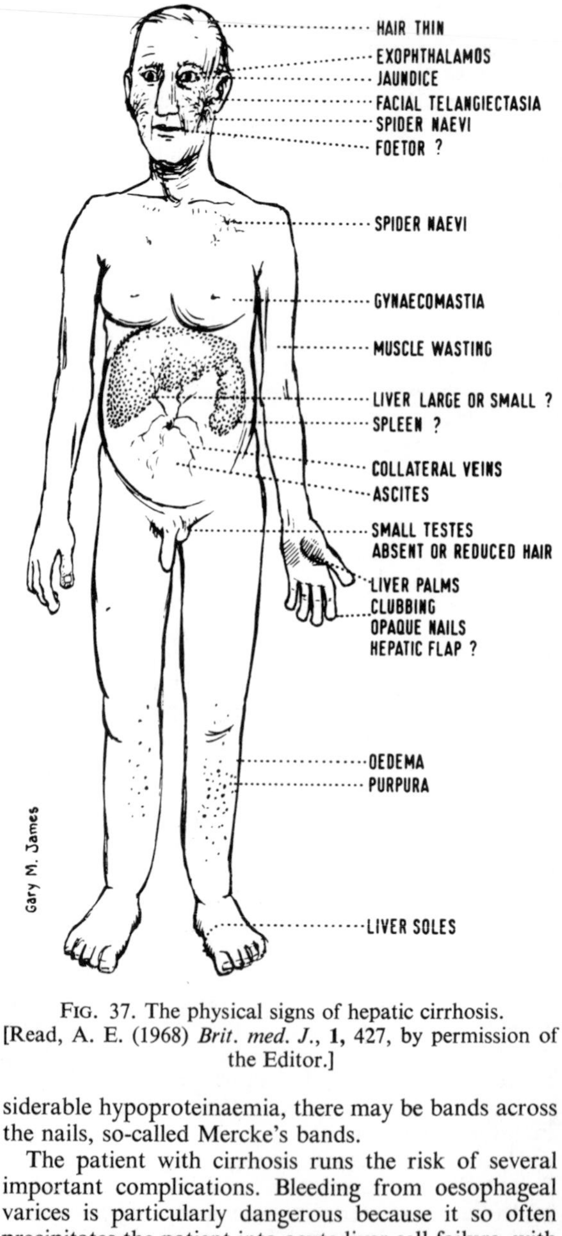

FIG. 37. The physical signs of hepatic cirrhosis. [Read, A. E. (1968) *Brit. med. J.*, **1**, 427, by permission of the Editor.]

siderable hypoproteinaemia, there may be bands across the nails, so-called Mercke's bands.

The patient with cirrhosis runs the risk of several important complications. Bleeding from oesophageal varices is particularly dangerous because it so often precipitates the patient into acute liver cell failure, with deepening jaundice, ascites and hepatic coma. This may be an extremely difficult situation to treat as the hypotension associated with the alimentary bleeding produces an increasing embarrassment to the already damaged liver.

Malignant Change ('Hepatoma'). In perhaps up to one fifth of patients with hepatic cirrhosis, the cellular regenerative activity in hepatic nodules becomes autonomous. One or several foci of neoplasia develop and a gradual deterioration of the patient's health leads to death [see p. 650]. The major types of cirrhosis will now be described, and the clinical features, pathology and treatment of these reviewed.

TYPES OF CIRRHOSIS

CRYPTOGENIC CIRRHOSIS

Aetiology

This is a disease of unknown cause in which the patient develops a macronodular cirrhosis. The disease is fairly common in this country where it principally effects middle-aged and elderly women. In about 30 per cent. of these patients there is a previous history of viral hepatitis and it is thought by many that the disease represents the continuing damage of the hepatitis virus in the liver.

Clinical Features

The disease may be discovered by accident or sometimes by the abnormalities it produces in blood tests, perhaps done for some other problem. The physical signs include the cutaneous abnormalities associated with chronic liver disease, namely spider naevi, palmar erythema and clubbing. The patient may also show hepatosplenomegaly. The liver may, on the other hand, be reduced in size. There may be ascites and ankle oedema. The patient is not markedly icteric. On some occasions the patient presents because of the onset of one of the complications of cirrhosis and particularly is this so of bleeding oesophageal varices, of ascites and of portosystemic encephalopathy.

Diagnosis

Laboratory investigation shows an abnormal blood count with a mild normochromic anaemia, a reduced total white count and thrombocytopenia. These latter are collectively the signs of 'hypersplenism'. The liver function tests usually show a normal or near normal serum bilirubin, a low serum albumin and raised globulins and usually some elevation of the alkaline phosphatase and transaminases. A barium meal may show the presence of varices and on biopsy with a needle the liver shows the characteristics of a macronodular cirrhosis with coarse bands of fibrous tissue separating large regeneration nodules and accompanying this there is an increased infiltration of cells in the portal triads. Important differential diagnoses are hepatomegaly due to secondary neoplasm, hepatic venous obstruction and fatty infiltration.

Treatment

No treatment is required or is effective in this disease but complications, such as bleeding from varices, ascites and hepatic encephalopathy are, however, treated in the usual way [see p. 643]. There is a 50 per cent. 2-year mortality once these complications have occurred.

CHRONIC ACTIVE HEPATITIS (LUPOID HEPATITIS, JUVENILE CIRRHOSIS)

Aetiology

This is a disease of unknown aetiology, though many people feel that it represents continuing and aggressive activity by the hepatitis virus and that autoimmune damage is a factor in its progression.

Clinical Picture

The patient is usually young and is more commonly female than male. The striking symptoms include icterus, and in female patients, amenorrhoea. On examination apart from scleral icterus there is usually florid evidence of chronic liver disease, spider naevi and palmar erythema. The spleen is often considerably enlarged, as is the liver. The patient's general health seems well maintained despite the obvious and gross evidence of liver cell disorder. Another interesting factor is that the disease is a multi-organ one and symptoms and signs of disease outside the liver are often found. These include:

1. Pleurisy and pneumonia, with pulmonary infiltration and in some cases interstitial fibrosis of the lungs.
2. Endocrine disturbances such as diabetes mellitus, myxoedema, and thyrotoxicosis.
3. Neurological disorders including depression, psychosis and in some patients evidence of pyramidal tract disease.
4. Renal involvement with hypertension, the syndrome of renal tubular acidosis, and glomerular nephritis.
5. Skin disorders. These include the rash of chronic or disseminated lupus as well as other various types of eruption.
6. Ulcerative colitis. This may in some cases precede the onset of the hepatic illness.
7. Arthritis; pulmonary hypertension.

Though all of the complications of cirrhosis may be seen in this disease they tend to occur late in the disorder and the clinical picture is overshadowed by the evidence of liver cell disorder. Jaundice in particular is almost universal.

Diagnosis

Liver function tests show, apart from a raised serum bilirubin, considerably elevated transaminases, and very high levels of beta and particularly gamma globulin, with some depression of the serum albumin level. Flocculation tests where they are used are markedly positive. The peripheral blood shows evidence of anaemia, the signs of hypersplenism and in a certain percentage of cases L.E. cells are found. Other abnormalities include a positive test for rheumatoid factor, a false positive W.R. and various other immunological abnormalities such as positive A.N.F. and smooth muscle antibody tests. The liver biopsy is helpful in diagnosis as not only is there an established cirrhosis in some cases but there is also considerable evidence of liver cell damage and, in particular, a heavy portal cell infiltrate rich in plasma cells and lymphocytes.

Treatment

The disease is usually treated with corticosteroid

drugs. This causes a fall in the serum bilirubin level and improvement in other liver function tests, together with a disappearance of icterus and a return of well-being on the part of the patient. If there are associated disorders such as arthritis, ulcerative colitis and skin rashes these are usually controlled as well. Corticosteroid drugs in patients with liver disease, however, are notorious for the fact that they readily produce complications. This is because of the slow breakdown of corticosteroids in liver disease so that even a relatively small dose of corticosteroid drugs is associated with fairly marked signs of corticosterone overdose. The side-effects therefore are often alarming and there is mooning of the face, acneiform rashes and a considerable danger of diabetes and systemic infections. Corticosteroid drugs such as prednisone, 30 mg. daily reducing to a maintenance dose of 5 mg. 2 or 3 times daily, is the sheet anchor of treatment and this is usually continued for about a year. The drugs are then stopped and only recommenced again if there is a return of activity of the liver cell lesion, as manifest by return of jaundice, elevation of the transaminases or a return of ill health on the part of the patient. Another recent approach has been the use of immunosuppressive therapy with azathioprine. This is useful where the disease seems to be resistant to corticosteroid drugs or where the side-effects of corticosteroids are so gross that they cannot be tolerated by the patient. A further indication is the presence of complications such as a haemolytic anaemia with a positive Coombs test.

Prognosis

The general prognosis in this disease for life is of the order of 4 years though liver cell dysfunction may disappear and the patient be left with a fully developed macronodular cirrhosis. At this stage of course the patient becomes susceptible to all the normal complications of cirrhosis such as bleeding varices, ascites and hepatic encephalopathy, but may survive 10–20 years.

PRIMARY BILIARY CIRRHOSIS (CHRONIC NON-SUPPURATIVE DESTRUCTIVE CHOLANGITIS)

Aetiology

This is a micronodular cirrhosis based on chronic biliary obstruction, the obstruction being at the level to the biliary ductules. The initial lesion is thought to be an immunological damage to these structures.

Clinical Picture

The disease is commonest in middle-aged and elderly women. It commences insidiously and the first symptoms noted are usually those of pruritus and malaise. At this time the patient is not usually icteric but on physical examination hepatosplenomegaly may be found. With progression of the disease obstructive jaundice becomes obvious but it is only of moderate depth. There is chronic pruritus, pale stools and dark urine, the liver is considerably enlarged and so is the spleen. Xanthomatous lesions may be seen on the eyelids, in skin creases and over pressure points. The patient is also pigmented and in these circumstances the jaundice often looks deeper than it actually is. Clubbing of the fingers is often found and the complications of obstructive jaundice of some duration may be seen. These include bone pain due to osteomalacia, a haemorrhagic tendency with epistaxis and skin bruising and in some patients there is a tendency for peptic ulceration to develop.

Diagnosis

Liver function tests show the presence of obstructive jaundice with a raised serum bilirubin, considerably raised serum alkaline phosphatase and an increase in the beta and gamma globulins. The blood lipids are raised, particularly the serum cholesterol which is usually over 400 mg. per 100 ml. With this evidence of obstructive jaundice there is also some evidence of liver cell damage and this is shown by the raised transaminases and the low serum albumin. Liver biopsy in the early stages shows granuloma formation around bile ductules and little evidence of either cirrhosis or cholestasis, but as the disease progresses both of these features may be seen. An important diagnostic test is the detection of mitochondrial antibodies in the patient's serum. The antibodies are demonstrated by a fluorescent technique using rat or other animal tissue. The mitochondrial antibody test, though positive in some other liver diseases is always negative in patients with extrahepatic biliary obstruction, so that it is a useful differentiating test. Barium X-rays show a malabsorption pattern and possibly oesophageal varices.

Treatment

There is no curative treatment for this disease. Patients who are suspected of having it should be thoroughly investigated and, in particular extrahepatic biliary obstruction must be excluded. For this purpose laparotomy is often required and operative cholangiography is essential. Bone disease must be prevented by the administration of regular monthly injections of vitamin D (100,000 Units by intramuscular injection) and by the giving of calcium supplements. Vitamin K is needed to prevent a bleeding tendency. The bile salt chelating agent cholestyramine is useful in preventing one of the most troublesome complications of this disorder, namely severe pruritus. Careful attention to make-up and the judicious application of cosmetics is often useful in disguising the icterus and pigmentation. Corticosteroids are valueless in this disease, not only do they *not* decrease the jaundice, but they may aggravate ulcer dyspepsia and thin already abnormal bones. A more recent drug to be used in this condition is azathioprine. The use of this drug is based on the theory that the initial damaging lesion is an immunological one and that azathioprine may be effective in arresting the activity of the harmful lymphocytic infiltration around the biliary ductules. This treatment has its own hazards and is only likely to be of any use in early cases prior to the onset of a true cirrhosis. The complications of ascites, encephalopathy and bleeding from oesophageal varices are dealt with in the usual way, but it should be pointed out that these features appear late in the disease, and their presence therefore is of grave significance.

Prognosis

The mean survival with this disease is about 5 years.

HAEMOCHROMATOSIS (BRONZED DIABETES)

Aetiology

This is a disease which appears in two main forms. The primary variety is probably associated with a congenital, and sometimes familial, increase of iron absorption. The secondary form occurs as a complication of a pre-existing alcoholic cirrhosis; in patients with thalassaemia and chronic hypoplastic anaemia treated by repeated blood transfusions in which large amounts of iron are deposited in the tissues; and it is seen in patients with sideroblastic anaemia [see Section 13]. On the whole the primary form is the most severe and in these patients the congenital abnormality of iron absorption results in widespread deposition of iron with resultant secondary damage in organs such as the liver, pancreas and testes. It is the only variety discussed in detail here.

Clinical Picture

The primary form develops insidiously. The patient is almost invariably male and has few of the features of chronic liver cell disease. He usually complains of general weakness, depression and lassitude, and accompanying this there is often upper abdominal discomfort and in some patients frank attacks of severe abdominal pain. The patient rapidly loses sexual drive and strength and may have the symptoms of diabetes. Examination at this stage reveals a slate-grey pigmentation of the skin with a large liver and sometimes splenic enlargement. The testes are small and there is atrophy of the axillary and pubic hair. The urine may contain sugar and on occasions the patient may even present in diabetic coma. Another important feature of the disease is that there is a tendency for cardiac complications to arise as a result of the infiltration of cardiac muscle by iron deposits. Cardiac failure, therefore, and disorders of cardiac rhythm are seen fairly commonly. Two other interesting features of the disease have been re-described recently. Firstly, there may be a troublesome arthritis which affects both the small joints of the hands and the larger joint such as the knee and wrist. Evidence of calcification of cartilage and of bone erosion may be seen on the X-ray. One other complication is of diagnostic importance. Attacks of abdominal pain with peritonism, shock and collapse are sometimes seen. The nature of this abnormality is unknown, but vasodilator material, perhaps allied to ferritin, may be released from the liver.

Diagnosis

Investigation in the early stages may show little abnormality of the liver function tests and the major diagnostic feature is the finding of deposits of iron in the tissues, but a high serum iron and fully saturated iron binding capacity are helpful. Iron can be found either in the liver after liver biopsy, in the skin following a skin biopsy, or in appropriate tissue from other organs such as the bone marrow. Deposits of haemosiderin are sometimes found in the urine. An ECG may show evidence of cardiac arrhythmia and T wave inversion, whilst a glucose tolerance test will either show evidence of abnormal glucose tolerance or may accompany frank glycosuria. Estimation of chelatable iron after desferrioxamine may be a valuable way of making the diagnosis and following the treatment.

Complications

An important complication of this disease is a hepatoma arising in the cirrhotic liver. Features of this include right upper abdominal pain and the appearance of one or several masses in the liver. The patient's general condition deteriorates and there is loss of weight and strength.

Treatment

Treatment of this disease is important for the following reasons. The successful removal of iron will result in a general improvement in well-being and strength; an improvement in diabetes, and an improvement in cardiac function. Treatment will not result in any significant alteration of the cirrhotic process in the liver, and certainly does not do away with the risk that is always present of hepatoma formation. As the patient with primary haemochromatosis has about ten times the normal amount of iron in the tissues, i.e. approximately 50 g. instead of 5, then venesection therapy to be successful must be continued for many months. A venesection of one pint per week for the first 6 months and then per fortnight for the next 2 years with frequent determination of the haemoglobin and serum iron are essential. This treatment is vigorous and a full explanation of its nature must be given to the patient. Usually the improvement in general well-being is enough to stimulate the patient to attend for further therapy, but doses of intramuscular testosterone propionate may act as a further stimulus if they are given at the same time. The treatment of diabetes is, of course, also essential and it is important having found one member of a family with primary haemochromatosis, to follow the other relatives in the family to make sure that they are not sufferers from this disease as well. In this case prophylactic treatment would be important. The use of oral iron chelating compounds such as desferrioxamine has added little to the treatment of this disease.

KINNIER WILSON'S DISEASE (HEPATOLENTICULAR DEGENERATION)

Aetiology

This is a rare congenital disorder of copper metabolism inherited as an autosomal recessive. The abnormality seems to consist of a deficiency of the serum copper-carrying protein caeruloplasmin. This means that the tissues become rapidly saturated with copper which is injurious to them. The most important tissues involved are the brain, liver and kidney.

Clinical Picture

The condition is first noted in childhood and the early symptoms are either neurological or hepatic but most patients show features of both. The neurological symptoms consist of the appearance of tremor and athetosis and other features of basal ganglion involvement. The speech may be slurred, the facies vacant and there may be fluctuating rigidity of the limbs. In the hepatic form of the disease the patient may present with jaundice and with bleeding from oesophageal varices, associated with portal hypertension. One other important cause of jaundice has been described recently and this is an acute haemolytic anaemia probably due to release of tissue copper into the blood stream. The classical physical signs includes the following:

A ring of copper deposited inside the corneo-sclerotic junction is called a *Kayser-Fleischer* ring. It is greenish-brown in colour and is best seen with transverse illumination or with a slit lamp. The liver is enlarged and there may be splenomegaly.

Diagnosis

The liver function tests may show evidence of liver cell disease and on liver biopsy increased amounts of copper can be found providing that the specific stain, 1 per cent. rubeanic acid, is used. The urine contains high levels of copper. The normal urinary excretion of copper is less than 100 μg. per day and in Wilson's disease this is increased up to twelve times. The most critical test is the estimation of the copper-carrying protein itself, caeruloplasmin; this is an alpha-2 globulin and its concentration in Wilson's disease is much decreased. It is estimated by a technique which measures its oxidase activity, and so copper oxidase activity is synonymous with caeruloplasmin. In patients with severe liver disease not due to Wilson's disease, or in malabsorption or nephrotic syndrome, this protein may on occasion be found in very low concentrations. Other tests of copper metabolism are then required. The urine may contain abnormal amounts of glucose, Phosphate and amino acids due to tubular damage from the copper deposition. It is most important that this disease is excluded in all young people with cirrhosis, particularly when there are bizzare features and this should include a clinical search for the Kayser-Fleischer ring as well as estimations of urine copper and serum caeruloplasmin.

Treatment

Though this disease is rare it is treatable and early diagnosis is important. The treatment these days is with penicillamine. This removes copper from the tissues, a fact which can be verified by estimating the copper excretion in the urine while the patient is on treatment. There are certain side-effects to this drug, such as drug rashes and nephrosis, which is given in a dose of 300 mg. of D penicillamine four times daily. The maximal improvement is seen in the central nervous system where speech and tremor may be so much improved that the patient is able to return to work or school. Treatment continues permanently. Osteomalacia is occasionally found with this disease and may require treatment with vitamin D.

Prognosis

Prognosis from the hepatic point is less favourable as most patients die in liver failure or from bleeding varices, which have precipitated liver failure. Discovery of a case of Wilson's disease should lead one to search for other patients with the disease in the family. Disease may occur in homozygous or heterozygous forms and it is only the first which needs treatment. Some help can be obtained from estimating the caeruloplasmin level, but more by doing a liver biopsy, noting any histological change and measuring liver copper. Even before there are clinical signs of the disease the patient with the latent homozygous condition shows abnormal ballooning of liver cells with fatty change, and a concentration of copper greater than 25 mg. per 100 g. dry weight. Such patients should commence immediate treatment with penicillamine however normal they may appear clinically. [See Section 15.]

ALCOHOLIC CIRRHOSIS

Aetiology

Alcoholic cirrhosis is due to the harmful effects of alcohol on the liver. Though some liver damage is guaranteed if the patient drinks enough, the actual factors which produce a true cirrhosis are unknown, and in fact only a tenth or so of heavy drinkers develop this change.

Clinical Picture

The patient is usually male and there may or may not be a history of a heavy alcohol intake either from the patient or from his relatives. In the early stages there may be no clinical symptoms apart from morning nausea, dyspepsia due to gastritis and the presence of an enlarged, firm liver. In some patients episodes of acute liver cell jaundice are seen which follow heavy bouts of drinking. These are related to acute necrosis of liver cells and are often accompanied by fever and general malaise (alcoholic hepatitis). With progression to cirrhosis the cutaneous signs of liver disease such as spider naevi, may develop; the patient may complain of increasing abdominal girth due to ascites or may present with bleeding from oesophageal varices or from an alcoholic gastritis. Other important symptoms are related to the complications, and include mental deterioration, paralysis and paraesthesiae due to peripheral neuropathy. Other changes include a high incidence of Dupuytren's contractures, and of enlarged parotid glands. Gynaecomastia is a not infrequent finding. Patients with this disease may also develop some of the features of haemochromatosis whilst others may be admitted in coma following acute alcoholism and with the features of severe malnutrition, and Wernicke's encephalopathy.

Diagnosis

The diagnosis of this disease is suggested by the history and by the physical signs of hepatic enlargement in a patient with a history of high alcoholic intake. Helpful diagnostic aids include liver function tests which usually show features of liver cell disease, at least in those patients who are progressing to cirrhosis. A blood count shows the presence of anaemia which is sometimes partly haemolytic in type. This feature combined with a raised serum cholesterol and triglyceride level is known as Zieve's syndrome and is only found in alcoholism. The white blood count is raised in patients with acute alcoholic hepatitis and a barium meal may show evidence of oesophageal varices or peptic ulceration. The most classical and helpful changes are found on liver biopsy. Here there is always fatty infiltration in patients who have been drinking recently. There also may be the features of a micronodular cirrhosis and increased deposits of iron. In a high percentage of patients there may be a hyaline change in the perinuclear cytoplasm of liver cells called Mallory's alcoholic hyaline. This is not pathognomonic of alcoholic liver disease, but is very helpful in a suspicious case. In patients with acute alcoholic hepatitis there may be the features of marked liver cell damage and focal necrosis of liver cells with polymorph infiltration. It seems likely that this type of lesion is liable to progress to a true micronodular cirrhosis.

Treatment

The treatment of this disease is unsatisfactory because of the risk that the patient will not be able to give up alcohol and if he does will return to it soon after he has left hospital. Hospital treatment, however, is necessary in order to withdraw alcohol, to suppress delirium tremens with chlorpromazine, and to provide a nutritious diet with high vitamin B and other supplements including magnesium. The long-term prognosis is uncertain. If drinking continues then it is likely that a percentage will go on to progressive liver failure or death from bleeding varices. The services of an expert social worker or the use of an organization such as 'Alcoholics Anonymous' may be valuable. Simple manoeuvres such as changing the occupation of the patient may also be helpful for there tends to be a high risk group in publicans, commercial travellers and in Service personnel.

REFERENCES

Hepatic Cirrhosis

Alcoholic Cirrhosis

SUMMERSKILL, W. H. J., DAVIDSON, C. S., DIBLE, J. H., MALLORY, G. K., SHERLOCK, S., TURNER, M. D., and WOLFE, S. J. (1960) Cirrhosis of the liver. A study of the alcoholic and non-alcoholic patients in Boston and London, *New Engl. J. Med.*, **262**, 1.

ZIEVE, L. (1958) Jaundice hyperlipaemia and haemolytic anaemia: a heretofore unrecognized syndrome associated with alcoholic fatty liver, *Ann. intern. Med.*, **48**, 471.

Chronic Active Hepatitis

READ, A. E., HARRISON, C. V., and SHERLOCK, S. (1963) Juvenile cirrhosis. Part of a system disease, *Gut*, **4**, 378.

Haemochromatosis

FINCH, S. C., and FINCH, C. A. (1955) Idiopathic haemochromatosis, an iron storage disease, *Medicine* (*Baltimore*), **34**, 381.

MACSWEEN, R. N. M. (1966) Acute abdominal crisis, circulatory collapse and sudden death in haemochromatosis, *Quart. J. Med.*, **35**, 589.

Wilson's Disease

WILSON, S. A. K. (1912) Progressive lenticular degeneration: a familial nervous disease associated with cirrhosis of the liver, *Brain*, **34**, 295.

DENNY-BROWN, D. (1964) Hepato-lenticular degeneration (Wilson's disease). Two different components, *New Engl. J. Med.*, **270**, 1149.

Primary Biliary Cirrhosis

SHERLOCK, S. (1959) Primary biliary cirrhosis (chronic intrahepatic obstructive jaundice), *Gastroenterology*, **31**, 574.

DONIACH, D., ROITT, I. M., WALKER, J. G., and SHERLOCK, S. (1966) Tissue antibodies in primary biliary cirrhosis, etc., *Clin. exp. Immunol.*, **1**, 237.

COMPLICATIONS OF CIRRHOSIS

PORTAL HYPERTENSION

This complication is an important one and it occurs in several types of liver disease. Portal hypertension may, however, be due as well to extrahepatic causes: the hepatic forms of portal hypertension may be classified as pre-sinusoidal and post-sinusoidal.

Pre-sinusoidal Portal Hypertension. This is the form produced by obstruction of the portal vein due to thrombosis or external pressure as from tumours (extrahepatic portal hypertension). It is also associated with various diseases where there is cellular infiltration in the liver. These include schistosomiasis and chronic leukaemia.

Post-sinusoidal Portal Hypertension. Here there is obstruction after blood has left the hepatic sinusoid. This type of portal hypertension is found in cirrhosis and in patients with Budd-Chiari syndrome. In cirrhosis it is due to the obstruction of hepatic venules by regeneration nodules.

Features of Portal Hypertension

The opening up of a circulation between the obstructed portal system and the systemic circulation results in the formation of varices at the lower end of the oesophagus and in the fundus of the stomach. These occur in all types of cirrhosis, but are commonest in the macronodular variety. The precipitating event which causes rupture is in most cases unknown, but the taking of aspirin and the importance of respiratory infection and tense ascites have been stressed by some investigators. The disorder begins either with haematemesis or melaena or with slower bleeding and the presence of positive occult blood tests in the stools. In severe cases the patient becomes shocked and may quickly pass into hepatic failure when the serum bilirubin rises and ascites rapidly collects and coma ensues.

Diagnosis

All patients with haematemesis or melaena must be examined closely for the presence of chronic liver disease and in particular splenomegaly must not be missed. The cutaneous signs of liver disease when they are present are suggestive and a history of jaundice or alcoholism or a previous diagnosis of cirrhosis is helpful.

Treatment

Strong sedative drugs such as morphine must be avoided. The patient must be treated in hospital with liberal blood transfusion. Neomycin should be given to prevent the onset of hepatic coma and the blood contained in the alimentary tract must be removed by purgation and bowel washouts.

When this treatment fails to control bleeding an intravenous infusion of vasopressin, 20 Units in a 5 per cent. dextrose given over half an hour may produce a cessation of bleeding. This acts by diminishing the inflow of blood into the portal system by causing arteriolar constriction. It should be avoided in patients with coronary artery disease and there is some evidence that it can produce deterioration in liver function by further compromising the precarious liver blood flow.

When these measures fail a decision must be made on the patient's fitness to withstand surgery. The operation can either be a localized attack on varices in the oesophagus, by variceal ligation or oesophageal or gastric transection, or in suitable patients some sort of shunt can be undertaken. It is essential that the patient is classified early on as suitable for an operation or not, because when there is evidence of gross liver cell failure with oedema, deep jaundice and encephalopathy surgery carries a prohibitive mortality. The only possibility in this situation is injection of oesophageal varices with sclerosant solutions through an oesophagoscope. If the patient is considered suitable for surgery then more energetic means of stopping any recurrent bleeding may be employed. This involves the use of a Sengstaken-Blakemore tube. This is a triple lumen tube with intragastric and intra-oesophageal balloons, both of which are blown up once the tube has been passed into the stomach. Traction on the apparatus with the gastric balloon inflated compresses the fundal veins which drain into the oesophageal varices therefore reducing variceal blood flow. The oesophageal balloon acts as a stabiliser for the apparatus and is also blown up to a pressure of about 25 mm. Hg. so that it can compress oseophageal varices. The apparatus is uncomfortable for the patient and there are numerous important complications, so that skilled nursing care is vital. These include aspiration pneumonia, and ulceration of the oesophagus and pharynx. On no account must this apparatus be used unless it is felt that the patient can, with some likelihood of success, be made fit for surgical therapy. The apparatus is used for a few hours until bleeding has ceased and in combination with vasopressin and blood transfusion. When there is good evidence that the intestinal bleeding has stopped from the fact that the aspirations from the stomach are free of blood, the apparatus can be deflated, traction taken off and, if all is well after 24 hours, it can be removed.

Once the bleeding has stopped a splenic venogram must be performed to assess whether the portal vein is patent [PLATE 1]. It will, of course, also outline any collateral vessels that are present. If the portal vein is patent, if the patient's serum albumin is reasonable (3 g. or more per 100 ml.) and if there is no icterus and no previous history of encephalopathy the patient should be considered for an elective portacaval anastomosis. Most surgeons require that the patient should not be more than 50 years of age, as there is undoubtedly a higher risk of post-operative encephalopathy in persons over this age. If the patient is thought to be unsuitable for a shunt operation a local 'attack' on varices may be indicated. It should be pointed out that the patient with liver disease does not withstand major thoracic surgery well, that operations of this type still carry a high mortality and that they are not guaranteed to prevent bleeding from varices in the future. A successful portacaval shunt operation is accompanied by cessation of bleeding, disappearance of varices and a decrease in the size of the enlarged spleen. Certain complications are seen after the operation; these include hepatic encephalopathy in about 30 per cent. of patients, and fluid retention due to the further deterioration in liver function, following reduction of hepatic blood flow by the operation.

ASCITES

The collection of fluid in the peritoneal cavity of the patient with cirrhosis is a common event. This may either occur chronically as a result of a gradual deterioration in liver function or more acutely, as for example after an intestinal haemorrhage. In the latter situation the deterioration of liver function due to intestinal bleeding is sufficient to cause an 'acute' ascites which disappears as soon as the intestinal bleeding or other causative insult to the liver ceases. There is, therefore, a difference both in aetiology and prognosis of these two types of ascites.

Aetiology

Ascites in cirrhosis of the liver is the result of a fall in the plasma colloidal osmotic pressure due to a reduction of the serum albumin. This, in combination with portal hypertension results in the exudation of fluid into the peritoneal cavity. Other factors which are important include an increased secretion of aldosterone which promotes sodium and fluid retention, this is said to be due to a fall in effective blood volume, possibly the result of splanchnic pooling of blood. Oestrogens and antidiuretic hormone are also concerned in fluid retention and the levels of these substances may be raised in patients with liver disease. Another important factor producing ascites is an increased production of hepatic lymph. This results from the increased resistance to blood and lymph flow associated with post-sinusoidal obstruction, resulting from regeneration nodules.

Clinical Picture

The patient with liver disease and ascites presents a striking picture. There is wasting of the limbs and a protuberant abdomen. The patient often complains of abdominal pain and discomfort, accompanied by anorexia and nausea. The physical signs of chronic liver disease are usually present and on examination there is a fluid thrill, shifting dullness in the flanks and often engorged veins on the anterior abdominal wall, either the effects of portal hypertension or of venacaval obstruction by tense ascites. The umbilicus is everted and there is often an umbilical hernia. Inguinal herniae and prolapse of the rectum or uterus are not unusual. There is often basal pulmonary collapse and on some occasions small collections of fluid in the pleural cavities. In patients with tense ascites it may be impossible to feel the liver but it may be possible to dip through and feel the enlarged liver underneath.

Diagnosis

Laboratory investigations show the abnormality of the liver function tests present in any chronic cirrhosis, but the serum albumin is usually less than 3 g. per 100 ml. The ascitic fluid in patients with chronic ascites is straw-coloured with a low albumin content (less than 2 g. per 100 ml.) and it contains epithelial cells. A blood-stained fluid or one with a high protein content suggests either neoplasia or the presence of hepatic vein obstruction. In many patients the serum sodium falls to below 130 mEq. per litre, there is reduction in the serum potassium and a mildly raised blood urea. The urinary sodium excretion is often less than 1 mEq. per 24 hours and the potassium excretion is increased.

The important other causes of ascites which have to be excluded include tuberculosis, which of course is not uncommon in patients with alcoholic liver disease, neoplasia, conditions of generalized fluid retention such as the nephrotic syndrome and ascites secondary to severe right heart failure such as complicates constrictive pericarditis. These can be excluded by careful physical examination and this can be supplemented by examination of the peritoneal fluid and urine.

Treatment

The treatment of ascites should be carried out in hospital and this usually requires sodium restriction to approximately 22 mEq. of sodium per day. Daily weighings and measurement of the abdominal girth, accurate collections of urine, and measurement of electrolyte excretion are also essential. Treatment is begun after 3 or 4 days of sodium restriction with an oral diuretic such as chlorothiazide, 0·5 G. twice daily, or frusemide, 40 mg. twice daily. If no response occurs then this can be reinforced with spironolactone (which is an aldosterone antagonist), 25 mg. three times a day. If a diuretic response does not occur after this combined therapy a further diuretic such as triamterine, 50 mg. three times a day, can be added. Failure of a response to this triple therapy is unusual but may occur, particularly in patients who have developed a low sodium state. In these patients the use of prednisone, 10 mg. three times a day, or intravenous mannitol therapy (500 ml. as a 20 per cent. solution) can be considered as may infusions of human salt-free albumin. On the whole, however, patients with a low serum sodium and gross ascites respond poorly to diuretic therapy and the hyponatraemia is normally a sign of terminal liver damage. Paracentesis should not be employed unless patients are resistant to a full hospital course of medical treatment. The only exception to this rule is if patients are admitted with very tense ascites which makes them severely short of breath or very uncomfortable from abdominal distension. In these circumstances a small paracentesis, say 1 or 2 litres, may be used prior to the administration of full diuretic regime.

The patient who responds to diuretic therapy loses oedema and gains flesh and makes a remarkable physical recovery. In many patients, however, the problem of underlying chronic liver disease is the over-riding one, and it is doubtful even in these days of full and successful diuretic therapy whether the patient's expectation of life is much improved.

Electrolyte abnormalities are common in patients with liver disease undergoing diuretic therapy, and they often manifest themselves as impending hepatic coma. One further complication is well recognized and this is infection of the ascitic fluid, usually with *Escherichia coli*; these patients have few signs of peritoneal infection, and present with hepatic encephalopathy, complicating severe ascites and other evidence of liver cell failure. It is therefore important in patients such as these to take specimens of ascitic fluid for culture.

HEPATOMA [see p. 650]

HEPATIC ENCEPHALOPATHY (HEPATIC COMA, PORTOSYSTEMIC ENCEPHALOPATHY)

Some patients with liver disease are known to develop neurological complications. In patients with acute liver failure this usually consists of progressive drowsiness or noisy delirium leading to coma. Hepatic coma may also occur in patients with chronic liver disease, particularly after some stressful situation which temporarily embarrasses already diminished liver function. It is therefore not unusual for hepatic coma to ensue after the following events in someone with chronic liver cell disease: (1) alimentary bleeding; (2) the use of certain drugs, particularly narcotics and diuretics; (3) systemic infections; (4) high protein feeding; and (5) surgical operations or paracentesis abdominis.

Prior to coma the patient goes through a number of stages where there may be important physical signs. First, the patient becomes confused, uncertain of his surroundings, and acts inappropriately. The speech may become slurred, the limbs hypertonic and there may be increased salivation. A most important physical sign at this stage is the presence of a tremor known as a 'hepatic flap', which is seen particularly in the outstretched hands, or on extending the wrists with the fingers full extended and separated. The flap is a coarse one, 2–3 beats per second, and may be more pronounced on one side than the other, though in gross cases it may involve the tongue, arms and legs. Another sign is the presence of a sweetish pungent odour to the breath, called hepatic foetor; it is quite characteristic of this condition and defies similes. In patients who are being treated with antibiotics the foetor may disappear. In recent years it has been recognized that patients with chronic liver disease may develop chronic neurological syndromes, and that hepatic coma, therefore, is not the only long-term neurological complication seen. In these patients there may be predominantly cerebellar, basal ganglion or mental symptoms, and another important group have shown paraplegia without sensory loss as a manifestation of the disorder.

Aetiology

The precise cause for the neurological syndromes that accompany liver disease is unknown. It depends on the precipitating events, but certainly in patients with a large shunt between the portal and systemic circulations, either naturally produced or as a result of portacaval anastomosis, it is likely that there is an intoxication of the brain by products of protein digestion which enter the portal circulation from the bowel and are not 'detoxified' in the liver. This has been shown to be true both in man and experimental animals for hepatic coma is aggravated by high protein feeding. In patients who develop chronic hepatic encephalopathy following diuretics it seems likely that ammonia production by the kidneys is increased as a result of the potassium deficiency and alkalosis. In the case of sedative drugs such as morphine and pethidine it is likely that the neurological complications result from increased brain sensitivity. It has been suggested recently that depletion of various neuroamines, particularly serotonin, in the brain could be responsible, but no single cause of hepatic coma has been consistently found.

Diagnosis

The diagnosis of hepatic encephalopathy is suggested when any neurological complication is found in a patient with liver disease. In acute liver disease the patient is usually jaundiced and has other evidence of hepatic failure. In chronic liver disease the syndrome may be confused with the neurological complications of chronic alcoholism and may simulate closely Wilson's disease. Diagnosis is verified by showing that the patient's condition is improved by protein restriction and by the administration of a broad-spectrum antibiotic such as neomycin. EEGs will often be helpful and show slowing, even before the patients show neuropsychiatric abnormality. The EEG slowing is a generalized one and again is affected by the factors which improve or worsen the patient's condition. Therefore, neomycin therapy and protein loading can be used diagnostically in conjunction with the EEG. The blood ammonia level is a reasonably good index of the presence of protein breakdown products from the gut in the systemic circulation. It also mirrors the inability of the liver to convert ammonia into urea. Blood levels of ammonia are difficult to measure and the samples have to be arterial ones taken in the fasting state. The technique is largely a research one.

Treatment

In all patients it is important to remove any precipitant cause, for example, in a patient with intestinal bleeding the blood loss must be replaced and blood, which is a source of protein for bacterial breakdown, must be removed from the alimentary tract by purgation and intestinal washouts. Sedative drugs and diuretics must be stopped and any electrolyte abnormality treated. Otherwise the treatment is protein restriction, the provision of nutrition with calories obtained from carbohydrate, usually given as a 20 per cent. solution of glucose or lactose by mouth, or in stuporose patients, by cannula into a large vein. Neomycin is given in a dose of 1 G. 6-hourly and supplements of potassium are important. It is also imperative that clinical examination to detect intercurrent infection and blood cultures should be performed as the patient with liver disease is susceptible to *Esch. coli* septicaemia. A non-absorbable sugar (lactulose) which causes an osmotic diarrhoea which is broken down by colonic bacteria to acid by products which prevent ammonia absorption may also be helpful. It is given orally in a dose of 45–60 G. daily as a 50 per cent. flavoured solution. In acute hepatic failure such as may complicate viral hepatitis recent workers have introduced various new techniques. These include exchange transfusion, in which the patient's blood is exchanged on one or several occasions, with the view to removing toxic products presumably responsible for the hepatic coma. Another method has been perfusion of the patient's blood through an isolated liver from a pig. Some dramatic responses have been recorded both from exchange transfusion and liver perfusion, but the over-all results as regards survival are not encouraging. If patients with chronic hepatic encephalopathy fail to respond to the regime of protein restriction and antibiotic therapy then some of them may be suitable for the operation of colonic by-pass. The theoretical basis of this operation is that the small bowel contents are diverted directly into the rectum so that the major site of bacterial protein breakdown, namely the colon, is excluded from the intestinal circuit. It should be remembered, however, that by the time the patient is considered suitable for this operation there may already be permanent neurological physical signs, and these are unlikely to be improved, and, moreover, the patient with liver disease is a poor operative risk. Certainly a recent double blind trial of this type of therapy compared with the routine medical therapy of chronic hepatic encephalopathy showed no long-term increase in the patient's length of survival.

REFERENCES

Ascites

Sherlock, S., Senewiratne, B., Scott, A., and Walker, J. G. (1966) Complications of diuretic therapy in hepatic cirrhosis, *Lancet*, i, 1049.

Sherlock, S., and Shaldon, S. (1963) The aetiology and management of ascites in patients with heptaic cirrhosis, *Gut*, **4**, 95.

Hepatic Encephalopathy

Read, A. E. (1967) Medical treatment of hepatic coma, in *The Liver*, Vol. 19 of the Colston Papers, p. 191, London.

Read, A. E., Sherlock, S., Laidlow, J., and Walker, J. B. (1967) The neuropsychiatric syndromes associated with chronic liver disease and an extensive portal collateral circulation, *Quart. J. Med.*, **36**, 135.

Portal Hypertension

Sherlock, S. (1964) Haematemesis in portal hypertension, *Brit. J. Surg.*, **51**, 746.

Walker, R. M., Shalden, C., and Vowles, K. D. J. (1961) Late results of portacaval anastomosis, *Lancet*, ii, 727.

VASCULAR DISORDERS OF THE LIVER

PASSIVE CONGESTION

A persistently raised central venous pressure due to right-sided heart failure, pericardial or myocardial constriction results in hepatic venous congestion and hepatomegaly. Pathologically the hepatic lesion is one of centrilobular congestion with surrounding fatty change (nutmeg liver). Clinically the lesion is of importance because hepatic congestion causes right upper abdominal pain and distension. Indeed there may be confusion as to the cause of these signs and symptoms unless a careful examination of the cardiovascular system is performed. The most common cardiac lesion is chronic right-sided heart failure often associated with tricuspid regurgitation. In this situation the liver may not only be enlarged and tender, but there may be systolic pulsation of the liver and in the jugular veins.

Ascites is commonly seen in this situation and because of the raised sinusoidal pressure splenomegaly is not unusual. Help may be obtained in diagnosis by examination of the liver function tests. The serum bilirubin is increased due both to liver cell dysfunction and the common accompaniment of pulmonary infarction, whilst the alkaline phosphatase and S.G.O.T. are also increased. In chronic cases the serum albumin may be low and in such cases cardiac 'cirrhosis' may be found on histological examination. In fact true cirrhosis with regeneration nodules due to cardiac failure is excessively rare and the picture is rather one of hepatic fibrosis without an upset in basic hepatic architecture.

Treatment consists of that of the primary cause and vigorous antibiotic therapy with agents effective against Gram-negative bacteria.

PORTAL VENOUS THROMBOSIS (EXTRAHEPATIC PORTAL HYPERTENSION)

Aetiology

Thrombosis of the portal vein is usually the result either of an ascending infection along the umbilical vein at birth, secondary to umbilical sepsis, or of sepsis within the abdominal cavity, causing a septic endophlebitis of the mesenteric and portal veins. This results in the development of portal hypertension with oesophageal varices though liver function and structure remain reasonably normal. Occasionally thrombosis occurs because of occlusion by a pancreatic neoplasm or in polycythaemia rubra vera.

Clinical Picture

The patient is usually young and in children there may be a history of umbilical sepsis at birth; the occasional young patient has had an exchange transfusion for rhesus incompatibility. These cases are unusual and in the older patient there is more often a history of intra-abdominal sepsis such as appendicitis or diverticular disease with abscess formation. Convalescence from this primary disorder may have been delayed by pyrexia and signs of intra-abdominal sepsis. There is sometimes no preceding history of such an event, though a rare patient may have a primary blood dyscrasia, such as polycythaemia rubra vera. The patient usually gives a history of haematemesis or melaena, and on examination has an enlarged spleen, but does not have the signs of chronic liver cell disease.

Diagnosis

Liver biopsy in these patients is normal as may be the liver function tests in the early stages. It is recognized, however, that as the disease process progresses abnormalities of liver function, particularly raised serum alkaline phosphatase and bilirubin levels may occur, and in these circumstances the patient may mimic closely the patient with cirrhosis and secondary portal hypertension. Ascites is not a feature of this disease unless the bleeding is severe and hypoproteinaemia extreme. On barium examination of the oesophagus, varices are seen but the most important investigation is a splenic venogram which shows occlusion either of the splenic or portal vein and the appearance of many collateral channels [Plate 1]. On occasions this may be associated with the appearance of a so-called 'cavernous transformation' (cavernoma) of the portal vein. This used to be thought a congenital abnormality of this vessel, but almost certainly represents the development of multiple collateral vessels secondary to a primary portal vein occlusion.

Treatment

The treatment of this disease is that directed towards stopping bleeding from varices as indicated on page 644.

In that these patients have a normal liver there is much less risk of the precipitation of hepatic failure, and most patients with this type of portal hypertension recover rapidly from their bleeding. The episodes of bleeding, however, tend to be repeated and consideration must be given to the possibility of surgical correction. For this portal venography is a prior essential. If this shows that there is a suitable length of portal vein available for anastomosis following high portal vein obstruction, then a portacaval anastomosis operation may be possible and curative. Often, however, this is impossible and though the occasional patient may be suitable for a superior mesenteric-caval anastomosis most patients are treated with some sort of direct surgical attack on the varices, i.e. an oesophageal ligation or transection or a gastric transection or gastrectomy. No operation is entirely satisfactory and unless the patient is likely to be away from good transfusion facilities multiple operations should be avoided unless the patient is in a serious condition and the haemorrhage cannot be controlled.

SUPPURATIVE PYLEPHLEBITIS

Septic venous thrombosis within the portal circulation may result in occlusion of the portal vein and give rise to extrahepatic portal venous occlusion. Spreading infection from an appendix or from acute colonic diverticular infection are the usual sites of commencement of this septic embolic process. Occasionally a systemic septicaemia may produce a similar result and ulcerative colitis (portal bacteraemia) is an occasional cause.

The acute phase of this disorder may produce fairly characteristic signs and symptoms. Apart from pyrexia and abdominal pain due to the causative lesion there may be obvious evidence of septic embolization to the liver. Right upper abdominal pain and tender hepatomegaly may be accompanied by mild jaundice and rigors. A polymorph leucocytosis and abnormal liver function tests—raised serum bilirubin, alkaline phosphatase and transaminases—may be found. Occasionally one or more large intrahepatic abscesses may form and the patient becoming more acutely ill with rigors, a swinging temperature, and a very tender hepatomegaly, possibly accompanied by signs at the right lung base.

BUDD-CHIARI SYNDROME

Definition

The Budd-Chiari syndrome is the name used to describe the clinical disorder which results when the hepatic venous outflow is obstructed.

Aetiology

The aetiology of this condition is variable and the lesions are best considered under those that affect the major hepatic veins at their entrance into the inferior vena cava, and those affecting the small central hepatic venules in the lobules of the liver. The former is caused by massive thrombosis of the hepatic veins. This can occur in blood dyscrasias such as polycythaemia, or from invasion of the hepatic veins from a tumour such as a carcinoma of the right kidney or retroperitoneal sarcoma. Lesions which affect the smaller hepatic venules include a disease called veno-occlusive disease, which is found particularly in the West Indies and in Africa and India, where it is thought that toxic substances consumed in the patient's diet produce an endophlebitis and secondary thrombosis of the central hepatic venules. In the West Indian cases this has been traced to various plant alkaloids of the species *Crotalaria.* An interesting new cause for the Budd-Chiari syndrome is the occasional case which is associated with the taking of the contraceptive pill. Another form of the disorder which has also been described recently is probably congenital in origin. Here a membranous obstruction of the inferior vena cava and of the hepatic veins is caused by a fold of endothelium. Antimitotic drugs may also be an occasional cause.

Pathology

The pathology of the condition is characteristic. The liver is enlarged and congested, and shows on sectioning a prominent nutmeg pattern with centrilobular haemorrhage and a surrounding yellow appearance of the rest of the hepatic lobule. On microscopy the centrilobular congestion is very obvious and the rest of the liver shows either fatty or other degenerative change and a commencing micronodular cirrhosis.

Clinical Picture

The symptoms are due to the accumulation of ascites which is likely to occur rapidly with enlarging abdominal girth and generalized abdominal pain. The cutaneous signs of cirrhosis are usually absent and the surface of the liver is smooth and tender. It is therefore unlike the hepatomegaly of neoplasia. Diagnosis is aided by the liver function tests which generally show a normal serum bilirubin, possibly some fall of the serum albumin level and a moderate rise in the serum transaminase levels. Considerable help may be obtained by performing a liver biopsy when the characteristic histological picture of centrilobular haemorrhage and congestion with surrounding liver cell degeneration will be found. The histology does not, however, usually indicate the cause of the lesion. Further evidence of Budd-Chiari syndrome may be obtained by scintillo, graphy, when a rather characteristic scan showing a high midline uptake of the radioactivity is sometimes seen. A diagnosis of Budd-Chiari syndrome must lead to a careful examination of the patient's dietary habits, particularly with respect to drugs and herbal medicines. It should also be a reason for examining the peripheral blood to detect any evidence of a tendency to thrombosis and, of course, in women an inquiry about the taking of the contraceptive pill. An intravenous pyelogram will not only help to exclude a retroperitoneal tumour, but will also indicate if there is any pathology such as renal carcinoma in the right kidney. An inferior venacavagram will be helpful in demonstrating patency of the major hepatic veins and in detecting a vena caval web obstruction. Hepatic vein catheterization is also valuable, particularly if accompanied by retrograde venography.

Treatment

The treatment of this disease depends on the cause. For example in the case of polycythaemia this must be energetically treated and the patient put on anticoagulant drugs. Usually, however, the treatment can only be symptomatic, but it must be stressed that the use of a diuretic regime with agents such as chlorothiazide and spironolactone may well control the patient's ascites and produce symptomatic relief. In some cases a portacaval shunt should be done in order to short-circuit the venous obstruction.

Prognosis

This depends on the cause, but in many patients there is a progression to chronic liver damage, cirrhosis and death from liver cell failure unless the obstruction is relieved. It should be remembered that patients who have evidence of the Budd-Chiari syndrome may develop portal hypertension with bleeding from oesophageal varices and this may further complicate the illness.

INFECTIONS OF THE LIVER

PYOGENIC INFECTION

ABSCESS

Pyogenic infection in the liver with resultant liver abscess formation results from entry of infected material either via the portal system (septic portal endophlebitis) [see p. 647], by the systemic circulation (septicaema) or by spread via the biliary tract (ascending cholangitis). The clinical picture is indistinguishable in these instances, though in patients with ascending cholangitis rigors, hepatic tenderness and features of obstructive jaundice may in particular suggest the biliary route of infection [p. 655].

Patients are ill and may in subacute cases mimic closely the appearances of carcinomatosis. Sometimes the illness develops acutely with fever, hepatomegaly and mild jaundice and a blood count showing leucocytosis. Diagnosis can be difficult and confusion with hepatic cancer, subphrenic abscess and a primary pulmonary infection may occur. Amoebic abscess of the liver is also an important diagnostic consideration in those who have been abroad in endemic areas.

Aids to diagnosis include estimation of the serum B_{12} level which is raised due to release from damaged liver tissue, whilst scintiscanning and ultrasonic scanning will demonstrate one or more space-occupying lesions within the liver. Ultrasound is particularly valuable in demonstrating the fluid-filled nature of the lesion. Occasionally coeliac axis angiography will be helpful in demonstrating an intrahepatic lesion but its ultimate nature may only be diagnosed by aspiration at laparotomy. A careful examination of the pus and abscess wall must be made to exclude amoebiasis though the characteristics of the abscess contents are helpful. Once a diagnosis of suppurative liver abscess has been made treatment consists of massive antibiotic therapy with aspiration or surgical drainage for large localizations of purulent material. Any acute suppurative lesion within the abdominal cavity must also be detected.

Supportive treatment in this disease—which carries a high mortality—must not be forgotten. Patients are often elderly, dehydrated, anaemic and poorly nourished. Intravenous fluid therapy, blood transfusion and parenteral feeding are often required.

TUBERCULOSIS

Tuberculous disease of the liver is rare, except for its involvement in miliary tuberculosis and in tuberculous peritonitis. Spreading tuberculous disease is occasionally seen when the picture is of jaundice of the liver cell variety, pyrexia, cachexia and hepatomegaly. There is invariably evidence of caseating disease elsewhere.

SYPHILIS

The liver is involved in congenital syphilis by a fine hepatic fibrosis but this is exceedingly rare. Though jaundice was common in patients with syphilis this was the result of the therapy and in most cases due to serum hepatitis or more rarely arsphenamine jaundice. In tertiary syphilis there may be one or more gummata in the liver causing coarse hepatic scarring without cirrhosis. In liver disease the W.R. may be anticomplementary and a treponemal immobilization test may be required to exclude syphilic infection. Male cirrhotics, however—presumably because of progressive serum hepatitis contracted at the time of therapy—may be found at presentation with cirrhosis either to have had proven syphilis or to have evidence of undiagnosed disease requiring treatment. A W.R. and treponemal immobilization test is therefore important in all cirrhotics, particularly males. Arsenic has also been shown to be a cause of cirrhosis and this may follow in patients given arsenical treatment.

HEPATIC AMOEBIASIS [see Section 2]

HYDATID DISEASE

The liver is the site of over two thirds of hydatid cysts —the cystic stage of the dog tape worm *Echinococcus granulosus* of which man and sheep are intermediate hosts.

Common in sheep-raising areas because of the fact that dogs have access to the carcass of this intermediate host, the disorder is associated in man with hepatic enlargement and occasionally the signs of a smooth rounded mass or masses exhibiting a third thrill. The patient is generally well and diagnosis is helped by radiology which may show calcification of the cyst wall either in the liver or elsewhere. Ultrasonic and scintiscanning are helpful whilst eosinophilia in the peripheral blood and serology (complement fixation test) are further diagnostic aids. The intradermal Casoni test indicates a *past* or present existence of a hydatid cyst and this fact must be borne in mind. Rupture of a cyst into the peritoneal cavity, lungs, etc., may be associated with dangerous anaphylaxis and secondary infection so that if possible surgical excision is required following cyst sterilization, avoiding the spilling of its contents. This may require partial hepatectomy or even hepatic lobectomy [see Section 2].

TUMOURS AND CYSTS OF THE LIVER

SCHISTOSOMIASIS [see Section 2]

LIVER FLUKES [see Section 2]

THE LIVER IN POLYCYSTIC DISEASE

The liver may be involved in three different ways as a result of this inherited disease.

POLYCYSTIC DISEASE OF THE LIVER

The liver is involved by cyst formation which produces a nodular hepatomegaly. The cysts are surrounded by fibrous tissue capsule and lined by columnar epithelium. About half the patients with polycystic liver disease have renal involvement. Usually there are no symptoms referable to the liver, but on occasions patients may complain of quite severe hepatic pain. Liver cell function is retained and liver function tests are normal. The most successful method of diagnosing this condition is ultrasonic scanning of the liver. No treatment is required, though on occasion aspiration of cysts may be helpful in the relief of pain.

CONGENITAL HEPATIC FIBROSIS

In this disorder where there may also be cystic involvement of the kidneys the liver is traversed by dense bands of fibrous tissue. Fibrous tissue contains bile-ducts and small intrahepatic portal venous radicals. Because of the disorganization of the portal venous system the disorder causes portal hypertension. Patients with this disease therefore show hepatosplenomegaly and may bleed from oesophageal varices. Liver function tests are often normal with the exception of the alkaline phosphatase which is often considerably raised. Liver biopsy is difficult because of the extreme toughness of the liver and for this reason needle biopsy often fails. Splenic venography demonstrates a patent portal vein and haemodynamic studies show that the portal hypertension is pre-sinusoidal. These patients do well as a result of a shunt operation because of the fact that liver function is well preserved and because they are predominantly of a young age group. The one exception to this rule is the danger that post-operative renal failure may be precipitated because of renal involvement by this polycystic disease.

DILATATION OF THE INTRAHEPATIC BILE-DUCTS

Partial or complete dilatation of the intrahepatic bile-ducts forms another example of the effects of polycystic disease in the liver. The cystic dilatation of the bile-ducts results in attacks of cholangitis and obstructive jaundice, and may be complicated by cholangiocarcinoma.

PRIMARY TUMOURS OF THE LIVER

HEPATOMA

This is a malignant neoplasm of the liver which can occur either with or without accompanying hepatic cirrhosis. About 20 per cent. of patients with hepatic cirrhosis develop such a tumour either at one or several sites. It may be of liver cell (hepatoma) or bile-duct (cholangioma) origin. The former is the commonest. In this country about 70 per cent. of primary hepatic tumours develop in cirrhotic livers.

Aetiology

The precise aetiology of this condition is unknown, and the factor responsible for transforming the proliferative cellular activity in a benign cirrhosis to that of a malignant tumour is uncertain. One important piece of evidence comes from the fact that in the experimental animal hepatic tumours can be produced by a variety of compounds obtained from the various moulds, notably *Aspergillus flavus*. These toxins collectively called aflatoxin consistently produce liver disease and/or hepatomata in various rodents and in poultry. It is perfectly possible that moulds such as *A. flavus* could contaminate cereal crops particularly when they are stored, and this may explain the high incidence of hepatoma in certain parts of the world, such as in tropical Africa. Another important fact which has been brought home recently is that a considerable proportion of patients who underwent contrast angiography with thorium dioxide have since developed malignant tumours of the liver and other organs, including hepatoma and malignant haemangio-endothelioma.

Clinical Picture

The patient with hepatic cirrhosis who develops one or more malignant tumours in the liver usually presents either with abdominal pain or with an enlarging mass due to malignant infiltration of a cirrhotic liver. Loss of weight, anorexia, vomiting and weakness accompany the abdominal pain. Signs of involvement of structures outside the liver are relatively late, though pulmonary secondaries and secondaries in the spine and ribs may cause pain. Ascites may occur due to peritoneal involvement or encroachment on the portal venous radicles. Bleeding from oesophageal varices may be the first sign of multiple deposits of hepatoma. Occasionally the hepatoma will rupture into the peritoneal cavity with profuse and fatal intraperitoneal haemorrhage. A number of unusual manifestations of hepatoma are now well recognized. These include polycythaemia, hypercalcaemia due to production of parathormone, and hyponatraemia due to the production of antidiuretic hormone. Various abnormalities of the serum proteins with a high lipoprotein level may also occur. In patients without cirrhosis the condition presents as a progressive enlargement of the liver.

Diagnosis

This is suggested by the picture of clinical deterioration in someone with known hepatic cirrhosis, and particularly is this important in patients with haemochromatosis or with macronodular cirrhosis. Diagnostic confirmation may either be obtained by needle biopsy if the mass presents as a tumour in the epigastrium or, on occasions, malignant cells may be found in the accompanying ascitic fluid. Occasionally plain abdominal X-rays show that the lesion is calcified. Hepatic angiography is a good way of demonstrating tumours in the liver for they have a predominantly arterial blood supply.

Recently it has been shown that about 70 per cent. of patients in Africa with a hepatoma have in the serum an alpha-1 feto-globulin, that is a protein found in the human foetus which normally disappears at birth. It reappears as a result of manufacture by the hepatic tumour. This seems only to be found in primary hepatoma as opposed to primary cholangioma. Whether or not this will be an equally useful test for hepatoma in this country is unknown—preliminary results suggest a positive test in only 30 per cent.

Treatment

Treatment of hepatoma is unsatisfactory. If the lesion is solitary, particularly if the patient has no accompanying cirrhosis then hepatic lobectomy is a possible, though massive, operation. In patients with multiple deposits throughout the liver there is, at present, no curative treatment with the possible exception of hepatic transplantation. Severe pain, however, when it occurs can be treated with intra-arterial infusions of antimitotic drugs [see Section 4]. There is always a risk with this type of therapy of producing further damage in an already chronically damaged cirrhotic liver.

OTHER TUMOURS OF THE LIVER

The other important primary tumours of the liver are the benign haemangioma which is usually symptomless though it may occasionally calcify or cause an audible bruit on auscultation and the highly malignant haemangio-endothelioma which has all the clinical features of a hepatoma in a non-cirrhotic liver though the course is generally more rapidly downhill. Treatment is by either X-irradiation, resection, or both.

SECONDARY TUMOURS OF THE LIVER

The liver is frequently the site of metastases from a primary carcinoma of the alimentary tract, bronchus, breast, pancreas, kidney and from skin and ocular melanomata.

Pathology

The liver may contain one or two small deposits or may be greatly enlarged and largely replaced by neoplastic tissue. Histology may often fail to reveal the site of the primary though there are exceptions such as oat-cell tumours of the bronchus or melanoma.

Clinical Picture

The patient may have the symptoms referable to a primary tumour of the gut, bronchus, breast, etc., or may give a history of previous surgical or radiotherapeutic treatment. Patients have generally lost weight and may complain of abdominal distension and pain. These two symptoms are usually due to hepatic enlargement. Anorexia, nausea and alteration of bowel habit—constipation or diarrhoea—may also be symptoms. On examination the patient is wasted and generally there is nodular hepatomegaly which may be tender. In these subjects the umbilicated pattern of individual superficial metastases may be detectable and in some an audible friction rub may be heard when the patient breathes, and a stethoscope is placed on the skin of the right upper abdomen. Palpable lymph nodes in the supraclavicular fossae and axillae, the presence of jaundice and ascites, or umbilical secondary deposits are further possible physical signs that may be present.

Diagnosis

The liver function tests are helpful for the alkaline phosphatase is often raised when there are only a few secondary deposits, whilst massive secondary tumour replacement of the liver may cause elevation of the serum bilirubin—a low serum albumin without a striking increase in total globulins and moderate elevation of the transaminases. A polymorph leucocytosis and mild anaemia are also common.

The presence of neoplastic deposits in the liver can be shown by scintillography or by coeliac axis angiography. This latter gives much better definition than portal venography because of the predominantly arterial blood supply of the deposits. Ultrasound is also useful but the abnormality may be difficult to tell from other hepatic lesions by this method. Precise diagnosis means liver needle biopsy either under direct vision (at laparoscopy) or into a palpable nodule (via the subcostal route). Laparoscopy is of value without biopsy as it allows inspection of much of the liver surfaces and recognition of superficial deposits.

Of the other diagnostic possibilities mention should be made of the importance of excluding carcinoid syndrome (estimation of urinary 5HIAA and 5HTP). This type of neoplastic infiltration is important to recognize as the prognosis is relatively good and some of the associated symptoms (particularly the diarrhoea) can be controlled. Hepatic cirrhosis and polycystic disease of the liver must also be excluded.

Treatment

There is no effective treatment, though on occasions a solitary secondary may be resected, though it does not guarantee freedom from others. It is important to determine whether the primary tumour is hormone dependent (breast, prostate) as treatment—hypophysectomy, adrenalectomy or hormone therapy—may be helpful in these cases.

Infusion of cytotoxic drugs via the hepatic artery plus hepatic artery ligation has been suggested as an aggressive therapy for some patients. The former may be helpful for severe pain but for most patients the treatment is supportive only.

RETICULOSES

The liver may be involved by reticulosis. In certain types (particularly Hodgkin's disease) this may be in the form of neoplastic expansion of portal zones with resultant biliary obstruction. In others larger masses of neoplastic tissue cause nodular hepatomegaly.

REFERENCES

Polycystic Disease of the Liver

COMFORT, M. W., GRAY, H. K., DAHLIN, D. C., and WHITESELL, F. B. (1952) Polycystic disease of the liver: a study of 24 cases, *Gastroenterology*, **20**, 60.

Congenital Hepatic Fibrosis

KERR, D. N. S., HARRISON, C. V., SHERLOCK, S., and WALKER, R. M. (1961) Congenital hepatic fibrosis, *Quart. J. Med.*, **30**, 91.

Hepatoma

MACDONALD, R. A. (1957) Primary carcinoma of the liver: A clinico-pathological study of 108 cases, *Arch. intern. Med.*, **99**, 266.

Aflatoxin

REES, K. R. (1966) Aflatoxin, *Gut*, **7**, 205.

Secondary Hepatic Tumours

SCHAEFER, J., and SCHIFF, L. (1965) Liver function tests in metastatic tumour of the liver: a study of 100 cases, *Gastroenterology*, **49**, 360.

THE GALL-BLADDER

INTRODUCTION

The liver secretes about 1 litre of bile a day. It is normally secreted at a pressure of 20 cm. of water and if the pressure within the biliary system rises because of obstruction secretion of bile will cease at a level of about 35 cm. of water. In addition to its pigment, bile contains bile salts as conjugates, hormones such as thyroxine and steroids, electrolytes and lipids. The lipids are kept in solution by the formation of micelles composed of bile salts, cholesterol and of phospholipid. These allow insoluble cholesterol esters to be kept in solution.

Bile salts are able to increase the flow of bile and the hormone, secretin, has a similar effect. Hepatic bile is stored in the gall-bladder. Gall-bladder bile differs from the hepatic variety in being concentrated ten times or so by the active removal of chloride, bicarbonate and sodium together with water. The gall-bladder contracts under the action of hormone called cholecystokinin, which is released from the upper small bowel into the blood stream. A fatty meal provokes the production of cholecystokinin. The sphincter of Oddi normally withstands a pressure of about 25 cm. of water and bile is therefore diverted into the gall-bladder where it is concentrated. It is only the active contraction of the gall-bladder by cholecystokinin which overcomes the sphincter's resistance. [Note. Cholecystokinin (CCK) and pancreozymin (PZ) are identical hormones, i.e. CCKPZ.]

CONGENITAL DISORDERS OF THE GALL-BLADDER

ATRESIA OF THE BILE DUCTS

Failure of union of the intra- and extrahepatic bile ducts results in biliary atresia. This manifests with progressive obstructive jaundice and pruritus in the newborn with the gradual production of hepatomegaly, secondary biliary cirrhosis, xanthomatosis and failure to thrive. The diagnosis may be difficult in the first two weeks and confusion with giant-cell hepatitis may only be resolved by needle biopsy of the liver and/or laparotomy with wedge biopsy and cholangiography. These techniques are difficult and dangerous in the newborn and pre-operative nutritional deficiency (particularly of vitamins D and K) must be corrected.

If the diagnosis is substantiated and operative cholangiography (using gall-bladder) demonstrates that the process is confined to a portion of the extrahepatic bile-duct system an attempt must be made to correct this by resection and re-anastamoses of normal duct to an uninvolved and dilated bile-duct above the obstruction. This type of surgery is extremely difficult and only one in six patients can be treated in this way. Examples of intrahepatic atresia which are inoperable may survive several years with a syndrome similar to primary biliary cirrhosis in the adult. Liver transplant may in the future be an answer to this otherwise fatal form of intrahepatic biliary atresia. Treatment in cases managed conservatively must include a low-fat diet—perhaps with medium chain triglyceride supplements, vitamins D and K and cholestyramine.

CHOLEDOCHAL CYST

This is a congenital dilatation of the common bile-duct of unknown cause. It presents clinically as attacks of obstructive jaundice usually in young females. There is often right upper abdominal pain and a cystic tumour. Following identification by intravenous or transhepatic cholangiography treatment is by internal anastomosis and subsequent drainage into the jejunum.

OTHER CONGENITAL ABNORMALITIES

These include absence of the gall-bladder, double gall-bladder and abnormal configuration of the duct system. The gall-bladder may also be contained within the liver substance, or kinked (Phrygian cup deformity). These abnormalities are not of great clinical importance.

CHOLECYSTITIS

ACUTE

An acute inflammation of the gall-bladder is usually associated with the presence of gall-stones, particularly where these produce obstruction of the cystic duct. On rare occasions the disease may occur without stone formation and then it seems likely that a previously abnormal gall-bladder is the site of blood stream embolization by pathogenic bacteria, particularly *Esch. coli.*

Clinical Features

Pain is of sudden onset referred to the right upper abdomen, right shoulder and angle of the right scapula. Though on occasions colicky, it is in fact often a steady pain accompanied by nausea, retching and pyrexia. The patient lies still and seeks relief from a hot-water bottle applied to the upper abdomen. Radiation of pain to the chest or to the left side of the abdomen may cause diagnostic confusion with myocardial infarction and left basal pneumonia.

Examination at this phase usually reveals a middle-aged obese woman (though not necessarily so) with right upper abdominal pain, with local tenderness over the gall-bladder or on deep palpation under the right costal margin on inspiration (Murphy's sign). Slight icterus may be present if bile-duct obstruction has resulted from gall-stones and in such situations pruritus with pale stools and dark urine may be noted.

Increasing toxaemia, swinging temperature and the presence of a localized mass in the right upper abdomen suggest the presence of an empyema of the gall-bladder.

Diagnosis

The differential diagnosis must include the major abdominal emergencies which present with epigastric and right-sided abdominal pain such as right-sided pneumonia or pleurisy, acute hepatitis, perforation of a peptic ulcer, pancreatitis and right-sided pyelonephritis. The distinction from cardiac pain has already been mentioned.

Further diagnostic proof is usually obtained after the patient has recovered from the attack—by the use of oral and/or intravenous opacification of the gall-bladder and bile-ducts.

In some patients where there is doubt as to the diagnosis, and where the clinical condition is deteriorating, it is worthwhile considering infusion and cholangiography as a way of making a diagnosis in the acute phase.

Complications

The complications of acute cholecystitis include perforation and gangrene of the gall-bladder and the closely related condition of empyema. All are associated with increasing upper abdominal pain and toxaemia, and in the case of perforation by the signs of localized and then spreading upper abdominal peritonitis. Gram-negative septicaemia associated with active infection of the biliary tree is a further complication usually associated with deepening jaundice and tender hepatomegaly. A falling blood pressure with warm extremities (warm shock) and obvious deterioration in the patient's clinical condition are then indications for blood culture and urgent supportive treatment with antibiotics, fluid replacement and possibly corticosteroids.

Treatment

The treatment is as indicated under the section on gall-stones, that is conservative, providing the patient is responding, and surgery after the acute phase has subsided. Tetracycline is the most usual antibiotic to prescribe but *Rifamide*, an antibiotic reaching very high concentrations in bile, may be useful in very ill patients. Difficulties arise when the patient is deteriorating despite treatment with antibiotics and in these circumstances emergency surgery, though carrying an appreciable risk, is indicated. Drainage of the infected gall-bladder—cholecystostomy—carries a lower risk than cholecystectomy provided necrosis of the gall-bladder wall has not occurred. Cholecystectomy is then performed when the acute situation has subsided.

CHRONIC

There is no doubt that this diagnosis is made more frequently than it should be. Certainly it should rarely be entertained if gall-stones are not found on radiological examination. The cause of flatulent dyspepsia is in many patients unknown and is certainly not always a sign of an unhealthy gall-bladder. Biliary regurgitation into the stomach, irritable colon syndrome, gastritis, hiatus hernia and lactose intolerance, and even ischaemic heart disease, must all be considered. All too often a patient with nondescript symptoms may opacify the gall-bladder poorly on oral cholangiography and there may be a poor contractile response to a fatty meal. A method for the diagnosis of chronic gall-bladder disease based on quantitation is much needed and until this happens the disease of chronic cholecystitis may be over diagnosed and treated. The cases of chronic bacterial cholecystitis will include the occasional carrier of *Salmonella typhi* and in these circumstances antibiotics and/or surgery may be required to eradicate the carrier state [Section 2].

GALL-STONES

Definition

The precipitation of the biliary constituents, bile pigment, calcium and cholesterol in the gall-bladder or bile-ducts gives rise to gall-stones. This is a common abnormality, more common in females than in males and its frequency increases with age, so that at the age of 70 about 30 per cent. of the population are affected. Various types of gall-stones have been described. These are:

1. Solitary stones composed of cholesterol and largely radio-translucent.
2. Bilirubin stones, found particularly where there is increased haemolysis, and also radio-translucent.
3. Mixed stones consisting of calcium, bile pigments and cholesterol; they are often radio-opaque.

Only about 20 per cent. of all gall-stones are radio-opaque. The rest can only be demonstrated by opacifying the gall-bladder with contrast medium. Though there has been a tendency to describe separate types of stones, in fact far less distinction is now thought to exist between them.

Aetiology

Gall-stones are likely to be present in patients who are forming excess amounts of bilirubin. This explains the bilirubin stones of patients with haemolytic anaemia. Infection, formerly considered the common cause of stone formation, is probably not important. It is nowadays thought that a primary abnormality of bile salt metabolism could at least play a part in gall-stone disease. The evidence for this is that hepatic bile from patients with biliary stones differs in its constituents from normal bile. The major differences include an alteration of the amount of trihydroxy to dihydroxy bile acids, with a reduction in the former. This probably results in defective micelle formation. Micelles are the minute combinations of bile salts, phospholipids and cholesterol which keep the latter in solution. If micelle formation is defective cholesterol precipitates out and forms a nidus for stone formation. Another abnormality which is present is an increase in the concentration of biliary mucus. This accelerates the formation of bilirubin and calcium complexes with precipitation and stone formation. It is unlikely that abnormalities of cholesterol metabolism are of particular importance and the reported relationship between multiple pregnancies and the formation of gall-stones is now questioned. Recently it has been demonstrated that gall-stones are found more commonly in those with ileal disease or ile-ectomy—a disturbance of bile salt metabolism seems likely. A similar explanation may hold for the increased incidence in chronic liver disease (cirrhosis).

Clinical Picture

The symptoms caused by gall-stones are variable. The disorder is commonest in females and a family history of the condition is not unusual. The disorder may start acutely with severe right upper abdominal pain and vomiting. The pain is usually felt in the epigastrium or under the right costal margin and it travels through to the angle of the right scapula or to the shoulder. The pain may be colicky, but not uncommonly it is severe, intense and constant. It is accompanied by nausea and vomiting and to get relief the patient often walks around or clutches a hot-water bottle to the appropriate part of the abdomen. There may be pyrexia and slight icterus. The urine may be dark due to the presence of bilirubin. On examination the only physical signs are right upper abdominal guarding and rigidity and the presence of pyrexia. In patients with chronic biliary disease the precise symptomatology is more difficult. There has been a tendency to assume that patients with chronic flatulent dyspepsia and right upper abdominal discomfort after meals are probably suffering from gall-stones. This is unlikely to be the case in many patients and gall-stones can only be diagnosed with confidence when there is an acute history such as has been previously described.

Diagnosis

The diagnosis of biliary stones can only be confirmed by radiological studies of the gall-bladder, but in patients with acute symptoms there may be transient jaundice if the stone obstructs the common bile-duct and an elevation of the alkaline phosphatase which may be helpful. Otherwise the investigation to confirm the diagnosis is an oral cholecystogram. The gall-bladder is shown to opacify with the contrast medium and any radio-translucent stones appear as a filling defects. Following visualization of the gall-bladder its ability to contract following a fatty meal is also noted. Adequate delineation of the bile-ducts is not always obtained in this way; if it is required or if there is no concentration of dye in the gall-bladder, intravenous cholangiography using *Biligrafin* should be considered. Although non-visualization of the gall-bladder may signify the presence of gall-bladder disease it must be remembered that there are other causes of this. These include non-absorption of the contrast medium due to vomiting or diarrhoea and the presence of liver cell disease. In this light it should be remembered that oral cholecystography is unlikely to produce a filling of the gall-bladder unless the serum bilirubin is less than 3 mg. per cent. A double dose of contrast should be given and the examination of the gall bladder repeated in all uncertain cases. Where there is further doubt intravenous cholangiography will not only demonstrate the bile-ducts but will also confirm whether or not the gall-bladder is functioning.

In any young person with gall-stones the possibility of haemolytic anaemia should be considered and the appropriate laboratory tests made [see Section 13].

The onset of right upper abdominal pain, icterus and pyrexia is suggestive of gall-bladder disease, but pain in this area may also occur as a result of hepatic congestion due to heart failure, or myocardial infarction. Pain may be referred to this area from the chest in lobar pneumonia and it may also result from a lesion of the right kidney such as acute pyelonephritis. In patients with hepatitis the onset may be acute with pain, so that this must be included in the differential diagnosis, and so must appendicitis.

Treatment

In a patient with acute cholecystitis the usual policy is to wait for the attack to subside. When the patient has improved, and providing cholecystographic evidence of gall-bladder disease is found, the patient should be sent for an elective cholecystectomy. There may be occasions when this policy is unwise, if for example, the patient has had only mild symptoms or if there is some other reason such as extreme age which mitigates against surgery. Although one attack of biliary colic may be rapidly recovered from there is no telling whether a patient will not have a more serious attack in the future, and generally prophylactic surgery after the acute attack is to be recommended. During the acute attack the patient should be given analgesics of which the most satisfactory appears to be phenazocine (*Narphen*) in a dose of 2 mg. by intramuscular injection. Oral fluids only are permitted and antibiotics are not usually considered necessary unless the patient is pyrexial or has signs suggesting an empyema of the gall-bladder. If a patient has symptoms which do not subside or if he becomes increasingly ill then blood cultures must be performed to exclude an *Esch. coli* septicaemia. In the ill patient not responding to conservative therapy and antibiotics there may be a place for operation during the acute phase. On the whole, however, this should be avoided if possible.

Complications of Gall-stones [FIG. 38]

The following are the chief complications of gall-stones:

Pancreatitis. There is an association between gall-bladder disease and pancreatitis. The precise cause of this relationship is unknown. Pancreatitis should be suspected if the attacks of pain are severe, localized to the epigastrium and radiate through to the back. In these circumstances the patient is usually very ill and the serum and urinary amylase levels are helpful in making diagnosis. The treatment is conservative, though a diagnostic laparotomy may, on occasions, be essential.

Obstructive Jaundice. A stone which migrates from the gall-bladder into the common bile-duct or which forms in the common bile-duct initially may cause obstructive

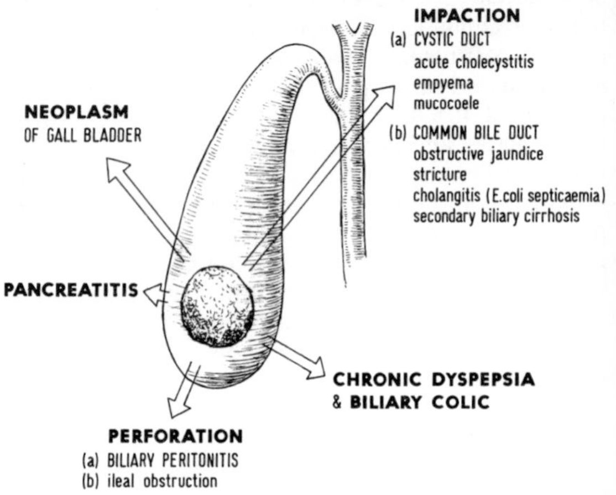

FIG. 38. The complications of gall-stones.

jaundice with a characteristic change in liver function tests. If this jaundice is not relieved either by spontaneous passage of the stone or by surgery, then an ascending infection and chronic biliary obstruction may cause secondary damage to the liver. In progressive cases this results in a secondary biliary cirrhosis.

Small Bowel Obstruction. An acutely inflamed gall-bladder containing a large solitary stone may rupture into adherent small bowel and produce intestinal obstruction when the stone impacts in the ileum. Patients will show the signs and symptoms of acute small bowel obstruction following an initial period of acute abdominal pain. The diagnosis can be suspected on plain X-ray of the abdomen which shows not only small bowel dilatation but the presence of gas in the biliary tree. The treatment is operative following fluid replacement and antibiotic cover.

Acute Ascending Cholangitis. [See p. 655].

Carcinoma of the Gall-bladder. [See p. 656].

POST-CHOLECYSTECTOMY SYNDROME AND BILIARY DYSKINESIA

POST-CHOLECYSTECTOMY SYNDROME

The physician is not uncommonly asked to see

patients with continuing or recurrent symptoms following cholecystectomy. Some of these patients will have other disorders in the alimentary tract such as hiatus hernia, peptic ulcer or irritable colon. Barium studies are essential to make the diagnosis. The surgeon will usually have excluded by intravenous cholangiography the biliary lesions which are known to be associated with symptoms such as bile-duct stricture or common duct stone (pain and recurrent jaundice) and a residual cystic duct stump—this latter lesion being of uncertain importance unless there is evidence of stone formation with it or subsequent stone migration into the common bile-duct.

Often difficulty is encountered in deciding whether a dilated common bile-duct is of significance or not. Here some knowledge of the state of the duct before cholecystectomy is required. A previously dilated duct may not decrease in calibre even if the pre-existing obstruction is removed. On the other hand, dilatation of a duct ($>$12 mm. diameter) on cholangiography known pre-operatively to have been of normal calibre obviously requires further investigation.

It is important to make sure that ischaemic heart disease is not the cause of the patient's symptoms and that recurrent pancreatitis has been excluded. Failure of the patient to obtain any relief at all from operation suggests improper pre-operative selection.

The physician also has the responsibility of making sure that the patient is not over-investigated, that further surgery is carried out only in the face of proper indications and that, for example, primary disease of the liver has been excluded. The physician must be able to explain in those cases where symptoms continue that serious organic disease has been appropriately excluded and in these circumstances firm reassurance to the patient and relatives can be given.

BILIARY DYSKINESIA

This term has been given to a variety of functional biliary disturbances, most important of all being sphincter of Oddi spasm. The basis of the existence of these disorders has rested on manometric studies which have demonstrated inappropriate pressures within the gall-bladder and biliary tree. It must be said straight away that biliary dyskinesia is a diagnosis which is rarely made in this country or the United States. In that it is impossible except under the highly abnormal conditions pertaining at laparotomy to obtain manometric studies on the human biliary tract it would appear of little value making this diagnosis to explain attacks of upper abdominal discomfort or symptoms following cholecystectomy, i.e. post-cholecystectomy syndrome when these are of unknown origin. This has been, however, a field for the trial of operations such as sphincterotomy or various operations to denervate the biliary system and as such the results do not on the whole stand up to critical review. Though spasm of the sphincter of Oddi may not be important in the pathogenesis of biliary symptoms, it is possible that fibrosis with resultant sphincter of Oddi stenosis may be more common than is usually realized and this may help to explain the more dramatic results of sphincter of Oddi surgery.

CHOLANGITIS

ACUTE 'ASCENDING' CHOLANGITIS

Definition

An acute infection of the extra- and intrahepatic biliary tract usually complicating gall-stones or other biliary obstruction.

Aetiology

The onset is usually sudden following impaction of a gall-stone in the common bile-duct. On occasions the cause of the biliary obstruction may be a traumatic or neoplastic stricture of the common bile-duct or it may complicate rare causes of such as these due to Ascaris or liver fluke infestation. An acute cholangitis may result from operations which allow free reflux of intestinal contents into the biliary tree such as sphincterotomy, cholecystenterostomy or choledochotomy with Roux en Y anastomosis.

Pathology

The bile-ducts above the obstruction are dilated and filled with purulent material. The liver is enlarged and may contain multiple abscess cavities related to the enlarged and acutely inflamed bile-ducts.

Clinical Picture

The onset of acute right upper abdominal pain, deepening jaundice, pyrexia and rigors is highly suggestive of this condition. The liver is enlarged and tender and if the infecting organism is an *Esch. coli* septicaemia peripheral circulatory failure may follow. The abdomen may show the scars of previous biliary tract operations and on occasions a plain X-ray of the abdomen will reveal gas in the biliary tree.

The liver function tests show evidence of obstructive jaundice—there is a polymorph leucocytosis in the blood and *Esch. coli* may be found on blood culture as well as in duodenal aspirate. Renal failure is an important complication in the jaundiced hypotensive patient.

Treatment

The basis of treatment is the use of massive doses of systemic antibiotics (tetracycline, ampicillin or *Rifamide*) to cure the acute infection. In patients with accompanying shock this may require fluid replacement, corticosteroids and the use of pressor amines. Providing the patient responds to this treatment investigation follows in the convalescent phase when any obstructive lesion in the biliary tree will, if possible, be dealt with surgically. In some cases of biliary stricture this procedure may entail difficult biliary tract surgery with excision of a stenosed area and re-anastomosis where this is possible. In this phase of treatment transhepatic cholangiography is an essential prerequisite investigation so that the cause and location of the obstructing lesion may be determined.

For patients not responsive to therapy in the acute phase, surgery is exceedingly dangerous but occasionally life saving. Drainage of the biliary tree above the obstructing lesion is followed in successful cases by later elective surgery of the causative stricture.

CHRONIC CHOLANGITIS (SECONDARY BILIARY CIRRHOSIS)

If biliary obstruction is not relieved and in particular if repeated attacks of cholangitis occur the liver may be irreversibly damaged. The infective process produces a fine micronodular fibrosis of the liver with inflammatory changes in the portal tracts and a fibrotic process linking the portal tracts with each other. Areas of hepatic necrosis result in regeneration and the presence of a true biliary cirrhosis. Accompanying this there may be evidence of portal hypertension and liver cell failure.

Clinical Picture

The patient has usually had biliary tract surgery and has mild obstructive jaundice with a history of attacks of cholangitis. The physical signs are of icterus, xanthomata and hepatosplenomegaly and in some patients evidence of liver cell failure (cutaneous stigmata—ascites, encephalopathy).

Helpful investigations include liver biopsy which will confirm the presence of an acute inflammatory process centred on the portal triads where there is polymorph infiltration. Evidence of cholestasis and cirrhosis may also be found. Liver function tests show a combined picture of biliary obstruction and liver cell disease whilst there are no antimitochondrial antibodies in the patient's serum (an important distinction from primary biliary cirrhosis). A transhepatic or operative cholangiogram is important for the demonstration of the extent and site of biliary obstruction.

Treatment

Treatment is based on the surgical relief of biliary obstruction wherever this is possible. By the time that hepatic fibrosis and cirrhosis have occurred the patient has usually undergone one or more operations. The resultant surgical problems are therefore considerable, the operation being made more difficult by multiple adhesions, increased congestion due to portal hypertension and damaged and fibrosed bile-ducts. In some cases corrective surgery may not be possible whilst in others biliary drainage can be achieved by bringing up a loop of bowel for anastomosis above the upper level of biliary obstruction, or even in some cases by T tube drainage of the common duct. In some cases where there is portal hypertension an initial portacaval shunt may make adhesions less vascular so that biliary surgery can then be attempted.

If no alleviation of biliary obstruction is possible treatment is conservative, with diuretic therapy for oedema or ascites and continuous antibiotics for the prevention of cholangitis.

It cannot be over-stressed that no patient should be labelled as primary biliary cirrhosis if there is any possibility that the lesion is due to common bile-duct obstruction. Liver biopsy, antimitochondrial antibody studies and cholangiography are helpful in making this distinction.

SCLEROSING CHOLANGITIS

Definition

A rare chronic obstructive disorder of the bile-ducts due to progressive fibrosis of the duct system.

Clinical Picture

This disease may complicate ulcerative colitis and also may be seen with other diseases known to be associated with abnormal fibrosis. These include retroperitoneal and mediastinal fibrosis, Riedel's thyroiditis and rarities such as pseudotumour of the orbit. The picture is one of intermittent obstructive jaundice with superadded attacks of cholangitis. The patient may be a known sufferer from ulcerative colitis and in any case it is always worthwhile X-raying the large bowel to see whether there is radiological evidence of this disease. The diagnosis is usually made at laparotomy when the bile-ducts are narrowed and thickened, and operative cholangiography shows a beaded appearance due to multiple strictures with intervening areas of dilatation. In the event of biopsy being possible this shows a chronic inflammatory process with fibrosis in the wall of the affected bile-ducts. Occasionally this spreads into the liver to affect the intrahepatic major bile-ducts and the gall-bladder which becomes chronically thickened.

Treatment

There is no satisfactory treatment for this disease which is thought to be of a generalized collagen variety with its maximal effect on the bile-ducts and certain other structures in the body. Antibiotics such as rifamycin are extremely useful when the patient has superadded infection and a trial of azathioprine may be useful as a way of preventing progression of the disease along the bile-ducts. Though the disease may be a chronic one there is always the possibility of death from secondary biliary cirrhosis and ascending sepsis with liver failure.

TUMOURS OF THE GALL-BLADDER AND BILIARY PASSAGES

CARCINOMA OF THE GALL-BLADDER

Aetiology

Carcinomata arising from the gall-bladder are usually (70–90 per cent.) associated with gall-stones so that chronic mucosal irritation and inflammation are important aetiological factors. However, whilst gall-stones are common (30 per cent. of routine post-mortems in subjects over 60 years of age show them) carcinoma of the gall-bladder is rare. It is commoner in women (as are gall-stones) and is usually an adenocarcinoma. It spreads by direct growth into liver and neighbouring structures as well as by lymphatic and possibly vascular routes.

Clinical Picture

The diagnosis is difficult simply because many sufferers are thought to have a pancreatic or bile-duct tumour. The early symptoms are often those of gall-stones and a carcinoma may be found at operation by accident. Rarely a tumour will show on cholecystography. The most important symptom is progressive obstructive jaundice often with severe right upper abdominal pain. Rarely ascites due to direct invasion of the peritoneum or portal vein is the first symptom, but the classical physical signs are obstructive jaundice, hepatomegaly and in severe cases a palpable mass due to the tumour. Helpful investigations include transhepatic cholangiography and on some occasions before the onset of jaundice, a cholecystogram. Peritoneoscopy is also worth considering as the diagnosis from the nodularity of the cirrhotic liver may be difficult and cirrhotic patients should not for obvious reasons be subjected to unnecessary laparotomy. Scintiscanning, particularly using ^{131}I Rose Bengal in those patients with obstructive jaundice, may show absence of gall-bladder concentration and obstruction of biliary flow into the gut.

Treatment

In many patients the diagnosis is made only at laparotomy in a patient with persistent obstructive jaundice—and with a chronically inflamed and thickened gall-bladder. The diagnosis may require frozen section facilities. The results of simple excision are bad (5 year survival 2–3 per cent.) and if the diagnosis is certain, and if there are no extrahepatic metastases, the modern approach, if spread is unequivocal and in a reasonably fit patient, would be right hepatic lobectomy. A local excision of the gall-bladder and hepatic tissue immediately adjacent to it suffices for less invasive growths.

CARCINOMA OF THE BILE-DUCTS; CARCINOMA OF THE AMPULLA OF VATER

A primary tumour of the bile-ducts may occur anywhere along the length of the major ducts, but is commonest either at the ampulla of Vater or at the junction of the two main hepatic ducts.

Pathology

The tumour is small and constricts the bile-ducts and is usually an adenocarcinoma with a variable stromal response. At the ampulla the tumour may have an origin either from the mucosa of the ampulla itself or from the adjacent pancreatic or biliary ducts. There is no relationship with the presence of gall-stones. Rare examples are known to occur in conditions of biliary obstruction and/or infection. They may complicate liver fluke obstruction of the bile-duct (*Clonorchis sinensis*) and the cholestatic syndrome of ulcerative colitis.

Clinical Picture

The clinical picture is of painless progressive obstructive jaundice with gradual development of hepatomegaly and splenomegaly. The patient may have few complaints apart from severe itching and icterus. There are few physical signs apart from hepatomegaly and splenomegaly though occasionally the gall-bladder may be palpable if the growth is in the ampullary region. The lesion is slow to metastasize, so that evidence of extension is not usually seen. If jaundice is chronic then xanthomata may appear together with a chronic bleeding tendency and there may be wasting due to steatorrhoea.

Diagnosis

In patients with ampullary neoplasms the occult blood test in the faeces may be positive. The liver function tests merely mirror the presence of obstruction without indicating its site. Radiological examination of the alimentary tract in some patients with ampullary growths may show a filling defect where the tumour invades the loop of the duodenal loop, a so-called 'reversed three' sign. In patients with lesions in the biliary ducts there are no changes in the barium meal apart from those of malabsorption. A tumour of the hepatic ducts is best demonstrated by a transhepatic cholangiogram [PLATE 2]. This is performed by inserting a needle through the liver aiming towards the major ducts at the hilum and aspirating to determine when it lies in a bile-filled duct. Contrast material is injected into the biliary tree after aspiration of bile. Bile can be sent to the laboratory for cytological examination for malignant cells and for bacterial culture. After the radiological procedure has been completed the patient is taken to the theatre for laparotomy and surgical treatment.

In the case of an ampullary growth the operation is a partial pancreatectomy, with removal of the duodenum and anastomosis of the stomach to the jejunum. In the case of a bile-duct neoplasm formal removal of the tumour is usually impossible, but some form of by-pass operation may be feasible. If this is not so the patient faces a long period of chronic obstructive jaundice. In these circumstances skin irritation can be relieved with cholestyramine and complications such as bone thinning and bruising prevented by the use of injections of fat-soluble vitamins D and K.

Survival for many months after the demonstration of hepatic duct carcinoma is well recorded and in patients who are successfully operated on for an ampullary carcinoma long-term survival is also occasionally recorded.

REFERENCES

Gall-stones

RAINS, A. J. H., (1968) Gall-stone disease, *Brit. med. J.*, **1,** 295.

BOUCHIER, I. A. D., and FRESTON, J. W. (1968) The aetiology of gall-stones, *Lancet*, i, 340.

Carcinoma of the Bile-ducts

WHELTON, M. J., PETRELLI, M., GEORGE, P., YOUNG, W. B., and SHERLOCK, S. (1969) Carcinoma at the junction of the main hepatic ducts, *Quart. J. Med.*, **38,** 211.

Sclerosing Cholangitis

THORPE, M. E. C., SCHEUER, P. J., and SHERLOCK, S. (1967) Primary sclerosing cholangitis of the biliary tree and ulcerative colitis, *Gut*, **8,** 435.

Atresia of the Bile-ducts

MILLER, S., FONKALSRUD, E. W., and LONGMIRE, W. P. (1966) Current concepts in the management of congenital biliary atresia, *Arch. Surg.*, **93,** 813.

Carcinoma of the Gall-bladder

RIVKIN, L. M. (1955) Carcinoma of gall-bladder. Report of 52 operative cases and resumé of the literature, *Arch. Surg.*, **70,** 128.

THE PANCREAS

INTRODUCTION

The pancreas is a gland with both exocrine and endocrine functions. The secretory tissue is composed of acini and these pour their digestive secretion into the pancreatic duct system. Amongst the secretory acini are islets of alpha and beta cells. The former secrete glucagon and the latter insulin. These two secretions are delivered directly into the blood stream. The exocrine or digestive secretion contains a high concentration of bicarbonate as well as electrolytes. The enzymes found in this juice are the product of the acini and they are amylase, lipase, trypsin, chymotrypsin and carboxypeptidase. These last three are secreted as inactive precursors and they only become active when they enter the duodenum. The activator is a locally produced duodenal enzyme enterokinase. This obviously prevents the gland from being digested by its own secretions. The control of pancreatic exocrine secretion is largely via the hormone secretin which is released from the duodenal mucosa when acid gastric juice enters the duodenum. It causes a profuse flow of pancreatic juice with a high bicarbonate concentration. Another hormone, pancreozymin, is also released from the duodenal mucosa in response to a large variety of foods. This causes pancreatic secretion with a juice rich in enzymes. It is identical in structure to cholecystokinin. The pancreas is also partially under the control of the central nervous system. The endocrine secretion, insulin, is stimulated by a rise in the blood glucose concentration. It has been shown that the insulin released is greater when glucose is given orally than when given intravenously. This suggests that a substance is released from the small bowel and secondarily stimulates the secretion of insulin. This substance is certainly an enzyme and may be secretin, pancreozymin or glucagon.

FIBROCYSTIC DISEASE

With the advent of effective chemotherapy the chances of sufferers from this disease surviving until adult life are of the order of 70 per cent. so that reference to it in a textbook of adult medicine is appropriate.

Aetiology

The disease which is inherited as an autosomal recessive and is characterized by a widespread disorder of mucus-secreting glands. The mucus is unduly viscid and this leads to retention of secretions secondary infection and fibrosis. This is particularly noticeable in the gut, bronchi, pancreas and liver. A basic abnormality of sodium reabsorption from the sweat glands is also found.

Clinical Picture

In the newborn intestinal obstruction due to impaction of viscid intestinal secretions may be a rare presentation. More commonly the young child fails to thrive, develops diarrhoea with loose bulky stools and suffers from repeated chest infections. The physical signs are of impaired growth, intestinal distension, wasting and often rectal prolapse. There may be enlargement of the liver due to secondary biliary cirrhosis due to bile-duct obstruction and this may be complicated by portal hypertension. In this event there is splenomegaly.

There is an excessive loss of sodium in the sweat and mucus-secreting glands and this may result in excessive sodium loss and fluid depletion in hot weather.

Diagnosis

The diagnosis rests on the basis of the discovery of malabsorption accompanied by chest infection whilst the simplest diagnostic test is the measurement of sweat concentration.

Sweat Sodium. There are various methods of collecting sweat for sodium estimation. The most convenient and simplest is by iontophoresis using pilocarpine. Sweat sodium levels (normal 60 mEq. per litre are elevated, figures varying from 70 to 140 mEq. per litre).

Malabsorption. Characteristically there is malabsorption only of fat as the intestinal mucosa is intact.

Lungs. A suppurative pneumonia and secondary bronchiestasis normally due to infection with *Staphylococcus aureus* is the usual finding. In time emphysema is an added complication.

Biopsy. Histological examination of the jejunal mucosa may be a useful way of demonstrating abnormal mucous glands but a simpler method is based on the fact that the rectal glands are similarly obstructed due to abnormal mucus and this can be a simple and non-traumatic diagnostic aid.

Treatment

The basis is the treatment of malabsorption and the treatment of chronic chest infection. The former is fairly easily achieved with a low-fat high-protein diet and pancreatic hormone replacement, e.g. with *Cotazym*, 2–3 capsules powdered over each main meal. The problem of lung infection is more difficult. Continuous or intermittent courses of antibiotics either given systemically or by aerosol inhalation are the basis of treatment. The part to be played by mucolytic agents such as methyl cysteine (bromhexine) and mist tents is less certain. Antibiotics, to be of value, must be effective against the infecting bacteria which are usually staphylococci, *Haemophilus influenzae* and pseudomonas. Penicillin, cloxacillin and cephaloridine are therefore amongst the most useful agents. Portal hypertension may also require treatment.

PANCREATITIS

ACUTE PANCREATITIS

Aetiology

This disease is of unknown cause. It is generally

accepted, however, that there is a connexion with biliary disease in some cases which may be associated with reflux of bile along the pancreatic duct. In others biliary infection may some how produce pancreatic damage. It seems likely that whatever initiates the acute injury, ischaemia and activation of protein-splitting enzymes are likely to increase the local pancreatic and tissue damage. Acute pancreatitis is also seen in acute alcoholism and after abdominal operations. The disease is commoner in this country in women, probably because of its association in about 30 per cent. of cases with gall-stones and biliary tract disease.

Pathology

There is an acute inflammatory and occasionally haemorrhagic process in the pancreas with destruction of glandular tissue, polymorph infiltration and necrosis. The surrounding tissues are also affected and there may be exudation of fluid into the lesser sac of the peritoneal cavity. Fat necrosis may be seen in the mesentery surrounding the inflamed pancreas and occasionally in subcutaneous or bone marrow fat. The presence of biliary tract disease and gall-stones may also be verified.

Clinical Features

The patient usually complains of severe upper abdominal pain, usually maximal in the epigastrium, which radiates to the back and which is accompanied by the signs of peripheral circulatory collapse. These are pallor, coldness, tachycardia and hypotension. The patient often looks cyanosed and on abdominal examination there are rigidity and signs of peritoneal irritation. Occasionally there is a discoloration of the skin in the loins (Grey Turner's sign) or around the umbilicus (Cullen's sign) where there is tracking of inflammatory and haemorrhagic exudate.

Diagnosis

The diagnosis is in some cases difficult but it should be considered in any patient with severe abdominal pain and collapse, but obviously perforation of a viscus, coronary thrombosis and acute cholecystitis are other possibilities. With reference to myocardial infarction it should be noted that alteration of the ECG with ST depression, probably due to electrolyte disturbances, is occasionally seen in patients with pancreatitis, and should not lead to confusion. The most helpful test is a serum amylase, the normal level being up to 150 Somogyi units per 100 ml. Elevation of the serum amylase to over 1000 Somogyi units is diagnostic of this condition. Serum lipase or urinary lipase and iso-amylase estimations may also be helpful. A plain X-ray of the abdomen may occasionally show gall-stones, or a dilated small bowel due to accompanying ileus. The blood count may show a polymorphonuclear leucocytosis, though the haemoglobin is usually normal or even increased due to vomiting and dehydration. Sugar may often be found in the urine and the blood glucose level may be raised or abnormally low. If hypotension is profound the picture of oliguric renal failure with a rising blood urea and serum potassium may occur. Serum calcium and the serum potassium may be low, the former due perhaps to precipitation in areas of fat necrosis and the latter due to the accompanying vomiting and fluid exudation into gut and peritoneum.

Treatment

The treatment should be conservative and laparotomy only considered where there is diagnostic difficulty or where there is biliary tract disease which needs urgent treatment. The latter would be suggested by the presence of jaundice and liver function tests showing an obstructive profile. Apart from this the patient is treated in bed and no fluids and solids are given by mouth. An intravenous drip is set up and the blood volume is restored. Fluid and electrolyte requirements are maintained by intravenous infusion. Accurate fluid balance recordings in this situation are essential. Because of the stimulatory effect of secretin on pancreatic function the stomach is aspirated and atropine, probanthine or other anticholinergic drugs are given. The important part probably played by activation of pancreatic enzymes has led to the use of inhibitors of the actions of trypsin and chymotrypsin. The agent most used has been *Trasylol*. This is a biological preparation extracted from bovine parotid tissue which has an inhibitory effect on pancreatic trypsin, but not lipase or amylase. Reports on the efficacy of *Trasylol* are not particularly encouraging. It is given by intravenous infusion, 200,000 units at once being followed by 80,000 units daily for 5 days.

In a favourable case the patient gradually improves with this conservative regime and the pain and peritoneal reaction subside. Following the remission the patient's biliary tract must be X-rayed to exclude disease in this organ.

Complications

The complications of acute pancreatitis are:

1. Intestinal obstruction due to ileus associated with pancreatitis.
2. Oliguric renal failure.
3. Hypotension and shock.
4. Hypo- or hyperglycaemia.
5. Hypocalcaemia.
6. Abscess formation.

Prognosis

The prognosis of acute pancreatitis must be guarded and there is an appreciable mortality of the order of 10 per cent. Patients who recover from the acute incident may develop relapsing pancreatitis with repeated acute attacks. There is a risk of addiction to strong analgesic drugs if this happens. It is now well recognized that patients with acute pancreatitis do not progress to the phase of chronic pancreatitis with complete destruction of the gland.

CHRONIC PANCREATITIS

Definition

Chronic pancreatitis is a disorder of the pancreas characterized by destruction of glandular tissue, the formation of fibrous tissue and calcification. As a result of this the pancreas is shrunken and thickened and there is dilatation of the pancreatic ducts. The end picture is one of failure of endocrine and exocrine pancreatic function.

Aetiology

The cause of chronic pancreatitis and of chronic relapsing pancreatitis is difficult to determine. Undoubtedly in some patients it is due to chronic alcoholism. Unlike acute pancreatitis biliary disease does not seem to be important.

A form of chronic destruction of the pancreas, often painless, is recorded in some tropical areas, particularly East Africa. The cause of this syndrome is unknown, though it seems likely that chronic protein malnutrition could at least be a factor.

Hyperparathydroidism may be associated with chronic relapsing pancreatitis, and a further form of this disorder has been described as a rare finding in some families where, apart from the pancreatic dysfunction, there is a urinary aminoaciduria.

Pathology

The gland is reduced in size, fibrosed and on sectioning may be calcified. The pancreatic ducts may be dilated, and may contain calculi. On microscopy there is destruction of the secretory apparatus and at least in the initial stages there may be preservation of the islets of Langerhans.

Clinical Picture

The course of chronic pancreatitis is usually punctuated by episodes of severe pain. The pain may be aggravated by a heavy meal or alcohol. It usually lasts for 24–48 hours and is not relieved by alkalis or the vomiting which accompanies it. The supine position may bring some relief. It is usually felt in the epigastrium but may travel widely in the abdomen and to the shoulders or to the back. Attacks of pain may be accompanied by diarrhoea with pale, greasy, bulky stools. Painful eructations are said to be characteristic symptom of involvement of the tail of the pancreas. On examination at this stage the patient may be found in a characteristic position sitting upwards, leaning forwards or supporting himself with his elbows on his knees. The abdomen is tender, but there is usually no frank peritonism. The stools are pale and there may be glycosuria.

Diagnosis

The diagnosis of chronic pancreatitis should be considered in any patient who has an unexplained malabsorption syndrome, particularly if associated with abdominal pain. It should be remembered that sometimes chronic pancreatitis runs a painless course and then the symptoms and signs may be only those of malabsorption of its complications or of mild diabetes. The following tests will be found to be of use in the diagnosis of this disease. A glucose tolerance test may show a diabetic curve, or there may be frank glycosuria. Examination of the stools may show the presence of steatorrhoea (passage of greater than 6 g. of fat per day) and there may be undigested muscle fibres on microscopy.

A plain X-ray of the abdomen may show calcification of the pancreas [PLATE 2], and a barium meal examination a non-specific pattern of malabsorption. Recent scanning techniques with selenomethionine labelled with ^{22}Se may demonstrate a failure of uptake of the material in patients with chronic damage to the pancreas. This technique, however, is relatively new and little experience of it has so far been obtained.

In patients with acute bouts of pain there may be elevation of the serum amylase or lipase values just as there are in the acute form of the disease. The presence of chronic irreversible destruction of the pancreas can, however, only be proven by the use of pancreatic function tests. The most satisfactory is the secretin or secretin-pancreozymin test. In this test the duodenum is intubated and the duodenal contents are quantitatively aspirated free from acid, whilst gastric secretion is removed by gastric aspiration. The characteristic response in chronic pancreatitis is a reduced total volume of secretion, a reduced maximal bicarbonate concentration, and in some cases, a reduced enzyme output following pancreozymin. The most important measurements are probably those of volume and bicarbonate. The secretin-pancreozymin test distinguishes chronic pancreatitis where there is gland destruction from recurrent acute pancreatitis where there is usually normal function between attacks. Recently it has been shown that where there is failure of exocrine function of the pancreas, iron absorption from the small bowel may be increased so that the patient may have increased tissue iron on biopsy.

Treatment

A distinction must be made on the basis of the history and of the response of the pancreas to stimulation as to whether the patient has chronic pancreatitis or the relapsing form. The latter is often associated with biliary disease and responds well to the removal of gall-stones or treatment of other biliary abnormalities. In chronic pancreatitis there is usually no biliary disease and the treatment is symptomatic in most patients. The acute attack is treated with analgesics, intravenous fluid and gastric aspiration. It therefore differs little from the treatment of acute pancreatitis, though the attacks are not generally so severe. Upon recovery the patient must be assessed for biliary tract disease, placed on a low-fat high-protein diet, and alcohol forbidden, even where alcohol does not seem to be a precipitating factor. Diabetes may need treatment by carbohydrate restriction or with insulin. It is unlikely that oral hypoglycaemic agents will be effective, for they depend on stimulating the pancreas to produce more insulin. If attacks of pancreatitis remain troublesome, then it is justifiable to seek surgical relief. This is usually done by exploring the pancreas, performing X-ray studies on the duct system, looking for obstruction due to stones or strictures, and alleviating it where this is possible. Another approach is excision of the diseased part of the pancreas and anastomosis of the more healthy tissue with its patent duct system to the jejunum. Sphincterotomy seems to be less successful and less widely practised than it was, and for this reason thorough radiological and surgical exploration of the duct system seems to be justified. It must not be forgotten that these patients are poor surgical risks; they are often debilitated and pulmonary tuberculosis is a not uncommon complication. Apart from treatment with a low-fat diet the addition of a potent lipase may bring about a significant improvement in fat absorption. Various preparations are obtainable and of these *Cotazyme* in a dose of 3 capsules four times a day with meals seems to be as effective as any.

TUMOURS AND CYSTS

PANCREATIC CYSTS AND PSEUDOCYSTS

True pancreatic cysts are uncommon and are usually due to retention of pancreatic secretions by impaction of duct calculi or they are associated with congenital cystic disease or hydatid disease.

A pseudocyst of the pancreas is due to a collection of fluid in the walled lesser sac of the peritoneum. It is the result of trauma or more usually acute pancreatitis. It can grow to a considerable size and present as a supra-umbilical cystic swelling which transmits aortic pulsation and with colonic resonance on percussion across it. Diagnosis is considerably helped by barium meal examination which shows characteristic forward displacement of the stomach, and also by coeliac axis angiography or ultrasound. Treatment is by surgical means which drains the cyst into the stomach or colon.

CARCINOMA OF THE PANCREAS

Aetiology

The tumour is usually an adenocarcinoma, but malignant change may also be seen in islet-cell tumours, and these will be discussed separately. It accounts for about 2 per cent. of all cancers.

Clinical Picture

The early symptoms of the patient with a pancreatic carcinoma may be minimal. They include pain in the abdomen, frequently related to meals, and sometimes radiating to the back or to the shoulders. It is dull, persistent and sometimes relieved by leaning forward. It may closely mimic that of peptic ulcer. There is loss of weight, and attacks of diarrhoea may occur associated in some cases with steatorrhoea. Some patients may complain of a vague ill health, depression and anxiety, and it is important to remember the association of psychological symptoms with carcinoma of the pancreas. With carcinoma of the body of the pancreas symptoms may be caused by the development of diabetes, and this is often unstable. A further important finding in some patients is multiple superficial venous thromboses which tend to be associated with cancer of the body or tail (thrombophlebitis migrans). Carcinoma of the head of the pancreas invariably causes one important further symptom; the development of progressive obstructive jaundice with pale stools, dark urine and pruritus. There may be an enlargement of the gall-bladder and of the liver. It is unusual for a pancreatic mass to be palpable except in very thin subjects. The patients usually have evidence of weight loss and there may be evidence of metastases at a distance, such as in the liver or in the lungs.

Diagnosis

The following tests are helpful in proving the diagnosis.

Examination of the blood may show mild anaemia and a raised sedimentation rate. The stools may give a positive occult blood reaction, particularly if there is invasion of the duodenal loop. The urine may contain glucose and bile and a glucose tolerance curve may show a diabetic response. The serum amylase is often raised when there is obstruction of the main pancreatic duct.

Radiological investigation may reveal deformity of the duodenal loop, or abnormal motility on screening. An intravenous cholangiogram is of no value in the icteric subject, but it may be possible by transhepatic cholangiography to show dilatation of the main bile-duct system due to a lesion of the head of the pancreas. Two further techniques may be of value. Scintiscanning of the pancreas with selinomethionine may show a filling defect. Estimation of pancreatic secretion following a secretin-pancreozymin injection, may reveal a reduced response but relatively normal bicarbonate and enzyme concentrations are found if the pancreatic duct is unobstructed.

The differential diagnosis in patients with obstructive jaundice includes jaundice due to gall-stones, malignant tumours of the ampulla of Vater, and of the hepatic ducts, as well as prolonged jaundice due to drugs and hepatitis. In patients who are not icteric the differential diagnosis can be extremely difficult, and includes ulcer dyspepsia, carcinoma of the stomach and of the colon, as well as the malabsorption syndrome and psychoneurosis.

Treatment

Treatment of malignant lesions of the body or tail of the pancreas is by formal pancreatico-duodenectomy. The long-term results of this type of surgery are poor, though no doubt they could be improved if the pancreatic carcinoma could be diagnosed earlier. Vitamin K is given by intramuscular injection before surgery. Postoperative renal failure is a hazard in those with a high serum bilirubin.

INSULINOMA OF THE PANCREAS (BETA-CELL ADENOMA)

Aetiology

This is a rare insulin-secreting tumour of the beta cells of the islets. It therefore causes symptoms due to hypoglycaemia.

Clinical Features

Patients with an insulinoma suffer periodic bouts of confusion, diplopia, faintness and sweating, or from frank epilepsy. The other significant feature is that these attacks are relieved by the taking of food or glucose. Diagnostic difficulties may occur with the mental symptoms which are often thought to be due to psychosis or psychoneurosis. The tumour produces few symptoms due to its size, though the tumour is malignant in about 15 per cent. of cases and may then metastasize. In progressive cases the patient may go into coma because of the profound hypoglycaemia. The diagnosis in the early stages is difficult, and many patients are diagnosed as having vasovagal attacks or of 'blackouts' and the true nature of the abnormality is often missed. Fluctuating neurological symptoms of many types may occur.

Investigation

The key investigation in these patients is the serum glucose, and if this is determined when the patient is in an attack then the level is less than 50 mg. per 100 ml. The diagnosis may be confirmed by the therapeutic response to intravenous 20 per cent. glucose. In patients who are seen between attacks confirmation can usually be obtained by fasting the patient for 12–24 hours or even longer. Monitoring the serum glucose level and also monitoring the EEG, which in hypoglycaemia becomes progressively slower, are helpful. A tolbutamide tolerance test (1 g. of sodium tolbutamide intravenously) may produce very profound hypoglycaemia and hyperinsulinaemia and its action should be monitored very carefully, and intravenous 50 per cent. glucose should always be available. Coeliac axis angiography may be helpful in diagnosis as these tumours are highly vascular and may show a tumour circulation. The differential diagnosis of this condition includes *functional hyperinsulism* where there is thought to be an excessive response to the normal stimulus for insulin secretion and *factitious hyperinsulism* due to injection of excessive amounts of insulin, and *organic hyperinsulism* due to the presence of a massive and often retroperitoneal tumours [see Section 4].

Treatment

The treatment of choice is an exploration of the pancreas and removal of the tumour. Some of these are multiple and therefore thorough mobilization and visualization is essential. A frozen section is helpful prior to enucleating the lesion under suspicion. In the difficult cases where no tumour is found in the pancreas or in the usual sites for ectopic pancreatic tissue it is probably worth while resecting the body and the tail of the gland. If surgical treatment is not possible, or if symptoms recur after operation then drugs can be used to combat further attacks of hypoglycaemia. These include corticosteroids and diazoxide, whilst a diet low in carbohydrate is also helpful in diminishing the stimulus to the abnormal source of insulin. The operative mortality for resection of lesions in the pancreas is about 8 per cent. It should be remembered that multiple tumours may make operative therapy unsuccessful and that multiple endocrine tumours of the parathyroid, pituitary and adrenal may occur and need treatment.

THE ZOLLINGER-ELLISON SYNDROME

This disorder is due to the presence of a non-β-cell adenoma or islet-cell hyperplasia of the pancreas which produces gastrin. The syndrome is therefore associated with excessive gastric secretion. It occurs at any age and one third of the tumours become malignant.

Pathology

The tumours are often multiple; they measure up to a centimetre in diameter and are composed of small cells in nests separated by a broad stroma. Though 90 per cent. are found in the pancreas and two-thirds of these are located in the body or tail it must not be forgotten that 10 per cent. of tumours are ectopic, in the spleen or in the wall of the stomach or duodenum, and these sites are of importance when surgery has failed to show an intrapancreatic lesion.

Clinical Picture

The disease is characterized by the presence of the symptoms of peptic ulceration which is atypical in the following ways. The symptoms are remarkably persistent; the ulcers are in unusual sites and classically occur in the jejunum; there is gastric hypersecretion so that a one hour unstimulated total of 40 mEq. of acid is not unusual, and the overnight gastric juice may be of the order of 2 litres in volume and may contain 200 mEq. or more of hydrochloric acid. The rate of secretion is uninfluenced by the giving of secretagogue drugs.

Further abnormalities are known to occur in this syndrome and the patient not infrequently complains of attacks of diarrhoea sufficiently severe to cause potassium deficiency and of wasting; on occasions there may be a frank steatorrhoea. The symptoms of ulcer dyspepsia are complicated by bleeding and perforation. Local resection of the ulcer is soon followed by recurrence of ulceration.

Diagnosis

The diagnosis should be suspected in any patient with multiple ulcers, particularly in abnormal situations such as in the jejunum and particularly, too, where there is a history of ulcer complications following gastric surgery.

Radiology may demonstrate ulceration in the small bowel as well as in the duodenum and stomach and may also reveal the presence of a malabsorption picture. Studies of gastric secretion performed overnight or after a secretagogue drug will show high volumes of gastric juice and high gastric acidity.

Techniques to identify gastrin, which is the responsible hormone, either in the blood stream or in the urine using a bioassay technique, are at the moment showing promise. It is not unknown for patients with the Zollinger-Ellison syndrome to develop other endocrine tumours in the pituitary, parathyroids, adrenals, etc. These patients are examples of the 'multiple adenoma syndrome' and this possibility should be borne in mind and estimations of serum calcium, pituitary and adrenal function tests made in suspicious cases.

Treatment

The only satisfactory treatment for this condition is surgical excision of the tumour with total gastrectomy. If tumour removal is complete then the gastric operation may not be necessary, but in fact tumours are often multiple and not infrequently malignant and the patient succumbs because of the troublesome gastric complications. It is also important that the surgeon should consider the diagnosis of Zollinger-Ellison syndrome in any patient with persistent peptic ulceration, particularly if there is a relapse following previous operation. In patients who are unsuitable or unwilling to have surgical treatment it is possible for there to be some control of the profound gastric hypersecretion with anticholinergic drugs, such as poldine sulphate (*Nacton*) in maximal doses. It is possible, too, that a gastrin antagonist may in time be suitable and effective enough for the medical treatment of some patients with this disorder.

REFERENCES

The Pancreas

Fibrocystic Disease of the Pancreas

Di Sant 'Agnese, P. A., and Talamo, C. (1967) Cystic fibrosis of the pancreas, *New Engl. J. Med.*, **277**, 1287, 1344.

Acute Pancreatitis

Fleming, L. B. (1968) Pancreatitis, *Brit. med. J.*, **1**, 813.

Trapnell, J. E. (1968) The pathogenesis of gall-stone pancreatitis, *Postgrad. med. J.*, **44**, 497.

Chronic Pancreatitis

Howat, H. T. (1968) Chronic pancreatitis; medical aspects, *Postgrad. med. J.*, **44**, 733.

Carcinoma of the Pancreas

Broadbent, T. R., and Kerman, H. D. (1951) One hundred cases of carcinoma of the pancreas; a clinical and roentgenologic analysis, *Gastroenterology*, **17**, 163.

Zollinger-Ellison Syndrome

Zollinger, R. M., and Ellison, E. H. (1955) Primary peptic ulceration of the jejunum with islet cell tumours of the pancreas, *Ann. Surg.*, **142**, 709.

Insulinoma

Howard, J. M., Moss, N. H., and Rhoads, J. E. (1950) Collective review: hyperinsulinism and islet cell tumours of the pancreas with 398 recorded tumours, *Surg. Gynec. Obstet.*, **90**, 417.

THE PERITONEUM AND MESENTERY

ASCITES

The accumulation of fluid within the abdominal cavity is known as ascites. When small in amount (less than one litre) this may cause no signs or symptoms but with progressive accumulation the abdomen distends and clinical signs are recognizable.

Clinical Features

The abdomen is distended with prominent elongation of its upper segment, i.e. increased distance from xiphisternum to umbilicus. In chronic cases, where abdominal muscles are lax, swelling causes bulging into the loins. There may be prominent veins on the abdominal wall even in patients without portal hypertension, and in cases of generalized fluid retention the abdominal wall shows pitting oedema.

On percussion there is a central area of gut resonance whilst the flanks and suprapubic region remain dull. This pattern of dullness shifts when the patient lies first on one then on the other side as the fluid is tipped away from raised loin. The amount of shift is conveniently measured in the supine and lateral position with the end of a skin pencil. This physical sign, if positive, is known as shifting dullness. It is essential for the diagnosis of ascites that the physical sign is found in *both* loins. If ascites is tense a fluid thrill may be transmitted through the ascitic fluid when the abdominal wall is flicked with the fingers.

Apart from these physical signs there may be others related to the particular cause of the ascites.

In Chronic Liver Disease. Ascites is due to portal hypertension, increased hepatic lymph production and a low serum albumin level. Icterus, cutaneous signs of liver disease and hepatosplenomegaly may be found. The latter may only be found when ascites is not tense. The ascitic fluid is of low protein content unless there is complicating hepatoma.

Hypo-albuminaemia. When due to malabsorption or nephrotic syndrome ascites is seen as part of a generalized oedema with fluid in other body centres. The fluid is of low protein concentration.

Neoplastic Disease. In neoplastic disease of the peritoneum the ascites is accompanied by nodular hepatic enlargement or other masses in the abdominal cavity. There is gross wasting and evidence may be found of lymph node enlargement or of pelvic tumour formation. The ascitic fluid may be of high protein content and contain malignant cells. One benign neoplasm is sometimes associated with ascites. This is a fibroma of the ovary. The resultant combination of ascites associated with this tumour is called Meigs' syndrome. It is of importance because it means that a pelvic examination by a gynaecologist is of great importance in female patients with ascites. This lesion, which is sometimes accompanied by pleural effusion, is easily correctable by surgery.

Tuberculous Peritonitis. [See p. 665].

Heart Failure. Ascites is rare in heart failure unless the latter is prolonged, severe and affects the right side of the heart. Lesions such as tricuspid valve disease, constrictive pericarditis, and in the tropics, endomyocardial fibrosis, are the important causes. Diagnosis is usually easy though a very high venous pressure in the neck may be missed by not examining the patient sitting up, and a secondary cardiac 'cirrhosis' may confuse by its association with abnormal liver function tests.

Budd-Chiari Syndrome. In Budd-Chiari syndrome ascites is always present though it can be controlled by diuretic therapy. The fluid is often of high protein content and it is usually accompanied by tender hepatomegaly.

Myxoedema. Ascites is rarely seen in myxoedema.

SPECIAL TYPES OF ASCITES

Ascites due to obstruction of the thoracic duct or other major lymphatics in the root of the small bowel vicinity may give rise to *chylous* ascites. This is milky on inspection and contains fat particles 'chylomicrons' which dissolve with fat solvents. The cause is usually a neoplastic one—lymphoma invading the para-aortic glands being the usual cause and in these cases the fluid may be both milky and haemorrhagic. In others the condition arises because of operative damage to the cisterna chyli or thoracic duct or is associated with a congenital abnormality of lymphatic vessels. Chronic ascites may be associated with milky opacification. This is chyliform ascites, the turbidity being due to cellular debris.

PARACENTESIS

Diagnostic paracentesis is indicated in *all* patients with ascites as examination of ascitic fluid may be extremely helpful in making a diagnosis. If ascites is tense, therapeutic paracentesis may be necessary but it should be pointed out that if hypoproteinaemia is the cause, e.g. nephrotic syndrome, liver disease, etc., paracentesis may rob the patient of valuable protein and in the patient with hepatic cirrhosis there is a real risk of hepatic coma and severe electrolyte imbalance. For treatment of ascites in liver disease see page 645.

PERITONITIS

ACUTE PERITONITIS

Aetiology

Acute primary peritonitis may be the result of perforation of a viscus, e.g. the stomach or gall-bladder, into the peritoneal cavity. The cause of this may be ulceration, trauma, either spontaneous or surgical, such as leakage from an intestinal anastomosis. Peritonitis may also result from spread of infection from inflamed abdominal structures such as the appendix or Fallopian tubes, and where there has been devitalization of tissue by ischaemia, as for example in an intestinal volvulus or following an embolus of the superior mesenteric artery. In certain cases peritonitis is the result of blood stream infection from a focus outside the abdomen, e.g. pneumococcal pneumonia or otitis media. Certain groups of patients with lowered body resistance may be susceptible to this type of peritonitis (secondary peritonitis). The contaminating fluid may be irritant largely because of its chemical properties, e.g. biliary peritonitis, whilst in others bacterial infection is of paramount importance even from the start. The patient with liver disease and ascites is probably prone to bacterial invasion of the peritoneal cavity where there is often very little in the way of signs and symptoms. The patient on high doses of corticosteroid drugs may also develop relatively silent peritonitis following rupture of a viscus, e.g. ulcerative colitis, whilst in the elderly and enfeebled the signs of peritonitis may also be atypical.

If the patient has some other serious disease, e.g. acute respiratory failure due to an exacerbation of bronchitis or myocardial infarction, similar confusion may occur.

Clinical Picture

The condition may be of acute or subacute onset, the former being classical of intestinal perforation. The symptoms include severe and generalized abdominal pain accompanied by vomiting (the latter due to intestinal paralysis—a consequence of spreading peritonitis). The patient may at this stage be pyrexial, the abdomen rigid and tender and silent on auscultation. There is rebound tenderness on releasing pressure and where there has been involvement of the pelvic peritoneum tenderness and induration of the rectovesical and rectovaginal pouch. In examples which arise from spreading infection from the uterus or Fallopian tubes there is tenderness and induration of the broad ligaments and manipulation of the cervix is painful.

With progression of the disease the patient becomes hypovolaemic due to vomiting and exudation into the gut and peritoneal cavity. The facies becomes pinched, the tissues lax, the blood pressure low, whilst the abdominal cavity distends. Death ensues from circulatory failure and toxaemia.

Diagnosis

The importance of this condition means that constant watchfulness is required in any patient with acute abdominal pain, in the elderly and in those on corticosteroids great care and caution must be exercised. Age may be helpful in suggesting the cause of peritonitis, the appendix and female genitalia being common in the young whilst diverticular disease of the colon may be responsible in the elderly. Primary pneumococcal peritonitis may be seen in young children.

Helpful investigations include a full blood count and electrolyte estimates with radiology to exclude intestinal perforation. In some cases 'four-quarter' aspiration of the abdominal cavity using a needle and syringe may make a diagnosis possible and examination of the aspirated fluid may allow differentiation from intra-abdominal haemorrhage (e.g. from an ectopic pregnancy) or from pancreatitis, etc. A tap showing purulent fluid with organisms proven on microscopy and culture can be helpful. The particular problem of the cirrhotic with ascites and peritoneal infection with few clinical signs can also be aided by diagnostic paracentesis and subsequent microscopy and culture.

Treatment

This is either conservative or operative or a combination of both depending on the cause, the duration of the disease and the presence of intercurrent illness.

Briefly, if the patient is seen soon after the onset, i.e. in the first 48 hours, and particularly if the history suggests rupture of a viscus or devitalization, the correct treatment is surgery with removal or repair of the cause and peritoneal toilet and drainage.

In patients where there has been delay before hospitalization and where there is walling-off of infection to form abscess cavities, operative treatment may produce spreading peritonitis so that in these circumstances surgery is best avoided until localization is well established. The basis of treatment is rest in a semi-Fowler position and complete rest to the alimentary tract so that food and fluid administration is stopped. Small bowel distension is prevented by intestinal suction either with a Levine tube or in severe cases using the Miller-Abbot technique. Electrolyte deficiency is carefully monitored and fluid and electrolytes given intravenously. Calorie supplements in the form of dextrose or intravenous lipid may also be required if protein depletion and ketosis are to be combated. Chemotherapy to combat the infective process in the peritoneal cavity is also required. This is given intravenously, either ampicillin or a combination of penicillin and streptomycin being suitable in most patients if the precise bacteriology is not known. Shock may also require treatment with intravenous fluid, possibly including dextrose, plasma or blood and large doses of systemic hydrocortisone may be helpful in those with severe shock—or where treatment with corticosteroids was being carried out for some other reason, e.g. rheumatoid arthritis.

If the patient responds to this therapy, surgery of abscesses or of the initial cause of the peritonitis, e.g. an appendix, may be required 10 days or so after the onset, and in those who fail to respond to conservative therapy, surgery, though carrying a considerable mortality, may be considered and employed at any time.

TUBERCULOUS PERITONITIS

Aetiology

Infection of the peritoneal cavity by the tubercle bacillus is from mesenteric lymph nodes, though occasionally peritonitis may be part of a generalized miliary, and therefore blood stream, dissemination of the organism. The disease is now uncommon in this country, but still occurs in those who are debilitated by alcoholism or malnutrition. It is usually seen in young adults when primary tuberculosis infection is most common.

Pathology

The end result of tuberculosis peritonitis is the production of ascitic fluid, with miliary tubercles scattered over the involved peritoneum or there may be more localized thickening and gradual obliteration of the peritoneal cavity by fibrous tuberculous peritonitis. There may also be caseous tuberculous disease in the mesenteric nodes as well as in other parts of the body.

Clinical Picture

The onset of this disorder is usually insidious. The early symptoms are non-specific and consist of abdominal pain, anorexia, and loss of weight. There may be alteration of bowel habit with constipation or diarrhoea. In patients with extensive disease of the bowel or mesenteric glands there may be steatorrhoea. In women amenorrhoea is a common symptom.

Occasionally the symptoms may be of acute onset with a high fever and severe abdominal pain. In those cases that go on to the production of ascitic fluid there may be generalized abdominal distention which is often accompanied by severe colicky pain. Such patients presenting with weight loss and ascites may be thought to have cirrhosis. Careful examination may reveal masses of thickened bowel on abdominal palpation as well as the signs of fluid. Enlarged nodes and evidence of tuberculous disease elsewhere must be sought.

It is particularly important to remember that this disease may attack malnourished patients, and in this respect the alcoholic with cirrhosis seems to be particularly at risk. When such a patient develops tuberculous peritonitis it may be wrongly assumed that the ascites is secondary to liver cell disease. Herein lies the danger of misdiagnosis of this condition.

Diagnosis

The diagnosis should be suspected in any patient with wasting and the signs of chronic peritonitis or ascites. Radiology of the chest and the abdomen may show evidence of tuberculosis. Examination of the ascitic fluid is important. Generally this is straw coloured with more than 2·5 g. of protein per 100 ml. and contains lymphocytes with a few polymorphs. The results of examination of the fluid for *Mycobacterium tuberculosis*, either on direct microscopy or on culture are disappointing, and only a third of cases show a positive result. Peritoneoscopy or laparotomy may be useful for patients who are suspected of having this disease. In a similar way liver biopsy may occasionally show tuberculous granulomata if the clinical picture is part of a miliary spread. The important point to remember, however, is that if the disease is suspected clinically a wait for confirmation of the diagnosis bacteriologically cannot be made, and treatment should be instituted quickly.

Treatment

The disease responds dramatically to antituberculous chemotherapy. If the organism has not been isolated then it is probably best to start therapy with daily injections of 1 G. streptomycin with oral para-aminosalicylic acid, 16 G. daily, and with isonicotinic acid hydrazide (INAH), 100 mg. three times daily. Once an organism has been obtained and its sensitivity assessed then appropriate long-term therapy is usually continued for a year. Any complicating chronic disease must also be treated and the patient's nutritional status must be improved with high protein feeding and liberal supplements of vitamins. One long-term result of tuberculous peritonitis may be the formation of bands and adhesions which constrict the bowel and later cause subacute intestinal obstruction or a blind loop syndrome.

Prognosis

The prognosis, providing the disease is diagnosed early, is excellent.

TUMOURS OF THE PERITONEUM

MESOTHELIOMA

This is a rare tumour identical to that which occurs in the pleural cavity and with the same important relationship to inhalation of asbestos dust. Pathologically the tumour which is initially confined to the peritoneum produces invasion of surrounding organs. Occasionally there may be several isolated plaques and the diagnosis from secondary carcinoma may be difficult. Histologically there is great structural variation with admixture of mesenchymal and epithelial elements which singly may either predominate or be mixed. Usually there is a tendency towards differentiation of tubular and glandular elements and in 25 per cent. of cases asbestos bodies will be found in the tumour on careful examination. The clinical picture is not distinctive, abdominal pain and distension is followed by ascites and a rapidly downhill path. The diagnosis is made at laparotomy or peritoneoscopy, whilst peritoneal biopsy is occasionally helpful, as obviously is chest X-ray, but the diagnosis of secondary carcinoma, often from an ovarian primary in females, is likely to be made unless a careful history and precise histology is possible. Treatment with intraperitoneal nitrogen mustard or with radioactive colloidal gold is disappointing. Death usually occurs within a few months of the diagnosis being made.

Tumour formation may be found from 20 to 40 years after exposure, which may have lasted for 1–30 years. The pulmonary features of asbestosis do not have to be present. The patients exposure may therefore be forgotten and it is in any case possible that some exposure, as, for example, in those living near asbestos works, is accidental rather than occupational.

In patients with asbestosis carcinoma of the bronchus is present in nearly a third at autopsy, whilst mesothelial tumours of the pleura are more common than those of the peritoneum so that a variety of neoplasms, perhaps including alimentary ones, are related to this disease. There is evidence that of the three commercially important types of asbestosis, crocidolite is in particular likely to be associated with mesothelial tumours. It would appear that the rich diaphragmatic lymphatic network allows asbestos particles to reach the peritoneum where they can initiate tumour formation.

REFERENCE

Enticknap, J. B., and Smither, W. J. (1964) Peritoneal tumours in asbestosis, *Brit. J. industr. Hyg.*, **21**, 20.

RETROPERITONEAL FIBROSIS

Definition

A disease of unknown cause in which a progressive inflammatory fibrosis of the retroperitoneal tissues occurs causing symptoms by strangulation of structures in the retroperitoneal space. Its commonest effect is ureteric obstruction.

Pathology

The gross pathological picture is that of a firm rubbery mass, several centimetres thick; of grey adherent fibrous tissue, this adherent mass is attached to the posterior peritoneal surface displacing it forward. The borders may be indistinct and although there is no invasion of muscle tissue the process surrounds and constricts the retroperitoneal structures. These include the ureters, vena cava, and occasionally the biliary tract, duodenum and colon. Microscopically it consists of fibrous tissue with a variable amount of fat and inflammatory change. Some areas show hyalinization. The process is usually maximal at about the level of the sacral promontory.

Clinical Picture

The symptoms are non-specific. The occlusion of one ureter may give rise to attacks of loin pain due to hydronephrosis and renal infection; as the process advances to involve both, the picture of obstructive uropathy with hypertension and uraemia develops. When the nerves of the lumbar plexus are involved in the fibrotic process there is low backache with pain in the thighs and occasionally in the testes. Obstruction of the duodenum or colon produces colicky abdominal pain and the signs of intestinal obstruction, whilst compression of the inferior vena cava may be responsible for the appearance of oedema, and of varicose veins in the lower extremities and collateral venous channels on the abdominal wall. Obstruction of the bile-ducts is associated with jaundice. Clinical examination is often unrewarding although a mass may be palpable on abdominal examination. Pelvic examination is also important because of the possibility of extension of the process into the pelvis. Rarely patients with this disorder show evidence of abnormal fibrosis in other regions such as in the mediastinum.

Diagnosis

Diagnostic help is given by a plain abdominal X-ray which may show blurring of the psoas shadow, or loss of the renal outline on one or both sides. An intravenous or ascending pyelogram sometimes shows a characteristic radiological picture. This consists of a medial displacement of both ureters usually at the level of the 4th or 5th lumbar vertebrae. The renal pelvis and ureters above the point of obstruction are dilated. In a lateral projection it may be possible to show the forward displacement of the viscera by the retroperitoneal tissue. The erythrocyte sedimentation rate is raised.

In difficult cases it may be essential to proceed to laparotomy, and even then it may be difficult to distinguish between this disorder and a diffuse malignant infiltration of the retroperitoneal tissues. Reticulosarcoma is perhaps the tumour most frequently encountered and the distinction can often only be made by biopsy.

Venography and lymphangiography may be useful in making the diagnosis, and it should be remembered that this disorder can produce obstruction of the duodenum, superior vena cava and azygos vein, together with hepatic venous obstruction, oesophageal obstruction and granulomatous change in the lungs. The patients are not infrequently thought to have a psychiatric illness, so bizarre and atypical are some of the early features.

Treatment

Treatment of this disease is difficult but where vital structures such as the ureters are involved then obviously surgical therapy to free and possibly re-implant them may be helpful. On occasions nephrostomy may be essential. Therapy other than surgical is not usually successful, and corticosteroid drugs, antibiotics and X-ray therapy are usually without effect. It should not be forgotten, however, that patients with this disease sometimes undergo spontaneous remission and the obstructive symptoms are then not progressive.

FAMILIAL RECURRING POLYSEROSITIS (PERIODIC PERITONITIS)

Aetiology

This is a rare disease which has been recognized in patients of Jewish, Arab or Armenian extraction. The disease has various names but in essence it is a disorder where there are attacks of inflammation of serosal surfaces. This produces acute and recurrent symptoms. The aetiology of the disease is unknown.

Clinical Picture

The disorder produces episodes of severe abdominal, chest or joint pain. The episodes are periodic but occur at irregular intervals with gaps of up to several months between them. The disease may commence in childhood but it is more usually seen in the second or third decade of life. Abdominal pain is the most important symptom and this is accompanied by vomiting, the whole episode lasting 24–48 hours. The patient is often pyrexial during this time. Other manifestations of the disease include attacks of pleurisy with dyspnoea and also attacks of pain and periarticular swelling, usually affecting the joints of the lower limbs. During these acute bouts other physical signs may occasionally be found. These include hepatomegaly, signs of renal failure and occasionally evidence of retinopathy.

Diagnosis

The most helpful diagnostic procedure includes intestinal radiology which shows ileus or delayed intestinal transit, while X-rays of the chest may show a small effusion in patients with pleurisy. Joint symptoms are not usually accompanied by X-ray changes. Help, of course, is also obtained in those patients where there is a family history and the patient's ethnic background is obviously of importance. Laboratory tests may show a high leucocyte count during the acute illness. It is important to exclude other causes of recurrent abdominal pain such as gall-stones, renal colic, peptic ulcer, haemolytic crises, porphyria and abdominal pain associated with hyperlipidaemia.

Treatment

There is no satisfactory treatment for this disease though there is some evidence that a low-fat diet, that is one containing 20 g. of fat per day, produces a reduced incidence of acute episodes. Corticosteroids and ACTH have not been useful and it should be borne in mind that it is possible that progression of the disease to involvement of the kidneys by renal amyloidosis may be accelerated by these drugs.

Complications

Renal amyloidosis not infrequently complicates this disease and usually presents either as a nephrotic syndrome or as renal failure. It is certainly a most serious complication of the disorder, which otherwise, apart from difficulties with the initial diagnosis, is a benign disorder.

MESENTERIC LYMPHADENITIS

Mesenteric lymphadenitis is a common disorder in childhood. The aetiology is obscure but many cases seem to follow an acute viral or bacterial upper respiratory infection. Pathologically the mesenteric lymph nodes are enlarged and histologically an acute inflammatory reaction is seen. In some cases there may be an exudation of fluid into the peritoneal cavity. The affected person is usually a young child, and the symptoms are identical to those of acute appendicitis, although the temperature is often higher. Almost invariably laparotomy is performed and even when the diagnosis is clearly one of mesenteric adenitis the appendix is usually removed. Infection with *Pasteurella pseudo-tuberculosis* is sometimes responsible for this syndrome.

REFERENCES

McDonald, J. C. (1963) Nonspecific mesenteric lymphadenitis, *Int. Abstr. Surg.*, **116,** 409.

Ward-McQuaid, J. N. (1951) Acute non-specific mesenteric adenitis, *Lancet*, ii, 524.

TUBERCULOSIS OF THE MESENTERIC LYMPH NODES

Tuberculous disease of the mesenteric lymph nodes is more common. The incidence, however, is falling with the universal adoption of pasteurization of milk (the source of the bovine tubercle bacillus).

The tubercle bacillus gains entry through the wall of the small bowel where it may occasionally cause ulceration or, more rarely, a chronic granulomatous induration of the bowel. Patients are usually children but the disease is still not uncommon in adult immigrants to this country. The symptoms are not distinctive and consist of attacks of central abdominal pain, nausea, vomiting and alteration of bowel habit (usually constipation). There are usually no physical signs unless there is associated hypertrophic granulomatous disease of the bowel present and then there may be a mass in the right iliac fossa due to involvement of the ileum and caecum. Patients with bowel disease of this type may be wasted and ill so that Crohn's disease or even a carcinoma of the caecum may be mimicked. Helpful investigations include abdominal X-rays which, however, only show enlarged glands when they are calcified, and a barium study of the bowel and examination of the faeces for tubercle bacilli when hypertrophic tuberculous ileocolitis is present. Usually the disease can only be diagnosed by noting the onset of symptoms in a child who has recently become Mantoux positive, or at laparotomy. Treatment following verification of the diagnosis by surgery is with a long course of antituberculous drugs. Apart from occasional cases of miliary spread due to rupture of the contents of a caseous gland into the blood stream and local rupture producing tuberculous peritonitis, the reaction to drug therapy is excellent.

TUMOURS OF THE MESENTERIC LYMPH NODES

Involvement of the aortic chain of lymph nodes by reticuloses such as lymphoblastoma, lymphosarcoma or reticulosarcoma is common due to the multicentric origin of these lesions. Though usually causing no specific symptoms they may be associated with pyrexia, anorexia, wasting and pruritus and when they are the only site of the disease, i.e. there are no apparent glands involved elsewhere, no hepatosplenomegaly and a normal chest X-ray, these symptoms should suggest such a possibility. Metastatic involvement of aortic lymph nodes also occurs from the small and large bowel and the pancreas, whilst the testis is also an important site for malignant spread to these lymph nodes.

Lymph nodes involved in either of these types of malignancy are seldom palpable unless the patient is thin and the nodes large. Occasionally a retroperitoneal tumour either of lymph node or neural or connective tissue origin will cause enlargement of the abdomen with symptoms not only related to its size but also symptoms due to pressure on neighbouring structures such as constipation, renal colic and breathlessness due to diaphragmatic elevation.

Ascites may occur from portal venous obstruction and when the cysterna chyli is involved the resulting ascitic fluid may be chylous, due to escape of intestinal lymph. Leg oedema is due to inferior vena caval obstruction. Hypoglycaemic attacks are an important feature of some retroperitoneal fibromata.

Helpful investigations in patients with retroperitoneal lymph node and other tumours include barium studies of the bowel which will demonstrate in some cases displacement of the gut without intrinsic tumour formation, whilst an intravenous pyelogram is occasionally very helpful for the demonstration of ureteric obstruction or indentation from lymph nodes. Most helpful of all, though not without some risk, is the technique of lymphangiography which not only detects lymph node enlargement but also can produce a fairly characteristic picture in reticulosis or secondary carcinoma which may be useful in view of the retention of contrast medium in the glands, as a means of following the effects of therapy.

REFERENCES

Tuberculous Peritonitis

BURACK, W. R., and HOLLISTER, R. M. (1960) Tuberculous peritonitis. A study of 47 cases encountered by a general unit in 25 years. *Amer. J. Med.*, **28**, 510.

Retroperitoneal Fibrosis

SAXTON, H. M., KILPATRICK, F. R., KINDER, C. H., LESSOF, M. H., MCHARDY-YOUNG, S., and WARDLE, D. F. I. (1969) Retroperitoneal fibrosis: A radiological and follow-up study of 14 cases, *Quart. J. Med.*, **38**, 159.

Periodic Disease

REIMANN, H. A. (1951) Periodic disease, *Medicine (Baltimore)*, **30**, 219.

Acute Peritonitis

MENZIES, T. (1961) The management of peritonitis, in *Modern Trends in Gastro-Enterology*, **3**, p. 127, London.

A. E. READ

SECTION 7

DISEASES OF THE GASTRO-INTESTINAL TRACT

DISEASES OF THE MOUTH

GENERAL

It is convenient to consider diseases of the tongue, gums and mouth separately, although in many cases all three are involved together. For the most part the aetiological factors are the same and therefore the main general causes are given first, followed by details of specific conditions.

Traumatic Causes

Badly fitting dentures (causing prosthetic ulcers), deposits of calcium in the gingival sulci, excessive brushing of the teeth or use of toothpicks, the habit of cheek-biting in nervous individuals, or the sharp edges of broken teeth may all cause traumatic lesions with often severe inflammation of gums, cheek or tongue. Burns from accidental ingestion of hot food or drinks are usually of trivial nature and rarely involve more than the anterior portion of the tongue and the palate.

Chemical Causes

Chewing of tobacco, betel-nut and the repeated ingestion of strong alcohol may cause irritation of the mouth, as may a number of drugs such as aspirin, strong peppermint, or antiseptics such as lysol swallowed accidentally or with suicidal intent. Certain occupations are especially liable to buccal disorders, especially chrome-plating and work involving strong acids or alkalis; welding, in which nitrous oxides formed in the process may combine with the saliva secretion, may be dangerous, and particularly occupations in which exposure to metallic mercury may occur. These include mining, the manufacture of barometers, or electric lamps, photo-engraving and certain pharmaceutical processes. In mercurial poisoning excessive salivation with swollen bleeding gums is an early manifestation, and only later as a rule does a dark 'mercurial' line, similar to the lead line of plumbism, appear on the gums.

Infection

Bacterial, viral or fungal infections of the mouth may occur, the latter often as a sequel of antibiotic treatment or in association with the use of corticosteroid drugs.

Allergic and Cryptogenic Causes

Angioneurotic oedema may cause intense swelling of the tongue, lips, buccal mucosa or glottis. Allergic reactions to drugs such as antibiotics, barbiturates, iodides or sulphonamides may be a cause of stomatitis medicamentosa, or the local reaction of the oral mucosa to mouthwashes or other drugs may less commonly cause erythema or vesicle formation (stomatitis venenata). Certain diseases which are possibly of allergic or infective nature are described below: the aetiology in these cases is uncertain and includes lichen planus, erythema multiforme, Stevens-Johnson syndrome, oral pemphigus and cancrum oris.

Deficiency States

Chronic iron deficiency leads to degenerative changes in the mouth; a lack of vitamin C (scurvy), folic acid, riboflavine, nicotinic acid, or cyanocobalamin (vitamin B_{12}) are other causes, which may occur in conditions of malabsorption or malnutrition.

THE TONGUE

Examination of the tongue should be directed to its colour, size, the distribution and appearance of the papillae, the degree of smoothness or coating on its surface and its muscle tone and movements. An abnormally furred or coated tongue is not an index of gastric or intestinal dysfunction, or of constipation, but results from drying of the mouth as in mouth-breathers, or from lack of the mechanical action of chewing with the proper flow of saliva. It occurs in conditions of dehydration such as fevers or renal failure, and often in patients fed on fluids only or parenterally. It occurs more frequently in tobacco smokers than in others. When the coating, which is made up of yeasts, microbes and desquamating epithelial cells, becomes infected with certain bacterial or fungal organisms, these may produce a dark pigment giving rise to the so-called 'black tongue'. Discoloration may also be caused by food, sweets or drugs and may follow the sucking of penicillin lozenges. It has no serious pathological significance.

GEOGRAPHIC TONGUE

This condition is also known as erythema migrans or benign migratory glossitis. It occurs most frequently in children, and more often in women than men. Areas of the tongue surface become denuded of papillae and bright red in colour, but as a rule cause no symptoms and are only noticed by chance if the tongue is inspected. The aetiology is unknown. Geographic tongue has no serious sequelae, requires no special treatment, and is usually transitory in duration.

ATROPHIC GLOSSITIS

The papillae of the tongue may undergo atrophy, the filiform papillae on the dorsum being as a rule most affected. The atrophy is due to lack of oxidase enzymes and occurs especially in deficiency states, particularly in iron-deficiency anaemia when the tongue becomes smooth, flabby and pale. In riboflavine deficiency it also becomes smooth and of a bright magenta colour. Lack of nicotinic acid is associated with a bright scarlet tongue as is seen in pellagra [p. 530], and a similar smooth red 'raw' tongue occurs in cases of steatorrhoea, sprue, chronic dysentery, and after gastro-enterostomy. Atrophic glossitis is a feature of the Plummer-Vinson syndrome and may be associated with excessive furrowing or fissuring of the surface (scrotal tongue), which is itself of little clinical importance. In some cases such an abnormally fissured tongue is familial, and the deep longitudinal fissure known as median rhomboid glossitis is due to a developmental failure of the two halves of the tongue to unite normally. This condition has been thought to be pre-cancerous but there is no definite evidence of this. In many cases of atrophic glossitis there are no symptoms. In others, particularly in pernicious anaemia, the tongue feels painful, with burning brought on by tobacco smoking or by hot or strongly flavoured food and drink. A painful tongue is often complained of by patients in whom no abnormal changes in the mouth can be found, and in these cases there is often a marked cancerphobia associated with a chronic anxiety state.

MACROGLOSSIA

The tongue may be enlarged in cases of cretinism, myxoedema or mongolism, and characteristically in the rare condition of primary amyloidosis.

STOMATITIS

APHTHOUS STOMATITIS

Synonyms. Vesicular stomatitis; Canker sore; Dyspeptic ulcers of the mouth.

Aetiology

The condition occurs more often in women than men, and mainly between the ages of 20 and 50. The ulcers often appear at times of emotional stress, or may arise in crops at irregular intervals. No virus has been found as a causative agent, in contrast to cases of true recurrent herpes simplex. Aphthous ulcers may first develop at the time of the menopause in women and rarely are present during pregnancy.

Symptoms

The aphthae consist of small raised vesicles, each surrounded by a red areola: the commonest sites are the buccal mucosal membrane and inside the lips, the tongue and less often the fauces. In about 10 per cent. of women patients, painful ulceration of the vulva and vagina may occur at the same time. The vesicles rapidly burst, leaving small grey ulcers which may be solitary or very numerous. There is no constitutional disturbance, but there may be dyspepsia and sometimes loss of weight owing to pain on mastication reducing the amount of food eaten, or to an anxiety neurosis.

Treatment

No specific treatment is known. Local application of steroids is only occasionally successful, and a suspension of tetracycline, 250 mg. in 10 ml. of water, may give relief. Local application of the silver nitrate stick to individual ulcers will relieve the pain, but the effect of suggestion or hypnotism may be very good and in many cases adjustments to domestic or environmental stress appear to result in cure.

Prognosis

Crops of ulcers may recur for many years but as a rule the condition gradually disappears after middle age. There are no serious complications.

VINCENT'S STOMATITIS

Synonyms. Ulceromembranous gingivostomatitis; Ulceronecrotic stomatitis; Trench mouth.

Aetiology and Pathology

Severe ulceromembranous stomatitis is a contagious disease, caused by infection with the same spirochaetes and fusiform bacilli which cause Vincent's angina [p. 680]. The disease is not easily transmissible and is especially liable to occur in cases of malnutrition, or blood diseases such as leukaemia. It is commonly found in young adolescents, especially where there is poor oral hygiene, dental caries or badly fitting dentures.

Symptoms

All parts of the mouth and pharynx may be involved but the margins of the gums are specially liable to be affected. The stomatitis is similar to that caused by mercury, and the gums may be so swollen and bleed so readily that scurvy is simulated. The breath has a characteristic foetid odour, and the tender gums may make mastication painful. The disease is sometimes acute, but more often runs a chronic course and may be followed by pyorrhoea alveolaris. It generally gives rise to but little constitutional disturbance though the ulceration may be very painful.

Treatment

Metronidazole (*Flagyl*), 200 mg. three times daily is usually curative.

Prognosis

Rapid relief of symptoms with treatment is usual, but the damaged areas of the gums may remain diseased and chronic stomatitis result. This may be very intractable and demands the continued co-operation of the patient in the care of the gums, and the elimination of any predisposing factors such as carious teeth.

GANGRENOUS STOMATITIS

Synonyms. Cancrum oris; Noma.

Aetiology

This rare disease occurs in children, especially girls between the ages of 2 and 5, who live under very insanitary conditions. It generally develops during convalescence from an acute fever, especially measles, and less frequently scarlet and typhoid fever. It also forms part of the clinical picture of agranulocytosis [see Section 13].

Symptoms

A sloughing ulcer develops in the inside of the cheek or on the gums; it rapidly spreads and leads to brawny induration of the skin of the cheek. Occasionally it heals spontaneously, but more frequently it perforates the cheek or spreads to the tongue, chin, jawbone or eyelid and eye.

Cancrum oris is accompanied by severe constitutional symptoms, the patient being prostrated with a high temperature and rapid pulse. Diarrhoea or broncho-pneumonia frequently follows, and death generally occurs between 7 and 10 days from the onset.

Treatment

The only adequate treatment for cancrum oris in children is to destroy the diseased part as completely as possible with the cautery. Intramuscular injections of penicillin should be given in massive doses related to the child's weight. For the treatment of agranulocytosis see Section 13.

THRUSH (MONILIASIS)

Aetiology

Thrush, an infection of the mucosae of the oro-pharynx by *Candida albicans*, is most common in weak, emaciated infants with gastro-intestinal symptoms who have been fed with an unsuitable diet and whose mouths have not been kept clean. It occurs in epidemic form in badly managed institutions, being spread by dirty feeding bottles, transmitted by the nipples or carried in the air. It may follow treatment by antibiotics, especially tetracyclines, or by corticosteroids. If the first are used for long periods their action in destroying bacteria in the gut leads to vitamin deficiency and stomatitis, and allows infection with monilia to take place [see Section 2].

Diagnosis

Adherent milk curds may superficially simulate thrush. In aphthous stomatitis the white patches are at first vesicles and then definite ulcers, and salivation is present in contrast to the dry mouth in thrush. The diagnosis from other lesions, particularly leucoplakia or lichen planus, can be made by examination of smears of the lesions which under the microscope show typical clusters of spores and filaments; the growth may be cultured on Sabouraud's medium.

Treatment

Thrush should be prevented by keeping the mouth clean and babies' bottles sterilized. It is important to improve the patient's general health as well as to give local treatment. Nystatin or amphotericin B mouthwashes 6-hourly will usually eradicate the infection.

OTHER DISORDERS ASSOCIATED WITH STOMATITIS

Some lesions in the mouth may be the first manifestation of erythema multiforme (Stevens-Johnson syndrome), pemphigus vulgaris and pemphigus erythematodes (Senear-Usher syndrome). Oral lesions are common in lichen planus. The many conditions in which cutaneous and buccal manifestations are combined are considered in Section 14.

THE GUMS

PYORRHOEA ALVEOLARIS; CHRONIC PERIODONTITIS

Aetiology and Pathology

Stagnation of food mixed with pyogenic organisms between the teeth leads to inflammation of the edge of the gums—marginal gingivitis. The attachment of the mucoperiosteum to the neck of the tooth is destroyed, and a pocket develops between the tooth and the gum. The margin of the alveolar process is then slowly eroded as a result of rarefying osteitis, until it may finally be replaced by granulation tissue. Stagnation of infective material in the pocket leads to gradual extension of the disease and aggravation of the gingivitis. Pus is produced, the condition at this stage being commonly known as pyorrhoea alveolaris.

Symptoms

In marginal gingivitis the edge of the gum of one or more teeth is red and swollen and bleeds with abnormal ease when brushed, the first part to be affected being usually the interdental papillae. When pyorrhoea alveolaris has developed, pockets are present round the teeth, and pus can generally be seen exuding from the edge of the gum. Even when none is seen on first examining the mouth, beads of pus appear if the edges of the gum are pressed. In chronic cases the teeth are often loose. Reflex salivation occurs, and an excessive quantity of mucus is secreted by the small mucous glands of the mouth. The accumulation of decomposing food, debris and pus in the pockets round the teeth produces an unpleasant taste in the mouth, most marked on waking in the morning, and is a common cause of foul breath. There is no pain, and the slight discomfort which may be present is generally insufficient to induce the patient to consult a dentist.

Treatment

In early cases the disease can be arrested by scaling and treatment of the pockets with strong antiseptics. When the supporting bone has been destroyed to more than half the depth of the root, extraction is necessary. In intermediate cases the gum should be cut away in order to eradicate the pockets. The patient should then be given instructions regarding oral hygiene. Stimulation of the gums and proper brushing of the teeth, with a diet requiring proper chewing, are points of importance.

PIGMENTATION OF THE MOUTH

Patchy pigmentation of the buccal mucosa or of the tongue is an important sign of Addison's disease. The pigmentation is of browny-black colour and is most often seen on the cheek. It may be difficult to distinguish from racial pigmentation. Pigmentation in the mouth is also seen in haemochromatosis and in cases of metallic poisoning with bismuth, arsenic, gold, silver and some other metals used in industrial processes.

PEUTZ-JEGHER SYNDROME

This condition is inherited as a Mendelian dominant and is characterized by the presence of melanin pigmentation of the lips and buccal mucous membrane associated with intestinal polyposis. The polyps may be single or multiple, and tend to arise in recurring crops. They are benign adenomata and in a few cases occur as a diffuse micropolyposis [see p. 720].

Symptoms

Bouts of severe recurring colic, due to transient intussusceptions, occur and are often relieved by passing flatus. Borborygmi sometimes with vomiting (which may ease the pain) are frequent, but between attacks the patient feels well and the bowels are regular. The colicky attacks are usually of short duration and are often regarded as hysterical.

Diagnosis

Radiology rarely gives definite evidence of the polyps. Occult blood may be present in the stools and sigmoidoscopy may show associated polyps in the colon. The pigmentation shows as small black or brown spots around the mouth, eyes or nose, and may be seen on the hands and fingers. The mucous membrane of the mouth is always affected but never the tongue. The skin pigmentation tends to disappear in adult life.

Treatment and Prognosis

The acute attacks of colic rarely require urgent operation, and can usually be relieved by enemata if they do not subside spontaneously. The polyps are usually multiple, so that the removal of one or two is unlikely to lead to permanent cure. Anaemia should be treated by oral iron. The genetic risks should be explained to sufferers, but the prognosis as regards life is good.

DENTAL CARIES

The immediate cause of dental caries is unknown, but two main theories have been put forward. The chemico-parasitic theory postulates that acid produced by bacterial fermentation of carbohydrates causes decalcification of the enamel and dentine, the acid being kept in contact with the tooth by a plaque of debris on its surface. The alternative theory is that the initial change is a degradation of the organic matrix of the enamel by bacterial enzymes and that the inorganic matrix subsequently disintegrates. It is generally agreed whichever theory is correct that caries is due to the activity of bacteria.

Symptoms

Carious teeth are tender, and their presence renders mastication painful. The patient therefore avoids using the affected teeth, and this favours the deposit of tartar and the stagnation of food. If many teeth are affected the food is bolted, so that indigestion is likely to occur owing to insufficient mastication, quite apart from possible infection of the alimentary canal caused by swallowing septic material from the mouth. The irritation produced by the decomposition of stagnant food around the teeth gives rise to marginal gingivitis and pyorrhoea alveolaris. Inflammation of the pulp spreads to the periodontal membrane and may finally produce an alveolar abscess.

Dental caries is the most common cause of toothache, and pain is often referred to various situations more or less remote from the teeth.

Prophylaxis

The incidence of caries can be significantly reduced by the addition of vitamin D, calcium and phosphorus to a diet which is deficient in these substances, and the improved dentition of British children in the post-war years was attributed to the war-time provision of extra milk and vitamin D. Calcium carbonate was also added to the flour and the vitamin D content of margarine was increased. Refinement of flour is detrimental because it removes phosphorus and increases the content of phytic acid, a substance which interferes with the absorption of calcium. Caries is especially prevalent in regions where there is a natural deficiency of fluorine and it has been shown that the artificial fluoridation of drinking water, to an optimal value of 1·0–1·2 parts per million significantly reduces its incidence. Concentrations above this level are liable to cause mottling of the teeth. Fluorides can also be applied directly to the teeth, and four applications of a 2 per cent. solution of sodium fluoride at weekly intervals will usually reduce the amount if not entirely prevent the onset of caries.

Oral Hygiene. The teeth should be brushed regularly vertically from the gums to the teeth, and wooden toothpicks used to clear and massage the gum spaces between them. Tincture of iodine may be applied on a wisp of wool on the end of the toothpick. The mouth should be well rinsed after meals. Ideally, sugar and sticky carbohydrates should be eliminated from the diet, and they should be replaced by natural unrefined vegetable foods.

Treatment

This is the province of the dental surgeon.

APICAL INFECTION

Aetiology

Infection of the apex of the root of a tooth can occur only if the pulp is dead, except in rare cases of extensive caries.

Symptoms

Apical infection may be acute or chronic. In the former an alveolar abscess forms, which gives rise to the usual symptoms and signs of inflammation. Chronic apical infection, on the other hand, frequently gives rise to no pain or discomfort, and no signs recognizable on ordinary examination. It can then be recognized only in a good radiograph.

Treatment

This is surgical.

LEUCOPLAKIA

Aetiology and Pathology

Oral leucoplakia occurs twice as often in men as in women and more often over the age of 40. It is especially frequent in heavy smokers and only rarely seen in those who do not smoke at all. At one time 10 to 20 per cent. of the cases were associated with syphilis. Bad teeth or badly fitting dentures are commonly found.

The lesion is one of hyperkeratosis and appears as white thickened areas on the tongue or other parts of the mouth. The edges of the diseased area are well defined and it is seen as a stiff white patch with—on the tongue—absence of papillae. Later the area may become inflamed and fissured and at this stage it is likely to have undergone malignant degeneration.

Symptoms and Diagnosis

There is usually no pain at the start, but later erosion of the plaque and painful fissuring develops. Biopsy of the area—or excision if it is small—is advisable both to differentiate the condition from lichen planus and to exclude malignant change. In lichen planus the lesions are more often bilateral and less white in colour than in leucoplakia; nor is there any rigidity or papillary atrophy as in this condition. In some cases the lesions are similar to those of herpetic stomatitis, being bullous at first and later red, painful and eroded.

Treatment and Prognosis

Careful treatment and observation is necessary since leucoplakia of the mouth is potentially a cancerous lesion. The dental state must be put into good order, a high vitamin diet prescribed and all tobacco smoking strictly forbidden. Surgical excision of the area is advisable if there is suspicion of malignancy on biopsy. Local applications to the lesion are of little value.

HALITOSIS (BAD BREATH)

An offensive odour to the breath is mainly of importance because it may give rise to serious feelings of inferiority and self-consciousness if the sufferer is made aware of his complaint. In most cases of halitosis the individual is, in fact, unconscious of any bad smell—on the contrary, when he is continually complaining of his breath it is often found to be due to an obsessional neurosis and that he has actually no odour at any time. A pungent heavy breath is frequently due to bad teeth, decaying food in dental cavities, pyorrhoea, or to cheesy putrefactive material in the crypts of the tonsils. Ozaena is a further local cause, as may, rarely, be infected accessory nasal sinuses. Decaying material on the back of the tongue may become offensive and pulmonary conditions, such as lung abscess or bronchiectasis, are other causes.

Hepatic or intestinal causes of halitosis can less easily be demonstrated and, though it is popularly believed that chronic constipation may be a cause, this is, in fact, very doubtful. The odour of garlic when swallowed in capsules may remain in the bile after it has disappeared both from the breath and the intestine, and it seems probable that liver dysfunction may play a part in some cases of halitosis. The sulphur-smelling mercaptan may be smelt strongly in the breath in cases of hepatic necrosis.

Treatment

Some cases of unexplained halitosis are improved by much reducing the amount of fats in the diet. Purgatives are of little use, though saline laxatives are often advocated. Attention must be paid to the mouth, teeth, throat and nose. Chlorophyll tablets taken orally are popularly supposed to remove the odour, although their efficacy is doubtful; but they may be ordered freely without ill effects. Proper hygiene of the mouth and a diet which requires good mastication are important, as well as the clearing of any periodontal pockets of food or debris.

DISEASES OF THE SALIVARY GLANDS

PTYALISM

Aetiology

The flow of saliva is increased by reflexes originating in the mouth and also in more distant situations. Thus all pathological conditions in the mouth and its neighbourhood, such as stomatitis, epithelioma of the tongue and carious teeth, especially if associated with pain, are accompanied by salivation. Trigeminal neuralgia, whatever its cause, is frequently associated with a reflex flow of saliva. Mechanical irritation of the oesophagus caused by the passage of a tube into the stomach or by the impaction of a foreign body causes salivation, which is a common symptom in achalasia of the cardia and in simple and malignant ulceration of the oesophagus. Reflex salivation is the cause of waterbrash associated with duodenal ulcer.

The salivation which may occur during menstruation and in the early months of pregnancy is also probably reflex in origin. Salivation is a common and sometimes very distressing symptom of paralysis agitans and post-encephalitic Parkinsonism. Ptyalism may result from excessive smoking. It is also caused by the specific stimulating action of certain drugs, such as pilocarpine, and by drugs such as the iodides and mercury, which are partially excreted by the salivary glands.

Symptoms

Every time saliva is swallowed air passes with it into the stomach. In neurotic individuals a spitting or swallowing tic may develop; the latter is always accompanied by aerophagy and the patient consequently complains of severe flatulence with excessive belching [p. 702].

Treatment

In order to cure ptyalism the primary cause must be discovered and removed. As purely symptomatic treatment, belladonna should be given, 0·3 ml. of the tincture, taken three times a day, half an hour before meals may be sufficient, but much larger doses are often required. The drug has the additional advantage of diminishing the secretion of gastric juice when gastric hypersecretion is also present.

XEROSTOMIA

Aetiology

The dry mouth, which is constantly present in fevers, is due mainly to deficiency in the physical, chemical and mechanical stimuli to salivary secretion. Depressing emotions and the loss or perversion of taste result in diminution in the physical secretion. The paralysis of the secretory nerve endings produced by belladonna, stramonium and their alkaloids sets the limit to the dose of these drugs which can be administered. The secretion of saliva is also diminished when excessive quantities of fluid are lost by other channels, as in severe diarrhoea or diabetes mellitus. Diseases of the salivary glands themselves, such as mumps, result in diminished secretion. Severe xerostomia occasionally develops without any obvious cause. A dry mouth is also a common result of sleeping with the mouth open.

Symptoms

Deficient secretion of saliva causes the mouth to become dry and septic, as particles of food remain between the teeth, where they undergo bacterial decomposition. The tongue is furred and dry, and there is often an unpleasant taste in the mouth. It is difficult to chew food sufficiently, and the appetite is impaired as a result of the condition of the mouth and the difficulty in tasting. The insufficiently chewed food is likely to irritate the stomach. In severe cases dysphagia occurs and speech becomes difficult. The loss of the digestion of starch by the ptyalin of the saliva is of no importance owing to the amylolytic activity of the pancreatic juice.

Treatment

A diet should be chosen which stimulates the flow of saliva; acids are most active, then salt and bitters, whilst sweet substances have very little action. The food should be given in as appetizing a form as possible and masticated very thoroughly. The taste of a bitter mixture taken immediately before meals may directly stimulate the flow of saliva, and pilocarpine may be tried, but it is rarely of much use, as a dose sufficiently large to increase the flow of saliva generally produces unpleasant symptoms, such as excessive sweating. It is, however, valuable in the treatment of paralysis agitans and postencephalitic Parkinsonism, as it counteracts the xerostomia (and also the paralysis of the intrinsic eye muscles) often caused by hyoscine and stramonium, without diminishing their effect on the tremor of paralysis agitans and the rigidity following encephalitis. Great care should be taken to keep the teeth clean, and the mouth should be washed after each meal. Local application of medicinal paraffin may temporarily relieve the dryness.

SPECIFIC PAROTITIS (MUMPS)

[see Section 2]

SJØGREN'S SYNDROME

[see Section 4]

MIKULICZ'S SYNDROME

Symptoms

There is symmetrical swelling of the salivary glands together with the lacrimal glands, and sometimes of the accessory glands in the tongue and hard palate. The enlargement is gradual and there is little or no constitutional disturbance. The swollen glands are firm, painless and mobile. The diminution in secretions causes dryness of the mouth and conjunctival irritation; the swollen parotids and protrusion of the eyeballs caused by the enlarged orbital glands with ptosis produces a characteristic facies. A similar syndrome may rarely occur in lymphatic leukaemia, lymphosarcoma [see Section 13], and uveoparotid fever which is a variant of sarcoidosis [see Section 9]. The syndrome occurs most frequently in adult males, but its cause is not known.

Treatment

Arsenic and potassium iodide are used, and X-ray therapy may also be given with diminution in size of the glands.

PAROTITIS

Aetiology

Parotitis is usually due to infection ascending Stensen's duct from the mouth. This is particularly apt to occur in the acute parotitis that not infrequently follows operations on the alimentary tract when the mouth has become septic owing to dehydration, the absence of chewing and normal salivation. It may develop secondarily to obstruction from a stone in Stensen's duct, or in the dry mouth of Sjøgren's syndrome or diabetes mellitus. It may also follow trauma of Stensen's duct by ill-fitting dentures. Subacute parotitis, which is often recurrent, may also occur in persons with apparently healthy mouths. The infection may be limited to Stensen's duct, when it is referred to as sialodochitis, or it may spread from the ducts to the tissues of the gland. Blood stream infection may also take place. The subacute recurrent type of infection is relatively common in children and occurs more frequently in women than in men. In children recurrent attacks tend to become less severe as adolescence is reached and usually clear up before adult life.

Symptoms

In acute parotitis following operation one or both

glands may be affected. The glands are enlarged and tender, the skin over them reddened, shiny and oedematous. In severe cases, suppuration takes place, the neighbouring lymph nodes enlarge, the temperature is high and severe constitutional symptoms are present. The mouth is dry and difficult to keep clean; the tongue is covered with a thick fur. The mouth of Stensen's duct is everted and forms a small, red nodule from which a bead of pus can usually be squeezed. In most cases the inflammation subsides with antibiotic treatment; abscess formation may occur; rarely the condition becomes chronic, the parotid glands remain permanently enlarged and excrete a reduced quantity of saliva.

In the subacute form swelling of one or both glands may occur on a single occasion or repeatedly at intervals of weeks or months, sometimes over a period of many years. The swelling usually lasts for several days but may persist for months. Fluctuation in the size of the swelling takes place, an increase usually accompanying or following mastication. The inflamed gland is tender to pressure and the overlying skin may be reddened and hot. Firm pressure over the gland often causes expulsion of pus or turbid saliva from the reddened orifice of Stensen's duct. The submandibular glands may be affected in the same way, either by themselves or in association with parotid swellings. In these patients radiographic examination of the ducts after injection of *Lipiodol* frequently shows beadlike dilatation of the terminal acini, or there may be irregular dilatation of the main duct and its branches. The condition must be differentiated from leukaemia with infiltration of the parotid and submandibular glands and from uveoparotitis or Heerfordt's disease which is a special form of sarcoidosis.

Microscopical examination of the parotid saliva shows degenerated leucocytes, epithelial cell debris and organisms. In acute parotitis *Staphylococcus pyogenes* is the organism usually responsible, while in the subacute and recurrent forms *Streptococcus viridans* and pneumococci are commonly found.

Treatment

In acute parotitis treatment with penicillin in full doses usually leads to resolution. Hot fomentations or application of an electric pad may ease the pain of the swollen gland. Mouth washes may be used and steps should be taken to overcome dehydration and to deal with local conditions in the mouth, if these exist. If abscess formation has occurred incisions of the gland will be necessary.

In subacute cases penicillin is also useful, local application of heat to relieve the pain and chewing-gum to assist drainage. When the active phase has subsided short-wave diathermy is often helpful. In long-standing cases with chronic infection and persistent swelling, deep X-ray therapy is sometimes justified, but this treatment, which destroys the secretory mechanism of the gland and induces fibrosis, should never be employed in children whose facial bones are still developing, since in such cases it may interfere with the growth of the mandible.

SALIVARY CALCULI

Calculi occur most frequently in Wharton's duct from the submaxillary gland, though they are not uncommon in the parotid duct. They are mainly composed of calcium oxalate associated with inspissated mucus and cellular debris. They are rarely bigger than 10–20 mm. in diameter. When they cause obstruction of the duct the patient notices swelling and pain in the gland as soon as he begins to eat, or thinks of food. With only partial obstruction they may cause no symptoms but can often be felt on digital examination. An X-ray may show calculi to be present, or sialography may demonstrate an obstruction in the duct. Calculous obstruction may cause secondary infection of the gland which, in a few cases, may require surgical removal.

NON-INFECTIVE RECURRENT SWELLING OF THE PAROTID GLANDS

Aetiology

This condition may occur at all ages. The cause is often uncertain, but the frequent association with allergic conditions in the patient himself or in his relatives has led to the suggestion that an allergic process is responsible. A number of cases have been described in which this pathogenesis has been demonstrated beyond doubt.

Symptoms

Eating may precipitate attacks, especially when the food is acid in character, and in some patients the parotid glands become swollen whenever food is taken over a period of many years. In others, the swelling is definitely associated with the eating of certain foods to which the patient is specifically sensitive. The swellings are more often bilateral than unilateral. They develop rapidly and are present for a short time only, often subsiding within half an hour and seldom persisting for more than 24 hours. Single isolated attacks may occur, but owing to their brief duration and the absence of after-effects they are seldom seen, and cases presenting themselves for treatment are usually recurrent. Signs of inflammation are absent, the parotid saliva contains no pus, and the swellings are seldom painful.

In most cases secretion can be expelled from the parotid duct by pressure during the attack. Globules of jelly-like mucus obstructing Stensen's duct may first be forced out, followed by 2 or 3 ml. of clear saliva. It is in this type of case that eosinophil cells have been observed both in the mucous plugs and in the pent-up secretion. This is sterile and contains no pus, but secondary infection may supervene in patients in whom swellings have recurred over a long period. In early cases saliva may be difficult to obtain.

Sialography may show gross fusiform dilatation of the main and branch ducts in long-standing cases; in others the appearance is similar to that seen in infective parotitis, with bead-like terminal dilatations. In early cases the appearance may be normal.

Treatment

Massage over the gland is of value, especially when mucous obstruction is present. In some cases injection of adrenaline subcutaneously leads to subsidence of the swelling. If specific foods cause the swelling, these must be avoided.

REFERENCES

BURKEL, L. W. (1962) *Oral Medicine*, 3rd ed., London.

SIRCUS, W., CHURCH, R., and KEELEHER, J. (1957) Recurrent aphthous ulceration of the mouth, *Quart. J. Med.*, **26**, 238.

SJØGREN, H. (1933) Keratoconjunctivitis sicca and polyarthritis, *Acta med. scand.*, **130**, 484.

A. M. DAWSON

DISEASES OF THE TONSILS

ACUTE TONSILLITIS

Aetiology

This common disease principally affects children and young adults. Children are particularly subject to the condition during their early school years. The infecting organism is usually a haemolytic streptococcus of Lancefield's Group A. The mode of spread is by droplet or dust infection and the disease flourishes in conditions of overcrowding and poor ventilation. Occasional outbreaks can be traced to infected milk supplies. The disease also occurs in scarlet fever, measles and many acute infections of the upper respiratory tract.

Symptoms

There is severe soreness of the throat and a marked general reaction. Children occasionally do not complain that their throat is sore but swallowing is obviously difficult for them and examination of the throat reveals the condition. The temperature may rise to 103° F. (39·5° C.) or more and there is a variable degree of malaise with headache, muscle and joint pains. The throat symptoms are made worse by swallowing, even liquids and saliva causing acute discomfort in many cases. The voice becomes thick and the breath foul and there is tender adenitis in the submandibular and upper deep cervical glands. Earache during the course of the disease is often a referred pain but it may be due to the development of acute otitis media as a complication so that inspection of the ear-drums is a wise precaution.

The tonsils are swollen and inflamed often with pus exuding from the crypts. This exudate may coalesce to cover most of the tonsil, it is soft and readily wiped away. The tongue is coated; the fauces, soft palate and uvula are inflamed and may be covered with sticky mucus.

Acute suppurative otitis media is the most frequent complication. Occasionally peritonsillar abscess or lung infection occurs and rarely acute nephritis or acute rheumatism may follow.

Diagnosis

Many conditions begin with a sore throat and fever and the differential diagnosis is important and may be difficult. Diphtheria, although rarely seen nowadays, should not be forgotten. This disease begins more insidiously than acute tonsillitis and the symptoms and general reaction are less marked while the adenitis is often very considerable. The diphtheritic membrane may cover the fauces and soft palate as well as the tonsil. It can only be removed with difficulty and leaves a raw bleeding surface. There is a characteristic musty odour easily recognized by those with previous experience of the disease. If there is any suspicion of diphtheria, a throat swab should be taken and antitoxin given immediately.

Nowadays the most common alternative diagnosis is the anginal type of glandular fever. Superficial ulceration may affect the tonsils and pharynx, but is not always present, while the cervical adenitis is more generalized than in acute tonsillitis and there may be lymphadenitis elsewhere, splenomegaly and hepatomegaly. Blood examination and a Paul-Bunnell reaction will confirm the diagnosis.

Agranulocytosis and acute leukaemia may also simulate acute tonsillitis though in these conditions ulceration in the pharynx is usually a marked feature. With adequate treatment acute tonsillitis should resolve within a week. If this does not occur suspicions of one of these alternative diagnoses should be investigated by means of a throat swab, full blood investigation, Paul-Bunnell reaction and a chest X-ray.

Treatment

With bed rest, most cases quickly recover. The appetite is poor and the patient should be encouraged to take ample bland fluids and can usually manage a semi-solid diet. Swallowing is made easier if a tablespoonful of aspirin mucilage is taken just before meals. A mild purgative may be required. Many types of lozenges are available but probably have very little beneficial effect, and penicillin lozenges are contra-indicated because of the severe stomatitis that they cause in susceptible subjects.

Although antibiotics are almost always prescribed for this condition it is doubtful if they speed recovery in many cases. Ideally their use should be reserved for severe cases with marked general reaction and adenitis and for those in whom a complication is suspected. Penicillin is still the first choice and should be given in adequate dosage for at least one week.

PERITONSILLAR ABSCESS OR QUINSY

Aetiology and Pathology

The abscess develops between the capsule of the

tonsil and the muscular bed of its fossa. The usual situation is above and lateral to the tonsil but in rare cases it develops behind it. Previous tonsillitis or peritonsillar abscess are predisposing causes. If untreated the abscess usually bursts and discharges through the supratonsillar cleft. Resolution of the infection and fibrosis of the abscess cavity then follows in most cases, but occasionally a chronic abscess develops which discharges intermittently.

Symptoms

The affection is almost always unilateral and develops during an attack of acute tonsillitis. The patient's condition suddenly worsens with increased pain radiating to the ear and enlarged tender glands on the affected side. Marked trismus develops and there is a sharp rise in temperature. Examination of the throat is difficult but if a good view is obtained the affected side shows a large red swelling of the soft palate with the tonsil pushed downwards and medially. Pus forms in 2–4 days and if spontaneous rupture occurs there is immediate relief of symptoms.

Diagnosis

Mixed salivary tumours developing in the soft palate adjacent to the tonsil produce similar physical appearances, but there is no acute illness, pain or trismus.

Complications

These are rare. If the abscess ruptures during sleep the pus may be inspirated and cause lung infections. Severe haemorrhage from the internal carotid artery has been reported. Suppuration in the cervical glands, pneumonia and blood infection may occur. Spreading inflammation in the pharynx may lead to laryngeal oedema and necessitate tracheostomy.

Treatment

The general treatment is the same as that for acute tonsillitis and antibiotics should be administered to reduce the risk of complications. Pus is probably present after four days and as soon as the swelling has assumed a well-defined rounded form, still more so if there is a boggy area in the centre. The abscess should be opened without delay, for this cuts short the attack and relieves the worst of the symptoms. The swelling should be incised at a point halfway between the last upper molar tooth on the affected side and the base of the uvula. This area is painted with 20 per cent. cocaine solution and the abscess incised with a special quinsy forceps or a scalpel with a half centimetre unguarded blade. Pus usually gushes forth and should be expectorated into a bowl; the patient should then use a hot mouthwash. Further hot mouthwashes used four times daily for the next few days aid drainage of the abscess. After the disease has subsided, removal of the tonsils is indicated in order to prevent recurrence.

RECURRENT TONSILLITIS IN CHILDREN

Symptoms

Some children are subject to frequent attacks of acute tonsillitis. These may start before the child begins school but the first few years of school life are the commonest period for these recurrent infections. They may occur without much evidence of infection elsewhere in the upper respiratory tract but more usually there is associated nasal and sometimes chest infection. The attacks are particularly frequent following one of the exanthemata.

The tonsils hypertrophy in most cases and may reach a very large size so that swallowing food becomes mechanically difficult and the child eats slowly. Associated adenoid hypertrophy and nasal infection is common and the child then presents the classical picture with a perpetually open mouth, nasal discharge and a history of snoring and nocturnal cough. Recurrent earache and suppurative otitis media often complicate this condition. Cervical adenitis accompanies the acute attack and enlargement of the glands often persists between the acute episodes. If this enlargement seems out of proportion to the throat symptoms, the glands may be tuberculous. Simple hypertrophy may occur without severe recurrent infection while in a few cases the tonsils become fibrosed at an early age and although the seat of severe recurrent infection, do not enlarge. Children with an allergic diathesis who have suffered from infantile eczema often develop considerable hypertrophy of the tonsils and adenoids and suffer from nasal obstruction and discharge.

Treatment

Each acute episode is treated as described already for acute tonsillitis. The problem is to decide when the condition warrants surgical removal of the tonsils which is combined in most cases with curettage of the adenoids.

If four or more attacks of severe tonsillitis have occurred during the preceding twelve months without the predisposing cause of an acute exanthem, and especially if there has been associated acute otitis media, the tonsils should be removed. They should also be removed if there is suspected tuberculous cervical adenitis or if it is considered that recurrent tonsillar infection is the cause of repeated attacks of rheumatic fever or acute nephritis. The operation should be avoided in an allergic child unless there is much infection associated with the hypertrophy of the tonsils and adenoids. The operation is also contra-indicated if the child has a bleeding diathesis and during an epidemic of poliomyelitis. Details of the operation may be found in surgical textbooks.

CHRONIC TONSILLITIS

Symptoms

Young adults are the usual sufferers. There may be a history of frequent attacks of acute tonsillitis, often dating from childhood or the condition may have developed recently. In others there are no severe acute exacerbations but a more or less constant discomfort and soreness in the throat without much general reaction, and sometimes accompanied by laryngeal infection. Chronic tonsillitis may be secondary to chronic sinusitis or dental sepsis.

Treatment

Any dental or sinus infection must be treated appropriately. Mandl's paint applied with a soft brush to the fauces and tonsils twice daily for two weeks may help, and smoking, alcohol and dusty atmospheres should all be avoided. If the symptoms are severe tonsillectomy is indicated.

VINCENT'S ANGINA

Aetiology

This affection is generally believed to be due to two organisms, the fusiform bacillus and *Borrelia vincenti* which are commonly found together in many ulcerative lesions of the mouth or throat, as well as in tropical ulcer, pulmonary spirochaetosis and certain ulcerative lesions of the genitalia. It has never been established beyond doubt that these two organisms are the cause of these lesions: it is quite possible that they are only secondary invaders. Affection of the throat is frequently secondary to periodontal infection. It occurs especially in debilitated persons and under insanitary conditions and was common during both World Wars.

Symptoms

The attack begins insidiously with malaise, general pains and a temperature of 100°–101° F. (37·8°–38·3° C.). The pain in the throat is often slight, but in some cases may be severe; the glands on the affected side become enlarged and tender, and the breath is characteristically offensive.

There is superficial ulceration which commonly involves the tonsils and fauces but may affect the inner surface of the cheek, pharyngeal wall or larynx. The ulcers vary in size; their base is covered with a yellowish-grey pseudomembrane which is not easily detached, and there is marked hyperaemia around the edges. By the end of a week the membranes cease to form, and the ulcers begin to heal. If dental hygiene is poor there may be recurrent attacks of ulceration.

Diagnosis

The disease may imitate diphtheria in its early stage, and syphilitic ulceration later. In both cases the discovery of numerous spirilla and fusiform bacilli in smear preparations—they are difficult to cultivate—will help to confirm the diagnosis. However, these organisms can be found in syphilitic ulcers and the Wassermann reaction is sometimes positive in Vincent's angina. The subacute onset, the raised temperature and the tenderness of the glands aid the differentiation from syphilis; and from diphtheria the milder constitutional symptoms, the soft pliable character of the membrane and the absence of the diphtheria bacillus. Ulceration of the fauces and tonsils also occurs in glandular fever, agranulocytosis and leukaemia and in the elderly it may be a tuberculous infection secondary to phthisis. Recurrent non-specific ulceration of the mouth, palate, fauces and tonsils is not uncommon. In most cases the cause is unknown, but some are due to herpes simplex while in rare instances it is a manifestation of Behçet's syndrome, pemphigus vulgaris, or pemphigoid.

Treatment

The lesions respond to parenteral penicillin in full dosage. Alternatively, adminster metronidazole, 200 mg. thrice daily for 3 days.

A paint of 5 per cent. neoarsphenamine in equal quantities of glycerin and water may be applied to the ulcers.

Attention to dental hygiene and a course of ascorbic acid and vitamin B complex will prevent recurrent attacks.

DISEASES OF THE PHARYNX

ACUTE CATARRHAL PHARYNGITIS

This is not a well-defined affection, and is usually accompanied by acute rhinitis on the one hand, and by laryngitis on the other; the tonsils also often participate in the inflammation.

Aetiology

The affection is generally the result of coryza, and it is a feature of various acute infectious fevers, such as measles, German measles, scarlet fever, influenza and typhoid.

Symptoms

The discomfort varies from a tickling sensation, or the feeling of a lump in the throat, to severe dysphagia. The voice is husky and thick, and the cervical glands tender and somewhat enlarged. There is slight fever and general malaise.

The pharynx is to a varying degree red and swollen, especially at the sides behind the posterior faucial pillars, where the swelling forms the so-called 'lateral bands'. The palate is swollen and relaxed, and the uvula elongated. The posterior wall is often covered by a film of tenacious mucus.

Treatment

The patient should stay in a warm room and avoid the irritation of smoking, talking, alcohol or irritating foods. Aspirin, or sodium salicylate, is helpful and it is important to treat any primary cause.

ACUTE SEPTIC PHARYNGITIS

This term includes a series of severe infective inflammations; oedematous, phlegmonous and gangrenous pharyngitis and laryngitis, and Ludwig's angina. Any classification must necessarily be a clinical one, based on the severity of the symptoms and their localization, for they can be produced by a variety of micro-organisms, though they are usually caused by a streptococcus. These severe inflammations are fortunately uncommon, and most often, though by no means invariably, occur in debilitated or alcoholic persons.

Symptoms

These vary greatly with the severity of the infection, which ranges from a mild inflammation to the most severe septic intoxication. They include malaise, sore throat, dysphagia, hoarseness and dyspnoea. The temperature in some cases rises to 105°–106° F. (40·5°–41° C.); but in many of the worst cases it is hardly raised at all, and may be subnormal. Pleurisy, pneumonia and pericarditis may ensue, or death may result from asphyxia; but the worst cases die from general toxaemia and heart failure, even within 24 hours of the onset of the disease.

The objective appearances, also, are very variable. The pharynx and palate are of a deep purplish-red, and there may be sloughy pseudomembranous patches. The entire mucosa may be enormously swollen, and the oedema may involve the upper aperture of the larynx and produce asphyxia. The sublingual region is sometimes occupied by a peculiar brawny swelling, of a hardness like wood, which spreads downwards into the neck to a variable extent, and is known as Ludwig's angina.

Treatment

The patient must be in bed and well nursed, and every care must be used to ensure that he takes as much nourishment as possible. Antibiotics must be administered in full dosage and a high fluid intake be assured. Oedema of the glottis may call for emergency tracheostomy. For Ludwig's angina it is now only rarely necessary to make an incision deeply into the neck in the hope of striking pus; the swelling will either subside or a fluctuating abscess will become apparent.

RETROPHARYNGEAL ABSCESS

There are two forms—(1) Acute, and (2) Chronic.

1. The acute form occurs in children up to the age of 3 or 4, but is far more frequently met with in the first 12 months. It is due to suppuration in the prevertebral glands situated behind the posterior pharyngeal wall; these glands disappear in later life. The abscess is secondary to nasal, nasopharyngeal or tonsillar infection and may occur during the course of an infectious fever.

Though rare the condition is an important one for it may easily remain unrecognized in a young infant and could then cause death either by rupturing with inspiration of the pus, or by spread to the mediastinum, or by general toxaemia and septicaemia. The symptoms are fever and restlessness, a hoarse cry and croupy cough, with difficulty in swallowing and dyspnoea. Such symptoms should arouse a suspicion of retropharyngeal abscess, which may be seen on inspection as a rounded swelling of the posterior pharyngeal wall.

As soon as the condition is recognized a broad-spectrum antibiotic should be administered in high dosage. Intramuscular penicillin is the first choice unless specifically contra-indicated. The abscess must then be incised and, as it is often large, care is needed to avoid aspiration of pus and blood. It should be opened widely over the most prominent and inferior part of the bulge. In a child under one year old this can be done without anaesthesia if the child is firmly held lying on its back with the head hanging almost vertically. Over one year old general anaesthesia with a cuffed endotracheal tube is used and suction should be available in all cases. A specimen of the pus should be sent for bacteriological examination and if the sensitivity reports indicate it the antibiotic must be changed. Antibiotic therapy should continue for at least one week after incision of the abscess. Recovery is usually rapid unless the child was severely debilitated before treatment commenced.

2. The chronic form also is found most frequently in children but generally after the third year. This is a tuberculous abscess forming behind the prevertebral fascia and is secondary to caries of the cervical spine. X-rays of the spine usually demonstrate the lesion well. It should not be opened through the mouth as this may lead to secondary infection of the diseased bone but is best drained via a vertical incision along the posterior border of the sternomastoid. General antituberculous chemotherapy is indicated and temporary support for the cervical spine may be necessary.

CHRONIC PHARYNGITIS

(Pharyngeal Hyperaesthesia)

Aetiology

Chronic pharyngitis is usually secondary to chronic infection in the nasal sinuses, tonsils or teeth. It is aggravated by mouth breathing, smoking and over-indulgence in alcohol. Excessive use or misuse of the voice perpetuates the condition which may be initiated by an acute pharyngitis which fails to resolve satisfactorily.

Symptoms

Discomfort may take the form of aching, fullness or feeling of a lump, a hair or a pricking. The voice has a dead tone, and there is usually much hawking and frequent swallowing. The sufferer often becomes depressed, and fears that he has cancer of the throat. The unpleasant sensations are markedly lessened after a meal.

The mucosa of the pharynx and palate is thickened, and there is a loss of the finer modelling of the faucial pillars; the uvula is elongated, often slightly oedematous at its edges and tip, and fails to retract on phonation. The posterior wall is covered by a film of mucus, which puckers up and becomes more obvious on touching it with a probe or swab. The wall of the pharynx is traversed by enlarged venules, and sometimes it is set with slightly raised pink lenticular nodules of lymphoid tissue, constituting a variety known as 'granular pharyngitis'. In other cases two elongated masses of lymphoid tissue appear behind and parallel to the posterior pillars; these are the 'lateral bands', and this form is called 'lateral pharyngitis'. Patients suffering from atrophic rhinitis may complain of dryness of the throat; the posterior pharyngeal wall presents a glazed desiccated appearance, sometimes alluded to as pharyngitis sicca.

Treatment

Any focus of infection elsewhere in the nose or mouth should be eradicated. Tobacco, alcohol, spiced foods and excessive use of the voice must be avoided. A warm alkaline saline nasal douche and throat spray may help, but local medication should be avoided when possible as it concentrates the patient's attention on his throat. In cases of chronic granular pharyngitis and those with enlarged 'lateral bands' of lymphoid tissue the hypertrophied lymph follicles may be reduced by painting them at weekly intervals for one month with a 5 per cent. solution of silver nitrate. It is most important to reassure these patients that there is no growth in their throat as many of them have an underlying cancer phobia and this reassurance will often cause their symptoms to abate.

KERATOSIS PHARYNGIS

In this condition a number of sharply defined white or yellow spikes project from the surface of the tonsils; they also occur, though less profusely, scattered over the lingual and nasopharyngeal tonsils and on any lymphoid granules in the pharynx. They occur at any age after childhood and the causation is unknown. The projections consist of heaped-up epithelium and detritus containing numerous micro-organisms of the kind ordinarily present in the mouth. On microscopical examination branching fungus mycelium can usually be demonstrated. They sometimes disappear quickly, in other cases they remain for many months, or they may recur. They produce no symptoms, or at most a slight discomfort, and are of interest chiefly because they are frequently mistaken for the exudation of chronic follicular tonsillitis. Once seen they can, however, be recognized at a glance, for they are hard and adherent, discrete and prominent, and occur beyond the limits of the tonsils, on the pharynx and base of the tongue. They are usually discovered accidentally by the patient, who is naturally alarmed at their appearance. They are quite harmless, and local treatment is useless, for they are removed with difficulty and usually recur; it is wise to reassure the patient by telling him these facts and, if any treatment be required, to trust to attention to the general health, a holiday and change of air. In rare cases when the condition is confined to the tonsils, marked symptoms and persistence of the condition may justify tonsillectomy.

R.F. McNab Jones

DISEASES OF THE OESOPHAGUS

ANATOMY AND PHYSIOLOGY

The oesophagus is a distensible, normally closed tube of approximately 25 cm. in length which connects the pharynx to the stomach. Its muscle layers comprise an outer longitudinal and inner circular coat; above, they are striated and fuse with the sphincter of the cricopharyngeus but lower down the muscle is smooth. The site of this transition varies and is usually at the junction of the upper and middle third. Although a physiological sphincter has been demonstrated over the lower 3 cm. of the oesophagus there is little anatomical basis for this. The lower 4 cm. of the oesophagus is known as the vestibule or cardiac antrum and is partly within the abdominal cavity where it is anchored by the phreno-oesophageal ligament. The innervation of the muscles is both from the sympathetic and parasympathetic nervous system, together with a particularly rich intrinsic innervation as shown by the presence of Auerbach's and Meissner's plexus in the lower third. The epithelium lining the oesophagus is mainly stratified squamous with scattered islets of submucous glands deep to the muscularis mucosae. Cardiac glands which are superficial to the muscularis mucosae occur in the upper and lower third of the oesophagus. The transition to columnar epithelium is abrupt but irregular and usually occurs in the intra-abdominal part of the oesophagus and above the junction of the oesophageal muscle with the cardia; the upper few millimetres of this columnar epithelium is usually devoid of parietal cells and known as the 'buffer zone'. The exact site of transition is variable and on occasions this junction takes place some centimetres above the diaphragm when it has pathological significance.

Swallowing is initiated by reflexes from inside the mouth and upper pharynx. There is compression of the tongue to the roof of the mouth and reflux of food into the nose is prevented by contraction of the upper pharyngeal muscles and elevation of the soft palate. As the bolus is pressed to the back of the pharynx the upper oesophageal lumen is enlarged by raising and pulling forward of the larynx. Peristaltic waves sweep down the oesophagus following closure of the cricopharyngeal muscle. At the start of swallowing there is a relaxation of the intrinsic lower oesophageal sphincter so that the oncoming bolus passes without hindrance into the stomach. The peristaltic sweep is mainly of importance when swallowing is not aided by gravity. The normal mechanism preventing reflux is still debated and must explain its absence under conditions of straining and coughing when there is a pressure difference between the stomach and the gullet of sometimes up to 100 or 200 mm. Hg, and also it must allow for the phenomenon of vomiting. One explanation is that the lower 2 cm. of this thin-walled collapsible tube is within the abdomen and is kept closed by the intra-abdominal pressure. This portion of the gullet acts as a flutter valve and increased intra-abdominal pressure increases the action of this valve and makes regurgitation difficult. Vomiting is accomplished by contraction of the longitudinal muscles of the oesophagus with the production of a small hiatus; this abolishes the intra-abdominal oesophagus. The relatively weak intrinsic sphincter is then overcome. Normally it has a pressure of more than 15 mm. of water. In patients with free oesophageal reflux the sphincter pressure is low, indicating its importance in preventing reflux. The acute angle of entry of oesophagus into stomach which acts as a flap valve is of doubtful importance as in experimentally-produced sliding hiatus hernias maintenance of an acute angle of entry does not prevent reflux.

REFERENCES

BENEDICT, E. B., and NARDI, G. L. (1958) *The Oesophagus*, Boston.

INGLEFINGER, F. J. (1958) Oesophageal motility, *Physiol. Rev.*, **38**, 533.

KRAMER, P. (1968) The oesophagus, *Gastroenterology*, **54**, 1171.

DYSPHAGIA

Dysphagia is the difficulty in the swallowing of food or drink. Oral and pharyngeal causes may either be painful when they are usually obvious to inspection or due to a disturbed innervation of the pharynx, when the patient may well complain of regurgitation of fluid through the nose and difficulty in getting the bolus to pass from the mouth into the gullet. This may occur in various neurological conditions, such as poliomyelitis or bulbar palsy. If the food can leave the throat and if the difficulty occurs during rather than after the act of swallowing it is extremely dangerous to ascribe the symptoms to other than an organic cause. So-called globus hystericus is not dysphagia but the sensation of a painful lump in the throat. When there is organic obstruction the site may be localized accurately by the patient but often there is false proximal localization, possibly due to retropulsive oesophageal contractions. When the condition is painful the pain may be substernal, it occasionally passes through to the back and may pass up to the throat and into the arms, when it can be mistaken for myocardial pain. The commonest oesophageal causes of dysphagia are carcinoma, oesophagitis with or without stricture formation and less commonly achalasia of the cardia.

CARCINOMA OF THE OESOPHAGUS

Aetiology

The aetiology is unknown but there is an unexplained wide geographical variation in frequency. For example, it is common in France and in the Chinese province of Hunan, where there is the extremely high incidence of 67·2 per 100,000. It is less frequent in England and among the white population of the United States, but whether this is due to environmental or genetic difference is unknown. The sex ratio varies in different countries. It affects men four times as commonly as women in the United States, while the ratio is 2:1 in England and 8:1 in Finland. This variation may be partly due to the association of upper oesophageal lesions with chronic iron deficiency which is more common in women. Other relatively uncommon predisposing factors are chronic irritation of the oesophagus by alcohol, tobacco and chronic oesophagitis occurring in untreated achalasia of the cardia and occasionally when caused by reflux. There is a rare genetic form of carcinoma occurring in some familes with tylosis, an affection of the skin of the hands and feet which is transmitted as a Mendelian dominant.

Pathology

Ninety per cent. of the lesions are squamous and 10 per cent. are adenocarcinomas which arise from the oesophageal glands; adenocarcinomas occurring in the lower third of the oesophagus may be difficult to distinguish from those arising in the gastric cardia. In men approximately 50 per cent. of the lesions are in the lower third, 40 per cent. in the middle third and only 10 per cent. in the upper third, while in women approximately equal proportions occur in each third, presumably due to the prevalence of iron deficiency anaemia in women.

Clinical Picture

The earliest symptom is usually dysphagia, typically with bread or meat. The patient will tend to wash down the food with liquids. This rarely occurs until the disease is advanced, for owing to the great distensibility of the gullet approximately three-quarters of the circumference has to be involved before swallowing is sufficiently impaired to cause dysphagia. Once dysphagia occurs it is nearly always progressive. In only 20 per cent. of patients is there pain initially. This may occur at the impact of the bolus, when there is muscular contraction or there may be a constant dull boring pain in the advanced case due to infiltration of mediastinal tissues. Occasionally with lesions of the lower gullet there is violent oesophageal pain which continues until there is regurgitation of the meal into the mouth. Not unnaturally, weight loss progresses to emaciation. If there is considerable ulceration of the lesion there is an associated iron deficiency anaemia. Eventually, when even liquids cannot be swallowed, dehydration ensues. Late local symptoms may be due to paralysis of the recurrent laryngeal nerve, when there are voice changes and laryngeal anaesthesia due to infiltration of the sensory supply of the larynx which allows inhalation of both saliva, which is excessively produced, and stagnating food. This together with direct infiltration of the bronchus may give rise to respiratory infection. Further disability may occur from mediastinitis, a haemorrhage from involvement of the large vessels and involvement of spinal roots. Occasionally the patient may present with an iron deficient anaemia, sudden dysphagia, when the partially occluded gullet is impacted by, for example, a fruit stone, recurrent laryngeal paralysis or glands in the neck. Presentation with distant metastases is rare. In patients with a lower oesophageal lesion the first symptom may be 'dyspepsia' before true dysphagia ensues.

Diagnosis

The most important investigation is the barium

swallow [Plate 3] and with increase in skill and improvement in technique its accuracy is high, only 2 per cent. of lesions being missed in a recent series of Franklin and his colleagues. However, this type of result can only be obtained when the radiologist has been specifically asked to look at the oesophagus. All too frequently in a routine barium meal the oesophageal examination is relatively perfunctory. Oesophagoscopy and biopsy is usually performed to confirm the nature of any lesion seen and always when the barium swallow is normal and the patient has persistent dysphagia. However, this investigation is not undertaken lightly for it carries the risk of oesophageal perforation in patients who are kyphotic or have cervical osteophytes. These reservations may well be obviated by the more general use of the flexible 'fibre optic' instrument. Exfoliative cytology of the oesophagus will give between 70 and 95 per cent. positive diagnosis, depending on the extent of the lesion and the skill of the cytology department.

Treatment

The results of treatment of this condition are disappointing and for most patients must be considered to be palliative. There is still no complete agreement as to the best form of treatment which may either be surgical when cure may be attempted or palliative measures only adopted; on the other hand radiotherapy may be used. For example, Franklin and his colleagues try always to do a radical resection and out of 129 cases 91 were deemed fit for exploration but only 58 underwent a radical resection and only 20 were alive one year after operation. The results of radiotherapy are equally depressing, although there have been some good results with the upper oesophageal lesions. Palliation is aimed at relieving dysphagia so that not only may nourishment be taken but inhalation of food and saliva be minimized. This may be attempted by intubation of the growth. The best method is to use the Gourevitch tube which consists of a wire spiral within a latex rubber tube. Unfortunately all intubation procedures are potentially dangerous for they are used in inoperable neoplasms which tend to split during intubation and so produce mediastinitis. If intubation is successfully accomplished the patient has to avoid pith and coarse food or the tube blocks. More recently by-pass procedures have been used, especially using a sling of colon which goes subcutaneously and is anastomosed to the upper oesophagus in the throat. This can be done on frail people, the mediastinum is not opened and the local lesion may then be treated by radiotherapy. It is probably not much more dangerous than intubation, while palliation is greater, there being no subsequent dietary restriction. It should be emphasized that feeding gastrostomies and feeding jejunostomies are not palliative; the patient is left with a severe disability and gradually chokes from aspirated saliva. Before embarking on any of the above procedures the patient has to be rehydrated and the standard of nutrition improved. These precautions together with improvement in technique of surgery and anaesthesia has decreased the appalling operative mortality of resection but this is still high, e.g. of the 58 patients in Franklin's series 38 per cent. were dead within one month of operation.

Course and Prognosis

The disease runs a nearly ineluctable course, the mean time of diagnosis after symptoms occur is 5 months; few patients live for a further year.

REFERENCES

Adams, C. L. (1966) The complications of endo-oesophageal tubes, *J. thorac. cardiovasc. Surg.*, **51**, 685.

Franklin, R. H., Burn, J. I., and Lynch, G. (1964) Carcinoma of the oesophagus: a review of 129 treated patients, *Brit. J. Surg.*, **51**, 178.

Sturdy, D. E. (1965) Surgical management of carcinoma of the oesophagus, *Brit. J. Surg.*, **52**, 245.

Tanner, M. C., and Smithers, D. W., eds (1961) *Neoplastic Diseases at Various Sites*, Vol. 4, Tumours of the Oesophagus, Edinburgh.

OTHER MALIGNANT TUMOURS OF THE OESOPHAGUS

These are rare, for example, sarcoma of the oesophagus makes up only 0·5 per cent. of all oesophageal malignant neoplasms.

BENIGN TUMOURS OF THE OESOPHAGUS

These are relatively uncommon and nearly 80 per cent. are myomas but the whole gamut of benign tumours has been described as clinical oddities. The symptoms may be similar to the early non-invasive symptoms of carcinoma. X-ray changes may show typical splitting of the barium stream round a sharply demarcated rounded swelling. When polypoid the lesions may change position and have been missed on X-ray or mistaken for an air bubble.

DIAPHRAGMATIC HERNIA

In a diaphragmatic hernia there is translocation of abdominal contents into the chest with or without a hernial sac. These may either be congenital or acquired, when occasionally they seem to be of traumatic origin. Non-traumatic hernias most frequently occur through the oesophageal hiatus and only rarely do other holes which occur from inadequate fusion of the diaphragm during foetal development allow the passage of abdominal contents into the chest. These latter may be anterior on either side of the attachment of the diaphragm to the sternum, posterior due to the failure of fusion of the pleuroperitoneal canal in the lumbar region or near the foramen of Bochdalek or elsewhere along the costal margin, when they are not related to an embryonic fusion line. These rare defects when occurring on the right side are usually blocked by the liver. Traumatic hernias usually follow a blunt injury as in a road traffic accident and must be considered in such patients who have respiratory distress. They are seldom missed when caused by penetrating wounds as these are explored surgically. Non-hiatal diaphragmatic hernias may be diagnosed in infancy and if very large cause respiratory embarrassment when they call for urgent treatment. However, smaller ones can escape detection into adult life and be found either incidentally on a routine chest X-ray or present with a catastrophe such as strangulation of a loop of bowel.

HIATUS HERNIA AND REFLUX OESOPHAGITIS

There are two main types of hernia through the oesophageal hiatus, the sliding and rolling. In the sliding type, which comprises at least 80 per cent. of patients, the gastro-oesophageal junction remains at the apex of the herniated stomach. In the rolling hernia the gastro-oesophageal junction remains at the level of the diaphragm and either a part of the stomach enters the chest beside the oesophagus, the para-oesophageal hernia, or the greater curvature of the stomach may pass into the chest through the hiatus. In approximately 5 per cent. of patients there is a mixture of these two types.

Aetiology

There is little reliable information as to the aetiology of the hiatal hernia. This will remain so until there is accurate knowledge of the incidence of the condition in the general population. With improved techniques to demonstrate this hernia it is realized that it is very common and a recent survey showed that 30 per cent. of an asymptomatic population had a hiatus hernia which in no way differed in size and sex distribution from a comparable series of symptomatic subjects. Symptomatic hernias are three times more common in women than men and the symptoms often start during pregnancy; these patients are frequently overweight.

Pathology

When there is a sliding hernia there is a disappearance of the intra-abdominal oesophagus and so loss of the flutter valve mechanism. When the lower oesophageal sphincter is weak there is reflux of acid and pepsin into the vulnerable squamous-lined oesophagus giving rise to oesophagitis. It is now realized that this sphincter incompetence can occur even in the absence of a hiatus hernia. The oesophageal mucosa may then become friable and bleed and also progress to stricture formation; a localized penetrating ulcer may occur. Reflux oesophagitis may also occur when the anti-reflux mechanism has been destroyed or by-passed following oesophagectomy or oesophagogastric resection, cardioplasty, oesophagogastric lateral anastomosis, Heller's operation and porto-azygos disconnection for oesophageal varices.

A short oesophagus may be due either to retraction of the oesophagus once the stomach has entered the chest due to the tonic state of the longitudinal muscles or to contraction of fibrous tissue during stricture formation, there being fixation of the hernia. A truly congenitally short oesophagus is rare.

In some patients an appreciable length of the lower gullet (e.g. 10 cm.) may be lined by columnar epithelium of the cardiac type. If this congenital anomaly is associated with a hiatus hernia and oesophagogastric reflux, reflux oesophagitis and stricture formation tend to occur proximal to the squamocolumnar junction as the columnar epithelium is relatively resistant to the erosive power of gastric juice. This anomaly accounts for most patients who have a peptic stricture proximal to the gastro-oesophageal junction. Very rarely the columnar-lined oesophagus contains abundant parietal cells which may secrete acid and cause peptic oesophagitis. Occasionally the columnar lined oesophagus itself is affected by a simple peptic ulcer (Barret's ulcer) prone to the complications of other gastric ulcers such as penetration, perforation and haemorrhage.

Clinical Features

There is too great a tendency to explain vague gastro-intestinal symptoms on the basis of a coincidental hiatus hernia when they are psychogenic or caused by some other organic disease. In a simple sliding hernia the symptoms are mainly due to reflux and subsequent oesophagitis. There is heartburn or regurgitation of gastric contents especially on stooping or lying, particularly on the right side. This is worse after food and may be eased by alkalis. The patient may be woken from sleep choking from inhalation of gastric contents. With the advent of oesophagitis there is typical lower substernal pain on eating which is aggravated by hot foods and alcohol and now the heartburn becomes more painful. Once stenosis sets in there is intermittent dysphagia which is usually painful but stenosis is relatively rare considering how frequent such hernias are in the population. If penetration of an ulcer occurs pain can be severe and only temporarily relieved by alkalis. Occasionally a major vessel is eroded causing an often fatal haematemesis, less commonly there is perforation which causes an acute mediastinitis, there being severe epigastric, retrosternal or pleuritic pain and usually surgical emphysema in the neck. This is more likely to occur in peptic ulcer of the columnar-lined oesophagus. Iron deficiency anaemia may be an important associated phenomenon due either to loss from oesophagitis or an associated peptic ulcer. Massive haematemesis is uncommon. In view of the frequency of such hernias one must emphasize that other causes of both acute and chronic gastro-intestinal blood loss must be excluded. There may also be symptoms and attendant complications of an associated duodenal or gastric ulcer; the latter often occurring in the neck of the sac as it passes the diaphragm.

In large para-oesophageal hernias symptoms may be aggravated after food when the loculus becomes distended. There may be a bursting substernal pain or fullness and gurgling which may be relieved by pacing round the room. Occasionally there is dysphagia due to pressure of the sac or when distended this may induce dyspnoea or palpitations. Rarely there may be torsion and strangulation of a loop of gut or volvulus of the stomach in the hernial pouch. These symptoms especially occur in the rolling type of hernia. Symptoms may be mysteriously intermittent and the cause of long remissions is obscure.

Diagnosis

This should depend on typical clinical features and be confirmed by a barium meal [PLATES 3 and 4] which is performed in association with various manoeuvres to raise the intra-abdominal pressure. The presence of a large phrenic ampulla should not be confused with a true hernia. Besides the presence of a hernia, the presence or absence of reflux is noted and any irregularity of the lower oesophageal mucosa.

In doubtful cases oesophagoscopy is useful to confirm the presence or absence of oesophagitis and, in addition, in the presence of dysphagia to exclude a coincidental carcinoma.

Occasionally it is difficult to decide whether the oesophagus or heart is responsible for substernal pain radiating into the throat and arms, especially if the patient has a coincidental hiatus hernia. Such pain can arise from oesophagitis and if the oesophagus is perfused with N/10 hydrochloric acid the pain can often be reproduced and the patient will recognize its nature. It is only to confirm that the pain is of oesophageal origin that the test is useful.

Differential Diagnosis

As has been previously stressed, the presence of a demonstrable oesophageal hiatus hernia does not mean that this is the cause of the patient's symptoms and unless the symptoms are typical, other causes must be sought. For example substernal and epigastric colic may be ascribed to oesophageal spasm when they are due to gall-stones, and similarly myocardial ischaemia may be misdiagnosed. Furthermore, heartburn can be produced experimentally not only by putting acid in the gullet but also by distending it with balloons, and therefore heartburn in itself does not mean that reflux is occurring. When dysphagia is present a coincidental carcinoma must be excluded. A stricture may also arise post-operatively or after prolonged intubation of the stomach, especially if the patient was unconscious and nursed lying flat. The sudden onset of painful dysphagia in a malnourished person or a patient on steroids raises the possibility of oesophageal moniliasis.

Treatment

Medical treatment is often satisfactory for a patient with a sliding hernia unless there is severe oesophagitis or stricture formation. This is aimed at weight reduction, taking small amounts of food rather than large meals, using antacids after meals and blocking the head of the bed nine inches to prevent reflux at night. If oesophagitis is present frequent antacids may help to control symptoms. As already stated, these symptoms tend to be intermittent. However, should the frequency or severity of reflux be intolerable, oesophagitis produce intolerable pain or there be a stricture surgical treatment is desirable. When there is no complicating factor, such as stricture formation, the aim of the operation is to reduce the oesophagogastric junction to its normal intra-abdominal position where it is anchored and to narrow the widened oesophageal hiatus. This may be done transthoracically or transabdominally. The results of this operation are reasonably satisfactory ir at least 80 per cent. of cases and many poor results are due to operation for symptoms such as vomiting not caused by the hernia. Once a peptic stricture has occurred there is much debate as to which operation to perform. Some surgeons suggest that simple reduction of the hernia when possible will suffice. This may not be technically feasible if there is a lot of para-oesophageal oedema and fibrosis. When resection of the stricture is undertaken the gullet is usually reconstructed by swinging up the colon as a graft. Many abdominal surgeons now advocate the less formidable operations of either a partial gastrectomy or even vagotomy and gastro-enterostomy combined with dilatation of the stricture; this is especially indicated if there is a complicating duodenal ulcer. With this conservative treatment many strictures gradually dilate and after 6 months swallowing can be normal. Simple dilatation alone does not usually help as this once again allows regurgitation of acid and pepsin into the gullet. Surgical treatment of a para-oesophageal hernia is successful and is advised when symptoms occur.

REFERENCES

EDMONDS, V. (1957) Hiatus hernia: a clinical study of 200 cases, *Quart. J. Med.*, N.S. **26,** 445.

EDWARDS, D. A. W., PHILIPS, S. F., and ROWLANDS, E. N. (1964) Clinical and radiological results of repair of hiatus hernia, *Brit. med. J.*, **2,** 714.

WINANS, C. S., and HARRIS, L. D. (1967) Quantitation of lower oesophageal sphincter competence, *Gastroenterology*, **52,** 773.

DISTURBANCE OF MOTILITY

ACHALASIA OF THE CARDIA (CARDIOSPASM)

Definition

A disturbance of swallowing and function of the oesophagus due to denervation mainly of the lower part of the body of the oesophagus with subsequent muscular hypertrophy.

Aetiology

This is unknown, the condition equally affects men and women and true achalasia has no particular geographical distribution.

Pathology

Manometric studies using open-tipped catheters or balloons show that there is no increase in the normal pressure of the lower oesophageal sphincter so that the term cardiospasm is misleading. If pressure recordings are taken simultaneously at various points down the oesophagus it may be shown that once swallowing is initiated there is no reflex relaxation of the lower oesophageal sphincter and that instead of a normal peristaltic sweep purposeless, often large, synchronous pressure changes take place in the body of the oesophagus. This disordered motility is due primarily to denervation of the body of the oesophagus. This has been shown both morphologically and functionally. Histologically degenerative, and on occasions inflammatory, changes may be seen in Auerbach's plexus. *In vitro* strips of muscle from the body of the oesophagus contract when acetylcholine is applied but are not stimulated by nicotine or electrical impulses which depend either on the presence of ganglia or nervous elements. Finally the oesophagus responds to a cholinergic stimulus like a denervated organ (Cannon's Law), for intravenous acetyl methylcholine produces severe substernal pain in patients with achalasia which may be shown both by manometric studies and on barium swallow to be associated with spasm throughout the length of the gullet; this does not normally occur. In addition it is thought that there is some abnormality in the sphincter zone. Normally there are two types of adrenergic endings, those which control contraction and the other relaxation of the transverse muscle. In achalasia of the cardia there is an absence of the adrenergic relaxing transverse fibres. Thus the failure of relaxation at the lower end is not only due to loss of the nervous reflex arc down the oesophageal wall but also the absence of the actual nerve endings in the sphincter itself. The aetiology of this myenteric disorder is unknown but Chagas' disease, endemic in South America, is associated with a destruction of the myenteric plexus by a toxin from *Trypanosoma cruzi* not only in the oesophagus but also in other parts of the intestinal tract.

Morbid Anatomy

As with denervated smooth muscle elsewhere the muscular wall of the oesophagus is hypertrophied. In long standing cases the gullet is dilated and also elongated and may take on a sigmoid shape. The mucosa is inflamed probably from irritation by stagnant putrefying residue in the gullet. In advanced cases 3–8 per cent. will have an associated carcinoma of the lower end of the oesophagus. In addition there may be changes in the lung from aspiration of liquifying gullet contents.

Clinical Picture

Symptoms may occur at any age and equally among men and women and although initially the patient may say that the onset is sudden subsequent questioning will show that there has been some disturbance in swallowing for many years. This has often been that the patient cannot eat quickly or has had some substernal discomfort. The common presenting feature is dysphagia which typically but not invariably is equally severe with either solids or liquids. Initially the symptoms are intermittent and periods of remission may last for many months. The attacks are often put down to fatigue or stress, so much so that it has even been suggested that this is a psychosomatic disorder. As dysphagia becomes more persistent, regurgitation sets in. Initially this is food of a recent meal but eventually there may be regurgitation of putrefying remnants of meals taken several days previously. This embarrassment at the regurgitation often of foul fluid in the advanced case together with the self-taught ability to improve the passage of food through the chest by tricks, such as a Valsalva manoeuvre, induce curious forms of behaviour and self-consciousness on the part of the patient. Pain may be present in up to 80 per cent. of patients and indeed can be the presenting feature in 15 per cent. This may be not only on swallowing but also there may be severe retrosternal spasms of pain passing up to the throat or down the arms. Once dysphagia has become permanent weight loss ensues and when fluids are unable to be taken the patient becomes dehydrated. The patient may also present with nocturnal coughing and recurrent chest infections due to the aspiration of the contents of the gullet into the chest. This has occasionally caused the presenting symptom to be a pyrexia of unknown origin. A routine chest X-ray may show a widened mediastinum, sometimes with a fluid level caused by the dilated gullet.

Diagnosis

Diagnosis may usually be made on a barium swallow which in the advanced case shows gross dilatation of the gullet, tertiary contractions especially present in the lower part of the gullet and the barium mixing with a stagnant column of liquid which has not been emptied into the stomach from the previous meal. In early cases, especially those that just present as pain, the dilatation may not be severe and the disordered motility may only be seen when the barium swallow is performed lying down so that the barium does not travel under the force of gravity. A ciné barium swallow will show the absence of co-ordinated peristalsis. If the oesophagus contains much food debris this may have to be aspirated and the oesophagus washed out before a satisfactory outline of the lower oesophageal mucosa is obtained. This is important to exclude a coincidental carcinoma of the oesophagus. If manometry is readily available it is a simple investigation with little discomfort to the patient. The absence of peristalsis and the synchronous activity is diagnostic and potentially helpful in the doubtful case. Oesophagoscopy should be performed when initially diagnosing achalasia, especially to exclude the presence of an associated carcinoma, but may be technically difficult in those patients with a sigmoid oesophagus as the distal oesophagus runs a horizontal course. Differential diagnosis includes all those conditions which give rise to dysphagia or to oesophageal pain.

Treatment

Drugs have little to offer in the treatment of these patients although occasionally inhalations of octyl nitrate can relieve the pain of oesophageal spasm and if used before a meal may help the dysphagia but generally speaking this is unsatisfactory. The rationale of other types of treatment is to destroy the circular fibres of the lower oesophageal sphincter so that under the effect of gravity food swallowed will pass into the stomach. This should be done in such a way as to prevent reflux of gastric contents with subsequent reflux oesophagitis. This procedure may be done under direct vision at thoracotomy when it is known as Heller's operation. The results are satisfactory, between 60 and 90 per cent. of patients getting benefit, although results may be disappointing in the advanced case and occasionally reflux oesophagitis occurs. The alternative is forced dilatation of the oesophageal sphincter by various instruments; either a radio-opaque balloon or metal dilator which is placed under fluoroscopic control may be suddenly expanded to rupture the circular muscle; this may be quite painful. It is difficult to be dogmatic about the choice of either procedure for the surgeons who claim that dilatation is of no value are usually treating patients in whom dilatation has failed. Dilatation does in many cases obviate the need for a thoracotomy and make hospital stay much shorter. Occasionally dilatation is associated with a rupture of the oesophagus but the mortality is no greater than with Heller's operation and such a complication would be treated by a thoracotomy. It should be pointed out that this forced dilatation in no way resembled dilatation by the original Hurst mercury bougies and the famous whale bone of John Willis. Both of these instruments passed through the lower oesophageal sphincter with little resistance and the dilatation was performed before eating. It seems most likely that by passing such an instrument through the oesophageal sphincter, the sphincter is opened and the gullet emptied. The empty dilated oesophagus is thus ready to receive the food of a next meal without too great a discomfort. This technique should not be used.

REFERENCES

Adams, C. W. M., Brain, R. H. F., Ellis, F. G., Kauntze, R., and Trounce, J. R. (1961) Achalasia of the cardia, *Guy's Hosp. Rep.*, **110**, 191.

Jekler, J., Lhotka, J., and Borek, Z. (1964) Surgery for achalasia of the oesophagus, *Ann. Surg.*, **160**, 793.

Misiewicz, J. J., Waller, S. L., Anthony, P. P., and Gummer, J. W. P. (1969) Achalasia of the cardia: pharmacology and histopathology of isolated cardiac sphincteric muscle from patients with and without achalasia, *Quart. J. Med.*, **38**, 17.

DIFFUSE OESOPHAGEAL SPASM

With advancing age the normal peristaltic waves in the oesophagus may be partly replaced by purposeless tertiary contractions. This becomes common after 50 years of age and when these contractions are very severe the disorder is known as 'curling' or a corkscrew oesophagus. This may be associated with no symptoms or, on the other hand, the patient may complain of substernal discomfort, occasionally dysphagia and regurgitation of fluid and food back into the mouth. Medical treatment is unsatisfactory and in a few patients where symptoms have been severe a myotomy has been performed.

Minor changes of this degree are so common that other causes of dysphagia must be sought in the individual patient.

REFERENCE

Craddock, D. R., Logan, A., and Walbaum, P. R. (1966) Diffuse oesophageal spasm, *Thorax*, **26**, 511.

MISCELLANEOUS OESOPHAGEAL DISORDERS

THE LOWER OESOPHAGEAL RING

These rings are of two types. Mucosal rings which occur at the squamo-columnal junction of the gullet, and muscular rings which are proximal to the mucosal rings and correspond to the lower oesophageal sphincter. They occur equally in men and women and increase in frequency with age. However, they are extremely common and in one series 10–20 per cent. of adult males are said to show this anomaly. The claim that they are associated with a hiatus hernia may be a spurious one in view of the frequency of both these conditions. If the diameter of the lumen is reduced to less than 12 mm. symptoms may occur characterized by recurrent bouts of dysphagia usually precipitated by such food as meat or bread. It is not usually associated with pain or heartburn or weight loss. Barium meal shows a typical X-ray picture and oesophagoscopy may show the ring especially if a large bore instrument is used.

REFERENCE

Goyal, R. K., Baver, J L., and Spiro, H. M. (1971) The nature and location of the lower oesophageal ring, *New Engl. J. Med.*, **284**, 1175.

SCLERODERMA

Sixty per cent. of patients with scleroderma may have changes in the oesophagus. The muscle of the oesophagus is replaced by inflammatory and scar tissue, normal peristalsis is disturbed, the oesophagus becomes dilated, the intra-abdominal oesophagus gradually disappears and there then may be reflux oesophagitis with subsequent dysphagia due to the inflammation or actual stricture formation. There is no peristaltic activity in the oesophagus. One may see a very similar type of picture in the rare condition of amyloid of the bowel [see Section 4].

REFERENCE

Alkinson, M., and Summerlong, M. D. (1966) Oesophageal changes in systemic sclerosis, *Gut*, **7**, 402.

OESOPHAGEAL WEBS

Occasionally dysphagia may be due to a post-cricoid oesophageal web which may be seen best on a lateral barium swallow film [Plate 4]. At one time this was thought to be always due to iron deficiency anaemia but now such webs have been described in otherwise normal persons. In iron deficiency the dysphagia is partly due to painful degenerative changes in the oesophageal mucosa similar to those occurring in the tongue. There is an increased incidence of carcinoma of the oropharynx or oesophagus in such patients; 16 per cent. were encountered in 58 patients described by Shamma'a and Benedict, while conversely in 250 patients with carcinoma of the mouth, pharynx and upper oesophagus the findings of iron deficiency and long-standing dysphagia were noted in 70 per cent. of cases.

REFERENCES

Elwood, P. C., Jacobs, A., Pitman, R. G., and Entwhistle, C. C. (1964) The epidemiology of the Paterson-Kelly syndrome, *Lancet*, ii, 716.

SHAMMA'A, M. H., and BENEDICT, E. B. (1958) Oesophageal webs, *New Engl. J. Med.*, **259**, 378.

MALLORY—WEISS SYNDROME

Haematemesis may be caused by a linear tear at the lower end of the oesophagus. This commonly occurs after prolonged retching and vomiting, typically in the alcoholic but also from such causes as migraine and pancreatitis. It also occurs with other causes of raised intra-abdominal pressure such as paroxysms of coughing and epilepsy. On occasions vomiting blood may be the presenting feature. Such tears may be produced experimentally in animals. It is probably a common cause of haematemesis in patients with a normal barium meal and may be seen on endoscopy. The haemorrhage often stops spontaneously; if it continues laparotomy and suture of the bleeding point may be needed. If no pre-operative diagnosis has been made the lesion may be missed unless a gastroscopy is performed and the oesophagogastric junction inspected.

If the laceration passes through the oesophageal wall spontaneous rupture of the oesophagus occurs with sudden onset of upper abdominal substernal or pleural pain, the patient is shocked and surgical emphysema appears in the neck. Treatment is surgical.

REFERENCE

British Medical Journal (1965) Mallory-Weiss syndrome, Leading article, **2,** 549.

DIVERTICULA

Diverticula of the oesophagus are uncommon and occur at three sites. Those at the oesophagopharyngeal junction and at the lower end of the oesophagus are said to be pulsion diverticula due to incoordinated activity of the oesophageal muscle. Those arising at the bifurcation of the trachea are said to be traction diverticula usually due to adhesion of a tuberculous gland.

The diverticula are often asymptomatic and when present they are often due to the underlying oesophageal abnormality but they may be inadvertently entered on endoscopy or intubation. The main symptoms are dysphagia, unpleasant breath from stagnant debris and inhalation of regurgitated food residue. When these symptoms are persistent surgery is the most efficient treatment. They are diagnosed on X-ray.

DISEASES OF THE STOMACH AND DUODENUM

NORMAL STRUCTURE AND FUNCTION

ANATOMY

Under the dissecting microscope the mucosa of the stomach has the appearance of a lattice caused by the opening of myriads of gastric glands. These comprise three types. The cardiac glands, which are present in a narrow band near the cardio-oesophageal junction and also to a variable extent in the lower part of the oesophagus, are coiled and lined by mucus-producing cells. The glands of the body of the stomach cover two-thirds to three-quarters of the gastric mucosa and contain two main types of cell, the oxyntic (parietal) cells present in the neck of the gland which secrete both hydrochloric acid and intrinsic factor. Most of the other cells in the glands are the chief or peptic cells which secrete pepsinogen. The antral and pyloric mucosa is thinner and the glands there secrete neither hydrochloric acid nor pepsinogen. They extend into the duodenum as Brunner's glands and secrete an alkaline viscous juice. Gastrin is produced in this area by recently demonstrated G cells. Mucus-secreting cells are found scattered throughout the gastric mucosa.

The muscular coat of the stomach comprises three layers. The deepest or oblique fibres are continuous with the circular muscle of the oesophagus, are present in two strips mainly on the front and back of the stomach and fade as the antrum is approached. The outer or longitudinal coat is continuous with the longitudinal muscles of the oesophagus as two broad bands along the greater and lesser curvature. The best developed is the middle or circular coat which increases in thickness distally where eventually it becomes the pyloric sphincter.

The innervation of the stomach is entirely from the autonomic nervous system. The vagus usually enters the abdomen as two or three main trunks, the anterior trunk giving off the hepatic branch which also supplies the pylorus. This hepatic branch is preserved in selective vagotomy. Many anatomical variations exist. Only 10 per cent. (approximately 3,000) of the fibres are motor, but many millions of ganglion cells exist in Auerbach's and Meissner's plexus which mainly mediate local reflexes and amplify the effect of impulses from the main trunks. The main effects of vagus stimulation are to increase gastric emptying and promote gastric secretion. The rich sympathetic supply has a less well-defined function.

SECRETION

Hydrochloric acid, pepsinogen and intrinsic factor are all produced by the gastric glands of the body of the stomach so that after partial gastrectomy much of the acid bearing area is still intact. The secretion of hydrochloric acid is partly mediated by the vagus nerve and partly by humoral mechanisms. Vagal action causes gastric secretion both by the direct action of the vagus on the gastric glands and also indirectly by initiating and potentiating the release of gastrin from the antrum. Gastrin is now regarded as the naturally occurring gastric secretogogue while the role of histamine is still uncertain. Gastrin is liberated from the antral mucosa when it comes into contact with food and also when it is stretched. This secretion is inhibited when the antral or duodenal pH falls. Gastric secretion is also inhibited by a humoral mechanism when fat is present in the duodenum. Both pepsin and intrinsic factor are secreted under the action of both the vagus and gastrin in a similar way to hydrochloric acid. There are various other moieties in gastric juice of unknown significance and plasma proteins, especially albumin, transude into the stomach in unknown quantities.

INVESTIGATIVE TECHNIQUES

The Assessment of Gastric Secretion

This has a time honoured place in medical investigations but is now performed less frequently and is rarely of routine clinical value. The indications for analysis of gastric acid are to demonstrate true achlorhydria in the diagnosis of pernicious anaemia, and to demonstrate the gross hypersecretion which is usually present in the Zollinger-Ellison syndrome. Some surgeons modify their choice of operation for peptic ulcer on the results of such tests—with dubious justification. Innumerable types of tests have been performed in the past but it is now usually considered that the most useful estimation is of basal secretion and also the maximum secretory capacity under the influence of pentagastrin (6 μg. per kg. body weight). Histamine is now rarely used as it has undesirable side-effects even in the presence of antihistamines. The normal basal secretion of acid is $2{\cdot}5 \pm 15$ mEq. per hour and the maximum secretion is 25 ± 15 mEq. per hour. The values are lower for women and decrease with age. Maximum output has been found to correlate with the number of parietal cells present in the stomach. Erroneous results are often obtained by inaccurate positioning of the tube in the stomach which must be checked by X-ray. Gastric secretion may also be induced by hypoglycaemia produced by insulin. This is mediated by the vagus and is used to test the completeness of vagotomy. There is no standard procedure but the blood sugar should fall below 50 mg. per 100 ml. and a positive response is indicated by the increase in acidity of more than 20 mEq. acid per litre. There are often technical difficulties in obtaining gastric juice uncontaminated with bile from the post-operative stomach.

Gastric Emptying

The control of gastric emptying allows time for peptic digestion to take place and prevents the small bowel being flooded by hypertonic fluid or large food particles. Emptying is inhibited by hypertonic material entering the duodenum, where there are osmoreceptors, and also by lipids. Emptying seems to be controlled by the pump-like action of the antrum rather than by the size of the pyloric opening, the closure of the latter being more important in preventing reflux of duodenal contents back into the stomach. The antral mechanism has a sieve effect so that liquid leaves the stomach more quickly than solids. Methods are being developed to assess gastric emptying by incorporating γ-emitting isotope into a meal and assessing its disappearance from the stomach by external scanning. This is a more physiological method than using a liquid meal and aspirating gastric contents at timed intervals.

Barium Meal Examination

This is the most important examination of the stomach but it must be emphasized this is not infallible and that both neoplasms and ulcers may be missed even by the most experienced radiologist.

Gastroscopy

Gastroscopy was introduced over 30 years ago. It became a fashionable mode of investigating gastric disease, led to erroneous conclusions concerning the nature of gastritis but was of help in deciding whether a lesion in the stomach was benign or malignant and occasionally showed chronic ulcers when a barium meal was negative. It also allowed the diagnosis of acute ulcers especially after a haematemesis. More recently with the introduction of fibre optic instruments to which are attached biopsy forceps this type of technique is gaining in importance, for using these instruments the procedure is far less uncomfortable, the ulcer under observation may usually be directly biopsied and previously blind areas in the antrum and the fundus may now be visualized. Newly developed instruments can enter the duodenum.

Exfoliative Cytology

Over 90 per cent. accuracy may be obtained in the diagnosis of gastric neoplasm by experts using this technique. Difficulties arise from inadequate collection of samples as much as from unskilled interpretation. A tyro produces very misleading results.

Miscellaneous

Antibodies to gastrin have now been produced experimentally so that an immunoassay of gastrin has now been developed. The application of the technique is still in its infancy but raised levels have been found in the Zollinger-Ellison syndrome and also in pernicious anaemia where there is no inhibition of gastrin secretion as the antral pH is always high.

REFERENCES

McGuigan, J. E., and Trudeau, W. L. (1970) Studies with antibodies to gastrin. Radioimmunoassay in human serum and physiological studies, *Gastroenterology*, **58,** 170.

Schade, R. O. K. (1960) *Gastric Cytology*, London.

Schnitka, T. K., Gilbert, J. A. L., and Harrison, R. C., eds (1967) *Gastric Secretion. Mechanism and Control*, Oxford.

GASTRITIS

This is an extremely confusing subject and the term was often loosely used to describe a gastroscopic picture or invoked to explain 'indigestion' especially if this followed some dietary excess. However, many of the changes of so-called hypertrophic gastritis seen on gastroscopy are now thought to be due to changes in mucosal blood flow, mucus production and tone of the muscularis mucosae. Indeed, when a comparison was made between gastric biopsy findings and endoscopic observation the correlation was extremely poor.

Gastritis should really be confined to the conditions where true inflammation is present in the mucosa. It may be either diffuse or localized. Diffuse gastritis may either be acute or chronic. Acute gastritis may be due to the ingestion of irritant substances, such as drugs, corrosives and alcohol. Once the irritation has stopped the mucosa rapidly regenerates and the condition does not continue into a chronic form. Clinically it has a brief course with abdominal discomfort and sometimes vomiting. Inflammatory changes may also occur in such infections as diphtheria and infective hepatitis, and are rarely associated with suppuration due to infection by streptococci or staphylococci.

Currently chronic gastritis is divided into superficial gastritis, atrophic gastritis, and also gastric atrophy, the latter condition being associated with pernicious anaemia, when beside complete achlorhydria there is a high titre of circulating antibodies to parietal cells and intrinsic factor. It may be shown that with increasing atrophic changes there is a decreasing gastric secretion. Although clinically patients are often told that their symptoms are due to inflammation of the stomach there is very little correlation between the presence or absence of inflammatory changes in the mucosa and the presence or absence of dyspeptic symptoms.

Localized forms of gastritis are the antral gastritis which occurs in duodenal ulcer patients, the zonal gastritis surrounding a gastric ulcer or gastric carcinoma and also the chronic gastritis which occurs in the gastric remnant following a gastro-enterostomy or partial gastrectomy.

REFERENCE

JOSKE, R. A., FINCKH, E. S., and WOOD, I. J. (1955) Gastric biopsy, *Quart. J. Med.*, **24,** 269.

GIANT RUGAL HYPERTROPHY OF THE GASTRIC MUCOSA (MÉNÉTRIER'S DISEASE)

This is an extremely rare condition and should not be confused with hypertrophic gastritis so frequently diagnosed by endoscopists and radiologists. There is a thickening of the wall of the stomach with proliferation of the mucosa with a constant enlargement of the gastric folds, especially on the greater curvature of the stomach. This diffuse or localized hyperplasia of the surface epithelium produces elongation and tortuosity of the glands which are occasionally dilated and in which the parietal cells may be replaced by mucus-secreting cells. This is not a true inflammatory disease and there is no increased secretion of hydrochloric acid. The clinical features may be atypical epigastric pain which is often dull and aching in character and may be made worse by food. There may also be anorexia, nausea, weight loss and occasionally gastric haemorrhage. On the other hand, the patient may present with ankle oedema due to hypoproteinaemia secondary to gastric loss of albumin (see protein losing enteropathy). The diagnosis may be radiological but in the early stage of the disease it may be difficult to distinguish the lesion from the coarse gastric folds associated with hypersecretion of acid in some patients with a duodenal ulcer. Gastric biopsy may not be helpful as the biopsy specimen may be too shallow and show little abnormality. In patients with a short history giant folds may also be caused by an infiltrating carcinoma or lymphoma.

REFERENCE

JONES, E. A., MORSON, B., YOUNG, W. B., and DAWSON, A. M. (1972) Hypertrophy of the gastric mucosa. In press.

PEPTIC ULCER

Definition

Ulceration of the gastro-intestinal tract due to the combined action of hydrochloric acid and pepsin. This occurs most commonly in either the stomach or duodenum but it may also occur in the oesophagus following gastro-oesophageal reflux or in a Meckel's diverticulum where gastric mucosa is found. It may also occur in the jejunum after a gastro-enterostomy or partial gastrectomy, and more rarely with the massive gastric hypersecretion of the Zollinger-Ellison syndrome.

Aetiology

Acute ulcers or erosions are defined as ulcers which do not penetrate the muscularis mucosae. They are most commonly diagnosed in the stomach for they can only be visualized by direct inspection, for example by gastroscopy and do not show up on radiology. The precise reason for the triumph of the aggressive forces of acid and pepsin over the defensive mechanism of the mucosa is unknown. On the one hand there is a tendency to greater acid secretion in patients with a duodenal ulcer and the normal noctural rise in pH does not occur in these patients. However, the overlap between such patients and normal controls is considerable. On the other hand, patients with a gastric ulcer tend to have a lower than normal acid secretion and also tend to have some degree of gastritis in the stomach so that impaired mucosal resistance is thought to be of importance. At least 15 per cent. of patients with gastric ulcers have or have had duodenal ulcers and these patients have the secretory pattern of duodenal ulcer patients. This difference in the aetiology of gastric and duodenal ulcer is further emphasized by genetic and blood group studies. Gastric ulcers occur three times more frequently in the relatives of patients with gastric ulcer. Relatives of patients with a duodenal ulcer have three times the likelihood of developing duodenal ulcers. A greater proportion of these patients are blood group O and fail to secrete ABH blood group substance in the saliva (non-secretor) than do the general population. Indeed, a person who is group O and a negative secretor has two and a half times the chance of developing a duodenal ulcer as compared with a group A, B or AB secretor and furthermore are more liable to develop a stomal ulcer after surgical treatment for a duodenal ulcer. Patients with a combined duodenal and gastric ulcer have similar blood group characteristics to those with an uncomplicated duodenal ulcer.

The incidence of the condition varies in different countries but probably up to 15 per cent. of the adult male population of Great Britain has been affected by a peptic ulcer by the age of 40. The relative incidence of gastric and duodenal ulcer also varies, the ratio being 1:3 in London and 1:9·5 in Scotland. Four times as many men as women have duodenal ulcers but this ratio is nearly equal for pyloric and chronic or acute gastric ulcers.

Stress is usually invoked as a cause of peptic ulcer and at the anecdotal level the association is very striking especially for duodenal ulcer patients. However, it is often difficult in surveys to demonstrate a greater degree of stress or any particular pattern of stress in such patients when compared with a control group. There is the same incidence of duodenal ulcers in all social groups, although gastric ulcers tend to occur more frequently in the poorer social class V. The concept that irregular meals and 'abuse' of diet predisposes to ulcer has little support. Although there is a tendency for gastric ulcers to heal on withdrawal of tobacco, and the mortality rate of patients with peptic ulcer is slightly higher among smokers than non-smokers, there is no impressive evidence that smoking is an important aetiological factor.

The role of steroid treatment in the production of ulcers is surprisingly controversial. Typically an antral ulcer is produced and it seems possible that the main danger is in patients with rheumatoid arthritis who are possibly taking other analgesics, such as aspirin and phenylbutazone, rather than in the population at large who are placed on steroid tablets.

It is always difficult to be sure of the causal relationship of peptic ulcer with any disease as it is such a commonly occurring condition and therefore extremely large groups of patients have had to be studied. However, there seems little doubt that there is a high incidence in primary biliary cirrhosis, there is probably an increased incidence in patients with hepatic cirrhosis of long duration and also in polycythaemia and chronic respiratory disease. Hyperparathyroidism is also associated with an increased incidence of peptic ulcer and it is now known that a raised serum calcium level in man stimulates gastric secretion. It is worthwhile routinely measuring serum calcium levels in all patients with duodenal ulcers although, of course, the yield of parathyroid adenomas will be small.

Symptomatology

Despite traditional teaching there is little difference in the symptomatology of patients with duodenal or gastric ulcers and they are not striking enough to allow one to make a pre-barium meal differentiation with any accuracy. The main symptom is pain which is usually localized to the epigastrium, is periodic with remissions lasting days, weeks, months or years. The pain typically comes on later in the morning, becomes worse towards the evening and rarely occurs before breakfast. It may wake the patient at night about 2.00 a.m. It may be eased or aggravated by food and is often improved within 10 minutes of taking alkalis. Occasionally the patient vomits acid which eases the pain. Other symptoms are waterbrash, which seems to be caused by an increased salivary secretion. Atypical features may be colonic-type pain in the lower abdomen which may, beside being altered by food and alkalis, also be altered by bowel action and it is not uncommon for patients with peptic ulcer to have an initial diagnosis of a spastic colon. Occasionally heartburn and waterbrash may predominate. On other occasions the patients will have a painless course and present with a complication.

When the ulcer penetrates through the intestinal wall and the area is sealed off by surrounding viscera, penetration is said to occur. If this happens posteriorly it often passes into the pancreas but any adherent viscera may be involved, giving rise to a fistula between the stomach, duodenum, colon, gall-bladder or bile-duct. The exact symptoms will differ in each case but typically the periodicity of the pain changes, relief by alkali and food disappears and in patients with a posterior ulcer the person may present with severe back pain and, in fact, first of all attend an orthopaedic surgeon or physiotherapist. On the rare occasion when a gastrocolic fistula occurs there is onset of diarrhoea suggestive of steatorrhoea and malnutrition due to anorexia and malabsorption secondary to bacterial contamination of the small bowel (stagnant loop syndrome, p. 711).

Physical examination is usually normal, occasionally there is localized epigastric tenderness but a definite diagnosis does depend upon the demonstration of an ulcer by a barium meal or endoscopy. Although a barium meal is the sheet anchor of our diagnostic techniques it is not infallible and small ulcers may be missed so that if a history is characteristic and the barium meal is negative, treatment should be instituted as though the patient had a peptic ulcer. If the duodenal cap has been shown to be deformed one does not need to see an ulcer crater to make the diagnosis of active peptic ulceration as such craters may be very difficult to demonstrate. The presence of typical symptoms with such radiological findings is adequate. The corollary of this is that once a duodenal ulcer is demonstrated there is usually no point in doing repeated X-rays of the duodenum unless symptoms change which suggest some complication has occurred.

Differential Diagnosis

The commonest differential diagnostic problem is whether any organic disease exists or whether the patient has 'functional' dyspepsia. Unfortunately, exacerbations of both conditions may be related to periods of stress. Another difficult differential diagnostic point is whether the gastric lesion is malignant. It is more likely to be so in an antral lesion but even the most benign looking gastric ulcers can turn out to be malignant ulcers; duodenal ulcers are always benign. The recent introduction of fibre optic endoscopy combined with direct biopsy may help to improve the accuracy of a diagnosis. This differential diagnosis may also be aided by cytological examination of the gastric juice but as there is always some doubt, however slight, it is routine to re-X-ray the patient after 4–6 weeks' medical treatment and demonstrate actual healing of a gastric ulcer.

Simple disappearance of symptoms does not exclude the possibility that the underlying lesion is malignant. Gall-stones and pancreatic disease may also mimic peptic ulcer especially if the latter has perforated. Recently a group of patients has been described who have typical ulcer dyspepsia, a tendency to a high gastric secretion and coarse duodenal folds. These patients may develop ulcers later.

Medical Treatment

The aims of treatment are twofold, to afford symptomatic relief and also to heal the ulcer and prevent its recurrence. Unfortunately achieving the first does not guarantee the second. This is underlined by the few studies published on the natural history of a peptic ulcer. For example, in one Scandinavian survey of 687 patients with peptic ulcers who had strict 'ulcer treatment' for 3 weeks in hospital comprising bed rest, frequent bland feeds and antacids, only 30 per cent. over the next 10 years were free of symptoms, 40 per cent. had a serious disability and 35 per cent. had periodic abdominal pain, 4 per cent. died. The outlook was much worse if symptoms had been present for more than 5 years before the treatment was given. The patients with duodenal ulcer fared as badly as those with a gastric ulcer.

By far the best study of factors affecting healing of an ulcer have been carried out by Doll on patients with gastric ulcers, for in these patients objective measurements of the size of the ulcer crater may be undertaken and, as previously mentioned, in patients with a duodenal ulcer this is often not possible. Until recently only two measures were known to increase the healing rate of a gastric ulcer. These were bed rest in hospital and giving up smoking. More recently carbenoxolone sodium (*Biogastrone*), which is normally present in liquorice extracts, given to ambulant patients in a dose of 100 mg. three times a day has been shown to be as effective as bed rest in healing gastric ulcers, giving a 90 per cent. reduction in the size of the ulcer crater. A lower dose was less effective. The disadvantages are the side-effects of salt retention and potassium loss which in the elderly may precipitate heart failure. An alternative liquorice preparation which is devoid of glycerizinic acid is incorporated into an antacid tablet, *Caved-S*, in a dose of two tablets three times daily, does not have these disadvantages and is probably as effective as carbenoxolone sodium. Other treatments such as anticholinergics, dietary manipulations, antacids and sedatives were found not to affect the rate of healing of the ulcer and, surprisingly, had very little affect on the symptoms. Other studies extended to patients with duodenal ulcers strongly support the contention that dietary restriction does not increase healing or prevent relapses. The results of treatment with liquorice extracts have been less convincing in duodenal ulcers. However, it seems sensible to advise the patient to avoid foods that he knows upset him, try to eat regularly, especially if food prevents pain, and to use antacids to anticipate pain rather than when it occurs. There are a vast number of alternative medicines with antacid formulae and the patient usually finds his favourite. It is usually more convenient to prescribe tablets than liquids for day use. Unfortunately the effect of antacids on antral and duodenal pH is very short lived and the theoretical assumption that the gastroduodenal pH may be adequately controlled by antacids and bland food have negligible factual support. The use of anticholinergics has not been very adequately investigated in clinical trials but possibly the most promising is poldine sulphate (*Nacton*), but to alter the gastric pH after a meal and possibly reduce relapse rates large doses are needed, the dose being increased until just below when side-effects are produced. The routine prescription of one tablet three times a day is valueless; sometimes 40 tablets a day are needed. There seems little evidence that patients should be forbidden to drink coffee or tea. Cocktails on an empty stomach often induce pain but it seems permissible to allow alcohol in moderate amounts with or after meals. There seems no evidence that gastric secretion is further increased by the addition of alcohol in this situation. Giving up smoking has been found to promote healing and where possible this should be done. Usually long descriptions are given as to how the patients must modify their life but this is often impossible, although it is often reasonable to suggest that the patient tries to cut down on social commitments during periods of professional stress and to rest as much as possible during the exacerbation of an ulcer. The main function of the physician is to help the patient control his symptoms by adequate antacid therapy and to keep him at work. Too often the ulcer treatment initiates as much invalidism as it cures; this is especially so in persons with a neurotic disposition.

The complications of treatment of peptic ulcers are neurosis and obesity from frequent feeds which may hinder subsequent surgery. At one time avitaminosis occurred when strict dietary regimens were employed, as also did the milk-alkali syndrome when large amounts of sodium bicarbonate combined with up to eight pints of milk a day were taken. In this latter condition the serum calcium rose giving rise to nephrocalcinosis and subsequently renal failure. On some occasions it has been difficult to distinguish this syndrome from hyperparathyroidism which has a high incidence in patients with peptic ulcer. Anticholinergic drugs also have their attendant disadvantages, especially retention of urine in the elderly male.

Surgical Treatment

In uncomplicated peptic ulcer the indications for surgery vary with the type of ulcer. This is advised for patients with a chronic gastric ulcer in whom no radiological evidence of healing is demonstrated after a four-week course of medical treatment or in whom there is a suspicion of a carcinoma. In patients with a chronic duodenal ulcer it depends on the degree of disability that the ulcer has caused the patient. This will partly depend on the stoicism of the patient and partly on the severity of the ulcer. Once a duodenal ulcer has been present for 5 years there is little chance of a permanent remission ensuing.

The operation performed for a chronic gastric ulcer is usually a partial gastrectomy, often a Billroth I type, which involves a gastroduodenal anastomosis. There has been, however, a change in the surgical treatment of chronic duodenal ulcers. At one time partial gastrectomy was the standard procedure but when it was realized that nutritional complications are a fairly common sequel vagotomy with preservation of the gastric reservoir was used. It was soon found that this had to be combined either with a pyloroplasty or a gastro-enterostomy to allow adequate gastric emptying. The relative merits of the different operations are still debated. On the one hand the patients undergoing partial gastrectomy have less recurrent ulcers but there is a slightly higher mortality. On the other hand, the over-all disability which entails a variety of gastro-intestinal complaints (as distinct from the nutritional disturbance) are very similar. Whether the more conservative vagotomy type of operation with either pyloroplasty, gastro-enterostomy or partial gastrectomy has been performed; although the type of symptom complained of differs in the two groups. More recently selective vagotomy which aims to denervate only the stomach has been put forward as the treatment of choice in that it may be associated with a less frequent incidence of post-vagotomy diarrhoea. One problem with vagotomy is that although apparently a simple operation it may on occasions be technically difficult to ensure sectioning of all the appropriate vagal fibres and one cannot be sure of the effectiveness of the operation in terms of altering gastric secretion until the patient has recovered from the operation. Some surgeons tailor their operation to the secretory status of the patient, e.g. patients with a high gastric acid undergo antrectomy as well as vagotomy. Although this is a theoretically satisfying exercise its importance has yet to be proved.

Complications of Gastric Surgery

It must be stressed that after gastric surgery 70–80 per cent. of patients have very good results but up to 10 per cent. have a serious disability.

Stomal Ulcer. This nearly always occurs following operations on a duodenal rather than a gastric ulcer. It is uncommon after a Polya gastrectomy, less than 2 per cent. in most series, but may occur in between 5 and 10 per cent. of patients having undergone vagotomy and a 'drainage' procedure. In that such patients have not been followed for so long as those undergoing partial gastrectomy the incidence may eventually be higher. The diagnosis of a stomal ulcer may often have to depend on the reappearance of typical peptic ulcer symptoms for the radiological diagnosis of this condition may be difficult as the stoma may often be distorted from this previous surgical manoeuvre. Endoscopy may be helpful but the site of the ulcer which is distal to the stoma may not be seen; it may also present as a gastro-jejuno-colic fistula with sudden onset of diarrhoea and features of malabsorption due to a stagnant loop syndrome. If the previous operation involved a vagotomy a stomal ulcer usually indicates that the vagotomy has been incomplete; this may be demonstrated using an insulin test meal.

The treatment of a stomal ulcer is usually surgical. If the initial operation has been a partial gastrectomy then a vagotomy is performed and rarely is it necessary to remove the offending ulcer. If the previous operation has been a vagotomy, re-vagotomy is a disappointing manoeuvre unless a large trunk can be found, and usually an antrectomy or partial gastrectomy is performed. Recurrent stomal ulceration may be a manifestation of the Zollinger-Ellison syndrome.

Epigastric Fullness. This is noticed soon after starting to eat and is aggravated by taking liquids with the meal. It is very frequent in the early postoperative period but persists to a mild degree in 20–50 per cent. of patients; on occasions this may be a severe disability. It may occur after any gastric operation and is more liable to occur in women.

Early Dumping. Soon after meals patients become weak and dizzy and wish to lie down. Mild forms are common in the early postoperative phase and persists in 10–15 per cent. of patients. The cause is open to debate. Symptoms are associated with a rise in haematocrit due to a fall in plasma volume and may be prevented or relieved experimentally by parenteral fluid. There must be an increased sensitivity to such changes as they occur in many patients who are symptomless. This disturbance occurs with comparable frequency after any of the operations. Surgical treatment is occasionally needed when the syndrome is disabling.

Late Dumping. This is a feeling of faintness approximately 2 hours after meals and is thought to be due to reactive hypoglycaemia. It occurs in between 1–5 per cent. of patients and can occur after any gastric operation.

Bilious Vomiting. During or soon after eating a meal the patient complains of epigastric fullness and vomits. The vomitus is usually pure bile and rarely contains the food which has just been eaten. The taste is particularly foul and bitter and leaves a burning sensation in the chest. It can occur after any gastric operation in 10–16 per cent. of cases and is more frequent in women. When frequent it is severely disabling and may warrant surgical treatment.

Diarrhoea. Diarrhoea may occur with up to 12 stools a day. There is usually urgency in call to stool and the attacks tend to be episodic. Some diarrhoea occurs in approximately one quarter of patients who have had a vagotomy but only in 6 per cent. of patients after partial gastrectomy, but is only severe in less than 5 per cent. of the vagotomy patients. The mechanism is unknown but is probably associated with rapid gastric emptying. The effectiveness of selective vagotomy in reducing this complication is still under trial.

Other symptoms are nausea, flatulence and heartburn but it must be remembered that 10–15 per cent. of a random group of people will complain of some indigestion. Sometimes patients do not present with the clear-cut symptoms described above. If symptoms occur after many years of apparent good health some other disease which is undermining the patient's health must be looked for. This may be organic, such as carcinoma of the lung, or psychiatric, such as depression.

Occasionally patients develop bolus obstruction of the ileum from matted vegetable fibre such as orange pulp. Presumably the absence of the sieving effect of the pylorus allows larger particles to enter the small bowel. Pulmonary tuberculosis is often cited as a complication; this mainly occurs in a group prone to the condition, i.e. middle aged to elderly men in social class V and who are underweight at the time of the operation.

Nutritional Consequences. After partial gastrectomy these are weight loss, anaemia and more rarely bone disease and protein deficiency. Weight loss is relatively common and is nearly always due to poor intake of food. It may be profound if dumping or bilious vomiting is disabling. Anaemia occurs in up to 40 per cent. of patients 5 years after operation. This is nearly always due to iron deficiency, the precise reason for which is unknown. There is no impairment of absorption of inorganic iron but it seems possible that patients after gastrectomy once rendered anaemic are unable to increase their iron absorption, such as occurs in other forms of iron deficiency anaemia. This defect is possibly due to hypochlorhydria associated with secondary gastritis in the gastric remnant. Vitamin B_{12} deficiency is important in the pathogenesis of anaemia in 10 per cent. of the cases and indeed after 10 years a subnormal B_{12} level is found in up to 40 per cent. of the cases. This is probably again due to secondary gastritis and impairment of intrinsic factor secretion. Very rarely folate deficiency is a contributory factor but this is nearly always when the dietary intake has been poor if there is an associated complication such as bilious vomiting and severe dumping. Frank osteomalacia may occur occasionally after gastrectomy but probably in only 1–2 per cent. of cases. However, a raised alkaline phosphatase may be found in nearly 40 per cent. of patients 10 years after partial gastrectomy and on X-ray of the spine and hands there may be some evidence of bone thinning. As with other nutritional disturbances such patients seem to remain in a balanced state of partial under-nutrition and rarely come to harm. Protein deficiency following uncomplicated partial gastrectomy is extremely rare and when present usually means there is a complicating factor such as an associated pancreatic deficiency or that a long afferent loop is acting as a nidus for bacterial infestation and allowing a stagnant loop syndrome to occur. Furthermore, should steatorrhoea be gross, for example over 20 g. a day, this type of associated disease is usually present. On the other hand, modest steatorrhoea of 7–12 g. a day is extremely common after any gastric operation if the patient is put on a high fat diet but can rarely account for weight loss which is usually due to anorexia. One of the reasons that vagotomy and 'drainage' procedures were introduced was to prevent these nutritional disturbances. Experience is not large enough yet to be sure whether this has been achieved and already patients who have undergone gastro-enterostomy and vagotomy have been found with a significant incidence of anaemia and in some cases alteration in alkaline phosphatase.

REFERENCES

DOLL, W. R. (1964) Medical treatment of gastric ulcer, *Scot. med. J.*, **9**, 183.

KRAG, E. (1966) Long term prognosis in medically treated peptic ulcer, *Acta med. scand.*, **180**, 657.

LANGMAN, M. J. S. (1968) Carbenoxolone sodium, *Gut*, **9**, 5.

MCCONNELL, R. B. (1966) *The Genetics of Gastro-intestinal Disorders*, London.

MCMILLAN, D. E., and FREEMAN, R. B. (1965) The milk alkali syndrome, *Medicine (Baltimore)*, **44**, 485.

STAMMERS, F. A. R., and WILLIAMS, J. A., eds (1963) *Partial Gastrectomy*, London.

WATKINSON, G. (1960) The incidence of peptic ulcer found at necropsy, *Gut*, **1**, 14.

WILLIAMS, J. A., and COX, A. G., eds (1969) *After Vagotomy*, London.

PERFORATED PEPTIC ULCER

Perforation is said to occur when an ulcer penetrates through the wall and is not sealed off by viscera. In men the chances of this being a duodenal as compared with a gastric ulcer is 5:1, in women the ratio is 2:1. The ulcer may be acute or chronic. The mortality from this condition is inversely proportional to the length of time between the occurrence of the perforation and its diagnosis and treatment and is also worse for gastric ulcers.

Clinical Picture

The diagnosis of classical acute perforation presents little difficulty. There is sudden onset of severe generalized abdominal pain which is aggravated by movement and in 50 per cent. of patients the pain is referred to the shoulder, while 75 per cent. will give a previous history of dyspepsia; there is often nausea and initial vomiting. On examination 75 per cent. of the patients will have board-like rigidity either diffuse or confined to the epigastrium and there will be absent bowel sounds, absent liver dullness and tenderness on rectal examination. After an initial phase of bradycardia there is pallor, sweating and tachycardia but true shock with a fall in blood pressure is relatively uncommon, probably occurring in only 5 per cent. of patients in the initial phase. One to four hours later there is symptomatic improvement which is short-lived. The patient then becomes toxic with a malar flush, tachycardia and signs of diffuse peritonitis. X-ray may show free gas under the diaphragm, in over 99 per cent. of cases the white count is raised, as also may be the serum amylase. The peritonitis which occurs is initially in effect a chemical burn. Once this has set in the exuded fluid in the peritoneal cavity causes a relative loss of intravascular fluid and a rise in the haematocrit. Bacterial contamination of the peritoneal fluid occurs in about 25 per cent. of patients, usually by oral organisms which enter the peritoneal cavity through the stomach or duodenum.

Diagnosis

This condition has to be distinguished from other causes of acute severe abdominal pain especially acute pancreatitis, coronary occlusion, but it may also be difficult to distinguish it from pleurisy, cholecystitis and diverticulitis. Difficulty in diagnosis also occurs when the perforation is relatively pain free. This may happen in patients receiving corticosteroid treatment, or in old and feeble patients when such misdiagnoses as pneumonia, unexplained heart failure, collapse or toxaemia are made.

Treatment

The patient has to be resuscitated with plasma expanders and the stomach intubated and aspirated to prevent further contamination of the peritoneum. Treatment is usually surgical. The operation usually comprises over-sewing of the perforated ulcer but may be combined with radical treatment of the ulcer. This course is especially advocated when a gastric ulcer is found, for 8 per cent. are carcinomas so that at least a biopsy of a gastric ulcer should routinely be performed. If there is a chronic duodenal ulcer a vagotomy and either pyloroplasty and gastro-enterostomy may be performed for there is little likelihood that the patient will remain in remission for long; thus in one series only 3 out of 75 patients who had had symptoms for more than 5 years before perforating remained in remission. These more radical procedures are only undertaken if the patient is relatively fit and the operation is not performed too long after the perforation. In very severely ill patients medical treatment may be used. This comprises restoration of the plasma volume, continual gastric suction to prevent soiling of the peritoneum combined with antibiotics, but if the treatment is confined to such patients the mortality is very high, for example 80 per cent. The mortality is much lower if used in fitter patients but in such patients even in expert hands the mortality is still unacceptably high at 3 per cent.

REFERENCES

DEAN, A. C. B., CLARK, C. G., and SINCLAIR-GIEBEN, A. H. (1962) The late prognosis of perforated duodenal ulcer, *Gut*, **3**, 60.

TAYLOR, H., and WARREN, R. P. (1956) Perforated acute and chronic peptic ulcer, *Lancet*, i, 397.

PYLORIC OBSTRUCTION

When this condition occurs in the adult it is nearly always due to a peptic ulcer which is usually in the duodenum but may be in the pre-pyloric region or antrum. On the other hand if dyspeptic symptoms have been present for less than one year a carcinoma should be suspected. Gross examples are now less frequent as patients tend to have surgical treatment earlier. In one series 92 per cent. of the patients had a duodenal ulcer. These are nearly always active and the stenosis is accounted for by the surrounding oedema together with scarring and distortion.

Clinical Picture

The cardinal symptom is vomiting large amounts of fluid admixed with undigested food which is bile free. Occasionally there is foul gaseous eructation and the vomitus is offensive due to bacterial action on the food residue. Typically the vomit occurs towards the end of the day and may contain residue of food eaten the previous day. Pain when present is cramp-like or may be an epigastric fullness and distension which is eased by vomiting. This is different from the typical pain of an uncomplicated ulcer which the majority of patients have previously experienced. This vomiting should be distinguished from the vomiting of acid secretions in uncomplicated peptic ulcer which may ease the typical ulcer pain. Anorexia occurs with consequent weight loss. Although constipation is common, up to 25 per cent. of patients have diarrhoea which is probably due to the irritation of the small bowel by putrefying gastric contents. Finally, there is weakness and lethargy due to dehydration, electrolyte depletion and rarely tetany from accompanying alkalosis. On physical examination there may be signs of dehydration and weight loss and otherwise the main sign is a gastric succussion splash. The diagnosis is confirmed by finding a resting gastric juice of greater than 250 ml. and gross gastric dilatation together with delayed gastric emptying on barium meal examination. The X-ray may also help to decide the nature of the obstructing lesion. Serum electrolytes are measured and typically there is a low sodium, chloride and potassium with a high bicarbonate, and in severe cases a raised blood urea and haematocrit. Severely affected patients may both be sodium and potassium depleted, for example in one series patients were depleted of 800 mEq. of potassium and 1,600 mEq. of sodium. The potassium deficiency is in part due to loss of potassium in gastric contents and in part to increased urinary excretion due to secondary aldosteronism. This is induced by loss of sodium in the gastric contents. Hypochloraemia may then be partly secondary to the potassium deficiency. There is relatively more water than electrolyte depletion, as no fluid is absorbed by mouth yet water is lost insensibly.

Treatment

This is initially aimed at repairing electrolyte disturbances, relieving the obstruction and feeding the patient. The best electrolyte fluid to use is normal saline, which is a relatively acidifying material, together with potassium chloride up to 40 mEq. per litre once urine is being secreted. Only very rarely are powerful parenteral acidifying solutions, such as hydrochloric acid, needed. Between 5 and 10 litres of parenteral fluid may be needed in the severely dehydrated patients. To counteract the relative water depletion every third bottle should be 5 per cent. glucose. A large bore stomach tube is passed, the stomach washed out with large volumes of fluid to get rid of mucus and debris and following this the patient is either placed on a liquid diet or a milk drip through a fine polythene tube is started. Progress is demonstrated by showing a decreasing gastric aspirate at a similar time each night.

In most cases the above medical treatment should be a prelude to surgery for even though the symptoms may settle the likelihood of recurrence and ultimate need for surgery is high.

REFERENCE

BLACK, D. A. K., and JEPSON, R. P. (1954) Electrolyte depletion in pyloric stenosis, *Quart. J. Med.*, **23**, 367.

HAEMATEMESIS AND MELAENA

The commonest cause of this acute gastro-intestinal emergency in the United Kingdom is peptic ulceration, for example in one series of 1,900 patients only 7 per cent. bled from another cause, there being 2 per cent. from carcinoma of the stomach, 2.7 per cent. from portal hypertension and 2·7 per cent. from a variety of rare disorders, such as a leiomyoma of the stomach, pseudoxanthoma elasticum, angiomatous malformations of the bowel, diverticula and blood dyscrasias. Occasionally the bleeding may be spurious or rarely due to vasculitis or anticoagulants. The type of peptic ulcers involved were 18 per cent. gastric ulcer, 30 per cent. chronic duodenal ulcer, 6 per cent. had undergone ulcer surgery in the past, 30 per cent. had an acute erosion and only 2 per cent. had a hiatus hernia, 5 per cent. were not classified due to incomplete investigation. It is possible that in this series the incidence of the Mallory-Weiss syndrome [p. 689] has been underestimated. There are known precipitating factors, such as aspirin and other analgesics which may account for up to 30 per cent. of the acute gastro-intestinal bleeds but also can account for some of the bleeding in patients with a duodenal ulcer who may have associated gastric erosions. Burns and surgical trauma may also induce gastric erosions.

A large gastro-intestinal haemorrhage causes a depletion of blood volume with a consequent shock-like state, although occasionally with chronic moderate-sized bleeds this situation does not obtain and anaemia may gradually occur. If the loss of blood is severe, besides shock there is extrarenal uraemia and the rise in urea is further aggravated by the absorption of a large amount of digestion products of the blood from the gastro-intestinal tract. The initial haemorrhage rarely kills but death occurs when haemorrhage is repeated especially in patients over the age of 50. The exact cause of death varies but may be an associated cerebrovascular accident, myocardial infarct, pulmonary embolus, uraemia or pneumonia. As death seems to be due to the effects of blood loss on an already depleted cardiovascular system the aim of treatment is rapid repletion of blood volume and adequate fluid replacement to that the patient is fit to withstand the effect of subsequent haemorrhage. On admission to hospital the fact that a gastro-intestinal haemorrhage has occurred should be confirmed. This may be done by demonstrating occult blood in faeces obtained at rectal examination—if no melaena is present. A previous history of dyspepsia is elicited, the previous use of aspirin is asked about and the presence of rare diseases is excluded. Furthermore, hepatosplenomegaly, jaundice and fluid retention suggesting the possibility of oesophageal varices are also looked for. The degree of shock is assessed, blood is drawn for cross-matching and an early barium meal arranged. This may easily be done in the X-ray department; when a patient has a chronic ulcer which has bled it is usually demonstrated. The patient is then sent to the ward and a blood transfusion started if there has been a considerable loss. The size of the transfusion needed may be estimated by measuring the central venous pressure. Sedation may be necessary if the patient is fearful. Once vomiting has stopped, and this is usually the situation by the time the patient reaches hospital, fluids are encouraged by mouth together with whatever food the patient desires. Pain is rarely present and if complained of an associated perforation must be suspected. The patient is kept on a pulse and blood pressure chart and the urine output checked. Ideally in patients with a negative barium meal, endoscopy should be performed to try to identify any bleeding point. There is probably no justification for keeping the patient in bed longer than 6 or 7 days. If a transfusion has not been given oral iron may be started. If a patient presents many days after the acute episode with anaemia he also should be treated with iron and not blood transfusion which is used to replace blood volume.

Indications for Surgery

The sharp drop in mortality over the last 35 years came not necessarily with the introduction of surgery but by the liberal use of blood (at one time it was considered that transfusion with the associated rise of the blood pressure would cause further haemorrhage) and ample fluid replacement (patients used to die of dehydration and parotitis). Some patients need surgical treatment but the indications vary in different centres. Age is an important factor. With medical treatment the mortality rate under the age of 60 is relatively low although in patients with demonstrable chronic gastric ulcer even then the mortality rate is nearly 7 per cent. but for a chronic duodenal ulcer only 1·2 per cent. Patients with acute lesions have a negligible mortality. On the other hand, over 60 years of age the over-all mortality rises to nearly 11 per cent., in the patient with a chronic gastric ulcer the mortality is 20 per cent. and with a chronic duodenal ulcer 11·6 per cent. The effect of age is mainly due to the ageing cardiovascular system being unable to withstand recurrent rapid changes in intravascular volume. From the figures quoted it would seem that anybody with a chronic gastric ulcer who has a gastro-intestinal haemorrhage should have early gastric surgery and that any person who re-bleeds over the age of 60 would be advised to have surgical treatment. However, in the very old, that is over 75 years, the dividends of surgery are not great. In assessing the results of surgery one must see what impact surgery has on the over-all mortality of all the patients entering a hospital unit rather than discussing the mortality of the individual surgically treated patients. It is of some interest that two groups in London, Central Middlesex Hospital and St. James' Hospital, Balham, specializing in the treatment of haematemesis, one predominantly surgical and one predominantly medical, have very similar mortality rates. These indications for surgical treatment only obtain when the surgical treatment is undertaken by an experienced surgeon and anaesthetist: it is not an exercise for a surgical tyro. At times this is difficult to ensure as the operations are usually emergency procedures. Partial gastrectomy is usually undertaken for a chronic gastric ulcer, but the less hazardous operation of oversewing the duodenal lesion and vagotomy with either pyloroplasty or gastro-enterostomy is often now performed for a chronic bleeding duodenal ulcer but the procedure has a high (10 per cent.) rate of re-bleeding.

REFERENCES

Jones, F. A. (1956) Haematemesis and melaena, *Gastroenterology*, **30**, 166.

JONES, F. A., READ, A. E., and STUBBE, J. L. (1959) Alimentary bleeding of obscure origin, *Brit. med. J.*, **1**, 1138.

CARCINOMA OF THE STOMACH

Aetiology and Pathology

Constitutional factors play some part as there is an association between blood group A and carcinoma of the body of the stomach and occasionally patients have a strong family history although the incidence among spouses is not increased. The incidence is high in Japan where it causes half of the deaths due to cancer but low in the United States and high in North Wales as compared with the rest of the United Kingdom. These latter differences are thought to be due to environmental factors for Japanese migrants in the United States show an incidence of gastric carcinoma comparable to the rest of the local inhabitants. The gastric atrophy of pernicious anaemia predisposes to gastric cancer as does atrophic gastritis which may account for the high incidence in patients with a benign gastric ulcer. It is likely that most gastric cancers arising in patients with a gastric ulcer are carcinomas *de novo* and that very few benign ulcers undergo a truly malignant change. Approximately half of the carcinomas occur at the pyloric end of the stomach. They may be polypoid, ulcerating or infiltrating, when the latter has a very gross fibrous reaction and infiltrates widely, it gives rise to a leathern-bottle stomach. The growth either spreads directly through the stomach wall, often involving other viscera or via the lymphatics to the regional nodes. It may also pass into the blood giving secondary deposits especially in the liver and across the peritoneum with the production of malignant ascites and pelvic deposits. Rarely there is a superficial invasive carcinoma which involves only the mucosa; this is difficult to feel at operation but important to diagnose for there is a very high (70 per cent.) 5 year cure rate following resection.

Clinical Picture

In the early stage the disease may be silent or produce such mild symptoms as to be overlooked or ascribed to psychoneurosis. The course may be protracted or rapid. Typically there is anorexia, epigastric discomfort or fullness after meals, loss of energy and eventually loss of weight. Initially it is impossible to distinguish the features from those due to a functional dyspepsia or peptic ulcer. The pain may become boring and pass through to the back. This condition accounts for less than 3 per cent. of patients with massive gastro-intestinal haemorrhage, but it may present with symptoms of anaemia due to chronic blood loss.

Growths in the fundus of the stomach often present as dysphagia and may be difficult to differentiate from other obstructive lesions of the lower oesophagus. Growths in the pylorus may produce pyloric obstruction when nausea and vomiting predominate. Diarrhoea may be prominent especially in patients with a leathern-bottle stomach. Occasionally the patient's first symptom is when he discovers a mass in his own abdomen. An acute perforation may also be the first symptom and 8 per cent. of perforated gastric ulcers are gastric cancers. Once spread occurs signs and symptoms will depend upon the organ affected, whether of a very hard enlarged liver, the presence of malignant ascites, the lymphatic infiltration of the lungs or enlargement of the ovaries in a woman.

Diagnosis

Diagnosis usually depends on the efficient demonstration of the tumour by a barium meal [PLATE 5]. Lesions near the cardia may occasionally be missed, deformities of the antrum found difficult to interpret and the presence of an ulcer gives rise to debate whether it is malignant or not. Further ancillary measures are gastric cytology, the efficiency of which depends on the frequency it is performed in the laboratory, and also endoscopy. With the introduction of flexible fibroscopes and an attached biopsy forceps the incidence of correct diagnosis may be considerably increased and it is gradually superseding the more old-fashioned gastroscope. In addition there may be anaemia, alterations in the E.S.R. and hypoproteinaemia if there is excessive loss of albumin into the stomach.

Treatment

Attempts at curative treatment are surgical. Radical surgery is still advised if the tumour is limited to the stomach and if the lesion is in the proximal stomach a thoraco-abdominal operation is needed. If there has been extension of the disease a limited operation to relieve symptoms, such as partial gastrectomy or even a gastro-enterostomy to relieve vomiting may be undertaken.

Course and Prognosis

This is bad. It depends partly on the type of tumour; for example, survival of 5 years when the diagnosis of linitis plastica is made is extremely rare but the proliferative type of tumour gives a better prognosis. Of those patients found to have involvement of the sub-pyloric glands at operation only 6 per cent. survive 5 years, while if only the lesser curve nodes are involved 65 per cent. survive for 5 years. Only about one quarter of patients have lesions which are considered to be resectable when first diagnosed and over-all only 15–20 per cent. of these patients are alive 5 years later. The duration of symptoms before operation may be misleading as in some cases the slowly growing tumour which has caused symptoms for many months may when resected have an extremely good prognosis. The prognosis for superficial carcinoma of the stomach is altogether different; 95 per cent. survive 5 years when there is no nodal involvement and 75 per cent. with nodal involvement but the diagnosis is only infrequently made before symptoms arise unless as the result of a mass screening programme.

REFERENCES

FRIESEN, G., DOCKERTY, M. B., and REMINE, W. H. (1962) Superficial carcinoma of the stomach, *Surgery*, **51**, 300.

REMINE, W. H., and PRIESTLEY, J. T. (1966) Trends in prognosis and surgical treatment of cancer of the stomach, *Ann. Surg.*, **163**, 736.

OTHER MALIGNANT TUMOURS OF THE STOMACH

These account for approximately 5 per cent. of gastric malignant tumours, they comprise lymphomas, leiomyosarcomas, sarcomas, carcinoids and secondary deposits.

LYMPHOMAS

These account for half the gastric sarcomas and include Hodgkin's disease, reticulum-cell sarcoma and lymphosarcoma. When isolated they are usually clinically thought to be carcinomas. They may present as ulcers—often multicentric or as a polypoid growth. When they infiltrate the stomach wall they may be mistaken for linitis plastica or giant rugal folds. The precise diagnosis depends on microscopy. Treatment is usually by resection and then either radiotherapy or chemotherapy. The prognosis is better than for cancer of the stomach.

LEIOMYOSARCOMAS

These account for approximately a quarter of gastric sarcomas. These are polypoid growths which ulcerate and often bleed. They may also present as epigastric pain or an epigastric mass. The diagnosis is suspected on barium meal and endoscopy but will only be made definitely histologically. Resection is possible in over 80 per cent. of patients when the 5 year survival is between 30 and 55 per cent. A large number of other connective tissue tumours have also been reported on occasions.

REFERENCE

Marshall, S. F., and Adamson, N. E. (1959) Malignant tumours of the stomach, *Surg. Clin. N. Amer.*, **39**, 699.

BENIGN TUMOURS OF THE STOMACH

These comprise adenomas arising from glandular proliferation which are usually single, leiomyomas arising from the smooth muscle of the stomach and also lipomas. They may present as a dyspepsia, or in the case of a leiomyoma more typically as gastro-intestinal haemorrhage due to ulceration on the surface of the tumour. The lesion is diagnosed by barium meal and/or endoscopy. Resection is advised for the presence of malignancy or subsequent malignant degeneration cannot be excluded.

HYPERTROPHIC PYLORIC STENOSIS

Pyloric stenosis in the adult is occasionally caused by hypertrophy of the pyloric muscle. This may be a congenital anomaly although most patients do not give a history of pyloric stenosis of infancy. The hypertrophy is usually associated with a peptic ulcer but this may be secondary to the gastric retention. The patient complains of recurrent bouts of upper abdominal fullness relieved by vomiting, and a barium meal shows a narrow, elongated pyloric canal. It may be difficult to distinguish this from a carcinoma. Treatment is surgical when either pyloroplasty of gastrojejunostomy is performed. Other rare causes of pyloric obstruction in adults are the presence of a mucosal diaphragm, the prolapse of a polyp through the pylorus and possibly the prolapse of antral mucosa through the pyloric canal. At one time the diagnosis of prolapsed mucosa was frequently made radiologically but it is now generally agreed to be a rare cause of illness.

REFERENCE

Du Plessis, D. J. (1966) Primary hypertrophic pyloric stenosis in the adult, *Brit. J. Surg.*, **53**, 485.

A. M. Dawson

CONGENITAL HYPERTROPHIC PYLORIC STENOSIS

Synonym. Congenital hypertrophy of the pylorus.

Definition

This is an important cause of vomiting which comes on between 2 weeks and 2 months of age. The essential abnormality is over-development of the muscle in the wall of the pyloric sphincter resulting in partial obstruction. The term congenital is perhaps inaccurate since the condition is not present at birth. Wallgren carried out radiological studies on 1,000 infants in the early neonatal period and was unable to demonstrate any signs of obstruction although five of these subsequently developed pyloric stenosis. It is suggested that spasm of the pylorus in response to the passage of food causes it to hypertrophy, and the fact that antispasmodic drugs are sometimes effective in its treatment is put forward in support of this view. Other investigations have demonstrated degenerative changes in the nerve cells of the myenteric plexus and have interpreted these as being a response to excessive vagal stimulation and resulting spasm.

Pathology

The pylorus appears as a greyish-white, hard, gristly mass which is increased in length to more than 2 cm. It ends abruptly at the duodenal end but tapers off gradually into the hypertrophied stomach. When cut across the muscle bulk may project into the luman of the duodenum and the appearance has been likened to the uterine cervix. Microscopic examination shows gross hypertrophy of the circular layer of muscle and to a lesser degree of the longitudinal fibres. The mucosa is often oedematous and infiltrated by inflammatory cells. Although the muscle bulk is increased it is otherwise of normal appearance. The mechanism whereby this overgrowth of muscle comes about is unknown but two factors, a genetic predisposition and an environmental stimulus would seem to be involved.

Aetiology

The condition is not rare and in North West Europe

is seen in 1 in 350 of all infants. There is a marked preponderance of boys with a sex incidence of 5:1 while the first child in a family appears to be more liable to be affected than subsequent children. On the other hand it was noted that if one member of a family had pyloric stenosis there was a 12 times greater risk of further children developing the condition. Until recently it was rare to find parents who had had pyloric stenosis giving birth to affected infants, but prior to the mid-1920s no effective treatment was available and survival was the exception. Now there are an increasing number of affected families and it is interesting that the risk in male infants born to the relatively fewer mothers who have had pyloric stenosis is in the region of 1 in 5. In twin studies less than half the identical co-twins have been affected, further emphasizing that although there is a strong genetic predisposition external factors are also involved.

Clinical Features

The baby is commonly a healthy, full-term infant born after a normal pregnancy who progresses well initially but begins to vomit when 3 weeks old. At first this is intermittent and usually results in the feed being changed, but after a few days the vomiting becomes more forceful and occurs immediately after the baby is fed. Towards the end of a feed the baby appears to be uncomfortable and this is followed by a massive projectile vomit; he is relatively unconcerned by this and will often resume feeding avidly. The vomitus rarely contains bile but may contain milk curds from previous feeds and sometimes this sets up a gastritis so that the vomit may contain blood. The other cardinal symptoms are constipation and weight loss. The reduction in the volume of food reaching the colon together with dehydration result in the passage of small, hard stools. Less often frequent stools consisting mainly of bile-stained mucus are passed.

By this time the baby has taken on the appearance of an anxious, hungry infant with considerable loss of subcutaneous fat. Weight loss may be in the region of 20 per cent. of the body weight yet the baby remains active and, unlike an infant with an infection, continues to feed vigorously. When the baby is examined after a feed three signs may be apparent; upper abdominal distension, visible gastric peristalsis and a palpable pyloric tumour. When the baby is watched during a feed waves of peristalsis arising in the hypertrophied stomach can be seen passing slowly towards the duodenum. They are best observed with a good horizontally-placed light and may be provoked by gently tapping the abdomen. Although similar less characteristic waves may be seen in thin premature babies they are rare in full-term infants and when present are highly suggestive of pyloric stenosis.

The most important diagnostic sign is palpation of the pyloric 'tumour'. With experience many believe that this is always possible, though not necessarily at the first attempt. This is easier if the stomach is empty, following a wash-out with normal saline if necessary. The examiner sits on the left side of the baby at a height at which he may comfortably palpate the upper abdomen. The hardened pylorus is felt 3–5 cm. below the right costal margin with the finger hooked around the rectus and directed towards the vertebral column. If a feed is begun the 'tumour' may be felt to contract actively under the examining finger and is then unmistakable.

Investigations

Sometimes the tumour is obscured by gastric distension or by enlargement of the liver and it is then that radiology is helpful in confirming the diagnosis. Erect and supine straight films may show a large, gas-filled stomach. Examination with contrast material shows elongation and narrowing of the pyloric canal with the base of the duodenal bulb indented and tipped superiorly. At fluoroscopy peristaltic waves can be seen, there is delay in gastric emptying and the pyloric canal is not distensible.

Vomiting results in a considerable loss of fluid and gastric acid so that the electrolytes show a low chloride and a raised bicarbonate, often associated with a raised blood urea secondary to dehydration. Gastric aspiration is often needed before surgery and the increased volume of fluid retained in the stomach 4–6 hours after a feed is further confirmation of pyloric stenosis.

Diagnosis

The onset of vomiting in the latter half of the neonatal period differentiates pyloric stenosis from hiatus hernia where regurgitation is present from birth and often occurs between feeds, with blood and mucus in the vomitus. Infection, particularly of the urinary tract may be associated with vomiting but it is rare for the infant to remain hungry and vigorous. Mismanagement, especially under-feeding, may mimic pyloric stenosis with weight loss and constipation in a hungry infant, but the vomiting is rarely projectile and no signs of obstruction can be elicited. Congenital adrenal hyperplasia of the salt-losing type with vomiting usually begins in the second week of life and can be confused with pyloric stenosis. There may be signs of virilization but in boys this may not be obvious and the diagnosis remains unsuspected until lethargy progresses to coma. By this time the characteristic electrolyte picture of an Addisonian collapse with low sodium, raised potassium and an acidosis helps to indicate the correct diagnosis.

Course and Management

In the infant with fully developed pyloric stenosis vomiting occurs after each feed, the weight loss is relentless and the picture of gross malnutrition is seen. If treatment is not provided a fatal outcome in 4–6 weeks is likely. Milder cases with incomplete obstruction may vomit with less regularity and less force, but their weight gain is often unsatisfactory. These infants are occasionally treated medically when the symptoms gradually abate over a period of 3–4 months. It is rare for symptoms of pyloric stenosis to persist beyond 6 months although the muscle hypertrophy may be distinguished in children dying from other causes many months later.

Providing adequate surgery and anaesthesia are available, medical treatment has little to recommend it. Even attempts to treat milder cases presenting at 6 weeks or later often end in delayed surgery, after much difficulty and increasing maternal anxiety. Medical treatment is directed at maintaining nutrition until the spontaneous opening of the pyloric canal is complete. This may involve washing out the stomach once or twice daily together with small feeds every 2–3 hours. Antispasmodics such as atropine methylnitrate (*Eumydrin*) are given usually in an alcoholic solution of 0·6 per cent. dropped on to the tongue before feeds. Response tends to be slow and the dosage has to be adjusted to the individual. Toxic effects such as flushing, fever and a dry mouth are controlled by omitting the next dose, though rarely more serious complications due to paralytic ileus may cause concern. Methyl scopolamine nitrate (*Skopyl*) is also used and is thought to act more by diminishing gastric tone than by action on the sphincter. Expert nursing care is needed if medical treatment is to succeed and not end in disaster from an infective gastro-enteritis in an already wasted infant.

Surgical Treatment

Ramstedt's operation of pyloromyotomy is the treatment of choice and now carries a mortality of about 1 per cent. Careful pre-operative rehydration and the correction of electrolyte balance is important, washing out the stomach with normal saline is also helpful in diminishing gastritis and preventing post-operative vomiting. The operation consists in splitting the pyloric tumour following longitudinal incision so that the submucosa can protrude into the opening and maintain the patency of the pyloric canal. Feeding after operation is started with glucose saline, 30 ml. being offered every 2–3 hours, and dilute milk feeds are gradually introduced so that it may be 3 days before normal strength feeds are given. In straightforward cases the baby may be discharged on the third or fourth postoperative day. Complications are uncommon but arise if the duodenum is perforated at operation or if division of the muscle fibres is incomplete. Rupture of the abdominal wound is also a well-recognized, though rare, postoperative hazard.

The long-term sequelae of infantile pyloric stenosis are not fully known. Scandinavian workers have demonstrated an increased incidence of peptic ulceration when these patients reach adult life. It is equally true that radiological studies in 40 children 1–14 years after operation, showed an abnormal pattern in all but six. Suffice that in the large majority the operation may be regarded as a cure and no long-term effects need be anticipated.

DENNIS COTTOM

VOLVULUS OF THE STOMACH

Volvulus may be a twisting about the axis anchored by the duodenum and oesophagogastric junction or about the long axis of the gastrohepatic omentum. It may be idiopathic but in approximately one quarter of patients there is a diaphragmatic defect or gastric lesion such as an ulcer or tumour.

ACUTE VOLVULUS

This is an abdominal emergency. There is an abrupt onset of severe upper abdominal pain, retching and vomiting which is not profuse on account of the occluded gastric lumen: this also prevents the passage of a nasogastric tube. The epigastrium rapidly becomes distended.

The treatment is surgical when reduction of the volvulus is only possible after the stomach has been decompressed.

CHRONIC VOLVULUS

This is more common than acute. Symptoms are minimal or coincidental. The role of surgery is disputed and unless severe symptoms or complications have occurred is best avoided.

CUP-AND-SPILL DEFORMITY

A cup-and-spill deformity occurs when the distended gastric fundus falls backwards forming a bilocular stomach once the patient is in the upright position. A large pocket of gas may be trapped in the fundus and liquid does not empty until its level has risen high enough to spill into the body of the stomach. This is a form of a partial rotation about the mesenteric axis which is often facilitated by gaseous distension of the colon. This is not an uncommon condition and may produce intermittent symptoms which are not usually severe. These are upper abdominal discomfort or pain which may radiate through to the back or up to the chest and neck; the pain may be aggravated by large meals or excessive fluid and eased by altering position. Attempts to relieve the pain by belching often increase the symptoms as the patient usually attempts to initiate the unsuccessful belching by swallowing air. Usually no special treatment is required except explanation and warning to prevent air swallowing. Very rarely when symptoms are severe operative treatment may be indicated.

GASTRIC DIVERTICULA

Over 80 per cent. of gastric diverticula occur posteriorly near the junction of the oesophagus and stomach, the remainder are juxtapyloric. This is a relatively rare anomaly and occurs in 0·1 per cent. of barium meals. The diverticula may be asymptomatic or cause intermittent and variable symptoms which typically are localized epigastric pain which may or may not be related to food and worse towards the end of the day when the diverticula become distended. The diagnosis is made by barium meal examination. Usually the disability is minimal; occasionally relief may be obtained by leaning forwards over a ledge after meals. Only rarely is surgery indicated.

REFERENCE

TILLANDER, H., and HESSELSJÖ, R. (1968) Juxta cardiac gastric diverticula and their surgery, *Acta chir. scand.*, **134**, 255.

ACUTE DILATATION OF THE STOMACH

Aetiology

Acute dilatation of the stomach may follow operation, particularly on the pelvic organs and the biliary tract. It sometimes occurs after childbirth, the application of a plaster cast or following injury and rarely during the course of an acute infection.

The mechanism of this disorder remains obscure, but the viscus rapidly becomes distended with gas and mucoid gastric secretion containing little hydrochloric acid. The raised pressure within the stomach leads to mucosal congestion which is responsible for the hypersecretion.

Clinical Picture

The onset is usually within three days of an operation. Within an hour or less there is immense abdominal distension; effortless vomiting is the rule and pain is trivial. The excessive gastric secretion leads rapidly to hypovolaemic shock and if not corrected the condition carries a high mortality.

Treatment

Treatment consists of emptying the stomach by passing a large gastric tube which is replaced later by a nasogastric or Ryle's tube. Water and electrolyte losses are made good in the usual way and the stomach emptied at the first suggestion of recurrence.

DUODENAL ILEUS

Duodenal ileus is a dilatation of the duodenum usually due to obstruction of a part of the duodenum. Most typically this is where the mesenteric arteries pass over the third part of the duodenum. Intractable examples of this phenomenon are rare but minor fluctuating examples are not uncommon. It is dangerous to ascribe symptoms such as vomiting to this anomaly and most patients who have undergone surgery to by-pass the 'obstruction' do not have permanent relief of their symptoms.

Very rarely a lesion in the myenteric plexus of the duodenum may give rise to duodenal dilatation.

FUNCTIONAL DISORDERS OF THE GASTRO-INTESTINAL TRACT

Disturbances of gastro-intestinal function may be caused by organic disease but similar symptoms may be present when there is no apparent disease. In such patients there may or may not be obvious psychogenic factors. Thus not only is the problem to exclude organic disease and to make a positive psychiatric assessment but also to assess whether the symptoms complained of by the patient can be explained by any organic anomaly discovered. For example, a common mistake is to ascribe the digestive symptoms of undiagnosed depression to a hiatus hernia.

COMMON DYSPEPTIC SYNDROMES

Nausea and vomiting may be reflexly induced by severe pain. They may occur when there is gastro-intestinal obstruction and also in association with disorders such as an intracranial lesion, gastric irritation from an excess of food, alcohol or drugs, or as an expression of such metabolic disturbances as hypercalcaemia, uraemia and hyponatraemia. However, the common cause of chronic nausea in a patient in whom there are no abnormal physical signs and who has a normal barium meal is tension. Some claim that the environmental situation is typically that of living with a person with whom they are out of sympathy but feel duty bound to look after, and also having been deprived of affection in childhood. Besides simple psychiatric treatment, metoclopramide (*Maxolon*), 10 mg. before meals, which partly acts by promoting gastric emptying, or an anti-emetic such as chlorpromazine, 25 mg. three times daily, may be prescribed.

DISTENSION AND GAS

Although a bloated sensation after meals, often associated with feeling full rapidly while eating a meal, may be a manifestation of organic gastric disease, usually none is found. Usually the patient complains of rapidly feeling full up after food, that his belly swells rapidly either in the upper or lower abdomen and that he may have to loosen his clothes. This he attributes to gas. Often on physical examination this explanation may easily be refuted when one asks the patient to demonstrate the changes which he can often produce at will by a contraction of the diaphragm and the lumbar muscles which forces the abdominal contents forward. Minor examples of this syndrome are an extremely common cause of functional dyspepsia, and gross examples occasionally occur, the most extreme causing pseudocyesis.

GAS SYNDROMES

Collections of gas trapped in pockets of bowel are a frequent cause of abdominal discomfort. This may be partly due to excessive swallowing due either to a nervous habit (over one pint of air is normally swallowed a day) or in an attempt to initiate a belch which it is hoped would relieve upper abdominal discomfort either induced by a functional disturbance or possibly some other organic lesion. Swallowed air may reach the colon in 30–60 minutes. The patient may present with upper abdominal discomfort and belching or one of the colon gas syndromes. Gas trapping may be aggravated by a cup-and-spill deformity of the stomach. The colonic gas syndromes due mainly to trapping of swallowed air but possibly also to excessive bacterial fermentation are caused by gas collecting either in the caecum, the hepatic flexure or the splenic flexure. The splenic flexure is the commonest; the patient complains of left upper abdominal pain passing through to the chest and often giving a bursting sensation. If gas is passed per rectum or the bowels are opened the pain is usually eased but the patient often swallows more gas in an attempt to belch, hoping that this manoeuvre will ease the situation. Gas trapped in the hepatic flexure giving chronic pain of a similar nature in the right upper quadrant is usually diagnosed as chronic gall-bladder disease, a condition which rarely in fact gives rise to chronic right hypochondrial pain. On some occasions the gas collects in the caecum giving rise to pain in the right iliac fossa of a chronic nature, often like a stitch. In all these symptoms it is important to explain the mechanism of the symptoms to the patient who must try and stop aerophagy and also to exclude obvious gas-forming foods such as beans and sprouts in the patients with the colonic syndromes. However, explanation, reassurance and treatment of tension is usually the most important.

FOOD INTOLERANCE

It is not unnatural that various digestive complaints have been ascribed to dietary indiscretion and that treatment in the past has been directed at prescribing fastidious dietary regimes. Some patients acquire a long list of foods of which they claim that they are intolerant. In adults this has rarely been found to have any immunological or chemical basis except in sugar intolerance and the malabsorptive states when very specific symptoms occur. On the other hand the patient with food intolerance will complain of a wide variety of symptoms ranging from nausea, vomiting, headache, abdominal distension, diarrhoea or constipation. It is often very difficult to wean them from their restricted life. It should be pointed out that the frequently suggested intolerance of certain foods in various organic conditions has not been borne out by surveys, thus fat intolerance is not indicative of gall-bladder disease.

REFERENCE

ALVAREZ, A. (1954) *Nervousness, Indigestion and Pain*, New York.

CONSTIPATION

Constipation may be defined as the infrequent passage of hard stools. Although most people have their bowels opened once a day the normal variation is great. Many people use the term constipation to denote abdominal discomfort, headache and general ill health which are widely held to be caused by this disorder; such views have given rise to the practice of regular purgation.

Organic causes of constipation may be abnormalities of the colon such as obstruction due to carcinoma, bands, or diverticular disease, a painful anal lesion and either intrinsic or extrinsic disturbed innervation of the bowel or abdominal wall. Metabolic disturbances such as hypothyroidism and hypercalcaemia may be at fault, both of which must be distinguished from a depressive illness where constipation may dominate the symptoms.

Functional causes are by far the most common. Symptoms may occur transiently in any person who becomes physically inactive or changes to a low roughage diet. It is also a feature of pregnancy. Chronic constipation, if not a manifestation of the irritable bowel syndrome, is usually considered to be due to faulty training and initiated by a failure to respond to a call to stool, either due to a painful anal lesion, uncomfortable facilities in the lavatory or socially unacceptable timing, the latter often occurs when people start to work, have to leave home immediately after breakfast and are travelling when the call to stool has to be repressed. Eventually rectal sensation is suppressed (dyschezia). Purgation may be indulged in which further aggravates the condition and also may be the cause of associated abdominal discomfort.

In treating such patients it must be explained that a daily bowel action is not necessarily normal or desirable, but previous training and the effect of folk-lore often precludes such advice being taken seriously. Any local cause should be dealt with, exercise encouraged and a diet high in roughage, such as fruit, vegetables, wholemeal bread and morning Allbran prescribed. The patient is advised to allow time after breakfast for a bowel action. Bulk may also be improved by prescribing a dehydrated cellulose preparation, such as *Isogel*, which swells in the bowel, initially in a dose of 1–2 teaspoonsful at night but this may be increased to three times daily if needed. Occasionally an osmotic purge may be needed, such as magnesium sulphate, this acts in a few hours; occasionally direct stimulation of the bowel wall by a senna preparation may be used but strong purgatives are to be avoided. Liquid paraffin is not prescribed indefinitely because of its possible carcinogenic properties but other stool softeners, such as dioctyl sodium sulphosuccinate (*Dioctyl forte*), 100 mg. up to six times daily, is occasionally of help. In severely disabled patients glycerine suppositories or self-administered isotonic phosphate enemas may be used.

CHRONIC DIARRHOEA

This is a frequent gastro-intestinal symptom. The term is usually used to describe fluid, frequent stools. Some patients may on the other hand use the symptom to describe the passage of frequent small amounts of mucus associated with a constipated stool such as occurs in granular proctitis. It is important always to inspect a specimen of stool when investigating a patient with this complaint. The commonest single cause in England is anxiety, but a list of some of the causes is shown in TABLE 42.

TABLE 42

CAUSES OF CHRONIC DIARRHOEA

1. Psychogenic.
2. Gastric disease: pyloric stenosis, Zollinger-Ellison syndrome, after gastric surgery (including vagotomy).
3. Small bowel disease: ±malabsorption [see TABLE 43].
4. Colonic disease: inflammation, e.g. ulcerative colitis and Crohn's disease, carcinoma.
5. Pancreatic disease: ±steatorrhoea.

6. Metabolic: thyrotoxicosis, uraemia, diabetes, Addison's disease, medullary carcinoma of thyroid, carcinoid tumour.
7. Irritants: post-antibiotics, drugs, e.g. quinidine sulphate, purgative abuse, beer.
8. Infection or infestation of bowel.

PURGATIVE ABUSE

This term is used to describe two situations. On the one hand the patient with chronic constipation who becomes addicted to increasing amounts of purgative, and the other the person who purges herself, induces diarrhoea and may present to the doctor asking for this symptom to be investigated. In the latter situation the patient is usually suffering from a personality disorder and is analogous to other self-induced gastro-intestinal disturbances such as surreptitious vomiting, factious rectal bleeding and oral bleeding. In adolescent young women it is often associated with the syndrome of anorexia nervosa.

The diarrhoea induced by purgative addiction may be so profound as to cause areflexia from potassium deficiency and there may be associated extrarenal uraemia. All investigations may be negative although a barium enema may show a thin colon with lack of haustral pattern. The stools of all patients with unexplained diarrhoea, especially if large faecal volumes are observed, must be undertaken by adding alkali to exclude phenolphthalein and other vegetable laxatives. If negative, the faecal magnesium is measured.

A. M. DAWSON

GASTRO-ENTERITIS

Synonyms. Epidemic diarrhoea; Summer diarrhoea; Acute enterocolitis.

Definition

Gastro-enteritis is not a single disease but a complex of symptoms caused by a wide variety of agents. It may be due to intestinal pathogens or secondary to a parenteral infection such as otitis media. Case-to-case transmission occurs in both types but is especially likely when the infant is excreting large numbers of pathogenic bacteria. It may occur at all ages but it is in infants and small children that it is most prevalent and dangerous.

Summer diarrhoea used to occur in epidemic proportions and in 1913 the infant mortality in England and Wales from gastro-enteritis was 91 per 1000 live births, more than four times the total infant mortality from all causes in 1969. Since in developing countries it remains the commonest single cause of death in childhood it is useful to analyse the progress that has lead to its control in Western countries. Many factors have contributed to this improvement, initially the encouragement of breast feeding, and improved hygiene in the collection and distribution of milk were all important; then better techniques for sterilizing or pasteurizing milk and the introduction of dried milk played a dominant role. Up to 1948 public health measures were responsible for most of the progress but over the last 20 years earlier recognition and better treatment have contributed more to the reduction in mortality.

Aetiology

The common organisms causing gastro-enteritis are: (1) Specific enteropathic *Esch. coli* (e.g. types 0.26, 0.55, 0.111, 0.119, 0.127, etc.). (2) Salmonella (e.g. *S. typhimurium*, *S. enteriditis*, *S. choleraesuis*). (3) Shigella (e.g. *Sh. sonnei*). (4) Staphylococci. (5) Enteroviruses (e.g. Echo Types 11, 14, 18).

Since the initial discovery by Bray in 1946, it has been established that certain types of *Esch. coli* are causal agents in gastro-enteritis and may be responsible for nursery epidemics of varying severity. In one infant the disease may be fulminating and fatal while in others anorexia, low-grade fever and vomiting may resolve without treatment. The incubation period is from 2–10 days and transmission is primarily by faecal contamination from an infected infant, though routine investigation often reveals the presence of specific *Esch. coli* in symptomless infants and nursery attendants. In one three-month study 20 per cent. of the infants and seven per cent. of the nurses harboured enteropathic coliforms though none exhibited clinical disease.

Shigella infection classically causes dysentery with blood and mucus in the stools. Within 4 days of becoming infected there is a sudden onset of abdominal pain, fever and vomiting. In infants this may cause rapid and life-threatening dehydration. Many strains are now sulphonamide resistant but respond to treatment with ampicillin or gentamicin.

Salmonellae of the food-poisoning type cause gastro-enteritis particularly in children between 6 months and 2 years. The organism may be present in water, eggs, milk and occasionally in pharmaceutical products of animal origin such as pancreatin or thyroid. In one nursery epidemic in Africa cockroaches acted as the carrier. Staphylococcal gastro-enteritis may occur as an epidemic with an abrupt onset 3–4 hours after eating uncooked foods containing the toxin or in previously ill patients as a pseudomembranous enterocolitis. The latter form is equally common in adults and may carry a significant mortality.

Pathology

The changes found after death may be surprisingly slight considering the severity of the disease. As a rule the mucosa of the stomach and intestines is diffusely oedematous with engorged blood vessels and petechial haemorrhages. The lymphoid tissue of the alimentary canal is often swollen, and in severe cases the solitary follicles in the colon and lower ileum may be ulcerated. The lungs are often congested and oedematous, with, in protracted cases, patches of bronchopneumonia in the lower lobes.

Clinical Features

Diarrhoea may occur in an infant who is already ill with an upper respiratory infection or pneumonia when it may begin insidiously. More often there is a rapid onset with fever, vomiting and abdominal distension. Feeds are commonly refused and, although diarrhoea may not be marked in the early stages, the baby appears to have colicky, abdominal pain and the bowel sounds are increased. The motions vary both in character and frequency, they may be green with bile and excess mucus or they may consist of profuse, partially digested material which is acid and causes excoriation of the buttocks.

Two factors influence the course of the illness, the passage of toxins and bacteria into the blood and, more important, the extent of fluid loss. As the diarrhoea increases dehydration becomes marked and will lead to circulatory collapse if not corrected. The baby appears restless with a grey appearance due to vaso-constriction, the mouth is dry and the fontanelle is depressed. The skin is inelastic and the eyes appear sunken, later there may be convulsions and stupor, sometimes associated with rapid respiration due to a progressive acidosis. There is oliguria with the presence of albumin and casts.

Management

A high standard of nursing care is vitally important in the management of infants with gastro-enteritis. Not only must the baby be barrier-nursed with meticulous regard for all measures to prevent the spread of infection, but careful in-put and out-put charts are essential. Frequent observation and management of intravenous infusions using very small volumes, together with skilled feeding make this a major nursing challenge.

Stool cultures, haematocrit and electrolyte estimations are needed and it is necessary that micro-methods are available so that venepunctures are not required. Accurate replacement of fluid and electrolytes is all important.

In the normal infant, although large volumes of fluid are secreted into the gut, most of this is reabsorbed so that the daily stool loss is only 50 ml. water. All intestinal excretions (except saliva) have the same osmolarity as plasma and with the exception of gastric juice have bicarbonate concentrations in excess of those found in plasma. In mild diarrhoea the water loss is 10–25 ml. per kg. body weight rising to 50 ml. per kg. in severe cases. The fluid is hypotonic with respect to plasma having an osmolarity in the region of 150 mOsm. per litre while it may contain 40 mEq. per litre each of Na^+, K^+, Cl^- and HCO^-_3. Consequently if the diarrhoeal losses exceed those from vomiting the baby is likely to be depleted of water together with potassium and bicarbonate since these electrolytes are present in plasma at lower concentrations than are sodium and chloride.

The replacement of fluid is oral or intravenous. Subcutaneous or intraperitoneal infusions have their advocates but play little part in normal treatment. The object is to provide sufficient fluid and electrolytes to restore renal function and a normal flow of urine. In the mildly affected baby, feeds of 5 per cent. glucose saline are given given by mouth at 1–2 hourly intervals, an indwelling intragastric tube being used if necessary. Volumes of 250–300 ml. in addition to the baby's maintenance requirements is often sufficient and milk feeds may be cautiously reintroduced after 24 hours, gradually increasing from quarter strength to normal full strength feeds.

Normal maintenance needs for each kg. body weight are calculated as 100 calories, 150 ml. water plus 3 mEq. each of sodium, potassium and chloride in each 24 hours. These quantities are required in addition to those needed for the correction of dehydration. When the baby is shocked or has lost more than 10 per cent. of its body weight, feeding by mouth is suspended and intravenous fluids are started immediately. Initially it is important to restore the blood volume so that normal saline or half normal saline with glucose is given at rates of 50 ml. per kg. for the first 3–4 hours or until urine is passed. When this has been accomplished infusion of one fifth normal glucose saline is continued at a slower rate. Potassium chloride or sodium bicarbonate are added to correct the calculated electrolyte depletion. Intravenous therapy alone is often desirable for 48 hours after which clear fluids by mouth may gradually be replaced by milk feeds.

The place of antibiotics is undetermined. If there is a parenteral infection it should of course be treated. In the case of intestinal pathogens, neomycin, 100 mg. per kg. a day in four doses, is often used and may be of importance in reducing the infectivity of the stool. There is conflicting evidence as to its effect in the individual patient. General measures such as the maintenance of body temperature, blood transfusion and skin care are important in emaciated, marasmic babies. Monilial infection is common both in the mouth and over the napkin area, treatment with nystatin, 100,000 Units per ml. is indicated.

Complications

Hypernatraemic Dehydration. In some infants water loss from the stool exceeds the loss of electrolytes, if at the same time oral feeding with milk or saline mixtures is continued hyperelectrolytaemia will result. Serum sodium values in excess of 160 mEq. per litre are often encountered and if rehydration is too rapid convulsions occur. This is similar to the disequilibration syndrome in renal dialysis when there is a marked difference between intracellular and extracellular osmolarity. A small number of infants suffer permanent brain damage with or without subdural haemorrhages.

Disaccharide Intolerance. It has long been known that following an infective gastro-enteritis infants may be intolerant of normal milk formulas. Partially digested milks used to be popular and it is likely that these acted by hydrolysing lactose and sucrose to monosaccharides. Mucosal damage after gastro-enteritis is associated with depletion of intestinal enzymes particularly those concerned in the digestion of carbohydrate. If lactase is absent, lactose remains unabsorbed and may be converted to lactic acid by bacteria in the colon. This causes further diarrhoea, not only by its osmotic effect but by irritating the gut wall. In any post-enteritis diarrhoea the stool pH should be checked and the presence of disaccharides determined. If present a milk preparation free from lactose and sucrose should be used together with additional vitamin supplements.

REFERENCES

LLOYD-STILL, J. (1969) Gastro-enteritis with secondary disaccharide intolerance, *Acta paediat. scand.*, **58,** 147.

MACAULAY, D., and BLACKHALL, MARGARET I. (1961) Hypernatraemic dehydration in infantile gastro-enteritis, *Arch. Dis. Childh.*, **36,** 543.

DENNIS COTTOM

FOREIGN BODIES

Anything which can pass the mouth has at one time or other been swallowed. Inappropriate objects are usually swallowed as an accident by children in professional acts and by the insane. Many small objects, such as buttons and marbles, once swallowed, pass through the pylorus and gastro-intestinal tract and out of the anus causing no trouble. If the object lodges anywhere it may give rise to local irritation and needles have been known to work their way through the blood stream and even become ejected at the knee. Acute obstruction may also occur; this is more likely to occur in patients who already have some narrowing of the bowel from any cause.

BEZOARS

Trichobezoars or hairballs are a medical curiosity for it seems that chewed hair has difficulty in passing the pylorus. They account for 55 per cent. of bezoars, the rest are phytobezoars due to vegetable matter. The patient presents with upper abdominal discomfort or pain and also vomiting; occasionally there is gastro-intestinal haemorrhage. The diagnosis is made on barium meal examination, when a large filling defect is found in the stomach, the surface of which remains impregnated with barium once the stomach has been emptied. On gastroscopy the bezoar appears as a black, tarry mass. Treatment is surgical removal. After gastrectomy or gastro-enterostomy the absence of a pylorus allows vegetable matter to enter the small bowel in a poorly divided form and occasionally the patient presents with obstruction of the ileum from inspissated vegetable pith.

MALNUTRITION AND MALABSORPTION IN GASTRO-INTESTINAL DISEASE

The small bowel is the only indispensable portion of the gastro-intestinal tract since almost all the digestive products of food are absorbed through its mucosa. It is therefore not surprising that a variety of nutritional disturbances may occur when it is diseased, although they may not necessarily be accompanied by gastro-intestinal symptoms such as diarrhoea and abdominal pain. Furthermore, steatorrhoea is not invariably present. Until recently, disturbed small bowel function was considered to be relatively uncommon in temperate zones but this view has changed with the advent of more precise ways of assessing the different functions of the small bowel together with the introduction of peroral biopsy of the intestinal mucosa as a safe routine procedure. It should be further stressed that though malabsorption may be an important cause of malnutrition, impaired intake of food due to anorexia associated with gastro-intestinal disorders and an increased requirement of a nutrient or an increased loss from the bowel may be of equal or greater importance. With the recent realization that small bowel function can frequently be disturbed, far too frequently a slight change of an absorption test has been erroneously taken as adequate evidence of malabsorption which is then assumed to account for weight loss or other nutritional disturbances which are present.

STRUCTURE OF THE SMALL INTESTINAL MUCOSA

The walls of the small bowel are thrown into folds by the valves of Kerckring. The lining of these folds consists of finger- or leaf-shaped projections called villi which comprise a central core of connective tissue together with lymphatics and vessels covered by a single layer of mucosal cells. At the base of the villi, projecting into the mucosa are the intestinal glands or crypts where proliferation of cells take place; as they mature they pass up the villus and then are lost into the lumen. The whole cycle of renewal probably takes 48 hours. It seems likely that the cells of the distal two-thirds of the villus are most active in the absorption process. The absorptive surface of the intestine is further increased by the presence of innumerable microvilli on the surface of the villous cell. Specimens of small bowel mucosa may be obtained by peroral biopsy using a variety of techniques, one of the simplest being the Crosby-Kugler capsule. Such specimens may be inspected for morphological abnormalities by using both the dissecting microscope and standard histological techniques. Furthermore, the estimation of enzymatic content (e.g. disaccharidases) and functional integrity may be undertaken.

ABSORPTION AND ASSESSMENT OF SMALL BOWEL FUNCTION IN MAN

CARBOHYDRATE ABSORPTION

The commonest dietary polysaccharide is starch which comprises a mixture of two types of glucose polymers. In one of these the glucose units are in straight chains (amylose) and in the other in branched chains (amylopectin). These molecules are both attacked by the alpha amylase of pancreatic juice and the resultant digestion products are disaccharides, trisaccharides and oligosaccharides. Very little free glucose is formed. Other dietary sugars are the disaccharides lactose (glucose + galactose) and sucrose (fructose + glucose). The final stage of digestion of these sugars takes place in or on the brush border of the mucosal cell by their respective enzymes which are in close proximity to the specialized transport process which pumps glucose and galactose efficiently across the cell membrane. Fructose is absorbed by a different and less efficient mechanism. Carbohydrate absorption has usually been tested by the glucose tolerance curve. This is now rarely used as the shape of the curve also depends not only on gastric emptying but upon the metabolism of the sugar. The glucose tolerance test has been superseded by the xylose test. This pentose sugar is poorly absorbed, little utilized and mainly excreted by the kidney. Mild damage to the intestine can be shown up as impairment of absorption giving rise to low blood levels and so to low excretion in the urine. This test is commonly used but it is not a test of carbohydrate absorption but rather a crude assessment of jejunal function and probably is of little importance clinically if one has the facilities to perform a small bowel biopsy.

More recently with the realization that disaccharidase deficiency can occur the sugar tolerance curves may be performed by feeding the appropriate disaccharide, especially sucrose or lactose. In the absence of the mucosal disaccharidase one gets a flat blood curve and the unabsorbed products often induce an osmotic-type diarrhoea. However, when the constituent simple sugars are fed a normal blood sugar rise occurs.

PROTEIN ABSORPTION AND LOSS FROM THE BOWEL

Protein is mainly degraded by the gastric and pancreatic proteases, but the final stage of digestion to amino acids is probably a mucosal function. The amino acids are pumped across the mucosa by specialized transport systems, of which there are at least three. Impaired absorption alone rarely accounts for protein deficiency for the normal requirement is very low, for example less than 30 g. of protein a day. Thus on a normal dietary intake of 70 g. a day impairment of absorption would have to be profound. If, on the other hand, there is associated impaired intake impaired absorption may assume some significance.

A frequent cause of hypo-albuminaemia is loss of plasma proteins from the bowel. This situation is analogous to the nephrotic syndrome. The exuded protein is digested and often completely reabsorbed so that the condition cannot be detected by estimating the faecal nitrogen. However, loss out-strips the liver's capacity to synthesize albumin and hypo-albuminaemia results. This condition differs from simple protein deficiency for hypoalbuminaemia dominates while other signs of protein deficiency, such as dry scaly skin, are not in evidence. The most frequent way of assessing the presence of this increased loss is by injecting chromium-labelled albumin which leaks through the sites of increased permeability into the bowel lumen where, although the albumin itself is degraded, the released chromium is poorly absorbed and appears in the faeces. This phenomenon of protein-losing enteropathy occurs in a wide variety of gastro-intestinal disorders ranging from gastric carcinoma to giant rugal hypertrophy of the stomach and congestive heart failure with lymphatic obstruction; other conditions will be mentioned specifically in the individual sections.

FAT ABSORPTION

The common dietary fat is triglyceride which consists of three long chain fatty acids esterified with glycerol. Pancreatic lipase splits this compound into monoglyceride and to fatty acids. These are the major forms which are absorbed from the intestine. These products are solubilized into small enough particles to enter the mucosal cell by being assimilated into aggregates of bile salts which are called micelles. Once these digestion products have entered the mucosal cell they are mainly incorporated into chylomicrons which are resynthesized triglyceride surrounded by an envelope of protein, lecithin and cholesterol ester. From here they pass via the lymphatics into the systemic circulation. A small and variable amount passes into the portal vein. Shorter chain fatty acids which are water soluble pass through the intestinal cell, remain unesterified and pass up the portal vein. Although the presence of bile salts is not absolutely essential for the absorption of dietary triglyceride it is almost obligatory for the absorption of sterols and fat-soluble vitamins.

The sheet anchor of assessment of fat absorption is the analysis of faecal fat and as daily excretion varies stools are collected over 3- or 5-day periods. The normal excretion is up to 7 g. a day and steatorrhoea may be diagnosed on a normal ward diet. If the result is borderline the estimation should be repeated on a high-fat (100 g.) diet which will stress the absorptive capacity of the bowel. Other indirect assessments of fat absorption, such as the radioactive triolein test and the vitamin A absorption test are rarely performed.

The major causes of steatorrhoea are impaired lipolysis due to pancreatic insufficiency, impaired solubilization by a decreased luminal bile salt concentration or impaired mucosal function due to destruction or resection of the bowel. Bile salt deficiency may occur in several ways. Normally bile salts are synthesized in the liver and immediately conjugated with glycine or taurine before being excreted in the bile. They pass down the lumen of the jejunum where a high concentration is maintained and are absorbed in the ileum by an active process which prevents loss into the faeces. It should be pointed out that only the conjugated bile salts have the power of solubilizing fat in the lumen of the bowel. The unconjugated form is very inefficient in this process. Luminal bile salt deficiency may therefore occur with impaired synthesis as in liver disease, impaired secretion into the bowel as in bile-duct obstruction, or with resection or disease of the ileum when a large amount of bile salt is lost from the body. Furthermore, a deficiency occurs in some patients with the so-called stagnant loop syndrome when aberrant colonic bacteria in the jejunum degrade the conjugated bile salts to their unconjugated form which are less efficient at forming micelles and can be absorbed by the jejunum.

MISCELLANEOUS TESTS

Other tests of most use in assessing intestinal function are those of B_{12} absorption, such as the Schilling test, performed with added intrinsic factors, which assesses ileal function, and also on special occasions bacteriological assessment of small bowel contents to determine whether there is a stagnant loop syndrome or not.

Further assessment of small bowel function is by radiology of the small bowel [PLATE 5]. This is to demonstrate the presence or absence of such anatomical defects as strictures, fistulas and diverticula rather than the presence of a flocculated malabsorption pattern. Other routine investigations should be to assess the presence or absence of malnutrition. This is most commonly manifested as anaemia which may be iron deficient or a mixed hypochromic and megaloblastic anaemia. The presence or absence of hypoproteinaemia and osteomalacia should be assessed, the latter being shown by a raised alkaline phosphatase and low serum calcium or phosphate.

CONSERVATION OF WATER AND ELECTROLYTES BY THE GASTRO-INTESTINAL TRACT

The gut is capable of reabsorbing large amounts of water and electrolytes. This is shown by the fact that normally we lose only up to 150 ml. of water and 30 mEq. of sodium in the faeces each day, while the combined amounts of diet and gut secretions comprise approximately 9 litres of fluid and 1100 mEq. of sodium together with 80 mEq. of potassium. The mechanisms of water and electrolyte absorption vary throughout the gastro-intestinal tract. It may be said that the duodenum is the area of osmotic equilibration so that fluid either rapidly enters or is absorbed to render its contents isotonic with plasma. Net absorption of sodium and water occurs in the jejunum and is coupled to the absorption of glucose and other actively absorbed sugars which are present in the gut lumen after a meal and is under negligible control from aldosterone. Absorption does not occur from a simple isotonic saline solution. An application of this coupling of glucose to sodium reabsorption in the jejunum is shown in the treatment of cholera. In this condition there is massive secretion of sodium-rich fluid into the bowel lumen, there is no morphological change in the mucosa, no impairment of glucose absorption and when glucose is absorbed a large amount of this secreted fluid is reabsorbed into the circulation. Thus treatment with oral unsterilized glucose saline mixtures may prevent or drastically reduce the need for intravenous treatment in such patients. In diseases such as adult coeliac disease there is secretion of water and electrolytes into the jejunum.

The ileum and colon act functionally as one. The absorption of sodium and water here is not potentiated by the presence of sugar. There is an active process which can absorb sodium and chloride against huge concentration gradients from the lumen to the plasma. Normally the jejunum and ileum are the major sites of reabsorption as can be seen from measurements of normal ileostomy output. These usually have a volume of 400–500 ml. with 60 mEq. of sodium and 13 mEq. of potassium. However, the ileum is not very adequate at regulating the amount of fluid and electrolyte lost so that the ileostomy sodium content is similar whether a patient is on a very low or very high sodium-containing diet. Thus on a low-sodium diet sodium depletion rapidly occurs in patients with an ileostomy and in countries where excessive sodium is lost through the sweat mild chronic sodium depletion may be frequently present in such patients. This may induce secondary aldosteronism and there may be a slight alteration in the sodium/potassium ratio in the ileostomy fluid and this is very marked in the urine. Thus secondary potassium depletion may occur due to this mechanism.

It is usually suggested that with diarrhoea potassium loss is primarily a result of colonic malfunction. This seems to be untrue. The nature of the faecal loss depends on the volume of faeces passed, which in turn is related to the rate of transit of the faeces passing through the colon. Throughout the colon there is a sodium potassium exchange and the more rapid the transit the less likely is the ileal effluent to be modified by processes in the colonic mucosa.

REFERENCES

British Medical Bulletin (1967) Intestinal absorption, **23,** No. 3.

MALABSORPTION SYMPOSIUM (1971) *J. clin. Path.*, **24,** Suppl. (Roy. Coll. Path.), No. 5, ed. Dawson, A. M.

THE MALABSORPTION SYNDROME

The patient may present with the clinical picture either dominated by gastro-intestinal symptoms or nutritional features with little or no gastro-intestinal disturbance. Diarrhoea is the commonest single symptom. Fatty stools which are pale, greasy, unformed and difficult to flush from the lavatory are typically described but are not invariably present. Occasionally the stool may be watery. The patient often complains of distension, bloating and flatulence and occasionally abdominal cramps are associated with excessive bowel action. Severe pain is unusual except when there is associated inflammatory bowel disease or ischaemia. The commonest nutritional manifestations are weight loss, which is probably due to a combination of anorexia as well as impaired absorption; anaemia, which is usually a mixed picture due to iron deficiency, combined with folate or B_{12} deficiency, depending on the underlying disturbance; bone disease due to a mixture of osteomalacia and osteoporosis and hypoproteinaemia. The causes of malabsorption are listed in TABLE 43.

TABLE 43

CLASSIFICATION OF MALABSORPTION STATES

I. *Disorders of Digestion*
   (1) Pancreatic Deficiency—cystic fibrosis, inflammation, carcinoma.
   (2) Bile Salt Deficiency—liver disease, biliary disease, ileal resection, stagnant loop syndrome, neomycin, cholestyramine.

II. *Disorders of Absorption*
   (1) Loss of absorptive surface.
      (a) Surgical—resection, by-pass.
      (b) Mucosal damage—coeliac disease, tropical sprue, radiation, drugs.
      (c) Infection—Whipple's disease, enteritis, hepatitis, tuberculosis.
      (d) Inflammation—Crohn's disease.
      (e) Infestation—hookworm, giardiasis, strongyloidiasis.
      *(f) Infiltration—amyloid, lymphoma.
   (2) Stagnant loop syndrome.
      Blind loops, strictures, fistulae, diverticula, scleroderma.

*(3) Lymphatic obstruction.
*(4) Vascular.
Mesenteric insufficiency, cardiac failure, constrictive pericarditis.
*(5) Endocrine.
Hypoparathyroidism, diabetes mellitus, Addison's disease, Zollinger-Ellison syndrome, thyrotoxicosis, carcinoid syndrome, systemic mastocytosis.
*(6) Miscellaneous.
(a) Drugs—neomycin, PAS, phenindione, cholestyramine.
(b) Hypogammaglobulinaemia.
(c) Pneumatosis cystoides intestinalis.
(d) Acrodermatitis enteropathica.
(e) Allergic gastro-enteropathy.

III. *Isolated Biochemical Abnormalities*
(1) Disaccharidase deficiency.
*(2) Monosaccharide malabsorption.
*(3) Abetalipoproteinaemia.
*(4) Cystinuria.
*(5) Hartnup disease.
*(6) Pernicious anaemia.

* Uncommon clinical causes of nutritional disturbances due to malabsorption.

PANCREATIC INSUFFICIENCY

Steatorrhoea is often gross and the diagnosis may be suggested by the presence of abdominal pain and diabetes. Provided the underlying cause is not debilitating the patients may retain their appetite and weight loss may not occur. Anaemia, osteomalacia and a bleeding tendency are uncommon. Xylose absorption and a jejunal biopsy are normal and the glucose tolerance may show a diabetic curve. There is calcification frequently on a plain abdominal X-ray and the diagnosis may be proven by intubating the duodenum and demonstrating a low trypsin on feeding a standard meal (a Lundh test). Treatment is by a low-fat (40 g.), high-protein (100 g.) diet; pancreatic extracts may be of some help but tend to be disappointing in adults. The most efficient seems to be *Cotazym forte*, 1–2 capsules with each meal.

RESECTION OF THE SMALL INTESTINE

Aetiology and Pathology

Massive resection of the small bowel is arbitrarily said to have occurred if more than two-thirds of the small bowel has been removed and is usually due to either infarction or volvulus. With proximal resection the ileum may take over jejunal function but the converse does not seem to be true. Thus more limited resections of the ileum which excise the absorbing sites of vitamin B_{12} and conjugated bile salts tend to produce more disability than comparable resections of jejunum.

Clinical Picture

Massive resection of the jejunum may give rise to steatorrhoea and osteomalacia due to loss of the absorbing site of fat and vitamin D. The steatorrhoea of distal resection is aggravated by bile salt depletion due to their interruption of the enterohepatic circulation. The excessive loss of bile salts into the large bowel prevents colonic water and electrolyte absorption and so aggravates or is the main cause of diarrhoea. Other evidence of malnutrition may occur if the resection is sufficiently severe.

Treatment

Steatorrhoea is controlled by a diet low in fat (less than 40 g.) and adequate calories are provided by a high carbohydrate and protein intake. Occasionally supplements of medium chain triglycerides (M.C.T.) which are easily absorbed forms of fat, are used as a calorie supplement or in small amounts to make a strict low-fat diet palatable. These are of especial nutritional use in children. The type and necessity of vitamin supplements will depend on the site and extent of the resection. Troublesome diarrhoea caused by unabsorbed bile salts interfering with colonic function may be improved by the bile salt binding resin cholestyramine.

REFERENCES

Dowling, R. H. (1970) Small bowel resection and bypass, in *Modern Trends in Gastroenterology*, ed. Card, W. I., and Creamer, B., Vol. 4, p. 73, London.
Jackson, W. P. U. (1958) Massive resection of the small intestine, in *Modern Trends in Gastroenterology*, Vol. 2, ed. Avery Jones, F., London.

COELIAC DISEASE

Synonyms. Non-tropical sprue; Gluten-induced enteropathy; Coeliac sprue; Idiopathic steatorrhoea; Primary malabsorption syndrome.

Definition

A disease of the small bowel mucosa affecting the jejunum more than the ileum, characterized by deformity of the normal villous pattern, a damaging of the absorptive cell which tends to revert to normal on withdrawal of gluten from the diet. It may present in either childhood or adult life.

Aetiology

The mucosa is sensitive to the effect of the gliadin fraction of gluten but whether this is due to an absence of a specific peptidase which prevents the complete breakdown of gluten and allows a toxic peptide to damage the cell or whether this represents an immunological disturbance is unknown; the latter seems by far the most likely and is supported by the improvement in the jejunal lesion following treatment with corticosteroids. There is a familial tendency but identical twins have been reported in whom an abnormal biopsy was present in only one of the pair.

In untreated coeliac disease there is an over-all reduction in the lymphoreticular tissue. This is suggested by the small spleen, reduction in peripheral lymphoid tissue, and an impaired lymphocyte transformation in one-third of patients. The serum IgM is reduced in 60 per cent. of patients due to a decreased IgM synthesis which returns to normal on successful treatment with a gluten-free diet. On the other hand the jejunal mucosa contains a predominance of IgM-producing plasma cells instead of the normal preponderance of IgA-producing cells. Similarly the jejunal juice contains an increased amount of IgM.

Circulating antibodies to gluten fraction and other food substances, especially milk proteins, are often found but they also occur in other intestinal diseases such as ulcerative colitis.

Pathology

The essential lesion is seen in the small bowel mucosa under the dissecting microscope. The normal leaf- or finger-shaped villi are deformed and the mucosa is either flat and featureless or merely shows ridges. Histologically most of the mucosa is taken up by the crypt region in which there is an increased mitosis count and the villi have either virtually disappeared when there is a flat biopsy (subtotal villous atrophy) or are grossly stunted (partial villous atrophy). There is an increase in inflammatory cells in the lamina propria. The absorptive cells themselves are no longer columnar but are of irregular shape and on electron microscopy the microvilli are damaged. The jejunum is more severely affected than the ileum, presumably because little gluten reaches the ileum, for it is known that the ileum is sensitive to the effect of gluten and an ileal lesion may be induced within hours of directly instilling gluten there.

Clinical Picture

This is the commonest form of generalized malabsorption in temperate climates and has an approximate incidence of 1 in 4000 of the population. It may present at any age. In childhood, symptoms often start soon after weaning when gluten is added to the diet. At this stage the children produce loose stools, become pot-bellied and may develop anaemia, general wasting, irritability and failure to grow. The adult may give no history of such childhood illness although on direct questioning may admit to mild ill health and stunting of growth in childhood or a sore tongue. Although gut symptoms may be present, the patient may often present with a megaloblastic anaemia with hypochromic features which is predominantly due to a combined folate and iron deficiency, but a refractory iron deficiency may predominate and mask the features of folate deficiency in the peripheral film. The peripheral film may be suggestive of splenic atrophy by containing target cells and Howell-Jolly bodies. The combination of these features with a dimorphic picture is almost diagnostic of coeliac disease. In about a third of the patients B_{12} deficiency is also present and usually indicates that the lesion is extensive with ileal involvement. Other patients may have hypoproteinaemia which may be due to protein loss into the bowel, together with a protein deficiency state, a bleeding tendency due to vitamin K deficiency, rarely night blindness due to vitamin A deficiency and more commonly osteomalacia due to vitamin D deficiency. Occasionally tetany ensues. Untreated female patients may be infertile but if they become pregnant the nutritional disturbance may deteriorate and coeliac disease is a cause of megaloblastic anaemia of pregnancy. Other complications are an eczematous rash and rarely a neuromyelopathy. These patients have a higher risk of lymphosarcoma of the bowel and also neoplasms of any part of the gastro-intestinal tract including the small bowel. Occasionally patients develop severe ulceration of the small bowel which is refractory to treatment.

Diagnosis

The *sine qua non* for diagnosing this condition is the demonstration of an abnormal small bowel biopsy and the improvement of a patient on a gluten-free diet. It is generally unwise to attempt the latter form of treatment, which is a life-long sentence without histological proof. Other diagnostic features are confirmatory but the assessment of the extent of nutritional deficit is of course important.

Treatment

The choice rests between the use of a gluten-free diet or the administration of nutritional supplements and symptomatic measures. A gluten-free diet is usually favoured and in most series has induced a remission in 80–90 per cent. of patients. Whether the patients who do not respond suffer from the same condition is at present unknown but some of them are probably not keeping strictly to the diet. Remission of symptoms usually starts within a few days but it may take up to a year for full benefit to occur and a tendency to slack stools, not indicative of malabsorption, may persist. The usual early changes noted are improvement in appetite and well-being, the lessening of gastro-intestinal symptoms and an increase in weight. The role of cereals other than wheat in perpetuating the condition has only been partly assessed but it seems that oats do not damage the mucosa. The use of the gluten-free diet is the usual choice of treatment for this restores the histological abnormality of the small bowel to normal and presumably helps to prevent the insidious onset of various nutritional deficiencies. The diet as now modified is palatable and membership of the Coeliac Society ensures that any improvement in technique of food preparation is immediately circulated to members. In some refractory cases a course of steroids, such as prednisone, 15 mg. three times daily, may be of benefit, while very rarely there is a secondary stagnant loop syndrome.

Course and Prognosis

In the untreated patient the symptoms fluctuate in intensity although the intestinal biopsy remains abnormal. Similarly the childhood coeliac patient who at puberty goes into apparent clinical remission when investigated has an abnormally flat intestinal biopsy and often subnormal serum folate level.

REFERENCES

Booth, C. C. (1970) Enterocyte in coeliac disease, *Brit. med. J.*, **3**, 725 and **4**, 13.

Cooke, W. T., Fone, D. S., Cox, E. V., Meynell, M. J., and Gaddie, R. (1963) Adult coeliac disease, *Gut*, **4**, 279.

Hamilton, J. R., Lynch, M. J., and Reilly, B. J. (1969) Active coeliac disease in childhood, *Quart. J. Med.*, N.S., **38**, 135.

Nilson, B., ed. (1970) *Coeliac Handbook*, Coeliac Society.

WHIPPLE'S DISEASE

This is a rare disorder predominantly affecting

middle-aged men and should be suspected if malabsorption is associated with arthralgia. Other features include fever, pigmentation, abdominal pain, polyserositis and peripheral lymphadenopathy. The diagnosis is made by jejunal biopsy or histological examination of a peripheral lymph node. The villi may appear distorted or even flattened due to the presence of large numbers of periodic acid Schiff (PAS) positive macrophages which are present in the lamina propria. The epithelial cells are relatively normal on light microscopy but on electron microscopy some patchy non-specific changes have been reported. The PAS positive material has been shown to be the end product of bacterial degradation and small rod-shaped organisms have been demonstrated in the mucosa. The condition responds to long-term treatment with antibiotics, for example tetracycline, 250 mg. four times daily for 2 years, but other antibiotics have been equally effective. The nature of the organism is unknown.

REFERENCE

HENDRIX, T. R., and YARDLEY, J. H. (1970) Whipple's disease, in *Modern Trends in Gastroenterology*, Vol. 4, ed. Card, W. I., and Creamer, B., p. 229, London.

THE STAGNANT LOOP SYNDROME

Synonym. Blind loop syndrome.

Definition

A condition in which there is an abnormal proliferation of colonic-type organisms in the small bowel which interfere with the absorption or metabolism of foodstuffs.

Aetiology

Normally the jejunum is relatively sterile. In conditions of stasis due to intestinal strictures, disturbed motility from infiltration by systemic sclerosis or lymphoma, the presence of fistulas between the colon and the small bowel or the presence of a long afferent loop after gastric surgery, stagnation of contents occur and colonic-type bacteria proliferate. This may impair absorption of at least three nutrients. There is nearly always impaired absorption of vitamin B_{12} even in the presence of adequate intrinsic factor. Fat absorption is often subnormal due to bacteria converting the normally conjugated bile salts to the free form which are poor at solubilizing lipid and also tend to be absorbed by non-ionic diffusion in the jejunum. Thirdly, the bacteria may themselves metabolize dietary constituents. This probably can account for the protein deficiency which occasionally occurs when dietary protein and amino acids are broken down to ammonia or amines. It must be stressed that within each bacterial species are many distinct types which have varying metabolic potential so that the incidence of the metabolic changes will vary from patient to patient.

Clinical Picture

This will depend on the underlying cause of the stagnation. On the one hand the patient may have no gastro-intestinal symptoms and present with a megaloblastic anaemia due to B_{12} deficiency. This not infrequently occurs in elderly patients with small intestinal diverticula. At the other extreme is the patient with a gastroje-juno-colic fistula who has gross diarrhoea, gross steatorrhoea, protein malnutrition and weight loss.

Diagnosis

This depends on the demonstration of the anatomical abnormality and the presence of functional abnormalities which can be improved by treatment with an antibiotic; tetracycline, 250 mg. four times daily, is usually the most efficient. Where possible the demonstration of abnormal numbers of bacteria in the jejunal and mid-bowel contents is confirmatory. This latter investigation is, unfortunately, extremely time consuming and at the moment is a research technique. Screening tests such as an increased urinary excretion of indican are not sufficiently sensitive to be of clinical use.

Treatment

Where possible this will be most effective if the anatomical defect can be corrected. If not, anaemia should be treated by intramuscular B_{12}, steatorrhoea by a low-fat diet, hypoproteinaemia by a high-protein diet. Intermittent antibiotics may also be used in a hope of suppressing bacterial proliferation.

Course and Prognosis

Course and prognosis will depend entirely on the nature of the underlying bowel condition.

REFERENCES

HAMILTON, J. D., DYER, N. H., DAWSON, A. M., O'GRADY, F. W., VINCE, A., FENTON, J. C. B., and MOLLIN, D. L. (1970) Assessment of significance of bacterial overgrowth in the small bowel, *Quart. J. Med.*, N.S., **39,** 265.

TABAQCHALI, S., and BOOTH, C. C. (1970) Bacteria and the small intestine, in *Modern Trends in Gastroenterology*, Vol. 4, ed. Card, W. I., and Creamer, B., p. 143, London.

DISTURBANCES OF THE LYMPHATIC CIRCULATION

Abdominal lymphatics are the predominant route by which fat and fat-soluble substances are transported to the systemic circulation after they have been absorbed. Any condition interfering with this transport may be associated with steatorrhoea and a disturbance of protein metabolism. One of these conditions is intestinal lymphangiectasia, a disease which tends to run in families and usually starts in childhood. It is caused by a sclerotic lesion of the abdominal lymphatics and lymph nodes. This causes dilatation of the proximal vessels including those within the serosa and mucosa of the bowel. Sometimes these lymphatics burst into the abdominal cavity causing chylous ascites and on occasions a chylothorax. On the other hand others may burst into the lumen of the bowel causing a protein-losing state, indeed, chyle has been occasionally aspirated from the gut lumen. There may be associated disturbances of lymphatics elsewhere such as lymphoedema. Biopsy of the small bowel may occasionally show dilated lymphatics in the villi but negative findings do not rule out the diagnosis. Hypoproteinaemia is frequent though phasic and due to loss of protein into the bowel lumen. Similarly plasma gamma globulin may also be low due to the loss into the bowel. Steatorrhoea is frequent and gross disorders of calcium metabolism may occur. Treatment is difficult and usually depends on the use of a low-fat diet which controls the steatorrhoea and may help the hypoproteinaemia by preventing the usually postprandial rise of lymph flow which in such patients would aggravate loss into the bowel.

A protein-losing state has been described in some patients with severe heart failure associated with a chronically high venous pressure such as constrictive pericarditis or a cardiomyopathy. This is rare and probably due to dilatation of lymphatics. Such dilatation has been produced experimentally by obstruction of the superior vena cava in animals which causes back pressure on the thoracic duct.

REFERENCE

Waldman, T. A. (1970) Protein losing enteropathy, in *Modern Trends in Gastroenterology*, ed. Card, W. I., and Creamer, B., Vol. 4, p. 125, London.

DRUGS AFFECTING ABSORPTION

Transient steatorrhoea has been reported to occur with large doses of neomycin (8–10 G. a day). Under these conditions the steatorrhoea is gross with a faecal fat content of 20–30 g. a day but other disturbances of intestinal absorption are relatively mild and changes in the intestinal mucosa are minimal. The result is probably due to the precipitation of fatty acids in the lumen of the small bowel from the mixed micelles of fatty acid and monoglyceride and bile salts. PAS may on occasions produce steatorrhoea and interfere with the absorption of B_{12}, as shown by the Schilling test; the mechanism is unknown. Phenolphthalein may be a cause of steatorrhoea as well as diarrhoea, while phenindione has also produced this condition. Cholestyramine used in the treatment of the pruritus of obstructive jaundice and the diarrhoea of ileal resection may induce or aggravate steatorrhoea.

DISACCHARIDASE DEFICIENCY

CONGENITAL DEFICIENCY

It is not surprising that children have been discovered who are lacking in one or other of the enzymes. The main clinical conditions result from absence of lactase or a combined sucrase-isomaltase deficiency. These children present in the neonatal period with acid diarrhoea, failure to thrive, dehydration and malnutrition. Treatment with a diet which excludes the offending disaccharide or its precursor improves growth and diminishes symptoms. In adult life such subjects can partly outgrow their symptoms, though they are still unable to absorb the disaccharide. Occasionally sucrase-isomaltase deficiency is a cause of diarrhoea in adults.

CONSTITUTIONAL HYPOLACTASIA (ACQUIRED DEFICIENCY)

Lactase deficiency in older children and adults is quite a different problem. The symptoms are variable and less severe. Diarrhoea, abdominal colic, borborygmi and distension may follow ingestion of milk. Similar symptoms may be present in other subjects who are unable to relate them to milk. A further group may be asymptomatic and some may even be able to tolerate large amounts of milk. The severity of the symptoms depends on the amount of lactose in the diet and the variable response of the colon to the stimulus of the unabsorbed free sugar and its fermentation products. When a large lactose load is ingested there is a high concentration of unabsorbed sugar in the small intestinal lumen, which attracts fluid by osmosis and so behaves like a bulk purgative, sweeping water, electrolytes and occasionally fat and protein down the intestine. Such an episode is uncommon on a normal diet, since the concentration of lactose in milk is not high (40 g. per litre). In most subjects lactose forms only a small proportion of the dietary carbohydrate and produces only recurrent minor symptoms throughout the day, which are probably the result of bacterial fermentation of lactose in the colon to produce short chain organic acids which irritate the large bowel.

Diagnosis is suggested by a flat lactose tolerance test (see above), which produces diarrhoea, borborygmi and abdominal pain in 70 per cent. of patients. Absorption of glucose and galactose is normal. Other screening tests of absorption and nutrition are normal. Jejunal biopsy shows no anatomical abnormality, and assay of the disaccharidase content of the specimen confirms the diagnosis.

Constitutional hypolactasia has now been found in many different parts of the world. There is a very high incidence (up to 90 per cent.) in certain racial groups such as Negroes and Greek Cypriots, although in Northern Europeans the incidence is probably about 10 per cent. In affected populations it seems that there is a gradual regression of lactase activity as maturation proceeds, since there is a normal lactase concentration in the neonatal period. This is comparable with most animal species, and it can be argued that it is those who retain lactase activity who are abnormal.

The clinical significance of lactase deficiency has probably been overstressed in the past few years. It must be very rare for lactase deficiency to be the sole cause of severe diarrhoea as a presenting symptom. Moreover, since hypolactasia is a common finding, it should not be used as an explanation for other major symptoms such as marked weight loss or nutritional disturbance, when another cause should be sought. Lactase deficiency has been described in association with a number of other diseases, including ulcerative colitis, Crohn's disease, infectious hepatitis, and febrile illnesses. This association probably reflects the high incidence of the defect in any population. However, the symptoms of these diseases may be made worse by dietary lactose, or the development of the disease may render a previously compensated subject intolerant of milk.

SECONDARY DEFICIENCY

This occurs when the intestinal mucosa is damaged by such conditions as coeliac disease, tropical sprue and infections. Depression of the activity of all enzymes of the mucosal cell occurs in proportion to the severity of the damage. The condition is reversible when the underlying disease heals. It is not usually functionally significant in adults, but in neonates and young children selective restriction of dietary sugars is often beneficial.

REFERENCE

DAWSON, A. M. (1970) The absorption of disaccharides, in *Modern Trends in Gastroenterology*, Vol. 4, ed. Card, W. I., and Creamer, B., p. 105, London.

A. M. DAWSON

TROPICAL SPRUE

Definition

Sprue is a primary intestinal malabsorption syndrome clinically characterized by steatorrhoea, glossitis and stomatitis, dyspepsia and abdominal distension and rapid weight loss occurring in individuals who inhabit or have lived in certain tropical areas. The clinical picture is subject to frequent remissions and to relapses. The cause is unknown.

Aetiology

Sprue has a regional rather than climatic distribution. It occurs most commonly in India, Pakistan, Burma, Ceylon, China, Indonesia and Puerto Rico. It has been reported in North and Central America, parts of the West Indies, Southern Europe, the Middle East and occasionally in the Pacific islands. Variants of the syndrome occur, for example, in hill diarrhoea which appears sometimes in high areas of India and the malabsorption diarrhoea of Hong Kong and other parts of the Far East. During the Second World War outbreaks of a sprue-like syndrome occurred in troops in India and Burma. It has not been reported from Africa.

Classical sprue is a disease of middle life. There is no sex or racial disposition and often no social background of either malnutrition or poverty. The patient is usually either living in the 'sprue area' or has lived there for some time, usually for years, occasionally for only a few weeks. The clinical picture may develop months or years after the patient has left the tropics for a temperate climate.

The primary physiological disturbance in sprue is defective absorption in the small intestine involving especially fats and certain carbohydrates.

The cause of this malabsorption has not been ascertained. There is general agreement that it is not infective or primarily derived from the deficiencies in essential substances which accompany it. These deficiencies are secondary and some of them are believed to arise from failure of biosynthesis following invasion of the relevant area of the small intestine by bacteria derived from the large intestine. The megaloblastic anaemia which is often a striking feature of the clinical picture in certain geographical areas but not in others is also secondary.

The digestion of foodstuffs in the gut is normal but absorption of fat and glucose is defective. The particulate absorption of fat is reduced and the triglycerides which remain are broken down normally into free fatty acids which are both absorbed and excreted in larger amounts than normal. This process is associated with excessive secretion of mucus. The more saturated fatty acids are less well absorbed and cause intestinal irritation. Insoluble soaps are formed with calcium, and excreted, leading to loss of this element.

Absorption of glucose is defective and delayed, as may be seen in a flat oral absorption curve. Other sugars, such as fructose and xylose, are often absorbed normally, suggesting that there may be some fault in phosphorylation. Bacterial action on the unabsorbed foods including glucose, together with the disturbances of fat absorption, result in flatulence and distension and the passage of bulky gaseous stools containing excess fat, most of which is 'split', i.e. in the form of free fatty acids and soaps.

Pathology

The pathogenesis of sprue, although still obscure, is probably related to that of other closely allied syndromes such as idiopathic steatorrhoea and coeliac disease. Sensitivity to gluten, however, does not occur in sprue.

Changes in the structure of the intestinal wall have recently been described in biopsies of the jejunum taken during the active phase of the disease. There is considerable decrease in the absorptive surface, some mucosal oedema, and alteration of the appearance of the villi which have apparently coalesced to become leaf-like, ridged and convoluted; the mucus-secreting goblet cells are increased and there is often an accompanying round cell subepithelial infiltration. This pattern is quite different from that of idiopathic steatorrhoea in which there is mucosal atrophy with 'flat featureless villi'. Autopsy changes not unlike the biopsy findings were described by Manson-Bahr but most observers have reported merely atrophy and thinning of the intestinal walls sometimes with perforation.

In the stool there is an excessive excretion of fat which comes partly from the fat ingested in the diet and partly from excretion into the gut. Absorption of vitamin A is concurrently impaired. The total blood and plasma particulate fat curves after a meal are low. Fasting blood glucose is normal or may be low. The oral absorption curve is delayed and flat. The disappearance of glucose injected intravenously is normal.

In advanced sprue dehydration may be severe, with relevant changes in plasma electrolytes including potassium. In cases exhibiting tetany serum calcium and sometimes magnesium may be considerably reduced.

Many cases have some degree of megaloblastic anaemia with corresponding changes in the bone marrow, arising from deficiency of folic acid and occasionally of vitamin B_{12}. There is often gastric hypo-acidity or achlorhydria, but the latter is rarely histamine-fast.

The macroscopic appearance of the fatty stool is characteristic in the fully developed syndrome [see signs and symptoms]. In the early and intermediate stages there may be only watery diarrhoea.

Signs and Symptoms

The patient is either living in or gives a history of having lived at some time in an area where sprue is endemic.

The onset is usually gradual and the patient may not seek help until the syndrome is well advanced. The presenting symptoms are nearly always gastro-intestinal, varying from diarrhoea to the full picture described below. Occasionally the anaemia may be a dominant factor.

There is commonly an early period of watery diarrhoea with urgent, pale, frothy and offensive stools discharged most frequently in the early part of the day and not so much at night. The syndrome may not develop beyond this stage as, for example in hill diarrhoea.

Remissions of varying duration occur, interspersed with increasingly lengthy attacks of diarrhoea or 'looseness' which gradually develop into the classical pattern of long episodes of looseness in which several motions are passed during the day, mainly in the morning. The need for passing the stool is urgent, especially on awakening. The motion is discharged explosively with large volumes of gas. The 'sprue stool' is characteristically bulky and soft or porridgy, full of tiny bubbles, greasy, light brown or grey in colour and extremely offensive. Its passage occurs without pain but is often preceded by abdominal colic. Even at this stage remissions are likely to occur, but they may be short and incomplete.

Dyspepsia occurs early and is severe and progressive. There is usually very uncomfortable flatulence especially after meals. The abdomen is distended in the lower central region corresponding roughly to the position of the small intestine. These symptoms become increasingly severe during the day and are at their worst in the early morning before the first stool is passed, after which there is temporary relief. In advanced cases the abdominal wall is very thin and the peristaltic movements of the distended intestine are often clearly visible. There is usually little tenderness, but the abdomen sometimes has the 'doughy' feel usually associated with tuberculosis.

Achlorhydria may be present but responds to histamine. In dyspeptic cases the ordinary barium emulsion clumps heavily and irregularly in the small intestine, producing the so-called 'deficiency pattern' due to excess mucus secretion. Normal 'feathering' of the barium occurs when non-agglutinable emulsions are used. Some cases show moderate dilatation and loss of radiological pattern in the large intestine, but megacolon, as seen in coeliac disease or idiopathic steatorrhoea, does not develop.

The appetite varies considerably. In some patients anorexia is persistent and the patient becomes highly selective in his diet, avoiding particularly hot and spicy foods which cause pain and discomfort of the mouth and tongue and exacerbate the dyspeptic symptoms. Sometimes there may be no loss of appetite or only occasional bouts of anorexia. The appetite commonly recovers early in treatment.

Changes in the tongue and mouth usually follow shortly after the establishment of diarrhoea and are pronounced in most well developed cases. They are essentially due to secondary vitamin deficiencies. The tongue is clean and patchily inflamed, with red raw areas of papillary denudation especially near the tip and sides. Small vesicles and ulcers develop in the tongue and buccal mucous membrane especially on the frenum of the tongue and floor of the mouth. The severity of these lesions varies in a given patient and from patient to patient; they cause most discomfort during the periods of active looseness or diarrhoea. Sometimes they persist or become increasingly severe, and are associated with excessive salivation. The oesophagus may become involved, with accompanying dysphagia. Cheilosis and angular stomatitis are common, especially in advanced cases.

As the syndrome progresses weight is steadily and sometimes rapidly lost and the patient becomes emaciated with loss of subcutaneous fat and with dry wrinkled sometimes scaly skin on which appear irregular light brown pigmented patches, usually on the face, back and buttocks. The nails become ridged and brittle. Avitaminotic skin changes may occur on the scrotum and legs but the symmetrical lesions of pellagra do not develop.

Anaemia appears in many cases but not in all and is probably secondary and associated with the dietary status of the patient. In its fully developed form it is megaloblastic and almost invariably responds well to folic acid administration. In most cases there is also an element of iron deficiency. The bone marrow response in anaemic cases is megaloblastic or may be mixed. Subacute combined degeneration of the cord does not occur.

Personality changes are invariable in the well established case. The patient becomes irritable, querulous and introspective. He is often frankly dishonest over such things as diet, particularly in the early stages of treatment if food is restricted.

Where there is deficiency of calcium and magnesium, or both, characteristic tetanic spasms of the hands and feet occur, especially during periods of exacerbation of the gastro-intestinal symptoms.

The final stages occur months or years after the onset, with signs of protein deficiency, severe dehydration and vascular failure. Death results from any or all of these conditions or from secondary infections.

The development is commonly progressive, with shortening periods of remission. The picture described above of watery diarrhoea gradually merging into looseness and the passage of 'sprue stools' is usual but sometimes these symptoms are preceded by those of deficiencies, and loss of weight, dyspepsia and sore tongue may be the first indications of the disease.

There are many variants. In the Burma campaign during the Second World War there were widespread outbreaks of diarrhoea with defective intestinal absorption of fat, associated with variable degrees of deficiency signs. Some of these cases went on to develop classical sprue. The syndromes appeared in both Indians and Europeans, usually after months of subsistence on restricted diets or 'rations'.

More recently cases of malabsorption with diarrhoea have been described in areas of the Far East including Hong Kong.

Diagnosis

The clinical diagnosis is made on the geographical history, the state of the patient and the demonstration of the malabsorption.

Conditions likely to cause confusion are other forms of steatorrhoea, vitamin deficiencies and megaloblastic anaemia.

Sprue is rare in children in whom coeliac disease may present a very similar clinical picture. In the latter megacolon is common, there is no response to sprue diet and excellent response to a gluten-free diet.

Idiopathic steatorrhoea may appear in sprue endemic areas but there is usually no relevant geographical history and cases respond to a gluten-free diet. Megacolon occurs occasionally, the anaemia is seldom severe, and osteoporosis is common.

Sprue may have to be distinguished from malabsorption caused by giardiasis and capillariasis (as seen in a recent outbreak in the Philippines).

Obstruction to lacteal flow from enlarged glands as in Hodgkin's disease or tuberculosis produces a syndrome not unlike sprue. Differentiation is made by discovery of the aetiological factor.

Surgical intestinal short-circuit operations and gastro-jejuno-colic fistula may have a similar effect.

Steatorrhoea occurs in diseases of the pancreas. In chronic pancreatitis the proportion of neutral to 'split' fat is high, the reverse of the case in sprue; the enzyme content in the duodenal juice is reduced and the glucose absorption curve is either normal or of the diabetic type.

The anaemia is a typical megaloblastic response to deficiency of folic acid or a block in the folic acid: folinic acid mechanism. It may be distinguished from pernicious anaemia by the response to folic acid and absence of response to administration of vitamin B_{12} and by the absence of histamine-fast achlorhydria. Changes in the spinal cord do not occur in sprue.

The laboratory diagnosis of sprue must include an estimation of fat excretion. This may be made by measuring the total faecal fat on several successive days or by a fat-balance test. In the latter, the patient is placed on a diet with a known content of fat (usually 50 G. per day) and is given a charcoal marker. A second marker is given three days later. All faeces passed between the appearance and disappearance of the charcoal in the stools are collected and the total quantity of fat estimated.

In the normal subject only about 5 G. fat per day is passed. The sprue case excretes considerably more.

An alternative is to carry out a vitamin A absorption test. In sprue the absorption is markedly reduced.

Faecal fat in sprue is composed of free fatty acids and soaps ('split' fat) and neutral fat in the ratio of 3:1 or higher. In normal faecal excretion of fat the ratio is seldom above 2:1 and in pancreatic steatorrhoea it may be 1:1 or less.

Microscopic examination of faeces may show fatty acid crystals, fat globules and undigested food.

Oral absorption of glucose is examined in the usual way by giving 50 g. and measuring the blood concentration half hourly. In sprue the curve is flat and the fasting blood sugar sometimes low. Absorption curves for xylose and fructose are usually normal.

Treatment

The patient should be treated in bed under careful supervision.

The basis of treatment is control of diarrhoea, adjustment of the diet with replacement of vitamins and minerals and control of complications such as dehydration. The anaemia responds to folic acid.

Diarrhoea in early cases responds well to antibiotics and insoluble sulphonamides. Tetracycline has been widely used, in doses of 250 mg. 6-hourly. Long-term treatment with antibiotics, sometimes for as long as 6 months, has had good results in the Far East and Caribbean, but not in India.

In advanced cases with intractable steatorrhoea calcium salts sometimes help by forming soaps and thus reducing the quantity of irritating split fat present.

In the past very good results in severe cases were often obtained by adjustment of the diet so as to provide high protein and relatively low carbohydrate and fat. The food intake was built up over weeks or months to a full balanced diet. Sources of protein were meat or milk. The addition of lightly cooked liver or crude liver extracts was found beneficial.

Present opinion is against this form of rigorous dieting. There is usually no evidence of fat intolerance, and low lactase levels in the jejunal mucosa occur as they do in kwashiorkor and render some individuals intolerant of lactose and therefore of milk.

The modern practice is, therefore, to allow the patient to take a normal diet, supplemented as needed to replace vitamin and mineral deficiencies which may be present. Where hypoproteinaemia is marked, a high protein diet is called for. After the patient has reached a full diet he must be given instructions regarding a maintenance diet and learn by experience and advice which foods he can manage and which he cannot. Most kinds of cooked meat, fish and poultry are well tolerated but fatty or fried meats or fish, spiced foods and vegetables containing excess roughage should be avoided. Bread, alcohol and sweets or sweet drinks are all likely to promote dyspepsia and distension.

Sprue patients do not respond to a gluten-free diet.

Folic acid has a rapid and remarkable effect on the anaemia and sometimes on the whole syndrome especially upon the gastro-intestinal symptoms. In spite of this it has little effect on the malabsorption itself.

In severely ill patients it is given parenterally in doses of 10–20 mg. daily for the first fortnight and then 10 mg. orally once or twice a week or a maintenance dose of 5 mg. daily for weeks or months.

In some patients, particularly in India, there may be some concomitant B_{12} deficiency, which can be treated by intramuscular injection of 1000 μg. cyano- or hydroxo-cobalamin once weekly. If there is suspicion of B_{12} deficiency, this vitamin and folic acid should be given together. Treatment may have to be continued for 2–3 months.

Vitamins must be added to the diet, including nicotinic acid and riboflavine, either as specific substances in the usual doses or as extracts and proprietary preparations.

The administration of vitamins leads to rapid

improvement of the deficiency signs such as the tongue and mouth lesions and often the gastro-intestinal symptoms. It will not, however, check the malabsorption or the ultimate progress of the syndrome.

Minerals also need replacement in some cases with low serum calcium levels. Tetanic episodes can be limited or prevented by administration of calcium lactate.

Where dehydration is present, oral administration of sodium chloride and water may be sufficient. In more severe forms of the disease, water absorption from the gut is often restricted and even a moderate degree of dehydration may require parenteral isotonic saline. Potassium may also be needed, either parenterally or orally. Where possible it should be given orally, e.g. as potassium chloride in doses of not more than 10 G. daily, otherwise with the parenteral saline, in amounts of not more than 200 ml. of a solution containing 15 mEq. per litre.

Prognosis

Response to treatment is usually good and progressive commencing with improvement in the diarrhoea and other gastro-intestinal symptoms. Spontaneous cure may sometimes occur without treatment.

The defect in absorption improves only slowly and may be still present after apparent cure. For this reason there may be relapses at any stage.

The co-operation of the patient is essential at all stages and often very difficult to obtain.

If improvement continues over three years without relapse the patient usually thereafter remains well. Prognosis is worse in older people.

In untreated cases in which the syndrome is well developed, the mortality rate is high.

REFERENCE

O'Brien, W. (1968) The diagnosis and treatment of tropical sprue, *Trans. roy. Soc. trop. Med. Hyg.*, **62**, 148.

Brian Maegraith

ACUTE INTESTINAL OBSTRUCTION

Definition

A failure of progression of intestinal contents due to physical obstruction of the bowel or impaired motor activity of the bowel (paralytic ileus).

Aetiology

Obstruction due to occlusion of the bowel lumen may be due to foreign bodies, such as gall-stones, bezoars, meconium, worms or enteroliths. Causes in the wall of the bowel are atresia, neoplasms, strictures and diverticular disease. Causes compressing the wall are obstructed hernias, adhesions or volvulus. The small bowel is involved in 80 per cent. of patients with acute intestinal obstruction. In the neonate the common causes are atresia, volvulus, meconium ileus and Hirschsprung's disease. In infants they are intussusception, a strangulated hernia and Hirschsprung's disease; and in the young adult and middle-aged adhesions and bands, and obstructed hernias; in the elderly a carcinoma, diverticulitis and faecal impaction are the common causes. Special forms of obstruction due to volvulus, mesenteric occlusion and paralytic ileus will be considered separately. There are geographic variations in the frequency of each cause. Thus volvulus of the sigmoid is very common in East Africa but uncommon in England. In Western countries the commonest single cause of obstruction is adhesions, which latterly has supplanted hernias.

Pathology

The effects of obstruction are related to the depletion of fluid and electrolytes and also 'toxaemia'; they are also modified by the underlying cause. Once the bowel is obstructed it dilates and although fluid is excreted into the lumen it is poorly reabsorbed, especially in the jejunum. Fluid thus collects in the bowel lumen and is lost from the circulating volume whether or not the patient vomits. The most important ion lost is sodium, the luminal fluid having a similar composition to plasma. Once sodium deficiency occurs there is secondary aldosteronism with consequent loss of potassium from the kidney. This latter mechanism is as important as potassium loss from the bowel in the genesis of potassium deficiency. Eventually extrarenal uraemia ensues. The bowel becomes dilated partly due to gas and probably 70 per cent. of this is derived from swallowed air. The distended abdomen impairs diaphragmatic movement and may facilitate the occurrence of pneumonia. When the pressure in the lumen increases there may eventually be ischaemic changes with necrosis of the bowel wall. This is associated with an increased permeability of the mucosa and so protein is lost into the bowel lumen. This phenomenon is more florid when there is strangulation and the blood supply to a segment of the bowel is compromised. The intestinal contents in such patients contain material which can induce profound shock in experimental animals which is probably of bacterial origin. The bowel above the obstruction becomes colonized with faecal type organisms which are probably ingested.

Clinical Picture

This is dominated by pain, vomiting, abdominal distension and constipation. The pain is colicky, often severe, and may coincide with loud borborygmi, heard with or without the stethoscope. There are periods of complete freedom intervening. Reflex vomiting is often caused by the severe pain but with high obstruction vomiting becomes profuse. So-called faeculent vomiting occurs when the stagnant contents of dilated bowel loops have been modified by faecal type organisms. Vomiting may be minimal in ileal obstruction and absent in large bowel obstruction. Constipation is often absolute even to the point of not passing gas. Distension of the upper abdomen tends to occur with upper small bowel obstruction, central abdominal distension with ileal obstruction, and the whole of the abdomen with large bowel lesions. On examination, besides the distension, there may be variable peritonism. Examination of the rectum and hernial orifices is mandatory. The presence of dehydration and shock will depend on the length of history as well as the nature of the underlying lesion. Local tenderness may point to the site of a lesion and a scar suggest an adhesion.

Diagnosis

The clinical findings are supplemented by a plain X-ray of the supine abdomen for the presence of gas in dilated bowel and the erect abdomen when fluid levels in either the small or large bowel are seen. A haemoglobin and PCV estimation together with plasma electrolytes and urea give an indication of the degree of dehydration. The syndrome must be differentiated from acute gastro-enteritis, pancreatitis, appendicitis, a perforated peptic ulcer and renal or biliary colic.

Treatment

This entails decompression of the bowel and preventing swallowed air entering the bowel by suction of an intragastric or intra-enteric tube. There must be rehydration with appropriate fluid and electrolyte mixture. In acute mechanical obstruction operation will nearly always be needed especially if the cause is unknown but, for example in Crohn's disease, an episode may settle with medical treatment. The great danger is missing a strangulated loop of bowel with the attendant high mortality and, unfortunately, this form cannot be differentiated with certainty clinically.

Prognosis

Over-all mortality varies in different series between 10 and 20 per cent. Beside the underlying lesion affecting the outcome the mortality is higher at the extremes of age, even so the single most important factor is whether a loop of bowel is strangulated. The ratio of mortality reported for strangulated to simple obstruction varies from two to tenfold.

REFERENCES

ELLIS, H. (1969) Acute intestinal obstruction, in *Abdominal Operations*, ed. Maingot, R., p. 1497, New York.

LEFFAL, L. D., QUANDER, J., and SYPHAX, B. (1965) Strangulated intestinal obstruction, *Arch. Surg.*, **91**, 592.

PARALYTIC ILEUS

Even with the most gentle handling of the bowel at operation there is usually some post-operative impairment of motor activity which always affects the stomach and large bowel. Paralysis of bowel movement is an invariable accompaniment of peritonitis from any cause and may also occur with retroperitoneal haemorrhage and in patients in plaster jackets. It may be seen in patients being treated with ganglionic blocking drugs and occasionally in such metabolic states as uraemia and diabetic coma and is aggravated by potassium depletion and severe infections such as pneumonia. A chronic form may also occur when the retroperitoneal tissue is infiltrated by a carcinoma. Treatment entails rehydrating the patient, decompressing the bowel by intubation and dealing with the underlying cause.

VOLVULUS

Definition

A twisting of a portion of the intestine about its mesenteric attachment.

Aetiology and Pathology

The twisting of the intestine about its mesenteric axis produces a closed loop type obstruction. In the acute fulminating form the blood supply becomes occluded and features of strangulation associated with enormous distension follow with the consequent danger of gangrene and perforation. In other cases the volvulus may be subacute and recurrent. The production of volvulus may be favoured by congenital anomalies such as a long mesentery or the presence of adhesions fixing a loop of gut. The common sites for it to occur are the small gut and sigmoid colon. The caecum is rarely affected unless there is an anomalous long mesentery. The wide geographical variation in the incidence of sigmoid volvulus, it being high in Africa, is possibly due to the high roughage content of the diet in such countries which is associated with a large stool weight (in Uganda the normal daily stool weight is 700–1000 g., in Western countries 50–150 g.).

Clinical Picture

When the small bowel is involved there is a fulminant intestinal obstruction and the common differential diagnosis is mesenteric occlusion or peritonitis. With sigmoid volvulus a small group of patients run an acute painful course similar to that of small bowel volvulus but the common form is that of recurrent mild attacks when the condition is reversible. There is a gradual onset often with a history of previous attacks and enormous distension of the abdomen; vomiting occurs late. On X-ray of the abdomen the segment of distended colon may be seen. If untreated, symptoms and signs of dehydration and extrarenal uraemia ensue.

Treatment

The acute form is treated by operation. For the chronic form, reduction of the torsion may be effected by a simple enema or passing a soft rubber flatus tube. This gives good results in 80 per cent. of cases. An operation is indicated if reduction does not occur or acute strangulation is suspected. It may also be advised once reduction has taken place to avoid a recurrence; partial resection of the sigmoid colon is then undertaken.

REFERENCES

HINSHAW, D. B., and CARTER, R. (1957) Surgical management of acute volvulus of the sigmoid, *Ann. Surg.*, **146**, 52.

PRATHER, J. R., and BOWERS, R. F. (1962) Surgical management of volvulus of the sigmoid, *Arch. Surg.*, **85**, 869.

ACUTE MESENTERIC VASCULAR OCCLUSION

Definition

An acute occlusion of the mesenteric artery or vein with subsequent impairment of bowel function or gangrene of the bowel.

Aetiology

The commonest causes of vascular occlusion are embolism or thrombosis, two-thirds of which affect the arterial tree. In approximately 40 per cent. of patients with an arterial obstruction this is caused by an embolus and in 40 per cent. by a thrombus complicating atheroma of the mouths of the main vessels. In 20 per cent. of patients no complete obstruction is found but it seems that the lesion is induced by a combination of partial occlusion to the main vessel combined with a condition which causes a low cardiac output, such as severe congestive heart failure or shock. Approximately 80 per cent. of patients suffering from embolism have auricular fibrillation, in other cases the emboli are derived from a variety of sources such as an atheromatous aorta or the heart valves in subacute bacterial endocarditis. Venous occlusion is always caused by thrombosis which may be secondary to septic pyelophlebitis or extrahepatic portal vein thrombosis. It sometimes occurs as a complication after splenectomy possibly due to a thrombus spreading from the splenic bed. The superior mesenteric artery is involved in 90 per cent. of cases, the inferior mesenteric in 10 per cent.

Pathology

Sudden occlusion of the main artery causes gangrene of the bowel when the superior mesenteric vessel is involved. This extends from the duodenojejunal flexure to the mid transverse colon. Lesser areas of bowel are involved if an embolus lodges past the first potential collateral vessels. If only one small segment is involved from a small embolus this may heal with stricture formation but retrograde thrombosis may affect proximal collateral vessels with subsequent spreading infarction. Occlusion of the inferior mesenteric vessel causes infarction of the left side of the colon. Occlusion of the veins causes a less spectacular effect as they occur slowly, gradually spread and give time for collateral vessels to open up. The lesion in the bowel takes the form of haemorrhagic infarction with eventual gangrene. Shock is induced by profound exudation of fluid both into the lumen and wall of the bowel and possibly by a humoral factor which is released from the bowel.

Clinical Picture

The condition can rarely be diagnosed with confidence before a laparotomy but typically there is severe pain which is out of proportion to abdominal tenderness, shock and abdominal distension associated with vomiting and loose stools both of which may be blood stained. The condition must be differentiated from any cause of an acute abdomen. Special investigations offer little help as an abdominal X-ray may merely show dilated bowel; there is frequently a pronounced leucocytosis.

Treatment

This is surgical and by the time laparotomy is performed irreversible gangrene is often present so that resection is necessary for cure but this may not be feasible in a frail elderly patient. If gangrene has not supervened various vascular surgical procedures may be used such as embolectomy, thrombo-endarterectomy or a by-pass graft which may re-establish the blood supply to the bowel. It must be pointed out that these can only rarely be performed.

Prognosis

This is bad. Probably only 5–10 per cent. of patients recover from such an episode of arterial occlusion. If patients do have extensive bowel resection they may present a problem in management of their malabsorptive state.

REFERENCES

Jackson, B. R. (1963) *Occlusion of the Superior Mesenteric Artery*, Springfield, Ill.

Laufman, H., Nora, P. F., Mittelpunkt, A. I. (1964) Mesenteric blood vessels: advances in surgery and physiology, *Arch. Surg.*, **88,** 1021.

APPENDICITIS

Definition

An acute inflammation of the vermiform appendix.

Aetiology and Pathology

Appendicitis occurs at any age but 70 per cent. of patients are between the age of 10 and 40 years. Dietary or environmental factors have been invoked because the condition is very common in Western countries, is rare in rural Africa, but more common in urban Africa, while there is no difference in the incidence in the White and Negro population of the United States. There is some suggestion that the incidence is now gradually declining. There is often some obstruction to the appendix either by a faecolith or the presence of a band or kink, while a variety of exotic foreign bodies have been found occluding the lumen. Transmural inflammation of the appendix wall is due to a variety of enteric and other organisms which may arrive possibly by the blood stream or from the bowel lumen. Once inflammation starts the oedema further produces occlusion and eventually the blood supply to the appendix, which is by an end artery, is compromised. Gangrene may then occur with perforation and either local abscess formation or diffuse peritonitis.

Clinical Features

Typically the patient presents with abdominal pain which is usually central and cramping. There is associated nausea, anorexia and even vomiting due to the obstructive phase of the disease. This is followed a few hours later by pain in the right iliac fossa when the peritoneal coat becomes inflamed. Very early in the disease signs may be minimal apart from some tenderness in the right iliac fossa. Later on the tongue may be furred, there may be tachycardia, a slight temperature, tenderness or rebound tenderness in the iliac fossa and much later signs of general peritonitis or a local mass due to abscess formation. Although this is said to be the typical clinical picture variants are extremely common. These are due on the one hand to the variation in site of the normal appendix and on the other to the fact that atypical features are common both in children and in older patients. For example, the commonly occurring retrocaecal appendix may have minimal tenderness in the right iliac fossa and pain referred to the back. If the appendix is in the pelvis this may irritate the bowel, cause diarrhoea and mimic salpingitis or some other gynaecological disorder. If touching the ureter it may give rise to symptoms suggestive of pyelitis. Occasionally a high temperature occurs early on in the disease and the condition may be misdiagnosed as a right lower lobe pneumonia.

Appendicitis in children may be difficult to diagnose and in a group of 100 children admitted to hospital with a provisional diagnosis of acute appendicitis, fewer than 40 in fact had an acutely inflamed appendix removed. This is partly due to children's difficulty in localizing pain. The pain is often aggravated by movement and the child's appetite nearly always vanishes, while vomiting occurs in four out of five. Diarrhoea is especially common in younger children but becomes less important with age and, of course, gives rise to the problem of misdiagnosis of gastro-enteritis in this age group; some children complain of headache. An unfailing physical sign is localized tenderness and often guarding.

Appendicitis in the aged may be difficult to diagnose due to a very poor history as well as the atypical clinical features. Initially it can start like simple intestinal obstruction with vomiting, cramp-like abdominal pains but no change in pulse rate. Eventually signs of toxaemia may appear together with those of peritoneal involvement. In one series the average delay in calling medical aid was 60 hours for patients over the age of 45 years but 13 hours for those below this age.

Diagnosis

Appendicitis is the commonest acute abdominal emergency and must be included in all differential diagnoses of episodes of acute abdominal pain, and on occasion it is impossible to make a precise diagnosis so that a laparotomy has to be resorted to. When the disease is advanced a leucocytosis is often present but a normal leucocyte count does not exclude the diagnosis which is made essentially on clinical grounds. Radiological and laboratory techniques have little to offer except to exclude such diseases as pneumonia or a urinary tract infection. Appendicitis may mimic all other causes of the acute abdomen.

Treatment

This is essentially surgical. If there is any doubt it is wise to operate early rather than risk the danger of perforation and peritonitis. Exceptionally conservative treatment may be indicated if, for example, at sea. Conservative treatment is also advised once a mass has formed; this is allowed to resolve and later on appendicectomy performed.

Course and Prognosis

The mortality rate depends on how soon after the onset of the disease operation is performed and also on the age of the patient but, as previously stated, these two are partly interrelated. Thus in one series the mortality rate of patients under 45 years of age was 0·2 per cent. and that over 45 years of age was 9·9 per cent. The incidence of gangrene and ruptured appendices was twice as great in the older age group. Generalized peritonitis was the usual cause of death, although, of course, older patients have many other degenerative conditions which reduce their chance of survival of such a severe complication. Once the acute episode resolves complications are rare. Occasionally adhesions with intestinal obstruction may occur. Chronic appendicitis is now not considered to be an entity but recurrent acute attacks of appendicitis may be a cause of recurrent bouts of abdominal pain and disability.

REFERENCE

MAINGOT, R. (1969) Acute appendicitis, in *Abdominal Operations*, 5th ed., ed. Maingot, R., p. 111, New York.

MECKEL'S DIVERTICULUM

This occurs in between 1 and 3 per cent. of the population although it rarely gives rise to symptoms. It is a diverticulum arising as a vestige of the vitelline duct on the antimesenteric border of the ileum. It may be the site of heterotopic gastric mucosa or pancreatic tissue. The associated anomaly may cause symptoms due to peptic ulceration such as haemorrhage or central abdominal pain. On the other hand the diverticulum may become infected or be the site of a volvulus or of an intussusception.

REFERENCE

RUTHERFORD, R. B., and AKERS, D. R. (1966) Meckel's diverticulum: a review of 148 paediatric patients with special reference to the pattern of bleeding and to meso-diverticular vascular bands, *Surgery*, **59**, 618.

DUODENAL DIVERTICULA

These typically occur in the second part of the duodenum just against the bile-duct. They are present in 2–4 per cent. of all barium meal examinations. They are nearly always asymptomatic and one should resist the temptation of ascribing various symptoms to their presence. However, occasionally true diverticulitis may occur and pancreatitis and obstructive jaundice have been described. In one series the incidence of diarrhoea was higher than the general population and occasionally they may cause a stagnant loop syndrome, when antibiotics may help symptomatically. Surgical treatment is rarely indicated and when the diverticula arise near the bile-duct is hazardous, there being a risk of postoperative pancreatitis for the diverticulum is embedded behind the head of the pancreas.

REFERENCE

NEIL, S. A., and THOMPSON, N. W. (1965) The complications of duodenal diverticula and their management, *Surg. Gynec. Obstet.*, **120**, 1251.

JEJUNAL DIVERTICULOSIS

The over-all incidence of this condition is unknown but is probably in the order of 0·5 per cent. of the population over the age of 40 years. The diverticula are usually associated with duodenal diverticula and are situated on the mesenteric border of the proximal jejunum. They represent pouches of mucosa through the jejunal wall at the entry of the nutrient artery. On occasions they are associated with hypertrophy of the jejunal muscle. They give rise to trouble either by becoming inflamed, by causing bouts of intestinal colic or by allowing a stagnant loop syndrome to develop. Inflammation may be associated with inspissated diverticular contents and give rise to bouts of abdominal pain with signs of peritoneal irritation and temperature; perforation or haemorrhage from the mouth of a diverticulum may also occur. Bouts of cramping abdominal pain with borborygmi and vomiting may be severe and are most likely to occur in patients who have jejunal muscle hypertrophy. Manifestations of the stagnant loop syndrome are discussed elsewhere. Many patients are asymptomatic and jejunal diverticula when found must not be assumed to explain atypical abdominal symptoms.

The treatment of recurrent inflammation or bouts of severe colic is surgical resection. The stagnant loop syndrome is usually treated by appropriate dietary supplements and antibiotics.

REFERENCE

COOKE, W. T., COX, E. V., FONE, D. J., MEYNELL, M. J., and CRADDIE, R. (1963) The clinical and metabolic significance of jejunal diverticula, *Gut*, **4**, 115.

TUMOURS OF THE SMALL BOWEL

These are relatively uncommon but examples of most benign and malignant mesenchymal and epithelial tumours have been described. Symptoms may be due to small bowel obstruction, to ulceration which may give rise to either pain or haemorrhage and also to bouts of intussusception. Occasionally in malignant tumours secondary deposits may be the herald. There is a greater incidence of adenocarcinomas of the small bowel in patients with coeliac disease.

THE PEUTZ-JEGHER SYNDROME

In this condition there is intestinal polyposis most frequently affecting the jejunum but occasionally affecting the stomach and large bowel. The polyps may be scanty or numerous. It is associated with spots of melanin pigmentation around the lips and on the buccal mucosa and occasionally this may occur around the eyes, ears, nostrils, fingers and toes. This pigmentation may also be sparse or profuse. The polyps are more in the nature of hamartomas and carcinomatous degeneration is rare [see p. 674].

REFERENCE

DORMANDY, T. L. (1958) Peutz-Jegher syndrome, in *Modern Trends in Gastroenterology*, 2nd Series, ed. Jones, F. A., London.

CARCINOID TUMOURS

Aetiology and Pathology

These are relatively uncommon and account for less than 1 per cent. of tumours of the gastro-intestinal tract. They usually arise from argentaffin cells which occur in the crypts of the gastro-intestinal glands and are most frequent in the ileocaecal region. The finding of an incidental carcinoid tumour of the appendix is not uncommon but how frequently these tumours, which are potentially of low grade malignancy, would in fact spread and grow large enough to cause the carcinoid syndrome is unknown. The metabolic effects of compounds produced by the tumour are usually apparent when there are large secondary deposits in the liver so that the metabolic products can be secreted directly into the systemic circulation and are not inactivated by liver tissue. Circulating tryptophan is converted in the tumour to 5-hydroxytryptamine (serotonin) and this is deaminated by amine oxidase to 5-hydroxyindoleacetic acid (5HIAA) which is then excreted in the urine. Atypical tumours which arise from argentaffin cells of the foregut (stomach and bronchus) tend to lack 5-hydroxytryptophan decarboxylase and so excrete 5-hydroxytryptophan in the urine.

In patients with the established disease the endocardium of the right side of the heart as well as the pulmonary valve may become thickened and stenosed. There is subsequently right-sided heart failure with tricuspid incompetence. This thickening is probably due to a humoral agent and it has occasionally been seen on the left side of the heart when there has been a right to left shunt. The cause of the flush and other features of the syndrome is unknown. Serotonin itself does not cause the flush but may be the cause of diarrhoea. A flush may be induced by adrenaline or noradrenaline infusions but the substance so liberated has not been identified although a kinin is a possible candidate.

Clinical Picture

Local symptoms of pain and distension due to chronic small bowel obstruction are rare and the patient usually presents with the systemic effects of the disease. These are diarrhoea with the passage of loose, watery stools and colicky abdominal pain together with attacks of flushing. These may be brought on by alcohol, food or emotion. The flush particularly affects the face, is of a purple violaceous colour and during the attack the patient may complain of wheezing dyspnoea. Eventually the dilatation of the facial capillaries is continuous and the patient is left with a permanent flush and telangiectasia of the face. When the heart is affected there is progressive dyspnoea and signs of right heart failure due to pulmonary stenosis and tricuspid incompetence. Abdominal examination nearly always shows a very large liver. Pellagra has been described due to utilization of a large amount of circulating tryptophan by the tumour so producing a niacin deficiency, especially when there has been a low intake of protein. The whole disease runs a very chronic course and eventually intractable heart failure and cachexia ensues.

Diagnosis

The condition is suspected in any patient with intractable diarrhoea especially if there have been attacks of flushing and if hepatomegaly has been found. The diagnosis is confirmed by estimating the urinary 5-

HIAA but it should be remembered that dietary intake of bananas may give a falsely high value.

Treatment

The possibility of surgery should always be considered and the sites of the secondary deposits in both lobes of the liver delineated by arteriography. Involvement of both lobes of the liver does not necessarily preclude surgery in that the tumour is very slow growing so that even incomplete excision leaving small deposits behind may control symptoms for a considerable time. Recently hepatic artery ligation and portal perfusion by cytotoxic drugs have been advocated. If surgical treatment is impossible the diarrhoea may be controlled by methysergide, 4 mg. four times daily, but to date treatment of the flush has been disappointing. Parachlorophenylalanine has also been used with some success. Once heart failure ensues symptomatic treatment with sodium restriction, diuretics and digitalis may be tried.

REFERENCES

GRAHAME-SMITH, D. G. (1970) The carcinoid syndrome, *Gut*, **11,** 189.

SHAMI, M., and SHEBA, CH. (1970) Parachlorophenylalanine treatment in carcinoid syndrome, *Brit. med. J.*, **4,** 784.

STAPHYLOCOCCAL ENTEROCOLITIS

This usually follows a gastric operation and is associated with massive secretion of fluid and electrolytes into the small bowel so that the patient may present with shock and dehydration before diarrhoea actually occurs. In this condition staphylococci invade the intestinal mucosa and are seen in the stools. Massive fluid and electrolyte repletion (up to 20 litres a day) is needed and also an appropriate oral antibiotic must be given. Although the condition has a high mortality recovery may occur with aggressive fluid replacement and antibiotic treatment.

PSEUDOMEMBRANOUS ENTEROCOLITIS

This severe inflammatory disease of the colon was at one time confused with staphylococcal enterocolitis. The inflammatory reaction is usually confined to the colon which is covered by a pseudomembrane reminiscent of diphtheria. The condition tends to occur in old arteriopathic or debilitated patients and may be precipitated by an operation or colonic manoeuvre, such as manual evacuation of the rectum or a barium enema. The patient has often had broad-spectrum antibiotics but the condition was described in the pre-antibiotic era. It may run an acute or relatively chronic course with intractable diarrhoea, often with fever and abdominal distension due to colonic dilatation; there may also be rebound abdominal tenderness. There is subsequent dehydration and protein depletion due to loss of protein in the stool. It is usually diagnosed circumstantially or at autopsy but may be confirmed by rectal biopsy. Treatment is to give adequate parenteral fluid and nutritional supplements, but the mortality is very high.

EOSINOPHILIC INFILTRATION OF THE GASTRO-INTESTINAL TRACT

This rare condition presents with symptoms and signs due to two main types of eosinophilic lesion. A polypoid lesion which usually affects the pyloric antrum and an infiltrative lesion which either affects the stomach or small bowel. In both types there is infiltration of the gut wall with sheets of eosinophils particularly in the perivascular region. Lymph nodes may be affected and if obstruction to the bowel has occurred there is muscle hypertrophy. There is usually an eosinophilia in the peripheral blood and there may be symptoms of asthma or infiltration of the pleura or pericardium. This is presumably an allergic disorder. One allergen is the larva of the herring parasite (*Eustoma rotundatum*) but others may well be involved. If symptoms are severe treatment with corticosteroids is indicated.

REFERENCE

SALMAN, P. R., and PAULLEY, J. W. (1967) Eosinophilic granuloma of the gastrointestinal tract, *Gut*, **8,** 8.

PNEUMATOSIS CYSTOIDES

This is a rare condition in which there are numerous endothelial-lined cysts in the mesentery, usually of the jejunum and ileum and far more rarely in the colon. The gas in the cyst is nitrogen. This is most frequently associated with chronic chest conditions, especially asthma, and it is thought that alveoli rupture and air tracks down the mediastinum into the mesentery. Occasionally the condition is associated with lesions of the bowel, especially with pyloric stenosis. It clinically presents as abdominal pain, diarrhoea and occasionally blood and mucus in the stool; steatorrhoea has been reported. Occasionally a pneumoperitoneaum occurs. The diagnosis is made by radiology when a plain X-ray may show numerous air-filled cysts in the abdomen and barium studies show indentation of these cysts into the lumen of the affected part of the bowel. Treatment is usually expectant, but occasionally resection of an obstructed segment of bowel has to be undertaken.

REFERENCE

HUGHES, D. T. D., GORDON, K. C. D., SWANN, J. C., and BOLT, G. L. (1966) Pneumatosis cystoides intestinalis, *Gut*, **7,** 553.

ENDOMETRIOSIS

Displaced endometrial tissue may be implanted in the rectum or colon and cause symptoms by inducing adhesions in the peritoneal cavity. This is relatively uncommon. Symptoms tend to occur before or at the menstrual period and these are mainly abdominal distension, nausea, cramping abdominal pains or rectal pain. The rectal mucosa is rarely involved so that rectal bleeding is uncommon. Eventually partial or complete intestinal obstruction may persist between menstrual periods. The diagnosis may be suggested by the relation of symptoms to the period, the fact that nodules may occasionally be felt on pelvic examination together with other evidence of endometriosis. A barium enema may show partial obstruction but this is not pathognomonic. The diagnosis is often made at laparotomy and even then may only be obvious on histological examination. If possible medical treatment with hormones should be undertaken, but occasionally the adhesions have to be divided. They tend to recur.

REFERENCE

MACAFEE, C. H. G., and GREER, H. L. H. (1960) Intestinal endometriosis, *J. Obstet. Gynaec. Brit. Emp.*, **67**, 539.

ISCHAEMIA OF THE GASTRO-INTESTINAL TRACT

INTESTINAL ANGINA

The gut is supplied by three main vessels, the coeliac axis, the superior mesenteric artery and the inferior mesenteric artery, between which are adequate collateral vessels so that after gradual occlusion of one major artery the blood supply to the gut is usually adequate. Indeed, it is usually conceded that before persistent symptoms due to disease of the large vessels of the bowel occur two of the three major arteries have to be occluded.

In intestinal angina there is typically abdominal pain which occurs 15–30 minutes after food. This leads to fear of eating and subsequent weight loss. In some patients there is diarrhoea but rarely is the small gut supply so compromised as to produce a generalized malabsorption syndrome. The condition may be suspected on hearing an abdominal bruit and often there are other signs of atherosclerosis. Most patients are past middle age. The diagnosis is proven by angiography. It is nearly always caused by atheroma. The criteria of the diagnosis have to be strict for abdominal bruits are heard frequently in elderly patients, while occlusion of one or more vessels and narrowing of the mouths of others are not infrequent. Furthermore, these physical and arteriographic findings may be present in the absence of any symptoms. The treatment is surgical, when various by-pass procedures may be used. Unfortunately, the generalized atheroma is often so severe as to preclude such an operation. This disorder may be a prelude to acute infarction of the bowel.

THE COELIAC COMPRESSION SYNDROME

It has recently been suggested that diffuse vague abdominal pain after food may be due to compression of the coeliac axis by a slip of diaphragm or the coeliac ganglion. The patients are often young women. The important physical sign is an epigastric bruit which changes with respiration and on aortography the lateral films show an anterior indentation of the coeliac axis. Although brilliant results have been claimed by surgical relief of this condition, it is difficult to understand the mechanism of the production of pain as only one vessel is intermittently obstructed and recent reports have tempered initial enthusiasm. This anomaly is common; whether it causes pain is still debatable.

TRANSIENT ISCHAEMIC COLITIS

In this form of segmental colitis which usually occurs in older people there is a sudden onset of cramping abdominal pain with tenesmus and the passage of blood and loose stools. The patient is often febrile, there is tenderness in the left iliac fossa and the symptoms usually settle in a few days. The rectum is not involved in the process and sigmoidoscopy is usually normal except that blood may be seen coming from above. The barium enema shows a segment of bowel, usually the splenic flexure and descending colon, to be abnormal often with so-called thumb-printing indentation. In mild cases the symptoms and signs resolve completely, in others stricture formation supervenes. A vascular cause for this syndrome is assumed especially as the splenic flexure is the place of the poorest vascular supply and probably represents a mild example of the process which leads to gangrene of the colon. The condition has often been confused with ulcerative colitis or Crohn's disease and many patients have been inadvertently treated with steroids in the past. In the early stage of the disease a carcinoma of the colon and diverticulitis have also to be excluded. Furthermore, if the patient is only seen after the acute episode a residual short stricture may be mistaken for a carcinoma.

VASCULITIS

Periarteritis nodosa may affect the abdominal viscera and patients present with either recurrent abdominal pain or even an acute abdomen. Furthermore, variants of polyarteritis nodosa or disseminated lupus may have a more chronic history of abdominal complaints which may mimic ulcerative colitis and Crohn's disease, the correct diagnosis only being apparent when other systems are involved.

ISCHAEMIC STRICTURES OF THE SMALL BOWEL

These most frequently occur after repositioning partially strangulated bowel in the abdomen. Non-specific ulcers of the small gut which may perforate, bleed and heal with stricture formation most probably arise from focal ischaemia. The so-called potassium ulcer and stricture is indistinguishable and probably is due to local high concentrations of potassium inducing local venospasm.

REFERENCES

BOLEY, S. J., SCHULTZ, L., KRIEGER, H., SCHWARTZ, S., ELGUEZABAL, A., and ALLEN, A. C. (1965) Experimental evaluation of thiazides and potassium as a cause of small-bowel ulcer, *J. Amer. med. Ass.*, **192**, 763.

EDWARDS, A. J., HAMILTON, J. D., NICHOL, W. D., TAYLOR, G. W., and DAWSON, A. M. (1970) Experience with coeliac axis compression syndrome, *Brit. med. J.*, **1**, 342.

MARSDEN, A., PHEILS, M. T., LEA THOMAS, M., and MORSON, B. C. (1966) Ischaemic colitis, *Gut*, **7**, 1.

Rob, C. (1969) Vascular diseases of the intestine, in *Modern Trends in Gastroenterology*, 4th ed., ed. Card, W. I., and Creamer, B., p. 252, London.

THE IRRITABLE COLON

Synonyms. Spastic colon; Mucous membranous colitis; Unhappy colon.

Definition

A disturbance of colon function in the absence of organic disease which consists of colon pain, disordered bowel habit and occasionally the passage of mucus rectally.

Aetiology and Pathology

It is an extremely common condition and probably accounts for nearly half of all patients who complain of gastro-intestinal symptoms. The aetiology is unknown but approximately half of the patients' symptoms follow on an attack of dysentery or food poisoning and so this condition accounts for many people with so-called chronic dysentery who return from abroad. Over 80 per cent. have obvious stress and attacks are precipitated when this increases, while there is objective evidence of irritability of the bowel for pressure recordings from the sigmoid colon show far greater rises of pressure after injections of neostigmine than in the control population.

Clinical Features

The patient complains of pain over any part of the colon so that although it is typically in the left iliac fossa it may also occur in the epigastrium, hypochondrium or on the sides of the abdomen. Occasionally there is hypogastric griping pain. Usually the pain is eased by bowel action or passing flatus; it may be aggravated by food, presumably due to an exaggerated gastrocolic reflex. Occasionally special foods are incriminated but this is rare. Bowel habits are those of alternating constipation, during which time the pain is aggravated, to be relieved by an attack of diarrhoea when occasionally an excess of mucus is passed, when the condition has been called 'mucous colitis'. The stool may either be pellety or thin and there may be an urgent desire to defaecate and occasionally a feeling that the bowels are not emptied. About 20 per cent. of the patients present with painless diarrhoea. There are frequently obvious psychiatric symptoms of anxiety and depression.

Diagnosis

Physical examination shows no abnormal physical signs apart from tenderness over the sigmoid colon. On sigmoidoscopy, although the rectal mucosa may have lost its vascular pattern and there may be an excess of mucus, there is no increased friability such as occurs in ulcerative colitis. On the other hand positive evidence that the pain is of colonic origin may be afforded by reproduction of the pain during sigmoidoscopy. Organic diseases such as carcinoma of the colon or diverticulitis have to be excluded by a barium enema, haemoglobin and E.S.R. and one of the most difficult diagnostic problems is the development of carcinoma in a person a life-long martyr to an irritable bowel. Occasionally a barium meal and follow through is called for to exclude Crohn's disease, while even a duodenal ulcer may mainly have colonic type pain. Despite its frequency the condition is often confused with all other conditions known to cause abdominal pain.

Treatment

The patient must be reassured that this is not a true colitis, does not give rise to complications and will not need surgery. The mechanism of the production of the pain and its relation to stress have to be explained. Any psychiatric disturbance is treated on its merit and pain itself may be helped by using mebeverine, 100–200 mg. four times daily, and for more severe spasms of pain propantheline, 15–30 mg. Occasionally the stool is made more regular by the use of *Isogel* in increasing doses up to 4 teaspoonfuls three times daily. Codeine phosphate, 30 mg. twice daily, may be used if painless diarrhoea is present.

Course and Prognosis

In one series 30 per cent. went into complete remission, 60 per cent. had mild symptoms which they came to accept, but 10 per cent. had intractable symptoms causing considerable invalidism.

REFERENCE

Truelove, S. C. (1965) The irritable colon syndrome, in *Recent Advances in Gastroenterology*, ed. Badenoch, J., and Brooke, B. N., p. 268, London.

CROHN'S DISEASE

Synonym. Regional ileitis.

Definition

A chronic, non-specific transmural inflammatory disease of the bowel typically affecting the terminal ileum and caecum but capable of attacking any part of the alimentary tract from mouth to anus.

Aetiology

The aetiology is unknown. No infective agent has been isolated. There is a slight familial tendency and also a greater proportion of patients among Jews. There is little evidence for the presence of disturbed delayed hypersensitivity as the incidence of positive skin tests to tuberculin and *Candida* do not differ from controls; but over 50 per cent. of patients have a positive Kveim test which at one time was said to be specific to sarcoidosis. As with any unexplained disease there is a tendency to seek for psychosomatic factors but it is doubtful if these are of great aetiological importance and the case is certainly not as good as in ulcerative colitis.

Pathology

The inflammatory reaction seems to start in the submucosa and is in essence transmural so that when it affects the colon it is usually quite distinct from ulcerative colitis. Ulceration may be superficial or go deep into the mucosa and may give rise to intramural abscess formation. In approximately 70 per cent. of cases there are epithelioid granulomata. Stenosis of the bowel typically occurs but is not related to ulceration. There is a tendency for fistulas to form between loops of bowel or between bowel and other organs such as the bladder or vagina while following operation they often connect with the abdominal wall. Lymph nodes are often enlarged, inflamed and contain granulomas.

Clinical Picture

The clinical picture is protean and the precise features will depend on the site, extent and activity of the lesion. Typically the history is of chronic abdominal symptoms with pain, diarrhoea, ill health, weight loss and often fever. A significant proportion of patients, for example a quarter in one series, presented with a clinical picture indistinguishable from acute appendicitis or an appendix abscess. These patients may be differentiated from those with acute ileitis in that the symptoms have lasted for one week or more. Pain may be that of hypogastric spasms occurring with bowel action or may follow meals and occasionally when there is intestinal obstruction small bowel colic will occur. On other occasions the pain may be ill defined or constantly present in the right iliac fossa, especially when abscesses or fistulas have formed, when there will be local tenderness. Diarrhoea of varying severity is frequent, affecting 70 or 80 per cent. of patients. Although the stool is usually unformed and watery there may be on occasions overt steatorrhoea or streaking with blood; only rarely does brisk gastro-intestinal haemorrhage occur. Anal lesions in the form of fistulas or fissures or both, are typically indolent, purplish and irregular with undermined edges, often being surprisingly painless and were diagnosed in the past as tuberculous. The disease may present as an anal lesion when abdominal symptoms may be mild or non-existent. Fever is frequently present and indeed the patient may present the problem of pyrexia of unknown origin; this may be either due to the disease itself or a secondary infected abscess. There may also be gynaecological complications, such as tubo-ovarian abscess, abscess of Bartholin's glands, dyspareunia and, of course, amenorrhoea. As with ulcerative colitis, various associated phenomena may be present. These are sacro-iliac sclerosis, flitting polyarthritis with a negative Rose-Waaler test, occasionally iritis and vasculitis of the erythema nodosum type.

Various nutritional disturbances may occur. These are often due to an impaired intake from depressed appetite associated with ill health or being afraid to eat because of pain after food. In addition malabsorption may occasionally be important. This can be due either to involvement of the bowel by the inflammatory process, resection of the bowel, or the complication of a stagnant loop syndrome due either to the presence of strictures in the small bowel or fistulas from large to small bowel so allowing bacterial overgrowth in its lumen. Finally, loss of nutrients from the inflamed bowel is also an important factor. The commonest nutritional disturbances are weight loss, anaemia and hypoproteinaemia. The weight loss is nearly always due to impaired appetite. The anaemia is extremely common and due to a combination of toxic depression of the marrow, iron deficiency secondary to blood loss from the bowel, and folate deficiency which seems to be associated with the inflammatory disease itself rather than malabsorption since it occurs just as commonly when the large bowel only is involved. This is aggravated by patients who are taking a low-roughage diet which is also low in folate. Mild B_{12} deficiency quite frequently occurs and is occasionally severe. Although this most commonly follows resection, it may also be due to inflammation of the ileum and very rarely to the stagnant loop syndrome. Hypoproteinaemia may be due to loss of protein from the bowel and in fact the patient may present with ankle oedema and minimal gastro-intestinal symptoms. The situation may be aggravated by inadequate intake due either to a poor diet or impaired absorption; in this case true generalized protein depletion will take place. Depletion of water and electrolytes may occur when there is gross diarrhoea. Steatorrhoea may be seen in these patients. The mechanism is partly due to bile salt deficiency as bile salts are normally reabsorbed by the terminal ileum. There may also be the additional factor of the stagnant loop syndrome and in the rare case where the jejunum is involved actual inflammation of the absorptive site. Occasionally Crohn's disease is complicated by amyloid disease but, unlike ulcerative colitis, carcinoma is an extremely rare complication. It is probable that both biliary and renal calculi occur more frequently.

Diagnosis

The small bowel disease is often diagnosed as an appendix abscess or recurrent appendicitis and the differentiation from hyperplastic tuberculosis is at times impossible. This condition, though rare in England, must be suspected in the immigrant population and is not excluded by a negative chest X-ray. Occasionally it is difficult to distinguish lymphosarcoma of the gut and it cannot always be assumed that all inert strictures of the small bowel are the end result of Crohn's disease. These may be caused by healing of non-specific ulcers or ischaemic lesions. The presence of fever, arthralgia and even erythema nodosum may dominate the picture so that the diagnosis of a collagen disease may be considered before that of a primary bowel disorder. Furthermore, Whipple's disease, characterized by fever, joint pains, wasting and diarrhoea, can initially be suspected. In spite of these organic conditions the biggest differential diagnostic problem is presented by the irritable bowel syndrome. It is not infrequent for emotional young women with diarrhoea to have normal results of investigations and to be said to have nervous diarrhoea. In retrospect it is often found that the terminal ileum has not been adequately demonstrated by the barium examination. It cannot be emphasized too much that the haemoglobin and sedimentation rate may be normal initially. Thus one of the sheet-anchors of diagnosis is the barium follow through examination. This is often technically not well performed and the irritable terminal ileum is often difficult to fill. Typical changes are narrowing of the lumen, a cobblestone-type appearance, fissuring due to deep ulcers and stricture and even fistula formation [PLATE 6]. The differentiation of Crohn's disease of the large bowel from ulcerative colitis depends on the relative sparing of the rectum, deeper ulceration of the colon, asymmetrical and discontinuous lesions and the greater tendency for stricture formation [PLATE 6]. Sigmoidoscopy and rectal biopsy findings may be diagnostic and patients with colonic Crohn's disease are more likely to have perianal lesions. Occasionally the differentiation is extremely difficult.

Treatment

There is little accurate information as to results of treatment in this condition. This is only undertaken when symptoms are present. Initially one of the main symptoms is that of diarrhoea which is often helped by codeine phosphate, 15–30 mg. up to four times daily, or dephenoxylate hydrochloride (*Lomotil*), 2·5–5 mg. up to four times daily, while *Isogel* or *Celevac*, 15–30 ml. up to four times daily, may also help to make the stool firm. If the diarrhoea is caused by steatorrhoea a low-fat diet (less than 50 g. daily) is indicated as this will cut down the fat loss and thus excessive loss of magnesium, calcium and nitrogen in the stool. Otherwise the diet should have a high nutritional value. The various dietary restrictions, including a low-roughage diet, have little to recommend them and, indeed, may aggravate the nutritional disturbance. Occasionally a low-milk diet may help to control diarrhoea because some patients with hypolactasia may tend to develop symptoms when the bowel is affected by some other disease.

Anaemia is often treated with oral iron and folic acid, 5 mg. twice daily, but usually does not respond until the inflammatory disease is brought under control. If on the other hand vitamin B_{12} deficiency is due to ileal resection or a stagnant loop treatment with the vitamin will produce a good haemopoietic response. Electrolyte depletion may be prevented by appropriate supplements. If the patient is toxic, rest in bed is indicated and treatment with corticosteroids prescribed. ACTH, 80 Units, or *Synacthen*, 2 mg. daily, is used initially. Once the patient has responded the treatment is changed to oral prednisone, 15 mg. three times daily. Often such patients will need long-term treatment with prednisone on a maintenance dose of approximately 5 mg. twice or three times daily. This is justified in this condition for, unlike ulcerative colitis, there is no curative surgical alternative. In addition antibiotics may be used if there is associated sepsis. Sulphasalazine is sometimes used but there is no evidence that this is effective. The use of immunosuppressive drugs, such as azathioprine, 2 mg. per kg. body weight, although promising is still in the experimental stage. Surgical treatment is obligatory when there are signs of intestinal obstruction or massive haemorrhage but is also indicated when there is an abscess or fistula formation or when the symptoms are otherwise disabling, especially when due to intractable pain. Treatment is usually that of excision of the affected part but occasionally the diseased bowel has to be by-passed.

Course and Prognosis

This chronic disease is characterized by relapses and remissions. No one can ever claim a cure for the inflammatory process never resolves completely. The fact that 5 years after surgical treatment between 20 and 68 per cent. of patients had recurrence of symptoms in different series, illustrates why one should be hesitant about suggesting surgery. It is impossible to be sure that all the microscopically affected tissue has been removed for even normal looking bowel may be affected. This fact is underlined by abnormal rectal biopsies being found in patients whose disease is apparently localized to the ileocaecal region.

REFERENCE

LENNARD-JONES, J. E. (1969) Crohn's disease, in *Modern Trends in Gastroenterology*, 4th series, ed. Card, W. I., and Creamer, B., p. 273, London

ACUTE TERMINAL ILEITIS

This probably is distinct from chronic regional ileitis. By definition, symptoms are present for less than a week before the operation and clinically the condition simulates appendicitis except that diarrhoea is more frequent and at operation an acutely inflamed ileum is found. Histologically the resected ileum occasionally shows giant cells but more usually there is an eosinophilic infiltration. It has recently been suggested that this is due to a specific infective agent (*Yersinia enterocolitica*). The importance in making the distinction from Crohn's disease is that this condition remits and does not tend to progress to chronic regional enteritis.

REFERENCE

WINBLAD, S., NILEHN, B., and STERNBY, N. H. (1966) *Yersinia enterocolitica* (*Pasteurella X*) in human enteric infections, *Brit. med. J.*, **2**, 1363.

ACUTE JEJUNO-ILEITIS

In a small group of patients who have diffuse involvement of the jejunum and ileum the condition seems to run a particularly malignant course. It has been suggested that such patients differ fundamentally from those with typical Crohn's disease and may in fact be suffering from a variant of polyarteritis nodosa.

ULCERATIVE COLITIS

Definition

A chronic non-specific inflammatory disease of the large bowel which is usually confined to the mucosa. It starts in the rectum and spreads by continuity towards the caecum. Clinically all grades of severity exist between mild rectal bleeding and a severe toxic syndrome similar to fulminating dysentery. Typically it is punctuated by relapses and remissions. There is no specific treatment.

Aetiology

This is unknown. No infective agent has been consistently isolated and allergy to food-stuffs is probably unimportant except possibly occasionally to milk. Psychological factors are frequently stressed but although they may aggravate the existing condition they cannot be invoked as a necessary cause. More recently auto-immune mechanisms have been suggested but claims that a serum factor cytopathic to colonic epithelium is of aetiological importance need to be kept in perspective. There is a familial tendency to the condition and a slightly increased incidence in Jews (1·5:1) compared with a comparable non-Jewish population. It is virtually unknown in the African and American Negro. It is not an uncommon disease and a recent survey in Oxford showed that 79·9 per 100,000 of the population were attacked, with a suggestion that the infrequency is increasing.

Pathology

The inflammatory process is confined to the mucosa with infiltration of lymphocytes, eosinophils and plasma cells. There are often abscesses round the crypts which probably result from secondary infection but these are not diagnostic of the condition. In the severe acute form transmural inflammation may occur when the mucosa is shed, laying bare the muscularis mucosae; this may be a prelude to perforation. In some patients with total colonic involvement 'backwash' ileitis may occur. This ileitis must be distinguished from Crohn's disease since after the excision of the colon it tends to resolve.

Clinical Picture

The severity of the attack depends to some extent on the amount of colon involved. It varies from a person with only partial rectal involvement (granular proctitis) who is otherwise well, apart from passing blood and mucus rectally with a constipated stool, to the patient with fulminating disease. In fulminant colitis there is extensive and often total colonic involvement, the patient looks ill, is febrile, has a tachycardia and passes frequent, e.g. up to twenty liquid, foul smelling stools admixed with blood and mucus per day. There may be abdominal pain and the abdomen may become distended and exhibit rebound tenderness, especially when toxic dilatation of the colon occurs. Anaemia may be a dominant feature due partly to blood loss into the colon; indeed, profuse rectal haemorrhage may occur and in the severely ill patient there is toxic depression of erythropoiesis such as occurs in any inflammatory disorder. Hypoproteinaemia which may cause oedema is largely due to loss of protein from the inflamed bowel into its lumen and may occasionally be aggravated by impaired intake. When the stool volume is great dehydration and electrolyte depletion may occur as in any diarrhoeal state. Weight loss, which may be profound in the untreated patient, is mainly caused by poor food intake due to anorexia or a fear of aggravating diarrhoea.

Local complications can be caused by local extension of the disease and include anorectal fistulas and strictures of the colon or rectum but these tend to be more frequent in Crohn's disease. Perforation of the bowel may occur and is often preceded by toxic dilatation of the colon when the usually mucosal inflammation becomes transmural. Polypoid lesions in the bowel are nearly always pseudopolyps of heaped up granulation tissue and are not thought to be premalignant. However, carcinoma of the colon which is often multifocal tends to occur with increased frequency especially in patients who have had total bowel involvement for 10 years; indeed, after 25 years of illness the cumulative incidence of this complication is over 40 per cent.

Systemic complications include a variety of skin manifestations such as erythema nodosum or, more rarely, pyoderma gangrenosum. The eyes may be affected by an episcleritis and there is a specific arthritis which affects large joints, there being no X-ray changes and a negative Rose-Waaler test. In addition the sacroiliac joints may become sclerosed but true ankylosing spondylitis is uncommon. There is an increased incidence of oral aphthous ulcers in these patients.

A high incidence of involvement of the liver is frequently manifest by a raised alkaline phosphatase and increased BSP retention, possibly due to pericholangitis. In addition there is an increased incidence (5–6 per cent.) of hepatic cirrhosis in which the liver function tests usually show a predominantly obstructive pattern, but some of the patients have the clinical features of chronic aggressive hepatitis. There is also a rare group of patients who have predominantly florid biliary obstruction in whom there is an increased incidence of sclerosing cholangitis and cholangiocarcinoma. Mild, non-specific fatty change and inflammatory cell infiltration also may occur in the severely ill patient.

Diagnosis

This is confirmed at sigmoidoscopy for over 95 per cent. of patients have rectal involvement, the crucial sign being increased friability of the rectal mucosa which bleeds when wiped with a swab. Discrete ulcers are rarely seen, while a mucosa which shows lack of vascular pattern and some increased mucus secretion may often occur in patients with any form of diarrhoea, including the irritable colon. The only two inflammatory disorders of the bowel with which ulcerative colitis may be confused are Crohn's disease of the rectum and amoebic colitis. Crohn's disease may be indistinguishable but may have associated discrete obvious ulcers, sometimes with relatively normal mucosa between or there may be a cobblestone appearance. Amoebic colitis is far less common in England; here typically the intervening mucosa between the ulceration is normal. The diagnosis may be confirmed by a rectal biopsy which is best taken with a suction-type instrument. Chronic inflammatory changes may be seen on the rectal biopsy but again the distinction between ulcerative colitis and Crohn's disease may be difficult. A barium enema is performed after sigmoidoscopy to define the extent of colonic involvement, and once the diagnosis is known may be performed without prior preparation as the affected bowel does not contain solid faeces (instant enema). Typically there is lack of haustration, an irregularity of the bowel outline said to look like torn blotting paper and indicating shallow ulceration, and enlargement of the post-rectal space due to perirectal oedema [PLATE 6]. The changes start in the rectum and are continuous and symmetrical. Occasionally pseudopolyps and rarely strictures may be seen. In the post-evacuation air-contrast picture abnormalities of the mucosal relief pattern are observed. It must be stressed that lack of haustration alone can occur in the irritable bowel syndrome, especially when associated with diarrhoea and is not diagnostic of ulcerative colitis.

Treatment

Medical treatment is aimed at trying to terminate the attack as quickly as possible, prevent a relapse and recognizing when surgery is indicated. A patient should never be allowed to become a bad surgical risk due to procrastination while under medical treatment.

In both the moderate and severe attack bed rest is helpful and if the attack is severe admission to hospital mandatory. Besides bed rest other general measures include an adequate intake of food to maintain adequate nutrition. The only dietary restriction is to prescribe a milk-free diet; this may help symptomatically if the patient has hypolactasia but may also actually help to induce a true remission. It should only be tried for 1–2 weeks. A low-roughage diet has no place in the treatment of this condition. In the patient with severe toxic dilatation all food may be stopped by mouth for 24 hours while medical treatment is being tried. If the haemoglobin falls below 9 g. per 100 ml. blood transfusions are given but oral iron should also be used should any anaemia be present. Potassium chloride in the form of *slow K*, 3 G. three times daily, is prescribed to prevent potassium depletion and if necessary parenteral fluids may be needed to prevent dehydration.

The diarrhoea may be symptomatically treated with varying success with *Isogel*, 15–30 ml. three times daily, and codeine phosphate, 15–60 mg. three times daily.

More specific treatment includes sulphasalazine in increasing doses up to 1 G. four times daily; this has been demonstrated both to improve the mild attack and to prevent relapses when the patient is in remission. Complications of sulphasalazine are indigestion with nausea or vomiting and occasionally Heinz-body haemolytic anaemia; this especially occurs if there is an inherent red cell abnormality, such as glucose-6-phosphate dehydrogenase deficiency. This drug does not act by its antibiotic properties; it is known to attach itself to elastic tissue and similar beneficial results are not obtained with other sulpha drugs. Other antibiotics are contra-indicated except if there is a specific septic condition; indeed, there is some suggestion that broad-spectrum antibiotics may aggravate the bowel condition.

Corticosteroids may be used locally or systemically. Local steroid treatment may be effected by using either prednisolone suppositories once or twice daily for patients with granular proctitis, or retention enemas containing 20 mg. prednisolone when more bowel is involved. The enemas are eventually self administered by the patient from disposable packs in the prone position and may reach the transverse colon if the bowel is inflamed. Retention of the enemas may be facilitated by giving propantheline bromide, 30 mg. half an hour beforehand. In the more severely affected patient, especially if systemic symptoms are present, systemic steroids are indicated. This is often best started using ACTH, 80 Units daily or *Synacthen*, 2 mg. daily, to produce a maximum adrenal response; once treatment takes effect this may be replaced by prednisone, 15 mg. three times daily. In contrast to sulphasalazine there is little evidence that long-term treatment with steroids is beneficial; it helps the acute attack but patients should be weaned completely off them where possible. If large doses of steroids are needed to maintain control of the symptoms surgery is preferable. The use of immunosuppressive drugs is to date experimental. It must be emphasized that during the medical treatment of ulcerative colitis the patient's general condition should always be maintained in such a state so that surgery may be safely undertaken at any time.

Surgical treatment is advised in the acute attack if there are signs of toxic dilatation of the colon with rebound abdominal tenderness which has not rapidly responded to treatment within 24–48 hours and in the severe attack which has not responded to treatment within 4–7 days. These are both immediately life-threatening situations. In addition it is indicated for chronic ill health when the illness dominates the patient's life, and also when there is a tight rectal stricture or perianal sepsis. Severe joint or skin manifestations may rarely be an important indication. Prophylactic surgery in patients who have total bowel involvement of more than 10 years' duration is being increasingly advised. The precise type of surgery, whether this is total proctocolectomy with permanent ileostomy or colectomy with ileorectal anastomosis, is still debatable but in some cases certainly the latter may be advised.

When ileostomy is undertaken it is of great help if the patient can discuss the problems involved with a patient of similar age and sex who has undergone the operation. If no such patient is available at the hospital the Ileostomy Association will readily help. With modern appliances the ileostomy causes surprisingly little disability. A proportion of patients have to have their ileostomy refashioned to overcome ileostomy dysfunction; in this condition there is a stricture as the ileum passes through the abdominal wall and the partially obstructed bowel reacts by secreting an excess of fluid. Any patient with an ileostomy is unable to conserve sodium efficiently so many patients in hot climates may be sodium depleted. Urine output is often low and there is an increased tendency to urate stone formation.

Course and Prognosis

The disease typically runs a course punctuated by relapse and remissions which in the individual patient are unpredictable, but different groups of patients are known to have different prognoses.

Factors affecting the prognosis of the first attack are the extent of the disease in the colon, the severity of the first attack (a severe attack is classified as one in which the patient has more than six stools a day which contain obvious blood, a fever of greater than 99·5° F. (37·5° C.), a pulse rate greater than 90 per minute, a haemoglobin of less than 11 g. per 100 ml., and an E.S.R. of greater than 30 mm. per hour) and also the age of the patient. There is a 10 per cent. death rate during a severe attack but no mortality when there are no systemic symptoms. Similarly the death rate is 12 per cent. when there is total bowel involvement and 15 per cent. for the patient over the age of 60, but nil under the age of 20. The effect of the extent of the disease in the initial attack on the subsequent course is debatable but there is little doubt when there is total bowel involvement the ultimate prognosis is poor with medical treatment alone, there being a 50 per cent. mortality at the end of 25 years.

REFERENCE

Goligher, J. C., de Dombal, F. T., Watts, J. McK., and Watkinson, G. (1968) *Ulcerative Colitis*, London.

HIRSCHSPRUNG'S DISEASE

Definition

A disorder in which chronic obstruction of the colon due to failure of peristalsis in a segment of large bowel, usually in the rectosigmoid region, is accompanied by great dilatation of the intestine proximal to the obstruction.

Aetiology and Pathology

There is a congenital absence of ganglion cells of the intrinsic nerve plexus of the distal colon which may reach below the rectosigmoid in 65 per cent. of patients but in 5 per cent. may involve the whole colon. On occasions the innervation of the genito-urinary tract is also involved. It occurs in between 1 in 5,000 to 1 in 10,000 births and affects boys thirteen times more frequently than girls. There is a familial tendency. The affected portion of the bowel is macroscopically normal but is a functional block to the passge of faeces. The colon above, which is dilated and hypertrophied, may occasionally be the site of stercoral ulceration.

Clinical Picture

The condition accounts for many of the patients with neonatal intestinal obstruction. In the neonates, apart from distension, constipation and vomiting, a dangerous complication is a severe colitis which may be of the pseudomembranous type. In milder cases there may be chronic constipation with failure to thrive. Occasionally the condition may remain undiagnosed into adult life, especially if there is only a very short abnormal distal segment.

Diagnosis

The condition has to be differentiated from intestinal obstruction or gastro-enteritis in the neonate. In the older child the commonest condition with which it may be confused is simple constipation due either to faulty training or a painful anal lesion; faecal soiling is common in this condition but rare in Hirschsprung's disease. A positive family history is of value. It is very easy to miss the adult with a very short segment of affected rectum whose only complaint is obstinate constipation.

A limited barium enema is aimed at outlining the distal contracted segment—attempts to fill the whole dilated colon are dangerous and may lead to water intoxication and faecal impaction. To prevent this latter complication a water-soluble contrast medium is often used. The definitive diagnostic procedure is biopsy of the contracted segment for identification of the intrinsic nerve supply; this usually must include the rectal muscle.

Treatment

This is essentially surgical and in severely affected patients should be undertaken quickly as medical treatment has little to offer, the child's general condition deteriorates and there is the danger of complicating enterocolitis. In much milder cases rectal washouts and laxatives may help to control symptoms. The usual operation procedure involves resection of the affected segment and anastomosis of the dilated segment of colon to the anorectal margin (the pull-through operation). This gives a good functional result in over 80 per cent. of patients.

REFERENCE

Nixon, H. H. (1964) Hirschsprung's disease, *Arch. Dis. Childh.*, **39**, 109.

MEGARECTUM AND MEGACOLON IN ADULTS

This is a relatively uncommon feature of constipation in the absence of organic obstruction and may occasionally be associated with a variety of conditions. It may occasionally be due to a short segment of Hirschsprung's disease. The neurotoxin of *Trypanosoma cruzi* may affect the colon as well as the oesophagus and Chagas' disease is a fairly common cause of megacolon in Brazil. Recently a group of patients with obstinate constipation and a dilated colon have been shown to have a denervated bowel which differs from Hirschsprung's disease and is similar to that occurring in achalasia of the cardia, for it is the dilated hypertrophied segment which is denervated. Occasionally there may be an intrinsic defect in relaxation of the anal sphincter. However, most patients seem to be extremely florid examples of simple constipation or dyschezia [Plate 6]. The treatment of the latter is medical but surgery may have to play a part in patients with proven denervation.

REFERENCE

Smith, B. (1970) Disorders of the myenteric plexus, *Gut*, **11**, 271.

DIVERTICULAR DISEASE OF THE COLON

Definition

Small pouches of mucous membrane which herniate through the wall of the colon and are covered by peritoneum.

Aetiology and Pathology

The aetiology is unknown. It is very rare in underdeveloped countries and may be produced experimentally in animals by feeding a low-roughage diet. It tends to occur in later life; over 50 per cent. of persons over the age of 60 years have colonic diverticula. Approximately 500 patients a year die of the disease in England.

Diverticula may either be generalized, isolated or most commonly localized to the sigmoid colon. In the sigmoid form of the disease the initial lesion seems to be hypertrophy of the longitudinal muscle of the colon. This muscle remains contracted, giving rise to a concertinering of the bowel. It is thought that the pockets of high intraluminal pressure increase the outpouching of mucosa through the areas of deficient longitudinal muscle beside the mesenteric taeniae where the nutrient arteries perforate the bowel wall. The mouths of the diverticula open at the bottom of the corrugated bowel lumen. Faecal material may become impacted and inflammation occur in the obstructed pouch. The resulting diverticulitis may give rise to a pericolic abscess, other viscera may adhere to the inflamed bowel allowing either a volvulus and obstruction to occur or fistula formation to ensue, for example between the colon and bladder or small bowel. Occasionally the inflamed bowel ruptures into the peritoneal cavity giving rise to diffuse peritonitis, or it may erode a vessel and cause a large haemorrhage from the colon.

Clinical Features

Uncomplicated diverticular disease may cause cramping, left-sided colonic type abdominal pain with irregular bowel action by virtue of the muscle hypertrophy. This is extremely difficult to distinguish from the irritable colon. Once true diverticulitis occurs the picture changes. In acute diverticulitis the patient experiences severe left-sided pain, he has a temperature with a high white cell count and there is local tenderness over the colon. The attack may resolve completely or he may develop a chronic diverticulitis with left-sided pain, tenderness and alteration of bowel habit and the passage of blood and mucus. At this stage a mass on the left side of the abdomen is often found. This may also be due to a pericolic abscess. The abscess may infiltrate backwards and cause a left-sided psoas abscess, and also the thickening of the bowel wall may give rise to chronic intestinal obstruction. Symptoms of fistula formation are those of urinary tract infection with occasional pneumaturia and diarrhoea when an enterocolic fistula occurs. Occasionally peritonitis occurs, when there is severe generalized abdominal pain often preceded by colicky abdominal pain as it is often secondary to an obstructed bowel. The tempo of this complication may initially be slower than that of a perforated ulcer and lead to an unfortunate delay in diagnosis for this complication has a high mortality. Rectal haemorrhage may be the only presenting feature.

Diagnosis

If there is a long pelvic colon, the inflammation is in a caecal diverticulum, or if there is peritonitis or ileus an acute attack may be misdiagnosed as appendicitis. In chronic cases it is important to distinguish the disease from carcinoma of the colon with which it may coexist and only be differentiated on barium enema examination. This is especially true when rectal haemorrhage is the only symptom of the disease. Sigmoidoscopy rarely reveals the mouth of the diverticula but when there is a chronically inflamed sigmoid colon it is often difficult to pass the sigmoidoscope beyond 15 cm. The barium enema shows diverticula and also the saw-tooth appearance which is now thought to be due to muscle hypertrophy rather than true diverticulitis. The inflammatory complication can only be diagnosed radiologically when a pericolic abscess or fistula is demonstrated.

Treatment

In the acute attack the patient is treated by rest and antibiotics, such as ampicillin, 250 mg. four times daily. Thereafter no dietary restriction is advised. If constipation is present methylcellulose, 15–30 G., may be prescribed at night. The indication for surgery is the acute emergency of a perforated diverticulum with peritonitis. A planned operation may be advised for the presence of urinary symptoms, if no other cause is present, recurrent bleeding from the colon, abscess formation, chronic intestinal obstruction and fistula formation. If acute attacks become frequent operation may also be undertaken. Although colonic resection is becoming increasingly safe it must be remembered that in elderly patients who often have other degenerative diseases and are over-weight there is still a definite mortality.

POLYPS OF THE COLON

FAMILIAL POLYPOSIS COLI

This rare hereditary disease is characterized by a large number of adenomatous tumours arising from the mucosa of the colon and rectum. It is transmitted as a Mendelian dominant and the tumours inevitably undergo malignant degeneration. The two most common symptoms are diarrhoea and rectal bleeding and the diagnosis is made on sigmoidoscopy and on double-contrast barium enema examination.

If malignant changes have already occurred in the rectum the treatment is by total proctocolectomy, otherwise colectomy with ileorectal anastomosis and fulgurization of the remaining rectal polyps should be advised.

SINGLE POLYPS OF THE COLON

Adenomatous polyps of the colon may present as rectal bleeding. There has been some discussion over whether they are pre-malignant but it is generally agreed that any lesion less than 1·5 cm. in diameter has very little chance of being a carcinoma and that the risk of operation is probably greater than the likelihood of developing a cancer. Therefore polyps of the colon should be removed if they are causing significant symptoms and if they are greater than 1·5 cm. in diameter, or if they are in the rectum and within reach of an operating sigmoidoscope. On the other hand, incidental findings of polyps less than 1·5 cm. in diameter does not call for operative treatment but the patient should be re-X-rayed in 6 months' time; if there has been an increase in size excision is then advised.

VILLOUS ADENOMAS

These uncommon tumours mainly occur in the upper rectum. They are sessile, have scant stroma and contain numerous goblet cells. They may secrete large amounts, for example 4 litres a day, of potassium-rich mucus and so the patients complain of diarrhoea and eventually suffer from weakness, oliguria and weight loss caused by prerenal uraemia and potassium deficiency. Tenesmus may occur but obstruction is rare. The tumour is so soft that it may be missed both on rectal examination and sigmoidoscopy, when the appearance may be misinterpreted as the colour is similar to that of rectal mucosa and the sigmoidoscope is offered little resistance. It may be demonstrated on barium enema examination.

The treatment is surgical after appropriate electrolyte repletion and consists of wide local excision to prevent local recurrence.

REFERENCES

Dukes, C. E. (1952) Familial intestinal polyposis, *Ann Eugen. (Lond.)*, **17,** 1.

Lockhart-Mummery, H. E., Dukes, C. E., and Bussey, H. J. P. (1956) The surgical treatment of familial polyposis of the colon, *Brit. J. Surg.*, **43,** 476.

Southwood, W. F. W. (1962) Villous tumours of the large intestine: their pathogenesis, symptomatology, diagnosis and management, *Ann. roy. Coll. Surg. Engl.*, **30,** 23.

CARCINOMA OF THE COLON AND RECTUM

Aetiology and Pathology

This neoplasm is slightly more common than carcinoma of the breast and causes approximately five and a half thousand deaths a year in Great Britain. There is a striking geographical variation, it being common where carcinoma of the stomach is rare and conversely rare where carcinoma of the stomach is prevalent. The rate per hundred thousand of the male population are 45·2 for the United States, 24·7 for Great Britain and 6·6 for Japan. Very similar figures obtain for women. Two-thirds of neoplasms affect the rectosigmoid area and in 4 per cent. of patients there are multiple neoplasms. There is a slight preponderance of women with proximal growths and men with distal growths. Predisposing diseases are chronic ulcerative colitis and familial polyposis, but simple solitary polyps of the colon rarely become malignant. There is possibly a genetic predisposition distinct from these predisposing diseases. The growths are predominantly adenocarcinomas, approximately only 15 per cent. being of the colloid variety. They may be papillomas which have ulcerated, secondarily infected and ooze blood or ulcerate. On the other hand, scirrhous lesions, especially on the left side of the colon leading to obstruction may occur. The growth may be graded histologically either by the degree of malignancy or by the Duke classification in which note is taken of the degree of spread. In a grade A tumour penetration of the bowel wall has not occurred, in a grade B tumour there is penetration through the bowel wall, in a grade C tumour lymph nodes are involved.

Clinical Picture

This varies with the site of the lesion but the disease must be suspected in any middle aged or elderly patient who complains of a change in bowel habit, unexplained iron deficiency anaemia or dyspepsia of recent onset. Abdominal pain occurs in more than half the patients with right-sided lesions and less than 5 per cent. of those with a rectal carcinoma. This is often misinterpreted as being due to a gastric lesion and when a barium meal is negative further investigation is deferred. Changes in bowel habit occur in less than one-third of patients with right-sided lesions but in 80 per cent. of those with a rectosigmoid growth. This change may be constipation, alternating constipation and diarrhoea or frequent passage of mucus often tinged with blood, the latter being most common in carcinoma of the rectum when the patient may have a call to stool as soon as he moves about in the morning once the mucus trickles into the anal canal. Frank bleeding is noted in two-thirds of the patients with a rectal growth and only 10 per cent. of those with a right-sided lesion, but an unexplained melaena or iron deficiency should always be investigated by a barium enema as caecal lesions may present in this manner. Approximately 30 per cent. of patients with a sigmoid lesion have symptoms of partial intestinal obstruction with abdominal distension and borborygmi, especially after food; this occurs before absolute obstruction supervenes. With further infiltration there may be tenesmus, invasion of the bladder and prostate or vagina. In advanced cases there is spread to the liver with an associated enlargement and occasionally jaundice. Once peritoneal spread has occurred there may be ascites so that abdominal distension may be due not only to partial obstruction and a mass but also to fluid. There is eventually weight loss, usually due to anorexia, and rarely fistulas may occur between the stomach, gall-bladder or other organs.

Diagnosis

Most rectal growths may be felt on rectal examination and two-thirds of colonic neoplasms may be seen on sigmoidoscopy. When seen the nature of the lesion must be confirmed by biopsy. A suspicious sign, even in the absence of an actual growth, is blood coming from above the sigmoidoscope. Following sigmoidoscopy a barium enema is performed to define the site of the lesion and also to exclude the presence of a second neoplasm. Growths may be missed in the caecum due to inadequate preparation of the bowel resulting in poor filling and missed in the rectosigmoid junction which may be obscured by overlying loops of bowel. The introduction of the Malmo double-contrast barium enema has improved the accuracy of the examination and smaller lesions may be diagnosed with certainty. It must be stressed that if the clinical picture is suggestive and there is any doubt about the technical adequacy of the barium enema examination this must be repeated. There is often a hypochromic anaemia but the faecal occult blood is not invariably positive. The E.S.R. may be raised and if the liver is involved there is usually an increase in the plasma alkaline phosphatase. Carcinoma of the rectum may be mimicked by invasion of the rectum by a neoplasm of the cervix or prostate, endometriosis, a solitary ulcer of the rectum and lymphogranuloma venereum. A caecal carcinoma must be differentiated from an inflammatory mass in the ileocaecal region either arising from a solitary caecal ulcer, diverticula, appendicitis, Crohn's disease, tuberculosis or an amoeboma. The most difficult diagnosis is in a patient with an existing colonic disorder such as the irritable bowel syndrome or diverticular disease when the symptoms may not alter until the neoplasm is advanced and in whom one cannot perform a barium enema examination with every exacerbation of symptoms. The problem of ulcerative colitis has been discussed elsewhere.

Treatment

This is surgical. Usually the lesion is resected and the continuity of the bowel restored, but with growths affecting the lower third of the rectum an abdominoperineal excision of the rectum with a colostomy is usually performed. Even if the growth cannot be completely eradicated palliative resection is often justified.

Prognosis

This depends on the malignancy and extent of the lesion at operation and is more favourable than with most other tumours. Between 50 and 75 per cent. of colonic cancers can be resected and 30 per cent. of patients are alive with no evidence of recurrence 5 years later. For patients with carcinoma of the rectum who have undergone an abdominoperineal resection 95 per cent. of patients with Duke's grade A, 72 per cent. of those with grade B and 25 per cent. grade C are alive after 20 years. Unfortunately the tumour is relatively insensitive to X-rays and cytotoxic drugs but if secondary deposits in the liver are the main cause of symptoms an intra-arterial infusion of 5-fluorouracil into the coeliac axis may induce a temporary remission.

REFERENCE

Muir, E. G. (1961) *Carcinoma of the Colon*, London.

A. M. Dawson

SECTION 8

DISEASES OF THE HEART AND BLOOD VESSELS

DISEASES OF THE HEART

GENERAL CONSIDERATIONS

The function of the heart and blood vessels is to supply all tissues of the body with adequate oxygenated blood. The cardiac output is the effective volume expelled by the heart in a minute, and it varies between 4 and 6·5 litres per minute at rest with an average of 5·3 litres. The output with each beat averages between 70 and 80 ml. when the heart rate is 72 per minute. An increase in heart rate or an increase in stroke volume causes an increase in cardiac output. Blood is ejected into the great vessels against peripheral resistance thus creating arterial pressure, and each separate ventricular systole causes a pulse pressure wave. The resistance offered in the systemic circulation is much higher than that in the pulmonary circulation; thus the arterial pressures differ in each circulation by a corresponding degree, although the output of the two ventricles is equal; the difference in the thickness of right and left ventricles reflects the difference in resistance against which each works.

The cardiac output varies greatly under physiological conditions; changes in venous return are largely responsible for significant changes in cardiac output, which are brought about by alterations in stroke volume and heart rate. Cardiac output decreases with a change to the upright position because of a fall in venous return; it increases with emotion and may increase fivefold or more on exercise in a trained athlete. The arterial pressure remains relatively constant because these physiological variations in cardiac output are balanced by reciprocal changes in the tone of the peripheral vascular system. The cardiovascular system functions as a whole; changes in one variable factor are offset by alterations in others and there is integration of the whole through the autonomic nervous system.

The heart beat is initiated at the sino-atrial node, from which the atria are activated by the stimulus which passes over them in a cephalocaudal direction to the atrioventricular node. The atria function as low-pressure receiving reservoirs and they augment ventricular filling by contraction at the end of diastole. Systole of the right and left atria is almost simultaneous, and the left functions at a slightly higher pressure than the right. The clinical manifestations of atrial contraction are an 'a' wave in the jugular venous pulse, a soft atrial sound formed by low frequency vibrations before the first heart sound, and the 'P' wave of the electrocardiogram.

The cardiac stimulus passes through the junctional tissues of the atrioventricular node and is conducted to the ventricles by the right and left branches of the bundle of His, and the Purkinje network. The function of the ventricles is to eject blood into the high-pressure arterial systems. In systole the atrioventricular valves are closed, and each ventricular chamber and its outflow tract to the aorta or pulmonary artery behaves as a smooth continuum; after the peak pressure is reached relaxation follows and the semilunar valves close, preventing the regurgitation of blood and thereby creating a diastolic arterial pressure. The clinical manifestations of ventricular systole are the arterial pulse wave, the 'c' wave in the jugular venous pulse, the lift of the apex beat, the first heart sound and the QRS complex on the electrocardiogram. The second sound which occurs at the end of systole is normally split into two sounds from asynchronous closure of the semilunar valves. When the intraventricular pressure has fallen low enough for the atrioventricular valves to open, ventricular filling starts and it is completed by atrial systole. Impulse formation and its conduction over the heart is further described in the section on arrhythmias [p. 754].

The normal basal systemic arterial pressure is between 100 and 145 mm. Hg in systole and between 60 and 90 mm. Hg in diastole. Considerably higher figures may be recorded in normal subjects at a casual examination, but after rest and reassurance the blood pressure falls. The elasticity of the normal aorta damps the initial systolic thrust so that as the aorta loses elasticity with increasing age, systolic pressures tend to rise. The normal pulmonary artery blood pressure is between 15 and 25 mm. Hg in systole and between 6 and 10 mm. Hg in diastole. The pulmonary capillary pressure may be obtained by passing a cardiac catheter into a branch of the pulmonary artery to the point of blockage, and in this wedged position the pressure and pulse wave forms appear to be a direct reflection of the dynamics of the left atrium which, however, may be investigated by direct methods [see cardiac catheterization, p. 745].

Symptoms in Heart Disease

There are relatively few symptoms of cardiovascular disease but it is most important to obtain a detailed account of each; in most cases this necessitates a searching inquiry by direct questions, the results of which can only be interpreted correctly when some assessment of the patient's emotional state and level of intelligence has been made. *Dyspnoea on effort* is the first and most sensitive indication of cardiac failure. It is due to diminished vital capacity, increased stiffness of the lungs from congestion of the pulmonary vascular bed and reflexes arising therein which abbreviate the depth of respiration and increase its rate. Dyspnoea may be due to primary lung disease or obesity, but a carefully taken history will often reveal a subtle but significant change when cardiac dyspnoea is superimposed on dyspnoea due to these other factors. Respiratory symptoms associated with psychoneurosis, such as sighing and tachypnoea, are readily distinguished from those due to organic disease. *Chest pain* in heart disease is mostly due to cardiac ischaemia, pericarditis or psychoneurosis. The type of pain, its site and radiation, provoking and relieving factors and natural history must be known before a diagnosis and full assessment can be made. *Palpitation* is an awareness of the heart beating due to an increase of rate, or force or an arrhythmia. It is a frequent symptom of neurotic ill health, but is common in heart disease and thyrotoxicosis. *Fatigue* and *weakness* are often symptoms of neurosis, but may also be due to a low cardiac output from chronic valvular disease. *Syncope* is loss of consciousness due to acute systemic arterial hypotension. An adequate history usually distinguishes syncope from unconsciousness due to primary cerebral causes. Simple fainting is vasovagal syncope which, like other symptoms of cardiac disease, may be associated with psychoneurosis. *Giddiness* is the term used by patients to mean various sensations such as vertigo, a sensation of dimmed vision, a pressure on the head, general weakness or even local weakness in the legs. This symptom thus always requires careful analysis with particular reference to near syncopal reactions and true vertigo.

Physical Examination in Heart Disease

Examination should include a general inspection of the patient, a detailed examination of the cardiovascular system and of any other systems indicated. Appearance and demeanour may reveal anxiety or depression; other signs such as dyspnoea, wheeziness, obesity, malnutrition, cyanosis, pallor, icterus and goitre may be observed whilst obtaining the history. The hands and skin should be inspected, structural abnormalities of the hands may be associated with congenital heart disease; coldness, pallor and blotchy cyanosis indicate peripheral vascular constriction, whilst hot moist hands, with pulsation of digital vessels may indicate anxiety or a state of high cardiac output: hyperidrosis is also a feature of the rheumatic state, when a diffuse swelling of digital joints and nodules may be found. Xanthomata on tendons indicate hypercholesterolaemia and are often associated with coronary diseases. Inspection of the nails may show such important signs as clubbing, undue pallor, capillary pulsation, koilonychia or splinter haemorrhages. Changes in texture of the skin are important pointers to disturbed water balance, endocrinopathy and collagen diseases. Skin rashes are obviously important and are often related to previous medication.

Examination of the Cardiovascular System

Arterial and venous pulses should be examined first, then the peripheral signs of heart failure should be sought and the examination is completed with inspection and palpation of the precordium and auscultation of the heart. *The venous pulse* should be examined with the subject reclining at approximately 45 degrees; in normal subjects it appears just above the clavicles in this position. The upper limit of a normal pulse wave is 3 cm. above the sternal angle. Normally there are three positive waves: a sharp 'a' wave due to atrial systole; a small 'c' wave due to ventricular systole and largely transmitted from the adjacent carotid; and at the height of atrial filling a blunt 'v' wave whose apex just precedes the opening of atrioventricular valves, signified by a steep trough in the venous pulse ('y' descent). The venous pressure may be generally elevated in heart failure, pericardial tamponade, constrictive pericarditis and mediastinal obstruction, or individual waves may be augmented, diminished or absent. The jugular venous pulse is distinguished from the carotid arterial pulse by the following features: (1) triple wave form; (2) the diffuse undulating nature of the pulse which is seen over a relatively large area; (3) an upper level of pulsation (which, however, may not be seen when the venous pressure is very high); (4) variation of the level of pressure with respiration and an increase in the distinctiveness of the separate waves with inspiration; (5) elevation of the level of the venous pulse in the neck by hepatic pressure; and (6) obstruction of the venous pulse by relatively gentle pressure at the root of the neck. The atrial 'a' waves have a sharp, 'flicking' form and are presystolic in time. They are augmented in conditions which cause atrial systolic hypertension and thus are largest in tricuspid stenosis and when atrial systole is obstructed by closed atrioventricular valves, as in the occasional coincidence of atrial and ventricular systole in heart block; 'a' waves are also augmented in conditions of right ventricular hypertension such as pulmonary stenosis and pulmonary hypertension. Large fused 'cv' waves coinciding with ventricular systole, having a large pulse volume, appearing to rise rather slowly and followed by a diastolic collapse, are characteristic of tricuspid incompetence and may be confused with a Corrigan pulse in the carotid arteries.

The arterial pulse is traditionally examined at the wrist, but both radial pulses and the brachial vessels should be palpated, and where there is any difference in these pulses, or if hypertension is present, the subclavian, carotid and femoral pulses should also be felt. The pulse pressure and volume determine the size of the pulse; the level of the blood pressure cannot be determined without a sphygmomanometer or other manometric method. Intra-arterial recording shows that the cuff sphygmomanometer is reasonably accurate except when the arm is excessively fat. Pulse volume is increased when the stroke output is increased in high cardiac output states, in aortic incompetence, and, to a lesser degree, in mitral incompetence. The pulse appears full and bounding and often pulsation can be felt as far as the digital arteries; the hands are warm and often moist. The pulse is diminished in low cardiac output states and when there are obstructive lesions such as aortic stenosis and mitral stenosis. Aortic valve disease causes a change in the pulse wave form, apart from an alteration in its volume; aortic stenosis causes a notched and flattened wave—the anacrotic pulse, whilst aortic incompetence (and other causes of a rapid leak from the arterial system such as patent ductus arteriosus or arteriovenous aneurysm) causes a water-hammer pulse. Combined aortic stenosis and aortic incompetence produce a deeply notched pulse—the pulsus bisferiens. An absent peripheral pulse may be due to very low pulse pressures from an arterial obstruction (e.g. peripheral embolism or coarctation of the aorta), but the diastolic pressure and the resting blood flow to the area concerned may be within normal limits. The state of vessel walls is assessed by digital examination; the brachial vessels are always thickened in established hypertension and further evidence of the state of the smaller vessels may be obtained by ophthalmoscopic examination.

Heart size and shape are most accurately determined by radiological methods. Percussion of the chest and palpation of the apex may be illusory; however, the position of the apex beat is a reliable guide to heart size when its displacement is not due to deformity of the thorax, fibrosis of lung, or pleural effusion, and when apparent displacement is not due to great over-activity as in thyrotoxicosis. Percussion of the precordium reveals relatively gross changes in size to right or left, and is helpful when the apex cannot be felt when emphysema is present, but many physicians now regard evidence from percussion of the heart with suspicion.

Abnormal *pulsations* of the heart may be detected by observation and palpation, and are of great significance in diagnosis. The hyperdynamic heart of anxiety, thyrotoxicosis and other high output states causes an increased pulsation of the whole precordium and apex. In conditions with a left to right shunt, such as atrial septal defect, the increased activity may become very great, affecting the whole precordium, or it may be more or less confined to the intercostal spaces over the right ventricle and pulmonary artery. Equally significant but much more difficult to appreciate is the quiet heart of a pericardial effusion, myxoedema or a primary cardiopathy. In left ventricular hypertrophy the apex beat is strong and appears to be sustained, but when ventricular dilatation develops the beat eventually loses its heaving quality. Right ventricular hypertrophy is characterized by a systolic heave or lift in the parasternal region and precordium; this is felt by placing fingers in the intercostal spaces or placing the flat hand along the parasternal region over the right ventricle and pulmonary artery; sometimes it is best appreciated by placing the fingers high in the epigastrium and directed towards the right ventricle. In right ventricular hypertrophy the apex beat is rather localized and is still formed by the left ventricle which appears to tilt forward on the enlarged right ventricle. Pulsation of the right ventricle merges into that of the pulmonary artery at the level of the third interspace. The vibrations caused by heart sounds and murmurs can be palpated when of sufficient intensity, and they are often superimposed on the pulsations described above. The tapping quality of the apex in mitral stenosis is due to left ventricular systole together with an appreciation of the loud and sharp first heart sound. In pulmonary hypertension the diastolic shock of valve closure may be felt as well as the systolic thrust of the tense pulmonary artery.

Heart sounds and murmurs are vibrations set up by the main events in the cardiac cycle and are essentially recognized by auscultation, but when of sufficient intensity they may be appreciated by palpation. Heart sounds and murmurs may be recorded by phonocardiography [see below]. *Technique of auscultation.* The stethoscope should have well-fitting earpieces and moderately thick tubing between 10 and 15 in. long. Chest pieces are of two types, bell and diaphragm, and available in a combined form; the bell-end is better for low-pitched sounds and murmurs, the diaphragm for high-pitched ones. On auscultation it is essential to listen to one sound or murmur at a time, and with practice the other sounds and murmurs may be actively excluded. The ear is more sensitive to higher frequencies than to the lower ones—low frequency vibrations must be of much greater intensity to bring them within the range of audibility. *Heart sounds.* The timing, pitch, intensity and site of maximal intensity should be noted for all sounds. The first heart sound is due to the closure of atrioventricular valves. It is best heard in the mitral area and is preceded by a soft sound due to atrial systole. Mitral closure and the slightly later tricuspid valve closure are often heard as physiological splitting of the first sound which is soft when the P-R interval is long, loud and short when the P-R interval is short, and when there is tachycardia; it also becomes very loud in mitral stenosis. Systole is normally silent, except in young children, and is terminated by the second heart sounds, which are due to the closure of the semilunar valves. Although usually referred to as the second heart sound, there are essentially two components, aortic and pulmonary, which are slightly asynchronous. The second heart sounds are best heard in the second left intercostal space, where slight splitting, increased by inspiration, is physiological. The aortic second sound is the first component, and, being louder, is widely heard, and is the second heart sound at the mitral area. The later component is pulmonary and is softer. It follows that augmentation of either component reflects a rise of pressure in the vessel concerned; conversely when the pressures are low, valve closure is delayed and less violent, i.e. in pulmonary stenosis P2 is significantly late and soft. Asynchronous contraction of the ventricles due to bundle branch block leads to wide separation of the second heart sounds which is proportional to the degree of delay of systole in the affected ventricle. Pathological splitting of the first sounds is more difficult to appreciate than splitting of the crisp second sounds. The third heart sound is the most important additional heart sound. It is associated with ventricular filling and occurs in early diastole. It is a low-pitched, soft thud, best heard at the mitral area (except in the case of right ventricular failure) and with light pressure of the bell-ended stethoscope. It is physiological in the young, its incidence diminishes up to the age of 30, and thereafter it is pathological; it occurs in all forms of heart failure, and when the heart rate is normal or slow it produces a protodiastolic gallop rhythm (triple rhythm). The third sound may become the loudest of the heart sounds in heart failure and when the heart rate is increased there is summation of the third heart sound and the next atrial sound, producing a presystolic gallop rhythm. In constrictive pericarditis the third heart sound is shortened and sharpened and occurs rather earlier in diastole than is usual; this may be due to the very high venous pressure and restriction of ventricular filling by the pericardium. In mitral stenosis rapid ventricular filling is prevented by the obstruction so that a third sound is not heard; however, in pure mitral reflux, there is a free and augmented flow to the ventricle so that a third heart sound is usual. An additional sound, the opening snap, is heard in mitral stenosis. It is due to the diastolic opening movement of thickened inelastic mitral valves, but it disappears when such valves are completely rigid and calcified. It is short and sharp and best heard above and inside the apex. Added sounds in systole are not uncommon; their significance is not well understood but it appears that most are of benign import. It has been shown, however, that a short sharp sound in early systole, the ejection click, is associated with dilatation of either aorta or main pulmonary artery just beyond the valves. A mid-systolic click often introduces the late systolic murmur of mild mitral reflux.

Murmurs are due to a more prolonged series of vibrations than sounds. The timing, duration, pitch, intensity, variations with posture and respiration, site of maximal intensity and radiation should be observed in all murmurs. *Systolic murmurs.* It is customary to classify systolic murmurs in the first instance as either innocent or organic. The distinction has been largely based on loudness, but this is not correct, since most loud organic systolic murmurs presumably start as soft ones; duration and quality are more important. Many systolic murmurs are related to deformities of the chest or very minor abnormalities in the heart, and as such they are of entirely benign significance but not necessarily innocent in the sense that there is no structural or haemodynamic cause for their existence.

Many children have a soft, mid-systolic, parasternal murmur, especially when there is tachycardia—this is of no significance and disappears in adult life. Soft, mid-systolic murmurs in the parasternal region and over the pulmonary artery are not uncommon in adults; some are due to an increased blood flow into the great vessels, e.g. in pregnancy, thyrotoxicosis and atrial septal defect, and others are associated with sternal depression or kyphoscoliosis. A soft, mid-systolic murmur may occur in the parasternal region without evidence of an hyperdynamic circulation or heart disease, and these often diminish greatly with a change from a reclining to an upright posture and are regarded as innocent. The systolic murmurs of aortic stenosis, aortic sclerosis and pulmonary stenosis are also of maximal intensity in mid-systole; those arising in the aortic valve are best heard in the second right intercostal space and radiate to the neck and downwards towards the apex; those arising in the pulmonary outflow tract are best heard in the third left intercostal space and radiate upwards to the left. The systolic murmurs due to regurgitation from the ventricles, i.e. mitral and tricuspid incompetence and ventricular septal defect, tend to be heard throughout systole (pansystolic). In the case of mitral reflux the murmur may be so loud and long at the apex that the second heart sound cannot be distinguished there, and it tends to radiate towards the left axilla. In tricuspid reflux the murmur is not usually as loud as in mitral reflux; it is heard best at the lower end of the sternum and it tends to get louder on inspiration.

Diastolic murmurs. All indicate heart disease. Incompetence of the aortic or pulmonary valves is shown by an early diastolic murmur which is high pitched and diminuendo, starting immediately after the second heart sound and often loudest in the third or fourth left intercostal spaces. These murmurs are best heard when the patient is in an upright position with the breath held in expiration. A diaphragm chest piece is superior to the bell for the detection of soft, early diastolic murmurs. The murmur of mitral stenosis is of much lower pitch and its onset is delayed well after the second sound; it is heard best at the apex and aptly described as a rumble. Presystolic murmurs, or more accurately atrial systolic murmurs, are short, brisk and tend to increase in intensity to the first heart sound. Mid-diastolic murmurs also occur in conditions associated with an increased flow through the atrioventricular valves, e.g. atrial septal defect, ventricular septal defect and patent ductus arteriosus. Mid-diastolic murmurs are best heard when the patient is reclining, and by using light pressure with a bell endpiece to the stethoscope. Continuous murmurs occur when the pressure on one side of a vascular fistula is higher than that on the other throughout the cardiac cycle. A continuous rushing noise is produced, usually loudest in systole.

Murmurs are often described in such terms as 'blowing', 'musical', 'harsh', 'machinery', 'seagull', etc. There is little place for such inaccurate and unsatisfactory adjectives if murmurs are described in terms of loudness, pitch, duration and site of maximum intensity. *Phonocardiography* is a graphic method of registration of heart sounds and murmurs. By means of sensitive microphones, valve amplifiers and multiple galvanometers, synchronous records from various sites on the precordium may be made and the characteristics of human hearing with the stethoscope may be represented. By this means permanent records of auscultatory findings at particular times in the natural history of the disease may be made, heart sounds may be accurately timed and identified, and the special features of various murmurs may be determined. At present the methods do not lend themselves to routine use, for considerable technical skill and care is required, and quiet undisturbed conditions are necessary in order to obtain useful records.

Electrocardiography

When heart muscle contracts the polarized state which exists between the cell membrane and its cytoplasm is disturbed and total depolarization follows; recovery is associated with repolarization. These phases of ionic reorientation are accompanied by minute potential changes which are conducted in the surrounding medium. At maximal activity and at complete rest there is no change and no current flows. The heart is thus the source of electrical activity which is conducted through the surrounding medium in all directions to the body surface, and an electrocardiogram is the graphic registration of the surface potential changes by means of a galvanometer. Since the heart is completely surrounded by a varying electrical field, it follows that the potential changes may be registered at any point on the body surface, and at such points (or lead positions) the record represents the resultant electrical forces in the axis of the electrode.

In practice the electrocardiographic lead connexions between the body and the galvanometer are of two types: (1) *Bipolar* when two electrodes are placed on different points of the surface and the resultant potential differences existing between them are recorded. The standard leads of Einthoven are bipolar and obtained by connecting the left arm and right arm to form lead I, the right arm and left leg to form lead II, and the left leg and left arm for lead III. The apices of the hypothetical Einthoven triangle are formed by connexions from the left arm, right arm and left leg, and the heart is considered to be lying in the centre and equidistant from each apex of the triangle. Bipolar chest leads are formed by connecting an exploring chest electrode and the right arm (CR leads). (2) *Unipolar* leads are formed by recording between an exploring electrode and an indifferent electrode which is formed by joining together three limb leads, each through 5000 ohm resistances (Wilson). The exploring electrode may be used to record and measure the voltages from any point on the surface (V leads).

The horizontal components of the heart's electrical field are explored anteriorly by means of chest electrodes (either CV or CR) at the following stations, which are conventionally designated 1 to 7: 1 and 2 are at the level of the fourth intercostal space on the right and left sides of the sternum, 4 is at the level of the fifth left intercostal space in the mid-clavicular line, and 3 is half-way between 2 and 4. Numbers 5, 6 and 7 are also in the fifth left intercostal space in the anterior, mid and posterior axillary lines. CR leads show slightly greater voltages than CV chest leads and when recording from the routine stations C_1 to C_7, the differences are insignificant. The components of the central electrical field in the frontal plane are recorded in Einthoven's standard leads and by means of the unipolar limb leads VR, VL and VF, referring to the right arm, left arm and left foot connexions of the exploring electrode.

The normal electrocardiogram consists of a series of waves arising from an isoelectric baseline and associated with each heart beat. By convention positivity is recorded above and negativity below the baseline. The recordings are standardized so that a current of one millivolt will cause a deflection of one centimetre, that is 10 of the lighter or 2 of the heavier horizontal lines. The heavier vertical lines are 0·2 seconds apart. In addition each of these intervals is divided into five equal intervals of 0·04 seconds by lighter vertical lines, which are not evident in all of the examples shown.

The P wave is caused by activation of the atria and is the first *wave*. It is upright in standard leads and in left-sided chest leads, but it is inverted in VR and often in V_1. The duration of the P wave is usually 0·10 seconds or less and its amplitude varies from 0 to 2·5 mm. P waves are followed by a small recovery wave (atrial T wave), but this is not usually recognizable in the ensuing isoelectric part of the P-R interval. The P-R interval represents the time taken by an impulse from the sinus node to reach the ventricles; it is measured from the beginning of the P wave to the beginning of the ventricular complex and varies normally from 0·12 second to 0·21 second.

The QRS complex is the second and major series of deflections of the electrocardiogram and is due to ventricular activation. Q refers to any initially negative wave. R waves are positive waves and S waves are negative waves following positive deflections. Left ventricular activity dominates the electrical field during the phase of ventricular activation and its resultant positive axis is directed downwards and to the left; the surface components of this field are thus positive over a wide area of the left chest and leads taken from this area are said to show left ventricular complexes. It is probable, however, that such deflections are the resultant effect of the electrical activity from the whole heart. Dominant 'left ventricular' complexes (QR pattern) may be obtained in any one of the standard leads, but mostly in lead I, and in left chest leads V_5, V_6 and V_7. Normally there is a small initial Q wave in leads I, II, V_6 and V_7; it does not exceed 0·04 second in duration and is usually less than 2 mm. in depth. R waves in left ventricular leads exceed 5 mm. and are usually more than 10 mm. high. The height of the R wave in the left chest leads added to the depth of the S wave in right chest leads should not exceed 35 mm. A short, brief S wave follows the R wave in leads I and V_7 and this wave deepens and widens as right-sided lead stations are approached. In right-sided chest leads V_1 to V_3, the ventricular complex is usually of an RS form, the height of R wave being from 1–5 mm. and the depth of the S wave from 5–15 mm. in V_1. The R waves gradually increase across the chest to V_6 or V_7 and the S waves progressively diminish. The total duration of the QRS complex is usually 0·08 second and should not exceed 0·10 second.

The direction of the greatest electrical potential in the frontal plane may be assessed from the direction of the main deflections in the standard leads. When the QRS is mainly positive in lead I, and mainly negative in lead III there is left axis deviation, which indicates a rather horizontal position of the electrical axis; this is found in thickset subjects with a high diaphragm, and often in patients with left ventricular hypertrophy. When the main QRS deflection in lead I is negative and in lead III is largely positive there is right axis deviation, which is associated with the vertical heart of tall thin subjects, with emphysema and with right ventricular hypertrophy.

The QRS complex is followed by the S-T interval and T wave. The S-T interval represents total activity of the myocardium and should thus be isoelectric; usually there is a slight upward curving slope from the end of the S wave to the T wave, but general deviation of the S-T segment from the baseline of 1 mm. or more is pathological, and smaller deviations than this may be significant when taken in conjunction with the clinical and other electrocardiographic findings. The T wave is associated with recovery of the myocardium. It is normally upright in all standard leads but it may be inverted in lead III when the heart is horizontal, as in patients with obesity, and a high diaphragm; on deep inspiration, which moves the heart to a more vertical position, such negative T waves tend to become upright. The T wave is also often negative in lead V_1, and in children the negativity of T waves from the right chest may extend to the left as far as V_4. T waves are normally positive when the ventricular complex shows a left ventricular QR pattern. The Q-T interval indicates the total duration of ventricular excitation and recovery; it is normally an inverse function of heart rate and varies from 0·39 to 0·41 seconds at 70 beats per minute. The Q-T interval is prolonged by carditis and hypocalcaemia and shortened by digitalis. The U wave is a small deflection which follows the T wave and is positive in left ventricular leads, where it is best seen.

The abnormal electrocardiogram shows abnormalities of two different kinds. First, disorders of the sequence of atrial and ventricular contraction and the time relations between successive cycles may be shown—these are the arrhythmias—and here the electrocardiogram confirms accurately abnormalities which may be detected by clinical examination [FIGS. 46–49]. The electrocardiogram in the arrhythmias is described in the section on this subject. Secondly, a different type of information concerning the qualitative changes of individual P, QRS and T waves may be shown; such changes are due to alterations in the relative order in which different areas of myocardium pass through stages of excitation and recovery, and the abnormalities referred to in this group are associated with various clinical conditions but they have no direct clinical counterpart, e.g. there is no physical sign corresponding to a negative T wave. *Abnormalities of the P wave.* P waves become tall (up to 5 mm.) and sharp in right atrial hypertrophy, and are best seen in leads II and III, and in V_1 to V_6, e.g. in congenital heart disease and pulmonary heart disease. Pathological P waves due to left atrial hypertrophy are seen in mitral stenosis; they are notched and widened and the two peaks correspond to right and left atrial activity respectively [FIG. 39]. When activation of the atrium starts at its caudal end, the direction of activation is reversed, and P waves become inverted in lead III, VF and left chest leads, e.g. in nodal rhythm [FIG. 47a].

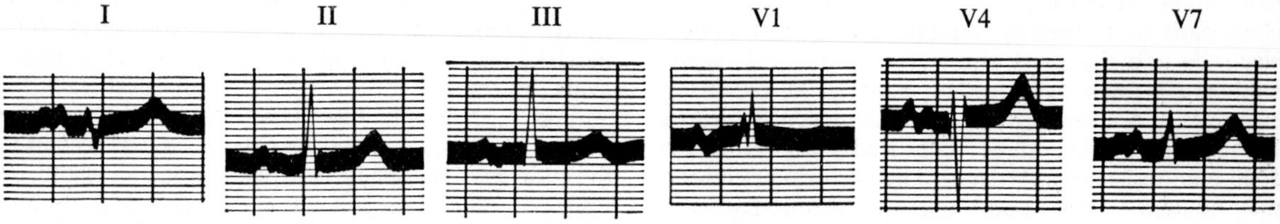

FIG. 39. *Right and left atrial hypertrophy in mitral stenosis.* P. mitrale seen in I, II, V4 and V7. First peak due to right atrial wave and second peak due to left atrial activity.

Abnormalities of the QRS-T complex—Left ventricular hypertrophy. The first electrocardiographic sign of left ventricular hypertrophy is an increased height of left ventricular R waves. At a further stage the duration of the QRS is slightly prolonged and the T waves in left ventricular leads become flattened; in more extreme degrees the S-T segment is depressed below the isoelectric line and it merges into an inverted T wave [FIG. 40a]. Ultimately when ventricular muscle is greatly damaged, the voltage becomes lower, the duration longer and a left bundle branch block pattern with inverted T waves may emerge. The changes of left ventricular preponderance are best seen in lead I, VL and left-sided chest leads. The tall R waves in I and deep S waves in III

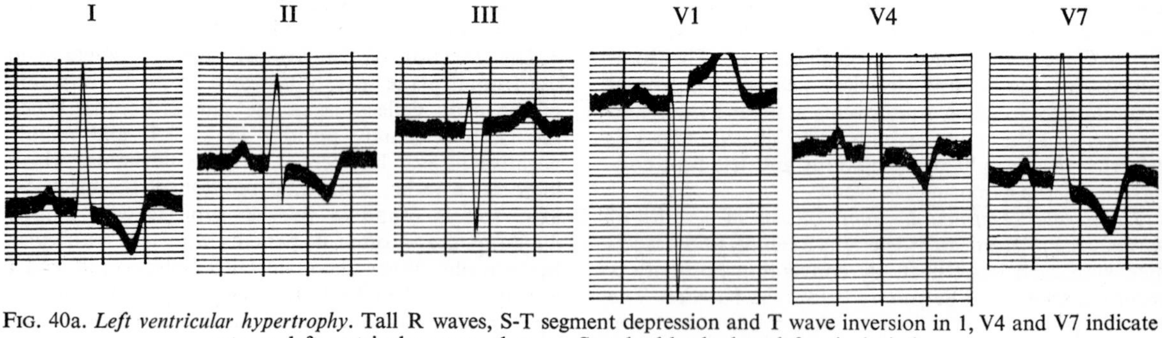

FIG. 40a. *Left ventricular hypertrophy.* Tall R waves, S-T segment depression and T wave inversion in 1, V4 and V7 indicate extreme left ventricular preponderance. Standard leads show left axis deviation.

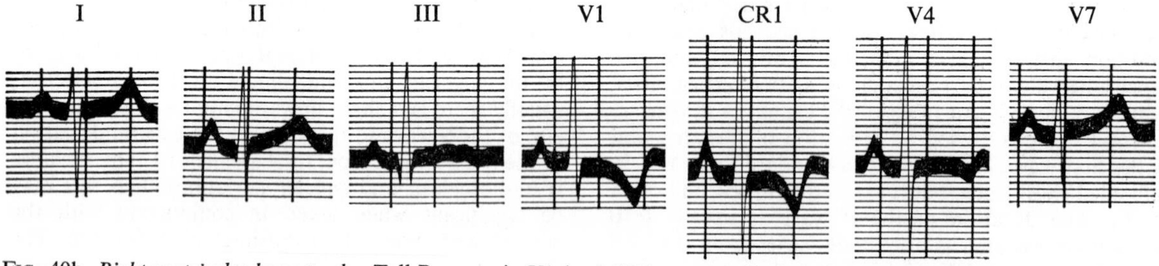

FIG. 40b. *Right ventricular hypertrophy.* Tall R waves in V1 (and CR1, note similarity). S-T segment depression and T wave inversion indicating right ventricular preponderance. There is right axis deviation.

are due to left axis deviation which is mostly present, but occasionally the electrical axis may be more vertical (especially in aortic stenosis) and then the QRS-T changes of left ventricular preponderance are best seen in leads II, III and VF. *Right ventricular hypertrophy.* The normal preponderance of the left ventricle masks early right ventricular preponderance which is often difficult to detect without additional leads taken from the right side of the chest. The R waves of right pectoral leads are of increased amplitude and S waves tend to diminish [Fig. 40b]. The R wave from hypertrophy of the right ventricle tends to occur slightly after the normal initial R wave in V_1, so that a positive secondary R wave, producing a notched complex, appears in V_1 to V_7 and resembles the pattern of right bundle branch block. Right ventricular hypertrophy is reflected in V_5 to V_7 by a deepening of normal S waves and the standard leads generally show right axis deviation [Fig. 41]. In extreme degrees of right ventricular preponderance the R wave is monophasic in V_1 to V_3 and followed by inversion of the T waves, and R in V_1 to V_3 usually exceeds R in V_5 and V_6.

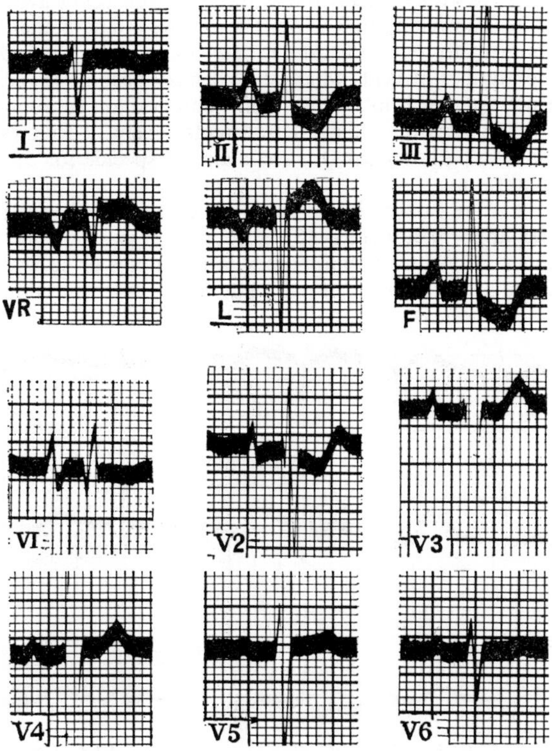

Fig. 41. *Right atrial and right ventricular hypertrophy in pulmonary heart disease.* Tall right atrial waves are best seen in II and V1. Late R waves in VR and V1 due to right ventricular hypertrophy which is responsible for the persistent S waves in left chest leads.

Bundle branch block (intraventricular block) [see also p. 764]. The essential feature of the electrocardiogram of bundle branch block is an increased duration of the QRS time; it is due to lesions of the intraventricular septum and also occurs as a transitory functional phenomenon in acute dilatation of the heart, e.g. in pulmonary embolism. Left bundle branch block is always associated with heart disease, whereas right bundle branch block may be innocent. *In left bundle branch block* the ventricular septum is stimulated from the right side, and activation of the left ventricle is delayed so that the normal initial Q wave of left ventricular leads (V_5 to V_6) is replaced by a small R wave from the septum, which is followed by a delayed R wave due to activation of the left ventricular muscle. This is reflected in late wide S waves after an initial R wave in right chest leads. The S-T segment is usually depressed below the isoelectric line and the T wave is secondarily inverted in leads showing the left-sided pattern [Fig. 42a]. *In right bundle branch block* the initial deflections of the QRS are normal since the septum is normally stimulated from the left side. Leads V_1 to V_3 show that the small initial R wave is followed by a second and taller R wave from the right ventricle. V_5 to V_6 show the normal QR pattern followed by a wide S wave which reflects delayed right ventricular activation [Fig. 42b].

Myocardial injury. Damage to the myocardium is shown in changes of the ventricular complex of the

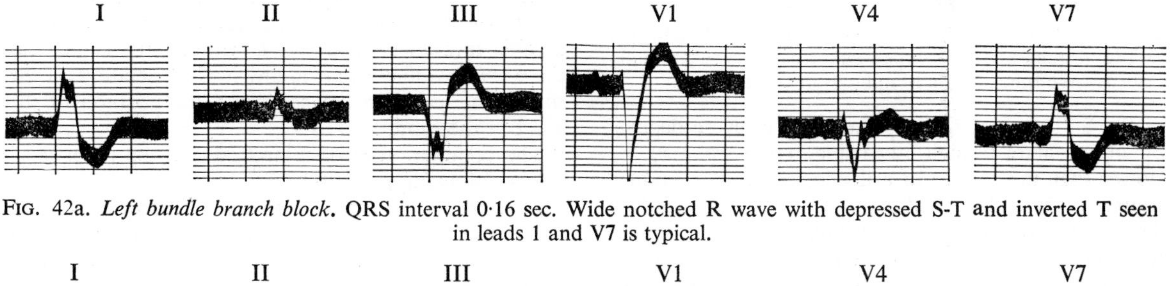

Fig. 42a. *Left bundle branch block.* QRS interval 0·16 sec. Wide notched R wave with depressed S-T and inverted T seen in leads 1 and V7 is typical.

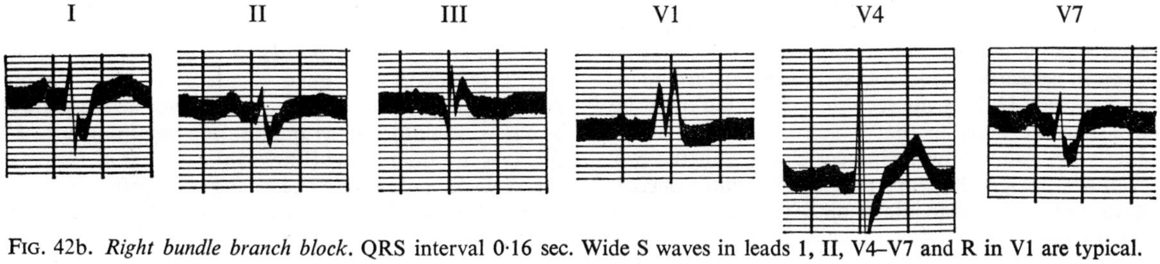

Fig. 42b. *Right bundle branch block.* QRS interval 0·16 sec. Wide S waves in leads 1, II, V4–V7 and R in V1 are typical.

electrocardiogram. The cause is commonly ischaemic heart disease with or without infarction, but inflammation, infiltration, intoxication and trauma may produce similar changes. The degree and extent of damage may be assessed approximately from abnormalities of the T wave, S-T and QRS deflections and from the leads in which these changes are seen to occur. *The T wave* may become flattened and inverted in left ventricular leads from ischaemia and other injurious processes. The change is non-specific and reversible. In coronary disease the T wave inversions tend to be sharp and form a symmetrical triangle below the isoelectric line. Inversion may be transient and produced only by effort in the first instance [FIG. 43], or a spontaneous transient inversion may be the only evidence of a small restricted infarction. *The S-T segment.* Deviation

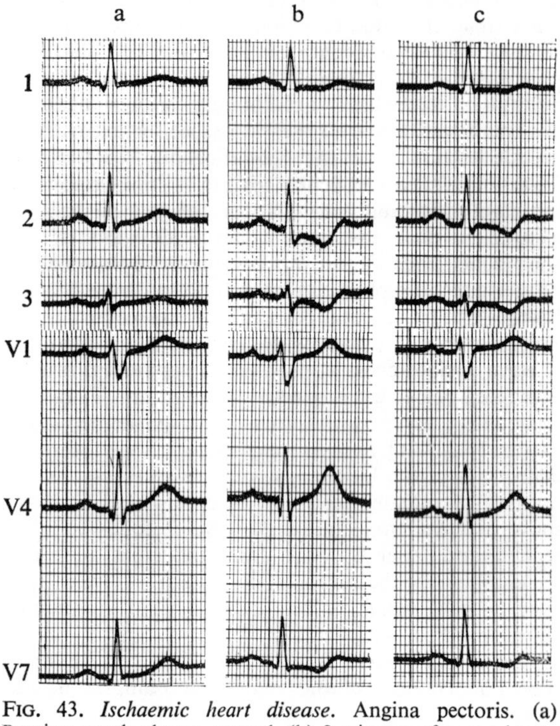

FIG. 43. *Ischaemic heart disease.* Angina pectoris. (a) Resting graph almost normal, (b) 2 minutes after moderate exercise S-T segment depression seen in I, II, III and V7, and (c) 4 minutes after exercise abnormality less, gradually returns to resting state at 10 minutes in this patient.

of the S-T interval may represent more severe degrees of injury and, though reversible, recovery may be slower than in the case of a fleeting T wave inversion. Injury to the endocardial layers of muscle causes S-T depression in surface leads 'facing' the lesion, whilst relatively superficial injury causes an S-T elevation; the former change is seen in severe attacks of angina pectoris and in coronary insufficiency and S-T elevation is seen in pericarditis [FIG. 44] and in recent cardiac infarction [FIG. 45a]. Leads recording from the opposite surface of the body to that which is adjacent to the underlying lesion show reciprocal changes in the S-T deviation, though these are usually of slighter degree, e.g. in posterior cardiac infarction S-T elevation is seen in lead III and VF, but precordial leads frequently show S-T depression. *The QRS deflection.* Potential changes are not produced by necrotic muscle so that an area of cardiac infarction does not contribute to the R wave and in leads 'facing' an area of infarction large negative waves (pathological Q waves) [FIG. 45] appear and are the result of positive potentials arising in remaining normal muscle and directed away from the exploring electrode. Pathological Q waves are of more than 0·04 second duration and usually more than 2 mm. deep, they may occupy the whole QRS time (QS waves) or be followed by an R wave. The Q wave is a permanent abnormality but with time it may become smaller and the number of leads which show it may become fewer. Since few conditions other than infarction are responsible for local muscle death and replacement, it follows that the pathological Q wave is almost specific for this condition.

In acute cardiac infarction S-T elevation is often the first abnormality [FIG. 45]; it soon regresses but may persist. Q waves may appear within minutes or several hours after the onset of pain, but the T wave inversion

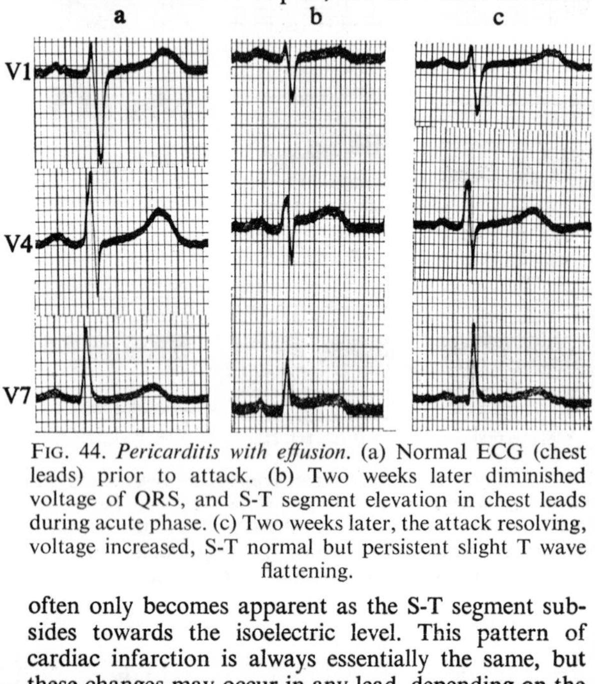

FIG. 44. *Pericarditis with effusion.* (a) Normal ECG (chest leads) prior to attack. (b) Two weeks later diminished voltage of QRS, and S-T segment elevation in chest leads during acute phase. (c) Two weeks later, the attack resolving, voltage increased, S-T normal but persistent slight T wave flattening.

often only becomes apparent as the S-T segment subsides towards the isoelectric level. This pattern of cardiac infarction is always essentially the same, but these changes may occur in any lead, depending on the site of the lesion in the heart and the position of the heart in the thorax.

The common sites of infarction may be recognized by the following patterns:

1. *Anterior cardiac infarction.* Characteristic Q waves and T wave inversion are present in leads V_3 to V_5 with more or less distinctive changes in leads I and VL [FIG. 45a].

2. *Posterior cardiac infarction.* The deep Q waves and T inversion are found in leads II, III and VF. Physiological Q waves in lead III are not accompanied by changes in other leads and on deep breathing normal Q waves are diminished [FIG. 45b].

3. *Lateral infarction.* The changes of infarction are found in leads I, VL and V_7 and may be combined with anterior or posterior patterns.

4. *Septal infarction.* Q waves are present in V_1, V_2 and V_3 (i.e. QS waves in these leads) and may be combined with either anterior or posterior patterns of infarction.

Radiology in Heart Disease

Three important methods are used in radiological diagnosis of heart disease; radioscopy (X-ray screening), teleradiography (films taken at a tube distance of 6 ft. or more) and angiocardiography. Less frequently used methods are electrokymography and roentgenkymography, by means of which pulsations may be recorded, and tomography, which is a method of investigating structures at various depths of the thorax.

The radiological silhouette of the mediastinum shows the following structures from above downwards: on the right border a soft straight line, the superior vena cava, joins the sternoclavicular joint to a gentle convexity due to the ascending aorta, at the lower end of which the hilar vessels protrude into the right lung shadow; below this a larger convexity due to the right atrium extends to the diaphragm below, where a soft straight line, due to the inferior vena cava, often interrupts the sharp angle between the atrium and diaphragm. On the left border the aortic arch forms a smooth, semicircular knob (diameter from 2 to 4 cm.) just below the sternoclavicular joint; this meets a second and somewhat longer convexity—the pulmonary arc, due to the main left branch of the pulmonary artery. Below this the short, flattish segment of the left auricular appendage joins the bold sweep of the left ventricle which meets the shadow of the diaphragm at a variable angle. On radioscopy all of these structures are moving. In systole the left ventricle moves sharply inwards and so does the right border formed by the right atrium, whilst the pulmonary artery and aorta above move outwards. Pulmonary vessels form the hilar shadows and on screening slight pulsation is normally seen in the main branches. Films taken at a fast exposure time are necessary to study the smaller lung vessels in detail —a fine arborization of vessels may be seen almost as far as the pleura.

The oblique views provide further useful information. After screening in the anteroposterior position, the patient is rotated to the left so that the right chest is applied to the screen (the first or right oblique), the right arm is moved backward and the left forward; these adjustments are made by the operator and, with experience, a satisfactory view is soon obtained. in this view the anterior border of the mediastinal shadow comprises the aorta (the circumference of the arch may be seen) and a gentle curve due to the pulmonary artery, the upper part of the right ventricle, and the border of the left ventricle below. The posterior border may be outlined by a barium swallow and comprises: aorta, a lighter region due to the left main bronchus, and below this a slight gentle curve due to the left atrium, and a variable small part of the right atrium followed by a short, straight line due to the inferior vena cava. The second oblique or left oblique position is obtained by rotating the patient so that the left shoulder and chest are pressed to the screen; the arms are moved again to give a clear view. The anterior border is formed of two bold convexities, that above being due to the ascending aorta and that below due to the right auricular appendage and the right ventricle. The ascending aorta may be followed in a continuous backward curve over the arch to the descending aorta behind. Below the arch of the aorta a second arch, due to the pulmonary artery and its left main branch, extends from the base of the heart shadow to intersect the shadow of the descending aorta. Below this there is a backward convexity due to left atrium above and left ventricle below—the latter extends backwards to reach the line of the descending aorta, and when the patient takes a deep breath the ventricle is separated from the anterior line of the dorsal spine by a short space. The point of intersection of the ventricle with diaphragm below is near the interventricular sulcus. In the frontal view the aortic valve lies almost in the centre of the heart shadow and slightly to the left of the midline, whilst the mitral valve lies somewhat lower and slightly farther to the left. During radioscopic examination it is most important to view the whole

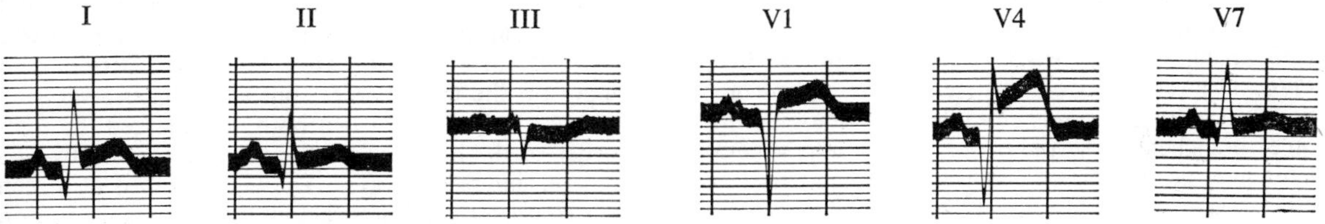

FIG. 45a. *Anterior wall infarction.* Deep and wide Q waves in I, II and V4 with S-T segment elevation indicating recent infarction.

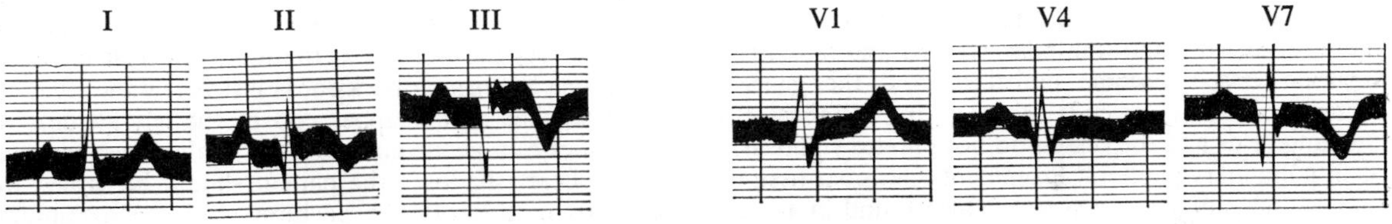

FIG. 45b. *Posterior (inferior) wall infarction.* Abnormal Q waves in II, III, V4 and V7 associated with S-T segment elevation indicate posterior cardiac infarction (with some lateral extension).

chest, noting any deformity of the thoracic cage which may influence an assessment of heart size through displacement of the heart within the thorax.

The apparent size and shape of the heart vary greatly in normal individuals. Deformities of the thorax such as funnel depression of the sternum and kyphoscoliosis often produce gross deviations (usually to the left) which may be mistaken for enlargement. Radioscopy in all views, however, usually indicates the nature of the condition. Minor degrees of apparent enlargement may be found when there is bradycardia, in obese subjects when the diaphragm is high and the heart tends to be horizontal, and when there is epicardial fat seen as a soft triangular-shaped shadow beyond the true apex. Very small hearts are seen in long, lean individuals and as a result of wasting disease.

Radiology of the Abnormal Heart. Investigation of cardiovascular disease by radiology is largely concerned with the assessment of enlargement of the whole heart or its separate chambers, with abnormal anatomy therein, with derangements of function and not least with changes in the vascular shadows of the lungs. *Pulmonary vessels.* Gross changes in the level of blood flow to the lungs are recognizable by radiology. Small, quiet branches of the pulmonary artery and generally light lung fields indicate a diminished blood flow (i.e. oligaemia); large, pulsating branches and a generally increased opacity of the lungs due to increased vascular markings indicate an increased blood flow (i.e. plethora or pleonaemia). In venous congestion of the lungs the upper lobe veins are the first to become prominent, in more advanced stages the hilar regions are dense, the separate vessels become indistinct, and the general increase of density extends for a varying distance into the lung fields and the vessels do not pulsate vigorously as in pulmonary plethora. Prominent interlobar fissures and effusions of varying sizes are also found in association with congestion. Short dense horizontal lines (Kerley lines) in the basal regions indicate chronic venous congestion.

The pulmonary artery. Enlargement of the main pulmonary artery shows as a bulge on the left border in the anterior view and as a large oval opacity below the aortic arch in the left oblique view. An enlarged main pulmonary artery may be associated with either plethora or oligaemia of the lung fields. In the young, in subjects with a vertical narrow heart, and in deformities of the thoracic cage with rotation of the heart, a normal pulmonary artery may appear enlarged.

The aorta. In the anterior view, enlargements of the aorta cause a widening of the superior mediastinum from bulging of the ascending aorta on the right or dilatation of the arch and descending aorta on the left side. A similar widening or localized bulging of the mediastinal shadow may be produced by unfolding of the aorta in hypertension, tortuosity of the aorta from degenerative changes and by mediastinal tumours. Calcification in the wall of the aorta is often helpful in diagnosis. A barium swallow outlines the posterior border of the arch and is an aid to assessment of its diameter. Irregularities of the descending aorta may also be outlined by deviation of the barium-filled oesophagus. Localized pulsation, though not expansile, is sometimes transmitted to tumours; on the other hand, an aortic aneurysm when filled with clot may show no pulsation. Excessive pulsation of the whole aorta is usually due to aortic incompetence, but may be due to a high cardiac output. When due regard is paid to the appearance in all views, it is usually possible to distinguish syphilitic dilatation from other conditions, but when doubt remains, angiocardiography can show clearly the course of the aorta and the calibre of its lumen. Coarctation of the aorta may be recognized by the absence of a normal aortic knuckle, rib notching and enlargement of the ventricle. Here also angiocardiography is necessary if accurate anatomical details are required.

The atria. The enlarged right atrium bulges from the lower half of the cardiac shadow into the right lung field and meets the diaphragm at a variable angle. The right atrium is often greatly enlarged in congestive heart failure, especially when there is tricuspid incompetence; it is usually associated with enlargement of other chambers but it is selectively enlarged in organic tricuspid valve disease. An enlarged left atrium also bulges on the right border, but at a higher level than the right atrium, and when both are enlarged the right border of the heart below the aorta is formed by two graceful, intersecting arcs. The left atrium is also seen as a characteristic hump below the pulmonary arc on the left border of the heart, and sometimes the whole contour of this chamber may be seen through the heart shadow. Its size and minor degrees of enlargement are best assessed in the right oblique view, with a barium swallow. As the barium is followed down, it changes its course by turning backwards just below the level of the bronchus at the upper end of the left atrium; it continues in a gentle curve almost to the lower margin of the heart shadow—the patient should be turned to and fro in this oblique position until the maximum backward displacement of the barium is best seen. A small left atrial curve is often seen in normal subjects, but this can be straightened with a deep inspiration. In some patients, when the barium-filled oesophagus appears as a straight line in the right oblique view, a large left atrium can be best seen in the left oblique view. Expansile pulsation of the left atrium in ventricular systole is seen in severe degrees of mitral incompetence. In the anterior view both right and left borders of the atrium are seen to protrude beyond the cardiac shadow when the ventricle moves inwards in systole. When there is aneurysmal dilatation of the left atrium the greater part of this chamber may be seen in the right hemithorax.

The ventricles. The right ventricle does not form a distinctive border of the heart in the anteroposterior view so that its enlargement is not easily recognized. With considerable right ventricular enlargement the heart may still appear relatively normal sized in the anterior view, but the apex is often high and the left border rather straight above and below it. In the left oblique view the angle between the aorta and the anterior border of the right heart is sharpened, producing a more globular heart shadow. The left ventricle enlarges backwards as well as outwards. In the anterior view the ventricular part of the left border develops a bold curve, and extends farther to the left; in the second oblique view the left ventricle extends backwards often well into the vertebral shadow. An acute angulation or local bulging on the left ventricular border indicates a ventricular aneurysm, and on screening the swelling may bulge outwards as the apex is withdrawn in systole.

Angiocardiography

Radiography of the heart chambers and great vessels after an injection of radio-opaque substance is known as angiocardiography. Various methods are used for exposing a series of cut films, large roll films or smaller sized but much faster ciné film. Furthermore, video tape recording devices may be used for storage and visual data retrieval. Lateral views in addition to antero-posterior films are necessary: the introduction of simultaneous two-plane exposure eliminates a second injection of dye and provides directly comparable pictures in the two planes. The most useful results are obtained by selecting the injection site after consideration of the probable diagnosis and the nature of the further information required (selective angiography). The dye is non-toxic and should be injected rapidly by mechanical means. The procedure is not without risk; a few deaths have occurred in severe cyanotic congenital heart disease.

The normal angiocardiogram shows the right heart chambers as a 'U'-shaped curve, and on the right side the column of dye in the superior vena cava is seen entering the right atrium, and in the centre the tricuspid valve may sometimes show as a notch. On the left side of the 'U' lies the right ventricle, a ragged chamber, the size of which will depend on whether the picture is taken in systole or diastole. The pulmonary outflow tract is well seen towards the periphery of the cardiac silhouette at the base of the right ventricle, as the terminal portion of the 'U'. The main pulmonary artery does not form the pulmonary arc. In the left anterior oblique view, the superior vena cava is superimposed on shadows of right atrium and right ventricle, which are seen anteriorly. The pulmonary artery curves backwards, forming an arch, the terminal downstroke of which is formed by its left main branch. The bifurcation of the pulmonary artery is usually seen about the centre of the arch. The pulmonary arteries and veins are well seen in both anterior and oblique views. In the anterior view, the pulmonary veins are seen draining into a central oval opacity, which is the left atrium. Superimposed upon the atrium is the base of the left ventricle; the apex of the ventricle projects downwards to the left. The left ventricular cavity varies considerably in size with the phase of the cardiac cycle. The root of the aorta is in the centre of the cardiac shadow; the dye-filled aortic arch is seen above it. The chambers of the left heart are best seen in the left anterior oblique view where the left atrium is seen above the shadow of the left ventricle. The aorta arises almost in the centre of the cardiac shadow and arches anteroposteriorly. At the origin of the aorta, which is deep in the heart shadow, the sinuses of Valsalva appear as a bulbous dilatation. In the normal adult the progress of the dye through the right heart and pulmonary arteries is seen in pictures taken between ½ and 4 seconds after the beginning of the injection of dye; and that through the left heart and aorta is seen in pictures taken after 6 seconds.

Angiocardiography can show abnormal anatomy of the heart chambers and great vessels, and if the passage of the dye is recorded with sufficient continuity some aspects of the dynamics of the circulation may be studied. Angiocardiography is especially valuable in congenital heart disease where shunts from the right to the left side are shown by premature opacification of the 'left side', but shunts in the reverse direction are not readily seen unless dye is injected directly into the left heart. In addition, the size, position and abnormalities of the aorta and its branches may be seen, information which is of value to the surgeon when planning operations for coarctation of the aorta or anastomotic operations for the treatment of cyanotic congenital heart disease. Aneurysms of the great vessels may be distinguished from other masses in the mediastinum. Visualization of the coronary arteries and their branches by coronary angiography is now an accepted technique. Specially designed catheters are manipulated via a limb artery to the coronary ostia, side holes maintain the circulation and dye is injected synchronously with sequential film exposures.

Cardiac Catheterization

Three kinds of information can be obtained by means of cardiac catheterization: (1) pressures may be measured in any heart chamber or in the great vessels; (2) samples of blood for gas analysis may be obtained from these sites; and (3) derangements of anatomy may be demonstrated by observing the passage of the radio-opaque catheter, by the injection of radio-opaque dyes or by the injection of other substances whose time-dilution curves may be detected at some other point in the circulation. Cardiac catheterization is safest and likely to provide the most useful information when carried out by an experienced team comprising an operator, with one assistant and technicians.

Technique. The plastic catheter is very flexible, radio-opaque, and has a slight curve a few centimetres from the tip: it is filled with heparinized saline from a 10 ml. syringe attached by an adaptor. The tip is introduced into the cubital vein which has been exposed and opened by a small cut after adequate infiltration of the skin and surrounding tissues by a local anaesthetic. Subsequent manipulations of the catheter should be checked by X-ray screening. The catheter is gently manoeuvred up the arm vein to the thoracic inlet where it curves into the superior vena cava to gain the right atrium. By various manoeuvres the operator may now move the catheter through the tricuspid valve to the right ventricle, the pulmonary artery and its branches. If observations on the pulmonary capillaries are required, the catheter may be pushed into the smaller lung vessels to the point of blockage. The left heart chambers may be investigated by the technique of trans-septal puncture which has proved to be a remarkably safe procedure. A special catheter and guide wire is introduced via a femoral vein to the right heart, the atrial septum is punctured and the catheter passed on to left atrium and ventricle. The left heart may also be studied by passing a catheter from the brachial, or other limb artery, to and through the aortic valves to the left ventricle. This procedure has proved to be safe and has replaced trans-septal catheterization in many centres.

Blood samples are withdrawn through the catheter at various points and preserved under paraffin for gas analysis with a Haldane or Van Slyke apparatus. Pressures should be measured by means of an electromanometer and an adequate device for recording graphically the pulse pressure curves.

Applications. The cardiac output may be calculated from the Fick principle as follows: cardiac output (litres per minute) = total oxygen consumption in ml. per minute divided by the arterial oxygen saturation minus the oxygen saturation of mixed venous blood in ml. per litre. Oxygen consumption is obtained by means of a spirometer, arterial samples are obtained by femoral artery puncture, and samples of mixed venous blood from the pulmonary artery by catheterization.

Intracardiac shunts may be detected by obtaining blood samples of high oxygen saturation from the right heart and pulmonary artery, e.g. in the septal defects and patent ductus arteriosus. X-ray visualization of the passage of the catheter or radio-opaque dye through these channels into the left heart or aorta is of diagnostic importance when the shunt is in the reverse direction.

Pressure measurements, pressure gradients and pressure curves help in the diagnosis and assessment of various conditions, especially pulmonary hypertension and valve stenosis. Cardiac catheterization has provided much information concerning the haemodynamics of heart disease during the past two decades.

CIRCULATORY FAILURE

In circulatory failure the body receives an inadequate supply of blood. There are two forms; one is acute, causing shock or syncope, and is sometimes due to heart disease but often to extracardiac causes; the symptoms are mainly due to low cardiac output and systemic arterial hypotension. The second form, generally known as heart failure or congestive heart failure, is almost always due to cardiac disease; the clinical picture is largely the result of secondary and compensatory effects of a chronically inadequate cardiac output, with the maintenance of a relatively normal blood pressure.

HEART FAILURE

The ultimate cause of heart failure lies in the physiology of heart muscle, but the clinical causes of heart failure include all the known forms of heart disease. More than one cause is often present—thus systemic hypertension and myocardial disease often coexist, whilst rheumatic valvular disease is often accompanied by active rheumatic myocarditis. The causes of heart failure may be classified as follows: 1. Primary myocardial disease (e.g. inflammation, ischaemia, etc.). 2. Increased resistance to systolic ejection (e.g. hypertension). 3. Increased stroke volume (e.g. aortic incompetence, mitral incompetence). 4. Dysrhythmia (e.g. prolonged tachycardia in infants). Generally loads due to increased volume are tolerated better than those due to increased pressure, and tachycardia is tolerated extremely well, but persistent fast rhythms over a long period may lead to failure.

The essence of heart failure lies in the inability of the heart to deliver an adequate blood supply to the tissues under all circumstances. In other words, the cardiac output is inadequate and fails to meet all requirements of the individual. The site of this failure may be primarily located in one or other ventricle or in the heart as a whole. Lewis emphasized that the level of cardiac output as a measure of circulatory efficiency is significant only when considered in relation to the demand on the circulation, e.g. in thyrotoxicosis or anaemia the cardiac output required for adequate oxygen transport at rest may be double that of the normal subject.

Under physiological conditions the heart responds to increased venous filling by a greater liberation of energy and increased output. At the level of the muscle fibre this means that increased stretching, resulting in increased surface area, results in more powerful contraction; more energy is stored in diastole and more is liberated on contraction. The isolated muscle strip or heart-lung preparation responds in this way up to a critical point beyond which a further load results in a diminished response (Starling's principle). This critical point is never reached in healthy man, but in heart failure it may be reached and passed; there is then an inadequate systolic ejection into the great vessels, some blood is retained in the chambers and dilatation and hypertrophy follow. Compensatory hypertrophy is a long-term adaptation to these adverse factors. The diastolic filling pressure rises and atrial contraction becomes more forcible. Up to a point output may be restored but ultimately this is permanently reduced. Incompetence of the atrioventricular valves, a consequence of dilatation of the ventricles, accounts for considerable reduction of forward output and is clearly partly responsible for the descending limb of the Starling curve in man. The difficulty of deciding what is cause or consequence dominates all the problems in heart failure. It is still not certain whether venous hypertension behind the failing chamber is a merely passive phenomenon or whether it is positive and compensatory. Haemodynamic changes occur very rapidly and an unstable equilibrium is soon established, so that the exact sequence of events is difficult to analyse.

Corvisart (1812) considered that the clinical phenomena of heart failure were due to the increased size of the heart pressing on the lungs and obstructing the circulation. Hope (1830) introduced the back pressure theory which has been elaborated and maintained to the present day. Starling's work with the heart-lung preparation appeared to support the back pressure theory but it should be remembered that there is no chronic dilatation or hypertrophy in the heart-lung preparation, no long-standing oedema and no elaborate system of reflexes in the central nervous system, whereas clinical heart failure is a relatively chronic process, often lasting years. In the back pressure theory venous congestion is paramount in the formation of oedema, but there is now much evidence to show that oedema formation depends on other factors. Mackenzie and Lewis assumed that the inadequate blood supply to the organs was the important abnormality; this theory of forward failure is supported by modern researches, but the older theories cannôt be abandoned lightly. It is probable that neither theory explains all the facts.

In all forms of heart failure the cardiac output is subnormal at rest in the late stages, but in the early stages output may be normal at rest and only inadequate during exercise; in other words, the cardiac reserve is diminished. An inadequate supply of blood results in its redistribution in the circulation as a whole. There is some evidence to show that the fall in renal blood flow is selective and relatively greater than the fall in cardiac output. Lowered renal blood flow results in diminished glomerular filtration and greater tubular resorption of water and salt; this appears to be a vital process and under circumstances other than congestive heart failure the mechanism has homeostatic features. The retention of water and salt leads to haemodilution, hypervolaemia and ultimately an increase of extravascular fluid volume and the accumulation of oedema. Oliguria results from the retention of water and urine analysis at this time shows a falling salt content. Man's habitual high intake of sodium chloride is of no consequence when renal excretion is normal and unlimited, but in heart failure a deteriorating situation is potentiated. Hydrostatic factors, increased capillary permeability, increased accumulation of tissue metabolites and malnutrition probably also play a part in accumulation of oedema. Whatever the true importance of the various factors in heart failure, the importance of salt retention is emphasized by the remarkable improvement which may be achieved by salt depletion using dietetic, diuretic or ion exchange methods. Any mechanism causing further salt retention aggravates heart failure.

Venous hypertension is the most important sign of heart failure. It is possibly due to a reflex venopressor mechanism together with increased circulating blood volume, but when venous hypertension occurs behind an insufficient or stenosed atrioventricular valve, this seems to be a true backward effect. In the early stages of failure and in high output states, it is possible that systemic venous hypertension is compensatory but later the adverse effects of increased venous hypertension in heart failure are shown by the effects of the recumbent posture and by blood transfusion, whilst the beneficial effects of a reduction in venous pressure are shown by venesection and change from a lying position to a more upright one. The elevation of systemic venous pressure in heart failure is responsible for the distension of the liver which must be considered of secondary importance. Even here there is some evidence that the damage to liver cells is the result of diminished blood flow rather than venous congestion.

When heart failure arises primarily on the left side, pulmonary venous hypertension develops. This is probably due to a temporary imbalance between the output of the left and right sides of the heart and this state is adversely affected by fluid retention. Pulmonary arterial pressure also rises in left heart failure and this is probably a direct consequence of the pulmonary venous congestion. Pulmonary oedema occurs when hydrostatic pressure in the capillaries exceeds the osmotic pressure of plasma. Dyspnoea is the most common symptom of heart failure and results from pulmonary congestion, cardiac dilatation which further reduces vital capacity, and an increased sensitivity of pulmonary reflexes.

There are many variable factors in the mechanisms which determine the passage from a normal circulation to one of unresponsive congestive heart failure and no one theory at present explains all of the facts. It appears that the clinical picture is produced by a series of relatively slow and only partially adequate adjustments to the diseased heart.

Clinical Features

From the clinical point of view it is convenient to assess cardiac failure in terms of left heart failure and right ventricular failure. Both conditions occur as isolated phenomena, or they may appear together, or more often right-sided failure follows left after a variable period when it is more satisfactory to use the general term congestive heart failure. Whilst most cases of left heart failure are due to ventricular failure, it should be noted that in pure mitral stenosis the left ventricle is unaffected, although the clinical picture is left-sided in the early stages.

Left Ventricular Failure

Dyspnoea refers to the distress accompanying increased effort in breathing. It is the essential symptom of left heart failure. Cough is also common and is sometimes accompanied by haemoptysis. Every grade of dyspnoea is encountered from the first detectable departure from physiological dyspnoea on effort to severest degrees which occur at rest and restrict all effort. Acute phases of dyspnoea, not necessarily provoked by effort, are common and range from orthopnoea, mild cardiac asthma, mild and severe paroxysmal nocturnal dyspnoea to pulmonary oedema.

At first *effort dyspnoea* occurs only with the more severe exertion; it is often only possible to detect a departure from the physiological by careful interrogation. Gradually the threshold of effort producing dyspnoea is lowered. It is often worse later in the day; undressing may provoke breathlessness, but a night's rest brings relief in the morning. Sooner or later breathlessness is present at rest and readily increased by speech, emotion and the slightest effort. Breathing is shallow, quick and obviously troublesome, being accompanied by much effort. It is never sighing and deep and is not relieved when attention is diverted. Obesity and diffuse pulmonary disease may produce a similar picture but it is rarely as severe. *Orthopnoea* commonly appears early in left heart failure. Here recumbency causes an increase of dyspnoea which is relieved by sitting or standing up. These patients sleep propped up by pillows or even prefer to spend nights in an armchair. It occurs in mitral stenosis and bronchial asthma as well as in patients with left ventricular disease.

Paroxysmal cardiac dyspnoea. Paroxysmal dyspnoea and *cardiac asthma* are synonymous. Although often occurring before effort dyspnoea and orthopnoea have appeared, paroxysmal attacks usually arise later in the natural course of the disease and they may be of any degree of severity. Most attacks occur at night and it is probable that change in posture to a more horizontal level is the immediate cause, although there is often a history of an anxiety dream immediately before the attack. A particularly strenuous day's work, large meals and a greater salt intake during the preceding day may be factors which precipitate an attack during the night. Attacks commence with a sense of suffocation and dyspnoea. The patient is compelled to sit up or often to get out of bed. Characteristically patients seek an open window. There may be a sense of constriction in the chest, cough, and the expectoration of blood-tinged watery mucus. Breathing may become extremely difficult, wheezy and accompanied by very great distress. Relief is mostly spontaneous and usually occurs within an hour. Anxiety is an especial feature of nocturnal attacks and the pressor response accompanying this probably increases the severity and duration of the attacks. *Pulmonary oedema* constitutes a more severe and acute stage of left ventricular failure. Dyspnoea is worse and there is often precordial pain, respiration is noisy and accompanied by coughing and expectoration of much watery mucus which is often pink with blood. Cyanosis develops from asphyxia caused by the transudate. Mental confusion may supervene and sometimes there is amnesia after the attack. After the pulmonary congestion has subsided, there is usually no deterioration in the patient's condition. *Cough* is a common symptom accompanying dyspnoea at any stage of left heart failure. Occasionally it is the dominant symptom and leads to erroneous diagnosis. *Haemoptysis* and staining of sputum occur commonly with the severe forms of congestion. Occasionally a large haemorrhage occurs.

Signs. *Examination of the lungs* may show the presence of adventitious sounds ranging from fine basal crepitations in the early stages, to extensive coarse crepitations over all of both lung fields in pulmonary oedema. The intensity of these signs parallels the level of dyspnoea. Unilateral or bilateral hydrothorax as shown by diminished air entry and dullness to percussion may occur in pure left heart failure. The pleura is drained by the pulmonary veins, as well as the systemic circulation. However, pleural effusions are more common in combined right and left heart failure. *Cheyne-Stokes respiration* frequently occurs in the late stages of left ventricular failure, especially in the elderly. Periods of heightened respiration alternate with depressed respiration or even apnoea. *Examination of the heart* may reveal the underlying cause of the heart failure, e.g. aortic incompetence, but of greater importance in relation to the question of heart failure *per se* is the presence of triple rhythm (or 'gallop' rhythm). *'Gallop' rhythm.* This is due to the addition of a third sound, similar in timing and quality to the third heart sound heard in children and young adults. It is intimately related to ventricular filling—it may be that filling becomes audible under the impact of atrial hypertension and in the presence of damaged ventricular muscle. It is heard as a low-pitched sound shortly after the second sound; it is most easily heard at or near the apex, and when using a bell-type stethoscope. These low-pitched vibrations can often be palpated and perhaps more often seen. If the apex is observed from one side, then the lift of systole may be seen to be followed by a small after-wave, coincident with the third heart sound. Tachycardia commonly accompanies heart failure. It will be readily appreciated that as diastole shortens with the increased heart rate, the third sound will approach the first heart sound; it may coincide with the sound of atrial systole which is thereby augmented and the gallop sound now appears late in diastole, giving rise to presystolic or summation gallop rhythm. Thus the essential feature of these triple rhythms, whatever the apparent cadence, is the addition of a filling sound. In some patients with early left ventricular failure the augmented systole of the hypertensive atrium can be appreciated by the presence of a loud atrial sound.

Cardiac enlargement accompanies heart failure. Left ventricular enlargement due to hypertrophy may be recognized by the apex which develops a sustained heaving character. As failure and dilatation increase, the apex beat becomes more diffuse and loses some of its force. These qualities of the beat are more important than its position in the chest. Murmurs are of no consequence in the diagnosis of heart failure but a systolic murmur often develops with increasing cardiac size and is due to functional incompetence of the atrio-ventricular valves.

During attacks of left ventricular failure (cardiac asthma, pulmonary oedema) the blood pressure is often elevated, and there may be alternation of the pulse, which is best detected by using the sphygmomanometer but may be felt at the radial pulse. Weak beats alternate evenly with the strong; this sign should not be confused with bigeminal pulse where the weak ectopic beat is close to the preceding strong beat. In attacks of left ventricular failure there is often intense peripheral constriction shown in pallor of the skin and coldness of the extremities.

Patients with great left ventricular enlargement occasionally present with the picture of right ventricular failure and are able to lie flat. This is due to mechanical embarrassment of the right ventricle, through bulging and hypertrophy of the interventricular septum which prevents the development of lung congestion (Bernheim's syndrome).

Right Ventricular Failure

The commonest cause of right heart failure is pulmonary hypertension and congestion due to left heart failure. Dyspnoea is therefore a prominent symptom in congestive heart failure, but its severity and paroxysmal nature tend to subside when right heart failure supervenes. In the relatively uncommon condition of pure right ventricular failure dyspnoea is not a prominent feature, although it may be severe when parenchymatous lung disease is responsible for the right heart failure. Patients with pure right heart failure do not have orthopnoea and are often able to lie flat.

Fatigue and exhaustion are common symptoms in

congestive heart failure; fatigue becomes a more prominent symptom when dyspnoea is relieved by the development of right heart failure and tricuspid incompetence. Generally dyspnoea is more incapacitating and unpleasant for the patient, so that fatigue is not noticed because of the limitations imposed by dyspnoea. Discomfort in the right hypochondrium from hepatic congestion is often present; it may become severe after effort and is rather slowly relieved by rest. This hepatic pain is not infrequently mistaken for gastro-intestinal disease and occasionally for cardiac pain. Anorexia usually accompanies congestive heart failure, nausea and vomiting sometimes follow; similar symptoms are sometimes caused by digitalis or morphine rather than the heart failure.

Severe heart failure may cause temporary amnesias and slight confusion, but the more serious psychotic reactions are rare. Slight jaundice is often present and is due to hepatic congestion or to haemolysis following extensive pulmonary infarction. Cardiac cirrhosis occurs in 2–5 per cent. of patients with heart disease and especially when there is chronic congestive heart failure with tricuspid incompetence.

Signs. *Systemic venous hypertension* with congestion of both venae cavae and their tributaries invariably accompanies right heart failure. The appreciation of raised jugular venous pressure is the most important sign of heart failure. A partial mechanical obstruction often leads to apparent congestion of the external jugular vein which is thus unreliable for estimating central venous pressure and it should not be used unless a free venous pulse is seen. Pulsation of the internal jugular veins can be seen when there is heart failure with the patient reclining at an angle of 45 degrees. The height of the venous pressure should be measured from the sternal angle. When the pressure is very high, congestion of veins is obvious even in the periphery. The recognition of jugular venous hypertension is difficult when there is tricuspid valve disease [p. 799]. In tricuspid incompetence a large 'cv' wave rises in the neck with each ventricular systole; although this is usually associated with congestive heart failure, it is not necessarily so. *Hepatic tenderness and enlargement* should be sought. Careful palpation of the abdomen usually reveals hepatic enlargement in congestive cardiac failure; systolic pulsation of the liver occurs when there is gross tricuspid incompetence. Gentle firm pressure over the liver will cause a further elevation of the jugular venous pressure; this manoeuvre may aid in the determination of the height and form of the venous pulse wave (hepatojugular 'reflux').

Oedema occurs in the dependent parts, at the ankles of ambulant patients, and over the sacrum, at the backs of the thighs and in the genitalia of those in bed. It is usually symmetrical—a gross difference between the degree of oedema of the ankles may indicate the presence of a local vascular lesion, particularly phlebothrombosis. Other manifestations of the dropsical state are pleural effusion, pericardial effusion and ascites. Oliguria and increased weight parallel the accumulation of oedema, and diuresis with a fall in body weight is a good guide to the effectiveness of therapeutic measures. *Cyanosis* is not an essential feature of heart failure, although *peripheral cyanosis* from peripheral arteriolar constriction and stasis is often the result of low cardiac output; the hands, feet, tip of the nose and lobes of the ears are cold and blue, but the arterial blood is normally saturated with oxygen. *Central* cyanosis, when present, is related more directly to the underlying cause of heart failure: it occurs when disease in the respiratory system causes anoxaemia and when anatomical abnormality (usually congenital) causes central mixing of the venous and arterial blood streams. Central cyanosis is generalized and the blueness is as obvious in the mouth, tongue and retinae as in the periphery. Arterial oxygen saturation is subnormal.

Radiology of Heart Failure [see also p. 744].

All degrees of vascular congestion of the lungs may be seen from a slight increase in the upper lobe veins in early left ventricular failure, to massive congestion which extends to the peripheral lung fields. In pulmonary oedema massive shadows extend from the hilar regions over the mid zones of the lung (resembling the wings of a butterfly) leaving the apices and bases relatively clear. In left heart failure small effusions may appear at the bases and in the interlobar fissures, and large effusions are commonly seen in congestive heart failure. Wedge shadows, linear shadows and other local opacities often show the presence of pulmonary infarction. The heart shadow is usually enlarged in heart failure and there is widening of the superior mediastinum due to distension of the great veins. Changes in the contour of particular cardiac chambers largely depends on the underlying disease which is responsible for the heart failure.

Other Tests

Urine analysis. Oliguria is related to the severity of heart failure. Urine is concentrated but the sodium chloride content is low. Slight albuminuria is usually present. *Blood chemistry.* Sodium and chloride ions tend to be subnormal but plasma potassium is usually normal unless lowered by over-zealous therapy. Blood urea may be moderately raised when urine output is low. Gross deviations of blood chemistry may be associated with excessive therapeutic salt depletion [p. 752]. The *erythrocyte sedimentation rate* is slowed in heart failure and is therefore not a reliable guide to the course of rheumatic carditis, bacterial endocarditis and other infections in the presence of heart failure.

Treatment of Heart Failure

Heart failure presents a clinical picture of varying severity which is largely independent of its underlying cause. Likewise the treatment of heart failure follows general principles which may be applied independently of the cause. Firstly the work of the heart must be reduced by physical and mental rest. Secondly the force of the heart beat should be improved by the use of digitalis, and thirdly the tendency to accumulate water and salt should be treated by diuretics, low salt diet and occasionally by the mechanical removal of fluid. Treatment of the underlying cause of heart failure is of fundamental importance; it is not always possible, but in many conditions such as valve disease, thyrotoxicosis, beriberi and anaemia, the cause may be removed or profoundly modified and this is described in the appropriate sections.

Rest. Physical and mental rest diminishes cardiac work and is the most important therapeutic measure in cardiac failure. The duration and degree of rest required for any patient depends on the severity of the illness. A single attack of cardiac asthma may require little more than a few days in bed, whilst 2 or 3 weeks of partial bed rest is advisable for the mildest cases of congestive heart failure; such patients should be allowed up for toilet purposes. In more severe degrees of congestive cardiac failure bed rest in a semi-upright position (obtained by pillows, a back rest or a special cardiac bed) should be maintained for at least 3 weeks or until the signs of congestion have subsided. Most patients may be allowed to feed themselves and receive visitors, but it is occasionally advisable to restrict all activities; continuous nursing care is then required. Mental rest should be promoted by reassurance, explanation and the use of sedatives.

Thrombosis in the deep leg veins with subsequent pulmonary infarction are hazards of prolonged strict bed rest in any condition, but they are especially common in patients with heart disease. Some physicians have advocated an armchair regime to overcome this and other adverse features of bed rest; the armchair position is good from the physiological point of view, but patients are tempted to increased physical activities and it seems best to reserve the armchair for a stage after a short period of initial bed rest.

The important considerations in deciding the mode of rest and its duration are the severity of circulatory failure and the patient's general physical and mental state; the domestic and economic circumstances of the patient usually determine the availability of nursing help and therefore the advisability of home or hospital treatment. It is better to err on the side of too little than too much rest in elderly patients, especially when the condition of the heart is such that little improvement can be expected.

Diet. One of the advantages of rest is that food requirements are less, so that cardiac work is further diminished. In severe heart failure anorexia limits food intake, but in other cases meals should be small and as attractive as possible, with a maximum daily intake of 1000 calories during the initial rest period. A *low salt diet* is a most effective method of relieving the symptoms of heart failure. Dietary sodium should be reduced to 500 mg. a day, but this is not always possible for psychological, gustatory or domestic reasons; it is impossible in unintelligent or unco-operative patients outside hospital, and attempts to reduce sodium should be abandoned in favour of other methods of producing hyponatraemia. It is not easy to achieve levels of 500 mg. of sodium daily and probably most patients on a well-managed low salt regime receive nearer 1 G. All food must be prepared and served without the addition of salt or soda. Foodstuffs must be carefully selected, bearing in mind that most protein foods (milk, eggs and red meat) have a relatively high sodium content. Certain proprietary foods high in protein and low in sodium are available if it is necessary to augment protein intake. The following rules should be observed. (1) Use salt-free bread (obtainable from many bakers), salt-free butter or margarine (if not obtainable it may be prepared by washing free of salt), salt-free fat or arachis oil for roasting and frying purposes. (2) Use plain flour and a special baking powder containing potassium bicarbonate instead of sodium bicarbonate for cakes, puddings and scones, which may help to vary the diet. (3) Restrict milk to half a pint daily and eggs to one per day. (4) Avoid the following foods with a high salt content: ham, bacon, sausages, tinned meat, meat extracts, smoked and salt fish, tinned fish, cheese, pickles, tinned vegetables and soup, chocolate, junket and dried fruits (except prunes). (5) Use vinegar, mustard, pepper and sodium-free salt substitutes for seasoning purposes. There is no necessity to restrict fluids on a low salt diet; water, tea, coffee and alcohol are allowed. Beer contains from 75 mg. to 130 mg. of sodium per pint (600 ml.). Many patients find that a low sodium diet is flat and monotonous, particularly in the first weeks of treatment, but most consider these unpleasant features worth while after experiencing relief from distressing symptoms. There are often difficulties in obtaining a regular low salt diet, especially for those who must feed in canteens and restaurants.

A diet of rice, sugar, fruit and water is worthy of trial in patients with intractable congestive heart failure, and especially where hypertension is the cause. Few patients keep to the diet for more than a few weeks, thereafter they are often happy to receive an otherwise unpalatable low sodium diet which may effectively maintain any improvement initially achieved by the rice diet. Obesity, which is almost invariably due to chronic habitual overeating, should be corrected in patients with heart failure by an appropriate reduction in the calorie value of the diet.

Tobacco should be discouraged except where its withdrawal causes much mental stress. Alcohol is permitted in moderation; it is a satisfactory sedative and diminishes anxiety.

Drugs. *Morphine* may be used in all forms of heart failure except in pulmonary heart disease, where its depressing effect on the respiratory centre may be fatal. Morphine is the drug of choice in acute left heart failure. It allays anxiety, reduces mental and physical tension, secures sleep and possibly causes a fall in venous pressure—all factors which tend to diminish cardiac work. Most patients with heart failure tolerate morphine well; it is better to err on the side of large doses than inadequate ones, and the drug should never be withheld when there is great distress in terminal heart failure. If, as in acute left ventricular failure, morphine is required urgently, it may be given intravenously (15 mg. in 5 ml. saline), but otherwise oral or subcutaneous doses (20–30 mg.) are effective and may be repeated in 2 hours if there is no improvement.

Digitalis. Withering published his *Account of the Foxglove and Some of Its Medical Uses* in 1785. Digitalis is still the most important drug in the treatment of heart failure. Many preparations are available and the pharmacological effects of the whole leaf or any of the glycosides are similar.

Mode of action. It is reasonably certain that the

beneficial effects of digitalis are mainly due to a direct action on heart muscle: stronger contractions of myocardium cause increased cardiac output and elevation of arterial tension, whilst congestion and high pressure in the venous or filling side of the heart are reduced. It is probable that a less important peripheral action also tends to lower the venous pressure. Digitalis also causes a beneficial slowing of the heart, particularly when there is tachycardia associated with heart failure and atrial fibrillation. Slowing is effected by direct central vagal stimulation and by a depression of the intracardiac conducting tissues. It is probable that even this slowing effect is largely due to a direct myocardial action which causes stronger contraction and increased refractoriness during recovery. Furthermore, as the cardiac output improves, reflex vagal action also causes slowing. Improvement of the circulation leads to a reversal of all the adverse factors accompanying heart failure. Thus renal blood flow is increased and diuresis follows. Congestion in the lungs subsides, heart size diminishes and vital capacity increases. All other organs, including the liver which becomes smaller, are relieved of congestion and there is a fall in circulating blood volume.

Administration. In most cases of heart failure it is advisable to obtain the greatest optimum effect of digitalis as soon as reasonably possible by giving large initial doses (digitalization). This may be achieved very rapidly by the intravenous route, but in most cases the oral method is satisfactory and it is safer. After digitalization the blood levels of digitalis are maintained by smaller doses.

Digoxin is a glycoside obtained from the leaves of *Digitalis lanata*; it should not be confused with digitoxin from *D. purpurea.* It is a pure substance and can be standardized by weight. Tablets contain 0·25 mg. and the daily maintenance dose is usually 0·5 mg. Rapid digitalization usually requires 2 mg. in 24 hours. It is available for intravenous use. One ml. contains 0·5 mg. of drug and this should be administered slowly after appropriate dilution. Lanatoside C is also derived from *D. lanata*; it acts quickly and excretion is very rapid; it may be given by mouth or intravenously. The powdered leaf of *Digitalis purpurea* (Digitalis folium) is effective but seldom prescribed: 60–200 mg. daily is required for maintenance. The tincture of digitalis has no advantages over tablets and dosage is less precise. The relatively pure glycosides of *D. purpurea*, digitoxin and Nativelle's digitaline, are not generally used in Great Britain; they are slow to act and elimination is prolonged. However, potency is relatively constant.

Ouabain (strophanthin) is derived from *Strophanthus gratus* and is usually reserved for emergency intravenous use. Its action and excretion are very rapid and digitalization should be maintained with a slower-acting oral preparation; 0·5 mg. should be injected slowly in the first instance.

Digitalis is indicated in all forms of heart failure whatever the cause and whatever the rhythm. It is as useful in cases of left heart failure as in those of congestive right heart failure, but the degree of therapeutic response varies and depends on many factors, the most important of which is the underlying cause. Care should be exercised when it is used in the presence of recent myocardial damage. Digitalis may be used with caution in the presence of complete heart block if failure supervenes, and is unresponsive to other drugs. Intravenous digoxin and ouabain have a pressor effect and should be used cautiously in acute left ventricular failure.

Overdosage of digitalis. The effects of excessive digitalis dosage are partly due to loss of potassium from cells; many of the powerful modern diuretics cause potassium depletion so that symptoms of digitalis poisoning are rather more common than in the recent past and their recognition is most important. The first and most common symptom is anorexia, which may progress to nausea and vomiting. Difficulty arises when these symptoms may be due to continuation of congestive cardiac failure. Arrhythmias of all sorts are common but extrasystoles are the most common sign of overdosage; they frequently follow each regular beat, producing pulsus bigeminus (coupled beats): digitalis should then be omitted for 1 day and thereafter reduced, but there is no necessity to change the form of digitalis or stop it altogether. Extrasystoles occurring before treatment is started are no contra-indication to digitalis. Excessive slowing of the heart is a common sign of digitalis overdosage. The vagal action of digitalis causes sinus bradycardia and even sinus arrest; nodal rhythm may appear and complete atrioventricular dissociation has been observed. Paroxysmal atrial tachycardia with block is not an uncommon complication of digitalis intoxication and other fast rhythms include nodal and ventricular tachycardia.

Toxic manifestations of digitalis require omission of the drug for from 1 to 5 days followed by cautious reintroduction in low dosage. Serum potassium levels should be checked. Dangerous arrhythmia and other toxic signs may be reversed by administration of potassium orally (or even intravenously in an emergency), but this is dangerous without continuous monitoring of blood pressure and the electrocardiogram). Propranolol, 1–10 mg intravenously, followed by an oral dose of 40 mg. eight-hourly, is effective in abolishing digitalis arrhythmia and is probably safer than potassium administration.

Digitalis causes profound changes in the electrocardiogram which may be indistinguishable from those produced by disease of the myocardium. These effects should not be regarded as an indication to reduce dosage for they are routine when a therapeutic effect is obtained and may occur when the heart is normal. The S-T interval is lowered and may become slightly coved, but it is more often depressed in a straight sloping form. The T waves may be blunted, lowered or even inverted. The P-R interval may be prolonged and in more serious levels of intoxication depressed conduction with or without extrasystoles may be seen.

Diuretics. The organic mercurial drugs have been largely replaced by thiazides, ethacrynic acid and frusemide. Chlorothiazide blocks the resorption of electrolytes in the tubules and is a mild carbonic anhydrase inhibitor. The oral dose is from 0·25 to 1 G. twice daily and potassium supplements are required.

Hydrochlorothiazide, bendrofluazide and cyclopenthiazide have the same action but are more potent and have superseded the original chlorothiazide member of the series. Ethacrynic acid causes a preferential excretion of chloride and sodium, thus although a useful diuretic in doses of 50–100 mg. a day hypochloraemic acidosis is a complication after long usage.

Frusemide, 40 mg., may be used by mouth or intravenously, 10–20 mg. It is a powerful diuretic with rapid action but potassium supplements are essential. Spironolactone, 100 mg. daily, is useful in resistant heart failure especially as potassium tends to be conserved.

The *toxic effects* of these diuretics are largely due to electrolyte depletion and excessive water loss. Weakness, malaise, apathy, cramps and vomiting are important symptoms. Accurate assessment requires serial biochemical investigation and may reveal hypochloraemia, hyponatraemia, hypokalaemia and even uraemia. Correction requires administration of the appropriate ion, a reduction of the diuretic and modification of a too strict dietary regime.

Oxygen. In most cases of heart failure the oxygen content of arterial blood is normal. If, however, this is lowered because of pulmonary insufficiency, oxygen is indicated. Oxygen is of great value in patients with anoxic pulmonary heart disease [p. 786] and when heart failure is due to other causes but complicated by pulmonary oedema, extensive pulmonary infarction, or bronchopneumonia. Various methods of administration are available: the Venturi mask is most satisfactory.

Venesection. This lowers venous pressure and relieves congestion. It is of value in congestive heart failure whatever the cause, but it should not be used when there is anaemia or severe hypotension. It is most effective in cases of acute left heart failure and should be used more often in this condition. In patients with chronic right ventricular failure with great venous congestion which is responding poorly to drug treatment, a venesection may 'break into' the vicious circle of failure and lead to a steady improvement with an increasing response to diuretics; 350–750 ml. should be removed from the antecubital vein with a wide-bore needle, using a sphygmomanometer cuff to increase the local venous pressure and enhance the flow. A similar effect to venesection can be produced by occluding the venous return from both legs by means of thigh cuffs inflated above the venous pressure but below the arterial pressure; symptoms may be relieved but they are likely to recur when the cuffs are released. This method is not advocated.

Acupuncture. This may be used to remove extensive oedema which is resistant to more usual therapy. The patient should be placed in an armchair position for 24 hours before puncture so that maximal accumulation of oedema occurs in the legs. Southey's tubes are introduced into subcutaneous tissues and small attached rubber tubes drain the fluid. Penicillin should be used to prevent sepsis which, however, should not occur if an adequate antiseptic technique has been used. *Paracentesis abdominis and thoracis.* Large effusions in the pleural sacs should be removed by tapping.

SYNCOPE AND SHOCK

Syncope is a transient interruption of consciousness due to acute failure of the circulation; shock is a more protracted form of acute circulatory failure resulting in a depression of all vital activity and having characteristic clinical features. Systemic arterial hypotension is an essential feature of both conditions. These hypotensive states are sometimes referred to as peripheral circulatory failure, but this term is misleading because the whole cardiovascular system is involved.

Arterial tension is the product of cardiac output and total peripheral resistance; changes in cardiac output are compensated by reciprocal changes in arteriolar tone so that arterial blood pressure remains relatively constant. When a fall in cardiac output, whether of physiological or pathological degree, is incompletely compensated by peripheral constriction the resultant hypotension leads to syncope, shock or sudden death.

SYNCOPE

Syncope is usually brief, transient and totally reversible, but when serious trauma or disease is the cause, shock or sudden death may follow. The cause of unconsciousness is sudden arterial hypotension with resulting loss of support to the brain substance and cerebral anaemia. A fall in cardiac output is the initiating event in most cases; this may be physiological, as occurs in the upright posture, but may remain uncompensated by an unstable vasomotor nervous system (vasovagal syncope) or rarely the autonomic nervous system may be diseased (see below). In other cases a severe pathological fall in output may be due to haemorrhage or heart disease (cardiogenic syncope) and remain uncompensated by relatively normal vasoconstrictor reactions.

Vasovagal Syncope (Fainting). Simple fainting is common and the clinical features are characteristic. The patient is usually in an upright posture and syncope is preceded by a feeling of 'faintness', rapidly developing pallor, sweating and tachypnoea. Bradycardia accompanies the sudden fall of arterial pressure. Unconsciousness is brief, but rarely convulsions may follow. Recovery occurs when the patient is recumbent; there is no mental confusion after the attack and there are no abnormal signs in the nervous system. Pallor and bradycardia may persist for an hour.

Many interacting factors cause fainting. The more important ones are: (1) the upright posture leading to venous pooling below the heart (functional haemorrhage), increased by prolonged quiet standing and lumbar lordosis; (2) an instability of vasomotor control leading to sudden vasodilatation in the muscles; (3) hot weather and a stuffy atmosphere which increase peripheral vasodilatation; (4) ill health—fainting is common during convalescence from illness; (5) psychic factors —intense emotional situations, fright and characteristically the sight of blood. Many subjects who have a tendency to recurrent fainting also show features of psychoneurosis. Fainting is common in pregnancy; lumbar lordosis and the tendency to increased venous pooling below the heart are probably causal factors. In late pregnancy fainting may occur in the recumbent posture when a sudden fall in venous return may be caused by the uterus pressing on the inferior vena cava; equilibrium is rapidly restored by turning to one side. Severe haemorrhage commonly causes syncope which has similar features to other forms of vasovagal fainting.

Postural hypotension severe enough to cause fainting occurs when the sympathetic system is paralysed by bilateral sympathectomy, spinal anaesthesia or one of the ganglionic blocking drugs. Nitrites are a potent cause of fainting which often leads to misdiagnosis in patients with ischaemic heart disease. It also rarely occurs in association with certain chronic diseases of the nervous system such as tabes dorsalis and syringomyelia. A rare form of syncope occurs in middle-aged males where the essential feature of postural hypotension is associated with anhidrosis and impotence. Faintness comes on shortly after standing and the blood pressure falls steeply. Normal vasoconstriction is lacking, and the disease appears to be due to a gradually developing paresis of the sympathetic nervous system possibly originating in hypothalamic centres; once the disease has reached a certain degree, there is no further deterioration and fatalities have not been recorded. The *carotid sinus syndrome* is rare. The carotid sinus is hypersensitive and pressure upon it caused by movement of the neck, external pressure, or a tumour, may lead to profound hypotension and loss of consciousness.

Cardiogenic Syncope. A transitory sudden loss of consciousness is not uncommon in heart disease and it is due to a sudden fall of cardiac output. The usual premonitory symptoms of vasovagal syncope are absent and in most cases the attack comes without warning. There is usually pallor and, if unconsciousness is prolonged, convulsions may occur. Consciousness is regained without confusion and incontinence is rare. The causes are: (1) a change of rhythm—syncope may occur at the onset of any arrhythmia; (2) heart block—see Stokes-Adams disease, page 763; (3) very rapid ventricular rates; (4) cardiac infarction; (5) aortic stenosis; (6) aortic incompetence (rarely); (7) severe pulmonary hypertension; (8) severe pulmonary stenosis; (9) ball-valve obstruction of the mitral valve. In obstructive conditions such as aortic stenosis and pulmonary hypertension syncope characteristically results from effort; this should not be confused with the syncope which may come on after the cessation of effort in hot weather, when the cause is extreme muscle vasodilatation. Syncope due to ball-valve thrombus or atrial myxoma in the mitral orifice is sudden, and produced characteristically by a change to the sitting or standing position; the prognosis is grave.

Treatment. Attacks of simple syncope are terminated by lying flat. The treatment of recurrent fainting depends on the cause and is described in the appropriate section. Chronic idiopathic postural hypotension is best treated by one of the sympathomimetic drugs given orally at least four times daily (ephedrine, 30 mg., or phenylephrine, 5–10 mg., should be tried).

SHOCK

The essential features of the shock state are arterial hypotension and a depression of all vital activities causing weakness, subnormal temperature, sweating and apathy. Consciousness is generally maintained without confusion, but syncope may occur when the patient attempts to sit up. The skin is pale and cold, the arterial pulse is weak and rapid, and the venous pressure may be low or high depending on the cause. Some patients are restless but most are quiet and lie still.

Aetiology. The fundamental cause of the shock state, whatever the immediate cause, is a relatively acute severe reduction in cardiac output. Intense sympathetic action causing vasoconstriction follows and maintains the perfusion pressure of arterial blood, although at subnormal levels, to the head and other vital organs. The pallor and sweating is the result of compensatory sympatheticotonia. It is probable that many homeostatic mechanisms are operative in the compensation of shock; the sympathetic nervous system and adrenal medulla are responsible for vasoconstriction; selective renal vasoconstriction causing a reduction in renal blood flow is responsible for fluid and electrolyte retention. Some degree of oliguria is always present in shock. If the shock state is prolonged it becomes irreversible and it is possible that the products of tissue anoxia are responsible for this.

The immediate causes of shock are severe external trauma and internal disasters to the major organs of the body. In the first category haemorrhage, crushing and burning are important factors causing loss of fluid and a fall in circulating blood volume; pain and possibly the products of tissue damage exert a further depressor action. The second category includes perforation of the gut, peritonitis, pancreatitis, acute severe diarrhoea and vomiting, overwhelming septicaemia and massive pulmonary embolism, but damage to the heart itself by cardiac infarction and acute pericardial tamponade is especially likely to cause shock because there are not only the factors of pain and tissue damage, but also the direct reduction of cardiac output through damage to the pump.

Treatment. Shock is a medical emergency, and treatment should be started as soon as the condition is diagnosed or before it occurs, if it can be anticipated. The immediate cause of the condition should be remedied if possible and as soon as possible, e.g. haemorrhage should be stopped or a perforated viscus repaired.

The patient should be kept warm but not hot, and sufficient morphine should be given to stop pain. Haemorrhage and all forms of traumatic shock are best treated by transfusion of blood, plasma or a plasma substitute. Saline or glucose saline solutions are useful but not as effective. The newer vasoconstrictor drugs such as L-noradrenaline raise arterial pressure and should be used if there is no sign of improvement after a few hours [p. 779]. Hydrocortisone appears to be effective in some cases, but its place in the treatment of shock is not yet established.

Prognosis depends on the nature and severity of the underlying cause, the response to treatment and upon the duration of the shock state.

REFERENCES

BRAUNWALD, E. (1965) The control of ventricular function in man, *Brit. Heart J.*, **27**, 1.

BURCHELL, H. (1964) A clinical appraisal of atrial transport function, *Lancet*, i, 775.

COURNAND, A. (1952) Discussion on the concept of cardiac failure in the light of recent physiologic studies in man, *Ann. intern. Med.*, **37**, 649.

DONALD, K. (1959) Exercise and heart disease, *Brit. med. J.*, **1**, 985.

EBERT, R. (1963) Syncope, *Circulation*, **27**, 1148.

HAYWARD, G. (1955) Pulmonary oedema, *Brit. med. J.*, **1**, 1361.

JACOBSON, E. D. (1968) A physiologic approach to shock, *New Engl. J. Med.*, **278**, 834.

KATZ, L. (1954) The mechanism of cardiac failure, *Circulation*, **10**, 663.

MACKENZIE, J. (1902) *The Study of the Pulse*, Edinburgh.

MCMICHAEL, J., and SHARPEY-SCHAFER, E. P. (1944) Cardiac output in man by a direct Fick method, *Brit. Heart J.*, **6**, 33.

MARSHALL, R. J., and SHEPHERD, J. T. (1968) *Cardiac Function in Health and Disease*, Philadelphia.

PAGE, A. (1964) Action of cardiac glycosides on heart-muscle cells, *Circulation*, **30**, 237.

PETERS, J. (1952) The problem of cardiac edema, *Amer. J. Med.*, **12**, 66.

RUSHMER, R., CITTERS, R., and FRANKLIN, D. (1962) Shock: a semantic enigma, *Circulation*, **26**, 445.

SPANN, J. F., MASON, W. T., and ZELIS, R. F. (1970) Recent advances in the understanding of congestive heart failure, *Mod. Conc. cardiov. Dis.*, **39**, 73.

WADE, D., and BISHOP, J. (1962) *Cardiac Output and Regional Blood Flow*, Oxford.

WEIL, M. H. (1967) *Diagnosis and Treatment of Shock*, Baltimore.

CARDIAC ARRHYTHMIA (DYSRHYTHMIA)

INTRODUCTION

Myocardium has an inherent rhythmicity, but certain specialized areas become dominant foci of stimulus formation. All myocardium has the capacity to conduct these stimuli and cause excitation of adjacent muscle, but this function is also carried out by specialized tissue bundles. This section is concerned with disorders of the rate and rhythm of impulse formation and disorders of stimulus conduction over the rest of the heart.

The cardiac impulse arises in the sino-atrial node which is situated in the right atrial muscle near the entrance of the superior vena cava and it produces normal heart rhythm known as sinus rhythm. The artery to the sino-atrial node arises from a coronary artery, usually the right one, near its origin from the aorta. The rate of impulse formation depends not only on spontaneous rhythmicity but also on neurogenic and humoral factors. Sympathetic cardio-accelerator fibres and vagal inhibitory fibres have a dominant influence. The natural rate of impulse formation at the sinus node (70 per min.) is rather higher than the inherent rhythmicity of lower centres. Excitation from the node spreads rapidly over the atria in all directions, inducing activity of the atrial myocardium which then stimulates the atrioventricular node. This focus is in the atrioventricular junctional tissues immediately to the right of the atrial septum, and is also influenced by the autonomic nervous system. Its own slower rhythm (60 per min.) is blocked normally by the higher frequency of the sino-atrial node. Conduction continues at a slower rate through the node and the ventricular muscle is reached by the bundle of His which divides into left and right bundle branches in the upper part of the septum. Each branch lies in the subendocardium of the septum and subsequently breaks up into a network of fine conducting fibres (Purkinje fibres) which remain in the ventricular subendocardium. Excitation of the ventricular muscle appears to spread from the endocardium to the epicardium. The inherent rate of impulse formation of foci in the ventricular muscle is 40 per min., but these are blocked by the higher rate of stimuli from supraventricular centres. The arrhythmias may be classified in various ways. The following order is adopted here:

1. Sinus rhythm:
   tachycardia, bradycardia, sinus arrest and phasic arrhythmia.
2. Ectopic beats and ectopic rhythm:
   atrial, nodal and ventricular.
3. Tachycardias; paroxysmal and otherwise:
   paroxysmal tachycardia (atrial);
   atrial flutter;
   atrial fibrillation;
   ventricular tachycardia;
   ventricular fibrillation.
4. Disorders of conduction.

SINUS RHYTHM

SINUS TACHYCARDIA

Tachycardia means a fast heart rate. Normal resting rates lie between 50 and 90 beats per minute. In sinus tachycardia the increased rate is due to increased rhythmicity of the sinus node and this is largely due to diminished vagal tone or sympathetic stimulation. Sinus tachycardia merges imperceptibly from the physiological response to effort, emotion and digestion into the pathological, which is only significant when considered in relation to its cause.

Aetiology

Tachycardia is found in all forms of heart failure, where it appears to be caused by the failure in some general way or by local damage to the myocardium. In some forms it may be compensatory in maintaining a higher than normal cardiac output but mostly it makes failure worse by diminishing the period of myocardial rest and recovery. Sinus tachycardia occurs in all conditions with a high cardiac output, such as thyrotoxicosis, arteriovenous aneurysm, aneamia, beriberi and anoxic cor pulmonale. Here it is a factor in maintaining the high output. Tachycardia occurs in most infectious diseases, especially those accompanied by carditis.

Tachycardia may be caused by excessive use of tea, coffee, tobacco, alcohol or certain drugs, especially those affecting autonomic activity, e.g. atropine and adrenaline. Simple tachycardia is a common symptom

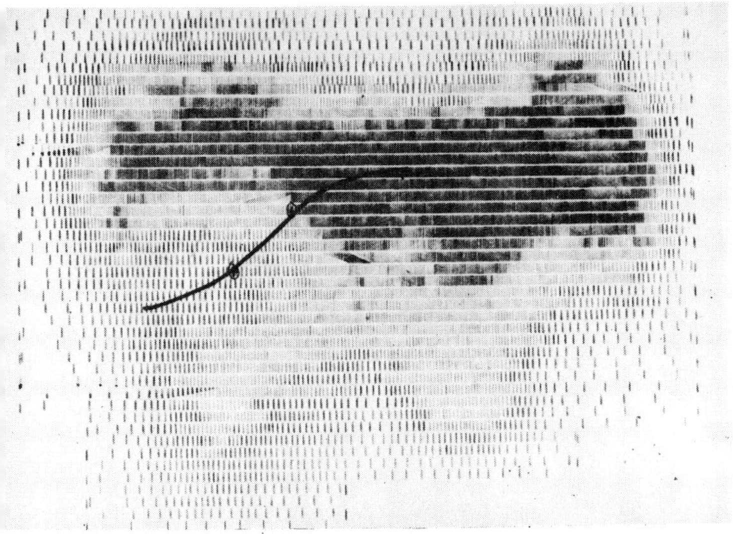

echnetium scan of liver containing multiple neoplastic deposits. The right costal argin is shown by the continuous line. The liver is much enlarged and a large art of the inferior part of both lobes is failing to take up the isotope due to he presence of neoplasm.

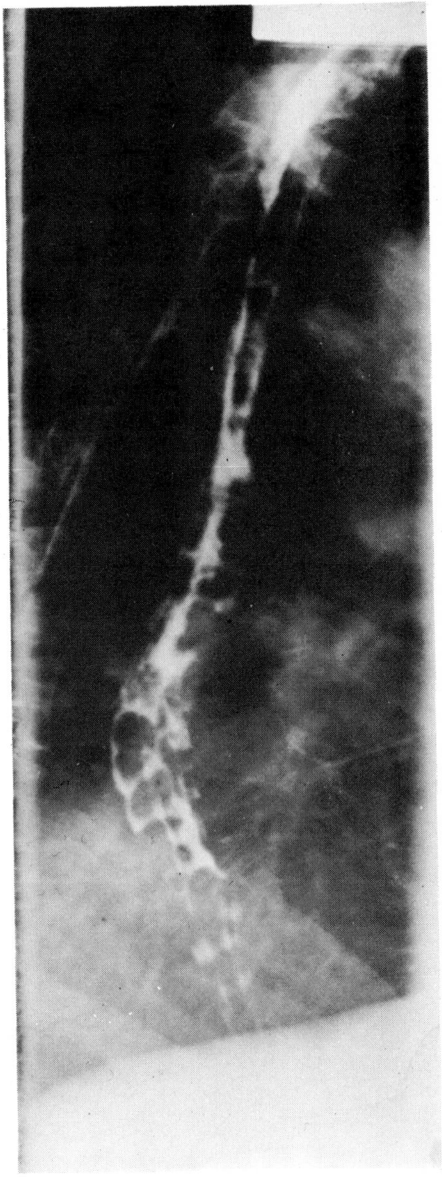

Barium swallow showing large oesophageal varices.

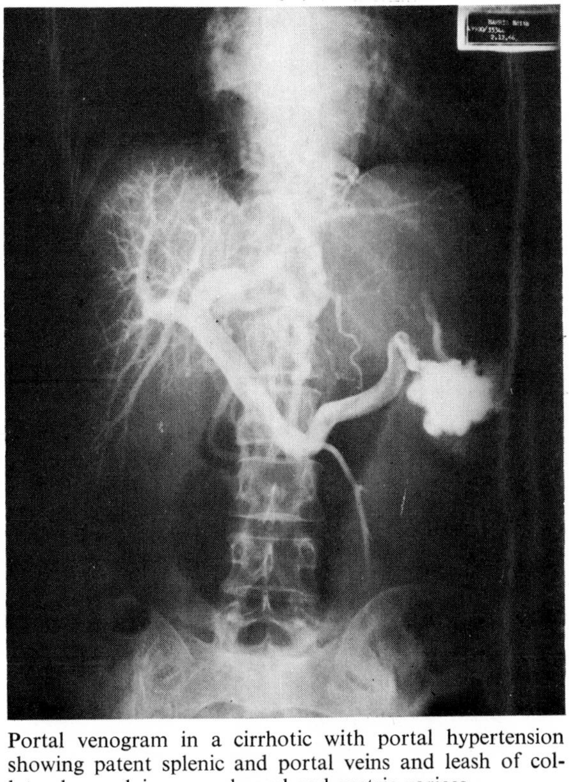

Portal venogram in a cirrhotic with portal hypertension showing patent splenic and portal veins and leash of collaterals supplying oesophageal and gastric varices.

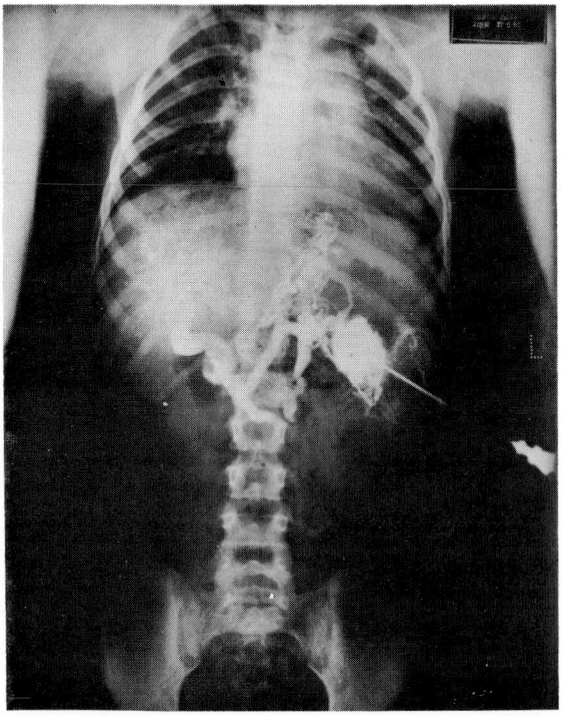

Portal venogram from a child with extrahepatic portal obstruction. There are many collaterals and the portal vein though appearing patent was occluded, the cavernomatous transformation around it consisting of large superficial and hepatic capsular veins.

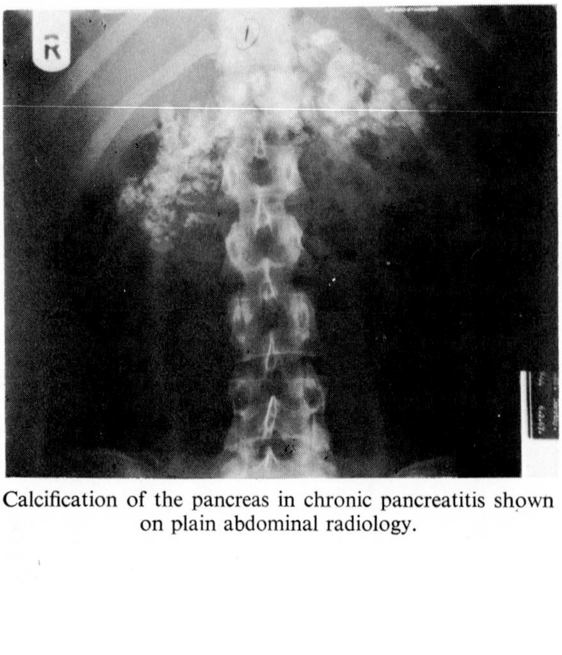

Calcification of the pancreas in chronic pancreatitis shown on plain abdominal radiology.

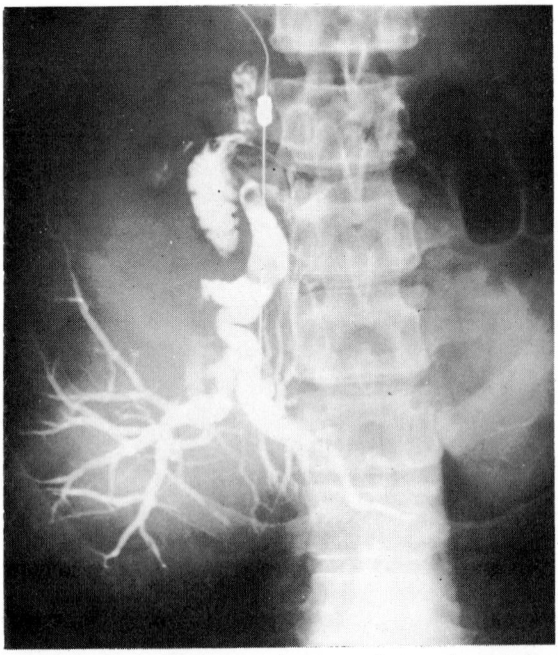

Transhepatic cholangiogram showing gall-stone impacted at the lower end of a dilated common bile-duct. Contrast has also entered the duodenum.

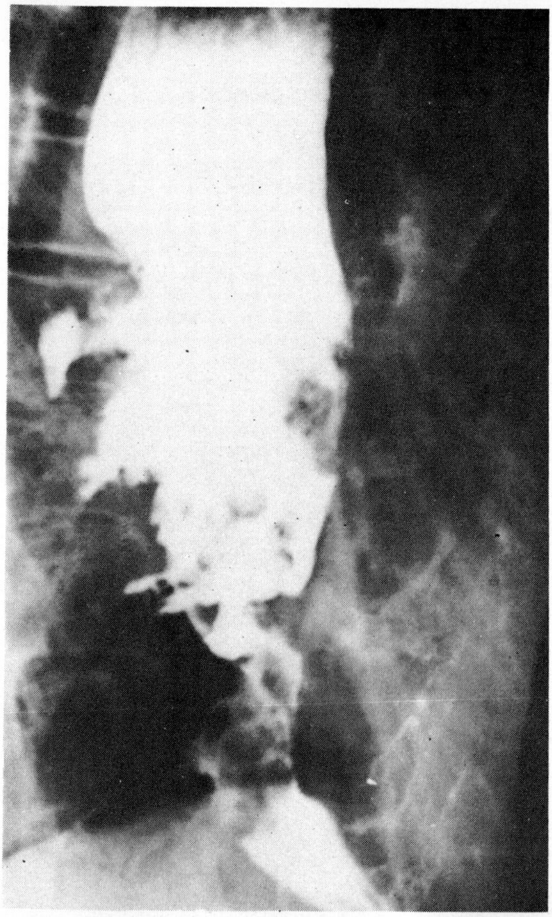

Large carcinoma of the oesophagus. This patient had had dysphagia for only 3 months.

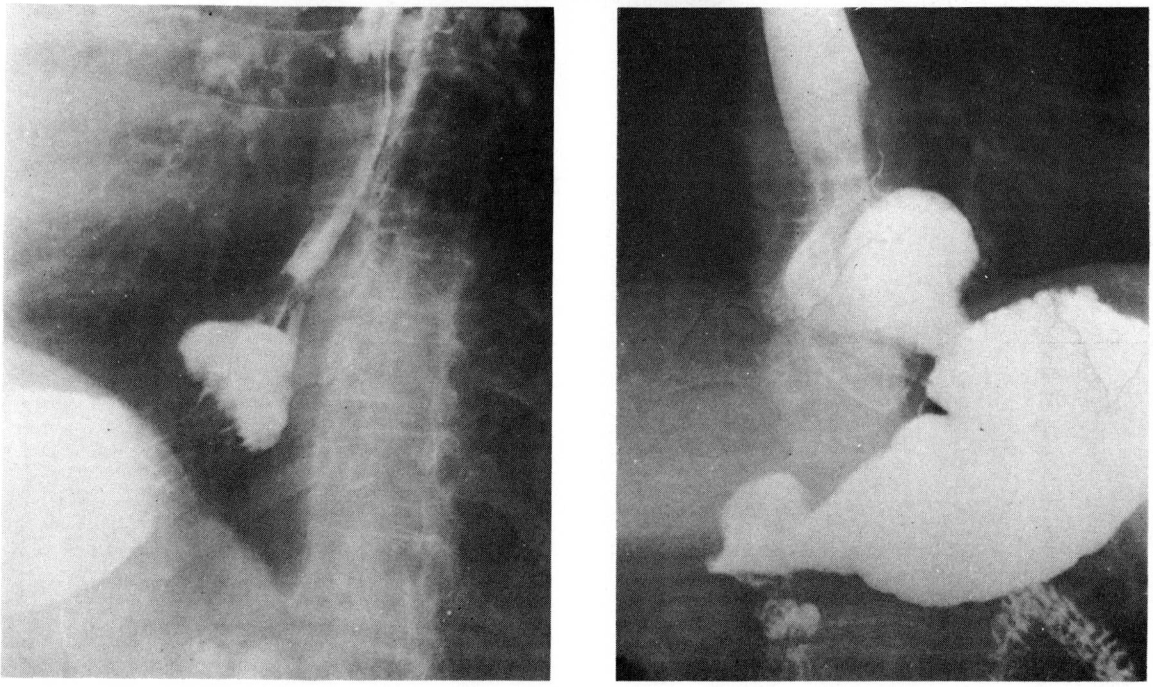

(a) (b)

Hiatus hernia. (a) Sliding hiatus hernia: note gastro-oesophageal junction above the diaphragm. (b) Para-oesophageal hernia: gastro-oesophageal junction below the diaphragm.

PLATE 4

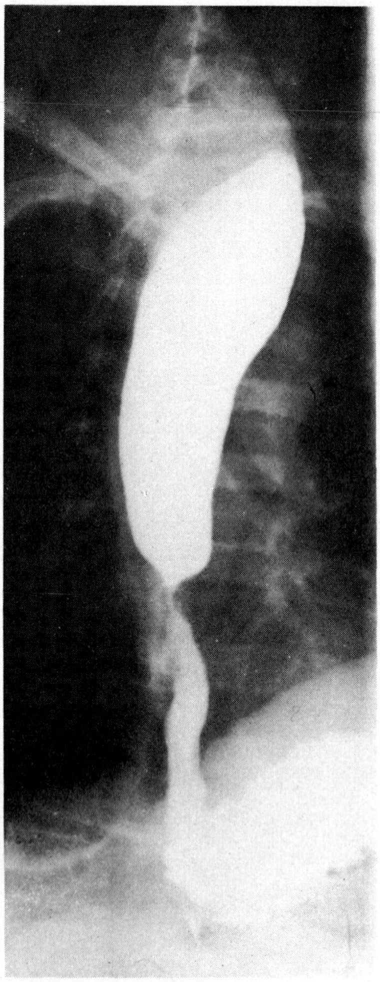

Benign oesophageal stricture associated with a sliding hiatus hernia.

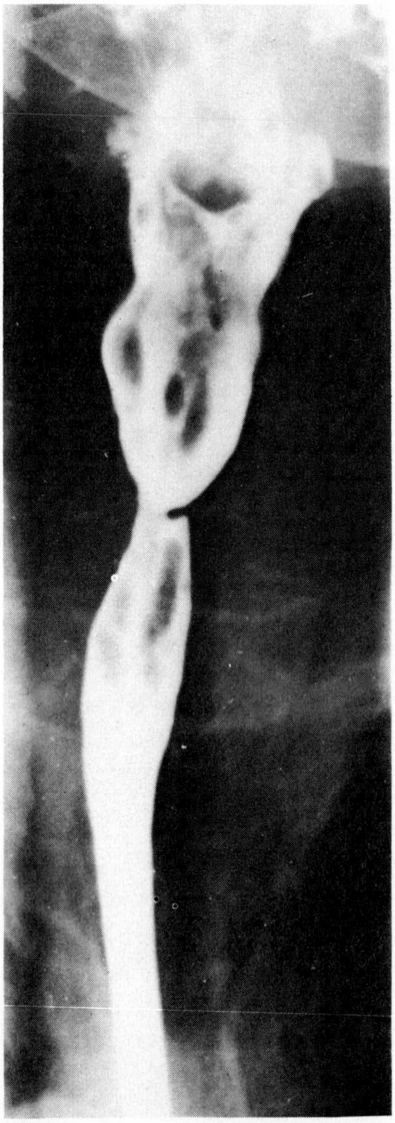

Barium swallow showing post-cricoid web. This patient had long-standing iron deficiency due to coeliac disease.

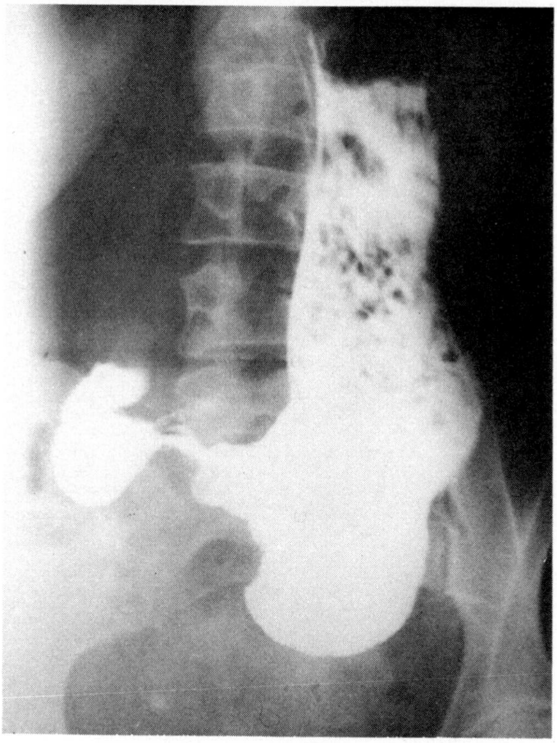

Prepyloric carcinoma of the stomach: food residue present.

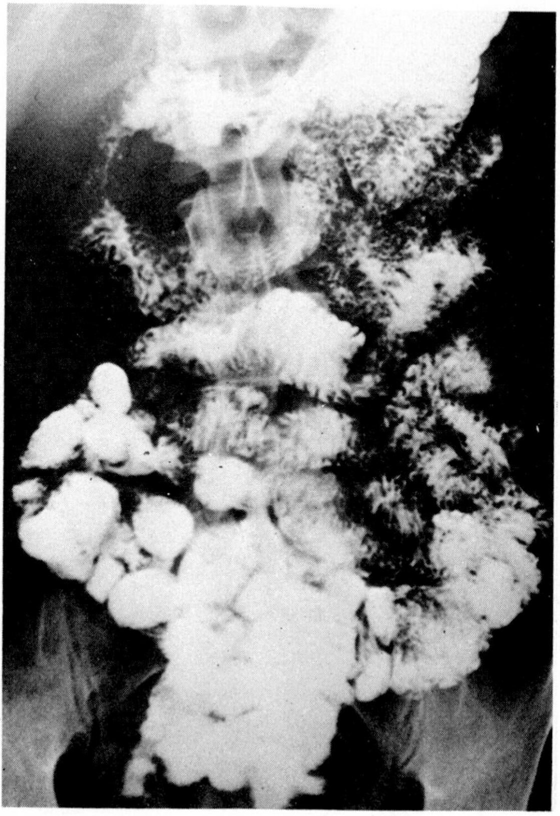

(a)

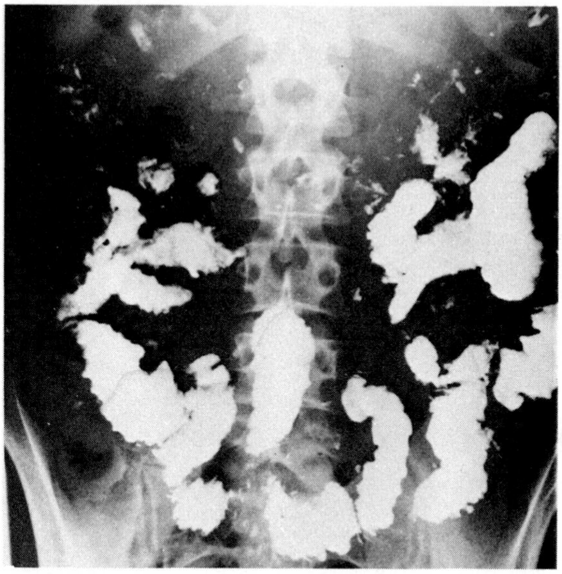

(b)

(a) Normal barium follow through. (b) Barium follow through in a patient with gross malabsorption. Note clumping of barium, dilated loops and loss of normal mucosal pattern.

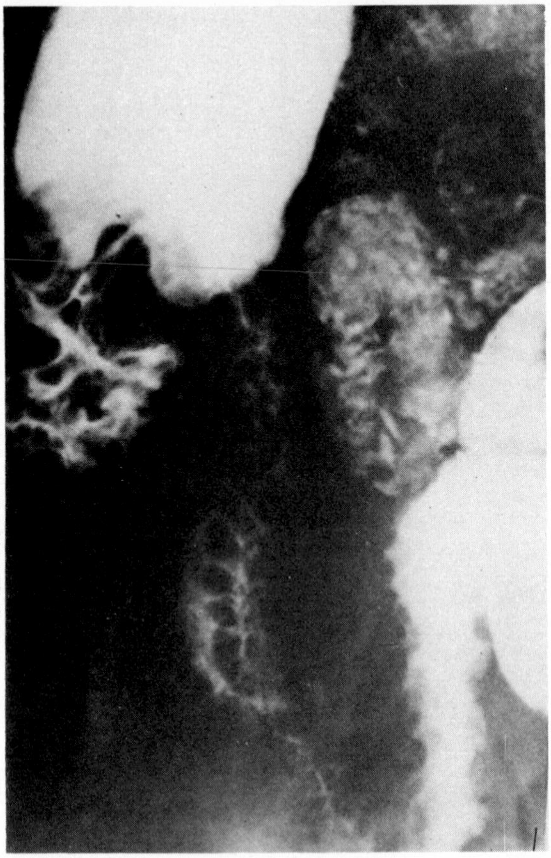

Crohn's disease—involvement of the ileum by ulcerative lesion; the terminal ileum has a cobblestone appearance.

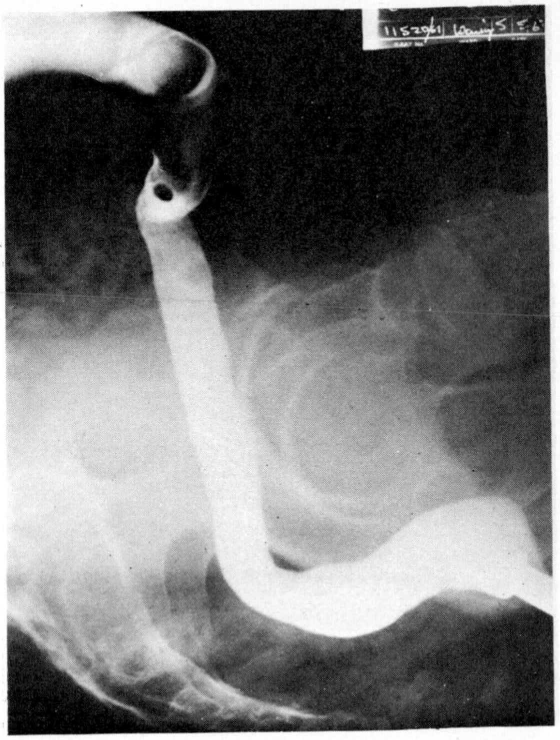

Ulcerative colitis with coincidental carcinoma. Lateral view of the rectum. Note enlarged presacral space, loss of haustration and mucosal pattern. A filling defect due to a carcinoma is shown at the rectosigmoid junction.

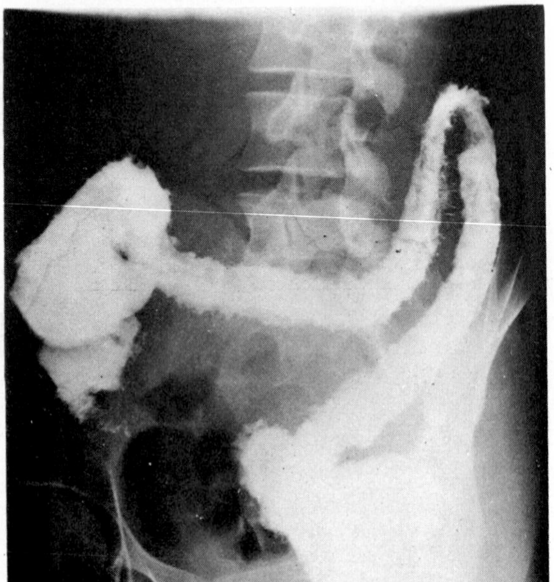

Crohn's disease of the colon. Note very deep ulceration. There is often rectal sparing, discontinuous and asymmetrical involvement of the colon. Fistulas and strictures may also be seen.

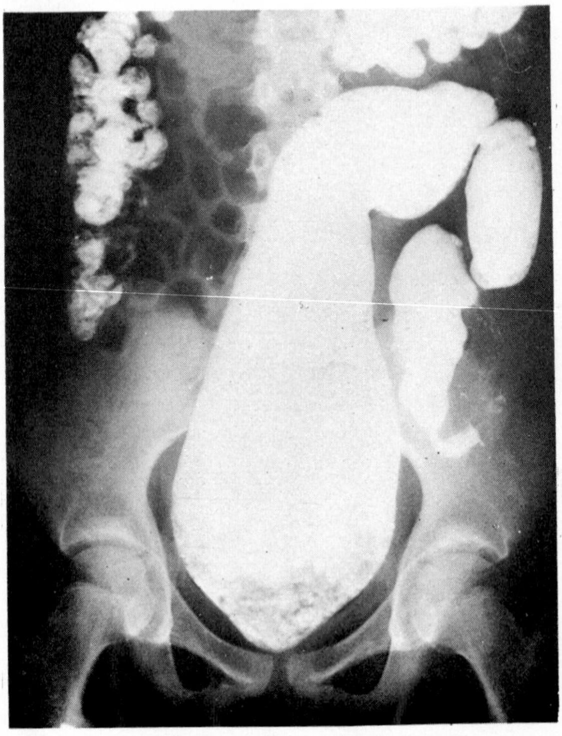

Megarectum due to dyschezia.

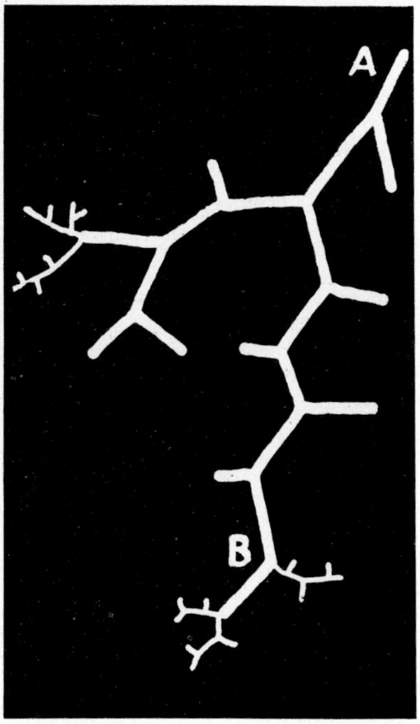

(a)

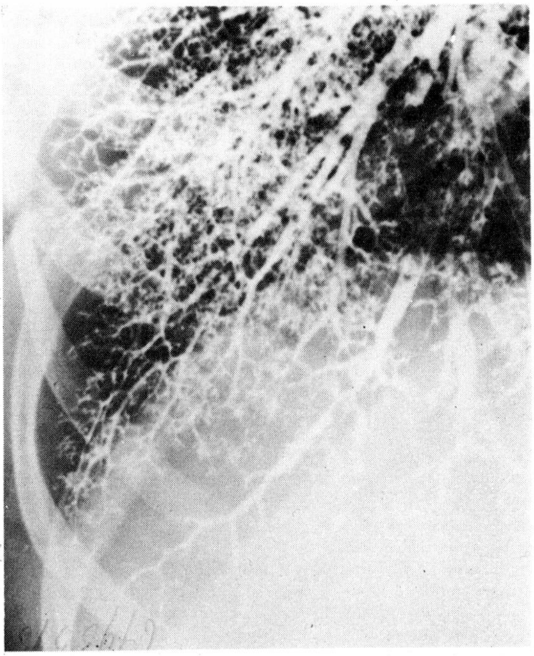

(b)

End of the bronchial pathway. (a) Diagram to show pattern of branching; at first the branches are at intervals of 0·5–1·0 cm., A–B, and beyond B they arise at intervals of approximately 2 mm. (millimetre pattern). (b) Anterior view of bronchogram of lower part of the right lung showing the short and fine ultimate lines, about 2 mm. long and arising at intervals of about 2 mm. (millimetre pattern).

(Reproduced by permission of the Authors and the Editor of *Thorax*.)

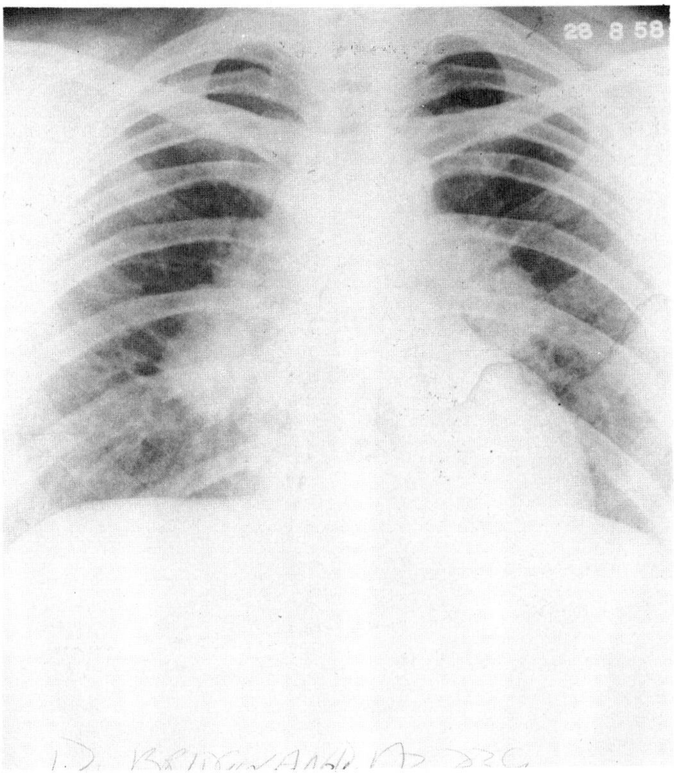

Sarcoidosis with bilateral hilar lymphadenopathy (BHL).

PLATE 8

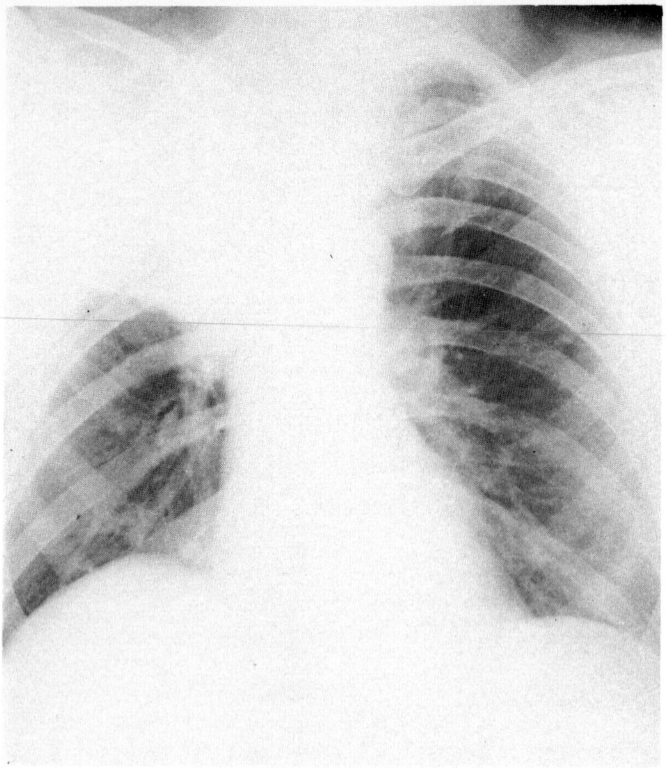

(a)

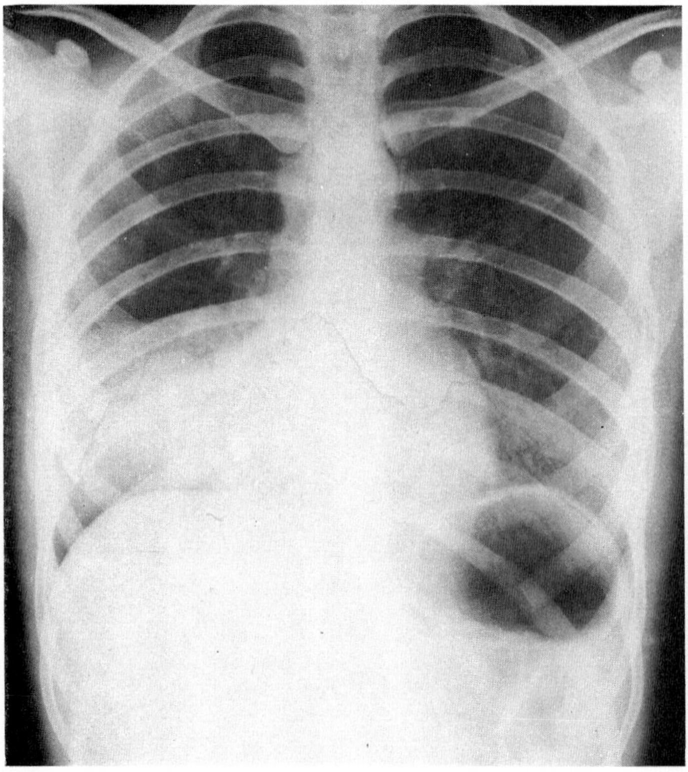

(b)

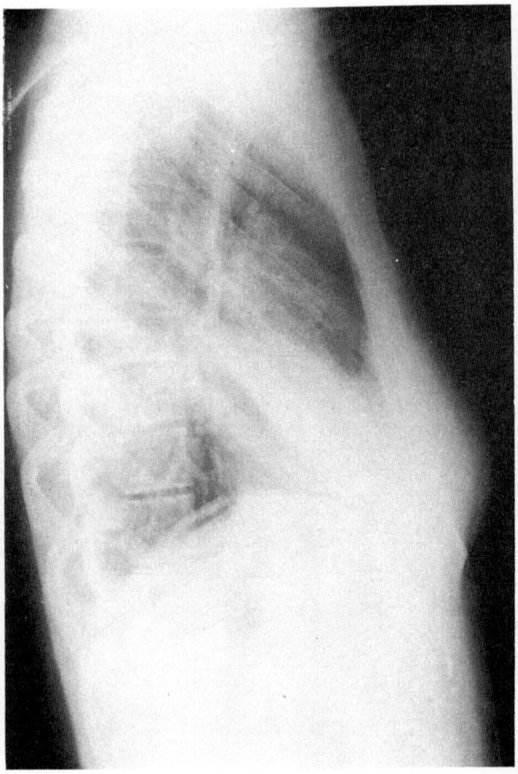

(c)

Homogeneous shadowing in pneumonia.
(a) Right upper lobe consolidation complete with a little shrinkage. (b and c) Right middle lobe. Complete consolidation seen in postero-anterior (b) and lateral (c) views.

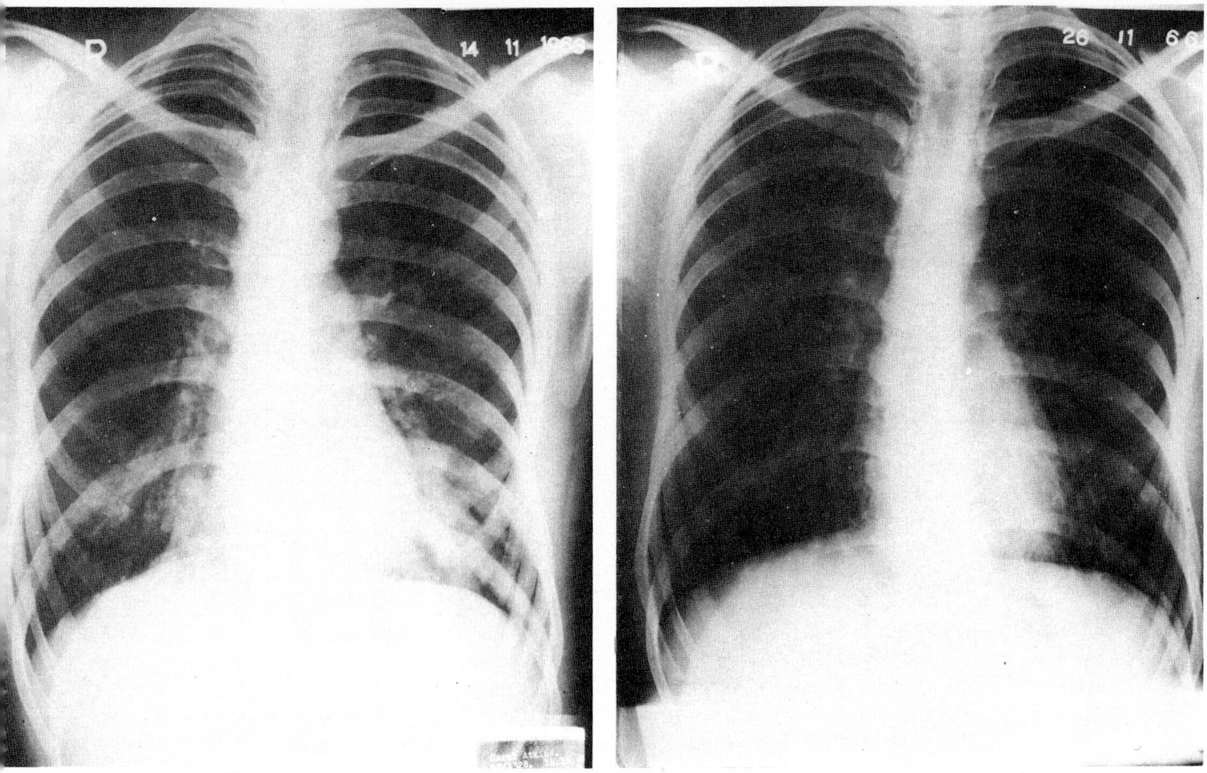

Plain chest radiograph of a patient with bronchiectasis before and after treatment.

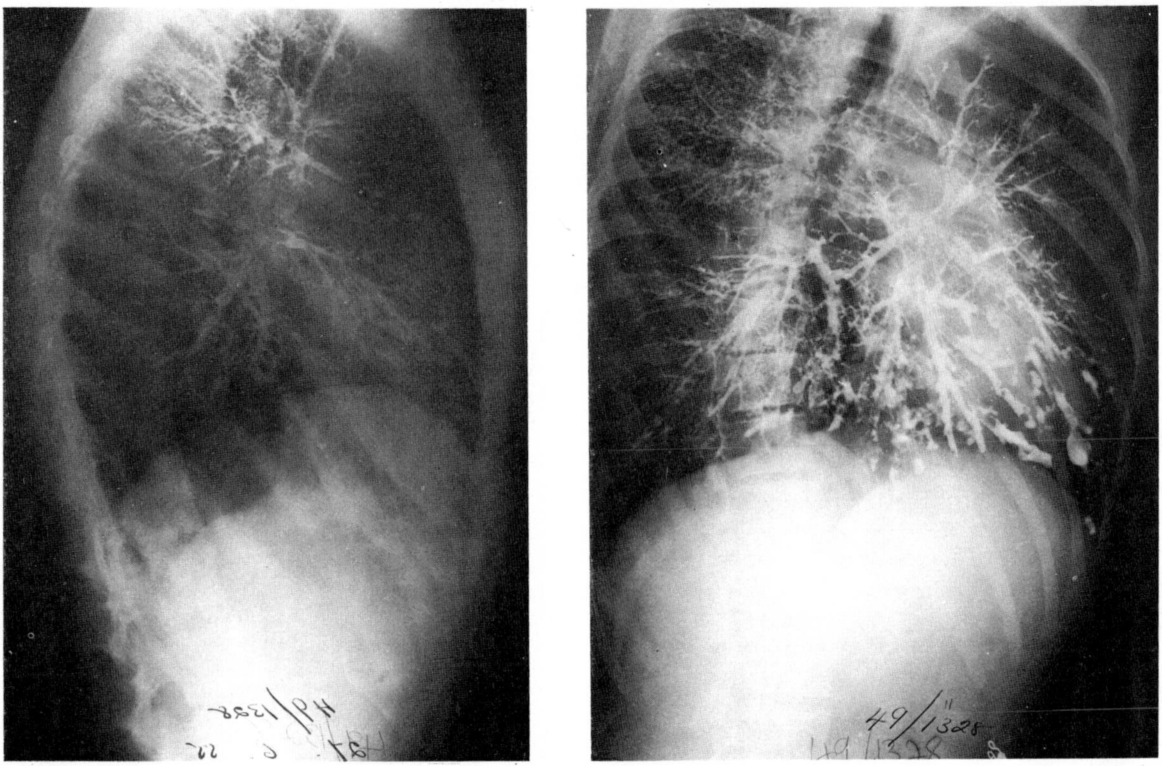

(a) (b)

Bronchogram of a patient with bilateral bronchiectasis. (a) Right lateral view showing abnormalities of the middle lower lobe bronchi. (b) Right anterior oblique view showing abnormal bronchi in the lingular segment of the left upper lobe and whole of the left lower lobe.

PLATE 10

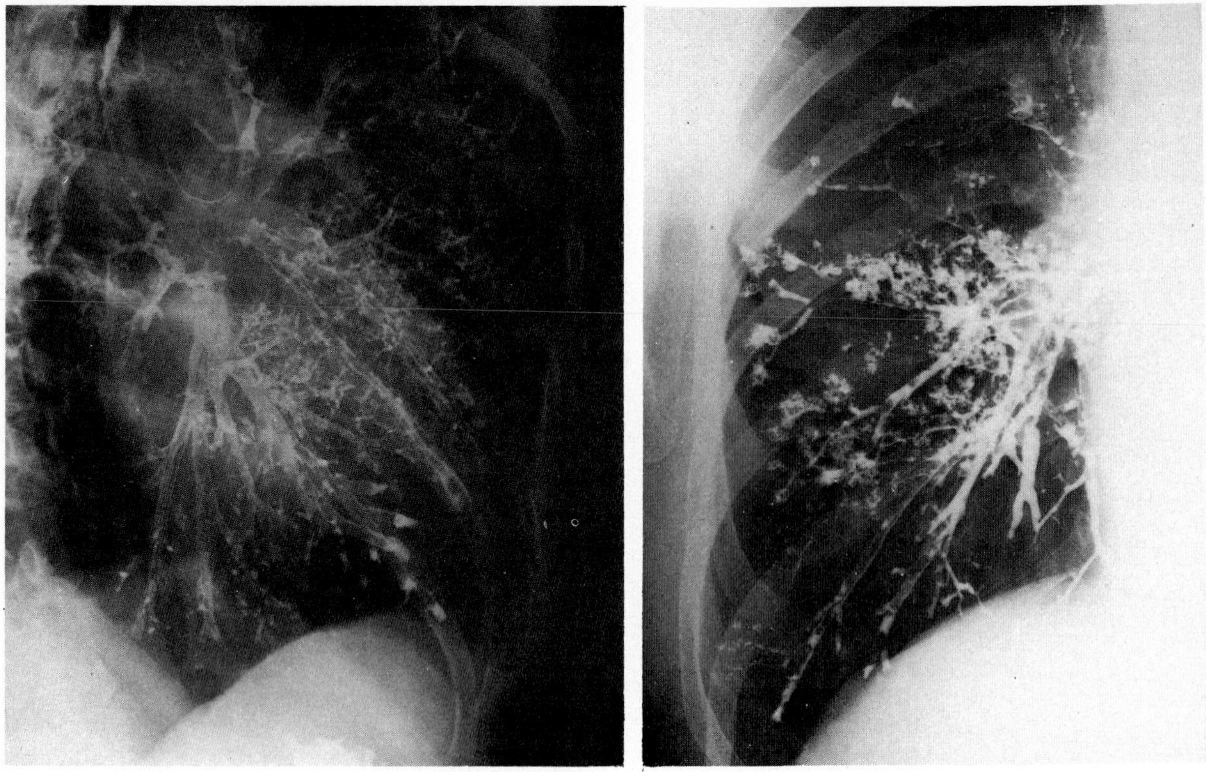

Characteristic bronchographic appearance in chronic bronchitis.

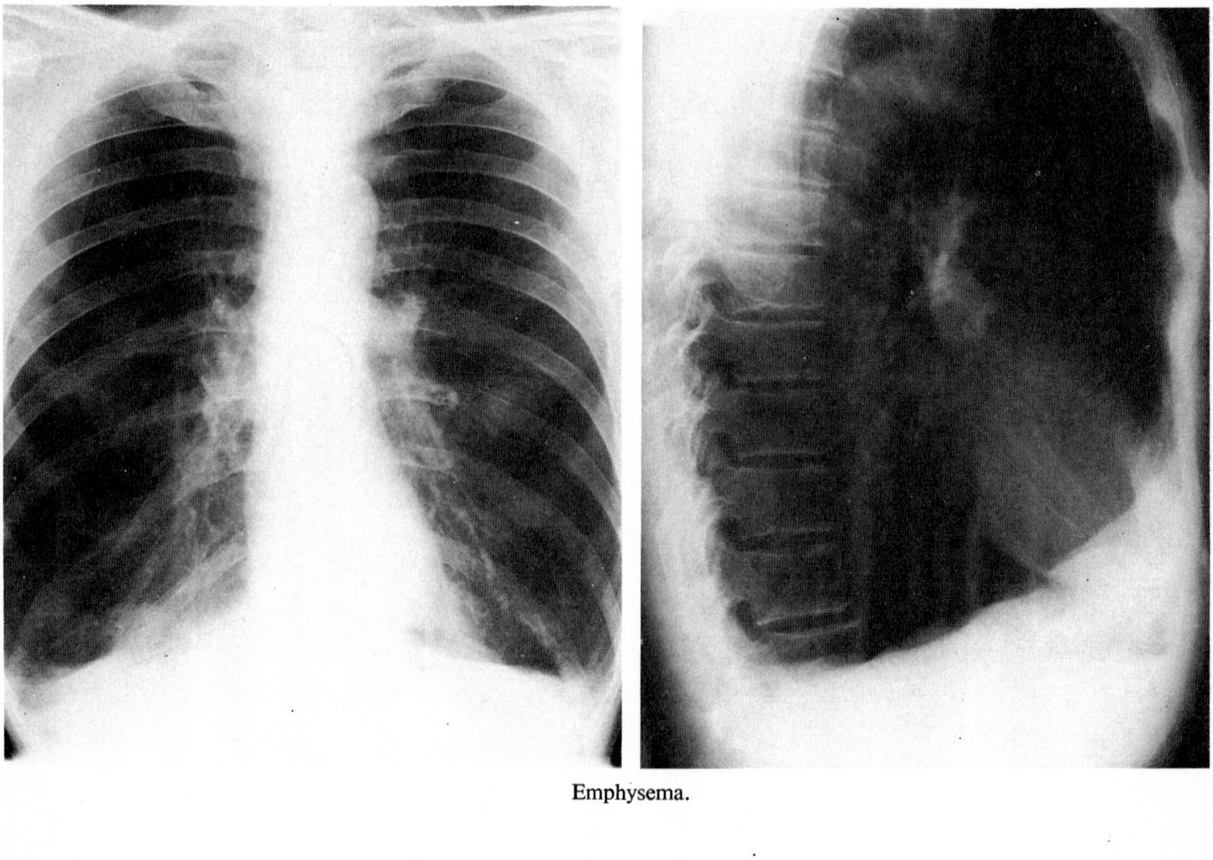

Emphysema.

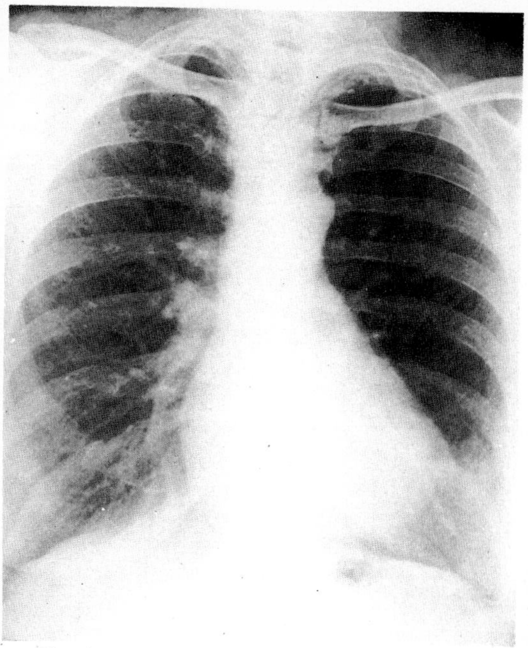

Emphysema of left lung (Macleod's syndrome).

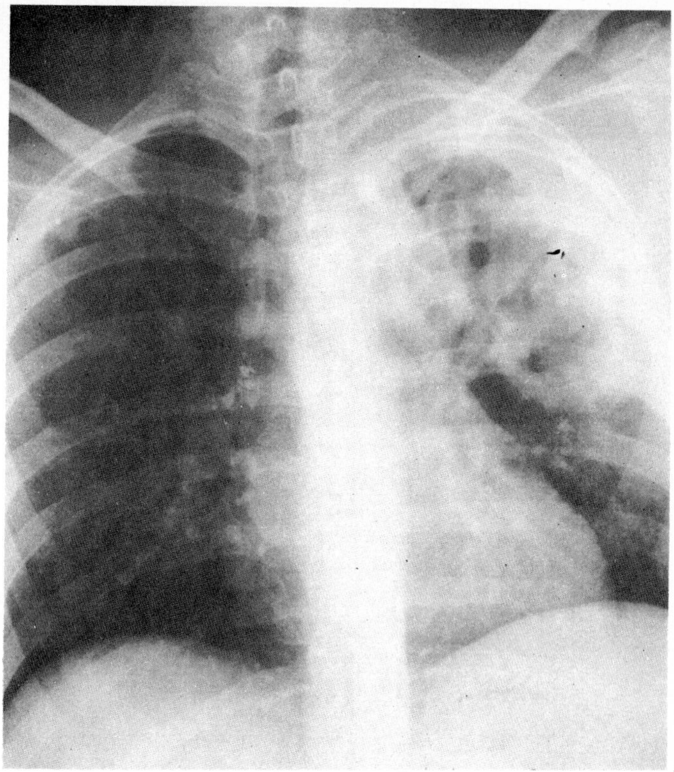

Massive shadowing and cavitation in Wegener's granuloma.

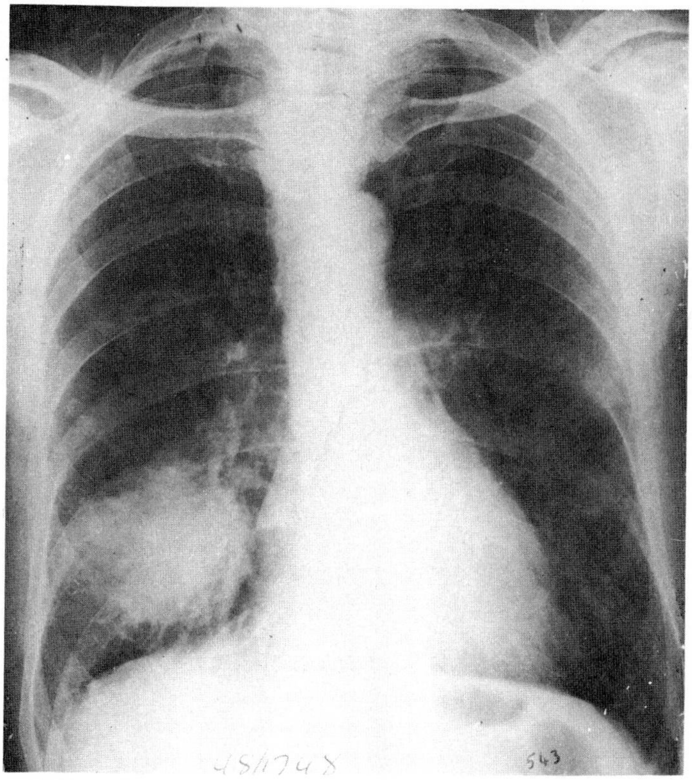

Massive round shadow due to carcinoma of the bronchus.

PLATE 12

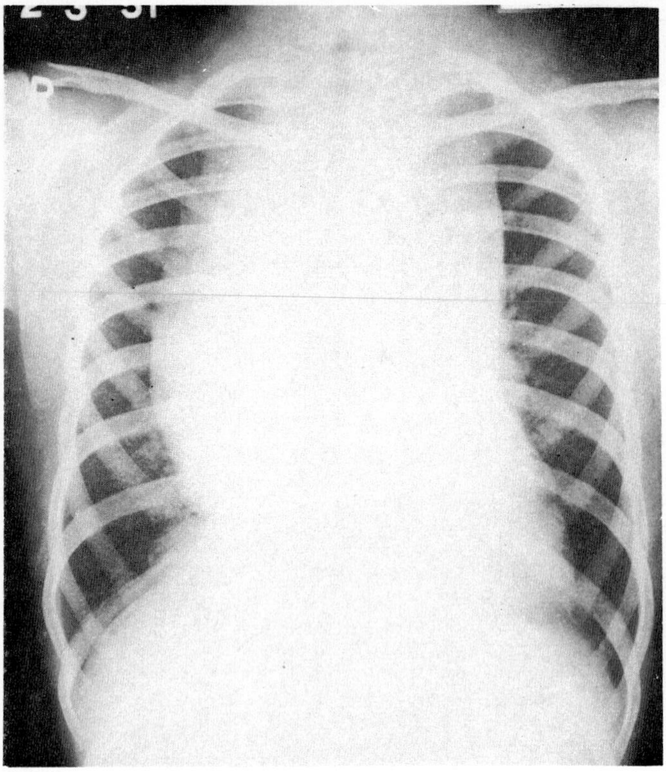

Shadow of enlarged mediastinal lymph nodes in Hodgkin's disease.

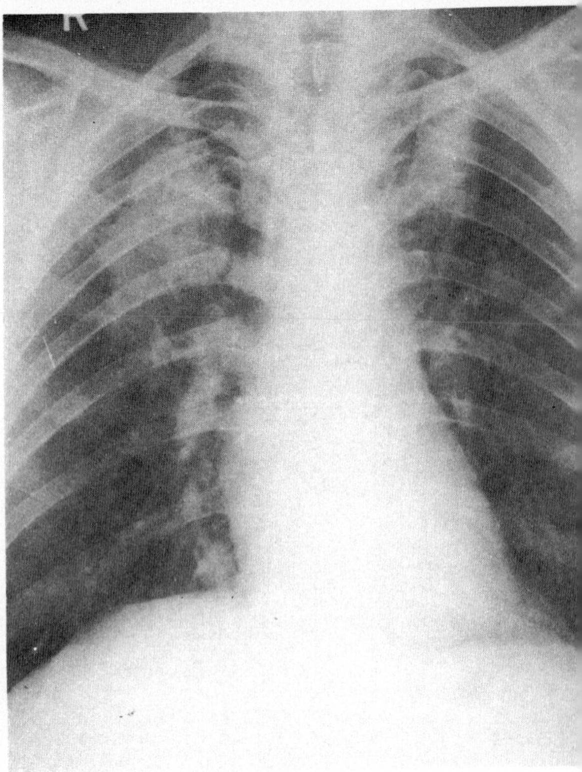

Characteristic upper zone shadows of progressive massive fi (P.M.F.) in pneumoconiosis.

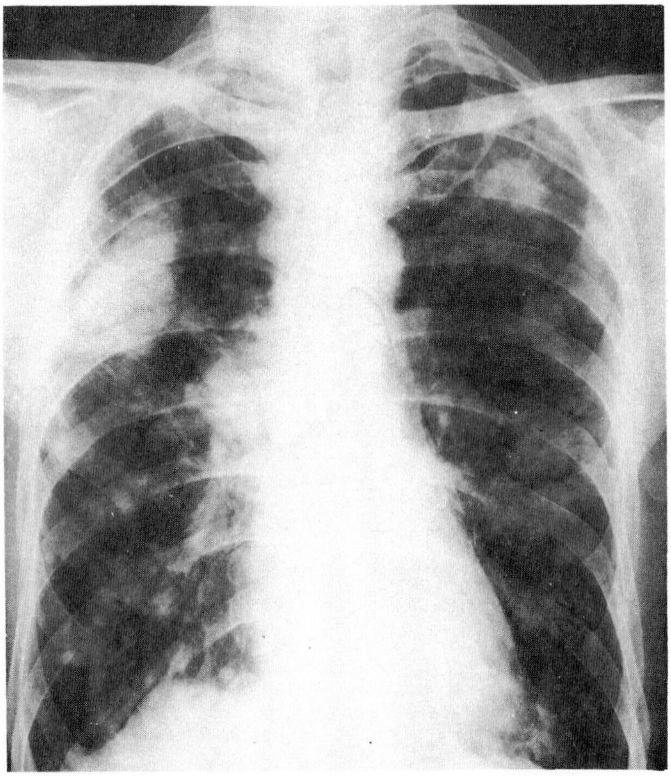

Rheumatoid pneumoconiosis (Caplan's syndrome); discrete shadows throughout the lungs.

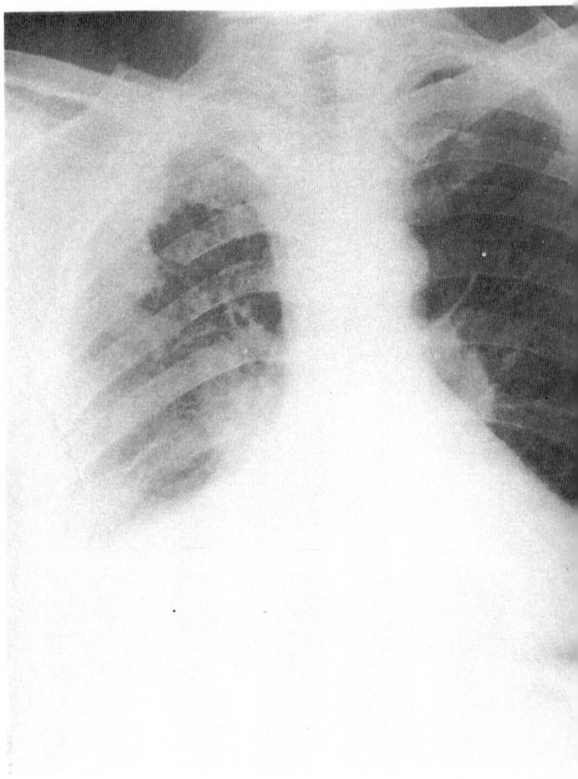

Asbestosis. Mesothelioma and pleural effusion (right)

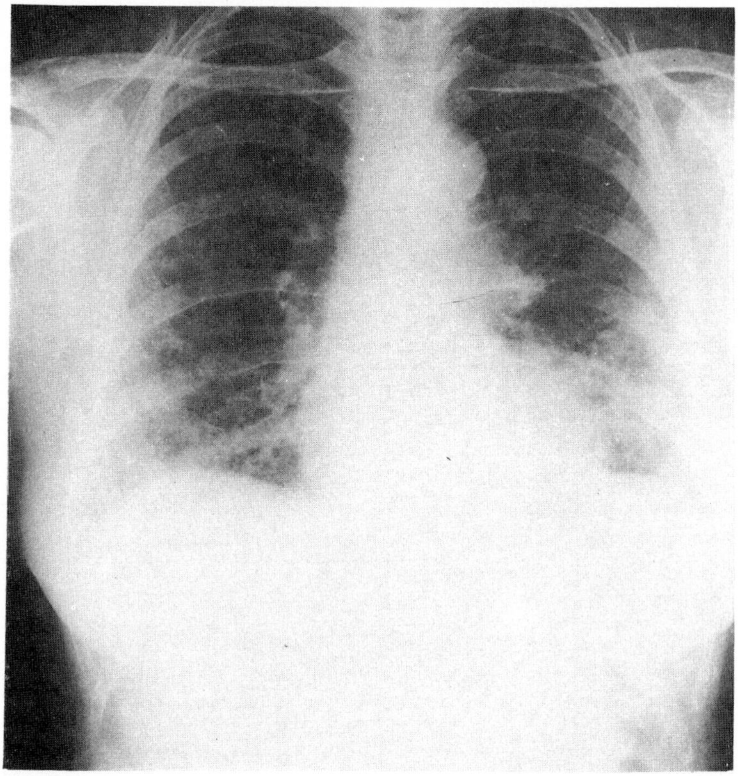

Fibrosing alveolitis with diffuse nodular and micronodular shadowing in middle and lower zones.

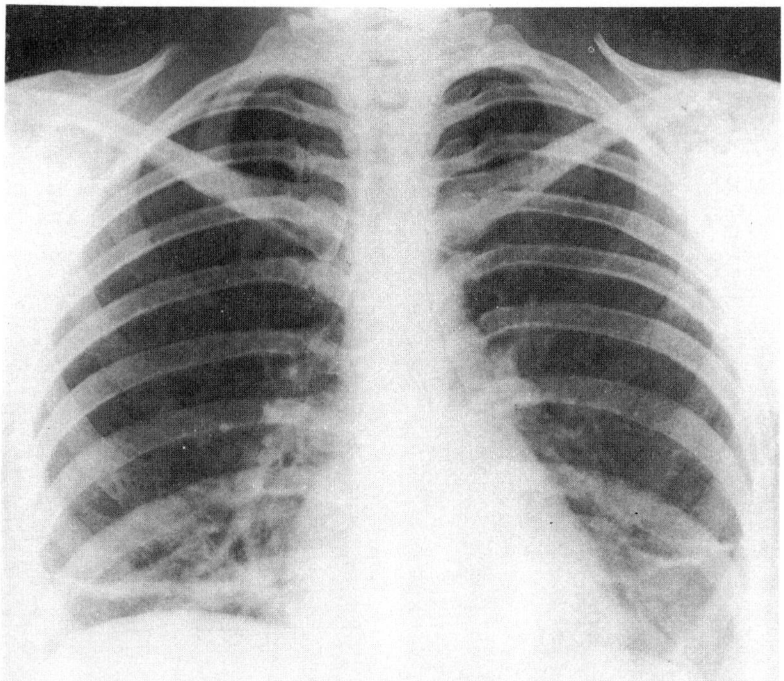

Systemic lupus erythematosus (S.L.E.) showing long basal linear shadows and elevated diaphragms.

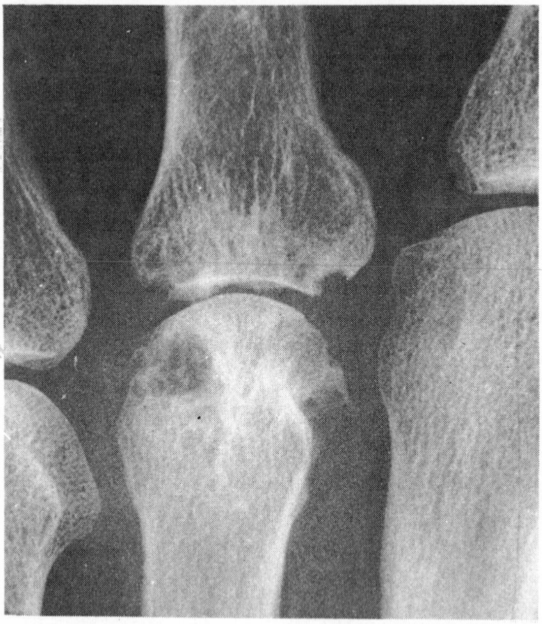

Rheumatoid erosions in metacarpophalangeal joint.

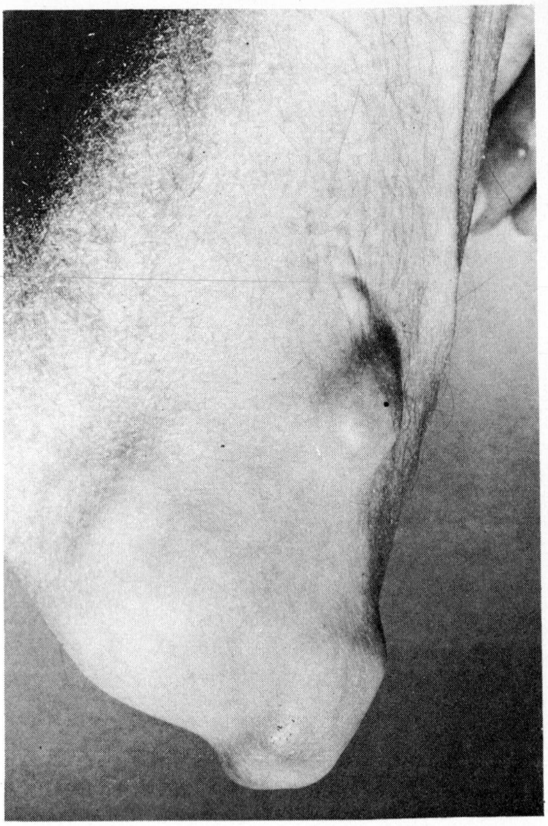

Subcutaneous nodules on extensor aspect of elbow in rheumatoid arthritis.

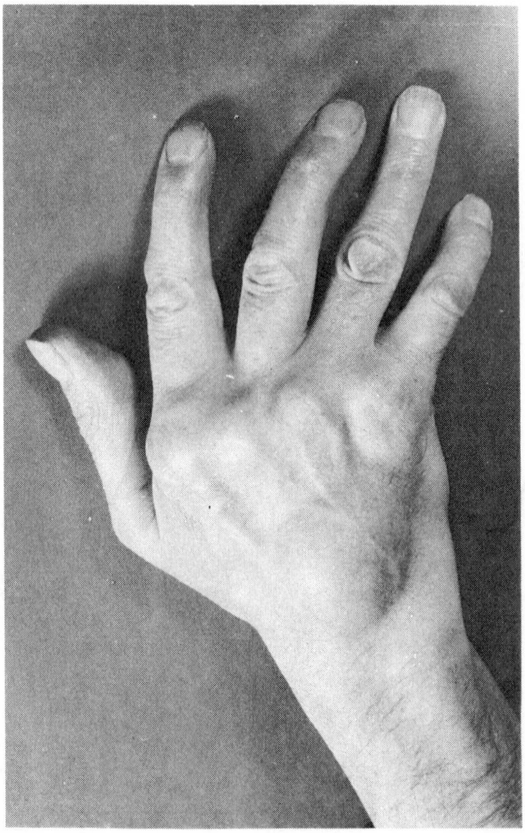

(a)

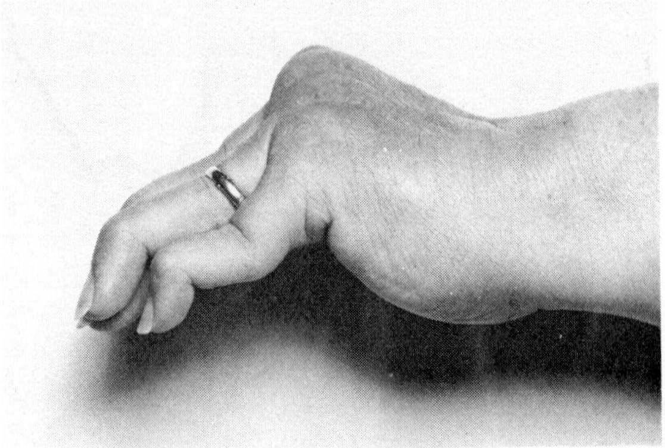

(b)

Two common deformities of the hand in rheumatoid arthritis.
(a) Ulnar deviation at the metacarpophalangeal joints. Note the synovial proliferation on the dorsum of the wrist.
(b) 'Swan-neck' deformity of the fingers.

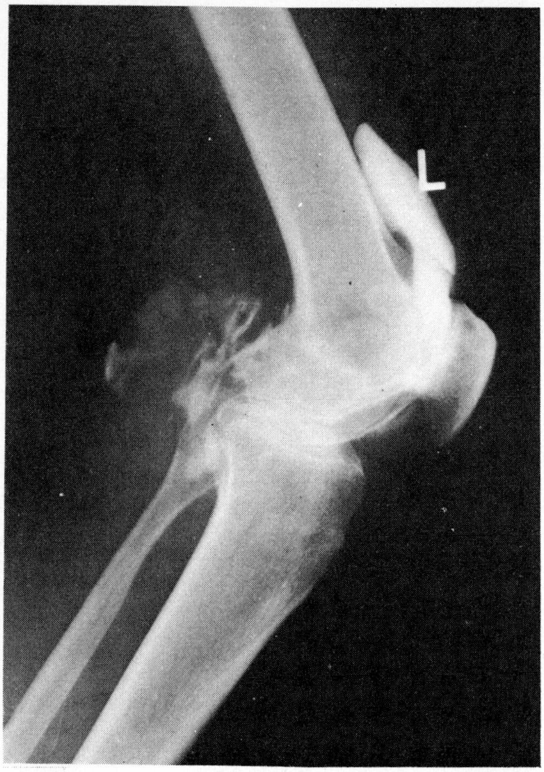

Arthrogram of knee joint in rheumatoid arthritis. The joint cavity communicates with a cystic swelling in the popliteal fossa.

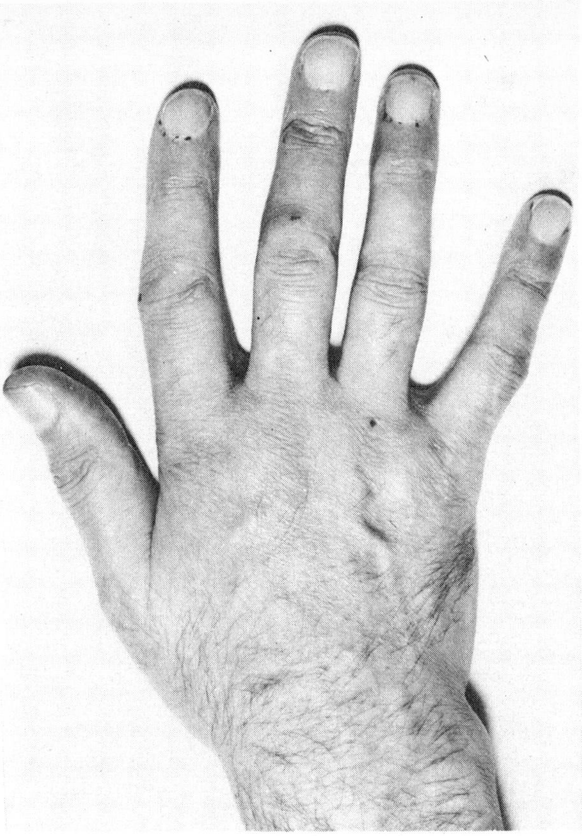

Arteritic lesions in rheumatoid arthritis. These often appear as small dark ischaemic areas around the nail folds.

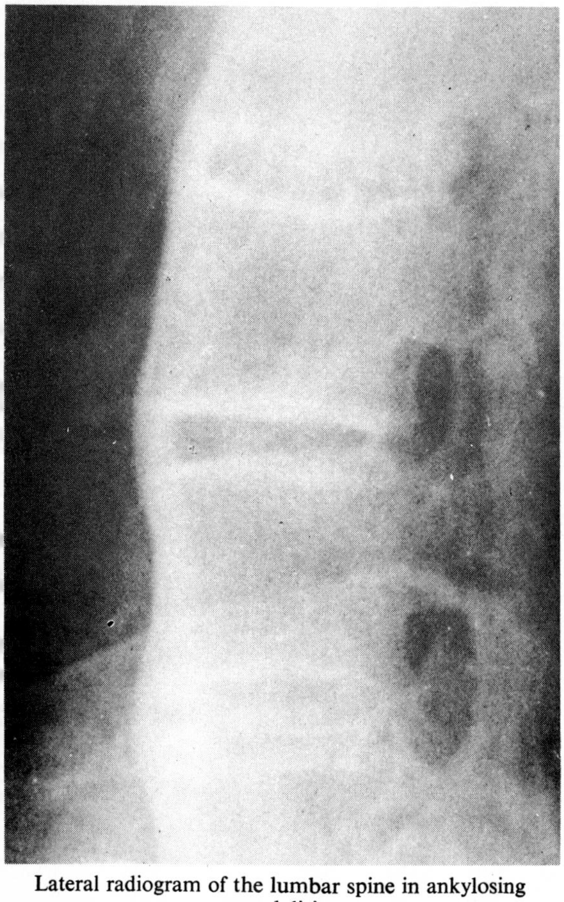

Lateral radiogram of the lumbar spine in ankylosing spondylitis.

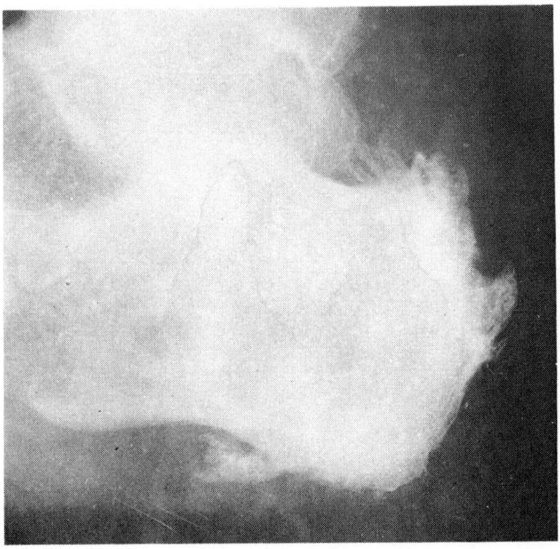

Reiter's disease. The characteristic florid periostitis associated with this condition is well shown around the os calcis.

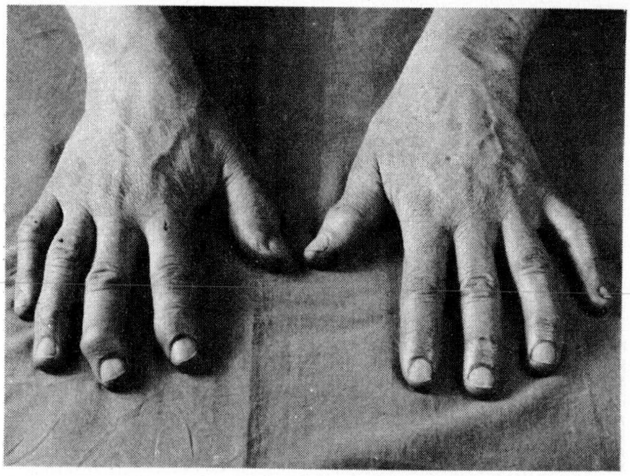

Heberden's nodes.

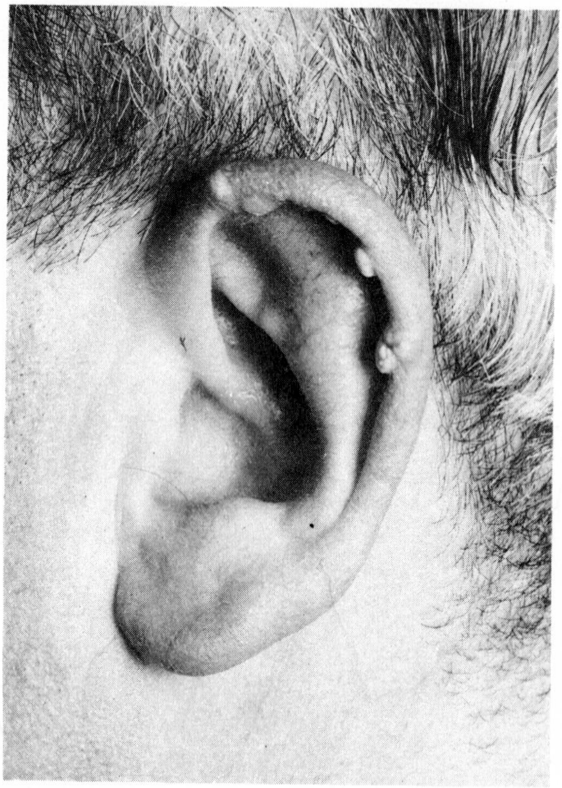

Tophi on the pinna of the ear in chronic gout.

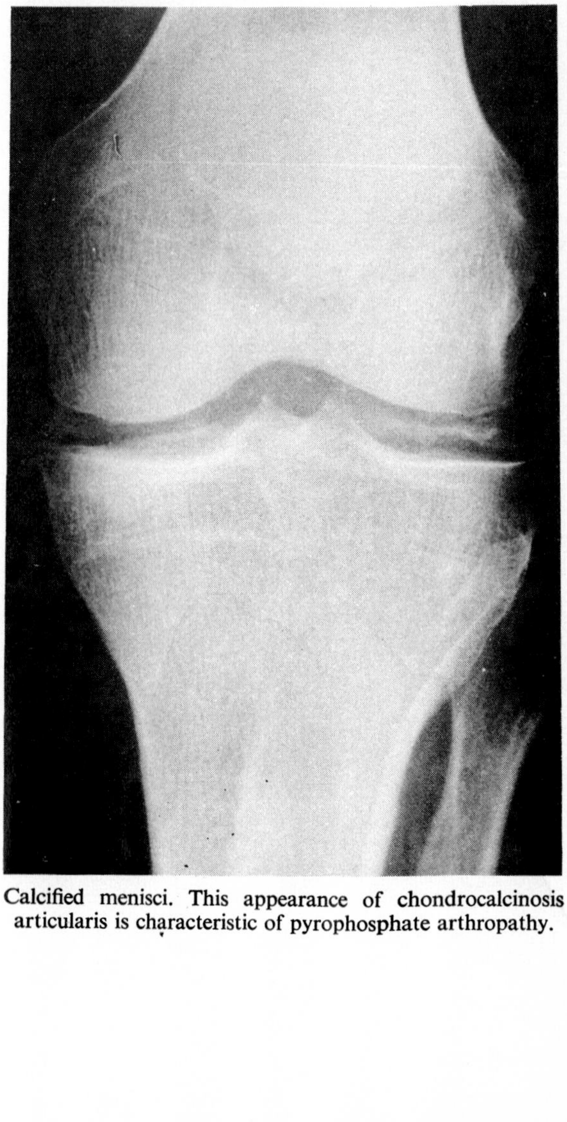

Calcified menisci. This appearance of chondrocalcinosis articularis is characteristic of pyrophosphate arthropathy.

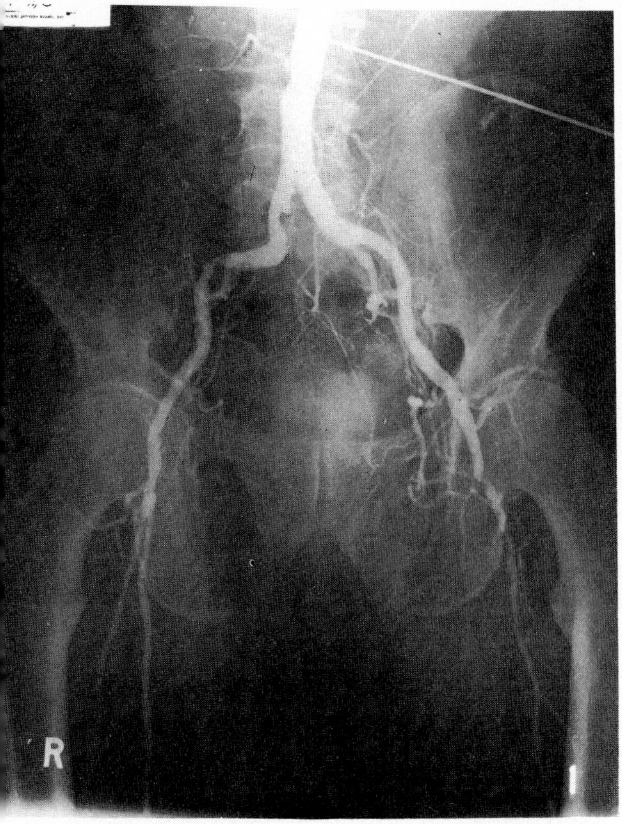

Aortogram showing irregularity of aortic outline and its branches due to severe atheroma, leading to peripheral arterial obstruction.

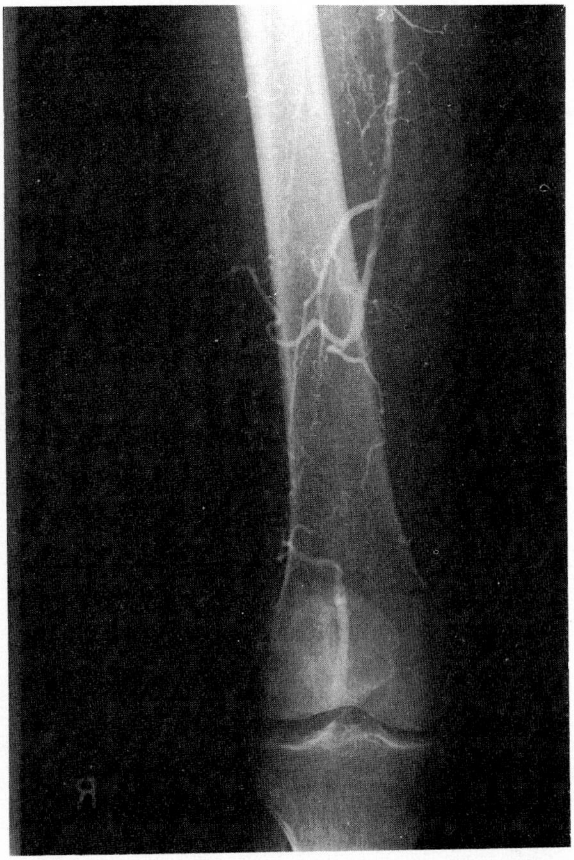

Femoral artery occlusion, showing well developed collateral circulation.

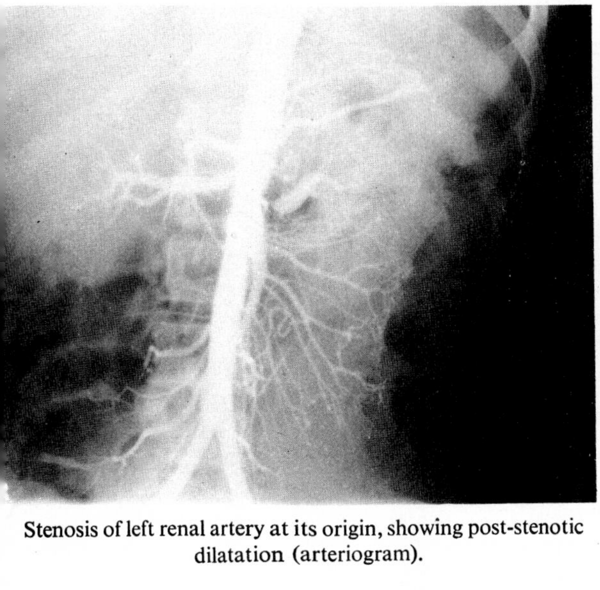

Stenosis of left renal artery at its origin, showing post-stenotic dilatation (arteriogram).

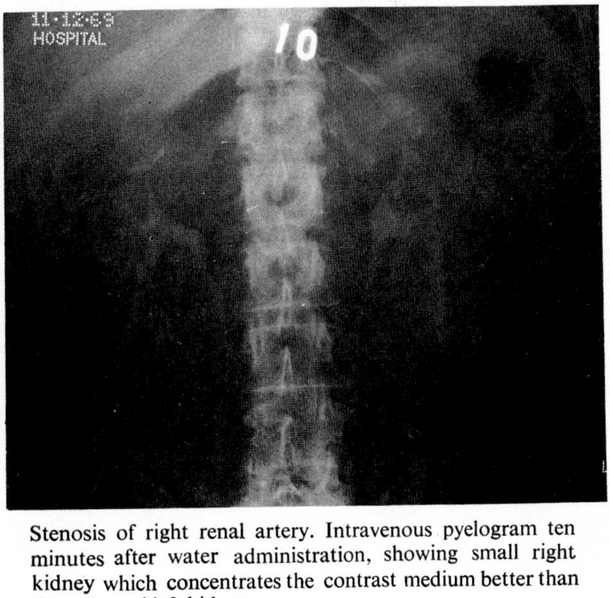

Stenosis of right renal artery. Intravenous pyelogram ten minutes after water administration, showing small right kidney which concentrates the contrast medium better than the enlarged left kidney.

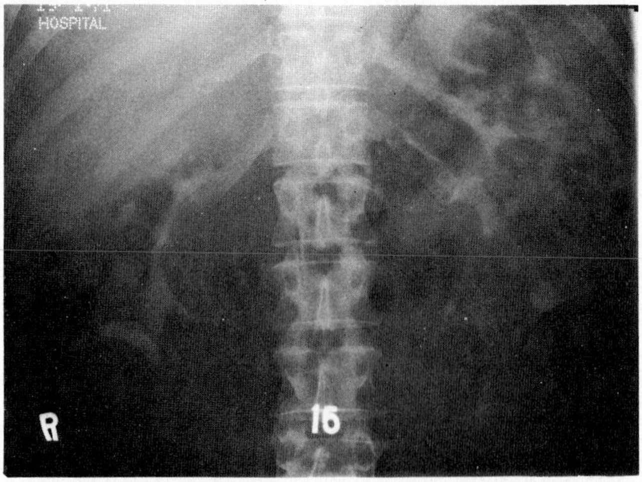

Congenital polycystic kidneys. Distortion and compression of renal pelves and calyces by cysts. Intravenous pyelogram.

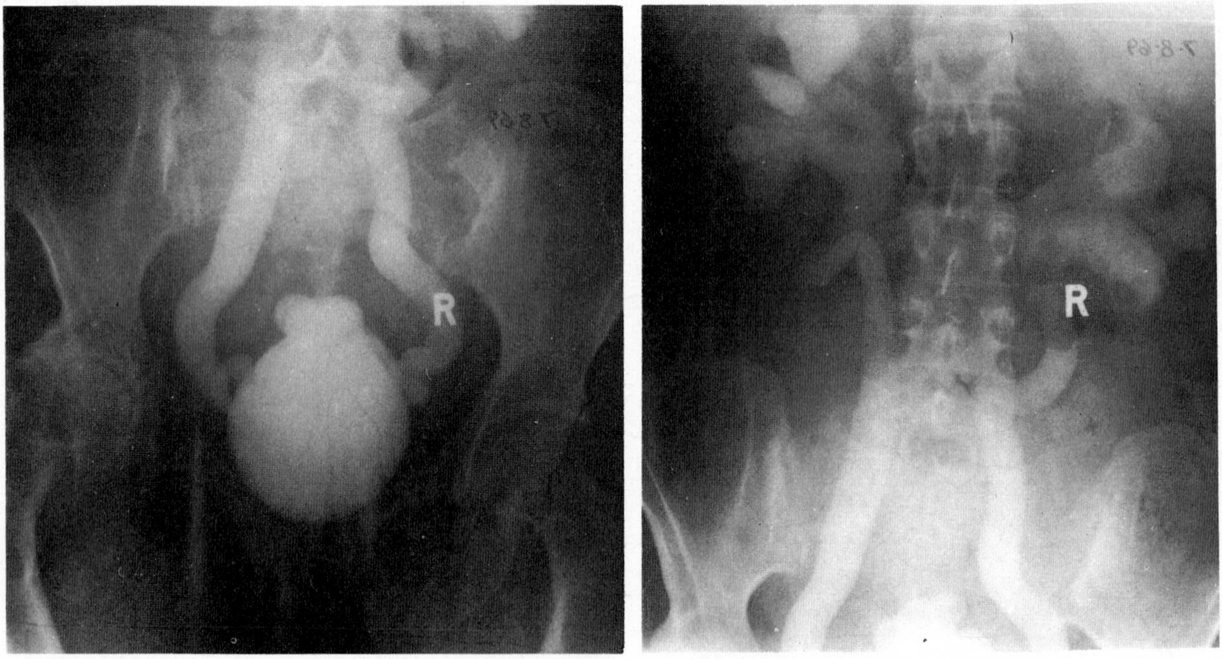

Micturating cystogram showing ureteric reflux of contrast medium into hydronephrotic kidneys.

Scanning electron micrographs (By courtesy of Dr. A. J. Salsbury, Brompton Hospital, and Dr. J. A. Clarke, St. Bartholomew's Hospital Medical College.)

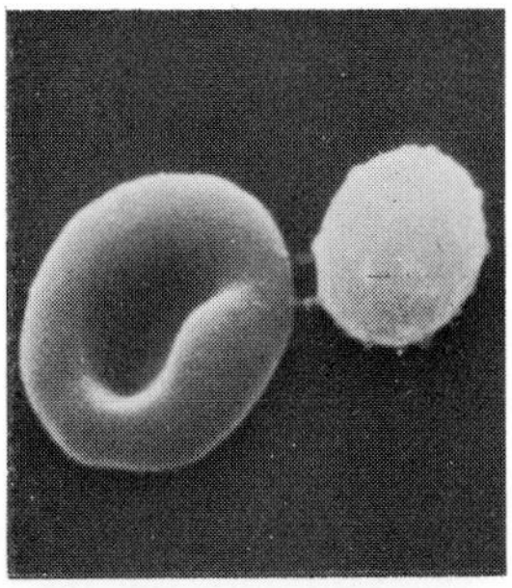

Right
Autoimmune haemolytic anaemia. A microspherocyte with a relatively normal red cell next to it. Magnification ×3,800.

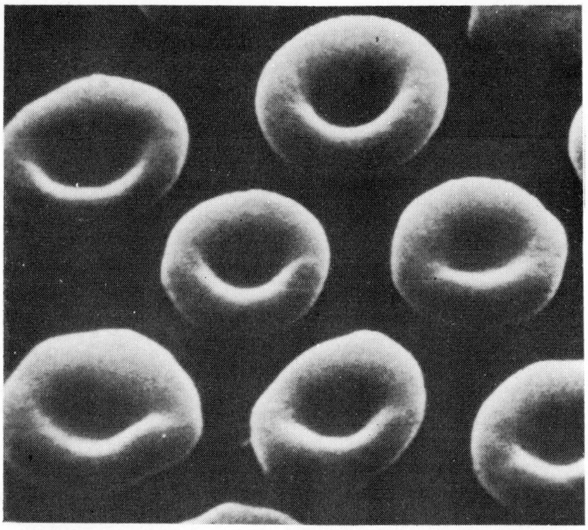

Left
Normal human red blood cells. Their characteristic shape of biconcave disks is clearly seen. Magnification ×3,800.

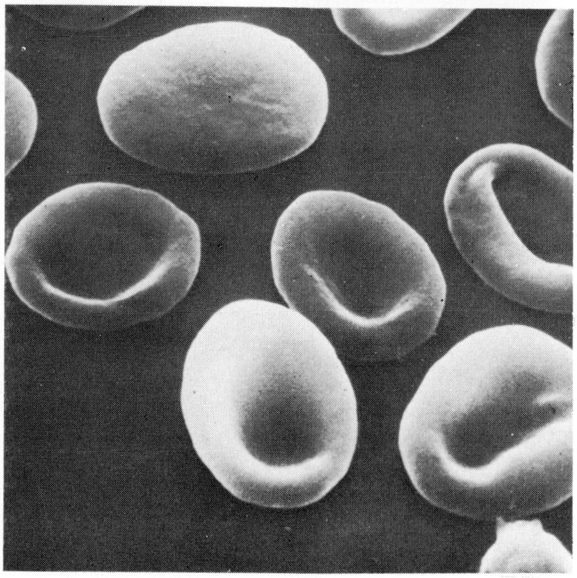

Megaloblastic anaemia due to folic acid deficiency. Several red cells are macrocytic and larger than normal. Magnification ×3,800.

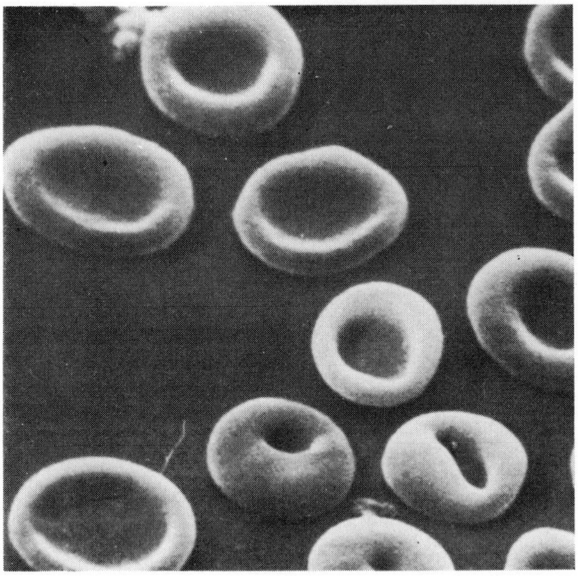

Iron deficiency anaemia. The red cells vary in size, but tend to be smaller than normal. Many possess a very narrow rim of haemoglobin. Magnification ×3,800.

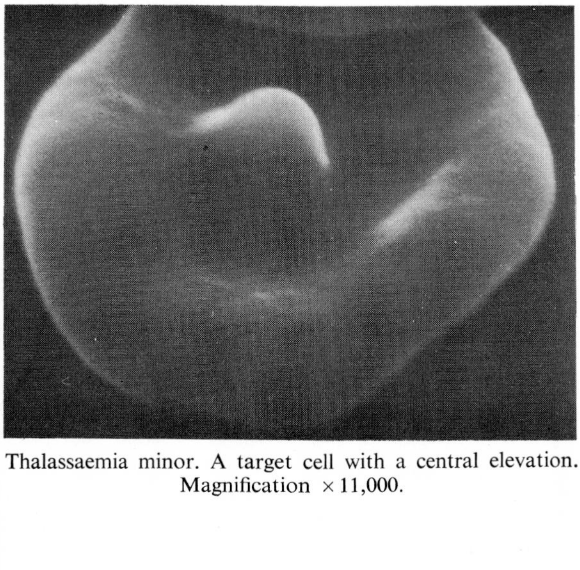

Thalassaemia minor. A target cell with a central elevation. Magnification ×11,000.

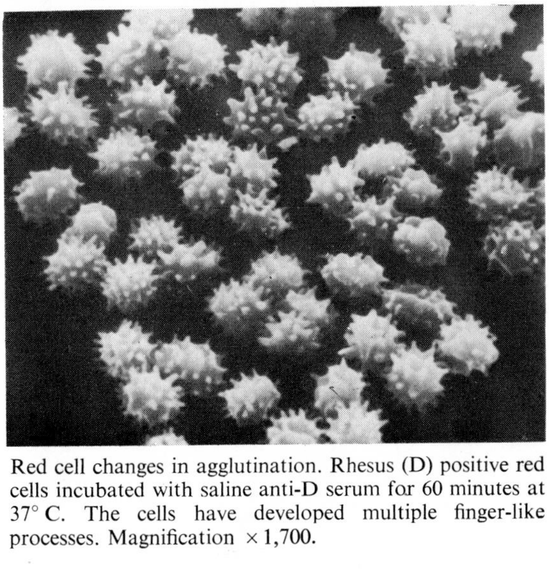

Red cell changes in agglutination. Rhesus (D) positive red cells incubated with saline anti-D serum for 60 minutes at 37° C. The cells have developed multiple finger-like processes. Magnification ×1,700.

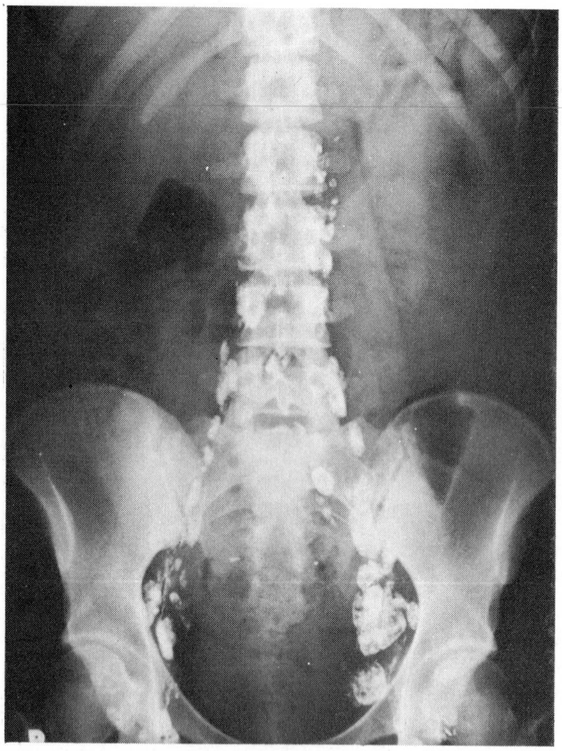

(a)

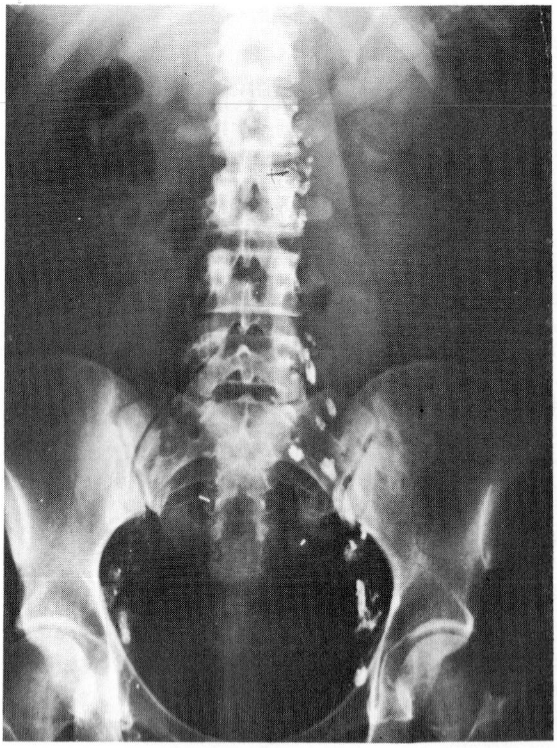

(b)

Lymphogram of a patient with Hodgkin's disease showing involvement of pelvic and para-aortic lymph nodes. (a) Before and (b) after radiotherapy. The dye may remain in the nodes for many months.

in patients who are convalescent after prolonged illness. Anxiety is a common cause of tachycardia especially when emotional disturbance is expressed through the cardiorespiratory system.

Symptoms

Sinus tachycardia is mostly symptomless but sometimes patients are conscious of the rapid heart action.

Treatment

This is not indicated apart from that of the underlying cause.

SINUS BRADYCARDIA

Bradycardia means a slow heart rate. Some people have a naturally slow pulse and the well-trained athlete may have a heart rate of 45–50 a minute. Sinus slowing is due to increased vagal tone and diminished sympathetic tone. It may be induced by carotid sinus massage.

Aetiology. Sinus bradycardia occurs: (1) during convalescence from some infectious fevers, especially influenza, diphtheria, typhoid and typhus; (2) in certain toxic conditions such as jaundice; (3) in hypothyroidism; (4) occasionally in organic heart disease; (5) as a result of certain drugs, e.g. digitalis, opium and its derivatives; (6) in increased intracranial pressure, especially in patients with cerebral tumours; (7) in vasovagal fainting-reactions.

Diagnosis. Sinus bradycardia may be distinguished from the various forms of heart block by clinical correlation of the arterial pulse, the venous pulse and heart sounds [p. 761]. The heart rate is increased by effort, emotion, fever, the nitrites and atropine in sinus bradycardia, but not in heart block. The electrocardiogram is diagnostic.

SINUS ARREST (SINO-ATRIAL BLOCK)

The sinus node may be inhibited by increased vagal tone so that the whole heart is stopped for one or more beats. These dropped beats may occur at irregular or regular intervals. If normal conduction is not soon resumed, nodal or ventricular escape beats occur. As in sinus bradycardia, carotid sinus pressure may induce the condition, and atropine abolishes it. Occasionally a transient dizziness or even syncope may occur.

This condition occurs in normal individuals and should be regarded as an extreme example of sinus bradycardia. It may be caused by digitalis or quinidine poisoning. Treatment is not usually indicated [see heart block, p. 761].

SINUS ARRHYTHMIA

The sinus node sometimes shows phasic activity, which is due to variations in vagal tone. The regular arrhythmia is most often related to respiration and the heart rate increases during inspiration and diminishes during expiration. Phasic arrhythmias are most apparent in the young, in the presence of sinus bradycardia and when digitalis is used.

Diagnosis is usually obvious. An electrocardiogram is confirmatory when there is doubt. This condition should be disregarded. Its significance is in the differential diagnosis from serious arrhythmia.

ECTOPIC BEATS

Definition

Ectopic beats or extrasystoles are premature contractions arising as the result of impulse formation at a site other than the sino-atrial node. They may arise in the atria, atrioventricular node or the ventricles. Most ectopic beats are followed by a diastolic pause which is longer than normal (compensatory pause) because the following sinus impulse falls on refractory tissues. Occasionally the ectopic beat occurs early in the cycle and muscle recovers in time for the next sinus beat to occur without a pause—this is then a true 'extrasystole' and is referred to as an *interpolated* beat.

Ectopic beats are the commonest cause of arrhythmia and those of ventricular origin are the commonest variety. They may occur at rare intervals or may be frequent and irregular, or regular. When premature contraction follows each normal contraction, coupling is produced and the pulse shows bigeminy. Ectopic beats may occur in short runs and occasionally an ectopic rhythm may be established. Premature contractions may be very frequent and arise from different foci in the same patient. The prematurity of the contraction results in subnormal filling so that the stroke volume is smaller than normal. Thus the ectopic pulse wave is smaller and often insufficient to be felt at the wrist, resulting in an intermittent pulse although the ectopic heart sounds may be heard on auscultation. Sometimes the premature contraction is so feeble that closure of the aortic valves is not heard; in this way a group of three sounds (two normal and one ectopic) is heard.

Atrial Extrasystoles. Here the ectopic focus is in the atrial myocardium and conduction to the ventricle follows a normal pathway thereafter. The compensatory pause is usually short. Occasionally the ectopic atrial sound may be heard preceding the first heart sound.

The electrocardiogram is diagnostic [FIG. 46a]. As might be expected, the P wave is abnormal and may be superimposed on the T wave of the preceding sinus beat. The premature ventricular complex has a normal or almost normal QRS; occasionally it is absent, the ventricle is refractory and the atrial ectopic stimulus is 'blocked'.

Nodal Extrasystoles. Here the ectopic focus is in the atrioventricular node and excitation passes in a retrograde fashion over the atrium and normally to the ventricle. The P wave is inverted in leads where it is normally positive and it may occur immediately before, during, or immediately after the ectopic QRS complex.

Ventricular Ectopic Beats [FIG. 46b]. The ectopic focus may lie anywhere in the ventricular muscle. The compensatory pause is long because the normal rhythm of the sinus node is not inhibited and the ventricle does not usually respond to the first stimulus after the ectopic beat; normal rhythm is resumed with the arrival of the second normal sinus impulse.

The electrocardiogram shows a premature and bizarre QRS complex often resembling bundle branch block. Right ventricular extrasystoles show a positive main deflection in left ventricular leads whilst left ventricular extrasystoles show the opposite.

Aetiology

Ectopic beats occur at any age in either sex, but they are rare in childhood and increase in frequency throughout adult life; they are more common in men than women.

Most patients with premature beats show no evidence of organic heart disease; however, the diseased heart shows an increased tendency to form ectopic beats. When there is ventricular disease ventricular ectopics are common, and when there is atrial disease as in mitral stenosis, atrial ectopics tend to occur and may herald the onset of atrial fibrillation, but the relationship is not a close one and all forms of premature contractions occur throughout the range of organic heart disease, particularly when the muscle is directly affected.

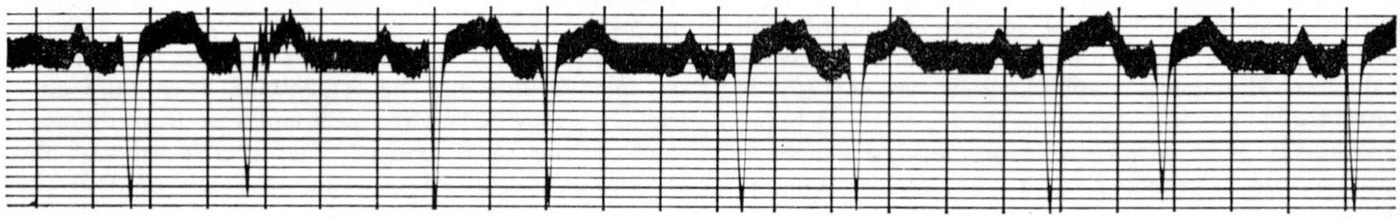

FIG. 46a. *Atrial premature beats* (*VI*). The rhythm is dominantly regular and each sinus beat is followed by an atrial extrasystole having the same QRS pattern as normal beat.

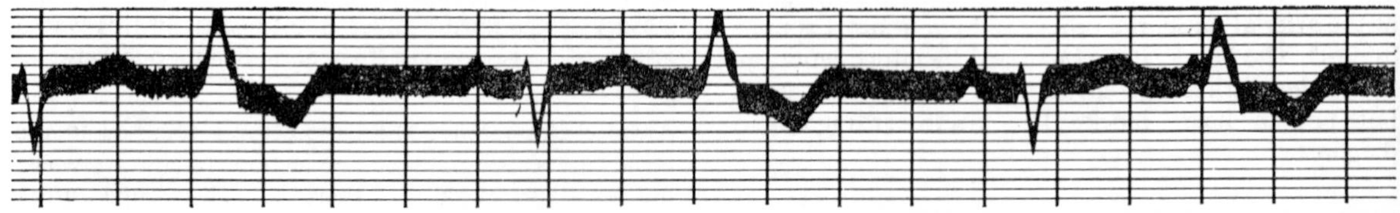

FIG. 46b. *Ventricular premature beats* (*VI*). Each normal sinus beat (preceded by normal P wave) is followed by bizarre QRS and inverted T wave of ventricular extrasystole.

It is unusual to detect any cause for ectopic beats in patients without gross organic heart disease, but mental and physical fatigue increase their occurrence, as does excessive use of tea, coffee, tobacco and alcohol. Emotional stress and unusual physical effort are also common provoking factors. Premature contractions are especially apt to occur during rest following physical exertion, soon after getting into bed, with change of posture and after large meals; they not infrequently occur in association with attacks of migraine and digestive disturbances. Premature contractions may be caused by digitalis and pressor amines, and they occur frequently during surgical anaesthesia and during cardiac catheterization.

Clinical Features

Many individuals are unconscious of ectopic beats, even when examination shows gross irregularity. Others experience palpitation, a sense of missing a beat, a large thumping in the chest or a sensation of the heart 'turning over', whilst some declare that the 'heart stops'. Occasionally more serious symptoms of faintness and even syncope may appear. The premature beat may be felt at the radial pulse or the pulse may be intermittent. When the ectopic pulse does not reach the wrist, auscultation reveals the sounds of premature contraction.

Diagnosis

In most patients a correct diagnosis can be made by palpation of the pulse and auscultation. The premature beat and following pause may be detected at the wrist. On auscultation the first and second heart sounds of the normal beat are followed in a rapid cadence by one or two sounds of the ectopic beat. When the pulse is interrupted by a long pause, partial heart block is excluded by palpating or hearing an ectopic beat at the apex. However, the occasionally inaudible or blocked ectopic beat necessitates an electrocardiogram for diagnosis. Sinus arrest may also confuse.

Coupled extrasystoles *pulsus bigeminus* may be confused with *pulsus alternans* and occasionally with *pulsus bisferiens*. In *pulsus alternans* the alternating weak and strong beats are equally spaced and the rhythm is quite regular, whereas in coupling the weak beat is clearly premature. In *pulsus bisferiens* the pulse wave is split, and rarely this bifidity may be enough to resemble two close but separate waves; auscultation reveals that a single heart beat is responsible and also reveals the presence of combined aortic stenosis and incompetence which causes a bisferiens pulse.

Frequent extrasystoles, especially if atrial in origin, may produce an extremely irregular pulse which may be difficult to differentiate from atrial fibrillation. Tachycardia induced by effort or drugs tends to diminish the frequency of ectopic beats but in all cases an electrocardiogram is diagnostic.

Treatment

As previously indicated, most premature beats are asymptomatic. When the arrhythmia is discovered in the course of examination, the patient should not be informed Patients who are aware of the condition should be reassured firmly and they should be dissuaded from feeling the pulse. Many respond to reassurance and require no other treatment. Where anxiety and the ectopic beats persist, a sedative should be used. Occasionally when there is much anxiety and distress due to frequent extrasystoles, more intensive therapy is indicated. Smoking should be avoided or diminished, sedation with phenobarbitone in doses of 30–60 mg. three times a day, should be given and quinidine sulphate in doses of 60–300 mg. three times daily may be tried with good effect. Propranolol sometimes suppresses ectopic beats but like quinidine it is rarely indicated for this purpose. When there is associated heart disease, this should be reviewed and treated.

Nodal rhythm occurs when the atrioventricular node becomes the pacemaker. The atrium is activated by a retrograde spread of the stimulus. The electrocardiogram shows the same changes in each complex as are seen in isolated nodal ectopic beats. This condition occasionally occurs in normal subjects, but it is more often associated with heart disease.

Prognosis

This depends on the nature of any associated heart disease.

ATRIAL TACHYCARDIA (PAROXYSMAL)

Paroxysmal tachycardia is commonly of atrial, auricular or supraventricular type, but it should be noted that other tachycardias may occur in paroxysms. In this condition there are repeated attacks of rapid beating. The onset and termination are sudden. The arrhythmia arises at a single ectopic focus which may be high or low in the atrium. The atrial rate is usually between 150 and 220 per min., and mostly there is 1:1 conduction to the ventricle which therefore contracts at the same rapid regular rate. The individual beats are essentially the same as isolated ectopic beats, which may precede or follow the termination of an attack. Paroxysms may last for a few minutes up to a few days. They may recur rarely or with great frequency.

Aetiology

The aetiology is unknown. As with extrasystoles, patients with normal or diseased hearts may be affected. Paroxysmal tachycardia may occur at any age; it is rare in infancy and increases in middle life, being less common after the sixth decade. Both sexes are equally affected. Paroxysmal tachycardia may occur in any form of heart disease but patients with mitral stenosis, hyperthyroidism and atrial septal defect are more commonly affected. It is not infrequently associated with anomalous atrioventricular conduction [see Wolff-Parkinson-White syndrome, p. 765].

Most attacks appear spontaneously but in some patients a sudden change of posture, excessive emotion, or physical exertion may provoke an attack. Tea, coffee, alcohol and tobacco may be aggravating factors.

Clinical Features

The common complaint is of severe palpitation commencing suddenly with little warning. Sometimes a 'heavy beat' or 'lunge' of the heart signifies an ectopic beat which precedes the main burst of palpitation. Although cessation is equally sudden, this change to normal rhythm is not appreciated so frequently as the sudden onset. The rapid heart beat may affect the whole body with pulsation; some patients will say that the bed appears to shake. Attacks may be accompanied by sternal discomfort and relative coronary insufficiency may develop, producing severe ischaemic pain. A sensation of faintness or giddiness is common and rarely syncope may occur. Many patients experience sensations of great anxiety and extreme exhaustion. There is often much flatulence and abdominal distension; vomiting may occur and this usually terminates the attack. Polyuria is common. Attacks of migraine are sometimes associated with paroxysmal tachycardia. With very fast rates a shock-like condition may appear, with coldness of the extremities, perspiration and extreme pallor and faintness. Rarely congestive heart failure may develop, especially in patients with pre-existing heart disease, in the very young and when paroxysms continue for long periods.

The physical signs are tachycardia (140–220) and those of any associated disease. If congestive heart failure develops, it rapidly improves with cessation of the attack, which is not infrequently followed by polyuria.

Diagnosis

Diagnosis depends mainly on a history of repeated sudden attacks of tachycardia without cause. An electrocardiogram in the attack is diagnostic [FIG. 47a]. Sinus tachycardia is distinguished by its slow onset, slow decline, variable rate and the knowledge of its cause. Carotid sinus pressure causes slight slowing in the sinus rhythm but in paroxysmal tachycardia there is either no effect or a sudden return to normal rhythm.

Atrial flutter causes a similar fast heart rate and should be distinguished [p. 758]. Clinical recognition is sometimes possible if two atrial venous pulse waves to each ventricular systole can be detected. Atrial flutter may continue for weeks or months, whereas simple paroxysmal tachycardia lasts for minutes or hours. Differentiation by the electrocardiogram may also be difficult. There is 1:1 conduction in atrial tachycardia but the alternate P waves in 2:1 atrial flutter may be buried in the QRS complex and therefore difficult to detect. When the pulse is irregular and fast, atrial fibrillation is the usual cause [p. 759]. Paroxysmal ventricular tachycardia is rare and associated with serious disease of heart muscle [p. 761].

Treatment

In most patients with paroxysmal tachycardia there is anxiety and attacks are often more frequent during phases of heightened emotional tension. Confident reassurance is thus essential, and it should be stressed that the heart is healthy and that sudden death is no more likely than in other people. In rare cases where the attacks are associated with serious organic heart disease and cardiac failure is present or a possibility, digitalis should be given indefinitely.

Many patients learn a simple method of terminating the attack, such as breath holding, drinking iced water or self-induced vomiting. Carotid sinus massage is, however, the most effective: with the neck extended in a reclining posture, the carotid sinus region is firmly massaged on one side only, and this procedure may be repeated on the opposite side; it should not be carried out in elderly, arteriosclerotic subjects. In severe, prolonged attacks, it is advisable for the patient to lie down and take 300 mg. of quinidine (repeated in 2 hours) together with a sedative. Most attacks cease during sleep or within 8 hours. Intravenous digoxin, 1 mg., or lanatoside C should be tried, and is usually effective in attacks which continue after quinidine has been used without success. Cholinergic drugs have unpleasant side-effects and are not advised unless sedation, quinidine and digitalis have failed. Patients having only occasional attacks need advice about the individual attack, but no long-term treatment other than reassurance and perhaps an occasional sedative. When attacks are frequent, 200–300 mg. of quinidine three times daily, should be given for a trial period of 2–3 months and if the frequency of attacks is reduced and the drug is well tolerated, it should be continued indefinitely.

Paroxysmal tachycardia in infancy is serious and may lead to congestive heart failure; digitalis is indicated and is almost always effective.

Prognosis

The outlook for individual attacks is good; cessation occurs spontaneously after a short period. However, when there is organic heart disease or when attacks are resistant to treatment and the tachycardia persists for a long time, congestive cardiac failure may develop. Persistent attacks occasionally cause coronary insufficiency and muscle damage. In infancy long attacks may be lethal from heart failure. From the long-term point of view, prognosis is very good for the vast majority of patients. Attacks may be infrequent and they rarely interfere with work and normal employment. They may cease as mysteriously as they started and the physician should invariably give an encouraging prognosis.

ATRIAL FLUTTER

Atrial flutter is a condition of rapid atrial pulsation at 180–360 beats per minute. The onset is sudden. In the majority of cases there is partial atrioventricular block varying from 2:1 to 5:1, the former being more common. Ventricular rates are usually from 160 to 180 per minute. Investigations by Lewis suggested that flutter was due to a continuous circus movement of excitation in the atrial myocardium; more recent work indicates that there is rapid stimulus formation at a single focus from which waves of activity spread through the atria in all directions.

The rate of stimulus formation in this condition is faster than in the atrial tachycardias and slower than in atrial fibrillation, but in each condition ectopic stimulus formation appears to be the fundamental disorder. Investigations by Prinzmetal showed that the ectopic focus tends to be at the caudal end of the atrium in flutter and at the cephalic end in atrial tachycardia. Atrial flutter is much less common than either atrial tachycardia or atrial fibrillation. Paroxysms of flutter usually last much longer than those of paroxysmal tachycardia (atrial) and conversion to atrial fibrillation occurs readily; there is much overlap between the two conditions.

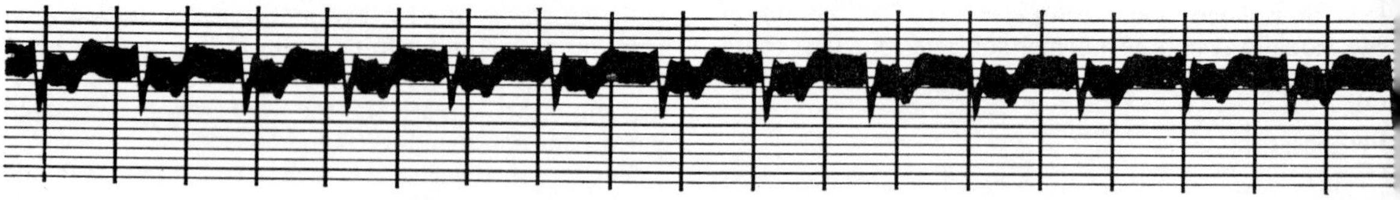

FIG. 47a. *Paroxysmal atrial (nodal) tachycardia (VI).* Regular ventricular rhythm (180). Atrial rate is the same. P waves best seen in this lead.

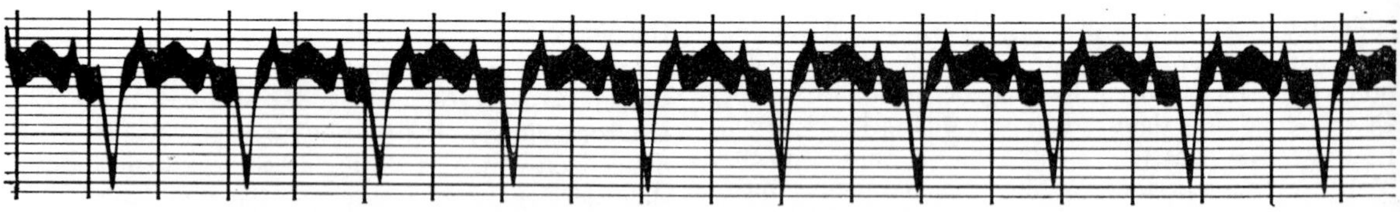

FIG. 47b. *Atrial tachycardia (flutter).* P waves readily seen in V1, rate 300. Regular ventricular response to alternate P waves. Ventricular rate 150.

Aetiology

Atrial flutter is almost always associated with organic heart disease. Men are most commonly affected. It may be responsible for tachycardia in infancy but otherwise is unusual under 40 years of age and most common after 60.

Clinical Features

Atrial flutter may cause the same symptoms as

paroxysmal tachycardia [p. 757]. Cardiac pain may occur and a persistent attack of atrial flutter may precipitate congestive cardiac failure.

Heart rate is usually rapid and regular, but there may be sudden changes in rate due to a variable degree of atrioventricular block. Exercise and emotional change leave the rate unaltered, but carotid sinus or eyeball pressure may result in a sudden rate change. When the degree of block is high (4:1) the ventricular rate may be normal. The loudness of the first heart sound may be variable when there is a varying degree of block. Sometimes 'a' waves may be seen in the neck, and their regular relationship to the less frequent ventricular pulse detected.

The electrocardiogram. P waves are regular at rates from 200 to 350 per minute [FIG. 47b]. They are most readily seen in leads II and III or right-sided precordial leads, especially CR1. The P waves often show a continuous undulating pattern without an isoelectrical interval; this appearance is due to the atrial T waves. P waves are also abnormal in form, depending on the site of ectopic impulse formation. The level of atrioventricular block determines the frequency of the QRS complex. When there is 1:1 conduction, P waves may not be distinguished and the appearance may be confused with ventricular tachycardia. Vagal stimulation leaves the P waves unchanged, whilst the QRS complexes may become irregular or recur at a regular slower rate.

Treatment

In all cases underlying heart disease should be reviewed and congestive heart failure treated by the usual methods. In the rare cases where natural heart block keeps the heart rate normal there are no symptoms and no treatment is indicated, but in others digitalis is the drug of choice. Digitalis is given to slow the ventricular rate and to produce atrial fibrillation which is more easily controlled than atrial flutter and more readily converted into normal rhythm. Many patients will remain in atrial flutter and in these the ventricular rate should be controlled by digitalis. Little is gained by using other anti-arrhythmic drugs, as in most cases underlying organic heart disease prevents the continuation of normal rhythm. Patients in whom atrial fibrillation has developed should be maintained on digitalis, but in some, where there is no serious organic heart disease, conversion to sinus rhythm should be attempted [see treatment of atrial fibrillation, p. 760].

Prognosis

Prognosis depends largely on the nature of any underlying heart disease. Prolonged attacks may precipitate heart failure when there is pre-existing heart disease, but when the heart is otherwise normal, atrial flutter may be tolerated well for years. Attacks of atrial flutter tend to recur, but they are extremely variable in duration and in frequency of recurrence.

ATRIAL FIBRILLATION

Atrial fibrillation is the most common persistent arryhthmia. Integrated atrial contraction disappears and is replaced by rapid irregular fibrillary twitching of the atrial muscle and there is irregular rapid ventricular contraction. Paroxysms may occur but mostly atrial fibrillation becomes a permanent condition.

As in the case of atrial flutter, Lewis came to the conclusion that atrial fibrillation was due to a single excitation wave travelling around a main circus path and giving rise to lateral 'daughter' waves. This circus theory has been generally accepted but recent investigations, particularly by Prinzmetal and his associates, have shown no evidence of circus movement, centrifugal waves or daughter waves. This work shows that atrial fibrillation is characterized by a chaotic disturbance of atrial muscle found only in this condition. There are asynchronous pulsations of minute segments of muscle, larger movements of larger areas of muscle and all intermediate varieties which may occur simultaneously or separately. It appears that the arrhythmia is initiated from a single ectopic focus but the larger movements arise from diverse foci and they pass over the atrium from 400 to 600 times a minute. These larger waves may pass in any direction during a given bout of fibrillation and they vary greatly in intensity of contraction.

With atrial fibrillation there is usually a degree of atrioventricular block. Stimulation of the ventricle is irregular and the rate is usually between 100 and 180 beats per minute. Some patients, especially when there is long-standing mitral stenosis, show a high degree of A-V block and the rate may be normal. Digitalis is, however, mostly responsible for slow ventricular rates accompanying atrial fibrillation.

Atrial fibrillation diminishes the efficiency of the heart but the importance of atrial transport depends on the nature of the underlying disease. There is good evidence to show that cardiac output rises when normal rhythm is restored; however, from the clinical point of view the circulation may show little evidence of inefficiency if the ventricular rate is controlled by digitalis. In those conditions in which ventricular filling is impeded by organic obstruction or diminished ventricular compliance atrial contraction is an important component in maintaining cardiac output; then atrial fibrillation may lead to severe heart failure.

The electrocardiogram. The characteristic feature of the electrocardiogram is the disappearance of P waves and their replacement by irregular waves of varying size called 'f' waves, and usually best seen in right chest leads [FIG. 48]. The ventricular complexes are irregular and vary slightly in contour, but have the same general form as those found when the patient is in normal rhythm. If they appear to be regular, measurement of successive R-R intervals reveals the underlying irregularity.

Aetiology

Atrial fibrillation is mostly associated with organic heart disease. However, in 7–10 per cent. of patients the heart muscle and valves are apparently normal; these patients have a good prognosis.

Any type of organic heart disease may be associated with atrial fibrillation. It occurs in the natural history of most patients with mitral stenosis, and the establishment of permanent arrhythmia may be preceded by frequent atrial ectopic beats or paroxysms of atrial fibrillation. Patients with great cardiac enlargement from mitral stenosis always have atrial fibrillation, but heart failure often occurs whilst there is still normal rhythm.

Atrial fibrillation may be continuous or paroxysmal in hyperthyroidism and its frequency increases with advancing years. Atrial fibrillation is common in chronic ischaemic heart disease and may be due to occlusion of the artery to the sinus node. Transient attacks are common in patients with recent cardiac infarction. Although many patients with hypertension develop heart failure with normal rhythm, atrial fibrillation sometimes occurs, particularly when coronary artery disease is also present. It is rare in malignant hypertension. Constrictive pericarditis is associated with atrial fibrillation in at least one-third of the cases, but in other forms of pericarditis, arrhythmia is rare. Atrial fibrillation is sometimes due to chest disease, especially carcinoma of the bronchus and other neoplasms which may damage cardiac nerves or directly invade adjacent pericardium or myocardium. Sudden physical or mental shock may precipitate the arrhythmia in some patients whilst in others there is no apparent cause. An excessive consumption of alcohol may precipitate atrial fibrillation [see nutritional cardiomyopathy, p. 810]. Atrial fibrillation may occur at any age but is much commoner after middle age whatever the aetiology.

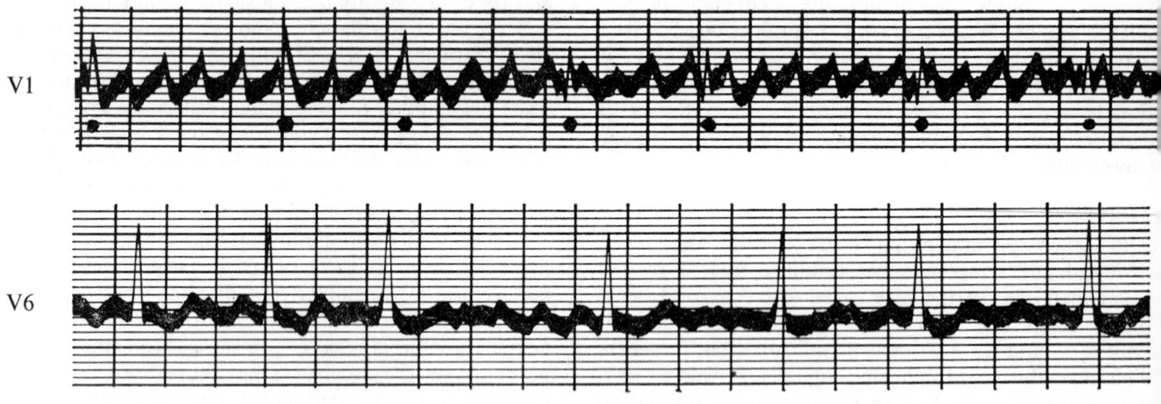

FIG. 48. *Atrial fibrillation* (V1 and V6). Coarse irregular 'f' waves seen best in V1 (rate approximately 400). Irregular ventricular response (marked in V1) is relatively slow due to digitalis.

Clinical Features

Some patients are unaware of any irregular heart action but many experience palpitation. Dizziness, syncope and cardiac pain sometimes accompany an attack of atrial fibrillation. Heart failure may develop, symptoms are then determined by its severity, and the nature of the underlying heart disease. Systemic and pulmonary emboli are common complications when atrial fibrillation is due to valvar disease.

Diagnosis

Atrial fibrillation is recognized by total irregularity of the pulse in rhythm and volume. Before treatment is given there is mostly tachycardia and some of the weaker beats may not reach the wrist so that a 'pulse deficit' is usual. Frequent irregular ectopic beats may resemble atrial fibrillation, but in most cases the basic regularity of sinus rhythm can be recognized and exercise tends to produce a more regular pulse. A slow ventricular rate in atrial fibrillation from natural heart block or digitalis therapy may result in an almost regular pulse. When there is doubt an electrocardiogram is confirmatory.

Treatment

The management of patients with atrial fibrillation depends mainly on its cause. When there is tachycardia, or any evidence of congestive cardiac failure, digitalis should be used [see p. 751]. Occasionally more rapid digitalization is necessary, when intravenous digoxin or lanatoside C may be used [p. 751].

Conversion of atrial fibrillation to normal rhythm must be considered in all cases where there is no evidence of serious organic heart disease. Conversion should also be attempted in successfully treated hyperthyroidism if spontaneous reversion has not taken place, it should also be attempted when atrial fibrillation persists after successful cardiac surgery. Quinidine is the anti-arrhythmic drug of choice; it should be combined with digitalis in all cases. It is traditional to give a test dose of quinidine, 120 mg. There are various recommended schedules for the oral administration of quinidine, the following one is satisfactory: 300 mg. four-hourly on the first day, 300 mg. two-hourly on the second day and repeated on the third day. The high dosage course is stopped when conversion to normal rhythm occurs or at the end of the third day, or if serious toxic effects occur. Toxicity is shown by vomiting, diarrhoea, hypotension and even syncope—the drug should be withdrawn if any one of these appears. Quinidine is an abortifacient drug and should not be used during pregnancy. If conversion to normal rhythm has occurred as a result of quinidine therapy a maintenance dose of 300 mg. three times a day should be continued for a few weeks. *Direct current shock* administered to the external chest wall under light anaesthesia is more effective and probably safer than drug therapy; it is the method of choice where facilities are available.

VENTRICULAR TACHYCARDIA

Ventricular tachycardia is a condition of rapid regular rhythm which is initiated from a focus in the ventricle. It may be paroxysmal or continuous and is almost invariably associated with serious organic heart disease affecting left ventricular muscle. Acute cardiac infarction is the commonest cause. Digitalis intoxication may be a precipitating or aggravating factor. Rarely there is no evidence of organic heart disease.

Symptoms

Symptoms are those of paroxysmal tachycardia; there may be little subjective disturbance or symptoms are submerged in those of cardiac infarction or heart failure. Ventricular tachycardia may be responsible for relatively sudden and rapid deterioration in the course of cardiac infarction. Examination shows a regular rapid heart rate between 150 and 300 per minute. Hypotension, peripheral constriction and sweating indicate shock; syncope is common.

The electrocardiogram shows abnormal QRS complexes which are widened and may resemble those of ventricular ectopic beats. There is slight irregularity of rhythm. P waves are rarely recognizable but during episodes of regular rhythm they are normal, whereas the QRS complexes usually show evidence of serious myocardial disease.

Diagnosis

Paroxysms of tachycardia occurring during the course of serious organic heart disease suggest a ventricular origin, particularly in cardiac infarction, hypertension or aortic valve disease. The diagnosis is confirmed by the electrocardiogram. In supraventricular tachycardia the QRS complexes are frequently normal and regular, whereas in ventricular tachycardia the QRS is obviously abnormal and not quite regular. The electrocardiogram of supraventricular tachycardia with functional bundle branch block may be difficult to distinguish from that of ventricular tachycardia.

Treatment

Lignocaine is probably the anti-arrhythmic drug of choice but if the clinical state of patient is poor and deteriorating, say in the course of acute cardiac infarction, then direct current counter-shock should be used. In less serious situations lignocaine should be given as a repeated bolus injection of 50 or 100 mg. intravenously at 2–3 minute intervals for a total dose of 5 mg. per kg. Suppression therapy with an intravenous infusion of lignocaine or procainamide in a dose of 1 mg. a minute may be required. Quinidine and magnesium sulphate have been largely superseded by the aforementioned drugs; however, oral quinidine in doses of 300 mg. thrice daily carried on for a few weeks is a useful alternate suppressive therapy when a tendency to ventricular dysrhythmia is indicated by frequent ventricular ectopic beats.

Although the above measures are not without danger of serious toxic effects the gravity of ventricular tachycardia in cardiac infarction demands effective and urgent treatment.

DISORDERS OF CONDUCTION

Conduction of the excitatory impulse may be delayed or interrupted at any point during its passage from the sino-atrial node over the rest of the heart. The site and degree of delay may be determined and forms a basis of classification as follows:

1. Sino-atrial block.
2. Atrioventricular block (usually known as heart block and including prolonged P-R interval, partial and complete heart block).
3. Bundle branch block and intraventricular block.

SINO-ATRIAL BLOCK

Sino-atrial block is a relatively rare condition in which there is no beat owing to failure of impulse formation at the sinus node or failure of atrial response to sinus activity. This condition is indistinguishable from sinus arrest [see p. 755].

ATRIOVENTRICULAR BLOCK (HEART BLOCK)

In atrioventricular block there is defective conduction in the atrioventricular node or the bundle of His or both. The condition may be transient, paroxysmal or permanent. There are three grades: (1) Delayed conduction of the impulse from atrium to ventricle, resulting in a prolongation of the P-R interval. (2) Partial heart block with dropped beats due to intermittent failure of atrioventricular conduction. (3) Complete heart block when there is complete atrioventricular dissociation.

Some authors group the first and second grades as partial or incomplete heart block, while other writers divide partial heart block into cases where there are irregular dropped beats and those where the conduction defect is regular [see FIG. 49].

Prolonged P-R Interval

When impulses are delayed in passage through the atrioventricular node and bundle there is a prolongation of the P-R interval on the electrocardiogram (normal is 0·12–0·22 sec.). A prolonged P-R interval may be transient, a stage in the development of more severe block, or permanent and non-progressive. The diagnosis is essentially electrocardiographic but the delay between atrial and ventricular events may be detected by clinical examination. Abnormal delay between jugular venous 'a' waves and 'c' waves or between atrial components and ventricular components of the first heart sound may be detected. As the P-R interval is prolonged the first heart sound becomes softer. In mitral stenosis a gap between the atrial systolic murmur and the first heart sound would indicate first degree block.

Aetiology. First degree heart block occurs in all conditions which produce complete heart block. It commonly occurs in the course of carditis, especially in rheumatic fever and diphtheria where a prolonged P-R interval is certain evidence of active carditis. A prolonged P-R interval may be a permanent result of scar formation.

Partial Heart Block

When the cardiac impulse fails to reach the ventricles, through intermittent failure of atrioventricular conduction so that dropped beats occur, the condition is spoken of as partial or second degree heart block. The dropped beats may be occasional, irregular or frequent and regular.

Wenckebach (1899) described a form in which the P-R interval becomes progressively longer after each dropped beat until conduction fails again. In other cases the ratio between atrial and ventricular beats may be steady and regular but each second, third or even fourth ventricular beat may fail, producing 2:1, 3:1 and 4:1 ratios; the pulse may then appear to be grouped in runs of twos or threes. Ventricular rate depends on the atrial rate and the degree of block; thus at normal atrial rates and 2:1 block the pulse rate is slow (34–40 beats per minute), whereas with an atrial tachycardia and partial heart block the pulse may be rapid (often the result of digitalis toxicity). Inspection of the jugular venous pulse may show an 'a' wave corresponding to the dropped ventricular beats and an atrial sound may be heard at the same time, but an electrocardiogram is necessary for confirmation.

The electrocardiogram shows the frequency of absent QRS complexes compared with the frequency of regular P waves. Lead II or a right-sided chest lead should be examined when P waves are not clearly shown in other leads. A progressive lengthening of the P-R interval followed by a dropped beat is the Wenckebach phenomenon.

Aetiology [see complete heart block].

Treatment depends on the nature of associated heart disease and the degree of disability caused by the heart block [see complete heart block].

Prognosis. Partial heart block nearly always indicates heart disease and implies damage to the myocardium. The condition may be transitional to complete heart block. Prognosis depends on the nature of the underlying heart condition.

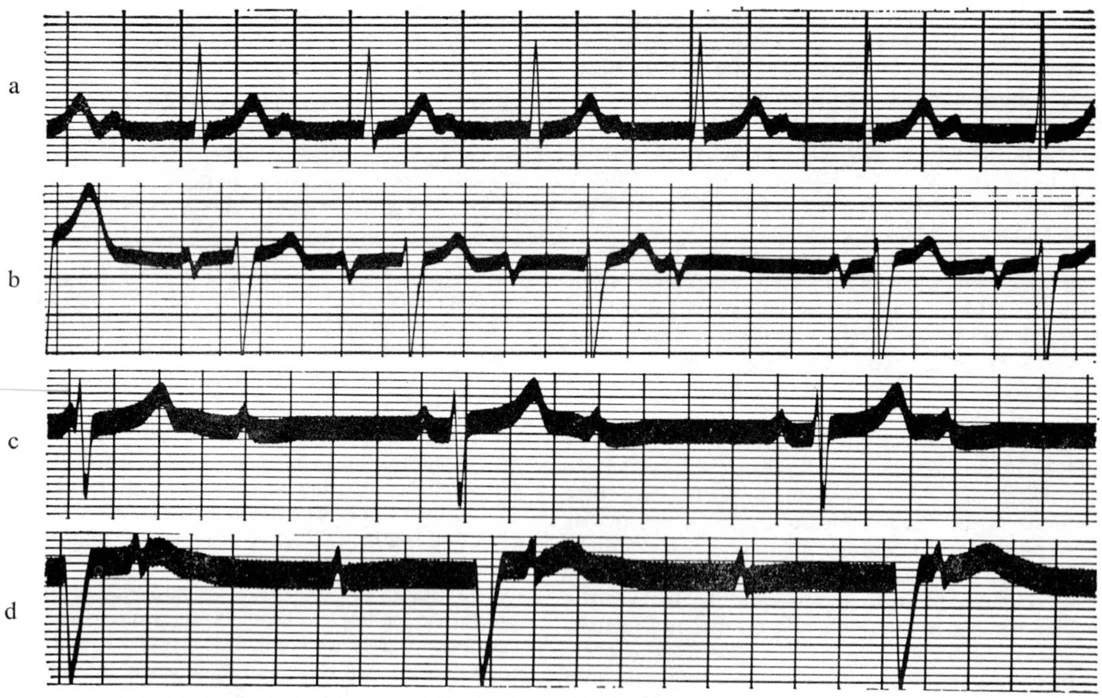

FIG. 49. *Various degrees of heart block.* (a) P-R interval prolonged to 0·3 sec. (b) Progressive increase in P-R interval followed by ventricular block (Wenckebach block). (c) 2–1 heart block. (d) Complete A-V dissociation. P waves regular and unrelated to ventricular rate (30 per min.) and rhythm shown by QS waves in V1.

Complete Heart Block

In complete atrioventricular block the cardiac impulse fails to reach the ventricles which continue to beat in response to a focus situated in the ventricular myocardium. The inherent rhythmicity of ventricular foci is slow and slightly irregular, being almost totally uninfluenced by external stimuli so that fever and effort leave the pulse rate unaltered. There is some evidence that vagal activity has a slight effect. The condition is spoken of as complete atrioventricular dissociation, and the ventricular beating as an idioventricular rhythm. The slow rate results in increased ventricular filling; the stroke volume is large and a near normal cardiac output may be maintained at rest.

Aetiology

There are many causes of delay in the conducting

system; the higher grades of atrioventricular block are usually associated with serious chronic heart disease, causing anatomical lesions of the conducting system, whereas in the lesser grades of block, which may be transient, the causative factors may be self-limiting, reversible and of a functional nature. The frequency of serious heart block increases with age and it is more common in men than in women. At necropsy many cases show no evidence of coronary or other known form of heart disease; histological examination showing only a selective degeneration of the bundle and its branches. Other causes are: *Coronary artery disease.* Occasionally extensive coronary occlusion is found in cases of chronic block, in others occlusion of the artery to the bundle occurs after its origin from the right coronary artery. Transient complete block is not uncommon in the course of acute cardiac infarction. *Calcific aortic stenosis* may be associated with various degrees of heart block. Calcification and fibrosis extend into the region of the bundle; associated coronary insufficiency is another factor in these cases. Rarely calcification may extend into the bundle from the mitral annulus in chronic mitral valve disease. *Rheumatic carditis* commonly causes first degree heart block, and less frequently severer grades of block. *Diphtheritic carditis* may cause any degree of conduction delay; complete block is more usual and indicates extensive and usually fatal myocarditis. *Syphilis* occasionally causes heart block; probably most cases are due to associated coronary insufficiency from coronary ostial stenosis, or coronary atherosclerosis; gummatous infiltration is a rare cause. Infiltration of the node and bundle by neoplasm occasionally produces heart block. Any one of the many forms of cardiomyopathy [p. 809] may cause heart block; cardiac amyloidosis and sarcoidosis seem to produce block more frequently than some other forms; myocardial fibrosis in Friedreich's disease and myotonia atrophica may damage the bundle of His causing an increase of the P-R interval and even complete heart block. *Digitalis* is perhaps the commonest cause of lesser degrees of heart block. The effect is due to vagal stimulation and a direct inhibition of the conducting tissues. Quinidine rarely causes conduction delay. *Congenital heart disease* may be associated with the various grades of heart block. Complete heart block is uncommon but occurs in some cases of ventricular septal defect, and occasionally where the septum is normal. It is rare in cyanotic congenital heart disease. The ventricular rates tend to be considerably higher than in cases of acquired heart block.

Clinical Features

The lesser grades of heart block do not usually produce symptoms. The dropped beats of partial heart block may produce unpleasant sensations in the chest; the long pause or the thud of the next beat may be felt and faintness may occur; however, it is with complete block that serious symptoms generally occur. Complete atrioventricular dissociation is mostly associated with a slow heart rate, usually from 30 to 40 per minute. At this rate symptoms may be completely absent but with slower rates faintness is common. Attacks of sudden syncope (Stokes-Adams syndrome) occur in nearly 50 per cent. of cases.

Stokes-Adams Syndrome [see syncope, p. 752]. This condition is characterized by sudden attacks of loss of consciousness associated with extreme bradycardia (10–20 per minute) or periods of ventricular asystole due to depression of the idioventricular focus. The atrium continues to beat at a normal rate whilst the ventricle is inactive.

Loss of consciousness is sudden and unaccompanied by any aura; attacks may last for a few seconds to 1 minute or more; recovery is unlikely after 2 minutes. As asystole continues extreme pallor develops and after some 10–12 seconds, movements commence and convulsions may follow. Breathing becomes stertorous and may be of the Cheyne-Stokes variety at the end of an attack. Ventricular fibrillation may supervene. When the ventricular beat is resumed consciousness returns, usually without any period of confusion, and flushing of the face is common.

Attacks may occur at infrequent intervals or in rapid succession. They are particularly likely to occur at an early stage when complete heart block develops from partial heart block. It appears that the idioventricular rhythm becomes more stable when complete heart block is permanent. Rarely complete heart block causing Stokes-Adams attacks may be paroxysmal so that between the attacks there is sinus rhythm. Lesser grades of the syncopal reaction such as giddiness and faintness may occur before and between attacks of complete unconsciousness.

Symptoms of circulatory insufficiency such as effort dyspnoea are common in heart block and depend on the nature and severity of the underlying heart disease. Less commonly complete block causes the development of florid congestive heart failure.

The most important sign of complete heart block is bradycardia. The rate is not influenced by effort, emotion, fever, nitrites or, as a rule, by atropine. The jugular venous pulse shows 'a' waves which are dissociated from the slow carotid pulse waves. From time to time atrial systole and ventricular systole happen to coincide, the atrium then contracts against closed valves, producing large regurgitant venous waves in the jugular veins (cannon waves). Auscultation may reveal soft atrial sounds between the sounds of ventricular systole. The intensity of the first heart sound varies depending on the proximity of atrial and ventricular systole. The peripheral arterial pulse wave is full and of a collapsing type; there is elevation of the systolic and a fall of the diastolic pressures. The apex beat usually indicates ventricular hypertrophy; however, the size and shape of the heart is essentially determined by the underlying pathology.

The electrocardiogram. P waves are regular or show slight variation and occur at a normal rate and are of normal form. The QRS complex occurs at a slow rate though usually at regular intervals; however, the P-R intervals are totally irregular because there is no relationship between the atrial and ventricular complexes. The QRS complex is usually abnormal, being widened and similar to that seen in bundle branch block and ectopic ventricular beats [FIG. 49].

Diagnosis

The diagnosis of all forms of heart block must be confirmed by the electrocardiogram. A prolonged P-R interval is not usually diagnosed by clinical methods. Second degree heart block may be diagnosed if attention is paid to ventricular activity as shown by the pulse, apex beat and the first heart sound, and to atrial activity by observing 'a' waves in the venous pulse. It should be remembered that sinus irregularity, sinus bradycardia and ectopic beats may be confused with the dropped beats of heart block when attention is only given to the wrist pulse. Although most cases with a ventricular rate of 36 or under are due to complete heart block, a 2:1 partial heart block may cause difficulty when the atrial rate is normal.

Congenital heart block should be diagnosed only when a slow pulse has been found at an early age or when there is other evidence of congenital heart disease.

Stokes-Adams attacks normally provide little difficulty in diagnosis when the presence of heart block is known. The suddenness of onset, absence of incontinence and absence of confusion afterwards help to differentiate from epilepsy. When heart block is paroxysmal, diagnosis is difficult between attacks and confirmation of the heart rate at the time of the attack is necessary.

Treatment

Isoprenaline (isoproterenol) has largely superseded ephedrine in the drug therapy of heart block. The long-acting form of isoprenaline (*Saventrine*) in doses of 30 mg. three or four times a day may abolish attacks of dizziness and even Stokes-Adams attacks in some cases. However, its vigorous stimulant effect on the heart may cause intolerable palpitation and even paroxysms of ventricular extrasystoles which prevent its continual use. A short trial of steroid therapy (say prednisone, 10–15 mg. thrice daily) for 10 days occasionally appears to raise the pulse and even restore sinus rhythm. However, drug treatment is generally unsatisfactory for persistent Stokes-Adams attacks and artificial pacemaking should be used.

There are several methods of bringing an electrical current to the heart for artificial pacemaking: external shocks are not practical for any situation other than the emergency treatment of ventricular asystole. This should not be confused with an external defibrillator which delivers a much higher voltage direct current for terminating a ventricular tachyarrhythmia.

An internal pacemaker delivering an impulse of small voltage and short duration should be used for long-term treatment of Stokes-Adams disease; its impulse is delivered by wire to the heart. The wires may be sutured to the myocardial surface or brought into contact with the right ventricular endocardium via the great veins using an electrode catheter. The selection of the best system in any patient, implantation, regular supervision, and replacement when necessary, necessitates referral to special units with facilities for dealing with this problem.

Patients with Stokes-Adams attacks should be warned against the common dangers of an open fireplace, the highway, electrified railways and high places.

Prognosis

The prognosis depends mainly on the nature of associated heart disease and severity of the conduction defect. Thus first degree heart block is common in rheumatic carditis and the outlook depends on other factors. Complete heart block in diphtheria, on the other hand, indicates very severe carditis which is usually fatal.

In chronic complete heart block, a life of moderately reduced activity may be pursued for many years. When Stokes-Adams attacks are frequent the outlook is poor, and apart from the risk of a fatal termination during an attack, death may occur from congestive heart failure. Transient block in acute cardiac infarction does not materially influence prognosis when compared with other factors such as shock and congestive heart failure. The progress of patients with congenital heart block depends almost entirely on the nature of the associated lesion. Treatment of chronic heart block by artificial pacing certainly improves symptoms and probably improves prognosis.

BUNDLE BRANCH BLOCK

Activation of both ventricles occurs simultaneously in the normal heart. When there is delayed conduction of the impulse to one ventricle asynchronous contraction results. Unilateral delay may occur in the left or right branch of the bundle of His due to disease in the ventricular septum. In some cases there is no demonstrable disease of the septum and the delay appears to be of a functional nature. There are no symptoms or significant haemodynamic effects of this asynchronous contraction, and bundle branch block should not be considered apart from the condition of the heart with which it is associated. Although bundle branch block is essentially recognized by the electrocardiogram, its presence may be inferred by clinical recognition of ventricular asynchrony.

The normal second heart sound contains the almost simultaneous sounds produced by the closure of aortic and pulmonary semilunar valves. Inspiration accentuates the normal slight delay of pulmonary valve closure. When there is bundle branch block the asynchrony of ventricular systole is shown by an increased time interval between these two components of the second heart sound so that wide 'splitting' results. This sign is most obvious in cases of right bundle branch block which exaggerates the physiological delay of pulmonary valve closure.

The electrocardiogram [FIG. 42]. Experimental work and clinical research has established clearly the cardiographic patterns associated with left and right bundle branch block. The P wave and P-R interval are normal, but the QRS complexes are prolonged to 0·12 sec. or more due to the delayed activity of one ventricle. The diagnosis of left or right bundle branch block is best made from the precordial leads.

In *left bundle branch block* the normal Q wave is absent from left-sided chest leads and is replaced by a small R wave, which is followed by a second R wave due to late excitation of the left ventricle. The complex tends to resemble an M. The initial R wave of right-sided chest leads is normal but there is a late S wave reflecting the delayed activity of the left ventricle.

T waves are usually inverted in left precordial leads [FIG. 42a].

In *right bundle branch block* right-sided chest leads show a delayed secondary R wave after the small normal initial R wave producing a characteristic RSR′ complex. Left-sided chest leads show a normal left-sided QR wave, followed by a delayed S wave which is a reflection of the delayed right ventricular activity. T waves are frequently inverted in the leads showing an RSR′ pattern [FIG. 42b].

Aetiology

Left bundle branch block tends to occur in conditions producing left ventricular hypertrophy and left ventricular disease so that it is not uncommon in hypertensive heart disease, ischaemia, aortic valve disease and cardiomyopathy. Cardiac infarction may produce right or left bundle branch block, which may be transient or permanent.

Right bundle branch block occurs in conditions particularly affecting the right heart. It occurs in some cases of mitral stenosis, chronic pulmonary heart disease and in 90 per cent. of patients with atrial septal defect. Massive pulmonary embolism may produce right bundle branch block. Bundle branch block often occurs as a functional phenomenon in association with paroxysmal tachycardia. Right bundle branch block occurs in a few healthy individuals but left bundle branch block is always associated with heart disease.

Clinical Features

Apart from the clinical recognition of asynchronous ventricular contraction described above, the clinical picture is determined by associated heart disease.

Prognosis and Treatment

Prognosis and treatment likewise depend entirely on associated heart disease.

WOLFF-PARKINSON-WHITE SYNDROME

Although there is no conduction delay in this condition it is conventionally described with bundle branch block. The diagnosis is essentially by electrocardiogram. The P-R interval is short (0·1 sec. or less) and is followed by a QRS complex resembling bundle branch block. The short P-R interval is compensated by the prolongation of the QRS complex so that the time between the P wave and the end of the QRS is normal. It appears, therefore, that there is premature ventricular excitation. This premature excitation wave probably travels by an anomalous pathway from atrium to ventricle. Anomalous bundles of tissue have been demonstrated occasionally by histological examination.

The condition may be permanent, transient or paroxysmal. Normal QRS complexes may alternate with pre-excitation ones. The heart is mostly normal but paroxysmal tachycardia occurs in 50 per cent. of cases.

REFERENCES

CAMPBELL, M. (1947) The paroxysmal tachycardias, *Lancet*, ii, 681.

EPSTEIN, S. E., and BRAUNWALD, E. (1966) Beta-adrenergic receptor blocking drugs, *New Engl. J. Med.*, **275**, 1106.

GIANELLY, R., GRIFFIN, J. R., and HARRISON, D. C. (1967) Propranolol in the treatment and prevention of cardiac arrhythmias, *Ann. intern. Med.*, **66**, 667.

HUDSON, R. (1960) The human pacemaker and its pathology, *Brit. Heart J.*, **22**, 153.

HUMPHRIES, J. O'N. (1964) Treatment of heart-block with pacemakers, *Mod. Conc. cardiov. Dis.*, **23**, 857.

LANDEGREN, J., and BIÖRCK, G. (1963) Clinical assessment and treatment of complete heart block and Adams-Stokes attacks, *Medicine (Baltimore)*, **42**, 171.

LOWN, B. (1964) 'Cardioversion' of arrhythmias, *Mod. Conc. cardiov. Dis.*, **33**, 863.

NAKAMURA, F., and NADAS, A. (1964) Complete heart block in infants and children, *New Engl. J. Med.*, **270**, 1261.

PANTRIDGE, J. F., and HALMOS, P. B. (1965) Conversion of atrial fibrillation by direct current countershock, *Brit. Heart J.*, **27**, 128.

PRINZMETAL, M. (1952) *The Auricular Arrhythmias*, Springfield, Ill.

CONGENITAL HEART DISEASE

About three children in each thousand are born with congenital heart disease, but a high mortality in the serious forms during early infancy reduces this proportion to 0·1 per cent. at 10 years of age. In about 2 per cent. of all patients with heart disease the condition is congenital.

The critical period of heart development lies in the first two months of foetal life and especially between the fifth and eighth weeks. During this period atrial and ventricular septa are forming, and rotation of the septum in the truncus followed by its fusion with cardiac septa takes place. Many defects arise from failure of development at this period, consequently such defects are often multiple. The cause of this failure is sometimes due to maternal environmental or uterine factors, and less frequently true genetic factors are the cause.

Maternal rubella in early pregnancy has been clearly shown to cause congenital defects. Possibly 4 per cent. of all cases of congenital heart disease, especially ventricular septal defect and patent ductus arteriosus, are due to rubella. Other maternal virus infections and possibly metabolic disorders at this critical stage in pregnancy may cause failures in foetal development.

Hereditary factors undoubtedly operate in some forms of congenital heart disease but their importance has not been determined so far. Clearly the most serious lesions which are incompatible with long survival make genetic investigation difficult, as does the absence of a powerful dominant trait. However, parent and child, or two sibs have congenital heart disease more often than would be expected by chance. Furthermore, some heart defects occur commonly in association with other defects, such as Marfan's syndrome, which are considered to have a genetic basis.

Classification

None is entirely satisfactory, but that proposed by Wood (1950) has the merit of ready application to those conditions which are of clinical importance. This classification is based on the presence or absence of an abnormal communication (a shunt) between the great vessels or between the two sides of the heart. When there is no communication anomalies may affect either the right or left heart (rarely both) and do not usually result in central cyanosis. When there is a communication between the two circulations the direction of shunting is the most important factor in determining the clinical features of the disorder.

Congenital heart disease can thus be divided into the following groups:

Group 1. Anomalies without an abnormal communication between the right and left sides of the heart:

(*a*) affecting the left heart and aorta;

(*b*) affecting the right heart and pulmonary artery;

(*c*) of a general nature.

Group 2. Anomalies with an abnormal communication and having a shunt:

(*a*) from the left to right side (acyanotic);

(*b*) from the right to the left side (cyanotic).

In the first group the most frequent and important abnormalities compatible with life cause obstruction to ventricular output either at the semilunar valve, above it or below it. On the left side (1*a*) aortic stenosis (and subaortic stenosis) and coarctation of the aorta are important whilst pulmonary valve stenosis and infundibular stenosis are common lesions on the right side (1*b*). Of the anomalies of a general nature (1*c*) those of the coronary circulation are relatively rare, some produce little or no disability and are compatible with a long life, whilst others cause death in infancy. Of the other abnormalities of a general nature isolated dextrocardia is unimportant; corrected transposition, though rare, may cause serious mitral incompetence. The inherited myopathies are considered elsewhere [familial cardiomegaly, p. 809; von Gierke's disease, p. 810; and Friedreich's disease, Section 15] as is congenital heart block [p. 763].

In Group 2*a* abnormal communications between the heart chambers or great vessels permit shunting of blood from the left to the right side because pressures are normally higher in the corresponding chambers of the left heart than those on the right. This results in the short circuiting of some blood to the right heart and its recirculation through the lungs (causing pulmonary plethora) at the expense of the systemic circulation. Such left to right shunts may be from pulmonary veins to venae cavae, from pulmonary veins to the right atrium, most commonly through an atrial septal defect, between the ventricles (ventricular septal defect), between the aorta and pulmonary artery (patent ductus arteriosus and aortopulmonary window).

When the abnormal communications are associated with another lesion (usually obstructive) which causes a rise of pressures on the right side sufficient to deviate blood from right to left, veno-arterial mixing occurs (Group 2*b*). Central cyanosis is the common feature of such conditions (morbus caeruleus). Important ones are tricuspid atresia, pulmonary stenosis and atrial septal defect, pulmonary stenosis and ventricular septal defect (tetralogy of Fallot), obstructive pulmonary hypertension with a right to left shunt at atrial, ventricular or aortopulmonary level (Eisenmenger syndrome).

GROUP 1. ANOMALIES WITHOUT AN ABNORMAL COMMUNICATION BETWEEN THE RIGHT AND LEFT SIDES OF THE HEART

BICUSPID AORTIC VALVES

These are not uncommon and may be unrecognized throughout a normal life. An ejection click may be the only physical sign pointing to this anomaly. Bicuspid valves may become incompetent and more frequently they become the site of calcific aortic stenosis. They are not infrequently associated with other congenital defects, particularly coarctation of the aorta and are prone to bacterial endocarditis.

AORTIC STENOSIS

Congenital aortic stenosis is usually valvar and often due to fusion of commissures between bicuspid valves. A minimal degree of regurgitation is common. Calcification of the valves is usual after middle life. The signs are the same as in acquired aortic stenosis [see rheumatic heart disease, p. 796]. Aortic valvotomy or aortic valve replacement is indicated for congenital aortic stenosis when there are symptoms, or evidence of significant left ventricular hypertrophy; however, this should not be an essential criterion because many children with significant obstruction (say, a gradient across the valve of more than 70 mm. Hg) do not show left ventricular hypertrophy on the cardiogram. Operative results are encouraging in this form of aortic stenosis and it is usual to obtain relief of symptoms and regression of the signs of left ventricular strain or hypertrophy. Subvalvar fibrous ring stenosis is congenital and very rare; the absence of post-stenotic dilatation of the first part of the aorta and the absence of an ejection click in the presence of other signs of aortic stenosis are pointers to the diagnosis, which may be proved by selective angiocardiography. Supra-aortic stenosis is also rare and associated with peculiar facies somewhat reminiscent of gargoylism.

COARCTATION OF THE AORTA

The aorta is obstructed by a localized constriction usually in the region of the junction of the arch and descending aorta. The narrowing varies in degree and may be proximal, opposite or distal to the ductus arteriosus, which may be patent or closed. The left subclavian junction usually lies just before the constriction but may be incorporated in it. The importance of coarctation of the aorta lies in its association with significant arterial hypertension, with medial arterial lesions especially in cerebral arteries, and with aortic valve disease.

The essential diagnostic feature of coarctation is the high pressure in the upper part of the body with a lower pressure and delayed or absent arterial pulsation in the arteries of the legs. If the femoral pulses are always felt in patients with high blood pressure, unexplained systolic murmurs, or unexplained aortic incompetence, the diagnosis should not be missed. Other physical signs include an excessive arterial pulsation at the base of the neck, visible or palpable pulsation of collateral vessels especially around the scapulae, minor degrees of retinal arteriopathy and palpable left ventricular hypertrophy. On auscultation there is an ejection systolic murmur over the upper sternum and this may be heard well over the dorsal spine. An ejection click (associated with dilatation of the aorta) preceding the murmur is common. An early diastolic murmur from aortic incompetence is also common; this is usually due to bicuspid aortic valves which occur in at least 25 per cent. of patients with aortic coarctation. Rarely a short mitral diastolic murmur due to thickening of the mitral cusps may be heard.

The electrocardiogram is often normal but left ventricular preponderance due to hypertension is usual in adults. Many also show right bundle branch block, the cause of which is unknown.

On X-ray there are four common features, rib notching due to tortuous collateral arteries, elongation and duplication of the aortic knuckle due to dilatation of the origin of the left subclavian artery, dilatation of the aorta immediately distal to the constriction and slight to moderate enlargement of the left ventricle.

Prognosis and Treatment

The average age at death is about 35; however, many patients live a normal life span. Death is usually due to heart failure, aortic rupture, bacterial endocarditis or cerebral haemorrhage. Coarctation of the aorta may be cured by surgical resection of the constriction and restoration of the tube by end-to-end anastomosis or the insertion of an aortic graft. The operative risk is low so that almost all patients under 30 years of age with uncomplicated aortic coarctation should be offered surgical treatment. An exception should be made when blood pressure is normal and femoral pulsation is good.

PULMONARY STENOSIS (WITH NORMAL AORTIC ROOT)

The majority of patients with this common form of congenital heart disease have pure valvar stenosis. The sexes are equally affected. When the obstruction is mild the pulmonary artery pressure and flow is normal and achieved by only a slight rise of right ventricular pressure. However, when the obstruction is severe the right ventricular pressures may rise to 150 mm.Hg or more and the cardiac output and pulmonary artery pressure is low; this great right ventricular load results in great right ventricular hypertrophy and secondary right atrial hypertrophy. Indeed, right atrial systole becomes vital in the maintenance of the circulation because of the greatly diminished compliance of the massive right ventricle.

The clinical features depend on the severity of the stenosis. Angina of effort, syncope on effort and severe dyspnoea may occur in the most severe cases but mild cases having a right ventricular pressure of 75 mm.Hg or less usually have no symptoms. An ejection systolic murmur loudest over the pulmonary artery and sometimes preceded by a click is common to all forms. The pulmonary second sound is variably delayed and soft. A right atrial gallop is audible in the more severe cases—when an atrial wave is also visible in the jugular venous pulse. Peripheral cyanosis is apparent when cardiac output is low (central cyanosis is not present unless a patent foramen ovale allows right to left shunting).

On X-ray there is post-stenotic dilatation of the pulmonary artery, and the vascular markings in the lungs are reduced to a variable degree depending on the severity of the stenosis.

The electrocardiogram shows some degree of right ventricular preponderance which depends on the degree of right ventricular hypertension. In the mildest cases it may be normal.

The diagnosis of isolated pulmonary stenosis is relatively easy in most cases; however, when great right ventricular hypertension results in the development of a reversed shunt through a patent foramen ovale the clinical features resemble those of atrial septal defect with pulmonary stenosis and Fallot's tetralogy. The diagnosis can then only be established by full haemodynamic investigation and angiocardiography.

Treatment

Mild cases may lead a normal life but extreme physical exertion (resulting in a great rise of right ventricular pressure) should be avoided. In all other cases pulmonary valvotomy is indicated. The operation is a satisfactory one, the risk relatively low and the results are excellent in the majority of cases. If the disease has progressed to the stage of great right ventricular hypertrophy diminished compliance of the ventricle continues to present a problem after successful relief of the obstruction.

Isolated infundibular pulmonary stenosis is uncommon. The effects are similar to those of valvular stenosis but post-stenotic dilatation is absent, the murmur is loudest at a lower level at the left side of the sternum and there is no ejection click.

RARER ANOMALIES

Congenital *pulmonary incompetence* is a very rare anomaly and results from agenesis of the pulmonary valves.

Ebstein's disease is a rare congenital disorder of the right heart in which the tricuspid valve is malformed and displaced downwards, dividing the ventricle into a proximal atrialized portion (greatly dilated atrium) and a distal portion functioning as the ventricle. The foramen ovale is open to varying degrees in many cases. Symptoms are often slight but paroxysmal rhythm changes may be troublesome. On auscultation a third heart sound and a tricuspid pansystolic murmur are common. The electrocardiogram usually shows some degree of right bundle branch block. On X-ray the heart appears remarkably large from great dilatation of the right heart. The X-ray appearances may be mistaken for those of pericardial effusion. Prognosis is often surprisingly good; there is no specific treatment.

GROUP 2. ANOMALIES WITH AN ABNORMAL COMMUNICATION BETWEEN THE RIGHT AND LEFT SIDES OF THE HEART

Congenital heart disease with abnormal communication between the right and left sides of the heart may be divided into acyanotic and cyanotic groups. Cases with left to right shunts (acyanotic) account for at least half of all forms of congenital heart disease surviving to adult life, whereas the blue ones with right to left shunts possibly total some 20 per cent. In adults atrial septal defect is the commonest left to right shunt, patent ductus arteriosus next, and ventricular septal defect next. Other sites of left to right shunt are rare. Fallot's tetralogy is the commonest cyanotic form surviving to adult life.

ABNORMAL COMMUNICATIONS WITH LEFT TO RIGHT SHUNT (GROUP 2A)

ATRIAL SEPTAL DEFECT (A.S.D.)

This is very common and often asymptomatic through adolescence and early adult life. Dyspnoea tends to develop gradually, or suddenly with the onset of atrial fibrillation. Palpitation from the hyperkinetic heart, extrasystoles or paroxysmal tachycardia are common. Bronchitis is prone to occur in older patients.

The physical signs depend mainly on the magnitude of the shunt (and thus on the size of the defect or on the existence of anomalous pulmonary veins draining into the right atrium). Patients with A.S.D. tend to be rather tall and thin. A small arterial pulse reflects the deviation of arterial blood to the pulmonary circulation. The jugular venous pressure is slightly raised. An increased pulsation over the pulmonary artery and at the left sternal edge and precordium may be seen or palpated in most cases. On auscultation a mid systolic murmur over the pulmonary artery is usual, and this is almost invariably followed by wide separation of the second sounds which remain 'fixed' on inspiration or expiration. A tricuspid diastolic murmur (heard best on inspiration at the fourth left intercostal space) occurs in cases with large shunts. When the picture is complicated by pulmonary hypertension the second pulmonary sound becomes very loud and may be followed by a pulmonary diastolic murmur. A systolic thrill over the pulmonary artery usually indicates complicating pulmonary stenosis.

On X-ray the most striking features are the large pulmonary arteries (pulmonary plethora or pleonaemia). Striking pulsation is visible on radioscopy. The right atrium is usually prominent and occasionally anomalous pulmonary veins may be seen entering the right atrium or superior vena cava. The electrocardiogram shows partial or complete right bundle branch block in nearly all cases. The diagnosis may be proved by cardiac catheterization when highly oxygenated blood may be obtained from the right atrium (when compared with samples from the venae cavae) and the defect crossed, where samples of blood from the left heart may be obtained and found to be normally saturated.

Uncomplicated cases of A.S.D. may live to middle life but dyspnoea gradually increases thereafter; the onset of atrial fibrillation usually causes a distinct deterioration in cardiovascular status. Important complicating factors are the development of pulmonary hypertension which may lead to central cyanosis from shunt reversal. The presence of pulmonary stenosis may have a similar effect but it is usually mild and does not materially alter prognosis in most cases. Mitral stenosis is occasionally associated with atrial septal defect (Lutembacher's syndrome) and tends to increase the left to right shunt.

The above description concerns ostium secundum defects: the *ostium primum* defect is much less common and may be distinguished by finding evidence of mitral incompetence (due to a cleft mitral valve), left axis deviation in the cardiogram and sometimes partial heart block.

Treatment

Treatment by operation is indicated for moderate to large shunts but is unnecessary for uncomplicated cases with shunts of less than 2 to 1 (i.e. a ratio of pulmonary to systemic blood flow of less than 2 to 1). Surgery is contra-indicated when there is severe obstructive pulmonary hypertension.

VENTRICULAR SEPTAL DEFECT (V.S.D.)

Defects in the membranous or muscular parts of the ventricular septum vary in size. The small ones produce no disability and are compatible with a normal life, and the term *maladie de Roger* should be reserved for this type. Larger defects may cause heart failure at any age, commonly in infancy and early adult life. The degree of shunt depends on the size of the defect and the resistance to increased flow in the right ventricle and pulmonary vasculature. The extra blood ejected from the right ventricle to the lungs is received by both left atrium and left ventricle; hence all chambers except the right atrium perform extra work.

The pulse is small and the jugular venous pressure is normal. Increased precordial and apical pulsation is usual and due to the biventricular volume load. On auscultation there is usually a loud pansystolic murmur in the mid precordium, and in some cases with a large shunt there is a functional mitral diastolic murmur. The second sounds are normal but the second component (pulmonary) is loud when there is pulmonary hypertension. X-rays demonstrate enlargement of the left ventricle and pulmonary plethora but the appearances may be normal in *maladie de Roger*. The electrocardiogram shows moderate degrees of left ventricular preponderance but when there is pulmonary hypertension a mixed pattern appears with added evidence of right ventricular hypertrophy. The diagnosis may be confirmed and the haemodynamic status assessed by cardiac catheterization.

The most important complications of ventricular septal defect are the development of pulmonary hypertension and bacterial endocarditis. Rarely, severe aortic reflux may develop with the prolapse of an aortic cusp into the defect. Infundibular pulmonary stenosis, like pulmonary hypertension, causes a reduction in the left to right shunt and eventually reversal with cyanosis may supervene.

Treatment

Pyogenic infections and dental procedures should be covered by penicillin to prevent bacterial endocarditis. Patients with a small shunt should lead normal lives, those with larger shunts should be advised to have surgical repair. The operative risk is greater than that for A.S.D. but with improving techniques in intracardiac surgery the mortality and morbidity is low.

PATENT DUCTUS ARTERIOSUS (P.D.A.)

This is due to the persistence of a foetal channel between the aorta and the main pulmonary artery. Perhaps the most readily recognized acyanotic congenital heart disease, this condition is not as common as A.S.D. but more so than V.S.D. Mild to moderate shunts through the ductus cause no symptoms, but when large, dyspnoea, bronchitis and palpitations are common as in the septal defects. The pulse is collapsing as in aortic reflux. The apex beat is of a left ventricular type and hyperkinetic. On auscultation there is a continuous murmur loudest in the first or second left interspace (machinery or Gibson murmur). As in V.S.D. there is a functional mitral diastolic murmur in the more severe cases. X-rays show a degree of pulmonary plethora depending on the size of the shunt and an enlarged left ventricle and first part of the aorta. The electrocardiogram shows left ventricular preponderance, though in the mild cases it remains normal and shows some evidence of right ventricular hypertrophy when there is pulmonary hypertension. In cases of doubt the diagnosis may be proved by cardiac catheterization and angiocardiography. The rare aortic septal defect presents a similar clinical and haemodynamic picture to patent ductus arteriosus.

The prognosis for patent ductus depends, as in other left to right shunts, mainly on the size of the shunt. The development of pulmonary hypertension and bacterial endocarditis are important complications. Death may occur in infancy from heart failure but this is rare in childhood and early adult life.

Treatment

This condition can be completely cured by operation which is best carried out in childhood. The mortality is less than 1 per cent. and the operation should be advised in all but the mildest cases. The ductus may be ligated or sectioned. Severe pulmonary hypertension is a contra-indication.

ABNORMAL COMMUNICATIONS WITH RIGHT TO LEFT SHUNT (GROUP 2B)

Patients look the same whatever the anatomical abnormality; the veno-arterial mixing results in arterial oxygen unsaturation which becomes visible as cyanosis, the capillary blood contains more than 5 g. per 100 ml. of reduced haemoglobin—usually detected when the arterial saturation falls below 85 per cent. Compensatory polycythaemia with a greatly increased haematocrit follows and heightens the appearance of cyanosis. Clubbing of the fingers and toes is usual and may reach a remarkable degree in those cyanotic conditions compatible with survival to adult life. The outlook for patients with morbus caeruleus is generally poor; only one in five reaches the age of 14, and less than one in ten reaches 21.

FALLOT'S TETRALOGY

The essential anatomical features of this condition are pulmonary stenosis, a high ventricular septal defect, an overriding aorta and right ventricular hypertrophy; all of these features were described by Peacock in 1858. It is the most common form of cyanotic congenital heart disease (66 per cent.). The stenosis is at the infundibulum of the right ventricle in half of the cases, at the pulmonary valve in a third and at both sites in the remainder. In the most severe cases the aorta may arise almost entirely over the right ventricle. Malformations of the aortic arch are commonly present, a right-sided aortic arch occurs in at least 25 per cent.

Cyanosis is present from the first few months of life. Squatting is a common attitude after effort. Dyspnoea becomes a serious problem in the more severe cases. Right ventricular hypertrophy sometimes causes a moderate increase in pulsation at the left sternal edge but this is not a conspicuous sign. There is always a systolic murmur over the right ventricular outflow tract and this is often loud enough to cause a thrill. This murmur may diminish during severe cyanotic attacks. The second heart sound is single and clearly arises from aortic valve closure.

The electrocardiogram shows prominent right atrial P waves in some cases and some degree of right ventricular preponderance is usual. On X-ray the lung fields are characteristically oligaemic and the main pulmonary artery shadow is absent or greatly diminished. In many cases the apex is uptilted giving the so-called *coeur en sabot* appearance.

The diagnosis may be made with confidence from the clinical features and confirmed by selective angiography or cardiac catheterization. Characteristically the pulmonary pressure is low, and there is a high right ventricular pressure which equals that in the left ventricle under changing haemodynamic circumstances.

The only important differential diagnosis is from *pulmonary stenosis with a right to left shunt at atrial level.* In this condition there is greater load on the right ventricle and right atrium, thus there is a right ventricular heave and great right preponderance on the electrocardiogram. There is an atrial gallop and large 'a' waves are visible in the jugular venous pulse.

Treatment

Complete surgical repair, i.e. resection of the infundibular or valvar stenosis and closure of the ventricular septal defect, is the treatment of choice. However, the mortality and morbidity is still on the high side so that mild cases can be left to await the inevitable fall in risk levels with improving techniques. Shunt operations of the Blalock-Taussig type are now rarely indicated because the risks for a later complete repair operation are considerably increased.

PULMONARY ATRESIA

This condition resembles the tetralogy of Fallot (it represents the extreme range of pulmonary stenosis). Life is sustained by collateral circulation of vessels from the aorta and small arteries in the lungs. These anastomoses are responsible for the continuous murmur which is a characteristic and distinguishing sign from the tetralogy of Fallot. Although a single great vessel leaves the heart this is unlike the true truncus arteriosus in which there is great pulmonary plethora.

TRICUSPID ATRESIA

In this condition systemic venous blood reaches the left heart through an atrial septum. The right ventricle is rudimentary. These patients are cyanosed from birth: the most important diagnostic feature is the presence of left axis deviation and left ventricular dominance in the electrocardiogram.

CYANOTIC HEART DISEASE WITH PULMONARY HYPERTENSION

Eisenmenger Syndrome. This term is used to describe the clinical picture of pulmonary hypertension with reversed shunt, and Eisenmenger's complex is used when the site of the reversed shunt is at ventricular level. Cyanosis is usual but when the shunt is through a patent ductus cyanosis may be confined to the lower extremities (differential cyanosis). High pulmonary resistance seems to be established at birth or very early in life in most cases of V.S.D. or P.D.A. However, in A.S.D. the high resistance may be acquired later in life (cyanose tardive).

Dyspnoea, pain or syncope on effort are important and serious symptoms. Haemoptysis is common especially in V.S.D. The signs apart from those of cyanosis are essentially those of severe pulmonary hypertension; left parasternal pulsation, an ejection click, a loud pulmonary second sound and a Graham Steell murmur are common features.

The electrocardiogram always shows some evidence of right ventricular preponderance but there may be some evidence of left preponderance in V.S.D. and P.D.A. X-rays show a large main pulmonary artery and peripheral oligaemia. Larger heart shadows occur in pulmonary hypertension with A.S.D. than in the other forms. Sometimes calcification in the region of P.D.A. may be observed and is diagnostic.

The prognosis is fair. Many live longer than anticipated from the degree of disability and their appearance. There is no remedial treatment.

REFERENCES

Abbott, M. E. (1936) *Atlas of Congenital Heart Disease*, New York.

Bedford, E. (1960) The anatomical types of atrial septal defect, *Amer. J. Cardiol.*, **6**, 568.

Bedford, E., and Holmes Sellors, T. (1960) Atrial septal defect, in *Modern Trends in Cardiology*, London.

Bedford, E., Papp, C., and Parkinson, J. (1941) Atrial septal defect, *Brit. Heart J.*, **3**, 37.

Bloomfield, D. (1964) The natural history of ventricular septal defect in patients surviving infancy, *Circulation*, **29**, 914.

Braunwald, E., Goldblatt, A., Aygen, M., Rokoff, D., and Morrow, A. (1963) Congenital aortic stenosis, *Circulation*, **27**, 426.

Campbell, M. (1961) Place of maternal rubella in the aetiology of congenital heart disease, *Brit. med. J.*, **1**, 691.

Ciba Foundation (1957) *Symposium on Congenital Heart Disease*, London.

Fyler, D. C., Rudolf, A., Wittenborg, M., and Nadas, A. (1958) Ventricular septal defect in infants and children, *Circulation*, **18**, 833.

Goldblatt, E. (1962) The treatment of cardiac failure in infancy. A review of 350 cases, *Lancet*, ii, 212.

Hudson, R. E. B. (1965) *Cardiovascular Pathology*, Vol. II, p. 1645, London.

Kjellberg, S., Mannheimer, E., Rudhe, U., and Jonsson, B. (1959) *Diagnosis of Congenital Heart Disease*, Chicago.

Morse, D. P., ed. (1962) *Congenital Heart Disease*, Philadelphia.

Scherlis, L., Koenker, R., and Yu Chen Lee (1964) Pulmonary stenosis, *Circulation*, **28**, 288.

Taussig, H. B. (1960) *Congenital Malformations of the Heart*, 2nd ed., Cambridge, Mass.

Wakai, C. S., and Edwards, J. E. (1958) Pathologic study of persistent common atrioventricular canal, *Amer. Heart J.*, **56**, 779.

Wood, P. (1958) The Eisenmenger syndrome, *Brit. med. J.*, **2**, 701 and 755.

ISCHAEMIC HEART DISEASE

Ischaemic heart disease includes all conditions which are due to a failure of the coronary circulation to meet the demands of cardiac muscle. As a rule the coronary arteries are diseased, so that the term is almost synonymous with coronary heart disease, and in most cases atheroma is the cause. Angina pectoris is a clinical syndrome comprising cardiac pain from effort or emotion due to coronary disease. Cardiac infarction indicates a clinical syndrome but also refers to pathology because it is essentially associated with necrosis of heart muscle. Coronary thrombosis refers to pathology and is almost synonymous with cardiac infarction, but occasionally either condition occurs without the other. Acute coronary insufficiency refers to an acute severe functional disturbance and may be recognized as a clinical syndrome having some of the features of angina pectoris and some of cardiac infarction. Such terms as coronary infarction, cardiac thrombosis, angina innocens, pseudo-angina and angina minor should never be used.

The clinical picture largely depends on the rate of development and extent of myocardial ischaemia. The main syndromes, angina pectoris, cardiac infarction and coronary insufficiency, may occur in any sequence, in combination, or as isolated events. The slow development of ischaemic heart disease may rarely lead to impaired function and heart failure without cardiac pain. The disease should be regarded as a continuous process with cardiac infarction as the outstanding event responsible for deterioration in circulatory efficiency.

Aetiology

All forms of ischaemic heart disease are manifestations of one disease process, the essentials of which are a discrepancy between the supply and demand for oxygen by the heart muscle. Occlusive disease of the coronary arteries, usually due to atheroma and associated thrombi, is the cause, but ischaemia may be increased by the abnormal requirements of muscle hypertrophy or greatly increased external work.

The cause of coronary atheroma and thrombus formation is unknown. There has been a great increase in the incidence of all manifestations of ischaemic heart disease during this century in modern Western states. This increase is real and cannot be accounted for by improved methods of diagnosis or a changing age distribution of the population. Ischaemic heart disease is the commonest single cause of death and probably accounts for 50 per cent. of all cardiac deaths in the British Isles.

Males are more commonly affected than females; when hypertension, diabetes and other endocrine disorders are excluded, coronary disease is rare in women below 60 years of age. This sex difference must have an important association with the cause. Coronary artery disease is more frequent in the higher age groups, but it is not uncommon under the age of 40 in men, and conversely many aged people show little evidence of atheroma; indeed the absence of atheroma is a prerequisite of attaining great age. It is doubtful whether coronary atheroma leading to ischaemic heart disease should be regarded in any way as a part of the normal ageing process. *Hereditary factors* may be important in the pathogenesis of coronary disease. There is a relatively high incidence of coronary disease, hypertension and degenerative vascular affections in the close relatives of patients with coronary disease; however, the relationship is by no means a close one and in general a common disease in the community is more likely to be due to environmental factors than genetic ones. There is no doubt that hypertension of any aetiology accelerates the process of atheroma; clinical coronary disease is thus more common in hypertensive subjects than normotensive ones.

There is considerable evidence that *abnormal lipid metabolism* is a factor in the development of atherosclerosis [p. 814]. There is a higher incidence of atheroma in modern states where diets contain much more animal fat than those of primitive peoples, in whom atheroma is almost unknown. It is obvious that many other factors may be operative, and it has not yet been shown that decreasing the dietary intake of fats and cholesterol influences the severity or incidence of ischaemic heart disease. Further evidence for the metabolic theory comes from the laboratory, where atheroma may be produced in rabbits and chicks by feeding large amounts of animal fats and cholesterol; the conditions are not comparable with those in man and the lesions produced, though closely resembling human atheroma, are not identical. Many patients with coronary disease show rather high levels of blood cholesterol and certain other lipid substances. The high incidence of coronary atheroma in diseases associated with high blood levels of cholesterol, e.g. diabetes, myxoedema and familial hypercholesterolaemia, strongly suggest that abnormal lipid metabolism is an aetiological factor in these conditions. Further evidence comes from the histopathology of the lesions in human atheroma, where deposits of cholesterol in the intima are invariably found. Excess cholesterol esters are thought to adhere to the intimal wall and to be deposited in it by macrophages, a connective tissue reaction is then provoked, with resultant scar formation.

When diseases such as coronary occlusion and peptic ulceration are not only common but especially prevalent in particular communities and groups within the community, it is probable that environmental factors play a considerable part in their aetiology. There appears to have been a fundamental change in the mode of life in civilized communities during the last half century. Coronary disease has shown a continuous tendency to increase during this period; it is possible that new conditions of stress especially affecting certain groups are an important aetiological factor. Those whose occupations are largely concerned with mental work, carrying responsibility, and whose lives are more individualized than the manual workers, are thought to be the special subjects of modern stress; they are the professional men, the managerial and executive classes who are often in tense competition with one another, and whose aims are set high yet are largely unattainable. These groups have numerically increased during the past century and coronary disease has selectively increased within these classes. Heavy cigarette smoking shows a positive correlation with sudden death from coronary heart disease and may accelerate progress of the disease. Improved diagnosis, increased longevity and the diminution of previously prevalent infectious diseases do not account for the present status of coronary disease, and its cause must account for an increasing incidence and the great prevalence amongst middle-aged men. There is some evidence to show that *diminished physical activity* predisposes to coronary disease or conversely that coronary disease is less likely to occur in those whose occupation necessitates a vigorous outdoor life. The various 'risk' factors mentioned above probably affect not only the disease process in the arterial wall but also the mechanisms of thrombogenesis. It is known that adhesiveness of platelets is increased by some of these risk factors.

Less common causes of ischaemic heart disease are syphilitic coronary ostial stenosis [p. 787], coronary embolism, periarteritis nodosa [see Section 4], thromboangiitis obliterans [p. 825] and congenital abnormalities of the coronary arteries. Trauma to the precordium is a rare cause of ischaemic heart disease; blunt, non-penetrating blows have been held responsible for coronary occlusion and infarction, but it is difficult to exclude pre-existing coronary atheroma even in young subjects. Penetrating injuries which damage the coronary circulation largely produce their effects through the development of haemopericardium.

Pathology

The Coronary Arteries. All degrees of atheroma are found in the coronary arteries from small, infrequent, yellowish plaques on the intima to extensive thickening of the whole vessel with irregular large plaques encroaching upon the lumen. Macroscopic calcification and ulceration of atheromatous plaques is common and the whole vessel may become a 'pipe stem'. Localized complete occlusion of the vessel may be due to large contiguous plaques of atheroma, fresh thrombosis on an ulcerated plaque, or more rarely to haemorrhage in the intima. The morphology of the coronary circulation may be demonstrated by radiography of the heart after the injection of opaque media into the coronary arteries. Complete occlusion occurs in any branch but the commonest sites are in vessels supplying the left ventricle at a point 2–3 cm. from their origin. Collateral channels in the vicinity of an occlusion are a common finding. In long-standing cases the normal homogeneous vascular pattern is lost and replaced by ischaemic areas with a fine lace-work of vessels between. The major arteries show gross irregularities and narrowing of the lumen.

Microscopical changes are principally found in the intima. The smallest lesions show large lipoid-containing mononuclear cells, whilst in larger lesions and presumably older ones, masses of cholesterol are found outside the cells. The adjacent intima and the margins of atheromatous plaques are supplied by numerous capillaries, but the larger lesions appear to undergo central necrosis where a mass of lipoid and cells may form an atheromatous abscess which tends to break down with resulting ulceration. The elastic and muscle coats may be completely absent and replaced by fibrosis. Microscopic sections through an area of thrombotic occlusion sometimes show layers of thrombus in varying states of organization, with a central fresh thrombosis responsible for the final obstruction.

The Myocardium. All degrees of damage to the left ventricular myocardium are found in ischaemic heart disease. The right ventricle and atria are rarely affected. When sudden death has occurred in the course of angina pectoris, the heart size and weight may be normal and the myocardium may show little macroscopic evidence of disease, whilst microscopic examination may show only an occasional patch of fibrosis. In other cases more widespread fibrosis is found either in frequent scattered patches or widely diffused throughout the muscle mass. This type of fibrosis probably represents a slow process of muscle death and replacement.

In recent cardiac infarction the heart may be of normal size, but it is usually dilated when there has been heart failure. A serofibrinous or serosanguinous pericarditis is common and occurs when the epicardium is involved. The pericardial sac is full of blood when cardiac rupture has occurred. The area of infarcted muscle varies in size but may involve a large part of the anterior wall and apical region, the septum, or postero-inferior wall. The infarcted area is pale, soft, friable and sometimes almost gelatinous. Haemorrhagic patches are frequently seen in the necrotic zone and recent thrombi may be adherent to the endocardium beneath the area of infarction, which is sometimes surrounded by a reddish zone of hyperaemia. When the ventricular septum is involved, rupture may occur, leading to direct communication between the right and left ventricles. The papillary muscles are sometimes involved in cardiac infarction and occasionally one or more of the mitral valve chordae may be fractured. In most cases of recent infarction a diligent search of the coronary vessels reveals a recent thrombus, but in some cases this is not so and it is presumed that intense prolonged ischaemia [acute coronary insufficiency, see p. 781] may result in necrosis. In such cases the necrosis is often patchy or in the subendocardial layers, which are usually preserved in massive cardiac infarction due to acute occlusion.

Microscopical examination of recent cardiac infarction shows that the nuclei of muscle cells disappear first, followed rapidly by the disappearance of the whole cell structure and surrounding vessels and connective tissue. The necrotic mass becomes surrounded by a zone of reactive inflammation, with abundant leucocytes and extravascular red cells. Organization involving resorption of necrotic cellular material and invasion by new vessels and fibroblasts begins within 7 days. Healing by fibrosis and contraction of the scar continues for many weeks. In long-standing cases of ischaemic disease and cardiac infarction the heart is frequently enlarged. Dilatation is present when there has been heart failure. Hypertrophy of the surviving good muscle is present in chronic cases especially when there is associated hypertension or valvular disease.

The pericardium is often thickened and adherent over areas of old infarction and the ventricular wall is thin, hard and pale, due to dense fibrous tissue. Layers of organized thrombus are frequently found lining the ventricular cavity beneath the damaged area. Aneurysm formation occurs when an area of old infarction stretches and bulges under the influence of ventricular pressure. The aneurysmal cavity is usually filled with layers of partially organized clot. Calcification occasionally occurs in the scar tissue.

ANGINA PECTORIS

Synonyms. Angina of effort; Heberden's angina.

Definition

Angina pectoris was described by Heberden in 1768, but its relationship to coronary disease was not appreciated until the present century. Angina pectoris is essentially a clinical syndrome of characteristic chest pain produced by increased cardiac work and relieved by rest. The underlying cause is occlusive disease of the coronary arteries, which is mostly atheroma, sometimes syphilitic coronary ostial stenosis, and very rarely coronary embolism or congenital anomalies of the coronary vessels. Cardiac pain identical with angina pectoris may also be caused by aortic stenosis and less commonly aortic incompetence; it also occurs in patients with severe pulmonary hypertension and rarely in pulmonary stenosis. Anaemia, if severe, may cause cardiac pain, but rarely of the severity met with in coronary atheroma. Angina pectoris may be associated with myxoedema, rarely with thyrotoxicosis and frequently with diabetes mellitus, and in these conditions coronary atheroma is the underlying cause.

Clinical Features

Paroxysmal chest pain caused by effort and other stimuli is the cardinal feature of angina pectoris. Although the pain varies in intensity, radiation, and the ease with which it is provoked, there is a constancy of the pattern which enables the disease to be recognized from the clinical history in the great majority of patients.

Anginal pain is usually situated in the front of the chest and mostly over the sternum. It tends to spread transversely from the sternum to the right and left pectoral regions. Occasionally the area of pain is small and it may be confined to the upper end of the sternum, or localized in the left pectoral region. It is more common on the left than the right side of the chest. Anginal pain tends to spread centrifugally to the arms, neck, jaws and epigastrium; the left shoulder and left upper arm are most often involved but frequently both arms are affected, and further spread down to the elbow, ulnar side of forearm and fingers is common. Many patients complain of numbness and a sense of great weakness in one or both arms. From the upper chest pain tends to spread to the neck, lower jaw, gums and teeth; occasionally it is experienced in the arm or jaws at first but in all cases the front of the chest is eventually involved. Less frequently pain is experienced in the epigastrium. Patients may feel that the pain is deep in the centre of the chest and often pain between the scapulae and across the shoulders accompanies the usual sternal pain. The extent of radiation of pain is roughly related to its severity. Ischaemic pain is characteristically described as constricting, crushing, vice-like or pressing. Sometimes there is a sensation of a weight on the front of the chest and some patients complain of a rawness or burning in the sternal region. The pain is steady during the attack, it does not stab, prick or shoot and is not related to chest movement or respiration.

Physical effort is the most common immediate cause of anginal pain. The first attack may be noticed with unusual effort, but sooner or later walking brings on the pain. An increase in pace, running or walking uphill diminish the threshold at which effort induces angina. A recent meal, cold air and worry also cause the pain to appear more readily. In some patients a meal, prolonged conversation, an argument, or any intense emotional situation may induce the pain without physical exertion. Rarely, and when ischaemia is severe, attacks of angina may be produced by lying down and, as with left ventricular failure, patients may be wakened from sleep. In such cases there is often a history of an unpleasant dream, but it would seem more likely that posture is responsible for these attacks, which are rapidly relieved by sitting up in bed. When physical exertion is the exciting cause, there is a remarkable constancy in the kind, rate or amount of effort which will probably, if not always, bring on an attack, and this also applies in a lesser degree to other exciting causes. Occasionally there is a clear history of a rapid increase in severity of the condition, threshold of onset is progressively lowered, pain becomes more severe and the frequency of attacks is greater. Such a history suggests impending cardiac infarction.

Attacks of angina rarely last for more than a few minutes. The pain rapidly reaches maximal intensity and subsides when the provoking stimulus is removed. In most cases the patient stops walking or slows below the critical point at which pain is produced. In very rare mild cases relief may come in spite of continued effort but in all severe cases pain brings the patient to a complete standstill—this immobility is enforced and is not a voluntary act to relieve pain. Even when pain has been largely abolished by a sympathectomy, a curious sensation is often experienced which demands immediate rest. With advanced disease the attacks may become very frequent, being evoked by the smallest effort. Although angina pectoris is essentially paroxysmal, sometimes a dull sternal ache persists between the attacks. Occasionally attacks are accompanied by a sense of anxiety out of all proportion to the severity of the pain and sometimes by a sense of impending dissolution.

The facial expression is often strained and anxious and there may be pallor at the time of the attack, but there are no important abnormal signs directly related to an attack of angina; the pulse rate may change—in some patients it is increased, while occasionally it is diminished. The arterial blood pressure is usually somewhat increased. A few patients show a general pressor reaction associated with the pain; there is flushing of the face, sweating and a sharp rise of systemic blood pressure. When angina pectoris is due to disease other than coronary atherosclerosis, there are associated symptoms and signs of the underlying cause.

The Electrocardiogram. The electrocardiogram should be obtained in all cases of suspected angina pectoris. There is no close agreement between various investigators concerning the frequency of a pathological electrocardiogram. However, if the electrocardiographic investigation includes standard leads, lead III on inspiration, unipolar limb leads and at least three precordial leads, it is probable that 85 per cent. of patients will show some abnormality of the tracing. Those patients showing a normal electrocardiogram at rest should have further tracings taken at 2-minute intervals for 6 minutes, after moderate exercise [FIG. 43]. The amount of exercise is graded to the patient's capacity and should never continue after pain has started. It is obviously unnecessary to proceed with exercise tests if the resting electrocardiogram is abnormal. In angina pectoris the electrocardiogram may show such gross changes as left bundle branch block [FIG. 42a] or old cardiac infarction [FIG. 45a, b], but more often the changes are slight and these are: (1) depression of the S-T segment by 1 mm. or more; (2) unusual coving or winging of the S-T segment; (3) flattening or inversion of T waves; (4) inversion of U waves in left ventricular leads. Any one or all of these changes may be present when the patient is at rest or they may be produced by effort and recede with rest, or be produced by induced anoxaemia.

Other Investigations. The ballistocardiogram is pathological in a high percentage of cases of angina pectoris but this has little to add to the electrocardiogram from the diagnostic point of view.

Radiography often shows a normal sized heart but radiographic screening should be routinely carried out. Coronary angiography may be used to localize the site of blockage and to evaluate the extent of disease.

Further investigations to assess the possible presence

and severity of metabolic abnormalities such as hypercholesterolaemia, hyperglycaemia, hyperuricaemia and myxoedema should be made. If hypertension is present a full investigation of this is required and serological tests for syphilis complete a reasonable minimal investigation of patients with angina pectoris when the disease is first diagnosed.

Diagnosis

1. *The symptom.* Angina pectoris is recognized by the clinical history, the most important features of which are the sternal site of pain, the relationship to effort and relief by rest. The constancy of the type, site and amount of effort required to cause the pain is an important feature of angina. Patients do not tell of other minor symptoms, their concern is with the one pain and they usually remember well the circumstances of a first attack, which is so often indelibly impressed on the mind. The relief of pain by nitrites may be misleading; many neurotics are relieved by drugs through suggestion and the relief of spasm of smooth muscle elsewhere, e.g. oesophagospasm, may be relieved by nitrites. The results of physical examination are not helpful except where the presence of hypertension, and organic heart disease known to be associated with angina, is detected. Even in such cases it is on the characteristic features of the pain that diagnosis is made. The presence of ischaemia of the myocardium is confirmed by an electrocardiogram.

2. *The cause.* A diagnosis of angina pectoris is insufficient; it refers only to a symptom and contains no information concerning aetiology. In all cases a cause other than coronary atherosclerosis should be sought; in males from the age of 30 onwards coronary disease is by far the commonest cause, but in women this is not so. Most of the other causes of ischaemic pain, i.e. aortic stenosis, syphilitic aortitis, anaemia, myxoedema and pulmonary hypertension may be diagnosed readily by clinical examination.

Other Causes of Chest Pain. There are many causes and types of chest pain. Few should be confused with angina pectoris after a comprehensive history has been obtained by the art of firm interrogation. Pain associated with anxiety or other manifestations of psychoneurosis is the most common source of confusion. Neurotic patients often have numerous symptoms and the pain is usually beneath the left nipple; occasionally it is over the sternum and related to effort, but careful questioning usually shows that the relationship is inconstant or that the pain lasts for hours and comes on after the effort is over. It is frequently related to fatigue, both sexes may be affected and there are often obvious signs of anxiety. The electrocardiogram is normal before and after exercise. Pain arising from the oesophagus may cause difficulty. Here there is rarely any relation to effort although oesophageal pain may have the same quality and distribution as angina pectoris. Hiatus hernia produces a similar spasmodic pain, but there is no relation to effort, although a particular posture or particular movement may produce this pain. Hiatus hernia is not uncommonly associated with angina pectoris; both conditions occur with increasing frequency after middle life. Oesophageal spasm, oesophageal arrhythmia and hiatus hernia are diagnosed by radiological investigation. Pain referred from musculoskeletal lesions may superficially resemble angina pectoris, especially if movement is confused with effort. Lesions of the cervical spine such as cervical spondylosis may cause pain over the upper chest and pain in the arms. Lesions of the upper dorsal spine may likewise cause neuritic pain in the front of the chest and a sudden movement of the chest or sneezing may produce it. Often there is no demonstrable musculoskeletal lesion, but occasionally there is spondylitis or a prolapsed intervertebral disc. In these referred skeletal pains the electrocardiogram is normal. Especial care must be taken in the diagnosis of shoulder pain associated with chest pain.

Gall-bladder disease is said to cause confusion with angina pectoris; these conditions often coexist and whilst gall-bladder disease may in some way lower the threshold for cardiac pain when there is coronary disease, it does not alone produce chest pain related to effort.

Treatment

Individual attacks of angina pectoris are relieved by rest. Most patients discover this in the first few attacks and all should be advised to cease exertion as soon as the first suggestion of pain is experienced.

Nitrites specifically relieve anginal pain by causing dilatation of coronary vessels; systemic arterioles are also relaxed, causing a fall in peripheral resistance. Therapeutic doses produce slight hypotension and tachycardia. Glyceryl trinitrate (trinitrin, trinitroglycerin) is the drug of choice; it is cheap, effective, administered in tablet form and is devoid of the more unpleasant side-effects caused by amyl nitrite. Fresh tablets of glyceryl trinitrate, 0·5 mg., act in about 2 minutes when chewed and take longer when retained under the tongue. The effect lasts from 15 to 30 minutes. One tablet chewed at the onset of pain is usually effective, more may be taken if necessary. There are no long-term toxic effects and patients with angina pectoris should always carry a supply of fresh tablets. When it is necessary to undertake effort which is known to produce pain, a tablet should be dissolved under the tongue in anticipation and is frequently effective in preventing the attack. Glyceryl trinitrate sometimes causes a throbbing in the head and rarely a sense of giddiness or faintness.

Amyl nitrite is supplied in silk-covered glass capsules, which must be broken, and the malodorous vapour is then inhaled—an altogether unpleasant procedure. This drug acts somewhat more quickly than glyceryl trinitrate, but the side-effects due to vasodilatation are more unpleasant. Octyl nitrite is volatile and acts quickly but suffers the disadvantages of amyl nitrite. The longer-acting organic nitrites should not be used for separate attacks but are said to diminish the intensity and frequency of attacks [see below].

General Management and Prevention of Attacks. Those situations which cause anginal pain are best avoided. Effort should be confined to levels below that which provokes pain, and if this is not possible, a tablet of trinitrin should be taken prior to the expected pain.

Hurry should be eliminated, arguments, excitement or situations charged with emotional tension should be avoided and a quiet, philosophic attitude to life developed. It is advisable to avoid the spectacle of highly competitive sport, but quiet personal exercise of a steady kind below the level at which pain is caused should be encouraged.

Large meals are best avoided and exercise should not be taken after meals. When there is obesity, weight reduction is advisable, and this should be carried out by a low-fat, low-calorie regime. Weight reduction is most effectively carried out during a period of supervised bed rest in the first instance, when a 1000 calorie diet may be used and salt restricted to 0·5 g. daily if there is associated hypertension: after an initial response the diet may be increased.

Problems concerning hours of work, type of work, leisure time and holidays can only be resolved having due regard for the severity of the illness and individual economic and social responsibilities of the patient. In general it is better to remain in employment, but to reduce the number of working hours and diminish the physical and mental loads where these are heavy.

Regular sleep, eight hours in bed per day and most of one day a week in bed may be beneficial. A period of prolonged partial bed rest up to 4 weeks is advisable for patients seen soon after the onset of angina pectoris. Bed rest is also indicated when the disease is increasing rapidly in severity, for this suggests impending cardiac infarction. In such cases when brief attacks of pain begin to occur at rest, anticoagulant therapy [p. 779] may be used with benefit.

Sedatives are advisable where emotional factors readily produce pain and for patients with secondary anxiety. It is especially important to ensure sound sleep and barbiturates should be freely used.

Tobacco smoking is best stopped altogether, if this can be done without causing too much mental stress.

Alcohol is not contra-indicated. It is a sedative and possibly a mild coronary vasodilator. The admissibility of alcohol can be used to offset the withdrawal of tobacco, and even in total abstainers the news that it may be taken comes as relief when it is expected that the physician's advice will be entirely restrictive. An optimistic reassuring attitude should be adopted by the physician at all times.

When attacks are frequent one of the so-called β blocking drugs such as propranolol should be used. The tachycardia caused by effort and emotion is diminished and in those patients where tachycardia and hypertonia is a particular feature associated with the pain propranolol is most effective. The dose should be slowly increased from 40 mg. thrice daily after one week to a maximum of 240 mg. a day. The long-acting nitrates such as erythritol tetranitrate and mannitol hexanitrate, 15–30 mg., may be tried, but the results are not impressive: many other long-acting so-called coronary vasodilators are available and widely used but true therapeutic effect is doubtful. The xanthine drugs, especially aminophylline, are often used in the treatment of angina pectoris. There is much disagreement about their value. It is certain that any effect is slight and xanthines, if used at all, should be invariably secondary to the nitrites. A suppository of aminophylline at night is well worth a trial for patients having frequent nocturnal attacks. When early left ventricular failure appears to be associated with angina pectoris, as in patients having nocturnal attacks of pain, sodium restriction, digitalis and diuretics should be used [see treatment of heart failure, p. 749].

Many physicians advocate the use of long-term anticoagulant therapy [p. 779] and there is some evidence that the risk of subsequent attacks of cardiac infarction is reduced thereby. Others consider that the hazards of anticoagulants outweigh any benefit. However, the drugs and methods available for reduction and control of coagulability of blood will gradually improve and these controversial problems may then be solved.

Antithyroid drugs, and in the past thyroidectomy, have been used to induce hypothyroidism and thereby lower the demands on the heart and circulation. It is doubtful whether the serious nature of the treatment is justified. However, in cases where disability is great and even slight effort is attended by pain, carbimazole (*Neo-Mercazole*) or propylthiouracil should be tried for a few months.

Surgical treatment has been attempted during the last two or three decades. One object has been to cut the sympathetic nerves which conduct pain sensation or to improve the coronary circulation by producing new vascular pathways. Pain fibres are cut by either dorsal ganglionectomy and stellate ganglionectomy or posterior rhizotomy of the upper five dorsal roots. Some 50 per cent. of patients obtain considerable relief, but many patients complain that pain is replaced by an equally unpleasant but indefinable sensation often associated with giddiness which demands immobility. The creation of an adhesive pericarditis has been carried out by introducing irritants into the pericardial sac in the hope that new vessels will develop between pericardium and epicardium and between end vessels of the coronary circulation. In practice either magnesium silicate or bone dust is used, and the procedure has a few advocates who claim considerable success.

The creation of an effective anastomotic circulation is a more rational procedure, but long-term results are unknown. Various methods have been used. Earlier attempts, notably by Beck and O'Shaughnessy, involved the suturing of pectoral muscle or omentum to the heart. More recently the internal mammary arteries have been directly implanted in the myocardium at an ischaemic site after an investigation of the coronary circulation by selective coronary angiography. Vein grafts between the aorta and coronary system have produced the best results so far. The indications for such operations are not yet fully assessed. Attempts to disobliterate coronary arteries have been made but have not met with much success.

Treatment of the Underlying Cause. Unfortunately this is rarely possible, but in all cases the aetiology should be reviewed. The treatment for syphilitic aortitis, anaemia, aortic stenosis, myxoedema, thyrotoxicosis and other causes of angina pectoris are described in the section concerned.

Prognosis

One of the features of angina pectoris due to coronary artery disease is the varied course and uncertainty of outlook. Sudden death or cardiac infarction may occur early in the disease; on the other hand, attacks may subside in frequency and intensity and even completely disappear for years. However, in most cases the malady tends to be slowly progressive and the average duration of life is 8 years, but many live for 15–20 years. Hypertension, arrhythmia, diabetes mellitus, excessive weight, heavy cigarette smoking, and a strong family history of degenerative vascular disease adversely influence prognosis. The outlook is worse when attacks are caused by relatively slight exertion or excitement and when the pain is severe, widespread and persistent. A history of increasing severity indicates impending cardiac infarction, and if this episode is survived, subsequent effort pain may be less severe or even absent. Sudden death or cardiac infarction may supervene even in the mildest cases. The outlook for women is better than for men.

Prognosis in angina pectoris is affected by the underlying cause; it is good when associated with conditions which can be treated, such as paroxysmal tachycardia, thyrotoxicosis and anaemia. Cholecystectomy may favourably influence the outlook in cases where gall-bladder disease appears to be related to the attacks. When angina pectoris is associated with pulmonary or systemic hypertension, the outlook is usually unfavourable. It is worse when syphilis is the cause of aortitis, coronary stenosis, aortic incompetence and ventricular hypertrophy. A good response to treatment in all cases of angina favourably influences prognosis, especially when life can be modified in such a way that attacks no longer occur.

CARDIAC INFARCTION

Synonym. Myocardial infarction.

Aetiology

The essential feature of cardiac infarction is necrosis of heart muscle. This is usually due to coronary occlusion which in most cases is due to coronary thrombosis, so that these terms have become almost synonymous by common usage. The aetiology of ischaemic heart disease and coronary atheroma has been discussed and similar factors are operative in cardiac infarction. There are no constant conditions which precipitate cardiac infarction; physical exertion and exceptional emotion do not appear to be important, and in many cases the onset is during sleep; it may occur at any time of the day or at any time of the year, but it is somewhat more frequent during winter months.

Cardiac infarction is said to be more common in short, obese individuals, but there is no doubt that it may occur in patients of any physical build or mental type. There are, in fact, no constant common features apart from the great preponderance of the disease in men. Coronary thrombosis is associated with coronary atheroma, but it is probably not the only aetiological factor, for advanced coronary atheroma is often found in patients who have never had manifestations of ischaemia; furthermore, there is evidence from necropsy studies that whilst cardiac infarction has increased in frequency during recent years, coronary atheroma has remained unchanged; it is thus probable that an altered state of blood coagulability may be concerned with the pathogenesis of coronary thrombosis in addition to the presence of coronary atheroma. Coronary embolism, usually due to bacterial endocarditis, is a rare cause of acute occlusion and cardiac infarction.

Hypertension is frequently associated with coronary disease and it appears that coronary atheroma is more likely to become manifest as ischaemic heart disease when hypertension is present. Hypertension is almost certainly a factor in the pathogenesis of coronary atheroma, but it is also possible that both conditions are the result of the same common factors, which remain unknown. Hypercholesterolaemia is another powerful determinant in the development of coronary atheroma but cardiac infarction often occurs in patients with normal levels of serum cholesterol.

Gall-bladder disease occasionally appears to precipitate ischaemic heart disease and it is possible that reflexes from the alimentary canal lower the threshold for cardiac pain. However, there is no evidence that gall-bladder disease or any other disturbance of the alimentary system is closely related to the cause of coronary occlusion.

Clinical Features

Pain is the most prominent symptom and it may be associated with shock or acute heart failure. There are prodromal symptoms in many cases. Brief attacks of pain may occur during the preceding 24–72 hours and sometimes there is a general feeling of malaise for a few hours before the major attack of pain. Patients having a long previous history of angina pectoris may recognize an increase in its severity during the preceding weeks and a few patients give a short history of angina pectoris which, from its onset, increases in frequency and intensity until brief attacks of pain at rest may herald a major attack of infarction. Many patients in this group seek medical advice before infarction occurs.

The onset of pain is usually independent of any exciting cause; it may occur at any time of the day or waken the patient from sleep. The maximal intensity of pain is soon reached; it is a steady pain and may be mild or of agonizing intensity—among the severest of pains experienced by man. Its site, radiation and quality is the same as occurs in angina pectoris [p. 772], but it tends to be more severe and lasts for hours or even days. Few patients remain motionless as in angina pectoris; most become restless and adopt various positions in an attempt to get relief; some walk about and I have known one patient who ran 'to work off' the pain, and another who proceeded to exercise in a gymnasium in order to relieve the 'acute rheumatism' in his chest. None of these manoeuvres brings relief from the steady intense pain. Painless cardiac infarction is probably very rare. In some cases extreme shock and unconsciousness may be responsible for the early absence of pain, which, however, appears when the syncopal state passes off. The pain of past cardiac infarction may be forgotten when there is advanced cerebral vascular disease.

Shock is a common feature of cardiac infarction and all degrees occur, from those with symptoms of dizziness, weakness or faintness, sweating and vomiting, to those with severe degrees of shock which dominate the whole clinical picture. A distinction should be made between true cardiogenic shock when extensive muscle damage causes a profound fall in cardiac output and simple vagal hypotension—a fainting reaction—possibly due to pain and not necessarily associated with more than minimal damage to the pump. In severe cases there is great weakness; postural syncope may be the first symptom and this may be recurrent unless the patient is recumbent. The skin is pale, cold and moist, the face is greyish, drawn and anxious, and the mind is often clear. The skin of the extremities shows extreme vasoconstriction, being white or patchily cyanosed. The blood pressure is low and the pulse pressure may be so diminished that a radial pulse cannot be felt, tachycardia is usual. Shock may persist for hours or even days. Pain, left ventricular failure or a general improvement may emerge as the shock state passes off. In the simple fainting reaction the patient is not so ill, the lesion is often small, bradycardia is usual and the whole episode is of brief duration.

Heart failure may occur alone or in combination with pain or shock at any time during the history of cardiac infarction. In the early stages of the disease heart failure usually appears as acute left ventricular failure; indeed the first symptom may be an acute attack of cardiac asthma or even pulmonary oedema. Pain is usually present but the patient is sometimes overwhelmed by dyspnoea and a history of pain may not be obtained until later. Congestive cardiac failure may develop at any time, but usually after an interval of a few days. Cheyne-Stokes respiration is often present.

Nausea and vomiting are common features of cardiac infarction and may be combined with upper abdominal discomfort or epigastric pain. Morphine is often responsible for gastro-intestinal symptoms. *Arrhythmias* frequently develop in cardiac infarction, extrasystoles and brief episodes of atrial fibrillation being the commonest, but most patients are unaware of the irregularity and few complain of palpitation. Atrial or ventricular tachycardia may be paroxysmal or persistent and are often responsible for serious deterioration. Transient heart block is not uncommon.

Abnormal physical signs are not a prominent feature of cardiac infarction; even with prolonged severe pain there may be no abnormal findings. *Fever* is common. It is of mild degree and lasts for a few days from the first or second day of the attack. A moderate leucocytosis and elevation of the erythrocyte sedimentation rate is usual. Within the first 48 hours of a cardiac infarction various enzymes escape from the damaged heart muscle and are found in increased concentration in the serum. The rise roughly parallels the extent of the injury and the increased serum levels provide confirmatory evidence of infarction. The glutamic oxalacetic transaminase (SGOT) rises in the first 48 hours from a normal of less than 40 units per ml., sometimes as high as 800 units per ml. The lactate dehydrogenase (LDH) and the α-hydroxybutyrate dehydrogenase (HBD), the normal levels of which are less than 500 and 300 units per ml. respectively, increase about the same time but fall more slowly. *Tachycardia* is often more than can be accounted for by fever and the *arrhythmias* mentioned above, including heart block, may be detected by examination of the radial arteries and jugular pulses.

Pericardial friction occurs early in some 10–15 per cent. of cases, especially in those with anterior infarction. It is often fleeting but may persist for days and indicates accompanying pericarditis. An atrial sound or triple rhythm due to the addition of a diastolic filling sound (third heart sound) is often audible depending on the degree of myocardial damage and heart rate. Either of these additional sounds indicates some degree of left ventricular dysfunction.

Shock is indicated by pallor, sweating, peripheral constriction and hypotension. When shock is absent, blood pressure may rise initially but tends to fall after 24–48 hours, and it may return to normal or near normal levels after a varying interval of days or weeks.

Heart failure is indicated by dyspnoea, orthopnoea, triple rhythm, a rise in jugular venous pressure and hilar congestion on X-ray of the chest. Any of the signs of heart failure may be encountered at any stage of the illness, but the signs of shock are early.

The Electrocardiogram. The electrocardiogram is of great diagnostic value. It is always abnormal in cardiac infarction although rarely it may remain normal for a few hours after the onset of pain. The ventricular complex is altered in three ways [FIG. 50]. (1) Large primarily negative waves (Q waves) appear in leads recording the main left ventricular potentials, i.e. where R waves existed before. These pathological Q waves are usually more than 0·04 sec. duration and may replace all of the QRS or be followed by the remnants of an R wave. The development of Q waves indicates muscle death, hence the change is usually permanent and is highly specific since coronary disease is the commonest cause of circumscribed myocardial necrosis. (2) Elevation and coving of the S-T segment in leads facing the damaged area (and reciprocal depression of the S-T segment in remote leads) are due to superficial injury involving the epicardium and pericardium. S-T elevation is maximal in the early phases of the attack and subsides after a few days. S-T changes are not as specific for cardiac infarction as Q waves, since the same changes occur in pericarditis from other causes. Persistent elevation of the S-T segment may be due to the development of a ventricular aneurysm. (3) Inversion of the T wave in leads where it is normally positive is usual in cardiac infarction. In the earliest days of the attack S-T elevation may be great and the isoelectric interval reached without the development of a separate T wave; however, sharp inversions of the T waves appear as the S-T elevation subsides. T wave inversion mostly occurs in combination with Q waves and with S-T changes in cardiac infarction. Isolated T wave changes are not specific and occur as the result of many varied physiological and pathological changes in the muscle; however, when assessed with the clinical features, flattening and inversion of the T wave have great diagnostic value.

The T waves may become positive after recovery and healing of cardiac infarction.

These pathological changes occur in leads related to the left ventricle and maximally in those 'facing' the area of infarction, so that it is often possible to determine approximately its site and size. *Anterior infarction* is indicated by Q, S-T and T wave changes in anterior chest leads and in lead I. When the septum is involved, complete Q waves also occur in right anterior chest leads [FIG. 50a]. *Posterior* (*or inferior*) *infarction* is indicated by the finding of Q, S-T and T wave abnormalities in leads from the left leg, i.e. in leads II, III and VF, which record potentials in the field facing the diaphragmatic surface of the heart [FIG. 50b]. *Lateral infarction* is diagnosed when changes are found in the extreme left chest leads, i.e. V7 CR7 and VL. These changes may occur alone or in combination with an anterior or posterior pattern.

Final diagnosis depends on radiological examination; a hump or bulge on the left ventricular silhouette which swells in systole is diagnostic and if surgical resection is contemplated the diagnosis may be further confirmed and the size and site of the aneurysm determined by left ventricular angiography. The electrocardiogram shows the changes of cardiac infarction and persistent S-T elevation is usual.

Rupture of the heart at the site of the infarct is not uncommon; haemopericardium follows and may cause sudden death. An internal rupture occasionally occurs, producing a left to right shunt or acute mitral reflux from rupture of the ventricular septum or a papillary muscle.

The so-called 'post-infarction syndrome' is a rare condition probably caused by hypersensitivity to damaged tissue. Delayed fever, joint pains, serositis—especially recurrent pericarditis and a raised E.S.R. are usual features. The condition responds to steroid therapy. The 'frozen shoulder' and 'the shoulder-hand syndrome' sometimes develop after cardiac infarction and are closely related to the post-infarction syndrome. Pain frequently occurs in either shoulder at variable periods from a few weeks to a few months after an attack of cardiac infarction, and in severe forms the shoulder may become stiff, painful and ultimately almost immobile. Less commonly the hand becomes stiff, swollen or shows trophic changes in the skin. The fingers become smooth and pale, resulting in a scleroderma-like condition. Spontaneous recovery after a variable period is usual.

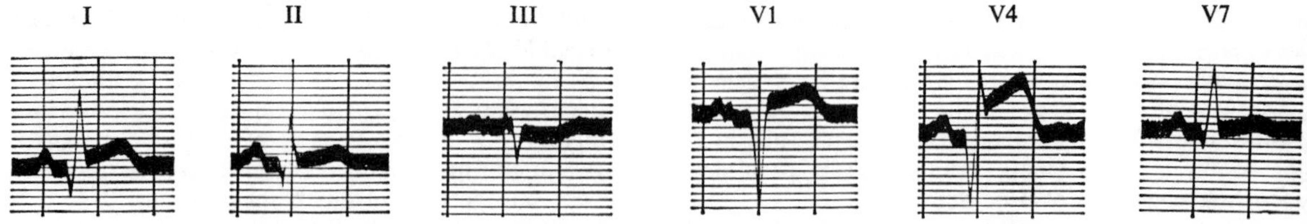

FIG. 50a. *Anterior wall infarction.* Deep and wide Q waves in I, II and V4 with S-T segment elevation indicating recent infarction.

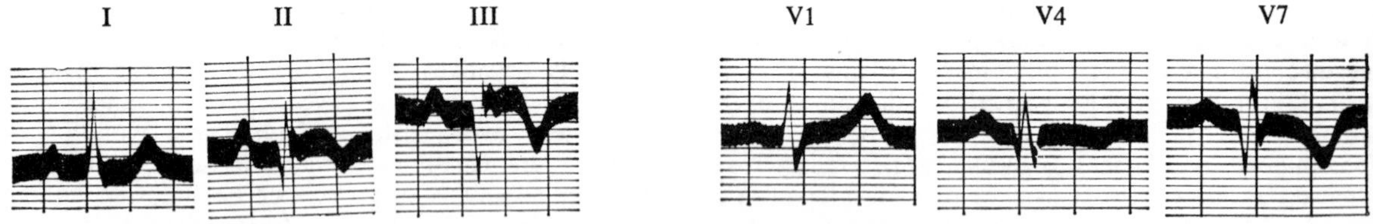

FIG. 50b. *Posterior* (*inferior*) *wall infarction.* Abnormal Q waves in II, III, V4 and V7 associated with S-T segment elevation indicate posterior cardiac infarction (with some lateral extension).

Complications

Thrombo-embolism is found in more than one-third of necropsy examinations and is a clinical problem in some 15 per cent. of cases. Phlebothrombosis in the leg is the most common and is responsible for episodes of pulmonary infarction and for massive pulmonary embolism. Systemic emboli may involve any organ and arise from ventricular mural thrombi; however, there is evidence to suggest that arterial thrombosis in the affected organ is sometimes responsible. Cerebrovascular episodes are uncommon.

The infarcted area of myocardium may bulge, producing a local ventricular aneurysm, which, if large enough, causes a diffuse pulsation of the chest wall. Occasionally there appears to be a double apex; that due to the aneurysm is usually above and internal to the true apex, and a see-saw like movement occurs between the two pulsations. Ventricular aneurysms develop soon after the episode of infarction, which is usually of the anterior variety, but they do not necessarily influence the outcome. The cavity of the aneurysm often becomes partially obliterated by organized clot which may become calcified and visible on X-ray.

Treatment

Treatment of cardiac infarction is based on four principles: (1) the relief of pain; (2) the treatment of shock and heart failure; (3) the reduction of cardiac work; and (4) the prevention and treatment of complications. This treatment is most effectively and successfully carried out in a special coronary care unit, staffed by trained medical and nursing personnel, equipped with apparatus for continuous monitoring of the ECG and other parameters and provided with special facilities for resuscitation. However, the same general principles of treatment apply whether the patient is in a special unit, the ward of a general public or private hospital or in the relaxed environment of home. Immediate bed rest is indicated and fluids only should be given for 24 hours followed by an 800 calorie diet.

Morphine is usually required to relieve the pain, but when the pain is slight a milder analgesic may be sufficient. Intramuscular injection of morphine, 10–20 mg., combined with *Phenergan*, 25 mg., is most effective. If pain is very severe 10 mg. of morphine in 5 ml. of sterile water should be given intravenously. *Amytal*, 100–200 mg., is useful for night sedation. Vomiting and disturbances of the bowel are sometimes due to morphine, but this symptom is often due to the attack of infarction.

Shock passes off under the influence of rest and morphine in many patients, but in some it is more severe and persistent. When acute hypotension is responsible for giddiness or syncope, patients must be nursed flat unless left ventricular failure appears when a more upright posture is necessary. Persistent shock carries a very high mortality; transfusions of glucose, plasma and blood have been advocated but they are of little value. Oxygen, 10 litres per minute by Venturi mask, is indicated and digoxin or ouabain should be given. If the venous pressure is below 10 cm. H_2O this should be elevated by an infusion of 5 per cent. dextrose. If hypotension persists, isoprenaline, 2 mg. per 500 ml., should be added to the intravenous therapy and maintained until and if recovery from hypotension occurs.

Heart failure of any type and severity should be treated with a low salt diet and diuretics. Aminophylline given as a suppository at night may help to control nocturnal attacks of dyspnoea. Digitalis should be used [for treatment of heart failure, see p. 749].

Arrhythmias are often transient and do not require special treatment unless persistent. When extrasystoles are frequent quinidine in doses of 200–300 mg. four times a day may abolish them but repeated injections of lignocaine, 50–100 mg. intravenously at three-minute intervals, are most effective. Ventricular tachycardia requires immediate treatment and lignocaine is the drug of choice [see p. 761 for details]. Ventricular fibrillation calls for immediate direct current counter-shock. Sinus bradycardia (less than 60 per minute) may be troublesome and atropine, 0·6 mg. intravenously, should be given as necessary. Persistent complete heart block carries a bad prognosis which is, however, improved by transvenous pacing [see p. 764].

Most patients require from 3 to 4 weeks' modified bed rest, depending on the severity of the attack. From the physical point of view, the difference between complete and modified bed rest is slight, but morale and mental rest are benefited by the less exacting regime. Complete bed rest also increases the risk of peripheral thrombo-embolism. The recognized hazards of prolonged complete bed rest have led to the advocation of armchair treatment during recent years. This method has its dangers and there appears to be no sound reason for abandoning bed rest provided that it is intelligently carried out. It is therefore recommended that: (1) all cases rest in bed for at least 3 weeks and ideally none should return to work before 12 weeks. (2) Mild and moderate cases with no shock, no heart failure, no cardiac enlargement are allowed to use a commode, feed, wash and shave themselves and sit out of bed for short periods. After the third or fourth week, activity should be steadily increased. (3) More seriously ill patients should be rested in bed for 4 weeks or more if necessary. (4) Shocked patients should be nursed recumbent until the arterial pressure rises, whilst those with heart failure should be nursed in a more upright position. It is emphasized that at all stages the clinical condition of the patient should determine the nursing regime, the length of rest and the rate of convalescence.

Diet. It is advisable to reduce the diet below 1000 calories daily for the first week in all cases. Thereafter more food is allowed but the separate meals should be small. Salt should be restricted to less than 1 g. daily in all patients with hypertension or any evidence of heart failure.

Constipation may become a problem and strenuous defaecation should be avoided by the use of liquid paraffin. Acute retention of urine is not uncommon in the elderly, and it is often advisable to allow elderly patients to sit out of bed for micturition during bed rest for cardiac infarction.

Anticoagulant Therapy. In a disease where intravascular clotting is an essential part of the pathology and where thrombo-embolism is responsible for most of the complications leading to a high morbidity and mortality, there are strong theoretical reasons for using anticoagulant therapy and there is now abundant evidence of its value in the treatment of thrombo-embolic disease. The aims of anticoagulant therapy in cardiac infarction are the prevention of peripheral venous thrombosis and consequent pulmonary embolism, the prevention of intracardiac mural thrombosis and consequent arterial embolism and the prevention of further thrombotic occlusion in coronary vessels. It is probable that these aims are in part achieved without undue risk of haemorrhage if anticoagulant treatment is correctly regulated in an institution with adequate pathological services. Anticoagulant therapy should be used for cases of cardiac infarction where there is continued shock, heart failure or evidence of extensive muscle damage as judged by fever, sedimentation rate and the electrocardiogram. It is not indicated in mild cases and when there is a possible pre-existing source of haemorrhage, e.g. peptic ulcer and cirrhosis of the liver. In most cases where urgent treatment is indicated, heparin is used for 48 hours and one of the oral preparations for reducing blood prothrombin is administered concurrently and then continued for 6–12 weeks. In less urgent cases the heparin may be omitted.

Heparin is the best anticoagulant drug available; it is effective within minutes of intravenous injection and when discontinued the coagulability of blood returns to normal in a short time. The necessity for frequent parenteral administration and its high cost are disadvantages. Administration is regulated by estimates of the coagulation time which should be prolonged to two or three times the normal. For short-term use before one of the coumarin drugs is effective, heparin is best given by intravenous infusion (the intravenous line being also useful for the administration of other parenteral drugs as necessary). 5000 Units every 6 hours is a reasonable dose. Overdosage with heparin may be corrected immediately by 50 mg. of protamine sulphate given intravenously or by a transfusion of whole fresh blood.

Courmarin drugs affect the production of prothrombin by the liver and thereby prolong the prothrombin time of plasma, but they do not materially alter the coagulation time of whole blood. These drugs have the great advantage of being effective when given by mouth. Disadvantages are the necessity for control of administration by frequent estimation of prothrombin time, their relatively slow action and slow elimination. These drugs should not be used in the presence of liver disease, kidney disease or a serious blood dyscrasia.

Dicoumarol has been superseded by ethyl biscoumacetate (*Tromexan*), phenindione (*Dindevan*), warfarin and nicoumalone (*Sinthrome*) which have a more rapid action and are more easily controlled. A daily estimation of prothrombin time should be made before the next dose is administered. Prothrombin time is estimated by the Quick method, in which oxalated blood plasma is mixed with an excess of calcium ion and an excess of thromboplastin. The clotting time is prolonged in proportion to decrease in concentration of prothrombin. In all cases the prothrombin time should be estimated before treatment, the normal is between 12 and 17 seconds and a safe therapeutic level is achieved when this is approximately doubled, which corresponds to a prothrombin level of 15–30 per cent. Average doses for patients of medium weight are as follows: Ethyl biscoumacetate, 1500 mg. first day and thereafter 300–900 mg., phenindione, 200 mg. on the first day and 50–150 mg. thereafter. Warfarin, 3–10 mg. a day. Division of the daily dose produces a more even lowering of the blood prothrombin.

Inspection of a daily urine specimen for red cells is a useful adjunct to control by prothrombin time. Haemorrhage due to overdosage is treated by transfusion if necessary. Vitamin K_1 oxide is an effective antidote; prolonged prothrombin time may be raised quickly by an intravenous dose of 20 mg. or more slowly by oral capsules (20 mg.). Some physicians advocate the use of anticoagulants over long periods with monthly estimations of prothrombin time. The results are difficult to evaluate.

Treatment of Complications. *Phlebothrombosis* in the legs, with or without accompanying pulmonary infarction, is an indication for anticoagulant therapy [see above]. The treatment of peripheral arterial embolism or thrombosis depends on the site and severity of the resulting ischaemia [p. 828]. There is no accepted treatment for ventricular aneurysm, but surgical excision has been successfully carried out in many patients.

Shoulder-hand syndrome causing pain and stiffness tends to become permanent but many mild cases recover spontaneously or with the help of physiotherapy. A short course of prednisone cures some more resistant cases; when this fails, procaine block of the stellate ganglion is indicated.

Management After the Acute Attack. Convalescence should be from 4 to 6 weeks. The degree of activity permitted thereafter depends entirely on the degree of physical and mental recovery. Many patients are able to return to their previous occupations and should be encouraged to do so. It is advisable to continue with small meals if there is a tendency to obesity. Smokers should reduce their tobacco consumption. Alcohol should not be prohibited. It is customary to advise moderation in all things and to reduce physical activities, but most patients are benefited by following their personal inclinations for work, exercise and leisure activities. There is evidence that restriction of activities beyond that imposed by diminished cardiac reserve not only fails to prevent further deterioration but may even hasten it. Angina of effort or heart failure require treatment and often cause permanent incapacity. The physician should maintain an attitude of optimism tempered by intelligent explanation and above all he should never cause unnecessary anxiety.

Prognosis

Cardiac infarction is an unpredictable disease. Sudden death may occur at any time and in the mildest cases, whilst others who are gravely ill during the acute stage may survive to live many years. There is no agreement about mortality rates but probably 25 per cent. die in the first attack; however, this figure is considerably lower for those receiving early, competent treatment. The greatest mortality occurs in the first 48 hours and remains high during the first 7–10 days. After 3 weeks there is an excellent chance of recovery from the immediate illness provided that there are no signs of heart failure or other complications.

Prognosis is adversely affected by increasing age, but sudden death from cardiac infarction under the age of 40 is not uncommon. The prognosis for patients with a mild attack is relatively better than for those with symptoms and signs in addition to pain. The persistence of the shock over 24 hours is a grave sign and few recover when shock continues for more than 2 days. The early development of congestive heart failure is serious; however, many patients show a slight rise in venous pressure or signs of mild left ventricular failure for a few days, which does not necessarily affect the outcome. The disappearance of triple rhythm during the early weeks indicates improving ventricular function and a better prognosis than in those patients with a persistent third heart sound. Transient arrhythmias are common and prognosis is not adversely affected, but a persistent irregularity, especially when due to multiple ventricular ectopic beats, ventricular tachycardia, heart block or atrial fibrillation, is of grave significance.

Pulmonary infarction and other thrombo-embolic manifestations often cause deterioration and may adversely affect the outcome at any time during the first 3 weeks.

Hypertension and preceding angina pectoris do not materially alter prognosis, but a history of previous cardiac infarction does. The site, duration and intensity of pain, unless associated with shock, do not affect prognosis; nor does the anatomical site of the cardiac infarction.

As in all forms of ischaemic heart disease, women do better than men. The outlook improves with each week that passes free of complications, but after recovery from the acute illness, the ultimate prognosis depends on many factors. Prognosis is favourable when heart failure, cardiac enlargement, triple rhythm, hypertension, diabetes mellitus, obesity and angina pectoris are absent, and when the electrocardiogram shows recovery of the S-T segments and T waves. Under such circumstances many years of good health are possible, but the development of a further attack of infarction is always possible and unpredictable.

ACUTE CORONARY INSUFFICIENCY

Acute coronary insufficiency is not a clearly defined clinical syndrome; the term is used to indicate an acute disparity between the supply of oxygen and the demands of the myocardium, which is more prolonged than in angina of effort. On the other hand, it excludes the clinical syndrome of acute coronary occlusion with cardiac infarction which is more severe and permanent. In acute coronary insufficiency the emphasis is on sudden abnormal increased demand or a sudden fall in blood supply due to factors other than complete coronary occlusion.

Pathology

There is coronary atherosclerosis of varying degrees but fresh thrombotic occlusion is not usually found. Subendocardial necrosis or small patches of necrosis in deep layers of the muscle are usual, but massive necrosis involving pericardium and endocardium is not seen. As indicated there is usually some restricted area of infarction; thus from the pathological point of view the differentiation of this condition (really a clinical syndrome) from coronary occlusion and salient cardiac infarction is hardly justifiable.

Aetiology

The sudden diminution of blood supply or greatly increased cardiac work required to produce acute coronary insufficiency is usually due to coronary disease associated with one or more of the following conditions: (1) haemorrhage and other causes of shock and hypotension; (2) acute heart failure; (3) asphyxia and especially carbon monoxide poisoning; (4) acute severe pulmonary disease; (5) pulmonary embolism; (6) unusually severe effort or great emotional stress; (7) paroxysmal tachycardia; and (8) acute hypertension.

Symptoms

Pain is the usual symptom as in other manifestations of cardiac ischaemia; it lasts longer than in angina pectoris and it may occur under a variety of circumstances depending on the immediate cause. Shock, heart failure, fever and leucocytosis are not present. There are no signs of acute coronary insufficiency *per se*, but the signs of an associated precipitating cause may be present.

The electrocardiogram. The electrocardiogram shows similar changes, but of greater magnitude than those found during an attack of angina pectoris. Great depression of the S-T segments in left ventricular leads is usual. T waves may remain flat or inverted for a few days after the attack. Pathological Q waves do not occur.

Treatment

During the attack trinitrin should be given as for angina pectoris [p. 774], but it is usually ineffective and morphine may be necessary for the relief of pain. Heparin, 50 mg., should be given intravenously and continued in similar doses every 4–6 hours for 48 hours. A full course of anticoagulant therapy should be given in those cases where a history of increasing angina precedes the attack of insufficiency and therefore suggests impending infarction. The precipitating cause, e.g. anaemia or hypertension requires treatment. A period of bed rest depending on the severity of the attack and subsequent progress is indicated.

Prognosis

Prognosis largely depends on the nature of the immediate cause and whether there is evidence of severe coronary artery disease. The same general factors determine prognosis as for angina of effort.

HYPERTENSIVE HEART DISEASE

Heart disease was the cause of death in approximately 75 per cent. of patients with established high blood pressure but there is increasing evidence that the widespread use of antihypertensive drugs has resulted in a great decline in the incidence of acute left ventricular failure from this cause; however, cardiac infarction continues to be a common complication. In the great majority of cases the hypertension is of the essential and so-called benign variety. The transition from asymptomatic systemic hypertension to compensated cardiovascular hypertrophy and final decompensation is slow and mostly insidious, though sometimes interrupted by more or less acute cardiac or cerebral episodes; the point at which the heart becomes diseased is usually indefinable. Cardiac infarction is the most important complication and a common cause of acute deterioration in the natural history of hypertensive disease. There is abundant evidence that high blood pressure accelerates the process of atheroma anywhere in the vascular system. The subject of hypertension is dealt with elsewhere [p. 815].

Aetiology and Pathology

The aetiology of hypertension is discussed on pages 815 and 816. Systemic hypertension is due to an increased total peripheral resistance with a normal cardiac output; the work of the left ventricle is increased, which leads to compensatory hypertrophy, and in the course of time dilatation of the ventricle occurs.

Disease of the heart in hypertension is essentially disease of the left ventricle. The ultimate failure of compensatory hypertrophy is probably due to failure of the coronary circulation to meet an increasing demand. Hypertension accelerates the development of coronary atheroma which is present in all cases of long-standing hypertensive heart disease.

At necropsy there is hypertrophy of the left ventricle and the whole arterial system. The myocardium shows varying degrees of ischaemic damage ranging from widespread fibrosis to more localized areas of infarction.

Clinical Features

Cardiac symptoms are absent during the compensated stages of hypertension unless coronary sclerosis causes angina pectoris [p. 772]. During the phase of decompensation the symptoms are those of left ventricular failure and congestive cardiac failure [p. 777]. The onset of heart failure may be shown by increasing effort dyspnoea or by paroxysmal dyspnoea which is frequently of the nocturnal variety. Cardiac pain is often present and symptoms suggesting cardiac infarction may precede those of heart failure.

Examination during the compensated phase of hypertension shows varying degrees of arteriopathy in the fundus oculi, thickening of radial and brachial arteries, an apical impulse suggesting left ventricular hypertrophy, a loud aortic second sound, sometimes an atrial gallop sound, occasionally an aortic diastolic murmur and always arterial hypertension. When heart failure has developed there is usually cardiac enlargement, a less forcible apex beat which, however, retains some of the sustained heave of hypertrophy, triple rhythm or a summation gallop, a variable apical systolic murmur due to functional mitral incompetence, together with the signs of pulmonary or systemic congestion in varying degrees. The blood pressure usually remains elevated, but as heart failure increases, the pulse pressure falls due to a greater drop in systolic pressure than in the diastolic level. Pulsus alternans may be present and Cheyne-Stokes respiration is common in the late stages. Atrial fibrillation occurs in about 25 per cent. of patients with hypertensive heart failure. In attacks of severe left ventricular failure and in the terminal stages of congestive cardiac failure, extreme peripheral constriction may occur.

Radiographic examination reveals varying degrees of pulmonary congestion when there are symptoms of left ventricular failure. The aorta tends to become 'unfolded', causing a widening of the superior mediastinum; the aortic 'knob' is unduly prominent and there are often scattered flecks of calcification in the wall. The left ventricle is enlarged and best seen in the left oblique view.

The electrocardiogram shows varying degrees of left ventricular hypertrophy associated with ischaemic changes. Characteristically the R waves in lead I, VL and V5 to V7 are tall and associated with some degree of S-T depression and T wave flattening or inversion in the same leads. In late stages left bundle branch block is common or the R waves become lower in voltage [see electrocardiogram of left ventricular hypertrophy, FIG. 40a, p. 740].

Diagnosis

Diagnosis depends on the finding of raised blood pressure together with the signs of cardiovascular hypertrophy. Gross hypertrophy of the left heart in the absence of the signs of valvar disease is often due to systemic hypertension. When the signs of heart failure have supervened diagnosis may be more difficult, since the arterial tension tends to fall and the powerful thrust of a hypertrophied left ventricle diminishes. However, in such cases the diastolic tension usually remains elevated, whilst retinopathy and thickened brachial vessels indicate long-standing hypertension. Systolic murmurs may suggest organic mitral incompetence but the raised arterial tension and the clinical and electrocardiographic evidence of gross left ventricular hypertrophy indicate the true nature of the condition. Similar criteria serve to distinguish the cause of an early diastolic murmur associated with severe hypertension from that due to organic aortic incompetence. Angina pectoris associated with hypertension must be differentiated from cardiac pain due to other causes.

Treatment

Treatment is required for the hypertension and for heart failure when this is present. The treatment of hypertension is discussed on pages 817 and 820. It is emphasized that attempts to lower blood pressure with the various hypotensive agents and a low salt diet are not contra-indicated by the development of heart failure or evidence of coronary disease. Heart failure should be treated on the lines indicated on page 749. Regular periods of rest are advisable and an attack of cardiac asthma should be followed by a few days of bed rest. A low sodium diet [p. 750] is helpful in controlling both hypertension and heart failure; the action of the hypotensive drugs is potentiated by a low sodium regime. Acute left ventricular failure is best treated with morphine, aminophylline, oxygen if there is central cyanosis, and a diuretic; a venesection of 250–500 ml. should be carried out if other methods are not rapidly effective; parenteral methonium halide has been tried with good effect in acute left heart failure, but this is rarely necessary. Digitalis should be given to patients with hypertensive heart failure as in other forms of heart failure and maintained indefinitely irrespective of rhythm.

Prognosis

During the compensated stage of hypertension the prognosis is worse in males than in females, and is adversely affected by high diastolic levels of pressure, evidence of myocardial disease and impaired renal function. When breathlessness develops the prognosis depends on the degree of cardiac damage; the presence of cardiac pain and evidence of ischaemia are adverse factors and triple rhythm, great cardiac enlargement, pulsus alternans and attacks of paroxysmal dyspnoea, occurring in spite of treatment, are of grave import.

REFERENCES

BIÖRCK, G. (1960) Some fundamental problems in coronary heart disease, *Acta med. scand.*, **168**, 245.

BIÖRCK, G., and WEDELIN, E. (1964) Return to work of patients with myocardial infarction, *Acta med. scand.*, **175**, 215.

COHEN, L. (1967) Contributions of serum enzymes to

diagnosis of myocardial injury, *Mod. Conc. cardiov. Dis.*, **36**, 43.
DAWBER, T. R., and KANNEL, W. B. (1962) The epidemiology of coronary heart disease—the Framingham enquiry, *Proc. roy. Soc. Med.*, **55** 265.
DOUGLAS, A. S. (1962) *Anticoagulant Therapy*, Oxford.
EDWARDS, J. E. (1961) *Atlas of Acquired Disease of the Heart*, Vol. 2, Philadelphia.
ELLIOT, W. C., and GORLIN, R. (1966) The coronary circulation, myocardial ischaemia and angina pectoris, *Mod. Conc. cardiov. Dis.*, **35**, 117.
FULTON, M., JULIAN, D. G., and OLIVER, M. F. (1969) Sudden death and myocardial infarction, *Circulation*, **50**, 182.
JAMES, T. (1961) *The Anatomy of the Coronary Arteries*, New York.
KILLIP, T., and KIMBALL, J. T. (1968) A survey of the coronary care unit: Concept and results, *Progr. cardiovasc. Dis.*, **11**, 45.
LOGUE, B. (1960) Treatment of intractable angina pectoris, *Circulation*, **22**, 1151.
McDONALD, L. (1962) Studies on blood coagulation and thrombosis and on the action of heparin in ischaemic heart disease, *Amer. J. Cardiol.*, **9**, 365.
MORRIS, J. (1964) *Uses of Epidemiology*, Edinburgh.
WOOD, P. (1961) Acute and subacute coronary insufficiency, *Brit. med. J.*, **1**, 1779.

PULMONARY HYPERTENSION AND PULMONARY HEART DISEASE

A raised pressure in the pulmonary arterial system above the normal level of 20–30/10–15 mm.Hg is caused by an increase of resistance or of blood flow or both. An increase in pulmonary vascular resistance is due to three main causes: (1) organic obstruction in the vascular bed thereby reducing its capacity by some two-thirds; (2) a sustained elevation of pulmonary venous pressure usually from disease in the left heart; and (3) pulmonary vasoconstriction. Increased flow in the pulmonary circulation of sufficient magnitude to raise the pressure is only found in large left to right shunts.

The clinical features of severe pulmonary hypertension are the same whatever the cause. Dyspnoea on effort rather than orthopnoea is usual, angina or syncope on effort may occur in the most severe forms. Right ventricular hypertrophy may be detectable as a parasternal heave, and pulmonary valve closure may be palpable. On auscultation the pulmonary second sound is loud and may be followed by the Graham Steell murmur of pulmonary incompetence when the pressure is very high, and in such cases there may be a right atrial gallop sound and large 'a' waves in the jugular venous pulse. An ejection click is present when the pulmonary artery is very large.

Pulmonary heart diseases are best divided on the basis of the dominant functional derangement into pulmonary hypertensive and hypoxic groups. This wide range of diseases is represented by idiopathic pulmonary hypertension (obstructive hypertension without parenchymatous lung disease) at one end of the range and hypoxic emphysema without hypertension at the other. There are many overlapping cardiopulmonary factors contributing to the clinical picture in almost all forms so that no classification is entirely satisfactory.

Hypertensive Pulmonary Heart Disease
- Primary or solitary pulmonary hypertension.
- Secondary pulmonary hypertension.
- Pulmonary embolism (acute and subacute).
- Schistosomiasis.
- Pulmonary arteritis.
- Carcinomatosis.

Hypoxic Pulmonary Heart Disease
- Chronic obstructive airway disease. (Bronchitis with or without emphysema.)
- Kyphoscoliosis, asthma, pneumoconiosis, bronchiectasis, fibroid tuberculosis and sarcoidosis.
- Fibrosing alveolitis (Hamman-Rich syndrome).
- Cystic lung disease.
- Massive obesity (hypoventilation syndrome).

PRIMARY PULMONARY HYPERTENSION

This is a rather rare disease mainly affecting young women. The aetiology is unknown. The symptoms and signs are those of severe pulmonary hypertension. The prognosis is bad when symptoms have appeared and pregnancy seems to have an especially adverse effect on the course of the disease. No effective treatment is known.

MASSIVE PULMONARY EMBOLISM

Synonym. Acute cor pulmonale.

Definition

Acute pulmonary heart disease may be defined as a cardiac and circulatory disturbance resulting from rapid obstruction of the pulmonary circulation by one or more massive emboli.

Aetiology

The immediate cause is sudden obstruction of the pulmonary artery by a large embolus which has become detached from its site of formation either in the systemic veins or the right heart. Prolonged bed rest predisposes to the formation of thrombi, particularly in the leg veins, which may be locally asymptomatic or give rise to only minor symptoms (phlebothrombosis) although sometimes there is local tenderness, swelling and oedema. Pulmonary embolism may occur after operations, especially pelvic and abdominal, fractures and other serious injuries, and is most common in the first three postoperative weeks. It may follow childbirth and may be associated with the use of the contraceptive pill. Chronic congestive heart failure may be complicated by pulmonary embolism, since the poor peripheral circulation encourages the formation of thrombi, but pulmonary embolism is also associated with heart disease without failure, where reduction of clotting time seems to be a predisposing factor. It may occur in patients with carcinoma, especially of the stomach, and with a variety of blood disorders.

Pathology

The deep veins of the calf muscles are the commonest source of pulmonary emboli. Less commonly the pelvic veins or the chambers of the right heart may be the source.

Pulmonary emboli causing severe cardiac and circulatory disturbance are large and obstruct the main pulmonary artery and its branches. The large size of the embolus is caused by coiling up of a long thrombus into a compact mass after detachment from its site of formation. A common site of lodgement is the bifurcation of the pulmonary artery with complete occlusion of one branch and partial occlusion of the other. The obstructing pulmonary embolus may or may not be all of the same age, being in some cases formed of repeated smaller emboli and in others enlarged by local thrombosis. Smaller pulmonary emboli, insufficient to obstruct the main pulmonary arterial trunk, seldom give rise to serious general cardiovascular disturbances unless repeated over a period of time, although they often cause pulmonary infarction.

If the patient survives initial pulmonary embolism, pulmonary infarction may follow, depending on the site and size of vessel obstructed and the collateral circulation to the segment of lung involved. Embolism is more likely to give rise to infarction in the presence of pulmonary venous congestion from heart failure. Acute pulmonary heart disease, however, usually occurs without the development of pulmonary infarction.

The cardiac and circulatory effects of massive pulmonary embolism are due to mechanical circulatory obstruction and to myocardial ischaemia. It has been estimated that, in order to cause circulatory embarrassment, 50–70 per cent. of the cross-sectional area of the pulmonary arterial tree must be cut off. When this occurs, the output from the right heart is diminished and consequently the left ventricular output also falls. At the same time, acute right heart strain develops with ventricular dilatation and a rise in systemic venous pressure. Myocardial ischaemia resulting in subendocardial necrosis, most severe in the left ventricle, is probably the result of diminished coronary flow (i.e. acute coronary insufficiency) resulting from a fall in left ventricular output and systolic pressure, associated with arterial anoxaemia; reflex coronary arterial spasm may also play a part.

Clinical Features

The onset of massive pulmonary embolism is sudden. In some patients, however, smaller emboli precede the massive embolism and in these premonitory symptoms may be present.

The patient often complains of chest pain, which may be similar in type and distribution to that of cardiac infarction. This is accompanied by acute dyspnoea or tachypnoea. Syncope is not uncommon. There may be faintness, dizziness, restlessness, mental apathy or convulsions. Sometimes the pain is abdominal rather than substernal. Occasionally there is haemoptysis and in some palpitation from an associated paroxysmal arrhythmia. The symptoms vary widely from case to case and may be relatively mild.

On examination there are usually signs of acute circulatory failure and shock, with a rapid, thready pulse, low blood pressure, pallor, coldness and sweating. In some cases deep cyanosis may be present. In contrast to the systemic hypotension, resulting from inadequate venous return to the left ventricle, in the right heart there are signs of pulmonary hypertension with systemic venous congestion. A right ventricular triple rhythm, best heard at the left sternal edge or in the epigastrium, is often present. The pulmonary second sound may be accentuated. There may be dilatation of the pulmonary artery, with a systolic murmur and thrill in the pulmonary area. The jugular venous pressure is raised and often associated with acute engorgement of the liver.

If the patient survives, signs of pulmonary infarction may develop. There is usually pyrexia and leucocytosis: there may be pleural pain on the side of the infarction; there may be cough with expectoration of bright red frothy sputum. Examination may reveal signs of consolidation over the infarcted area, sometimes accompanied by a pleural rub and there may be a pleural effusion, which on diagnostic aspiration is found to be blood-stained. The clinical picture, however, varies considerably and neither pain, cough nor haemoptysis is necessarily present.

The electrocardiogram in massive pulmonary embolus usually shows a shift in frontal plane axis to the right. There may be deep S waves in standard lead I and a Q wave with inversion of the T wave in lead III. In the V leads there is frequently inversion of the T wave from V1 to V4, while in some cases transient right bundle branch blocks may develop. These signs may persist for days or weeks. With smaller emboli, on the other hand, the electrocardiogram usually remains normal.

Radiography. The hilar shadows may be prominent and the main pulmonary artery large whilst peripheral areas of the lung appear oligaemic. In addition there may be evidence of pulmonary infarction with a triangular, ovoid or irregular shadow in the lung fields, often accompanied by a pleural effusion. Transient cardiac enlargement, especially of right heart chambers, is usual.

Diagnosis

Collapse, precordial pain, dyspnoea, tachycardia and cyanosis in a patient confined to bed after an operation, delivery or during a medical illness should at once suggest the diagnosis of massive pulmonary embolus. The diagnosis becomes even more probable if signs of phlebothrombosis or thrombophlebitis are present in the veins of the calf muscles. If, added to this, there are signs of right heart strain with elevation of the jugular venous pressure and characteristic electrocardiographic changes, then the diagnosis of acute pulmonary heart disease is established.

The differential diagnosis from cardiac infarction may be difficult, since pulmonary embolus may complicate cardiac infarction and since either may occur postoperatively. The electrocardiogram is usually diagnostic, but some cases of posterior cardiac infarction may be difficult to differentiate in the electrocardiogram from acute pulmonary heart disease. The development of localizing signs in the lung may help to establish the diagnosis. Other conditions, which must be excluded, are pneumonia, pleurisy, postoperative shock and an acute abdominal emergency. Selective pulmonary angiography may be indicated when diagnosis is uncertain and may show the site and extent of pulmonary arterial obstruction. Radio-isotope injection and lung scanning has proved useful in diagnosis and indicates the site and extent of pulmonary oligaemia.

Treatment

The most important aspect of treatment in massive pulmonary embolus and acute pulmonary heart disease is prophylactic. Unnecessarily prolonged periods of bed rest should be avoided and frequent changes of posture with leg exercises encouraged in chronic bed-ridden patients. In surgical cases, gentle handling at operation of the veins draining the lower extremities and avoidance of tight bandages obstructing the venous return are desirable. Since heart failure seems to predispose to venous thrombosis and pulmonary embolism, energetic and prompt treatment of failure may ward off these complications. When calf vein thrombosis develops two main forms of treatment are available, medical and surgical, in order to avoid pulmonary embolism. Anticoagulants should be given in order to prevent extension of the venous thrombus, or in cases where pulmonary embolus has already occurred, to prevent growth of the embolus by local thrombosis. The principles and details of anticoagulant therapy have already been discussed [p. 779], and treatment should be continued for many weeks. Surgical treatment is by ligation of the femoral or common iliac veins or even of the inferior vena cava. This treatment should be reserved for cases of recurrent embolism where anti-coagulant treatment is contra-indicated or where it has failed.

Treatment of pulmonary embolism itself largely consists of supportive measures to tide the patient over the acute emergency. The patient should be nursed flat in order to encourage cerebral circulation in the presence of a low blood pressure. Oxygen should be given either by mask or in an oxygen tent. Papaverine hydrochloride, 30 mg. intravenously, has been recommended, but it is doubtful if it dilates the pulmonary artery. Venesection is contra-indicated, since reduction in systemic venous pressure does nothing to relieve the cause, namely obstruction to right ventricular output. Surgical removal of embolus from the main pulmonary artery and branches is indicated if there is no improvement in cardiac function after a few hours or when a fatal termination appears imminent. Surgery is likely to be successful only when cardiopulmonary by-pass and a highly trained team are available. Results of treatment with fibrinolytic agents may be comparable with those of surgery but so far have not been fully evaluated.

Prognosis

The prognosis after massive pulmonary embolism resulting in acute pulmonary heart disease is extremely unfavourable and death occurs in over 80 per cent. of patients. Death is usually delayed for a number of hours or days, but may take place within a few minutes. Smaller emboli seldom cause death, but these may precede larger emboli, which may prove fatal. In patients who survive a massive pulmonary embolus, the thrombus may undergo lysis or fibrosis and recanalization.

CHRONIC PULMONARY EMBOLISM (REPEATED PULMONARY EMBOLISM)

Repeated small emboli may gradually produce a condition of severe irreversible obstructive pulmonary hypertension. Early diagnosis is difficult but important, as anticoagulant therapy may arrest the disease and even restore deranged haemodynamics to normality. A history of repeated attacks of pleural pain or brief periods of faintness and dyspnoea are suggestive symptoms. Examination may show the signs of early pulmonary hypertension. A swollen leg may indicate the origin of thrombo-emboli.

FAT EMBOLISM

Acute pulmonary heart disease may rarely be caused by fat embolism, resulting from the entrance of fat globules into the systemic veins. The commonest cause of fat embolism is fracture of a long bone; orthopaedic operations, blast injuries and burns may sometimes be responsible. Usually the fat globules are small and obstruct the smaller pulmonary or cerebral arteries. Sometimes, however, a large amount of fat may obstruct the main pulmonary artery with the production of acute pulmonary heart disease.

AIR EMBOLISM

The sudden entrance of air in large quantities into the systemic veins may result in death from heart failure. The commonest causes of air embolism are operations on the neck, diagnostic or therapeutic procedures involving air insufflation, such as tubal insufflation or pneumoperitoneum. The air entering the right heart impedes the action of the right ventricle and may block the main pulmonary artery or result in widespread embolism of the pulmonary arteries and arterioles. Death results from acute right heart failure with low cardiac output and anoxaemia.

SCHISTOSOMIASIS

In this disease an obliterating pulmonary endarteritis may arise from the embolic impaction of ova of either *Schistosoma haematobium* or *S. mansoni.* Extreme pulmonary hypertension may develop leading to great dilatation of the main pulmonary arteries, and enlargement of the right heart chambers. Haemoptysis is common and death occurs from heart failure within 2 years of the onset of symptoms.

PULMONARY ARTERITIS

In the *collagen diseases* both hypertensive and hypoxic cor pulmonale are rare. Dyspnoea is mainly due to pulmonary fibrosis and pleural disease. However, a subacute pulmonary arteritis leading to pulmonary hypertension and right heart failure has been observed in most of the forms of collagen disease particularly polyarteritis nodosa.

CARCINOMATOSIS

In *metastatic carcinomatosis* both subacute hypertensive and hypoxic cor pulmonale may arise. The vascular bed may be reduced by malignant occlusive arteritis, compression of vessels and by secondary thrombi (lymphangitis carcinomatosa). Approximately

50 per cent. of the reported cases are secondary to carcinoma of the stomach.

CHRONIC PULMONARY HEART DISEASE

Aetiology

Chronic bronchitis is largely a disease of middle-aged men and hence heart disease due to chronic bronchitis and emphysema (chronic airway obstruction) shows a similar sex and age incidence. Sufferers from chronic cor pulmonale are almost invariably inveterate smokers and the highest incidence of the disease is amongst industrial town dwellers.

Pathogenesis

Pulmonary hypertension. Fixed structural changes in the pulmonary vascular bed, which increase its rigidity or reduce its cross-sectional area, have previously been considered to play the major part in the production of high pulmonary arterial pressure in lung disease. However, haemodynamic studies have shown that the high resting pressures recorded during cardiac failure are transitory and reversible. Permanent structural changes, therefore, cannot alone be responsible for the high pressure, although they almost certainly play some role in maintaining the moderate pulmonary hypertension seen at rest in patients not in congestive cardiac failure.

Functional factors must therefore be considered in the mechanism of production of pulmonary hypertension in chronic bronchitis and emphysema. It is probable that anoxia is an important factor causing acute pulmonary hypertension: arterial oxygen saturation is decreased when patients are in congestive cardiac failure and have raised right ventricular pressures, but the saturation returns to a higher level as the pressure falls with recovery. The blood volume increases during congestive failure and decreases on recovery and it is possible that this may contribute to the production of transient pulmonary hypertension. The pulmonary arterial pressure rises during exercise as the cardiac output increases, whereas in normal subjects, little alteration in pulmonary arterial pressure results from changes in blood flow. At rest, however, it is unlikely that levels of flow are high enough to be directly responsible for the production of pulmonary hypertension. The extent to which neurogenic activity influences circulation through the pulmonary vascular bed remains uncertain. Compensatory polycythaemia is always present and presumably the increased blood viscosity also increases resistance to blood flow through the lungs.

Cardiac output. Normal or even increased cardiac output is present in heart failure secondary to lung disease and is one of the features distinguishing it from left ventricular failure [p. 747]. The arteriovenous difference usually remains normal and the cardiac output is therefore appropriate to the raised level of oxygen consumption present in these breathless patients.

Symptoms

The clinical diagnosis of the onset of cardiac complications in chronic bronchitis and emphysema is often difficult, since symptoms due to heart disease are gradually superimposed upon those of the obstructive airways disease.

Three patterns of pulmonary symptoms occur in patients with this disease. There are those who have been subject to repeated episodes of winter 'bronchitis' which gradually increase in severity and begin to recur each year. Some date their symptoms from a specific respiratory illness, usually described as 'pneumonia'. Others give a long history of asthma with the gradual development of a persistent cough. Regardless of the type of onset, the symptoms become similar in all patients with increasing severity of their pulmonary disease and the gradual development of cardiac complications. They have a round-the-year cough, usually productive of sputum, and dyspnoea on exertion. Cold weather, fog and minor respiratory infections all increase their dyspnoea, but patients subject to asthma may be most incapacitated in the summer. Owing to interference with the normal oxygenation of the blood, they gradually become cyanosed. As the disease progresses, recurrent acute exacerbations of bronchitis incapacitate them more, until each exacerbation is attended by an attack of severe anoxia and frank congestive cardiac failure.

Examination of the heart by palpation and auscultation is often unrewarding because of the thickened chest wall and deep barrel shape of the thorax. Adventitious sounds from bronchial catarrh add to the difficulty. It is thus difficult to recognize pulmonary hypertension but forceful pulsation in the epigastrium, suggesting right ventricular hypertrophy, is often present and it is sometimes possible to detect the triple rhythm of right heart failure.

These patients are often plethoric with a dusky blue cyanosis and in some cases mild curvature of the finger nails is present. Obvious clubbing usually signifies more pulmonary pathology than mere chronic bronchitis, e.g. bronchiectasis or fibroid changes. On auscultation of the lungs, there may be signs of bronchial obstruction with widespread râles and rhonchi, and expiration is always prolonged. In attacks of congestive cardiac failure, there is marked cyanosis, the neck veins are distended and there is often considerable oedema. In cases with severe anoxia there may be drowsiness and delirium. Papilloedema may be present, without localizing signs of intracranial disease.

Radiography. Radiography of the chest may show right ventricular and pulmonary artery enlargement in addition to the changes of emphysema. Cardiac enlargement is usual in the presence of congestive cardiac failure.

Electrocardiogram. The development of cardiographic evidence of right ventricular hypertrophy is often relatively late in the course of pulmonary heart disease. Special points to be looked for are the development of an RSR′ pattern in right chest leads accompanied by a deep S wave in left chest leads. In some cases tall spiked P waves are seen in standard lead II.

Diagnosis

The diagnosis of chronic pulmonary heart disease rests on the recognition of right heart enlargement with or without cardiac failure in the presence of emphysema and bronchitis. The disease is usually difficult to diagnose with certainty until definite evidence of right-sided heart failure develops, since the symptoms of dyspnoea and cyanosis may be due to respiratory disease alone and since radiological and electrocardiographic evidence of right heart enlargement may be absent in the early stages of the disease. When frank congestive cardiac failure with a rise in jugular venous pressure, hepatomegaly, oedema and triple rhythm have developed, the diagnosis is clear. Other causes of right heart failure must be excluded.

Treatment

Although no 'curative' treatment is available for the underlying lung disease, much can be done to help the patient in attacks of congestive heart failure. Except where facilities for complete bed rest and skilled nursing are available at home, admission to hospital is desirable. It is probable that acute or subacute respiratory infection plays the most important role in the production of pulmonary hypertension and heart failure in these patients, thus antibiotics, selected according to the flora in the sputum, should always be given. Treatment with bronchodilators is also useful. Oxygen therapy is of great value in combating hypoxia, but is not without danger, since it may induce carbon dioxide narcosis and should therefore be given intermittently or in relatively low concentration, e.g. with a Venturi mask which delivers 25–29 per cent. of oxygen.

The response to diuretics during episodes of congestive failure is often excellent. A low salt diet may be helpful. The value of digitalis is probably not as great as in other forms of heart failure, but there is evidence that it improves myocardial function and it should be tried in all patients.

Prognosis

Once congestive cardiac failure supervenes, the prognosis is poor, and, in spite of treatment, some patients die within a year. The outlook is, however, considerably improved by energetic treatment of attacks of respiratory infection and heart failure.

OTHER CAUSES OF CHRONIC PULMONARY HEART DISEASE

Kyphoscoliosis. Severe kyphoscoliosis may lead to pulmonary heart disease and is an important adverse factor when combined with any of the other causes of cor pulmonale.

Fibroid Lung. Advanced pneumoconiosis, bronchiectasis, widespread fibrocaseous tuberculosis, sarcoidosis and scleroderma may cause chronic pulmonary heart disease.

Cystic Lung Disease. Honeycomb lung may lead to either chronic hypoxic pulmonary heart disease or the dominant derangement may be of obstructive pulmonary hypertension.

Cardiopulmonary Syndrome of Obesity (also called the Hypoventilation or Pickwickian Syndrome). Extreme obesity may lead to chronic anoxia and ultimately right heart failure. Cyanosis with polycythaemia and somnolence are additional features. Respiratory function tests show decreased lung volume and decreased expiratory reserve. Weight reduction may be followed by remarkable improvement with complete recovery from heart failure, restoration of normal arterial oxygen saturation and normal lung function. This disease in its pure form emphasizes the adverse effects which extreme obesity may have on other forms of heart and lung disease.

REFERENCES

Burchell, H. B. (1959) Studies in pulmonary hypertension in congenital heart disease, *Brit. Heart J.*, **21**, 255.

Estes, E. H., Jr., Sieker, H. O., McIntosh, H. D., and Kelser, G. A. (1957) Reversible cardiopulmonary syndrome with extreme obesity, *Circulation*, **16**, 179.

Evans, W., Short, D. S., and Bedford, D. E. (1957) Solitary pulmonary hypertension, *Brit. Heart J.*, **19**, 93.

Hanley, T., Platts, M. M., Clifton, M., and Morris, T. L. (1958) Heart failure of the hunchback, *Quart. J. Med.*, **27**, 155.

Harris, P., and Heath, D. (1962) *The Human Pulmonary Circulation*, Edinburgh.

Harvey, R. M., and Ferrer, M. I. (1960) A clinical consideration of cor pulmonale, *Circulation*, **21**, 236.

Heath, D., and Edwards, J. E. (1958) The pathology of hypertensive pulmonary vascular disease. A description of six grades of structural changes in the pulmonary arteries with special reference to congenital cardiac septal defects, *Circulation*, **18**, 533.

Neal, R. W., and Nair, K. G. (1968) A pathophysiological classification of cor pulmonale with remarks on therapy, *Mod. Conc. cardiov. Dis.*, **37**, 107.

Short, D. S. (1957) The arterial bed of the lung in pulmonary hypertension, *Lancet*, ii, 12.

Stuart-Harris, C. H. (1959) A hospital study of congestive heart failure with special reference to cor pulmonale (Compiled by C. H. Stuart-Harris with the assistance of Drs. R. S. H. Twidle and M. Clifton and a group of physicians of the Sheffield Hospital Region), *Brit. med. J.*, **2**, 201.

SYPHILITIC HEART DISEASE

Syphilis indirectly affects the heart by causing an aortitis, which is a late manifestation of syphilis. However, it may occur as early as 5 years after primary infection; clinically it is rarely detected in under 10 years and often not until 30 years after infection. Aortitis occurs in a large proportion of patients with syphilis, treated or otherwise, and in 80 per cent. of patients with neurosyphilis.

During recent decades there has been a decline in the incidence of cardiovascular syphilis, which is probably due to a fall in the incidence of primary infection coupled with more effective early treatment. There is a higher incidence of all forms of the disease in males; for uncomplicated aortitis the ratio of men to women is 3:1, but for aortic aneurysm the ratio is 10:1. This difference is probably related to physical effort and occupation; similar factors probably explain the higher incidence of complicated aortitis amongst heavy manual workers when compared with sedentary workers. Congenital syphilis rarely affects the cardiovascular system.

Pathology

Aortitis is the fundamental lesion in almost all cases

of cardiovascular syphilis; a true spirochaetal myocarditis and syphilis of medium-sized vessels are both rare and are not considered further.

Syphilitic aortitis begins as an obliterating endarteritis and periarteritis of the vasa vasorum, especially in the ascending aorta; ischaemic changes follow and the media undergoes a slow necrosis with resulting loss of elastic tissue and replacement by fibrosis. The underlying intima is damaged and may ulcerate, but more often it becomes scarred in a characteristic linear fashion. Other areas of the intima undergo thickening from hyalinization and the development of secondary atheroma with calcification is common. This process of chronic inflammation results in dilatation and irregularity of the aorta which, under the influence of arterial pressure, tends to bulge locally or generally with resultant aneurysm formation. Saccular aneurysms may occur in more than one place and they are often filled with layers of partially organized clot. Surrounding structures are frequently damaged by pressure and adjacent bone is eroded.

The ascending aorta suffers most and aortitis usually extends down to the level of the aortic valve ring, causing dilatation which is the most important factor in the production of aortic incompetence. Valvulitis contributes to the incompetence by thickening of the free upper edges and intimal thickening of the commissures.

If the mouths of the coronary arteries are situated above or near the upper margin of the sinus of Valsalva, they tend to be taken up in the aortitis and partially closed. Ischaemic changes of the myocardium follow and histologically a widespread diffuse fibrosis is not uncommon; such changes have been confused with syphilitic myocarditis, which is extremely rare. Gummata in the heart are also very rare.

Clinical Features

The clinical features of syphilitic aortitis are due to aneurysm formation, or to coronary ostial stenosis and aortic incompetence.

Uncomplicated syphilitic aortitis presents no diagnostic symptoms, but a dull aching substernal pain which is constant and localized has been described. In patients known to have latent syphilis a loud second sound over the aorta or an aortic systolic murmur in the absence of hypertension suggests the possibility of aortitis. Radiological examination should be carried out in all cases of late syphilis and widening or irregularity of the aorta may be discovered before the clinical features of aortitis have developed.

Angina pectoris commonly develops in syphilitic aortitis. It is due to stenosis at the origins of the coronary arteries and is mostly accompanied by incompetence of the aortic valves which are also damaged by the aortitis. Coronary ostial stenosis produces cardiac pain on effort indistinguishable from angina pectoris due to coronary atheroma. However, syphilitic cardiac pain tends to last longer and often comes on at rest, especially at night; it is not readily relieved by trinitrin and a dull, substernal ache tends to persist between the attacks. Coronary ostial stenosis occasionally causes acute coronary insufficiency, but massive cardiac infarction is rare. As in all conditions producing cardiac ischaemia, sudden death is not uncommon.

Aortic incompetence due to aortitis is more common in males than in females, in the ratio of 3:1. There are no symptoms until pathological dyspnoea indicates early heart failure or cardiac pain indicates involvement of the coronary ostia.

The physical signs are as in rheumatic aortic incompetence [p. 798]. A mid-systolic murmur is usually present in addition to the early diastolic murmur and both are heard best at the 'aortic area' or in the left parasternal region. The systolic murmur, though similar to that found in aortic stenosis, is not loud enough to cause a thrill and does not indicate stenosis. The incompetence soon becomes well established with gross signs in the peripheral vessels and the murmur takes on a 'to and fro' character. There are no accompanying signs of mitral valve disease, but when the leak is severe a functional presystolic murmur may develop [see p. 798].

Left ventricular failure, as shown by effort dyspnoea or cardiac asthma, appears early in the disease, and thereafter deterioration is relatively rapid, especially when cardiac pain indicating myocardial ischaemia is also present.

Aneurysms of the Aorta. Diffuse fusiform dilatation and localized saccular bulging of the aorta are common in syphilitic aortitis. Radiological examination is essential to the diagnosis of both conditions but a saccular aneurysm often produces characteristic symptoms and signs which depend on its anatomical site. Some aneurysms remain symptomless for many years, but others cause severe pressure pain, and rupture may occur after a relatively short period.

Aneurysm of the ascending aorta. Aneurysm in this situation may present a local bulge in the anterior chest wall, usually to the right of the sternum. Those skilled in percussion may detect dullness to the right of the sternum before superficial bulging occurs. The second sound due to aortic valve closure is often sonorous and is usually heard widely in the right chest. Aortic incompetence and angina pectoris tend to develop with aneurysms in this situation. Sometimes the right bronchus is compressed with the development of partial atelectasis, and occasionally a medial extension of the aneurysm leads to deviation of the trachea. Death may be due to external rupture of the aneurysm, or more commonly to rupture into the pleura, pericardium or bronchus.

Aneurysm of the arch of the aorta produces symptoms and signs by pressure on adjacent structures in the superior mediastinum. The orifices of vessels arising from the aorta are frequently involved and cause differences in the pulse pressures in the two arms. Compression of the great veins leads to a pulseless distension of the veins of the neck and upper chest wall. The bloated facies of superior mediastinal obstruction are characteristic. Pressure on the trachea produces stridor and an unproductive cough, whilst damage to the recurrent laryngeal nerve causes changes in the voice and cough. Haemoptysis may be due to congestion of the tracheal mucosa, or a leak from the aneurysm which not uncommonly ruptures into the trachea. A tracheal 'tug' may be detected with each heart beat by placing the tip of a finger under the cricoid ring. Upward and backward extension of an aneurysm into the paravertebral sulcus may lead to severe brachial neuralgia and a Horner's syndrome from sympathetic paresis. The phrenic nerve is sometimes damaged with resulting paralysis of the diaphragm. Death from rupture of the aneurysm into trachea, pleura, mediastinum or pericardium is usual.

Aneurysms of the descending aorta may develop to a large size without producing symptoms. They almost never occur below the origin of the coeliac vessels and rarely below the diaphragm. Erosion of vertebrae may cause a severe constant pain in the back and occasionally large aneurysms present in the posterior chest wall. Aneurysms in the abdominal aorta are usually symptomless but may be palpated in the epigastrium; they rarely cause pressure symptoms on the viscera.

Patients with syphilitic aortitis may have evidence of syphilis elsewhere; neurosyphilis is present in approximately 25 per cent., and evidence of past gummatosis and of leucoplakia of the tongue is not infrequent.

Radiology of Syphilitic Aortitis. Radiological examination is most important. Uncomplicated aortitis may show a diffuse dilatation of the aorta which is often particularly prominent in the ascending portion and well shown in the left oblique view, where the anterior border of this part of the aorta may bulge beyond the level of the ventricle below it. The calibre of the arch of the aorta may be assessed in the right oblique position, and a barium swallow in this position outlines the posterior circumference. Irregularities in the calibre of the vessel are usual in aortitis and best detected by following the course of the aorta in the left oblique or left lateral views. Thin linear calcification in the wall is common in aortitis, and is very strong evidence of aortitis when seen in the ascending portion of the vessel.

Angiocardiography can show more clearly the calibre of the lumen and its irregularities. Aneurysms show as large local bulges in the three main regions described above. Pulsation is often absent but may be clear and expansile, or transmitted from the adjacent aorta and heart. Erosion of bone is commonly seen. Angiocardiography is valuable in doubtful cases and is essential if surgical treatment is being considered. Tomography and roentgenkymography help in the assessment of the anatomy and pulsations of the mass but are rarely necessary. It is emphasized that these more elaborate radiological methods are no substitute for careful clinical assessment, and good X-ray films in the postero-anterior and oblique views, together with radioscopy and a barium swallow.

The Electrocardiogram in syphilitic aortitis may be normal if the lesion is uncomplicated, but when there is ischaemia from coronary ostial stenosis or ventricular hypertrophy from aortic incompetence the tracing is always abnormal. When cardiac pain indicates ischaemia the electrocardiogram usually shows varying degrees of S-T depression and inversion of T waves in lead I and left-sided chest leads. The changes are similar o those found in ischaemic heart disease due to oronary atheroma.

Serological Tests are positive in some 80 per cent. of patients with syphilitic aortitis [see Section 2]. Past treatment often modifies these tests without having influenced the development of aortitis. In some cases blood reactions are negative whilst the cerebrospinal fluid may show a positive reaction. The erythrocyte sedimentation rate is frequently raised and is related to the degree of activity of syphilitic aortitis in some cases.

Diagnosis

Isolated aortic incompetence in an adult over 30 may be due to syphilis and serological tests are always indicated in such patients; the possibility of syphilis is greatly increased by the presence of cardiac pain. The association of aortic incompetence with signs of neurosyphilis or positive serological reactions confirm the diagnosis of syphilitic aortitis. Radiological examination is the most important aid and should be carried out in all suspected cases; dilatation of the aorta, irregularity of its calibre and calcification in the wall of the ascending portion are diagnostic points, but should not be confused with the smooth aortic unfolding and tortuosity which occur with hypertension and with atherosclerosis in the elderly.

The presence of lesions at other valves practically excludes syphilis; rheumatic aortic incompetence is usually less severe and there is often a history of rheumatic fever, and on radiological examination the aorta is not dilated or calcified although the aortic valves are usually calcified when there is aortic stenosis.

The diagnosis of aortic aneurysm is essentially radiological. Aneurysm should be suspected when there are signs of superior mediastinal obstruction with cough, a pathological aortic second sound, differences in the pulses of the arms and other signs of syphilis. The differential diagnosis from mediastinal tumours and bronchial carcinoma is sometimes difficult; angiocardiography is confirmatory when simpler methods are inadequate.

Positive serological tests are strong evidence that the clinical findings in question are due to syphilis, but this is not always so; conversely, in aortitis, tests do not exclude syphilis, for in some 15–20 per cent. of cases they are negative.

Treatment

The management and treatment of syphilitic heart disease consists of the treatment of syphilis and of the sequelae of aortitis.

All untreated cases of syphilitic heart disease should receive a course of antiluetic treatment after the cerebrospinal fluid has been examined. The course of advanced disease is probably not materially altered by this treatment, but the prognosis of uncomplicated and mild cases is improved since there is active syphilitic inflammation in all untreated cases [see Section 2].

The risks of treatment are slight, but an acute exudative reaction (Jarisch-Herxheimer reaction) accompanied by fever may occur within 24–48 hours. In patients with coronary ostial stenosis this may be serious and lead to acute coronary insufficiency. Rarely, contracting scar tissue may result in the therapeutic paradox of increased aortic incompetence or increased cardiac pain. In general there is no element of urgency in treatment of the luetic condition, so that a course of bismuth or iodides, which diminish the risk of severe reactions from the more powerful antiluetic drugs, should be given first. Various schedules of treatment are recommended and may be modified to suit individual cases [see also general article on syphilis in Section 2].

Cardiac pain should be treated as described [p. 774], but the nitrite drugs are not as effective as in angina pectoris due to coronary atheroma. Surgical treatment may be indicated [see below].

Heart failure in aortitis should be treated as in other cases of left ventricular failure [p. 749]. A prophylactic low salt regime is advisable as soon as effort dyspnoea is present.

Treatment of aortic aneurysm. Pain may necessitate the frequent use of analgesic drugs. Various operative procedures have been devised to treat aneurysms of the aorta, but none has had great success. Cellophane wrapped around the aneurysm induces a fibrous tissue reaction which may limit further extension and strengthen the wall. Excision of the aneurysm has been performed but the pathological state of the remaining aorta is not conducive to effective reconstruction and grafting.

Aortic incompetence, when severe, should be treated surgically by replacement of the damaged valve with an aortic valve homograft or prosthesis. If cardiac pain from ostial stenosis is a problem then the narrowed openings of the coronary arteries may be enlarged at the same operation.

Prognosis

The history of patients with syphilitic aortitis is extremely variable. Some pursue a rapid downhill course, whilst others live long and die of another malady. Consequently prognosis is difficult. In aortic insufficiency there is often a long asymptomatic period, and after the appearance of symptoms many patients live from 5 to 10 years, but few live more than 2 years after signs of heart failure have appeared. Cardiac pain indicating coronary ostial stenosis is an adverse factor in all cases and sudden death is not uncommon. The prognosis for cases of aortic aneurysm is also variable. Some appear to progress rapidly whilst in others the condition appears to be stationary. Heavy physical work is an unfavourable factor and probably women do better than men. Antisyphilitic treatment carried out in the asymptomatic stages appears to improve the outlook, but it is doubtful whether treatment other than surgical replacement of the aortic valve has much influence in the later stages of the disease.

CHRONIC VALVAR DISEASE

MITRAL VALVE DISEASE

Chronic mitral valvulitis is the commonest form of rheumatic heart disease. The valve may be narrow, thereby offering an obstruction to the circulation (mitral stenosis) or it may be incompetent. Mitral stenosis with some degree of regurgitation is the commonest form of organic mitral valve disease, but all grades of the combination occur and either lesion may occur alone.

Aetiology

Mitral stenosis is almost always due to rheumatic heart disease although only some 60 per cent. of adult patients give a history of rheumatic fever. In the majority of patients with acute rheumatic carditis the mitral valve is damaged and it is affected in some 85 per cent. of cases of chronic rheumatic heart disease examined at necropsy. During the first attack of acute rheumatic carditis, mitral valvulitis causes incompetence but this is a transitory lesion and many patients ultimately develop stenosis. Mitral stenosis is more common in females in the ratio of 3:1. Pure organic mitral regurgitation in adults is relatively rare and is probably due to rheumatism in most cases, but only 25 per cent. give a past history of rheumatic fever; mitral incompetence also differs from pure mitral stenosis in the sex incidence since men are affected rather more commonly than women. Endomyocardial fibrosis, common in Africa and some other parts of the world frequently damages the mitral valve causing severe incompetence [p. 808].

Functional mitral regurgitation is common; it develops when ventricular dilatation from any cause results in dilatation of the valve ring and stretching of the chordae tendineae and papillary muscles. Bacterial endocarditis may cause ulceration of mitral valve cusps or rupture of chordae tendineae producing acute mitral regurgitation or an increase of pre-existing regurgitation. Occasionally fracture of chordae tendineae may occur at the junction with papillary muscles as a result of cardiac infarction. Congenital lesions of the mitral valve are rare but a few cases of congenital mitral stenosis have been reported, and mitral reflux occurs in ostium primum A.S.D. [see p. 768].

Pathology

In chronic rheumatic mitral valvulitis the valve cusps are thickened and deformed to varying degrees. The chordae are also shortened and thickened by fibrosis. In stenosis the orifice of the valve is narrowed by fusion of the cusp margins whilst rigidity and thickening of the cusps and chordae holds the valve in a relatively fixed position so that a narrow slit is formed. The whole ring, cusps and chordae may be fused into a narrow rigid funnel. Incompetence results from deformity of the cusps, and from shortening and sclerosis of the chordae. In pure incompetence the valve ring is thickened and immobile and the chordae are shortened, but there is no fusion of the commissures. Calcification in the valve ring and adjacent cusps is not uncommon. Microscopic examination shows vascularization of the cusps and thickening from fibrosis.

The left atrium is dilated and its walls are thickened in mitral stenosis and incompetence. The mural endocardium is often scarred and a thickened patch is especially likely to occur above and adjacent to the valve ring when there is incompetence. The lumen of the auricular appendage is sometimes obliterated by clot and layers of partially organized clot may line the atrial chamber. In mitral stenosis the left ventricle tends to be small (except when there are aortic valve lesions or systemic hypertension), whereas in mitral regurgitation the left ventricle is dilated and moderately hypertrophied. In mitral stenosis the right ventricle is hypertrophied and dilated to varying degrees. The lungs are especially damaged in mitral stenosis, they become brownish, indurated and inelastic; the small branches of the pulmonary artery are thickened and project from the cut surface of the lung. Pulmonary infarcts of varying size are common. On microscopic examination the alveolar walls are thickened, the capillaries dilated and the alveolar cavities tend to contain cellular debris and large 'heart failure' cells containing iron pigment.

MITRAL REGURGITATION

In mitral regurgitation the left atrium receives a regurgitant stream of blood during ventricular systole in addition to the inflow from the pulmonary veins. The atrial pressure rises with ventricular systole, but the absence of obstruction at the mitral orifice prevents the development of diastolic hypertension in the atrium. The left ventricle is overfilled in diastole by the augmented volume, and an effective output into the aorta is maintained by rapid ejection. The increased stroke volume is expelled at relatively normal pressures and compensation is thus maintained by the left ventricle at the expense of only a slight increase in cardiac work.

Pressures do not rise greatly above normal in the left heart except for a systolic peak in the atrium, so that pulmonary congestion and pulmonary hypertension are not prominent features. The hypervolaemic state of the left heart is well tolerated if the muscle is good; hypertrophy is not great, and heart failure tends to develop late in the disease.

Clinical Features

Symptoms. There are no symptoms peculiar to mitral incompetence. The pure lesion is well tolerated and many patients remain active to the sixth or seventh decade. Palpitation due to extrasystoles is common. Some patients complain of fatigue and weakness rather than breathlessness, which tends to appear late. Many die of an intercurrent disease. Patients with severe mitral incompetence develop heart failure which does not respond well to treatment and when rupture of the chordae causes acute mitral incompetence, severe heart failure tends to occur.

Signs. The pulse is normal or rapidly rising—almost waterhammer in some patients. In cases where regurgitation is considerable, ventricular overfilling may be appreciated at the apex which is hyperdynamic; after the lift of systole, which is never as forceful as in left ventricular hypertension, a small diastolic filling wave may be seen or palpated. Many patients have minor degrees of incompetence which do not alter the pulse or apex beat, and a systolic murmur is then the only sign.

Auscultation provides the most significant signs of mitral regurgitation. The first sound is normal or soft and it is immediately followed by a systolic murmur which is loudest at the apex and radiates towards the axilla; very loud murmurs may be palpated as an apical systolic thrill and are widely heard in proportion to their loudness. The murmur is pansystolic and tends to be crescendo in late systole; occasionally the murmur appears to be confined to late systole but phonocardiograms show that vibrations start early in systole. The second sound is often inaudible at the apex, being buried in the murmur. A third heart sound, related to augmented ventricular filling is frequently present. In pure cases the first heart sound is not loud, there is no opening snap and no mid-diastolic murmur, and usually no signs of pulmonary hypertension. Extrasystoles are common, and atrial fibrillation may occur late in the disease.

Radiology. Radioscopy shows a varying degree of left atrial enlargement, but the most important change is in the dynamics of the atrium which may be seen to expand during ventricular systole. In the anterior view the left atrium expands laterally in systole, appearing as a momentary bulge high up on the left border and as a less obvious bulge in the upper part of the right border. In the oblique views the barium-filled oesophagus is moved backwards by the left atrium during ventricular systole. Systolic expansion indicates a considerable degree of mitral regurgitation and the absence of this sign does not mean that there is no regurgitation. Slight to moderate enlargement of the left ventricle is also seen.

Ciné angiography, using a selective left ventricular injection of dye, is the most satisfactory method of demonstrating the extent and site of mitral reflux.

The electrocardiogram may show the presence of arrhythmia. The standard leads tend to show normal or left axis deviation. Left-sided chest leads may show the signs of slight to moderate left ventricular hypertrophy.

Complications

Bacterial endocarditis may occur on the scarred valve in mitral incompetence, and it is not an uncommon complication in mild cases when a mitral systolic murmur is the only evidence of abnormality. Systemic embolism is uncommon compared with its frequency in mitral stenosis.

Diagnosis

Mitral regurgitation should not be diagnosed lightly on the finding of a systolic murmur. A pansystolic murmur or a late systolic murmur which is loudest at the apex and engulfs the second sound is highly suggestive of mitral incompetence. A hyperdynamic apex beat is further evidence. Expansion of the left atrium in ventricular systole seen on radioscopy is confirmatory. The diagnosis of mitral regurgitation in dominant mitral stenosis is suggested by the presence of an apical pansystolic murmur in addition to the signs of mitral stenosis. Furthermore, mitral incompetence in this combination is frequently associated with calcification of the mitral valve seen on screening. The sudden appearance of a pansystolic murmur at the apex during the course of cardiac infarction or bacterial endocarditis suggests acute mitral incompetence due to the fracture of chordae tendineae or perforation of a cusp.

The murmur of ventricular septal defect is also pansystolic (a separate mid-systolic murmur may be heard over the pulmonary artery) and may be heard easily at the mitral area, but is loudest near the sternum. A functional mid-diastolic murmur may be present in ventricular septal defect and adds to the difficulty of differentiation from mitral valve disease, but on radiography there is pulmonary plethora with but little left atrial enlargement.

Other conditions causing a systolic murmur at the apex must be differentiated. Innocent murmurs are soft and most are short and parasternal or over the pulmonary artery. When a murmur is the only indication of mitral disease (i.e. when there is no cardiac enlargement) the prognosis is good, the patient should live a normal life and be reassured, and the only added risk is the remote possibility of bacterial endocarditis.

Mid-systolic murmurs arise from ejection and flow into the great vessels. The murmur of aortic stenosis may be loud at the mitral area, but the second sound is audible and the murmur is also heard at the aortic area, and the pulse is characteristic. Anaemia, thyrotoxicosis, pregnancy, kyphoscoliosis and sternal depression may also produce mid-systolic murmurs, but these are usually soft, loudest in the parasternal region and the cause is usually obvious.

Treatment

The great majority of patients with organic mitral incompetence have only slight symptoms or none at all; they require no treatment and they should be reassured. However, prophylactic penicillin should be given before undergoing dental extraction or other operation in a septic field. Heart failure is treated by routine methods.

In patients with severe organic mitral incompetence, surgical repair of the valve is now possible; various types of valve for replacement are in use but none is yet wholly satisfactory. Open operation is essential.

Prognosis

The prognosis in mitral regurgitation depends on its cause and severity, the state of the myocardium and presence or otherwise of complicating factors such as hypertension. In acute rheumatic carditis mitral incompetence is a product of valvulitis and cardiac dilatation; immediate prognosis depends on the severity of the rheumatic process and the remote prognosis is variable; a few recover completely, many develop mitral stenosis and a few are left with organic incompetence only. In established organic mitral incompetence the prognosis is excellent in mild cases and a normal life span can be expected. In moderate cases with enlargement, heart failure may supervene after middle life, and this tends to be fairly rapidly progressive. Heart failure responds to prolonged rest and the usual treatment. Bacterial endocarditis may occur in any patient with mitral incompetence, whether the lesion is mild or severe. Early treatment may cure, but further deterioration is likely if treatment is delayed or ineffective; fracture of chordae tendineae causing a greater degree of mitral incompetence is common. Embolism and atrial fibrillation occur later in the natural history of mitral incompetence than in mitral stenosis. Successful valve replacement relieves symptoms and improves immediate prognosis but long-term results await further evaluation.

MITRAL STENOSIS

The essential feature of mitral stenosis is obstruction to blood flow through the valve orifice during diastole. Symptoms are not produced until the area of the orifice is reduced from normal (8·5 cm^2.) to approximately 2·5 cm^2., although the signs are present with lesser degree of stenosis. Increasing haemodynamic disorder and a resulting increase in severity of symptoms occurs with greater degrees of stenosis, and most patients are bed-ridden when the valve orifice is less than 1 cm^2.

In significant mitral stenosis the blood flow to the left ventricle is diminished and the pressure and volume of blood in the left atrium rises. The high atrial pressure and increased contraction of the atrium, which shows compensatory hypertrophy, result in an increased pressure gradient across the valve which partially compensates for the obstruction. The increased left atrial pressure is transmitted to pulmonary veins, pulmonary capillaries and the pulmonary arterial system to a variable degree. Pulmonary hypertension develops in the majority of patients with severe mitral stenosis, and in some the pressure rises to very high levels; the raised pulmonary vascular resistance appears to be due to arteriolar spasm and secondary changes in the vessel walls. Pulmonary hypertension causes right ventricular hypertension and secondary hypertrophy.

Compensation occurs at the expense of muscular hypertrophy and increased work of the left atrium and right ventricle. Decompensation may occur in the left atrium for its walls are relatively thin; atrial fibrillation is common; this produces the syndrome of left heart failure. Decompensation of the right ventricle produces the features of right heart failure. The raised tension and congestion throughout the pulmonary circulation causes severe secondary damage to the fine structure of the lung.

Clinical Features

Some patients with mild mitral stenosis are asymptomatic and may remain so throughout a long life, but this is unusual. Sooner or later most patients develop symptoms, and ultimately congestive heart failure.

Dyspnoea. Breathlessness on effort tends to occur during early adult life in most patients with mitral stenosis. Effort tolerance gradually diminishes unless episodes of pulmonary infarction, pulmonary oedema, atrial fibrillation or bronchitis cause relatively rapid phases of deterioration. Sudden paroxysmal attacks of cardiac asthma are not uncommon and may even appear in apparently mild cases before effort dyspnoea is noticed; cardiac asthma may occur during the day, but is more common at night and often occurs for the first time during pregnancy; some attacks are more severe and reach the stage of pulmonary oedema.

Pulmonary oedema tends to occur in those patients

with slight or only moderate pulmonary hypertension rather than in those with very high levels of pressure; it is characterized by extreme respiratory distress, expectoration of pink frothy sputum, cyanosis, hypotension and peripheral vasoconstriction. The various forms of dyspnoea due to left atrial failure tend to subside when right heart failure develops.

Right heart failure. The signs of congestive cardiac failure may develop slowly or appear rapidly after a variable period during which dyspnoea has been the dominant symptom. Oedema appears at the ankles, the jugular venous pressure is raised, and the liver becomes palpable and tender. In some patients this phase brings relief from the symptoms of pulmonary congestion, but in many it does not. During the early stages of right heart failure, discomfort and even pain in the right hypochondrium and epigastrium may accompany effort and are due to hepatic congestion. Right heart failure steadily increases, but with treatment improvement occurs and many episodes may recur before a chronic unresponsive stage is reached, which is characterized by a low fixed cardiac output. Activity is then severely restricted by dyspnoea and fatigue, appetite is poor and weight loss is evident, tricuspid incompetence is often gross but saves the patient from paroxysmal dyspnoea, the liver becomes large, firm and pulsatile. Slight icterus from cardiac cirrhosis is usually present.

Haemoptysis is a common symptom at various stages of the natural history of mitral stenosis. There are three main types: pink staining of the sputum with relatively small quantities of blood due to pulmonary congestion, occasional massive haemoptysis, and blood-stained sputum associated with pleural pain which indicates the presence of pulmonary infarction. Haemoptysis may be repeated many times over a span of years.

Pain in the chest in mitral stenosis is not a prominent feature, but there are three types: a submammary discomfort which is probably psychogenic and reflects anxiety about the heart condition; a dull precordial discomfort when there is great cardiac enlargement, and true ischaemic cardiac pain which is due to failure of the coronary circulation when there is a low cardiac output, pulmonary hypertension and anoxaemia. Most patients, however, do not complain of pain.

Dysphagia, a dry persistent cough or hoarseness of the voice may occur from pressure on adjacent mediastinal structures by an enlarged left atrium which may cause paresis of the left recurrent laryngeal nerve. Very rarely aneurysmal enlargement of the left atrium appears to be the cause of erosion of the vertebral bodies giving rise to severe pain between the scapulae.

Signs. Mitral stenosis presents a pattern of characteristic signs, some of which are directly related to the valve lesion and others to the secondary haemodynamic disturbance. The most constant and important one is the apical diastolic murmur set up during the passage of blood through the obstruction.

There is often a slight bulging in the left precordium, the cardiac impulse may be seen in the parasternal intercostal spaces (right ventricle) and the apex beat (left ventricle) is seen as a separate pulsation farther to the left. On palpation the apex beat is localized and it has a sharp, tapping quality due to the loud first heart sound; an apical diastolic or presystolic thrill is common. Over the parasternal region there may be a strong pulsation due to right ventricular hypertrophy, indicating pulmonary hypertension, which is also suggested by a palpable second sound over the pulmonary artery.

On auscultation the first sound is mostly sharp and loud; it can be heard over the whole precordium but is loudest at the apex. A soft systolic murmur is common at the apex but in pure mitral stenosis systole may be significantly silent. The second heart sound is loud at the pulmonary area and its second component due to pulmonary valve closure is especially loud when there is pulmonary hypertension. An additional sound, the 'opening snap', occurs shortly after the second heart sound, which it resembles in pitch and brevity, but it is loudest just internal to the apex. The 'opening snap' is audible in most cases of mitral stenosis but, like the first heart sound, it is soft when there is gross calcification of the mitral valve. The opening snap is distinguished from the second component of a widely split second sound by timing and by the area where they are best heard: the third heart sound is distinguished by its low-pitched quality, but this sound does not occur in dominant mitral stenosis. The 'opening snap' appears to be essentially related to the pathological state of the valve itself.

A low-pitched, rumbling, mid-diastolic murmur follows the opening snap. This murmur is best heard through a bell stethoscope placed lightly on the apex, with the patient reclining and slightly tilted to the left side. The mid-diastolic murmur may be short in mild cases, but in all others it continues throughout diastole. When the rhythm is normal, the diastolic murmur merges into a sharp, crescendo murmur—the presystolic or atrial systolic murmur, which is most readily heard after exercise. When there is severe pulmonary hypertension, atrial fibrillation and a very low cardiac output, there may be no murmurs and the opening snap may be the only sign of mitral stenosis.

The arterial pulse tends to be small in mitral stenosis and the blood pressure is often low. The venous pulse may show prominent 'a' waves when there is pulmonary hypertension if the rhythm has remained regular. A general rise in the level of venous pressure occurs when there is right heart failure.

Atrial fibrillation occurs in the great majority of patients with mitral stenosis. Its onset marks a definite stage of deterioration and it is responsible for further diminution of cardiac reserve. A phase of changeable rhythm, when atrial ectopic beats are frequent or short periods of atrial fibrillation alternate with normal rhythm, often precedes the establishment of permanent atrial fibrillation. The change to abnormal rhythm may be associated with symptoms of palpitation, increased dyspnoea and fatigue, and sometimes congestive cardiac failure first appears at this time. Atrial fibrillation is usually responsible for tachycardia, but when the heart is very large there is often a high degree of block, causing a slow heart rate.

Mitral Stenosis and Incompetence. The signs of the common combined lesion depend on the relative dominance of regurgitation or obstruction. The signs of mitral stenosis are modified by additional incompetence, as follows. The apex tends to be less localized, the tapping quality is less obvious and it tends to become more hyperdynamic and left ventricular in character. The signs of pulmonary hypertension may or may not be present. The first sound and the opening snap are softer when there is calcification of the mitral valve, which is commonly associated with a mixed lesion. A pansystolic murmur is usually present—the absence of an apical systolic murmur means there is no significant incompetence. When mitral incompetence is great, the opening snap is replaced by a third heart sound.

Radiology. Asymptomatic patients with mild mitral stenosis show no abnormalities apart from slight backward bulging of the left atrium in the right oblique view. In all of the more severe degrees of mitral stenosis the enlarged left atrium may be seen as a hump below the pulmonary arc and as a bulge below the right hilum, and when penetrating films are taken the contour of the whole atrium may be seen through the heart shadow. The barium-filled oesophagus is deviated backwards in a characteristic curve, usually best seen in the right oblique view, but in some patients the oesophagus is deviated to the left, and left oblique views then show the large left atrium surmounting a small left ventricle. The left atrium may be 'aneurysmal' and seen bulging across the right hemithorax almost to its lateral wall. In advanced cases the right atrium is also large. The aorta tends to be small and the pulmonary artery tends to be large. The heart shadow develops a rather triangular shape.

The lungs show varying degrees of venous congestion. The hilar shadows are large and the clear outlines of vessels are often blurred. The peripheral lung fields lose normal translucency, show a fine reticulation and occasionally large miliary shadows due to haemosiderosis are seen. Wedge shadows of pulmonary infarcts are common, and small effusions frequent. The lung parenchyma in the costophrenic angle shows horizontal thread-like lines in cases of long-standing congestion (Kerley's lines).

Cardiac catheterization and *selective angiocardiography* is indicated when a full haemodynamic assessment is required or when the diagnosis is uncertain. The pressure gradient across the obstructed valve is determined by measuring: (1) the left atrial pressure directly (transeptal puncture) or indirectly from the pulmonary wedge pressure; and (2) the left ventricular diastolic pressure from retrograde arterial catheterization of the ventricular cavity. The pulmonary artery pressure and pulmonary vascular resistance is determined at the same time. The valve movement and the pressure or otherwise of mitral reflux is best assessed by ciné angiography using a left ventricular injection of dye.

Echocardiography appears to be a useful non-traumatic method of assessing valve thickness and movement. However, the exact status of this method in the armoury of diagnostic techniques awaits further evaluation.

The Electrocardiogram. P waves are characteristically widened and notched, especially in lead II and left-sided chest leads. The second peak of the notch is due to delayed left atrial activation. The P waves may be single and tall when there is severe right heart hypertension. The QRS complex shows varying degrees of right axis deviation in cases with pulmonary hypertension. The chest leads show increased positivity on the right side depending on the degree of right ventricular hypertrophy.

Complications

Haemoptysis, cardiac asthma, pulmonary oedema and pulmonary infarction are sufficiently common to be considered a part of the natural history of the disease. The most important complications are due to peripheral emboli arising from clot in the left atrium. Embolism may occur in patients with mild mitral stenosis and normal rhythm, but patients having atrial fibrillation are more commonly affected. Emboli are of varying sizes. Medium-sized cerebral and limb vessels are frequently occluded; aphasia with hemiplegia is a common sequel to middle cerebral arterial embolism and may be transient or permanent. Multiple emboli in the kidneys may cause systemic hypertension. Splenic infarction and mesenteric infarction sometimes occur. Many patients have repeated attacks of arterial occlusion. A massive clot may even occlude the aorta at its bifurcation with resulting severe pain in the legs, buttocks and abdomen, and peripheral signs of arterial insufficiency. Occasionally massive clot in the left atrium may become free and occlude the narrow mitral orifice causing sudden death. Rarely recurrent attacks of syncope, characteristically relieved by a change of position, are due to intermittent occlusion of the mitral orifice by a ball-valve thrombus. Bacterial endocarditis is a very rare complication of pure mitral stenosis.

Diagnosis

The diagnosis of mitral stenosis depends on auscultation and radiology. A loud and sharp first heart sound, usually palpable, is strongly suggestive, but a low-pitched mid-diastolic murmur at or near the apex is the essential evidence of mitral stenosis; the opening snap is further evidence when there is doubt about the presence of a mid-diastolic murmur. Rarely, when the flow through the valve is greatly reduced, the mid-diastolic murmur may become inaudible and then the opening snap and sharp first heart sound are the only auscultatory signs. Left atrial enlargement determined by radioscopy confirms the clinical diagnosis.

The diagnosis of mitral stenosis is incomplete without an assessment of the functional state of the circulation. Particular attention should be paid to effort intolerance, paroxysmal dyspnoea, haemoptysis, history of embolism, rhythm, the signs of pulmonary and systemic congestion, and the presence and approximate level of pulmonary hypertension which is recognized by the degree of right ventricular hypertrophy and the loudness ot the pulmonary second sound. Difficulties in the assessment of the state of the pulmonary circulation are likely to arise in some patients when mitral stenosis is combined with mitral incompetence or with pulmonary disease; in such cases the pulmonary artery pressure, pulmonary capillary pressure and the pulse pressure tracings should be obtained by cardiac catheterization. Diagnosis in mitral stenosis must include an assessment of the state of other valves which are often affected.

Differential diagnosis of the signs: on casual auscultation a normal split first heart sound may be mistaken for a presystolic murmur, but in mitral stenosis the mid-diastolic murmur, loud first sound and opening snap, as well as the radiological signs are present. In pure aortic incompetence a presystolic murmur (Austin Flint) may be present, but the other signs of mitral stenosis are absent and the aortic lesion is always severe. Functional diastolic murmurs also occur in atrial septal defect and ventricular septal defect, but in these conditions also attention to the detailed findings of auscultation show that the other signs of mitral stenosis are absent, whilst the signs of a left to right shunt are present on clinical examination and on radiography. A *left atrial myxoma* (or other tumours) may partially or intermittently obstruct blood flow causing pulmonary venous hypertension and signs referable to the mitral valve. This condition tends to produce low-grade fever, a raised sedimentation rate and abnormal serum proteins: thereby suggesting bacterial endocarditis which, however, does not occur in pure mitral stenosis.

Differential diagnosis of symptoms: haemoptysis and dyspnoea may suggest pulmonary disease, paroxysmal dyspnoea may suggest left ventricular disease or bronchial asthma, and embolism may cause symptoms referable to any organ, but when the physical signs of the mitral valve lesion are recognized the aetiology of these symptoms is usually clear.

Treatment

Asymptomatic patients with mild mitral stenosis having no evidence of pulmonary congestion or pulmonary hypertension do not require treatment. All other patients with dominant mitral stenosis must be considered as possible subjects for mitral valve surgery unless the severity of the disease and great enlargement of the heart are obvious contra-indications. Surgery offers the only cure of the disease.

General. Exercise in patients without heart failure should not be unduly restricted but it should be kept within the limits imposed by symptoms. Occupation, though largely dictated by economic and social factors, should be regular and not of the manual variety. In pregnancy there should be medical supervision and regular hours of extra daily rest. A period of 2 week's partial bed rest is advisable before delivery, which is best conducted in hospital or a similar institution. Mitral valvotomy may be performed during pregnancy if symptoms are severe and increasing in severity.

The symptoms of mitral stenosis are largely due to heart failure, which should be treated by routine methods [p. 749 *et seq.*]. Digitalis may be given at any stage, whether rhythm is regular or not, preferably early rather than late in the natural history of the disease. Sodium restriction is advisable and may prevent attacks of pulmonary oedema; thiazide diuretics are very useful in the long-term management. Haemoptysis rarely requires special treatment but if it is severe, bed rest is necessary. Bacterial endocarditis requires treatment with appropriate antibiotics [p. 807] but is extremely rare in pure mitral stenosis. The treatment of embolic episodes depends on the site of embolism and severity of ensuing ischaemia. Embolectomy is almost never necessary in the arm, but is advisable if the site of embolism can be accurately located in the femoral or popliteal vessels. A saddle embolism at the aortic bifurcation should be removed. Atrial fibrillation marks a definite stage in the deterioration of patients with mitral stenosis and attempts to restore sinus rhythm are useless unless mitral valvotomy has been performed. Indefinite anticoagulant therapy is indicated when there is atrial fibrillation and when surgery, for one reason or another, is contra-indicated.

Surgical treatment. Surgical relief of the stricture is indicated in all patients in whom obstruction to the flow of blood through the valve is serious enough to cause symptoms. An accurate assessment of the degree of dyspnoea is quite a good guide to the degree of obstruction when mitral stenosis is the only lesion. Indeed, in pure mitral stenosis selection of patients for surgery can usually be made by clinical examination, with electrocardiography and chest radiographs without recourse to cardiac catheterization or angiocardiography. When, however, there are complicating factors such as valve calcification, mitral reflux, other valve lesions and pulmonary hypertension, a full investigation by the aforementioned techniques is indicated.

Surgery should be deferred in mild asymptomatic patients because there is significant, though low, mortality (1–2 per cent.) and even in mild cases there is an embolic risk at operation. Furthermore, there is a small postoperative morbidity risk from mitral reflux, post-cardiotomy syndrome, atrial fibrillation in some who were in sinus rhythm before, and more remotely there is the possibility of re-stenosis.

There are two types of operation for patients with mitral stenosis: 'closed' operation when simple splitting of the stricture (mitral valvotomy) is carried out, and 'open' operation using cardiopulmonary by-pass when the valve may be split, repaired, or replaced under direct vision. In the author's opinion the closed operation remains the operation of choice in pure mitral stenosis without valve calcification or other complicating factors. The most effective method is by the transventricular technique in which a dilator is passed to the valve through the ventricle and guided into the valve orifice by a finger introduced through the left atrium. The valve orifice may be split to a diameter of 3·5 cm. and relief of the stenosis is satisfactory for 7–12 years in most correctly selected cases. All other 'complicated cases' require operation under direct vision followed by valvotomy or valve replacement with a homograft or a prosthesis.

Course and Prognosis

A minority of patients live a normal life span and a minority deteriorate progressively from attacks of rheumatic fever in childhood and adolescence. Most die of the disease between the ages of 30 and 50, the average age at death being 35; most of these have had a symptom-free period in early adult life, followed by the development of increasing effort dyspnoea and then congestive heart failure. The prognosis in an individual case depends on a full assessment of many factors; the presence of recurrent rheumatic activity, severe pulmonary hypertension and right heart failure are serious adverse factors. Patients with atrial fibrillation may live for several years but many die within 3 years of its onset and peripheral embolism is, at any time, an additional hazard. Pregnancy is tolerated moderately well, but it is noticeable that many patients have their first symptoms or a first attack of heart failure at this time. Favourable factors in prognosis are a continued absence of symptoms in the third decade, absence of rheumatism, a small heart with no signs of pulmonary hypertension on clinical examination and the absence of right ventricular preponderance on the electrocardiogram. A short and soft mid-diastolic murmur with a normal pulse volume, together with the factors mentioned, suggests that the valve has an area greater than 2 cm^2. and that the obstruction is slight and prognosis correspondingly good. Successful mitral valvotomy reverses much of the symptomatology, diminishes pulmonary hypertension and may restore some patients to a relatively normal life.

Postoperative Complications. Atrial fibrillation may occur for the first time in the immediate postoperative period and is commonest during the first 14 days. Reversion to sinus rhythm may be attempted with quinidine or by electrical defibrillation (D.C. converter); in some cases this reversion occurs spontaneously.

A traumatic pericardial effusion sometimes develops and this may give rise to subacute pericardial tamponade during the first or second postoperative week. Pericardial effusions are less frequent if local intrapericardial procaine is avoided at operation and adequate dependant drainage into the pleural cavity allowed for, when the pericardium is sutured. Postoperative mitral regurgitation, where none was present pre-operatively, is rarely produced when the finger alone splits the commissures of the valve at their line of fusion. After the use of a valvotome, postoperative regurgitation has been reported more frequently, although it is seldom of any serious functional significance.

Cerebral emboli or emboli elsewhere, originating from particles of clot detached from the intra-atrial thrombus or from calcified masses on the valve itself, may occur at the operation or in the immediate postoperative period.

Results. In most reported series of patients treated by mitral valvotomy results are classed as excellent in about a quarter of cases; in about a half they are good, while in the remaining quarter improvement, if any, is poor. The mortality rate is less than 2 per cent. for 'good risk' patients. Mortality is higher when operation is performed under cardiopulmonary by-pass for there is risk (now small) attending the procedure and the more seriously affected patients with complicated lesions are treated by this method.

Re-operation is required in a considerable proportion of patients in 7–10 years after valvotomy. It is too soon to assess the outlook for patients who have received graft or prosthetic valve replacement.

AORTIC STENOSIS

Narrowing of the aortic orifice to one-quarter or less of its normal size causes symptoms and signs from the decreased cardiac output, decreased coronary flow, and left ventricular hypertrophy which eventually results in failure of the myocardium.

Aetiology

Aortic stenosis is rheumatic in many patients when it is frequently combined with aortic incompetence and mitral stenosis. Many cases of pure or predominant aortic stenosis are of a congenital origin and in these the valve is often bicuspid. There is a striking predominance of males (about 3 to 1) compared with the female dominance in mitral stenosis. With the development of more accurate criteria for diagnosis aortic valve stenosis appears to be more common than was formerly thought. Congenital subaortic stenosis is rare and is difficult to distinguish clinically from the valvular variety.

Pathology

The aortic cusps are thickened and deformed and joined together. In severe cases the identity of the cusps is lost and only a narrow crescentic or triangular orifice is left. Extensive calcification is almost invariable in the older age groups. Beyond the obstruction the aorta often shows a local area of dilatation: the aorta and the coronary arteries are sometimes strikingly free of atheroma. There is usually considerable hypertrophy of the left ventricle and the heart may weigh between 500 and 900 g. Dilatation of the ventricle is usual, though late, and some interstitial fibrosis of the myocardium occurs.

Symptoms and Signs

Slight or moderate aortic stenosis causes no symptoms. Severe aortic stenosis causes striking and characteristic symptoms which tend to appear in middle life, and late in the course of the disease. Shortness of breath on exertion is usually the first symptom and gradually progresses until left ventricular failure causes paroxysmal nocturnal dyspnoea [see left ventricular failure, p. 747]. Cardiac pain on effort is caused by the diminished coronary flow and is indistinguishable from angina pectoris due to coronary disease. The reduced cardiac output is responsible for attacks of dizziness, 'blackout', or even syncope characteristically provoked by effort; these symptoms may occur as a result of changes in posture, or peripheral vasodilatation and sometimes no provoking cause can be discovered. Syncopal attacks may be severe and frequent.

Characteristic abnormalities are found on examination of the pulse, on palpation of the heart and on auscultation. All these abnormalities are required for the firm diagnosis of aortic stenosis. The pulse is small and rises slowly, and pulse tracings frequently show a notch on the ascending limb (anacrotic pulse). The blood pressure is normal or low. The venous pulse is normal in form and in pressure. Palpation may indicate hypertrophy of the left ventricle and there may be a systolic thrill at the base. On auscultation there is an obvious systolic murmur in the aortic area which may be loud enough to produce a thrill and is well transmitted to the neck. The same murmur is transmitted to the apex where it may be as loud as in the aortic area, and occasionally the murmur is loudest at the apex. In many cases the systolic murmur is no more than moderately loud; it starts at the moment of ejection, rises to a crescendo in mid-systole and diminishes as the flow diminishes, ceasing before the second sound. This mid-systolic pattern, which can be detected with the stethoscope, is common to all systolic murmurs produced during ejection through the aortic (or pulmonary) valve and does not mean stenosis unless accompanied by the abnormal pulse and hypertrophy of the left ventricle. This murmur is frequently preceded by an ejection click. The aortic component of the second sound may be soft or absent, but it is frequently normal and can be clearly heard at the apex where the pulmonary component of the second sound is not normally transmitted. Physiological splitting of the second sound in the pulmonary area, due to inspiratory delay of the pulmonary component, is seldom heard in aortic stenosis. This may be due to prolongation of left ventricular systole making the two sounds coincide, or to reversal of the normal order of valve closure making the earlier pulmonary component difficult to detect in the systolic murmur. A faint aortic diastolic murmur indicating a minor degree of aortic incompetence is not uncommon.

The electrocardiogram is useful in assessing the degree of left ventricular hypertrophy and therefore the severity of the aortic obstruction. Deep S-T depression and T wave inversion are a feature in chest leads taken over the left ventricle, and this pattern with a tall R wave is frequently transmitted to both the left arm and left leg, making all three standard limb leads of a similar pattern. There may be left bundle branch block. The rhythm is usually normal, but prolonged atrioventricular conduction and dissociation are not uncommon. *On radiography* the left ventricle may be enlarged but evidence of hypertrophy is usually found earlier by electrocardiography and by palpation. The ascending aorta can usually be seen to be dilated immediately distal to the valve. Calcification of the aortic valve can be detected by fluoroscopy in a very high proportion of the older patients.

Left-heart catheterization [p. 745] is indicated when surgery is considered or when diagnostic problems are unsolved. By such means the pressure gradient across the valve may be demonstrated and radio-opaque dye injected for direct visualization of the left ventricular outflow tract and valvar anatomy.

Complications

Bacterial endocarditis may occur at any time in the course of the disease, even in the early stages when the only physical sign is a mid-systolic murmur. Sudden death is not infrequent once symptoms have developed.

Diagnosis

A diagnosis of aortic stenosis is made by finding a slow rising pulse, an aortic systolic murmur and evidence of left ventricular hypertrophy. In hypertension with aortic dilatation there may be left ventricular hypertrophy and a soft aortic systolic murmur but no stenotic pulse. In dilatation of the aorta from atheroma alone there may be a soft aortic systolic murmur but no abnormal pulse or left ventricular hypertrophy. Perhaps the most difficult and most important diagnostic problem concerns the differentiation of classical aortic valvar stenosis, with which this section is concerned, from subaortic stenosis and subaortic obstructive myopathy: in this condition an ejection click, valvular calcification and post-stenotic aortic dilatation are absent [see cardiomyopathy, etc., p. 809].

In active rheumatism with aortic valvulitis without stenosis there is a soft or moderately loud aortic systolic murmur but no abnormal pulse or evidence of left ventricular hypertrophy. In aortic incompetence there is usually an aortic systolic murmur, and when associated with aortic dilatation as in syphilis, there may be a loud systolic murmur and even a thrill, but the pulse is waterhammer and the left ventricle feels hyperdynamic as well as hypertrophied. Differentiation from mitral incompetence may be difficult since in both conditions there may be a loud apical systolic murmur. The systolic murmur in mitral incompetence is always pansystolic, often with a crescendo in late systole obliterating the second sound at the apex, though this sound is clear enough elsewhere. The mitral systolic murmur is not loud in the aortic area and is frequently better conducted to the axilla and back. In mitral incompetence the pulse is not anacrotic unless there is associated aortic valve disease.

Treatment

No treatment is necessary for cases of mild or moderate aortic stenosis except to avoid hard physical effort, especially competitive games. In severe aortic stenosis with ischaemic pain, syncopal attacks and/or evidence of left ventricular failure surgery is indicated. Left ventricular failure is treated with digitalis, a low sodium diet and diuretics [p. 750]. Closed aortic valvotomy has not been as successful as mitral valvotomy and has been replaced by open heart techniques; in the vast majority of cases excision of the damaged valve and its replacement by an aortic homograft or ball-valve prosthesis is necessary. Both types of replacement valve have met with considerable success, and the operation carries a reasonably low mortality.

Course and Prognosis

The course of patients with aortic stenosis may be long and benign. A systolic murmur may have been heard in childhood and passed as innocent, and the stenotic pulse and left ventricular hypertrophy may not develop until middle age. Once symptoms of cardiac failure have been noticed, the course is usually downhill. Shortness of breath on exertion is succeeded by paroxysmal nocturnal dyspnoea from left ventricular failure; pulmonary congestion and congestive heart failure ensue. In some cases raised jugular venous pressure and oedema may appear without preceding symptoms of left ventricular failure (Bernheim's syndrome) and this is probably due to interference with filling of the right ventricle owing to encroachment by the massive hypertrophy of the left ventricle. Angina pectoris and syncope on effort adversely affect prognosis and sudden death is not uncommon. The long-term results of valve replacement surgery await the passage of time but it is clear that successful operations are followed by relief of symptoms and the regression of unfavourable signs.

AORTIC REGURGITATION

Damage to the aortic cusps, a dilated valve ring or a combination of these circumstances leads to aortic incompetence. The magnitude of the backflow varies from a small fraction to half of the stroke output when the cusps are totally deficient; this regurgitated blood increases the residual left ventricular volume and stretches the myocardium, causing a more vigorous contraction of the left ventricle and a steep rise of intraventricular pressure resulting in early ejection of an increased volume of blood. This steep rise of pressure imparts a 'hyperdynamic feel' to the apex beat, which is transmitted to the carotid arteries where it is known as Corrigan's sign, to the peripheral arteries causing a waterhammer pulse, and to the capillaries where the increased pulsation may be seen. The increased left ventricular volume causes dilatation, and the increased work causes hypertrophy of the left ventricle which may reach an enormous size.

Aetiology and Pathology

Rheumatic valvulitis is by far the commonest cause of aortic incompetence in Great Britain, and in most cases there is additional involvement of the mitral valve. Syphilitic aortic incompetence is now less commonly seen [p. 788]; here the main damage is in the aorta, causing dilatation of the aortic ring, and severe involvement of the cusps is much less common. Syphilitic aortitis also results in aneurysm formation, coronary ostial stenosis leading to cardiac ischaemia and, rarely, cardiac infarction. In severe hypertension stretching of the aortic ring may cause a minor degree of incompetence. Damage to the aorta from a dissecting aneurysm occasionally causes aortic incompetence. Bacterial endocarditis is rarely the primary cause, although it may increase pre-existing damage and is the commonest cause of a ruptured aortic cusp. Congenital bicuspid aortic valves, or rarely, quadricuspid valves, tend to be incompetent when associated with hypertension or atheroma. A minor degree of incompetence from a bicuspid valve is frequently found in patients with coarctation of the aorta. Congenital abnormalities of the aortic valve causing incompetence are occasionally associated with other forms of congenital heart disease: in patients with a high ventricular septal defect a valve cusp may prolapse into the defect thereby partially replacing left to right shunt with aortic incompetence. Aortic reflux is not uncommon in cystic medial necrosis of the aorta (a feature of Marfan's disease). It is occasionally seen in association with ankylosing spondylitis and ulcerative colitis.

Symptoms and Signs

A slight or moderate degree of aortic incompetence does not produce symptoms for many years. Shortness of breath on exertion is usually the first symptom and, as with aortic stenosis, paroxysmal nocturnal dyspnoea and cardiac asthma tend to follow rapidly if left ventricular failure is not treated. Ischaemic pain is not uncommon, especially in the syphilitic group with coronary ostial stenosis; pain tends to occur during attacks of paroxysmal nocturnal dyspnoea as well as on effort.

The pulse of aortic incompetence rises steeply in systole and gives a characteristic tap to the palpating finger which is described as a 'waterhammer'. The rapid fall of pressure produces a collapsing quality. These signs are best appreciated by palpating the radial and brachial arteries with the flat of the fingers when the arm is elevated. The same pulsation can be seen in the carotid arteries (Corrigan) and in the capillaries especially of the nail bed. The compensatory rise in systolic pressure and the low diastolic pressure from the aortic backflow and peripheral vasodilatation produce a wide pulse pressure. There may be difficulty in estimating the diastolic pressure, and persistence of the diastolic sound down to zero does not indicate a diastolic pressure at this level. The apex is heaving from left ventricular hypertrophy and the sudden steep lift in systole combined with a second small wave in diastole gives the apex a hyperdynamic quality. *The apex* is displaced downwards and to the left. On auscultation there is an early diastolic murmur commencing immediately after the aortic component of the second sound. This murmur is high pitched and best heard with a diaphragm stethoscope. It is usually loudest to the left of the sternum in the third and fourth left spaces, but when the ascending aorta is dilated, especially in syphilitic aortitis, the murmur is often loudest to the right of the sternum. Early diastolic murmurs may be very soft and then they are more easily heard on expiration, in the sitting position, and when the heart is slowing after exertion. An aortic systolic murmur is usually heard, and is of the same quality as in aortic stenosis but is not so loud. Occasionally the systolic murmur may be loud, and even associated with a thrill when the first part of the aorta is greatly dilated from syphilitic aortitis. Apparent splitting of the first heart sound is not unusual, and is due to the addition of an extra ejection sound in early systole from dilatation of the aorta. In some patients with isolated free aortic incompetence a short mid-diastolic murmur, or a pre-systolic murmur, may be heard at the mitral area (the Austin Flint murmur). It has been ascribed to the regurgitant stream from the aortic valve pushing back the aortic cusp of the mitral valve in diastole, causing some obstruction to the mitral orifice.

The electrocardiogram shows left axis deviation, tall R waves, depression of S-T segments and T wave inversion in leads over the left ventricle when this is hypertrophied, but it is normal when the aortic incompetence is slight. On *radiography* there is great enlargement of the left ventricle in severe cases, and obvious uncoiling of the aorta even in the rheumatic cases. Aortic pulsation is greatly increased. There is no calcification of the aortic valve.

Complications

Bacterial endocarditis may occur at any time in the rheumatic group but is extremely rare in the syphilitic cases. Rupture of a damaged aortic cusp is usually due to superimposed bacterial endocarditis, and tends to be a serious complication owing to the increase in strain on the left ventricle. Recurrence of active rheumatic carditis may precipitate heart failure.

Diagnosis

The diagnosis of aortic regurgitation is made by hearing an aortic diastolic murmur, and in mild cases this may be the only physical sign. It may be difficult to distinguish from a pulmonary diastolic murmur but the latter is almost confined to patients with great pulmonary hypertension with its characteristic physical signs. In severe aortic incompetence the combination of a waterhammer pulse, enlarged left ventricle and early diastolic murmur are characteristic. It may be much more difficult to decide the aetiology. Syphilitic aortic regurgitation is favoured by an age of over 35 years, a positive history of infection, ischaemic cardiac pain, a positive Wassermann reaction and by signs of syphilis elsewhere. An aortic aneurysm indicates luetic aetiology, but it must be remembered that free rheumatic aortic incompetence may cause great dynamic unfolding of the aorta; this always appears symmetrical and involves the ascending part, arch and upper descending aorta equally, while syphilitic dilatation is irregular [p. 788]. An incorrect diagnosis of additional mitral stenosis, and therefore of a rheumatic aetiology, may be made by hearing an Austin Flint murmur and by seeing apparent enlargement of the left atrium in the right oblique view, on the X-ray screen; this is due to enlargement of the left ventricle which displaces the atrium backwards. When heart failure has ensued, left atrial and right-sided enlargement may further simulate the effect of additional mitral stenosis. Rheumatic aortic incompetence may be diagnosed with confidence when there is additional mitral stenosis recognized by a loud first sound, an opening snap and a mid-diastolic murmur. A pansystolic murmur at the apex, with systolic backward movement of the left atrium, favours additional organic mitral valve disease, but when there is great left ventricular enlargement from aortic valve disease, a mitral systolic murmur may be due to functional incompetence. Calcification of the mitral valve indicates a rheumatic aetiology. Occasionally the murmurs of aortic incompetence may be simulated by pericardial friction in acute pericarditis. The peripheral signs of aortic incompetence are present in patent ductus arteriosus, and occasionally the murmur of this condition may be confused with the 'to and fro' murmur of aortic incompetence. However, in patent ductus arteriosus the characteristic continuous murmur is best heard in the second left intercostal space. The left ventricle is usually not greatly hypertrophied, and on X-ray screening there is pulmonary plethora. In occasional cases cardiac catheterization is necessary to establish the diagnosis of patent ductus arteriosus. Rupture of a sinus of Valsalva into any one of the heart chambers produces the peripheral signs of aortic regurgitation, an early diastolic murmur and other signs which depend on the site, magnitude and direction of the leak.

Aortic Stenosis with Incompetence. A combination of stenosis and incompetence is frequent when the aetiology is rheumatic, and incompetence in the younger age groups may change to dominant stenosis in later years. The physical signs of both valve lesions may be present and the pulse frequently has a double impulse (pulsus bisferiens).

Treatment

Treatment is the same as for aortic stenosis except that surgical repair may be more difficult when there is great dilatation of the ascending aorta; however, various types of reconstruction operation, and insertion of homograft valves and plastic metal prostheses, have met with great success. The onset of breathlessness indicating left ventricular failure should be taken seriously; a full 3 weeks' rest in bed is advisable, together with intensive treatment of left ventricular failure [p. 749], followed by surgery after an interval of weeks or months depending on response to treatment.

Prognosis

Minor degrees of aortic incompetence are compatible with a long and full life. Severe aortic incompetence causes great strain on the left ventricle and once symptoms have started, the downhill course is usually rapid as in aortic stenosis. Heart failure occurs with normal rhythm. Prognosis depends on the degree of incompetence as judged by peripheral signs and cardiac enlargement. The outlook of patients with rheumatic aortic incompetence is better than those with syphilitic aortitis. Successful valve replacement is followed by relief of symptoms; it is probable that a competent replacement valve will lead to greatly improved prognosis.

TRICUSPID VALVE DISEASE

Functional tricuspid incompetence is a common condition: it results from dilatation of the right heart and thus usually accompanies congestive heart failure. Organic tricuspid valve disease is mostly due to chronic rheumatic valvulitis. It is much less common than chronic mitral valve disease with which it is usually associated. Some degree of tricuspid valvulitis is present in about one-third of cases of chronic rheumatic valvulitis at necropsy. Tricuspid stenosis is rarely due to congenital malformation, but tricuspid incompetence may result from a curious congenital malformation (Ebstein's disease) in which the cusps of the valve are incompletely formed or displaced into the right ventricular chamber. In general, the pathological findings in organic tricuspid valve disease are the same as in mitral valve disease: in the rare, pure tricuspid valve lesions, however, the left heart and the lungs are relatively normal.

Symptoms and Signs

The *symptoms* are those of progressive right heart failure, but as most cases are associated with mitral stenosis, there is dyspnoea on effort in addition to weakness. Tricuspid valve disease tends to prevent all forms of paroxysmal dyspnoea; indeed when functional tricuspid insufficiency develops in left ventricular disease or mitral stenosis, the patient is often relieved of cardiac asthma. In tricuspid valve disease severe symptoms may develop from extreme congestion of all organs; dyspepsia, pain in the right hypochondrium and insomnia are common features.

Signs. In advanced chronic tricuspid valve disease, wasting, slight icterus, peripheral cyanosis, hepatomegaly and recurrent ascites are commonly present. *Tricuspid incompetence* causes an increased venous pulse wave which is coincident with ventricular systole ('cv' wave); it appears to rise rather slowly in the neck veins in contrast with augmented atrial waves; this systolic venous pulse wave is associated with systolic expansile pulsation of the liver, elicited by bimanual examination of the liver, when tricuspid incompetence is great. Various murmurs are frequently present from associated valve lesions, but the systolic murmur of tricuspid incompetence may be distinguished; it is pansystolic, heard best inside the apex or at the lower end of the sternum and its intensity varies with respiration, being louder in inspiration.

Tricuspid stenosis causes an augmented atrial wave ('a' wave) in the venous pulse—this wave is short, quickly rising, of variable amplitude and presystolic in time. A tricuspid diastolic murmur may be present; it is best heard at the lower end of the sternum and is loudest in inspiration, but as the lesion is mostly associated with mitral stenosis, it is not always possible to distinguish with certainty the right and left heart murmurs.

The outstanding feature of tricuspid valve disease on radiography of the heart is right atrial enlargement—in some cases the right atrium may appear to occupy most of the enlarged heart shadow. Radiographic screening sometimes shows systolic pulsation of the right atrium, but more often the atrium is so large that the regurgitant stream produces little movement; however, appropriate atrial or ventricular pulse waves may be seen in the superior vena caval shadow. The lungs are frequently clear in spite of the degree of heart disease.

Diagnosis

Careful observation of the venous pulse is the key to diagnosis in tricuspid valve disease. Tricuspid incompetence is frequently overlooked because of the dominant signs of associated organic heart disease. Tricuspid stenosis is relatively rare: it should be considered in chronic rheumatic heart disease when there are signs of right heart failure, recurrent ascites and hepatomegaly: if the heart rhythm is regular, large atrial waves in the neck veins and presystolic hepatic pulsation are diagnostic signs.

Treatment

The treatment of functional or organic tricuspid incompetence is the treatment of heart failure. The rare cases of pure or dominant tricuspid stenosis should be treated by tricuspid valvotomy, but tricuspid incompetence is the usual sequel.

Prognosis

The prognosis in functional tricuspid incompetence is essentially that of the causal disease. In organic tricuspid disease prognosis also largely depends on the degree of associated chronic mitral valvulitis and its effect on the whole heart.

REFERENCES

BRIGDEN, W., and LEATHAM, A. (1953) Mitral incompetence, *Brit. Heart J.*, **15**, 55.

BROCK, R. C. (1952) Surgical and pathological anatomy of the mitral valve, *Brit. Heart J.*, **14**, 489.

DORFMAN, A. (1964) Treatment of rheumatic pancarditis, *Circulation*, **24**, 811.

GIBSON, R., and WOOD, P. (1955) The diagnosis of tricuspid stenosis, *Brit. Heart J.*, **17**, 552.

GOODWIN, J. F. (1967) Indications for surgery in mitral valve disease, *Proc. roy. Soc. Med.*, **60**, 1009.

HUDSON, R. E. B. (1970) *Cardiovascular Pathology*, Vol. 3, p. 564, London.

LEATHAM, A. (1951) The phonocardiogram of aortic stenosis, *Brit. Heart J.*, **13**, 153.

MOUNSEY, P. (1953) The opening snap of mitral stenosis, *Brit. Heart J.*, **15**, 135.

ROSS, D. N. (1966) Aortic valve replacement, *Lancet*, ii, 461.

SHORT, D. (1955) The radiology of the lung in mitral stenosis, *Brit. Heart J.*, **17**, 33.

SYMPOSIUM ON CARDIOVASCULAR SURGERY (1964) *Circulation*, **24**, Suppl. 4.

WERKÖ. L. (1964) *Mitral Valvular Disease*, Stockholm.

WOOD, P. (1954) An appreciation of mitral stenosis, *Brit. med. J.*, **1**, 1051 and 1113.

WOOD, P. (1958) Aortic stenosis, *Amer. J. Cardiol.*, **1**, 553.

DISEASES OF THE PERICARDIUM

Inflammation of the pericardium may be acute or chronic and occurs as a primary disorder or as part of a general disease. The acute form may be dry (fibrinous) or accompanied by effusion (serous). Chronic pericarditis occurs as constrictive pericarditis, adhesive mediastinopericarditis and rarely as a chronic effusion. The aetiology and the effect of the disease process on circulatory dynamics are the two important considerations in all types of pericarditis.

ACUTE PERICARDITIS

Aetiology

The age and sex incidence in acute pericarditis depends on the nature of the cause. In most cases of acute isolated pericarditis—so-called idiopathic or benign pericarditis—the aetiology is obscure although a virus infection is usually assumed and sometimes proved; the Coxsackie group being most frequently detected. Pyogenic infections and tuberculosis are sometimes the cause but these have become uncommon in recent years. The collagen diseases including rheumatic fever, rheumatoid arthritis and systemic lupus are often associated with acute pericarditis. Other causes include uraemia, hyperuricaemia, trauma, invasion by neoplasm, and cardiac infarction. Occasionally dissection of the aorta presents with acute pericarditis.

Pathology

The morbid anatomical findings largely depend on the aetiology. The acute fibrinous forms may be local or general in distribution. In the early stages the pericardium loses its smooth, shiny appearance because of a surface exudate of lymph, fibrin and inflammatory cells. This exudate may become thick and irregular, resulting in a ragged, honeycomb appearance—the so-called 'bread-and-butter' pericardium'. In many cases the superficial layers of the myocardium also show an inflammatory reaction. Organization takes place, leaving varying degrees of slight pericardial thickening, often with adhesions. In other forms the fibrinous reaction may be associated with a large effusion of serous or serosanguinous or seropurulent fluid, and occasionally the sac may be full of pus.

Clinical Features

1. *Acute fibrinous pericarditis* (*i.e. without effusion*). In many cases there are no symptoms; in others the symptoms are submerged in those of associated disease, e.g. rheumatic carditis or cardiac infarction, whilst in others distinctive features are present.

Pain varies in intensity and is situated across the front of the chest, sometimes radiating to the neck and shoulders; it may occasionally be confined to the epigastrium. Pericardial pain may be indistinguishable from the pain of cardiac infarction, but sometimes it is made worse by moving the chest, especially into the hyperextended position, on deep breathing and frequently worse on swallowing; it is always aggravated by lying flat. It is generally agreed that the visceral pericardium is insensitive and the pain of pericarditis appears to arise from the parietal pericardium and its area of continuity with the diaphragm and pleura. Some degree of dyspnoea is usual, but this is not a prominent feature unless there is pericardial effusion.

There is often moderate fever, sweating and a leucocytosis, depending on the aetiology of the pericarditis. The characteristic physical sign is a friction rub which occurs in systole and diastole, giving it a 'to and fro' character, which sometimes resembles the murmur of aortic stenosis and incompetence. Friction rubs are best heard towards the base.

2. *Pericarditis with effusion.* The clinical picture varies with the amount of fluid and the rate at which it accumulates. If the amount is small there may be no symptoms. If, on the other hand, it is large and the accumulation is rapid, pain is usual and the patient is often anxious, restless and pale. Dyspnoea and orthopnoea develop in proportion to the size of the effusion and appear to be due to a direct compression of adjacent lung and diminution of vital capacity. An irritating cough occurs with large effusions. Cardiac asthma sometimes occurs, but is probably due to underlying myocardial disease.

A friction rub is sometimes heard towards the base of the heart. The apex beat becomes weak and may disappear, and the heart sounds are soft at the apex. The extent of cardiac dullness increases and is said to vary with the posture of the patient. In large effusions dullness to percussion and bronchial breathing occur posteriorly over the left lower lobe, due to partial or complete atelectasis.

The interference with cardiac function known as *cardiac tamponade* which occurs in many cases is related to the size of the effusion and its rate of development. The clinical features of tamponade are due to restriction of diastolic filling and consequent reduction in cardiac output, a rise in atrial pressure above the pericardial pressure, and peripheral vasoconstriction which maintains blood pressure in the presence of a falling cardiac output. Tamponade is recognized by a rising jugular venous pressure and this should be carefully assessed in all cases of suspected pericardial effusion. The systemic blood pressure tends to fall and the radial pulse may become very small—occasionally it fades during inspiration (pulsus paradoxus). A paradoxical rise of venous pressure with inspiration may be observed in the jugular veins. Tachycardia is usual. Rapidly developing tamponade may lead to shock, whilst a slowly increasing pericardial effusion may produce widespread venous congestion resembling congestive heart failure.

The radiology of acute pericarditis. Radiological changes in acute pericarditis occur when an effusion collects in the sac. The important signs are: (1) an enlargement of the heart shadow and a decrease in size with recovery shown by serial films; (2) a rounding of the heart shadow, becoming almost globular in some cases, with obliteration of the normal angulation along the left border, sharpening of the pericardiophrenic angles and a bulging into the retrocardiac space best seen in the right oblique view; (3) diminution of cardiac pulsation seen on radioscopy—in extreme cases the shadow appears quite still; (4) on cardiac catheterization there is a space between the catheter lip lying against the right atrial endocardium and the outer border of the heart. This increase in thickness of the wall due to fluid may be clearly demonstrated by angiocardiography —a small quantity of dye introduced through a catheter is sufficient for diagnostic purposes.

The electrocardiogram in acute pericarditis tends to show pathological changes in all leads due to the widespread nature of the injury. The time relations of various complexes remain normal. P waves are unaffected. The QRS complex remains normal in form but the voltage is frequently diminished in all leads in pericardial effusion. The important pathological changes in pericarditis are due to epicardial injury, and are found in the S-T segment and T waves. The S-T segment is slightly elevated in all leads, showing more in some leads than in others [FIG. 51]. Usually the S-T is concave upwards, in others it is straighter and occasionally coved with a convexity upwards, as is found in myocardial infarction. These changes fluctuate, tend to be transient and rarely last for more than 10 days. The T waves tend to become flattened and inverted. A small inversion of T waves in all standard leads and chest leads is sometimes seen—the widespread nature of such a change is strong evidence of pericarditis. Occasionally the T wave is tall and sharp at the termination of a raised concave S-T segment.

The electrocardiogram of cardiac infarction is partly due to epicardial disease so that differentiation from pericarditis is sometimes difficult. The changes in pericarditis are more diffuse and are never associated with Q waves. An isolated steep inversion of T waves occurring in only one or two leads is not due to pericarditis.

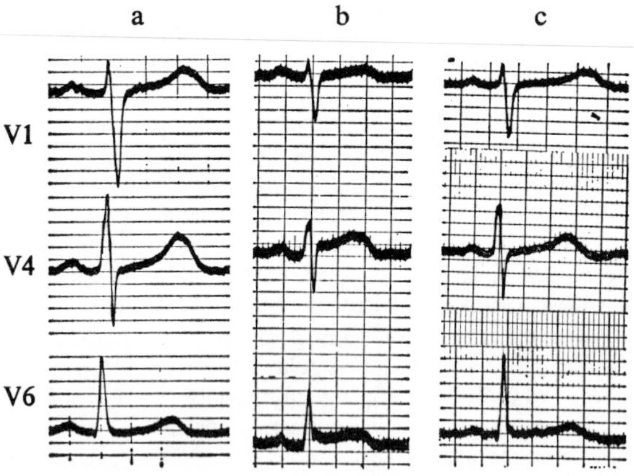

FIG. 51. *Pericarditis with effusion.* (a) Normal ECG (chest leads) prior to the attack. (b) Two weeks later diminished voltage of QRS, and S-T segment elevation in chest leads during acute phase. (c) Two weeks later, the attack resolving, voltage increased, ST normal but persistent slight T wave flattening.

Paracentesis of the pericardium is indicated when diagnosis remains in doubt, when examination of the fluid is required for diagnosis of the cause, and as an urgent therapeutic measure when cardiac tamponade is great or increasing rapidly.

The skin and underlying tissues should be anaesthetized down to the pericardium. The needle should be inserted just beyond the apex beat, or high in the angle between the ensiform cartilage and the left margin of the sternum and then passed upwards, backwards and slightly to the right; the needle should be withdrawn a little when pulsation of the heart is felt on reaching the epicardium. Sufficient fluid is withdrawn for diagnostic purposes or to relieve symptoms. This procedure is not indicated unless there is evidence of a considerable quantity of fluid or severe tamponade.

Special Types of Pericarditis. 1. *Acute benign pericarditis* (idiopathic pericarditis, non-specific pericarditis or virus pericarditis) is almost certainly due to virus infection. (Coxsackie and Echo viruses have been recovered from pericardial fluid in a few cases.)

This condition is possibly the commonest cause of acute pericarditis. Adults of either sex may be affected but males preponderate. The symptoms may resemble those of cardiac infarction from which it must be distinguished because of the difference in management and prognosis. A moderate-sized effusion may develop, friction may appear and fever may last a few days. The condition lasts for days or weeks, but relapse is not uncommon; however, recovery is invariable and apparently complete. No specific treatment is indicated but if frequent relapse becomes a problem this may be prevented by steroid therapy which should be continued (a small maintenance dose of prednisone, say 5–10 mg. twice daily, is sufficient) for at least 10 weeks.

2. *Tuberculous pericarditis.* This is a relatively rare clinical condition. It usually appears to be the primary manifestation of tuberculosis, but in most cases it is secondary to an obscure lesion elsewhere. The onset is often insidious, with general symptoms rather than local ones due to pericarditis. Chest pain usually develops, but may be transitory, cough is common and fever is high and irregular, but may be completely absent in elderly patients. Signs of tamponade develop and cardiac arrhythmias are common. The tuberculous aetiology may be confirmed by examination of aspirated pericardial fluid. The prognosis is bad without treatment; mortality rate in the first year after the onset of symptoms being approximately 50 per cent. Surviving patients, whether treated or untreated, may develop constrictive pericarditis later.

Prolonged bed rest similar to sanatorium regime is necessary. The prognosis is greatly improved by the concurrent administration of intramuscular streptomycin, sodium aminosalicylate and isoniazid [see general article on tuberculosis in Section 2]. When pericardial aspiration is possible and indicated by the size of the effusion, 1 G. of streptomycin in saline should be injected into the sac. This procedure may be repeated at weekly intervals and good results have been obtained. There is some evidence that early surgical drainage after treatment with streptomycin may be beneficial. The progress of treatment is assessed from the degree of fever, improvement in general symptoms, the erythrocyte sedimentation rate, radiological heart size and the electrocardiogram.

3. *Pericarditis in collagen disease.* Some degree of transient fibrinous pericarditis probably occurs in a majority of cases of rheumatic carditis and its significance is subordinate to the whole disease. In some cases, however, usually the more serious ones, an effusion develops and this adversely affects the course of the disease. Acute pericarditis is very common in systemic lupus erythematosus, and it tends to be recurrent; however, constriction does not seem to occur. Acute pericarditis also occurs with rheumatoid arthritis and several cases of chronic constrictive pericarditis have been reported in association with this condition.

4. Acute pericarditis is a feature of both the *postinfarction syndrome* and the *postcardiotomy syndrome.* In these conditions pericarditis tends to be acute, recurrent and associated with generalized joint discomfort and pleuritis. There is evidence that the aetiology is concerned with hypersensitivity to damaged heart tissue.

5. *Purulent pericarditis* is fortunately rare now that the pyogenic conditions which cause it are treated with antibiotic agents or chemotherapy. Surgical drainage together with the appropriate chemotherapy is indicated.

Diagnosis

Chest pain, a friction rub, fever and widespread S-T elevation and T wave changes in the electrocardiogram are the diagnostic features of acute pericarditis, but these features do not always occur together. Pain is often absent, friction rubs are often fleeting, fever may be absent or due to associated disease and the electrocardiogram may be pathological only for a brief period. When pain, friction or electrocardiographic changes occur in the course of a disease known to be complicated by pericarditis, such as rheumatic fever, septicaemia, chest neoplasm and uraemia, the diagnosis is readily made.

The accumulation of pericardial fluid is recognized by radiographic change in heart shape, softening of the heart sounds, electrocardiographic changes and the signs of developing tamponade. The withdrawal of pericardial fluid by paracentesis is diagnostic and helps in the investigation of its aetiology. Repeated physical examinations, serial electrocardiograms and chest films are of great importance, not only for observing the progress of the disease, but for diagnostic purposes.

The important differential diagnosis of acute virus pericarditis is cardiac infarction [see above]. Congestive cardiac failure must be differentiated from pericardial effusion causing tamponade. Here a knowledge of the underlying aetiology, the radiographic features, serial electrocardiograms and special investigations mentioned above for pericardial effusions are of diagnostic importance. The prognosis and treatment of acute pericarditis depend on the underlying cause.

CHRONIC CONSTRICTIVE PERICARDITIS

Synonym. Pick's disease.

Definition

This condition is essentially one of great thickening of the pericardium, which imposes a restrictive action on the heart so that diastolic filling is impeded, systolic ejection is diminished and venous congestion develops. It was known long before a series of cases were described by Pick in 1896. There are descriptions by Lower and by Lancisi over a century before, and Chevers discussed the pathophysiology of the condition in 1842.

Aetiology

Constrictive pericarditis occurs in men more often than in women and mostly between 15 and 50 years of age.

It is not surprising that the aetiology is difficult to find since it is not until healing and organization of previous inflammation have taken place that the condition comes into existence. Probably many cases are due to tuberculosis, but a definite history of previous pericarditis is rare and tuberculosis can only be demonstrated in some 16–20 per cent. of biopsy or necropsy specimens by histological and bacteriological methods. Rarely inflammation with pyogenic organisms may produce constrictive pericarditis, it may also occur as a result of organization of haemopericardium, and occasionally in rheumatoid arthritis.

Pathology

The heart is encased in pericardium which is thickened from 2 to 10 mm. This scar tissue shows varying degrees of hardness from an heterogeneous fibrocaseous mass to hard homogeneous hyalinized tissue or dense fibrosis with extensive calcification. This compression scar usually encases most of the heart and sometimes extends up to the great vessels, but occasionally it is more localized. The heart muscle is essentially normal, but the superficial myocardium is frequently involved in the overlying pericarditis so that a line of cleavage cannot be found.

The serous cavities usually contain effusions and the peritoneum is often thickened, sometimes to the extent of producing a so-called 'sugar-icing' appearance. The liver shows the results of long-standing venous congestion; it may be large or normal sized with a nutmeg appearance, or shrunken and fibrotic. It appears that the cirrhotic process continues after surgical relief of the constrictive pericarditis in the more long-standing severe cases.

Clinical Features

The clinical features are the result of restricted diastolic filling which causes a reduction in cardiac output; this leads to sodium and water retention. The resulting hypervolaemia means an increased venous return which, however, cannot be accommodated by the constricted ventricles so that exteme venous congestion results.

Constrictive pericarditis develops quietly and symptoms are not usually prominent until the signs are well developed. The patient may first complain of dyspnoea on effort or swelling of the abdomen. Sometimes cough is a prominent feature and occasionally faintness on bending down or coughing may be troublesome.

The most important physical sign is congestion of the cervical veins—this may be so great that the top level of venous pulsation is well above the ears and cannot be seen (20–30 cm. above the right atrium is usual). The venous pulse wave form appears continuously high with sharp descents in early diastole (y) and a paradoxical rise in venous pressure with inspiration is usually present. Constrictive pericarditis does not occur without venous hypertension. The arterial pulse tends to be small and often shows a diminution with inspiration (pulsus paradoxus). The blood pressure is usually low; peripheral arterial constriction shown by peripheral cyanosis and coldness of the extremities is sometimes present. Atrial fibrillation is not uncommon.

The apex beat is small or absent. The heart sounds tend to be soft but a cadence of three sounds is heard. The additional sound occurs in early diastole and is rather shorter, higher pitched and earlier than the physiological third sound. It is related to the high pressure of ventricular filling.

Ascites is usually present and is a prominent feature of the disease. Its extent is in contrast to the smaller amount of peripheral oedema. Ascites is persistent and peritoneal tapping is followed by recurrence. The liver may be small or moderately enlarged; it is hard but cannot always be felt through the ascites. Pleural effusions of varying extent are often present. The disease runs a long chronic course with gradually increasing venous congestion, diminishing cardiac output and hepatic failure.

Radiology. The heart is not greatly enlarged and on radioscopy the pulsations are seen to be diminished and the angulations of the left border are smoothed out. The most conspicuous finding in many cases is extensive calcification of the pericardium. This is often best seen in oblique views and sometimes appears to encase the heart excepting the origin of the great vessels. Small pleural effusions are common. The lungs do not usually appear congested.

The Electrocardiogram. The P waves may show abnormal forms or they are absent when there is atrial fibrillation. The QRS complex tends to be of low voltage, but is otherwise normal. The S-T segment is isoelectric but T waves are usually flattened or inverted in several leads. Occasionally the electrocardiogram is surprisingly normal and there is some evidence that the pericarditis has not involved the underlying myocardium in such cases.

Other investigations are not usually indicated. Liver biopsy shows the degree of cirrhotic change. Catheterization of the right heart shows the high level of the right atrial venous pressure and the right ventricle shows a characteristic pressure curve. Diastolic filling causes a very rapid rise of pressure which then reaches a plateau presumably when the restrictive forces prevent further change. Haemodynamic studies of the left heart show that the left atrial pressure and pulse wave form are usually similar to those of the right.

Diagnosis

The diagnostic features of constrictive pericarditis are jugular venous congestion, ascites and a quiet small heart with an additional heart sound in early diastole. The radiological features are important and calcification of the pericardium is diagnostic in the presence of venous hypertension; however, calcified plaques may occur in the pericardium without pericardial constriction. The electrocardiogram provides important additional evidence, but the diagnosis is essentially based on the clinical findings.

Congestive heart failure is differentiated from constrictive pericarditis by the presence of extensive oedema, lower levels of jugular venous pressure, cardiac enlargement and the recognition of a cause for the heart failure. Other causes of ascites are not usually difficult to differentiate because of the absence of severe venous congestion.

The greatest problem in differential diagnosis is cardiomyopathy, e.g. myocarditis, amyloidosis and endomyocardial fibrosis [p. 809]. The haemodynamics may be similar, for diastolic filling may be restricted and the heart pulsations diminished. Dyspnoea is a more prominent feature of cardiomyopathy and this reflects a greater frequency of left heart disease. In cardiomyopathy left atrial pressures are usually higher than right: calcification does not occur and the QRS complex of the electrocardiogram usually shows evidence of myocardial involvement. An inspection of the pericardium at operation may in the last resort be the diagnostic method of choice so that pericardectomy can be performed if constriction is present. Experience has shown that if there is no calcification the problem may prove to be myopathic.

Treatment

Decompression of the heart by surgical removal of the pericardium is indicated. It is advisable to reduce ascites before operation, and pre-operative treatment with streptomycin or other appropriate antibiotics is indicated if there is any evidence of active infection. Thickened pericardium is gradually removed from the left ventricle, and increased movement of the underlying heart or herniation through the area of removal indicates that decompression is being effective. It is often necessary to carry the decortication process over the right heart and the right atrium. Haemorrhage and infection are dangers, but in expert hands and with the use of antibiotics the mortality rate is low. An indifferent result from pericardectomy may mean that resection has not been sufficiently extensive or that the underlying cause is myocardial rather than pericardial. The results of operation are satisfactory and it should be advised in all cases of constrictive pericarditis other than the very mildest ones.

Prognosis

Untreated patients with constrictive pericarditis steadily deteriorate, become bedridden and die of the long-term effects of low cardiac output and hepatic failure. Surgical treatment entirely alters the outlook and patients are now living reasonably active lives several years after operation.

CHRONIC ADHESIVE PERICARDITIS

In this condition there are fibrous adhesions between the parietal layer of the pericardium and adjacent mediastinal structures, the chest wall, the pleura or the diaphragm. Various symptoms and signs have been attributed to this condition, but none is reliable and most are due to other changes such as chronic valve disease, cardiac enlargement or even true constrictive pericarditis. Although much has been written on this condition in the past, there is no evidence that it has any adverse effect on the function of the heart. No treatment is indicated.

PNEUMOPERICARDIUM

Air in the pericardial sac is a rare condition and occurs as a result of chest wounds and erosion by malignant growths from the bronchus or oesophagus. It is invariably associated with serous or purulent effusion. The symptoms and signs depend on the presence or otherwise of cardiac tamponade, its rate of development and the nature of the causal condition. Diagnosis is essentially radiological. Treatment depends on the cause, but severe tamponade requires relief by paracentesis of the sac.

HYDROPERICARDIUM

Transudation of excess fluid into the pericardium occurs in cardiac failure, renal disease, myxoedema and malignant hypertension. It is of entirely secondary importance and no special management or treatment is indicated other than for the causal disease.

TRAUMATIC PERICARDITIS

Haemopericardium may result from stab wounds and various missiles which have not caused fatality by complete penetration of the heart. Cardiac tamponade tends to develop and indicates surgical evacuation of blood clot and repair of the wound. Foreign bodies lodging in tissues adjacent to the pericardium may lead to a recurrent sterile fibrinous pericarditis. Non-penetrating injuries to the precordium may lead to contusion of the heart with the development of a transient pericarditis, detected by a friction rub and electrocardiographic signs of pericarditis. No treatment other than rest until signs and symptoms have disappeared is necessary [see traumatic heart disease, p. 811].

REFERENCES

BRADLEY, E. (1964) Acute benign pericarditis, *Amer. Heart J.*, **67**, 121.

EVANS, W., and JACKSON, F. (1952) Constrictive pericarditis, *Brit. Heart J.*, **14**, 53.

GIMLETTE, T. (1958) Constrictive pericarditis, *Brit. Heart J.*, **21**, 9.

JOHNSON, R., PORTNOY, B., ROGERS, N., and BUESCHER, E. (1961) Acute benign pericarditis, *Arch. intern. Med.*, **108**, 67.

ROBINSON, J., and BRIGDEN, W. (1963) Immunological studies in the post-cardiotomy syndrome, *Brit. med. J.*, **2**, 706.

ROBINSON, J., and BRIGDEN, W. (1968) Recurrent pericarditis, *Brit. med. J.*, **2**, 272.

WOOD, P. (1961) Chronic constrictive pericarditis, *Amer. J. Cardiol.*, **7**, 48.

DISEASES OF THE ENDOCARDIUM

The endocardium may be affected by any disease process which damages the myocardium. Inflammatory reactions of the endocardium are common in the collagen diseases especially rheumatic fever and systemic lupus erythematosus. Direct infection of the endocardium is almost confined to bacterial endocarditis.

BACTERIAL ENDOCARDITIS

This disease occurs in two main clinical forms—acute and subacute—which are largely determined by the nature of the infecting organisms; there is much overlap, but the distinction is justified on clinical grounds. The early diagnosis and effective treatment of bacterial endocarditis and of the serious septic conditions from which acute bacterial endocarditis arises make this distinction less important than formerly. Acute bacterial endocarditis is usually due to virulent pyogenic organisms, e.g. Gram-positive cocci, and the source is usually some obvious septic lesion associated with pyaemia. In the commoner subacute form the organism is of relatively low virulence, e.g. *Streptococcus viridans*, and it is the low virulence of these organisms which explains the insidious nature of the disease, chronicity, apyrexial periods and the absence of any obvious focus of infection.

SUBACUTE BACTERIAL ENDOCARDITIS

Aetiology

Infection occurs on a heart which is already damaged. The infecting organism is an α-haemolytic streptococcus (viridans) in about 80 per cent. of cases; non-haemolytic streptococci occur in about 5 per cent. and a variety of organisms occur in the remainder. The route and mode of infection is not definitely known, but subacute bacterial endocarditis not infrequently develops in patients with heart disease after the extraction of a septic tooth and after other relatively minor operations. A transient bacteraemia frequently follows such procedures and bacteria presumably settle on the damaged endocardium at this time. Bacterial endocarditis is especially associated with certain types of heart disease. (1) Rheumatic heart disease is present in more than half of the cases. Occasionally bacterial endocarditis develops in the presence of active rheumatism, but this is rare. Bacterial endocarditis does not usually develop on the grossly damaged rheumatic heart; it rarely occurs on the severely stenosed mitral valve and for this reason is almost never associated with atrial fibrillation; it commonly occurs in organic mitral reflux and in aortic valve disease. (2) Patients with congenital heart disease are commonly affected, but here also bacterial endocarditis shows a strange predilection for certain abnormalities and never occurs in others. Patent ductus arteriosus, coarctation of the aorta, bicuspid aortic valve and ventricular septal defect are sometimes infected; it is perhaps significant that these lesions are in the high pressure and arterialized blood streams. Fallot's tetralogy and other lesions with right to left shunts are rarely affected and atrial septal defects are immune. (3) The aortic valves are occasionally affected in syphilitic aortitis; and (4) an atherosclerotic aortic valve ring rarely appears to be the site of infection. In recent years endocarditis has proved to be a serious complication of the more prolonged and elaborate cardiac operations. Furthermore, infection of homograft, autograft and prosthetic valves is not uncommon.

The sexes are equally affected. The majority of cases occur between 15 and 55 years of age. Bacterial endocarditis is extremely rare in infancy and childhood.

Pathology

The primary lesions of bacterial endocarditis are in the heart; the secondary ones are due to peripheral arterial emboli, toxaemia and heart failure.

In the heart the lesions are proliferative and destructive. Small friable vegetations form at the site of endocarditis. They tend to form at the contact margins of valves, but may spread over the whole valve and extend to the adjacent mural endocardium. Ulceration may occur and rupture of valve cusps and chordae is not uncommon. Microscopically the vegetations surmount the endocardium and the valve beneath may show only a moderate cellular reaction. The vegetations consist of a more or less compact mass of platelets and fibrin which enmesh clumps of organisms.

The heart lesions are mainly valvular but the sites of congenital anomalies are also affected, e.g. the patent ductus and the interventricular septum. Myocarditis and pericarditis are not important features compared with the endocardial lesions. The myocardium shows accumulations of cells (Bracht-Wächter bodies) but it is not as severely affected as in rheumatic carditis.

Arterial emboli may produce infarction of varying degrees in the kidney, spleen, brain, retina, gut, and limbs; when the right heart is affected, pulmonary infarction may occur. Bacterial embolization of medium-sized arteries may produce a local arteritis with mycotic aneurysm formation; there is local medial necrosis and bulging of the damaged vessel. The kidney is almost invariably affected and shows three types of lesion: (1) large wedge infarctions from embolic occlusion of medium-sized vessels; (2) focal glomerulonephritis in which a varying number of glomeruli show an occluded vessel with surrounding reaction and organization; the surface of the kidney shows petechial spots and has been called the 'flea-bitten kidney' (deriving from the days when flea bites were 'physiological' and did not cause a brisk surrounding allergic response); (3) a diffuse glomerulonephritis is not uncommon and has been found in patients dying after penicillin treatment has cured the active endocarditis. Heart failure is not a prominent feature until late in the disease.

Clinical Features

The symptoms and signs are due to toxaemia, septicaemia, emboli in various organs and cardiac failure. The onset is gradual so that it is rarely possible to determine accurately when the disease began, but occasionally the onset is sudden, with high fever and rigors. The initial symptoms are general weakness and anorexia, with frequent sweats. Fever is usual and variable, there may be brief apyrexial periods, but it is mostly continuous and rarely rises above 102° F. (39° C.). Rigors are not uncommon and occur especially when there are crops of petechial haemorrhages. Headache and pain in the joints and limbs are common. Anaemia develops from the start and tends to be progressive; splenomegaly appears early in the disease.

The Heart. In the great majority of cases there are definite signs of heart disease at the onset. Often the signs are slight at first; a pansystolic murmur at the apex with no cardiac enlargement indicating a minimal mitral valve lesion is common. On the other hand, there may be obvious signs of extensive aortic valve disease or the signs of a congenital defect. As the disease progresses it is common to find evidence of spread to other valves, especially the aortic valve when the mitral valve was originally involved. Undue importance has been attached to changes in the character of murmurs from day to day. The sudden appearance of a loud or a musical murmur in systole or diastole may be due to the rupture of a cusp or fracture of one of the chordae tendineae. Atrial fibrillation is most unusual in the early stages of the disease, but it occasionally develops later.

Embolic Phenomena. Arterial emboli cause important signs of the disease. Lesions range from multiple microscopic ones to single large ones and may affect any organ of the body. The skin shows a variety of lesions. Petechiae are commonest, there may be no more than two or three or there may be vast numbers; they are commonly seen under the nails as splinter haemorrhages, at the base of the neck, in the conjunctiva, in the fundus oculi and the buccal mucosa. Petechiae may recur in showers, but in the early stages a diligent search is often required to find one. Larger areas of ecchymosis are not uncommon and may be tender. Osler's nodes are small, tender, swollen areas, usually a few millimetres in diameter, occurring commonly on the pulp of the fingers or toes; they are usually discoloured and transient, the patient complains of a sudden tender spot and often the examiner finds no signs a few days later. Osler's nodes appear to be almost specific for the disease.

The spleen enlarges early in the disease and is generally rather soft. Episodes of sudden severe left hypochondriac pain suggest splenic infarction; the spleen is then tender and a friction rub due to perisplenitis may be heard. Sudden loin pain may indicate renal infarction which sometimes causes macroscopic haematuria. Microscopic haematuria is common and is the result of focal embolic nephritis. Renal failure is a late manifestation of the disease.

Cerebral embolic episodes with resulting hemiplegia are not uncommon. Rarely diffuse cerebral damage may produce a meningitic or encephalitic picture. Central retinal arterial embolism occasionally occurs and causes sudden blindness, and optic atrophy may cause a more insidious loss of vision. The mesenteric vessels and those of the limbs are frequently involved. Mycotic aneurysm may develop, leading to fatal haemorrhage or gangrene. Sudden pain in a joint is probably due to endarterial embolism; repeated attacks of joint pain may cause confusion with rheumatic fever. Coronary embolism may cause cardiac infarction, resulting in heart failure or sudden death.

When bacterial endocarditis complicates a congenital lesion with left to right shunt, e.g. patent ductus arteriosus and ventricular septal defect, there may be few, if any, manifestations of systemic embolization; the clinical features are then largely pulmonary; the lungs may show repeated infarction and rarely abscess formation.

Cachexia with a *café au lait* complexion, gross finger clubbing, severe anaemia, haemorrhagic lesions, heart failure and renal failure are late features of the disease. The clinical picture and natural history of bacterial endocarditis have been changed by antibiotic drugs and chemotherapy. In early cases the disease may be completely cured; however, this is by no means invariably the case. When treatment is started late in the disease infection may be eradicated, but extensive valve lesions may lead to progressive heart failure. In some cases progressive renal failure from diffuse nephritis continues after sterilization of the infection.

Investigations. The blood shows a progressive anaemia averaging between 8 and 12 g. of haemoglobin per 100 ml.; the red cells rarely fall below three million per mm^3. The white cell count is variable, most cases show a slight to moderate leucocytosis but leucopenia sometimes occurs. Large monocytes are usually increased. The sedimentation rate is usually raised but this is not invariable.

Blood cultures are positive in some 75 per cent. of cases. Several samples of 10–20 ml. of blood should be examined, and several days must elapse before culture can be accepted as negative. When cultures are attempted after penicillin therapy has started they are likely to be negative unless treated with penicillinase.

Radiological and electrocardiographic examinations aid the assessment of the cardiac condition but are not specifically altered by bacterial endocarditis.

Diagnosis

Early diagnosis is imperative if antibiotic therapy is to prevent further irreparable damage to the heart. Any patient with an organic heart murmur who has vague ill health or prolonged fever should at once be considered as a possible case of bacterial endocarditis and appropriate investigations undertaken. The main features which lead to clinical diagnosis are: (1) heart disease; (2) fever; (3) embolic features, particularly petechiae and Osler's nodes; (4) splenomegaly; (5) anaemia; and (6) haematuria. Positive blood cultures confirm the diagnosis but in some 10–15 per cent. of cases the blood culture remains negative. The diagnosis is rarely tenable when the haemoglobin concentration and the sedimentation rate are normal.

Differential diagnosis. If bacterial endocarditis is kept in mind when considering patients with an organic heart murmur, confusion with other conditions rarely arises. However, bacterial endocarditis which is characterized by prolonged fever and the involvement of many organs must obviously be distinguished from many other conditions. Fever, endocarditis and anaemia due to active rheumatism in adolescents and young adults may resemble bacterial endocarditis, and in any case these conditions may coexist. The presence of Osler's nodes, petechiae, clubbing, splenomegaly and positive blood cultures do not therefore exclude rheumatic fever but indicate the existence of bacterial infection. Other causes of fever such as malignant reticulosis, tuberculosis and the enteric fevers should be considered but are readily excluded by the absence of signs of endocarditis described above. Malignant reticulosis with fever, splenomegaly and anaemia may cause difficulty but investigations usually reveal the true nature of the condition and signs of endocarditis are absent. Tuberculosis and the enteric fevers causing pyrexia and wasting are usually excluded on clinical grounds, but in cases of doubt the blood culture, Widal reaction, Mantoux test and a search for tubercle bacilli are decisive. Systemic lupus erythematosus and other collagen diseases, if associated with a heart murmur may resemble bacterial endocarditis, but clubbing, Osler's nodes and positive blood cultures are absent, and in systemic lupus erythematosus the presence of L.E. cells can be demonstrated in the blood [Section 4]. If the presenting feature of bacterial endocarditis is due to embolism, such as hemiplegia, haematuria, pulmonary infarction, the nature of the underlying disease may not be immediately apparent but continued fever and other features soon reveal the presence of infection and endocarditis.

Infected ventricular septal defect causing repeated episodes of pulmonary infection and infarction may be confusing, but if the possibility of superadded endocarditis is always kept in mind when dealing with patients with an organic murmur the diagnosis is readily made.

Treatment

Prophylactic. Any patient with rheumatic heart disease (especially organic mitral incompetence, or lone aortic valve disease) or with congenital heart disease should receive penicillin before undergoing any operative procedure, particularly dental extraction, tonsillectomy or any sort of endoscopy; 300 mg. (500,000 Units) of benzylpenicillin should be given 1 hour before operation, and the blood level maintained for 3 days thereafter by oral penicillin, 250 mg. four times daily. Larger doses for a longer period before or after operation are indicated if this is for a known septic lesion.

Curative. Bed rest, a good diet and added iron are indicated, but the essential part of treatment is the early and adequate administration of penicillin. The sooner it is started the better is the outlook, and a delay of 24 hours may result in the development of serious complications. If the clinical diagnosis is reasonably certain, penicillin therapy should be started after several samples of blood have been withdrawn for culture during the first 24–48 hours; there is no justification for awaiting a positive culture which may take several days, and indeed negative culture does not invalidate a sound clinical diagnosis. The positive blood culture provides confirmation of the diagnosis, and the infecting organism should be tested for sensitivity to penicillin and other antibiotics. Penicillin should be given in a minimum daily dose of 1·2 G. (2,000,000 Units) for 6 weeks. A continuous intravenous infusion for the first 4 weeks is safest and often the most comfortable. In patients who have responded quickly and well further treatment may be given by oral penicillin. A larger daily dose should be given if the resistance of the infecting organism is four or more times that of the Oxford staphylococcus, or if clinical improvement is not apparent in the first week. On such grounds it may be necessary to give 6 G. (10,000,000 Units) daily. In other cases, depending on the bacteriology and clinical response, it may be advisable to combine penicillin with streptomycin or other antibiotic drugs.

The effectiveness of treatment is shown by remission of fever, improved appetite and well-being, and a gain in weight; anaemia improves and the sedimentation rate falls. It should be noted that petechiae may continue to appear for some time after the temperature is normal. Failures of treatment are due to delay in starting treatment through delay in diagnosis, inadequate dosage and the development of resistant organisms.

Surgical Treatment. In cases of patent ductus arteriosus it is advisable to ligate the ductus when treatment and convalescence are completed. Occasionally ligation should be advised whilst infection is still present if this is resistant to antibiotic therapy. Mycotic aneurysms require removal and grafting of the affected vessel where this is possible.

Prognosis

Prognosis without treatment is hopeless. Antibiotic therapy has completely changed the outlook which is now good, provided that treatment is applied early in the disease. Relapse may occur and when this happens it usually does so within one month of the cessation of treatment. Resistant strains of organisms may develop, but by increasing dosage and with the wide range of antibiotics now available this problem can be overcome. In spite of sterilization of the infection some cases continue to deteriorate from heart failure, renal failure, or as the result of infarction of vital organs. Heart failure is the commonest cause of death, and tends to occur during treatment or within 6 months after treatment. Other adverse prognostic factors are increasing age, severe primary valve lesions and poor nutrition of the patient; the most important factor in prognosis is the duration of infection prior to the start of treatment.

Ninety per cent. of patients with bacterial endocarditis may be cured if treated within 6 weeks of the onset of the disease, but if treatment is delayed until after the third month, only 50 per cent. are cured.

ACUTE BACTERIAL ENDOCARDITIS

There is much overlap with subacute bacterial endocarditis and now that serious septic conditions are treated effectively with antibiotic drugs, the differentiation of these conditions is of doubtful value.

Acute bacterial endocarditis is now rare. It is mostly due to one of the pyogenic organisms, and is incidental to the course of an acute pyogenic illness. The primary lesion is generally obvious, such as suppurative pneumonia, puerperal fever, osteomyelitis, a carbuncle or gonorrhoea. An undamaged heart may be affected. Vegetations develop on the valvular and mural endocardium, and there is a greater tendency to ulceration and destruction than in subacute bacterial endocarditis.

Clinical Features

The onset is rapid, but it cannot always be detected against the background of the severe septic primary disease. The symptoms are largely septicaemic; swinging fever, rigors and sweats are usual; pain and swelling of joints together with cutaneous ecchymoses are common. Finger clubbing is rare, but petechial haemorrhages and a soft enlargement of the spleen are usual. Embolic phenomena occur as in the subacute variety, but tend to produce metastatic abscesses. Meningitis, pericarditis, pleurisy and peritonitis are possible complications.

Treatment

Treatment is essentially that of the primary condition and otherwise the same as for subacute endocarditis.

Prognosis

This disease was invariably fatal in a few days or weeks, but treatment of the aetiological condition with antibiotic drugs is preventive, and curative if the endocarditis has not progressed too far.

RHEUMATIC ENDOCARDITIS (ACUTE AND SUBACUTE)

Endocarditis involving the valves (valvulitis) is present in the majority of cases of rheumatic fever and is always present as the principal manifestation of rheumatic carditis [see Section 2]. The valves are inflamed and their surfaces become roughened from exudates and adherent platelets; small beady vegetations develop, the valve becomes vascular and infiltrated with cells and Aschoff bodies. Mitral and aortic cusps are mainly affected. The earliest signs of mitral valvulitis are the development of a pansystolic murmur at the apex with or without a short mid-diastolic murmur (Carey Coombs). Aortic valvulitis is shown by the development of a basal systolic murmur which ends before the second heart sound and it is confirmed by the development of an early diastolic murmur. These valve murmurs are variable in the acute stages and may disappear with recovery [see rheumatic fever, Section 2].

OTHER FORMS OF ENDOCARDITIS

Endocardial fibro-elastosis is a rare condition occurring especially in infancy and mostly associated with other congenital lesions. It should not be confused with endomyocardial fibrosis which is common in African children and young adults (E.M.F.)—this condition is essentially a disease of the myocardium.

Endomyocardial fibrosis is one of the more common forms of myocardial disease found in the central and most humid areas of Africa. Either or both ventricles may be 'silted up' with thrombosis sited on organized endomyocardial disease. Ventricular filling is greatly reduced, pulmonary hypertension and atrioventricular valve incompetence are common features. There is no specific treatment.

Systemic lupus erythematosus (Libman-Sacks disease, atypical verrucous endocarditis). Endocardial vegetations are sometimes found in this condition. The valves are not affected so that heart murmurs are not a prominent feature. The vegetations are large and fleshy but do not appear to fragment, for embolism is uncommon [Section 2].

Tuberculosis of the endocardium is extremely rare. Granulomatous verrucae and ulcers due to tubercle have been described. *Non-bacterial mural thromboses* are not uncommonly found at necropsy after prolonged cachectic illnesses such as nephritis, carcinomatosis and chronic pulmonary suppuration. These lesions develop in the terminal stage of these illnesses and are non-specific platelet agglutinations on the mural endocardium.

REFERENCES

Ball, J. D., Williams, A. W., and Davies, J. N. P. (1954) Endomyocardial fibrosis, *Lancet*, i, 1049.

Cates, J. E., and Christie, R. V. (1951) Subacute bacterial endocarditis. A review of 442 patients, *Quart. J. Med.*, **20**, 93.

Meade, R. (1959) Staphylococcal bacteraemia and endocarditis, *Circulation*, **19**, 440.

Morgan, W., and Bland, E. (1959) Bacterial endocarditis in the antibiotic era, *Circulation*, **19**, 753.

Vogler, W. R., Dorney, E., and Bridges, H. A. (1962) Bacterial endocarditis, *Amer. J. Med.*, **32**, 910.

Williams, A. W., and Somers, K. (1960) The electrocardiogram in endomyocardial fibrosis, *Brit. Heart J.*, **22**, 311.

DISEASES OF THE MYOCARDIUM

CARDIOMYOPATHY

All forms of heart disease eventually affect the heart muscle and in some, such as coronary disease and rheumatic fever, the myocardium is directly damaged from the onset by ischaemia or inflammation. This section deals with those conditions in which the disease process is mainly confined to the myocardium. The term cardiomyopathy is used to describe the whole group of primary myocardial diseases. Most of the known pathological processes, including congenital disorder, infection, metabolic, allergic and nutritional disorders are represented. However, it must be emphasized that in the majority of patients with primary myocardial disease there is no evidence concerning aetiology.

As the clinical features are largely independent of the cause these are considered for the whole group and comment on the aetiological types follows.

Clinical Features

Non-coronary myocardial disease most commonly presents as heart failure. Although a sudden attack of paroxysmal dyspnoea may be the first indication of left ventricular myopathy, in most patients symptoms develop slowly with increasing dyspnoea on effort and fatigue. In such patients chronic heart failure with a low cardiac output is shown by a small pulse, a low systolic and a raised diastolic pressure (hence the error of fallen hypertension) and signs of peripheral vasoconstriction. The jugular venous pressure is elevated and there may be oedema and ascites. Pain from hepatic congestion is common and, as it may be increased by effort, it is sometimes confused with cardiac pain. Patients presenting with these features are conveniently considered to have *congestive cardiomyopathy*.

When the nature of the myocardial disease is such that the heart is not greatly dilated in spite of great elevation of venous pressure (as in cardiac amyloidosis) the physical signs may closely resemble those of *constrictive pericarditis*. A similar picture may result from occlusion of the right ventricular cavity by extensive thrombus formation as in endomyocardial fibrosis.

In a large group the essential problem concerns unexplained general or localized hypertrophy of the myocardium referred to as *hypertrophic cardiomyopathy*. In this group patients may have no symptoms or may present with dyspnoea, true cardiac pain, syncope or pathological fatigue. Localized hypertrophy may produce signs suggesting inflow or outflow tract obstruction on either or both sides of the heart. Incompetence at the atrioventricular valves is not uncommon.

Palpitation from arrhythmia is a common symptom. It may be the first indication of myocardial disease. Any type of irregularity may occur and sometimes leads to syncopal attacks.

The electrocardiogram always shows evidence of myocardial disease. It indicates the extent and localization of the disease process rather than its nature. In many cases abnormalities are present in all leads, indicating a diffuse abnormality rather than a local one as in cardiac infarction. T wave abnormalities are the commonest, but the QRS is often bizarre and pathological Q waves are not uncommon so that an erroneous diagnosis of cardiac infarction may be made.

Chest X-rays reveal varying degrees of cardiac enlargement; this tends to be general rather than localized to one of the chambers. The silhouette is often remarkably clear because of diminished ventricular movement, and the possibility of pericardial effusion often arises. In many cases the relative absence of lung congestion is in contrast to the heart size, presumably because of the presence of biventricular failure. The aorta is often small, especially when, as in familial cardiomegaly, the disease has been present since childhood.

SPECIAL TYPES OF CARDIOMYOPATHY

It is known that many different disease processes may affect the myocardium but it is often impossible to determine the aetiology in life and even at necropsy. However, after appraising all of the evidence from a comprehensive past history, the family history, the nutritional history, a full clinical examination of all systems and laboratory investigations, it is often possible to recognize one of the following types.

CONGENITAL (OR FAMILIAL) CARDIOMYOPATHY

This disease is inherited as a Mendelian dominant. Several members of two or three generations in one family may be affected. Palpitation due to arrhythmia and syncopal attacks from the same cause are common, but the most striking feature of this grim disease is the tendency to sudden death which often overtakes a young adult who has usually appeared to be healthy. Males and females are equally affected. At necropsy the heart is very large and there is extensive fibrosis and hypertrophy. No treatment, preventive or otherwise, is known for this condition.

Myocardial disease is often associated with specific inherited neurological disorders such as *Friedreich's ataxia* and *myotonic dystrophy*. Furthermore, isolated cardiomyopathy has been found in members of an affected family although free of the neurological manifestations of disease.

INFLAMMATORY CARDIOMYOPATHY

The term, myocarditis, should be reserved for myocardial disease which is clearly due to an infection. It is known that myocarditis may occur in the course of many viral, bacterial, protozoal and even metazoal generalized infections. Diagnosis depends upon the relatively easy recognition of the general illness and an awareness of the possibilities of myocarditis in the particular infection. An isolated myocarditis or myocarditis in the course of an otherwise unimpressive infection, however, may be extremely difficult to recognize. The disease may be revealed by the pain of an associated pericarditis, severe dyspnoea from heart failure, or an arrhythmia. It is probable (as in the case of mild hepatitis or nephritis) that recovery is complete in most mild cases, whilst in others scar tissue and an accompanying hypertrophy result in organ failure much later in life. In some of the severest forms of myocarditis, such as that associated with diphtheria or with poliomyelitis, recovery may also be complete. The great diagnostic difficulty lies in the recognition of isolated myocardial infection. Even at necropsy and when histological examination has revealed an intense cellular reaction in the myocardium due to infection, the organism is usually not isolated. No doubt the frequency of a post-mortem bacteriological diagnosis depends to a not inconsiderable extent upon the intensity and thoroughness of the search for an organism.

The *Coxsackie virus* may invade the heart as part of a generalized infection but occasionally there is only an isolated myocarditis. There have been reports of this disease causing heart failure in neonatal infants. Myocarditis is common in the *rickettsial fevers*. In some epidemics it appears that the heart is involved in all cases, but isolated rickettsial myocarditis does not appear to occur. Protozoal myocarditis may arise from invasion of the heart by *Trypanosoma cruzi* (Chagas' disease): it occurs in South America and death from heart failure is usual. *Toxoplasma gondii* has also been found in the myocardium in myocarditis. In *diphtheria* some degree of myocarditis probably occurs in the majority of patients. The muscle fibres are diffusely damaged and histological examination may show little in contrast to the findings in interstitial myocarditis. In some it produces serious clinical features and may be fatal. Where recovery occurs it is usually complete, but occasionally there are permanent electrocardiographic changes. The first clinical signs tend to appear in 7–10 days. Arrhythmias occur early and heart block is common. Other signs of myocarditis may develop and are followed by those of congestive heart failure in severe cases. The haemodynamic state may be complicated by toxic depression of the vasomotor system so that the shock state is associated with central failure. The outlook for diphtheritic carditis which is causing symptoms and signs is poor, but if there is recovery from the acute illness, it is usually complete. Prophylaxis is essential and consists of the early diagnosis and treatment of diphtheria with adequate antitoxin and bed rest for 1 month. There is no active curative treatment for carditis when this has developed. Patients should be kept at complete rest for at least 6 weeks. If there is congestive heart failure a diuretic should be given, but digitalis is contra-indicated.

NUTRITIONAL CARDIOMYOPATHY

Starvation does not appear to cause myocardial disease; the heart merely undergoes atrophy along with other organs. When deprivation of food is associated with a disturbed balance of foods over a long period of time, however, myocardial disease may result as in oriental beriberi. In the myocardial diseases which are prevalent in Africans the aetiological factors are probably numerous and varied, but it is possible that the myocardium is especially vulnerable to infections and other noxious processes when there has been a long-standing problem of nutritional anaemia, liver disease and metabolic disturbance.

In the occident, *alcoholism* is the only important cause of nutritional cardiomyopathy. A very high consumption of alcohol over a long period of time may lead to *beriberi heart disease*, or, more commonly, to an isolated myocardial disease which does not respond to thiamine. Common symptoms are palpitation, sweating and dyspnoea. Arrhythmia is common in patients with alcoholic cardiopathy and atrial fibrillation occurs in 50 per cent. Heart failure tends to be episodic, mild at first and recovering spontaneously with the withdrawl of alcohol; in the late stages, however, severe low-cardiac-output failure is irreversible.

Treatment consists of total abstinence, a trial of thiamine which is usually ineffective, together with digitalis and diuretics.

METABOLIC AND ENDOCRINE CARDIOMYOPATHY

Certain metabolic and endocrine disorders, including amyloidosis, haemochromatosis, myxoedema, hyperthyroidism and acromegaly, may primarily affect the heart and cause death from chronic heart failure. *Primary amyloidosis* of the myocardium is an uncommon condition. In this form of amyloidosis there is no associated chronic suppuration and the heart is mainly affected, but amyloid may be found elsewhere, e.g. in vessels of the tongue and gums. At necropsy the heart is dilated and the muscle feels firm, but histological examination shows extensive replacement of the muscle cells by amyloid material. There are no symptoms or signs apart from those due to progressive heart failure and cardiac enlargement. The disease runs a long course, often with signs of heart disease for 3–5 years. The electrocardiogram shows signs of extensive myocardial damage. Bundle branch block or pathological Q waves in several leads may occur. The electrocardiogram may be indistinguishable from the pattern of myocardial infarction, but the changes tend to be more widespread in amyloidosis. Radiological examination shows cardiac enlargement. Histological examination from biopsy may show deposits of amyloid material in the walls of small vessels. There is no specific remedy but heart failure requires the usual treatment.

Von Gierke's Disease. This condition is due to a congenital error of metabolism resulting in abnormal glycogen storage. Both sexes are affected and the condition may be familial. Abnormal glycogen storage occurs in various organs including the liver, kidneys and the heart. Involvement of the heart causes cardiomegaly and sudden death may occur. Diagnosis is suggested by the combination of unexplained cardiomegaly and hepatomegaly. No treatment is known.

In endocrine disease the myocardium is often involved but it is rare for the disorder to present as a primary myocardial problem. In *myxoedema*, however, cardiac enlargement and even frank heart failure may dominate the clinical picture although in some cases apparent cardiac enlargement may be due to pericardial effusion. Histological examination does not show any striking abnormality of the muscle; presumably the disorder is at a biochemical level. Heart failure and cardiac enlargement in myxoedema cannot be accounted for by the anaemia which is often present. Diagnosis is especially important as treatment with thyroid hormone is so effective. Myxoedema should be considered in all cases of obscure cardiac failure. Important pointers to recognition are the sluggish personality and the sluggish heart with a low-voltage electrocardiogram.

In *hyperthyroidism* elevated basal metabolism is responsible for functional changes in the circulation, but the high incidence of atrial fibrillation in thyrotoxicosis suggests that the heart may be directly affected by toxaemia. Increased tissue demands for oxygen are met by an increased cardiac output, which is characteristic of thyrotoxicosis. Circulating blood volume is increased, and peripheral vasodilatation, amounting to extensive arteriovenous shunting, leads to an increased venous return. The increased cardiac output is achieved largely by an increase in heart rate, although there is some evidence that stroke volume is also elevated. The circulation becomes hyperdynamic and there is a greatly diminished circulation time. Tachycardia, hypervolaemia and increased circulation velocity are well tolerated by the heart in young subjects with thyrotoxicosis, although the metabolism of the myocardium is presumably pathological. The manifestations of thyrotoxic heart disease are atrial fibrillation and cardiac failure; these occur almost exclusively in the older age groups, suggesting that degenerative changes in the heart are the cause of breakdown in the circulatory compensations for hyperthyroidism. The clinical features of congestive cardiac failure develop in spite of the high cardiac output. This apparent paradox is characteristic of thyrotoxic heart failure. Although the cardiac output is often higher than normal, it is inadequate for the demands of the thyrotoxic state.

Symptoms. Palpitation, weakness and dyspnoea are common symptoms in thyrotoxicosis but these do not indicate heart disease. Palpitation may be continuous and regular and without apparent cause, or it may be paroxysmal or continuous and irregular when due to multiple ectopic beats or atrial fibrillation. Palpitation may occur in young patients, but it is more common in older patients with toxic adenoma. Dyspnoea and weakness are present in uncomplicated thyrotoxicosis, but true cardiac dyspnoea develops only with the onset of cardiac failure, which is confined to the older age groups. Ischaemic cardiac pain may also occur in patients after middle life, and is probably due to latent coronary disease which is revealed by the increased cardiac work.

In thyrotoxic heart disease the general signs and symptoms of thyrotoxicosis may be obvious or they may be slight and easily overlooked. In particular the thyroid gland may not be visibly enlarged and only careful examination may reveal a small adenoma, or radiography may show an intrathoracic gland.

The signs of a hyperdynamic circulation are present; there is tachycardia, an increased pulse pressure with a moderately elevated systolic pressure and palpable digital arteries. The apex beat is increased in force and rate and the whole precordium may pulsate with the heart beat. The first heart sound is loud, and it is usually followed by a systolic murmur which is best heard over the pulmonary artery. The second heart sound is not remarkable, and there are no murmurs in diastole unless there is associated valvular disease.

Atrial fibrillation is common in patients over the age of 45. It may be paroxysmal or permanent and is characteristically associated with chaotic high ventricular rates in untreated patients. Paroxysmal tachycardia and atrial flutter occur occasionally in hyperthyroidism. Congestive cardiac failure occurs when there is atrial fibrillation in the older age groups; but the circulation remains hyperdynamic in spite of failure. Other forms of organic heart disease, especially hypertension, coronary disease or chronic valvar disease, are sometimes associated with thyrotoxicosis.

Radiology. Cardiac enlargement is not present unless there is cardiac failure or associated heart disease. An intrathoracic extension of the thyroid gland may be shown.

The electrocardiogram is not characteristic. Arrhythmia is confirmed when present. Changes associated with ventricular hypertrophy or ischaemia, such as T wave flattening or S-T depression, are present if there is additional organic heart disease.

Treatment. The primary object of treatment is the correction of hyperthyroidism [Section 5]. After correction of hyperthyroidism, congestive heart failure subsides and atrial fibrillation tends to be replaced by sinus rhythm. If the arrhythmia persists, conversion should be attempted [p. 760].

In *acromegaly* the heart may be greatly enlarged, and death not uncommonly results from heart failure. It has been suggested that less obvious forms of pituitary disorder may be responsible for some obscure cases of idiopathic cardiac hypertrophy.

COLLAGEN DISEASE

The heart may be affected in any of the so-called collagen diseases, but in most cases myocardial disease is only a small part of disseminate organ damage and often passes unrecognized. In hypersensitivity myocarditis there may be little general disturbance in other organs. Many drugs have been thought to cause this condition but proof is usually lacking. A previous history of allergy, an eosinophilic leucocytosis, a raised erythrocyte sedimentation rate and a brisk response to corticosteroids suggest the allergic nature of the disorder. Isolated myocardial disease does not appear to result from polyarteritis or from systemic lupus erythematosus although severe myocardial disease leading to heart failure may occur in both conditions. *Scleroderma* is one of the collagen diseases in which some patients present with heart failure from cardiac myosclerosis when the general features, such as cutaneous thickening, Raynaud's phenomenon, pulmonary fibrosis and intestinal disorder, are unimpressive. It is probable that the rare cases of sarcoid myocarditis and giant cell myocarditis should be considered as diseases of a hypersensitivity or collagen type [Section 4].

TRAUMATIC HEART DISEASE

The heart may be injured by direct penetrating

wounds or by non-penetrating blows to the precordium. *Penetrating wounds* are mostly caused by stabbing, gunshot or shell fragments, and rarely by fracture of adjacent sternum or ribs, the passage of a foreign body from the oesophagus, or paracentesis of the pericardium. Most deep, penetrating injuries are rapidly fatal, but recovery occurs in a considerable proportion when the injury is relatively superficial, especially when due to stabbing. Any part of the heart may be damaged. Penetration of the myocardium results in haemopericardium and cardiac tamponade [p. 801]. Wounds adjacent to the heart or grazing the pericardium tend to cause a serous pericarditis which is recurrent if a foreign body remains imbedded in adjacent tissues. The symptoms and sign are those of pericarditis, with or without an effusion [p. 801].

Treatment. The possibility of injury to the heart should be considered in all cases of penetrating chest injury. Haemopericardium with tamponade requires urgent paracentesis followed by surgical evacuation of clot and repair of the wound as soon as possible. Deep, penetrating wounds may damage any structure of the heart and death is the usual result.

Non-penetrating injuries of the heart sometimes present difficult medico-legal problems. A history of trauma to the chest followed by cardiac symptoms, which may be due to neurosis or natural heart disease, should be interpreted with the greatest caution. Blunt injuries to the anterior chest wall by heavy blows or crushing may injure the heart by causing sudden arrhythmia, contusion of the pericardium, myocardium or coronary arteries, and rarely by causing rupture of one of the valves, one of the cardiac chambers or the aorta. A previously diseased heart is more likely to be damaged by blunt trauma than a normal heart which, however, is not immune.

Arrhythmia. Palpitation and tachycardia is common after injury and is due to emotional disturbance, not infrequently associated with the possibilities of compensation. However, serious arrhythmia may be precipitated by blows of varying severity and by sudden immersion in cold water. Arrhythmia is probably induced by reflex action in most cases, but when the trauma is over the precordium, contusion of the myocardium may be the cause. Transient atrial fibrillation is the commonest disturbance; sometimes it occurs in young subjects with a normal heart. Ventricular tachycardia and sudden death from ventricular fibrillation have been recorded after relatively trivial injury. Elderly subjects and those with coronary artery disease are probably the most vulnerable. Transient heart block may follow indirect trauma; the cause is presumably contusion of the conducting tissues but reflex inhibitions cannot be excluded.

Contusion. Bruising of the pericardium and epicardium may result in transient pericarditis, pericardial effusion or haemopericardium. Spontaneous recovery is usual. Contusion of the myocardium causes varying degrees of muscle damage with or without damage to the coronary vessels; the right atrium, right ventricle, septum or left ventricle may be involved. The clinical features and electrocardiographic changes may be similar to those of cardiac infarction; cardiac pain of all degrees from a dull precordial ache to severe widespread pain associated with fever and leucocytosis may result. Angina pectoris occasionally follows blunt injury which has involved the coronary vessels.

The electrocardiogram shows various changes in the ventricular complex, ranging from transient T wave flattening or inversion, and S-T elevation or depression, to the development of pathological Q waves when there is extensive muscle necrosis. These changes are best seen in precordial leads, but occasionally injury to the precordium results in electrocardiographic changes indicating isolated damage to the septum or posterior wall of the ventricle.

Valve rupture may follow blunt injury or excessive effort in subjects with pre-existing heart disease. The aortic valve is most likely to be damaged in patients with syphilitic aortitis. The resulting acute aortic incompetence causes severe chest pain and left ventricular failure. Rupture of the mitral valve chordae with resulting acute mitral incompetence has been recorded but it is also extremely rare.

Treatment of disorders following non-penetrating injury. Arrhythmia is usually of brief duration but if prolonged the appropriate anti-arrhythmic drugs should be used [p. 757]. Patients with cardiac contusion require bed rest for 3–6 weeks, depending on the severity of the damage. In rare cases where there is cardiac tamponade, paracentesis is indicated.

REFERENCES

ABRAHAMS, D. G. (1962) Endomyocardial fibrosis, *Quart J. Med.*, **31**, 1.

BRAUNWALD, E., LAMBREW, C., ROCKOFF, S., ROSS, J., and MORROW, A. (1964) Idiopathic hypertrophic subaortic stenosis: a description of the disease based on an analysis of 64 patients, *Amer. Heart Assoc. Monograph*, No. 10.

BRIGDEN, W. (1957) Uncommon myocardial diseases, *Lancet*, ii, 1179, 1243.

BRIGDEN, W. (1964) Cardiac amyloidosis, *Progr. cardiovasc. Dis.*, **7**, 2.

BRIGDEN, W., BYWATERS, E., LESSOF, M., and ROSS, I. (1960) The heart in systemic lupus erythematosus, *Brit. Heart J.*, **22**, 1.

BRIGDEN, W., and ROBINSON, J. (1964) Alcoholic heart disease, *Brit. med. J.*, **2**, 1283.

CIBA FOUNDATION (1964) *Symposium on Cardiomyopathies*, London.

EVANS, W. (1944) The heart in myotonia atrophica, *Brit. Heart J.*, **6**, 41.

EVANS, W. (1949) Familial cardiomegaly, *Brit. Heart J.*, **11**, 63.

GOODWIN, J., GORDON, H., HOLLMAN, A., and BISHOP, M. (1961) Clinical aspects of cardiomyopathy, *Brit. med. J.*, **1**, 69.

HUDSON, R. E. B. (1970) *Cardiovascular Pathology*, Vol. 3, Classification of cardiomyopathy, London.

SAPHIR, O. (1959) Myocarditis, *Amer. Heart J.*, **57** ,639.

WALLACE BRIGDEN

DISEASES OF THE BLOOD VESSELS

Diseases of the blood vessels are closely related to diseases of the heart, and combined cardiovascular disorders now form the largest group of fatal diseases. Arterial degeneration, mainly by its effects on the heart and brain, is the commonest underlying factor. With advancing years there is a steadily rising incidence of ischaemic heart disease and cerebral vascular disorders, of the same order as the incidence of cancer. Examination of the Registrar General's returns over the past 20 years does not indicate any increase in deaths due to arterial disease apart from the greater incidence in the later decades due to longer survival, largely resulting from more effective treatment of infectious disease.

The mechanisms involved in the production of arterial degeneration are obscure, but advancing age, diabetes and high blood pressure are the chief contributory causes. High blood pressure may be produced by increased cardiac output in the presence of normal peripheral resistance, or increased peripheral resistance in the presence of normal cardiac output. The latter is by far the commoner situation. It may be secondary to renal disease or more rarely to endocrine dysfunction; but in the great majority of cases of arterial hypertension no organic cause for the increase in arteriolar resistance can be demonstrated. High blood pressure, whatever its origin, is a major factor in determining the age of onset and severity of atheroma, and coronary atheroma is the commonest cause of heart disease. Hypertension, therefore, not only increases the work which the heart must perform to overcome the increased peripheral resistance, but also leads to steady deterioration in the blood supply to the myocardium owing to coronary artery degeneration. Since atheroma is a generalized disorder, peripheral vascular disease, by which is usually meant occlusive arterial disease of the limbs, will frequently be associated with ischaemic heart disease and with the effects of arterial degeneration in other organs.

Maintenance of circulatory function involves the peripheral vessels no less than the heart. For example, after severe haemorrhage or fluid loss, the blood pressure is maintained by peripheral vasoconstriction. Failure of this compensatory vasoconstriction leads to a fall in blood pressure and is a major factor in the production of shock.

CLASSIFICATION OF ARTERIAL DISEASE

Pathological processes in the arteries can be classified as follows:

Congenital

This group of arterial diseases is relatively small. It includes a number of developmental defects such as congenital aneurysm of the cerebral arteries, coarctation of the aorta and arteriovenous fistulae.

Traumatic

Injuries to the peripheral vessels by penetrating wounds, particularly in the lower limbs, may lead to arterial obliteration, to a false aneurysm, or to arteriovenous aneurysm.

Inflammation

The arteries are particularly resistant to specific bacterial infections. Syphilis is exceptional in producing inflammation of the media of the aorta (mesaortitis) with destruction of elastic tissue; it also involves the cerebral vessels, producing endarteritis and thrombosis. Tuberculosis is also a cause of endarteritis. Arteritis may result from obstruction by infected emboli in bacterial endocarditis and weakening of the wall leads to mycotic aneurysm. Non-specific arteritis is a feature of a large and diverse group of disorders which are classified as allergic or collagen diseases. Sensitization to some bacterial or chemical antigen is probably the common aetiological factor, and histologically, necrotic changes in the capillaries, arterioles or arteries are associated with a degeneration of collagen which leads to widespread changes throughout the body. Rheumatic fever, rheumatoid arthritis, periarteritis nodosa, temporal arteritis, systemic lupus erythematosus, scleroderma and dermatomyositis are all diseases of this type. Vascular disorders due to these diseases are described in the section on collagen disease [Section 4].

Necrotizing arteriolitis and endarteritis are also the characteristic lesions of malignant hypertension. Although morphologically there is a close similarity with the vascular lesions of the collagen diseases, the mechanism of their production in hypertensive states is quite different, being most probably related to excessive intravascular pressure which leads to acute ischaemia of the vessel wall.

Degeneration

By far the commonest and most important arterial degeneration is atheroma. This is a primary degeneration of the intima. Arterial stress or 'wear and tear' is the chief predisposing factor, so that the maximum incidence is seen in old age and chronic hypertension. Disordered cholesterol metabolism may also play a part, and patients with diabetes and hypercholesterolaemia are particularly prone to develop atheroma. Medial degeneration is less common. It is a disorder of old age and is usually associated with atheroma.

Neoplasm

True neoplasms of the arteries are rare. Angiomata affect the capillaries and are commonly found in the skin. Larger tumours, so-called cavernous angiomata, occur in the liver. Capillary angioma (haemangioblastoma) occurs in the cerebellum in association with similar lesions elsewhere.

Local Disorders of Vascular Tone

Excessive vasoconstrictor response to cold or mechanical stimuli produces digital asphyxia (Raynaud's phenomenon). Arterial spasm may also complicate arteriosclerosis. Other disorders of peripheral tone are erythromelalgia and erythrocyanosis. Disturbances of vascular tone may occur as premonitory symptoms in the collagen disorders.

ATHEROSCLEROSIS

Atheroma has already been mentioned as the commonest form of arterial degeneration. Although a strictly localized lesion may cause disease in a particular organ in young subjects, e.g. coronary occlusion or renal artery stenosis, atheroma is a generalized disease and is found *post mortem* to have a widespread distribution. The arteries of the heart, brain and kidneys, the aorta and its branches, and the peripheral arteries, particularly of the lower limbs, are almost always affected in some degree, which increases progressively after about the age of 40. While serious interference with blood supply may be due to an atheromatous plaque obstructing a small or medium-sized artery, the process of vascular occlusion usually involves not only atheroma, but thrombosis at the site, and reduction of blood flow is often a cumulative process due to repeated thrombosis with fibrosis and calcification. This combination of atheroma and organized thrombosis finds its most dramatic and typical manifestation in coronary occlusion.

Aetiology

On clinical grounds alone there is evidence of a variety of factors which influence the development of atherosclerosis; nevertheless the pathogenesis of the lesion itself remains obscure. In recent years much attention has been paid to the *role of lipids*, particularly cholesterol. The atherosclerotic lesion contains cholesterol and phospholipids, and it seems likely that these are derived from the β-lipoproteins of the plasma. The evidence for this is indirect, but epidemiological studies seem to show that, at any rate for coronary artery disease, the severity of atherosclerotic damage is related to the blood cholesterol level, and when this is high, the β-lipoprotein fraction is elevated. These observations have naturally led to a search for the causes of elevated blood cholesterol. The diseases in which hypercholesterolaemia occurs, particularly diabetes, are well known to have a high incidence of atherosclerosis. In healthy subjects the blood cholesterol level is related to the unsaturated fatty acid content of the diet. The more industrialized and prosperous nations consume a diet with a high animal fat content, which contains a large proportion of saturated compared with unsaturated fatty acids. Under these circumstances blood cholesterol levels, and the incidence of coronary thrombosis, are significantly higher than in the less developed countries whose diet contains a high proportion of vegetable fats, rich in unsaturated fatty acids. It is thus possible that an important factor in the production of atherosclerosis is the high dietary content of animal fats, leading to increase in blood cholesterol and lipoproteins.

The mechanism by which the blood lipids accumulate in the intima of the arterial wall is the real problem, and it is at this point that the second factor, ***vessel trauma***, may be important. The sites of election for atheroma formation are at points of maximum stress, e.g. where arteries bifurcate or branch, or where movement is greatest. The role of arterial hypertension in accelerating the development of atherosclerosis is presumably of the same nature. On this basis the β-lipoproteins would gain access to the subendothelial space of the intima as a result of increase in vessel wall permeability due to some mechanical or pressure effect. In the vessel wall, the lipoproteins break down and the various soluble components are absorbed leaving behind cholesterol and lipoprotein. In this way the atheromatous plaque evolves and enlarges, and a sequence of reactive and degenerative changes, including fibrosis and calcification, contribute to the final lesion.

The third process involved in the atherosclerotic lesion is *thrombosis*, and this seems to depend on additional aetiological factors, for epidemiological studies indicate that the increasing frequency of coronary heart disease is due to a greater incidence of thrombosis rather than increasing atheroma. The factors which determine thrombosis are obscure, but mental stress, the blood lipid level, 'platelet stickiness' and fibrinolysins may all play a part, and these are the present directions of investigation. Undoubtedly enlargement of the atheromatous plaque, with projection into the lumen and ulceration of its surface, are usual preliminaries to thrombosis, which starts with platelet deposition, followed by accumulation of leucocytes and red cells, and later incorporation of fibrin. Organization leads to fibrosis, while secondary degenerative changes result in further deposition of fat and fibrin within the substance of the lesion. Repeated thrombotic episodes produce a laminated structure, the constituent layers of which reflect the age and evolution of the process.

In the individual patient, therefore, it is likely that multiple factors contribute to the clinical consequences of atherosclerosis. The blood cholesterol level and the height of the blood pressure are probably the most potent. When both are high it has been shown that the risk of coronary thrombosis is increased some eight times. Nevertheless other factors may have an overriding effect, for example, the incidence of atherosclerosis is much lower in women before the menopause than in man, but after the menopause the sex incidence is equal. These widely differing aetiological factors have not unnaturally stimulated a variety of therapeutic experiments in patients and have suggested possible lines of prevention; but at the present time there is no indication that a solution of this, the major problem of vascular disease, is in sight.

REFERENCES

BREST, A. N., and MOYER, J. H., eds (1968) *Atherosclerotic Vascular Disease*, London.

CONSTANTINIDES, P. (1965) *Experimental Atherosclerosis*, Amsterdam.

FLOREY, H. (1960) Coronary artery disease, *Brit. med. J.*, **2**, 1329.

HILDITCH, T. P., and JASPERSON, H. (1959) *Lipids in Relation to Arterial Disease*, Liverpool.

MORRIS, J. N., and CRAWFORD, M. D. (1958) Coronary heart disease and physical activity of work, *Brit. med. J.*, **2**, 1485.

SANDLER, M., and BOURNE, G. H. (1963) *Atherosclerosis and Its Origin*, New York.

SYSTEMIC ARTERIAL HYPERTENSION

The Normal Blood Pressure

There is a wide range of blood pressure in healthy subjects varying usually from 100–145 mm. Hg systolic and 60–90 diastolic. The average normal is about 125/75 and a figure of 140/90 in an otherwise healthy adult may be taken as the upper limit of normal. A slight increase tends to occur with age. In the same individual, transient variations in blood pressure are common; nervousness, excitement, exertion, fatigue, cold and smoking may raise the normal level 20 or 30 points or more, but in these conditions the systolic pressure is affected more than the diastolic.

The systolic blood pressure is chiefly determined by the force of contraction of the left ventricle. The diastolic pressure is regulated by the arteriolar resistance, which converts the intermittent output of the heart into a continuous capillary blood flow. During systole the large musculo-elastic arteries are distended and during diastole their elastic recoil helps to maintain the arterial pressure.

Systolic Hypertension

A raised systolic pressure may be associated with a low, normal or high diastolic pressure. Increased emptying of the arterial system during diastole, either centrally as in aortic incompetence or peripherally due to vasodilatation as in thyrotoxicosis or severe anaemia, tends to lower the diastolic pressure and this is compensated by increase in systolic pressure. In such conditions, therefore, the pulse pressure is greatly increased. If the diastolic pressure falls considerably the pulse has a large volume and may be 'waterhammer' in type. It is found, too, with extreme bradycardia as in complete heart block. A high systolic pressure with a normal diastolic pressure is seen in elderly patients in whom arteriosclerosis has impaired the elastic properties of the large arteries. Maintenance of the diastolic pressure then requires the production of a higher systolic pressure by the heart.

Diastolic Hypertension

Apart from the various disorders enumerated above, systolic hypertension is always associated with elevation of the diastolic pressure and increased arteriolar resistance. The common forms are essential hypertension and renal hypertension; less frequently diastolic hypertension results from endocrine disease.

Essential Hypertension. This is by far the commonest type of high blood pressure. The term essential hypertension is used to indicate the absence of any discoverable extravascular cause such as renal or endocrine disease. In benign essential hypertension (hyperpiesia of Allbutt) clinical evidence of renal involvement is nearly always lacking. In malignant essential hypertension, secondary arterial damage leads to rapidly progressive renal destruction; hypertensive encephalopathy and retinopathy develop as a result of vascular disturbance in the brain and retinae.

Renal Hypertension. The great majority of patients with renal disease develop high blood pressure. The usual cause is acute or chronic glomerulonephritis. Hypertension may be encountered in chronic pyelonephritis, congenital cystic kidney, tumours of the kidney, hydronephrosis and amyloid disease. Unilateral renal disease may also produce high blood pressure, the underlying lesion usually being pyelonephritis or obstruction to a main renal artery [see Section 12].

Endocrine Hypertension. High blood pressure is a feature of adrenal cortical hyperfunction (Cushing's syndrome). This syndrome may be due to a tumour or simple hyperplasia of the adrenal cortex, or to cortical hyperfunction, without discoverable organic lesion. In severe progressive cases malignant hypertension may develop. Administration of cortisone or corticotrophin sometimes causes a sharp rise in blood pressure. Primary aldosteronism due to a tumour of the adrenal cortex (Conn's syndrome) may also give rise to hypertension. Phaeochromocytoma of the adrenal medulla or of ectopic medullary tissue may lead to attacks of paroxysmal hypertension. Eventually in this condition the hypertension becomes fixed at a high level and may pass into the malignant phase. The blood pressure may be raised in hyperthyroidism; usually the systolic pressure alone is raised, but there may be an associated benign essential hypertension. High blood pressure is a frequent complication of diabetes and in this disease renal arterial and glomerular sclerosis may be an important contributory factor.

Other Causes of Diastolic Hypertension. In coarctation of the aorta the blood pressure may be considerably raised in the arms. In the lower limbs the systolic pressure is low but there is commonly slight diastolic hypertension which is probably due to renal ischaemia.

Organic disease of the brain may give rise to acute elevation of blood pressure. This is particularly encountered with rapidly expanding lesions, e.g. haemorrhage into cerebral tumours, and with sudden increase in intracranial pressure such as occurs after subarachnoid haemorrhage. Hypertension in renal disease is discussed in Section 12. Further reference to endocrine disorders which produce hypertension will be found in Section 5.

ESSENTIAL HYPERTENSION

The nomenclature of this condition is somewhat confused owing to the common use of the term essential hypertension in different senses. Thus it is sometimes applied to benign hypertension or it may be used to cover all forms of non-renal hypertension. This confusion will be avoided if the term essential hypertension is restricted to those patients in whom no primary cause for the hypertension can be discovered. Such a definition would exclude primary renal and endocrine causes of all kinds. It would, however, include the malignant as well as the benign phase of the disease.

Aetiology

The cause of essential hypertension is unknown. There is no evidence that it is referable to organic disease of the renal arteries or arterioles. There are, however, certain facts concerning the development and incidence of essential hypertension which are important. There is a clearly recognized hereditary factor or more probably a combination of factors. The incidence is highest in the sixth decade and the disease is slightly more common in women, but more severe in its course and complications in men. There is some racial variation, hypertension being rare in Chinese and in Negroes in rural circumstances, although under western civilization and in urban life it may be more common in and more severe than in Whites. In the benign phase hypertension is often labile and large variations may be produced by nervousness, emotion or activity. Later in the disease the level of blood pressure tends to become fixed even at rest, fluctuations diminishing in size and finally disappearing. There is evidence to suggest that transient hypertension occurring in times of stress may later become persistent, and that the change from benign to malignant hypertension may in certain individuals be preceded by episodes of severe emotional or nervous tension. Nevertheless, no consistent psychogenic factor can be demonstrated in patients with high blood pressure particularly when this is of the more severe type. The fact that sympathectomy may bring the blood pressure back to normal is not evidence of a neurogenic origin. Similar lowering of the blood pressure is often observed after non-specific operations and the blood pressure frequently returns to a high level after sympathectomy. Estimation of circulating adrenaline or noradrenaline in essential hypertension shows a tendency to high values in a minority of cases, but this has not been correlated with either emotional stress or high blood pressure levels. Obesity is undoubtedly an aggravating factor in essential hypertension and the blood pressure is usually observed to fall with weight reduction.

BENIGN HYPERTENSION

Synonyms. Hyperpiesia; Benign nephrosclerosis.

Pathology

The only morbid anatomical changes found in essential hypertension are secondary to the high blood pressure. They are of two main types: cardiovascular hypertrophy, which is a direct response to the increased strain imposed on the heart and blood vessels, and arterial degeneration. In benign hypertension the degenerative process takes the form of fatty hyaline change in the arterioles with homogeneous swelling of the wall, but without necrosis. This is characteristically seen in the afferent arterioles to the renal glomeruli. In larger arteries a combination of medial hypertrophy and intimal thickening is seen, the latter being characterized by proliferation of elastic and fibrous connective tissue. In medium and large arteries atheromatous degeneration occurs in the intima and the atheromatous plaques may ulcerate or calcify and may be the site of arterial thrombosis. Occlusion of the lumen may lead to infarction, or embolism may occur from an arterial thrombus and lead to obstruction of more peripheral vessels. The cerebral, coronary, mesenteric and the peripheral arteries of the limbs are the sites of election for atheromatous degeneration and its sequelae. Progressive narrowing of arteries may lead to slow ischaemia of tissues such as the myocardium, brain and kidney; obliteration of small arteries may lead to repeated focal parenchymal lesions as in cerebral arteriosclerosis and arteriosclerotic retinopathy. Atheromatous narrowing of a main renal artery or its branches, or renal infarction due to thrombosis, may lead to sudden aggravation of pre-existing hypertension or even to development of the malignant phase. The pathological changes in malignant hypertension are described later.

Symptoms

Benign hypertension may be symptomless for many years, particularly if the patient is unaware of its existence. The various clinical syndromes of the disease are in fact related to the degenerative changes in the organs resulting from arterial degeneration. Before manifestations of organic vascular disease appear, however, it is not uncommon for symptoms such as headaches, giddiness, nervousness and palpitations to arise. These may, on the one hand, be due to awareness of the high blood pressure and a fear of its consequences, particularly where there is a family history of vascular catastrophes. Or again these symptoms may be part of a general anxiety state, particularly in women at the menopause, for hypertension is likely to be discovered when menopausal symptoms first lead the patient to seek medical advice. Apart from these circumstances there is no doubt that some patients with benign hypertension develop headaches which are often severe, intractable and apparently related to the high blood pressure. They are often present when the patient wakens in the morning and may last for the greater part of the day. They may be associated with morning nausea or even vomiting. Not infrequently they are migrainous in type and in such patients there may be a long history of migraine. There is no evidence that these headaches are due to organic cerebral vascular disease. The condition is not severe enough to warrant the diagnosis at this stage of hypertensive encephalopathy which is so common in malignant hypertension. If the level of the blood pressure is reduced by administration of sympatholytic drugs or by sympathectomy, dramatic relief of these headaches is usually obtained.

The majority of patients with benign essential hypertension will have no premonitory symptoms before the onset of organic complications. Breathlessness on exertion or, in more severe cases, paroxysmal nocturnal dyspnoea, indicates the development of myocardial insufficiency. Blurring of vision or sudden blindness in one eye may be due to haemorrhage or from thrombosis in one of the main retinal veins or arteries. Hemiplegia results from cerebral thrombosis or from haemorrhage, commonly into the internal capsule due to rupture of the lenticulostriate branch of the middle cerebral artery; or subarachnoid haemorrhage may result from escape of blood into the ventricular system. Isolated paralyses occasionally occur, giving rise to diplopia, facial palsy or aphasia. Repeated attacks of paresis in one or more limbs may occur as the disease advances, and in older patients, progressive cerebral arteriosclerosis may lead to focal or generalized convulsions and steady deterioration of intellectual power, ending in progressive dementia. Haemorrhagic manifestations outside the brain are not common, but occasionally attacks of haemoptysis, haematemesis or haematuria are attributable to benign hypertension.

There are few physical signs until the advent of complications. The appearance may be plethoric and obese, or thin and pale. The radial and brachial arteries are usually thickened due to medial hypertrophy, and may be tortuous. The heart is often enlarged on clinical examination, the apex beat being forcible, the first sound at the apex loud or duplicated and the second aortic sound accentuated. Yet many patients, particularly women, continue with a high level of blood pressure for decades without appreciable evidence, clinical or radiological, of cardiovascular hypertrophy.

The Fundi. Hypertensive retinopathy is a general term which covers a variety of retinal changes encountered in different types of hypertension. The retinopathy of benign essential hypertension represents the basic picture found in all forms of chronic hypertension and on this may be superimposed more severe lesions, for example, in malignant hypertension or diabetes. The most constant features are tortuosity of the arteries and nicking of the veins at the arteriovenous crossings. Very rarely the arteries are narrowed and threadlike but more often there is an obvious irregularity in calibre. The so-called 'silver-wire' appearance of the retinal arteries is very inconstant and has no real diagnostic value. The veins usually appear congested. Superficial flame-shaped or small discrete deep haemorrhages may be seen in any part of the fundus, but are most frequent in the macular region; there are often associated but scanty grey or creamy exudates. Massive haemorrhages may result from retinal vein thrombosis or the retina may be pale due to thrombosis in the central artery. Resolution of these lesions leads to sclerosis of obstructed vessels and neighbouring parts of the retina; pigment usually remains at the site of old haemorrhages. When haemorrhages or exudates occur near the optic disc some swelling of the disc margin may be observed. This is usually distinguishable from the papilloedema of malignant hypertension, since it is almost invariably unilateral.

As Allbutt pointed out, clinical evidence of renal involvement is rare, but nocturnal polyuria occasionally develops in severe benign hypertension. The presence of albumin in the urine is again rare and is usually attributable to advanced renal arteriosclerosis, renal congestion due to heart failure, renal infarction or coincident diabetes. In elderly patients with long-standing benign hypertension and severe arteriosclerosis a slight to moderate degree of renal impairment may lead to reduction in tubular concentrating power and moderate elevation of the blood urea.

Treatment

In any individual it is impossible to prognosticate the course of the disorder or to prescribe a mode of life which will prevent complications. The introduction of active treatment by antihypertensive drugs has therefore aggravated rather than simplified the problem of treatment. To submit a patient to a life of maintenance drug therapy with its attendant side-effects, is a heavy premium to pay for a doubtful insurance against uncertain hazards. On the other hand, when complications have arisen reduction of the blood pressure may be highly beneficial and may not only accelerate recovery, e.g. in heart failure, but may prevent further recurrences, e.g. of subarachnoid haemorrhage. In deciding on treatment various aspects of prognosis discussed above must be borne in mind. Hypertension is likely to run a more severe course, with cardiac and cerebral complications, in men than in women. The malignant change is rare, probably affecting less than 1 per cent. of patients, but a progressively rising diastolic pressure, exceeding 120 mm., is a warning sign. An occupation or mode of life involving excessive physical or mental stress is likely to have an unfavourable effect on prognosis. It is also axiomatic that the possibility of any primary cause for the hypertension must be excluded before active treatment is started.

In asymptomatic benign hypertension, i.e. when the high blood pressure is discovered accidentally on routine medical examination, the fact should not be disclosed to the patient if it can be avoided, or if this is not practicable he should be advised that the condition is benign. Obesity should be treated by dietary restriction. In the present status of therapy there is no justification for attempting to lower the blood pressure by drugs as a routine measure in the absence of symptoms. An exception may be made in young subjects, especially men, with a high fixed level of blood pressure (e.g. diastolic exceeding 120 mm.). In such cases it may be felt that complications are likely to occur sooner rather than later and for this reason some reduction of the pressure with hypotensive drugs is justifiable. The level may be regarded as fixed when residual hypertension persists after 7 days' complete rest in bed with adequate sedation.

The second grade of severity includes those patients with symptoms which are not referable to organic vascular disorders. This is a miscellaneous group and for the most part the symptoms will be anxiety, headaches, dizziness, palpitations, various aches and pains, spots before the eyes and even breathlessness. As already explained, many of these patients will be women at the menopause and appropriate hormone therapy will often relieve the symptoms; otherwise reassurance, weight reduction and a placebo are indicated. In a minority of this group severe headaches occur, especially on waking and may be associated with nausea. Such headaches will often respond to aspirin or codeine, but failing these, benefit is sometimes obtained from ergotamine tartrate, 1 mg. at half-hourly intervals until the headache passes off, but not exceeding three or four doses. If in spite of this treatment headache is incapacitating, associated with a high relatively fixed pressure and unaccompanied by other anxiety symptoms, administration of hypotensive drugs is justifiable.

The third therapeutic group consists of those patients with benign hypertension in whom early evidence of arterial damage is found. Such evidence may be the appearance of superficial retinal haemorrhages, a transient paresis, a mild attack of encephalopathy or the onset of dyspnoea on exertion. Only a minority of these patients progress to the fully developed stage of malignant hypertension with papilloedema and renal failure. Nevertheless various other arterial complications may occur, especially in men, and it is justifiable to give at least a limited course of hypotensive drug therapy. The aim should be to produce an appreciable lowering of blood pressure which is sustained throughout the day without excessive swings and with minimal side-effects.

The fourth grade of severity is characterized by obvious complications which result from arterial degeneration. Such are cardiac infarction, hypertensive heart failure, cerebral vascular accidents and severe grades of retinal vascular damage leading to impairment of vision; the latter include extensive haemorrhages or exudates in the macular region, or thrombosis of main branches of the retinal vessels, but without papilloedema. Therapeutic control of the blood pressure is essential in this group and should be carried out in hospital, since special precautions are necessary.

Regime of Drug Therapy for Hypertension. Blood pressure lowering drugs are best used in combination since their synergic effects make blood pressure control possible with smaller doses of the more potent agents, which diminishes the incidence of side-effects. In general, effective treatment means reduction of the standing blood pressure to around 160/90 for the greater part of the day. Reserpine (*Serpasil*) alone, 0·25 mg. three times a day, sometimes produces satisfactory results although it may take 2–3 weeks to achieve its full action; depression, nasal obstruction and weight gain due to fluid retention are the chief side-effects. If reasonable control is not obtained, chlorothiazide (*Saluric*), 0·5 G. daily, or a similar diuretic should be added. Reserpine and methyldopa (*Aldomet*), 250 mg. twice a day starting dose, provide an alternative combination, but are usually ineffective when hypertension is severe. In such cases the addition of guanethidine (*Ismelin*) is necessary, starting with 10–20 mg. in a single morning dose, increasing by 10 mg. on alternate days, until postural hypotension leads to slight faintness on standing. Whether a thiazide diuretic is used with guanethidine depends on the patient's response, but in general this combination produces a satisfactory postural fall in blood pressure with a lower dose of guanethidine; it also avoids unpalatable salt restriction. Bethanidine sulphate (*Esbatal*) given in the same dosage as guanethidine is a quicker and shorter acting drug and should be tried when rapid control of hypertension is required or if guanethidine produces diarrhoea. Ganglion blocking drugs have varied side-effects, chiefly constipation, impotence, dry mouth and impaired accommodation. Guanethidine is less objectionable in that bowel disturbance is less severe and its depressing effect on sexual performance is limited to failure of ejaculation; moreover tolerance does not readily develop. Since the effectiveness of guanethidine treatment depends largely on postural hypotension, the patient must be warned against the risk of faintness on prolonged standing, and the danger of driving a car. Muscle weakness, especially in the morning, and drowsiness, are sometimes troublesome. Potassium supplements may be needed if thiazide diuretics are used. More recently the beta-adrenergic blocking drugs have been used in the treatment of hypertension. Of these propranolol has proved effective although the dose required varies greatly, limits of 10–4000 mg. being observed. Results with oxprenolol and practolol have been inconsistent.

The maintenance of effective drug therapy in severe hypertension is a trial for both patient and doctor. Hospital admission is highly desirable when the decision is made to start treatment, so that full investigation can be carried out, and the optimal combination and dosage of drugs can be decided by hourly blood pressure determinations throughout the day. Reduction of blood pressure to normal levels should not be attempted in elderly patients with evidence of atherosclerotic disease, and an electrocardiogram must always be obtained. After cerebral vascular episodes only moderate blood pressure reduction should be attempted. In renal failure, ganglion blocking drugs are best avoided since their poor excretion leads to a risk of paralytic ileus. If the patient is severely ill with acute heart failure or encephalopathy, as is often the case in malignant hypertension, parenteral administration is the most effective treatment, e.g. intramuscular or intravenous guanethidine, until the acute condition improves, and oral therapy can be substituted.

Course and Prognosis

Benign essential hypertension is compatible with a long life and freedom from symptoms; nevertheless in most patients complications occur which shorten the expectation of life. Whilst the height of the blood pressure, particularly the diastolic pressure, is an obvious pointer to the severity of the disease, there is no method of forecasting if or when complications will occur. At any time, either for no obvious reason or during periods of severe mental or physical strain or in pregnancy, the blood pressure may rise to serious levels; periodic exacerbations may lead to repeated or progressive vascular damage in the heart, brain, retinae or kidneys. Coronary thrombosis or a cerebral vascular accident may considerably lower the level of blood pressure and may so alter the patient's habits of life that the menace of the hypertension is greatly diminished. The prognosis is then that of the residual vascular complication.

MALIGNANT HYPERTENSION

Synonyms. Malignant essential hypertension; Malignant nephroslcerosis.

The term malignant hypertension was first used to describe a syndrome consisting of very high blood pressure, transient cerebral attacks (hypertensive encephalopathy) and retinopathy with papilloedema, occurring in a variety of disorders such as acute and chronic nephritis, eclampsia and essential hypertension. Subsequently a number of writers applied the term exclusively as a clinical synonym for the malignant nephrosclerosis of Volhard and Fahr. Clinical and pathological studies have demonstrated, however, that the renal changes of malignant nephrosclerosis are not the cause of the hypertension, but develop during the course of the disorder. Furthermore, experimental observations in animals have provided convincing evidence that the renal changes of malignant hypertension are directly attributable to severe elevation of blood pressure. It is now recognized, therefore, that malignant hypertension (with its associated nephrosclerosis) is a syndrome which may occur in any patient with severe hypertensive disease whether essential, renal or endocrine in origin. The clinical features and the hypertensive renal lesions which result are very similar whatever the origin of the hypertension.

Incidence and Pathology

It is not known what determines the transformation from the benign to the malignant form of essential hypertension. It is a feature of severe hypertensive disease that sudden exacerbations periodically occur. During these phases of very high blood pressure focal vascular damage may be produced in the brain, retinae, kidneys and other viscera. The mechanism of this vascular damage is not clear, but there is strong experimental evidence that sudden increase in intravascular pressure may cause intense focal vasoconstriction and that this may lead to both vascular necrosis and perivascular tissue damage. In essential hypertension successive episodes of this character, manifested by attacks of encephalopathy, retinal haemorrhage, heart failure or haematuria may be followed after a variable interval of months or years by the establishment of malignant hypertension which, in the absence of treatment, progresses steadily without remission. This change from the phasic to the fixed stage of the disease may be due to progressive renal vascular damage maintaining and even aggravating the initial hypertension.

Two clinical groups have long been recognized; in the larger group the patients present with malignant hypertension in the fourth or fifth decades without a previous history of long-standing benign hypertension. The smaller group comprises patients, usually in the sixties, in whom long-standing benign hypertension changes to the malignant type. The progress of the disease tends to be much slower in the older age group and the development of renal failure may take several years. Owing to the growing frequency of routine blood pressure determination in young subjects there is increasing evidence that even in the first group symptomless hypertension may be present for many years before the malignant termination. It is uncertain what proportion of patients with essential hypertension pass into the malignant phase. Estimates from hospital practice are almost certainly too high and it is probable that the figure is not more than 1 per cent., possibly much less.

Malignant hypertension differs from benign hypertension essentially in the intensity of secondary vascular changes. Arteriolar degeneration is more acute and characteristically takes the form of fibrinoid necrosis of arterioles with endarteritis in the larger vessels. These changes are most prominent in the kidney, the afferent arterioles of the glomeruli undergoing necrosis whilst the interlobular arteries show endarteritis. The resulting acute ischaemia produces focal necroses in the glomeruli and haemorrhage into the capsular space. Organization of these acute ischaemic changes leads to gross distortion of the glomerular tufts, capsular adhesions, occasional epithelial crescent formation and chronic fibrotic thickening and occlusion of the arterioles. In addition there may be chronic ischaemic lesions of the glomeruli due to long-standing benign hypertension and for the same reason the larger renal vessels may show intimal fibrosis and elastosis together with medial hypertrophy. Hyaline droplet degeneration of the tubular epithelium is almost invariably present in the acute phases. Recurrent episodes of acute hypertensive damage lead to progressive involvement of the kidney and the final stage is that described as malignant nephrosclerosis. Here the architecture of the kidney is grossly disorganized, areas of interstitial fibrosis and tubular atrophy alternating with zones of dilated tubules. This focal destruction is presumably related to the arterial origin of the lesions. The histological picture of malignant nephrosclerosis may present a mixture of acute and chronic lesions of the renal parenchyma. Occasionally acute arteriolar necrosis may be absent and the histological appearances may represent stages of organization of the acute lesions.

The most diagnostic feature which differentiates malignant hypertension from chronic Type 1 nephritis is the relatively small reduction in the number of glomeruli and the large proportion of normal looking glomeruli relative to the degree of interstitial and tubular damage. This is consistent with the natural history of the disorder. Acute fibrinoid necrosis of arterioles and endarteritis is common in other organs, particularly in the adrenal glands, pancreas and small intestine, less frequently in the brain, retina, liver and testis. As in the kidney, vascular lesions may lead to destruction of parenchyma, particularly in the pancreas. The rest of the body may, of course, show changes referable to severe benign hypertension and chronic vascular degeneration, such as cerebral haemorrhage, cardiac infarction and pulmonary oedema.

Symptoms

Malignant hypertension usually presents acutely with severe disabling symptoms in a previously healthy middle-aged adult. An analysis of a series of 100 cases showed headache as a presenting symptom in 76, dyspnoea in 54 with nocturnal attacks in 14, visual impairment in 51, frequency of micturition in 49, vomiting in 44, dependent oedema in 23, weight loss in 19, haematuria in 17, giddiness in 15 and organic paralysis in 11. Epistaxis, haemoptysis, haematemesis, mental confusion, convulsions, abdominal pain and pain in the loin were occasional symptoms.

Headache, the commonest early manifestation, usually occurs on waking in the morning and is frequently associated with nausea or vomiting. It may last for a few hours or throughout the day and is generally localized in the frontal region or vertex. The attacks are sometimes limited to one day of the week, usually Sunday, when the patient breaks his normal early morning routine. Severe suboccipital headache should suggest the possibility of subarachnoid haemorrhage. Paroxysmal nocturnal dyspnoea may be a prominent symptom before there is any complaint of dyspnoea on exertion; these attacks of pulmonary oedema are often accompanied by a distressing cough with frothy blood-stained sputum. Signs of right heart failure are almost always inconspicuous and if present at the onset should suggest an independent cardiac lesion. Polyuria, especially at night, may be sufficient to cause severe thirst and considerably increased fluid intake. Haematuria may be a solitary symptom and because of its painless, profuse character may suggest a surgical lesion of the urinary tract; intense necrotizing lesions in the kidney are usually found in such cases. The characteristic visual disturbance is blurring of vision which is due, not to papilloedema, but to the presence of exudates or haemorrhages, or both, in the region of the macula. Although transient paralysis or a mild convulsive attack may occasionally be an early symptom, fully developed hypertensive encephalopathy is not usually seen until later in the disease. The characteristic features of these attacks are disorientation, often with mental excitability and gross abnormalities of behaviour; there may be severe headaches, convulsions, complete blindness and coma. All these symptoms may be reversible and rapid improvement usually follows administration of hypotensive drugs. Organic cerebral vascular lesions may, however, occur in the course of an attack, leaving permanent paralysis. In occasional patients episodes of abdominal pain may be extremely severe and give rise to anxiety. There is no doubt that such symptoms can be produced by vascular necroses in the gut, and intestinal obstruction due to this cause has been described. Testicular and gall-bladder pain may be due to acute vascular lesions in these organs.

On examination the clinical signs are unmistakable. In the early stages there is a striking contrast between the apparent physical well-being of the patient and the grave prognosis. Hypertension is severe, with systolic pressure over 220 mm. and diastolic over 120 mm. in the majority of cases. During the course of the disease there is little fluctuation in blood pressure even in response to prolonged rest or after the development of heart failure; in fact there may be a progressive rise. Cardiac arrhythmia is rare. There is marked cardiovascular hypertrophy with obvious thickening of the radial and brachial arteries and enlargement of the heart. Papilloedema is the diagnostic sign of malignant hypertension. It is bilateral and is usually associated with retinal oedema, haemorrhages and exudates. Retinal oedema or exudates may produce a 'star figure' radiating from the macula. Other retinal lesions occasionally seen are thrombosis of a large retinal artery or vein, subhyaloid haemorrhages and retinal detachment. Pulmonary oedema produces fine inspiratory crepitations at the lung bases and in paroxysmal dyspnoea these may be widespread and associated with rhonchi.

In early cases of malignant hypertension there may be no evidence of renal involvement. In most cases, however, there is albuminuria, which varies from a trace to as much as a third volume on boiling; obvious or microscopic blood may be found, but urinary casts are not commonly present. The specific gravity of the urine is usually fixed at 1·010 to 1·012 when the patient is first seen and renal function tests show diminished tubular concentrating power. Nitrogen retention is, however, usually absent and in many cases the disease runs its whole course without the development of more than moderate elevation of the blood urea. In the active stages the blood count frequently shows a polymorphonuclear leucocytosis and rapidly developing anaemia, which is occasionally haemolytic. In some cases the serum potassium is depressed and it has been shown that aldosterone secretion is often raised in malignant hypertension due to over-secretion of renin. Renal infarction and thiazide diuretics also cause hypokalaemia.

Diagnosis

The presence of papilloedema is the all important diagnostic sign which differentiates malignant from benign hypertension. The separation from chronic nephritis and from other types of renal disease in which the hypertension has become malignant may in the late stages be extremely difficult. In general, papilloedema does not develop in primary renal disease until the patient has reached an advanced stage of renal failure. In chronic uraemia the urine is usually colourless due to absence of urochrome, whereas in malignant essential hypertension the urine is usually well coloured. When renal function tests are unimpaired it is important to exclude unilateral renal disease. Intravenous pyelography may show such an abnormality either in the form of a non-functioning kidney or a grossly contracted kidney with deformity of the renal calyces. In unilateral renal artery stenosis there may be only a slight difference in size of the kidneys, but characteristic differences in excretion are seen. The 3-minute pyelogram shows delayed appearance of the contrast medium, whilst in the 20-minute film it is more concentrated than on the normal side. If there is contraction of the ischaemic kidney, this is uniform in main renal artery stenosis with reduction in size of the calyces; in branch occlusion there may be a localized thinning of the cortex. The full investigation of renal artery stenosis is discussed in Section 12. A further problem is the differential diagnosis between malignant hypertension and intracranial tumour. Both conditions may present with papilloedema and focal neurological signs. Cerebral tumour may occur in a patient with benign hypertension or more rarely may itself cause hypertension. If marked albuminuria is present, and particularly if there is renal impairment, a diagnosis of malignant hypertension should be made. In the absence of renal involvement full investigation for a space-occupying lesion should be carried out. The finding of hypokalaemia may require differential diagnosis from primary aldosteronism due to adrenal cortical tumour (Conn's syndrome). Papilloedema very rarely occurs in this condition and an adrenal tumour may be demonstrable by special techniques such as angiography.

Treatment

Malignant hypertension is an absolute indication for

hypotensive drug therapy. In acutely ill patients this should at first be given parenterally, and then maintained orally with close supervision, as described on page 818. Severe acute pulmonary oedema and hypertensive encephalopathy may need prompt venesection, but in this case sympathetic blocking drugs must be given with care, since with a reduced blood volume they may produce sudden and serious hypotension, which may cause cerebral thrombosis. Potassium depletion if present should be corrected. Lumbodorsal sympathectomy may still be indicated in the rare drug resistant case, or in non-cooperative subjects; even though it may produce only slight lowering of blood pressure, the response to hypotensive drugs is much greater after reduction in sympathetic vasoconstriction by this operation. When the stage of renal failure is reached, blood pressure control is more difficult to achieve, and treatment must be directed to relief of symptoms by appropriate measures, or regular dialysis therapy may be instituted as for terminal renal failure due to other causes [see Section 12].

Course and Prognosis

In the absence of treatment malignant hypertension is a progressive disorder and there may be rapid deterioration with a fatal outcome within a few months of the first symptom. In most series of cases the average prognosis is given as 1–2 years, the expectation of life being rather longer in women than in men. Very occasionally the disease appears to pass into an inactive phase which may continue for several years before a further deterioration sets in. During this period there may be no evidence of new vascular lesions, papilloedema may subside and exudates resolve; the margins of the optic disc often remain indistinct with filling in of the optic cups, but there is no true swelling. This appearance is sometimes called secondary optic atrophy. Albuminuria may diminish and even cerebral symptoms and breathlessness may improve. Nevertheless in most cases the rapid deterioration, and the distressing nature of the later symptoms due to a combination of pulmonary oedema, renal failure, hypertensive encephalopathy and retinopathy, justify beyond any terminological scruple the name malignant hypertension. With effective hypotensive drug therapy the expectation of life may be increased to 5 years or more. Papilloedema, retinal haemorrhages and exudates resolve slowly and vision may improve considerably, but the hazards of cerebral vascular accidents and acute heart failure remain.

REFERENCES

British Medical Journal (1963) Hypotensive drugs, current practice, **1**, 1006, 1073.

Byrom, F. B. (1954) The pathogenesis of hypertensive encephalopathy and its relation to the malignant phase of hypertension, *Lancet*, ii, 201.

De Graeff, J., ed. (1963) Hypertension, in *Boerhaave Symposium*, Leiden.

Fishberg, A. M. (1954) *Hypertension and Nephritis*, 5th ed., Philadelphia.

Gowenlock, A. H., and Wrong, O. (1962) Hyperaldosteronism secondary to renal ischaemia, *Quart. J. Med.*, **55**, 323.

Pickering, G. W. (1955) *High Blood Pressure*, London.

Platt, R. (1961) Essential hypertension; incidence, course and heredity, *Ann. intern. Med.*, **55**, 1.

Wilson, C., and Byrom, F. B. (1941) The vicious circle in chronic Bright's disease, *Quart. J. Med.*, **10**, 65.

PULMONARY HYPERTENSION

Systemic hypertension is not associated with a rise in pulmonary arterial pressure. Pulmonary hypertension is due to a variety of lesions all of which produce either increased peripheral resistance in the lungs or increased output of the right ventricle or both. Mitral stenosis, emphysema, pulmonary fibrosis due to any cause, primary pulmonary endarteritis and certain types of congenital heart disease are the common aetiological factors [p. 768].

HYPOTENSION

There is no arbitrary limit which supplies a satisfactory definition of hypotension, but in adults 100 mm. may be regarded as the lower limit of the systolic pressure. The reading may be slightly lower in the supine than in the erect position.

Aetiology and Pathology

Abnormally low blood pressure may be due to myocardial infarction or reduction in cardiac output due to terminal heart failure. Reduction in cardiac output may also be due to diminished venous return in oligaemic states, e.g. following haemorrhage, loss of fluid due to burns or acute gastro-enteritis. Severe toxaemia may also produce an abnormally low blood pressure and so may heat exhaustion. In vasovagal syncope hypotension is a usual feature. Low blood pressure is a characteristic of Addison's disease. Postural hypotension is a specific variety which will be described separately.

Symptoms

In acute hypotension due to oligaemia the skin is cold and clammy, the pulse is usually rapid and small in volume; the blood pressure may be unrecordable or the sphygmomanometer may register the systolic but not the diastolic pressure. Hypotension with bradycardia, nausea and sweating suggests a vasovagal attack. In shock there will usually be evidence of a primary cause and the blood pressure is chiefly important as an index of deterioration or recovery.

Prolonged hypotension is sometimes associated with states of unconsciousness following head injury or operations on the brain. In these and in other patients with prolonged hypotension, renal function may be considerably impaired and elevation of the blood urea may be associated with hyperchloraemic acidosis.

Treatment

This depends upon the cause. Hypotension following haemorrhage is a grave sign and usually indicates a loss of at least 25 per cent. of the blood volume. Transfusion of whole blood should be given until the systolic pressure reaches 100 mm. After this point, a further 2 pints are usually necessary to restore the blood volume.

POSTURAL HYPOTENSION

Postural hypotension is present if the systolic pressure in the erect posture after 3 minutes' quiet standing, with the arm at heart level, is 50 mm. or more below the systolic pressure in the supine position.

Aetiology

This disorder is due to impairment of the carotid sinus reflex. It may follow bilateral denervation of the carotid sinus or may be associated with neurological or endocrine disease, particularly tabes dorsalis, syringomyelia, diabetic neuropathy, Parkinsonism, Addison's disease or hypoparathyroidism. It may follow extensive sympathectomy or the administration of drugs paralysing the vasoconstrictor nerves. In many cases, however there is evidence of widespread disorder of the autonomic nervous system unaccounted for by any organic lesion. To this condition the term idiopathic postural hypotension has been given. The central lesion in such cases is above the spinal reflex level and is probably a specific autonomic degeneration. It is rare before the age of 40 and less common in women.

Symptoms

The cardinal symptom is syncope, usually preceded by dizziness. It rarely occurs while the patient is sitting and never while lying down. Attacks are usually more frequent early in the day, during hot weather and on standing still after moderate activity. They are often first noticed while standing in queues or at the kitchen sink. In most cases, especially of the idiopathic type, the pulse rate is unchanged despite great variations in blood pressure. There may also be patchy or total anhidrosis, nocturnal polyuria and, in males, loss of libido and potency. Pigmentation of the skin is sometimes observed and hyperhidrosis has been reported. There may be absence of pupillary reaction to light.

Diagnosis

Epilepsy is usually suspected until the postural variation in blood pressure is discovered. The presence of pigmentation may suggest Addison's disease, but again the demonstration of a gross fall in blood pressure on standing still, establishes the diagnosis.

Treatment

Elastic stockings and an abdominal binder are useful measures to diminish pooling of the blood. Symptoms may be improved by avoiding the supine position at all times during the day and elevating the head of the bed 18 inches at night. Treatment with vasoconstrictor drugs usually produces little if any permanent relief of symptoms, but is worthy of trial. The administration of salt and a synthetic electrocorticoid, e.g. 9-alpha-fluorohydrocortisone, will lead to fluid retention and may diminish the postural fall.

Prognosis

Postural hypotension may persist unchanged for very many years with minor disability or it may progress to a disabling affliction which confines the sufferer to a wheel-chair. Remissions rarely occur. The postural hypotension which follows dorsolumbar sympathectomy usually passes off in 6–9 months. More extensive sympathectomy may be followed by a permanent, disabling, postural hypotension.

REFERENCE

Barraclough, M. A., and Sharpey-Schafer, E. P. (1963) Hypotension from absent circulatory reflexes, *Lancet*, i, 1121.

PERIPHERAL VASCULAR DISEASE

The term peripheral vascular disease includes a number of obliterative arterial diseases of the limbs and a group of less common functional disorders of the small peripheral vessels. It also includes a variety of conditions affecting the venous and lymphatic pathways.

There are two main types of obliterative arterial disease:

1. *Chronic vascular occlusion* due to arterial degeneration or vascular spasm, or both processes in combination. The commonest variety of peripheral vascular disease is atheromatous degeneration which may be complicated by vascular spasm and by thrombosis. Detachment of thrombus from an atheromatous area may give rise to embolism in a more peripheral artery. Raynaud's phenomenon is an example of vasospastic peripheral arterial disease, but this also may in the later stages be complicated by thrombosis.

2. *Acute obstruction* to the vessel lumen by embolism or acute thrombosis. Systemic emboli usually arise from the valves of the left side of the heart or from mural thrombi in atrium or ventricle or from thrombosis over atheromatous areas of the larger arteries. Acute thrombosis, causing acute arterial obstruction, usually occurs at the site of atheromatous ulceration, but it may occur as a primary lesion.

Peripheral vascular disease of all kinds leads to ischaemic manifestations in the limbs, the chief of these being muscle pain and gangrene.

Methods of Investigation

Since peripheral vascular disease is most commonly due to generalized arterial degeneration a complete examination of the cardiovascular system is essential in all cases. This involves examination of the peripheral arteries of the head and neck, upper and lower limbs, retinoscopy, examination of the heart and the blood pressure. Electrocardiographic investigation and radiography of the heart and aorta should be carried out, and the urine should be tested for sugar and albumin. The Wassermann reaction must be tested in all patients with indolent ulceration of the limbs. Radiographic examination of the affected parts for arterial calcification is of value. In all cases of deep ulceration, radiography of the underlying bones and joints is essential for the detection of osteomyelitis or destructive arthritis.

Local examination of an affected limb should be directed first to the colour of the skin, which is determined by the filling of the subpapillary venous plexus and by the proportion of reduced haemoglobin in the blood. Pallor is usually due to arterial occlusion or vasoconstriction, cyanosis to slowing of the blood flow, redness to increased blood flow, which may be persistent or may be transient if due to inflammation or reactive hyperaemia. Engorgement of the superficial veins should be looked for. Inspection will also reveal the presence of oedema which may be inflammatory or may indicate venous obstruction. Oedema is sometimes present in the chronic ischaemic limb, especially where there is undernutrition of the tissues and muscular atrophy due to disuse. In the severely ischaemic limb, especially with rest pain, dependency is a common cause of oedema. Trophic lesions should be observed in their general extent and for the presence of sinuses indicating involvement of deep tissues. Associated eczema or fungus infections between the toes should be noted. The skin temperature is regulated by rate of blood flow and the comparison should be made of normal and abnormal limbs. Lowering of skin temperature indicates arterial occlusion or vasoconstriction, while increase is usually due to inflammation. Pulsation should be looked for in all the main arteries of the limb, e.g. in the lower limb the femoral, popliteal, posterior tibial and dorsalis pedis arteries, the two sides being compared. If there is a marked difference in pulsation the blood pressure should be compared on the two sides.

Special investigations may be carried out to determine the extent and severity of the vascular occlusion. A simple test is to elevate the lower limb and then measure the time taken for the circulation to return to the toes after hanging the leg downwards. In the normal limb, provided it is warm, this should take a few seconds, but in vascular occlusion it may be increased to half a minute or longer. The amplitude of pulsation at different points in the main arteries may be measured by the recording oscillograph.

Exercise tolerance under standard conditions, as indicated by claudication time and maximum walking distance, provides a useful assessment of response to treatment. More sophisticated measures of muscle or total tissue blood flow by plethysmographic or isotope clearance techniques, and blood flow velocity profiles by ultrasonic methods, may be of value in general assessment. Clinical examination and angiography remain, however, the most important methods of investigation.

The use of angiography in degenerative arterial disease of the lower limbs should be reserved for cases where reconstructive surgery is contemplated. It gives an accurate picture of the extent of the disease before operation, and after operation distal arterial filling is a reliable guide to prognosis. Complications such as haemorrhage, thrombosis and fistula formation may occur and emphasize the need for care and selection in this investigation.

Measurement of skin temperature can be used to determine whether ischaemia can be relieved by sympathetic vasodilatation. In the reflex vasodilatation test the patient is placed in a hot chamber with the affected limbs outside. Alternatively, reflex vasodilatation may be produced by putting the arms in hot water (when the skin temperature of the feet is to be tested) until general vasodilatation and sweating occur. With the room temperature about 68° F. (20° C.) reflex vasodilatation should produce in the normal subject a rise in skin temperature over the hand or foot to at least 86° F. (30° C.). Sympathetic release may also be obtained by spinal anaesthesia and this method is preferable if sympathectomy is being considered as a form of treatment. In all these investigations, if only one limb is affected, the sound limb should be used as a control.

PERIPHERAL ARTERIOSCLEROSIS

Aetiology and Pathology

The all-important pathological lesion in peripheral arteriosclerosis is atheroma, usually occurring as part of a generalized condition. The aetiology and pathology of atheroscleross ha ve already been discussed. Medial degeneration (Mönckeberg's degeneration) is a much rarer form, which leads to ring-like calcification of the media and this may be recognized radiologically. It occurs in elderly patients and atheroma is almost always present. The lower limbs are most commonly affected by arterial degeneration, the lower abdominal aorta and distal third of the superficial femoral artery being the vessels most frequently involved [PLATE 17]. Occasionally atherosclerosis in the proximal arteries of the upper limb produces ischaemic pain, numbness and blanching of the digits.

Symptoms

Peripheral arteriosclerosis is five times as common in men as in women. The two cardinal manifestations are pain and ischaemic necrosis of the tissues. The usual type of pain is *intermittent claudication* (angina cruris). This consists of cramp-like pain in the calf, produced usually by a constant amount of exercise, and relieved promptly by rest. This distribution of pain is due to femoro-popliteal artery occlusion. Less frequently the obstruction is in the iliac arteries or at the aortic bifurcation (Leriche's syndrome), and claudication pain may then occur in the thigh or gluteal region. Claudication may first affect one side and later, as improvement occurs with the development of collateral circulation, the other limb may in turn be affected. As the disease progresses effort pain is characteristically brought on by diminishing amounts of exercise, until the patient may be unable to walk more than 10 or 20 yards. *Rest pain* is a continuous type of pain which affects the distal portions of the feet or toes. It usually comes on at night when the patient gets warm in bed, and relief may only be obtained by hanging the foot downwards out of bed. The ischaemic lesion is in general very severe in these cases and gangrene is a common sequel. Rest pain may also be produced by inflammatory changes associated with gangrene, especially if there is considerable oedema or deep necrosis with involvement of bone or joints.

Gangrene due to arteriosclerotic occlusion is common in the lower limb but rare in the upper. It may involve one or more toes, or the distal part of the foot according to the particular arterial branch which is obstructed. Trauma is a frequent precipitating factor, bruising of the foot leading to oedema and thereby depressing the local circulation to a point below which effective nutrition cannot be maintained. In other cases gangrene may appear or extend suddenly in a manner which indicates either embolism or acute extension of a thrombotic lesion. Gangrene may also occur over pressure points, especially the ball of the heel and the malleoli. Trophic ulceration may be observed in the absence of massive tissue necrosis. This may take the form of ulceration around the nails or between the toes and the condition may be aggravated by fungus infection or an eczematous eruption. All forms of infection tend to aggravate ischaemia by producing oedema, but the introduction of antibiotic therapy has made it possible to combat moist, spreading gangrene with satisfactory delimitation of the lesion. Vascular spasm is sometimes a prominent feature of peripheral arteriosclerosis and the appearances may resemble Raynaud's phenomenon due to other causes. Sometimes individual digits are affected (so-called 'dead fingers') particularly after exposure to cold. The combination of arterial degeneration with secondary vasoconstriction may lead to symmetrical peripheral gangrene of the fingers or toes.

The physical signs which may be present in obliterative vascular disease have been discussed under methods of investigation. Pallor or cyanosis of the skin will depend on the degree of arterial occlusion. Skin temperature is lower on the abnormal side unless inflammation is present. The femoral pulses will usually be diminished in amplitude and the posterior tibial and dorsalis pedis pulses are frequently absent. It should be noted, however, that dorsalis pedis pulsation is absent in about 10 per cent. of normal young adults. Popliteal pulsation is sometimes difficult to feel in normal subjects and this sign is equivocal unless there is a definite difference between the two sides.

Diagnosis

The diagnosis of obliterative arteriosclerosis is indicated by the age of the patient, generalized signs of arterial degeneration and evidence of predisposing factors such as hypertension or diabetes. The radiological demonstration of calcification is a conclusive sign of arterial degeneration. Difficulty arises over the occasional young patient in whom localized atheroma produces obliteration of a large artery in one of the limbs. The differentiation from thrombo-angiitis in these cases is difficult; the absence of recurrent episodes and of associated venous thrombosis are the most important diagnostic points in favour of arteriosclerosis.

Treatment

The most essential treatment in patients with peripheral arteriosclerosis is prophylaxis. The foot should be kept clean and warm and at all costs trauma should be avoided. Thus special shoes should be fitted if necessary and warm, woollen socks should be worn. Exposure to cold and wet should be carefully avoided. When vascular occlusion gives rise to definite ischaemic changes, complete rest in bed is necessary, extremes of heat or cold should not be permitted to the affected part and bed socks should be worn. The treatment depends on the nature of the disorder. Intermittent claudication may gradually improve with the passage of time as collateral circulation develops. Planned daily exercises may improve calf muscle blood flow and increase exercise tolerance. Vasodilator drugs are of little or no benefit but some improvement may follow minor surgical procedures such as calf muscle denervation, tendo Achillis tenotomy and lumbar sympathectomy. The skin temperature response to sympathetic release gives no reliable indication of the muscle blood flow. Arterial surgery has a definite though limited place in treatment. The best results are obtained from relief of obstruction in the lower abdominal aorta and common iliacs, 70 per cent. of patients remaining symptom free for five years. In distal femoro-popliteal disease the results of surgery are much less favourable. Endarterectomy and synthetic grafts are widely used, but in superficial femoral artery occlusion autogenous vein by-pass operations give the best results. Patients should be carefully selected for arterial surgery, the worst results being obtained in elderly patients and those with associated coronary disease. Diabetics are unsuitable if there is generalized involvement of small arteries but reconstructive surgery should be considered when a major vessel is obstructed.

Rest pain is treated by putting the patient to bed and giving analgesic drugs. Intermittent venous occlusion may be tried; occasionally this kind of pain, particularly if of sudden onset, may gradually improve with the development of collateral circulation. In intractable cases, unless reconstructive arterial surgery is undertaken, amputation is inevitable. All patients with ischaemic pain should be investigated by arteriography.

Gangrene is now treated conservatively in the majority of cases. Rest in bed and use of antibiotics quickly lead to the subsidence of inflammation and demarcation of the area of gangrene. Necrotic tissue may then be removed and healing accelerated by means of pinch grafting. Where gangrene is superficial and when considerable improvement in the skin circulation follows reflex vasodilatation, sympathectomy may be the most effective treatment particularly when secondary vasconstriction is a prominent feature. In resistant cases, particularly in elderly subjects with generalized arteriosclerosis or diabetes, mid-thigh amputation may be the only effective form of treatment.

Course and Prognosis

Peripheral arteriosclerosis produces a permanent and usually progressive obliteration of the arteries. After an initial attack of intermittent claudication or gangrene, considerable improvement may occur over a long period of time with establishment of collateral circulation. The treatment of infection with antibiotics, with subsidence of oedema, frequently leads to considerable healing and makes local surgery a practical measure. It is common for both lower limbs to be involved in sequence although, of course, intermittent claudication occurs only in the more affected limb. The individual prognosis is frequently determined by the consequences of arterial degeneration elsewhere in the body. Thus relief of angina cruris is sometimes followed by the onset of angina pectoris as the patient returns to normal activity.

REFERENCES

DARLING, R. C. (1969) Peripheral arterial surgery, *New Engl. J. Med.*, **280**, 26, 84 and 141.

FRIEDMAN, S. A., HOLLING, H. E., and ROBERTS, B. (1964) Etiologic factors in aorto-iliac and femoro-popliteal vascular disease, *New Engl. J. Med.*, **271**, 1382.

STRANDNESS, D. E., and BELL, J. W. (1965) Peripheral vascular disease; diagnosis and objective evaluation, *Ann. Surg.*, Suppl **161**, 3.

WESLER, S. (1955) Intermittent caudication, *Circulation*, **11**, 806.

PULSELESS DISEASE

Synonyms. Takayasu's disease; Constrictive arteritis.

Definition

Chronic progressive arteritis of the aorta and its branches causing absent peripheral pulses.

Aetiology

The cause is unknown. The disease is most common in the Far East, especially Japan. It is rare in men and chiefly affects women from 18–40 years of age. Sex incidence and histology suggest a form of collagen disease resembling temporal arteritis.

Pathology

There is diffuse arteritis affecting the arch of the aorta and its branches, but sometimes involving the thoracic and abdominal aorta. In the latter case renal artery stenosis may lead to hypertension. All coats of the arteries are involved by inflammatory reaction (sometimes with giant cells) and the lumen is narrowed by intimal proliferation and thrombosis. Carotid stenosis may lead to cerebral and retinal damage, coronary stenosis to cardiac ischaemia.

Symptoms

Giddiness and syncope are the usual symptoms due to cerebral ischaemia. Hemiplegia, visual impairment, coldness and paraesthesiae of the arms may be present. The peripheral pulses are commonly absent or diminished. The blood pressure may be unmeasurable in the arms but raised in the lower limbs. Symptoms of hypertension or cardiac ischaemia may occur.

Diagnosis

The age, sex and country of origin are important, although the disease has been described in Europeans. Intravenous aortography will reveal the site and extent of the constriction. Differential diagnosis is from other causes of 'aortic arch syndrome' such as atherosclerosis with thrombosis, dissecting aneurysm and syphilitic aortitis.

Treatment

Long-term anticoagulant therapy has been used to prevent extension of thrombosis. Surgical resection and grafting has been employed in selected cases with success.

REFERENCES

MCKUSICK, V. A. (1962) A form of vascular disease relatively frequent in the Orient, *Amer. Heart J.*, **63**, 57.

VINISCHAIKUL, K. (1967) Primary arteritis of the aorta and its main branches (Takayasu's arteriopathy). A clinicopathologic study of eight cases, *Medicine (Baltimore)*, **43**, 15.

THROMBO-ANGIITIS OBLITERANS

Synonym. Buerger's disease.

Definition

A disease characterized by acute inflammation with thrombosis affecting both arteries and veins.

Aetiology

The disease has been recorded in all countries and races, and usually presents between the ages of 25 and 40 years. Men are affected almost exclusively although there is some evidence that the incidence in women is rising. A history of smoking is present in 99 per cent. The cause is unknown. Attempts to demonstrate an infective cause or an allergy to nicotine have been inconclusive. The association of non-specific inflammation of arteries and veins suggest a relationship to periarteritis nodosa and the other collagen diseases. Some patients develop visceral vascular lesions and the relationship to the collagen disorders is even more marked in these cases. For these reasons and because of the non-specific pathological changes doubts have arisen on the existence of this condition as a separate entity.

Pathology

Any vessel may be affected, but the medium-sized arteries and veins of the lower limbs are most commonly involved. It is likely that the earliest change is a proliferation of the intima and inflammatory infiltration. When thrombosis has occurred there is a marked intimal proliferation with a few foci of lymphocytes. The other coats show the usual changes associated with thrombosis, fibroblastic response in the media and capillary dilatation with fibroplasia in the adventitia. As the lesion ages, fibrosis occurs in the thrombus and recanalization follows. Characteristically only a short length of the vessel is affected and lesions in all stages, with intervening normal areas, may be found.

Symptoms

These depend on the vessel involved. The most usual symptom is intermittent claudication, but patients may present with superficial venous thromboses, Raynaud's phenomenon, gangrene of the extremities or a visceral catastrophe. Venous thrombosis commonly affects the lower limb and characteristically produces episodic attacks of localized, superficial, painful swelling, particularly in the calf. Peripheral gangrene may affect the toes, or a larger part of the extremity if a main artery is obliterated. Pain in the feet at night is not uncommon, and is characteristically eased by hanging the leg downwards out of the bed, or by walking about. Paraesthesiae may occur. Ischaemic pain in the arms is rare but may be severe enough to prevent the patient from following his usual employment. Cardiac infarction or cerebral thrombosis may occur.

The physical signs depend on the site and age of the lesions. When a main artery to a limb is involved the skin beyond the lesion is cold, and the peripheral pulses absent. If ischaemia is induced by elevating the limb for some minutes, the return of the circulation to the skin on lowering the limb is delayed. When the flush does appear it is usually more intense than on the normal side due to reactive hyperaemia. Occasionally in bilateral disease the skin of the calf is warmer and the leg blood flow is increased on the symptomatically more affected side.

Diagnosis

The disease must be distinguished from other causes of arterial occlusion including generalized atheromatous disease and isolated arterial lesions such as 'idiopathic' thrombosis of the popliteal artery. The finding of obliterative arterial disease with or without gangrene in a male under 50 strongly suggests thrombo-angiitis obliterans. The association of arterial disease with superficial painful swellings due to venous thrombosis is diagnostic. Radiological demonstrations of calcified vascular lesions is strong evidence against Buerger's disease as is the finding of a raised blood cholesterol. Lesions restricted to the upper limbs should suggest the possibility of some anatomical abnormality causing compression of the subclavian artery. In an early case diagnosis may be impossible until further scattered venous or arterial lesions appear.

Treatment

Complete abstinence from tobacco should be advised, but the patients are often compulsive cigarette smokers. Vasodilator drugs may help to relieve pain. Sympathectomy may assist healing of ischaemic ulcers but the results are often disappointing. Progressive gangrene may require amputation which should be as conservative as possible.

Course and Prognosis

The course of the disease is episodic with recurrent attacks of venous thrombosis, intermittent claudication or gangrene involving several sites in succession. The outcome is unpredictable. Cardiac infarction may cause sudden death early in the disease, or the condition may progress steadily over many years with recurrent episodes of thrombosis. Although there may be considerable improvement between attacks due to partial restoration of the circulation some residual disability is usual. In many cases the disease becomes inactive after a succession of attacks.

REFERENCES

BUERGER, L. (1908) Thrombo-angiitis obliterans: a study of the vascular lesions leading to presenile spontaneous gangrene, *Amer. J. med. Sci.*, **136**, 567.

CRAVEN, J. L., and COTTON, R. C. (1967) Haematological differences between thromboangiitis obliterans and atherosclerosis, *Brit. J. Surg.*, **54**, 862.

MCKUSICK, V. A., HARRIS, W. S., OTTESON, O. E., GOODMAN, R. M., SHELLEY, W. M., and BLOODWELL, R. D. (1962) Buerger's disease. A distinct clinical and pathologic entity, *J. Amer. med. Ass.*, **181**, 5.

RAYNAUD'S PHENOMENON

Definition

Intermittent pallor or cyanosis of the extremities brought on by cold, with return of skin colour to normal between attacks.

Aetiology

Very great changes in the calibre of the digital vessels occur in normal subjects in response to variations in temperature. The resulting changes in blood flow are greatest in the finger tips (where the blood flow may be a hundred times greater in the hot finger than in the cold) and diminish progressively towards the wrist. Raynaud's phenomenon is the result of a temporary, complete occlusion of the digital arteries due to an excessive vasoconstrictor response to cold. It may occur over many years without evident cause and without any demonstrable structural changes in the vessels; it is then usually referred to as Raynaud's disease. It may be well to recall, however, that Raynaud's original description was entitled 'local asphyxia and symmetrical gangrene of the extremities', so that many of his cases were due to varying types of organic vascular disease. Bilateral gangrene of the digits rarely, if ever, occurs in the condition we now term Raynaud's disease (*vide infra*). On the other hand, the phenomenon of digital asphyxia (what we now call Raynaud's phenomenon) frequently complicates organic vascular disease (atheroma, thrombo-angiitis obliterans, thrombosis and embolism), repeated trauma (in workmen using vibrating tools), intoxication with heavy metals and ergot, and shoulder-girdle compression syndrome. It may occur in the presence of cold haemagglutinins or cryoglobulins which lead to blood sludging in the cold. It is also an early manifestation in many cases of the collagenoses, particularly scleroderma, often before other signs of the disease have appeared.

Young women frequently suffer from Raynaud's phenomenon. The explanation in these patients was shown by Lewis to be an excessive reaction to cold in otherwise normal vessels. The term Raynaud's disease is usually reserved for this type of digital asphyxia, which is five to ten times commoner in women than in men.

Symptoms

Attacks may be brought on by any stimuli which cause digital vasconstriction. These include handling cold objects, the heat conservation response to a cold environment, sudden fright or emotional tension. In those who work with vibrating tools the attacks are usually brought on by cold but may occur in a warm environment, for example, while in bed. In these patients there are usually signs of sensory loss.

The colour of the fingers during an attack depends upon the state of venous tone. Commonly it is a pale bluish white, often white with small blue patches. In a prolonged and severe attack the fingers become waxen and shiny. If the spasm relaxes momentarily and the venules fill, the fingers may be deeply cyanosed. In this stage the fingers feel dead and often tingle. If cut, they do not bleed, or only a little dark blood oozes out.

After a period, which may be from a few minutes to 20 minutes or more, the arteries relax and the circulation returns. Pinkish patches begin to appear at the base of the finger, and whole digits become cyanosed. Finally the skin changes to a bright red (reactive hyperaemia) and paraesthesiae are felt. There may be an unpleasant, numb, aching sensation. After several years of severe attacks, the fingers become thickened and the skin atrophic, a condition termed 'acrosclerosis'. Superficial ulceration of the finger tips is sometimes seen but extensive gangrene of the digits rarely, if ever, occurs unless there is some underlying organic vascular disorder.

Diagnosis

Raynaud's phenomenon should be distinguished from chilblains, acrocyanosis, erythromelalgia and from the numbness and tingling sometimes found in erythrocyanosis. Diagnosis is certain if immersion of the hands in cold water provokes an attack. When the water is warmed the characteristic changes associated with returning circulation are seen. The localization to the fingers is characteristic. In early scleroderma Raynaud's phenomenon may be the most prominent feature of the disease. Nevertheless characteristic skin changes are, as a rule, present at this stage, and affect parts of the body other than the fingers. In Raynaud's disease sclerotic changes are usually confined to the fingers and develop only after many years of intermittent digital asphyxia. In scleroderma, radiological examination of the oesophagus (barium swallow) may reveal the typical functional disturbance. Whenever digital asphyxia occurs in men or in middle or old age, a more intensive search for the precipitating causes mentioned above should be made. Attacks of localized vasoconstriction in the fingers ('dead fingers') may be a symptom of atherosclerotic narrowing of the arteries of supply.

Treatment

Protection against exposure of the hands to cold should be provided by gloves or mittens, and the general vasoconstrictor response to a cold environment prevented by warm clothing. Where occupation or the severity of the disease makes these measures ineffective oral tolazoline or phenoxybenzamine (*Dibenyline, Dibenzyline*) may be tried. Where medical treatment fails in Raynaud's disease, cervical sympathectomy is of great value. It prevents reflex vasoconstriction, and keeps the hand warm. Marked local cooling, however, will still provoke attacks. Relapse after sympathectomy is usually associated with return of vasomotor activity.

Superficial ulcers heal slowly and careful treatment with suitable antibiotics is necessary. Sympathectomy may produce dramatic improvement of these trophic lesions, but treatment with vasodilator drugs is often disappointing.

Prognosis

In Raynaud's phenomenon secondary to organic arterial disease the prognosis depends upon the cause. When there is partial obstruction in the digital arteries, for example, due to embolism secondary to brachial artery compression, relief of the latter will arrest the condition, but improvement is unlikely. In tool workers the attacks do not occur during work and a change of occupation does not usually prevent attacks; indeed the condition may progress. Raynaud described remissions in young women during pregnancy. In these patients the disease may remit spontaneously for many years, to return at the menopause in a milder form.

REFERENCES

GIFFORD, R. W., Jr., and HINES, E. A., Jr. (1957) Raynaud's disease among women and girls, *Circulation*, **22**, 13.

LEWIS, T. (1929) Experiments relating to the peripheral mechanism involved in the spasmodic arrest of the circulation in the fingers; a variety of Raynaud's disease, *Heart*, **15**, 7.

RAYNAUD, M. (1889) On local asphyxia and symmetrical gangrene of the extremities, trans. Thomas Barlow, in *Selected Monographs*, the New Sydenham Society, p. 29, London.

RITZMANN, S. E., and LEVIN, W. C. (1961) Cryopathies: a review, *Arch. intern. Med.*, **107**, 754.

ERYTHROMELALGIA

Definition

Pain, heat and redness of the extremities due to excessive dilatation of the skin vessels in response to heat, i.e. the functional disorder is the reverse of Raynaud's phenomenon.

Symptoms

The disease may occur at any age but is commonest after middle life. There may be no obvious predisposing factor or the condition may be secondary to organic nervous disease such as spastic paralysis, or to polycythaemia vera. The hands or feet, or both, may be affected and the symptoms usually come on when the patient gets warm in bed or after exercise. The pain is a distressing, burning sensation which may last several hours and relief is only obtained by leaving the feet exposed to the cold air. On examination the skin of the affected parts is red and hot; there may be swelling of the extremities due to vasodilatation.

Diagnosis

The condition is to be distinguished from other forms of pain and redness of the extremities, so-called erythralgia, in which the skin is cold. This occurs, for example, in arteriosclerotic vascular occlusion and thrombo-angiitis. Relief of symptoms by cooling and elevation of the limb is diagnostic. The possibility of some primary cause such as polycythaemia should be investigated.

Treatment

In an attack the pain is relieved by raising and cooling the affected part. Aspirin often produces considerable benefit. The condition is persistent but leads to no serious complication, hence prophylactic measures are the main form of treatment. Hot environments, over-warm clothing, excessive walking or standing and anything else which provokes vasodilatation must be avoided.

REFERENCE

LEWIS, T. (1933) Clinical observations and experiments relating to burning pain in the extremities, and to so-called erythromelalgia in particular, *Clin. Sci.*, **1**, 175.

ERYTHROCYANOSIS

Erythrocyanosis crurum puellarum frigida is the full name of this condition. It is a recurrent state of capillary stasis occurring in young girls, affecting the lower limbs, and provoked by exposure to cold. The skin is blue in patches, uniformly cold and there is usually oedema of the ankles. Chilblains are a common association and ulceration may develop. In fact this condition is not separable from chronic perniosis. At first attacks occur only in cold weather but later the discoloration and swelling become permanent. The ulcers are painful and take several weeks to heal, leaving behind a brown pigmentation.

Treatment

Exposure to cold must be minimized and in severe cases it may be worth while to move to a warmer district. Warm clothing, especially woollen stockings, should be worn in cold weather. Exercises and massage may be beneficial. Sympathectomy is not an appropriate form of treatment.

ACROCYANOSIS

Definition

Persistent cyanosis of the hands, usually in women, without evidence of organic arterial disease.

Aetiology

The condition is persistent, but is worse in cold weather. The lesion is due to dilatation of the small vessels of the skin, but there is no venous obstruction; hence it has been suggested that the primary fault is increased arteriolar constriction with secondary dilatation of capillaries and venules. There may be a familial incidence.

Symptoms

The disease is almost entirely confined to women. The fingers are noticed to be cold and blue especially in cold weather. There may be swelling and tenderness but no trophic disturbances occur.

Diagnosis

The condition is distinguished from erythromelalgia by the coldness of the skin and the fact that pain is inconspicuous. Raynaud's disease differs in the sequence of events during attacks, particularly the pallor due to digital asphyxia. The cyanosis of obliterative arterial disease commonly affects the feet, and the underlying obstructive lesion usually produces other more prominent symptoms or signs.

Treatment

The condition is benign and the only necessary treatment is protection from the cold.

ARTERIAL EMBOLISM AND THROMBOSIS

Blockage of a systemic artery by an embolus is due to detachment of a portion of clot from a thrombus in the heart or a large atheromatous vessel or of vegetations from the heart valves in subacute bacterial endocarditis. In pulmonary embolism [p. 783] the clot is derived from a thrombus in one of the veins of the lower extremity or from the right atrium or right ventricle (mural thrombosis). Very rarely a portion of clot from the right side of the heart may pass to the left side through a septal defect and may cause so-called 'paradoxical embolism' in a systemic artery.

The common sites for systemic embolism are the cerebral arteries, especially the middle cerebral [see Section 15], the arteries of the limbs, especially the femoral, and the mesenteric arteries [see Section 7]. Infarction of the spleen, kidney and retina also occurs. Occasionally a clot lodges astride the bifurcation of the aorta (saddle embolus of the aorta). It may later move into one or other common iliac artery and thence to the femoral, or it may cause symptoms of bilateral femoral obstruction.

Femoral embolism is typical of obstruction to the main artery of a limb. The embolus may be detached from the left atrium in a patient with rheumatic carditis after the institution of quinidine therapy for atrial fibrillation or during the stress of labour. Embolism is still an occasional feature of resistant or untreated bacterial endocarditis. In elderly subjects the embolus may be derived from a ventricular mural thrombus secondary to cardiac infarction or chronic heart failure, or from thrombosis in an atheromatous or syphilitic aorta. The onset is usually sudden with acute pain in the limb which rapidly becomes numb, cold and useless. Occasionally the signs of obstruction develop gradually over several hours without much pain. On examination the limb is pale and pulsation is absent below the level of obstruction. Sensation may be lost in a few hours, but hyperaesthesia develops later. If the embolus is not removed gangrene is likely to occur, its extent depending on the age of the patient and the amount of collateral circulation. Relaxation of spasm may be the reason for the gradual improvement which is commonly seen during the first 12 hours, but it is unwise to delay surgical intervention to evaluate the improvement which may derive from this.

Diagnosis

The onset of pain in the leg in a patient with cardiovascular disease should lead to careful examination of the limb for venous thrombosis or arterial occlusion. The distinction is easy since oedema is prominent in venous thrombosis, the limb is warm and arterial pulsation can usually be felt. Differential diagnosis between arterial thrombosis and embolism depends on the primary disorder. Arteriosclerosis is the common cause of thrombosis and there will usually be evidence of this process elsewhere. Moreover, the superficial femoral artery at the site of the adductor hiatus is the common site of thrombosis in the lower limb. The symptoms of obstruction are usually less acute and less severe after thrombosis than after embolism, since previous incomplete arterial narrowing will have produced some degree of collateral circulation.

Treatment

The patient is nursed in a warm room to encourage vasodilatation. No attempt should be made to warm the affected limb. The leg should be lowered by blocking the head of the bed. Analgesics are given as required. Any lowering of systemic blood pressure must be avoided. Anticoagulant therapy should be given at once, a suitable regime being 50 mg. heparin intravenously every 4 hours and a coumarin derivative by mouth, the dosage being regulated by the prothrombin time. If improvement in the circulation takes place, this treatment is continued for a week. *Should no improvement be observed in two hours*, embolectomy must be undertaken. This may be performed in most cases under local anaesthetic and since the introduction of the Fogarty embolectomy balloon catheter it is a relatively minor operation. Delay in surgical treatment may jeopardize the survival of the limb. Embolism complicating rheumatic mitral valve disease is an indication for subsequent prophylactic valvotomy or long-term anticoagulant therapy.

Arterial thrombosis is usually a complication of atheroma or thrombo-angiitis obliterans. The femoral, popliteal or posterior tibial arteries may be involved in the lower limb, or the subclavian, axillary, brachial or radial arteries in the upper limb. The symptoms and signs resemble those produced by embolism but the onset is usually more gradual and gangrene is less common and less extensive. Medical treatment as described for arterial embolism should be carried out. Since underlying arterial disease is usually present, operative interference is not advisable if the diagnosis is unequivocal.

Course and Prognosis

Most patients may be expected to recover with medical treatment alone; with prompt resort to surgery where necessary, gangrene should rarely occur. The prognosis depends very considerably on the age and general condition of the patient. Since severe cardiovascular disease is usually present, active treatment may be impracticable or death may supervene from other causes.

REFERENCES

DARLING, R. C., AUSTEN, W. G., and LINTON, R. R. (1967) Arterial embolism, *Surg. Gynec. Obstet.*, **124**, 106.

EDWARDS, E. A., TILNEY, N., and LINDQUIST, R. R. (1966) Causes of peripheral embolism and their significance, *J. Amer. med. Ass.*, **196**, 133.

VENOUS THROMBOSIS (THROMBOPHLEBITIS)

Thrombophlebitis may be suppurative or non-suppurative, the latter being the common form.

SUPPURATIVE THROMBOPHLEBITIS

This condition may be due to the introduction of infection into a vein, usually during prolonged infravenous infusion of blood or saline. There are usually general symptoms—malaise, fever and shivering. Pyaemia may follow if the condition is not treated promptly and effectively. Locally there is redness and pain, with swelling of the affected limb, and the thrombosed vein, if superficial, may be hard and tender. An abscess may form and local incision may be necessary. Treatment is by local application of heat and administration of an antibiotic to which the infecting organism is sensitive.

Suppurative thrombophlebitis may complicate pyogenic infection anywhere in the body. Thus mastoid infection may lead to suppurative thrombosis of the lateral sinus or jugular vein; pyogenic infection of the bowel may be followed by suppurative pylephlebitis [see Section 7].

NON-SUPPURATIVE (SIMPLE) THROMBOPHLEBITIS

Aetiology

Simple thrombophlebitis is a not infrequent complication of a variety of conditions which lead to venous stasis. The usual predisposing causes are chronic congestive failure, immobilization after abdominal operations and childbirth. Thrombophlebitis complicates ½–1 per cent. of labours. Hysterectomy and other pelvic operations, herniorrhaphy, gastrectomy, cholecystectomy and prostatectomy are the operations commonly followed by thrombophlebitis. The veins of the calf, the femoral vein or the long saphenous vein are most frequently involved, in that order. It has been assumed that venous stasis due to relative immobilization is the primary cause of the thrombosis. This is almost certainly not the whole explanation. Other factors such as associated infection, or changes in blood coagulability due to the primary disease or to operative trauma are probably involved, but the exact mechanism is still obscure.

Thrombophlebitis occurs in other conditions where venous stasis is not a prominent feature. It may complicate polycythaemia, leukaemia, carcinomatosis, collagen disease, or Behçet's disease. It may develop in any severe infection, especially typhoid fever. The oestrogen-containing contraceptive pill may predispose to peripheral venous thrombosis and thrombo-embolism. Finally, venous thrombosis is frequently encountered in otherwise healthy subjects who present no evidence of any predisposing factor although in about 15 per cent. there is a history of minor injury to the limb. In such patients recurrent attacks may occur (thrombophlebitis migrans) and this condition may be so extensive as to produce chronic invalidism.

Pathology

Venous thrombosis rapidly leads to inflammation of the vein. As a result of invasion by fibroblasts the clot becomes adherent to the vessel wall. The head of the thrombus is composed of leucocytes and fibrin (white thrombus) but the tail is lamellated due to layering of red and white clot. The tail itself becomes firmly adherent in a few hours and detachment to produce embolism rarely occurs after this interval and certainly not after 3 days. Canalization in the organized thrombus results in partial restoration of blood flow.

Symptoms

The characteristic picture is seen in so-called ileofemoral thrombosis, in which the obstruction usually involves both external iliac and femoral veins. The whole limb becomes swollen; pain is variable and not usually conspicuous. There is congestion of superficial veins and frequently the thrombosed vein may be palpated as a tender, hard cord. Fever, malaise and tachycardia may be present at the onset. Occasionally the limb may become massively swollen with signs of arterial insufficiency—so called 'phlegmasia caerulea dolens'. The arterial insufficiency may be due to arterial spasm or to sudden development of massive oedema. There is a frequent association with malignant disease, trauma or surgical operations. Where gangrene is threatened venous thrombectomy should be performed, combined with anticoagulant therapy. Thrombophlebitis secondary to abdominal operation usually starts in the deep veins of the calf and is observed between the fourth and fourteenth postoperative days in most cases. Local tenderness may be the only sign, although the circumference of the calf may be increased due to oedema. Passive dorsiflexion of the foot may elicit pain in the absence of other signs.

Thrombosis of the axillary or subclavian vein produces similar changes in the upper limb. It commonly follows trauma such as carrying an unaccustomed weight on the shoulder.

Thrombosis of the inferior vena cava may occur under the same conditions as peripheral vein thrombosis. Special causes are the pressure of abdominal masses such as liver abscess, ascites or retroperitoneal tumours, or thrombophlebitis migrans extending from the femoral veins. Swelling of both legs may be present due to associated iliac or femoral thrombosis. Distension of the venous collaterals over the lower abdomen develops later.

Diagnosis

The early diagnosis of thrombosis of the calf veins after operation, described above, is particularly important. In cases without obvious precipitating cause full investigation is essential to rule out any underlying lesion, such as pelvic carcinoma involving the iliac veins or abdominal neoplasms compressing the inferior vena cava. Venography and ultrasonic devices may be of value in localizing the site of thrombosis. After operations, thrombus formation may be detected in the early stages by the use of radioisotope-labelled fibrinogen.

Treatment

Preventive measures against postoperative thrombophlebitis include early ambulation, leg exercises and massage, avoidance of tight bandages and pressure on the calves, and the adequate treatment of dehydration and infection. After operation and in congestive heart failure anticoagulant therapy, as described on page 779, is given at the earliest intimation of venous thrombosis to prevent extension and pulmonary embolism. Ligation of the femoral vein or even of the inferior vena cava has been performed as a prophylactic measure against pulmonary embolism after thrombophlebitis has occurred, but these measures have not been justified by the results.

In the treatment of femoral thrombosis the patient should be kept at rest in bed until all oedema, tenderness and constitutional signs have subsided. The limb should be elevated to about 30 degrees on an inclined plane. Analgesics are given as required. After 3 days, active movements at all joints are encouraged. Should there be any return of oedema when the patient is allowed up, knee-length elastic stockings should be fitted; these are worn during the day and removed at night until the venous circulation returns to normal.

Successful treatment of recent ileofemoral thrombosis has been reported by venous thrombectomy or the use of fibrinolytic therapy. Both aim at removal of thrombosis in order to preserve the venous valves which otherwise may be destroyed, leading to late symptoms such as venous claudication, chronic oedema and ulceration. The risk of pulmonary embolism may also be diminished.

Course and Prognosis

In the uncomplicated case oedema, pain and constitutional signs subside in 2–3 weeks and recovery is complete. Pulmonary embolism is the most serious complication of thrombophlebitis [p. 783]. *Chronic venous obstruction* may follow femoral or axillary vein thrombosis, the chief manifestations being persistent or recurrent oedema and aching pain in the limb when standing or walking. Chronic venous distension leads to varicosities and varicose ulceration. Induration of the limb due to persistent oedema and recurrent cellulitis may produce lymphatic obstruction which greatly aggravates the swelling and further impairs the nutritional state of the tissues. Obesity, varicose veins and inadequate treatment in the early stages predispose to chronic venous obstruction.

THROMBOPHLEBITIS MIGRANS

This condition has already been mentioned as a recurrent form of idiopathic thrombophlebitis. Attacks of venous thrombosis occur over a number of years and the veins of the legs, arms, trunk and the inferior vena cava may be involved. Chronic venous congestion of the legs may lead to widespread varicosities and indolent ulceration. In a subacute form it is commonly associated with visceral malignant disease, particularly carcinoma of the pancreas. It is probable that some varieties are a manifestation of a collagen disorder, but many remain unexplained. In a rapidly progressive case it may be justifiable to give a course of anticoagulant therapy, but this is only a temporary measure and does not halt the progress of the disease.

REFERENCE

SHERRY, S., GENTON, E., BRINKHOUS, K. M., and STENGLE, J. M., eds (1969) *Thrombosis*, Washington.

LYMPHATIC OBSTRUCTION

Synonym. Lymphoedema.

Aetiology, Pathology and Symptomatology

Lymphatic obstruction may be congenital (developmental or hereditary), traumatic, inflammatory or neoplastic. An idiopathic type (lymphoedema praecox) is not uncommonly seen, chiefly in girls or young women, coming on around puberty and aggravated by menstruation and a hot environment. There is often a family history. A similar but rarer type, occurring after the age of 35, is described as lymphoedema tarda.

Congenital lymphoedema may be present at or soon after birth. In the heredofamilial type (Milroy's disease) the condition occurs in successive generations and is usually present at birth. It may be unilateral or bilateral and the lower limbs are the more commonly affected. The fundamental abnormality appears to be stasis and dilatation (lymphangiectasis) in valveless lymphatics. The subcutaneous fat is replaced by a sponge-like mass of dilated lymph spaces and fibrous connective tissue.

Inflammatory lymphoedema may be due to pyogenic or non-specific chronic lymphadenitis and lymphangitis. Recurrent attacks of inflammation accompanied by malaise, fever and sometimes cellulitis, lead to progressive lymphatic obstruction and brawny swelling due to a combination of oedema and subcutaneous fibrosis. Severe lymphoedema (elephantiasis) is a feature of chronic filariasis [see Section 2].

Infiltration or compression of lymphatics by new-growth may cause lymphoedema, although this type of obstruction more commonly affects the abdominal lymphatics to produce *chylous ascites*. Operative removal of lymph nodes, e.g. of the axillary lymphatics for carcinoma of the breast is a common cause of lymphatic oedema, and radiotherapy may have a similar effect.

Diagnosis

Although pitting oedema is usually present, lymphoedema has a characteristic solid or brawny consistency due to its chronicity, which leads to proliferation of connective tissue and inflammatory fibrosis. The age and circumstances of onset, rate of development and presence or absence of primary lymphangitis make the diagnosis of the cause fairly obvious.

Treatment

Attempts should be made to reduce the oedema by elevation of the limb and elastic bandaging. A well-fitting elastic stocking may keep the swelling down in less severe cases. Intermittent use of diuretics may be helpful. If lymphangitis, cellulitis and ulceration are present every effort must be made to reduce oedema; the infection is treated by appropriate antibiotics and local application of a non-adherent (oily) dressing. Hereditary lymphoedema, if severely disabling, is best treated by superficial lymphangiectomy, the oedematous subcutaneous tissue being removed and the muscles covered with free skin grafts.

Prognosis

Lymphoedema is a chronic disorder which increases gradually or by successive attacks according to the aetiology. Although partial remissions occur in the early stages, irreversible changes due to inflammation and connective tissue thickening eventually lead to permanent enlargement of the limb. Recurrent attacks of cellulitis and ulceration are then liable to aggravate the symptoms still further.

ARTERIAL ANEURYSM

An aneurysm is a permanent dilatation of an artery due to destruction of its wall. Since the strength of the arterial wall lies in the muscular or musculo-elastic tissue of the medial coat the causes of aneurysm formation are pathological lesions affecting the media. These may be congenital, traumatic, inflammatory or degenerative.

Congenital aneurysm is almost entirely confined to the arteries at the base of the brain. The cause is a congenital defect of the media, leading to the formation of a 'berry' aneurysm usually at some point on the circle of Willis. More than one aneurysm may be present. Pressure effects due to enlargement of the sac, and rupture, leading to intracerebral or subarachnoid haemorrhage, are responsible for the various clinical manifestations [see Section 15]. The so-called cirsoid aneurysm is a developmental anomaly in which greatly dilated arteriovenous communications form a large vascular tumour, particularly in the brain.

Traumatic aneurysm. This results from a penetrating injury, commonly a gunshot wound, which injures a main artery and gives rise to aneurysmal swelling. The sac may connect with the neighbouring vein, producing a so-called arteriovenous aneurysm. The main arteries of the limbs, especially the popliteal, are most frequently affected. A bruit is commonly heard over the sac. If an arteriovenous fistula is large, the pulse may be collapsing and increased cardiac output leads to cardiac enlargement. Treatment lies in closing the anastomosis and restoring continuity of the artery by local excision or grafting.

Inflammatory causes. The common inflammations producing aneurysms are syphilis, bacterial endocarditis and polyarteritis nodosa. The last may affect any artery, particularly the abdominal branches of the aorta, the cerebral and the limb arteries [see Section 4]. Syphilitic aneurysms are almost entirely confined to the aorta and its large branches [p. 788]. Mycotic aneurysms in bacterial endocarditis are due to blockage of arteries by infected emboli arising from valvular vegetations. The femoral, brachial, retinal and cerebral arteries are particularly affected. Rupture of the last causes subarachnoid haemorrhage. Mycotic aneurysms are becoming less common as a result of antibiotic therapy but may still arise when the causative organism is resistant to antibiotic control. Rupture of a mycotic aneurysm in a limb vessel may produce a large intramuscular haematoma, followed by great pain and swelling of the limb and even gangrene. Surgical release of tension by evacuation of clot may be necessary.

Degenerative lesions causing arterial aneurysms are atheroma and mucoid degeneration of the media. Medial degeneration is the usual cause of dissecting aneurysm. Atheroma is the common cause of aneurysmal dilatation of peripheral arteries. The aorta may be affected at any site but particularly in the abdominal segment below the origin of the renal arteries. The subclavian, common femoral and popliteal are the most frequent peripheral sites of aneurysmal dilatation. Complications at any site include rupture, thrombosis and peripheral embolism.

ABDOMINAL AORTIC ANEURYSM

As indicated above the common cause is atherosclerosis and the common site below the origin of the renal arteries.

Symptoms

Pain may be felt in the epigastrium or hypogastrium and may be confused with a variety of gastro-intestinal or biliary disorders. It may be referred to the lower dorsal or lumbar spine and radiate to the loin, buttocks or thighs. Anorexia and weight loss occur with an expanding aortic aneurysm and abdominal pulsation may keep the patient awake at night. Acute onset of pain at any site may be due to leakage and may indicate the risk of imminent rupture. Rarely an abdominal aneurysm may bleed into the gastro-intestinal tract, form a fistula communicating with the inferior vena cava, or cause left ureteric obstruction by involvement in peri-aneurysmal fibrosis.

Signs

An expansile pulsating tumour at the site of the abdominal aorta is the diagnostic sign, but must be distinguished from a tortuous abdominal aorta in a thin lordotic subject, and from transmitted pulsation in a tumour overlying the aorta. Associated aneurysms in peripheral arteries should be looked for.

Abdominal X-ray, including a lateral film, may show the typical curvilinear calcified shadow outlining the margin of the aneurysm. Intravenous pyelography should always be performed, but angiography is rarely necessary.

Treatment

The most successful surgical procedure is aneurysmectomy with synthetic graft-replacement. For elective surgery, operative mortality is 6–18 per cent., whereas emergency surgery when rupture has occurred carries a mortality of 35–85 per cent.

Prognosis

This is greatly influenced by the fact that abdominal aortic aneurysm is only one manifestation of a generalized atherosclerosis which may lead to fatal cerebral and cardiac complications. A variety of studies suggest a five-year survival after diagnosis and before rupture of 17–36 per cent. in untreated cases. Size of the aneurysm is more important, and where this is over 7 cm. diameter surgical treatment is indicated unless there are other serious complications.

DISSECTING ANEURYSM OF THE AORTA

Incidence

Dissecting aneurysm is a not uncommon cause of sudden death. The subjects are almost always elderly and the incidence is reported to be five times as high in men as in women.

Aetiology and Pathology

The primary cause is mucoid degeneration of the media. This is common in Marfan's syndrome (arachnodactyly) and accounts for the relatively high incidence of dissecting aneurysms in this condition. Rarely it is a complication of pregnancy. Atheroma is invariably present but is not itself a cause of the dissection; other pathological changes in the aorta have been described. Hypertension is a predisposing factor. The dissection occurs down the centre of the medial coat, forming a false channel between the two layers. The tear usually starts in the ascending aorta, less commonly in the descending thoracic or abdominal aorta. By rapid extension the aneurysm may reach the bifurcation of the aorta, occluding one or both renal arteries *en route*. Extension towards the heart may lead to rupture into the pericardium and sudden death. External rupture into the mediastinal or retroperitoneal tissues is less common. Very rarely the dissection may be arrested before any main arteries are involved and over a period of years there may be recurrent attacks. In most cases, however, death occurs in the first attack.

Symptoms

The common presenting symptom is agonizing pain in the abdomen, chest or back together with shock. The pain is persistent and may change in site as the dissection spreads. Obstruction of the renal vessels leads to pain in the loins and anuria. Occlusion of one or both common iliac arteries produces pain, numbness or coldness of the affected extremity. The patient is grey and collapsed, the pulse rapid and small, but the blood pressure is often maintained, hypertension being present in many cases. Involvement of the carotid or spinal arteries may produce paralyses, or the limbs may be pulseless and cold due to arterial obstruction. Dissection in the region of the aortic valve may interfere with its function, and the sudden appearance of basal systolic or early diastolic murmurs is most suggestive. There may be some degree of improvement for a few hours, after which rupture into the pericardium may lead to a sudden attack of pain in the chest and fatal collapse. It is impossible to determine what proportion of cases die suddenly, for in many of these the diagnosis is never made. In those surviving several hours and coming under medical care, some three-quarters succumb in two weeks and 90 per cent. in the first year.

Diagnosis

The condition is most commonly mistaken for coronary thrombosis or an acute abdominal emergency such as perforation of a peptic ulcer. Diagnosis can only be made with certainty if signs of occlusion of specific arteries, e.g. renal, femoral, spinal or carotid can be detected. More often the diagnosis may be suspected in life but is only confirmed *post mortem*. In patients surviving the acute attack of pain, the persistence of hypertension, a high sedimentation rate and leucocytosis, together with a rapid fall in haemoglobin, strongly suggest the diagnosis. There may be irregular persistent fever.

Treatment

Treatment is largely symptomatic, but there is a limited place for surgery in selected cases.

REFERENCE

HIRST, A. E., JOHNS, V. J., and KIME, S. W. (1958) Dissecting aneurysm of the aorta, *Medicine* (*Baltimore*), 37, 217.

ARTERIOVENOUS FISTULA

Definition

An abnormal arteriovenous communication, bypassing or replacing the normal capillary circulation in some area of the body.

Aetiology

Arteriovenous fistula may be congenital or acquired. The acquired form is almost invariably traumatic and is caused by the opening of an artery into a vein by a penetrating wound. Surgical trauma is occasionally the cause; aorto-caval shunts have followed operations for prolapsed intervertebral disc. Intravenous rupture of an aneurysm may very occasionally produce a fistula.

Pathology

Traumatic shunts usually involve a single artery and vein. Dilatation of both artery and vein results, and there may be an aneurysm at the site of communication. Congenital fistulae more often lead to multiple small vessel communications which are known by a variety of names, including cirsoid aneurysm, cavernous haemangioma, plexiform angioma and aneurysmal varix. Whilst the limb vessels are the commonest site in both cases, fistulae may occur in any organ, especially brain, lung, kidney and bones. The effects are both structural and functional. Structural changes include dilatation of the veins, varicose ulceration, oedema, and increased size of the limb, partly due to increased growth in congenital lesions or in traumatic fistulae arising before puberty. Gangrene of the extremities may occur. Functional changes are the result of increased blood flow through the fistula due to lowered resistance. The skin temperature rises, and if the communication is large enough, diastolic pressure falls, the pulse is collapsing and cardiac output is increased, with enlargement of the heart due to both dilatation and hypertrophy. Bacterial endarteritis at the site is a rare complication.

Symptoms

These will be obvious from the above pathological changes and their nature will depend on the site of the fistula. The lower limb is the usual site and increased length and girth, venous distension, ulceration, oedema and raised skin temperature may be present. The classical signs are a palpable thrill and loud bruit at the site of the fistula, the latter being continuous but with systolic accentuation. Occlusion of the fistula leads to marked slowing of the pulse and rise in diastolic pressure. Collapsing pulse and cardiac enlargement are found only with large arteriovenous shunts.

Diagnosis

Arteriovenous fistula will be suspected when the above vascular and trophic changes occur in a limb following a penetrating wound, or in the absence of trauma, develop during growth. The discovery of a thrill and bruit are diagnostic. Venous pressure will be raised in the limb as will the oxygen saturation of the venous blood. With large fistulae blood volume is increased. Arteriography will demonstrate the site, extent and character of the arteriovenous communication.

Treatment

Traumatic fistulae involving a single vascular shunt should be excised at an interval after the injury sufficient to allow collateral vessels to open up. Congenital fistulae are usually multiple and are then rarely benefited by attempts at excision or ligation. Amputation may be necessary if ulceration does not respond to conservative measures or if gangrene supervenes.

CLIFFORD WILSON

SECTION 9

DISEASES OF THE RESPIRATORY TRACT

DISEASES OF THE NOSE AND NASOPHARYNX

EPISTAXIS

Aetiology

The causes are classified as (1) local and (2) general. Local causes include trauma, acute infection, ulceration which may be due to non-specific or specific infection or to neoplasm, separation of crusts as in rhinitis sicca or atrophic rhinitis, and hereditary haemorrhagic telangiectasia.

General causes include hypertension, venous congestion of the head and neck from any cause, bleeding diseases and leukaemia. It often occurs during the prodromal stages of any of the acute infectious fevers and may rarely be due to overdosage with drugs, such as quinine or salicylates.

In the majority of epistaxes the bleeding arises from Little's or Kiesselbach's area on the front of the septum just beyond the mucocutaneous junction of the nasal vestibule.

In children and young adults trauma or repeated bleeding from dilated vessels in Little's area are the common causes. In later life the majority of severe haemorrhages are due to hypertension. Hereditary haemorrhagic telangiectasia causes severe repeated epistaxes which are difficult to control and many of these patients eventually die from the effects of an epistaxis or intestinal haemorrhage.

Treatment

Severe epistaxis should always be treated, though it is of comparatively little importance in healthy young people. In older patients with hypertension the loss of blood may be beneficial, but the occurrence is so distressing and alarming to the patient that steps must be taken to stop the bleeding. The patient should be sat upright bending slightly forwards over a bowl and should breathe through the open mouth. If the end of the nose is firmly squeezed and the pressure maintained for five minutes, bleeding from Little's area will be controlled. If bleeding persists after this time the anterior two-thirds of the affected nostril should be firmly packed with well-lubricated ribbon gauze (B.I.P.P. gauze is suitable for the purpose). Sedation is important as many epistaxes are perpetuated by the patient's alarmed and excited state. Occasionally blood transfusion is also required. These measures control the great majority of epistaxes but a few persistent cases may require postnasal packing or even ligation of the anterior ethmoidal or maxillary arteries. A postnasal pack demands antibiotic cover to reduce the risk of otitis media and it should never be left *in situ* longer than two days.

Recurrent epistaxes should always arouse suspicions of an underlying bleeding disease or blood condition such as leukaemia, but if the bleeding is arising from dilated vessels in Little's area it can be stopped by electric cauterization.

Treatment with high dosages of sex hormones, which causes squamous metaplasia of the nasal mucosa, has reduced nasal bleeding in some cases of hereditary haemorrhagic telangiectasia.

ALLERGIC AND VASOMOTOR RHINITIS

Although a distinction is usually drawn between these two conditions, allergic rhinitis being attributed to a specific sensitivity reaction and vasomotor rhinitis to vasomotor imbalance in the blood vessels of the nasal mucosa, the symptomatology of the conditions is similar. Both produce the triad of nasal obstruction, bouts of sneezing and excess nasal discharge which is usually watery, but occasionally thick and mucoid. Some patients also suffer from conjunctival irritation with itching and watering of the eyes. On examination the nasal mucosa is oedematous and often pallid or slightly bluish in colour and is coated with excess secretion. Mucous polypi may be present in the middle meatus and if sinus infection complicates the picture mucopus will be visible in the middle meatus and postnasal space. Transillumination of the sinuses is often poor and X-rays usually show thickening of their lining membranes. Other allergic conditions, particularly asthma, may be present. There may be an excess of eosinophils in nasal smears and in the blood.

The disease can commence at any age. Infants who suffer from eczema often develop rhinitis in childhood, but in these patients the condition usually improves in early adult life. Males and females are equally affected. Causative factors include a hereditary and racial tendency, a specific allergy, hormonal and vasomotor imbalance, and psychosomatic effects. More than one of these factors may be present in a particular case.

An allergic tendency is hereditary and Jews seem particularly susceptible.

Specific allergy is usually due to sensitization of the nasal mucosa to some inhalant allergen. The allergen-antibody reaction occurs in the mucosa and causes oedema, excess secretion and eosinophil concentration. The commonest and best example of this is pollenosis or hay fever where the patient only gets symptoms during the pollen season. If the condition is perennial it may be due to sensitivity to such things as house dust, mould spores, animal hair or feathers and to many other inhaled substances which have been incriminated in various patients. Rarely a food or bacterial allergy is the basic cause of the condition.

Hormonal imbalance may cause these symptoms. They are manifested in some patients during pregnancy and the menopause and occur as side-effects with some contraceptive pills, particularly those containing norethisterone. The symptoms in pregnancy usually disappear within a few hours of delivery.

Direct upset of the vasomotor control of the nasal blood vessels sometimes follows cervical sympathectomy and results in nasal congestion and excess secretion. Very troublesome nasal obstruction can complicate hypotensive medication.

Finally emotional causes are obviously present in some cases where symptoms are initiated, or exacerbated, by stress.

Investigation and Treatment

Satisfactory investigation of these patients is time-consuming and requires detailed history taking, skin-testing, blood examinations and sinus X-rays; it is best conducted at a separate clinic. If a specific allergy is discovered avoidance of the allergen is the best treatment, but this is rarely practicable. Mild and intermittent symptoms can be controlled with antihistamines and, as the individual response to these drugs is variable, experimentation with several different compounds may be necessary to discover the one most suitable for a particular patient. Improved symptomatic relief is obtained in many cases when ephedrine is combined with the antihistamine. When the symptoms are severe, if not controlled by antihistamines, desensitization to the specific allergen may be attempted and is most likely to be successful in pollenosis cases. Severe cases with associated asthma will be improved by steroid therapy.

Correction of any hormonal imbalance usually produces a rapid improvement in the nasal condition.

Surgical measures, include removal of polypi and drainage of infected sinuses. Submucosal diathermy of the inferior turbinates gives long-lasting relief in cases of persistent nasal oedema.

Eye symptoms may be controlled by using a simple lotion such as Compound Zinc Sulphate Eye Lotion, B.P.C.

ACUTE SINUSITIS

Aetiology

Transient inflammation of the lining of the nasal sinuses occurs in most acute infections of the upper respiratory tract. If the infection is severe and the host's resistance inadequate, one or more sinuses may become acutely inflamed. Oedema of the lining membrane narrows the ostium and the ciliary activity may fail to clear the sinus of inflammatory exudate. If the ostium becomes completely blocked, pus collects under pressure in the sinus. The disease may also result from bathing in 'fresh' water when infected material is driven into a sinus and this often causes especially acute and dangerous frontal sinusitis.

Symptoms

Mild symptoms are a feeling of heaviness in the face and head, made worse by bending forwards, and copious nasal discharge. If the ostium is blocked the pain becomes intense and continuous while the nasal discharge diminishes. Acute antral infection often causes generalized toothache in the upper jaw on the affected side and incorrect diagnosis can lead to the extraction of healthy teeth. Ethmoid and frontal sinusitis cause pain above, around and behind the eye and in severe infections, oedema of the lids may completely close the eye.

On examination there is tenderness over the inflamed sinus and pus can usually be seen in the middle meatus of the affected side and in the postnasal space. Transillumination of the sinus is poor and X-rays show thickening of the lining membrane and either a fluid level or, if the ostium is blocked, complete opacity.

Complications

Although not common these may be dangerous and especially in ethmoidal and frontal sinusitis which can lead to osteomyelitis of the frontal bone, meningitis, cerebral abscess, orbital cellulitis or cavernous sinus thrombosis. Gross oedema of the lids, restricted ocular movements and any impairment of vision are danger signs, while osteomyelitis of the frontal bone produces a tender fluctuant swelling of the forehead. It is important to realize that the great majority of infections of the orbit originate in the nasal sinuses.

Treatment

If the patient rests indoors, uses a nasal decongestant spray or drops such as ephedrine hydrochloride, 0·5 per cent. in normal saline solution every four hours, and follows this 15 minutes later with a steam inhalation, most infections quickly subside. Analgesics are required in most cases to allow proper rest, but antibiotics should be reserved for severe cases and those in which complications are suspected. Penicillin is the first choice unless there is some special contra-indication to its use.

Antral infections which fail to respond to these measures after 5 days' adequate treatment, require puncture and lavage of the sinus under local anaesthesia and this should be repeated every 5–7 days until the infection resolves. In resistant frontal infections the floor of the sinus should be trephined and a tightly fitting polythene tube inserted through which the sinus is washed out thrice daily until the fluid passes easily into the nose, indicating reopening of the frontonasal duct.

CHRONIC SINUSITIS

Aetiology

This follows an acute sinus infection which fails to resolve and the cause of failure is usually some anatomical or pathological narrowing of the middle meatus which prevents adequate drainage. Common causes of such narrowing are septal deviations, enlargement of the middle turbinate, chronic generalized oedema of the nasal mucosa due to allergic or vasomotor rhinitis and mucous polypi. Chronic frontal sinusitis is usually secondary to antral or ethmoidal infection and a dental abscess can cause a particularly severe and foul infection of the maxillary antrum.

Symptoms and Complications

Local symptoms are often slight so that the disease can easily be overlooked. There is intermittent nasal obstruction and discharge with a feeling of dullness or heaviness in the face and head. These symptoms are made worse by a coryza and the patient often suffers from nasal catarrh for a long time after each cold. Recurrent or chronic tonsillitis, pharyngitis or laryngitis is often the complaint which makes the patient seek medical advice and sinus infection should always be looked for in such cases. Chronic sinusitis is often present in bronchiectasis and chronic bronchitis.

There is no tenderness over the sinus as in acute infection and nasal examination often shows no obvious infection but will reveal the narrowing of the middle meatus. X-rays are particularly useful in revealing the condition and the state of the lining membrane.

Spread to the orbit or anterior cranial fossa may occur as in acute infections.

Treatment

This is mainly surgical and is directed in the first instance towards improving the natural drainage route. Straightening of the nasal septum, amputation of an enlarged turbinate and the removal of polypi may be necessary and suitable treatment for any allergic or vasomotor rhinitis is important as this is a common underlying cause of chronic sinusitis. Any dental abscess must be drained.

Should the sinus fail to recover in spite of these measures surgical drainage will be required either by an intranasal or external approach. Antibiotic treatment is rarely effective in this condition because the basic cause is poor drainage.

ADENOIDS

Aetiology and Pathology

The nasopharyngeal tonsil or adenoids is a collection of lymphoid tissue on the posterior wall and roof of the nasopharynx, which normally atrophies and disappears in early adult life. Hypertrophy and infection of this lymphoid tissue commonly occurs during childhood as a result of repeated infection of the upper respiratory tract. In some children this enlargement becomes permanent with resultant deleterious effects on the nasal passages, middle ears, pharynx and chest. Chronic hypertrophy and recurrent infection of the tonsils often, but not invariably, accompanies these adenoid changes.

Symptoms

The child with a large pad of infected adenoids partially, or in some cases totally, blocking his post-nasal airway suffers from nasal obstruction and consequent mouth breathing. There is chronic nasal discharge and often associated sinusitis and the child finds it difficult to blow his nose satisfactorily. Snoring and nocturnal cough are common and in some cases the voice becomes slightly hoarse with a thick 'nasal' intonation. There is usually marked cervical lymphadenitis. Some of the most serious direct consequences of enlarged adenoids are those affecting the middle ear cleft. While recurrent acute otitis media is not uncommon, less dramatic but important effects result from interference with the proper function of the Eustachian tube. These are intermittent earache, the collection of seromucinous fluid in the middle ear and variable conduction deafness. In such children the tympanic membranes may appear pink or dull, retracted or slightly full, but even when fluid is present in the middle ear the changes in the drum may be slight compared to the degree of deafness. Persistent or recurrent bronchitis may be aggravated by adenoids. Enlarged adenoids are present in a few infants shortly after birth and can cause serious feeding difficulties by interfering with sucking. Similar feeding difficulties arise in the rare condition of bilateral congenital choanal atresia. In older children adenoids, especially when associated with enlarged tonsils, interfere with the child's general development. The appetite is poor and the child eats slowly.

Disturbed sleep, the discomfort of nasal obstruction and sinusitis and impaired hearing make the child appear physically and mentally slow and unresponsive.

Adenoids have also been described as causing gastro-intestinal upsets, enuresis, night terrors and stammering but their aetiological role in these conditions, which are rarely improved by adenoidectomy, is dubious.

Diagnosis

Adenoids can be seen on mirror inspection of the postnasal space and placid children readily permit this examination. In others soft tissue radiography will demonstrate the condition or the postnasal space can be palpated under anaesthesia and if the adenoids are grossly enlarged they can be removed.

Treatment

A damp climate, poor nutrition and overcrowding all aggravate the condition so that children from poor homes who have suffered several severe upper respiratory tract infections during the winter benefit considerably from a few weeks of seaside convalescence. Others will be helped if a period of open air schooling can be arranged for them.

Local medication is rarely helpful but in mild cases instillation of silver proteinate, 5 per cent. solution, three drops into each nostril at night, for ten days may cause regression of the adenoids. When an allergic background is suspected diphenhydramime hydrochloride as an elixir in suitable dosage at nights for one month may produce a marked improvement.

When the enlargement is persistent and is producing marked effects and especially if the middle ear cleft is affected, then adenoid currettage is indicated. In most cases this is combined with removal of the tonsils and if the maxillary antra are infected they should be washed out at the same time. Postoperatively these children often benefit from a course of breathing exercises to correct their habit of mouth breathing and to improve their physique.

MALIGNANT TUMOURS OF THE NASOPHARYNX

Pathology

Most varieties of malignant neoplasms as well as deposits of the reticuloses may occur in the nasopharynx but the majority of the growths are squamous-cell carcinomata, sarcomata or lympho-epitheliomata.

Symptoms

Malignant disease in the postnasal space is rare in this country but is one of the commonest neoplasms affecting the Chinese race. The presentation can be misleading because the initial symptoms are more likely to be in the ear, eye or neck than in the nose. The most common presenting symptom is enlargement of the upper deep cervical lymph nodes and a growth in the postnasal space should always be suspected when there is malignant disease of these glands without an obvious primary source. These growths may also cause pain or anaesthesia in one or more divisions of the trigeminal nerve and obstruction of the Eustachian tubes with conductive deafness. Invasion of the skull base, usually via the foramen lacerum, may cause paralysis of the external ocular muscles. Local effects are nasal obstruction and epistaxis and impaired mobility of the palate.

Treatment

This is mainly by radiotherapy and the prognosis is poor, the over-all cure rate being less than 35 per cent.

DISEASES OF THE LARYNX

ACUTE LARYNGITIS

Aetiology

This affection most often occurs during the course of a cold, the inflammation spreading downwards from the nose and nasopharynx. Over-use of the voice will precipitate an attack, especially if voice production is faulty. It arises in the course of acute infectious fevers such as influenza, measles or scarlatina. Predisposing causes are nasal obstruction, infection of sinuses, tonsils or teeth and sedentary occupations in ill-ventilated overheated rooms. Acute laryngitis of a non-tuberculous nature is not uncommon in patients with pulmonary tuberculosis.

Symptoms

The symptoms consist of hoarseness, local discomfort varying from dryness or tickling to a burning sensation or actual pain, and irritating cough. There is little expectoration, unless the trachea and bronchi are involved. At the onset there may be slight feverishness and malaise. The degree of hoarseness is by no means proportionate to the objective appearances; the voice may be quite good in cases of decided hyperaemia, and may be completely lost when little abnormal is to be seen. A muscular man may retain a strong voice with a degree of inflammation which would render a weakly woman almost aphonic—indeed some women lose the voice with every slight cold, so that it becomes difficult to differentiate between laryngeal catarrh and 'functional aphonia'. On the other hand, in some voice-users redness of the cords appears to be the normal condition and causes no interference with function. This variable effect on the voice is to be observed in all forms of laryngeal disease. In children, acute laryngitis is a serious affection. They show a far greater tendency to oedema and to spasm and, as the glottis is not only absolutely but relatively smaller than in adults, dangerous dyspnoea may ensue with great rapidity. The larynx is reddened, and this is most obvious on the parts usually pale—the epiglottis and vocal cords, the vessels on the former being unduly prominent. The cords may be red or salmon pink, or may merely have lost their bright pearly lustre. A small amount of mucous secretion is generally present, but there are no large accumulations or strings of mucus, such as are seen in chronic laryngitis.

Treatment

The patient should be confined to a warm, well-ventilated room, preferably in bed, and must not attempt to use the voice. Steam inhalations are of value and may be scented with pine. The correct temperature of water is obtained by mixing boiling water 2 parts with cold tap water as 1 part. The patient must not go outside for at least an hour after the inhalation. If cough is severe it should be controlled by a simple linctus to reduce the traumatic effect on the larynx. A suitable antibiotic should be administered if the condition fails to respond to the above measures after 2 days' treatment, or it may be given initially where there is a marked general reaction and chest infection.

OEDEMATOUS LARYNGITIS

Synonym. Oedema of the larynx.

Aetiology

Oedema of the larynx is a pathological condition due to a variety of causes. Non-inflammatory oedema may be mentioned here for the sake of completeness; it occurs, though rarely, as part of the general anasarca of renal or cardiac disease. Angioneurotic oedema sometimes occurs in the larynx, in which event it produces rapid and sometimes fatal dyspnoea. The swelling which occasionally results from administration of potassium iodide in susceptible subjects may be placed in the same category.

Inflammatory oedema seldom results in adults from a simple catarrh, but it may do so in children; it more often occurs as part of an acute infection of the pharynx, trachea and bronchi, 'acute fulminating laryngotracheobronchitis' [p. 841]. Oedema may follow various forms of trauma, the drinking of corrosive poisons, inhalations of irritating vapours such as the poison gases of warfare, the lodgment of foreign bodies or rough or unduly prolonged bronchoscopy. Scalding, from attempts to drink from a kettle-spout, is a common cause among children. In other cases it is a sequel of typhoid fever, pneumonia, scarlet fever or smallpox, and is a local complication of syphilitic, tuberculous, cancerous or traumatic ulceration. Persistent oedema is sometimes a sequel of X-irradiation of the larynx.

Symptoms

If part of a septic pharyngolaryngitis, the general symptoms are severe. The chief local symptom is dyspnoea with inspiratory stridor and the associated symptoms of asphyxiation; there is hoarseness or aphonia, local discomfort and tenderness and sometimes dysphagia. The aryepiglottic folds are enormously swollen, appearing as pale or purple translucent flask-shaped masses; if the epiglottis is oedematous it forms a sausage-shaped swelling of the same appearance. The mucosa of the vocal cords is too adherent to permit much swelling, and 'oedema of the glottis' is therefore a misnomer. The subglottic region is lax and may become swollen; indeed, the oedema may be confined to this region and then appears as a red swelling below each vocal cord. In children oedema may be inferred from the steadily increasing dyspnoea without the rapid increase and decrease typical of spasmodic laryngitis.

Treatment

Patients should be nursed in a semi-sitting position. In slight cases, the swelling may be reduced by sucking ice and by the application of an ice-bag to the neck; the latter is inadmissible in young children. A spray of adrenaline, 1 in 1000, may be used. If the oedema is due to streptococcal infection, penicillin in full dosage should be administered immediately.

Angioneurotic oedema usually responds to antihistamines and adrenaline sprays but if necessary steroid therapy can also be given. Large doses of bicarbonate of soda are recommended for the oedema produced by iodides. In a few cases tracheostomy is necessary and this should be performed before respiratory embarrassment is too great. Introduction of an endotracheal tube can be used to relieve respiratory obstruction but should not be left *in situ* longer than 2 days.

STRIDOR IN INFANTS

This alarming symptom is common in infancy and may arise from a variety of causes, the most important of which are considered below in clinical groups.

CONSTANT STRIDOR FROM BIRTH

This is likely to be due to a congenital abnormality of the larynx and direct laryngoscopy may be necessary to establish the exact cause.

Laryngeal webs cause inspiratory and expiratory stridor and occasionally are large enough to require surgical treatment; the stridor improves as the child grows and the web becomes smaller relative to the increased size of the larynx.

Cysts of the aryepiglottic fold cause inspiratory stridor and should be incised and drained via the direct laryngoscope.

STRIDOR ASSOCIATED WITH EXERTION

Some infants whose respiration is quiet at rest, develop stridor, mainly inspiratory, when crying or otherwise exerting themselves. The symptom becomes worse during any respiratory infection and causes much concern.

On direct inspection the larynx shows the usual infantile appearances in exaggerated form. The epiglottis is folded upon itself so that the two halves are almost touching while the aryepiglottic folds are tall and flaccid. As a result the laryngeal orifice is narrower than normal at rest and on inspiration the aryepiglottic folds can be seen to be drawn together and the epiglottis is pulled backwards and downwards so that the laryngeal inlet becomes markedly narrowed and stridor results. As the child grows the larynx enlarges and muscular tone improves so that by the age of three years the stridor disappears.

Treatment

Any respiratory infection should be treated with especial care. General measures to improve the child's muscular tone are important and the parents should be reassured regarding the eventual prognosis.

STRIDOR ASSOCIATED WITH ACUTE INFECTION

The infantile larynx is relatively smaller than the adult and is more subject to oedema and spasm during acute inflammation. Consequently stridor (often referred to as 'croup') is not uncommon in infants during any respiratory infection or exanthem. The stridor is usually more noticeable at night and disappears as the infection subsides. Two acute conditions of serious import, namely acute laryngotracheobronchitis and laryngeal diphtheria, are considered separately.

Treatment

The causative infection must be treated energetically and this usually necessitates antibiotic therapy. Humidification of the air in the patient's bedroom will help most cases and a few require nursing in an oxygen tent. Tracheostomy is rarely necessary in these cases.

ACUTE LARYNGOTRACHEOBRONCHITIS

Aetiology

This is a serious infection of the respiratory tract affecting children under two years of age and usually occurring during the winter months. The infection is probably of virus origin with secondary bacterial invasion. The main pathological changes are marked oedema of the larynx, trachea and bronchi and the production of an especially viscid bronchial secretion which is difficult to expel. Many of the smaller bronchi become occluded by a combination of oedema and retained secretions.

Symptoms

The onset is often sudden so that a child may be seriously ill within a few hours of the commencement of the disease. The initial symptoms are general malaise and a weak 'croupy' cough. Respiratory embarrassment soon develops, the breathing is rapid and difficult and the child becomes prostrated. Fever is not marked but the pulse is rapid and weak and there is marked general muscular weakness. Slight cyanosis is followed, as the disease progresses, by a greyish pallor, and increasing toxaemia and anoxia reduce the respiratory efforts to a minimum. If the child survives the critical period during the first 2–3 days of the disease gradual recovery takes place during the next 7–10 days.

Treatment

Where possible these cases should be treated in hospital. Antibiotics must be given in full dosage and, if the child is severely ill when first seen, they should be administered intravenously. The child must be nursed in an oxygen tent with effective humidification of the air inside the tent. Bronchoscopic suction may be necessary to clear the viscid mucus from the lungs. If this has to be repeated often it is less upsetting to the patient to perform tracheostomy whence suction clearance of the trachea and bronchi via a soft rubber catheter can be repeated as often as is necessary.

These cases require much devoted nursing and skilled medical supervision.

LARYNGEAL DIPHTHERIA

This once common lethal disease of childhood is now a rarity but should be considered in any child developing respiratory obstruction during the course of an acute infectious illness, The obstruction is due to the development of diphtheritic membrane in the larynx and trachea and if similar membrane is visible covering the fauces the diagnosis is obvious. Antitoxin should be given immediately the diagnosis is suspected and not withheld pending bacteriological confirmation. Tracheostomy is usually necessary and should be done early rather than late.

CHRONIC LARYNGITIS

Aetiology

The causation is similar to that of acute laryngitis; indeed, chronic laryngitis is often the result of recurrent acute attacks. The principal factors which predispose to chronicity are nasal obstruction and discharges, dental infections and chronic tonsillar sepsis, dusty occupations and lack of fresh air, over-use of the voice and faulty voice production, and the abuse of alcohol or tobacco; consumptives are particularly liable to non-specific catarrhal laryngitis. Almost any cause of general ill health may be included among the predisposing causes.

Symptoms

The only constant symptom is impairment of the voice, which is hoarse, easily tired or, rarely, almost completely lost. It is sometimes weakest when tired in the evening, but is often at its worst on rising in the morning or after a rest. There is frequently a sensation of aching, dryness, tickling or of a lump in the throat, and there is usually some cough, but little expectoration unless the trachea and bronchi are involved.

The objective appearances vary with the severity of the affection. The larynx generally is of a deeper red than usual, and the vocal cords have lost their normal pearly lustre and are pink; they are usually somewhat thickened at the edges, and enlarged vessels may be visible on their surface; the vocal processes are often prominent and may be reddened or show up white against the hyperaemic cord. Strings of sticky secretion may stretch between the cords, or a little globule of mucus may form on the centre of the cord during phonation; adduction is frequently imperfect. When the epiglottis is reddened, its yellow edge stands out clearly and enlarged vessels are visible; the ventricular bands are often swollen so as to hide the outer part of the cords. The mucous membrane in the inter-arytenoid space is seen to be thrown into folds on adduction of the cords, and may form a mass large enough to prevent their complete approximation. The general picture is one of symmetry, a useful point in diagnosis from neoplasm and tuberculous laryngitis.

In a few cases, nearly always males, areas of hyper-keratinization develop on the vocal cords appearing as irregular raised white patches which in rare instances become large enough to cause respiratory difficulty and have to be 'stripped off' with forceps under direct vision. This condition, known as keratosis laryngis, can persist for many years and occasionally malignant change occurs.

Singers' nodes are small swellings on the middle third of the vocal cord which cause peristent hoarseness. Usually bilateral and symmetrical they are organized subepithelial haematomata and result from vocal trauma especially when the voice is over-used during an attack of acute laryngitis. The majority of cases occur during early adult life and both sexes are equally affected.

Treatment

The detection and correction of the aetiological factors are the most important part of treatment. Any constitutional disturbance should receive attention. Over-indulgence in tobacco or alcohol, lack of ventilation and exposure to dust must be considered; with teachers the blackboard chalk is a common source of irritation.

Incorrect voice-production is a factor of great importance and a good speech therapist can often provide substantial help.

Elimination of any infection in the nose, sinuses, tonsils or teeth is an important part of treatment.

Local treatment must begin with rest of the voice which should be absolute in the case of professional voice-users. It may even be necessary to admit a few cases to hospital, to ensure that this part of the treatment is enforced. Where there is much secretion a saline lotion may be used in a spray.

Sodium bicarbonate .	1·5 g.
Sodium borate . .	1·5 g.
Sodium chloride . .	1·5 g.
Glycerin . . .	1·5 ml.
Water to . . .	100 ml.

Direct laryngoscopy and biopsy may be necessary to exclude neoplasm especially in cases of keratosis laryngis. Singers' nodes which fail to resolve with voice rest must be removed via the direct laryngoscope.

TUBERCULOSIS OF THE LARYNX

Tuberculous infection of the larynx is secondary to open pulmonary tuberculosis and is due to direct infection of the laryngeal mucosa by the sputum.

The lesions are either superficial ulcers or patches of granulation tissue. Although the inter-arytenoid region and posterior half of the true and false cords are the common sites for these lesions any part of the larynx may be affected.

The earliest laryngeal symptom is weakness of the voice, which may be attributed to functional aphonia; later there is marked hoarseness with severe pain on swallowing.

The earliest changes visible in the larynx are not very noticeable. These may be patchy redness or injection of the cords or a slightly granular appearance of the inter-arytenoid mucosa. Later, ulceration and granulation tissue become more obvious, but the laryngeal appearances are not diagnostic so that chest X-ray and sputum examination are important investigations in any suspicious case. Nowadays the condition is seen most commonly in the elderly or destitute, in whom it may draw attention to a previously unsuspected pulmonary infection.

Treatment

The laryngeal lesions respond well to antituberculous chemotherapy and usually heal completely after 3–4 weeks' treatment.

PARALYSIS OF THE VOCAL CORDS

Aetiology

This results from a lesion of the vagus or recurrent laryngeal nerve and may be unilateral or bilateral. There are a considerable number of possible causes as the vagus may be affected in the brain stem, the posterior fossa, base of skull or upper cervical region, while the recurrent laryngeal nerve may be affected in the lower cervical region and on the left side in the thorax as well. A lesion in the brain stem, posterior fossa or base of skull is likely to involve other cranial nerves besides the vagus, particularly the ninth, eleventh and twelfth nerves.

The larynx is represented bilaterally at cortical level so that laryngeal paralysis cannot be due to lesions above the nucleus ambiguus. Among the causes of paralysis in the brain stem and posterior fossa are virus or bacterial infections, particularly neurosyphilis, vascular accidents, degenerative and demyelinating diseases and neoplasm. The vagus may also be affected at the base of the skull and in the upper deep cervical region by penetrating wounds or neoplasms.

Either recurrent laryngeal nerve may be affected in the neck by penetrating wounds, thyroid surgery and thyroid or other tumours, while the left recurrent may be damaged in the thorax by bronchial or oesophageal carcinoma, mediastinal tumours or aneurysm.

The largest single group of cases are described as idiopathic paralysis. If carefully followed up many of these recover full function and it is assumed that they are due to peripheral neuritis or anterior poliomyelitis.

Effects of Unilateral Paralysis

On mirror examination the paralysed cord can be seen lying immobile just lateral to the midline in the paramedian position. The arytenoid cartilage on the affected side frequently becomes displaced anteriorly and the vocal process and posterior attachment of the cord lie at a lower level than on the normal side. On phonation there will be a gap between the cords making the voice weak and giving it a characteristic 'break'.

When the vagus is involved above the origin of the superior laryngeal nerve there is also anaesthesia of the laryngeal opening on the affected side, and a tendency to a 'spilling over' of fluids into the trachea, which however improves with time. The superior laryngeal nerve supplies the cricothyroid muscle which tenses the vocal cord. Removal of this tensor effect makes the paralysed cord more flaccid than it is in recurrent nerve paralysis.

Gradually the normal cord compensates so that on phonation it crosses the midline and approximates closely to the paralysed cord and the voice becomes stronger. The airway is adequate except in extreme exertion.

Effects of Bilateral Paralysis

Both cords lie immobile near the midline and the airway is restricted especially on inspiration when the paralysed cords tend to be drawn together. The degree of respiratory embarrassment is variable, being worst in cases of bilateral recurrent nerve paralysis. Here the paralysed cords are still tensed by the cricothyroid muscles and therefore lie nearer the midline than is the case in bilateral lesions of the vagus or its nuclei when the cricothyroids are also paralysed. The 'glottic chink' enlarges in some of these cases as the intrinsic muscles of the larynx atrophy and become fibrosed. For this reason no attempt to enlarge the airway by surgery should be made until eighteen months or more after the onset of paralysis for the eventual position of the cords may provide an adequate airway. Speech is usually adequate in these cases.

Bilateral lesions of the vagus above the origin of the superior laryngeal nerve are fortunately rare because they cause paralysis of the pharynx and larynx and anaesthesia of the laryngeal orifice with constant 'spill over' into the trachea. Both cords are immobile and 'flaccid' due to lack of cricothyroid tensing effect so the voice is weak and the airway adequate for a quiet existence.

Treatment

The cause of the paralysis should be treated or removed as adequately as possible. In many cases there is no recovery of movement. Speech therapy may improve compensation by the normal cord during phonation in cases of unilateral paralysis. Some cases of bilateral paralysis have an adequate airway but many will require a tracheostomy which may have to be permanent but this is not a great disability providing a speaking valve is fitted to the inner tube. Several types of operation are practised to enlarge the laryngeal airway in cases of bilateral paralysis.

FUNCTIONAL APHONIA

This condition usually afflicts young or middle-aged women and is particularly common at the menopause. The patient either loses the power of speech completely or can only communicate in a weak whisper. However, the cough remains normal thus showing that voluntary closure of the cords is still possible.

Mirror examination shows full movement of the cords on coughing but on phonation adduction either does not occur at all or the cords are drawn tightly together and then suddenly abducted without any sound being produced.

While the condition may originate during an acute respiratory infection the basic cause is psychological. There is usually some real or imagined social worry and if this can be corrected, or the patient's anxiety relieved by a sympathetic listener, the voice usually returns to normal. There is a tendency for the condition to recur if further worries arise.

Treatment

In the first instance reassurance that no serious disease is present and that the voice will certainly return may be all that is necessary. Speech therapy is effective in most cases but if this fails it is best to obtain psychiatric advice.

CARCINOMA OF THE LARYNX

Middle-aged or elderly men are the usual victims. In many cases there is no obvious causative factor but it may develop in a larynx which is already the site of chronic inflammation and the early diagnosis of malignant change may be particularly difficult in these cases.

Histologically these growths are squamous cell carcinomata with wide variations in their degree of differentiation.

The commonest site of origin is the anterior half of one vocal cord but subglottic and supraglottic growths also occur.

The dominant symptom is hoarseness of the voice and it is fortunate that this occurs early in all carcinomata of the vocal cord itself. It is a later symptom in subglottic and supraglottic growths. Therefore, hoarseness in an adult which lasts longer than six weeks with adequate treatment demands skilled laryngeal examination. Early symptoms in supraglottic growths are slight discomfort in the throat made worse on swallowing, repeated 'clearing' of the throat, and 'plumminess' of the voice.

As the growth develops it causes fixation of the affected half of the larynx and eventually there will be respiratory obstruction. Pain in the ear is another late symptom. Growths of the vocal cord only metastasize to the cervical lymph nodes at a late stage in the disease but in subglottic, and especially supraglottic, growths, it is an earlier feature and a lump in the neck may be the presenting symptom.

Mirror examination reveals the growth as an ulcer, wart or cauliflower mass and the diagnosis is confirmed by endoscopy and biopsy.

Treatment

The majority of cases are treated initially by radiotherapy. This cures 80 per cent. of early cordal cancers with return of normal function. Advanced cordal cancers and subglottic and supraglottic growths do not respond so well to radiotherapy. Cases in which radiotherapy fails or cases which are very advanced when first seen are usually treated surgically by total laryngectomy which is often combined with a block dissection of the neck on the affected side.

REFERENCE

Williams, R. G. (1959) Idiopathic recurrent laryngeal nerve paralysis, *J. Laryng.*, **73**, 161.

R. F. McNab Jones

DISEASES OF THE LUNGS AND BRONCHI. GENERAL CONSIDERATIONS

LUNG STRUCTURE

The lungs comprise two main zones—the first or *conducting zone* in which gas and blood are transported to and from the second or *respiratory zone*, where a gaseous interchange takes place between the air in the alveolus and the blood in the alveolar capillary. These two zones are separated by a small transition zone where conducting and respiratory elements are mixed. The conducting zone consists of an irregular dichotomous branching system of air passages from the trachea to the terminal bronchiolus. This zone also carries the branches of the pulmonary artery and veins.

The Conducting Zone

The trachea and main bronchi are supported by 'C' shaped bands of cartilage open posteriorly. The gap is spanned by muscle and dense longitudinal elastic strands. As the main bronchi enter the lung, the cartilagenous plates become irregular in shape and together with muscle they surround the large intrapulmonary bronchi. The main bronchi divide into lobar branches to supply the lobes of the lung of which there are three on the right and two on the left and then the segmental branches [Fig. 52a] and the lung segments which they supply [Fig. 52b]. Within the segments the airways diminish in size at each division, those pursuing the longest course to the periphery are called axial or conducting pathways and from them arise the lateral or distributing pathways. The number of branches or generations of airways from the segmental hilum to the periphery varies in different parts of the lung from fifteen to twenty-five [Fig. 53].

Bronchi are defined as airways proximal to the last

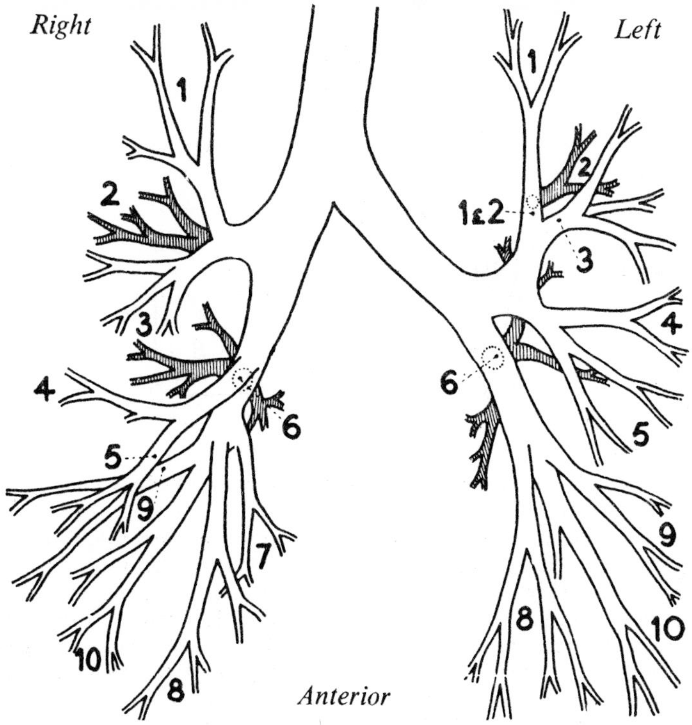

UPPER LOBE
1. Apical segment
2. Posterior segment
3. Anterior segment

Right	*Left*
MIDDLE LOBE	LINGULA
4. Lateral segment	4. Superior segment
5. Medial segment	5. Inferior segment

LOWER LOBE

Right	*Left*
6. Apical segment	6. Apical segment
7. Medial basal (cardiac)	
8. Anterior basal segment	8. Anterior basal segment
9. Lateral basal segment	9. Lateral basal segment
10. Posterior basal segment	10. Posterior basal segment

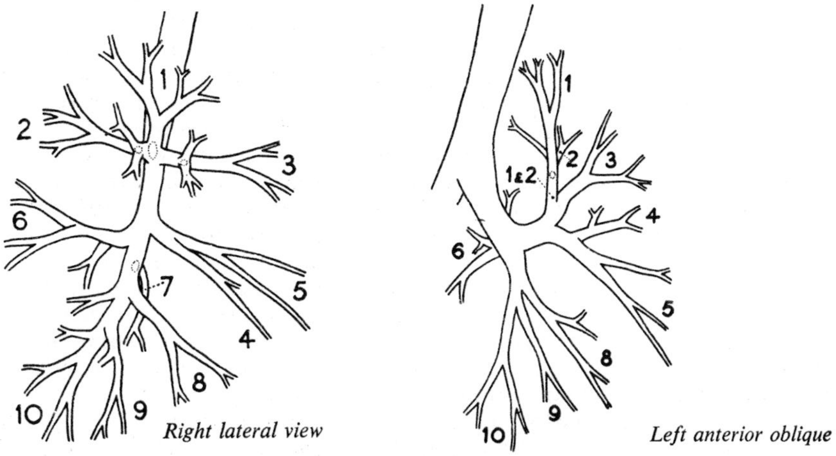

FIG. 52a. Segmental bronchi.
[Reproduced by permission of the Authors and the Editor of *Thorax*.

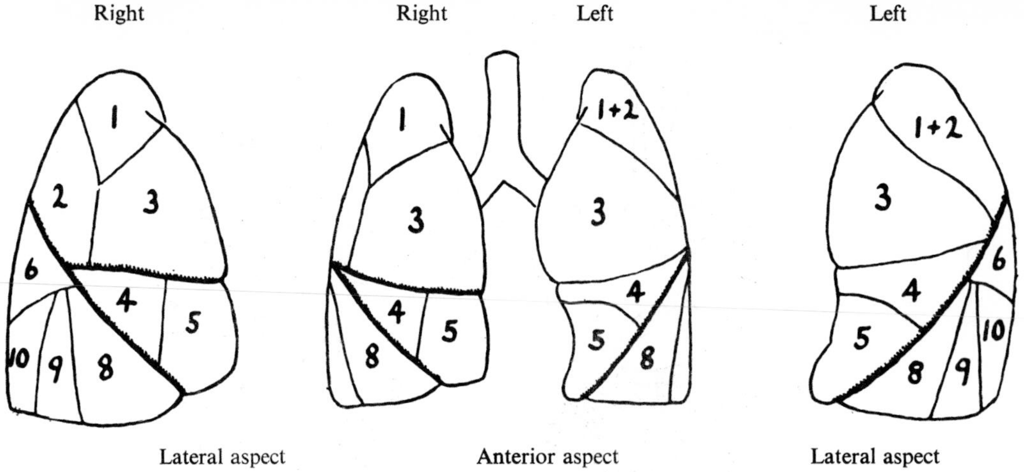

FIG 52b. Segmental anatomy of the lungs seen from the surface.

plate of cartilage and contain mucous glands in their walls. The walls of large bronchi are completely supported by cartilage whereas those of small bronchi are not and are collapsible. Bronchioli are those airways peripheral to bronchi and therefore normally contain no cartilage or mucous glands in their walls. The most distal or respiratory bronchioli are recognized by the gas exchanging tissue or alveoli opening into the lumen [FIG. 53]. Terminal bronchioli are immediately proximal to respiratory bronchioli, have a complete epithelial lining and no gas exchanging tissue in their walls. Recently communications have been demonstrated between these smallest bronchioli and adjacent alveoli. The total cross-sectional area of the conducting zone increases from 2·54 cm.^{2} in the adult trachea to 180 cm.^{2} at the level of the terminal bronchioles which themselves number about 65,000. The site of maximum resistance to airflow in the normal bronchial tree is not known but is probably at the level of the medium size bronchi. The trachea and bronchi have an internal lining of ciliated columnar epithelium. More distally this epithelium becomes non-ciliated and more flattened.

Respiratory Zone

This consists of alveoli and alveolar capillaries which are contained in the functional units of the lung distal to the terminal bronchiolus called the *acinus* [FIG. 54]. Mass movement of air ceases beyond the terminal bronchiolus and molecules of gas move through the respiratory bronchioli and alveolar ducts to and from the alveoli by diffusion. The *secondary lobule* consists of a cluster of two to five terminal bronchioli with their acini.

Alveoli. These air sacs are like tiny bubbles whose walls contain numerous capillaries and in them gas exchange takes place. By electron microscopy elastic, collagen and reticulin fibres can be seen to separate the capillary endothelium from the alveolar lining epithelium [FIG. 55]. The alveolus is completely lined by a continuous epithelial layer which consists of flattened epithelial cells—type I. Epithelial cells of type II are less numerous and protrude more into the alveolar space—they contain osmophilic inclusions which may be the source of the lipoprotein surface-active material which lines the alveolar wall. This reduces surface tension, prevents collapse of the tiny, tight bubble-like air spaces and is probably vital in maintaining the structural integrity of the gas-exchanging tissue. Whereas development of the airways is complete by birth, new alveoli form during the first eight years of life when their number increases from twenty million to three hundred million. After this age alveoli increase in size with the growth of the thoracic cage. The average diameter of an adult alveolus is 250 micra and the total surface area about 75 m.^{2}. The alveolar size varies with age and body surface area (which is itself related to oxygen consumption). Alveoli are larger at the top of the lung and become smaller in the dependent parts.

SEGMENTAL STRUCTURE

Each segment of the lung of which there are nine or ten on either side is roughly pyramidal in shape and bronchi, arteries, veins, lymphatics and nerves enter at its hilum or apex. Adjacent segments may share venous drainage and the lymphatics may cross-communicate. Occlusion of a bronchus or bronchiolus would always lead to absorption of air and collapse of the distal respiratory units if there were no free communications of air between adjacent units in the lung. Such communications do exist: those between adjacent alveoli are known as alveolar pores (of Kohn) and those between terminal bronchioli and adjacent alveoli have recently been described (by Lambert). These communications allow *collateral ventilation* or air drift across segmental boundaries and may prevent segmental collapse when the bronchus is blocked. Connective tissue accompanies blood vessels and bronchi. It also occasionally forms septa which arise from the pleura and pass for varying distances into the segments. These septa are particularly frequent at the margins and sharp edges of the lung. Where present they limit collateral ventilation and predispose the middle lobe and the inferior segment of the lingula in particular to collapse. This localization of the septa may also explain the frequency with which bullae are found in the sub-

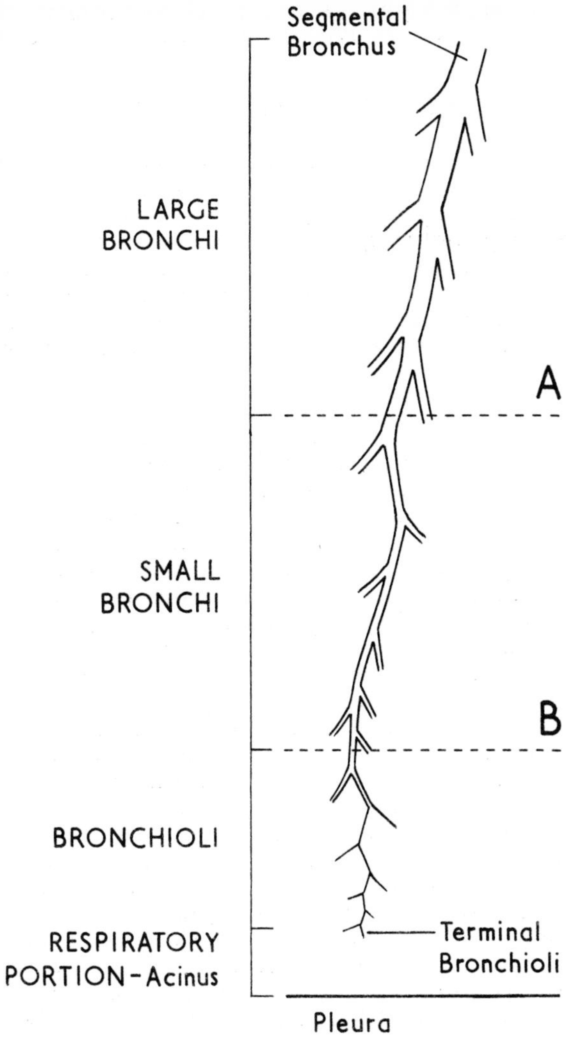

FIG. 53. Diagram of axial pathway.
A. Point at which large bronchi, six in number and with abundant cartilage, give way to small bronchi, seven in number, with only occasional plates of cartilage.
B. Point at which cartilage is lost and the bronchiolus starts —there are eight of the latter.

pleural region on the anterior edge of the lung, at the apex, and on the diaphragmatic surface where the absence of collateral ventilation may encourage over-inflation.

The branching of the bronchial tree continues from the segmental bronchi to the acinus where the respiratory bronchioli are continuous with the alveolar duct and alveoli. The smallest bronchi can be seen in the normal bronchogram forming the 'centimetre pattern' and the terminal bronchiolus about 1 mm. in diameter can be seen forming the 'millimetre pattern' [see PLATE 7].

PULMONARY BLOOD VESSELS

The Bronchial Arteries. These arise usually from the aorta and run within the bundle containing the bronchi and pulmonary arteries and supply the capillary bed

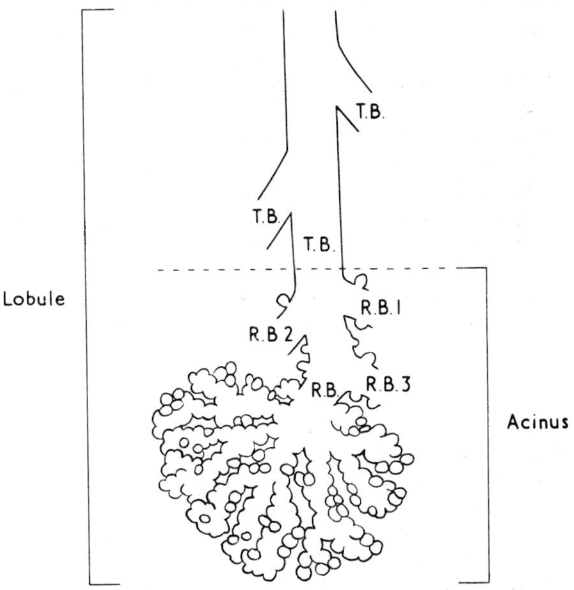

FIG. 54. Simplified diagram of the acinus. TB = terminal bronchiolus; RB = respiratory bronchiolus of which there are four orders.
[Reid, Lynne (1967) *The Pathology of Emphysema*, Lloyd-Luke (Medical Books) Ltd., London.]

of this bundle as far as the terminal bronchiolus. Bronchial veins drain only the small region of the lung around the hilum into the systemic venous system.

Pulmonary Arteries. These run in the bronchial/arterial bundle and divide with the bronchi to supply the respiratory zone beyond the terminal bronchiole. Proximally the media of the vessels contain concentric elastic laminae with muscle in between. Distally, in vessels of 2 mm. diameter or less, the media is predominantly muscular and it is in these vessels that

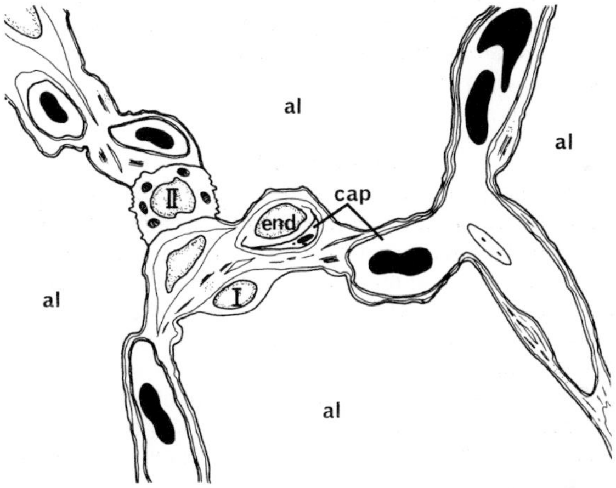

FIG. 55. Diagram to show structure of the alveolar wall as revealed by electron microscopy.

al Alveolar space
I Type I pneumonocyte } Epithelial cells
II Type II pneumonocyte }
end Endothelial cell
cap Capillary

pulmonary blood flow is controlled by alteration in lumen size. In disease, anastomoses may open up between the bronchial and the pulmonary arteries: in general, however, any lesion whether inflammatory or neoplastic will be supplied primarily by bronchial arteries unless it be very small and intra-acinar.

Pulmonary Veins. Those which drain the respiratory tissue and most of the bronchial tree pass around the periphery of the lung units. The larger veins run in the intersegmental boundaries. Communications or anastomoses between pulmonary arterioles and pulmonary veins have only been clearly demonstrated in disease, e.g. hereditary telangiectasia and cirrhosis of the liver.

PULMONARY LYMPHATICS

One group of lymphatics starts peripherally around the alveolar ducts and passes centrally along bronchi (peribronchial). The other group forms in the pleural plexus of lymphatics and passes round the periphery of the lobules with the veins (perivenous). Anastomoses pass between the peribronchial and perivenous channels in the connective tissue sheaths.

The lymphatics contain valves and flow is directed to the lymph glands. Although aggregations of lymphoid tissue are found as far out as the respiratory bronchiolus, the bronchopulmonary lymph nodes are found around the lobar bronchi (the hilar nodes) and their first divisions. The tracheobronchial lymph nodes lie around the tracheal bifurcation, the lower ones in the angle of bifurcation. Further up the trachea on either side lie the paratracheal nodes. The aorta separates a few para-aortic nodes from the bronchopulmonary group on the left side and the lymphatics of the apical segment of the left upper lobe pass to them. The remainder of the left upper lobe lymphatics drain into the left bronchopulmonary nodes and thence to the thoracic duct. The lymphatics from the left lower lobe and the right lung drain to the bronchopulmonary and tracheobronchial nodes on the right side and thence mainly into the right lymphatic duct. Other lymph nodes in the chest are to be found along the internal mammary artery and the heads of the ribs.

NERVE SUPPLY

The main innervation of the lung is by the vagus nerve which contains both efferent and afferent fibres. The vagal efferents contract bronchial smooth muscle, stimulate bronchial mucous glands to secrete, and dilate pulmonary arterioles. The vagal afferents carry fibres from cough receptors in the trachea and extrapulmonary bronchi and from baroceptors and other receptors in the pulmonary blood vessels. From stretch and irritant receptors in the airways and probably from some receptors in the alveoli arise afferent fibres which subserve reflexes which may affect bronchial calibre and the rate and depth of ventilation. There is also a sympathetic nerve supply to the bronchopulmonary tree which is mainly bronchodilator in function.

REFERENCES

Hayek, H. von (1960) *The Human Lung*, New York.

Miller, W. S. (1947) *The Lung*, 2nd ed., Springfield, Ill.

Reid, L. (1967) *The Pathology of Emphysema*, p. 319, London.

RESPIRATORY FUNCTION

In other fields of medicine disorders of function are commonly recognized, e.g. congestive cardiac failure raised intracranial pressure, etc. Now that simple tests of respiratory function are generally available, distinctive disturbances of function can be recognized in respiratory disease, not only to correlate with the clinical state and pathology and to assist in diagnosis but to measure progress of disease and response to treatment.

VENTILATION

Air flows into the lung when intrathoracic pressure falls due to contraction of the inspiratory muscles of which the diaphragm is the most important. Accessory muscles (e.g. the scalenes and the sternomastoids) are reflexly activated when larger intrathoracic pressure changes develop, for example when larger volumes of air are shifted on exercise or when resistance to air flow or expansion of the lung increases.

Expiration in quiet breathing is a passive process and the intrathoracic pressure rises due to recoil of the elastic lung: the recoil of the lung is as much due to changes in surface tension in the air spaces as it is to interstitial elastic tissue. The volumes of air moved in and out of the lung can be measured with a spirometer, and a typical trace is shown in Figure 56. The *tidal volume* in quiet breathing is about 450 ml. and this mixes with the *expiratory reserve volume* (about 1,500 ml.) and the *residual volume* (about 1,500 ml.) which together constitute the *functional residual capacity* (FRC). 150 ml. of the tidal volume fills the conducting airways which constitute the anatomical dead space and take no part in gas exchange. The rate of flow of gas entering the lung falls as the cross-sectional area of all the airways increases so that mass movement of air ceases at about the level of the respiratory bronchiolus. Molecules of gas reach the blood-gas interface in the alveolar wall by diffusion.

Even in the normal lung inspired air is not distributed uniformly: in the erect posture ventilation per unit volume of lung is greater in the lower than the upper parts. Gravity influences blood flow so that there is a gradient in blood flow to the alveoli from the upper to the lower parts of the lung. These gradients of ventilation and blood flow are not matched so that normally there is a slight over-all non-uniformity of ventilation and blood flow.

The additional volume of air that can be inspired after a normal inspiration is termed the *inspiratory reserve volume* and that volume that can be completely expelled from a maximum inspiratory position is the *vital capacity* (VC), see Figure 56. The *forced vital capacity* (FVC) is measured during a maximum expiratory effort from the point of maximum inspiration. When air is trapped in the lungs, e.g. by premature closure of the small airways, the FVC may be less than the VC. All lung volumes can be measured by the spirometer except the residual volume which requires more complicated methods which either depend on the dilution of an inert insoluble gas such as helium, the concentration of which is measured in a re-breathing circuit, or on the compression of intrathoracic gas which can be measured with a body plethysmograph.

Various measurements can be made of expiratory and inspiratory flow rate, but the most useful and most discriminating is the forced expiratory volume in one second (FEV_1). This is the fraction of the FVC that is expired in the first second, from a maximum inspiration. Normally more than 75 per cent. of the FVC can be expelled in one second so that the FEV_1/FVC ratio is greater than 75 per cent. For ease of measurement, portability and reproducability the Wright Peak Flow Meter can be used. This apparatus consists of a vane and ratchet which holds the pointer in the position of maximum deflection during a forced expiration from the peak expiratory position. This is the peak expiratory flow rate (PEF). The values for FEV_1 and PEF are higher in men than in women and they rise in childhood to reach adult levels during adolescence. If smokers are excluded the fall in expiratory flow rate that occurs with age is small. While simple measurements of flow rate are of practical value in assessing airways obstruction more complicated methods are required to measure airways resistance which entail the use of apparatus such as a whole body plethysmograph.

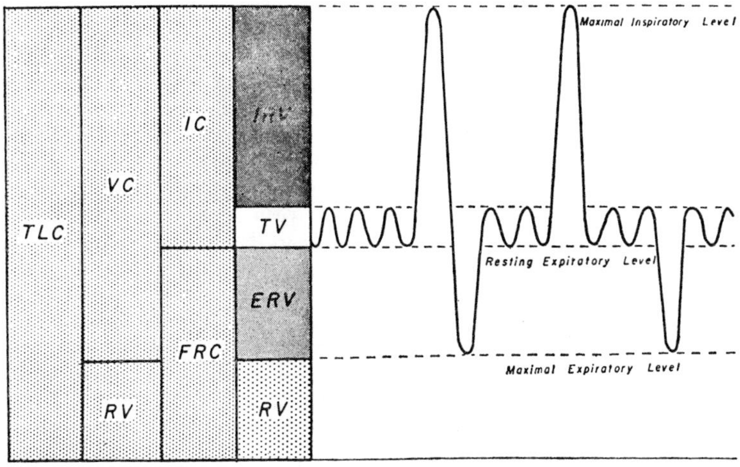

FIG. 56. Ventilatory Function.

TLC	Total Lung Capacity
VC	Vital Capacity
RV	Residual Volume
IC	Inspiratory Capacity
FRC	Functional Residual Capacity
IRV	Inspiratory Reserve Volume
TV	Tidal Volume
ERV	Expiratory Reserve Volume
RV	Residual Volume

Defects in Ventilatory Capacity

These defects can be divided into two: (1) obstructive; and (2) non-obstructive.

Obstructive Defects of Ventilatory Capacity. Generalized airway obstruction may be fixed or variable. Fixed airways obstruction is due to:

1. Widespread organic narrowing or occlusion of airways which is found in chronic obstructive bronchitis.

2. Premature closure of the airways due to an increased pressure gradient across the wall of the small collapsible bronchi (air-trapping). This pressure gradient may be the result either of loss of elastic support in the surrounding lung which develops in widespread emphysema or of narrowing of the smaller airways with increase in the surrounding alveolar pressure and this is found in obstructive bronchitis and asthma.

Variable airway obstruction will result from: (1) bronchial secretion, particularly mucus; (2) oedema of the bronchial mucosa; or (3) active contraction of bronchial smooth muscle (bronchoconstriction). These are the hall marks of bronchial asthma.

Measurement of Obstructive Ventilatory Defects. Airway obstruction leads to increased resistance to airflow. Provided that a maximum effort (the highest possible alveolar pressure) is generated, then the maximum expiratory flow rate which can be achieved will vary inversely with the airway resistance. Measurements therefore such as the FEV_1 and the PEF are valuable in order to assess the severity of airway obstruction and the changes which take place from time to time either spontaneously or in response to treatment. In airways obstruction the fall in the flow rate is proportionally greater than is the reduction in the vital capacity. Thus the FEV_1/VC ratio, normally greater than 75 per cent., tends to fall below 50 per cent. [FIG 57].

Non-obstructive Defects of Ventilatory Capacity. These defects may be restrictive or hypodynamic.

Restrictive Defects. These may result from: (1) stiffness of the lung (reduced compliance) which tends to develop in diffuse infiltrations, fibrosis, and oedema of the lung; (2) stiffness of the pleura or the chest wall, e.g. pleural thickening, kyphoscoliosis, etc.; and (3) diminished volume of ventilatable lung, e.g. after resection, or with large space-occupying malignant tumours, pneumothorax, pleural effusions, etc.

Hypodynamic Ventilatory Defects. These develop with failure of central respiratory drive, e.g. with depressant drugs, anaesthetics, or cerebrovascular accidents. They are also found with neuromuscular failure, for example in poliomyelitis, polyneuritis and after muscle relaxant drugs.

Measurement of Non-obstructive Defects. In non-obstructive ventilatory defects the vital capacity (VC) may be reduced often very severely. The VC, however, varies widely in health so that a fall of more than 20 per cent. of the predicted normal value is necessary to achieve any significance. Usually more than 75 per cent.

of the VC will be expired in the first second so that the FEV_1/FVC ratio will remain normal [FIG. 57]. There are various ways of measuring the compliance or stiffness of the lung and chest wall, though these are not usually necessary in the routine assessment of patients. By measuring the change in volume of the lung (spirometrically) per unit change in intrathoracic pressure

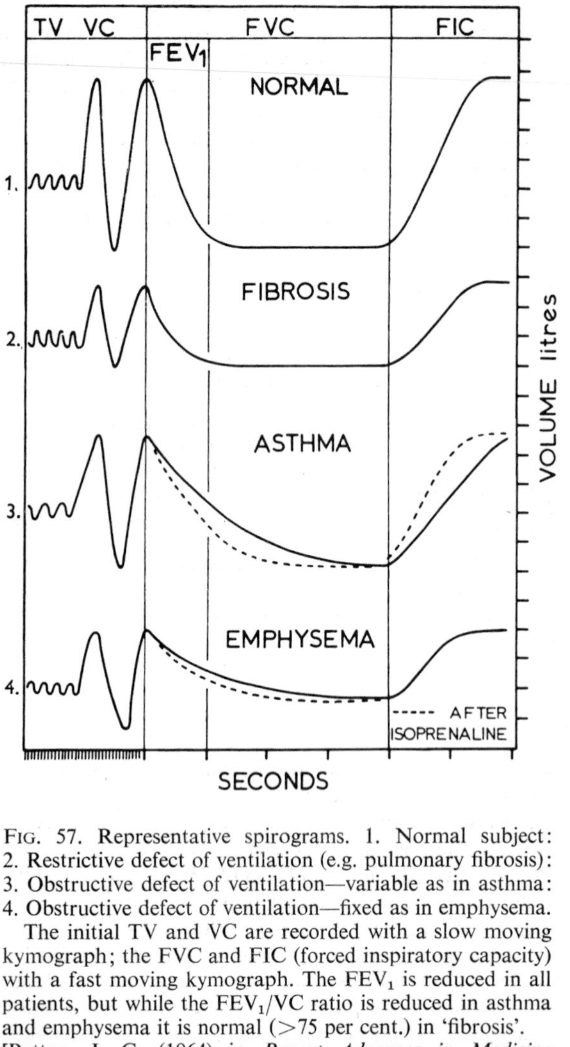

FIG. 57. Representative spirograms. 1. Normal subject: 2. Restrictive defect of ventilation (e.g. pulmonary fibrosis): 3. Obstructive defect of ventilation—variable as in asthma: 4. Obstructive defect of ventilation—fixed as in emphysema.

The initial TV and VC are recorded with a slow moving kymograph; the FVC and FIC (forced inspiratory capacity) with a fast moving kymograph. The FEV_1 is reduced in all patients, but while the FEV_1/VC ratio is reduced in asthma and emphysema it is normal (>75 per cent.) in 'fibrosis'. [Batten, J. C. (1964) in *Recent Advances in Medicine* (Beaumont and Dodds), 14th ed., p. 250, Churchill Livingstone, London.]

(by means of an intra-oesophageal tube) a value can be obtained for lung compliance—this is about 150 ml. per cm. of water change in intrathoracic pressure. When the lung becomes stiffer or less compliant this value falls.

Obstructive and non-obstructive ventilatory defects may co-exist and changes in other aspects of lung function which may accompany them are described below.

GAS TRANSFER

Transfer of molecules of oxygen from alveolar space to capillary blood and of carbon dioxide in the opposite direction, depends on:

1. An even distribution of an adequate volume of inspired air to the air spaces. This depends on the integrity of the airways and of the air spaces through which oxygen and carbon dioxide diffuse so that the molecules in the gas phase can reach equilibrium with those molecules in the capillary blood.
2. A similar even distribution of capillary blood to the air spaces.
3. A permeable alveolar wall and a normal capillary blood volume.

If there is normal ventilation of, but reduced blood flow to, the gas exchanging tissue, there is the equivalent of a 'dead space'. This is known as the physiological dead space. If ventilation is reduced but blood flow normal there is the equivalent of a 'shunt'. This is known as the physiological shunt.

Defects in Gas Transfer. Impaired diffusion across the alveolar wall and abnormalities of capillary blood volume play a relatively minor role in defects of gas transfer. Uneven distribution of ventilation and blood flow is the dominant defect in disease and most diffuse disorders of the lung of any severity may be responsible. Physiological dead space is wasted ventilation. Physiological shunting is the major cause of defective gas transfer. Transfer of oxygen is more severely impaired than of carbon dioxide so that arterial oxygen tension falls and the arterial blood eventually become desaturated, particularly on exercise. Arterial carbon dioxide tension tends to remain within normal limits or even to fall because increased ventilation of the better ventilated air spaces will remove additional carbon dioxide and compensate for the poorly ventilated parts. The blood leaving the well ventilated spaces is already fully saturated with oxygen and cannot compensate for undersaturation of the blood emerging from the poorly ventilated parts. The final composition of pulmonary venous blood and expired air is a resultant of the flow to and the function within millions of acini.

Measurement. Defects in gas transfer are most readily measured with carbon monoxide. It is necessary to estimate the uptake of carbon monoxide and to obtain a representative value for the alveolar concentration and pressure of the gas. From these values the transfer factor for carbon monoxide (T_{CO}) can be calculated. Normally 15–25 ml. of carbon monoxide are transferred per mm. Hg pressure difference per minute at rest and this value doubles on exercise (25–50 ml. per mm. Hg per min.). While of use in diagnosis and prognosis, serial estimations of T_{CO} are of value in assessing response to treatment of various diseases of the lung.

BREATHLESSNESS

Breathlessness or dyspnoea is an unpleasant awareness of difficult breathing or the need for a deeper breath. The sensation, which is visceral, is aroused with a considerable degree of variation from one person to another according to their age, physical training, and mode of origin. The mechanisms concerned with breathing and breathlessness are complex and largely speculative at present.

The respiratory centre, the precise site of which is uncertain, can be considered as a device for computing the rate and depth of ventilation required on the basis of information received from two sources—one is *chemical* and gives the total ventilation needed from moment to moment, i.e. the P_{O_2}, P_{CO_2} and pH.: the other is *neural* and this originates in a variety of the receptors in the lung concerned with inflation, deflation, irritation and vascular patency (mediated by the vagus nerve) and other receptors in the chest cage, in joints, muscles and ligaments (somatic)—all these allow the required ventilation to be achieved with the minimum work (optimal rate and depth of breathing). The higher centres can assess and modify normal breathing but only within certain limits, e.g. the breath can only be held voluntarily for a certain length of time.

When respiratory work is excessive for the ventilation achieved (or the ventilation excessive for the degree of exercise undertaken) then the information derived from the lung and chest wall is carried to higher centres where disparities enter awareness as dyspnoea. The threshold for this sensation and its magnitude depend on many factors which may be inherited and acquired—amongst the latter are blood gas tensions, drugs and neuropsychiatric disorders, e.g. depression, hysteria and organic nervous conditions, which may be vascular, neoplastic, etc.

That dyspnoea is not a single sensation is clear from the different but normal sensations aroused by breath holding, by rebreathing into a bag (hyperventilation) and exercise, particularly at high altitude. In fact dyspnoea can conveniently be subdivided into 3 groups:

1. Awareness of ventilatory *excess*: often physiological as in exercise or at high altitude. Ventilatory excess may occur with nervous disorders such as hysteria or reflexly with pulmonary embolism. It may have a metabolic origin, e.g. with anaemia, metabolic acidosis, thyrotoxicosis.

2. Awareness of ventilatory *need*: physiologically this is encountered with breath holding. It develops with respiratory paralysis in poliomyelitis or polyneuritis.

3. Awareness of ventilatory *difficulty*: with obstructive ventilatory defects, e.g. chronic bronchitis, emphysema, and asthma—restrictive ventilatory defects encountered in widespread infiltration, fibrosis, or oedema of the lung.

It is important to note that deviations of blood gases from normal do not of themselves cause breathlessness —they may modify the sensation or indirectly create conditions which arouse breathlessness.

REFERENCES

Bates, D. V., and Christie, R. V. (1964) *Respiratory Function in Disease*, Philadelphia.

Comroe, J. H., Forster, R. E., Dubois, A. B., Briscoe, W. A., and Carlsen, E. (1962) *The Lung: Clinical Physiology and Pulmonary Function Tests*, 2nd ed., Chicago.

Cumming, G., and Hunt, L. B. (1968) *Form and Function in the Human Lung*, Edinburgh.

Howell, J. B. L., and Campbell, E. J. M. (1966) *Breathlessness*, Oxford.

Scadding, J. G. (1966) Patterns of respiratory insufficiency, *Lancet*, i, 701.

CONGENITAL ABNORMALITIES OF THE LUNG

Minor variations in the anatomy of the bronchopulmonary tree are common—thus a separate subapical segmental bronchus may arise from the right lower lobe bronchus below the origin of the apical segmental bronchus to that lobe—the left upper lobe bronchus may divide into three branches (rather than two) so that there is no common bronchus of origin for the lingular and anterior segmental branches. Other variations are less common.

An interesting rarity is *bronchial atresia*, in which there is no communication between a lobar bronchus and the main bronchus proximally. This most commonly affects the left upper lobe bronchus. The lobe supplied by the abnormal bronchus is hypoplastic and emphysematous [p. 889].

In about 0·1 per cent. of people the azygos vein loops over the apex of the lung and pulls in a fold of pleura as the apical segment of the right lung grows round it. An azygos lobe functions normally and is revealed on the chest radiograph by a hairline passing from the apex to the azygos vein at the upper part of the right hilum.

Very rarely and for reasons unknown, part of a lung, e.g. a lobe, may be small, i.e. hypoplastic, or absent—*agenesis* of a whole lung is seen more often however: diagnosis in infants may be difficult. Although there is normally a small hemithorax on the affected side and mediastinal shift to the abnormal side, congenital heart disease coexists in one third of cases and this and other gross congenital disorders are usually responsible for death in infancy. Pure pulmonary agenesis is compatible with long survival. It has to be differentiated from congenital lobar emphysema, pneumothorax especially with staphylococcal pneumonia, dextrocardia and congenital diaphragmatic hernia. The latter condition may be very rarely associated with *dysgenesis of the lung* on the same side in which there is hypoplasia not only of alveoli but also of the bronchial tree—it is likely that the hernia interferes with development of the foetal lung from a very early stage.

A more common but still rare abnormality is *sequestrated segment*. This is usually found within a lobe, most often the posteromedial part of the lower lobes, rather more often on the left than the right (3:2). This is called *intralobar sequestration*. There is no bronchial communication between the normal part of the segment and the abnormal part which usually receives its blood supply directly from the lower thoracic or upper abdominal aorta. It may be asymptomatic, but infection of the sequestrated segment may lead to recurrent pneumonia, pleurisy or empyema at any age although most often in the second decade. Haemoptysis is a not infrequent symptom. Tuberculous infection in a sequestrated segment has been reported. The chest radiographs show dense homogeneous shadows or cystic spaces which may change in appearance quite rapidly. Communication must exist with the normal part of the lobe if a cystic appearance or a fluid level exist, but these communications may be difficult to demonstrate. Lung abscess due to other causes or staphylococcal pneumonia must be differentiated. An infected intralobar sequestrated segment should be treated as a lung abscess [p. 866]. Chemotherapy will be used. Infection or haemoptysis arising in or from a sequestrated segment usually requires surgical intervention. The diagnosis should be suspected by the position of the abnormal segment: tomography and/or aortography do not necessarily reveal the abnormal blood vessel supplying the segment.

In *extralobar sequestration* (accessory lung) there is complete anatomical separation of the abnormal lung tissue from the normal lung and the abnormal element may lie above or below the diaphragm.

Truly *congenital cystic lung* is very rare and may be limited or widespread in extent. It may appear as honeycombing [see p. 883]. It is found in infants and may arise within terminal airways with multiple air spaces sometimes in association with dilated lymphatics (lymphatic cysts).

REFERENCES

BOYDEN, E. A. (1955) *Segmental Anatomy of the Lungs*, New York.

EADE, A. W. T., and STRETTON, T. B. (1961) Clinical features of intralobar sequestration of lung, *Brit. med. J.*, **1,** 774.

EVERLEY JONES, H., and HOWELLS, C. H. L. (1961) Pulmonary agenesis, *Brit. med. J.*, **2,** 1187.

DISEASES OF THE LUNGS AND BRONCHI

RESPIRATORY FAILURE

Definition

Respiratory failure exists when the blood gases are abnormal at rest as a result of a disorder of respiration or its control.

Pathogenesis

There are two patterns of respiratory failure in both of which there is a fall in arterial oxygen tension (arterial P_{O_2}), but they may be distinguished by the arterial carbon dioxide tension (arterial P_{CO_2}):

Type I—in which there is a normal or low arterial P_{CO_2} with a low arterial P_{O_2}.

Type II—in which there is a high arterial P_{CO_2} together with a low arterial P_{O_2}.

RESPIRATORY FAILURE WITH A NORMAL OR LOW ARTERIAL P_{CO_2} (TYPE 1)

A normal or low arterial P_{CO_2} is found in respiratory failure when the low arterial P_{O_2} is due to a defect in gas transfer. The most common cause of this is uneven distribution of inspired air and pulmonary blood flow. Thus respiratory failure will be encountered in:

1. Non-obstructive restrictive defects of ventilation found in pulmonary oedema, infiltration or fibrosis.

2. Pulmonary vascular disease: particularly thrombo-embolic disease.

3. In disorders causing obstructive defects of ventilation when the latter is adequate to maintain total overall alveolar ventilation, but in which a low arterial pO_2 may be found at rest. This may be transient as in severe asthma or with acute bronchial infection, or permanent, and if severe, then the second type of ventilatory failure will develop.

Clinical Picture. This form of respiratory failure is seen most strikingly in severe restrictive disorders of ventilation when the lung is stiff (less compliant) as a result of widespread oedema of the lung, infiltration (e.g. lymphangitis carcinomatosa) or fibrosis (e.g. chronic fibrosing alveolitis). The patient is usually very breathless indeed. On the slightest exertion he may become centrally cyanosed and this cyanosis will be prevented by breathing 30 per cent. oxygen. The breathing tends to be rapid and shallow. Chest expansion is limited and the lower sternum and ribs indrawn on inspiration. The patient may be so restricted as to be unable to take a deep breath or yawn. The signs are otherwise of the *disease*. The condition will be suspected by the development of cyanosis on exertion and severe breathlessness and confirmed by the estimation of the arterial blood gases.

Treatment

This must be directed at the cause which may be reversible, e.g. left heart failure, acute fibrosing alveolitis, etc. Whatever the cause the symptoms may be relieved by oxygen breathing.

RESPIRATORY FAILURE WITH A HIGH ARTERIAL P_{CO_2} (TYPE II)

A high arterial P_{CO_2} is due to deficient total aveolar ventilation and it is accompanied by a fall in arterial P_{O_2}. It will be encountered:

1. In severe obstructive ventilatory defects due to chronic obstructive bronchitis, emphysema and asthma.
2. Hypodynamic defects of ventilation due to disorders of the central control mechanism, e.g. when the respiratory centres are depressed by drugs, anaesthesia or structural defects of a vascular or other nature. Similar functional disorders may occur with neuromuscular failure, e.g. poliomyelitis, polyneuritis, myasthenia, and chest injury.
3. The terminal stages of type I respiratory failure.

Clinical Picture

Respiratory failure of this type may remain unsuspected as the physical signs of hypercapnia are non-specific—thus restlessness, sweating, and flapping tremor associated with a warm periphery with dilated veins over the forearm and hand, tachycardia and systemic hypertension may all be present. Occasionally headache is prominent and is due to an increased intracranial tension. This rise in pressure is due to a direct effect of the elevated P_{CO_2} on cerebral blood flow and may lead to papilloedema. The respiratory centre may become insensitive to changes in arterial P_{CO_2} and may be responsive only to hypoxia. Under these circumstances the symptoms and signs may be worsened by oxygen breathing and the patient may even become sleepy, stuporose, or frankly comatose, while the cyanosis may be relieved by the oxygen breathing. This sequence of events is diagnostic of this type of respiratory failure. When airway obstruction is lacking and a hypodynamic defect such as barbiturate overdosage or polyneuritis is responsible then respiratory failure may not be obvious and cyanosis may be absent or difficult to detect. Restlessness is usually apparent and if respiratory failure is a possibility the diagnosis should be confirmed by measuring the blood gas tensions, especially the arterial P_{CO_2}, which will be considerably elevated, often above 100 mm. Hg.

Treatment

The aim of treatment is to restore arterial oxygen saturation to normal and to diminish the arterial P_{CO_2} by increasing alveolar ventilation. The underlying cause must receive attention, e.g. infection will require chemotherapy, bronchoconstriction will require bronchodilators, etc.

The general measures are directed at: (1) hypoxia; (2) clearance of the airways; and (3) ventilation.

1. If the patient is cyanosed (and the arterial oxygen saturation reduced below 85 per cent.) oxygen must be given continuously. The minimum concentration of oxygen to restore a pink colour or a saturation above 85 per cent. should be given. The concentration in the inspired air should be increased gradually and this is best achieved by a series of simple Venturi type masks delivering from 23 to 30 per cent. oxygen. The smallest increment in oxygen which achieves an oxygen saturation of about 85 per cent. may allow adequate ventilation.

2. If the airways are obstructed clearance may be achieved by reducing infection by appropriate chemotherapy and by the use of physiotherapy including postural coughing. If the patient becomes sleepy or stuporose he must be awakened if necessary by the use of nikethamide, 2–10 ml. of 5 per cent. solution intravenously, and made to cough frequently. Nikethamide and other respiratory stimulants are effective only because they wake the patient and facilitate cough. They have no useful action on the respiratory centre and of themselves do not lower arterial P_{CO_2}.

In non-obstructive hypodynamic failure cough may be assisted by simple measures to relieve pain after injury to the chest, e.g. with pethidine, 50 mg. intramuscularly, or pentazocine, 30 mg. intramuscularly.

If effective coughing and clearance of the airway cannot be achieved by simple medical measures then resort may have to be made to bronchoscopy or endotracheal intubation or even tracheostomy. Tracheostomy should not be considered in chronic respiratory cripples. It allows repeated suction in those unable to cough effectively and diminishes the anatomical dead space. Scrupulous care should be paid to the technique of nursing to reduce infection around the tube and in the respiratory tract and to avoid such complications as herniation and obstruction by the inflatable cuff.

3. Mechanical ventilation. If ventilation remains inadequate, and the arterial P_{CO_2} high and the arterial P_{O_2} continues to fall despite the measures mentioned above then ventilation must be assisted. When respiratory failure is acute and likely to be short lived, e.g. in severe bronchiolitis or pneumonia in previously healthy individuals or with an overdose of barbiturate drugs, then ventilation can be carried out through an endotracheal tube with inflated cuff. If ventilation will require assistance for more than 48 hours or so it will be necessary to carry out a tracheostomy and to introduce a cuffed tracheostomy tube. There are a number of machines available for assisting ventilation, either pressure or volume cycled. Each has its relative merits and drawbacks but it is best for those that use this type of apparatus to familiarize themselves with one or other type of machine so that they are accustomed not only to its mechanism and maintenance but are alive to its difficulties. They should also supervise its disinfection. There is need to manage the volume, frequency and rates of inflation and the pressure at which it is performed. Rapid shallow inflation tends to stiffen the lungs but in general a tidal volume adequate to maintain the arterial P_{CO_2} within the normal range should be achieved with respiratory rates varying from 16 to 20 per minute. A negative phase on deflation assists systemic venous return and thereby augments the cardiac output, but this will accentuate air trapping when there is severe airways obstruction. Proper nursing and general management are of great importance and the patient should be reassured constantly. Pain and any anxiety should be relieved if necessary with such drugs as morphine or diamorphine and careful attention paid to fluid and electrolyte balance. It is easier to manage patients when there are facilities for repeated measurements of arterial gas tensions and pH.

LOCALIZED AIRWAY OBSTRUCTION AND ATELECTASIS

Obstruction of the larger airways may arise from conditions within them or outside. With complete obstruction of a main or lobar bronchus there is usually atelectasis (collapse) of the lung distally—with occlusion of a segmental bronchus atelectasis depends on whether or not there is collateral ventilation to the distal segment.

TRACHEAL OBSTRUCTION

Aetiology

The trachea may be obstructed by a foreign body within the lumen, by stenosis, by a growth arising in the wall, or by external pressure.

Foreign Body. A great variety of foreign bodies may obstruct the trachea—they may be inhaled or aspirated while vomiting. A large blood clot in haemoptysis may obstruct the trachea temporarily. Unless they are impacted, foreign bodies are usually coughed up or pass lower down the bronchial tree. If they are not, there will be sudden death in asphyxia. After intense breathlessness and alarm during passage through the larynx, tracheal foreign bodies may cause breathlessness which is mainly inspiratory and accompanied by stridor together with paroxysmal cough and cyanosis. The foreign body should be removed as rapidly as possible by bronchoscope.

Stenosis and External Pressure. Stenosis of the trachea most commonly follows tracheostomy at the site of the cuff of the tube and is due to ischaemia of the tracheal wall with or without infection and loss of support from the excised cartilagenous rings. Stenosis is rarely the result of trauma or a chronic granulomatous process, e.g. tuberculosis. Obstruction by external pressure on the trachea arises from enlargement of the thyroid, pressure of cervical lymph nodes, e.g. in Hodgkin's disease or malignant disease, or below the neck by an aneurysm of the aorta, retrosternal goitre, enlarged thymus or other tumour or cyst in the superior mediastinum.

Clinical Picture

Breathlessness and stridor develop usually quite insidiously and become severe when there is gross reduction in the size of the lumen. A paroxysmal dry metallic cough which is often croupy in childhood is sometimes prominent and the voice becomes weak. Intermittent obstruction may lead to alarming and suffocating breathlessness and cyanosis. While the stridor is very loud on auscultation over the trachea the breath sounds in the lung are diminished. If evidence of an external cause is not apparent on clinical examination it will usually be revealed by radiography.

Treatment

Tracheal stenosis which gives rise to symptoms requires either surgical repair which is difficult or a permanent tracheostomy tube fitted with a valve to permit an effective cough and voice. Treatment is directed at any lesion which is causing external pressure where this is practicable. Anxiety should be allayed by sedation. Airway resistance may be temporarily reduced using a gas mixture of helium and oxygen which is less dense than air and which reduces turbulence. It may be possible to introduce an endotracheal tube and pass it beyond the obstruction.

BRONCHIAL OBSTRUCTION

Aetiology

A wide variety of solid or semi-solid objects may obstruct the bronchi. They may be exogenous, e.g. articles of food, or endogenous such as teeth, pieces of tonsil at surgery or broncholiths. A foreign body is particularly liable to be aspirated when the cough reflex is dulled by anaesthesia, sleep, drugs or alcohol. This allows the foreign body to be inhaled and impacted in one of the bronchi. Carelessness is otherwise the most frequent cause and children are most often at fault.

Pathology

The effects of impaction of a foreign body in a bronchus depend on its nature, the duration of its impaction, the size of the bronchus and the degree of obstruction. If the foreign body is smooth and uninfected and removed quickly there may be no untoward effects whatsoever. On rare occasions such foreign bodies may remain for years in the bronchus if it is not completely obstructed. If the foreign body remains and occludes a bronchus then the lung beyond will usually collapse and become totally airless or partially filled with non-inflammatory oedema fluid. If the obstruction is incomplete on inspiration than a valve-like mechanism may cause obstructive or ball valve emphysema of the lung beyond. If the foreign body is infected or the obstruction partial and progressive, a secondary pneumonia may develop beyond the obstruction which may proceed to suppuration and lung abscess. Foreign bodies of vegetable origin, especially peanuts, may cause an acute inflammatory reaction with gross swelling of the bronchial wall which may render the foreign body invisible at bronchoscopy and therefore obscure the cause.

Other causes of bronchial obstruction may have similar consequences: for example plugs of mucus or blood clot, strictures due to chronic granulomata (e.g. endobronchial tuberculosis) or past trauma, and adenoma or carcinoma of the bronchus.

Clinical Picture

Inhalation of a foreign body may be accompanied by gagging or choking and great distress which ceases when the object enters the bronchi. Aspiration, however, may pass quite unnoticed. A variable latent interval may follow impaction lasting days or weeks before symptoms such as cough develop. Sputum may become copious and purulent if infection intervenes distally. Haemoptysis is not uncommon. Breathlessness and discomfort follow occlusion of a larger bronchus particularly in patients in whom lung function was previously impaired. With causes of bronchial obstruction other than foreign body the onset of these symptoms is either insidious or rapid if a secondary pneumonia intervenes. External pressure on the bronchus, e.g. with tuberculous lymph nodes will have similar effects. The physical signs will be either absent or those of atelectasis of a lobe together with fever and malaise if there is infection. Constitutional upsets are common with impacted peanuts in children. If the occlusion is partial a persistent rhonchus may be heard and more rarely the signs of obstructive emphysema may be elicited—in which case there is a shift of the mediastinum away from the area of diminished chest expansion and breath sounds. Rarely a pneumothorax complicates the picture. Further complications of a bronchial occlusion are suppuration with or without lung abscess or empyema, and later bronchiectasis.

Diagnosis

Chest radiography is essential to the diagnosis except in the obvious case where the inhalation of a foreign body was observed and it has lodged in a major airway causing distressing symptoms. The development of the signs and radiological changes of atelectasis, with or without consolidation, with or without lung abscess formation or of obstructive emphysema should arouse suspicion of a bronchial occlusion. Difficulties arise in the case of foreign bodies where a history of inhalation is absent: it may well have been forgotten or not even noticed. A specific pneumonia is most likely to be confused with local airways obstruction and infection and in case of doubt bronchoscopy should be performed. The radiograph may reveal a dense foreign body such as a tooth or metallic object or evidence of a lesion such as a neoplasm or lymphoma which may be occluding the bronchus by external pressure.

Treatment

The cause of the bronchial occlusion must be removed if possible: foreign bodies in the bronchi should be removed as quickly as possible by bronchoscopy as spontaneous expulsion is rare. Peanuts and other vegetable matter may present great difficulties because of gross local oedema. Impacted mucus will probably be dislodged by assiduous physiotherapy. In other cases treatment should be directed to the cause whether it be tuberculous, benign or malignant neoplasia or lymphoma. With infection, chemotherapy is necessary and benzylpenicillin, ½–1 mega Unit 6-hourly intramuscularly, is usually the most effective. If other methods fail thoracotomy may be necessary with resection of the damaged part of the lung and occluded bronchus.

Prognosis

Prognosis is poor with a foreign body unless it is removed, for complications usually develop. Otherwise the prognosis depends on the condition causing the bronchial occlusion.

ATELECTASIS OR COLLAPSE

Definition

A condition in which the volume of the lung is diminished due to failure of, or reduction in, aeration.

Pathogenesis

Atelectasis may be congenital or acquired.

Congenital Atelectasis. Exists when the foetal lung fails to inflate at birth and remains totally or partially airless. This is commoner with prematurity and when incomplete may give rise to the respiratory distress syndrome or hyaline membrane disease. Absence or reduction of the surface-active lipoprotein film which lines the air spaces is the usual cause of this disorder. The lungs are extremely stiff and high pressures are needed to inflate them. Mechanical ventilation, oxygen therapy and correction of metabolic and respiratory acidosis may on occasions be successful.

Acquired Atelectasis. This is of two types:

1. *Relaxation collapse* arises when air is expelled from the lung by elastic retraction when the pleural space is enlarged by a pneumothorax or effusion or with large space-occupying lesions like diaphragmatic hernia.

2. *Absorption collapse* is usually due to bronchial obstruction after which air will always be absorbed distal to the obstruction unless there is collateral ventilation of the distal segment or subsegment [p. 844]. Air is absorbed because the total gas tension of venous blood is about 50–60 mm. less than atmospheric or trapped air. Oxygen breathing provides a greater pressure gradient from air in the trapped air spaces to capillary blood and absorption becomes even more rapid. This is one factor responsible for rapid collapse of parts of the basal segments of the lung in oxygen-breathing pilots exposed to extreme gravitational pull (high G) in high speed aircraft on the turn. Collapse after bronchial occlusion proceeds over a few hours in lungs previously containing air. Complete obstruction of a main bronchus always leads to collapse of the whole lung (massive collapse) and the lobe to lobar collapse. The pathological state of the lung or lobe distal to the occlusion varies: while it is airless it may contain a variable amount of exudate or oedema fluid. Moreover, the bronchus distal to the occlusion often distends with mucus secreted within its lumen. Sometimes in pneumonia and infarction varying degrees of shrinkage of the lung accompanies consolidation without necessarily any bronchial occlusion (non-obstructive atelectasis). Segmental or subsegmental collapse will be prevented by collateral ventilation through alveolar pores and communications between terminal bronchioles and adjacent alveoli. Such communications are limited by connective tissue septa which are more frequent in the middle lobe and lingula segment of the left upper lobe. These segments are therefore more liable to collapse. Oedema and exudation also interferes with collateral ventilation and this may predispose to atelectasis.

Clinical Picture

There may be no symptoms at all if atelectasis is slow in developing. If, however, underlying function is impaired or parts of lung larger than segments suddenly collapse then breathlessness may be a feature. Shunting of blood through a collapsed lung or lobe may cause cyanosis but this is usually only temporary because of rapid adjustments in blood flow by reflex mechanisms. Signs of atelectasis of lobes and segments may be difficult to elicit but if a large lobe is involved and is adjacent to the surface then signs of consolidation appear and the shift of the mediastinum towards the abnormal side may be detected. Sudden collapse of a lobe may resemble more closely the clinical picture of massive collapse. In the *middle lobe syndrome* (Brock's syndrome) there is obstruction of the middle lobe bronchus usually by tuberculous hilar lymph nodes or occasionally mucus plugs that lead to atelectasis which is usually partial. This usually develops in childhood. Subsequently recurrent pneumonia, cough and sputum may be a feature. Recurrent haemoptysis from the damaged branches of the middle lobe bronchus is the other presenting feature.

Massive collapse of the lung is usually sudden in onset and often follows anaesthesia and surgery. There is pain in the lower thorax behind the sternum, severe dyspnoea, cyanosis and restlessness. Tachypnoea, tachycardia and fever may ensue. The affected side is immobile, the trachea and mediastinum are displaced to the same side and there is dullness to percussion. Breath sounds are either diminished or there are frank signs of consolidation (bronchial breathing, bronchophony and whispering pectoriloquy). Massive collapse may be complicated by infection and suppuration and respiratory failure may be precipitated especially if function in the other lung had been previously impaired.

In any atelectatic portion of lung there is bronchial dilatation due initially to distension with mucus secreted beyond the obstruction: if this is relieved then bronchial calibre may be restored to normal. If unrelieved or if infection develops then permanent bronchiectasis ensues even though the obstruction may later be relieved.

Diagnosis

A characteristic homogeneous shadow of the shrunken atelectatic lung, lobe or segment is usually seen on the chest radiograph. The shape and position of the shadow will of course depend on which part is collapsed. Its extent will depend on the amount of exudate within the collapsed part or on other pathology also present and its general configuration will be modified by pleural adhesion. Displacement of the fissures, elevation of the diaphragm and deviation of the trachea and heart towards the side of the collapse will also be helpful. If the bronchial occlusion has been removed and the collapse persists then tubular shadows (an air bronchogram) will be seen within the abnormal shadow.

Atelectasis of the lung or lobe must be distinguished from other massive lesions in the chest such as pleural effusion, pneumothorax and lobar pneumonia or infarction. Proper attention to the clinical and radiological findings usually allows easy differentiation.

Treatment

Careful attention should be given to the physical state of the patient before operation; smoking, tight bandages, and surgery with acute respiratory infection should be avoided. He should be encouraged to mobilize and cough as soon after operation as possible and when necessary, postural drainage and percussion are best carried out by a physiotherapist. These measures usually dislodge the obstructing mucus. Cough may be stimulated by nikethamide, 3–5 ml. intravenously, if the obstruction cannot be dislodged and in other cases where the nature of the obstruction is in doubt, bronchoscopy should be performed to determine the nature of the cause and to remove it if possible. Infection will require chemotherapy and benzylpenicillin, 2 mega Units 6-hourly intramuscularly, is usually the most appropriate. Respiratory failure will be treated with oxygen and other measures outlined on page 853. A permanently collapsed lobe in which recurrent infection or haemoptysis recur should be resected if lung function is satisfactory.

Course and Prognosis

Sudden massive collapse of the lung is usually relieved rapidly and the lung restored to normal. Otherwise the prognosis depends on the underlying cause and complications such as suppuration and pre-existing respiratory function.

REFERENCE

SIMON, G. (1971) *Principles of Chest X-ray Diagnosis*, 3rd ed., London.

ACUTE BRONCHOPULMONARY INFECTION

Anatomical classification of acute bronchopulmonary infection has not proved satisfactory. Many of the commoner infections may affect parts or the whole of airways or gas exchanging tissue and infection may pass from one site to another in the course of the illness. The matter has to some extent been simplified by the Medical Research Council suggestion in 1965 for the classification of syndromes of *acute respiratory infection.* As this is not comprehensive *acute tracheobronchitis* will be described.

ACUTE TRACHEOBRONCHITIS

The further down the bronchial tree the main impact of the infection lies, the more severe the illness becomes. Viruses are by far the most common cause. Amongst the most frequent of these primary invaders are the rhinovirus, the influenza and para-influenza viruses, the respiratory syncytial virus, the enteroviruses and the adenoviruses. In children, particularly, acute tracheobronchitis may be a feature in measles and pertussis. Less commonly it is found in typhoid and diphtheria.

In the common forms of tracheobronchitis, secondary bacterial infection with the pneumococcus, *Haemophilus influenzae*, and the staphylococcus are the more serious pathogens but not infrequently normal inhabitants of the upper respiratory tract may be responsible for pus formation.

Both acute tracheitis and bronchitis are common disorders which most frequently affect children and the aged, and males more frequently than females. They are particularly common in the winter and in epidemics due to one or other of the viruses already mentioned. They are more severe and perhaps more frequent in cigarette smokers, patients with established bronchitis and in industrial societies.

Pathological changes vary from simple catarrhal inflammation to intense destructive changes with ulceration. When the acute inflammatory process spreads to the bronchioli healing may occur with some patchy fibrosis and leave residual organic obstruction of the smallest airways. This is uncommon.

Clinical Picture

The onset of acute tracheitis is usually quite sudden with mild constitutional symptoms and the temperature in the range 37–38·8° C. Retrosternal irritation gives way to soreness and on occasion severe pain which is aggravated by the harsh dry cough. The voice may be hoarse or absent if the larynx is also involved. The rawness behind the sternum tends to be short lived as the cough becomes productive.

When bronchitis is dominant and the illness severe the temperature may be higher, even up to 103° F. (39·5° C.). Usually, however, the illness is mild and the fever either trivial or absent. The initial dry irritating cough is painless but there may be a tightness in the chest. The cough becomes productive, usually of purulent sputum which on rare occasions may be blood stained. While the constitutional signs rapidly abate the cough and sputum may persist for one to two weeks, sometimes even longer and it is usually worse on lying in bed and waking in the morning. The patient is often flushed, the breathing usually normal. On auscultation widespread inspiratory and expiratory wheezes may be heard. These together with coarse crepitations are modified by coughing.

Acute bronchiolitis occasionally produces a much more severe illness which merges into the broad clinical group of pneumonias. Bronchiolitis may develop in previously normal patients or those with chronic bronchitis. It is characterized by cough which becomes productive of purulent sputum which follows the onset of constitutional symptoms. Dyspnoea is a feature and may become severe. It may be accompanied by central cyanosis and widespread crepitations may be heard all over the chest. There is a tachypnoea and tachycardia.

When acute bronchitis complicates chronic bronchitis, a common occurrence, the patient is usually more severely affected and breathlessness with wheezing is a more striking feature. Previously established airways obstruction will become more severe and respiratory failure may develop. Prolonged hypoxia and the rise in the arterial P_{CO_2} may be responsible for a rise in the pulmonary vascular resistance and right ventricular failure may follow. Acute tracheobronchitis may be complicated by pneumonia [p. 860].

Diagnosis

The clinical picture is usually straightforward and sufficient to establish the diagnosis. A chest radiograph is usually normal even in bronchiolitis but in the latter condition there may be quite faint but widespread shadows of micronodular size.

Treatment

When febrile or with constitutional symptoms the patients should be kept in bed. An even temperature should be maintained in the room between 59° and 64·5° F. (15 and 18° C.) if possible. Inhalation of steam is comforting and the vapour of benzoin (1 per cent. mixture of benzoin in water) may give relief of the retrosternal discomfort. Codeine, pholcodeine or other sedative cough preparations may be helpful. When the sputum is purulent if chemotherapy is given early the course of the disease may be shortened. Chemotherapy is important when acute bronchitis complicates chronic bronchitis or heart disease. Either tetracycline, 250 mg. four times a day, or ampicillin, 500 mg. four times a day, are usually the most appropriate agents to use. When respiratory failure complicates the picture then treatment should be given as outlined on page 853. Persistence of purulent sputum should lead to the suspicion that other organisms such as the staphylococcus or *Klebsiella* sp. are present. The sputum should be cultivated and the pathogen isolated. Acute tracheobronchitis occurring in the course of such diseases as diphtheria or typhoid should receive treatment specific to those diseases.

ACUTE RESPIRATORY INFECTION
(Medical Research Council, 1965)

A group of acute disorders primarily affecting the upper and lower respiratory tract with characteristic symptoms usually due to viruses.

INTRODUCTION

Acute respiratory infection comprises a number of symptom complexes which are usually due to certain respiratory viruses. Those disorders referred to as the *common cold*, *febrile cold*, *sore throat* and *influenza* chiefly affect the upper respiratory tract: whereas in *croup* or *laryngotracheobronchitis*, *acute bronchitis*, *acute bronchiolitis and pneumonia*, the lower respiratory tract is mainly involved. Some of the viruses so far isolated in these syndromes are shown in TABLE 44. It will be seen that there are several main groups of respiratory viruses, the myxoviruses, picornaviruses, the adenoviruses, and the corona-viruses. The broad clinical pictures produced by each of the viruses is not clear cut but in FIGURE 58 is shown the relative frequency of each symptom complex amongst patients infected with each of these viruses. As evidence for infection with one or other of the viruses can at present be found in only about 30 per cent. of cases, a random sample of patients with characteristic symptoms, but in whom no evidence

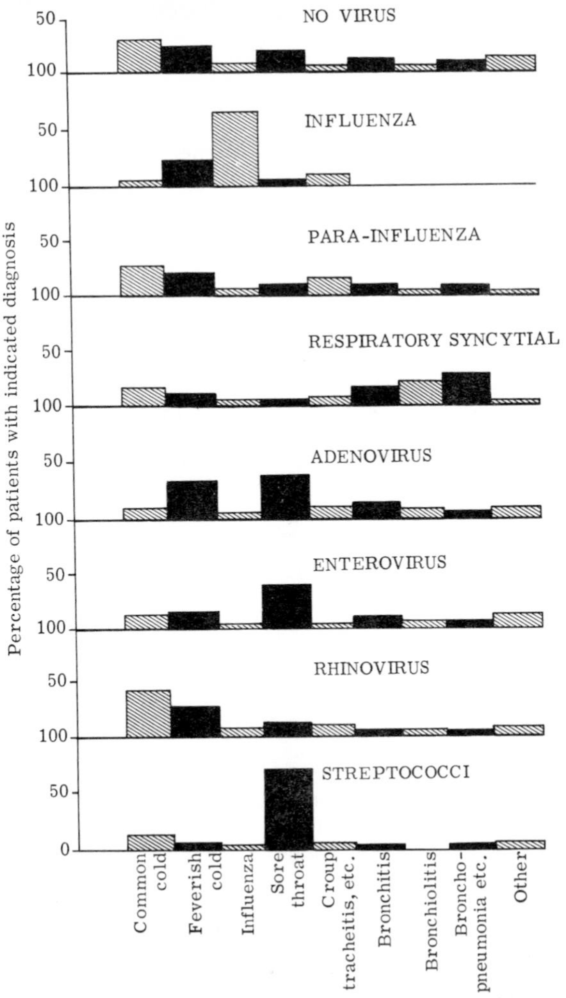

FIG. 58. Relative frequency of the clinical syndromes amongst patients infected with respiratory viruses and streptococci (also a 10 per cent. random sample of patients from whom no pathogens were isolated. 1278 of the 1888 patients were under 10 years of age [Medical Research Council (1965) *Brit. med. J.*, **2**, 324, by permission of the Author and Editor.]

TABLE 44

AGENTS ASSOCIATED WITH ACUTE RESPIRATORY DISEASE SYNDROMES

VIRUS	NUCLEIC ACID	CLASSIFICATION	SEROTYPES
Influenza	RNA	Myxovirus	A, B, C (subgroups within A)
Para-influenza	RNA	Paramyxovirus	1, 2, 3, 4
Respiratory syncytial	RNA		1 (or ? 2)
Rhinovirus	RNA	Acid-labile } Picornavirus	About 100
Coxsackie	RNA	Enterovirus Acid-stable } Picornavirus	A: 1–24 B: 1–6
ECHO	RNA	Enterovirus Acid-stable } Picornavirus	30
Adenoviruses	DNA	Adenovirus	>28
Coronaviruses	RNA		3 or more

of virus infection could be found, is included in TABLE 44, together with a group of cases from which a streptococcus was isolated.

In temperate climates colder periods of the year favour outbreaks of illness due to the influenza and respiratory syncytial virus (RSV) which tends to disappear from the population between times. On the other hand infection with para-influenza type 3 virus is endemic. Infections with the enteroviruses are more prevalent in the warmer months. Rhinovirus infections are perennial with some increase during the autumn and spring.

The incidence and severity of all these clinical syndromes are greater in infants and children and males are more susceptible than females. The incidence is similar in all social groups in the United Kingdom but severe disease is ten times greater in social group V than social group 1. Recurrent attacks are frequent in children. Over 50 per cent. of children will suffer three to seven episodes each year and some even more. The incidence falls after the first 3 years and increases again during the first 2 years of school and then falls sharply thereafter. Prevalence of infection may be higher in families that include a patient with chronic respiratory disease, e.g. chronic bronchitis.

The common cold, sore throat, febrile cold and influenza are fully described earlier [see Section 2].

CROUP

Synonym. Laryngotracheobronchitis.

Aetiology and Pathology

The most common pathogen is the para-influenza virus but many other viruses have been isolated in children with croup. It is most prevalent in infancy and is four times more frequent in boys than girls. There is inflammatory oedema of the larynx and airways with mixed mucoid and mucopurulent secretion.

Clinical Picture

The onset is often quite rapid with malaise, 'croupy cough' which may progress to stridor and severe breathlessness due to respiratory obstruction. The infant may display weakness and restlessness with central cyanosis. The temperature may be a little elevated but the pulse is rapid and of poor volume and the respirations rapid, difficult and accompanied by stridor and intercostal recession.

Diagnosis

Croupy cough or stridor is common during any respiratory infection or exanthem in infancy when the larynx is relatively small.

Bacterial infections such as *acute epiglottitis* due to *H. influenzae* may closely simulate the above disorder. The fiery-red oedematous epiglottis is characteristic and may cause respiratory obstruction with prostration and collapse. Rarer bronchial infections which cause croup and respiratory obstruction are diphtheria in which the membrane may form in the larynx and trachea, typhoid and scarlet fever. *Laryngeal oedema* must be differentiated. It may be a reaction to an ingested or inhaled allergen or a manifestation of angioneurotic oedema and is rare especially in infancy but may cause stridor and respiratory obstruction. *Congenital abnormalities* such as cysts and webs may cause stridor but usually improve as the larynx grows.

All children with croup and laryngotracheobronchitis should be carefully examined and in particular the larynx should be inspected so that a more accurate clinical impression can be formed and specimens taken for microbiological diagnosis.

Radiographs of the chest will usually be normal.

Treatment

All but the mildest cases should be admitted to hospital. They should be nursed in a warm humid environment and in an oxygen tent if there is cyanosis or restlessness. In severe cases of laryngeal obstruction or where repeated suction is necessary to keep the airways clear, tracheostomy should be performed, particularly with severe dyspnoea, rib recession, diminished breath sounds, restlessness or tachycardia. Chemotherapy with a tetracycline, 30 mg. per kg. per day, is necessary if there is a possibility of epiglottitis due to *H. influenzae*. Restlessness and sleeplessness may be helped by chloral hydrate, 0·3–0·5 G. to infants, and convulsions should be treated with diazepam or some other sedative drug like paraldehyde.

Prognosis

This is worst in infants but the over-all prognosis is good, especially after the second and third day of illness.

ACUTE BRONCHIOLITIS AND PNEUMONIA IN INFANTS

ACUTE BRONCHIOLITIS

Aetiology and Pathology

This syndrome tends to occur in epidemics in winter and spring and infection is particularly liable to spread in families. There is a degree of either bronchitis or pneumonia in most cases: in mild forms bronchitis tends to dominate the picture. Respiratory syncytial virus is most often isolated; in some epidemics in as many as 70 per cent. of cases. The airways are acutely inflamed with excessive tenacious mucus. There are catarrhal changes in mucous glands and ducts. Pus may form and the secretion becomes less viscous. Then *H. influenzae*, *Staphylococcus aureus* or *Streptococcus pyogenes* may be grown from the secretions and are presumably secondary invaders. In fatal cases the lungs do not collapse and are just firm to the touch—the alveoli are filled with oedema fluid and macrophages and are often collapsed. There may be an alveolar membrane. There is striking dysplasia of cells lining the airways with destruction of cilia. Immunity probably depends more on local than circulating antibody (IgA). Respiratory function is impaired as a result of airways obstruction with air trapping, diminished compliance together with inequality of ventilation and blood flow leading to hypoxia with cyanosis. This respiratory failure may in turn precipitate convulsions.

Clinical Picture

Acute bronchiolitis in infants and children usually begins with deceptively mild symptoms such as nasal discharge, slight cough and loss of appetite.

There is a sudden increase in the severity of the symptoms with respiratory distress, harsh or irritating unproductive cough and wheeze—fever is notable for its absence or brief duration. The child may become restless and cyanosed. The pulse and respiration rates are rapid and there is intercostal recession with hyperinflation of the chest. The breath sounds may be diminished, and there are widespread rhonchi and crepitations, most frequently over the lower zones. The spleen is occasionally palpable. With cardiac failure the liver will also enlarge.

Diagnosis

The wheeze and other signs of primary involvement of the airways helps to differentiate between pneumonia in infants in which it may be difficult to discern signs in the respiratory tract—the chest radiograph in bronchiolitis shows hyperinflation especially in the lateral view and little or no opacity.

PNEUMONIA IN INFANTS

Aetiology and Pathology

In epidemic form viruses are responsible for most pneumonias in infancy especially the respiratory syncytial virus (RSV) but also adenovirus type 21, para-influenza virus, enterovirus (e.g. Coxsackie) and rhinovirus. In some epidemics RSV may be isolated from as many as 70 per cent. of cases by direct immunofluorescence. Mild respiratory infections are often prevalent in the family. Measles and influenza virus also cause pneumonia—the former may be severe, especially in infants.

Pneumonia is not often bacterial in origin in infancy but in more than 50 per cent. of cases the infecting organism is *Staph. pyogenes*: this organism infrequently causes a specific pneumonia but may be a secondary invader in measles, influenza and other virus infections. Pathologically the lung changes are localized with areas of consolidation.

Clinical Picture

This may be similar to acute bronchiolitis but fever is more pronounced and the child is more ill in relation to the physical signs in the chest. Pallor and cyanosis, tachycardia and tachypnoea are prominent while vomiting and diarrhoea may be misleading. With increasing severity of the disease restlessness and prostration may develop. Wheezes are less than in bronchiolitis while crepitations and signs of consolidation may be found. Complications such as tension cyst, empyema, pyopneumothorax and tension pneumothorax are encountered in bacterial infections, especially staphylococcal. Delayed resolution is unusual and should lead to suspicion of mycoplasma, adenovirus, pertussis, tuberculosis or a foreign body.

Diagnosis

The chest radiograph is vital to the diagnosis and either dense opacities of segmental or lobar distribution, or disseminated shadows of lesser size will be found. Ring shadows due to tension cysts, pleural effusions (empyema) and pneumothorax suggest a bacterial component. The blood count may help to differentiate a viral from a bacterial infection, for a polymorph leucocytosis is more likely in the latter. The infecting organism should be sought from the upper respiratory tract or from blood cultures while special techniques will be needed for virus isolation.

The possibility of underlying disease should be considered, e.g. *congenital heart disease* with pulmonary venous congestion and secondary infection—apart from the physical signs of the cardiac abnormality, the heart is more obviously enlarged on chest radiography, the liver more likely to be enlarged from congestive failure and the cyanosis less likely to be relieved by oxygen breathing if there is a right to left shunt. *Cystic fibrosis* should be suspected if *Staph. pyogenes* is isolated: evidence of pancreatic insufficiency should be sought and the diagnosis confirmed by estimation of the sweat sodium concentration: if this is more than 70 mEq. per litre it will confirm the diagnosis in infants. When collapse dominates the clinical picture meningitis and septicaemia must be eliminated.

Treatment

The child must be admitted to hospital in all but the mildest cases and especially when cyanosis, or restlessness, tachycardia and convulsions are evident. The infant should be handled as little as possible except for feeds. It should not be overcovered or constricted. The environment should be cool and the infant given glucose saline feeds (500 ml. water with 5 G. glucose, 6·5 G. salt). Serum electrolytes should be determined, the state of hydration assessed and deviations from normal corrected. Restlessness and sleeplessness may be alleviated with chloral hydrate, 15 mg. per kg. given three times a day, or 250–750 mg. as a hypnotic. While chemotherapy will not affect the course of a pure virus infection, if there is uncertainty about a bacterial component to the infection, methicillin, cloxacillin or cephaloridine should be given. It is doubtful whether adrenocorticosteroids are of any value. If possible the blood gases should be measured to assist in the management of severe cases and to assess progress. Oxygen should be given by an oxygen tent or hood if there is a fall in arterial oxygen saturation. Fine aerosol mists of saline should be tried when secretions are causing respiratory difficulties. With heart failure digoxin should be added.

Course and Prognosis

Mortality from bronchiolitis and pneumonia is greatest in infants from 6 to 8 weeks old. It then declines gradually during the first year of life and remains low after that. There is an over-all mortality of about 5 per cent. The majority of cases, however, recover rapidly after just 3 days or so of illness to become well again in 7–10 days. Signs of improvement include disappearance of cyanosis and restlessness and return of the appetite.

REFERENCES

Medical Research Council (1965) Report of the M.R.C. Working Party on Acute Respiratory Virus Infections. A collaborative study of the aetiology of acute respiratory infections in Britain 1961–4, *Brit. med. J.*, *2*, 319.

The College of Pathologists Symposium on Acute Respiratory Diseases (1968) ed. Tyrell, D. A. J., *J. clin. Path.*, **21**, Suppl. No. 2.

THE PNEUMONIAS

Synonym. Pneumonitis.

Definition

Inflammatory consolidation of the lung.

Aetiology

While anatomical and other features may be characteristic an aetiological basis of classification is the most satisfactory. Pneumonia is usually due to infection. The definition, however, also includes those rare pneumonias due to chemical and physical agents. Diffuse inflammatory consolidation may also be encountered in allergic or collagen disorders but these are described elsewhere.

Infections which cause pneumonia may be *specific* or *non-specific*. In specific pneumonias the micro-organism invades the lung in which local defences are usually intact, i.e. the cough reflex and the ciliary-mucus mechanisms. Micro-organisms which may specifically cause pneumonia are listed in Table 45. In non-specific pneumonias, the micro-organism—often a common inhabitant of the upper respiratory tract or alimentary tract—is able to invade the lung because these local defence mechanisms are impaired.

A generalized impairment of immune mechanisms may lead to pneumonias in which the invading micro-organism is an unusual virus, fungus or protozoon—a so-called *opportunistic* infection. Such immune deficiencies are found in primary hypo- or dysgammaglobulin-anaemia or in those that occur with the leukaemias, lymphomata and myeloma, or in the rare granulomatous disease of childhood. Immunosuppressive and cyto-toxic drugs, radiation and corticosteroid therapy are also contributory factors. Those micro-organisms more likely to be found in opportunistic infections of the lung are indicated in Table 45.

Specific pneumonias may develop in the course of a systemic infection, e.g. typhus, typhoid, infectious mononucleosis, chickenpox and smallpox. These pneumonias form only a part of the total clinical picture and may be relatively unimportant.

THE BACTERIAL PNEUMONIAS

Aetiology

The prevalence and severity of bacterial pneumonias and the relative frequency of pathogens causing them varies from country to country. Amongst hospital patients in New Zealand, for instance, the pneumococcus was found in no more than 8 per cent. of all cases of pneumonia, while the staphylococcus accounted for 38 per cent. of cases. On the other hand in North America and in Africa more than 80 per cent. of pneumonias are attributed to the pneumococcus. In the United Kingdom there is an increasing proportion of pneumonias which are thought to be of bacterial origin from which the organism is not recovered and in one series this amounted to half of all hospital patients with pneumonia. It is assumed that this was because of previous chemotherapy. While specific bacterial pneumonias appear to be less common, those of the non-specific type are more so. Bacterial pneumonias are frequently secondary to virus infections such as influenza: they complicate chronic bronchitis and even pulmonary oedema. In these pneumonias the bacterial flora may be nondescript or pathogens such as the *Staphylococcus pyogenes* may predominate. In 5 per cent. of cases Gram-negative organisms were thought to be responsible for pneumonia in a large series of cases; a quarter of these cases were due to *Escherichia coli*. Care, however, must be exercised in interpretation

TABLE 45

MICRO-ORGANISMS WHICH CAUSE PNEUMONIA

COMMON	UNCOMMON	UNCOMMON
BACTERIA		YEASTS AND FUNGI
Streptococcus pneumoniae	*Klebsiella pneumoniae*	*Actinomycosis israeli*, etc.
Staphylococcus pyogenes	*Streptococcus pyogenes* and *viridans*	**Nocardia asteroides*
Mycobacterium tuberculosis	*Escherichia coli*, *Pseudomonas aeruginosa*	**Aspergillus fumigatus*
	Haemophilus influenzae	**Mucor rhizopus*
	Salmonella typhi and *paratyphi*	*Coccidioides immitis*
	Brucella abortus and *melitensis*	*Histoplasma capsulatum*
	Pasteurella pestis	**Cryptococcus neoformans*
	Bordetella pertussis	
MYCOPLASMA		
Mycoplasma pneumoniae		
	Coxiella burnetii (Q fever)	
	Rickettsia prowazeki (typhus)	
VIRUSES		PROTOZOA
Myxovirus: influenza, para-influenza and respiratory syncytial virus	*Psittacosis-ornithosis* group	*Entamoeba histolytica*
	Varicella, *variola*	**Pneumocystis carinii*
	Herpes zoster	**Toxoplasma gondii*
Adenovirus	*Infectious mononucleosis*	
Measles virus	*Lymphocytic choriomeningitis*	
Picornavirus	*Cytomegalovirus*	

* Indicates micro-organisms sometimes found in *opportunistic* infections of the lung.

of sputum flora. Gram-negative organisms frequently replace the true pathogens particularly when the latter have been eradicated by earlier chemotherapy, and play no pathogenic role. It is often very difficult to establish a causal relationship between such Gram-negative organisms as *Esch. coli*, *Pseudomonas aeruginosa*, *H. influenzae*, *Bordetella pertussis* and pneumonia.

In specific pneumonias there may be an antecedent injury to the respiratory mucosa by virus infections, e.g. the rhinovirus, but this has yet to be established. There is clinical and experimental evidence to suggest that aspiration of mucus with the pathogen is necessary for the invasion by the micro-organism. In specific bacterial pneumonias due to the pneumococcus it is types 1, 3, 7, 2, 8, 4, 9, and 10 and 14 in children that are the most common invaders. *Staph. pyogenes* is also common but *Klebsiella* and streptococci are rare. *Mycobacterium tuberculosis* is becoming a less frequent cause of pneumonia in developed countries: tuberculous pneumonia is described on page 869.

Specific pneumonias of bacterial origin occur at all ages, that due to the pneumococcus is most prevalent between the ages of ten and forty whereas those due to the staphylococcus are more severe in infants and the aged.

Pathology

There is clinical and experimental evidence to suggest that aspiration of mucus in which the pathogen is transported to the periphery of the bronchial tree is necessary for the initiation of infection. Alternatively, obstruction or impairment of the ciliary mechanism may prevent clearance of aspirated material and favour the growth of micro-organisms peripherally.

In pneumonia there is exudation of fluid into the alveoli which spreads to adjacent acini and segments. The fluid is invaded by neutrophils and red cells which give rise to consolidation. The alveoli are first filled with red cells and fibrin and the pulmonary capillaries are widely dilated (*red hepatization*). The red cells are then replaced by neutrophil leucocytes which phagocytose the bacteria and the capillaries become less congested (*grey hepatization*). The intensity of this process of exudation of inflammatory oedema probably depends on the virulence of the pathogen and is a particular feature of influenzal pneumonia whether this is complicated by staphylococcal or streptococcal infection or not.

Necrosis may accompany a severe inflammatory reaction and proceed to the formation of small abscesses or of tension cysts, particularly in staphylococcal pneumonia. Less commonly the inflammation may develop into diffuse suppuration and abscess formation —especially with infection due to the staphylococcus and *Klebsiella*.

Clearance of the inflammatory debris is in part non-cellular by enzymes and in part cellular by macrophages derived from the alveolar epithelium and the pulmonary capillaries.

The pneumonic process may be confined to a segment or lobe or may be patchy. The distribution is not characteristic of any particular micro-organism. The initial acute inflammatory process may be associated with bacteraemia which is more common with pneumococcal pneumonias than with others. The inflammation may spread directly to invade the pleura or less commonly the pericardium. The resolution of the inflammatory process in pneumococcal pneumonia is usually complete. The process however, may be delayed or arrested by intense fibrosis—this is called organized pneumonia.

The reason for this is not usually clear but it may follow necrosis of the lung particularly with staphylococcal pneumonia or *Klebsiella* pneumonia.

Pneumonia causes a restrictive defect of ventilation with a reduction in vital capacity and lung compliance. The work of breathing is diminished by a small tidal volume and a rapid rate of breathing. This pattern of breathing is encouraged by pleuritic pain if it is present. Ventilation of the alveoli is also grossly impaired by inflammatory oedema. On the other hand, the blood flow is maintained. Physiological shunting ensues and is the cause of the reduction in arterial P_{O_2}. If this is considerable then the arterial oxygen saturation is reduced with development of cyanosis. The arterial P_{CO_2} usually remains normal unless the pneumonia complicates a disorder associated with severe airways obstruction (e.g. chronic obstructive bronchitis).

Clinical Picture [PLATE 8]

Symptoms and physical signs are notable for their great variability and may be considerably modified by previous chemotherapy. An acute onset is characteristic of pneumococcal pneumonia in which 80 per cent. of patients experience a rigor. On the other hand an insidious onset following a previous upper respiratory infection is characteristic of a staphylococcal pneumonia. Seventy per cent. of patients with primary pneumonias experience chest pain at the onset which is of a pleuritic nature. The pain strikes the patient on the affected side and may be referred to the abdomen or shoulder if the diaphragmatic pleura is involved. Upper abdominal pain and rigidity may simulate an abdominal emergency. Cough at first is usually dry and irritating and may cause distress because it aggravates the pain. At this stage sputum is scanty and tenacious, but it becomes less viscid and more abundant later. It is often frankly blood-stained particularly at the onset, but it may appear rusty or pink in colour. The sputum is particularly viscid with certain types of pneumococcal pneumonia (Type 3) and with *Klebsiella* infection. Sleeplessness, headache, delirium and confusion with much weakness are manifestations of toxaemia.

The physical signs are also variable and they depend on the severity of the infection and the degree of lung involvement. The patient is frequently extremely ill and apprehensive with a rapid progression of manifestations. There is characteristically a high fever and a temperature as high as 102°–105° F. (38·9°–40·6° C.) may be found. This high fever may be continuous, for example, with pneumococcal pneumonia, or remittent, for example with staphylococcal pneumonia. With the severest toxaemias the body temperature may not be so high. The skin tends to be hot and moist and may be pale due to peripheral vasoconstriction with systemic hypotension. There is often central cyanosis and active contraction of the alae nasi muscles with breathing. The breathing tends to be rapid and shallow at a rate of 30–60 or more per minute. Herpes simplex may erupt round the lips. Jaundice is sometimes apparent early in the disease and the onset may be punctuated by convulsions particularly in younger people who also may have neck stiffness (meningism). Physical signs may be almost absent at the onset but diminished chest movement on the affected side is frequently found if the disease is unilateral. Then localized crepitations appear and spread and then usually give way to the signs of gross consolidation of the lung, i.e. an impaired percussion note, bronchial breathing, bronchophony, and whispering pectoriloquy. A pleural friction rub is frequently heard over the consolidated area and may be early in its appearance. As the disease regresses the physical signs of consolidation tend to be replaced once again by crepitations during the ensuing days. After 7 days or so high continuous fever in pneumococcal pneumonia is characteristically abruptly terminated by crisis with sudden fall to normal. This characteristic pattern is no longer seen for chemotherapy causes a rapid fall in temperature over 2 to 3 days by lysis. A similar and gradual fall in body temperature may occur naturally in other non-pneumococcal pneumonias. With the fall in temperature to normal there is a rapid relief of symptoms but the physical signs are slower to clear.

Pneumonia is most frequently complicated by a *pleural effusion*. Physical signs of pleural fluid will replace the pleural rub early in the disease or later when the signs of consolidation are resolving. The volume of fluid is usually small, serous in nature and sterile on culture as a result of the chemotherapy that has usually been given. Even so there may be a slight persistence of fever with such a sterile effusion. If, however, chemotherapy is delayed or inappropriate an *empyema* may develop with persistent remittent, or intermittent fever. At the same time the patient remains ill. A *spontaneous pneumothorax* or *pyopneumothorax* is an occasional complication of staphylococcal pneumonia and is usually produced by rupture of a tension cyst through the pleura. This complication is seen most frequently in infants. *Pericarditis* is a less common complication and should be suspected when the patient becomes less well, develops precordial pain affected by posture as well as coughing, together with a pericardial friction rub. Pericardial tamponade would be indicated by pulsus paradoxus and an elevated systemic venous pressure. *Meningitis*, *endocarditis*, and *suppurative arthritis* may complicate a bacteraemia.

Toxaemia may precipitate *congestive cardiac failure* with a rise in systemic venous pressure, enlargement of the liver and oedema. This is often associated with atrial fibrillation. The development of systemic *hypotension* and *oliguria* or *anuria* are serious complications. A fall of systolic blood pressure below 90 mm. Hg may result simply from toxaemia and may be aggravated by dehydration, electrolyte disturbance and anoxia. Oliguria or anuria are due to toxic changes in the kidney with or without tubular necrosis. These are very serious developments and may complicate as many as one third of patients with staphylococcal pneumonia but rather less often with other bacterial pathogens. *Paralytic ileus* and *jaundice* are further manifestations of severe toxaemia. Jaundice is usually 'obstructive' in type.

Diagnosis

Usually the clinical picture of pneumonia is characteristic but occasionally an onset with meningism particularly in children may simulate meningitis. The reference of pleuritic pain to the upper abdomen or renal angle may simulate an abdominal emergency such as a perforated viscus, subphrenic abscess or acute pyelonephritis. A rapid respiration rate is characteristic of pneumonia and when other conditions are in doubt the *chest radiograph* will usually be helpful. It is important for lateral views to be taken as well as the conventional postero-anterior view to exclude involvement of the posterior basal segments of the lower lobes. In the chest radiographs the shadows may be segmental or lobar, complete, or partial but usually homogeneous. On the other hand, the shadowing may be non-homogeneous, patchy clouding. There may be a little shrinkage of the affected lobe or segment. Bacterial pneumonias may be unilateral or bilateral and their extent or distribution is not diagnostic of any bacterial pathogen. Ring shadows, which may be large, are usually due to infection with the staphylococcus or *Klebsiella*. The radiological appearances are not helpful in distinguishing bacterial pneumonias from those due to other micro-organisms. It is necessary for the *sputum* to be examined by microscopy and culture to identify the pathogen. Large numbers of pneumococci or staphylococci may be seen on a Gram stain of the sputum. Large numbers of acid-fast bacilli indicate a tuberculous aetiology. *Blood cultures* should be taken and from these pneumococci or other bacteria may be cultivated. A neutrophil leucocytosis with a count of twelve to fifteen thousand is usually found. Counts as high as forty thousand neutrophils are not common but such leukaemoid responses are more frequently encountered with pneumococcal pneumonias. A neutrophil leucocytosis, however, is unreliable evidence of a bacterial cause for the pneumonia. On the other hand the absence of such a response with pneumococcal, staphylococcal and streptococcal pneumonias is considered a poor prognostic sign.

It is important to distinguish *pulmonary infarction* from pneumonia, and the predominance of haemoptysis, the absence of purulent sputum with pleuritic pain and haemodynamic evidence of right ventricular strain or failure with a low cardiac output, and the peripheral evidence of venous thrombosis should raise the suspicion of pulmonary infarction.

Treatment

The patient should be nursed in bed. Tepid sponging may be required for high fever and sweating which readily cause dehydration. Three to four litres of fluid will be required in the 24 hours in whatever form pleases the patient most. A high salt intake is necessary as well (5–10 g. per 24 hours) provided that there has been no sodium retention beforehand, e.g. with congestive cardiac failure. Serum electrolytes should be measured if there is any doubt, and fluid and electrolytes given intravenously if they cannot be taken by mouth. The urinary output must be measured and fluid therapy guided by this and the specific gravity when renal function is otherwise normal. Concern for calorie intake and solid food can await defervescence.

In previously normal patients with an acute, severe pneumonia, sleeplessness, restlessness, pleuritic pain and irritating cough are best relieved by diamorphine hydrochloride, 5 mg., or morphine sulphate, 10 mg. subcutaneously. Drugs which depress respiratory drive should be avoided in patients with severe airways obstruction in whom the arterial P_{CO_2} may be elevated. In these cases pethidine, 50 mg., or methadone hydrochloride, 5–10 mg., might be used instead. Restlessness and sleeplessness alone may be relieved by diazepam, 5–10 mg., or paraldehyde, 10 ml. by deep intramuscular injection. Hypoxaemia with cyanosis requires correction by oxygen breathing. This should be given by a plastic mask, nasal catheter or oxygen tent in a concentration adequate to raise the arterial oxygen saturation above 90 per cent. and abolish central cyanosis.

Chemotherapy. In established pneumococcal or streptococcal pneumonia and in other bacterial pneumonias in which penicillin-sensitive organisms are known to be the causal agents (e.g. penicillin-sensitive staphylococci) benzylpenicillin remains the drug of choice. It should be given in a dose of one million Units (1 mega Unit) intramuscularly six-hourly for at least a week, for relapse will occur in a proportion of patients if treatment is curtailed. Staphylococcal pneumonia requires rather longer treatment—at least 10–14 days or even longer if there has been a bacteraemia or metastatic spread. In staphylococcal pneumonias where the sensitivity of the organism is unknown, treatment should be instituted with penicillinase-resistant penicillins, e.g. cloxacillin, 1 G. intramuscularly followed by 0·5 G. six-hourly by mouth. In more severe cases methicillin may be given in a dose of 8–12 G. intravenously in the first 24 hours. The subsequent treatment of such a staphylococcal pneumonia should be guided by the sensitivities of the organism and by the response to treatment. Chemotherapy should be changed to benzylpenicillin if sensitivity tests reveal the organism to be sensitive. With *Klebsiella* pneumonia, chemotherapy with streptomycin sulphate, 1 G. daily or twice daily, or gentamycin, 4 mg. per kg. per day in three divided doses, in combination with a sulphonamide is probably the treatment of choice. With *Esch. coli* pneumonias, kanamycin, 0·5–1 G. intramuscularly daily together with chloramphenicol, 500 mg. six-hourly, or tetracycline, 250 mg. six-hourly is the treatment of choice. Treatment of these pneumonias should be continued for at least 10 days. In a rare pneumonia due to pseudomonas, carbenicillin should be given in a dose of at least 6 G. given rapidly intravenously four to six-hourly together with gentamycin, 4 mg. per kg. per day in three doses intramuscularly.

In severe pneumonias where the causal organism is unknown, treatment should be started with parenteral methicillin or cloxacillin together with gentamycin, streptomycin, or cephaloridine. When the results of sputum culture and sensitivities of organisms are obtained then treatment can be modified. In mild pneumonias where the organism is unknown treatment may be started with tetracycline, 250 mg. four times a day or ampicillin, 500 mg. four times a day.

With hypotension it may be necessary to give plasma or saline intravenously while carefully observing the systemic venous pressure, arterial pulses, blood pressure and urinary output. The use of adrenergic drugs to increase peripheral vascular resistance has proved of little value. It is claimed that adrenocortical steroids in very high doses may help to counteract some of the severe toxaemic manifestations and for this hydrocortisone is given intravenously in a dose of 1 G. in the 24 hours. The treatment of oliguria and anuria is discussed in Section 12 but it may be necessary to undertake dialysis if medical measures are inadequate to control such effects of anuria as arise in serum potassium and urea, etc.

Prognosis

The prognosis of untreated pneumonia depends upon the resistance of the host and is therefore worse when cellular or humoral immunity is impaired: of equal importance is the nature of the infecting organism—thus in pneumococcal pneumonia, the mortality before the advent of chemotherapy was about 25 per cent. Since the discovery of penicillin this mortality has been reduced to about 5 per cent. The mortality with staphylococcal pneumonias is much higher at 25 per cent. and with *Klebsiella* pneumonia higher still at about 40 per cent. The prognosis is worse in infants and the aged and is adversely affected by delayed treatment, extensive pneumonia, bacteraemia, jaundice, hypotension and oliguria. The outcome is usually fatal if anuria develops.

REFERENCES

KELLAWAY, G., and LE GRICE, H. (1962) Hypotension and oliguria in staphylococcal pneumonia, *Brit. med. J.*, **1**, 426.

MORROW, G. W., OLSEN, A. M., and MARTIN, W. J. (1962) Infectious pneumonia, a continuing process in diagnosis and management, *Proc. Mayo Clin.*, **37**, 151.

SATHAVARA, S., and FLIPPIN, H. F. (1956) Klebsiella in respiratory disease, *Ann. intern. Med.*, **45**, 1010.

TILLOTSON, J. R., and LERNER, A. M. (1967) Characteristics of pneumonias caused by *Escherichia coli*, *New Engl. J. Med.*, **277**, 115.

TILLOTSON, J. R., and LERNER, A. M. (1968) *Hemophilus influenzae* bronchopneumonia in adults, *Arch. intern. Med.*, **121**, 428.

WEISS, W., EISENBERG, G. M., SPIVACK, A., NADEL, J., KAYSER, H. L., SATHAVARA, S., and FLIPPIN, H. F. (1956) Klebsiella in respiratory disease, *Ann. intern. Med.*, **45**, 1010.

PNEUMONIA DUE TO SMALLER MICRO-ORGANISMS
(Mycoplasma, Rickettsia and Viruses)

The pneumonias due to these agents vary widely in severity and in their clinical presentation. Thus, in infectious mononucleosis, the illness is usually mild, whereas in influenza it may be devastating and rapidly fatal. Many of the pneumonias, however, pursue a somewhat common clinical pattern, especially those due to mycoplasma, rickettsia (Q fever) and certain viruses, e.g. adenovirus and para-influenza virus, which may have given rise to trivial respiratory illness in contacts. Mycoplasma pneumonia is described in more detail as an example. Pneumonias associated with infection due to rickettsia (Q fever), the ornithosis group of viruses (psittacosis) and other viruses such as influenza, variola, varicella and certain other viruses are described in Section 2.

PNEUMONIA DUE TO MYCOPLASMA PNEUMONIAE

Synonyms. Primary atypical pneumonia; Eaton agent pneumonia.

Aetiology

In a number of community studies *Mycoplasma pneumoniae* was found to be responsible for 10–35 per cent. of lower respiratory infections and is world wide in prevalence. It is often the cause of such illness in the summer and autumn, though it is perennial in its attack. Spread of infection is often observed within families or institutions with an interval of about 16–23 days between cases. The infection has a high attack rate, especially in children over five and young adults and usually causes minor or trivial respiratory illness: only about one in thirty infected persons develops pneumonia. The organism continues to be secreted for a long time, i.e. 10–13 weeks.

Clinical Picture

The illness of mycoplasma pneumonia varies considerably in severity. The onset is usually characterized by general symptoms such as malaise, fever and headache 1–5 days before development of respiratory symptoms. Occasionally there are sore throat and coryza. The cough at first is dry, later becoming productive of mainly mucoid sputum. These symptoms may persist as long as 4 weeks. Pleurisy is unusual. The fever is usually remittent at first and then intermittent, lasting from 10 to 14 days. Physical signs such as crepitations or those of consolidation develop after the fourth day or so. A pleural friction rub may be heard in about 5 per cent. of cases. The illness is usually uncomplicated but on rare occasions a haemolytic anaemia may occur, even less commonly erythema multiforme, erythema nodosum, otitis media, pericarditis, arthralgia and meningo-encephalitis.

Diagnosis

This is difficult on clinical grounds but is easier if some of the rarer complications accompany the clinical picture. Chest radiographs most commonly show patchy, mainly basal shadows and one fifth of cases are bilateral. Any lobe, however, may be completely consolidated and small pleural effusions may be seen in 20 per cent. of cases. The hilar lymph nodes may be enlarged. Cold agglutinins appear early and are found in about 50 per cent. of cases. The development of complement fixing antibodies occurs in 90 per cent. of patients and a high level of this antibody or a change in level provides the most satisfactory confirmation of the diagnosis. *M. pneumoniae* can be grown in artificial media but this is a slow process.

Treatment

Patients who are ill with this type of pneumonia should generally be treated along the lines recommended in bacterial pneumonias. Chemotherapy with the tetracyclines (i.e. demethylchlortetracycline, 300 mg. two to three times a day for 6 days) have been shown to reduce duration of the fever, clinical signs and radiological abnormalities. This favourable response, however, is not commonly encountered in clinical practice and *M. pneumoniae* may be grown from sputum during and after treatment with tetracyclines or erythromycin to which the organism is sensitive.

Course and Prognosis

The illness normally pursues a slow course and cough with abnormal signs and radiological shadows may persist for several weeks. In one series 13 per cent. of cases suffered clinical relapse. The prognosis is very favourable.

REFERENCES

CHANOCK, R. M. (1965) Mycoplasma infections of man, *New Engl. J. Med.*, **273,** 1199 and 1257.

LAMBERT, H. P. (1968) *M. pneumoniae* infections, in Symposium on Acute Respiratory Diseases, *J. clin. Path.*, Suppl. No. 2, 52.

OTHER PNEUMONIAS

CHEMICAL

Inflammatory consolidation of the lung may be due to inhalation of irritant gases, smokes and fumes. They may develop after exposure to dust which contains beryllium, manganese, etc. Aspiration of petrol or paraffin (kerosene) may cause a severe pneumonia, usually in children, in addition to widespread systemic toxic effects. If the initial poisoning is survived then the pneumonia usually resolves.

Inhalation of vegetable, mineral or animal oils leads to the development of *exogenous lipoid pneumonia.* This is most common in the young or aged and is most often due to inhalation of nasal drops or laxatives which contain liquid paraffin. The lesions may be diffuse or localized in which case they may resemble a carcinoma. Inquiry concerning oil-containing preparations should always be made in suspicious cases. The finding of oil or fat-laden macrophages in the sputum is not specific. *Endogenous lipoid pneumonia* is a rare chronic granulomatous lesion in which there are macrophages filled with cholesterol, the cause of which is unknown, but it may complicate carcinoma of the lung, lung abscess, etc. Equally obscure are the cases of focal granulomatous lesions with macrophages laden with fat and cholesterol which have been described in association with pulmonary hypertension of diverse origin.

REFERENCES

British Medical Journal (1969) Cholesterol granuloma of the lung, Leading article, **1,** 396.

WEILL, H., FERRANS, V. J., GAY, R. M., and ZISKIND, M. M. (1964) Early lipoid pneumonia, *Amer. J. Med.*, **36,** 370.

PHYSICAL

Diffuse lymphocytic infiltration, organizing alveolar exudate and fibrosis with consolidation may complicate radiotherapy, e.g. to the breast. The extent of this pneumonia depends on the radiation dose and the amount of lung irradiated. A restrictive defect of ventilation develops at a variable rate, but is usually maximal about a month after radiation and if extensive causes severe breathlessness. Massive shadowing may be seen in the chest radiograph in the acute stage which resembles pulmonary oedema. This gives way eventually to linear shadowing and distortion of fibrosis and sometimes to rib necrosis with fractures. Symptoms may be relieved by oxygen breathing, and adrenocortical steroids (e.g. prednisone, 50 mg. daily at first). If the process is severe and widespread it may prove fatal.

REFERENCE

WHITFIELD, A. G. W., BOND, W. H., and KUNKLER, P. B. (1963) Radiation damage to thoracic tissues, *Thorax*, **18,** 371.

NON-SPECIFIC PNEUMONIAS AND LUNG ABSCESS

Synonyms. Aspiration pneumonia; Suppurative pneumonia.

Definition

Non-specific pneumonias are those due to micro-organisms not primarily pathogenic in the lung and that develop as a result of impaired local bronchopulmonary defence mechanisms.

Pathogenesis

Aspiration of mucus and other material into the bronchial tree and impairment of the cough reflex and ciliary mechanism allow micro-organisms normally non-pathogenic in the lung to flourish and cause inflammatory change. Aspiration is particularly likely to happen with infections of the upper respiratory tract, with oral or dental infection, with neurological disorders affecting swallowing, e.g. pseudobulbar palsy and myasthenia gravis, and with obstructive lesions of the oesophagus. These predisposing factors together with the reduction of the cough reflex during sleep, anaesthesia, stupor or coma allow material to be lodged in the lung most commonly in the posterior and axillary segments of the upper lobes and apical segments of the lower lobes. Gravity usually determines which lung is involved. Material for aspiration may come from suppurative conditions within the lung itself such as bronchiectasis or lung abscess. Progressive inflammation with suppuration is especially liable to develop in weak and debilitated patients who are unable to cough and in those with diabetes mellitus. The airways may be blocked not only by aspirated mucus and vomit but also by external pressure of lymph glands and by pathological processes involving the wall or lumen of the bronchus such as a fibrous stricture or benign and malignant neoplasms.

As a result of the impaired clearance of the blocked airway, the lobe or segment of lung distal to the block may partially collapse and become the site of an acute inflammatory process due to organisms which lie normally outside the lower respiratory tract. These organisms may be aerobic or anaerobic. The inflammatory process may be mild and unnoticed and produce a trivial illness: it may be moderate to severe and present as a suppurative pneumonia or progress to lung abscess. Presentation, however, may be that of a solitary lung abscess with little or no surrounding pneumonia. Acute suppurative pneumonia with or without lung abscess may resolve if the cause is removed but this process is accelerated by chemotherapy. Otherwise the suppurative process may persist as a chronic non-specific suppurative pneumonia with or without abscess formation. The incidence of trivial non-specific pneumonias is not known but suppurative pneumonia and lung abscess which may develop at any age are now very uncommon.

LUNG ABSCESS

Lung abscess may develop under circumstances other than those in which the bronchopulmonary defence mechanisms are impaired. Thus lung abscesses are found:

1. As a complication of certain specific bacterial pneumonias, particularly those due to *Staph. pyogenes* and *Klebsiella pneumoniae* which themselves may develop into a subacute or chronic suppurative pneumonia.
2. As a result of invasion of the lung from below the diaphragm. An example of this is the spread through the diaphragm from a liver abscess due to *Entamoeba histolytica* which causes suppuration in the adjacent lung and sometimes rupture of the abscess into the bronchus.
3. With emboli derived from septic systemic thrombophlebitis (pyaemia) in which suppuration develops in one or more infarcts in the lung which then proceeds to abscess formation.

The lung abscess may be only a minor factor in a severe systemic illness; but in children particularly a subpleural abscess of this type may rupture into the pleura with the formation of a pyopneumothorax. In these cases the organism is usually a staphylococcus. The same organism may be found in septic emboli introduced by intravenous injection in drug addicts in which cases there may be multiple small septic infarcts which may cavitate without severe illness. Endocarditis or endaortitis of a patent ductus arteriosus may be the site of origin of septic emboli. It is unusual for a sterile pulmonary infarct to become secondarily infected and suppurate. Such a development should be differentiated from a cavitated sterile infarct which may be associated with a systemic infection.

Clinical Picture in Non-specific Pneumonia and Lung Abscess

The severity of illness produced by the non-specific pneumonias varies widely and is often trivial with mild non-specific infections. Suppurative pneumonia with or without lung abscess may be sudden or gradual in onset. A latent period may follow aspiration and the incident in which aspiration occurred may be forgotten. There is increasing fever and cough. Purulent sputum is expectorated from the start and is often copious in volume (i.e. 50–200 ml. or more per day). Sputum is sometimes offensive or foetid. Pleuritic chest pain and haemoptysis are frequent. If the illness is inadequately treated the symptoms may settle, and the patient feel relatively well. Then sputum is retained and expectoration diminishes, but over the succeeding week or two fever returns to 38° or 39° C. Sputum expectoration may then suddenly increase in volume with further amelioration of the illness. Such remissions and exacerbations may continue for months. Clubbing of the fingers may develop quite rapidly but pulmonary osteoarthropathy rarely develops. Signs of consolidation may be found in the chest. As suppurative pneumonia and abscess may be complicated by aspiration of pus into other parts of the lung the signs may be more widespread.

Suppurative pneumonia and lung abscess may be complicated by the spread of the inflammatory process locally to affect the pleura or pericardium, or distally via the blood stream to cause, for instance, a cerebral abscess. If the suppurative process is inadequately controlled amyloidosis may result. Resolution is accompanied by fibrosis and bronchiectasis.

Diagnosis

This is usually straightforward in the classical case with fever and copious purulent sputum which follows an event such as an operation under general anaesthesia with dental sepsis or following alcoholic excess. Underlying oesophageal obstruction, e.g. achalasia of the cardia, stricture or carcinoma, may pass unnoticed and should always be considered in the absence of any other cause. Carcinoma of the lung is frequently associated with the development of suppurative pneumonia and abscess. The growth itself may undergo necrosis and cavitate, particularly if it is a well differentiated squamous cell variety. In this case, however, the presentation is usually so mild that it may be discovered on routine chest radiography or following a haemoptysis.

Chest radiography is essential in the diagnosis. Suppurative and non-suppurative pneumonias should be suspected when a homogeneous opacity affects the apical segment of the lower lobe or posterior and axillary segments of the upper lobes, but it may be lobar in extent. Fluid levels may appear early or late and indicate abscess formation. Shadows arise elsewhere in the lung from aspiration of pus. Multiple fluid levels may on occasion be found in extensive suppurative pneumonia. In necrotic, cavitated carcinoma the radiograph usually shows an irregular or ragged margin to the airspace. Secondarily infected bullae, cysts both bronchogenic and hydatid, and sequestrated lung segments may mimic lung abscess. Barium swallow or oesophagoscopy should be considered if oesophageal obstruction is suspected.

Bronchoscopy is always necessary to exclude obstruction of the bronchus. A carcinoma is the commonest intrabronchial finding in adults and a foreign body in children. With inflammatory change and a segmental site of origin the causal lesion may be difficult to see. From the *sputum* a variety of organisms is usually found in non-specific suppurative pneumonia with or without abscess, e.g. *Str. viridans*, haemolytic or non-haemolytic, aerobic or anaerobic streptococci, pneumococci, Vincent's organisms, *Mycobacterium tuberculosis* should always be sought by microscopy to exclude cavitating tuberculosis. If a carcinoma is a possibility cytology of the sputum should be investigated—occasional false positive findings are found in suppurative pneumonia. Pure growth of organisms such as *Staph. aureus*, *Kl. pneumoniae*, *Str. pneumoniae* or fungi such as *Actinomycosis israeli* would indicate a specific pneumonia that has proceeded to suppuration.

A neutrophil leucocytosis of more than 12,000 and often more than 20,000 is usually found.

Treatment

Removal of the cause if such exists is the most important aspect of treatment and to this end physiotherapy with postural coughing and percussion of the chest, bronchoscopy and oesophagoscopy are important means of obtaining bronchial clearance.

Chemotherapy. Intramuscular benzylpenicillin remains the drug of choice in non-specific infections for the wide variety of micro-organisms are nearly always penicillin sensitive. According to the severity of the infection, one or two mega Units should be given intramuscularly every 4–6 hours for 4–6 weeks. A predominant growth of other organisms resistant to penicillin, e.g. *Klebsiella* and other Gram-negative bacteria, would demand appropriate chemotherapy. Medical treatment is usually successful unless bronchial drainage remains impaired.

If this treatment fails and if suppuration and abscess formation remain localized and contained then surgery has to be considered. The affected lobe should be resected together with the causal lesion, e.g. the carcinoma if this is possible.

Prognosis

The prognosis for mild non-specific pneumonias properly treated with chemotherapy is excellent and recovery without lung damage is expected. Sometimes there is open healing of an abscess which becomes epithelialized. Half to three-quarters of patients recover satisfactorily and are restored to good health. Unfavourable factors in recovery are delayed treatment, very large abscesses, permanent pre-existing bronchial disease and diabetes mellitus. When bacteriological control is not obtained or where underlying disease cannot be removed then the disease may progress and prove fatal.

REFERENCES

BROCK, R. C. (1952) *Lung Abscess*, Oxford.

FIFER, W. R., HUSEBYE, K., CHEDISTER, C., and MILLER, M. (1961) Primary lung abscess—analysis of therapy and results in 55 cases, *Arch. intern. Med.*, **107**, 668.

NICHOLSON, H. (1950) Suppurative pneumonia, *Lancet*, ii, 605.

THE LUNG IN THROMBO-EMBOLIC DISEASE

Peripheral venous thrombosis, embolism to and thrombosis within pulmonary arteries and the haemodynamic consequences of thrombo-embolism are discussed in Section 8. Treatment of massive and recurrent embolism is also discussed in that section.

Pulmonary veno-occlusive disease of unknown aetiology is a very rare condition which presents with the picture of subacute pulmonary oedema without evidence of primary alveolar abnormality or of any disorder of the left side of the heart on clinical examination or detailed investigation, including cardiac catheterization.

PULMONARY INFARCTION

Definition

Haemorrhagic necrosis of the lung distal to an occlusion of the pulmonary artery.

Pathogenesis

Pulmonary infarction does not always follow occlusion of a branch of the pulmonary artery—presumably because of collateral supply from other branches of the same artery or because of the bronchial artery supply. Conditions required for infarction to develop are not known, but an important factor is an elevated pulmonary venous pressure, e.g. with mitral stenosis or left ventricular failure. The commonest form of occlusion leading to infarction is thrombotic, usually embolic from a peripheral venous source or the right heart, e.g. right atrium in atrial fibrillation. Sometimes the thrombosis is local, occurring *in situ* in a branch of the pulmonary artery in which atheroma has developed as a result of long-standing chronic pulmonary disease or heart disease, e.g. pulmonary hypertension, which may be primary or secondary to congenital heart disease, mitral stenosis, pulmonary fibrosis or chronic bronchitis. Local obstruction of pulmonary vessels is also encountered in polycythaemia and sickle-cell disease. Other forms of embolism are rare, e.g. fat embolism, which may follow severe trauma. This causes symptoms and signs due to obstruction of small pulmonary vessels, but infarction is not usually found. Pulmonary infarction is most commonly seen in the lower parts of the lung, due probably to streaming of emboli and greater blood flow to the dependent parts of the lung. A pulmonary infarct consists of a wedge of haemorrhagic necrotic lung, one side of which usually lies along the pleura. The pleura becomes inflamed and frequently an effusion develops (a pleural exudate). The pleurisy is painful if inflammatory changes involve the parietal pleura. Pulmonary infarcts are frequently multiple and bilateral and rarely cavitate or become infected. However, septic thrombotic emboli may originate in an infected peripheral vein, commonly in drug addicts.

Infarcts are most commonly encountered in middle-aged or elderly people with or without evidence of peripheral venous disease. Conditions known to predispose to thrombo-embolism or primary thrombosis and infarction are often found, e.g. immobilization, surgery, pregnancy, the contraceptive pill, malignancy and evidence of left heart disease or pulmonary hypertension.

Clinical Picture

This varies greatly, for there may be no symptoms at all or the onset may be quite dramatic, with pleuritic chest pain. Breathlessness may be due to the pain. Alternatively, it may be more an unpleasant awareness of hyperventilation induced by reflexes arising in afferents in the small pulmonary vessels. About half the patients with symptoms will have haemoptyses, which while not profuse may persist for a few days. There may be a fever up to 102° F. (38·9° C.), but this is frequently absent. Tachycardia and arrhythmias in general are not infrequent if there have been multiple emboli. Tachypnoea is variable. A pleural friction rub, localized crepitations or frank signs of consolidation are often detected either on one or both sides. If pulmonary infarction has been superimposed on widespread pulmonary artery occlusions there may be central cyanosis, signs of a low cardiac output with a cold periphery and systemic hypotension, right ventricular stress or failure with a right ventricular filling sound and a high systemic venous pressure. Clinical evidence of a peripheral venous thrombosis will be found in less than half the patients.

Pleural effusion often develops and may be the presenting clinical feature. It is usually of limited size, but may persist for weeks, especially if there is left heart disease. Effusions may, of course, be bilateral. The diaphragm may be considerably elevated with basal infarction and may mimic the signs of an effusion or give a false impression of a large effusion. With septic infarction due to pyaemia, the clinical picture will resemble lung abscess and an empyema may be present.

Diagnosis

The chest radiograph is important in diagnosis and may show one or more shadows, 1–3 cm. in size or larger, well demarcated or hazy, usually occupying part or whole of a segment, but rarely a lobe. Occasionally the shadows are wedge shaped or even rounded. This shadowing may be obscured by the shadows of a pleural effusion. The pulmonary shadows may condense to a linear form, up to 3 mm. wide and frequently horizontal, usually just above the diaphragm. The latter is often elevated. The radiographic appearances of a high diaphragm with linear shadows above is characteristic of pulmonary infarction and is to be differentiated from the radiological changes seen in systemic lupus erythematosus and basal atelectasis. The line shadows usually resolve in a week or two or leave a residual scar. A shift of the frontal plane axis of the QRS complex on the electrocardiogram to the right is a useful indication of changes in pulmonary vascular resistance and right ventricular function.

There may be a transient neutrophil leucocytosis (up to 20,000 per mm^3.) and the blood picture may be of further assistance in rare instances where the red cell count and packed cell volume show evidence of polycythaemia. Sickling may be observed.

The lactate dehydrogenase and serum bilirubin are sometimes elevated, particularly when infarction is superimposed upon cardiac cirrhosis resulting from a prolonged rise in systemic venous pressure. Then frank jaundice may be seen. Aspiration of pleural fluid will reveal an exudate—blood-staining of the fluid or an excess of mesothelial cells is evidence in support of the diagnosis.

Bacterial pneumonia or segmental collapse are most frequently confused with infarction. With bacterial pneumonia the sputum is usually purulent while the X-ray usually shows shadows of segmental or lobar distribution and systemic upset is rather more pronounced. With atelectasis, on the other hand, the patient had difficulty in coughing and rarely has chest pain. As with infarction, pneumonia and atelectasis may complicate immobilization in both medical and surgical patients, especially in the post-operative period, but the clinical findings (especially haemoptysis), radiological and electrocardiographic changes will establish one or other as the cause—infarction is by far the most common. A high index of suspicion is required and the diagnosis should be considered in any patient, especially one who is old who develops fever, breathlessness, confusion, cardiac dysrhythmia, pleurisy with or without effusion, even when peripheral venous signs are absent. Unexplained pleural exudate causes considerable difficulty in diagnosis when evidence of infarction is lacking. Carcinoma of the lung may cause such a blood-stained exudate and evidence for this should be sought.

Treatment

Anticoagulation and other aspects of management of thrombo-embolic disease are considered in detail in Section 8. Prevention is of the greatest importance, i.e. mobilization after injury and surgery. The patient with pulmonary infarction is rested in bed until the thrombotic process is well controlled and then he may be mobilized.

The pleuritic pain of infarction may require pethidine, 50–100 mg. intramuscularly, pentazocine, 25–100 mg. intramuscularly, or even morphine, 10–15 mg. subcutaneously or intramuscularly. Morphine or pethidine should not be given if there is marked hypotension. Septic infarcts require appropriate chemotherapy, but otherwise this is not required in ordinary uncomplicated infarction, which rarely becomes infected.

PULMONARY TUBERCULOSIS

Synonym. Phthisis.

Definition

Disease of the lung due to infection by *Mycobacterium tuberculosis* (*Myco. tuberculosis*).

Aetiology

Pulmonary tuberculosis due to *Myco. tuberculosis* of the human and bovine strains is world-wide and is most prevalent in less developed areas such as India, China, Africa and South America. In 1964 there were about 10 million cases of infectious tuberculosis mainly in those areas. The incidence of pulmonary tuberculosis has fallen progressively for more than 50 years in the highly developed countries, particularly in North America and Europe. Thus in England and Wales between 1900 and 1950 the death rate from pulmonary tuberculosis fell from 125 per 100,000 to 43 per 100,000. This change was initially due to host resistance and an improvement in social and economic factors which reduced overcrowding and cross infection. Since 1950 the reduction in morbidity and mortality has been accelerated by chemotherapy and B.C.G. vaccination. In England and Wales the mortality has fallen from an over-all rate of 43 per 100,000 in 1950 to 4·6 per 100,000 in males, and 1·6 per 100,000 in females in 1968: 1,548 persons are reported to have died in England and Wales from pulmonary tuberculosis in that year.

Host resistance to tuberculosis may be affected by *genetic* factors but the high rate of tuberculosis observed in monozygotic twins (about three times that found in dizygotic twins) and the apparent increase in susceptibility of the Irish compared with the English and the East African compared with the West African, are probably the result of environmental factors. *Age and sex* have a definite influence on susceptibility to infection with *Myco. tuberculosis.* Under the age of 3 years the human is highly susceptible to infection and particularly liable to haematogenous spread (miliary tuberculosis and meningitis); there follows a relative resistance to infection which lasts until puberty. Up to adolescence progressive pulmonary disease is rare. During adolescence and early adult life the susceptibility of the two sexes is about the same but progressive pulmonary disease is much more common than haematogenous tuberculosis. After the age of forty the male remains much more susceptible than the female both in terms of morbidity and mortality. Since 1950 and the advent of chemotherapy the morbidity and mortality in males over forty has declined far less than other groups. Most males over 40 years were infected in their youth and such factors as tobacco smoking may be responsible for the activation of the disease. Younger age groups have not been exposed to infection and have been vaccinated by B.C.G. Pregnancy is not thought to have an important effect on susceptibility.

Of *environmental factors* which may affect host resistance, nutrition and housing conditions, alcohol and cigarette smoking may all have an adverse effect. Silicosis and asbestosis lower resistance to the infection but there is no good evidence that any other occupation has the same effect.

Pulmonary tuberculosis is usually due to infection with the human or rarely the bovine strain of *Myco. tuberculosis.* These organisms are of similar virulence in the experimental animal but strains do vary in virulence from one part of the world to another. The least virulent strains have been isolated from patients in South India. Man is the major source of tubercle bacilli and sputum in which acid-fast bacilli can be seen on microscopy is by far and away the most common vehicle of cross infection. Tubercle bacilli can survive for long periods in sputum not exposed to sunlight. In developed countries bovine tuberculosis has largely disappeared with the elimination of infected cattle. Cats and dogs are also a possible source. Less virulent strains of *Myco. tuberculosis*, e.g. the avian and murine, and atypical tubercle bacilli are rare causes of disease and are considered later.

Pathology

Only small numbers of organisms are required for the initial and primary infection which may develop at any site where the bacillus can gain entrance. Most commonly, however, the organism is inhaled by droplet or aerosol, lodges in the peripheral lung parenchyma, usually subpleural, and then multiplies. The organism survives phagocytosis by polymorphonuclear leucocytes. If the tubercle bacillus survives phagocytosis by macrophages, there is aggregation of mononuclear cells, epithelioid cells and typical giant cells which are formed in response to the lipoid fraction of the organism. Avascularity and direct toxic action of the protein component of the tubercle bacillus cause necrosis or caseation in the centre of the developing lesion. There are attempts at localization and repair by fibroblasts at the periphery. Calcium may be deposited in the caseating tissue. The dynamics of the process are determined by the relative strength of bacterial virulence on the one hand, and of the inborn and developing acquired immunity on the other. Tubercle bacilli are carried to the adjacent lymph nodes via the lymphatics where a similar tissue reaction develops and the parenchymal lesion together with the lymph node component is called the *primary complex* (Ghon focus).

During the early weeks of infection the development of hypersensitivity to the protein component of the tubercle bacillus is an important factor in the outcome of the infection. This is a delayed type allergic reaction mediated by lymphocytes (type 4 of Gell and Coombs). This can be demonstrated in the skin by the Mantoux reaction to antigens from the tubercle bacillus. Old Tuberculin (O.T.) was the original extract of *Myco. tuberculosis* used for skin testing and one Tuberculin Unit (TU) is defined by the World Health Organization as that quantity of O.T. contained in 0·00001 ml. of International Standard Old Tuberculin. There are various purified protein derivatives of tuberculin (P.P.D.) in use today. Skin reactions vary considerably in intensity so that various concentrations of P.P.D. are used, but for standard testing either 1, 2 or 5 TU are used in 0·1 ml. which is injected into the skin on the anterior aspect of the forearm. A positive reaction is indicated by a central area of induration which should be measured. If the reaction exceeds 10 mm. 48–72 hours after injection, then it is probably of tuberculous origin. Smaller reactions may be non-specific and in some cases may be due to non-tuberculous mycobacteria. P.P.D. derived from the protein of other mycobacteria may help to clarify these non-specific reactions which vary from one part of the world to another. Skin testing may also be carried out by the multiple puncture method (Heaf test) in which concentrated P.P.D. is inoculated into the skin by six needles which penetrate to a depth of 1–2 mm. Grade 1 reactions show separate papules, Grade II reactions are those in which the papules coalesce to form a ring, and in Grade III reactions the induration spreads centrally and peripherally. This is well tolerated by children.

A positive skin reaction indicates that the host has at some time in the past developed an active parenchymal lesion with multiplication of tubercle bacilli and liberation of the protein component. The stronger the skin reaction the more recent is the infection likely to have been. The acquisition of hypersensitivity has two broad effects on the host-parasite reaction. It tends to localize the reponse in the tissues so that the lymphatic spread is diminished; at the same time the local response is considerably intensified.

The primary infection usually heals by fibrosis with or without calcification in the lesion. The process, however, may progress to involve larger units of lung and if this is a rapid process then *tuberculous pneumonia* will result. A central caseous area may evacuate into a bronchus and give rise to a *cavity* and spread of the infection via the bronchopulmonary tree in the same or to the other lung.

The glandular component of the primary complex at

the hilum may occlude a bronchus and cause collapse of the lung peripherally. It may evacuate its caseous contents into the bronchus and cause disease peripherally by aspiration. The gland may penetrate a pulmonary blood vessel, in which case the tubercle bacilli are carried via the blood stream (*haematogenous*). This is accepted as the common mode of spread of the disease to distant organs, e.g. the brain, meninges, the genito-urinary tract, the adrenal gland, bones and joints. This mode of spread is usually subclinical and the tubercle bacilli may lie dormant for varying periods of time and then multiply later and manifest as active tuberculosis, e.g. tuberculous meningitis, pyelonephritis, etc. Tissues vary in their resistance to bacterial growth—thus aggressive tissue damage in the liver, spleen and voluntary muscle is unusual. If the haematogenous spread is massive or the host resistance is low, then clinical *miliary tuberculosis* develops. Subclinical haematogenous spread from the primary lesion may originate in the lymphatics of the primary complex from which organisms gain access to the systemic veins and pulmonary circulation.

The predilection of the disease for the upper and posterior parts of the lungs in *post-primary tuberculosis* has not been fully explained. It is unlikely to be due to mechanical streaming of the bacilli in the pulmonary arteries and is more likely to be due to biochemical advantages in the tissue environment in those parts of of the lung. As in tissues elsewhere the organisms may lie dormant in the lung for years after their redistribution and then resume growth when the tissue environment becomes favourable. Such factors as age are possibly significant and hormone differences may explain the differences between the sexes. Malnutrition, cigarette smoking, pneumoconiosis, uncontrolled diabetes, adrenocortical steroids and the post-gastrectomy state may diminish host resistance. Characteristically, focal or confluent lesions are produced in the lung, with or without caseation and cavitation. Repair is brought about by various degrees of fibrosis and calcification.

The primary infection may develop at sites other than the lung and from the primary complex there may be haematogenous spread to the lung. This explains the post-primary pulmonary tuberculosis due to bovine strains which gain access via the alimentary tract. This form of tuberculosis has become rare in developed countries with pasteurization of milk and eradication of infected cattle. During the early stages of infection manifestations due to acquisition of hypersensitivity may develop, e.g. erythema nodosum, phlyctenular conjunctivitis, lichen scrofulosorum. A tuberculous pleural effusion is also an early complication but this is due to direct spread of infection to the pleura; hypersensitivity is an accesory factor.

Clinical Picture

The symptoms of pulmonary tuberculosis depend upon the site and intensity of the inflammatory process and the amount of lung involved. Usually the onset is insidious and cough, sputum, haemoptysis and breathlessness usually develop only as the disease becomes advanced. Systemic symptoms such as weight loss, fever and sweating also reflect advanced disease. Rigors are unusual. Pulmonary tuberculosis is often revealed by screening procedures such as routine chest radiography and in these circumstances the disease is usually asymptomatic. Chest pain, other than that due to pleurisy, is uncommon and should raise the suspicion of other disease such as neoplasia. Cough may be stimulated by mucoid or purulent sputum in the airways, by endobronchial disease, or by pressure of tuberculous glands. It may be troublesome with tuberculous laryngitis but then hoarseness and discomfort are the prominent features. Haemoptysis may be minimal with speckling of the sputum and on occasions occurs early in the disease. Bleeding from a large vessel in a cavity may cause a profuse or even fatal haemoptysis. Breathlessness develops with widespread fibrosis or infiltration and is due to a restrictive ventilatory defect. Pulmonary tuberculosis sometimes presents as an acute pneumonia: it should always be considered when any pneumonia fails to resolve within a short period of time.

The physical findings are as variable as the symptomatology. The general condition of the patient may be very good but occasionally with far advanced disease there may be extreme weight loss. In such advanced cases there may be remittent or intermittent fever. Classically the morning temperature may be higher than that in the evening. In most cases, however, there is little or no fever and little change in pulse or respiration rate. Clubbing of the fingers is unusual in pulmonary tuberculosis unless there is widespread fibrosis with bronchiectasis. The signs in the lung in all but the advanced forms of the disease are minimal, the most characteristic being the presence of fine or medium post-tussive crepitations. With the grossest forms of the disease signs of consolidation, fibrosis or cavitation may be elicited. With very large cavities the breath sounds may be cavernous or amphoric. All these physical signs are more often encountered in the upper and posterior parts of the lung where the disease most often occurs.

Pulmonary tuberculosis may be *complicated* by severe haemoptysis, tuberculous laryngitis, intestinal tuberculosis and amyloid disease, but these are rare and tend to be associated with advanced forms of the disease.

Miliary tuberculosis and *meningitis* may complicate pulmonary tuberculosis at any stage though they are more common during the primary or early post-primary forms in children under 3 years. This disease may be *insidious* in onset with fever, malaise and weight loss; sometimes it is sudden in onset with high fever and tachycardia. In either case physical signs are unusual in the chest though there may be diffuse crepitations. The spleen may be enlarged; on retinoscopy choroidal tubercles are particularly likely to be seen in children and are most helpful in the diagnosis. An insidious onset is most common in the middle-aged or elderly and if miliary tuberculosis is not considered it usually proves fatal: in this age group there may be a considerable fall in the serum potassium.

Spread of pulmonary tuberculosis to the pleura may result in pleurisy with effusion. This may progress to a tuberculous empyema—a pyopneumothorax may also develop if a caseating tuberculous process ruptures into the pleura. Pulmonary fibrosis, bronchiectasis and spontaneous pneumothorax are late complications of healing. Mycetoma (fungal balls) due to growth of the mycelia usually of the *Aspergillus* species are encountered in about 11 per cent. of healed tuberculous cavities. These may give rise to haemoptysis. Healing of a bronchial lesion may give rise to a tuberculous bronchostenosis.

Diagnosis

The declining incidence of pulmonary and other forms of tuberculosis reduces suspicion of this as a cause not only of disease in the chest but elsewhere—so much so that the diagnosis may be overlooked.

In any acute pneumonia the possibility of infection with *Myco. tuberculosis* should be considered, especially when response to treatment is tardy and resolution is incomplete. Chronic pulmonary tuberculosis which presents with localized massive lesions in the lung, with or without cavitation must be distinguished from other chronic granulomatous processes. Non-specific granulomata in the lung and granulomata due to other bacteria such as the staphylococcus, *Klebsiella*, and granulomata due to mycoses, such histoplasmosis, coccidioidomycosis, actinomycosis, nocardiosis are all uncommon possibilities. Sarcoidosis and pneumoconiosis may be difficult to distinguish at times. Lymphomata and neoplastic processes are occasionally difficult to differentiate from tuberculosis, particularly carcinoma of the bronchus which is so common and which may present in so many ways that resemble tuberculosis. This is particularly the case in the older age groups especially in males in which the two diseases may coexist. Attempts must always be made to establish an unequivocal diagnosis of tuberculosis by appropriate investigation.

Examination of the Sputum. Smears of the sputum should be examined directly by the Ziehl-Neelsen technique in which acid- and alcohol-fast bacilli should be sought, and by fluorescence microscopy. If these are seen in the sputum they are usually pathogenic, i.e. *Myco. tuberculosis*. In some cases, however, these organisms are 'atypical' or even non-pathogenic. From cultures of the sputum the characteristic colonies of *Myco. tuberculosis* may be grown: other biochemical studies can be carried out to establish the true nature of the organism and its pathogenicity (e.g. catalase, niacin and peroxidase activity, etc.). Inoculation of guinea-pigs may be necessary to isolate the tubercle bacillus if all other methods fail. If sputum cannot be produced then early morning gastric washings, bronchial washings, or laryngeal swabs should be cultivated after suitable preparation. In general at least three specimens should be examined. Bacteriological proof of the diagnosis by microscopy and culture should always be established by examination of material that might be available, e.g. pleural fluid, pleural tissue removed by biopsy and biopsy material obtained from other tissues such as lymph node, lung, liver or bone marrow.

Supporting Evidence. Absence of *cutaneous sensitivity* to tuberculin (a negative Mantoux reaction) makes a tuberculous aetiology improbable. The more florid the response to 1 or 5 Tuberculin Units the more active the disease is likely to be if the disease is tuberculous. Skin reactivity, however, may be suppressed by adrenocortical steroids and also by very severe infection. The *chest radiograph* is of great importance in diagnosis, in defining the extent of the disease and determining the activity. In general, shadows are usually in the upper zones, are often bilateral and may persist unaltered for many weeks or longer. They are often patchy or nodular with linear shadows due to fibrosis. They are often associated with calcification or cavitation. Soft shadows, cavitation, or a recent increase or decrease in size of shadows suggests an active process. On the other hand, 'hard' shadows, calcification and contraction due to fibrosis tend to favour chronicity and even inactivity.

Shadows of segmental or lobar extent or of a patchy nature associated with lymph node enlargement at the hilum, extending occasionally to the paratracheal nodes would be in favour of a primary tuberculous process and would be more common in children. Pressure of glands or obstruction of the bronchial lumen by granulation tissue or caseous material produce various degrees of atelectasis. This may be followed by bronchiectasis.

The evenly distributed micronodular shadows of miliary tuberculosis may be faint, or if slightly larger, more dense. They may be seen throughout both lung fields; but early in the disease the shadows may be very difficult to see.

In pulmonary tuberculosis *tomography* is useful in detecting cavitation, calcification and subtle changes that might not be seen on a straight X-ray film. In the investigation of solitary single shadows in the lung satellite shadows may be seen only on tomography and tend to support a diagnosis of tuberculosis.

The *haematological* findings in pulmonary tuberculosis are variable. There may be a slight normocytic anaemia. Changes in the white blood count are unusual. A raised E.S.R. may be found in active disease. With miliary tuberculosis and other severe forms of the disease extraordinary blood pictures may be encountered. Thus pancytopenia, agranulocytosis or leukaemoid reactions may be found. Thrombocytopenia and polycythaemia have also been described. Differentiation from primary blood disorders may be difficult: miliary lesions may not be apparent in the lungs on chest radiography and the Mantoux reaction may be negative.

Treatment

Prophylaxis and Prevention. While social and economic factors are important in prevention, removal of sources of infection are of the greatest importance. Thus tuberculous cattle should be eliminated and healthy herds checked by regular tubercular testing. Pasteurization of milk removes *Myco. tuberculosis* from milk. Human sources of infection ('open' cases of tuberculosis) should be detected by skin testing and chest radiography in contacts or people with symptoms: sputum testing may be used when X-rays are not available. Mass X-ray screening of large populations is very expensive and limited in value. Immediate treatment of active cases by correct chemotherapy rapidly renders them non-infective to contacts. It is preferable to segregate those patients with positive sputum by direct examination and those that will not accept treatment or who have organisms resistant to chemotherapy.

Vaccination with B.C.G. confers a measure of protection and the relevance of its use depends upon many factors in a community. Thus, where skin reactors are rare no advantage is to be gained by mass vaccination and cutaneous reactivity should be preserved for diagnosis. When tuberculosis is common in a community vaccination should be carried out as soon after birth as possible. In the United Kingdom present policy is to offer B.C.G. vaccination to school-children aged 12–14 years. This has been shown to reduce significantly the chance of acquiring active tuberculosis after leaving school. The policy for mass B.C.G. vaccination in any community should be reviewed from time to time as the incidence of tuberculosis and skin reactivity of the population changes.

B.C.G. should be offered to tuberculin-negative persons of all ages who are contacts or who are at special risk, such as those who work in hospitals or schools.

Chemoprophylaxis. This is usually carried out with isoniazid. Chemoprophylaxis may be *primary*, i.e. when chemotherapy is given to negative cutaneous reactors to tuberculin or, in other words to those who have at no time been infected with *Myco. tuberculosis*. This does not prevent implantation of tubercle bacilli in the tissues but it does prevent disease. No immunity develops so that organisms may multiply when the drug is stopped. The indications for use of primary chemoprophylaxis are few. Isoniazid, 5 mg. per kg. in one dose daily, may be given to children under the age of three who have had close contact with an infectious mother. This treatment can be given in association with vaccination using isoniazid-resistant B.C.G. The multiplication of isoniazid-resistant B.C.G. confers immunity so that chemoprophylaxis can be discontinued after 6 months or so.

Secondary chemoprophylaxis is given to prevent active disease developing in highly susceptible people who are found to be tuberculin positive, i.e. those who have been at some time infected with *Myco. tuberculosis*. Thus, isoniazid, 5 mg. per kg., should be given once daily for at least a year to all tuberculin-positive infants under the age of 3 years to prevent miliary and meningeal tuberculosis. It should also be considered in those who have recently converted from a negative to a positive tuberculin reaction, or who have inactive tuberculosis and have to receive adrenocortical steroids or who have undergone gastrectomy.

Chemotherapy. When properly given chemotherapy is so successful that the need for bed rest, surgery and other measures has largely been eliminated in the management of tuberculosis. Bed rest is required only for those who are weak and ill or who have had a severe haemothorax or a pneumothorax. Indications for surgery are discussed below.

The frequency with which drug resistant mutants of *Myco. tuberculosis* appears in a growing population varies from about 1 in 100,000 to about 1 in 10,000,000 according to the drug. The number of tubercle bacilli in a tuberculous cavity usually far exceeds that number—therefore mutants resistant to one or other of the antituberculous drugs are likely to be present at the start of treatment in the majority of cases. To overcome this, drugs are used in pairs because the chance of emergence of a mutant resistant to two drugs at the same time is extremely small (i.e. of the order of $1/10^{12}$). A variable proportion of patients are infected *de novo* with *Myco. tuberculosis* resistant to one or the other primary drugs, isoniazid, streptomycin and para-aminosalicylic acid (PAS). In the United Kingdom about 5 per cent. of cases have such primary drug resistance. In some parts of the world, however, particularly in India, parts of Africa and the Far East the incidence of primary drug resistance is much higher. At the start of treatment, therefore, when the drug resistance pattern of the infecting tubercle bacillus is unknown three drugs are given to allow the possibility of there being strains resistant to one agent from the start. Isoniazid should be given once daily at a dose of 300 mg. by mouth, streptomycin sulphate is given once daily intramuscularly as a dose of 1 G., and PAS 12 G. (sodium salt) daily by mouth. If the tubercle bacillus is found to be fully sensitive by *in vitro* tests of drug sensitivity the treatment can be modified, and continued with two drugs in combination, e.g. isoniazid with either streptomycin or PAS in the same dosage. Antituberculosis drug treatment should be continued for at least 18 months but with all but minimal disease the period should be extended to 2 years. This standard drug regimen is successful in more than 95 per cent. of cases treated—tubercle bacilli are eliminated from the sputum, abnormal radiological shadowing becomes stabilized and subsequent relapse of the disease is prevented. The commonest cause of failure is refusal or failure to take the prescribed treatment: irregular treatment is more common than generally supposed. Treatment with drug combinations containing intramuscular streptomycin given together with oral isoniazid can be supervised and is thereby gaining favour when it is possible to organize it.

Modification of the Standard Drug Regimen. 1. Patients between 45 and 60 years: 0·75 G. of streptomycin sulphate should be given daily intramuscularly. Because renal clearance of streptomycin is reduced after this age, higher doses may cause damage to the eighth cranial nerve.

2. Patients over 60 years of age or patients with renal failure (blood urea elevated above 40 mg. per 100 ml.): streptomycin should be withheld or the dose controlled by estimation of blood levels, which should not be allowed to rise above 2 μg. per ml. 24 hours after injection.

3. Drug toxicity, intolerance or hypersensitivity: reactions to one or more of the commonly used drugs develop in about 15–20 per cent. of patients treated [see TABLE 46]. Minor gastro-intestinal upsets can usually be tolerated. With hypersensitivity reactions desensitization may be attempted. Fever and rashes may be suppressed by adrenocortical steroids (e.g. prednisone, 10–20 mg. daily) and withdrawal of the steroid gradually may be accompanied by desensitization. This should only be attempted if the infecting organism is sensitive to the antituberculosis drugs used. With serious toxicity

the offending drug or drugs should be discontinued and alternative drugs given.

4. Initial drug resistance: acquired resistance may be suspected if the patient has received incorrect treatment in the past or primary drug resistance if he has been in contact with a case of tuberculosis known to have been infected with drug-resistant organisms. In these instances the standard drug regimen should be modified from the start. Subsequently when *in vitro* tests of drug resistance become available, the treatment can be changed to the most appropriate drugs. A combination of drugs should be given to which the organism is susceptible. When reserve drugs are given it is advisable to treat with at least three drugs, for by so doing at least 80 per cent. success can be achieved in patients even with far advanced tuberculosis if the regimen is tolerated and taken regularly. The reserve drugs have varying degrees of antituberculosis activity: where possible two of the three drugs should be of high potency—a widely used regimen comprises ethionamide, pyrazinamide and cycloserine. In TABLE 46 are listed the alternative drugs at present available, their dose and toxic manifestations. In place of streptomycin or isoniazid it is reasonable to give either ethionamide, pyrazinamide, ethambutol, capreomycin, viomycin or kanamycin. There is good evidence to suggest that rifampicin will prove to be a highly active drug: at present it is expensive but is probably of the same order of activity as isoniazid or streptomycin. In many developing countries PAS has been replaced by thiacetazone. Whatever drug regimen is most appropriate for a given patient it should be continued for at least 18 months, preferably 2 years.

5. Alternative regimens: there is increasing interest in intermittent drug regimens. Streptomycin, 1·0 or 0·75 G. intramuscularly, and high dosage isoniazid, 14 mg. per kg., given twice weekly proved rather more effective than daily isoniazid and PAS in conventional dose in Indian patients in Madras. Similar trials in other less developed countries have confirmed the value of such intermittent supervised chemotherapy. Not only may such intermittent regimens be supervised but they are cheaper and more pleasant for the patient. Studies in Great Britain and elsewhere in Europe have also confirmed the value of intermittent treatment, but it is preceded by a period of continuous daily treatment. This period of daily treatment should probably last

TABLE 46

ANTITUBERCULOSIS DRUGS

DRUG	DAILY DOSE (ADULT)	TOXICITY
STANDARD		
Isoniazid	200–300 mg.	Neuropathy (prevented by 10 mg. pyridoxine daily). Impaired concentration and fits. Jaundice.
Streptomycin	0·75–1·0 G. intramuscularly	Fever, rashes, etc. Giddiness (VIII cranial nerve). Jaundice.
PAS Sodium	10–12 G.	Nausea, vomiting and diarrhoea. Fever, rashes, lymphadenopathy and splenomegaly. Jaundice. Goitre. Blood dyscrasias.
RESERVE		
Capreomycin (Kanamycin) (Viomycin)	1 G. intramuscularly	Deafness, giddiness (VIII cranial nerve). Nephropathy.
Cycloserine	0·75–1 G.	Confusion, depression and psychoses. Convulsions.
Ethambutol	25 mg./kg. for 2 months 15 mg./kg. thereafter	Optic neuritis.
Ethionamide (Prothionamide)	0·5–1 G.	Nausea, jaundice, neuropathy.
Pyrazinamide	20–40 mg./kg.	Jaundice, arthropathy (gout), fever, rashes.
Rifampicin	450–600 mg.	Jaundice, purpura, etc.
Thiacetazone	150 mg.	Nausea, rashes, jaundice, bone marrow dyscrasia.

from 2 to 3 months. Rifampicin and ethambutol will probably prove to be extremely useful in intermittent regimens.

Adrenocortical steroids may be given to patients with active tuberculosis provided that the infecting organism is sensitive to the antituberculosis drugs. The steroids are indicated in severely ill patients, in slowly resolving pleural effusions and in drug hypersensitivity. During their administration radiological improvement is accelerated but the ultimate effect of antituberculosis chemotherapy is not modified so their routine use is not indicated.

During chemotherapy microscopy and culture of the sputum is the most important way of judging progress. Persistence of *Myco. tuberculosis* in the sputum should arouse suspicion that the organism may be drug resistant or the patient irregular in his treatment. Normally the sputum is 'sterilized' in 3–6 months after the start of treatment. Occasional chest radiography is helpful in following progress. The aim of treatment is to eliminate *Myco. tuberculosis* permanently from the sputum but also to obtain maximum resolution of the disease. Persistence of cavitation is not followed by relapse provided that the tubercle bacillus is eliminated from the sputum. Cases of pulmonary tuberculosis are usually followed for 5 years after the start of treatment if circumstances allow.

Surgery. While the treatment of pulmonary tuberculosis is essentially medical, surgery should be considered and the lesion resected if:

1. Cavitation persists with a positive sputum despite standard and reserve drug treatment. Under these circumstances the infecting organisms are nearly always resistant to many drugs and the prognosis is poor. Resection should be carried out if the disease is not too widespread and the respiratory function is adequate.
2. The development of multiple drug toxicity so that no suitable long term chemotherapy can be achieved—this is rare.
3. The patient is unco-operative or where supervision of treatment cannot be given at all.

Course and Prognosis

The natural history of pulmonary tuberculosis if untreated is uncertain. It depends on so many factors which affect host resistance. Useful data are now no longer available in developed countries. With proper chemotherapy, however, the prognosis is excellent. With standard drug regimens in newly treated patients the disease is usually arrested, the sputum sterilized and subsequently relapse prevented in more than 95 per cent. of patients treated. This is so provided the treatment is taken properly. Following a course of proper treatment life expectancy is almost certainly normal. If these conditions are fulfilled, the extent of the disease does not affect the outcome. With reserve drug regimens and with disease due to drug-resistant organisms the outcome of treatment becomes less certain and other factors such as bed rest may influence the prognosis. Properly applied triple drug regimens in the treatment or re-treatment of far advanced cavitating disease due to drug-resistant organisms (to the standard drugs) is successful in about 70 per cent. of patients treated. In these cases the outcome is largely dependent upon the mental stability of the patient and the tolerance and patience of the physician.

REFERENCES

BARRY, V. C. (1964) *Chemotherapy of Tuberculosis*, London.

CROFTON, J., and DOUGLAS, A. D. (1969) *Respiratory Diseases*, p. 163 et seq., Oxford.

FOX, W. (1968) Changing concepts in the chemotherapy of pulmonary tuberculosis, *Amer. Rev. resp. Dis.*, **97**, 767.

RICH, A. R. (1951) *The Pathogenesis of Tuberculosis*, 2nd ed., Oxford.

PULMONARY DISEASE DUE TO OTHER MYCOBACTERIA

Disease due to avian, murine and other strains of *Myco. tuberculosis* are exceptionally rare.

'Atypical' (anonymous or unclassified) mycobacteria have been isolated in pulmonary disease and should be considered as the cause when they are repeatedly found in the sputum. The incidence of infection (cutaneous sensitivity) with these organisms varies in different parts of the world. Disease is uncommon because the organisms are of low virulence and cause a very chronic form of pulmonary tuberculosis with cavitation. Bacilli of Group I, the *photochromogens* (*Myco. kansasii*) and of Group III, the *non-chromogens* (Battey) may be found in pulmonary disease. These organisms and those of Group II, *the scotochromogens* may cause lymphadenitis. Group IV bacilli, the *rapid growers* (*Myco. smegmatis*, *fortuitum*, *phlei*, *balnei*, etc.) do not cause pulmonary disease but they may affect the skin [see Section 14].

Atypical mycobacteria of Group I may be sensitive to isoniazid, streptomycin, and other antituberculosis drugs. Bacilli of the other groups are usually resistant to most or all of these drugs. Prognosis of pulmonary disease is poor.

REFERENCE

GOLDMAN, K. P. (1968) Treatment of unclassified mycobacterial infection of the lungs, *Thorax*, **23**, 94.

JOHN BATTEN

SARCOIDOSIS

Synonyms. Lymphogranulomatosis benigna; Besnier-Boeck-Schaumann disease; Uveoparotid fever of Heerfordt; Osteitis multiplex cystica vel cystoides of Jüngling; Lupus pernio; Löfgren's syndrome.

Definition

Sarcoidosis is a disease of undetermined causation characterized by the presence in all affected tissues of epithelioid cell tubercles without caseation.

Aetiology

The incidence of sarcoidosis is unknown, but since pulmonary lesions are believed to be present in 94–100 per cent. of patients, it may be assumed that the frequency of characteristic radiographic changes is much the same as that of the disease itself. Mass radiography surveys in which 70 per cent. of the population in defined areas were examined showed appearances regarded as those of sarcoidosis in 5·9 per 100,000. In volunteers from the general public the figures were 14·4 in males and 19·6 in females; in the Swiss Army 13; and in Sweden 30 in males and 50 in females.

The disease occurs at all ages, but 50 per cent. when first seen are between 21 and 30 years and 75 per cent. between 21 and 40 years. Females outnumber males by 3 to 2 and their preponderance is greater at the lower ages. In the United States, Negroes are affected 16 times more frequently than those of other races. It is rare in the tropics, especially in Chinese, Indians and African Negroes. There are numerous examples of two cases in one family, and the chance of both identical twins being affected is greater than for both of a binovular pair which may indicate the operation of a genetic factor.

The causation of sarcoidosis is unknown. The plentiful hypotheses advanced include suggestions that it is a neoplasm, a collagen disease, a granuloma due to a specific but unidentified micro-organism and an abnormal form of tuberculosis. This last drew support from the resemblance between the sarcoid tubercle and that due to *Mycobacterium tuberculosis*, although efforts to isolate this organism from sarcoid tissue are almost always unavailing. The view which accords best with current thinking regards sarcoidosis as due to an immunologically determined alteration in tissue reactivity. In persons thus predisposed, it is postulated, sarcoidosis occurs as a reaction to certain specific agents; one of these may be *Myco. tuberculosis*, but this does not exclude the possibility of others. Indeed, many causes of non-caseating epithelioid cell granulomata have been recognized and of these the most interesting is chronic beryllium poisoning which in sensitized persons leads to a syndrome sharing many of the features of the disorder under discussion. Moreover, the frequency of erythema nodosum, the depression of delayed cutaneous hypersensitivity and the raised level of immunoglobulin in the serum are all compatible with a deeper immunological disturbance.

Pathology

Clinical estimates of the anatomical distribution of the disease are fallacious, reports of autopsies are few and selection by death in such a benign disorder clearly distorts the picture. Figures for 92 cases examined *post mortem* show the organs most frequently affected to be the lungs (86 per cent.), the lymph nodes (86 per cent.), the liver (65 per cent.), the spleen (63 per cent.), the heart (20 per cent.), the kidneys (19 per cent.), the bone marrow (17 per cent.) and the pancreas (6 per cent.). Evidence of disease of the skin, the eyes and the nervous system is often clinically obvious: indeed, the suprarenal glands are said to be the only tissues never affected.

The characteristic lesion is the epithelioid cell granuloma or tubercle formed by a sharply defined collection of epithelioid cells, arranged concentrically about giant cells of Langhans type which may contain inclusion bodies. Lymphocytes are scanty, but plasma cells may be plentiful around the perimeter and older lesions may be encircled by fibroblasts. Occasionally central necrosis occurs, but the reticulum is always preserved and there is never caseation. Sarcoid tubercles may resolve without trace, but when they have persisted for more than a year their disappearance usually leaves an acellular hyaline scar.

Clinical Picture

The clinical picture of sarcoidosis defies succinct description, because the lesions are so widely scattered in time and space. The cutaneous infiltrations were the first noted and were only recognized many years later as relatively uncommon manifestations of a systemic affection. In the interval several syndromes, such as Schaumann's disease, osteitis multiplex and the uveoparotid fever of Heerfordt, later shown to be clinical variants of sarcoidosis, had been described.

Onset and Course. The true frequency of the presenting symptoms is difficult to assess because they are so diverse that the advice of different specialists is sought and their different interests are inevitably reflected in their reports. Nevertheless, it is undoubtedly the respiratory system which first draws attention to the disease in the majority. The mildness, or even absence, of symptoms contrasts with the objective evidence of extensive disease and 25–45 per cent. are first revealed by a routine radiograph of the chest. Others record 20–70 per cent. presenting with respiratory symptoms, of which dyspnoea is the commonest.

The second most frequent mode of onset is with erythema nodosum and bilateral hilar lymphadenopathy (BHL), a combination sometimes called Löfgren's syndrome. In addition to the typical cutaneous lesions and the radiographic changes, there is often fever and arthralgia. This pattern accounts for 10–15 per cent. of cases in the United Kingdom, 25 per cent. in Sweden, but only 2 per cent. in the United States, for it is rarely seen in Negroes. It is considerably more common in females than in males.

Other common presenting symptoms are ocular (10–15 per cent.), cutaneous eruptions other than erythema nodosum (5 per cent.), and enlargement of lymph nodes (4 per cent.). A few patients seek advice on account of general ill health, and an occasional one for cardiovascular or neurological reasons.

Individual lesions have a strong tendency to resolve. If this occurs within two years, no trace may be left but the more chronic are replaced by fibrous tissue. Further lesions may appear and these in their turn heal. The cycle may continue irregularly over many years, but at any time the disease may become inactive. With some clinical patterns resolution with apparently complete recovery is common, with others rare. Since the lungs are the only organs commonly affected in which scarring causes disastrous impairment of function, the extent of pulmonary disease usually determines the issue.

The Respiratory System. The frequency of intrathoracic sarcoidosis is unknown, for it commonly exists without symptoms and sometimes without radiographic changes. Two broad clinical groups may be recognized: BHL and diffuse infiltration of the lungs with or without BHL [PLATE 7].

The combination of BHL and erythema nodosum as a presenting feature has been noted. In 45 per cent. of patients the first evidence of disease is BHL revealed by routine radiography. Symptoms are rare, but there is occasionally breathlessness, cough or fever. Extra-thoracic manifestations are found in 15 per cent. of those with BHL.

Although some develop diffuse pulmonary infiltration without preceding BHL, in most patients with lung involvement the two are associated when first seen. At this stage symptoms are limited to minor grades of cough, breathlessness, loss of weight and lassitude. With fibrosis, breathlessness is frequent and may become severe with a day of productive cough. Physical signs are scanty: crepitations are rarely heard and clubbing of the fingers is confined to those with superimposed infection. Respiratory insufficiency develops later with or without recurrent bronchial infection: the right ventricle will then often hypertrophy, although it rarely fails.

Sarcoidosis occasionally gives rise to stenosing lesions of one or more major bronchi.

Pulmonary sarcoidosis may occur with normal lung function, but when diffuse, tends to cause progressive impairment shown by diminished compliance with reduced total lung and vital capacities. The FEV_1/FVC ratio is normal, for widespread airways obstruction is unusual. Gas transfer (T_{CO}) is impaired, failure to rise on exercise being the earliest change, due to ventilation/perfusion irregularity. It may cause respiratory failure. Progressive widespread fibrosis leads to hypoxaemia and cyanosis, particularly on exercise. P_{CO_2} rises only as a terminal event. There is no correlation between the clinical, radiographic and physiological changes.

The Lymph Nodes. Enlargement of superficial lymph nodes is reported in 70 per cent. of American patients, but is only half as frequent in Europeans. This is due to the different pattern of the disease in the North American Negro. The cervical (70 per cent.), the axillary (40 per cent.) and the epitrochlear (20 per cent.) groups are most commonly affected. Individual nodes seldom exceed 3–4 cm. in diameter; there is no tenderness, fluctuation, nor periadenitis and they share the tendency to spontaneous remission.

The Spleen. Palpable splenomegaly is variously reported as occurring in 6–40 per cent. of patients. It is usually of minor grade but occasionally large enough to cause the patient to seek advice, when a hypersplenic blood picture is not uncommon.

The Liver. Notable enlargement of the liver is rare although infiltration is common and puncture biopsy reveals sarcoid lesions in 60 per cent. Symptoms referable to the organ are unusual, although liver function, judged by bromsulphthalein retention, is often impaired. Occasional instances are on record of hepatic cirrhosis apparently resulting from sarcoidosis.

The Skin. The cutaneous lesions of sarcoidosis enjoy historical seniority but are, in fact, relatively uncommon. In the United Kingdom they occur in 15 per cent. of patients; their frequency in Negroes makes them commoner in the United States (29 per cent.).

Numerous morphological varieties are described: the more superficial (*sarcoids of Boeck*) are found on the face, shoulders and arms. They may be raised, dome-shaped nodules with an apple-jelly appearance on diascopy, or purple or red plaques with fine vessels coursing over the surface (*angio-lupoid of Brocq and Pautrier*). Subcutaneous lesions (*Darier-Roussy sarcoids*) appear on the face and extensor aspects of the limbs. Erythrodermic, lichenoid, annular and serpiginous forms occur.

The most striking variety is *lupus pernio*. It occurs, particularly in women, as a diffuse livid, purple-red infiltration on the nose, ears, cheeks, hands or feet.

Old standing scars on the skin have a peculiar liability to infiltration by sarcoid tissue.

Lupus pernio and the larger infiltrative lesions show little tendency to remit and are usually associated with pulmonary sarcoidosis which progresses to fibrosis. The small lesions are often ephemeral and have no prognostic import.

The Eyes. Ocular changes are seen in 15–20 per cent. of patients: in half they are the reason for seeking advice. The lesion is a uveitis, commonly anterior (iridocyclitis), but sometimes affecting, too, the posterior part of the uveal tract. Mild acute iridocyclitis is common in the opening stages of the disease and usually resolves completely: chronic uveitis, especially when posterior, is commonly associated with visual sarcoidosis. The formation of posterior synechiae with secondary glaucoma, vitreous opacities and choroidoretinal scarring may leave gross visual impairment.

When carefully sought, sarcoid nodules are often to be found in the conjunctival fornices.

The Salivary and Lacrimal Glands. These may be affected together or severally and sarcoidosis is one cause of Mikulicz's syndrome. Uveoparotid fever (Heerfordt's syndrome) is an occasional mode of presentation: in its complete and rarely seen form it consists of enlargement of parotid and submaxillary glands, uveitis and facial palsy. It usually resolves within a year.

Enlargement of lacrimal glands is rare, but deficient lacrimal secretion with keratoconjunctivitis sicca is often found when specifically sought.

The Bones, Joints and Muscles. Infiltrations in the phalanges of the hands and feet have long been known as osteitis multiplex of Jüngling. Although they may cause no symptoms, cutaneous lesions are almost constantly associated, and the skin of the affected phalanges is often the site of lupus pernio. Occasionally lesions occur in other bones, especially those of the nose, the forearm and the leg.

A febrile arthralgia affecting the larger joints, and usually fleeting, often accompanies the onset with erythema nodosum and BHL. The interphalangeal joints may be affected by neighbouring osteitis multiplex and occasionally a chronic monarticular or polyarticular arthritis occurs.

Sarcoid tubercles are probably common in voluntary muscle in the early febrile stage of the disease, but symptoms are rare and complete resolution seems the rule. Rarely the process extends to cause a polymyositis. In an occasional patient there is painless, progressive muscular wasting.

The Heart. The heart usually suffers indirectly as a

result of pulmonary fibrosis, although myocardial infiltrations are reported in 20 per cent. of autopsies. Clinical evidence of heart disease is rare, but conduction defects, paroxysmal ventricular tachycardia, congestive heart failure and cardiac arrest are all recorded.

The Nervous System. The commonest neurological lesion is facial palsy. It is usually transient and not invariably accompanied by parotid gland enlargement. Peripheral neuropathy is an occasional finding. In neither is the cause certain.

In the central nervous system meningeal infiltrations and tumour-like deposits of sarcoid tissue occur: they may affect the brain, the spinal cord or both. A multiplicity of clinical pictures may result. Nervous symptoms are seen in only 1–3 per cent. of patients.

Other Lesions. There are few tissues or organs which have not at some time been affected by sarcoidosis. The breast, the upper air passages, the hypophysis, the testis and the gastro-intestinal tract are among the less rare.

Diagnosis

The diagnosis of sarcoidosis is reached by a consideration of the clinical picture and the radiographic changes: it is confirmed by histological study of excised tissue. Individual lesions may raise problems of differential diagnosis, but the complete symptom-complex can be confused with nothing but chronic beryllium disease which can logically be regarded as 'sarcoidosis due to beryllium'.

Radiology. The Thorax. The symmetrical discrete enlargement of the bronchopulmonary, and often paratracheal lymph nodes described as BHL, gives a radiographic picture typical of sarcoidosis and if widespread mottled shadowing is seen as well, the appearances are diagnostic. Tomography will display the discrete nature of the nodal enlargement which has to be distinguished from tuberculosis, lymphoma, metastatic carcinoma, histoplasmosis and coccidioidomycosis.

With *pre-fibrotic sarcoidosis* there are widespread nodular (greater than 2 mm.) or micronodular (less than 2 mm.) shadows. Individual opacities rarely exceed 5 mm. in diameter and may be associated with cloudy shadowing. The changes are usually symmetrical and total, but if not the mid-zones are predominantly involved. These diffuse lung shadows must be differentiated from those seen in miliary tuberculosis, miliary carcinomatosis, pneumoconiosis, extrinsic allergic and other forms of fibrosing alveolitis, histiocytosis X and myodermal dysplasia.

In *fibrotic sarcoidosis* the shadowing becomes denser in the mid-zones and lessens elsewhere. Linear opacities radiate from the dense hila and fibrotic contraction elevates the pulmonary artery shadows. Scarring causes bullous emphysema, shown by apical and basal transradiancy. Shadows may fuse to form large localized opacities. Less commonly there is a fine homogeneous linear or reticular shadowing usually associated with some breathlessness. Cavitation, calcification and involvement of the pleura are rare; they do not necessarily imply a tuberculous aetiology, although whenever sarcoidosis is suspected every effort must be made to exclude this infection. Distinction must also be made from mycoses, pneumoconiosis and chronic fibrosing alveolitis.

The Bones. In osteitis multiplex the cancellous pattern of the affected phalanges is changed to a lace-like network with small irregular areas of rarefaction separated by bone of increased density.

Biopsy. The diagnosis can only be established with certainty when the characteristic histological picture is demonstrated. Enlarged lymph nodes provide the most suitable material, and 90 per cent. show diagnostic changes. With disease confined to the thorax, scalene node biopsy gives positive results in 80 per cent. Liver puncture biopsy is diagnostic in about 60 per cent. and more likely to be helpful in the early stages. Skin lesions are excellent for this purpose, and sarcoid tubercles have been demonstrated in conjunctival follicles, excised tonsils and material obtained by biopsy of nasal mucosa, bronchial mucosa and lung tissue.

Immunological Changes. Delayed hypersensitivity reactions are depressed in sarcoidosis and increasingly so as the disease progresses. This is thought to be due to inability to form cell-borne antibody and is commonly revealed by a negative intradermal tuberculin test (Mantoux test); 45–70 per cent. of patients with sarcoidosis have a negative reaction to 100 TU, compared with an average of 20 per cent. in the general population. A similar failure to react is shown to other antigens such as those prepared from *Candida albicans* and *Trichophyton*. The Mantoux test is of little practical value, although a negative reaction to 100 TU supports and a positive to 1 TU makes unlikely a diagnosis of sarcoidosis.

The production of humoral circulating antibody is unimpaired or even enhanced. This accords with the moderate rise in serum gamma globulin levels, due to an increase in IgG immunoglobulin, often found in the active phase, which explains the finding of a positive latex test for rheumatoid factor in 18 per cent.

The Kveim test is carried out by the intradermal injection of 0·1–0·2 ml. of a 10 per cent. saline suspension of sarcoid lymph node or spleen which has been heated to 56°–60° C. for 1 hour on two consecutive days. A positive result is shown in 4–6 weeks by the appearance at the site of injection of a nodule with the histological pattern of sarcoid. The test is positive in 70 per cent. of active subacute, 64 per cent. of active chronic and 17 per cent. of inactive cases. False positive reactions are less than 2 per cent. The test is said to be negative in beryllium disease.

The substance responsible for the Kveim reaction is probably a lipoprotein and it appears to detect a peculiar reactivity in the patient rather than a specific infective agent.

Haematological Changes. Mild normochromic anaemia with raised E.S.R. is usual in the active stage, often with eosinophilia. Thrombocytopenia and haemolytic anaemia are recorded usually in association with notable splenomegaly. In 50 per cent. of patients with the second submitted to splenectomy, the excised organ has shown no sarcoid tubercles.

Biochemical Changes. Hypercalcaemia, usually of moderate degree, occurs in 25 per cent. Hypercalciuria and a low faecal excretion of calcium prove it due to increased absorption from the gut and this results from an unexplained hypersensitivity to vitamin D. Patients with sarcoid become hypercalcaemic when photosynthesis of the vitamin is stimulated by exposure to sunlight.

The acute hypercalcaemic syndrome may occur, particularly after medication with vitamin D. Renal calculus, nephrocalcinosis with renal failure and calcinosis in soft tissues have all been recorded.

Treatment

The long-term results of treatment are hard to assess in a benign disease of such chronicity as sarcoidosis, when there is a strong tendency to spontaneous remission. The only agents known to influence local lesions are the corticosteroids, although some claims are made for chloroquine.

The effects of the corticosteroids are purely suppressive, and although they bring about resolution the lesions recur and progress immediately treatment ceases. The problem is to define the indications for their use.

Anterior uveitis often responds to instillation of hydrocortisone, but if it fails to improve or if there is posterior uveitis, systemic treatment is essential. Hypercalcaemia is an indisputable indication. If skin lesions cause unacceptable disfigurement and resist treatment with chloroquine sulphate, 200 mg. twice daily, systemic corticosteroids must be given. Myocardial infiltration if detected, should be treated: neurological lesions respond poorly, but corticosteroids are inevitably prescribed.

Systemic corticosteroids should be given in pulmonary sarcoidosis, even in the fibrotic stage when symptoms are severe enough to demand relief. The same is true in the active phase when radiographic changes remain or progress after 2 years' observation, particularly when there are also extrathoracic lesions. The aim of preventing fibrosis is by no means always achieved, and there is no general agreement that corticosteroid treatment brings any great advantage. The rare stenosing lesions of the bronchi respond well and provide an absolute indication for treatment.

Prednisolone should be given initially in a dose of 20–30 mg. daily, being slowly reduced after 6 weeks if there is a satisfactory response, until the lowest effective dose is found. Treatment must be continued for 1–2 years. Final withdrawal must be slow, the daily dose being reduced by 1 mg. every 4 weeks.

There is no evidence that antituberculous drugs are beneficial, but some authorities use them prophylactically when patients with sarcoidosis and a strongly positive tuberculin test are given corticosteroids.

Preliminary reports on the use of chlorambucil and methotrexate in sarcoidosis are encouraging.

Prognosis

Occasionally patients die from renal failure or heart disease, but in the overwhelming majority the outcome depends upon the state of the lungs. BHL is benign: in 55 per cent. the lungs remain inviolate and when the onset is with erythema nodosum the outlook is even better. In another 20 per cent. lung changes develop and resolve spontaneously. In the remainder, lung changes and BHL persist; in 12 per cent. fibrosis develops, but only in a few is it progressive and disabling.

If lung infiltration is taken as the starting point, 28 per cent. will develop pulmonary fibrosis in 5 years; if it be present when first seen, 25 per cent. will die in this period. If there are associated skin lesions, the prognosis is worse, but it is unaffected by uveitis.

The case mortality from sarcoidosis in the United Kingdom is about 7 per cent. The outlook is less favourable in the United States, where Negroes form a high proportion of the cases. The long-term prognosis is unaffected by pregnancy. The recovery rate is probably 80–85 per cent. A few are disabled by blindness or pulmonary fibrosis.

REFERENCES

Anderson, R., James, D. G., Peters, P. M., and Thompson, A. D. (1963) The Kveim test in sarcoidosis, *Lancet*, ii, 650.

James, D. G. (1957) Dermatological aspects of sarcoidosis, *Quart. J. Med.*, **28**, 109.

Longcope, W. T., and Freiman, D. G. (1952) A study of sarcoidosis, *Medicine (Baltimore)*, **31**, 1.

Scadding, J. G. (1967) *Sarcoidosis*, London.

Smellie, H., and Hoyle, C. (1960) The natural history of pulmonary sarcoidosis, *Quart. J. Med.*, **29**, 539.

John Batten
R. Bodley Scott
Brian Russell

CHRONIC SPECIFIC BRONCHOPULMONARY INFECTION (OTHER THAN TUBERCULOSIS)

While *syphilis* of the lung, both congenital (interstitial pneumonia) and acquired (e.g. gummata), is exceptionally rare [Section 2] mycotic infections are less so. Mycotic or fungal infections are generally discussed in Section 2 in which reference is made to bronchopulmonary involvement in particular with *actinomycosis*, *nocardiosis*, *cryptococcosis* (torulosis), *histoplasmosis*, *coccidioidomycosis*, *North* and *South American blastomycosis*, *aspergillosis* and *mucormycosis*.

BRONCHOPULMONARY ASPERGILLOSIS

Bronchopulmonary aspergillosis is due to infection with *Aspergillus* species—usually *Aspergillus fumigatus*. There are three types of disease:

Saprophytic

A. fumigatus may colonize and flourish in both closed and open lesions of the lung, e.g. pneumonia, infarction, neoplasm and air spaces which may be found in bronchiectasis, healed tuberculous cavities, and abscesses. The pleura may be involved via a bronchopleural fistula or externally by injury or surgery. This fungus is particularly liable to grow in debilitated patients.

Mycetoma (fungal ball or aspergilloma): Mycelia of *A. fumigatus* (or rarely other species) may proliferate to form dense masses or balls within cavities in the lung.

These may be old healed tuberculous cavities usually in the upper zones, or less commonly in cavities associated with bronchiectasis, necrotic neoplasms or infarcts, cysts, etc. These cavities may be wholly or partly epithelialized.

Mycetomata are usually asymptomatic. They may present either as a radiological curiosity in which a translucent halo is seen round a dense shadow or with haemoptysis which may be considerable. Mycetomata may be multiple. They usually grow slowly and sometimes spontaneously disappear. The diagnosis is established by the characteristic radiological appearance which may be clarified by tomography. In more than 90 per cent. of cases precipitating antibodies to the relevant fungus are present in the serum.

Treatment is required if there is severe or recurrent haemoptysis. If the respiratory reserve is adequate and surgery seems feasible then the lesion should be resected. Success has been claimed for direct intracavitary instillation of antifungal agents (e.g. nystatin or amphotericin in a semi-fluid base). This may result in arrest of haemoptysis and regression of the lesion with ultimate disappearance of precipitating antibody.

Allergic

While *Aspergillus* sp. may be significant allergens in the genesis of extrinsic asthma [p. 891] they are of greater importance as the cause of recurrent localized pulmonary infiltrations with eosinophilia in the peripheral blood—allergic bronchopulmonary aspergillosis [p. 226]. Segmental and subsegmental bronchi may be obstructed by plugs which often contain fragmented mycelia of *A. fumigatus*. There is an immunologically determined inflammatory reaction with eosinophilic infiltration in the adjacent part of the lung. This is an Arthus Type III sensitivity reaction (Gell and Coombs). The reaction in the skin to an intracutaneous injection of *A. fumigatus* antigen probably reflects the changes in the lung: this is a dual reaction which consists of an immediate Type I wheal and flare reaction followed by a delayed precipitin mediated Arthus reaction 3–6 hours later. Precipitating antibodies to *A. fumigatus* can be demonstrated in the serum in about 70 per cent. of cases. The inflammatory reaction in the bronchial wall leads to permanent damage with characteristic bronchiectasis in which the proximal bronchi are dilated while the peripheral airways are spared and can be seen to fill normally on bronchography.

Allergic aspergillosis is usually found in atopic subjects who have mild asthma and there may be constitutional symptoms such as mild fever with the pulmonary infiltrations. In some patients brown plugs are expectorated containing the fungal fragments which stain with silver stains. The fungus may be grown from these plugs. Patients with cystic fibrosis are prone to develop allergic aspergillosis. While recurrent infiltrations in the lung with eosinophilia are most commonly due to allergic aspergillosis in the United Kingdom, these should be differentiated from atelectasis due to obstruction by a plain mucus plug which not infrequently occurs in asthma. Recurrent infiltration with eosinophilia is also a feature in non-atopic subjects with intrinsic type asthma, the most striking form of which is a manifestation of presystemic polyarteritis nodosa. In this rare form of pulmonary infiltration the shadows are more widespread and are not usually segmental. The eosinophilia is often greater than 2000 per mm^3.

Treatment with antifungal agents (e.g. nystatin, brilliant green) whether by mouth or by aerosol has been largely unsuccessful. Although disodium cromoglycate (*Intal*) inhibits immediate and late bronchoconstriction after challenge with an aerosol of *Aspergillus* antigen it is yet uncertain whether it will always inhibit clinical allergic aspergillosis. If infiltrates recur and bronchial wall damage becomes a possibility then allergic aspergillosis should be suppressed by adrenocortical steroids (prednisone, 10–20 mg. daily by mouth followed by the smallest dose required to prevent pulmonary infiltration).

Invasive

A. fumigatus may invade the lung in a widespread fashion when there is impaired immunity, e.g. with lymphomata, leukaemias, etc. especially in patients on steroid or immunosuppressive drugs. Such an opportunistic infection may spread via the blood stream to many organs where metastatic abscesses develop, e.g. in brain, kidney, skin, etc.

REFERENCES

CAMPBELL, M. J., and CLAYTON, Y. M. (1964) Bronchopulmonary aspergillosis: a correlation of the clinical and laboratory findings in 272 patients investigated for bronchopulmonary aspergillosis, *Amer. Rev. resp. Dis.*, **89**, 186.

PEPYS, J. (1969) *Hypersensitivity Diseases of the Lung due to Fungi and Organic Dust*, Basel.

BRONCHIECTASIS

Definition

Dilatation of the bronchi.

Aetiology

Bronchiectasis may arise in congenital disorders. Thus, dilated bronchi may be associated with dextrocardia and absent or poorly developed frontal sinuses (*Kartagena's syndrome*). Bronchiectasis may also develop in *sequestrated lung segments*, and in the rare condition of *bronchial atresia*.

Bronchiectasis, however, most commonly results from *infection* and *obstruction* and usually develops in childhood.

Obstruction. Bronchiectasis and collapse of the lung follow obstruction of a large bronchus by foreign bodies, a stricture, neoplasm or by pressure from without, e.g. large lymph nodes, etc. Elastic retraction round the bronchi in the collapsed lobe or segment and pressure of retained mucus cause dilatation which will become permanent if the obstruction is unrelieved or infection increases the intraluminal secretion and damages the musculo-elastic wall. Bronchial obstruction and associated lung collapse due to mucus may persist when the mucus is aspirated peripherally, in which case the proximal bronchial lumen will not be subjected to the pressure of intraluminal secretion but to the forces of elastic retraction and possibly further damage by bronchial infection. In either case the bronchi may regain their normal calibre if the obstruction is relieved and the lung re-expands. Such temporary ectasia of the bronchus is not uncommon in pneumonia.

Infection. This may cause bronchiectasis without bronchial obstruction in childhood pneumonia. This may accompany measles, pertussis and tuberculosis. In the latter there is a glandular component which may obstruct the bronchus proximally.

Two broad clinical types of bronchiectasis have been described in Australia in which specific causes were recognized. In one type, which affected children under 3 years of age, there was insidious *bronchiolitis* without pyogenic infection but often associated with upper respiratory infection. There was usually irreversible involvement of mainly peripheral bronchi and the process was often widespread. Chronic upper respiratory disease was found in about one third of cases. The other type, *subacute pyogenic collapse*, developed more rapidly without family predisposition in children between the ages of 2 and 6 years. Pyogenic organisms were isolated from the sputum and there was no association with upper respiratory infection. The process was usually localized and involved mainly the larger bronchi. It was often non-progressive and often reversible. Symptoms tended to disappear within 2 years or so.

Bronchiectasis is also caused by *fibrosis* complicating tuberculosis, unresolved or suppurative pneumonia with lung abscess, mycotic infections, sarcoidosis, etc. Bronchiectasis is a feature of certain well-defined clinical states in which there is bronchial infection or atelectasis to a varying degree. It is a feature, for example, in *cystic fibrosis* (mucoviscidosis, p. 881), *hypogammaglobulinaemia*, congenital and acquired [see Section 4], *allergic bronchopulmonary aspergillosis* in which larger segmental or subsegmental bronchi are dilated while the peripheral airways may be quite normal [p. 226].

Pathology

Bronchiectasis may be localized to a segment or lobe or it may be widespread and patchy—in 30–50 per cent. it is bilateral. Upper lobe disease is often a sequel to pulmonary tuberculosis. Lower lobe disease is often associated with involvement of either the lingular segment of the left upper lobe or the middle lobe. Cylindrical, fusiform and saccular dilatations are found in the larger bronchi: these are purely descriptive terms which indicate the shape of the bronchial dilatation. Peripheral bronchial ectasia is often cystic.

The bronchial epithelium may be squamous or columnar or replaced by ulcerated granulating tissue. The bronchial wall may be partially destroyed and there may be pneumonia, collapse or fibrosis in the adjacent lung. These changes may lead to distortion and variable obliteration of the bronchi and their branches (bronchitis or bronchiolitis obliterans). A patchy distribution of obliterative bronchitis or bronchiolitis in childhood may lead to alveolar hypoplasia and emphysema which is often unilateral and may involve the whole lung or a lobe (Macleod's syndrome) [p. 889].

The abnormal bronchus is supplied by the bronchial artery branches which may enlarge and anastomose with the pulmonary arteries and veins and on occasion lead to a sizeable shunt of blood.

Infection of the abnormal bronchial tree is common as a result of the impaired defence mechanisms. *H. influenzae*, pneumococci, staphylococci (especially in cystic fibrosis) and streptococci may be encountered but a wide variety of usually non-pathogenic organisms are found. Anaerobic infection was frequent in pre-chemotherapy days.

Impairment of pulmonary function depends on the degree of obstruction (peripheral or central) and lung involvement. If this is extensive there will be a restrictive ventilatory disorder. The presence of generalized airways obstruction is usually due to associated chronic obstructive bronchitis. Ventilation and blood flow are often equally reduced in the affected parts: changes associated with unilateral emphysema or transradiancy of the lung are described on page 889.

Clinical Picture

Cough and sputum are usually of long-standing and are variable in severity. Sputum is usually purulent and may be scanty with a tendency to increase with acute respiratory infections and to diminish with chemotherapy. Often the purulent sputum is considerable in quantity (even up to 200 ml. or more a day) and before chemotherapy was often not only copious but foetid. Blood-streaking of the sputum is not infrequent and there may be frank severe haemoptysis. There may be haemoptysis in so-called dry bronchiectasis, in which there is no sputum or bronchial secretion; the bronchiectasis may be quite limited in extent. Dyspnoea is usually due to associated chronic obstructive bronchitis unless the bronchiectasis and associated lung damage with fibrosis are so widespread that ventilation is restricted.

Physical signs depend on the extent of the bronchiectasis and the amount of secretion. The physical condition of the patient is usually quite good. Clubbing of the fingers and even pulmonary osteoarthropathy may be present, usually with more extensive disease. Medium and coarse crepitations localized to the major sites of disease are a characteristic physical sign: these crepitations persist and may be accompanied by widespread rhonchi if there is associated bronchitis. Other signs of consolidation, collapse and fibrosis of the lung may be present.

Bronchiectasis is complicated by *pneumonia*, which may develop in the surrounding lung or at a distant site due to aspiration of pus (a spill-over infection). The pneumonias are usually non-specific and often follow an acute respiratory infection. With bronchiectasis *infected sinuses* are frequently encountered. The inflammation may spread to the pleura to give rise to either *dry pleurisy* with pain or less commonly to a *pleural effusion*, which may be a simple exudate or empyema. Bronchiectasis is a recognized cause of acute benign *pericarditis* due to direct spread of infection. *Brain abscess* may result from septic emboli, and *amyloidosis* is a rare complication when infection is uncontrolled.

Diagnosis

While the clinical picture of long-standing cough and sputum, often going back to childhood, with persistent crepitations on auscultation of the chest and clubbing of the fingers is strongly suggestive of the diagnosis, these manifestations may be absent. Chest radiography is necessary to establish the diagnosis. The plain X-ray may be normal, but associated atelectasis, patchy clouding (localized pneumonia), hypertransradiancy (lobar or the whole lung) may be seen. Shadows may be cast by dilated bronchi full of secretion which may disappear with treatment, leaving linear shadows of the bronchial walls. Ring shadows with or without fluid levels may be seen in saccular or cystic bronchiectasis.

Bronchography is often necessary to establish the diagnosis and to define the extent of disease [PLATE 9]. In addition to the dilated bronchi, organic distortion or obliteration are often seen, together with the changes of chronic bronchitis. When haemoptysis or recurrent pneumonia are the presenting symptoms and when the chest X-ray is normal between times, bronchography will be needed to discover the cause.

Treatment

Bronchiectasis may be prevented by adequate treatment of those infections in childhood which may lead to bronchiectasis and by the removal of causes of bronchial occlusion before bronchial walls become permanently damaged.

Physical Treatment. Bronchial clearance is impaired in bronchiectasis and purulent secretions are retained unless gravity is used to assist drainage. Postural coughing and if necessary percussion of the chest is carried out with the patient in such a position that the affected segment or lobe is uppermost. Bronchography may be necessary to recognize all the affected segments. This treatment should be carried out after waking up in the morning and before retiring to bed at night as a minimum. With copious secretion or with exacerbations then the treatment should be given more frequently. The patient is best taught by a physiotherapist how to maintain each position by the use of pillows or simple apparatus for elevating the foot of the bed, etc.

Chemotherapy. The aim of chemotherapy is to eliminate infection and this is frequently unsuccessful. It should be tried if sputum is purulent in association with physiotherapy. If the sputum becomes mucoid with treatment, then physiotherapy should be continued alone. Usually purulent sputum persists although the treatment may have reduced the quantity of the sputum and restored well-being to the patient. In these cases physiotherapy should be continued and chemotherapy perhaps reserved for exacerbations due to acute respiratory infection with or without pneumonia. Sometimes pus in the sputum is eliminated by treatment only to return a short time after finishing the chemotherapy. In these cases chemotherapy should be resumed and continued on a long-term basis if it suppresses bronchial infection and keeps the patient well.

A wide variety of micro-organisms (normally non-pathogenic) are usually cultivated from the sputum. These organisms are usually sensitive to penicillin, and benzylpenicillin, 1 mega Unit intramuscularly two to four times a day, remains the most effective preparation. Sometimes treatment can be continued successfully with an oral penicillin (phenoxymethylpenicillin, 500 mg. four times a day). Other organisms, such as *H. influenzae*, *Staph. pyogenes*, *Strep. pneumoniae* and *Klebsiella sp.* may be found and will require appropriate antibiotics. As with chronic bronchitis, the routine culture of the sputum may not reveal the true pathogen and trials have shown that tetracycline, 0·5 G. four times a day given on 2 days each week, significantly reduces the quantity of sputum and the loss of time from work. Tetracycline given in this fashion or in a dose of 0·5 G. twice a day every day may be the most convenient way to control infection in bronchiectasis.

Medical treatment with physiotherapy and chemotherapy has very considerably reduced the need for surgery. Surgery should be considered, however, in patients in whom copious and purulent sputum persists despite medical treatment, in those with recurrent pneumonia and in cases of severe or recurrent haemoptysis. For surgery to be successful the disease should be localized and respiratory function of the remaining lung should be adequate. The results are best in children and young adults and are unsatisfactory when there is widespread bronchitis and in patients over forty. In expert surgical hands about half the patients in whom resection is carried out become symptom free and about another 25 per cent. are much improved with only minimal symptoms. The results are better with unilateral cases. Surgery of childhood bronchiectasis should be deferred because of the frequency of postoperative complications in young children. At least 6 months and preferably one year's proper medical treatment should be given to all cases before a decision is made.

Prognosis

With proper medical and surgical treatment the prognosis is now excellent and most patients may be rendered symptom free or the disease may be adequately controlled. The prognosis becomes less certain when there is associated chronic obstructive bronchitis or widespread lung damage.

REFERENCES

BORRIE, J., and LICHTER, I. (1965) Surgical treatment of bronchiectasis: Ten year survey, *Brit. med. J.*, **2,** 908.

CLARK, N. S. (1963) Bronchiectasis in childhood, *Brit. med. J.*, **1,** 80.

WILLIAMS, H., and O'REILLY, R. N. (1959) Bronchiectasis in children: Its multiple clinical and pathological aspects, *Arch. Dis. Childh.*, **34,** 192.

CYSTIC FIBROSIS

Synonyms. Fibrocystic disease of the pancreas; Mucoviscidosis.

Definition

Cystic fibrosis is a symptom complex which comprises pancreatic insufficiency, chronic bronchopulmonary infection and a high sweat sodium concentration.

Pathogenesis

Cystic fibrosis is transmitted as a recessive gene with a frequency of about 1 in 20 in most populations. In Europe and North America about 1 in 2,000 live births is homozygous for the gene and the majority of these infants manifest as overt cystic fibrosis in the first few weeks of life. Cystic fibrosis is one of the commonest inherited disorders of childhood.

The basic defect is unknown, but its major effect is to impair cell membrane function so that electrolyte transport is abnormal, e.g. there is diminished reabsorption of sodium from the primary secretion in the ducts of the parotid and sweat glands. The disorder is not confined to exocrine glands for there is also defective function of the pupil, which dilates more slowly in the dark in patients with cystic fibrosis than in the normal. This cannot be observed clinically. There is also a serum globulin component which impairs ciliary action *in vitro*. The concentration of this component is said to be high in homozygotes, low in heterozygotes and absent in normals. The structural consequences of this functional defect vary greatly from one exocrine gland to another. In some, e.g. the pancreas, liver, sublingual salivary gland, prostate and testes, the ducts are blocked completely by solidified secretion with severe effects from birth. On the other hand there appears to be excessive activity of the mucus secreting glands of the respiratory and gastro-intestinal tracts, which are hypertrophied—the mucus itself, however, is qualitatively normal. Measurements of sputum viscosity have shown this to be normal, although the flow characteristics are probably abnormal. The sweat and parotid glands are structurally normal. The high concentration of sodium, however, in sweat is affected little by such changes as salt depletion and aldosterone.

In rare cases the functional and structural defects are for reasons unknown delayed or reduced so that pancreatic insufficiency may be minimal, even absent, and respiratory disease mild or delayed—to manifest in late childhood or adult life.

Pathology

The *pancreas* is usually lobulated and fibrotic. The ducts are occluded and the acinar tissue atrophied soon after birth. There is cystic dilatation of the small ducts together with interstitial fibrosis—sometimes all the exocrine tissue is replaced by fat, leaving the islets of Langerhans intact. Diabetes mellitus is encountered in older patients with a frequency rather greater than expected in a normal population.

In 10 per cent. of cases obstruction of the small intrahepatic bile ducts may lead to *cirrhosis* with portal hypertension.

The *lung* is normal at birth and often in neonates who present with meconium ileus. There is, however, progressive hypertrophy and hyperplasia of the bronchial mucous glands and goblet cells which starts at the time of the initial infection, which in 50–70 per cent. of cases is due to *Staph. pyogenes*. Suppurative bronchitis, bronchiolitis and focal, segmental or lobar pneumonia with necrosis are followed by progressive obstructive purulent bronchitis or bronchiolitis. *H. influenzae* and *Ps. aeruginosa* may be important pathogens as well. Hypoplasia and scarring of the lung with irregular emphysema and limited bronchiectasis and honeycombing may follow.

The physiological consequences are often more severe than routine laboratory testing may reveal. Initially there is an increase in the physiological dead space without there necessarily being any detectable evidence of an increase in airways resistance. Later obstructive and restrictive defects of ventilation develop, with falls in PEF, FEV_1, FVC and VC, while the RV (residual volume) increases. The TLC tends to remain normal. As the mechanical defect becomes more severe so the arterial P_{O_2} tends to fall and in the more severe cases respiratory failure will be present at rest. The arterial P_{CO_2} rises only as a terminal event—right ventricular hypertrophy and right ventricular failure are likewise late manifestations.

Clinical Picture

Cystic fibrosis affects the sexes equally and in 10 per cent. of cases presents as meconium ileus.

Usually the infant, normal at birth, fails to thrive in the first weeks despite a good appetite. The abdomen distends and later, with change in diet, diarrhoea with steatorrhoea becomes apparent, sometimes with rectal prolapse. Cough is usually the presenting respiratory symptom. It usually persists after the first infection and is often distressing. If the disease is not recognized there is progressive bronchopulmonary infection with expectoration of sputum which may be basically mucoid with plugs of pus or frankly purulent. Haemoptysis is a late complication and breathlessness is often less than would be expected from the observed changes in function. With increasing severity of the disease, growth (both weight and height) is impaired. Clubbing of the fingers and toes is usually prominent. The chest appears hyperinflated. With exercise or with infection the breathing becomes rapid, cyanosis may develop and intercostal recession may be seen. Other signs in the chest are usually minimal, but there may be evidence of consolidation, especially in infants, or localized crepitations. The liver and spleen become palpable in about 10 per cent. of cases. Puberty and the growth spurt at that time are usually delayed and in males the vas deferens may be absent. On the other hand, females may remain fertile and conceive.

Structural damage to the lung is prevented by early diagnosis and energetic treatment. Then all the respiratory manifestations may be prevented or delayed and growth and development may proceed almost normally, even with pancreatic insufficiency, provided this is corrected. The major impact of the disease falls on the lungs and the most frequent and terminal complication is *respiratory failure*. *Spontaneous pneumothorax*, often bilateral, may develop in about 10 per cent. of adolescent or older patients. Empyema is unusual and amyloidosis has not been reported. Less common complications are *nasal polyposis* (in about 8 per cent.), while *allergic bronchopulmonary aspergillosis* is seen with a rather lesser frequency. *Portal hypertension* may be complicated by bleeding from oesophageal varices, or hepatic failure [see Section 6].

Diagnosis

Cystic fibrosis should be suspected in any child which fails to thrive with malabsorption or rectal prolapse; with chronic or recurrent cough with sputum; or with cirrhosis and portal hypertension. Difficulties arise where there is little involvement of either the pancreas or lung or when manifestations appear in older children or even later.

Evidence should be sought for pancreatic insufficiency [p. 658]. The high concentration of sodium in sweat and parotid secretion is of major diagnostic value. The normal sweat sodium concentration rises from a mean value of 22 mEq. per litre in infancy to 55 mEq. per litre in adults. Values above 70 mEq. per litre are diagnostic in infants, but not so in adolescents and adults. In cystic fibrosis, however, the fall in sweat sodium concentration after 9α fluorohydrocortisone (1–5 mg. daily by mouth for 3 days) is usually less than 10 per cent., whereas in normals the fall is much greater.

With respiratory infection there is usually a *polymorphonuclear leucocytosis*. The *chest radiograph* may show only parallel line shadows cast by bronchial walls in the more peripheral parts of the lung. Ill-defined nodules or patchy clouding up to 1 or 2 cm. in size may appear—these shadows may cavitate. Ring shadows (honeycombing), segmental or lobar consolidation with or without atelectasis (usually under one to two years of age) and enlarged hilar nodes are also seen. None of these shadows are diagnostic alone, but in the aggregate they are very characteristic.

Treatment

The general condition and growth improve following the correction of the malabsorption due to pancreatic insufficiency by the administration of pancreatin in powder or tablet form with all feeds or meals. Protein and vitamin supplements are necessary and fat may need to be limited in the diet if steatorrhoea persists. Salt supplements are only required with excessive sweating in hot climates or heat waves.

Effective treatment of the respiratory disease from the earliest possible moment is the single most important factor in preventing disability and in the prognosis. Treatment is aimed at bronchial clearance and prevention or eradication of infection. Bronchial clearance is promoted by vigorous physiotherapy. Postural coughing and percussion even in infants should be applied three or four times a day. This should be carried out initially by the physiotherapist, but subsequently by the parents after instruction by a physiotherapist. Physical exercise is also good physiotherapy and swimming, games and exercise should be encouraged. Simple aerosols of saline or water may encourage cough and bronchial clearance. High density aerosols created by ultrasonic apparatus in mist tents may ease bronchial clearance, but firm evidence is lacking. Many mucolytic agents may cause inflammatory change in the bronchial mucosa and some inactivate antibacterial drugs. Enzymatic preparations may give rise to hypersensitivity. Saline aerosols should therefore be tried and may incorporate bronchodilators, such as isoprenaline, salbutamol or orciprenaline if they are shown to be effective.

Oral chemotherapy should be directed at the infecting organisms. As the first infection is so frequently staphylococcal some advocate the administration of cloxacillin from the moment of diagnosis to prevent established infection. Once infection with *Staph. pyogenes*, *H. influenzae* or *Ps. aeruginosa* is established, it is unusual for infection to be eradicated and it can then only be suppressed by appropriate chemotherapy. Chemotherapy by aerosol may limit the bronchial spread of infection or help to suppress it (e.g. carbenicillin in Pseudomonas infection, methicillin or neomycin in staphylococcal infection.).

Prevention

Siblings of patients with cystic fibrosis should be screened by estimation of sodium concentration in sweat or parotid secretion. Those found to have high values, i.e. homozygotes, and patients who present with gastro-intestinal manifestations, even in the absence of respiratory symptoms, may be treated with cloxacillin thereafter to prevent staphylococcal infection. There is as yet no reliable way to detect heterozygotes. Measles, pertussis and influenza vaccine should be given.

Prognosis

If cystic fibrosis is untreated, 80 per cent. of patients will die in the first year of life, usually from staphylococcal bronchopulmonary infection. With prompt treatment applied in special centres so that lung damage is prevented, about 75 per cent. of patients at present reach adolescence. The mean survival from diagnosis in the best centres in the United Kingdom and North America is about 12 years.

REFERENCES

ANDERSEN, D. H. (1938) Cystic fibrosis of the pancreas and its relation to coeliac disease. A clinical and pathological study, *Amer. J. Dis. Child.*, **56**, 344.

DI SANT'AGNESE, P. A., and TALMARO, R. C. (1967) Pathogenesis and physiopathology of cystic fibrosis of the pancreas, *New Engl. J. Med.*, **277**, 1287, 1344 and 1399.

LAWSON, D., ed. (1969) *Proceedings of the Fifth International Cystic Fibrosis Conference*, London, Cystic Fibrosis Research Trust.

DISEASES ASSOCIATED WITH GENERALIZED AIRWAY OBSTRUCTION

CHRONIC BRONCHITIS

Definition

Simple chronic bronchitis is a condition in which there is chronic or recurrent increase in the volume of mucoid bronchial secretion sufficient to cause expectoration. Throat clearers who swallow their sputum should also be included within the definition but it is not possible to diagnose chronic bronchitis with confidence in the presence of other cardiopulmonary diseases which may themselves give rise to expectoration.

Chronic bronchitis may be complicated by infection giving rise to *chronic* or *recurrent mucopurulent bronchitis* in which the sputum is persistently or intermittently mucopurulent (in the absence of localized bronchopulmonary disease). On the other hand chronic bronchitis may be further complicated by persistent widespread narrowing of the airways, at least on expiration, which causes airways obstruction. It may then be termed *chronic obstructive bronchitis*.

Aetiology

Mucus hypersecretion in the respiratory tract in chronic bronchitis is due to cigarette smoking, and atmospheric pollution and may be reversible. Other possible factors whether they be genetic, social, occupational or infective are less clearly defined.

Tobacco smoking. Ten per cent. of eleven-year-old school-children in certain parts of the United Kingdom who admit to cigarette smoking have simple chronic bronchitis. The prevalence and death rate for chronic bronchitis in the United Kingdom is higher in cigarette smokers than ex-smokers, or non-smokers, and increases with the amount smoked. The prevalence in pipe and cigar smokers is less.

Atmospheric Pollution. Smoke and sulphur dioxide are the major known factors in air pollution. The prevalence and mortality of chronic bronchitis are higher with urbanization. There is a correlation between the seasonal peaks in atmospheric pollution (e.g. fog) and mortality and between atmospheric pollution and loss of time from work due to exacerbations of chronic bronchitis.

The role of infection in the natural history of bronchitis is uncertain. Infection with respiratory viruses, *Mycoplasma pneumoniae* and bacteria (especially *H. influenzae*) undoubtedly cause acute exacerbations in chronic bronchitis but they are not a primary cause of the disease. Significant infection with *H. influenzae* detected by the presence of precipitating antibody, appears more likely with increasing degrees of pre-existing structural damage within the bronchial tree. Whether persistent infection with *H. influenzae* or any other micro-organism affects the rate of deterioration or not, is unknown. Some of the pathological changes found in the acini described below are probably attributable to infection.

In *occupations* in which there is exposure to dust and fumes, e.g. coal miners, steel and flax workers, there appears to be an increased prevalence of chronic bronchitis.

Chronic bronchitis is more common in men and the incidence increases with age. About 17 per cent. of males and about 8 per cent. of females between the ages of 40 and 60 years have chronic bronchitis in Great Britain. The incidence of chronic bronchitis in other developed countries is probably similar but disabling forms of the disease (chronic mucopurulent and obstructive bronchitis) are more prevalent in Great Britain than elsewhere and are much more prevalent in males than females. The mortality of chronic bronchitis is much higher in the United Kingdom than elsewhere and in 1964 amounted to 90 per 100,000 of the population. The mortality is greater in towns, in winter and in lower social classes (i.e. it is five times higher in a social group 5 than in social group 1).

Pathology

The bronchial mucous glands are hypertrophied. This hypertrophy can be measured in sections of the bronchial wall: the thickness of the gland layer is related to the thickness of the bronchial wall (Reid index). The gland/wall ratio in normals is 0·26, in chronic bronchitis it is 0·59. The mucus-secreting goblet cells proliferate in the surface epithelium most dramatically in the bronchioles where normally only an occasional goblet cell is seen, while in chronic bronchitis almost every cell may be transformed to one distended with mucus. The mucus is histochemically altered so that there is a higher concentration of fucose and sialic acid.

Normally the respiratory tract is sterile but in simple chronic bronchitis a wide range of micro-organisms is found in bronchial mucus. Respiratory virus infections, trivial in the healthy, increase secretion and encourage secondary bacterial growth. *H. influenzae* is the dominant pathogen though *Strep. pneumoniae* may occasionally be found. It is unusual to find *Staph. pyogenes*. With these infections the airways become acutely inflamed and the sputum purulent. Recovery from acute infection may be complete but *H. influenzae* in particular may persist in the sputum and it is possible that it may cause permanent damage, particularly with repeated acute episodes. Ulceration, granulation tissue and fibrosis may cause irregularity, narrowing or dilatation of the smaller airways. Distally the acinus may be collapsed or scarred: on the other hand the air spaces may be enlarged by a process of destruction or distension. This increase in size of the air spaces distal to the terminal bronchiole is termed *emphysema* and is discussed later [p. 887].

Organic narrowing and mucus impaction in chronic bronchitis cause airway obstruction. This obstruction may be further potentiated by the destruction and distension of alveolar walls (emphysema). Many years must elapse before airway obstruction becomes detectable: impaired airflow, however, can be detected as early as 5 years of age in children with adverse environmental, social and infectious aspects.

Airways less than 3 mm. in diameter in a normal adult contribute little to total airways resistance simply because the flow of air within them is so small. It is therefore possible for a considerable proportion of the smallest airways to be obstructed without detecting any impairment of air flow by methods which measure flow rate (peak expiratory flow rate, FEV_1) or airways resistance. Thus, obstruction in chronic bronchitis may be advanced when impaired air flow or an increased resistance is manifest. Reduction in PEF correlates well with the number of cigarettes smoked. As airway obstruction becomes more severe the PEF and the FEV_1 diminish and the FEV_1/FVC falls below 75 per cent. The work of breathing increases and breathlessness may develop. There is, however, a poor correlation between the degree of airway obstruction and this symptom.

Gas transfer (T_{CO}) is only moderately impaired in chronic bronchitis. This is mainly due to uneven distribution of inspired air to the alveoli and only becomes important in severe obstructive bronchitis. When there is this severe mismatch of ventilation and blood flow arterial oxygen saturation falls and the patient may become cyanosed. If over-all alveolar ventilation is inadequate then there is an increase in the arterial P_{CO_2}. Infection increases airway obstruction and the mismatch of ventilation and blood flow with further deterioration of the blood gases. Prolonged deviation of the blood gas tensions from the normal, especially the arterial P_{O_2}, and other factors as yet unknown may eventually be associated with an increase in pulmonary vascular resistance. This in turn may lead to right ventricular hypertrophy. Right ventricular failure with oedema is usually provoked by a transient rise in pulmonary vascular resistance due to hypoxia which results from acute respiratory infection.

Clinical Picture

The onset of chronic bronchitis is extremely insidious, so much so that the majority of patients with chronic bronchitis regard themselves as normal. Throat clearing and the swallowing of mucus may be the only symptom. There is usually expectoration of mucus with cough after waking but if more than 2 ml. of sputum are produced each day then expectoration will tend to continue through the waking hours. Over the years the cough may become more troublesome. The sputum at first is just mucoid but it may contain black specks of carbon particles from smoke. Later the sputum may become yellow or green with acute respiratory infections and the purulence may sometimes persist. Haemoptysis is rare. After varying periods of time, usually many years, there may be disabling respiratory infection which keeps the patient away from work, usually during the winter. In these episodes not only are cough and sputum more troublesome but he may become breathless for the first time. Breathlessness may first become apparent very gradually on exertion and then, or with infection, it may be accompanied by a wheeze. Progression of breathlessness is usually protracted, but sometimes there is a sudden deterioration which persists following a respiratory infection.

There may be no physical signs but with increasing mucus secretion rhonchi may be heard which clear on coughing. With increasing airways obstruction wheezing may become persistent and expiration prolonged: the accessory muscles of breathing come into use even at rest and the chest may appear hyperinflated—but (unless emphysema is present) although chest expansion is limited the outward movement of the lower ribs persists for the diaphragm retains its curvature. Clubbing of the fingers is exceptional and should give rise to suspicion that other disease may be present, e.g. carcinoma of the lung, or bronchiectasis.

The plethoric cyanosed patient with advanced chronic bronchitis with suffused conjunctivae and stocky build is a characteristic clinical picture. There is no doubt then that he is in respiratory failure. The detection of right ventricular hypertrophy due to elevated pulmonary vascular resistance is more difficult. There may be loud closure of the pulmonary valve and an atrial sound but actual detection of the right ventricular hypertrophy may be prevented by hyperinflation. With hypercapnia the periphery is usually warm and the superficial veins dilated. When right ventricular failure supervenes then the systemic venous pressure is elevated, the liver is enlarged and there is peripheral oedema. There may be evidence of gross tricuspid incompetence. The right ventricular filling sound may be audible. With all these late developments the patient may make little complaint about breathlessness.

Diagnosis

The chest radiograph is usually normal in chronic bronchitis. When obstructive bronchitis is severe and right ventricular hypertrophy and failure ensue then the cardiac shadow will enlarge, particularly with acute respiratory infection. When polycythaemia supervenes then there may be an increase in size of the pulmonary vessel shadows. The bronchogram [PLATE 10] may show striking changes. Wide ducts of mucous glands are clearly seen in the large bronchi. The smaller airways are irregular in diameter and may be cut off peripherally by mucus or organic obstruction [PLATE 10A]. There may be loss of smaller side branches and pooling of the radio-opaque material due to bronchiolectasis giving a mimosa pattern [PLATE 10B].

Although pathogens, in particular *H. influenzae*, are found in the sputum, special culture techniques are required for consistent results. Random sampling of the sputum is of little value. If pus persists or recurs despite chemotherapy aimed at *H. influenzae*, it is important to exclude less common but nevertheless important pathogens such as *Strep. pneumoniae*, *Staph. pyogenes*, *Ps. aeruginosa* and *Klebsiella* sp. While many viruses and *Mycoplasma pneumoniae* have been found in association with exacerbations of chronic bronchitis, this knowledge has contributed little to the management.

Simple measurements of ventilatory capacity (PEF and FEV_1) and of effective over-all ventilation (arterial P_{CO_2}) are of value in assessing the severity of airways obstruction, the response to treatment and the progress of the disease. Those tests of respiratory function which tend to discriminate between pure chronic bronchitis and emphysema are shown in TABLE 47.

In severe obstructive bronchitis the ECG may show evidence of right ventricular hypertrophy. The blood count is usually normal but polycythaemia may develop with prolonged hypoxaemia; in this case the haemoglobin and packed cell volume and red cell mass will be increased without any change in the white cell count or platelets.

Differential Diagnosis. Chronic bronchitis is so common that other disease should be excluded if new symptoms develop. If purulent expectoration is persistent bronchiectasis may be present and it is particularly likely if there is haemoptysis, clubbing of the fingers and persistent crepitations on auscultation. If mucropurulent bronchitis develops in childhood or adolescence, cystic fibrosis should be excluded [p. 881].

Treatment

Cigarette smoking should be forbidden in all cases and when possible the patient should be removed from a heavily polluted or dusty environment. He should remain indoors during fog. Adverse factors such as obesity and heart disease should be treated. Influenza is the only infection which can be prevented at present and provided that the vaccine contains the prevalent strain of influenza virus then at least 50 per cent. of patients may be protected during an epidemic. Vaccines should therefore be given when an epidemic threatens.

Antibacterial drugs should be used at the onset of acute respiratory infections with the aim of preventing development of purulent sputum or of eliminating it. As *H. influenzae* is the most likely pathogen a tetracycline, 250 mg. four times a day by mouth, is the antibiotic of choice and the cheapest preparation should be given, for the differences between the effectiveness of the various tetracyclines is marginal. If tetracycline is not successful after 4–5 days' treatment then ampicillin, 500 mg. four times a day by mouth, should be tried. Although less convenient, benzylpenicillin, 2 mega Units, and streptomycin, 0·5 G. given intramuscularly twice daily for a week, are sometimes more effective in reducing sputum purulence and keeping the sputum mucoid thereafter. Trimethoprim, 80 mg., which acts synergistically with sulphonamides (e.g. sulphamethoxazole, 400 mg.) may be given by mouth twice daily if the above chemotherapy is unsuccessful. If pus remains despite these measures the sputum should be cultivated for less common pathogens and appropriate chemotherapy given. While such treatment shortens the period of disability, the affect on the long-term natural history of the disease remains doubtful.

If purulent sputum returns after the cessation of treatment then a trial of long-term chemotherapy should be considered, perhaps during the winter, but should only be continued if it is successful. In general the treatment of acute exacerbations is the more rewarding and economical and the patient may be given a supply of antibiotic so that treatment may be started right at the onset of an acute respiratory infection.

When sputum is copious then postural drainage and percussion of the chest may give considerable relief. If there is variable airways obstruction as revealed by wheezing and a significant increase in airflow (PEF or FEV_1) with isoprenaline, then bronchodilators may help, e.g. isoprenaline, orciprenaline or salbutamol by mouth or aerosol. Small but significant increases in airflow with bronchodilators often gives considerable relief to the patient with severe obstructive bronchitis. Adrenocorticosteroids are usually ineffective in the relief of airways obstruction in chronic bronchitis but just occasionally considerable relief may be gained especially if there is a sputum eosinophilia. A trial of prednisone (starting with 40 mg. a day and reducing the dose over a period of ten days or so) is justifiable in any patient with severe breathlessness due to airways obstruction —the treatment should be withdrawn if no improvement in ventilatory capacity is achieved. Subjective improvement should not be taken as a measure of success. Expectorant and mucolytic agents are usually without objective benefit though mixtures containing iodides or a hot saline drink may help bronchial clearance in the morning. For the treatment of respiratory failure and right ventricular failure see Section 8.

TABLE 47

CHRONIC BRONCHITIS AND EMPHYSEMA

SUMMARY OF THE DIFFERENCES BETWEEN THE FINDINGS IN EMPHYSEMA AND SEVERE CHRONIC OBSTRUCTIVE BRONCHITIS

	EMPHYSEMA	BRONCHITIS
Rhonchi	Usually absent	Present
Right ventricular hypertrophy	Unusual	Frequent
Oedema or heart failure	Unusual	Frequent
Total lung capacity	Increased	Normal
Gas transfer (T_{CO})	Decreased	Normal
Arterial oxygen saturation	Usually more than 90 per cent.	Often less than 90 per cent.
Arterial P_{CO_2}	Normal (or Low)	Raised

Prognosis

The prognosis of simple chronic bronchitis is good, especially in females. When, however, infection becomes established or, more important, when airways obstruction develops then the life span may be reduced. If there is severe airways obstruction with a PEF of less than 100 litres per minute or of FEV_1 less than 1200 ml. there is a tendency to increasingly severe disability: 50 per cent. of patients over the age of fifty who are breathless will be either significantly worse or dead 5 years later. Respiratory failure with a rise in the arterial P_{CO_2} is the single most important indicator of a poor prognosis. Episodes of right ventricular failure, and polycythaemia are also untoward signs.

REFERENCES

REID, L. (1938–1959) Chronic bronchitis and hypersecretion of mucus, *Lect. sci. Basis Med.*, **8,** 235.

STUART-HARRIS, C. H. (1968) Chronic bronchitis. *Abstr. Wld Med.*, **42,** 649, 2135.

EMPHYSEMA

Definition

A condition of the lung characterized by increase beyond the normal in the size of the air spaces distal to the terminal bronchioles arising either from dilatation or from destruction of their walls.

Aetiology and Pathogenesis

While *hypoplasia* (failure of alveolar development in childhood), *atrophy*, *over-inflation* and *destruction* may be important factors in the genesis of emphysema, the ultimate cause is unknown. The distribution of emphysema within the acinus distal to the terminal bronchiole may be: (1) central, i.e. *centri-acinar* (or centrilobular); (2) peripheral, i.e. periacinar or *paraseptal*; (3) total or *panacinar*; or (4) *irregular*. All forms of emphysema can be seen with the naked eye in sections of the lung and are depicted in diagrammatic form in FIGURE 59.

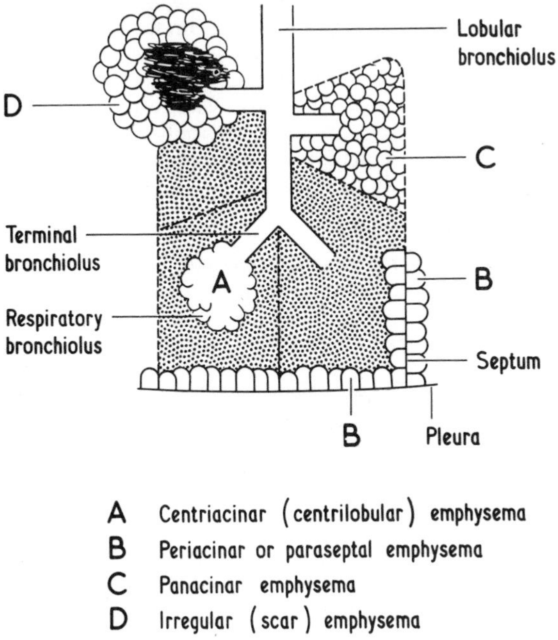

FIG. 59. Types of emphysema.

Emphysema in all these forms may exist without air trapping and it is due either to alveolar atrophy or hyperinflation and is not necessarily associated with impaired function in life. In the *aged lung* (senile emphysema) the lungs are normal in size but the alveoli are larger than in youth: their outline is smoother and simpler and the capillaries are reduced in number. The total lung volume is reduced and the functional residual capacity (FRC) increased. There is no airways obstruction and the chest radiograph is normal. *Paraseptal emphysema* is rare and itself causes no symptoms but may give rise to a spontaneous pneumothorax. Dilated air spaces may be seen radiographically along the edges of the lung. In *centriacinar* (*centrilobular*) *emphysema* the alveoli in the centre of the acinus, chiefly those arising from the respiratory bronchiole are enlarged, but those at the periphery are normal. It may be widespread and an incidental finding at autopsy without any previous history of lung disease. Centriacinar emphysema may be found in association with deposition of dust (simple pneumoconiosis of coal workers), or with chronic bronchitis but no causal relationship has been established between them. Moreover, it is uncertain that any disturbance of function results from this lesion: some claim that distribution of the inspired air may be impaired by the large air space which might interfere with diffusion of gas into the small peripheral air spaces or alveoli. It might thus be a major cause of abnormal gas exchange in chronic bronchitis. Pure centriacinar emphysema gives rise to no radiological abnormality.

When part of a lung is collapsed or removed there is enlargement by over-inflation of the air spaces in the remaining lung to fill the space—this is called *compensatory emphysema*. Contrary to current thought there may be no increase in transradiancy in the chest radiograph in compensatory emphysema in a perfectly normal lobe, nor is the diaphragm necessarily elevated. The larger pulmonary blood vessels although normal in calibre are necessarily more widely separated. These radiological appearances are to be contrasted with *ball-valve emphysema* in which a ball-valve obstruction causes over-inflation of the lung beyond. Transradiancy is increased, the blood vessels are normal and dispersed and the diaphragm often depressed—the heart is displaced to the opposite side. This form of emphysema is reversible.

PRIMARY EMPHYSEMA

Primary emphysema is characterized by widespread panacinar emphysema of unknown cause in which there is failure of the lung to collapse at autopsy and in which there is no associated disease of the airways. In life there is airways obstruction with air trapping.

Aetiology

The cause of primary emphysema is unknown. It is not common in the United Kingdom and it is difficult to find cases of widespread panacinar emphysema without chronic bronchitis. In striking contrast to those cases associated with chronic bronchitis, however, females are equally affected and the disease may become manifest in early middle age. It is occasionally encountered in association with deficiency in serum alpha$_1$-antitrypsin. This is genetically determined and about half those homozygous individuals with antitrypsin deficiency (about 1 in 5000 births) will also have emphysema. Primary emphysema has also been observed to follow in the wake of a diffuse infiltration of the lungs, e.g. histiocytosis X.

Pathology

The lungs are large and do not deflate after removal from the chest. The air spaces of most of the lung can be seen to be enlarged and to retract below the airways and blood vessels on the cut surface. Bullae are often found. In primary emphysema the bronchi are normal on microscopy but the alveoli are large, their walls thin and often interrupted and the capillaries few in number. Atrophy results in a considerable reduction in the number of alveoli.

Clinical Features

Breathlessness is the cardinal symptom and may be insidious or quite rapid in onset without previous history of any respiratory disease. It is progressive and may rapidly become incapacitating on the slightest exertion. Cough is usually trivial and sputum may develop sometime after the onset of breathlessness. There may be considerable loss of weight. On physical examination the patient presents a striking appearance. He is often thin and has an anxious drawn expression. The chest is hyperinflated and the accessory muscles are actively used. Breathing is often laboured at rest and frequently the patient indulges in lip pursing and grunting in expiration which is prolonged. Breathlessness is induced by the very slightest exertion and persists for some time after. This is in striking contrast to the pinkness of the mucosae. The flattened diaphragm may draw the lower ribs inwards on inspiration and expansion of the thorax is limited. Clubbing of the fingers is unusual. Percussion is clearly resonant and the breath sounds often much diminished in volume. Expiration is usually prolonged and expiratory wheeze may be heard. Heart sounds are usually distant but normal.

Primary emphysema may be complicated by *spontaneous pneumothorax* which is usually painless but severely aggravates the breathlessness. It may prove fatal. *Respiratory failure* is usually late and may be precipitated by infection. Some patients develop oedema without a rise in systemic venous pressure or other obvious cause. The right ventricle hypertrophies less than with chronic obstructive bronchitis and right ventricular failure is unusual except as a terminal event. Polycythaemia and a rise in the red cell mass are also less common than in chronic obstructive bronchitis.

Diagnosis

The *chest radiograph* is characteristic in widespread panacinar emphysema and is essential to the diagnosis [PLATE 10]. There is excess of air in the lungs which causes a low flat diaphragm (usually below the 7th rib anteriorly), the diaphragm moves less than 3 cm. from maximum inspiration to expiration: there is a large retrosternal translucent space which may be seen in the lateral view reaching within 3 cm. of the diaphragm. The heart shadow is normal in size (often less than 11·5 cm. across and vertical in position). The main pulmonary artery tends to be large and the majority of the larger intrapulmonary vessels are strikingly small—in at least four of the six zones seen on the postero-anterior view of the chest radiograph. Bullae are found in about a third of cases. Whole lung tomography at hilar level may help to demonstrate the vascular changes. The peripheral airways (terminal bronchioli) remain unfilled in the bronchogram.

With significant panacinar emphysema as shown by the chest radiograph there is always gross impairment of air flow which can be simply measured with a peak flow meter or spirometer. The peak expiratory flow rate (PEF) is usually less than 120 litres per minute and the FEV_1 less than 1200 ml. Air trapping is inferred when the forced vital capacity (FVC) is less than the vital capacity (VC). The total lung capacity (TLC), the functional residual capacity (FRC) and residual volume (RV) are usually increased whereas the factor for gas transfer (obtained with carbon monoxide (T_{CO})) is diminished often to 5–7 ml. per mm. Hg per minute. This value increases very little on exercise. While there must be some uneven ventilation and blood flow, the sensitivity of the respiratory control mechanism is preserved and respiratory drive is often excessive. The reason for this is unknown but it manifests as a preservation of the arterial P_{O_2} at a normal or low value. The low P_{CO_2} which may be around 30 mm. Hg may be confused with that which is encountered in psychogenic hyperventilation unless the case is fully assessed. Arterial oxygen saturation is usually within the normal range but the arterial P_{O_2} falls on exercise. The pulmonary vascular resistance rises little: this may be because of the relatively normal arterial P_{O_2} or because of loss of small muscular pulmonary arterioles. The right ventricle therefore hypertrophies little so that the ECG tends to remain normal. Pressures within the right ventricle and pulmonary artery are usually normal at rest but may rise on exercise. The cardiac output is usually within normal limits. The systemic venous pressure is difficult to assess clinically because of the accessory muscle activity: if it is required it should be measured directly.

Treatment

Primary emphysema is irreversible. Acute respiratory infection must be treated with chemotherapy and measures outlined for management of chronic obstructive bronchitis adopted if this complicates the emphysema.

Oxygen by light weight portable apparatus may increase exercise tolerance. Response to oxygen is unpredictable and should be tried. By graded exercise and gradual training, patients with emphysema may marginally increase their ventilatory efficiency and improve their exercise tolerance. Weight reduction (where appropriate) may also help. Patients readily become exhausted by the effort of breathing and are often helped by a day or two of complete rest each week. A spontaneous pneumothorax requires immediate treatment usually with an intercostal tube to an underwater seal. Surgery has no place in the treatment of primary emphysema. Breathing exercises have yet to be shown to be beneficial.

Prognosis

Although patients with severe widespread emphysema are grossly incapacitated and are usually unable to work at least 50 per cent. of patients will survive for 5 years. This is significantly better than patients with severe chronic obstructive bronchitis. Respiratory failure, oedema, or right ventricular failure are bad prognostic signs.

CHRONIC BRONCHITIS WITH EMPHYSEMA

Widespread panacinar emphysema which resembles the primary form in every particular may complicate chronic bronchitis. The clinical and functional findings may then be a mixture of those features characteristic for the two conditions outlined in TABLE 47. The assumption that the destructive changes due to chronic bronchitis which may damage the small airways and bronchioles may lead to panacinar emphysema is as yet unproven: the two disorders may have developed independently. They both give rise to fixed airways obstruction but the mechanisms by which this develops are different. The part which widespread centriacinar emphysema and the aged lung may play in the disability associated with chronic bronchitis is uncertain but widespread panacinar emphysema significantly affects function and the prognosis in chronic bronchitis.

OTHER FORMS OF EMPHYSEMA

There are rare developmental causes of emphysema with obstruction of the airways without bronchial disease, e.g. *congenital lobar emphysema* and *bronchial atresia*. The former is a condition which occurs in infants and appears to be obstructive distension of one lobe due to mucosal swelling, a plug of mucus or an abnormality of bronchial cartilage. The condition presents with breathlessness and displacement of all the other intrathoracic contents with bulging of the over-distended lobe. The treatment is surgical. In *bronchial atresia* there is complete atresia of the proximal bronchus usually of the left upper lobe which is hypertransradiant, hypoplastic and ventilated by collateral ventilation. The dilated bronchus distal to the atresia may be seen as a small circular shadow and the distal airways are usually distended with mucus. This condition gives rise to no symptoms and requires no treatment.

Unilateral Emphysema of a Lobe or Lung (Macleod's Syndrome)

Patchy obliterative bronchitis and bronchiolitis in childhood may give rise to emphysema because of subsequent impairment of alveolar growth which normally takes place up to the age of 8 years. The affected parts which contain far too few alveoli therefore occupy a smaller space than the normal. Ventilation of the affected lobe or lung is mainly by collateral air drift and air is trapped therein. Although there is vascular hypoplasia, this is probably secondary to the hypoventilation: the circulation may be further impaired by air trapping. Involvement of a whole lung presents a striking radiological appearance of hypertransradiancy of one lung in which the hilar and intrapulmonary vessels are very small [PLATE 11]. The mediastinum tends to be drawn to the affected side and X-ray films taken in expiration show deviation of the structures away from the affected side with failure of the diaphragm to rise because of gross air trapping on that side. Bronchograms show poor peripheral filling due to distal occlusion and absence of suck or air. Sometimes the proximal bronchi are dilated and the contrast medium ends in a distorted airway or a dilatation or 'pool'. There are usually no symptoms and the striking diminution of breath sounds is usually the only physical sign. The condition is unmasked by routine radiography. Special investigations by bronchospirometry, angiography or radioactive gases (i.e. ^{133}Xe) clearly demonstrate the striking reduction in ventilation and blood flow of the affected lobe or lung. The condition is rare: the prognosis is excellent provided that there is no other lung disease.

REFERENCES

FLETCHER, C. M., HUGH-JONES, P., McNICOL, M. W., and PRIDE, N. B. (1963) The diagnosis of pulmonary emphysema in the presence of chronic bronchitis, *Quart. J. Med.*, **32,** 33.

REID, L. (1967) *The Pathology of Emphysema*, London.

SCADDING, J. G., DUNNILL, M. S., CUMMING, G., and FLETCHER, C. M. (1969) Emphysema, *Proc. roy. Soc. Med.*, **62,** 1023.

EMPHYSEMATOUS BULLAE

Definition

A bulla is an emphysematous space greater than 1 cm. in diameter.

Aetiology

The cause of bullous change in the lung is unknown but bullae may be found with many types of emphysema, most commonly with panacinar emphysema associated with chronic bronchitis. Alternatively there may be little disease in the remaining lung. Bullae are of three types, all of which project beyond the surface of the exposed lung:

Type I. Represents a small amount of lung grossly overdistended with a narrow neck—bullae of this type are usually apical.

Type II. Represents a shallow but wide layer of lung greatly over-inflated with a broad neck—these bullae are found anywhere on the lung surface.

Type III. Represents a large volume of lung, often a whole lobe, slightly over-inflated—the tissue in this type of bulla usually exhibits severe panacinar emphysema.

If a bulla is ventilated the residual volume will be increased but studies of regional lung function will demonstrate a large poorly or non-ventilated space. Frequently associated panacinar emphysema with or without chronic bronchitis will cause airways obstruction. When patients with bullae are breathless the airways obstruction is usually severe with a low PEF and FEV_1. Impaired gas transfer with a low T_{CO} and reduced arterial oxygen tension are also found usually when there is associated lung disease. It is difficult to determine the relative contribution of large bullae and the generalized lung disease to the breathlessness and impaired function.

Clinical Picture

Large bullae may be found at routine chest radiography and may not produce symptoms. These are usually in the upper zones. Giant bullae may cause breathlessness but airways obstruction due to chronic bronchitis and emphysema are usually partly or mainly responsible for the symptom. Spontaneous pneumothorax is a recognized complication. Chest radiography with Type I bullae shows an obvious line of demarcation. With the other types of bullae lines of demarcation are usually partial or absent but may be seen best in the lateral view. Bronchography and tomography sometimes help to determine the extent of lung involved.

Treatment

Patients without symptoms require no treatment. Patients with large bullae causing breathlessness require surgical removal of the bullae. If the cause of the breathlessness is obstructive bronchitis and emphysema surgery is best avoided. When breathlessness is the result of both the bullae and the generalized lung disease it is usually extremely difficult to judge which is the major factor as no clinical, radiological or physiological changes are able to discriminate. Relatively little cough and sputum and few physical signs with large bullae will tend to make surgery feasible. Surgery should not be undertaken unless there is severe breathlessness after a period of medical treatment. Improvement can be expected in about 70 per cent. of cases; in some it is dramatic. On the other hand, symptomatic improvement does not extend beyond 2–3 years and there is a poor correlation between symptomatic improvement after surgery and changes in lung function.

REFERENCES

Pride, N. B., Hugh-Jones, P., O'Brien, E. N., and Smith, A. L. A. (1970) Changes in lung function following the surgical treatment of bullous emphysema, *Quart. J. Med.*, **39**, 49.

Reid, L. (1967) *The Pathology of Emphysema*, p. 211, London.

BRONCHIAL ASTHMA

Definition

A condition in which there is variable breathlessness due to widespread narrowing of peripheral airways which varies in severity over short periods of time, either spontaneously or with treatment.

Aetiology and Pathogenesis

Variable narrowing of the peripheral airways (bronchoconstriction) is due to one or all of the following: (1) contraction of bronchial smooth muscle; (2) oedema of the mucous membrane; and (3) mucus within the lumen.

Bronchoconstriction is a normal response to noxious stimuli such as cigarette smoke and sulphur dioxide—also to alterations in the concentration of oxygen and carbon dioxide in the lumen. These responses are either direct or mediated reflexly by the vagus nerve. Normal bronchial 'tone' can be demonstrated in bronchial musculature by a decrease in airway resistance after administration of atropine or isoprenaline. All these physiological responses are very small in degree and are not felt by a normal individual.

The pathogenesis of bronchoconstriction in asthma is not yet fully understood. While it is known that various agents such as histamine, bradykinin, slow reacting substance in anaphylaxis (SRS–A) and 5-hydroxytryptamine are liberated, there are other as yet unidentified substances which are released in the bronchial wall probably from mast cells too—all of these agents both known and unknown cause bronchoconstriction, and their relative importance is uncertain. Many factors appear to be responsible either directly or indirectly for release of these mediators amongst which are exercise, allergy, infection, but the actual mode of release is conjectural. Other factors, for instance psychological or pharmacological, may potentiate bronchoconstriction.

Exercise. This frequently brings about bronchoconstriction in asthma and this may be detected by simple tests of ventilation in patients many years after a complete clinical remission. There is often a delay of about 2–3 minutes after the end of exercise before the onset of constriction: this may be prevented by adrenergic agents (e.g. isoprenaline) or by disodium cromoglycate though not by adrenocortical steroids. The mechanism of exercise-induced bronchoconstriction is unknown but it is common with exercise such as running, particularly after 5 minutes or so. Oddly enough it is much less likely to be provoked by exercise on a static bicycle ergometer or by walking on a treadmill.

Allergy. Hypersensitivity reactions in the bronchial wall may provoke the release of bronchoconstricting agents. In the case of asthma this is usually the end result of an immediate hypersensitivity response (Type I of Gell and Coombs) to one or more allergens (antigens) to which the patient has become sensitized. Entry of the allergen is usually by inhalation but on occasion by ingestion (e.g. milk, aspirin, *Toxocara canis*). Reaginic antibody formed in response to this stimulus becomes fixed to cells in the lining of the respiratory tract, most importantly the mast cells. Inhalation of the allergen provokes an antigen-antibody reaction in which the mast cells are damaged with release of bronchoconstrictor agents. The tissues in close proximity become infiltrated with eosinophils and there is an increase in mucus secretion. The counterpart of this reaction in the respiratory tract is the immediate wheal and flare response which may be provoked in the skin when the same or other allergens are introduced by a prick or intracutaneous injection. Although reaginic antibodies have not been satisfactorily demonstrated in man their presence has been inferred by the passive transfer of reactivity. Recent evidence suggests that circulating reaginic antibody is mainly to be found in the IgE component of the immunoglobulins. Capacity to produce IgE is widespread but concentrations are very small compared with the other circulating immunoglobulins. About 10 per cent. of the population produce more than five times the amount of IgE in response to allergens, particularly when mucosal surfaces are affected. These individuals have one or more allergic manifestation, e.g. asthma, hay fever or eczema. They have multiple skin reactions to common allergens and frequently have a family history of allergy—they are called *atopic*. The disposition of reaginic IgE antibody may to some extent be governed by the route of entry of the allergen which is mainly produced on the surfaces of the respiratory and gastro-intestinal tracts—thus in asthma, provided that the allergen is of the right particle size its inhalation into the bronchopulmonary tree may determine the local production and concentration of IgE which becomes fixed to the cells. This can only be part of the explanation of the individual variation in response to exposure to allergens. Inflamed tissue, however, may play a part in this localization and genetic factors may also be important for they may determine not only the capacity to produce IgE but also the tendency of smooth muscle to react to the allergic process.

Asthma is broadly divisible into two groups: *extrinsic* in which there is an external factor which can be detected or inferred and *intrinsic* (non-extrinsic). Extrinsic asthma is much more common. These two forms of asthma differ characteristically as follows:

Extrinsic	*Intrinsic*
IgE raised in at least 70 per cent.	IgE normal or low.
Usually atopic subjects.	Non-atopic subjects.
Onset in early years.	Onset in middle age.
Often intermittent.	Usually constant.
Family history of allergies.	Family history of asthma.

This distinction is of practical value because the prognosis of intrinsic asthma is much less certain.

Rare Forms of Hypersensitivity. There is a rare form of extrinsic asthma in non-atopic subjects after long sustained exposure to inhaled antigenic dusts often at work, e.g. redwood cedar; bronchoconstriction may be provoked by a precipitin mediated reaction in the bronchiolar wall (Type III of Gell and Coombs). There may be skin reactivity and delayed bronchoconstriction on inhalation of the antigen on formal testing. Such a delayed type bronchoconstriction may occur in association with an alveolar reaction—also a Type III sensitivity response, an example of which is farmer's lung.

In allergic aspergillosis [p. 226] on the other hand both immediate and delayed bronchoconstriction are usually provoked by *A. fumigatus* antigen. Asthma is usually a feature of this syndrome in which pulmonary infiltration with eosinophilia is found in atopic subjects. Immediate and delayed reactions are observed in the skin on testing with the fungal antigen and precipitating antibody is detected in the peripheral blood. It is assumed that hypersensitivity reactions of both Type I and Type III are taking place in the bronchial wall.

Infection. Bacterial or viral infection may be an important factor at the onset and in the course of asthma. The mechanism by which the infection may provoke or prolong asthma remains unknown though allergy to bacterial protein as well the direct effect of inflammatory reactions in the bronchial mucosa are possible. Circulating precipitating antibody to bacteria such as *H. influenzae*, *Ps. aeruginosa* and *Klebsiella sp.* are found in about 8 per cent. of patients with asthma, which is not much greater than that found in a random sample of the population. More refined studies have shown, however, that precipitating antibodies to *H. influenzae* may be found in 17 per cent. of infected asthmatics and in only 3 per cent. of non-infected asthmatics, though the role of these antibodies is uncertain. Infection in asthma adversely affects the prognosis.

Psychological Factors. Families of asthmatics have a higher than normal incidence of neurosis and psychiatric illness as do the asthmatics themselves. In about 40 per cent. of asthmatics psychological factors are present but their mode of action is unknown. Almost certainly they merely intensify the asthma rather than exert any causal influence.

Pharmacological Factors. Beta-adrenergic blockade causes bronchoconstriction in asthma but not in normal subjects. This implies that there is enhanced adrenergic activity in asthma. Drugs such as propranolol should be avoided.

Chronic chest diseases as well as asthma, hay fever and eczema are more common in families which contain asthmatics. The incidence of asthma in first-degree relatives approaches 40 per cent. after the age of sixty-five. The mode of inheritance is unknown.

The incidence of bronchial asthma in the general population is in the order of 1–2 per cent. and it affects social classes equally. No race is exempt. In Birmingham in 1961 asthma was observed to be twice as common in boys (2·58 per cent.) at 5 years of age as in girls (1·02 per cent.) of the same age. The prevalence in boys fell with age so that the sex difference was abolished by early adult life.

Physiological Changes

Variable narrowing of the peripheral airways is the characteristic physiological change in asthma. This airways obstruction usually gives rise to an increase in airways resistance which may be diminished by bronchodilator drugs. These drugs may be adrenergic (e.g. isoprenaline, adrenaline, salbutamol), anticholinergic (e.g. atropine) and others, e.g. aminophylline. Thus, simple tests of ventilatory capacity may show a rise in the FEV_1 or PEF after a bronchodilator drug. The maximum resistance to air flow resides in the larger bronchi. It is thus possible for many of the smaller airways to be narrowed or even totally occluded without increase in airways resistance or necessarily any reduction in the FEV_1 or PEF. Usually, however, with increasingly severe airways obstruction and falls in tests of ventilatory capacity, the lung tends to over-inflate reflexly and the residual volume (RV) and FRC increase. In the severest forms of asthma the FRC may increase to such an extent that it exceeds the normal TLC. This extreme inflation of the lung increases the elastic retraction on the smaller airways and permits air to flow more readily within them. At the same time, of course, it greatly increases the elastic work of breathing. This increase in elastic work is probably responsible for the unpleasant tightness of the chest in asthma and of the tachypnoea. As the patient improves the lungs tend to deflate with relief of this tightness in the chest but without apparent improvement in air flow for the elastic retraction round the small airways is diminished. With further improvement in the clinical state the airways dilate and tests of ventilatory capacity return towards normal.

Gas transfer is characteristically normal in asthma but ventilation and blood flow become uneven with increasing severity of the disease. This is responsible for the fall in arterial P_{O_2} and eventually in arterial oxygen saturation. Arterial P_{CO_2} tends to remain normal or even low. This is evidence of preservation of an adequate respiratory drive and is a good prognostic sign. If, however, the P_{CO_2} rises then the prognosis for the attack becomes less certain. Occasionally a metabolic acidosis develops in severe asthma which is due to excessive muscular work of breathing at a reduced arterial P_{O_2}.

Tests of ventilatory capacity are not only essential in the diagnosis and the assessment of severity of asthma but also in management from day to day.

Clinical Picture

The dominant symptom in bronchial asthma is *breathlessness*—an unpleasant awareness of difficulty in breathing which may be sensed not only in expiration but also in inspiration especially when there is marked hyperinflation. *Tightness in the chest* is then also a component of the dyspnoea. *Wheezing* usually accompanies both inspiration and expiration unless the asthma is so severe that the reduced air flow is unable to create the sound. The pattern of wheezy breathing varies considerably. It may be episodic in which the episodes are short or long or it may persist for very long periods.

In *extrinsic asthma* the attacks are usually episodic with periods of complete freedom between times. This form of asthma usually starts in childhood. Characteristically there is an allergic background of infantile eczema or hay fever. The wheezing may be seasonal at first. Attacks vary in frequency and duration. Wheezing is often provoked by exercise and is usually worse during the night. Attacks may be precipitated by inhaled allergens such as pollens or dust of animal danders or hair. Asthma may occur at times of emotional stress or with acute respiratory infection. Sometimes no precipitating factors can be found on questioning but psychological factors may be obscure. With *intrinsic asthma* on the other hand wheezy breathlessness although episodic at first tends to be much more persistent. The illness usually starts later in life, often in the late twenties or thirties but no age is exempt. A frank allergic background is not found but perennial rhinitis is not uncommon. Aspirin sensitivity is sometimes a feature and nasal polyps not an infrequent finding. The onset of intrinsic asthma is often related to an acute respiratory infection and persistence of infection is a serious matter.

Asthma may be associated with acute bronchitis in childhood (acute wheezy chest) or with chronic bronchitis in adults. In these cases wheezy breathlessness usually develops at the time of acute infection and may even persist and dominate the clinical picture.

Frequently the clinical type of asthma is not characteristic. An irritating cough, productive of a little viscid mucus often accompanies the wheeze and at times may dominate the picture. Sputum is variable in quantity and is often more copious after the attack. Bronchial casts may be expectorated often with a very distressing cough. These casts may have a worm-like appearance. There is a rare form of asthma in which there is copious expectoration of frothy mucoid sputum which may exceed 100 ml. per day. Asthma in this case is usually of the intrinsic variety and the excessive secretion is called bronchorrhoea. The sputum in asthma may be purulent either as the result of an infection, less commonly to a gross excess of eosinophils. Whereas bronchial casts and plugs are usually mucoid, with allergic aspergillosis brown plugs are expectorated: these contain mycelial fragments.

Physical examination during an attack usually reveals an apprehensive agitated patient. The breathing is not only difficult but is often rapid and associated with a wheeze. The body temperature is usually normal but the pulse rate is often raised and in severe asthma there may be a pronounced tachycardia exceeding 150 per minute. The chest is hyperinflated but diaphragmatic function is usually preserved so that the lower ribs move outward normally. The shoulder girdle is elevated and the accessory muscles are active. Expiration is prolonged and both inspiratory and expiratory rhonchi are audible.

Status asthmaticus is prolonged asthma, unrelieved by treatment, which may threaten life. In status asthmaticus there is increasing obstruction of the smaller airways by tenacious mucous plugs infiltrated with eosinophils. These plugs tend to be laminated due to successive layering of mucus. Sometimes the mucus is aspirated peripherally and in fatal cases there is detachment of the superficial lining of the mucous membrane together with thickening of the basement membrane.

A *spontaneous pneumothorax* or massive collapse due to a mucous plug should be suspected with any sudden deterioration but the physical signs may be difficult to detect. A chest radiograph should be taken at once to establish the diagnosis. *Respiratory failure* with a rise in the arterial P_{CO_2} is usually a late event in severe asthma but may complicate the clinical picture earlier if asthma is superimposed upon chronic obstructive bronchitis. A rise in pulmonary vascular resistance is rare in asthma so that right ventricular hypertrophy and failure are unusual even in the severest forms of the disease. Respiratory failure with hypoxia may precipitate ventricular arrhythmias though the frequency of this complication as a cause of death is uncertain.

Diagnosis

The diagnosis of asthma is usually straightforward and is based on the history and examination and established by simple tests of ventilatory capacity (i.e. FEV_1 or PEF) before and after a bronchodilator. *Obstruction of the trachea* or *main bronchi* may be difficult to distinguish—absence of a history of asthma and the presence of a stridor rather than a wheeze usually helps to distinguish: if there is any doubt bronchoscopy should be carried out.

Cardiac asthma due to left heart failure and pulmonary venous hypertension which occur, for example, with mitral or aortic valve disease, systemic hypertension or myocardial infarction tends to be sudden in onset and to develop rather more frequently during the night when the patient slips down in bed. Wheezing may accompany the breathlessness due to exudation into the airways but crepitations are usually heard, tachypnoea due to lung stiffness is more obvious and there is nearly always evidence of left heart disease. A rise in the systemic venous pressure and radiographic evidence of pulmonary venous hypertension or oedema may help in the differential diagnosis. *Renal asthma* is much less likely to present difficulties in diagnosis: hyperventilation rather than airway obstruction can usually be seen on examination of the patient with renal failure. The nature of this disorder is clarified by a clinical examination and tests of renal function.

Chest radiographs are usually normal in asthma

although over-inflation may be suggested by a low diaphragm. The appearance of the pulmonary vessels is usually normal and the diaphragm retains its rounded shape. Transient shadows may be observed in asthma and are of three types. First, the shadows may be well demarcated and due to lobar, segmental or subsegmental collapse which results from mucus impaction. The radiograph returns to normal when the plug is expectorated. Secondly, the shadows may be more dense, may be segmental or partially so or even lobar together with a blood eosinophilia (more than 500 per mm^3.)—this is characteristic of allergic aspergillosis [p. 226]. The allergic process damages the bronchial wall and may cause a unique type of bronchiectasis in which there is dilatation of the segmental or subsegmental bronchi with preservation of the normal peripheral airways. Thirdly, more widespread shadowing may be associated with intrinsic asthma: in these cases the eosinophilia is usually greater (more than 1000 per mm^3.). These shadows may be early manifestations of polyarteritis nodosa in which case there is a persistent rise in the erythrocyte sedimentation rate [see p. 431].

The *blood count* in asthma may be normal or there may be an eosinophilia either in intrinsic or extrinsic asthma (more than 500 eosinophils per mm^3.). Eosinophil counts in excess of 1500 per mm^3. should lead to a suspicion of *tropical eosinophilia* [see Section 2].

Sputum may contain excess of eosinophils and characteristic casts of the smaller airways may be expectorated (Curschmann's spirals). Brown plugs or casts are usually produced in allergic aspergillosis and contain mycelial fragments of the fungus which stain with silver.

Tests of Hypersensitivity. Skin testing by prick or intracutaneous methods using allergens of animal, vegetable, or microbiological origin may reveal specific, immediate, wheal and flare reactions to one or more of these agents. Approximately 10 per cent. of a random population will react to one or more of these allergens—that is they are atopic subjects. Skin testing is chiefly of value in assessment of the type of asthma—extrinsic asthmatics are usually atopic and react to more than one of these agents whereas patients with intrinsic asthma tend to be non-atopic and to react to one allergen or frequently to none. Skin tests do not correlate absolutely with bronchial reactivity to inhaled allergens but the results of skin testing are helpful in clarifying those allergic factors which may be responsible for the asthma—the history obtained from the patient remains the most important guide to these factors.

Tests of Respiratory Function. In particular those of ventilatory function (FEV_1, FVC and PEF) are important in the diagnosis, for variability of the airways obstruction is characteristic. A rise of more than 20 per cent. in the FEV_1 or PEF may be expected to follow the inhalation of an aerosol of an adrenergic agent such as isoprenaline in all but the most refractory cases. The response is greater than with atropine. (0·6 mg. subcutaneously.) In chronic obstructive bronchitis the response to atropine is as great or greater than that to isoprenaline. If the diagnosis of asthma remains in doubt particularly with refractory asthma the patient should be admitted to hospital and twice daily measurements made of FEV_1 and FVC (or PEF if a spirometer is not available) during administration of prednisone, 40 mg. reducing to 20 mg. over 7–10 days. A rise of more than 20 per cent. in these measurements would confirm that asthma is a major cause of the airways obstruction. These tests of ventilatory capacity and the measurement of blood gas tensions in severe asthma are essential guides to the management.

Treatment

Attacks of asthma usually respond to simple bronchodilator drugs. Adrenergic drugs that stimulate alpha and beta-receptors in the bronchial wall are the most valuable agents—particularly those with mainly beta action (they relax bronchial smooth muscle). Isoprenaline, orciprenaline, and salbutamol are the agents of choice. Orciprenaline and salbutamol are preferable because they exert less effect on the heart rate and contraction. Adrenaline, ephedrine and phenylephrine exert mainly alpha action, therefore in theory should affect vessels in the bronchial mucosa reducing oedema as well. It is unusual, however, to observe an additional effect due to this action. Other drugs that relax bronchial smooth muscle are the theophylline derivatives, e.g. aminophylline and choline theophyllinate, and cholinergic drugs such as atropine and its derivatives.

Many of these drugs bring about a fall in the arterial P_{O_2} by increasing blood flow to poorly ventilated parts of the lung. Reports that some bronchodilators are safer because they do not exert this effect have yet to be substantiated.

Adrenergic drugs may be given by mouth, e.g. salbutamol, 2 mg., or orciprenaline, 20 mg.: isoprenaline may be given sublingually in a dose of 10–20 mg. A more convenient way is to administer these agents by metered aerosol—salbutamol and orciprenaline act for longer following inhalation than isoprenaline—the latter drug exerts more undesirable effects upon the heart, giving rise to palpitations. Excessive use of these drugs, particularly by aerosol, must be avoided for there is a danger of ventricular fibrillation particularly with isoprenaline and adrenaline when the oxygen tension is reduced. Dangers of aerosol administration can be avoided if it is made clear to the patient that only one to two puffs should be taken at no more than three-hourly intervals. Failure to obtain relief is the indication to abandon the use of the aerosol and either seek medical advice or turn to further treatment such as the adrenocortical steroids.

Alternative treatment for the rather more severe attack of asthma may be to give adrenaline, 0·5 ml. of 1/1000 solution subcutaneously or intramuscularly. A further 1–2 ml. may be given over the next 7–10 minutes and the effect on the patient's breathing, pulse rate and blood pressure observed. If this is not successful aminophylline should be given intravenously (500 mg. very slowly). If all these agents have been given properly and do not abort an attack then the patient can be considered to be in *status asthmaticus*—particularly when respiratory distress has been prolonged, central cyanosis has developed and the pulse rate continues to rise. It is then urgently necessary to give adrenocortical steroids. These should be given earlier if patients have been known to have been in status asthmaticus before.

Hydrocortisone, 300 mg. intravenously in the first 24 hours, may be a life-saving measure. If prednisone is given at the same time as the hydrocortisone—in a dose of 50 mg. by mouth—the intravenous hydrocortisone may be stopped after 24 hours and the daily dose of prednisone continued until improvement occurs and then reduced gradually until the patient recovers. Steroids do not begin to take effect for at least 12 hours and their mode of action is unknown. Previous administration of adrenocortical steroids may have suppressed adrenocortical function—therefore corticotrophin should be avoided.

Oxygen should be given to correct any fall in the arterial P_{O_2}. If the arterial P_{CO_2} rises and the arterial P_{O_2} falls despite all these measures, mechanical ventilation should be introduced and if this is inadequate, bronchial lavage using saline or bicarbonate solution by bronchoscope may prove life-saving. A severe metabolic acidosis should also be corrected by intravenous bicarbonate: this may help to re-establish sensitivity to adrenergic drugs.

Treatment between the Attacks. Between attacks of asthma, precipitating factors should be eliminated as far as possible. *Allergens* will have been discovered by careful history-taking and skin tests. Environmental sources of allergens such as bedding, dust, domestic animals, etc., which precipitate attacks should be eliminated or controlled. Specific desensitization by injection of increasing doses of allergens is of value only in some cases of pollen-induced asthma. It has been shown that crude extracts of house dust are no better than control injections in preventing asthma when there was established hypersensitivity to the dust. The discovery of the house dust mite (*Dermatophagoides culinae*) may lead to the preparation of an effective means of desensitization to house dust, but in general, specific desensitization is of little or no value in the management of asthma.

Infection should be sought particularly when there is a clear history of attacks precipitated by acute respiratory infection. Appropriate chemotherapy should be given and future episodes of respiratory infection treated immediately at their onset. Infestation with filariae which may cause asthma in association with tropical eosinophilia should be eradicated by injection of diethylcarbamazine, 6–8 mg. per kg. in three doses by mouth each day for 7–10 days. Other infestations, e.g. toxocariasis, hypersensitivity to which may be associated with asthma and eosinophilia, should be treated appropriately.

Psychogenic factors should be assessed and if possible remedied. Studies have shown that removal of children with asthma to a completely new environment may often relieve their symptoms. When anxiety or panic accompany the onset of an attack of asthma autohypnosis may help to ameliorate it—this treatment, however, is uncertain in its benefit and should be used with caution.

Chronic Asthma. Ephedrine, 30–60 mg., salbutamol, 2–4 mg., or orciprenaline, 10–20 mg., are useful preparations when given by mouth: the most effective should be given after trial. Aminophylline given by suppository is often helpful at night and mild sedation may also assist sleep—the most convenient preparation is promethazine, 25–50 mg. by mouth. Other hypnotics may be given in mild asthma, e.g. butobarbitone or chloral hydrate. In severe asthma, however, sedatives and hypnotics should be avoided—morphine may be lethal because it depresses the respiratory centre.

Disodium Cromoglycate. The discovery of a group of compounds derived from khellin has opened a new approach to the prevention and treatment of asthma—the most effective compound so far available is disodium cromoglycate (*Intal*). This is poorly absorbed from the gut and rapidly excreted in the urine and has to be given as a finely dispersed powder by inhalation. So far it appears to be without important side-effects. Cromoglycate probably prevents the release of bronchoconstricting agents from mast cells in the bronchial mucosa and to be fully effective has to be inhaled in doses of 20 mg. four to five times in the 24 hours through a propeller device. Asthma induced by inhalation of allergens, exercise or histamine is prevented by previous inhalation. In bronchial asthma which is manifest as chronic or frequent recurrent attacks which are uncontrolled by simple bronchodilators, a trial of cromoglycate should be given—preliminary reports suggest that it is of particular value in extrinsic asthma and it is often effective in children. A good response can be judged by the return of appetite and uninterrupted sleep, diminished wheezing and need for bronchodilators. Frequently there is a rise in the FEV_1 or PEF. Success is to be expected in about 50 per cent. of patients treated, but the results of double-blind controlled trials are awaited. If asthma is inhibited by 20 mg. four times a day the frequency of the inhalations can be reduced. Cromoglycate should be given without added isoprenaline for improvement noted by the patient is often due to the bronchodilator. If a bronchodilator drug is needed with cromoglycate it should be given separately.

Adrenocortical Steroids. These should be reserved for more severe or protracted asthma that does not respond to the proper use of all other measures outlined above. Their mode of action in the relief of the airway obstruction is unknown but they take effect in 12–24 hours after they are first given. They should not be withheld in status asthmaticus and indeed should be given immediately in those cases already known to develop very rapid and severe episodic asthma, particularly in the high risk group aged 10–15 years. Their use should be considered in the long term management of children whose schooling is frequently interrupted and whose growth and development are impaired by the asthma—and in adults who cannot pursue their occupation or perform their housework as a result of their asthma. Interruption of sleep and loss of appetite are other relative indications for their use. The aim of treatment is to restore and maintain well-being, a good appetite and sleep and the ability to work, with the smallest possible dose. Patients are best admitted to hospital to institute treatment, for a change in environment and detailed assessment of the case may bring about such an improvement that the need for steroids is eliminated. The patient and his relatives should be thoroughly reassured about the lack of side-effects of this treatment in asthma. Prednisone is the steroid of choice and should be given initially in a dose of 25–50 mg. daily according to the severity of the symptoms. Daily measurements of PEF and FEV_1 should be made to guide subsequent dosage which is reduced by 5 mg. a day and then 2·5 mg. alternate days to 15 mg. If the asthma is relieved and the patient well, with a return of ventilatory capacity towards normal values, the dose of prednisone can be reduced slowly and the drug withdrawn if the patient is well. Prednisone should be reserved for severe attacks in the future.

If the attacks are frequent or if further reduction in dose is accompanied by a fall in PEF or FEV_1 then the dose should be reduced from that which is clinically satisfactory by 1 mg. amounts every week or so to a level that keeps the patient well. This is often quite critical so that 11 mg. in 24 hours may be satisfactory whereas 10 mg. may be inadequate. It has been suggested that intermittent steroid therapy may have the advantage not only of reducing the total weekly requirement and therefore the likelihood of untoward side-effects but also eliminating adrenal suppression. This treatment may be tried and continued if successful, e.g. prednisone in 10–30 mg. doses every other day or every third day. Whatever method of long-term treatment is applied it is necessary to have the patient under close supervision during the first few months. Some patients are able to make minor adjustments in their dosage from time to time according to their symptoms provided that they understand and keep the dose as small as possible. Where sudden severe episodes occur the patient may be instructed to increase the dose to 40–50 mg. in the 24 hours if he has warning of the onset of such an attack. Where close supervision is difficult, the patient may keep his own record of PEF as a more sensitive index of response to treatment. More than 75 per cent. of patients are much improved or improve on this regimen without any serious side-effects. In cases where 15 mg. or more of prednisone are required each day then occasionally a switch to another adrenocortical steroid may be of benefit, e.g. betamethasone, triamcinolone, etc. Alternatively, corticotrophin may be tried either as the long-acting gel (40 Units daily intramuscularly) or as the synthetic substance tetracosactrin depot preparation (1 mg. daily of the zinc preparation intramuscularly). When control of the asthma has been achieved the daily dose should be reduced or intervals between doses extended to once or twice weekly if necessary. Intervals between doses of more than one day may preserve adrenal response to endogenous corticotrophin. This hormone may be used in the same fashion in children but claims that it preserves normal growth and development of children in contradistinction to adrenocortical steroids have to be substantiated. Where doses of steroids equivalent to 15–20 mg. of prednisone a day or more are required then side-effects emerge, the most serious of which is osteoporosis with vertebral collapse. Unfortunately there are no certain ways of preventing this.

Immunosuppressive drugs such as azathioprine are under trial in the treatment of asthma but so far no reliable information is available.

Asthma in Pregnancy. Pregnancy may be associated with an improvement or a deterioration of asthma. While no harm can come to the mother or child from the simple treatment outlined, there is some doubt as to the effects of adrenocortical steroids during pregnancy. There is some evidence to suggest that there is an increased risk of stillbirth and risk to the foetus due to placental faults induced by steroids. During pregnancy, therefore, adrenocortical steroids should be given in the minimum dose compatible with maternal health, although they should be avoided if possible they must be given if asthma in the mother requires this treatment. The effect of disodium cromoglycate on pregnancy and the foetus is so far unknown.

Prognosis

The prognosis for extrinsic asthma starting in childhood is good. The attacks usually cease later in childhood or adolescence, twice as often in boys. Adults free of asthma for years, however, may show a reduction in PEF or FEV_1 or other tests of ventilatory capacity after exercise—this indicates a persistence of the increased reactivity. After periods of many years freedom from asthma attacks may start again in later life. The prognosis for extrinsic asthma is less certain in those that react to a larger number of allergens.

The prognosis for intrinsic asthma which starts later in life is much less certain. Over-all, 3 per cent. of asthmatics die with increasingly severe asthma despite all measures. Bronchial infection, if it becomes established, adversely affects the prognosis too.

In the United Kingdom there has been a recent increase in the mortality due to bronchial asthma in all age groups (from 1214 cases in 1959 to 2040 in 1966—an increase in death rate from 2·7 to 4·2 per 100,000 of the population). This increase was most striking in the age group 10–14 years and amounted to an eightfold increase. The reason for this increase in mortality was unknown but could not be attributed to the use of steroids. A later report indicated a fall in mortality after 1966—while this fall in mortality coincided with a drop in the sale of aerosol bronchodilators it is yet too early to be certain of the link between these two observations. Severe asthmatics, particularly in adolescence require close supervision and rapid modifications of their treatment when attacks of asthma develop.

REFERENCES

CROFTON, J., and DOUGLAS, A. (1969) *Respiratory Diseases*, p. 394, Oxford.

SPEIZER, F. E., DOLL, R., and HEAF, P. (1968) Observations on recent increase in mortality from asthma, *Brit. med. J.*, **1**, 335.

PULMONARY DISEASE WITH EOSINOPHILIA, POLYARTERITIS NODOSA AND WEGENER'S GRANULOMA

Synonyms. Pulmonary infiltration with eosinophilia; Loeffler's syndrome.

Definition

Disease of the lung associated with eosinophilia in the peripheral blood.

Aetiology and Pathogenesis

This heterogeneous group of disorders of the lung associated with eosinophilia may vary greatly in severity but in all there is abnormal radiological shadowing with an eosinophil count in excess of 500 per mm³. Some are associated with disease elsewhere. There are three broad clinical types:

Pulmonary Infiltration with Eosinophilia (without Asthma). This is worldwide and mainly a hypersensitivity reaction in the alveoli in which focal areas of eosinophilic infiltration may be seen. Loeffler's original description included only those cases of a benign asymptomatic nature but sometimes the hypersensitivity reaction may be more severe and prolonged and symptomatic. The reaction may be to *parasites* such as *Ascaris*, *Toxocara*, *Ankylostoma*, etc., to *pollens* including privet (e.g. *Ligustrum vulgare*)—privet cough or to *drugs* including para-aminosalicylic acid, sulphonamides, penicillin, aspirin, and nitrofurantoin.

There may be cough which may be dry or accompanied by pale yellow sputum containing large numbers of eosinophils. In more severe cases there may be systemic symptoms such as fever, malaise, etc. Hay fever, angioneurotic oedema and other hypersensitivity states may coexist. A wide variety of shadows may be seen on the chest radiograph—from homogeneous shadows of any size to nodular or micronodular. In mild cases the shadows may come and go in one or more parts of the lung and usually disappear in a few weeks. In severe cases the shadows may persist longer. The radiological appearances need to be differentiated from tuberculosis, infarction and mild pneumonia. The transient nature of the shadows and the high eosinophil count, usually between 500–1500 per mm³., sometimes above 10,000 per mm³. usually serve to differentiate this condition. A cause should be sought and either removed or treated, whichever is appropriate.

Asthma with Eosinophilia. Eosinophilia is frequently found with asthma. Infiltration of the lung with eosinophilia in asthma is less common—it is, however, the commonest form of pulmonary disease with eosinophilia. It is usually encountered with *extrinsic asthma*. In the United Kingdom 95 per cent. of cases are manifestations of hypersensitivity to *A. fumigatus* (allergic bronchopulmonary aspergillosis, see p. 226). Outside the United Kingdom the cause of the Arthus type hypersensitivity reaction which damages the bronchial wall is less certain.

Widespread peripheral radiological shadows are encountered with *intrinsic asthma* in which evidence of an immunological basis is lacking. The eosinophilia is often considerable, the onset is often very acute and followed by asthma. There may be pulmonary vasculitis but not all cases are variants or precursors of polyarteritis nodosa.

Tropical eosinophilia due to infestation with filariae is usually associated with asthma. It is most common in patients of Indian stock. There is usually a dry cough and wheeze, and sometimes fever. The chest radiograph shows bilateral rather vague nodular or micronodular shadowing which may coalesce; sometimes there is a pleural effusion. There are focal alveolar collections of eosinophils and macrophages and granulomata including large giant cells and after a time there is fibrosis [see Section 2].

Polyarteritis Nodosa. [See Section 4.] The lung is involved in about a third of cases of polyarteritis nodosa and of those with lung involvement about a half have an eosinophilia and many have asthma. Intrinsic asthma usually of late onset with eosinophilia and a high E.S.R. may be a pre-systemic manifestation of polyarteritis—there may be a latent interval of more than a year before development of renal, gastro-intestinal, neurological, cardiac or other manifestations of systemic disease. Polyarteritis nodosa with lung involvement is rare, it involves both sexes equally and is of unknown aetiology.

Polyarteritis nodosa restricted to the lung may cause severe illness with or without asthma or eosinophilia. Cough, weight loss, weakness, high fever and pleurisy may be encountered with widespread signs of consolidation in the lung. The clinical manifestations and radiological changes, often dense homogeneous shadows representing infarcts or consolidation, may come and go or progress. Pleural effusions may be seen. For treatment and prognosis see Section 4.

Wegener's Granuloma. This is probably a variant of polyarteritis and is characterized by ulcerating nasal granulomata, necrotic lesions in the lungs which may cavitate, and renal involvement. The pathology resembles polyarteritis nodosa, is more common in middle life, affects both sexes equally and is accompanied by fever, cough, and often haemoptysis and pleurisy. Single or multiple, large or small round dense opacities are seen on the chest radiograph [PLATE 11]. These may cavitate. As with polyarteritis renal involvement usually determines the prognosis and when untreated the disease usually progresses rapidly. The progress of the disease may be favourably influenced by adrenocortical steroids —daily doses as high as 50–75 mg. of prednisone may be required. Immunosuppressive drugs may prove to be more effective [see Section 4].

REFERENCES

BAKER, S. J., RAJAN, K. T., and DEVADATTA, S. (1959) Treatment of tropical eosinophilia. A controlled trial, *Lancet*, ii, 144.

CROFTON, J. W., LIVINGSTONE, J. R., OSWALD, N. C., and ROBERTS, A. T. M. (1952) Pulmonary eosinophilia, *Thorax*, **7**, 1.

LEAK, D., and CLEIN, G. P. (1967) Acute Wegener's granulomatosis, *Thorax*, **22**, 437.

ROSE, G. A., and SPENCER, H. (1957) Polyarteritis nodosa, *Quart. J. Med.*, **26**, 43.

DRUG INDUCED LUNG DISEASE

Many drugs are capable of inducing lung disease either by direct toxic action, by idiosyncrasy (a genetically determined reaction), or by hypersensitivity.

Apart from drug reactions which may be associated with asthma, pulmonary infiltration with eosinophilia, polyarthritis nodosa and systemic lupus erythematosus (hydralazine), reactions to drugs may take the form of extrinsic allergic alveolitis (e.g. due to pituitary snuff), a variant of fibrosing alveolitis (e.g. due to busulphan, hexamethonium, pentolinium, mecamylamine, chlorambucil, imipramine, chlorpropamide, or mephenesin). For an account of drug induced lung disease the reader is referred to the review by Davies (1969).

POISONING WITH PARAQUAT

A devastating form of intrabronchiolar and alveolar haemorrhage may follow some days after accidental ingestion of small quantities of the herbicide paraquat. Bronchiolar epithelial proliferation, thickening of alveolar walls, fibroblasts and inflammatory cells are found together with central hepatic and renal tubular necrosis and myocarditis. Respiratory failure and death usually occur within 3 weeks or so. Recovery is unusual.

REFERENCES

DAVIES, P. D. B. (1969) Drug induced lung disease, *Brit. J. Dis. Chest*, **63**, 57.

MATTHEW, H., LOGAN, A., WOODRUFF, M. F. A., and HEARD, B. (1968) Paraquat poisoning—lung transplantation, *Brit. med. J.*, **3**, 759.

CARCINOMA OF THE BRONCHUS

Synonyms. Bronchial carcinoma; Carcinoma of the lung.

Definition

This is a carcinoma which has originated in the epithelium of the bronchial tree.

Aetiology

In 1968 28,826 persons died of carcinoma of the bronchus in England and Wales—the mortality for males was 1·01 per 1000 and for females 0·197 per 1000. This is about one-third of all deaths from cancer. The number of deaths in the United Kingdom is expected to rise so that in the 1980s between thirty-five and forty thousand people are expected to die annually. Unless new factors have appeared, the trend is then expected to level off. The death rate of lung cancer rises from a very low level after the fourth decade and this rise is greater in males than females. There is also a rising death rate for each successive cohort; thus cancer of the lung was not a major cause of cancer death in males born in 1871 but lung cancer accounted for about half of all cancer deaths in fifty-year-old males born in 1901. Only a small part of this change can be ascribed to improved diagnosis: environmental and genetic changes must be responsible. While environmental factors have definitely been established, genetic factors have not. There is a greater mortality in towns and industrial regions, and cigarette smoking is now recognized as the most important contributory factor. There are also occupational hazards.

Death rates from carcinoma of the bronchus vary from one country to another—in 1951–1953 the death rates from bronchial carcinoma varied from 0·617 per 1000 in England and Wales and 0·419 per 1000 in Finland to 0·263 per 1000 in the United States and 0·204 per 1000 in Australia (these figures have only superficial value because of differences in definition, etc.). Another factor affecting mortality is social status, for there is some evidence to suggest that the death rate amongst males aged twenty to sixty-four is higher in social Group 5 (the poorest) than in social Group 1 (the richest).

Aetiological Factors

Occupation. There is an increased liability to develop bronchial carcinoma in certain occupations. These include the mining of radioactive ores, e.g. uranium, the refining of nickel, the manufacture of chromates, and asbestos and coal-gas production. Amongst occupations which carry a possible risk are certain processes involving inorganic arsenic, the mining of haematite and the manufacture of iron products.

The latent interval between first exposure and appearance of the disease is between 15 and 30 years.

Radiation. Radiotherapy itself has been shown to increase the risk of lung cancer, e.g. in patients who have been treated for ankylosing spondylitis. Amongst the Japanese subjected to more than 90 rads of atomic radiation during the Second World War the observed incidence of carcinoma of the bronchus was approximately twice the expected.

Atmospheric Pollution. There is definite increase in mortality in large towns and therefore airborne carcinogens are a possible factor.

Cigarette Smoking. This is now established as the most important known cause of bronchial carcinoma—not only is the incidence higher in cigarette smokers but it is directly related to the number of cigarettes smoked. The death rate amongst heavy smokers is twenty times that of non-smokers. The incidence diminishes the longer the period after giving up cigarette smoking—it is also less in pipe smokers. Smoking habits may explain the increase in incidence in the last 50 years and the difference between the sexes. The differences in the duration of cigarette smoking, in the way cigarettes are smoked and in the curing of tobacco may explain the high incidence in the United Kingdom and Finland compared with the relatively low incidence in, for example, the United States and Australia.

Other Possible Factors. There is some evidence to suggest that scars and fibrosis within the lung may play a part in the genesis of neoplasia and explain the not infrequent finding of lung cancer in healed tuberculosis and other fibrotic lesions. The association with chronic bronchitis is probably due to factors common to the cause of both conditions, e.g. cigarette smoking and atmospheric pollution.

Pathology

Carcinoma of the bronchus arises in the epithelium or mucous glands which line the airways. An origin from the alveolar epithelium itself is uncertain. There are several cell types:

1. *Squamous cell*, about 56 per cent. approximately of bronchial carcinomas have a characteristic histology with cell nests, intracellular bridges, with keratinization and epithelial pearls and much stroma. Necrosis is common.

2. *Adenocarcinoma*, about 6 per cent of lung carcinomas are of the tubular or glandular type and mucin may be formed. Sometimes cells can be seen to spread along the surface of the alveolar wall, resembling bronchiolar carcinoma.
3. *Undifferentiated*, this type of growth comprises about 37 per cent. of bronchial carcinomas and is characteristically pleomorphic. The oat-cell variety, however, contains uniformly small cells with little stroma and deeply staining ovoid nuclei which almost fill the cells. This tumour probably originates in the basal layer of the bronchial epithelium.

Bronchial carcinoma may be central or in the periphery of the lung. Squamous- and oat-cell tumours are more often central in origin while adenocarcinomas are usually peripheral. Forty-five per cent. of growths are in the upper lobes, 30 per cent. in the lower lobes and 25 per cent. involve the main bronchi.

Most growths extend beyond the bronchus of origin and infiltrate the surrounding lung. The pleura tends to act as a barrier except at the apex. The growth may obstruct the bronchus causing retention of secretion and infection: pneumonia may be suppurative and proceed to abscess formation. More peripheral growths, especially the squamous-cell variety may cavitate. Direct spread may involve the pericardium, intrathoracic nerves, oesophagus, thoracic duct and the veins.

Lymphatic spread to hilar nodes is most common and important and occurs via peribronchial and perivenous lymphatics. The growth then tends to spread from tracheobronchial to paratracheal glands and then outside the thorax, most commonly up into the neck and even the axillae, rarely via the para-aortic glands to the inguinal region. Lymphangitis carcinomatosa due to wide-spread infiltration of the pulmonary lymphatics is described on page 902.

Blood stream spread. Microscopic tumour emboli leave the primary site and travel via the pulmonary veins to the systemic circulation and may lodge in most tissues. Undifferentiated tumours and adenocarcinomas are more invasive than squamous-cell tumours. Subsequent growth of the distant metastases depends on the local tissue environment. Thus, deposits in the liver (40 per cent.), adrenal (30 per cent.), brain 20 (per cent.), bone (15 per cent.), and kidney (15 per cent.) grow at different rates. Deposits in brain, liver and bone are more likely to give symptoms than kidney and adrenal, whilst growth in the skin, ovary, spleen and thyroid are unusual, accounting for less than 10 per cent. of cases. Deposits in voluntary muscles are insignificant.

The incidence of metastases bears no relation to organ size or blood flow, but there is some evidence to suggest that the distance from the lungs is relevant and therefore, lymphatic, rather than blood stream is the more likely channel of spread. In about a quarter of patients dying with lung cancer no distant metastases can be found.

Growths in the lung, may, when large enough, or particularly when infiltrating the lymphatics impair function of the lung by restriction of ventilatory capacity. Invasion of the pleura causing an effusion or collapse of part or whole of the lung will also restrict ventilation. As chronic obstructive bronchitis so often accompanies bronchial carcinoma an obstructive ventilatory defect will often predominate. Lymphangitis carcinomatosa produces the grossest defect in lung function due to widespread infiltration—there is diminished compliance and severe breathlessness and later cyanosis due to unequal ventilation and blood flow.

Clinical Picture

The mode of presentation is influenced by the site of the tumour but little by its histology: presentation with metastases, however, is more common with undifferentiated tumours and adenocarcinoma. Adenocarcinoma is almost as common in females as in males and this is probably because it bears little relation to cigarette smoking. It is also found in younger people and is more often in the periphery of the lung; therefore it is more often picked up on mass radiography and with a longer history of illness.

Carcinoma of the bronchus presents in very many ways either with manifestations within the thorax or as a result of distant effects which may be metastatic or biochemical. More than 10 per cent. of growths first manifest with disorders outside the thorax. In the United Kingdom a considerable proportion of new cases is found in asymptomatic patients at routine chest radiography—that is about 5 per cent. of all cases.

Suspicion of carcinoma of the bronchus should be aroused when cough, haemoptysis, breathlessness or chest pain develop, especially in cigarette smoking males between the ages of forty-five and sixty-five. The pain may be pleuritic or of a dull boring quality due to involvement of the mediastinum or thoracic cage. Alcohol may induce pain in lymph nodes invaded by growth. Suspicion should also be aroused when pneumonia resolves slowly or not at all. Weight loss, malaise, hepatic pain, sudden development of a hoarse voice, dysphagia or obstruction of the superior vena cava are less common modes of presentation. The development of an intracranial space-occupying lesion, a pathological fracture, anaemia due to bone marrow involvement, hypertrophic pulmonary osteo-arthropathy, myopathy, endocrine abnormalities or recurrent thrombophlebitis may be the presenting features.

On physical examination the patient is characteristically a late middle-aged male who has been a heavy cigarette smoker and he may well be rather wasted in appearance. There is often clubbing of the fingers and there may be palpable lymph nodes, especially in the supraclavicular fossae.

When the growth involves a large bronchus there may be impaired movement of the chest on that side with a fixed rhonchus indicative of a partial occlusion, or signs of collapse of a lobe or lung when the occlusion is total. Occasionally the tumour is itself big enough to impair the percussion note and impair the breath sounds. Otherwise the physical signs may indicate an unresolved pneumonia, a pleural effusion or a paralysed diaphragm. Stridor may be detected if mediastinal spread involves the trachea or main bronchi. Superior vena caval obstruction can be recognized when the face and upper extremities are oedematous, cyanosed and the eyes suffused—the superficial veins over those areas are dilated and there is fixed engorgement of the superficial and deep veins of the neck. Frequently, however, the physical signs are absent or minimal.

Irregular enlargement of the liver, hard palpable lymph nodes and neurological signs are the common manifestations of spread outside the thorax.

Complications by Direct Effect of the Growth. Pneumonia, often of the non-specific or suppurative variety, may develop as a result of obstruction to a major bronchus: it may develop into a *lung abscess*. *Pleural effusions* may follow either direct invasion of the pleura or underlying infection of the lung: in the first instance the effusion may be a serous exudate or it may be blood stained or even a frank *haemothorax*. More rarely a *chylothorax* develops if the tumour has invaded the thoracic duct or the other main lymphatic channels. Symptoms and signs may arise when the bony thoracic cage, the nerves of the brachial plexus, the intercostal, and the phrenic nerves and the recurrent laryngeal nerves are invaded. Direct invasion of the pericardium may cause a *pericardial effusion* and of the myocardium, *dysrhythmias* such as atrial fibrillation.

Indirect Effects of the Growth. Metastases to the central nervous system, bone, liver, adrenal and skin may produce symptoms and signs as a direct effect of growth, pressure or destruction. Carcinoma of the bronchus, however, not infrequently causes distant effects not by metastases but by the synthesis of a number of substances, e.g. amines (e.g. 5-OH tryptamine), amino acids (5-OH tryptophane) or peptides (e.g. antidiuretic hormone). In many cases the mechanism, whether it be humoral or neurohumoral, is unknown particularly in neuropathic, myopathic, and haematological complications and in clubbing and in pulmonary osteo-arthropathy. A number of intrathoracic growths may cause dysfunction in this manner but oat-cell carcinoma seems to be the most versatile. In TABLE 48 are listed many of the extrathoracic, non-metastic disorders induced by carcinoma of the bronchus [see Section 4].

Hypertrophic Pulmonary Osteo-arthropathy. This occurs in 5 per cent. of patients, sometimes precedes all other manifestations of the tumour and may mimic an acute arthropathy. The wrist and ankles are particularly likely to be involved and are painful, warm, swollen and tender and there may be soft tissue swelling of the hands and feet and effusions into the knee joints. Clubbing of the fingers is invariably present. The cause of this osteo-arthropathy is unknown but as it may be relieved by removal of the tumour, stripping of its nerve supply or by resection of the branches of the vagus nerve to that lung, it is probably of a complex neurohumoral nature. Circulating levels of oestrogens are raised and in some cases gynaecomastia is found as well. There is subperiosteal new bone formation which can usually be seen on radiographs of the long bones adjacent to the ankle or wrists. Relief of pain may also be obtained by the use of adrenocortical steroids.

TABLE 48

SOME EXTRATHORACIC DISORDERS DUE TO BRONCHIAL CARCINOMA (NON-METASTATIC)

Neurological	Venous thrombosis (thrombophlebitis migrans)
Encephalomyelopathy	Venous gangrene
Cortical cerebellar degeneration	Haematological
Peripheral neuropathy	Anaemia – normoblastic
Sensory, motor or mixed	Red cell aplasia
Myopathy – often central	Erythrocythaemia
Myasthenic syndrome	Thrombocythaemia
Dermatological	Endocrine
Pruritus	Carcinoid syndrome (5-OH tryptamine, etc.)
Herpes zoster	Parathormone-like activity – hypercalcaemia
Acanthosis nigricans	Corticotrophin-like activity – adrenal hyperfunction (Cushing's syndrome)
Dermatomyositis	
Erythema gyratum perstans	Inappropriate antidiuretic activity
Clubbing and pachydermoperiostosis	(A.D.H.-like substance – low serum sodium, high urinary sodium with hyperosmolarity)
Gynaecomastia	
Pulmonary osteo-arthropathy	

Diagnosis

Carcinoma of the lung should be considered in any patient over forty with new and persistent respiratory symptoms, especially if they are cigarette smokers or have chronic bronchitis. Whilst the diagnosis is usually straightforward when radiological and cytological evidence is available the major difficulties encountered are:

1. An isolated round shadow in the lung due to a carcinoma is easily confused with that cast by a secondary tumour, a benign tumour, e.g. hamartoma, tuberculoma or a cyst, e.g. hydatid. The presence of satellite shadows or of calcium within the shadows make a primary carcinoma less likely.

2. Coexisting shadows of fibrosis and collapse may conceal the presence of a neoplasm which itself may have arisen in the scar tissue, e.g. healed tuberculosis or pneumoconiosis.

3. Pneumonia or suppuration with lung abscess may obscure the underlying carcinoma.

4. Chronic inflammatory disease with granuloma formation which may be specific, e.g. staphylococcal or chemical or non-specific, may resemble a carcinoma radiologically.

5. Unexplained pleural effusions may conceal the underlying growth.

The chest radiograph [PLATE 11] is vital to the diagnosis and all manner of abnormal shadowing may be encountered. An isolated shadow may be small or large, solid or cavitated, sharply demarcated or serrated at its margin. Primary carcinomas do not calcify. Massive lobar or segmental shadows often show some reduction in volume due to accompanying collapse but do not reveal an 'air bronchogram'. Cavitation may represent a necrotic tumour or abscess in the lung distal to the tumour. Associated hilar or mediastinal shadows usually indicate neoplastic spread but on occasions may represent inflammatory change only. A high diaphragm due to phrenic nerve involvement, or a large heart shadow due to a pericardial effusion are suggestive of invasion. Secondary deposits in bone with rarefaction or fracture indicates metastatic spread. *Tomography* may add discrimination to the routine radiograph and is particularly useful in defining patency of the main airways, detecting shadows of calcium density and involvement of the central lymph nodes. A barium swallow showing displacement of the oesophagus is useful in the detection of enlarged mediastinal lymph nodes.

Histological evidence is invaluable in the diagnosis of bronchial carcinoma and the discovery of the cell type is important in the management and prognosis. *Sputum cytology* is laborious and requires skill if it is to be reliable. In expert hands it is more likely to confirm the diagnosis than any other method and will do so in about 60–80 per cent. of cases. Fresh specimens, especially those which contain blood and white opaque streaks are best studied by wet preparations which are stained by methylene blue. Clumps of cells can be seen in depth and occasionally the cell type can be specified. The chief value of this method is in the diagnosis of tumours beyond bronchoscopic vision: bronchoscopy itself may dislodge sheets and clumps of cells which may resemble oat cells—so search for neoplastic cells should be avoided for 10 days or so after bronchoscopy. Chronic inflammatory disease, especially tuberculosis in the elderly, may cause difficulty but otherwise 'false positive' findings are rare.

Tissue may be obtained at *bronchoscopy* or *mediastinoscopy* when the tumour or evidence of lymph node involvement may be seen. Furthermore, bronchoscopy may reveal paralysed vocal cords or abnormalities of the carina and main bronchi which will help in assessment of operability. In *pleural fluid* due to invasion by growth, while mesothelial cells are usually abundant, neoplastic cells are rarely found. Inflammatory and red blood cells are often numerous. The fluid itself is usually an exudate, but has no other special features. *Biopsy of the pleura* should always be performed when effusions are aspirated—positive results, however, are more often found with metastases, especially from the breast. *Biopsy of lymph* nodes, either scalene, supraclavicular or distant but hard nodes may give histological evidence as may nodules in the liver or skin.

Scanning of the lung using radioactive isotopes: macroaggregated serum albumin labelled with ^{131}I or ^{99}Te is injected intravenously and defects in perfusion of the lung are found with tumours more than 2 cm. in diameter which range in size from the tumour mass to almost absent perfusion of the lung. The larger the defect in perfusion the greater the involvement of the mediastinum. This is often much greater than would be suspected on clinical or radiological grounds. Scanning of bone or liver is of great value in detecting metastases.

Treatment

Prevention. The current epidemic of lung cancer in the United Kingdom and to a lesser extent in other technologically advanced countries, is due mainly to cigarette smoking. If all cigarette smoking was stopped the incidence of lung cancer would probably fall to about 10 per cent. of the present incidence. Reduction in cigarette smoking by doctors from 1952 to 1961 reduced the mortality by 7 per cent. If carcinogens cannot be removed from cigarettes, individuals must be persuaded by propaganda and every possible means to avoid the temptation of smoking or to give it up. Penal taxation and simple propaganda so far devised have had little impact. Reduction of atmospheric pollution and occupational hazard should also make a contribution.

Surgery and Radiotherapy. These constitute the main radical and palliative measures for treating bronchial carcinoma. Of the 5140 patients attending the Brompton and Royal Marsden Hospitals in London between 1951 and 1963, resection was carried out in 1092, i.e. 21 per cent.; radiotherapy was carried out in 2008 cases, i.e. 39 per cent. Radiotherapy was combined with resection or was given for metastases in 318 cases and 1721 patients were untreated. These data, while similar to those of other large series, are of course highly selected: amongst these cases there was a higher proportion of patients suitable for surgery and radiotherapy and of those who presented difficult diagnostic and therapeutic problems.

Surgery. Pneumonectomy or lobectomy with or without sleeve resection of the main bronchus was carried out whenever there was a reasonable chance of eradication without causing respiratory insufficiency. About 30 per cent. of all patients underwent surgery in this series, but in 7 per cent. who had a thoracotomy the growth was too advanced to be resected—thus about 23 per cent. had the growth removed. Open thoracotomy was precluded in 70 per cent. on the following grounds:

1. Clinical, radiological or other evidence of metastases—37 per cent.
2. Cachexia—5 per cent.
3. Involvement of the pleura and chest wall and other structures which made the growth inoperable—11 per cent.
4. Inadequate respiratory function, advanced age, or other disease—17 per cent.

Younger patients can adapt to loss of functioning lung better than the aged. People over sixty-five withstand pneumonectomy poorly and especially if there is any limitation of lung function. In all patients considered for surgery, function of the lungs must be assessed, bearing in mind the amount of functioning lung that may be removed by surgery and the possibility of post-operative morbidity. Occasionally it is difficult to assess operability where function is impaired, particularly when there are moderate degrees of airways obstruction, whatever the cause—it is usually due to associated chronic obstructive bronchitis. Simple observation of the patient during and after exercise is often a valuable adjunct to more detailed tests of respiratory function in assessment for operation. Patients with respiratory insufficiency are not suitable for thoracotomy and withstand radiotherapy well without deterioration in their function.

Of the 1092 patients who had a resection, 62 per cent. survived one year, 39 per cent. survived 3 years, and 27 per cent. survived 5 years. Those who had lobectomy fared better than those that had a pneumonectomy. Prognosis was better for squamous-cell growths but age and sex and site of the tumour had little effect on survival after surgery which has remained almost unchanged over the last three decades.

Radiotherapy. This was given mainly by X-rays to about 30 per cent. seen with bronchial carcinoma in this series. This form of treatment was given chiefly to relieve symptoms such as cough, bone pain, breathlessness, haemoptysis, dysphagia and superior vena caval obstruction. The latter condition is certainly the most important indication for radiotherapy and is usually rapidly relieved. While the use of radiotherapy to relieve symptoms is unquestioned and valuable, its ability to effect a radical cure remains largely unknown. Tumours vary in their susceptibility to radiotherapy and in general undifferentiated and oat-cell carcinomas are more responsive than squamous and adenocarcinomas. Radiotherapy offers slightly longer survival than resection of central oat-cell carcinomas when the diagnosis has been established by bronchial biopsy. In general, however, about 19 per cent. of patients survived one year with radiotherapy and 1·5 per cent. were alive about 5 years after concluding treatment.

This surgical and radiotherapeutic experience in London is representative of the general experience in the management of carcinoma of the bronchus by these methods.

Radioactive seeds (*Radon*) can be implanted locally into tumours with often useful reduction of tumour size and delay in growth.

Chemotherapy. While mustine and other cytotoxic agents do not prolong life and offer little in symptomatic relief they are occasionally of value in relieving superior vena caval obstruction and in large airway compression if radiotherapy is unavailable.

Symptomatic Treatment. This is of the greatest importance with patients suffering from carcinoma of the bronchus. Pain should be relieved. In certain cases, especially those with involvement of bone or mediastinum this may be achieved with radiotherapy. Simple analgesics like paracetamol, 0·5–1 G. three to four times a day, may be successful; if not, more potent drugs such as dihydrocodeine, 30–60 mg. by mouth, methadone, 5–10 mg., pentazocine, 25–100 mg. by mouth or injection, diamorphine, 2–5 mg. by injection, or morphine, 15–30 mg. by injection, may be tried. The headache of cerebral metastases is often relieved by large doses of adrenocortical steroids such as prednisone, 20–60 mg. daily. Distress and anxiety may be relieved by sympathetic and understanding conversation with the patient and by the use of drugs such as chlorpromazine, 25–100 mg. three to four times a day: this drug may potentiate analgesics too. Prednisone in high doses may exert a euphoric effect and in the terminal stages a sweet linctus containing morphine, 15 mg., cocaine, 10 mg., and alcohol may give considerable relief.

Course and Prognosis

The bad prognosis of carcinoma of the bronchus is widely known and advances in surgical technique and high voltage radiotherapy have, as yet, brought no improvement. In general, in the United Kingdom the over-all survival rate at 5 years is less than 7 per cent. Whereas with surgery of selected cases 62 per cent. of patients survive one year and 27 per cent. 5 years: when left untreated 14 per cent. of patients survive for one year and 0·3 per cent. for 5 years. The survival of a large group of patients untreated is, of course, unknown. The majority of patient deteriorate slowly and less than 20 per cent. are distressed with pain. About one in seven patients dies of cerebral metastases and often suffer very little. Sudden death is uncommon and terminal haemoptysis, superior vena caval obstruction, dysphagia or tracheal obstruction are unusual.

REFERENCES

BIGNALL, J. R. (1958) *Carcinoma of the Lung*, Edinburgh.

BIGNALL, J. R., MARTIN, M., and SMITHERS, D. W. (1967) Survival in 6086 cases of bronchial carcinoma, *Lancet*, i, 1067.

MEDICAL RESEARCH COUNCIL (1966) Comparative trial of surgery and radiotherapy for the primary treatment of small cell or oat cell carcinoma of the bronchus, *Lancet*, ii, 979.

METASTASES IN THE LUNGS

Many tumours metastasize to the lungs via the systemic venous system either directly or indirectly via the thoracic duct. They produce solitary or multiple tumours which on chest radiography are usually well demarcated round shadows of various sizes. On rare occasions they may cavitate or calcify. Sometimes a miliary appearance is seen and in these cases the myriad shadows may not be clearly demarcated.

The commoner sites of origin are breast, gastro-intestinal tract and pancreas, genito-urinary tract, especially hypernephroma, prostate, bone and thyroid. Symptoms are notable for their absence but when metastases are massive and widespread in the lung there may be breathlessness. Haemoptysis is rare. The pleura is not infrequently involved especially with metastases from the breast, and effusions are frequent.

Usually the primary site is known, but if not the diagnosis may be difficult. With solitary shadows, usually from a hypernephroma, primary carcinoma of the bronchus, benign tumours, e.g. hamartoma, tuberculoma, or a cyst, e.g. hydatid cyst, have to be considered in the differential diagnosis. Widespread shadowing has to be differentiated from disseminated or miliary tuberculosis, sarcoidosis, pneumoconiosis, histiocytosis X, alveolitis, lymphomata, haemosiderosis, etc. [see TABLE 50].

Careful physical examination, including that of the

pelvis and thyroid, examination of the sputum for malignant cells and *Myco. tuberculosis*, for evidence of hydatid infection, and if necessary an intravenous pyelogram which may reveal the primary tumour. Further search for a primary source is usually unrewarding and if the diagnosis remains uncertain biopsy of lymph node, liver or even of the lung may be necessary. Resection of solitary primary metastases is justifiable —removal of a primary hypernephroma has been followed by spontaneous regression of metatases in the lung. Metastases from tumours which are hormone dependent (e.g. breast or prostate) may respond dramatically to the appropriate treatment and secondaries from a thyroid may be successfully treated with radioactive iodine. Metastases from choriocarcinoma may respond dramatically to chemotherapy (methotrexate and 6-mercaptopurine).

Metastases to the lungs, however, are frequently a terminal event and seldom merit any other than symptomatic treatment.

SPECIAL FORMS OF CARCINOMATOSIS OF THE LUNGS

Bronchiolar Carcinoma (Alveolar-cell Carcinoma). In about 1 per cent. of bronchial carcinoma there are sheets of neoplastic cells often only one cell thick which spread through the acini lining the alveolar walls. They are derived from adenocarcinoma. This process may be seen even at the edge of a solitary adenocarcinoma of the lung on microscopy or may be the chief component of a small solitary pulmonary lesion detected on chest radiography. The most striking form appears to be multicentric in origin with shadows throughout one or both lungs which are usually of variable size—reaching massive proportions as the disease advances. The patient then develops a cough, sometimes with copious mucoid sputum which may be streaked with blood, and breathlessness, weight loss, and fever. This diagnosis should be considered when multiple lung shadows, usually ill-defined and of variable size, are found on chest radiographs and confirmed by examination of the sputum in which malignant cells almost invariably are found. The pleura is not usually involved.

Although bronchiolar carcinoma is probably of pulmonary origin some pathologists regard this as a metastasis from adenocarcinomata of the pancreas or gastro-intestinal tract which remains undetected. Treatment of generalized bronchiolar carcinoma is of no avail and should be symptomatic, but solitary lesions should be resected with a prognosis rather better than that of bronchial carcinoma—which is strongly suggestive that the growth is usually primary in the lung.

Lymphangitis Carcinomatosa (Lymphatic Carcinomatosis). Carcinoma derived from the bronchus or extrathoracic sites such as pancreas, stomach and breast may spread to mediastinal glands, then grow along the peribronchial and perivenous lymphatics—if the pleural plexus of lymphatics is permeated a fine network of channels may be seen over the surface of the lung. This condition may be unilateral or bilateral and in the early stages appears as linear shadows radiating from the mediastinum which is usually enlarged by glands.

Progressive breathlessness may become extremely severe as the process permeates and stiffens the lungs and produces not only a linear but a reticular pattern on the chest radiograph. Cough and haemoptysis with weight loss are usually overshadowed by the breathlessness. Infiltration along the broncho-arterial bundle may initiate widespread thrombosis within the smaller branches of the pulmonary artery with an increase in pulmonary vascular resistance.

Treatment can only be symptomatic.

REFERENCES

Bagshawe, K. D., and McDonald, J. M. (1960) Treatment of choriocarcinoma with a combination of cytotoxic drugs, *Brit. med. J.*, **2**, 426.

Harold, J. T. (1952) Lymphangitis carcinomatosa of the lungs, *Quart. J. Med.*, **21**, 353.

Hewlett, T. H., Gomez, A. C., Aronstam, E. M., and Steer, A. (1964) Bronchiolar carcinoma of the lung. Review of 39 patients, *J. thorac. cardiovasc. Surg.*, **48**, 614.

OTHER PULMONARY TUMOURS

Tumours other than carcinoma of the bronchus are rare and include bronchial adenoma, hamartoma, papilloma, cystadenoma, fibroma, lipoma, myxoma, chondroma, myoblastoma and sarcoma of diverse origin: neurofibroma and neurogenic sarcoma, haemangiopericytoma, histiocytoma, plasmacytoma.

BRONCHIAL ADENOMA

These tumours may be benign or of low grade malignancy and comprise about 2 per cent. lung tumours. There are two main types *carcinoid* and *cylindroma*—muco-epidermoid and mixed tumours of the bronchus are extremely rare.

Carcinoid Tumours. Ninety per cent. of adenomata of the bronchus are of this type and the majority arise in the walls of the larger bronchi. The cells are small and are arranged in an orderly fashion, e.g. in columns or rosettes. The cells are pleomorphic and mitoses are unusual. This tumour may on occasion metastasize sometimes many years after discovery of the primary growth. There is a cover of epithelium and the thin stroma is often very vascular and may degenerate, calcify or even ossify.

Cylindromata. These infiltrate the walls of larger bronchi and also the trachea and the surrounding tissue. The cells are pleomorphic, darkly staining and are arranged in tubular fashion with interspersed fibrous tissue and mucin. Mitoses are seen and local invasiveness, and metastases are more common than with the carcinoid variety. Both may spread to local lymph nodes and occasionally to the liver.

Clinical Features

Adenomata may present with:

1. Repeated haemoptysis with or without cough.

2. Obstruction of a main, lobar or segmental bronchus with atelectasis or with obstructive emphysema if the occlusion is partial. Breathlessness may then be the presenting symptom.

3. Recurrent infection with non-specific pneumonia

or suppurative pneumonia and lung abscess, or bronchiectasis in the distal parts of the lung.

4. With carcinoid syndrome: this is a rare manifestation of carcinoid tumours in the lung and resembles in every particular the classical carcinoid syndrome [see Section 7] except that lesions of the left side of the heart may develop, e.g. mitral valve disease.

5. With multiple endocrine tumours (pluriglandular syndrome) [see Section 5].

The chest radiograph may be normal, may show partial or complete atelectasis of a segment or lobe or obstructive emphysema. There may be a rounded or ovoid shadow cast by the tumour itself peripherally which may contain specks of calcium or bone.

Diagnosis

The diagnosis, except with peripheral tumours, is usually established by bronchoscopy: the appearances of the tumour are often absolutely characteristic—if not biopsy should be undertaken. Carcinoid varieties may secrete 5-OH tryptamine or 5-OH tryptophan and excessive amounts of 5-OH indole acetic acid (greater than 10 mg. in the 24 hours) may therefore be found in the urine even in the absence of the carcinoid syndrome.

Treatment

This is mainly surgical. Endoscopic resection of the tumour is palliative for it is usually followed by recurrence. The tumour may be removed by sleeve resection but usually this is not feasible and resection of a segment, lobe or even lung may have to be undertaken, particularly if permanent damage has been sustained by the lung distal to the tumour. Enlarged nodes should be excised. Sometimes the progress of infiltrating cylindromata may be arrested by radiotherapy. For treatment of carcinoid syndrome see Section 7.

Prognosis

The prognosis of carcinoid tumours is excellent; if the growth is removed 75 per cent. survive 4 or more years and recurrence is unusual. Survival without treatment even with metastases may be prolonged for years. The prognosis for cylindromata is much less satisfactory for recurrences are frequent and the mortality is high.

HAMARTOMA

This tumour is composed of normal tissue elements in a disorganized form. Hamartomata may grow anywhere in the lung, or much less frequently in the bronchus or even the trachea. They are usually detected after adolescence, they vary in size from a centimetre or less upwards but most are between 1–3 cm. in size. They grow at a variable rate. They consist of rounded even slightly lobulated masses of cartilage, a framework of connective tissue with scattered clefts of epithelium and fat. Calcification may be seen. They are asymptomatic unless they happen to occlude a bronchus and are found usually on routine chest radiography. A well demarcated round or slightly lobulated shadow is seen and specks of calcium may be demonstrated particularly on tomography. Unless the shadow has been known to exist for many years and if the condition of the patient allows the lesion will usually be resected for it may not be possible to reach a diagnosis or to exclude a carcinoma. These tumours are almost always benign and recurrence is rare.

REFERENCES

ABBEY-SMITH, R. (1969) Bronchial carcinoid tumours, *Thorax*, **24**, 43.

British Medical Journal (1962) Bronchial adenoma and serotonin, Leading article, **2**, 249.

LE ROUX, B. T. (1964) Pulmonary hamartomata, *Thorax*, **19**, 236.

SPENCER, H. (1962) *Pathology of the Lung*, London.

THOMAS, C. P. (1954) Benign tumours of the lung, *Lancet*, i, 1.

INTRATHORACIC LYMPHOMATA

The lymphomata are a group of disorders characterized by neoplasia primarily of lymph nodes. This group includes Hodgkin's disease (lymphadenoma) [PLATE 12], lymphosarcoma and reticulum-cell sarcoma. Intrathoracic manifestations are very common—they are more common in generalized disease than with disease localized to the thorax [see Section 13].

THE PNEUMOCONIOSES

FATE OF INHALED AEROSOLS (INCLUDING DUST)

Definition

An aerosol consists of dispersed solid particles or liquid droplets or a mixture of both in which the particles or droplets are small enough to give a stable aerial suspension.

General Considerations

The maximum size of a particle or droplet in an aerosol is 50 microns, but the majority of aerosols contain particles of less than 20 microns in size. These have a settling velocity which varies with the square of the particle diameter—when this falls below 0·1 of a micron, however, particles move by diffusion rather than gravitation. In general, therefore, particles or droplets of a size less than 50 microns in diameter are deposited in the respiratory tract. They may consist of organic or inorganic (mineral) dusts, fumes, mists, smokes, pollens, bacteria, fungi or viruses.

Retention of particles will vary according to many physical factors such as particle size, solubility, stability, but a proportion of an inhaled aerosol may be exhaled, as can be clearly seen after the inhalation of cigarette smoke. Droplets containing water change in size almost instantaneously in the nasal passages and largest airways, where they encounter the dead space air which is 100 per cent. saturated. Deposition of particles in relation to their size is shown in FIGURE 60.

1. Particles greater than 10 microns are retained in

the nasal passages, pharynx and larynx (e.g. chromate particles are arrested in the nose where they give rise to ulceration).

2. Particles between 2 and 10 microns are mainly deposited in the airways.

3. Particles 0·1–2·0 microns reach the acinus, where a proportion are retained. Maximum retention occurs with particle size about 1 micron. When particles are half this size only about 25 per cent. are retained and 75 per cent. remain freely moving as aerosols and return with the expired air.

4. Particles 0·1 microns or less diffuse into the alveoli, where they remain. Gases behave likewise.

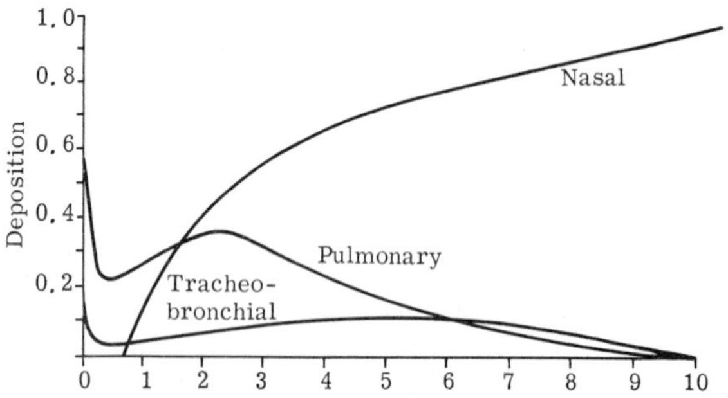

Particle size in micra

FIG. 60. Deposition of inhaled particles as a function of size. Respiratory frequency, 15 per minute; tidal volume, 750 ml.

Retention in the alveoli thereafter depends upon such factors as density, viscosity and solubility

The deposition of aerosols is minimal at respiration rates between 15 and 20 per minute.

Clearance of the Lungs

The bronchopulmonary tree is continuously exposed to aerosols and gas from the environment and is very efficient at removing all but the most nocuous. A very small reduction in efficiency from 99 to 98 per cent., for example, leads to the long-term retention of dust and may be an important factor in the genesis of pneumoconiosis. The majority of particles retained in the airways are cleared by the ciliary-mucus mechanism at a rate of 1 cm. per hour in health. This function is impaired by alcohol, anaesthetics, certain drugs, dehydration and excessive mucus secretion, for example with cigarette smoking. Micro-organisms are usually removed from a normal bronchial tree without any reaction on the part of the host. Excessive secretion stimulates cough receptors in the larger airways, but normally the ciliary mechanism is a continuous process and the escalated mucus reaches the larynx and is swallowed. Excessive concentrations of particles settling on the bronchial wall will cause reflex bronchoconstriction mediated by the vagus. Many soluble and diffusible substances in the aerosol, e.g. drugs and antibiotics are rapidly absorbed from the larger airways.

Distal to the ciliary mechanism retained particles are cleared:

1. By solution and absorption via the pulmonary capillaries or lymphatics, e.g. gases and aerosols of the smallest particle size.

2. By phagocytosis and transport by alveolar macrophages either to the lymphatics across the alveolar wall, or to accumulate in the alveolar space as tiny plaques, or they may be carried to the respiratory bronchioles from whence they pass up the bronchial tree. Under certain circumstances, probably with excessive amounts of dust, laden macrophages may be trapped at the level of the respiratory bronchiolus.

The rate of clearance by these mechanisms is very slow and dependent on the nature of the material. Thus noxious materials, e.g. silica, are liberated from macrophages and may travel freely in the lymphatics. This may result in slower clearance than is the case with particles remaining within the macrophage.

The site and nature of bronchopulmonary disease due to inhalation of aerosols depends ultimately not only on the *size* and *concentration* of the particles and their *mode of retention* and clearance and on the *physical state* of the particle, but also upon the *reactivity of the host*. The development of allergic response with antibody production and hypersensitivity will considerably modify the reaction to inhaled organic particles (including micro-organisms). Inert dust particles such as coal or iron do not affect the function of macrophages unless they are present in high concentration. On the other hand even a few silica (quartz) particles may immobilize macrophages and disrupt the cells. The liberated cellular debris modified by the silica may be fibrogenic.

Other responses on the part of the host include *hypersecretion of mucus*, which may be stimulated by aerosols not only of polluted air in general and of cigarette smoke, but also of occupational dusts, and *neoplasia*, which may result from the prolonged inhalation of aerosols such as tobacco smoke or asbestos.

REFERENCE

HATCH, T. F., and GROSS, P. (1964) *Pulmonary Deposition and Retention of Inhaled Aerosols*, New York.

PNEUMOCONIOSIS

Synonym. Occupational lung disease.

Definition

Deposition in the lung of inorganic or organic dusts.

General Considerations

The pneumoconioses are usually the result of inhalation of dust particles at work. The industrial processes which produce aerosols of this nature are more and more complex and diverse and there is now much greater awareness of the potential hazards which each new process may bring. Inhalation of aerosols created by time honoured occupations such as farming, milling and malting has been found relatively recently, with the help of new immunological, microbiological and physiological techniques, to be associated with bronchopulmonary disease. The occupations most frequently associated with the pneumoconioses in the United Kingdom, however, are coal miners, asbestos workers, foundry and pottery workers and other occupations involving mining and quarrying. The general effects of aerosol inhalation have been considered already. In addition to *deposition of dust*, however, other factors have to be taken into account when the pathogenesis of the pneumoconioses is considered. First, *mucus hypersecretion* leading to chronic bronchitis. Secondly, the *bronchoconstriction* that occurs, for example, with the inhalation of cotton dust (byssinosis) and toluene diisocyanate. And thirdly, *pulmonary* or *bronchopulmonary oedema* due to an acute inflammatory response to inhaled gases and fine particles, e.g. ammonia, chlorine, phosgene, nitrogen and sulphur oxides.

The diagnosis of a pneumoconiosis is often difficult and this has caused much anomalous legislation in the past. The diagnosis must take into account the occupational history, the clinical findings, and the results of radiological and physiological investigation. The radiological appearances of the lung alone are an inadequate assessment. Not only can the shadows seen in the pneumoconioses be closely mimicked by other diseases (e.g. tuberculosis, sarcoidosis, etc.), but the shadows themselves will vary greatly according to the amount of dust and its radio-density. There is no correlation between the degree of radiological abnormality and the development of symptoms, signs and physiological impairment. Thus, small amounts of iron or tin particles will give dense shadows and yet produce no impairment, while asbestos may produce minimal or no shadowing and gross disturbance of function. A table showing the categories of the radiological appearances in the pneumoconioses is shown on page 906. The assessment of symptoms, especially of breathlessness, must always take note of cigarette smoking and its duration, for chronic obstructive bronchitis is a common disorder which may be partly or wholly responsible.

Many of the pneumoconioses may be complicated by *progressive massive fibrosis* (P.M.F.) or a *rheumatoid pneumoconiosis* (Caplan's syndrome), both of which are probably host determined immunological responses to tissue, injured or conditioned by the dust.

PROGRESSIVE MASSIVE FIBROSIS
(P.M.F. or Complicated Pneumoconiosis)

The development of massive lesions, usually in the upper lobes in association with the pneumoconioses is known as progressive massive fibrosis (P.M.F.).

Pathogenesis

P.M.F. develops in response to a variety of dusts including coal, silica, graphite, kaolin, etc. but it is independent of the amount of dust inhaled. There is a concentric deposition of collagen around a central necrotic zone which may soften and cavitate by evacuation into a bronchus. There is increasing evidence to suggest that this process is the result of an immunological response on the part of the host to tissue modified by dust deposition, although the mechanism is unknown. The fact that 25 per cent. of miners with the more advanced forms of P.M.F. (Category B and C) have significant titres (greater than 1 in 80) of rheumatoid factor is of interest in this respect. At one time it was thought that the tissue response was conditioned by tuberculous infection; this is now considered unlikely because:

1. *Mycobacterium tuberculosis* is rarely found in the sputum (less than 2 per cent. of cases).
2. The proportion of coal miners with cutaneous reactivity to tuberculin (positive Mantoux reaction) is similar whether they have simple pneumoconiosis, P.M.F. or no evidence of pneumoconiosis at all.
3. Antituberculosis drugs do not influence the progress of the lesions.

The possibility remains, however, that pneumoconiosis, especially P.M.F., may reduce host resistance to infection with *Myco. tuberculosis* in general and the anonymous forms of *Myco. tuberculosis* in particular. The sputum should always be examined in cases of P.M.F. for acid fast bacilli and cultivated for *Myco. tuberculosis*. Anonymous forms if they are found carry an adverse prognosis because of their resistance to the antituberculosis drugs.

The incidence of P.M.F. in pneumoconiosis varies greatly from one region to another and depends at least to some extent on the composition of the dust—in some areas the incidence may be as high as 50 per cent. of those workers with pneumoconiosis. The severer forms of P.M.F. produce a restrictive disorder of ventilatory capacity with breathlessness. There is also uneven ventilation and blood flow with impaired gas transfer and in the most severe cases there is respiratory failure. *Haemoptysis* is a feature of P.M.F. There may also be diffuse *fibrosis* and *bronchiectasis* and in the more severe cases a rise in pulmonary vascular resistance with right ventricular hypertrophy and failure.

In the *chest radiograph* [PLATE 12] dense, rather rounded shadows are seen, which may be single or multiple and more concentrated in the upper than the lower zones. They may be up to several centimetres in diameter and the large shadows may coalesce or cavitate. They may also be calcified. They are classified according to their size into categories A, B and C [see TABLE 49].

P.M.F. must be differentiated from *carcinoma of the lung*, especially when the shadow is single; rapid changes in the radiograph favour carcinoma, in which characteristic cells may be seen on cytological examination of the sputum. *Pulmonary tuberculosis* may present difficulties, but the diagnosis of tuberculosis in the presence of the pneumoconiosis requires the finding of *Myco. tuberculosis* in the sputum.

RHEUMATOID PNEUMOCONIOSIS
(Caplan's Syndrome)

The development of round, well demarcated lesions throughout the lungs 0·5–5 cm. in diameter after exposure to a variety of dusts such as those encountered in coal mines, potteries, sand blasting, iron foundries and even asbestos industries should raise the suspicion of a rheumatoid pneumoconiosis. In such cases there is usually a significantly raised titre of *rheumatoid factor* (sheep cell agglutinating factor)—thus, about 75 per cent. of patients with typical rheumatoid pneumoconiosis have titres of 1 in 640 or above. The remainder are negative at all titres. This form of pneumoconiosis

TABLE 49

ILO/UICC CLASSIFICATION OF RADIOGRAPHIC APPEARANCES OF PNEUMOCONIOSES

		CODES	DEFINITIONS
SMALL OPACITIES	*Rounded* Profusion	0/– 0/0 0/1 1/0 1/1 1/2 2/1 2/2 2/3 3/2 3/3 3/4	The category of profusion is based on assessment of the concentration of opacities in the affected zones. The standard films define the mid categories. Category 0—small rounded opacities absent or less profuse than in category 1. Category 1—small rounded opacities definitely present but relatively few in number. Category 2—small rounded opacities numerous. The normal lung markings are usually still visible. Category 3—small rounded opacities very numerous. The normal lung markings are partly or totally obscured.
	Type	p q r	The nodules are classified according to the approximate diameter of the predominant opacities. p—rounded opacities up to about 1·5 mm. diameter. q—rounded opacities exceeding about 1·5 mm. and up to about 3 mm. diameter. r—rounded opacities exceeding about 3 mm. and up to about 10 mm. diameter.
	Extent	Lung zones	The zones in which the opacities are seen are recorded. Each lung is divided into thirds—upper, middle, lower zones. Thus a maximum of 6 zones can be affected.
	Irregular Profusion	0/– 0/0 0/1 1/0 1/1 1/2 2/1 2/2 2/3 3/2 3/3 3/4	The category of profusion is based on assessment of the concentration of opacities in the affected zones. The standard films define the mid categories. Category 0—small irregular opacities absent or less profuse than in category 1. Category 1—small irregular opacities definitely present but relatively few in number. The normal lung markings are usually visible. Category 2—small irregular opacities numerous. The normal lung markings are usually partly obscured. Category 3—small irregular opacities very numerous. The normal lung markings are usually totally obscured.
	Type	s t u	As the opacities are irregular, the dimensions used for rounded opacities cannot be used, but they can be roughly divided into three types. s—fine irregular or linear opacities. t—medium irregular opacities. u—coarse (blotchyl) irregular opacities.
	Extent	Lung zones	The zones in which the opacities are seen are recorded. Each lung is divided into thirds—upper, middle, lower zones—as for rounded opacities.
LARGE OPACITIES	Size	A B C	Category A—an opacity with greatest diameter between 1 cm. and 5 cm., or several such opacities the sum of whose greatest diameters does not exceed 5 cm. Category B—one or more opacities larger or more numerous than those in category A, whose combined area does not exceed one third of the area of the right lung. Category C—one or more large opacities whose combined area exceeds one third of the area of the right lung.
	Type	wd id	As well as the letter 'A', 'B' or 'C', the abbreviation 'wd' or 'id' should be used to indicate whether the opacities are well defined or ill defined.
OTHER FEATURES	*Pleural thickening* Costophrenic angle	Right Left	Obliteration of the costophrenic angle is recorded separately from thickening over other sites. A lower limit standard film is provided.
	Other sites	1 2 3	Grade 0—not present or less than grade 1. Grade 1—up to 5 mm. thick and not exceeding one half of the projection of one lateral chest wall. A lower limit standard film is provided. Grade 2—more than 5 mm. thick and up to one half of the projection of one lateral chest wall *or* up to 5 mm. thick and exceeding one half of the projection of one lateral chest wall. Grade 3—more than 5 mm. thick and extending more than one half of the projection of one lateral chest wall.
	Diaphragm Ill defined	Right Left	The lower limit is one third of the affected hemidiaphragm. A lower limit standard film is provided.
	Cardiac outline Ill defined (shagginess)	1 2 3	Grade 0—up to one third of the length of the left cardiac border or equivalent. Grade 1—above one third and up to two thirds of the length of the left cardiac border or equivalent. Grade 2—above two thirds and up to the whole length of the left cardiac border or equivalent. Grade 3—more than the whole length of the left cardiac border or equivalent.

	CODES	DEFINITIONS
Pleural calcification Diaphragm Walls Other sites	1 2 3	Grade 0—no pleural calcification seen. Grade 1—one or more areas of pleural calcification, the sum of whose greatest diameters does not exceed 2 cm. Grade 2—one or more areas of pleural calcification, the sum of whose greatest diameters exceeds 2 cm. but does not exceed 10 cm. Grade 3—one or more areas of pleural calcification, the sum of whose greatest diameters exceeds 10 cm.

OTHER SYMBOLS

OBLIGATORY

- ca —suspect cancer of lung or pleura.
- co —abnormality of cardiac size or shape.
- cp —suspect cor pulmonale.
- es —eggshell calcification of hilar or mediastinal lymph nodes.
- tba—opacities suggestive of active clinically significant tuberculosis.
- od —other significant disease. This includes disease not related to dust exposure, e.g. surgical or traumatic damage to chest walls, bronchiectasis, etc.

OPTIONAL

- ax —coalescence of small rounded pneumoconiotic opacities.
- bu—bullae.
- cn —calcification in small parenchymal opacities.
- cv —cavity.
- di —marked distortion of the intra-thoracic organs.
- em—marked emphysema.
- hi —marked enlargement of hilar shadows.
- ho—honeycomb lung.
- k —Kerley (septal) lines.
- px—pneumothorax.
- rl —pneumoconiosis modified by rheumatoid process.
- tb —inactive tuberculosis.

[Reproduced by permission of the Director-General, International Labour Office, Geneva.]

The ILO (Geneva 1958) description of X-ray appearances is being replaced by the ILO/UICC (1971) classification. Besides recording their opinions observers should also record whether they considered any other categorization, for example 1/2 means that the observer categorized the appearance as simple pneumoconiosis in category 1 but considered category 2. Difficulty is most likely to occur in distinguishing normal films. 0/– is a 'barn door' normal, with exceptional clarity of normal architecture. 0/0 is a film with small opacities absent or less profuse than in category 1 and in 0/1 but within the bounds of normality the film is normal, but category 1 was considered. If 3 observers of equal competence read each film of a series, interobserver differences can be used to distinguish degrees of normality (or abnormality) falling within a given category: for example, films read as 0/0, 0/0, 0/0; 0/0, 0/0, 0/1; 0/0, 0/1, 0/1, though all normal, differ in a subtle way. Statistical treatment can be applied. The description p, q and r replace p, m and n, and indicate small rounded opacities in simple pneumoconiosis, s, t, u are descriptions applied to small irregular opacities (such as seen in asbestosis).

may precede, coincide with, or follow the development of rheumatoid arthritis.

Radiologically, the shadows are more circular than is the case with straightforward P.M.F. Further, they are distributed throughout the lungs rather than in the upper zones and develop in crops, often more rapidly than is the case with P.M.F. There is less evidence of the underlying pneumoconiosis.

Histologically, there is a peripheral zone of active inflammation with polymorphs in necrotic collagen and disintegrating macrophages containing the original dust around concentric rings of previous activity. Around the lesions there are aggregates of leucocytes and plasma cells; rheumatoid factor with immunoglobulin (IgM) may be demonstrated by immunofluorescence intra- and extracellularly. These lesions may remain static or progress, cavitate and calcify and even coalesce into much larger masses resembling P.M.F. The relationship of this particular tissue response in dust-conditioned lung to the development of pneumoconiosis in general remains obscure. Speculation would suggest that two variables may be responsible for the final tissue response —first, the ability of the dust to modify and impair macrophages with liberation of fibrogenic material, and secondly immunological factors of the same nature as rheumatoid factor [see Section 10].

COAL WORKERS' PNEUMOCONIOSIS

Synonym. Anthracosis.

Definition

Pneumoconiosis due to inhalation of coal dust. This may be simple or complicated (P.M.F.).

Pathogenesis

Fine particles of coal dust, mainly 1–5 microns in diameter, are deposited in the smallest airways and the alveoli. In the latter they are ingested by macrophages and either pass through the alveolar wall to the lymphatics or are transported to the respiratory bronchiolus. From thence most of the dust is removed up the airways. Clearance is slowest from alveoli adjacent to the pleura, the interlobular septa and blood vessels and dust particles in excess inside and outside macrophages tend to clog the alveoli around the respiratory bronchioli, where, on histological section, aggregates or plaques of dust can be seen. Coal dust is not particularly toxic to macrophages and reticulin formation and fibrosis are minimal. There is experimental evidence to suggest that if silica (quartz) is mixed with coal dust in the same particle size in a ratio of more than 1 to 50 then fibrosis is more likely to develop. The ability of coal dust to cause structural damage such as centri-acinar (centrilobular) emphysema is not established and there is no evidence that the incidence of carcinoma of the lung is increased in this disorder.

The over-all incidence of P.M.F. among working miners is about 1 per cent., with an incidence of 4 per cent. in South Wales. The proportion of cases of the simple form of coal workers' pneumoconiosis which develops P.M.F. varies considerably from 5 to 50 per cent. [p. 905]. The incidence of rheumatoid pneumoconiosis (Caplan's syndrome) as a complication is variable. Although there is no strict relationship to the amount of dust inhaled, P.M.F. tends to develop more often in miners with category 2 and 3 pneumoconiosis than category 1.

TABLE 50

SOME LUNG DISEASES WITH WIDESPREAD MICRONODULAR AND NODULAR SHADOWS

Bronchiolitis Some pneumonias, e.g. virus mycoplasma Miliary tuberculosis Mycoses, e.g. histoplasmosis coccidioidomycosis blastomycosis Sarcoidosis Histiocytosis X Mesodermal dysplasia { tuberous sclerosis Lymphomata, e.g. Hodgkin's disease Carcinomatosis: miliary bronchiolar	Pneumoconiosis (*Mineral dust*) e.g. coal, silica, mixed dust, talc, beryllium, iron (siderosis), tin (stannosis), barium (*Organic dust*) e.g. extrinsic allergic alveolitis: → farmer's lung, bagassosis { see TABLE 51 p. 913 Alveolitis → cryptogenic → with rheumatoid arthritis polyarteritis nodosa, other connective tissue disorders Idiopathic haemosiderosis Pulmonary alveolar proteinosis

There is difference of opinion as to the degree and nature of the *physiological impairment* which can properly be attributed to the deposition of dust. Undoubtedly, normal function is frequently found with advanced simple pneumoconiosis. Symptoms and impaired ventilatory capacity are as likely to be the result of cigarette smoking, which is so common in coal miners, as any other factor. The excess incidence of physiological impairment may be attributable to inhalation of coal dust, which itself may be an accessory cause of mucus hypersecretion (chronic bronchitis). From large-scale studies in the United Kingdom it is claimed by some that ventilatory capacity is little affected by simple pneumoconiosis, but by others that the ventilatory capacity is slightly but significantly impaired in advanced forms (category 3). The residual volume of the lung (RV) has been found to be greater in coal workers than in non-miners with a similar degree of airways obstruction, but this did not correlate with the degree of radiological shadowing. Studies of lung compliance have been inadequate and conflicting, but gas transfer may be impaired, especially in patients whose radiographs show pinhead (less than 1·5 mm.) as opposed to micronodular shadows (1·5–3 mm.).

Coal workers' pneumoconiosis is by far the most common occupational lung disease in the United Kingdom. The number of cases reported annually, however, is falling. Thus, 3279 cases were reported in 1960 and by 1964 this had fallen to 1213. This fall can be attributed as much to a drop in the total population of miners as to improved control of coal dust. There is a great variation from region to region in the incidence of coal workers' pneumoconiosis: thus, while the average rate in the United Kingdom was about 2·4 per 1,000 active miners in 1964, that for South Wales was 7·5 per 1,000 and for Northumberland 0·2 per 1,000. These differences are assumed to be due to varying concentrations of dust in the pits and to differences in composition of the coal—both physical (hardness, etc.) and chemical (e.g. content of minerals other than carbon).

Clinical Picture

Simple pneumoconiosis is not associated with symptoms or physical signs. When these are present they indicate that the pneumoconiosis is complicated by chronic bronchitis [p. 883], or progressive massive fibrosis (P.M.F.). Cough, sputum and breathlessness are most likely to be due, therefore, to chronic bronchitis, while haemoptysis and breathlessness occur with P.M.F. Grosser forms of P.M.F. will produce distortion of the lung with production of the physical signs of pulmonary fibrosis [PLATE 12].

Diagnosis

Chest radiography is essential in the diagnosis of simple pneumoconiosis of coal workers and the appearances must be differentiated from the large numbers of disorders that can produce widespread pinhead, micronodular or nodular type shadows [see TABLE 50]. The occupational history and the absence of clinical evidence of other disease are of the greatest importance.

An international classification of the radiological changes in coal workers' pneumoconiosis is shown in TABLE 50. Although this was based on a study of coal miners, it is a valuable classification for description of many of the pneumoconioses due to inhalation of mineral dusts.

Treatment

Prevention is all important, for there is no treatment of the established condition. Prevention consists in the proper application of methods to suppress dust formation and dissemination in the mines. Miners should be screened clinically, radiologically and where possible physiologically and where pneumoconiosis is suspected the diagnosis should be confirmed and the miner's case reviewed. Where progression from minimal change is detected, alternative employment should be considered. In the United Kingdom benefits can be claimed under the National Insurance (Industrial Injuries) Act of 1946.

SILICOSIS

Definition

A pneumoconiosis due to inhalation of dusts containing silica.

Pathogenesis

Particles of silica, mainly from 1 to 5 microns in size, when inhaled may cause silicosis. Varieties of silica in the form of silicon oxide (free silica) are usually responsible and of these quartz is the most important. Others, such as tridymite, cristobalite and vitreous silica are less so. These forms are equally soluble but vary in their ability to cause fibrosis. Silicates, such as stericite and mica, talc and kaolin are less fibrogenic.

The industries in which significant concentrations of silica may be found are:

1. Mining in which there is a high proportion of silica-containing rock together with the mineral under exploitation, especially gold, copper, tin, graphite and less often coal.
2. Quarrying of granite, slate, etc.
3. Trimming and crushing of stone with a high quartz content.
4. Sand blasting and metal casting.
5. Pottery and ceramics.
6. Trimming of refractory bricks and boiler scaling.

The particles of silica dust are taken up by macrophages, to which they are more lethal than coal dust. The tissue reaction consequent upon disruption of the cell is mainly collagenous and the fibrous tissue caused by silica dust is very much less than that produced by an equivalent amount of coal dust. The nature of the response is almost certainly immunological, although the composition of the silica 'antigen' is unknown. Evidence suggesting that this is an immunological reaction is: (1) about 60 per cent. of the nodule is composed of beta and gamma globulin; (2) serum globulin is increased; and (3) plasma cells are found in excess. The immunological theory for the development of silicosis is now preferred to the silica solubility theory, in which silicic acid, formed by the very slow solution of silica, was thought to have a direct action on tissues causing fibrosis. This acid may well impair enzyme systems within macrophages. Rheumatoid pneumoconiosis may complicate silicosis, in which case there is an accelerated immune response, but the basic tissue response is similar.

Silicotic nodules vary from microscopic size to 1 cm. in size and are composed of concentric layers of collagen fibres embedded in an amorphous matrix with a high globulin concentration. Around the lesion there are particles of silica with or without carbon. Calcification occasionally develops, often at the periphery. Some particles are transported by the lymphatics to the lymph nodes, where characteristic collagenous nodules may be found. Extensive fibrosis may develop round the pulmonary blood vessels, bronchi and lymphatics and progressive massive fibrosis (P.M.F.) may complicate the picture [p. 905].

The effects of silicosis on pulmonary function are uncertain and widespread lung involvement may be associated with normal function. In the later stages of the disease, with more extensive fibrosis but without P.M.F., then a restrictive defect of ventilatory capacity may be found together with impairment of gas transfer. Inequality of ventilation and blood flow with physiological shunting also develop, particularly with progressive massive fibrosis.

Clinical Picture

Rapid development of breathlessness and constitutional symptoms some months after exposure to the millstone grit component of abrasive soaps was a rare form of silicosis, which has been abolished by the substitution of carborundum. Patients frequently died in respiratory failure within weeks of the onset.

The classical chronic form of the disease has no symptoms or signs until late in the course of the disease when fibrosis is advanced or P.M.F. has developed. Then breathlessness and haemoptysis may occur and the physical signs are those described for progressive massive fibrosis. Silicosis was also frequently associated with an indolent form of tuberculosis which might add to the symptoms and signs.

Diagnosis

This rests upon a careful occupational history in association with chest radiography, for physical signs are so frequently absent.

The *chest radiograph* shows widespread pinhead, micronodular or nodular shadows throughout both lungs. These evolve slowly and are often more marked in the upper and middle zones. These underlying appearances may be complicated by P.M.F. or rheumatoid pneumoconiosis. The radiological differential diagnosis is to be found in TABLE 49 on page 906, but the occupational history on the one hand and careful clinical appraisal on the other help to clarify the diagnosis. In all cases sputum should be examined for *Myco. tuberculosis*, the miliary form of which may simulate silicosis, as may sarcoidosis.

Management

There are no measures for treating silicosis. Prevention, notification and regular observation are the same as for coal workers' pneumoconiosis.

Course and Prognosis

Silicosis develops many years after initial exposure to the dust and usually progresses after removal from exposure. Complications such as progressive massive fibrosis and pulmonary tuberculosis demand careful follow-up. The incidence of carcinoma of the lung or any other neoplasm is not increased in silicosis.

ASBESTOSIS

Definition

A pneumoconiosis due to inhalation of dust containing asbestos.

Pathogenesis

Asbestos fibre occurs naturally in rock form and is mined in many parts of the world. There are six chief varieties of the mineral which are composed of various silicates of magnesium, iron and calcium, nickel and aluminium.

1. Crysotile (Canada, Rhodesia and U.S.S.R.) and anthophyllite (Scandinavia) contain mainly magnesium. Crysotile is soft and silky and is easily woven into heat and acid resistant material. It is the most widely used form.
2. Amosite (South Africa) and crocidolite (South

Africa, Bolivia and Australia) contain mainly iron. Amosite is used mainly for heat insulation, crocidolite for acid resistant material, mainly in the chemical industry. They both contain traces of 3:4 benzpyrene.

3. Tremolite and actinolyte (Italy) contain calcium and are used in filters, paper, etc.

The filaments of the fibrous rock vary in length from millimetres to centimetres and are stronger than steel. They also resist fire, water, acid and alkalies. Because of these properties the demand for asbestos has grown vastly. World production has risen from 300,000 tons in 1934 to 3 million tons in 1967. It has innumerable uses in ship building, electrical and heat insulation, refrigeration, the paper, textile, engineering and plastics industries and many others.

The mining, manufacture and disposal of asbestos create dust which may be inhaled and retained not only by people at work but also by those living nearby. As there is a lag of 20–40 years for the pathological effects of inhaled asbestos to become manifest, the sharp increase in its use in recent years may see a considerable increase in the incidence of disease in the next few decades. From 1959 to 1967 the number of cases of asbestosis notified in the United Kingdom rose from 37 to 168. The control of asbestos dust in manufacture, use and waste becomes more and more difficult as its use is diversified. About half the cases of asbestosis at the present time are discovered in *unscheduled* occupations, such as lagging, brake lining and spraying.

The microscopic fibres in the inhaled and retained dust are up to 50 microns long and 0·5 microns wide. Because the diameter of the fibre is very narrow the settling velocity is slow. This probably allows the particle to reach the smallest conducting airways and even the respiratory bronchioles. Its long and narrow shape may determine its distribution mainly down the axial pathways of the lung to the lower zones.

The relative ability of the various types of asbestos to cause fibrosis in man is not yet known and the pathogenesis unclear: that is, whether it causes damage by direct chemical or physical injury, or whether the process has to be mediated by an intracellular stage, as is thought to be the case with silica and coal dust.

Apart from the development of *fibrosis*, asbestos particles in the lung may be associated with:

Asbestos Bodies. The coating of microscopic asbestos fibrils with protein material often with a bulbous thickening over the sharp point of fracture gives rise to characteristic asbestos bodies. The asbestos body is less fragile and more flexible than asbestos alone and may disintegrate over the years. In this form asbestos is less fibrogenic in the guinea-pig than in the uncoated form. Asbestos bodies in smears and sections of the lung are a reliable and useful indication of the degree of exposure to dust containing asbestos. Asbestos bodies are found in sections and smears of lung in a considerable proportion of routine necropsies—reports vary from about 10 to 50 per cent. In one report from London asbestos bodies were found in section in 28 of 115 specimens routinely examined at autopsy. There is evidence to suggest that asbestos bodies are found with a higher frequency in the lungs of town dwellers than country folk.

Pleural Plaques. Discrete elevated greyish hyaline plaques are found chiefly in the parietal pleura of men between the ages of 50 and 60. They vary in size and shape and are often bilateral. There is often focal calcification in the laminated hyaline collagen. There is good evidence to support the association of this type of pleural plaque with asbestos, although how the asbestos fibril gains access to the serosa and then causes a tissue reaction is unknown. In one large series of pleural plaques found at necropsy, 85 per cent. were radiologically invisible in life. In the majority of these cases no histological evidence of pulmonary fibrosis could be found, whereas those with radiological evidence of pleural plaques (which at necropsy were large and often calcified) were found to have pulmonary fibrosis. In all 56 cases with hyaline plaques, asbestos bodies were found in sections of the lung (compared with 24 per cent. of the controls). There was a significant history of exposure to asbestos in those with pleural calcification seen in the chest X-ray. Thus, there may be a dose response relationship between on the one hand the degree of asbestos exposure (from no close contact with a known source of asbestos to close contact with a major source); and on the other hand, the number of asbestos bodies in the lung, the extent and the degree of calcification of pleural plaques and therefore their radio-density and histological fibrosis. Pleural plaques may be due to other causes, e.g. tuberculosis and in some parts of the United Kingdom and elsewhere in Europe, e.g. Czechoslovakia, pleural thickening and calcification have been found on chest radiography where asbestos could not be implicated.

Carcinoma of the Lung. While there is no histological or epidemiological evidence to suggest that asbestos is an important factor in the genesis of carcinoma of the lung in general, the incidence of carcinoma of the lung is eight times that expected in workers heavily exposed to asbestos in certain textile mills. Workers less heavily exposed for the same length of time show no increased incidence. The variation in reported incidence of carcinoma in association with asbestos dust may be the result therefore of differing periods and degree of exposure as well as to qualitative differences in the dust itself, e.g. its content of chromium, nickel, cobalt and benzpyrene. Pulmonary fibrosis is usually found as well (for other aspects of carcinoma of the lung, see page 897).

Mesothelioma. There is strong evidence linking asbestos exposure to the development of mesothelioma of the pleura and peritoneum. The number of reports of this association are increasing from many parts of the world, including South Africa, the United Kingdom and the United States. In the United Kingdom the incidence of mesothelioma is highest in London and in ship building towns. No cases, however, have been reported from Finland, where men have been exposed to *anthophyllite* for more than 3 months between 1935 and 1967. In Canada, where *chrysotile* alone is produced, no excess of incidence of mesothelioma has been found. Furthermore, while there has been a large number of proven cases of mesothelioma in those mining and milling *crocidolite* in the North West Cape area of South Africa (or indeed resident there), no cases have been found, using the same criteria and methods of investigation, in similar groups in the Transvaal, where large quantities of *crocidolite* are mined. The relationship, therefore, of specific types of asbestos to the development of mesothelioma remains speculative. It is possible that only limited exposure to asbestos may be sufficient to produce this growth up to 30 or 40 years later, but the association of rare cases of mesothelioma to environmental pollution with asbestos dust in persons not clearly exposed to asbestos also remains speculative. Mesothelioma of the pleura may develop with pleural plaques as well and like pleural plaques may appear without underlying pulmonary fibrosis [PLATE 12]. On the other hand all of the eleven cases in a series of peritoneal tumours reported in 1964 had histological evidence of asbestosis in the lung. The diagnosis of mesothelioma is often difficult, even with histological material available. This is particularly so for carcinoma of the lung may spread diffusely to the pleura and resemble a mesothelial tumour. (For clinical aspects, see page 897).

PULMONARY FIBROSIS

Pathology

Commonly, *pulmonary fibrosis* develops from reticulin laid down in relation to disintegrated macrophages, asbestos fibrils and dust particles within the respiratory bronchioli. A fibrotic network develops mainly in the lower lobes, in which asbestos bodies may be found. 'Honeycomb' changes may develop. This fibrous network usually involves the adjacent pleura as well. Tuberculosis is probably more prevalent in asbestosis than in otherwise normal people and in 1955 30 per cent. of deaths in those exposed to asbestos were reported to be complicated by tuberculosis. On the other hand, 13 per cent. had neoplasia of the lung or pleura.

Fibrosis may exert a profound effect on function of the lung before radiological changes can be seen. The earliest change is a reduction in gas transfer (T_{CO}). With further impairment of function lung compliance is reduced and a restrictive defect of ventilatory capacity becomes measurable (reduction in vital capacity and total lung capacity), together with the effects of inequality of ventilation and blood flow. Respiratory failure and terminal right ventricular failure may develop.

Clinical Picture

The first symptom is breathlessness, which may become extremely severe. This tends to be accompanied by a dry cough, weight loss and fatigue. On examination, finger clubbing is commonly found and crepitations are characteristically heard at the bases of the lungs. Respiratory failure may be manifest as cyanosis, at first on exertion. The signs of right ventricular failure are a late manifestation. Other physical signs in this pneumoconiosis include those due to *pleural effusion* and *pleural thickening*. When the latter is gross, mesothelioma should be suspected. Signs of *tuberculosis* and *carcinoma of the lung* might also coexist.

Diagnosis

Asbestos bodies are an irregular finding in the sputum, and their presence can only be taken as evidence of exposure. The radiological appearances of the lungs vary from pinhead and micronodular shadows, mainly in the lower parts of the lungs, to gross linear shadowing with distortion of the lung and pleura. This gives a characteristic puckered and tattered appearance round the heart shadow, diaphragm and lower pleura. Calcification may be seen in the pleura. A history of exposure to asbestos, the physical signs of clubbing of the fingers and crepitations together with the physiological findings of defective gas transfer with or without a restrictive defect of ventilatory capacity which may precede the radiological changes usually make the diagnosis. Asbestosis, however, must be differentiated from other forms of pneumoconiosis, fibrosing alveolitis and honeycomb lung, etc.

Treatment

As with other pneumoconioses, no treatment has been found to influence the course of the disease and this includes adrenocorticosteroids.

Prevention is fraught with difficulty for two reasons: (1) the very diverse nature of handling of asbestos in industry; and (2) the unknown effects of limited exposure to asbestos.

The maximum practicable reduction of dust liberated in any industry where it is used should be the aim. Meanwhile, patients who have any of the manifestations of disease due to asbestos should be removed from exposure. Superimposed tuberculosis should respond to chemotherapy as described on page 871.

Course and Prognosis

Asbestosis usually progresses even after removal from exposure and over a period of years may terminate in respiratory and right ventricular failure. A proportion of patients (up to one third) will develop superimposed pulmonary tuberculosis but with treatment this should not affect prognosis. Carcinoma of the lung will develop with eight to ten times the expected incidence, but it is reported to be rare in this pneumoconiosis when the worker is a non-smoker. Mesothelioma of the pleura or peritoneum is a very real threat in those with established pulmonary and pleural fibrosis, although the exact incidence is not known. With either growth the prognosis is usually hopeless.

BERYLLIOSIS

Definition

A pneumoconiosis due to inhalation of dust containing beryllium.

Pathogenesis

Beryllium causes disease not only in the lung but contact with this substance also causes disease of the skin. Beryllium is of low density and possesses many physical properties that are valuable in the manufacture of alloys (e.g. mixture containing 2 per cent. of beryllium with copper), in atomic reactors, ceramics, fluorescent lighting, etc. The latter use has ceased since the toxicity was encountered by workers in the industry. Poisoning has been reported in those living near a beryllium plant and in those laundering contaminated clothes.

Beryllium is biologically very active and exposure to dust containing the metal, its oxide, salts or silicates may provoke an acute inflammatory response in the skin or a chronic granulomatous process involving tissues other than the skin and lung which resemble sarcoidosis.

The host response to beryllium suggests a hypersensitivity reaction for the following reasons:

1. The onset of the acute process occurs 10 to 14 days after exposure.
2. Involvement of small proportions of those exposed.
3. Considerable variation in degree of exposure required to produce disease.
4. The presence of skin hypersensitivity and sensitization of individuals by small amounts of intracutaneous beryllium.

Although experimental neoplasia (skin and bone) has been induced by beryllium in animals, there is no evidence of such a link in man, either in the lung or elsewhere.

Acute Berylliosis. Usually within 10–14 days of exposure certain individuals develop skin lesions—an acute dermatitis in the exposed parts—and this is followed by acute laryngotracheobronchitis dominated by a pneumonitis with severe breathlessness, cough and cyanosis. There is diffuse miliary micronodular shadowing in the chest radiograph. This rare illness may cause death in the acute stages, but the majority recover and only about 1 in 10 progress to a chronic form of the disease.

Chronic Berylliosis. This has been chiefly reported from the United States and has been seen only rarely in the United Kingdom or elsewhere. The onset is extremely insidious and may develop many years after quite limited exposure. The disease process, a sarcoid-like granulomatous reaction with fibrosis, continues after exposure has stopped. The lungs are diffusely involved, usually with enlargement of the hilar nodes, but the lesions may involve the liver, spleen and other lymph nodes. Skin lesions resemble those of sarcoidosis too and implantation of beryllium particles in the skin may give an ulcerating granulomatous lesion. Involvement of the eye, parotid gland or bone has not been reported. Complaints of breathlessness, cough, weight loss, fatigue and anorexia may be noted. Clubbing of the fingers is reported in one third of cases, but physical signs are not usually found in the chest.

The chest radiograph is usually striking, with diffuse miliary shadowing varying from pinhead to nodular (1–5 mm. in size). The shadowing is often profuse without coalescence or cavitation and calcification is rare. Diffuse reticulation may also develop with or without hilar node enlargement. The hilar nodes are usually less conspicuous than in sarcoid and do not enlarge without lung shadowing. There is often a rise in the gamma globulin fraction of plasma proteins and even hypercalciuria has been reported. Disturbance in lung function resembles that in sarcoidosis.

Differentiation from sarcoidosis can clearly be very difficult. An occupational history is of the greatest importance. Beryllium can be detected in tissues and urine of normal people and conversely it may be absent in affected individuals. A patch test with beryllium fluoride (1 per cent.) or sulphate (2 per cent.) applied for 48 hours and read at 72 hours is usually but not always positive in affected individuals in whom the Kveim test is negative. Unfortunately, this skin test with beryllium may sensitize subjects and exacerbate symptoms.

Treatment

Prevention should be achieved by reducing environmental concentration of beryllium to safe levels. This is reported from the United States Atomic Energy Commission in 1948 to be as follows:

1. An average concentration less than 2 μg. per mm^3. during 8 hours (peak not to exceed 25 μg. per mm^3.).
2. Average monthly concentration of less than 0·1 μg. per mm^3. in the neighbourhood of plants.

These levels are practicable and can be achieved by the proper control of the processing of beryllium. Handling of contaminated clothing must be avoided. Masks and respirators must be used with concentrations above 25 μg. per mm^3.

Acute berylliosis requires immediate treatment with oxygen and adrenocortical steroids (300 mg. of hydrocortisone intravenously in the first 24 hours with prednisone, 50 mg. daily). As control of the disease is achieved, the dose of prednisone should be gradually reduced. Corticosteroids such as prednisone are given in doses of from 10 to 20 mg. a day in chronic berylliosis in an attempt to reduce the development of fibrosis. This treatment may need to be continued for long periods, even for years. Inactivation of beryllium in the tissue with chelating agents, such as aurintricarboxylic acid, although effective in animals has not been proved successful in man.

Course and Prognosis

The disease may remain stationary for years or may progress slowly or quite rapidly over 1–15 years, terminating in cardiorespiratory failure.

OTHER PNEUMOCONIOSES

Aluminium

Pneumoconioses due to aluminium develop under two different conditions:

1. In those exposed to aluminium powder in which the metal is uncoated with lubricants such as stearin. Pulmonary fibrosis due to this dust was reported in the explosives industry in Germany during the Second World War and from the fireworks industry and others using aluminium powder elsewhere. The fibrosis may be quite rapid and cause severe breathlessness with a high incidence of spontaneous pneumothorax. On the other hand the progress of the fibrosis may be slow and found incidentally. In the United Kingdom no evidence of respiratory disease was found in an extensive survey of workers in industries preparing or using aluminium.
2. In those exposed to aluminium oxide (bauxite) during the manufacture of abrasive wheels (Shaver's disease). Bauxite is ground and intimately mixed with iron and coke and then fused at 2,000° C. between car-

TABLE 51

OTHER INHALED OCCUPATIONAL DISEASES

SUBSTANCES	COMMON NAME	PROCESS	PATHOLOGICAL FINDINGS	RADIOLOGICAL CHANGES
MINERAL DUSTS Tungsten and other carbides (silicon) Cobalt	Hard metal disease	Manufacture of cutting tools, bonding tungsten and other carbides with cobalt and shaping with silicon or diamond.	Pulmonary fibrosis	Micronodular shadows Linear shadows
Iron oxide	Siderotic lung disease (a) Silver polisher's lung	Iron oxide powder – in manufacture of silverware	No fibrosis	Pinhead or micronodular shadows
	(b) Arc welder's lung	Welding and oxyacetylene cutting Pure iron oxide fume → Impure iron (+ silica, etc.) →	No fibrosis Fibrosis	Pinhead or micronodular shadows (reversible)
	(c) Haematite miners U.K., Belgium, Sweden, N. America	Mining of iron oxide ore without silica → with silica →	No fibrosis Fibrosis (siderosilicosis) Increased incidence of bronchial carcinoma	Pinhead or micronodular as in silicosis
Tin oxide Antimony, emery, etc. Barium	Stannosis (benign pneumoconiosis due to tin oxide) Baritosis	Smelting	Deposition of dust No fibrosis No dysfunction	Dense pinhead shadows micronodular shadows
ORGANIC DUSTS	Farmer's lung Bagassosis	See p. 914 and TABLE 52	Extrinsic allergic alveolitis	
Cotton, hemp, flax, sisal dust	Byssinosis (world wide)	See p. 916	Bronchoconstriction Chronic bronchitis	
FUMES AND GASES Ammonia, chlorine phosgene Sulphur di- and trioxides		Chemical manufacture	Pulmonary oedema ?chronic bronchitis	Pulmonary oedema
Oxides of nitrogen (esp. NO_2 and N_2O_4)	Silo filler's disease	Decomposing corn ($\rightarrow NO_2$)	Acute broncho-pulmonary oedema	Pulmonary oedema
	Mining Chemical industry Welding	Oxidation of nitrogen from atmosphere Plastics and nitro-cellulose	Obliterative bronchiolitis Pulmonary fibrosis	Fibrosis
Cadmium		Copper alloys, electro-plating, welding, atomic reactor control rods	Acute bronchopulmonary oedema Emphysema	Pulmonary oedema Emphysema
Toluene di-isocyanate		Manufacture of plastic foam	Bronchoconstriction (hypersensitivity) (purpura)	

bon electrodes. Dense white fumes are emitted which contain 7 per cent. silica, an aluminium oxide, ferric oxide and traces of other constituents. Six per cent. of men exposed to this process in Canada developed respiratory symptoms within months due to oedema, followed by interstitial fibrosis and emphysema. Spontaneous pneumothorax occurred in about a third of these people and about the same proportion died. Silica and aluminium were found in the ash of the lungs at post-mortem.

Other Inhalational Occupational Diseases

These are summarized in TABLE 51.

EXTRINSIC ALLERGIC ALVEOLITIS

Definition

A diffuse inflammatory process involving the gas exchanging tissue of the lung with cellular thickening of the alveolar walls with a tendency to fibrosis, and large mononuclear cells in the alveolar spaces, due to inhalation of organic dusts.

Pathogenesis

Inhalation of organic dusts, often of vegetable or microbial origin, may cause an immunologically determined inflammatory response in the peripheral gas exchanging tissue of the lung in sensitized individuals. Characteristically an allergic response in the *airways* manifests as bronchoconstriction (e.g. extrinsic allergic asthma) in atopic subjects and is mediated by a non-precipitating reaginic antibody, probably the immunoglobulin IgE (type 1 hypersensitivity of Gell and Coombs): *alveolar* reactions to a wide variety of organic dusts are mediated by *precipitating* antibody (Arthus type 3 hypersensitivity of Gell and Coombs). The subjects of this reaction are usually non-atopic, and a more intense antigenic stimulus is required than is the case in atopic asthma. Nevertheless, on occasion an organic dust may provoke both a bronchial and alveolar response in the same individual.

Conditions Required for the Development of Allergic Alveolitis:

1. Particle size of the organic dust must permit adequate concentration reaching and remaining in the alveoli (i.e. size 1–5 microns approximately).

2. The concentration of the dust in the alveoli must be sufficient to provoke an immune response in the form of precipitating antibody—detection of such antibody can be taken as evidence of exposure to the dust. These antibodies tend to disappear when exposure ceases.

3. The development of hypersensitivity—only a proportion of those exposed to organic dusts and in whom precipitating antibodies can be detected develop the clinical and other features of allergic alveolitis—thus, while 15–20 per cent. of farmers have antibodies to farmer's lung hay antigenic extracts, only a proportion develop farmer's lung. Similarly with bird fanciers, malt workers, etc. In the case of some organic dusts, e.g. coffee, sisal, etc. those exposed often develop antibodies, but so far allergic alveolitis has not been observed.

While evidence of hypersensitivity may be inferred from immediate and delayed type reactions to intradermal injections of the extracts of the relevant organic dusts (e.g. in bird fancier's lung) this evidence may be unreliable or absent, e.g. in farmer's lung. To establish a causal relationship between a suspected inhaled organic dust and a hypersensitivity or allergic alveolitis, it is necessary to perform inhalation tests. In such tests, 5–6 hours after inhalation of an aerosol of a suitable dilution of the organic dust containing the antigen, there are systemic symptoms, such as malaise, aches and pains and fever, breathlessness, cough and tightness in the chest. Crepitations may be heard in the lung. A transient dominantly neutrophil leucocytosis is found in the blood. Tests of lung function show a reduction of lung compliance with a fall in vital capacity, without change in airway resistance, most easily measured by spirometry (VC, FVC, and FEV_1)—together with an impairment of gas transfer (T_{CO}). There is sometimes diffuse patchy but transient radiological shadowing. These manifestations are similar to the clinical state after heavy exposure to dust.

4. The clinical presentation of allergic alveolitis depends on the concentration and duration of exposure. Thus, there may be:

(a) Acute episodes similar to that described after inhalation testing which follows 6–8 hours after intermittent heavy exposure to the dust, e.g. in pigeon fanciers after clearing out a loft.

(b) An insidious development of respiratory symptoms and clinical evidence in those with frequent but limited exposure, e.g. budgerigar fanciers. In this latter group, the insidious onset may obscure the nature of the disorder and make diagnosis difficult.

(c) There may be a combined onset which may further be confused by the development of an immediate bronchial response with wheezing and breathlessness on exposure to the dust.

Some organic dusts known (or strongly suspected) to cause alveolitis and situations in which they are encountered are listed in TABLE 52.

Management in general is concerned with removal of the cause of the dust from the environment, e.g. birds must be removed, even though this may cause distress to the owner with bird fancier's lung; or of the individual patient from the dust-containing environment.

FARMER'S LUNG

Definition

Extrinsic allergic alveolitis due to inhalation of the dust of mouldy hay or mouldy vegetable products.

Aetiology

Although the actual prevalence is unknown, the peak incidence is between January and March, when stored hay is usually used. If this has been stored wet (more than 30 per cent. water) the temperature within the hay may rise to 140° F. (60° C.) or thereabouts. This encourages the growth of certain thermophyllic actinomycetes (*Micropolyspora faeni* and *Thermoactinomyces vulgaris*) and it is the inhalation of the dust-containing products of these fungi (e.g. the spores) and the mouldy hay which may cause farmer's lung.

Pathology

In the acute stages of farmer's lung variant of allergic alveolitis there is a vasculitis of pulmonary capillaries and arterioles with thickening of the alveolar walls due to infiltration with lymphocytes, plasma cells and histiocytes; compact lymphoid follicles develop. The alveolar spaces are found to harbour many large histiocytes with foamy cytoplasm and inflammatory cells. Epithelioid cell granulomata may be found early in the natural history with Langhans type giant cells and foreign body material, some of which is doubly refractile. Reticulin then gross fibrous tissue form interstitially in relation to the granulomata and may become dense and diffuse. In about 25 per cent. of cases obliterative bronchiolitis is also seen. These structural defects are accompanied by diminished compliance of the lung (a restrictive ventilatory disorder) and impaired gas transfer.

100°–102° F. (37·8°–38·9° C.) with cyanosis. Diffuse crepitations can usually be heard on auscultation of the lungs, which persist with the symptoms up to 2–3 weeks. With an insidious onset the signs are those of pulmonary fibrosis and clubbing of the fingers develops only in the later stages of the disease. Ultimately the clinical picture is complicated by respiratory failure and after many years death is usually in combined cardiorespiratory failure.

Diagnosis

The chest radiograph is abnormal in about two-thirds of patients and then shows widely scattered micro-nodular or nodular shadows, mainly in the middle and lower parts of the lung. Later the changes of fibrosis develop, often with honeycombing, especially in the upper parts of the lung.

The blood picture in the acute episode shows a leucocytosis mainly neutrophilic—eosinophilia is not a feature. Serum precipitating antibodies to farmer's lung hay antigen (F.L.H. antigen), which contain extracts of mouldy hay, *M. faeni* and *T. vulgaris* are found in about 80 per cent. of patients with farmer's lung and they tend to disappear when exposure ceases. They are not diagnostic, for about 15–20 per cent. of farm workers exposed to dust but who have no disease have similar antibodies to the F.L.H. antigen. Skin tests are unsatisfactory and inhalation tests with mouldy hay antigens are usually unnecessary, but may be used to confirm the diagnosis in cases of difficulty. Usually, the combined history of exposure to the dust with the clinical picture, radiological and serological evidence, supported by the physiological findings of a restrictive ventilatory defect (reduced vital capacity and lung compliance) with impaired gas transfer are adequate for the diagnosis. Other causes of alveolitis or pulmonary fibrosis, including such conditions as sarcoidosis and honeycomb lung have to be differentiated.

TABLE 52

EXTRINSIC ALLERGIC ALVEOLITIS

	SOURCE OF ANTIGEN	PRECIPITINS PRESENT AGAINST
Farmer's lung	Mouldy hay	*Micropolyspora faeni* *Thermoactinomyces vulgaris*
Bagassosis	Mouldy bagasse	*T. vulgaris*
Mushroom worker's lung	Mushroom compost	*M. faeni* and *T. vulgaris*
Fog-fever in cattle	Mouldy hay	*M. faeni*
Suberosis	Mouldy oak-bark, cork dust	Mouldy cork dust
'New Guinea' lung	Mouldy thatch dust	Thatch of huts
Maple-bark pneumonitis	Mouldy maple-bark	*Cryptostroma* (*Coniosporium*) *corticale*
Malt worker's lung	Mouldy barley, malt dust	*Aspergillus clavatus* *Aspergillus fumigatus*
Bird fancier's lung	Pigeon/budgerigar/parrot/hen droppings	Serum protein and droppings.
Pituitary snuff-taker's lung	Heterologous pituitary powder	Serum protein/pituitary antigens
Wheat weevil disease	Infested wheat flour	*Sitophilus granarius*
Sequoiosis	Mouldy sawdust	*Graphium* *Aureobasidium pullulans* (Pullularia)

Clinical Picture

The patients have usually spent many years farming and are predominantly male. About half the patients present with the characteristic clinical picture of episodic attacks which develop some 6–8 hours after working with mouldy hay. These symptoms subside quite rapidly and then recur with re-exposure. Breathlessness and cough are the most frequent symptoms—in half of them there is expectoration of sputum, which may be blood-stained. About a third feel tight in the chest or are wheezy. Systemic symptoms, such as malaise, generalized aches and pains, chills and fever are noted in about half the patients.

The other half of patients with farmer's lung may develop the same symptoms insidiously. A small proportion, i.e. about 10 per cent., later develop a rapid asthmatic response to the inhaled dust and this is followed some hours later by the systemic reaction.

During acute episodes there is usually a fever of

Treatment

The prevention of farmer's lung is achieved by reducing the moisture content of the hay, which must be kept to a minimum to discourage growth of thermophyllic actinomycetes. Masks are not able to prevent inhalation of spores, which may be as small as one micron in size. Otherwise, patients with farmer's lung must be removed from the source of dust.

Adrenocortical steroids may suppress the acute manifestations of the disease and prednisone may be given in a dose of 30 mg. daily, reducing to 10 mg. daily over 10–14 days. No other medical treatment is of value except in the advanced stages of pulmonary fibrosis [p. 918].

Course and Prognosis

The insidious form carries a worse prognosis as fibrosis is usually well established before the diagnosis is made. Progress of the disease is halted if the patients are removed from the source of dust.

REFERENCES

CROFTON, J., and DOUGLAS, A. (1969) *Respiratory Diseases*, p. 469, Oxford.

PEPYS, J. (1969) *Hypersensitivity Diseases of the Lungs due to Fungi and Organic Dusts*, Basel.

BYSSINOSIS AND OTHER DISEASES DUE TO COTTON, FLAX AND HEMP DUSTS

A high proportion of people exposed to cotton, hemp or flax dust for the first time may experience mild fever, headache, sneezing and coughing, which lasts a few days and then disappears despite continued exposure—a presumed hypersensitivity response (mill fever, cotton cold, etc.). Weavers' cough occurs in epidemics in weaving sheds and is caused by inhalation of fungal spores in mouldy cotton—it clears quickly after leaving the shed.

BYSSINOSIS

Byssinosis is found in a large proportion of those who have worked for some years in card rooms and blow rooms in the cotton industry and is world wide in prevalence. It begins as a tight feeling in the chest some hours after exposure, characteristically at 3 p.m., after a weekend away from work (Monday fever). At first symptoms disappear for the rest of the week, only to reappear the following Monday. Gradually symptoms persist for longer periods of the week. Tightness and breathlessness are associated with a fall in FEV_1 and P.E.F., which at first improve during the week and particularly at the weekend.

Byssinosis therefore is a slowly acquired, delayed bronchoconstriction due to exposure to an unknown constituent of cotton, hemp, flax or sisal dust. The long period of exposure before development of symptoms would favour a form of hypersensitivity, but symptoms can be produced by inhalation of cotton dust in those not previously exposed. Furthermore, the rapid tolerance displayed after Monday fever is not a feature to be expected in hypersensitivity.

Chronic obstructive bronchitis (not necessarily due to cigarette smoking) progresses hand in hand with the bronchoconstriction and may give rise to severe disability.

Dust should be reduced to a minimum and simple tests of ventilation (FEV_1) should be carried out regularly in all those exposed to detect the earliest changes. Workers who react after exposure should be removed from contact with the dust to avoid permanent lung changes.

REFERENCE

SCHILLING, R. S. F. (1956) Byssinosis in cotton and other textile workers, *Lancet*, ii, 261 and 319.

FIBROSING ALVEOLITIS

Synonyms. Diffuse interstitial pulmonary fibrosis; Interstitial pneumonitis; Desquamative interstitial pneumonia; Hamman-Rich syndrome.

Definition

A diffuse inflammatory process involving the gas exchanging tissue of the lung with cellular thickening of alveolar walls with a tendency to fibrosis and large mononuclear cells in the alveolar spaces.

Pathogenesis

A wide variety of causal agents may be associated with this definitive pathological picture, or it may be just one part of a systemic connective tissue disorder. Thus, fibrosing alveolitis may be:

1. The extrinsic allergic type [p. 914].
2. Drug induced: hexamethonium and other ganglion blocking agents, busulphan, chlorambucil, etc.
3. Associated with connective tissue or auto-immune disorders, such as rheumatoid arthritis, systemic sclerosis, Sjøgren's syndrome, systemic lupus erythematosus, biliary cirrhosis.
4. Cryptogenic.

CRYPTOGENIC FIBROSING ALVEOLITIS

Definition

Fibrosing alveolitis of unknown cause and not associated with a definite systemic disease.

Although this disease is rare, it is now recognized with increasing frequency and is reported from all over the world. It may develop at any age, but most commonly occurs in the middle or later years. It affects both sexes about equally and is occasionally familial.

Pathology

There is wide variation in the description and interpretation of the pathological findings in this condition. On the one hand some would separate those cases in which there is filling of the air spaces with large alveolar cells, considered to be granular rather than phagocytic pneumocytes associated with giant cells and foci of lymphocytes and called *desquamative interstitial pneumonia*, from those cases called by others *diffuse interstitial fibrosis*. In the early stages of this latter disorder there is inflammatory thickening of the alveolar walls with increase in the reticulin and fibrous tissue and later exudation of a fibrinous fluid into the air spaces where macrophages congregate. Finally, there is condensation of fibrous tissue with irregular destruction of alveoli and bronchioles with formation of cystic spaces (honeycomb lung).

On the other hand, others would regard these as differing manifestations of one broad category of disease, i.e. *fibrosing alveolitis*, which has two essential features—cellular thickening of the alveolar walls with a strong tendency to fibrosis and the presence of mononuclear cells in the alveoli—those cases with dominant thickening of alveolar walls are described as the 'mural' type of alveolitis, while those cases with many intra-alveolar granular cells and relatively little alveolar wall thickening the 'desquamative' type. There is no gross difference between these two types of fibrosing alveolitis in the clinical manifestations or physiological disturbance (i.e. a restrictive ventilatory defect with impaired gas transfer), but widespread well-defined micronodular shadows usually exist in the chest radiograph with the mural type, whereas, the desquamative type more often had opacities of uniform density above elevated diaphragms or irregular patchy consolidation at the bases, with widespread ill-defined mottling. The latter or desquamative type is more likely to respond to steroids.

Aetiology

No uniform causation is implied in this distinction, for the cause or causes remain obscure.

1. An immunological basis for cryptogenic fibrosing alveolitis is suggested by the finding of non-organ specific antibodies in a proportion of cases: about a third have significant titres of rheumatoid factor (D.A.T.), and antinuclear factor (A.N.F.) is found in about a quarter. These findings suggest a relationship to the connective tissue disorders in which auto-immune factors may be present and in which fibrosing alveolitis similar to the cryptogenic form may be found, i.e. rheumatoid arthritis, systemic sclerosis, Sjøgren's syndrome, systemic lupus erythematosus and dermatomyositis. It has also been reported in association with biliary cirrhosis. Speculation further suggests a parallel between the relationship on the one hand of cryptogenic alveolitis to allergic alveolitis, and on the other hand between extrinsic and intrinsic asthma in which immune factors may be playing a part.

2. External factors may occasionally be responsible. There is the known association of fibrosing alveolitis with orally administered drugs such as busulphan: inhaled substances such as a mixture of tungsten and carbide and cobalt may cause diffuse fibrosis—reports that hair sprays may cause fibrosing alveolitis have not been confirmed.

The physiological defect varies considerably and does not correlate well with the degree of radiological change. The restrictive ventilatory defect is manifested by a reduced total lung capacity (TLC) and vital capacity (VC), the latter often severely diminished while there is no airways obstruction (FEV_1 and FEV_1/FVC ratio remain normal): lung compliance is reduced. Gas transfer (T_{CO}) is usually severely reduced and this change may precede the change in ventilatory capacity. Hyperventilation at rest (greater than 10 litres per minute) and on exercise is usually striking and the arterial oxygen tension (P_{O_2}) is usually low, often falling precipitately on exercise. The arterial carbon dioxide tension (P_{CO_2}) is normal or low.

Clinical Picture

The course of this disease varies from an acute rapidly fatal form to that which is extremely chronic.

In the acute form cough is as marked as breathlessness and tightness in the chest. Sputum may be minimal and occasionally purulent, but pleuritic pain is rare. Fever may be prominent (greater than 39° C.). Tachypnoea, cyanosis, widespread striking crepitations on auscultation and clubbing of the fingers may develop rapidly and these manifestations usually mimic a severe pneumonia.

The chronic form presents with gradually increasing breathlessness on exertion. Normally, this is a striking symptom, although it may take 2 or 3 years before medical advice is sought. Sometimes it is much more rapid in onset and in other cases it remains mild. There is usually a cough, which is usually dry but occasionally productive of a little mucoid sputum. Sometimes fleeting pains are felt in the large joints. Clubbing of the fingers is common and is found in about 75 per cent. of cases and in some it is reversible. Hypertrophic pulmonary osteoarthropathy is unusual. Cyanosis develops at first on exercise and at rest when the disease is advanced. Physical examination often reveals hyperventilation at rest and there may have been some weight loss, but the general condition of the patient is usually good, and fever is unusual. On auscultation, showers of characteristic fine or medium inspiratory crepitations are heard. They may be audible only over parts of the lower lobes, but they may extend to involve the middle and lower zones completely. They persist after coughing and from day to day. With extensive confluent disease signs of basal consolidation may be elicited and accentuated by the high diaphragm. The disease is occasionally complicated by a pneumothorax. Progression of the acute form of the disease leads to respiratory failure and of the chronic form to respiratory failure with or without right ventricular hypertrophy and right ventricular failure.

Diagnosis

The symptoms and signs in middle-aged to elderly patients previously well without signs of cardiovascular disease present a striking and characteristic picture which is almost diagnostic of fibrosing alveolitis.

Chest Radiography. The appearances are variable and changes may be minimal even when breathlessness is established. In the acute form there is usually extensive patchy clouding, mainly in the lower zones. In the chronic form there may be micronodular or nodular shadowing which may be so concentrated as to give a ground glass appearance. Small ring shadows, mainly basal and about 2 mm. in diameter, are often seen and are a form of honeycombing. With micronodular, ground glass or patchy clouding there is often a striking rise in the diaphragm with a considerable reduction in the volume of the middle and lower lobes. These changes are potentially reversible. Linear shadows and bullae may cause considerable distortion of the radiological pattern with reduction of lung volume. Involvement of the pleura is rarely seen [PLATE 13].

The blood count is usually normal. The E.S.R. and serum globulins are often raised.

Thus, the clinical, radiological, immunological and physical defects are strongly suggestive but must be differentiated from those connective tissue disorders which may themselves be complicated by fibrosing alveolitis and other conditions which cause similar diffuse radiological change. These can often be distinguished by their extrathoracic manifestations (e.g. barium swallow in systemic sclerosis), and other investigations may assist in the differentiation. Left heart failure and other conditions such as those due to the inhalation of mineral and organic dusts, including extrinsic alveolitis, will be brought to light by careful history and examination. Such conditions as lymphangitis carcinomatosa, bronchiolar carcinoma, histiocytosis X (e.g. eosinophilic granuloma), sarcoidosis, tuberous sclerosis and alveolar proteinosis and idiopathic haemosiderosis all have to be considered and where the diagnosis is in doubt and careful clinical and other investigations have not revealed a cause, it may be necessary to proceed to a *lung biopsy*. If this is essential a portion of lung showing slight mottling only should be selected, for only the early pathological changes are characteristic. Honeycombed areas are unsatisfactory.

Treatment

Adrenocortical steroids are the only agents so far known to affect the course of the disease, but the response to them is unpredictable. The results of treatment are unimpressive in at least half the patients and the course of the disease remains unaffected. The acute disease, or that form with uniformly dense shadows or patchy clouding in which desquamative changes are likely to be present respond best. Improvement is not confined to this type of disease, however, and if the process appears to be active and progressive or symptoms are moderate or severe the adrenocortical steroids should be tried and their effect measured by clinical response and by radiological and physiological changes. The E.S.R. may also be helpful. Spontaneous remissions or arrest of progress make it more than usually difficult to assess the effects of treatment. Exacerbations also develop if the steroids are withdrawn too hastily. It is preferable in the chronic cases to start with a dose of 10–20 mg. a day by mouth and to increase the dose every 2–4 weeks if necessary. If there is improvement this treatment should be continued for months, even years, and the drugs should always be withdrawn as slowly as possible for fear of relapse. In the acute cases, 40–50 mg. of prednisolone will be needed daily to control the disease initially. The effects of immunosuppressive drugs, such as azathioprine, are at present uncertain. Respiratory failure with hypoxaemia requires oxygen therapy and terminal right ventricular failure should be treated on conventional lines with digoxin and diuretics.

Course and Prognosis

The acute form, especially in the young, is usually rapidly progressive and may be fatal within weeks or months unless arrested by treatment. The chronic disease is usually, but not always, progressive. In about 10 per cent. of patients symptoms and X-ray changes persist unaltered for years and in small numbers there is a spontaneous and permanent remission. Development of finger clubbing, radiological progression to honeycombing and a mural type of disease are unfavourable. The majority of cases, however, progress but the rate of progress is usually slower in the older patient. About one half of patients will die in about 2–6 years with superimposed bronchopulmonary infection or with respiratory failure with or without right ventricular failure. A few patients succumb with bronchial carcinoma, the incidence of which is probably increased in this condition. A favourable response to steroids improves the prognosis: in a small number of patients all symptoms and signs, including clubbing of the fingers and crepitations in the lung, may disappear.

REFERENCES

LIEBOW, A. A., STEER, A., and BILLINGSLEY, J. G. (1965) Desquamative interstitial pneumonia, *Amer. J. Med.*, **39,** 369.

LIVINGSTONE, J. L., LEWIS, J. G., REID, L., and JEFFERSON, K. E. (1964) Diffuse interstitial pulmonary fibrosis, *Quart. J. Med.*, **33,** 71.

SCADDING, J. G., and HINSON, K. F. W. (1967) Diffuse fibrosing alveolitis—correlation of histology at biopsy with prognosis, *Thorax*, **22,** 291.

TURNER-WARWICK, M., and DONIACH, D. (1965) Autoantibody studies in interstitial pulmonary fibrosis, *Brit. med. J.*, **1,** 886.

THE LUNGS IN DISORDERS OF CONNECTIVE TISSUE AND AUTO-IMMUNE DISEASE

THE LUNGS IN RHEUMATOID ARTHRITIS

As rheumatoid arthritis is a common condition (it affects 1·4 per cent. of men and about 3·3 per cent. of women in an urban population) coincidental respiratory disease may sometimes be found. Rheumatoid arthritis, however, predisposes to bronchopulmonary infection for this was found to be more common in men with rheumatoid arthritis than in an equivalent population of men with degenerative arthritis. Rheumatoid arthritis is linked with three conditions of the lung or pleura.

Nodules. Nodules of the lung and pleura have the histological structure of subcutaneous nodules seen in rheumatoid arthritis and take two forms in the lung and pleura:

1. Rheumatoid pneumoconiosis (Caplan's syndrome) [p. 905].

2. Single, or more usually multiple rheumatoid nodules similar to those found in rheumatoid pneumoconiosis are *rarely* found in patients with rheumatoid arthritis without a history of dust exposure or radiological evidence of pneumoconiosis. They are more

common in men than women, are usually subpleural, but may involve the pleura or pericardium. They vary from about 1 to 7 cm. in diameter, may cavitate and may precede or follow the onset of the arthritis. They are usually asymptomatic.

Pleural Changes. While pleural adhesions are an inexplicably common autopsy finding in rheumatoid arthritis (about two-thirds of cases), pleural effusions are less common and pleural exudates develop in the course of rheumatoid arthritis in about 8 per cent. of males and 1·6 per cent. of females. The fluid may have a low glucose content (below 20 mg. per cent.). There may be associated pleural or subpleural rheumatoid nodules. Needle biopsy of the pleura may on occasion reveal histological changes reminiscent of the nodules. Rheumatoid factor may be found in the cells of the pleural fluid.

Fibrosing Alveolitis. This may accompany rheumatoid arthritis, but it is a rare complication. It resembles in every way the cryptogenic form described on page 916. Taking all cases of fibrosing alveolitis, rheumatoid arthritis is found in about 15–20 per cent. It is slightly more common in males, but affects the same age range as the chronic form of fibrosing alveolitis (20–60 years). The lung changes may precede the development of arthritis, but rheumatoid factor is usually found in titres normally associated with arthritis. The pathology of the underlying lung tends to more of the mural type of fibrosing alveolitis and it is unusual for rheumatoid nodules to be found as well. Thus, the radiological appearances are of the micronodular type or nodular type, progressing to fibrosis with honeycombing. Restrictive defects of ventilation due to shrinkage of the lung and reduced compliance are more prominent than reduction in gas transfer (T_{CO}). The course is prolonged and response to corticosteroids poor.

REFERENCE

SCADDING, J. G. (1969) The lungs in rheumatoid arthritis, Philip Ellman Lecture, *Proc. roy. Soc. Med.*, **62**, 227.

THE LUNGS IN SYSTEMIC LUPUS ERYTHEMATOSUS (S.L.E.)

The lungs and pleura may be involved in systemic lupus erythematosus in which widespread manifestations are usually found in other systems, often with evidence of auto-immune disease [see Section 4]. The disease is more common in women than men in a ratio of 3 to 1 and may occur in families. It is characterized by the finding of structureless ovoid or spindle-shaped bodies with fibrinoid change in the tissues accompanied by L.E. cells in the peripheral blood or pleural fluid. L.E. cells may, however, be found in rheumatoid arthritis and lupoid hepatitis.

The lungs may be involved in one or more ways.

Pleurisy. Pleurisy and pleural exudates may occur in from 20 to 60 per cent. of patients with systemic lupus erythematosus. They are often bilateral and may be accompanied by a pericarditis. L.E. cells may be found in the effusion, which is usually small or moderate in size, and responds to treatment with corticosteroids.

Pneumonia. Massive shadowing in the lung, sometimes dense, multiple and bilateral may represent true infection of bacterial or viral nature, but may be due to S.L.E. itself. In the latter case the shadows may persist for several weeks. There may be no symptoms, but breathlessness is usual with dry cough and even cyanosis. Crepitations may be heard.

More commonly, long, almost horizontal linear shadows are found in the lower zones of the lung that transgress segmental boundaries [PLATE 13]. The pathology of these shadows is unknown, but the appearance may be reminiscent of infarction—the shadows, however, in S.L.E. are usually of greater length. The diaphragms are usually considerably elevated and the patient is often breathless.

A restrictive defect of ventilation will be found with impaired gas transfer. All these lesions usually respond to corticosteroid drugs. They are not usually important in the prognosis of the disease.

Fibrosing alveolitis is rarely associated with systemic lupus erythematosus.

OTHER CONNECTIVE TISSUE DISORDERS

Systemic Sclerosis. In addition to fibrosing alveolitis, which develops in about one third of cases [see Section 4], breathlessness in systemic sclerosis may be due to rigidity and restriction of the thoracic cage due to direct involvement by the sclerotic process.

Dermatomyositis, *Sjøgren's syndrome* [see Section 4] and *biliary cirrhosis* [see Section 6] may be associated with the development of fibrosing alveolitis.

REFERENCES

HARVEY, A. MCG., SHULMAN, L. E., TUMULTY, P. A., CONLEY, C. L., and SCHOENRICH, E. H. (1954) Systemic lupus erythematosus: A review of the literature and clinical analysis of 138 cases, *Medicine (Baltimore)*, **33**, 291.

WEAVER, A. L., DIVERTIE, M. B., and TITUS, J. L. (1967) The lung in scleroderma, *Proc. Mayo Clin.*, **42**, 754.

IDIOPATHIC PULMONARY HAEMOSIDEROSIS

Synonyms. Lung purpura; Goodpasture's syndrome.

Definition

This is a condition characterized by recurrent haemorrage into the lung in which there is degeneration, excessive shedding and hyperplasia of the alveolar epithelium and cytoplasmic vacuolation of unknown cause. In some cases there is associated proliferative glomerulonephritis (Goodpasture's syndrome), although the link between the disease which involves the lung alone and that in which the kidney is involved too remains obscure.

Clinical Picture

In the majority of cases the onset is in childhood, usually less than 7 years of age; 15 per cent. of patients are over 15 and then glomerulonephritis is frequently found as well. Haemoptysis is the outstanding symptom. It is intermittent, often severe, and this may be associated with anaemia of the iron deficiency type (the haemoglobin may fall below 7 g. per 100 ml.) and non-specific haemosiderin-laden macrophages may be found in the sputum. There may be dyspnoea, cough, malaise, fever and weight loss. At times of haemorrhage crepitations may be heard in the lung. Enlarged lymph nodes, liver and spleen and even clubbing of the fingers may sometimes be found. Diffuse, fine or coarse, often confluent opacities are seen on the chest radiograph in one or both lungs—they may disappear if bleeding lessens or ceases. After months or years with intermittent symptoms discrete, fine pinhead micronodular shadows may appear on the chest radiograph throughout both lungs. Fibrosis is not a feature. This condition must be differentiated from haemosiderosis of the lung secondary to mitral stenosis in which pinhead or micronodular shadows are seen.

The course is extremely variable—about one third of patients die within 3 years and in about one third of patients the disease becomes apparently inactive. Progressive glomerulonephritis usually declares itself within 1–8 months of the first haemoptysis with protein, red cells and pus in the urine. The blood pressure is initially normal. In the majority of these patients renal failure develops and is the usual cause of death within weeks or years of the onset.

Diagnosis

It may be difficult to differentiate this condition from *polyarteritis nodosa*—indeed, a generalized arteritis may be found in patients manifesting all the characteristics of pulmonary haemosiderosis. Without evidence of a generalized arteritis or of systemic polyarteritis nodosa, pulmonary haemosiderosis should be considered as a separate entity.

Treatment

Treatment with adrenocortical steroids (prednisone, 15–40 mg. per day) may be associated with remissions, but such remissions may be spontaneous and steroids are unlikely to affect the long-term course of the disease. The anaemia will respond to iron by mouth (e.g. ferrous sulphate, 200 mg. thrice daily). Acute severe blood loss may require blood transfusion.

REFERENCES

RUSBY, N. L., and WILSON, C. (1960) Lung purpura with nephritis, *Quart. J. Med.*, **29**, 501.

SOERGEL, K. H., and SOMMERS, S. C. (1962) Idiopathic pulmonary hemosiderosis and related syndromes, *Amer. J. Med.*, **32**, 499.

PULMONARY ALVEOLAR MICROLITHIASIS

This is a very rare disease of unknown cause, often familial, in which there is an extensive alveolar deposition of calcium-containing nodules which manifest throughout both lungs as very fine but very dense shadows of pinhead size on the chest radiograph. At first there are no symptoms, but dyspnoea becomes slowly progressive and death may ensue in cardio-respiratory failure after many years.

REFERENCE

VISWANATHAN, R. (1962) Pulmonary alveolar microlithiasis, *Thorax*, **17**, 251.

PULMONARY ALVEOLAR PROTEINOSIS

This is a rare pulmonary disorder of unknown cause in which the alveoli are filled by P.A.S. positive (periodic acid-Schiff stain), proteinaceous material which is lipid: that this is a reaction to an inhaled dust is unproven: alveolar epithelium sloughs into the lumen where the cells necrose and add granular and laminated bodies to the alveolar material.

This disorder has been found in North America, Europe and Australia and is three times more common in men, especially those between the ages of 20 and 50. In some cases there may be antecedent febrile episodes, but normally the illness is insidious, afebrile and dyspnoea, chest pain, cough dry or productive with sometimes blood-stained sputum, lassitude and weight loss are the chief symptoms. Crepitations and clubbing are the exceptions rather than the rule. The radiographic findings are strikingly uniform and consist of fine diffuse, perihilar, radiating feathery or vaguely nodular, soft density shadows which often resemble in their butterfly distribution the pattern seen in severe pulmonary oedema.

The diagnosis depends on lung biopsy and must be differentiated from sarcoidosis (in which a lymph node component is usually found), extrinsic and other forms of alveolitis and other forms of pulmonary infiltration with eosinophilia. In pneumonia due to *Pneumocystis carinii*, the protozoon should be demonstrated in the biopsy and an inflammatory reaction with many plasma cells will usually be seen.

Treatment has been largely of no avail, but success has been claimed for repeated washouts of the lung through a Carlens catheter (7·5 Units of heparin per ml. of 0·5 per cent. buffered normal saline). About 25 per cent. of patients progress and die in respiratory failure, while another 25 per cent. seem to recover.

REFERENCE

ROSEN, S. H., CASTLEMAN, B., and LIEBOW, A. A. (1958) Pulmonary alveolar proteinosis, *New Engl. J. Med.*, **258,** 1123.

BRONCHOPULMONARY AMYLOIDOSIS

Amyloidosis of the lower respiratory tract is exceptionally rare. Amyloid deposits may be found in the lung presenting as silent tumours or in the bronchus presenting as an obstructive lesion or with cough—these forms are benign. Generalized submucosal infiltration of the trachea and bronchi produces narrowing of the airways and is the most common form. The prognosis, however, becomes unfavourable with increasing obstruction and secondary infection.

REFERENCE

PROWSE, C. B. (1958) Amyloidosis of the lower respiratory tract, *Thorax*, **13**, 308.

DISEASES AFFECTING THE PLEURA

GENERAL CONSIDERATIONS

The pleura is a mesodermal serous membrane covering the surfaces of the lobes of the lungs (visceral pleura) and the inside of the thoracic cage (parietal pleura). These two membranes are continuous and form a potential space which is lubricated by a small volume of fluid: they consist of a layer of simple squamous epithelium resting on the connective tissue and are supplied on the one hand by branches of the pulmonary and bronchial arteries and on the other by the branches of the intercostal and internal mammary arteries. The visceral pleural lymphatics drain into the hilar lymph glands and the parietal to the lymph nodes along the internal mammary artery and the heads of the ribs and from the diaphragm to the anterior and posterior mediastinal nodes.

The visceral pleura has no somatic nerve supply. The parietal pleura is innervated in the main by branches of the intercostal nerves, but that part over the central aspect of the diaphragm is innervated by the phrenic nerve. The parietal pleura is sensitive to painful stimuli, which are localized accurately except from the diaphragm, involvement of the central part of which causes pain referred by the phrenic nerve to the shoulder and of the peripheral part to the abdomen along the corresponding intercostal nerve.

The pressure in the pleural space is below atmospheric pressure because of the elastic retraction forces within the lungs and in normal quiet breathing varies between −2 cm. of water in expiration and −6 cm. of water on inspiration: gravity exerts an effect on intrathoracic contents so that the pressure at the top of the pleural space is 5 cm. of water higher than at the most dependent part. With increase in depth of ventilation (e.g. on exercise), or with the increased work of breathing in restrictive or obstructive defects of ventilation the variations in pressure between inspiration and expiration increase and the accessory muscles of respiration are reflexly brought into play (e.g. scalenes, sterno-mastoids).

Normally, there is a dynamic equilibrium between formation and resorption of pleural fluid. Water and electrolyte are exchanged rapidly, whereas protein is absorbed slowly via the lymphatics, mainly of the mediastinal pleura. Formation of pleural effusions may be the result of impaired resorption of protein or of excessive formation due to changes in hydrostatic pressure or osmolarity within the capillary. The pleura, following inflammatory lesions often heals by fibrosis and obliteration of the pleural space sometimes in a patchy fashion. Repair, however, may occur without fibrosis with restoration of the potential space.

PLEURISY

Pleurisy is an inflammation of the pleural membranes. If the inflammatory process leads only to fibrinous deposit it is described as *dry pleurisy*. If in addition much serous fluid is produced the condition of *pleurisy with effusion* results, while if pus is formed the condition is described as a *purulent pleurisy* or *empyema*. While this distinction is convenient from a clinical standpoint, the three conditions are in reality only stages or degrees in the pleural response to irritation, whatever the cause. The form which occurs in any given case depends on the nature of the cause, the extent of the inflammatory process and the degree of resistance on the part of the individual affected.

DRY PLEURISY

Synonyms. Fibrinous pleurisy; Fibrinous pleuritis.

Definition

Dry pleurisy is inflammation of the pleura without an increase in pleural fluid.

Aetiology

Inflammation of the pleura is usually secondary to adjacent disease of the lung, chest wall or subphrenic region. The commonest lesion leading to dry pleurisy is pneumonia, either specific (e.g. bacterial, particularly pneumococcal, mycoplasma, viral, etc.), or non-specific (e.g. aspiration pneumonia). However, dry pleurisy may occur in association with pulmonary infarction, carcinoma of the bronchus, pulmonary tuberculosis, bronchiectasis and less common lung infections.

Lesions of the chest wall, resulting from injury, tuberculous osteitis of a rib, or epidemic myalgia (Bornholm disease), as well as subphrenic abscess or amoebic hepatitis may be responsible for the inflammatory change. On rare occasions systemic disorders such as rheumatoid arthritis or systemic lupus erythematosus may be complicated by dry pleurisy.

Pathology

The area of inflammation may be localized or generalized in the pleura, which is hyperaemic. The membrane loses its shiny appearance and becomes dull. Fibrin is deposited on the roughened pleural surface. Adhesions between the visceral and parietal pleura may form during resolution, but this is not invariable and thickening without adhesions may be the ultimate result.

Clinical Picture

The onset is often quite sudden with a stitch-like pain in the side. The pain is aggravated by inspiration, by coughing and sometimes by movements of the trunk. The pain may become extremely severe and knife-like and limit ventilation, particularly inspiration. There may be a dry cough which is ineffective and distressing. There may be a slight fever, 100°–101° F. (37·8°–38·3° C.), but this is not invariable. Breathing tends to be rapid and shallow and the impaired ventilation may aggravate hypoxia, particularly in pneumonia. Movement of the chest is usually reflexly depressed on the affected side and a pleural friction rub is usually heard except when the diaphragmatic pleura is involved. In these cases pain is referred to the shoulder or the abdomen. In the latter case the reflex rigidity and guarding of the relevant upper quadrant of the abdomen may simulate an abdominal emergency. Dry pleurisy more often than not is followed by a pleural effusion; otherwise it regresses and the rate of resolution depends on the nature of the adjacent primary cause.

Diagnosis

The characteristic pain and pleural rub are diagnostic of pleurisy and a careful search should be made for the primary condition. Chest radiography will be most helpful in determining the cause. Pain due to herpes zoster, epidemic myalgia (Bornholm disease), fibrositis, fractured rib, and other lesions of the chest wall may simulate pleurisy but will not be associated with a pleural rub.

Treatment

Obviously treatment should be directed to the primary lesion, but local heat, splinting and analgesics may help. Severe pain may require relief with dihydrocodeine, 30–60 mg. by mouth, pethidine, 50–200 mg. orally, or even morphine, 5–15 mg. subcutaneously, in the most severe cases. Care should be taken to avoid sputum retention as a result of these measures.

PLEURAL EFFUSION

Definition

A collection of fluid within the pleural space.

Aetiology

Pleural effusions are broadly divisible into two types, *transudates* and *exudates*.

Transudates. (Synonym: hydrothorax.) The fluid may increase in the pleural space by transudation from capillaries due to osmotic changes associated with hypoproteinaemia or to an increase in hydrostatic pressure which may occur in heart failure or constrictive pericarditis. Sometimes a transudate may develop in the presence of a pneumothorax due to interference with resorption. A transudate or hydrothorax is often bilateral, although in heart failure it may start on one or other side. The fluid is pale yellow and clear and has a specific gravity less than 1015 and a protein content less than 3 g. per 100 ml. Transudates should be suspected when one or other of the underlying causes are found on routine clinical examination. Transudates are sometimes localized in the interlobar fissures and then may appear on the chest radiograph as rounded or massive shadows: they rapidly disappear on treatment (phantom or pseudotumours).

Exudates. Pleural fluid may increase by exudation from the subepithelial capillaries, particularly when these are involved in an inflammatory or neoplastic process. As these are usually unilateral so pleural effusions of this nature are usually unilateral. The fluid is straw or amber coloured and may clot rapidly after collection. The protein content is usually greater than 3 g. per 100 ml. and the specific gravity more than 1015.

The most common causes of pleural exudates are pneumonia, pulmonary infarction, pulmonary tuberculosis, malignant disease including lymphomata and bronchiectasis. Less commonly pleural exudates are found with fungal infections, connective tissue diseases (especially systemic lupus erythematosus), subphrenic abscess, amoebic abscess and pancreatitis. Rare causes are asbestosis, ovarian tumours of various types (Meigs' syndrome), myxoedema and myelomatosis. Very occasionally no cause can be found to account for unilateral or pleural exudates which may recur over long periods of time.

Pleural effusions may be blood-stained or consist of frank blood (*haemothorax*). They may be milky or chylous (*chylothorax*) or purulent (*empyema*) [p. 924].

PLEURAL EFFUSION ASSOCIATED WITH PNEUMONIA

Before chemotherapy pleural exudates associated with specific or non-specific bacterial pneumonias usually became purulent (empyema). With chemotherapy, however, the fluid frequently remains amber coloured and translucent or perhaps slightly cloudy. Although the patient is usually recovering, clinically the fever may persist or recur with the advent of the effusion: the fluid usually contains an excess of neutrophil granulocytes, but may be sterile on culture. The fever disappears with removal of the fluid which rarely re-accumulates: if it does the possibility of tuberculosis or underlying neoplasia should be considered. Pleural effusions complicating mycoplasma or viral pneumonias are unusual: they are usually small and incidental and clear during the course of the pneumonia.

PLEURAL EFFUSION ASSOCIATED WITH PULMONARY INFARCTION

Pleural exudates with pulmonary infarcts are frequently blood-stained and often bilateral. They are usually quite small in volume and rarely an important factor in the pathogenesis of breathlessness. Apart from large numbers of red cells seen in the fluid, mesothelial cells are often plentiful as well. Effusions with pulmonary infarcts are usually short-lived except in patients with a high pulmonary venous pressure (e.g. mitral valve disease), in which case the fluid may persist for weeks. The diagnosis of effusions of this nature should be particularly suspected whenever there is evidence of thrombo-embolic disease.

PLEURAL EFFUSIONS ASSOCIATED WITH MALIGNANT DISEASE AND LYMPHOMATA

1. *Primary pleural tumours.* These may be benign, e.g. fibromata, or malignant, e.g. mesothelioma, or fibrosarcomata.

All these tumours are rare and are often accompanied by clubbing of the fingers or pulmonary osteo-arthropathy. Mesothelioma is a malignant tumour which may diffusely involve the pleura and may invade the thoracic cage to cause a visible mass. The accompanying pleural effusion is often blood-stained. It is usually associated with asbestosis. Fibrosarcomata of the pleura are very rare tumours that may secrete hormones, e.g. insulin.

2. Malignant effusions are usually secondary to underlying *carcinoma of the lung*. They may be due to metastatic spread from such primary sites as the breast, stomach, pancreas or uterus: in these cases the effusions may be unilateral or bilateral. With carcinoma of the lung the exudate is usually unilateral. It may be due to inflammatory change in the lung distal to the tumour, to direct invasion by the growth itself, or to lymphatic obstruction. There may be no obvious involvement of the lung when the primary growth is outside the lung and occasionally massive pleural deposits may be seen radiographically, especially after aspiration of fluid. The primary site of growth may defy detection or have been removed many years beforehand without evidence of local recurrence. Pleural effusions with lymphomata, including Hodgkin's disease, and lymphosarcoma, resemble those of metastatic carcinoma but there is usually clinical evidence of the underlying disease.

Clinically, malignant effusions are characteristically recurrent and are often massive. They frequently lead quite rapidly to breathlessness due to restriction of ventilation.

The diagnosis of a malignant effusion is straightforward when the site and nature of the primary tumour are known. Further investigation is often required to establish the cause when the underlying tumour is not recognized. Examination of the fluid usually reveals an exudate with an excess of mesothelial cells and often inflammatory cells, particularly if there has been an underlying infection. Occasionally neoplastic cells may be seen in a smear of the fluid. Biopsy of the pleura, however, is more likely to give unequivocal histological evidence of neoplasia.

Treatment

While surgery and radiotherapy have little to offer in the treatment of malignant pleural effusions, chemotherapy, particularly in the lymphomata, when given systemically may affect the formation of pleural fluid. Instillation of chemotherapeutic agents or radioactive materials into the pleural space, however, may prevent or diminish reaccumulation of fluid. Thus, in effusions due to invasion of the pleura by carcinoma of the lung, a need for repeated aspiration to relieve breathlessness may be abolished by instillation of mustine, 30 mg., after aspiration almost to dryness. Thiotepa, radioactive gold (^{198}Au) or ytrium (^{90}Yt) are no more effective. Prednisone, 20 mg. daily by mouth, may also delay reformation of pleural fluid. Chemical pleurodesis with iodized talc may eliminate the need for repeated chest aspiration. Prolonged suppression of metastatic growth and pleural effusion may be obtained when the primary tumour is sensitive to hormone therapy. Thus, pleural effusions with post-menopausal carcinoma of the breast may respond to oestrogens, as may those from carcinoma of the prostate.

PLEURAL EFFUSION ASSOCIATED WITH TUBERCULOSIS

This may occur at any age and at any stage in the natural history of pulmonary tuberculosis. In the United Kingdom it was an uncommon complication of primary tuberculosis in childhood (about 7 per cent. of cases). It classically occurred in adolescents and young adults after their primary infection. Tuberculous pleural effusion has become much less common with the reduction in frequency of primary tuberculous infection and with B.C.G. vaccination. At a later age and stage in the natural history, pleural exudates may follow direct invasion of the pleura by a caseating process in the underlying lung, less commonly from an adjacent tuberculous node, or active tuberculosis of bone, either in a vertebra or rib. Chemotherapy, particularly in the developed countries, has reduced extension of active tuberculosis to the pleura to an insignificant incidence.

Clinical Picture

The onset of a tuberculous pleural effusion is similar to that of dry pleurisy, but the constitutional symptoms are usually more pronounced. Pleuritic pain and dry cough are usually the earliest symptoms, but there may be a preceding period of malaise, when constitutional signs, however, may be absent. When the effusion develops the pain is often relieved. If a large quantity of fluid accumulates rapidly the patient may become severely breathless due to a restrictive defect of ventilation, which may be aggravated by a shift of the mediastinum to the contralateral side, impeding the ventilation of that lung also. In more slowly developing effusions there is usually little or no breathlessness except on exertion. Fever is of moderate degree and may reach 39·5° C. or more. At the onset of the illness there may be an audible friction rub, but this usually rapidly disappears as fluid accumulates. There are then obvious signs of a pleural effusion.

Tuberculosis effusions usually resolve with little residual fibrosis but occasionally gross pleural fibrosis, perhaps with contraction and restriction of the hemithorax, occurs. If left untreated, all clinical and radiological signs of a tuberculous pleural effusion usually disappear within a few months, but are followed by active tuberculosis in about 25 per cent. of cases, usually within 5 years. Tuberculous empyema is a rare complication.

Diagnosis

A tuberculous cause for a pleural exudate should be considered with any unexplained effusion, particularly when there is a positive cutaneous tuberculin reaction with or without radiographic evidence of underlying pulmonary tuberculosis. A sample of fluid should be withdrawn—analysis will reveal lymphocytes predominating on microscopy and usually few or absent mesothelial cells. Acid and alcohol fast bacilli are rarely seen in the fluid, but may be cultivated. The diagnosis is established in more than 75 per cent. of cases by pleural biopsy, in sections of which typical caseating tubercles can be seen, often with visible acid fast bacilli. Biopsy of the pleura should be repeated if necessary several times if the diagnosis remains unproven.

Treatment

Antituberculosis chemotherapy should be instituted and given for at least 18 months, as described on page

871. Subsequent pulmonary or extrapulmonary disease will be prevented. If the patient is febrile and ill he would prefer to be rested in bed and pain should be relieved by analgesics. After the institution of chemotherapy the tendency for re-accumulation of fluid to occur after total aspiration rapidly diminishes. Adrenocortical steroids, e.g. prednisone, 20 mg. orally daily, may hasten the absorption of pleural fluid and relieve constitutional symptoms if they are troublesome. If prednisone is used the dose should be gradually reduced after two weeks' treatment. Adrenocortical steroids also diminish pleural fibrosis. Neither steroids nor chemotherapy need be given locally.

PLEURAL EFFUSIONS ASSOCIATED WITH RHEUMATOID ARTHRITIS

Pleural exudates may occur with or without any underlying disease in the lung and may anticipate the arthritis. They more commonly accompany the nodular form of rheumatoid arthritis. They are associated with a rise in titre of rheumatoid factor in the serum and are most commonly encountered in middle-aged men. They are usually unilateral and often persist for periods of weeks or more. They may be associated with pericardial effusion due to the same cause. They are found in just under 1 per cent. of men with rheumatoid arthritis and occur with a significantly higher frequency than in degenerative forms of arthritis. The fluid is often pale yellow with a high protein content (greater than 3 g. per 100 ml.), sometimes with a low glucose content (less than 20 mg. per 100 ml.). It is unusual for pleural biopsy to provide specific histological evidence, but occasionally granular leucocytes may be seen in the fluid containing cytoplasmic inclusions which liberate rheumatoid factor.

PLEURAL EFFUSIONS WITH OTHER CONNECTIVE TISSUE DISORDERS

Pleural exudates are rarely associated with rheumatic fever, polyarteritis nodosa, and systemic sclerosis but are more common in systemic lupus erythematosus (S.L.E.), in which they may be bilateral and recurrent. Underlying lesions in the lung may or may not present. Extrathoracic manifestations of S.L.E. may be minimal, e.g. joint pains. L.E. cells may be found in the peripheral blood or pleural fluid. Other diagnostic evidence should be sought [see Section 4] but high titres of antinuclear factor should be found.

EMPYEMA

Synonyms. Purulent pleural effusion; Pyothorax.

Definition

An empyema is a pleural exudate which is frankly purulent or contains a gross excess of pus cells. It may be total or localized to part of the pleural cavity (loculated).

Aetiology

Empyema almost always results from a spread of infection or inflammatory process from the lung or some other adjacent structure. Thus, it may complicate a pneumococcal, staphylococcal, tuberculous or some other specific pneumonia or follow a non-specific aspiration pneumonia, a suppurative pneumonia, lung abscess or bronchiectasis. Where the pneumonia is of a non-specific nature underlying occlusive lesions of the main bronchi should be considered, such as neoplasm and foreign body. Empyema may follow lesions in the mediastinum such as lymphadenitis, perforation of the oesophagus which may be spontaneous or associated with a lesion such as a carcinoma. A mediastinal infection may have spread down from the neck. Empyema not uncommonly follows penetrating wounds or infection may be introduced at aspiration or surgery. It may spread from an osteomyelitis involving a rib. Infection under the diaphragm, such as a subphrenic abscess or an amoebic abscess or perinephric abscess should also be considered if the underlying process is obscure. Occasionally empyema is a direct complication of a septicaemia.

The organisms most commonly associated are bacteria, e.g. *Strep. pneumoniae*, *Staph. pyogenes*, *Strep. pyogenes*, *Myco. tuberculosis*. *H. influenzae*, *Salmonella typhi*., *Esch. coli* and *Klebsiella sp.* and other Gram-negative organisms are less common bacterial invaders. Mycotic infections, such as actinomycosis and nocardiosis and protozoal infections, e.g. *Entamoeba histolytica*, are rare in the United Kingdom. Chemotherapy has made empyema a relative rarity in developed countries and frequently renders the purulent exudate sterile. Empyema, however, remains a common complication of pneumonia in less developed countries. Empyema occurs at all ages from infancy onwards and the staphylococcus is the commonest cause of empyema in childhood.

Pathology

The developing empyema is usually turbid and translucent and is rich in protein and in neutrophil leucocytes. It may become frankly purulent with thick, opaque creamy pus. The colour varies from pale yellow to green or grey. The fluid may be odourless or foul smelling. The pleura may be covered with a shaggy fibrinous exudate which may be thick, e.g. with pneumococcal infection. Adhesions may then cause loculation of the pus and considerable fibrosis may develop and prevent expansion of the lung and interfere with its function. When a fibrinolysin is produced by the infecting organism, e.g. beta haemolytic streptococcus, loculation is prevented or delayed, and the fluid is usually less viscous. In long-standing cases amyloid disease may develop.

Clinical Picture

The onset of an empyema may be masked by the symptoms of the primary infection. Failure of a pneumonia to respond adequately to treatment should raise the possibility of an empyema, but increasing malaise with pleuritic pain, high fever up to 103° F. (39·5° C.), possibly with rigors, are suggestive; however, fever may be absent. The signs are those of a pleural effusion but when pleural empyemata are prolonged then weight loss, pallor and clubbing of the digits may all develop. The pus may track intercostally and appear as a fluctuant subcutaneous swelling (*empyema necessitatis*). Resonance will be found above the fluid if a *bronchopleural* fistula develops; the patient may then produce large amounts of sputum if the empyema drains through the fistula. The cough and expectoration is often accompanied by a vile smell to the breath. Occasionally evacuation of the empyema in this fashion results in a spontaneous cure. The signs will be considerably modified if the empyema is loculated or localized, e.g. between the lobes (*interlobar empyema*). The pleural infection may spread to the pericardium, but rarely to the mediastinum, subphrenic space or ribs. Persistence of pus in the pleura (*chronic empyema*) may be due to mechanical factors such as fibrosis or contraction of the pleura or lung or bronchopleural fistula with inadequate drainage or foreign bodies in the pleura. Persistent suppurative pneumonia with or without abscess formation, bronchiectasis, or carcinoma of the lung may also prolong the pleural suppuration. Chronic empyema otherwise may be due to the nature of the infection itself, e.g. *Myco. tuberculosis* or fungi such as actinomycosis. A sinus may persist if there is drainage to the exterior: organization of the pleural space may give contraction of the thorax and scoliosis, especially in children. Hypertrophic pulmonary osteo-arthropathy and amyloid disease are further complications of chronic empyemata.

Diagnosis

Empyema will be suspected when there is recrudescence of fever and especially when there is a neutrophil leucocytosis of 15,000 per mm^3. in the presence of signs of effusion. The onset, however, is often insidious and may be misleading and the clinical picture may be obscured by the underlying disease. In all cases *chest radiography* is essential and lateral as well as postero-anterior views are necessary to localize the abnormality. In all cases it is necessary to aspirate some fluid from the pleura to establish the diagnosis. Failure to obtain pus from the empyema may be due to blockage of the aspirating needle by thick viscid pus. Chest radiography is of great importance: it may show the characteristic but rather dense shadow of pleural fluid, or it may help to demonstrate unsuspected fluid in patients with systemic symptoms who have not developed characteristic signs of fluid. Shadows of fluid localized to the apex, to an interlobar region, or below the lung above the diaphragm may be revealed. Recovery of pus from these sites will establish the diagnosis. In all cases the pus should be examined microbiologically, bearing in mind the possibility of mycotic and mycobacterial as well as of more common infections.

Treatment

Treatment required by an empyema must depend on the general condition of the patient and the condition of the underlying lung. Pus must be removed for the best chance of a good functional recovery. The primary source of infection must be sought and treated, e.g. by bronchoscopy if carcinoma of the lung is a possibility. In septicaemic conditions other sites of infection, such as endocarditis, meningitis and osteomyelitis must be sought, particularly in children.

Acute Empyemata. When the pus is thin repeated aspiration is usually adequate. Some empyemata complicating bacterial pneumonias which themselves have been treated by chemotherapy often resolve spontaneously, but this resolution may be hastened by aspiration. When an organism has been recovered the appropriate chemotherapy should be applied and may be given into the pleura as well as systemically. If these measures are inadequate and the pus remains thin, then an intercostal tube may be used to drain the fluid to an underwater seal.

Chronic Empyemata. The pus is usually much thicker. If the patient is ill the drainage is best effected by rib resection and a large bore drainage tube inserted into the most dependent part. When the patient's condition allows, a chronic empyema with thick pus should be resected and the lung decorticated. It is necessary beforehand, however, to determine the condition of the underlying lung and as far as possible bronchiectasis, carcinoma of the lung and foreign body should be excluded by such investigations as bronchoscopy and bronchogram. Chemotherapy appropriate to the organism isolated on culture should be continued for several weeks. In the case of amoebic infection systemic emetine, 60 mg. per day for 10–12 days, is required as well as repeated aspiration: mycotic empyemata due to actinomycosis may respond to penicillin, 10–20 mega Units per day, together with drainage.

REFERENCE

LE ROUX, B. T. (1965) Empyema thoracis, *Brit. J. Surg.*, **52,** 89.

CHYLOTHORAX

Definition

A collection of chyle or lymph in the pleural space.

Aetiology and Pathology

Chylous effusions due to leakage of lymph from the thoracic duct, right lymphatic duct, or broncho-mediastinal lymphatic trunk, into the pleura are rare. They usually result from surgical trauma, but very rarely injuries in which there is hyperextension of the spine, severe compression of the trunk due to blows or blasts, or penetrating wounds, may cause the leak. Congenital anomalies of the lymphatic ducts, malignant infiltration of the thoracic duct in the thorax or round the subclavian vein, aneurysms, tuberculosis, filariasis may be even rarer causes.

Over two litres of chyle may leak into the pleural cavity daily and if this is removed the patient may rapidly become depleted of protein, fat, electrolytes and fat-soluble vitamins.

Clinical Features

For varying periods after trauma or quite spontaneously the patient becomes breathless and the physical signs of a pleural effusion are elicited. The milky fluid rapidly reforms after removal and the loss of essential protein, fat and fluid with electrolyte gives rise to rapid weight loss and dehydration. With healing there is often gross pleural fibrosis, with contraction of the hemithorax and scoliosis, particularly in children.

Diagnosis

On chest radiography the appearances are those of a pleural effusion, which on aspiration is characteristically milky, opalescent or oily and must be differentiated from pus and from pseudochylous effusions. The latter contain an excess only of cholesterol crystals (these may be deposited in any long-standing effusion) or fat globules due to degenerate cells in chronic effusions which have usually a tuberculous or neoplastic cause. The fluid in a chylothorax will alter its appearance in relation to meals and will become coloured after ingestion of fat stained with a dye.

Treatment

In about half the cases of traumatic chylothorax there is spontaneous closure of the leak. Local repeated aspiration is justified initially. If this is not successful after an arbitrary period determined by the nutrition of the patient, exploration with repair or ligation of the thoracic duct after lymphangiography should be considered. Insufflation into the pleural space of iodized talc followed by suction drainage early after diagnosis may result in obliteration of the space.

REFERENCES

Roy, P. H., Carr, D. T., and Payne, W. S. (1967) The problem of chylothorax, *Proc. Mayo Clin.*, **42,** 457.

Schmidt, A. (1959) Chylothorax: Review of 5 years' cases in the literature and report of a case, *Acta chir. scand.*, **118,** 5.

PNEUMOTHORAX

Definition

A collection of air in the pleural space.

Aetiology

A pneumothorax may be spontaneous, traumatic, or artificial. Whatever the cause may be the collection of air may be localized by adhesions or generalized, in which case the whole pleural space contains air. A pneumothorax is either *closed*, i.e. air-tight, or *open* in which there is a free communication with the bronchial tree (a bronchopleural fistula). A *tension pneumothorax* may develop when a valve mechanism allows air to enter the pleural space during inspiration, especially during the inspiratory phase of coughing, and prevents escape of air during expiration. This causes progressive and often rapid shift of the mediastinum to the normal side, which impedes ventilation not only on the affected side but of the contralateral lung and may obstruct the venous return.

Traumatic Pneumothorax. Both penetrating and non-penetrating injuries may be associated with a pneumothorax. In the latter case there are usually fractured ribs. There is often an associated bleeding into the pleural space—*haemopneumothorax*. Severe non-penetrating injuries to the chest may be complicated by rupture of a bronchus and escape of air into the pleura. Surgical procedures in the neck are not infrequently complicated by a pneumothorax, but simple aspiration of pleural effusions or biopsy is a frequent cause.

Artificial Pneumothorax. While this was commonly used for the treatment of pulmonary tuberculosis, it is now induced only for diagnostic purposes in order to determine whether a lesion is in the lung or in the parietal pleura or chest wall.

SPONTANEOUS PNEUMOTHORAX

Definition

A pneumothorax due to spontaneous escape of air into the pleura as a result of disease, usually of the lung, pleura or oesophagus.

Aetiology

In the United Kingdom and North America spontaneous pneumothorax most commonly results from the rupture of an apical subpleural bleb or bulla. In the majority of cases this is a congenital defect. This has its highest incidence in tall and otherwise healthy young men; it is five times more common in men than in women and has an incidence of about 0·5 per 1,000 of the population. It occurs on either side with equal frequency. The actual mechanism is not known, but neither physical activity nor preceding infection are necessary. In older patients, usually over 40, spontaneous pneumothorax usually results from rupture of bullae with or without emphysema usually of the widespread panacinar type. Scar emphysema, e.g. with healed tuberculosis, may be the cause.

Other factors known to predispose to spontaneous pneumothorax are bronchial occlusion such as may complicate asthma, or bronchial carcinoma; necrosis with rupture of the pleura in staphylococcal pneumonia or acute caseating tuberculosis. In the former case tension cysts are common, particularly in infants and it is the cyst which ruptures. Spontaneous pneumothorax is also associated with congenital cysts, with pneumoconioses, particularly that associated with aluminium (bauxite), honeycomb lung, cystic fibrosis, fibroid sarcoidosis of the lung. A rare form complicates menstruation. This manifests as a recurrent right-sided pneumothorax during the first 2 days of menstruation and usually in females in their fourth decade. Endometriosis and a perforated right diaphragm may be the cause in some cases. There is some evidence that adrenocortical steroids and intermittent positive pressure respiration may precipitate a pneumothorax.

A simple closed pneumothorax initially restricts ventilation of the affected lung more than it impairs the blood flow. This may result in a fall in arterial oxygen tension, but there is a rapid adjustment and P_{O_2} rapidly returns to normal. Even a large pneumothorax is well tolerated unless patients have already impaired function of the lung, e.g. in chronic bronchitis with or without emphysema or severe pulmonary fibrosis, etc

Clinical Picture

In the common form of spontaneous pneumothorax due to rupture of an apical bleb the patient is often tall and rather underweight but is otherwise a healthy individual. There is sudden pleuritic chest pain and breathlessness. The pain is usually short-lived for a few hours only. Much less commonly the moment of the development of a pneumothorax is preceded by central chest pain due to rupture of interstitial air in the lung into the mediastinum before secondary rupture into the pleura. This central chest pain may be severe and mimic myocardial infarction.

If the lung remains partially inflated the breathlessness usually diminishes rapidly. In older patients, however, with chronic bronchitis or emphysema the breathlessness may become severe even with modest deflation of the underlying lung and in these patients pleuritic pain is usually lacking—cyanosis is much more likely to develop with progressive respiratory failure. Serious and distressing breathlessness may often develop if a spontaneous pneumothorax is superimposed upon status asthmaticus. This complication must always be borne in mind if there is deterioration in patients with severe asthma. Breathlessness may also become severe if the pneumothorax is bilateral or if a tension pneumothorax develops. In the latter case there is severe restlessness with anxiety and breathlessness. There is cyanosis, tachycardia, hypotension and cold extremities due to a fall in cardiac output. The jugular veins are distended and there is usually a marked shift of the trachea and mediastinum to the normal side. If this condition is not immediately relieved, cardiorespiratory failure may rapidly cause death.

The physical signs of a spontaneous unilateral pneumothorax may be difficult to interpret, especially if there is only a small volume of air. The shift of the mediastinum to the normal side, the diminished breath sounds and movement with preservation of resonance on the affected side are the most common findings. With a large pneumothorax, breath sounds of an amphoric type and coin sounds may be heard. With very shallow pneumothorax, almost always on the left side, a clicking or crackling sound may be heard. On occasions it may be so loud that the patient himself is aware of the noise. This sound occurs with the frequency of the heart beat, which is thought to generate the sound by close proximity to the free medial border of the lung. The sound is often modified by movement or a shift in position of the patient. When this sound is heard following the sudden onset of left chest pain, it may lead to the erroneous diagnosis of pericarditis and it may on occasion be simulated by mediastinal emphysema.

A spontaneous pneumothorax may be complicated by an effusion. This is usually a small exudate which absorbs spontaneously. However, it may be a large collection and if adhesions rupture the fluid may be a frank haemothorax. A large accumulation of fluid follows spontaneous rupture of the oesophagus. When the effusion is large a splash may be detected in addition to the signs of the basal collection of fluid. With underlying staphylococcal or tuberculous pneumonia infection may spread to the pleura as well, giving rise to a pyopneumothorax.

Diagnosis

The clinical picture is usually quite typical and confirmation of the diagnosis is obtained by chest radiography in which a clear zone without lung markings can be seen separating the lung margin from the chest wall. This is seen more clearly on expiration. Indeed, a shallow pneumothorax may only be seen on an expiratory film. Line shadows within the lung may indicate the presence of bullae; with large collections of air the underlying lung collapses down to a small opacity adjacent to the hilum and the mediastinum tends to shift to the normal side, especially when there is a tension pneumothorax.

The symptoms may on occasion resemble myocardial infarction or pulmonary embolism with infarction, but the physical signs and radiological shadowing clarify the diagnosis. A large air space within the lung, such as a bulla or cyst, with or without obstructive emphysema, or a large diaphragmatic hernia may resemble a pneumothorax but careful radiological studies usually differentiate these causes.

Treatment

Smaller spontaneous pneumothoraces in which the lung remains more than 70 per cent. inflated are left alone. The ambulant patient should be seen regularly to ensure the lung re-expands over the ensuing 2–4 weeks. With persistent symptoms or with considerable deflation of the lung an intercostal tube should be inserted in the axilla and attached to an underwater seal. The lung usually re-expands rapidly within 12–24 hours. After expansion of the lung the tube should be clipped and if the chest radiograph shows that the lung has remained re-expanded the tube should be removed. Thoracotomy is necessary if the lung fails to re-inflate.

A tension pneumothorax demands immediate insertion of any needle or tube and this should be connected if possible to underwater drainage. This should be replaced as soon as possible by an intercostal catheter. If a pneumothorax complicates severe chronic bronchitis with emphysema or asthma the patient will require oxygen supplements.

Twenty-five per cent. of spontaneous pneumothoraces recur and then recurrences become more probable thereafter. On rare occasions the pneumothorax becomes chronic if there is a persistent bronchopleural fistula.

After two or more recurrences of the pneumothorax, artificial pleurodesis should be considered. In the case of air-crew or patients who travel frequently by air, then this should be considered even after a single pneumothorax. Chemical methods are either painful (silver nitrate) or potentially neoplastic (talc). Ten millilitres of a 1 per cent. solution of camphor in oil can be inserted into the pleural cavity and then the air removed. This treatment, however, is often unsuccessful. With recurrent pneumothorax pleurectomy should be considered. This is the treatment of choice for a chronic pneumothorax. Stripping of the parietal pleura is most likely to obliterate the pleural space permanently and in expert hands is remarkably free of complications and discomfort to the patient. This is the method of choice in air-crew with bilateral pneumothorax and if there is progressive underlying lung disease such as cystic fibrosis.

Course and Prognosis

The prognosis for a simple spontaneous pneumothorax is good for in 70–80 per cent. of cases there is a rapid absorption of the fluid and no recurrence. The prognosis is much less certain in chronic pneumothorax, especially when this complicates chronic respiratory disease. In the latter case the pneumothorax may be a terminal event. Tension and bilateral pneumothoraces are rare and on occasions may prove rapidly fatal, but provided the condition is recognized and dealt with immediately the prognosis is good.

REFERENCES

KILLEN, D. A., and GOBBEL, W. G. (1968) *Spontaneous Pneumothorax*, Boston.

LENNOX, S. C. (1970) Treatment of spontaneous pneumothorax, *Brit. J. hosp. Med.*, **3,** 893.

PLEURAL TUMOURS

Primary pleural tumours are rare and may be benign, e.g. fibroma, or malignant, e.g. mesothelioma or sarcoma. Fibromata and sarcomata arise from the visceral pleura and either displace or invade the lung—the origin from the pleura may be difficult to establish, especially when the tumours arise in the interlobar pleura. Both these tumours may be associated with gross clubbing of the fingers and pulmonary osteo-arthropathy and the sarcomata with the production of 'hormones' which cause hypoglycaemia, usually due to inhibition of glucose release from the liver rather than to an insulin-like substance. A pleural fibroma gives a well-defined shadow on the X-ray and usually gives rise to no local symptoms.

The pathogenesis of mesothelioma of the pleura is considered in the section on asbestosis [p. 910]. Primary pleural tumours often cause pleural effusion—but secondary or metastatic tumours which have arisen from the lung, breast, etc. are much more commonly encountered in the pleura with or without effusion [p. 902]. These metastases may cause single or multiple opacities arising from the pleura when seen on the chest radiograph.

Clinically malignant pleural tumours often cause persistent pain in the chest wall, weight loss, and breathlessness when they are large or associated with an effusion. The physical signs frequently resemble a pleural effusion, but vocal fremitus is usually retained with solid masses. A coarse friction rub may be heard and sometimes a visible firm or hard swelling develops in the chest wall, which may be tender. Haemoptysis and cough often follow direct invasion of the lung.

The condition has to be differentiated from a primary carcinoma of the bronchus which is invading the pleura, from chronic empyemata particularly those associated with tuberculosis or actinomycosis and from unilateral pleural effusions [p. 922]. The diagnosis should be established by aspiration of pleural exudate, which is often blood-stained, and pleural biopsy which usually reveals the nature of the growth.

Pleural fibromata should be resected for fear of malignant change or for relief of pulmonary osteo-arthropathy. Malignant tumours of the pleura are rarely amenable to surgery. Some relief of pain may be achieved by radiotherapy but symptomatic treatment with analgesics will usually be required. The prognosis for malignant pleural tumours is uniformly bad. Treatment of malignant pleural effusions is discussed on page 923.

REFERENCES

MANFREDI, F., ROSENBAUM, D., and CHILDRESS, R. H. (1965) Diffuse mesothelioma of the pleura, *Amer. Rev. resp. Dis.*, **92,** 269.

PRICE THOMAS, C., and DREW, C. E. (1953) Fibroma of the visceral pleura, *Thorax*, **8,** 180.

DISEASES OF THE MEDIASTINUM

The mediastinum is the interpleural space which extends from the thoracic inlet above to the diaphragm below and is divided into four parts. The *superior mediastinum* lies above the manubriosternal joint anteriorly and the lower border of the fourth thoracic vertebra posteriorly and contains the aortic arch and its main branches, the innominate vein and part of the superior vena cava, the thymus, trachea, oesophagus and thoracic duct, the vagus, recurrent laryngeal, cardiac and phrenic nerves. The other three parts lie below; the *anterior mediastinum* is limited by the sternum anteriorly and pericardium posteriorly and contains connective tissue; the *posterior mediastinum* lies behind the pericardium and in front of the lower eight thoracic vertebrae and contains the descending aorta, intercostal arteries, the azygos and hemiazygos veins, the thoracic duct, oesophagus and vagus nerves; the *middle mediastinum* comprises the heart and pericardium, the ascending aorta, the lower part of the superior vena cava and the phrenic nerves and lies between the anterior and posterior parts. All parts contain some lymph nodes.

MEDIASTINITIS

Infection of the mediastinum is rare and may be acute or chronic. Infection may gain access either from direct spread from outside with trauma, from adjacent structures (e.g. from bone or along the fascial planes from the neck, from the pleura, pericardium or lung), or from structures contained within the mediastinum such as the oesophagus or lymph nodes.

Acute suppurative mediastinitis usually follows perforation of the oesophagus and may be spontaneous (following vomiting), with carcinoma or foreign body or after endoscopy or dilatation. There is generally a rapid onset of severe pain behind the sternum which radiates to the back, followed by toxaemia, restlessness and high fever with leucocytosis (more than 10,000 neutrophils per mm^3.). Inflammatory oedema and pus may press on the trachea with cough, stridor or breathlessness, on the oesophagus with dysphagia, on nerves, e.g. the left recurrent laryngeal with hoarseness, on veins with obstruction to venous return. Mediastinal emphysema will also follow rupture of the oesophagus or trachea and the air and infection most commonly gain access to one or other pleural cavities with effusion or empyema (pyopneumothorax). The diagnosis is usually clear from the clinical findings. The chest radiograph may show widening of the mediastinal shadow with displacement of the trachea or oesophagus in either the postero-anterior or lateral view—there may be also air and fluid levels in the mediastinum or pleura. Treatment consists of chemotherapy and supportive measures (intravenous fluid and feeding if necessary). Abscess formation requires surgical intervention, as does pyopneumothorax.

Chronic mediastinitis is even more rare: it may be tuberculous, having spread from an infected lymph node or even more rarely be due to histoplasmosis. *Idiopathic mediastinal fibrosis* is characterized by the deposition of dense collagen most often in the superior mediastinum—this resembles retroperitoneal fibrosis and in fact the two conditions may rarely coexist. They are usually of unknown cause, but in some cases fibrosis has followed the use of methysergide, which is used in the treatment of migraine. The clinical picture is usually one of slowly developing obstruction of either the superior vena cava or the pulmonary veins, but oesophageal obstruction may develop. Radiography is usually unhelpful in the diagnosis, which has to be confirmed by biopsy (to exclude malignancy). This is usually undertaken by formal thoracotomy, at which time partial resection of the fibrous tissue may be achieved with some relief of symptoms. The development of collateral venous channels in some cases allows a very slow improvement.

MEDIASTINAL EMPHYSEMA

Air may gain access to the mediastinum by rupture of the oesophagus spontaneously or as a result of trauma, foreign body, or new growth, by rupture of the trachea and bronchi due to external or surgical trauma, by interstitial rupture of air spaces in the lung and rarely through the diaphragm after perforation of the bowel, following pneumoperitoneum or perirenal insufflation of air.

Rupture of alveoli and interstitial escape of air to the mediastinum may be due to sudden intrathoracic pressure change when there is small airways obstruction, as may be found in whooping cough, asthma, bronchiolitis, etc. It is particularly liable to occur in the neonatal period with congenital anomalies of the lung, e.g. lobar emphysema or cyst and with intermittent positive pressure respiration. It may develop 'spontaneously', (spontaneous mediastinal emphysema). Air may spread up to the neck in deep or superficial planes, rarely below the diaphragm (retroperitoneal) and to the pleura giving rise to a pneumothorax (a mechanism by which spontaneous pneumothorax sometimes develops). Mediastinal emphysema is often asymptomatic, but may cause severe central chest pain like that of myocardial infarction. On examination there may be subcutaneous emphysema in the neck and face, and characteristic crackling sounds over the mediastinum, usually heard over the heart with the patient sitting up. This sound may be similar to that heard with a shallow left pneumothorax. Breathlessness, cyanosis, distension of the jugular veins may all develop if the mediastinal air is under tension. Physical signs of a pneumothorax or a hydropneumothorax may be detected. On chest radiography a separate linear shadow may be seen along the line of the mediastinum and round the heart border, usually on the left side. Air may also be seen in the cervical region. A pneumothorax or hydropneumothorax may be seen on the radiograph, too. The air is usually absorbed spontaneously without any special measures. Although obstruction to venous return and fall in cardiac output may require surgical intervention, this rarely proves necessary.

Treatment should be directed at the causal condition and associated pneumothorax or empyema should be treated appropriately.

MEDIASTINAL TUMOURS (CYSTS AND NEW GROWTHS)

A wide variety of tumours, both primary and secondary, lymphomata and cysts are encountered in the mediastinum; many are of developmental origin. Many of the tumours are benign but all these lesions may compress, displace or interrupt function of many of the vital structures within the mediastinum—the symptoms and signs created depend on the site of the tumour or cyst and the direction and rate of growth. Thus, pressure on the major airways will result in breathlessness and stridor, harsh brassy cough and sometimes sputum which may be blood-stained. There may be collapse of the lung or invasion of the lung and of the pleura with effusion. There may be deep pain with rapidly growing mediastinal tumours or pain from invasion of the bone anteriorly or posteriorly. There may be superior vena caval obstruction, hoarseness due to recurrent laryngeal nerve palsy, Horner's syndrome or diaphragmatic paralysis from phrenic nerve involvement. Dysphagia will result from pressure or invasion of the oesophagus. A mediastinal tumour may deform the chest wall anteriorly or may bleed suddenly. Special effects of these mediastinal lesions are mentioned below. Large mediastinal lesions may be detected on examination posteriorly, where they may be signs of paravertebral consolidation.

The site of origin of tumours, cysts or lymphomata of the mediastinum is to be found in TABLE 53, together with the disorders from which they have to be differentiated. Hydatid cyst, rare as it is, has to be considered in any of these sites.

The majority of the mediastinal tumours and cysts are found on routine radiography—these and those presenting with symptoms will need to be differentiated from other lesions such as aortic aneurysm, pericardial effusion, intrathoracic thyroid. Careful physical examination may often provide the evidence on which to base the diagnosis, but usually tomography, barium swallow or angiography, bronchoscopy or mediastinoscopy will be needed to arrive at a definitive diagnosis. This may not prove possible before thoracotomy, which is required to remove all but the inoperable malignant tumours and lymphomata. The latter may yield to radiotherapy.

Tumours and cysts of the mediastinum are encountered infrequently compared with carcinoma of the bronchus, which is about 30 times more common and that of the oesophagus, which is about seven times more common. The most common tumours are neurogenic, followed by cysts, teratomata, thymic tumours and lymphomata—the remainder are extremely rare.

Neurogenic Tumours

These arise from the sympathetic nerve trunk and spinal nerves and therefore lie in the paravertebral gutter and posterior mediastinum. They comprise: (1) *neurilemmoma* which may lie partially within the intervertebral foramina and compress the spinal cord (dumb-bell tumour) and is the commonest; (2) *neurofibroma* which usually originates from an intercostal nerve but may grow into intervertebral foramina—it may become malignant and is sometimes found with generalized neurofibromatosis (von Recklinghausen's disease); (3) *benign ganglioneuroma* which arises from the sympathetic ganglia and may also enter the intervertebral foramina: it is more common in childhood than the other neurogenic tumours; (4) *neuroblastomata* are malignant tumours which arise from the sympathetic nerves; they occasionally calcify and are commoner in children.

These neurogenic tumours are usually symptomless unless they compress the spinal cord, become very large, or undergo malignant change. Neurofibromata will sometimes be associated with widespread cutaneous neurofibromata and pigmentation. These tumours usually cast well circumscribed homogeneous shadows in the upper posterior mediastinum on the chest radiograph—there may be splaying and thinning of the ribs posteriorly or erosion or broadening of the foramina and spinal pedicles—the shadows may sometimes contain calcium. The benign tumours should be removed for they grow slowly and cause symptoms or undergo malignant change—in any case the diagnosis may be in doubt. The prognosis is good. With malignant tumours the prognosis is less satisfactory, but surgery and radiotherapy may be successful.

Mediastinal Cysts

These are uncommon and apart from hyatid cysts, which are very rare, they are congenital and arise from the pericardium, foregut or thymus.

Pleuropericardial cysts are simple congenital cysts with a thin fibrous outer wall and an inner lining of flattened mesothelial cells—they are filled with clear colourless fluid (spring water cysts). They are usually found anteriorly in the cardiophrenic angle, more often on the right, and they may be circular or lobulated, casting a rounded homogeneous shadow on the X-ray. They seldom become very large or cause symptoms—they may communicate with the pericardium. They are most likely to be confused with a hernia of the foramen of Morgagni, which will be revealed by barium studies. These cysts may be left *in situ*.

Most cysts which originate in the developing embryonic foregut are either *bronchogenic* (in or around the trachea or major bronchi) or *gastro-enterogenous* (around the oesophagus). They arise in the circular

TABLE 53

SITE OF MEDIASTINAL TUMOURS, CYSTS AND OTHER LESIONS

	TUMOURS AND CYSTS	OTHER MEDIASTINAL DISORDERS
SUPERIOR	Intrathoracic thyroid Thymic tumours and cysts Teratomata Cystic hygroma Haemangioma Lymphomata	Aneurysm of aorta and innominate artery Oesophageal } lesions Tracheal } Enlarged lymph nodes, e.g. sarcoid, tuberculosis, metastases
ANTERIOR	Thymic tumours and vsts Teratomata Intrathoracic thyroid Pleuropericardial cyst Cystic hygroma Lymphomata	Hernia Enlarged lymph nodes
MIDDLE	Cardiac tumours Lipoma Bronchogenic cyst	Aneurysm of aorta Congenital defects of heart and vessels
POSTERIOR	Neurogenic tumours and cysts Enterogenous and bronchogenic cysts Meningoceles, posterior thyroid	Oesophageal lesions Aneurysm of aorta

muscle coat and are lined by ciliated columnar or stratified squamous epithelium and may become infected and rupture. Gastro-enterogenous cysts may have gastric mucosal elements in the wall and secrete gastric juice. Bronchogenic cysts may contain cartilage. In either case they may be accompanied by other congenital anomalies, such as spina bifida, etc., and they should be resected.

Teratomata

These tumours may be benign (dermoid cysts) or malignant and contain some tissue from all the germinal layers. They usually lie in the anterior mediastinum. The benign variety is mainly composed of ectodermal tissue, e.g. skin, hair, teeth, nervous tissue, bone, exocrine gland, etc., and is usually cystic. The malignant variety on the other hand usually comprises all three germinal layers, is solid and may be large—there may be evidence of either adenocarcinoma or a pleomorphic tumour as well as many other varieties of tissue. Choriocarcinoma is a very rare variant.

Infection and malignant change produce symptoms; in the former case there may be rupture into a bronchus or the pleura. Cough, dyspnoea, stridor, and sternal pain are the most likely symptoms. On radiography, clearly demarcated, dense homogeneous shadows may be seen in the anterior mediastinum which may sometimes contain teeth or calcium. Teratomata should be excised and radiotherapy may be helpful in malignant varieties in which the prognosis is uncertain.

Thymic Cysts and Tumours

The thymus is relatively large at birth. It increases in size in the first 2 years of life, often unduly so, giving a wide mediastinal shadow in the anterior mediastinum. It rarely causes symptoms, however, and after the age of two its growth much diminishes and it involutes after puberty. The thymus may enlarge in thyrotoxicosis and systemic lupus erythematosus. Hyperplasia or tumour may be associated with *myasthenia gravis* [p. 1322], *red cell aplasia, haemolytic anaemia* and other immunological disorders. Aplasia may be associated with generalized lymphoid aplasia and hypogammaglobulinaemia.

Cysts of the thymus are rare and often multiple. They are usually asymptomatic and only exceptionally cause sternal pain or cough.

Thymoma may be solid or cystic, well demarcated or invasive or calcified. The varieties of cell type encountered are numerous but most thymomata are malignant, invading locally and the adjacent lymph nodes but distant metastases are unusual. In the absence of *myasthenia gravis* (15 per cent. of cases have a thymic tumour), thymomata present with pressure effect, e.g. dyspnoea, stridor, or sternal pain. They may be an incidental radiographic finding, if not in the postero-anterior view then they will be seen in the lateral view in the anterior part of the upper mediastinum as a rounded or elongated homogeneous shadow.

Cysts and tumours of the thymus should if possible be treated surgically for fear of malignancy whether myasthenia gravis is present or not. For the role of thymectomy in myasthenia gravis, see page 1324.

REFERENCES

Barrett, N. R. (1958) Idiopathic mediastinal fibrosis, *Brit. J. Surg.*, **46,** 207.

Cloutier, C. T., Payne, M. L., and Gaensler, E. A. (1966) Mediastinal emphysema, *Med. Thorac.*, **23,** 183.

Holmes Sellors, T., Thackray, A. C., and Thomson, A. D. (1967) Tumours of the thymus: a review of 88 operation cases, *Thorax*, **22,** 193.

Morrison, I. M. (1958) Tumours and cysts of the mediastinum, *Thorax*, **13,** 294.

Oosterwijk, W. N., and Swierenga, J. (1968) Neurogenic tumours with an intrathoracic localization, *Thorax*, **23,** 374.

DISORDERS OF THE DIAPHRAGM

The diaphragm is the most important muscle in ventilation of the lungs. It is subject to a number of disorders, both congenital and acquired.

In congenital *eventration of the diaphragm* there is gross deficiency of muscle, usually on the left-hand side, which results in an elevated thin fibrous diaphragm which moves paradoxically. There are usually no symptoms, but when first discovered eventration has to be differentiated from acquired paralysis. Sometimes eventration may be partial and is then usually found anteriorly on the right side, when the localized bulge contains liver and resembles either a pleuropericardial cyst or a hernia through the foramen of Morgagni. If no cause is found for an elevated diaphragm or if it has been known to be present for a long time eventration may be assumed.

Unilateral diaphragmatic paralysis is usually the result of interruption of the phrenic nerve, most commonly by tumours, especially bronchial carcinoma. Birth trauma or surgical interference in the neck or thorax or gross displacement by other lesions, neurological disorders, e.g. myelitis or other cervical spinal cord lesions, herpes zoster, lead poisoning, poliomyelitis, or diphtheria may be responsible. Paralysis may rarely follow measles, typhoid fever, rheumatic fever and tetanus antitoxin. It is a rare occurrence in pulmonary tuberculosis, especially primary tuberculosis, and sometimes it develops without any known cause—idiopathic diaphragmatic paralysis is more common in males, affects both sides with equal frequency and in about 75 per cent. of cases is permanent.

Unilateral paralysis is usually asymptomatic—bilateral paralysis, e.g. with myelitis or after tetanus antitoxin, causes breathlessness and distress due to ventilatory failure; it is worse on lying down. With eventration and paralysis the diaphragm is not only elevated but can be seen to move paradoxically upwards further on sniffing. Paralysis may be distinguished from eventration by possession of a previously normal radiological appearance or may be assumed in the context of the clinical state. It must also be differentiated from *displacement* by disease above or below. Elevation of the diaphrgam accompanies atelectasis or fibrosis of a lobe or lung or resection. It is also found with pulmonary infarction and in certain cases of systemic lupus erythematosus—it also develops with lesions below the diaphragm, e.g. subphrenic abscess, liver abscess (often amoebic), tumours and cysts of the liver. Pregnancy, obesity, ascites and large abdominal masses will cause both diaphragms to rise.

Herniation through the diaphragm may be *congenital* through foramina of Morgagni (retrosternal) or Bochdalek (posterolateral) and anterolateral defects—these may present as emergencies in infancy or later. *Acquired herniation* is most commonly spontaneous through the oesophageal hiatus and may be para-oesophageal, sliding, or mixed. This and other forms of diaphragmatic hernia (e.g. traumatic) are discussed in Section 7, but they may produce shadows on the chest radiograph which may be confusing, especially in the posterior mediastinum where a hiatus hernia may produce a variable-sized shadow often with a fluid level or in anterior herniation through the foramen of Morgagni which resembles a pleuropericardial cyst. If the hernia contains gut then the diagnosis will be established by barium studies.

Cysts may develop within the diaphragm which in their structure resemble pleuropericardial cysts. *Primary tumours* of the diaphragm are very rare. The pleura or lung in relation to the diaphragm is usually the site of origin of a tumour. Fibroma, myoma and other benign tumours are exceptionally rare, but sarcoma is a little more common.

Hiccup is due to sudden involuntary contraction of the diaphragm with closure of the glottis, usually due to local reflex stimulation via the phrenic by excessive gastric distension after food or drink. In more serious causes, such as pericarditis, uraemia, or neurological disorders such as encephalitis or cerebrovascular accident or cerebral tumours, it may be difficult to control even with chlorpromazine, 25–50 mg. three to four times a day; hiccup may then prove extremely distressing and exhausting.

Tonic contraction of the diaphragm may be encountered in tetanus, rabies, etc. as part of a generalized disorder. Pain and respiratory distress may result and will require relief by those measures usually adopted in the treatment of tetanus and rabies, but may require muscle relaxants and mechanical ventilation.

Flutter of the diaphragm is very rare and the rate of contraction of the diaphragm exceeds 100 per minute. It is usually of unknown cause and may require phrenic paralysis by local anaesthesia or crush.

REFERENCES

Bonham Carter, R. E., Waterston, D. J., and Aberdeen, E. (1962) Hernia and eventration of the diaphragm in childhood, *Lancet*, i, 656.

Lancet (1962) Idiopathic diaphragmatic paralysis, Annotation, i, 1225.

John Batten

SECTION 10

DISEASES OF JOINTS

DISEASES OF JOINTS

INTRODUCTION

Pathological changes in joints may arise from a wide variety of causes (known and unknown) and no satisfactory or systematic classification of joint disease can be devised on an aetiological basis. Joint structures may be the site of some primary disturbance, e.g. local infection, trauma or new growth, but in addition joints may participate to an extent varying from transient and mild arthralgia to the most prominent and presenting symptom of some generalized systemic or connective tissue disease. Conversely, in many of the diseases in which arthropathy is often the only, and usually the most important, feature of the disease there may be involvement of other systems which are important from the clinical and therapeutic points of view. In general, joint disease can be considered under four major headings:

Inflammatory Arthropathy. This group contains those forms of arthritis in which joint inflammation of unknown cause is the main feature—the prototype being rheumatoid arthritis.

Degenerative Joint Disease. Osteoarthrosis (hitherto loosely called osteoarthritis). Here, as the name implies, the cause is degenerative.

Metabolic Deposition Arthropathy. In this group metabolic products are deposited in the joint, e.g. gout, in which sodium biurate crystal deposition is the cause of the acute and of the chronic arthritis. Other metabolic deposits, both crystalline and non-crystalline, are now recognized.

Miscellaneous. Other types of arthropathy lend themselves less easily to classification but include bacterial, virus and fungal infections, coagulation defects, sensitivity reactions, neuropathic arthropathy and various other well recognized clinical syndromes in which joint disease occurs to a greater or lesser extent.

INFLAMMATORY ARTHROPATHY

The term inflammatory arthropathy is used to describe those forms of joint disease that are characterized by synovial inflammatory changes which tend to become chronic and lead to destructive (erosive) changes in the joints. It does not include the specific forms of joint infection such as staphylococcal, tuberculous or fungal arthritis. An important and convenient development in the recognition of these various arthropathies has been the identification of IgM antiglobulins known as rheumatoid serum factor (RSF). The presence or absence of these serve to divide the inflammatory arthropathies into two groups, those in which RSF is present being called *sero-positive* arthropathy, and the group of arthropathies in which it is not found being classified as *sero-negative*.

Unfortunately such a classification is imperfect for a number of reasons. The sensitivity and specificity of tests for RSF vary. Thus the test in which human globulin is attached to Latex (polystyrene) particles appears to be the more sensitive than those in which rabbit gamma globulin (IgG) is attached to sheep cells. The latter, however, seem to be more specific. However, positive tests may occur in systemic lupus erythematosus, progressive systemic sclerosis, dermatomyositis, dysproteinaemias, subacute bacterial endocarditis, hepatocellular disease, chronic pulmonary tuberculosis and leprosy. Studies in the normal population show that some 4 per cent. of apparently healthy people give positive tests with a tendency for these to be found more frequently in the older age groups. Finally, tests for RSF may remain negative throughout the course of what in all other respects appears to be rheumatoid arthritis.

RHEUMATOID ARTHRITIS

Synonym. Rheumatoid disease.

Definition

Rheumatoid arthritis is a symmetrical peripheral polyarthritis characterized by inflammation of the synovium which leads to destructive joint change. It is often associated with the presence of rheumatoid nodules occurring in the subcutaneous tissues over pressure points and occasionally in tendons. Whilst arthritis is the most prominent manifestation many other systems may be involved so that it can be more correctly called *rheumatoid disease*. The clinical picture is variable, and incomplete forms of the disease are common.

Aetiology

The cause of rheumatoid arthritis is not known. In general, females are affected three times as commonly as males, although the sex differential diminishes with increasing age of onset and with more precise diagnostic criteria. The peak age of onset is between 35 and 50 years, but no age is exempt and ranges from childhood [see Still's disease, p. 941] to the age of over 75 years. Rheumatoid arthritis is a common disease, the over-all prevalence in the United Kingdom being approximately 2 per cent. in males and 5 per cent. in females—a prevalence which increases in the older age groups, some 16 per cent. of females over 65 showing evidence of past or present rheumatoid arthritis. The general belief that the prevalence of rheumatoid arthritis is influenced by climate has not been substantiated by population surveys, and there appears to be no consistent correlation between clinical rheumatoid arthritis or the presence of rheumatoid serum factor with latitude. Such minor differences as do appear in various populations relate to the severity rather than the prevalence of the disease. The role of genetic and environmental factors is not at present understood and no race or continent is apparently spared. Familial aggregations of the disease have been observed. This is associated with more severe disease (sero-positive and erosive), the prevalence in the first degree relatives of such patients being three to five times greater than in normal controls. This contrasts with the finding that the prevalence in the consorts of patients with rheumatoid arthritis is similar to that of the general population, and suggests that genetic factors are more important than environmental.

The role of infection as an aetiological factor is still undetermined. It is clear that the hypothesis that 'focal infection' is a factor can no longer be sustained. Whilst a number of claims have been made that *Mycoplasmata* and diphtheroids have been identified within rheumatoid synovial cells the role of these groups of organisms in the aetiology remains unproven. Evidence of overactivity of immune processes is more substantial. Rheumatoid serum factor is an immunoglobulin and is produced by immunologically competent cells which are also present in the synovium; complement levels are diminished in the synovial fluid and immune complex particles can be identified within the synovial fluid cells. It is possible that these are formed within the joint and that they are phagocytosed by the leucocytes which become damaged as a result releasing lysosomal enzymes which set up a further inflammatory response. The nature of the antigen is not known—it might, of course, be produced by a microbial agent such as has already been mentioned.

Pathology

Synovitis occurs in joints, tendon sheaths and bursae. No pathognomonic features are found but the presence of lymphocytes and plasma cells occurring in clumps is characteristic. In the joint the proliferating synovium erodes the cartilage of the joint margin invading the subchondral bone, producing the characteristic erosive change, visible radiologically [PLATE 14]. Once the bone cortex is breached the pumping action of synovial fluid when the joint is used may enlarge this to produce a cystic appearance. The proliferating synovium also spreads over the surface of the cartilage forming a pannus. In the advanced stages absorption of bone ends may take place, and in weight-bearing joints trabecular collapse may occur. Such changes, with involvement of periarticular soft tissues, lead to subluxation, instability and deformity.

Subcutaneous nodules occur in 25 per cent. of patients with rheumatoid arthritis, being found only in those with positive tests for RSF. They commonly appear in pressure areas—over the olecranon, sometimes within the bursa at this site, and on the extensor aspect of the forearm [PLATE 14]. Similarly they may be found over the sacrum or ischial tuberosities. Not infrequently they occur in association with tendon sheaths, particularly in the hand, especially in relation to the flexor tendons in the palms. They are also found in relation to the Achilles tendon. Such nodules are characterized by the presence of a central area of fibrinoid necrosis, surrounded by a palisade of epithelioid cells. Lymphocytes and plasma cells are prominent in the outer layers.

Arteritis is an important feature and accounts for many of the systemic features of rheumatoid arthritis. This may involve the smallest vessels where intimal hyperplasia results in local ischaemia. In the larger vessels necrotic changes in the arterial wall resemble those seen in polyarteritis nodosa.

Clinical Picture

The fully developed picture of rheumatoid arthritis is easily recognized. Difficulty arises, however, when the patient presents with only a few features of the disease. Whilst this is commonest early in the course of the arthritis in some cases the full expression of the disease never appears. Spontaneous remissions are common (often, of course, attributed to therapy) or the disease may pursue an episodic course.

Typically the onset is insidious with a gradually progressive symmetrical peripheral polyarthritis. The pattern of joint involvement is one that includes the proximal interphalangeal and metacarpophalangeal joints of the hands, the wrists and the lateral four metatarsophalangeal joints of the feet. New joint involvement develops irregularly to include the larger limb joints, ankles, knees, elbows and shoulders, and often later the hips. The temporomandibular joints may be affected, usually transiently. The spinal joints are usually spared with the important exception of the cervical spine where involvement of the atlanto-axial joint, and of the facetal joints of the upper cervical spine (in contrast to degenerative joint disease which affects the lower cervical spine), is characteristic. Involvement of the crico-arytenoid and of the joints of the middle ear has been described. Tendon sheath involvement with tenosynovitis may be a significant cause of symptoms, especially in the hands and wrists. The arthritis is accompanied by synovial swelling and joint effusions, and tendon sheath proliferation with swelling may be observed.

A characteristic complaint is of morning stiffness which, when it lasts more than half an hour, is a highly significant index of inflammatory joint disease. Not only are the joints painful on movement but spontaneous pain may become an important feature causing, in particular, loss of sleep. Systemic symptoms, malaise, loss of weight and fever are common. Nodules may appear at any stage and, if present, are very important for the diagnosis from other forms of inflammatory arthropathy. Bursitis, occasionally with nodular walls to the bursae, may develop, most frequently in the olecranon bursa. Tendon nodules in the flexors in the palms may cause triggering of the fingers. Synovitis of the wrist is a frequent cause of carpal tunnel syndrome which may cause symptoms of median neuritis—this syndrome develops in two-thirds of patients with rheumatoid arthritis at some stage. It is an important cause of functional impairment and easily overlooked. Lymphadenopathy may be present especially in the drainage area of active joints. The rate of progression of the polyarthritis is extremely variable. The fully developed picture may appear within days or may take many years. With persisting synovitis, anatomical changes gradually appear in the joints and joint laxity, subluxation, and deformity develop. The symptoms are now partly those due to the synovitis but increasingly due to the resulting structural changes.

The deformity which results from these structural changes is usually characteristic and most easily observed in the hands where three patterns may develop: (1) ulnar deviation at the metacarpophalangeal joints often associated with palmar subluxation of the proximal phalanges; (2) 'swan-neck' deformity of the proximal interphalangeal joints—hyperextension of this joint with fixed flexion of the metacarpophalangeal and of the terminal interphalangeal joint [PLATE 14]; and (3) boutonnière (buttonhole) deformity of the proximal interphalangeal joint—flexion deformity of this joint with extension contracture of the metacarpophalangeal and of the terminal interphalangeal joint. In the feet the toes may develop subluxation of the metatarso-phalangeal joints with clawing, causing them to be prominent dorsally and exposing the metatarsal heads to present unprotected weight-bearing surfaces. At the same time progressive hallux valgus develops. A valgus deformity of the feet and ankles then follows. Elsewhere flexion deformities are common, such a deformity developing particularly in the knees, hips and elbows. Subsequent development of deformity depends largely on the mechanical features of the joints—in the knees, for example, both anterior and lateral laxity allows the development of posterior subluxation of the tibia and a valgus or varus deformity. In the hips flexion deformity is usually accompanied by adduction and external rotation. The shoulder is held adducted and internally rotated. Three special complications may develop as a result of these structural changes in the joints: (1) tendon rupture—this commonly occurs in the extensor tendons to the fingers, usually affecting the 5th at the wrist and causing a complete failure to extend the affected finger. Later the 4th and sometimes the remaining tendons become similarly affected. Such ruptures result either from attrition where the tendon passes over an exposed area of bone as it crosses the arthritic wrist, or from invasion of the tendon by synovial granulation tissue. (2) Posterior rupture of the knee joint, the weakened peri-articular structures being unable to sustain the high intra-articular pressures of this joint [PLATE 15]. Posterior rupture may then occur with tracking of synovial fluid into the calf, sometimes becoming encysted and often giving rise to a picture similar to deep vein thrombosis and often misdiagnosed as such. (3) Atlanto-axial and upper cervical subluxation causing spinal cord pressure and long-tract involvement.

Systemic Features

Whilst the arthropathy may be an important part of the clinical picture of rheumatoid arthritis, most other systems of the body may be affected and may make an important contribution to the clinical picture. *Arteritis* is a feature of severe sero-positive disease, usually with nodules. Commonly this presents with ischaemic skin lesions appearing as dark brown areas 1–2 mm. in diameter in the nail folds [PLATE 15]. The development of these is often the first sign that the disease is assuming a more widespread form. Larger areas of necrosis or skin ulceration result from involvement of medium sized arteries; rarely peripheral gangrene or mesenteric occlusion may develop. *Neuropathy* in the form of a mononeuritis probably results from such an arteriopathy comparable to that seen in polyarteritis nodosa. It usually affects the lower limbs, e.g. the lateral popliteal nerve, but the upper limbs may later be involved. Sensory symptoms with paraesthesiae are associated with objective sensory loss and appear first. Motor weakness may follow. Multiple nerve involvement—mononeuritis multiplex—may give rise to a picture indistinguishable from a peripheral neuropathy. *Entrapment neuropathy* may also occur. Median neuritis from carpal compression (carpal tunnel syndrome) has already been mentioned [p. 936] but similar entrapment of the ulnar nerve at the elbow, of the lateral popliteal nerve at the knee and of the posterior tibial nerve behind the medial malleolus (tarsal tunnel syndrome) may be recognized. *Pleurisy with effusion* is not uncommon in men with sero-positive rheumatoid arthritis. It is usually unilateral and develops at the onset or in association with an exacerbation. Exclusion of other coincidental causes of pleural effusion is mandatory and may require pleural biopsy when a modified rheumatoid granulomatous lesion may be seen. The fluid is sterile, containing lymphocytes, and often has a characteristic low content of glucose (less than 20 mg. per 100 ml.). It may take many months to clear. Fibrosing alveolitis may cause dyspnoea due to a reduced diffusing capacity. Whilst this is regarded as part of rheumatoid disease it may be no more than a reflection of an increased susceptibility to pulmonary disease generally. Frank *rheumatoid nodules* may, however, develop both in the pleura and in the lung parenchyma. They are usually found incidentally on routine radiography and may give rise to considerable difficulty in diagnosis, not least when they develop, as they may do, as the first manifestation of rheumatoid disease before the arthropathy is apparent. Tests for rheumatoid serum factor are always positive but tuberculosis and carcinoma in particular require exclusion. Central necrosis may occur, but the lesions may disappear spontaneously more frequently than the commoner superficial nodules over pressure areas already mentioned. Where pneumoconiosis is associated these opacities may become large and confluent (Caplan's syndrome) [see Section 9].

Cardiac involvement is rarely apparent clinically but rheumatoid nodules may be discovered *post mortem* in some 10 per cent. of cases. Pericarditis is evidently not uncommon, being observed in up to 40 per cent. of patients coming to autopsy. Pericardial effusion and pericarditis are occasionally manifest clinically.

Rheumatoid disease of the eye is relatively common and more easily recognized. Reduced lacrimal secretion is associated with a dry irritable eye—keratoconjunctivitis sicca (Sjøgren's syndrome). Episcleritis and scleritis, sometimes associated with the presence of rheumatoid nodules in the sclera and occasionally progressing to scleromalacia perforans, is a feature of severe rheumatoid arthritis.

Anaemia is an almost invariable feature. This may be due to iron deficiency or simply the 'anaemia of chronic inflammation'. Occasionally a megaloblastic anaemia occurs attributable to the disease itself, or the anaemia may be associated with hypersplenism—Felty's syndrome [see below]. Iron deficiency commonly arises from occult gastro-intestinal tract bleeding as a result of prolonged aspirin consumption. The anaemia of chronic inflammation is found in patients with chronic active inflammatory joint disease—it is normochromic and is not only associated with a low plasma iron level (as occurs in the iron deficiency group) but also with a low total binding capacity. Some 20 per cent. of patients will be found to have a mild megaloblastic anaemia. This can usually be attributed to folic acid deficiency.

The association of rheumatoid arthritis with splenomegaly and neutropenia, often with lymphadenopathy, skin pigmentation and leg ulceration, is known as *Felty's syndrome* and merits brief special discussion. This syndrome commonly develops late in the course of severe disease. Not only is it associated with positive tests for rheumatoid serum factor in 90 per cent. of cases but tests for antinuclear factor and for L.E. cells are also usually positive. The neutropenia may be profound and secondary infection is a common and critical complication, which may influence therapy. Thrombocytopenia and haemolytic anaemia may also develop. Spontaneous remissions occasionally occur.

Rheumatoid myopathy rarely occurs and can be responsible for muscle weakness and wasting over and above that resulting from the arthropathy. Electromyography may be necessary to establish its presence. More commonly myopathy results from corticosteroid therapy.

Complications

These many systemic manifestations can all be regarded as part of rheumatoid arthritis. Secondary *amyloidosis* and *septic arthritis* may, however, occur as complications of the disease. Other common complications result from treatment and are dealt with under that heading. *Amyloid disease* is found in some 25 per cent. of patients at post-mortem examination but is rarely diagnosed in life. Clinically it usually presents as persistent albuminuria, sometimes progressing to a nephrotic syndrome; alternatively hepatosplenomegaly and occasionally a malabsorption syndrome may draw attention to the diagnosis which can be confirmed by biopsy of kidney or liver or more simply by rectal or gingival biopsy. *Septic arthritis* may supervene in a rheumatoid joint and presents an easily missed phenomenon, especially if the patient is under treatment with corticosteroids when the inflammatory reaction may be suppressed. Alertness to the possibility of this complication is always necessary, especially in a patient who is more ill than the clinical situation seems to require, and an apparent exacerbation in an individual joint should not routinely be accepted as being due to rheumatoid arthritis. Joint aspiration and examination of the fluid should be considered as an essential procedure to be carried out wherever joint infection is considered a possibility.

Diagnosis

Special Investigations. The ESR is one of the most reliable indications of inflammatory joint disease but it is, of course, quite non-specific. Rarely an anomalous normal ESR may persist despite active disease. Tests for rheumatoid serum factor have already been discussed—they are positive in 80 per cent. of patients with classical rheumatoid arthritis and in all patients with rheumatoid nodules. In about 20 per cent. of patients, tests for L.E. cells or antinuclear factor will be positive, usually in the more severe examples with a greater tendency for multisystem involvement; their presence does not necessarily invalidate the diagnosis, although clearly they call for reappraisal. Anaemia is common and may reflect disease activity, but has no diagnostic features.

Radiography is of prime importance in the diagnosis. Whilst soft tissue swelling is visible clinically and osteoporosis and loss of joint space are liable to observer error the presence of erosions should be carefully sought. These are best seen in the small joints of the hands and feet (especially the latter even when asymptomatic), and straight views of both hands, including the wrists, and feet, should be routinely carried out. Erosive change can often be seen, especially in the metatarsal and metacarpal heads [see PLATE 15], and occasionally in the ulnar styloid. Radography of the larger joints has much less diagnostic value since small erosions may not be seen. In younger patients a periosteal reaction may be seen in relation to actively inflamed joints.

These simple measures enable a patient to be diagnosed as having nodular or anodular, sero-positive or sero-negative, erosive or non-erosive disease. With the presence of each feature in turn the diagnosis becomes more certain. Where the disease is sero-negative and anodular then other types of sero-negative arthropathy have to be considered. These are discussed under this heading elsewhere in this chapter. The presence of definite erosions, however, serve to differentiate this group from other connective tissue diseases with arthropathy, especially rheumatic fever, systemic lupus erythematosus, dermatomyositis, progressive systemic sclerosis and polymyalgia rheumatica. The cystic changes occasionally seen in degenerative joint disease do not normally cause difficulty. Difficulty may, however, arise in monarticular disease when synovial biopsy may be necessary to exclude tuberculosis, sarcoid, pigmented villo-nodular synovitis and synovioma, even though the histological picture of the synovium in early rheumatoid arthritis may be quite non-specific. Examination of the joint fluid may be helpful in excluding septic arthritis and the presence of crystals of urate or calcium pyrophosphate should be looked for specifically. Chest X-ray is necessary to exclude carcinoma or the bilateral hilar lymphadenopathy characteristic of sarcoidosis which will also be associated with a negative Mantoux test. The differential diagnosis from rheumatic fever more commonly arises in children (see Still's disease) but an antistreptolysin titre estimation is occasionally useful. Rheumatoid nodules are always associated with positive tests for rheumatoid serum factor, except in the rare case of hypogammaglobulinaemia. Where nodules are present whilst tests for rheumatoid factor are negative then biopsy of a nodule is mandatory to determine the diagnosis.

Treatment

In the absence of a known cause prophylaxis is not possible and no preventive measures can be taken. Treatment is designed to modify the course of the inflammatory joint disease and to reduce the structural consequences of this leading to deformity and consequent disability. Close collaboration between physician and surgeon from the earliest stage is invaluable and should always be developed where possible. *Rest* is traditional but requires careful prescription. The prescription of rest removes the patient and her joints from a traumatic environment and may produce immediate improvement. When prolonged unduly it leads to muscle wasting, weakness and often to deformity. Rest of a joint, the site of inflammatory arthropathy, reduces trauma, splinting prevents deformity and is likewise invaluable in relieving symptoms, but, again, if over-prescribed leads to osteoporosis and disuse atrophy of the joint and supporting muscles. Rest and splinting should always be supervised and combined with skilled physiotherapy to prevent deformity and maintain musculature. Early admission to hospital appears to have a beneficial effect on the outcome, probably because it provides rest and physiotherapy under skilled supervision. *Analgesics* provide relief of pain as a background to more specific treatment, and are essential. Chronic, often spontaneous, pain has a profound effect on the psyche and morale and the achievement of complete co-operation in what may be a prolonged, sometimes lifetime, programme of treatment cannot be successful without symptomatic relief. The salicylates remain the mainstay—aspirin in some form is the most useful substance and should be prescribed in sufficient doses—some 4 G. daily being ideal if tolerated. Occult blood loss may require supplementary iron. Paracetamol may occasionally be preferred but is usually less effective. Phenacetin or phenacetin-containing compound tablets should be avoided absolutely because of the risk of phenacetin nephropathy, one of the iatrogenic causes of death in rheumatoid arthritis. Many other analgesics are available and may occasionally be preferred. Most have their particular potential toxic effects. Phenylbutazone (*Butazolidin*) or oxyphenbutazone (*Tanderil*) are well established but require haematological monitoring because of occasional marrow toxicity. Indomethacin may cause headache, mental confusion and gastro-intestinal tract irritation. The fenamates—mefenamic (*Ponstan*) and flufenamic acid (*Arlef*)—or ibuprofen (*Brufen*) are sometimes preferred. Indeed, a wide variety of analgesics are available to suit every individual and permit variation in the course of time. The more potent analgesics—codeine, or dextropropoxyphene—may occasionally be required but the more habit forming and more potent analgesics should be rigorously avoided. None of these substances appears to have any significant effect on the disease and should be used only for symptomatic control.

Treatment with gold salts, sodium aurothiomalate (*Myocrisin*), should be instituted once the diagnosis is firmly established, when conservative treatment with rest and salicyclates is not associated with clinical remission, and when there is evidence of progressive disease, for example when radiological erosive changes are observed to be developing. The presence of positive tests for rheumatoid factor is an added indication. Whilst the mode of action of gold is not known its efficacy has been established by at least one adequate clinical trial. The usual dose regime is an initial test dose of 10 mg. by intramuscular injection followed a few days later by 20 mg. and thereafter 50 mg. weekly, to a total dose of 500 mg. This is approximately the therapeutic dose and a response should now be observed. The injections can then be spaced out to once every fortnight until a total of 1 G. has been administered. The dose can now be reduced to 50 mg. monthly (approximately the rate of excretion) and maintained at this rate for as long as necessary in the hope of maintaining remission. If there is no response after 0·5–1 G. the treatment should be abandoned. Toxic effects include nephrosis, skin rashes, stomatitis, gastro-intestinal disturbance and bone marrow aplasia. Rarely an acute sensitivity reaction follows the initial dose—hence the need for a small test dose. Each injection should be preceded by inquiry for appropriate symptoms. A blood count, including platelets, is necessary before starting treatment and this should be carried out at least monthly when weekly injections are being given and later three monthly. Most toxic reactions disappear gradually on prompt discontinuation but occasionally corticosteroid therapy is necessary. D-penicillamine may rarely be required to produce rapid elimination of gold salts. This regime may be modified to suit individual cases but once a remission is achieved prolonged maintenance therapy, if necessary for 2 or 3 years, is desirable in an endeavour to prevent relapse. An arbitrary minimum requirement for discontinuation should be 6 months of complete remission.

Chloroquine compounds appear to have a similar clinical effect in inducing remission. Again their mode of action is not known. Chloroquine sulphate (*Nivaquine*) is commonly used in a dose of 200 mg. twice daily. Several other chloroquine salts are available. Toxic effects include drug eruptions, loss of hair pigment, dyspepsia and corneal deposits. These are reversible on discontinuation. Retinal deposits may also occur, causing an irreversible retinopathy with permanent visual impairment. For this reason the drug should only be administered with expert ophthalmological supervision and should not be continued for more than 12 months continuously. This hazard has greatly reduced the value of this form of therapy, but occasionally satisfactory remissions may follow administration.

Corticosteroid drugs will predictably suppress the inflammatory activity of the disease. A wide variety of preparations are available and considerable experience in their use has been amassed. Their effect is to produce suppression of the pituitary-adrenal axis and, in sufficient dosage, all the phenomena of Cushing's syndrome. Dose levels must, therefore, be restricted to those which will produce some degree of suppression without, even over a prolonged period, causing the patient to develop unacceptable features of overdose. Prednisone or prednisolone are the most satisfactory preparations since, being relatively less potent, they can be given in larger doses. This allows for more accurate dose adjustment. In ordinary circumstances a dose of 10 mg. of prednisone or its equivalent should not be exceeded, and the use of 1 mg. tablets enables accurate tailoring of the dose to the patient's requirements, balanced against the hazards of overdosage. Abrupt dose reduction should be avoided and dose modification is required for periods of increased stress, e.g. surgical operation. There is no place for a short course of these drugs in a chronic disease such as rheumatoid arthritis, since their effect is purely suppressive. Initial doses should be small rather than large since, again, there is no advantage in producing a temporary suppression by doses which cannot be maintained over the long term.

Corticosteroid administration is indicated in the following circumstances: (1) in the patient whose rheumatoid arthritis continues to be remorselessly progressive despite conservative measures; (2) in the patient threatened with complete dependence, especially in the elderly who may become rapidly bedbound; (3) occasionally for the breadwinner or the housewife at a critical point where they are no longer able to maintain their economic or domestic responsibilities and whose social situation may be destroyed; (4) as a nightly dose of 5 mg. on retiring to overcome crippling morning stiffness. No patient should be allowed to become totally disabled without corticosteroid therapy receiving careful consideration and we should never simply preside over the destruction of any patient's joints by rheumatoid arthritis. Corticosteroid injections into individual joints may provide some temporary palliation. This may be of value for a specific purpose to 'buy time' or to enable some deformity to be corrected, for example a flexion deformity of the knee, which, when corrected, can be prevented by appropriate splinting. But it is never a substitute for other systematic treatment and never the prime line of treatment. Full aseptic precautions are, of course, essential. Adrenal stimulation with ACTH or *Synacthen* is sometimes preferred. It has the disadvantage of the necessity for regular injections and a greater tendency for salt retention. There is often more difficulty in accurate dose adjustment.

The *cytotoxic* and *antimetabolic drugs* appear to suppress immune responses and, on the assumption that rheumatoid arthritis is due to some perversion of immune mechanisms, these substances have been subjected to clinical trial in this disease. Evidence is accumulating that they may be of value. Azathioprine, 2·5 mg. per kg. body weight daily, and cyclophosphamide, 50–100 mg. daily, have both been claimed to be effective. Chlorambucil has also been used. At the present time these substances should be regarded as still on trial and only to be used under experimental conditions.

Supplementary drugs—haematinics, hypnotics, antidepressives and diuretics are often required. The frequent need for supplementary iron has already been mentioned. Occasionally the normochromic anaemia of chronic inflammation will respond to full doses of parenteral iron. Folic acid deficiency, if established, merits treatment. Many patients also require hypnotics, antidepressives and diuretics, which may be invaluable, although selectivity is required to prevent the patient's drug regime becoming too complex.

Surgery

Many orthopaedic procedures from synovectomy to arthroplasty and arthrodesis provide enormous scope in treatment and management. Operations represent only incidents, albeit often of critical importance, in the treatment programme. The closest co-operation between orthopaedic surgeon and physician should be maintained from the outset. Surgical operations are not simply salvage procedures to be considered late in the course of the disease. Early operation may serve to prevent later disability and may modify the drug regime. The choice and timing of operation requires regular, careful and time-consuming consideration throughout the whole course of a patient's disease.

Course and Prognosis

A major difficulty in the diagnosis and treatment of rheumatoid arthritis is the extreme variability of the onset and in the course of the disease. The onset may be acute so that the patient can recall the day and the exact time of the onset. It may be monarticular or polyarticular. It may be episodic, so-called 'palindromic' rheumatism. The onset may indeed be non-articular with malaise and fever, the diagnosis being obscure until the arthropathy develops.

The natural history has largely been observed in patients whose disease is sufficiently severe to cause them to present as hospital out-patients. Population studies indicate, however, that the disease is more common and milder than is indicated by such data, thus some 16 per cent. of females over the age of 65 years in the general population have evidence of past or present rheumatoid arthritis, and about half of these had never even consulted their family doctor. A working approximation of the natural history in patients attending hospital is as follows: about half the patients will remit leaving no or minimal residua; some 10 per cent. will develop severe crippling disability causing them to become totally dependent; the remainder require prolonged treatment and supervision and will become partially disabled, some of them partially dependent. Death may result from arteritis, amyloid disease, atlanto-axial subluxation, secondary infection (especially in Felty's syndrome) and as a result of therapy—salicylates or indomethacin producing gastro-intestinal bleeding; marrow suppression from phenylbutazone, oxyphenbutazone or gold therapy; phenacetin neuropathy and corticosteroid therapy producing Cushing's syndrome or adrenal insufficiency. It is wise to remember, however, that death may also be coincidental. The prognosis is thus difficult to assess but the following features can all be regarded as suggesting that remission is unlikely to occur spontaneously: an insidious onset (by contrast an acute onset often carries a good prognosis), persisting active disease of more than one year's duration, the presence of nodules, strongly positive tests for rheumatoid serum factor, positive tests for ANF, progressive erosive changes on radiography. A high sedimentation rate during the first 12 months of the disease is not of significance, but a high sedimentation rate late in the disease is a bad prognostic sign. Similarly anaemia as such is a bad prognostic sign late in the course of the disease. On the whole, men carry a better prognosis than women although occasionally men suffer from the most severe form of the disease with multisystem involvement and death from some complication.

REFERENCES

DUTHIE, J. J. R. (1971) Infection in the aetiology of rheumatoid arthritis, in *Modern Trends in Rheumatology*, ed. Hill, A. G. S., p. 78, London.

EMPIRE RHEUMATISM COUNCIL (1961) Gold therapy in rheumatoid arthritis, *Ann. rheum. Dis.*, **23,** 15.

OSMOND-CLARKE, Sir HENRY, and MASON, R. M. (1969) Combined medical and orthopaedic management, in *Textbook of the Rheumatic Diseases*, ed. Copeman, W. S. C., 4th ed., p. 775, Edinburgh.

PALLIS, C. A., and SCOTT, J. T. (1965) Peripheral neuropathy in rheumatoid arthritis, *Brit. med. J.*, **1,** 1141.

SCADDING, J. G. (1969) The lungs in rheumatoid arthritis, *Proc. roy. Soc. Med.*, **62,** 227.

TURNBULL, A. (1971) The blood in arthritis, *Rheumatol. phys. Med.*, **11,** 53.

STILL'S DISEASE

Hitherto this has been regarded simply as a form of juvenile rheumatoid arthritis. It is preferable, however, to define it less precisely as a chronic polyarthritis of children under the age of 16 years, of at least 3 months' duration, and affecting at least four joints. Such a definition includes more than one arthropathy: (1) a polyarthritis resembling rheumatoid arthritis but which is sero-negative and usually remits in adolescence, leaving variable residua and on the whole causing considerably less disability than adult rheumatoid arthritis; (2) rheumatoid arthritis beginning in childhood which may develop into adult rheumatoid arthritis, often with nodules and positive tests for rheumatoid factor; (3) ankylosing spondylitis of the type which begins with a peripheral arthropathy (see ankylosing spondylitis below) and which develops in adult life into classical ankylosing spondylitis. Since a distinction often cannot be made between these during childhood the term Still's disease remains a useful clinical diagnosis.

The peak age of onset is between 1 and 3 years. There is no marked difference in sex incidence. The onset commonly occurs as a polyarthritis sometimes accompanied by systemic manifestations. In about 10 per cent. of patients the onset is monarticular, usually affecting the knee. Occasionally the disease may commence as a severe systemic disturbance with malaise, a high remittent fever, often accompanied by a characteristic intermittent maculopapular rash and sometimes pericarditis, splenomegaly, lymphadenopathy and a marked leucocytosis, joint symptoms only appearing weeks or months later.

The pattern of the arthritis is similar to that of adult rheumatoid arthritis, but differs in that involvement of distal interphalangeal joints is common; cervical spine involvement occurs frequently and early, often progressing to fusion of apophyseal joints; radiological changes of sacro-iliitis are frequently present. Unlike adult rheumatoid arthritis iridocyclitis is an important manifestation occurring in some 10 per cent. of patients. If this is left untreated it may progress to blindness. The uveitis tends to be chronic with an insidious onset, and a course not apparently related to the activity of the arthritis. All patients therefore need regular slit lamp examinations despite the absence of symptoms or obvious eye signs. Growth in general may be impaired and local defects may occur due to involvement of epiphyses. Short metacarpals or metatarsals, asymmetrical limb length, hypoplasia of the mandible and cervical vertebrae may occur and persist into adult life. As in adult rheumatoid arthritis, amyloidosis occurs occasionally and has a similar course and prognosis eventually leading to death. Otherwise the prognosis is considerably better than that of the adult disease. However, this is not so in the small group described as type (2) above (about 15 per cent.) who have erosive nodular sero-positive polyarthritis which has the prognosis of adult rheumatoid arthritis. About 10 per cent. of the boys belong to type (3) and later develop ankylosing spondylitis.

Treatment is modified by the patient's age but is otherwise similar to that of the adult disease. Prevention of flexion deformities of involved joints by night rest splints is particularly important and a regular supervised exercise programme to maintain full range of movement of all joints is essential. As in adult rheumatoid arthritis aspirin forms the back-bone of drug therapy. Corticosteroid therapy should be avoided if possible, particularly since it causes further stunting of growth. However, chronic iridocyclitis or severe systemic illness may dictate the necessity for administration of these drugs. With severe active disease, particularly in those with positive tests for rheumatoid factor, gold therapy, sodium aurothiomalate (*Myocrisin*), should be given, modified for the patient's age and weight—injections of 20 mg. weekly for those over the age of 10 years, 10 mg. weekly over 5 years, and 5 mg. weekly for the younger, with the usual precautions [see p. 939], for a total of 20 weeks. Thereafter if improvement has occurred, fortnightly or monthly injections should be given as maintenance therapy according to disease activity.

The differential diagnosis is from rheumatic fever usually distinguished by the flitting nature of the arthropathy and evidence of recent streptococcal infection. Henoch-Schonlein purpura is recognized by the characteristic purpuric rash, renal and abdominal involvement in addition to the polyarthritis. Rarer connective tissue diseases such as systemic lupus erythematosus and dermatomyositis may present with a similar polyarthritis. Psoriatic and colitic arthropathy must be considered. Occasionally virus infections such as rubella may be associated with an arthropathy but this usually occurs in recognized epidemics. Acute leukaemia and neuroblastoma may simulate arthritis due to bone involvement. In these cases bone marrow or blood examination may reveal the diagnosis. With a systemic type of onset septicaemia must always be considered in the differential diagnosis. Finally, in monarticular disease examination of the joint fluid and synovial biopsy is necessary for the exclusion of acute septic arthritis and tuberculosis.

REFERENCE

Ansell, B. M., and Bywaters, E. G. L. (1969) Juvenile chronic polyarthritis or Still's disease, in *Textbook of the Rheumatic Diseases*, ed. Copeman, W. S. C., 4th ed., p. 323, Edinburgh.

SERO-NEGATIVE ARTHROPATHY

ANKYLOSING SPONDYLITIS

Synonyms. Marie-Strümpell disease; Von Bechterew's disease; Spondylose rhizomélique; Spondylarthritis ankylopoietica; Spondylitis deformans; Pelvospondylitis ossificans; Rheumatoid spondylitis.

Definition

Ankylosing spondylitis is an erosive inflammatory arthropathy affecting the sacro-iliac joints and the spine with a marked tendency to ankylosis. The peripheral joints may sometimes be affected. It commonly affects young men in the third decade but women may also develop the disease.

Aetiology

The aetiology is unknown. It is a relatively rare form of arthritis affecting no more than 0·5 per cent. of the male population at risk. It is less common in females, the sex incidence being 4 males to 1 female. Two factors are, however, recognized: (1) Sacro-iliitis (which may be symptomless) is found in some 9 per cent. of relatives of known sufferers. Thus a genetic factor would seem likely and a careful family history and, if necessary, a clinical and radiological examination of close relatives may be helpful in the diagnosis of a doubtful case. (2) Urogenital inflammation is invariably present in patients with ankylosing spondylitis, manifested by evidence of prostatovesiculitis. No organism has regularly been identified. It seems probable, therefore, that both genetic and environmental factors are important in the aetiology.

Pathology

Knowledge of the earliest changes in the sacro-iliac and spinal joints is scanty because of their inaccessibility. It is, however, an inflammatory arthropathy characterized by the formation of granulation tissue, which, in the spine, usually arises at the anterior corners of the vertebrae. These lead to erosive changes with periosteal reaction and new bone formation with the formation of syndesmophytes. The later changes show a marked tendency to ankylosis. The joint fluid shows no characteristic change but rheumatoid factor is invariably absent. Rheumatoid nodules are never found.

Clinical Picture

In the classical case the first symptom is of low backache beginning insidiously and characterized by morning stiffness, often awaking the patient. Rarely the onset may be acute and following trauma when misdiagnosis is common. The onset may be prepubertal (in 10 per cent. of cases), and the schoolboy with low backache requires careful examination of the spine for the characteristic physical signs. In some 10 per cent. of patients the onset is in a peripheral joint, nearly always in the lower limb, e.g. the knee, ankle, or foot, occasionally with a 'painful heel syndrome', or plantar fasciitis. When the onset is in a peripheral joint before puberty this may be an example of so-called Still's disease [see p. 941]. Iritis occurs at some time in 40 per cent. of patients and when this is the presenting symptom it may draw attention to the diagnosis. Routine screening of all patients with iritis will reveal many examples of the disease. The disease tends to spread gradually upwards to produce an increasingly rigid spine. Usually proximal limb joints are affected thereafter and the disease may then spread peripherally. The most important joint is the hip, ankylosis of which leads to severe disability. The physical signs are characterized by loss of mobility of the lumbar spine in all directions and these can be observed only by careful clinical examination, with the patient fully undressed, when the loss of lumbar lordosis is often also apparent. Forced movements of the sacro-iliac joints, when these are the site of inflammatory change, are painful. The most useful test is with the patient lying prone when firm, sharp pressure on the sacrum with the flat of the hand instantly reproduces or exacerbates the patient's backache. Restricted movement in the dorsal spine in rotation follows and the respiratory excursion is diminished below 5 cm. due to the involvement of the costo-vertebral joints. Loss of movement in the cervical spine is readily observed. A dorsal kyphosis may develop so that the patient is unable to see the ceiling above his head and in the advanced stages he may no longer be able to see straight ahead. Multisystem involvement occurs less commonly in ankylosing spondylitis than in rheumatoid arthritis. *Iritis* (which does not occur in adult rheumatoid arthritis) occurs in some 40 per cent. of patients. It is often associated with severe disease but can also be a feature of mild forms, the diagnosis only becoming apparent when the iritis draws attention to the possibility. The attacks are usually self-limiting and permanent loss of vision is rare with appropriate treatment. Conduction defects and *lone aortic incompetence* occur, the latter affecting 1 per cent. of patients. Routine electrocardiographic examination may reveal minor defects of conduction. *Ulcerative colitis* and *regional enteritis* occur more frequently in patients with ankylosing spondylitis than in the general population. The relationship of these conditions to ankylosing spondylitis is not clear (see colitic arthropathy). *Secondary amyloidosis* may occur and should be suspected in any patient with severe spondylitis and a high sedimentation rate with proteinuria.

Diagnosis

The E.S.R. is usually raised but is an unreliable index of disease activity. There may be a mild anaemia but no pathognomonic changes are found in the blood. Serological tests for rheumatoid factor are invariably negative. Prostatic massage will reveal a purulent smear but no organisms are identifiable. Radiography is an essential for definitive diagnosis. Evidence of bilateral sacro-iliitis is mandatory. These joints appear blurred with patchy areas of osteoporosis and sometimes erosive changes can be made out. In later stages the joint becomes obliterated as ankylosis takes place. Interpretation of radiographs of the sacro-iliac joints in children is difficult and cannot be relied upon. In the lumbar spine the vertebrae appear squared with filling-in of the anterior concave surfaces and small erosions may be seen in the upper and lower corners. These changes are followed by the formation of syndesmophytes due to calcification in the annulus which gradually unite with their partner on the next vertebra to form a vertical line of calcification [PLATE 15]. These syndesmophytes must be distinguished from osteophytes which are usually horizontal in direction and denote degenerative disc disease. Extension of these calcified areas through the spine leads eventually to the 'bamboo spine'.

Treatment

The whole emphasis in treatment should be on active mobilization. Immobility rapidly leads to ankylosis. Patients should be encouraged to lead an active, even, athletic life with due attention to posture. Special precautions are necessary if the patient develops some intercurrent illness requiring hospitalization when regular physiotherapeutic supervision should be insisted upon, since prolonged bedrest may have irreversible effects on mobility. Regular analgesics should be employed, and in the more severe case phenylbutazone (*Butazolidin*) or oxyphenbutazone (*Tanderil*), 100–300 mg. daily, appear to have an almost specific effect in reducing stiffness and permitting mobilization. Small doses are often sufficient but routine haematological supervision is necessary. Indomethacin (*Indocid*), 25–100 mg. daily, may have a similar effect. Corticosteroid administration is seldom effective and rarely indicated. The role of immunosuppressive or cytotoxic drugs has not been determined. Radiotherapy has fallen into disrepute because of the increased risk of the development of leukaemia in later life, and because there is no real evidence that it has anything other than a palliative effect. Irradiation of the spine may, however, still be indicated in those cases uncontrolled by conservative measures. Irradiation of the hip joint may be indicated where this becomes involved and is threatening function. Gross deformity of the spine may rarely require osteotomy to improve posture. Crippling disability, as a result of hip joint involvement, may now be corrected by the operation of total hip replacement, especially in the older age groups.

Course and Prognosis

The natural history is commonly benign and self-limiting and may amount to no more than asymptomatic sacro-iliitis. Rarely does a 'poker back' develop with a rigid spine and severe deformity. In a recent series from the Royal Air Force 60 per cent. were able to continue with a full service career.

REFERENCES

BALL, J. (1971) Enteropathy of rheumatoid and ankylosing spondylitis, *Ann. rheum. Dis.*, **30,** 213.

SHARP, J. (1965) in *Progress in Clinical Rheumatology*, ed. Dixon, A. St. J., Chap. 11, London.

WYNN PARRY, C. B. (1966) Management of ankylosing spondylitis, *Proc. roy. Soc. Med.*, **59,** 619.

PSORIATIC ARTHROPATHY

Definition

Psoriatic arthropathy is an erosive arthropathy occurring in patients with psoriasis and associated with this condition. It commonly affects the terminal interphalangeal joints of the fingers in which nail involvement has occurred. Occasionally the arthropathy may precede the development of psoriasis by many years. The condition should be distinguished from rheumatoid arthritis with coincidental psoriasis but it may affect many joints in a similar manner, although with a somewhat different pattern of joint involvement.

Aetiology

The aetiology is unknown, but relatives with patients suffering with psoriatic arthropathy are found to have psoriasis at least four times as frequently as the general population. Rarely keratoderma developing during an attack of Reiter's disease [see p. 151] may become chronic and then become indistinguishable from psoriasis, suggesting the possibility of an infective as well as a genetic factor.

Pathology

There are no specific features. Tests for rheumatoid serum factor are negative and nodules never occur.

Clinical Picture

Usually the psoriasis precedes the onset of the arthropathy. Occasionally it may be absent for many years when the diagnosis must remain presumptive. The pattern of joint involvement is characteristic, involving the terminal interphalangeal joints of the fingers, the interphalangeal joint of the thumb and of the big toe, and the interphalangeal joints of the toes themselves, but all peripheral and spinal joints may be affected. Sacro-iliitis and spondylitis may occur, the latter being difficult to distinguish from ankylosing spondylitis. Systemic complications such as occur in rheumatoid arthritis are not seen, but secondary amyloidosis may be a feature.

Diagnosis

The diagnosis depends on the finding of psoriasis in the presence of a characteristic arthropathy with a typical pattern of joint involvement. The arthropathy is sometimes associated with the development of an exacerbation of the psoriasis, but it may occur in the absence of psoriasis when the diagnosis remains presumptive, and is based on the absence of rheumatoid nodules and negative tests for rheumatoid serum factor. The presence of psoriasis may, however, require a careful search with special attention to the scalp, flexor surfaces, natal cleft, umbilicus and genitalia. A positive family history may be helpful, bearing in mind that psoriasis affects 1 per cent. of the general population. The sedimentation rate is raised but there are no specific changes in the blood and the histology of the synovium is non-specific. A mild degree of hyperuricaemia is common and often misleading. Radiological examination shows an erosive arthropathy with little osteoporosis and a tendency for florid periosteal proliferation.

Treatment

The treatment is similar to that of rheumatoid arthritis except that chloroquine compounds are contraindicated since they may exacerbate the psoriasis. Gold therapy may be given along similar lines, however, although evidence that it is effective is lacking. Cytotoxic and antimetabolic drugs are under trial. The folic acid inhibitor methotrexate is claimed to be effective for psoriasis and it is hoped that it may be equally effective for the arthropathy. It is administered intramuscularly, 25 mg. every 7–14 days, or orally 2·5–5 mg. daily. Toxic effects are common—stomatitis, gastro-intestinal disturbance and agranulocytosis in particular. The role of azathioprine, cyclophosphamide and chlorambucil are not yet established. Corticosteroid therapy may occasionally be justified but dose reduction may be associated with an exacerbation of the psoriasis. Orthopaedic surgical treatment is indicated as in rheumatoid arthritis.

Course and Prognosis

The course of the disease tends to be either mild with minimal residua or, rarely, to develop into a severe destructive arthropathy causing gross joint damage—arthritis mutilans. The characteristic slowly progressive arthritis of rheumatoid arthritis is rare. The prognosis is extremely difficult to determine in an individual case and prolonged observation is necessary.

REFERENCE

WRIGHT, V. (1969) Psoriatic arthritis, in *Textbook of the Rheumatic Diseases*, ed. Copeman, W. S. C., 4th ed., p. 632, Edinburgh.

COLITIC ARTHROPATHY

Synonym. Colitic arthritis.

Definition

Ten per cent. of patients with ulcerative colitis develop a sero-negative peripheral arthropathy. A similar percentage of patients with ankylosing spondylitis will be found to have ulcerative colitis. Colitic arthropathy may therefore be of two types: (1) a mild peripheral arthropathy usually affecting few rather than many joints asymmetrically and leaving no or minimal residua; (2) an arthritis of the spine indistinguishable from ankylosing spondylitis.

Aetiology

This is unknown. The hypothesis that the disease results from invasion by organisms through the damaged intestinal wall is not established. Alternatively, the arthritis may represent an immune response to some antigen in the gut. Type 1 arthropathy is usually associated with frank ulcerative colitis, whilst in type 2 the colitis may be asymptomatic or the arthritis may precede the development of ulcerative colitis by many years.

Pathology

There are no distinctive features. The synovium shows non-specific inflammatory changes. The E.S.R. is elevated. Tests for rheumatoid serum factor are negative. The colitis may be symptomless in type 2 arthropathy and require barium enema, sigmoidoscopy or biopsy to establish the diagnosis.

Clinical Picture

Type 1. The symptoms of ulcerative colitis usually precede the onset of the arthropathy which may develop in association with an exacerbation. The arthritis affects both sexes equally, in contrast to ankylosing spondylitis, and type 2 colitic arthropathy which affects predominantly males. The arthritis is usually an oligo-arthropathy with a pattern of joint involvement affecting larger joints characteristically—knee, ankle, wrist or elbow in an asymmetrical manner, but occasionally the small joints of the hands may be affected when it may resemble rheumatoid arthritis. The synovitis is mild and causes no or minimal erosive change, usually tending to remit without residua. Involvement of the sacro-iliac joints is common, especially in women when the disease may merge into type 2 colitic arthropathy. Erythema nodosum frequently develops. Iritis and mouth ulcers also occur.

Type 2. This is indistinguishable from ankylosing spondylitis. The spondylitis may precede the development of ulcerative colitis which may be symptomless and only found on special investigation. Men are more commonly affected as in ankylosing spondylitis.

Diagnosis

When the arthritis is associated with the onset or with an exacerbation of ulcerative colitis the diagnosis may be obvious, but such patients are not immune from developing rheumatoid arthritis. However, investigation for ulcerative colitis may be necessary to establish the diagnosis in any sero-negative arthropathy of the type described. Radiography will show no or minimal erosive changes in the affected joints. Bilateral sacro-iliitis is common. The radiological changes of spondylitis are indistinguishable from those of ankylosing spondylitis.

Treatment

Effective treatment of the ulcerative colitis will relieve type 1 arthropathy. In particular colectomy is invariably associated with relief of the joint symptoms. Ileostomy alone is less reliably effective. Treatment of the colitis does not influence the course of the spondylitic type, the treatment of which is that of ankylosing spondylitis. Phenylbutazone, oxyphenbutazone and indomethacin may be tolerated and, if they do not exacerbate the colitis, are indicated. As in ankylosing spondylitis prolonged immobilization will lead to increased stiffness.

Course and Prognosis

The peripheral arthritis is usually mild and remits

spontaneously leaving no or minimal residua. The course of the spondylitis is variable and resembles that of ankylosing spondylitis.

REFERENCE

WRIGHT, V., and WATKINSON, G. (1965) The arthritis of ulcerative colitis, *Brit. med. J.*, **2**, 670.

REGIONAL ILEITIS (Crohn's disease)

This may be associated with a peripheral arthritis indistinguishable from that of colitic arthropathy type 1. Sacro-iliitis is common. Treatment of the ileitis usually relieves the arthritis.

DIFFERENTIAL DIAGNOSIS OF SERO-NEGATIVE ARTHROPATHY

Whilst these sero-negative arthropathies have all been described as if they were separate entities they have so many common features that in clinical practice patients may be seen who cannot be so clearly categorized. In the absence of any known aetiological agent, differential diagnosis on such a basis is at present impossible. *Rheumatoid arthritis* is, however, distinguished by the presence of nodules and positive tests for rheumatoid serum factor. When these are both absent the diagnosis should be carefully reviewed. Rheumatoid arthritis, however, affects females more commonly than males and the arthritis is symmetrical and erosive. Iritis, conjunctivitis and urethritis do not occur and sacro-iliitis is uncommon, mild and asymptomatic. In *ankylosing spondylitis* the sacro-iliitis is usually early and causes a prominent complaint of low backache and stiffness, whilst in *Reiter's disease* sacro-iliitis is a late development and always associated with a peripheral erosive arthropathy [PLATE 15]. Genital inflammation is often a presenting complaint in Reiter's disease but if present in ankylosing spondylitis it is symptomless. *Psoriatic arthropathy* is associated if not with psoriasis at the onset with a positive family history. Genital inflammation, buccal ulceration and iritis do not occur. *Colitic arthropathy* requires the presence of ulcerative colitis except in the case of the spondylitic type when it may develop late in the course of the disease. *Gonococcal arthritis* is rare in the United Kingdom and is usually monarticular or oligo-articular. Gonococci can be identified in the joint fluid and there is a prompt response to antibiotic therapy. *Rheumatic fever* may occasionally give rise to difficulty. Erythema marginatum may be found. Genital inflammation and iritis do not occur. A history of sore throat and elevation of the ASO titre may be helpful.

OSTEO-ARTHROSIS

Synonyms. Osteo-arthritis; Hypertrophic arthritis; Degenerative joint disease.

Definition

Degenerative changes take place in joints *pari passu* with similar changes in all other systems. They begin in the third decade of life. Where they occur at a physiological rate of development symptoms do not arise and the changes hardly qualify as pathological. If, however, the degeneration is excessive joint symptoms develop and the diagnosis of osteo-arthrosis becomes tenable.

Aetiology

The transformation from physiological to pathological degeneration is determined by many factors; these depend on a disproportion between the forces imposed on the joint and the mechanical properties of that joint. Two aetiological factors are concerned: (1) the variability of the cartilage itself; and (2) the anatomical or 'biomechanical' state of the joint. Arthrosis arising from abnormality of the cartilage itself may be termed primary osteo-arthrosis, and that caused by a disturbed biomechanical situation secondary osteo-arthrosis. *Primary osteo-arthrosis* is due to an inherited predisposition; it usually affects multiple joints and is commonly associated with involvement of the terminal interphalangeal joints of the fingers—Heberden's nodes. This type of arthrosis is thus correctly termed nodal multiple osteo-arthrosis. *Secondary osteo-arthrosis* may have many causes. Trauma is often important, either single such as a fracture through the joint, or multiple and minor as occurs in obesity or in certain occupations. In hypermobility syndromes, sometimes due to inherited connective tissue disease, e.g. Marfan's syndrome, the joints are subject to excessive trauma from this quality alone. Anatomical disturbances such as congenital dislocation of the hip, slipped epiphysis, Perthes' disease or in association with developmental disorders such as chondro-osteo-dystrophy (Morquio-Brailsford disease) may also cause secondary osteo-arthrosis. Inflammatory joint disease may damage a joint sufficiently to render it liable to later osteo-arthrosis. Metabolic disease, such as crystal deposition disease (e.g. gout) and ochronosis may damage the cartilage and render it liable to degenerate. Kashin-Beck syndrome due to the eating of cereals infected with fusaria, or lathyrism from eating sweet peas, are rare examples of acquired cartilage abnormality. Endocrine disturbances such as acromegaly cause softening of the cartilage. Neurological deficit with impairment of sensory appreciation of joint pain can give rise to gross osteo-arthrosis—the Charcot joint. In brief, any factor which causes excessive joint trauma may lead to secondary osteo-arthrosis.

Pathology

The cartilage becomes softened due to loss of mucopolysaccharide ground substance—chondroitin sulphate. Superficial layers of cartilage, often, but not always, in areas of stress become fragmented and fibrillated. As this progresses ulceration of the joint surface develops. New bone formation occurs on the joint margins and osteophytes form. Altered mechanical stress may now produce micro-fractures in trabeculae and cyst formation due to breaches in the cortical bone. These changes are followed by increasing mechanical inefficiency of the joint, which in turn stimulates further degenerative change. Similar changes occur in the spinal joints as in the peripheral joints, facetal and intervertebral joints behaving in the same manner, modified only by the local biomechanical situation.

Clinical Picture

Nodal Multiple Osteo-arthrosis. This is a familial condition affecting women much more commonly than men, being inherited characteristically from mother to daughter. Heberden's nodes develop in the terminal interphalangeal joints of most fingers, together or in turn. New bone formation occurs on the dorsal aspect of the proximal end of the distal phalanx, causing a characteristic bony swelling [PLATE 16]. This may be acutely painful at the onset with cyst formation. Aspiration will reveal a thick clear glairy or jellified content. The acute painful phase passes off after months and discomfort disappears sometimes after years, leaving a bony swelling often with some deviation of the joint. Whilst these nodes are pathognomonic of nodal multiple osteo-arthrosis many other joints may be similarly affected and the pattern of joint involvement includes the carpometacarpal joint at the base of the thumb [PLATE 16], occasionally the other finger joints, the first metatarsophalangeal joint of the foot, the knees, the cervical and lumbar spines. The wrist joint is never affected but any other joint may participate. Spontaneous pain may be considerable but morning stiffness does not occur. Functional disability in the hands is remarkably slight despite considerable deformity. Soft tissue swelling of tendons and their sheaths is not a feature. Symptoms of pain and stiffness are worse after use and will be related to the anatomic situation of the affected joint.

When the spinal joints are affected neurological symptoms may arise. Osteo-arthrosis of the spinal joints—spondylosis—may give rise not only to local stiffness and pain but to symptoms of nerve root irritation with pain and paraesthesiae and occasionally neurological signs in the appropriate distribution. In cervical spondylosis, neck and shoulder-girdle pain may be accompanied by peripheral symptoms of paraesthesiae—a common cause of acroparaesthesiae. In lumbar spondylosis sciatic pain and paraesthesiae may also occur in the appropriate distribution. Dorsal spondylosis is less common but may give rise to dorsal backache. Disc degeneration renders the discs more liable to prolapse into the intervertebral foramina causing increased root pressure or interfering with the vascularity of the nerve, and causing neurological deficit. Posterior disc protrusion may, in the cervical spine, cause cord compression. Disc degeneration itself may be responsible for a transverse bar forming along the posterior margin of the disc which may of itself produce cord compression with long-tract symptoms and signs. The affected joints are characterized by absent or minimal signs of synovitis or effusion, but loss of range and crepitus are found and careful examination may reveal evidence of bony enlargement with palpable osteophytes at the joint margins. Involvement of the patellofemoral joint gives rise to typical painful grating on rubbing the patella against the lower end of the femur. With increasing disturbance of joint mechanics deformity may develop especially in weight-bearing joints.

Secondary Osteo-arthrosis. This may be multiple where the aetiology, as mentioned above, is appropriate. The pattern of joint involvement is that of the underlying cause. Thus a past attack of inflammatory arthropathy may be a cause of multiple osteo-arthrosis in the same pattern, e.g. an old mild attack of rheumatoid arthritis may cause secondary osteo-arthrosis later in the proximal interphalangeal and metacarpophalangeal joints of the hand. These symptoms and signs in the joints will be those described above. Monarticular osteo-arthrosis is determined by some local bio-mechanical disturbance. Osteo-arthrosis of the hip joint is an important problem since the mechanical forces acting on the hip are large. Severe disability may result. Pain is prominent on weight-bearing, and disturbs sleep. Walking is limited. Loss of range occurs and a flexion adduction and external rotation deformity develops.

Diagnosis

The diagnosis of osteo-arthrosis is suggested by the characteristic pattern of joint involvement. There are no symptoms or signs of inflammatory arthropathy and morning stiffness is strikingly absent. Synovitis and soft tissue involvement is not a feature. The E.S.R. is normal and no changes occur in blood chemistry. Radiography reveals sclerosis, cartilage loss and new bone formation. Erosions are absent although cystic changes may be observed. Examination of the joint fluid reveals a clear viscous fluid with a low cell count. Serological tests for rheumatoid serum factor are negative. In the spine the presence of spondylosis is invariable beyond middle life and it must not be assumed to be responsible for symptoms. Other space-occupying lesions must be considered and bony disease excluded as far as possible. Estimations of sedimentation rate, plasma alkaline phosphatase and plasma proteins are valuable screening tests to exclude secondary deposits or multiple myeloma. Radiography may reveal secondary deposits or Paget's disease of bone.

Treatment

In general, treatment is essentially symptomatic. Careful explanation to the patient and reassurance is often all that is required. The prognosis for function in nodal osteo-arthrosis is excellent. Analgesics are sometimes necessary especially for the spontaneous pain which occurs at night. Phenylbutazone or indomethacin are often more effective than aspirin. Osteo-arthritic joints respond well to reduction in trauma and to rest. Splinting of appropriate joints may be invaluable, e.g. a plastic splint for the first carpometacarpal joint, a soft cervical collar or a lumbosacral corset. Modification of activities with reduction of the patient's demands on the joints may be possible. Weight reduction may be helpful but not as helpful as might be expected, and often a waste of effort. Reduction in the load on the hip by the use of a walking-stick in the opposite hand reduces the load by a factor of four times and is perhaps the most important single measure in the treatment of osteo-arthrosis. Orthopaedic surgery offers great scope when the mechanical situation is irreversible and includes excision of the trapezium for osteo-arthrosis of the first carpometacarpal joint, osteotomy, arthrodesis and occasionally arthroplasty of the knee, osteotomy of the hip joint or total replacement of the hip. Spinal fusion may be indicated in severe spondylosis. Systemic corticosteroids have no place in the treatment of osteo-arthrosis, but occasionally local injections may be helpful especially when minor capsular strains are the cause of symptoms. Physiotherapy may be invaluable in re-educating wasted muscles serving mechanically disturbed joints. The place of manipulation in the relief of symptoms of minor spondylosis is controversial but supported by popular belief. It is contra-indicated when neurological complications have developed.

Course and Prognosis

Nodal multiple osteo-arthrosis has an entirely benign course and leaves little disability. The course of osteo-arthrosis in an individual joint is determined, however, by the local biomechanical situation. If the joint mechanics are insufficiently retained to sustain the demand made on it progressive disability will follow, the disability being in its turn determined by the function of that joint. In general non-weight-bearing joints never become a source of gross disability, whereas in weight-bearing joints the tendency is for progressive disability to occur. This applies particularly to the hip joint. Curiously the knee joints very rarely cause serious disability unless valgus or varus deformity becomes prominent when orthopaedic correction may be necessary. In general also no joint should be beyond orthopaedic correction unless some other systemic disease makes operation impossible.

REFERENCE

Ansell, B. M., and Wigley, R. A. D. (1964) Arthritic manifestations in regional enteritis, *Ann. rheum. Dis.*, **23**, 64.

METABOLIC DEPOSITION ARTHROPATHY

Two types of crystal may be deposited in joints: (1) monosodium biurate; (2) calcium pyrophosphate dihydrate. The joint disease produced by urate deposition is gout; that by calcium pyrophosphate deposition is best termed pyrophosphate arthropathy, although it has been popularly called 'pseudo-gout' because of its resemblance to its better known partner.

GOUT

Synonym. Podagra.

Definition

Gout is an acute or chronic arthropathy which results from the formation of urate crystals in the joint fluid causing acute arthritis; later, deposition of crystals in the joint structures causes chronic arthropathy characterized by the formation of tophi in the joint, in avascular structures elsewhere, and in the renal tract. It results from an elevated level of uric acid in the tissue fluid. Hyperuricaemia may be defined as a level in excess of 7 mg. per 100 ml. in the plasma. The joint symptoms are merely one, often dramatic, manifestation of the underlying metabolic abnormality.

Aetiology

The causes of hyperuricaemia are many. Man is almost unique in lacking the enzyme uricase which converts uric acid to allantoin, so that the end product of purine metabolism is the relatively insoluble uric acid. The renal handling of this substance remains, however, as if uricase was present. Thus uric acid is filtered through the glomerulus and completely reabsorbed by the proximal tubule—a mechanism which would serve to protect the renal tract from carrying fluid containing the insoluble urate and permitting uricase to operate in the liver. However, excretion of urate in man takes place in the distal tubule by a process of active secretion and is usually sufficient to maintain the plasma level below the critical concentration of 7 mg. per 100 ml. This mechanism is only just adequate and hyperuricaemia may readily result from disturbances of production or excretion of urate, the production depending upon the rate of endogenous purine metabolism, the intake of purine in the diet, and on the rate at which the kidney is able to excrete urate. Thus either over-production or insufficient excretion of urate may cause hyperuricaemia and subsequent clinical gout.

Secondary Gout. This may result from any factor influencing either of these mechanisms. Excessive purine intake or any of the myeloproliferative disorders or neoplasia may cause an excessive turnover of purines, e.g. leukaemia or polycythaemia (primary, secondary to cyanotic heart disease) may cause sufficient hyperuricaemia to precipitate clinical gout. Psoriasis with proliferation of epidermal cells may be sufficient to cause a mild hyperuricaemia (leading incidentally to diagnostic difficulties since psoriasis itself may cause an explosive arthropathy resembling gout). Alternatively, impaired renal tubular function, e.g. lead nephropathy, will produce a similar effect. Certain drugs modify the renal handling of urate—these include salicylates in small doses (less than 4 G. daily), thiazide derivatives, pyrazinamide and pempidine. Alcoholic excess probably acts in a similar manner and accounts for the traditional association between gout and alcoholism. Ketosis also reduces urate excretion—thus starvation and glycogen storage disease may cause secondary hyperuricaemia. Thyroid deficiency and hyperparathyroidism may cause a reduction of renal output of urate sufficient to precipitate gout.

Primary Gout. Where no cause for the hyperuricaemia can be found it is legitimate to classify this as primary gout. In these cases a family history of gout is often found, and a genetic determination seems likely, resulting commonly in a tendency to over-produce uric acid, but a similar inherited tendency to excrete urate at a lower level may also operate. Over-production may be due to a partial deficiency of the enzyme—hypoxanthine-guanine-phosphoribosyl-transferase — a complete loss of which produces the Lesch-Nihan syndrome. Primary gout occurs in post-pubertal males and post-menopausal females. Partly for this reason it is much commoner in males. There seems some association with social class and the disease is commoner in the higher income groups—it 'affects more rich than poor, more wise than fools'. There is no evidence that chronic alcoholics have gout more frequently than teetotallers. It is rare amongst the Scots but common amongst certain Polynesian races and in the Maori when it is associated with obesity, hypertension and diabetes. Patients with rheumatoid arthritis almost never develop gout and vice versa. Eunuchs, unless treated, do not suffer from gout.

Pathology

The acute attack of gout results from the appearance of crystals of urate in the joint fluid. It is not clear what precipitates their development although in general this is associated with plasma levels above 7 mg. per 100 ml., or occurs at a time when the plasma level is changing rapidly—upwards or downwards. A rapid fall in plasma levels (e.g. therapeutically induced) as readily precipitates acute attacks as a rapid rise. The presence of crystals induces an invasion of the joint fluid by leucocytes which ingest the crystals which can be regularly seen lying within the cell. Many of the leucocytes fail to digest the crystals, die and release lysosomal enzymes which add to the inflammatory reaction. Thus an acute synovitis develops. This is determined solely by the particular nature of the crystals and their size, and is independent of their chemical constitution. Thus the mechanism of acute pyrophosphate arthropathy (pseudo-gout) [p. 950] (q.v.) is identical. Both conditions produce a similar *crystal synovitis*. With long-standing disease urates become deposited in the cartilage and bone ends. Deposition in cartilage leads to osteo-arthrosis, occasionally with ankylosis especially in the mid-tarsal joints, and in the bone, tophi give rise to cystic changes readily seen on radiography. Tophi are also deposited in the helix of the ear and in the renal tract. Urate stones form in some 20 per cent. of subjects. Hypertension and hyperuricaemia appear to be related. Over 25 per cent. of untreated patients with hypertension will be found to have hyperuricaemia. This is due to diminished uric acid clearance with near normal glomerular filtration rates, suggesting an abnormality of tubular function.

Clinical Picture

The acute attack is characteristic. Classically it affects the first metatarsophalangeal joint (podagra) but any distal joint of the body may be involved. Involvement of the hip and shoulder joints is extremely rare and never occurs in a first attack. The onset is usually acute, perhaps with a brief prodromal period of irritability, malaise or vague joint discomfort recognizable to the experienced sufferer. Within a few hours the joint is acutely painful and exquisitely tender so that the patient cannot bear it to be touched and even the weight of the bed sheets cannot be tolerated. Redness and a shiny appearance of the skin is usual with peripheral joint involvement, but in a large joint such as the elbow or knee redness may be absent and the diagnosis thus missed. The skin over the affected joint remains dry. Within a few days the attack subsides and in the earlier stages leaves no residua. Attacks occur sporadically, traditionally in the spring, and are usually monarticular at first, but later becoming polyarticular. The rate of development of the disease is extremely variable and intervals between attacks may vary from months to 20 or more years. Gradually the attacks become more prolonged and tophaceous deposits develop in affected joints. Chronic gouty arthritis now develops with secondary osteo-arthrosis. Tophi begin to appear in the ear [PLATE 16], over the olecranon and in the neighbourhood of affected joints. These may become massive occasionally with necrosis of the overlying skin and secondary infection with sinus formation. Gross joint deformity may follow in the untreated patient. At this stage the acute attacks often diminish in frequency and severity, although they may still occur. Renal colic or the passage of gravel may occur and frank urate urolithiasis occurs in 20 per cent. of patients. Renal impairment and hypertension may follow. Some patients recognize precipitating factors for the acute attacks—alcoholic excess, certain foods or wine, stress anxiety and fatigue, all being familiar to some individuals.

Diagnosis

The diagnosis of gout is of great importance since the arthropathy is treatable and indeed preventable. Misdiagnosis is common both in that patients with gout are diagnosed as suffering from some other arthropathy, e.g. septic arthritis or occasionally rheumatoid arthritis, and conversely patients with some other inflammatory arthropathy are frequently diagnosed as having gout. This may be supported by a mildly raised plasma uric acid level as a result of small doses of aspirin, and occasionally from psoriasis which causes, likewise, some degree of hyperuricaemia. The character of the attack as described above is highly suggestive. The acute tenderness of the joint is an important clue, only rheumatic fever or septic arthritis requiring consideration. In both of these conditions the skin overlying the joint is moist. This is in contrast to the dry skin of the gouty joint. A finding of dry skin with exquisite tenderness is thus almost pathognomonic. A finding of a plasma uric acid level in excess of 7 mg. per 100 ml. is mandatory and repeated estimations should be carried out if there is doubt. The definitive diagnosis is made, however, by aspiration of joint fluid and identification of urate crystals (especially intracellular crystals) by polarized light microscopy. If the fluid, removed under aseptic conditions, is placed in a sterile bottle without anticoagulants it will be suitable for examination for several days. When tophi are present, urate crystals can be identified from biopsy material or the *murexide test* carried out. Radiography should never be required for the diagnosis—if there are bone tophi causing cystic changes these will be apparent on careful clinical examination. Whilst a positive family history may be helpful this is only present in 50 per cent. of cases of primary gout. The possibility of secondary gout should always be excluded by appropriate investigations.

Treatment

Acute Attack. Colchicine, 0·5 mg. every 2 hours, is effective but so often produces profound gastro-intestinal tract disturbance that it has now been superseded by phenylbutazone (*Butazolidin*), 600 mg. daily for 2 or 3 days, with gradual dose reduction thereafter, or by indomethacin (*Indocid*), 100–200 mg. daily in a similar manner. The choice between these two drugs is one of personal preference and patient tolerance. The former may be given by intramuscular injection (500 mg.), the latter by suppository (100 mg.) if there are contra-indications to administration by mouth, e.g. a history of peptic ulceration. If a large joint, e.g. the knee, is affected aspiration of the fluid (useful for polarized light microscopy for the presence of urate crystals) and the injection of appropriate corticosteroid will give very rapid, even dramatic, relief. Corticosteroid administration is effective but very rarely required, and ACTH or *Synacthen* administration likewise, but they may be useful in the rare resistant attack. *An acute attack should never be treated with uricosuric or xanthine oxidase inhibitor drugs.* These will only exacerbate or prolong the attack. The affected joint should be protected from trauma by a bed-cage if necessary. Hot poultices or applications of ice are sometimes soothing. Analgesics may be necessary but aspirin or other salicylate should be avoided.

Long Term and Preventive Treatment. The acute attack of gout serves to draw attention to the underlying metabolic disorder. This remains and may require treatment. Uricosuric drugs, by modifying the renal handling of urate, cause an increased elimination of uric acid in the urine. Salicylates in a dose in excess of 4 G. daily are effective but the large doses required will not be maintained; smaller doses cause uric acid retention, and moreover they reduce the effect of other uricosuric drugs, so that it is best to withdraw the salicylates permanently from the patient's regime. Probenecid (*Benemid*) and ethebenecid (*Urelim*) are both effective uricosuric drugs in a dose of 500 mg., two to four times daily. Sulphinpyrazone (*Anturan*), 100 mg. two to four times daily, is equally effective. The choice between these drugs is again one of personal preference and patient tolerance. These rarely cause gastro-intestinal disturbance or drug rash. It is necessary to commence treatment with small doses and at a time when the patient is free of an acute attack. The dose can be titrated over the months against the plasma level of uric acid, aiming to achieve and maintain a level below 7 mg. per 100 ml. Continuous indefinite administration is, of course, essential, since discontinuation will allow hyperuricaemia to reappear. These drugs increase the concentration of uric acid in the urine, with the risk of renal colic or passage of gravel. If renal urolithiasis is present uricosuric therapy is contra-indicated and allopurinol should be used [see below]. Similarly these substances may be ineffective in the presence of renal failure. Care must therefore be taken to maintain the fluid output, especially in hot climates, and the urine may, if necessary, be made alkaline by the administration of sodium bicarbonate by mouth. Acute attacks may be precipitated during the first few weeks or months of therapy. This is often avoided by initiating treatment with relatively small doses and thus producing a gradual fall in plasma urate levels. However, it is wise to give colchicine as prophylaxis, 0·5 mg. twice daily for the first few months, and, if necessary, indefinitely. In these doses toxic effects rarely occur. Phenylbutazone or indomethacin may be used in a similar manner, the former requiring regular supervision of blood counts. The recent introduction of allopurinol (*Zyloric*) in the treatment of gout represents a major advance in therapy. As an effective inhibitor of xanthine oxidase it blocks the final stages of purine metabolism reducing the production of uric acid at the stage when hypoxanthine and xanthine is produced. These substances have the advantage of being more soluble than uric acid. Administration lowers the urate concentration in the urine and thus reduces the likelihood of urolithiasis. Moreover, it is effective in the presence of renal failure. It is also of special value in situations which may produce a significant renal overload of urate, e.g. in leukaemia or neoplasia being treated with irradiation or radiomimetic drugs. In a dose of 100 mg. twice daily up to 600 mg. daily, it effectively lowers plasma uric acid levels. As with the uricosuric drugs any rapid reduction in plasma uric acid levels is likely to precipitate acute attacks, and if treatment is initiated during an episode of acute gouty arthritis it usually exacerbates or prolongs the attack. *Thus allopurinol is never indicated in the treatment of the acute attack.* Prophylactic colchicine should be used in the same manner as with the uricosuric drugs. Clinical experience to date has not suggested that toxic effects are common or serious. Occasionally drug rash or gastric intolerance may occur.

The decision as to when metabolic control should be instituted depends on a judgement of each individual case. It involves a lifetime of therapy to which the patient should not be committed lightly. At the same time these drugs bid fair to correct an important underlying metabolic abnormality. In general frequent disabling attacks of gout, or a persistent plasma uric acid level above 8 mg. per 100 ml. merit metabolic control. Hypertension is a further indication. Severe clinical gout, the presence of tophi or urolithiasis demand treatment. The patient must understand that continued treatment is necessary and that short courses are worthless. The choice between uricosuric drugs and allopurinol is often an individual one. The former have the merit of much experience (over 20 years) whilst allopurinol has only been in general use since 1966. However, increasing experience with allopurinol is increasingly reassuring, and reports of significant toxicity are impressively lacking. The risk of urolithiasis with uricosuric drugs may be an important factor to be considered. Clearly, in a patient with a history of renal colic, the passage of gravel or of urolithiasis allopurinol is the drug of choice. Intolerance or ineffectiveness of uricosuric drugs and significant renal failure are other indications. In patients whose 24-hour output of uric acid exceeds 1 g., allopurinol would seem to be rational. In patients whose hyperuricaemia cannot be controlled by either uricosuric drugs or allopurinol alone, both substances may be administered concurrently. This combined therapy may also be indicated in gross tophaceous gout when either alone may lead to very slow resolution of the tophi. With these drugs dietary restrictions are rarely required since strict reduction in foods of high purine content will only produce about a 1 mg. fall in plasma uric acid levels. Similarly restrictions on alcoholic intake are now much less severe than hitherto. Surgical excision of prominent and troublesome tophi may occasionally be desirable.

Course and Prognosis

Untreated gout is likely to be progressive with increasing frequency and severity of attacks, tophaceous deposits and, if the patient survives long enough, renal failure. With these measures gouty arthritis should be entirely preventable, and the tophus should become as fare as the gumma. Whether these measures will prevent renal failure is not yet determined, but it seems likely that gouty nephropathy should become less frequent.

REFERENCE

Barnes, C. G., and Mason, R. Michael (1967) The treatment of gout, 1967, *J. roy. Coll. Phys. Lond.*, **1,** 427.

PYROPHOSPHATE ARTHROPATHY

Synonyms. Pseudo-gout; Chondrocalcinosis articularis.

Definition

Pyrophosphate arthropathy is one form of crystal deposition disease which resembles gout in that acute attacks of crystal synovitis occur as a result of the formation of crystals of calcium pyrophosphate dihydrate in the joint fluid. Chronic arthrosis may result. It is characterized by calcific radio-opaque deposits in both hyaline and fibrocartilage, most easily seen in the knee menisci. It may occasionally be associated with recognizable metabolic disease but commonly no such disturbance can be recognized.

Aetiology

The disease does not show the sex preference for males characteristic of gout. It is equally distributed between the sexes, commonly affecting the middle-aged and elderly. It may occasionally be recognized in early adult life when it appears to be familial although the familial tendency of true gout is otherwise absent. Hyperparathyroidism, haemochromatosis, and true uric acid gout can occasionally be associated, but the mechanism whereby these conditions cause pyrophosphate arthropathy is not yet clarified.

Pathology

In the acute attack crystals of calcium pyrophosphate dihydrate can be observed in the joint fluid by polarized light microscopy. The crystals are often intracellular as in urate gout. An acute crystal synovitis occurs. Deposition of calcium pyrophosphate dihydrate occurs in both hyaline and fibrocartilage, especially in the knee menisci, but may affect the hyaline cartilage of many other joints. In the average case some three sites are affected. Analysis of the radio-opaque material in the menisci shows that this is apatite.

Clinical Features

The clinical course is very variable. Acute attacks may result although the gouty tendency to affect the first metatarsophalangeal joint (podagra) is rarely seen. The knee joint is most commonly affected. The acute episodes are associated with fever, malaise and often a high sedimentation rate with a leucocytosis, so that the clinical picture resembles septic arthritis (and may be misdiagnosed as such—see Diagnosis). Acute attacks may be absent and the patient may slowly develop chronic osteo-arthrosis. In such cases the diagnosis is only made by radiography. Rarely the arthropathy may resemble rheumatoid arthritis.

Diagnosis

The diagnosis depends on the recognition of chondrocalcinosis articularis on radiography, commonly in the knee menisci [Plate 16]. Routine screening of patients with arthrosis should include an anteroposterior view of the knee joint to exclude this finding. Calcification of single menisci in elderly subjects may not be significant. Chondrocalcinosis articularis may be observed in many other joints including the symphysis pubis and the small joints of the hands. Unlike gout, the hip and the shoulder are not spared. Calcification of the triangular ligament in the wrist is not uncommon and may give the clue to the diagnosis. Definitive diagnosis, as in gout, depends on identification of the crystals in the joint fluid by polarized light microscopy. Uric acid crystals are negatively birefringent whilst those of calcium pyrophosphate are weakly positive birefringent. Determination of the optical properties of these crystals therefore provides a valuable distinguishing factor. Biochemical abnormalities are uncommon. Occasionally a raised alkaline phosphatase has been found but the significance of this is not known. Hyperparathyroidism is occasionally found but it must be remembered that hyperparathyroidism may of itself also produce an arthropathy as a result of the metabolic bone disease which allows subchondral trabecular fractures to take place, leading to a widespread traumatic synovitis. Haemochromatosis is an important cause of pyrophosphate arthropathy occurring in up to 50 per cent. of cases. The arthropathy tends to be chronic and to affect the small joints of the hands. True (uric acid) gout may also occur and be associated with chondrocalcinosis articularis. The most important differential diagnosis is from septic arthritis and it is mandatory that all patients suspected of having septic arthritis should have the joint fluid examined, not only for bacteria but for intracellular crystals, using polarized light microscopy.

Course and Prognosis

A chronic secondary osteo-arthrosis usually develops in affected joints. When other metabolic diseases are present the outcome is that of the underlying disease. Correction of hyperparathyroidism will usually relieve the arthropathy.

REFERENCES

Currey, H. L. F. (1970) Pyrophosphate arthropathy and calcific periarthritis, *Clin. Orthop. rel. Res.*, **71,** 70.

Hamilton, E., Williams, R., Barbour, K. A., and Smith, D. M. (1968) The arthropathy of idiopathic haemochromatosis, *Quart. J. Med.*, **37,** 171.

OCHRONOSIS

Synonym. Alkaptonuria.

Definition

Ochronosis may be regarded as an example of metabolic deposition disease in joints causing arthropathy. The mechanism is different from that of crystal deposition disease in that the material deposited is not crystalline. Homogentisic acid, however, accumulates in cartilage causing it to become leathery and rigid, and thus prone to rapid degeneration. A characteristic osteo-arthrosis follows, affecting particularly the spinal joints, the disc spaces becoming thin and ragged and a painful arthropathy developing. Any peripheral joint may also be affected and severe disability may result.

Diagnosis

The diagnosis is usually obvious, homogentisic acid appearing in the urine causing it to go black on exposure to the light or on alkalinization. The deposits in the cartilage of the ear or in the sclera also become blackened when exposed to light.

Treatment

The treatment is that of osteo-arthrosis but in the absence of the capacity to correct the underlying metabolic abnormality it is largely ineffective.

REFERENCE

O'Brien, W. M., LaDu, B. N., and Bunn, J. J. (1963) Biochemical, pathologic and clinical aspects of alcaptonuria, ochronosis and ochronotic arthropathy. Review of world literature (1584–1962), *Amer. J. Med.*, **34,** 813.

ACROMEGALIC ARTHROPATHY

This arthropathy is a result of the growth hormone stimulus which causes overgrowth of bone, cartilage and connective tissue. The joints become hypermotile with a tendency to subluxation. Traumatic effusions develop and later marked new bone formation may occur with osteo-arthrosis developing. The latter is characterized, however, by an increased thickness of joint cartilage which is apparent on radiography. Osteoporosis rather than sclerosis also serves to distinguish this arthropathy from primary osteo-arthrosis. Carpal tunnel syndrome is common.

REFERENCE

Bluestone, R., Bywaters, E. G. L., Hartog, M., Holt, P. J. L., and Hyde, S. (1971) Acromegalic arthropathy, *Ann. rheum. Dis.*, **30,** 243.

Kellgren, J. H., Ball, J., and Tutton, G. K. (1952) The articular and other limb changes in acromegaly, *Quart. J. Med.*, **21,** 405.

ANAPHYLACTOID (HENOCH SCHOENLEIN) PURPURA

This condition may be associated with a transient synovitis, usually of the knee. It commonly occurs in children under the age of 6 years. The rash is usually diagnostic. Glomerulonephritis with haematuria and intussusception may occur [see Section 4].

REFERENCE

Bywaters, E. G. L., Isdale, I. C., and Kempton, J. J. (1957) Schönlein-Henoch purpura, *Quart. J. Med.*, **26,** 161.

BEHCET'S SYNDROME

Behçet's syndrome may present as an uncommon form of arthropathy. It is of importance for it resembles many of the other sero-negative arthropathies. Major features are painful buccal ulceration, genital ulceration and skin lesions, especially erythema nodosum or multiforme involvement of the eye with corneal ulceration, uveitis or retrobulbar neuritis. Less common features include thrombophlebitis and pericarditis, ulcerative colitis and central nervous system degenerative change. When some or all of these features are associated with a sero-negative non-erosive inflammatory arthropathy there may be considerable difficulty in diagnosis unless this condition is considered.

The aetiology is not known. No treatment appears to influence the natural history favourably. Corticosteroid therapy is indicated to preserve sight but does not influence the arthritis which remits spontaneously without residua [see Section 4].

REFERENCE

Mason, R. Michael, and Barnes, C. G. (1969) Behçet's syndrome with arthritis, *Ann. rheum. Dis.*, **28,** 95.

CLUTTON'S JOINTS

One manifestation of congenital syphilis may be a painful synovitis of both knees. Occasionally the elbows are affected. The arthropathy is benign. The age of onset is similar to that of Still's disease and this should be considered in the differential diagnosis. Other features of congenital syphilis will usually be present [see Section 2].

REFERENCE

Scott Gray, M., and Phelp, T. (1963) Syphilitic arthritis. Diagnostic problems with special reference to congenital syphilis, *Ann. rheum. Dis.*, **22,** 19.

COAGULATION DEFECTS

An important complication of both haemophilia and Christmas disease is a tendency to acute haemarthrosis either spontaneously or as a result of, often minor, trauma. Immediate treatment is indicated to prevent joint damage which leads to severe disability in later life. The immediate administration of cryoprecipitate for haemophilia or fresh plasma or concentrations for Christmas disease is necessary. Joint aspiration may be required but its value is not established. Ice packs to the affected joints may give symptomatic relief and splinting may be necessary to prevent deformity [see Section 13].

REFERENCE

Webb, J. B., and Dixon, A. St. J. (1960) Haemophilia and haemophilic arthropathy. An historical review and a clinical study of 42 cases, *Ann. rheum. Dis.*, **19,** 143.

ERYTHEMA NODOSUM

Arthritis is a common feature of erythema nodosum. Synovitis with effusion may develop, usually affecting the knees and ankles but occasionally the hands. The arthropathy is non-erosive, self-limiting and leaves no residua. The E.S.R. may be considerably raised. Salicylates usually provide effective relief but corticosteroid therapy may occasionally be necessary. The cause of the erythema nodosum should be determined if possible [see Section 14].

REFERENCE

TRUELOVE, L. H. (1966) in *Modern Trends in Rheumatology*, ed. Hill, A. G. S., Chap. 25, London.

FAMILIAL MEDITERRANEAN FEVER

A synovitis of the knees is often a prominent feature of familial Mediterranean fever. The joints may be acutely involved with marked pain and swelling but usually remit completely without specific treatment. Secondary osteo-arthrosis may occasionally result in later life. The disease is restricted to Sephardic Jews and is familial. The onset is commonly in childhood or early adult life. It is associated with fever and attacks of abdominal pain lasting 1–3 days due to a non-specific peritonitis. Secondary amyloidosis is a well recognized complication [see Section 4].

REFERENCE

EHRLICH, G. E. (1968) Arthritis in familial Mediterranean fever, *Clin. Orthop. rel. Res.*, **57,** 51.

JESSOP, J. (1969) Familial Mediterranean fever, *Proc. roy. Soc. Med.*, **62,** 199.

FUNGAL INFECTIONS

Fungal infections of joints rarely occur. *Actinomycosis* commonly affects the mandible but involvement of vertebrae occasionally occurs from local spread. Bone abscesses develop. *Blastomycosis* may cause punched out lesions in the neighbourhood of joints or in the vertebrae with vertebral collapse. The organisms can be identified in the joint fluid. *Coccidioidomycosis* may cause a benign polyarthritis occasionally associated with erythema nodosum. A chronic arthritis occasionally develops. *Histoplasmosis* may also be associated with erythema nodosum and a monarticular destructive arthritis has been described. *Sporotrichosis* may also affect joints causing disruptive local lesions [see Section 2].

HAEMOGLOBINOPATHIES

The haemoglobinopathies may affect the joints causing haemarthrosis, infarction of bone ends and synovitis. The latter is a feature of sickle-cell disease which may also cause periostitis, especially of the phalanges, and is sometimes associated with osteomyelitis due to *Salmonella typhimurium* [see Section 2].

REFERENCE

SILVER, H. K., SIMON, J. L., and CLEMENT, D. H. (1957) Salmonella osteomyelitis and abnormal hemoglobin disease, *Pediatrics*, **20,** 439.

HYPERCHOLESTEROLAEMIC ARTHROPATHY

Primary familial hypercholesterolaemia may be associated with a migratory polyarthritis. Xanthomata may produce tendon nodules and involve bone with the formation of para-articular bone cysts which may on radiography resemble the changes seen in gout or rheumatoid arthritis. The condition is recognized by the presence of cutaneous xanthomata and the presence of a marked arcus senilis. The plasma cholesterol is greatly increased. Beta-lipoproteins and phospholipids are also increased but the plasma triglycerides are normal.

REFERENCE

KHACHADURION, A. K. (1968) Migratory polyarthritis in familial hypercholesterolemia (Type II hyperlipoproteinemia), *Arthr. and Rheum.*, **11,** 385.

HYPERMOBILITY SYNDROMES

Hypermobility of the inherited connective tissue disorders such as Ehrlers-Danlos and Marfan's syndromes renders joints liable to secondary osteo-arthrosis. Otherwise normal individuals sometimes show a tendency to hypermobility and these patients are more liable to develop secondary osteo-arthrosis [see Section 4].

REFERENCES

BEIGHTON, P., PRICE, A., LORD, J., and DIXON, E. (1969) Variants of the Ehrlers-Danlos syndrome. Clinical, biochemical, haematological and chromosomal features of 100 patients, *Ann. rheum. Dis.*, **28,** 228.

KIRK, J. A., ANSELL, B. M., and BYWATERS, E. G. L. (1967) The hypermotility syndrome. Musculoskeletal complaints associated with generalised joint hypermobility, *Ann. rheum. Dis.*, **26,** 419.

HYPERTROPHIC PULMONARY OSTEO-ARTHROPATHY

An arthropathy of peripheral joints may be associated with clubbing of the fingers or toes from whatever cause, most commonly bronchial carcinoma. It is characterized by a periostitis readily visible on radiological examination, usually at the lower end of the radius and ulna. These areas should always be included in routine radiograms of the hands. The arthritis may be the first indication of the presence of bronchial carcinoma or pleural neoplasm. Resection of the carcinoma or vagotomy immediately relieves the symptoms.

HYPOGAMMAGLOBULINAEMIA

Patients with hypogammaglobulinaemia, congenital or acquired, may develop a non-erosive inflammatory arthropathy strikingly resembling rheumatoid arthritis. It is, however, characterized by absence of rheumatoid serum factor. Subcutaneous nodules are occasionally found. These, however, are distinct from rheumatoid nodules in the absence of plasma cells. The arthritis remits spontaneously without residua. Patients with hypogammaglobulinaemia are also prone to develop a septic arthritis.

REFERENCE

BYWATERS, E. G. L., and ANSELL, B. (1969) in *Textbook of the Rheumatic Diseases*, ed. Copeman, W. S. C., 4th ed., Chap. XIX, pp. 535 and 536, Edinburgh.

MALIGNANT SYNOVIOMA

Malignant synovioma is a rare tumour affecting young males more commonly than females usually in a lower limb joint. It presents as a painless swelling arising from synovial tissue. The tumour is a sarcoma and highly malignant. Treatment is by excision usually involving amputation and irradiation but the survival rate in 5 years is less than 50 per cent.

NEUROPATHIC JOINTS

Synonym. Charcot's joints.

Any loss of joint sensation renders that joint liable to develop a gross osteo-arthrosis with prolific new bone formation and marked instability. In practice Charcot's joints are seen in association with tabes dorsalis, syringomyelia and diabetes mellitus. They may also occur in association with paraplegia, Charcot-Marie-Tooth disease, myelomeningocele and leprosy.

REFERENCE

SCOTT, J. T. (1969) in *Textbook of the Rheumatic Diseases*, ed. Copeman, W. S. C., 4th ed., pp. 690–6, Edinburgh.

PIGMENTED VILLO-NODULAR SYNOVITIS

This is usually a monarticular arthropathy commonly affecting the knee which becomes spontaneously painful and swollen. Effusion is present and aspiration shows a heavily blood-stained fluid. Synovectomy may give relief although relapse is common. The synovium is greatly hypertrophied and histologically shows many giant cells containing haemosiderin. The aetiology is unknown.

RELAPSING POLYCHONDRITIS

Articular cartilage may be affected in relapsing polychondritis, giving rise to joint pains resulting from loss of cartilage which is due to intrinsic inflammatory change in the cartilage itself. Peripheral joints may be affected. The symphysis pubis and manubriosternal joint are sometimes involved. The condition is recognized by involvement of the cartilage of nose and ear, collapse of which is readily apparent. The disease is associated with fever and a raised sedimentation rate. Involvement of the tracheal cartilage with collapse is a common cause of death. The cause is unknown. Corticosteroid therapy may reduce the inflammatory changes in the cartilage.

REFERENCE

DOLAN, D. L., LEMON, G. B., and TEITELBAUM, S. L. (1966) Relapsing polychondritis. Analytical literature review and studies on pathogenesis, *Amer. J. Med.*, **41,** 285.

RETICULOHISTIOCYTOSIS

This is a rare disease producing a synovitis with a marked excess of histiocytes and abnormal beta-lipoproteins in the blood. Glycolipoprotein accumulates in the synovium and causes gross joint destruction sometimes amounting to arthritis mutilans.

REFERENCES

DIXON, A. ST. J. (1960) 'Rheumatoid arthritis' with negative serological reaction, *Ann. rheum. Dis.*, **19,** 209.

WARIN, R. P., EVANS, C. D., HEWITT, M., TAYLOR, A. L., PRICE, C., and MIDDLEMISS, J. H. (1957) Reticulohistiocytosis (lipoid dermato-arthritis), *Brit. med. J.*, **1,** 1387.

SARCOIDOSIS

Joint involvement may be the presenting feature of sarcoidosis associated with erythema nodosum and hilar lymphadenopathy (Löfgren's syndrome). The arthropathy may precede the development of erythema nodosum. This is a polyarthritis which may affect the ankles, knees, wrists and hands commonly. It is a synovitis and is associated with morning stiffness and may resemble rheumatoid arthritis. The development of erythema nodosum and the finding of hilar lymphadenopathy will usually reveal the diagnosis. A negative Mantoux test is characteristic. The arthritis is benign and responds to salicylates or, if necessary, to corticosteroid therapy. *Sarcoid dactylitis* with painful swollen fingers may also resemble rheumatoid arthritis but is distinguished by the characteristic X-ray appearance of diffuse osteitis of the phalanges. Cystic changes may arise in bone from granulomatous deposits. The response to corticosteroid therapy is poor. In some cases sarcoid granulomata may form in the synovium giving rise to attacks of hydrarthrosis [see Section 9].

REFERENCE

SPILBERG, I., SILTZBACH, L. E., and MCEWEN, C. (1969) The arthritis of sarcoidosis, *Arthr. and Rheum.*, **12,** 126.

SERUM SICKNESS

A generalized polyarthritis may be associated with serum sickness usually following the injection of foreign serum for therapeutic purposes. After some 10 days an acute reaction may develop resulting from widespread vascular damage associated with the development of an immune antigen-antibody complex. The arthropathy recovers spontaneously without residua.

REFERENCE

HART, F. D. (1969) *Tex tbook of the Rheumatic Dieases*, ed. Copeman, W. S. C., 4th ed., pp. 602–5, Edinburgh.

SUPPURATIVE ARTHRITIS

The most common bacteria to invade joints are staphylococci, and haemolytic streptococci, but pneumococci, gonococci, meningococci, *Escherichia coli* and many others including salmonellae and brucellae may do so likewise. Tuberculous arthritis presents a somewhat separate problem and is dealt with below. Section 2 should be referred to for the more general aspects of bacterial infection. Only certain special features will be dealt with here. Although septic arthritis is now rare prompt diagnosis and treatment is of paramount importance.

Clinical Features

Septic arthritis may occur at any age and affect either sex, but is particularly common under the age of 15 years and in the elderly. It is usually monarticular, affecting knee or shoulder joint particularly and of acute onset. The joint is acutely inflamed and exquisitely painful. When the organism is the gonococcus a migratory polyarthritis may precede localization in a single joint. Fever and rigors frequently occur. If the patient is on corticosteroid therapy, e.g. for rheumatoid arthritis, then the signs of inflammation may be greatly suppressed. The diagnosis depends on aspiration of the joint fluid for bacteriological examination. This essential investigation must be carried out prior to the administration of antibiotic therapy. The joint fluid will be purulent with a high cell count over 100,000 cells per mm^3., predominantly neutrophils. Blood cultures may also be useful. A search must be made for a primary focus, particularly in the nasopharynx and in the genito-urinary system.

Differential Diagnosis

Acute rheumatic fever, crystal synovitis (gout or pyrophosphate arthropathy), rheumatoid arthritis or Still's disease or any other inflammatory arthropathy may present in an acute manner resembling septic arthritis.

Treatment

Once the diagnosis is established appropriate antibiotic therapy should be promptly initiated. If the diagnosis seems probable it may be initiated whilst awaiting definitive bacteriological information, giving penicillin, 10–20 million Units daily, and streptomycin, 0·5 G. twice daily. It is often helpful to instil 100,000 Units of crystalline penicillin into the joint at the time of aspiration. The limb should be splinted in a good functional position. Surgical drainage may occasionally be required. Adequate analgesics with pethidine or morphine may be necessary. Early mobilization should be undertaken once the infection is controlled.

REFERENCE

Argen, R. J., Wilson, C. H., and Wood, P. (1966) Suppurative arthritis. Clinical features of 42 cases, *Arch. intern. Med.*, **117,** 661.

TUBERCULOUS ARTHRITIS

This is rare in the United Kingdom but the possibility of the diagnosis should always be considered in any monarticular arthropathy. When, however, as is most frequent, the spine is affected, the diagnosis may be difficult but it is then characterized by local tenderness and destructive radiological changes affecting the disc space. In a peripheral joint the hip or knee is most commonly affected with a gradual onset of a slowly developing monarticular arthropathy. The diagnosis is established by synovial biopsy, by the demonstration of tubercle bacilli in a smear of joint fluid, by culture or by guinea-pig inoculation. A negative Mantoux test usually excludes the diagnosis but a positive test is of less significance. Radiography of the chest may show a primary focus and of the affected joint destructive changes gradually developing. Treatment is by conventional antituberculous chemotherapy with immobilization of the joint under orthopaedic supervision.

VIRAL INFECTIONS

RUBELLA AND MUMPS

Occasionally other virus infections such as glandular fever and smallpox may be associated with a true arthritis. This may be polyarticular and superficially resemble rheumatoid arthritis or rheumatic fever. However, when this occurs in the presence of an epidemic the diagnosis is usually clear. The arthritis is self-limiting, lasting a few days to a few weeks. Complete recovery takes place. Treatment is symptomatic but this is one situation where, if the symptoms are severe enough, a brief course of steroid therapy is justified.

REFERENCE

Smith, J. W., and Sanford, J. P. (1967) Viral arthritis, *Ann. intern. Med.*, **67,** 651.

WHIPPLE'S DISEASE

Arthritis may be a feature of this disorder. It is a non-erosive intermittent oligo-arthropathy commonly affecting the knees but often migratory. The disease is almost entirely restricted to males. The periodic acid-Schiff staining bodies observed in the lymph nodes and endocardium are not regularly seen in the synovium [see Section 7].

REFERENCES

Farnan, P. (1959) Whipple's disease, *Quart. J. Med.*, **28,** 163.
Kelly, J. J., and Weisiger, B. B. (1963) The arthritis of Whipple's disease, *Arthr. and Rheum.*, **6,** 615.

Michael Mason

SECTION 11

GENERAL DISEASES OF THE SKELETON

GENERAL DISEASES OF THE SKELETON

OSTEOPOROSIS

Definition

Many aspects of osteoporosis have been subject to considerable controversies for the last twenty years or so. The definition of the condition, however, has never been controversial and has generally been accepted as a skeletal disease with reduction in bone mass without change of chemical composition of the remaining bone. This reduction in bone mass may be either local as a result of immobilization of a particular part of the body, or generalized as is usually the case. Although the definition given is simple and not controversial, it begs the question of what constitutes too little bone and of whether the commonly seen rarefaction of bone with age should be regarded as pathological or physiological. It is to be particularly noted that the term osteoporosis is not synonymous with rarefaction of bone. The latter may occur in other conditions such as osteomalacia and osteitis fibrosa cystica whereas the term osteoporosis should be restricted to cases where it can be shown that this clinical entity is truly present.

Aetiology

The main causes of osteoporosis are listed systematically in TABLE 54. It should be noted, however, that this table does not include some of the very rare causes and the causes are by no means listed in order of frequency. The most common cause of osteoporosis is undoubtedly senility, with postmenopausal osteoporosis coming a good second. Whether there is any true difference, apart from that of age, between these varieties of osteoporosis and 'pregnancy' osteoporosis remains a moot point. It has been suggested that all these varieties might be classified as 'idiopathic osteoporosis' presenting at different ages. A case for including juvenile osteoporosis in this idiopathic category is not quite so strong since spontaneous remission may occur after the disease has progressed for a few years, and this is quite unlike the course of other forms of 'idiopathic osteoporosis'.

TABLE 54

THE MAIN CAUSES OF OSTEOPOROSIS

1. Endocrine disturbances
    (a) Hypogonadism
    (b) Hyperadrenocorticalism
        (1) Natural; Cushing's syndrome
        (2) Iatrogenic; steroid administration
    (c) Acromegaly
    (d) Thyrotoxicosis
2. Nutritional disturbances
    (a) Scurvy
    (b) Calcium deficiency
    (c) Protein deficiency
    (d) Alcoholism
3. Idiopathic
    (a) Juvenile
    (b) Pregnancy
    (c) Postmenopausal
    (d) Senile
4. Inherited
    (a) Osteogenesis imperfecta
5. Immobilization
6. Loss of gravity

The endocrine causes of osteoporosis are important in as much as the underlying cause can often be removed. Although acromegaly and thyrotoxicosis are included under this heading, it should be noted, first that in thyrotoxicosis the main bone lesion is not osteoporosis but osteitis fibrosa cystica, and secondly that it has recently been suggested that osteoporosis is rather uncommon in acromegaly.

The nutritional disturbances, although of great theoretical interest as causes of osteoporosis, are probably rather uncommon causes of the condition. Thus, although calcium deficiency in animals can certainly lead to osteoporosis, there is almost no evidence that an analogous situation ever arises in growing children.

One of the long-term effects of immobilization is undoubtedly osteoporosis and the onset of bone rarefaction is indicated in the immobilized patient by a rise in urinary calcium which occurs within a week of onset of immobilization. The rate of bone rarefaction is very great while the rate of excretion in children of urinary calcium is limited so that hypercalcaemia may result. It might well be expected that the loss of gravity experienced by astronauts might also lead to hypercalciuria with the possibility of osteoporosis occurring in space flights of long duration. Unhappily, there is still no reliable and accurate information about what happened to the urinary calcium in the space flights undertaken so far. Although there is good histological evidence that, in the long-term, immobilization causes osteoporosis, there is still doubt about the precise histology in the short-term.

Pathology

The bone loss of osteoporosis is accompanied by little or no significant changes other than the bone loss itself and micro-fractures which may be seen in many of the trabeculae. Thus there is no increase in osteoid seams as occurs in osteomalacia and there is no increase in numbers of osteoblasts or osteoclasts as in osteitis fibrosa.

While there is no doubt that osteoporosis is common in old age, there is still controversy over whether it should be regarded as an inevitable part of the ageing of the whole body, or as a disease which happens to occur commonly in the elderly. It seems that bone loss commences at an early age in certain parts of certain bones, but only after the menopause or even later in other bones. Trabecular bone is generally affected before the cortical bone, and this explains why osteoporosis frequently affects the axial before the peripheral skeleton. In the vertebral bodies, which are especially affected, the transverse trabeculae are removed before the vertical trabeculae.

Albright and Reifenstein thought that osteoporosis was due to a reduction in the rate of osteoblastic activity and the consequent reduction in the rate of formation of bone matrix. Studies with isotopic and tetracycline labeling, however, have revealed that absorption rate of bone is increased in relation to the amount of bone remaining. Certain groups, both before and after Albright, have suggested that osteoporosis is due primarily to mineral deficiency, and indeed it has been shown that animals reared on a calcium-deficient diet can develop osteoporosis, sometimes reversible with a high calcium intake. There is no evidence, however, that human osteoporosis as usually seen can be attributed to calcium deficiency.

Clinical Features

Osteoporotic bones are brittle and therefore fracture easily. The bone is not tender except at the sites of recent fractures. Consequently, osteoporosis may give rise to no symptoms at all in the early stages. The next stage is shortening of the trunk height which may be a gradual process passing unnoticed even by the patient. This is due in part to a dorsal kyphosis and in part to a series of fractures of different vertebral bodies. Each fracture leads to sudden onset of pain, which is severe and may cause the patient to take to bed or a wheel-chair at least for a time, but which gradually diminishes over a period of some four to eight weeks. During this period the fracture will heal well and the patient will become quite pain-free until the next fracture occurs. These fractures may occur in response to obvious stress such as lifting a heavy weight like a bag of cement or a baby, but at other times may occur without any clear predisposing stress. Constant backache is a late feature of osteoporosis and may well be due in fact to osteo-arthritis, possibly made worse by the forward curvature of the spine which often accompanies osteoporosis. While idiopathic osteoporosis tends to be central, affecting the spine especially, fractures do occur at other sites, and the pelvis, ribs, and long bones are not infrequently affected, while fractures of the sternum occasionally have been reported, and fractures of the femoral necks are quite common in senile osteoporosis. The skull appears to be virtually immune from osteoporosis.

Since the spine is especially affected in osteoporosis, the loss of height can be demonstrated in the following ways. First, the crown to pubis dimension is shorter than the pubis to heel dimension instead of approximately equal as is usually the case. Secondly, there may be a transverse skin crease across the abdomen at about the level of the umbilicus. Thirdly, a diminution of the normal gap between the lower ribs and the iliac crests can be observed. This narrowing can itself give rise to symptoms due to the rubbing of the lower ribs on the iliac crests. None of these signs of height loss above the pubis are specific for osteoporosis, since they may occur in other conditions accompanied by vertebral compression as in osteomalacia, Paget's disease or malignancy.

Characteristically, the symptoms of osteoporosis in women develop in the sixth and seventh decades of life and since the condition is generally irreversible but consistent with life, it may last for up to thirty or forty years. The period of progressive height loss and repeated fractures, however, is generally limited to some ten or fifteen years. On the other hand the condition may start at a much younger age and progress much more rapidly, when there is some underlying cause such as cortisol administration or immobilization. In juvenile osteoporosis there seems to be a severe and probably progressive phase for a limited period of a few years followed by a recovery phase strongly suggesting that a specific cause has come into play for a limited period and then ceased to operate.

Diagnosis

The diagnosis of osteoporosis is based on the demonstration of bone rarefaction in the presence of no demonstrable cause for this other than osteoporosis. As previously mentioned, osteoporosis is characterized by a lack of observable biochemical abnormalities. Thus the plasma calcium is normal, except in those cases (usually children) where immobilization has led to so rapid a process of bone demineralization that hypercalcaemia develops. Plasma phosphate is normal for the age and sex of the patient unless this has been lowered by cortisol administration or raised by acromegaly. Plasma alkaline phosphatase is normal unless slightly raised due to recent fractures. Urinary calcium is generally normal in idiopathic osteoporosis but may be raised if the patient has been immobilized and may also be raised in steroid-induced osteoporosis and thyrotoxicosis.

Radiology plays an important part in the diagnosis of osteoporosis. It must be noted, however, that the observation of bone rarefaction is a very crude indicator of osteoporosis, since about a third of the bone must be lost before it is recognizable on an ordinary X-ray plate. Furthermore, the recognition of rarefaction does not necessarily imply osteoporosis, since very similar results can be produced by osteomalacia. Again, however, the characteristic of osteoporosis is the fracture. These occur in an apparently random fashion in the spine and best seen in a lateral view. The compression fractures are then seen, at least in the early stages, to be irregular not only in distribution but in kind, different vertebral bodies being compressed in different ways. This is demonstrated in FIGURE 61 which also contrasts the findings of osteoporosis with those of osteomalacia. Fractures may of course also be found at the other sites mentioned above. While these radiological generalizations are extremely useful, certain important exceptions must be noted. First, an 'osteoporotic spine' may be found in multiple myelomatosis and secondary carcinoma. Secondly, the 'osteomalacic spine' may be seen in juvenile osteoporosis. Thirdly, it must be remembered that osteomalacia may lead to immobilization which may then be accompanied by osteoporosis.

Treatment

He who sets out to treat osteoporosis should be modest in his ambitions. The literature of the past thirty years is strewn with therapies which have been hailed enthusiastically as cures for osteoporosis but which have subsequently been unsubstantiated, and in many cases completely forgotten. Indeed, so far, osteoporosis in the human subject has proved to be substantially irreversible. This has been most strikingly demonstrated in the osteoporosis of Cushing's syndrome, where removal of all hyperfunctioning adrenal cortex has not been followed, even in long-term follow-up studies, by any improvement in the osteoporosis.

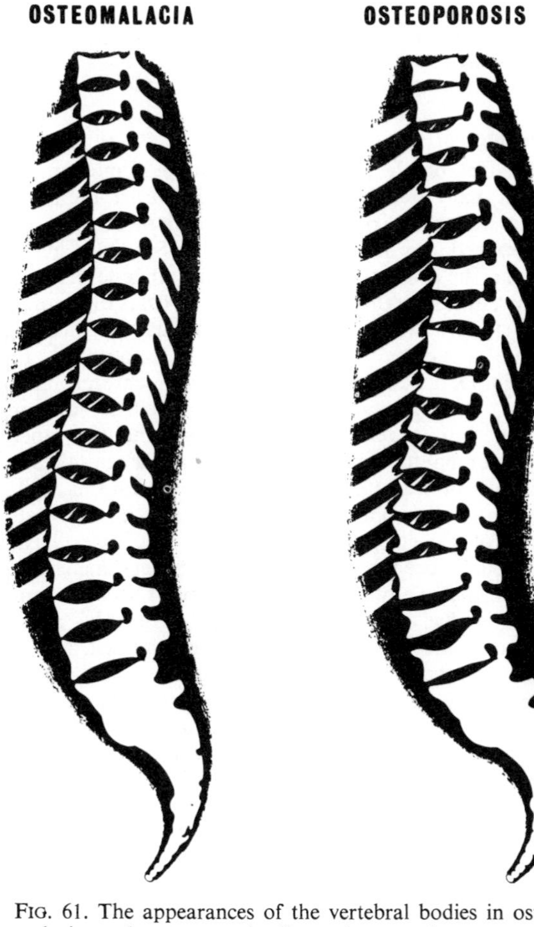

FIG. 61. The appearances of the vertebral bodies in osteomalacia and osteoporosis. In each case the appearance characteristic of the condition is shown, but the important exceptions mentioned in the text must be remembered. [Reproduced with kind permission from *Clinical Surgery*; Orthopaedics, ed. Rob, C. and Smith, R., Butterworth and Co. (Publishers) Ltd., London, 1966.]

The best that is to be hoped for, therefore, would appear to be an arrest or slowing down of the rate of bone demineralization. An important part of the treatment is a search for any underlying condition such as an endocrine disorder or a nutritional disturbance which can be treated in its own right. Otherwise the condition will have to be treated as idiopathic osteoporosis in which case two main types of drug therapy are available, namely hormonal and by high calcium intake. In the case of the female, stilboestrol in the dose of 1–3 mg. per day in repeated courses of 4–5 weeks on and 1 week off can be given to both pre- and post-menopausal women. In the case of males, methyltestosterone, 25–50 mg. per day, can be taken sublingually continuously. Jaundice is a risk, but apparently only a very slight one. With the hormonal treatment, urinary calcium may show a slight fall and faecal calcium is virtually unchanged and the negative calcium balance therefore slightly diminished. It should be noted, however, that the possible benefit will be greatest when the urinary calcium is high rather than low. High calcium intake has had a temporary vogue in the last twenty years. It used to suffer from the disadvantage that calcium lactate and other similar salts taken by mouth were rather unpleasant. Nowadays there are effervescent tablets commercially available with very high calcium content and which are quite pleasant to take. With these tablets the calcium intake can quite easily be raised from the normal 1 up to 4 or more grams per day. In deciding which of these two treatments to use, it is perhaps legitimate to consider the urinary calcium level prior to treatment. If this is high then hormonal treatment may be advocated, but if it is low, it would seem more sensible to use a high calcium intake.

Perhaps even more valuable than the therapy prescribed is the common sense advice which can be given at the same time. Thus any unnecessary immobilization, either local or general, is to be resisted and indeed calculated risks may be sometimes warranted in order to gain early mobility following a fracture. On the other hand unnecessary stresses of a type that have been shown to induce fractures in a particular patient should be avoided. Finally one should ensure that the patient's diet is adequate with regard to calcium, protein, vitamins C and D. With such a regime of treatment many osteoporotic patients will in fact stop fracturing or fracture less frequently and lose height less rapidly than before. It is uncertain, however, whether this is due to the specific therapy, or to the common sense already referred to above.

Albumin or plasma infusions, strontium, and fluoride have all been advocated but probably have no place in the treatment of established osteoporosis at the present time. Calcitonin is under active investigation in various centres, but no definite place has been established for it at the time of writing.

OSTEOMALACIA

Definition

Classical osteomalacia may be defined as the condition which arises when the vitamin D intake, both from normal dietary and solar sources, is deficient in the adult. When the same cause operates in children or in growing animals, then the same abnormal biochemical and physiological processes give rise to the condition of rickets. This definition, however, is not entirely adequate, as will be shown below, since in many types of osteomalacia and rickets, the vitamin D intake may be at a normal level. A histological definition may therefore be considered more appropriate and the presence of abnormally wide osteoid seams has been taken to signify osteomalacia. Even this definition is not infallible since the biochemical osteomalacia may ante-date histological osteomalacia, biochemical osteomalacia being defined as a low plasma calcium times phosphate product in the plasma simultaneous with a raised plasma alkaline phosphatase. This biochemical definition also breaks down occasionally since histological osteomalacia can occur without biochemical osteomalacia. Despite these exceptions, in practice there is very little difficulty in saying when osteomalacia is or is not present in particular cases.

Aetiology

The maximum normal requirement for vitamin D is 400 International Units per day (equivalent to 10 μg. calciferol) for growing children. Adults require very much less but a precise figure cannot be given.

The vitamin D-rich foods are few in number. The fish-liver oils are the richest sources but relatively few people indulge in them. The oily fishes such as salmon and herrings come next, but again these foods are not to everybody's taste. Margarine is next in this country since vitamin D is added to it by law. Some people, however, refuse to eat margarine and insist on butter which only contains vitamin D during the summer months. Eggs also contain a small amount of vitamin D in the yolk but this, too, is seasonal depending on the exposure of hens and hen food to sun-light. Since the only other source of vitamin D in large quantities is sunlight itself, it requires, in northern climates where sunshine is not a large contributor, only a few food fads to allow a state of vitamin D deficiency to arise. Thus vitamin D deficiency may arise by chance even in the midst of an adequate supply of the vitamin D-rich foods. It has also arisen in immigrants to this country from countries with hot climates, Pakistan amongst them, who by continuing with their old dietary habits, avoid vitamin D-rich foods. It is thought that these immigrants had been obtaining vitamin D by exposure to sunshine in their countries of origin, and that this source has proved inadequate in this country. A second factor suggested, however, is that the pigmented skin of these immigrants is less efficient in synthesizing vitamin D than the fairer skin of the indigenous population.

Osteomalacia and rickets not infrequently occur in patients who have had an amount of vitamin D which would normally be considered adequate. These patients are said therefore to be vitamin D-resistant or vitamin D-insensitive. The causes of such resistance form a very large and confusing group, some of which are listed in TABLE 55.

TABLE 55

THE CAUSES OF OSTEOMALACIA AND RICKETS

1. Vitamin D deficiency
   - A. Infancy
   - B. Food fadism
2. Vitamin D resistance or insensitivity
   - A. Hereditary pseudo-vitamin D deficiency rickets
   - B. Chronic renal failure
   - C. Steatorrhoea (any cause)
   - D. Renal tubular disturbances:
     - i. Phosphate leak only
       - (a) Familial
       - b) Sporadic
     - ii. Phosphate and glucose leaks
     - iii. Renal tubular acidosis
       - (a) Sporadic in infancy
       - (b) Familial in adolescents and adults
     - iv. 'Fanconi' syndrome with:
       Renal tubular glycosuria, aminoaciduria, acidosis, and loss of water, sodium and potassium
       - (a) Familial in children with cystinosis
       - (b) Familial in adults, without cystinosis
       - (c) Sporadic, due to toxic substances, e.g. copper, degraded tetracyclines, and myeloma protein
3. Urinary diversion
   Ureterocolic anastomosis, colocystoplasty, ileal conduit
4. Anticonvulsant therapy
5. Phosphorus depletion (aluminium hydroxide therapy)

Pathology

The lack of effect of vitamin D may be demonstrated at four main sites. First, in the intestinal tract, there is a failure to absorb dietary calcium, and faecal calcium may exceed it by some 200 mg. per day. Secondly, in the plasma, the calcium or inorganic phosphate levels may be low, although this need not apply in cases of chronic renal failure where plasma calcium may be normal despite a normal or raised plasma phosphate. In vitamin D deficiency, steatorrhoea and chronic renal failure, the plasma calcium may be either low or normal, but in renal tubular acidosis and the other forms of renal tubular osteomalacia, the plasma calcium is always normal unless there is renal failure as well. Plasma alkaline phosphatase is generally raised in all forms of rickets and osteomalacia, but cases have occasionally been described in which this parameter has been normal. Thirdly, the osteoid seams of bone, as seen in histological sections, are enlarged. Fourthly, phosphate clearance by the kidneys may be increased. This is always the case in the renal tubular types of osteomalacia and is sometimes so in the other types. This results in hypophosphataemia unless renal failure is present. Despite a great deal of work in the last twenty years it is still not clear whether this increased phosphate clearance is due directly to a failure of vitamin D to act on the renal tubule, or whether it is due to secondary hyperparathyroidism.

Secondary hyperparathyroidism undoubtedly occurs in some cases of osteomalacia due to vitamin D deficiency, steatorrhoea and chronic renal failure, and it is due to a tendency to a low plasma calcium. Radiological techniques are generally required to demonstrate secondary hyperparathyroidism since the only other practical techniques generally available at present are by viewing the parathyroids at surgery or autopsy.

Clinical Features

Rickets and osteomalacia are characterized by hypotonia, bony deformities, and tetany in those cases accompanied by severe hypocalcaemia. The results of the hypotonia and bony deformities are dependent on the age at which the disease occurs but not upon the cause. Rachitic children show widening of the epiphyses of the long bones at the growing points, so that the wrists, knees, ankles and costochondral junctions are especially affected, the latter giving rise to the 'rickety rosary'. The ribs become drawn in under the pull of the diaphragm giving rise to Harrison's sulcus. Antero-lateral bowing of the tibia and knock-knees or bow-legs may be present. The skull may show softening (craniotabes) with platybasia between 6 and 12 months of age, and beyond this age there may be bossing of the frontal bones.

The softened bones of osteomalacia give rise to aches and pains which have certain characteristic features which enable them to be distinguished from other types of 'rheumatism' with which they might be confused. First, these aches and pains begin in the spine and thighs, but later spread to affect the arms and ribs and possibly many other bones. Secondly, on close inquiry these pains are frequently referred to the bones themselves rather than the joints, although exceptions do occur. Thirdly, the pains are frequently symmetrical and do not radiate. Fourthly, the bones are tender to palpation, quite unlike the case in osteoporosis and other types of 'rheumatism'. Muscular weakness is frequently a marked feature of adult osteomalacia. It specially affects the proximal muscles of the limbs and leads to difficulties with stairs, in rising from the sitting position without the use of the arms, and to the characteristic waddling gait. This muscular weakness frequently occurs simultaneously with the aches and pains, but at other times the weakness may ante-date any aches or pains by an appreciable period. The deformities in osteomalacia may be due either to the action of gravity, as in the case of the triradiate pelvis which interferes with childbirth, and the spinal kyphosis, or to the muscular pull as in the case of the ribs (see above) and deformities of the arms.

Diagnosis

If the condition is suspected, it is helpful to seek an underlying cause. Thus inquiry should be made about dietary and family history, about bowel habits in cases of steatorrhoea, and about micturition in cases of renal failure. Signs of pre-tetany should be sought. Confirmation of the diagnosis may be obtained by laboratory tests on plasma (see above) and by radiology. In the case of children the X-rays should include the wrists, knees and ankles which may show the characteristic rachitic changes, with enlargements of the metaphyses, irregularities of the ends of the shafts with loss of definition and cupping. In the case of adults the X-rays should include postero-anterior views of the chest, pelvis, knees and hands, and lateral views of the skull and lumbar spine, and any other bones which appear to be especially affected. The characteristic radiological feature of osteomalacia in the adult is the Looser zone, consisting of a ribbon-like zone of decalcification occurring in bone which appears otherwise perfectly normal. These zones tend to be symmetrical and to occur at certain sites of which common examples are the femoral necks, the rami of the pubic and ischial bones, the ribs and axillary edge of the scapula. In the case of the long bones, these zones may go right across the bones giving the appearance of complete fractures. In fact a fracture is not demonstrable clinically, since the gap is bridged by osteoid tissue and this gives rise to the alternative name of 'pseudo-fracture'. The lateral view of the spine shows bi-concave or 'codfish' vertebrae as illustrated in FIGURE 61. These radiological signs of osteomalacia may be partly or completely replaced by those of hyperparathyroidism when they exactly mimic those found in primary hyperparathyroidism as discussed in Section 5.

Treatment

As indicated above, vitamin D deficiency is easily preventable either by simple dietary means, or by exposure to sunlight, or by supplementation of baby foods, or by administration of vitamin capsules. For prophylaxis, not more than 1,000 I.U. per day of vitamin D should be given, either in the form of calciferol (vitamin D_2), or vitamin D_3. In the treatment of established vitamin D deficiency, the same drug should be administered in a dose of not more than 10,000 I.U. per day. It is important to note that vitamin should be contained in an oily suspension containing an anti-oxidant, and preferably in capsule form, although oily drops may be useful for infants. In the case of vitamin D resistance, much larger doses are required and the size of the dose varies very much from patient to patient so that it is necessary to experiment, gradually increasing the dose and learning the chemical and clinical response. In cases of gluten-sensitive steatorrhoea, doses of up to 15 mg. per day may be required. It must be especially stressed, however, that in chronic renal failure particular care is required to avoid giving an over-dose of vitamin D which might cause hypercalcaemia and worsening of the renal failure. In these cases doses of 1–5 mg. per day might be appropriate. In cases of vitamin D resistance, vitamin D_2 and vitamin D_3 are both effective, but dihydrotachysterol (DHT) is advantageous since it acts slightly faster and appears to cease acting somewhat faster than the other forms of vitamin D. It is also very important to note that the dose of vitamin D which is sufficient to heal osteomalacia in cases of vitamin D resistance, will be sufficient to cause hypercalcaemia once the osteomalacia is healed, and therefore the dose should be gradually reduced as the plasma alkaline phosphatase falls to normal and the radiological signs regress.

Tertiary Hyperparathyroidism. When secondary hyperparathyroidism has persisted for a long time, one or more parathyroids may become an autonomous adenoma and this state of affairs has been described as 'tertiary' hyperparathyroidism. This diagnosis may be suspected when one of the causes of secondary hyperparathyroidism, i.e. steatorrhoea or chronic renal failure, is accompanied by raised plasma calcium. It may then be necessary to treat the tertiary hyperparathyroidism surgically as for primary hyperparathyroidism, and also to treat the secondary hyperparathyroidism medically as described above. The advent of successful renal transplantation has created interesting and important diagnostic problems in this field. Following a successful transplantation the plasma calcium, which may have been normal or subnormal prior to the transplantation, may become persistently raised. This may be due to the presence of tertiary hyperparathyroidism and require surgical treatment, but there may be an alternative explanation, namely the inability of enlarged parathyroids immediately to stop secreting excessive amounts of parathyroid hormone. This latter explanation may be revealed by a gradual fall in the plasma calcium to normal over a period of up to six months.

Footnote

In this section the term 'phosphate' is used as an abbreviation for 'inorganic phosphate'.

REFERENCES

DAVIES, D. R., DENT, C. E., and WATSON, L. (1968) Tertiary hyperparathyroidism, *Brit. med. J.*, **3**, 395.

DENT, C. E. (1969) Rickets (and osteomalacia), nutritional and metabolic, 1919–1969, *Proc. roy. Soc. Med.*, **63**, 401.

FOURMAN, P., and ROYER, P. (1968) *Calcium Metabolism and the Bone*, Oxford.

ROSE, G. A. (1967) A critique of modern methods of diagnosis and treatment of osteoporosis, *Clin. Orthop.*, **55**, 17.

G. A. ROSE

OSTEITIS DEFORMANS

Synonym. Paget's disease.

The name of Sir James Paget is used throughout the world as an eponym for this familiar condition which was given the title of osteitis deformans by Czerny in 1873. Its cause is unknown, but there is now extensive evidence of dominant inheritance. Because the disease appears usually so late in life it is difficult to produce conclusive evidence of inheritance over more than two generations, and certainly many sporadic cases occur. It is a common condition in Great Britain, and apparently even more common in Australia, and extremely rare among the Chinese.

Pathology

Almost every bone in the body can be affected, but involvement of the hand and foot is exceptional and of the facial bones very rare. The pelvis is the most commonly involved part of the skeleton, followed closely by the upper ends of femur and tibia, vertebral bodies, the skull and humerus. The changes are asymmetrical; a single bone may be affected and sometimes only a small part of a bone. The earliest changes consist of irregular osteoporosis at the same time accompanied by new bone formation. At first the former predominates, the bone is softened and tends to bow, and there is often marked hyperaemia of new connective tissue filling the narrow spaces. Later, new bone formation overtakes the osteoporosis and the bones become hard and brittle. The microscopic appearance with its mosaic of new cement lines is characteristic. In the later stages the bone as a whole is markedly thickened, the cortex itself being also wider with a rough external surface, while the marrow cavity is increased in size and may appear heavily trabeculated.

Joints adjacent to affected bone are more liable to osteo-arthritis, particularly the hip and the knee. It is remarkable that if an arthritic knee with either femur or tibia alone affected by Paget's disease be arthrodesed, the disease does not spread across the fusion plane to the previously unaffected bone. A severely affected and bowed tibia can apparently increase in length as well as thickness, for in such cases neither end of an unaffected fibula subluxates. Impingement on the cranial foramina is fortunately rare, but optic atrophy may occasionally occur. Deafness is quite common but is due usually to otosclerosis.

Clinical Manifestations

Paget's disease typically affects the elderly; rarely noted before the age of fifty, it can certainly occur in the thirties and very rarely even earlier. Both sexes are almost equally affected. In many instances the disease is completely asymptomatic and the diagnosis is made on radiographs taken for some independent condition. In others it may cause deep continuous bone pain, usually worse at night and unrelieved by change of posture. In others, bowing of the limbs, loss of height and enlargement of the skull—the classical triad—may bring the patient to the physician. The tibia usually bows forwards, the femur outwards and forwards, and the spine becomes kyphotic as much from disc degeneration as from vertebral collapse. The anterior margin of the tibia becomes rounded as well as bowed, and the surface temperature is raised. In rare instances, when there is very widespread involvement of the skeleton, the hyperaemia and the accompanying medullary arteriovenous shunts may lead to high output heart failure.

Pathological fractures are common; in most cases union takes place rapidly, but if the affected bone is very sclerotic union may be delayed and set the surgeon a formidable problem. Paraplegia occasionally results from the spinal changes.

Malignant change in Paget's disease has an evil reputation and the prognosis is dismal indeed. Its true incidence is unknown because so many cases of Paget's disease remain undiagnosed throughout life, but has been placed as high as 10 per cent. Most series, however, suggest a much lower figure. Osteogenic sarcoma is the commonest, but chondrosarcoma and osteoclastoma (giant-cell tumour) are also seen. Any bone can be affected and multiple tumours can occur. Any increase of pain in a patient with known Paget's disease should give rise to immediate suspicion of this complication.

Diagnosis

The radiological appearance of the cortex itself is very variable: it may appear streaky or honeycombed, sometimes with quite large cavities, and partial fracture lines may cross part or all of one cortex. Only the outer cortex of the skull is affected so that the size of the cranial cavity is not diminished.

The serum alkaline phosphatase may reach very high levels but this is, of course, not diagnostic and is evidence of no more than rapid new bone formation. Serum calcium and phosphorus are usually normal, but if the disease is extensive and osteoporosis progressing rapidly there may be some rise in urinary excretion of these elements. This situation is particularly liable to arise during the period of immobilization after a fracture, and if the kidneys are unequal to their task a dangerous hypercalcaemia may result unless a low calcium diet and a high fluid intake are prescribed.

Treatment

The aetiology being unknown it is not surprising that no effective medical treatment has been discovered. Sodium fluoride in doses of 20–40 mg. daily may relieve pain, and recently calcitonin, mithramycin and actinomycin D have all been tried with encouraging results, lowering the rate of bone calcium turnover, alkaline phosphatase, and urinary hydroxyproline excretion and reducing bone pain. Aluminium salts have failed to live up to their early promise, and radiotherapy is often disappointing. Paget's disease is so common that the physician must always beware of attributing to it pain which is in fact of another origin, but pain in the long bones, if severe enough to warrant what can be a very haemorrhagic procedure, can be relieved by surgical 'guttering' of the bone, while an osteotomy is sometimes required for severe bowing, particularly in those cases where bilateral bowing of the femora accompanied often by bilateral osteo-arthritis of the hip joints with fixed adduction has led to a cross-leg deformity.

OSTEOGENESIS IMPERFECTA

Synonym. Fragilitas ossium.

Definition

This disease is a hereditary disorder of connective tissue, which although involving the tissue throughout the body produces its most important defect in the bone matrix, resulting in slender brittle bones. Bone fragility, blue sclerotics, and later otosclerosis are the major manifestations.

Aetiology

Probably all cases are hereditary in origin. Many are due to a casual mutation, but in 25 per cent. of cases the defect is inherited through an autosomal dominant gene; many family trees covering several generations have been published. There is some doubt whether there are closely linked, but separate, genes responsible for the blue sclerotics and otosclerosis or whether these and bone fragility are all caused by a single gene with pleiotropic effect. The sexes are almost equally affected.

Clinical Manifestations

The disease varies widely in severity: although there is no clear-cut division three types can be recognized. There is a severe pre-natal type where the baby is stillborn or only lives for a few days, with scores of fractures affecting almost every bone in the body; the limbs are stunted, the long bones being short, thickened and deformed from the multiplicity of fractures *in utero*.

In the second group the baby survives but suffers repeated fractures from the most trivial injuries. The fractures heal normally but the child is left with limb deformities both from malunion and from bowing of the bones, which are soft as well as brittle. Even with suitable braces walking may be impossible without fractures occurring, and in the past a spinal carriage existence was the fate of these children until their death from intercurrent infection.

Lastly there is a milder group where fractures occur with undue frequency during childhood but the bones become stronger, although never completely normal, after adolescence.

Other important freatures result from the generalized connective tissue disorder. Blue sclerotics are common but not universal; thus variation may occur even within the affected members of a single family. The blue is a slaty blue, an exaggeration of that seen normally in the eyes of the newborn. Otosclerosis does not usually produce deafness before the third decade, often later still, and rarely earlier. Laxity of ligaments and hypotonia of muscles are common features. The muscles are wasted and feeble but this may partly be due to relative disuse and frequent fractures.

The bones of the cranial vault are slow to develop; in a baby the fontanelles stay open unduly late and the suture lines are widely spaced. The soft skull tends to bulge laterally above the small face which, with its turned down ears, large eyes, and pointed chin, give a somewhat elfin appearance.

Although epiphysial development is not affected in this condition growth is stunted, and this with the bowing and shortening of the limb bones, and frequently curvature of the spine as well, makes dwarfism a feature of all but the mildest cases.

Intelligence is normal.

Diagnosis

This is usually obvious on clinical grounds; in severe cases in the newborn there may be confusion with achondroplasia, but the radiological findings are usually characteristic. In older children the epiphyses are of normal size but thin in texture; the metaphysis tapers rapidly to an attenuated diaphysis with a thin but smooth cortex. Bowing of these soft bones or deformity from old fractures is very common. The bone density throughout the skeleton is poor, and in severe cases the medullary cavity is obliterated, the fibula being represented by no more than a faint white line on the radiograph.

There are no diagnostic biochemical abnormalities.

Treatment

No known treatment affects the underlying defect. The use of intramedullary rods by the method introduced by Sofield has dramatically improved the prospects of enabling the more severe cases to walk without their bones giving way.

POLYOSTOTIC FIBROUS DYSPLASIA

Synonym. Albright's syndrome.

Definition

This condition is considerably less common than the monostotic variety where only a single bone or part of one bone is affected by an apparently similar process. It is probably congenital, but as yet there is no evidence of a hereditary factor. In about half of the patients bone lesions are restricted to one side of the body and sometimes to a single limb. Very commonly associated, and indeed almost universally in severe examples, are patches of skin pigmentation, and in this type sexual precocity in girls may be seen in the syndrome to which the name of Albright is usually applied.

Aetiology

The aetiology is unknown. Girls are affected at least twice as commonly as boys. Any bone in the body may be affected but even in the most severe cases some bones will escape. The femur, tibia, humerus, ribs and skull are the most commonly affected, the whole or only part of a bone being involved. There is no predilection for the metaphyses, and epiphyses may be affected too.

Pathology

Pathologically the interior of the bone is filled with loose fibrous tissue containing a variable quantity of bone trabeculae. There may be islands of cartilage and often large cysts, either haemorrhagic or degenerative in origin, with bony trabeculae giving a polycystic appearance on the radiograph. The cortex is eroded from within and replaced on the exterior so that the bone is usually expanded and is left with a thinned and weakened cortex leading to bowing and often to pathological fractures.

Clinical Manifestations

Many patients remain asymptomatic, minor bone changes being diagnosed on a radiograph taken for other purposes, e.g. an affected rib seen on a chest film.

The condition is most commonly diagnosed in childhood or adolescence, rarely before the age of two, often not until adult life. The patient may present because of deformity of a limb from bowing, a pathological fracture, or a localized swelling on a limb, face or rib. Bone pain is unusual—unlike hyperparathyroidism with which the disease was at one time confused. Bowing may lead to shortening of a limb, but in fact bone growth is somewhat precocious and the children may be at first tall for their age. However, because of early closure of the epiphyses they are usually shorter than average when mature. Involvement of the bones of the face or cranial vault may cause facial asymmetry and sometimes nasal obstruction or proptosis. Localized fibrous dysplasia is one of the causes of so-called congenital pseudarthrosis of the tibia.

Areas of pigmentation, pale yellow to dark brown in colour without thickening of the skin, are common and rarely absent in cases of any severity. They vary in size from little more than freckles to areas large enough to cover the whole of one buttock. The lower part of the trunk and thighs are other common sites. The pigmentation is asymmetrical in distribution and although in some it is confined to the limb or limbs with affected bones more commonly its distribution appears random. These patches may be seen in babies who later develop bony lesions.

In a small proportion of the more severe cases, probably much smaller than the literature would suggest, there is sexual precocity. Menstruation may start even in infancy, and there is early development of the secondary sexual features. This precocity is almost confined to girls but has been reported in a few boys. No hormonal abnormalities have been found in the urine. The occasional occurrence of other endocrine abnormalities, such as hyperparathyroidism, acromegaly, gynaecomastia and diabetes mellitus, as well as the skeletal precocity, are suggestive of pituitary involvement, perhaps secondary to bony changes in the base of the skull.

Diagnosis

Biochemical examination of the blood reveals no abnormality except that the alkaline phosphatase may be moderately elevated in some instances, especially after a fracture.

Diagnosis is primarily radiological and in severe cases present few problems. Hyperparathyroidism, Ollier's disease, or multiple enchondromatosis, and Gaucher's disease can easily be differentiated. Localized lesions may, however, need a biopsy to exclude a variety of possible neoplasms. The facial lesions are markedly similar to those of leontiasis ossium; some examples at least of this condition are certainly due to localized fibrous dysplasia.

Treatment

Treatment is that of the complications. Fractures unite readily but may need bone grafting to strengthen the weakened areas after curettage. This procedure may need repeating as the grafts are often absorbed. Osteotomy may be required to correct bowing. Symptomatic localized lesions amenable to total resection, e.g. in a rib, are best so treated. Partial resection for cosmetic reasons or to relieve nasal obstruction and other pressure symptoms may be required in the face.

Course and Prognosis

The bone lesions may remain static but more commonly progress steadily until growth is complete when further expansion ceases. This is not always so, however, and new areas of bone involvement can appear occasionally during adult life. Some degree of mental impairment is said to be common in severe cases. Expectation of life is not affected, except that sarcoma can rarely complicate this condition.

INFANTILE CORTICAL HYPEROSTOSIS

Synonym. Caffey's disease.

Clinical Manifestations

This is a rare condition of unknown aetiology affecting the skeleton and adjacent soft tissues. The patient is an infant usually less than 6 months old, more commonly male than female, in whom firm tender swellings appear suddenly over the lower part of the face, thorax or extremities. There is no increase in local heat, nor any lymphadenitis. These swellings may appear before there are any visible radiological changes, and with the exception of the scapula are often bilateral.

The baby is pale and irritable, the temperature is raised, and there may be signs of pleurisy. Pseudoparalysis may be present, as use of the affected limbs causes pain. Proptosis occasionally occurs. Leucocytosis is uncommon but the erythrocyte sedimentation rate is raised, as is the alkaline phosphatase. In many instances the platelet count has been notably high.

Diagnosis

Radiologically all parts of the skeleton with the exception of the phalanges and vertebral column may be affected, including the pelvis and cranial vault. The lower jaw is almost always involved and the clavicles and ulnae commonly. The first change is the appearance, within a week or so of the onset, of a subperiosteal shadow along part or the whole of the diaphysis, sometimes one surface only being affected at first. Usually smooth, it may be lumpy, but never spicular. The shadow becomes progressively denser, until its density exceeds that of the underlying cortex with which it eventually blends. Within a year or two the bones are completely normal again.

The differential diagnosis includes scurvy, rickets, multiple osteomyelitis, trauma, neoplasm, and hypervitaminosis A. The first of these is only relevant in older babies. A skeletal survey revealing widespread changes will usually exclude multiple osteomyelitis, although it must be noted that in small babies the latter disease may produce surprisingly little constitutional upset. Although infantile cortical hyperostosis has been reported in the foetus, birth trauma rarely produces a problem, but the physician must always beware of the 'battered baby' syndrome.

Treatment

Response to steroid therapy is rapid, but because of the high platelet count, and the occasional evidence of venous thrombosis, some caution is indicated. There may be recurrence of swellings when therapy ceases.

Prognosis

Complete recovery is the rule, although a few fatal cases have been reported. The swellings regress spontaneously over a few weeks or months, but they may recur or new swellings appear in the course of the disease.

THE 'BATTERED BABY' SYNDROME

This sad condition is probably more common than would appear in that many cases are missed because the suspicions of the physician are never aroused. The baby has been maltreated by one or other parent.

The trauma suffered by the baby may be of any type from simple bruises to fatal cerebral injury, or even a ruptured liver from violent shaking. The injuries are characteristic in that they are multiple, repeated, and inadequately accounted for. Apart from a story that the child 'bruises easily' no explanation is forthcoming, and any history of injury is usually stoutly denied. It is often pressure from neighbours as well as panic on the part of the parents that leads to the child being brought to hospital with some unexplained swelling, usually of a limb.

Although fractures of the shafts of the long bones are commonly seen, the diagnostic lesion radiologically is to be found in the region of the epiphysial plate. Macroscopic displacement of the epiphysis is rarely seen, but flakes of bone may be detached from the margin of the metaphysis and local soft part swelling is visible. A subperiosteal haematoma spreads up the shaft of the bone, sometimes for its whole length, and within a week or so of injury this haematoma starts to ossify. It is thickest at the metaphysis and a characteristic rim of bone appears to overlap the epiphysis. A skeletal survey is essential and usually diagnostic in revealing evidence of bony injury elsewhere in varying stages of recovery. As Caffey has said, 'the bones tell a story the child is too young to tell'.

In hospital no further lesions occur; the early slight pyrexia and leucocytosis rapidly settle; all other investigations prove negative. The child should not be allowed to return home until the difficult parental problem has been resolved.

THE HEREDITARY CHONDRODYSPLASIAS

This term (Hobaek 1961) which the writer prefers to hereditary chondrodystrophies as used by Lamy and Maroteaux (1961), has been coined to cover all the conditions where disturbances of the development of cartilage appear to be the major defect. The subject is bedevilled not only by the multiplicity of different names applied to even the most clear-cut of these affections, but also by the high proportion of cases seen, and often individually reported, which are atypical in one or more respects. There is no doubt that there can be considerable overlap between some of the conditions, and that in time further sub-grouping will become justifiable. Unfortunately, histological and biochemical changes are too limited in variety to be of much help, except in differentiating the mucopolysaccharidoses. The whole subject remains one of considerable confusion.

Although individually most of the conditions are rare, *in toto* they make up the majority of skeletal developmental abnormalities, especially if the many mild variants are included. The diseases which various authors have put into this group include amongst others achondroplasia, dyschondroplasia (Ollier's disease), diaphysial aclasis or multiple extoses, chondro-osteodystrophy, Leri's pleonosteosis, spondylo-epiphysial dysplasia, dysplasia epiphysialis multiplex and dysplasia epiphysialis punctata. The major features of the more important of them are described below.

ACHONDROPLASIA

This condition was so named by Parrot in 1878, and this title has always remained more popular in the English-speaking world than chondrodystrophia foetalis. It is the commonest cause of dwarfism of the short-limbed type (hence the old name of micromelia) and is due to an autosomal dominant gene. About three-quarters of cases are due to a casual mutation and the incidence is about 1 in 10,000 births.

Clinical and Radiological Features

It affects chiefly the process of endochondral ossification and therefore the bones developed from cartilage, and is characterized by short limbs, the proximal segments being more severely affected than the distal, a relatively normal trunk, and a large head with a short base to the skull due to early fusion of the participant bones. The cranial vault is brachycephalic and the frontal region bulges above the depressed bridge of the nose. In a lateral radiograph of the skull the occiput appears to hang down over the back of the neck and the angle between ethmoid and clivus is reduced from the normal 120 degrees to 90 degrees. The fingers are short, stubby and divergent, the so-called 'trident hand', and scarcely reach to the greater trochanter.

Achondroplasia is recognizable at birth, when the only condition with which it might be confused is the severe pre-natal form of osteogenesis imperfecta, from which radiographs will differentiate it at once. There is said to be a high mortality during the first year of life when hypotonia may be present sometimes resulting in a lumbar kyphosis, but the survivors become robust children with a normal expectation of life and assume the appearance familiar to all in the dwarf circus clown. Intelligence, dentition and sexual development are normal, and the musculature well developed, so that the subjects are often capable of surprising acrobatic feats.

The patient walks with a waddling gait; the legs are often bowed and the knees hyperextended. The buttocks are prominent and there is a marked lumbar lordosis. The pelvis is rotated forwards so that the sacrum lies nearly horizontally and the acetabula are situated more posteriorly than usual. The range of movement of elbows and shoulders may be slightly restricted. The skin and subcutaneous tissue are thickened and may form folds as if too big for the underlying structures.

The large head of these babies may cause obstetric trouble, and because of pelvic deformity pregnant achondroplasiacs must almost always be delivered by Caesarean section. In older patients paraplegia may develop due to vertebral anomalies, with accompanying disc lesions and spondylosis.

In the older child a differential diagnosis must be made from osteochondrodystrophy, dysplasia epiphysialis multiplex, and the various other forms of spondylo-epiphyseal dysplasia. The important radiological points, apart from those already mentioned in the skull, are the stoutly built but shortened long bones, sometimes with the medullary cavity almost obliterated, flaring rapidly to a relatively wide metaphysis with a V-shaped notch in the case of the lower end of the femur, coxa valga, horizontally lying acetabula, and the wings of ilia broad, short, and appearing to face forwards. The bony protuberances for muscular attachments are very well developed. The bony epiphyses are almost normal, but appear to lie very closely against the metaphyses. In the spine the vertebral bodies are rather short from back to front—not low and flat—with short pedicles and a tendency for the interpeduncular space as seen in the anteroposterior view to diminish in the lower lumbar spine. Very rarely is a wedged vertebra in the upper lumbar spine to be seen.

No treatment is available, but a watch should be kept on older patients for the onset of paraplegia which can be treated by suitable decompression.

DIAPHYSIAL ACLASIS

Diaphysial aclasis (Keith, 1919), a not uncommon condition of autosomal dominant inheritance with rather greater penetrance in males, is characterized by the formation, apparently from nests of cartilage cells 'left behind' from the margins of the growth plate, of lumps of bone covered with a cartilage cap from which they grow and which usually disappears when body growth is completed. The more actively growing ends of long bones are chiefly affected and the metaphyses become thickened and distorted by outgrowths which tend to point away from the adjacent epiphysis. Growth in length is little affected and any dwarfism quite minor. Inflamed bursae may arise from local pressure, movements at ankles and wrists may be disturbed, and very occasionally pressure on peripheral vessels and nerves, and even on the spinal cord, may give rise to symptoms. Exostoses on the pelvis have an evil reputation for developing into chondrosarcomata. The condition is usually bilateral but not necessarily symmetrical; the number of exostoses varies widely; the medullary cavity is not affected, and surgical removal is not followed by recurrence if the cartilage cap is removed completely.

DYSCHONDROPLASIA

Synonyms. Ollier's disease; Multiple enchondromatosis.

Definition

This disease is not uncommon. As the name given by Ollier (1900) implies, it is a disorder of cartilage growth and affects therefore only those bones preformed in cartilage. Parts or the whole of the shafts of the bones become filled with masses or columns of cartilage. Bowing of the bones may occur but this is due rather to irregular growth at the bone ends than to softening of the shafts. There is a strong tendency for bone lesions to be unilateral or at least for one side of the body to be much more affected than the other. Growth of affected bones is limited, so that shortening of the limb is universal in the more severe cases.

Aetiology

The aetiology is unknown. Almost all cases are sporadic, and the few examples reported with another member of the family affected suggest possible dominant inheritance with low penetrance.

Pathology

Any bone preformed in cartilage can be affected, but involvement of spine, carpus and tarsus is rare, and of the facial bones only occasionally seen. The elbow region usually escapes. Otherwise all the limb bones are liable to the disease, and especially the metacarpals and phalanges. Sometimes only a single bone in hand or foot may be attacked. A single lesion in a metacarpal is radiologically very similar to a solitary enchondroma, which may indeed be looked on as a *forme fruste* of dyschondroplasia, but a skeletal survey will reveal occult lesions elsewhere, and histologically it is more cellular than the solitary type.

Pathologically it appears that cartilage cells from the epiphysial plate get 'left behind' within the metaphysis as growth proceeds, and then multiply to form irregular masses or long columns of cartilage which expand and distort first the metaphysial region and later the more central parts of the shaft. The whole diaphysis may be affected, but much more commonly only one end of the major bones. In the hands (to a lesser extent in the feet) the metacarpals and phalanges may be involved from end to end with gross expansion and distortion of the original bony outlines.

Clinical Manifestations

Males and females are almost equally affected with a slight male preponderance. Rarely shortening of the limb may call attention to the condition in the newborn, but the diagnosis is seldom made before the age of 2 years when local swelling, bowing of a bone, or perhaps knock-knee are noticed. Limb length disparity increases with age and in severe cases may even reach 25 cm. in the lower limbs. The radius tends to bow outwards and, as so often seen in developmental abnormalities of the skeleton, the ulna may be markedly shortened at its lower end, and this with the radial bowing may lead to dislocation of the head of the radius. Bone pain is rare and pathological fractures seldom occur; fractures through affected regions heal normally. Anaemia is unusual and there is no alteration in blood chemistry.

Bone lesions tend to progress inexorably until adult life when they usually become static. Some of them, however, may continue to develop throughout life and this is unfortunately often seen in the hands, the fingers being rendered stiff and useless by the grossly expanded and distorted bones. Surprisingly the thin, tight skin covering the monstrous digits rarely ulcerates.

Particularly in those with severe bone involvement there may be *multiple haemangiomata* (Maffuci's syndrome), an association first noted by Maffuci (1881). Most of them lie in the subcutaneous tissues but muscles and deeper organs have been implicated. They are soft, lobulated and non-pulsatile, with a bluish discoloration if sufficiently superficial, and may reach a diameter of 5 cm. or more. There is only rarely any apparent anatomical relation between them and the bone lesions. Phleboliths are often formed within them and there may be also overlying phlebo-ectasia.

Diagnosis

Radiological diagnosis is usually easy if a skeletal survey is done. The irregular areas of translucency often arranged in long bands or longitudinal stripes with slightly sclerosed margins, the distortion of the bones, the stippling to be seen from patches of calcification in the larger cartilage masses and the distribution of the lesions are so characteristic that biopsy is seldom required. Although growth at the epiphysial plate is so often retarded or irregular the epiphyses themselves usually escape till growth has ceased.

Treatment

Suitable osteotomies may be required for knock-knee or severe bowing of a bone, and occasionally epiphysial arrest performed on the longer side to reduce severe disparity in the lower limbs. No general treatment has any effect, and the surgeon's most useful function is often to reduce the size of metacarpals and phalanges by intermittent *ad hoc* curettage operations.

Course and Prognosis

Chondrosarcomatous change in the cartilage masses of this condition has been frequently reported. Its incidence is uncertain; at one time considered a rarity, Jaffe (1958) goes so far as to suggest that it may be as high as 50 per cent. if all cases were to be followed into old age. This disastrous complication rarely occurs in childhood and seldom before middle age.

CHONDRO-OSTEODYSTROPHY

The group of conditions to which this title has been applied are genetic in origin, and with the exception of Morquio-Brailsford disease they are associated with an inborn error of metabolism affecting mucopolysaccharides. They are also considered in Section 4.

The cause of the abnormality appears to be an inability of the body to link these mucopolysaccharides with proteins to form the basic material of connective tissues. The resultant changes are therefore widespread; not only is the composition of the ground substance affected but there are intracellular abnormalities affecting tissues from all the embryonic layers. In accordance with the particular mucopolysaccharides involved they are sometimes referred to as mucopolysaccharidosis I, II, III, etc., although perhaps more familiar to us under their eponyms, and analysis of the mucopolysaccharides excreted in the urine, both quantative and qualitative, is essential in their differentiation. In the case of Morquio-Brailsford disease, however, no such abnormality has yet been detected, but the skeletal changes are so strikingly similar to those found in the Morquio-Ullrich type, which is clearly one of the mucopolysaccharidoses, that it seems reasonable to include it in this section. It must be stressed that all these conditions are rare, there is probably some overlap between them, and the considerable differences between affected members of the same family in any instance suggest that there may be marked variation in expressivity.

THE MORQUIO-BRAILSFORD TYPE

This is a condition due almost certainly to an autosomal recessive gene. The diagnosis is not often made before the age of 4 years; the child is dwarfed, the trunk being affected more than the limbs, with knock-knees, flat feet and a thoracolumbar kyphosis. The short neck lets the head sink between the shoulders, the hips and knees often have flexion deformities, and the child tends to waddle like a duck. Whereas the proximal joints are stiff, the distal joints of the limbs may be hypermotile. The chest is narrow, the sternum projecting unduly forwards; intelligence is normal. The epiphyses are enlarged and their ossification centres irregular in shape and often fragmented, particularly in the hip joints where radiographs commonly show coxa vara but sometimes coxa valga. The wings of the ilia may appear to face forwards, a condition reminiscent of the ape's pelvis. The radiographic changes in the spine are the most important diagnostically; there is flattening of the vertebral bodies with irregularity of the upper and lower surfaces and increase in the anteroposterior diameter, particularly in the lower thoracic and upper lumbar regions, and commonly in this region a tongue of bone is visible in the lateral view projecting from the middle of the shallow anterior surface. In about one third of patients one vertebral body, usually the first lumbar, is much smaller than its fellows, and the spine above it is sharply tilted forwards to produce a kyphosis above the markedly lordosed lumbar spine. No biochemical changes have so far been defined in the urine, no corneal opacities are to be found, and intelligence is usually normal.

In the more severe cases progressive crippling occurs, and probably not more than half reach adult life.

THE MORQUIO-ULLRICH TYPE

This type has only been clearly defined in the last few years. Radiologically the condition is almost indistinguishable from the Morquio-Brailsford type, but coxa valga is almost universal, there may be more than one of the small misshapen lumbar vertebrae, the lower ends of the radius and ulna are tilted towards each other, and the bases of the metacarpals are often cone-shaped. In other respects, however, this type bears similarities to gargoylism in that corneal opacities can be seen with the slit lamp, hearing defects often develop, there is commonly enlargement of the spleen, liver, or both, and Reilly granules, i.e. azurophil inclusion bodies in the cytoplasm of the polymorphonuclear leucocytes, may be seen. The condition is apparently due to an autosomal recessive gene and histologically all three embryological layers are involved. Analysis of the urine reveals an excess of keratosulphate and of chondroitin sulphate A or C or both, and it is probably this condition that should be labelled mucopolysaccharidosis IV instead of the Morquio-Brailsford type to which it has hitherto been applied.

GARGOYLISM

Synonyms. Hurler's syndrome; Mucopolysaccharidosis I.

This disease is usually called dysostosis multiplex on the Continent. Inheritance is autosomal recessive. The condition is recognizable within a year or two of birth; the child becomes increasingly dwarfed and the important features are mental deficiency, cloudiness of corneae and a characteristic appearance. The head is large, the features coarse and ugly; the eyebrows are bushy on prominent supra-orbital margins, the hair thick but fine and silky in texture. The tongue is enlarged and protrudes from the ever-open mouth; the child snuffles and dribbles. The neck is short, there is almost always a thoracolumbar kyphosis, and the muscles are weak. The fingers are short and stiff and sometimes clawed. The abdomen is protuberant, both liver and spleen are enlarged, and herniae are very common. Cardiac murmurs from valvular involvement are often to be heard. Corneal opacities, and later deafness, tend to become worse. Perhaps fortunately almost all these patients die during childhood, usually from intercurrent infection.

Differential diagnosis must be made from the Morquio-Brailsford type of chondo-osteodystrophy and from cretinism. In the former corneal opacities rarely if ever occur, and the radiographs of spine, pelvis and skull are quite different. In gargoylism the vertebral bodies are deep and rounded on their upper and lower surfaces in the lateral views, instead of shallow and flat, and any 'beaking' projects from the lower margin rather than from the middle of the anterior surface. Both conditions may reveal the angular deformity above a small misshapen vertebral body; it is much more common in gargoylism. In gargoylism there is coxa valga, not coxa vara. The epiphyses are more nearly normal, and in most instances radiographs of the skull show enlargement of the sella turcica with an anterior pocket, the so-called 'shoe-shaped' sella.

In gargoylism the metabolic defect can affect structures of all three embryological layers, the cells becoming distended with a complex mucopolysaccharide and a glycolipid. Urine analysis reveals excessive quantities of chondroitin sulphate B and of heparin monosulphate. Water-soluble metachromatic granules can be found in the lymphocytes as well as Reilly granules in the polymorphonuclear white cells.

A milder form of this condition, Hunter's syndrome or mucopolysaccharidosis II, occurs where inheritance is X-linked recessive. The onset is later, the corneae are said to be normal but an atypical retinitis pigmentosa may be present, the lumbar gibbus is absent, and the mental deterioration less marked. Deafness is, however, more common, and the biochemical changes in the urine are similar to those in Hurler's syndrome.

DYSPLASIA EPIPHYSIALIS MULTIPLEX

This condition, so named by Sir Thomas Fairbank, and at one time confused with achondroplasia, bears a host of eponyms and in France the title of *dysplasie poly-épiphysaire*. It is variable in its manifestations, but in its typical form is due to an autosomal recessive gene. There is also a variety usually diagnosed later in childhood where platyspondyly is the main feature and involvement of the limb epiphyses minor or absent and in which inheritance is X-linked recessive, while to add to the confusion yet another spondylo-epiphysial dysplasia has been described with autosomal dominant inheritance.

The diagnosis is most commonly made between the ages of five and ten. Difficulty with walking or joint stiffness are the commonest complaints. Some dwarfism of the short limb type is usually present but rarely severe. There may be fixed flexion in the elbows and knees and restriction of movement in hips and shoulders. The hands are often helpful diagnostically, the fingers being short and blunt. Intelligence and facies are unaffected and no abnormalities are to be detected in the blood or urine.

Radiographically the essential feature is multiple involvement of the epiphyses, although mild examples are not uncommonly seen in which perhaps only the upper femoral epiphyses are affected, giving rise to confusion with Perthes' disease. The bony centres may appear early, or more commonly late. They are fragmented and often irregular in shape and density, being reminiscent of mottled mulberries. The humeral and femoral heads are often flattened, the upper tibial epiphysis is often irregular and apparently underdeveloped on the inner side, and the ankle joint line lies obliquely. Platyspondyly is most unusual and the skull is normal.

The limited growth in the limbs results in some shortness of stature, but symptoms not uncommonly regress until in later life osteo-arthritis in the malformed joints inevitably supervenes.

REFERENCES

ALBRIGHT, F., SCOVILLE, B., and SULKOWITCH, H. W. (1938) Syndrome characterised by osteitis fibrosa disseminata, areas of pigmentation and a gonadal dysfunction. Further observations including a report of two cases, *Endocrinology*, **22,** 411.

BARRIE, H., CARTER, C., and SUTCLIFFE, J. (1958) Multiple epiphysial dysplasia, *Brit. med. J.*, **2,** 133.

BECKER, P. E. (1964) *Humangenetik*, Band II, Stuttgart.

CAFFEY, J. (1957) Some traumatic lesions in growing bones other than fractures and dislocations. Clinical and radiological features, *Brit. J. Radiol.*, **30,** 225.

CAFFEY, J. (1961) *Paediatric X-Ray Diagnosis*, 4th ed., Chicago.

CONDON, J. R., REITH, S. B. M., NASSIM, J. R., MILLARD, F. J. C., HILB, A., and STAINTHORPE, E. M. (1971) Treatment of Paget's disease of bone with mithromycin, *Brit. med. J.*, **1,** 421.

FAIRBANK, SIR THOMAS (1947) Dysplasia epiphysialis multiplex, *Brit. J. Surg.*, **34,** 225.

FAIRBANK, SIR H. A. T. (1951) *An Atlas of General Affections of the Skeleton*, Edinburgh.

FENNELLY, J. J., and GROARKE, J. F. (1971) Effect of actinomycin D on Paget's disease of bone, *Brit. med. J.*, **2,** 423.

FRASER, G. R., FRIEDMANN, A. L., MAROTEAUX, P., GLEN-BATT, A. M., and MITTWOCH, U. (1969) Dysplasia spondyloepiphysialis and related generalised skeletal dysplasias among children with severe visual handicap, *Arch. Dis. Childh.*, **44,** 490.

GOIDANICH, I. F., and LENZI, L. (1964) Morquio-Ullrich disease, *J. Bone Jt Surg.*, **46A,** 734.

GRIFFITHS, D. LL., and MOYNIHAN, F. J. (1963) Multiple epiphysial injuries in babies ('battered baby' syndrome), *Brit. med. J.*, **2,** 1558.

HOBAEK, A. (1961) *Problems of Hereditary Chondrodysplasias*, Oslo.

LAMY, M., and MAROTEAUX, P. (1961) *Les Chondrodystrophies Génotypiques*, Paris.

McKUSICK, V. A. (1966) *Hereditable Disorders of Connective Tissue*, 3rd ed., St. Louis.

MAROTEAUX, P., and LAMY, M. (1965) Hurler's disease, Morquio's disease and related mucopolysaccharidoses, *J. Pediat.*, **67,** 312.

SOFIELD, H. A., and MILLAR, E. A. (1959) Fragmentation, realignment, and intramedullary rod fixation of deformities of the long bones in children. A ten-year appraisal, *J. Bone Jt Surg.*, **41A,** 1371.

WOODHOUSE, N. J. W., BORDIER, PH., FISHER, M., JOPLIN, G. F., REINER, M., KALU, D. N., FOSTER, G. V., and MACINTYRE, I. (1971) Human calcitonin in the treatment of Paget's bone disease, *Lancet*, i, 1139.

T. J. FAIRBANK

SECTION 12

DISEASES OF THE URINARY TRACT

DISEASES OF THE URINARY TRACT

NORMAL RENAL FUNCTION

The prime function of the kidney is to maintain homeostasis, i.e. the constancy of the internal environment. It is in fact the main executive organ of the body in this respect, acting in some directions under the influence of the endocrine system, in others through complex physical and chemical regulatory mechanisms. Thus the excretion of waste products such as urea, although an essential role of the kidney, is of minor biological importance compared with its contribution to homeostasis. These various regulatory functions include volume control of body water, osmotic control of the extracellular fluid, acid-base balance, body concentration of individual electrolytes, arterial blood pressure and possibly erythropoiesis.

THE MECHANISM OF URINE FORMATION

The kidney in health elaborates a urine appropriate in volume and composition to the needs of the body at all times. A few statistics are useful in grasping the size and complexity of the problem. There are approximately 1 million nephrons in each kidney. The glomerular filtration area is about 1·5 m^2., the length of each tubule is 1½–2 inches (3·5–5 cm.), giving a total tubular length of about 45 miles (72 km.). Renal blood flow is about 1·3 litres per minute, i.e. one-third to one-quarter of the cardiac output. Glomerular filtration rate is 120 ml. per min. or 180 litres in 24 hours, which is 60 times the total plasma volume. Of this, only 1·5 litres appears as urine, so that approximately 178·5 litres of water must be re-absorbed each day by the tubules. A simple example will demonstrate the importance of these relative quantities. A patient during recovery from anuria may pass 5 litres of urine daily and yet die in uraemia. The explanation is that tubular re-absorption is still in abeyance and the urine may be virtually unchanged glomerular filtrate—i.e. a urine output of 5 litres daily may represent little more than 5 per cent. recovery of glomerular filtration.

Glomerular filtration is a purely physical process determined by the glomerular capillary pressure. Reduction in filtration pressure, as in shock or severe dehydration, will reduce the glomerular filtration rate (G.F.R.). In composition the filtrate is identical with plasma without its protein content, substances of molecular weight over about 60,000 being unable to pass the filtering membrane. There is indeed a minute quantity of low molecular weight protein in glomerular filtrate, which in health is re-absorbed by the tubules. Since non-colloid substances have the same composition in glomerular filtrate and plasma, the amount of any constituent cleared from the blood will depend on the G.F.R. and its plasma concentration, assuming no re-absorption or secretion by the tubules. The clearance of substances wholly excreted by filtration, e.g. inulin and creatinine, may be used to measure G.F.R. The renal clearance, which is the volume (ml.) of blood cleared of the substance in question per minute, is calculated as UV/P (where U and P are the urine and plasma concentrations and V the urine volume per minute), and is expressed as ml. per minute. The clearance of substances such as urea, which are partially re-absorbed by the tubules, provides an inaccurate measure of G.F.R. Since filtration rate depends on renal perfusion pressure it follows that reduction in G.F.R. may be caused not only by organic damage to the glomeruli, but also by purely functional circulatory disturbances of the kidney, and elevation of blood urea of this nature is termed extrarenal uraemia.

Tubular function modifies the glomerular filtrate both by re-absorption and secretion. Substances may be secreted into the tubular lumen or into the interstitial fluid. The term tubular excretion is used to indicate the former. Unlike glomerular filtration these are usually active processes, using energy and activated by specific enzymes. Consequently tubular re-absorption and secretion are highly selective, and it is in this way that excretory function is adapted to the special demands of the organism. In general, water and useful substances are absorbed and waste products are rejected. The essential functions of the tubule are therefore conservation and concentration. Many factors influence these processes, including hormones such as antidiuretic hormone (ADH), aldosterone and parathormone, concentration gradients and competition for secretion pathways, congenital enzyme deficiencies, chemical substances such as diuretics, and internal autoregulatory factors both chemical and circulatory, which for example have a profound effect on the counter-current exchanges between the medullary interstitium and the loop of Henle. For example glucose, which is normally completely re-absorbed in the proximal tubule, appears in the urine in diabetes because the filtered load exceeds the maximal tubular re-absorptive capacity. On the other hand glycosuria may occur with a normal blood sugar due to congenital enzyme deficiency (renal glycosuria). About 80 per cent. of water is re-absorbed from the glomerular filtrate in the proximal tubules. This accompanies active re-absorption of solutes (chiefly sodium) so that the re-absorbed fluid is isotonic. Other ions such as glucose and amino acids are actively re-absorbed at this site. In the distal tubule, there is a variable and independent relationship between the absorption of water and electrolytes. It is here that highly selective re-absorption produces the wide variations in urine concentration and composition according to body needs. ADH acts at this point and controls water re-absorption so as to maintain the osmolarity of the extracellular fluid, which in turn is the regulating factor in ADH secretion. Aldosterone increases sodium re-absorption in the distal tubule. This is an over-simplification; recent work indicates the presence of a third factor regulating sodium handling and of other controlling mechanisms for ADH release.

Concentration of the urine increases progressively from the cortex through the medulla to the papilla. The basic condition for urine concentration is medullary hypertonicity. This is chiefly brought about by the active transfer of sodium from the ascending loop of Henle across the interstitial fluid to the descending loop. This 'counter-current' transfer leads to progressive increase in interstitial fluid tonicity, which is augmented by passive diffusion of urea. Concentration takes place in the distal nephron, particularly in the collecting tubules, under the influence of ADH. This renders the tubular membrane permeable to water, which is then passively re-absorbed into the hypertonic interstitial fluid. The hypotonic urine leaving Henle's loop may remain hypotonic in the absence of ADH (e.g. in water diuresis) or become more hypotonic due to sodium re-absorption under the influence of aldosterone. Osmotic diuresis may be caused by increased solute load as in uraemia and diabetes, or by enlargement of the remaining functioning nephrons in organic renal disease. In either case a larger volume of isotonic urine per nephron is delivered to the distal tubules and concentration is impaired. This is made worse by reduced medullary hypertonicity; hence urine specific gravity becomes fixed in organic renal disease, leading to polyuria which first manifests itself as nocturnal frequency. Failure of urine concentration with excretion of hypotonic urine is sometimes a prominent and early feature of certain forms of renal disease, e.g. chronic pyelonephritis, in which interstitial fibrosis of the medulla is severe. This again may be due to loss of medullary hypertonicity.

Tubular excretion of a substance may be recognized when its clearance is greater than that of inulin. A number of important homeostatic functions depend on this process. Hydrion is excreted throughout the tubule but chiefly in the distal tubules. Filtered potassium is largely re-absorbed and urinary potassium is derived from tubular excretion. Hydrion and potassium are excreted reciprocally in exchange for re-absorbed sodium and must therefore share a common pathway. Ammonia is formed in the tubule cells by deamination of glutamine and is excreted into the tubular lumen where it combines with hydrion to form ammonium. Certain foreign substances, e.g. diodone or *p*-aminohippurate (PAH) may be so rapidly excreted by the tubules that they are completely cleared from the blood by a single passage through the kidney. Their clearance rate (UV/P) can therefore be used as a measure of renal blood flow. Iodinated contrast media used in intravenous pyelography are excreted by the proximal tubule so that failure to visualize the dye is due to reduced tubular excretion as well as to impaired concentrating power.

HOMEOSTATIC MECHANISMS

Body Water

The kidney regulates both the volume and osmolarity of the extracellular fluid and therefore indirectly the volume of intracellular fluid. Increase in extracellular and plasma volumes will, in health, increase glomerular filtration and vice versa. This direct method of volume control is, however, supplemented by the action of aldosterone on tubular re-absorption of sodium. Changes in plasma volume produce alterations in intravascular pressure and these in turn stimulate pressure receptors in various parts of the circulation. The most important of these is the juxtaglomerular apparatus of the kidney which responds to a fall in renal perfusion pressure by secretion of renin. This enzyme acts on a plasma globulin substrate to produce the octapeptide angiotensin, which is now known to be a potent stimulus to aldosterone secretion. Reduction in plasma volume by haemorrhage or sodium depletion, or loss of fluid into the tissue spaces in severe oedema, will therefore lead to sodium retention. The restoration of the isotonicity of the extracellular fluid by ADH will require a corresponding water retention and the extracellular fluid volume is thereby brought back to normal. Other mechanisms, as yet obscure, probably influence the response of tubular sodium re-absorption to changes in plasma volume. When water depletion occurs, the raised osmotic pressure of the tissue fluid stimulates osmoreceptors in the hypothalamus, ADH secretion is increased, and the distal tubules become more permeable to water which diffuses out into the hypertonic interstitial fluid of the medulla. The urine is thereby decreased in volume and is highly concentrated. The reverse occurs when body water is in excess, as after water drinking, when the tubular fluid, which is hypotonic in the distal tubule, becomes even less concentrated as sodium is re-absorbed without water.

Acid-Base Balance

The urine is normally slightly acid compared with plasma (pH 7·4) since acids formed during metabolic oxidation are being continually excreted. Carbonic acid is excreted as CO_2 by the lungs but the anions, sulphate, phosphate and organic acids are excreted in the urine. The kidney maintains acid-base balance by excreting hydrion and conserving sodium. The exchange of hydrion for sodium occurs in the distal tubule and is brought about by several mechanisms. Under the action of carbonic anhydrase, CO_2 and water in the tubule cell form carbonic acid and this liberates hydrion into the tubular fluid in exchange for sodium, which returns to the blood as bicarbonate. The excreted hydrogen ion combines with phosphate buffer which is converted into the acid phosphate, releasing sodium for re-absorption. The hydrion taken up by phosphate (and other buffers) forms the 'titratable acidity'. In addition hydrion combines with ammonia, and ammonium ion is excreted, thereby conserving further sodium. The titratable acidity is about 30 mEq. daily and the ammonium excretion 30–50 mEq. In severe metabolic acidosis, both can be increased many times. The minimum pH attainable by the urine is about 4·5 and this is a limiting factor to the amount of hydrion which the kidney can excrete as titratable acid for a given excretion of buffer.

Other Electrolytes

The excretion of potassium is increased by aldosterone but it is also reciprocally affected by hydrion excretion, and the elimination of both potassium and hydrion is dependent on sodium re-absorption. The renal clearance of phosphate is increased by parathormone, probably due to reduced tubular re-absorption. The various factors which influence electrolyte homeostasis are further discussed in relation to renal failure.

The Blood Pressure

The kidney undoubtedly plays a role in blood pressure regulation, although its nature still remains obscure. The pressor activity of the renal enzyme renin was discovered by Tigerstedt and Bergman in 1898. It has long been known that this powerful vasoconstrictor effect is brought about by the peptide angiotensin. Nevertheless, there is so far no convincing evidence that this substance plays a role in blood pressure regulation. The importance of angiotensin as a stimulus to aldosterone secretion is well established. In the hypotension of haemorrhage, shock, or sodium depletion, renin secretion is increased, and the restoration of plasma volume which results from enhanced aldosterone production undoubtedly contributes to the return of the blood pressure to normal. Further reference to this subject is made under renal hypertension.

Erythropoiesis

Although there are many causes of anaemia in renal disease it is probable that the kidney contributes a specific factor to erythropoiesis ('erythropoietin'). Although this active principle has not yet been defined as a single substance, biological assay has shown that its activity in plasma increases in all forms of anaemia except the hypoplastic anaemia of renal failure, i.e. a renal factor appears to be necessary for normal blood regeneration. Failure of erythropoietin production is not related to the degree of nitrogen retention. In certain forms of renal disease, especially renal carcinoma, polycythaemia may occur, and high levels of erythropoietin have been demonstrated both in plasma and in tumour extracts. The stimulating effect of anoxaemia on erythropoiesis appears to act via renal production of erythropoietin rather than directly on the bone marrow [see Section 13].

INVESTIGATIONS IN RENAL DISEASE

RENAL FUNCTION TESTS

In view of the many regulatory activities of the kidney, a wide variety of tests of renal function have been devised. Some of these estimate glomerular function, some determine general or specific disorders of tubular function. Others are based on recognition of the over-all biochemical disturbances in the body fluids. Specific tests have been devised to measure the kidneys' response to metabolic loading, e.g. the acid load test. Others are designed to study the function of the kidneys separately.

Blood Levels of Metabolites

The blood urea provides a rough guide to glomerular function, although it does not distinguish between organic renal damage and circulatory (extrarenal) causes of diminished clearance. In advanced organic disease it is the best guide to progress since clearance tests are severely impaired and unreliable at this stage. Factors which increase formation of urea must be taken into account in interpreting the results, for example, fever, catabolic steroids and tissue trauma all increase the rate of urea formation, while high protein intake and increased absorption of protein after gastro-intestinal haemorrhage increase the blood level. The normal limits of blood urea are taken as 20–40 mg. per 100 ml., but this depends on standardization of the above factors. Plasma creatinine is derived largely from endogenous sources and its level is less dependent on variations in protein intake. Under certain circumstances, however, creatinine may be both excreted and reabsorbed by the tubules and plasma chromogens may lead to false high values for plasma creatinine. Blood levels of sodium, potassium, chloride and bicarbonate are important indicators of electrolyte or acid-base disturbance, whilst calcium and phosphate are necessary estimations when there is any suggestion of osteodystrophy, nephrocalcinosis or hyperparathyroidism.

Clearance Tests

Inulin clearance is the most accurate measure of glomerular filtration rate, but for routine purposes the endogenous creatinine clearance is a useful approximation and easier to perform. The blood level, urine volume and creatinine concentration are estimated in a 3-hour specimen in the fasting state. Errors may arise due to failure of complete bladder emptying and timing errors in collecting specimens. Special care is needed therefore in patients with urinary retention, hypertensive subjects under treatment with ganglion blocking drugs, and in small children. For research purposes more accurate and technically simpler methods for G.F.R. estimation have made use of labelled substances such as cobalt-labelled vitamin B_{12}, and I^{131}-labelled sodium diatrizoate (*Hypaque*). As with blood urea levels, clearance tests do not distinguish between renal and extrarenal causes of reduced glomerular filtration. They do, however, give an early and relatively sensitive indication of impaired renal function if proper precautions are taken. As already described, clearance of diodone or PAH may be used to estimate renal plasma flow.

Tests of Concentrating Power

Measurement of urine specific gravity is one of the simplest and most informative tests of renal function. The first specimen passed on waking should be tested, and in ward practice daily observation provides useful evidence of impaired concentrating power. A more reliable test of concentration is based on examination of the early morning urine after 24 hours' fluid deprivation, when the specific gravity should register 1·020 or over. Errors are introduced if protein or sugar is present, 1 per cent. albumin in the urine raising the specific gravity by 3 points. A still more accurate test of concentrating power, independent of variations in fluid intake or loss, is the pitressin test. Pitressin tannate in oil (5 Units) is given intramuscularly at night and free access to water is allowed. This test is unsuitable for infants. The urea concentration test and phenolsulphonphthalein (P.S.P.) excretion are still widely used as tests of tubular function. Whilst they are somewhat inaccurate they give a useful indication of the progress of renal impairment over long periods in chronic renal disease. At this stage, urine specific gravity may be fixed and therefore gives no information on progressive deterioration of function. After ingestion of 15 g. of urea in 100 ml. of water in the fasting state, the urine concentration should reach at least 20 g. per litre. Three separate hourly specimens should be examined since the first is liable to be diluted by osmotic diuresis. As in the case of the blood urea, a variety of extrarenal factors may affect concentrating ability. These include protein starvation, heavy drinking, heart failure and sodium or potassium depletion.

Specific Tests of Tubular Function

The acid loading test is of value in estimating hydrion excretion, especially in distinguishing between acidosis in chronic renal disease and renal tubular acidosis. It may indeed differentiate these conditions before systemic acidosis develops. In renal tubular acidosis, ammonium excretion is normal or high for the pH of the urine, which, however, remains at a high level owing to reduced total hydrion excretion. In organic renal disease, e.g. glomerulonephritis, urine acidification is normal (and pH is therefore low) but ammonium excretion is reduced. The ratio of phosphate to creatinine clearance may be helpful in the diagnosis of hyperparathyroidism. Renal glycosuria is detected by lowering of the renal threshold, as indicated by glucose excretion in the urine, with normal blood glucose levels. Amino-acid excretion should be tested by paper chromatography whenever specific tubular dysfunction is suspected.

Differential Renal Function Tests

Estimation of renal function of the kidneys separately is of special diagnostic value in unilateral renal artery stenosis. The 'ischaemic pattern' of excretion in the abnormal kidney is due to excessive tubular reabsorption of sodium and water from a reduced filtrate volume. The urine from the abnormal kidney will therefore be reduced in volume and sodium concentration, and increased in its concentration of other substances such as creatinine and PAH, relative to the urine from the unaffected kidney. These differences can be accentuated by osmotic diuresis produced by administering urea or mannitol. In branch renal artery stenosis, the difference between the two sides is smaller and the test is less reliable. In unilateral renal disease due to other causes, e.g. chronic pyelonephritis, creatinine and inulin clearance are reduced on the affected side, but their concentration in the urine is diminished instead of being increased. The intravenous pyelogram reflects the ischaemic excretory pattern in unilateral renal artery stenosis. Owing to reduced renal blood flow the 3-minute pyelogram shows delay in appearance of the contrast medium on the affected side, whilst in the later films the shadow is more dense owing to greater concentration.

REFERENCES

Black, D. A. K. (1970) Diagnosis in renal disease, *Brit. med. J.*, **2**, 315, 387.

Dahl, D. S., O'Conor, V. J. Jr, Walker, C. D., and Simon, N. M. (1967) The morbidity of differential renal function studies: Analysis of 271 studies, *J. Amer. med. Ass.*, **202**, 857.

Kim, K. E., Onesti, G., Ramirez, O., Brest, A. N., and Swartz, C. (1969) Creatinine clearance in renal disease. A reappraisal, *Brit. med. J.*, **4**, 11.

EXAMINATION OF THE URINE

Proteinuria

Postural (orthostatic) proteinuria may continue for some time after adopting the supine position, so that in testing for it the bladder should be emptied after a period of recumbency and a further specimen collected after an hour. Postural proteinuria may be present in organic renal disease, hence a difference in protein content between the early morning and midday specimens is not necessarily sufficient to exclude organic disease. Tubular proteinuria occurs in syndromes of tubular dysfunction such as the Fanconi syndrome and after heavy metal poisoning. The protein excreted consists largely of α- and β-globulins with relatively little albumin. Bence-Jones protein is a low molecular weight protein, immunologically related to γ-globulin and identifiable on electrophoresis. Albuminuria due to organic renal disease is often present in myelomatosis, and can be separated by heat precipitation and filtration. The Bence-Jones protein will then precipitate as the filtrate cools to about 122° F. (50° C.). Paper strip tests (*Albustix*) give false positive results in infected urine, in the presence of mucoprotein, and in pregnancy. Positive results should therefore be checked by the boiling or sulphosalicylic acid tests.

Microscopy

Microscopy of the urinary deposit is the most reliable test for haematuria and pyuria. Red cell casts, epithelial and granular casts are of great importance in recognizing nephron damage, especially as a criterion of recovery in nephritis, and in differentiating glomerular haemorrhage from bleeding elsewhere in the urinary tract. Granular casts may, however, be found after exercise, in renal congestion, or in association with postural proteinuria. Hyaline casts are formed by combination of albumin with another protein present in small traces in normal cells and urine; their significance is therefore no greater than that of albuminuria alone. Cells and casts disintegrate in urine which is left standing for some hours or on centrifuging at high speed. They should, therefore, be looked for in freshly passed urine, after low speed centrifuging. Crystalluria may be due to phosphates, urates or uric acid, oxalates or cystine, and if excessive may lead to calculus formation.

Other Urinary Abnormalities

Abnormal pigments or their precursors in the urine include haemoglobin, urobilin, bilirubin, porphyrins, melanin and homogentisic acid. The latter is found in alkaptonuria due to an inborn error of metabolism and causes the urine to darken on standing, or on addition of alkalis. Myogloblinuria occurs after extensive muscle injury and may be a feature in acute anuric uraemia. Haemoglobinuria is due to intravascular haemolysis [see Section 13].

RENAL BIOPSY

Percutaneous renal biopsy has made a considerable contribution to knowledge of renal structural pathology, and to the development of renal electron microscopy. It is not entirely without risk, haematuria and perirenal haematoma occurring in a proportion of cases, and fatalities have been recorded. It is contra-indicated in chronic renal failure, malignant hypertension, haemorrhagic states, during anticoagulant therapy, in patients with a single kidney and in the presence of renal infection. While scientific advance has undoubtedly come from this technique, the benefit to the individual patient is not so obvious. It can be used in anuria to clarify the extent and nature of the structural lesion, a finding of intense glomerulonephritis usually precluding haemodialysis [p. 984]. It may be the only means of indicating the underlying lesion in the nephrotic syndrome, e.g. amyloid disease which is not always detected by rectal biopsy, and systemic lupus erythematosus which is usually identified by other tests. Biopsy will, however, indicate the presence of minimal glomerular damage in the nephrotic syndrome, which may be taken as a criterion for the use of steroid therapy; but the decision can be made on clinical grounds in the absence of renal impairment, hypertension, and of inflammatory cells and casts in the urine deposit. In unilateral renal disease renal biopsy may reveal the presence of secondary vascular disease or pyelonephritis in the opposite kidney, and this may be considered to contra-indicate nephrectomy, but if renal function is normal it is doubtful if such a contra-indication is valid. Biopsy may disclose structural abnormalities to account for asymptomatic proteinuria, but this rarely adds very much to prognosis or treatment. Before carrying out renal biopsy therefore, the investigator should be clear in his mind whether the result is likely to benefit the patient, or only to add to knowledge.

REFERENCES

BLACK, D. A. K. (1967) *Renal Disease*, 2nd. ed., Oxford.
DE WARDENER, H. E. (1968) *The Kidney*, 3rd ed., London.
HAMBURGER, J., and WALSH, A. (1967) *Nephrology*, Vols. 1 and 2, London.

DISORDERS OF RENAL FUNCTION

Failure of renal function may be discussed in terms of defects in the glomerular and tubular functions described above. Alternatively it may be dealt with in terms of the over-all biochemical disturbance in the body, i.e. disorders of homeostasis. From the clinical point of view it can be described in terms of the various syndromes of uraemia which are encountered in different forms or renal disease.

DISORDERS OF GLOMERULAR AND TUBULAR FUNCTION

Impaired glomerular function results in reduced glomerular filtration and increased glomerular permeability to protein. The *causes* of reduced glomerular filtration may be structural or functional. Structural renal disease causes disorganization of the glomerular tufts, as in acute nephritis, with eventual destruction and loss of filtering glomeruli in the chronic stages of the disease. The reduction in filtrate volume may be so extreme that oliguria or even complete anuria result. Functional causes reduce filtration owing to fall in blood pressure. This occurs for example in shock, haemorrhage, or sodium depletion due to a variety of causes which include vomiting, polyuria, excessive use of diuretics, and Addison's disease. Sodium depletion is always accompanied by reduced plasma volume and this may depress glomerular filtration even in circumstances where severe oedema is present, e.g. in the nephrotic syndrome. The G.F.R. is also depressed in severe heart failure. Gross reduction in filtration results from two other causes, namely rise in intrapelvic pressure due to complete ureteric obstruction, and acute cortical ischaemia. These disorders give rise to the syndrome of acute oliguric renal failure, the causes and effects of which are discussed later. *The results* of reduced glomerular filtration are due to retention of water and metabolites, and all degrees of this occur, from the slight nitrogen retention of congestive heart failure to the complete suppression of excretion in the anuria syndrome. Progressive elevation of blood urea occurs; sodium and potassium are retained, the latter being more serious since it may produce cardiac arrest. It is obvious that the increased blood concentration of urea and other metabolites will increase the solute load presented to the tubules and osmotic diuresis will follow. This serves as a compensatory measure, the blood urea becoming stabilized at a high level at which production and clearance are in balance.

Abnormal glomerular permeability leads to loss of proteins which are normally unable to pass the glomerular filter, i.e. those with molecular weight over 60,000. This applies to the bulk of the plasma proteins although the small albumin molecules will be lost in greater amounts than the globulins. The factors responsible for increased permeability are obscure, but from the practical point of view we can recognize a functional and reversible lesion, and a structural and irreversible one. The former is present in postural proteinuria, renal congestion and the nephrotic syndrome; the latter in structural glomerular damage as in glomerulonephritis. In general, the greater the degree of structural damage, the larger the protein molecules which pass through the glomerular membrane. In the nephrotic syndrome with diffuse glomerulitis both types of increased permeability will be present. When the glomeruli are severely damaged, erythrocytes and leucocytes will also pass through the filtering membrane.

Impaired tubular function may affect either re-absorption or tubular excretion, and both may be increased or diminished. Defective tubular re-absorption causes a wide variety of disorders and is best classified as selective or unselective. Unselective impairment of tubular re-absorption is present during osmotic diuresis. It affects all solutes and greatly restricts the homeostatic function of the kidney. This impairment of tubular function will increase as the total functioning nephrons are progressively destroyed by structural damage, until water and electrolyte balance become almost entirely dependent on the filtered load, with little adaptability to varying conditions of intake and loss of water. Selective defects of tubular re-absorption are much less common, but comprise an interesting group of specific tubular anomalies in which the usual cause is inherited enzyme deficiency. Fanconi syndrome, renal tubular acidosis and renal glycosuria are typical examples. Similar selective tubular defects may be produced by metabolic disorders such as potassium depletion, or by chemical poisons such as lead, cadmium and copper (in hepatolenticular degeneration), by diuretics, or occasionally in chronic renal disease, the so-called 'sodium-losing' or 'potassium-losing' nephritis. Of a quite different nature are the absorption defects due to endocrine disease. Hyperaldosteronism, primary or secondary, leads to potassium depletion, adrenal cortical failure causes impaired sodium re-absorption, and hyperparathyroidism impaired phosphate re-absorption. Diabetes insipidus is due to failure of water re-absorption in the distal tubule which normally occurs under the influence of pituitary ADH.

Increased tubular re-absorption is largely due to hormonal activity acting in the reverse direction to these tubular absorption defects, e.g. potassium retention in Addison's disease, sodium retention in secondary aldosteronism, increased re-absorption of phosphate in hypoparathyroidism. A syndrome of water retention and hyponatraemia has been described due to inappropriate secretion of ADH by tumour cells.

Abnormalities of tubular excretion largely affect the elimination of hydrion, potassium and ammonium by the distal tubule. These are best discussed under disorders of acid-base regulation and potassium depletion. A number of solutes may compete for the same tubular excretion pathway, hence the phenomenon of excretion blockage, e.g. of penicillin by probenecid.

DISORDERS OF HOMEOSTASIS

In renal disease, abnormalities of glomerular and tubular function usually occur together and interact on one another, so that the clinical manifestations are most clearly explained by examination of the over-all biochemical disturbance. This is a composite picture arising from varying degrees of failure or impairment of the homeostatic controls described under normal renal function. One of the most important features of renal failure is the frequency with which disorders of homeostasis themselves interfere with renal function. This on the one hand often leads to progressive deterioration due to the establishment of vicious circles, and on the other hand holds out the prospect of therapeutic benefit if these vicious circles can be broken. A typical example is the production of sodium and water depletion by polyuria and vomiting in organic renal disease, which superimposes reversible 'extra-renal' nitrogen retention on irreversible uraemia due to the primary disease. Similarly heart failure, hypertension, potassium depletion and anaemia are all consequences of renal disease which themselves adversely affect renal function, and are amenable to corrective treatment. In fact, the therapy of chronic renal disease is largely based on the recognition of this reciprocal relationship between primary renal disease and its secondary manifestations. Whilst these disorders of homeostasis will be described separately, it must be recognized that this is an artificial separation, since they are closely interrelated, and disturbance of one homeostatic mechanism sets in train adaptive or secondary changes in others. Finally there is a very variable correlation between failure of homeostatic control and renal structural damage. Gross hypoproteinaemic oedema may occur in the nephrotic syndrome with minimal histological changes in the kidney; severe biochemical disturbances may be due to specific tubular defects without any obvious structural lesion. Secondary structural damage may, moreover, result from the functional disorder, e.g. tubular atrophy and renal fibrosis occur in potassium depletion, and progressive renal vascular disease is caused by severe hypertension. These effects lead to difficult problems of diagnosis, e.g. between primary and secondary aldosteronism, or between essential hypertension and renal hypertension in the malignant phase.

Body Water and Sodium—Dehydration and Oedema

Sodium and water are considered together since they are the main constituents of the extracellular fluid and most disturbances of body water are due to sodium depletion or retention. Sodium and water depletion may be renal or extrarenal in origin. Renal salt loss is due to failure of tubular re-absorption of sodium, either due to osmotic diuresis or to specific tubular damage in predominantly medullary lesions such as pyelonephritis. Extreme sodium wasting may lead to a picture resembling Addison's disease. Excessive or prolonged diuretic therapy, especially if supplemented by a low salt intake, may produce severe sodium and water depletion. The extrarenal causes of sodium depletion include vomiting, polyuria, diarrhoea and aldosterone deficiency in adrenal cortical hypofunction. The resulting hypovolaemia reduces renal blood flow and leads to rise in blood urea, as already described under impaired glomerular filtration.

Sodium and water retention lead to *oedema* in renal disease and this again may be of renal or extrarenal origin. Renal causes arise from reduced filtration, either due to diffuse glomerular damage as in acute nephritis or to cortical ischaemia as in the anuria syndrome. Fluid retention in acute nephritis may lead to hypervolaemia and the haemodilution produces apparent anaemia. In both acute and chronic renal disease albuminuria leads to hypoproteinaemia and the reduced colloid osmotic pressure favours retention of fluid in the tissues, while extrarenal factors such as heart failure aggravate sodium retention and will contribute to oedema formation. When plasma volume is low, as in the nephrotic syndrome, secondary aldosterone production will cause tubular sodium retention, thereby increasing and perpetuating the oedema, since in the presence of hypoproteinaemia, the retained sodium and water are rapidly transferred from the vascular compartment to the tissues. The features of oedema in the nephrotic syndrome will be discussed under that heading.

Renal Acidosis

Renal acidosis occurs in chronic renal failure, in acute oliguric renal failure and in primary tubular disorders. The mechanism depends on the cause. In organic renal failure, ability to excrete hydrion is usually unimpaired but ammonia formation is deficient and titratable acidity is low owing to reduced excretion of phosphate buffer, which is the principal hydrion acceptor in the tubular fluid. The urine is very acid therefore, i.e. pH may fall to low levels. The accumulation of fixed acids in the blood depletes plasma bicarbonate, which is therefore not available in the tubular fluid to combine with hydrion and so prevent the pH from falling. In renal tubular acidosis, tubular hydrion excretion is impaired but ammonia excretion may be little affected. The urine pH remains high therefore even when acidosis develops. In the metabolic acidosis of diabetes the tubular excretion of ammonia and titratable acidity may increase 5 times or more, and free excretion of keto-acids occurs. Nevertheless in severe cases these are retained in high concentration in the blood with corresponding reduction in plasma bicarbonate. Hyperchloraemic acidosis occurs in a variety of conditions, an example of which is uretero-colic anastomosis. Here excessive chloride absorption from the bowel reduces the plasma bicarbonate, and the ability of the kidney to correct this situation is often impaired by tubular damage resulting from ascending pyelonephritis. When the kidney no longer compensates adequately in metabolic acidosis, the respiratory centre is stimulated and acidotic (Kussmaul) breathing occurs. The resulting washing out of CO_2 partly relieves the acidosis, but at the same time reduces the plasma bicarbonate, so that a proper assessment of the state of acid-base balance can only be made by estimating the blood pH. The reciprocal relationship of potassium and hydrion excretion will lead to potassium depletion when hydrion excretion is deficient as in renal tubular acidosis. Acetazolamide, which reduces hydrion excretion by inhibiting carbonic anhydrase, will similarly produce potassium depletion.

Other Disorders of Electrolyte Homeostasis

Potassium. In previous sections the factors which regulate and vitiate potassium excretion have been discussed. In renal disease both potassium retention and depletion occur. Potassium retention of renal origin arises when there is severe reduction in glomerular filtration rate, as in acute nephritis and the anuria syndrome. Increased tissue breakdown due to infection or muscle damage (crush syndrome) aggravate hyperkalaemia. So also does acidosis, which causes transfer of potassium from cells to extracellular fluid, a process which can be temporarily reversed by glucose and insulin. Potassium depletion due to primary renal disease is always due to defective tubular re-absorption, e.g. in the severe diuresis which occurs in the recovery phase of acute anuria or during relief of chronic retention of urine. Severe potassium depletion is a feature of the various specific tubular defects [p. 987] whether these are congenital or acquired, and the resulting muscle weakness may be a presenting symptom of the disease. Extrarenal causes producing increased potassium excretion include primary or secondary aldosteronism, diuretics such as chlorothiazide and glucocorticoid administration or overproduction. Potassium depletion exemplifies the secondary effects which disordered homeostasis may have on the kidney. Even moderately severe potassium loss leads to vacuolar degeneration of the epithelium of the convoluted tubules. These lesions disappear if the potassium deficiency is corrected, but otherwise tubular atrophy and interstitial fibrosis occur and renal failure eventually ensues. Extrarenal potassium loss, e.g. in severe chronic diarrhoea, leads to similar renal damage. Apart from these structural changes potassium depletion adversely affects renal function, the most obvious change being polyuria with defective urine concentration—the urine specific gravity may be as low as 1·002. Sodium retention may occur and contribute to oedema formation, e.g. in the nephrotic syndrome. Extracellular alkalosis with raised plasma bicarbonate is a frequent finding and is associated with intracellular acidosis. Acidification of the urine is defective, titratable acidity being low, although ammonia formation is relatively high. There is therefore little fall in urine pH (which is usually about 6–7) when an acid load is administered.

Calcium. Disturbances of *body calcium* in renal disease are extremely complex and very gross forms of osteodystrophy may occur. These are described under chronic uraemia [p. 982] and specific tubular disorders [p. 987]. Plasma calcium is often low in chronic uraemia, but there is no consistent abnormality. While phosphate retention is the rule in chronic uraemia, excessive loss of phosphate occurs in primary tubular disorders. Secondary hyperparathyroidism, which is a common result of long-standing uraemia, is probably a homeostatic response to depression of ionized calcium, representing an attempt to maintain normal or high serum calcium levels. Hypercalcaemia of varied origin has marked secondary effects on renal function. G.F.R. may be depressed leading to rise in blood urea; ADH resistance develops giving rise to polyuria and polydipsia; hypercalciuria occurs but tends to diminish as renal failure develops. Deposition of calcium in the renal parenchyma (nephrocalcinosis) is seen in renal tubular acidosis and conditions leading to hypercalcaemia. It can lead to renal fibrosis and uraemia.

Magnesium. In many cases with uraemia serum magnesium levels are increased. In health the kidney conserves magnesium effectively under conditions of deficient intake or excessive loss (as in intestinal malabsorption). Failure of this conservation may be due to osmotic diuresis or it may be due to tubular damage.

Anaemia in Renal Disease

The common cause of anaemia in renal disease is defective 'erythropoietin' response to anoxia by the kidney, and the anaemia is hypoplastic. Severe renal failure is usually present, and may be due to chronic nephritis, pyelonephritis or congenital cystic kidneys, but a similar anaemia develops in acute oliguric uraemia, and in severe acute nephritis. There is no clear evidence that metabolite retention plays a part, indeed the blood urea need not be excessively high, and severe uraemia may be present without anaemia. Other factors leading to anaemia are discussed under chronic uraemia [see also Section 13].

RENAL HYPERTENSION

The discovery by Goldblatt that constriction of the renal arteries in the dog leads to persistent hypertension, suggested a humoral origin of the high blood pressure, since it was shown to be independent of the nervous connexions of the kidney. Renal hypertension was also found to be dependent on the presence of the adrenal cortex, although salt and desoxycortone could act as substitutes in this role. The discovery of the renin-angiotensin system at first appeared to provide a satisfactory basis for the humoral mechanism. The shortcomings of this solution were, first, the failure to find an excess of circulating renin in established hypertension, either in man or in experimental animals, although an increase was reported in malignant hypertension. Secondly, it did not explain the undoubted role of salt and the adrenal cortex in the maintenance of high blood pressure. The discovery that angiotensin stimulates the adrenal cortex to produce aldosterone has provided a physiological function, hitherto unrecognized, for renin. This enzyme is apparently an essential link in the feedback mechanism which regulates plasma volume, and recently improved methods of renin assay indicate that its secretion is highly sensitive to sodium depletion and reduced plasma volume. There is also increased production of renin in the juxtaglomerular apparatus following renal artery constriction, i.e. like reduction in plasma volume, this manoeuvre apparently stimulates the pressure receptors by which fall in blood volume is registered. There is some evidence that expansion of extracellular fluid and plasma volumes takes place in acute hypertension, e.g. in acute nephritis and after renal artery constriction, and this might theoretically increase cardiac output and raise the blood pressure. In established renal hypertension, however, E.C.F. and plasma volumes (and cardiac output) are normal. At the present time it can only be said that there is no good evidence that blood volume control (via renin and aldosterone) and blood pressure control share a common mechanism, or that the peripheral resistance in hypertension is increased by the direct vasoconstrictor action of angiotensin. Nevertheless blood volume and blood pressure changes are in some ways related. It is well recognized that when renal function is impaired, the blood pressure is very sensitive to blood volume changes. For example, in acute nephritis hypertensive encephalopathy may be dramatically relieved by venesection. In anuria, very small increase in blood volume occurring during haemodialysis may cause a steep rise in blood pressure.

Of particular interest is the change in physiological mechanism when hypertension changes from the benign to the malignant phase. The clinical manifestations of malignant hypertension—papilloedema, hypertensive encephalopathy and left ventricular failure, are associated with progressive renal damage, due to fibrinoid necrosis of small arteries and arterioles. Experimental observations have proved that the fibrinoid arterial necrosis is the result of malignant hypertension and not its cause. The functional disturbances in the brain and retina have been shown to be associated with intense regional vasoconstriction which can be abolished by lowering the blood pressure. It is possible that this intense vasoconstriction causes the vascular necrosis, and it is of great interest that malignant hypertension is apparently the one form of high blood pressure in which increase in aldosterone secretion (and renin formation) can be regularly demonstrated. Here again we have an example of a vicious circle arising in renal disease, since the secondary vascular lesions in the kidney lead to progressive renal damage, which maintains and aggravates the hypertension. If this vicious circle is broken by hypotensive drug therapy, the progressive course of the disease can often be arrested for several years.

REFERENCES

BLACK, D. A. K. (1960) *Essentials of Fluid Balance*, Oxford.

PLATT, R. (1951) Renal failure, *Lancet*, i, 1239.

ROBINSON, J. R. (1961) *Fundamentals of Acid-Base Regulation*, Oxford.

SMITH, H. W. (1951) *The Kidney: Structure and Function in Health and Disease*, New York.

STRAUSS, M. B., and WELT, L. G. (1963) *Diseases of the Kidney*, Boston.

ULLRICH, K. J., KRAMER, K., and BOYLAN, J. W. (1962) Mechanism of urinary concentration, in *Renal Disease*, ed. BLACK, D. A. K., Chap. 3, Oxford.

WESSON, L. G. JR. (1969) *Physiology of the Human Kidney*, New York.

CLINICAL SYNDROMES OF DISORDERED RENAL FUNCTION

While all forms of renal failure have much in common due to disturbances of metabolite excretion and homeostatic control, there are several widely differing clinical syndromes. These are, chronic uraemia due to progressive organic renal disease, acute oliguric uraemia (the anuria syndrome), extrarenal uraemia, the nephrotic syndrome and disordered renal function due to specific tubular anomalies.

CHRONIC URAEMIA

This is the commonest form of renal failure and arises from any chronic bilateral renal disease. The most frequent causes are chronic pyelonephritis, chronic glomerulonephritis, urinary tract obstruction and ischaemic renal atrophy, including diabetic nephrosclerosis. Less common are renal tuberculosis, congenital cystic disease, amyloid disease, interstitial nephritis due to nephrotoxic agents, such as lead and phenacetin, chronic gouty nephritis and myelomatosis. In many of these conditions the prominent clinical features are due to hypertension rather than to the biochemical disturbances of excretory failure. In others, hypertension is slight or absent and this permits a very chronic course which may lead to long-standing metabolic acidosis and various forms of renal osteodystrophy. In some patients, progress is rapid and symptoms are severe due to continued activity of the original disease or to secondary complications such as ascending pyelonephritis or malignant hypertension; in others, renal failure progresses slowly over decades, and for most of this time the patient may be asymptomatic and capable of living a useful and active life. In general the disabling symptoms of excretory failure mercifully come as a terminal event, whose significance is often masked for the patient by clouding of insight due to metabolite retention. Many of the manifestations of excretory failure are unexplainable but symptoms may be dramatically relieved when the biochemical lesion is corrected by haemodialysis.

It is useful to divide the natural history into the stages of renal impairment and renal failure, i.e. before and after the blood urea persistently exceeds the normal level. In the stage of renal impairment there may be no symptoms, and the basic disturbance is reduction of urine concentrating power. Diluting power is retained until the late stages. At first there is narrowing of the limits of specific gravity, then fixation around 1·010–1·012. Polyuria may be noticed, at first nocturnal due to failure of night concentration, and on direct questioning the patient may admit to increased thirst. In this stage albuminuria will be constantly found except in some cases of pyelonephritis where the infection has become inactive. Hypertension is usually moderate in degree but may lead to the development of cardiac failure in patients with atherosclerosis. In general, other symptoms of cardiac ischaemia seem to be unusual in patients with chronic renal disease. Further deterioration of renal function is often associated with rising blood pressure. Hypertensive heart failure, retinopathy, cerebral vascular lesions, and in untreated cases malignant hypertension with papilloedema and hypertensive encephalopathy, may be the presenting features. Extrarenal factors such as infection, vomiting, heart failure, anaemia or sodium depletion may cause further elevation of blood urea and retention of other metabolites responsible for uraemic symptoms, so that these factors should be identified and treated. Eventually progressive excretory failure leads to irreversible uraemia, but this may be of long duration or late development, since as already pointed out, increased filtered load of metabolites and osmotic diuresis may maintain clearance at a high and steady blood urea level. Various systems of the body are affected by excretory failure.

Gastro-intestinal symptoms are often prominent and refractory to treatment. A dry foul tongue, anorexia, hiccough, nausea and vomiting are common, stomatitis and diarrhoea are rare. These symptoms have been attributed to urea excretion and ammonia formation in the gastro-intestinal tract, but if so the stimulation threshold must be variable since they may resolve while the blood urea remains unchanged. Wasting is chiefly due to reduced appetite, but sodium depletion due to vomiting and polyuria, is a contributory cause and leads also to general weakness. Endogenous protein breakdown is increased by starvation and further aggravates nitrogen retention.

Neuromuscular symptoms are late in appearing and are presumably related to disturbance of cation balance, although the nature of this is obscure. Neuromuscular irritability is diminished by potassium and magnesium retention and increased by low plasma concentration of ionized calcium. Coarse muscle twitching, tremors and muscle cramps are the usual manifestations; latent tetany is occasionally demonstrable. Specific uraemic peripheral neuropathy may occur and appears to be due to the toxic effect of protein metabolites. This complicates regular dialysis therapy and may be cured by increased efficacy of dialysis. Convulsions may be metabolic in origin or may be due to hypertensive encephalopathy; they may be precipitated by fluid retention or by blood transfusion. Potassium depletion (in chronic uraemia) is rarely sufficient to produce muscular weakness except in so-called potassium-losing nephritis. Lassitude, mental depression and mental confusion result from acidosis or sodium depletion, and anaemia and heart failure may be contributory. Increasing drowsiness and coma are the eventual results of metabolite retention.

Blood disorders. The refractory anaemia of renal disease has already been discussed; other causes of anaemia include infection, deficient iron intake, achlorhydria, haematuria and rarely haemolysis. Haemorrhagic manifestations include bleeding gums, purpura, haemarthrosis and bleeding from the gastro-intestinal tract. These are not due to thrombocytopenia, although this occurs, but capillary fragility is increased, apparently due to defective platelet function.

Skin changes. Sallow pigmentation is usual and is partly due to anaemia. A yellowish tinge may be present, especially in outdoor workers, and is probably due to urochrome retention. Urea excretion in the sweat may form a 'urea frost'. In addition to purpura, pruritus and skin rashes are common but of obscure origin. The skin is lax and dry due to dehydration unless oedema is present.

Cardiovascular disorders. Heart failure is a common feature of chronic uraemia. Hypertension is the prime cause, but anaemia, infection and fluid retention often contribute. When excretion is restricted to osmotic diuresis the patient has little adaptability to raised fluid intake or impaired cardiac function. Oedema is often aggravated by hypoproteinaemia. In the malignant phase of hypertension visual impairment results from macular haemorrhages and exudates. Hypertensive encephalopathy may give rise to headaches, disorientation, blindness, convulsions and coma. Acute pulmonary oedema usually presents with paroxysmal nocturnal dyspnoea; renal vascular and glomerular necroses may produce frank haematuria. These symptoms are often dramatically relieved when the blood pressure is lowered. Acute non-infective, sometimes haemorrhagic, pericarditis, with or without tamponade, is a common complication in terminal uraemia, but localized pericarditis may recover if renal function improves. There is a reduced tolerance for digitalis in uraemia; heart block, nausea and vomiting may occur, and this drug is best avoided.

Respiratory manifestations include acidotic breathing which is deep, harsh and unaffected by exercise; exertional and nocturnal dyspnoea due to heart failure; and acute pulmonary infections. Protracted pulmonary congestion may give rise to fibrinous oedema (uraemic lung).

Renal osteodystrophy. Osteodystrophy occurs in two distinct types of renal disease, namely, in chronic uraemia and as a result of specific tubular enzyme defects. The former, so-called glomerular or azotaemic osteodystrophy, occurs typically in very long-standing renal failure, usually without hypertension, for example in congenital renal disease, especially with hydronephrosis, chronic pyelonephritis, or more rarely in chronic glomerulonephritis. The commonest form of osteodystrophy is renal rickets, or osteomalacia in adults, which in its morphological characteristics is identical with that produced by vitamin D deficiency. It appears that chronic uraemia produces resistance to vitamin D, and in fact administration of large doses of calciferol leads to healing of the active lesion. The required dosage is variable and unpredictable. A starting dose of 1·25 mg. vitamin D increasing to 2·5 mg. daily is usually effective, but with increasing dosage there is a risk of vitamin D intoxication. The other bone lesion of chronic uraemia is osteitis fibrosa due to secondary hyperparathyroidism, which leads to osteoclastic resorption and fibrous replacement of the bony trabeculae. These two forms of osteodystrophy coexist in varying degrees and may be associated with other bony changes including osteosclerosis and osteoporosis. Increased mobilization of calcium from bone may lead to its deposition in other tissues, including the kidneys, arteries and subcutaneous tissue (metastatic calcification). At present we can go little further than to ascribe the pathogenesis of azotaemic osteodystrophy to vitamin D resistance and secondary hyperparathyroidism.

In brief the syndrome of chronic uraemia presents a variable picture due to hypertension, metabolite retention and failure of homeostatic regulation. The physiological reserve of the kidney maintains excretory function and electrolyte homeostasis in a remarkable way in spite of gross structural damage, and the final rapid deterioration is often attributable to extraneous factors such as pulmonary infection, acute ascending pyelonephritis, cerebral vascular lesions or heart failure.

Treatment

As the foregoing summary indicates, the functional disorders in chronic uraemia are both variable and complex, and accurate diagnosis of their nature in the individual patient is essential for effective treatment. The pattern and sequence of events will to some extent differ according to the cause, e.g. the chronic anhypertensive uraemia leading to renal osteodystrophy will present different therapeutic problems from progressive glomerulonephritis terminating in malignant hypertension.

The appropriate adjustment of treatment according to the stage and complications of the particular disease is illustrated under glomerulonephritis [p. 989]. In general terms the treatment of irreversible terminal uraemia has been dramatically transformed by recent advances in regular dialysis therapy (R.D.T.) and renal transplantation. In patients with chronic uraemia peritoneal dialysis is chiefly of value to bring about rapid and effective correction of water and electrolyte imbalance, thereby improving the clinical state so that an accurate diagnosis of the cause of the renal failure may be made, e.g. by pyelography or renal biopsy. Where facilities for R.D.T. are not immediately available it may be possible to maintain the patient in reasonable balance for some weeks, or even a few months, by repeated peritoneal dialysis. Such continued treatment, with the risk of infection, has obvious disadvantages if renal transplantation is to be carried out subsequently.

The official recognition of centres for R.D.T. and renal transplantation has raised a wide variety of problems both social and medical—not least being the great difficulties in providing the highly trained staff, medical, nursing and technical, to meet the clinical need—it being estimated that of the 7,000 patients in this country dying in uraemia each year at least one third could obtain considerable benefit from these modern methods of treatment. The problem has been aggravated by the occurrence in most R.D.T. units of infective hepatitis among patients and staff. One answer to this serious development has been to increase home dialysis therapy which in turn makes increasing demands on the community, the patient's relatives, and the hospital technical staff. In spite of its many disadvantages R.D.T. linked with a renal transplantation programme must be regarded as the most promising therapeutic approach to terminal renal failure. In selecting patients for R.D.T. it is highly desirable that they should accept and be suitable for home dialysis and if possible for renal transplantation at some future date. Age, the presence of complicating diseases such as diabetes, pulmonary tuberculosis and cerebral or cardiovascular disease must be taken into account, and social conditions, particularly family co-operation and stability, are of paramount importance. The main argument in favour of R.D.T. is that with careful selection and supervision the majority of patients may return to full-time employment. The disadvantages are the dietary regulation, especially of protein and fluids, the psychological strain on the patient and his relatives and various complications which have become more apparent with increasing length of treatment. The main problems arise from 'shunt failure' which may be due to clotting, vascular closure or infection. These have been greatly minimized by the recent introduction of the Cimino-Brescia direct internal arteriovenous shunt in place of the external Quinton-Scribner teflon-silastic arteriovenous cannula. The Cimino shunt is suitable for home dialysis and allows the patient much greater freedom of action with much diminished risk of shunt failure. Long-term complications of R.D.T. include osteodystrophy, in the form of osteoporosis, osteomalacia and secondary hyperparathyroidism, metastatic calcification which may lead to occlusive vascular disease, and peripheral neuritis. These risks may be minimized by reducing the calcium content of the dialysate and by more frequent or prolonged dialyses. In the early stages of R.D.T. the refractory anaemia was treated by frequent blood transfusions. It was subsequently found that spontaneous rise in haemoglobin to about 11 g. per 100 ml. occurred in the absence of transfusion and this form of treatment has been discontinued. A further contra-indication to transfusion is the transmission of tissue antibodies which may increase the risk of rejection of a subsequently transplanted kidney.

Improvements in the results of renal transplantation have been brought about by advances in immunosuppressive therapy and by more effective pre- and post-transplantation haemodialysis. Further improvements will largely depend on more successful patient-donor matching. This in turn will depend on more accurate tissue typing and the development of co-operative schemes for the formation of large recipient pools so that cadaver kidneys can be transplanted into best-match recipients. Present evidence indicates a 40 per cent. 2-year survival of cadaver transplants rising to 75 per cent. with kidneys from living sibling donors.

ACUTE OLIGURIC URAEMIA

Causation

The syndrome of acute oliguric uraemia is essentially the result of gross reduction of glomerular filtration, usually accompanied by failure of tubular function. Suppression of urine (anuria) occurs in extreme cases. The three common causes are acute cortical ischaemia (so-called acute tubular necrosis), severe acute diffuse nephritis and bilateral ureteric obstruction. Rarer causes are massive cortical necrosis, bilateral medullary (papillary) necrosis, and as a manifestation of acute scleroderma. The pathogenesis of *acute cortical ischaemia* is obscure, and the provoking causes are numerous and varied. It first attracted general attention as the 'crush syndrome' complicating crushing injury of the limbs in air raid casualties. It may complicate acute hypotensive shock in infected abortion, obstetric haemorrhage and after surgical operations. It may develop in severe infections such as blackwater fever and Weil's disease. A massive hypersensitivity reaction is suggested by its occurrence after incompatible blood transfusion, sulphonamide therapy or heavy metal poisoning, and it has been reported after intravenous pyelography. It may follow instrumentation of the urinary tract, such as ureteric catheterization, and it has occurred as a complication of aortography when contrast medium has been injected into the renal arteries. Tubular blockage may be a contributory factor as in sulphonamide therapy (crystals), haemolytic anaemia (haemoglobin casts) and the crush syndrome (myoglobin casts). In heavy metal poisoning there appears to be diffuse toxic damage to the renal tubules, whilst in other types of anuria, patchy necrosis in the distal tubules (tubulorrhexis) is the characteristic lesion. Nephron dissection studies suggest that, in both, acute cortical ischaemia is probably the basic disorder, and this is supported by the occurrence of massive cortical necrosis in some instances. In fact, a wide variety of structural lesions, ranging from minimal focal tubular necrosis to diffuse cortical necrosis may occur in oliguric uraemia, and its frequent reversibility suggests that the primary disorder is intense cortical vasoconstriction, which according to its extent and duration leads also to a wide variety of structural damage.

The Biochemical Disturbance and Clinical Features

Renal functional changes depend on the stage of the disorder. There is an initial stage of shock, followed by oliguria or anuria, which in recovering cases is succeeded by diuresis. In the stage of shock, renal blood flow is reduced to a greater extent than cardiac output, suggesting renal vasoconstriction. In the stage of oliguria there is gross reduction of glomerular filtration, although total renal blood flow may be 30–50 per cent. of normal. There is some preservation of tubular function, since sodium conservation and potassium excretion still occur, and the urine pH may fall to 5·5 or lower. In the diuretic stage, glomerular filtration recovers before tubular re-absorption. Hence gross polyuria with excessive loss of sodium and potassium may occur. The U/P ratio of urea and creatinine may show that the urine in this stage consists of relatively unchanged glomerular filtrate, so that the blood urea may continue to rise in spite of massive diuresis. Subsequent impairment of renal function, especially of concentrating power, may persist for many months even when clinical recovery appears to be complete.

Gross disturbance of homeostasis occurs in this condition unless corrective therapy is continuously applied. The chief effects of continuing protein catabolism, in the absence of renal excretion, are azotaemia, hyperkalaemia and acidosis. If tissue breakdown is increased by trauma, infection or fever, these effects will be exaggerated, e.g. in post-traumatic anuria the blood urea may rise by 40–100 mg. per day compared with 20–30 mg. in other cases. Rise in serum potassium above 8 mEq. per litre may cause cardiac arrest or arrhythmia, and acidosis aggravates these effects. The latter is indicated by fall in plasma bicarbonate, and clinically by acidotic respiration; in severe acidosis periodic breathing, lassitude and mental confusion develop. Water retention occurs unless fluid balance is strictly maintained. Water produced from oxidation of fat and protein amounts to about 350 ml. daily, to which must be added about 250 ml. from cell breakdown; insensible loss is about 1 litre, so that if anuria is complete about 400 ml. water is required to maintain fluid balance. Fluid retention due to excessive sodium and water administration may cause subcutaneous and pulmonary oedema, raised venous pressure, hypertension and convulsions. Excessive water intake alone may lead to water intoxication. Neurological abnormalities include hyperreflexia, ankle clonus and asymmetrical weakness of the limbs suggesting cerebral vascular lesions, but are usually transient. Haemorrhages from the gums and purpura occur in severe cases, and resistance to secondary infection is lowered. Refractory, normocytic (renal) anaemia appears in severe cases. In the diuretic phase there is a risk of sodium and potassium depletion.

Treatment

The essentials of treatment are to maintain the patient in water and electrolyte balance. Potassium retention and acidosis are the most serious risks, and will increase in severity with the rate of protein catabolism. Endogenous protein breakdown is kept to a minimum by administration of a 20 g. protein diet, whilst, as already indicated, fluid balance is maintained by 400 ml. of water (plus volumes lost in urine and vomit), which is increased if fever or hyperpnoea are present. The indications for *dialysis* are clinical deterioration, including mental confusion, muscle twitching and acidotic breathing, or any of the following criteria, blood urea over 300 mg. per 100 ml., serum potassium above 7·0 mEq. per litre, serum bicarbonate below 12·0 mEq. per litre. Patients should therefore be transferred to a dialysis unit before this stage is reached, since irreversible damage may occur if treatment is delayed. The need for careful observation and investigation of patients with oliguria cannot be over-emphasized. A fluid balance chart must be kept and all urine saved for estimation of urea, potassium and sodium concentrations. The blood group should be determined. Daily clinical examination should be made with special attention to mental state and neurological signs, hypertension, cardiac arrythmia and venous congestion, pulmonary oedema, uraemic dyspnoea, evidence of infection or diarrhoea, and haemorrhagic manifestations. Careful palpation of the loins and presence of loin pain may suggest obstructive anuria requiring surgical intervention. Daily electrocardiograms give the best indication of hyperkalaemia (high T wave and broad QRS). Blood analysis for urea, sodium, potassium, bicarbonate, chloride and haematocrit should be made at least on alternate days. *Conservative treatment* will be successful in many patients and should always be instituted in non-traumatic cases when the rise in blood urea is not more than 40 mg. per 100 ml. daily. A 20 g. protein diet is given. Hyperkalaemia can be temporarily improved by insulin (10 Units 6-hourly) and glucose. Much more effective is the rectal administration of 50 G. sodium polystyrene sulphonate (*Resonium-A*), a cation exchange resin which exchanges sodium for potassium in the bowel, in 200 ml. tap water. The risk of excessive sodium retention may be avoided by *Calcium Resonium* which exchanges calcium for potassium, but the possibility of hypercalcaemia must then be considered. Severe acidosis cannot be corrected by measures other than dialysis.

Antibiotic therapy is frequently required in renal failure and special precautions are needed to avoid toxicity since these drugs are variably excreted by glomerular filtration. In general the penicillins can be safely given but dosage should be reduced with methicillin and cloxacillin. Tetracyclines have a cumulative effect and should be given in reduced doses (250–500 mg. daily). Sulphonamides are safe except in the presence of oliguria. Nitrofurantoin, streptomycin and kanamycin are dangerous in renal failure and should be avoided. Concomitant liver failure may induce toxicity by drugs which are normally poorly absorbed, e.g. neomycin. In all cases of doubt blood levels should be estimated frequently and the dose adjusted accordingly.

The effect of haemodialysis or peritoneal dialysis on blood concentration depends on the molecular size of the drug, its protein binding and serum concentration. Nephrotoxicity is obviously not of serious importance in patients on R.D.T. but loss of antibiotic in the dialysate will affect serum levels.

Peritoneal dialysis is the treatment of choice when the oliguria is not relieved by conservative treatment in 2–3 days. It consists of alternate instillation and removal, in 2-litre quantities, of approximately 75 litres of appropriate dialysing fluid across the peritoneal cavity, over 36 hours. It has the advantage of economy in time, apparatus and personnel, it corrects the renal failure gradually, and heparinization and transfusion are avoided. The chief dangers are protein depletion and peritoneal infection.

Haemodialysis is indicated in more urgent cases, where there has been abdominal trauma or infection, or at a later stage when failure of recovery of renal function necessitates a change to regular dialysis therapy

In nontraumatic anuria (excluding acute nephritis and ureteric obstruction) the recovery rate with conservative therapy, supplemented by dialysis if necessary, is 50–75 per cent. In traumatic cases it is 40 per cent. or below. Too rapid dialysis or excessive reduction of blood urea produces an osmotic gradient between blood and brain cells, which may lead to serious mental symptoms and neurological lesions, a further reason for early treatment before nitrogen retention is severe. The frequency with which dialysis must be carried out depends on the rate of protein catabolism, and is determined by the criteria already given. In the average case, once or twice at 3–7 days intervals usually suffices. Renal biopsy will indicate the degree of structural damage and the desirability of repeating the dialysis. It should be carried out only when anuria persists and not as a routine measure. The presence of severe diffuse glomerulonephritis with marked epithelial crescent formation or glomerular necrosis, makes recovery unlikely, but cases with extensive cortical necrosis have been reported to survive. Haemodialysis is an effective measure for treatment of poisons if these are freely dialysable. Alcohol, salicylates, barbitone and phenobarbitone, and certain tranquillizer drugs are readily cleared from the blood, but the shorter-acting barbiturates are not dialysable.

REFERENCES

BERLYNE, G. M. (1968) *Nutrition in Renal Disease*, Edinburgh.

BERLYNE, G. M., BAZZARD, F. S., BOOTH, E. M., JANABI, K., and SHAW, A. B. (1967). The dietary treatment of acute renal failure, *Quart. J. Med.*, **36**, 59.

BLAGG, C. R., HICKMAN, R. O., ESCHBACH, J. W., and SCRIBNER, B. H. (1970) Home dialysis: Six years' experience, *New Engl. J. Med.*, **283**, 1126.

CURTIS, J. R. (1968) Recent position and future prospects in the management of chronic renal failure, *Abstr. Wld Med.*, **42**, 561.

KUNIN, C. M. (1967) A guide to the use of antibiotics in patients with renal disease, *Ann. intern. Med.*, **67**, 151.

MERRILL, J. P. (1955) *The Treatment of Renal Failure: Therapeutic Principles in the Management of Acute and Chronic Uraemia*, New York.

OLIVER, J., MACDOWELL, M., and TRACY, A. (1951) The pathogenesis of acute renal failure associated with traumatic and toxic injury. Renal ischaemia, nephrotoxic damage and the ischemuric episode, *J. clin. Invest.*, **30**, 1307.

ROSENHEIM, M. L., and ROSI, E. J. (1967) Chronic renal failure, in *Renal Disease*, ed. Black, D. A. K., Oxford.

SCHWARTZ, W. B., and KASSIRER, J. P. (1968) Medical management of chronic renal failure, *Amer. J. Med.*, **44**, 786.

STEWART, J. H., TUCKWELL, L. A., SINNETT, P. F., EDWARDS, K. D. G., and WHYTE, H. M. (1966) Peritoneal and haemodialysis: A comparison of their morbidity and of the mortality suffered by dialysed patients, *Quart. J. Med.*, **35**, 407.

WILSON, C., and BYROM, F. B. (1939) Vicious circle in chronic Bright's disease, *Quart. J. Med.*, **10**, 65.

EXTRARENAL URAEMIA

Renal failure due to extrarenal factors is conveniently considered at this point since it usually arises from circulatory deficiency and therefore has much in common with acute cortical ischaemia. The difference may be one of degree, i.e. the circulatory impairment is not so severe that failure of glomerular and tubular function persist when the blood pressure is restored. The fall in glomerular filtration rate is due to reduced renal perfusion pressure and this may be due to primary *fluid loss*, as in haemorrhage, burns, vomiting and polyuria, *sodium depletion* as in diarrhoea, vomiting and Addison's disease, primary circulatory *shock* due to trauma, surgical procedures and cardiac infarction, or *congestive heart failure*. Several of these factors may be present, e.g. in diabetic coma, Addison's disease and postoperative states. The most obvious disorder of renal function is elevation of the blood urea. The urine volume is reduced but concentration is usually high, in keeping with normal tubular function. Of special importance is the frequency with which extrarenal uraemia complicates organic renal disease. Polyuria, vomiting, sodium depletion and heart failure may all aggravate renal uraemia. They are, however, for the most part reversible and treatment should be so directed.

THE NEPHROTIC SYNDROME

Causation

The primary cause of the nephrotic syndrome is hypoproteinaemia due to excessive proteinuria. The other features are generalized oedema and elevated blood cholesterol. The syndrome may therefore occur in a variety of renal diseases. The commonest of these is Type 2 nephritis, and in the London Hospital series of 130 cases of nephrotic syndrome this condition was diagnosed in 100, or 77 per cent. The less common causes include rapidly progressive Type 1 nephritis, amyloid disease, diabetic glomerulosclerosis and collagen disease, particularly systemic lupus erythematosus. Severe renal congestion may precipitate or aggravate the nephrotic syndrome, for example in chronic right heart failure, constrictive pericarditis or renal vein thrombosis but it is difficult to exclude the co-existence of Type 2 nephritis in such cases. Many specific aetiological factors of an allergic nature (poison oak, bee sting, pollens and serum sickness) or toxic action (mercury and its compounds, bismuth, gold, troxidone) have been incriminated as provoking causes. All these substances may act as antigenic agents and it is impossible to distinguish the renal lesion (histological or functional) in such cases from Type 2 nephritis, where as a rule no antigenic cause can be discovered. The occurrence and severity of the nephrotic syndrome bears no relationship to the structural lesions in the kidney, at any rate as revealed by light microscopy. There may be minimal or no discoverable glomerulonephritis, while other cases show wide variation in glomerular damage. There may be diffuse membranous glomerulitis, proliferative glomerulitis, lobulo-hyaline degeneration, or a mixture of these types, without any particular correlation with the clinical features. In general, however, the more severe types of glomerular damage are associated with excretion of a larger proportion of high molecular weight proteins (i.e. globulins), a greater frequency of erythrocytes, leucocytes and granular casts in the urine deposit, and more severe hypertension and impairment of renal function. These features are, however, characteristics of the glomerulonephritis rather than of the nephrotic syndrome, which is essentially a functional disorder, often rapidly reversible, indicating that the alteration of glomerular capillary permeability which leads to the proteinuria is itself functional and reversible, in contrast with the irreversible permeability change associated with progressive structural glomerular lesions. There is no evidence that reduced tubular re-absorption of protein contributes to the proteinuria of the nephrotic syndrome.

The Biochemical Lesion

Protein loss in the urine may amount to 30 g. daily. Most of this is albumin owing to the smaller size of its molecule, and the reduction of plasma proteins chiefly affects the albumin fraction, with a proportionately large reduction in the colloid osmotic pressure. The oedema level is usually about 2 g. albumin per cent., but values below 1 per cent. are not uncommon. The globulins are increased in the blood and there may be a high lipoprotein fraction associated with the elevation of blood lipids. The latter is probably responsible for lipid deposition in the tubular epithelium and interstitial tissue of the kidney, which led originally to the use of the term 'lipoid nephrosis'. The plasma protein level is not the absolute determinant of oedema in the nephrotic syndrome, since rapid reversal of oedema may occur without significant change in the protein level. There is in fact evidence of a complex homeostatic disturbance in body water with multiple factors playing a variable role in the maintenance of the syndrome. Hypoproteinaemia leads to hypovolaemia and this in turn stimulates renin and aldosterone production with resulting sodium retention and potassium depletion. Increased protein catabolism, present in most hypovolaemic states, contributes further to potassium depletion and causes nitrogen retention; gross tissue wasting in these patients is obvious when oedema disappears. Hypovolaemia also gives rise to elevation of blood urea due to reduced glomerular filtration. Creatinine clearance and urine concentration may be impaired, but if this is more than slight, irreversible structural damage is the likely cause. The secretion of antidiuretic hormone is increased and this is partly responsible for hyponatraemia and oliguria. There is also evidence for depression of protein synthesis which may explain the indifferent response of the plasma albumin level to high protein intake. This complex series of disturbances undoubtedly accounts for the variability of the nephrotic syndrome and the unpredictability of its response to treatment. The instability of body water control is shown by the well recognized phenomenon of massive diuresis, which may occur spontaneously or may be triggered off by a variety of stimuli such as diuretics, infection, subcutaneous drainage or steroid therapy.

Clinical Features

Oedema is the outstanding feature of the nephrotic syndrome. It is generalized in distribution and in severe cases the face, arms, abdominal wall and genitalia are affected, and pleural and peritoneal effusions are present. Cerebral, retinal and pulmonary oedema are rare but may occur, particularly in children. Secondary infection is common, especially peritonitis, pleurisy pneumonia, and pyoderma; rapidly spreading cellulitis is occasionally seen especially in patients treated with steroids. Renal vein thrombosis should be suspected if the condition suddenly deteriorates, with fall in urine volume and increase in proteinuria, and especially if there is loin pain or tenderness, or if pain in the calf or haemoptyses suggest peripheral thrombosis or pulmonary embolism. Renal vein thrombosis is usually unresponsive to treatment and leads to progressive renal failure. Persistent elevation of blood cholesterol may lead to severe widespread atheroma, and malignant hypertension has been observed in association with atheromatous renal artery occlusion. The course and prognosis of nephrotic syndrome depend on the severity of the associated structural lesion and the response to treatment. Thus in amyloid disease, diabetic glomerulosclerosis, systemic lupus erythematosus and severe Type 1 or Type 2 nephritis there may be persistent oedema and progressive deterioration. The outcome is most favourable when renal biopsy demonstrates minimal glomerular damage. In children there is in such circumstances at least a 50 per cent. spontaneous recovery, but less than this in adults. Many such cases gradually improve over 6–18 months after wide fluctuations in the state of oedema. Proteinuria lessens, the plasma proteins rise and there may be apparently complete remissions, followed by further episodes of proteinuria and oedema over many years. Other patients become incapacitated by severe intractable oedema which persists until the progress of the nephritis leads to renal failure.

Treatment

At the onset patients should be confined to bed and an assessment made of the functional and structural lesion. The condition often improves over 1–2 weeks without active therapy. A protein intake of 100 g. daily should be ensured, with restriction of added salt. Excessive sodium restriction makes the diet unpalatable and is made unnecessary by modern diuretic therapy. Chlorothiazide and *Aldactone* are the most effective drugs and, if necessary, should be used in conjunction with potassium supplements. If potassium depletion is present, its repletion will often produce a considerable diuresis and will certainly improve the clinical state. In resistant cases, drainage of effusions and subcutaneous oedema, under antibiotic cover, is usually effective and may itself lead to a diuresis, either spontaneous or induced by diuretics which previously were ineffective. The danger of sodium depletion must be constantly borne in mind, for it may lead to an irreversible shock-like state. It is wise, therefore, to give sodium supplements before and during subcutaneous drainage. Cation exchange resins may be extremely effective and can be continued as long-term therapy when the patient is ambulant. The problem of steroid therapy is a difficult one. Undoubtedly some patients respond with a reduction in proteinuria and oedema, which may lead to clinical remission. This obvious benefit is much more common in children than in adults, probably because the nephrotic syndrome with minimal glomerular damage is more usual in children. Recent trials, controlled by renal biopsy studies, indicate that good response to steroids is limited to cases with this mild type of nephritis, whilst the results in those with proliferative or membranous glomerulitis are usually poor. A useful method of distinguishing between cases with minimal and severe glomerular damage is to measure the selectivity of the proteinuria. The former have a highly selective excretion pattern, i.e. the urine protein is almost exclusively albumin, whereas with more severe types of glomerular lesions albumin is found in urine in association with variable amounts of higher molecular weight proteins. Even in cases with minimal glomerular damage there is as yet no evidence that steroids effect a cure, in the sense that the renal lesion is permanently or more rapidly healed. It is probable that if steroids are going to be effective, a response will be obtained within a fortnight with 20 mg. prednisone daily, and if this fails it is better to discontinue the drug and repeat it at a later date. There is in most patients a threshold dose of steroid below which proteinuria increases and oedema returns. Unfortunately tolerance tends to develop, and the appearance of side-effects, especially 'Cushingoid' facies or skin infection, necessitates withdrawal of the drug. At this point substitution of a combination of diuretics such as chlorothiazide and *Aldactone*, may bring about a satisfactory improvement. Potassium supplements and antibiotic therapy are important during prolonged steroid therapy, but even so this form of treatment should be avoided in most cases and withdrawn as soon as possible. Claims have been made of successful results with various immunosuppressive or anti-inflammatory drugs in the nephrotic syndrome associated with a wide variety of structural renal lesions. Substances used include cyclophosphamide, azathioprine, chlorambucil and indomethacin, either alone or in combination with steroid therapy. The rationale of these forms of therapy is the generally accepted view that the underlying renal lesions (in most cases glomerulonephritis) is an immunological disorder.

This is supported by the finding, in certain types of nephritis, of abnormal levels of serum complement or circulating immune globulins, as well as the demonstration by immuno-fluorescent techniques of antigen-antibody complexes deposited on glomerular basement membrane. The use of immunosuppressive drugs is at present quite empirical in that any effect on the nephritis, real or imagined, cannot be related to these immunological phenomena. Claims must therefore be regarded with caution, particularly in view of the toxic effects of these drugs on the bone marrow and other undesirable side-effects. Controlled therapeutic trials are at present being carried out and only when the results are available will it be possible to evaluate this form of treatment.

REFERENCES

Black, D. A. K., Rose, G., and Brewer, D. B. (1970) Controlled trials of prednisone in adult patients with the nephrotic syndrome, *Brit. med. J.*, **3**, 421.

Kark, R. M., Pirani, C. L., Pollak, V. E., Muehrcke, R. C., and Blainey, J. D. (1958) The nephrotic syndrome in adults: a common disorder with many causes, *Ann. intern. Med.*, **49**, 751.

Sharpstone, P., Ogg, C. S., and Cameron, J. S. (1969) Nephrotic syndrome due to primary renal disease in adults: I. Survey of incidence in South East England. II. Controlled trial of prednisolone and azathioprine, *Brit. med. J.*, **2**, 533, 535.

Squire, J. R., Blainey, J. D., and Hardwicke, J. (1957) The nephrotic syndrome, *Brit. med. Bull.*, **13**, 43.

SPECIFIC TUBULAR DEFECTS

Aetiology and Classification

Specific tubular defects leading to failure of re-absorption of certain constituents of glomerular filtrate may be inherited or acquired. The deficiency is probably due to absence or inactivation of the enzymes which are essential for ionic transfer across the tubule cell. Both multiple and isolated defects occur, but in the genetic forms the pattern is usually constant in members of the same family. Acquired causes include metallic poisons such as copper (in hepatolenticular degeneration), lead, cadmium or mercury, and organic tubular damage due to the nephrotic syndrome or pyelonephritis. Some defects such as failure of absorption of glucose, amino acids and phosphate, are localized in the proximal tubule and in these cases nephron dissection has shown a typical 'swan-neck' deformity near the glomerulus, with flattening of the tubular epithelium. Other defects occur in the distal tubule and include failure of acidification of the urine and potassium depletion, without any discoverable structural change. Both groups of defects may be present in the same patient. Furthermore renal tubular acidosis is often accompanied by nephrocalcinosis and stone formation, whilst chronic potassium depletion may lead to tubular atrophy and interstitial nephritis. Although, therefore, uraemia is not a primary feature of the specific tubular anomalies, it may develop as a result of these secondary structural changes.

ADULT FANCONI SYNDROME

Both Lignac and Fanconi described two distinct types of familial disease due to selective tubular defects. In both, the proximal and distal tubular anomalies described above occur, but in one type (which occurs in adults as well as in children and is therefore distinguished by the name 'adult Fanconi syndrome') the defects appear to be due to primary deficiency of tubular enzymes; whereas in the other (which is confined to children) the inherited abnormality is a defect in cystine metabolism which leads to accumulation of cystine in the tissues, and the tubular defects develop (possibly as a result of deposition of cystine in the tubules) some months after birth. This condition is described, therefore, under cystine storage disease. In adult Fanconi syndrome there is defective absorption of glucose, amino acids and phosphate, and failure of excretion of hydrion with consequent increased potassium loss. The clinical picture consists therefore of glycosuria, rickets, acidosis and weakness due to potassium depletion. The rickets, or osteomalacia in adults, is identical in appearance with vitamin D deficiency rickets and there is evidence that absorption of phosphate may be defective in the gut as well as in the kidney. A broad spectrum (up to 20) of amino acid is excreted, with a constant pattern in members of the same family, some of whom may show the biochemical defects without clinical manifestations. Cirrhosis of the liver may occur, but its cause is unknown.

RENAL TUBULAR ACIDOSIS

This is a congenital distal tubular defect, occurring in infants and in adults, in which failure of hydrion excretion may be associated with potassium depletion, osteomalacia and nephrocalcinosis. It presents in infants under one year with wasting, dehydration, acidotic breathing and weakness due to hypokalaemia. Plasma bicarbonate is low and plasma chloride high. The urine pH remains high (about 7·0) owing to defective hydrion excretion, but ammonia excretion may be increased. Nephrocalcinosis develops and renal failure may result. If diagnosed early, there is a good response to treatment with large doses of sodium bicarbonate and permanent recovery occurs. A similar lesion is found in adults, but osteomalacia and renal stone formation tend to be more advanced, so that uraemia may be present when the disorder is first diagnosed. The renal failure may be due to a combination of organic renal damage due to potassium depletion and nephrocalcinosis.

CONGENITAL CYSTINURIA

This is a hereditary, proximal tubular defect in which cystine production and blood cystine are normal, but its tubular re-absorption is deficient. Three other amino acids, lysine, arginine and ornithine, which presumably share the same excretion pathway as cystine, also appear in the urine in a constant concentration pattern. Cystine calculi develop (the other amino acids are soluble) and lead to progressive renal destruction. Ingestion of large amounts of water at night may help to reduce stone formation by preventing night concentration of the urine. Administered penicillamine combines with part of the cystine molecule and has been shown to reduce the amount of free cystine in the urine. This may prove an effective means of preventing stone formation, but at present it is too early to accept it as routine therapy.

OTHER CONGENITAL PRIMARY TUBULAR DEFECTS

Renal glycosuria may occur as an isolated absorption defect and leads to glycosuria with normal blood sugar levels. *Renal hyperphosphaturia* may also occur as an isolated defect and leads to low serum phosphate, and rickets or osteomalacia. It may be associated with renal glycosuria. *Congenital renal diabetes insipidus* occurs in children, usually males, and causes polyuria with hypotonic urine which is unresponsive to *Pitressin.* There may be hydronephrosis and physical retardation. *Pseudohypoparathyroidism* is characterized by excessive phosphate absorption which has been attributed to unresponsiveness of the proximal tubule cells to parathormone. The bones are dense and tetany may occur. *Idiopathic hypercalciuria* is a condition in which calcium excretion is high but the blood level normal, suggesting a defect of calcium re-absorption; renal calculi frequently result.

TUBULAR DEFECTS DUE TO METABOLIC DISORDERS

Cystine storage disease (Lignac-Fanconi syndrome, cystinosis) is characterized by deposition of cystine in the tissues, and this can be observed in the cornea. The tubular defects may be due to reduction in available thiol groups (due to presence of cystine) which are necessary for enzyme function. Administration of BAL and penicillamine, which increase the available thiol groups, has been shown to produce rapid improvement. The tubular lesion resembles that in the adult Fanconi syndrome, i.e. leads to mixed proximal and tubular defects, but it always presents in early life, usually a few months after birth, when polyuria, thirst, weakness and signs of rickets appear. There is mental retardation and early death. *Galactosaemia* is a metabolic disorder in which galactose is not metabolized and accumulates in the tissues causing various enzyme deficiencies. It produces proximal nephron absorption defects, chiefly amino-aciduria and occasionally glycosuria and hyperphosphaturia. Symptoms appear in infancy and include wasting, cirrhosis of the liver and cataracts. Treatment with a galactose-free diet corrects the defect. *Hartnup disease* is a rare congenital disorder in which there appears to be delayed absorption of tryptophan in the intestine, leading to excessive production of indole derivatives which are excreted in the urine. Gross amino-aciduria occurs due to a proximal tubular absorption defect. Clinically a pellagra-like skin rash is associated with cerebellar ataxia and other neurological manifestations. *Hepatolenticular degeneration* is due to deficient synthesis of caeruloplasmin, a plasma globulin to which copper is normally bound. In its absence copper is deposited in the tissues and excreted in the urine in large amounts. Its deposition in the tubular epithelium leads to proximal tubular defects including amino-aciduria, glycosuria and hyperphosphaturia. These usually develop late in the disease. *Heavy metal poisoning.* Lead, cadmium, uranium and mercury may produce amino-aciduria and glycosuria. Osteomalacia and rickets have also been reported in the first two types of poisoning.

REFERENCES

Chisholm, J. J., Jr., and Harrison, H. E. (1958) Clinical patterns of tubular dysfunction, *Amer. J. Med.*, **24**, 785.

Harris, H. (1962) Genetic aspects of renal disease, in *Renal Disease*, ed. Black, D. A. K., Chap. 26, Oxford.

Stanbury, S. W. (1958) Some aspects of disordered tubular function, *Advanc. intern. Med.*, **9,** 231.

HYPERTENSION DUE TO UNILATERAL RENAL DISEASE

It is well recognized that unilateral renal disease may produce high blood pressure of all grades of severity, including malignant hypertension. Unilateral pyelonephritis, hydronephrosis, renal tumours and cysts, tuberculosis, renal infarction due to embolism or thrombosis, X-irradiation to one kidney, congenital malformation and renal trauma may be the underlying lesion. Unilateral renal artery stenosis is an important variety since (as also occurs in the experimental model in animals) there may be little or no structural damage in the 'ischaemic' kidney, so that surgical relief of the stenosis may be a feasible alternative to nephrectomy [Plate 17]. The frequency of renal artery stenosis as a primary cause of hypertension has been exaggerated, and it is probable that less than 1 per cent. of cases of hypertension 'without apparent cause' are of this nature. An even smaller number can be permanently cured by vascular surgery. The commonest cause of renal artery stenosis is atheroma. Since this is a generalized arterial degeneration, surgical correction may be difficult owing to involvement of the aorta or the opposite renal artery, and recurrence may occur. Furthermore, hypertension predisposes to atheroma, so that in older subjects renal artery stenosis may be secondary rather than primary. In young subjects, especially women, fibromuscular hyperplasia, a rare and possibly congenital disorder, causes renal artery constriction. This also may be bilateral, and it may extend into the branches of the main renal artery, making surgical relief impossible.

In view of the possibility of surgical cure of hypertension due to unilateral renal disease, all patients under 50 with apparent essential hypertension should be screened by intravenous pyelography (IVP) for inequality of renal size and other features described on page 977. If the IVP presents strong diagnostic evidence of renal artery stenosis this may be confirmed by aortography. Differential renal function tests [p. 976] provide the most certain indication that the hypertension is due to renal artery stenosis and is likely to be cured by surgical correction. Nevertheless, the performance of these tests involves complete collection of urine from each kidney by ureteric catheterization which at present carries considerable hazards, and it is doubtful whether these are justified by the over-all results of surgical treatment. More recently it has been shown by renal vein catheterization that venous blood from a kidney with stenosis of its renal artery has a high renin content relative to the opposite kidney. If this investigation is available it may have considerable diagnostic value. It is often difficult to exclude essential hypertension even where obvious unilateral renal abnormality is present. A family history of hypertension is in favour of essential hypertension and it is even more valuable to measure the blood pressure in parents and siblings. At the present time the most appropriate action is to consider surgery only in subjects under 50 with severe hypertension but good renal function, in whom the IVP strongly suggests renal artery stenosis, confirmed by aortography. If the ischaemic kidney is contracted it should be removed; if not, renal vascular surgery may be attempted. If the IVP shows one kidney to be contracted, but there is no clear evidence of renal artery stenosis, nephrectomy is justifiable in severe (especially malignant) hypertension in a patient under 40 with no evidence of familial hypertension. In about half such cases, however, the high blood pressure will persist after nephrectomy. This may be due to unrecognized pyelonephritis or secondary hypertensive vascular damage in the opposite kidney, or to essential hypertension as the primary cause of the high blood pressure. When, in unilateral renal disease, surgical treatment is either not indicated or is unsuccessful, treatment with anti-hypertensive drugs is usually effective.

BRIGHT'S DISEASE

Bright's 'disease' is in fact a syndrome, consisting of albuminuria, oedema and (usually) high blood pressure associated with organic kidney disease. The majority of patients presenting with this clinical picture are suffering from glomerulonephritis in its acute or chronic forms. Other diseases which may produce the syndrome are amyloid nephrosis, chronic pyelonephritis, malignant hypertension and diabetic glomerulosclerosis.

CLASSIFICATION OF BRIGHT'S DISEASE

A. NEPHRITIS

1. GLOMERULONEPHRITIS
   - DIFFUSE. Type 1 (syn. acute nephritis, acute diffuse nephritis, acute haemorrhagic nephritis).
     Type 2 (syn. subacute and chronic parenchymatous nephritis, membranous glomerulonephritis, lipoid nephrosis).
   - FOCAL. Acute focal nephritis.
2. PYELONEPHRITIS. Acute and chronic. Unilateral and bilateral.
3. INTERSTITIAL NEPHRITIS. *Exogenous*. Lead, phenacetin, cadmium (nephrotoxic agents). *Endogenous*. Gout, myeloma.

B. RENAL CIRCULATORY AND VASCULAR DISEASE

- ACUTE. Acute cortical ischaemia (acute tubular necrosis).
  Massive cortical necrosis.
  Renal papillary necrosis.
  Renal vein thrombosis.
- CHRONIC. Benign nephrosclerosis } in essential
  Malignant nephrosclerosis } hypertension.
  Renal atherosclerosis.
  Diabetic glomerulosclerosis.

C. OTHERS

Renal amyloidosis.
Congenital disorders, structural and metabolic.
'Toxaemia' of pregnancy.

GLOMERULONEPHRITIS

In describing glomerulonephritis most of the confusion in the past has arisen because names have been given to cross-sections of the disease at different stages. Hence glomerulonephritis running a contінous course in the same patient might at different times be labelled acute haemorrhagic nephritis, subacute parenchymatous nephritis, chronic interstitial nephritis, azotaemic nephritis. This cross-sectional terminology can only be avoided by a long-term study of nephritis from both its clinical and pathological aspects. When this approach is followed we arrive at a classification of the natural *courses* of the disease, such as was introduced by Volhard and Fahr in 1914. In addition, recent information derived from experimental pathology and physiology of the kidney has made it possible to relate various disorders of function such as hypertension, oedema and uraemia to different organic lesions of the kidney. A long-term clinical and pathological study of some 600 cases of Bright's disease by Ellis and his colleagues at the London Hospital showed that the many clinical syndromes of glomerulonephritis were related to two main types of pathological process which were termed Type 1 and Type 2 nephritis. Type 1 is usually preceded by a streptococcal infection. Its onset is acute, with haematuria as a prominent feature. The prognosis is good, 80–90 per cent. of patients recovering completely. In the remainder, according to the severity of the glomerulonephritis, death may occur in the acute stage or after a rapidly progressive course running a period of months, or a slowly progressive course lasting from years to decades. Type 2 nephritis has an insidious onset with oedema, which tends to increase and persist for months or even years. This is the commonest cause of the nephrotic syndrome. Haematuria is not usually a prominent feature, but albuminuria is severe and is associated with gross depletion of plasma proteins. Recovery is rare and is practically limited to cases without hypertension. The great majority of patients continue with albuminuria and recurrent oedema for many years before renal failure develops. The morbid anatomical changes correspond closely with these clinical courses. In Type 1 nephritis the lesion is diffuse and severe at the onset, but in most cases resolves completely. In Type 2 nephritis there is a less intense diffuse glomerulonephritis which gradually progresses in severity and in the fully developed stage presents a characteristic involvement of the glomerular capillaries, with varying degrees of basement membrane thickening.

The development of knowledge in recent years on the collagen diseases and the reaction of the tissues to antigenic substances in general, has helped to clarify some of the problems of pathogenesis, classification and clinical-histological correlation in nephritis. Reference has already been made to a variety of immunological abnormalities in glomerulonephritis which have been invoked as a justification for the use of immunosuppressive drugs, especially in the nephrotic syndrome. The aetiological significance of these abnormalities, and even more so their relationships to the well established clinical and histological patterns of disease, are still in most cases unclear. Certain interesting relationships are, however, beginning to emerge. The fact that antigen-antibody complexes or complement can be localized on glomerular basement membranes would seem to be related to the frequent structural and functional changes which so often affect the glomerular capillaries in glomerulonephritis. Cases can be identified in which the antigen appears to be bacterial, e.g. streptococcus antigen, or some component of basement membrane. In a large proportion of cases, however, the specific antigen cannot be recognized and in these it seems likely that a state of non-specific hypersensitivity may underlie chronic or recurrent glomerulonephritis. Therapeutically these findings have important implications since they may lead the way to the discovery of specific forms of treatment aimed at various components of the abnormal immune response. There are many antigenic agents which provoke inflammatory reaction, but the tissues have a limited number of inflammatory responses. Moreover, under different conditions and in different subjects the same antigen may provoke different tissue reactions. More often than not the provoking antigen cannot be identified, and sometimes a hypersensitivity reaction may lead to gross functional disturbance with a minimum of obvious structure damage, e.g. in the nephrotic syndrome. Thus many different aetiological agents may produce the same functional and structural disorder, whilst the same antigenic agent may produce a variety of abnormal structural patterns. Moreover, there will be many transitional types of lesion which cannot be conveniently fitted into a well-defined category—as in the various forms of collagen disease. Glomerulonephritis is one of the group of collagen diseases, and Type 1 nephritis, Type 2 nephritis and focal nephritis may occur in the course of systemic lupus erythematosus and polyarteritis nodosa.

TYPE 1 NEPHRITIS

Synonyms. Acute haemorrhagic nephritis; Acute diffuse nephritis.

Aetiology

Most cases of nephritis presenting with acute onset are of this type. The disease is commonest in children and adolescents, but may occur at any age.

Scarlet fever and streptococcal tonsillitis are the common preceding infections. There is a limited number of nephritogenic streptococcal strains and the majority of cases are due to Type 12 Group A streptococcus. Sometimes the patient complains of a 'cold' or a chill without sore throat. Less frequent preceding infections are otitis media, pneumonia, peritonitis, erysipelas, impetigo, boils and pyogenic dermatitis. This type of nephritis may occur in subacute bacterial endocarditis and in the collagen diseases, especially as a presenting feature of polyarteritis nodosa. Severe burns may be followed by nephritis, possibly due to secondary infection. In time of war nephritis may occur in epidemic form, for example, the 'trench nephritis' of the First World War. In these outbreaks the nature of the primary infection may be obscure.

Pathology

Microscopically the characteristic feature in the acute stage is increase in cellularity of the glomerular tufts due to proliferation of endothelial cells and infiltration with polymorphonuclear leucocytes. Haemorrhage into Bowman's capsule is common, and collections of red cells and leucocytes may be seen in the tubules. In severe cases, fibrinoid necrosis of the glomerular arterioles and even of the glomerular capillaries occurs. In the rapidly progressive course the main feature is epithelial crescent formation (proliferative capsulitis). Vascular necroses may occur and the tubules may show hyaline droplet degeneration; the interstitial tissue is infiltrated with acute inflammatory cells. In the slowly progressive course, damaged glomeruli become organized and disappear, interstitial fibrosis is extensive and in the later stages acute and chronic lesions of the glomeruli and vessels are found—focal necroses, capsular adhesions, necrotizing arteriolitis—which are the result of severe hypertensive damage. This ultimately leads to focal scarring of the kidney with marked tubular atrophy, dilatation and hypertrophy of the intervening tubules, and hyaline cast formation. The final stage is sometimes termed secondary contracted kidney or chronic interstitial nephritis.

Symptoms

The onset is usually acute, with oedema, haematuria and moderate hypertension, often with a history of sore throat 1–3 weeks previously; occasionally it may be insidious. In the latter instance the patient may complain of biliousness, nausea, vomiting and abdominal pain, with headache and sometimes diarrhoea before the onset of renal symptoms. There may be no oedema in cases which present with anuria. When the onset is abrupt. there may be pain in the back or abdomen, and oedema soon develops. It usually starts in the face; the legs and scrotum are generally involved next, and the swelling soon spreads all over the body. Occasionally the dropsy is curiously localized and fugitive. Though dyspnoea is not regarded as a common feature of acute nephritis most patients admit to it on direct questioning, and if cardiac failure occurs it may be a prominent symptom. There is usually only slight fever, though occasionally a temperature of 102° or 103° F. (38·9° or 39·5 C.) may be reached; this may be due to persistence of the original infection. The pulse rate is increased and the blood pressure is generally raised. The skin may be dry and itching, with occasionally a papular or erythematous eruption. Retinal haemorrhages may occur, but very rarely.

The urine is greatly reduced in volume, and may be entirely suppressed. It is dark in colour and usually contains obvious blood. This may render the urine as dark as porter, but it may be bright red or merely smoky. Sometimes the blood forms a flocculent, reddish-brown precipitate. The urine is usually loaded with albumin, and casts are observed on microscopical examination. At first blood casts and epithelial casts will be found; but at a later stage, granular casts appear. Leucocytes are present, often in large numbers. Isolated renal cells, transitional epithelium and squamous cells from the lower urinary tract are also commonly found. The urine is sterile on culture. A sudden increase in urine output after a few days is a sign of definite improvement due to elimination of oedema fluid.

Slight impairment of renal function is common, the blood urea being moderately raised. Some degree of impaired concentrating power is found in the more severe cases. The disorder of renal function in acute nephritis is usually that described above under impaired glomerular function, but in severe cases with suppression of urine the disorder is that of acute oliguric renal failure [p. 983].

If recovery fails to occur the disease may run a rapidly progressive or slowly progressive course. These are described on page 992.

Complications

1. *Acute heart failure*. Shortness of breath may be a presenting feature, and in severe cases acute pulmonary oedema may occur. This complication may be associated with a marked rise in blood pressure and demands urgent treatment. Hypervolaemia is present in most cases and indeed may be the prime cause of the venous congestion rather than true 'heart failure'. Cardiac output is increased and is probably an important factor in producing the hypertension.

2. *Hypertensive encephalopathy*. The symptoms are sudden in onset and include convulsions, blindness, mental excitement, severe headache, vomiting and transient palsies. Coma sometimes develops. Severe hypertension is present but the renal function in these patients is good. With adequate treatment recovery is the rule. There is now good evidence that these symptoms are due to cerebral vasoconstriction and that cerebral oedema occurs only in the later stages. Fluid retention is probably an important factor in the production of encephalopathy, and of the acute rise in blood pressure which often precedes the symptoms.

3. *Infections*. Not infrequently a flare-up of the primary infection or the incidence of a new one may produce a recrudescence of the nephritis. Antibiotic therapy has lessened the risk of these infections, which were previously often fatal.

4. *Oliguria*. Diminution in the urine output may be due to: (1) actual suppression in severe cases, or (2) extrarenal factors such as vomiting, gross oedema, acute heart failure or therapeutic fluid restriction. Marked oliguria may be present in the absence of oedema or hypertension although these may appear later.

Diagnosis

The combination of dropsy, hypertension, albuminuria, haematuria, granular casts and scanty urine usually makes the diagnosis obvious. The differential diagnosis of acute nephritis from an exacerbation of chronic nephritis may be difficult. Definite evidence of cardiac hypertrophy and arterial changes are in favour of the latter. In cases presenting with anuria, without oedema or hypertension, the diagnosis is presumptive if the anuria persists, but can only be confirmed by renal biopsy. In acute pyelitis, pyuria with bacteriuria, especially of *Esch. coli* in pure culture, is typical; although haematuria may be present there is usually dysuria and frequency due to cystitis, and local pain and tenderness over the kidney are present. Moreover, constitutional disturbance, particularly high fever, with rigors and vomiting, is common. Acute focal nephritis usually occurs at the height of an acute infection rather than after an interval, and oedema and hypertension are absent. In polyarteritis nodosa, fever, leucocytosis, and variable signs due to arterial necrosis may be found. Bacterial endocarditis may present with nephritis, but evidence of a primary cardiac lesion, fever, clubbing and embolic manifestations are the differential signs. In haemorrhage from the lower urinary tract, there are no tubular casts in the urine deposit.

Treatment

Acute Stage. In the acute stage the patient should be put to bed. Daily observations of the blood pressure should be made, the fluid intake and urine output recorded and the urine examined for specific gravity, albumin and blood. Microscopic examination of the deposit for red cells, leucocytes and casts should be made twice weekly. Renal function tests and plasma protein examination should be made. It is important to search for any residual primary infection such as tonsillitis and for evidence of streptococcal infection by bacterial culture from the fauces and estimation of antistreptolysin O (A.S.O.) titre in the blood. In any case penicillin should be given in the hope of avoiding recrudescences which may otherwise lead to serious relapse of nephritis during the recovery period. A low-protein, low-salt, high-carbohydrate diet should be given to minimize retention of urea, potassium and sodium. Diuretics, and particularly potassium salts, should not be given. The patient must be kept in bed until pitting oedema has disappeared, the blood pressure has returned to normal and the urine is free from albumin. If, after a period of at least 4 weeks from the onset, the only residual urinary abnormalities are a faint trace of albumin and a few red cells per high power field on microscopic examination of the deposit, the patient may be allowed up, but periodic examination of the urine deposit for erythrocytes is advisable until these disappear; in children, particularly adolescents, this may take up to 12 months. Tonsillectomy is not advised until the nephritis has resolved and should then only be undertaken if the tonsils are obviously chronically inflamed or there is a past history of repeated sore throats.

Secondary infection should be treated with an appropriate antibacterial agent, penicillin being the most useful. Pyelonephritis frequently occurs in kidneys damaged by glomerulonephritis. Culture of the urine and frequent examination for pyuria is therefore essential and if active infection is present it should be treated with tetracycline or other appropriate antibiotic therapy as discussed under acute oliguric uraemia. Heart failure is a definite risk when there is marked hypertension. In severe cases with acute pulmonary oedema venesection is the treatment of choice. If the blood pressure is very high, it should be reduced by antihypertensive drugs of which guanethidine is the most reliable. Digitalis is of questionable value and in the majority of patients spontaneous improvement occurs as the nephritis subsides. The most serious complication is anuria. The essence of treatment is to maintain the electrolyte and fluid balance, as described under acute oliguric uraemia [p. 983]. If there is no response to treatment after 7–10 days, renal biopsy should be carried out in order to decide whether repeated dialysis is justifiable. Improvement may follow in cases with severe glomerulitis with epithelial crescent formation or glomerular necroses.

Hypertensive encephalopathy occurs with about the same frequency as heart failure in patients with very high blood pressure. Prompt venesection with removal of 300–500 ml. of blood will sometimes produce dramatic improvement. The blood pressure should be reduced as described above. In severe cases lumbar puncture should be performed. The C.S.F. pressure is usually normal in the early stages, but later, cerebral oedema may occur. Intravenous sucrose solution, 100 ml. 50 per cent., may then be given with benefit. Hypertensive encephalopathy and heart failure may occur together, but. fortunately, reduction of the blood pressure will often relieve both conditions. Anaemia in acute nephritis does not usually require treatment. It is in part due to haemodilution, since the haematocrit rises as oedema diminishes.

Rapidly progressive course. In these patients the nephritis is severe, and haematuria, hypertension and oedema persist. Treatment is continued as in the acute stage, and complications such as heart failure and hypertensive encephalopathy should be dealt with promptly. The patient should be kept at rest for at least 3 months, since recovery may occur even after this prolonged course. Diuretics must not be given or fluids restricted if renal failure is present. Tonsillectomy is to be avoided as it may aggravate the nephritis in this active stage.

Slowly progressive course (chronic Type 1 nephritis). In the long intermediate stage before the development of renal failure and severe hypertension, it is most important that the patient should not be made an invalid by unnecessary or even harmful treatment. There are frequently no symptoms during this time, the only findings being residual albuminuria and perhaps slight variable hypertension. The old practice of protein starvation is thoroughly bad as it leads to protein deficiency, iron deficiency anaemia, malnutrition and the conviction of invalidism. A normal diet should therefore be allowed so long as the renal function tests are normal. Iron should be prescribed if there is any degree of anaemia, and the only necessary medical attention is a periodic examination at 3 to 6-monthly intervals, when the urine and blood pressure should be tested and renal function tests occasionally carried out. In the later stages the blood pressure tends to rise progressively and renal impairment develops. It is essential to give antihypertensive drug treatment in this stage in an attempt to prevent secondary renal damage, hypertensive retinopathy and malignant hypertension. Reserpine, 0·25 mg. three times a day, should be tried first as some patients respond remarkably well if treated early, but if necessary this should be supplemented by chlorothiazide diuretics and guanethidine. By this means deterioration in renal function may be prevented for a considerable time, largely depending on the severity and activity of the nephritis. If increase in hypertension is due to an exacerbation of the nephritis the blood pressure may fall again as this recovers. When renal impairment appears, the fluid intake should under no circumstances be restricted; protein in the diet should not be reduced until the blood urea rises considerably above the normal, e.g. to 100 mg. per 100 ml. And then only when symptoms of uraemia such as lassitude, weakness, nausea or vomiting appear. Restriction of protein intake to 30–40 g. daily is usually satisfactory but if the blood urea continues to rise, further restriction along the lines of the 'Giovanetti' diet may be helpful for a time. Where facilities for regular dialysis therapy are available dietary treatment should, however, be regarded as an interim measure and the patient's general condition should not be allowed to deteriorate by over-prolonged protein restriction. In the late stages of uraemia electrolyte disturbances must be corrected, especially acidosis and sodium depletion. Sodium bicarbonate or citrate by mouth, or normal saline with sodium lactate intravenously, will correct both disturbances, the amount being judged from the urine output, plasma bicarbonate and particularly the clinical state. The common 'uraemic' symptoms of weakness, lassitude, loss of appetite, nausea and vomiting are usually dramatically relieved when sodium depletion is corrected by intravenous saline infusions. Persistent vomiting may be controlled by small doses of barbiturate or by cyclizine or chlorpromazine. Anaemia should be treated by iron preparations, but when uraemia is present it is usually refractory and the only beneficial treatment is blood transfusion. This is best avoided if there is a prospect of renal transplantation. It is well to remember that uraemia may in part be due to heart failure or anaemia or to severe hypertensive crises, and some improvement may be expected if these complications are adequately treated. Reference has already been made to the use of peritoneal dialysis in the treatment of chronic uraemia. In severe cases this technique may be invaluable in effecting rapid correction of fluid and electrolyte disturbances, e.g. where heart failure or severe acidosis is present. By this means the clinical state may be sufficiently improved to enable a more accurate diagnosis to be made, not only of the cause of the uraemia but also of the extent to which reversible factors such as sodium depletion, ascending infection and hypertension are contributing to the renal failure.

Prognosis and Progressive Courses

The prognosis in Type 1 nephritis is good and 80–90 per cent. of patients recover completely. Second attacks after complete clinical recovery are extremely rare. In the early stage, suppression of urine is the most serious prognostic symptom and death in the acute stage is most commonly due to persistent anuria. If this lasts more than a week the outlook is very grave, but recovery has been known to occur after 14 days' anuria. In such severe cases persistent vomiting may lead to extrarenal uraemia, the blood urea rising as high as 300 mg. per 100 ml. Severe hypertension (around 200 mm. mercury systolic) may also be a bad prognostic sign in the acute stage in terms of immediate complications, i.e. left ventricular failure and hypertensive encephalopathy. Heart failure as a complication has a much more serious significance than encephalopathy. Persistent haematuria is usually evidence of a progressive lesion, but recovery may occur even after visible blood has persisted in the urine for three months. Microscopic haematuria has a less serious significance particularly in younger subjects since it may be orthostatic in origin, and complete recovery may occur after red cells have persisted in the urine for a year or more. The same is true of a persistent trace of albumin in the urine. Recrudescences, usually marked by return of haematuria during the first few weeks, often following recurrence of the initial infection, may greatly prolong convalescence or lead to chronic nephritis. Recovery tends to be slower in the elderly than in young subjects. About 5 per cent. of patients with acute nephritis die in the acute stage, the causes being anuria, pulmonary oedema due to heart failure, or infection.

1. *Rapidly progressive course.* This occurs in about 5 per cent. of patients and is due to a severe irreversible glomerulonephritis characterized by epithelial crescent formation. Clinically there is persistent haematuria, hypertension and oedema which is often severe and generalized. Progressive renal failure occurs over a period of 6 months to 2 years and there may be a malignant hypertensive termination with papilloedema, encephalopathy and left ventricular failure.

2. *Slowly progressive course.* In a series of cases of acute nephritis studied by Ellis only about 5 per cent. followed this course. Nevertheless, in any clinic for renal disease there will be a large proportion of patients with chronic Type 1 nephritis, since the disease may last for decades. Moreover, about half these patients will give no history of acute nephritis, but first present with symptomless albuminuria or hypertension often discovered on routine examination; or hypertensive symptoms or uraemic manifestations later in the disease. The natural history and prognosis is decided by two factors, the severity of the residual nephritic lesions and the incidence of hypertension. Where the nephritic damage is severe there is no hard-and-fast demarcation from cases running a rapidly progressive course. There is severe destruction of the kidney, and uraemia may develop insidiously in 5–10 years, with or without marked hypertension. Polyuria may appear when concentrating power becomes impaired, but as destruction of nephrons progresses, urine output returns to normal and in the final stages there is usually oliguria. Anaemia is not likely to be present before the onset of uraemia, unless there is an independent cause, such as iron deficiency. In chronic renal failure refractory anaemia develops and this is in some patients the presenting feature of the disease. Further symptoms are described under chronic uraemia [p. 981].

With less severe degrees of residual renal damage the patient may continue for 30 years or more and during this stage may be free from symptoms, but regular examination of the urine shows persistent albuminuria. During this long stage, inflammatory elements are usually absent from the urine unless recurrent attacks of nephritis occur. These have been observed in 25 per cent. of our cases, commonly preceded by acute tonsillitis. At any time the blood pressure may be observed to rise, often over a period of months, and rapid deterioration in renal function may then follow. About 50 per cent. of patients develop the malignant hypertension syndrome. This complication may be the first manifestation of renal disease and it may be very difficult, if there is no past history of acute nephritis, to decide whether the hypertension is nephritic or essential. In general, patients with malignant essential hypertension are found to have only slight impairment of renal function when papilloedema is first discovered, whereas in chronic nephritis renal failure is usually advanced at this stage. Although the ultimate prognosis is poor in both conditions the results of treatment by blood-pressure lowering drugs are somewhat better in malignant essential than in malignant renal hypertension. The clinical features of the malignant termination in chronic Type 1 nephritis are identical with those of malignant essential hypertension [see Section 8] except that symptoms of renal failure are more pronounced. Attacks of hypertensive encephalopathy, producing headaches, blindness, convulsions, disorientation and coma may occur; as in acute nephritis this condition is reversible and improves after the blood pressure is lowered by hypotensive drugs. In chronic nephritis, however, the improvement is usually short-lived because of the associated irreversible uraemia.

Other Forms of Acute Nephritis. *Acute focal nephritis* is characterized clinically by an attack of haematuria occurring in the course of a variety of acute infections. Hypertension, oedema and renal failure are absent and recovery usually takes place after a few days. Occasionally, however, attacks of focal nephritis recur at intervals and in such patients albuminuria may persist, indicating residual renal damage. If the attacks continue, hypertension and renal impairment eventually appear and the histological picture in this late stage is indistinguishable from that of chronic Type 1 nephritis.

In *subacute bacterial endocarditis*, nephritis, when it occurs, is characteristically focal but may be diffuse. Histologically the focal lesion consists of glomerulitis with haemorrhage into Bowman's capsule, which leads to epithelial crescent formation and later to characteristic 'boat-shaped' collagen crescents. Although this lesion was at one time thought to be embolic, it is doubtful whether there is any aetiological difference between the focal and diffuse forms of glomerulonephritis in bacterial endocarditis. A similar state of affairs occurs in *Henoch-Schönlein purpura* where renal involvement may take the form of haematuria alone or the full picture of nephritis may develop with hypertension, oedema and renal failure. In the latter case the prognosis is usually poor. This form of nephritis is probably allied to that occurring in *polyarteritis nodosa*, which may present with a typical attack of acute nephritis and purpura. In both conditions acute necrotizing arteriolitis may be found in the kidney and in other organs. Acute nephritis has recently been described in young, usually male patients, suffering from repeated haemoptyses. This condition, which is usually fatal, bears some resemblance to the nephritis of Henoch-Schönlein purpura, and the name 'lung purpura with nephritis' or Goodpasture's syndrome has been given to it. The lung shows no evidence of inflammatory disease and the pulmonary lesion is probably related to that of pulmonary haemosiderosis. Acute nephritis is occasionally seen in patients with acute rheumatic carditis but so rarely that the association may be fortuitous.

TYPE 2 NEPHRITIS

Synonyms. Subacute and chronic parenchymatous nephritis; Membranous glomerulonephritis; Lipoid nephrosis.

Aetiology

Type 2 nephritis is less common than Type 1 nephritis, but its incidence ranks high in a clinic for renal diseases since in the majority of patients it follows a chronic course of many years' duration. The incidence is more uniformly distributed over the first six decades of life than that of Type 1 nephritis. In young children and occasionally in adults, hypertension and haematuria may be absent. It is in these circumstances that renal biopsy usually shows minimal renal damage. The term lipoid nephrosis is still sometimes applied to such cases, but long-term clinical and histological study reveals no clear dividing line from the more severe cases of Type 2 nephritis, and if the condition persists diffuse nephritis usually develops.

In most cases no aetiological factor is established and it is rare to obtain a previous history of acute streptococcal infection. This is no doubt partly due to the fact that albuminuria (and therefore the onset of the disease) may precede the oedema by months or years. In such cases symptomless albuminuria is usually found on routine medical examination and the later development of oedema may be precipitated by an acute infection or by pregnancy, which presumably lower the plasma albumin below the oedema level. Occasionally Type 2 nephritis with the nephrotic syndrome follows exposure to vegetable antigens, such as pollen dust, or chemical toxins such as mercury or troxidone. From the rarity of his occurrence it is presumably a hypersensitivity response in a susceptible individual. As previously stated, the clinical and histological features cannot be distinguished from those in other cases of Type 2 nephritis without apparent cause.

Pathology

The kidney is large and pale and may or may not be oedematous. The kidney pattern and the demarcation of cortex from medulla are blurred, and fatty changes in the tubules and interstitial tissue may appear as white streaks on the cut surface. The microscopic picture depends on the stage of the disease and its severity. In cases with little or no hypertension there are minimal changes in the glomeruli, consisting of bland focal necroses, together with deposition of lipoid in the tubular epithelium and interstitial tissue; slight interstitial cellular infiltration may be present. Even when light microscopy reveals no structural glomerular damage electron microscopy shows constant changes in the epithelial cells of the tufts, with loss of 'foot processes'. In more severe cases there is a diffuse proliferative glomerulitis with accentuated lobulation of the tufts and swelling of the capillary basement membrane. As this lesion progresses, deposits of hyaline material appear in the glomerular tufts and the glomerular capsule undergoes fibrous thickening, but epithelial crescent formation is almost always absent. Glomerular hyalinization gradually increases so that even after 10 years' duration the characteristic glomerular lesion may still be recognizable. The tubules undergo fairly diffuse atrophy and a uniform interstitial fibrosis develops, but it is unusual for more than a moderate degree of renal contraction to result. Vascular lesions are not conspicuous although occasional arteriolar necroses may be observed in those cases with a malignant hypertensive termination.

Symptoms

It has already been stated that albuminuria, discovered on routine examination, may provide the first indication of the disease, months or years before the appearance of oedema or other symptoms. In most patients, however, Type 2 nephritis presents with gradual or rapid onset of oedema, which steadily increases and tends to become massive. The oedema may be generalized, affecting the face, hands, trunk and legs. It is often first noticed as puffiness of the eyelids, or it may first appear as a swelling of the feet and ankles extending up the legs. The patient may feel quite well apart from the disability caused by oedema. On the other hand, there is more usually complaint of malaise and fatigue, loss of appetite and nausea, and sometimes of epigastric pain. There may be cough and slight shortness of breath due to bronchial catarrh, oedema of the lungs or hydrothorax. A pericardial effusion may develop. Swelling of the abdomen may be the result of oedema of the abdominal wall or ascites. The face is pale and the eyelids and cheeks are puffy, but the mucous membranes are of a good colour, and the blood count is usually normal. The urine is reduced in quantity, its specific gravity is normal, and it contains a large amount of albumin, usually between 10 and 30 g. daily. In mild cases the urinary deposit contains only a slight excess of cells and few or no casts, while red blood cells are generally absent. In the more severe cases leucocytes, red blood cells and granular casts are regularly found. The blood pressure may be normal or moderately raised. There is no retinitis in the early stages. Characteristic changes are found in the blood; these are fully described under the nephrotic syndrome [p. 985]. Occasionally Type 2 nephritis is diagnosed histologically by renal biopsy, or *post mortem*, in patients dying in uraemia, without evidence of oedema having been present at any time in the course of the disease.

Complications

These are:

1. Pulmonary oedema and cerebral oedema which occur only in cases with gross anasarca. Cerebral oedema is very rare but has been observed in children after rapid generalized increase in swelling.
2. Pyogenic infection—the common ones being pneumococcal peritonitis, pneumonia and erysipelas.
3. Hypertensive encephalopathy. Owing to the moderate degree of blood pressure elevation, this complication is not often seen, but it may develop in the subacute stage when, especially in adult males, severe hypertension is sometimes encountered. The symptoms are identical with those described under Type 1 nephritis.
4. Renal vein thrombosis. This may or may not be associated with thrombophlebitis elsewhere, but the presence of the latter may be suggested by haemoptysis due to pulmonary embolism. Sudden deterioration with oliguria, increase in proteinuria and oedema, and impairment of renal function, especially if accompanied by pain and tenderness over the kidney, strongly suggest the occurrence of this complication.

Diagnosis

The insidious onset with oedema, gross albuminuria and hypoproteinaemia is so characteristic of Type 2 nephritis that there is usually no problem of diagnosis. There may be some difficulty in the early stages in distinguishing it from Type 1 nephritis running the rapidly progressive course. Here also there is often gross generalized oedema and heavy albuminuria, but the acute onset and greater degree of haematuria, hypertension and renal impairment enable the separation to be made in most cases. Amyloid disease of the kidney also produces generalized oedema, albuminuria and hypoproteinaemia. Some underlying cause such as bronchiectasis, rheumatoid arthritis or chronic pyogenic infection may be found, but the nephrotic syndrome does occur in primary amyloidosis. The spleen may be enlarged and the Congo red test is of value. The nephrotic syndrome occasionally arises in the later stages of diabetic glomerulosclerosis. Although Type 2 nephritis may occur in the diabetic, the appearance of albuminuria in the course of chronic diabetes is usually due to focal and diffuse glomerular hyalinization characteristic of this condition. The finding of diabetic retinopathy is strongly confirmatory. Disseminated lupus erythematosus may be complicated by any of the histological forms of Type 2 nephritis but the membranous variety (wire loop hyalinization) is more usual, and clinically the nephrotic picture may develop. The associated features of disseminated lupus erythematosus are, however, diagnostic. Renal biopsy has an obvious value in the differentiation of these causes, but is rarely necessary as the diagnosis can be made on clinical grounds with the aid of laboratory investigations.

Treatment

In the early stages, particularly if examination of the urinary deposit reveals evidence of active nephritis (i.e. red cells, leucocytes and granular casts), treatment should follow the regime advised in acute Type 1 nephritis. As a rule, however, the disease is in its subacute or chronic stage when the patient is first seen. Even then it is advisable to insist on rest in bed so that a full assessment of the condition can be obtained. Observations on the blood pressure, urine, renal function and plasma proteins should be made as in Type 1 nephritis and it is of value to record the patient's weight daily as this gives a useful index of changes in oedema. The objectives are to rest the patient, treat or prevent secondary infection, counteract plasma protein depletion by a high protein diet, and encourage the removal of oedema fluid. Very severe generalized oedema may present an urgent problem since, particularly in children, fatal pulmonary oedema or cerebral oedema may result. In the average case, however, no heroic measures are required, and since the oedema is a manifestation of nephritis it cannot be expected to resolve completely until the nephritis subsides. It is wise, therefore, to maintain complete rest, and during the first week or two treatment should consist in restriction of salt intake, the sodium content of the food being reduced to 0·5 g. daily. The diet should otherwise be adapted to please the patient. Under this regime oedema will gradually diminish in most instances. If, however, there is no response to this 'expectant' treatment the therapeutic measures described under the nephrotic syndrome [p. 985] should be instituted. The use of steroids is fully discussed in this section.

Pulmonary oedema and the much rarer complication of cerebral oedema occur only when subcutaneous swelling is gross, and both should be avoidable if diuretic therapy is used in appropriate combinations and in good time. Should either of these complications develop, direct subcutaneous drainage should be started immediately. Infections should be treated by antibiotics.

Chronic Type 2 nephritis. After the initial stage, continued supervision is necessary. When the patient first becomes ambulant it is common for some oedema of the legs to return and this can usually be controlled by fitting full-length elastic stockings, which should be worn only during the day. In some cases oedema continues for many months and can only be satisfactorily controlled by maintenance diuretic therapy or cation exchange resins. A high-protein, low-salt diet should be continued, but the use of chlorothiazide or similar oral diuretics has reduced the need for severe salt restriction, which makes the diet unpalatable. The serum potassium should be measured periodically and potassium supplements given as required. The main point, however, is to encourage the patient to lead a normal life and return to work, with the obvious precautions of avoiding chills and excesses of any kind. It is in the nature of the disease that relapses tend to occur. If these are mild, and unaccompanied by more than slight oedema, rest in bed at home is often sufficient, but if oedema increases, the patient should be admitted to hospital and treated as described above. In the later stages of the disease when hypertension and uraemia develop, treatment is the same as in chronic Type 1 nephritis.

Course and Prognosis

Complete recovery is rare in Type 2 nephritis, particularly in adults. Clinical resolution does, however, occasionally occur, sometimes after many years of persistent or recurrent oedema. In children, recovery is not uncommon, particularly when hypertension and haematuria are absent. In the great majority of patients, however, the disease runs a steadily progressive course and the prognosis is closely related to the degree of hypertension which develops. With no hypertension or a moderate degree which subsides under treatment, good health often continues for many years, whereas with marked elevation of blood pressure the course may be rapidly progressive. Hypertension is generally more severe, and the course correspondingly shorter, in men than in women. Thus in men, Type 2 nephritis usually continues with variable oedema, moderate hypertension and considerable albuminuria; after 2 or 3 years, progressive renal impairment sets in and leads to uraemia 3–6 years from the onset of oedema, often with the development of the malignant hypertension syndrome. In less severe cases (more commonly women) the disease runs a slower course; oedema may subside very gradually over the course of months or may recur at intervals, but in the absence of hypertension the patient may lead a useful and symptom-free existence for 10 or 20 years. In this group the degree of albuminuria tends to diminish, and the plasma proteins to rise, at a variable interval after the onset. Intercurrent infection may occur at any time and this is particularly serious in children with generalized oedema. Occasionally intercurrent infection is associated with an exacerbation of the nephritis and there may be frank haematuria during such episodes; in other patients infection may precipitate a massive diuresis with subsequent reduction in the degree of albuminuria.

REFERENCES

BOOTH, L. J., and ABER, G. M. (1970) Immunosuppressive therapy in adults with proliferative glomerulonephritis, *Lancet*, ii, 1011.

DAVSON, J., BALL, J., and PLATT, R. (1948) The kidney in periarteritis nodosa, *Quart. J. Med.*, **17**, 175.

ELLIS, A. (1942) Natural history of Bright's disease. Clinical, histological and experimental observations, *Lancet*, i, 1, 34, 72.

JENNINGS, R. B., and EARLE, D. P. (1961) Post-streptococcal glomerulo-nephritis: histopathologic and clinical studies of the acute, subsiding acute, and early chronic latent phases, *J. clin. Invest.*, **40**, 1525.

MUEHRCKE, R. C., KARK, R. M., PIRANI, C. L., and POLLAK, V. E. (1957) Lupus nephritis: a clinical and pathological study based on renal biopsies, *Medicine (Baltimore)*, **36**, 1.

ROSS, J. H. (1960) Recurrent focal nephritis, *Quart. J. Med.*, **29**, 391.

RUSBY, N. L., and WILSON, C. (1960) Lung purpura with nephritis, *Quart. J. Med.*, **29**, 501.

WILSON, C. (1962) Natural history of nephritis, in *Renal Disease*, ed. BLACK, D. A. K., Chap. 9, Oxford.

PYELITIS AND PYELONEPHRITIS

In recent years new diagnostic techniques have led to a much clearer understanding of the frequency, natural history, aetiology and consequences of pyelonephritis. Renal biopsy studies have shown that in all probability extension of the infection into the kidney occurs in most cases of acute pyelitis. The frequent persistence or recurrence of infection in the absence of symptoms is now apparent, and the role of anatomical and functional defects in the urinary tract, particularly vesico-ureteric reflux, has been demonstrated by new radiological techniques.

Incidence

In post-mortem series, pyelonephritis, as a histological finding, has been reported in some 10 per cent. of cases, and as a major renal lesion in 3–5 per cent. The majority of these have been undiagnosed during life, and urinary symptoms have often been absent. Chronic pyelonephritis is therefore the commonest cause of renal failure. It frequently complicates other forms of chronic renal disease. In childhood and in adult life it is far commoner in the female, although in infants the sex incidence is equal. After childhood, clinical episodes of active infection increase in frequency after about the age of 16 and are commoner in married than in unmarried women.

Aetiology

Infection is usually by the intestinal bacteria, *Escherichia coli* being the most common. Others include *Proteus vulgaris*, *Pseudomonas pyocyanea*, *Streptococcus faecalis* and *Staphylococcus albus* or (rarely) *aureus*. Bacteria other than *Esch. coli* are particularly common when anatomical abnormalities are present in the urinary tract. Infection with yeasts may occur in diabetes and in patients undergoing treatment with steroids or immunosuppressive drugs. Infection is frequently introduced and reactivated in women by sexual intercourse ('honeymoon' cystitis). Until its dangers were recently recognized, the use of the catheter in obtaining diagnostic specimens of urine was a common method of introducing bacteria into the bladder. The equality of sex incidence in infants suggests haematogenous infection, but in older subjects, the greater frequency in the female, the effects of urinary tract obstruction, and the common finding of ureteric reflux, all suggest ascending infection from the bladder along the ureters to the kidney. In animal experiments, foci of medullary scarring act as areas of lowered resistance for the development of pyelonephritis when organisms are introduced intravenously, and urinary tract obstruction has a similar predisposing effect. Pyelonephritis is often classified as primary, when the urinary tract appears to be otherwise normal, and secondary when some obstructive factor or other cause of urine retention is present. In so-called primary cases however ureteric reflux is frequently found. This may be intermittent and only demonstrated after repeated examination. The common causes of obstruction are, renal, vesical and ureteric calculi, urethral stricture and prostatic enlargement, neoplasms (within or outside the urinary tract) and in children bladder neck obstruction (usually in boys) and other congenital malformations. Vesico-ureteric reflux is revealed by the micturating cystogram in a high proportion of patients, both children and adults, with recurrent infection. It may develop secondarily as a result of infective damage to the ureteric orifices or obstruction to bladder outflow, but it seems likely to be a primary lesion, possibly congenital, in most cases. In the last trimester of pregnancy and in the puerperium, ureteric dilatation is frequent and results in imperfect drainage which predisposes to urinary infection. Catheterization at the time of labour is also likely to produce infection.

Pathology

One or both kidneys may be affected. In acute pyelonephritis the lining of the pelvis is swollen and congested and there is acute inflammatory infiltration of the subepithelial tissue. Irregular 'streaks' of acute inflammatory cells extend upwards through the medulla to the cortex and the collecting tubules are distended with pus and debris. In chronic pyelonephritis the characteristic picture is one of irregular contraction with focal tubular atrophy and interstitial fibrosis. Active infection may or may not be present, and in many cases of atrophic pyelonephritis no histological evidence of pyelitis is found. The surface of the kidney often shows broad depressed scars, and arteries of all sizes may be very prominent and may show gross intimal thickening (obliterative endarteritis). The glomeruli are relatively normal in less affected areas, but in others show a variety of lesions including periglomerulitis, capsular fibrosis and dilatation, ischaemic atrophy and focal necroses with capsular adhesions. Hyalinized glomeruli may form large aggregates in scarred areas. The tubules show focal zones of atrophy or dilatation, and are often distended with hyaline casts, presenting an appearance resembling thyroid tissue. Fibrinoid arteriolar necroses and glomerular necroses may be found when malignant hypertension has supervened. Papillary necrosis (necrotizing papillitis) is a serious and often fatal complication. It is probably due to acute medullary ischaemia.

Symptoms

Acute pyelitis or pyelonephritis may occur with no symptoms or there may be only frequency and dysuria due to associated cystitis. In the typical acute attack, however, there is severe malaise with high fever, rigors, vomiting, headache and constipation. Dull aching or colicky pain in the loin or anteriorly, is associated with marked renal tenderness and guarding. The kidney may be palpably enlarged. Recurrent attacks usually present with similar but less marked symptoms, frequency and dysuria indicating the presence of cystitis, while loin pain and tenderness point to renal involvement. Chronic pyelonephritis may be without symptoms between the attacks and is often asymptomatic throughout its course until hypertension or uraemia develop. Many cases, probably the majority, have little or no hypertension; a few present with malignant hypertension, the clinical features being those described under chronic Type 1 nephritis. Since atrophic pyelonephritis is common in the elderly, the high blood pressure is probably essential rather than renal in many patients, but there seems no doubt that unilateral pyelonephritis can cause hypertension, since removal of the diseased kidney may restore blood pressure to normal [see hypertension due to unilateral renal disease, p. 988]. Owing to the predominance of medullary and tubular damage, impairment of concentrating power, polyuria and electrolyte depletion may be out of proportion to nitrogen retention, and (rarely) sodium loss may be so severe that the picture closely resembles Addison's disease ('salt-losing nephritis'). In the absence of hypertension, uraemia may be very long-standing and various forms of azotaemic osteodystrophy may develop. The clinical and biochemical manifestations in the late stages are similar to those described under chronic uraemia.

Diagnosis

The diagnosis of acute pyelonephritis is obvious on clinical grounds in severe cases and is confirmed by the finding of high bacterial counts in the urine. A count of over 100,000 colonies per ml. indicates active infection, while less than 10,000 per ml. is usually due to contamination. Between these figures repeat examination shows high counts in about half the cases. Since these high urine counts are due to multiplication of bacteria within the bladder, rapid emptying of the bladder due to frequency, polyuria due to high fluid intake, or administration of antibacterial agents may give false negative results in active infection. False positive counts are avoided by thorough cleansing of the vulva and by immediate refrigeration of specimens. In doubtful cases the presence of bacteria in urine obtained by suprapubic aspiration (a simple and safe procedure in both adults and infants) is diagnostic of infection. Pyuria is usually present in acute cases but its absence does not exclude active infection. A prednisolone provocation test may be used to increase leucocyte excretion but is neither reliable nor specific for pyelonephritis. Tuberculous infection should always be suspected where persistent pyuria is associated with negative cultures on ordinary media.

In the absence of clear-cut symptoms and signs (i.e. loin pain and tenderness) it may be difficult to prove renal involvement in urinary tract infection. Positive bacterial cultures and the presence of leucocytes in ureteric urine constitute the best evidence. The finding of raised antibody titres to the infecting bacteria has been claimed to indicate renal infection but this is not generally accepted. The diagnosis of chronic pyelonephritis should be suspected in patients who have had frequent episodes of acute infection. Where however, no such evidence is present, chronic pyelonephritis is likely, particularly in women, when renal failure develops insidiously, especially if hypertension is slight, and where failure of concentrating power and polyuria occur in the early stages. Albuminuria is usually less than in glomerulonephritis, and may be absent. Before the onset of renal failure the diagnoses may be confirmed by intravenous pyelography which may reveal unequal contraction of the kidneys, irregular thinning of the renal substance and clubbing of the calyces. When renal failure is too advanced for this investigation, straight X-ray of the kidneys may show unequal renal contraction and irregularity of outline.

Treatment

Personal and sexual hygiene should be directed to reducing the risks of faecal contamination of the urethra and it should be a part of health education to impress on young girls and newly married women the need to seek early treatment when urinary symptoms first appear. When infection is diagnosed it is essential to treat it adequately in the initial stages, with subsequent follow up, including urine cultures. In infants and young children the presentation may be atypical, including P.U.O., febrile fits, enuresis, painless frequency and failure to thrive. Urine culture and microscopy in antenatal clinics forms an essential part of preventive therapy, since the treatment of asymptomatic bacteria will greatly reduce the risk of acute pyelonephritis later in pregnancy.

When chronic pyelonephritis is established there is no method of cure, and recurrent infection with progressive renal damage is likely to occur. The greatest possible emphasis should therefore be placed on preventive treatment. Anatomical lesions leading to urine retention should be looked for in all cases, and intravenous pyelography is the minimal investigation; a micturating cystogram should be performed especially in children, and whenever there is a history of recurrent attacks. In many cases however no structural abnormality will be found in the early stages. This so-called primary ascending pyelonephritis is largely a disease of the female, both in childhood and during early adult life, and the majority of infections are due to the faecal organisms *Esch. coli* and *Strep. faecalis*. Co-operative studies from general practice have shown that after childhood, acute episodes are related to the period when sexual intercourse is commonest, and that the incidence in nulliparous married women is no less than in those who bear children. Most initial urinary infections are due to sulphonamide-sensitive *Esch. coli* and 1 G. sulphadimidine 6-hourly should be commenced, after taking urine culture, and continued for at least ten days. Infections resistant to sulphonamides should be treated by the most appropriate agent according to sensitivity tests. Ampicillin, *Septrin* or tetracycline produce adequate blood concentrations by oral administration, but nitrofurantoin and nalidixic acid produce high urine concentrations, with insignificant blood concentrations. The latter should therefore not be used in acute pyelonephritis which is frequently accompanied by bacteraemia. Sensitivity tests should be repeated twice weekly during treatment and urine cultures should be made one week, six weeks and six months after treatment is completed. Recurrence of bacteriuria calls for a further course of treatment as well as radiological investigation for anatomical abnormalities in the urinary tract. The latter are a likely cause for the appearance of Proteus or Pseudomonas in urine cultures. Prolonged follow-up and repeat courses of treatment are particularly important in infants and young children to prevent progressive renal destruction. Repeated infection may be treated by continuous nitrofurantoin in low dosage, e.g. 100 mg. nightly so long as renal function is normal. *Pseudomonas pyocyanea* infection may be difficult to eradicate; short courses of carbenicillin, gentamicin or colistin by injection may not fully sterilize the urine but may result in replacement of Pseudomonas by other bacteria more amenable to long term therapy. When renal failure develops certain drugs produce toxic side-effects by accumulation. Nitrofurantoin may lead to irreversible peripheral neuropathy and should not be given when the G.F.R. falls below 60 ml. per minute. Sulphonamides and the penicillins are safe and effective so long as urine output is adequate. Surgical measures should be undertaken where anatomical defects or obstruction are present. Vesico-ureteric reflux may disappear when infection is treated but its persistence may indicate the need for ureteric transplantation or relief of bladder neck obstruction.

RENAL PAPILLARY NECROSIS

Synonyms. Medullary necrosis; Necrotizing papillitis.

Aetiology

Acute papillary necrosis arises as a complication of acute or chronic pyelonephritis, or of chronic interstitial nephritis due to nephrotoxic agents. It is now most commonly encountered in phenacetin nephritis, less frequently in patients with urinary tract obstruction, e.g. due to prostatic enlargement, or in diabetes with pyelonephritis. The necrosis is believed to be ischaemic in origin, and although the majority of cases are associated with pyelonephritis, it may occur in the absence of such infection.

Pathology

The necrosis involves one or more papillae which may separate and subsequently calcify, forming pelvic calculi.

Symptoms

The condition may present as a fulminating terminal infection with rigors, or with symptoms of acute pyelonephritis. Renal colic may be due to passage of necrotic medullary fragments and these may be recognizable on microscopy of the urine deposit. The urine may be infected but is occasionally sterile, with scanty leucocytes; it may contain blood. If extensive, papillary necrosis may cause anuria.

Diagnosis

Papillary necrosis should be suspected in patients with chronic pyelonephritis or diabetes, or a history of phenacetin addiction, if acute renal failure occurs. High fever, oliguria, renal colic, or sudden development of coma are highly suggestive. In the non-fulminating cases intravenous pyelography may indicate the diagnosis from the filling defects due to cavitation of the papillae, or the soft shadows of separated papillae in the pelvis. In surviving cases calcification of the detached papillae produces characteristic ring shadows in the plain X-ray.

Treatment

This is as for pyelonephritis or for anuria if this complication develops.

REFERENCES

BAILEY, R. R., and LITTLE, P. J. (1969) Suprapubic bladder aspiration in diagnosis of urinary tract infection, *Brit. med. J.*, **1**, 293.

CATTELL, W. R., CHAMBERLAIN, D. A., FRY, I. K., MCSHERRY, M. A., BROUGHTON, C., and O'GRADY, F. (1971) Long-term control of bacteriuria with trimethoprim-sulphonamide, *Brit. med. J.*, **1**, 377.

KIMMELSTEIL, P., KIM, O. J., BERES, J. A., and WELLMAN, K. (1961) Chronic pyelonephritis, *Amer. J. Med.*, **30**, 589.

KLEEMAN, C. R., HEWITT, W. L., and GAZE, L. B. (1960) Pyelonephritis, *Medicine (Baltimore)*, **39**, 3.

LAULER, D. P., SCHREINER, G. E., and DAVID, A. (1960) Renal medullary necrosis, *Amer. J. Med.*, **29**, 132.

LINDVALL, N. (1960) Renal papillary necrosis: a roentgenographic study of 155 cases, *Acta radiol. (Stockh.)*, Suppl., 192.

ROSENHEIM, M. (1963) Problems of chronic pyelonephritis, *Lancet*, i, 1433.

WEISS, S., and PARKER, F. (1939) Pyelonephritis: its relation to vascular lesions and to arterial hypertension, *Medicine (Baltimore)*, **18**, 221.

CHRONIC INTERSTITIAL NEPHRITIS DUE TO NEPHROTOXIC AGENTS

Aetiology

The insidious development of renal fibrosis due to chemical agents is being increasingly recognized. Owing to the similarity of the histological lesion to atrophic pyelonephritis, many such cases may have been missed in the past, but the widespread occurrence of phenacetin nephritis has emphasized the importance of the condition and the need for preventive measures. Chronic lead poisoning, cadmium and uranium are other chemical causes. Endogenous renal damage of a similar nature occurs in gout and in myelomatosis, and possibly in potassium depletion. X-irradiation to the kidney may also be placed in this category although it has certain special features. Acute medullary necrosis (necrotizing papillitis) is a feature of some of these conditions.

Pathology

The essential features are focal or diffuse interstitial nephritis leading to fibrosis in the later stages. Tubular atrophy is severe in the fibrotic areas and may indeed be the primary lesion; glomerular involvement is relatively slight, being limited to ischaemic capsular thickening and glomerular atrophy. The periglomerular fibrosis of ascending pyelonephritis is absent and in uncomplicated cases there is no evidence of chronic pyelitis. The arteries are often prominent and show elastosis and obliterative endarteritis. The changes of secondary pyelonephritis or acute papillary necrosis may be superimposed.

Clinical Features

Phenacetin nephritis has in recent years been reported to occur on a large scale in Denmark and in Switzerland, where phenacetin is the common analgesic in use. It is virtually a drug of addiction, several kilogrammes having been taken over the course of many years by patients developing renal damage. The symptoms are those of slowly developing renal failure in patients with a long-standing history of headaches, often of migrainous character. The addiction is aggravated by the fact that persistent taking of phenacetin itself produces headache. Acute and chronic pyelonephritis and papillary necrosis are frequent complications.

Chronic lead poisoning. Lead nephropathy is usually a late sequel of ingestion of lead-containing paint by young children. Various types of renal lesion occur, the commonest being a diffuse interstitial nephritis with severe hypertension. The kidney is greatly contracted and in some cases this may occur with relatively normal renal architecture. The tubulo-toxic action of lead is indicated by tubular absorption defects which may be seen in the early stages, but the progressive renal fibrosis is predominantly ischaemic in origin, as chronic vascular renal lesions and hypertension are prominent features.

The kidney in gout. Renal involvement of some degree is present in the majority of patients with gout, and uraemia is a cause of death in about one-quarter of the cases. Uric acid deposits in the tubules and interstitial tissue produce the renal damage, leading to surrounding giant cell inflammation, tubular atrophy and interstitial fibrosis. Secondary pyelonephritis is common, and calculi are often present. Attacks of haematuria may occur and renal colic or loin pain may be associated with passage of gravel. These symptoms may be precipitated by uricosuric drugs. Proteinuria is present and renal failure develops slowly, with or without high blood pressure. In some cases hypertension is a marked feature and may become malignant. It seems likely that hyperuricaemia and hypertension may be inherited as separate genetic factors, since either or both may occur in members of the same family. Urinary excretion of uric acid may be more rapid in gouty subjects than in normal individuals, suggesting over-production as the cause of hyperuricaemia rather than defective re-absorption. Although secondary hyperuricaemia occurs in renal failure it rarely gives rise to clinical gout. This has, however, been reported in chronic lead poisoning.

Irradiation nephritis. Severe chronic renal fibrosis occurs after exposure of the kidneys to X-irradiation, usually in the wide-field treatment of seminoma of the testis or carcinoma of the ovary. Albuminuria, oedema, hypertension and renal failure may result. The blood pressure usually rises about six months after irradiation, and in most cases renal damage is complicated by hypertensive vascular lesions. Malignant hypertension is common and has been reported after unilateral renal irradiation. In other cases the course may be very protracted due to the gradual progression of interstitial fibrosis, with associated tubular degeneration and ischaemic glomerular atrophy.

REFERENCES

ABEL, J. A. (1971) Analgesic nephropathy: A review of the literature 1967–1970, *Clin. Pharmacol. Ther.*, **12**, 583.

LINDENEG, O., FISCHER, S., PEDERSEN, J., and NISSEN, N. I. (1959) Necrosis of the renal papillae and prolonged abuse of phenacetin, *Acta med. scand.*, **165**, 321.

MURRAY, R. M., LAWSON, D. H., and LINTON, A. L., (1971) Analgesic nephropathy: Clinical syndrome and prognosis, *Brit. med. J.*, **1**, 479.

SPUHLER, O., and ZOLLINGER, H. U. (1953) Die chronisch-interstitielle nephritis, *Z. klin. Med.*, **151**, 1.

TALBOTT, J. H., and TERPLAN, K. L. (1960) The kidney in gout, *Medicine (Baltimore)*, **39**, 405.

RENAL VASCULAR DISEASE

BENIGN ESSENTIAL HYPERTENSION

Synonym. Benign nephrosclerosis.

In this form of hypertension, renal vascular changes rarely produce clinical symptoms, the disorder being one of chronic arterial and arteriolar degeneration, and it will be necessary to make only a brief reference to it here.

Pathology

The chief kidney changes are in the smaller arteries and arterioles. They are described in detail in Section 8. In contrast with malignant nephrosclerosis, renal arterial lesions rarely produce more than slight parenchymal damage. In long-standing cases, however, arteriolar and arterial degeneration may be severe with consequent irregular contraction and fibrosis of the renal parenchyma. In some cases this condition is marked and a granular contracted kidney results. There is then a patchy fibrosis of glomeruli with tubular atrophy and secondary interstitial changes. This fibrotic atrophy is secondary to the arterial narrowing, and it is because of its patchy distribution that renal function is usually intact.

Symptoms

See benign essential hypertension [Section 8]. The urine may contain albumin, but this is confined to long-standing cases with severe ischaemic fibrosis. The differential diagnosis from chronic nephritis is then made on the absence of a past history of acute nephritis and of renal failure. In a small proportion of cases (probably not more than 1 per cent.) benign hypertension may progress to malignant hypertension and terminate in uraemia.

Treatment

See that of benign hypertension, and of hypertensive heart disease in Section 8, and of uraemia on page 982.

MALIGNANT ESSENTIAL HYPERTENSION

Synonym. Malignant nephrosclerosis.

As in benign hypertension, the renal changes are secondary to the vascular lesions. This disease is called malignant nephrosclerosis because the kidneys are severely affected, so severely in fact that fatal uraemia is the usual outcome.

Pathology

The chief kidney changes are in the smaller arteries and arterioles. They are described in Section 8. In contrast with benign nephrosclerosis, there is, in addition, fibrinoid necrosis, especially of the arterioles.

Symptoms

These are described in Section 8.

Diagnosis

The differential diagnosis of malignant nephrosclerosis from chronic nephritis depends on the fact that in the former there is no past history of acute or chronic nephritis, nor is there renal oedema. Further, in malignant nephrosclerosis papilloedema usually appears whilst renal function is fairly good; in fact it may be normal in the early stages and there may be no albuminuria. In chronic nephritis, however, renal failure is usually advanced by the time papilloedema develops.

Treatment

See that of malignant hypertension, and of hypertensive heart disease in Section 8, and of uraemia on page 982.

RENAL ATHEROSCLEROSIS

Synonym. Ischaemic renal atrophy.

In this form of kidney disease also the vascular changes are of greater importance than the renal.

Pathology

The kidneys show depressed red areas, which are due to contraction of fibrous tissue along the distribution of particular interlobular arteries and, therefore, tend to be conical in form, with their base to the surface of the organ. There is absence of cardiac hypertrophy. The glomeruli in scarred areas shrink, and the connective tissue around them becomes condensed and thickened. The degenerate glomerulus and its capsule fuse together and undergo fatty and fibrotic changes. The atheromatous kidney is, therefore, contracted due to atrophy following insufficient circulation, with consequent fibrosis.

Symptoms and Diagnosis

Symptoms are more likely to arise from atherosclerosis in other organs, particularly the heart, brain or lower limbs, than from renal disease. There may, however, be albuminuria and impairment of renal function, which is often partly extrarenal due to congestive heart failure. Atheroma of a main renal artery or its branches, on one or both sides may give rise to hypertension [p. 988] and this may develop suddenly due to renal artery thrombosis. Infarcts from this cause produce localized, sunken scars with thinning of the renal cortex, which can be identified on intravenous pyelography or angiography. Severe diffuse ischaemic glomerular damage may occasionally result in heavy proteinuria, and this may possibly, as in diabetic glomerulosclerosis, be sufficient to produce the nephrotic syndrome. In ischaemic renal atrophy the clinical diagnosis from chronic Type 1 nephritis or atrophic pyelonephritis may be impossible when renal function is impaired.

REFERENCE

MEANEY, T. F., DUNSTAN, H. P., and MCCORMACK, L. J. (1968) Natural history of renal arterial disease, *Radiology*, **91**, 881.

RENAL LESIONS IN DIABETES MELLITUS

Renal disease is now one of the commonest fatal complications of diabetes. This is due to the fact that control of hyperglycaemia and ketosis by insulin has greatly prolonged life so that the vascular complications are becoming increasingly prominent. The gradual change in the natural history of diabetes over the past 20 years has brought to light a specific form of renal involvement which is closely related to chronic vascular degeneration in other organs. This condition, first described by Kimmelstiel and Wilson in 1936 and named by them *intercapillary glomerulosclerosis*, is the commonest renal lesion in diabetes. Electron microscope studies have shown that the hyaline deposits in the glomerular tuft are not derived from the capillary basement membrane but are intercapillary. Ischaemic atrophy of the kidney tends to be very severe in the diabetic; furthermore, ascending pyelonephritis may occur in a particularly intense form leading to papillary necrosis. The diabetic patient is therefore particularly liable to these three forms of renal damage. In addition, other types of renal disease such as glomerulonephritis are occasionally encountered [see Section 4].

DIABETIC GLOMERULOSCLEROSIS

Incidence

It is probable that diabetic glomerulosclerosis occurs in 10–20 per cent. of all cases of diabetes. In long-standing cases, starting before the age of 15, the incidence is much higher and may reach 50 per cent.; i.e. its occurrence is related to long duration of diabetes rather than to the age of the patient. Although it may be discovered within a few years of the onset of glycosuria, the average duration of diabetes when clinical evidence of renal lesion appears is about 10 years. Thus the majority of patients present evidence of this renal disorder in middle age. The incidence is higher in females than in males. Neither severity of diabetes nor insulin treatment plays any essential role in its pathogenesis, since the lesion is found in patients who have never received insulin, and it is not uncommon in those who have a mild, easily controlled diabetes with little or no tendency to ketosis. It would thus appear that, as with the other vascular complications of the disease, there is little relation between the incidence and severity of diabetic glomerulosclerosis on the one hand and the disturbance of carbohydrate metabolism on the other. Apart from these factors, nothing is known about the aetiology of the process.

Pathology

As its name implies, diabetic glomerulosclerosis consists of a degeneration of the glomerular tuft. This takes the form of progressive hyalinization, but it is possible to recognize several distinct histological features. The first is a nodular deposit of hyaline material in the intercapillary stroma of the glomerular tuft which resembles amyloid material but does not take amyloid stains; this lesion is peculiar to diabetes. In addition the majority of affected glomeruli show a diffuse hyaline change which is seen to be an extension into the glomerular tufts of a similar hyaline degeneration in the afferent arterioles. An identical, but much less conspicuous hyaline degeneration may result from simple atherosclerosis of the kidney. Thirdly, lipohyaline deposits and occasional capillary aneurysms occur within the glomerular tuft and contribute to its disorganization; focal glomerular necroses may also be found, particularly if the blood pressure has been very high. It will be seen, therefore, that diabetic glomerulosclerosis is closely associated with severe degenerative changes in the arterial system of the kidney; furthermore, the association is equally close with severe atheromatous change elsewhere in the body, especially in the heart, brain and retina. Because of the severe ischaemic atrophy the kidney is usually considerably contracted and the arteries are seen to be extremely prominent.

Clinical Features

Albuminuria may for a period of many years be the only manifestation of diabetic glomerulosclerosis. It is variable in amount and is not usually accompanied by inflammatory elements in the urinary deposit. The further development of the clinical syndrome is due not so much to the specific diabetic lesion, but to other complications resulting from generalized arterial degeneration. Hypertension, heart failure and progressive ischaemic damage to the kidney are the most important of these. Impairment of renal function is the rule, although its development is very gradual. In the later stages albuminuria may increase to a degree which leads to a considerable reduction in the plasma protein level. When this occurs, and particularly when myocardial failure due to coronary disease supervenes, severe generalized oedema may appear. Hypertension is usually, but not invariably, present and is moderate in degree; malignant hypertension is only rarely encountered. The final picture is one of combined heart failure and renal failure, and there is often severe mental disturbance due to cerebral vascular degeneration. Diabetic retinopathy will be found in practically all patients with diabetic glomerulosclerosis, and diabetic peripheral neuropathy, usually mild in degree, is also commonly present. During the later stages of the disease it is not infrequently found that the insulin requirement falls. This is probably accounted for by the diminished food intake and restricted activity of the patient due to increasing incapacity.

Diagnosis

When the usual investigations have excluded focal lesions such as calculus, tuberculosis, neoplasm, cystitis and pyelonephritis, albuminuria in a diabetic patient is almost certainly due to glomerulosclerosis with associated renal ischaemic damage. The presence of retinopathy strongly supports the diagnosis as does evidence of arterial degeneration in other organs. There is no specific test for the disease. The association with retinopathy is so close that if renal failure is discovered in a diabetic patient in the absence of retinal changes it is highly probable that some other form of kidney disease is the cause.

Treatment

Apart from control of the diabetes, treatment is the same as in other patients with chronic hypertensive renal disease [see chronic nephritis, p. 992].

Prognosis

As already indicated, glomerular hyalinization and ischaemic atrophy develop very slowly and albuminuria may be present for 10 years before the late complications supervene. The prognosis in fact depends rather more on the extent of vascular degeneration elsewhere in the body than on the presence of glomerulosclerosis.

REFERENCES

Gellman, D. D., Pirani, C. L., Soothill, J. F., Muehrcke, R. C., and Kark, R. M. (1959) Diabetic nephropathy: a clinical and pathological study based on renal biopsies, *Medicine (Baltimore)*, **38,** 321.

Kimmelstiel, P., and Wilson, C. (1936) Intercapillary lesions in the glomeruli of the kidney, *Amer. J. Path.*, **12,** 83.

CONGENITAL RENAL DISEASES

Many errors of development resulting in abnormalities of the shape or position of otherwise normal kidneys occur but are of little clinical importance. They are unlikely to give rise to symptoms or to progressive renal impairment, although there is evidence that such kidneys have an increased tendency to infection. Specific renal tubular disorders of genetic origin are described on page 987. The terms agenesia or congenital hypoplasia, have been applied to small kidneys with relatively normal renal architecture, i.e. where there is no apparent gross structural disease which might have led to contraction. However, the kidney always contains the adult number of nephrons at birth and there is no evidence that congenital disorders are associated with reduction in this number. It is likely, therefore, that the renal contraction in these cases is due to acquired disease occurring either *in utero* or in infancy.

CYSTIC DISEASE OF THE KIDNEY

Solitary cysts of the kidney may present as renal tumours but rarely give rise to clinical symptoms unless they become infected. Multiple small cysts are common in contracted kidneys, either as a result of ischaemic atrophy, or chronic nephritis or pyelonephritis.

Congenital polycystic disease is a condition in which multiple cysts cause great enlargement of both kidneys. There are infantile and adult types. In the former the cysts are present at birth and the condition is not usually compatible with long survival. The cysts do not communicate with other parts of the nephron and inheritance is thought to be as a Mendelian recessive character. In the adult type the condition may present in any decade but is usually diagnosed between 40 and 50. It is inherited as a Mendelian dominant, and the cysts may communicate with the collecting tubules. In a much rarer form, multiple small cysts are present in the medulla (congenital 'sponge kidney') and are readily diagnosed radiologically.

ADULT POLYCYSTIC DISEASE

Pathology

The cysts project from the surface and form the mass of the organ. They are lined by a layer of flattened cells, and are filled with fluid, which is clear or turbid, colourless or yellowish, and is sometimes blood-stained. Urea has been found in the fluid, which may also contain fat globules, cellular debris, cholesterol and triple phosphate crystals. On microscopic examination compressed renal parenchyma is found in the septa between the cysts; the tubules are distorted and exhibit varying degrees of atrophy, degeneration and dilatation, while the glomeruli show changes due to chronic ischaemic or hypertensive damage. The blood vessels of the kidney undergo sclerotic changes and there is interstitial fibrosis. In some cases cysts are also found in the liver, ovaries, broad ligament, uterus, pancreas and spleen; but they are rare in any organ other than the liver.

The disease is nearly always bilateral. When the tumours develop to large size in the foetus, difficulty in labour may result. In the adult there may be no symptoms, or any of the symptoms of chronic hypertensive uraemia may develop, including cerebral haemorrhage or cardiac failure. On the other hand, the condition may reach an advanced stage and fatal termination without appreciable hypertension or cardiac hypertrophy. In a third group bilateral renal tumours are the most striking features, associated with general malaise, dull aching pain in the loins and recurrent haematuria. The kidney may become acutely painful due to haemorrhage into a cyst which may be very tender on palpation. In the late stages hypoplastic anaemia develops. The urine is of low specific gravity and large volume, and commonly contains albumin.

Diagnosis

The finding of albuminuria in association with large, irregular, bilateral renal enlargement should suggest polycystic disease. Hydronephrosis produces a smooth rounded renal swelling. Renal neoplasms are nearly always unilateral. Intravenous pyelography often shows characteristic 'bat's wing' shadows due to distortion of the calyces by the cysts [PLATE 18]. A positive family history confirms the diagnosis.

Treatment

The treatment is symptomatic as described under chronic Type 1 nephritis. Surgical puncture of distended superficial cysts has been recommended especially if these are painful, but the value of this procedure is doubtful.

Course

This closely resembles that of chronic nephritis, with slowly progressive uraemia usually associated with hypertension and hypoplastic anaemia.

REFERENCES

MONGEAU, J. G., and WORTHEN, H. G. (1967) Nephronophthisis and medullary cystic disease, *Amer. J. Med.*, **43**, 345.

SIMON, H. B., and THOMPSON, G. J. (1955) Congenital renal polycystic disease (a clinical and therapeutic study of three hundred and sixty-six cases), *J. Amer. med. Ass.*, **159**, 657.

RENAL AMYLOIDOSIS

Aetiology

Amyloid disease is usually secondary to some chronic disease such as rheumatoid arthritis, bronchiectasis, leprosy, pulmonary tuberculosis or myelomatosis. The once common causes such as osteomyelitis and tertiary syphilis are now rarely found as the provoking lesions. In certain cases no cause is found and the term primary amyloidosis is used. This involves the kidneys less often than secondary amyloid, and even in the latter renal amyloidosis is absent in about 30 per cent. of cases. A rare hereditary form of primary amyloidosis occurs in association with familial Mediterranean fever.

Pathology

In uncomplicated cases the affected kidneys are large and pale, with a smooth surface and a capsule that strips easily. On section, the cortex is thicker than normal and has a yellowish-white appearance; the glomeruli may be visible as minute translucent spots. The pyramids are dark red, in contrast to the pale cortex. If a solution of iodine in potassium iodide is poured over the surface, some of the glomeruli stand out as mahogany-brown spots. Glomerular involvement is at first focal both in distribution and in the involvement of the tufts. The afferent arterioles, vasa recta and capillary plexus are next affected; in more advanced cases there is amyloid deposition in the basement membrane of the tubules and in the interstitial tissue. In some cases there is an associated glomerulonephritis.

Symptoms

Proteinuria may be the only manifestation of renal amyloidosis but albumin loss may lead to hypoproteinaemia and the nephrotic syndrome. Hypertension is usually slight, but if there is associated glomerulonephritis it may be moderate. Renal failure may be absent or may progress rapidly according to the degree of renal damage. Renal vein thrombosis is a complication and may lead to oliguric renal failure.

Diagnosis

Amyloidosis is suspected when severe proteinuria occurs in any of the provoking diseases mentioned above, particularly if the nephrotic syndrome is present. Enlargement of the liver or spleen supports the diagnosis. In primary amyloidosis, involvement of the heart or tongue by amyloid change is not uncommon. Rectal biopsy although simpler and safer than renal biopsy is a less reliable method of establishing the diagnosis of amyloid disease.

Treatment

The treatment is that of the primary disease, together with treatment of the nephrotic syndrome and renal failure as already described.

Course and Prognosis

This depends on the primary cause. If the latter is unchecked, the disease is slowly progressive and death occurs from the effects of the original disease, or from uraemia. Where the original disease can be cured, improvement may occur. If there is an associated glomerulonephritis the outcome is less favourable and deterioration may be very rapid.

RENAL ABSCESS AND PERINEPHRIC ABSCESS

Aetiology

Renal abscess is usually due to the *Staphylococcus pyogenes*, which reaches the kidney via the blood stream from a skin infection following trauma, or boils and carbuncles. It is, therefore, one of the varieties of metastatic infection resulting from staphylococcal bacteraemia. Perinephric infection may arise by direct extension from a renal abscess to the perinephric tissues, or it may arise, like a subphrenic abscess from neighbouring sepsis in the intestine, liver or gall-bladder.

Symptoms

The onset is generally gradual, with fever and malaise. There may be no local symptoms for the first 7–14 days, and during this period there is increasing toxaemia, general abdominal discomfort or pain, and slight fullness and resistance, with deep tenderness, in the affected loin. As the abscess forms, pain and tenderness increase, there is induration and later, redness of the skin and oedema in the lumbar region. The swelling first tends to spread backwards, obliterating the normal hollow in the loin, and then as pus collects it may spread forwards, forming a tender tumour palpable from the front, with resistance or rigidity of the abdominal wall on the affected side. A high swinging fever with rigors may develop at this stage and may indeed be the presenting feature. There is an increasing polymorphonuclear leucocytosis up to 20,000 or even 40,000 per mm^3. The urine does not contain pus unless the abscess ruptures into the renal pelvis.

Diagnosis

The diagnosis rests on localized pain and tenderness associated with a visible or palpable swelling in the loin, high fever and leucocytosis. Blood culture may be positive. The presence of a primary skin lesion, or recent operation for appendicitis or cholecystitis will suggest the source of infection. A perinephric abscess may obliterate the shadow of the psoas muscle in the straight X-ray of the renal area.

Treatment

When the signs of abscess formation are present, surgical drainage should be carried out. If the blood culture is positive appropriate antibiotic therapy should be given.

RENAL TUBERCULOSIS

Aetiology and Pathology

Tuberculous infection reaches the kidney via the blood stream from an active focus in the lungs or lymph nodes. Both kidneys are affected, but as a rule the initial miliary lesions persist only on one side and a focus is formed in one papilla which gradually enlarges and ulcerates into a calyx. The infection spreads to the bladder via ureteral lymphatics and may extend to the opposite kidney. Lesions more deeply situated in the renal substance may form single or multiple closed tuberculous abscesses, unilateral or bilateral, which later undergo calcification. Involvement of the bladder or ureter may lead to tuberculous hydronephrosis.

Symptoms

Frequency of micturition is often the earliest symptom; it is first noticed by day and later at night. Urgency and painful micturition develop next, due to tuberculous cystitis. The urine may show no other abnormality than a trace of albumin in the early stage; characteristically it is pale and a little turbid from the presence of pus; it is acid in reaction, it may contain epithelial cells, and it is sterile on routine culture. By appropriate staining, tubercle bacilli may be demonstrated in the deposit. Haematuria may be the first symptom, or the disease may develop insidiously with lumbar pain.

Diagnosis

Culture of the urine for tubercle bacilli should always be carried out in patients with unexplained proteinuria, and particularly if pus is present, but no growth is obtained on routine culture. X-ray of the kidneys may reveal calcification and the IVP sometimes shows ulceration of one or more calyces. Cystoscopy may show oedema and even tubercles round a ureteric orifice, or early evidence of tuberculous cystitis. Specimens of urine should be obtained from both kidneys for culture to determine whether active bilateral infection is present.

Treatment

If one kidney is grossly affected, nephro-ureterectomy should be carried out. Localized infections are treated with streptomycin, isoniazid and para-aminosalicylic acid for an initial period of 6 months, followed by the two latter drugs for at least 18 months, the treatment being regulated according to the progress of the disease, as indicated by the symptoms, urinary findings and X-ray appearances. Tuberculous cystitis may heal by dense fibrosis leaving a grossly contracted bladder for which corrective surgery may be necessary.

Course

Untreated, closed lesions may heal, leaving caseous or calcareous masses in one or both kidneys. Open lesions progress rapidly or insidiously, often over many years, with gradual development of uraemia in bilateral cases.

RENAL CALCULI (NEPHROLITHIASIS)

Renal calculi are commonly composed of calcium oxalate or phosphate or both. Phosphate stones tend to develop when infection is present. Uric acid or urates, and cystine stones are less frequent.

Aetiology

Certain specific factors are known to play a role in particular varieties of stone formation, such as hyperparathyroidism, congenital cystinuria and oxaluria, gout, and infection of the renal tract. The reasons for formation of the common oxalate or mixed oxalate and phosphate stones is, however, obscure. Concentration of the urine as in hot climates, recumbency and prolonged high calcium intake, are predisposing factors but do not explain the individual predisposition to stone formation. Uric acid stones occur when the urine is persistently acid. Many stone formers have 'idiopathic' hypercalciuria with a normal serum calcium, or constantly excrete an excessive amount of oxalate, factors which are likely to favour precipitation in the tubules or renal pelvis. Hyperparathyroidism is frequently unsuspected in patients with recurrent calculi, and all such cases should have repeated measurements of serum calcium in the fasting state, as slight elevation above normal (10·5 mg. per 100 ml.) may be significant. In *congenital oxaluria* (oxalosis) urinary oxalate amounts to 100–400 mg. daily (normal 45 mg.). This is due to an inborn error by which the normal metabolism of glycine is diverted to formation of oxalate. The latter is deposited in various tissues of the body, including the kidneys, which become grossly disorganized and contracted, death occurring in childhood from uraemia. Ascending pyelonephritis is commonly present.

Symptoms

Renal calculi may cause symptoms due to obstruction, ulceration and haemorrhage, or infection. Stones in the kidney may cause loin pain, especially on jolting. Stones in the ureter cause renal colic and if retained, produce hydronephrosis, infection and ureteric stricture. Ascending pyelonephritis and pyonephrosis may occur. The diagnosis is usually made by X-ray demonstration except in the case of uric acid stones which are translucent. Crystals in the urine deposit may be significant, especially in ureteric colic which may be due to very small oxalate stones.

Treatment

Ureteric colic should be treated by morphine and free fluid administration, the urine being strained to intercept any solid matter which is passed. A stone impacted at the lower end of the ureter requires surgical intervention. The risk of infection and obstruction makes it desirable to remove renal calculi unless these are small and asymptomatic, or very large (staghorn calculi) and bilateral. The latter may cause considerable impairment of renal function which may remain static for many years. A unilateral staghorn calculus with a badly damaged infected kidney calls for nephrectomy. The possibility of specific metabolic disorders such as hyperparathyroidism requires thorough investigation in all cases, and appropriate surgical treatment when indicated.

REFERENCES

McGeown, M. G., and Bull, G. M. (1957) The pathogenesis of urinary calculus formation, *Brit. med. Bull.*, **13**, 53.

Scowen, E. F., Stansfeld, A. C., and Watts, R. W. E. (1959) Oxalosis and hyperoxaluria, *J. Path. Bact.*, **77**, 195.

HYDRONEPHROSIS

Definition

A condition in which the pelvis and calyces of the kidney are distended by non-infected urine due to ureteral or urethral obstruction.

Aetiology

Congenital. The condition may be congenital, due to an abnormality of the ureter or urethra; congenital defects may be present in other organs. Ureteral stricture is usually at its upper or lower end, the former due most commonly to an aberrant renal artery. Hydronephrosis is sometimes found *post mortem* in infants and children without evidence of organic obstruction to the outflow of urine. In these cases the condition is presumed to be due to a bladder-neck obstruction comparable to congenital hypertrophic stenosis of the pylorus and often associated with ureteric reflux.

Acquired. Bilateral hydronephrosis results from stricture of the urethra, phimosis, enlarged prostate, obstruction within the bladder, or from a pelvic tumour. Unilateral hydronephrosis is due to ureteral obstruction from obstruction of the lumen by a stone or growth, stricture of the ureter, or pressure from without by growths. In the latter case the ureter is usually infiltrated.

Pathology

Two types of hydronephrosis are recognized, namely, the pelvic type due to upper urinary tract obstruction, and the renal type from obstruction to the lower tract. In the former the pelvis of the kidney is dilated and there is less marked atrophy of renal parenchyma. In the latter the calyces are more dilated and there is considerable destruction of kidney substance. It is generally held that hydronephrosis results from intermittent obstruction. Complete obstruction is more usually followed by atrophy of the kidney.

Symptoms

Many cases give rise to no symptoms. The tumour may be discovered accidentally, or there may be complaint of pain in the flank or back. The onset is insidious. Haematuria may occur or there may be symptoms of ascending pyelonephritis. In intermittent hydronephrosis the swelling may become evident and more painful after heavy drinking, and may then subside with the passage of a large volume of urine.

Diagnosis

This may be obvious clinically from the finding of a cystic renal swelling. More usually it is diagnosed by intravenous pyelography [Plate 18].

Complications

Infection is the chief complication, massive haemorrhage and rupture are rare. Pyelonephritis may arise in unilateral or bilateral hydronephrosis while pyonephrosis is usually unilateral. The latter gives rise to high fever, sweats and rigors, loin pain, malaise, rapid wasting and anaemia. Since ureteric obstruction may be present, pus may be absent from the urine.

Treatment

When the hydronephrosis is mild or moderate in degree the cause may be remediable, for example, by division of an aberrant renal artery, removal of a ureteric calculus, re-implantation of the ureter, relief of prostatic enlargement or of bladder neck stenosis. In advanced cases, nephrectomy is necessary.

PERIURETERIC FIBROSIS

This is a rare condition caused by chronic retroperitoneal fibrosis of unknown aetiology; recently this lesion has been reported following methysergide administration. One or both ureters may be obstructed, usually just below the pelvi-ureteric junction or at the pelvic brim. Hydronephrosis results, which if bilateral leads to renal failure. Other structures may be compressed including the inferior vena cava or spinal nerve roots, and biliary obstruction has been reported.

Symptoms

These usually appear in middle-aged men, and their nature depends on the structures involved. Severe and persistent backache of varying localization may occur, and may typically be relieved by adopting the kneeling posture, suggesting a diagnosis of carcinoma of the pancreas. All investigations may prove negative unless an intravenous pyelogram is performed, and the condition is often labelled as hysteria or psychoneurosis. In other cases inferior vena caval obstruction leads to oedema of the legs and greatly dilated veins over the legs and abdomen. Ureteric involvement may cause renal colic or loin pain, and loss of appetite, nausea and vomiting may be present. Renal function is impaired, anaemia develops and anuria may occur.

Diagnosis

Diagnosis is based on the above clinical manifestations supported by pyelographic evidence of high ureteric obstruction. It can be confirmed only by operation.

Treatment

Improvement may result from ureterolysis, but recovery is usually incomplete. Steroid therapy may be beneficial.

REFERENCES

RAPER, F. P. (1956) Idiopathic retroperitoneal fibrosis involving the ureters, *Brit. J. Urol.*, **28**, 436.

SAXTON, H. M., KILPATRICK, F. R., KINDER, C. H., LESSOF, M. H., MCHARDY-YOUNG, S., and WARDLE, D. F. H. (1969) Retroperitoneal fibrosis: A radiological and follow-up study of 14 cases, *Quart. J. Med.*, **38** 159.

RENAL TUMOURS

Pathology

Benign renal tumours are small and of little clinical importance. They include adenoma, fibroma and angioma, and may cause haematuria when situated in the pelvis.

Malignant tumours include *Wilms' tumour*, usually occurring in children under the age of 3 and sometimes bilateral. The tumour consists of undifferentiated foetal connective tissue resembling spindle-cell sarcoma. Unilateral Wilms' tumour has been known to cause hypertension. *Adenocarcinoma* (Grawitz tumour, hypernephroma) arises from the renal tubular epithelium. These tumours vary considerably in size, vascularity and rate of growth. They are fairly well circumscribed by a capsule of compressed renal tissue, and on section are yellowish in colour due to lipoid material. Rapidly growing tumours may extend along the renal vein and cause inferior vena caval obstruction. Metastases occur in the lungs, bones, brain and skin and may be responsible for the presenting symptoms.

Symptoms

Pain, haematuria and a palpable renal swelling are the characteristic features. Pain may be in the loin, or in the form of renal colic due to haematuria. Bleeding may be intermittent. Albuminuria is often present and may be gross if vena caval obstruction occurs; oedema of the legs may be due to the same cause.

Diagnosis

Grawitz tumour is suspected when a renal swelling is associated with haematuria. It is confirmed by intravenous pyelography which shows distortion, elongation or compression of the calyces. Renal angiography may demonstrate the tumour owing to its vascularity, and is particularly valuable in differentiation from a solitary cyst.

Treatment

Treatment is by nephrectomy, and in a well encapsulated tumour which has not metastasized, survival up to 10 years may occur.

CLIFFORD WILSON

SECTION 13

DISEASES OF THE HAEMOPOIETIC ORGANS

DISORDERS OF HAEMOSTASIS

DISEASES OF THE HAEMOPOIETIC AND RETICULAR ENDOTHELIAL SYSTEMS

DISORDERS OF HAEMOSTASIS

INTRODUCTION

THE HAEMOSTATIC MECHANISM

In health, the haemostatic mechanisms have two functions: the arrest of blood loss from injuries and the maintenance of vascular integrity. The importance of this second becomes apparent only when it is defective. An example is the patient with haemophilia who suffers a haemarthrosis without obvious injury. In health it is probable that bleeding into a joint occurs as a consequence of the physiological stress of walking or running, but this breach of vascular integrity will be so immediately and efficiently sealed that no evidence of bleeding is apparent. Effective haemostasis will depend on normal vascular function, normal platelet function and normal deposition of fibrin by the blood coagulation system; furthermore, this fibrin should not be removed by the fibrinolytic mechanism until it has served its purpose.

THE ARREST OF HAEMORRHAGE

Haemostasis in Response to Injury

The mechanism by which bleeding is arrested from injured vessels is threefold; the blood vessels themselves react by transient constriction; around their edges platelets adhere and aggregate to form a plug which stops further blood flowing. It may be that exposure of collagen or the release of adenosine diphosphate from injured tissues initiates this process, but once started, there is a mechanism within the platelets which encourages their aggregation. The platelet plug is reinforced by deposition of a firm fibrin clot. By itself it is insufficient to maintain haemostasis, and this is readily observed in bleeding after extraction of a haemophiliac's tooth. Abnormal bleeding may not be immediately evident, but only after some hours when the platelet plug has failed to be reinforced by fibrin and vascular constriction has worn off, does the haemostatic failure become clinically apparent.

Physiological Haemostasis

It is probable that protection against physiological haemostatic stress occurs at the capillary level, and that the platelets have a major part to play in maintaining their integrity. Normal platelets, however, are not sufficient in themselves to prevent this type of bleeding, because it is seen in haemophilia. Platelet aggregation occurs under the influence of thrombin, and the failure to produce thrombin at normal rates in a condition such as haemophilia may be the cause of haemostatic failure.

BLOOD COAGULATION

Prothrombin Conversion to Thrombin

It has been known for over a century that blood coagulation consists in the formation of the insoluble fibrin from a soluble plasma precursor, fibrinogen. This conversion of fibrinogen to fibrin occurs under the influence of the proteolytic enzyme thrombin; thrombin is not present in circulating blood but arises from a precursor, prothrombin, by the action of a thromboplastin system. In FIGURE 62 it will be seen that prothrombin is converted to thrombin by thromboplastin in the presence of calcium, and that thrombin converts fibrinogen to fibrin. This is the so-called classical theory as postulated by Morawitz in 1905; provided the term 'thromboplastin' is given a wider meaning than originally intended, it is still valid.

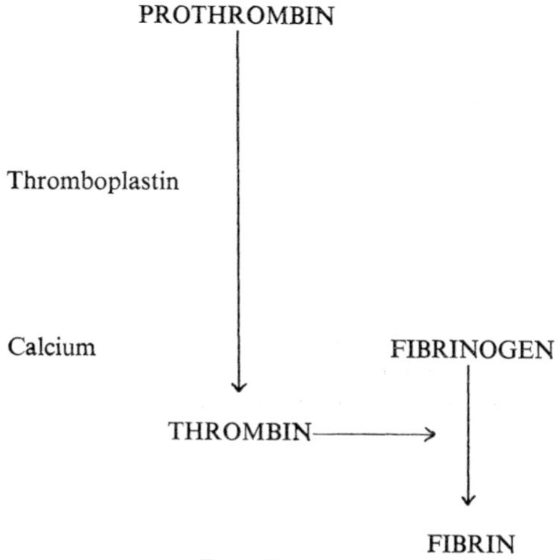

FIG. 62

If blood obtained by clean venepuncture is delivered to two glass tubes, one containing macerated tissue, and the second empty, that in each tube clots, albeit at differing rates. The blood in the tube containing tissue clots in 10 seconds, whereas that in the other may take 10 minutes. The components of the thromboplastin system responsible for the conversion of prothrombin to thrombin in the tube without tissue, are all contained within the blood itself and this mechanism of prothrombin conversion is therefore referred to as the intrinsic thromboplastin system. The other is spoken of as the extrinsic system. Both require to be intact to ensure physiological haemostasis.

It is now appreciated that there are many components as shown in FIGURE 63 which make up both systems. The extrinsic system requires in addition to the tissue factor, three others: Factors V, VII and X—to make up the prothrombin-converting principle. In the intrinsic system, the factors required are V, VIII (the plasma factor missing in haemophilia), IX (the factor missing in Christmas disease), X, XI and XII and the phospholipids obtained from the platelets.

There has been much interest in recent years in attempting to establish the sequence of the reactions involved in the formation of blood thromboplastin. The so-called 'cascade scheme' suggests that it is a series of pro-enzyme/enzyme transformations and that the whole process acts as a biochemical amplifier resulting in explosive production of thrombin from prothrombin.

A study of FIGURE 63 will show that Factors V and X are required for the formation of both blood (intrinsic) and tissue (extrinsic) thromboplastin. Factor VII is

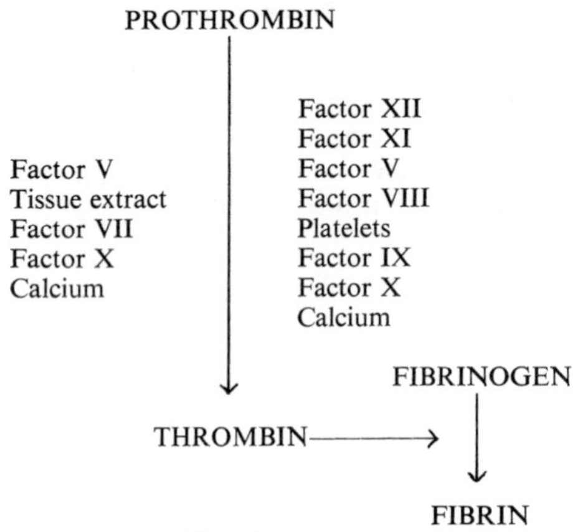

FIG. 63

needed only in a tissue system; Factors VIII and IX (the factors missing in haemophilia and Christmas disease respectively) and Factors XI and XII are needed only in the intrinsic system. In TABLE 56 is shown a list of coagulation factors with the internationally agreed numbers.

TABLE 56

FACTOR	
I	Fibrinogen
II	Prothrombin
III	Tissue extract
IV	Calcium
V	Labile factor
	Proaccelerin
VII	Proconvertin
	Stable factor
VIII	Antihaemophilic globulin (A.H.G.)
	Antihaemophilic factor (A.H.F.)
	Antihaemophilic factor A
IX	Christmas factor
	Plasma thromboplastin component (P.T.C.)
	Antihaemophilic factor B
X	Stuart-Prower factor
XI	Plasma thromboplastin antecedent (P.T.A.)
XII	Hageman factor
XIII	Fibrin stabilizing factor (F.S.F.)

Fibrinogen Conversion to Fibrin

Thrombin acts on fibrinogen as a proteolytic enzyme splitting off specific fibrinopeptides to form the smaller molecule, fibrin monomer, which undergoes polymerization to soluble fibrin. In the presence of calcium ions and a further coagulation factor, Factor XIII, the soluble fibrin polymer is converted to the final product, insoluble fibrin [see FIG. 64]. The biochemical characteristics of Factor XIII activity suggest it is a transglutaminase.

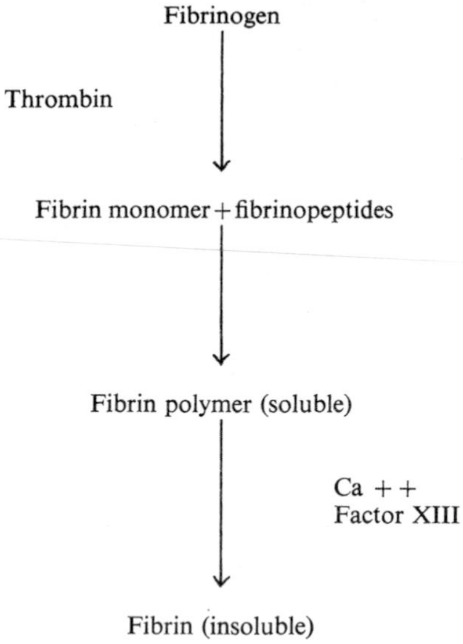

FIG. 64

PLATELETS

Platelets contain a phospholipid which is an essential component of intrinsic thromboplastin. They have, however, another important role in haemostasis. When a vessel is injured, bleeding is arrested by the formation of a platelet mass occluding the gap in the vessel wall. This plug normally becomes stable and no further bleeding is observed unless it is forcibly dislodged. Its stability is in part due to the formation of fibrin binding the platelet mass and reinforcing its base; the thrombin, which has caused the fibrin to form, is also important in the aggregation of platelets.

One of the first steps in the formation of the haemostatic plug is the interaction of platelets with collagen, with release of adenosine diphosphate which leads to further platelet aggregation. As well as this substance, contact of platelets with collagen induces release of other factors which influence vessel permeability and contraction of smooth muscle; serotonin and histamine are important in this aspect of haemostasis.

Initiation of Haemostasis

It is not known for certain what triggers the formation of fibrin as part of the haemostatic plug, but in patients with a defect of the intrinsic system the platelet plug may disintegrate and renewed bleeding may occur. Platelet plugs in patients with defective blood coagulation contain less fibrin than normal, and show little evidence of the structural changes which usually accompany the production of thrombin. The number of circulating platelets necessary to provide an adequate haemostatic plug is probably far less than that normally present in blood issuing from the wound. It is common experience that thrombocytopenia has to be severe to produce abnormal haemorrhage.

It will be seen that the interaction of platelets with connective tissue, particularly collagen, is important in the formation of the haemostatic plug. There is evidence that some of the drugs in common use, for example, aspirin, inhibit this platelet-collagen reaction and impair haemostasis.

FIBRINOLYSIS

Fibrinolysis is mediated by the proteolytic enzyme, plasmin, normally arising from an inactive precursor, plasminogen. The latter, a plasma globulin, widely distributed in blood and other body fluids, is converted to plasmin in the presence of activator. Plasmin is capable of digesting not only fibrin, but also fibrinogen and other coagulation factors [see FIG. 65]. Plasminogen activators are found in most tissues of the body and exist in especially high concentrations in the uterus, lung, prostate and thyroid. Although plasma normally contains only traces of activity which is responsible for its physiological fibrinolytic activity, the level rises sharply in response to physical and mental stress, adrenaline injection and other stimuli.

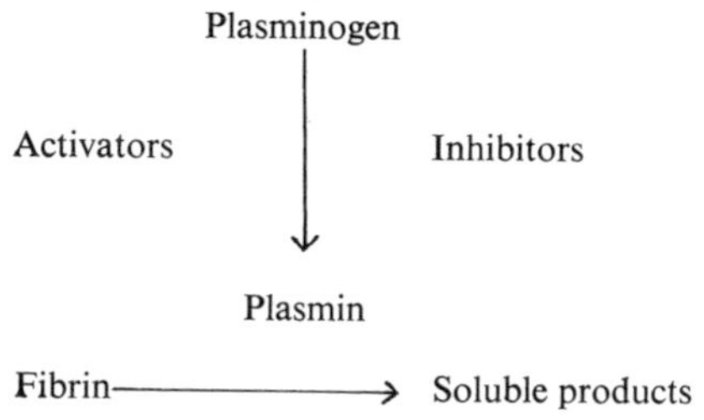

FIG. 65

Plasminogen has an affinity for fibrin which carries with it sufficient to ensure its subsequent lysis whenever it is deposited. This appears to be achieved primarily by the direct diffusion or incorporation of activator from the circulation on to the fibrin of the haemostatic plug. In physiological circumstances there is an inhibitory mechanism in the circulation which neutralizes any free plasmin. If a large amount of plasminogen activator is released into the circulation, this inhibitory mechanism may be temporarily overwhelmed and free plasmin appear. When this happens, fibrinogen is attacked and the resulting breakdown products interfere with normal fibrin polymerization. As a result, fibrin formation is delayed and defective and that formed is friable and unstable.

DIAGNOSIS OF HAEMOSTATIC DEFECTS

Each of the haemostatic defects has its own particular pattern of clinical presentation, and clinical appraisal of the individual is of vital importance, for it may provide a major diagnostic lead as well as indicate the line laboratory investigation should take. Although the laboratory can now provide screening tests for most of the haemorrhagic disorders, the ultimate proof may well be the patient's response to haemostatic challenge such as the extraction of a tooth. Faced with a patient with a suggestive history, one should always remember that past events may well be the best guide to the future. The patient's history should be treated with appropriate respect and subsequent management planned accordingly.

Acute haemostatic failure in previously normal persons may follow thoracic operations or open heart surgery, using the heart-lung bypass machine. It may occur, too, in obstetrics, particularly with abruptio placentae. The clinical circumstances are likely to indicate the abnormality, and although the nature of these defects is complex, the common denominator is a reduced fibrinogen concentration.

Other recognized disease associations will often permit clinical suspicion of the cause. Patients with chronic liver disease and those with chronic renal failure often have abnormal haemorrhage. These are less acute, acquired haemorrhagic disorders.

Differentiation between Acquired and Congenital Disorders

The time of onset of symptoms may help to differentiate between an acquired and a congenital disorder. The family history may also be of value, since the genetic haemorrhagic disorders have characteristic modes of inheritance, although they are not excluded by a negative family history. For example, in at least one-third of the patients with haemophilia it is not possible to obtain a positive family history. These details are not only important in understanding the problem in an affected person and his family, but the pattern of inheritance may be a guide to its nature and permit exclusion of the condition in certain relatives. For example, the sons and daughters of an unaffected male in a family with haemophilia, cannot suffer from the disease although the daughters will all be potential transmitters.

Differentiation between Disorders of Blood Coagulation and 'Platelet-Capillary' Defects

A careful history and physical examination may enable the clinician to distinguish between a patient with a coagulation abnormality and one with a 'platelet-capillary' defect. Bleeding from superficial scratches and abrasions is unusual in coagulation defects, although often profuse and prolonged in platelet capillary abnormalities. Haematomata in coagulation defects are often enormous and spread widely. In the platelet-capillary group, bruises are small, multiple and usually superficial. Haemarthrosis is common in severe coagulation defects, but unusual in platelet-capillary disorders. In coagulation defects bleeding from deep cuts or after tooth extraction is often delayed in onset, not permanently controlled by local measures and continues for many days. With platelet capillary defects, such wounds cause immediate bleeding and local haemostatic measures may often be successful. In the coagulation defects, the characteristic abnormality is a deep haematoma either spontaneous or traumatic, and there is prolonged and dangerous bleeding, often difficult to control by local measures, after injury. In the platelet capillary group, mucosal bleeding is the feature. It should be appreciated, of course, that the distinctions are not absolute.

Diagnostic Relevance of Time of Onset

The appearance of bleeding in the early days of life will, in most cases, leave little doubt of the congenital nature of the disorder, although of course a reversible situation such as haemorrhagic disease of the newborn or neonatal thrombocytopenia must be considered.

Bleeding after Significant Haemostatic Challenge

The history obtained from the patient may indicate that there is haemostatic failure only after significant trauma. The patient with mild haemophilia or mild Christmas disease comes into this category. It is not uncommon for normal people to bleed from dental extraction for 24–36 hours, but if this has continued intermittently for as long as 3 or 4 days, then it is likely to be abnormal, particularly if repeated. It is not the amount of blood but the duration of the bleeding which matters. In coagulation disorders, bleeding may appear to have stopped only to start again some hours later and continue intermittently for days or weeks. In disorders affecting the platelets and blood vessels, there is usually no such temporary arrest and it continues from the moment of injury. Of all the various injuries which can be inflicted on the patient, tooth extraction, because it is common and often repeated, provides a particularly important area of interrogation.

Apart from dental extraction, inquiry should be made about circumcision and tonsillectomy. Both of these represent major haemostatic challenges. Prolonged bleeding after circumcision may be the first symptom of the hereditary bleeding disorders such as haemophilia, and may be the only one until the child starts to walk. Tonsillectomy may present a serious hazard to a patient with a coagulation defect. If it is unaccompanied by excessive bleeding, then a genetic haemorrhagic disease is most unlikely.

Spontaneous Bleeding

A patient with a history of spontaneous bleeding is unlikely to present a major diagnostic problem. Such patients have no protection against physiological haemostatic stress as defined above. All normal people notice occasionally a small bruise for which they cannot account. In women of menopausal age and in children they are particularly common; they are usually not more than 2–3 cm. in diameter, occur most frequently on the legs and are unassociated with other evidence of a bleeding disorder. In normal people the area of bruising is only two or three times the size of the area of impact. If it is much greater a coagulation defect must be suspected. An occasional purpuric spot may be seen in normal people, but more extensive purpura usually indicates an abnormality of the platelets or of the small vessels.

Epistaxis, Haematuria and Menorrhagia. Inquiry should be made about epistaxis, which is a common symptom of a platelet-capillary type of disease. Haematuria occurs in coagulation defects and in platelet-capillary disorders, and may be a presenting feature in thrombocytopenic purpura and occasionally occurs in von Willebrand's syndrome.

Haemarthrosis. Spontaneous bleeding into the joints (haemarthrosis) is the most characteristic symptom of haemophilia and Christmas disease. It is exceptional in platelet disorders.

Bleeding from the Gums. This is a characteristic feature of thrombocytopenia, but also occurs in patients with haemophilia, particularly in children. It is often the presenting symptom in macroglobulinaemia. In congenital disorders bleeding may occur from the site of shedding of the deciduous teeth.

Gastro-intestinal Bleeding. This occurs in platelet disorders, and in coagulation defects. In haemophilia and Christmas disease it may be difficult to know whether it is simply a manifestation of a haemostatic defect or whether there is a complicating local lesion. Duodenal ulceration, for example, appears to have at least the same incidence in a haemophiliac as in the population at large. In infants, haemorrhagic disease of the newborn may manifest with gastro-intestinal bleeding.

Bleeding into the Respiratory Tract. Haemoptysis is rarely a presenting feature in haemorrhagic states. Interstitial bleeding in the lungs may occur in coumarin drug therapy, and in severe genetic coagulation defects.

Bleeding from the Umbilical Stump. This is a symptom of haemorrhagic disease of the newborn and of neonatal thrombocytopenia; Factor XIII deficiency characteristically presents in this way, and it is occasionally the first symptom of haemophilia or Christmas disease.

Bleeding into Other Sites. Retroperitoneal bleeding is a particular feature of haemophilia and Christmas disease. Amongst other sites commonly affected is the plane along the ileopsoas muscle resulting in femoral nerve palsy; such haematomata are large, and if on the right-hand side may arouse suspicion of an appendix abscess. Bleeding into the wall of the small bowel occurs in haemophilia and Christmas disease; it may happen with coumarin overdose and lead to intestinal obstruction. Intracranial haemorrhage may result from a birth injury of a haemophilic child, and is not an uncommon cause of death in the elderly with this disease as it may be in thrombocytopenia.

LABORATORY TESTS

A general physician may well have to seek specialized haematological guidance in the laboratory investigation of the haemostatic mechanisms, although the clinical features will often give a pointer to the aspects which should be explored.

Platelet-Capillary Disorders

The platelet count is the most important single test in the investigation of these disorders. The bleeding time is a useful technique, but to be of value must be carried out under rigidly standardized conditions. It may be prolonged in von Willebrand's syndrome when the platelet count is normal. A capillary resistance test adds little to the information these two give.

Coagulation Disorders

The *whole blood coagulation time* may be of value

if carried out under strictly standardized conditions; if the result is prolonged, there is a defect of coagulation, but a normal reading does not exclude it. The blood collected for the whole blood clotting time may be studied an hour after coagulation to determine whether the prothrombin has been converted to thrombin at a normal rate, that is whether the intrinsic thromboplastin system has functioned normally. This is the *prothrombin consumption test*. If this is abnormal, there is a defect in the intrinsic thromboplastin system, but it is not a very sensitive technique.

When plasma is collected after venepuncture and added to a suitable anticoagulant, it can be studied for the rate of clotting on the addition of tissue extract. This is the *one stage prothrombin time*. From the information shown in FIGURE 63, it will be seen that deficiencies of Factors V, VII, X or prothrombin itself may lead to a prolongation of the clotting time in this test. However, it will not reveal deficiencies and Factors IX, VIII and XI or of platelets; it is a test only of the extrinsic thromboplastin system.

A more sensitive screening test of the intrinsic thromboplastin system is the *kaolin-cephalin clotting time*, in which the patient's plasma is clotted by re-calcification in the presence of kaolin to provide an optimal surface and platelet lipid in adequate concentration. A prolonged result will occur in deficiencies of any of the plasma factors required to make up intrinsic thromboplastin, namely, Factors V, VIII, IX, X, XI, XII. Deficiencies of Factors V and X will have previously been detected by the one-stage prothrombin time. In the presence of a normal one-stage test, the commonest abnormalities will be deficiencies of Factors VIII or IX and then specific assays for these Factors should be made. This can be done by adding the test plasma to plasma obtained from a high-grade haemophilic or a high-grade Christmas factor defect. The correction obtained is tested against the ability of normal plasma to correct these known defects.

Deficiencies of Factors XI and XII require to be detected by other methods. These involve the contact activation of the test plasma and a normal plasma with celite and demonstration of the ability of this celite-surface activated plasma to reduce the clotting time of plasma which has been collected and tested in silicone, after the addition of celite treated plasma. These are tests of the contact activation mechanism of blood coagulation.

Clinical situations are recognized in which patients develop inhibitors of blood coagulation. These are so-called 'circulating anticoagulants', and can be demonstrated by a technique such as the kaolin-cephalin clotting time by showing that a small addition of the patient's plasma will prolong the clotting time of normal plasma.

Disorders of Fibrinogen and of the Fibrinolytic Enzyme System

Fibrinogen may require to be measured and biochemical techniques for this are available. Plasminogen is measured by conversion to plasmin by streptokinase and the plasmin assayed by proteolysis of casein. The activator of plasminogen can be measured by studying the rate of lysis of fibrin formed in diluted blood or by making the euglobulin precipitate which contains fibrinogen, plasminogen and blood activator and studying the lysis time of the euglobulin-fibrin once clotted. Factor XIII can be detected by studying the solubility of the patient's fibrin in 5-molar urea. Fibrin formed in the absence of Factor XIII is soluble in 5-molar urea while stabilized fibrin is insoluble.

GENETIC HAEMORRHAGIC DISORDERS

Despite the large number of genetic disorders mentioned, in clinical practice only the following require to be considered, for the others are excessively rare:

- Haemophilia, or deficiency of Factor VIII
- Christmas disease, or deficiency of Factor IX
- von Willebrand's syndrome
- Hereditary telangiectasia

HAEMOPHILIA AND CHRISTMAS DISEASE

The appreciation that the syndrome of haemophilia was made up of two diseases, haemophilia and Christmas disease, resulted from the observation that occasionally two clinically identical patients had blood which was mutually corrective. The two are clinically indistinguishable and occur in grades from mild to severe. Within each affected family the nature and the severity of the bleeding defect breed true.

Patients with mild haemophilia or Christmas disease have a normal whole blood clotting time, and only bleed abnormally after events such as tonsillectomy or tooth extraction. They usually lead an otherwise normal life. A severely affected patient has a life of chronic invalidism with no protection from physiological haemostatic stress, with spontaneous bleeding into tissue planes and joints.

Incidence

These conditions occur approximately once in 10,000 of the population in Britain. Haemophilia is about five times as common as Christmas disease. Approximately 50–60 per cent. suffer from the severe grade. All major racial groups are known to be affected.

Inheritance

Both haemophilia and Christmas disease are inherited as sex-linked recessives. Thus all the daughters of an affected man will be transmitters, and all his sons will be unaffected and there is a 50 per cent. chance that the daughters of a transmitter female will in turn be transmitters. For genetic counselling, the points to remember are that the daughter of a haemophilic man will be a transmitter, but it is difficult to be certain whether her daughters will be. Occasionally the transmitter female may have an abnormally low level of the relevant clotting factor, but a normal value does not exclude the possibility that she is a transmitter. The mother of more than one haemophilic son or more than one transmitter daughter, can confidently be labelled as a transmitter.

Clinical Picture

In severe haemophilia the earliest manifestations may be prolonged bleeding following circumcision or from the umbilical stump; more often the first symptom is abnormal haemorrhage from a cut on the forehead or lip, or from a bitten tongue when the child first starts to walk, crawl and fall. Bruising is excessive. Haemarthrosis, commonly of the knees and ankles, may occur when the severely affected child begins to walk; the shedding of deciduous teeth may lead to prolonged bleeding from the gums; epistaxis and haematuria are common and may continue for days or weeks; retroperitoneal haemorrhage can be a problem; bleeding from the gastro-intestinal tract is uncommon, but in some adult haemophiliacs may occur with or without evidence of peptic ulceration. Haemorrhage into the central nervous system is rarely spontaneous, but may be disproportionately serious after injury. Intracranial haemorrhage, although uncommon, is becoming an increasingly frequent cause of death in elderly haemophiliacs as advances in treatment increase their life span. Extradural haematomata may cause compression of the brain or cord.

Surgical procedures such as tooth extraction and tonsillectomy will inevitably be followed by abnormal bleeding, but it is not uncommon to find the mild haemophiliac who has some years previously had an appendicectomy without the diagnosis becoming apparent. In the case of a wound, immediate haemostasis may occur, but bleeding starts some hours later and continues for days or weeks.

Repeated haemarthroses result in increasing damage to the affected joints and flexion deformities of the knees and elbows are common in severe haemophilia. Incomplete reabsorption of the intra-articular blood is followed by chronic damage to the synovial membranes, thickening of the joint capsule, destruction of the cartilage and underlying bone and finally by chronic osteo-arthritis with irregular new bone formation and often with loose bodies in the joint. Bleeding may also occur into the adjacent bone, causing localized areas of rarefaction and sometimes leading to the gradual development of a cystic 'haemophilic pseudotumour'.

Major haematomata may threaten life by their mechanical effects. Bleeding into the neck, for example, may lead to respiratory obstruction; haematomata in the limbs may result in paralysis of peripheral nerves; when haemophilic blood cysts occur, they may infiltrate muscle planes, erode bones and cause necrosis of overlying skin.

Haematuria is not an uncommon manifestation and there is evidence that permanent renal damage may result from it.

Diagnosis

Laboratory tests will in general correlate with the clinical degree of severity. Anaemia is the result of bleeding, but the haemorrhage may be exclusively internal and, indeed, the haemophilic patient may bleed to death without any external loss of blood. The mild haemophiliac and the patient with Christmas disease will have a normal whole-blood clotting time. Where the plasma concentration of the missing factor is 1 per cent. of normal or less, the disability will be severe with many spontaneous bleeding incidents. At the other end of the scale, mildly affected patients will have levels of the relevant factor between 15 and 30 per cent. of normal; these patients only bleed after severe haemostatic challenge and the diagnosis may not become apparent until early adult life following the first extraction of permanent teeth.

Patients often insist that they have periods with repeated bleeding and others with relative freedom from symptoms. The explanation of this impression is unknown, for there is no evidence of any cyclical alteration in the degree of coagulation defect. There is surprising variation in the levels of these coagulation factors amongst the general population; in health the value should lie above 50 per cent. of the mean normal level.

Treatment

There is at present no curative treatment available for haemophilia or Christmas disease, and the management of patients must be based on two principles—the avoidance of injury and the provision of supportive treatment when injuries or spontaneous bleeding do occur and when surgical procedures are necessary. The severely affected haemophiliac appears to have less spontaneous bleeding as he grows older, but this is probably due to conscious or unconscious avoidance of minor injuries. The degree of restriction of activity which the affected individual will find it wise to impose upon himself varies greatly from patient to patient, but all with these diseases, even if mildly affected, must be made aware of the dangers of serious injury or of surgical and dental procedures.

It is more difficult to stop haemorrhage once it has occurred than to prevent it, and the aim should be to achieve normal haemostasis, not merely to reduce the amount of blood loss. Treatment consists of local measures at the site of bleeding, appreciating the limited role of these manoeuvres and the correction of the blood defect by replacement with appropriate intravenous preparations.

The haemophiliac's veins may well be his life-line and due respect must be paid to them. It is unwise to leave the setting up of infusions to an unskilled operator, and unless the veins have been exhausted, 'cut-downs' should be avoided. Where there is evidence of phlebitis and therefore risk of thrombosis, the needle should be inserted in another vein. Problems may also arise with repeated venepunctures necessary to obtain samples for determination of the Factor VIII level.

Principles of Replacement Therapy

The aim of replacement therapy is to raise the recipient's plasma concentration of Factor VIII or Factor IX sufficiently to enable him to meet the haemostatic challenge anticipated or received, and to maintain it at this level as long as necessary. The precise figure depends upon the extent of the challenge. A useful guide is the mild haemophiliac in whom the level may be between 15 and 30 per cent.; the normal range is between 50 and 200 per cent. If it is possible, therefore, to raise the level to 50 per cent. and maintain it at this, haemostasis is likely to be achieved. This level is required, for example, to stop bleeding from the tonsil bed after tonsillectomy.

For the treatment of a closed tissue haemorrhage, a lower level—say in the range of 5–20 per cent. for 24–48 hours—is usually sufficient to stop further increase in the size of the haematoma. It is important to appreciate that half the dose of infused Factor VIII disappears from the circulation in 10–12 hours. For this reason infusion once every 24 hours is likely to be required to maintain the level, and in order to attain a level of 50 per cent. it may be necessary to give the Factor VIII from 3 to 5 litres of plasma. It is for this reason that concentrates of Factor VIII have become necessary

Available Materials for the Management of Bleeding in Haemophilia

1. *Whole blood* is used for the replacement of blood loss and is not an effective method of raising the recipient's Factor VIII level. Factor VIII is relatively labile on storage, and thus the content of bank blood is variable.

2. *Fresh plasma or fresh frozen plasma.* Fresh plasma is a satisfactory form of therapy for lesser haemostatic problems, but there are few centres which can provide a constant supply, and for this reason fresh frozen plasma is commonly used. It is separated from the red cells and maintained frozen at $-20°$ C. There is gradual loss of activity, but in most centres it is used within 3 months and by this time the level of Factor VIII may have fallen to 50 per cent. The Christmas factor is more stable than Factor VIII and is well preserved both in frozen plasma and in bank blood.

3. *Cryoglobulin precipitate.* For the preparation of this material blood is collected in a two plastic bag system. It is centrifuged, the plasma transferred into the secondary bag which is then snap frozen, and both it and the plastic bag containing the red cells are put in a refrigerator at 4° C. After standing overnight at this temperature, a cryoglobulin precipitate forms in the secondary pack; the bulk of the plasma is then returned to the red cells, re-constituting the blood for routine transfusion purposes. The cryoglobulin precipitate is re-suspended in the small amount of plasma left in the secondary pack and stored frozen until used. Up to thirty packs may require to be infused daily to maintain a haemostatic level.

4. *Human Factor VIII—lyophil dried preparations.* These are expensive to prepare and involve the sacrifice of plasma. The process is complicated and there is a risk of loss of potency unless meticulous care is used in production. It is likely that as the technique improves, it will become the method of choice.

5. *Animal (bovine and porcine) preparations.* These are powerful preparations of Factor VIII made from porcine or bovine blood. They can be used for a ten-day period in the management of a specific episode in a haemophiliac, but it must thereafter be assumed that the patient is sensitized and that fatal anaphylaxis might result from further injections. The clinician must decide, therefore, to use this material only in episodes of extreme gravity. These preparations are commonly available in the United Kingdom, but are expensive.

Reactions to animal Factor VIII are not uncommon, and include pain along the infusion vein, back pain and rigors. Reactions may lessen after the first few injections; 10 mg. of chlorpheniramine should be given intravenously as a routine in an attempt to reduce the reaction, and procaine injections into the drip may ease the pain along the course of the vein.

Management of Episodes of Bleeding

The site of haemorrhage should be rested as efficiently as possible; oral analgesics are required to relieve pain and appropriate infusion is indicated.

The choice of preparation for replacement therapy depends upon which is most readily available. It is likely to be fresh frozen plasma or cryoprecipitate. If it is thought that a modest rise in Factor VIII is likely to meet the patient's needs, a litre of fresh frozen plasma should be given over a period of about an hour. Many of these patients have had plasma in the past and are liable to sensitivity reactions. Thus wise precautions are pre-infusion oral administration of 25 mg. of promethazine hydrochloride and 100 mg. of oral cortisone or 100 mg. intravenous hydrocortisone.

Whole blood will be needed where a fall in haemoglobin has occurred. The haemoglobin level must be followed at least once daily and blood replaced as required. A falling haemoglobin provides the best evidence of continuing haemorrhage. Usually no attempt should be made to drain the haematoma. Iron is seldom needed unless there has been external blood loss.

A common site for bleeding is around the air passages into the neck and at the root of the tongue, and because of the risk of respiratory obstruction such patients should be given the most powerful source of human Factor VIII available.

Epistaxis should be treated by replacement of Factor VIII and packing with Vaseline gauze or an absorbable pack. Cauterization is contra-indicated in haemophilia, because the subsequent slough causes more problems. Haematuria, either painless or accompanied by renal colic, is common and because renal damage may result, adequate replacement therapy should be given. The fibrinolytic inhibitor, epsilon aminocaproic acid (EACA), may well stop the bleeding because it inhibits the action of the urokinase in the urinary tract, but it should only be used as a last resort because there is a risk of unlysable fibrin occluding the ureter. However, this material may be useful in haemophiliacs with haematuria who have developed Factor VIII inhibitors.

With small open injuries on the skin surface, the bleeding can often be controlled by local pressure. This should not be excessive, otherwise the blood may track backwards into the tissues and cause a greater problem. Russell's viper venom and topical thrombin can be applied, but it should be appreciated that they are of limited value because they cannot produce haemostasis at the point of exit of the blood from severed vessels. Dressings should be left undisturbed unless there is some major reason for inspecting the wound. Bleeding is likely to recur from any haemophilic wound until healing is complete.

Bleeding in relation to the central nervous system can be very serious. Intracranial or spinal extradural haematomata may follow recognized trauma. Whatever else is done in the investigation and management, adequate replacement is required.

The management of acute haemarthrosis is often difficult. Aspiration of the joint even after haemostatic level of Factor VIII in the blood has been reached is often disappointing, because the blood is clotted within the joint. Moreover, in some instances the bleeding is subchondral or even intra-osseous. Appropriate replacement therapy should be given, and the joint splinted with a plaster slab. Occasionally aspiration of a tense knee joint may be indicated, but should only be attempted after adequate replacement therapy. Encasing the whole limb in plaster carries the risk that if bleeding continues, arterial obstruction may result. It is now customary to encourage haemophiliacs to come to hospital as out-patients to receive a plasma infusion as soon as the earliest symptoms of haemarthrosis become apparent. As soon as discomfort permits, gentle active exercises should be instituted under the guidance of an experienced physiotherapist. Weight bearing on the affected limb should not be allowed until the muscles around the joint are strong enough to protect it from further injury. Quadriceps exercises are particularly important. When a patient is put to bed for haemarthrosis of one joint, appropriate measures should be taken to keep the others active. The correction of joint deformities after contractures is a skilled orthopaedic problem, requiring much patience and adequate replacement therapy.

Surgery in the Haemophiliac

In the operative management of the haemophiliac, the objective is to maintain a level of 50 per cent. Factor VIII until the area in question has healed. It is an important rule not to embark on elective surgical procedures unless a 2 weeks' supply of material for replacement therapy can be set aside for this purpose. Before an elective operation, it is essential to determine whether the patient has a Factor VIII inhibitor (circulating anticoagulant); Factor VIII inhibitors develop in a proportion treated with any of the preparations of the human antihaemophilic globulin including fresh frozen plasma. It is a specific inhibitor to the administered Factor VIII. They can be detected by demonstrating that the patient's plasma destroys the Factor VIII when incubated *in vitro* with normal plasma.

It is important to stress to the surgeon operating on a haemophiliac, that meticulous haemostasis is essential and should be carried out by ligature rather than cautery. Once a decision has been taken to operate, it is usually wise to complete it in one stage rather than two because the same degree of Factor VIII cover is required. Intramuscular and subcutaneous injections should be avoided in a haemophiliac. If, for some special reason, subcutaneous injection is necessary, then the area must be supported afterwards with a crepe bandage. This applies, too, to venepuncture sites. Premedication should be given by mouth, and so should analgesics and antibiotics. Aspirin and compounds which contain it should be avoided, because of the increased risk of haemorrhage, particularly into the alimentary tract.

Management of Patients in Intervals between Episodes

A degree of limitation of physical activity proportional to the severity of the defect is essential. One important issue which must be arranged is the conservative care of the haemophiliac's teeth. It carries no particular hazard if adequate care is observed. Nerve block must be avoided and if possible, fillings should be done without analgesia; if necessary, anaesthesia should be local around the tooth. Dental extractions must, of course, be carried out in hospital and the grade of Factor VIII replacement depends on the severity of the haemophilia and on the number of teeth to be extracted. Local dental splints are useful in protecting the socket; their aim is not to exert pressure. The mild haemophiliac needing several extractions may require splints, and management with plasma; the severe haemophiliac needing many extractions will require splints and cover with cryoprecipitate. Replacement therapy will be necessary for a week. Skilled dentistry is essential to minimize trauma. *Calgitex* or other absorbable dressing is placed in the socket soaked in topical thrombin or Russell's viper venom and the splint inserted. An oral antibiotic should be given to cover the period of extraction, for infection adds to the risk of bleeding.

CHRISTMAS DISEASE

In Christmas disease the principles of management are essentially the same as in haemophilia. Fresh frozen plasma is likely to be a more powerful source of Factor IX than of Factor VIII. On the other hand, the Christmas disease patient is at a disadvantage in that there are no generally available concentrates, either human or animal, with which to treat his haemorrhagic episodes. In the United Kingdom probably only one centre can provide replacement therapy for major surgical procedures.

HEREDITARY DISORDERS CHARACTERIZED BY PROLONGED BLEEDING TIME

VON WILLEBRAND'S SYNDROME

Von Willebrand's syndrome affects males and females and is inherited as an autosomal dominant.

It is characterized by a prolonged bleeding time and a deficiency of Factor VIII. The deficiency differs from that in haemophilia in that plasma from a haemophiliac infused into a patient with von Willebrand's syndrome will result in a rise of Factor VIII in the recipient. Furthermore, when normal plasma is infused into a patient with von Willebrand's disease, not only is there the immediate anticipated rise in the Factor VIII level, but a further sustained increase lasting for 24–36 hours; this differs from the response in haemophilia, where the level declines immediately the peak has been reached. The explanation is likely to be that the von Willebrand's patient can create Factor VIII from some precursor material present in the haemophiliac and in the normal plasma. In von Willebrand's disease there may be a deficiency of another factor, for purified Factor VIII preparations may not correct the prolonged bleeding time although normal blood will. The nature of the defect in von Willebrand's syndrome is even more complex, in that under certain specifically standardized conditions the platelets in this disease have impaired adhesiveness to glass.

The incidence of this condition is approximately one in 150,000 of the population in the United Kingdom. It is characterized by bleeding from mucous membranes, particularly of the nose and gastro-intestinal tract, and by menorrhagia. Where access to wounds is available, local measures tend to be more successful in control of bleeding than in haemophilia. In the management of the menorrhagia, epsilon aminocaproic acid may have a role. Pregnancy in these patients can be hazardous at the time of delivery. Replacement therapy with whole blood, fresh frozen plasma or cryoprecipitate may be needed.

OTHER DISORDERS WITH PROLONGED BLEEDING TIME

If we restrict the term 'von Willebrand's syndrome' to patients with a prolonged bleeding time, a deficiency of Factor VIII and a normal platelet count, there is another genetic disorder in which the only demonstrable feature is a prolonged bleeding time.

Recently developed techniques in the study of platelet behaviour are revealing hereditary forms of functional platelet abnormality.

HEREDITARY HAEMORRHAGIC TELANGIECTASIS (OSLER-RENDU-WEBER SYNDROME)

This disorder is inherited as an autosomal dominant, and is characterized by telangiectasis on the nasal mucosa, on the tongue, on the lips and face, on the fingers and in the alimentary tract. The lesions increase in number with the years, and bleeding from them is seldom a serious problem before adult life, when it becomes progressively more troublesome. Because of repeated epistaxis or chronic blood loss into the alimentary tract, patients often present with iron-deficiency anaemia which may be alleviated by constant oral iron therapy. Throughout their later years they are liable to prolonged and troublesome epistaxis. There is no demonstrable laboratory abnormality except a prolonged bleeding time if a telangiectatic area is punctured.

In individual families the pattern tends to be constant. In some, pulmonary arteriovenous aneurysms are common and increase in frequency with advancing years. Aneurysms of other visceral vessels have also been recorded.

There is no curative treatment. Local measures, as for haemophilia, should be used but individual lesions should not be cauterized. Where epistaxis is the main symptom, oestrogens may be of value; they act by inducing a squamous metaplasia of the columnar epithelium of the nasal mucosa, which provides a protective layer over the lesion. Ethinyloestradiol, 0·25 mg., is given daily and increased to 0·5 mg. per day at the end of 4 weeks.

OTHER GENETIC HAEMORRHAGIC DISEASES

Of the coagulation defects, Factor IX deficiency is probably the next most common. This causes a mild haemorrhagic disease affecting males and females with an autosomal recessive type of inheritance. It is most commonly seen in Jews. Factor V deficiency is a rare autosomal recessive defect with a relatively mild haemorrhagic state. Isolated deficiencies of Factors II (prothrombin), VII and X (vitamin K coagulation factors) all occur and do not respond to vitamin K; the inheritance again is autosomal recessive. Factor XII deficiency (or Hageman trait) usually produces no haemostatic problems and the patients are discovered incidentally when it is observed that blood collected without anticoagulant fails to clot. These patients have a major abnormality in their intrinsic thromboplastin system concerned with a failure to respond to contact with foreign surfaces. The absence of a haemorrhagic state is strange and totally unexplained. Factor XIII deficiency (fibrin stabilizing factor) also produces a relatively mild haemorrhagic disease, often presenting soon after birth with bleeding from the umbilical stump. A number of combined deficiencies of these coagulation factors have been reported, the most common one being a combination of Factor V and Factor VIII.

The Ehlers-Danlos syndrome [see Section 4] is a genetically determined connective tissue disorder in which there is a structural defect in the vessel walls which may result in spontaneous haemorrhage. It is inherited as an autosomal dominant.

ACQUIRED HAEMORRHAGIC DISORDERS

THERAPEUTICALLY INDUCED

Heparin

The use of intravenous heparin may occasionally be associated with a haemorrhagic state. When it becomes necessary urgently to neutralize its effect, protamine sulphate should be given intravenously. Heparin and protamine vary in potency, but the usually accepted dose is protamine sulphate, 1–1·5 mg. per 1 mg. (100 Units) of heparin. With intravenous heparin, the quantity of protamine required for neutralization falls rapidly with the lapse of time after the injection of heparin. Heparin neutralization may be required for haemorrhage or before surgery in a heparinized patient.

Coumarin and Indanedione Drugs

The reported incidence of haemorrhage depends on how closely the patients are studied for evidence of bleeding. Minor haemorrhage, for example microscopic haematuria, epistaxis, rectal bleeding, small bruises and subconjunctival haemorrhage, is two or three times as common as major incidents such as gross haematuria or melaena.

Provided the physician in charge of the patient is experienced in the use of the drug of his choice, then it is probable that none of this group carries a greater or a lesser risk of haemorrhage than any other. Inexperience and divided responsibility in the control of therapy increase the occurrence of haemorrhage. Neglect of established contra-indications will again result in an increased incidence of bleeding as does concomitant administration of certain other drugs, especially salicylates. The more ill the patient, the greater the risk of haemorrhage and the liability also increases with advancing years. Certain specific complications of coumarin or indanedione therapy require mention:

1. *Renal.* Microscopic or macroscopic haematuria is probably the commonest form of haemorrhage in patients on coumarin therapy.

2. *Gastro-intestinal.* Twenty-five per cent. of all deaths occurring as a direct consequence of anti-coagulant therapy have been due to massive gastro-intestinal bleeding from a previously unsuspected peptic ulcer. Intestinal obstruction is a well documented complication due to bleeding into the wall of the bowel. Rectal bleeding is usually from haemorrhoids and seldom serious. If alimentary bleeding occurs when the drug effect is not excessive, an occult tumour should be sought.

3. *Pulmonary.* Pulmonary interstitial haemorrhage may occur, and the clinical and radiological features may resemble those of pulmonary embolus.

4. *Neurological.* Subdural haematoma is a recognized complication and should always be considered in patients on treatment who develop headache, mental or neurological abnormalities. Patients on anti-coagulants who receive head injuries should be followed with this possibility in mind.

5. *Ophthalmic.* Subconjunctival haemorrhages are common and usually harmless.

6. *Skin.* Minimal skin purpura and small spontaneous bruises are not uncommon. The platelet count should be checked to exclude thrombocytopenia, especially if the drug administered is phenindione which may produce this change as a toxic reaction. Haemorrhagic cutaneous necrosis is a complication which usually affects the breast. There is extensive haemorrhage into the skin with ensuing necrosis, and the skin may slough leaving an ulcerated area which needs grafting.

7. *Muscle.* Haemorrhage into muscle is unusual, but of all the possible sites bleeding into the rectus sheath is the most common and may cause the patient to present to the surgeon as an abdominal emergency.

8. *Pregnancy, puerperium and menstruation.* Coumarin drugs given to the pregnant patient carry a significant risk to the foetus. Intra-uterine death due to haemorrhage has often been reported. If anticoagulant treatment must be given during pregnancy, only heparin should be used. Oral anticoagulants do not cause a haemostatic problem in the puerperium or in relation to menstruation. At the beginning of the puerperium, the child should not be breast fed because the drug is excreted in the milk.

Treatment. When it is necessary to counteract the coumarin and indanedione drugs, vitamin K_1 should be administered; this is the only vitamin K preparation which can be relied upon to be efficacious. It is given orally or intravenously, depending on the clinical situation. When there is frank haemorrhage and a firm decision is taken that anticoagulants will not be re-introduced, a dose of 25–50 mg. should be given. This will render the patient resistant to further coumarin treatment for about 2 weeks. When there is frank haemorrhage but it is intended to continue treatment later, 15 mg. should be given to reduce the drug effect without cancelling it. When the routine test shows an excessive effect but the patient is not bleeding, a dose of 5 mg. should be prescribed.

Arvin

A purified fraction of the Malayan pit viper venom is now commercially available for the management of thrombo-embolic disease. This is a coagulant venom but the fibrin which forms is unstable and defibrination of the blood results, without obvious clinical evidence of vascular occlusion. *Arvin* is proteolytic to fibrinogen in a different way from thrombin and the polymer which forms is unstable. The fibrinogen breakdown products which are released have an inhibitory effect on the response of platelets to adenosine diphosphate. In other respects the coagulation mechanism is believed to be intact and the action of the venom can be reversed by giving an antivenom and if need be thereafter raising the fibrinogen level by infusion of fibrinogen. Although oozing from venepuncture sites and some bruising have been recorded under the influence of *Arvin*, the haemorrhagic risk in so far as experience has allowed to date, has been small.

Salicylates and other Analgesic Preparations

Salicylates cause a depression of the vitamin K dependent coagulation factors, but probably of more relevance to haemostasis is the effect on the platelets which alters the response to adenosine diphosphate (ADP), preventing secondary ADP release. Other analgesic drugs, for example, phenylbutazone, have a like effect. These platelet changes may well provide an explanation for the haemorrhage which occasionally occurs after the ingestion of salicylates.

Thrombolytic Enzymes

It has been known for more than a century that in certain circumstances clots may undergo spontaneous lysis, but it is only in the last 20 years that detailed knowledge of the enzyme system responsible has become available. There is now evidence that the intravascular administration of plasminogen activators will bring about the lysis of preformed thrombi in man. When plasminogen activation occurs in plasma there is no effect on fibrin or fibrinogen, provided it is not unduly rapid, because the plasma antiplasmin readily inhibits plasmin as it is formed. On the other hand, within a mass of fibrin the intimate spatial relationship of plasminogen and fibrin produces thrombolysis.

The plasminogen activators which are currently in therapeutic use in man are streptokinase and urokinase. Streptokinase is a streptococcal exotoxin prepared from cultures of streptococci. Urokinase is present in human urine and can be extracted from this source, but its recovery is extremely costly. When these activators are given by rapid intravenous infusion, plasminogen activation can temporarily overwhelm the antiplasmin mechanism with the appearance of free plasmin in the circulation. This results in a haemorrhagic state. Thrombin converts fibrinogen to fibrin by splitting off specific fibrinopeptides from the fibrinogen molecule to form a fibrin monomer [see FIG. 64]; fibrin monomer then polymerizes to form a fibrin polymer which gels to form a visible clot. When free plasmin is present in the circulation, the fibrinogen is digested and the ensuing breakdown product becomes incorporated with fibrin monomer as it polymerizes, resulting in delayed and defective polymer formation and hence either a total failure of clot production or the formation of friable, unsound fibrin. Other factors in the genesis of the haemostatic failure in hyperplasminaemia are digestion of the coagulation factors required in the production of blood thromboplastin and the accelerated lysis of such fibrin as does form.

If serious haemorrhage should develop during thrombolytic therapy, then fibrinolytic inhibitors, in particular epsilon aminocaproic acid (EACA), may be required. EACA prevents plasminogen activation and in high concentration it also inhibits the action of plasmin. In taking the decision to use EACA, however, the clinician must appreciate that any fibrin laid down while EACA is in circulation will be resistant to subsequent lysis. Accordingly, if bleeding occurs during thrombolytic therapy, initial reliance should be placed on blood transfusion and if necessary termination of the infusion. EACA should be given only if severe haemorrhage fails to respond to these measures. In such circumstances EACA should be given intravenously, a priming dose of 5 G. followed by 1 G. per hour for 5 hours.

HAEMORRHAGE DUE TO LOCAL FIBRINOLYSIS

Fibrinolysis may contribute to local haemostatic defects without any significant systemic proteolytic activity and without defibrination of the blood. The commonest example of this is continuing bleeding from the prostatic bed after prostatectomy due to the action of urokinase in the urine dissolving fibrin at the site. This blood loss can be markedly reduced by giving EACA orally or intravenously. When this is excreted in the urine it inhibits the action of urokinase. A similar type of local inhibition of fibrinolysis may be attained in certain patients with menorrhagia.

DEFIBRINATION SYNDROME

A description of two situations where defibrination occurs has already been given: after the administration of *Arvin* and after the use of thrombolytic enzymes. Other causes of the defibrination syndrome are listed in TABLE 57. It is probable that the entry into the circulation of thromboplastic tissue factors at the placental site in the obstetrical patient and at the operation site when there is extensive dissection or handling of tissues, explains these two categories. In giant haemangioma, static blood probably coagulates in the large cavernous channels. With an extracorporeal circulation, the haemorrhagic state is complex but an important feature may be intravascular coagulation, although there is also excessive fibrinolytic activity. In carcinomatosis again, intravascular coagulation is likely to be the abnormality although excessive fibrinolytic activity is reported in metastatic carcinoma of the prostate. The bite from a snake with a coagulant venom is a clear-cut example of intravascular coagulation. About 30 years ago Schwartzman showed that in animals the intravenous administration of two consecutive doses of bacteria or their products was followed by wide-spread but localized parenchymatous haemorrhages and cortical necrosis of the kidneys. This generalized Schwartzman phenomenon is due to intravascular coagulation with thrombocytopenia, the platelets presumably being caught up in the fibrin. The haemorrhages are due to local necrosis rather than to haemostatic failure. The clinical syndrome of purpura fulminans is thought to have a similar basis.

TABLE 57

CLINICAL SITUATIONS ASSOCIATED WITH GENERALIZED DEFIBRINATION

1. Obstetrical
   - Abruptio placentae
   - Retained dead foetus
   - Amniotic fluid embolism
   - Septic abortion
2. Surgical
   - Operations (especially on the thoracic viscera) when there is much handling of the lungs, or in other areas involving much dissection of tissue, e.g. excision of the rectum, excision of malignant glands.
   - Giant haemangiomata
3. Mismatched blood transfusion
   - Extracorporeal circulation
4. Carcinomatosis
5. Snake-bite by coagulant snake venoms
6. Schwartzman phenomenon—purpura fulminans

The haemostatic failure in this group of patients with presumed intravascular coagulation, should be managed by blood transfusion, preferably fresh, and fibrinogen. Although the fibrinolytic inhibitor drugs, particularly EACA, have been used in the management of the above conditions, their use should be confined to situations in which increased fibrinolytic activity has been clearly demonstrated.

The value of heparin as an anticoagulant in treatment of some of the above situations is difficult to assess and has as yet been inadequately investigated. The author and his associates have used it in a chronic defibrination syndrome complicating carcinomatosis, and there followed a rapid rise in the fibrinogen. If troublesome bleeding does occur in such a situation, then the use of heparin merits a trial.

BLEEDING FOLLOWING MASSIVE BUT COMPATIBLE BLOOD TRANSFUSION

Generalized haemostatic failure has been observed following massive compatible blood transfusion. The predominant feature is thrombocytopenia, presumably due to loss of the patient's own platelets and failure of those transfused to survive. Other coagulation factors may similarly be reduced; the logical treatment is to give fresh whole blood.

Citrate overdosage has occasionally been blamed, but is unlikely to be responsible because the cardiac effects of hypocalcaemia would long precede any interference with haemostasis. However, 10 ml. of a 10 per cent. solution of calcium gluconate should be administered for every litre of citrated blood given, above a calculated rate of 2 litres of blood per 20-minute period.

A bleeding tendency has occasionally been found after plasma volume expanders, particularly dextran.

CIRCULATING ANTICOAGULANTS

An acquired haemophilia-like disease may be due to the development of circulating anticoagulants, and occurs in certain well documented clinical situations:

1. In patients with haemophilia or Christmas disease treated with the appropriate missing factor, in any of the available preparations; presumably this is an antigen-antibody response. It is not known why this should develop in some patients and not in others.
2. In female patients following completion of a pregnancy.
3. As a complication of systemic lupus erythematosus where the characteristic feature, in addition to the presence of the inhibitor, is a deficiency of prothrombin.
4. In otherwise healthy people, often elderly, who develop a clinical condition indistinguishable from severe haemophilia and where the inhibitor present is a specific inhibitor of Factor VIII.

There is no known specific treatment for these inhibitors. When one develops in haemophilia or Christmas disease, infusion of the missing factor must, if at all possible, be avoided as this merely stimulates further production. Where the titre of the inhibitor is not excessively high, it may be possible temporarily to overwhelm it with large doses of Factor VIII or Factor IX.

DEFICIENCY OF VITAMIN-K DEPENDENT COAGULATION FACTORS

These factors, prothrombin (Factor II), Factors VII, IX and X have much in common. They are reduced in concentration when the patient becomes vitamin-K deficient or receives coumarin or indanedione drugs, and share certain laboratory properties. Furthermore, deficiency of Factor VII, Factor X, and to a lesser extent prothrombin, is reflected in a prolongation of the one-stage prothrombin time.

Haemorrhagic Disease of the Newborn

This is due to a coagulation defect in which the vitamin-K dependent factors are deficient. The blood of a normal newborn infant is by adult standards usually slightly deficient in these factors. Their concentrations fall immediately after birth, reaching their lowest level on the third day. Thereafter they rise steadily, reaching adult levels within a few weeks. Body levels of the vitamin are low at birth, and particularly in premature infants or when the mother has been undernourished. The lack of gut flora during the first few days of life may be an important cause in the development of this disorder. Immaturity of the newborn liver, especially in the premature infant, is also likely to be a factor.

Bleeding may arise from the gastro-intestinal tract, the umbilical stump, the nose or mouth or into the skin. Intracranial haemorrhage has occasionally occurred.

It is questionable whether routine administration of vitamin K to all mothers of newborn infants is justifiable, but it should be given prophylactically in prematurity, difficult or instrumental delivery, birth injury, foetal distress or anoxia. The appropriate dose for the mother is 5 mg. of vitamin K_1 parenterally as soon as possible after labour has started; for the infant 1 mg. of vitamin K_1 should be given intramuscularly on the first day of life. In the treatment of fully developed haemorrhagic disease, 1–2 mg. of vitamin K_1 should be given by intramuscular injection daily until the one-stage prothrombin time is corrected. Transfusion may be necessary to manage the blood loss and will also help temporarily to correct the coagulation defect. Particularly in premature infants, the liver may not respond fully to vitamin K_1 by production of the missing coagulation factors. Synthetic water-soluble analogues of vitamin K_1 should not be used in the treatment of haemorrhagic disease of the newborn, in view of the risk of producing haemolytic anaemia, bilirubinaemia and kernicterus. Vitamin K_1 is believed to be without this danger.

Vitamin K Deficiency in Obstructive Jaundice or Intestinal Malabsorption

The prophylactic administration of vitamin K_1 prior to biliary surgery is an almost invariable routine, and thus haemorrhage in obstructive jaundice is now seldom seen. A dose of 10–25 mg. intravenously is effective in correcting this type of abnormality within a few hours. Other malabsorption states and protracted diarrhoea may occasionally be associated with vitamin K deficiency.

The practising clinician should become familiar with the use of vitamin K_1 as this meets the needs of all the relevant clinical situations. Although the water-soluble and other analogues may be effective in obstructive jaundice, their limitations in other situations are such that their over-all usefulness is limited.

LIVER DISEASE

Parenchymal liver disease may be associated with a haemorrhagic state which is of multifactorial origin. Frequently these patients have portal hypertension and hypersplenism with thrombocytopenia. They may have a deficiency of any of the coagulation factors, but the antihaemophilic globulin (Factor VIII) is often surprisingly well maintained. In addition they have an excessively active fibrinolytic state possibly due to failure to remove activator from the circulation. Apart from replacement therapy, which is often disappointing, there is little effective treatment. Vitamin K_1 and epsilon aminocaproic acid have both been used, but their value is uncertain.

URAEMIA

Patients with uraemia usually have a platelet-type haemorrhagic state with purpura and bleeding from mucous membranes, particularly epistaxis and menorrhagia. Defects in their platelets have recently been defined, in particular the pattern of the response of the platelets to adenosine diphosphate may be abnormal. The treatment is clearly the management of the uraemia where this is possible; local measures such as packing in the nose and endocrine therapy to suppress menstruation may be needed.

THE PURPURAS

Definition

This term includes all of those conditions characterized by multiple spontaneous capillary haemorrhages chiefly in the skin and mucous membranes.

VASCULAR PURPURAS

There are a number of non-thrombocytopenic purpuras, the majority of which are not described here. With a few exceptions, these do not represent significant haemostatic failure.

Mechanical compression of small vessels may lead to purpura over the presenting part in newborn infants or over the face and neck following prolonged spells of coughing or vomiting or after a convulsion. Orthostatic purpura may develop on the legs of elderly people, particularly in association with varicose veins.

A variety of skin diseases may have a purpuric element. The purpuric lesion of the Henoch-Schönlein syndrome [see Section 4] has an inflammatory component and is easily distinguished from the simple petechia.

Non-thrombocytopenic purpura may follow the administration of drugs. In the United Kingdom carbromal is a common cause; others sometimes responsible are penicillin, sulphonamides, salicylates, barbiturates, meprobamate, and iodides. On other occasions some of these drugs appear to cause thrombocytopenia by an immune mechanism and, if there is an antigenic relationship between capillary endothelium and platelets, it is possible that these lesions could be similarly explained.

Senile purpura is seen in both sexes and especially from the seventh decade of life. The platelet count is normal. The lesions are almost always confined to the extensor surface of the forearms and backs of the hands, but sometimes occur on the face in relation to spectacle frames. The individual haemorrhages are often 2 or 3 cm. across; the affected skin is usually thin, inelastic and pigmented. The blood spreads more widely and is absorbed more slowly than in the skin of younger subjects. Similar lesions may be seen in middle-aged patients on steroid therapy.

SCURVY [see Section 4]

DYSPROTEINAEMIAS

A bleeding tendency is a feature of a variety of conditions where the common denominator is an abnormal increase in plasma globulins; these include hypergammaglobulinaemia, macroglobulinaemia and cryoglobulinaemia. Haemorrhages in such patients may be both purpuric and ecchymotic. Various explanations for haemostatic failure have been put forward but there is no universal agreement and it is likely that several factors may be responsible. Increased viscosity of the blood may lead to slowing and stagnation in the capillary circulation with resulting impairment of nutrition, hypoxia and increased capillary permeability. There may be infiltration of the vascular wall with abnormal protein or with the responsible underlying tumour. The abnormal globulins may interfere with platelet function. An increased level of fibrinogen breakdown products has been described. Thrombocytopenia may be present as a consequence of marrow infiltration.

THROMBOCYTOPENIC PURPURA

The bleeding in this condition is usually into the skin as petechiae and below the skin as small bruises. Bleeding from mucous membranes is characteristic, particularly epistaxis, gastro-intestinal bleeding and menorrhagia. Microscopic haematuria may occur but seldom is the only feature. Intracranial haemorrhage does undoubtedly occur, but is probably much rarer than many of the accounts of this disease would indicate. Retinal haemorrhages occur in many thrombocytopenic patients; they are surprisingly rare in idiopathic thrombocytopenic purpura, but common in severe pernicious anaemia, leukaemia, aplastic anaemia or marrow replacement by tumour.

There is no simple relationship between the number of platelets and the severity of bleeding but it is seldom significant unless the platelet count is lower than 50,000 per mm.^{3} and usually with frank haemorrhage it is much lower. Knowledge of the factors which influence production of platelets, their release from the marrow and their utilization is scanty. The lifespan of the normal human platelet is probably 8–14 days, but it is uncertain whether they perish through a normal ageing process or by random removal from the circulation, perhaps in the course of physiological haemostasis.

The causes of thrombocytopenia are listed in TABLE 58.

TABLE 58

CAUSES OF THROMBOCYTOPENIA

THROMBOCYTOPENIA PROBABLY DUE TO FAILURE OF PLATELET PRODUCTION

(Megakaryocytes usually reduced in number)

- Aplasia or hypoplasia of megakaryocytes:
  - Idiopathic aplastic anaemia
  - Drugs, chemicals and ionizing irradiation
- Neoplastic disease of the marrow:
  - Leukaemia
  - Malignant lymphomata
  - Myelomatosis
  - Secondary carcinomatosis
  - Myelofibrosis
- Megaloblastic anaemia
- (Vitamin B_{12} or folic acid deficiency)

THROMBOCYTOPENIA PROBABLY DUE TO EXCESSIVE DESTRUCTION OF PLATELETS IN THE PERIPHERAL CIRCULATION

(Megakaryocytes in the marrow—at least normal in number and possibly increased)

- Probably due to immune mechanisms:
  - Drug sensitivity
  - Following acute infections

Idiopathic thrombocytopenic purpura
Association with disseminated lupus erythematosus
Neonatal thrombocytopenia
Probably due to other causes:
Defibrination syndrome
Thrombotic thrombocytopenic purpura
Giant haemangioma
After extracorporeal heart-lung bypass
Probably due to dilution with platelet-poor blood:
Massive blood transfusion
Thrombocytopenia of uncertain aetiology:
Thrombocytopenia in patients with splenomegaly-hypersplenism
Paroxysmal nocturnal haemoglobinuria
Burns; heat stroke

THROMBOCYTOPENIA DUE TO FAILURE OF PRODUCTION OF PLATELETS BY THE MARROW

Aplasia or Hypoplasia of the Marrow

In so-called idiopathic aplastic anaemia, thrombocytopenia is a constant feature. In the recovery phase the megakaryocytes may lag behind other marrow elements and the patient be left with a normal haemoglobin and white cell count although still markedly thrombocytopenic. In the hypoplastic and aplastic states following drugs and chemicals a distinction must be made between cytotoxic drugs used as antineoplastic agents which will constantly cause thrombocytopenia [see Section 4], and those to which some individual sensitivity is responsible.

As an occasional effect in susceptible individuals the following drugs may cause thrombocytopenia: chloramphenicol, tetracyclines, streptomycin, sulphonamides, thiosemicarbazones, methoin, troxidone, phenylbutazone, meprobamate, carbimazole, potassium perchlorate. This list is not exhaustive.

No particular form of therapy can be relied upon to restore marrow function, and the chief principles of treatment should be to avoid further exposure to possible toxic substances and to keep the patient in reasonable health by transfusion of fresh platelet-rich blood or plasma platelet concentrates. Antibiotics should be used when infections occur but not in long-term prophylaxis; they should be given orally, for intramuscular injections in any form of haemostatic failure are inadvisable. Steroid therapy deserves a limited trial and some control of the bleeding may occur even when the platelet count is unaffected. If there is no improvement in 4 weeks the question arises of whether the risks of continuous steroid therapy are greater than any possible gain. It is doubtful whether a small maintenance dose of steroid has any non-specific tonic effect on the vascular component of capillary haemostasis and it is only indicated when there is an apparent relationship between administration of steroids and maintenance of platelet count. Other hormone preparations such as testosterone and oxymetholone have been used but their roles are ill defined. The question of splenectomy may arise, but it is usually the last resort in a therapeutically destitute situation and the chances of any significant response are remote. Marrow transplantation has not been shown to be of value except possibly in identical twins.

Neoplastic Disease of the Bone Marrow

The therapeutic issue here is obviously that of the underlying problem and need not be dealt with further in this section.

Megaloblastic Anaemia

In thrombocytopenia associated with megaloblastic anaemia the marrow will respond with a brisk outpouring of platelets at the same time as the reticulocyte response occurs. Where folic acid deficiency is present it is important to remember that it may be due to malabsorption and that deficiency of vitamin K may contribute to the haemostatic failure.

THROMBOCYTOPENIA, PROBABLY DUE TO THE EXCESSIVE DESTRUCTION OF PLATELETS IN THE PERIPHERAL CIRCULATION

DRUG SENSITIVITY

There are two main mechanisms whereby drugs cause thrombocytopenia. In addition to direct damage to megakaryocytes the drug's action may be directed against circulating platelets. In this case the drug appears to act as a hapten to the platelets and the resulting antigen causes an antigen-antibody reaction. An initial dose sensitizes the patient and thereafter he rapidly becomes thrombocytopenic whenever the drug is taken and as soon as it is stopped the platelet count returns to normal. When the patient has recovered from the drug his platelets studied *in vitro* can be shown to aggregate on addition of the drug. This mode of action has been established as the cause of thrombocytopenia due to apronal (*Sedormid*), quinine, quinidine, antazoline (an antihistamine) and sulphamethazine (a sulphonamide). It is probable that other drugs including the barbiturates, thiazide diuretics and some of the antidiabetic compounds, particularly chlorpropamide, produce thrombocytopenia in the same way.

The onset of thrombocytopenic purpura due to drug sensitivity is usually sudden and will follow a single dose of the drug which the patient had received on a previous occasion, or develop after a week of continuous therapy. No treatment is usually required apart from withdrawal of the drug.

FOLLOWING ACUTE INFECTIONS

Thrombocytopenia is seen in the acute phase of some infections; examples are smallpox, typhoid fever, epidemic haemorrhagic fever and infectious mononucleosis. More often, particularly in childhood, it may follow almost any of the common infective illnesses, such as measles, rubella, chickenpox or mumps. The purpura is usually seen 10 days to 3 weeks after the onset of the preceding infection, suggesting a hypersensitivity reaction to the causative agent. Some of these patients are labelled as having idiopathic thrombocytopenic purpura and it may well be that in others the infecting agent has not been recognized. The management is better considered under acute idiopathic thrombocytopenic purpura; this condition is thrombocytopenia without alteration in the red cells or white cells except in so far as bleeding might explain these. The bone marrow should contain at least a normal number and often has an increased number of megakaryocytes.

IDIOPATHIC THROMBOCYTOPENIC PURPURA (I.T.P.)

Definition

Thrombocytopenic purpura for which no cause can be found, accompanied by no changes in the red or white blood cells other than those due to haemorrhage and associated with normal or increased numbers of megakaryocytes in the bone marrow, many of which appear to be inactive.

Clinical Picture

Before making this diagnosis all recognized causes of thrombocytopenia, including drugs, current infections, infections in the recent past and disseminated lupus erythematosus, must be excluded. In the clinical management of these patients it is important to differentiate between acute and chronic I.T.P.

The *acute form* is most often seen in childhood. The sexes are affected with equal frequency and the onset is sudden, commonly following an infective illness. Apart from the purpura, physical examination is usually negative. It is unusual for the spleen to be palpable; indeed, splenomegaly is a point against a diagnosis of idiopathic thrombocytopenic purpura. This condition usually runs a self-limiting course, ending in spontaneous and permanent remission after a period of 10 days to a few months. If remission has not occurred after 3 months it is unlikely and the condition should be regarded as chronic I.T.P.

A well defined but poorly understood form of idiopathic thrombocytopenia occurs in Africa and is called 'onyalai'. It is characterized by haemorrhagic bullous formation on the buccal mucosa in addition to the more conventional features.

Chronic I.T.P. usually starts insidiously and is predominantly a disease of young adults, affecting women three times more often than men. There usually is a history of easy bruising for some months with crops of petechiae and menorrhagia.

Untreated, this condition runs a fluctuating course often with long periods of freedom from symptoms although the platelet count may never return to normal. Correlation between the platelet count and the clinical manifestations may be poor. These patients may have serious mucous membrane haemorrhage from the nose, the alimentary tract or the uterus, but bleeding is seldom profuse except at the onset. Death from cerebral haemorrhage is rare after the first few weeks of the disease.

Diagnosis

There is constant, if variable, thrombocytopenia and such platelets as are seen may be giant or otherwise irregular in morphology. The bone marrow contains normal or increased numbers of megakaryocytes, but there is little evidence that they are actively engaged in the production of platelets. The red blood cells and haemoglobin level show no changes other than those due to haemorrhage. The white blood cells are quantitatively and qualitatively normal. Special techniques may allow the demonstration of antibodies against platelets in the sera of about 50 per cent. of patients with I.T.P. The erythrocyte sedimentation rate is normal.

It is important that the tests necessary to exclude systemic lupus erythematosus be carried out in every such patient.

Treatment

Blood transfusion will be required where significant blood loss has occurred; if there is evidence of continuing bleeding, fresh blood should be given. In discussing the management of this condition one can only lay down certain general guide-lines and the appropriate treatment for each case must be decided on its own merits. It is usual to give 40–60 mg. of prednisone daily when the patient is first seen, but such doses should not be maintained for long periods. If the platelet count rises to normal the dosage of steroids should be gradually reduced and withdrawn completely, if possible. In some patients the raised platelet count is maintained after withdrawal. In another group the platelet count falls when the steroid therapy is discontinued and here, provided at least 3 months have elapsed since the onset of symptoms, steroid therapy should be re-introduced and splenectomy carried out. In a third group there will be no rise in the platelet count and, when the 3-month period has passed, one should proceed to splenectomy. If, for some reason, splenectomy cannot be carried out or if thrombocytopenia persists afterwards a decision must be taken whether the continuing thrombocytopenia or the continuing administration of steroid drugs is the greater risk; in the author's experience it is the continued steroid therapy. Many patients live for years with a reduced number of platelets and experience nothing more alarming than occasional subcutaneous haematomata or skin purpura. This does not deny that intracranial haemorrhage or gastro-intestinal bleeding may occur, but it is exceptional in long-standing chronic I.T.P.

If a point in time, 3 months after the onset of symptoms, has passed then the following situations indicate that the patients should be offered splenectomy:

1. There has been no rise in the platelet count.
2. The platelet count can only be maintained so long as steroid therapy is continued.

In proceeding to splenectomy the chances of success or failure should be clearly explained to the patient or the relatives. In general one can say that approximately half the patients in the situations indicated above, subjected to splenectomy have an immediate and sustained rise in the platelet count. In about a quarter there is no rise in the platelet count and he is no better off as a consequence of his splenectomy, although there is a suggestion that symptoms are fewer after operation. In the remaining one-quarter the platelet count rises after splenectomy, but the rise is not sustained, symptoms and platelet count subsequently pursuing a fluctuating course.

The operation must be carried out under full steroid cover, intravenous steroid administration being used for the oral doses missed on account of the anaesthesia.

The platelet count is followed in the immediate post-operative phase and if there is a significant rise within 24 hours a satisfactory response is likely. In those responding well the platelet count may rise well above normal before settling down at about the normal level. When this occurs the steroid therapy can be 'tapered off' starting 2 or 3 days after the operation unless there is some new complicating feature. When a satisfactory platelet response has not been obtained, the issue is more difficult but it is the author's policy to maintain steroids until the wound has healed. Thereafter, even if the platelet count has not risen, it is our practice to reduce and discontinue steroids believing that in the long term the risk of the steroid is greater than the risk of bleeding. Good results can be forecast in those patients in whom the platelet count rises well above the normal by the third or fourth day after operation. There is no way, unfortunately, of predicting pre-operatively which patients will respond well to splenectomy. In many accounts of this topic the question of an accessory spleen causing the failure of the response to splenectomy is raised. This issue can be decided by the technique of injecting the patient's own heat-treated tagged red cells and attempting to detect evidence of splenic tissue. Unless this is found, there is no justification for re-exploration of the abdomen.

On follow-up of patients with apparent idiopathic thrombocytopenic purpura a small proportion later develop unequivocal evidence of systemic lupus erythematosus. For this and other reasons these patients should be placed on long-term outpatient follow-up.

Idiopathic thrombocytopenic purpura during pregnancy can be a problem. If clinical manifestations are severe steroids may have to be given as previously indicated. If it persists, splenectomy may be performed in late pregnancy, possibly combined with Caesarean section. In coming to a decision it should be recalled that many patients with thrombocytopenia have been delivered without undue bleeding.

ASSOCIATION WITH SYSTEMIC LUPUS ERYTHEMATOSUS

Idiopathic haemolytic anaemia and thrombocytopenic purpura may co-exist without concurrent evidence of systemic lupus erythematosus or they may be accompanied by clinical and laboratory criteria of this disorder. When thrombocytopenia is the presenting problem in systemic lupus erythematosus then the management should be as described above for idiopathic thrombocytopenic purpura in spite of suggestions that splenectomy may aggravate the underlying disease. It should always be remembered that in systemic lupus erythematosus there may be other causes, such as circulating anticoagulants, for haemostatic failure.

NEONATAL THROMBOCYTOPENIA

Infants born to mothers with idiopathic thrombocytopenic purpura are more likely than not to be thrombocytopenic at the time of birth, even though the mother's thrombocytopenia may be in remission following splenectomy. The probability is that this form of neonatal thrombocytopenia is due to the transfer of a platelet antibody across the placenta from the mother to the infant.

Occasionally thrombocytopenia has occurred in the otherwise healthy infant of mothers who have never suffered from thrombocytopenic purpura and it has been suggested that this might represent iso-immunization of the mother against the infant's platelets. Haemolytic disease of the newborn is occasionally complicated by thrombocytopenia and it is possible that such infants have received maternal antibodies produced against the infant's platelets as well as against the red cells. Alternatively the thrombocytopenia might result from intravascular haemolysis. Exchange transfusion may cause transitory thrombocytopenia but it is doubtful if this has ever led to significant bleeding.

The child with neonatal thrombocytopenia may be observed to have skin petechiae and sometimes more extensive ecchymosis, gastro-intestinal bleeding and bleeding from the umbilical cord. It should be remembered, of course, that some petechiae are common in normal infants at birth particularly over the presenting part and are likely to be due to mechanical compression of the veins during delivery.

Although death has been known to occur in this condition, the majority of the infants recover, the disease process 'burning itself out' over a period of 10 days to 3 weeks. The most dangerous time for the infant is during delivery and in the first few days of life. Intracranial haemorrhage is the chief cause of death. The condition is self-limiting and there is no specific therapeutic issue. Platelet transfusions may be indicated.

THROMBOTIC THROMBOCYTOPENIC PURPURA (MICROANGIOPATHIC THROMBOCYTOPENIA; MICROANGIOPATHIC HAEMOLYTIC ANAEMIA)

This is a condition characterized clinically by fever, jaundice, thrombocytopenia, haemolytic anaemia, with transitory and fluctuating neurological manifestations [see p. 1033]. It is usually a fatal disease within days or weeks. The blood film, in addition to the reduction in platelet numbers, usually shows distorted, fragmented red cells. In view of the similarity to the generalized Schwartzman reaction there is at least a theoretical case for giving heparin and this has been reported favourably by some. The thrombolytic enzyme urokinase is another theoretical alternative.

It may be that the thrombocytopenia and haemolytic anaemia reported as an occasional association with eclampsia is caused in the same way.

THROMBOCYTOPENIA ASSOCIATED WITH HAEMANGIOMA

Giant cavernous haemangiomata may be associated with thrombocytopenia and fibrinogen depletion. It is likely that this condition is due to continuous intravascular coagulation either within the haemangioma itself or throughout the circulation. Regression of the haemangioma will often be followed by cure of the haemostatic problem. Surgical excision of the tumour, however, is often very hazardous and radiotherapy may be the treatment of choice. A considerable proportion of these haemangiomata tend to become relatively smaller as the child grows and the haemostatic defect may disappear. Some have used anticoagulants in the management of these patients and have shown that this is associated with a reversal of the fibrinogen depletion and the lowered platelet count.

THROMBOCYTOPENIA IN PATIENTS WITH SPLENOMEGALY (HYPERSPLENISM)

The term 'hypersplenism' is often used to describe patients who are anaemic, neutropenic and thrombocytopenic. In the case of hepatic cirrhosis and portal hypertension there is a well established relationship in this context in that removal of the spleen results in the correction of the neutropenia, the thrombocytopenia and to some extent of the anaemia. Splenectomy is both the treatment and the ultimate diagnostic test for hypersplenism. In many cases, however, the clinical effects of the anaemia, neutropenia and thrombocytopenia are not sufficiently severe to justify splenectomy and any question of splenectomy in portal hypertension has to be considered together with the question of a shunt procedure for relief of the portal hypertension.

In other pathological conditions causing splenomegaly the relationship is often less clear-cut although it undoubtedly may coexist. For example, malignant lymphomata may be associated with anaemia, neutropenia and thrombocytopenia and the same form of hypersplenism may indeed be present. In these circumstances, however, it may be difficult to dissociate this component of the haematological problem from other causes such as marrow infiltration.

PAROXYSMAL NOCTURNAL HAEMOGLOBINURIA

Purpura and bleeding are uncommon in this condition and indeed thrombosis is a common feature. Thrombocytopenia, however, is characteristic. It may often be a manifestation of bone marrow hypoplasia.

REPLACEMENT THERAPY IN THROMBOCYTOPENIA

Human platelets are thought to survive as long as 10 days in the circulation, but the haemostatic value of platelet transfusion seldom lasts more than a few days. Transfused platelets are probably removed from the circulation much more rapidly than normally either by immune mechanisms or by utilization for haemostatic purposes. Furthermore, even with the most concentrated platelet preparations it is extremely difficult to raise the recipient's count to normal levels. There is also evidence that many patients who receive multiple platelet transfusions develop iso-antibodies against the donor platelets with progressive shortening of survival time.

The viability of transfused platelets is largely dependent upon the storage time before infusion and upon the degree of manipulation to which they have been subjected. The smallest loss of viable platelets results from the use of whole blood within about one hour of bleeding from the donor or platelet rich plasma prepared by slow centrifugation and transfused without delay. Clearly, blood withdrawn for the purpose of giving platelets should have the minimum of agitation and frothing. Platelet concentrates have theoretical attractions but their preparation demands centrifugation and loss of platelets from aggregation and reduced viability are inevitable. Despite the extensive use of platelet concentrates in many large transfusion services, there is little firm information on their role.

HAEMORRHAGIC THROMBOCYTHAEMIA

Paradoxically, not only does thrombocytopenia cause haemorrhage but thrombocythaemia may also do so; thrombocythaemia, of course, may also be associated with thrombosis. Thrombocythaemia may occur as one feature of the myeloproliferative syndrome [see p. 1037] when red cells and white cells are normal. It may be a feature in chronic myeloid leukaemia or polycythaemia vera. The commonest manifestations are gastro-intestinal bleeding, epistaxis and bleeding from the gums and mouth. Purpura is very rare but extensive ecchymoses are common. The spleen may be enlarged; on the other hand a condition of hyposplenism with splenic atrophy may be found or thrombocythaemia may be a consequence of splenectomy. The platelet count is usually over 1,000,000 per $mm.^3$ and the platelets are often morphologically abnormal with giant and irregular forms. There may be accompanying anaemia due to gastro-intestinal bleeding. The marrow shows marked hyperplasia of the megakaryocytes. It can be shown even with normal platelets artificially concentrated in a test system, that there is interference with blood thromboplastin formation. It could be that, in the presence of an excessive amount of phospholipid from the platelets, the final prothrombin converting principle does not form normally because there is so much lipid that the appropriate other relevant coagulation components do not all react with the same lipid molecule. The condition may be compatible with many years of active life and may indeed be surprisingly benign. When thrombocythaemia is associated with chronic myeloid leukaemia or myelofibrosis and polycythaemia vera then the prognosis is that of the associated condition. The treatment of choice is the use of radioactive phosphorus in a dosage of 3–4 millecuries, but more may be needed when there is accompanying polycythaemia vera. Splenectomy is contra-indicated as this may aggravate the problem.

REFERENCES

Biggs, R. (1969) The treatment of haemophilia, *J. roy. Coll. Physns (Lond.)*, **3**, 151.

Biggs, R., and Macfarlane, R. G. (1962) *Human Blood Coagulation and its Disorders*, Oxford.

Biggs, R., and Macfarlane, R. G. (1966) *Treatment of Haemophilia and Other Coagulation Disorders*, Oxford.

Dormandy, K. M. (1969) Von Willebrand's disease, *J. roy. Coll. Physns (Lond.)*, **3**, 211.

Douglas, A. S. (1962) *Anticoagulant Therapy*, Oxford.

Hardisty, R. M., and Ingram, G. I. C. (1965) *Bleeding Disorders: Investigation and Management*, Oxford.

Poller, L., ed. (1969) *Recent Advances in Blood Coagulation*, London.

Ratnoff, D. D. (1968) *Treatment of Hemorrhagic Disorders*, New York.

A. S. Douglas

DISEASES OF THE HAEMOPOIETIC AND RETICULO-ENDOTHELIAL SYSTEMS

The blood is of great importance in clinical medicine because it is so easy to examine and provides vital information for the diagnosis and treatment of many diseases. This chapter will include those diseases which involve the cellular elements of the blood produced by the bone marrow—the red cells, granulocytes and platelets; those produced primarily in the lymph nodes and spleen—the lymphoid cells and monocytes, and the haemorrhagic disorders.

TABLE 59 shows the normal values of the common haematological investigations.

The red cells, whose primary function is the transport of oxygen, are biconcave discs. This is difficult to appreciate on ordinary light microscopy, but is shown well by three-dimensional pictures obtained with the stereoscan as shown in PLATE 19, which also shows various abnormal cells. There are many morphological changes which may occur, and these are discussed when the different diseases are considered.

The leucocytes produced by the bone marrow (granulocytes) are the neutrophils which are phagocytic and essential for combating infections; eosinophils which are associated with allergic diseases, but whose precise function is not clear; and basophils whose function is completely unknown. Until quite recently the function of lymphocytes, which are formed in the lymph nodes and spleen, was unknown, but it is now established that they have a key role in immune mechanisms. Lymphocytes are the direct mediators of cell-mediated immunity, as shown by delayed hypersensitivity reactions and graft rejection. They are also indirectly involved in the formation of circulating antibodies, since plasma cells are derived from lymphocytes. The third leucocyte, the monocyte, is a phagocytic cell and probably plays an essential part in modifying antigens prior to stimulation of lymphoid cells to initiate an immune reaction.

The platelets are concerned with the prevention of haemorrhagic phenomena and will be considered under haemorrhagic diseases.

REFERENCE

DACIE, J. V., and LEWIS, S. M. (1968) *Practical Haematology*, 4th ed., London.

ANAEMIA

This is without doubt the commonest blood disorder in clinical medicine, and is defined as occurring when the haemoglobin concentration in the blood falls below the lower limit of normal [TABLE 59].

The best classification of the different forms of anaemia is by aetiology, for the essential procedure on finding a patient to be anaemic is to determine the cause.

Anaemia may be due to:

1. Blood loss in the form of acute or chronic haemorrhage.
2. Lack of essential factors for the formation either of haemoglobin itself or the red cell stroma (dyshaemopoietic anaemias). Such factors include iron, vitamin B_{12}, folic acid, vitamin C, protein, and thyroxine.
3. Bone marrow failure (hypoplastic anaemia) due to lack of erythropoietin, the action of drugs or irradiation, and unknown causes (idiopathic).
4. Infiltration of the bone marrow with malignant cells, e.g. secondary carcinoma, leukaemia, myelomatosis, or with fibrous tissue or bone as in myelosclerosis.
5. Increased red cell destruction (haemolytic anaemia).
6. Miscellaneous anaemias occurring in the course of other diseases (secondary anaemias).

Clinical Manifestations of Anaemia of any Cause

The symptoms of anaemia depend not only on the severity, but also on the speed at which the anaemia has developed. For example, with haemorrhage, acute blood loss will produce much greater disturbance than will chronic loss. The symptoms are due to the decreased oxygen-carrying capacity of the blood and include dyspnoea on exertion, palpitations, fainting attacks and oedema of the ankles. In the elderly, ischaemic muscular pain both from the heart (angina pectoris) and legs (intermittent claudication) may occur. The signs include pallor, particularly of the mucous membranes of the mouth, the conjunctiva, the nail beds and palmar creases, and in the cardiovascular system a high output state with tachycardia, a high pulse pressure, oedema and heart failure may be present.

Diagnosis

Once anaemia is suspected this is confirmed by measuring the haemoglobin concentration in the peripheral blood. It is then necessary to determine which type of anaemia is present, and subsequently why that type of anaemia should be present in the patient. In the first instance this is done by studying the morphology of the red blood cells and the other cellular elements of the blood, determining the red cell indices, and where indicated carrying out appropriate additional tests. The significance of these investigations will be discussed under the different varieties of anaemia.

HAEMORRHAGE

The anaemia of acute blood loss presents no diagnostic problem. The source of the loss is obvious and the clinical state is one of peripheral circulatory failure. It is important to remember that in haemorrhage whole blood is lost and the haemoglobin will only begin to

TABLE 59

NORMAL HAEMATOLOGICAL VALUES

VARIATION IN HEALTH

Red cells	
Men	4·5–6·5 × 10^6/mm³.
Women	3·9–5·6 ,,
Infants (full-term, cord blood)	4·0–5.6 ,,
Children, 3 months	3·2–4·5 ,,
Children, 1 year	3·6–5·0 ,,
Children, 10–12 years	4·2–5·2 ,,
Haemoglobin	
Men	13·5–18·0 g./100 ml.
Women	11·5–16·5 ,,
Infants (full-term, cord blood)	13·6–19·6 ,,
Children, 3 months	9·5–12·5 ,,
Children, 1 year	11·0–13·0 ,,
Children, 10–12 years	11·5–14·8 ,,
Packed cell volume (PCV; haematocrit value)	
Men	40–54%
Women	35–47%
Infants (full-term, cord blood)	44–62%
Children, 3 months	32–44%
Children, 1 year	36–44%
Children, 10–12 years	37–44%
Mean corpuscular volume (MCV)	
Adults	76–96 μm³.
Children, 3 months	83–110 ,,
Children, 1 year	77–101 ,,
Children, 10–12 years	77–95 ,,
Mean corpuscular haemoglobin (MCH)	
Adults	27–32 pg.
Children, 3 months	24–34 ,,
Children, 1 year	23–31 ,,
Children, 10–12 years	24–30 ,,
Mean corpuscular haemoglobin concentration (MCHC)	
Adults	30–35%
Children, 3 months	27–34%
Children, 1 year	28–33%
Children, 10–12 years	30–33%
Mean corpuscular diameter (dry films)	
Adults	6·7–7·7 μm.
Reticulocytes	
Adults and children	0·2–2·0%
Infants (full-term, cord blood)	2–6%
Blood volume	
Red cell volume, men	26–33 ml./kg.
women ..	22–29 ,,
Plasma volume	40–50 ,,
Total blood volume	60–80 ,,
Leucocytes	
Adults	4,000–11,000/mm³.
Infants (full-term, at birth) ..	10,000–25,000 ,,
Infants (1 year)	6,000–18,000 ,,
Children, 4–7 years	6,000–15,000 ,,
Children, 8–12 years	4,500–13,000 ,,

Differential leucocyte count

Adults:	Neutrophils	40–75%	2,500–7,500/mm³.
	Lymphocytes	20–45%	1,500–3,500 ,,
	Monocytes	2–10%	200–800 ,,
	Eosinophils	1–6%	40–440 ,,
	Basophils	<1%	0–100 ,,

Platelets	150,000–400,000/mm³.
Bleeding time (Ivy's method) ..	Up to 11 min.
Coagulation time (Lee and White's method, 37° C.)	5–11 min.
Prothrombin time (brain-thromboplastin time, 1-stage (Quick))	10–14 seconds
Prothrombin consumption index ..	0–30%
Plasma fibrinogen	150–400 mg./100 ml.

Osmotic fragility (at 20° C. and pH 7·4)

%NaCl	Before incubation % lysis	After incubation for 24 hours at 37° C. % lysis
0·20	100	95–100
0·30	97–100	85–100
0·35	90–99	75–100
0·40	50–95	65–100
0·45	5–45	55–95
0·50	0–6	40–85
0·55	0	15–70
0·60	0	0–40
0·65	0	0–10
0·70	0	0–5
0·75	0	0
0·80	0	0
0·85	0	0
Median corpuscular fragility (MCF) (% NaCl)	0·40–0·445	0·465–0·590

Autohaemolysis (37° C.)	
48 hours, without added glucose	0·2–2·0%
48 hours, with added glucose ..	0–0·9%
Cold-agglutinin titre (4° C.) ..	<64
Serum iron	80–180μg./100 ml.
Total iron-binding capacity ..	250–400 ,,
Serum vitamin B_{12}	160–925 pg./ml.
Serum folate	6–21 ng./ml.
Red cell folate	160–640 ng./ml.
Plasma haemoglobin	1–4 mg./100 ml.
Serum haptoglobins	30–200 mg. Hb-binding per 100 ml.
Sedimentation rate (method of Westergren) (at 20±3° C.)	
Men	0–5 mm. in 1 hour
Women	0–7 mm. in 1 hour
Heterophile (anti-sheep red cell) agglutinin titre	<80
After absorption with guinea-pig kidney	<10

[Dacie, J. V., and Lewis, S. M. (1968) *Practical Haematology*, 4th ed., J. &. A. Churchill, London.]

fall when the blood volume is restored by the formation of more plasma, a process which takes many hours. The haemoglobin concentration under these circumstances is no guide to the amount of blood lost, which is assessed by the degree of peripheral circulatory failure.

Chronic blood loss is the commonest cause of iron deficiency anaemia which is considered in the next section.

DYSHAEMOPOIETIC ANAEMIAS

These are due to a deficiency in one of the essential factors for the synthesis of haemoglobin or the manufacture of normal red cell stroma.

IRON DEFICIENCY

This is the commonest form of anaemia in Britain, and is usually due to chronic blood loss, although inadequate iron intake and malabsorption account for a number of the cases.

Haematological Findings

The initial diagnosis of iron deficiency anaemia is suspected by finding a hypochromic microcytic anaemia. The basic defect is in the formation of haem for haemoglobin, and hence red cells are produced which contain a lower concentration of haemoglobin than normal; the MCHC is therefore reduced [see TABLE 59]. The red cells also show anisocytosis and poikilocytosis and in severe forms target cells may even be seen. Although iron deficiency is the commonest, it is not the only cause of a microcytic hypochromic anaemia, as other conditions in which haemoglobin synthesis is defective may give this blood picture, e.g. thalassaemia and sideroblastic anaemia. It is therefore necessary to confirm the diagnosis either by establishing the common cause, chronic haemorrhage, or by further investigation. The two most useful tests are first the serum iron and iron binding capacity, the former being low and the latter increased in iron deficiency; and secondly staining particles obtained on aspiration of the bone marrow for iron and assessing the iron stores in this way. The normoblasts in the marrow frequently present a ragged appearance.

Special Clinical Features

In addition to the symptoms and signs of anaemia, there are special manifestations which suggest the presence of iron deficiency. Koilonychia, a spoon-shaped deformity of the nails, is diagnostic of iron deficiency. Glossitis may be present, and in middle-aged women there may be dysphagia due to atrophic changes in the post-cricoid region—the Plummer-Vinson or Paterson-Kelly syndrome—which shows a web on barium swallow, and which is a pre-malignant condition leading to post-cricoid carcinoma. The spleen is sometimes palpable, but seldom grossly enlarged.

Aetiology of Iron Deficiency Anaemia

There are several causes of iron deficiency anaemia which may be summarized as follows:

1. *Inadequate iron intake.* This is particularly likely in infancy and old age.
2. *Inadequate absorption of iron from the gut.* This occurs with gastric lesions particularly following gastrectomy and with lesions of the small bowel such as that due to gluten-sensitivity (idiopathic steatorrhoea).
3. *Increased demand for iron.* At certain times in life, particularly in menstruating women and during pregnancy, increased amounts of iron are required.
4. *Chronic haemorrhage.* This is obvious unless the bleeding is coming from the gastro-intestinal tract, the common lesions being carcinomas of the stomach or large bowel, hiatus hernia, peptic ulceration, regional enteritis, ulcerative colitis, diverticulitis and haemorrhoids.

Inadequate Iron Intake. The iron deficiency anaemia of infancy (previously called the nutritional anaemia of infancy or the anaemia of prematurity) is now rare in Britain but is still common in the developing countries. The haemoglobin at birth ranges between 14 and 19 g. per 100 ml., but falls steadily to reach a level of 11–12 g. per 100 ml. at 2–3 months and then slowly climbs to reach a maximum at the age of 14 years. In the early months, since breast milk does not contain adequate amounts of iron, although it contains more than dried cow's milk, the infant uses its iron stores and anaemia is therefore commoner in twins and premature babies. The reason that iron deficiency in infancy is now becoming rare in Britain is that iron deficiency is corrected in the mother, and that many proprietary dried milks and baby foods contain iron supplements. Another recently discovered contributory factor is gastro-intestinal haemorrhage due to sensitivity to cow's milk.

If overt iron deficiency anaemia is present the infant should be treated with iron by mouth in the form of ferrous sulphate or ferrous fumarate syrup, the latter being the more palatable. There is rarely any need for parenteral iron, the use of which should be avoided if possible.

Inadequate intake of iron at other ages is uncommon except for the very poor and elderly who may have a diet not only lacking sufficient iron but also folic acid and vitamin C, thus presenting a complex haematological state.

Inadequate Absorption of Iron. The role of the stomach in the absorption of iron is not completely understood, but there is no doubt that patients with achlorhydria do not absorb iron as well as those who produce gastric acid, and there is some evidence to suggest that the stomach produces other factors which may promote the absorption of iron from the upper part of the small intestine. Other factors which control the absorption of iron include the degree of iron deficiency, the lower the body iron the greater the absorption; the form of the iron, ferrous salts being better absorbed than ferric; and the presence of lesions in the small intestine, particularly those of gluten-sensitivity. Under some circumstances, e.g. in haemochromatosis and in alcoholism particularly when pancreatitis is present, excessive iron absorption may occur, and since iron is only excreted in minute amounts iron overload results. This also occurs in patients with refractory anaemia who receive multiple blood transfusions.

From this it is clear that iron deficiency anaemia may arise following the different forms of gastrectomy, and the situation may be further complicated by chronic haemorrhage from anastomotic or recurrent ulceration. Iron deficiency due to malabsorption may occur in patients with chronic gastritis, and parietal cell antibodies may be found although their significance is uncertain. Similarly malabsorption of iron may occur as part of the malabsorption syndrome [see Section 7] but it is commonest in gluten sensitivity. Again, some causes of malabsorption such as regional ileitis may be accompanied by bleeding as well. Iron absorption is probably best assessed by giving ^{59}Fe by mouth and then measuring the residual radioactivity using a whole-body counter.

Increased Demand for Iron. This occurs particuarlly in menstruating women and during pregnancy. The chronic blood loss of menstruation means that women require more iron than men, and it is sometimes difficult to assess in a woman with iron deficiency whether the menstrual loss is sufficient to explain the anaemia or whether a search must be made for another cause, such as bleeding from elsewhere, inadequate diet, or malabsorption. The anaemia of pregnancy is more complex. Certainly a considerable amount of iron is required for the foetus, but this is partially offset by amenorrhoea. In addition there is an increase in plasma volume causing a fall in haemoglobin (the physiological anaemia of pregnancy), and there is also an increased demand for folic acid which may cause a mild macrocytic anaemia or occasionally an overt megaloblastic anaemia as well. It is now established practice to give both iron and folic acid prophylactically during pregnancy. Rarely, a megaloblastic anaemia may arise in pregnancy due to vitamin B_{12} deficiency [see p. 1030].

Chronic Blood Loss. It cannot be overemphasized that iron deficiency anaemia must be presumed to be due to blood loss until proved otherwise. Various malignant diseases of the gut, in particular the caecum and colon, may present with an iron deficiency anaemia without any abdominal symptoms. All patients with unexplained iron deficiency anaemia should be investigated for gastro-intestinal blood loss, by looking for occult blood in the stools either chemically or by injecting ^{51}Cr labelled red cells and by barium studies.

Treatment

If there is acute blood loss, or the haemoglobin is very low, blood transfusion is required, but usually the anaemia is best corrected by giving oral iron. The British National Formulary lists only four preparations of oral iron but there are over sixty proprietary preparations. Ferrous sulphate is the cheapest, and is usually satisfactory given in a dose of 200 mg. three times a day. Occasionally this causes gastro-intestinal symptoms, nausea, vomiting, diarrhoea or abdominal pain, in which case other preparations may be tried including ferrous gluconate, fumarate, or succinate or ferric ammonium citrate. Occasionally when there is impaired absorption of iron, or if oral preparations cannot be tolerated, parenteral iron may be required. This can be given by the intramuscular route as an iron sorbitol injection (*Jectofer*), or intravenously as saccharated iron oxide (*Ferrivenin*) or iron dextrin injection (*Astrafer*). It is important that only the correct amount should be given and this is calculated from the severity of the anaemia and the weight of the patient. A recent technique has been to use a total-dose infusion, but this carries the risk of systemic reactions, particularly acute hypersensitivity, which may be very severe. Similar reactions may occur with the other parenteral methods of administration.

DEFICIENCY OF VITAMIN B_{12} AND FOLIC ACID

Deficiency of either of these factors leads to a megaloblastic anaemia.

Haematological Findings

Since the basic defect in megaloblastic anaemia is in the maturation of the erythrocyte and not in the synthesis of haemoglobin, fewer red cells are produced but they contain full amounts of haemoglobin and tend to be large, i.e. the peripheral blood shows a macrocytic normochromic anaemia with an increased MCV and a normal MCHC [see TABLE 59]. The production of leucocytes and platelets is also affected, leading to leucopenia and thrombocytopenia. The neutrophil leucocytes may show hypersegmented polymorphonuclear cells. The bone marrow is characteristic, with marked hypercellularity; the red cell series show megaloblastic changes, the most striking feature being that the development of the nucleus is delayed so that the nucleated red cells become filled with haemoglobin while the nucleus remains primitive, with an open chromatin pattern. In the granulocyte series, in addition to hypersegmented polymorphonuclear cells, giant metamyelocytes are present.

Aetiology

As with any vitamin deficiency there may be inadequate intake, inadequate absorption, excessive demand, and in the case of folic acid inability to utilize it properly.

Inadequate Intake. Vitamin B_{12} deficiency due to inadequate dietary intake is excessively rare, and only occurs in the rigid vegetarians who will not consume animals or animal products (Vegans). This is not true of folic acid, of which the major source is fresh vegetables and which is easily destroyed in cooking. In Britain this type of folic acid deficiency is most commonly found in the elderly poor with an inadequate diet. It is also an important factor in the anaemia of alcoholism.

Inadequate Absorption. *Lesions of the stomach*—the commonest form of megaloblastic anaemia in temperate climates is Addisonian pernicious anaemia. Vitamin B_{12} (the extrinsic factor) cannot be absorbed from the terminal ileum unless Castle's intrinsic factor produced by the stomach is also present. In pernicious anaemia there is failure to produce intrinsic factor. Other lesions of the stomach leading to vitamin B_{12} deficiency are total gastrectomy, and sometimes partial gastrectomy with consequent atrophy of the gastric cells in the stomach remnant. It is important to remember that a normal individual has two to five years' supply of vitamin B_{12} stored in the liver so there may be considerable delay following gastrectomy before vitamin B_{12} deficiency becomes apparent.

Lesions of the small bowel—apart from the diseases which specifically affect the terminal ileum, e.g. Crohn's disease or following surgical resection, most of the small bowel lesions which cause a megaloblastic anaemia do so because of deficiency of folic acid, which is largely absorbed in the jejunum. These include tropical sprue, gluten-sensitive enteropathy (non-tropical sprue, coeliac disease) and the blind-loop syndrome, details of which are considered on pages 709 and 711. An unusual cause of vitamin B_{12} deficiency occurs in Scandinavia due to the fish tapeworm *Diphyllobothrium latum* which lives in the duodenum and consumes the ingested vitamin B_{12}.

Increased Demand. The major example is in pregnancy, where mild folic acid depletion is the rule unless there is additional dietary intake. For this reason folic acid is given together with iron to all pregnant women. Increased amounts of folic acid are also required when there is increased haemopoiesis, as occurs in haemolytic anaemia.

Inability to Utilize Folic Acid. This occurs with the folic acid antagonists, methotrexate and pyrimethamine, and also in patients receiving continuous anti-epileptic treatment with phenytoin, primidone, and phenobarbitone. Trimethoprim prevents the conversion of folic acid to the biologically active derivative folinic acid by antagonizing the action of folic acid reductase.

Pernicious Anaemia. (Addisonian Anaemia). Of all the causes of megaloblastic anaemia pernicious anaemia needs special mention. The fundamental abnormality is an atrophic gastritis with failure of the stomach to produce intrinsic factor, which is usually accompanied by achlorhydria as well. Antibodies to both intrinsic factor and gastric parietal cells may be present.

A family history of pernicious anaemia is quite common, and relatives of patients with this disease may show low vitamin B_{12} levels, impaired absorption, and antibodies to intrinsic factor. There is also a racial incidence, being commoner in those of Northern European stock, less frequently found in Southern Europe, and very rare in Negroes and Asiatics. The other interesting thing about patients with pernicious anaemia is that they are more likely to develop gastric carcinoma than the normal population.

Clinical Manifestations

Apart from symptoms due to the underlying cause, both folic acid and vitamin B_{12} deficiency produce glossitis, and a megaloblastic anaemia with leucopenia and thrombocytopenia. However, only vitamin B_{12} deficiency causes the neurological changes of peripheral neuropathy, and subacute combined degeneration of the spinal cord, with both posterior column and pyramidal tract lesions [see Section 15]. The neurological picture may therefore be confusing, but it is essential always to keep the possibility of vitamin B_{12} deficiency in mind, because if treated early the lesions are reversible, but if left may become irreversible.

Diagnosis

The diagnosis of megaloblastic anaemia is made by the changes in the blood and bone marrow already described. Further tests have to be carried out to determine which variety of megaloblastic anaemia is present. These include:

Serum Folate and Vitamin B_{12} Level. These will be reduced below the lower limit of normal in folate and vitamin B_{12} deficiency respectively, except when trimethoprim is responsible.

Tests of Vitamin B_{12} Absorption. This is carried out by giving vitamin B_{12} labelled with radioactive cobalt by mouth together with a large intramuscular injection of unlabelled vitamin B_{12} (1000 μg.) to raise the blood level above the renal threshold. The amount of radioactivity in the urine over the ensuing 24 hours is a measure of the absorption. This is the Schilling test, which can be used to distinguish malabsorption of vitamin B_{12} due to lack of intrinsic factor, from that due to lesions of the terminal ileum, by giving the oral dose with and without intrinsic factor. The older tests for gastric acidity have been replaced by the Schilling test, because it is possible, particularly in juvenile pernicious anaemia, to have lack of intrinsic factor without complete achlorhydria.

Tests for Folic Acid Deficiency. The two tests in clinical practice are folic acid clearance, and the histidine loading test. In the folic acid clearance test the rate of removal of folic acid from the blood following the intravenous injection of a standard quantity of folic acid gives an index of folate deficiency, the faster the removal the greater the deficiency. Also, in folic acid deficiency histidine is not completely converted into glutamic acid, with the result that formiminoglutamic acid is excreted in the urine following a histidine loading dose (the FIGLU test).

Differential Diagnosis

Once it has been established that deficiency of either folic acid or vitamin B_{12} exist, the appropriate investigations to discover the causes (as already discussed) should be carried out. One difficulty which arises is when a macrocytic anaemia is discovered without megaloblastic changes in the bone marrow. This may occur in haemolytic anaemia, liver disease, hypothyroidism, scurvy, protein malnutrition, and anaemias associated with marrow infiltration from any cause. Another difficulty which occurs, particularly in pernicious anaemia, is when neurological manifestations are present, suggesting vitamin B_{12} deficiency, but the patient is not anaemic. This, in fact, does not exclude the diagnosis and a serum vitamin B_{12} level and marrow examination may well confirm the presence of B_{12} deficiency.

Treatment

Deficiency of folic acid can be corrected by giving the compound by mouth in a dose of 5 mg. thrice daily. Vitamin B_{12} deficiency can be corrected by giving the vitamin in the form of cyanocobalamin, or hydroxycobalamin by intramuscular injection. In patients without neurological involvement an initial dose of 200 μg. followed by 100 μg. twice weekly for 2 weeks will restore both the blood and body stores to normal. Thereafter 100–200 μg. once a month if sufficient for maintenance, and injections have to be continued for the rest of the patient's life. If neurological manifestations are present, weekly injections of 100 μg. may be needed for up to 6 months. Oral preparations of vitamin B_{12} with intrinsic factor are not yet satisfactory. Folic acid should not be given to patients with vitamin B_{12} deficiency, as this may precipitate subacute combined degeneration of the spinal cord.

DEFICIENCY OF OTHER ESSENTIAL FACTORS

These include vitamin C, protein and thyroxine. In uncomplicated deficiency of these factors there is either a macrocytic or normocytic anaemia, although on rare occasions vitamin C deficiency has been associated with megaloblastic changes. However, with both protein and vitamin C deficiency there are usually other deficiencies such as iron and folic acid as well which complicate the blood picture.

HYPOPLASTIC ANAEMIA

Synonym. Aplastic anaemia.

Definition

A form of anaemia due to hypoplasia of the bone marrow, and usually accompanied by failure to produce normal granulocytes and platelets, resulting in pancytopenia.

Aetiology

Hypoplasia of the bone marrow may be caused by many factors which may be classified as follows:

Congenital Red Cell Aplasia (Diamond-Blackfan syndrome). This is a rare congenital erythroid hypoplasia, possibly due to an abnormality in tryptophan metabolism. It usually becomes apparent about the 2nd or 3rd month of life, and may respond to corticosteroids. Some cases remit at puberty but in others it proves fatal in early childhood.

Familial Hypoplastic Anaemia (Fanconi's anaemia). This is a rare form of pancytopenia, occurring in families, and usually associated with other congenital abnormalities, such as skeletal deformities particularly involving the radius and thumb together with dwarfism, testicular hypoplasia and pigmentation of the skin. Treatment with androgens and corticosteroids may be beneficial (see below) but rarely affects the white cells or platelets.

Chemical Agents. Two types of hypoplasia due to chemical agents may be recognized:

1. Drugs which regularly cause marrow depression. These include all the cytotoxic agents used in the treatment of malignant disease [see Section 4].

2. Drugs which rarely cause marrow depression. The hypoplasia here is due to an idiosyncrasy and may occur with many compounds including anti-epileptic drugs (e.g. methoin, troxidone), antibacterial agents (chloramphenicol, sulphonamides), antirheumatic drugs (phenylbutazone and gold), antithyroid drugs (methyl thiouracil) and many others. For a full list see de Gruchy (1970). Under this heading may be included certain industrial poisons, such as benzene, trinitrotoluene, insecticides, aniline dyes and hair dyes containing paraphenylenediamine.

In these patients there is no strict relationship between the dose and the development of the hypoplasia. As far as drugs are concerned chloramphenicol and phenylbutazone may both produce a severe hypoplasia from which recovery may not occur.

Ionizing Radiation. This is an obvious cause of marrow hypoplasia and is dose dependent.

Post-viral. Hypoplastic anaemia may follow virus infections, particularly viral hepatitis, but may respond well to androgens (see below).

Pure Red Cell Aplasia. This is a rare form of hypoplasia of the bone marrow in adults which may be associated with a thymoma and/or abnormalities in immunoglobulin, such as hypogammaglobulinaemia. It affects only the red cell series, and the leucocytes and platelets are normal. When a thymoma is present the anaemia may respond to thymectomy.

Lack of Erythropoietin. In chronic renal disease failure to produce erythropoietin leads to red cell hypoplasia and contributes to the anaemia of uraemia.

Idiopathic. Many cases of hypoplastic anaemia occur for no apparent reason.

Haematology

Except for the cases of pure red cell aplasia, there is a pancytopenia with granulocytopenia, thrombocytopenia and a normocytic normochromic anaemia. The red cells may show morphological abnormalities and have a shortened survival contributing further to the anaemia. Occasionally the white cells are chiefly affected (agranulocytosis) and sometimes the platelets are the only elements affected. In other instances granulocytopenia or thrombocytopenia appear first and is followed by pancytopenia. The bone marrow may be difficult to aspirate but is predominantly hypocellular. Sometimes the diagnosis is difficult due to the occasional hypercellular particle and a bone-marrow trephine is needed.

Clinical Manifestations

The clinical features are very similar to those seen in acute leukaemia with infections due to granulocytopenia, haemorrhage due to thrombocytopenia, and anaemia. The spleen and liver are not usually enlarged and lymphadenopathy is not a feature.

Treatment

Obviously a careful social, occupational and past history must be taken to exclude any of the known aetiological agents, exposure to which must be stopped. Supportive measures to correct the anaemia, by blood transfusion, to treat infections immediately by antibiotics, and to lessen haemorrhage by limiting trauma and if necessary giving platelet transfusions, must be used. For many years both androgens and corticosteroids have been used and have produced remissions in some cases. At first testosterone was used, but better results have been obtained with oxymetholone. Both have to be used in large doses (oxymetholone, up to 300 mg. daily for an adult). Corticosteroids, such as prednisone, 40 mg., may be useful and can act synergistically with androgens. Androgens should be tried for at least 3 months before being abandoned.

Course and Prognosis

Between 10 and 20 per cent. of patients may recover completely. Some die rapidly, but others can live for many years supported by regular blood transfusions. They usually die of overwhelming infection, haemorrhage or heart failure due to iron overload following multiple transfusions.

INFILTRATION OF THE BONE MARROW

Infiltration of the bone marrow with malignant cells or fibrous tissue produces either a pancytopenic or a leuco-erythroblastic anaemia. This is fully discussed under the heading of myelofibrosis.

HAEMOLYTIC ANAEMIA

This form of anaemia is due to a shortened survival of red cells, due to premature destruction in the blood (intravascular haemolysis), or the reticulo-endothelial system. There are certain features shared by all forms of haemolytic anaemia.

First, excessive red cell destruction leads to an increased production of unconjugated (pre-hepatic) bilirubin, which may rise to a level causing clinical jaundice. Faecal and urinary urobilinogen are increased, but bilirubin does not appear in the urine unless pigment gall-stones are formed. These may lodge in the common bile-duct, resulting in obstructive jaundice.

Secondly, marrow hyperplasia occurs with an increase both in red cell production and in the premature release of reticulocytes into the peripheral blood. The degree of anaemia depends on the balance between the rates of destruction and production of red cells.

Thirdly, if there is any increase in plasma haemoglobin, this will combine with an $alpha_2$ globulin, haptoglobin, which is then removed from the circulation. In florid intravascular haemolysis the excess of haem in the blood combines with albumin to form methaemalbumin, and free haemoglobin and methaemoglobin may be found in the urine. Chronic intravascular haemolysis leads to haemosiderinuria due to the deposition of iron in the tubular cells of the kidney, which are subsequently shed into the urine.

The degree of haemolysis can be assessed by labelling the red cells with an isotope, usually ^{51}Cr, and following the radioactivity in the blood. This technique can also be used to determine the sites of red cell destruction by external counting; this can show, for example, whether cells are being destroyed chiefly in the spleen, in which splenectomy may be beneficial.

Many other investigations are required to determine which type of haemolytic anaemia is present, and these will be considered in detail below. There are many causes of haemolysis which may be classified as follows:

Haemolysis due to Intrinsic Red Cell Abnormalities

Inherited:

Abnormalities of shape—spherocytosis and elliptocytosis.

Abnormalities of haemoglobin synthesis—thalassaemia, sickle-cell anaemia, etc.

Enzyme defects—glucose-6-phosphate dehydrogenase, pyruvate kinase.

Acquired:

Paroxysmal nocturnal haemoglobinuria.

Abnormalities External to the Red Cell

Mechanical trauma--burns, microangiopathic haemolysis, following the use of teflon in heart surgery, and march haemoglobinuria.

Chemicals—phenylhydrazine, lead, sulphones, snake venom, etc. (see below).

Infections—malaria, Oroya fever and *Clostridium welchii.*

Antibodies—incompatible blood transfusion, haemolytic disease of the newborn, and auto-immune haemolytic anaemias.

Hypersplenism—this can occur with an enlarged spleen from many causes.

HEREDITARY SPHEROCYTOSIS

Synonym. Familial acholuric jaundice.

Definition

A hereditary disease in which the red cells are formed as spheres [PLATE 19], not as biconcave discs, due to abnormal lipid metabolism in the cell membrane. It is inherited as a Mendelian dominant and chiefly affects the European races. The abnormality is present from birth, although it may not become apparent until childhood or even later in life.

Haematological Findings

The peripheral blood will show the presence of many microspherocytes together with polychromasia due to an increased number of reticulocytes. Spherocytes can accommodate more haemoglobin than normal red cells, and the M.C.H.C. may therefore be raised. The red cells show increased osmotic fragility due to the inability of spherocytes to accommodate any more water without rupturing. The fully oxygenated corpuscles show gross haemolysis in 0·45 per cent. solution of sodium chloride, and lesser degrees of haemolysis in stronger solutions, sometimes even as high as 0·8 or 0·85 per cent. solution. The normal values for osmotic fragility are shown in TABLE 59. Anaemia may or may not be present, depending on the balance between red cell production and destruction, but occasionally haemolytic crises may occur in which the patients become profoundly anaemic.

Clinical Manifestations

The clinical manifestations consist of anaemia and jaundice, both of varying intensity. The severity of the anaemia varies from time to time and from patient to patient. Sometimes crises occur in which erythropoiesis fails due to marrow aplasia. The cause of these is unknown, but possibly infection is a factor. Since the jaundice is haemolytic there is no bilirubin in the urine, hence the term 'acholuric jaundice'. In addition, the spleen is almost invariably palpable, pigment gall-stones may occur and leg ulceration may be present.

Diagnosis

This usually presents no problem. The presence of a haemolytic anaemia with spherocytes in the peripheral blood, a palpable spleen, and increased osmotic fragility of the red cells, together with a family history, makes the diagnosis virtually certain. The only other major cause of spherocytosis is auto-immune haemolytic anaemia, and in this condition the direct antiglobulin (Coombs) test is positive, whereas it is always negative in hereditary spherocytosis.

Treatment

Since the red cells are selectively destroyed in the spleen, splenectomy cures the anaemia and prevents jaundice and the formation of pigment stones, but does not, of course, affect the basic abnormality, and spherocytes continue to be produced. Splenectomy is best avoided in the first few years of life if possible, because if it is done at this time there is an increased incidence of infections.

HEREDITARY ELLIPTOCYTOSIS

Like hereditary spherocytosis this is an inherited abnormality in which the cells are elliptical in shape. In the majority there are no signs of excessive haemolysis, but when there is a haemolytic anaemia it is completely controlled by splenectomy, which is the treatment of choice.

HEREDITARY ENZYME DEFICIENCIES

GLUCOSE-6-PHOSPHATE DEHYDROGENASE

Synonym. Primaquin-sensitive anaemia.

This is commoner in Negroes, and of the European populations in Italians, Greeks and Sephardic Jews. It is inherited by an incompletely dominant sex-linked gene with variable expressivity. Most of the time these patients are not anaemic, but if exposed to certain chemical compounds haemolysis (which can be very severe) can result. The major precipitating factors include the antimalarial drugs, particularly primaquin and pamaquine; the sulphonamide group; the antipyretics and analgesics, particularly aspirin and phenacetin; the nitrofurantoins, and the fava bean, *Vicia fava* (favism).

PYRUVATE KINASE DEFICIENCY

This is one of the causes of hereditary non-spherocytic haemolytic anaemia. It is transmitted as a recessive and only homozygotes have the overt disease.

The anaemia which may appear in infancy varies greatly in severity from patient to patient. Splenomegaly is usual. Splenectomy is not curative but often reduces transfusion requirements.

PAROXYSMAL NOCTURNAL HAEMOGLOBINURIA

Synonym. Marchiafava-Micheli syndrome.

This is a rare disease which in its classical form consists of paroxysms of haemoglobinuria, particularly at night, but some patients never in fact develop frank haemoglobinuria. However, there is always persistent haemosiderinuria due to chronic intravascular haemolysis. It is an acquired defect of adult life in which the red cells become exquisitely sensitive to the action of complement and are much more readily haemolysed in an acid serum than normal red cells. This forms the basis for the diagnostic test (the acid haemolysis or Ham test). The white cells and platelets are also affected in this disease, and there is an accompanying leucopenia and thrombocytopenia presenting the picture of pancytopenia. As a result of this, patients may suffer from infections as well as haemolytic anaemia, but the most serious complications are due either to haemorrhage or to thromboses which may occur both in the arterial system, such as the cerebral arteries, or in the venous system, for example in the pelvic veins or portal vein. The only treatment is by blood transfusion, preferably with 'washed' red cells, and many patients die within the first few years from vascular lesions, particularly thromboses.

HAEMOLYSIS DUE TO MECHANICAL TRAUMA

Haemolysis may result from the traumatic destruction of red cells within the blood stream. In *march haemoglobinuria*, intravascular haemolysis may occur following marching or running, particularly on hard surfaces for long periods of time in apparently fit young adults. It can be prevented by placing sorbo rubber inside the shoes, and is thought to be due to some vascular abnormality in the blood vessels of the feet. It is a completely harmless condition, although the passage of red urine following violent exercise of this type naturally causes alarm.

In burns intravascular haemolysis may occur for two reasons. First, the red cells may actually be destroyed during the process of burning, and secondly the passage of red cells through the abnormal arterioles and capillaries in burnt tissue leads to the fragmentation of the red cells.

The same phenomenon is found in the condition of *microangiopathic haemolytic anaemia*, which may occur in acute renal disease with hypertension. Once again the passage of red cells through the abnormal arterioles leads to fragmentation of the red cells with haemolysis.

Finally, the use of teflon in heart surgery has produced a few cases of chronic intravascular haemolysis, because if the patch in the heart fails to be covered with endocardium the red cells are forced directly on to the raw teflon leading to severe damage to the cells. Similar consequences have followed prosthetic valve replacements and have even been reported with calcific aortic stenosis.

HAEMOLYTIC ANAEMIA DUE TO DRUGS AND CHEMICALS

These may be divided into three groups. First those

which regularly cause haemolysis due to their direct action on the red cells; these include phenylhydrazine, naphthalene and nitrobenzine, lead, the sulphones such as dapsone, and large doses of phenacetin and acetanilide. It has recently become apparent that patients receiving large doses of phenacetin develop intravascular haemolysis with fragmentation of the red cells, and this is frequently difficult to diagnose because the patients will not admit to taking large quantities of phenacetin daily.

Secondly, there are various drugs which only occasionally cause haemolysis, either due to a lack of the enzyme glucose-6-phosphate-dehydrogenase (which has already been considered), or to hypersensitivity. The drugs chiefly involved here being antimalarials, para-aminosalicylic acid (PAS), and phenacetin. Quinine was particularly likely to cause haemolysis when used in the treatment of malignant tertian malaria.

Thirdly, an immune-type haemolytic anaemia is rarely induced by drugs. In one variety intravascular haemolysis occurs when the drug is administered after the patient has received an initial 'sensitizing' dose some 10 days or more previously. This has been recorded with penicillin, stibophen and sulphonamides. In a second variety a chronic haemolytic state with a positive antiglobulin test has appeared after months or years of exposure to the drug. This has been reported with methyldopa and mefenamic acid.

HAEMOLYSIS DUE TO INFECTIONS

Anaemia may occur in many bacterial infections, presumably due to bone marrow depression, but there are three infections in which frank haemolysis occurs.

First, *Clostridium welchii* infection, which arises most commonly in Britain following abortion, produces severe intravascular haemolysis and the features of profound toxaemia with pyrexia.

Secondly, malaria, in which the parasites undergo division in the red cells with the disruption of the cells at regular intervals, producing tertian or quartan fever [see Section 2].

Thirdly, Oroya fever due to *Bartonella bacilliformis*, which is a disease occurring in South America transmitted by the sand fly, with direct invasion of the red cells by the organism producing haemolysis [see Section 2].

HAEMOLYSIS DUE TO ANTIBODIES

This type of anaemia is characterized by the presence of antibodies directed against the red cell, which can invariably be detected by the direct antiglobulin (Coombs) test, and which are sometimes present in the serum as well. Such antibodies may be introduced into the body either by the administration of incompatible blood or in haemolytic disease of the newborn, or they may arise *de novo* in the so-called auto-immune haemolytic anaemias. The principles of the antiglobulin test are represented diagrammatically in FIGURE 66.

INCOMPATIBLE BLOOD TRANSFUSION

The most obvious example of haemolytic anaemia due to antibodies is incompatible blood transfusion. In 1900 Landsteiner and his colleagues showed that iso-antibodies existed in human sera and that basically there were four main blood groups as shown in TABLE 60. The naturally occurring agglutinins will agglutinate and haemolyse red cells containing antigens against which they are directed. For example, if a group B recipient is given group A blood, the A cells will be destroyed by the anti-A in the recipient's plasma. This discovery led to the establishment of blood transfusion as a routine procedure in clinical medicine, with blood grouping and cross-matching as prerequisites. Since then many other blood groups have been discovered, particularly the Rhesus group, but with these systems iso-antibodies do not exist, so that prior stimulation with incompatible cells has to be given before antibodies develop. With modern techniques of cross-matching, incompatible blood should never be given, and in dire emergency group O Rhesus negative blood can be given with considerable safety to patients who have never been transfused or pregnant in the past. Most of the mistakes in which incompatible blood has been given have in fact been due to administrative errors such as failure to check the label of the donor bottle before it is given, or the placing of an incorrect label on the bottle. Should incompatible blood be given the clinical syndrome is one of acute intravascular haemolysis with fever, severe lumbar back pain, followed by haemoglobinuria, and even severe oliguria due to renal tubular necrosis.

REAGENTS:

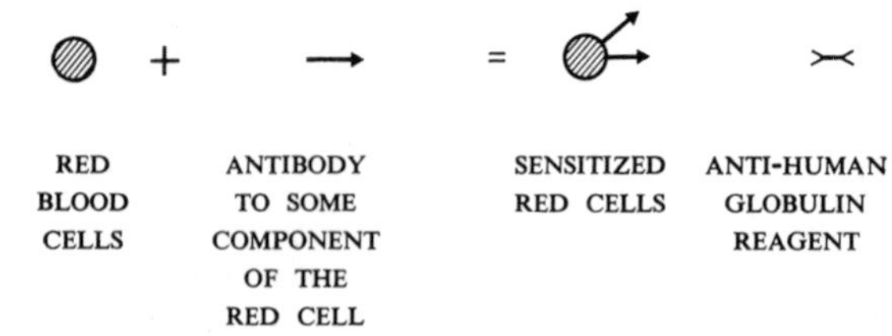

The addition of the anti-human globulin reagent to sensitized red cells causing agglutination is the basis of the antiglobulin test.

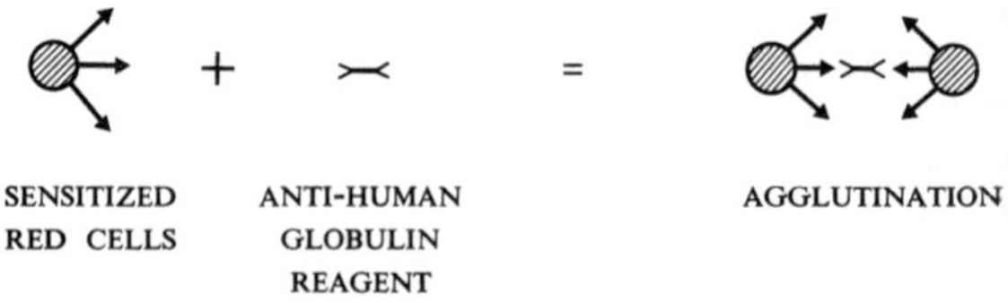

FIG. 66. Antiglobulin test (Coombs test). If the red cells are already sensitized, as in haemolytic disease of the newborn and auto-immune haemolytic anaemia, the anti-human globulin is simply added to the cells. This is the Direct Coombs Test.

Searching for free antibody in the serum means that two stages are necessary; first the serum is incubated with normal red cells for the antibody to become attached to the membrane, and then the anti-human globulin is added. This is the Indirect Coombs Test, and is used for detecting anti-Rh antibodies in the sera of pregnant women and in patients with auto-immune haemolytic anaemia. [Modified from Gell and Coombs (1968)]

Febrile reactions, which usually occur in those who have had previous transfusions, are probably due to antibodies against white cells, and may be lessened by using intravenous hydrocortisone and antihistamines at the time of transfusion. Other hazards include the transmission of infection, e.g. malaria, virus hepatitis, syphilis, etc., circulatory overload, air embolism, transfusion haemosiderosis and local thrombophlebitis.

TABLE 60

ABO BLOOD GROUPS

GROUP	ANTIGEN IN THE CELLS	AGGLUTININ IN THE SERUM	PER CENT. OF POPULATION IN BRITAIN
A	A	Anti-B or β	42
B	B	Anti-A or α	9
AB	A and B	Neither α nor β	3
O	Neither A nor B	Both α and β	46

HAEMOLYTIC DISEASE OF THE NEWBORN

This occurs when there is incompatibility between the blood of the foetus and the mother. The commonest group to be involved is the Rhesus blood group, in which a Rh-negative mother has a Rh-positive child, and the cells of the baby stimulate the mother to form anti-Rh (usually anti-D) antibodies, which then cross the placenta and become attached to the baby's red cells causing haemolysis. There is usually a history of previous pregnancies or miscarriages, and at birth the baby's cord blood shows a positive direct Coombs test. There is recent evidence that the principal release of foetal red cells into the maternal circulation occurs at the time of parturition, and this is presumably when the mother is most likely to be immunized. For this reason the injection of anti-D Rh-antibody at birth may prevent immunization of the mother by destroying the sensitizing red cells, and lessen the risk of haemolytic disease of the newborn in subsequent pregnancies. The same situation arises when a Rh-negative woman receives a blood transfusion of Rh-positive blood.

This disease may be fatal with hydrops foetalis, or may lead to the birth of an apparently normal child who rapidly develops haemolytic jaundice and who requires exchange blood transfusion as soon as possible.

AUTO-IMMUNE HAEMOLYTIC ANAEMIA

Antibodies against red cells may occur without prior immunization in various diseases or as a primary event. In Dacie's series of 175 patients, 108 were 'idiopathic', and 59 occurred as part of some other disease, the principal ones being neoplastic disorders of lymphoreticular tissue, particularly chronic lymphocytic leukaemia; lymphosarcoma and reticulum-cell sarcoma; connective tissue disease, particularly disseminated lupus erythematosus and more rarely rheumatoid arthritis; infections such as mycoplasma pneumonia, infectious mononucleosis, hepatitis and a number of other diseases in which auto-immune phenomena may occur, such as ulcerative colitis.

There are three major forms of this disease: the first due to 'warm' antibodies; the second due to 'cold agglutinins'; and the third, which is very rare, due to a cold haemolysin giving paroxysmal cold haemoglobinuria.

In the *warm antibody disease* the antibody is a 7S (IgG) protein which is active at room temperature. The direct Coombs test is positive and free antibody may be present in the sera in fulminating cases. The peripheral blood may show spherocytosis as a result of coating the red cells with antibody, as well as the other features of haemolytic anaemia. Clinically, in addition to anaemia and haemolytic jaundice, the spleen is nearly always palpable, though rarely greatly enlarged.

This form of auto-immune haemolytic anaemia usually responds well to corticosteroids such as prednisone, but should these fail, immunosuppressive drugs like azathioprine may be used as well. Splenectomy sometimes is of benefit, particularly if there is marked spherocytosis with excessive splenic destruction of red cells.

The *cold agglutinin syndrome* is quite different. Here the antibody is a complement-binding 19S macroglobulin (IgM); there is free antibody in the serum; the direct Coombs test is positive; but unlike the 'warm' type it is complement on the surface of the cells which reacts with the antiglobulin serum giving the so-called 'non-gamma' reaction. Clinically this syndrome may cause haemolysis on exposure to cold with frank haematuria. There is persistent chronic intravascular haemolysis with haemosiderinuria, and the patients frequently present with Raynaud's phenomena; actual agglutination of the cells can be observed in the capillaries of the nail beds. The spleen may be enlarged and the disease runs a long course. It usually occurs in late life, as with other types of macroglobulinaemia. Unlike the 'warm' type, corticosteroids and splenectomy are usually unsuccessful, and attempts to destroy the protein *in vivo* with penicillamine have failed. In some instances it is associated with a lymphoproliferative disease and in these continued treatment with chlorambucil may help.

In mycoplasma pneumonia cold agglutinins may be found, but they rarely cause a haemolytic anaemia and are only a transient event.

Paroxysmal cold haemoglobinuria is a rare disease, usually associated with syphilis, and is due to a cold haemolysin detected by the Donath-Landsteiner test.

HYPERSPLENISM

Whenever the spleen is enlarged it may overact and destroy red cells, white cells or platelets, or any combination of these cells. This is, therefore, a convenient point at which to discuss the causes of splenomegaly and the medical indications for splenectomy.

Splenomegaly may occur in a variety of diseases, which may be summarized as follows:

Infections

Viruses, e.g. infectious mononucleosis, viral hepatitis, and any other viraemia.

Rickettsiae, e.g. typhus.
Bacteria, e.g. typhoid, brucellosis, tuberculosis, subacute bacterial endocarditis, and any bacteraemias.
Spirochaetes, e.g. secondary syphilis.
Protozoa, e.g. malaria, kala-azar.
Trematodes, e.g. schistosomiasis.

Proliferative Diseases of Lymphoreticular Tissue

Splenomegaly may occur in any of the myelo- or lympho-proliferative diseases, and may reach giant proportions in chronic granulocytic leukaemia and myelofibrosis. Sarcoidosis may be included here.

Haemolytic Anaemia

Splenomegaly occurs in many forms of haemolytic anaemia, with massive enlargement occurring in thalassaemia major.

Other Blood Diseases

Splenomegaly may occur in any other form of anaemia, particularly in pernicious anaemia. It is often marked in leuco-erythroblastic anaemia due to skeletal metastases or Albers-Schönberg disease.

Connective Tissue Diseases

Systemic lupus erythematosus, rheumatoid arthritis (Felty's syndrome) and polyarteritis nodosa.

'Storage' Diseases

Gaucher's, Niemann-Pick, Hurler's and Hand-Schüller-Christian syndromes.

Chronic Venous Congestion

Due to portal hypertension (this used to be called Banti's syndrome).

Usually when the spleen overacts it causes a pancytopenia, but occasionally one cell type is destroyed more than the others, e.g. in Felty's syndrome the neutrophils are often selectively destroyed leaving the platelets unaffected.

Splenectomy is only likely to be effective when there is evidence that cell destruction is occurring in the spleen, and when the marrow is functioning normally or excessively to compensate for this. This may involve studies using labelled red cells or platelets, and the use of ^{59}Fe to determine marrow function. Only when these criteria are present should the spleen be removed, and even then there are hazards, e.g. it is dangerous to remove the spleen in portal hypertension unless the portal pressure is also reduced by a shunt operation, because there may be a dramatic rise in the platelet count causing thrombosis in the portal system. It may be required for purely mechanical reasons when its enlargement is prodigious.

Splenectomy is the treatment of choice in some blood diseases, such as hereditary spherocytosis and elliptocytosis, and may be of benefit in some others, particularly idiopathic thrombocytopenic purpura. These are discussed under the headings of the individual diseases.

SECONDARY OR SYMPTOMATIC ANAEMIAS

Apart from the conditions already mentioned, anaemia may arise in the course of many other diseases, such as chronic infections and infestations, the connective tissue diseases such as systemic lupus erythematosus and rheumatoid arthritis, generalized malignant disease, and renal failure. However, as the mechanisms for these anaemias become clearer they are slowly being placed in one of the above categories; for example the anaemia of uraemia may result from lack of erythropoietin and also from haemolysis; the anaemia of rheumatoid arthritis is due to ineffective erythropoiesis; the anaemia of advanced malignant disease may be due to marrow infiltration, bleeding, and in the terminal stages a shortened red cell survival as well.

However, there still remains a small group of anaemias, sometimes referred to as 'refractory anaemia', which fail to respond to haematinics and the aetiology of which remains obscure. These patients frequently have to be maintained with regular blood transfusions until such time as a more definitive diagnosis is made. There is one form of 'refractory anaemia' in which there is inability of the normoblasts to utilize iron and which results in the formation of a number of nucleated red cells with iron arranged in a circle around the nucleus. This is called *sideroblastic anaemia*, and it may result from pyridoxine deficiency often caused by treatment with INAH used in the treatment of tuberculosis. Some cases respond to pyridoxine and folic acid, but others remain refractory and the only treatment is blood transfusion.

REFERENCES

BEUTLER, E., FAIRBANKS, V. G., and FAHEY, J. L. (1963) *Clinical Disorders of Iron Metabolism*, New York.

BITHELL, T. C., and WINTROBE, M. M. (1967) Drug-induced aplastic anaemia, *Seminars in Hematology*, **4,** 194.

BRAIN, M. C. (1969) The haemolytic-uraemic syndrome, *Seminars in Hematology*, **6,** 162.

CARTWRIGHT, G. E. (1966) The anaemia of chronic disorders, *Seminars in Hematology*, **3,** 351.

CHANARIN, I. (1969) *The Megaloblastic Anaemias*, Oxford.

DACIE, J. V. (1960–67) *The Haemolytic Anaemias*, Parts I–IV, London.

DACIE, J. V., and LEWIS, S. M. (1968) *Practical Haematology*, 4th ed., London.

DACIE, J. V., and WORLLEDGE, S. M. (1969) Auto-immune haemolytic anaemias, in *Progress in Hematology*, Vol. VI, ed. BROWN, E. B., and MOORE, C. V., New York.

DE GRUCHY, G. C. (1970) *Clinical Haematology in Medical Practice*, 3rd ed., Oxford.

GELL, P. G. H., and COOMBS, R. R. A. (1968) *Clinical Aspects of Immunology*, 2nd ed., Oxford.

GOLDBERG, A., and BRAIN, M. (1970) *Recent Advances in Haematology*, London.

GROSS, F., ed. (1964) *Iron Metabolism. An International Symposium*, Berlin.

MOLLIN, D. L., and HOFFBRAND, A. V. (1967) Sideroblastic anaemia, in *Recent Advances in Pathology*, ed. HARRISON, C. V., p. 273, London.

WITTS, L. J. (1969) *Hypochromic Anaemia*, London.

WORLLEDGE, S. M. (1969) Immune drug-induced haemolytic anaemias, *Seminars in Hematology*, **6,** 181.

MALIGNANT DISEASES OF LYMPHORETICULAR TISSUE

Synonyms. Reticuloses; Leukaemias and Lymphomas.

In recent years, largely due to the work of Dameshek and Gunz, the concept that many of the primary malignant disorders of the bone marrow are interrelated has been accepted; and the same applies to those involving the lymph nodes and lymphoreticular tissue elsewhere. This classification is based on that of Dameshek and Gunz.

PRIMARY MALIGNANT DISEASES OF THE BONE MARROW (MYELOPROLIFERATIVE DISEASES)

Acute

1. Acute leukaemia (proliferation of the different forms of 'blast' cell; myeloblastic, lymphoblastic, or monoblastic leukaemia).
2. Acute erythraemia (proliferation of primitive erythroblasts).

Chronic

1. Chronic granulocytic leukaemia (proliferation of all forms of developing granulocytes).
2. Polycythaemia vera (proliferation of the erythroid series with the excessive production of mature red cells).
3. Essential thrombocythaemia (proliferation of megakaryocytes with excessive platelet production).
4. Myelofibrosis (proliferation of connective tissue within the bone marrow).

PRIMARY MALIGNANT DISEASES OF LYMPHOID TISSUE (LYMPHOPROLIFERATIVE DISEASES)

1. Hodgkin's disease (proliferation of many forms of cell within the lymph nodes, the essential feature being the presence of Reed-Sternberg giant cells).
2. Reticulum cell sarcoma (proliferation of reticulum cells).
3. Giant follicular lymphoma (proliferation of lymphoid cells in which a pattern of giant pseudofollicles is present).
4. Lymphosarcoma (proliferation of primitive or mature lymphoid cells).
5. Burkitt's lymphoma (proliferation of lymphoid cells with characteristic histological and anatomical features).
6. Chronic lymphocytic leukaemia (proliferation of 'mature' lymphocytes in the bone marrow with or without a lymphocytosis in the peripheral blood. When the lymph nodes are also involved they usually show the changes of giant follicular lymphoma or lymphosarcoma).
7. Myelomatosis (proliferation of plasma cells within the bone marrow, and occasionally plasmacytosis in the peripheral blood (plasma-cell leukaemia), associated with the abnormal production of immunoglobulin other than IgM).
8. Macroglobulinaemia (proliferation of cells of the lymphocyte-plasma series, associated with the abnormal production of macroglobulin (IgM)).

There are several reasons why this classification is valuable. First, it enables one to appreciate that these diseases are interrelated. For example, in the myeloproliferative diseases polycythaemia vera frequently progresses to myelofibrosis: chronic granulocytic leukaemia almost invariably ends with uncontrolled proliferation of myeloblasts (i.e. acute leukaemia). In the lymphoproliferative diseases giant follicular lymphoma and lymphosarcoma, the disease at first may not involve the bone marrow or blood but can do so later, i.e. chronic lymphocytic leukaemia may develop. Secondly, it helps to understand why some of the diseases are not purely proliferations of one type of cell. For example, in chronic granulocytic leukaemia the platelet count may be considerably increased, and in polycythaemia vera there may be both thrombocythaemia and leucocytosis before treatment. Thirdly, it helps to rationalize the treatment of these disorders. For example, in the lymphoproliferative diseases chronic lymphocytic leukaemia, lymphosarcoma and giant follicular lymphoma, all respond well to the nitrogen mustard drugs such as chlorambucil and cyclophosphamide, while in the myeloproliferative disorders busulphan is effective in chronic granulocytic leukaemia and polycythaemia.

ACUTE LEUKAEMIA

Synonym. Acute leukosis.

Definition

An acute proliferative disease of the bone marrow characterized by infiltration with the most primitive form of white cell precursor, the blast cell. Three different forms may be recognized, depending on the morphology of the blast cell—lymphoblastic, myeloblastic, and monoblastic. Sometimes it is difficult to be sure which variety is present and then the term stem-cell leukaemia is used.

Aetiology

It is now clearly established that in many animals leukaemia can be transmitted by a virus, and that irradiation may also cause leukaemia although this may work by activating a latent leukaemia virus. In man there is a definite correlation between irradiation and acute leukaemia and chronic granulocytic leukaemia. Evidence from Japan following the atomic bomb explosion, and from patients with ankylosing spondylitis treated with radiotherapy has shown that the incidence of these forms of leukaemia is greatly increased following irradiation. There has also been some evidence that irradiation of the foetus *in utero* produces an increased incidence of acute leukaemia in children, and unnecessary irradiation should be avoided in pregnant women.

Definite proof of a virus causing leukaemia in man is lacking, although viral particles have been seen in leukaemic cells. However, unless human leukaemia is quite different from animal leukaemia, a virus may be one of the aetiological factors and evidence for this may well be forthcoming in the near future.

Acute leukaemia is commoner in Down's syndrome (mongolism) than in normal children and it is interesting that the chromosomal abnormality in chronic granulocytic leukaemia the Ph′ chromosome occurs in the same chromosome as the abnormality in mongolism.

It is also possible that exposure to chemicals, in particular benzene, may cause acute leukaemia.

Acute leukaemia is becoming commoner in Britain; the Registrar General's figures for England and Wales showed that 722 died of this disease in 1949, 939 in 1957, and 1495 in 1967. Some, but certainly not all of this increase could be due to better diagnosis.

The age incidence varies with the different forms of acute leukaemia. Lymphoblastic leukaemia is much commoner in children and adolescence than in adult life though it can occur at any age. Myeloblastic leukaemia is spread evenly throughout the whole life-span, and monoblastic leukaemia affects chiefly the middle-aged. The male/female ratio is 3:2.

Clinical Manifestations

Usually the presenting features of acute leukaemia are due to a failure of the bone marrow to produce the normal cellular elements of the blood resulting in anaemia, a haemorrhagic state due to thrombocytopenia, and infections due to neutrophil leucopenia. Frequently when first seen the patient is pale, ill, febrile, sometimes with obvious infection such as pharyngitis or pneumonia, with purpura, or overt haemorrhage from the gums or lower in the gastro-intestinal tract. The spleen is usually, but not invariably palpable. In lymphoblastic leukaemia there may be marked local or general lymphadenopathy, and sometimes in the so-called Sternberg variety in children the initial presentation is of a large mediastinal mass, and only subsequently do the marrow and the blood show the presence of leukaemic cells; some authorities classify this as an acute form of lymphosarcoma with marrow involvement, but it is best regarded as acute lymphoblastic leukaemia for purposes of treatment.

During the course of the disease infiltration may occur in many organs. Particularly common is involvement of the central nervous system causing meningeal leukaemia with the symptoms and signs of meningitis, intracerebral deposits, or infiltration of cranial or peripheral nerves. Other sites include the skin, testes, ovaries, kidneys, liver, the gut, particularly the stomach, ileum and colon, and serous membranes such as the pleura and peritoneum. In lymphoblastic leukaemia in children overt bone lesions usually in the metaphases may cause pain and show on radiography as lytic areas in the bone. In adult leukaemia joint pains are common but usually not associated with radiological changes.

Infiltration of the gums is particularly characteristic of monoblastic leukaemia. Enlargement of the salivary and lacrimal glands may occur giving rise to Mikulicz's syndrome. Occasionally large tumours develop near the orbit and elsewhere and may on section be green in colour (chloroma).

Diagnosis

The combination of anaemia, haemorrhage, and infection with or without splenomegaly and lymphadenopathy suggests the diagnosis of leukaemia, which is confirmed by examination of the blood and bone marrow. The total white count varies widely from gross leukaemic infiltration of the blood (over 50,000 blast cells per mm^3.) to severe leucopenia (less than 1,000 white cells per mm^3.) in the so-called aleukaemic form. The percentage of patients presenting with a normal or low white cell count has increased in recent years, and if there are no blast cells in the blood the diagnosis will rest on examination of the bone marrow. This is the essential diagnostic procedure. The marrow will be hypercellular due to infiltration with blast cells, and normal erythropoiesis, granulopoiesis and thrombopoiesis will be depressed. The diagnosis of the type of acute leukaemia is based on the morphology and special staining properties of the leukaemic cells. In lymphoblastic leukaemia the nuclei are round, the cells are smaller, the nuclear/cytoplasmic ratio higher, and the number of nucleoli fewer than in myeloblastic leukaemia; the PAS stain is usually positive and Sudan Black negative. In myeloblastic leukaemia the cells are larger, the nuclear/cytoplasmic ratio lower and nucleoli more numerous than in lymphoblastic leukaemia; Auer rods and granules may be present in the cytoplasm and the nucleus may appear folded in appearance. This is particularly apparent with monoblastic leukaemia. Staining with Sudan Black may be positive but the PAS stain is negative.

Treatment and Prognosis

Since acute lymphoblastic leukaemia responds to treatment so much better than acute myeloblastic or monoblastic leukaemia it will be considered first.

Acute Lymphoblastic Leukaemia. The first essential in the treatment of this disease is to obtain a complete remission, which is defined as a complete return to normal of the blood and bone marrow, no abnormal signs such as splenomegaly, and no evidence of disease elsewhere. One of the most remarkable events in malignant disease is that this is now possible in about 95 per cent. of children with lymphoblastic leukaemia. The most commonly used regime is prednisolone or prednisone, 40 mg. per m^2. per day in children, and 40 mg. per patient in adults (although much higher doses are used in other countries, particularly the United States), together with vincristine, 1·4 mg. per m^2. weekly by intravenous injection. Usually three injections are required. If these drugs fail to produce complete remission others should be used as shown in TABLE 61. Once complete remission has been obtained it is necessary to give further chemotherapy to delay the onset of relapse, and the drugs commonly used are also shown in TABLE 61. It is probably desirable at this time to give prophylactic radiotherapy to the meninges in the skull and spinal canal to prevent or delay the occurrence of meningeal leukaemia. Following this period of chemotherapy other varieties of treatment are given, the two current forms being intermittent methotrexate, and either specific or non-specific immunotherapy [TABLE 61]. When relapses occur attempts are made to induce remission again with vincristine and prednisone, and failing this the other drugs shown in TABLE 61.

TABLE 61

SCHEME FOR THE TREATMENT OF ACUTE LYMPHOBLASTIC LEUKAEMIA

INDUCTION OF REMISSION →	CONSOLIDATION OR CYTO-REDUCTION →	MAINTENANCE
1. Vincristine	6-Mercaptopurine	Immunotherapy
+		
Prednisone	Methotrexate	Methotrexate
Failing this	Cyclophosphamide	
other drugs	+	Repeated courses
2. Cytosine	I.T.Methotrexate	of combination
arabinoside	±	chemotherapy
3. Daunorubicin	Prednisone	
4. Asparaginase	and other drugs	
5. BCNU	used for induction	

Quite deliberately no attempt has been made to give a specific regime for the treatment of this disease, for two reasons. First, knowledge is advancing so rapidly that the details will have changed within the next year although the principles will almost certainly be the same. Secondly, these patients are best treated in close collaboration with special units, which will be able to advise on the latest forms of treatment and the complications arising from them. The more intensive the treatment the greater have to be the supporting facilities of red cell and platelet transfusion, and in the future possibly leucocyte transfusions, and to deal with the infectious complications. If meningeal leukaemia occurs, intrathecal methotrexate and/or cytosine arabinoside should be given and radiotherapy to the spinal canal and skull may be effective. Radiotheraphy may also be of value in relieving the bone pain of osteolytic lesions and dissolving large glandular masses in acute lymphoblastic leukaemia.

In the past there have been many who have been critical of subjecting patients to intensive chemotherapy with all its accompanying toxicity in what is regarded as an inevitably fatal disease. However, an aggressive approach to the treatment of acute leukaemia is justified by the results of Burchenal (1968) who has collected from the entire world 157 cases of proven acute leukaemia of all types who are alive at 5 years, and of whom 103 are free from disease 5 to 17 years later. Even in the absence of any 'cures' modern intensive chemotherapy has greatly improved the prognosis; the median survival in children with acute lymphoblastic leukaemia was less than 5 months when there was no specific treatment, but is now more than 3 years using intensive combination chemotherapy. Now the *aim* is to cure the disease, although it may only rarely be achieved.

Acute Myeloblastic and Monoblastic Leukaemia. Even with modern chemotherapy the results of treatment in

TABLE 62

SCHEME FOR THE TREATMENT OF ACUTE MYELOBLASTIC LEUKAEMIA

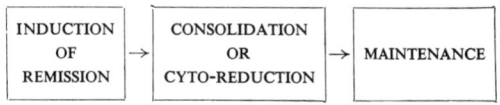

INDUCTION OF REMISSION →	CONSOLIDATION OR CYTO-REDUCTION →	MAINTENANCE
METHOD		
1. 6-Mercaptopurine	6-Mercaptopurine	Methotrexate
+		
Cytosine arabinoside	Methotrexate	? Immunotherapy
or	Any other drug shown in TABLE 61	
2. Cytosine arabinoside		
+		
Daunorubicin		
±		
Prednisolone		

this disease are much worse than in lymphoblastic leukaemia. Complete remissions are only obtained in about 50 per cent. of the patients, and many of them are shortlived. However, the principles are the same as for lymphoblastic leukaemia, though there is some difference in the drugs used as shown in TABLE 62.

ACUTE ERYTHRAEMIA

Synonyms. Di Guglielmo's disease; Acute erythromyelosis.

This is an acute myeloproliferative disease characterized by infiltration of the bone marrow and often the blood with primitive normoblasts many of which are binucleate and bizarre in appearance. The disease clinically presents in the same way as acute myeloblastic leukaemia and frequently terminates with myeloblastic infiltration of the marrow. The response to treatment is poor, and the prognosis very bad, as remissions are extremely rare. It is best treated in the same way as acute myeloblastic leukaemia.

Another rare acute myeloproliferative disease is acute myelofibrosis, which is best treated with prednisone, and which is discussed on page 1042.

CHRONIC GRANULOCYTIC LEUKAEMIA

Synonyms. Chronic myeloid leukaemia; Chronic myelogenous leukaemia; Chronic myelocytic leukaemia.

Definition

Malignant proliferation of the bone marrow involving principally all the developing cells of the granulocyte series.

Aetiology

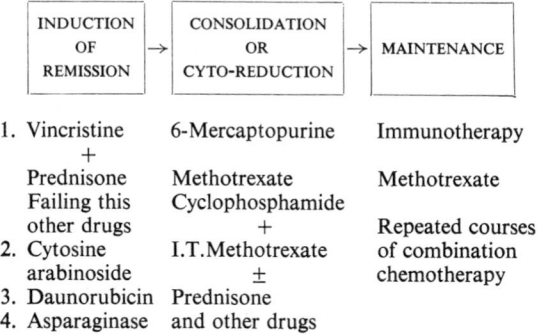

As with acute leukaemia the only proven aetiological factor is irradiation; the incidence being greatly increased following exposure to nuclear explosions, radiotherapy for other diseases (particularly ankylosing spondylitis), and in patients who were repeatedly screened in the past during maintenance of artificial pneumothoraces. The disease occurs in both sexes in approximately equal numbers, is rare in children and the very old, 70 per cent. of the patients developing the disease between the ages of 30 and 60.

Clinical Manifestations

The most frequent presenting symptoms are general malaise, lassitude and weakness, abdominal swelling or pain due to splenomegaly with or without splenic infarction, weight loss, symptoms of anaemia, or purpura. Occasionally the disease is discovered by chance when a blood count is done for some other reason. Examination of the patient almost invariably reveals an enlarged spleen which may be massive, and the signs of anaemia or a haemorrhagic state may be present. Lymphadenopathy is rare and is usually a bad prognostic sign. Priapism, bone lesions and skin infiltrations are uncommon but well documented features.

Diagnosis

In most cases the diagnosis presents no problem. The combination of splenomegaly, anaemia, a greatly raised white blood count frequently above 100,000, with all forms of developing granulocytes from blast cells through to mature polymorphonuclear cells, involving not only the neutrophil series but sometimes also eosinophils and basophils is diagnostic. (Eosinophilic leukaemia may be regarded as a form of chronic granulocytic leukaemia.) There is a normal or raised platelet count. The white cells show a similar differential count in the blood and in the marrow. Prior to treatment chronic granulocytic leukaemia is not aleukaemic, but in the early stages when the disease is developing and the white count only slightly raised it may be confused with myelofibrosis or with a leukaemoid reaction. Under these circumstances aspiration bone marrow biopsy, or failing this, a bone marrow trephine, will exclude the presence of myelofibrosis. Two additional investigations may also be helpful. The finding of an abnormal chromosome (the Philadelphia or Ph′ chromosome) in the cells of the peripheral blood or bone marrow is diagnostic of chronic granulocytic leukaemia, but is not present in every case, although so far it has not been found in any other disease. The neutrophil polymorphonuclear cells usually show an increased staining reaction for alkaline phosphatase in leukaemoid reactions and myelofibrosis, but reduced or absent staining in granulocytic leukaemia.

Treatment

Specific Treatment. In the past both radiotherapy and chemotherapy have been used to control the chronic phase of the disease, but a recent trial by the Medical Research Council has proved conclusively that the treatment of choice is busulphan. This is given by mouth, the initial dose being 4 mg. daily, and the haemoglobin concentration, white blood cell and platelet counts are carefully observed over the first 4 weeks whilst the white cell count is falling. Once the white cells reach a total of around 10,000 cells per mm^3. the dose required to keep the cells at this level will have to be determined for each patient, the usual maintenance dose being between 0·5 and 2 mg. daily. It is vital not to give too much busulphan, for should the marrow be rendered aplastic by this drug, it rarely recovers. For the other toxic effects of busulphan see Section 4. With this treatment the spleen usually shrinks dramatically and may become impalpable, the haemoglobin rises and the patient feels fit. Occasionally patients are refractory to busulphan, and then other forms of treatment including hydroxyurea, dibromomannitol, pipobroman or radiotherapy to the spleen may be used.

Once the blastic phase has occurred treatment with busulphan is discontinued, and the drugs used in the treatment of acute myeloblastic leukaemia, such as prednisolone, 6-mercaptopurine or vincristine may be tried. In some patients worthwhile remissions are obtained, but most are refractory to all forms of treatment, and progressive anaemia, thrombocytopenia causing a haemorrhagic state, granulocytopenia with resulting infections, progressive splenomegaly and occasionally leukaemic infiltrations elsewhere lead to death.

Supportive Measures. The usual supportive measures of blood transfusion for anaemia, platelet infusions for thrombocytopenia, and appropriate antibiotics for infections may be required. In addition, during the early stages of specific treatment when large numbers of leukaemic cells are being destroyed, the serum uric acid may rise dramatically and allopurinol, 100 mg. three or four times a day should be given to control this. However, great care must be taken with patients also receiving 6-mercaptopurine as allopurinol greatly potentiates the action of this drug.

Prognosis

Chronic granulocytic leukaemia is invariably fatal, and although the quality of life during the chronic stage improved greatly following the introduction of busulphan, the length of life has remained almost unchanged. With modern treatment the patients should be able to lead symptom-free normal lives until the onset of the blastic phase. So far there are no reliable signs indicating when this terminal phase will start, though the prognosis is probably worse in patients who do not possess the Ph′ chromosome. The mean survival from the time of diagnosis is between 2 and 3 years.

POLYCYTHAEMIA

This is a condition in which there is an excessive production of mature red cells, resulting in an absolute increase in the red cell volume so that the haemoglobin concentration and packed cell volume are persistently raised. Polycythaemia may be a primary myeloproliferative disease, or secondary to an excessive production of erythropoietin or decreased arterial oxygen saturation. There is also a type of apparent polycythaemia in which the haemoglobin and packed cell volume are increased but the red cell mass is in fact normal (stress polycythaemia; Gaisbock's disease). For convenience secondary polycythaemia will be considered first.

SECONDARY POLYCYTHAEMIA

INCREASED PRODUCTION OF ERYTHROPOIETIN

This enzyme is formed in the kidney, and polycythaemia due to overproduction is usually due to the presence of a hypernephroma, although other renal lesions including cysts and pyelonephritis may on rare occasions cause polycythaemia. Tumours elsewhere in the body including uterine fibroids, cerebellar angiomas and hepatoma may also on rare occasions produce excessive amounts of erythropoietin. This type of polycythaemia only involves the red cells; the white cells and platelets are normal and there is no splenomegaly. The diagnosis is established by finding increased levels of erythropoietin in the blood and urine, and the polycythaemia is cured when the tumour is removed.

POLYCYTHAEMIA DUE TO DECREASED ARTERIAL OXYGEN SATURATION

It is well known that people living at high altitudes have persistently raised haemoglobin and PCV levels. In addition any disease leading to chronic arterial oxygen desaturation may also cause polycythaemia. The two major causes are cyanotic congenital heart disease, and chronic cyanotic lung disease, particularly chronic bronchitis and emphysema, pulmonary fibrosis and arteriovenous fistulae in the lung. Once again this type of polycythaemia only affects the red cells; the other cellular elements of the blood are normal and the spleen is not enlarged. The polycythaemia can only be satisfactorily controlled by treating the underlying lesion.

POLYCYTHAEMIA VERA

Synonyms. Primary polycythaemia; Osler-Vaquez disease.

Definition

This is a primary proliferative disease of the bone marrow involving chiefly the red cell series, but frequently also showing an increased number of circulating granulocytes and platelets together with splenomegaly.

Aetiology

As with the other myeloproliferative diseases, this is unknown. It is a disease of the second half of life and occurs in both sexes.

Clinical Manifestations

The commonest presenting features are vascular. The increased viscosity of the blood may produce disturbances of cerebral circulation with headache, lack of concentration, vertigo, transient disturbances of vision, dysphasia, and hemiplegia. Permanent neurological damage may occur. The tendency to thrombosis involves both the veins and arteries. Common sites for venous thrombosis are, of course, the lower limbs and pelvis, but unusual sites such as the hepatic veins causing the Budd-Chiari syndrome may be involved. Arterial thrombi may form in the coronary and cerebral arteries as well as in the peripheral blood vessels to the limbs.

In addition to the tendency to thrombosis these patients may also develop a haemorrhagic diathesis, presumably due to the abnormal platelets, as occurs in essential thrombocythaemia, and a common site for bleeding is the gastro-intestinal tract. Other manifestations include a plethoric appearance sometimes with peripheral cyanosis, gout due to the raised serum uric acid, generalized pruritus and splenomegaly.

Diagnosis

This is suspected from the clinical signs of plethora and splenomegaly, and confirmed by the finding of a raised haemoglobin concentration and PCV. The presence of a thrombocytosis, granulocytosis with an increased leucocyte alkaline phosphatase, and splenomegaly confirm the diagnosis. In borderline cases the diagnosis should be established by measuring the red cell volume using ^{51}Cr labelled red cells and the plasma volume using ^{131}I labelled albumin. A raised red cell volume distinguishes true polycythaemia from so-called 'stress polycythaemia', which is due to a shrinkage of plasma volume and tends to occur in middle-aged obese men with hypertension. The bone marrow usually shows hyperplasia of all cellular elements particularly the erythroid series.

Treatment

The immediate danger with uncontrolled polycythaemia is that one of the major vascular complications may occur and sometimes prove fatal. For this reason the disease must be controlled. There are two major factors contributing to the vascular lesions, the increased red cell volume with resultant high viscosity, and the increased platelet count. The red cell volume can be controlled by venesection, but this alone is not enough as it may lead to a rise in the platelet count. For this reason either ^{32}P or chemotherapy, usually in the form of busulphan, is necessary. There has recently been some controversy about the use of ^{32}P on the grounds that it may cause acute leukaemia. There has been much confusion in the past about leukaemia in this disease. No matter what treatment is given a blood picture resembling chronic myeloid leukaemia may develop, and the disease may progress to myelofibrosis or hypoplastic anaemia, but only if ^{32}P has been given does the disease end with infiltration of the bone marrow with blast cells (i.e. acute leukaemia). However, there is much evidence to suggest that patients treated with ^{32}P live as long as, if not longer, than those treated with chemotherapy. Furthermore, the disease is easier to control with ^{32}P than with chemotherapy. For this reason it is probably best to control the red cell volume with venesection and the platelet count with ^{32}P using the smallest dose possible, with chemotherapy held in reserve if it proves difficult to control the disease with ^{32}P. If the serum uric acid is raised allopurinol should be given (see Section 10).

Prognosis

Before any treatment was available half the patients died within the first 18 months; treatment with venesection alone prolonged this to 3½ years; and the introduction of ^{32}P and chemotherapy lengthened it to 12 years.

ESSENTIAL THROMBOCYTHAEMIA

This myeloproliferative disease is characterized by marked thrombocythaemia, the platelet count varying between 500,000 and 2,000,000 per mm^3. This frequently produces a haemorrhagic state, hence the synonym, haemorrhagic thrombocythaemia, with bleeding from the gastro-intestinal tract as a common presenting feature. The spleen is usually enlarged, and once the haemorrhagic state has been controlled by treatment, preferably with ^{32}P, the clinical course is very similar to polycythaemia vera ending with myelofibrosis.

MYELOFIBROSIS

Synonym. Myelosclerosis.

Definition

This is a primary myeloproliferative disease in which the predominant feature is a proliferation of connective tissue within the marrow.

Aetiology

Myelofibrosis may follow one of the other chronic myeloproliferative diseases, particularly polycythaemia vera and essential thrombocythaemia, or it may arise *de novo*. Like polycythaemia it is a disease of middle-age and occurs in both sexes.

Clinical Manifestations

The usual presenting features are those of anaemia coupled with an enlarged spleen, which may reach enormous proportions and cause pain particularly when infarctions occur. The liver may also be enlarged. Occasionally actual myelosclerosis can be seen on radiographic examination of the skeleton. The disease usually runs a chronic course ending with bone marrow failure either with aplasia or infiltration with blast cells (acute leukaemia). There is also an acute form of myelofibrosis which is rapidly fatal, resistant to treatment and may progress quickly to acute myeloblastic leukaemia.

Haematological Investigations

Myelofibrosis produces a type of anaemia which may occur whenever there is infiltration of the bone marrow with abnormal cells—a leuco-erythroblastic anaemia. This is characterized by anaemia, a total white cell count which may vary widely (10,000–30,000 per mm^3.) but which shows the presence of some primitive cells of the granulocyte series, myeloblasts, promyelocytes, myelocytes and metamyelocytes together with circulating normoblasts. The morphology of the red cells is abnormal with poikilocytosis and anisocytosis, and polychromasia due to an increased number of circulating reticulocytes. The platelet count is usually reduced. It is usually difficult to aspirate bone marrow, but histological examination of a trephine biopsy of the iliac crest reveals the diagnosis.

The cause of the anaemia is complex. Clearly the infiltration of the marrow disrupts normal erythropoiesis, but this may be compensated to some extent by extramedullary erythropoiesis due to myeloid metaplasia in the spleen and liver. The situation can be assessed by ^{59}Fe studies. However, there is also a haemolytic element, some of the haemolysis occurring in the spleen, and this can be assessed by ^{51}Cr labelled red cells.

Diagnosis

The presence of a leuco-erythroblastic anaemia with splenomegaly denotes marrow infiltration but this does not always mean myelofibrosis. The other common cause of this syndrome is malignant infiltration of the bone marrow with carcinoma of the prostate, breast, bronchus, kidney and thyroid, or occasionally other malignant processes such as myelomatosis. These are usually suggested by manifestations of the primary tumour, radiological evidence of bone metastases, and the finding of the malignant cells in the bone marrow. Also with carcinomatous infiltration of the marrow the spleen may be palpable but is not grossly enlarged as in myelofibrosis.

Another but rare cause of marrow infiltration causing a leuco-erythroblastic anaemia is the congenital disease characterized by increased density of the bone, spontaneous fractures and splenomegaly (Albers-Schönberg or marble-bone disease). The disease presents in childhood and the radiographic appearance of a reduced medulla due to a thickened cortex of the bones is diagnostic.

The other conditions with which myelofibrosis may be confused are chronic granulocytic leukaemia, or a leukaemoid reaction if the total white cell count is very high. Chronic granulocytic leukaemia is distinguished by the appearance of the bone marrow, the frequent occurrence of the Ph′ chromosome and a reduced alkaline phosphatase content of the granulocytes. In both leukaemoid reactions and myelofibrosis the Ph′ chromosome is not present and the leucocyte alkaline phosphatase is normal or raised.

Leukaemoid reactions may be defined as high white cell counts in the peripheral blood, accompanied by the presence of early cells of the granulocyte series, particularly myelocytes and metamyelocytes due to some other disease process. Leukaemoid reactions are rare but may occur in severe infections such as miliary tuberculosis and acute haemorrhagic smallpox.

Treatment

The two major problems in the management of myelofibrosis are the anaemia, and the progressive splenomegaly. For the anaemia blood transfusions are usually necessary, but stimulation of the bone marrow with androgens, particularly oxymetholone in large doses of up to 300 mg. daily for an adult may be helpful, together with the administration of folic acid, as the patients are sometimes folate deficient. Splenectomy may both relieve the abdominal discomfort or severe pain if splenic infarction is occurring, and also reduce the blood transfusion requirements. The theoretical danger of removing one of the sources of extramedullary erythropoiesis is seldom of practical importance, and some authorities recommend removing the spleen early in the course of the disease before it becomes so large that the technical difficulties of splenectomy increase the post-operative complications, particularly subphrenic abscess.

However, splenectomy is not free from risk even early in the disease as it may be followed by a marked thrombocythaemia requiring treatment with ^{32}P. If the white count becomes very high busulphan may be given, but with great caution, starting with 2 mg. daily and watching the blood very carefully.

Prognosis

In most patients the disease runs a chronic course, but eventually terminates with marrow failure in the form of hypoplasia or acute leukaemia.

HODGKIN'S DISEASE

Synonyms. Lymphadenoma; Lymphogranulomatosis.

Definition

A primary malignant disease of lymphoreticular tissue characterized by the presence of Reed-Sternberg giant cells.

Aetiology

This is completely unknown, although various theories have been propounded in the past, some authors regarding it as some sort of infection and others as an overt neoplastic process. Most authorities now classify it as a malignant disease, the malignant change occurring in a reticulum cell with a tendency to form giant cells. It is commoner in males than females, and the curve of the age incidence is bimodal with a peak at the age of 25 and another at the age of 70.

Clinical Manifestations

In most cases the first manifestation is painless enlargement of lymph nodes, usually in the neck, but sometimes in the axillae, and more rarely in the inguinal regions. Other presenting signs may be enlargement of lymph nodes in the chest revealed by a chest X-ray, a palpable abdominal mass, a palpable spleen or hepatic enlargement. The disease may also involve other tissues, e.g. the bones which sometimes show sclerotic deposits on diagnostic radiography (ivory vertebrae); extradural deposits may cause spinal cord compression, and infiltrations elsewhere may give rise to local symptoms such as compression of major bronchi, pleural effusions, obstructive jaundice, and ascites. In the later stages the disease may spread to involve almost any organ in the body including the skin, gastro-intestinal tract, lung and more rarely the kidneys, but direct involvement of the central nervous system is very rare. Leuco-encephalopathy and peripheral neuropathy may occur. Classically the lymph nodes are painless but pain can occur particularly after taking alcohol even in small quantities.

In addition to these local signs there may be systemic symptoms, which consist of generalized pruritus; fever which may be undulant in type (Pel-Ebstein) or irregular; general malaise, weakness, weight loss and anaemia. The presence of these symptoms usually denotes generalized disease and a poor prognosis. The anaemia in Hodgkin's disease may be due to haemolysis, hypersplenism, ineffective erythropoiesis with or without definite bone marrow infiltration, and haemodilution due to an expanded plasma volume. Prior to treatment the white blood count may be normal, or slightly reduced with only occasionally a mild lymphopenia, but sometimes there is a marked leucocytosis due to increased numbers of neutrophils or eosinophils. Occasionally marrow infiltration causes thrombocytopenia in the later stages of the disease.

Infections are not uncommon in Hodgkin's disease, partly due to impairment in cellular immunity which occurs when the disease is active, and partly to lack of normal granulocytes as a result of bone marrow infiltration or intensive chemotherapy. Herpes zoster is particularly common in patients in Britain and in some other parts of the world tuberculosis may occur quite frequently. Sometimes rare fungal diseases such as torula meningitis [see p. 1205] may complicate the course of the disease. It is important to exclude infection as a cause of fever before attributing it to the disease.

Diagnosis

This can only be made by finding Reed-Sternberg cells in biopsy material, usually from a lymph node but occasionally from the liver, bone marrow or from the extradural space when a laminectomy is done for the relief of spinal cord compression. The older division of Hodgkin's disease into three main varieties has now been superseded by the classification of Lukes which has been modified in TABLE 63 to show the relationship between the two.

TABLE 63

HISTOLOGICAL CLASSIFICATION OF HODGKIN'S DISEASE (1969)

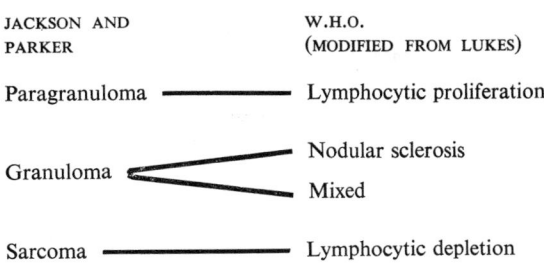

JACKSON AND PARKER	W.H.O. (MODIFIED FROM LUKES)
Paragranuloma	Lymphocytic proliferation
Granuloma	Nodular sclerosis
	Mixed
Sarcoma	Lymphocytic depletion

The significance of this classification is discussed under Course and Prognosis.

Treatment

Until comparatively recently Hodgkin's disease has been regarded as invariably fatal, but it is now clear that if the diagnosis is made when the disease is still localized, and the correct treatment given, many patients may be cured, and others may have many years of happy useful life. The change in prognosis has occurred for two reasons; first it is now possible to determine with much greater accuracy the anatomical extent of the disease; and secondly, there have been considerable advances in the use of both radiotherapy and chemotherapy.

Once the diagnosis has been established the anatomical

distribution of the disease is determined by clinical examination and by special investigations including tomography of the hilar regions of the lungs, lymphangiography to outline the pelvic and para-aortic lymph nodes [PLATE 20], liver function tests, liver biopsy, liver and spleen scans, and a bone marrow examination. The disease can then be staged as shown in TABLE 64.

TABLE 64

RYE METHOD OF STAGING HODGKIN'S DISEASE

Stage I	Disease limited to lymph nodes of one anatomical region.
Stage II	Disease confined to lymph nodes on one side of the diaphragm.
Stage III	Disease on both sides of the diaphragm but limited to involvement of lymph nodes and spleen.
Stage IV	Involvement of bone marrow, lung, pleura, liver, bone, skin, kidneys, gastro-intestinal tract or any tissue other than lymph nodes and spleen.

If the systemic symptoms of fever, sweating, pruritus and weight loss are absent the patients are classified as 'A', and if present as 'B'.

There is now absolutely no doubt that the correct treatment for localized diseases (Stages I and II) is radiotherapy. The best results are obtained using big doses of radiotherapy not only to the area involved, but also to the adjacent lymph node areas. Over 80 per cent. of such patients survive 5 years and if they are free of disease at that time they are almost certainly cured.

Chemotherapy is used in two ways in Hodgkin's disease, first as an adjuvant to radiotherapy; for example, with a large mass pressing on the spinal cord or a major bronchus, a reduced dose of mustine hydrochloride, 0·2 mg. per kg., can be given into a fast running intravenous infusion to relieve the immediate dangers of compression by the tumour, at the same time as a course of radiotherapy is started. Secondly, chemotherapy may be used as the definitive treatment in patients with generalized disease. All authorities would agree with its use in Stage IV disease, but with Stage III some would give radiotherapy to all lymph node areas above and below the diaphragm, while others would treat with chemotherapy.

Three main groups of cytotoxic agents have been found to be beneficial in Hodgkin's disease. First, the nitrogen mustard group—mustine hydrochloride itself, chlorambucil, and cyclophosphamide; secondly, the vinca alkaloids–vincristine and vinblastine; and thirdly, the methyl hydrazine derivative—procarbazine. These drugs used singly and in conventional dosage will control the disease in most patients, and will produce complete remission in 25 per cent., and partial remission in a further 50 per cent. The use of corticosteroids, such as prednisone, in Hodgkin's disease is sometimes of value, particularly in controlling fever, pruritus and anaemia, but the effect is often of short duration and the dose required may be 40 mg. prednisone daily by mouth, or even more. However, by giving intensive combination chemotherapy using these four agents simultaneously, 90 per cent. of the patients derive benefit, and 80 per cent. will return completely to normal. There are several possible regimes, which originated at the National Institute of Health, Bethesda, Maryland. The one most extensively used is described under reticulum-cell sarcoma. We have made some slight alterations, and our present regime is as follows:

Prednisolone	40 mg. per day	Orally on days 0–14 inclusive
Procarbazine	100 mg. per m^2. per day	Orally on days 0–14 inclusive
Mustine hydrochloride	6 mg. per m^2. intravenously on days 0 and 7	
Vinblastine	10 mg. intravenously on days 0, 7 and 14	

Each course of treatment lasts 2 weeks, and an interval of at least 4 weeks is left between the end of one course and the beginning of the next. This regime may cause marked leucopenia and thrombocytopenia, particularly if the patients have been given previous chemotherapy, and regular blood counts are essential. Full details are discussed by Goldberg and Brain (1970).

Course and Prognosis

The prognosis of Hodgkin's disease depends on three factors: first the histological type, for Lukes has shown that patients with lymphocytic and/or histiocytic proliferation or nodular sclerosis have a much better prognosis than those with mixed cellularity and lymphocytic depletion; secondly, the stage of the disease at the time of treatment; and thirdly, the immediate institution of the correct treatment. Under these circumstances many patients with localized disease may be cured, and even in those with generalized disease the quality as well as the duration of life has improved by the use of intensive combination chemotherapy.

RETICULUM-CELL SARCOMA

Synonym. Reticulosarcoma.

Definition

This is a malignant proliferation of reticulum cells usually arising in lymphoreticular tissue in the lymph nodes or spleen.

Aetiology

This is unknown. As with lymphosarcoma it may occur at any age, but is commoner in middle and late life, and there is a higher incidence in males than in females.

Clinical Manifestations

Like Hodgkin's disease the first manifestation may be enlargement of lymph nodes or spleen, but the disease may spread rapidly to involve other organs; skin lesions are relatively common [see Section 14]; isolated tumours may arise in the tonsil, or elsewhere in the gut including the stomach, small and large bowel causing obstruction or intussusception, and widespread involvement can cause steatorrhoea; infiltration of the lung, pleura, peritoneum, meninges and central nervous system produces symptoms depending on the organ involved. Other tissues which have been recorded as infiltrated on rare occasions include the thyroid gland and the gonads. Indeed, no tissue is immune from this malignant process. Anaemia may arise for the same reasons as in Hodgkin's disease, but pruritus is uncommon and fever is more likely to be due to infection than to the disease.

Diagnosis

This is made on histological examination of biopsy material showing loss of the normal architecture and replacement by reticulum cells, which in the case of lymph nodes may have infiltrated outside the capsule. Other organs are frequently involved as mentioned above, including the bone marrow which may lead to anaemia, thrombocytopenia and leucopenia.

Treatment

The principles of treatment are those already described for Hodgkin's disease. Radiotherapy should be used for localized (Stages I and II) and chemotherapy for generalized (Stages III and IV) disease. The chemotherapy used is similar to that in Hodgkin's disease, the most effective drugs being those of the nitrogen mustard series (mustine hydrochloride, cyclophosphamide, chlorambucil), the vinca alkaloids (particularly vincristine) and to a lesser extent procarbazine. Prednisone may be helpful particularly when anaemia or pancytopenia are present. The use of four agents in combination (mustine, vincristine, procarbazine and prednisone) is beginning to improve the prognosis which in the past has been very bad. There are many suggested regimes, but the one in use at the National Institute of Health, Bethesda, is as follows:

[1]Prednisolone	40 mg. per m^2. per day	Orally on days 0–14 inclusive
Procarbazine	100 mg. per m^2. per day	
Mustine hydrochloride	6 mg. per m^2.	Intravenously on days 0 and 7
Vincristine	1·4 mg. per m^2.	

[1] Only given with some courses.
(Carbone *et al.*, 1967)

After 2 weeks of treatment there is a rest period of 2–4 weeks before the next course is given. Further details are given by Goldberg and Brain (1970).

Prognosis

This disease has the worst prognosis of any of the lymphoproliferative disorders, but it is difficult to give an accurate prognosis as the disease varies considerably from patient to patient. Most patients are dead within 2–3 years of diagnosis but occasionally there is a long survival, particularly if the disease is localized at the time of the first treatment.

GIANT FOLLICULAR LYMPHOMA

Synonyms. Follicular lymphoma; Lymphoid follicular reticulosis; Brill-Symmers disease.

Definition

A primary malignant disease arising in the lymph nodes or spleen, characterized by the presence of giant pseudofollicles.

Aetiology

This is unknown, but it is clearly related to the other lymphoproliferative disorders in that marrow and blood infiltration may occur giving the picture of chronic lymphocytic leukaemia, and it frequently terminates as frank lymphosarcoma. It is slightly commoner in males than in females and may occur at any age, although most cases fall into the same age group as chronic lymphocytic leukaemia, the average age being about 50 years.

Clinical Manifestations

Initially the commonest manifestation is either localized or generalized lymphadenopathy, which may be accompanied by splenomegaly. In some patients splenomegaly may be the only presenting feature. Providing the disease is correctly treated at this stage there are often no signs of recurrence for many years. However, most patients eventually relapse with splenomegaly or lymphadenopathy, sometimes with local pressure symptoms such as obstructive jaundice, superior vena caval obstruction, or spinal cord compression. Occasionally blockage of the thoracic duct causes a chylous pleural effusion and ascites. Once the disease progresses to involve the bone marrow and peripheral blood the clinical picture becomes that of chronic lymphocytic leukaemia. Frequently, late in the course of the disease, the disease becomes frankly lymphosarcomatous and invades other organs with massive pleural effusions, ascites, lung involvement, and infiltration of the gut. It is a rare cause of the malabsorption syndrome. Generalized lymphosarcoma is a common terminal event.

Anaemia may occur, due to infiltration of the bone marrow, or excessive haemolysis with or without a positive direct antiglobulin (Coombs) test.

Diagnosis

This is invariably made by histological examination of biopsy material, usually from a lymph node. It can almost be diagnosed naked-eye or with a hand lens because the giant pseudofollicles can readily be seen. At the onset the blood is usually normal, but later lymphocytosis (chronic lymphocytic leukaemia) may occur, and thrombocytopenia or anaemia may be found, as already discussed.

Treatment

As with the other lymphoproliferative disorders, if the disease is localized the treatment should be local, either by irradiation of the lymph nodes, or in the case of isolated splenomegaly, the spleen is removed in order to make the diagnosis. It may be many years before recurrence occurs, and some cases have apparently been cured by splenectomy alone. If the disease is generalized, chemotherapy should be given and the same principles apply to this disease as in chronic lymphocytic leukaemia, reticulum-cell sarcoma and lymphosarcoma. However, the disease is so sensitive to orthodox doses of chlorambucil that it is probably best to try this before proceeding to combination chemotherapy.

Prognosis

This is extremely variable, with some cases apparently cured by splenectomy, others surviving many years before clinical recurrence, but some follow a more rapid course. About 65 per cent. of patients are alive at 3 years and 40 per cent. at 5 years.

LYMPHOSARCOMA

Definition

This is a lymphoproliferative disease characterized by infiltration of lymph nodes, spleen and other organs with lymphoblasts or lymphocytes.

Aetiology

Lymphosarcoma occurs at all ages and in both sexes, but is commoner in males. The cause is unknown, although a virus may be associated with one particular form, the Burkitt lymphoma, which is considered in the next section.

Clinical Manifestations

Lymphosarcoma encompasses a range of lymphoproliferative diseases from conditions very similar to, and sometimes accompanied by, acute lymphoblastic leukaemia at one extreme and chronic lymphocytic leukaemia at the other. In the absence of infiltration of the blood or bone marrow the disease resembles reticulum cell sarcoma in its clinical manifestations.

Diagnosis

This is made by the histological appearance of biopsy material showing infiltration with lymphoblasts or lymphocytes.

Treatment

The principles are those already outlined in the treatment of reticulum-cell sarcoma, chronic lymphocytic and acute lymphoblastic leukaemia. Radiotherapy is used for local lesions but with chemotherapy what really matters is the type of malignant cell involved. If the infiltration is purely lymphocytic it should be treated like chronic lymphocytic leukaemia and giant follicular lymphoma with chlorambucil. If it is predominantly lymphoblastic then the drugs used in acute lymphoblastic leukaemia should be used.

Prognosis

As with reticulum-cell sarcoma the prognosis is very variable, and depends on whether the disease is localized when first treated. Most patients are dead within 2–3 years, but occasionally long-term survival occurs.

BURKITT LYMPHOMA

Definition

A particular form of lymphosarcoma occurring chiefly in Africa with a special histological appearance and anatomical distribution.

Aetiology

This tumour occurs chiefly in children in the malarious areas in Africa. A herpes virus (the Epstein-Barr or EB virus) has been isolated from the tumour cells grown in tissue culture, and antibodies against both this virus and the cell membranes of Burkitt lymphoma cells have been found in the sera of patients with this disease. However, an identical or very similar virus has also been incriminated as the cause of infectious mononucleosis; hence its role in the pathogenesis of the Burkitt lymphoma remains obscure. The disease has also been found in Europe and North America although it is very rare.

Clinical Manifestations

The clinical manifestations of this disease differ from other forms of lymphosarcoma. The commonest presenting feature is a tumour of the jaw, and the other organs frequently involved are the kidneys, ovaries or retroperitoneal tissue giving rise to abdominal masses. Other methods of presentation include paraplegia due to spinal cord compression and bone lesions other than in the jaw. The disease terminates as a generalized invasive lymphosarcoma, sometimes with a leukaemic phase, and sometimes with meningeal infiltration with malignant cells in the cerebrospinal fluid.

Diagnosis

This is made by histological examination of biopsy material showing infiltration with lymphoid cells together with large phagocytic cells giving the 'starry-sky' appearance.

Treatment

This is one of the most remarkable of all malignant diseases, in that there may be a dramatic response to a single injection of a cytotoxic drug, such as cyclophosphamide, vincristine or methotrexate, with complete remission occurring in many patients. Recent work from Uganda has shown that relapses are more likely to occur if no further chemotherapy is given, and maintenance treatment is therefore recommended.

Prognosis

This is very variable and depends on the stage of the disease when it is first treated. With localized tumours confined to the jaw the prognosis may be very good with remissions lasting many years and some patients definitely seem to have been cured. If the disease is generalized when first treated, the prognosis is much worse, but remarkable remissions may occur following chemotherapy.

CHRONIC LYMPHOCYTIC LEUKAEMIA

Synonyms. Chronic lymphatic leukaemia; Lymphatic leukaemia.

Definition

Malignant proliferation of lymphocytes with infiltration of the bone marrow, and frequently the blood.

Aetiology

Unlike acute and chronic granulocytic leukaemias irradiation is not an aetiological factor. The disease occurs in both men and women in the ratio of 2:1, and becomes commoner with advancing years, 80 per cent. of the patients being aged 40–70 at the time of diagnosis. It is very rare under the age of 30 years. There is an interesting geographical difference in that it is common in Europe and North America but very rare in China, Japan and the Western Pacific sea border. It appears to be unduly common in Jews.

Clinical Manifestations

The most frequent presenting features are lymphadenopathy, which may be localized or generalized, malaise and lassitude, and anaemia, but unlike chronic granulocytic leukaemia although the spleen is often enlarged it rarely causes symptoms. About 15 per cent. of the patients are diagnosed on a routine blood count. Purpura may be present. Patients with chronic lymphocytic leukaemia fail to form antibodies to foreign antigens, which renders them more prone to infections, particularly of the respiratory tract, with bronchitis and pneumonia, and the skin with multiple boils, cellulitis, and herpes zoster. Another complication is haemolytic anaemia, with or without a positive antiglobulin (Coombs) test, and this may be a presenting feature. Infiltration of any organ in the body may occur, usually late in the course of the disease, with involvement of the skin where the infiltration may be nodular or diffuse (*l'homme rouge*), serous membranes such as the pleura and peritoneum causing pleural effusion or ascites, salivary glands (it is one of the causes of Mikulicz's syndrome), the gastro-intestinal tract and indeed any tissue of the body. Unlike chronic granulocytic leukaemia, this disease does not become transformed into acute leukaemia as a terminal event. The patients die either of leukaemic infiltration of other organs, infection or uncontrolled haemolysis, or associated carcinomas to which these patients are more prone than the general population.

Diagnosis

This is established by the presence of a persistent lymphocytosis, either in the peripheral blood (>5000 lymphocytes per mm^3.) or the bone marrow (>40 per cent. of the nucleated cells) or both. The haemoglobin concentration and platelet count may be reduced and the direct antiglobulin (Coombs) test may be positive. Another common pathological finding is hypogammaglobulinaemia which is present in 60 per cent. of the patients and which becomes more severe as the disease advances. Occasionally hypergammaglobulinaemia occurs and a monoclonal increase particularly of IgM may be found.

Treatment

There are three main forms of treatment for chronic lymphocytic leukaemia; radiotherapy, cytotoxic drugs, and corticosteroids, each of which may be used under different circumstances. First, it must be emphasized that it may be quite unnecessary to give any treatment, and there is no indication simply to reduce the number of lymphocytes in the blood if this is the only abnormality.

The best group of drugs for the treatment of this disease is the nitrogen mustard group, and the one most commonly used is chlorambucil, although cyclophosphamide is also effective. As with chronic granulocytic leukaemia the aim is to control the disease rather than attempt radical cure, and most authorities use conventional doses of these drugs: in the case of chlorambucil, starting with 0·2 mg. per kg. per day by mouth, and slowly reducing the dose as the disease becomes controlled. Some authorities now recommend using larger doses intermittently. In addition to reducing the number of lymphocytes in the blood and bone marrow, these drugs usually cause reduction in the size of the lymph nodes, liver and spleen, but have less effect on anaemia and thrombocytopenia.

If anaemia and thrombocytopenia are present, corticosteroids should be used, and may prove rapidly effective. It is probably best to start with a large dose (prednisone, 40 mg. daily by mouth) and to reduce this as soon as the haemoglobin concentration and platelet count improve. It is often desirable to treat the patient first with prednisone and later with chlorambucil.

Radiotherapy has been used in the past in the form of ^{32}P to control the disease, but is now reserved for the local treatment of large glandular masses, which may be very sensitive, responding to much lower doses than are required in Hodgkin's disease and reticulum-cell sarcoma.

General supportive measures such as blood transfusion may be required, and a special watch must be kept for the presence of infections, particularly in patients receiving prednisone. Appropriate antibiotics must be given as soon as possible. Attempts to correct the deficiency of gammaglobulin by the regular injection of gamma globulin may be successful, but this is an expensive regime and probably has only a slight advantage over the use of antibiotics.

Course and Prognosis

The course of this disease is very variable, some patients living for many years with little trouble, while others may die within the first few years, the median survival being about 5 years, and 15 per cent. of the patients survive 10 years.

MYELOMATOSIS AND MACROGLOBULINAEMIA

This group of diseases is characterized by the abnormal production of a homogeneous immunoglobulin or part of an immunoglobulin (hence the term monoclonal gammopathy). They are distinguished from other types of hypergammaglobulinaemia because the abnormal protein migrates in a discrete band on electrophoresis, and can be shown to be a homogeneous protein on immuno-electrophoresis.

MYELOMATOSIS

Synonyms. Multiple myeloma; Kahler's disease; Plasma-cell leukaemia.

Definition

This is a malignant proliferation of plasma cells within the bone marrow with the excessive production of immunoglobulin in the form of IgG, IgA, IgD, IgE or as light chains (Bence-Jones protein).

Aetiology

This is unknown. In the past 30 years it appears to have become more common but this is probably the result of better diagnosis and ageing of the population. It affects both men and women and occurs late in life, some 80 per cent. of cases being over the age of 50. It is rare under the age of 40.

Clinical Manifestations

There are five major manifestations of this disease. The first, and probably the commonest mode of presentation is due to the osteolytic bone lesions produced by the malignant plasma cell. These may occur throughout the skeleton, and are particularly marked in the skull, ribs, vertebrae, pelvis and long bones. They appear radiographically as discrete punched-out osteolytic areas, and pathological fractures, associated with great pain, are common. Secondly, bone marrow infiltration may cause anaemia, which is sometimes accompanied by leucopenia and thrombocytopenia (pancytopenia) or sometimes presents as a leuco-erythroblastic anaemia. Thirdly, renal failure may occur, particularly if there is Bence-Jones proteinuria, and this can be quite rapidly fatal. Fourthly, hypercalcaemia, presumably due to excessive resorption from bone, may cause abdominal pain, vomiting and constipation. Fifthly, a haemorrhagic state may occur as in macroglobulinaemia due to large amounts of circulating immunoglobulin in the plasma. It is also a cause of generalized amyloidosis.

Patients with myelomatosis are particularly prone to infection, because of their inability to form antibodies against foreign antigens, as well as neutropenia due to marrow infiltration or treatment.

Diagnosis

In order to make the diagnosis of myelomatosis several of the essential criteria must be present. The reasons for this are, first, that solitary plasma cell tumours in bone do occur, and if treated may never become disseminated, or it may be many years before generalized disease ensues; secondly, a 'monoclonal' increase in immunoglobulin may be present for many years before the other features of myeloma become apparent, and treatment is not required for this alone. The three essential criteria for establishing the diagnosis therefore are multiple osteolytic lesions; infiltration of the bone marrow with normal, and frequently abnormal, plasma cells, and the presence in the serum and/or urine of an abnormal immunoglobulin which migrates in a narrow band on electrophoresis. Additional findings may also include hypercalcaemia, uraemia, anaemia with pancytopenia or a leuco-erythroblastic blood picture. Occasionally plasma cells are seen in the peripheral blood (plasma-cell leukaemia) and this is often accompanied by splenomegaly. The E.S.R. is very high (over 100 mm. in the first hour) if the serum contains the abnormal immunoglobulin. Occasionally the abnormal protein has the property of precipitating in the cold (cryoglobulinaemia) but it is not specific for myeloma protein, as this phenomenon may occur with any form of hypergammaglobulinaemia.

Treatment

Prednisone, starting with a dose of 40 mg. daily by mouth, is of value in the presence of anaemia and uraemia, and has the dramatic effect of lowering the serum calcium, particularly if a high fluid intake and a low calcium diet are given at the same time.

There is no doubt that the best treatment for the relief of bone pain is radiotherapy. It acts much faster than chemotherapy, but of course it has no effect on the disease in other parts of the body and is purely palliative. Chemotherapy for myelomatosis has proved disappointing in the past, although both cyclophosphamide and melphalan have produced a definite increase in survival. One of the best regimes appears to be the use of intermittent melphalan and prednisone although a special danger exists in using melphalan if uraemia is present, and under these circumstances the dose should be reduced. Melphalan, 10 mg. daily is given concurrently with prednisone, 40 mg. daily, for periods of 4–7 days, the courses being separated by intervals of 4–6 weeks. The dose of melphalan is halved if the blood urea level exceeds 60 mg. per 100 ml.

Prognosis

This is very variable; patients presenting with renal failure have a very poor prognosis, many dying within the first weeks or months. Other patients may survive for several years. It is hoped that the more recent treatment with intermittent combination chemotherapy will improve the prognosis.

HEAVY-CHAIN DISEASE (FRANKLIN'S DISEASE)

Immunoglobulins are made of light chains, which constitute Bence-Jones protein in myelomatosis, and heavy chains, which may on rare occasions be produced without the light chains. This was first described in middle-aged Negroes in the United States. The clinical syndrome resembles lymphosarcoma with enlarged lymph nodes, rather than myelomatosis. The disease tends to run a rapid course, the patients dying of generalized lymphosarcoma.

MACROGLOBULINAEMIA

Synonym. Waldenström's macroglobulinaemia.

Definition

A group of diseases characterized by the presence in the serum of a high concentration of macroglobulin (IgM) accounting for more than 10 per cent. of the total serum proteins.

Aetiology

This is unknown. The excessive production of IgM may occur as an isolated event, but most frequently is associated with a lymphoproliferative disorder (lymphosarcoma or chronic lymphocytic leukaemia) of low malignancy. It affects both men and women, particularly the elderly, having the same age distribution as chronic lymphocytic leukaemia. Macroglobulinaemia is sometimes classified with myelomatosis because they are both characterized by a monoclonal increase in immunoglobulin, but clinically there are important differences between the two conditions (see below).

Clinical Manifestations

Like myelomatosis, macroglobulinaemia may present with anaemia or a haemorrhagic disorder; unlike myelomatosis, osteolytic bone lesions and pathological fractures are not present, renal failure and hypercalcaemia are not usually prominent features, but lymphadenopathy and splenomegaly are commonly present.

The clinical manifestations may be subdivided into those of the primary underlying lymphoproliferative disease (lymphosarcoma and chronic lymphatic leukaemia, discussed elsewhere) and those due to the presence of the circulating macroglobulin which increases the viscosity of the blood. This leads to congestive cardiac failure and to retinopathy with papilloedema, engorged retinal veins, haemorrhages and exudates, closely resembling the appearance of retinal vein obstruction. A haemorrhagic state with bleeding gums and bruising may occur. Occasionally the abnormal IgM acts as a cold agglutinin causing the cold agglutinin syndrome with a haemolytic anaemia.

Treatment

Treatment for the underlying lymphoproliferative disease is the same as for chronic lymphocytic leukaemia, but treatment with one of the alkylating agents (chlorambucil or cyclophosphamide) has to be given for many months in conventional dosage before the level of IgM becomes significantly reduced. Emergency measures to relieve heart failure, retinopathy or the haemorrhagic state may be necessary, and plasmapheresis, removing the patient's own plasma and returning his red cells plus fresh frozen normal plasma, may be life saving.

Prognosis

Macroglobulinaemia even when accompanied by an overt lymphoproliferative disease may run a very long course, and patients can live for a number of years, many of them dying of associated conditions such as cardiac failure. Some, however, succumb with generalized lymphosarcoma.

REFERENCES

Brodsky, I., and Kahn, S. B., eds (1967) *Cancer Chemotherapy*, New York.

Burchenal, J. H. (1967) Long-time survival in Burkitt's tumor and in acute leukemia, *Cancer Res.*, **27**, Part 1, 2616.

Carbone, P. P. (1967) Hodgkin's disease: Combined clinical staff conference at the National Institutes of Health, *Ann. intern. Med.*, **67**, No. 2, 424.

Dameshek, W., and Dutcher, R. M., eds (1968) *Perspectives in Leukemia*, New York.

Dameshek, W., and Gunz, F., eds (1964) *Leukaemia*, 2nd ed., New York.

de Gruchy, G. C. (1970) *Clinical Haematology in Medical Practice*, 3rd ed., Oxford.

de Vita, V. T., Serpick, A., and Carbone, P. A. (1969) Combination chemotherapy of advanced Hodgkin's disease, *Proc. Amer. Ass. Cancer Res.*, **10,** 19.

Goldberg, A., and Brain, M. (1970) *Recent Advances in Haematology*, London.

Hayhoe, F. G. J., Quaglino, D., and Doll, R. (1964) The cytology and cytochemistry of acute leukaemias, *Spec. Rep. Ser. med. Res. Coun.* (*Lond.*), No. 304.

Hobbs, J. R. (1969) Immunochemical classes of myelomatosis, *Brit. J. Haemat.*, **16,** 599.

Kaplan, H. S. (1966) Clinical classification of Hodgkin's disease, *Cancer*, **19,** 371.

Lawrence, J. H. (1955) *Polycythemia: Physiology, Diagnosis and Treatment Based on 303 Cases*, New York.

Lukes, R. S., Butler, J. S., and Hicks, E. B. (1966) The natural history of Hodgkin's disease as related to its pathological picture, *Cancer*, **19,** 317.

M.R.C. Working Party for Therapeutic Trials in Leukaemia (1968) Chronic granulocytic leukaemia: Comparison of radiotherapy and busulphan therapy, *Brit. med. J.*, **1,** 201.

M.R.C. Leukaemia Committee and the Working Party on Leukaemia in Childhood (1971) Treatment of acute lymphoblastic leukaemia, *Brit. med. J.*, **4,** 189.

McCallister, B. D., Bayrd, E. D., Harrison, E. A., and McGucken, W. F. (1967) Primary macroglobulinemia: review with a report of 31 cases and notes on the value of continuous chlorambucil therapy, *Amer. J. Med.*, **43,** 394.

Molander, D. W., and Pack, G. T. (1968) *Hodgkin's Disease*, Springfield, Ill.

Szur, L., and Lewis, S. M. (1966). The haematological complications of polycythaemia vera and treatment with radioactive phosphorus, *Brit. J. Radiol.*, **39,** 122.

MISCELLANEOUS DISORDERS OF THE RED AND WHITE BLOOD CELLS

METHAEMOGLOBINAEMIA AND SULPHAEMOGLOBINAEMIA

Definition

Cyanosis due to the presence of methaemoglobin or sulphaemoglobin in the circulating red cells.

Aetiology

Most cases are due to the administration of drugs, particularly phenacetin, phenazone, acetanilide, sulphonamide, sulphones, primaquine, potassium chlorate and nitrites. Some cases may also occur due to industrial poisoning with dinitrobenzene and aniline dyes. Methaemoglobinaemia is due to the direct action of these chemicals, which increase the rate of auto-oxidation of haemoglobin in the red cells. Sulphaemoglobin is an abnormal sulphur-containing haemoglobin derivative, allied to methaemoglobin, and therefore arises in patients with methaemoglobinaemia, particularly in constipated patients where it is thought that increased amounts of hydrogen sulphide are absorbed from the bowel. There are also rare congenital and familial forms due to congenital metabolic defects of the red cell.

Clinical Manifestations

The most striking feature is cyanosis in the absence of any obvious cause, and frequently there are no other symptoms. However, in chronic cases the patients may complain of weakness, palpitations, headache, fainting and constipation.

Diagnosis

This is suggested by the presence of cyanosis without obvious heart or lung disease, and confirmed by the spectroscopic examination of the blood for methaemoglobin or sulphaemoglobin.

Treatment

Most cases are due to long self-medication with analgesics tablets containing phenacetin, although often patients deny that they are doing this. Removal of the causative agent enables methaemoglobin to be converted back to haemoglobin in a few days, and the cyanosis can be promptly relieved by the intravenous injection of methylene blue, 1·5 mg. per kg. Large doses of ascorbic acid are also effective. Sulphaemoglobinaemia is not reversible and the sulphaemoglobin persists in the affected red cells until the end of their normal life span.

LEUCOCYTOSIS AND LEUCOPENIA

NEUTROPHIL POLYMORPHONUCLEAR CELLS

An increase in the number of circulating neutrophil polymorphs is the commonest cause of leucocytosis, and may occur in a number of diseases. The most important is, of course, infection with a variety of bacteria, particularly the pyogenic cocci; following haemorrhage and trauma, e.g. surgical operations, fractures, crush injuries and burns; following pulmonary or myocardial infarction; in malignant disease particularly when there is involvement of the liver; in Hodgkin's disease, and, of course, in the myeloproliferative syndromes of chronic granulocytic leukaemia, polycythaemia vera and sometimes myelofibrosis. Not only is there an increase in the number of circulating neutrophil polymorphs, but frequently there is a 'shift to the left' with the appearance of blood of metamyelocytes and even myelocytes, particularly if the white count is very high.

Leucopenia, due to the decrease in the number of circulating neutrophils, may also occur for a variety of reasons [see TABLE 65].

TABLE 65

CAUSES OF NEUTROPHIL LEUCOPENIA

INFECTIONS:
- Bacterial—typhoid fever, paratyphoid fever, brucellosis.
- Viral—influenza, measles, rubella, infective hepatitis, atypical virus pneumonia.
- Rickettsial—typhus, scrub typhus.
- Protozoal—malaria, kala-azar.
- Overwhelming infections—miliary tuberculosis, severe infections in elderly or debilitated persons.

ACUTE LEUKAEMIA (sub-leukaemic variety)

DRUG-INDUCED NEUTROPENIA:
- Selective neutropenia.
- As part of an aplastic anaemia.

APLASTIC ANAEMIA

HYPERSPLENISM

IDIOPATHIC NEUTROPENIA:
- Acute.
- Chronic.

BONE MARROW INFILTRATION OR SCLEROSIS—secondary carcinoma, malignant lymphomas, myelosclerosis, multiple myeloma.

MEGALOBLASTIC ANAEMIAS

DISSEMINATED LUPUS ERYTHEMATOSUS

IRON DEFICIENCY ANAEMIA

MISCELLANEOUS—anaphylactoid shock, myxoedema, thyrotoxicosis, hypopituitarism, cirrhosis of the liver, paroxysmal nocturnal haemoglobinuria.

(Modified from de Gruchy (1970) *Clinical Haematology in Medical Practice.*)

The term 'neutropenia' is used when the number of neutrophils falls below the lower limit of normal [see TABLE 59], and the term 'agranulocytosis' is reserved for severe neutropenia accompanied by infection, which usually occurs when the neutrophil count falls below 1000 per mm^3. The symptoms of severe neutropenia are those of infection, particularly of the oral cavity with sore throat and ulceration in the mouth, which may later involve other parts of the gastro-intestinal tract. Infection of the lung, skin and urine are common and the temperature may become very high. Apart from bacterial infection, secondary infection with *Candida* may occur, particularly in the mouth and oesophagus.

Of the varieties of leucopenia shown in TABLE 65 two deserve special mention: the drug-induced neutropenia, and idiopathic neutropenia. Many of the drugs which cause neutropenia also affect the production of red cells and platelets, and are discussed under the heading of hypoplastic anaemia. However, some frequently affect the granulocytes more than the other cellular elements, in particular the antibacterial agents chloramphenicol and sulphonamides, the analgesics amidopyrine and phenylbutazone, the anti-epileptic drugs phenytoin and troxidone, the phenothiazine group such as chlorpromazine, and the antithyroid drugs methylthiouracil and carbimazole. In some cases, as with amidopyrine, antibodies to white cells can be detected, while other cases appear to be due to a failure of production of granulocytes. Clearly these drugs should be avoided if suitable alternatives are available.

The treatment of drug-induced neutropenia is, of course, to stop the drug immediately; to treat any existing infections as rapidly as possible, and to remove the patient from an environment in which he may become infected. In severe cases the patient should be barrier nursed in a single room, or even transferred to a special centre where he can be placed in a sterile environment.

Unfortunately it is not yet practicable to maintain the neutrophil count at a satisfactory level by giving infusions of white cells, but this may become possible in the future. There is controversy about the use of corticosteroids because they may have a deleterious effect on infection, but there is some evidence also to suggest that they may have a beneficial effect on the bone marrow. However, if there is no spontaneous recovery within a week of stopping the drug, prednisolone, in a dose of 40–80 mg. daily, should be given, and it is possible that the newer androgenic hormone, oxymetholone, may prove to have an effect on the white cell as well as the red cell series (see hypoplastic anaemia).

There is a rare condition of *chronic idiopathic neutropenia*, resulting in chronic infections, the pathogenesis of which is unknown but some cases appear to be due to defective production of granulocytes while others may be due to increased destruction, possibly as a result of antibodies against the white cells. Some cases show a periodic or cyclical neutropenia which may persist for many years. There is no specific curative treatment, and the essentials of management are to prevent and treat infections. Splenectomy, and the administration of corticosteroids are usually without benefit.

EOSINOPHILS

An increase in the number of circulating eosinophils occurs in many diseases, particularly those associated with allergic reactions. Eosinophilia may be found in asthma, hay fever, drug allergy, serum sickness and urticaria. It is also frequently, but not invariably, present in parasitic infestations such as intestinal worms, hydatid cysts, schistosomiasis, and filariasis. It also occurs in some skin diseases, such as eczema, pemphigus, dermatitis herpetiformis, and prurigo. Under some circumstances eosinophilia occurs in association with pulmonary infiltrations with or without asthma (pulmonary eosinophilia). Many of these are associated with the passage of larvae from worm infestations through the lungs, particularly *Ascaris lumbricoides* (Loeffler's syndrome). Other causes include tropical eosinophilia [see Section 2] and polyarteritis nodosa. In many forms of malignant disease eosinophilia may occur, but it is particularly common in Hodgkin's disease. Eosinophilia may also be a feature in some patients with chronic granulocytic leukaemia. There is also a very rare familial disorder in which the ratio of eosinophils to neutrophils is reversed (hereditary eosinophilia).

Eosinophilic leucopenia occurs whenever there is an increase in circulating adrenocortical hormones, and therefore occurs during treatment with these drugs, in Cushing's disease, following 'stress' in the form of haemorrhage or trauma, and as part of hypoplastic anaemia.

BASOPHILS

An increase in the number of circulating basophils is almost invariably due to a myeloproliferative disease, in particular chronic granulocytic leukaemia. Very occasionally it may occur in haemolytic anaemia and other chronic anaemias, but the increase is usually small.

LYMPHOCYTES

As shown in TABLE 59 the total white cell count is higher in infants and children than in adults, and the absolute lymphocyte count is partly responsible for this until about the age of 12, when it becomes the same as in adults. Lymphocytosis may occur in many of the acute infectious diseases of childhood, particularly in whooping cough (pertussis) with very high counts (up to 80,000 per mm^3.). Milder lymphocytosis may be present in viral infections like mumps, measles, rubella, chickenpox, influenza, infectious mononucleosis, viral hepatitis, etc. and some bacterial infections such as typhoid, brucellosis, tuberculosis, and in secondary syphilis. Occasionally slight lymphocytosis occurs in hyperthyroidism, myasthenia gravis, and hypopituitarism. In adult life the commonest cause of lymphocytosis is chronic lymphocytic leukaemia, and levels remaining persistently above 5000 lymphocytes per mm^3. are diagnostic in this country. However, in Africa a marked lymphocytosis is found in 'big spleen disease' [see Section 2].

Lymphopenia occurs in any form of pancytopenia, and also in some of the rare congenital immune-deficiency diseases [see Section 4].

MONOCYTES

The monocytes are increased in some patients following acute infections, in infectious mononucleosis and subacute bacterial endocarditis, as well as in monocytic or monoblastic leukaemia.

REFERENCES

ADAMS, E. B., and WITTS, L. J. (1949) Chronic agranulocytosis, *Quart. J. Med.*, **18,** 173.

BRAUNSTEINER, H., and ZUCKER-FRANKLIN, D. (1962) *The Physiology and Pathology of Leukocytes*, New York.

CRONKITE, E. P., and FLEIDNER, T. M. (1964) Granulocytopoiesis, *New Engl. J. Med.*, **270,** 1347, 1403.

DONOHUGH, D. L. (1966) Eosinophils and eosinophilia, *Calif. Med.*, **104,** 421.

ELVES, M. W. (1967) *The Lymphocyte*, London.

FREDERICKS, R. E., and MOLONEY, W. C. (1959) The basophilic granulocyte, *Blood*, **14,** 571.

HUGULEY, C. M., LEA, J. W., and BUTTS, J. A. (1966) Adverse haematologic reactions to drugs, in *Progress in Hematology*, ed. BROWN, E. B., and MOORE, C. V., Vol. V, p. 105, New York.

SHILLITOE, A. J. (1950) The common causes of lymphopenia, *J. clin. Path.*, **3,** 321.

WOLF-JURGENSEN, P. (1968) The basophilic leukocyte, *Series Haemat.*, **1,** No. 4, 45.

MISCELLANEOUS DISEASES OF LYMPHORETICULAR TISSUE

LYMPHADENOPATHY

Enlargement of lymph nodes is a common physical sign in clinical medicine, and is due either to inflammation or neoplasia, the infecting agents or neoplastic cells reaching the nodes either through the lymph or via the blood stream, the former causing localized and the latter generalized lymphadenopathy.

LYMPHADENOPATHY DUE TO INFECTION

In any infected area of the body, the organisms may pass in the lymph to the drainage lymph node causing enlargement. If the defence mechanisms within the node are effective the infection may pass no further, but if not spread may occur to other nodes or the blood stream. This is well illustrated by septic lesions of the hand which can give rise to painful lymphangitis, the inflamed lymph vessels being visible, followed by epitrochlear and then axillary lymphadenopathy.

Many organisms can therefore give rise to local lymphadenopathy: viruses in lymphogranuloma venereum, and cat scratch fever; rickettsiae in scrub typhus; bacteria with staphylococci, streptococci, tubercle bacilli and in diphtheria and plague; spirochaetes in primary syphilis; protozoa in trypanosomiasis; and worm infestation in filariasis. In lymphadenopathy due to pyogenic organisms the glands are obviously inflamed, tender and painful, but with other organisms such as tuberculosis and syphilis the enlargement is painless.

Generalized lymphadenopathy may occur with many infections due to transmission via the blood stream. With viruses these include infectious mononucleosis and rubella; bacteria in typhoid, brucellosis and tuberculosis; spirochaetes in secondary syphilis; and protozoa in kala-azar and toxoplasmosis. Generalized lymphadenopathy may also accompany some of the connective tissue diseases, particularly rheumatoid arthritis in children (Still's disease) and systemic lupus erythematosus, and is common in sarcoidosis.

LYMPHADENOPATHY DUE TO MALIGNANT DISEASE

As with infections, this may be localized due to the passage of malignant cells via the lymph to the regional drainage nodes, or generalized due to spread beyond this either via lymph or blood. It is the carcinomas rather than the sarcomas which spread via lymphatics, and sometimes for anatomical reasons the lymph node may be some distance from the primary tumour. For example, in carcinoma of the stomach, spread may occur to the supraclavicular nodes via the thoracic duct. In addition to secondary involvement of the nodes in malignant disease, there are primary malignant diseases of lymph nodes which may be localized or generalized, and which are considered under the heading of lymphoproliferative diseases [see p. 1037].

With localized lymphadenopathy it is essential to search for a primary infective or malignant lesion in the area drained by the involved lymph nodes. Sometimes the cause is obvious, but occasionally it is difficult to find. This occurs in infections particularly with dental abscesses, sepsis between the toes, and in venereal diseases such as syphilis and lymphogranuloma venereum when the primary lesion may be very small. Similarly, with malignant disease, small primary tumours in the nasopharynx can easily be missed. With generalized lymphadenopathy appropriate investigations for the causes already mentioned may reveal the diagnosis, but in both the localized and generalized forms lymph node biopsy may be required.

LIPOID STORAGE DISEASES

GAUCHER'S DISEASE

Synonym. Lipoid histiocytosis of kerasin type.

Definition

This is a rare disorder of metabolism characterized by the accumulation of lipid in the form of cerebroside (kerasin) in the cells of the reticulo-endothelial system.

Aetiology

This is a familial disease, particularly affecting Jews, which is thought to be due to an autosomal recessive gene. Very occasionally it is transmitted as an autosomal dominant. It occurs both in adult and infantile forms.

Clinical Manifestations

In the adult form the disease is usually recognized in late childhood or early in adult life. The common manifestations are splenomegaly which is progressive; hepatomegaly; bone pain, due to infiltration of the bone marrow with Gaucher cells, which may expand the bones, particularly the lower ends of the femora giving the 'Erlenmeyer' flask deformity; pathological fractures; pigmentation of the skin; pingueculae, which are yellow-brown wedge-shaped thickenings of the conjunctiva at the lateral margin of the cornea, and occasionally trivial lymphadenopathy may occur. In the infantile form occurring within the first 6 months of life, in addition to the features already mentioned, widespread neuronal degeneration occurs with muscular wasting leading to death by the age of one year.

Haematological Investigations

The blood changes are due to two different mechanisms, marrow infiltration and hypersplenism. Both may result in a normochromic normocytic anaemia, leucopenia and thrombocytopenia. The bone marrow shows Gaucher cells which are large, pale cells 20–40 μ in diameter with pale cytoplasm showing a wavy pattern of fine fibrils.

Treatment

There is no specific treatment, but radiotherapy

relieves the bone pain, and splenectomy may correct the pancytopenia if this is due to hypersplenism.

Course and Prognosis

Providing that the effects of hypersplenism and the bone lesions can be controlled patients may live for many years.

REFERENCES

GROEN, J. J. (1964) Gaucher's disease, *Arch. intern. Med.*, **113,** 543.

MATOTH, Y., and FRIED, K. (1965) Chronic Gaucher's disease, *Israel J. med. Sci.*, **1,** 521.

NIEMANN-PICK DISEASE

Synonym. Lipoid histiocytosis of phosphatide type.

Definition and Aetiology

This is due to a rare familial autosomal recessive genetic defect in which large amounts of phospholipid (especially sphingomyelin) are deposited in the cells of the reticulo-endothelial and nervous systems. Like Gaucher's disease it is common in Jews.

Clinical Manifestations

The onset is in the first year of life with weight loss, vomiting, abdominal distension due to hepatosplenomegaly and with neurological lesions leading to weakness, spasticity, blindness and deafness. The diagnosis is established by finding large cells similar to Gaucher cells, but containing hyaline droplets in the bone marrow. There is no treatment and the disease is fatal within months of onset.

REFERENCE

CROCKER, A. C., and FARBER, S. (1958) Niemann-Pick disease, *Medicine (Baltimore)*, **37,** 1.

HAND-SCHÜLLER-CHRISTIAN DISEASE

Synonym. Histiocytosis X.

Definition

There are three rare clinical syndromes, all showing a proliferation of histiocytes, which contain cholesterol, and which progress to fibrosis and scarring—Letterer-Siwe disease, Hand-Schüller-Christian disease, and eosinophilic granuloma.

Clinical Manifestations

Letterer-Siwe disease is a rapidly progressive fatal disease of the reticulo-endothelial system occurring in infancy and untreated ends in death within a few weeks or months. *Hand-Schüller-Christian* disease is characterized by the triad of skull defects, exophthalmos due to lesions in the orbit, and diabetes insipidus due to involvement of the hypophysis. It most commonly begins about the age of 5, and apart from the classical triad may show hepatosplenomegaly, yellow-brown maculopapular skin lesions, petechiae, honeycomb lung and skeletal defects elsewhere. *Eosinophilic granuloma* is the term used to describe isolated bone lesions of the same pathology.

Diagnosis

The diagnosis is established by the characteristic histology on biopsy material.

Treatment

Until recently there was no effective treatment but the disease may be controlled by the use of corticosteroids such as prednisone, and if this fails alkylating agents such as chlorambucil may be used as well.

The other lipoid storage diseases—hypercholesterolaemia, xanthomatosis and Tay-Sachs disease are considered elsewhere.

REFERENCES

AVIOLI, L. V., LASERSOHN, J. T., and LOPRESTI, J. M. (1963) Histiocytosis X, *Medicine (Baltimore)*, **42,** 119.

LEWIS, J. G. (1964) Eosinophilic granuloma and its variants, with special reference to lung involvement, *Quart. J. Med.*, N.S. **33,** 337.

INFECTIOUS MONONUCLEOSIS

Synonym. Glandular fever.

Definition

This is an acute infection characterized by abnormal mononuclear cells in the blood, and the presence of a heterophile antibody against sheep red cells detected by the Paul-Bunnell reaction.

Aetiology

The causative organism is almost certainly a virus. Following infectious mononucleosis, antibodies are formed which react against the cell membranes of Burkitt lymphoma cells and the herpes virus (Epstein-Barr virus) present in them. Furthermore, a similar if not identical virus has been isolated from glandular fever cells in tissue culture. The disease occurs chiefly in children and young adults, particularly in those living in institutions such as hospitals and residential colleges. The incubation period is uncertain but is probably several weeks.

Clinical Manifestations

The usual symptoms of fever, malaise and headache occur as with any infection. Pharyngitis, lymphadenopathy which may be localized or generalized, and splenomegaly are common features. Jaundice due to hepatitis occurs in 15 per cent. and liver function tests are abnormal in 90 per cent. Less commonly erythematous skin rashes, conjunctivitis, myocarditis, meningitis, pneumonia, haemolytic anaemia and thrombocytopenic purpura may occur. Palatal petechiae and periorbital swelling with oedema of the eyelids are common early features.

Haematological Investigations

The total white cell count may be normal or slightly raised, but there is neutrophil leucopenia associated with the presence of large lymphoid cells with eccentric oval or lobulated nuclei with basophilic cytoplasm, which sometimes presents a 'foamy' appearance. These cells are usually present by the third or fourth day, may persist for several weeks, or may disappear quite rapidly within a few days. The Paul-Bunnell reaction usually becomes positive by the end of the first week, but may not be present until the second or third week in some cases. This reaction depends on the presence of a heterophile antibody active against sheep red cells. The antibody is not absorbed by guinea-pig kidney, but is absorbed by ox red cells. Other heterophile antibodies which may be present in some diseases such as the reticuloses are absorbed by guinea-pig kidney and not by ox red cells; but the antibody in serum sickness or following injections of horse serum is absorbed by both.

Diagnosis

This disease must be distinguished from acute leukaemia, and from other virus infections which produce similar cells in the blood. There is usually no difficulty in telling the difference between the mononuclear cells of glandular fever and those of leukaemia, and the presence of a positive Paul-Bunnell reaction will settle the diagnosis. There is, however, a group of diseases which has many of the characteristics of infectious mononucleosis, although the Paul-Bunnell reaction remains negative. It is difficult to classify these, but with advances in virology the aetiological agents will probably be discovered shortly. It has been possible to recognize one syndrome due to cytomegalovirus infection.

Treatment

There is no specific treatment, but antibiotics should be given if secondary bacterial infection occurs and corticosteroids have been advised in the seriously ill.

Course and Prognosis

This is a benign disease, in most cases the illness only lasting for 1 or 2 weeks. In some patients this is followed by general malaise, tiredness, weakness and depression, which may persist for a variable period of time ranging from a few weeks to many months. Patients with hepatitis and meningitis may become severely ill, but recovery is the rule, the only deaths in this disease being due to splenic rupture which is excessively rare.

REFERENCES

BENDER, C. E. (1967) The value of corticosteroids in the treatment of infectious mononucleosis, *J. Amer. med. Ass.*, **199**, 529.

CARTER, R. L., and PENMAN, H. G., eds (1969) *Infectious Mononucleosis*, Oxford.

HOAGLAND, R. J. (1967) *Infectious Mononucleosis*, New York.

RIFKIND, D. (1968) Cytomegalovirus mononucleosis, *Ann. intern. Med.*, **69**, 840.

G. HAMILTON FAIRLEY

THE HAEMOGLOBINOPATHIES

The inherited disorders of haemoglobin synthesis, the haemoglobinopathies, are by far the largest group of congenital anaemias. Although these conditions are most frequently found in the Mediterranean region, Africa and parts of Asia, they have now been encountered in every racial group.

The clinical classification of the haemoglobinopathies is based on the structure and genetic control of normal haemoglobin. Furthermore, the clinical manifestations of these disorders are best appreciated if examined in terms of a breakdown of these control mechanisms and of the normal oxygen-carrying properties of haemoglobin.

NORMAL HUMAN HAEMOGLOBIN

Structure and Function

Normal adult haemoglobin, haemoglobin A, is a spherical protein with a molecular weight of 68,000. It consists of a protein part, globin, and four haem groups, each consisting of a protoporphyrin ring containing one iron atom.

The globin fraction of haemoglobin A is made up of two pairs of peptide chains, α and β-chains, each associated with one haem. The α-chains consist of 141 amino acids, or residues, while the β-chains are 146 amino acid residues long. The chains consist of eight coiled or helical areas, designated A to H, separated by non-helical zones, AB, BC, etc. Because of the properties of the side chains of the constituent amino acids the globin chains are further folded into a complex configuration with each haem group occupying a deep crevice on the surface of the molecule. Each α-chain is in contact with both β-chains, these contacts being designated $\alpha_1\beta_1$ and $\alpha_1\beta_2$. During the taking up and liberating of oxygen the β-chains rotate on the α-chains at these contact areas, the distance between the haem units of the β-chains widening by about 7 Å during deoxygenation. The production of a physiological oxygen dissociation curve requires that when one haem unit takes on oxygen the rate of oxygenation of the others is greatly facilitated. This haem-haem interaction almost certainly depends on the rotational movements between the α and β-subunits which occur during oxygenation.

In adult life human haemoglobin is a mixture of proteins, consisting of a major component, haemoglobin A, and a minor fraction which makes up about 2·5 per cent. of the total, haemoglobin A_2. In intra-uterine life foetal haemoglobin is the main respiratory pigment while in the embryo, up to about 9 weeks, a distinct embryonic haemoglobin makes up a variable proportion of the total haemoglobin. At birth foetal haemoglobin synthesis ceases and by the age of one year haemoglobins A and A_2 are fully established. The mechanisms which control this remarkable series of adaptive changes have not yet been worked out.

All the human haemoglobins have a pair of α-chains. In adult life these are paired with β-chains to form haemoglobin A ($\alpha_2\beta_2$) and with δ-chains to form haemoglobin A_2 ($\alpha_2\delta_2$). In foetal life α-chains are combined with γ-chains to form haemoglobin F ($\alpha_2\gamma_2$) and with ϵ chains to form embryonic haemoglobin ($\alpha_2\epsilon_2$).

The Genetic Control of Haemoglobin Synthesis

The sequence of amino acids in any peptide chain is determined by the length of DNA which constitutes the 'gene' for that particular chain, i.e. there is a 'one gene—one peptide chain' relationship. The sequence of amino acids in the chain is determined by the sequence of bases, thymine (T), cystosine (C), guanine (G) and adenine (A) which constitute the DNA. Each amino acid is coded by a series of three bases, e.g. the sequence CGA is the code word or codon for arginine.

Studies of families with abnormal haemoglobins have provided a clear picture of how the genetic control of normal haemoglobin is organized [FIG. 67]. Separate pairs of allelomorphic genes control the structure of the α, β, γ and δ-chains. In intra-uterine life the α and γ-chain genes are active, α-chains combining with γ-chains to form foetal haemoglobin ($\alpha_2\gamma_2$). After birth the γ-chain genes are repressed and the β and δ-chain genes activated; α-chains now combine with β-chains and δ-chains to form haemoglobins A ($\alpha_2\beta_2$) and A_2 ($\alpha_2\delta_2$), respectively. This explains why inherited disorders of the α-chains affect both foetal and adult haemoglobin whilst abnormal β-chain production only affects adult haemoglobin.

The globin chains are synthesized on groups of ribosomes in the cytoplasm of the red cell precursors. A form of ribonucleic acid (RNA) called messenger RNA, with a sequence of bases exactly complementary to those of the DNA upon which it is copied, acts as the cytoplasmic template for globin chain synthesis. Each haemoglobin gene produces a separate messenger RNA which diffuses into the cell cytoplasm. The constituent amino acids are carried to the ribosomes attached to a form of RNA called transfer RNA, which has three bases, the anticodon, complimentary to those of the messenger RNA. The correct amino acid is put into the growing chain because the anticodon of the transfer RNA finds the correct codon in the messenger RNA. The ribosomes act as a carrier or jig, carrying the growing chains and moving across the messenger RNA from one end to the other as the message is 'translated', by appropriate transfer RNAs. As each amino acid is put into position it forms a peptide bond with the preceding amino acid and the chain is thus lengthened by one amino acid, the transfer RNA being released to carry further amino acids to the template. When the chain is finished it is released from the ribosome and combines with other chains to form a haemoglobin molecule.

A more detailed account of the genetic control of haemoglobin production will be found in several recent reviews (Huehns and Shooter, 1965; Lehmann and Huntsman, 1966; Weatherall and Clegg, 1969).

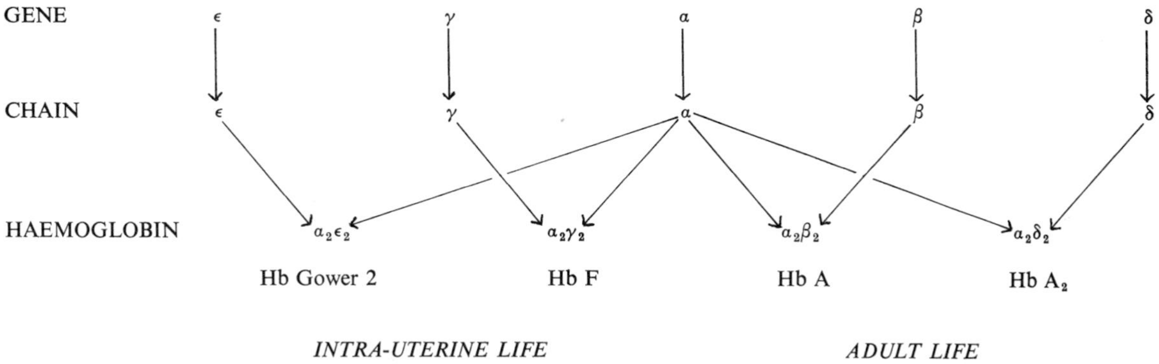

FIG. 67. The genetic control of haemoglobin synthesis. The single genetic locus directing α-chain synthesis in foetal and adult life explains why α-thalassaemia is associated with defective synthesis of foetal and adult haemoglobin while β-thalassaemia is only manifest after the neonatal period. For the sake of simplicity the fact that some of these loci, e.g. γ and probably α-loci, consist of multiple structured genes has been omitted.

THE HAEMOGLOBINOPATHIES

There are three groups of inherited disorders of haemoglobin synthesis [TABLE 66]. First there are those conditions which result from a genetically determined alteration in the structure of haemoglobin. A second and larger group is comprised of disorders which result from an inherited defect in the *rate* of synthesis of one of the globin chains. These are known collectively as the thalassaemia syndromes. In the thalassaemias such globin as is synthesized has a normal chemical structure. Finally there is a heterogeneous group of congenital and acquired alterations of the haemoglobin pattern characterized by the persistence of foetal haemoglobin synthesis into adult life or the reactivation of foetal haemoglobin production in response to disease.

TABLE 66

CLASSIFICATION OF THE HAEMOGLOBINOPATHIES

1. Structural haemoglobin variants:
   a. α-chain
   b. β-chain
   c. γ-chain
   d. δ-chain

2. Defects in the rate of globin production:
   a. α-thalassaemia
   b. β-thalassaemia
   c. δ-thalassaemia

3. Developmental changes in haemoglobin production:
   a. hereditary persistence of foetal haemoglobin
   b. chromosomal abnormalities

There are several extensive reviews of the structural haemoglobin variants (Huehns and Shooter, 1965; Itano, 1965; Lehmann and Huntsman, 1966; Weatherall, 1971).

THE STRUCTURAL HAEMOGLOBINOPATHIES

Most of the structural haemoglobin variants differ from haemoglobin A by the substitution of a single amino acid in one of the globin chains. These alterations are all in agreement with a single base change in a codon of the gene for the affected chain [FIG. 68], i.e. they result from a mutation or alteration of a single base in the genetic code. A few haemoglobin variants have one or more amino acids missing or deleted, probably the result of unequal crossing over during meiosis. All these disorders are inherited in a Mendelian co-dominant fashion.

ABNORMAL HAEMOGLOBIN	AMINO ACID ALTERATION	POSSIBLE CHANGE IN GENETIC CODE
S	β^6 glutamic acid ↓ valine	G*A*A or G*A*G ↓ ↓ G*U*A or G*U*G
C	β^6 glutamic acid ↓ lysine	*G*AA or *G*AG ↓ ↓ *A*AA or *A*AG
I	α^{16} lysine ↓ glutamic acid	*A*AA or *A*AG ↓ ↓ *G*AA or *G*AG

FIG. 68. Abnormal haemoglobins and the genetic code. The code is degenerate, i.e. there is more than one code word per amino acid. In all the abnormal haemoglobins there is a single altered base which results in the amino acid substitution.

The majority of haemoglobin variants have been discovered by electrophoresis, the amino acid substitution so altering the charge of the molecule that it moves differently from haemoglobin A in an electric field. Originally letters of the alphabet were used to designate a new haemoglobin variant, but since these have long been used up, the place of origin of the affected individual is now used. The heterozygous carrier state for a haemoglobin variant is called the 'trait', e.g. haemoglobin S trait, while the homozygous condition is designated 'disease', e.g. haemoglobin S disease.

Many of the haemoglobin variants have no clinical significance and have been found during population surveys. However, some amino acid substitutions, presumably because they occur at critical areas of the molecule, result in lack of molecular stability or abnormal oxygen transport, and hence disease. The clinical disorders which result from structural haemoglobinopathies are summarized in TABLE 67. The sickling disorders and haemoglobin C disease are very common in parts of Africa while haemoglobin E disease occurs frequently in South East Asia. The other structural haemoglobin variants are rare, occur in all racial groups and are associated with conditions such as familial polycythaemia, congenital methaemoglobinaemia and congenital non-spherocytic haemolytic anaemia.

TABLE 67

CLINICAL DISORDERS RESULTING FROM STRUCTURAL HAEMOGLOBIN VARIANTS

1. Haemolytic anaemia
   a. Haemoglobin S disorders
   b. Haemoglobin C disease
   c. Haemoglobin D disease
   d. Haemoglobin E disease
   e. The unstable haemoglobin disorders
2. Congenital methaemoglobinaemia
   The haemoglobin M disorders
3. Congenital polycythaemia
   Haemoglobins with increased oxygen affinity
4. Congenital hypochromic anaemia
   Haemoglobins with a reduced rate of synthesis
   The haemoglobin Lepore syndromes

THE SICKLING DISORDERS

Synonyms. Sickle-cell disease; Sickle-cell anaemia; Drepanocytic anaemia; Meniscocytic anaemia.

Definition and Distribution

The sickling disorders are those which result from the inheritance of haemoglobin S, either alone or in combination with other abnormal haemoglobins [TABLE 68]. They consist of homozygous sickle-cell anaemia and the heterozygous states for haemoglobin S and other structural haemoglobin variants or thalassaemia. Sickle-cell anaemia is most frequently encountered in Africa where it occurs in a broad belt across the middle third of the continent. The carrier rate in this area is 10–30 per cent. of the population and the disease accounts for approximately 80,000 infant deaths per year. It also occurs with a much lower incidence in parts of Italy, Greece, the Middle East and India. The high frequency of this gene in Africa has arisen because heterozygous carriers are more resistant than normal individuals to falciparum malaria during early childhood.

Aetiology

Haemoglobin S differs from haemoglobin A by the substitution of valine for glutamic acid in the sixth position along the β-chain [FIG. 68]. This alteration results in fundamental differences in the physical properties of sickle haemoglobin as compared with haemoglobin A. Thus in conditions of reduced oxygen tension haemoglobin S is relatively insoluble, the haemoglobin molecules forming linear stacks or tactoids. These produce the typical sickled deformity of the red cell which has two main consequences. First, small vessels become blocked by aggregations of sickled erythrocytes resulting in tissue infarction. Secondly, the deformity of the sickled cells results in their shortened survival and hence a severe haemolytic anaemia. Because haemoglobin S has a reduced oxygen affinity oxygen is easily released from the red cells of patients with the sickling disorders. This results in a poorly compensated haemolytic anaemia since tissue anoxia is the main drive to increased red cell production.

It is still not certain how the substitution of valine for glutamic acid results in sickling. It is possible that it causes an alteration in the physical properties at the surface of the β-chain. In this altered state the end of the chain may find a complementary site on an adjacent molecule produced by the conformational changes which occur during deoxygenation. This process leads to 'molecular stacking' and hence to tactoid formation.

The clinical severity of the sickling disorders depends on the number of cells capable of sickling, the level of haemoglobin S in each red cell, the amount of interaction between haemoglobin S and other haemoglobin variants which may be present, and the packed-cell volume.

Symptoms occur if the number of sickle cells form 50 per cent. or more of the total red cell mass. The higher the level of haemoglobin S in each cell, the more severe the clinical disorder. Thus in sickle-cell trait where there is only 30–40 per cent. haemoglobin S, symptoms are rare. Haemoglobin S interacts with haemoglobin C and D to produce a severe clinical disorder, whereas large amounts of haemoglobin F appear to protect against sickling. The blood viscosity in sickle-cell anaemia increases as deoxygenation occurs, due to the sickling phenomena. This effect is much more marked when the packed cell volume rises above 30 per cent.

TABLE 68

THE SICKLING DISORDERS

DISORDER	GENOTYPE	CLINICAL FINDINGS
Sickle-cell disease	$\alpha\alpha\ \beta^S\beta^S$	Severe haemolytic anaemia
S-C disease	$\alpha\alpha\ \beta^S\beta^C$	Moderate haemolytic anaemia
S-D (Punjab) disease	$\alpha\alpha\ \beta^S\beta^D$	Moderate haemolytic anaemia
S-J (Baltimore) disease	$\alpha\alpha\ \beta^S\beta^J$	No clinical abnormality
S-K disease	$\alpha\alpha\ \beta^S\beta^K$	No clinical abnormality
S-hereditary persistence of Hb F heterozygosity	$\alpha\alpha\ \beta^S\beta^-$	No clinical abnormality
S-E disease	$\alpha\alpha\ \beta^S\beta^E$	Moderate haemolytic anaemia
Haemoglobin Memphis-S	$\alpha^{mem}\alpha\ \beta^S\beta^S$	Mild haemolytic anaemia
Haemoglobin G (Philadelphia) S	$\alpha\alpha^G\ \beta^S\beta^S$	Mild haemolytic anaemia
S-O disease	$\alpha\alpha\ \beta^S\beta^O$	Moderate haemolytic anaemia
S-D (Ibadan) disease	$\alpha\alpha\ \beta^S\beta^D$	No clinical abnormalities
Sickle-cell β-thalassaemia	$\alpha\alpha\ \beta^S\beta^{thal}$	Variable – depending on type of associated thalassaemia gene
Sickle-cell α-thalassaemia	$\alpha^{thal\ 1}\alpha^{thal\ 2}\beta^S\beta^S$	Mild anaemia. No sickle crisis

SICKLE-CELL ANAEMIA; HOMOZYGOUS HAEMOGLOBIN S DISEASE

Clinical Picture

The disease usually presents after the third month of life when adult haemoglobin synthesis is fully established. The earliest symptom is often that of symmetrical, painful swelling of the hands and feet, the so-called 'hand and foot' syndrome. At about this stage of development the child is noticed to be pale and slightly icteric. Other symptoms during early childhood include those of chronic anaemia with an increased tendency to infection. This chronic ill health is interspersed with acute episodes or crises which are described in detail below.

On clinical examination affected children are pale, icteric and may show the 'sickle-cell habitus', i.e. a disproportionately long lower segment and arms with narrow shoulders and hips. Recurrent leg ulcers may leave characteristic scars over the anterior tibial regions. Splenomegaly is commonly observed during early childhood but, due to repeated episodes of infarction, it rapidly regresses and it is quite exceptional to find a palpable spleen at puberty. The heart is commonly enlarged and a variety of murmurs may be heard.

The blood picture in sickle-cell anaemia is very characteristic. There is nearly always a marked degree of anaemia, the packed cell volume usually being in the 20 per cent. range. The peripheral blood film is characterized by marked variations in size, shape and colour of the red cells and usually sickled forms are present. The reticulocyte count is elevated in the 15–20 per cent. range. The serum bilirubin level is raised, haptoglobins are absent and the Schumm's test for methaemalbumin positive. The white cell count is normal except in crises where it may be markedly elevated. There is usually a moderate elevation in the platelet count. Sickling can be demonstrated by incubating the cells in 2 per cent. sodium metabisulphite under a coverslip sealed by Vaseline. The diagnosis is confirmed by haemoglobin electrophoresis which shows only haemoglobin S with an elevation of foetal haemoglobin usually in the 5–10 per cent. range, and by finding the sickle-cell trait, i.e. haemoglobins A and S, in both parents.

Complications

Patients with sickle-cell anaemia are very susceptible to all types of infection. They are particularly prone to pneumococcal infections including meningitis and to Salmonella infections of bone. Infection is the usual precipitating factor in the production of crises.

Several types of crises occur in the sickling disorders. Frequently a crisis is characterized by severe pain in the back, limbs and abdomen associated with a high fever and prostration. In severe crises generalized sickling may occur and death result from massive hepatic, cerebral or pulmonary infarction.

In children during severe crises massive sequestration of sickled erythrocytes in the liver and spleen may result in rapid enlargement of these organs associated with a dramatic fall in the packed cell volume. In some crises there may be severe intravascular haemolysis resulting in a rapid fall in the haemoglobin level. Another mechanism for sudden worsening of the anaemia is that of erythroid hypoplasia. Such 'aplastic' crises commonly occur in more than one family member at the same time, have a distinct seasonal and geographical incidence and hence are thought to follow infections, probably viral. Exacerbation of the anaemia may also be brought about by folic acid deficiency resulting from a rapid turnover of erythroid precursors.

The complications which result from repeated infarctions during crises may involve practically any organ. Thus repeated splenic infarcts result in severe pain in the left hypochondrium and ultimately in autosplenectomy. Aseptic necrosis of the femoral heads may occur in sickle-cell anaemia but is commoner in haemoglobin S-C disease. Similar changes may occur in the upper ends of the humerus. Bone infarction may also result in sequestra formation, sometimes associated with osteomyelitis, the organism usually being of the Salmonella group. The gradual cardiac enlargement which occurs in sickle-cell anaemia probably results from a combination of factors including multiple small infarcts, chronic anaemia, siderosis of the myocardium and pulmonary hypertension secondary to multiple small pulmonary thrombotic episodes. Focal neurological signs, recurrent attacks of haematuria and priapism also result from small vessel blockage.

Ocular manifestations occasionally occur in sickle-cell anaemia and take the form of a remarkable tortuosity of the retinal vessels. These changes are more marked in haemoglobin S-C disease where there is often a gross proliferation of the retinal vessels with a tendency to intra-ocular haemorrhage and permanent visual disturbance.

Pregnancy in sickle-cell anaemia is associated with a high incidence of folic acid deficiency and also, in some cases, an increased frequency of crises. There is an increased incidence of foetal mortality and morbidity.

Treatment

The treatment of sickle-cell anaemia presents two distinct problems. First there is the management in between crises, including their prevention, and there is the management of the established crisis.

In between crises patients should be maintained on folic acid supplements and iron should be avoided. They usually manage quite well with a packed cell volume in the 20–25 per cent. range and on no account should they receive blood transfusions to try and raise the haemoglobin to a higher level. Transfusions that raise the packed cell volume into the 30 per cent. range bring the blood viscosity up to a dangerous level without reducing the number of sickle cells and tend to precipitate crises. Malarial prophylactics should be taken regularly in tropical areas and there is some evidence that the taking of prophylactic antibiotics in the winter months may be helpful for sicklers who live in Europe or North America. Certainly many crises are precipitated by mild upper respiratory tract infections and the patient should be warned of this danger.

Crises should be managed by adequate analgesia, warmth, oxygen and antibiotics with frequent estimations of the packed cell volume. It should be remembered that these patients can become profoundly anaemic over the period of a few hours. Transfusion should be withheld unless the packed cell volume falls to a dangerously low level but sometimes the use of a plasma volume expander may be helpful. Regimes using alkalis, magnesium, low molecular-weight dextrans, phenothiazines, hyperbaric oxygen, urea and many other forms of therapy have been advocated for the treatment or prevention of crises. Because of the natural tendency for crises to settle, it has been extremely hard to assess the value of such regimes, and where they have been exposed to a double blind trial none has been shown to be of any benefit.

If there are repeated crises over a short period of time or if major surgery is contemplated for such complications as chronic leg ulceration or osteomyelitis, exchange transfusion is the most reliable method of management. This should aim to lower the number of sickle cells to less than 50 per cent. of the total cell mass. Once this is achieved it is possible to maintain the patient in this state by frequent small transfusions which depress the patient's own red cell production. It is possible to prevent crises for many months using this technique.

Anaesthesia is hazardous in patients with sickling disorders unless a high oxygen concentration is maintained. Nitrous oxide anaesthesia for minor operations is particularly dangerous. All Negro patients should have a sickle-cell preparation performed before being anaesthetized.

Pregnancy in sickle-cell anaemia is associated with increased risk to both mother and foetus. Although the sickling disorders are not an indication for termination, affected mothers require careful antenatal care. Folic acid supplements are vital and if frequent crises occur exchange transfusion is indicated.

Prognosis

The prognosis in sickle-cell anaemia depends on the socio-economic background of the patient. In Africa it has been unusual for patients with this disorder to survive early childhood. With earlier treatment of infection and anaemia and improved facilities for diagnosis this picture is changing and there are increasing numbers of adult patients with sickle-cell anaemia in Africa. In the United States it is quite common for patients to reach adolescence and adult life although few of them survive over the age of 50. The commonest cause of death at all ages is infection. In addition many adult sicklers in the United States develop progressive cardiac failure.

OTHER SICKLING DISORDERS

This sickle-cell trait does not usually cause any symptoms. There is an increased incidence of haematuria and serious organ infarction, e.g. spleen, may follow exposure to very low oxygen tensions such as occur in unpressurized aircraft.

The features of the other sickling disorders are summarized in TABLE 68. These conditions result from heterozygosity for the sickle-cell gene and for another haemoglobin variant. The clinical picture depends on the degree of interaction of the particular haemoglobin variant with haemoglobin S. Thus haemoglobins C and D interact with haemoglobin S to produce a variable degree of haemolytic anaemia with sickling crises, while haemoglobin J shows no such interaction and haemoglobin S-J disease is a very mild disorder. The nature of this variable interaction is unknown but it probably depends on the physical properties of the particular haemoglobin variant and its ability to potentiate or reduce the rate of tactoid formation.

Haemoglobin S-C disease results from the inheritance of both haemoglobin S and C genes. It is characterized by a mild haemolytic anaemia associated with splenomegaly and a variable number of sickling crises. The blood film shows numerous target cells, sickled erythrocytes and intracellular crystals. This condition is important because it may present for the first time in adult life with serious thrombo-embolic episodes particularly during pregnancy. Massive pulmonary infarction occurring in late pregnancy is a particular hazard. If symptoms suggestive of a sickling crisis occur in a pregnant woman with this disorder exchange transfusion is indicated. Patients with haemoglobin S-C disease are also prone to aseptic necrosis of the femoral heads and haematuria.

Haemoglobin S-D disease is usually associated with a clinical picture indistinguishable from that of sickle-cell anaemia. Sickle-cell thalassaemia is of variable severity depending on the type of thalassaemia gene. In the most severe cases the clinical picture is very similar to homozygous sickle-cell anaemia.

All these variants of sickle-cell anaemia can be diagnosed by haemoglobin electrophoresis combined with a family study. The treatment, where required, is similar to that of sickle-cell anaemia.

OTHER HAEMOGLOBINOPATHIES ASSOCIATED WITH HAEMOLYTIC ANAEMIA

The other common haemolytic haemoglobin disorders are haemoglobin C, D and E diseases and the familial non-spherocytic haemolytic anaemias due to unstable haemoglobins.

Haemoglobin C disease occurs commonly in West Africa, the carrier rate being highest in North Ghana with an incidence of 16–28 per cent. The homozygous disorder is characterized by a mild haemolytic anaemia associated with splenomegaly. This disorder can be recognized by examination of a blood film which shows 100 per cent. target-cell formation with intracellular crystals. The diagnosis can be confirmed by haemoglobin electrophoresis.

Haemoglobin D disease has been found in several racial groups. The clinical picture is that of a moderately severe haemolytic anaemia with splenomegaly. The blood film usually shows moderate numbers of target cells. There are several different types of haemoglobin D, all of which have the same rate of electrophoretic migration as haemoglobin S but do not result in sickling. Haemoglobin D (Punjab) is the one which is associated with the most marked clinical symptoms.

Haemoglobin E disease is extremely common in South East Asia, and also occurs in India, Burma and Pakistan. It is characterized by a very mild haemolytic anaemia, occasionally associated with splenomegaly. The blood film shows evidence of haemolysis with target-cell formation. Haemoglobin E is easily recognized on haemoglobin electrophoresis, migrating in the same position as haemoglobin A_2.

Congenital non-spherocytic haemolytic anaemia with Heinz-body production after splenectomy usually results from an unstable haemoglobin. A list of these haemoglobins is shown in TABLE 69. Many of them have an amino acid substitution near the haem pocket which causes molecular instability.

The clinical picture is that of a mild to moderate haemolytic anaemia, present from birth, and often associated with intermittent attacks of jaundice with the passage of dark urine. Haemolytic episodes may be precipitated by infection or oxidant drugs such as the sulphonamides. The haematological findings are those of chronic low grade haemolysis. The blood film shows a moderate degree of anisopoikilocytosis with macrocytosis and Heinz-body formation, particularly after splenectomy. The absence of spherocytes distinguishes these conditions from congenital spherocytosis.

All the unstable haemoglobins are precipitated by heating the haemoglobin solution to 50° C. and this 'heat denaturation test' provides a useful screening procedure. This is particularly important because haemoglobin electrophoresis may fail to separate the unstable haemoglobins, many of them having amino acid substitutions which do not alter the charge of the molecule. If haemolysis is mild no particular treatment is required for these patients but it is important to avoid the use of drugs with an oxidant action. In the presence of severe haemolysis, or if hypersplenism develops, splenectomy may be helpful.

ABNORMAL HAEMOGLOBINS CAUSING CONGENITAL METHAEMOGLOBINAEMIA

Congenital cyanosis due to methaemoglobinaemia is inherited in either a dominant or recessive pattern. In the dominant group there is usually an underlying structural abnormality of the haemoglobin while the recessive cases result from a deficiency of one of the methaemoglobin-reducing enzyme systems of the red cell.

There are a number of structural haemoglobin variants, all designated haemoglobin M, which cause congenital methaemoglobinaemia. These result from different amino acid substitutions near the attachment of the haem groups. These substitutions, which may occur in either the α or the β-chains, form permanent bonds with the iron of the haem unit in the oxidized state and thus continuous methaemoglobinaemia. If the abnormality is in the α-chain, cyanosis is present from birth, whereas if it is in the β-chain, cyanosis only appears when adult haemoglobin synthesis is fully established at about the third month. Thus a careful history determining the type of inheritance and the time of onset of cyanosis can provide an accurate diagnosis, not only of the type of methaemoglobinaemia, but which particular globin chain is involved if it is due to an abnormal haemoglobin. The haemoglobin Ms can be further characterized by electrophoresis under special conditions (Gerald and Scott, 1966).

No particular treatment is required and apart from the continual cyanosis these patients do not have any clinical disability. The cyanosis is not responsive to ascorbic acid or methylene blue, a fact which is helpful in distinguishing this form of methaemoglobinaemia from those due to chemicals or enzyme deficiency.

TABLE 69

THE UNSTABLE HAEMOGLOBINS

HAEMOGLOBIN	AMINO ACID SUBSTITUTION	HELIX	CLINICAL PICTURE
Zurich	β63 His->Arg	E7	Drug haemolysis
Köln	β98 Val->Met	FG5	Mild Heinz body anaemia
Hammersmith	β42 Phe->Ser	CD1	Moderate Heinz body anaemia
Freiburg	β23 Val->O	B5	Haemolytic anaemia. Cyanosis
Genova	α28 Leu->Pro	B10	Haemolytic anaemia
Sydney	β67 Val->Ala	E11	Haemolytic anaemia
Kansas	β102 Asp->Thr	G4	Haemolytic anaemia
Torino	α43 Phe->Val	CD1	Haemolytic anaemia
Bibba	α136 Leu->Pro	H19	Haemolytic anaemia
Santa Ana	β88 Leu->Pro	F4	Haemolytic anaemia
Sabine	β91 Leu->Pro	F7	Haemolytic anaemia
Wein	β130 Tyr->Asp	H8	Haemolytic anaemia
Gunhill	β91–95 or 92–96	F7–FG_2	Mild haemolytic anaemia
	deleted	F8–FG_3	Mild haemolytic anaemia
Philly	β35 Tyr->Phe	C1	Mild haemolytic anaemia
Seattle	β76 Ala->Glu	E20	Haemolytic anaemia
Tacoma	β30 Arg->Ser	B12	Haemolytic anaemia

This table shows a selection of some of the unstable haemoglobin syndromes. For references see Lehmann and Carrell (1969).

POLYCYTHAEMIA RESULTING FROM STRUCTURAL HAEMOGLOBIN VARIANTS

Familial polycythaemia sometimes results from an abnormal haemoglobin (Weatherall, 1969). The structural haemoglobin variants which have been associated with congenital polycythaemia are summarized in TABLE 70. All these haemoglobin variants have abnormal oxygen-binding properties resulting in increased oxygen affinity. This causes a shift to the left in the oxygen dissociation curve and so each red cell gives up less oxygen to the tissues. This results in tissue anoxia leading to stimulation of erythropoietin production and an increased red cell mass.

These patients have a moderate elevation of the packed cell volume in the 50–60 per cent. range and an associated increase in the red cell mass. There is no elevation of the white cell or platelet counts and there are no abnormal clinical findings, the spleen and liver not being palpable. The diagnosis can be confirmed by the finding of other affected family members, oxygen dissociation studies on blood samples, and haemoglobin electrophoresis. It is important to distinguish these disorders from other causes of pure red cell polycythaemia such as respiratory disease and renal and posterior fossa neoplasms.

THE THALASSAEMIA SYNDROMES

Synonyms. Cooley's anaemia; Mediterranean anaemia; Thalassaemia; Target-cell anaemia; Hereditary leptocytosis; Haemopathic Mediterranean syndrome; Familial microcytic anaemia.

Definition

The thalassaemias are inherited abnormalities of the rate of synthesis of the globin chains of haemoglobin.

Thalassaemia was first described by Thomas Cooley of Detroit in 1925. He described a series of children with severe anaemia and splenomegaly who usually died within the first years of life. The term 'thalassaemia' from 'θαλασσα', 'the sea', was invented when it was noted that all these children came from the Mediterranean region. Some years later it was realized that thalassaemia is inherited and that Cooley's anaemia is

TABLE 70

THE HAEMOGLOBINS WHICH ARE ASSOCIATED WITH FAMILIAL POLYCYTHAEMIA

HAEMOGLOBIN	SUBSTITUTION	HELIX	CONTACT	CLINICAL FEATURES
Chesapeake	α92 Leu->Arg	FG4	$\alpha_1\beta_2$	Polycythaemia
Capetown	α92 Leu->Gln	FG4	$\alpha_1\beta_2$	Mild polycythaemia
Yakima	β99 Asp->His	G1	$\alpha_1\beta_2$	Polycythaemia
Kempsey	β99 Asp->Asn	G1	$\alpha_1\beta_2$	Polycythaemia
Rainier	β145 Tyr->Cys	HC2	—	Polycythaemia
Hiroshima	β146 His->Asp	HC3	—	Polycythaemia
Malmö	β 97 His->Gln	FG4	$\alpha_1\beta_2$	Polycythaemia

(References in Weatherall, 1971.)

the homozygous state for a partially dominant Mendelian gene. This became known as 'thalassaemia major' and the heterozygous carrier state, 'thalassaemia minor'. It is now known that the clinical picture of thalassaemia can result from several different inherited abnormalities of haemoglobin synthesis which are now grouped together as the thalassaemia syndromes [TABLE 71] (Weatherall, 1965). Furthermore, thalassaemia is not localized to the Mediterranean. It occurs with a high frequency, i.e. a carrier rate of 2–10 per cent., in the Far East, parts of India, Burma and Pakistan, and in the Middle East and North Africa. Sporadic cases have been described in practically every racial group. It has been estimated that there are more than 100,000 children with homozygous thalassaemia in the world population.

Aetiology

Thalassaemia can result from an inherited defect of either α or β-chain production and therefore there are two main types of thalassaemia, the α-thalassaemias and the β-thalassaemias [TABLE 71].

The exact cause of the reduced rate of globin chain production is still uncertain although current work points to a deficient production of messenger RNA for the affected chain. A deficiency of one chain results in an excess of the unaffected chain, e.g. in β-thalassaemia there is a large excess of α-chains produced. These tend to be unstable and to form intracellular precipitates or inclusion bodies. It is this denatured globin and its deleterious effect on the red cell membrane which causes the haemolytic component in thalassaemia.

The anaemia of thalassaemia is thus the end result of both defective haemoglobin production and shortened red cell survival following excess production of unstable globin. Because free α-chain is less stable than free β-chain the anaemia of β-thalassaemia tends to be more severe than that of α-thalassaemia.

TABLE 71

THE THALASSAEMIAS

TYPE	HOMOZYGOUS STATE	HETEROZYGOUS STATE
β-thalassaemia (with haemoglobin A production)	Classical Cooley's anaemia. High level of haemoglobin F	Increased level of haemoglobin A_2
β-thalassaemia (with no haemoglobin A production)	Similar clinical picture to above Haemoglobin consists of F and A_2 only	As above
β-thalassaemia (with no haemoglobin A production). Milder type—probably genetically separate from above	Mild anaemia. Haemoglobin consists of F and A_2 only	Increased level of haemoglobin A_2. Haemoglobin F in 8 per cent. region
δ-β-thalassaemia	Moderate anaemia. Haemoglobin consists of F only	Normal level of haemoglobin A_2. Haemoglobin F in 5–20 per cent. range
Haemoglobin Lepore thalassaemia	Classical Cooley's anaemia. Haemoglobin consists of Lepore and F only	Low level of haemoglobin A_2. Haemoglobins F and Lepore present
α-thalassaemia	Genetics uncertain. Homozygous state for two severe α-thalassaemia genes probably always results in intra-uterine death. Heterozygosity for two α-thalassaemia genes produces haemoglobin H disease. Heterozygosity for a single α-thalassaemia gene probably silent.	

β-THALASSAEMIA

Clinical and Haematological Features

The homozygous state for β-thalassaemia results in the clinical picture first described by Thomas Cooley. Affected children are well at birth but become anaemic from about the third month of life. There is increasing hepatosplenomegaly and retardation of growth. Characteristic bone changes develop which include 'bossing' of the skull, overgrowth of the maxillary regions and a tendency for spontaneous fracture. The skull changes cause the typical Mongolian facies which characterize this entire group of anaemias. X-rays of the skull may show a typical 'hair on end' appearance. Many of these children require regular blood transfusion if they are to survive. They are particularly prone to infection, folic acid deficiency and iron overload, and if they survive early childhood, usually die during the second decade of cardiac failure following iron deposition in the myocardium.

The blood picture is characterized by anaemia, gross hypochromia and variation in size and shape of the red cells with variable numbers of target cells and nucleated red cells. The reticulocyte count is only moderately elevated but the bone marrow shows striking erythroid hyperplasia. Erythropoiesis is 'ineffective' with a large amount of haemoglobin, i.e. excess chain, destroyed in the bone marrow. After staining the red cells with methyl violet many irregular inclusion bodies can be demonstrated, particularly after splenectomy. The haemoglobin pattern is characterized by a variable increase of foetal haemoglobin ranging from 20 per cent. to over 90 per cent. of the total. Electrophoresis on starch gel demonstrates free α-chains. The diagnosis is confirmed by finding thalassaemia minor in both parents.

β-Thalassaemia minor or heterozygous β-thalassaemia is associated with very variable clinical abnormalities. In some cases there is no anaemia and mild morphological changes of the red cells are the only indication of the presence of a thalassaemia gene. In others there may be a moderate degree of anaemia and splenomegaly. The anaemia of thalassaemia minor is made worse by infection or stresses such as pregnancy. The haematological findings are characterized by variation in size and shape of the red cells with variable hypochromia. Haemoglobin electrophoresis shows an increase in the level of the minor haemoglobin component, haemoglobin A_2, from the normal range (1·5–3·3 per cent.) to a level of about 5 per cent. Foetal haemoglobin is slightly elevated (2–5 per cent.) in about half the cases.

There are certain well-defined variants of β-thalassaemia. In some cases there may be a deficiency of both β and δ-chain production and the haemoglobin pattern of heterozygotes is characterized by high levels of haemoglobin F without any increase in the amount of haemoglobin A_2. The clinical findings are the same as in true β-thalassaemia.

β-Thalassaemia may occur in association with structural haemoglobin variants, i.e. thalassaemia is inherited from one parent and the haemoglobin variant from the other. The commonest of these combinations are sickle-cell thalassaemia, haemoglobin C-thalassaemia and haemoglobin E-thalassaemia. The clinical findings in sickle-cell thalassaemia vary, in some cases being as mild as those in thalassaemia minor, in others resembling sickle-cell anaemia. This variability depends on the severity of the associated thalassaemia gene. Haemoglobin E-thalassaemia is extremely common in South East Asia and the clinical picture is very similar to homozygous β-thalassaemia. The condition can be distinguished from the latter by the finding of one parent with thalassaemia minor and the other with haemoglobin E.

The Course, Complications and Prognosis of β-Thalassaemia

Children with homozygous β-thalassaemia are profoundly anaemic from the first few months of life and the course of the illness depends on whether adequate transfusion facilities are available. If this is the case and if the repeated infections which occur in early childhood can be controlled, many of them survive to the second decade. At this time death due to cardiac failure following siderosis of the myocardium is common. At puberty there is usually retardation of growth and secondary sexual development, with multiple endocrine deficiencies. Pancreatic insufficiency with diabetes is particularly common. Some children with β-thalassaemia major run a much milder course requiring fewer transfusions and, when adolescence is reached, may not require further transfusion. It is difficult in early childhood to anticipate which children will fall into this group.

During the course of the illness the spleen may become grossly enlarged with resultant hypersplenism leading to worsening of the anaemia and a haemorrhagic tendency. Due to expansion of the bone marrow cavity pathological fracture is not uncommon and massive extramedullary erythropoiesis may result in tumour-like masses. If these occur in the chest the diagnosis of bronchial neoplasm may be made while similar deposits in the spinal meninges may result in cord compression.

A few patients with heterozygous β-thalassaemia run almost as a severe a course as those with the homozygous disorder. This condition, which may be a separate entity, has been called 'β-thalassaemia intermedia'. The prognosis in haemoglobin E-thalassaemia is very similar to that of homozygous β-thalassaemia. In sickle-cell thalassaemia the outlook depends on the severity of the associated thalassaemia gene. In the severe form the prognosis is very similar to homozygous sickle-cell anaemia while in the mild form the life expectancy is normal.

Management of β-Thalassaemia

Patients with severe β-thalassaemia require constant hospital supervision in a centre with a special experience of this disease. The parents must be interviewed as soon as the diagnosis is properly established and the whole problem fully explained to them. It is unwise to give a totally hopeless prognosis and they should be encouraged in the hope that, if the child can be seen through early childhood, there may be some improvement with the onset of adolescence. The need for complete co-operation must be emphasized and genetic and eugenic aspects must be discussed as soon as the diagnosis is established.

The children's haemoglobin should be maintained at a level of about 10–12 g. per 100 ml. by repeated blood transfusions. The intervals between transfusions vary greatly but are usually about 6–8 weeks. Although it has been claimed that, with more frequent transfusions, there is better all-round growth and development, the danger of transfusion siderosis is probably increased with this type of regime. Similarly, it is unwise to transfuse only when symptoms develop since children treated in this way develop poorly and often come into hospital in cardiac failure due to severe anaemia. Despite careful cross-matching, transfusion reactions are common and include transient pyrexias, urticarial rashes, the development of antibodies against minor blood groups and serum hepatitis. The use of washed or frozen red cells, white cell filters and corticosteroids may be helpful. Regular folic acid supplements should be given, but other haematinics, particularly iron, should be avoided. If hypersplenism develops, splenectomy is indicated but not until after the age of 5 years because of the risk of infection. A guide to whether splenectomy is likely to help can be obtained by measuring the plasma volume and by splenic sequestration studies using ^{51}Cr-labelled red cells. If there is persistent leucopenia, thrombocytopenia or a sudden worsening of the anaemia, splenectomy should certainly be considered.

The use of chelating agents to prevent iron overload is still under study. A regime using desferrioxamine by daily intramuscular injection combined with 4–6 G. of diethylenetriamine-penta-acetate (DTPA) in each blood transfusion will remove almost as much iron as is administered with an average transfusion regime. The parents can be taught to give the desferrioxamine injections. It is important to study iron excretion patterns from time to time to see how well the chelating agents are working. At the present time it is not possible to say whether this type of regime is really helpful in thalassaemia major. It is, however, the only approach to the problem of iron overload and so far has not been associated with any serious side-effects.

α-THALASSAEMIA

Definition and Aetiology

α-Chains are shared by both foetal and adult haemoglobin. For this reason inherited abnormalities of α-chain synthesis result in defective haemoglobin synthesis both in foetal and adult life and a severe defect in α-chain synthesis is incompatible with foetal survival.

In the presence of a deficiency of α-chains an excess of γ-chains and β-chains are produced in infancy and adult life respectively. In infancy the excess of γ-chains form molecules with the formula γ^4 . This haemoglobin migrates more rapidly than haemoglobin A and is called haemoglobin Bart's. Similarly excess β-chains form molecules with the formula β^4. This haemoglobin, designated haemoglobin H, is also separable by electrophoresis. Thus the α-thalassaemias are disorders which are characterized by a thalassaemia-like blood picture associated with the presence of haemoglobins Bart's and/or H.

As in β-thalassaemia the reason for the defective production of α-chains in α-thalassaemia is not yet known. Since haemoglobins Bart's and H are unstable the α-thalassaemias are characterized by the production of intracellular inclusion bodies with a resultant haemolytic anaemia.

THE HAEMOGLOBIN BART'S-HYDROPS SYNDROME

This condition probably represents the homozygous state for a severe type of α-thalassaemia gene. It is characterized by intra-uterine death, usually at about the 34th week although affected infants may survive until term and live for a few hours. The condition is common in South East Asia and has been observed in Cyprus.

The clinical picture is that of severe hydrops foetalis with massive oedema and enlargement of the liver rather than the spleen. The blood picture is characterized by severe anaemia with gross abnormalities in size and shape of the red cells and numerous nucleated red cells in the peripheral blood. The haemoglobin pattern consists almost entirely of haemoglobin Bart's with no haemoglobins F, A or A_2. This finding indicates that these children have a total deficiency of α-chain synthesis and that the haemoglobin is made up entirely of the γ-chains of haemoglobin F. There is no treatment for the infants who do survive until term.

The parents usually show very mild abnormalities in size and shape of the red cells with no abnormalities on haemoglobin electrophoresis.

HAEMOGLOBIN H DISEASE

Haemoglobin H disease is a milder form of α-thalassaemia which is compatible with survival into adult life. The clinical severity is very variable ranging from an incapacitating anaemia rather like that of homozygous β-thalassaemia to a very mild disorder associated with low grade haemolytic anaemia. The clinical findings are those of anaemia and splenomegaly. The haematological changes are similar to those of a β-thalassaemia of intermediate severity. Incubation of the red cells with brilliant cresyl blue results in ragged inclusion bodies which consist of precipitated haemoglobin H. The diagnosis can be confirmed by haemoglobin electrophoresis which shows the presence of a rapidly migrating haemoglobin component. The findings in the parents and relatives are variable, and the inheritance is not fully understood. Usually one parent shows evidence of mild thalassaemia and the other is normal. It is thought, therefore, that this condition results from the simultaneous inheritance of two genes for α-thalassaemia, one being almost completely 'silent'.

Haemoglobin H disease should be managed like β-thalassaemia minor unless the spleen enlarges enough to cause hypersplenism when it should be removed. Oxidant drugs should be avoided since their administration results in the precipitation of haemoglobin H.

THE HETEROZYGOUS STATES FOR α-THALASSAEMIA

It is probably not possible to recognize the carrier states for α-thalassaemia with certainty. Affected persons show very mild thalassaemia-like changes of their red cells, sometimes with the presence of small quantities of haemoglobins H or Bart's. α-Thalassaemia has been found in association with structural haemoglobin variants. The clinical disorders, haemoglobin I α-thalassaemia and haemoglobin Q α-thalassaemia resemble an intermediate form of thalassaemia. These conditions can be diagnosed by the characteristic electrophoretic pattern.

DEVELOPMENTAL AND ACQUIRED ABNORMALITIES OF HAEMOGLOBIN PRODUCTION

There are several well-defined developmental abnormalities of haemoglobin production. These are not of great clinical importance but may be mistaken for such disorders as thalassaemia because they are usually associated with elevated levels of foetal haemoglobin after the neonatal period.

HEREDITARY PERSISTENCE OF FOETAL HAEMOGLOBIN

This disorder is characterized by a genetic persistence of foetal haemoglobin synthesis beyond the neonatal period. For this reason it is usually called 'hereditary persistence of foetal haemoglobin' or the 'high F gene'. It is inherited in a simple Mendelian dominant fashion. The haemotological picture varies considerably from race to race and has been best defined in the Negro and Greek populations.

Heterozygous carriers in the Negro population carry about 25 per cent. foetal haemoglobin in adult life while homozygous individuals have 100 per cent. foetal haemoglobin and no haemoglobin A or A_2. These individuals have no clinical abnormality except that the homozygotes have slight morphological abnormalities of the red cells and a tendency to a high packed cell volume. The distinguishing features between these disorders and thalassaemia are summarized in TABLE 72.

In the Greek population the findings are similar to those in the African Negro except that the levels of the foetal haemoglobin in the heterozygotes are lower. There is another form of hereditary persistence of foetal haemoglobin, described first in Switzerland, in which affected persons have an inherited elevation of foetal haemoglobin in the 1–2 per cent. range. This is of no clinical importance except that again it may be mistaken for a thalassaemia carrier state. It occurs in about 2 per cent. of northern Europeans.

HAEMOGLOBIN F AND CHROMOSOMAL ABNORMALITIES

Increased levels of haemoglobin F and persistence of embryonic haemoglobin are regularly found in infants with the D_1 trisomy syndrome. This is not the case with the other syndromes resulting from chromosomal abnormalities.

ACQUIRED ABNORMALITIES OF HAEMOGLOBIN PATTERN

Haemoglobin pattern may be altered in various acquired disorders of the haematopoietic system. The most common alteration is that of an increase in foetal haemoglobin but alterations in the levels of haemoglobin A_2 and the presence of an abnormal haemoglobin may also be encountered in acquired disorders.

A slight elevation in foetal haemoglobin is commonly seen in haemolytic anaemia and also in children with various forms of leukaemia. In one form of childhood leukaemia, juvenile myeloid leukaemia, foetal haemoglobin levels may rise to 50 per cent. or more and the haemoglobin pattern resemble that of umbilical cord blood. At the same time as the foetal haemoglobin level rises the haemoglobin A_2 level falls and red cell enzymes assume a foetal pattern. The level of foetal haemoglobin is sometimes elevated in the megaloblastic anaemias of vitamin B_{12} or folic acid deficiency.

Haemoglobin A_2 values are reduced in iron deficiency anaemia and in patients with thalassaemia who are also iron deficient. The diagnosis may be masked due to the reduction of the haemoglobin A_2 level. Small amounts of haemoglobin H have been occasionally encountered in patients with erythroleukaemia.

THE DIAGNOSIS OF THE HAEMOGLOBINOPATHIES

An approach to the diagnosis of the abnormal haemoglobin disorders is summarized in TABLE 72. These conditions must be suspected from the clinical history,

TABLE 72

AN APPROACH TO THE DIAGNOSIS OF THE HAEMOGLOBINOPATHIES

1. History
   Race. Familial incidence. Developmental landmarks. Age of onset. Jaundice. Crisis. Spontaneous fractures. Recurrent infections. The passage of dark urine.

2. Physical findings
   Anaemia. Jaundice. Body habitus. Skull and facial changes. Leg ulcers. Splenomegaly. Bronzing of skin.

3. Haematology
   Blood film. Haemoglobin. P.C.V. Red cell indices. Reticulocytes. W.C.C. Platelets. Red cell fragility. Bilirubin. Haptoglobins.

4. Other investigations
   Biochemical indications of haemolysis. X-rays of long bones and skull. E.C.G. Serum iron. Serum folate.

5. Haemoglobin studies
   Haemoglobin electrophoresis. Haemoglobin F and A_2 estimation. Sickling test. Slide test for foetal haemoglobin (homogeneous distribution would indicate the 'high F' gene). Heat precipitation test. Incubation of red cells in brilliant cresyl blue for Hb. H bodies. Isolation and chemical characterization of haemoglobin variant.*

All laboratory techniques are standard except that marked*.

racial background of the patient and physical examination with particular reference to such features as anaemia, icterus, cyanosis, polycythaemia, splenomegaly, abnormal body habitus, bone and joint deformities and the presence of scars from leg ulcers. The skull and facial deformities of thalassaemia are easily overlooked, particularly in the Oriental races.

Examination of a stained blood film is the single most useful laboratory investigation. Morphological appearances of a blood film can be diagnostic in thalassaemia, the various sickling disorders and in the haemoglobin C disorders. The standard investigations for haemolysis and red cell osmotic fragility should be carried out. Methaemoglobinaemia can be recognized by spectroscopic examination of the blood. In those haemoglobinopathies associated with polycythaemia it is necessary to rule out the myeloproliferative disorders and pure red cell polycythaemia secondary to renal disease or neoplasia. This will require platelet and white cell counts, a bone marrow biopsy to assess the amount of reticulin, a leucocyte alkaline phosphatase score and radiological examination of the long bones and kidneys.

Structural haemoglobin variants are recognized by their electrophoretic behaviour on either filter paper, cellulose acetate or starch gel. Most haemoglobin variants separate on these media although a few have the same migration rate as haemoglobin A. The latter group, which are often associated with Heinz body anaemias, can be recognized by their tendency to precipitate at 50° C. It may be necessary to perform haemoglobin electrophoresis in series of buffers of different pH values since some haemoglobins will only separate at an acid pH.

The diagnosis of thalassaemia can be confirmed by measuring the level of haemoglobins F and A_2. If α-thalassaemia is suspected the red cells should be incubated in brilliant cresyl blue and haemoglobin electrophoresis performed on an acid pH, both procedures being designed to demonstrate haemoglobin H.

If a haemoglobin variant is found it can be partially identified by its rate of migration as compared with known standards. However, this is insufficient to characterize completely a new haemoglobin and it should then be referred to a special centre for chemical studies designed to identify the altered amino acid residue. If it has not been described before it should be named after the place of origin of the propositus of the affected family.

REFERENCES

GERALD, P. S., and SCOTT, E. M. (1966) The hereditary methemoglobinemias, in *Metabolic Basis of Inherited Disease*, ed. Stanbury, J. B., Wyngaarden, J. B., and Fredrickson, D. S., 2nd ed., New York.

HUEHNS, E. R., and SHOOTER, E. M. (1965) Review Article: Human haemoglobins, *J. med. Genet.*, **2,** 1.

ITANO, H. A. (1965) The synthesis of normal and abnormal haemoglobins, in *Abnormal Haemoglobins in Africa*, C.I.O.M.S. Symposium, ed. Jonxis, J. H. P., Oxford.

LEHMANN, H., and CARRELL, R. W. (1969) Variations in the structure of human haemoglobin with particular reference to the unstable haemoglobins, *Brit. med. Bull.*, **25,** 14.

LEHMANN, H., and HUNTSMAN, R. G. (1966) *Man's Haemoglobins*, Amsterdam.

WEATHERALL, D. J. (1965) *The Thalassaemia Syndromes*, Oxford.

WEATHERALL, D. J. (1971) The abnormal haemoglobins, in *Recent Advances in Haematology*, ed. Goldberg, A., and Brain, M. C., p. 194, London.

WEATHERALL, D. J., and CLEGG, J. B. (1969) The control of human hemoglobin synthesis and function in health and disease, in *Progress in Hematology*, *VI*, ed. Brown, E. B., and Moore, C. V., p. 261, New York.

D. J. WEATHERALL

SECTION 14

DISEASES OF THE SKIN

DISEASES OF THE SKIN

STRUCTURE AND FUNCTIONS

The skin varies greatly in structure and function from one region to another. There are contrasting hairy and hairless areas, warm humid flexures and dry cool convexities, oily head and chest and less oily limbs, and variations in pigmentation, thickness, elasticity and mobility over the underlying structures as between one part and another.

The structure of the skin from without inwards consists of a stratified cellular avascular epidermis, a fibrous, elastic and vascular dermis and a fibrous and fatty hypoderm.

The epidermis is not uniform in thickness. The epidermo-dermal junction is not straight because epidermal cells dip down forming a network, the rete ridges, into the meshes of which the papillary processes of the dermis protrude. As a result the surface area of the epidermo-dermal junction is greater than the surface area of the outer aspect of the epidermis, thus providing for efficient heat exchange.

There are marked regional variations in the thickness of the epidermis. The palms, soles and sites subject to pressure or friction have a thicker epidermis than the flexures, where physical effects are less.

The basal cells of the epidermis are the parent cells from which the more superficial cells develop, starting with prickle cells and proceeding to granular cells (and on palms and soles, clear cells) before the end product, non-nucleated horn cells, are formed at which stage the formation of the insoluble protein keratin is complete.

Scattered among the basal cells are the melanocytes, relatively clear cells with small nuclei, which form melanin pigment and convey it by their dendritic processes to the more external cells of the epidermis, where it is deposited as a protective supranuclear cap or, when abundant, more diffusely in the cytoplasm. Melanocytes are also present in the hair matrices. Thus there are two pigmentary systems in the skin, one serving the surface skin and the other the hairs, and they sometimes work independently of each other.

The melanocytes are derived from the neural crest and form melanin from the amino acid tyrosine after a complex series of chemical changes. The melanin-synthesizing capacity of the skin is regulated by the melanocyte-stimulating hormone (MSH) of the anterior pituitary. Adrenocortical hormones have a counter-balancing suppressive action on the pigmentary system.

The prickle cell layer undergoes hyperplasia and thickens (acanthosis) when the skin is subjected to repeated friction (lichenification). It is also irregularly thickened in psoriasis, a condition in which the turnover of epidermal cells is accelerated. In other conditions, for example lichen planus, it may be thinner than usual. In atrophic skin it is conspicuously thinned.

The prickle cell layer is also the scene of intercellular and intracellular oedema in eczema (spongiosis).

The granular layer becomes thinner in conditions in which the cellular division is accelerated, for example, psoriasis. It is also thin in ichthyosis but thicker than usual in lichen planus.

The outer horny layer consists of non-nucleated cells which are constantly shed from the surface as invisible scaling. In some inflammatory skin conditions, for example psoriasis, the turnover of the cells is too fast and immature horn cells retaining their nuclei reach the surface (parakeratosis). The scaling is then visibly abnormal and excessive.

When an area of skin is subjected to repeated pressure the horny layer undergoes hyperplasia (hyperkeratosis) forming local condensations (corns) or more diffuse calluses. These may develop on the hands from repeated occupational traumata or on the feet from malfitting shoes, or from faulty weight-bearing from high heels and cramped-in toes, or from obesity.

The horny layer also plays a part in protecting the underlying cells from sunlight by thickening up slightly from this stimulus. The deeper cells of the horny layer also form the main barrier against the penetration of chemicals. The main route of penetration of substances through healthy skin is via the hair follicles and sebaceous glands. Water penetrates hardly at all but fat-soluble substances pass more easily. Fat-soluble alkaloids pass through easily, as does phenol and its derivatives, including salicylic acid, resorcin and hydroquinone. Damage to the epidermal cells or a break in their continuity predisposes to greater penetration.

Fat-soluble vitamin D is synthesized in the surface film of the skin and absorbed through the epidermis. The intact epidermis is resistant to common bacterial infections. The surface film of fat originates from the desquamated epidermal cells as well as from the sebaceous glands and is emulsified and spread over the surface by the sweat. It acts as a protectant against some of the bacteria likely to be encountered on the surface. It is acid (pH 4·2–5·6). In particular it protects against *Streptococcus haemolyticus* but not against *Staphylococcus pyogenes*, or Gram-negative bacilli.

Before the era of industrial development and synthetic chemistry the skin was only exposed externally to a few natural chemical irritants and sensitizers of animal or vegetable origin. The epidermis reacts to external noxae by oedema and exudation or by exfoliation of its superficial cells.

The skin has no effective protection against ionizing radiation, but individual variations of reaction are marked.

The smooth skin of the palms and soles is patterned on its surface by individually unique ridges and grooves in the form of loops, whorls and triradii. The sweat ducts open on the ridges of these dermatoglyphics.

The dermis also varies in thickness and structure depending on the needs of different regions. It consists mostly of fibrous protein known as collagen (because it has been the source of animal glue). The collagen is embedded in a ground substance of mucopolysaccharides. Elastic fibres are also present in smaller numbers. Other cells include fibroblasts, histiocytes and mast cells, all derived from the primitive mesenchymal cell. The fibroblasts are precursors of collagen and elastin; the histiocytes are scavenger cells, concerned with phagocytosis; the mastocytes manufacture and release heparin and histamine into the surrounding tissue. Melanophores are histiocytes which engulf melanin which has passed down from the epidermis.

The dermis has a rich blood supply which enables it to carry out its thermostatic functions efficiently. The deep arterial plexus supplies the skin appendages and the intermediate subpapillary plexus from which smaller vessels pass to the papillary bodies. Corresponding veins convey the blood away. There are arterio-venous anastomoses which provide shunt systems enabling blood to be passed into superficial vessels or retained in deeper vessels depending on the thermostatic requirements of the moment.

The skin is also well supplied with lymphatic channels which drain by lymphatic vessels to the regional lymph nodes.

The sensory nerves of the skin link up with the dorsal spinal roots and the central nervous system. Beneath the epidermis of the volar aspects of the hands and feet there are encapsulated sense organs which provide fine temperature discrimination and touch perception. The nose, lips and finger tips are particularly sensitive and at the other extreme the skin of the trunk is particularly insensitive. Injury to the epidermis or dermis causes a sense of pain, but minor injury causes itching, the desire to scratch. In hairy areas a complex of free nerve endings around each follicle represent the equivalent of the encapsulated sense organs. There are also free nerve endings beneath the epidermis concerned with touch, pain and temperature discrimination and some specialized end organs, the Pacinian corpuscles and the Meissner corpuscles, are found in areas of high tactile sensibility.

On the motor side the eccrine sweat glands, the apocrine sweat glands, the musculature of the arterioles and the arrectores pilorum muscles are all innervated from the sympathetic ganglia of the autonomic nervous system. The sebaceous glands have no motor nerves, being controlled by endocrine stimuli.

The dermis provides toughness and at the same time elasticity to the skin. Its blood vessels react to a large number of noxae arriving in the blood stream from animate (infective) sources and from drugs and probably some food sophisticants. A simple redness (erythema) may result or there may be wealing, a transient pink or blanched swelling with surrounding red flare, resulting from the release of histamine. The skin of the face and upper part of the chest may also undergo a transient flush without wealing from embarrassment. The blood supply of the skin varies from one region to another as does its histamine content which is greatest on the face.

The hypoderm (panniculus adiposus) is a connective tissue layer between the dermis and the deep fascia specially adapted to the formation of aggregates of fat. Connective tissue strands run between the fat cells. The dermo-hypodermal junction is often indistinct. The thickness and distribution of the panniculus varies according to age, sex, race, site and feeding habits. As man is a relatively hairless animal the panniculus serves as an alternative method of heat conservation. It also makes an effective cushion, spreading and mitigating physical stresses from without. It also acts as a reserve depot of calories. It provides for greater mobility of the overlying skin on the underlying structures. (Compare the mobile skin of most of the body surface to the tethered skin of the palms and soles.)

The skin appendages consist of eccrine sweat glands, pilosebaceous units, apocrine sweat glands, hair and nails. Both types of sweat glands and the pilosebaceous units are situated in the hypoderm but developmentally they are invaginations of the surface epithelium.

An eccrine sweat gland consists of a secreting coil in the deeper part of the dermis and in the hypoderm. There are large clear secreting cells and smaller dark cells of uncertain function. From the coil a duct leads to the surface. It has two layers of cells and a layer of longitudinally arranged myoepithelial cells outside the basement membrane the contractile peristaltic properties of which allow a rapid delivery of sweat on the surface. The sweat glands are innervated from the hypothalamus and sweat is actively secreted as a result of thermal or emotional stimuli, the latter in particular causing sweating of the forehead, axillae, palms and soles. The eating of spicy foods may cause sweating of the face. Colicky pain is characteristically associated with sweating. Axon-reflex sweating may occur around skin lesions, particularly on the feet.

Sweat normally has a pH of between 4·5 and 5·5, but when it is retained on the surface the pH may approach neutrality at 7. The electrolytes of the plasma are present in the sweat in lower concentrations. The chief constituents are sodium chloride, urea and lactates, but the prime function of sweating is to secrete water for evaporative cooling of the body. On the palms and soles the eccrine ducts open on the ridges of the dermatoglyphics where they can be seen through a hand lens, actively secreting. In these situations there are no accompanying pilosebaceous units or apocrine glands.

Adjustment to temperature variations in the environment or in the body itself are made by alterations of blood flow in the upper dermis, variations in sweating and surface evaporation and to a small extent in man by erection of the hair follicles. Failure of thermostasis is most likely to occur in conditions of humid heat or in extreme cold.

The sweat also acts as an emulsifying agent and in so doing helps to spread the skin fats, formed in the sebaceous glands and from decomposition of surface epidermal cells, over the body surface. Thus the sweat protects the surface of the skin both from dehydration and from defatting. Failure may result from an inborn lack of development of sweat or sebaceous glands or from ageing, sometimes accompanied by an excessive use of soap.

Hair-bearing skin is relatively thinner and is penetrated both by pilosebaceous units and by sweat ducts. There are no encapsulated sense organs in the dermis but there are free nerve endings around the follicles which probably have a similar function.

A pilosebaceous unit consists of a dermal papilla from which a hair grows and a sebaceous gland lying beside the follicle and secreting into it. Most pilosebaceous units lie obliquely in the skin. An arrector pili muscle under autonomic nervous control runs from the deeper part of the wall of the follicle up to the under surface of the epidermo-dermal junction and by its contraction pulls the hair up from an oblique to a vertical position. Individual follicles are developed more towards hair formation (scalp, brows, beard), while others (forehead, cheeks, chest) are differentiated more towards sebum formation, the hair component being vestigial and fine. It is in the latter areas that acne vulgaris tends to develop.

The sebaceous glands secrete by complete disintegration of their cells into the lumen (holocrine secretion). The sebum passes into the main duct and thence into the follicle whence it oozes to the surface alongside the hair shaft. The secretion is activated at puberty and not under nervous control but results from androgenic stimulation from testicular, adrenal or (probably) ovarian sources. It is suppressed by oestrogens. Sebum is a complex mixture of lipids. After secretion it becomes mixed with epidermal lipids which are formed during keratinization and with the spreading and emulsifying action of sweat forms the surface film. Insolation of these lipids leads to the formation of vitamin D, which is re-absorbed.

Sebaceous glands are largest and most numerous on the forehead, the face, at the external auditory meatus and in the anogenital region. They are less numerous on the backs of the hands and feet and are absent on the palms and soles. In some situations they open directly on the surface, for example the Meibomian glands on the eyelids, the Fordyce brown spots on the lips or buccal mucosae, glands of the external genitalia of both sexes and glands of the areolae of the nipples. Owing to the lack of positive secretory pressure and owing to the vulnerability of pilosebaceous orifices to trauma, these units are particularly susceptible to infection from the surface. Their funnel-like orifices tend to accumulate both surface bacteria and extraneous matter which may have irritant properties.

Human hair is under different hormonal influences, depending on site, age and sex. The lanugo hair of the foetus is shed and replaced by the vellus hair of childhood and adult life. These hairs are short, soft, unmedullated and often unpigmented. Individual follicles may change from vellus to terminal hair formation under the influence of androgens. Terminal hairs are long, coarse, medullated and pigmented. Scalp, brow and lash hairs are asexual in origin. With ageing, regression often takes place at the frontal region of the scalp and at the pubis to vellus hair formation.

Axillary and pubic hair is bisexual in origin, whereas beard, trunk and limb hair and the male pattern pubic escutcheon are androgenic, although genetic influences are also relevant. The coarse hairs in the nostrils (vibrissae) and external auditory meati (tragi) of elderly males are thought to be under androgenic control, and the bifrontal hair loss, so characteristic of many males and of some elderly women is similarly controlled.

Hair growth is cyclic. A stage of active growth (anagen), lasting 3 years or more is followed by catagen lasting about 2 weeks. In this stage the hair is released from its papilla with the formation of a club-shaped end. This is followed by a resting stage (telogen) lasting for 3 or 4 months, during which the follicular invagination shrinks towards the surface and remains as a nipple-like downward projection until the next cycle starts, when the 'secondary germ' extends downwards again, becomes invaginated by a papilla and forms a new bulb. The newly formed hair subsequently emerges alongside the old club hair which is drawn to the surface with it and shed. The rate of growth of scalp hair is 0·35 mm. a day.

The hair cycle in the human is not seasonal as in many animals but is of the mosaic type, with each follicle acting independently of its neighbours. At any one time approximately 4–24 per cent. of hairs are in telogen, less than 1 per cent. in catagen and the remainder in anagen. There may be a disproportional increase of catagen during and after pregnancy or after prolonged and continuous fever as in typhoid.

In some regions, particularly at the external auditory meatus, the nipples, the axillae and the anogenital region there are apocrine sweat glands. They are much larger than eccrine sweat glands (the lumen may be up to ten times the diameter of an eccrine gland lumen). They secrete continually, if slowly, whereas eccrine glands only secrete as a result of thermal or emotional stimuli. The secretory coil and duct are similar to those of eccrine glands apart from the difference in size, but secretion takes place by a process of nipping off of part of the cytoplasm (hence 'apocrine'). The duct opens into a pilosebaceous follicle above the sebaceous gland and there is a common orifice on the surface usually without any accompanying hair.

Apocrine glands develop at puberty and undergo atrophy after the climacteric. Their role in man is uncertain, they would appear to be analogues of odoriferous libido-stimulating glands of certain animals. They also secrete actively as a result of any emotional stress which causes adrenergic sympathetic discharge, for example fear, pain or anger.

Each nail is formed from its matrix in a fold of epidermis on the dorsum of the distal phalanx of a digit. The fold is lined by a soft keratin layer, the eponychium, which with the cuticle, an anterior extension of the posterior nail fold, helps to form a protective barrier against entry of organisms into the paronychial fold. It is uncertain how much the nail bed beyond the exposed part of the nail participates in the formation of the under surface of the nail plate. The area covered by the lunula represents the anterior portion of the nail matrix. Nails grow between 0·5 and 1·2 mm. a week.

As has already been mentioned, the skin is an organ of emotional display, as shown by sweating, flushing or blanching and horripilation. It may also be subjected to self-inflicted violence, in the form of scratching, picking, excoriating, rubbing, pinching, even chewing. Similarly the hair may be subjected to tractional or frictional trauma and the nail folds may be picked or chewed or the free borders of the nails bitten away.

The skin, the hair and the nails are also used extensively in all races and in both sexes in order to attract attention. Defects in the appearance of the skin of exposed parts, too little hair in the right places or too much in the wrong places may all cause anxiety and feelings of inferiority.

AETIOLOGY

The aetiology of many skin diseases remains obscure. Hence the continued use of morphological descriptive terms which avoid the pitfall of attaching hypothetical aetiological concepts which may subsequently be proved incorrect. These terms also facilitate communication and are applicable particularly to different types of cutaneous reaction, such as eczema, urticaria and psoriasis.

Genetic predisposition is clearly of the greatest importance in the development of dry or greasy skin, acne vulgaris, atopic dermatitis, psoriasis, alopecia, vitiligo, and many other conditions.

Anomalies in the course of development cause various naevi—haemangiomata, benign melanomata (moles), linear epidermal naevi and many more.

Acquired influences include the numerous gradual effects of ageing which may be hastened at sites exposed to ionizing radiation or, in Caucasians, at sites repeatedly and excessively exposed to the sun.

Physical effects include pressure and friction, heat and cold, humidity and dryness and insolation.

Chemicals encountered on the surface may affect the skin by direct irritant action or by inducing an allergic response. Exposure to hazards of this nature may occur during the course of work or recreation; from antiseptics, antihistamines, local anaesthetics, antibiotics and other drugs applied externally; from sensitivity to metals, rubber antioxidants, formalin, dyes, matchboxes or match heads, cosmetics, plants, even articles of clothing, or lanolin.

Similarly, many drugs taken internally may cause changes in the skin of erythema, urticaria or vasculitis. Others may induce pruritus, disturb keratinization or aggravate existing dermatoses through various mechanisms. Antibiotics taken by mouth may so disturb the intestinal flora as to encourage *Candida albicans* infections.

It is possible that some food additives in the form of colouring or flavouring agents and other chemicals may be the cause of some unexplained eruptions. Urticaria induced by food proteins is relatively rare.

Bacterial infection is a common sequel to any break in continuity of the epidermis. Chinks in the cutaneous horny armour include the pilosebaceous follicles, the body flexures and the nail folds. Other infections, for example tuberculosis, may reach the skin from breaking down infection in deeper organs, or by the lymphatics or the blood stream. The type of reaction in the skin depends in syphilis, tuberculosis, leprosy and other infections on the immunological status of the host.

A number of virus infections also cause skin lesions.

Infestation with mites or lice or the bites of insects cause typical skin lesions, while in some tropical countries worm infestations causing skin lesions, pruritus or urticaria are common.

The epidermis is also often invaded by fungi, some of which may also penetrate hair or nail. Deep fungal infections are rarer, particularly in temperate climates.

The skin is affected by malnutrition, whether caused by insufficiency, excessive demands, dietetic imbalance or malabsorption. It is also affected by endocrine and metabolic disturbances, including disordered activities of the pituitary, thyroid and parathyroids, pancreas, suprarenals and gonads. Abnormal metabolic deposits occur in gout (sodium urate) xanthomatosis (cholesterol), calcinosis (mostly calcium phosphate), myxoedema (mucin) and amyloidosis (amyloid). Disturbed porphyrin metabolism of hepatic origin, genetically determined and often activated by drugs or alcohol has manifestations which include light sensitivity. Biliary cirrhosis or renal failure may present as general pruritus.

Diseases classed as autoimmune processes, such as lupus erythematosus, rheumatoid arthritis, nodular vasculitis, scleroderma and dermatomyositis may all have manifestations in the skin. Sometimes they are conspicuous, sometimes minimal or even absent.

Disorders of the haemopoietic system and of the reticulo-endothelial system may reveal themselves in the skin as pruritus or thromboses (polycythaemia), non-specific rashes, nodules or ulcers (Hodgkin's disease), infiltrated plaques and obtuse nodules (lymphomas), purpuric obtuse nodules (monocytic leukaemia), to give examples.

Severe zoster, extensive staphylococcal or extensive fungal infection may be a manifestation of Hodgkin's disease, reticulosis or leukaemia.

Visceral malignancy may present in the skin as secondary deposits, conveyed by lymphatics or the blood stream; or as pruritus, acanthosis nigricans or dermatomyositis.

Peripheral vascular disease is responsible usually in part, sometimes wholly, for a number of skin conditions, including eczema and ulcers of the legs, gangrene or near gangrene (necrobiosis), painful necrotizing purpura and ulceration (nodular vasculitis), some forms of panniculitis, erythema induratum, erythema nodosum, perniosis, Raynaud's phenomenon, calcinosis circumscripta and nail dystrophy.

Owing to the common ectodermal source of the skin and the nervous system, genetic and developmental anomalies of one often also affect the other. Examples include tuberous sclerosis and neurofibromatosis. In a number of these conditions there is some degree of mental deficiency. In mongolism, if scabies infestation occurs the picture is of severe and extensive crusted scabies owing to imperfect sensory appreciation of itching.

Involvement of peripheral nerves causing impaired sensation of touch, heat discrimination and pain may lead to neurotrophic (perforating) ulcers of the feet, burns and other traumata in leprosy, tabes dorsalis, diabetes mellitus, syringomyelia, peripheral nerve injury or disease, including facial ulcers following alcohol injections into the Gasserian ganglion. Anaesthesia of the trigeminal nerve in tuberculoid leprosy puts the eye at risk. Last, but not least, emotional disturbance has to be considered as a factor in the direct causation, activation or aggravation of some dermatoses. Delusions of parasitosis, syphilophobia, morbid anxiety about trivial lesions, dermatitis artefacta, neurotic excoriations, nail biting and trichotillomania are all clear manifestations of emotional disorder having an outlet through the skin.

Dermatoses in which emotional factors are important include lichen simplex and excoriated acne, hyperidrosis of axillae, perineum, palms and soles, anogenital pruritus, rosacea, atopic dermatitis, pompholyx and infective flexural dermatitis. The threshold of reaction may be lowered and the disease activated by feelings of anxiety or aggression in many patients with eczema, urticaria, or psoriasis. There is a much looser, less established association in some cases of lichen planus, alopecia areata, acne vulgaris, vitiligo, oral aphthosis and herpes simplex.

It is clear that many skin diseases have a multifactorial aetiology, operating sequentially or simultaneously.

DIAGNOSTIC METHODS

A comprehensive history and clinical examination is adequate for the diagnosis of most skin diseases. Complementary investigations may be necessary because of the nature of the skin condition itself or because of incidental findings in other organs or systems during the examination.

Complementary investigations include direct microscopy of epidermal material for fungi or sarcoptes, dermal snippings for onchocerciasis, superficial incisions and scrapings for leprosy bacilli, fungal culture, bacteriology, biopsy, patch testing and intradermal testing, and such other haematological, immunological and biochemical investigations as seem necessary. Electrocardiograms, electromyograms, electroencephalograms, muscle or lymph node biopsy may all be necessary in selected cases. The help of a medical social worker is invaluable for patients with social problems.

THE HISTORY

It is necessary first to determine the age, marital status, country of origin and past places of residence of the patient. The ethnic background is usually apparent.

The essential questioning discloses:

1. The duration of the condition.
2. Its site of onset.
3. The appearance of the original lesions.
4. Their subsequent manner of spread.
5. The presence or absence of itching.
6. Whether there has been any previous similar condition.
7. Past treatments and their effects.
8. Any information suggesting a possible cause for the condition.

Further questioning depends on the answers and on the morphology of the dermatosis.

It is important to know the exact nature of the patient's occupation, both at the time of examination and at the time the dermatosis began. Inquiry also has to be made about leisure activities and hobbies, in particular gardening and domestic decoration and repair. The effects of climate, seasons, holidays and weekends may give useful clues.

Under 'habits' the diagnostician is concerned with bathing habits and the nature of soaps and additives used, the use of cosmetics, feeding habits, and the amount of alcohol consumed. Inquiry about drugs is best made by asking about the use of aperients, analgesics, hypnotics, sedatives, euphoriants and contraceptives, and any medicine that is being taken for some other condition. It is as well also to ask about quinine taken as a bitter drink or Alka-Seltzer, with its aspirin content, taken to relieve the after-effects of alcoholic excess.

Under 'past health' information is obtained about illnesses, operations and accidents which may be relevant to the present condition.

Present 'general health' gives information of any current disease, physical or psychosomatic and the nature of the treatment the patient is receiving for it.

The family history is most important for evidence of a genetic basis for the condition under review. It is also important when a contagious condition such as scabies or impetigo is suspected.

The social history helps to assess the effects of the environment, and the adjustment of the patient to his family, neighbours and working conditions which may be relevant to the dermatosis.

During the taking of the history the diagnostician should be able to assess the patient's personality, stable or neurotic, unconcerned or hypochondriacal.

The history is at least as important as the physical examination in arriving at a diagnosis and sometimes, for example in urticaria and pruritus, it may be all there is to go on because all physical signs in the skin may be absent at the time of examination.

THE EXAMINATION

The general appearance, estimated age, height, weight and ethnic group are immediately apparent. Facies, mannerisms and choice of words may indicate something of the patient's personality.

Except when a lesion is obviously only of local significance examination is made in orderly fashion from head to foot, although it may first be advisable to examine the lesion which is the reason for the consultation. Attention is paid to the state of the hair and scalp, the eyes, ears, nose and throat, the lips, mouth, teeth, palate and tongue, the face, neck, body and anogenital region and finally the limbs, including the nails. The presence of any enlargement of the thyroid, liver, spleen or lymph nodes is observed, the presence of any vascular anomaly noted and the urine examined.

MORPHOLOGICAL CLASSIFICATION

It is necessary to determine the morphology of the lesions, and when a dermatosis is widespread to note the distribution, local arrangement, patterning and shape of the lesions and their more detailed morphology, sometimes with the aid of a hand lens, with particular attention to primary unmodified lesions which may perhaps be present at the margin of the main eruption.

Primary lesions are defined as follows:

A macule is an impalpable discoloration due to an increase or decrease of melanin, due to blood or blood pigments or due to some extraneous matter. The term is usually applied to lesions 1 cm. in diameter or less, larger lesions being described as patches. Erythematous macules are differentiated from purpuric ones by diascopy, in which glass pressure is applied and the lesion fades if the blood is intravascular (erythema) but does not if it has been extravasated (purpura). Paradoxically in haemangiomata it may not be possible to bring about more than partial blanching on diascopy, owing to blood being trapped in individual vessels when pressure is applied.

A papule is a solid, skin-coloured or pink elevation up to 1 cm. in diameter. Larger elevations are spoken of as plaques.

A vesicle is a circumscribed collection of translucent fluid within the epidermis often surmounting a papule. Its diameter is up to about 0·5 cm. above which the expression bulla is used. Bullae may be intra-epidermal or at the epidermo-dermal junction but this fact is often only determinable at biopsy.

A pustule is a circumscribed collection of opaque fluid of similar size to a vesicle. Many pustules are follicular. A combination of papules, vesicles and pustules may occur.

Scales are visible accumulations of partially detached horn, indicative of imperfect keratinization.

A weal is a pale or pink oedematous papule or plaque with a surrounding red flare.

A comedo is a dark follicular plug of horn, sebum and extraneous matter with coiled up vellus hairs within it.

A burrow is a linear fine epidermal elevation which contains an acarus.

A nodule is a circumscribed soft or firm solid elevation larger than a papule, involving the dermis and sometimes the hypoderm. A large area of nodulation may be described as a plaque.

Secondary lesions include scratch marks and deeper excoriations. Erosions are superficial losses of tissue involving only the epidermis whereas ulcers extend into the dermis and often into the hypoderm. Fissures are linear cracks extending into the dermis. Crusts are dried exudates from erosive or ulcerative lesions. They may consist of serum, blood or pus. Lichenification results from repeated friction applied to an area of the skin, usually the nape, behind the ears, the supraclavicular region, the antecubital or popliteal fossae, the extensor aspects of the forearms or the shins, the vulva, scrotum or the anal region. Usually there is an oval area fading off at the edges into normal skin and lying in the long axis of a limb. The thickened plaque shows reddish-brown discoloration with accentuation of the diamond-shaped epidermal elevations with corresponding increase of depth of the surrounding superficial creases. Sometimes there are discrete flat-topped papules around the edge, resembling lichen planus, the so-called pebbly lichenification. On the palms lichenification presents as ill-defined dyskeratotic thickening. On the transitional skin of the vulva it presents as leucoplakic thickening.

A cyst is a spherical nodule containing liquid or semisolid material. It may be of epidermal or of dermal origin.

Scars are the sequel to any destructive process affecting the dermis.

Sclerosis is a term used to describe diffuse smooth hardness of the hypoderm and dermis due to thickening and condensation of the collagen either secondary to inflammation, or primary as in scleroderma in which the collagen extends down to and around the sweat glands.

Atrophy may be primary, or secondary to a number of skin conditions. The surface is wrinkled, resembling tissue paper, thin and relatively translucent, inelastic, anhidrotic and with loss of hair follicles. The term poikiloderma is applied to a form of atrophy which shows reticulate macular pigmentation and hypopigmentation with telangiectasia.

Although some dermatoses are monomorphic, for example vitiligo, erythema, papular urticaria, folliculitis, pemphigus, ichthyosis, others may show several types of elementary lesion, either in sequence, as with eczema-dermatitis, or coexisting, as with acne vulgaris, and varicella. The dynamic nature of skin disease is well portrayed by eczema which may pass through erythematous, erythemato-papular, papulo-vesicular, pustular, crusted, eroded and fissured, scaly and perhaps lichenified stages before resolution. The diagnostician has to visualize the changes that have occurred up to the time of examination.

Placing a dermatosis into its correct category of primary lesion greatly reduces the differential diagnostic possibilities.

MACULAR CONDITIONS

Some of the commoner macular conditions are indicated below:

Paler Areas

Vitiligo (idiopathic depigmentation).

Leucoderma (depigmentation secondary to inflammatory processes).

Leucoderma colli (secondary syphilis, around neck).

Leprosy (hypopigmentation and sensory loss).

Tinea versicolor (in pigmented races or at sun-tanned areas in white individuals); scaling may only be apparent on grattage.

Morphoea and lichen sclerosus et atrophicus (the change in substance may be difficult to determine at certain stages).
Sutton's naevus (around central hyperpigmented zone).
Naevus anaemicus.

Darker Areas

Pink. Erythema, morbilliform, scarlatiniform or erythema multiforme-like (specific fevers, other virus infections, drug eruptions). Lesions blanch on pressure. Erythema also occurs in the earliest stage of eczema-dermatitis and in secondary syphilis. In early psoriasis, parapsoriasis, pityriasis rosea and tinea versicolor the scaling may be inconspicuous and only revealed by grattage.

Red or purple. Haemangioma (port-wine stain)—made patchily paler by pressure. Extravasation—not made paler by pressure, as in purpura, ecchymosis, capillarosis, fading erythema nodosum. Fixed drug eruptions.

Pale brown. Ephilides (freckles, on exposed areas). *Café au lait* spots. Tinea versicolor (peeling inconspicuous).

Darker brown. Local and guttate. Lentigines (not confined to sun-exposed areas). Urticaria pigmentosa (urtication on friction). Chloasma (face). Peutz-Jegher syndrome (perioral and dorsa of hands). Pellagra (sharply limited to sun-exposed areas). Berloque dermatitis (linear, necklace-like streak running down from behind the ears due to a light sensitizer in a perfume). Reticular pigmentation of the face from light-sensitizing cosmetics. Local effects from heat, ultra-violet light or ionizing radiation. Resolving lichen planus. Xeroderma pigmentosum (exposed areas, with atrophy and keratoses or epitheliomata). Segmental pigmentary naevus, etc.

More generalized pigmentation occurs in Addison's disease, thyrotoxicosis, rheumatoid arthritis, Hodgkin's disease, abdominal tuberculosis, malignant disease, biliary cirrhosis, haemochromatosis, malnutrition, vagabonds' disease, acromegaly, scleroderma, acanthosis nigricans, Albright's syndrome (hyperpigmentation, polyostotic fibrous dysplasia and precocious puberty in girls), Darier's disease, after treatment with mepacrine, and in rain-drop form after prolonged treatment with liquor arsenicalis. Argyria causes a battleship grey pigmentation. Bismuth, gold and mercury may do the same.

Dark brown or black macules occur after inflammatory processes in the skin of pigmented persons, particularly after lichen planus, the active lesions of which may also be extremely dark. Lentigo undergoing malignant change may be barely palpable and dark brown. Blue macules occur as Mongolian spots in the lumbosacral region and as blue naevi, also with pediculosis pubis as maculae caeruleae. Accidental tattooing is often blue-black. Deliberate tattooing may be blue-black (carbon), red (mercuric sulphide), blue (cobalt) or green (chromium oxide). Other extraneous pigments include carotene (orange-yellow) and picric acid (yellow).

PAPULAR CONDITIONS

These include early eczema, psoriasis (topped with silvery scale), lichen planus (flat-topped, violet with 'waxy glance'), lichen nitidus (micropapular lichen planus) lichen scrofulosorum (a rare tuberculide) papular urticaria, urticaria pigmentosa, syphilis, acne vulgaris, acne agminata (acuminate), early boils, rosacea, scabies (itchy, follicular and associated with burrows), ingrowing hairs (below chin line), warts, molluscum contagiosum (umbilicated), pityriasis rubra pilaris, parapsoriasis guttata, Darier's disease, halogen eruptions, moles and warty naevi. Necrotizing papules occur with papulonecrotic tuberculides, pityriasis lichenoides acuta, vasculitis and polycythaemia (capillary thrombosis).

VESICULAR CONDITIONS

Vesicles (localized collections of clear fluid up to 0·5 cm. diameter) occur in eczema-dermatitis, cheiro- and podo-pompholyx (hands and feet, eccrine areas), tinea pedis, erythema multiforme (target lesions), halogen eruptions, early impetigo, virus infections (variola, varicella, herpes simplex, herpes zoster, Kaposi's varicelliform eruption due to herpes simplex or vaccinia), papular urticaria, dermatitis herpetiformis, herpes gestationis, lymphangioma circumscriptum.

BULLOUS CONDITIONS

Bullae (local collections of clear fluid larger than 0·5 cm. in diameter) occur from burns and scalds, frost-bite, friction, sunburn, incipient necrosis (haemorrhagic), halogen drugs, contact irritants and sensitizers, insect bites (legs), staphylococcal pemphigus neonatorum (palms and soles spared), syphilitic pemphigus neonatorum (palms and soles affected), erythema multiforme, dermatitis herpetiformis, herpes gestationis, pemphigoid, various forms of pemphigus and epidermolysis bullosa. Bullae rarely occur in lichen planus or in morphoea.

PUSTULAR CONDITIONS

Pustules (local collections of opaque fluid) occur in folliculitis both superficial and deep, prickly heat, boils, acne vulgaris, rosacea, scabies, fungal infections, pustular psoriasis, infected eczema, variola, halogen eruptions and subcorneal pustular dermatosis.

SCALY CONDITIONS

Scaling occurs after any inflammation which involves the epidermis but not after urticaria. Widespread scaling occurs in chronic or resolving eczema-dermatitis, in erythroderma and in ichthyosis, inherited or acquired. It is a feature of psoriasis (silvery and centrifugal) and parapsoriasis, also pityriasis rubra pilaris and in low-grade infective (seborrhoeic) dermatitis (irregular, greasy, grey). Scaly plaques are a feature of mycosis fungoides before the tumour stage. After scarlet fever widespread fine scaling occurs, with coarse 'glove and stocking' peeling of the hands and feet. More localized scaling also occurs in eczema-dermatitis, pityriasis rosea (centripetal), tinea versicolor (trunk, inconspicuous), fungal infections (centripetal), and psoriasis. On the scalp it occurs as simple scurf (diffuse, barely palpable), psoriasis (localized, red, palpably elevated, sometimes with white scales extending up the hairs), and fungal infections (local or diffuse, with short broken hairs with brush-like ends).

NODULAR CONDITIONS

Nodules (soft or firm swellings in the epidermis or dermis, and sometimes also in the hypoderm, of more than 0·5 cm. diameter) may have a number of causes. They may be hamartomata (tumours of developmental anomaly), simple hyperplasias, benign neoplasms, malignant neoplasms, cysts, vasculitides, granulomata or due to metabolic infiltrates.

Hamartomatous nodular conditions are numerous and include epidermal naevus, naevus sebaceus, naevi of apocrine origin, trichoepithelioma, haemangioma simplex, lymphangioma, neurofibroma, leiomyoma, tuberous sclerosis, benign melanomatous naevus and others.

Hyperplasias include calluses, rhinophyma, elephantiasis neuromatosa in neurofibromatosis, and elephantiasis nostras secondary to chronic lymphoedema.

Benign neoplasms include papilloma, fibroma, keloid, keratoacanthoma, fibroepithelial polyp, lipoma and histiocytoma.

Borderline and precancerous conditions ('carcinoma in situ') include keratoma (on exposed parts), some examples of keratoacanthoma and 'tar warts', leucoplakia (transitional surfaces), Bowen's disease (persistent papulosquamous plaque), Queyrat's erythroplasia (velvety plaque on glans penis) and lentigo maligna (tangentially-spreading melanoma), also Kaposi's angiosarcoma, and dermatofibrosarcoma protuberans.

Malignant neoplasms include basal-cell epithelioma, squamous-cell epithelioma, melanoma, malignant lymphoma, monocytic leukaemia, Hodgkin's disease, mycosis fungoides, secondary deposits of epithelioma or melanoma, and rarer conditions such as fibrosarcoma.

Cysts include epidermal cysts (milia) (secondary to acne vulgaris or subepidermal bullae), sebaceous cysts, implantation cysts, dermoid cysts, lymphangioma, myxomatous degeneration cysts (near interphalangeal joints), and cystic acne vulgaris.

Vasculitic nodules occur in erythema nodosum (shins), erythema induratum (backs of legs), polyarteritis nodosa and various forms of nodular vasculitis.

Granulomatous nodules occur in syphilis and other treponematoses, tuberculosis and other acid-fast infections, leprosy, leishmaniasis, sarcoidosis, halogen drug eruptions, from foreign bodies, in actinomycosis, sporotrichosis and blastomycosis, from beryllium and in some chronic coccal infections, also in granuloma annulare and necrobiosis lipoidica.

Metabolic infiltrates causing nodulation include cholesterol (elbows, knees, buttocks, palms, tendons), calcium (ears, hands, feet, elbows, some tumours), sodium urate in gout (ears, metatarsophalangeal and other joints), mucin in circumscribed myxoedema, and amyloid.

ULCERS

Ulcers due to degenerative arterial disease usually occur on the anterolateral aspect of the lower third of the leg or on the foot, whereas venous (hypostatic) ulcers usually occur below and behind the medial malleolus. Mixed forms occur. Perniones and areas of nodular vasculitis may break down and ulcerate. Similarly, foci of panniculitis may break down and discharge fatty material. Ecthyma is a deep, ulcerative coccal infection, or may be a form of cutaneous diphtheria. Syphilitic ulcers tend to arise higher up on the leg and are characteristically steep walled, sometimes kidney shaped and with slough on the base. Tuberculous ulceration occurs in erythema induratum, usually around the back of the lower third of a somewhat perniotic leg. Lupus vulgaris, actinomycosis, sporotrichosis and blastomycosis may ulcerate. Ulcers may be a feature of cutaneous amoebiasis. Rodent ulcer is common on the face but may also occur on the body or limbs sparing only the palms and soles. Nodules of Hodgkin's disease may ulcerate as may the tumours of mycosis fungoides and malignant lymphomata. Artefactual ulcers are sometimes made with applications of heat or caustics or an ulcer may be maintained by remote control by constricting the limb above with a bandage as a tourniquet. Neurotrophic ulcers mostly occur as perforating ulcers beneath the first metatarsal head but are sometimes seen in the trigeminal area. Late effects of radiation with X-rays or radium include poikilodermatous atrophy proceeding to ulceration.

Phagedenic, spreading, undermining ulcers may develop in ulcerative colitis. Ulcers may also occur on the legs in rheumatoid arthritis and after poliomyelitis, from defective muscle pump action. Sickle-cell anaemia causes chronic indolent ulcers from intravascular agglutination of sickle cells. Hypochromic anaemia predisposes to leg ulcers or causes chronicity. The lesions of necrobiosis lipoidica may ulcerate when they occur, as they usually do, on the legs. Decubitus ulcers are ischaemic pressure sores, associated with immobility, insensibility, vascular disease, incontinence, chronic illness, malnutrition, senility and creased or debris-contaminated sheets.

CHARACTERISTIC DISTRIBUTION OF DERMATOSES

There are many exceptions to the characteristic patterns of skin diseases but a knowledge of them is a help to diagnosis and also enables the diagnostician to know where to look for likely supporting evidence of a tentative diagnosis.

Examples are as follows:

Acanthosis nigricans. Lips, neck, axillae, submammary, umbilical, anogenital, palms and soles.

Acne vulgaris. Vellus hair areas of face more than terminal hair areas, sides and back of neck, shoulders, upper part of trunk.

Atopic dermatitis. Face, brows, supraclavicular, antecubital, hands, popliteal, feet, widespread.

Contact dermatitis. Depending on nature of agent and whether volatile, liquid, solid or particulate.

Dermatitis herpetiformis. Scalp, shoulders, elbows, buttocks, knees. Widespread.

Dermatomyositis. Periorbital, elbows, knees, knuckles.

Discoid eczema. Extensor aspects of forearms, arms, thighs, legs, trunk.

Drug eruptions. Symmetrical, mimicking other dermatoses. Fixed eruption is an exception.
Erythema induratum. Around legs in their lower thirds.
Erythema multiforme. Mouth, face and neck, external genitalia, hands and feet. May be extensive.
Erythema nodosum. Fronts of legs. Occasionally on forearms.
Folliculitis. Beard area, forearms, thighs, legs.
Fungal infections. Varies with type. Scalp, hair, beard, hands, finger nails, genitocrural folds, buttocks, legs, soles, toe webs and flexures and toe nails.
Candida albicans infections. Angles of mouth, within mouth, body flexures, nail folds, vagina and vulva perianal, glans and prepuce, finger and toe webs and flexures.
Herpes simplex. Perioral, digits, external genitalia.
Herpes zoster. Unilateral in dermatome supplied by one or two dorsal ganglia.
Infective ('seborrhoeic') dermatitis. Scalp, aural meatus, postauricular, follicles, flexures, presternal and spinal 'sweat grooves'.
Leprosy; Lepromatous—symmetrical, face, widespread.
Leprosy; Tuberculoid—Asymmetrical, few, face, limbs or trunk. Indeterminate forms exist.
Lichen planus. Buccal mucosa, lips, front of wrists, lumbosacral, external genitalia, ankles. On legs, lesions may be hypertrophic.
Lichen simplex. Nape, supraclavicular, extensors of forearms, anogenital, calves.
Lupus erythematosus. Scalp, forehead, nose, malar ridges, ears, temples, buccal mucosa, dorsa of phalanges, periungual, finger tips.
Napkin area eruptions. In folds if of infective origin, or convexities if of chemical irritant nature.
Parapsoriasis. Trunk and limbs.
Pemphigoid. Extensor surfaces of limbs, widespread. Mouth, vulva.
Pemphigus. Depends on type. Face, mouth, periungual, vulva, widespread.
Pityriasis rosea. Trunk and proximal parts of neck and limbs.
Pityriasis (tinea) versicolor. Chest and back, abdomen and arms.
Psoriasis. Guttate type, widespread. Nummular type, scalp, elbows, lumbosacral, knees, nails. Flexural type, widespread and universal forms.
Rosacea. Between brows, nose and centre of face, cheeks, chin.
Scabies. Adults—anterior axillary folds, medial elbows, wrists, finger webs, breasts, abdomen, buttocks, penis and scrotum, ankles, widespread.
Scabies. Children—as above, and palms and soles.
Scabies. Infants—as above and face.
Stasis dermatitis. Lower third of leg, particularly medially.
Syphilis. Mouth, forehead, perioral, palms and soles, anogenital, widespread.

SIZE, SHAPE AND LOCAL ARRANGEMENT OF LESIONS

Lesions may be single or multiple, sharply or ill defined, discrete or confluent, grouped or uniformly disposed.

For descriptive purposes guttate lesions are rain-drop size, nummular lesions are coin sized and discoid and plaque forms are larger still. Large 'geographical' map-like areas may develop. Lesions may resolve in one part and spread elsewhere, giving an arcuate or festooned effect. Oval lesions may be described as petaloid, ash-leaf, etc.

Circinate (ringed) lesions occur in a large number of conditions, including impetigo, fungal infections, secondary or tertiary syphilis, lupus vulgaris, leprosy, psoriasis, lichen planus, erythema multiforme, erythema annulare centrifugum, purpura annularis telangiectodes, lupus erythematosus, granuloma annulare, pityriasis rosea, sarcoidosis, mycosis fungoides, porokeratosis and superficial basal-cell epithelioma of cicatrizing type. Fusion of rings results in polycyclic lesions, as in psoriasis.

Grouped lesions occur in papular urticaria due to insect bites, in syphilis (corymbose), lupus vulgaris, herpes simplex, herpes zoster, dermatitis herpetiformis, contact eczema, lichen planus, lichen nitidus, lichen scrofulosorum, warts, lymphangioma and leiomyoma.

Linear lesions occur with naevi, incontinentia pigmenti, morphoea, lichen striatus, contact dermatitis, particularly when the contactant has light-sensitizing properties as in Berloque dermatitis and phytophotodermatitis, in lichen planus and psoriasis from local trauma (Koebner effect), and in warts and molluscum contagiosum from autoinoculation. Artefacts made with caustic liquids may show a characteristic gravitational streak. Thrombophlebitis causes a linear redness and induration.

Cleavage line patterning occurs in pityriasis rosea and in parapsoriasis en plaque, sometimes also in morphoea, the lesions lying parallel to the ribs.

Nodules are described as sessile (broad based), semipedunculated or pedunculated, with smooth or irregular flat-topped, domed or umbilicated surfaces, verrucoid or polypoid, and with infiltrated or non-infiltrated bases.

EFFECTS OF RACE, AGE AND SEX

Race. In pigmented races erythema is partially or totally obscured. Slight pallor may occur with wealing. The pigmentary system is easily disturbed causing dark brown or black lesions in lichen planus, pityriasis rosea, lupus erythematosus and other inflammatory conditions or depigmentation may occur causing more pronounced colour contrasts than when the same thing happens in white skins, as after herpes zoster, syphilis, lichen simplex. Similarly the hypopigmentation of tuberculoid leprosy is far more conspicuous than in a white person. Mongolian pigmented spots often occur in Negroes as well as in mongoloids. Pigmentation of the oral mucous membranes or linear streaky pigmentation of the nails is common.

Some diseases, for example syphilis, may run a more florid course in Negroes. Skin diseases to which Negroes are prone include keloids and multiple basal-cell papillomas (dermatosis papulosa nigra), and carcinoma in scars. Psoriasis, pompholyx, prickly heat and alopecia areata are rare, and basal-cell epithelioma in sun-exposed areas is extremely rare.

In Asians the incidence of light-provoked basal cell

epitheliomas and of psoriasis is less than in Europeans but more than in Africans. Vitiligo causes great social concern but it is uncertain whether it is more common.

Age. The skin of the infant is especially susceptible to coccal infections and forms blisters (pemphigus neonatorum) when the same organisms would only cause impetigo in an older child and inconspicuous lesions in an adult or possibly none at all. Similarly, syphilis causes severe and extensive bullous lesions and herpes simplex virus may cause a severe local mucocutaneous and systemic reaction and, in the presence of infantile eczema, Kaposi's varicelliform eruption. Accidental or deliberate vaccination may cause a similar condition in eczematous infants.

Similarly, urine and stool burns may cause bullous reaction in the napkin area. Children and infants are rarely affected by contact eczematous reactions. On the other hand atopic dermatitis causes a papular eczematoid condition in infants whereas it later causes lichenification and excoriation. Scabies in infants may affect the face which it does not do later in life. The palms are often affected in childhood, rarely in adult life.

The common forms of tinea capitis affect only children, becoming self-limited at puberty. Papular urticaria is also commoner in childhood. Psoriasis in childhood is often of the guttate type at the onset and has a poor prognosis regarding chronicity, especially in girls.

The ageing skin is subject to atrophic changes predisposing to asteatosis and winter itch or frank dermatitis and to malignancy particularly at parts exposed to sunlight. Other changes include basal-cell papillomata, pigmentary anomalies and changes secondary to circulatory defects or diabetes.

Sex. Sex differentiations in skin disease are also marked. Acne vulgaris tends to be a more severe condition in males. Folliculitis, boils and tinea cruris are commoner in males. Females are more susceptible to contact irritants, although, outside the home males are more exposed to them, and atopic dermatitis tends to persist more in females. Systematic lupus erythematosus is about eight times more common in females than in males. In discoid lupus erythematosus females are affected twice as often as males. Similarly systemic sclerosis is at least three times commoner in females than in males. Perniosis and Raynaud's phenomena are also commoner in women, also hypostatic dermatoses.

COMPLEMENTARY INVESTIGATIONS

Diascopy is the examination of a lesion through glass applied so as to compress the superficial vessels. It helps to differentiate between erythema, telangiectasia, purpura and melanosis and it reveals the 'apple jelly' nodule of lupus vulgaris.

Grattage is the examination of a scaly lesion by scraping it with a wooden spatula (not a finger nail!). It reveals the fine branny scales of tinea versicolor, the silvery centrifugal scaling of psoriasis, the slight scaling of parapsoriasis, the single scutuliform scale of pityriasis lichenoides, the centripetal scaling of pityriasis rosea and the irregularly disposed scaling of 'seborrhoeic' dermatitis.

Dermographism is an exaggerated wealing produced by firmly stroking the skin with a blunt instrument. It occurs in about 5 per cent. of individuals, and is important in that it reveals traumatic urticaria which may confuse the diagnosis in scabies or other pruritic conditions or temporarily fog patch test readings.

White dermographism is blanching in the line of stroke starting after about 15 seconds, rising to a maximum and fading after about 2 minutes. It is a feature of atopic dermatitis and indicates high vasoconstrictor tone and temporary exhaustion of the histamine content of the mast cells as a result of chronic friction. It may also be seen in lichen simplex.

Nikolsky's sign is the sliding off of a superficial portion of the epidermis on applying tangential pressure with the pad of a digit. It is positive in pemphigus vulgaris, pemphigoid, benign familial pemphigus, epidermolysis bullosa, toxic epidermal necrolysis and genetic porphyria cutanea tarda. A similar test may be made by applying lateral pressure on an intact bulla and observing it creep before the pressure. Negative results are obtained with thermal blisters, insect bites, erythema multiforme and dermatitis herpetiformis.

Tzanck Test. This consists of scraping the floor of a bulla and examining the material microscopically for acantholytic cells. It is positive in pemphigus vulgaris.

Hess's test of capillary fragility is made by applying a sphygmomanometer cuff to the arm at a pressure above the diastolic pressure and below the systolic, usually at 80 mm. Hg for 5 minutes. Below the cuff an area 5 × 5 cm. is marked out and the number of petechiae counted before (if any) and after.

Fluorescence under Wood's Light. Ultra-violet light transmitted through Wood's glass (barium silicate containing nickel oxide) causes fluorescence in a number of conditions and is of great diagnostic assistance:

Microsporum canis and *Microsporum audouini*—broken hair shafts fluoresce a brilliant green.

Trichophyton schoenleini hairs (favus) fluoresce light green. The hairs may be of normal length.

Erythrasma, due to a diphtheroid (*Corynebacterium minutissimum*), affects axillae, perineum, genitocrural folds and toe webs. It fluoresces coral pink.

Pityriasis versicolor, due to *Malassezia furfur*, fluoresces a golden brown.

The vesicles of porphyria cutanea tarda may show a pink fluorescence. The urine fluoresces pink during an attack and the faeces during a remission.

Fluorescent contact sensitizers and many photosensitizers can be detected on the skin. Tetracycline can be detected in milk teeth and mepacrine in nails.

Pigmentary disorders can be rendered more obvious and fading dermatoses revealed.

Direct microscopy is used for the detection of fungal and *Candida albicans* infections, scabies and demodex infestations, and onchocerciasis infestations. In fungal infections a blunt scalpel is used to take scrapings of scales, or the roof of a blister is removed with cuticle scissors. The material is transferred to a slide, liquor potassii and a cover-slip added and heat is applied short of boiling the liquid. This makes the keratin less opaque and the mycelial elements are more easily seen.

The same technique applies to *Candida albicans* infections and to tinea of hair and nails except that with the latter a scraping is made of nail with the edges of a microscope slide. It is also advisable to take a full thickness snippet of nail and to digest it overnight in liquor potassii in a test tube, as a negative finding from a nail scraping cannot be accepted as final.

Specimens to be used for culture must be taken dry, without the use of liquor potassii, and caught on a folded piece of coloured paper to help subsequent recognition and manipulation of the particles in the laboratory.

In suspected scabies a fine needle is passed along a burrow. The mite becomes attached to the point and is removed. Sometimes burrows are hard to find and an alternative method of scraping suspected lesions, moistened with liquor potassii, is used. In this way adult females, nymphae, developing eggs or empty egg shells may be revealed. In infestations with animal scabies discovery of a mite is not easy.

Demodex folliculorum can be demonstrated by gently scraping the mucoid material from a follicular orifice in rosacea or extracting an eyelash in blepharitis.

For information on mycological techniques the reader is referred to a mycological textbook. Briefly, the specimen is inoculated on to Sabouraud's maltose peptone or similar medium in a test tube or Petri dish at 28°–30° C. A recognizable growth may be obtained in between 3 and 14 days of inoculation.

Histopathology

The microscopic examination of biopsy specimens plays an important role in the diagnosis of many skin conditions. For the best results collaboration between clinician and histopathologist is essential and, ideally, this should consist of a full clinical description on the form accompanying the specimen of the age, sex and race of the patient, the site from which the specimen came and a concise description of the history and appearance of the dermatosis. It is unreasonable to expect a pathologist to give a useful report without such information. Mutual examination of the stained specimen is a further advantage. Useful advice may be obtained beforehand from the pathologist about the preparation of specimens for culture or with special fixatives. Suggested diagnoses may indicate special staining methods.

Knife biopsy is usually preferable to punch biopsy. A specimen of up to 1·5 × 0·5 cm. is removed under local anaesthesia with lignocaine. The specimen should include normal as well as pathological tissue, and should be pressed gently on to a small square of blotting paper in order to maintain its shape and discourage it from curling up. It is then dropped into a specimen jar containing 10 per cent. formalin. One or more stitches are usually inserted but with ulcerating neoplasms this may be unnecessary. It is important to remove sufficient depth of tissue, particularly from neoplasms and in nodular conditions. When possible, incisions should be made along Langer's lines and, when there is a choice, biopsy from the lower part of the leg should be avoided. If punch biopsy is performed the skin should be stretched at right angles to Langer's lines in order to make best use of this natural phenomenon.

Biopsy is of the greatest value in nodular conditions, including neoplasms, hamartomata, granulomata, cysts, vasculitis, metabolic infiltrates; also in bullous eruptions, urticaria pigmentosa, and various other persistent lesions. It is often uninformative in more transient reactions, and the diagnostician may be left in these circumstances with no increase in knowledge but with a patient with an ugly biopsy scar and a resolved dermatosis. Clearly clinical acumen should be used to the full before resorting to biopsy except in the special indications shown above.

Patch Tests

Patch testing is a method of finding specific outward contact causes for eczematous reactions. The causal agent may be volatile, liquid, solid or particulate. Patch testing is called for in the presence of eczematous type dermatitis but not when primary irritant dermatitis is diagnosed.

The selection of the test substances and the concentration at which they are applied to the skin depends on the history, and knowledge of the appropriate concentrations from experience and reference to the experience of others.

A positive reaction to a test substance means that the individual concerned has a contact sensitivity to that substance but it does not prove that the dermatosis being investigated has of necessity been caused by this substance. Individuals may react to more than one test substance and false positives may occur if the strength of a test substance which has both irritant and sensitizing properties is too great.

A drop or portion of the test substance is applied on a square of linen, fine mesh gauze or white blotting paper measuring 1 × 1 cm. The outer part of the square is not covered with the test substance, in order to prevent confusion should there be any irritant or eczematous reaction to the surrounding adhesive with which the patch is applied. As each patch is applied to the back or arm it is given an identifying mark which is also recorded on a card. Patches are removed after 48 hours and the results recorded as negative, E1 = erythema, E2 = papular erythema and E3 = vesicular erythema or crusting exudate. False positives arise from poral occlusion (miliaria), folliculitis, or diffuse irritant effect. Dermographic urticaria may occur. The sites of the patches are marked with a skin pencil and re-examined at 4–7 days after the original application to reveal any delayed reactions. Ready-made patches for testing are now commercially available.

Patch test substances are mostly incorporated in Vaseline and may be kept ready for instant use in nozzle-protected syringes on a frame.

A useful range to be selected from for routine purposes is the following:

		Nature of Contact
Nickel sulphate	1%	Nickel, coins, metal-plated objects
Potassium dichromate	0·5%	Chromium, cement, leather, metal-plated objects

		Nature of Contact
Cobalt chloride	1%	Cobalt
Copper sulphate	1%	Copper coins
Finsen rubber	as in	Rubber antioxidants
Mercaptobenzthiazole	1%	Rubber antioxidant
Tetramethylthiuram monosulphide	1%	Rubber antioxidant
Tetramethylthiuram disulphide	1%	Rubber antioxidant
Colophony	50%	Adhesive plaster mass
Formalin	4%	Plastics, drip dry clothing
Paratertiary butyl phenol	10%	Shoe glue
Tricresyl phosphate	1%	Synthetic chair fabrics
Araldite F	2%	Synthetic glues
Primula leaf	'as is'	
Balsam of Peru	10%	Cosmetics, perfumes
Turpentine	10%	
Lanolin	as in	Many topical applications, cosmetics
Paraphenylene diamine	2%	Hair dyes, hair nets, clothing
Parabens	3%	Vehicle for Aureomycin, etc.
Parachlormetaxylenol	1%	Dettol
Neomycin	1%	
Soframycin	1%	
Vioform	1%	
Procaine	1%	
Phosphorus sesquisulphide	1%	Red match heads
Santolite	as in	Nail varnish resin

For other substances reference should be made to larger texts which recommend the appropriate dilution [see References].

Patch tests should only be applied to skin of normal appearance and not while eczema is active. The best sites are the upper back and the outer arms.

Photopatch tests are carried out with substances believed to be causing a light-sensitizing reaction. If the conventional test is negative the site is irradiated with a first degree erythema exposure from an ultra-violet source. An area of skin which has not been patch tested is similarly irradiated as a control. The reaction is read at 12–24 hours.

Intradermal Tests

Intradermal tests are carried out in the search for hypersensitivity to animal danders, tree, shrub and grass pollens, household dust, *Dermatophagoides culinae*, etc., up to 0·1 ml. of the test substance being injected intradermally or pricked in along the anterior aspect of the forearm, with controls. After 20 minutes to half an hour measurements are made of the widths of weals and flares, the former being more significant than the latter. From a practical point of view the results are disappointing.

A similar technique may be used with penicillin and streptomycin, the results being significant and of practical value.

Intradermal tests also are carried out to detect delayed sensitivity to bacterial antigens. With the tuberculin test, if hypersensitivity is suspected a start is made with a 1 in 10,000 concentration. Otherwise a 1 in 1,000 concentration is first used and if the result is negative a 1 in 100 concentration. Sometimes tests at 1 in 100,000 or 1 in 1,000,000 are made. A 5 mm. diameter or more infiltrated papule is regarded as a positive reaction. It does not imply active infection, only of past exposure and reaction to the organism, a positive at 1 in 10,000 indicating hyperergy, 1 in 1,000 normergy, 1 in 100 hypoergy, and a negative reaction, anergy.

The lepromin test is also not diagnostic of leprosy but places a proven infection in its immunological category. Thus lepromatous leprosy gives a weak or negative reaction and tuberculoid leprosy a strongly positive one. Indeterminate forms give weak positive reactions if they are leaning towards the tuberculoid end of the spectrum.

Intradermal tests are also sometimes performed with brucella antigen, candida antigen, cat-scratch fever antigen, coccidioidin, Frei antigen, histoplasmin, toxoplasmin, psittacosis antigen and trichophytin.

The results are significant when a disease is rare in the community, otherwise sometimes irrelevant.

In the Kveim test an antigen prepared from human sarcoidal tissue is injected intradermally. A reddish-brown infiltrated nodule appears at 7–10 days and is biopsied and studied histologically. A sarcoidal type granuloma is regarded as positive, a non-specific or foreign-body giant-cell reaction is regarded as negative.

Bacteriological Investigations

These are made by taking swabs from lesions, from the anterior nares, the aural meatus, flexures and the paronychial folds, according to individual indications. Wet swabs dipped in sterile normal saline are advisable when taking specimens from suspected carrier sites or from dry lesions. In suspected tuberculosis or atypical acid-fast injections a portion of a biopsy specimen is sent for culture. In suspected leprosy superficial scratches are made in the alae nasi and ear lobes, a fold of skin being squeezed up to render it avascular and a scraping made of tissue juice with the least possible admixture with blood. A smear is made on a slide and stained by the Ziehl-Neelsen method. In lepromatous leprosy positive findings may be made extensively on the surface of the skin. Some borderline cases give positive findings but tuberculoid cases are negative.

Parasitic Infestations

In suspected onchocerciasis, skin snips are taken, minced or teased out and examined for microfilariae. A needle point is inserted tangentially into the skin of a buttock, the skin lifted and a snip shaved off briskly with a scalpel.

In suspected oxyuriasis the adhesive side of a portion of scotch tape is applied radially to the anus and perineum: or it may be wrapped around a spatula, adhesive outwards, and similarly applied. The adhesive tape is subsequently applied to a microscope slide and examined for ova. The hands should subsequently be washed as the performance of this test carries some degree of occupational risk.

In all the above tests the clinician is wholly or partly concerned in taking the specimen and sometimes in examining it. There are a large number of complementary tests carried out in the laboratory which the dermatological diagnostician may wish to employ. They include haemoglobin estimations, white cell and platelet counts, investigations of clotting, erythrocyte sedimentation rate, serological tests for syphilis, antistreptolysin titre, antinuclear factor, serum proteins and electrolytes, examination for L.E. cells, liver function tests, serum blood urea, serum blood uric acid, serum blood cholesterol and phospholipids, sugar tolerance tests, sometimes cortisone provoked, serum calcium and phosphorus, serum transaminases, phosphocreatine kinase, aldolase and lactic dehydrogenase, plasma B_{12} and vitamin B_{12} absorption tests, serum folate, protein bound iodine, xylose tolerance, urinary oxogenic steroids and oxosteroids, faecal fat estimations, radiography particularly of the chest.

Clearly the diagnostician must be selective in deciding which tests to ask for and not perform 'battery' investigations.

GENODERMATOSES AND DEVELOPMENTAL ABNORMALITIES

An hereditary predisposition is a conspicuous feature of several dermatoses, including acne vulgaris, atopic dermatitis, alopecia areata, psoriasis, hirsutism and vitiligo. But as postnatal environmental influences often play an important part in activating or exacerbating them they are not usually classified as genodermatoses, this term being restricted to conditions which are primarily genetic in origin with environmental factors operating only in a secondary capacity.

In the space available only a brief summary can be given of the genodermatoses, their modes of inheritance and their clinical manifestations.

Non-sex linked (autosomal) dominant inheritance occurs in the following conditions (about half of the children will be affected):

Benign familial pemphigus—Vesicles, erosions, crusting, resembling flexural infective dermatitis, but affecting friction sites around neck, anterior axillary folds and genitocrural folds.

Bullous ichthyosiform erythroderma—Bullae, redness, hyperkeratosis with warty streaks in flexures, rough dry skin.

Cylindroma—Multiple nodules on scalp, 'turban tumours', of sweat gland origin, starting in adolescence or early adult life.

Darier's disease (keratosis follicularis)—Light brown, greasy crusted papules forming warty plaques on scalp, face, flexures. Minute pits on palms and soles.

Dupuytren's contracture (palmar fibromatosis) is sometimes associated with plantar fibromatosis, knuckle pads, keloids, plastic induration of the penis.

Ehlers-Danlos syndrome. [See Section 4.]

Familial hypercholesterolaemia—Xanthomata at elbows, knees, on tendons, xanthelasma palpebrarum, atheroma leading to cardiovascular calamities.

Gardner's syndrome—Epidermal cysts, osteomas, fibromas, lipomas, gastric, ileal or retroperitoneal leiomyotomata and colonic polyposis.

Hereditary haemorrhagic telangiectasia (Osler-Rendu-Weber disease. [See Section 13.]

Hidrotic ectodermal dysplasia—Thickened, striated, discoloured slowly growing nails, paronychia, diffuse hyperkeratosis of palms and soles, universally sparse hair. Squamous epithelioma may develop on palms or soles.

Ichthyosis vulgaris—Starts at 1–4 years, extensor surfaces, small white scales, keratosis follicularis. Also scalp, face, back; flexures spared; increased palmar markings. Atopic dermatitis may coincide.

Milroy's disease—Primary lymphoedema of legs, arms, face or genitalia, due to hypoplasia of lymphatics.

Monilethrix—Horny follicular papules with sparse, brittle, beaded hairs on scalp, and sometimes eyebrows, eyelashes, axillary and pubic hair.

Nail-patella syndrome (Osteo-onychodysplasia)—Grossly dystrophic small nails particularly of the thumbs, patellae hypoplastic or absent, dislocation of the radial heads, bony spines on iliac bones.

Neurofibromatosis (von Recklinghausen's disease)—Five or more *café-au-lait* spots and darker macules, sessile, domed and pedunculated fleshy tumours (molluscum fibrosum), pigmented macules in domes of axillae, pseudoherniations of skin, nodules on nerves, plexiform neurofibromata, and many associated anomalies. Extreme form is elephantiasis neurofibromatosa. [See Section 15.]

Pachyonychia congenita—Finger nails and toe nails yellow and thickened, subungual keratosis, keratoderma of palms and soles, keratosis pilaris, leukoplakia of mouth and anus, hair may be sparse.

Peutz-Jeghers syndrome—Pigmented macules in and around the mouth, on hands and feet associated with gastro-intestinal polyposis [see Section 7].

Tuberous sclerosis (epiloia)—Discrete brown fibrous papules near nasolabial folds, cheeks, chin ('adenoma sebaceum'), para-ungual fibromata, thickened area of 'shagreen' skin in lumbosacral region, fibromata, premature greyness of hair, *café-au-lait* spots and other anomalies [see Section 15].

Tylosis—Diffuse palmar and plantar keratoderma, with fissuring and hyperidrosis.

Non-sex linked (autosomal) recessive inheritance occurs in the following conditions (about one quarter of children of heterozygous parents will be affected):

Acrodermatitis enteropathica—Alopecia, diarrhoea, and a vesicobullous eruption around the orifices and on the extremities, psoriasiform lesions, secondary infection with *Candida albicans*. May be fatal. *Diodoquin*, 400–600 mg. per day may control the condition but may have to be maintained for years.

Albinism—Tyrosinase defect with white hair and skin and pink irides, excess of vellus hair, photophobia and nystagmus, early solar degenerative changes in the skin. Incomplete forms are commoner.

Ataxia telangiectasia (Louis-Bar syndrome)—Ataxia, telangiectases and recurrent respiratory infections, with absent thymus, hepatosplenomegaly and defective formation of immunoglobulin A.

Bloom's syndrome—Telangiectatic erythema and stunted growth. Mode of inheritance inconclusive.

Chondroectodermal dysplasia—Defective teeth, nails and sometimes hair with achondroplasia and dwarfism.

Dyskeratosis congenita—Mostly males with atrophy and pigmentation of the skin, nail dystrophy and leucoplakia, upon which epithelioma may develop.

Dystrophic epidermolysis bullosa—Large, flaccid bullae at birth and developing spontaneously; Nikolsky's sign positive; atrophic scars and miliaria; pseudowebbing enclosing digits; squamous epithelioma may develop; mucosae involved; bullae in mouth, larynx, oesophagus, teeth malformed; epidermolysis bullosa lethalis may be a variant and can occur in a sibling. Infant may survive for up to 3 months.

Ichthyosiform erythroderma—Widespread ichthyosis with redness also affecting scalp, neck and flexures where it persists though other areas may improve, with diminution of erythema; ectropion, corneal dystrophies. A severe form is the harlequin foetus.

Phenylketonuria—Phenylananine deficiency. Fair-haired, fair-skinned infant, mentally retarded with eczema sometimes atopic in type.

Poikiloderma congenitale (Rothmund-Thomson)—Commoner in females; redness and oedema followed by atrophy, telangiectasia and pigmentary variations, face, hands, legs; light sensitivity, keratoses and epithelioma, cataracts, sparse hair.

Werner's syndrome—Premature ageing, greying of hair, shiny tense skin, small stature, hypogonadism, cataracts, malignancy common.

Xeroderma pigmentosum—Increased sensitivity to sunlight, leading to acute sunburn or freckling on exposed parts, becoming permanent, with telangiectasia, atrophy, keratoses and squamous epitheliomata, photophobia and ectropion; mental deficiency; many die before adult life. A particulate light screen is necessary as a protective.

Sex-linked recessive inheritance, transmitted by females and affecting males, occurs in the following conditions:

Angiokeratoma corporis diffusum. (Fabry's disease)—Telangiectatic macules or papules on abdomen, thighs, scrotum, or widespread: inconspicuous keratosis on papules; lipid deposits in small vessels, causing cerebral, cardiac or renal manifestations; vasomotor disturbances in limbs and neuritic pains relieved by elevation or cooling; corneal opacities.

Anhidrotic ectodermal dysplasia—Generalized anhidrosis causing intolerance of heat, absent or defective teeth, sparse hair, defective nails, atrophic rhinitis, xerostomia, central nervous manifestations. Partial forms occur.

Sex-linked ichthyosis vulgaris (ichthyosis nigricans)—Large brown scales on abdomen, widespread, involving scalp, face, neck, axillae and sometimes the antecubital and popliteal fossae, patchy hair loss.

Wiskott-Aldrich syndrome—Eczema, thrombocytic purpura and immunological deficiency.

DEVELOPMENTAL ABNORMALITIES

The cause of these conditions remains a matter for conjecture, possibilities including ionizing radiation, drugs, virus infections, and nutritional disturbances affecting women early in pregnancy.

Some of the commoner naevi (hamartomata) affecting the skin are considered below. A naevus is not necessarily a birth mark as these circumscribed lesions may develop after birth and even in adolescence.

Haemangiomata

Telangiectatic naevus (naevus flammeus, port wine stain). Not all telangiectatic naevi present at birth persist. Those between the brows and on the eyelids fade within the first year or soon after but those on the nape of the neck often persist throughout life.

A port wine stain is commonest on the face and neck but may be extensive. They are usually asymmetrical and may be unilateral. The mouth may be involved. Naevus flammeus in the trigeminal area may be accompanied by angiomatosis of the meninges and eye (Sturge-Weber syndrome). Epilepsy is common and hemiplegia may develop. Some degree of mental retardation is usual. X-ray examination of the skull, angiography and electroencephalography may help in the localization of the angiomatosis.

Treatment of port wine stains is unsatisfactory. Cosmetic cover preparations are effective in females but impractical in males. Vascular excrescences may develop in adult life. They can be flattened by cautery destruction.

Cavernous Naevus (Strawberry Mark Haemangioma)

These soft vascular tumours start to develop during the first month after birth although occasionally they are visible at birth. They enlarge upwards and outwards for about 9 months after which they start to regress, as shown by central streaky pallor and shrinkage. The smaller lesions disappear by about 5 years of age but the larger ones with deeper vascular components only regress to soft skin-coloured fleshy swellings by this time and may not finally become inconspicuous before adolescence. Nevertheless, there is rarely any necessity for surgical intervention, and even when there is this should be deferred until the vascular component has disappeared.

Three clinical types are seen, namely the simple red raised strawberry mark, the strawberry mark with a bluish surround of deeper involvement resembling a poached egg; and an entirely deeper pale blue type sometimes with visible venules. The second and third types are those with the slower resolution.

The commonest complication is ulceration, particularly when the haemangioma is over the extensor surface of a joint or on the buttocks or in the anogenital area. Haemorrhage from trauma is rare, but occasionally cavernous haemangiomata occur with thrombocytopenia, and deposition of platelets in thrombi within the haemangioma. Purpura, ecchymoses, visceral haemorrhages and anaemia may develop. This type is rare.

Cavernous naevus is best left to run its natural course unless its situation near the eye, or on the nose, lip or in the anogenital region makes action necessary. The eyeball may be displaced, breathing embarrassed and feeding or attention to bowel function rendered difficult.

In these circumstances or if the lesion is enlarging rapidly, threatening to ulcerate or is accompanied by thrombocytopenia, radiotherapy is the treatment of choice [see Section 13]. Radiotherapy is inadvisable in most simple haemangiomata particularly when the lesion is near a joint, because its epiphyseal development may be interfered with, or when it is near the nipple in a girl, as subsequent pubertal breast development may be prevented. A useful practice is to photograph the lesion and make a natural size print for subsequent comparison. Reassurance of the parents is helped by the demonstration of a series of photographs showing the natural course of events in a previous similar patient. In the absence of photographic control, simple recorded measurements are adequate. Ulceration is best treated with chlortetracycline ointment and a firmly applied dressing. The rare serious cases with haemorrhage may need transfusion of whole blood.

Haemangiectatic Hypertrophy (Klippel-Trénaunay-Weber Syndrome)

Cavernous naevus with hypertrophy of a limb, venous varicosities and sometimes lymphangectasia. The area of the haemangioma is warmer than the same site on the opposite limb, and arterial pulsation or a bruit may be present, from arteriovenous anastomosis. Ulceration may occur on the foot. Some are relatively localized and in the deep fascia, others are more diffused, perhaps with multiple communications and involvement of muscle by the haemangiomatous proliferation. The condition calls for angiography and the advice of a vascular surgeon.

Senile haemangiomata (Campbell de Morgan's spots) and angiokeratomata of the scrotum are degenerative conditions with capillary dilatation. They have no systemic significance.

Epidermal Naevi

These are organoid hamartomata, differentiated towards surface epidermal cells, sebaceous glands, apocrine glands, hair follicles, or to a combination of these structures. Linear, warty or hard naevi and unilateral forms are examples of the first group, sometimes needing surgical help if the hand or foot is involved. Basal cell epithelioma is a rare complication. Naevus sebaceus occurs on the scalp or face as a brown soft warty plaque. Present at birth it undergoes no change in childhood but in adult life warty proliferation or basal-cell epithelioma may develop. Hence excision is advisable prophylactically in early adult life, especially as the affected area is also hairless and unsightly. Naevus syringocystadenomatosus papilliferus is an apocrine naevus with sebaceous components. Comedo naevus may be localized, linear or extensive and unilateral.

Melanotic Naevi

These are hamartomata of melanocytes and sometimes of Schwann cells. The commonest form is the lentigo macule, a lesion differing clinically from ephelis in that the latter only develops after exposure to sunlight whereas the former occurs extensively on covered parts as well as on light-exposed areas and does not darken after solar irradiation. The melanocytes are at the epidermo-dermal junction but are not proliferating.

The cellular, fleshy, hairy pigmented naevus, mole or benign melanoma is a brown firm nodule, sometimes with coarse hairs protruding. A compound naevus is sometimes diagnosed clinically, sometimes only at histological examination. It may be warty or mulberry-like. Histologically, the melanocytes are in places dermal and elsewhere junctional. These lesions are benign in childhood though potentially malignant in adults.

A junctional naevus is brown, somewhat speckled and flat or slightly raised. The diagnosis may be clinical or histological. Although the melanocytes are in the junctional zone, these lesions are benign in childhood, sometimes converting to compound naevi. In adults they are potentially malignant.

Large melanocytic naevi are sometimes present at birth which may involve a whole limb or a large area on the trunk. This rare form may undergo malignant change even in childhood.

Connective Tissue Naevi

The commonest of these is the pale, soft slightly rough-surfaced plaque (shagreen skin) which may occur in the lumbosacral region in epiloia.

EFFECTS OF PREGNANCY AND OF AGEING

EFFECTS OF PREGNANCY

Skin changes occurring in pregnancy may be directly related to it or coincidental.

Generalized increase of pigmentation of already pigmented parts is usual, particularly the areolae of the nipples, the linea nigra and the genital skin. Pigmentation of forehead, cheeks and temples (chloasma uterinum) often occurs, particularly with women of dark complexion.

Atrophic striae, vascular 'spiders' and palmar erythema are often present. Sweating may be increased.

Pruritus may occur during pregnancy for no recognizable cause and has to be differentiated from scabies coinciding with pregnancy. Urticaria in pregnancy is often of undetermined cause.

Herpes gestationis (q.v.) is the classical dermatosis of pregnancy and impetigo herpetiformis is a very rare, serious pustular condition, with fever, related to hypocalcaemia of pregnancy and possibly a variant of pustular psoriasis.

The effects of pregnancy on existing dermatoses is

variable. Psoriasis and atopic dermatitis may improve, remain unchanged or worsen. Systematized lupus erythematosus is not usually aggravated. Acne vulgaris usually improves. *Candida albicans* and virus wart infections of the vulva become much worse. Lentigines may become visibly more numerous and neurofibromatosis may worsen.

Puerperal telogen effluvium is not uncommon in various degrees of severity; in due course recovery is usually complete.

EFFECTS OF AGEING

In some inherited conditions, for example progeria, premature ageing of the skin occurs, while in others, for example xeroderma pigmentosum, the intolerance of ultra-violet light leads to early degenerative changes and malignancy.

The dry, wrinkled, relatively hairless, yellowish skin of the aged indicates the lessened action of the sweat and pilosebaceous units, the epidermal atrophy and the degeneration of the collagen and elastica. Disturbed pigmentary function is shown by lentigines which appear on exposed parts, and by greying of the hair. Nail growth is slowed and the nails become brittle and ridged.

The commoner conditions in the ageing skin for which treatment is asked include pruritus hiemalis (winter itch); discoid eczema and eczéma craquelé related to asteatosis; increased susceptibility to contact with irritant substances; xanthelasma palpebrarum; 'senile haemangiomata; basal-cell papillomata (seborrhoeic keratoses or seborrhoeic warts); freckling of face and hands; solar keratoses; Bowen's disease; squamous or basal-cell epitheliomata; and lentigo maligna or malignant melanoma.

Conditions in the skin secondary to diseases which are more common in the elderly include the manifestations of diabetes mellitus, of malignancy or other visceral disease and of arterial or venous insufficiency in the extremities.

THE SKIN AND VISCERAL MALIGNANCY

SECONDARY DEPOSITS

These may reach the skin from visceral foci of malignancy by the blood stream or by the lymphatics. Blood-borne metastases may arise from the breast, lung, stomach, intestines, liver, kidney (hypernephroma), uterus, ovary, prostate or bone. They may also originate from unrecognized malignant melanoma or from a lesion previously removed, possibly years earlier.

Secondary deposits present as single or multiple, often vascular nodules or plaques with a varying amount of inflammation. On the scalp, thickened bald areas may form, resembling morphoea.

Direct lymphatic spread occurs mostly from a breast cancer, causing a hard, red, pitting area of skin with a clearly marked border (carcinoma erysipelatoides, cancer *en cuirasse*).

PAGET'S DISEASE

This is a destructive condition of a nipple due to spread of malignant cells from a ductal carcinoma. There is scaling and pinkness of the skin around the nipple, with slight palpable thickening. The nipple may be partly or totally destroyed or it may be retracted. There may be a clear or blood-stained discharge. Lymph nodes are not usually palpable in the axilla and no other abnormality can be found in the breast.

Diagnosis is from eczema of the nipple. This is usually bilateral and due to atopic dermatitis, scabies, maceration from lactation or allergy to rubber in a brassiere. In eczema there is no infiltration or retraction and the nipple remains intact and equal in size to its fellow.

Rarely, extramammary Paget's disease occurs in the axilla or anogenital region from an underlying sweat gland adenocarcinoma. There is a demarcated, red, scaly, lightly crusted or eroded patch.

BOWEN'S DISEASE

This is an intra-epidermal carcinoma, potentially invasive. It may occur anywhere on the skin or mucosal surfaces and may be single or multiple. There is a persistent, flat, brownish-red, scaly or lightly crusted plaque which slowly extends. There is a statistically significant relationship with carcinoma of the bronchus, gastro-intestinal tract or genito-urinary tract. There may be a past history of treatment with arsenic in the form of Fowler's solution. Others may have been exposed to trivalent arsenic in the course of agricultural or industrial work or even in contaminated water supplies. An histologically similar condition of the glans penis (Queyrat's erythroplasia) presents as a well demarcated red, glistening, velvety plaque. It is not known to be associated with visceral malignancy.

ASSOCIATED CONDITIONS

Skin conditions which are sometimes associated with visceral malignancy in varying degrees of probability include the following:

A high incidence of carcinoma of the oesophagus has been reported in some families with palmo-plantar keratoderma (tylosis).

Acanthosis nigricans in adults is often associated with an adenocarcinoma, usually of the stomach. Dark velvety folds occur in the flexures. In severe cases the lips, gums, tongue, oesophagus, palms and soles may also be affected. It has to be differentiated from pseudo-acanthosis nigricans, which may occur in the flexures of the obese.

The gastro-intestinal polyposis of the Peutz-Jeghers syndrome may undergo malignant change.

Signs of past treatment with inorganic arsenic indicate a liability to develop visceral malignancy, particularly in the bronchus. The signs include 'rain drop' hypopigmentation with patchy hyperpigmentation, keratoses, Bowen's disease and epitheliomata.

Dermatomyositis occurring in adults is often associated with visceral malignancy of breast, bronchus, stomach, kidney, rectum, uterus, ovary or testis or with a reticulosis.

Much less certain and occasional associations with malignancy in internal organs are generalized pruritus, bullous pemphigoid, urticaria and figurate erythema (erythema annulare centrifugum).

Systemic reticuloses (malignant lymphomas and leukaemias) may present with pruritus, herpes zoster, furunculosis, extensive fungal infection, oral ulceration and infections, erythroderma, figurate erythema, ichthyosis or acanthosis nigricans.

DISTURBANCES OF FUNCTION

Itching is the desire to scratch, a normal phenomenon when it can be relieved by a rub or a scratch. Pathological itching or pruritus occurs when the desire to scratch is morbidly persistent, disturbing well-being by day and sleep by night.

GENERALIZED PRURITUS

Itching is initiated in the skin by the release of proteolytic enzymes. From the practical point of view the clinician is concerned with finding and, if possible, removing or suppressing the primary cause, whether it be local or remote. It is first necessary by questioning to exclude urticaria which often shows no physical signs at the time of the examination. Infestation with scabies or pediculi must also be excluded. A patient with scabies complains of widespread itching, worse at night, but does not necessarily mention the presence of a rash. The sites most affected are the finger webs, wrists, medial aspects of the elbows, axillary folds, breasts, abdomen, buttocks, penis and scrotum (highly diagnostic), and the lower limbs. The palms and soles are often affected in childhood and even the face may be affected in infancy. Bedfellows or other members of the family may also be itching. Scabies is an occupational hazard for nurses and physiotherapists.

Pediculosis should be suspected when person and clothing are dirty. Linear scratch marks are present on the trunk, particularly the shoulders, and pediculi and ova are found in the seams of the underwear or on coarse body hairs. A combination of pediculosis with nutritional deficiency produces pigmentation, scars and scratch marks (vagabonds' disease). Pediculosis capitis may also present with itching and scratch marks around the shoulders and the diagnosis is confirmed by finding glistening ova attached to the hairs, particularly in the occipital region. (Scurf is dull and amorphous but particles of hair lacquer may resemble ova.) It is unusual to find many lice but in extreme cases the hair may be matted and entangled. *Phthirus pubis* may spread to other areas where there is coarse hair. In hairy males the body and limbs may be infested and in children the eyelashes. The diagnosis may be missed unless a hand lens is used.

Insect bites can cause widespread itching but examination usually reveals characteristic grouped urticarial papules, some with central puncta, or there may be varicelliform papulovesicles.

Dermatitis herpetiformis has to be excluded, particularly in young or middle-aged adults. The lesions predominate on the scalp, at the shoulders, elbow tips, buttocks and knees but vesicles or bullae may be inconspicuous or absent owing to their rapid destruction by scratching. There is often hyperpigmentation in the affected areas.

A personal or family history of atopy should be inquired into. Lichenification, with white dermographism may be relatively inconspicuous during partial remissions. Xeroderma may also be present.

Itching in the elderly occurring or worsening in the winter is often a manifestation of dehydration and defatting of the skin by a combination of cold, low humidity, and sometimes the excessive use of soap and water on the ageing skin which is naturally becoming more atrophic and drier.

In patients coming from the tropics itching may be symptomatic of infestation with hookworm, round worm or onchocerciasis.

The commoner systemic causes of pruritus are as follows:

It may be the first symptom of biliary cirrhosis, preceding the onset of jaundice or xanthomata by several months. In all forms of obstructive jaundice itching may be a troublesome symptom.

Chronic renal failure may cause general pruritus but this is usually overshadowed by other manifestations.

Diabetes mellitus is not a cause of generalized pruritus but is a common cause of localized anogenital pruritus. Myxoedema may present with itching of the 'winter itch' type and pruritus has been described as 'the lisping of the gout'.

Iron deficiency anaemia, polycythaemia, Hodgkin's disease when the para-aortic glands are involved—lymphatic leukaemia, mycosis fungoides and lymphosarcoma may all present with widespread pruritus. In mastocytosis the urticating pigmented papules may be relatively inconspicuous.

It is difficult to assess the relationship of pruritus to visceral malignancy as both conditions tend to affect similar age groups. Drug-induced pruritus must always be borne in mind. In particular, morphine and its derivatives, belladonna and cocaine, are suspect, and morphine derivatives are contra-indicated in the management of itchy skin conditions owing to their histamine-releasing properties. Chlorpromazine, testosterone and other drugs may cause generalized pruritus by inducing intrahepatic biliary obstruction.

Psychogenic generalized pruritus is uncommon,

emotional disturbances more often causing localized pruritus with lichenification in the anogenital region, at the nape of the neck, in the forearms or on the legs (lichen simplex). There is worsening after tension-provoking episodes. The underlying drive is more likely to be aggressive than libidinous and in this respect the favoured use by many patients of the expression 'irritation' (Latin irritare = excite to anger) instead of itch (Latin prurire = to be wanton) is perhaps significant.

As generalized pruritus has so many possible causes it is often necessary to supplement the clinical examinations with a number of laboratory investigations including a haemoglobin estimation, total and differential white cell count, urine analysis, blood urea, blood uric acid, liver function tests and an X-ray examination of the chest. In selected cases, skin snippets for onchocerciasis, and stool examinations for worms are necessary.

Treatment

Sudden changes of temperature should be avoided. Baths should be tepid and 120 g. of bicarbonate of soda may be added to a 100 litre bath. Woollen underclothing should not be worn in direct contact with the skin. Mental and physical occupation may help to distract attention from the skin. Condiments, strong hot tea or coffee and excess of alcohol should be proscribed. For sedation barbiturates or promethazine hydrochloride are useful but opiates should not be prescribed when there is pruritus. Methyltestosterone in a dose of 5–10 mg. thrice daily may relieve the pruritus of biliary cirrhosis.

If the skin is dry emulsifying ointment is useful, both as a local application and as a substitute for soap in the bath.

Prognosis

In the idiopathic senile variety the prognosis as regards permanent relief is poor though longevity is not affected. When defatting of the skin is the cause treatment with refatting applications is usually effective. In other varieties the prognosis depends on the cause.

LOCALIZED PRURITUS

This may occur without physical signs or friction may produce lichen simplex (q.v.). The commonest sites are the scalp, the back of the neck, the eyelids, behind and above the ears, just distal to the tips of the elbows, the wrists, the palms, the external genitalia and the anal region, the anteromedial aspects of the thighs, the calves and the feet. In every case a contact cause should be excluded before diagnosing lichen simplex.

ANOGENITAL PRURITUS

This may occur as pruritus ani in either sex, as scrotal and perineal pruritus in the male, or as vulvar pruritus in the female.

PRURITUS ANI

This often occurs without physical signs; when signs are present they may be those of a causal condition or secondary to scratching.

Aetiology

The cause may be some cutaneous, anal or rectal condition or the effect of a drug. Proctitis with irritating discharge is an occasional cause. More common is pruritus due to thread worms passing through the anal canal for oviposition. Piles and anal fissures are other common causes but cutaneous tags resulting from fibrosed piles should not be removed in an attempt to give relief. On the skin, lack of cleanliness, infection with *Candida albicans* or with pathogenic fungi, or *Phthirus pubis* infestation may be causal. Local applications containing benzocaine or antihistaminic drugs may cause or aggravate pruritus ani. Phenolphthalein taken internally can cause it and wide-spectrum antibiotics taken by mouth may encourage *Candida albicans* infection. Sometimes local skin conditions such as viral warts or lichen planus are responsible. There may be local hyperidrosis which aggravates the discomfort and encourages bacterial or fungal infection. In resistant cases either without physical signs or with simple lichenification an emotional cause may be operating. There may be inadequate expression of aggression or exhibitionism and a passive homosexual tendency. Sometimes there is cancerphobia.

Clinical Picture

The skin may appear normal or there may be scratch marks and lichenification or some recognizable local skin pathology. Microscopic examination of material taken with a scotch tape swab from the perianal skin may reveal ova of *Oxyuris vermicularis*, or scrapings may reveal *Candida albicans* or fungal elements.

Treatment

If no local cause can be found and dealt with treatment has to be symptomatic with bland local applications and sedatives. Cleanliness is important but medicated soaps or antiseptics should not be used. After bathing, the skin should be dabbed dry without friction. Topical corticosteroids are often effective even when diluted.

Candida albicans infection responds to magenta paint, nystatin ointment or *Fungilin* cream (amphotericin B). *Tri-Adcortyl* cream, containing antibacterial, anti-candidal and anti-inflammatory components, is often effective. Relapse may occur unless the overabundance of *Candida albicans* in the gut is brought under control with nystatin, 500,000 Units thrice daily by mouth.

A barbiturate or promethazine hydrochloride makes a useful antipruritic sedative. Aperients, particularly phenolphthalein and aloes, may aggravate, but liquid paraffin is safe. Strong coffee and condiments should not be taken.

Patients with insight into their personality problems may benefit from discussion, but those with homosexual tendencies are often not amenable to psychotherapy.

SCROTAL AND PERINEAL PRURITUS

Candida albicans or fungal infection may be present. There may be hyperidrosis. Friction from clothing may aggravate the condition or sensitization to dyed material may start it. Pruritic scrotal dermatitis may arise from a diet deficient in protein, iron and vitamin B complex. There may be lesions of lichen planus, psoriasis or lichen simplex or abnormal physical signs may be absent.

Treatment

This is much the same as for pruritus ani, except that patients with fungal infections may be treated with half strength salicylic acid and benzoic acid ointment and, if this fails to clear the condition, a course of griseofulvin, 500 mg. daily for 6 weeks.

PRURITUS VULVAE

Aetiology

The causes include pregnancy, oral contraceptives, wide-spectrum antibiotics and other causes of *Candida albicans* infection, with or without vaginal discharge. There may be nutritional deficiency, threadworm infestation (in children), glycosuria, psychosexual difficulties, contact sensitization to contraceptives or vaginal douche solutions, lack of cleanliness or the abuse of antiseptics, or *Phthirus pubis* infestation. Fungal infection of the genitocrural folds is rare in Caucasian women but may occur in Asians and Africans. Local skin conditions include psoriasis, infective (flexural) dermatitis, lichen planus, atrophic senile vulvovaginitis, lichen sclerosus et atrophicus and Bowen's precancerous dermatosis.

Clinical Picture

There may be no abnormal physical signs or there may be lichenification, excoriations, boils or impetiginous lesions, or a superimposed mixed contact and infective dermatitis resulting from inappropriate treatment. In *Candida albicans* infection there is centripetal peeling, with non-suppurative satellite lesions.

Treatment

This depends on the cause. Control of diabetes, relief of an emotional conflict, avoidance of an offending drug, or contact irritant, and an adequate diet may, one or other, be helpful. Phenolphthalein may cause a pruritic fixed erythema at the vulva, as may sulphonamides, barbiturates and other drugs. *Candida albicans* infection responds to magenta paint, nystatin powder or ointment, or *Fungilin* lotion. (amphotericin B) Mixed *Candida albicans* and bacterial infection is common and this may respond well to a combination of nystatin with neomycin, gramicidin and triamcinolone (*Tri-Adcortyl* cream). For staphylococcal infection, with pustules and boils, chlortetracycline ointment, 0·25 per cent., is suitable. A 1 per cent. solution of cetrimide is useful for cleaning the skin. Hip-baths of potassium permanganate 1 in 8000 are also useful for infected lesions.

In non-infective pruritus with or without lichenification, psoriasis or lichen planus a topical corticosteroid is usually effective.

General sedation is often necessary in the form of a barbiturate or promethazine hydrochloride.

For Bowen's disease, after biopsy confirmation, surgical excision is advisable.

Psychogenic forms may respond to open discussion of conflict situations, but sometimes the pruritus serves as a means of avoiding coitus.

PRURIGO

This term is used for a group of intensely itchy conditions in which the predominant physical signs are lichenification and excoriated papules. Lichenification is produced by friction and presents as dusky thickened skin with accentuation of the diamond-shaped ridges and intervening furrow. Prurigo papules are ill-defined obtuse elevations with excoriated tops, caused by trauma from the finger nail.

Aetiology

Itching in this condition is usually central in origin. The scratching is an outlet for inadequately expressed feelings of resentment. Sometimes a local irritant initiates the itching but the emotional state results in the formation of a vicious circle in which friction and scratching perpetuate the condition.

Thus, lichenification may develop on contact dermatitis, when an industrial compensation claim remains unsettled.

Clinical Picture

A patch of lichen simplex is usually oval and, if on a limb, lies in its long axis. The colour is reddish-brown and the edge fades off gradually into the normal skin with no outlying 'satellites'. The surface shows an accentuation of the normal skin pattern, creases being increased in both depth and width and intervening elevations being more conspicuous than usual. The areas may be shiny and resemble grouped papules of lichen planus. There may be a fine scaling or warty thickening. There may be scabbed excoriations and usually there is hyperpigmentation. Being thickened and inelastic, lichenified skin tends to become cracked and secondarily infected, causing cellulitis, impetigo or boils. The sites most characteristically affected are the back and sides of the neck, the supraclavicular regions, the extensor aspects of the forearms just distal to the elbows, the hands, the external genitalia, the perianal region, the anteromedial and lateral aspects of the thighs and the anterolateral aspects of the calves.

Lichen simplex is modified in appearance in certain situations. On the scalp scabbed excoriations may be seen, or diffuse redness and profuse, coarse scaling, sometimes with asbestos-like scaling for a few millimetres up the hair shafts—the so-called 'tinea amiantacea'. At the nucha an oval area is usually superficially excoriated, with grey scales and light crusting. A mild infection may be superimposed. On the brows the hairs are broken off short. On the palms, dyskeratosis dominates the picture and accentuation of the skin pattern is inconspicuous. In the genitocrural folds and natal cleft the skin may become fissured, sodden and whitened, resembling leucoplakia. The patient may start to rub the lesions during the interview, if relevant personal matters are touched upon.

Diagnosis

The resemblance to lichenified dermatitis of external origin may cause difficulty. With lichenified dermatitis there is usually a history of a more widespread eruption which has become localized, for example in the antecubital region.

In lichen planus there are usually some discrete, flat-topped papules with a shiny surface which can be found in the course of a general examination of the skin. On the legs in particular, lichenoid plaques may be due to lichen simplex, lichen planus (often hypertrophic) or lichen amyloidosus (rare); differentiation may only be possible by biopsy.

At the nucha, lichen simplex may resemble infective (seborrhoeic) dermatitis or psoriasis, but the circumscribed pattern is not typical of the former and the absence of psoriasiform silvery scaling or psoriasis elsewhere makes the latter diagnosis improbable. The presence of pediculosis or of hair dye or hair net dermatitis has to be excluded.

On the palms, psoriasis and dyskeratotic contact dermatitis have to be excluded on the evidence of the history and the presence or absence of psoriasis elsewhere.

At the flexures, leucoplakia can be excluded because it only occurs on transitional epithelial surfaces; but lichen simplex of the medial aspects of the labia majora and the labia minora may be accompanied by leucoplakia.

Treatment

It is important to direct attention to the relief of any related tension state as well as to the skin lesions themselves. Barbiturates, promethazine hydrochloride and trimeprazine tartrate are useful from their sedative, hypnotic and antipruritic effects. Locally, topical corticosteroids are usually effective or tar may be used, either alone in the form of a paste, or in combination with a corticosteroid. Tar should not be prescribed for use in the flexures. For very resistant lesions a corticosteroid preparation applied beneath polythene film at night may succeed, apparently because, by hydrating the surface of the skin and increasing the surface temperature, it increases percutaneous absorption. Occlusive paste dressings, containing a corticosteroid or tar, are sometimes effective when all else fails. They are usually changed once a week but are not always tolerated. Hot baths and proximity to fires should be proscribed.

Course and Prognosis

This depends upon adjustments to the life situation as well as to management of the skin lesions themselves.

ATOPIC DERMATITIS

Synonyms. Besnier's prurigo; Flexural prurigo; Asthma-hay-fever-prurigo syndrome; Pruriginous facial eczema.

This is an intensely itchy condition affecting in particular the face and the flexures; it usually begins in infancy and often alternates with, or is accompanied by, asthma or vasomotor rhinitis.

Aetiology

Inheritance and the early environment are both important factors in the aetiology. There is an instability of the autonomic nervous system of unexplained mechanism. Without obvious cause or as a result of emotional tension, asthma, vasomotor rhinitis or intense itching develops. Excessive tone of unstriped muscle shows as blanching from vasoconstriction and as horripilation (goose flesh). Sweating is sometimes excessive and this may coincide with pruritic episodes. Electroencephalographic tracings are often abnormal.

Very high serum immunoglobulin IgE levels occur in atopic dermatitis, with or without asthma or vasomotor rhinitis. The presence of reagins is also a feature of atopy but they are of doubtful importance in atopic dermatitis, having more a genetic association than a direct cause and effect link. Thus, most cases have reagins to a wide range of allergens but these only indicate the antigens to which the patient has been exposed and they do not indicate aggravating factors.

Atopic individuals are often above average intelligence but are excitable and prone to feelings of insecurity. There may be an unsatisfactory relationship with their parents, particularly the mother (the so-called 'maternal rejection factor'). Threats to security may coincide with exacerbations, at times of detachment from parents, changes of school or occupation, marriage or bereavement. Other factors include changes of temperature or of humidity, airborne, ingested or injected allergens, contact with rough clothing, drugs and infections. The atopic individual reacts to everyday stimuli with a mechanism designed for use in emergencies. Thus, pollens, danders and household dust (including *Pteronyssimus culinae*) may cause asthma, vasomotor rhinitis and, possibly, atopic dermatitis. Stroking the affected skin causes a white line to develop in the line of stroke in 15 seconds. The normal red line with adjoining white band develops if this procedure is carried out at non-lichenified sites, suggesting that white dermographism indicates that the mast cells in the lichenified areas have discharged their granules and liberated histamine as a result of repeated past trauma and have now temporarily become refractory.

Staphylococcal infections are remarkably rare in atopic dermatitis, considering the gross scratch trauma that takes place; but when it does occur the staphyloderma may be extensive and severe, particularly in patients receiving systemic treatment with corticosteroids. Virus infection with herpes simplex or vaccinia is a serious complication. A generalized eruption may result (eczema herpeticum, eczema vaccinatum). The former may be fatal in infancy.

Clinical Picture

Atopic dermatitis may start as early as the second month as a papulovesicular and erythematosquamous condition involving parts most easily rubbed by the infant—the face, neck, antecubital regions, wrists, hands, popliteal spaces, calves, ankles and feet. The trunk may escape or it may show a patchy, ill-defined, faintly pink papular and scaly eruption. The lesions may be exudative, infected or lichenified.

The infant periodically indulges in bouts of rubbing, particularly in the evening, when bored, frustrated or tired, and with determination overcomes any attempt to check its activity. The condition usually becomes milder when the child starts to walk and to do things for itself.

Scratching may cease for several years but there is usually a recurrence at puberty, when the condition is localized more to the bends of the elbows and of the knees, the wrists and hands, the face and neck and sometimes to the genitocrural region and the feet. The affected areas show lichenification and excoriations. The severity may be less when adult life is reached but in some patients there is indefinite persistence and in others it may start in adult life.

Xeroderma is often present and modifies the picture. Cataracts are a serious complication in some persistent cases. They are believed to be congenital but friction applied to the eyelids probably plays a part in their maturation.

Diagnosis

Atopic dermatitis has to be differentiated from contact eczematous dermatitis, especially when the latter is complicated by lichenification. In atopic dermatitis the primary lesion is not a papulovesicle but is a prurigo papule, an obtuse elevation of a reddish-brown colour, often with an excoriated top; or if these elementary lesions are not discernible, lichenification and excoriations dominate the picture.

Atopic dermatitis involving the face (pruriginous facial eczema) has to be differentiated from actinic dermatoses and from eczematous dermatitis of the face caused by airborne or hand-transferred agents. The latter affects particularly the eyelids and the skin of the neck just above the collar line. Actinic dermatoses affect the forehead, nose and malar ridges and other parts exposed to light. In atopic dermatitis the whole face may have a thickened leathery or terracotta appearance, unless the patient has recently been rubbing it in which case there may be marked pallor due to white dermographism. The eyebrows are often broken off short, causing a very characteristic facies.

Treatment

The treatment of atopic dermatitis is that of the whole patient with his characteristic personality and problems, rather than the management of the skin condition by itself. Co-operation on the part of the parents is important. A steady level of affection in a calm home atmosphere is ideal. Sometimes removal from the home environment is advisable for a time. For some patients a period in a residential school offers the best solution. Owing to the risk of infection with herpes simplex, admission to hospital is inadvisable for infants with atopic dermatitis.

Medicinal treatment is largely symptomatic, with topical antipruritic and anti-inflammatory agents and with general sedatives in ample dosage, bearing in mind that sufferers from atopic dermatitis usually need larger than average doses of sedative drugs to bring about quiet and sleep and freedom from scratching. Promethazine hydrochloride (*Phenergan*), 25 mg. twice a day and 50 mg. at night, or amylobarbitone, 100 mg. twice a day and 200 mg. at night, may be prescribed alone or in combination, for adults, with proportional doses for children. The atopic patient needs to be kept fully occupied, either with suitable toys in childhood or by mental and manual distraction in adult life.

For the worst cases or during severe exacerbations in-patient treatment is necessary. Sedation can then be used in larger doses and the patient gets temporary relief from the home environment or any other source of agitation.

Systemic treatment with corticosteroids should only be used in the worst cases and then only after full consideration of the possible complications that may ensue and the difficulty of weaning the patient from this form of treatment. As a short-term measure intramuscular injections of corticotrophin gel, 20–40 I.U. daily or at longer intervals, may prove helpful.

Warm baths may be taken, using simple soap, a 'baby soap' or, when there is xeroderma, emulsifying ointment or a superfatted soap. A 10 per cent. urea cream, e.g. *Calmurid*, may be helpful when there is conspicuous xeroderma. Corticosteroid applications are helpful, but the large area of skin to be covered makes it advisable to dilute them, otherwise absorption may be enough to cause untoward symptoms. Chronic patches sometimes do well with tar paste, thickly applied.

Course and Prognosis

This varies considerably from one patient to another and may depend, *inter alia*, on the patient's adjustment to the life situation.

DISSEMINATED NEURODERMATITIS

This term is used for extensive and severe examples of atopic dermatitis and other widespread lichenified and pruriginous eruptions in which no contact, toxic or reticulotic cause can be discovered and in which the condition is thought to represent a maladjustment to the environment, particularly from loss of work, bereavement, sexual frustration and a general sense of unwantedness. It affects adults of all ages.

PRURIGO NODULARIS

This is a rare condition of large obtuse, dome-shaped nodules affecting the extensor surfaces of the forearms and legs. It is resistant to many local applications but may respond to local intralesional injections of triamcinolone, 1–2·5 mg. in 0·1–0·25 ml.

HYPERIDROSIS

Generalized excessive sweating (often worse at night) is a function of body thermostasis controlled from the hypothalamus and is a feature of infections including tuberculosis and malaria or of toxicity from alcohol or tobacco. It also occurs in hyperthyroidism. It may persist for a while after fever has subsided.

Emotional sweating is worse during the waking hours and when performing difficult tasks or at social contacts and interviews. It is usually limited to the forehead, axillae, groins, palms and soles, but there may also be a degree of generalized hyperidrosis. Disturbed mental states are apparent in some but in others the phenomenon appears to be only borderline excessive physiological activity. There may be an accompanying vasomotor instability causing 'symmetrical lividity' of the soles which are cold blue and clammy. Treatment is unsatisfactory. Acetylcholine-blocking drugs are sometimes effective, but their side-effects in the dose necessary to give relief may include paralysis of visual accommodation, dryness of the mouth, glaucoma, hyperthermia or convulsions—a state of affairs much worse than the condition for which they are administered. Propantheline has a good reputation, at 15 mg. thrice daily, or more, up to the limit of tolerance but not beyond 150 mg. per day. Similarly ganglion-blocking drugs may be effective but also cause side-effects, in particular hypotension. Sedatives and tranquillizer drugs are often a better solution.

Local treatment is also relatively ineffective or impractical. Aluminium acetate lotion is helpful.

Sympathectomy is usually only temporarily effective. X-ray suppression of the sweat glands can only be performed at the risk of subsequent chronic radiodermatitic changes and possible epithelioma. Undercutting or excision of the sweat glands in the dome of the axilla may be successful.

Gustatory sweating around the mouth occurs particularly after eating hot, spiced food, but is rarely a matter for concern. It may also occur after injuries involving the autonomic nerves in the head or neck.

Asymmetrical sweating may arise from lesions of the autonomic nervous system, centrally or peripherally. It has also been described in association with visceral disturbances.

ANIDROSIS

Anidrosis or at least hypoidrosis can occur from local skin conditions in which ductal obstruction occurs; for example prickly heat (miliaria) and in varying degrees when there is an inflammatory condition involving the epidermis, for example pompholyx, eczema, atopic dermatitis and psoriasis. It also occurs in scleroderma and in atrophic conditions of the skin and sweat glands or when there is eccrine aplasia as in ichthyosis and some forms of ectodermal defect. Organic lesions affecting brain, spinal cord or peripheral nerves (sympathectomy, neural leprosy, syringomyelia) may cause it as may the use of ganglion-blocking and anticholinergic drugs. Diminished sweating occurs in senile skin, myxoedema, diabetes mellitus, renal disease and cachectic states. Extensive anidrosis may cause hyperpyrexia.

SEBORRHOEA

This is an endocrine (androgen) controlled condition affecting males and is genetically determined but more a feature of some races than of others. Females as well as males may be affected in disease states, e.g. Cushing's syndrome and virilism. Parkinson's disease, particularly the post-encephalitic variety, is accompanied by marked seborrhoea as are some forms of epilepsy. Acne is accompanied by seborrhoea in both sexes, the male being more affected than the female.

ASTEATOSIS

This is a feature of the aged skin, and presents as winter itch, and discoid eczema with eczéma craquelé, a crazy paving or dried-out mud at low tide appearance. It also occurs in xeroderma. Loss of water by evaporation may be as important as asteatosis in the production of chapped skin, hence the aggravation in cold dry weather.

HIRSUTISM

The growth of coarse terminal hair in the male adult sexual pattern is described as hirsutism when it occurs in women. It results from androgenic stimuli and has to be differentiated from hypertrichosis which is excess of hair not in adult sexual pattern and not resulting from androgenic stimuli. Examples are lumbosacral hypertrichosis (faun tail), often associated with diastematomyelia, and hairy moles.

In hirsutism there is excess of hair at sites other than the scalp, axillae and pubis. There is no rigid pattern, some overlapping occurring between the sexes. For example, the suprapubic escutcheon does not always have a horizontal border in women who are otherwise 'normal'. The androgens originate from the testes, the adrenals (weak) and (probably) the ovaries, possibly also from other sources.

Testosterone is the physiological androgen in both sexes, some being found in the plasma of women. Hirsutism occurring at puberty is more likely to be constitutional whereas when it occurs in childhood or in adult women it is more likely to have an organic basis. The constitutional or idiopathic variety is by far the commonest, those afflicted showing no clinical or biochemical evidence of endocrine disorder of a masculinizing type.

Hirsutism with conspicuous elevation of 17-oxosteroid urinary excretion occurs in corticotrophin-secreting tumours of the pituitary, in congenital adrenal hyperplasia (manifested at puberty, sometimes with increased pregnanediol excretion), bilateral adrenal hyperplasia of later life and adrenal cortical tumours. There is slighter elevation of 17-oxosteroid excretion in masculinizing tumours of the ovary (arrhenoblastoma, Leydig and hilum-cell tumours).

The administration of androgens causes hirsutism. Many anabolic steroids have androgenic activity and progestogens occasionally show similar effects.

HYPOTRICHOSIS

Sparseness of hair is a feature in several hereditary conditions, including ectodermal dysplasias, monilethrix, pili torti, progeria, Rothmund-Thomson syndrome and Werner's syndrome. Fine sparse hair may be familial, at one end of the spectrum of 'normality'. Post-menopausal hair loss is of masculine pattern.

Diffuse sparseness arises as an acquired condition in telogen effluvium, in which there is premature transference of anagen follicles to the telogen phase, with shedding of an increased number of long club hairs. Causes include prolonged fever (particularly enteric fever), cachexia, pregnancy, systematic lupus erythematosus, erythroderma and emotional disturbances. Diffuse hair loss also occurs in hypothyroidism and to a less extent in hyperthyroidism; also in hypopituitarism, hypoparathyroidism and in imperfectly controlled diabetes. It may also occur after oophorectomy. It may be a feature of protein deficiency or of iron deficiency. Drugs capable of causing it include antimitotic agents, anticoagulants, thyroid antagonists, excess of vitamin A, amphetamine, and thallium salts used as pesticides and inadvertently contaminating food.

Trauma to the hair from traction due to wearing rollers at night, the use of nylon brushes or even excessively vigorous massage may cause or aggravate diffuse hair loss. Habitual tugging or twisting the hair may cause relatively local loss. Inflammation of the scalp, either infective or chemical, may cause diffuse hair-fall. Moth-eaten sparseness may occur in secondary syphilis. There remains a proportion of patients in whom no cause can be found.

Trichorrhexis (fractured hair shafts) has to be differentiated from hypotrichosis. It is a feature of some developmental abnormalities, e.g. monilethrix, pili annulati and pili torti (the hair is also sparse in these conditions). Trichorrhexis nodosa is a condition of brittleness of the hair arising at nodal swellings on their shafts. There may be an inherited predisposition and physical causes (friction, tension, heat) or chemical agents (bleaches, thioglycollates) account for the fractures.

ALOPECIA

This term is best limited to local circumscribed areas of partial or more often total loss of hair, without visible scarring. In alopecia areata one or more circular or oval smooth bald patches are present. When multiple there may be polycyclic patches. The hair margin may be affected, frontally, temporally or occipitally, a form in which the prognosis is often poor. When the disease is active short club-shaped hairs can be seen at the margin of the lesions. Alopecia areata tends to run in families. It may first appear in childhood or in adult life. Regrowth often occurs after the first attack but recurrences, perhaps several years later, are common and each makes the ultimate prognosis worse, the hair follicles gradually undergoing atrophy. Alopecia totalis is a term applied to total involvement of the scalp and alopecia universalis to loss of all hairs including brows, lashes, axillary, pubic, body and limb hairs. Alopecia areata is sometimes limited to the beard. Sometimes the nails are involved, with pitting.

Differential Diagnosis

Alopecia areata has to be differentiated from localized traumatic sparseness (sparse, fine shortish hairs, some with twisted or broken ends) and tinea capitis (brush-like swollen short hairs with scaling). It also has to be differentiated from the numerous causes of cicatricial alopecia. These include epidermal naevi, physical damage (mechanical, thermal, ionizing radiation). X-ray damage shows as scarring atrophic baldness, with patchy hyperpigmentation and telangiectasia. Other causes include chemical damage, fungal infections, e.g. favus, also lupus vulgaris, syphilis, leprosy, leishmaniasis, boils and carbuncles, folliculitis, acne necrotica, herpes zoster, variola and varicella, lichen planus, lupus erythematosus, scleroderma (linear morphoea—'coup de sabre'), necrobiosis lipoidica, sarcoidosis, and epithelioma, either primary basal-cell lesions or metastatic deposits. Pseudopelade is a form of cicatricial alopecia superficially resembling alopecia areata, but atrophic with scarring, no exclamation mark hairs, somewhat angular lesions and tufts of hair remaining in the scarred areas. It may be a sequel to lichen planus, lupus erythematosus or folliculitis.

Treatment

Local intradermal injections of triamcinolone are often effective or can be used to test the responsiveness of the affected follicles. They are best given by dermojet, needle injections being painful, and more difficult to place within the dermis without hypodermal involvement. This treatment is only practicable for relatively small lesions. The injections are given at intervals of 2–3 weeks and the responsiveness can usually be determined 3 weeks after the second treatment. A temporary dimpling often occurs due to atrophic changes in the collagen. Occasionally, when there is sudden widespread loss with a large number of exclamation hairs, it is justifiable to give a short course of oral steroid therapy. General and local ultra-violet irradiation and counter-irritant applications are sometimes used, also sedatives in those cases where emotional tension seems relevant.

Course and Prognosis

Recovery is usual from the first attack and with localized lesions but the prognosis worsens with each recurrence or if the condition is extensive. Alopecia totalis and alopecia of the margins of the scalp have a poor prognosis.

PIGMENTARY ANOMALIES

The colour of the skin depends on the melanin content of the epidermis and dermis, haemoglobin and oxyhaemoglobin in the blood vessels and carotene in the horny layer and in the subcutaneous fat.

Abnormal pigmentation arises from extravasated blood (haemosiderosis), abnormal haemoglobins—methaemoglobin, sulphaemoglobin and carboxyhaemoglobin, degraded haemoglobin (bilirubin) or haem (biliverdin), metals, drugs, tattooed materials and chemicals, including dinitrophenol, tetryl, picric acid, trinitrotoluene, santonin and acriflavine. Neglected dirty skin can deceive the unwary as can local applications including potassium permanganate, dithranol, tar and mercury.

Yellow coloration can be caused by excessive ingestion of food with high carotene content (carrots, tomatoes, egg yolk, etc.), jaundice, mepacrine (sparing the sclerae), and chemical stains such as picric acid and acriflavine. It has also been reported from high blood levels of *Salazopyrin* (sulphasalazine).

Haemosiderosis is brick red as opposed to the brown of melanosis, but the two may coexist and clinical differentiation can be difficult. Causes include hypostasis, capillaroses, drugs, haemochromatosis and haemolytic anaemia.

Silver, gold and bismuth cause blue grey discoloration.

Accidental tattooing is usually with carbon. Deliberate tattooes are made with carbon (black), mercuric sulphide (red), chromic oxide (green), cobalt aluminate (blue), cadmium sulphide (yellow) and iron oxides (brown).

MELANOGENESIS

This is considered at two levels: the hormonal controlling influences on the melanocytes and the biochemical changes within the melanocytes.

The melanocytes are activated by the melanocyte-stimulating hormone of the pituitary. Increased activity of the pituitary in pregnancy results in hypermelanosis (chloasma uterinum), affecting particularly the face, nipples, linea nigra and flexures. There is increased pigmentation in hyperpituitarism (acromegaly, gigantism) and diminished pigmentation in hypopituitarism. Pigmentation sometimes occurred in the early days of ACTH therapy, possibly from M.S.H. content. Oestrogens and progesterones stimulate melanogenesis.

Stimulation of the melanocyte leads to a complex chain reaction in which tyrosine becomes converted by oxidation into dihydroxyphenylalanine (DOPA), dopaquinone, a number of intermediates, reduced melanin (melanoid) and finally by polymerization and linkage with protein to melanin. A copper-containing aerobic oxidase is essential for tyrosinase and dopa-oxidase activity in melanogenesis, which is also increased following exposure to ultra-violet rays, heat or friction. Ascorbic acid by redox action inhibits melanin formation as do sulphydril (-SH) groups, which bind copper. This binding effect is lost by their oxidation to -S-S-groups, as in chronic inorganic arsenical intoxication.

DEFECTS OF PIGMENTATION

In vitiligo DOPA positive melanocytes are absent but DOPA negative cells (? Langerhan's cells, ? effete melanocytes) are present. The absence of DOPA positive melanocytes may be total or partial or weakly positive cells may be present. Vitiligo may be inherited as an irregular dominant trait and is sometimes associated with endocrine disorders, particularly hyperthyroidism, Addison's disease or pernicious anaemia. Alopecia areata may coexist.

Differential Diagnosis

The differential diagnosis is from acquired leucoderma, from tinea versicolor, and from a hypopigmented patch of tuberculoid leprosy.

Acquired leucoderma occurs at sites of eczema or psoriasis or as 'pityriasis alba' on the faces of blonde individuals, particularly children after exposure to the sun. Repigmentation usually occurs in all forms but in blonde individuals care should be taken to avoid further excessive insolation.

In pigmented races hypopigmentation (or for that matter hyperpigmentation) may be extreme after inflammatory processes in the skin.

Tinea versicolor causes slight hyperpigmentation on the covered skin of white individuals but hypopigmentation on the skin of pigmented individuals or on sun exposed areas of the white skin. Peeling may only be discernible by grattage. Diagnosis is confirmed by microscopic demonstration of fragments of mycelium and spores resembling bunches of grapes. Examination is made either by scraping off scales or by applying transparent adhesive tape and subsequently applying this to a microscope slide.

In tuberculoid leprosy there is hypopigmentation rather than depigmentation, the patch may be hairless and anhidrotic and there is impaired sense of temperature discrimination and touch, although on the face this may not be discernible. Thickened nerves may be felt. The histological appearance is usually diagnostic.

Treatment

The treatment of vitiligo is unsatisfactory. If hairs (vellus or terminal) in the patch are also unpigmented, then the prospect of bringing about repigmentation is slight. If, however, the hairs in a depigmented patch of skin remain pigmented then there is, theoretically at least, the possibility of bringing about some perifollicular repigmentation if the melanocytes at the hair papilla can be encouraged to migrate by setting up an inflammatory process, as with the application of phenol liquefactum or of a light-sensitizing substance, such as furocoumarine in bergamot oil (as in eau-de-Cologne). Some repigmentation may also occur when there is partial vitiligo from the administration of methoxypsoralen, 10–20 mg. daily, 2 hours before carefully graduated exposures to ultra-violet light. If there is no response after 2 months or if nausea, vomiting or depression develops, the treatment should be stopped. Blistering without repigmentation is also an indication for withdrawal.

Piebaldism is a condition of locally unpigmented patches of skin and hair present at birth. It is unrelated to albinism which is a recessive genetic anomaly in which there is a lack of pigment owing to the absence of tyrosinase. Albinism may be total, with white skin and hair and pink irides, or more often partial, with pale skin, hair and irides. Photophobia is usual. Solar atrophic changes occur on exposed parts and squamous epithelioma may result.

In phenylketonuria there is pale skin and hair, eczema of the atopic type and mental retardation. It is caused by a deficiency of tyrosine due to a metabolic block in the conversion of phenylalanine to tyrosine.

INCREASED PIGMENTATION

This occurs from endocrine causes, as in pregnancy (face, nipples, linea nigra and anogenital region), Addison's disease (widespread, especially light-exposed areas, sites of pressure and friction, flexures, creases of palms and soles, within the mouth, sometimes conjunctival and vaginal), acromegaly (widespread), Cushing's syndrome (Addisonian), malignant phaeochromocytoma (Addisonian, with hypertension, headaches, sweating, palpitations, apprehension), from ACTH in some patients and from progestational steroids taken as contraceptives (chloasmal).

Widespread pigmentation is sometimes a feature of chronic infections, as in tuberculosis, malaria, kala-azar and subacute bacterial endocarditis.

Increased pigmentation may occur with malignancy. An ectopic M.S.H. compound is formed in some cases of carcinoma of the bronchus. Pigmentation may also be present in severe malnutrition either from widespread deficiencies or from deficiency of vitamin A, vitamin C, or nicotinic acid.

Acanthosis nigricans is a condition of excessive pigmentation accompanied by epidermal hyperplasia causing velvety elevations and dark warty lesions particularly in the flexures, at mucocutaneous junctions and sometimes on the palms and soles. The juvenile form is generally determined and benign as far as systemic effects are concerned, but the adult form is often accompanied by malignancy, particularly adenocarcinomata of stomach, intestines, ovary, uterus, also sometimes with carcinoma of the breast or of the bronchus, and with epithelial neoplasia, e.g. of cervix uteri and sometimes with lymphoma. Acanthosis nigricans has also been described with endocrine disorders, including acromegaly, Addison's disease and diabetes mellitus, but in such cases the possibility of malignancy involving the endocrine system must be considered, or the possibility of benign pseudo-acanthosis which may occur in the flexures in obesity. These different types cannot be differentiated histologically.

Malignant melanoma with hepatic metastases may cause increased pigmentation and the urine may be dark brown.

Chronic renal failure is often accompanied by increased pigmentation and it may be a feature of polycystic renal disease. Pigmentation is also often increased in rheumatoid arthritis and in Still's disease. Hepatolenticular degeneration and some other diseases of the central nervous system (Schilder's disease, post-encephalitic Parkinsonism, etc.) are often accompanied by increased pigmentation.

Excessive pigmentation occurs, mostly in middle-aged women, in xanthomatous biliary cirrhosis and to a less extent in other forms of cirrhosis. In haemochromatosis there is slaty-grey or bronzed pigmentation, hepatomegaly, diabetes mellitus and a raised serum iron level. It is mostly seen in middle-aged men.

Several drugs can cause increased pigmentation. The classical example, inorganic arsenic, is rarely used today. It causes hyperpigmentation with guttate 'rain drop' macules of hypopigmentation. Other drugs with hyperpigmentary properties include chloroquine and hydroxychloroquine, hydantoin and chlorpromazine.

Certain skin diseases produce pigmented lesions. These include lupus erythematosus, scleroderma, dermatomyositis, lichen planus, lichen simplex, dermatitis herpetiformis, erythroderma, urticaria pigmentosa and 'vagabonds' disease' (malnutrition and louse infestation).

Localized forms of hyperpigmentation include the following:

Exposed parts. Occupationally from exposure to coal tar products, with or without poikiloderma, keratoses and malignant changes. Also from drugs taken internally or applied locally with light-sensitizing properties. *Phytophotodermatitis*—from contact with plants containing furocoumarins, including cow parsley, giant hogweed, parsnips, dill, angelica, fennel, anise, carrot and celery. Similar reactions may occur after contact with essential oils containing furocoumarins, as in Berloque (necklace) dermatitis from bergamot oil in Eau-de-Cologne and other cosmetic preparations.

Melanosis affecting the face and neck is sometimes of undetermined perhaps multiple causation, e.g. cosmetics, excessive light exposure or average exposure when there is light sensitivity, and in some cases dietetic imbalance.

Chloasma uterinum affects the forehead and cheeks and is usually seen in pregnancy, sometimes also from progestational drugs. A very similar pattern of pigmentation can occur in either sex with liver disease (chloasma hepaticum). Pigmentation is conspicuous in 'fixed' drug eruptions.

NAIL ANOMALIES

Nails may be absent from birth in congenital ectodermal syndromes, the nail-patella syndrome or in more widespread defects.

Hypoplastic nails also occur as a developmental abnormality or, in acquired form, as a manifestation of iron deficiency. There may be thinning or spoon-shaped depressions. Thin atrophic nails also occur in lichen planus, epidermolysis bullosa and in peripheral vascular disease.

Hypertrophy of the nails occurs in pachyonychia congenita but is more often a result of trauma. The nails are hard and thick. In psoriasis the thickening of the nails is softer and dystrophic. Similarly, in fungal infections the nails are discoloured, thickened, honeycombed and crumbly.

In clubbing of the fingers the nails are curved both longitudinally and transversely and the distal phalanx is enlarged. Although it occasionally occurs as a developmental abnormality, clubbing is usually related to chronic lung disease or cyanotic heart disease, or occasionally to disorders of the thyroid, liver or intestines.

EFFECTS OF PHYSICAL AGENTS

Differentiation has to be made between normal and abnormal reactions to physical agents.

MECHANICAL EFFECTS. PRESSURE AND FRICTION

The normal response to repeated or continual pressure is hyperkeratosis (callosities, corns) but pressure suddenly applied may cause bruising. Continual pressure at one site, as from a truss, may cause pigmentation and atrophy, or in chronic illness, with immobility and impaired sensation, may cause decubitus ulcers.

Sudden friction may cause blister formation whereas continual or recurrent friction may cause callus formation at sites where the skin is tethered, and lichenification where it is more mobile. Suction applied to the skin may cause ecchymoses.

In pathological states, e.g. keratoderma of the palms and soles, thickening occurs from minor stimuli; similarly in epidermolysis bullosa and in pemphigus blistering occurs from stimuli normally insufficient to have this effect. In the Ehlers-Danlos syndrome the defective collagen predisposes to tearing of blood vessels from minor trauma. In delayed pressure urticaria wealing occurs 4–6 hours after the pressure is applied, possibly from kinin release.

Foreign bodies may cause local infections, granulomatous reactions, or keloid formation. The carbon in accidental or deliberate tattoos is inert, but metallic dyes may cause reactions, either allergic (mercury, chromium, cobalt) or sarcoidal (chromium).

Accidentally introduced vegetable matter may cause urticaria, local infections or granulomata. Similarly, animal matter, for example sea-urchin spines, can cause granulomata. Silica and beryllium can also cause sarcoidal granulomata.

Implantation of one's own hair or nail is the commonest foreign body in the human skin. Very close shaving may result in the hair shafts ingrowing through the walls of the follicles. Near the orifice of the follicle this causes non-suppurative follicular papulation; deeper it causes keloid formation. At the nucha the condition known as folliculitis keloidalis nuchae results. In individuals with curly hair the sharp cut ends may re-enter the skin forming the 'croquet hoop' type of ingrowing hairs. In Negroes multiple keloids may result.

Barbers sometimes suffer from implantation of fragments of hair between the fingers, and some examples of pilonidal sinus are due to hairs working their way into the skin from repeated friction, as in 'jeep disease'.

Ingrowing toenails nearly always affect the great toes and arise from tight footwear and imperfect cutting which leaves a marginal spike of nail.

Hairs are very susceptible to injury. Friction or twisting may cause fracture of the shafts, and continual traction may cause an effluvium. This may occur with some hair styles, from curlers worn at night or from habitual manipulation. Similarly nails may be shortened by repeated nibbling, deformed by chewing or picking at the nail folds or worn flat and smooth at their free borders from repeated friction on the itchy skin.

OIL GRANULOMATA

Paraffin oil injected with intent to cause cosmetic improvement of lax skin has caused grotesque fibrous granulomatous masses. A similar result may follow the injection of other mineral oils (grease gun injury), animal oil, vegetable oil or silicone.

DERMATITIS DUE TO HEAT

Acute Heat Effects. These are caused by dry heat (burns) or moist heat (scalds) and are dealt with at length in surgical textbooks. Suffice it here to say that a first degree burn (erythema only) arises when the heat causes drying of the surface but insufficient damage to cause exudation into the skin. The treatment consists of the application of a bland animal fat such as lanolin, preferably mixed with mineral oils, as in the ointment of wool alcohols.

In a second degree burn there is erythema and blistering, with a risk of infection if the blisters become broken and of loss of protein and electrolytes if the blistered area is extensive. Large intact blisters should be punctured under aseptic conditions, allowed to collapse and then covered with a gauze dressing. Chlortetracycline ointment is a safe application for ruptured blisters. Tulle-gras dressings enable healing to proceed with the minimum of trauma to the young granulation tissue.

The treatment of third degree burns is a surgical matter.

Electric Burns. Electric burns are often painless, aseptic and dry, but slow in healing. The treatment is similar to that of other burns.

Effects of Repeated Exposure to Warmth. This causes the condition known as erythema ab igne. There is a pigmentary network corresponding with the sites of anastomoses between adjoining vascular areas where the blood supply is minimal.

DERMATITIS DUE TO COLD

Prurigo Hiemalis. An itching eruption occurring only in the winter, usually confined to the legs, sometimes affecting the forearms and thighs. The patient is usually elderly, with skin lacking the sebum content of younger days. In such individuals the defatting action of soap and hot water may, if too frequently applied, cause itching. The itchy episodes occur on exposure to changes of temperature, for example on undressing, taking a hot bath or sitting near the fire. The lesions are inconspicuous, patchy, with mild lichenification, and may show scratch marks and marked dryness of the skin.

Treatment consists of the avoidance of extremes of temperature and of the excessive use of soap. Baths should be warm, not hot. Emulsifying ointment should be used as a soap substitute on the affected parts.

Livedo Reticularis. The legs show a livid network of venules, corresponding to the anastomoses between adjoining vascular areas. It may also occur in a persistent form in cutaneous arteriolitis due to polyarteritis nodosa, syphilis, tuberculosis or with hypertension.

Chilblains. A chilblain is a static dilatation of venules secondary to anoxia caused by arteriolar spasm.

Immersion Foot (Trench Foot). This is due to prolonged exposure to cold water, insufficient to cause frostbite. The feet are cold and livid. The patient complains of numbness and cramp. Minor injuries may cause gangrene. On removal from the cold, a red, swollen, blistery hyperaemic stage develops unless the parts are very slowly warmed. Chronic circulatory insufficiency of the perniotic type may follow.

Treatment is by gradual warming, cleansing and elevation of the limb, followed by exercise and the application of zinc and salicylic acid dusting powder.

Frostbite (Dermatitis Congelationis). This is due to

freezing of the soft tissues with cessation of the blood flow. On thawing, there is an erythematous, a bullous or a gangrenous reaction.

Treatment is by very gradual defrosting and treatment of the damaged tissue on recognized surgical lines.

Cryoglobulinaemia. This causes purpura at exposed parts, cold urticaria and haemorrhages from the nose or eyes or in the retina. Causes include myeloma, leukaemia, collagen disease, rheumatoid arthritis, subacute bacterial endocarditis, liver disease, carcinomatosis and kala-azar.

Cold agglutinins may cause Raynaud's phenomenon, acrocyanosis or gangrene. They may occur in virus infections, systematized lupus erythematosus, lymphomas, haemolytic anaemias and trypanosomiasis.

Cold Urticaria. This may be familial or acquired. The latter type may be associated with atopy, or occasionally with cryoglobulins or cold haemolysins, which have been described as a manifestation of syphilis, with haemoglobinuria and fever.

HUMIDITY

Low humidity can cause dryness and cracking of the horny layer (eczéma craquelé) or fissuring ('chaps'). A high barometric pressure may aggravate the effect.

High humidity predisposes to prickly heat (miliaria), aggravates acne vulgaris and hydradenitis and encourages staphylococcal folliculitis or *Candida albicans* infection. High humidity at the surface of the skin encourages percutaneous absorption.

DERMATITIS DUE TO ACTINIC RAYS

Acute Solar Dermatitis. This arises from excessive exposure to the sun and may occur in all degrees of intensity as with heat burns. It is treated on similar lines.

Chronic Solar Dermatitis. Repeated exposures to the sun cause premature ageing of the skin. The physical signs consist of atrophy with telangiectasia, patchy pigmentation and depigmentation, and a tendency to form keratoses. It is sometimes called 'farmers skin' or 'sailors skin' and is seen on the face, on the backs of the hands and sometimes also on bald heads. Another condition of solar-induced elastotic degeneration of the collagen occurs on the back of the neck in the form of lozenge-shaped, pink, thickened areas of skin. It has been called 'peasant skin'.

Solar Eczema. This condition of hypersensitivity to light may present in many forms: hence the term 'polymorphic light eruption'. The same individual in one attack may show eczematous features and in another pruriginous ones. The lesions are on the forehead, cheeks, ears and exposed parts of the neck and limbs. Many substances applied to the skin have a light sensitizing effect. These include tar, bergamot oil, acriflavine, sulphonamides and eosin. Dermatitis bullosa striata pratensis is a bullous dermatitis of exposed parts coming on after contact with a light-sensitizing plant followed by exposure to the sun (phytophotodermatitis). Various plant juices including lime, figs, rue, wild parsnips, may have this effect. Some drugs also have light-sensitizing effects, particularly sulphonamides, chlorpromazine, antibiotics including penicillin, tetracycline and griseofulvin, barbiturates, gold, phenothiazines, chloroquine, diphenhydramine, chlordiazepoxide and others. Photosensitivity has been classified as phototoxic or photo-allergic. The former is an exaggerated sunburn with pigmentation occurring after a single exposure to a substance. The latter occurs after 7–21 days or more rapidly after repeated exposure and is eczematous, nodular or urticarial, with little pigmentation.

Light sensitivity can be hereditary as in xeroderma pigmentosum, and congenital poikiloderma (cause undetermined), due to absence of melanin (albinism, phenylketonuria), due to nutritional deficiency (pellagra, Hartnup disease), due to porphyria (genetic, idiopathic, alcoholic or due to drugs), due to contact sensitizing agents (plants, drugs, tar, tetrachlorsalicylanilide, etc.), due to drugs taken internally or due to unknown causes. Lupus erythematosus is the classical example of an existing dermatosis aggravated by light.

Erythropoietic Protoporphyria. This is a familial condition of light sensitivity with the presence of a hyaline carbohydrate-protein complex in the skin and the presence of protoporphyrin in the red cells.

Porphyria Cutanea Tarda. This is a scarring, pigmented condition of areas of skin which are exposed to sunlight, usually occurring in chronic alcoholics or with liver disease from other causes.

Xeroderma Pigmentosum. In this rare disease there is an inborn over-sensitivity to ultra-violet and visible rays and, as a result, senile atrophic changes resembling radiodermatitis develop at an early age and the sufferer may in adolescence begin to develop keratoses and skin cancers on the face, backs of the hands or on the legs.

Treatment

The skin can be protected from ultra-violet irradiation by *Uvistat* cream containing 4 per cent. of mexenone, or by *Spectraban* lotion containing 2·5 per cent. of isoamyl-p-N, N-dimethylaminobenzoate in ethyl alcohol. Alternatively a particulate screen can be provided against ultra-violet and visible rays by the compound paste of titanium dioxide. Oily calamine lotion helps to soothe any severe reaction. In most of these conditions reaction only occurs to the ultra-violet range. Reaction to visible light is rare and usually of the urticarial type. Patients sensitive to ultra-violet light are protected by window glass, whereas those sensitive to visible rays are not. Sophisticated testing requires special filters or a monochromator.

DERMATITIS DUE TO IONIZING RADIATION

X-rays and radium may cause acute changes in the skin, which may result from one large exposure or from repeated small exposures. Repeated exposures may also cause chronic changes.

Acute Effects. Kienboeck classified X-rays burns as:

First degree: latent period 3 weeks; no visible inflammation; temporary shedding of hair.

Second degree: latent period 2 weeks; redness and swelling of the skin lasting 1 or 2 weeks; falling of the hair.

Third degree: latent period 10 days; redness, superficial erosion and vesiculation; parts restored to normal in 3–4 weeks.

Fourth degree: latent period under a week; necrosis with ulceration; healing takes 6 weeks or longer.

Treatment of X-ray burns is similar to that of other burns.

Chronic Effects. These are similar to those of repeated and long-continued over-exposure to the sun. There is atrophic scarring with a mixture of pigmentation, depigmentation and telangiectasia (poikiloderma). Keratoses develop and squamous epithelioma may follow. Atrophy and ulceration is also common and must be differentiated from epithelioma by biopsy.

DERMATITIS ARTEFACTA

Blisters, ulcers, necroses and other lesions are sometimes self-produced by physical or chemical means with intent to gain sympathy, to escape responsibilities or for pecuniary gain. The lesions may be produced by sharp instruments, friction, constricting bandages, hot coins, cigarette ends, caustic liquids, subcutaneous injections and in various other ways.

Clinical Picture

The condition is commoner in women. Usually there is a trivial wound or burn which does not heal as soon as might be expected but extends with blistering or sloughing ulceration. The lesions are bizarre, discoid or linear, sometimes with straight edges. Hot coins cause round blisters, cigarette ends cause small burns or ulcers and caustic liquids cause linear discoloration, dermatitis or sloughing, often with a gravitational trickle where the caustic has flowed over the surface. The lesions are at sites easily reached by the hand; usually the face, breasts, forearms, hands or legs.

The patient shows the characteristic belle indifférence and examination may reveal Charcot's triad of anaesthesia of the cornea and pharynx, with suggestion anaesthesia of the skin, perhaps in a glove and stocking distribution.

When compensation claims remain unsettled, occupational dermatitis may continue as lichenified dermatitis long after the patient has been removed from the irritant.

In several other skin reactions, particularly pompholyx, eczematous dermatoses, pruritus vulvae, infective dermatitis, and psoriasis, the persistence of the dermatosis or its exacerbation may serve the purpose of enabling the patient to avoid some distasteful task or action and to receive care and attention.

Treatment

Treatment is difficult. It is one thing to understand the psychological mechanism but quite another to help the patient towards a better and more positive attitude to life. It is useless to accuse the patient: it will be indignantly denied. A reasonable level of self-esteem must be maintained. Immediate relief may be obtained by occlusive dressings but new lesions may develop unless the patient can be encouraged to adjust better to the life situation.

VASOMOTOR DISORDERS

ERYTHEMA PERNIO

Synonyms. Chilblains; Erythrocyanosis; Perniosis; Acrocyanosis.

A condition of bluish cold skin of exposed parts with swelling and itching, caused or aggravated by exposure to cold.

Aetiology

Cold acting on a susceptible skin causes arteriolar spasm and anoxaemia in the affected parts, at first intermittent, later more persistent and with secondary changes. The blood stagnates in dilated venules, leading to oedema, degeneration and fibrotic thickening of the connective tissue and of the vascular endothelium itself.

Aetiological factors include personal predisposition, lack of exercise or defective muscle pump as in poliomyelitis, insufficient clothing to the body as a whole and to the extremities in particular and attempts to rewarm chilled parts too rapidly by the application of heat.

Clinical Picture

Perniosis may affect any part of the skin that is exposed to cold, particularly the distal parts of the limbs, the nose and the ears. Involvement of the upper limbs is usually confined to the digits but on the lower limbs the lower parts of the calves are affected as often as the feet.

Chilblains are far commoner in females than in males, a fact only partly explained by their more scanty clothing. Sedentary tasks in cold, draughty or even damp surroundings may be relevant. Adolescents and young adults are affected most.

Chilblains present as cold, bluish, swollen, non-pitting areas of skin. There may be blotchy redness or this can be induced by gently massaging an affected area from the periphery. Itching may be severe and the skin may feel warm to the touch when red and swollen after rubbing. Sometimes the blueness is most marked around hair follicles. If oedema is severe, bullae may develop, which, on rupturing leave ulcerated, possibly secondarily infected chilblains. Fissures ('chaps') form on the fingers and hands and infection may lead to cellulitis. On the ears calcinosis may later occur.

Diagnosis

On the hands chilblains have to be differentiated from lupus erythematosus (lupus pernio of Hutchinson). This may be difficult, except after a period of observation. Lupus erythematosus persists in warm weather, chilblains do not. Chilblains on the fingers affect in particular the skin over the knuckles, or there may be sausage-like swellings of the whole digits. In lupus erythematosus the finger tips, the paronychial folds and the skin over the phalanges are most affected, the knuckles often being spared. The involvement is more patchy than in perniosis. In difficult cases, biopsy may clarify the diagnosis.

On the face and hands chilblains also have to be differentiated from sarcoidosis (lupus pernio of Besnier), a persistent, doughy, bluish swelling of the nose, ears or digits. The histology is distinctive.

On the legs perniosis has to be differentiated from Bazin's disease and from Darier-Roussy subcutaneous sarcoids. Both of these conditions occur in individuals with perniotic circulations, but in addition there are extensive areas of hard, bluish nodulation. In Bazin's disease the lesions may ulcerate.

Erythema multiforme may cause lesions resembling chilblains on the fingers but the palms are also usually affected and characteristic 'target' lesions may be seen.

Treatment

Suitably warm clothing should be worn all over the body as well as on the affected parts; this may necessitate non-adherence to the strictest requirements of fashion. Chilled areas should not be warmed suddenly by hot water bottles or immersion in hot water. Bad housing conditions need correction, as by draught control, duck-boarding on stone floors, etc. Adequate exercise and the avoidance of prolonged standing or sedentary work are necessary. Diffuse and continuous warmth is needed, as by central heating, electric blankets, etc.

Drugs have a minor place in the treatment of chilblains. It is important to make the patient realize that there is no easy cure in this way and that alleviation depends much more on the correction of faulty habits than on medicines. Thyroxine should only be prescribed if there is definite evidence of hypothyroidism. A temporary increase in the blood flow to the extremities may be brought about by tablets of nicotinamide, 50 mg., with acetomenaphthone, 10 mg., or of tolazoline hydrochloride (*Priscol*), 25 mg. Phenoxybenzamine hydrochloride (*Dibenyline*), 10 mg. has a more prolonged action. The accompanying drop in blood pressure may cause faintness. Thymoxamine hydrochloride (*Opilon*), 40 mg., is also worthy of trial. Calcium has been reputed to help and is best prescribed with vitamin D. General ultra-violet and infra-red irradiation are worthy of trial.

For unbroken chilblains massage may be applied from the periphery using oily calamine lotion. For fissures, the ointment of wool alcohols or emulsifying ointment is useful, with appropriate antibiotics for any secondary infection.

Course and Prognosis

Individual attacks resolve with warmer weather, but repeated attacks leave progressively more connective tissue changes of doughy swelling.

ROSACEA

Aetiology

In rosacea there is a tendency to blush easily from emotional stimuli, exposure to heat or the ingestion of hot foods and drinks. Persistent static dilatation of the facial blood vessels may ultimately develop. Often follicular papules form (acne rosacea), with inflammation which may end in discharge of glairy fluid. Hyperplasia of the pilosebaceous units may result (rhinophyma).

Usually rosacea affects the centre of the forehead, the nose and the fronts of the cheeks and the chin. Atypically lesions appear elsewhere. The rosaceous patient tends to be obsessional and anxious. Excessive activities (often self-imposed) and hurried meals may be habitual. The condition has been described as one of hurry, flurry and worry, though some authors deny this.

A seasonal exacerbation in the spring has been noted.

Clinical Picture

Rosacea is slightly more common in women than in men. Most patients are between 30 and 50 years of age, though occasionally young adults are affected. The patient complains of a sense of heat (not of itching) and of redness and usually pimpling of the face, with aggravation from exposure to extremes of temperature, from hurry, anger, anxiety or from social activities. Hurried meals, hot drinks or indigestible foods or spices may all aggravate the condition as may the premenstrual tension phase. There may be a flatulent dyspepsia. A tendency to blush is followed by persistent redness and telangiectasia and, usually, red papulation, which may become crusted and leave pitted follicular scarring. Direct microscopical examination of the glairy exudate from the follicles often reveals a heavy infestation with *Demodex folliculorum*. Acne vulgaris rarely coexists but sometimes acne vulgaris in adolescence is followed by rosacea some years later. Conjunctivitis, blepharitis, keratitis and corneal ulceration may all complicate rosacea. The eye-lash follicles may also be infested with *Demodex folliculorum*.

Rhinophyma mostly affects middle-aged or elderly males. There is often no history of previous rosacea. Skin-coloured or bluish irregular fleshy masses develop on the distal two-thirds of the nose, with patulous, enlarged follicular orifices and dilated venules.

Diagnosis

Diagnosis is from acne vulgaris, lupus erythematosus, contact eczematous dermatitis, polycythaemia and flushing due to a carcinoid tumour. In acne vulgaris the distribution of the lesions is different, the face is pale and comedones are present. In the rosaceous form of lupus erythematosus, atrophy can be discerned on careful inspection and the eruption is characteristically worsened by exposure to the sun. Contact eczematous dermatitis may coexist; it presents with ill-defined itchy areas of redness and peeling at various sites on the face, particularly the eyelids, around the mouth and on the neck. In polycythaemia the whole face is persistently plum-coloured. From carcinoid the differentiation may be extremely difficult and reliance has to be placed on other manifestations such as diarrhoea, an abdominal tumour, a right-sided valvular cardiac lesion and increased urinary excretion of 5-hydroxyindole acetic acid (5-HIAA).

Treatment

Flush-provoking stimuli must be avoided as far as possible. This means the avoidance of environmental heat, emotional heat and hot drinks. Hot tea-drinking is a commoner cause of exacerbations than alcohol, condiments or indigestible food. The patient should be encouraged to modify obsessional traits and allow ample time for meals and relaxation. Sedation, e.g. with amylobarbitone, 30–45 mg. twice a day, may be helpful. Bromides and iodides should be avoided as they may grossly aggravate the condition.

The face should be washed twice a day with soap and water and not with 'cleansing' creams. The application of sulphur is often very helpful. It may be applied in a 2 per cent. strength in aqueous cream or in a diluted steroid cream. The prolonged use of powerful fluorinated steroid creams has been reported to induce or aggravate telangiectasia. If local treatment in itself is not effective, a course of oxytetracycline is indicated, with gradual withdrawal until the minimum effective dose is attained. Ocular complications are best dealt with by an ophthalmologist, there being a risk of corneal opacities. For immediate use homatropine or cortisone drops may be indicated. The excrescences of rhinophyma are responsive to surgery, excellent cosmetic results often occurring.

DERMATITIS DUE TO CHEMICAL SUBSTANCES

Chemical substances may cause dermatitis by coming into contact with the skin in gaseous, liquid, particulate or solid form. Contact dermatitis may be caused by primary irritants or by sensitizers.

Primary irritant dermatitis is caused by substances that affect all who are exposed to them in sufficient concentration or for sufficient time. They cause physicochemical alterations in the structure of the skin and act in various ways, mechanical, physical or chemical. They may abrade the surface, destroy keratin or stimulate its excessive formation, abstract fat or mix with skin fat, macerate or desiccate, denature protein, oxidize or reduce, hydrolyse or form toxic nitro derivatives.

Primary irritants include caustics, alkalis and acids, skin cleansers with and without abrasives, detergents, surface acting and wetting agents, emulsifiers and sulphonated oils; cutting oils (which may contain oil, water, emulsifier, antioxidant and anticorrosive agents, preservatives and antiseptics, metallic particles and bacteria); organic solvents, oxidizing and reducing agents, cytotoxic substances, e.g. formaldehyde, some plants and medicaments applied in excessive concentrations, e.g. potassium permanganate; even water acts as an irritant once the surface is eroded.

The effect of primary irritants and sensitizers is greatly increased by occlusion, for example beneath a rubber glove, because of the increased hydration of the surface cells and resultant greater absorption.

Sensitization dermatitis (contact eczema) is caused by substances which provoke allergic skin reactions in a proportion of individuals after repeated or prolonged exposure.

They consist mainly of complex organic chemicals, many of which are synthetic, certain vegetable and animal products, and a few inorganic chemicals which are able to take on sensitizing properties when they are combined with protein. They include plants, woods, balsams, turpentine, colophony, wood preservatives, dyes, photographic chemicals, rubber accelerators and antioxidants, certain metals, cosmetics, perfumes, flavouring agents, items of clothing, pesticides, plastics, glues, coal tar derivatives, drugs (antibiotics, chemotherapeutic agents, local anaesthetics, antihistamines), antioxidants, formaldehyde, hydrazones, hydroxyquinolines, thiuram sulphide, phosphorus sesquisulphide, and many others.

Some chemicals and plants have a photosensitizing effect on the skin, e.g. tar, eosin, acriflavine, sulphonamides and various plants including wild parsnips, figs, rue and others. Some substances can act both as primary irritants and as sensitizers. For example, cement may have a primary irritant effect from its alkalinity, while traces of chromium in it may be responsible for sensitization dermatitis. Turpentine and formaldehyde have primary irritant effects in concentration and may sensitize even in considerable dilution.

Aetiology and Pathology

Predisposing causes such as race, complexion, sex and age all modify the tendency to dermatitis. White races are, on the whole, more susceptible than dark races, and blondes more than brunettes. Women are more susceptible than men, and children and the aged are more susceptible than young or middle-aged adults. But there are exceptions to these generalizations. Sweating may leach out irritants from solids; hairiness may carry with it some follicular vulnerability; a greasy skin may enable a person better to withstand contact with degreasing agents but it also may expose him to greater peril from irritants that are miscible with skin fat. Seasonal effects of sweating in the summer and chapping in the winter may be important. Constitutional xeroderma, lack of cleanliness or careless methods of cleaning up after work, fatigue, emotional instability or an anxious, obsessional temperament and malnutrition, may all play a part.

The primary irritants most commonly responsible include soda and alkaline soaps, cement and lime, paraffin oil, petrol, turpentine or turpentine substitutes, cooling and cutting oils, glue, formalin, phenol, ultraviolet or X-irradiation, or friction from gritty particles. The sensitizers are many and include medicaments, sulphonamides, benzocaine, chloramphenicol, neomycin, antihistamine drugs, penicillin, flavine, streptomycin, formalin, phenol, Dettol, lanolin and adhesive dressings; plants, particularly *Primula obconica*, chrysanthemums and many others, teak, ebony and other woods; cosmetics including paraphenylenediamine hair dye, eosin in lipsticks, nail varnish, hair lacquers, bergamot oil and orris root powder; clothes and jewellery including dyed furs, leather and rubber garments, texturized shirts, dyes and adhesives in shoes, chromium and nickel plating; occupational hazards involving work with mercury, chromium or nickel, dyes and explosives, flour improvers, rubber anti-oxidants and very many others. Occupations with more than average dermatitis hazards include bakers, carpenters, cleaners, dustmen, dyers, florists, french polishers, garage hands, gardeners, housewives, labourers, machine hands, miners, painters, photographers, platers, rubber workers and tar workers. Bacteria, fungi and animal parasites may also cause, predispose to or complicate occupational dermatitis.

The development of dermatitis from primary irritants depends, *inter alia*, on the possession of skin secretions with poor alkali-neutralizing properties; on some degree of xeroderma, with insufficient sebum production to replace that removed by fat solvents and emulsifiers and on thinness of the horny layer.

The cause of eczematous eruptions is the combination of an allergen with skin or serous protein and sensitization of lymphocytes which are subsequently disseminated via the lymphatics, lymph nodes and blood stream. Breaks in the continuity of the surface of the epidermis predispose to the development of contact dermatitis or eczema. The prickle cells are normally protected from external noxae by an intact horny layer and they react violently if they are exposed to primary irritants or to sensitizing substances.

In the acute stage there is spongiosis (intercellular and intracellular oedema) in the prickle cell layer, causing microscopic or macroscopic vesicles and a variable degree of disintegration of the epidermis. In the dermis a lymphocytic infiltrate surrounds the dilated vessels, the sweat glands and the pilosebaceous follicles. In the subacute and chronic forms there is parakeratosis (nucleated horn cells), acanthosis and a chronic inflammatory infiltrate in the dermis.

The histopathology of dermatitis due to primary irritants differs from that of sensitization dermatitis in that the infiltrate is more polymorphonuclear in the former and lymphocytic and eosinophilic in the latter.

Clinical Picture

In the most acute forms due to caustics there is destruction of the epidermis before an inflammatory reaction can develop. In less acute forms there is smarting, redness and swelling, followed by vesiculation and blistering, and a raw surface. In subacute forms there is papulovesiculation with abnormal scaling. Milder and chronic forms present as redness and pathological scaling with lichenification, increase of pigmentation and a tendency to fissuring.

The reaction usually remains localized to the site of contact. But if the irritant or sensitizer is in liquid or semisolid form, as often applies with outwardly applied medicaments, the dermatitis tends to spread up to and just beyond the limits of each application. If the irritant or sensitizer is miscible with sebum, the reaction may be mainly follicular and discrete follicular papules may develop beyond the zone of confluent dermatitis.

Dermatitis varies in appearance according to the stage at which it is seen. Erythema, papulation or vesiculation predominate in the earlier states; later, according to the degree of secondary infection or of rubbing and scratching, it may proceed to pustulation with moist infected scabs on an exuding surface, or to lichenification and blood scabbing. If neither complication develops, resolution follows on the moist exuding surface by serous scabbing, finer scaling, diminution of redness and a return to the original state. If at any stage a further contact with the causal agent takes place, the whole process may recur.

Diagnosis

Diagnosis of primary irritant and sensitization dermatitis on the face has to be made from solar dermatitis, atopic dermatitis, urticaria, infective dermatitis and erysipelas; on the body from ringworm, seborrhoeic dermatitis, pityriasis rosea, lichen planus, psoriasis and parapsoriasis; on the hands from nummular eczema, mycides, erythema multiforme and pompholyx.

Solar dermatitis affects the forehead and malar ridges and other sites most exposed to light; contact dermatitis more characteristically affects the eyelids, lips and neck; atopic dermatitis is often accompanied by hay fever, asthma or flexual dermatitis; urticaria is not accompanied by peeling; erysipelas has a brawny, spreading edge and there are constitutional symptoms; on the body the other diseases and reactions are usually more circumscribed; nummular eczema affects the backs of the hands, but adjoining areas escape entirely, whereas with dermatitis the finger webs or knuckles are more typically affected and the eruption is more diffuse. Pompholyx is symmetrical, whereas eczematous dermatitis of the hands may be asymmetrical. Dermatitis caused by liquid affects particularly the webs of the fingers and the ulnar and anterior aspects of the wrists, whereas dermatitis caused by contact with solid objects (gloves, plants, metals) tends to affect convex surfaces, such as the knuckles. At all sites frictional dermatoses (lichenification) have to be differentiated from eruptive ones (eczema dermatitis).

The diagnosis 'contact (eczematous) dermatitis' having been made on the basis of the morphology of the lesions, the more difficult task remains of trying to find the cause. For this purpose it is necessary to know the ways in which sensitizing substances may come in contact with the skin and the likelier causes of eczematous dermatoses affecting various parts of the body. The history is all-important, with possible seasonal fluctuations, relief at weekends or on holiday, and other significant evidence that the patient alone can supply. Leading questions are necessary concerning work, hobbies, hygienic practices, clothing, cosmetics, jewellery, plants, volatile agents, day-by-day contacts and past treatment. Sometimes the history can be supplemented by a diary kept by the patient of daily contacts, after which patch tests can be performed with suspected sensitizers. The distribution suggests the more likely causes.

On the scalp the possible causes include paraphenylenediamine hair dye, permanent-waving solution, brilliantine and perfumes, hair lacquers, hatbands and, occasionally, medicaments. On the face, airborne and inadvertently hand-transferred substances have to be considered, also topical medicaments and cosmetics including hair lacquer on another's hair. The eyelids are particularly affected by volatile substances and by substances transferred by the hands; thus, formalin vapour and streptomycin are possible causes, also eye lotions, drops and ointments, and occasionally nail varnish and other hand-transferred agents including nickel from plated objects. On the neck, hair dyes, necklaces, fur collars and other dyed materials are suspect; also hand-transferred substances and dusts having a primary irritant action such as lime or cement. Dusts also affect sites of pressure from clothing such as the waistline, also the skin within the socks, as well as the hands. Clothing, e.g. texturized materials, tends to affect the neck, the axillary folds, the belt line, the buttocks, hips and perineum. Perfumed dusting powders may give a rash of similar distribution. The sock areas and the dorsa of the feet are affected when footwear is responsible. Nickel-plated fittings and jewellery may affect many sites, including the neck, lobes of ear, midline of back and wrists.

The accurate recognition of sensitizers depends to some extent on patch tests. These are helpful provided the results are interpreted correctly. For success there should be adequate control, suitable concentrations of the suspected sensitizers, no patch testing with primary irritants, inspection at 48 hours and re-inspection at 96 or 120 hours. Contact eczematous responses (erythematovesicular) must be differentiated from follicular obstructive effects (follicular-papulopustular) and from the trauma of removal of the adhesive material (erythematous and follicular-papular). The conditions of patch testing and those in which the sensitizer is met in everyday life can never be identical (site, sweating, abrasions, fissures, friction, etc.) and allowance has to be made for this. A positive patch test does not of necessity prove that the dermatitis was produced by this substance, and a negative patch test does not completely exonerate the tested substance as the cause of the original dermatitis. Patch tests are best performed on the upper part of the back. The patient should not know which patch is which, but suitable identification marks should be made on the adhesive dressings. Patch testing should not be performed in the presence of active dermatitis; and if the dermatitis has been severe, patch testing should only be performed after complete clearance and with expert supervision, the patient being instructed to remove the patches at once if a severe reaction occurs. If this is not done, an acute relapse or exacerbation may result at the sites of the original eruption.

Prevention and Treatment

The essentials in the prevention of occupational dermatitis are selection of the most suitable workers, their protection at work, their periodic inspection and supervision to see that precautionary measures are conscientiously carried out, and the provision of adequate washing facilities. Selection includes rejection of hyperidrotic, seborrhoeic or xerodermatous individuals or those with atopic dermatitis, tinea pedis or acne vulgaris as far as certain trade procedures are concerned. Protection includes good ventilation, abatement of humidity, exhaust draughts, suitable clothing, gloves and goggles, and barrier creams which may have either water-repellent or oil-repellent effects and also emollient properties. Too much reliance must not be placed on barrier creams, their chief function being to prevent excessive soiling of the skin so that it is easier to clean. Inspection should include not only the working conditions and the proper use of protective appliances but also medical inspection of the workers for minor injuries and infections that may be the precursors of something more serious. Washing facilities should include hot and cold running water, soap and towels and the worker must be discouraged from travelling home in soiled working clothes or from using paraffin, petrol, scouring agents and other primary irritants for cleaning the skin. In some industries these are the cause of more sickness than the industrial hazards themselves.

Desensitization can occasionally be performed, for example, in streptomycin cutaneous sensitivity, by graduated injections. This procedure is most valuable when the sensitivity interferes with the work of a sister in charge of a tuberculosis unit; for a nurse in training it is better to rely on minimizing further exposures.

Attempts at 'hardening' by continuing to expose the worker to an occupational sensitizer are more likely to bring about ever-increasing sensitivity, ending in generalized eczema, than to succeed in enabling him to continue in the work.

Local treatment in the acute phase consists of rest and elevation of the affected part and the application of a corticosteroid preparation if the reaction is eczematous, or oily calamine lotion, aqueous or oily cream if the condition is due to a primary irritant. Tubular gauze dressings make the most comfortable covering; fine mesh gauze may also be used. The dressings are changed once a day, a bland vegetable oil or liquid paraffin being used gently to remove debris from the surface of the skin before another application of lotion or cream is made. For any infection that may develop soaks in 1 in 8000 solution of potassium permanganate are helpful, with applications of the appropriate antibiotic depending on the cultural findings.

As the condition gets less acute calamine cream or aqueous cream may be used and when it becomes scaly or cracked Lassar's paste, salicylic acid ointment or wool alcohol ointment is useful. If lichenification develops a 2 per cent. tar paste or a corticosteroid application is indicated, but the use of tar should be abandoned at once if there is any tendency to develop folliculitis. At no stage should benzocaine local anaesthetics or antihistamines be applied as they are liable to cause severe eczematous dermatitis.

General treatment consists of bed rest in severe or extensive cases. Exposure to sunlight, heat and cold should be avoided. Ample sedation to relieve the pruritus should be given, e.g. amylobarbitone (*Amytal*), 50 mg. twice a day and 100–200 mg. at night, or promethazine hydrochloride (*Phenergan*), 10–25 mg. twice a day or 20–50 mg. at night.

Course and Prognosis

This depends on the discovery of the cause and the possibilities of its subsequent avoidance. Sometimes a trade irritant can be replaced by something harmless; sometimes a process can be modified so as to lessen the exposure of a workman; sometimes protective clothing, better ventilation and washing facilities are all that are needed. 'Hardening' by continuous re-exposure is not likely to be successful. With some specific sensitizers (e.g. streptomycin) desensitization can be carried out; with others there may be a group sensitivity to chemically similar substances (e.g. sulphonamides, flavine, benzocaine, paraphenylenediamine) or there may be a non-specific broadening of sensitivity to many substances. In this last form the prognosis is poor.

INFECTIVE (SEBORRHOEIC) DERMATITIS

This term applies to many dermatoses, differing in situation and pattern, but in all of which the patient's skin is unduly susceptible to bacterial and *Candida albicans* infection, chemical and physical injury and emotional stress.

Aetiology and Pathology

The organisms recovered from the lesions of infective dermatitis are, alone or in combination, *Staph. aureus*, *Strep. pyogenes*, other streptococci, *Candida albicans* and Gram-negative bacilli.

The 'seborrhoeic' individual is sometimes obese and may indulge in fats and carbohydrates to excess, while taking insufficient exercise. The diet is often deficient in foods rich in protein and vitamins. Some drugs taken internally, some chemicals applied externally and emotional disturbances may activate or aggravate the condition.

Clinical Types

The sites commonly affected by infective dermatitis, either alone or in combination, are the scalp, brows, lashes, eyelids, conjunctivae, medial and lateral canthi, nasolabial folds, the vestibule of the nose, post-auricular folds, outer ears, aural meatus, angles of the mouth, beard, sweat grooves of centre of trunk, submammary region, axillae, navel, pubis, glans penis and coronal sulcus, vulva, genitocrural folds, inter-gluteal cleft, toe webs and, in discoid form, on hairy areas of arms, forearms, thighs and legs, as well as on the trunk.

The possibility of an underlying infective dermatitis has to be considered in many cases of contact dermatitis. The converse also applies, the diagnosis of infective dermatitis should not be made lightly without giving thought to possible contact factors.

On the scalp there may be simple scurf (pityriasis simplex) on skin of normal colour or there may be profuse and widespread greasy scaling (pityriasis steatoides) on a reddened itchy skin, the condition often extending a little on to the forehead as the 'corona seborrhoeica'. The hair tends to fall more rapidly. When the scalp becomes further infected with pathogenic cocci, purulent crusting results.

On the ears there may be a scaly and inflammatory condition of the meatus (meatitis), perhaps with exudation or with folliculitis and perifolliculitis of the ceruminous glands, with pain and varying degrees of meatal stenosis and deafness, or the skin of the external ears may be inflamed (otitis externa) and scaling or exuding. Above, behind and beneath the ears the inflamed skin is very liable to crack, and the painful fissures may form a portal of entry for streptococci, causing cellulitis (erysipelas). The ears are often contaminated with Gram-negative faecal organisms as well as with pathogenic cocci, the infection being conveyed by digital transference from the anal region due to a coexisting pruritus ani or to imperfect hygiene.

The eyes may be affected in various ways—folliculitis of the brows or of the lashes (blepharitis) or styes; inflammation of the skin and folds of the upper lids; conjunctivitis with chemosis and a slight sticky discharge, or scaling and fissuring of the lateral canthi.

The nose may have greasy scales and follicular crusts on the nostrils and at the nasolabial folds. There may be a vestibular folliculitis, or fissuring at the nares. The nose is the most important reservoir of staphylococci and sometimes of other organisms.

At the mouth angular stomatitis with fissuring is common. This may be due to infection with *Candida albicans* or with cocci.

The beard area may be affected with a frank folliculitis or there may be patchy or diffuse redness and exudate or scaling.

On the trunk, pityriasis simplex and steatoides are common in the midline 'sweat grooves'. In the obese, intertriginous dermatitis may occur in all grades of severity in the axillary domes, under the breasts, at the navel, in the genitocrural folds and natal cleft or under pendulous abdominal folds of fat. Satellite follicular papulopustules are grouped around the main lesions in staphylococcal infections and there are white, flaking non-suppurative satellites in *Candida albicans* infections. On the penis inflammation may develop in the coronal sulcus or on the glans causing infective balanoposthitis. *Candida albicans* is often the causal organism in balanitis and also in vulvitis. Glycosuria may be present, or, rarely, hypoparathyroidism. Folliculitis of the pubis, in varying degrees of intensity, is present in the most intractable forms.

Discoid or petaloid lesions of infective dermatitis may occur on the trunk and on the limbs, particularly across the scapular region and on the extensor aspects of the limbs and the backs of the hands or feet. These lesions may be scaly, sharply demarcated discs and ovals with a few discrete guttate papular lesions, or in the more acute form, there may be eczematous papulovesicular discs proceeding to exudation and crusting (seborrhoeic, nummular or discoid eczema, staphylococcide).

Intertiginous dermatitis between the toes provides an ideal medium for the growth of *Candida albicans* and staphylococci and is a common cause of 'foot rot'.

In addition to all these patterns of infective dermatitis, there are 'seborrhoeides' or 'eczematides', conditions in which the use of one or other of various topical remedies sets off an explosive outburst of a papulovesicular nature, at first near the site of application, later contralaterally, and finally, in widespread fashion. This condition is thought to be due to the development of sensitization to bacterial or fungal products or to the patient's own disintegrating epidermal cells, or to the topical agent used. It occurs when there is profuse exudation or maceration at the site primarily affected.

Diagnosis

On the scalp, the diagnosis is made from ringworm in children by examination for broken hairs, microscopy and Wood's light examination. Psoriasis of the scalp causes palpable discoid lesions, with heavy scaling, and no loss of hair, whereas in seborrhoeic dermatitis the lesions are impalpable except when impetiginized and there is conspicuous hair fall. On the trunk, the diagnosis is from pityriasis versicolor, pityriasis rosea, ringworm, psoriasis and parapsoriasis.

Treatment

The general treatment consists of dietetic adjustment, the withdrawal of any possible harmful contact or drug and attention to any emotional disorder.

The diet should be well balanced.

For local treatment of the scalp and other affected areas a 1 per cent. solution of cetrimide is useful.

For pityriasis simplex, Salicylic Acid Lotion, B.P.C., is useful, rubbed in daily and gently with the finger-tips.

For pityriasis steatoides of the scalp, Salicylic Acid and Sulphur Ointment, B.P.C., is useful, but the strength should be reduced to 1 per cent. when the patient is a child.

For impetiginous lesions, it is advisable to have a culture made and to use the appropriate antibiotic according to the findings. Pending the report a clioquinol application or chlortetracycline ointment offers the best prospects of relief.

For milder lesions salicylic acid and sulphur cream or oily calamine lotion may be used with the addition of 1 per cent. of sulphur or of ichthammol. If there is more obvious infection clioquinol cream is often helpful.

For intertriginous dermatitis magenta paint, nystatin ointment or powder, or amphotericin B lotion is effective for simple candida infection. *Triadcortyl*, a preparation containing neomycin, gramicidin and nystatin with triamcinolone, is effective in itchy mixed infections. Brilliant green, 1 per cent. in zinc paste, sometimes succeeds when other remedies have failed. When the moist phase has passed zinc oxide and salicylic acid dusting powder is appropriate, the opposing skin surfaces being kept apart by light gauze dressings, up-lift brassieres, etc.

Course and Prognosis

Course and prognosis are uncertain, owing to the constitutional factors concerned. If the causal factors (dietetic, drug, contact, emotional) can be dealt with, there is a reasonable prospect of success; when this is impossible for reasons of age, environment or disposition the outlook is proportionately bad.

OTHER FORMS OF ECZEMATOUS DERMATITIS

The term 'eczema' implies a 'boiling over' of the skin, and its use should be confined to spontaneous eruptions characterized clinically by papulovesiculation and microscopically by spongiosis. This definition excludes all primarily frictional dermatoses such as lichen simplex (neurodermatitis circumscripta) and disseminated neurodermatitis (atopic dermatitis).

NUMMULAR (DISCOID) ECZEMA

Nummular (discoid) eczema is an outbreak of papulovesicles, often confined to the extensor surfaces of the limbs, particularly the forearms and legs, but sometimes becoming more generalized. Discrete shotty vesicles may also develop. A chemical contactant cannot be incriminated and the causal factors seem to be xeroderma, defatting of the surface and sensitization to bacteria on the surface.

Infectious eczematoid dermatitis is a disorder closely related to nummular eczema. In it the discharge from an area of infective dermatitis produces a mixed eczematous and infectious (impetiginous) reaction wherever it touches.

Treatment

Nummular eczema responds best to non-sensitizing bacteriostatic and fungistatic remedies, such as chlortetracycline or clioquinol in combination with a corticosteroid cream or ointment, or one part of clioquinol cream with 3 parts of tar paste may be used. Symptomatic treatment should also be given to relieve insomnia from itching by barbiturates or promethazine hydrochloride in the evening.

POMPHOLYX

Synonym. Dysidrosis.

This is a vesicular eruption of the palms, and of the palmar and lateral aspects of the digits and of the under-surfaces of the feet. It may recur indefinitely.

Aetiology and Pathology

It may be secondary to fungal infection of the feet (mycide); it may be a manifestation of eczematous dermatitis, exogenous or endogenous; or it may be of psychogenic origin or caused by heat and humidity.

Clinical Picture

There are vesicles of uniform size, resembling frog spawn in the skin of the palms and fingers and on their lateral aspects. The backs of the hands may be quite normal. The feet may show a similar condition in a comparable distribution. The affected areas do not sweat. There is considerable itching until the fluid is either absorbed or discharged by rupture of the vesicles. Coarse peeling follows and resolution may occur, or the whole process may be repeated.

Diagnosis

Diagnosis is from pustular psoriasis, erythema multiforme and tinea pedis. The former presents with creamy pustules and brown macules scattered in a scaly red patch, whereas in pompholyx the vesicles are skin coloured.

In erythema multiforme there may be large bullae and 'target' lesions and there is also erythema, which is absent in pompholyx.

Tinea pedis presents with large bullae in the roofs of which mycelial threads may be found on microscopy; but the same foot may also have on it many small vesicles of pompholyx type (mycide) in which fungus cannot be found. Tinea pedis is often asymmetrical, its mycide symmetrical; other forms of pompholyx are symmetrical, but contact eczematous dermatitis is often asymmetrical.

Treatment

Treatment is with bland and supportive applications, e.g. Zinc and Salicylic Acid Paste, B.P., or oily calamine lotion, while the fungal infection is being controlled, while irritants and sensitizers are being avoided, or while the patient is receiving sedation therapy. If infection occurs, with purulent blebs, lymphangitis and lymphadenitis the part should be elevated and kept at rest. Soaks for 10 minutes in a 1 in 8000 solution of potassium permanganate are useful and a sulphonamide, e.g. sulphadimidine, penicillin or tetracycline may have to be used systematically. Many patients need sedatives and antipruritics (amylobarbitone or promethazine hydrochloride) to enable them to sleep.

Course and Prognosis

The form due to fungal infection clears when the infection is controlled. Other forms tend to recur unless a sensitizing substance can be found and subsequently avoided, or unless the patient can be brought into better adjustment with life situations.

AUTOLYTIC ECZEMA

Synonym. Eczematide.

This is a widespread papulovesicular eruption caused by absorption from an area of erosion or of ulceration. The absorbed products may originate from organisms on the skin or from the breakdown of epidermal cells. The phenomenon has been observed mostly after the use on the skin of sulphonamides, flavine, paraphenylenediamine, benzocaine, mercurials, etc.; but it may even develop from the occlusion of a moist area by soft paraffin, which suggests that the substances applied are not primarily responsible but that they hasten cellular disintegration or encourage infection. Autolytic eczema typically arises from faulty treatment of ulcers or eczema on the legs but it also occurs from overtreatment of extensive abrasions, second degree burns, herpes simplex, eczematous or infective dermatoses.

Prevention and Treatment

There should be avoidance of the sensitizers mentioned above, also of occlusive soft paraffin dressings over moist areas.

It is best treated by steroid applications, combined with an antibiotic if infection is present. The secondary eruption subsides briskly, as soon as the primary focus is brought under control.

ENDOGENOUS ECZEMA

This is a widespread papulovesicular eruption for which no immediate contact cause can be found. Sometimes the epidermal sensitization has arisen from the administration of a drug (e.g. sulphonamide) previously used topically; but often the most careful history fails to elicit any cause in the form of a focus of infection, drug, food or metabolic disorder.

Treatment

This is largely symptomatic. Bed rest is advisable in the more severe forms. The intake of fats and carbohydrates, alcohol, coffee and condiments is reduced. Sedatives are given by mouth and bland local applications are used.

INFANTILE ECZEMA

The term covers infective eczema of infants and the earliest papulosquamous stages of the condition usually called atopic dermatitis later in life.

In the infective variety there is greasy scaling of the scalp and sometimes of the face, chest and flexures. The child is often overweight.

In the pruriginous form there is a widespread erythematopapulosquamous rash with exudation and crusting affecting particularly the face (eczema larvale) and parts of the limbs and body most accessible to the infant's efforts at scratching and rubbing, that is the shoulders, elbows, wrists and hands, knees, legs and feet. The trunk is less affected, with a blotchy erythematopapular eruption.

Aetiology

In the infective form, an excess of fat or carbohydrate in the diet is often an important factor. This may occur because the child is weaned at an early age on to a full cream milk because of failure of lactation. It may also occur at about 6 months because the child is given an excess of cereal foods. The skin as a result becomes susceptible to infection by *Candida albicans* or by pathogenic cocci.

In the rare allergic form, milk (lactalbumin) or cereal products are usually responsible.

The more common pruriginous form (atopic dermatitis) is in part due to an inherited predisposition and in part often due to an unsatisfactory mother-child relationship, in which an emotionally labile mother, who is unable to give the child the steady and unselfish affection it needs, clashes with a child of higher than average intelligence, peculiarly prone to itching and frenzied rubbing and scratching whenever deprived of pleasurable activities or of affection. Xeroderma often coexists and congenital cataracts are occasionally present. Electroencephalographic tracings are abnormal in a higher than normal proportion of these patients.

Diagnosis

The affixment of the label 'eczema' offers no difficulty; the problem is to apportion blame to inheritance, environment, diet and infection, and this depends on consideration of the history and signs.

Treatment

In the infective form, the protein, vitamin and mineral content of the diet should be rendered adequate but fats and carbohydrates should be reduced.

Local treatment depends on the degree of infection. If this is severe, the most suitable antibiotic should be applied. If milder, the skin should be cleaned with a 1 per cent. solution of cetrimide, and 1 per cent. of salicylic acid and of sulphur in an emulgent base applied. Later, oily calamine lotion can be substituted.

The diagnosis of allergic eczema is made by elimination diets. Cow's milk is first omitted. If there is improvement lactalbumin of milk is suspected as the cause. If there is no improvement, cow's milk is given alone for 24 hours and then one item is added each day until any aggravating factor or factors are found. These are then omitted from the diet. If cow's milk is the cause, goat's milk can be substituted or a lactalbumin-free product (e.g. *Allergilac*).

Pruriginous eczema depends for its control on adjustments in the mother-child relationship as well as on all the physician can do by bland local applications and sedatives. The parents should be encouraged to generate a calm and unselfishly affectionate atmosphere; at the same time some children use eczema as a weapon for getting their own way. The child should be kept fully occupied with suitable toys on which he can relieve his aggressive urges. Eczematous children tolerate sedatives such as phenobarbitone in higher doses than the more normal child, and a dose of 15 mg. three or four times a day for a child 12 months old is nothing unusual. In milder cases the elixir promethazine hydrochloride (*Phenergan*) may be sufficient.

Local applications should be bland and free from sensitizing properties; steroid lotions and creams give most relief but fluorinated steroids should be used in dilution to minimize the risk of cutaneous atrophy which may occur from their prolonged application undiluted. When xeroderma is present aqueous cream or emulsifying ointment may subsequently be applied.

Where treatment is not proving successful at home, a period in hospital is sometimes of great value but this has to be balanced against the risk arising from the fact that children with eczema are especially susceptible to virus infections (herpes simplex or vaccinia) which may cause severe generalized eruptions (Kaposi's varicelliform eruption). Generalized herpes in infancy may be fatal.

Course and Prognosis

The infective type tends to clear up with suitable dietetic adjustments and local treatments, but it may relapse.

The allergic form responds to the withdrawal of the proven allergen but this may prove to be only one factor.

The pruriginous form tends to get better at 1½–3 years when the child can do more for itself in exploration of its environment. There is, however, often a recrudescence at puberty, this time with a preponderance of facial and flexural involvement (atopic dermatitis).

ERYTHEMA INFANTUM

Synonym. Napkin eruption.

Erythema of the napkin area may be due to infection or to chemical irritation. The infective form involves the depths of the folds of skin. It may be a part of pemphigus neonatorum. The chemical irritative form affects the convex summits between the folds of skin, on the buttocks, thighs and external genitalia. The cause is a urea-splitting organism in the infant's faeces (*Bacillus alkaligenes*). The resultant ammoniacal urine causes a contact dermatitis (Jacquet's erythema) sometimes with granulomatous foci of ulceration. In other cases, excesses of fat or sugar in the infant's diet may result in stools that burn the skin. Occasionally, insufficient rinsing of the napkins after they have been washed is responsible for an alkaline or detergent dermatitis.

Treatment

In all forms the infant should be kept whenever possible with the napkin area uncovered.

In the infective form cleansing with 1 per cent. cetrimide and the application of an inert dusting powder is often sufficient, or the appropriate antibiotic can be applied after cultural examination.

In the chemical irritant form, treatment depends on the cause but further aggravation must be prevented by the application of zinc and castor oil cream or Dimethicone Cream, B.P.C., to the infant's buttocks; a cream of neomycin and bacitracin is often effective by eliminating urea-splitting organisms.

Dietetic adjustments may be necessary, or greater care in rinsing the napkins. In Jacquet's erythema soaking the napkins in a quaternary ammonium compound before use is effective. After these procedures the napkins must be rinsed thoroughly before use.

HYPOSTATIC ECZEMA AND ULCERS ON THE LEGS

Defective venous return of blood from the legs leads to a gradual deterioration of the vitality of the skin of the lower parts of the calves and ankles, resulting in the various clinical conditions known as hypostatic eczema. Minor wounds of the legs take longer to heal than similar wounds on the upper limbs, even in healthy youths. This tendency to poor healing is accentuated if there is any deficiency of the veins either through incompetent valves or deep thrombosis, each of which may be responsible for the development of varicosities. But varicosities in themselves are not the cause of eczematous and ulcerative changes; eczematous changes are usually due to the combined effects of trauma, lack of compression support, unsuitable applications and low grade infections of the itchy anoxic skin, while ulceration is due to superficial venous thrombosis causing a focal necrosis in the dermis.

Ulcers may develop from minor traumata. The skin below and behind the medial malleolus is specially vulnerable in part because of downward pressure on the venous blood from the pumping action of the calf muscles when the valves are defective and in part from the poor support and lack of rest supplied by the underlying tendons. Stasis and local oedema are the most important factors in the non-healing of ulcers of the leg, and secondary infection is usually a minor feature; but sometimes healing is prevented by a heavy mixed infection of cocci, *Ps. pyocyanea* and *Proteus*, or streptococci may gain entry and cause cellulitis, followed by chronic solid oedema of the part (elephantiasis nostras).

Diagnosis

Most ulcers on the legs are hypostatic and related to thromboses, varicosities or chilblains, but some are due to arterial insufficiency. They tend to form on the anterolateral aspect of the lower third of the leg and may be associated with diabetes mellitus.

Gummatous ulcers tend to occur higher up the leg and are serpiginous in outline, ham-coloured and appear as if punched out. Lupus vulgaris, erythema induratum, sporotrichosis, sickle-cell anaemia, hereditary spherocytosis, polycythaemia, perniosis, and halogen granulomata can all cause leg ulcers. Factitious ulcers are sometimes seen.

Rodent ulcers occasionally form on the legs, and nodes of Hodgkin's disease or lymphosarcoma may break down in that situation.

Pseudo-epitheliomatous hyperplasia is a warty condition clinically and histologically resembling carcinoma but due to intolerance of a local application. It clears up when the irritant is withdrawn.

Ecthymatous ulcers due to coccal infection are moist, with dirty sloughs and without granulations.

Treatment

Treatment of hypostatic eczema is by support with elastic hose or bandages, and with bland, non-absorbable local applications, e.g. oily calamine lotion. The patient needs to wear a support to the leg indefinitely, or in suitable cases, provided the deep veins are patent, the varicose veins may be given surgical attention by injections or ligations. Bandages impregnated with pastes of zinc oxide, ichthammol, coal tar, *Vioform* or hydrocortisone are useful in selected cases. Elastic adhesive bandages are sometimes applied over paste bandages but should not be applied direct to the eczematous skin because of the risk of exacerbation of the eczema. They may, however, be tolerated when applied with the adhesive surface outwards.

Treatment of hypostatic ulcers aims at reducing local oedema. Tulle gras is applied to the ulcerated area with an overlying gauze, orthopaedic felt or sponge rubber pad covering the ulcer and the skin around the whole leg being firmly bound with an elastic bandage. The patient is encouraged to take exercise and is warned about the bad effects of prolonged standing, but recommended to rest with the leg elevated whenever possible. Massage to the surrounds of the ulcer and to the limb as a whole is helpful. Any infective element is controlled by the appropriate antibiotic, but often a dressing of eusol and liquid paraffin is as effective as any other. Excessive granulations are reduced by a silver nitrate pencil.

THE COMMON COCCAL, BACILLARY AND CANDIDA INFECTIONS

THE NORMAL FLORA

The common resident organisms are micrococci, diphtheroids and *Propionebacterium acnes*. A great variety of transient organisms may be deposited upon the skin from the environment but usually they do not obtain a lodgement and are removed by desquamation, desiccation and washing.

In the nasal vestibule of about half the population *Staph. pyogenes* occurs as a resident and *Strep. pyogenes* may also be carried there, hence the importance of this site as a source of infection both personally and in the community. The face and hands often become colonized or invaded by these nasal organisms and they can also often be recovered from the umbilicus of neonates.

At the anogenital region enterococci and coliforms are residents and gut organisms including *Staph. aureus*, *Ps. pyocyanea*, Proteus and *Candida albicans* are likely to obtain lodgement when there is any local disease. They may be transferred elsewhere either digitally or on underclothing, particularly to the aural meatus, the nostrils, the paronychial and body folds and to leg ulcers. This particularly applies when there is any pruritic anogenital condition or when hygienic standards are poor.

In health the intact skin resists invasion by organisms arriving on the surface. Infection results either from breaks in the surface or from damage to hair follicles or nail folds. The natural 'acid mantle' has protective properties against streptococci but these organisms thrive in the serous exudates from fissures or exuding or eroded dermatoses. Staphylococci survive the 'acid mantle' and also thrive in serous exudates and within the pilosebaceous follicles.

Fissures result from defatting and dehydration of the epidermis. On the other hand the relative dryness of the surface of the skin especially on convex surfaces is an important factor preventing infection. In obesity, sweat retention in body folds induces maceration of the surface and encourages infection with *Candida albicans* (intertriginous dermatitis).

Skin infections develop more easily and are more severe in uncontrolled diabetes mellitus, renal failure, nutritional deficiency and leukaemia. Immunological deficiency states may in particular cause candida or virus infections. They should be suspected in the presence of telangiectasia, eczema with purpura, connective tissue disease and lymphoreticular malignancy.

As a general rule the organisms responsible for different types of infected skin lesions are as follows:

Staphylococcus pyogenes: Pemphigus neonatorum, impetigo, ecthyma, vestibulitis, folliculitis, furuncle, carbuncle, abscess, otitis externa, flexural dermatitis, hydradenitis suppurativa.

Streptococcus pyogenes: Impetigo, ecthyma, erysipelas, cellulitis, vestibulitis, otitis externa, flexural dermatitis, infected fissures and infected exuding dermatoses.

Candida albicans: Angular stomatitis, stomatitis (tongue, palate, cheeks), otitis externa, paronychia, onychia, intertriginous dermatitis, non-suppurative folliculitis, balanoposthitis, vulvovaginitis, perianal dermatitis.

Pseudomonas pyocyanea, proteus and enterococci: Intertriginous dermatitis, secondary infection of diseased tissue including leg ulcers and foci previously infected with cocci.

In severe or widespread coccal infections local causes such as infestations and itchy dermatoses must be excluded, also general causes such as diabetes mellitus, uraemia, leukaemia or anxiety neurosis, and search should be made for a site of carriage of pathogenic staphylococci, especially in the nasal vestibule and on the perineum, particularly when there is pruritus ani.

IMPETIGO CONTAGIOSA

Impetigo is a coccal infection of the epidermis, sometimes involving the ostia of the pilosebaceous follicles (follicular impetigo of Bockhart) or of the sweat ducts (infected miliaria rubra).

Aetiology and Pathology

Impetigo vulgaris is usually a disease of children but may occur in a milder form in adults. It usually follows some break in the skin's surface, caused by insect bites, scratching or the rupturing of herpetic bullae. Purulent discharges from the nose, ears or eyes are often responsible, or the infection may be transferred to the face and other exposed parts from a painless cuticular whitlow. The nasal vestibule may be a site of carriage of staphylococci without any abnormal physical signs. Nasal diphtheria may be complicated by impetigo.

Clinical Picture

When impetigo is caused by streptococcal or mixed streptococcal and staphylococcal infection the lesions consist of yellowish-brown 'stuck on' crusts, discoid, polycyclic or annular, scattered over the face, scalp or limbs on areas of normal skin. Even when streptococci are present in the early stages *Staph. pyogenes* usually predominates later. In staphylococcal cases there are intact bullae containing thin pus. Crusting may be present in the nostrils. At the angles of the mouth, or behind and beneath the ears, fissures may form with exuding red, sodden or crusted skin nearby.

Diagnosis

Impetigo has to be differentiated from herpes simplex, from eczematous dermatitis and, sometimes, from primary bullous diseases.

In herpes simplex the vesicles often remain intact for a while and they are hemispherical, grouped, of uniform size and contain clear fluid. Ruptured herpes vesicles may become impetiginized.

In eczematous dermatitis the lesions at first spread in continuity from the site of application of the sensitizer, but later they may erupt symmetrically. In impetigo the spread is more irregular and impetuous, skipping areas of normal skin. Individual lesions develop rapidly by peripheral spread at several sites of skin inoculation. Primary bullous conditions are erosive and blood scabbed and the bullae contain clear fluid.

Treatment

If pediculosis or scabies is present it is dealt with first. Any residual infection is then treated.

With a rapidly spreading disease such as impetigo treatment cannot wait on bacteriological culture and the usual practice is to apply the antibiotic which the prescriber believes will prove most effective. Nevertheless, culture and antibiotic sensitivity tests should be made if rapid improvement does not occur. No antibiotic should be persisted with for more than 3 days if it is not giving satisfactory results.

Failure to respond implies resistant organisms or a wrong diagnosis and continuing with the use of the antibiotic may lead either to a spread of infection or to the development of eczematous hypersensitivity. Chlortetracycline ointment, 0·25 per cent., is usually effective or *Genticin* cream or a combination of neomycin and bacitracin. Clioquinol cream, 1 per cent., or crystal violet paint, 0·5 per cent., are useful alternatives.

Loose crusts and the roofs of intact bullae should be removed before any remedy is applied. For this purpose normal or slightly hypertonic saline, 3 per cent. hexachlorophane, or 1 per cent. cetrimide solution are useful.

Course and Prognosis

Without treatment, impetigo may continue for several weeks. Any precipitating cause must first be dealt with, e.g. pediculosis, otorrhoea, rhinorrhoea or scabies, because once this is under control the elimination of the coccal infection is a simpler matter. Use of the appropriate antibiotic then leads to clearance in a few days. Impetigo due to certain strains of streptococci may be complicated by acute glomerulonephritis. Impetigo should be investigated epidemiologically in order to control the outbreak in a family or school. Contacts should be examined for banal lesions, septic fissures, running noses, etc.

PEMPHIGUS (IMPETIGO) NEONATORUM

This is a form of staphylococcal impetigo affecting new-born infants, highly infectious and having a considerable mortality rate.

Aetiology

The infection is usually introduced from a skin or nasal infection or carrier state in a medical or nursing member of a maternity unit, a visitor, a lay worker or one of the patients. One attendant may infect several infants.

Clinical Picture

Large bullae containing thin pus cover the body surface, and pink, shiny, moist areas indicate where bullae have ruptured. The flexures are most severely affected. The widespread, severe and often fatal form of the condition resembles exfoliative dermatitis (dermatitis exfoliativa neonatorum of Ritter).

Diagnosis

Diagnosis is from congenital syphilis in which the blisters occur on the palms and soles as well as elsewhere. Other signs of congenital syphilis may be present, including rhagades, snuffling, etc.

Treatment

Treatment is by the appropriate antibiotic locally, also systematically if there is fever or constitutional disturbance. Good nursing is essential and protection of the child from chilling when dressings are being done.

Course and Prognosis

Premature and inadequately treated infants may succumb to the infection but, as a rule, there is a good response to antibiotic therapy. A careful search must be made for the primary source, for carriers and possible conveyance by fomites. All in attendance on new-born infants should wear efficient surgical masks.

IMPETIGO PITYROIDES (PITYRIASIS ALBA)

This consists of scaly, often faintly depigmented discs which usually occur on the faces of fair-skinned children. The lesions are not infective but are thought to be due to exposure to sun and wind sometimes combined with the excessive use of soap and water.

Treatment

The lesions usually respond to the application of the ointment of wool alcohols (Hydrous Wool Fat Ointment, B.N.F.) or to a light screening cream such as mexenone.

ECTHYMA

This is a coccal infection, originating from the surface and affecting the dermis, leading to necrosis, ulceration and scarring. Trauma and poor hygienic standards are important predisposing factors.

Clinical Picture

Ecthyma is more common in undernourished, ill-cared for children and in individuals of low intelligence. It usually affects the legs, where one or several areas of dirty grey crusting may be seen, with a purulent discharge and red surrounds. Later, the crusts become detached, leaving shelving ulcers with an inflammatory rim and a seropurulent base. There may be regional lymphadenopathy. Ecthyma may also occur with pediculosis or from infection of traumatized legs (e.g. desert sores).

Diagnosis

An ecthymatous syphilide must be excluded.

Treatment

Having excluded parasitic infestation, attention is directed to any malnutrition and uncleanliness that may exist.

For local treatment, cleansing with 1 per cent. cetrimide or 3 per cent. hexachlorophane is indicated, followed by application of the antibiotic most suitable according to the cultural findings. Gentamicin is useful both for simple and mixed infections. The nails should be kept closely trimmed and attention paid to any infective foci in the nostrils or paronychial folds.

FOLLICULITIS

Coccogenic folliculitis is one form of sycosis barbae (folliculitis profunda), the other being mycotic folliculitis. Staphylococcal folliculitis may also be superficial (ostiofolliculitis, Bockhart's impetigo).

FOLLICULITIS BARBAE

Aetiology and Pathology

Shaving trauma and staphylococcal infection usually secondary to nasal carriage.

Clinical Picture

Folliculitis barbae is a chronic staphylococcal inflammation of the depths of the hair follicles in the beard region. Folliculitis profunda may also occur at other sites, e.g. the nucha and the pubis.

Discrete follicular papules and pustules are present and from them hairs protrude. The lesions may be grouped or widespread all over the beard area. Tender nodules may form.

Diagnosis

Diagnosis has to be made from impetigo, mycotic folliculitis, foreign body reactions due to ingrowing hairs, pustular acne and syphilis. In impetigo the lesions are superficial and not necessarily follicular. In mycotic folliculitis the patient usually gives a history of contact with cattle, the lesions are much more acute, fig-like (hence 'sycosis') and oedematous, and hairs can easily be pulled out from the follicles; mycelium and spores of fungus may be found on microscopic examination of infected hairs.

Foreign body reactions due to ingrowing hairs are most common in Africans with coarse curly hair which bores its way back into the skin producing a croquet hoop effect. This especially occurs on the sides of the neck under the chin line but may also occur on the face. In all races hairs can also ingrow through the walls of the follicles if shaving has been too close with the skin held tense. If the hair grows into the epidermis a banal folliculitis results; but if it grows into the dermis keloid scarring may develop. Embedded hairs are visible on inspection with a hand lens and their free ends can be extracted with a needle. Culture in such a case usually grows saprophytic organisms or coliforms.

Folliculitis cheloidalis nuchae is a similar condition at the back of the neck due to close shaving.

Pustular acne occurs in the skin adjoining the beard area but may coexist with folliculitis barbae. The presence of comedones is an essential feature in the diagnosis of acne.

Secondary syphilis may present with pustulation and framboesiform crusts at the cleft of the chin. Its presence should be suspected from any atypicality of the lesions and any signs of syphilis elsewhere.

Treatment

Treatment consists of the application of the appropriate antibiotic to the lesions and to the nostrils twice a day. This treatment should be persevered with for a fortnight after apparent clinical cure. A chlortetracycline ointment or a combination of neomycin and bacitracin is usually effective. An electric razor does not necessarily prove better than wet shaving. Growing a beard is the last resort in resistant cases.

Course and Prognosis

Relief can usually be obtained with one antibiotic or another, but it is always wise to have a culture made and the antibiotic sensitivity of the organisms investigated before starting treatment. Sometimes two different strains of staphylococci are present.

If folliculitis relapses a fresh strain of organisms may be responsible with different antibiotic sensitivities from the previous ones and it is therefore advisable to repeat the culture. It is also advisable to take a swab from the nasal vestibule and to treat any carriage of staphylococci with the appropriate antibiotic.

Organisms recovered from a lesion are not necessarily the cause of it. They may be secondary invaders of devitalized tissue which has been caused by some non-infective process.

OSTIOFOLLICULITIS (BOCKHART'S IMPETIGO)

This is a staphylococcal infection of the orifices of the follicles.

Aetiology

Ostiofolliculitis is caused by stimulation of the epidermis by oil, tar, adhesive plasters or other surface irritants. It is often a complicating feature of prickly heat (miliaria rubra). Poor hygiene is often a factor.

Clinical Picture

Discrete, superficial pustules are present at the orifices of hair follicles. Hairs penetrate the pustules. On rupture, superficial erosions are left. The lesions are often grouped but may be extensive. There is often an associated keratosis follicularis or acne because the irritants causing the folliculitis also stimulate epithelial proliferation at the ostia. The sites usually affected are the forearms and thighs.

Treatment

Parasitic infestation must be excluded. A culture should be made and the appropriate antibiotic used. Clioquinol cream is sometimes effective and crystal violet paint may succeed after antibiotics have failed.

Course and Prognosis

This depends on the avoidance of further contact with irritants such as oil, adhesive plaster, powerful degreasers and dehydrators. The worker should be provided with facilities to change his clothes and wash parts exposed to oil immediately after work is finished; he should be discouraged from postponing washing until he gets home, perhaps after a considerable journey.

BOILS AND CARBUNCLES

A boil (furuncle) is a staphylococcal infection of a pilosebaceous unit forming a perifollicular abscess, with sloughing of the whole unit and its replacement by scar tissue.

Furunculosis is a condition of multiple boils which may be confined to the face, limbs or trunk or widespread. A carbuncle is a localized group of boils which by their mutual pressure cause sloughing of an extensive area of skin and subcutaneous tissue with much constitutional disturbance.

Aetiology and Pathology

Boils are usually due to some local breakdown in the skin's protective mechanism. Carbuncles are usually due to some general lowering of resistance. Thus, boils may be secondary to scratch damage in an itchy skin condition, whether it be parasitic infestation, dermatitis or prurigo, or they may result from local damage arising from shaving or haircutting, rough clothing, oil or dirt. A carrier site of staphylococci in the nose or on the perineum is often the source from which the skin is inoculated and furunculosis may set a problem in domestic epidemiology in which the sharing of face flannels, towels, etc., may prove to be responsible for the spread of infection within the family. Attention should be directed to the possible presence of anaemia, malnutrition, diabetes, renal disease, leukaemia or nutritional deficiency, either of insufficiency or of imbalance.

Clinical Picture

A boil begins as a painful, red nodule which enlarges and becomes hard and tender. At its centre a small papule or papulopustule is visible, penetrated by a hair. Induration and pain cause difficulty in moving the affected part. After 36–48 hours the centre softens, a small scab or slough detaches and a purulent discharge begins. In another 36–48 hours the 'core' or pilosebaceous slough is extruded, the purulent discharge and induration lessens and the boil heals with a varying amount of scar formation.

A carbuncle begins with a greater constitutional disturbance. There may be fever, malaise and prostration. Instead of a nodule there is a brawny plateau in which several follicular pustules can be seen. The mass enlarges and a shelving induration with oedema extends for some way around. Softening and liquefaction of the mass may take days or even a week or two, but sooner or later a large slough forms and is gradually detached, or many points of suppuration develop with subsequent extensive scarring. Smaller boils and follicular pustules often form around the main lesion as a result of auto-inoculation.

Diagnosis

A boil or carbuncle has to be diagnosed from a malignant pustule (anthrax). In the latter, the onset is more rapid and the constitutional symptoms are more marked, while the history of exposure to wool or hides makes the diagnosis likely. Culture or even a direct smear will usually reveal the bacilli but treatment should be started on clinical grounds alone, without awaiting cultural confirmation.

The primary tuberculous complex resembles an indolent boil but the chronicity, history of contact, liquefactive lymphadenopathy draining the site of inoculation and resistance to antistaphylococcal measures should arouse suspicion.

Treatment

Glycosuria or albuminuria, malnutrition, anaemia or leukaemia should all be excluded. If itching preceded the boils, search should be made for its cause. Occupational hazards, unsuitable clothing and faulty hygiene should receive attention. A swab should be taken from the nasal vestibule for evidence of staphylococcal carriage.

Severe boils and carbuncles are best dealt with by systemic penicillin or some other antibiotic depending on organismal sensitivity tests.

Smaller and single lesions are better treated by local

remedies. Local treatment should aim at resolution of the lesions with minimal discomfort and with the avoidance of further contamination of the skin by the pus coming from the boils. Softening or maceration of the skin must be avoided and boracic fomentations, kaolin poultices and glycerin and magnesium sulphate dressings often do more harm than good. Dry heat may be applied with precautions to prevent burning, or hot hypertonic saline bathing may be used. The use of a hexachlorophene soap or application all over the skin is useful for destroying bacteria on the surface.

Once the boil is discharging, dry dressings, frequently changed, are used, and chlortetracycline cream, 1 per cent., Brilliant Green and Crystal Violet Paint, B.N.F., or 75 per cent. industrial spirit, applied to the skin around.

It is rarely necessary to incise boils, whereas in subcutaneous abscesses this procedure is often essential.

Boils on the nose and upper lip need especial care because of the risk of infection spreading by communicating veins to the interior of the skull, with possibly fatal results. On no account should they be subjected to pressure. The patient should be put to bed and systemic antibiotic treatment started at once. Locally, the gentle application of warmth is justifiable.

Course and Prognosis

These depend on the cause and the ease or difficulty of its removal. In all cases it is essential to treat the sites of carriage (nose and/or perineum) as well. A carbuncle in a debilitated patient is a serious and sometimes fatal complication.

HYDRADENITIS SUPPURATIVA

This is an infection of apocrine glands in the axillae or perineum, often giving rise to deep abscesses which tend to track beneath the skin.

Aetiology

The condition is more common in women than in men. The apocrine glands are susceptible to psychosexual and endocrine stimuli. Infection may be initiated by scratching caused by chemical irritation from depilatories, deodorants, or the rubber of dress protectors.

Clinical Picture

In one or both axillae or at the perineum are oblong tender swellings, firm or fluctuant. Pus may be discharged from sinuses and there is a marked tendency to tracking, irregular scarring, chronicity and recurrence.

Treatment

Any chemical irritation of the region should be avoided. Culture and use of the appropriate antibiotic in a cream is usually effective, or 75 per cent. industrial spirit may be applied. In the most severe and chronic forms excision of the affected tissue may be necessary with subsequent plastic repair.

PYODERMA GANGRENOSUM

This is a rare condition of burrowing colliquative necrosis and ulceration of the skin, of undetermined cause occurring with ulcerative coiltis or rheumatoid arthritis. There may be hypogammaglobulinaemia. A similar condition has rarely been reported in extensive cachectic states with varicella. There is leucopenia due to marrow depression.

Treatment

Treatment is of the primary condition. Replacement of fluid and electrolytes, blood transfusions and antibiotics are necessary. Treatment with gammaglobulins and systemic corticosteroids is also advisable. With control of the loss of fluid and electrolytes, healing usually begins spontaneously.

CELLULITIS

Infection of the cellular tissues with streptococci usually occurs through a fissure in the skin. The patient experiences malaise, fever, headache, perhaps vomiting and in children convulsions and a red, tense, painful oedematous swelling which gradually extends from the site of origin, sometimes with vesicles at the advancing edge. Lymphangitis and lymphadenitis are usual. The condition subsides rapidly after treatment with penicillin but recurrent attacks are common and each attack further impairs lymphatic drainage resulting ultimately in solid oedema (elephantiasis nostras), and a disfiguring condition of the face or disability of a limb. Common sites are the face and the lower limbs, portals of entry usually being in the region of the nose, ears, mouth, toe webs, or sometimes the perineum. An inherited deficiency of lymphatics often predisposes, as does oedema of renal origin or due to disease of lymphatics or their surgical removal.

Treatment

It is essential to bring about healing of fissures. Chlortetracycline ointment, 0·25 per cent., is useful for this purpose and may prevent further attacks. Individual attacks respond well to penicillin and sometimes it is justifiable to administer this drug prophylactically. Elephantiatic distortion of the face or lips is sometimes amenable to surgery.

ERYSIPELOID

An infection of the cellular tissues of the fingers or hands with the organism of swine erysipelas resulting from injury to the skin arising during the handling of animal or vegetable matter.

Clinical Picture

This is essentially a disease of food handlers. It starts as an erysipelas-like swelling on a finger or on the hand. The swelling advances with a well demarcated border and may travel up one finger, on to the hand and down an adjoining finger. Constitutional disturbance is slight. If untreated, the condition persists for several weeks.

Erysipeloid spreading to a diffuse generalized involvement of the skin is rare. It may be accompanied by fever and arthritis. Even rarer is the septicaemic form in which purpura, joint pains and endocarditis may develop, sometimes with a fatal outcome.

Treatment

It quickly responds to intramuscular injections of penicillin.

CUTANEOUS DIPHTHERIA

This is rare. Wounds (for example desert sores) may become infected with *Corynebacterium diphtheriae* and occasionally lesions develop on the skin of children suffering from nasopharyngeal diphtheria. The skin may also be affected without mucosal involvement.

Clinical Picture

There may be one lesion or several. There may be a blister which ruptures, leaving an ulcer with an adherent membrane on its floor. The flexures may be affected or whitlows may be simulated. Paronychia may occur. In children with eczema there may be multiple lesions. Constitutional symptoms are often slight, but serious myocardial or neurological complications may occur.

Diagnosis

Differential diagnosis is from infected eczema, impetigo and ecthyma. Direct smear and cultural examination for *Corynebacterium diphtheriae* confirms the suspicion.

Treatment

Diphtheria antitoxin, 20,000–50,000 Units, should be administered intramuscularly immediately the condition is suspected without waiting for a bacteriological report. The patient should be kept at rest, and isolation is necessary. Penicillin should also be administered. Locally, the area should be cleared with cetrimide, 1 per cent., and an antibiotic applied.

FUNGAL INFECTIONS

Mycotic infections of the skin may be superficial (epidermal) or deep (dermal). In the United Kingdom the former type is common, the latter rare.

SUPERFICIAL FUNGAL INFECTIONS

Pathogenic fungi are classified according to their morphological and cultural characteristics, macroscopically and microscopically, into Microsporum, Trichophyton and Epidermophyton. For the clinician it is more convenient to classify fungal diseases according to the region of the body they are affecting. The chief groups are tinea capitis, tinea barbae, tinea glabrosa, tinea axillae et cruris, tinea pedis and tinea unguium. Two or more regions on one patient can be affected by a fungus concurrently, the zonal terminology being arbitrary. For example *Trichophyton rubrum* may affect the nails, the hands, the feet and the groins at one time.

Fungal eruptions, particularly if infected with cocci or if over-treated, may give rise to secondary eruptions or mycides which, depending on the nature of the fungus, are described as microsporides, trichophytides, epidermophytides, favides or moniliides (levurides).

TINEA CAPITIS

Synonym. Tinea tonsurans.

Ringworm of the scalp in over 90 per cent. of cases is due to microsporum species, either *M. audouini* (the human form) or *M. canis* (the animal type). A much rarer form acquired from soil or animals is *M. gypseum*. All forms mainly infect children, the skin at puberty acquiring fungistatic properties.

Aetiology and Pathology

The human form is believed to be spread by direct contact and by indirect contacts, e.g. hair clippers and caps; it may also be airborne. The animal form is acquired from kittens and puppies and may spread from child to child, for two or three transferences, before it loses its vitality, which is re-established after infection of an animal host once more.

The organisms invade the stratum corneum and the mycelium grows down the hair follicles and thence passes to the hair shafts, forming a mosaic of spores around them and mycelial threads within them. The hair shafts become fibrillated and break off about 3 mm. above the surface of the skin.

Clinical Picture

As a general rule, *M. audouini* causes less severe reactions than *M. canis*, and is less likely to be associated with tinea of the glabrous skin. The history of animal contacts in the latter, and of a school or institutional epidemic in the former, may also help to suggest the nature of the fungus.

Characteristically there are circular areas of short, bent or broken hairs with frayed ends and having thicker shafts than those of the unaffected hairs around. The scalp itself shows a dirty scaling, without redness, or there may be slight papulopustulation. Rarely there are numerous follicular pustules with much oedema, causing a boggy, dusky, dome-shaped swelling, a condition known as kerion. This is more common with trichophyton infections.

Sometimes the circular or annular arrangement is inconspicuous or absent, and casual inspection may suggest a diagnosis of infective dermatitis, if the whole or most of the scalp is affected, until closer inspection shows broken hairs which are not found in infective dermatitis.

Examination with Wood's light is a great help in the diagnosis and management of these disorders. It consists of ultra-violet rays passed through a nickel glass filter. With microsporum, but not with trichophyton infections there is a brilliant green fluorescence of the affected hairs. As the infection persists, the fluorescence tends to become less brilliant. With Wood's light the diagnosis can be made of microsporum ringworm, affected hairs can more easily be removed for microscopy and culture, and the follow-up of patients until cure is greatly facilitated. It is often noted under the lamp that single outlying hairs are affected and even that small patches are present which were not suspected on examination by daylight. Direct microscopy is not essential if examination under Wood's light is positive. It is carried out by extracting a hair and placing it on a slide with potassium hydroxide. Heat is applied to hasten the keratolytic action of the potassium hydroxide. Microscopy then reveals a mosaic of small spores surrounding the hair shaft.

Diagnosis has now reached the stage of microsporum infection, since small spored ectothrix infection, due to *T. mentagrophytes* does not fluoresce. Further differentiation is made by culture, using Sabouraud's medium. Usually the macroscopic and microscopic features of the culture are characteristic but occasionally dysgonic forms are seen.

Diagnosis

In alopecia areata there are smooth bald patches with exclamation mark hairs at the periphery. In traumatic alopecia there are areas of broken-off hairs and sparseness, usually at one temporofrontal region. Infective dermatitis causes redness and scaling and loss of hair but no breaking of the hairs. Impetigo of the scalp is more exuberant and lesions are usually present elsewhere, or there is some other cause for it such as pediculosis.

Treatment

Scalp ringworm is a problem in epidemiology. With *M. audouini* it is necessary to examine the contacts and to trace the infection to its source, if possible. A Wood's light makes this much easier. In residential institutions tracing the source and quelling the infection is relatively simple. In day schools it may be difficult because siblings of all the school contacts should be examined as well. Fortunately, as small-spored ectothrix ringworm is almost unknown after puberty, it is not necessary to examine children over 14 years of age.

Treatment is by the oral administration of griseofulvin in a dose of up to 0·5 G. daily of the finely divided product, taken in a single dose, after the meal which has the greatest fat content of the day.

This antibiotic inhibits the growth of fungus from one cell into another. After it has been administered for 4–6 weeks it becomes possible to cut off the infected distal portions of the hairs, after which the scalp is shampooed and the child is free of infection.

Course and Prognosis

The natural history differs in the two types of infection. *M. audouini* tends to persist indefinitely or until puberty, whereas *M. canis* usually dies out after about 3 months. It follows that local applications may be sufficient in the latter but not in the former.

OTHER FORMS OF SCALP RINGWORM

Small-spored ectothrix ringworm of the scalp may be due to *Trichophyton mentagrophytes* and presents as an inflammatory reaction. Large-spored ectothrix infection may also affect the scalp—*T. verrucosum* (*T. discoides*). These two fungal infections are contracted from animals, *T. mentagrophytes* from many species and *T. verrucosum* from cattle. Four endothrix forms, all of human origin, are *T. sulphureum*, *T. tonsurans*, *T. violaceum* and *T. schoenleini* (favus). None of these forms of scalp ringworm cause fluorescence under Wood's light, except favus, which gives a pale bluish-green fluorescence throughout the length of the hairs which often remain unbroken.

Microscopically the endothrix ringworms show filaments and spores within the hair shafts. Favus may be recognizable at this stage by its polymorphic filaments and oval spores, with areas having the appearance of air spaces within the shafts.

Clinically the trichophyta of animal origin usually cause kerion but the endothrix forms cause much less violent reactions, perhaps some scattered broken hairs with thick scurf. With *T. violaceum* the hairs break off flush with the surface of the skin (black dot ringworm), giving an appearance that can easily be confused with alopecia areata. Microscopy, after careful removal of a hair, reveals the fungus as mycelial threads and oval segments. Favus may resemble infective dermatitis, mousey-smelling, yellow, scutuliform scales may be present, or in long-standing cases where the scalp has been kept clean it may present as a slowly extending cicatricial alopecia. Favus may also affect the glabrous skin with scutuliform lesions in which bright yellow cups form massive crusts, and it may cause nail deformity. Favus is usually acquired in childhood but it persists into adult life if untreated.

Treatment of scalp trichophyta is with griseofulvin. At the same time, infected hairs should be removed with forceps. It is wise to give warning of the probability of some degree of scarring. The boggy swelling of kerion should not be incised. With favus it is important to examine all close contacts under Wood's light, particularly children, to find if any clinically undetectable early cases exist.

TINEA BARBAE

Ringworm of the beard is nearly always caused by *T. mentagrophytes* or *T. verrucosum* (*T. discoides*) infections of animal source: hence it is found mostly amongst grooms and farm workers. It presents as irregular areas of follicular papulopustulation in the beard area, with considerable perifollicular swelling which gives rise to the fig-like nodular appearance of mycotic sycosis. Microscopy of an extracted hair often fails to reveal the fungus because of a secondary coccal infection, as in kerion celsi.

Treatment

Treatment is by manual epilation and the administration of griseofulvin.

TINEA GLABROSA

Tinea of the glabrous skin may be classified for clinical purposes as: tinea circinata of body and limbs; tinea axillae et cruris and tinea pedis.

TINEA CIRCINATA

This form of ringworm affects children or adults and may be due to microsporum or trichophyton. The former may occur in children with tinea capitis due to *M. canis*, or in adults coming into contact with them. The latter may be of human or animal source. In nearly all forms the infection spreads peripherally and heals centrally with the result that the early macular or papulovesicular lesion becomes a ring with a scaly or vesicular border and a central zone of normal or discoloured skin. In infections by *T. verrucosum* ('cattle ringworm') groups of papulopustules occur on the forearms or on the backs of the hands; but the endothrix trichophyta tend to form large rings.

Diagnosis

Diagnosis is from pityriasis rosea, patchy infective (seborrhoeic) dermatitis, nummular eczema and pustular psoriasis.

Pityriasis rosea begins with a herald patch followed by a general eruption, but microscopy reveals no fungus. Discoid infective dermatitis has greasy scales, a sweat area distribution and signs of infective dermatitis elsewhere. Nummular eczema presents with papulovesicular discs on the forearms and hands, thighs, calves and feet.

In pustular psoriasis the affected area is red and scaly, with creamy pustules and brown macules.

Treatment

Tinea circinata is usually eliminated easily with fungistatic agents such as Whitfield's ointment, magenta paint or weak tincture of iodine. If the patient is a child, it is important to examine the scalp under Wood's light even in the absence of clinical evidence of scalp involvement.

In the pustular form, it is advisable to carry out manual removal of any hairs present. Resistant forms should be treated with griseofulvin.

TINEA AXILLARIS ET CRURIS

This presents as extensive areas of erythema in the flexures, with festooned polycyclic edges showing some scaliness or slight vesiculation, from which mycelium can be recovered. The anal region, the perineum, the scrotum and the buttocks may be affected as well as the genitocrural folds. The responsible organism is usually either *T. rubrum* or *Epidermophyton floccosum*: either may also affect the hands, feet and nails, but *E. floccosum* does not affect the hair.

Diagnosis

In infective dermatitis of the flexures there are numerous follicular erythematous 'satellite' lesions. In ringworm of the axillae and groins (eczema marginatum) these are not present. In doubtful cases microscopy should make the diagnosis clear. In flexural dermatitis due to cocci the intensity of inflammation is much greater and in flexural dermatitis caused by *Candida albicans* the white, sodden epidermis overlying the moist, reddened surface with fissuring in the depths of the folds makes the diagnosis clear. Contact dermatitis due to textiles is recognized by its situation in the folds of the axillae rather than in their domes.

Treatment

Treatment is with a topical fungicide. If this fails to clear the condition a course of griseofulvin, 500 mg. daily for 6 weeks, is indicated.

TINEA PEDIS

This is usually due to *T. mentagrophytes*, *T. rubrum* or *E. floccosum*. Cultural differentiation is important because eradication of *T. rubrum* is a far more difficult matter than eradication of *T. mentagrophytes* or *E. floccosum*.

Aetiology

Foot ringworm is most easily spread where people mix in bare feet; hence its designation 'athlete's foot'. Changing rooms, swimming baths and bathrooms are probably the commonest sources of contagion but individual susceptibility, because of variations in immunological response, hyperidrosis, crowded toes and minor foot deformities, is also important. Other factors include climatic and working conditions of heat and humidity, and faulty footwear, in particular thick shrunken socks and impervious footwear.

Clinical Picture

With *T. mentagrophytes* and *E. floccosum* infections skin-coloured bullae and vesicles are present, mostly on the medial surface of the foot spreading on to the sole. Other parts of the sole and heel may also be affected, also the toe webs and flexures. Secondary infection may cause opalescence of the vesicles. When there is only white, sodden skin, with fissuring of the fourth toe webs, intertriginous dermatitis caused by candida is a more likely diagnosis.

In the presence of secondary infection or over-treatment, a secondary eruption (mycide) of vesicles often develops symmetrically on the hands and feet. These vesicles do not contain fungus and the hand condition is in no way contagious. Infection may, however, spread to the nails of hands and feet.

T. rubrum infections behave in a different fashion. It is not unusual to find simultaneous infection of the hands, feet, nails and groins. The hands and feet usually show a diffuse, fine peeling and some redness only, perhaps with hyperkeratosis and fissuring but without vesiculation; the condition is sometimes unilateral on hand or foot. One or more nails may be affected as well. On the calves there may be discrete deep follicular lesions resembling a deep coccal folliculitis, tuberculide or even erythema nodosum.

Fungal infections may extend and intensify in patients taking oral corticosteroids and in patients with leukaemia or reticulosis. Their appearances may be masked by the use of topical corticosteroids making them difficult of recognition.

Diagnosis

Microscopic confirmation by removing the roofs of suspected vesicles is essential if errors are to be avoided, as a very similar, if not identical picture can arise in pompholyx (dysidrosis) and in contact dermatitis. Contact eczematous dermatitis of the feet usually arises on the dorsa but may itself be due to over-treatment of tinea pedis. Tinea pedis is often asymmetrical whereas pompholyx is symmetrical. Sodden toe clefts may be due to excessive sweating and maceration or to *Candida albicans* infection. Pustular psoriasis of the feet presents as reddened areas with excessive scaling and creamy and brown 'pustules' which are sterile on culture and microscopically show no fungus.

Treatment

Footwear should be well fitting; socks should be of cotton and changed daily, or a fresh pair of white cotton in-socks can be worn each day. Shoes with sponge-rubber soles should not be worn. The feet should be washed twice a day and magenta paint applied at night and zinc oxide and salicylic acid powder liberally shaken into the socks and between the toes each morning. If any secondary infection is present foot soaks in potassium permanganate, 1 in 8000, for 10 minutes twice a day are useful. In cases due to *T. rubrum* and in other resistant forms treatment with griseofulvin is necessary for 6 weeks.

TINEA UNGUIUM

Ringworm of the nails may be due to trichophyton or epidermophyton infection. It may pick out one nail, one hand or foot, or both. It is unusual for all the nails to be affected and the distribution is usually asymmetrical. Extensive disease is usually due to *T. rubrum.*

Clinical Picture

The nails are usually affected from their free edges and become grey or brown, thickened, rough, dull, friable and honeycomb-like. They are sometimes easily shed. To make a microscopic examination for fungus a microscope slide is used; by scraping with its edge, fine flakes of nail can be detached. The more superficial ones are discarded; the deeper ones are caught on another slide covered with potassium hydroxide and a cover-slip, and heated to hasten the keratolytic action of the potassium hydroxide. It is usually easy to find mycelium by this method but subsequent attempts at culture often fail.

Diagnosis

Ringworm of the nails has to be differentiated from psoriasis, eczema, lichen planus, syphilis and nail dystrophies. Psoriasis usually affects many nails in symmetrical fashion. Thimble-like pitting may be present or the nails may be thickened and yellow. In tinea unguium there may be only one or two nails affected and the discoloration is dirty grey rather than yellow. Microscopic examination for mycelial filaments is the deciding factor in doubtful cases, in addition to the presence or absence of psoriasis or fungal disease elsewhere. Paronychia is rarely caused by fungi but is often in part or wholly due to candida infection.

Treatment

Griseofulvin, 500 mg. daily of the fine particulate form, is effective in ringworm of the nails. It is necessary to take the drug for at least 6 months for treatment of the finger nails and for more than a year for the toe nails. Recurrences are common both in toe nails and in the fourth toe webs.

CANDIDIASIS

Synonyms. Moniliasis, Candidosis.

Candida albicans may affect the mucosae and the skin in several ways causing stomatitis (thrush), angular cheilitis, vulvovaginitis, balanoposthitis, intertriginous dermatitis or paronychia. Stomatitis occurs as thrush in infants, with white, easily detached shreds overlying the mucosae. Angular stomatitis is often caused by *Candida albicans,* and detachable white plaques may also form on the palate, cheeks or tongue. Candida vulvovaginitis is a common cause of pruritus vulvae and vaginal discharge. There is a shiny flexural erythema with a heaping up of white sodden epidermis at the margin. Flexural dermatitis has a similar appearance at other sites, chiefly under pendulous breasts or abdominal folds, at the umbilicus, at axillary and genitocrural flexures and between the fingers in the form known as erosio interdigitalis blastomycetica. *Candida albicans* is a common cause of sodden skin in the toe clefts.

In all forms of *Candida albicans* infection it is important to test for glycosuria, look for dietetic imbalance and exclude hypoparathyroidism. Rarely, Addison's disease, immunological deficiency, pernicious anaemia or hypothyroidism are implicated. Pregnancy or the taking of contraceptive pills predisposes to it, and wide-spectrum antibiotics, particularly when taken orally, may disturb the intestinal flora in favour of candida, causing anogenital dermatitis and pruritus.

The primary cause of chronic paronychia is a break in the epidermal barrier due to the effects of alkalis, detergents, cuticle removers, habitual picking or biting of the nail folds or excessive manicuring. Once this barrier is broken down cocci and Gram-negative bacilli or *Candida albicans* gain access to the folds. As a result pyogenic cocci cause acute paronychia and less virulent organisms, especially candida, cause chronic paronychia.

Treatment

Treatment of *Candida albicans* infections consists of attention to the general health; attention to the local anatomical condition predisposing to this infection; and the application of a *Candida albicans* antagonist.

Unbalanced nutrition, obesity and any associated diabetes must be controlled. Opposing skin folds should be prevented from rubbing against one another by means of suitable dressings, up-lift brassières and abdominal supports, well-fitting socks and shoes. The affected areas should be kept clean with an unscented toilet soap and after its use a talcum dusting powder should be liberally applied to the less active areas and magenta paint to the more active ones.

Nystatin dusting powder is effective against most strains of *Candida albicans.* It may be advisable to treat the gut infection as well. Alternatively, amphotericin B cream may be used. Griseofulvin is ineffective against *Candida albicans.*

Chronic paronychia can only be relieved with full co-operation on the patient's part. Wet work must be kept to a minimum and exposure to washing soda, alkaline soaps and detergents avoided. Magenta paint is applied beneath the nail folds using a camel-hair brush. The patient must be reminded of the possibility of recurrence and advised how to take especial care to avoid the known hazards. Rubber or plastic gloves should be worn for wet work but preferably for only 10 minutes at a time. In some cases the infection is secondary to intestinal candidiasis with angular cheilitis and anogenital pruritus. Special hygienic precautions must be taken in these circumstances to prevent re-infection of the paronychial folds, and a course of oral nystatin is advisable.

TINEA VERSICOLOR

Malassezia furfur is the organism responsible for this condition, which presents as brown, slightly scaly plaques on the body and to a lesser degree on the proximal parts of the limbs. If the skin has been exposed to sunlight the affected areas may be paler than the normal areas adjoining (achromia parasitica). The affected areas are also paler than the surrounding normal skin in pigmented races.

Diagnosis

In tinea versicolor in the white man, the brown areas are 'islands' in a 'sea' of white and the edges of the brown are outwardly convex. In vitiligo the converse applies. In tinea versicolor there is slight scaling, made more apparent by scraping. Microscopic examination of these scales reveals fragments of mycelium and many spores, sometimes in clusters resembling bunches of grapes. Examination may be made either of scraped off scales or of scales removed by the application of transparent adhesive tape. This fungus will not grow on artificial media. Another diagnostic feature is a golden fluorescence when the patient is examined under Wood's light.

Treatment

Tinea versicolor is encouraged by hyperidrosis or sweat retention: hence it is wise to look for any tuberculosis, hyperthyroidism or other condition which might be responsible for the sweating. Insufficient bathing and the wearing of the same underclothing day and night is occasionally to blame. Bad habits of this sort must be corrected and porous underclothing worn and changed daily if the condition is to be cured. The application of 10 per cent. sodium thiosulphate lotion is effective; or the 3 per cent. ointment of sulphur and salicylic acid may be applied. Treatment should be continued for 2 weeks after apparent cure. The bed linen and underclothes should be disinfected by laundering. The organism is not sensitive to griseofulvin.

TRICHONOCARDIOSIS AXILLARIS

This is a fungal infection around hairs in the axillae, producing dark-reddish concretions and caused by *Nocardia tenuis* in symbiosis with a coccus which forms red, yellow or black pigment. The causative organism may be re-classified as a corynebacterium species.

Treatment is by shaving the axillae, cleaning with cetrimide solution, 1 per cent., and the application of salicylic acid compound dusting powder.

ERYTHRASMA

This is a superficial skin infection believed to be caused by *Corynebacterium minutissimum*. It causes brown, slightly scaly areas in axillae and groins, or scaly skin in the toe webs, usually the fourth. Under Wood's light a coral fluorescence is seen. On culture the causative organism can be isolated and it fluoresces similarly.

Treatment is by the application of salicylic acid compound dusting powder.

MYCIDES

These may take the form of vesiculation of the hands (pompholyx) or lichenoid, horny, follicular papules in groups on the trunk (lichen trichophytide). Erythematous, urticarial, erythema multiforme and erythema nodosum types have been described.

Treatment is by bland local applications while the primary focus is brought under control.

CUTANEOUS TUBERCULOSIS

The skin may be invaded by tubercle bacilli or it may be the site of reactions of hypersensitivity to these organisms (tuberculides). When the skin is invaded by tubercle bacilli its manner of response depends on the immunological state of the host at the time. If the individual has suffered no previous tuberculous infection at any site, the Mantoux reaction is negative (primary anergy) and the response will be the primary tuberculous complex; but if there has been a previous tuberculous infection in the skin or elsewhere, and the Mantoux reaction is positive, the response will be lupus vulgaris (normergy). It is believed that if a secondary anergy develops, any subsequent tuberculous infection causes the condition known as sarcoidosis, although this reaction may also be non-tuberculous. Some individuals develop an excessive sensitivity to tuberculin. In them, tuberculous infection at any site may be followed by some form of tuberculide (hyperergy).

THE PRIMARY TUBERCULOUS COMPLEX IN THE SKIN

This consists of a tuberculous chancre on some exposed part of the body such as the face, eye, hands or knees, and enlargement of the lymph node draining the area. The chancre resembles a boil, but instead of suppurating it persists as a crusted indurated patch with a little blood-stained discharge. The lymph node draining the site enlarges, softens and breaks down through the skin, leaving an irregular scar. Subsequently the primary chancre slowly heals up, or it may form the focus from which a patch of lupus vulgaris develops. The Mantoux reaction changes from negative to positive with the development of the primary complex. A primary lesion may also develop within the mouth or throat, with lymphadenopathy as in the cutaneous form.

Diagnosis has to be made from a low-grade coccal infection.

LUPUS VULGARIS

Aetiology and Pathology

Infection of the skin causing lupus vulgaris may take place by inoculation, by lymphatic spread, by the breaking down of some underlying tuberculous focus or by the blood stream. Either human or bovine bacilli may be responsible.

Inoculation through the skin may occur from abrasion with contaminated dust. Thus an infant crawling on the floor may be infected indirectly by an adult with open pulmonary tuberculosis. Lupus usually begins in the first decade but occasionally starts much later in life. The face is the commonest site of infection, particularly around the orifices, but the elbows, hands, knees, buttocks and perianal region are sometimes affected. Local spread then proceeds by the lymphatic channels or these vessels may be the route by which an infection primarily infecting the nose reaches the skin. Involvement of the skin by spread from underlying tuberculous foci takes place in scrofuloderma (King's evil) from the breaking down of cervical tuberculous lymph nodes and also from sinuses draining tuberculous kidneys, bones or joints. Spread by the blood stream only occurs in states of extreme debility, which may arise with measles or pertussis. In this form, multiple foci may occur on widely separated parts of the skin. In its extreme form of severity, blood dissemination causes the rare and often fatal condition of tuberculosis cutis miliaris acuta or lupus miliaris, in which the multiple miliary areas of tuberculosis are only the outward signs of a miliary tuberculosis of internal organs.

Clinical Picture

The nodule of lupus vulgaris is a flat, semitranslucent area with slight scaling—the 'apple-jelly' nodule described by Jonathan Hutchinson. Subsequently the lesion may have exudative or fibrotic characters. In the former, there is some swelling and redness and no tendency to heal spontaneously; ulceration may occur. In the fibrotic form, the lesions are flat and ulceration does not occur but healing with scar formation and extension go on side by side. As a result, multiple foci of activity may remain amongst extensive areas of scarring.

Lupus around the nose and mouth is often complicated by mucosal lupus in the nose or on the gums, cheek, tongue, palate, pharynx or larynx. Mucosal lesions are different from the cutaneous ones, being dusky, granular infiltrations which bleed easily.

Lupus vulgaris may destroy cartilage but not bone. The resultant deformities that may arise include simian or parrot-bill deformities of the nose, due to destruction of the alae and septum respectively, septal perforation and stenosis or occlusion of the anterior nares. The mouth may be narrowed by scarring (microstomia) or the upper lip may be retracted, permanently exposing the gums. Contracture of scarring below the eye may cause ectropion. The pinnae may be destroyed, irregularly or completely, or they may, as a result of the inflammatory process, become adherent to the skull. Some of these deformities are in part due to secondary infection or to the use of caustics and X-rays in treatment. Lesions on the limbs and body may be very extensive. Ulceration may be followed by scarring and contractures or lymphatic obstruction may lead to elephantiasis.

Complications of lupus include secondary infection, particularly in the nose, contractures, elephantiasis and the development of keratoses, squamous cell epithelioma and fibrosarcoma. This is particularly likely to happen in patients who have received X-ray treatment for the lupus, but it may also occur in patients who have had much treatment by ultra-violet irradiation and other locally destructive procedures.

Lupus vulgaris may be associated with phlyctenular keratitis, tuberculosis of the upper respiratory tract, of bones, joints or kidneys and, more rarely, of the lungs.

Diagnosis

The earliest lesion may resemble a juvenile melanoma, but on diascopy (inspection through a piece of glass firmly applied to the skin) it is clear that the brown colour is due to an exudative process and of apple-jelly appearance, whereas with moles and freckles it is duller and without translucency. More advanced lesions have to be differentiated from syphilis, tuberculoid leprosy, sarcoidosis, lupus erythematosus, leishmaniasis, a drug granuloma, lupoid sycosis and rodent ulcers. Lupus vulgaris usually starts in the first decade, affects the skin and cartilage and takes years to develop, showing characteristic apple-jelly nodules. Syphilitic gummata develop much more rapidly, usually in the 30–50 age group, and may ulcerate and destroy in weeks or months to an extent that would take lupus several years. Bone may be destroyed as well as cartilage and skin, and it is not unusual for a gumma to form deeply and to ulcerate rapidly with the formation of a large cavity. Tuberculoid leprosy may closely mimic lupus but there is anaesthesia to light touch, and impaired temperature discrimination; the nerves in the area may be thickened and tender and a history of residence in an area of endemic leprosy. Leishmaniasis is suspected when the patient has come from an area where this disease is endemic, and histological examination reveals Leishman-Donovan bodies. A drug granuloma, usually due to iodides, is exuberant and often accompanied by bullae and purpuric lesions.

Sarcoidosis presents as raised, pinkish-yellow, translucent nodules about the face or on the shoulders and arms, or as indurated erythematous lesions on the legs. Histological study may be necessary for differentiation.

Lupus erythematosus is often symmetrical and involves the 'bat's wing' area of the face, the scalp (which is seldom affected by lupus vulgaris), the vermilion surface of the lips and perhaps the backs of the fingers. There is redness with follicular plugging, scaling and central atrophic scarring but without apple-jelly nodulation. A very important differential point from lupus vulgaris is that lupus erythematosus never involves cartilage, so that no matter how long it has been present there is no serious deformity of nose or ears, and no loss of tissue other than the skin.

Rodent ulcer may be simulated by ulcerated lupus but it has a hard pearly edge, whereas ulcerated lupus is ragged. Lupus vulgaris may be complicated by squamous cell epithelioma.

Ancillary aids to differential diagnosis include biopsy, culture for tubercle bacilli, the Wassermann reaction, the Mantoux reaction, the Kveim test and the lepromin test.

Treatment

Isoniazid in a dose of 300 mg. a day leads to disappearance of the nodules and of scaling within 2–6 months; the drug is usually administered for a total of up to eighteen months. There is no evidence of the development of drug-resistant organisms. Toxic reactions are rare. Under an 'umbrella' of isoniazid a surgeon can carry out plastic repairs with complete confidence. Combined treatment with isoniazid and streptomycin or sodium aminosalicylate is unnecessary unless the lungs or other organs are affected.

The general health, domestic and occupational surroundings, and nutrition should always receive attention. The diet should include ample milk, butter and eggs. General ultra-violet irradiation helps to hasten recovery. Coexistent tuberculosis in other organs is not uncommon, particularly in lymph nodes, bones, joints and kidneys but it is rare in the lungs.

LUPUS VERRUCOSUS

Synonym. Tuberculosis verrucosa cutis.

This is due to inoculation of the skin of an adult with tubercle bacilli. It usually occurs on the hands or buttocks as a violaceous, warty excrescence, with a reddish surround and a slight seropurulent discharge. One form of it is the verruca necrogenica, the anatomical tubercle or post-mortem wart, acquired from a human or bovine cadaver, but the infection can also occur from a patient's own tuberculous sputum. The lesions may be secondarily infected but they do not ulcerate. Dissemination of tubercle bacilli may occur causing subcutaneous abscesses in the course of the lymphatics and in the lymph node draining the area.

Diagnosis

Diagnosis is from warts, lichen planus verrucosus, syphilis, vegetating pyoderma, sporotrichosis and blastomycosis. Warts do not show dusky discoloration. Lichen planus verrucosus usually occurs on the shins or on the forearms, and itches intensely. Syphilis is much more actively inflammatory than the indolent lupus verrucosus. Vegetating pyoderma, sporotrichosis and blastomycosis can only be differentiated by histological and cultural methods.

Treatment

Treatment is with isoniazid, when the source of infection is external and with isoniazid combined with streptomycin or sodium aminosalicylate when the infection is autogenous (from the patient's own sputum).

TUBERCULOSIS COLLIQUATIVA

Synonym. Scrofuloderma.

This is tuberculosis of the skin secondary to tuberculosis of underlying lymph nodes, joints or bones.

Clinical Picture

The commonest form is in the neck (scrofuloderma), secondary to tuberculous cervical adenitis. Subcutaneous nodules become attached to the skin which becomes dusky and indurated. Finally the mass breaks down and a crusted sinus is exposed or ragged, undermined ulcers form with intercommunicating sinuses. When the condition heals, irregular scarring is left.

Diagnosis

Diagnosis from syphilis, actinomycosis and sporotrichosis is on clinical grounds and by cultural, serological and histological methods.

Treatment

Treatment is by attention to good feeding, housing and fresh air, general ultra-violet irradiation and isoniazid by mouth with sodium aminosalicylate or streptomycin. Surgical intervention is sometimes necessary.

TUBERCULOSIS CUTIS ORIFICIALIS

This is a form of painful tuberculous ulceration in or around the orifices, usually secondary to tuberculosis of internal organs. Thus tuberculous ulcers of the nose, palate, tongue, floor of mouth or the lips arise from infection by sputum from a pulmonary or laryngeal focus; ulceration of the external genitalia in both sexes may occur from tuberculosis of the genital or urinary tracts. Perianal ulcers may occur in persons with intestinal tuberculosis. The ulcers are painful, shallow and ragged, with undermined edges and dirty grey bases from which there is a mucopurulent secretion.

Diagnosis is from chancre or chancroid by bacteriological examination from the base of the ulcer and from epithelioma by biopsy.

Treatment is with isoniazid and streptomycin or sodium aminosalicylate.

TUBERCULIDES

These are skin reactions which are due to hypersensitivity (hyperergy) to tuberculin. In some forms this relationship is clearly established; in others it is suspected but not proven.

ERYTHEMA NODOSUM

This is a non-specific reaction of hypodermal vascular hypersensitivity, one of the causes of which may be a tuberculous infection.

ERYTHEMA INDURATUM

Erythema induratum or Bazin's disease is a condition of dusky, painful nodulation usually occurring on the lower halves of the legs in young women with perniotic 'billiard-table' legs. A faulty peripheral circulation predisposes to it. The indurated areas are painful and tender and may break down and form ragged ulcers with undermined edges; secondary coccal infection may follow. The condition is usually bilateral.

The Mantoux reaction is usually positive at 1 in 10,000.

Clinical Picture

The legs are bluish and have, particularly on the

posteromedial and posterolateral aspects of the lower thirds, irregular, hard, dusky, painful, plaque-like nodulations which often necrose centrally and leave depressed scars. There may be no other sign of tuberculosis or there may be a history of a pulmonary infection or of the presence of tuberculides elsewhere, for example of the papulonecrotic variety.

Diagnosis

Diagnosis is from subcutaneous (Darier-Roussy) sarcoids, erythema induratum of Whitfield (nodular vasculitis) and syphilitic gummata. In sarcoidosis there are often other lesions elsewhere on the skin, ulceration is unusual, and the Mantoux reaction is often negative at 1 in 100. In Whitfield's erythema induratum middle-aged women are mostly affected and the lesions are multiple and recurrent. Syphilitic gummata cause painless, often single, ham-coloured, serpiginous or reniform 'punched-out' ulcers.

Treatment

Treatment is by elastic supports, good food, adequate housing, fresh air and isoniazid with streptomycin or sodium aminosalicylate. Ulcerated lesions need appropriate antibiotics to control secondary infection: apart from this they should be treated in the same way as hypostatic ulcers.

Course and Prognosis

The changes in the hypoderm are, to some extent, irreversible, and some degree of scarring is inevitable.

LICHEN SCROFULOSORUM

This is a rare form of tuberculide, consisting of lichenoid papules, which usually occurs in children with tuberculous lymph nodes, bones or joints.

Clinical Picture

There are brownish-red, lichenoid papules scattered or grouped, sometimes with spiny tips, slight scaling, crusting or even pustulation. The lesions mostly appear on the trunk and there is slight itching. The Mantoux reaction is strongly positive.

Diagnosis

Diagnosis is from lichen planus and from lichen trichophytide. Lichen planus is rare in children and usually causes severe itching. The lesions are violaceous, polygonal papules with a waxy surface. In doubtful cases the histology is diagnostic, the papules of lichen scrofulosorum having a tuberculoid structure. In lichen trichophytide a primary focus of fungal infection is to be found.

Treatment

Treatment is of the underlying tuberculous condition.

PAPULONECROTIC TUBERCULIDES

Papulonecrotic tuberculides have various forms and distributions: some are truly tuberculous but others may in fact be virides. Superficial forms have been called 'folliclis', deeper ones 'acnitis'. Papulonecrotic tuberculides of the extremities consist of discrete, inflamed papules which undergo central necrosis, ulcerate, form scabs and heal with scarring. They occur on the trunk and limbs. The whole process may take some 8 weeks but there may be successive crops. The Mantoux reaction is usually positive at 1 in 10,000.

Lupus miliaris disseminatus faciei consists of multiple, pinhead-sized, flat, discrete, semitranslucent lesions which occur symmetrically on the cheeks. It may be a late form of acne agminata, a condition in which acneiform, apple-jelly-like nodules occur on the nose, eyelids and face, often grouped together. They may also occur on the genitalia. After a variable persistence they may disappear, with slight pock-like scarring. The Mantoux reaction is usually hypo- or anergic and the condition is not proven to be tuberculous: it may be of viral origin and does not usually react to antituberculous drugs.

HISTOPATHOLOGY OF THE TUBERCULIDES

All these lesions show a tuberculoid structure, but this does not of necessity prove a tuberculous aetiology, as a tuberculoid structure is also often seen in acne vulgaris and in rosacea.

OTHER CUTANEOUS MYCOBACTERIAL INFECTIONS

[See Section 2.]

SARCOIDOSIS [see Section 9]

VIRUS INFECTIONS

KAPOSI'S VARICELLIFORM ERUPTION

There are two forms, eczema herpeticum and eczema vaccinatum. The first is a generalized infection with the virus of herpes simplex, the second a generalized infection with vaccinia pox virus officinale, a mutant of cowpox virus.

Eczema herpeticum occurs in infants with eczema who have been exposed to a sufferer from herpes simplex. Eczema vaccinatum occurs in atopic individuals who have been vaccinated deliberately or accidentally. It may also occur with other widespread inflammatory dermatoses. It may be less severe than eczema herpeticum.

Clinical Picture

There is a generalized eruption of umbilicated varicelliform lesions, high fever and general malaise occurring usually about 10 days after exposure.

Treatment

Isolation and good nursing are necessary. Secondary infection is common and the use of antibiotics both systemically and topically is advisable. The lesions may be dressed with chlortetracycline ointment. Corticosteroids should not be used either systemically or topically. Hyperimmune vaccinal γ-globulin should be administered in eczema vaccinatum. The use of hyperimmune globulin in eczema herpeticum is of uncertain value but it should be administered.

OTHER COMPLICATIONS OF VACCINATION

These include secondary infection, non-infective necrosis, non-specific eruptions of erythema multiforme, exanthematous, urticarial or purpuric type and progressive vaccinia.

WARTS AND MOLLUSCA CONTAGIOSA

These are not discussed here.

HAND, FOOT AND MOUTH DISEASE

This is an enterovirus infection, mostly affecting children in epidemics. It is a relatively mild and transient condition with no general malaise but with painful ulcerating vesicles in the mouth and oval pearly vesicles on the hands and feet, sometimes elsewhere. Other coxsackie viruses and echoviruses may cause macular, maculopapular and petechial exanthems usually loosely designated 'toxic erythema'. Pox viruses may cause epidermal necrotic lesions.

ORF

Synonym. Contagious pustular dermatitis of sheep.

Aetiology

Orf is due to a pox virus infection and may affect all handlers of sheep's heads and carcasses—shepherds, meat porters, butchers, cooks and housewives. The histological picture resembles that of cowpox, but virological studies differentiate the two conditions.

Clinical Picture

The lesion usually occurs on a finger, on the hand or on the face as an oedematous inflammatory nodule which becomes haemorrhagic and pustular. The conjunctiva may be infected. The inflammation attains its maximum intensity after 7–10 days, some central necrosis occurs and the lesion gradually shrinks, disappearing after several weeks, leaving a scar. Lymphadenitis and constitutional symptoms are slight.

Diagnosis

Diagnosis is from vaccinia and milkers' nodules.

Treatment

No treatment is effective in shortening the course. Topically applied antibiotics are helpful to control secondary infection.

MILKERS' NODULES

These are red nodules, single or multiple, occurring on the hands of milkers and due to a pox virus similar to orf. Brownish-red or purple nodules develop after an incubation period of 5–7 days and reach maximal size within 2 weeks. They are painless unless there is secondary bacterial infection. Lymphadenopathy may develop.

COWPOX

This virus is similar to that of vaccinia but antigenically distinct. Papules develop on exposed parts and become vesicopustular, with malaise, fever and lymphadenitis.

LYMPHOGRANULOMA VENEREUM

[See Section 2.]

GRANULOMA VENEREUM VEL INGUINALE

[See Section 2.]

PARASITIC INFESTATIONS

SCABIES

Definition

Scabies is an acarine parasitic infestation of the stratum corneum caused by *Sarcoptes* (*Acarus*) *scabiei.*

Aetiology

The adult female is about 0·4 mm. long, just visible to the naked eye, oval in shape, with two anterior pairs of limbs which bear suckers and two posterior pairs which bear trailing bristles. The gravid female burrows in the horny layer where she deposits up to 30 eggs and then dies. The larvae hatching from the eggs have only two hind limbs until, by repeated moulting, they develop to mature males and females. The larvae and males live in the orifices of hair follicles, the males dying after impregnation of the females. The complete cycle takes 10 days. Infestation is by intimate skin contact; the infestation is either a familial and household one or a complaint of bedfellows. It may rarely spread by more casual contacts, as in the handling of an infested patient by a nurse. In the first attack itching begins about 2 weeks after infestation, apparently due to the development of allergic hypersensitivity.

Clinical Picture

Scabies may present as pruritus, widespread eczema or infected dermatitis, urticaria, impetigo or furunculosis. Itching may be intolerable or inconspicuous, depending on the integrity of the sensory tracks and on the mental alertness of the individual. Thus, in the presence of leprosy, mental deficiency (e.g. mongolism) or senile dementia there is no obvious discomfort from itching in heavily infested individuals. Secondary infection may then produce a picture resembling infective dermatitis or exfoliative dermatitis (Norwegian or crusted scabies). Nurses are very liable to become infested as a result of attending to these patients whose scales and even nails show an enormous acarine population.

A history of familial incidence or of venereal exposure makes the diagnosis probable. In any widespread itchy eruption, the physician should examine for scabies. The sites involved and the presence of burrows should make the diagnosis clear. Scabies affects thin skin areas below the collar line; thus, the anterior axillary folds, the medial sides of the elbows, the ulnar sides of the wrists and hands, and the clefts of the fingers are sites commonly affected on the upper limbs. On the trunk the sites most affected are the female breasts, the abdomen, male external genitalia and the buttocks; and on the lower limbs the thighs, ankles and feet; in infants, palms and sole are characteristically affected, and in neonates lesions may also occur on the face.

The burrow is a linear, slightly sinuous elevation in the skin, at one end of which a darker speck marks the site of the parasite. In cleanly individuals the burrows may be inconspicuous and it is best to search for them by oblique lighting with the aid of a lamp in order to make minor elevations in the skin more obvious. In less cleanly persons, accumulations of dirt beside the burrows make their recognition easier. Skin-coloured or red follicular papules are also observed at the characteristic sites. Both these types of lesion may be masked by scratching, secondary infection or eczematous dermatitis. In doubtful cases the diagnosis can often be made by finding adult parasites, larvae or ova. This is best done by scraping open suspect burrow-like lesions with a Harrison's scarifier or blunt scalpel, through potassium hydroxide. Microscopic examination may then reveal one or more adult parasites, larvae, unhatched eggs or eggshell fragments. An alternative method is to lift out a female mite from a burrow with a fine-pointed needle.

Animal scabies may be caught from cats and dogs, but the parasites do not burrow and establish themselves, there are only itchy papules and the disease dies out if there is no further contact with the animal.

Diagnosis

Diagnosis is from pediculosis and from other causes of widespread itching eruptions associated with urticaria, eczema-dermatitis, furunculosis and impetigo. A history of itchy contacts is very suggestive. The manual lesions by themselves may suggest a contact dermatitis and a more general examination should be made in all such cases if there is the least cause for suspicion. The diagnosis of scabies is made from consideration of the history and the distribution and nature of the lesions, and from microscopic examination. Involvement of the penis and scrotum with itchy red papules is characteristic.

Pediculosis corporis mostly affects the upper trunk and shoulders with scratch marks, excoriations and patchy pigmentation. Pediculosis capitis may also cause scratch marks on the shoulders. Parasites are found on the seams of underclothing and eggs attached to coarse body hairs or to underclothing.

Treatment

The patient and all members of the household should be treated concurrently. Self-treatment is difficult and the treatment of patients by each other is best. In extensive family infestations and in epidemics, or if home facilities are inadequate, treatment at special cleansing stations is sometimes preferable.

The full course of treatment takes 3 days. On the first day the patient takes a warm bath and lathers and scrubs the body and limbs, thoroughly all over, with particular attention to the sites known to be most heavily infested. After the bath, the skin is not dried but a solution of 25 per cent. benzyl benzoate is applied all over from the neck downwards, using a paint brush 2 or 3 inches wide. Having made certain that every square inch of skin has been covered, including the genitalia, perineum and toe clefts, the patient dries in front of a fire, puts on the previously worn nightwear and goes to bed between the previously used sheets. On the second day another application of benzyl benzoate is made, but without a preceding bath; then the patient dries before a fire and puts on clean underwear. That night clean nightwear is worn and the patient goes to bed between clean sheets. On the third day the patient takes a bath and the treatment is then at an end. An alternative treatment is with 1 per cent. gamma benzene hexachloride application on two occasions. Crotamiton lotion, 10 per cent., is another effective sarcopticide and also has antipruritic properties.

If there is any further itching, calamine lotion is applied and on no account must further applications of benzyl benzoate be made. Patients sometimes give themselves repeated applications because itching often persists for a while after the two treatments, and they interpret this as meaning that the infestation persists. Repeated applications of benzyl benzoate may cause dermatitis medicamentosa. For infants under 2 years of age, a half-strength emulsion may be used. Sulphur Ointment, B.P. (it is 10 per cent., but 2½ per cent. should be used for infants), may be used instead of benzyl benzoate emulsion, but is more liable to irritate the skin. Underclothing, nightwear and sheets are best dealt with by laundering and ironing. Sarcoptes essentially lives on and in the epidermis and does not, like the louse, move away from the host; hence it is unnecessary to disinfest bedding, blankets and the outer clothing.

Course and Prognosis

If untreated, scabies infestations go on indefinitely. This is only likely to occur in individuals of low intelligence in whom itching may be slight or absent. By concurrent treatment of all members of the household, scabies can be eliminated quickly; but if any one member of the household remains untreated, or is treated at some other time, recurrences are likely.

PEDICULOSIS

Three forms of lice live on man: *Pediculus capitis*, *Pediculus corporis* (*vestimenti*) and *Pediculus* (*Phthirus*) *pubis*.

PEDICULOSIS CAPITIS

Clinical Picture

The parasite is about 3 mm. long with an oval head having two antennae, a powerful mandible and a proboscis. The narrow thorax supports three pairs of legs, each of which has a hook-like extremity. The abdomen is much wider than the thorax. The eggs (nits) are laid on hairs, being affixed by a cement-like substance. The larvae hatch out from the egg by means of a movable lid. *P. capitis* may be asymptomatic and found during the course of routine examination of the scalp, or it may present as itching of the scalp, neck or shoulders, with scratch marks, or as impetigo or pyoderma of the scalp.

On examination, ova are found, obliquely attached to hair shafts, especially in the occipitoparietal region. In light infestations there may be eggs on a few hairs, but in heavy infestations several eggs may be seen attached to one hair shaft. The discovery of adult parasites on clinical examination is difficult except in heavy infestations. Secondary infection causes matting of the hair, an offensive odour, pyoderma, cervical lymphadenitis and sometimes oedema of the orbital tissues causing closure of the eyes.

Treatment

Infestation may affect the family and it is no use treating the individual without at the same time treating all other cases in the house. All infested individuals should be treated concurrently.

The hair is combed thoroughly with a fine-mesh comb to remove the nits (ova). In severe infestations it makes things easier if the hair is cut short. Dicophane Application, B.P.C. (containing 2 per cent. dicophane), is then rubbed into the scalp and not washed out for the next 24 hours; the parasites are not killed immediately and may survive for a few days; Gamma Benzene Hexachloride Application, B.N.F. (contains 0·1 per cent. gamma benzene hexachloride), may be used in a similar way, or *Quellada* lotion which contains 1 per cent. of gamma benzene hexachloride. Benzyl Benzoate Application, B.P. (contains 25 per cent. benzyl benzoate) can also be used and is said to make it easier to remove the nits. Any coccal infection that remains is dealt with afterwards by an antibiotic application. Heat disinfestation of the bedding and headwear should be carried out.

Prophylaxis

Of great importance in the prevention of scalp infestation is daily brushing and combing of the hair and a weekly shampoo. A low intelligence is common in adults with scalp infestations and in the parents of infested children.

PEDICULOSIS CORPORIS

The parasite is structurally similar to *P. capitis* but slightly larger (4 mm. long). Infestation with *P. corporis* is rare in peacetime, except among vagrants and inhabitants of common lodging-houses. In war conditions of overcrowding with poor hygienic facilities, it tends to become more widespread.

Clinical Picture

Itching of the body and scratch marks, excoriations and patchy pigmentation with areas of eczematization and lichenification, sometimes with secondary infection, suggest the diagnosis. Exposed parts escape and the trunk is mostly affected, especially the backs of the shoulders, the waist and the buttocks and the proximal parts of the limbs. The parasites visit the skin to feed and to deposit eggs on coarse hairs, but spend most of their existence on the underclothing and bedding, a completely different mode of life from sarcoptes. Eggs are also affixed to fibres of underwear. If the host is pyrexial the parasites move to the outer clothing and occasionally transference takes place of louse-borne typhus in this way. More common is transference from one person to another under overcrowded and unhygienic conditions.

Diagnosis

Diagnosis is from scabies, senile or general pruritus, and dermatitis herpetiformis. Scabies has a different distribution, pathognomonic signs in the form of burrows, and sarcoptes or ova may be found on scraping. Senile pruritus may present with scratch marks and excoriations but parasites are not found on inspecting the clothing. To exclude pediculosis it is just as important to examine the underwear, particularly at the seams, as it is to examine the skin. Dermatitis herpetiformis affects the shoulder and pelvic girdles chiefly, also the genitalia, elbows and knees. The physical signs are flaccid vesicles, easily ruptured, excoriations and patchy pigmentation. There is a characteristic histology and a brisk response to treatment with dapsone.

Treatment

Dicophane Dusting-powder, B.N.F. (contains 10 per cent. dicophane) liberally dusted on the patient's skin beneath the underwear is effective in controlling the personal infestation. The underclothes and bedding should be heat disinfested and the seams of more superficial garments run over with a hot iron.

Course and Prognosis

Pediculosis is important not only in itself but also as the means of spread of more serious conditions, such as typhus.

PHTHIRIASIS PUBIS

Phthiriasis pubis or crab louse infestation is usually acquired venereally. *Phthirus pubis* is a short, wide, almost triangular louse 1·5 mm. long and about the same width, with three pairs of legs having hook-like ends. Infestation may also take place in the axillae, on coarse hairs covering the body and limbs and, rarely, on the eyebrows, eyelashes or beard. The brownish parasite hides in follicular orifices attached to hair shafts, or suspends itself from two hairs, and the females deposit ova on the hairs. The bites of these parasites may cause blue stains known as 'maculae caeruleae'.

Clinical Picture

There is itching of the pubis and the sufferer often recognizes the presence of the lice. Bluish macules are observed in old cases but few, if any, scratch marks can be seen.

Treatment

Shaving the pubis is a great help. Then Dicophane Application, Gamma Benzene Hexachloride Application, B.N.F., or Benzyl Benzoate Application, B.P., may be applied. Parasites on the eyelashes should be removed with forceps.

INSECT BITES AND STINGS

The flea (human or dog), bed bug, mosquito, gnat or midge may cause urticarial papules with central puncta, tending to be in groups and lines, especially on the limbs, or large blisters may develop, particularly on the legs. Bee, wasp and ant stings may cause more violent allergic reactions in susceptible individuals.

Treatment

The cause must be looked for (in bedding, wall paper and furniture, pets, static water tanks, etc.) and eliminated when possible. Calamine lotion or a diluted steroid cream may be applied and an antihistamine taken by mouth. Attempt should be made to extract a bee sting. If there is a generalized reaction with collapse, a subcutaneous Injection of Adrenaline, B.P. (1 in 1,000), 0·5–1 ml. should be given, followed, if necessary, by 50 mg. of prednisolone-21-phosphate intramuscularly. There are several insect repellent creams available, e.g. dimethyl phthalate.

Myiasis is infestation of the skin with larvae of Diptera, causing maggots in wounds or ulcers, boil-like lesions or creeping eruptions [see Section 2].

ERYTHEMATOUS CONDITIONS

Erythema is a transient redness of the skin due to vasodilatation.

SIMPLE ERYTHEMA

A transient redness of the skin from physical causes such as heat, cold and friction.

INTERTRIGO

A shiny, pink condition of opposing skin surfaces due to erosion of the superficial cells of the epidermis by mutual friction. Secondary infection with *Candida albicans* and cocci is common, giving rise to intertriginous (infective) dermatitis, often with fissuring.

Treatment of intertrigo is by suitable clothing, uplift brassières, etc., to prevent friction of the opposing surfaces and maceration from retention of sweat. For simple intertrigo a dusting powder such as boracic talc powder is suitable. If candida infection is superimposed, Magenta Paint, B.P.C., or nystatin powder is often helpful and if coccal infection develops, the appropriate antibiotic. Silver nitrate solution (2 per cent.) is a useful application to persistent fissures at the depths of the folds.

'TOXIC' ERYTHEMA

A widespread reddening of the skin due to toxic agents: of viral origin in measles and rubella and some coxsackie infections; of streptococcal origin in scarlatina; due to drugs in morbilliform and scarlatiniform drug eruptions and some examples of urticaria, erythema multiforme, etc., or due to unknown causes.

Diagnosis depends on a careful history and examination; on the presence of fever, coryza, photophobia and Koplik's spots in measles; occipital lymphadenopathy in rubella; fever, tachycardia, headache, vomiting, circumoral pallor, exfoliation of the tongue and sore throat in scarlatina; drug eruptions and idiopathic toxic erythemata may occur with or without fever; they do not spread over the body surface in the same order as the exanthemata, and some areas may escape. In scarlatiniform toxic erythema the pattern may be coarse and the peeling more marked than in scarlatina, but mouth lesions may be absent. Milian's ninth-day erythema is a scarlatiniform rash thought to be due to activation of a latent infection by a drug, e.g. arsphenamine or sulphonamides. The phenomenon is known as 'biotropism'. Roseolar syphilides may be mimicked by drug rashes.

Treatment is symptomatic.

FIXED ERYTHEMA

A localized and circumscribed recurrent erythema erupting in the same situation every time one particular drug is taken.

URTICARIA

A transient redness and swelling of the skin, causing weals in the dermis or large hypodermal swellings.

Aetiology

Urticaria is caused by dilatation and increased permeability of the capillaries and small arterioles. Capillary dilatation may arise from the release of histamine from mast cells and arteriolar dilatation from the release of acetylcholine or other activating substances including kinins and globulins.

Urticaria may arise from external or internal causes. The external causes include nettle stings, insect or jellyfish bites, contact with 'wooly bear' caterpillars, or infestation with scabies. In some individuals friction causes wealing (dermographism or factitious urticaria), and any itching condition may then present as urticaria. In others, heat, excitement or exertion cause urtication (cholinergic urticaria). Urticaria from cold or from light (the violet or yellow bands of the spectrum) are both rare.

Internal causes include certain foods and drugs, foci of infection, intestinal parasites and hydatid cysts, cutaneous reticuloses and emotional causes, particular states of resentment and masochism.

Dermal urticaria presents with itchy papules or weals of varying size up to large plaques; hypodermal urticaria presents with large, non-itchy swellings (giant urticaria, angioneurotic oedema, Quincke's oedema). These swellings particularly affect the eyelids, lips and external genitalia and may cause alarm because of their sudden development and gross nature. The tongue and larynx may be involved, necessitating adrenaline injections or even tracheostomy. In the large familiar form the onset is in childhood, abdominal symptoms may occur and the threat to life from laryngeal obstruction may be so great as to render permanent prophylactic tracheostomy essential. In these patients dental procedures may initiate the swellings.

Clinical Picture

Clinically urticaria occurs in two forms: acute or subacute single attacks and chronic or recurrent attacks.

The acute form presents as itchy, pink papules and weals—elevated pink areas with blanched centres brought about by the obliteration of the dermal vessels by the pressure of the exudate. The lesions appear suddenly with intense itching, and disappear just as rapidly, with the result that when the patient attends for examination wealing may be inconspicuous or absent. Urticaria from nettle stings may have pseudopodia, apparently from lymphatic spread of the injected histamine and acetylcholine. Non-itchy hypodermal skin-coloured or pink swellings may also appear, particularly around the eyes or mouth. Swellings within the mouth are rare but potentially lethal at the back of the tongue or on the larynx, from respiratory obstruction. The lesions may recur at intervals for a few hours or days and then cease. Constitutional symptoms are usually slight or absent but anxiety and depression may result from disturbance of sleep due to itching and uncertainty as to the cause. Nervous tension may lower the threshold of reaction to an antigen. Sometimes a gastro-intestinal disturbance precedes the eruption, or foods such as shellfish, strawberries or mushrooms may have been eaten. Other suspect foods include egg, fish, meat, chocolate, nuts and bananas. Urticaria with hay fever may be caused by inhalation of mould spores, grass pollens or animal danders. Acute local urticaria is usually caused by nettle stings or insect bites; it may also occur around sites of injections, e.g. of insulin. Dermographism also tends to be localized to sites where clothes press or rub. Even the removal of adhesive plasters may initiate it, causing, e.g., temporary fogging of patch test readings.

Chronic or recurrent urticaria presents as itchy papules and weals and subcutaneous swellings which usually occur more in the evening. Food and drugs are only occasionally implicated. Drugs such as aspirin or penicillin may activate urticaria or aggravate existing urticaria. The most thorough search for foci of infection or infestation is often unrewarded with success. Rarely, virus infections, malignant foci, reticuloses or collagen disease are responsible. Suppression of intense emotions may cause or aggravate urticaria and fatigue often seems to be the immediate precipitant.

Diagnosis

The recognition of urticaria is usually easy; even if there are no physical signs at the time of the examination the history of transient swellings, perhaps with itching, can only mean urticaria. Dermatitis herpetiformis presents with vesicles, excoriations, crusts and pigmentation. The lesions of erythema multiforme are more persistent than those of urticaria but less itchy.

Giant urticaria is differentiated from erysipelas and contact eczematous dermatitis by the absence of fever and a dusky, brawny swelling which are found in erysipelas, and by the absence of vesiculation and peeling which occur in eczematous dermatitis. Discovery of the cause is another matter. This is often simple in the acute form but in chronic cases it necessitates the most careful history and examination directed towards the discovery of allergens, toxic foci, infestations, physical causes or disturbed attitudes of mind. The urticarioid lesions of the reticuloses must also be borne in mind.

Treatment

Treatment consists of removal or avoidance of the cause; and symptomatic relief by means of antihistaminic drugs while looking for the cause. The patient should be instructed to stop taking any drugs that are not essential. Suspected foods should be avoided and foci of infection treated. Of the antihistaminic drugs, promethazine hydrochloride (*Phenergan*), 25 mg. in the evening or twice a day, is perhaps most useful owing to its powerful soporific effect, but sometimes this action is not desired and then chlorpheniramine (*Piriton*), 4–8 mg. 8-hourly, or mepyramine maleate (*Anthisan*), 100 mg. up to three times a day, may be more suitable, or triprolidine hydrochloride (*Actidil*), 2·5 mg. thrice daily, or 10 mg. daily in the long-acting form (*Pro-Actidil*). The dose of any antihistaminic drug should be adjusted so as to give the best control with a minimum of unwanted side-effects: the dose is reduced and the drug finally withdrawn as the symptoms are relieved. This particularly applies to urticaria from injected drugs such as penicillin. An aperient is sometimes useful. In severe forms rest in bed is advisable. Patients receiving antihistaminic drugs should be warned that these drugs may have a soporific effect and that they should not take them before driving a vehicle or while taking an alcoholic drink.

In laryngeal crises an immediate subcutaneous injection of adrenaline, 0·5 ml., is called for.

In the psychogenic variety, barbiturates or bromides may be as useful as antihistaminic drugs, but if the urticaria is believed to have an allergenic basis it is wise to avoid all drugs except the antihistamines. Relief of the psychogenic type depends on helping the patient to understand the significance of the symptoms in relation to his attitude of mind. Local treatment consists of calamine lotion.

PAPULAR URTICARIA

Synonym. Lichen urticatus.

Aetiology and Pathology

This form of urticaria is commoner in children than in adults and tends to occur most in the summer with recurrences for some years. Insect bites are responsible in most cases.

Clinical Picture

Itchy, skin-coloured or pink, shotty papules appear in crops, mostly on the extensor surfaces of the limbs, sometimes also on the face, buttocks and trunk. The papules often acquire vesicular tops which may become crusted and excoriated.

Diagnosis

Diagnosis is from scabies and varicella. Scabies mostly affects the flexor surfaces and the elementary lesions are burrows and follicular papules. Penile, scrotal and mammary lesions are characteristic. The history may reveal other cases in the family. Varicella presents with a polymorphic eruption of macules, papules, vesicles and crusts. The scalp is often affected and the trunk more than the limbs. Flexures, such as the domes of the axillae, may be involved. There are often vesicles on the buccal mucosa. Insect bites show central puncta but these are often absent in older lesions. Bullae may occur on the legs.

Treatment

The environment of the patient should be examined, often with the help of local authority health officials and veterinary surgeons. Bedding, furniture and wall paper should be examined for bugs; pets and their habitats (rugs, chairs) for infestations; water butts for mosquito larvae; and the patient warned about the greater risk of being bitten by biting insects in the open at dusk. Treatment of the patient consists of calamine lotion and a sedative antihistamine orally. Topical insect repellents are useful for prevention of further lesions.

URTICARIA PIGMENTOSA

Synonyms. Xanthelasmoidea; Telangiectasia macularis eruptiva perstans.

Definition

A macular pigmented eruption with urtication.

Aetiology and Pathology

Most forms represent a mast cell naevoid state but the systemic variety is more akin to a reticulosis. Histologically there are numerous mast cells in the upper dermis.

Clinical Picture

There is a range of conditions from the solitary mast cell urticating naevus through cutaneous mastocytosis to a systemic mastocytosis with involvement of bone marrow, liver and spleen. The infantile form may be maculopapular or nodular. In the commoner maculopapular form, which occurs in the first year after birth, brown macules, urticating papules and small weals are seen. The lesions appear anywhere on the skin in crops, each lesion starting as a maculopapule or weal and proceeding to pigmentation. The pigmented areas urticate on friction. There may be telangiectasia with red maculation and very slight pigmentation as in the form described by Parkes Weber.

Diagnosis

Diagnosis from papular urticaria may be difficult on clinical grounds alone, although the pigmentation usually provides the clue. Firmly stroking a macule reveals the urtication. Biopsy is an important diagnostic aid, revealing mast cells in the dermis. The adult form may be mistaken for secondary syphilis but is recognizable by the urtication.

Treatment

This is symptomatic.

Course and Prognosis

In the infantile form the lesions may disappear after several years.

In the adult form they may be more persistent and the telangiectatic form may proceed to a mast cell reticulosis.

ERYTHEMA MULTIFORME

An eruption with a marked tendency to recurrence, of well-defined, reddened areas of skin, sometimes with blister formation, mostly appearing on the distal parts of the limbs and around the orifices.

Aetiology and Pathology

Erythema multiforme is a reaction of hypersensitivity to known and unknown causes, including bacterial and viral infections and drugs. It is characteristically recurrent and is often preceded by herpes simplex or sometimes by vaccinia. It sometimes follows radiotherapy for Hodgkin's disease or for carcinoma mammae.

Clinical Picture

Erythema multiforme usually affects young adults. There is no obvious seasonal incidence but a marked tendency to recurrence. The distal parts of the limbs and the face are most affected and often the vermilion and mucous surfaces of the lips and the mucosae of the mouth and genitalia are also involved. Lesions on the trunk are less common. There may be malaise for 48 hours before the characteristic outbreak occurs.

The lesions are polymorphic; maculo-erythematous, papulovesicular, bullous and haemorrhagic varieties occur. They persist in one situation throughout an attack and do not show the evanescent properties of urticaria. The central part of the lesions may be paler or darker than the periphery; the former indicates early bulla formation; the latter is due to haemorrhage or to brown pigmentation. In either case the picture of erythema iris results.

When the exudate in these cutaneous lesions has been absorbed they take on a dry, superficially fissured and scaly, brownish-red discoloration, followed by peeling and resolution. The mucosal orogenital lesions differ from those of the skin in that erosion occurs more easily, with the result that a moist ulcerative, pseudomembranous condition results along the vermilion surface of the lips, in the mouth, or on the glans penis or mucosa of the vulva. There may also be pain and swelling of joints, fever and albuminuria; but usually subjective symptoms, including itching, are slight.

The Stevens-Johnson syndrome is a severe variant of erythema multiforme with fever and malaise and with exudative, bullous and erosive cutaneous lesions, extensive and distressing involvement of the mouth, and lesions on the conjunctiva and cornea of the eye which may go on to pannus and blindness. There may also be ulcerative genital lesions and urethritis.

Diagnosis

Diagnosis is from other bullous and erythematous conditions. Thus, pompholyx, dermatitis herpetiformis, pemphigus and pemphigoid, lupus erythematosus and urticaria, may all, at one time or another, have to be excluded. Pompholyx may present with large bullae, but there is no marked erythematous component unless secondary infection occurs. Dermatitis herpetiformis presents with intensely itchy vesicular and eroded lesions on the shoulders, buttocks, elbows, knees or elsewhere, but there is little or no erythematous halo to the lesions. In pemphigus the bullae are flaccid and extend when lateral pressure is applied to them (Nikolsky's sign). They may arise from normal-coloured skin. In pemphigoid the bullae are tense, but Nikolsky's sign is also positive. There may be pink areas around the bullae. Pemphigoid may, in fact, so closely conform to the clinical and histological pattern of erythema multiforme as to be regarded as senile erythema multiforme perstans. Subacute and cutaneously disseminated lupus erythematosus may resemble erythema multiforme but the distribution is more on the face and upper part of the chest. In doubtful cases, a positive antinuclear test, a raised erythrocyte sedimentation rate, leucopenia and increased serum globulins will support the diagnosis of lupus erythematosus. Urticaria is characterized by the short-lived and recurrent nature of its lesions which come and go, first at one site, then at another.

Treatment

Treatment is supportive, by rest (in bed in severe forms) and bland local applications such as calamine lotion or Zinc and Salicylic Acid Paste, B.P. (Lassar's paste). Internally antihistaminic drugs such as mepyramine maleate or promethazine hydrochloride may prove helpful. In the severe Stevens-Johnson form, the administration of prednisone is urgently needed to prevent serious ocular complication. The initial dose should be at least 40 mg. in the first 24 hours, with gradual reductions.

Course and Prognosis

Attacks of erythema multiforme usually clear spontaneously after 2 or 3 weeks, but the recurrence after intervals of months or years are common. The milder form leaves no sequelae but the severe form may lead to dimness of vision or blindness.

ERYTHEMA ANNULARE CENTRIFUGUM (DARIER)

This is believed to be a variant of erythema multiforme, though some examples have seemed to be more akin to dermatitis herpetiformis. There are large annular and polycyclic, pinkish-grey lesions with slightly scaly borders usually with a free edge centripetally. The lesions may slowly extend in one direction and fade out in another.

Treatment

Search should be made for a remote bacterial or fungal focus of infection, for visceral carcinoma, for a blood dyscrasia or for a possible drug cause. Apart from this treatment is symptomatic.

ERYTHEMA MARGINATUM RHEUMATICUM

This condition occurs in about 10 per cent. of patients with acute rheumatism, mostly in children. There are pink or red rings, arcs, segments or polycyclic figures, flat or just palpable. It is usually associated with rheumatic carditis.

PURPURA

There are many causes for the extravasation of blood into the skin; one of three pathological conditions is usually responsible. There may be a defect in the vessel walls due to bacterial or chemical toxins, malnutrition, hepatic or renal disease; there may be a deficiency of platelets or some defect in the complex process of clotting; or there may be an increase of capillary pressure.

In the first group is purpura in meningococcal septicaemia or subacute bacterial endocarditis; also the purpura of fulminating exanthemata—scarlet fever, measles, smallpox, typhus, etc. Certain drugs, e.g. iodides, barbiturates, sulphonamides, phenylbutazone, quinidine and others may cause purpura. The purpura of scurvy is due to a lack of support to the vessels owing to a deficiency of the ground substance between the endothelial cells.

Henoch-Schoenlein purpura or 'allergic' purpura is caused by damage to the capillary endothelial cells [see Section 4].

Thrombocytopenic purpura is considered in Section 13.

Dysproteinaemia is a rare cause of purpura. With cryoglobulinaemia there is purpura on exposed parts in cold conditions. In hyperglobulinaemia itchy red papules may develop, proceeding to purpura, transient or persistent.

Purpura may also occur on the legs from increased capillary pressure as in hypostatic conditions. Eczema on the legs may become purpuric. Senile purpura, due to degeneration of connective tissue occurs on areas of skin which have been most exposed to sunlight. Irregular patches occur mostly on the supinator aspects of the forearms and on the backs of the hands. In steroid purpura there is a similar condition not limited to sun-exposed areas.

Diagnosis

Purpura is differentiated from erythematous lesions by the persistence of the dark red colour on diascopy—examination through a glass spatula, slide or watch-glass with which pressure is applied so as to expel blood from the vessels. Discovery of the cause of the purpura depends on a full and careful clinical investigation with particular attention to the diet, drugs, fever, enlargement of the spleen and manifestations of non-cutaneous allergy or purpura, such as joint swellings, haematuria, intestinal colic, etc. A full blood and platelet count is essential and an estimation of the clotting and bleeding times. In the rare cryoglobulinaemic purpura, the plasma undergoes gelification at room temperatures. It chiefly affects exposed parts.

Treatment

Treatment is of the cause. This is dealt with more fully elsewhere [see Section 13].

THE CAPILLAROSES

In addition to frank purpura the skin may be affected by pigmentary and telangiectatic conditions which have been given various clinical descriptions but which all show a similar histological picture suggesting some damage to the endothelium of the vessels.

Aetiology and Pathology

In all types the cause is unknown.

Clinical Picture

This varies according to the type of capillarosis.

In *Majocchi's disease* (purpura annularis telangiectodes) the patients are usually young women and the eruption consists of discs or rings of telangiectasia with brown discoloration due to slight extravasations of blood. The lesions form on the thighs or legs, and very slowly extend peripherally and heal centrally with a slight residuum of atrophy.

In *Schamberg's disease* (progressive pigmentary dermatosis) men are usually affected, on the legs more often than elsewhere, but sometimes at sites of pressure. Dark, reddish-brown puncta 'cayenne pepper' spots, are visible in a zone of brownish skin. The lesions may itch and they slowly enlarge but may ultimately resolve spontaneously, leaving some pigmentation. A similar condition is sometimes seen on the legs of patients with varicosities.

The pigmented lichenoid *purpuric dermatitis of Gougerot and Blum* presents with discrete and agglomerated papules, with petechiae, pigmentation and telangiectasia. The lesions may appear on the trunk or on the limbs.

Angioma serpiginosum (Hutchinson) presents with telangiectasia which by clearance at one site and spread at another comes to acquire an annular or a serpiginous arrangement. The body or limbs may be affected.

Treatment

As no cause is at present known for these conditions, only supportive treatment can be offered. The patient should be investigated for foci of infection, diabetes and vascular hypertension. Inquiry should be made about drugs, particularly carbromal, which may cause a fine brick-coloured and purpuric dermatosis affecting mostly the dependent parts.

COLLAGEN DISEASES AND CUTANEOUS VASCULITIS [see Section 4]

DRUG ERUPTIONS (DERMATITIS MEDICAMENTOSA)

Many drugs can cause skin eruptions but some do so more than others. Some individuals, for inherited or acquired reasons, are unduly susceptible to drugs. Ill effects may arise from the external application or the internal administration of drugs or from external application followed by the internal administration of the same or a chemically similar substance.

External Use: Drugs used externally may cause contact eczematous dermatitis after repeated applications; some drugs cause sensitization to light; others have toxic effects on internal organs after absorption.

Internal Use: There may be direct toxic effect on the skin (overdosage, genetic intolerance, impaired metabolism or excretion, accumulation); there may be cutaneous vascular reactions from direct histamine-releasing drugs or from antigen-antibody histamine-releasing drugs; there may be toxic effects on bone marrow, liver, kidneys, thermostatic centre, etc., causing purpura, skin infections, nutritional deficiency, haematuria, albuminuria, fever, etc.; platelet-drug antigens may be formed; indirect toxic effects may result from the destruction of bacteria and the release of their toxins; organisms capable of synthesizing vitamin B in the gut may be destroyed, absorption may be interfered with, or competitors of *Candida albicans* may be eliminated, causing candidiasis; there may be competition for enzymes essential for cellular welfare; no doubt, many other mechanisms exist.

External and Internal Cross-Effects

Eczematoid eruptions may occur after the systemic administration of a drug which has previously applied to the surface.

Clinical Picture

Many drugs cause non-specific eruptions while only a few have specific effects.

Non-specific eruptions include morbilliform and scarlatiniform erythemata, erythema multiforme, with or without bulla formation, urticaria and purpura. More specific effects include pruritus, fixed eruptions, erythroderma, epidermal necrolysis, pigmentation, eczematoid, psoriasiform, acneiform, lichenoid, seborrhoeic or pityriasis rosea-like eruptions, granulomata, stomatitis and urethritis. Systemic effects include fever and granulocytopenia. Usually there is something atypical about a drug eruption which differentiates it from the disease it mimics. There are many unexplained eruptions where a drug cause is suspected but not proven. Some are due to virus infections, others may be due to food additives. Table salt fortified with iodide or drinks containing quinine are occasionally responsible; phenolphthalein has been used as a substitute for cochineal! It is speculative how much synthetic dyes, flavourings, sweeteners, preservatives and other chemical 'sophisticants' of food are responsible.

The commoner manifestations and some of the drugs that may cause them are indicated below. Clearly this list needs constant review.

ACNEIFORM OR PUSTULAR: androgens, bromides, corticosteroids, corticotrophin, iodides, isoniazid, sulphonamides. Phenobarbitone may aggravate.

ALBUMINURIA: bismuth, calciferol, gold, mercury, sera, sulphonamides.

ALOPECIA (CICATRICIAL): gold, mepacrine. (NON-CICATRICIAL): diffuse hair loss—aminopterin, amphetamines, antimitotic agents, arsenic, colchicine, heparin, progestogens, salicylates, thallium acetate, vitamin A when taken in large doses.

BULLOUS: arsenicals, barbiturates, bromides, chloral, cinchophen, dapsone, iodides, phenazone, phenolphthalein, phenytoin, quinacrine, quinine, salicylates, streptomycin, sulphonamides.

CYANOSIS: dapsone, phenacetin, sulphonamides.

ECZEMATOID: (drug externally applied and subsequently taken internally), antihistamines, arsenic, gold, halogens, hydroxyquinolines, mepacrine, mercury, penicillin, streptomycin, sulphonamides; also topical aromatic benzenes of the para-amino group and systemic sulphonamides, local anaesthetics of the benzocaine group, thiazides and chlorpropamide; topical neomycin and systemic streptomycin or kanamycin; topical hydrazine and systemic isoniazid, *Apresoline* or *Nardil*; topical Balsam of Peru and systemic cinnamon; topical formaldehyde and systemic *Mandelamine*; topical thiuram and systemic Antabuse; topical chlorbutanol and systemic chloral hydrate.

EPIDERMAL NECROLYSIS: dapsone, hydantoin, penicillin, phenolphthalein, phenylbutazone, sulphonamides.

ERYTHEMA, FIXED (LOCALIZED AND RECURRENT): phenolphthalein most commonly; also arsenic, amidopyrine, barbiturates, bismuth, bromides, cinchophen, dapsone, gold, iodides, mercury, penicillin, phenazone, phenytoin, quinine, quinidine, salicylates, sulphonamides, tetracycline.

ERYTHEMA, MORBILLIFORM OR SCARLATINIFORM: most drugs mentioned elsewhere, particularly barbiturates and sulphonamides; also antibiotics, antihistamines, atropine, belladonna, chloral hydrate, digitalis, ephedrine, gold salts, insulin, ipecachuanha, isoniazid, organic mercurials, para-aminosalicylic acid, phenothiazines, phenylbutazone, procaine, quinine, quinidine, rhubarb, salicylates, santonin, thiazides.

ERYTHEMA MULTIFORME: acetanilide, barbiturates, bismuth, bromides, dapsone, gold, iodides, phenazone, quinine, salicylates, sera, sulphonamides, thiouracil.

ERYTHEMA NODOSUM: iodides, salicylates, sulphonamides thiouracil.

ERYTHRODERMA: arsenic (organic), barbiturates, bismuth, gold, mepacrine, mercury, para-aminosalicylic acid, phenolphthalein, phenylbutazone, phenytoin, quinine, streptomycin, sulphonamides.

FEVER: arsenic, barbiturates, para-aminosalicylic acid, quinidine, sulphonamides, streptomycin.

GENITAL LESIONS: phenazone, phenolphthalein, quinine.

GINGIVITIS: bismuth, mercury, phenytoin (hypertrophy).

GRANULOCYTOPENIA: amidopyrine, antihistamines, arsenic, barbiturates, chloramphenicol, cytotoxic drugs, isoniazid, phenazone, phenylbutazone, sodium aminosalicylate, sulphonamides, thiouracil.

GRANULOMATOUS, VEGETATING, ULCERATIVE: halogens.

GYNAECOMASTIA: oestrogens, ACTH, monoamine oxidase inhibitors.

HERPES SIMPLEX: arsenic.

INFECTIVE (SEBORRHOEIC) DERMATITIS: arsenic, gold, mepacrine, mercury, penicillin, sulphonamides.

KERATOSES, EPITHELIOMATA: arsenic (inorganic).

LICHENOID: amiphenazole, arsenic, bismuth, chloroquine. chlorothiazide, gold, mepacrine, methyldopa, phenothiazine, quinine, quinidine.

LIGHT SENSITIZATION: arsenic, chlorpromazine, gold, mercury, quinine, sulphonamides.

LUPUS ERYTHEMATOSUS: antibiotics, anticonvulsants, some ganglion-blocking drugs, griseofulvin, hydantoin, hydralazine, phenylbutazone, sulphonamides, thiouracil.

PIGMENTATION: antimalarials, arsenic, barbiturates, chlorpromazine, corticotrophin, hydantoin, phenazone, phenolphthalein, quinine; also bismuth, gold and silver deposited in the skin.

PITYRIASIS ROSEA-LIKE: antihistamines, arsenic, gold, mepacrine.

PRURITUS, ANOGENITAL: wide-spectrum oral antibiotics, codeine, phenolphthalein, quinine.

PRURITUS, GENERAL: belladonna, codeine, morphine, opium; also amidopyrine, arsenic, bismuth, gold, mepacrine, penicillin, phenobarbitone, phenolphthalein, sulphonamides, etc.

PSORIASIFORM: arsenic, gold, mepacrine.

PURPURA: amidopyrine, antihistamines, arsenic, aspirin, barbiturates, belladonna, bismuth, carbromal, chloral hydrate, chloramphenicol, chlorothiazide, chlorpromazine, corticosteroids, diethylstilboestrol, glyceryl trinitrate, gold, halogens, isoniazid, menthol, meprobamate, mercury, novobiocin, para-aminosalicylic acid, penicillin, phenazone, phenytoin, piperazine, quinine, quinidine, reserpine, salicylates, *Sedormid*, sera, snake venom, sodium aminosalicylate, sulphonal, sulphonamides, thiourea, tolbutamide.

STOMATITIS: antibiotics, arsenic, barbiturates, bismuth, gold, halogens, mercury, phenacetin, phenazone, phenolphthalein, quinine, salicylates, sulphonamides (and see granulocytopenia).

TINNITUS: Quinine, salicylates (also nasal congestion and lacrimation).

TUBERCULIDES (EXACERBATION): calciferol.

URTICARIA: most of the drugs in the list; arsenic, aspirin, barbiturates, bromides, iodides, isoniazid, nicotinic acid, organ extracts, penicillin, phenacetin, phenolphthalein, pollen vaccines, procaine, quinine, salicylates, sera, sulphonamides, thiouracil and toxoids are some of the commoner causes.

VESICULATION (VARIOLIFORM): halogens, sulphonamides.

VISUAL DISTURBANCES: chloroquine—haloes (reversible) or retinitis (rare, irreversible).

ZOSTER: arsenic.

Diagnosis

The possibility of drug causation or aggravation has to be borne in mind in many dermatoses, particularly if there is something atypical in the eruption, and questioning has to be directed accordingly. Analgesics, aperients, hypnotics, sedatives and antibiotics are particularly suspect. Withdrawal of a suspected drug may be followed by immediate improvement. With non-specific eruptions and when the patient has been taking more than one drug, a test dose is sometimes justifiable. This should only be given when the dermatosis has subsided and one-tenth of the previous therapeutic dosage should be given in the first instance because if the full dose is given an unnecessarily violent reaction may result.

Prevention and Treatment

The history may indicate sensitivity to one or more drugs. Some drug eruptions result from neglecting to inquire into this possibility. Potent drugs are sometimes used without sufficient justification. In every case it is a useful self-discipline to ask oneself, 'Do the advantages likely to be obtained by giving this drug outweight its possible ill effects?' Whenever there is a choice, a drug of lesser toxicity and sensitizing potential should be used. Especial care is necessary when there is albuminuria.

To make treatment easier, it is as well to tell the patient of possible side-effects of a drug. This encourages discontinuation of the drug immediately untoward symptoms develop and prevents further toxicity. For most drug eruptions, withdrawal of the drug is all the treatment that is necessary or, in fact, possible. An aperient or an enema is sometimes useful when there is reason to think that some of the drug remains in the bowel. Specific treatments are indicated in a few conditions. For halogen eruptions, sodium chloride or ammonium chloride may be given in a dose of 5–10 G. daily. In severe cases with toxaemia, intravenous normal saline infusions should be given daily, 100 ml. on each occasion, for a week.

Heavy metal intoxications (gold, bismuth, mercury) are treated with Dimercaprol, B.P. (BAL), 2 ml. four-hourly, gradually reduced to 2 ml. daily, in a course lasting a week. The pigmentation of argyria is permanent. The effects of inorganic arsenic (raindrop pigmentation, keratoses, carcinomata, hepatitis) are irreversible. The keratoses are best treated with carbon dioxide snow application and the epitheliomata by X-irradiation, excision or carbon dioxide snow, depending on their size, depth and situation. Toxic effects from organic arsenic need treatment with dimercaprol.

Rest in bed is advisable for the more severe eruptions. Plenty of fluid should be given. Repeated urine examinations should be made and haemoglobin deficiency, leucopenia or thrombocytopenia should be excluded. Vitamin C in large doses is indicated and multiple vitamin supplements are justified. Blood transfusions may tide the patient over a period of marrow depression. Antihistamines are helpful in urticaria but in other conditions can only help by their sedative and antipruritic actions; in certain circumstances they may even aggravate, e.g. an antihistamine of phenothiazine structure is likely to aggravate a chlorpromazine reaction. Local treatment of drug rashes usually consists of the application of calamine lotion or a diluted steroid preparation. Systemic steroids may have to be administered for the more severe types of reaction, including erythroderma, vasculitis, bullous eruptions, severe serum sickness or anaphylactic shock (preceded by adrenaline therapy) and epidermal necrolysis.

Course and Prognosis

Many eruptions are transitory, clearing rapidly after withdrawal of the drug; but penicillin urticaria may persist for several weeks and halogen eruptions may continue to worsen for a time after the drug has been withdrawn. Vasculitis has prolonged effects. Some drugs are cumulative in their effects; for example gold may cause a dermatosis that steadily worsens although administration of the drug has ceased. Inorganic arsenic has delayed effects, the first sign often appearing some years after the drug was first taken, possibly even several years after its use has been abandoned.

The prognosis depends on the possibilities of inducing elimination of the drug and on the degree of reversibility of its effects on cells of the skin, vasculature, liver, kidneys, bone marrow, etc.

ERYTHRODERMA

Synonym. Exfoliative dermatitis.

Erythroderma is a persistent redness of the skin, with a varying amount of exfoliation (as opposed to erythema, which is transitory).

Aetiology and Pathology

There are numerous causes for this type of reaction. It may develop as a result of over-treatment of eczema-dermatitis, infective dermatitis or psoriasis. A number of drugs can cause it. It may be a manifestation of malabsorption. It also occurs in an idiopathic form as lymphadenopathic erythroderma, a condition which is probably toxic and sometimes recurrent, with much pigmentation (lipomelanic 'reticulosis').

Another form of erythroderma is associated with lymphoblastomatous reticulosis (*l'homme rouge*), sometimes preceding or following the clinical phenomenon of mycosis fungoides and ultimately being accompanied by an increase of circulating lymphocytes. An erythrodermatous form of sarcoidosis also occurs. The more superficial variety of pemphigus (pemphigus foliaceus) presents as erythroderma. Biopsy is often helpful in the differential diagnosis of the erythrodermata but sometimes repeat biopsies are necessary at intervals of several months to establish the diagnosis of a reticulosis, the histology in the early stages often being non-specific.

Clinical Picture

In the over-treatment form there is a history of a preceding more localized dermatosis and of its extension to the condition observed following the application of one or more known irritants or sensitizers. There is coarse peeling with moderate redness and sometimes a greasy texture to the scales particularly in the flexures. In the toxic forms the exfoliation develops uniformly during or after a course of treatment with one of the drugs mentioned elsewhere. In both types fissuring and secondary infection may develop and there may be considerable enlargement of the regional lymph nodes.

In the idiopathic lymphadenopathic erythroderma the skin is dark brown and shiny and the exfoliative element is often less marked. The lymph nodes are enlarged and rubbery and those at the axillae and the groins may be seen bulging the skin.

In lymphoblastoma with erythroderma the skin is red and coarsely peeling. The lymph nodes, liver and spleen may all be palpably enlarged.

In all forms of erythroderma, heat loss is excessive and care must be taken not to expose the patient unduly during examination. Cardiac embarrassment may arise from the greatly increased cutaneous blood flow. There may be diffuse loss of hair and thickening of the nails.

Diagnosis

Psoriasis universale can develop without any over-treatment and may resemble erythroderma of the *l'homme rouge* type. The history, the redness and the mica-like scales should make the diagnosis clear. Pemphigus foliaceus (pemphigus erythematodes) is often patchy and has a distinctive histological appearance. In infants, extensive staphylococcal pemphigus may have erythrodermatous characteristics (Ritter's disease).

Treatment

Bland applications should be used and they should not be occlusive. Oily calamine lotion, oily cream or aqueous cream are all useful. Bed rest and sedation may be necessary. The skin may be cleaned with a bland vegetable oil. When malabsorption is present treatment is directed to the special dietetic requirements of minerals, vitamins and protein.

In the toxic form Dimercaprol, B.P., is valuable when arsenic, gold, mercury or bismuth is believed to be responsible. It is best given in a 6-day course, 2 ml. 4-hourly on the first day, 2 ml. twice daily on the second, third and fourth days, and 2 ml. daily on the fifth and sixth days.

In severe or resistant forms systemic treatment with a corticosteroid is indicated, starting with a dose of 30 mg. of prednisone daily. Prednisone may also give symptomatic relief in the lymphomatous form, without objective relief beyond a slight diminution of scaling. Cytotoxic drugs may give temporary relief.

Course and Prognosis

The over-treatment form resolves with suitable bland treatment. The toxic form persists longer, depending on the intensity of the damage caused by the toxic agent and the speed of its elimination from the system. The worst forms may be fatal from bronchopneumonia, hepatic or renal failure. The idiopathic form tends to clear up after some months, with a tendency to recur even after an interval of years. The lymphomatous form is steadily progressive, with a fatal outcome.

SQUAMOUS DERMATOSES

PSORIASIS

Definition

Psoriasis is a common condition of sharply marginated reddened areas of skin with abnormal scaling. It is most variable in its intensity and course, remissions, recurrences and exacerbations being a characteristic feature.

Aetiology and Pathology

The fundamental abnormality appears to be a biochemical fault in epidermal cell formation, with a too rapid turnover of cells resulting in abnormal horn cells. The fault is inherited and psoriasis occurs in 1 in 5 on the average, of children of a psoriatic parent. The first signs are usually noted in the second or third decades but it may first appear in children under 10 or in persons over 30 or even in old age.

Precipitating factors are the hereditary predisposition, infections, an unfavourable environment, emotional stresses and trauma to the skin.

Clinical Picture

From the clinical standpoint, psoriasis can be divided into seven types:

1. Guttate psoriasis, often in childhood.
2. Localized extensor psoriasis.
3. Flexural psoriasis.
4. Widespread or universal psoriasis.
5. Pustular psoriasis of the palms and soles.
6. Widespread pustular psoriasis.
7. Psoriasis of the nails.

GUTTATE PSORIASIS

This may have no obvious precipitant but often there is a history of an infection, particularly a streptococcal throat infection, some ten days to three weeks before the onset of the rash. It may begin after scarlet fever or varicella, measles or mumps, suggesting that the malady is a type reaction of certain individuals to various infections.

The lesions are raindrop-sized, pink, flat-topped papules, with scaling which is at first inconspicuous. Itching is slight or absent. The scaling is made more obvious by scraping (grattage) a papule with a spatula (not a finger nail!). This makes visible the silvery mica-like delicate scales, and pin-point bleeding indicates the presence of dermal papillae very near the surface. The lesions are widespread, even generalized in distribution, but the face and hands tend to be less affected.

Diagnosis

Guttate psoriasis has to be differentiated from a secondary papulosquamous syphilide. In psoriasis there is no lymph node enlargement or mucosal involvement. The skin lesions are not infiltrated or ham-coloured in psoriasis and, although the scalp may be affected, there is no loss of hair.

Infective (seborrhoeic) dermatitis presents with dirty grey scales of greasy texture beginning as follicular papules which affect by preference the face, sweat grooves and flexures; the scalp is involved, with loss of hair.

In pityriasis rosea the lesions are oval, pink or fawn-coloured, with a centripetal free border to the collarette. They occur on the trunk and proximal parts of the limbs.

Lichen planus presents with itchy, violaceous, polygonal papules with a waxy glance, mostly on the flexor surfaces.

Treatment

Oily calamine lotion is a useful local application. All measures directed towards improving the general well-being are likely to help, including a holiday, vitamin supplements and (if under skilled observation) ultra-violet irradiation with a suberythema exposure daily. It is advisable to make an X-ray examination of the chest before starting this treatment.

Course and Prognosis

Provided the condition is not over-treated, this form of psoriasis often gradually clears in about 3 months. In others, it may persist, with enlargement of some of the lesions to coin-like (nummular) or discoid areas. At any time in life there may be recurrences, usually of the discoid type, the guttate form rarely returning.

LOCALIZED EXTENSOR PSORIASIS

This may exist from the beginning and may persist. with fluctuations, for the remainder of the patient's life, without any obvious disturbance in the general health. This type may begin in childhood or in adult life and is most common at and just below the tip of the elbows and over the patella and patellar tendon. Other sites, often affected, include the lumbosacral region, the calves, the forearms and the scalp, or any of these areas may be affected alone. The lesions may be nummular, circular rather than oval, circinate, polycyclic or irregular in shape (psoriaris geographica). There is usually no itching.

Diagnosis

Nummular eczema may resemble a nummular psoriasis but the lesions are papulovesicular, exuding or crusted. A single chronic patch of psoriasis has to be differentiated from lichen simplex, lupus vulgaris, tuberculoid leprosy, tertiary syphilis, Bowen's disease and superficial basal cell epithelioma [p. 1084].

The patient is encouraged to accept the lesions as blemishes which are not contagious and which do not interfere with the general health. A pessimistic attitude can only aggravate the condition. It is true that psoriasis is incurable as far as removing the basic cause is concerned. Nevertheless, the active manifestations can largely be suppressed and activating or aggravating factors can be alleviated.

Treatment

Localized lesions may respond well to daily applications of solution of coal tar with a camel-hair brush, followed by soft paraffin ointment to any cracked or excessively dry areas. Solution of coal tar may also be applied in a 6–12 per cent. concentration in emulsifying ointment, simple ointment or soft paraffin ointment. 2–4 per cent. of salicylic acid may be added. Emulsifying ointment mixes with skin fats and so brings the tar into more intimate contact with the skin. Simple ointment, and to a greater extent soft paraffin ointment, mitigate the action of the tar but they are often more effective because of their greater soft paraffin content.

The application of one or other of the more powerful corticosteroid ointments is often highly effective when used with polythene film occlusion by night. Treatment may have to be stopped if folliculitis develops. Remissions induced by this treatment are often of short duration.

FLEXURAL PSORIASIS

Flexural psoriasis is most commonly seen in the obese, and friction between opposing surfaces of skin plays an important part. The axillae, submammary folds, umbilicus, genitocrural folds and intergluteal cleft may be affected. Secondary infection may occur, particularly with *Candida albicans*. Sometimes diabetes mellitus coexists. Psoriasis of the genitocrural region may be either the result of friction or the cause of pruritus vulvae. The lesions are sharply marginated, smooth, shiny salmon-red areas, without satellites.

Diagnosis

The presence of psoriasis elsewhere usually helps in differentiation from infective dermatitis and from intertrigo. The absence of satellite lesions and the sharply demarcated salmon-pink involvement of opposing surfaces is characteristic of psoriasis.

Treatment

Obesity, diabetes mellitus and various causes of flexural and anogenital pruritus need attention. Topical corticosteroid preparations are often effective, even in dilution.

WIDESPREAD OR UNIVERSAL PSORIASIS

This may develop *de novo* or it may follow guttate psoriasis or localized psoriasis of the extensor or flexor surfaces. The reason for the extension may be some infection, over-treatment, intoxication, bad environmental conditions or emotional stress, due either to environmental or to personal difficulties. There may be no constitutional disturbance but mental depression is common. A persistent widespread rash may easily induce that feeling of ostracism often called the 'leper complex' and this accounts for the depression in some cases but, in others, the variation of mood coincides with changes in the state of the skin, neither preceding nor following them, and suggests that fluctuations in intensity of the psoriasis and mood changes are often due to a common cause. The involvement may be widespread, subtotal or universal. The lesions may be nummular, discoid, figurate, polycyclic or annular. The Koebner phenomenon may be present, in which scratching the skin causes the development of psoriasis in the line of scratch. The skin in the centre of annular lesions may not show this reaction, having become refractory for a time to this stimulus. The sites commonly affected include the scalp (where the scales may be in several diminishing layers giving a limpet-like appearance—rupioid psoriasis), the trunk, particularly the lumbosacral region, the extensor surfaces of the limbs and the nails. Sometimes the flexures are also affected. The face and hands usually escape except in severe cases. Arthropathy mostly affecting the smaller joints is often associated with excessive psoriasis. [See Section 10.]

Treatment

Admission to hospital is often advisable for investigation and treatment. Infective, metabolic and emotional disorders need attention. If a topical corticosteroid is to be used it is advisable to treat the upper limbs on one occasion, the trunk on a second and the lower limbs on a third. This lessens the risk of excessive absorption, and makes the treatment more tolerable. The corticosteroid should be diluted 1 in 5 for extensive use. Polythene jackets, roll, gloves and foot-bags are worn at night in order to increase the efficacy of the corticosteroid application.

Often it is better to treat the patient with the more old-fashioned Goeckerman regime which has stood the test of time well. The patient's skin is cleansed of ointment with liquid paraffin each morning and general ultra-violet irradiation is given in a sub-erythema exposure. The patient next takes a warm bath to which is added 60–120 ml. of solution of coal tar to 100 litres of water. The skin is washed with a toilet soap but forcible removal of scales is inadvisable. After the bath 6 per cent. solution of coal tar in soft paraffin is rubbed in, except at the flexures where 2 per cent. of coal tar solution in simple ointment or simple ointment alone may be used. For the scalp equal parts of Teepol and water with 1 per cent. of glycerin makes an effective shampoo. Corticosteroid preparations in special vehicles for use on the scalp are available. Coal tar and Salicylic Acid Ointment, B.P.C., is a useful alternative.

Dithranol is effective, being especially useful for the management of thickened plaques on the extensor surfaces and on the trunk. Except for patients who are experienced and can be trusted the treatment is best carried out under supervision. Starting with dithranol, 0·1 per cent. in Lassar's paste, the strength can gradually be increased as desired even up to 1·0 per cent. Injudicious use can aggravate and even initiate exfoliative dermatitis. Dithranol stains the skin a violet-brown colour. Its daily application is continued until the lesions look paler than the surrounding skin. It is then withheld and soft paraffin ointment used instead. Dithranol causes a severe conjunctivitis if it gets inadvertently transferred to the eyes.

Oral systemic treatment with corticosteroids is inadvisable, because of the risks of habituation, side-effects and withdrawal exacerbations.

Methotrexate, a cytotoxic drug with folic-acid antagonistic properties, is sometimes used for inveterate psoriasis. Its use should be limited to males not wishing to procreate and to women past the child-bearing age. There should be no evidence of impaired function of bone marrow, liver or kidneys and before each injection there should be a routine check on the blood count, liver function tests and blood urea. The initial dose by injection is 30 mg.

Sedation may be necessary, or euphoriants for depressed patients. Emotional factors are best dealt with by open discussion. Complete clearance of lesions is the ideal but often the physician has to encourage the patient to learn to live with partial clearance.

The treatment of psoriasis is no routine matter but consists of dealing with each individual according to his needs.

A holiday in pleasant surroundings with relaxation and isolation from the telephone may be as effective as any of the above measures.

Course and Prognosis

This is uncertain and often unfavourable unless causal factors can be controlled.

PUSTULAR PSORIASIS OF THE PALMS AND SOLES

Synonyms. Acrodermatitis perstans; Pustular bacteride.

Clinical Picture

The 'pustules' are creamy from the beginning, proceeding to brown macules. There is no vesicular phase. The lesions occur on palms and soles, sometimes on fingers or toes, in areas of red scaly skin. Psoriasis may also occur on the palms as ill-defined areas of redness and scaling. Either form may occur with or without lesions of psoriasis elsewhere.

Diagnosis

This is from tinea pedis, in which there are translucent vesicles or irregular centripetally peeling patches; also from eczema, in which there is usually uniform 'frog-spawn' vesiculation.

Treatment

Soft paraffin ointment is often helpful, controlling any tendency to fissuring. The stronger corticosteroid ointments, applied beneath polythene film, may be effective, if tolerated. Often the condition persists in spite of all treatment.

Course and Prognosis

Chronicity is the rule but some cases gradually resolve.

WIDESPREAD PUSTULAR PSORIASIS

This develops in psoriatic individuals as an acute pustular eruption, with fever, malaise and leucocytosis. The pustules appear in crops and the prognosis is poor. Fortunately it is a rare condition. Arthropathy is common. The sterile pin-head pustules develop either on existing lesions of chronic psoriasis, on erythroderma or on normal skin. The flexures are worst affected. The nails are thickened or detached from their beds by collections of pus. The inside of the mouth may be affected, also the external genitalia. Reiter's disease is probably a variant.

Aetiology

Aetiological factors include infections, metabolic disorders particularly hypocalcaemia, possibly activated by pregnancy as in impetigo herpetiformis, also with diabetes mellitus. The systemic use of corticosteroids for psoriasis or some other condition may precipitate an attack, and various drugs including antimalarials, iodides and salicylates have been reported to cause it.

Treatment

Any infection or metabolic disorder should be treated. A course of tetracycline may be helpful. Systemic corticosteroids are contra-indicated. In the absence of any contra-indication cytotoxic drugs, e.g. methotrexate, may be helpful. Local treatment should be bland. If topical corticosteroid applications are used they should be diluted.

Course and Prognosis

Some patients die from infection, toxicity or exhaustion. Others slowly recover to the original milder psoriatic state or to erythrodermatous psoriasis.

PSORIASIS OF THE NAILS

This usually occurs with psoriasis elsewhere but occasionally it is the only evidence of the disease.

Clinical Picture

The mildest form is a thimble-like pitting of the nail plate. This may vary in extent from a single pit on one nail to extensive involvement of several nails. Pitting is strongly diagnostic of psoriasis. It occasionally occurs also in alopecia areata and in eczema.

With worse involvement there is brown or yellow discoloration of parts or all of the nail plates, without thickening. When the nail beds and matrices are affected the nail plates become dull, discoloured, thickened, hard and opaque. Paronychial involvement causes deformity with longitudinal or transverse ridging and grooving.

Diagnosis

Psoriasis unguium has to be differentiated from tinea unguium, and eczema-dermatitis affecting the nail folds. Rarer possibilities include syphilis, lichen planus and idiopathic nail dystrophies.

Ringworm usually affects one or a few nails of the hands and feet in asymmetrical fashion and is often associated with ringworm elsewhere in toe clefts, on the feet or hands or in the groins. Microscopic examination of nail shavings removed with the edge of a glass microscope slide reveals fragments of mycelium. The nails in ringworm are usually a dirty grey colour, with irregular deformity, a honeycomb texture and a powdery friable surface.

Syphilis or lichen planus are recognized by evidence of the presence of these diseases elsewhere. The affected nails in lichen planus are markedly atrophic. Rarely, with alopecia areata, the nails are pitted. Idiopathic nail dystrophy is a discoloured and deformed condition of the nails without evidence of psoriasis or of other skin disease elsewhere.

Treatment

Paronychial psoriasis may respond to the application of a corticosteroid, with occlusion. Paronychial injections of triamcinolone, preferably by a dermojet, may help other forms.

PARAPSORIASIS

This is a descriptive term for some forms of persistent scaling. They are relatively rare and of unknown cause but are probably distinct conditions.

PITYRIASIS LICHENOIDES CHRONICA

Synonym. Parapsoriasis guttata.

There are guttate grey-brown scaly lesions, the scales being single and concave (scutuliform) without the mica-like appearance on grattage so characteristic of psoriasis. They are distributed on the trunk and limbs and itching is usually slight and adjoining redness inconspicuous. The lesions may persist for several months, without constitutional disturbance. Young or middle-aged adults are usually affected.

Diagnosis

Secondary syphilis, lichen planus, drug eruptions and pityriasis rosea must be excluded. The prolonged course rules out syphilis and pityriasis rosea. In syphilis, mucosal changes, condylomata, enlarged lymph nodes and traces of a primary lesion may be found and the lesions tend to be ham coloured. In pityriasis rosea, the herald patch, characteristic distribution, cleavage line patterning and centripetal peeling are characteristic. Lichen planus is usually very itchy, the lesions give a 'waxy glance', have a characteristic distribution and often involve the mouth and external genitalia.

Treatment

This is ineffective.

Course and Prognosis

The condition usually persists for several months but spontaneous remissions may occur. It is sometimes the precursor of a cutaneous reticulosis.

PITYRIASIS LICHENOIDES ET VARIOLIFORMIS ACUTA

This is more sudden in onset, presenting with lichenoid and varioliform lesions, necrotizing and crusting. It is a form of cutaneous vasculitis, and may resolve spontaneously after weeks or months, leaving depressed scars. The palms, soles and mucosae escape. The lymph nodes may be enlarged.

Diagnosis

This is from variola and varicella, secondary syphilis, drug eruptions, pityriasis rosea and lichen planus.

Treatment

This is symptomatic, and supportive.

PARAPSORIASIS DISCOIDES

Synonyms. Parapsoriasis en plaques; Xantho-erythroderma perstans.

Clinical Picture

This presents as fawn to pink discs and ovals, some with finger-like extensions, non-itchy, on the trunk and limbs, usually in adults of 30 years or more.

The lesions tend to lie with their long axes parallel to lines of cleavage, e.g. in the line of the ribs. There is fine scaling and often slight atrophy. There is no constitutional disturbance.

Treatment

The condition is unresponsive to treatment and tends to progress slowly.

Course and Prognosis

A benign form persists for years without any change to a reticulosis. Others develop poikiloderma (telangiectasia, atrophy, hyperpigmentation and hypopigmentation). This sign is prognostic of the development of a reticulosis in due course, in one of its many guises, such as erythroderma or mycosis fungoides. These changes may take years to develop and it may be necessary to perform periodic biopsies in order to determine whether a reticulosis is developing.

PITYRIASIS ROSEA

Pityriasis rosea is a scaly disease of limited duration, characterized by the appearance of a herald patch followed by a widespread eruption.

Aetiology and Pathology

The cause is unknown. It often follows an upper respiratory infection or slight fever and may be a viride. Second attacks are rare.

Clinical Picture

Children and young adults are most affected. There is often a history of malaise, coryza and of sore throat a week or two before the onset. The first change in the skin is the herald patch, somewhere on the trunk, near the axilla or hip, occasionally more distally on a limb. The lesion is an oval, fawn to pink plaque with scaling, the free edges of the scales being centripetal. Itching is slight or absent as a rule. The herald patch may be missed. The generalized eruption begins a week or two later and is usually confined to the trunk and proximal parts of the limbs. It often extends up the neck and down the arms and forearms, but the face, lower thighs and legs are seldom affected.

Two types of generalized eruption are seen, the more usual macular and plaque form and the follicular papular form, in which, however, a few plaques are always present as well. The plaques start as pink macules which extend to become oval 'medallions' which, on the trunk, lie parallel to the ribs; they vary in size from 0·5 to 2 cm. or more. Scaling is not apparent at first but, after a week or 10 days, the lesions become fawn-coloured and scaling begins from their centres, causing a centripetal arrangement of the free border of the scaling. In the early stage, when this feature is not apparent, it can be demonstrated by scraping a lesion so as to detach the looser scales. There are no mucosal changes and the lymph nodes are not enlarged. The follicular papular variety is more difficult to recognize, but the manner of onset and the distribution should give rise to suspicion, and the discovery of medallions makes the diagnosis clear.

Diagnosis

This is from secondary syphilis, drug eruptions, tinea circinata and infective dermatitis. In secondary syphilis, the examination of the anogenital region, mucous surfaces and lymph nodes reveals other evidence of that disease. Pityriasis rosea-like drug eruptions are usually in some way atypical. Tinea circinata is usually more acute; the lesions are circular rather than oval; they are few in number and may appear on the face; the scalp, too, may be affected with scaling and short broken hairs. Microscopy reveals mycelia and spores. Infective dermatitis is recognized by its grey greasy scales and sweat area distribution.

Treatment

Reassurance, explanation and calamine lotion are usually all that are required. The patient need not be isolated. Warm but not hot baths may be taken. If any doubt exists, the Wassermann reaction should be tested. Over-treatment must be avoided.

Course and Prognosis

The total course is usually 6–8 weeks, but it may last longer or shorter. The appearance may be modified in xerodermatous or seborrhoeic individuals. Misdiagnosis and treatment with fungicides may cause a distressing, very itchy, papulovesicular change.

PITYRIASIS RUBRA PILARIS

This is a rare chronic condition characterized by red follicular papules with horny spines, keratoderma of the palms and soles and psoriasis-like plaques of a bright pink colour.

Aetiology

It may be a follicular variant of psoriasis.

Clinical Picture

There are widespread groups of pink or red follicular papules, with keratotic tips, on the body and limbs. The hairy backs of the proximal phalanges show follicular keratoses. There is marked thickening and dirty discoloration, with fissuring of the horn on the palms and soles, and the nails become deformed and brittle. The plaques are pink or red scaly areas, having a resemblance to psoriasis on the one hand, and lichen simplex on the other, but they differ from both these conditions in that central circles or polycyclic areas of normal skin are present. Ectropion may occur. The mucous membranes are not affected. There is no obvious constitutional disturbance.

Treatment

There is no evidence that the administration of vitamin A shortens the duration. Treatment is symptomatic, with applications of Salicylic Acid Ointment, B.P., or a mixture of this with an equal part of glycerin of starch.

Course and Prognosis

The onset is insidious and the course unpredictable. A spontaneous remission may occur after several months.

DYSKERATOSIS FOLLICULARIS

Synonym. Darier's disease.

A rare condition of inherited abnormality of horn formation, it has an autosomal dominant inheritance.

Clinical Picture

The lesions first appear in late childhood or adolescence. Firm dirty grey or brown papules appear with crusted or warty tops. The face and flexures are affected most. Vegetating, malodorous lesions may develop in the flexures. Punctate keratoses and minute pits are present on the palms and soles. Exposure to sunlight may aggravate the lesions.

Diagnosis

This is from acanthosis nigricans, in which there are velvety, hyperpigmented folds and wartiness, also from pemphigus vegetans, arsenical keratoses and dermatitis vegetans.

Treatment

Ten per cent. salicylic ointment may help to soften the lesions. Vitamin A in a dose of 200,000 Units daily for an adult is worthy of trial.

Course and Prognosis

The course is prolonged. There is often mental retardation, small stature and genital hypoplasia.

LICHENOID DERMATOSES

This is a group of flat-topped papular conditions.

LICHEN SIMPLEX

This is a common condition in which oval areas of reddish-brown, thickened skin develop at sites of repeated friction [see p. 1093].

LICHEN PLANUS

This is a disorder of unpredictable duration in which itchy, flat-topped, shiny, violaceous papules appear on various parts of the body.

Aetiology and Pathology

The cause is unknown. It is suspected to be of viral origin and to be activated by varied noxae, including drugs, physical stimuli and emotional stresses.

Clinical Picture

Lichen planus most characteristically affects the buccal mucosae, the fronts of the wrists, the lumbo-sacral region, the external genitalia, the medial aspects of the thighs, the shins, calves and ankles: it may appear on the palms or soles and anywhere on the body, though rarely, if ever, on the face. Scratching sometimes causes linear lesions (Koebner's phenomenon) or exposure to sunlight may localize the rash. Involvement of the scalp with lichen planopilaris may end in the picture of pseudopelade [p. 1147] and rarely the nail matrices are affected and the nails atrophic and deformed as a result.

The elementary lesion of lichen planus as seen on the skin is a violaceous, polygonal, flat-topped, shiny papule. Sometimes the papules are only a shade darker than the surrounding skin. Often Wickham's striae and spots can be seen upon them—grey streaks and spots of pseudoscaling, thought to be colour changes caused by the thickened stratum granulosum. The individual papules often enlarge or coalesce to form extensive plaques.

Central healing, often somewhat atrophic, is common, resulting in lichen planus annulare. On the penis and scrotum this is most characteristic and the lesions here are often non-itchy. Resolution of lichen planus is nearly always accompanied by a great deal of pigmentation. It is not unusual for all the lesions to clear except those on the legs which may, on the contrary, become verrucose and persist indefinitely.

Lichen planopilaris presents as shiny follicular papules with a violaceous rim, the papules often being grouped. The process ends in atrophic scarring and in patchy baldness.

Lichen planus of the mouth gives rise to white, slightly raised polygonal spots and white streaks and delicate web-like, arborate, foliate or feathery patterns. Erosion or redness is unusual and the lesions are either symptomless or give rise to a sensation of slight roughness.

Involvement of the nail matrices is rare and causes grey, rough, atrophic nails.

Diagnosis

Diagnosis is from psoriasis, parapsoriasis guttata, syphilis, plane warts, lichen simplex, lichen nitidus, lichen sclerosus et atrophicus and lichen amyloidosis [p. 1135]. The diagnosis depends on a careful consideration of the elementary lesions, their 'waxy glance', their distribution, and the presence of orogenital lesions. Lichen planus may be non-itchy and in the early stage of evolution the lesions may be atypical. Hence it is sometimes necessary to re-inspect a patient after a week's interval, with a view to coming to a firm diagnosis. It may also be necessary to perform biopsy, a very useful procedure because of the highly characteristic histology in lichen planus. Diagnosis by clinical methods alone is difficult when, as occasionally happens, there is only one lesion in an atypical situation.

Treatment

The choice of treatment depends upon the amount of disturbance with sleep and general well-being which results from the itching. If severe and with widespread lesions it is advisable to admit the patient to hospital for a short course of suppressive treatment with prednisone, starting with 30 mg. a day and reducing the dose so as to withdraw the drug after 3 or 4 weeks. In milder cases adequate relief may be obtained from the local application of the more powerful steroid ointments, with or without polythene occlusion.

The oral lesions are more resistant but local corticosteroid applications are worthy of trial.

Sedation is often necessary, with promethazine, 25–50 mg., or a barbiturate.

Course and Prognosis

The course varies from case to case. New lesions may appear while others are fading, after first converting into hyperpigmented macular remnants. Leg lesions tend to be particularly persistent and the lesions may here become hypertrophic or bullous. Relapses may occur months or even several years later.

Lesions on transitional surfaces such as the mouth and the external genitalia have very rarely been reported to undergo malignant change.

LICHEN NITIDUS

This rare eruption consists of grouped lichenoid papules and may be a micropapular variant of lichen planus.

Clinical Picture

Itchy or non-itchy, skin coloured to light brown or pink, shiny, flat-topped papules occur in close set groups, particularly on the penis, the flexor surfaces of the wrists and forearms, on the abdomen and on the ankles and feet, occasionally there are white patches within the mouth like those of lichen planus.

Diagnosis

Diagnosis is made from lichen planus by the smallness of the papules, their light brown colour, their grouping and the absence of pigmentation. Biopsy reveals a distinctive histology.

Treatment

This is as for lichen planus.

Course and Prognosis

The lesions persist for an indefinite period but ultimately fade without residual pigmentation.

LICHEN SCLEROSUS ET ATROPHICUS

A condition of lichenoid papules, ending in atrophy or sclerosis, affecting both sexes; commoner after 30 years of age and rare in childhood.

Aetiology

This is unknown.

Clinical Picture

It presents with genital and extragenital lesions. In both sexes the latter consist of roughly circular or polygonal pinkish-grey atrophic parchment-like patches with some follicular keratoses. At flexural sites there may also be white lichenoid papules and scleroderma-like plaques without follicular keratoses.

In the male the genital lesions may be similar to those already described if they are on the shaft of the penis. A fibrous constriction of the prepuce may develop causing phimosis. On the inner surface of the prepuce, at the coronal sulcus, and on the corona and glans, there may be a variable degree of atrophy and sclerosis. Atrophy may be confined to the penile meatus and this may later cause some urethral stenosis; or the whole surface of the glans may be irregularly thickened, dry, white and hard, a condition known as balanitis xerotica obliterans. In the female the atrophic and sclerotic changes may affect the labia minora or majora and the adjoining skin of the perineum and perianal region. Itching is variable but may be intense. Secondary changes include fissuring and leucoplakia. The severest cases may have bullous lesions sometimes containing blood.

Diagnosis

This is from localized scleroderma (morphoea), macular atrophy, leucoplakia and atrophic vaginitis with kraurosis.

Morphoea presents as an oval, firm, ivory, shiny plaque with a lilac halo. There may be hyperpigmentation. Atrophy is not marked except sometimes in the later stages. There are no follicular keratoses. Nevertheless, morphoeic lesions may occur in a patient with lichen sclerosus et atrophicus and it is possible that the latter is a superficial form of morphoea. In macular atrophy there are soft bulgings, giving a hernia-like feeling on palpation. Leucoplakia only affects transitional epithelial surfaces. Lichen sclerosus of the vulva may be complicated by leucoplakia. Atrophic vaginitis presents as shrinkage (kraurosis) of the vaginal orifice with patchy hyperpigmentation, depigmentation, atrophy and telangiectasia of the transitional epithelium. The labia minora are often atrophic.

Treatment

This is symptomatic. Oily cream or aqueous cream may be comforting. Topical corticosteroids relieve the pruritus. In the male meatal stenosis or phimosis may develop. Periodic examination of women with lichen sclerosus et atrophicus is necessary in order to recognize early the development of leucoplakic or epitheliomatous change which may necessitate surgery to the vulva.

Course and Prognosis

It continues indefinitely but a patch may undergo central resolution while extension persists peripherally. Extragenital lesions remain uncomplicated.

LICHEN STRIATUS

This rare condition usually occurs in children. A band of lichenoid papules erupts, usually in the long axis of a limb, and after a few weeks or months resolves spontaneously. Itching is slight or absent.

Diagnosis is from lichen planus linearis on the clinical and histological features.

Treatment is symptomatic.

LICHEN SPINULOSUS

Synonym. Keratosis follicularis.

Widespread or grouped horny, follicular papules are present, most conspicuously on the extensor surfaces of the limbs and trunk (phrynoderma). The cause is a deficiency of vitamin C and possibly A. Children are mostly affected. A similar picture may occur in follicular xeroderma (keratosis suprafollicularis).

An eruption of oval areas of lichen spinulosus may occur on the trunk and limbs with fungal infections of the feet (lichen trichophytide).

Diagnosis is from lichen planopilaris in which the papules have violaceous rims and on the scalp cause a form of folliculitis decalvans.

Treatment

Avitaminosis, fungal infection, xeroderma or lichen planus needs appropriate treatment. Locally salicylic acid ointment may be helpful, or a cream containing 10 per cent. of urea, e.g. *Calmurid.*

LICHEN SCROFULOSORUM

This eruption, today rare, consists of skin-coloured or pink, lichenoid papules, usually occurring on the trunk in childhood. There is often also tuberculosis of lymph nodes, bones, joints or elsewhere, a strongly positive Mantoux reaction and a tuberculoid histology. Treatment is of the primary condition.

LICHEN AMYLOIDOSIS

This is a localized cutaneous form of amyloidosis, presenting as very itchy papules and plaques, mostly on the limbs, particularly on the shins where they resemble lichen planus hypertrophicus. Biopsy and staining for amyloid confirms the diagnosis. Treatment is symptomatic, as for lichen simplex. The course is often prolonged. There are no systemic implications.

LICHEN URTICATUS

This is papular urticaria (q.v.), usually occurring in childhood. The lesions are more varicelliform than lichenoid.

LICHENOID ERUPTION OF AXILLAE (FOX-FORDYCE DISEASE)

It usually occurs in women, but is rare. Pink or brown, dome-shaped, grouped papules are present in the axillae, also sometimes at other apocrine sites, the areolae of the nipples, the umbilicus, pubic region and the perineum. Itching may be severe. The aetiology is uncertain, the treatment symptomatic, with topical corticosteroids. Oral contraceptive drugs may help. In the worst cases excision is necessary.

ACNEIFORM DERMATOSES

These are eruptions in which acuminate papules provide the most characteristic feature.

ACNE VULGARIS

A papular condition with hyperkeratotic plugging of the pilosebaceous follicles, diffuse hyperkeratosis of the skin and hyperplasia of the sebaceous glands.

Aetiology

Acne is brought about either by an androgen-oestrogen imbalance or by excessive reactivity of the pilosebaceous and apocrine units to circulating androgens. Resultant hyperkeratosis causes a muddy complexion and obstruction of pilosebaceous orifices. In glabrous areas this causes retention both of sebum and vellus hairs, while the sebaceous hyperplasia causes an increased secretion of sebum which is retained within the follicle. A blackhead (comedo) is a hyperkeratotic follicular plug, discoloured through oxidation and the addition of a certain amount of sebum and extraneous matter. The obstruction leads to inflammatory changes (papular acne), the keratin and sebum having a foreign body effect when retained. The inflammation may end in resolution or suppuration (pustular acne), but the pustules are usually sterile. Some fibrosis may result. If the pus is deeply situated it may form fluctuant swellings in the hypoderm (acne conglobata). Burrowing tracks may form in extreme cases, with epidermal bridges and tunnels lined with epidermis having one or more openings.

Severe acne may end in keloid formation, particularly if lesions are habitually manipulated by the patient. Keloids form particularly at the nucha, over the sternum and on the face and neck (acne keloid).

Epidermal cysts (milia) of pinhead size may be interspersed among the acne lesions ('white acne').

There is doubt about the role of the acne bacillus. This lipophilic organism thrives in the follicles and it is possible that some product of its metabolism stimulates keratin formation at the follicular orifices. Acne can become secondarily infected with staphylococci (acne sycosis); in these circumstances the pustules are more superficial and painful, with liquid pus.

Clinical Picture

Slight degrees of acne at puberty are so common as to be regarded as physiological. It usually begins at about 12–14 years of age and diminishes in severity at 18–20. In girls it often coincides with the menarche. Occasionally acne persists into adult life and may even last throughout life. As a rule, males are more severely affected than females.

Acne affects the face and neck, the upper trunk and, to a lesser degree, the lumbar region, buttocks and limbs.

A comedo (blackhead, acne punctata) is a grey, pinhead-sized, hard speck at a pilosebaceous orifice, and is often enclosed beneath a thin film of epidermal horn cells. In uncomplicated acne punctata there is no redness or swelling, but when an inflammatory reaction occurs an acne papule results, acuminate, firm and comedo-topped; liquefactive changes lead to a deep-seated pustule. This may resorb or break spontaneously or be broken by the patient's manipulations, and a funnel-like, depressed scar results. Lesions of acne conglobata are obtuse, dome-shaped, bluish-grey nodules. It is not unusual to see comedones, papules, pustules, small epidermal cysts, cystic swellings and scars, often keloidal, in the same patient.

The complexion in acne is greasy and muddy, the thickened epidermis diminishing transmission of colour from blood flowing in the superficial vessels of the dermis. Visibly enlarged patulous follicles are present and excessive sebum formation may be visible especially at the alae nasi. There may be pityriasis capitis but this is by no means the rule. The acne patient of either sex is usually somewhat hirsute and in females the pubic hair often has a masculine distribution. There may also be hyperidrosis.

Diagnosis

Diagnosis is from folliculitis barbae, acne agminata, syphilides, drug eruptions and rosacea.

In folliculitis barbae, involvement is of coarse hair-bearing areas, whereas acne involves areas of glabrous skin and the borderline between coarse hair-bearing areas and glabrous skin. The two conditions may coexist.

Acne agminata presents as grouped brown translucent papules, particularly on the eyelids, nose and penis.

Acneiform syphilides are papulopustular but without comedones; but syphilis may also aggravate a pre-existing acne vulgaris.

Halogens, too, particularly iodides, may cause acneiform eruptions without comedones, or aggravate pre-existing acne vulgaris. Halogen acne is usually more exuberant than acne vulgaris. Occupational acne often affects the forearms and thighs as much as the face.

Rosacea usually occurs in an older age group than acne vulgaris. The lesions involve an oval area of the centre of the face. They are erythematopapular and pustular but there are no comedones, though scars of previous acne may remain. There is marked vasolability and the face is bright red in patches, not the muddy colour of acne vulgaris.

Treatment

This depends on control of the primary cause and of the aggravating factors. The primary cause is a relative excess of androgens or an excessive response of the skin to androgens. The aggravating factors are numerous. They include a familial predisposition, dietetic errors, certain drugs, contact irritants, imperfect hygiene, insufficient weathering and emotional tension related in particular to conflicts with parental authority and difficulty in psychosexual adjustment to adult life, the acne sufferer often being somewhat retarded in emotional development while intellectually adequate and physically mature.

Treatment aims at diminishing sebaceous overactivity and at maintaining patency of the pilosebaceous follicles.

It is inadvisable to use oestrogens in the male: with the dosage necessary to give relief emotional changes and gynaecomastia may result. In females oestrogens may justifiably be given if there is oligomenorrhoea, irregular menstruation, male type hirsutism or marked aggravation of the acne before the menses, but it is inadvisable to use them even in these circumstances for the first few years after the menarche; it is better to allow time for the endocrine changes of adolescence to proceed naturally.

When prescribing oestrogens for acne, the patient should be asked to estimate the expected first day of the next menstrual period and to begin the treatment 10 days before this date and continue until menstruation begins. In this way there is no interference with ovulation. If menstruation is markedly irregular, it is not possible to adopt this procedure and the patient is instructed to start treatment a fortnight after the last day of the previous menstrual flow and continue for a fortnight or until the next period begins, whichever is the shorter. This treatment is continued for 3–6 months. Women taking oral contraceptives often report improvement of any acne they may have.

The diet should be adequate in protein and vitamin content. Excess of fats and carbohydrates must be avoided. In particular, chocolate, cocoa, cream pastries, nuts, butter, eggs and cheese in excess, are liable to aggravate.

Bromides and iodides can cause severe aggravation and other drugs, for example aspirin, occasionally aggravate acne.

The skin should be washed at least twice a day with a good toilet soap. Tangential friction is important, using a rough face flannel or a 'complexion brush'. Medicated soaps are best avoided. If cosmetics are used they should be of the lotion type, not creams. The patient should be discouraged from experimenting with local applications. Irritant or sensitizing substances incorporated in a base capable of mixing with fat and water may cause a chemical folliculitis. Similarly, exposure to brine, pitch, tar, organic chlorine compounds, paraffin or petroleum oils (cutting oils, greases, waxes) may cause or aggravate acne.

Woollen underclothing should not be worn next to the skin.

The acne patient should be encouraged to take outdoor exercise in all weathers. The fine exfoliation that follows sun-bathing is beneficial as is, to a lesser extent, exposure to wind and rain.

Pustular acne may be improved by a course of a wide-spectrum antibiotic, for example oxytetracycline, starting with 1 G. daily for a few days and then dropping to 500 mg. and later to 250 mg. daily, a dose which may have to be maintained for several weeks or even months.

When emotional factors seem relevant, the acne patient has to be encouraged to get out and about socially and not to shun company because of the disfigurement.

Local Treatment. This mainly aims at bringing about a fine peeling of the skin. A weekly exposure to a second degree (fine peeling) irradiation with ultra-violet rays is very helpful. Natural sunlight is much better than an ultra-violet lamp in this respect and the mercury vapour lamp does not stimulate pigmentation, causing only redness, with peeling. It is advisable first to make a radiographic examination of the chest in order to exclude an asymptomatic focus of tuberculosis which might be activated by this treatment. For more severe cases a third degree reaction (coarse peeling) may be desirable.

Medicaments for local application should be in the form of lotions or pastes, creams and ointments being potentially harmful. Zinc Sulphate Lotion, B.P.C., Sulphur Compound Lotion, B.N.F., and Calamine Lotion, B.P., with added 2 per cent. of sulphur are all useful. A flesh-tinted paste can serve the double purpose of treatment and cosmetic coverage. Resorcinol and Sulphur Paste, B.P.C. (tinted), can be used in this way and there are several proprietary preparations. In the comedone and papular form an abrasive preparation, e.g. *Brasivol* paste is often helpful; or the patient may be encouraged to apply friction with a 'cosmetic brush' and soap and water to the lesions.

Squeezing must be discouraged as it is probably the cause of much funnel-like pitted scarring of the follicular orifices.

In selected cases with steep 'ice-pick' scarring the appearance can be improved by dermabrasion.

Nodules and cystic swellings can be reduced by

intralesional injections of 0·1 per cent triamcinolone at fortnightly intervals.

Course and Prognosis

Acne vulgaris usually clears up or improves considerably after adolescence. When it persists there may be a special reason, endocrine, psychological, occupational or therapeutic which accounts for it. The amount of residual scarring is extremely variable. There may be little or none; rarely it is gross.

EXCORIATED ACNE OF YOUNG WOMEN

In this condition there are numerous excoriated papules and scars, particularly at the forehead, temples, cheeks and chin. Comedomes are difficult to find. There is an associated psychological conflict. Local treatment is ineffective unless the compulsive urge to pick the spots is controlled. A flesh-tinted application such as Titanium Dioxide Paste, B.N.F., may be helpful. Psychological investigation is necessary.

ACNE IN INFANCY

This is rare but may occur in the following ways:

1. Neonates often have numerous small papulo-pustules on the face for a few days. They may be due to androgenic influences (progesterone) from the mother.
2. The use of camphorated oil, olive oil or tallow as an embrocation may cause an acneiform eruption on the face or chest (grouped comedones).
3. Excessive and occlusive wrapping of the child's body may cause increased sweating of the face and follicular papulation.
4. Excess of cod-liver oil or of fats by mouth may cause acneiform papules.
5. One type of unilateral naevus consists of grouped comedones.
6. Adrenocortical neoplasms are accompanied by acne. The administration of corticotrophin may have a similar effect.

ACNE NECROTICA

Synonym. Acne varioliformis.

This is a relatively rare condition of discrete papulo-pustulation on the forehead, scalp and temples going on to necrosis and scarring.

Aetiology

It is a necrotizing folliculitis in which coagulase-positive staphylococci probably play a role.

Clinical Picture

The patient is usually a middle-aged man or woman. Near the hair margin across the forehead, at the temples and on the neck are discrete, brownish papules, pustules and scabs, with depressed scars. Lesions may also appear on the face, limbs and trunk. Itching may cause picking of the lesions, which are present in all stages at the same time.

Diagnosis

Folliculitis, acne vulgaris, syphilis and variola have to be considered, but the distribution, duration, itching and polymorphic nature of the lesions with scarring suggest the correct diagnosis.

Treatment

Bacteriological culture and the application of the appropriate antibiotic is indicated. Alternatively a clioquinol application may be used or zinc and copper lotion (eau d'Alibour).

Course and Prognosis

It may be persistent or relapse after treatment is stopped. Any carrier site of staphylococci should be treated concurrently.

ACNE URTICATA

This is an eruption of itchy urticarial papules on the scalp, face or elsewhere. Excoriations often result. The cause is not known.

ACNE AGMINATA

Synonyms. Acnitis; Lupus miliaris faciei.

Clinical Picture

This is a papular eruption affecting the forehead, eyelids, nose and cheeks and sometimes the penis. The papules are brown and translucent, giving a lupoid apple-jelly appearance on diascopy. The lesions are all at the same stage of development. Necrosis subsequently occurs, and when the scabs separate, depressed scars are left.

Aetiology and Pathology

The condition has been thought to be a tuberculide but the Mantoux reaction may show normergy or hypo-ergy to tuberculin and it has been suggested that the condition is a viride.

Treatment

Treatment is supportive and non-specific.

Course and Prognosis

The lesions are usually resistant to treatment with antituberculous drugs but tend to undergo spontaneous resolution after several months, leaving scars.

CHRONIC BULLOUS ERUPTIONS

The chronic bullous eruptions are a group of reactions of unknown cause, the recognition of which is most important because of their differing prognoses and treatments. In their differentiation reliance has to be placed on the history and physical signs, and in particular on the presence or absence of Nikolsky's sign. The Tzanck test also is a simple and useful diagnostic procedure, and biopsy is indispensable.

Nikolsky's sign can be demonstrated in two ways. If there is an intact bulla an attempt is made to push this along in the skin with a thumb, while anchoring the adjacent skin with the other hand. Nikolsky's sign is positive if the bulla can be moved along in the skin. The other method is to apply tangential stress to the apparently normal skin. The skin over the collar-bone or tibia is anchored with the left thumb and forcible lateral pressure is applied with the right thumb. The sliding off of the superficial layers indicates a positive Nikolsky's sign. The sign is positive in pemphigus vulgaris, pemphigus erythematodes, pemphigoid, benign familial pemphigus and epidermolysis bullosa. It is negative in dermatitis herpetiformis and in erythema multiforme.

The Tzanck test is performed by removing the roof and scraping the floor of a bulla. The material thus obtained is spread on a slide, stained and examined under the microscope for acantholytic cells (epidermal cells which have lost their prickles). Alternatively, lateral stress may be applied to a portion of skin and biopsy subsequently performed. The Tzanck test is positive if slit-like clefts are apparent within the epidermis and if within them single acantholytic cells or groups of them are seen. The presence of acantholytic cells indicates pemphigus vulgaris or pemphigus erythematodes, whereas the absence of them and the presence of leucocytes, particularly eosinophils, indicates dermatitis herpetiformis, bullous pemphigoid or erythema multiforme.

DERMATITIS HERPETIFORMIS

Synonym. Duhring's disease.

Dermatitis herpetiformis is a disorder in which grouped, itchy vesicles and small bullae arise on normal or reddened skin.

Aetiology

The cause is unknown. In some patients there is evidence of malabsorption, apparently from gluten-induced enteropathy, as confirmed by impaired absorption tests and jejunal biopsy. Dermatitis herpetiformis is most common between the ages of 30 and 50 years. It is rare in early adult life and in childhood.

Histologically the bullae are at the epidermo-dermal junction; they tend to be oval in shape when seen in sections; they contain blood cells, with many eosinophils but no abnormal epidermal cells.

Clinical Picture

The patient complains of an intensely itchy eruption which, though often widespread, shows a marked tendency to grouping. The sites most commonly affected are the shoulder blades, the elbows, the buttocks and genitalia, and the knees, but no area is immune, and the face may be involved. The eruption is polymorphic. The individual lesions are flaccid or tense, vesicles 2–5 mm. in diameter arising from skin which may either be apparently normal or reddened. Owing to the severe itching it is rare to see many intact vesicles and the physical signs usually consist more of excoriated and scabbed papules, erosions, scars and patchy pigmentation. The mouth, pharynx and larynx are very rarely affected. Nikolsky's sign is negative and the Tzanck test shows blood cells, particularly eosinophils, but no acantholytic epidermal cells. Biopsy shows a subepidermal bulla containing neutrophil and eosinophil leucocytes. The administration of potassium iodide by mouth or a patch test with potassium iodide causes an increased vesiculation. There is usually eosinophilia. The general health suffers little, if at all, apart from the disturbing effects of the intense itching.

Diagnosis

Diagnosis is from other bullous eruptions, erythema multiforme, urticaria, prurigo, general pruritus and infestations. The other bullous eruptions are in no way so itchy as dermatitis herpetiformis. Pemphigus often affects the mouth and leaves extensive raw areas, the patient, if untreated, becoming gravely ill. In erythema multiforme bullosum itching is less, the blisters are always within erythematous areas, superficial epidermal necrosis may occur, and excoriations are absent. Urticaria is evanescent, though possibly recurrent. In prurigo lichenification and excoriation are the predominant features and vesicles are not seen. In pruritus there may be excoriations and scratch marks but no vesicles. In infestations there are scratch marks on the shoulders and around the waist and an examination of the scalp, skin of the trunk and underclothes should disclose the cause.

Dermatitis herpetiformis in infancy may be mistaken for an exanthem such as varicella or variola. A carefully taken history and the absence of fever or malaise makes this mistake unlikely.

Treatment

A gluten-free diet partly or completely controls the condition in some patients. In others, dapsone in the smallest effective dose up to 100 mg. a day is the drug of choice. Slight cyanosis due to methaemoglobin formation is common in patients taking this drug but does not necessitate its withdrawal. It is advisable to check the haemoglobin level and white cell count of patients taking this drug at regular intervals, particularly when they are on large doses. Additional iron therapy may be necessary. On larger doses of dapsone haemolytic anaemia or leucopenia may develop. An alternative drug is sulphamethoxypyridazine and, if all else fails, prednisone may have to be used, but it is not always effective.

Course and Prognosis

It may persist for several years, with variations of intensity. Sometimes it slowly improves and may even disappear. In childhood the eruption is more florid and affects in particular the buttocks and external genitalia. Children tend not to tolerate dapsone as well as adults. The prognosis as regards life is good.

HERPES GESTATIONIS

This is a rare condition, occurring once in about 5000 pregnancies. It resembles dermatitis herpetiformis or erythema multiforme, and starts during the third trimester as a rule, or sometimes even as late as the puerperium. It usually recurs in subsequent pregnancies.

It usually clears after delivery but monthly relapses may occur for a while. Its histology is similar to that of dermatitis herpetiformis.

Treatment

Dapsone is ineffective. Prednisone, in the minimum effective dose should be given, with withdrawal, if possible, as term approaches.

PEMPHIGUS VULGARIS

Definition

This is a bullous eruption with an irregular course, ending fatally if untreated. In the flexures vegetations form (pemphigus vegetans).

Aetiology

There is a lack of cohesion between the epidermal prickle cells of undetermined cause. It usually occurs after the age of 30 and there is an increased incidence in Jews.

Clinical Picture

Flaccid bullae are present on seemingly normal areas of skin. Extensive red, raw areas of ruptured bullae are present with considerable serous exudate. The raw areas tend to spread peripherally and show no tendency to heal spontaneously. Itching is slight or absent. The general health steadily deteriorates. Secondary infection is common, particularly in the flexures where malodorous soft, moist, warty elevations or vegetations develop. The disease may at first be localized, but ultimately the whole surface may be patchily affected. At pressure sites such as the elbows, scapulae, sacrum, buttocks and heels, deep sores are liable to form. The mucous membranes of the mouth and vulva or penis are usually affected, causing increased discomfort. The vermilion surface of the lips and the mucous surface of the tongue, cheeks and roof and floor of the mouth are extensively denuded, giving an appearance of rawness covered by a white exudate and with loose tags of epidermis at the edges. Nikolsky's sign and the Tzanck test are both positive. Biopsy shows intra-epidermal bullae with acantholysis. The serum proteins are often markedly diminished, particularly the albumin, owing to the severe serous loss from the raw areas. Severe hypochromic anaemia and salt depletion also occur. Ulceration of the mouth interferes with swallowing and may further weaken the patient from nutritional deficiency.

Diagnosis

Diagnosis from other bullous eruptions is made from a consideration of the history and physical signs, with confirmation by skin biopsy.

Treatment

A high standard of nursing care is essential until the condition is brought under control. Prednisone in a massive dose of 60–100 mg. a day usually brings about a remission but some patients need up to 180 mg. daily in the first instance. The dose is subsequently reduced, at first rapidly but gradually tailing off until the minimal effective maintenance dose has been reached. Corticotrophin is administered intramuscularly for a while towards the end of the reduction phase. Mucous lesions respond less satisfactorily than skin lesions as a rule. Systemic treatment with an antibiotic may also be necessary at first to control any secondary infection. A high protein diet should be prescribed.

Locally, the skin lesions should be dressed with an easily removed, non-adherent application such as chlortetracycline ointment diluted one part with nine parts of soft paraffin ointment. Normal saline or glycerol and thymol makes a useful mouth wash.

Course and Prognosis

The natural course is one of worsening with occasional partial remissions, usually followed by more severe relapses, ultimately leading to death from general infection or pneumonia, complicated by protein and electrolyte deficiencies.

Corticosteroids give the patient several additional years of life, often interrupted by the side-effects of prolonged dosage, such as infections, peptic ulceration, glycosuria or osteoporosis.

PEMPHIGUS FOLIACEUS AND PEMPHIGUS ERYTHEMATODES

In these forms of pemphigus exfoliation is the most prominent feature, diffuse in the former, localized in the latter, bullae rarely being seen because they are superficial (at the granular cell layer), and easily ruptured. The course is irregular but usually much more benign than pemphigus vulgaris. Remissions and relapses occur. It is uncertain whether the condition can develop into pemphigus vulgaris.

Clinical Picture and Differential Diagnosis

In pemphigus foliaceus the picture resembles erythroderma, perhaps with some secondary infection, but Nikolsky's sign is positive in pemphigus foliaceus and negative in erythroderma. There is crusting and a tendency to wartiness, with pigmentation. In pemphigus erythematodes (Senear-Usher syndrome) the condition resembles infective dermatitis because the superficial lesions become secondarily infected; or with single or few lesions on the face there may be a resemblance to lupus erythematosus but the moistness of the lesions and the looseness of the overlying skin rule out this diagnosis. Biopsy shows acantholysis, either subcorneal or in the granular layer.

There is a variable degree of general disability.

Treatment

This is as for pemphigus vulgaris with prednisone and antibiotics in the more severe cases and with topically applied corticosteroids in the milder and more localized forms.

Course and Prognosis

The natural course is a slow worsening with remissions and recrudescences.

SENILE DERMATITIS HERPETIFORMIS OR PEMPHIGOID

Definition

An eruption of tense bullae, often with considerable

erythema around, with much itching usually occurring in the seventh or eighth decades, sometimes earlier, and sometimes ending fatally if untreated.

Aetiology and Pathology

The cause is unknown.

The bullae are at the epidermo-dermal junction and contain blood cells including many eosinophils.

Clinical Picture

Large tense bullae, some containing straw-coloured fluid, others containing blood or even pus, are present in the skin, particularly on the limbs. The mucous membranes of the mouth are sometimes affected with blisters and raw areas but the vermilion surfaces of the lips escape. There is intense itching but less constitutional upset than in pemphigus vulgaris. Nikolsky's sign is positive but the Tzanck test shows eosinophil and other blood cells but no acantholytic cells. The bullae do not rupture easily and if they are broken they tend to heal and do not spread spontaneously as in pemphigus vulgaris. Small white cysts (milia) may form in the process of healing.

Diagnosis

Diagnosis from erythema multiforme may be difficult. In erythema multiforme Nikolsky's sign is negative and spontaneous resolution usually occurs in a few days or weeks.

Pemphigus vulgaris differs from pemphigoid by its more flaccid and easily ruptured blisters with severe involvement of the mouth and lips and a heavy loss of electrolytes and protein. Senile dermatitis herpetiformis differs from dermatitis herpetiformis in its larger tense bullae, positive Nikolsky's sign, mucosal involvement and more serious course.

Treatment

Treatment is as for pemphigus with prednisone. After obtaining a remission the ambulant patient can be treated with gradually reduced doses until in some cases the drug can be withdrawn and recurrence does not occur. In others, mild or severe recrudescence necessitates further treatment with prednisone. Local treatment consists of aseptic puncture and collapse of the large tense bullae and antibiotic or emollient dressings.

Course and Prognosis

The natural course is chronicity with occasional remissions, sometimes of long duration.

BENIGN PEMPHIGUS OF THE MUCOUS MEMBRANES

Synonym. Ocular pemphigus.

Definition

A bullous eruption in which the eyes and mouth are mostly affected and the skin slightly or not at all.

Pathology

The blisters are at the epidermo-dermal junction; there is no acantholysis but a heavy inflammatory infiltrate and later fibrosis.

Clinical Picture

The conjunctivae become inflamed and fibrous adhesions form between the palpebral and ocular surfaces or between the upper and lower palpebral surfaces. The conjunctival sacs become shallow and the palpebral fissures narrow and the eyeballs limited in their range of movement (essential shrinkage of the conjunctivae). The cornea may be damaged by entropion, xerosis or pannus, with loss of vision. Vesicles form in the mouth and by coalescence form large red, denuded areas. The vermilion surface of the lips escapes but the mouth may be narrowed by adhesions. Lesions may form anywhere in the mouth, nose or throat; in the oesophagus, causing dysphagia; on the glans penis or prepuce, causing phimosis; or on the vulva or vagina, causing narrowing (kraurosis). The skin of the scalp or face is affected in about half the patients with erythema, flaccid bullae and erosions, going on to scarring.

Diagnosis

Diagnosis is from pemphigus vulgaris, pemphigoid, severe erythema multiforme and aphthosis, including Behçet's syndrome.

In pemphigus the lesions are in the epidermis and the vermilion surfaces of the lips are often affected. In pemphigoid the eyes usually escape and the skin lesions, which predominate, consist of large tense bullae. In severe erythema multiforme the onset is abrupt, the patient is a child or young adult and the skin involvement is extensive. In Behçet's disease there are erosions and ulceration of the eyes, mouth and genitalia, often with some destruction of tissue.

Treatment

Cortisone eye drops are invaluable and a corticosteroid in large dosage, as in pemphigus, may help to alleviate the other manifestations.

Course and Prognosis

The malady is slowly progressive, with remissions and recurrences.

BENIGN FAMILIAL PEMPHIGUS (OF GOUGEROT AND HAILEY-HAILEY)

Definition

This is a chronic erosive condition of friction sites occurring in many members of the same family, benign in its course and with a tendency to spontaneous remissions.

Aetiology and Pathology

This inherited disorder is possibly a bullous variant of dyskeratosis follicularis.

Histologically there is acantholysis, the detachment occurring in the stratum mucosum.

Clinical Picture

Benign pemphigus resembles a very resistant infective dermatitis. The lesions are flexural or at sites of friction such as the collar line, axillary folds and groins; and they consist of erosions covered by greasy scaling. The patient complains of a tendency to chafing of the skin at sites of pressure from clothes and there is a history of a similar condition in other members of the family.

Diagnosis

From infective dermatitis the condition is recognized by its chronicity and by the characteristic histology.

Treatment

Clothing should be soft and smooth and loosely fitting. A dusting powder containing zinc oxide and zinc stearate may, by giving 'slip', help to prevent the development of further lesions. Active eroded lesions may be controlled, partly or completely, by the local application of a corticosteroid cream.

Course and Prognosis

The course is chronic, with occasional remissions which bear no relation to treatment, seasons or any other known cause. Regarding length of life the prognosis is good.

EPIDERMOLYSIS BULLOSA

Definition

This inherited disease occurs in two forms, the simple and the dystrophic. The skin is vulnerable to minor traumata and to sunlight.

Aetiology and Pathology

The cause is a genetic fault.

The histology differs in the two forms. In the simple form, clefts occur in the epidermis but in the dystrophic form they are in the dermis and scarring and loss of tissue often result, with the formation of epidermal cysts.

Clinical Picture

In the simple form the infant blisters easily at sites of minor trauma, especially the hands and feet, elbows and knees, shoulders and buttocks. In milder forms this phenomenon may not be apparent until later in life.

In the dystrophic form the disruption of the dermis is so severe that scarring and deformity often result. In particular the nails are likely to be shed, and the new nails are dystrophic and irregular. Ectodermal defects of the hair and teeth may also be present and erosions occur on mucous surfaces as well as on the skin.

Treatment

The aim should be the avoidance of traumata likely to cause blistering. Special care is necessary in the choice of clothing, particularly shoes, and the sufferer cannot take part in rough and tumble. Blisters should be dealt with by careful puncture and antibiotics applied if infection occurs. In the severe form it is justifiable to attempt suppression of the lesions with systemic corticosteroid treatment.

Course and Prognosis

Untreated, no remission occurs.

ATROPHY AND HYPERTROPHY

ATROPHY OF THE SKIN

This occurs in the ageing skin but, to a greater extent in areas exposed to light than in those not so exposed. In its simplest form, in covered areas, there is thinning and loss of elasticity, giving a yellowish, wrinkled and tissue-papery appearance and texture. At sites which have been subjected to prolonged exposure to the sun, particularly the face and the backs of the hands, the skin is atrophic with patchy variation of pigmentation, telangiectasia and the tendency to form rough grey elevations, solar keratoses, which in time may undergo malignant change.

Senile elastosis ('peasant's skin') is a leathery thickening with marked furrowing, occurring especially on the back of the neck (cutis rhomboidalis nuchae).

'Glossy skin' (atrophoderma neuriticum) occurs in conditions such as leprosy where there is interference with the nerve supply to a part.

Pressure atrophy occurs at sites of continuous pressure, for example under the pads of trusses.

Vulvar atrophy (senile vulvitis) may cause stenosis of the vaginal orifice (kraurosis vulvae). The mucosa is dry, shiny, smooth and pale, or there may be patchy telangiectasia and pigmentation. Leucoplakia (transitional cell hyperkeratosis) and squamous epithelioma may be the final outcome.

Macular atrophy (round and oval atrophic patches, particularly on the trunk) may be an idiopathic condition or a manifestation of past secondary syphilis. It may also occur in leprosy, lupus erythematosus, as a later stage of morphoea, or as a part of the condition known as acrodermatitis chronica atrophicans. The idiopathic form has two varieties, one preceded by inflammation (Jadassohn), the other (Schweninger-Buzzi) having no earlier inflammatory stage. Diagnosis is from von Recklinghausen's disease. In both conditions there are hernia-like weaknesses and grape-like swellings in the skin but in macular atrophy the other features of von Recklinghausen's disease [see Section 15] are absent.

Macular and striate atrophy is seen in the condition sometimes called 'striae cutis distensae', or 'striae gravidarum'. This linear form of atrophy chiefly affects the breasts, abdomen and thighs of pregnant women but is also seen in Cushing's syndrome and in some fat young people of either sex. It is probable that in all cases an endocrine factor is responsible, distension by itself not causing this condition, as is clear from observation of fat persons. The atrophic areas may be pink or purple when fresh: skin-coloured and more fibrotic when older.

Atrophoderma reticulatum is a condition of genetically determined, pinhead-sized atrophic areas separated by narrow ridges of normal skin. It occurs on the cheeks, is of unknown cause and is untreatable except by cosmetic coverage.

Acrodermatitis chronica atrophicans is a disease which is rare in the British Isles and more common on the Continent of Europe. As the name implies, it mainly affects the extremities where the skin is brownish-red and swollen, later becoming atrophic and wrinkled, with subcutaneous veins clearly visible. One or more limbs may be affected. Usually fibrotic nodules and bands are present over the subcutaneous surface of the ulna or of the tibia. The hypodermic fat is also atrophic. The cause of the disease is unknown. It goes on from an early inflammatory and swollen stage to a later atrophic stage but it has no effect on longevity. Diagnosis is from the 'main succulente' of syringomyelia (by the absence of neurological signs); from erythromelalgia (by the absence of pain and warmth). Treatment is empirical. Systemic treatment with penicillin may induce an early remission.

Poikiloderma. This is a condition of the skin in which telangiectasia, pigmentation, depigmentation and atrophy are intermingled. It is an atrophic pre-epitheliomatous or prereticulotic process.

It occurs after excessive solar irradiation or after repeated exposures to X-irradiation. It also occurs in an idiopathic form (poikiloderma vasculare atrophicans of Jacobi-Lane) which may terminate in cutaneous reticulosis with tumour formation. Poikilodermatomyositis is an atrophic end stage of certain cases of dermatomyositis.

All cases have to be watched for the development of keratoses or squamous epitheliomata, or in the idiopathic form for reticulosis or mycosis fungoides.

The irradiation forms are usually easy to recognize from the history and situation. The idiopathic form may occur with lichenoid papules on the trunk and with parapsoriasis-like patches in addition to the poikiloderma.

Treatment is by bland local applications, for example, the ointment of wool alcohols, and by appropriate action if malignancy occurs.

Poikiloderma vasculare atrophicans (Jacobi-Lane). This is a rare disorder of lichenoid papules, with poikiloderma. The skin is dry and itchy. The disorder is slowly progressive and may end in cutaneous reticulosis with tumour formation.

Diagnosis is from radiodermatitis, systematized lupus erythematosus and dermatomyositis. In radiodermatitis there is a history of irradiation; in lupus erythematosus [Section 4] there are cytological and serological changes; and in dermatomyositis there are muscle pain, weakness, creatinuria and increased serum aldolase, serum glutamic oxalacetic transaminase and serum creatine phosphokinase.

Lichen sclerosus et atrophicus [p. 1134].

Pseudoxanthoma elasticum [see Section 4].

Cutis hyperelastica (Ehlers-Danlos syndrome) [see Section 4].

HYPERTROPHY OF THE SKIN

A corn (clavus) is a localized reactive hyperplasia, the result of intermittent pressure and friction. Under the dermis a bursa may develop—a lymph space containing serous fluid. Abacterial or bacterial inflammation may occur, the latter sometimes with suppuration. Corns most commonly occur on the upper surfaces of the toes, particularly the small toes. Sometimes they occur between the toes and owing to maceration are known as 'soft' corns. In this situation, exostosis and fungal infection should be excluded. Diagnosis is from warts by the fact that the latter either have a papillated surface or at least show a break in continuity of the epidermal lines of the skin. (Plantar warts may, however, become buried under a hyperkeratotic cap.) Prevention depends on wearing suitable footwear. Treatment consists of well-fitting shoes and hose, and paring of the excessive horny matter. A salicylic acid plaster previously applied renders this procedure easier. Recurrence is likely unless further pressure or friction is avoided.

Callosities are diffuse thickenings of the horny layer. They are due to excessive weight-bearing, as in obesity or from unnatural stresses as in pes planus. They may also arise from roughened shoe linings, and at innumerable sites in different occupations from intermittent friction and pressure (for example, in gardeners, boatmen, housewives, cobblers, etc., as occupational stigmata). Bursae may form beneath the thickened, firm, inelastic skin which has a yellowish appearance with a shelving edge, and is painless. Callosities are liable to undergo fissuring from which infection may result.

Tylosis is a congenital hyperkeratosis of the palms and soles, dominant in its inheritance. The hard, thickened skin cracks easily in the winter and becomes macerated and offensive in the summer. The condition can be alleviated by 10 per cent. salicylic acid ointment.

Keratoderma climactericum affects the palms, soles and heels, and sometimes the knees of menopausal women, usually obese. There is much horny thickening at these sites and painful fissures tend to form around the heels. It is necessary to encourage the patient to lose weight by a stone or two in the course of a few months.

Keratoderma punctatum occurs in two forms, one hereditary but occurring in early adult life, the other apparently acquired and caused by keratin stimulants operating around the sweat ducts. On the palms (and sometimes on the soles) are discrete conical or rounded excrescences of dense keratin with central puncta. The condition is resistant to treatment but a 10 per cent. salicylic acid ointment may help to soften the lesions.

Arsenical keratosis (due to the ingestion of Fowler's solution) affects the palms with pinhead lesions although the soles may show larger excrescences. Dirty grey keratoses, Bowen's disease and basal cell or squamous cell epitheliomata may be present on the trunk and there may be raindrop depigmentation and hyperpigmentation.

Keratoderma blenorrhagica is a parakeratotic condition of the palms and soles [see Reiter's syndrome, Section 2].

Porokeratosis of Mibelli is a congenital hyperkeratosis affecting in particular the sweat duct ostia.

The lesions are skin-coloured or grey, warty elevations which spread peripherally, leaving a gutter and a depressed, scaly, atrophic centre. Treatment is by cryotherapy or dermabrasion.

A warty, hard or epidermal naevus usually presents as linear bands of itchy, brown, warty, cracked and bleeding skin. It is a unilateral condition, affecting the whole or part of a limb, one side of the external genitalia or the side of the neck or trunk (ichthyosis hystrix, naevus unius lateralis, linear naevus). Warty naevi are present at birth or develop at any time up to adolescence. They persist indefinitely. Epithelioma may become superimposed. Treatment is by protective dressings but if there is severe itching and resultant excoriation and secondary infection it is best to arrange excision and grafting.

Lichenification is hypertrophy of the stratum mucosum.

Cutis laxa is a hypertrophy of the skin and subcutaneous tissue with lax attachment to the deeper structures with the result that the skin hangs in folds. One variety is cutis gyrata, a cerebriform folding of the scalp, sometimes congenital and sometimes occurring in acromegaly.

METABOLIC DISORDERS

XANTHOMATOSES

Xanthomatosis is the presence of visible deposits of cholesterol in the skin. Deposition may also occur in deeper structures.

PRIMARY HYPERCHOLESTEROLAEMIC XANTHOMATOSIS

In this relatively common inborn error of cholesterol metabolism autosomal dominant inheritance is probable. Yellow papules and nodules (xanthoma tuberosum) appear in childhood or in adult life on the extensor aspects of the elbows and knees, the buttocks and the backs of the heels, also as yellow thin streaks in the palmar and plantar skin creases. Xanthelasma palpebrarum and corneal arcus may also be present. Nodules also occur in tendons, ligaments, fascia and periostia.

The serum is clear, the cholesterol and cholesterol esters are greatly increased, the triglyceride is normal or slightly increased. The serum albumin is reduced but the serum gamma-globulin fraction is increased. Paper electrophoresis shows greatly increased beta-lipoproteins and pre-beta-lipoproteins normal or slightly increased.

Because of the deposition of cholesterol in the endocardium and in the intima of blood vessels, cardiovascular phenomena often occur from involvement of coronary, cerebral or renal vessels or of those supplying the limbs. A family history of events of this sort is common. When the liver is affected xanthomatous biliary cirrhosis and cholesterol gall-stones may result.

Treatment consists of a low calorie, low cholesterol, diet and clofibrate, up to 1 G. daily.

SECONDARY XANTHOMATOSIS

This may occur as an incidental finding in biliary cirrhosis, lipid nephrosis, diabetes mellitus, chronic pancreatitis, hypothyroidism or haemochromatosis. Nodular, tuberous or eruptive lesions occur and both plasma cholesterol and plasma triglycerides may be raised. Treatment is that of the primary condition. Clofibrate is contra-indicated in the presence of hepatic or renal disease.

HYPERLIPAEMIC XANTHOMATOSIS

In this relatively rare familial, fat-induced hyperlipaemia a deficiency of lipoprotein lipase leads to increased lipoprotein absorption. It occurs in children or adults, in males more often than in females. Papular and tuberous xanthomata are present, eruptive xanthomatosis may occur and cardiovascular complications are common. Diabetes mellitus and pancreatitis may be present. The liver and spleen are enlarged and attacks of upper abdominal pain may occur. The serum is milky, the plasma cholesterol is normal or slightly raised and the plasma triglycerides are greatly increased. Paper electrophoresis shows chylomicrons (beta-lipoproteins synthesized in the intestine during fat absorption) greatly increased while all other lipoproteins are decreased. Treatment consists of a diet with small animal fat content.

CARBOHYDRATE-INDUCED HYPERLIPAEMIA

This form starts in adult life with tuberous xanthomata, eruptive xanthomata or palmar crease deposits. The serum is turbid, the plasma cholesterol normal or raised, the plasma triglyceride raised. Paper electrophoresis shows increased pre-beta-lipoproteins. Sugar tolerance tests may be slightly abnormal or frankly diabetic. A low carbohydrate diet controls the condition.

XANTHELASMA PALPEBRARUM

Flat or slightly raised yellow plaques of cholesterol in the skin of the eyelids occur as a result of degenerative changes in the tissues or from a raised blood cholesterol. (See secondary xanthomatosis.) Corneal arcus may also be present. Lesions of xanthelasma can be destroyed with the cautery under local anaesthesia with good cosmetic results.

JUVENILE XANTHOMA

This benign condition (naevo-xantho-endothelioma) presents as one or several yellowish, obtuse nodules on the neck, limbs or trunk of infants in the first year or two after birth. The blood cholesterol is normal and the lesions regress spontaneously after a few years.

NORMOCHOLESTEROLAEMIC XANTHOMATOSIS

See histiocytosis-X.

GRANULOMA ANNULARE

This non-itchy nodular condition is of undetermined cause but an occasional association with latent or overt diabetes mellitus has been noted. It may be necessary to perform a cortisone-provocation sugar tolerance test to demonstrate this link. Children and young adults are most affected. The mildest forms occur on the pinnae, elbows, knuckles or ankles and feet as skin coloured or slightly blue painless and non-itchy nodules without epidermal change. The nodules become annular or crescentic. Sometimes there are multiple lesions on the trunk and limbs in addition to the characteristic sites. The lesions may persist or fade spontaneously and recurrences are common.

Diagnosis is from polyarteritis nodosa, leprosy, tinea circinata and necrobiosis lipoidica. In polyarteritis nodosa the lesions are painful and tender. Annular sarcoid is usually erythematous and not characteristically situated on the knuckles. Tuberculoid leprosy lesions are anaesthetic to temperature discrimination and light touch and the histology is distinctive. Tinea circinata is an epidermal, ringed eruption with centripetal scaling.

Granuloma annulare tends to disappear after minor trauma has been applied. Adhesive dressings, carbon dioxide snow or slush applications, or biopsy may all have this effect. The lesions can also be suppressed by local injections of triamcinolone acetonide. Treatment is unnecessary except on cosmetic grounds. There is no effective systemic treatment.

ERYTHEMA ELEVATUM DIUTINUM

Erythema elevatum diutinum occurs as the Bury type or as the Hutchinson type. The Bury type is a firm, raised, dusky disc or ring of erythema. It may represent the end stage of granuloma annulare. The Hutchinson type consists of many firm nodules in a dusky background, scattered widely over the trunk and limbs. The lesions urticate on friction, heat or excitement. They persist indefinitely and end up as fibrous nodules. The cause of both conditions is unknown. The Hutchinson type behaves as if the persistent effects of an urticariogenic antigen lead to a refractory phase of the vessels so that damage occurs to the vessel walls.

Both conditions are chronic, but the Hutchinson type is of more serious import because of the distressing itching and smarting.

Treatment is symptomatic and largely ineffective. In the Bury form, carbon dioxide snow is worth a trial. In the Hutchinson form, antihistamine drugs may reduce the itching and urtication.

NECROBIOSIS LIPOIDICA

Necrobiosis lipoidica is a condition in which lipoid deposition occurs in areas of degenerate or necrobiotic collagen. Diabetes mellitus is often present or may subsequently develop.

The lesions usually appear on one or both shins but are occasionally seen at the ankles, on the feet or hands, on the forehead or elsewhere. They consist of slightly depressed plaques of shiny atrophic, waxy yellow skin, with well-defined margins and dilated venules showing clearly. Ulceration may occur.

The condition often becomes inactive after a time but it rarely regresses. Diagnosis is from other atrophic conditions, from sarcoidosis and from granuloma annulare. Biopsy is often diagnostic. There is no effective treatment.

DIABETES MELLITUS

The association of diabetes mellitus with xanthomatosis, granuloma annulare and necrobiosis lipoidica has already been mentioned. There are several other skin manifestations which suggest the possibility of diabetes. Candidiasis may occur, causing pruritus ani, balanoposthitis, vaginitis with pruritus vulvae, paronychia or intertrigo, including erosive interdigital dermatitis, and angular cheilitis. Generalized pruritus is not a feature of diabetes mellitus.

Staphylococcal infections may cause boils, carbuncles or styes, and streptococcal infections may cause recurrent cellulitis, sometimes secondary to fissuring caused by flexural foci of *Candida albicans* infection. Arterial disease may cause gangrene of digits or ulcers on leg or foot. Peripheral neuropathy may cause neurotrophic ulcers, Charcot's joints or polyneuropathy. Carotinaemia may result from a diet high in carotene.

Associated general disorders include acromegaly, Cushing's syndrome, haemochromatosis, porphyria cutanea tarda and Werner's syndrome.

Antidiabetic drugs occasionally cause allergic reactions and injections of insulin may cause localized or generalized urticaria, keloid scarring or fat dystrophy, usually atrophy, sometimes hypertrophy.

AMYLOIDOSIS

The skin is rarely affected in systemic amyloidosis secondary to chronic inflammatory disease.

In the rare primary systemic amyloidosis non-itchy waxy, semi-translucent papules, nodules and plaques occur on the face, lips and tongue [see Section 4].

Primary cutaneous amyloidosis. See lichenoid diseases.

CALCINOSIS

The deposition of insoluble calcium may be localized and due to injury, degeneration, inflammation or neoplasia. The serum calcium is not elevated (dystrophic calcinosis). Thus, it may occur in haematomata, perniosis of the pinnae, varicosities, arterial disease, systemic sclerosis, dermatomyositis, lupus erythematosus, sebaceous cysts, etc.

In metastatic calcinosis the serum calcium is raised. The cause may be hyperparathyroidism, either primary or secondary to renal disease, excessive dosage with vitamin D, the milk-alkali syndrome and sarcoidosis, Destructive bone disease can also cause it, for example carcinoma, reticulosis, leukaemia, osteomyelitis or Paget's disease of bone. The skin is rarely affected, most deposits occurring in the lungs, stomach or kidneys.

Skin deposits mostly occur in the fingers, hands, elbows and feet and can be felt as hard masses bulging the skin, often white and sometimes ulcerating, with a milky granular discharge. Deposits may also occur in the hypoderm, tendons and muscles.

Calcium deposits are radio-opaque, a feature which differentiates them from other abnormal metabolic deposits.

Treatment is of the primary condition.

MUCINOSES

In generalized myxoedema the skin is dry, pale and thickened and the hair is fine, sparse and dry. The non-pitting oedema is caused by mucinous deposits around the blood vessels and follicles.

In circumscribed (cutaneous) myxoedema, which occasionally develops with thyrotoxicosis, firm, raised, waxy, skin-coloured or purplish nodules or plaques form, mostly on the fronts of the legs ('pretibial myxoedema'), rarely also on the face, arms or abdomen.

Lichen myxoedematosus is a are condition of unknown cause in which diffuse papular deposits of mucin occur without any evidence of endocrine disorder.

PORPHYRIA

[see Section 4]

PORPHYRIA VARIEGATA

In this condition there are all the symptoms of acute intermittent porphyria and in addition light sensitivity, furrowing of the forehead, bullae, and scarring of parts exposed to light or to other physical traumata, also hypertrichosis. The epidermis on the backs of the hands detaches when tangential stress is applied (Nickolsky's sign). Porphobilinogen is present in the urine during an attack but is absent during remissions. Coproporphyrins and protoporphyrins are increased in the faeces.

PORPHYRIA CUTANEA TARDA

This is an acquired condition occuring in alcoholics or in individuals taking barbiturates, sulphonamides, griseofulvin, chloroquine or oestrogens. There is light sensitivity with blistering, scarring and increased pigmentation of exposed parts. Hypertrichosis and a positive Nickolsky's sign may be present. The liver is enlarged, uroporphyrin is present in the urine and the serum iron is increased.

ERYTHROPOIETIC PROTOPORPHYRIA

This is a dominant, genetically determined condition. Attacks of light sensitivity occur, with burning discomfort, oedematous urticarioid or eczematoid areas, with blistering, often leaving linear crusts and pitted areas on light-exposed parts. In remissions there is pock-like scarring of exposed parts. The erythrocyte protoporphyrin is raised.

HAEMANGIOMATA OF SYSTEMIC SIGNIFICANCE

ENCEPHALOTRIGEMINAL ANGIOMATOSIS (STURGE-WEBER SYNDROME)

[see Section 15]

HAEMANGIOMA WITH THROMBOCYTOPENIA

[See Section 13]

STELLATE HAEMANGIOMA

These small 'spider' naevi appear on the face or hands of healthy children and adults. They may become more numerous during pregnancy and in the presence of liver disease. There is a central venule with radiating capillaries. Treatment, when requested, consists of a touch with the galvanocautery [see Section 6].

MULTIPLE FAMILIAL HAEMORRHAGIC TELANGIECTASIA (RENDU-OSLER-WEBER SYNDROME)

Numerous discrete haemangiomata and telangiectases occur on the skin and mucous membranes; the latter may cause haemorrhages from the nose, mouth, stomach, kidneys, vagina or rectum [see Section 13].

KAPOSI'S IDIOPATHIC HAEMORRHAGIC SARCOMA

This is a relatively benign haemangiomatosis and lymphangiomatosis which occasionally becomes sarcomatous. Brown or purple nodules develop, usually on the feet, sometimes on the hands or elsewhere. Visceral lesions are common, particularly in the lymph nodes, lungs and abdominal organs. The lesions first appear in middle age, slowly enlarge and then become static or regress. Ulceration may occur. Treatment is by radiotherapy.

It is probably a proliferation of pericapillary fibroblasts, and uncertainty remains as to whether it is a multifocal reticulotic condition or a metastasizing one.

CUTANEOUS RETICULOSES

When malignancy occurs in the reticulo-endothelial system the term malignant lymphoma is applied. This covers lymphosarcoma, reticulum-cell sarcoma, Hodgkin's disease and mycosis fungoides if the abnormal cells are not present in the blood stream, and leukaemia (monocytic, lymphatic, myeloid) if they are.

Skin manifestations of reticuloses may be non-specific or specific.

Non-specific manifestations, which occur particularly in Hodgkin's disease, include widespread pruritus, sometimes with histologically non-specific itchy papules (prurigo lymphatica), acquired ichthyosis, erythroderma, diffuse loss of hair, extensive pigmentation, purpura, and susceptibility to widespread skin infections. There may be severe necrotizing and ulcerating zoster, with disseminated lesions of varicella, widespread furunculosis or widespread fungal infection. The histology of lymph nodes removed for biopsy is often non-specific at first in erythroderma which ultimately proves to be a manifestation of a reticulosis. Hence repeat biopsies at intervals of 6 months or more may be necessary to establish the diagnosis.

Specific lesions depend on the type of reticulosis. In monocytic leukaemia, which is the commonest type of leukaemia to have skin lesions, papules, dusky, obtuse, dome-shaped nodules or plaques may form with histology indicative of the nature of the condition. The hair of the scalp may be shed and the face may have a leonine appearance. Erythrodermatous plaques may show a specific histology. In acute cases purpura is common and the skin may show increased fragility. Plaques on the legs may ulcerate.

In multiple myeloma (plasma cell leukaemia) amyloidosis is the dominant feature. Waxy papules or plaques may appear on the face and at the flexures, with involvement of the lips and tongue, sometimes with haemorrhagic lesions and macroglossia. Cardiac involvement may lead to failure and laryngeal, hepatic, renal, and gastro-intestinal deposits may occur. The urine may contain Bence-Jones protein, the blood increased γ-globulin and cryoglobulins, and marrow biopsy shows plasma cell hyperplasia.

In Hodgkin's disease widespread pruritus is often the first symptom. Specific lesions (nodules and ulcers) are rare. The diagnosis often depends on lymph node biopsy.

In reticulum cell sarcoma skin lesions are much commoner than in lymphosarcoma. There are firm, skin coloured or dusky, obtuse dome-shaped nodules and plaques, sometimes grouped. Ulceration may occur.

Mycosis fungoides is a cutaneous reticulosis with a long course, sometimes up to 20 years or more, and with pre-infiltrative, infiltrative, and tumorous stages. In the pre-infiltrative stage the type of lesion varies from one patient to another. One form is *parapsoriasis-en-plaque*; non-itchy or slightly itchy, pale pink, somewhat atrophic, scaly, round, oval or elongated lesions are present, tending to lie with their long axes parallel to lines of cleavage. Another form is parapsoriasis guttata, a variety of pityriasis lichenoides; guttate lesions occur with a single scutuliform scale. A third form, poikiloderma, is most characteristic and diagnostically significant. There is atrophy, with telangiectasia, patchy reticulate hyperpigmentation and hypopigmentation in extensive plaques particularly on the trunk and near the axillae and groins. This condition clinically resembles chronic X-irradiation damage.

Not all cases of *parapsoriasis-en-plaque* or parapsoriasis guttata proceed to infiltrate mycosis fungoides, but in view of the long natural course of the latter it often remains uncertain for years whether the condition represents a benign or potentially malign variant. Poikiloderma, on the other hand, is a particularly significant sign, suggesting the development, sooner or later, of infiltrative or tumorous mycosis fungoides.

Erythroderma may be an early or a late manifestation of a reticulosis. The differential diagnosis is from idiopathic erythroderma with extensive lymphadenopathy, the latter being reactive to the former. This has been called 'lipomelanic reticulosis' because of the histological appearance of the lymph nodes at biopsy, but 'reticulosis' is a misnomer, the condition being benign, sometimes persistent, sometimes resolving, perhaps with recurrence some years later. Erythroderma of reticulosis may be bright red (*l'homme rouge*) and accompanied by total loss of hair. Lipomelanic erythroderma is brown or slaty.

Sometimes mycosis fungoides presents with infiltrated plaques or even with tumours ('tomato tumours', *tumeur d'emblée*). The infiltrated plaques are itchy, pink or red and scattered amongst non-infiltrated lesions, including areas of poikiloderma. The tumours may ulcerate, or may take bizarre forms, with arciform or polycyclic configurations. Terminally, the lungs or some other internal organ may be invaded. Death usually occurs from intercurrent infection, anaemia or terminal leukaemia.

Treatment of cutaneous reticuloses is by topical corticosteroid applications for the non-infiltrated lesions, thorium-X applications or Grenz-ray therapy later, and ultimately X-irradiation of individual plaques or tumours. Finally, cytotoxic drugs, systemic steroids or total body irradiation with electron beams may be indicated [see Section 13].

HISTIOCYTOSIS-X

This is a general term for a group of proliferative histiocytic diseases in which secondary xanthomatosis occurs (normocholesterolaemic xanthomatosis) [see Section 13].

FOLLICULAR LYMPHOCYTOMA

Synonyms. Lymphadenosis benigna cutis; Spiegler-Fendt sarcoid.

This occurs as one or more dome-shaped nodules in the scalp, face, ears, nose, breasts, genitalia or elsewhere.

Pathology

The nodules consist of nests of lymphocytes.

Treatment

The lesions usually flatten and disappear after two or three X-ray exposures of 250 r each at weekly intervals.

Course and Prognosis

Although relatively benign, some forms develop into a progressive malignant reticulosis after some years.

DISEASES OF THE HAIR

CONGENITAL CONDITIONS OF THE HAIR

These include pili torti (spiral twisting of the hair); monilethrix (beaded hair, the shaft being constricted, with absence of the medulla at regular intervals, as a result of which the hair breaks off short); congenital ectodermal defects in which the scalp hair may be delicate and fine, or woolly or absent (congenital alopecia). In albinism, the hair is white.

ACQUIRED CONDITIONS OF THE HAIR

CANITIES

Synonym. Whiteness of the hair.

This may be physiological from the age of about 40 years onwards. It may also be pathological and premature in endocrine disorders including hyperthyroidism and Simmonds' disease. There may be partial or general whitening of the hair that regrows after alopecia areata or in the involvement of hairy areas by vitiligo. The hair may also become white after severe emotional disturbance.

Treatment is by suitable dyes which may be of the harmless type, for example, henna; or potentially harmful, for example, paraphenylenediamine. Before using the latter, a patch test should be performed to determine the presence or absence of sensitivity to the chemical. It should never be applied to a scalp on which any cuts, abrasions, scabs or redness exist.

NON-CICATRICIAL ALOPECIA

Synonym. Baldness.

This may be local or general; all the hair may be lost from a given area or there may be sparseness of the hair (alopecia diffusa).

ALOPECIA AREATA

See Hypotrichosis.

CICATRICIAL ALOPECIA

Scarring baldness has a large number of causes, including:

Physical traumata—wounds, burns, X-rays, radium.
Chemical traumata—caustics, etc.
Exanthemata—variola, varicella, zoster.
Drug intoxications—lichenoid mepacrine eruption.
Fungus infections—kerion, favus.
Granulomata—syphilis, lupus vulgaris, sarcoidosis, leprosy, halogen eruptions.
Reticuloses—lymphocytomata or lymphoblastomata; Hodgkin's disease.
New growths—rodent ulcers.
Naevoid conditions—naevus sebaceus, hydrocystadenoma papilliferum (both present as bald areas with yellowish papillomatous outgrowths).
Skin diseases—lupus erythematosus, lichen planopilaris, morphoea, folliculitis decalvans, acne varioliformis, pseudopelade.

A few of these will be described in some detail.

Radiogenic alopecia presents as poikiloderma, that is, a polymorphic and patchy picture of atrophy, telangiectasia, depigmentation and hyperpigmentation. It is occasionally seen in patients who have been treated by X-rays for ringworm of the scalp in childhood. The condition is irreversible and, after several years, keratoses and squamous epithelioma may develop.

Varicella, variola and zoster may show macular bald areas at the sites previously occupied by the vesicles.

The lichenoid mepacrine dermatosis presents as one of its features a patchy folliculitis of the scalp, beard, eyebrows and lashes, which is followed by baldness. The history of drug treatment and the lichenoid features elsewhere help to supply the correct diagnosis.

Favus may present with scutuliform crusts with an offensive odour or as folliculitis decalvans. Affected hairs fluoresce pale blue under Wood's light and spores and mycelium are visible within the hair shafts on microscopic examination.

Syphilis, in addition to the 'moth-eaten' alopecia at the secondary stage already mentioned, may in the tertiary stage cause cicatricial alopecia at the sites of gummata which, in this situation, often develop a heavy secondary infection.

Leprosy may give rise to baldness in its lepromatous and in its maculo-anaesthetic (tuberculoid) forms.

Lupus vulgaris rarely involves the scalp, and when it does the face is usually heavily affected as well with the characteristic 'apple-jelly' nodulation.

Reticuloses may cause obtuse skin- or plum-coloured, dome-shaped swellings, with baldness on the scalp, or occasionally more diffuse pink infiltrated nodulation.

Rodent ulcer, when it affects the vertex, differs considerably from the button-like lesions seen on the face. The scalp lesions are flat or even slightly depressed, scleroderma-like plaques, perhaps with some patchy crusting. The edges have a slight translucency and pearly appearance. Ulceration may not occur for years.

Lupus erythematosus causes red, bald patches, with central atrophic scarring and marginal infiltrated redness with follicular plugging and adherent scales.

Lichen planopilaris causes irregular angular areas of baldness and itchy, acuminate, violaceous, follicular papules with shiny tops.

Morphoea causes an oval or linear waxy, shiny, bald area with a lilac halo.

Folliculitis decalvans is a coccal folliculitis causing atrophy of the follicles and atrophic scarring with baldness. Often the central area is bald apart from a few scattered hairs but shows no active inflammation; towards the margin of the bald area are scaly follicular papules and sometimes a few pustules. The condition can be controlled to some extent by local treatment with antibiotics.

Acne varioliformis leaves depressed, hairless scars around the hair margin.

Pseudopelade presents as irregular and angular areas of scarred baldness with tufts of hair remaining amidst the bald patches. It may be the end stage of lichen planopilaris of the scalp.

Ulerythema ophryogenes is a rare, scarring folliculitis of the eyebrows of uncertain aetiology. Sometimes it may be a manifestation of lupus erythematosus, sometimes of coccal folliculitis profunda (sycosis).

Perifolliculitis capitis abscedens et suffodiens is a rare condition of fluctuant swellings on the scalp with sinuous tracks, multiple sinuses and considerable loss of hair. Culture may be sterile. The condition is a form of hydradenitis suppurativa, and is most difficult to relieve. It may be necessary to open up the tracks and allow them to heal by granulation.

HYPERTRICHOSIS

Hirsutism [see p. 1090].

DISEASES OF THE NAILS

The nails may be affected by local or general conditions, congenital or acquired.

PARONYCHIA

This is caused by micro-organisms gaining entry to the nail fold through a break in the cuticular barrier. It may be acute or chronic.

ACUTE PARONYCHIA

The acute form (paronychial whitlow), due to coccal infection, presents as a red, tender, cushion-like swelling on one or both sides of the nail fold. Yellowish discoloration, due to pus formation, is soon apparent. A painless epidermal variety may be the unsuspected source of various staphylococcal infections of the skin.

Treatment

Systemic antibiotic treatment may be effective in the earliest stage; avulsion of the nail and a paronychial flap may be necessary at the later stage. The epidermal variety is easily dealt with by removal of the overlying portion of epidermis and cleansing with 1 per cent. cetrimide.

Hutchinson's melanotic whitlow (onychia maligna) is a melanoma masquerading as an infection and necessitating amputation.

CHRONIC PARONYCHIA

Chronic paronychia, like the acute form, is due to destruction of the protective cuticle on the nail plate. This happens following the use of powerful detergents, strong alkalis and soaps, constant exposure to water, the use of cuticle removers, and clumsy manicures or habitual chewing or picking the nail folds. Through the gap thus made pass detergents, soaps, alkalis and water which cause a chemical paronychia with alkalinity of the fold; this predisposes to infection with *Candida albicans*, cocci or Gram-negative bacilli. Contamination often arises from the anal region.

Chronic paronychia presents as a persistent, reddened cushion-like swelling around the nail fold, with a space between the fold and the nail into which a probe can be passed for a few millimetres. There may be occasional exacerbations with a slight discharge of thin pus. The nail plate is usually deformed (onychia) by irregular transverse ridging and grooving, with some discoloration. Sometimes a nail becomes detached from its bed. There may be a history of Raynaud's phenomenon, chilblains or chapping. Painless whitlows may draw attention to the presence of a sensory disturbance in syringomyelia, leprosy, etc.

Treatment

Wet work and the use of detergents and alkalis must be reduced to a minimum. Prolonged wearing of rubber gloves may also aggravate. Cuticle manicure must be forbidden.

Active treatment depends on the cultural findings. When *Candida albicans* predominates nystatin or amphotericin B is indicated. Magenta paint or cetrimide solution are other valuable applications. When there is a heavy mixed infection the appropriate antibiotic or combination of antibiotics should be selected, preferably in a water-miscible vehicle.

As many patients with paronychia also suffer from Raynaud's phenomenon and chapping, attention should also be paid to protection against cold by appropriate clothing.

INGROWING TOE-NAIL

Synonym. Unguis incarnatus.

The reader is referred to a surgical textbook.

SUBUNGUAL CONDITIONS

Hyperkeratosis beneath the free border of a nail may be due to psoriasis, fungal infection, wart, callus or subungual exostosis.

DISORDERS OF THE NAIL PLATE

Affections of the nail plate are often secondary to disease of the matrix. The nails may undergo atrophy or complete destruction (acquired anonychia), or hypertrophy, the latter either as a simple thickening following trauma (onychauxis) or as ram's-horn-like masses (onychogryphosis or 'claw nails'). Removal is followed by regrowth of a thickened nail. Excision of the nail beds is sometimes advisable but it is a delicate surgical procedure to remove all the bed proximally and laterally without opening the distal interphalangeal joints.

Congenital abnormalities include absence of the nails (anonychia), rudimentary nails, ectopic nails (onychoheterotopia), spoonshaped nails (koilonychia), extreme thickening (pachyonychia congenita).

Habitual interference with the nail and its surrounds include nail biting (onychophagia) and picking (onychotillomania), one form of hangnail, and knuckle chewing.

Dystrophy (dullness and roughening) of the nails may be due to ringworm, psoriasis, dermatitis, lichen planus, syphilis, tuberculosis, leprosy or unknown causes. Ringworm should always be suspected when one or a few nails are discoloured, irregular, friable or honeycombed. Microscopy, repeatedly if necessary, enables the diagnosis to be confirmed and an attempt to be made to identify the organism by culture.

Psoriasis of the nails usually occurs with psoriasis elsewhere so that the diagnosis is simple, but it may affect the nails alone. It presents as 'thimble pitting' of the nails, there being anything from a single pit to uniform involvement of all the nails. In its more severe forms, it causes yellow opaque, brittle thickening of the nails, usually distally or laterally, sometimes over the whole plate. The nails may be raised and shed by psoriasis of the nail bed.

Dermatitis around and in the nail folds leads to pitting and transverse or longitudinal grooving of the nails.

When dystrophy of the nails is not explicable as of fungal, psoriatic or dermatitic origin, the Wassermann reaction should be tested and examination directed especially to evidence of syphilis or of lichen planus elsewhere.

Median canaliform dystrophy is a permanent thickened groove running along the centre of the nail and due to previous chemical or physical trauma to the part of the matrix supplying this portion of nail. It sometimes occurs on the thumb nails as a result of habitual picking with the middle finger nail.

Splitting of the nail tips into lamellae (onychoschizia) is usually caused by detergents or alkalis; occasionally, nail manicure preparations, particularly cuticle removers, are responsible.

Transverse groovings and ridgings of the nails are spoken of as Beau's lines. They may arise in one or more nails from dermatitis, psoriasis and other skin conditions, or they may indicate some recent illness, for example pneumonia, which has led to a temporary impairment of the nutrition of the nail. They take about 6 months to 'grow out' and, from their situation on the nail, the date of previous ill-health can be roughly estimated.

Longitudinal grooving and ridging of the nails is very common and of no significance in minor degrees; but when severe and accompanied by splitting of the nails it is dignified by the name of onychorrhexis and attention should be paid to the avoidance of degreasing and dehydrating substances.

White spots on the nails (canities unguium or leuconychia) are of no diagnostic significance or import, except that they indicate areas of imperfect cornification, possibly the result of injury.

Slowly growing yellow nails occur in association with lymphoedema.

Fungal and monilial infections of the nail plate cause brown discoloration and *Ps. pyocyanea* causes a blue-black discoloration.

Longitudinal bands or variation in colour, either lighter or darker, may result from local pigmentary changes in the matrix, including moles.

Koilonychia may be congenital and of no serious import. When acquired, it often indicates a chronic malnutrition of the matrices from iron and vitamin B deficiency. A general cause cannot always be found and local ischaemic processes are sometimes responsible. Damage to one or more fingers may cause a somewhat similar deformity, except that the nails are not thin as they are in nutritional koilonychia.

Clubbing of the fingers includes an increased curvature of the nails, both in the longitudinal and transverse axes, and an increased springiness of the nails on their beds. It is associated with suppurative lung conditions and cyanotic congenital heart disease, etc. There is often also hypertrophy of the distal phalanx (hypertrophic pulmonary osteo-arthropathy).

Detachment of the nail from its bed may start proximally (onychoptosis) from haematoma or paronychia, or distally (onycholysis) as in psoriasis. Onychomadesis is a term applied to shedding of all the nails (sometimes recurrently), starting proximally. The causes of this phenomenon include epidermolysis bullosa, vasospastic states, skin diseases beneath the nails, for example exfoliative dermatitis or psoriasis, chemical contact, injury, syphilis, diabetes or scarlet fever in its peeling stage.

Usure des ongles is a term applied to wearing away of the free border of one or more nails as the result of occupational friction or persistently rubbing an itchy skin with the finger tips.

CONDITIONS OF THE NAIL BED

Conditions of the nail bed observed through the plate include the 'splinter haemorrhages' of subacute bacterial endocarditis and lupus erythematosus, purpura, haematoma, cyanosis, stains of various chemicals and racial pigmentation. A pigmented mole (lentigo) at the nail matrix may cause a linear band of brown pigmentation in the nail plate from the nail fold to the free border.

THE SKIN AND OTHER SYSTEMS

There follows a description of some of the commoner conditions which may affect other organs and systems as well as the skin. Clearly, such a list cannot be complete. Rarer and new-found associations may have to be added from time to time.

THE PSYCHE

Opinions differ as to the significance of psychological factors in the genesis of skin conditions. A psychogenic basis should only be assumed from positive evidence and never because no material cause can be found for a condition. The positive evidence should be that of a disturbed personality or relevant provoking circumstances in the life situation, coinciding in time with the development of the dermatosis.

Emotional disturbance may show in the skin as sweating, flushing, blanching, horripilation or as self-directed injury to the skin, hair or nails, usually with the finger nails, occasionally with the teeth.

While emotional disturbance may display itself in the skin, the opposite also applies. A skin condition may, by its very nature cause great anxiety and depression and set up a vicious circle of morbid introspection, sometimes leading to aggravation of the condition.

Rarely, for example in systemic lupus erythematosus or in Behçet's syndrome, the pathological process in the nervous system may in itself disturb behaviour and mood.

Life situations causing anxiety and resentment are the ones usually related to exacerbations or activations of dermatoses. In a small minority libidinous conflicts seem relevant.

Dermatoses exclusively emotional in origin include:

Dermatitis artefacta.
Neurotic excoriations.
Delusions of parasitosis or of infections.
Cutaneous hypochondriasis (obsessional anxiety over trivial lesions).
Habit tics (physical traumata by nails or teeth to hair, cheeks, lips, knuckles, nails or nail folds, or elsewhere).
Hyperidrosis of face, axillae, palms or soles.
Lichen simplex.

Existing dermatoses may be aggravated by self-inflicted trauma in:

Lichenified contact dermatitis (pending settlement of a claim for compensation).
Excoriated acne.
Atopic dermatitis.

Some dermatoses have a multifactorial, partly genetic, partly acquired aetiology and in them emotional factors may be of major or minor importance. Examples include:

Anogenital pruritus.
Atopic dermatitis.
Acne vulgaris.
Pompholyx.
Rosacea.
Psoriasis.
Infective ('seborrhoeic') dermatitis.
Eczema.
Urticaria.
Lichen planus.
Alopecia areata.
Oral aphthosis.
Herpes simplex.

In forming an opinion as to the relevance of emotional factors it is necessary to assess the personality of the patient, to inquire into childhood circumstances and into the domestic, social and occupational conditions preceding or coinciding with the development of the dermatosis in question and to assess the degree of adjustment of the patient to the life situation.

THE NERVOUS SYSTEM

Itching may be of central origin, arising in the nervous system. It may be a feature of G.P.I. or of thalamic tumours and segmental itching sometimes occurs in tabes dorsalis. Intoxication by cocaine or morphine may cause pruritus and sometimes other drugs cause it before overt urticaria develops.

GENETIC AND DEVELOPMENTAL ABNORMALITIES

The common origin of the nervous system and the epidermis from the ectoderm makes it clear why a number of genetic and developmental abnormalities have both neurological and cutaneous manifestations. Examples include:

Anhidrotic ectodermal dysplasia. Mental deficiency, with anhidrosis, defective teeth, hair and nails and xerostomia.
Atopic dermatitis. Abnormal electroencephalograms in a significant proportion. Cutaneous vasoconstriction from physical trauma (white dermographism).
Hartnup disease. Pellagroid light sensitivity with cerebellar ataxy and psychic disturbances.
Neurofibromatosis. Skin neurofibromata and *café-au-lait* patches, sometimes with gliomata, mental deficiency, epilepsy, and cranial nerve or spinal cord tumours.
Phenylketonuria. Eczema, mental retardation and extrapyramidal lesions, causing athetosis.
Sacral hypertrichosis (faun tail) with diastematomyelia.
Sturge-Weber syndrome. Port-wine stain type of haemangioma in part or all of the trigeminal area with angiomatosis of the leptomeninges, sometimes with calcification, and causing focal epilepsy, hemiplegia and mental retardation.
Tuberous sclerosis. Adenoma sebaceum, para-ungual fibromata, connective tissue naevi, epilepsy, mental deficiency. Nodules of glial proliferation in the cortex, basal ganglia, ventricular walls and retina.
Xeroderma pigmentosum. Mental retardation with sensitivity to light, patchy pigmentation of exposed parts and, later, epitheliomata.

Acquired conditions in which both the nervous system and the skin are affected include:

VIRUS INFECTIONS

Herpes simplex, vaccinia, eczema herpeticum and eczema vaccinatum may all be complicated by encephalitis.

Postencephalitic Parkinsonism is often accompanied by seborrhoea.

Herpes zoster may be activated by local spinal deposits of lymphoma, Hodgkin's disease, leukaemia or carcinoma. It may be activated by injury or X-irradiation. It may occur with tabes dorsalis.

TROPHIC LESIONS

Burns, ulcers and other results of injury occur, mostly on the extremities, in tabes dorsalis, diabetic neuropathy, leprosy, syringomyelia, hereditary sensory neuropathy and other peripheral neuropathies due to injury or disease. Neuropathic arthroses (Charcot's joints) may also occur in these conditions.

Pick ulcers develop on the nostril, cheek or forehead

as a result of injury or disease (e.g. leprosy), alcohol injections or operations involving the trigeminal nerve. Paraesthesia causes the patient to pick at and damage the nostril and ulceration results. There may also be corneal insensitivity.

THROMBOTIC AND VASCULITIC CONDITIONS AND COLLAGENOSES

Behçet's syndrome may be accompanied by meningo-encephalitis with various intracranial symptoms in addition to the more familiar triad of oculo-orogenital lesions.

In many of the collagen diseases cutaneous lesions and systemic conditions are associated [see Section 4].

OTHER CONDITIONS

Hodgkin's disease sometimes presents with pruritus, a non-specific itchy rash, nodules or ulcers.

THE EYES

The eyebrows. These may be hypertrophic, hypoplastic or aplastic in a number of inherited anomalies. Acquired conditions include alopecia areata, leucotrichia, lateral sparseness in hypothyroidism, leprosy and secondary syphilis, or with short, broken hairs in atopic dermatitis. Hairs may be plucked deliberately or as an habitual tic. Scarring loss of eyebrows may follow folliculitis, late syphilis, lupus vulgaris or lupus erythematosus. The eyebrows may be affected in widespread seborrhoeic dermatitis or psoriasis.

The eyelids. The eyelids, particularly the upper ones, may become inflamed as a result of contact with an air-borne or hand-transferred irritant or sensitizing substance. The history is usually clear when a primary irritant has caused it but much questioning and patch testing may be necessary to find the cause of an eczematous reaction. The eyelids are swollen, reddish-brown and scaly, or lichenified and fissured, and there may be periorbital oedema. Likely causes include nail varnish (examine also cheeks, neck, lips and anogenital region), nickel, plants, eye lotions and ointments or even preparations prescribed for use at sites remote from the eyes, such as legs. Airborne causes include pollens, wood dusts, formalin, and chemicals in propellant packs. Lichenification of the eyelids may also occur in atopic dermatitis and in lichen simplex.

The eyelids may be swollen because of local infections, tumours or cavernous sinus thrombosis. Swelling may also be caused by infection of the scalp, secondary to pediculosis, hair-dye dermatitis, trauma, insect bites or from recurrent cellulitis causing lymphoedema; also from antral infections, mediastinal obstruction, cardiac failure, nephrosis, hypoproteinaemia, hypothyroidism or thyrotoxicosis, or worm infestations (onchocerciasis, trichiniasis, filariasis). In dermatomyositis the swollen eyelids are characteristically heliotrope in colour. Intermittent swelling of the eyelids without subsequent peeling occurs in urticaria. The absence of peeling differentiates urticaria from dermatitis of the lids and from recurrent cellulitis, in the second of which there are also usually fever, malaise, headache and vomiting.

Other dermatoses that sometimes affect the eyelids include psoriasis, lichen planus and lupus erythematosus. Fungal, bacterial and viral infections may occur. Xanthomatous plaques (xanthelasma), giant comedones, hamartomata, benign tumours, basal-cell epitheliomata and Bowen's disease may all occur thereon.

The eyelashes. These are rarely absent at birth and are more often lost in alopecia areata, from chronic infection (ulcerative blepharitis), or from lupus erythematosus. A stye (ciliary furuncle) is usually secondary to nasal carriage of staphylococci. Squamous blepharitis is a milder condition which occurs as part of infective (seborrhoeic) dermatitis. Psorasis also occasionally affects the lid margins. *Demodex folliculorum* infestation may affect the cilia, particularly in rosacea in which these parasites may also be found in large numbers in the facial papules. Head lice and pubic lice are sometimes transferred to the eyelashes.

Partial or total leucotrichia may occur as an inherited phenomenon, as a part of vitiligo or in sympathetic ophthalmia.

A Meibomian cyst is a swelling of the lid margin originating from a specialized sebaceous gland which discharges directly on the conjunctival surface, just within the lash margin.

The conjunctivae. Contact dermatitis of the eyelids may also affect the conjunctivae or the latter may be mainly or solely affected, as sometimes with streptomycin sensitivity. Infection of the conjunctivae is common and may be part of a widespread cutaneous infection. *Pseudomonas pyocyanea* may cause a simple conjunctivitis, but when there is existing eye disease or after operations on the eye it is a potential cause of destructive keratitis or uveitis. Conjunctivitis also occurs in primary herpes simplex infections, ophthalmic herpes zoster, rosacea, sarcoidosis (phlyctenular, non-specific, or as keratoconjunctivitis sicca, from involvement of the lacrimal glands), Reiter's disease (often transient) and Behçet's syndrome. Blisters may develop in the eyes in erythema multiforme, epidermolysis bullosa, benign mucous membrane pemphigoid, pemphigus vulgaris and hydroa aestivale (hydroa vacciniforme). Shrinkage of the conjunctivae with thickening and opacity of the cornea occurs in benign mucous membrane pemphigoid.

The lacrimal glands. Keratoconjunctivitis sicca occurs from involvement of the lacrimal glands in collagen disease, be it lupus erythematosus, systemic sclerosis, polyarteritis nodosa, polymyositis, dermatomyositis or rheumatoid arthritis. It may also occur in sarcoidosis. In Sjögren's syndrome there are also xerostomia, xeroderma and, often, rheumatoid arthritis.

The cornea. This is dystrophic in many hereditary cutaneous anomalies, including one form of epidermolysis bullosa, ichthyosis vulgaris, pityriasis rubra pilaris, Darier's disease, keratoderma palmaris et plantaris, anhidrotic ectodermal dysplasia and angiokeratoma corporis diffusum. Keratoconus (conical deformity of the cornea) is common in atopic dermatitis and may be, in part, responsible for the development of cataracts in that condition. Corneal arcus is due to deposits of cholesterol around the cornea and may be a degenerative phenomenon or a part of hypercholesterolaemic xanthomatosis.

Keratitis is a serious complication of rosacea. Starting as vascularization it may proceed to ulceration and scarring with impairment of vision. Keratitis with ulceration can also occur in Reiter's disease, ophthalmic herpes zoster, herpes simplex and in polyarteritis nodosa.

Corneal deposits causing visual haloes may develop in patients being treated with chloroquine. They disappear when the drug is withheld.

The lens and uvea. Congenital cataracts occur in several inherited skin anomalies. The incidence of cataracts is increased in atopic dermatitis and in alopecia universale.

Uveitis occurs in sarcoidosis, Behçet's syndrome and Reiter's syndrome.

The retina. Retrobulbar neuritis may follow posterior uveitis complicating skin diseases. The retina and the choroid may also be affected in lupus erythematosus as a part of a widespread vasculitis, also in polyarteritis nodosa, in which hypertensive changes may be seen. Retinopathy is also rare but a very serious complication of the treatment of lupus erythematosus with chloroquine.

In pseudoxanthoma elasticum the characteristic angioid streaks due to changes in Bruch's membrane are diagnostic. Retinal haemorrhages and choroiditis may also occur. Angioid streaks may also be seen in some examples of the Ehlers-Danlos syndrome.

THE EARS

The commonest aural developmental defects are the preauricular sinus in front of the anterior attachment of the helix and the accessory auricle, a soft or firm, hemispherical nodule in front of the tragus. Infection of a preauricular sinus may necessitate excision of its track.

In the folds of skin above, behind and below the ears infective dermatitis is common, with fissuring and a risk of streptococcal infection and cellulitis.

The fold above and behind the ears may also be the site of contact eczema from hair dye, hair nets and spectacle frames. The ear lobes may be affected in the same way by the metal of ear clips and the surface of the ears by hair dyes, hair lacquers, medicaments and light-sensitizers which, with certain hair styles may only affect the lower part of the ears. The whole surface of the external ears may be affected in widespread eczema, particularly when there is secondary infection.

The pinnae may be distorted by trauma (cauliflower ear) and it is vulnerable to perniosis and to frostbite. Calcinosis may occur.

Impetigo often affects the external ear and may originate from an aural discharge. Chronic infections (lupus vulgaris, syphilis, leprosy and fungal infections) may involve the ear. Lupus erythematosus may affect any part of the external ear (pinna, concha, lobe or meatus). Psoriasis may also appear on pinna, concha, lobe or meatus.

Otitis externa is inflammation of the meatus and it is often bilateral. The most important factors in its causation are itching and digital transference of organisms from elsewhere. The cause of the itching is often obscure; it may, in fact, be due to habitual manipulation of the meatus. Sometimes, inadvertent digital transference of an irritant or sensitizing substance occurs, with subsequent trauma from finger nails, match heads or hair clips used to reach the site of itching. Thus, nail varnish, phosphorus sesquisulphide, chrome or nickel may be introduced.

When infection occurs the nature of the organisms present often indicates the anogenital region as the source, either because of co-existing anogenital pruritus or because of imperfect hygiene. Organisms recovered include *Staphylococcus pyogenes*, *Streptococcus haemolyticus* and *Streptococcus pyogenes*, *Pseudomonas pyocyanea*, Proteus, enterococci, *Escherichia coli* and *Candida albicans*. A relationship to nasal carriage is less common.

Nodules on the ear include metabolic deposits in gout and in calcinosis, inflammatory lesions in granuloma annulare or sarcoidosis (painless) and perichondritis (very painful on light touch, usually in middle-aged men, involving the rim of one or both helices), basal cell papilloma, basal cell epithelioma (concha or meatus), Bowen's disease, keratosis or squamous epithelioma (helix or concha).

Rare inherited skin conditions are associated with deafness. In Tietz's syndrome piebaldism, normal eye colour and deaf-mutism are present. In another syndrome, urticaria, deafness and amyloidosis are associated.

THE NOSE, PHARYNX AND MOUTH

THE NOSE

Epistaxis is often the presenting symptom in hereditary haemorrhagic telangiectasia. It may also occur in Wegener's granulomatosis.

The nares are the major site of staphylococcal carriage. There may be boils, crusting or fissuring at the vestibule, or no abnormal sign. *Streptococcus pyogenes* may also be carried in the anterior nares and secondary digital spread of *Pseudomonas pyocanea*, Proteus and *Candida albicans* may take place from other sites to the nares.

Lupus vulgaris may affect the nose, causing, in time, perforation of the cartilaginous septum and parrot-bill deformity or collapse of the bridge of the nose with simian deformity. Sometimes the alae nasi are eroded away.

In late syphilis gummatous perforation may occur of the bony part of the nasal septum or of the hard or soft palate.

Lupus erythematosus and sarcoidosis may affect the nostrils but without any accompanying cartilaginous destruction.

The nostrils and other parts of the nose are often the site of basal cell epitheliomata.

Wegener's granulomatosis (midline granuloma) causes ulceration of the nose, mouth, pharynx, larynx or trachea. There is also polyarteritis, with involvement of the kidneys.

Fibroma is one of the commoner benign tumours on the nose.

Rhinophyma is an irregular sebaceous hyperplasia causing considerable disfigurement of the nose.

THE PHARYNX

The tonsils may be a carrier site of streptococci relevant to episodes of infected fissures and recurrent cellulitis, scarlatiniform erythema or exacerbations of psoriasis.

The pharynx and larynx may be affected in bullous eruptions including epidermolysis bullosa, pemphigus, benign mucous membrane pemphigoid, erythema multiforme and, rarely, in dermatitis herpetiformis.

The pillars of the fauces and the uvula may be mutilated by ulceration in Behçet's syndrome, and the pharynx, uvula and larynx may be ulcerated in Wegener's granulomatosis.

Laryngeal tuberculosis may coexist with orificial tuberculosis (tongue, floor of mouth, lips); all being secondary to an open pulmonary focus.

THE LIPS AND MOUTH

THE LIPS

Commissural cheilitis (angular stomatitis) presents with redness, light crusting and fissuring of the corners of the mouth. It is a form of infective flexural dermatitis due to *Candida albicans* or pathogenic cocci. Deficiencies of iron or vitamin B occasionally contribute. Another factor may be a falling in of the angles of the mouth with a resultant extension of the moist surface to the skin. The cause may be lack of teeth or dentures which are too narrow and shallow. Occasionally excessive salivation is present, arising from hypersensitivity to denture materials, tooth paste, mouth wash or fruit juice. Framboesiform syphilides may develop in this situation or at the cleft of the chin. Conditions which encourage *Candida albicans* infections may be relevant, including diabetes mellitus, the oral use of wide-spectrum antibiotics, pregnancy, contraceptive pills, calcium deficiency or deficiency of iron, riboflavin and protein.

Exfoliative cheilitis is a peeling condition of the vermilion surface of the lips, sometimes caused by habitual sucking or biting, sometimes by contact sensitivity to lip cosmetics or, occasionally, to citrous fruits, tooth paste, mouth wash, nail varnish, essential oils, nicotine, mentholated cigarettes or chemicals handled at work. In severe forms oedema, vesiculation and crusting may occur, followed by fissuring. The lower lip alone may be affected by substances with light-sensitizing properties, for example, eosin in a lip stick; also in lupus erythematosus.

Glandular cheilitis is a rare condition of undetermined cause. The mucous glands are enlarged and there is a glairy exudate, with crusting.

Granulomatous cheilitis is also rare. There is swelling and chronic inflammation of a lip and biopsy reveals a sarcoidal type of histology.

Macrocheilia may be congenital or acquired. The latter is due to persistent lymphatic obstruction secondary to streptococcal cellulitis, the organisms gaining entry through a fissure. Syphilis and tuberculosis in this region can also be complicated by macrocheilia.

The lips may, *inter alia*, be affected in lichen planus, lupus erythematosus, psoriasis, urticaria, erythema multiforme and recurrent herpes simplex. They are the characteristic sites of brown maculation in the Peutz-Jeghers syndrome and of telangiectases in hereditary haemorrhagic telangiectasia. The vermilion surfaces may be the sites of haemangioma, granuloma telangiectaticum, papilloma, keratosis, leucoplakia or epithelioma. On the mucosal aspect mucous implantation cysts may occur.

THE ORAL CAVITY

Inflammation within the mouth may cause diffuse redness, erosions, blisters, submucous haemorrhages or ulcers. The tongue may be similarly affected or it may exfoliate. In more chronic conditions redness may be inconspicuous and there is leucoplakia.

Oral lesions may occur in syphilis, tuberculosis, streptococcal, *Candida albicans* and Vincent's angina infections, herpes simplex, zoster, varicella, variola, warts, coxsackie and other virus infections. Lesions also occur from intoxication by some drugs and heavy metals. Nutritional deficiency (scurvy, pellagra) may cause haemorrhages and inflammation. Blood disorders, including leukaemia, agranulocytosis, pernicious anaemia and haemophilia may cause oral lesions, as may metabolic disturbances including diabetes mellitus and uraemia.

Skin diseases which often have oral lesions include lichen planus, lupus erythematosus, erythema multiforme, pemphigus, epidermolysis bullosa, Behçet's syndrome, zoster, Darier's disease and acanthosis nigricans.

Syphilis. Primary lesions may occur on the lips, tongue, palate or tonsil. In early syphilis mucous patches and 'snail track' ulcers may develop anywhere within the mouth. In late syphilis gummata may develop in the palate or tongue or there may be a syphilitic glossitis with irregular lobulation, fissuring, and leucoplakia.

Tuberculosis. See Section 2.

Streptococcal stomatitis. This may complicate tonsillitis. There is a patchy or generalized cherry-red and swollen condition of the gums. *Candida albicans* produces soft, white, detachable, rapidly spreading raised patches (thrush). Vincent's angina, due to symbiosis between a spirochaete and a fusiform bacillus, causes grey patches in a red, raw, bleeding surface. It particularly affects the gingival sulci and the gingivobuccal margin. Gangrenous stomatitis (cancrum oris) is Vincent's angina as it affects severely debilitated and malnourished children.

Recurrent aphthous stomatitis (*aphthosis*). This relatively common condition is of undetermined cause and is probably not an infective but a vascular allergic condition. It is unrelated to herpes simplex. The recurrent, painful, superficial ulcers measure less than 5 mm. in diameter and occur, single or multiple, anywhere within the mouth and occasionally on the transitional surfaces of the external genitalia. Tetracycline suspension, 250 mg. in 5 ml., may give relief. Topical corticosteroid preparations may help to abort lesions, if applied early, but later may do more harm than good.

Herpetic stomatitis usually affects infants 2–3 years old, as a primary infection. The painful erosions, up to

5 mm. diameter on the cheeks, tongue, gums or lips, are accompanied by malaise, fever and headache. Culture confirms the diagnosis. In some individuals recurrences of herpetic stomatitis occur at times of general debility.

Zoster. [See Section 2.]

Varicella. [See Section 2.]

Variola. [See Section 2.]

Hand, foot and mouth disease. This coxsackie infection presents, usually in children, with slight fever, vesicles scattered anywhere within the mouth, and grey vesicles, up to 5 mm. diameter, on the fingers and toes.

Drugs may cause haemorrhages, erosions, bullae, ulcers or lesions resembling lichen planus or erythema multiforme. Mercury may cause salivation with gross swelling of the gums and tongue, often accompanied by nephritis. Lead causes a blue-black discoloration of the gums opposite areas of marginal gingivitis. There may also be ulceration. Silver deposits cause blue-grey pigmentation or may stimulate melanogenesis, causing brown discoloration. Bismuth may cause similar hyperpigmentation and gold may cause stomatitis and hyperpigmentation. These metallic pigmentations have to be differentiated from that of Addison's disease and from racial pigmentation which may occasionally be seen in the gums and cheeks of individuals of mixed ancestry as well as in the mouths of dark-skinned persons.

Scurvy causes swelling, redness and friability of the gums and purpura or haemorrhage. In pellagra the tongue is centrally stippled, beefy and raw at the narrow tip and sides.

In leukaemia and agranulocytosis there may be purpura, haemorrhages and secondary infection with ulceration. In pernicious anaemia the tongue is smooth and glazed or it may have a cobble-stone appearance. In haemophilia intraoral haemorrhages may occur.

In untreated diabetes mellitus the tongue is large, red, dry, glazed and fissured and there may be gingivitis. In uraemia the tongue is dry and foul and stomatitis may occur.

Behçet's syndrome presents with painful, large, persistent and mutilating ulceration of the lips, tongue, floor of the mouth, cheeks or pillars of the fauces. The external genitalia (mostly vulva or scrotum) may also be affected and in the eyes there may be conjunctivitis, keratitis or hypopyon iritis. One site may be affected alone or there may be progression from one to another. There may also be acuminate papules or nodules in the skin and a tendency to suppuration from minor trauma. Massive venous thromboses and neurological manifestations of various kinds may occur.

Skin diseases with oral lesions described elsewhere include lichen planus, lupus erythematosus, erythema multiforme, pemphigoid, benign mucous membrane pemphigoid and epidermolysis bullosa.

LEUCOPLAKIA

This is a chronic, non-specific inflammation of transitional epithelial surfaces.

Aetiology

It may be caused by physical or chemical irritation, or it may be the result of various diseases within the mouth, including lichen planus, lupus erythematosus, syphilis and drug intoxications.

Histologically there is hyperkeratosis, parakeratosis and slight acanthosis.

Clinical Picture

Leucoplakia may be smooth, irregular or verrucose. The smooth type is common on the buccal mucosa and is relatively benign, but on the lower lip it may be the precursor of epithelioma. The irregular form is often syphilitic and precancerous. It occurs especially on the tongue and within the angles of the mouth. The verrucose form is potentially malignant.

Diagnosis

White patches within the mouth are occasionally due to oral epithelial naevi (white and spongy), more often to lichen planus (white macules or delicate cobweb, feathery or foliate traceries on the cheeks, gums, tongue or mucous or vermilion surfaces of the lips), occasionally with red, eroded areas. Lupus erythematosus produces coarser white patches, mostly on the cheeks, with conspicuous redness, erosion and scarring. *Candida albicans* infections (thrush) cause white detachable plaques from which the diagnosis can be confirmed by direct microscopy and culture. Leucoplakia is a coarser, thickened, plaque-like condition, sometimes with fissuring. It may affect the lips, cheeks, tongue, or floor of the mouth. A cheek-biting habit presents as an irregular rough, white area, often triangular in shape just within the oral commisure, or in a band, on one or both sides where the cheek has repeatedly been sucked between the teeth and chewed. Lichenification of anogenital flexural skin surfaces may resemble leucoplakia but is benign.

Treatment

There is no effective treatment. Smoking, hot drinks, spiced foods and condiments are best avoided. Dental hygiene is important. Periodic inspection is necessary for the earliest possible detection of any epitheliomatous change. If there is hardness and thickening excision is advisable, preceded, if in doubt, by biopsy.

MUCOSAL PIGMENTATIONS

Yellow spots on the mucosal aspects of the lips or on the cheeks occur in the common physiological 'Fordyce condition'. They represent ectopic sebaceous glands. Misinterpretation of them as pathological sometimes causes unnecessary alarm.

Brown patches of melanin occur normally in many individuals of pigmented races, or of mixed ancestry, also in Addison's disease, Peutz-Jeghers syndrome, acanthosis nigricans, argyria, from antimalarial drugs or bismuth injections and in lead poisoning (on the gums, in the presence of sepsis).

THE TONGUE

Atrophic glossitis occurs in iron-deficiency anaemia, sometimes with dysphagia and koilonychia. Pernicious anaemia may present with soreness of the tongue, atrophy of the papillae and, sometimes, with a cobble-stoned appearance. Painful, vivid red patches may be present on the tip and sides of the tongue (Hunter's glossitis, Möller's glossitis).

Other factors in the aetiology of glossitis include alcohol, smoking and condiments. Glossitis may occur in diabetes mellitus, sprue and pellagra. A rare cause is electrogalvanism from metals of different electro-potentials in dental prostheses. A salty or metallic taste may be complained of or tingling sensations may occur.

'Burning tongue' (glossodynia) may be symptomatic of irritation from heat, alcohol or trauma; of avitaminosis, pernicious anaemia, leukaemia, drug intolerance (especially phenolphthalein), electrogalvanism, Sjögren's syndrome, gastric reflux from hiatus hernia or cancerphobia. It may also occur from changes in the temporomandibular joints, usually due to abnormal stresses arising in these joints from a lack of teeth. In many patients with glossodynia, particularly in middle-aged women, no material cause can be found.

Geographical tongue is a benign wandering rash of the tongue, usually asymptomatic and often discovered fortuitously. There is no predisposition to the later development of carcinoma. A wandering superficial exfoliation slowly travels over the surface, producing reddened denuded areas. It tends to persist indefinitely but no treatment is necessary, apart from reassurance.

Black tongue presents in two varieties. Black 'hairy' tongue is an hyperkeratotic condition of the filiform papillae which gives the centre of the tongue in its anterior third an appearance like a black dog's matted coat. It may be caused by smoking, antibiotic treatment, a soft diet and other undetermined causes. The non-hairy black tongue may be caused by chewing tobacco or tooth paste, dyed sweets, certain drugs, chromogenic bacteria, fungi or metallic sulphides.

The tongue may also be darker than usual in Addison's disease.

Median rhomboid glossitis is a benign nodular condition in the midline of the dorsum of the tongue, lozenge shaped, well defined anteriorly but fading posteriorly into the circumvallate papillae. It may be discovered accidentally and cause alarm, but it has no serious significance, being a persistence of the tuberculum impar.

Scrotal tongue (lingua plicata) is a congenital malformation of deep sulci running in various directions. Food debris may collect in the folds. Careful hygiene is necessary to keep the sulci clear.

Macroglossia occurs in primary systemic amyloidosis.

Lingual keratoses are present in some cases of Darier's disease.

Lingual tumours include haemangioma, lymphangioma, lipoma, fibroma, chondroma, mucous cysts, papilloma, carcinoma and sarcoma.

THE GUMS

Pigmentation occurs from bismuth and in lead poisoning. Lichen planus causes white spots and streaks, diphenylhydantoin causes hyperplasia, gingivitis arises from drugs, in blood dyscrasias and from Vincent's infection. Soft, bleeding gums occur in scurvy. Epulis is a fibrous tumour of the gums.

THE RESPIRATORY SYSTEM

The lungs and the skin may be affected concurrently in tuberculosis, sarcoidosis, systemic sclerosis, dermatomyositis, polyarteritis nodosa, lupus erythematosus, carcinoma and in rarer conditions including pyocyanea infections secondary to antibiotic treatment (lung abscess), tularaemia (pneumonia), and histoplasmosis (granuloma in skin), with or without pulmonary symptoms.

Pulmonary tuberculosis is rarely associated with lupus vulgaris but is more common in patients with lupus than in the general population. Ulcerative orificial tuberculosis of the nose or mouth usually originates from a pulmonary or laryngeal focus. Tuberculosis verrucosa may also arise from self-inoculation from an open pulmonary focus as well as from an infected human or animal cadaver. Cutaneous tuberculides may be secondary to a pulmonary focus or to an extrapulmonary one. Similarly, erythema nodosum may indicate hypersensitivity to a primary tuberculous focus in the lungs, upper respiratory tract or skin.

When sarcoidosis presents in the skin pulmonary involvement is shown by radiography as hilar lymphadenopathy, parenchymatous mottling, miliary infiltration or coarse nodulation. In the skin sarcoidosis presents in papular or nodular forms (cutaneous or subcutaneous) or as annular or circinate lesions. Other forms are lupus pernio of the nose (Besnier's lupus pernio) and, rarely, erythroderma. When sarcoidosis presents with erythema nodosum there is a relatively favourable prognosis, resolution often occurring within 18 months.

Systemic sclerosis affects the lungs in the majority of patients as shown by radiographic examination and pulmonary function tests. There is dyspnoea and, perhaps, cough, and reticular or nodular radiographic changes are found. Pulmonary function may be found to be impaired in the absence of any radiographic evidence of abnormality. The significant finding is an impaired diffusing capacity.

Dermatomyositis may be accompanied by respiratory distress owing to involvement of the intercostal muscles and the diaphragm. Heart failure may result or infection may supervene. In adult patients with dermatomyositis the condition may be secondary to visceral carcinoma, sometimes bronchial.

Polyarteritis nodosa often affects the lungs and occasionally the skin. There may be asthma, patchy pneumonia, or fibrosis radiologically resembling miliary tuberculosis, sarcoidosis or carcinomatosis. There may be pleurisy, with or without effusion. The diffusing capacity is impaired.

Systemic lupus erythematosus may present with, or be complicated by, pleurisy, with or without effusion. The diffusing capacity may be impaired and radiography may show mottled infiltration.

Carcinomatosis. Secondary deposits may occur in the skin from carcinoma of the bronchus as a number of skin-coloured or reddish painless nodules or morphoea-like plaques on the trunk or scalp. Other tumours which produce cutaneous metastases include malignant melanoma and carcinomata arising from breast, lung, stomach, kidney (hypernephroma), liver, large intestine, prostate, uterus and ovary; also osteosarcoma. Dermatomyositis or acanthosis nigricans may be skin manifestations, *inter alia*, of bronchial malignancy.

Bowen's disease of the skin is sometimes accompanied by visceral malignancy, including bronchial carcinoma. Patients with skin signs of chronic inorganic arsenical intoxication (pigmentation, rain-drop depigmentation, keratoses and epitheliomata) are also liable to develop carcinoma of the bronchus.

Hodgkin's disease and other reticuloses which may present with cutaneous nodules or ulcers may also have lymph node involvement in the mediastinum or pulmonary infiltrations or nodules.

THE CARDIOVASCULAR AND LYMPHATIC SYSTEMS

Disease of the peripheral vessels is more often associated with disease of the skin than is heart disease.

THE HEART

Familial hypercholesterolaemic xanthomatosis carries with it a risk of vascular catastrophes, including coronary thrombosis, cerebral or peripheral thromboses or haemorrhages. There may be a family history of similar happenings.

Arteriovenous anastomoses and angiomatosis in the Klippel-Trénauny-Weber syndrome cause haemangiectatic hypertrophy of a limb with hyperidrosis and varicosities. Ulceration may develop. If the shunt is extensive cardiac embarrassment may result.

In pseudoxanthoma elasticum defective elastic fibres in the media and intima of arteries may cause coronary, cerebral, renal, intestinal or peripheral vascular manifestations.

In the Ehlers-Danlos syndrome the collagenous deficiency may cause dissecting aneurysms or cardiac defects.

The increased blood flow in the skin in erythroderma may embarrass the heart.

Erythema marginatum, a pale pink, non-scaly arciform or polycyclic erythema is the characteristic skin manifestation of rheumatic fever. Other patients present with erythema multiforme, erythema nodosum or purpura.

The heart is often affected in the collagenoses. In systemic lupus erythematosus pericarditis may occur, with or without effusion, and it is commoner than Libman-Sacks endocarditis. The valves or the myocardium may be affected, with systolic or diastolic murmurs, atrial fibrillation or heart block. There may be hypertension. In systemic sclerosis the myocardial involvement may cause dyspnoea, and disturbances of rhythm are common. Similar changes may occur in dermatomyositis. Abnormalities may only be detected by electrocardiography. In polyarteritis nodosa the coronary arteries may be affected and the accompanying hypertension or myocardial disease may cause heart failure.

Sarcoidosis may involve the myocardium, causing disturbances of rhythm or heart failure.

In tertiary syphilis aortic disease is common (aneurysm, aortic valvular incompetence, coronary insufficiency), and all patients with late syphilis of the skin should be investigated accordingly.

PERIPHERAL VASCULAR DISEASE

Venous insufficiency results from incompetent valves in the veins or from increased pressure in the superficial plexus secondary to deep vein thrombosis or from both these conditions. There may be varicosities, eczema on the lower third of the leg and on the foot, areas of pigmented induration secondary to thrombosis or recurrent cellulitis, and ulcers, usually below and behind the medial malleolus. Any accompanying discomfort is eased by elevation of the foot.

Perniosis (chilblains) may develop on the digits (acrocyanosis), legs (erythema pernio), also on the ears, nose, knees or elsewhere. There is abnormal reactivity to cold, with arteriolar and venular constriction. Stagnation of blood in small venules then causes blueness and coldness. Massage of the affected part from the periphery causes a temporary colour change to red. There may be ulceration and secondary infection. Fissures (chaps) may also be present. Differentiation has to be made from lupus pernio of Besnier in sarcoidosis and from lupus pernio of Hutchinson in lupus erythematosus.

Venous thrombosis has many causes including trauma, infections in or near the vein, chemical toxins, smoking, local stasis, diseased valves, varicosity, haemorrhage, shock, blood dyscrasias, pregnancy or oral contraceptives with a high oestrogen content. It is a feature of Behçet's syndrome. In thrombophlebitis migrans multiple thromboses occur and there is a clear link with visceral malignancy. Thromboses often occur in varicose veins, causing firm, tender, sometimes elongated areas of induration. More diffuse induration results from recurrent attacks of low grade cellulitis following secondary infection of exuding hypostatic eczema.

Thromboangiitis obliterans is clinically similar to nodular vasculitis, with tender nodules on the legs and feet. There is a link with cigarette smoking. There may also be claudication, Raynaud's phenomenon, gangrene and phlebitis.

Arterial insufficiency causes pain in the calf on exertion, relieved by rest (angina cruris). There may be white, slightly depressed areas of atrophy on the ankle or foot when small, superficial vessels are affected or there may be painful ulceration, usually on the anterolateral aspect of the ankle or foot. Slow necrobiotic gangrene may occur with the slough taking a long time to detach or, with adequate treatment, to heal. The pain of arterial leg ulcers is relieved when the foot is held slightly dependent.

Combined arterial and venous insufficiency is not uncommon.

Arterial disease may present with ischaemic ulcers containing adherent sloughs, as nodular vasculitis with tender nodules and foci of necrosis, necrotizing papules, haemorrhagic bullae or purpura, depending on the size of the vessels affected and on the intensity of the pathological process and the amount of occlusion resulting from it. Arterial ulcers may occur in blood dyscrasias, including haemolytic anaemia, sickle-cell anaemia, polycythaemia, thrombocythaemia, dysglobulinaemia and coagulation disorders.

Whereas polyarteritis nodosa is a systemic condition affecting, in one patient or another, the lungs, cardiovascular system, kidneys, gastro-intestinal tract, peripheral nerves, muscles and joints, there is another form of vasculitis which affects either the skin alone or the kidneys in addition, usually sparing other organs. It presents with tender nodules, which may ulcerate, usually on the legs. Larger arteries may also be affected causing angina cruris. Reticular livedo may be present and there may be albuminuria, microscopic haematuria and biochemical evidence of impaired renal function.

Functional arteriolar vasoconstriction occurs in the digits in Raynaud's phenomenon, causing pallor followed by cyanosis. There may be no obvious cause (Raynaud's disease) or it may be caused by accidental or occupational trauma. It occurs in the collagenoses, rheumatoid arthritis, occlusive arterial disease or with paroxysmal haemoglobinuria, cold haemolysins, cold agglutinins or cryoglobulins, in diseases of the nervous system and in poisoning by ergot. Functional vasoconstriction is also responsible for the changes of perniosis and for some examples of livedo reticularis, particularly cutis marmorata.

Arteriovenous anastomoses may occur from penetrating injuries or from congenital anomaly as in the Klippel-Trénauny-Weber syndrome. The affected part of the limb is swollen and warm, with a localized or diffuse haemangioma presenting as dusky nodular excrescences. There may be a systolic bruit and thrill. Ulceration often occurs. The whole limb may be enlarged and longer than the other. Arteriography reveals the extent of the vascular abnormality and the feasibility of surgery. Progressive cardiac embarrassment may occur in the worst cases.

Ulceration of the legs. This has many causes, the commonest being venous stasis. Other causes include injuries (minor in the presence of stasis), self-inflicted injuries (artefacts), radiation atrophy, perniosis, arterial disease, arteriovenous anastomoses, coccal, mycobacterial, corynebacterial, spirochaetal, mycotic and leishmanial infections (rarely from brucellosis, cat-scratch disease, glanders, tularaemia, reticulosis, Hodgkin's disease, leukaemia, blood dyscrasias and coagulation disorders, necrobiosis lipoidica, pyoderma gangrenosum, polyarteritis nodosa, systemic sclerosis and other collagenoses, with or without calcinosis, epithelioma and others. Tropical ulcers are caused by malnutrition and a large number of organisms, including atypical mycobacteria and *Corynebacterium diphtheriae*.

Capillary disorders present as purpura. This may be caused by chemicals or drugs, infections (meningococcal, typhus, bacterial endocarditis, etc.), cryoglobulinaemia, hyperglobulinaemia, kidney or liver disease, carcinomatosis, amyloidosis, malnutrition, thrombocytopenia, raised local intravascular pressure, ageing and corticosteroid treatment. In the Ehlers-Danlos syndrome the fragile hyperelastic skin exposes subcutaneous vessels to traction trauma and rupture with the production of purpura and haematomas and later, some tumours of degenerate connective tissue.

There is also a group of benign purpuric capillaroses (of Schamberg, Majocci, Gougerot and Blum). Henoch-Schönlein purpura is an allergic phenomenon, usually accompanied by painful, swollen joints and abdominal symptoms (vomiting, colic, diarrhoea, melaena). Renal involvement is common, presenting as macroscopic or microscopic haematuria from glomerulitis.

TELANGIECTASIA

This occurs in a number of skin conditions including xeroderma pigmentosum, solar dermatitis, radiodermatitis, rosacea, poikiloderma, with varicosities, in the collagenoses and in Raynaud's disease. Telangiectasia macularis eruptiva perstans is a variety of mastocytosis in which the telangiectasia makes it difficult to see the pigmented maculation. 'Spider' telangiectases are present in many healthy individuals, children and adults. They may become more numerous during pregnancy and in the presence of liver disease. The lesions of hereditary haemorrhagic telangiectasia occur on the skin and lips, also in the nasal septum, mouth, nasopharynx, gastro-intestinal tract, kidneys and retina. Aneurysms may occur or arteriovenous fistulae in the lungs, causing dyspnoea, cyanosis and clubbing. Epistaxis is the commonest presenting symptom. Lesions also occur in the liver, sometimes with cirrhosis. Various haemangiomata are, partly or wholly, telangiectatic.

THE LYMPHATICS

Lymphoedema results from lymphatic insufficiency either due to hypoplasia or to obliteration or obstruction of lymphatics. In the fully developed condition there is rough warty thickening of the epidermis overlying a firm fibrotic thickened dermis—elephantiasis. Fissuring and secondary infection occur. Pitting is absent at this stage but may be present in the early stage in which there is swelling due to connective tissue hyperplasia and sometimes a characteristic yellow discoloration of the nails.

Congenital hypoplasia of the lymphatics predisposes to defective drainage of an area and to infection with streptococci which gain entry through fissures in the skin. These may be obvious, but often none can be found. Other predisposing causes include oedema of renal origin, malignant deposits in lymph nodes or surgical removal of lymph nodes, filariasis, tuberculosis or syphilis, probably with secondary streptococcal infection. Dysgammaglobulinaemia is sometimes a factor.

In the common streptococcal form each attack of cellulitis causes a further loss of functioning lymphatics, so increasing the lymphoedema and predisposing still more to further attacks of cellulitis. The sites most often affected are the face, lower limbs and external genitalia. Attacks of recurrent cellulitis are ushered in with increase of local swelling, redness and pain. A red streak of lymphangitis may be visible running up the limb and the regional lymph nodes may be swollen and tender. There is general malaise, fever, headache and, perhaps, vomiting. A brisk improvement results from treatment with penicillin and further attacks may sometimes be prevented by the treatment of any fissures with chlortetracycline ointment and, in more intractable cases, with penicillin systemically. Distortion of the face (often the lip) can sometimes be alleviated by the excision of excessive tissue, but, in general, the treatment of elephantiasis is unsatisfactory, namely supporting bandages, exercise, diüretics and prophylactic antibiotics.

Lymphangitis occurs with streptococcal infections of the skin and sometimes with other coccal infections. There may also be conspicuous enlargement of lymph nodes with many extensive itchy dermatoses, particularly erythroderma. In this condition lymph node biopsy may be the only means of differentiating between a reactive dermatopathic lymphadenopathy and one due to a reticulosis. Extensive lymphadenopathy may also be a feature of lupus erythematosus, Hodgkin's disease and sarcoidosis. In early syphilis lymphadenopathy is common; enlarged epitrochlear nodes are suggestive of this diagnosis but they may also be present with infected conditions of the hands.

Liquefactive lymphadenopathy is characteristic in the drainage area from a primary tuberculous complex in the skin.

Lymph node metastases occur from malignant melanoma or from squamous epithelioma, especially when it arises from transitional epithelium of the mouth or external genitalia, from atrophic scar tissue or from sites of thin skin once the hypoderm has been invaded. Metastasis from basal cell epithelioma is a great rarity.

Lymphangioma circumscriptum presents as a localized tumour of 'frog spawn' vesicles, some containing altered blood, on the skin or tongue. It may be accompanied by more extensive deeper anomalies locally in the lymphatic system and excision is often followed by a recurrence. Deeper defects in the lymphatics may show as more diffuse lymphangiomata which exude an opalescent fluid. There may also be hypertrophy of part of a limb. Cystic hygroma usually occurs in the neck as a swelling discovered in infancy. It is a developmental anomaly arising from the thoracic duct. Lymphangiosarcoma (Stewart and Treves) is a rare complication of chronic lymphoedema. It usually follows radical mastectomy for carcinoma and presents as rapidly growing and metastasizing bluish nodules clinically resembling those of Kaposi's sarcoma in the arm on the same side as the amputated breast.

THE GASTRO-INTESTINAL TRACT

THE OESOPHAGUS

A rare familial association has been noted between keratoderma of the palms and soles starting late in childhood and carcinoma of the oesophagus at 40–60 years of age. An autosomal dominant inheritance has been established.

The oesophagus is atrophic in the Plummer-Vinson syndrome (sideropenic dysphagia), the other manifestations being burning soreness of the tongue with diffuse papillary atrophy, angular cheilitis and koilonychia.

The oesophagus is often affected in systemic sclerosis. Radiographic changes may be present before symptoms develop, hence radiographic investigation may provide supporting evidence for a tentative diagnosis of systemic sclerosis. The changes may be of gastro-oesophageal reflux or of atonia, causing dyspepsia with heartburn or dysphagia. Dysphagia also occurs occasionally in systemic lupus erythematosus.

The oesophagus may undergo blistering, erosion or ulceration in some bullous conditions, including epidermolysis bullosa of the polydysplastic type (when stricture, pneumonitis or carcinoma of the cardia may follow), benign mucous membrane pemphigoid and (rarely) in pemphigus and pemphigoid.

THE STOMACH

A relationship between rosacea and gastro-intestinal disorder has long been suspected but not proven. Flatulent dyspepsia is not uncommon and habitual rush, with hurried meals and a fondness for hot tea in large quantities, may be relevant.

The stomach may be involved in the polyposis of the Peutz-Jeghers syndrome.

Some patients with systemic sclerosis have impaired gastric motility.

Acanthosis nigricans, when related to visceral malignancy, is most commonly associated with adenocarcinoma of the stomach. Other skin conditions which may suggest gastric cancer include dermatomyositis, pemphigoid (doubtful), figurate erythemas and secondary deposits (skin-coloured or inflamed nodules or morphoea-like areas, for instance on the scalp).

THE SMALL INTESTINE

Nutritional deficiency may arise from an inadequate or unbalanced diet, malabsorption, defective transport or utilization or increased requirements. Single vitamin deficiencies may arise from genetic causes or from drug antimetabolites.

Deficiencies are more often multiple than single, hence the clinical picture is often mixed. Single vitamin deficiencies cause:

Vitamin A. Dryness of the skin, follicular keratoses and xerophthalmia.

Vitamin B. Aneurine—peripheral neuritis, oedema, heart failure.
Riboflavin—cheilitis and glossitis (smooth, dusky, red tongue), infective dermatitis.
Nicotinic acid—dermatitis at sites exposed to sunlight or to physical trauma, gastro-enteritis and mental depression or dementia.

Vitamin C. Gingivitis, perifollicular purpura, ecchymoses, follicular keratoses, anaemia, apathy, depression.

Vitamin D. Rickets. Impaired resistance to cutaneous tuberculosis.

Vitamin K. Ecchymoses.

Jejunal malabsorption causes iron, folic acid and vitamin C deficiency, hypoproteinaemia and impaired fat absorption. There may be hyperpigmentation, oedema, acquired ichthyosis, often of follicular pattern, and defective hair and nails.

Severe protein deficiency in children causes the syndrome kwashiorkor, with mental and physical retardation, oedema, muscle wasting, reddish-brown scaly patches, dry, lustreless, discoloured hair, patchy hyperpigmentation and hypopigmentation, xerophthalmia, cheilitis, vulvovaginitis, apathy and defects of the nails. Degenerative changes occur in the liver, pancreas and gut. The hyperpigmentation of malnutrition and malabsorption may be a direct effect or post-inflammatory.

Hypervitaminosis can occur with fat-soluble vitamins. Acute overdosage of vitamin A causes increased intracranial pressure, optic neuritis, headache, dizziness, nausea and vomiting, followed by extensive peeling of the skin. Chronic vitamin A overdosage causes dry skin, diffuse loss of hair, keratoses, purpura, hyperpigmentation and tender bony swellings due to cortical hyperostosis.

Vitamin D in high dosage may cause headache, vomiting, diarrhoea and albuminuria with raised blood urea and metastatic calcification, particularly in the kidneys and the skin, resulting from hypercalcaemia.

Gluten sensitive enteropathy has been found in some examples of extensive eczema of 'seborrhoeic' type and in some cases of dermatitis herpetiformis.

Malignant atrophic papulosis (Degos) is a rare condition of crops of pruritic papules with central umbilication on the trunk and limbs. The lesions may coalesce and they take on an atrophic appearance. The patient has no other symptoms at first but after an interval of weeks, months or even years abdominal pains, weakness, fatigue, loss of weight and, possibly, diarrhoea develop. Multiple intestinal perforations may occur, either simultaneously or sequentially. These are due to foci of arteriolitis in the gut similar to those in the skin. There may be arteriolitis in other organs. Death results from gut perforations or from cerebral infarcts.

Acrodermatitis enteropathica is a severe, genetically determined condition of disordered tryptophan metabolism in which there is an extensive bullous eruption particularly affecting the skin around the orifices and in the flexures. Crusting and secondary infection with *Candida albicans* follow. The hair is sparse, there is diarrhoea and growth may be retarded. *Diodoquin*, 400–600 mg. daily, is often effective. For long-term treatment the dose should be kept down to the minimal effective level.

Carcinoid tumours (argentaffinomas which secrete an excess of 5-hydroxytryptophan) may occur in the lung, intestine, appendix or ovary. Flushing, resembling rosacea, is a feature when the intestines are involved, with or without hepatic metastases. There may be diarrhoea and dyspnoea. The urine contains an excess of 5-hydroxyindole acetic acid.

Small intestinal changes may occur in systemic sclerosis, with impaired motility, dilatation, colic and diarrhoea or constipation.

In the blue rubber-bleb naevus syndrome haemangiomata are present both in the skin and in the intestines, particularly the small intestine. Melaena and anaemia may result.

Regional ileitis (Crohn's disease) may occur with erythema nodosum, perianal granulomata, fissuring or ulceration, or maceration and erosion around ileostomy or colostomy, pyoderma gangrenosum, manifestations of malabsorption or remote sarcoid lesions.

In the Peutz-Jeghers syndrome lentigines on the face and lips, within the mouth or on the extremities are accompanied by intestinal polyposis affecting most the small intestine. There may be attacks of abdominal pain with or without intussusception or haemorrhage causing haematemesis or melaena.

In pseudoxanthoma elasticum intestinal arterial involvement may cause haemorrhage, with haematemesis or melaena.

THE COLON

This is often involved in systemic sclerosis, causing constipation or diarrhoea, and diverticula which may perforate.

Polyposis in Peutz-Jeghers syndrome may involve the colon.

Ulcerative colitis may be accompanied by various cutaneous manifestations of malabsorption. It is also associated with a condition resembling erythema nodosum excepting that the nodules may be recurrent and may ulcerate. Fever and joint swellings also occur. Pyoderma gangrenosum may develop from the erythema nodosum-like lesions or from papulopustules. The colliquative necrosis spreads, forming ulcers with undermined edges. The ulcers may reach several inches in diameter.

THE ANUS

Pruritus ani, with or without perianal dermatitis, may be caused by oxyuriasis, in children more than in adults. *Candida albicans* infections (non-suppurative) or coccal infections (suppurative), stool or urine chemical burns in infancy, haemorrhoids, fissures, sensitivity reactions to anaesthetic, antihistamine or antibiotic applications, fungal infections (rare in European women), psoriasis, lichen planus, lichen sclerosus et atrophicus, simple lichenification or Bowen's disease.

Pruritus ani without physical signs may be due to thread worms or it may have a psychogenic basis.

Virus warts (condylomata acuminata) may involve the anal canal as well as the perianal skin. They may occur in homosexual individuals and have to be differentiated from syphilitic condylomata lata.

Perianal ulceration may occur in Behçet's syndrome, in regional ileitis and in ulcerative colitis.

Ulcerating or verrucose tuberculosis of the perianal skin may arise from an intestinal focus of tuberculosis.

THE KIDNEYS AND GENITO-URINARY TRACT

THE KIDNEYS

Chronic renal disease with uraemia may cause general pruritus and a light brown diffuse pigmentation of the skin. There may be purpura and susceptibility to cutaneous infections.

The kidneys and urinary tract may be involved in a number of hereditary anomalies which also affect the skin. For example, in neurofibromatosis lesions may occur in the genito-urinary tract causing obstruction or infection. In tuberous sclerosis renal tumours may present with haematuria. In angiokeratosis corporis diffusum renal failure may occur from lipid infiltration of the glomerular vessels. In pseudoxanthoma elasticum the arterial involvement may affect the kidneys, causing haematuria and in hereditary haemorrhagic telangiectasia haematuria may occur.

The kidneys are also involved in metabolic disorders, particularly calcinosis and primary systemic amyloidosis.

Impetigo of streptococcal origin due to certain strains may be complicated by acute glomerulonephritis and this may also occur with scarlatina.

In drug eruptions, for example from gold, examination should always be made for coexistent albuminuria.

In all collagenoses and vasculitides renal vascular involvement may occur and seriously affect the prognosis. This applies to Henoch-Schönlein purpura, allergic vasculitis, polyarteritis nodosa, lupus erythematosus, systemic sclerosis, dermatomyositis and Wegener's granulomatosis.

THE EXTERNAL GENITALIA

Urethritis is a feature of Reiter's disease, often with circinate balanitis. It may also occur in severe erythema multiforme, accompanied by balanitis or vulvovaginitis.

Balanoposthitis is usually infective, from *Candida albicans* or a mixed flora of intestinal organisms. A mild form may develop from trichomonal infestation. It can also arise from contact irritants or sensitizers or from trauma.

Plasma cell balanitis is an histological diagnosis of resistant plaques of inflammation in elderly men, probably of mixed, partly infective aetiology. It has to be distinguished on histological grounds from Queyrat's erythroplasia, a single velvety red lesion of carcinoma *in situ*.

Vulvovaginitis is usually infective (*Candida albicans*, mixed coccal and Gram-negative bacillary infections), gonococcal, syphilitic, tuberculous or viral infections, the latter due to herpes simplex, zoster or vaccinia.

Non-infective causes include vaginal foreign bodies, artefact lesions, oxyuriasis, contact irritants and sensitizers and Bowen's disease.

Penile or vulval blisters occur in herpes simplex, pemphigus, pemphigoid, erythema multiforme and fixed drug eruptions.

Penile or vulval ulcers occur in syphilis, chancroid, gonorrhoea, tuberculosis orificialis, granuloma inguinale, histoplasmosis, virus infections, erythema multiforme, Behçet's disease, polyarteritis nodosa and epithelioma. Artefact lesions may be produced by emotionally disturbed individuals.

Skin disorders often affecting the penis or vulva include psoriasis, lichen planus, lichen sclerosus et atrophicus (from which, on the penis, balanitis xerotica obliterans may arise), lichen simplex, contact eczema and warts.

THE ENDOCRINE AND EXOCRINE GLANDS

THE PITUITARY

In acromegaly excessive somatotrophin secretion causes diffuse thickening of the skin and increased periosteal bone growth. The skin is oily and sweaty and may be furrowed on the scalp. The hair is coarse. Indirect effects from stimulation of other endocrine glands may include increased pigmentation, hirsutism, hyperthyroidism and diabetes mellitus.

In Cushing's syndrome overaction of the adrenal glands or their stimulation by the pituitary causes excessive glucocorticoid production.

The administration of corticosteroids can cause moon facies, 'buffalo hump', obesity of the trunk, striae atrophicae, a tendency to bruising and, secondarily, increased pigmentation and hirsutism. Similar changes may arise from neoplasms which produce corticotrophin-like substances, particularly oat-cell carcinoma of the bronchus, thymic or pancreatic neoplasms or carcinoids.

In pituitary atrophy lassitude and wasting are accompanied by partial or total loss of hair on the scalp and in the axillary and pubic regions, with atrophy of the skin.

In patients receiving large doses of corticosteroids the clinician must be on the alert for possible developments, including psychoses, mood changes, activation of tuberculosis, susceptibility to infections whether bacterial, viral or fungal and lack of adequate response to them, activation of peptic ulceration, aggravation of existing diabetes mellitus or activation of latent diabetes, thromboses, hypokalaemia, cardiac or renal failure, osteoporosis or the skin changes mentioned above.

THE THYROID

In hyperthyroidism there may be hyperidrosis, hyperpigmentation, either diffuse or chloasmal, vitiligo, alopecia areata or sparseness and fineness of the hair, pretibial myxoedema and acropathy. Patients with hyperthyroidism may present with periorbital oedema before other signs make the diagnosis obvious.

In hypothyroidism there may be generalized pruritus with cold, dry skin, oedema of the eyelids, wrists and hands, loss of hair, intolerance of cold, slowness of speech and movement and increase in weight.

THE PARATHYROIDS

Hyperparathyroidism may be primary, or secondary to renal disease. See calcinosis.

Hypoparathyroidism may cause xeroderma, sparseness of the hair, brittle and deformed nails and manifestations of candidiasis including angular cheilitis, paronychia, greenish discoloration of the nails, anogenital pruritus, etc. There may be cataracts, tetany, neurological manifestations and psychological disturbances.

Impetigo herpetiformis is a rare pustular condition occurring especially in pregnancy. It is associated with hypoparathyroidism and with hypocalcaemia. It may be a variant of pustular psoriasis.

THE THYMUS

Hyperplasia of the thymus or thymoma has been found in association with lupus erythematosus. Thymectomy for myasthenia gravis has been followed by the development of lupus erythematosus.

THE BREASTS

Supernumerary nipples are common and may be mistaken for pigmented fleshy moles. They usually occur along the course of the embryological milk lines, between the anterior axillary folds and the medial aspect of the thighs.

Eczema of the nipples may be a manifestation of scabies, atopic dermatitis, contact dermatitis or maceration from lactation. It is usually bilateral and has to be differentiated from Paget's disease (intraductal carcinoma), which is usually unilateral, with scaling, crusting or exudation and deformity of the nipple or some loss of its substance. Biopsy is often necessary to confirm the diagnosis.

Gynaecomastia (enlargement of the male breast, often temporary), occurs in many conditions. It may be genetic, physiological and temporary, drug induced (oestrogens, ACTH, monoamine oxidase inhibitors), due to endocrine disorders (orchitis, testicular tumours), suprarenal tumours, pituitary tumours, hyperthyroidism) or metabolic (in liver disease and starvation).

THE LIVER

Pruritus may occur in liver disease, with or without jaundice, particularly in biliary cirrhosis. Palmar erythema may also be present and stellate haemangiomata may erupt on the face, scalp and hands or become more numerous. There may be gynaecomastia and loss of axillary and pubic hair. Increased pigmentation occurs with biliary obstruction and in haemochromatosis. Xanthomatosis may also occur with biliary obstruction.

THE PANCREAS

DIABETES MELLITUS [See Section 4.]

In pancreatitis or carcinoma of the pancreas subacute fat necrosis may occur, causing subcutaneous lumps which later ulcerate, mainly on the lower limbs and near the joints.

When thrombophlebitis is associated with visceral malignancy a common site for the visceral lesion is the pancreas.

THE GONADS

Androgens are formed in the testes, the adrenal cortices and the ovaries. In women they cause hirsutism, deepening of the voice and enlargement of the clitoris.

Oestrogens are formed in the ovaries. They cause effemination in males.

Progesterones formed in the corpus luteum antagonize oestrogens and are weakly androgenic.

Combined oestrogens and progestogens, as in oral contraceptives may improve acne vulgaris, cause chloasma or encourage *Candida albicans* infection. In higher doses they also cause an increased tendency to thrombosis.

THE ADRENALS

ADDISON'S DISEASE [See Section 5.]

CUSHING'S SYNDROME [See Section 5.]

THE ADRENALS AND GONADS IN RELATION TO HIRSUTISM

Most patients with hirsutism (females with coarse terminal hair growth in the male sexual pattern) show no evidence of endocrine disorder by any methods of examination which are available at present. In fact it is difficult to define the boundary between physiological and pathological hairiness as racial standards vary in this respect. Hirsutism tends to increase with ageing. Much anxiety and depression may result from it because of social embarrassment and feelings of sexual inadequacy.

In the minority of hirsute patients in whom endocrine disorders are present either the adrenals or the ovaries may be at fault. In the adrenals congenital hyperplasia, Cushing's syndrome or adrenal tumours may be responsible. In the ovaries arrhenoblastoma, adrenal-rest tumours or hilus-cell tumours may be responsible or the large cystic and fibrotic ovaries of the Stein-Leventhal syndrome.

Medically administered androgens and, to a much lesser extent, progestogens may also cause hirsutism.

The investigation of hirsutism necessitates consideration of the race, age at onset and speed of development of the condition, the menstrual history and a comprehensive examination with particular reference to any signs of Cushing's syndrome, hypertension, glycosuria, abdominal or pelvic tumours and the condition of the external genitalia. Further investigations include the 17-oxosteroid and 17-oxogenic steroid excretion in the urine, ACTH stimulation and adrenal suppression tests.

Treatment

Even when an adrenal or an ovarian condition amenable to treatment is present the hirsutism rarely regresses although its further development is usually checked. In most cases electrolysis or diathermy for coarser hairs and depilatory applications for finer hairs are all that can be offered. When electrolysis is impractical because of the extent of the condition shaving is the only alternative. It does not stimulate hair growth but, of necessity the regrowing hairs are more stubbly.

THE MUSCULOSKELETAL SYSTEM

THE MUSCULATURE

Dermatomyositis is not the only type of collagen disease in which muscle disease may occur. In systemic lupus erythematosus there may also be weakness. An association with myasthenia gravis has been reported. In systemic sclerosis degenerative changes may be found in the muscles comparable to those found in dermatomyositis. Sometimes it is difficult to distinguish between these two conditions. The musculature of the oesophagus and gut is particularly affected in systemic sclerosis. In dermatomyositis the muscles of the shoulder and pelvic girdles and the proximal muscles of the limbs are affected most and there may also be involvement of the ocular muscles, the tongue and pharynx and the intercostal muscles. The heart muscle and the gut musculature may also be affected. In polyarteritis myopathy may occur as one of the numerous manifestations of a widespread vascular disorder.

Myopathy induced by large doses of corticosteroids may develop in the course of treating chronic idiopathic bullous eruptions or collagen disorders. In dermatomyositis it may be difficult to differentiate between a natural exacerbation and a corticosteroid-induced myopathy.

THE JOINTS

The arthropathy of psoriasis occurs in about 7 per cent. of patients with overt psoriasis. It usually affects the terminal interphalangeal joints and there may be psoriatic nail dystrophy in the affected fingers or toes. The Latex test is negative. Less common is a rheumatoid type of arthritis but with a negative Latex test. A third form is severe deforming polyarthritis with atypical psoriasis sometimes of a pustular type or a picture closely resembling or identical to Reiter's disease. In Reiter's disease a characteristic feature is plantar pain and tenderness resulting from involvement of the calcanean ligament. The symmetrical arthritis selects the sacro-iliac joints, the knees, the ankles and the small joints of the feet.

Rheumatoid arthritis may present with skin lesions, including subcutaneous nodules and bands, arteritis causing transitory painless, para-ungual infarcts, bullae, purpura or necrosis, particularly of the digits. Peripheral motor or sensory neuropathy may occur. Leg ulcers may develop from defective muscular pump action. Pyoderma gangrenosum is a rare complication. *Candida albicans* erosive dermatitis between opposed, ulnar-deviated digits is occasionally seen.

Joint pains are the commonest presenting symptom of systemic lupus erythematosus. Arthritis may occur, sometimes migratory. A rheumatoid arthritic type of deformity may develop. Similar joint pains and arthritic changes may occur in systemic sclerosis and in morphoea. Joint pains also sometimes occur in polyarteritis.

Osteoarthritis may develop in one or other knee from sparing of weight bearing, due to painful conditions of the ankle or foot, such as leg ulcers.

In sarcoidosis multiple joint pains may accompany erythema nodosum. The Latex test is negative.

Clutton's joints are due to painless synovitis of the knees in late congenital syphilis. Charcot's joints are a form of painless, destructive and deforming neurogenic arthropathy occurring in neurosyphilis, leprosy or other conditions of sensory loss.

In bacteraemic gonococcal infections arthritis of wrists, knees or ankles is accompanied by fever and a rash of haemorrhagic vesicopustules.

THE SKELETON

Osteoporosis from depletion of calcium and phosphorus is a feature of long continued treatment of skin diseases, such as bullous eruptions or collagenoses with corticosteroids. It may present with backache, collapse of vertebrae, spontaneous fractures, avascular necrosis of the femoral condyle or osteoarthrosis and is more likely to develop in elderly patients, particularly if confined to bed and depleted for any reason of protein. It may be prevented or deferred by exercise and a high protein and high calcium diet. Anabolic drugs are of doubtful value. Children on long-term corticosteroid treatment may suffer from retarded growth.

Periostitis and osteomyelitis can develop from deep pressure sores.

Congenital syphilis may affect the bones, causing osteochondritis or dactylitis in the early stage or periostitis of the long bones (e.g. sabre tibiae) in the later stages. Gummata may destroy the palate or the nasal septum in late congenital syphilis or in acquired syphilis.

Osteitis deformans is sometimes complicated by leg ulcers.

Subungual exostoses often mimic subungual warts or keratoses. Mucinous degeneration cysts related to osteoarthritis of a terminal interphalangeal joint may cause guttering of a nail and a local soft translucent swelling just proximal to the nail.

Radiographic examinations of the skeleton may be diagnostically helpful in suspected psoriatic arthropathy (hands), osteitis deformans (skull, pelvis), urticaria pigmentosa if systemic mastocytosis is suspected, myeloma, sarcoidosis, particularly lupus pernio (cysts and trabeculations of phalanges, swellings of interphalangeal joints), histiocytosis-X and many hereditary conditions including tuberous sclerosis (skull, hands and feet for cortical thickening and cyst-like swellings), Klippel-Trénauny-Weber syndrome and congenital lymphoedema.

THE HAEMOPOIETIC SYSTEM

Iron-deficiency anaemia may present with glossodynia, the tongue being dry and smooth. In the Plummer-Vinson syndrome (sideropenic dysphagia) there are also angular cheilitis, dysphagia and koilonychia. Leucoplakia within the mouth and subsequent erosion and, possibly, carcinoma may develop in untreated patients. Iron deficiency is sometimes a factor in hypostatic ulcers, diffuse hair loss in women and pressure sores.

In pernicious anaemia glossodynia may also be an early symptom and the tongue may have a smooth red or cobble stone appearance. In untreated cases the skin may have a lemon tint and there is an increased incidence of vitiligo and canities.

In haemolytic anaemias there may be hyperpigmentation of the legs from melanin or haemosiderin and arterial leg ulcers may occur. This also applies to sickle-cell anaemia.

Dapsone treatment of skin disease, for example dermatitis herpetiformis, may be complicated by haemolytic anaemia with Heinz body formation. For this reason dosage should be kept to the minimal level which gives adequate relief and regular blood counts should be made. Dapsone is poorly tolerated by children.

The anaemia of lupus erythematosus may be of iron deficiency type, due to haemolysis or due to renal failure. Leucopenia and thrombocytopenia may also occur.

Thrombocytopenia also occurs in a rare form of cavernous haemangioma, causing local haemorrhages, anaemia and purpura.

Polycythaemia rubra vera may present with swollen gums, arterial leg ulcers or necrotic infarcts at other sites in the skin. Erythromelalgia may occur.

Acute leukaemias characteristically present with ulcerated and necrotic, bleeding, swollen gums and ecchymoses within the mouth, Skin infections may occur and be severe. Monocytic leukaemia is the form of leukaemia most often associated with skin infiltrations, usually obtuse nodules, sometimes purpuric.

Similarly agranulocytosis presents with fever and gingivitis, ulcers and necroses with offensive sloughs within the mouth. It occasionally arises from treatment with dapsone, amidopyrine, phenindione, imipramine, antihistamines and other drugs.

CRYOGLOBULINAEMIA

This presents as cold urticaria, purpura of exposed parts and haemorrhages from the nose or in the eyes. It occurs in a large number of conditions including collagen diseases, rheumatoid arthritis, myeloma, leukaemia, liver disease, carcinomatosis, subacute bacterial endocarditis and kala-azar. It may also be idiopathic.

PAINFUL BRUISING SYNDROME

This condition, peculiar to middle-aged women, consists of pain followed by bruising and resolution. There is no serious associated systemic condition but sometimes there is hypersensitivity to red blood cells in the tissues, confirmed by intradermal injection of the patient's own red blood cells. Dermatitis artefacta must be considered in the differential diagnosis.

REFERENCES

Emmons, C. W., *et al.* (1963) *Medical Mycology*, London.

Garrod, L. P., and O'Grady, F. (1968) *Antibiotics and Chemotherapy*, Edinburgh.

Lever, W. F. (1967) *Histopathology of the Skin*, London.

Maibach, H. I., and Hildick-Smith, G. (1965) *Skin Bacteria and their Role in Infection*, New York.

McCarthy, P. L., and Shklar, G. (1964) *Diseases of the Oral Mucosa*, New York.

Montagna, W. (1960) *Advances in Biology of Skin*, Vol. 1, Cutaneous Innervation, New York.

Montagna, W., and Ellis, R. A. (1961) *Advances in Biology of Skin*, Vol. 2, Blood Vessels and Circulation, New York.

Montagna, W., Ellis, R. A., and Silver, A. F. (1962) *Advances in Biology of Skin*, Vol. 3, Eccrine Sweat Glands and Eccrine Sweating, New York.

Montagna, W., Ellis, R. A., and Silver, A. F. (1963) *Advances in Biology of Skin*, Vol. 4, The Sebaceous Glands, New York.

Montagna, W., and Billingham, R. E. (1964) *Advances in Biology of Skin*, Vol. 5, Wound Healing, New York.

Montagna, W. (1965) *Advances in Biology of Skin*, Vol. 6, Ageing, New York.

Montagna, W., and Dobson, R. L. (1966) *Advances in Biology of Skin*, Vol. 7, Carcinogenesis, New York.

Montagna, W., and Hu, F. (1967) *Advances in Biology of Skin*, Vol. 8, The Pigmentary System, New York.

Montagna, W., and Dobson, R. L. (1969) *Advances in Biology of Skin*, Vol. 9, Hair Growth, New York.

Pillsbury, D. M., Shelley, W. B., and Kligman, A. (1966) *Dermatology*, Philadelphia.

Rook, A., Wilkinson, D. S., and Ebling, J. G. (1968) *Textbook of Dermatology*, Oxford.

Samman, P. D. (1965) *The Nails in Disease*, London.

Schwartz, L., Tulipan, L., and Birmingham, D. J. (1957) *Occupational Diseases of the Skin*, London.

Simon, R. D. G. Ph., and Marshall, J. (1969) *Essays on Tropical Dermatology*, Amsterdam.

Turk, J. L. (1969) *Immunology in Clinical Medicine*, London.

Urbach, F. (1969) *The Biological Effects of Ultraviolet Radiation*, London.

Brian Russell

SECTION 15

DISEASES OF THE NERVOUS SYSTEM

DISEASES OF THE NERVOUS SYSTEM

INTRODUCTION

Diagnosis in neurology involves two questions: Where is the lesion?, and What is the lesion? The topographical diagnosis is made first and then the pathological.

Where is the lesion? The central nervous system cannot be examined directly, but we can observe its functions. The first step is to find what disturbances of function there are, and then inferences can be drawn as to what structures in the brain, the spinal cord, or the nerves are affected. This readily leads to recognition of the site of the lesion. Further information is obtained from special techniques such as contrast radiology, and electroencephalography, and sometimes these methods may provide the only evidence of localization.

What is the lesion? In determining the nature of the disease we depend more upon information obtained from the history, general examination, and special investigation, than upon examination of the nervous system itself.

1. In no branch of medicine is history-taking more important, for the same physical sign may have a very different significance if it has come on suddenly, fairly quickly, or gradually.

2. General examination of the patient should never be omitted: disorders of the lungs, heart, blood vessels, blood, liver, and abnormalities of the skin may all have great diagnostic significance.

3. Of the special tests, ophthalmoscopy usually comes first, and is performed with the examination of the nervous system; it often provides evidence of the nature of the disease. Then, special biochemical and biophysical investigations are used to increase knowledge of the disorder.

Symptoms and their Modification

There are two ways in which lesions of the nervous system may disturb its function—they may be stimulated to over-activity or be diminished. There are 'irritative' or 'excitatory' symptoms and 'paralytic' symptoms, a Jacksonian fit being an example of the first, and hemiplegia of the second. Impairment or abolition of one function may cause disturbance of another. For instance, a lesion of the posterior columns of the cord will give rise not only to impairment of position sense, but also to disorder of motor functions, but the ataxia which results is obviously produced by a normal motor system having to depend upon an inadequate sense of position; it is therefore an indirect or secondary effect of the lesion.

'Release phenomena' constitute an important group of symptoms. At the time of a stroke the patient has flaccid hemiplegia, but after a few weeks the paralysed limbs become spastic, the tendon jerks increase, and ankle clonus makes its appearance. These signs which are produced by over-action of intact nervous mechanisms freed by the lesion from the normal control of physiologically superior mechanisms are called 'release' signs. They may persist indefinitely and dominate the clinical picture.

The symptoms produced by a lesion depend mainly upon its localization on the nervous structures damaged by it, and from this point of view they are considered later on. The symptoms may of course be profoundly influenced by the pathological nature of the lesion. One of sudden onset, such as arterial occlusion, will probably produce a much more severe and definite local disorder of function than a slowly developing one. Indeed, it is surprising to see the degree to which the brain can adapt to gradual structural changes. Thus the intracranial cavity may accommodate a large tumour which compresses and deforms the brain without any symptoms or any abnormal physical signs.

Again, a tumour within the brain, whilst it may cause symptoms of increased intracranial pressure such as headache and vomiting, may show few or no localizing signs, not necessarily because it is in a 'silent area' but simply because the essential nervous elements have not been seriously damaged by it. For instance, a glioma, which is a tumour of the interstitial elements, may cause a minimal disturbance of nervous function even when large areas of the brain with specific functions are directly involved by it.

Another example of the modification of symptoms by the nature of the lesion is the general disturbance which may follow the effect of a local lesion. An example of this is the stage of cerebral shock where a vascular disaster will produce coma with flaccidity and inability to move, resulting from the upset to the whole nervous system by the local disaster. Symptoms of this sort are usually transient.

Finally, space-occupying lesions within the skull or brain may cause local disorder of function of parts remote from the lesion. These are false localizing signs and are caused by oedema, 'contrecoup' pressure, or interference with the circulation of blood or cerebrospinal fluid. From what has been said it will be apparent that whilst the first step in neurological diagnosis is the recognition of the disorders of function which are present, the localization of a lesion and the determination of its nature are usually something more than a simple essay in the applied anatomy and physiology of the nervous system, and that the complete diagnosis calls for a knowledge of the natural history of the different disease processes, and it also calls for clinical experience.

DISORDERS OF THE CRANIAL NERVES

THE OLFACTORY NERVE AND TRACT

The commonest cause of loss of smell (anosmia) is usually nasal disease, and it is not often of diagnostic value in disease or damage of the central nervous system. It occurs with head injury, usually from tearing of the fine nerve endings themselves with or without fracture of the cribriform plate, and then the anosmia is usually permanent. It may result from anterior tumours pressing on the cribriform plate, and may be unilateral with a meningioma or a frontal glioma. It is more often bilateral in patients with raised intracranial pressure. When smell is lost then flavour is affected, so that the patient may think that he has lost his sense of taste, but if taste is preserved he will be able to recognize the primary flavours—salt, sweet, bitter, and acid.

OPTIC

The optic nerve head or disc can be seen with the ophthalmoscope, and is the only part of the central nervous system which can be directly observed. Congenital abnormalities of the optic disc are fairly common, the most usual being the presence of opaque nerve fibres. By ophthalmoscopy a bundle of these fibres shows as a white streaky oval mass which streams out from the nerve head into the adjacent part of the retina. They are usually limited to a small area but may surround the disc. Common acquired disorders of the disc are papilloedema, due to raised pressure, retrobulbar neuritis, which is inflammation of the nerve head, and optic atrophy.

PAPILLOEDEMA

This is almost invariably due to raised intracranial pressure; and is its only directly observed sign. First, the disc veins and those of the retina become distended, and then the disc becomes redder than normal. The margin of the disc then becomes blurred in its upper and inner part, and this extends around the disc whilst the physiological cup becomes filled up. As it becomes redder the disc becomes almost indistinguishable from the retina. The swelling continues, and can be measured in terms of dioptres with the ophthalmoscope. As it increases, the disc margins become even more blurred, and haemorrhages and exudates may appear. With chronic papilloedema the disc assumes a greyish quality.

In the early stages there is little disturbance of vision, but when the swelling becomes severe there is blurring of vision, and intermittent brief severe disturbances (amaurosis fugax) which are associated with bending or straining.

If the high intracranial pressure is not relieved, sight begins to fail, the disc goes pale, and atrophic. This consecutive or post-neuritic atrophy can be recognized by the irregularity of the edges of the atrophied disc because of the preceding swelling and exudation.

OPTIC NEURITIS AND NEURORETINITIS

When due to arterial disease and hypertension this may mimic the papilloedema due to raised intracranial pressure. The disc is blurred and swollen, but the swelling rarely exceeds two dioptres whilst the changes in the retina are much more pronounced and widespread. These consist of albuminuric retinopathy shown by hard white patches of exudate, and small and large haemorrhages often having a flame shape around the disc. In this condition there is of course also evidence of retinal arteriosclerosis.

RETROBULBAR NEURITIS

This is due to demyelination of the optic nerve, and the appearance resembles that of papilloedema but the changes are usually less severe. Sometimes the disc looks normal, but when the demyelination is just behind the disc, there is redness, and diffuse swelling. In marked contrast to papilloedema, visual failure is early and severe, and central vision is affected first. There is often pain on movement of the eyeball, and also an ache above and behind the eye. The pupil is usually dilated, and though it reacts to light it does not maintain the reaction for long. Recovery is usual, and it may be complete.

Disseminated sclerosis is the commonest cause of acute retrobulbar neuritis, about one patient in five showing evidence of the disease later. The eyes are usually affected one at a time, and recovery of vision is common. It may be complete, or there may be some residual central disturbances. Mild degrees of this disorder account for the characteristic pallor of the optic disc in this condition.

Bilateral retrobulbar neuritis occurs from toxic causes, but in most cases no cause is found, and there may be no sequels, though in these cases the assumption is that the cause has been demyelinating. Less severe toxic causes include tobacco, methanol, arsenical compounds and, now largely disused, lead and quinine. There has been interest recently in the relationship of disorder of cyanate metabolism to optic atrophy. This seems to be a factor in tobacco amblyopia which occurs in heavy smokers who are the subject of intercurrent infections. Leber's optic atrophy is a familial form of retrobulbar neuritis, males only being affected, and the symptoms make their appearance after puberty and before the age twenty-five. There may be recurrent attacks and severe optic atrophy and loss of vision. This is known to be related to cyanate disorder. A particularly acute and severe form of demyelination called neuromyelitis optica, or Devic's disease, may cause permanent blindness through bilateral involvement of the nerves.

OPTIC ATROPHY

Here, there is a peculiar whiteness and flatness of the disc with marked contrast between it and the surrounding retina. The lamina cribrosa shows clearly, the retinal vessels are small, the disc edge is sharply seen, in contrast to the atrophy which follows papilloedema, and there is associated visual loss. Optic atrophy is called primary or consecutive, depending upon whether it was the first change seen, or whether it had followed papilloedema or retrobulbar neuritis. This division is purely one of convenience.

Aetiology

Primary optic atrophy will follow any direct damage to the nerve by injury or disease. Some of the main causes are:

1. Injury to the retina or optic nerve.
2. Demyelination in the optic tract, as in disseminated sclerosis and retrobulbar neuritis.
3. The heredofamilial diseases with primary degeneration of neurones, especially the hereditary ataxias. In amaurotic family idiocy and retinitis pigmentosa, both of which are familial, optic atrophy follows degeneration of the retinal neurones.
4. Disease of the optic chiasma and optic nerve, and pressure upon them. Here the causes may be tumours of the pituitary gland, or in the neighbourhood of the chiasma, aneurysms, or bony injuries behind or involving the optic foramen. Glioma of the optic nerve found in children presents with lowering of visual acuity and primary atrophy too.
5. Chemicals, such as methanol, quinine, and triorthocresyl phosphate.
6. Massive haemorrhage or severe anaemia causing ischaemia to the nerve.
7. General medical diseases such as diabetes mellitus, arterial disease with or without thrombosis of the central artery of the retina, for instance in giant-cell arteritis, and from glaucoma.

Consecutive optic atrophy. This follows:

1. Severe papilloedema and is due to pressure upon the optic nerve fibres by the oedema in the first place, and by the cicatrization subsequently. Even severe papilloedema may recover perfectly without atrophy or impairment of sight, however.
2. The late stages of the neuroretinitis following arterial disease and hypertension.

THE OCULOMOTOR NERVES

The third (oculomotor) nerve supplies all the intraocular muscles, and all the extra-ocular, except for the superior oblique (fourth or trochlear) and the external rectus (sixth or abducens). A complete third nerve palsy gives a dilated and inactive pupil, complete ptosis, and loss of upward, downward and inward movements of the eye; the eye looks downwards and outwards. As a rule, diplopia is not noticed because of the ptosis. Many third nerve palsies are, however, gradual, and the muscles innervated by the nerve may be affected in different degrees. When diplopia is present it is crossed because the strabismus is divergent, and there is false projection of the image in the opposite direction.

Paresis of the fourth (trochlear) nerve gives no obvious squint, but when the patient looks out and down there is a rotary movement of the eye. The diplopia is disturbing because it happens especially on looking down; it is uncrossed, the false image is lower than the true image, and its top is tilted towards it.

A sixth (abducens) nerve palsy causes a convergent squint and uncrossed diplopia.

The oculomotor nerves may be affected singly or in various combinations, and paralysis may be complete or partial. In some cases the lesion is in the brain stem where it can affect either the nuclei or the nerve fibres in their intramedullary course. More often it is peripheral within the cranium, in the neighbourhood of the sphenoid fissure, or within the orbit. Internal and external ophthalmoplegias are very common and they may have great diagnostic value. There is no point in listing all the causes.

The syndrome of the sphenoid fissure. In the sphenoid fissure are all the oculomotor nerves entering the orbit, branches of the first division of the fifth, and the ophthalmic vein. When there is aneurysm of the internal carotid artery at the anterior end of the cavernous sinus, or when a tumour blocks the fissure, all these structures are affected. There is usually pain in the eye, and a headache which is increased by pressing upon the eye, which may show proptosis. In its complete form there is total ophthalmoplegia with anaesthesia over the eye, the forehead and cheek, but the syndrome is often incomplete. When due to an aneurysm the condition may resolve in a few months. The oculomotor nerves are involved in thrombosis of the cavernous sinus and when there is an aneurysm of the internal carotid artery within it.

Gradenigo's syndrome is paralysis of the sixth nerve, and pain in the trigeminal area. It is uncommon now because it used to be associated with middle-ear disease, which is now so readily controlled by antibiotics. When the oculomotor nerves are affected within the brain stem due to any cause, there may be contralateral hemiplegia (*Weber's syndrome*) and when the red nucleus is also affected there will be tremor of the limb contralateral to the third nerve palsy (*Benedikt's syndrome*).

CONJUGATE PARALYSIS

Bilateral lesions involving the upper parts of both third nerve nuclei cause loss of vertical movement of the eyes, the horizontal movements being retained. The lower parts of the nucleus concerned together with the sixth nerve in conjugate lateral movement when involved in a lesion will cause total paralysis of horizontal movement, the vertical movements being retained. Conjugate paralysis on one side is not usual in brainstem lesions but is caused by disturbance of oculomotor centres within the hemispheres. Conjugate disturbances of vision, either lateral or vertical, may be difficult to distinguish from supranuclear palsies.

SUPRANUCLEAR PALSIES

Sometimes, although the patient cannot make certain eye movements, the muscles concerned are not paralysed, but eye movements can be made reflexly. For instance, the patient may be unable to deviate his eyes to order, but deviation may be produced by labyrinthine stimuli. More commonly, although the patient may have defect of lateral gaze, say to the left, if he fixes on an object and the head is passively rotated to the right, the gaze will remain fixed upon the object and the eyes will consequently take up a position of deviation which is impossible voluntarily. These disturbances are called supranuclear palsies, and they are in effect pyramidal disturbances of eye movement, movements being possible through the invocation of lower reflex mechanisms whilst voluntary movement is absent. Usually, the lesions are in the brain stem above the third nerve nuclei, or in the pathways above. Conjugate lateral defects of movement may sometimes occur in frontal lobe lesions involving the oculomotor mechanisms.

PUPILLARY ABNORMALITIES

Myosis: abnormally small pupils are found in paralysis of the cervical sympathetic chain above the first thoracic level with syphilis of the nervous system, and with central brain-stem lesions. It can be produced by the local action of eserine and related substances. It is also produced by morphine, codeine and their synthetic analogues.

Mydriasis: dilatation of the pupil comes in association with lesion of the third nerve, and it is readily induced by atropine alkaloids and their homologues. Spasmolytics used in the treatment of Parkinsonism also cause it. Cocaine, whether taken internally or used as eye drops, also causes mydriasis. Homatropine is used ophthalmologically for this purpose.

Anisocoria: inequality of the pupils is common. It may be produced by disturbances which have been described in either eye, it is common in brain-stem lesions, especially injuries, and in association with infections such as syphilis. It can be caused by lesions in the eye, the orbit, the oculomotor nerves, or the brain stem itself. There are obviously many causes.

Irregularity of pupillary shape is less common than inequality. This may be due to local disease of the irides, but it is also found with brain-stem disorder in the same way as is inequality of the pupils.

THE ARGYLL ROBERTSON PUPIL

A normal pupil reacts briskly to light and also to accommodation and convergence. These reflex responses may be lost independently. The Argyll Robertson pupil: (1) does not react to light; (2) is small; (3) does not dilate fully with a mydriatic; but (1) it reacts normally to accommodation-convergence; and (2) vision is preserved. This set of phenomena almost invariably is caused by central nervous system syphilis, especially tabes dorsalis. It is often bilateral, but the pupils differ in size, and they are irregular in outline. There is atrophy of the iris. The fully developed Argyll Robertson pupil is permanent.

THE HOLMES-ADIE SYNDROME

The myotonic pupil is an abnormal state in which the pupillary reactions are all slow, though the reaction to light is slower than that to convergence. The pupil may be normal in size, or larger than the unaffected one. No reaction can be obtained with the light of a torch, but if the patient sits for some minutes in a bright diffused light, the pupil is seen gradually to contract. If he sits in a dark room it equally slowly dilates. During accommodation-convergence, contraction of the pupil takes place slowly, and continues through an abnormal range of movement, so that as convergence is maintained the myotonic pupil finally becomes smaller than its fellow. After relaxation of convergence the pupil takes many minutes to dilate to its former size. The pupil responds rapidly to mydriatics. The phenomenon is often unilateral, and the iris of the affected eye does not show degenerative changes such as are seen with the Argyll Robertson pupil. Accommodation may be involved in the disturbance, and then the patient complains of inability to focus with the affected eye.

THE TRIGEMINAL NERVE

As the fifth cranial nerve is mainly a sensory one, the most common symptom which arises when it is involved in disease is pain. The sensory root with its small motor part leaves the pons for the Gasserian ganglion in Meckel's cave near the apex of the petrous bone. The first division supplies the sensation of the anterior part of the scalp, the forehead, the eye, including the cornea and conjunctiva. The maxillary division, having emerged through the foramen rotundum, enters the orbital canal and supplies the cheek. It is important that it impinges upon the territory of the second cervical root in the cheek to give the so-called trigeminal notch, which is useful in diagnosis. The mandibular division leaves the cranium through the foramen ovale to reach the infratemporal fossa with the motor root which unites with it to form a single trunk. It supplies the lower lip, chin, and lower part of the cheek, and its auriculotemporal arch supplies a part of the ear and the temporal area. It also supplies the inside of the mouth and two-thirds of the tongue, and its lingual branch contains taste fibres from the anterior two-thirds of the tongue which, however, leave it by the chorda tympani nerve to reach the facial. The motor root supplies the temporal muscle, the masseter, buccinator, internal and external pterygoids, the mylohyoid, the anterior belly of the digastric and also the tensor tympani and tensor veli palatini.

It is clinically important that the recurrent branch of the fifth nerve supplies the whole of the dura mater above the tentorium, which is why frontal headaches are such a common symptom of so many disturbances of the face, scalp, and intracranial structure. Pain in the face, including the disabling and unexplained trigeminal neuralgia, loss of sensation in the territory supplied by the nerve, degenerative changes in the eye due to sensory loss, and weakness of the muscles supplied by the fifth nerve are all symptoms of disorder of it, and of course the nerve can be affected within the cranium, in the cavernous sinus and Meckel's cave, as well as in the face itself. Its close relationship to the seventh and eighth nerve and to the temporal bone involves it in disease of these structures too, as is the case with a neurofibroma of the eighth nerve which may compress it. When the muscles are involved the jaw deviates to the side of the paralysis when the mouth is opened because of the action of the unopposed external pterygoid muscle of the unaffected side. When there is wasting of the muscles, the masseter and temporal muscles do not harden on biting and the wasting can be seen. The floor of the mouth does not stiffen on the paralysed side when the mouth is forcibly opened.

TRIGEMINAL NEURALGIA

Synonym. Tic douloureux.

Definition

A disorder confined to paroxysms of intense pain in the distribution of the trigeminal nerve only, without sensory loss or other evidence of organic disease of the nerve.

Aetiology

The cause of trigeminal neuralgia in most cases is unknown. Nearly all the patients are over 50 years of age, and like the subjects of other stereotyped recurring disorders of function of the nervous system without associated disturbances of structure—such as spasmodic torticollis—they often tend to show rigidity of temperament with compulsive features. Women are more often affected. A number of cases in younger people are due to disseminated sclerosis, and there is also a form different from the chronic trigeminal neuralgia of elderly people which occurs temporarily in young subjects from exposure to cold, and may recur.

Symptoms

The chief feature of the disorder is pain, which may be general throughout the distribution of the nerve, but which is more commonly confined to one of its three divisions and often to one branch of a division. It is characteristic for the pain of neuralgia to start locally, to spread in each attack and gradually, in the course of the disease, permanently to invade a larger area. Two different kinds of pain occur, the sharp and paroxysmal and the dull continuous pain. The paroxysmal pains are sudden in onset and in cessation. They have a lightning-like character and are described as piercing, knife-like or as if the affected region were penetrated by red-hot wires.

Though often quite spontaneous, these pains may be brought on by movements of the face and jaw, by touching the surface or by a cold wind. Eating may become so difficult as to make feeding a matter of anxiety. The paroxysms are brief, seldom lasting longer than one or two minutes, but they may recur frequently, and the patients usually describe different degrees of liability to them at different times.

When the paroxysms are occurring in a severe case the patient remains for a period, which may be from a few minutes to several hours, paralysed under the fear of pain, unable to move a muscle lest a spasm more dreadful than the last should occur. The paroxysmal pains are usually followed, if severe, by a more lasting dull continuous pain often of a boring character, and sometimes such pain becomes continuous. The skin over the affected region is sore and tender after the paroxysm, and the patient may be unable to bear brushing the hair or shaving the face. The pain may be of every degree of severity, from mild momentary starts to continuous incapacitating pain, interrupted only by excruciating attacks of agony.

The distribution of the pain is usually in one or two divisions of the nerve. The first division is rarely affected primarily, but pain may spread into it from the second division. If the pain begins in the second division it may, after a time, affect the third, and vice versa. The lightning-like onset of the agony often causes convulsive spasms of the face and of the body and limbs. The tender points or 'trigger zones' are constantly present during the attack and for some time afterwards. When the second division is affected a little oedema develops under the orbit when paroxysms are frequent. When the third division is affected unilateral furring of the tongue occurs. Fortunately the attacks usually cease at night.

Diagnosis

The quality of the pain is characteristic, and when trigeminal neuralgia is present the diagnosis is not often missed, especially if a paroxysm is witnessed. The usual mistake is to regard as trigeminal neuralgia pain that is due to some other cause, and since there are very many conditions that give rise to pain in the face the opportunities for error are numerous. Unless the pain is brought on by eating and talking and washing the face, it is almost certainly not due to trigeminal neuralgia. Pain that is constant or of a continuous character is not due to trigeminal neuralgia, and some other cause should be sought. Disease of the frontal sinus and glaucoma should be kept in mind. Local painful neuroses or 'psychogenic' pains are continuous though subject to fluctuation, and when at their worst they often spread to the other side of the face and beyond the territory of the trigeminal nerve.

A similar neuralgia occurs in the glossopharyngeal nerve, but is much rarer; the pain is induced by the movement of swallowing and is felt in the ear or throat.

Course

In the early stages remissions lasting months or years are usual, but in old patients remissions if they occur are likely to be brief. In all cases the remissions become shorter as time goes on and without treatment the neuralgia persists for the rest of the patient's life. In occasional cases the disease is bilateral.

Treatment

In the first place it is essential to look for evidences of organic lesions which may be irritating the nerve, and it is important to remember that in its early stages there may be quite long and complete remissions. These remissions do indeed tend to get shorter after some years, but their recurrence suggests that in planning treatment each case should be considered individually. Thus if a patient who may be expected to have a long period of freedom from pain can be tided over the present attack by medical means, it is clearly not wise to give an alcoholic injection immediately. The correct course today is to use carbamazepine (*Tegretol*), 200 mg. three or five times a day. Until its use the only medical help to be given for this distressing condition was the use of sedatives and analgesics. Patients vary in their response, but it may make previously distressed life into a normal one with either complete control or long periods of remission.

If carbamazepine is not successful, or if the patient does not tolerate it, whether or not an injection of the ganglia should be undertaken depends upon the whole history of the case as has been mentioned previously. Operative section of the nerve should not be undertaken until successful alcoholic injection of the ganglion has been achieved. This is a skilled procedure, which should only be undertaken by an expert, who with dexterity may be able to limit the analgesia to the part affected by the pain and the 'trigger zone' which induces the pain, sparing for instance the eye if the first division is not involved in the pain. The permanence of the relief gained by a successful injection varies, but relief is less prolonged if the peripheral roots are injected. The effects last longer when the second division is injected peripherally. The persisting analgesia and dysaesthesia which occurs in some people may be troublesome, and when the first division has been involved in the anaesthesia there may be trophic keratitis which calls for urgent treatment to the eye.

In elderly people the fifth nerve is prone to involvement in herpes zoster, the first division being most vulnerable, to cause the distressing disorder of ophthalmic herpes [see Section 2].

THE FACIAL NERVE

The seventh nerve is entirely motor, though it is joined by the chorda tympani carrying taste, and as well as supplying all the muscles of the face and forehead it also supplies the platysma. The distinction of facial paralysis caused by damage to the seventh nerve and that caused by disorder of its upper motor neurone may be difficult. It can be made by recognition of the fact that the muscles in the upper part of the face have a bilateral innervation from the hemispheres, so that movements of the forehead are relatively spared compared with those of the mouth. There is no loss of tone when the upper motor neurone is affected, except in the first few days, so that the face does not sag in the unsightly way as it does when there is complete peripheral facial palsy.

The nerve is vulnerable as it takes its long intracranial course to the facial canal, and as this canal passes over the attic on its way to the stylomastoid foramen. Like the trigeminal nerve, it is involved in tumours of the eighth nerve, it used to be commonly affected with middle-ear disease, and it is also likely to be involved in herpes of the geniculate ganglion. Swelling and consequent compression of the nerve just within the stylomastoid foramen is thought to be the cause of the common Bell's palsy. The nerve is unusual in having such a long bony canal, which renders much more severe the effects of local inflammation and swelling of it. When the nerve is affected within the pons or just outside it, the sixth nerve is likely to be affected also, so that there is failure of abduction of the eye on the affected side. When the lesion is near the attic of the ear, then taste is lost on the affected side, but more peripherally when the fibres from the chorda tympani have left it this is not so.

BELL'S PALSY

This is the name given to paralysis of the facial nerve which comes on quickly and is not associated with any other lesion. It is the result of local neuritis of the nerve within its bony canal, and operative studies show that the swelling of the nerve is just within the stylomastoid foramen. The swelling causes pressure neuritis of the nerve at this site, so that immediate operative intervention is urged by some, though the early use of steroids might reduce the swelling. Often, as well as the facial palsy there is also loss of taste on the affected side.

Bell's palsy may occur at any age, but it is commonest between twenty and fifty, the sexes being equally affected.

Symptoms

The onset is rapid, with pain of a neuralgic kind just below the ear, behind the mastoid process, or referred to the occipital region, but this pain only lasts a few days and may be mild or occasionally absent. There is tenderness on deep pressure between the ramus of the jaw, and a little swelling may be seen here occasionally. The face first feels stiff on attempted movement, then the paralysis comes on quickly and the face is drawn over to the opposite side. The paralysed side may be completely immobile, the eye cannot be closed, and there is epiphora. As the corner of the mouth is weak there is difficulty in articulation, and escape of fluids on drinking. When partial the lower part of the face is the more affected, and when this is so recovery is rapid. Taste is usually lost on the anterior part of the tongue in severe cases.

There are two forms of recovery, the first within a few weeks, and the other which may progress steadily after a matter of months. There should not be any attempt at operative repair of the facial muscles until after at least 7 months have gone by, to allow for complete growth, as there has been a lesion in continuity.

When there has been a typical paralysis, recovery is usually complete, and contracture may occur later so that the corner of the mouth ceases to droop, and at rest the asymmetry of the face is not marked, though on movement the limited action of the affected side is apparent. The secondary contracture may be sufficiently severe to cause some deformity. Rarely the condition may recur, but when bilateral facial palsy is seen other causes should be considered such as acute infective polyneuritis.

Treatment

It is difficult to advise upon treatment in any one case, for recovery may begin in about 3 weeks, or there may be permanent weakness of the face. The use of the electromyogram is valuable here, for if there is any sign of response to voluntary movement in the first few days then recovery is going to be virtually complete, and no special action need be taken. Theoretically, the use of steroids will reduce the oedema of the nerve and so help to prevent the pressure palsy from developing. Their use should be limited to days and no longer than a week. Otological surgeons have advised decompression of the stylomastoid foramen, but although swelling of the nerve has been demonstrated at this point, there is no convincing evidence that immediate operation does improve the prognosis. This really is the difficulty in seeing a patient with a Bell's palsy within the first few hours of the paralysis. In the absence of evident cause, there is no curative treatment for the condition. The eye should be protected with a shade and with paraffin drops, and when paralysis is complete undue stretching of the muscles may be reduced by supporting the corner of the mouth by a wire loop covered in plastic, or by strapping support from the temporal area. I tell patients to massage the side of the face upwards themselves, for it gives them something to do about it if nothing else. There is no evidence that faradic stimulation helps at all. When there is unsightly permanent facial palsy, then plastic surgical repair to the muscles may be undertaken, with great benefit in skilled hands.

FACIAL PALSY FROM HERPES OF THE GENICULATE GANGLION
(The Ramsay Hunt Syndrome)

Herpes zoster affecting the geniculate ganglion causes an immediate total facial palsy with severe local pain in and around the external auditory meatus, as well as within the throat. Injection and small ulcers may be seen in the affected fauces, and in the ear. The pinna may swell, the patient is ill and febrile, and facial palsy appears early and is complete in about 12 hours. There may be intense vertigo, some deafness and tinnitus. The cases vary in severity very much. As herpes zoster may affect sensation and indeed movement in any part of the body, there is not much to be gained in stressing the identity of this syndrome. Prognosis for recovery of movement in the face is worse than in Bell's palsy, but treatment is the same.

FACIAL HEMISPASM

This is a unilateral disturbance of the facial nerve, in which intermitting spasm of the facial muscles occurs, exactly like that caused by faradism of the facial trunk. It is associated with a slowly oncoming facial paralysis. Though it used to be called peripheral facial spasm its cause is evidently that of central dysfunction. A disorder like it may follow a facial paralysis due to injury. It occurs in adults, generally in middle-aged women, and the onset is usually insidious and without known cause.

Symptoms

It begins with twitching of some part of the facial musculature, which occurs at first at rare intervals, and subsequently becomes more and more frequent, so as in some cases to be almost continuous. Starting locally, usually around the eye, it spreads slowly over years so as to involve the whole face in a sudden contortion. The attacks of facial spasm may at first glance resemble a Jacksonian fit of the face. The spasms may be severe and continuous as to keep the eye closed for long periods together, and to interfere greatly with the work and enjoyment of life. It is associated with no other symptoms. Cases exist in all degrees of severity, from the mildest, in which an occasional flicker of the face occurs, to the most severe incapacitating and unsightly contracture.

Treatment

In severe cases the only way to help is by selective division or alcoholic injection of some of the branches of the facial nerve in the pes anserinus. As long as the spasm is mild such treatment is obviously worse than the disease. No other treatment has any effect on the spasm, but sedatives may enable the patient to bear it with less distress.

THE AUDITORY AND VESTIBULAR NERVES

The eighth nerve consists of two groups of fibres, different in their functions and in their origins and terminations; one group, arising in the cochlea and terminating in the cochlear nuclei in the pons, is called the auditory or cochlear nerve; the other, arising from the labyrinth and ending mostly in the vestibular nuclei, is called the vestibular nerve.

Lesions of the auditory nerve (as well as diseases of the cochlea) give rise to two symptoms, nerve deafness and tinnitus.

Nerve, or conductive, deafness is distinguished from deafness due to middle-ear disease by the fact that hearing is diminished or lost whether the sound is conveyed by air-conduction or by bone-conduction, whereas in middle-ear deafness the hearing by bone-conduction is increased. In Weber's test a vibrating tuning fork is placed on the middle of the forehead, the patient being asked in which ear the sound seems the louder; with middle-ear deafness the sound is heard better on the affected side, while with inner-ear or nerve deafness the opposite is the case or the patient does not appreciate any difference between the two sides. For Rinne's test the fork is applied first to the mastoid process, and when the patient ceases to hear it, it is held at the external auditory meatus; in nerve deafness the sound may be heard by air-conduction after it has become too feeble to be heard by bone-conduction, while in middle-ear deafness the opposite obtains. Quantitative audiometry has replaced these simple clinical tests in the detailed investigation of patients with disordered cochlear function.

Tinnitus is a subjective sensation of noise in the ears or in the head. It accompanies disease of the cochlea or auditory nerve of a slow degenerative nature, and though at first intermittent, it usually becomes continuous before long. It may also be produced temporarily by certain drugs, of which quinine and salicylates are the commonest. The sounds, at first faint, may be perceived only in stillness and silence at night, later become louder, more persistent, and often continuous. The noise may be high-pitched or low-pitched, a whistle or a hiss, or even a rumble; in some cases it is more elaborated and is described as 'like machinery', or again, 'bell-like'.

Division of the eighth nerve does not cure the tinnitus for it comes to have a central component with the passage of time.

The most prominent symptom which results from lesions of the vestibular nerve (as well as from disorders of the labyrinth) is *vertigo*. The word by derivation means 'a turning', and with vertigo of labyrinthine and vestibular nerve origin there is usually a sense of rotation, either of the surroundings or of the patient himself; the room may seem to rotate about a vertical or a horizontal axis and there is often a disorder of projection so that when the patient falls it seems to him that the floor has come up to strike his head. Sometimes there is no sense of rotation, but a sense of being pushed in the lateral or anteroposterior planes.

It must be noted that the vast majority of patients who complain of giddiness or dizziness do not have true vertigo. Those who have functional nervous disturbances complain of what they call dizziness, by which they mean a momentary sensation of unsteadiness; objectively such a patient is not unsteady and this sensation never causes him to fall. Patients suffering from generalized cerebral arteriosclerosis complain of a similar sensation, as also do those who are suffering from the after-effects of head injuries.

With true vertigo, unless it is minimal, nystagmus is present while the vertigo is experienced. Usually the nystagmus is seen with deviation of the eyes towards the side of the lesion, but with irritative lesions of the labyrinth, e.g. for a day or two after operations on the ear and with labyrinthitis the nystagmus is towards the opposite side.

Tests for Vestibular Lesions. 1. Barany's caloric test is made by irrigating the external auditory meatus with either hot or cold water or air. With an intact vestibular mechanism this causes irritation of the vestibular apparatus with the appearance of nystagmus on lateral deviation of the eyes. When the vestibular mechanism is impaired this test fails relatively or completely.

2. If the patient is rotated either by placing him in a special rotating chair, or by turning him round several times in the standing position, lateral conjugate deviation of the eyes immediately after the rotation will show nystagmus in the opposite direction to the rotation, if the labyrinth on that side is intact. It will not appear if the functional activity of the vestibular mechanism is deficient. Labyrinthine testing has been elaborated, quantitated and its results explained by the researches of Hallpike. Reference of the patient to a special department is required for his full investigation. Here labyrinthine function is tested by the response to controlled stimulation at known temperatures, by changes in head position, by audiometry, and by study of optokinetic nystagmus produced by viewing vertical lines on a drum revolving in either direction.

Vertigo may be peripheral or central in origin, due to disease of the labyrinth itself or its nuclei and their connexions within the brain stem. The form of the vertigo is the same in each but the associated symptoms differ and help in their recognition.

RECURRENT VERTIGO

There are two sorts of recurrent vertigo; *peripheral* due to disease of the labyrinth itself and *central*, caused by involvement of the vestibular nuclei or the temporal lobe in disease. The commonest causes of vertigo are within the middle ear, but all vertigo is caused by disorder of the labyrinth. Ménière's disease, otosclerosis, otitis media, or hydrops of the labyrinth are familiar examples. Central causes may include structural disease of the brain stem involving the vestibular nuclei and their connexions and, in the past few years, the importance of reductions in the rate of blood flow through the basilar artery in patients with atherosclerosis, arterial hypotension or occlusion or stenosis of the vertebral or basilar arteries has been recognized. This vascular mechanism offers an explanation for much of the intermittent vertigo of later life, in the absence of overt disease of the middle ear.

MÉNIÈRE'S DISEASE

This is a chronic disease of the labyrinth in which paroxysmal attacks of vertigo occur at irregular intervals, associated with tinnitus and progressive deafness. According to Hallpike the essential lesion is a gross distension of the endolymph system together with degenerative changes in Corti's organ and the presence of albuminoid coagula throughout the endolymph spaces. He regards these changes as incompatible with an infective origin, and as probably primarily degenerative in nature. Ménière's syndrome, so called, is intermittent vertigo without deafness and without evident cause. It is interesting that Ménière's case was that of a young woman with leukaemia, with a haemorrhage into the middle ear.

The precipitating causes of the attacks are unknown, and in the absence of precise knowledge disturbance of fluid balance, allergy and migraine have all been incriminated; in some instances the attacks are associated with diarrhoea.

Symptoms

The attacks begin suddenly with a buzzing noise in the ears, followed immediately by intense vertigo. It may be so severe that the patient feels he is hurled to the ground, but he usually has time to assume the sitting or lying position, before the vertigo reaches its height. Rarely consciousness may be impaired for a few moments. Spontaneous nystagmus occurs to the side of the lesion, and unilateral cerebellar signs on the side of the lesion. The patient becomes nauseated and often vomits repeatedly. The skin is pale and covered with a clammy sweat. The patient lies perfectly still, and in terror lest the least movement should bring on more vertigo. The duration of the attack is usually between 15 minutes and an hour, but the patient may take several hours to recover completely. Sometimes the attacks are excited by sudden movement, such as coughing or sneezing, but they are usually without any such antecedent. They may occur during sleep, and wake the patient. In the milder cases the vertigo is not infrequently present when the patient wakens in the morning and becomes apparent to him as soon as he moves. It is not spontaneous but is brought on by movements of the head, and it is also influenced by the posture of the head, being worse when the affected ear is on the pillow. The vertigo passes off within half an hour or an hour or two.

Ménière's disease is characterized by a slow onset of nerve deafness and by the time the first attack of vertigo occurs an impairment of hearing and some tinnitus are usually present. If the disease is persistent there is a gradual deterioration both of vestibular and of auditory function in the affected ear, and in some cases the labyrinth becomes defunct and the attacks cease.

Diagnosis

This presents no peculiar difficulty for the symptoms are highly characteristic, and although variable in degree are usually quite definite in the first attack. The rapid disappearance of the vertigo is striking. Vertiginous attacks from all other causes must be excluded. In acute cerebellar lesions (including thrombosis of the posterior inferior cerebellar artery) the symptoms are very like those of labyrinthine vertigo, but they are not transitory in a few hours. A careful search of the nervous system for signs of organic nervous disease should in every case prevent any mistake. Vertiginous attacks due to epilepsy rarely cause difficulty in the differential diagnosis because the loss of consciousness and probably the convulsive and other features of the epileptic attack are apparent.

Treatment

Sedatives have a pronounced palliative effect. The most commonly used drug is phenobarbitone; 30 mg. taken three or four times daily usually brings about prompt amelioration. Other measures include a salt-free diet, careful regulation of the bowel to prevent diarrhoea and the use of antihistamine drugs. Dimenhydrinate, 50 mg., and prochlorperazine (*Stemetil*), 5 mg., give symptomatic relief.

When medical treatment of vertigo fails surgery may be considered, the principal operations employed being division of the vestibular nerve, partial removal of the membranous labyrinth and total destruction of the labyrinth of one side. Operation is, however, reserved for those in whom there is no useful hearing in the affected ear, and in whom the side responsible for the vertigo is known, for deafness ensues on the operated side. As Ménière's disease affects both ears, operation is rarely recommended.

Prognosis

Most patients have infrequent mild attacks with slight impairment of hearing, or have long periods of remission. Some go from bad to worse and progressive deafness ensues with eventual disappearance of the attacks.

VESTIBULAR NEURONITIS

Vestibular neuronitis has been advanced as the explanation of cases with the following characteristics: There is no disturbance of hearing and in a large proportion there is an associated infection in the nasal sinuses or elsewhere, or the onset is associated with some febrile illness. The disorder affects chiefly patients in the age group 30–50 years, without preference for sex. Further study will no doubt show that the disorder is not homogeneous, but that reduction in central blood flow to the vestibular nuclei is causal in many cases, and that a direct infective cause upon the nucleus is less important than has been thought.

The attacks of vertigo are similar to those of Ménière's disease but are in general less severe.

Treatment is as for Ménière's disease, and the removal of any local or general infection which can be discovered. With these measures the liability to vertigo usually passes off in the course of a few months.

Epidemic Vertigo. Small epidemics of vertigo occurring in the spring months have been described, but whether or not these are true epidemics caused by one organism is extremely doubtful. Undoubtedly doctors do recognize several cases in a row, but vertigo is quite a common symptom of many virus infections. Treatment is symptomatic and quick recovery usual.

A common cause of intermittent vertigo is *transient ischaemia of the vestibular nuclei*, constituting part of the syndrome of basilar insufficiency. In this disorder, fairly common in older people, vertigo and blurring of vision are the commonest symptoms.

POSITIONAL VERTIGO (POSITIONAL NYSTAGMUS)

In this variety the vertigo always occurs when the head is put in a particular position, and in most instances the exciting position is with the head back and somewhat tilted to one side. Many follow head injury.

The condition can usually be identified by the patient's complaint that he becomes dizzy when he turns his head (face) upwards, but specialized tests are necessary to confirm the diagnosis.

Treatment is that of the other forms of vertigo and in most cases the symptoms pass off completely in 3–12 months.

THE GLOSSOPHARYNGEAL NERVE

Lesions of this nerve involve loss of taste over the posterior one-third of the tongue with some unilateral paresis of the pharynx. It is rarely involved alone; in association with the other nerves taking origin in the neighbourhood, it may be affected by tumours of the lateral region of the medulla, and by syringomyelia.

GLOSSOPHARYNGEAL NEURALGIA

This is a rare form of neuralgia within the distribution of the glossopharyngeal nerve. It is strictly comparable with trigeminal neuralgia in the quality and severity of the pain, its paroxysmal incidence, the remissions in its course, its provocation by special stimuli and finally by the absence of any discoverable lesion in, or loss of function of, the nerve.

Nothing is known of its aetiology. It is most often seen in middle-aged or elderly males. A symptomatic neuralgia of the same distribution is occasionally found with carcinoma of the tongue or oesophagus in which the growth invades the faucial region.

Symptoms

When fully developed, there are paroxysms of shooting pain of great severity in the throat and ear. The exciting stimulus is commonly the act of swallowing. But just as in trigeminal neuralgia the pain may at first be confined to a single branch of this nerve, so in glossopharyngeal neuralgia, the pain may for long be confined to the tympanic branch, the pain being felt deep in the ear, but not in the lobe. In other cases, pain in the faucial region predominates, the pharyngeal branches being affected. As in trigeminal neuralgia, the patient may enjoy long intervals of freedom from pain. During a paroxysm the patient screws up his face and may hold his head in his hand as does the subject of trigeminal neuralgia.

Diagnosis

The presence of neuralgic pain of great severity, provoked by the act of swallowing, and in its general characters and behaviour resembling the familiar and characteristic paroxysms of trigeminal neuralgia, but different from these in its restriction to the ear and throat, occurring also in the absence of objective signs of a lesion of the cranial nerves; these together are the features which make a diagnosis of glossopharyngeal neuralgia possible and easy.

Treatment

In the early attacks, the treatment is the same as that used in trigeminal neuralgia. The most effective substance available at present is carbamazepine (*Tegretol*). If the attacks of pain persist then surgery is needed and the operation usually performed is avulsion of the nerve high in the neck.

THE VAGUS NERVE

This is a mixed nerve. The motor fibres supply the voluntary muscles of the soft palate (except the tensor palati), pharynx and larynx in conjunction with the accessory fibres, and also the non-striped muscles of the respiratory and alimentary tracts.

The sensory fibres of the vagus supply the respiratory tract, the pharynx and oesophagus. Its visceral fibres supply the lungs, heart and abdominal viscera. No sensibility seems to be supplied to the abdominal viscera by this nerve, since with division of the spinal cord above the offshoot of the splanchnic nerves all sensibility in the abdomen is lost.

LESIONS OF THE VAGUS

The important signs of lesions of this nerve and its nuclei are pharyngeal and laryngeal paralysis and loss of sensibility. Symptoms indicative of lesions of its complicated and mysterious visceral supply are neither well marked nor well understood, and in unilateral lesions seem to be entirely absent; they are therefore not considered.

Lesions of the vagus in the medulla are common. Syringomyelia, when affecting that region, usually involves the nucleus ambiguus, causing unilateral palsy of palate, pharynx and larynx. Thrombosis of the posterior inferior cerebellar artery which supplies that region of the medulla containing the nucleus ambiguus is likely to produce vagal paralysis of the same side. Progressive muscular atrophy, in the form of progressive bulbar paralysis, may affect its cells. Lesions of the nerve roots often occur from tumours of the lateral region of the medulla, and growths outside the medulla arising from nerve roots or meninges, and here the lesion of the vagus roots is associated usually with those of the glossopharyngeal, spinal accessory and hypoglossal. In the neck penetrating wounds and growths may implicate the nerve, and in the thorax tumours, particularly aneurysms and new-growths, are apt to cause paralysis of the muscles supplied by its recurrent branch.

Unilateral Pharyngeal Paralysis. This is characteristic of all unilateral lesions of the vagus high up. It is recognized by the low-lying, motionless palate and the loss of sensibility of one side of the pharynx, with loss of the pharyngeal reflex on that side. There is no impairment whatever of deglutition. When the soft palate is elevated as in saying 'Ah!', it is pulled over to the sound side.

Bilateral Pharyngeal Paralysis. This results from lesions of the nucleus ambiguus on both sides, and from diphtheritic neuritis, myasthenia gravis and progressive muscular atrophy. The whole palate is low and paretic or paralysed, the voice is nasal, there is nasal regurgitation of liquids, the cheeks cannot be forcibly blown out, and there is difficulty in pronouncing final 'k' and 'g', the words 'kick' and 'egg' becoming 'kich' and 'enck'.

Total Unilateral Laryngeal Paralysis. Since the superior laryngeal nerve which supplies the cricothyroid muscle (the chief tensor and adductor of the vocal cords) is given off high in the neck from the ganglion of the trunk of the vagus, it follows that total paralysis of the larynx on one side can only result from a lesion of the vagus between the ganglion of the trunk and the nucleus ambiguus in the medulla. The vocal cord on the paralysed side becomes motionless in the cadaveric position—that is, midway between the abduction and adduction. The larynx is insensitive on the same side. There is some loss of vocal tone but no stridor.

Unilateral Abductor Paralysis or Recurrent Laryngeal Paralysis. This occurs from all lesions of the trunk of the vagus below the ganglion of the trunk, and from lesions of the recurrent laryngeal branch. The vocal cord on the side of paralysis lies close to the midline; it fails to abduct when the patient takes a deep breath; there is no change of voice, but there may be slight stridor on inspiration. The sensibility of the larynx is not affected.

Bilateral Abductor Paralysis. This may be a complication of thyroidectomy and of carcinoma of the thyroid gland. It occurs also in bilateral lesions of the recurrent laryngeal nerves in the thorax, which may result from tumour or aneurysm. It is the most dangerous form of laryngeal palsy, as the vocal cords cannot be abducted, and they tend to be sucked together during inspiration; for this reason bilateral abductor paralysis may cause death from asphyxia and necessitates tracheostomy.

THE SPINAL ACCESSORY NERVE

The eleventh nerve may be caught with the vagus by lateral lesions outside the medulla, or by lesions in the region of the jugular foramen; but it is more often damaged by injuries to the neck and by operations for the removal of cervical glands. The spinal accessory nerve, as it crosses the posterior triangle of the neck, is liable to injury, either from blows or from sudden strains, and most of the isolated trapezius palsies happen like this.

When the sternomastoid is paralysed there is neither complaint by the patient of weakness, nor deformity, nor peculiar attitude of the neck, other muscles compensating for its paralysis. The muscle does not harden when the head is turned to the side opposite to the paralysis.

Paralysis of the trapezius, on the other hand, causes great disability in raising the arm above the horizontal level of the shoulder and also difficulty in shrugging the shoulder or approximating the scapula to the middle line behind and therefore also in carrying the extended arm backwards. But the only part of the trapezius that is completely paralysed by disease of the spinal accessory nerve is the highest portion. Instead of its normal nearly straight contour, the neck presents on the affected side a concave curve, and the difference between the two sides is brought out more strongly by a deep inspiration. The other parts of the trapezius are weakened but not paralysed, since they receive additional innervation from the cervical nerves. In consequence of the weakness the shoulder falls a little, the scapula moves slightly laterally, and by the unopposed action of the rhomboids and levator anguli scapulae it is rotated, the lower angle moving medially.

THE HYPOGLOSSAL NERVE

The twelfth nerve supplies all the muscles of the tongue, both intrinsic and extrinsic.

A lesion of one hypoglossal nucleus in the medulla gives rise to fasciculation and eventual atrophic paralysis of one half of the tongue. When the hypoglossal nerve is divided the fasciculation is usually not apparent but the atrophy occurs more quickly and there is a loss of faradic excitability. True fibrillation can also be seen in the denervated tongue—the only muscle in the body where this is so, since there is no subcutaneous tissue to obscure it. The tongue becomes sickle-shaped with the concavity on the paralysed side. There is little impairment of movement within the mouth and no defect of articulation, but the tongue turns to the paralysed side when protruded. Tumours and injury are the commoner causes.

Atrophic paralysis of the whole tongue occurs when both hypoglossal nuclei are affected, and is commonly seen in progressive bulbar paralysis. Protrusion of the tongue is impossible and articulation is greatly impaired, but this may be partly due to other paralyses which are usually associated.

Upper motor neurone paralysis of the tongue is often seen, as in motor neurone disease. A patient suffering from motor aphasia is commonly unable to protrude his tongue, and in bilateral hemiplegia and the condition known as pseudobulbar palsy, the tongue is in a state of spastic paralysis; neighbouring parts are similarly affected, and dysarthria and dysphagia are frequent. The tongue appears contracted but there is no real wasting and no loss of electrical excitability.

REFERENCES

Adie, W. J. (1931) Argyll Robertson pupils true and false, *Brit. med. J.*, **2**, 136.

Atkinson, M. (1941) Observations on the aetiology and treatment of Ménière's syndrome, *J. Amer. med. Ass.*, **116**, 1753.

Brodal, A. (1947) The hippocampus and the sense of smell, *Brain*, **70**, 179.

Brodal, A. (1959) *The Cranial Nerves*, Springfield, Ill.

Brodal, A. (1969) *Neurological Anatomy in Relation to Clinical Medicine*, 2nd ed., New York.

Campbell, A. M. G., and Lloyd, J. (1954) Atypical facial pain, *Lancet*, ii, 1034.

Carbone, F. (1968) Étude électromyelographique de la paralysie de Bell, *J. neurol. Sci.*, **7**, 219.

Carmichael, E. A., Dix, M. R., and Hallpike, C. S. (1956) Pathology, symptomatology and diagnosis of organic affections of the eighth nerve system, *Brit. med. Bull.*, **12**, 146.

Cawthorne, T. (1957) Aural vertigo, in *Modern Trends in Neurology*, 2nd Series, ed. Williams, D., London.

Cawthorne, T., and Haynes, D. R. (1956) Facial palsy, *Brit. med. J.*, **2**, 1197.

Chawla, J. C., and Falconer, M. A. (1967) Glossopharyngeal and vagal neuralgia, *Brit. med. J.*, **3**, 529.

Cogan, D. G. (1956) *Neurology of the Ocular Muscles*, 2nd ed., Springfield, Ill.

Dix, M. R., and Hallpike, C. S. (1952) The pathology and treatment and diagnosis of certain disorders of the vestibular system, *Proc. roy. Soc. Med.*, **45**, 341.

Eccles, J. C. (1957) *The Physiology of Nerve Cells*, Baltimore.

Fitzgerald, G., and Hallpike, C. S. (1942) Studies in vestibular function, *Brain*, **65**, 115.

Freeman, A. G., and Heaton, J. M. (1961) The aetiology of retrobulbar neuritis in Addisonian pernicious anaemia, *Lancet*, i, 908.

Harris, W. (1937) *The Facial Neuralgias*, London.

Harrison, M. S. (1962) 'Epidemic vertigo'—'vestibular neuronitis', a clinical study, *Brain*, **85**, 613.

Henderson, W. R. (1967) Trigeminal neuralgia: the pain and its treatment, *Brit. med. J.*, **1**, 7.

Hierons, R., and Lyle, T. K. (1959) Bilateral retrobulbar optic neuritis, *Brain*, **83**, 56.

Holmes, G. (1952) *Introduction to Clinical Neurology*, 2nd ed., London.

Hughes, B. (1954) *The Visual Fields*, Oxford.

Jefferson, G. (1931) Glossopharyngeal neuralgia, *Lancet*, ii, 397.

Jefferson, G. (1931) Observations on trigeminal neuralgia, *Brit. med. J.*, **2**, 879.

Leigh, A. D. (1943) Defects of smell after head injury, *Lancet*, i, 38.

Mathew, N. T., and Chandy, J. (1970) Painful ophthalmoplegia, *J. neurol. Sci.*, **11**, 243.

Matthews, W. B. (1961) Prognosis in Bell's palsy, *Brit. med. J.*, **2**, 215.

Mayo Foundation (1963) *Clinical Examinations in Neurology*, 2nd ed., London.

Morris, W. M. (1938) Surgical treatment of Bell's palsy, *Lancet*, i, 249.

Paton, L. (1909) A clinical study of optic neuritis and its relationship to intercranial tumours, *Brain*, **32**, 65.

Penman, J. (1950) The differential diagnosis and treatment of tic doloureux, *Postgrad. med. J.*, **26**, 627.

Rasmussen, P., and Riishede, J. (1970) Facial pain treated with carbamazepin (*Tegretol*), *Acta neurol. scand.*, **46**, 385.

Renfrew, S. (1962) *An Introduction to Diagnostic Neurology*, London.

RUSSELL, G. F. M. (1956) The pupillary changes in the Holmes-Adie syndrome, *J. Neurol. Neurosurg. Psychiat.*, **19**, 289.

SYMONDS, C (1958) Recurrent multiple cranial nerve palsies, *J. Neurol. Neurosurg. Psychiat.*, **21**, 98.

TAVERNER, D. (1955) Bell's palsy, a clinical and electromyographic study, *Brain*, **78**, 209.

TAVERNER, D., KEMBLE, F., and COHEN, S. B. (1967) Prognosis and treatment of idiopathic facial (Bell's) palsy, *Brit. med. J.*, **4**, 581.

TRAQUAIR, H. M. (1957) *Introduction to Clinical Perimetry*, 7th ed., London.

WALSH, E. G. (1964) *Physiology of the Nervous System*, 2nd ed., Edinburgh.

WALSH, F. R. (1957) *Clinical Neuro-ophthalmology*, 2nd ed., London.

WALSHE, F. M. R. (1942) The anatomy and physiology of cutaneous sensibility: a critical review, *Brain*, **65**, 48.

WILLIAMS, D., and GASSEL, M. M. (1962) Visual functions in patients with homonymous hemianopia, *Brain*, **85**, 175.

THE SIGNS OF LOCAL LESIONS WITHIN THE SKULL AND BRAIN

In this chapter we must be content with a brief consideration of the signs and symptoms upon which we depend for the localization of cerebral lesions. We may take first the various regions of the brain, and secondly, as we have to deal not only with lesions within the brain, but also with lesions within the skull that may be outside the brain itself, we will consider the symptomatology peculiar to lesions in the three cranial fossae.

THE CEREBRAL HEMISPHERES

GENERAL LATERALIZING SIGNS

A lesion within or involving one cerebral hemisphere may reveal by the signs it produces whether it is right- or left-sided without affording further evidence of its localization. Such signs are unilateral loss or diminution of the abdominal reflexes, unilateral accentuation of the tendon reflexes, an extensor response or just perceptible unilateral paresis of movement of the lower part of the face. Fits starting unilaterally, or with turning of the head and eyes to one side may be of similar significance.

Those posterior include motor hemiplegia on the contralateral side, but anterior lesions may produce no symptoms or signs, so that unilateral amputations of the frontal pole, for the relief of epilepsy, for instance, may be undertaken with impunity. The feature of distortion, or massive deprivation of frontal lobe function is personality change, with thoughtless introversion and lack of insight.

THE FRONTAL LOBES

These consist of the portions of the hemispheres anterior to the coronal sulci (*fissures of Rolando*) and thus include the ascending frontal convolutions and the portions of the hemispheres anterior to them (*the prefrontal areas*). The lesions encountered in the prefrontal areas include injury, tumour, abscess and thrombosis of the anterior cerebral artery, the last named being comparatively rare.

The Syndrome of the Anterior Cerebral Artery. There is a spastic weakness of the opposite leg, especially in its distal part, with the appropriate changes in its reflexes. Sometimes there is slight weakness of the corresponding arm which may be associated with forced groping and grasping in the arm on one or both sides. The face is seldom affected. Apraxia of the left arm has been described and there is an unusual mental state with confusion.

The Syndrome of Frontal Lobe Tumour. The area of the frontal lobes anterior to the ascending frontal convolutions (the prefrontal areas) comprises a considerable portion of the cerebrum and is often the site of tumours. The symptoms vary with the rapidity of growth of the tumour and with other factors imperfectly understood. As a rule, an early, if not the initial symptom, is a change in the patient's mental state. He becomes apathetic and lacking in initiative. The association and flow of ideas tend to fail. He sits about idly, lacks attention and becomes indifferent to cleanliness and other aspects of personal behaviour. He is apt to permit the unhindered passage of urine and even of faeces, and to be totally insensitive to the embarrassments such conduct normally involves. This form of 'incontinence' is, in fact, a diagnostic symptom of great value in frontal lobe tumours. Rarely, the patient develops an abnormal facetiousness and euphoria—the so-called 'Witzelsucht'. These early symptoms may gradually give place to a profound dementia.

Movement is often disordered by the development of apraxia and sometimes by that of forced groping and grasping which, when unilateral, is a useful sign of frontal lobe involvement. When bilateral it is of less localizing significance. This grasping and groping has been shown to consist of two components: (1) Volitional grasping movements made by the conscious patient when some object is felt by him in his palm, or is seen by him to approach his hand. These movements wane and cease when consciousness is failing, or when attention is defective. (2) A true tonic reflex grasp of any object held in the hand, if this object is pulled away so as to put the flexors of the fingers on the stretch. The flexors tighten as the pull is maintained and their contraction may attain great force, such indeed that sometimes the patient can be pulled out of bed by this involuntary grasp which he is unable voluntarily to relax. This reflex may persist even after consciousness is lost but is abolished by injection of procaine into the appropriate afferent nerves.

Fits are a common feature of frontal tumours and may be generalized from their onset, or start with turning of the head and eyes to the opposite side, 'frontal adversive fits'. Other focal attacks include sensations and movements of the mouth and pharynx when the insula is involved and vasomotor and other visceral disturbances arising from the orbital frontal cortex. If the orbital lobule is affected there may be unilateral anosmia, or direct pressure on the optic nerve causing unilateral failure of vision associated with primary optic atrophy. This, when combined with papilloedema in the opposite eye has been described as Foster Kennedy's syndrome. These symptoms will be further considered in connexion with the syndrome of the anterior cranial fossa.

As the tumour expands it is likely to encroach upon the projection pathway from the motor cortex with a resulting contralateral hemiparesis, and when left-sided it is commonly associated with a predominantly executive disturbance of speech. Tumours in the medial portions of the frontal lobes may come to involve the corpus callosum and frequently spread through it to the opposite hemisphere. Then the patient becomes completely apathetic, silent and immobile, lying with open eyes, but displaying no initiative of any kind.

SYNDROMES OF THE CENTRAL REGION (REGION OF THE 'MOTOR CORTEX')

Hemiplegia is the characteristic symptom of a paralytic lesion in this portion of the hemisphere, and the Jacksonian fit that of an irritative lesion.

The Jacksonian fit most commonly originates in the face, thumb or big toe, and thence spreads with varying rapidity until much or all of the corresponding side of the body is affected. It may then become generalized. Consciousness is commonly preserved in attacks which remain unilateral. Such a fit may be accompanied by conjugate deviation of the head and eyes away from the side of the lesion and may be followed by a transient hemiparesis, Todd's paralysis, or in the case of a tumour by a progressive and permanent hemiplegia. The hemiparesis resulting from a destructive lesion near the surface will affect face, arm or leg predominantly according to the site of the lesion. The more deeply this extends into the underlying white matter, the more will the weakness affect the whole half body, since the pyramidal fibres converge from the cortex towards the capsule. Disturbances of cortical sensibility corresponding in distribution to the motor defect are not infrequent and result from simultaneous involvement of the neighbouring postcentral convolution.

PARIETAL LOBES

Irritative lesions in this area may cause focal fits heralded by subjective sensory disturbances on the opposite side, consisting of a numbness, tingling, or pins and needles, spreading in an orderly manner to other parts of the affected side of the body in the same way as the muscular spasm in discharging lesions of the motor cortex. Destructive lesions in this neighbourhood may be marked by a characteristic series of sensory disturbances. These include defective localization of tactile stimuli, defective appreciation of two simultaneous contacts, and defective appreciation of three dimensional space (i.e. size and form). There are, in addition, defect in differentiating minor differences in painful or thermal stimuli, and a ready fatigue of sensory functions. The simple recognition of such stimuli may be relatively intact. It will be seen that the defects in spatial discrimination which result from these modes of sensory loss lead to that inability to recognize and identify objects held in the hand, or to describe their size, shape or texture which is known as astereognosis. The appreciation of movement and of position is apt to be faulty, and some ataxy commonly results. Disturbances of attention may also occur on the contralateral side of the body together with failure of spatial orientation and of recognition of the body image. In left-sided lesions there may in addition be disorders of the visual speech function, resulting in dyslexia, agraphia and acalculia [see p. 1186]. Trophic changes, particularly decrease in size of the muscles, may be seen in the periphery of the limbs, and this may be so marked as to amount to true muscular wasting.

OCCIPITAL LOBES

Lesions of the cuneus and in the region of the calcarine fissure on the medial aspect of the occipital lobe result in hemianopia of the opposite field, but central vision escapes. Gordon Holmes showed that if the lesion is above the calcarine fissure a quadrantic hemianopia of the lower field results, and if below the quadrantic defect is of the upper field. Since central vision is represented at each occipital pole, a lesion of either pole causes contralateral, central, homonymous hemianopic scotomata, vision in the periphery of the field remaining intact. Similarly a bilateral lesion involving both occipital poles will result in bilateral central scotomata, and a bilateral lesion of the calcarine region will produce blindness of both peripheral fields, central vision remaining intact. If the lesion extends deeply into the occipital lobe so as completely to sever the optic radiation to the occipital cortex, complete hemianopia, affecting both the peripheral and central parts of the visual fields will result. The hemianopias resulting from a lesion of the occipital lobes have been distinguished from those due to lesions of the optic tracts by the fact that in the former the pupils react to light thrown on to the blind part of the field (Wernicke's hemianopic pupil phenomenon). To be of practical value this test needs to be made with a very narrow pencil of parallel rays to avoid the effects of dispersal of light within the eye.

On the outer surface of the occipital lobe, a lesion on the left side may sever the connexions between the visual centres and the speech centres, and so produce word blindness. Bilateral lesions in this region may be associated with visual disorientation.

Jacksonian attacks are often of great value in the localization of occipital lobe lesions. When the lesion is posterior there are undifferentiated visual hallucinations such as flashes of light or coloured figures, and when more anterior they may take the more elaborate form of visions of people, animals or places. In either case the hallucinations may be accompanied or followed by a transient hemianopia.

TEMPORAL LOBES

The considerable portion of the cortex comprised by the temporal lobes includes the cortical representation of the functions of smell, taste and hearing and on the left side, in right-handed persons, the function of speech.

The uncinate and hippocampal regions of these lobes are the cortical seats for taste and smell, and the localizing symptoms which are rarely absent when lesions in these regions exist are Jacksonian attacks of hallucinations of taste and smell of an unpleasant character. The hallucination is often associated with or immediately followed by a 'dreamy state' in which the patient may experience a feeling of strangeness or of intense familiarity. This state of altered consciousness may be accompanied by smacking of the lips, or champing of the jaw. The senses of taste and smell are not lost from a unilateral lesion of this region since they are bilaterally represented in the cerebral hemspheres. Epileptic discharges from the outer surface of the temporal lobes are associated with elaborately organized psychic experiences, 'temporal lobe epilepsy'. This loosely based morphological term is more satisfactory than its precursors 'epileptic equivalents' and 'psychomotor epilepsy'. In these states the patient may experience strange emotions, especially fear, disturbances of time perception (déjà vu), disorders of spatial integration and a miscellany of visceral sensations and activities. Quasi-purposive movements also occur. Long-standing lesions of the temporal lobes, with associated electroencephalographic changes are accompanied by disturbances of social behaviour, often of an aggressive sort, and they represent the physiogenic substate of the disturbed activity of the aggressive psychopath. Researches in this field are proving to be an advancing edge in our knowledge of the 'brain-mind relationship'.

The outer surfaces of the temporal lobes are concerned with hearing. Lesions here may result in fits which are heralded by crude auditory hallucinations, but owing to the complete semi-decussation of the auditory path unilateral lesions never produce detectable deafness. Bilateral lesions may, however, produce cortical deafness.

In right-handed subjects lesions of the left temporal lobe commonly give rise to serious disorders of speech function. With lesions situated far forward towards the insula the disturbance is predominantly one of spoken speech. With those situated in the posterior portion of the lobe the defect is predominantly one of the reception of speech. Deeply situated lesions of the temporal lobe commonly produce 'jargon aphasia'. Transitory disturbances of speech may occur in focal attacks originating from lesions in this area.

On account of the wide excursion which the optic radiation makes into the deep part of the temporal lobe in its course from the thalamus to the calcarine cortex, homonymous field defects, especially of the upper quadrants, are common in deep-seated lesions of the temporal lobes. Such lesions may also produce a paresis for emotional movements of the opposite half of the face which is relatively greater than the loss for voluntary movements.

INTERNAL CAPSULE

In this region, the chief motor tract is condensed into a small space, and is situated immediately in front of a narrowly localized sensory tract, while not much farther, posteriorly, the visual path emerges from the thalamus. Lesions of this region therefore produce severe and widely spread hemiplegia of the opposite side, often associated with hemianaesthesia and with hemianopia. From the proximity of the thalamus and corpus striatum, there is often involvement of these structures in a capsular lesion, with involuntary movements and sensory loss.

THE REGION OF THE FALX CEREBRI

Lesions of this region are likely to affect both hemispheres equally and to cause bilateral crural monoplegia with disturbances of cortical sensibility in the feet if the postcentral area is involved. Focal fits starting in one foot may occur. Disturbances of sphincter control are occasionally seen. Tumours arising from the posterior region of the falx may result in bilateral hemianopia. Parasagittal meningiomas are associated with these changes. Thrombosis of the superior longitudinal sinus may produce widespread bilateral lesions of the hemispheres, with double hemiplegia in which the face and hands are usually spared.

BASAL GANGLIA

OPTIC THALAMUS

Destruction of the thalamus by thrombosis causes the 'thalamic syndrome' of Dejerine; there is hemiparesis with spontaneous involuntary movements on the side of the body opposite to the damaged hemisphere. These may be tremor, intention tremor, choreic, athetotic, dancing or irregular. There is also hemianaesthesia, with hypersensitivity to painful, thermal or other stimuli, such as tickling or rubbing which may produce agonizing distress. Sometimes spontaneous, constant and unrelievable pain occurs on the affected side of the body. Emotional movement of the face may be impaired more than voluntary movement. The thalamic syndrome is found with vascular lesions but is rarely seen when the lesion is a tumour. In such cases the symptom-complex varies according to whether the growth primarily arises in the thalamus or invades it from its lateral aspect. In the former case it arises in the subependymal glia and spreads laterally. Such tumours cause early mental deterioration, with conjugate ocular palsies and sensory changes are absent or only terminal in appearance. In the case of tumours secondarily invading the thalamus from its lateral side, sensory changes of the order described under the 'thalamic syndrome' are seen.

CORPUS STRIATUM AND PUTAMEN

A bewildering feature of disease of the basal ganglia has been that no constant relationship has been established between the site and extent of morphological damage and the nature of the resulting disturbances of movement. The two aspects of dysfunction are those of spontaneous involuntary movement and of tone. The movements are rhythmic—tremors as in Parkinsonism—and arrhythmic as in chorea, athetosis, ballismus and torsion spasm. Usually in the quiet periods between the involuntary movements muscle tone is reduced, but the syndrome of Parkinsonism is the noticeable exception to this rule for here rigidity in some degree is invariable.

The chance discovery by Irvine Cooper that vascular damage in the territory of the anterior choroidal artery modified the syndrome of Parkinsonism led to further surgical researches by him and to the development of stereotactic devices to produce small lesions in known parts of the brain. This work, in addition to relieving many of the symptoms of Parkinsonism, is beginning to reveal the functional integration of the corpus striatum, globus pallidus and the lateral nuclei of the thalamus. Thalamectomy is dealt with later (see Parkinsonism).

With the uncommon exceptions of acute vascular lesions, causing for instance apoplectic chorea, most syndromes of the basal ganglia are chronic and degenerative in nature.

THIRD VENTRICLE AND HYPOTHALAMUS

Lesions occupying this cavity are usually neoplastic and may produce symptoms of localizing value in addition to those resulting from obstruction of the cerebrospinal fluid circulation (hydrocephalus). The most important of these are hypersomnia, diabetes insipidus, obesity and alteration in primary and secondary sexual functions of a more variable character than those which occur in lesions of the pituitary body. In the case of the rare 'colloid cysts' of the third ventricle, which hang suspended from its roof by a short pedicle, the symptoms, including the obstructive hydrocephalus, may be noticeably intermittent. Where the posterior end of the ventricle is affected there may be disturbance of the pupillary light reflex.

BRAIN STEM

THE MIDBRAIN

This portion of the brain stem consists of a small dorsal area, the quadrigeminal plate or tectum and a large ventral area, the cerebral peduncles or crura cerebri.

At the level of the corpora quadrigemina the oculomotor nuclei lie on either side of the aqueduct of Sylvius, and lower down on either side of the middle line, in the floor of the upper part of the fourth ventricle. Lesions of this region cause nuclear ophthalmoplegia—that is, paralysis of both eyes in terms of the conjugate movements upwards, downwards or laterally. From above downwards, lesions of this column of oculomotor nuclei will produce reflex iridoplegia, loss of convergence, paralysis of upward, downward and lateral movements respectively.

Immediately ventral to the third nerve nucleus and decussating below it lie the superior cerebellar peduncles passing to the red nuclei. Involvement of these structures causes ataxia of the limbs and trunk.

A lesion of the tectal region of the midbrain produces a characteristic syndrome of nuclear ophthalamoplegia with bilateral ataxia, which is *Nothnagel's syndrome.*

In the ventral portion of this region of the brain stem are the crura cerebri with the third nerve perforating each crus to emerge on its inner side, and the optic tract running round the crus as it passes back from the optic chiasma to the lateral geniculate body. A lesion of one crus will cause hemiplegia of the opposite side, and paralysis of the third nerve on the same side. This pathognomonic localizing combination is *Weber's syndrome.*

Situated a little more dorsally, a lesion of the crus will produce ophthalmoplegia of one eye with tremor and inco-ordination of the opposite limbs. This is *Benedikt's syndrome.*

Extension of a lesion outwards from the crus may cause tract hemianopia, in which the half fields are completely involved and the light reflex lost from the blind fields. Interference with the fillet may cause hemianaesthesia on the opposite side.

PONS AND MEDULLA

Here the motor and sensory tracts, the middle and inferior cerebellar peduncles, the cranial nerve nuclei and the outgoing cranial nerves are closely packed together, and the signs resulting from destruction of these will be various combinations of spastic paralysis, ataxia and sensory loss in the body and limbs—from interference with the long conducting tracts—together with nuclear and peripheral nerve palsies and anaesthesia in the distribution of the cranial nerves.

If the lesion is unilateral the body and the structures innervated by the cranial nerves will be affected on opposite sides, causing the 'crossed paralyses' or 'alternate paralyses' characteristic of lesions of the brain stem. Of these, facial palsy of lower motor neurone type with contralateral hemiplegia is the most frequently encountered, trigeminal palsy and anaesthesia and vagoglossopharyngeal palsy with contralateral hemiplegia being less common. Lesions of the brain stem below the oculomotor nuclei cause small pupils (pontine myosis) by cutting off those nuclei from the spinal cord, whence the tonic dilators of the pupils—the cervical sympathetic system—emerge. Lesions in the upper part of the pons commonly lead to loss of conjugate lateral movement of the eyes. If the connexions of the vestibular nerve are involved intense vertigo will result together with nystagmus. Glycosuria may occur in lesions in the neighbourhood of the fourth ventricle and the respiratory centre may be involved.

The common lesion involving the medulla is infarction of the lateral portion from thrombosis of the posterior inferior cerebellar artery or its branches, the so-called cerebellar apoplexy [see p. 1220]. Owing to the smallness of the brain stem, lesions of an inflammatory or neoplastic character commonly involve both sides of the structure and bilateral symptoms result.

CEREBELLUM

When lesions of the cerebellum develop suddenly they are apt to produce more striking disturbances of function than when gradual, a point which it is important to remember when the presence of an abscess or a tumour within the cerebellum is suspected. These disturbances are all due to disintegration of the central control of muscle 'tone', and the several different components of cerebellar ataxia are to be regarded not so much as special disorders of different cerebellar functions, but as expressions of this single disorder, which owe their varying appearance to the difference in the clinical tests employed.

Hypotonia. This is particularly marked in acute lesions, but can also be detected in those of slow evolution. It shows itself by marked flaccidity and extensibility of the limb muscles which permit of undue mobility of the joints and leads to a modification of the normal posture of the limbs and, when marked, to the 'pendular' form of knee-jerk. The hypotonia is largely responsible for the symptom of *dysmetria.* If the patient is asked to extend the arm and pick up some object, such as a glass, or to touch a fixed point, the limb is shot forward with undue force and may overshoot the mark. Similarly the hypotonia may give the *rebound phenomenon.* If the arms be extended horizontally by the patient, and the observer smartly strikes them downwards by a blow on the hand, the arm on the normal side is quickly brought to rest in its original position with the minimum of recoil. On the side of the lesion, however, the hand and arm 'bounce' freely and may oscillate two or three times before being brought to rest.

Dysdiadochokinesis. This absurd term has been used for the slowness, clumsiness and irregularity with which alternating movements (e.g. pronation-supination of the forearm) are carried out although the simple movement can be performed normally. In carrying out this test it is common to see adventitious movements in the proximal segments of the limb from disturbance of the normal co-ordinated contraction of the adjuvant muscles. To correct this disturbance the patient tends to break up complex movements into their several components, which are carried out successively instead of simultaneously—the 'movement by numbers'.

Tremor. This is not a resting tremor, but an unsteadiness which develops during movement, and in purposive movements tends to increase in range and severity as the climax of the movement is reached. It is thus essentially an 'intention' tremor caused by breakdown in tonal relationships. Similarly if the arms are outstretched, they may show a tendency to droop, which is corrected by a series of jerks which gives the form of a tremor. Again, in standing there may be irregular oscillations of the trunk and head or 'titubation'.

Gait. In bilateral lesions the gait has a reeling, staggering character and in unilateral lesions there is a tendency to sway and deviate towards the side of the lesion. The disorder may vary in severity from a slight unsteadiness to a complete inability to walk or stand unaided. There is a tendency to walk with the legs abnormally separated to lessen the tendency to overbalance and the feet are brought down irregularly with a stamp.

Speech. The articulatory musculature shares the incoordination of the other voluntary muscles with a resulting characteristic dysarthria. The defect is known as 'scanning' or 'staccato' speech. It consists of slowness of articulation, and a tendency to say each syllable of a word as though it were a separate word. The rhythm of speech becomes irregular, some syllables being slurred over, others being enunciated with almost explosive violence.

Nystagmus. Nystagmus is particularly frequent in those lesions of the cerebellum which involve its connexions with the brain stem and the neighbouring vestibular nuclei. In unilateral lesions there is coarse nystagmus on deviating the eyes to the side of the lesion with a finer and more rapid movement on deviation away from the side of the lesion. The drift of the eyes from the point of fixation is due to hypotonia. In bilateral lesions the nystagmus may be symmetrical and if the lesion is confined to the superficial areas of the cerebellar hemispheres nystagmus may be entirely absent. Rarely—usually after acute lesions such as gunshot wounds or operative interference—the phenomenon of 'skew-deviation' may appear temporarily: the eye on the side of the lesion being displaced downwards and inwards, the opposite eye upwards and outwards. A slight degree of skew-deviation on lateral deviation of the eyes may be seen in deeply seated tumours of the cerebellum.

The cerebellum forms part of the non-sensory afferent nervous system and is concerned with the co-ordination of voluntary movement. It is not a sensory organ and there is no disturbance of any form of sensibility in cerebellar lesions.

THE ANTERIOR FOSSA OF THE SKULL

This part is often damaged in head injuries but the lesion giving the characteristic syndrome is a meningioma arising from the dural covering of the cribriform plate and growing upwards into the olfactory groove. The earliest sign is anosmia from pressure on the olfactory bulb and tract, unilateral at first and later often bilateral. Unilateral loss of vision associated with primary optic atrophy may later be associated with papilloedema in the opposite eye as an expression of the general rise of intracranial tension. Such a tumour gradually displaces the overlying frontal lobe and may then give rise to mental deterioration and fits, but only in tumours of exceptional size is a crossed hemiparesis observed.

Aneurysm of the anterior cerebral or anterior communicating arteries may cause similar early symptoms, but owing to its limited size papilloedema and the remote pressure effects are not seen.

THE MIDDLE FOSSA OF THE SKULL

A rich variety of lesions may arise in or invade this fossa, and the syndromes vary according to their situation. Those in the midline include pituitary adenomata, tumours of the pituitary stalk, and meningioma of the sellar diaphragm (parasellar and suprasellar tumours). In the lateral parts of the fossa, passing from medial to lateral, we have to consider lesions in the cavity or walls of the cavernous sinus, and tumours arising from the sphenoidal ridge in its middle and outer parts. Finally, reference must be made to growths invading the base of the skull and either occluding its foramina and producing cranial nerve palsies, or actually invading the cranial cavity. Secondary deposits of carcinoma and epitheliomata of the nasopharynx are the common lesions of the last-named group.

REGION OF THE OPTIC CHIASMA AND THE PITUITARY BODY

The most common lesion in this region is tumour of the pituitary, usually an adenoma. The earliest symptoms of such a tumour are of an endocrine disturbance and vary according to the nature of the tumour. If this is composed of eosinophil cells acromegaly or gigantism will result, if chromophobe the endocrine disturbance will take the form of hypopituitarism. Basophil adenomata although producing a characteristic group of endocrine symptoms, commonly described as Cushing's syndrome [see Section 5], do not attain a size sufficient to produce symptoms as space-occupying lesions.

When a pituitary tumour extends outside the cavity of the sella turcica it distorts the optic chiasma and produces one of a variety of visual disturbances. The commonest is a bitemporal hemianopia, sometimes starting as bitemporal paracentral scotomata which gradually increase in size till the entire temporal fields are lost. This results from the stretching of the decussating fibres of the chiasma derived from the nasal halves of each retina. If the extension of the tumour is forward, uniocular scotoma, hemianopia or blindness may result; if it is backward homonymous hemianopia may follow involvement of the optic tract. The form of the visual field defect in pituitary tumours is determined by the position of the local pressure upon the visual pathway and that whilst a bitemporal hemianopia is the most usual and characteristic defect the others which have been mentioned are frequently seen. Primary optic atrophy in the affected eye is the rule in pituitary tumours, and papilloedema is not seen unless, as rarely happens, the tumour has attained such a size as to obstruct the third ventricle.

Meningeal tumours arising from the sellar diaphragm, aneurysms extending backwards from the anterior communicating artery and cystic arachnoiditis may produce identical pressure symptoms, but without the endocrine disorders of pituitary tumours.

Cysts derived from vestiges of Rathke's pouch cause endocrine and local pressure symptoms comparable to those of primary intrasellar tumours, but in addition give rise to papilloedema and internal hydrocephalus from obstruction of the third ventricle [see also p. 1193].

SYNDROMES OF THE CAVERNOUS SINUS

The commonest acute lesion of this cavity is thrombosis. Of the slowly developing lesions saccular aneurysm of the carotid artery is the most common, though the cavity may be encroached upon by tumours originating from the medial end of the sphenoidal ridge. Symptoms consist of paresis of the third, fourth and sixth cranial nerves often leading to complete ophthalmoplegia, anaesthesia in the distribution of the ophthalmic division of the trigeminus and proptosis of the corresponding eye with oedema of the orbital tissues and conjunctiva from congestion of the ophthalmic veins. In rapidly developing lesions unilateral papilloedema may occur, but in those of slow development optic atrophy from pressure on the neighbouring optic nerve is more often seen.

SYNDROMES OF THE SPHENOIDAL RIDGE

The dural sinus, which runs along the sphenoidal ridge (sinus sphenoparietalis), is one of the sites of election of the development of meningiomata. From the point of view of localizing diagnosis this ridge may be divided into three parts, the inner (or clinoidal), the middle and outer.

A meningioma arising from the inner part gives rise in its early stages to a syndrome similar to that of a lesion of the cavernous sinus. Later symptoms of pressure on the temporosphenoidal lobe may occur (uncinate fits, personality changes and crossed hemiparesis). Papilloedema may result from general increase of intracranial pressure.

A meningioma of the middle part of the ridge may remain for long without clear localizing signs, and radiography and ventriculography may be necessary to establish its position.

At the outer end of the ridge a meningioma may produce as its localizing syndrome unilateral exophthalmos without squint, some fullness of the temporal fossa with local tenderness on pressure, speech disturbances if the lesion is left sided, together with the general symptoms and signs of raised intracranial tension. The tumour may, however, reach a large size before it is recognized, its effects being a change in personality and social behaviour which may well appear to be psychogenic. The X-ray picture usually reveals densification of bone or even hyperostosis of a part of the ridge and adjoining bone.

SYNDROMES OF THE BASE OF THE SKULL

The characteristic signs of such lesions are palsies of the cranial nerves, often in groups anatomically close to one another, without any evidence of intracerebral damage or rise in intracranial tension. The common cause is malignant growth, either secondary deposits from remote carcinomata, the lung and breast being the most important, or direct invasion from the nasopharynx.

THE POSTERIOR FOSSA OF THE SKULL

Lateral Recess. The angle formed by the posterior surface of the petrous temporal bone and the tentorium (cerebellopontine angle) is a common situation for neurofibromata which grow usually from the eighth nerve, but occasionally from the fifth or seventh. Rarely a meningioma may occupy the same position. They press into the lateral lobe of the cerebellum and the side of the pons and a characteristic clinical picture results, of slowly progressive nerve deafness and tinnitus, facial weakness, often with peripheral facial spasm, impairment of sensibility in the area of the fifth nerve with diminution or loss of the corresponding corneal reflex and signs of ipsilateral cerebellar involvement. Such tumours are of slow growth, and headaches and papilloedema are often absent or occur late in the clinical picture.

REFERENCES

ADIE, W. J., and CRITCHLEY, M. (1927) Forced grasping and groping, *Brain*, **50**, 142.

ALLEN, I. M. (1930) A clinical study of tumours involving the occipital lobe, *Brain*, **53**, 194.

ANDREW, J., and NATHAN, P. W. (1964) Lesions of the anterior frontal lobes and disturbances of micturition and defaecation, *Brain*, **87**, 233.

BARNETT, H. J., and HYLAND, H. H. (1952) Tumours involving the brain stem, *Quart. J. Med.*, **21**, 265.

BIEMOND, A. (1951) Thrombosis of the basilar artery and vascularization of the brain stem, *Brain*, **74**, 300.

BLAU, J. N., and HINTON, J. M. (1960) Hypopituitary coma and psychosis, *Lancet*, i, 408.

BRAIN, W. R., and WILKINSON, M. (1959) Observations on the extensor plantar reflex and its relationship to the functions of the pyramidal tract, *Brain*, **82**, 297.

CLARK, G. (1948) The mode of representations in the motor cortex, *Brain*, **71**, 320.

CRITCHLEY, M. (1930) The anterior cerebral artery and its syndromes, *Brain*, **53**, 120.

CRITCHLEY, M. (1953) *The Parietal Lobes*, London.

DENNY-BROWN, D. (1951) *The Frontal Lobes and Their Function*, London.

DENNY-BROWN, D. (1960) Diseases of the basal ganglia, *Lancet*, ii, 1099, 1155.

EDWARDS, C. H., and PATERSON, J. H. (1951) A review of the symptoms and signs of acoustic neurofibromata, *Brain*, **74**, 144.

HARRIS, G. W. (1955) *Neural Control of the Pituitary Gland*, London.

HENSON, R. A., CRAWFORD, J. V., and CAVANAGH, J. B. (1953) Tumours of the glomus jugulare, *J. Neurol. Neurosurg. Psychiat.*, **16**, 127.

HOLMES, G. (1917) Croonian lectures. The clinical symptoms of cerebellar disease and their interpretation, *Lancet*, i, 1177, 1231, and ii, 59, 111.

HOLMES, G. (1931) A contribution to the cortical representation of vision, *Brain*, **54**, 470.

HUBBLE, D. (1961) The endocrine orchestra, *Brit. med. J.*, **1**, 523.

KELLY, R. (1951) Colloid cysts of the third ventricle, *Brain*, **74**, 23.

KUBIK, C. S., and ADAMS, R. D. (1946) Occlusion of the basilar artery, a clinical and pathological study, *Brain*, **69**, 73.

MAGOUN, H. W. (1958) *The Waking Brain*, Springfield, Ill.

MARTIN, J. P. (1968) *The Basal Ganglia*, London.

MCKISSOCK, W., and PAINE, K. W. E. (1958) Primary tumours of the thalamus, *Brain*, **81**, 41.

MORUZZI, G. (1950) *Problems in Cerebellar Physiology*, Springfield, Ill.

NORTHFIELD, D. W. C. (1957) Rathke pouch tumours, *Brain*, **80**, 293.

RANDALL, R. V., and CHARLES, E. C. (1961) Treatment of chronic diabetes insipidus, *Postgrad. Med.*, **29**, 94.

RIDDOCH, G. (1938) The clinical features of central pain, *Lancet*, i, 1093, 1150, 1205.

RUSSELL, D. S., and RUBINSTEIN, L. J. (1963) *Pathology of Tumours of the Nervous System*, London.

SAWYER, W. H. (1961) Neurohypophyseal hormones, *Pharmacol. Rev.*, **13**, 225.

VAN BUREN, J. M., and BALDWIN, M. (1958) The architecture of the optic radiation in the temporal lobe of man, *Brain*, **81**, 15.

WALSHE, F. M. R. (1951) On the interpretation of experimental studies of cortical motor function, *Brain*, **74**, 249.

WILLIAMS, D. (1969) The temporal lobes, in *A Handbook of Neurology*, Ch. 22, Part II, Amsterdam.

WILLIAMS, D., and GASSEL, M. M. (1962) Visual functions in patients with homonymous hemianopia, *Brain*, **85**, 175.

WILLIAMS, D., and WILSON, T. G. (1962) The diagnosis of the major and minor syndromes of basilar insufficiency, *Brain*, **85**, 741.

APHASIA AND OTHER DEFECTS OF SPEECH

Speech is the most highly developed and recently evolved function of the human being which is capable of direct analysis. Of all man's endowments it is the one which marks him off most clearly from his closest neighbours in the animal world. While in its final expression speech consists of sensorimotor activities of many mechanisms, each simple in comparison with the whole, its roots strike deeply into the texture of the mind and it constitutes the symbolic currency of thought itself; indeed it is doubtful if without speech in this wider sense any but the simplest thoughts are possible. So it is that we find that profound disturbances of speech function are invariably accompanied by disorder of the mind.

Speech in its simplest form is a means of communication of thought between individuals by the production and perception of sounds; it is an elastic function, capable of indefinite extension and elaboration both in the race and in the individual. We find an almost infinite variation between the simple language of a primitive people and the highly elaborate language of a civilized race; between the speech of an uneducated peasant, for whose simple needs a few hundred words suffice, and that of a master of prose who may use thousands of words to express shades of meaning far beyond the scope of an uncultured person; between the speech of a child and that of the same individual grown to maturity. The growth of speech proceeds *pari passu* with the growth of the mind which employs it for its needs. Furthermore, upon the foundation of the initial symbolic expression of thought in spoken language has been erected in all but primitive races, the further edifice of written speech in which visual symbols replace those of sound. The evolution of speech in the different races of mankind is the province of the science of philology, but its growth in the individual in health and its dissolution in disease make up one of the most fascinating and complex chapters of medicine. As would be expected in a function of such complexity the disorders of speech are many and varied. At one end of the scale are disturbances purely psychological in their origin such as hysterical mutism; at the other are those due to the defects of the executive structures such as the tongue and larynx, and the neuromuscular mechanisms which control them. To disturbances of this order the term *dysarthria* is applied. Between these extremes lie a group of speech disorders which depend upon physical disturbance of the portions of the cerebrum which form the anatomical substratum of the speech function and to these the terms *aphasia* or *dysphasia* are applied. Thus aphasia may be defined as loss of symbolic expression or understanding.

APHASIA

General Considerations

Few subjects have suffered more from attempts at over-simplification than the study of aphasia. Many attempts have been made by the creation of hypothetical 'centres' connected with one another by supposedly well-defined tracts, to explain the manifold and often apparently conflicting facts which may be observed in an aphasic patient. Such diagrammatic analyses have been based upon individual cases of aphasia in which particular aspects of speech function have been predominately affected and in which post-mortem examination has revealed damage to a circumscribed area of the brain. Thus, Broca's centre in the cortex of the posterior part of the left third prefrontal convolution was the motor centre for spoken speech, while Exner's centre in a similar position in the second left prefrontal convolution was the motor centre for written language. The 'auditory word centre' in which auditory memories of words were stored was in the cortex of the first and second temporal gyri, while the 'visual word centre' in which visual memories for words were impressed was in the cortex of the angular gyrus. These various centres were connected together by to-and-fro pathways which could be separately affected by a lesion. But the attempts to explain the multitudinous and varied phenomena which occur in lesions of the speech centre by assuming damage to one or other of these hypothetical 'word centres' or to their connecting paths proved highly unsatisfactory, and the validity of such clinico-pathological correlations was usually undermined by the fact that the majority of cases of aphasia result from vascular lesions in which multiple areas of disease are present or from tumours of wide extent. Head stigmatized those who thought of the mechanisms underlying speech in this naïve way as 'the diagram makers'.

Clinical observation shows that as the function of speech in health evolves *as a whole* from more simple to more complex by a process of gradual elaboration, so in disease it undergoes dissolution as a whole from more complex to more simple. The more critically cases of so-called 'pure motor aphasia' or 'pure word deafness' are examined the more clear it becomes that, while one particular aspect of spoken speech is particularly affected, the level of speech function as a whole is lowered. Furthermore, in a given case of aphasia the defect of function is not constant, but may vary widely with the activity of the brain as a whole in response to such factors as fatigue, attention, anxiety and the general level of health of the whole individual.

A moment's introspective thought makes it clear that when we make an intelligent statement we have relied on the incoming observations of others, on stimuli of other sorts from our immediate and past life, on experience and education, that we have comprehended and elaborated the idea, perhaps reduced its complexity to a polished statement, and then uttered it. How we uttered it, to whom and with what emotional content in turn depended upon a host of internal and external events relying upon the past, and modified by the present and future. In short we had used all of both hemispheres in achieving that statement.

These considerations must constantly be borne in mind in the examination of aphasic patients and in our attempts to generalize from such individual observations and to obtain a clear understanding of aphasia as a whole.

Anatomical Considerations

The function of speech seems to be concerned with the left hemisphere of the brain alone in right-handed persons, and this is explained by the major potential of the left hemisphere for receptivity and education associated with the major use of the right hand through the countless ages of humanity. True left-handedness is often associated with a transfer of the speech function to the right hemisphere, but there are exceptions to this rule. The possibilities of transfer of the speech function from the left to the right hemisphere is great during childhood, to the extent that no lesion of the speech region of the left hemisphere, however extensive, causes lasting loss of speech in a child under the age of 6 years, provided that sufficient intelligence remains to permit of re-learning. After this age the possibility of such compensation by the right hemisphere from lesions in the left hemisphere gradually diminishes.

When the operation of hemispherectomy was introduced to treat epilepsy associated with congenital hemiplegia it was found that though the left (major) hemisphere played little part in controlling bodily movement, because of extensive damage to it, aphasia resulted from the operation. Further researches have made it clear that in some patients transfer of the function of speech to the other hemisphere does not occur. Careful investigations are therefore essential before any part of the left hemisphere is removed. These may include slow injections of amylobarbitone into the left carotid artery to see if temporary aphasia results.

Within the left hemisphere speech function has as its anatomical substratum a region of the cerebral convolutions having its centre a little behind the middle of the first and second temporal convolutions. It is limited above by the posterior limits of the Sylvian fissure, occupies probably most of the external convexity of the left temporal lobe, and spreads backwards into the supramarginal and angular gyri, while anteriorly it extends forward, deep to the Sylvian fissure, over all the convolutions of the insula and to the posterior ends of the second and third left frontal gyri.

This 'speech area' comprises the cortex and the subcortical white matter which carries the paths between the speech area and other portions of the brain.

Posteriorly it receives an important tract from the visual region of the cortex. An interruption of this tract causes 'pure word blindness', in which the most conspicuous feature is an inability to appreciate written speech. Upon its deep aspect the speech region of the convolutions receives the temporal projection of fibres conveying auditory impressions, and destruction of this system by a lesion undercutting the convolutions in the centre of the temporal lobe causes serious speech disturbance in which 'word deafness', or inability to appreciate spoken language, is the most important component. In this same region another set of fibres impinges upon the speech area which conveys the muscular sense impressions and other sensory impressions which are produced in the movements of articulation, and which are the only guidance which the 'deaf mute' has in the knowledge of correct execution of his articulation. A lesion deep in the temporal lobe may interrupt the paths and so isolate the speech region from any appreciation of correct execution, with the result that spoken language becomes unshapen and degenerates into a voluble jargon or 'jargon aphasia' which is invariably associated with serious mental deterioration and confusion. There is today revived interest in these 'disconnexion syndromes'.

In the anterior half of the speech area a tract of fibres gathers by degrees to pass forwards to constitute the bulk of the 'temporal isthmus' beneath the middle and inferior frontal convolutions from whence it is connected with the pyramidal path of the left side, and by way of the corpus callosum with the pyramidal path of the right side. This is the executive outgoing path for speech movements, and a complete lesion of this path will result in inability to exteriorize spoken or written speech with relatively little impairment of comprehension of speech—the so-called 'pure motor aphasia' or 'pure agraphia'. Within the speech area of the brain thus limited, little is known of any localization of function, but it is generally held that there is a gradual passing over from receptive functions (appreciation of spoken and written language) in the posterior regions, to executive functions (exteriorization of spoken and written language) in the anterior regions.

In so far as the phenomena of 'word-blindness' and 'word-deafness' as well as 'motor aphasia' and 'agraphia' result from lesions of the speech area, they seem to result from lesions of the tracts concerned rather than from damage to the cortex itself. Lesions confined to the cortex and sparing the subcortical white matter, unless they are extensive, do not give rise to permanent disorder of speech.

Physiological Considerations

Speech is the ability to use language, not mere words, and discrete words are not the units of language, for the same sound or shape can mean different things in different contexts, as in 'bear' or 'arm'.

Within a short time after birth the child begins to recognize the nature and uses of some of the objects in the world around it, and to express its simple conscious processes by gestures, and it early appreciates the 'gesture language' of those around it. The 'mimesis', or gesture language, thus early impressed and expressed, remains throughout life the most stable, the least vulnerable and the longest lasting of the methods of receiving and communicating ideas. Long before it is able to utter any articulate sound, the infant learns to connect certain sounds which it hears with certain objects and with certain events, and the memories of these auditory patterns first implanted serve by far the most important function in the processes and expressions of thought throughout life. Whereas we rely upon our visual memories for our remembrance and intelligence in general matters almost exclusively, yet as regards speech we rely upon auditory memories to a very large extent, and of course those who have never learned to read do so exclusively. The process of recall, both in silent thought and in speaking, is the revival of auditory patterns. From the original connexion with hearing, the memories of speech patterns come to be located in that part of the brain associated with the auditory function—in and around the temporal lobe. Later, guided by the auditory memories, the child begins to express himself in articulate speech and he does so by the revival of auditory memories.

All living motion is sense-originated, sense-guided and sense-governed, and a motor process of itself has no proved conscious concomitant. Our consciousness is that of the sensations which accompany the movement, or which result from the movement. The knowledge of correct execution so gained fortifies and increases the functional stability of the speech area, and is of immense importance in the speech function. If it is absent owing to a lesion isolating the speech area on the incoming side, speech degenerates into a jargon and soon becomes impossible, just as in tabes the walking becomes irregular from loss of the muscular sense conveyed in the posterior columns, and ultimately standing becomes impossible.

When at a considerably later age the child learns to read and write, certain visual patterns (letters, words, sentences) become connected with certain objects and ideas, and become linked on to the already well-established auditory memories of speech. The meaning of the visual symbols is learned by the child from the meaning of the word or pattern spoken, which he already knows well, and the already developed auditory speech function serves as the instructor of the visual speech function, and throughout life remains the more potent, more dominant and less vulnerable function of the two.

Later still, in learning to write, the child relies upon his visual memories, and as his knowledge of correct execution in writing is largely visual and only in minor degree common sensory from the movements of the hand in writing, it follows that the function of exteriorizing speech by writing becomes intimately connected with and a part of the visual speech function, and is usually depressed or lost with the visual speech function as the result of disease. It will thus be seen that there are not separate regions of the speech area in which the auditory memories of language and the execution of spoken speech on the one hand, and the visual memories of language and the execution of written language on the other hand, are represented, but that there are four functions intimately coupled in pairs, which have their seat in the same anatomical substratum. As has already been pointed out, it is a general principle that when the speech area is damaged the speech function becomes depressed as a whole, with the result that function is lost in order of its depth of impression.

Pathological Considerations

By far the most common cause of aphasia, in all its degrees and varieties, is ischaemia caused by reduction of flow or vascular occlusion. Injury to the speech areas of the left hemisphere may cause a wide range of aphasic disturbances. Cerebral tumour is the usual lesion causing aphasia of gradual onset, and is much the commonest cause of 'jargon aphasia' for there are few other lesions which can undercut and, therefore, isolate the temporal convolutions without otherwise interfering with their function.

Symptoms

Small lesions of the cortex seldom if ever produce lasting disturbances of speech. This indicates that within the speech area there is no narrow localization of cortical function and there must be capacity for compensation for such small lesions in the surrounding undamaged cortex. With larger lesions of the cortex, and in proportion to their extent, mutilation of the patterns of speech, slowness of utterance, inability to find the words (inability to recall), especially nominals and above all isolated nominals, occur, in that order.

Stammering may sometimes be noticed in the mutilated speech of the dysphasic. This condition is at once distinguishable from true jargon aphasia, since the former is slow and halting whereas the latter is facile and voluble. Misplacement of words and the use of wrong words are common and are called 'paraphasia'. A tendency to repeat a word once pronounced is sometimes present and is designated perseveration of speech. The same faults occur also in writing, as faulty spelling, misplacement of letters and words and the use of wrong words. Much defect of general intelligence always accompanies severe damage to the speech area, especially if comprehension of spoken speech is involved, and this will be readily understood from the large role which speech patterns play in the working of thought. Difficulty in the recall of words and speech patterns, which has been termed 'verbal amnesia' or amnesic dysphasia, is a characteristic feature of lesions of the speech area. This difficulty is greater with spontaneous revival than with recall, which is brought about by direct sensory stimulation. For example, an aphasic person who is unable spontaneously to utter a word, may repeat the word at once when it is spoken to him, when he sees it in writing or when the corresponding object is shown to him. It is important in this connexion to remember that we do not speak in the letters of the alphabet, nor in the words of our dictionary, but in a running pattern of sound. The pattern or context provides the meaning, while the individual words are negligible and have no meaning. The power of the pattern in aiding revival is great both from sequence rhythm and musical quality. As an example, an aphasic who has no spontaneous utterance is told to count with his interlocutor. The interlocutor begins counting, the aphasic joins in. The interlocutor then stops, but the aphasic continues counting, carried by the sequence rhythm.

The confusional defects of speech function are found in extensive damage to the speech area, and are usual as immediate and transient phenomena in all suddenly occurring lesions of the speech area. There is general mental dullness, with varying degrees, usually severe, of depression of speech function and much confusion, both on the receptive and expressive sides, when any of these functions remain, and the results of the examination of the speech faculty are apt to vary from moment to moment, for attention is difficult to hold and the patient is easily fatigued and bored. Severe degrees of this form of defect may be associated with inability to recognize objects—'object-blindness', and with loss of ability to convey ideas by gesture—'amimia'.

Method of Examination

A dysphasic person fatigues readily and is often anxious so he should be examined quietly and only for short periods at a time. Dysphasia, like all manifestations of disordered cortical function, varies in severity and quality from hour to hour and almost from minute to minute in response to such varied factors as attention, fatigue and general bodily well-being. It follows that the best record of an examination of a dysphasic patient is an objective and factual one, a statement of what the examiner said or did, and what the patient said or did in reply.

Before any detailed investigation is attempted certain facts should be established and, when possible, confirmed from a relative. (1) Is the patient right- or left-handed and, if the latter, did he write with the right hand? (2) What was his state of education as regards reading, writing and knowledge of foreign languages? (3) Is he deaf? If so, to what extent? (4) Is his sight good or bad? Is there hemianopia? (5) Can he understand pantomime or gesture and express his needs thereby? (6) What is his state of consciousness? (7) To what extent is propositional speech preserved and to what extent can he convey a narrative in words? What defects are evident, e.g. perseveration, paraphasia or jargon utterances? (8) Can he name objects seen, both simple and familiar and unfamiliar? (9) Can he obey spoken commands? (10) Can he select correctly a test object from a number of them in response to the spoken word? (11) Can he write spontaneously and to dictation and what mistakes does he make? (12) Can he copy printed or written words? (13) Can he obey written commands? (14) Can he write figures and carry out simple arithmetic calculations? (15) Can he understand the significance of pictures? (16) Can he draw such simple objects as a bicycle, a flower or the façade of a house.

The examiner should have in mind a simple scheme relating motor (executive) and sensory (receptive) speech to their three aspects—written, spoken and drawn—and to the capacity for expression of ideas in movement. For instance, the subject who cannot speak may be asked in simple words or in writing to carry out non-verbal tasks, and so the examiner can assess his capacity to understand.

Having obtained some insight into the patient's speech defect in a preliminary survey it is essential to assess the degree of mental deterioration (if any) that is present by the battery of tests employed to investigate a case of organic dementia since dysphasia and global mental deterioration each in its way increases and distorts the severity of the other.

Treatment

The recovery of speech after a lesion causing dysphasia has much in common with the original acquisition of speech in a child. The preservation of a certain degree of intelligence is essential to recovery and the younger the patient the greater the prospect of a successful outcome. It is an unfortunate fact that the majority of cases of dysphasia occur in elderly subjects with arterial disease or in those with infiltrating tumours in whom a gradual deterioration of cerebral function must be expected. The most hopeful group are the young adults and children suffering from traumatic lesions of the brain, from transient cerebral lesions due to ischaemia without occlusion and from removable causes such as subdural haematomas and benign tumours. In such cases spontaneous recovery of speech occurs gradually, but it can be accelerated by a careful and patient system of re-education at the hands of a speech therapist carried out either individually, or in groups.

Testamentary Capacity

No rule can be laid down upon the capacity of a person with aphasic speech defects to exercise civil rights and to make a will, and each case must be judged upon its merits. The first consideration is the degree of intelligence, and when this is high it is essential for such capacity that there should be some mode of cognition and of expression left. In cases of uncomplicated executive aphasia either for spoken or written speech there is complete civil capacity, but when, as usually happens, the two conditions coexist, though intelligence and the receptive side of speech may be little impaired, if the expressive side of speech is reduced to gesture, there will be extreme difficulty in ascertaining the patient's wishes. Defects in the comprehension of spoken and written speech interfere seriously with testamentary capacity and with capacity for exercising civil rights.

Prognosis

In attempting to estimate the degree of recovery which is likely to occur in cases of aphasia, it is necessary first to bear in mind that sudden cerebral injury is apt at first, by the process which has here been described as functional depression or 'diaschisis', to cause very wide loss of function, though the lesion may not be very extensive. Total aphasia, for example, is often the immediate result of a lesion of moderate size. Such phenomena last usually not longer than a week, and until they have passed off it is impossible to make a definite statement, either as to the extent of the lesion or the likely degree of recovery. Speech may be regained by two entirely separate processes—either by recovery of function in partly damaged and functionally depressed areas, or by compensatory activity in the undamaged portions of the brain. The possible recovery of function will depend upon the nature of the lesion and upon its extent. It will be greater when a lesion is one of pressure rather than of actual destruction and if removable, as in subdural haemorrhage, and least when the cause is a thrombosis, or an irremovable tumour. The greater the extent of a vascular lesion, the less is the chance of functional restitution for there is then little hope of restoration of the circulation through collateral vessels. In young children unilateral lesions produce no permanent speech defects, provided sufficient intelligence remains, but even to this rule some exceptions have been recorded. When adult life is reached, transference occurs less readily, yet in a few instances destruction of the posterior half of the speech area has been followed by an almost complete restoration of speech function.

The study of speech and its defects, and indeed of the whole phenomenological basis of communication makes up a major part of the cultural background of clinical neurology. The actual form or degree of dysphasic disorder present does not have any precise value in localization, however. It is a reasonable aphorism that we use the whole of both hemispheres in speech, and it must be evident to the reader that the higher the level of intellectual performance which has been disturbed, the less localizing value in topographical neurology has that disturbance. This applies in a major degree to disorders of speech. There is, however, value in careful assessment of speech disorder in advising the patient and family on prognosis. This varies of course with the association of other disorders, and it also varies with the intellectual capacity of the handicapped person.

The clinician is usually surprised by the degree of restitution of speech function which can occur over the months and even years after, for instance, a major cerebrovascular disaster. He will judge his prognosis upon the time which has elapsed between the disaster and the patient's ability to use words correctly, then phrases, and then short sentences. There is, however, no set of rules to lay down, and it is probably true to say that there is no branch of neurology—a specialty in which assessing prognosis is particularly difficult—in which anticipating events is so unrewarding.

DYSARTHRIA

The conversion of mentally formulated speech symbols into spoken language requires the correct use of several mechanisms, concerned respectively with the production of the voice by the passage of a stream of air through the aperture between the vocal cords and the articulation of words by movements of the lips, tongue, palate and jaws. The term dysarthria is now applied for defects of speech dependent upon disorders of these executive processes. The neuromuscular mechanisms responsible for these movements are built upon the same principles as those which control other highly co-ordinated voluntary movements, for example those of the hand. Impulses originating in the appropriate areas of the cerebral cortex are transmitted through the pyramidal tracts to the lower motor neurones (in the case of speech the various bulbar nuclei), and from these a further relay of impulses proceeds through the various peripheral nerves to the muscles concerned. As in other movements the co-ordination of these impulses depends upon the simultaneous reception of afferent impulses from the muscles and organs themselves and upon the activity of the cerebellum and other subcortical centres. Thus the varieties of dysarthria are strictly comparable with the disturbances of voluntary movement encountered in the limbs.

As impulses from the executive zones of the speech area pass to the lower centres through both pyramidal tracts, speech disturbances do not result from unilateral lesions of the pyramidal tract. If, however, both pyramidal tracts are damaged, as commonly occurs in diffuse vascular degeneration, double hemiplegia, degenerative lesions of the pyramidal system, diplegia, tumours of the brain stem and in advanced cases of disseminated sclerosis, the characteristic disturbance known as *spastic dysarthria* results. Here the speech is slow, stiff and laboured. Words are squeezed out with great effort as if through a rigid mechanism and are poorly formed on account of the stiffness and paucity of movement of the lips, tongue and palate. This is 'pseudobulbar palsy'.

When the lower motor neurones subserving the speech mechanisms are bilaterally affected *flaccid or atrophic dysarthria* results. The speech is slurred, indistinct and often slightly nasal. Labial and dental sounds are especially affected, but the laboured character of spastic dysarthria is absent. Atrophic dysarthria is found in lesions of the medulla in motor neurone disease, myasthenia gravis and in some cases of myopathy. Diphtheria, the classical cause of 'bulbar palsy', no longer operates.

Ataxic dysarthria is most characteristically heard in cerebellar disease especially when both sides are damaged as in Friedreich's ataxia, disseminated sclerosis, cerebellar degeneration and extensive vascular or neoplastic lesions of the cerebellum and pons. In mild cases speech becomes slow and deliberate with faulty spacing and accentuation of syllables, the so-called 'scanning' or 'staccato' speech so common in disseminated sclerosis. When more severe, speech becomes 'explosive', some syllables being slurred and almost inaudible, others being produced with a gush of uncontrolled sound. This coarse form of cerebellar dysarthria is most often met with in Friedreich's ataxia and in acute vascular lesions of the cerebellum and brain stem. Dysarthria resulting from loss of afferent impulses from the periphery is rare, but is occasionally met with in severe cases of peripheral neuritis and of tabes. Conditions associated with involuntary movements may result in severe speech disturbance. This variety of dysarthria is most commonly found in cases of chorea and athetosis, but may occur in other varieties of striatal disease, or as a sequel of encephalitis lethargica. In Wilson's disease [p. 1239] dysarthria results from muscular rigidity and goes on to complete anarthria. A characteristic variety of dysarthria occurs in general paresis; speech is slow, slurred and tremulous and there is a tendency to repeat or reverse the order of the syllables in polysyllabic words. A very similar disorder may be met with in cases of chronic alcoholism and in some varieties of drug intoxication, especially barbiturate poisoning.

OTHER DEFECTS OF SPEECH

STAMMERING OR STUTTERING

Stammering is a spasmodic defect of articulation leading to a sudden check in the utterance of words or to a rapid repetition of the consonantal sounds in connexion with which the difficulty arises. To the trouble of articulation are often added spasmodic movements of face and head or indeed of any part of the body.

Except in the rarest instances this condition is not associated with any structural change in the nervous system, or in the organs of articulation, but it has been observed as the end result of a lesion of the speech areas. It occurs with a greater frequency than can be attributed to coincidence in naturally left-handed persons who have been trained to behave as if they were right-handed. It may occur in more than one member of a family, but whether this implies an hereditary or environmental influence is uncertain. The stammerer often shows signs of neurotic instability such as abnormal timidity and excitability, nocturnal enuresis, night terrors and habit spasms, and though these symptoms may recede or disappear with time he remains more liable than normal individuals to develop neurotic manifestations under circumstances of stress.

The disorder seems to consist of a lowering of the functional stability of the executive mechanism of speech by the effect of embarrassment either at a conscious or unconscious level. It is begotten of shyness and self-consciousness, and probably for this reason is infinitely commoner in boys than in girls, for the latter are much less liable to self-consciousness. It is never present in infancy or early childhood but arises at the age when shyness and self-consciousness first manifest themselves. Its onset sometimes follows a debilitating illness such as measles or whooping cough, and it often appears after a sudden fright, or an experience causing severe emotional strain or embarrassment. Indeed it is the historical utterance of fright and of those surprised '*in flagrante delicto*'.

Like other manifestations of anxiety in childhood it is more likely to occur in homes where there are disturbing factors such as parental discord, favouritism and jealousy, over-indulgence or over-strictness and frequent changes of teachers and surroundings.

The stammerer never stammers in the speech of thought nor when talking aloud to himself alone, nor at any time when singing, for in the two former cases the embarrassment of self-consciousness is absent, and in the last case the element of rhythm and music greatly increases the stability and confidence of the function of speech. In rebellious cases this element of self-consciousness, as well as the more overt evidences of psychological instability, may gradually disappear while the stammer remains unaltered as an ineradicable habit.

In articulate speech three muscular mechanisms are concerned: (1) the respiratory mechanism for supplying the blast of air; (2) the larynx for producing the voice; and (3) the muscles of the lips, tongue, jaw and palate for articulation. For distinct speech there must be absolute co-ordination of these mechanisms one with another. Consonants are in nearly all cases the source of the difficulty in stammering, and while these are buccal sounds, yet some begin with a laryngeal sound, while others are purely buccal. The former are termed 'voiced consonants', and are B, W, V, Zh, Z, Th (as in 'thus'), D, L, R, G, Y; and the latter, 'voiceless consonants', and are P, F, Th (as in 'thin'), S, Sh, T, K; while N, M and Ng terminal are 'voiced nasal resonants'. If one articulates these consonants it becomes at once clear, and it is the presence of the initial laryngeal element or 'voicing' which makes the difference between B, V, Z, D, G, and P, F, S, T, K, respectively.

A careful attention to the manner in which the letter sounds are produced is absolutely essential in the investigation and treatment of stammering. The difficulty occurs most commonly with the explosive consonants, P, B, T, D, G, K, and nearly always where these occur as initial letters—that is, in starting the articulatory mechanism; and to avoid this difficulty which arises after every pause, most stammerers speak in a rapid monotonous fashion. The fault chiefly lies in the direction of energy to articulation rather than to phonation. The patient held up by his stammer usually remains silent, but occasionally having produced the first sound, he continues to repeat it—the reduplication stammer, which has been the origin for the names 'stammer' or 'stutter' by which the malady is known. Often the patient uses a trick or contortion to prevent the stutter or to relieve the feeling of nervous tension and embarrassment in consciousness which the defect causes, and these tend to become engrafted on him, as (1) associated sounds—whooping, grunting, crowing, etc.; (2) habit spasms—contortions of the face, limbs or body, which sometimes take a complicated form and exactly resemble the co-ordinated form of tic.

Treatment

The development of confidence and self-reliance is everything in the treatment of stammering. The skilled speech therapist first gains the liking, respect and submission of his patient. He then assures him that his defect will disappear, and that he can cure himself, and demonstrates to him by correcting the faults that he can speak normally. In adult stammerers also first place in treatment is to be given to speech re-education. Even prolonged psychotherapy is seldom effective, although the stammer may become less pronounced by the lessening of the patient's state of anxiety and the general improvement in mental health.

Prognosis

The majority of the cases tend to a spontaneous cure, and recovery is hastened in all cases by systematic treatment. In every class of case the results of treatment may come slowly at first, but perseverance will in almost every case bring success.

REFERENCES

Brain, W. R. (1961) *Speech Disorders*, London.

Brain, W. R. (1961) *Aphasia, Apraxia and Agnosia*, London.

Ciba Foundation (1964) *Symposium: Disorders of Language*, London.

Geschwind, N. (1965) Disconnexion syndromes in animals and man, *Brain*, **88**, 237.

Head, H. (1926) *Aphasia and Kindred Disorders of Speech*, Cambridge.

Penfield, W., and Roberts, L. (1959) *Speech and Brain-Mechanisms*, Princeton, N.J.

Russell, W. R. (1963) Some anatomical aspects of aphasia, *Lancet*, i, 1173.

Travis, L. E. (1959) *Handbook of Speech Pathology*, London.

Zangwill, O. L. (1960) *Cerebral Dominance and its Relation to Psychological Function*, Springfield, Ill.

APRAXIA AND AGNOSIA

APRAXIA

Definition

A disorder of cerebral function, characterized by inability to perform certain familiar purposive movements, in the absence of motor and sensory paralysis and ataxia. This disorder does not depend upon defective perception (agnosia) nor upon general reduction of intelligence.

Aetiology

Apraxia may result from both general and local disease of the brain. It occurs in its purest form from local lesions, and may then be confined to one region of the body. It may result from lesions of the posterior part of the prefrontal area of the left side, the so-called 'motor or verbal' aphasia and agraphia being good examples of apraxia of speech and writing respectively, and lesions in this region may also cause apraxia of the limbs on one or both sides. Lesions of the anterior half of the corpus callosum have been associated with conspicuous apraxia, as have bilateral lesions in the posterior parts of the hemispheres. In the latter cases, the apraxia is likely to be associated with some degree of lack of recognition of an object, and of its uses (agnosia), and this causes apraxia from a loss of correct comprehension of the act required. Apraxia is sometimes found with hemiplegia in which, notwithstanding the complete recovery of motor and sensory paralysis, the performance of familiar acts—from the highest skilled movements, such as the fingering of the pianoforte or of the violin, or the use of his tools by a craftsman, to the simplest act—may be no longer possible.

Symptoms

The features of the condition may be well demonstrated by the consideration of left-sided hemiapraxia. There is neither loss of power nor loss of sensibility in the left upper extremity, but in many of these cases there is a diminished awareness of the left side of the body. When such a patient is asked to perform some familiar act with the right hand, he at once does so correctly, but when ordered to perform the same act with the left hand he is unable to do so. Either he makes aimless wandering movements with the left hand, or he may succeed in making movements somewhat resembling those required of him, with much slowness and clumsiness. Sometimes he may perform some act which is entirely different from that required of him, and this phenomenon is called parapraxia. When the apraxia is partial, the patient may be able to perform some acts and not others, his inability usually, but not always, increasing with the complexity of the act required. Or he may be able sometimes to perform an act in which he commonly fails. Sometimes such a patient, wearied with the unsuccessful attempts of his left hand, will abruptly perform the act correctly with his right hand, to get rid of it. And he will define his defect by saying, 'I know quite well what you want me to do, but I cannot do it'. Spontaneous volitional movement is similarly affected, and this leads invariably to a marked loss of initiative in the use of the affected limb—the patient will not try to use it. The apraxic patient is often to an astonishing degree unaware of his disability, and frequently becomes conscious of it for the first time when it is pointed out to him by another person.

Diagnosis

Apraxia may be confused with astereognosis, with agnosia and with cortical ataxia. A correct conception of the nature of the two former conditions will exclude the possibility of error In cortical ataxia the patient obeys the word of command at once and succeeds more or less with the act required, the defect being clumsiness of execution. The clinical examination of patients for apraxia must include: (1) the general intellectual state including the level of consciousness; (2) psychometric testing of attention; concentration, memory and reasoning; (3) an inspection of sensory appreciation for defects of simple perception in the regions of smell, sight, hearing, taste, cutaneous sensibility and muscular sense; defects of recognition of sensory impressions in these regions (agnosia); and (4) an examination of executive power for any defects in the movements determined by visual, auditory, tactile and kinaesthetic stimuli. What response does the patient make to objects held in front of him or to gestures made to him? Can he imitate movements? Can he, when requested, make simple and purposive movements, with and without the objects in his hands? When given an object, how does he hold it and use it?

AGNOSIA

In disease of the hemispheres the patient, having apparently normal sensation, may be unable to integrate the results of sensory stimulation, which thus fail to arouse an intelligent perception of the object exciting them. This inability to recognize the import of a sensory stimulus is called agnosia. Those patients who present apraxia and agnosia, often show other interesting phenomena which are of importance; these are: (1) inattention; (2) defective capacity for retaining recent impressions; (3) lack of initiative; and (4) perseveration. Agnosia is most commonly associated with lesions involving one or both parietal lobes.

It can affect any sensory understanding: difficulty in telling right from left—right-left agnosia; in recognizing fingers—finger agnosia; or in recognizing the relationship of objects in space—spatial disorientation or agnosia.

THE CEREBROSPINAL FLUID AND DISORDERS OF ITS CIRCULATION

The cerebrospinal fluid fills the cerebral ventricles, the subarachnoid cisterns and the general subarachnoid space. It is formed by the choroid plexuses of the lateral, third and fourth ventricles and, escaping through the foramina of Magendie and Luschka, passes over the convexities of the brain and through the whole extent of the spinal subarachnoid space to be reabsorbed into the venous blood stream through the arachnoid villi, particularly those contained in the Pacchionian bodies in relation to the sagittal sinus. It is produced by active secretion and corresponds accurately to a protein-free filtrate of the plasma varying in composition with changes in the circulating blood.

The total quantity of the cerebrospinal fluid in a healthy adult varies from 90 to 150 ml. Its rate of production under natural conditions is unknown, and is influenced by the composition of the blood plasma, the capillary pressure in the choroid plexus and the permeability of the cells of the plexus, as well as by the pressure of the fluid in the ventricles. Although the cerebrospinal fluid does not circulate in the sense that the blood circulates, there is a steady flow in health from its site of origin in the ventricles to that of its absorption in the arachnoid villi.

The normal cerebrospinal fluid is a clear, colourless fluid indistinguishable in appearance from water and it has a remarkably constant composition. As obtained by lumbar puncture it contains from 0 to 5 cells (endothelial cells and lymphocytes) per mm^3. Its chemical composition is as follows:

Protein (mainly albumin). 20–40 mg. per 100 ml.

Glucose . . . . 50–90 mg. per 100 ml.
Chlorides (as NaCl) . 720–750 mg. per 100 ml.

In health the globulin content is insufficient to give a positive Nonne-Apelt or Pandy test.

Pressure of the Cerebrospinal Fluid. This can only be ascertained by actual measurement with a manometer; estimates based upon the rate of flow are fallacious. When it is necessary to measure the pressure, a three-way needle with manometer attachment should be employed, and before the readings are taken the patient must be lying relaxed and comfortable, with easy respirations. The normal pressure of cerebrospinal fluid varies from 60 to 150 mm. of water, and will be seen to rise and fall over a distance of 5 to 10 mm. with the respiratory movements. Coughing and straining give rise to an abrupt increase in the pressure of from 30 to 50 mm. A pressure of over 150 mm. is evidence of increased intracranial pressure, and readings of over 300 mm. are common in the presence of intracranial tumours, meningitis and other conditions characterized by raised intracranial pressure. When the cerebrospinal pressure is found to be 300 mm. or more, fluid should be withdrawn slowly and in the minimum quantity necessary for pathological investigation (5 ml.), as the rapid withdrawal of a large quantity of fluid may result in sudden death from the formation of a medullary pressure-cone or from uncinate herniation.

Queckenstedt's Phenomenon. In the normal subject the pressure of the fluid in the lumbar sac directly reflects the pressure within the cerebral subarachnoid spaces and the ventricles; any change in the intracranial pressure is immediately transmitted through the patent subarachnoid space and causes a change in the level of the fluid in the manometer. This forms the basis of the valuable test for patency of the subarachnoid space known as Queckenstedt's test.

If, with the lumbar puncture needle and manometer in position, the right jugular vein is firmly compressed, an immediate rise in the level of the fluid in the manometer will be noted in the normal person, the pressure rising rapidly from the normal 80 to 120 mm. to 300 mm. or more. On releasing the compression the pressure rapidly returns to its former level. If there is any block in the spinal subarachnoid space, such as may be caused by extradural compression, or a spinal tumour, or if there is interference with the escape of fluid from the cranial cavity, there will be no rise in the pressure of the lumbar fluid on jugular compression (complete block), or only a small rise (incomplete block). In the latter case release of the jugular compression will be followed by a very slow return of the meniscus to the former level or the level may remain unaltered, indicating a ball-valve type of obstruction. Again, if the withdrawal of a small quantity (4–8 ml.) of fluid is followed by a persistent fall in the pressure of about 50 per cent., there is probably obstruction to the normal flow of cerebrospinal fluid. These two tests afford valuable evidence of any occlusion of the spinal subarachnoid space.

Appearance of the Cerebrospinal Fluid. The normal cerebrospinal fluid looks like water. The fluid may be freely blood-stained in cases of recent subarachnoid or cerebral haemorrhage, or of trauma to the brain. In such cases the blood is usually present in large amounts, and is intimately mixed with the cerebrospinal fluid in all specimens removed. Blood contamination resulting from faulty technique in withdrawing the fluid can usually be recognized, as it is usually scanty in amount and varies in intensity in different specimens. If the blood has been mixed with the fluid for more than a few hours before withdrawal, it assumes a slightly orange tint on account of the breakdown of the blood pigment. Such a specimen if centrifuged or allowed to stand will give a bright canary-yellow supernatant fluid, a condition known as *xanthochromia*. Several days after a severe subarachnoid haemorrhage, the fluid may be thick and brownish-orange in colour. In addition to cases of resolving subarachnoid haemorrhage, xanthochromia may be present in cases of long-standing spinal blockage, subdural haemorrhage, some cases of polyneuritis, and occasionally in cases of cerebral tumour. It is often associated with a great increase in protein content of the fluid, which may thus undergo spontaneous clotting on withdrawal.

The combination of xanthochromia with greatly increased protein content of the cerebrospinal fluid, and evidence of spinal block is known as *Froin's syndrome* (*loculation syndrome*), and is characteristic of severe spinal compression.

Turbidity of the cerebrospinal fluid is caused by the presence of a great excess of cells, and is thus characteristic of meningitis. It may vary in degree from slight opalescence to a frankly purulent fluid.

Increase of Protein Content. This is of great importance, and occurs in many pathological conditions of the central nervous system. As has already been stated, it may result from occlusion of the subarachnoid space from any form of spinal block. It occurs in all cases of bacterial, but not necessarily in viral, meningitis. An isolated increase in protein content occurs in many cases of intracranial tumour, particularly where the tumour impinges upon the surface of the brain or the walls of the ventricles. It may be met with after vascular lesions of the brain, even though there has been no escape of blood into the subarachnoid space, and also in cases of acute infective polyneuritis. Examination by paper chromatography offers a detailed and simple method of fractional protein study for differential diagnosis.

Increase in Cell Content. An increase in the cell count of the cerebrospinal fluid is found in almost all inflammatory diseases of the nervous system. In pyogenic meningitis an enormous excess (20,000 or more per mm^3.) is the rule, the vast majority being polymorphonuclear leucocytes. A small number of lymphocytes may also be present, and the proportion of these gradually increases as recovery takes place. A lymphocytosis is characteristic of tuberculous and syphilitic meningitis, and of most virus infections of the nervous system. In tuberculous meningitis a mixed cytosis often occurs, at first with as high a proportion as 40 per cent. of polymorphonuclear cells, but as the disease progresses the proportion of lymphocytes steadily rises until they represent 90 per cent. or more of the total cell count. A mixed pleocytosis is also seen in cases of cerebral and extradural abscess, in sinus thrombosis, and after extensive cerebral softenings.

Decrease in Glucose Content. The glucose content of the cerebrospinal fluid is decreased in varieties of meningitis, particularly in those due to pyogenic organisms. It is almost invariably reduced in tuberculous meningitis but only rarely in meningitis due to viruses [see Section 2]. It is present with spontaneous hypoglycaemia.

Alteration of Chloride Content. The chloride content of the cerebrospinal fluid is lowered in all cases of purulent or tuberculous meningitis, largely as a result of the diminution of the plasma chlorides, which occurs in these as in other acute febrile illnesses. This change is of particular value in the diagnosis of tuberculous meningitis, levels as low as 600 to 650 mg. per 100 ml. may be found early, in contrast to the relatively normal chloride content in the case of other diseases causing a lymphocytic pleocytosis.

An increase in the chloride content as well as that of non-protein nitrogen is found in uraemia and other conditions of salt retention.

Lange's Colloidal Gold Reaction. In neurosyphilis and in many cases of disseminated sclerosis, the globulin fraction of the total protein of the cerebrospinal fluid increases and may almost equal the albumin fraction. The high globulin content gives the fluid a power of precipitating colloids from suspension. The estimation of this power in relation to colloidal gold is the basis of Lange's test. To 10 dilutions of cerebrospinal fluid (from 1 in 10 to 1 in 10,000) constant amounts of colloidal gold are added, and the mixtures allowed to stand for 24 hours. The form of the precipitation curves has a differentiating value. Thus in general paralysis the first 6 dilutions are precipitated (paretic curve), in tabes dorsalis, the third and fourth dilutions show the maximal precipitation (luetic curve); in meningitis, the sixth to eighth dilutions are precipitated (meningitic curve). In disseminated sclerosis the combination of negative Wassermann reactions in blood and fluid and a paretic curve in the fluid is frequently found.

Electrophoresis. Electrophoresis of the cerebrospinal fluid shows the presence of normal and abnormal globulins, of value in the study of biochemical diseases involving the central nervous system.

Lipoid and Amino Acid Content. Microchemical methods of estimating the fluid content of such substances as sphingomyelin, cerebroside, cephalin and lecithin have been introduced. They are of diagnostic value since the presence and concentration of these and similar substances reflect structural breakdown within the brain.

Bacteriology. The bacterial flora of the fluid is studied by culture and by the examination of films made from the deposits yielded by centrifugation.

The Wassermann Reaction. This is positive in all conditions of recent syphilitic disease impinging upon the meninges, and always in general paralysis. Though often positive in tabes, it may be found negative.

Radioisotope Encephalography. By injecting a labelled salt into the spinal theca, the pattern of flow and of absorption of the cerebrospinal fluid can be studied, hydrocephalus showing as two large clear areas in the anteroposterior scan.

HYDROCEPHALUS

Definition

In hydrocephalus there is an abnornal accumulation of cerebrospinal fluid within the skull. This may be confined to the ventricular cavities, internal hydrocephalus; or it may involve both the ventricular and the general subarachnoid spaces—communicating hydrocephalus. This distension is associated in children with an expansion of the cranial bones and enlargement of the skull.

General Considerations

Theoretically this abnormal increase of fluid may be caused by: (1) excessive production of fluid; (2) interference in the normal flow of fluid; and (3) defective absorption.

Of the causes of hydrocephalus the most important and the one of which we have the most precise knowledge is obstruction of the normal cerebrospinal flow, and it is evident that this obstruction may occur at several different points and be produced by a great variety of pathological causes. Some of these are known and some remain obscure. Thus hydrocephalus is the end result of a variety of causes and until our knowledge is more complete, it is most satisfactorily classified on a clinical basis as: (1) congenital hydrocephalus; (2) chronic acquired hydrocephalus; and (3) acute acquired hydrocephalus.

In diseases in which general atrophy of the cerebral tissues occurs, fluid accumulates both in the ventricles and in the subarachnoid space; but such a compensating enlargement is not to be regarded as true hydrocephalus. It is found in cerebral diplegia, general paralysis of the insane, cerebral arteriosclerosis, and chronic alcoholism, and also in the brains of old people. It is merely the result of wasting and shrinkage of the brain tissue, and the accumulation of fluid takes place in order to fill the space within the rigid skull which is thus vacated. The physiology of 'low pressure hydrocephalus', which may happen without absorption of brain tissue, has recently caused much interest.

CONGENITAL HYDROCEPHALUS

Aetiology

Hereditary influences are important in the causation of congenital hydrocephalus and it may even appear as a striking familial disease, affecting members of several generations of the same stock. Spina bifida, meningocele and hydromyelia are often associated with the condition, and irregular or arrested development of the brain stem and cerebellum, particularly the Arnold-Chiari malformation [see p. 1195], are common. Commonly associated abnormalities are hare-lip, cleft palate, talipes, rectal and testicular ectopia and imperforate anus. In a few cases syphilitic lesions of the ependyma of the brain stem in the region of the aqueduct or fourth ventricle have been found. In many cases the aetiology remains unknown.

Pathology

The quantity of fluid which is found in the ventricles after death varies greatly, usually being 400–600 ml. In long-standing cases with great cranial enlargement, large quantities have been found. The character of the fluid does not usually differ from that of normal cerebrospinal fluid. Its specific gravity varies from 1·008 to 1·010. It is clear and colourless, or occasionally slightly yellow. It contains a small quantity of albumin and a normal quantity of chlorides. The dilatation of the lateral ventricles is more extensive than that of the third and fourth ventricles, and is usually symmetrical upon the two sides. It affects the body more than the cornua of the ventricles, so that the central cortex is most thinned. The foramina of Monro are greatly enlarged and the anterior pillars wasted. The convolutions are flattened and the sulci indistinct. The thickness of the cerebral substance is much reduced. In advanced cases the cerebral hemispheres have the appearance of thin-walled sacs, which collapse entirely when the contained fluid is allowed to escape. In a few cases the aqueduct has been found closed as if by an antecedent ependymitis.

Symptoms

In congenital hydrocephalus the enlargement of the head is the first noticeable feature. It may take place during intra-uterine life, and it may be so great as to make delivery impossible without destruction of the head. More frequently the cranial enlargement, not noted at the time of birth, becomes evident during the first weeks of life. The increase usually affects all the diameters of the cranial cavity, and is most marked at the vertex and least at the base. The forehead is large, rounded, and projects forward, the temporal fossae are obliterated and the parietal eminences carried backwards. The vertex is often somewhat flattened, as also may be the occipital region. The direction of the external auditory meatus alters with the increasing size of the head; normally directed obliquely forwards it comes to look directly inwards or even obliquely backwards in severe cases. The head is often asymmetrical. The sutures may be widely open, and then there is bulging along these lines and at the fontanelles. In untreated cases the face is characteristically triangular, contrasting markedly with the forehead. Wasting of the facial subcutaneous tissues and retarded development of the maxilla and mandible often render the contrast still more striking. Bulging of the orbital plates of the frontal bones presses down the eyeballs, so that the pupils become more or less covered by the lower lids, and a band of the sclerotic may be visible between the iris and the upper lid. The hydrocephalic child often uses his hands to depress the cheeks, and so draws down the lower lids out of the position which they impair the line of vision. The hair of the head becomes scanty, the subcutaneous veins of the scalp are often distended and sometimes a vortex of distended veins radiates from the region of the anterior fontanelle. Percussion of the skull gives a characteristic, hollow, 'cracked-pot' note.

The general nutrition is poor, and bodily development retarded in proportion to the severity of the effect of the hydrocephalus upon the nervous system. The nervous symptoms which appear during the course of untreated congenital hydrocephalus are both variable and inconstant, depending upon the severity of the condition and the rate at which it progresses. They may be summed up in the following list in order of frequency: convulsions, mental failure, spastic paralysis of the limbs, optic atrophy, deafness, nystagmus, headache, papilloedema and vomiting. There is no constancy regarding these symptoms. Convulsions may be absent, and mental acuity may be unimpaired. Spastic weakness occurs in less than half the cases, optic atrophy still more rarely and papilloedema is distinctly unusual.

Diagnosis

Because of the shape of the skull this seldom presents difficulty, though in childhood only a careful history will differentiate the congenital from the chronic acquired type of hydrocephalus. The enlarged skull of rickets is recognized by its different conformation, by the absence of nervous signs, with the possible exception of convulsions, by the absence of the characteristic percussion note and by the presence of other rachitic signs. The rare condition of macrocephaly is not associated with any distortion of the relative proportions of the skull. It should be remembered that a large head is hereditary in some families.

Treatment

Treatment is surgical by the use of ventriculo-ventricular or ventriculo-jugular shunts (see below in the treatment of chronic acquired hydrocephalus). Palliative dehydration with diuretics and dehydrating agents like glycerol and mannitol may be needed as a preoperative step only.

Prognosis

In all severe and progressive cases the prognosis is hopeless. In some of the milder cases the process becomes arrested, and the patient may reach adult life in possession of all his faculties. When the condition has been reversed by ventriculo-ventricular or ventriculo-jugular shunting, the prognosis for mental capacity and the continuance of recurring convulsions has to be considered. If the mental capacity at the time of the arrest is fair, it is not likely to deteriorate further. When mental reduction is marked at the time of arrest, any appreciable degree of improvement cannot reasonably be expected. A certain number of cases of mild congenital hydrocephalus cease to progress and the symptoms decrease and disappear permanently.

CHRONIC ACQUIRED HYDROCEPHALUS

Aetiology

Hydrocephalus, usually of the internal type secondary to obstruction in the cerebrospinal fluid pathway, may result from a variety of causes. Foremost among these is meningitis, including tuberculous meningitis, in which recovery from the initial disease takes place. It is caused by occlusion of the foramina of Luschka and Magendie, and results in a uniform distension of the entire ventricular system. Another group of cases depends upon a primary, non-neoplastic stenosis of the aqueduct of Sylvius. Some of these cases show a proliferation of the subependymal glia with constriction of the lumen of the aqueduct. In others the ependyma may undergo proliferation with the development of tufts which project into the lumen of the canal and form valve-like obstructions to the flow of fluid. Again, in others the lumen itself may be split up into a number of minute channels hardly visible to the naked eye. The ultimate cause of this aqueductal atresia is unknown. In a third group acquired hydrocephalus results from the presence of neoplasms of slow growth which obstruct the cerebrospinal fluid channels; of these the slowly growing cerebellar astrocytomata of early childhood are the most important. Other causes are cysts and slowly growing tumours of the third and fourth ventricles, suprasellar cysts and pineal or other tumours of the midbrain.

Symptoms

The symptoms of chronic acquired hydrocephalus depend largely upon the age of onset: if in early infancy the picture is similar to that of congenital hydrocephalus; if in early childhood before the sutures of the skull have become fused and the bones of the vault indistensible, it is that of moderate hydrocephalus combined with the symptoms and signs of raised intracranial pressure.

Pressure symptoms often begin abruptly after the signs of hydrocephalus have been present a long time. These are headache, usually paroxysmal in character, vomiting, strabismus and double vision. Papilloedema is common and if left leads to failure of vision from consecutive optic atrophy, which may come on quickly. In long-standing cases mental failure may occur, and weakness and inco-ordination of movement from a combination of disturbances of the pyramidal and cerebellar systems. There may be arrest of development, with delayed puberty and even infantilism.

Treatment

In some cases of acquired hydrocephalus the cause, such as a cystic tumour, can be removed by operation. Various methods of re-establishing the cerebrospinal fluid flow have been devised in cases of stenosis of the aqueduct or occlusion of the meningeal foramina. The most successful of these is Torkildsen's operation of ventriculo-ventriculostomy, in which the aqueduct is by-passed by means of a plastic catheter introduced into the posterior horn of one of the lateral ventricles and passing under the scalp to enter the spinal subarachnoid space through the atlanto-occipital membrane. A ventriculo-jugular shunt may also be established—an intermediary valve preventing reflux of venous blood.

ACUTE ACQUIRED HYDROCEPHALUS

This condition results from rapid and severe obstruction to the flow of cerebrospinal fluid in subjects whose skulls are no longer capable of expansion, or in the case of children when the expansion of the skull cannot keep pace with the ventricular distension. Therefore, unlike the congenital and the chronic forms of hydrocephalus there is little or no enlargement of the head and the clinical picture is that of raised intracranial pressure, usually without localizing signs.

Aetiology

The commonest cause is a midline tumour, particularly in the posterior fossa, obstructing the flow of cerebrospinal fluid at the third ventricle, in the aqueduct or in the fourth ventricle. Medulloblastomas and cerebellar cysts do this. Acute obstruction of the foramen of Magendie can occur by a thin curtain of arachnoid forming a valve, and diffuse arachnoid adhesions following meningitis or arising with no evident cause may obstruct the flow of fluid over the convexity or at the tentorial hiatus. Finally, after infection, absorption may be impaired at the Pacchionian villi in the sagittal sinus.

Symptoms

These are the general symptoms of increased intracranial pressure of rapid onset and great severity. The majority of cases present themselves with the symptom-complex of headache, vomiting and papilloedema without necessarily signs of local lesion of the hemispheres or cerebellum. Radiological examination may reveal a mottled appearance of the vault resembling that of beaten silver, and there may be some decalcification of the posterior clinoid processes and general flattening of the cavity of the sella turcica. The diagnosis is confirmed by ventriculography or angiography.

Treatment

This is surgical and is essentially that of the underlying cause.

BASILAR IMPRESSION AND THE ARNOLD-CHIARI DEFORMITY

Basilar impression is a disorder of the skull in which the bones surrounding the foramen magnum become invaginated into the cranial cavity. This leads to deformity of intracranial structures, particularly in the posterior fossa. This may be the result of bony disease such as osteoporosis or tumour, but can also be developmental in origin. When this latter is the case then there may be associated congenital anomalies of the brain stem (the Arnold-Chiari deformity) and of the cervical vertebrae (the Klippel-Feil syndrome) although both may occur without deformity of the base of the skull.

Congenital malformation of the base of the skull, the upper cervical vertebrae and of the brain stem prevent the circulation of cerebrospinal fluid and cause hydrocephalus. In these anomalous states there is insufficient room for the deformed structures in the posterior fossa, which are pushed down into the foramen magnum. The result is the development of cranial nerve palsies, ataxia and disorders of gait and station in addition to the hydrocephalus. Treatment is by surgical decompression in the upper cervical and occipital region.

REFERENCES

CHANDRASEKARAN, S., and REYNOLDS, R. E. (1970) Occult hydrocephalus in the elderly. *J. Amer. Geriat. Soc.*, **18**, 481.

CIBA FOUNDATION (1958) *Symposium: Cerebrospinal Fluid: Production, Circulation, Absorption*, London.

DAWSON, H. (1956) *Physiology of Ocular and Cerebrospinal Fluids*, London.

FOLEY, J. (1955) Benign forms of intercranial hypertension—'toxic' and 'otitic' hydrocephalus, *Brain*, **78**, 1.

FOLEY, J. (1957) Physiology of increased intracranial pressure, in *Modern Trends in Neurology*, 2nd Series, ed. WILLIAMS, D., London.

KUPER, S., MEDELOW, H., and PROCTOR, N. S. F. (1958) Internal hydrocephalus caused by parasitic cysts, *Brain*, **81**, 235.

LOCOGE, M., and CUMINGS, J. N. (1958) An analysis of results from the examination of 12,000 C.S.F.'s from various disorders, *Brit. med. J.*, **1**, 618.

MACFARLANE, A., and MALONEY, A. F. J. (1957) The appearance of the aqueduct and its relationship to hydrocephalus in the Arnold-Chiari malformation, *Brain*, **80**, 479.

MERRITT, H. H., and FREMONT-SMITH, F. (1939) *The Cerebrospinal Fluid*, Philadelphia.

OJEMANN, R. G., FISHER, C. M., ADAMS, R. D., SWEET, W. H., and NEW, F. P. S. (1969) Further experience with the syndrome of 'normal' pressure hydrocephalus, *J. Neurosurg.*, **31**, 279.

RUSSELL, D. S. (1949) Observation on the pathology of hydrocephalus, *Spec. Rep. Ser. med. Res. Coun.* (*Lond.*), No. 265.

SPILLANE, J. D., PALLIS, C., and SONAS, A. M. (1957) Developmental abnormalities in the region of the foramen magnum, *Brain*, **80**, 1.

SWEET, W. H. (1957) Formation, absorption and flow of cerebrospinal fluid, in *Modern Trends in Neurology*, 2nd Series, ed. WILLIAMS, D., London.

INTRACRANIAL TUMOURS

Under this heading are grouped all new formations which encroach upon the intracranial space and which produce the familiar pressure and local symptoms of tumour, though some of them are not, strictly speaking, neoplasms.

Aetiology

Cerebral tumour may occur at any age, but it is relatively rare in the very young and in the very old. There is no significant difference in its incidence in the two sexes. The relation between head injury and the first symptoms of cerebral tumour is one that has often been pointed out, though it is likely that in most cases where this relation exists, the blow on the head has simply served to bring a pre-existing tumour into symptomatic prominence, by causing either oedema or haemorrhage in its substance or vicinity. It must be remembered in this connexion that a cerebral tumour may exist for a long period without definite symptoms.

Pathology

The pathological classification of intracranial tumours has a practical importance for when the nature of a new growth can be determined clinically, some idea of its future behaviour can be formed and the surgeon can make his plans to meet the problems which each variety of tumour presents.

The chief varieties of intracranial tumour are as follows:

- Tumour of the brain substance—Glioma.
- Tumour arising in the meninges or nerve sheaths { Meningioma. Neurofibroma.
- Secondary carcinoma and sarcoma.
- Blood vessel tumours.
- Tumour of the pituitary body and stalk.
- Infective granuloma.
- Parasitic and other cysts.

The commonest intracranial tumour is a glioma. These are three times as common as meningiomas. About a quarter of all cerebral tumours are secondary carcinomas. The commonest extracerebral tumour is a meningioma, and the next common is a pituitary adenoma.

Glioma. The glioma is a tumour arising in the glial or supporting tissue of the brain. There are many types but they have certain important characteristics in common. They originate within the substance of the nervous system and all infiltrate the surrounding nerve tissue. They are thus locally malignant. They do not invade tissue outside the nervous system nor cause metastases in other parts of the body, though in some, fragments may become detached and be carried in the cerebrospinal fluid to distant parts of the subarachnoid space and there continue their growth as distinct implantation tumours. Gliomas may undergo degeneration and necrosis. If this is rapid it may lead to cyst formation; if it is slow it may lead to calcification within the tumour.

Many types of glioma have been described, but these classifications are ephemeral and largely artificial, for more than one pathological type may be represented within a single tumour and the same tumour may present different features at successive periods of its course. But with this reservation it is useful to recognize certain common and relatively well-defined clinical and pathological varieties.

Astrocytoma is the commonest of all gliomas and is a diffusely infiltrative tumour of the white matter which occurs at all ages and in any part of the brain. They are now simply divided into four grades of malignancy, grade I being slowly growing and grade IV the most malignant, formerly called the glioblastoma multiforme.

This last is a tumour of the cerebral hemispheres, and although it may occur at any age, is commonest in middle life or later and usually causes death within a year of its first symptoms. Because of its invasive nature it is, of all gliomas, the least amenable to surgical removal.

Medulloblastoma is a highly cellular and rapidly growing tumour almost confined to the roof of the fourth ventricle and cerebellum. It is commonly found in children and is in the form of glioma most often spread by implantation across the subarachnoid space.

Other varieties of glioma are described in relation to the ependyma, choroid plexus and oligodendroglia.

Meningioma. These are connective tissue tumours found in the neighbourhood of the venous sinuses, especially the superior longitudinal, the sphenoparietal, the petrosal and circular sinuses. They do not invade the brain but compress and displace it, and may become deeply embedded in it. They may infiltrate the overlying bone which may become so thickened that a visible or palpable boss is present on the surface of the skull. Meningiomata are highly vascular and large nutrient vessels may be present in the neighbouring skull and scalp. Calcification in their substance is common.

Neurofibroma. This also is a connective tissue tumour arising from the sheaths of the cranial nerves. The vast majority grow from the sheath of the auditory nerve and constitute the common tumour of the lateral recess —the acoustic neurofibroma. Occasionally they grow from the fifth or other cranial nerves. The neurofibroma may be solitary or may appear as part of a generalized neurofibromatosis when it is often bilateral on the acoustic nerves. It is a firm, nodular tumour which gradually buries itself in the side of the brain stem and often erodes the bones of the internal auditory meatus. It is usually of very slow growth but may undergo necrosis and cyst formation.

Secondary Carcinoma. Secondary carcinoma is a common intracranial tumour. It is particularly frequent in lung cancer and it is not uncommon for symptoms of secondary involvement of the brain to precede those of the primary growth. Indeed, in all adult cases presenting the signs and symptoms of intracranial tumour the possibility of carcinomatous metastasis should be explored, particularly in a patient who is losing weight or deteriorating. Less common sources of metastatic tumours are the breast, prostate and gastro-intestinal tract.

Carcinomatous deposits are blood-borne and multiple, and may undergo necrosis, cyst formation and haemorrhage. Rarely they may reach the brain by direct invasion from the nasopharynx. In exceptional cases there may be a diffuse infiltration of the subarachnoid space with carcinoma, and when it occurs alone this 'meningitis carcinomatosa' may be very difficult to diagnose.

Blood-vessel Tumours. Tumours and congenital anomalies of the blood vessels are relatively common in the brain compared with other organs. They take two principal forms: (1) angiomatous malformations consisting either of arteriovenous varices or telangiectases. These are most often found in the hemispheres but may occur in the brain stem or cerebellum. They involve the brain diffusely, particularly on its surface, and may present themselves as tumours or as cases of cerebral haemorrhage. (2) True angiomatous neoplasms or haemangioblastomata which commonly occur in the cerebellum and give rise to blood cysts. They may be associated with similar tumours in the retina and may be familial—a combination often known as Lindau's disease.

Pituitary Tumours. These arise from the glandular elements of the pars anterior. They usually take the form of an adenoma and may be composed of any of the three types of cell found in this body.

The commonest is the chromophobe adenoma; it is associated with symptoms of hypopituitarism. The less common variety is composed chiefly of eosinophil cells. This type is associated with the clinical picture of acromegaly. Both the foregoing varieties of adenoma commonly attain a sufficient size to expand the sella turcica, and to escape from it to cause neighbourhood symptoms by involving the optic chiasma or the oculomotor nerves. The rarest type of adenoma is that composed of basophil cells and associated with Cushing's syndrome. This is a tumour of small size and never causes expansion of the sella or symptoms of involvement of neighbouring structures. Rarely pituitary adenomata may undergo malignant degeneration, and occasional examples of tumours of mixed cell type occur.

Another tumour arising in association with the pituitary body is the craniopharyngioma or cyst of Rathke's pouch. These are commonly situated above the sella turcica but may be partially or wholly intrasellar. They are partially solid, partially cystic; they frequently undergo degeneration and subsequent calcification, and may reach the size of a golf-ball, penetrating into the floor of the third ventricle and so producing hydrocephalus.

Among the rarer tumours of the brain may be mentioned dermoid tumours, cholesteatomata, teratomata, chordomata, which arise from rests of the anterior end of the primitive notochord and are found below the base of the brain, lipomata, fibromata, neuromata, neuroblastomata, consisting actually of undifferentiated nerve cells, and enchondromata.

Cysts. Cysts occur on the surface or in the substance of the brain: (1) Serous cysts of the arachnoid. These may occur as part of a diffuse arachnoiditis or without any known cause. (2) Porencephalic cysts. These are unexplained but result from softening after embolism or thrombosis or severe brain injury in early childhood. They may lose all trace of their origin and form thin-walled cavities, containing colourless fluid, which often extend from the ependyma to the pia mater and involve the whole thickness of the pallium. (3) Cysts derived from tumours—especially gliomata and secondary carcinomata. The tumour with such a cyst may be small and may appear as a small nodule in one part of the circumference. Such cysts contain a highly albuminous fluid which is often yellow in colour. (4) Blood cysts, which are usually derived from highly vascular tumours but may follow trauma or intracerebral haemorrhage from any cause. (5) Cysts following the breakdown of infarcted areas of the brain. (6) Cysts of the septum pellucidum. (7) Colloid cysts of the third ventricle. (8) Cysts derived from remnants of the developing pituitary body and described in connexion with pituitary tumours. (9) Dermoid cysts. (10) Parasitic cysts of which the more common is the bladder worm of the tapeworm, *Taenia solium*, which is called, on account of the thickness of its wall, *Cysticercus cellulosae*. These are usually multiple, and grow in the folds of the pia mater in the depths of the sulci and occasionally in the fourth ventricle. It is usual for these cysts to shrink and become calcified in from 3 to 6 years. Less commonly the hydatid, or cyst of *Echinococcus granulosus*, is found. It is usually single, may reach a large size and present the signs of a slowly growing tumour with eosinophilia.

Infectious Granulomata. Tuberculoma is now exceedingly rare, gumma virtually non-existent, and actinomycetoma and other streptothrix infections of the brain curiosities in Great Britain. Toxoplasmosis, also rare, forms calcified areas within the hemispheres of young people and may be mistaken for tumours.

Symptoms

The rates of growth of the different kinds of tumour vary widely. Some cases run their course from onset of symptoms to death in a few weeks, while in others there is evidence of gradual growth over years. In these it may be only in the final stage that the true nature of the illness becomes clear, and only in retrospect that earlier symptoms assume their real significance. This is especially so in the case of those tumours which for months or years have shown their presence only by generalized convulsions. In yet other cases, an intracranial tumour may remain latent during life, being unexpectedly found at post-mortem examination.

Between these two extremes a great variety of symptom-complexes may be presented by an intracranial tumour. Thus, it may first show itself by signs of raised intracranial tension alone—that is, by general signs, or by signs of a gradually progressive local lesion alone—that is, by focal signs. Whichever of these two is initially lacking will probably appear later. A third way in which a tumour may first start to give trouble is by generalized fits in the absence of any other symptoms and signs. In this instance, also, general and focal signs will probably ultimately appear. Again, the sudden onset of symptoms from degeneration in a glioma, or from oedema of surrounding brain, may determine the clinical course of a tumour within the skull.

The age of the patient influences the course. Thus, in childhood the early appearance of greatly raised intracranial tension—that is, of general symptoms, is the rule. This is mainly because at this age the tumour is commonly in the fourth ventricle, and is thus placed to produce internal hydrocephalus. In the old, on the other hand, the picture of a tumour is apt to be blurred, general signs are late in development, and focal signs are indistinct. Possibly the presence of a background of cerebral arterial degeneration and its associated cerebral changes are responsible for this.

General Manifestations. These symptoms are the result of an increase in intracranial pressure and are therefore absent in cases where the pressure remains normal. The degree to which a cerebral tumour causes an increase in intracranial tension is variable and depends upon a number of factors. The growing tumour by its bulk occupies a portion of available the intracranial space, which is a constant, and, therefore, after displacing cerebrospinal fluid and venous blood, the tumour causes directly a rise in pressure. Many tumours, from their position, interfere with the free flow of fluid through the ventricular system and thus produce an obstructive hydrocephalus. This accounts for the rapid increase of pressure seen in tumours of the cerebellum, midbrain and third and fourth ventricles. Other tumours may interfere with the normal venous return from the hemispheres and so produce oedema of the brain tissue with a proportionate increase in its bulk. These different factors often reinforce one another and thus set up a complex vicious circle. This in large measure explains the fact that a tumour of rapid growth gives rise to greater increase in intracranial pressure than does one of similar size and position which has developed slowly.

The evidences of increased intracranial pressure are: papilloedema, headache, vomiting, mental drowsiness and loss of vivacity, double vision, alterations in the pulse rate, blood pressure and respiration, giddiness, nasal irritation, stiff neck and occasionally generalized convulsions. Transient obscuration of vision, 'amaurosis fugax', is a striking but uncommon symptom of raised pressure.

Papilloedema. This is the most constant of all the general manifestations. It depends upon the relationship between intravascular and intracranial pressures. Papilloedema is oedema of the nerve-head owing to the increased intracranial pressure forcing the cerebrospinal fluid into the meningeal sheath which invests the optic nerve, and into the perivascular spaces which accompany the central vessels of the nerve. The nerve sheath becomes distended, and venous stasis occurs. On ophthalmoscopic examination the earliest changes are increased redness of the disc, with disappearance of the physiological pit. As the process increases the whole margin of the disc becomes lost. It enlarges in area, and becomes visibly swollen and presents the appearance of a mole-hill as seen from above. The point of emergence of the vessels, at the centre of the disc, becomes buried by white exudation, which occurs also all over the disc, and taking a form determined by the radiating nerve fibrils, gives the disc the appearance of being striated in a radial fashion. A similar exudate may rupture the membrana limitans interna in little droplets at the macula, and coagulating as it comes in contact with the vitreous humour, produces the characteristic radially arranged macular figure or 'macular fan', exactly similar to that seen in renal disease. The venous congestion of the retina leads to haemorrhages which infiltrate along the radially arranged nerve fibres, and for this reason are flame-shaped. In time the haemorrhages become white flame-shaped scars, the whole disc contracts, the swelling disappears, and the disc becomes white, flat and atrophic, and distinguished only from that of primary optic atrophy by the scarred remains of the exudate at its edge, producing a fluffy outline like that of torn cotton wool, along the vessels and at the centre. In the early stages of papilloedema, even though there is considerable swelling of the disc, vision is little impaired. As the process increases, however, in proportion to the degree of the swelling, to the amount of exudate and to the length of time the papilloedema has lasted, consecutive optic atrophy sets in, vision becomes impaired and blindness results. Peripheral constriction of the visual fields, large pupil and dimness of vision are the signs that, if the papilloedema be not speedily relieved, blindness will certainly result. Perfect vision may be retained for a time, even with a high degree of papilloedema. So important is papilloedema in the diagnosis of tumour of the brain, that it is necessary to bear constantly in mind all other conditions which may cause it.

Papilloedema may occur in general conditions such as arterial hypertension, where the presence of papilloedema means that the disorder has entered the malignant phase; profound anaemia, especially when of rapid evolution; with emphysema, particularly when there is secondary polycythaemia; with compression of the uppermost part of the cervical cord and occasionally with hyperparathyroidism.

The retinal changes in diabetes mellitus are always, and those in hypertension often, distinguishable from papilloedema resulting from increased intracranial pressure. In diabetes the change is essentially a haemorrhagic retinitis due to degeneration of vessels, sometimes with waxy-looking exudation in circinate patches; and in hypertension it is often a general oedema of papilla and retina, with haemorrhages and white patches far away from the disc. Although the papilloedema resulting from raised intracranial pressure may appear in one eye before the other, it always becomes bilateral unless there is local pressure upon one optic nerve, which always delays or prevents papilloedema appearing in that eye. Otherwise, an earlier commencement upon one side is of no localizing value.

Headache. This may vary from a mere feeling of fullness of the head to the most agonizing pain. It is more often remittent than continuous, and may be absent for long periods together; it often occurs on first waking in the morning or after a period of recumbency or stooping. It is rarely localized, except when the growth involves the bone, or when pressure has caused local thinning of the bone, when local pain and tenderness on pressure may occur. Usually it is referred indefinitely to the frontal or to the occipital or to the vertical region. When occipital it may be associated with pain and stiffness of the neck, and head retraction. This is due to a general pressure effect, and does not indicate any localization. Headache may be entirely absent, even in the presence of severe papilloedema. It may precede the development of papilloedema even by a long period, or may be later in its appearance.

Vomiting. This rarely occurs in the absence of the two chief signs of increased intracranial pressure, papilloedema and headache. When the headaches are severe, they may be associated with much nausea, and the attacks are often referred to by the patient as 'bilious attacks'. Usually a result of increased pressure, it may be directly produced by lesions of the cerebellum, irritation of the vestibular nerve and the visual disorientation resulting from diplopia. As a symptom of intracranial tumour it hardly deserves the cardinal importance which has been assigned to it in most descriptions of this disease.

Loss of Vivacity, and Drowsiness. Even when intellectual capacity is not impaired there is slowness and a loss of vivacity. It is almost unheard of for a patient with cerebral tumour to suffer from insomnia. As the symptoms increase, so do heaviness and drowsiness, though slow cerebration may persist.

Double Vision. Diplopia is common and due to weakness of one or both external rectus muscles. It may be associated with an obvious convergent squint.

Blood Pressure, Pulse Rate and Respiration. In many cases of intracranial tumour of slow growth these remain unaltered, but if the diagnosis is not made and pressure is rising the pulse rate will slow to around 40 per minute. Less common is a rise in blood pressure occurring *pari passu* with the fall in pulse rate. It is most often seen in cases of rapid cerebral compression and is characteristic of extradural haemorrhage. Respiration tends to be slow and shallow, and when cerebral compression is severe it is often irregular and may become grouped and may show the wax and wane of movements—Cheyne-Stokes or periodic respiration.

Giddiness. This symptom is reported by some patients with intracranial tumour, particularly if it is situated below the tentorium. It usually consists of a feeling of faintness and general unsteadiness, particularly on stooping, but may amount to true vertigo.

Nasal Irritation. This curious symptom is common enough to mention. The cause is unknown.

Convulsions. As will be stressed later, fits of all types, like those of idiopathic epilepsy, are among the commonest early symptoms of tumours originating above the tentorium. Their focal nature may suggest other evidence of localization of the lesion. Convulsions occur with posterior fossa lesions but are four times as common when the lesion is above the tentorium.

Focal Signs. These have been described in the section upon the localization of lesions of the brain, but certain points need emphasis. Of all the early symptoms of tumours above the tentorium the most common are fits. These may be focal or general, and may precede any other manifestation of intracranial tumour by many years. Any person developing fits for the first time after the age of 25 should be looked upon as a tumour suspect. Although in all cases of intracranial tumour the symptoms and signs of raised intracranial pressure ultimately make their appearance, they may be late in doing so, and in this event the clinical picture is that of a progressive local destruction of brain tissue.

In examining patients with intracranial tumour signs may be observed which appear to be conflicting or mutually contradictory. It should be remembered that symptoms and signs which appear early in the clinical course are of greater localizing value than those which appear late, and that signs which only make their appearance in the presence of a severe rise in intracranial pressure should be treated with great reserve. Of these so-called 'false localizing signs' the most notorious is the abducens paresis seen in most cases of raised intracranial pressure. It probably results from shifting of the brain stem and stretching of the nerve in its course through the subarachnoid space, and should always be disregarded as a localizing sign. To a less extent the same is true of the third, fifth and seventh pairs of cranial nerves, whose functions may show slight impairment in the presence of greatly increased pressure without any direct involvement of their fibres in the tumour. On the other hand, cranial nerve palsies occurring early in the course of the disease, before there is any increase in intracranial tension, may be valuable evidence of direct involvement of these nerves, either in the brain stem or in their courses through the subarachnoid space or foramina of exit.

The presence of papilloedema may modify the localizing information to be obtained through the function of vision. Less severe degrees of papilloedema may cause irregular constrictions of the fields of vision, which may be mistaken for an incomplete bitemporal or homonymous hemianopia. When intracranial hypertension is severe, particularly in the case of posterior fossa tumours, deafness may be noticed.

Proptosis occurs in tumours of rapid growth or in the presence of rapidly developing internal hydrocephalus. It is caused by venous congestion of the orbital contents, and may be more marked on one side than on the other. In women, amenorrhoea may occur with tumours elsewhere than near the pituitary body. It is particularly common in mid-cerebellar tumours which cause severe hydrocephalus.

Especial mention may be made of tumours of the pituitary body and stalk. Their signs consist of a combination of endocrine disturbance and symptoms due to damage of surrounding nerve structures, and have been described in a previous section. The effects of these slowly growing tumours upon surrounding structures do not depend so much upon their pathological type as upon chance physical characteristics, so that their differential diagnosis largely depends upon ancillary methods including angiography, ventriculography and the ultra-sonogram.

Diagnosis

The differential diagnosis of intracranial tumour has to be made from: (1) other conditions causing papilloedema; (2) other conditions causing headache; and (3) other local lesions causing symptoms and signs of local diseases of the brain.

Any disorder, such as internal hydrocephalus or chronic abscess, which is causing a rise in pressure may suggest a cerebral tumour.

The diagnosis of intracranial tumour is not complete when a decision is reached that such a lesion is present within the skull. In the majority its presence will be obvious, but the evidence will be insufficient to determine its position and nature. In a few a local lesion may be diagnosed with certainty, but there may be doubt whether it is a tumour or some other destructive lesion. In either case special investigations are needed. Radiographs of the skull may show the changes of longstanding increased intracranial pressure, areas of local absorption of bone, abnormal vascular channels or areas of abnormal calcification. Examination of the cerebrospinal fluid should be avoided until the patient is in a special centre because of its dangers in the presence of raised intracranial pressure.

At this stage electroencephalography may give valuable information, whether or not abnormality is found. Signs in the records indicating local or general disturbance may suggest by their distribution and nature the position, extent and some physical characteristics of the lesion. Like other clinical methods of investigation its results should be related to all the other evidences of the lesion if its full usefulness is to be gained. Similarly the ultra-sound and isotope methods of locating deformity of the brain should be used in special diagnostic centres to elicit further information to add to that available by other techniques. The diagnosis of intracranial disease is so difficult that all ancillary aids are welcome, for the clinicain's aim is to 'visualize' the lesion as completely as possible without actually seeing it.

At about this stage of study the patient who may have a cerebral tumour must become the responsibility of the neurosurgeon. It is the writer's practice to ask neurosurgical help early rather than late in the diagnostic course, so that the interpretation of the results of special investigations including air encephalography, gamma encephalography and ventriculography can be shared. If the tumour can be lateralized, arteriography should follow study by electroencephalography and ultra-sound and precede introduction of air.

Treatment

The natural termination of a case of intracranial tumour is death.

In respect of the radical, surgical treatment of tumours, it will be remembered that probably more than half of the cases (if we include glioma and secondary carcinoma) are infiltrative tumours in the brain substance and thus not amenable to complete removal. In such, it is clearly improper to carry out mutilating operations which can at best only serve to prolong for a time a life which is a burden both to the patient and his relatives. On the other hand, successes can be obtained in the case of meningiomata, tumours of the auditory nerve and the pituitary body and some cystic astrocytomata, particularly of the cerebellum. It will therefore be seen how important it is to be able to determine the nature of the tumour present in any case. When this is not possible, an exploratory operation is often justified. But it would be a mistake to suppose that surgical intervenion is a matter of routine in every case in which intracranial tumour is diagnosed. Each case must be considered on its merits.

In cases in which complete removal has proved impossible radiotherapy may be employed. The results are variable and fatal recurrence occurs in most instances of invasive tumours two years or so after treatment. Statistical studies of the irradiation of gliomata show most disappointing results. Some types of tumour, notably the medulloblastoma, respond favourably at the time, but usually recur after an interval of ten years or so. No chemotherapy exists for any form of primary intracranial tumour, though the use of isotopes is advancing.

Relief of Pressure by Dehydration. There are circumstances in which it may be desirable and necessary to reduce the brain volume and the intracranial pressure; for example, to relieve pressure headache, to avert impending coma or death, to render the patient capable of co-operating in his examination and thus facilitating a localizing diagnosis, and finally to make surgical procedures more easy. This may be achieved by giving dehydrating agents as diuretics, by hypertonic dehydration or by steroids (dexamethasone). These methods are used to facilitate operation or to relieve symptoms after it.

Course and Prognosis

An untreated intracranial tumour usually causes increasing symptoms, which progress with exacerbations and remissions until papilloedema ends in blindness and until the pathological intracranial condition becomes incompatible with even a vegetative existence. Death usually comes in one of two ways. More commonly the patient sinks gradually into stupor and from this into deepening coma, in which he dies from respiratory infection. In a minority it occurs suddenly by an abrupt cessation of respiration, due to failure of the medullary centres. Although tumours are now recognized before pressure has reached a dangerous level, and are consequently treated, the physician is often faced with the terminal care of the patient, for except in the most unusual case a second operation or application of radiotherapy is quite unwarranted.

REFERENCES

BRAIN, W. R., and HENSON, R. A. (1958) Neurological syndromes associated with carcinoma, *Lancet*, ii, 971.

CLARKE, E. (1954) Cranial and intracranial myelomas, *Brain*, **71**, 61.

CROWE, F. W., SCHULL, W. J., and NEEL, J. V. (1956) *A Clinical, Pathological and Genetic Study of Multiple Neurofibromatosis*, Springfield, Ill.

CUSHING, H. (1932) *Intracranial Tumours*, Springfield, Ill.

CUSHING, H. (1938) *Meningiomas: Their Classification, Behavior, Life History and Surgical End Results*, Springfield, Ill.

EDWARDS, C. H., and PATTERSON, J. H. (1951) A review of the symptoms and signs of acoustic neurofibromata, *Brain*, **74**, 144.

MONDKAR, V. P., MCKISSOCK, W., and RUSSELL, R. W. R. (1967) Cerebellar haemangioblastomas, *Brit. J. Surg.*, **54**, 95.

OLIVECRONA, H. (1967) Acoustic tumours, *J. Neurosurg.*, **26**, 6.

RUSSELL, D. S., and RUBINSTEIN, L. J. (1963) *Pathology of Tumours of the Central Nervous System*, 2nd ed., London.

STRONG, R., and AJMORE-MARSON, C. (1961) Brain metastases, *Arch. Neurol. Psychiat.* (*Chic.*), **4**, 8.

WALSHE, F. M. R. (1931) Intracranial tumours, *Quart. J. Med.*, **24**, 587.

CLOSED HEAD INJURIES

The medical management of patients with head injuries received encouragement in the last war when there was close co-operation between physicians and surgeons in large head injury centres. In any patient who has had a head injury, once the associated wounds have healed the management depends entirely upon medical and psychiatric methods. The consequences of a closed head injury referred to as 'the post-traumatic state' vary in their pattern, intensity and duration from patient to patient, but in general have a common form. How quickly a person recovers from the effects of an injury depends upon the kind of person who is injured and the circumstances in which the injury occurs, as well as upon its severity. It is therefore usual in obtaining a history to carry out a short psychiatric interview with emphasis upon personality characteristics, previous strains in life, and the physical and emotional circumstances in which the injury happened. In planning for recovery from the injury once the patient has passed through the surgical phase of his management, attention to the patient's attitude, to his understanding of his shortcomings, and to the arrangement of his life within his capacity is of supreme importance. The complications of the injury which may include the effects of local brain damage such as diplegia, or weakness of a limb, must receive appropriate management, and the possibility of the development of post-traumatic epilepsy must always be borne in mind.

CONCUSSION

The basic disorder in all head injuries is concussion. In this state there is invariably amnesia. The amnesia before the accident (pre-traumatic or retrograde amnesia) is usually brief, consisting of seconds or minutes, whilst the post-traumatic, or postgrade amnesia, is invariably longer. The post-traumatic amnesia is a useful rough guide to the severity of the concussion, although why this should be so is not understood. Other circumstances being equal, it is likely that anyone who has suffered concussion with amnesia of minutes or hours will make a rapid recovery, whilst amnesia of up to a week may lead to a convalescence extending into months, and amnesia of more than four weeks is often associated with some permanent psychological disability. Here, it must be borne in mind that the more severe the head injury the more likely are there to be associated neurological disabilities resulting from local tearing or destruction of brain tissue, so that the blame for failure to recover cannot be laid at the door of the syndrome of concussion alone. The greater the violence the worse the concussion, and the more numerous and extensive are the associated injuries to the brain. The abnormal physiology of concussion appears to be due to damage to the midbrain, and in all fatal cases of head injury small haemorrhages may be seen here. The brain stem reticular formation which is responsible for the maintenance of the alert state is involved in the acceleration or deceleration which results from a blow to the head, and there is a critical speed below which concussion does not supervene. This is why falling on soft material might cause injuries elsewhere but does not usually lead to loss of memory (amnesia) or unconsciousness. During the phase of amnesia the patient may appear to be normal with no lowering of consciousness, although it is usual to find that there is some disturbance of cerebration. In more severe instances there is obvious confusion, and in many there is, of course, unconsciousness too. The period of amnesia is always longer than the period of unconsciousness.

In the absence of complications, patients with concussion make a full physical recovery but there may be transient or prolonged psychological disturbances.

THE POST-TRAUMATIC STATE

This condition is really a reversible neurosis which arises from the circumstance that a previously competent person has a sensorium rendered inefficient as a result of diffuse injury. The patient returning to work finds that he is unable to concentrate, that his memory is not as it was, and he finds that his mood is disturbed too. Depression, anxiety and irritability are the rule, and when the necessity to work too soon increases the strains, the emotional disturbances become more evident and there is subsequent further deterioration in cognitive function, so that the disorder is self-perpetuating. In association with this neurosis there are usually the direct physical effects of injury, namely intermittent headaches affected by posture and by worry, postural vertigo which may be vasomotor in origin or be the result of associated damage to the labyrinth, and other neurological symptoms resulting from local injury. The management of the post-traumatic state is that of the patient as a whole, and is largely psychiatric. The cardinal rule which governs management is to be guided by the patient's symptoms, a full physical life being encouraged so long as this does not give rise to headache or vertigo; on the emotional and intellectual side however, life should be kept as simple as possible with absence of responsibilities or cares. A difficulty which the patient experiences is in understanding his symptoms, for the subject of a post-traumatic state has so often been psychologically robust, and is bewildered by the nature of his disorder. Therefore frank explanation and encouragement of co-operation in a steady programme of rehabilitation is of first importance. Symptomatic treatment with the use of sedatives and tranquillizers is the same as in any other anxiety state with depression.

POST-TRAUMATIC EPILEPSY

The likelihood of the occurrence of epilepsy after an injury is directly related to the site and severity of the injury, the frontal and parietal lobes being most vulnerable, and penetrating wounds being more likely to cause fits than closed head injuries. It is unusual for traumatic epilepsy to make its appearance within 3 months of the injury, but from then to 18 months there is a sharp increase in the incidence, with a steady fall afterwards through the next 2 years, although convulsions may occur even 20 years after a severe injury. There is no difference between traumatic epilepsy and any other form of symptomatic epilepsy, and it is only in a small minority of people who have head injuries that fits of any kind supervene.

REFERENCE

FAHY, T. S., IRVING, M. H., and MILLAC, P. (1967) Severe head injuries: a six year follow-up, *Lancet*, ii, 475.

THE ELECTROENCEPHALOGRAM

The electroencephalogram is now used routinely in the study of patients with epilepsy, and with head injuries, and it has great value in the recognition of local or general disorders of the brain resulting, for instance, from tumour or infection. Nevertheless, the electroencephalogram is simply a clinical tool to be integrated with all the other clinical evidence, and should never be interpreted in isolation.

There has been a tendency in the 30 years that this procedure has been utilized by clinicians to rely upon it too much, and to think that it gives an absolute answer to any questions. That is not the case. Unlike the electrocardiogram, the pattern of an individual's electroencephalogram changes from moment to moment, there is a wide range of normal, at least 12 per cent. of normal people show abnormalities in the electroencephalogram, and many people with abnormalities in the brain have normal electroencephalograms. Furthermore, there is a very wide range of abnormal waves, wave patterns and rhythms in epilepsy, and there is no close relationship between the abnormalities which might be seen in patients with physical disease of the brain, and the nature of the disease process. The student should see the electroencephalogram in relation to his examination of the patient, and should refer to one of the many large atlases of records which are now available. The habit which has arisen of decorating a section of neurology with two or three samples of the electroencephalogram in epilepsy or with a brain tumour gives a false impression of the complexity of this neurophysiological subject.

There are a large number of excellent textbooks and atlases of electroencephalography in all the major languages, ranging from the elementary to the very sophisticated. References to a few of the more suitable for readers of this textbook are given below. As electroencephalographic records change steadily ('mature') from birth to adult life, their interpretation is even more difficult in childhood, and as more abnormalities are of degree than of kind, technical as well as clinical experience is required. This point is emphasized because a poor recording or inexperienced interpretation is much less satisfactory than no record at all; indeed, either may be disastrous and lead to a self-perpetuating misdiagnosis of epilepsy, for instance. In order to realize that its expertise is beyond the range of textbooks of clinical medicine, one has only to appreciate that on the technical side the waves are measured in microvolts, as contrasted with the millivolts of the electrocardiogram; one has only to understand the moment-to-moment variations in the same place and in different places of the electroencephalogram compared with the relative stereotypy of the electrocardiogram; and one has only to observe the inconstant relationship of the electroencephalographic changes to the nature of cerebral lesions, and to know that the electroencephalogram rarely reflects pathology.

REFERENCES

GIBBS, F. A., and GIBBS, E. L. (1964) *An Atlas of Electroencephalography*, 3 vols, London.

HILL, D., and PARR, G. (1963) *Electroencephalography*, London.

KOOI, K. A. (1971) *Fundamentals of Electroencephalography*, London.

KUGLER, J. (1964) *Electroencephalography in Hospital and General Consulting Practice*, London.

INFECTIONS OF THE MENINGES AND THE NERVOUS SYSTEM

MENINGITIS

Definition

These infective processes usually have their seat in the leptomeninges—the pia arachnoid. A true inflammatory lesion of the dura matter, that is pachymeningitis, is much less common, and is usually a localized process due to the direct spread of infection from adjacent bone.

Acute leptomeningitis, on the other hand, is usually generalized, and even when it arises from a local focus of infection it spreads rapidly throughout the subarachnoid space, this spread being facilitated by the cerebrospinal fluid and also by the negligible bactericidal potency of this fluid. Further, the inflammation not only produces its characteristic changes in the pia arachnoid, but also greatly changes the composition of the cerebrospinal fluid. These changes reflect with accuracy the nature and cause of the meningitis, and it is thus that the examination of this fluid has so great a diagnostic value. Acute leptomeningitis may be caused by invasion of the leptomeninges by organisms carried in the blood stream, as in septicaemic conditions, meningococcal meningitis, tuberculous meningitis and many cases of pneumococcal meningitis. Alternatively, the organism may reach the meninges by direct spread from a neighbouring focus of infection, of which suppuration in the middle ear and nasal sinuses, infections of the scalp, skull, face and eye, and cerebral abscesses are the most common. It may also gain direct access by penetrating wounds of the head and as a complication of fracture of the base of the skull.

Pachymeningitis may be cranial or spinal, and is usually secondary to tuberculous disease of bone, middle ear suppuration or syphilis. The condition formerly known as 'pachymeningitis haemorrhagica interna' is traumatic and not inflammatory, and is described under the heading of chronic subdural haematoma [see p. 1227].

The fine infiltration of the pia arachnoid by the cells of secondary carcinoma, of glioma, of lymphosarcoma, or of acute leukaemia may be called meningitis but although it may cause symptoms like meningitis, the term is not accurate, though it is well to remember that this form of new-growth does occur and gives a picture of meningeal irritation.

The most useful classification of the varieties of meningitis is according to the nature of the micro-organism producing the inflammation, namely: (1) pyogenic: meningococcal, pneumococcal, others (e.g. staphylococcal, streptococcal, *Haemophilus influenzae*); (2) tuberculous; (3) aseptic; (4) yeasts; (5) others, including syphilitic.

The clinical picture differs little with different causative organisms. These features of meningitis are described in Section 2, under Meningococcal Meningitis.

PYOGENIC MENINGITIS

Aetiology

Bacterial infection of the meninges almost always follows a similar infection elsewhere in the body, for instance empyema or otitis, while pneumonia, abdominal infection, abscess and joint infection are less common.

Apart from meningococcal and pneumococcal infections, suppurative meningitis may result from the invasion of the meninges by staphylococci, gonococci, *H. influenzae*, coliform bacilli, *Bacillus anthracis* and streptothrix.

Pathology

The pathology is similar in all cases. The exudation is purulent, and in the meningitis due to *B. anthracis* it is of a red colour, due to concomitant blood effusion. The cerebrospinal fluid contains large numbers of polymorphonuclear leucocytes, together with the micro-organism responsible for each variety. Suppurative meningitis resulting from bone disease and from wounds of the meninges may be localized by the formation of meningeal adhesions, and an intrameningeal abscess may result. Such an abscess situated upon the upper surface of the temporal bone is not an uncommon result of caries of the middle ear.

The clinical aspect is that common to all forms of acute meningitis, high pyrexia, rigors and delirium being conspicuous. The course is rapid, and, before the introduction of modern chemotherapy, led to an almost invariably fatal termination. In the localized form where drainage can be ensured and extension of the infection prevented, recovery should take place.

Diagnosis

This depends upon the presence of the clinical signs of meningitis and of a cerebrospinal fluid containing polymorphonuclear leucocytes in large quantities, and upon the recognition in this fluid of the several micro-organisms responsible, by microscopic examination and culture. The sensitivity of the organism should be established before treatment with antibiotics which should start as soon as possible. The recognition of *H. influenzae* requires that cultures should be made upon a blood medium, for otherwise the organism may be easily overlooked and the fluid reported as sterile. Further, the presence of some well-known cause for suppurative meningitis, such as ear disease, staphylococcal infection, etc., suggests the diagnosis.

Acute otitis media may cause symptoms like those of meningitis, such as headache, pyrexia, vomiting, head retraction and delirium. Examination of the ear, which should be made a routine in all cases where meningitis is suspected, will show tympanic distension, the relief of which is followed by disappearance of the symptoms. In this connexion it must be remembered that meningitis and intracranial abscess seldom follow directly upon acute otitis but are usually sequels of chronic otitis with caries of the temporal bone. When evidences of caries of the middle ear are present with cerebral symptoms, distinction has to be made between meningitis and abscess of the brain. Here localizing symptoms, either temporal or cerebellar, and papilloedema may suggest an abscess. Electroencephalography and other 'neurosurgical' investigations [see p. 1200] may be urgently needed to exclude an abscess. In cases of abscess in which cells and organisms are found in the cerebrospinal fluid, these exist in small numbers only, as compared with the copious cells and organisms present in the fluid of suppurative meningitis [see Section 2].

Treatment

This is that of pyogenic infections anywhere, with immediate and prolonged use of the appropriate antibiotic such as tetracycline, to which the organism is sensitive, maintenance of fluid intake, control of electrolytes, and treatment of symptoms, including headache and restless distress. In cases of meningitis secondary to mastoid disease, the source of infection should be at once cleared out by surgical procedure. Sulphonamides and penicillin remain the agents of choice in meningococcal meningitis; for others a broad-based antibiotic should be used immediately without awaiting a report on the sensitivity of the organism.

TUBERCULOUS MENINGITIS

This disease results from the general invasion of the cerebrospinal leptomeninges by blood-borne tubercle bacilli. Occurring at all ages, it is by far most common in childhood and early adult life, but its incidence is now very low in Britain.

Pathology

No patient with tuberculous meningitis should die of it. If he does tubercles and adhesive meningitis are found, with secondary hydrocephalus.

Symptoms

The onset is usually gradual, with signs of vague and slight illness. In children, general apathy and neglect of amusements and play, headache, loss of appetite, constipation, dullness, fretfulness, restlessness at night with grinding of teeth during sleep, headache, vomiting and pyrexia are common symptoms. The diagnosis should be suspected as early as this because immediate treatment is imperative. These slight and vague symptoms may last from a few days to several weeks in unrecognized and so untreated cases. Early disappearance of the knee- and ankle-jerks, and retention of urine are common and should be looked for in suspected cases and early lumbar puncture with diligent search for the bacillus instituted. The search is not complete until several hours' examination of spinal fluid fails to show a stained bacillus. In those cases which are said to begin acutely, careful inquiry will generally reveal that some symptoms such as the above have preceded the acute onset.

Diagnosis

The difficulty is to recognize the disorder soon enough, for every day matters to prognosis after treatment. The diseases liable to be confused with tuberculous meningitis at its commencement are other forms of meningitis, virus diseases of the nervous system, especially acute poliomyelitis, cerebral abscess, the exanthemata—especially enteric fever—and pneumonia. It must be borne in mind that in children convulsions, strabismus, head retraction and stiffness of the neck, with pyrexia, may be symptomatic of many maladies apart from meningitis, especially of apical pneumonia. When signs of meningeal irritation are unmistakable the condition has to be distinguished from the various forms of pyogenic meningitis. In these the degree of meningism is usually more intense and the cerebrospinal fluid is turbid or purulent with a predominantly polymorphic pleocytosis and the causative organism can usually be cultured.

Virus infections of the nervous system can look like tuberculous meningitis and it is in such cases that the retention of the cerebrospinal fluid chlorides and glucose at their normal level can help diagnosis.

The meningeal reaction apt to arise from time to time in cases of cerebral abscess may closely resemble tuberculous meningitis and may be associated with a mixed pleocytosis and a sterile fluid.

In suspected tuberculous meningitis a lumbar puncture should be carried out immediately and the whole laboratory occupied in search for the organism, for every hour of treatment wasted will affect the prognosis for function if not for life. The characteristic features of the fluid are, that it is usually under considerable pressure, it is clear or only slightly turbid, has no visible deposit before centrifuging, but it often forms a fine flocculent clot. It contains an excess of albumin. The normal sugar is reduced or absent, and a value over 50 mg. per 100 ml. practically excludes the diagnosis. It is sometimes between 40 and 50 mg. per 100 ml., but in the majority values under 30 mg. are obtained. In other forms of non-purulent meningitis such as poliomyelitis and benign lymphocytic meningitis the glucose content of the cerebrospinal fluid is almost invariably normal. Early reduction of the chloride content below 700 or even 650 mg. per 100 ml. is of value in distinguishing tuberculous meningitis, especially from virus diseases of the nervous system. There is a pleocytosis with a high proportion of lymphocytes, 70–80 per cent. being of this nature, and the rest being polymorphonuclears. In some cases the polymorphonuclear leucocytes may be in excess, but these cases are at once distinguished from other forms of meningitis by the presence of numerous lymphocytes, by the absence of the meningococcus and of the other pyogenic organisms and by the presence of the tubercle bacillus. It is wise to assume that the organism will be found with diligent search in every case and to appreciate that its recognition by culture or guinea-pig growth does not help the patient. In doubtful cases, when the diagnosis is not confirmed by bacteriology, the writer institutes full treatment with streptomycin, isoniazid and PAS, to withdraw it, without any feeling of guilt if the rapid decline of signs makes the diagnosis improbable in a couple of days.

Course and Treatment

Before the advent of streptomycin, tuberculous meningitis was invariably fatal and usually ended in the patient's death in from 3 to 8 weeks of the onset of symptoms.

Today, provided early diagnosis is achieved, the vigorous use of streptomycin with sodium aminosalicylate (PAS) and isoniazid (INH) should result in complete recovery in more than 50 per cent. of cases.

Streptomycin is administered intramuscularly and sometimes intrathecally and either sodium aminosalicylate or isoniazid by mouth continuously for the initial period of 8 to 12 weeks. If general improvement as measured by appetite, weight, subsidence of fever and loss of drowsiness is satisfactory and is confirmed by a gradual return of the cerebrospinal fluid towards normal, a rest of 1 month in intrathecal treatment alone should be given. At the end of this period a further course should be given and thereafter a gradual withdrawal of treatment may be achieved provided always that improvement is maintained. Good results are being obtained using isoniazid (e.g. 100 mg. thrice daily) combined with streptomycin administered only by the intramuscular route (e.g. 1 G. daily), thereby avoiding the need for daily intrathecal injections. The addition of cortisone to this regime is valueless.

Careful observation at increasing intervals must be maintained over a period of 5 years.

Prominent among the complications which may arise if treatment is delayed are chronic hydrocephalus from the development of a plastic meningeal fibrosis around the base of the brain and leading in its turn to double hemiplegia, convulsions, blindness and imbecility and deafness from the degeneration in the cochlear nerves resulting from the use of intrathecal streptomycin. A postmeningitic syndrome just like the post-traumatic syndrome, with convulsions, may persist in well-treated cases, the result of diffuse mild brain damage.

Sarcoidosis [see Section 9] rarely causes chronic meningitis or meningo-encephalitis. The tubercles invade the brain to cause, in some instances, the clinical picture of a cerebral tumour, with local paresis and convulsions. More often cranial nerves or peripheral nerves are involved in the quietly advancing granulomatous condition. When it invades the spinal theca, paraplegia results. The diagnosis, management and treatment with corticosteroids is that of the generalized and pulmonary condition.

VIRUS MENINGITIS

This is discussed in Section 2, under Virus Infections of the Nervous System.

YEAST MENINGITIS

These conditions are rare, and they present with evidence of chronic meningitis, raised intracranial pressure and of brain stem disorder.

Pathology

The condition macroscopically is similar to that of tuberculous meningitis, with extensive infiltration or the structures at the base of the brain with gelatinous purulent material and consequent obstructive hydrocephalus.

As with other fungal infections, the infestation is facilitated by alteration in the natural saprophytic relationship which occurs during chemotherapy or steroid therapy.

Symptoms

The patients are usually young adults who may have complained of double vision and who proceed to headache or lowering of intellectual efficiency and then drowsiness. The signs are those for low-grade meningitis, with stiff neck, damage to the upper cranial nerves and evidences of raised pressure including nausea, a furred tongue and papilloedema. The diagnosis is invariably made by examining the cerebrospinal fluid after the diagnoses of intracranial tumour and tuberculous meningitis have been entertained. The large yeast cells are seen, for instance *Torula* or *Blastomyces*, others are *mucormycosis* and *Cryptococcus neoformans*. The clinical picture may be complicated by the existence of a granulomatous mass which produces effects like those of an intracranial tumour.

The cerebrospinal fluid shows raised pressure, a marked pleocytosis, protein raised to about 200 mg. per cent. and lowering of sugar and chlorides due to the presence of the yeast, which is easily recognized after culture for which a special medium developed by Sabouraud is used.

Treatment

The conditions are fatal without treatment and even with appropriate chemotherapy mortality is high. The substances at present developed to arrest development of the organisms are given by intravenous infusion: 0·25 mg. increasing to 1 mg. per kg. body weight of amphotericin B (*Fungizone*) is slowly infused daily until a week after symptoms of infection have fully subsided.

SYPHILITIC MENINGITIS

Meningitis due to infection by *Treponema pallidum* may occur at any time after infection, but one-half of the cases occur during the first 4 years. In a few cases the symptoms have been noticed coincidently with syphilitic roseola. It is now rare.

Pathology

The process is an infiltration of the meninges with lymphocytes and plasma cells, spreading from the perivascular spaces where the treponemes multiply freely, and it may lead to scarring and opacity of the membranes, with consequent stricture of the nerves and vessels and occlusion of the arachnoid space, or to massive gummatous formation in the meninges. It is essentially a chronic form of meningitis, though it may result in the production of acute symptoms. A marked feature is that the meningeal changes may be found actively progressive in one spot, and equally regressive in another. The disease may be local or diffuse, and it may attack the dura (pachymeningitis) and involve the overlying bone, or it may spread from the pia arachnoid into the sublying nervous tissue (meningo-encephalitis).

The cerebrospinal fluid is usually under increased pressure, is clear and colourless with lymphocytes and no other cells. The number of the lymphocytes present is in direct proportion to the activity of the meningeal syphilis. The treponeme has rarely been found in the fluid, yet inoculation of apes with the fluid has proved successful.

Symptoms

Apart from those conditions of nervous syphilis in which meningitis is associated with arterial disease, the formation of massive gummata and neuronic degeneration, syphilitic meningitis may cause:

1. *Headache.*
2. *Hydrocephalus* [see p. 1193].
3. *Infantile syphilitic meningitis.* This is a rare chronic reaction beginning in the first few months of life, with signs of general nervous deterioration. The signs of meningitis are obvious and those of congenital syphilis may be present. There is an excess of lymphocytes in the cerebrospinal fluid, and a positive Wassermann reaction.
4. *Adult syphilitic meningitis*, with a symptom-complex closely resembling that of tuberculous meningitis, used to be reported [see p. 1208].
5. *Paralysis of cranial nerves.* This isolated symptom of nervous syphilis may result from sclerosing basal meningitis or from the presence of a gumma in the course of the nerve. Several of the nerves may be involved in one patch of meningitis. Any of the cranial nerves may be affected from the olfactory to the hypoglossal, but the third or oculomotor nerve is by far the most frequently attacked.

Treatment

Treatment with penicillin is appropriate for nervous syphilis in general [see Section 2]. Iodide of potassium is, however, still of great value in the treatment of gummatous syphilis, although its effect is still unexplained.

MENINGISM

The term 'meningism' is used for a group of cases which present symptoms of meningitis and in which no pathological change can be found either in the cerebrospinal fluid, or, if death occurs, in the meninges or cerebral tissue. It is met with in children in association with acute febrile diseases, and is presumably due to the toxin present. Recovery is usually rapid and complete.

NEUROSYPHILIS

Early in the century 'syphilis was responsible for far more cases of organic nervous disease than any other single factor' in the British Isles. Now, new cases of neurosyphilis are uncommon, the appearance of patients with old tabes dorsalis or the effects of meningovascular syphilis in clinics and examinations making the disease seem more irequent than is the case. Although the use of penicillin has so greatly reduced the occurrence of the disease, there was a steadily falling incidence during the half century before its introduction.

There has been an increase of primary syphilis in the 1960s, so further instances of syphilis of the nervous system will be appearing before long.

The nervous system is involved in congenital and in acquired syphilis and it seems that the *T. pallidum* invades it early in the secondary stage. After an interval of from 2 to 30 years symptoms may develop. The resulting diseases are divided into three forms, which may coexist.

1. General paralysis of the insane, in which the organism is found within the central nervous system.
2. Tabes dorsalis caused by degeneration of sensory roots and pathways.
3. Meningovascular syphilis, in which the neurological symptoms are secondary to gummatous changes.

As the classical Wassermann reaction of the cerebrospinal fluid is invariably positive in general paralysis only, other serological reactions such as the Kahn test have been devised but absolute certainty in diagnosis is now available in the *T. pallidum* sensitivity test. Lange's colloidal gold test is most valuable in helping to differentiate the three forms of syphilitic disease of the nervous system.

GENERAL PARALYSIS OF THE INSANE

Synonyms. Dementia paralytica; General paresis.

Definition

This is a progressive disease of the brain due to syphilis, causing mental and physical deterioration and finally dementia and paralysis.

Aetiology

The disease usually begins between 8 and 20 years after infection with *T. pallidum.* The incidence is much greater among males, and the onset is usually between the ages of 30 and 50. It may appear in adolescence as the result of congenital infection. It formerly represented about 10 per cent. of all cases of neurosyphilis and nearly a quarter of those treated as hospital in-patients. The reduction in the incidence of neurosyphilis is reflected in the fact that there were no cases of general paralysis among 3000 admissions to the National Hospital, Queen Square, London, in the 3 years to 1971.

Pathology

The essential changes are in the ganglion cells of the cerebral cortex, many of which appear while those that remain are arranged irregularly. The cells are often shrunken, and their nuclei stain deeply. In addition there is a marked reaction of the glial cells and histiocytes (rod cells). The subpial lamina of glia tissue is increased. The histiocytes proliferate and hypertrophy and contain iron in their cytoplasm—a pathognomonic finding. Many of the cortical blood vessels are surrounded by a perivascular 'cuff' of lymphocytes and plasma cells, and the vessels often show proliferative changes in their endothelium.

T. pallidum can be demonstrated in the nervous tissue.

Symptoms

For months before intellectual defect becomes apparent the patient has usually shown some impairment of emotional control. He has become excitable, moody, liable to outbursts of temper and easily moved to tears by music or the cinema. Thereafter he begins to show a lack of concentration and persistence; he ceases to pursue his old interests and adopts new ones in rather rapid succession. At this stage he begins to show deficiency of judgement, becomes forgetful, inattentive to business and careless. The classical delusions of grandeur are now rare. The psychiatric aspects of general paralysis of the insane are considered in greater detail in Section 17.

In many other cases the symptoms are merely those of simple dementia with gradual reduction of interests and of mental and physical activity. The patient is often depressed in the early stages but as the disease progresses he lies in his bed showing little sign of mental activity, indifferent to his surroundings, incontinent and more or less paralysed.

Diagnosis should always have been achieved at this stage, and the full-blown picture of 'classical' G.P.I. is now very uncommon, for penicillin arrests the symptoms by curing the disease.

The first of the physical changes accompanying the mental deterioration is almost always tremor. Usually, it begins by affecting the voice, and when the tongue, lips and cheeks become tremulous, the irregularity of articulation is pronounced. The typical tongue tremor is a backward and forward 'trombone' movement. Speech, at first, is merely hesitant; later it becomes indistinct and irregular, syllables are omitted, interpolated or slurred, and the voice becomes feeble, jerky and slurred. Elision of syllables or of words, and attacks of aphasia are common. As the memory fails, confusion arises in the construction of long sentences, proper names are forgotten, the choice of adjectives and verbs becomes more and more limited, and the vocabulary diminishes until only interjections are left. Written language suffers in the same way, and may show defects of execution and of ideation before spoken speech is noticeably altered. Tremor becomes marked in the hands and other parts of the body and, because of the unsteadiness of the hand the writing deteriorates.

Apart from tremor there are at first no physical signs. Pupillary abnormalities are common, but they simply indicate central nervous syphilis and have probably been present for some time before the onset of general paralysis. The complete Argyll Robertson phenomenon is not common, but incomplete forms of it and inequality and irregularity of the pupils are usual. Signs of disturbance of the pyramidal system—extensor plantar reflexes and exaggeration of the tendon-jerks—usually occur before long. If any of the tendon-jerks are absent, as is not uncommon, it is because of the presence of an element of tabes dorsalis. Incontinence of urine often occurs early, but it is more often due to lack of attention than to any failure of the sphincter reflexes. At a later stage control of both bladder and rectum is always lost. Sexual impotence is present in most cases for several years before mental symptoms appear.

Paralytic features thus become more pronounced. In the so-called 'congestive attacks', hemiplegia or monoplegia appears, with or without an initial Jacksonian fit. Recovery occurs in the course of a few days or weeks, but the limbs gradually become weak.

Generalized convulsions are common and death may occur in coma following a fit: a fit may be the first sign. When the patient is examined he is found to be tremulous. Such cases are among the most favourable for treatment, because the disease may be arrested before mental deterioration has become apparent. Insomnia is frequent in the prodromal period, but in the early stages sleep is often excessive. Later, sleeplessness and motor restlessness are often troublesome symptoms.

Taboparesis. This is a combination of certain features of general paralysis with some of tabes. The mental symptoms are, as a rule, relatively mild, tremor and the speech disturbances are moderate, the knee-jerks and ankle-jerks are absent, and there is usually some sensory impairment of tabetic type and distribution; the pupil reactions are likely to be of the Argyll Robertson type, and optic atrophy may be present. Many cases of nervous syphilis in which optic atrophy is the first recognized feature develop taboparesis.

Serological Reactions. If the patient has not had a course of penicillin, his blood will almost certainly give a positive Wassermann reaction. A negative result, however, should not be accepted as conclusive evidence against the presence of general paralysis of the insane. The cerebrospinal fluid in an untreated case usually shows an increase in the number of lymphocytes and in the protein content, with excess of globulin; the Wassermann reaction is invariably strongly positive, and Lange's colloidal gold test almost always gives a paretic type of curve. The Wassermann reaction may remain positive, even after a full course of penicillin, so that a *T. pallidum* sensitivity test should be requested.

Diagnosis

The diagnosis depends on the combination of mental deterioration with pupillary changes, tremor and typical alterations in the cerebrospinal fluid. The non-syphilitic conditions which cause similar gradual mental changes are rare with the exception of arteriosclerotic dementia, which usually occurs later and is associated with less tremor.

In rare cases chronic alcoholism gives rise to an 'expansive' mental state and tremulousness, which cannot with confidence be distinguished from general paralysis without examination of the cerebrospinal fluid. With delirium tremens visual hallucinations are a prominent symptom. Alzheimer's disease which comes on in middle age and causes gradual mental deterioration associated with tremor. Pupillary abnormalities are absent [see Section 17]. In the absence of pupillary or other clinical signs of nervous syphilis it may be impossible to distinguish the depressed form of general paralysis of the insane from other states of depression.

In many cases the tremulousness may suggest the correct diagnosis, but some tremor may also be seen in cases of depression with agitation due to other psychoses.

Treatment

One mega Unit of penicillin given daily for 10 days will destroy the organisms. Repeated courses, or the concomittant use of outmoded therapy by malaria or heavy metals is unnecessary and reactionary. The patient's recovery after the infection is over is gradual, and the changes in the cerebrospinal fluid are also delayed, the lymphocytes falling first, then the protein content, next the Lange gold curve becomes normal, and finally the Wassermann reaction may be reversed. In a follow-up since the Second World War the author has not needed to repeat treatment once, but a repeated course of penicillin is a small price to pay for safety and peace of mind.

The effect of antibiotics is to arrest the active disease, and the clinical results depend chiefly on the degree of mental deterioration that had occurred before treatment was instituted. The most satisfactory cases are those in which convulsions or other acute phenomena have brought the patient under care before mental impairment has become obvious. In cases of slower evolution, with evident mental impairment, arrest of the disease may leave the patient incapable of useful mental work and unfit to hold any position of responsibility. It is, however, remarkable what a degree of recovery can take place over many months.

MENINGOVASCULAR SYPHILIS

Aetiology

Meningovascular syphilis as distinct from general paralysis of the insane occurs in about 4 per cent. of all persons with syphilis. The onset of symptoms is commonest from 1 to 5 years after infection, but it may be as early as 2 or 3 months or as late as 30 or 40 years. Characteristically, the patients are young men, but a 'stroke' due to syphilitic vascular disease may occur at any age and at any interval after infection. The condition is a rare cause of neurological disease in the British Isles now, accounting for 0·1 per cent. of admissions to the National Hospital, Queen Square, London.

Pathology

Both the meninges and the cerebral blood vessels are always affected, but the degree of involvement of each is subject to great variation. When the disease falls chiefly upon the meninges it most frequently causes a diffuse, subacute or chronic, gummatous leptomeningitis at the base of the brain.

In cases where the main incidence is upon the blood vessels, the arteries at the base of the brain, forming the circle of Willis or arising from it, with their branches are most often affected causing obliterative endarteritis.

Gumma of the brain is not seen in this country now. Its clinical results are like those of a quickly growing intracranial tumour.

Symptoms

The symptoms of meningovascular syphilis depend first on the preponderance of cellular reactions or upon vascular occlusion, and secondly upon the chance involvement of intracranial structures in the disease processes. They, therefore, vary greatly from case to case.

The symptoms of basal meningitis are partly general and partly local from involvement of some of the cranial nerves. The general symptoms are headache, lethargy and impairment of intellect and memory. Any of the cranial nerves may be affected. With occular symptoms, pupillary changes are the rule and external ocular palsies common. Mild papilloedema is also common and optic atrophy may occur in one or both eyes. Involvement of the hypothalamus or of the pituitary causes obesity and diabetes insipidus. In severe cases convulsions are common and attacks of aphasia may occur. In all the more severe cases some mental impairment is the rule.

When the blood vessels are predominantly affected premonitory symptoms often occur before there is any stroke. There are transitory weakness of one arm or other part of the body or of local twitching with hemiplegia. In addition there may be sensory loss in the limbs and complete or partial hemianopia. Aphasia usually accompanies right-sided hemiplegia. The Wassermann reaction is usually strongly positive in the blood.

Treatment

One mega Unit of penicillin intramuscularly for 10 days as for general paralysis, is given with confident expectation of cure of the infection. Potassium iodide, 1 G. daily for 2–4 weeks, should be used if local disorder of function suggests gummatous activity, and this treatment may be dramatically effective in reversing signs.

Prognosis

With treatment, recovery is the rule but some mental impairment, headaches and occasional fits are common residual phenomena. The local effects of vascular disease may in some degree persist.

ACUTE SYPHILITIC MENINGITIS

This is rare. It used to be almost confined to young men and occurred within a year or two of infection.

Symptoms

The clinical picture was indistinguishable from that of other kinds of acute meningitis. Headache was intense, the temperature might rise to 102° or 103° F. (38·9° or 39·4° C.), the patient was delirious and might have maniacal outbursts, and stiffness of the neck was present, but Kernig's sign was not usually pronounced. The cerebrospinal fluid might contain 1000 or 1500 cells per mm^3., of which as many as 30 per cent. or even more might be polymorphonuclear. The Wassermann reaction was strongly positive both in the cerebrospinal fluid and in the blood.

Treatment

This is as for other forms of meningovascular syphilis.

TABES DORSALIS

Synonym. Locomotor ataxia.

Definition

This is a disease of syphilitic origin with ataxia and numerous other signs due to degeneration of the posterior columns of the spinal cord.

Aetiology

Nothing is known of the contributory factors which determine the occurrence of tabes dorsalis in some persons with syphilis and not in others. Males are affected a good deal more often than females. The onset is usually between the ages of 30 and 45 years, and usually between 5 and 15 years after infection.

Tabes dorsalis was once the commonest form of neurosyphilis, but only two new cases were seen in the National Hospital, Queen Square, London, in 1970.

Pathology

The most evident change is deterioration in the posterior columns of the spinal cord. It is, however, generally believed that this is not primary but results from disease affecting the fibres, of which these columns are composed, before they enter the cord. As a secondary change the neuroglia around the degenerated fibres increases in amount and density. Hence the characteristic feature in sections of the cord in tabes is shrinkage and sclerosis of the posterior columns. The sclerosis usually appears earliest in the posterolateral columns of the lower lumbar and upper sacral regions, but in advanced cases when the dorsal and cervical sensory roots are also affected the posterior columns are sclerosed throughout.

Atrophy of the optic nerves commonly occurs, and seems to be the result of a combined interstitial gummatous inflammation and primary degeneration of the nerve fibres.

Symptoms

Few diseases cause so many different symptoms. The most common features are: (1) 'lightning pains'; (2) objective disturbances of sensation; (3) loss of tendon reflexes; (4) ataxia; (5) disturbance of pupillary reflexes, especially the Argyll Robertson pupil, and (6) impairment of bladder control. Less frequent are: (7) visceral 'crises', i.e. acute disturbances of function of certain viscera, of which gastric crises are the most common, but rectal, vesical and laryngeal crises also occur; (8) atrophy of the optic nerves; (9) trophic changes—(i) Charcot's disease of joints, (ii) perforating ulcers of the skin; and (10) loss of vigour.

The usual syndrome is that of degeneration of the posterior spinal nerve roots, or of the corresponding nerve cells in the posterior root ganglia and, in fact, of the afferent elements of the nervous system in many parts of the body.

Sensory Disturbances. *Subjective.* Lightning pains are usually the first symptom—sudden intense stabbing pains which seem to shoot into parts of the lower limbs. They occur at irregular intervals and usually in bouts, vary greatly in severity, and are often mistaken for 'rheumatism' or 'neuritis'.

Objective. With these subjective disturbances, objective impairment of pain appreciation develops. This hypalgesia has a strongly selective incidence, the areas at first affected being as follows: (1) a patch across the chest and the back of 'cuirass' distribution; (2) over the lower halves of the shins; (3) on the nose; and (4) on the ulnar borders of the forearm. This odd distribution is because the longest fibres of the primary divisions of the sensory nerves, especially those between the limb dermatomes, are the most vulnerable to the tabetic process.

Reflexes. Simultaneously with the involvement of the pain fibres, the fibres which subserve reflex activities are affected, with consequent gradual interruption of the reflex arcs. The ankle-jerks and knee-jerks disappear. Loss of the ankle-jerks is an early sign in tabes, and often precedes loss of the knee-jerks by many years.

Hypotonia. Muscle tone gradually becomes reduced at a time when lightning pains are the only symptom of tabes, and loss of skin sensation the only other manifestation. It is shown by flaccidity of the muscles, and by an abnormal range of active and passive movement of the limbs.

Ataxia. At a slightly later stage the coarser fibres in the posterior roots which are concerned with sense of position suffer in the same way as the pain and reflex fibres. The patient then becomes unable to appreciate exactly the position of his extremities.

Sphincter Troubles. These are the result of lowering of pain sensation in the bladder which is the afferent element in the reflex of micturition. Difficulty in starting micturition and nocturnal incontinence are common. Acute retention of urine is sometimes the symptom which first brings the patient under observation. Impotence is usual.

Ocular Disturbances. Abnormalities in the reactions, size and outline of the pupils, and pupillary disturbances of some kind are often the first signs of tabes. The Argyll Robertson pupil is the most characteristic abnormality, but it is not common in its pure form [see p. 1170]. Absence of the light reaction in one or both pupils, with or without retention of the convergence reaction, is usual, and atrophic changes in the irides are common.

Partial bilateral ptosis usually come on later, and it is compensated for by elevation of the eyebrows. In addition there are a general flabbiness of the facial musculature and a greyish pallor of the skin. All these features combine to give the patient a somewhat distinctive facial appearance—the tabetic facies.

Optic atrophy. Optic atrophy is found in about one case in ten. It may be the first indication of neurosyphilis. The peripheral portion of the visual field is lost first, and charts of the fields at this stage have a most irregular outline. Central vision is the last to fail, and as long as it persists the impairment of sight may escape notice. The disc becomes white and flat, and is sharply outlined. Cases of tabes which begin with optic atrophy do not, as a rule, develop much ataxia, but they often develop mental disturbances and become cases of taboparesis.

Visceral Crises. Occasionally attacks of intractable vomiting occur, each lasting a few days. It may be associated with epigastric pain or just discomfort. Tabetic pains in the back are commonly associated with or precede the crisis. When the attack is over the patient is quickly well again, but such attacks continue to occur at intervals of months or weeks. They often take place before other symptoms of tabes and the vomiting may be attributed to intestinal obstruction, or to perforation of the stomach. Rectal crises consist of painful and prolonged tenesmus; vesical crises of severe dysuria and laryngeal crises of prolonged spasm of the larynx causing stridor, cough and dyspnoea.

Trophic Changes. *Charcot's disease of joints* (*neuropathic joints*). In chronic cases severe disease leading eventually to articular disorganization, occurs in one or two joints. The first sign is usually rapid swelling in and around a joint, with effusion and oedema. The effusion, in slight cases, subsides slowly and the joint recovers, but more often the enlargement is followed by destruction of the cartilages, wasting of the ends of the bones, periarticular new-bone formation and destruction of the ligaments. The joint becomes disorganized, the range of movement is increased and crepitations of startling coarseness are heard and felt when the part is handled. The characteristic feature is the complete absence of pain. The joints most often attacked, and in order of frequency are knee, hip, ankle, small joints of the hands and feet, the spine, shoulder and elbow.

Perforating ulcers of the skin. Changes in the skin give rise to chronic painless ulcers, usually on the sole of the foot, which gradually increase in depth until the foot may be perforated.

Tabes dorsalis in some races in the tropics, especially India, presents a somewhat different picture in which the features of a peripheral neuropathy predominate, other symptoms of a classical kind being present in sufficient degree to establish the diagnosis.

Diagnosis

Tabes dorsalis is diagnosed by its clinical features. Examination of the blood and cerebrospinal fluid may not provide any evidence of syphilis; the Wassermann reaction is negative in one or the other in about 30 per cent. of cases and completely negative in both in about 15 per cent. The *T. pallidum* sensitivity test will be positive. The diagnosis rests on: (1) lightning pains; (2) characteristic sensory signs; (3) the Argyll Robertson pupil in one or both eyes; (4) absence of one or both ankle- or knee-jerks, or a definite diminution in one of them; and (5) evidence of syphilis.

There are two groups of cases between which the diagnosis is especially difficult, and, in an individual case, may be impossible. On the one hand, there are rare cases of mild tabes occurring in adults but due to congenital infection, in which the blood Wassermann reaction is negative and the cerebrospinal fluid is completely normal; and on the other, the more common group of non-syphilitic cases in which the patients have spastic pupils and absent tendon-jerks, usually referred to as the Holmes-Adie syndrome [see p. 1170].

Treatment

Prophylactic. When tabes dorsalis is associated with a positive Wassermann reaction in the blood or in the cerebrospinal fluid, the treatment is the same as that described for general paralysis [p. 1208]. If in doubt give a course of penicillin: 1 mega Unit a day for 10 days.

Course and Prognosis

In many patients the disease remains stationary in an early stage and causes no disability. If untreated, incoordination may appear after a pre-ataxic stage of 10 or 20 years. Some become ataxic within 5 years of the onset of pains, a few within a year. The cause of the illness is arrested at any stage by antibiotic treatment.

The course of the other symptoms is variable.

Without treatment the prognosis for life is variable. Untreated tabetics die of intercurrent illness or of some cardiovascular complication; with treatment the disease is arrested, but arrest may also be found in benign cases in persons who have at no time had treatment.

SYPHILITIC MYELITIS

ACUTE TRANSVERSE MYELITIS

This condition is now very rare in Britain. The patients are almost invariably males between 30 and 45. Over a segment of the spinal cord there is intense infiltration with small round cells and red cells and small areas of softening; the meninges show similar local infiltration.

The symptoms are those of acute transverse myelitis due to other causes [see p. 1276] and the aetiological diagnosis depends on the discovery of syphilis. A course of 10 mega Units of penicillin is sufficient for the infection, but much of the damage to the spinal cord is permanent.

ERB'S SYPHILITIC SPASTIC PARAPLEGIA

This is a slowly developing condition which comes on many years after syphilitic infection. The spinal cord shows degeneration of the pyramidal tracts and some marginal degeneration involving particularly the direct cerebellar tracts.

Spasticity of the legs becomes pronounced, with corresponding weakness and typical reflex abnormalities. Sensory changes, if any, are slight, but vesical disturbances are the rule. Pupillary abnormalities may or may not be present.

PACHYMENINGITIS HYPERTROPHICA CERVICALIS

In rare cases the dura mater in the cervical region undergoes a gummatous and subsequently fibrous thickening, and the arachnoid and pia also become thickened and fused with it. The new tissue compresses the nerve roots, and weakness, wasting and sensory loss gradually develop in the arms. After a time the spinal cord is compressed and spastic paraplegia results.

SYPHILITIC AMYOTROPHY

This closely resembles idiopathic progressive muscular atrophy [see motor neurone disease, p. 1282]. The spinal cord shows degeneration of the anterior horn cells, most pronounced in the cervical region, and also some syphilitic changes in the meninges and blood vessels.

The pupillary changes of neurosyphilis are absent in

most of the cases. The muscular atrophy usually begins in the arms, and, as a rule, the tendon jerks are absent; the legs may be normal, become spastic, show wasting, or may merely lose their tendon jerks, but in some cases the wasting muscles retain their tendon jerks. There may be some sensory loss of the tabetic type, and vesical disturbances are common. It is arrested by treatment.

CONGENITAL SYPHILIS OF THE NERVOUS SYSTEM

The nervous system is much less often affected in congenital syphilis. Viewed broadly, the pathological changes and the clinical manifestations are the same in both congenital and acquired infections. Regarding the first, meningitis, endarteritis and gummata are common to both forms; but while *softening* from arterial disease is characteristic of acquired syphilis, *cortical cell atrophy and subsequent sclerosis* are prominent features in congenital cases. Mental defects, with convulsions and spastic weakness of the limbs, are typical of congenital syphilis in contrast to the hemiplegias and monoplegias, with or without convulsions, which occur in the acquired form. The combination of obvious visceral and skin lesions, with parenchymatous degeneration of the nervous tissue, is common in the congenital, but not in the acquired disease. New cases hardly ever occur in Great Britain today, but they are quite common in some underdeveloped countries.

Symptoms

Syphilitic infants may have convulsions in the first 2 years and these may be given as the cause of death. In those who survive, fits may continue or begin again towards the end of childhood, this being more common. They may continue throughout life without the addition of symptoms suggesting local brain disease. In another group, convulsions are followed by symptoms of hemiplegia or of spastic diplegia. The same defects may appear apart from convulsions. Hydrocephalus may develop.

Mental impairment is one of the common features of the disease. Idiocy is rare. More often the defect is first noticed between the ages of 5 and 15 years. The child may merely cease to learn, and retain any acquirements he possesses, or he may lose his memory and become slowly demented.

Vision is often defective because of atrophy of the optic nerve, of choroidoretinitis or simply of interstitial keratitis, and bilateral deafness is not uncommon. Affections of the remaining cranial nerves are rare.

Juvenile general paralysis appears most often between the ages of 10 and 17 years. It has been seen as early as the eighth, and as late as the thirtieth year. In some cases it results from congenital syphilis, in others from syphilis acquired in childhood. The physical signs are the same as in the adult form. The mental symptoms, as might be expected, differ from those in adults, because of the age of onset. Optic atrophy is common in juvenile cases, and signs of tabes are often present.

Juvenile tabes has the same features as in adults. It is, however, uncommon in its pure form because most cases begin with optic atrophy and go on to taboparesis. Diagnosis rarely causes any difficulty.

One or more courses of penicillin should be given until the cell content of the cerebrospinal fluid becomes and remains normal, but there is always persisting disability.

REFERENCES

ADAMS, R. D., and MERRITT, H. H. (1944) Meningeal and vascular syphilis of the spinal cord, *Medicine (Baltimore)*, **23**, 181.

BEERMAN, H., NICHOLS, L., SCHAMBERG, I. L., and GREENBERG, M. S. (1962) Syphilis, *Arch. intern. Med.*, **109**, 323.

GARSON, W. (1959) Recent developments in the laboratory diagnosis of syphilis, *Arch. intern. Med.*, **51**, 748.

HASSIN, G. B. (1929) Tabes dorsalis, *Arch. Neurol. Psychiat. (Chic.)*, **21**, 311.

LORBER, J. (1960) Treatment of tuberculous meningitis, *Brit. med. J.*, **1**, 1309.

MCKENDRICK, G. D. W. (1954) Pyogenic meningitis, *Lancet*, ii, 510.

MERRITT, H. H., and MOORE, M. (1935) Acute syphilitic meningitis, *Medicine (Baltimore)*, **14**, 119.

NICOL, W. D. (1948) Neurosyphilis, *Postgrad. med. J.*, **24**, 25.

NICOL, W. D., and HUTTON, E. L. (1935) Some clinical aspects of general paralysis, *J. ment. Sci.*, **81**, 804.

TUCKER, H. A., MOHR, C. F., HAHN, R. D., and MOORE, J. E. (1949) Syphilis, *Arch. intern Med.*, **83**, 77, 197.

ENCEPHALITIS

Inflammation of the brain happens under widely different clinical conditions. It may be a primary disease or a complication of known infective processes, affecting the system locally or generally, or seen as an associated event in diseases of the meninges. As a primary condition it is found in a variety of virus diseases of the nervous system. It is found as the result of infection of the brain with pyogenic organisms, either from local sources of infection in the neighbourhood of the brain or from pyaemia, and it may then be either suppurative (brain abscess) or non-suppurative. It may occur as a complication of many of the acute specific fevers, especially measles, vaccinia and mumps. In these the encephalitis may only be a part of a general inflammation of the nervous system—an encephalomyelitis. Acute encephalitis may be found in rare cases as the sole manifestation of cerebral syphilis.

In all forms of meningitis there is some degree of extension of the inflammation into the brain tissue, and this is marked in tuberculous meningitis and in some cases of meningococcal meningitis.

When the clinical evidences suggest disorder of the hemispheres alone the term 'encephalitis' is properly applied, but, such qualifications as 'meningo-encephalitis', 'encephalomyelitis' or 'meningo-encephalomyelitis' are often more accurate. It is wise to remember that the infection is invariably more widespread than appears—in acute anterior poliomyelitis, for example, although the effects are seen in the anterior horn cell destruction, changes are widespread in brain and cord.

A practical division of encephalitis is into;

1. Local (abscess or thrombophlebitis).
2. Generalized.
   (a) Suppurative.
   (b) Non-suppurative (virus): specific (of known type); non-specific.
   (c) Unknown nature, e.g. inclusion body encephalitis.

Non-specific encephalitis or encephalomyelitis may follow upper respiratory infections. The primary illness will be quite mild and unremarkable, the encephalitis appearing within a week of its peak. It is most unusual for a virus to be identified, and the question is unanswered whether the brain is involved in a related virus infection or whether there is, rather, a tissue reaction of a specialized kind of the central nervous system to the chemical consequences of the illness. In short, it is not known whether unspecific encephalitis is due to an unidentified virus or not.

When a virus is identified, the timing of the reaction of the central nervous system to it suggests that parenchymal damage occurs because of the intense antigen-antibody reaction within the cell rather than to the virus particles *per se*.

The symptoms common to all forms of encephalitis are the general symptoms of severe intracranial disease —headache, somnolence, coma, irritability, delirium, convulsions and vomiting; and, in addition, local symptoms of irritation and paralysis, the precise nature of which is determined by the position and extent of the lesions.

CEREBRAL ABSCESS

Synonym. Suppurative encephalitis.

Aetiology

Suppuration within the brain is never primary, but is the result of extension of infection from neighbouring tissues or through the blood stream from foci of infection in distant organs. In rare cases, the original focus of infection is undiscoverable.

The following are the important causal factors:

1. *Direct infection* from infected regions in the immediate vicinity. The important cause is any form of infective disease in the bones or soft tissues of the head and neck. From 60 to 70 per cent. of all cerebral abscesses arise in this way. The most common cause is infection of the nasal and aural structures. Infections of the bones of the skull, of the sinuses, of the scalp, orbital cellulitis, carbuncles of the neck and face are other causes. The organisms responsible are commonly streptococcus, pneumococcus or staphylococcus. The infection may be mixed. Other pyogenic organisms may be found, and rare cases are caused by streptothrix and other organisms.

2. *Pyaemic states*. Abscesses resulting from blood-borne infection make 20 to 25 per cent. of the total. They commonly arise as a complication of chronic suppuration in the chest, such as bronchiectasis, empyema or lung abscess. Less often they are a complication of chronic bone disease, puerperal septicaemia, acute infective endocarditis or other septicaemic conditions. Subacute bacterial endocarditis may lead to multiple embolic foci of encephalitis but not to actual abscess formation.

Metastatic abscesses are commonly multiple but may be solitary. The organisms responsible are streptococcus, staphylococcus and pneumococcus, and mixed infections may occur.

3. *Trauma*. Traumatic abscesses may result from penetrating wounds of the skull, particularly when fragments of metal, clothing, bone and scalp are carried into the brain. Fracture of the base of the skull may permit infection to gain access to the brain from the middle ear or nasopharynx. Fractures involving the inner wall of the frontal sinuses or cribriform plate may be followed by the development of a cerebral abscess after a long latent interval.

Pathology

Cerebral abscess—whether adjacent or metastatic in origin—usually starts at the junction of the cortex and the subcortical white matter. As it increases in size the surrounding brain tissue is displaced and severe distortion of the brain and ventricular system results. The commonest site is the temporal lobe, and approximately half of all abscesses are found here, a reflection of the importance of middle-ear disease as an aetiological factor. The frontal lobes and the cerebellum are other areas frequently affected.

The earliest stages of the development of a cerebral abscess seldom come under direct observation but the initial lesion is in an area of encephalitis around the nidus of invading organisms. The process can be reversed at this stage by the early use of antibiotics. Gradually liquefaction and pus formation take place in the centre, while a fibroblastic reaction at the periphery gives rise to the abscess wall. Outside this again is a neurological proliferation together with a diffuse inflammatory infiltration of the brain substance and perivascular spaces.

Symptoms

A cerebral abscess constitutes, when developed, a foreign body within the skull. Death may result from the effects of continually increasing intracranial pressure and wide interference with cerebral function, or from the spread of the infection from the abscess to the meninges and general subarachnoid space. The symptoms are: (1) those of local suppuration; (2) those of increased intracranial pressure; (3) localizing signs dependent upon the position of the abscess; and (4) those of the terminal extension of the infective process.

The onset is insidious and is apt to be overshadowed by those of the preceding disease. The usual sequence is that a case of mastoid suppuration or frontal sinusitis does not progress quite as well as it should do as judged by the local condition, and gradually the picture of cerebral abscess makes its appearance without it ever being possible to state with certainty where the original illness ended and the complication began. Similarly with blood-borne infections it is seldom possible to decide when an abscess began to form.

The first and most constant symptom is frontal and occipital headache, irrespective of the site of the abscess, especially on rising in the morning and made worse by coughing, sneezing or stooping. Occasionally, whilst a slowly developing abscess is forming, there may be periods lasting a day or two of intense occipital pain, nuchal rigidity, vomiting and fever. Vomiting is early and usually occurs with the headaches but, especially in cases of cerebellar abscess, it may arise suddenly and with great violence in the absence of any other symptoms. Mental changes are common. These vary from slight lassitude and a vague feeling of unwellness to drowsiness and ultimately coma. Double vision, usually an intermittent uncrossed diplopia on lateral deviation of the eyes, results from weakness of one or both external recti.

Symptoms of focal disturbance of the nervous system are less constant and usually later in occurrence than those of general intracranial disorder. Fits, focal or general, may occur. There may be weakness on one side of the body or in one limb, or sensory disturbances of a similar distribution. Hemianopia and disturbances of speech are common. Where the cerebellum is involved the patient may be aware of awkwardness of voluntary movement, particularly with regard to standing and walking, and there is intense giddiness.

The patient usually has a sallow complexion with a slightly cyanotic tint about the lips and nose. The tongue is coated, the breath offensive, the lips dry. The temperature is often raised but seldom higher than 100° F. (37·8° C.) and is often subnormal for a day or 2 days at a stretch. When above 101° F. (38·3° C.) it will usually be found that this rise is coincident with symptoms of meningism. The pulse is slow and in no intracranial condition with the possible exception of extradural haemorrhage is this depression so constant as in cerebral abscess. With the bradycardia is a less striking fall in the respiration rate.

The mental state is one of irritable drowsiness. Left alone the patient will remain quiet with eyes closed, only rousing to cry out with intense headache.

Papilloedema may come on with great rapidity and attain 3 to 4 dioptres of swelling with numerous haemorrhages during the course of a few days. It may continue to increase in severity for some days after the abscess has been drained or even appear for the first time during this period. Some degree of neck rigidity and a weakly positive Kernig's sign are usual, particularly when the abscess is situated in the cerebellum or when an appreciable degree of meningeal reaction is present. Local tenderness of the skull to firm pressure or percussion is a common finding and may afford valuable help in localizing the abscess in doubtful cases. The patient almost always looks very ill.

Localizing signs will naturally vary with the position of the abscess. Temporal abscess usually begins in the inferior portion of the lobe and extends upwards and forwards. When on the left side one of the earliest focal disturbances to occur is disorder of speech. At first this takes the form of difficulty, then of inability to name objects correctly; later, difficulty in understanding spoken and written language and paraphasia make their appearance. Naturally speech disturbances are not found in right-sided temporal lobe abscesses except in strongly left-handed persons. Another early sign of temporal abscess is disturbance of the contralateral fields of vision. This nearly always takes the form of a congruous upper quadrantic hemianopia which gradually spreads to involve the lower quadrants until a complete hemianopia is present. As the abscess extends forward towards the motor projection fibres weakness of the opposite side of the face of a supranuclear type develops, to be followed by similar weakness of the contralateral arm and then of the leg until a complete hemiparesis may be present with characteristic increase in the tendon reflexes, diminution or loss of the abdominal reflexes and an extensor plantar response. Contralateral sensory disturbances are late and uncommon. Fits may occur.

Abscesses in the frontal lobes are, on the whole, more silent than those in the temporal lobes. Whether adjacent or metastatic in origin they are prefrontal and may attain a large size without producing any localizing signs. Mental changes of the kind already mentioned may be a conspicuous feature. Apathy and forgetfulness are marked and early incontinence common. As the abscess extends backwards a contralateral hemiparesis develops involving face and arm before the leg, and if the lesion is on the left side, an increasing degree of executive aphasia may be in evidence in normal persons.

Abscesses are rare in the parietal and occipital lobes. Except as a complication of osteomyelitis of the skull they are almost invariably metastatic. The most important local signs that they cause are contralateral sensory loss of a cortical type in the case of parietal lobe abscesses and defects in the contralateral fields of vision in those situated in the occipital region. In either case epileptic attacks may occur.

Cerebellar abscesses often present great difficulties in localization. The general symptomatology is much the same as in cases where the abscess is situated above the tentorium, though on the whole the mental alteration is less and the vomiting and occipital pain more marked in cerebellar cases. Nystagmus is almost invariable and weakness of lower motor neurone type on the same side of the face is often present. Both these signs, however, may be found in cases with a localized area of meningitis in the posterior fossa without any abscess within the cerebellum itself. The most reliable sign is hypotonia and inco-ordination of movement of the limbs on the same side. In bed these changes are most readily detected in the arms but, if the patient is well enough to walk, the inco-ordination may be evident in the gait. It is by no means unusual for a cerebellar abscess to be present for many weeks without producing any detectable localizing signs while the general condition of the patient leaves little room for doubt as to the presence of an abscess somewhere.

Although the cerebrospinal fluid is always abnormal, lumbar puncture should never be undertaken. It is likely to be fatal, because the very high pressure forces the brain stem down into the foramen magnum. The localization of the abscess follows the same course as that of a tumour, clinical signs being supplemented by electroencephalography, angiography, and gamma encephalography, but the abscess is ultimately localized by blunt needles introduced through anterior and posterior burr holes on both sides if necessary. Sensitivity testing of the organism isolated and appropriate antibiotic therapy are essential.

Diagnosis

The diagnosis of cerebral abscess has to be made from other complications of suppuration in the vicinity of the brain, and from other expanding intracranial lesions, particularly cerebral tumour.

The varieties of intracranial complication of neighbourhood suppuration most likely to be confused with cerebral abscess are:

1. Acute spreading meningitis.
2. Localized meningitis, with or without an extradural abscess.
3. Infective venous sinus thrombosis.

1. *Acute spreading meningitis*. This differential diagnosis is not difficult. The high, sustained fever, rapid pulse, delirium and marked neck rigidity all make the recognition of acute meningitis easy. Difficulty arises when a cerebral abscess is causing a brisk meningeal reaction and actual infection of the subarachnoid space is imminent. Then the symptoms and signs of the two diseases are likely to be superimposed on one another.

2. *Localized meningitis*. This affords a difficult problem in diagnosis from a cerebral abscess. An acute infection on the outer aspect of the dura, especially if there is also an extradural abscess, causes a brisk local inflammatory reaction of the leptomeninges on its inner aspect. This local area of meningitis may produce the same symptoms and signs as an abscess and if it involves the base of the brain may also cause all the signs of raised intracranial pressure by obstructing the normal circulation of cerebrospinal fluid. In otitic cases this is particularly likely to occur in the posterior fossa. The condition tends to be more acute than an abscess and the symptoms and signs are more fluctuant; the temperature is usually higher and the pulse rate more rapid, and the signs of meningeal irritation more marked. The central nervous signs are those which might be expected from a lesion on the surface, rather than in the substance of the brain; for example there will probably be cranial nerve palsies. This localized meningitis can undergo complete resolution with antibiotics, but on the other hand, it may be the prelude of a general meningeal spread. Fortunately a favourable response to a broad-based antibiotic may simultaneously cure the patient and exclude an abscess.

3. *Infective venous sinus thrombosis*. This condition causes a high, swinging fever with frequent rigors, intense toxaemia and the other evidences of a pyaemic but probably viral state. There are no signs of raised intracranial pressure or of local disturbance of brain function. It happens especially in young children and may complicate specific fevers, for instance measles, as well as other pyogenic infections.

Treatment

The treatment of cerebral abscess is inevitably surgical and antibiotic. The condition is one of the greatest urgency, as death may occur at any moment. Transfer to a neurosurgical unit is, of course, desirable because of the need for full diagnostic facilities; but without them exploration with a brain needle may localize the abscess. Recovery is rarely complete for there is general local damage, and about half the patients develop epilepsy later.

OTHER INFECTIONS

Many organisms which infest the brain secondarily to invasion elsewhere have been dealt with in the appropriate section of the text. Those which need special mention are *malaria* [Section 2] which may cause an acute encephalitis (cerebral malaria) which may be fatal. There is a meningeal reaction, coma and convulsions. *Schistosomiasis* [Section 2] may cause granulomatous deposit to give a syndrome like that of a chronic abscess, whilst the myositic illness of *trichinosis* [Section 2] is rarely associated with acute encephalitis. An unusual form of infestation of the brain is that of *toxoplasmosis* [Section 2]. This widespread minute protozoon very rarely infests the foetus and invades the eye and the brain especially, to cause granulomatous masses which fibrose and calcify. Blindness is caused by chorioretinitis and optic atrophy, and mental defect, epilepsy and hydrocephalus by the intracranial masses, which are often apparent radiologically. The disease may be evident at birth or appear in early childhood, death being usual in months or a few years. *Behçet's syndrome*, a rare disease of unknown nature, is mentioned here because the central nervous system is occasionally involved [see Section 4]. Behçet described this disorder in 1937, but since then many examples with polyneuritis, cranial nerve palsies and meningo-encephalitis have been described. Though the disease itself often remits, when the brain is involved death is usual.

ENCEPHALITIS ASSOCIATED WITH ACUTE SPECIFIC FEVERS

Aetiology

Acute encephalitis may occur as a rare complication of a number of acute specific fevers, especially of the exanthemata. In some cases the brain alone may be involved but in others the nervous system may be more widely affected and the picture is rather that of an encephalomyelitis. The fevers most commonly associated with this complication are measles (about 1:3,000) and vaccinia (about 1:10,000) but it occurs also with variola, scarlatina, mumps and varicella and many other acute febrile disorders. The incidence of encephalitic complications of these diseases varies noticeably from time to time.

The relationship of the encephalitis to the preceding infection is not clear, nor the cerebral complications of the different exanthemata identical. The hypothesis that the exanthem merely serves to activate some unknown causative agent, such as a latent virus, is without confirmation. It must also be borne in mind that all cerebral complications of acute fevers are not necessarily encephalitic but may result from vascular occlusion by thrombosis or embolism, or from haemorrhage, or from meningitis.

There is increasing evidence that these encephalitides are the result of a specific tissue reaction of the central nervous system to the invading virus. An antigen-antibody reaction in turn causes widespread changes in parenchymal and supporting tissue alike. This tissue reaction can be mimicked by introduction of tissue protein into monkeys.

Pathology

A number of cases of encephalitis following measles and vaccinia have been subjected to pathological examination and have shown a constant condition of the nervous system, and the much rarer examples following other fevers have generally conformed to this picture. The brain and spinal cord show diffuse congestion, particularly of the white matter, sometimes causing petechial haemorrhages. Numerous areas of acute demyelination occur, particularly in the perivascular zones. These are so constant as to have suggested the title 'perivascular myelinoclasis' for this group of disorders. In addition there is a marked perivascular infiltration with round cells, and a more diffuse cellular reaction in the nervous tissue with mobilization of microglia and proliferation of the astrocytes.

The upper brain stem, the medial temporal lobes and the limbic system are especially involved in this reaction.

Symptoms

The time of onset of encephalitic symptoms is fairly constant in each exanthem. In measles it is commonest towards the end of the first week, in vaccinia from 10 to 14 days after the vaccination, and in variola during the second week of the eruption. Common symptoms are drowsiness or stupor, increasing in severe cases to coma, headache, convulsions, cranial nerve palsies, dysarthria and dysphagia, and in some cases myoclonic or choreiform movements. One of the most striking features of these disorders is the patient's mental state. He appears to be conscious but is unresponsive and shows no spontaneous movement. This state of akinesis with mutism or stupor is due to diffuse involvement of the midbrain and is often accompanied by supranuclear disturbances of eye movement. Slight signs of meningeal irritation, such as neck rigidity, irritability and photophobia, may occur and there may be an increase in the fever. Papilloedema may develop. In cases associated with myelitis marked weakness in the legs with patchy sensory loss and retention of urine is common. Loss of the abdominal and tendon reflexes and extensor plantar responses are frequent. The cerebrospinal fluid is commonly under increased pressure, and may show an increase in protein content with a mild lymphocytosis (10–50 per mm^3.) although the absence of pleocytosis does not exclude the diagnosis. The Lange colloidal gold reaction may be strongly positive and sometimes paretic in character. The content of sugar and chlorides is normal.

Diagnosis

The occurrence of symptoms of this order in childhood and early adult life at the significant period of the different diseases makes the diagnosis, in most cases, clear. It should be remembered, however, that acute fevers in children may determine the moment of onset of tuberculous meningitis, and that vascular disorders may occur in a similar setting.

Treatment

This is usually symptomatic, for antibiotics are only of use for infectious complications. Corticosteroids have been widely used but in any one case it is difficult to assess their efficiency, for in the great majority recovery will take place spontaneously. Trials suggest that the time to that recovery is shortened by the use of steroids. There is also evidence that ACTH may be more effective than corticosteroids. The general practice is to use ACTH, 40 Units intramuscularly, during the acute reaction of almost a week, and then slowly to reduce the amount and cease treatment.

Prognosis

In patients who do not die in coma or convulsions during the first week, recovery is the rule and usually remarkably complete. Residual paralyses are exceptional. In a small number of cases some residual intellectual impairment may result and in other cases a liability to fits. The mortality in vaccinal cases is from 25 to 40 per cent.; that in measles and the other common exanthemata very much lower.

ENCEPHALITIS DUE TO KNOWN VIRUSES

Epidemics of encephalitis and of encephalomyelitis happen in the summer especially, and more usually in hot climates. From time to time a virus is isolated, studied, and transmitted to animals. Some of these viruses such as the ECHO, a Coxsackie and herpes simplex are endemic, but others, such as those causing Japanese B encephalitis, St. Louis or equine encephalomyelitis are not. They are dealt with in Section 2, and the syndromes they produce, which vary greatly in severity from case to case, are the same as the encephalitides and encephalomyelitides.

ENCEPHALITIS DUE TO 'SLOW' VIRUSES

There is accumulating evidence that some diseases of the nervous system, long believed to be of degenerative origin, are due to a peculiar form of viral infection. The usual histological features of inflammation are lacking, and in all the incubation period is long and the clinical course protracted.

Interest in this possibility was first aroused when scrapie, a disease of sheep with histopathological similarities to disseminated sclerosis, proved transmissible to goats and certain rodents. No virus has yet been isolated from these animals.

There is now established proof that subacute inclusion body encephalitis in man is due to a 'slow' virus infection with measles virus, and it seems likely that kuru and Creutzfeldt-Jakob disease may be included in this group.

Kuru is an endemic disease of certain tribes of the central highlands of New Guinea, affecting particularly women and children. There is a gradual onset of cerebellar ataxia, followed by dementia with death in 3–6 months.

The cerebrospinal fluid remains normal and the pathological changes are a diffuse neuronal degeneration with proliferation of astrocytes. Inoculation of brain tissue from patients dying of kuru into chimpanzees is followed, after an incubation period of 18 months to 4 years, by a similar disease. Passage to other chimpanzees has been accomplished.

The disease has virtually disappeared since the suppression of ritual cannibalism in the tribes formerly affected, and there is good reason to suppose that this was the mode of transmission.

Creutzfeldt-Jakob disease is a rare disorder of middle life in which rapidly progressive dementia is accompanied by symmetrical myoclonic spasms and sometimes by cerebellar ataxia. It is usually fatal within a year. Inoculation into chimpanzees of brain tissue from patients dying of this disease causes a like disorder and similar histopathological changes in the nervous system. The incubation period is about a year.

Subacute inclusion body encephalitis or *subacute sclerosing leuco-encephalitis* has only been observed in children and adolescents and has been reported by Dawson, Van Bogaert, Foley and Williams.

Pathologically it is characterized by the presence of inclusion bodies in the nerve cells, regarded as the hallmark of virus diseases together with polioclasis and neuronophagia. Together with this is a degree of demyelinization and sclerosis of the white matter reminiscent of the leuco-encephalitides of the Schilder type. With the electron microscope virus patterns identical with those of measles have been identified within brain neurones, and the antibody titre against measles virus is found to rise steadily throughout the illness. The identification of this subacute or chronic degenerative disease with persisting infection with measles has now been proved by the isolation of measles virus from brain biopsies.

Clinically the disorder runs a progressive acute or subacute course towards a fatal termination. The earliest symptom is usually mental deterioration often associated with epileptic manifestations. Later, involuntary movements of various kinds occur and the child gradually develops dementia with the picture of bilateral rigidity of extrapyramidal type with relatively few pyramidal signs until death occurs at a stage of profound dementia with akinesis and contractures. The clinical course is a phasic one with episodes of myoclonus especially in response to being startled. The electroencephalogram shows dramatic phasic changes, too, and the cerebrospinal fluid always has a 'paretic' Lange gold curve, though the Wassermann reaction is negative.

NON-SPECIFIC ENCEPHALOMYELITIS

A clinical picture of encephalitis or encephalomyelitis identical in its presentation and in its pathological nature to that following acute exanthemata, just described, may occur sporadically, and especially after upper respiratory infections. In late childhood and in early adult life acute bronchitis, bronchopneumonia and even chronic bronchitis, may be followed by an acute neurological illness in which the association of mental changes with lowering of consciousness, and brain stem or spinal cord signs will suggest widespread and patchy disorder of the central nervous system. The condition must be differentiated from other acute infections, from meningitis and from intoxications. It may resemble disseminated sclerosis, but in that condition it is rare to find such severe disorder of consciousness or the absence of tendon jerks. The course and management of these non-specific encephalitides is identical with those of the specific group already described.

REFERENCES

BOGAERT, L. VAN (1959) Acute encephalitis in childhood, *Brit. med. J.*, **1**, 1201.

EVANS, A. D., PALLIS, C. A., and SPILLANE, J. D. (1957) Involvement of the nervous system in Behçet's syndrome. Report of three cases and isolation of the virus, *Lancet*, **ii**, 349.

FOLEY, J., and WILLIAMS, D. (1953) Inclusion encephalitis and its relation to subacute sclerosing leuco-encephalitis, *Quart. J. Med.*, **22**, 157.

GREGORY, D. H., MESSNER, R., and ZINNEMAN, H. H. (1967) Metastatic brain abscess: A retrospective appraisal of 29 patients, *Arch. intern. Med.*, **119**, 25.

HORNABROOK, R. W. (1968) Kuru. A subacute cerebellar degeneration—the natural history and clinical features, *Brain*, **91**, 53.

JOHNSON, R. T., and JOHNSON, K. P. (1969) Slow and chronic virus infections of the nervous system, in *Recent Advances in Neurology*, ed. Plum, F., Philadelphia.

KERR, F. W. L., KING, R. B., and MEAGHER, J. N. (1958) Brain abscess, *J. Amer. med. Ass.*, **168**, 868.

LYON, G., DODGE, P. R., and ADAMS, R. D. (1961) The acute encephalopathies of obscure origin in infants and children, *Brain*, **84**, 680.

METZ, H., GREGORIOU, M., and SANDIFER, P. (1964) Subacute sclerosing panencephalitis. A review of 17 cases with special reference to clinical diagnostic criteria, *Arch. Dis. Childh.*, **39**, 554.

MEYER, J. S., BAUER, R. B., RIVERAOLMOS, V. M., NOLAN, D. C., and LERNER, A. M. (1970) *Herpes virus hominis* encephalitis. Neurological manifestations and use of idoxuridine, *Arch. Neurol.*, **23**, 438.

MILLER, H. G., STANTON, J. B., and GIBBONS, J. L. (1956) Para-infectious encephalomyelitis and related syndromes, *Quart. J. Med.*, **25**, 427.

MILLER, J. D., and ROSS, C. A. C. (1968) Encephalitis: A four year survey, *Lancet*, **i**, 1121.

NORTHFIELD, D. W. C. (1942) The treatment of brain abscess, *J. Neurol. Psychiat.*, **5**, 1.

PENNYBACKER, J. B. (1948) Cerebellar abscess, *J. Neurol. Neurosurg. Psychiat.*, **11**, 1.

THIRUVENGADAM, L. V. (1959) Disseminated encephalomyelitis after influenza, *Brit. med. J.*, **2**, 1233.

WADIA, N., and WILLIAMS, E. (1957) Behçet's syndrome with neurological complications, *Brain*, **80**, 59.

VASCULAR DISORDERS OF THE NERVOUS SYSTEM

ISCHAEMIA AND HAEMORRHAGE

There has been a remarkable revival of interest in, and research into, cerebrovascular disease. Previously cerebral thrombosis, haemorrhage and embolus causing 'strokes' were regarded as the inevitable consequence of disease of the heart or blood vessels, and their results were accepted in a fatalistic way. The results of a stroke in the living were equated with the disorder of structure seen in the post-mortem room and in fixed pathological specimens, and the attitude to these disasters was as fixed as the specimens upon which it had been based. The change in this attitude, from a passive non-dynamic one, was due to a number of simultaneously evolving techniques. Probably the most evocative was arteriography which showed that the basis of many firmly held views was faulty. Then there was the opportunity to pursue cerebrovascular surgery in a controlled way through the time gained for the surgeon by the use of hypothermic techniques, and the associated development of positive pressure anaesthesia, and lastly there was the stimulus provided by the hopes for therapy with anticoagulants.

The most important advance was the discovery of marked discrepancies between what actually happens in life and what had been thought to happen on the basis of morbid anatomical study. It was, for instance, discovered that the obstructive lesion might be remote from its central effects, that the obstructions found might not be the immediate cause of those effects, and that complete occlusion of one or more of the great vessels in the neck was compatible with normal function within the central nervous system.

VASCULAR INSUFFICIENCY

From a static idea of cessation of neural function as the result of cessation of blood flow (complete ischaemia) due to thrombosis or embolus, there rapidly grew up the idea of reduction of flow occurring as a result of several dynamic factors operating together. Inherent in this change in attitude was the rediscovery of the importance of collateral flow, not only in the circle of Willis, but also through small peripheral vessels within the territory of the diseased parent artery. There was, too, the rediscovery of the high frequency of anomalies—that is to say deviations from the formal pattern of vessels stylized in textbooks—within the cerebrovascular tree.

In practice, for instance, disturbance of function resembling that of thrombosis of the middle cerebral artery may result from stenosis of the common carotid artery within the neck, or even from atheroma at its origin from the aorta or subclavian trunk. Again, a varying right hemiplegia may result from increasing stenosis of the right internal carotid artery in a patient who had for years been living with complete occlusion of the left, the collateral flow from the homolateral side being ultimately inadequate for the needs of both hemispheres.

In the days when it was presumed that all vascular disasters within the central nervous system were the result of thrombosis, embolus or haemorrhage, clinicians were perplexed by the rapid recovery of some from severe strokes. To account for this they postulated a state of vascular spasm of a transient nature but there is no pathological support for this hypothesis. The view is now held that transient ischaemia of the cerebral hemispheres and of the brain stem is a common event in the second half of life, and that a reduction in the speed of blood flow below a critical level offers an adequate explanation for many of the transient though severe disorders of neural function which are encountered in practice. Active thrombosis of cerebral vessels is much less common than diminished flow through them, although of course this diminished flow may be the result of stenosis or occlusion of a large vessel between the heart and the brain. Contributory factors in the development of these symptoms include essential hypotension; hypotension due to disturbance elsewhere in the body, aggravated by such states as fatigue, sleep, postprandial deviations, dehydration, postural change or pain; anaemia and the blood diseases; and cardiac insufficiency including coronary artery ischaemia. Finally relative hypotension due to treatment of hypertension by the use of hypotensive agents is a fruitful source of these syndromes. Whereas the cardiologist may wish to lower the blood pressure to protect the heart, the neurologist may wish to keep it high to maintain adequate flow of blood to the brain and brain stem.

The word insufficiency, linked as in 'carotid artery insufficiency' or 'basilar insufficiency' reflects the wish to imply a dynamic event resulting in diminished blood flow, rather than a static and continuing one. As the results of insufficiency of flow through peripheral vessels are similar to, though more transient than the effects of their occlusion through thrombosis, the more static syndromes of thrombosis will be described first.

Another explanation for the transient disturbances of function caused by alteration in blood flow is the circulation of minute emboli, sometimes made up entirely of platelets, which break off from the tip of a mural thrombus. These may be seen in the retina, and it has been shown that because of the effects of streaming of flow that emboli from the same source may repeatedly end up in the same small cerebral artery.

Aetiology and Pathology

Cerebral ischaemia and thrombosis are almost always the result of atheroma. Syphilis, once a common cause, is now a great rarity. Polyarteritis nodosa and other unusual arterial diseases are occasionally responsible. Cerebral haemorrhage is almost constantly associated with arterial hypertension and arteriosclerosis, and is much less often due to the rupture of an aneurysm or angiomatous formation; occasionally it occurs in the course of a generalized haemorrhagic state, particularly acute leukaemia and acute idiopathic thrombocytopenic purpura.

Both haemorrhage and thrombosis occur in association with rapidly growing cerebral tumours, with diffuse or localized inflammatory disease of the brain, and with head injuries.

Thrombosis is a much more common cause of strokes than is haemorrhage, but it is not nearly so often fatal. Many spontaneous intracerebral haemorrhages cause death within a few hours. In many cases, however—perhaps the majority of those which are clinically ascribed to cerebral thrombosis—actual thrombosis does not occur, but cerebral tissue to which the circulation has been inadequate for a long time eventually undergoes softening rather abruptly. There is little essential difference between the two groups of cases, and it used to be customary to apply the term cerebral thrombosis to all.

A stroke due to thrombosis may have an ingravescent onset, especially when clotting occurs in distal branches of an artery and extends towards the main vessel; or it may have a sudden onset when the clotting occurs primarily in a large artery. The immediate effect of the thrombosis is a condition of infarction with oedema, which causes the loss of consciousness so commonly seen a few hours after the apoplexy has occurred. The oedema tends to pass off in a few days, and the area bereft of circulation becomes narrowed by collateral flow from surrounding regions, which speeds recovery of function. The affected area becomes soft and shrunken. Finally, much of the softened tissue becomes necrotic and is absorbed, leaving one or several cystic cavities. An arterial thrombosis occurring at an early age may result in a porencephaly. Cavities found in cases of apoplexy after years have elapsed, are too often attributed to haemorrhage; in reality they are nearly all due to thrombosis. The cerebrospinal fluid in recent thrombosis is never found to contain blood, but a little later it is often coloured yellow or yellowish-brown from escape of changed blood pigments, when the lesion has reached the surface of the convexity or the surface of the ventricle, and pleocytosis may be found.

Haemorrhage, which is usually described as apoplexy of sudden onset, may be so when the escape is from a large artery. When the bleeding is from a smaller vessel, the symptoms are not sudden in their onset, but gather rapidly. Such a haemorrhage is much like an avalanche. Starting from a small vessel the haemorrhage tears a small cavity, and in so doing opens up fresh bleeding points, and with increasing destruction more and more bleeding occurs from every piece of torn tissue, until the haemorrhage reaches such a size as to burst, commonly into the ventricle, or much more rarely on to the surface. Indeed, it is difficult to conceive how a haemorrhage into such a soft and vascular tissue as is the brain should ever stop. As a matter of fact, it rarely does so, but causes death in the first attack of haemorrhagic apoplexy, within from a few hours to a few days after the onset.

Haemorrhage may occur anywhere within the nervous system, but its common seat of origin is in the centrum semiovale, and the vessel which bursts is one of the perforating arteries, of which the lenticulostriate—the 'artery of haemorrhage'—is the most common. Such bleedings are often called 'capsular haemorrhages' referring to the region outside the corpus striatum or external capsule, and not to the compact internal capsule as it converges to the crus cerebri. The cerebrospinal fluid in cases of haemorrhage contains blood within a very short time of the onset.

While both thrombosis and haemorrhage may occur in any part of the brain, the centrum ovale, the calcarine region and the pons are the common sites of both of them in that order of frequency. Haemorrhage is rare except in these regions, while thrombosis is seen elsewhere.

Symptoms and Diagnosis

The carotid system. The features of a stroke will depend upon the site of the vascular lesion and upon its nature—whether due to reduction in flow, complete occlusion by thrombus or embolus, or the result of haemorrhage. As the centrum ovale is the commonest site, and as many arteries supply the fibres of the pyramidal tract in different parts of its course, hemiplegia is the common result: if the lesion is in the left hemisphere some degree of aphasia is commonly associated.

Thrombosis of the *anterior cerebral artery* which is uncommon in its distal portion causes paralysis and postural sensory loss in the contralateral leg, but if the vessel is thrombosed proximal to the origin of the artery of Heubner—which supplies part of the anterior limb of the internal capsule—the contralateral arm and face are also affected, so that hemiplegia results.

The *middle cerebral artery* becomes thrombosed as commonly as all the other cranial vessels put together but it is rarely thrombosed as a whole. Thrombosis of the whole of this artery causes such extensive destruction in the corresponding cerebral hemisphere that the most severe hemiplegia, with postural loss and hemianopia results, accompanied by severe aphasia if the lesion is on the left side.

Both of these arteries may be involved when thrombosis occurs in the *internal* or *common carotid artery*. The frequency of this condition has been disclosed by arteriography. In such a large artery the clot is at first mural and portions of it may break off and cause emboli in branches of the derived arteries. When the lumen of the internal carotid artery becomes completely obstructed the anterior and middle cerebral arteries continue to receive blood by the circle of Willis, and even the ophthalmic artery receives enough blood to prevent blindness. While the middle and anterior cerebral arteries may remain patent the blood supply to them through the circle of Willis may be inadequate and, especially in elderly subjects, successive softenings of greater or less degree may therefore occur in the hemisphere of the affected side. It is fairly common for two or more incidents of partial hemiplegia to occur, with intervals of days or weeks, or even months, between them. The severity of the clinical pictures which may result from carotid thrombosis is therefore very variable, but often the paralysis is surprisingly slight, and it is only by arteriography that the condition can be confidently diagnosed. In the worst cases, however, all the arteries derived from the internal carotid may be thrombosed and it may be fatal in the acute stage. In some instances both internal carotid arteries have been found to be occluded, to cause dementia. There is evidence that the thrombosed carotid artery may become recanalized. Many patients who suffer from carotid thrombosis are men in the first half of life and trauma to the neck may be an important aetiological factor; in older patients the condition is usually associated with atheroma. When collateral flow from the homolateral carotid artery through the circle of Willis has compensated for the occlusion there may be from time to time transient ischaemic episodes depending upon changes in the subject's general state, alluded to in the Introduction. Thus fluctuating hemiplegic or monoplegic symptoms may appear to be called 'stuttering hemiplegia'.

In the common stroke where the lesion is in the area of the middle cerebral artery and the local sign of the lesion is hemiplegia, it will be obvious that when the rise in general intracranial pressure becomes severe and the coma deep, the hemiplegia becomes less apparent, or masked by the universal condition of paralysis consequent upon the general intracranial condition. The physician often sees the patient for the first time when there is deep coma, and he must determine upon which side the lesion is situated, and what is its prime cause.

The following points help to localize the lesion side: (1) The paralytic conjugate deviation is towards the side of the lesion. (2) The corneal reflex, when any is present, is diminished or lost on the hemiplegic side. (3) Painful stimulation will give less response upon the hemiplegic side (hemianaesthesia). (4) The patient may respond by blinking to a feint made with the observer's hands towards the patient's eyes upon the sound side, and not on the hemiplegic side (hemianopia). (5) The limbs on the hemiplegic side when raised and allowed to fall passively, do so in a more lifeless, inert and flaccid fashion than upon the sound side. (6) And when there is any difference between the knee-jerks, abdominal reflexes and plantar reflexes, the former tend to be diminished and lost on the hemiplegic side while the plantar reflex will be of the extensor type on the hemiplegic side.

The severity of the lesion may be judged: (1) from the depth of the coma; (2) from the degree to which the patient responds to any form of stimulation and from the general signs of nervous depression present—for example, a condition of complete bilateral flaccidity with complete loss of all reflex action and of all response to stimulation indicates a most severe lesion; and (3) from signs of failure of respiration as shown by irregular, grouped or Cheyne-Stokes breathing. Vomiting may occur before coma becomes deep. Hyperpyrexia, which is especially common in pontine apoplexy, heralds death.

Hemiplegia is the commonest sequel of vascular lesions of the brain. After cerebral ischaemia the initial hemiplegia may completely recover but unless improvement begins early and progresses rapidly it is not likely to be complete. The essential feature of hemiplegia is flaccid weakness of one side followed by hypertonus, increased tendon jerks and associated movements. It may be transient and completely reversible with carotid artery insufficiency.

The restoration of movements follows a certain order. Deviation of the tongue and facial asymmetry clear up early; next the leg begins to recover; and finally—and often very incompletely—the arm. The return of movements in the limbs is selective. In both upper and lower limbs, movement at the proximal joints recovers first and most completely. In the leg, extension and plantar flexion recover more completely than flexion and dorsiflexion. As a result, the patient can often stand when he cannot lift the foot and leg to step properly, and has instead to circumduct the limb when walking. In the arm, flexion movements recover first and best, while the fine skilled movements of the hand and fingers are frequently lost for ever.

The development of hypertonus, or spasticity, is as selective as the return of movements. In the leg, the extensor group of muscles becomes spastic; in the arm, the flexor group. Thus, the arm tends to take up a position of adduction, with flexion at elbow, wrist and digits. The leg is always spastic in extension, and does not go into flexion contracture, as may happen in spastic paraplegia from spinal cord lesions. The degree of hypertonus varies, and is greatest when the loss of movement is greatest.

The so-called associated movements are involuntary changes of posture of the paralysed limbs which accompany forceful voluntary movements, or such involuntary movements as yawning.

The tendon-jerks are exaggerated, and there is clonus in the affected limbs. The extensor plantar response persists, but the abdominal reflexes, which are initially lost on the affected side, sometimes return after a period of months.

The forced immobility of shoulder and distal joints in the arm may lead to the formation of adhesions and to much pain, the so-called frozen shoulder.

The *vertebrobasilar system* is a common site of embarrassed flow, due to the long and vulnerable course of the vessels from the thorax through the bones of the cervical spine to the posterior fossa of the skull. As there are two parallel vertebral arteries, and as in ideal circumstances collateral flow can be developed when the whole basilar artery is occluded, fluctuating symptoms due to insufficiency of flow are common. Indeed as sudden occlusion of the basilar artery by thrombosis or embolus is as likely to cause death as is haemorrhage into the brain stem, the majority of syndromes with survival are due to basilar artery insufficiency, the acute thrombotic lesions compatible with survival being in the terminal branches, such as the posterior cerebral, superior cerebellar or posterior cerebellar arteries.

The common syndromes of *basilar artery insufficiency* include intermittent vertigo, aggravated by neck movement; visual disturbances including teichopsia (fortification spectra), scotomata or hemianopic field defects, often occurring with vertigo; diplopia; disorder of sensation in the face; fluctuating weakness of the legs and 'drop attacks'; and disorders of consciousness. The occurrence of groups of symptoms which can be explained by patchy ischaemia of the brain stem accompanied by visual perceptual changes, especially if they are intermittent, strongly suggests this cause. Total thrombosis of the basilar artery is usually fatal, though cases of survival are well recognized. They teach a lesson that if occlusion advances slowly enough, astonishing collateral circulation can be developed through an intact circle of Willis, the large branches of the vertebrobasilar system and the smaller pial vessels.

It is common to find that the artery responsible for a stroke is narrowed or occluded by a fibrosed, organized clot. This means that occlusion, though being ultimately responsible, could not possibly have been the immediate cause of the sudden stroke. There must have been operative factors responsible for failure of blood flow at the time.

When the *posterior cerebral artery* is thrombosed the outstanding sign is contralateral hemianopia with sparing of the fixation point. There may be no other symptoms.

Pontine ischaemia produces motor and sensory hemiplegia—first on one side and then on the other with the onset of coma; involvement of cranial nerve nuclei, e.g. with loss of lateral movements of the eyes—may be the first sign.

Cerebellar thrombosis and thrombosis of the *posterior inferior cerebellar artery* produce acute ataxia with forced movements, vertigo and vomiting.

Conjugate deviation of the eyes is a common feature of strokes. At its onset, there may be active conjugate deviation, the eyes being turned away from the side of the lesion, but this lasts a short while and is followed by a paralytic conjugate deviation in the opposite direction, both eyes being directed away from the paralysed side and towards the side of the lesion.

The pupils are often unequal; they may be contracted, or dilated widely, and may be insensitive to light. In severe apoplexy, the pupils are widely dilated and insensitive. In pontine lesions, the pupils are often contracted to pin-point size, and this condition is of important localizing significance.

In proportion to the severity of the disturbance, respiration tends to be hurried, noisy and stertorous, and with increasing pressure to become irregular, grouped or of the Cheyne-Stokes type. The blood pressure tends to be raised and the pulse full in all strokes. Swallowing is often impossible, and the sphincters may be relaxed or retention may occur.

Thrombosis of the *posterior cerebellar artery*, which is a branch of the vertebral artery, presents a classical clinical picture. The patient has sudden intense vertigo. Incessant vomiting and forced movements follow, the forced movements rotating the patient, so that he comes to rest prone, with that side of the face corresponding with the side of the cerebellar lesion in contact with the pillow. There is intense ataxia and the patient is unable to lift his head, or to maintain the sitting or standing position. Nystagmus with the long slow movement to the side of the lesion, and the skew deviation of the eyes is sometimes seen. There is general hypotonia of limbs and trunk which soon becomes limited to the side of the lesion. Head retraction, pain and stiffness of the neck and opisthotonos may occur. When the patient recovers enough, all the signs of a unilateral cerebellar lesion will be found. Consciousness is not often lost. Since the posterior inferior cerebellar artery also supplies the lateral region of the medulla, signs of disturbance of this region are present, and may dominate the clinical picture. These are analgesia and thermanaesthesia of the face and head, due to implication of the quintothalamic path, and of the limbs and body upon the opposite side, due to involvement of that part of spinothalamic tract which has crossed below this level. Between these two areas of sensory loss there is often a gap where sensibility is normal, corresponding with that part of the spinothalamic tract which is crossing obliquely at this level, and, therefore, is too near the middle line to be affected. Paralysis of the motor vagus is often found from involvement of the nucleus ambiguus, and, from the extension of the lesion or of consecutive oedema towards and across the middle line, it sometimes causes severe dysphagia and dysarthria. Extension of the thrombosis to the medulla may embarrass respiration. When occlusion is not complete the most remarkable recovery may take place.

Diagnosis

The Nature of the Lesion. It is difficult to tell at the time of the event if a stroke is the result of ischaemia or haemorrhage, and even more difficult to decide if the ischaemic event is caused by transient reduction in the speed of blood flow on the basis of an old stenosis, to recent narrowing by thrombosis or atheroma, to complete occlusion of the vessel, or to embolus. Of course, the sudden onset of a disastrous stroke complicating heart disease with arrhythmia warrants a diagnosis of embolism. In retrospect a dense hemiplegia which develops over a few hours and persists with little improvement over minutes suggests a cerebral thrombosis, while a severe hemiplegia which recovers in hours or days makes transient ischaemia likely. When haemorrhage is the cause the patient is ill, collapsed, sweating and pale, with fixed dilated pupils and increasing coma. Nevertheless, at the time diagnosis of the cause is so difficult that it presents a major obstacle to the choice of management. Clinical features which may help to differentiate an ischaemic episode from intracerebral haemorrhage are that with haemorrhage the onset is more likely to be dramatically sudden; the syndrome to be severe; fits are more likely; intense headache, nausea and vomiting are experienced; there may be meningism; there may be bilateral extensor plantar responses and conjugate deviation of the eyes; there is cardiorespiratory disorganization and increasing coma. Lumbar puncture may differentiate haemorrhage by the presence of free blood and by raised cerebrospinal fluid pressure, and in a special centre angiography and ventriculography may confirm the diagnosis by evidence of distortion of structures.

Differential Diagnosis

Strokes are so common, and such a frequent cause of sudden unconsciousness that their diagnosis is generally easy.

The diagnosis of *coma* due to a cerebrovascular lesion is usually made without difficulty from the history, and from the presence of unequivocal signs of local lesion of the brain. In a patient without history, and when the coma has become so deep as to remove the unilaterality of physical signs, the diagnosis from other causes of coma such as uraemia and diabetes mellitus, poisoning by barbiturates or coal-gas may be difficult, and search should be made for the usually obvious signs of these conditions. Uraemia may present especial difficulties, for it is often associated with a cerebrovascular lesion, and transient hemiplegic attacks may occur. This is true also of the crises of essential hypertension, which are described in more detail in Section 8. Sudden death is usually due to cardiac infarction, not a stroke; with a stroke it is rare for it to occur in less than 2 hours. Other conditions causing hemiplegia with coma must be considered. Epilepsy, especially when the convulsion is unilateral, may be followed by marked unilateral paralysis (Todd's paralysis) which may last for 4 hours. Here the history of recurring attacks and the complete recovery will prevent confusion.

Space-occupying lesions, particularly subdural haematomas, spontaneous intrafrontal haematomas and extradural clots may be recognized by angiography and ventriculography.

Cerebral malaria and heat-stroke may resemble a stroke, and should always come to mind when rapid coma follows the development of cerebral symptoms in circumstances where these causes are likely. The congestive attacks of general paralysis of the insane, now rare, are difficult to diagnose from apoplexy.

In all cases of coma without history, especially when there are signs of local cerebral damage, a careful examination of the head should be made for traces of recent injury. If coma is increasing and a certain diagnosis of the cause has not been made, localizing investigations —electroencephalography, angiography, gamma scanning and perhaps ventriculography should always be carried out, lest a removable haematoma is present inside or outside the cerebrum.

Treatment

General. Often there has been no opportunity to treat the cause of the cerebrovascular accident because the development of a hemiplegia is the first evidence of the prime arterial disease. The stroke has happened and that is it; management is of the effects, for there has been no time to institute curative treatment. When the subject is known to be arteriopathic or hypertensive the management is that outlined in Section 8. When hypotensive agents are being used the physician should be on his guard against the development of neurological symptoms due to their efficiency in reducing blood pressure and therefore cerebral flow, and should realize how many of the 'toxic' effects of these agents arise from this effect. At the other extreme apoplexy may arise from haemorrhage resulting from imperfectly controlled anticoagulant therapy.

Central Ischaemia. Having as far as possible obviated the causes of arterial hypotension the question will arise whether angiography should be undertaken. There is little purpose in using it unless there is likelihood of vascular surgery or neurosurgery being employed as a result of the discovery of stenosis or vascular anomaly. Two points are appropriate here: the first that the causal lesion may be in the thorax, the neck or the cranium so that very elaborately integrated teamwork is needed; and the second that restitution of the flow through an occluded vessel is by no means synonymous with restitution of function. In patients with hemiplegia technically perfect results of carotid disobliteration rarely improve the hemiplegia.

The later medical care of the patient is directed towards maintenance of a steady blood pressure, perhaps at a high level. Many people who are 'normotensive' for their age, or even hypertensive, are hypotensive for their cerebral needs. No agent maintains blood pressure at a higher level for long, but methylamphetamine, 5 mg., may be used for a while. Phenobarbitone, 50 mg., and other sedatives help to prevent fluctuations in the pressure. Physical means, including elastic stockings and belts, and attention to exercise and daily hygiene, also help. Fortunately if the central ischaemia is affected by obvious changes in blood pressure the outlook is better than when it is the result of gross stenosis due to atheroma.

Thrombosis. When a patient is seen as the neurological signs are developing the first problem is to try to find the cause. When the lesion seems to be thrombotic the first question to be answered is whether anticoagulants should be used. If they are to be, obviously their use must precede the development of further disability so the decision is an immediate one, which can be resolved by the statement that there is little evidence of their efficacy in the results of the carefully controlled therapeutic trials that have been made. Anticoagulants do not dilate arteries, increase blood flow, establish collateral flow or reduce viscosity, nor can they travel distal to an occlusion. Theoretically the problem is similar to that of coronary artery occlusion, with the important exception that there is little effective collateral flow in the brain unless the obstruction is in one of the great vessels in the neck or base of the skull. Here, as has been said, even complete occlusion is compatible with normal health because of the adequacy of flow from alternative vessels via the circle of Willis, if this is intact.

The dilemma can be resolved by advising that when the thrombosis is recent and the syndrome of occlusion is incomplete it is best to carry out carotid angiography in a special therapeutic unit to allow a cerebrovascular surgeon the opportunity of arteriectomy. Unless the thrombus is very recent and there is still some flow the results of removal of the recent thrombus and the obstruction from which it is arising are poor. Vertebral angiography in these circumstances is dangerous, and pointless at present. With the development of units where teams of vascular, thoracic and neurological surgeons collaborate, and of techniques for total angiography via the aorta, hopes of prevention of the disaster grow, but at present, even in the most advanced countries, surgical triumphs often re-establish flow but seldom function.

The only circumstance in which anticoagulants may help is when disturbance of function is incomplete, fluctuating or recurrent and where there is no evidence of a stenosis which can be relieved surgically.

When a hemiplegia has become established the patient should be mobilized early, sitting in a chair 2 days after the disaster. When his general state permits the affected limbs must be put through the full range of active and of passive movements twice each day. When not being exercised muscles which may contract should be stretched in a light splint. The fingers especially should be kept extended on a padded wire frame. Sustained improvement depends on attention to details of general management, of bowel and bladder, and upon encouragement of the use of every function as it re-emerges. In the aphasic patient speech therapy should await enough return of the function of speech to justify its use.

Haemorrhage. There is no treatment that can arrest the disaster of apoplexy ; the less done the better. If the patient survives and his age, general state and the condition of his arterial system allow, neurosurgical removal of the resulting clot, as if it were a tumour, should be considered. In young subjects the haemorrhage may be the result of rupture of an aneurysm or of a vessel in an angioma, and this constitutes a neurosurgical emergency. After the lesion has been recognized by angiography it is as a rule dealt with during the use of hypothermic and hypotensive anaesthetic techniques. Slowly advancing haematomas—probably venous in origin occur in the frontal lobe particularly and follow injury. These are amenable to surgical removal.

It follows that in all but the most obviously arteriopathic subject, in whom apoplexy is the result of generalized disease, carotid angiography should be entertained.

CEREBRAL ARTERIOSCLEROSIS

Aetiology and Pathology

For the aetiology and pathology of arteriosclerosis articles in Section 8 should be consulted. In many subjects the cerebral arteries are affected at an earlier age and more severely than any others in the body. Men are the victims of generalized cerebral atheroma more often than women, and the symptoms, though most common in the sixties and later, are recognizable in the more severe cases soon after the age of 50. The brain is the seat of innumerable minute vascular lesions. There are many small softenings on its surface, and the cerebral cortex becomes thinned in consequence of degenerative changes. In the central parts of the brain, especially in the basal ganglia, small cysts develop from the softenings and eventually a mesh-like condition—the status lacunatus—may result.

Symptoms

The onset is insidious and its course steadily progressive. Mental or physical changes may predominate and both are liable to abrupt exacerbations due to small cerebral vascular lesions. The mental symptoms are often noticeable first. The patient's range of interests becomes reduced and intellectual activities of all kinds are gradually discarded. Memory for recent events becomes faulty, while that for events long past remains unimpaired. Confusion is liable to occur and the patients become unable to adapt themselves to new circumstances and are obstinately conservative. Emotional control becomes impaired, and affective response may fluctuate. Previously existing tendencies to anxiety, or depression or paranoid traits become exaggerated. Confusion and lack of attention may lead to incontinence and disorders of dress. Dysphasia is common and apraxia may also occur [see also p. 1190].

The physical symptoms take the form of a slowly developing muscular rigidity which has been called 'pseudo-Parkinsonism'. The facies becomes 'set', movements become less free and in walking the step becomes gradually shortened until it may be only a few inches; this *marche à petits pas* is very characteristic. The patient becomes unable to relax his muscles and if as he lies in bed passive movements of the limbs are attempted by the examiner, great resistance is encountered. The grasp reflex may be discovered in one or both hands. The tendon-jerks are exaggerated and the plantar reflexes indefinite or weakly extensor.

In some instances the most pronounced physical feature is a spastic paralysis of the muscles innervated from the pons and medulla and hence called 'pseudobulbar palsy'. The physical basis of this syndrome is the presence of bilateral spasticity due to involvement of both pyramidal tracts above the level of the pons. This is caused by the multiple cerebral lesions which involve the pyramidal cells and tracts. The facies become set, voluntary movements of the lips are restricted, the tongue is spastic and looks small and cannot be protruded beyond the teeth, and movements of the palate, pharynx and vocal cords are all similarly limited. The result is dysarthria of a degree which may render the patient's speech unintelligible, together with difficulty in mastication and in swallowing. There is no muscular wasting. The jaw jerk is exaggerated. The lips may be held apart and the saliva trickles from between them. Emotional movement temporarily inhibits the rigidity of the facies and is exaggerated because of the pyramidal impairment. Uncontrolled laughter or crying may occur, and there is usually a tendency towards one or the other so that the patient who suffers from uncontrolled laughter may laugh even on hearing bad news, and the patient who suffers from uncontrolled crying may weep when he is amused.

Pathological laughing and crying is really spasticity of emotional expression, caused by loss of control due to damage to both pyramidal tracts.

Diagnosis

Other forms of pre-senile dementia [see Section 17] are not associated with the same degree of motor disturbance as in atherosclerotic dementia. Signs of pyramidal disorder and of early dementia, and usually the absence of tremor, differentiate the condition from Parkinsonism. If mental symptoms dominate the early stages general paralysis of the insane must be ruled out. When pseudobulbar palsy is present, the diagnosis from motor neurone disease may be difficult, but the absence of wasting and the presence of rigidity in the facies and upper limbs are usually sufficient to make the distinction. When arterial tension is high and changes in the optic fundi are present the picture may closely resemble one of cerebral tumour, and the differentiation depends largely on the presence of arterial hypertension and the extensive retinal lesions, which distinguish hypertensive neuroretinopathy from the papilloedema of raised intracranial pressure.

Treatment

This can only be symptomatic, and the patient should be kept up and about as long as possible. It is unfair and unwise to put too much dietary restriction on him, and if he is a small or moderate eater no further limitation is required. Anticoagulants should not be given, and the blood pressure should not be lowered unless there are reasons to the contrary in cardiac or renal failure. The subject's life must be simplified and regulated to his capacity.

Prognosis

The course of the disease is gradually downward and may at any time end in a severe 'stroke', but in general the patients survive for years and severe cerebral vascular accidents are uncommon. In the end the patient becomes bed-ridden and dies from an intercurrent infection.

HYPERTENSIVE ENCEPHALOPATHY

In a preceding paragraph on the differential diagnosis of strokes sudden and transient cerebral symptoms associated with arterial hypertension were mentioned. It is known that the subjects of hypertension may have cerebral haemorrhage, but they are also liable to 'hypertensive crises'. Attacks of this kind occur in all forms of hypertension regardless of its cause. The attack is precipitated by a further rise in the already high blood pressure, and develops with intense headache, sickness and sometimes drowsiness or even semi-coma. There is hypertensive retinopathy in most cases, often with papilloedema with haemorrhages and exudate. There may also be hemiparesis, hemianopia, focal or generalized fits, or other indications of a local cerebral lesion. The crisis is brief, lasting from a few hours to several days, and usually ends in recovery, but recurrence is likely, and finally many subjects develop evidence of advancing cerebrovascular disease. Intervals of several months may intervene between succeeding crises.

The presence of papilloedema probably means that cerebral oedema is complicating the situation. The transient nature of the crisis, and particularly the rapid appearance and disappearance of such symptoms as hemiparesis, exclude the possibility of arterial thrombosis, and spasm of the arteries has been invoked to account for the symptoms, but there is no conclusive evidence that this occurs. It can be induced with experimental hypertension in animals.

Differential Diagnosis

The transient character of the symptoms excludes gross vascular lesions or intracranial tumour. In intracranial tumour, the systolic blood pressure is rarely above normal limits, the history is longer and the condition progressive. Uraemia can usually be excluded, since in essential hypertension the blood urea is within normal limits, and the only abnormality in the urine may be a trace of albumin. Plumbism in children, whilst very rare today, may develop with headache, vomiting, convulsions and focal signs, papilloedema, sometimes also with high blood pressure and albuminuria, and search for other indications of lead poisoning and careful history-taking are necessary to exclude this condition.

Treatment

The prime treatment is that of the arterial hypertension [see Section 8]. This must be intensified. Dehydration, maintaining fluid intake and controlling electrolytes, must be used. As a measure of urgency from 50–60 ml. of a 50 per cent. solution of dextrose or sucrose may be given intravenously. For less urgent cases and as a measure that can be repeated for the relief of headache, 150 ml. of a 20 per cent. solution of magnesium sulphate may be given per rectum at 6-hourly or less frequent intervals or glycerol, 50 ml. in 50 ml. of water, given in a nasal tube. Intravenous infusion of urea should be avoided in view of the probability of renal damage, mannitol being safe. The convulsions may be treated by rectal paraldehyde, 15–20 ml. in water, intramuscular paraldehyde, 10 ml., 200 mg. of soluble phenobarbitone or diazepam (*Valium*), 40 mg.

CEREBRAL EMBOLISM

Massive cerebral embolism is an uncommon form of catastrophe.

Aetiology

The embolus may be: (1) a fragment of blood clot; (2) a vegetation or detached portion of one of the cardiac valves or in rare instances an atheromatous plaque; (3) air bubbles; or (4) globules of fat.

1. The commonest cerebral embolus is a fragment detached from a clot in the left atrium in a case of atrial fibrillation complicating mitral stenosis. Less often it comes from a clot in the dilated auricular appendage in a case of mitral stenosis without fibrillation, or from one on the inner surface of the ventricular wall after myocardial infarction. It occurs as an immediate sequel of the operation of mitral valvotomy in about 5 per cent. of cases. Other sources of clot emboli are aneurysms of the large vessels between the heart and the brain, a clot covering an atheromatous ulcer in the first part of the aorta, and clots which may form in the pulmonary veins and even in the left heart in suppurative conditions of the lungs. In exceptional cases a congenital heart lesion may provide a route by which emboli from the systemic veins can reach the brain without passing through the lungs—paradoxical embolism [see Section 8].

2. The emboli of the second group are most commonly small portions of infected vegetations from the cardiac valves in cases of subacute bacterial endocarditis. In other instances larger emboli are formed by vegetations from acute bacterial endocarditis.

3. Air emboli are usually multiple. They may occur in association with operations on the lungs during pleural paracentesis, and in the course of almost any operation in which a vein of medium or large size is opened. While emboli of more solid character will not pass through the pulmonary capillaries it is probable that air emboli do so, and consequently air emboli from almost any part of the body may reach the cerebrum. It may follow insufflation of air into the vagina, it may occur in association with retained placenta, and even as a result of division of veins during the operation of Caesarean section.

4. Fat emboli are a cause of cerebral complications after fracture of one of the long bones, and may cause death. Like air emboli, some fat globules pass through the pulmonary filter.

Emboli usually pass into the middle cerebral arteries or their branches, because these are the direct continuation of the carotid arteries. Very rarely the internal carotid is obstructed, but if it is the circulation in its branches is usually maintained by the circle of Willis. Next in frequency is the posterior cerebral artery, and then the vertebral. Because of the mode of origin of the left carotid artery, emboli affect the left half of the brain more frequently than the right. In a case of subacute bacterial endocarditis, the cumulative effect of innumerable minute infected emboli may cause extensive softening in the left hemisphere at a time when the right hemisphere is little affected.

Small platelet emboli may also be fragmented from the tip of mural thromboses, as already described, to cause recurring and stereotyped disabilities—one of the causes of 'little strokes'.

Symptoms

The onset is immediate. A stroke due to embolism is the most suddenly occurring of all and there are no prodromal cerebral symptoms. Unless a large vessel such as the middle cerebral artery is occluded, consciousness is usually not lost, but a stuporose state may occur either with the onset or after a few hours, and may last several days. Hemiplegia is the common physical syndrome and it may be of all degrees of severity, according to the size of the cerebral lesion. When emboli are numerous and of small size, and particularly when they are infected, as in subacute bacterial endocarditis the development of hemiplegia may be gradual.

Diagnosis

Embolism should not be diagnosed unless there is evidence of cardiac disease, aneurysm or some other recognized cause, but in their presence and especially with atrial fibrillation, it is the usual cause of any stroke which may occur.

Treatment

In most cases the condition responsible for the embolism calls more urgently for treatment, and in cases of atrial fibrillation complete rest for several weeks and appropriate treatment of the cardiac disorder usually combined with anticoagulant therapy [see Section 8] is essential, in order to diminish the risk of further emboli occurring. Rehabilitation is the same as in other forms of cardiovascular disaster.

Prognosis

In cases of atrial fibrillation, the hemiplegia is in many cases not severe and good recovery is common, but when a large vessel is occluded the hemiplegia is usually severe, and remains so. Further embolism is likely to occur eventually. In other cases the prognosis depends largely on the course of the causal condition which is responsible, and whether the emboli are affected or not. In cases of bronchiectasis, for example, the emboli, being infected, generally give rise to multiple cerebral abscesses. Puerperal cases of cerebral embolism in the absence of cardiac and other disease usually do well.

INTRACRANIAL ANEURYSM

By far the most serious and common effect of aneurysms within the head is a subarachnoid haemorrhage. Aneurysms here are common and may be considered in four groups although their presence may be suspected clinically, their recognition is almost always by angiography.

1. Minute atheromatous aneurysms of the arteries at the base of the brain are common in old people, but they rarely cause symptoms. They occasionally cause bleeding or pressure on adjacent ocular nerves. Then the effects are similar to those of the more important group which follows.

2. Of the remainder, the great majority are 'berry' aneurysms situated on or near the circle of Willis. An aneurysm of this kind develops at a bifurcation of an artery because of a congenital defect of the elastic lamina. It is thus not really congenital, but develops at the site of a congenital weakness. The importance of berry aneurysms is that the first evidence of their presence is rupture, causing subarachnoid haemorrhage. Otherwise only a small proportion of them give any evidence of their presence. Aneurysms on the posterior or lateral portions of the circle may interfere with the third cranial nerve, causing paralysis, which is, as a rule, partial, and which may be either gradual or sudden in its outset. Less commonly aneurysms situated laterally on the circle compress the optic tract just behind the chiasma, and so produce homonymous defects in the visual fields, and aneurysms on the anterior communicating artery cause pressure on the optic chiasma with consequent disturbance in the central or temporal parts of the visual fields (see subarachnoid haemorrhage, below).

3. Aneurysms of the internal carotid artery are usually situated within the cavernous sinus. They may develop gradually, or, more commonly, after an initial period of slow development, they may dilate rapidly until they come into contact with the wall of the sinus; or, again, may rupture into the sinus, becoming an arteriovenous aneurysm [see also Section 8]. The oculomotor nerves and the branches of the trigeminal nerve in the wall of the sinus become affected. There is severe pain in one side of the forehead, or in

the forehead and cheek. Double vision may proceed to complete paralysis of the third, fourth and sixth cranial nerves, but the paralysis is more often partial. Ptosis is always a feature. The affected eye may become proptosed. When the lid is raised the patient may find that vision in the affected eye is impaired, but in some cases within a few days the vision improves greatly and the pain passes off, some ocular paralysis and proptosis usually remaining. If the aneurysm is above the cavernous sinus (supraclinoid carotid aneurysm), the optic nerve is affected by direct pressure, with progressive visual loss. By suitable radiographic technique erosion of the great wing of the sphenoid, or of some part of the sella turcica may be seen, or calcification may be seen in the wall of the aneurysm. When there is an arteriovenous communication a bruit may be heard with the stethoscope, either over the affected eye, or over the carotid artery in the neck.

The surgical treatment of intracranial aneurysm depends upon the special circumstances of the case, such as the patient's age, the state of his cardiovascular system, and the intensity of his illness, and also upon the site and size of the aneurysm seen by angiography. If operation is performed it either involves tying the bleeding vessel outside the cranium or clipping the neck of the aneurysm, or in some other way occluding it by intracranial operation. In general, the anterior aneurysms are treated by extracranial ligation and the others by direct intracranial occlusion. Though the ultimate results of surgical treatment of subarachnoid haemorrhage due to an aneurysm are better than conservative medical management, there is still a high mortality. Most surgeons prefer to wait two or three days after the haemorrhage before operating.

4. Angiomatous Malformations. The frequency of angiomas of the racemose or cirsoid type has been shown by angiography. They occur most often in the territory of the middle cerebral artery and are almost invariably arteriovenous racemose aneurysms—that is to say, instead of a capillary bed, a tangle of blood vessels is interposed between the arterial and venous systems: the arteries feeding the malformation are hypertrophied and dilated, and the veins draining it are dilated and pulsating and contain arterial blood. As most of the arteries enter the cerebral hemispheres from the surface these angiomata typically appear on the surface and extend in a sector, often with a roughly pyramidal shape, deeply into the hemisphere and may reach to the ventricle. Cerebral tissue is found between the vessels of the mass, and cerebral tracts evidently pass through it without being affected until haemorrhage or thrombosis occurs. They enlarge gradually. The vessels composing the angioma are vascular channels of imperfectly differentiated structure; with thin walls composed of fibrous tissue with some fragmentary and irregularly distributed muscular coat.

These angiomas may leak, and the haemorrhage may be either intracerebral, extracerebral (subarachnoid) or both. It may occur at any stage and it is uncommon for the patient to reach middle age without having a haemorrhage. In many cases fits, local or general, precede signs of haemorrhage by many years. A symptom which is typical, but by no means constant, is a systolic bruit; it may be heard with the stethoscope all over the head or only over the carotid arteries or through the orbit, and may be audible to the patient. Headaches are common and occasionally migrainous; in others they are associated with a feeling of stiffness in the neck suggesting a slight leak. Until haemorrhage or thrombosis occurs there are usually no abnormal physical signs. Carotid angiography is essential.

Many of these malformations are amenable to surgical removal, palliative ligation of vessels, or occlusion by deep X-ray therapy.

In rare instances similar malformations occur in the brain stem and recurrent small haemorrhages give a clinical course a little like that of disseminated sclerosis.

In a special group of cases there is an external as well as an internal angioma, the external manifestation being usually situated in the territory of the trigeminal nerve (Sturge-Weber syndrome). Here the angioma is a capillary one, the skin lesion being a 'port wine stain'. Epilepsy is usual, and mental retardation common.

SUBARACHNOID HAEMORRHAGE

Pathology

Bleeding into the subarachnoid space may be an accompaniment of head injuries and it may also follow intraventricular haemorrhage, but the usual cause of uncomplicated, or, 'spontaneous' subarachnoid haemorrhage, is rupture of a cerebral aneurysm on the circle of Willis or on one of its component arteries. What has been called the 'berry' aneurysm may rupture suddenly and freely, with the production of fatal apoplexy, or there may be recurrent leaking of blood in small amounts causing repetitive meningeal irritation. Whereas with cerebral haemorrhage the bleeding occurs into the substance of the brain which is severely and irrevocably damaged, with subarachnoid haemorrhage the blood is effused outside and over the surface of the brain, though intramedullary bleeding often occurs too, to cause hemiplegic symptoms and signs. Less than a quarter of the cases are due to other causes, including angiomas and arteriosclerosis without a berry aneurysm.

Symptoms

The Apoplectic Syndrome. The patient may have been subject to headaches, or the episode may be quite unheralded until a sudden intense headache, rapidly followed by lapse into unconsciousness, signals the free rupture of the aneurysm. It may be thought that an ordinary cerebral haemorrhage has occurred when the comatose patient is first seen, but when hemiplegic symptoms occur with subarachnoid haemorrhage they are not usually severe. Bilateral extensor plantar responses will be obtained and there will be marked neck rigidity. At first both pupils may be small and sluggish, but in fatal cases the pupils ultimately dilate. Examination of the optic fundi may reveal subhyaloid haemorrhage or papilloedema. Lumbar puncture produces a fluid that resembles pure blood. Two specimens should be taken and allowed to stand to see if the supernatant fluid is xanthochromic, to try to exclude accidental contamination with blood at the time of puncture.

Almost a third of the patients will die in the first attack. In fatal cases death commonly ensues within 24–36 hours or at some time during the first fortnight from fresh bleeding. If this period is safely passed the prognosis as to recovery becomes good. The course of the illness may, however, be prolonged. The patient gradually recovers from coma, taking possibly many days to regain full and continuous consciousness. The temperature may rise after 24 hours and remains at 99·5° or 100° F. (35·3° or 37·8° C.) for about a week, and the urine may contain abundant albumin and some sugar—either of which may lead to an erroneous diagnosis if the possibility of its occurrence is not known.

Headache is intense and may last for 2 or 3 weeks, with irritability and some stiffness of the neck. The knee-jerks or ankle-jerks, or both, are commonly abolished a few days after the onset, but they return after a further week or two and in slighter cases sooner. The patient who has recovered from his coma shows at first little intellectual activity, but answers rationally and briefly when questioned.

There is amnesia of days or weeks with slow recovery of intellectual function. Focal damage may be caused, either by the haemorrhage or by subsequent clotting. If the aneurysm lies close to, or partly embedded in, the brain, its rupture may cause considerable cerebral laceration, which if not fatal may leave partial hemiplegic weakness. If the aneurysm is at the bifurcation of the basilar artery, there may be motor or sensory hemiplegia of the opposite side of the body, associated, possibly, with oculomotor paralysis on the side of the new lesion.

The Meningitic Syndrome. In this case, the haemorrhage is less abundant and therefore consciousness may not be lost. There is violent headache, restlessness, delirium, rigidity of neck and spine, Kernig's sign, bilateral extensor plantar responses and sometimes diplopia and squint. Within a few hours, or somewhat later, ophthalmoscopic examination may reveal flame-shaped haemorrhages in the retina, or massive haemorrhage in the subhyaloid space. Low-grade papilloedema may also be seen.

In small leaking haemorrhages the cerebrospinal fluid is more or less heavily bloodstained, and may for 2 or more weeks be discoloured, yellow or brownish according to the amount of blood originally present.

The Lumbago-Sciatica Syndrome. This uncommon variant begins with pain and stiffness in the lumbar region, followed by pains in the legs, and sometimes the leg-jerks are absent. Pyrexia is the rule. The diagnosis depends upon the characteristic cerebrospinal fluid of subarachnoid haemorrhage. In some cases at least the source of the haemorrhage is in the spinal canal—spinal subarachnoid haemorrhage.

Differential Diagnosis

The recognition of subarachnoid haemorrhage is an easy matter in those cases in which the train of symptoms calls at once for the examination of the cerebrospinal fluid and blood is found in the fluid. Before lumbar puncture the distinction from other varieties of cerebral haemorrhage can often be made: (1) by the age of the patient, practically all haemorrhagic apoplexy in the first half of life being the result of ruptured aneurysm; and (2) by the history of preceding symptoms, such as headache, diplopia, ophthalmoplegia and migrainous phenomena. Angiography may show an aneurysm or angioma.

A distinction may be made of subarachnoid haemorrhage of arterial from that of venous origin. Those from angiomas are much milder in their course.

In a quarter of cases neither aneurysm or angioma is found by angiography, and in these cases the prognosis is much better.

Treatment

Every case of subarachnoid haemorrhage should at first be considered to be a neurosurgical emergency. The patient should no longer be allowed to remain at absolute rest in bed in the hope of recovery, for the condition has changed from a medical emergency to a surgical one.

When the diagnosis of subarachnoid haemorrhage is made the patient should be transferred to a neurosurgical centre for investigation. In the search for the causal lesion carotid angiography on one side and then the other, followed by vertebral angiography may be necessary. When an aneurysm or angioma is found —which will include about threequarters of all cases— the surgeon will decide, upon the age of the patient, his general condition, and the nature and site of the lesion, if surgical intervention is possible. He will try to remove all significant angiomas of moderate size and to clip the neck of aneurysms in the carotid, middle cerebral or posterior communicating arteries, but may well decide to tie the internal carotid artery if an anterior communicating aneurysm is present. In doing so he will use hypothermic and hypotensive techniques. Sometimes, if the causal lesion is inaccessible or of great size he may think it wise to handle the problem conservatively. Fortunately the prognosis is very much better when no causal lesion can be seen radiologically. There remain cases where operation is not prescribed for general or local reasons. Their conservative management consists of absolute rest in bed with sedation. Promazine, 25 mg. 8-hourly, with a nocturnal barbiturate, and analgesics are needed to keep the patient relaxed. An hypotensive agent such as guanethidine (*Ismelin*) should be used to keep the blood pressure steady at a level of, say, 120/80 mm. Hg in a young adult, bearing in mind that the blood pressure may be raised by the intracranial catastrophe itself. The prognosis is very bad if the patient is in coma, but if so, then control of fluid and electrolyte intake is needed, a nasal catheter being used. The medical care of the patient must be as detailed and punctilious as the surgical, and must be maintained for several weeks, absolute rest for 6 weeks being usual.

Prognosis

When the subarachnoid bleeding is caused by arteriosclerotic weakness of a vessel, or by an angiomatous malformation, the outlook is better than when an aneurysm has ruptured. Taking all sites of aneurysm into account, when one ruptures about a third of the patients survive the first haemorrhage, but there will be a recurrence in a high proportion of the survivors within 2 years. The chance of survival from a second haemorrhage is again about one in three, so that the likelihood of survival of a third is small indeed. It is against this prognosis that treatment must be considered. In a proportion of patients persistent arterial spasm within the skull leads to permanent mental change.

CHRONIC SUBDURAL HAEMATOMA

Aetiology

This is caused by venous bleeding and is traumatic in origin in about half the cases; falls, especially those on the forehead or occiput, not at the time apparently serious, may tear cortical veins as they pass from the surface of the brain to enter the dural sinuses. The tear is commonly in the subdural space on one or both sides of the vertex. Thereafter blood leaks from the torn veins and collects on one or both sides of the vertex, external to the arachnoid membrane. Though by no means unknown in young subjects, this type of lesion is much commoner in patients over 50 years of age.

Pathology

The periphery of the clot formed tends to organize so that a fine capsule is built up round the haematoma which remains liquid in its centre, and may reach a large size by a process of osmosis. The underlying cerebral hemisphere collapses downwards and medially, and the brain stem is pushed over so that the margin of the crus, which contains the pyramidal tract, may be indented by the free edge of the tentorium. As a result of this hemiparesis may be caused on the side of the haematoma. The intracranial pressure is often low, and bearing in mind that usually the pressure of the cerebrospinal fluid is higher than that of the intracranial venous bed, it may well be that people with low intracranial pressure select themselves for subdural bleeding, because in them tearing of a vein will cause blood to flow out of instead of fluid into the vein. Support for this is that the aged, the debilitated, dehydrated, alcoholic and diabetic are particularly prone to subdural haematomas.

Symptoms and Diagnosis

It must be emphasized that subdural haematoma may follow an apparently trivial head injury, that essentially its symptomatology is that of a space-occupying lesion, with a feature characteristic of haematoma: namely, a remarkable fluctuation in the course and severity of the symptoms; that owing to the frequently bilateral nature of the lesion the signs are apt to be difficult to interpret; and finally that with such a blurred picture a history of head injury some time before the illness should give rise to the suspicion of haematoma.

There is a latent period in the development of a subdural haematoma. This may vary from days to weeks or months; with young people the latent period is shorter and the symptoms more severe and of more rapid evolution. In young subjects, too, there is usually no difficulty in getting a history of head injury, either a fall upon the head or a blow sustained at sport or in some other way. The initial symptom is usually headache, fluctuating in intensity, most severe on awaking in the morning or on physical exertion. With the passage of days or weeks this becomes more severe and soon other symptoms are added to it. The patient has days on which he is drowsy. He may pass rapidly into stupor or even coma, emerging again to become almost normal. Transient diplopia with squint may be noted. There may sometimes be papilloedema, the plantar responses may be extensor with inequality of tendon jerks, the abdominal reflexes may be diminished or absent. Periods of mental confusion may also occur.

The fluctuation in symptoms, the fugitive character of the physical signs and the generally downhill tendency of the illness, are amongst the characteristic features of subdural haematoma and help to differentiate it from that of intracranial new growth. When the syndrome develops rapidly, it is common to meet a marked slowing pulse.

Simple radiographic examination of the skull usually shows nothing more than marked displacement of the pineal shadow to one side or laterally and downwards, but angiography or ventriculography give a characteristic deformity of structures which will confirm the diagnosis. The ultrasonogram will also show deviation of midline structures.

There is a great liability to a rapid development of coma with a fatal issue. Yet, the occasional finding at necropsy of what is clearly a subdural haematoma of very long standing, unsuspected during life, shows that from time to time the described sequence of events fails to develop.

Treatment

The features which should make clinical diagnosis possible have been described, but in the absence of angiography certainty can be obtained only by an exploratory operation. This consists in bilateral trephine holes and repeated tapping of the subdural space, and if necessary the turning down of an osteoplastic flap and the evacuation of the haematomas. No patient should be allowed to die in coma without full investigation for the presence of a subdural haematoma for unrecognized subdural haematoma is fatal, whilst recognition and treatment are usually followed by full recovery.

THROMBOSIS OF CEREBRAL SINUSES AND VEINS

Cerebral thrombophlebitis may occur as a primary condition, or it may be secondary to infective processes spreading to the sinuses from contiguous infected regions.

Aetiology

Primary thrombosis is a rare condition. It is said to affect the superior longitudinal sinus most commonly. It is more common in the first year of life than at any other period, when it may follow diarrhoea, bronchitis marasmus or acute diseases, such as measles. It may also occur at any age, in the terminal stages of cancer, and other chronic diseases. It happens in the puerperium, the antecedent confinement usually having been quite normal, and it may occur after abortion.

Secondary cerebral sinus infection is now very uncommon. The bacterial flora are often mixed, but the common organisms present are streptococcus, pneumococcus, and *Esch. coli.* The sinus may become infected as a part of a general pyaemia, or infection may spread directly through its wall from a focus of local disease, most commonly from an extradural abscess due to ear disease or frontal sinusitis. In most cases, however, the sinus becomes infected from a local spreading septic thrombosis of the veins which open into the sinus, from an infected spot at a distance. Thrombosis of sinuses may also occur from injury, as by bullet wounds and fractures of the skull, and may also result from surgical procedures in the region of the sinuses.

Pathology

Thrombosis of a vein causes intense congestion of the convolutions which it drains, and a moderate degree of subarachnoid haemorrhage due to rupture of the small tributary veins. The underlying brain softens on its surface and, later, a saucer-shaped depression is left at the site. The cavernous and lateral sinuses do not drain the brain directly, and blocking of one of them does not cause so much cerebral disturbance as obstruction of the superior longitudinal sinus. Thrombosis of the cavernous sinus may, however, extend to the ophthalmic veins and cause blindness, and at the same time the nerves which lie in its outer wall—the third, the fourth, the ophthalmic division of the fifth and the sixth nerves—may be paralysed.

In the infective forms, when untreated, the clot quickly breaks down into pus, and general pyaemia results, or the spread of infection along a tributary vein may give rise to a cerebral abscess. With prompt and efficient use of antibiotics this train of events should never be allowed to develop.

Symptoms

Many cases are infective and the clinical picture is greatly complicated by (1) the presence of infective disease in relation to the cranium, e.g. in the ear; and especially by (2) the onset of pyaemia. The symptoms due to thrombosis of individual sinuses or of cerebral veins are more easily recognized in the non-infective or primary cases.

Superior Longitudinal Sinus. This sinus has two functions: (1) it is a channel into which drain the veins from the upper and medial surfaces of the cerebral hemispheres; and (2) by the Pacchionian bodies associated with it, it forms part of the mechanism by which the cerebrospinal fluid is absorbed into the blood stream. Complete obstruction of the sinus by a clot causes: (1) extensive bilateral venous thrombosis on the surface of the brain, with resulting spastic paralysis of the legs and upper arms, the hands and face being spared; and (2) increased intracranial pressure, and in most cases some degree of papilloedema. In many cases, however, the clot does not obstruct the sinus. Mural clot may obstruct one or more of the entering veins and thus cause hemiplegia, which may or may not be ushered in by convulsions; or again, bilateral paralytic phenomena of any degree may occur. There may be associated drowsiness or coma. On the other hand, the veins may not be obstructed and the clot may be so situated as to interfere with the absorption of cerebrospinal fluid through the Pacchionian bodies; paralytic phenomena are then absent, and the disturbance is limited to the manifestations of raised intracranial pressure—headaches, papilloedema and, in some cases, vomiting.

Lateral Sinus. It is doubtful whether aseptic thrombosis of one lateral sinus gives rise to any symptoms, provided the other one is of normal size and communication at the torcula is free. Since the superior longitudinal sinus usually turns into the right transverse sinus, obstruction of the right lateral sinus may produce a moderate degree of hydrocephalus with headaches and papilloedema. In most cases of lateral sinus thrombosis, however, the clot is infected and signs of pyaemia rapidly ensue. Meanwhile the clot may extend into the jugular vein. and cause pain and stiffness in the side of the neck, and occasionally the thrombosed jugular vein may be felt beneath the anterior border of the sternomastoid as a tender solid cord. There may be tenderness and swelling over the region of the mastoid emissary vein, and the cervical lymph nodes may be enlarged. If when Queckenstedt's test is performed the jugular veins are compressed separately, compression of the vein on the side of the obstructed sinus causes little or no rise in the manometer, whereas compression of the other gives a normal result.

Cavernous Sinus. Thrombosis of this sinus follows septic spots or injuries on the face, sepsis in the frontal sinus or orbital cellulitis. Ordinarily the thrombus is infected. There is oedema of the orbit, with proptosis and oedema of the conjunctiva, forehead and face. Amblyopia or blindness is the rule, but the appearance of the fundus of the eye usually remains normal until the late stages. Paralysis of the ocular muscles and anaesthesia of the eye may also occur. The condition usually becomes bilateral within a day or two.

Diagnosis

These conditions are now sufficiently uncommon as to be forgotten and so overlooked. They occur in the presence of some of the conditions with which sinus or venous thrombosis is known to be associated. The possibility of clot in the superior longitudinal sinus and related veins should always be considered: (1) when any convulsive or paralytic phenomena come on within a month of childbirth or abortion; (2) when in an elderly or debilitated patient disabilities, which may include alexia and visual disorientation, suggesting vascular lesions on the two sides of the brain occur within a few days of each other; (3) when signs of hydrocephalus appear in association with or soon after an attack of otitis media, and there are no other indications of cerebral abscess; and (4) when paralytic or convulsive phenomena occur soon after an injury near the vertex of the skull.

Lateral sinus thrombosis is almost exclusively associated with ear disease, and its presence can usually be confirmed by Queckenstedt's test. Thrombosis of the cavernous sinus presents such a characteristic picture that if an exciting cause is present the diagnosis is seldom in doubt.

Treatment

In the non-infective cases convulsions should be controlled with phenytoin, 100 mg., and phenobarbitone, 50 mg., three times daily. Anticoagulants should be used to prevent the spread of thrombosis; as an immediate effect is needed treatment should begin with heparin. For the paralytic phenomena, the treatment is identical with that of cases of cerebral arterial thrombosis.

The infective cases should be treated immediately with antibiotics as cases of septicaemia, and if the local exciting conditions are likely to involve any collection of pus, such as an epidural abscess, appropriate prompt surgical measures should be taken.

Prognosis

In non-infective cases the prognosis for life is good. The paralytic phenomena generally make great recovery within a few weeks, but in the severe cases spasticity in the legs and upper arms may be left. Blindness or impairment of vision may follow cavernous sinus thrombosis. In the infected cases the prognosis, formerly ominous, has been revolutionized by sulphonamides and antibiotics. With lateral sinus thrombosis, recovery usually follows prompt operation.

REFERENCES

BAKER, R. N., RAMSEYER, J. C., and SCHWARTZ, W. S. (1968) The prognosis in patients with transient cerebral ischemic attacks, *Neurology (Minneap.)*, **18**, 1157.

BRAIN, W. R. (1957) Order and disorder of the cerebral circulation, *Lancet*, ii, 857.

BYERS, R. K., and HASS, G. M. (1933) Thrombosis of the dural venous sinuses in infancy and in childhood, *Amer. J. Dis. Child.*, **45**, 1161.

BYROM, F. B. (1954) The pathogenesis of hypertensive encephalopathy, *Lancet*, i, 201.

CARTER, A. B. (1957) The immediate treatment of cerebral embolism, *Quart. J. Med.*, **26**, 335.

CARTER, A. B. (1960) Ingravescent cerebral infarction, *Quart. J. Med.*, **29**, 611.

CARTER, A. B. (1965) The prognosis of cerebral embolism, *Lancet*, ii, 514.

COOKE, W. T., CLOAKE, P. C. P., GOVAN, A. D. T., and COLBECK, J. C. (1946) Temporal arteritis: a generalized vascular disease, *Quart. J. Med.*, **15**, 47.

DU BOULAY, G. H. (1965) Some observations on the natural history of intracranial aneurysms, *Brit. J. Radiol.*, **38**, 721.

DUVOISIN, R. C., and YAHR, M. D. (1964) Posterior fossa aneurysms, *Neurology (Minneap.)*, **15**, 231.

ECHLIN, F. A., SORDILLO, S. V. R., and GARVEY, T. Q. (1956) Acute, subacute and chronic subdural haematoma, *J. Amer. med. Ass.*, **161**, 1345.

EDWARDS, C. H., GORDON, N. S., and ROB, C. (1960) The surgical treatment of internal carotid artery occlusion, *Quart. J. Med.*, **29**, 69.

FALCONER, M. A. (1951) The surgical treatment of bleeding intercranial aneurysms, *J. Neurol. Neurosurg. Psychiat.*, **14**, 153.

GOLDNER, J. C., PAYNE, G. H., WATSON, F.R., and PARRISH, H. M. (1967) Prognosis for survival after stroke, *Amer. J. med. Sci.*, **253**, 129.

HENSON, R. A., and CROFT, P. B. (1956) Spontaneous spinal sub-arachnoid haemorrhage, *Quart. J. Med.*, **25**, 53.

HILL, A. B., MARSHALL, J., and SHAW, D. A. (1960) A controlled clinical trial of long term anticoagulant therapy in cerebro-vascular disease, *Quart. J. Med.*, **29**, 597.

HUTCHINSON, E. C. (1962) The circle of Willis today, in *Modern Trends in Neurology*, 3rd Series, ed. WILLIAMS, D., London.

HUTCHINSON, E. C., and YATES, P. O. (1957) Cortico-vertebral stenosis, *Lancet*, i, 2.

JEFFERSON, G. (1937) Compression of the chiasma, optic nerves and optic tracts by intercranial aneurysms, *Brain*, **60**, 444.

LASCELLES, R. G., and BURROWS, E. H. (1965) Occlusion of the middle cerebral artery, *Brain*, **88**, 85.

LHERMITTE, F., GAUTIER, J. C., and DEROUESNÉ, C. (1970) The nature of occlusions of the middle cerebral artery, *Neurology (Minneap.)*, **20**, 82.

LOGUE, V. (1951) Chronic subdural effusions, in *Modern Trends in Neurology*, 1st Series, ed. FEILING, A., London.

LOWE, R. D. (1962) Adaptation of the circle of Willis to occlusion of the carotid or vertebral artery: its implications in corticovertebral stenosis, *Lancet*, i, 395.

MARSHALL, J. (1964) The natural history of transient ischaemic cerebro-vascular attacks, *Quart. J. Med.*, **32**, 309.

MARTIN, J. P. (1941) Thrombosis in the superior longitudinal sinus (following childbirth), *Brit. med. J.*, **2**, 537.

MCDONALD, D. A. (1960) *Blood Flow in Arteries*, London.

MCDONALD, D. A., and POTTER, J. M. (1951) The distribution of blood to the brain, *J. Physiol. (Lond.)*, **114**, 356.

MCKISSOCK, W. (1961) Primary intracerebral haemorrhage. A controlled trial of surgically and conservatively treated in 180 unselected cases, *Lancet*, ii, 221.

MCKISSOCK, W., RICHARDSON, A., and WALSH, L. (1960) Spontaneous cerebellar haemorrhage, *Brain*, **83**, 1.

MCKISSOCK, W., and PAINE, K. W. E. (1959) Sub-arachnoid haemorrhage, *Brain*, **82**, 356.

MCKISSOCK, W., TAYLOR, J. G., BLOOM, W. H., and TILL, K. (1957) Extradural haematoma. Observations on 125 cases, *Lancet*, ii, 167.

NEVIN, S., and WILLIAMS, D. (1937) The pathogenesis of multiple aneurysms, *Lancet*, ii, 955.

PATERSON, J. H., and MCKISSOCK, W. (1956) A clinical survey of intracranal angiomas with special reference to their mode of progression and surgical treatment. A report of 110 cases, *Brain*, **79**, 233.

ROB, C., and WHEELER, E. B. (1957) Thrombosis of internal carotid artery treated by arterial surgery, *Brit. med. J.*, **2**, 264.

ROBINSON, R. W., DEMIREL, M., and LE BEAU, R. J. (1968) The natural history of cerebral thrombosis. Nine to nineteen year follow up, *J. chron. Dis.*, **21**, 221.

SEVITT, S. (1960) The significance and classification of fat-embolism, *Lancet*, ii, 825.

SHAW, D. A. (1962) Release of anti-coagulants in neurology, in *Modern Trends in Neurology*, 3rd Series, ed. WILLIAMS, D., London.

SYMONDS, C. P. (1924) Spontaneous subarachnoid haemorrhage, *Quart. J. Med.*, **18**, 93.

SYMONDS, C. P. (1944) Venous thrombosis in the central nervous system, *Proc. roy. Soc. Med.*, **37**, 387.

TATSUMI, T., and SHENKIN, H. A. (1965) Occlusion of the vertebral artery, *J. Neurol. Neurosurg. Psychiat.*, **28**, 235.

WALTON, J. N. (1956) *Subarachnoid Haemorrhage*, London.

WILKINS, R. H., ALEXANDER, J. A., and ODOM, G. L. (1968) Intracranial arterial spasm: A clinical analysis, *J. Neurosurg.*, **29**, 121.

YATES, P. O., and HUTCHINSON, E. C. (1961) Cerebral infarction: The role of stenosis of the extracranial arteries, *Spec. Rep. Ser. med. Res. Coun. (Lond.)*, No. 300.

THE DEMYELINATING DISEASES

DISSEMINATED SCLEROSIS

Synonyms. Multiple sclerosis; Insular sclerosis.

Aetiology

After intracranial new-growths and cerebrovascular disease, disseminated sclerosis is now the commonest incapacitating disease of the nervous system. It has its highest incidence in northern Europe, is less common in North America and relatively rare among the white population of the Southern hemisphere. It is very rare indeed in Africa and Asia. Where the disease is widespread, as in Scandinavia and the British Isles, it is most common in the wet, western and rural areas—in the Western Isles, the West Wales mountains and in Ireland. Here there has been interest in its high incidence in sheep farming areas, particularly because sway-back, a demyelinating disease of sheep, is pathologically similar. This condition is caused by copper deficiency in the maternal ewe, but research has failed to show any aetiological link between this disease and disseminated sclerosis.

Febrile illness may be followed by increase in the symptoms, and many patients with disseminated sclerosis relate that they became much worse after an attack of influenza. In most cases there is no family history but familial disseminated sclerosis is well recognized, and its occurrence in a parent and child or in two siblings is too frequent to be due to chance. In these cases the disease is the same as in others. Interesting topographical studies of the occurrence of the disease in towns and districts, at present continuing, show a distribution suggesting an environmental factor in its aetiology.

The onset is most frequent between the ages of 18 and 30, the sexes being affected equally. It is rare for the disease to begin after the age of 55.

The cause is still wholly unknown. There is no sure evidence that any of the demyelinating diseases of the nervous system are directly due to the action of a filtrable virus. The signs of inflammatory reaction in this disease are compatible with the view that it is infective in origin, but it behaves like no known infective disease. The intensive research into its nature indicates that there are factors inherent in the subject as well as in his environment and the present generalization is that the plaques represent a tissue reaction of sensitized parenchyma to mitochondrial substances, analogous to the allergic reactions. The brevity of this statement reflects the limits of reasonable deduction from a mass of experimental, genetic, geographical and clinicopathological studies.

Pathology

The disease has been described by Nageotte and Riche as 'an affection constituted by multiple inflammatory foci, varying greatly in size and number, disseminated irregularly throughout the length of the cerebrospinal axis'. The chief features of these foci are: (1) their sharp outline; (2) their irregular and capricious shape; and (3) the fact that they do not interrupt the axis cylinders, which are only demyelinated and deformed as they traverse the focus, hence the absence of Wallerian degeneration. The abundance of neuroglia in the foci justifies the name sclerosis which has been given to the process.

These foci are visible on naked-eye examination, the fresh ones as greyish translucent patches, the older ones as greyish or pinkish shrunken areas. Grey and white matter are both affected, the foci having some predilection for the walls of the ventricles. The foci bear no necessary relation to blood vessels.

Under the microscope the older patches are found to contain proliferated neuroglia and nerve fibres which have lost their myelin sheaths. The axis cylinders in the sclerosed areas escape destruction for a long time. For this reason secondary degenerations do not occur in the spinal tracts, and sections of the cord between lesions at different levels present normal appearances. Ganglion cells are also spared; hence wasting of the muscles supplied by the affected segments is not a feature of the disease. In recent patches, oedema is present, with infiltration by lymphocytes, plasma cells and compound granular corpuscles around the blood vessels, especially in the adventitial sheath of the veins. It is highly probable that these inflammatory changes represent the initial lesion, and that the alterations in the nerves and in the neuroglia are secondary to them.

Symptoms

In the early stages the axis cylinders in the diseased areas are not interrupted completely, but suffer partial and temporary impairment, which alters in intensity with the severity of vascular and other inflammatory changes in the tissues around them. Moreover, as the inflammation subsides in one patch a new one develops and produces a different set of symptoms. Hence it is not surprising that the earliest symptoms are often slight and fleeting, or that they may first appear now in one part and now in another. In spite of this, however, certain symptoms and physical signs appear with remarkable regularity and render disseminated sclerosis, in the more advanced stages at least, one of the most distinctive and most easily recognized diseases of the nervous system.

It is remarkable that though the demyelinating lesions, which are often of considerable size, occur anywhere in the central nervous system and commonly involve the fillet, the lateral fillet, the spinothalamic paths, the peripheral neurones in their intermedullary course and the visual path, yet usually quite transient loss of function occurs in connexion with them. On the other hand, the phylogenetically newer systems—the pyramidal paths and the proprioceptive system often suffer permanent damage. The optic nerve is a common site for the development of an area of the disease. This may be situated anywhere between the globe and the optic chiasma and produce the characteristic picture of acute unilateral retrobulbar neuritis.

Motor Symptoms. Weakness in the legs is the symptom for which many patients first seek relief. Beginning with a feeling of heaviness or stiffness in one or both limbs, the weakness, which may be limited at first to one group of muscles, increases, in some uniformly, in a large number with remissions or with periods of apparent recovery, until at last, after a time which varies from a few weeks to many years, it ends in spastic paraplegia. The physical signs are those of pyramidal lesions in general—increased tone in the muscles and exaggeration of the tendon reflexes, diminution or loss of the abdominal reflexes and extensor plantar responses. They are of extreme importance, for some or all of them may be present when the patient's complaints are still trivial, and they are found so constantly in all stages of the disease that the diagnosis of disseminated sclerosis is rarely made in their absence.

The paralysis can often be distinguished from that of other pyramidal affections by the variations in its severity from time to time, and by the occurrence of remissions or of apparent recovery, the improvement sometimes lasting for weeks or months, and, in rare cases, for many years. In most cases, moreover, examination will reveal some other sign—nystagmus, intention tremor or pallor of the disc—which betrays the cause of the paralysis. In one large group of cases, particularly common when the disease begins after the age of 35, the symptoms are those of a steadily increasing spastic paraplegia without remissions and without any indication, either in the physical signs or in the history of extrapyramidal disease. The gait may be only slightly altered, even when the tendon reflexes are greatly exaggerated and the plantar responses are 'extensor'. Later, it becomes spastic or spastic and ataxic. Sometimes ataxia makes walking very difficult, when the power in the limbs is only slightly impaired. In the arms there is often loss of power associated with exaggeration of the tendon reflexes. In some cases the arms are affected before the legs, when astereognosis and loss of sense of position from a lesion in the course of the corresponding posterior column of the cord produce one of the commonest of the early symptoms —the 'useless arm'.

Tremor. The characteristic tremor in the arms appears on voluntary movement only, and increases in rate and amplitude as the goal is approached. For these reasons it is called intention tremor. It may be noticed first in writing or in performing other delicate movements, such as threading a needle. Later, the rate and amplitude of the movements increase, and the tremor, although still greatest at the end, appears almost as soon as a voluntary movement begins. The arms are affected earliest and most often, but nodding of the head is common, and any part of the body may be affected. Beside intention tremor, other types of incoordination of the limbs are occasionally seen, such as those characteristic of lesions of the optic thalamus or of the midbrain or of the cerebellum.

Sensory Symptoms. *Subjective.* Numbness and tingling in the extremities and alterations in the sensation of various parts are common complaints. They are often transient, and may be the only symptoms during the premonitory period. Severe pains are rare, but many patients complain of stiffness or of aching in the limbs and in the back. Occasionally intense neuralgic pain of trigeminal nerve distribution is found.

Objective. Cutaneous sensory loss is not common, but careful examination will often reveal areas of skin in which sensation is impaired. Occasionally the loss is severe, and may show so sharp an upper level as to suggest the presence of a spinal tumour. In many cases the sense of position and passive movements in the limbs is seriously affected, in others loss of vibration sense is the only sensory sign. Like the other signs, the sensory disturbances often show considerable variations in extent and degree at different examinations.

Ocular Symptoms. Attacks of *double vision* are common, and characteristic of the disease. Double vision in a young person should always arouse the suspicion of disseminated sclerosis, and if it is associated with signs of pyramidal tract disease, the combination makes the diagnosis almost certain.

Strabismus is uncommon. Even when the patient is seen whilst complaining of double vision it is unusual to detect any limitation in the range of the ocular movements. *Ptosis* is rare.

Nystagmus is present in more than half the cases, but not so often as an early sign. It is usually fine, rapid and horizontal, appearing only when the eyes are directed to the side. In some cases the eyes oscillate constantly whatever their position. Except in rare cases, there is no apparent movement of objects, even when the oscillations are of wide range.

Visual failure. Diminution of visual acuity due to lesions in the optic nerves—*retrobulbar neuritis*—occurs sooner or later in many cases. It may precede all other symptoms by a period of several years. As in the case of the other symptoms, it is subject to exacerbations and periods of improvement. A young healthy person complains of rapidly increasing mistiness of vision, usually in one eye, sometimes in both or in one after the other, reaching its maximum in a few hours or days; this is often preceded or accompanied by pain about the orbit, which is increased on moving the eye. In the common unilateral case the signs are those of a lesion in one optic nerve; the pupil on the affected side is larger than its fellow; its direct reaction to light is impaired, but it contracts well consensually. Tests with a small object, preferably coloured, reveal a central scotoma. At the onset the disc is usually normal, but in a few instances the inflammation reaches the nerve head, in which event the disc is blurred and swollen. Later the disc may be pale or normal. Rapid improvement of vision is the rule. Special tests may reveal a persistent slight loss of visual acuity, and a partial central scotoma or, rarely, a complete central scotoma. Subsequent acute attacks are common. In some cases the onset of visual failure is gradual. Usually the defect is slight, but it may be serious, although complete blindness never occurs. In these cases the disc is pale, especially in its temporal portion, and the field shows a central scotoma or narrowing at the periphery.

Mental Symptoms. Defective memory and slight impairment of intellectual power are common but are late symptoms. Dementia as a presenting symptom of disseminated sclerosis is rare. Some of the patients are morose and subject to fits of depression, but the majority are surprisingly cheerful, and do not seem to suffer mentally even when their physical state is most pitiable. In many cases there is loss of emotional control, and ready laughter or weeping is common. More often there is merely a tendency to laugh at trivial things. Although a great deal is made of the euphoria of the patient with demyelinating disease, the physician should remember that this state entails lack of insight, and that many patients who appear to make light of their misfortune are really showing fortitude and may readily be misunderstood.

Sphincter Disturbances. These troubles arise from interference with the long paths in the spinal cord by which volitional consent and inhibition are held upon the act of micturition. Therefore, lack of control in the form of hesitancy and precipitancy are common, and retention may occur. In rare cases, control over the rectal sphincter is lost.

Other Symptoms. Deafness, giddiness and tinnitus, sometimes with repeated vomiting, are common. Convulsions are rare. In most instances the distribution of the signs will indicate that the lesions are multiple; but sometimes, although the patches are numerous, the signs are those of a single lesion, say of the internal capsule, of the midbrain or of the cerebellum.

Cerebrospinal Fluid. In many cases, even when the disease is in an active phase, the fluid is normal. In others there may be a moderate increase in protein, not usually more than 80 mg. per cent. and a lymphocytic pleocytosis of 10–30 per mm^3. The Lange colloidal gold test is negative in about half the cases. In the other half it may be of the luetic or paretic type. The latter variety may be strongly marked, and when occurring in association with a negative Wassermann reaction is very suggestive of disseminated sclerosis. Microchemical estimation shows the presence of sphingomyelin, due to damage of the long tracts. Electrophoretic changes are non-specific.

Diagnosis

The combination of spastic weakness of the legs with 'Charcot's triad' of symptoms—namely, intention tremor, nystagmus and scanning speech—which is so widely and so erroneously regarded as characteristic of the disease and as necessary to its recognition, is rarely seen except in the later stages of disseminated sclerosis. As this disease usually presents itself to us in its initial stages, when it may and should be diagnosed, it commonly consists in a group of signs of involvement of the pyramidal tracts: namely, increased tendon jerks, extensor plantar responses, absent abdominal reflexes, a little weakness of dorsiflexion of one or both feet, possibly also some weakness of flexion of the proximal segments of the lower limbs, and usually a degree of impairment, or loss, of vibration sense over the malleoli. In many cases, this is all we can find, but in an otherwise healthy young adult, it is a syndrome more likely to be due to disseminated sclerosis than to any other pathological process.

Perhaps there may be confirmatory signs, such as a little nystagmus, slight intention tremor or sensory ataxia of an arm; it may be pallor of the temporal half of one or both discs—a pathognomonic sign. If some or all of these signs persist after a fluctuating course so typical of most cases of disseminated sclerosis, then diagnosis can be no longer in doubt, and it is comparatively seldom that pathological examinations of blood or cerebrospinal fluid are really necessary.

At whatever stage disseminated sclerosis comes under observation, a careful inquiry into the history of the illness is important, and to elicit this needs a knowledge of the natural history of this disease as it has been outlined here.

Disseminated sclerosis has to be diagnosed from various diseases, of which we will consider the following:

Compression of the cord. When the signs in disseminated sclerosis are purely spinal, the diagnosis from *spinal tumour* presents real difficulties. The first may be mistaken for the latter, when the paralysis increases steadily without remissions and is associated with sensory loss extending upwards to a definite level, while the reverse error may be made when the symptoms caused by a tumour are purely motor, or vary in intensity, or are associated with nystagmus.

Cervical spondylosis in middle-aged and elderly subjects may give rise to a fluctuating lesion of the cervical cord causing an advancing spastic paraplegia closely resembling the course of disseminated sclerosis in middle life. There is some evidence indeed that the damage to the cord caused by the vertebral lesion may produce demyelination.

Friedreich's ataxia. This may be suggested by the presence of ataxia in a young patient with disseminated sclerosis. The distinction can be made at once, for in the latter disease the tendon reflexes in the lower limbs are exaggerated, whereas they are lost early in Friedreich's disease.

Subacute combined degeneration of the cord. In the rare cases where disseminated sclerosis has its onset in middle-aged subjects, the combination of signs of involvement of the posterior and lateral columns of the cord together with the presence of paraesthesia may closely stimulate subacute combined degeneration. Investigation of the blood for changes of pernicious anaemia and estimation of the level of vitamin B_{12} in the serum will render the differential diagnosis certain.

Treatment

The behaviour of disseminated sclerosis makes the assessment of any mode of treatment extremely difficult, and a failure to appreciate the wideness of its fluctuations and the length and completeness of some of its remissions is responsible for many unsupported therapeutic claims. When relapses have an acute onset and course they may respond dramatically to ACTH gel, 40 I.U. daily by intramuscular injection, but it is without effect in the more chronic forms.

The most important general considerations in treatment are to provide complete rest in bed during an acute relapse, and to arrange for a sheltered life during periods of remission or when the disease has become established. Re-education in walking and in limb movement by the use of Fraenkel's exercises will improve function, and the patient should be encouraged to be ambulant and to use inco-ordinate limbs. Well-directed physiotherapy has benefit.

The fact that disseminated sclerosis is sometimes adversely affected by a confinement may justify terminating pregnancy. The whole circumstances of each case must be considered, bearing in mind, too, that the operation of termination may modify the course of the disease. Further, women suffering from the disease in an active phase should be advised against becoming pregnant.

In the later stages of the disease much can be done by the provision of special walking appliances, by organization of the home with ramps and rails and by the use of special utensils for eating. Chlorpromazine, 25 or 50 mg., is used to help to reduce marked tremors, and intrathecal injection of 1 per cent. phenol in aqueous solution is used to reduce spasticity in the legs. Diazepam (*Valium*) in doses short of those causing drowsiness sometimes reduces the spasticity too while nitrazepam (*Mogadon*), 2·5 mg., helps intention tremor a little.

Of great importance is the right ordering of the patient's life, when practicable, and the avoidance of fatigue in the early stages of the disease.

Course and Prognosis

Despite the fluctuations which may mark its course, the disease ultimately disables the sufferer and is the cause of his death. Nevertheless, it is important to remember that after the initial outbreak of symptoms, such patients regain normal physical capacity, lose all abnormal physical signs and lead a normal life for several years; 5, 10 and 15 year periods of this kind are by no means rare, and in general it may be said that the period of evolution of the disease is longer than is generally supposed. On the other hand, a few cases run a rapidly downhill course from the onset. The later in life disseminated sclerosis makes its first appearance, the more benign its course, and sufferers may be found who have reached old age without gross disablement. When the disease appears in middle life it often takes the form of a very slowly advancing paraplegia with late involvement of bladder function. Commonly, after two or three fresh exacerbations with intervening recoveries of greater or less completeness, a slowly increasing permanent disability sets in. This may take years, and indeed the prognosis for continuation of work, for instance, in most cases of disseminated sclerosis, is much better than a general survey of the disabilities which may arise, suggests. But there are certain factors which appear to influence its course unfavourably; thus intercurrent illness, especially if it be febrile, injuries which disable the patient for a short period, all surgical interventions and prolonged or recurrent physical exhaustion.

NEUROMYELITIS OPTICA

This condition, also called Devic's disease, is really a rare presentation of disseminated sclerosis, in which severe retrobulbar neuritis is associated with acute paraplegia. It happens in adult life. The pathological picture is that of severe demyelination. In general the pathological changes are more intense than those of typical disseminated sclerosis and show less evidence of partial remission.

The blindness which indicates the optic nerve lesion may precede or may follow the appearance of paraplegic symptoms but the paraplegia generally occurs within days of the visual loss. It develops rapidly and may spread upwards until sensory loss and muscular weakness reach the upper thoracic level. Blindness, with some swelling of the optic disc, and central scotoma may ensue.

The paraplegia is that characteristic of a diffuse spinal lesion in that there is sensory loss, paralysis and loss of sphincter control.

Anything may happen from rapid and complete recovery to permanent paraplegia and blindness; it is most unpredictable. There is general awareness that steroids sometimes benefit acute and severe demyelination, and little harm at any rate will accrue if ACTH is used during the acute stage of this dramatic disease.

OTHER DEMYELINATING DISEASES OF THE NERVOUS SYSTEM

There are other diseases of the central nervous system having pathological affinities with disseminated sclerosis in that they depend upon a demyelinating process predominantly of the white matter, which may be either diffuse or localized and predominantly cerebral or spinal in incidence.

Of these disorders, acute encephalomyelitis associated with acute specific fevers [p. 1214], the incidence of which may be on either the brain or spinal cord or upon the two together, has already been considered in the article on encephalitis.

SCHILDER'S DISEASE

Synonym. Encephalitis periaxialis diffusa.

Definition

A diffuse disease of the brain with progressive and massive demyelination of the white matter, proceeding from a single focus or from two symmetrical foci, and producing the clinical picture of progressively increasing failure of cerebral function, local at first, but advancing in terms of the functions of the contiguous regions which are next affected, by the spread of the disease from its starting-point.

Aetiology

Nothing is known of the essential nature of the disease, nor is it certain that all cases included under this heading form a homogeneous group. Originally regarded as an inflammatory, probably an infective, disease, the increasing evidence of its familial incidence suggests that it may be primarily degenerative. It has also been suggested that those cases in which an inflammatory reaction is present may be infective, and those in which it is absent—as it may be—degenerative. Many of the reported cases have occurred in childhood, even as early as the second year. The oldest patient was in the fifth decade of life. The sexes are equally affected.

Pathology

The characteristic lesion consists of: (1) A primary demyelination and, later, destruction of the axis cylinders of the central white substances of the cerebral hemispheres, which till late spares the subcortical zone of white fibres and the radial cortical fibres, and produces a translucent jelly-like appearance of the centrum ovale. (2) An early and perhaps primary overgrowth of the neuroglia, forming a feltwork, which is particularly intense round the vessels. (3) A general infiltration of the white matter of the brain with round cells, most of which are engaged in the removal of altered myelin or in the formation of neuroglial fibres.

The process begins most commonly as asymmetrical patches of demyelination, in either occipital white centre, less often in both temporal lobes or in both prefrontal white centres and spreads directly thence until the whole of the central white matter becomes demyelinated. The corpus callosum is involved, and the demyelination spreads downwards through the crura into the brain stem. Sometimes, especially in the central regions, the disease starts on one side. Other patches of the disease may be scattered throughout the central nervous system. The massive character of the lesions together with their mode of spread and their distribution, its incidence in childhood and its entirely different symptomatology, separate Schilder's disease sharply from disseminated sclerosis.

Symptoms

In many of the cases cortical or central blindness—by which is meant blindness without any change in the optic disc and with pupils reacting normally to light—has been the first symptom, and is the result of the symmetrical demyelination of the occipital white matter. As the disease spreads forwards into the temporal regions, bilateral deafness appears; and, later, bilateral ataxia and astereognosis—due to partial involvement, bilateral spastic paralysis—the result of central involvement, and complete amentia—due to callosal and prefrontal involvement, develop.

In those cases in which the initial seat of the disease is in the temporal, central or frontal regions, the first symptom to appear is obviously determined by the location, and the order of development of symptoms will be changed, but the mode of progress is the same in all. Where the disease starts on one side only, hemianopia or hemiplegia is the first symptom, and these are followed by the train of added signs produced by the extension of the disease into other regions. Complete mindlessness and paralysis always dominate the clinical picture in the end. The disease process within the brain sometimes causes swelling with increase of intracranial pressure, and signs of the latter may appear in the form of headache, vomiting and papilloedema. Such cases are not common, and most of them have been regarded in life as cases of intracranial tumour. Fits occur sometimes early and may be local or general. Fever is usually absent, but there may be irregular pyrexia and some of the more acute cases have been pyrexial throughout. The cerebrospinal fluid is normal in the majority of the cases, but sometimes there is an increased protein content and a small excess of lymphocytes.

Diagnosis

The onset with cerebral blindness or with bilateral deafness, followed by signs of progressive cerebral destruction, is so rare in any other disorder as at once to suggest the diagnosis of Schilder's disease, indeed no less than two-thirds of the reported cases have shown this picture. When the disease begins unilaterally, and more particularly when headache, vomiting and papilloedema are present, the distinction from intracranial tumour is difficult or even impossible, for in both diseases the local commencement and the progressive destruction occur. No treatment is known to influence the course of this disease.

Course

In most cases Schilder's disease is regularly progressive to a fatal termination. In some, however, periods of standstill have been noted, while in a few others marked improvement for a time has occurred. The duration has varied from 7 days to 36 months, with an average of 9 months.

REFERENCES

Adie, W. J. (1932) The aetiology and symptomatology of disseminated sclerosis, *Brit. med. J.*, **2**, 997.

Allison, R. S. (1961) Epidemiology of disseminated sclerosis, *Proc. roy. Soc. Med.*, **54**, 1.

Collier, J., and Greenfield, J. G. (1924) The encephalitis periaxialis of Schilder, *Brain*, **47**, 489.

Farraro, A. (1937) Primary demyelinating processes of the central nervous system, *Arch. Neurol. Psychiat.* (*Chic.*), **37**, 1, 100.

Lumsden, C. E. (1957) Aspects of the chemistry of the myelin and sheath cell complex, in *Modern Trends in Neurology*, 2nd Series, ed. Williams, D., London.

McAlpine, D., and Compston, N. (1952) Some aspects of the natural history of disseminated sclerosis, *Quart. J. Med.*, **21**, 135.

McAlpine, D., Compston, N. D., and Lumsden, C. E. (1955) *Multiple Sclerosis*, London.

Miller, H., Newell, D. J., and Ridley, A. (1961) Multiple sclerosis. Treatment of acute exacerbations with corticotrophin (ACTH), *Lancet*, i, 20.

Scott, G. I. (1952) Neuromyelitis optica, *Amer. J. Ophthal.*, **35**, 755.

Stewart, T. G., Greenfield, J. G., and Blandy, M. A. (1927) Encephalitis periaxialis diffusa, *Brain*, **50**, 1.

Symonds, C. P. (1924) The pathological anatomy of disseminated sclerosis, *Brain*, **47**, 36.

HEREDITARY AND FAMILIAL DISEASES

FRIEDREICH'S ATAXIA

Synonym. Hereditary ataxia.

Definition

An hereditary disease characterized clinically by a progressive ataxia, and pathologically by the degeneration in the spinal cord of the posterior columns, lateral columns and spinocerebellar tracts and in the cerebellum of a number of the Purkinje cells.

Aetiology

Transmission occurs as a dominant through both sexes. Indirect heredity is the most common, because the subjects are usually afflicted in childhood and incapacitated by the time adult life is reached, and so do not procreate, but direct heredity does occur. Isolated cases in which no heredity can be traced are not rare. The first signs of the disease usually appear before the sixth year, but in many the onset is delayed until puberty, while in a few it may not be until after the age of 30. As a rule the age incidence is approximately the same in each child-rank of the same family; but sometimes the phenomenon of anticipation is well marked, the disease appearing at an earlier age in each succeeding generation. The disease is said to be slightly more common in males.

Pathology

The spinal cord is usually small, and the posterior roots tend to be small, grey and poorly myelinated. The essential change is a primary degeneration of neurones in the dorsal columns, of the pyramidal tracts and of the spinocerebellar tracts, both dorsal and ventral.

The spinocerebellar tracts are constantly degenerated, the direct cerebellar tract being the most seriously involved. The cells of Clarke's column, however, degenerate and disappear, as does also the network of collaterals which surrounds these cells. Secondary to this degeneration neuroglial proliferation or sclerosis occurs. The cerebellum may be normal, or it may show varying degrees of atrophy of Purkinje cells, or of any other of its cell elements, and of tracts connected therewith.

Symptoms

The onset is always insidious, and physical signs of abnormality usually precede any complaint on the part of the patient or his relatives. The first symptoms are generally felt between the sixth and the tenth year of childhood; but if a careful examination is made of the younger members of the families, physical signs of the disease, especially the extensor response in the plantar reflex, the retraction of the great toe and some degree of pes cavus may often be found before the sixth year.

Ataxia is always the first sign to appear, and this is shown by an awkwardness of gait and a tendency to stumble and fall readily. Sometimes it is obvious that it dates from infancy when it is said that the child was never strong on his legs from the time of learning to walk. As the disease progresses, the gait slowly becomes more irregular and clumsy. The patient walks with his feet upon a broad base, and reels from side to side; but, notwithstanding this, he keeps a fairly direct line of progression. He takes short steps which are unequal, and irregular, and the movement of each foot as it is raised is poorly co-ordinated.

In standing, the body oscillates from side to side in slow and clumsy fashion, and coarse tremors of the head and trunk are constant features in advanced cases (titubation). Sometimes Romberg's sign is present; but this is never so well marked as in tabes, and it is frequently absent. The ataxia invades the arms, as a rule, later than the legs. There is first clumsiness with the finer movements, and then little by little with all the movements. It closely resembles the ataxia due to gross disease of the cerebellum, and differs from that which occurs in tabes. That irregular breaking of a movement towards the end of its accomplishment, 'intention tremor', is often seen.

Irregular involuntary movements occur in advanced cases, and are most often seen in the head and neck as nodding movements and jerky tremors. Nystagmus is usual. Dysarthria is almost constant, and is gradually progressive. At first the speech is of the slurred 'cerebellar' type, but with increasing ataxia it becomes scanning or drawling.

The strength of movements is at first little impaired; but as the disease advances and the pyramidal degeneration increases, the power is gradually lost in proportion to the degree of the pyramidal degeneration, which varies greatly in different cases. The legs are affected first and most, and later the arms, and in severe cases at a late stage paralysis may be almost universal.

The condition of the muscular tone depends upon the relative degree of degeneration in the posterior roots and in the pyramidal tracts respectively, the former tending to abolish and the latter to increase it. As a rule the influence of the posterior root degeneration is preponderant and, therefore, the limbs are flaccid and hypotonic, but occasionally they are rigid. Contractures are the rule, but these are confined to the legs. The most constant of these produces the characteristic pes cavus. Moderate wasting of the small muscles of the feet and hands is seen. Sensibility is little affected, but in most cases minute examination reveals slight relative loss to touch, pain and temperature, most marked at the periphery of the limbs and diminishing upwards. Similarly there may be slight loss of sense of position in the limbs, and diminished vibration sense.

The ocular movements are almost intact apart from nystagmus. In rare instances strabismus, diplopia and ptosis have been recorded. The pupils are not affected. Optic atrophy is a rare phenomenon in Friedreich's disease, yet it has been reported in quite a number of otherwise typical cases.

Mental symptoms are usually not conspicuous, but some of the patients are of poor mentality from the first, while others show a tendency to severe mental degeneration in the later stages of the disease. Emotional instability, irritability and outbursts of temper may occur.

Absence of the tendon reflexes is a most characteristic feature, and is often the first objective sign of the disease, but in cases in which there is a major degeneration of the pyramidal tracts, the knee-jerks may persist or even be brisk into the advanced stages of the disease. The abdominal reflexes gradually disappear. The plantar reflex is invariably extensor. The sphincters usually escape. The cerebrospinal fluid presents no abnormality.

Spinal curvature is very common, and may reach a severe degree. It consists of a scoliosis of the dorsal region, and often with some kyphosis, and with a compensatory reverse lumbar curve. The cause of this deformity is probably the defect in the postural tone of the muscles.

Diagnosis

In uncomplicated cases the diagnosis is a matter of no great difficulty on account of the strikingly distinct nature of the symptoms. Friedreich's disease can hardly be mistaken for tabes, since the history of heredity, the peculiar deformity of the feet and spine, the extensor plantar reflex, the speech affection and the nature of the ataxia contrast strongly with the loss of pain sensibility and of deep sensibility, the pupillary changes, the sphincter trouble, the abnormal Wassermann reaction and the abnormal cytology of the cerebrospinal fluid in tabes. The distinction from disseminated sclerosis presents more difficulty; but in this disease the onset never occurs in childhood, there is no heredity, the deep reflexes are never lost and the spinal deformity does not occur.

Treatment

No treatment is known. Re-educational training of the limbs and trunk in the form of Fraenkel's exercises are most beneficial. Properly designed boots to ensure the most advantageous use of the deformed feet must be provided.

Course and Prognosis

The course is progressive in slow and irregular fashion, and the prognosis is therefore in every case serious; but the average duration of the disease is over 30 years, and in some cases it seems to have no tendency to shorten life. The prognosis is worse and the course more rapid in those patients who have shown disability from the time of learning to walk. In some cases the disease appears to become arrested. Intercurrent febrile illnesses cause deterioration. Confinement to bed from any cause has a bad influence upon the ataxia.

DELAYED CEREBELLAR ATROPHY

It may be said of all the primary atrophies of the cerebellum that their aetiology is unknown but the cause is probably endogenous. In some forms there is clear evidence of heredofamilial factors but not in all. Some of them appear in early infancy while others show themselves in later life and are hence called 'delayed'. The infantile forms are extremely rare. Of the delayed varieties the most common is an atrophy of the cerebellar cortex—*Marie's delayed cortical cerebellar atrophy*.

Aetiology and Pathology

This disease affects both sexes, and shows itself at any age from 45 onwards. The lesion is bilaterally symmetrical, and is most marked on the upper anterior parts of the cerebellum. It is essentially a cortical atrophy, with disappearance of the Purkinje cells as its characteristic feature. Familial incidence has been described. A clue to the biochemical nature of these disorders may well be found in the examples of Purkinje cell degeneration which are associated with carcinoma of the lung [see Section 9].

Symptoms

The clinical picture is that of a slowly developing ataxia of gait, accompanied by a disorder of articulation; ataxia of the arms develops later, but nystagmus rarely occurs. In many cases the tendon-jerks are increased, indicating an element of spinal degeneration.

Diagnosis

It is natural that the disease may be mistaken for disseminated sclerosis. The later age-incidence, the absence of nystagmus, of disc changes, of spasticity and of loss of sense of position and the steady progress should make the diagnosis of disseminated sclerosis untenable; while the reeling character of the ataxia and the sibilant instead of staccato quality in the articulation disclose the real nature of the disease. In tabes dorsalis, with which it may be confused because of the ataxia, numerous characteristic signs are present by the time ataxia becomes pronounced, and nystagmus rarely occurs. In many cases the tendon-jerks are increased and dysarthria is not a feature of tabes. It is likely that in the past many cases of carcinomatous neuropathy causing cerebellar atrophy have been mistaken for this rare disorder. There is no treatment.

FAMILIAL SPASTIC PARALYSIS

Aetiology

This rare disease is sometimes hereditary, but is more commonly familial and incident upon several children of the same parents. Sporadic cases also occur. The onset is gradual in early life, and usually occurs after the sixth year.

Pathology

The pathological changes consist in a primary degeneration of the pyramidal neurones related to the fibre length; those supplying the lumbosacral region, being lower and longer, are earliest affected; those supplying the brain stem, being shortest, are the last to be affected. Degenerative changes in the neurones of the posterior columns of the spinal cord are often present, showing the transition to the pathological type of the hereditary ataxias.

Symptoms

The clinical aspect consists in the slow development of spasticity and weakness, first and most in the legs, which gradually increases and progresses to the trunk and upper extremities, and involves the face last and least. The usual signs of pyramidal involvement are present in the loss of abdominal reflexes, increased deep reflexes and extensor type of plantar reflex. The disease is progressive, increasing to complete paralysis, and in its course contractures of the spastic muscles occur, that of the foot and leg producing some degree of pes cavus, while, above this, flexor contracture at hip and knee is met with. Optic atrophy is by no means uncommon. Mental symptoms do not occur in uncomplicated cases, neither is epilepsy observed.

Diagnosis

It is most easily confused with cerebral diplegia; but the latter disease appears much earlier, as soon after birth, in fact, as defective movement in the child can be ascertained. Further, cerebral diplegia is not a progressive disease in the majority of the cases, and it it often associated with mental deficiency and recurring convulsions.

Treatment

The management is the same as that of Friedreich's ataxia except that the purpose of exercises, if given, should be to secure the best use of the spastic lower limbs instead of to overcome ataxia.

THE LIPIDOSES

The lipidoses form a group of diseases in which the characteristic feature is an accumulation of lipid substances within the various cells. These accumulations are mainly to be found in the lymphoreticular tissue [see Section 13] but may occur within the cells of the nervous system when they lead to progressive failure of cerebral function. The commonest member of the group is Gaucher's disease where the lipid in question is kerasin: in this disorder the nervous system escapes except in the rare acute infantile form. In Tay-Sachs disease the abnormality is limited to the nervous system and the accumulated lipid is a ganglioside and in Niemann-Pick disease both the nervous system and lymphoreticular tissues throughout the body are affected; the cells in this instance containing sphingomyelin. At one time it was believed that Tay-Sachs disease was a variant of Niemann-Pick disease in which the changes were limited to the nervous system, but chemical analysis of the tissues has shown that the accumulated lipid differs in the two.

It seems justifiable to group these diseases together although their aetiology is not understood. A genetic basis for them seems certain for more than one member of a sibship is commonly affected. Parental consanguinity, however, is rare. It is impossible at present to localize the defect beyond saying that the accumulation appears to be due to a breakdown of intracellular metabolism possibly associated with deletion of one or more enzymes required for normal lipid turnover.

TAY-SACHS DISEASE

THE INFANTILE FORM

Synonyms. Amaurotic family idiocy; Cerebromacular degeneration.

Definition

A rare family disease of infancy occurring chiefly, but not entirely, in Jews, affecting children during the first year of life, who are apparently quite healthy when born, and characterized by: (1) progressive mental impairment, ending in absolute idiocy; (2) progressive paralysis of the whole body; (3) progressive diminution in sight, ending in absolute blindness. Retinal changes are constantly present, consisting of a large and conspicuous cherry-red spot in the region of the macula, and optic atrophy; and (4) a fatal termination in the marasmic state before the age of 2 years.

Aetiology

Nothing is known of the aetiology of the disease apart from its familial and racial incidence. It is due to an inborn error of lipid metabolism.

Pathology

There is a progressive degeneration of the nerve cells from the highest to the lowest, and ultimately there may be no normal cells remaining anywhere in the nervous system. The degenerating nerve cells contain granules of a lipid identified as a ganglioside. Vacuoles caused by lipid droplets in the lymphocytes are seen in less than half the cases, and similar lipid changes are seen in cells of the mucosa of the gut removed by rectal biopsy.

Symptoms

There are few diseases in which the clinical manifestations are so perfectly uniform. The children have all been born at full term, and in perfect health. They thrive well during the first 3–6 months of life, when they gradually become listless and apathetic, cease to take interest in the surroundings, and begin to show signs of the visual failure which ends in blindness. Later, the child is unable to sit up, or to hold up its head. The limbs, which may be slightly spastic at first, become flaccid and motionless. There is a gradual increase of all these signs. The mental defect becomes more and more noticeable, the paralysis more extreme, complete blindness follows and the patient sinks into a condition of marasmus, in which he dies. Convulsions occur but characteristically there are myoclonic attacks, especially in response to startle, and frequent attacks of petit mal with flaccidity, causing the body to drop forward in 'salaam' movements. These may happen hundreds of times a day. The electroencephalogram shows widespread changes, with 2-a-second spike and wave discharges.

The retinal changes are pathognomonic and are due to a degeneration and disappearance of the nerve cells of the retina and their processes, which constitute the fibres of the optic nerve. This change is most intense in the region of the fovea centralis, where the retina thins and disappears over a circular area, exposing the vascular choroid. This causes characteristic appearance of a cherry-red spot in the region of the macula. This spot is actually a hole in the retina exposing the choroid. The optic disc shows progressive atrophy.

Diagnosis

Distinction has to be made between this and other forms of progressive diplegia. The symptoms are so distinct that a physician who is acquainted with the disease, and able to recognize the retinal picture, can hardly fail to make the correct diagnosis. Other aspects of this disease are discussed in Section 13.

Treatment

Some patients respond to the use of corticosteroids but there is no guide to prognosis, and even when response occurs it is either temporary or partial.

JUVENILE AND ADULT FORMS

In addition to the classical infantile form described in the preceding article, two other forms are well known in which the pathological changes are similar but much less severe than in Tay-Sachs disease, and there is also a similar familial incidence, but the onset occurs later in life, the course is less rapid and the result far less serious. The later the onset in life the slighter and less progressive are the symptoms. The cherry-red spot at the macula, so constant in the infantile form, does not occur in the later forms. The characteristic retinal change is a disturbance of the retinal pigment commencing in the macular region, rather like retinitis pigmentosa, accompanied by honeycomb changes at the macula and sometimes by optic atrophy. The *juvenile* form occurs in later childhood and is characterized by the association of the retinal changes and visual defect with some degree of mental deterioration and myoclonic epilepsy. The *adult* form is the least progressive of any, and the clinical manifestations are the visual defect and retinal changes in the absence of mental deterioration. As in the infantile form corticosteroids may be tried guardedly.

NIEMANN-PICK DISEASE

This is a rare disorder of lipid metabolism in which the intracellular accumulations are of the diaminophosphatide, sphingomyelin. It is three times more common in Jews than in other races and fives times more common in girls than boys.

The onset is in infancy usually between the 1st and 5th months. Affection of the lymphoreticular tissue is shown by splenic and hepatic enlargement with anaemia and the presence in bone-marrow smears of typical Niemann-Pick cells. Neurological features are almost invariable. There is muscular weakness and the child is unable to hold up his head. Moderate pyramidal tract defect is the rule and early mental dullness progresses rapidly to complete idiocy. The macular cherry-red spot, once thought pathognomonic of Tay-Sachs disease, is to be seen in 60 per cent. of cases and nerve deafness is usual. It is also considered in Section 13.

No treatment alters the course of disease. By the end of the first year of life one-third of the patients are dead; only one-quarter survive the 2nd year; and all, except a rare exception, are dead by the age of 6.

GAUCHER'S DISEASE

This is a lipidosis in which the accumulated material is kerasin. Its onset is usually in later childhood or adolescence when neurological symptoms do not occur. An acute form is seen in infants with onset about the 3rd month. The child is normal at birth but starts to lose weight and to show signs of physical and intellectual failure. The spleen and liver enlarge; opisthotonos develops; there is trismus, laryngeal spasm and attacks of cyanosis. Death results from cachexia after 2–6 months. Gaucher's disease is considered more fully in Section 13.

LEUCODYSTROPHIES

Whereas in the lipid disorders just described, which present a wide selection from the very severe forms in infancy to the chronic forms in adult life, the disturbance of lipid metabolism is evident in the cell bodies, there is another group of diseases in which the changes are seen in the myelin of the cell fibre. They are disorders of white matter and so are called leucodystrophies. Sporadic as well as familial forms occur. The differentiation of many types which have been described, and which have eponymous names, is entirely pathological and in life depends mainly upon histological studies of brain biopsy material, though discovery of metachromatic material in the urine is pathognomonic. Some of the forms described are the metachromatic leucodystrophy of Norman; Krabbe's globoid cell leucodystrophy; and the Pelizaeus-Merzbacher disease. They all present in early life, and except that they do not lead to blindness or show the retinal changes of cerebromacular degeneration, are otherwise very similar to it in their clinical characteristics. There is dementia, personality disorder, epilepsy with myoclonus, and diffuse involvement of pyramidal and extrapyramidal systems, with consequent profound disorganization of movement. The course is a progressive one, with uncertain and temporary response to corticosteroids.

There cannot be a logical classification of the leucodystrophies. Norman, who attempted it, merely divided them into the familial ones—metachromatic 'globoid cell' (Krabbe), Sudanophil (Pelizaeus-Merzbacher and Löwenberg types) and the sporadic even more rare mixed forms, the Alexander type or Canavan type, and distinguished them from the lipidoses, such as Tay-Sachs disease and Gaucher's disease. The diagnosis is an histobiochemical one, rather than clinical.

REFERENCE

WILSON, J., LAKE, B. D., and DUNN, H. G. (1970) Krabbe's leucodystrophy. Some clinical ,genetic and pathogenetic considerations, *J. neurol. Sci.*, **10**, 563.

HEPATOLENTICULAR DEGENERATION

Synonyms. Progressive lenticular degeneration; Wilson's disease.

Definition

A rare progressive disease of the nervous system, often familial, due to a disorder of copper metabolism. It is characterized by involuntary movements, rigidity and hypertonicity, with contractures without signs of pyramidal disease; and by dysarthria, dysphagia, emotionalism and progressive emaciation. Several closely related clinical forms of the disease bear distinctive names: *tetanoid chorea* (Gowers), *pseudo-sclerosis* (Westphal), *progressive lenticular degeneration* (Wilson) and *torsion spasm*, and *dystonia musculorum deformans* (Thomalla). Cirrhosis of the liver occurs in all forms. The Kayser-Fleischer zone of corneal pigmentation occurs in the first three forms, but has not yet been recorded in torsion spasm. The most constant nervous lesions are found in the corpus striatum.

Aetiology

The disease often occurs in children of the same parents, but there is no evidence that it is congenital or hereditary. The age of onset has been as early as 7 years and as late as 26 years. The primary disorder is that of copper metabolism with consequent failure to synthesize the component of neurones, caeruloplasmin.

Pathology

A portal cirrhosis is always found after death. It has caused death in some members of the affected families before nervous symptoms appeared. The nervous lesions are degenerative. In Wilson's cases they were almost confined to the lenticular nucleus, especially the putamen. Every degree of degeneration is seen, from discoloration and sponginess of the nucleus in rapidly fatal cases, to shrinkage and atrophy, and even to complete disintegration and excavation of the ganglion. There are lesions in other parts of the nervous system. The lesions are often most intense in the corpus striatum, but the disorder has no strictly selective action on any one anatomical group of ganglion cells, or on any limited area of the nervous system. The degenerate basal ganglia contain excessive amounts of copper compounds and there is a persistent excess of this element in the urine as well as an increased urinary excretion of amino acids. This is caused by an inborn error of metabolism of unknown ultimate aetiology which fails to utilize the copper available for the manufacture of the molecule of the protein caeruloplasmin. The associated excess of copper in the tissues which is found by microchemical methods is reflected in the excretion of copper and in the effects upon the liver, which ultimately leads to liver failure. This process can largely be reversed by encouragement of the release of copper from the tissues by dimercaprol (BAL) and by penicillamine. Disorder of copper metabolism can be discovered in apparently unaffected siblings. The importance of the disease does not depend upon its frequency but upon its chemopathological significance.

Symptoms

In many cases there are no symptoms of disorder of the liver during life. In other cases an account is obtained of symptoms referable to acute hepatitis before the onset of nervous symptoms—attacks of diarrhoea and vomiting, pyrexia, jaundice, migrainous headaches, haematemesis and sometimes definite ascites.

The first nervous sign to appear is usually involuntary movement of the limbs, which may be of several kinds. In progressive lenticular degeneration, rhythmical tremors, increasing on voluntary movement, furnish the most common symptom. This is followed by rigidity of the face, the muscles of the neck and later of the trunk, which increases steadily until the patient becomes helpless. The rigidity of the face and neck muscles gives rise to a peculiar expressionless appearance interrupted by a characteristic slow and rather fatuous smile. Still later, extensive contractures, usually in the flexed position, in the upper and lower extremities, follow; but sometimes there is extensor contracture of the latter. During sleep the tremors cease, but the contractures do not relax. Dysarthria, of a slurring type, results from affection of the muscles of speech, and may end in complete anarthria. Without treatment progressive muscular weakness and general emaciation follow; and the patient becomes emotional, facile, docile and childish. The optic discs and pupillary reactions are normal. There is an absence of nystagmus, cerebellar symptoms and impairment of sensation. The reflexes are not altered, as is the case in pyramidal disease. The Kaiser-Fleischer ring can be seen on the limbus of the cornea by oblique lighting as a green-brown iridescence (just like lubricating oil). It is seen as a circular opacity by slit-lamp illumination.

Treatment

Previously fatal, the disease can now be partly or completely controlled by intramuscular injection of dimercaprol (BAL), 2 ml. weekly, or by penicillamine, 1 G. given orally, daily. Discontinuation leads to relapse. The effect of treatment is observed by estimating the level of copper excreted in the urine. While penicillamine remains the most efficacious treatment it remains extremely expensive.

Prognosis

The untreated disease always ends fatally in a few months or years; the average duration is about 4 years. The disease has now been completely controlled, with no evident deterioration, in a few cases, for about a decade.

KERNICTERUS

Definition and Aetiology

A yellow pigmentation of the basal ganglia, associated clinically with extrapyramidal motor disorders and found as a rare phenomenon in children who, normal at birth, develop jaundice within the first 3 days of life.

In neonatal jaundice the brain may be diffusely pigmented, or more rarely the pigmentation may be confined to the putamen, subthalamic and dentate nuclei, the hippocampus and fascia dentata. To the latter variety of jaundice of the brain the name 'kernicterus' has been given by Schmorl. The nerve cells in the affected masses of grey matter show destruction and degeneration, while the nerve fibres are demyelinated. The degeneration is a direct result of an excess of circulating unconjugated bilirubin in the blood, levels of more than 20 mg. per 100 ml. being dangerous. The presence of this breakdown product in sufficient quantity for a sufficient time in adults has been found to cause analogous changes.

Symptoms

The child, usually the second in a sibship, is healthy at birth, but within a few days develops intense jaundice due to *haemolytic disease of the newborn* [see Section 13] from Rhesus incompatibility between the parents, though kernicterus has been found in association with septic jaundice. The onset of jaundice is followed within 24 hours by tonic and clonic movements, muscular rigidity and opisthotonos, alternating with periods of flaccidity. If the child survives, involuntary movements of choreo-athetoid form develop within a few weeks. Emotional instability and mental retardation appear as the child grows older. The ultimate survival of treated cases is not yet known.

Diagnosis

Athetosis and comparable forms of involuntary movement seen in children are usually not associated with kernicterus, but the parents should be questioned about jaundice in infancy. Again, the development of marked symptoms of organic nervous disease immediately after the appearance of severe jaundice in a newly born infant should lead to a consideration of this condition.

Treatment

There is no curative treatment, so education and training in co-ordinated movements in a special centre should be arranged. Here, where sufficient intelligence exists, much can be done by patient training. Prevention of maternal iso-immunization should bring about the disappearance of haemolytic disease of the newborn but when it has occurred other siblings can be protected by the prompt and energetic treatment of its consequences [see Section 13].

Prognosis

These patients tend to die during infancy or childhood of intercurrent disease, but a minority survive to adult life with a varying degree of mental impairment and disorder of movement.

NEUROFIBROMATOSIS

Synonym. Von Recklinghausen's disease.

Definition

A developmental defect of ectoderm. The skin develops pigmented areas and a miscellany of tumours, the nervous system neurofibromata, in its peripheral and central components. Other abnormalities are associated with this disorder.

Aetiology

The disease is both hereditary and familial, though isolated cases occur. *Formes frustes* are common. Although the characteristic features evolve during the life of the patient, the disease undoubtedly results from congenital abnormality. It is often associated with other congenital and developmental anomalies of the nervous system with tumour formation.

Pathology

The cutaneous lesions comprise fibromata, many of which are degenerate, naevi and areas of pigmentation. In the nervous system multiple fibromata occur in the peripheral and cranial nerves and in addition meningeal tumours and gliomata of the brain and spinal cord may be found. The characteristic tumour is a neurofibroma of the acoustic nerve, which sometimes is bilateral. The disease may coexist with tuberose sclerosis, which is, however, distinct from it.

Symptoms

Of the essential features of the disease, the cutaneous lesions are usually the first to appear. Some may be present at birth, others develop during childhood, adolescence or adult life. They present a great variety of forms and are fully described in Section 14.

The tumours on the nerve trunks are also fibromata but usually firmer than those in the skin. They may occur on any of the peripheral nerves, the limb plexuses, or the intraspinal portions of the nerve roots. Those peripheral are usually painless and seldom interfere with the function of the nerve on which they grow. They are occasionally painful on pressure. Those which originate on the spinal nerve roots produce the picture of spinal compression, commonly preceded by a long period of root pain. They are often multiple. Within the cranial cavity neurofibromata are most often met on the acoustic nerves, but they may occur on any of the cranial nerves, and produce symptoms characteristic of their position.

Von Recklinghausen's disease is often found in association with other congenital anomalies, such as spina bifida, meningocele, cervical rib, syringomyelia, mental deficiency and epilepsy. Other tumours such as rhabdomyomata and phaeochromocytomata may develop.

The tumours are liable to undergo malignant degeneration and it is not uncommon to find other tumours, such as meningiomata and gliomata in patients with this disorder.

Treatment

Nothing is known to modify the natural course of

the disease. Central tumours should be removed surgically as they arise, and cosmetic improvement can often be achieved for the cutaneous and subcutaneous lesions.

Course and Prognosis

In many cases the condition is compatible with a long and relatively normal life, though there is a generally slow progression. Danger to life results only from central lesions in the cranial or spinal cavities, or from the rare malignant degeneration in the peripheral tumours.

TUBEROSE SCLEROSIS

Synonyms. Adenoma sebaceum; Epiloia.

Definition

A condition recognized clinically by the symptom triad of multiple cutaneous tumours of the cheeks and face, mental deficiency, and epilepsy, and pathologically by the presence in the brain of areas of gliosis of a peculiar type.

Aetiology

Hereditary and familial incidence is common, but many isolated cases occur. No other factors are known. The sexes are equally affected.

Pathology

The characteristic lesions of the brain consist of nodular tuberous masses, which are most plentiful under the ependyma of the ventricles, into which they project like candle-gutterings. Similar nodules can be seen and felt scattered throughout the cortex, and rarely in the cerebellum or spinal cord. They consist of dense tangles of neuroglia cells, many of markedly pathological type. The cutaneous tumours consist of an overgrowth of the sebaceous glands embedded in naevoid and fibrous tissue. Tumours also occur in other tissues, namely rhabdomyomas in the heart and kidneys, and the 'phakoma' in the retina.

Symptoms

These usually appear in early childhood. Varying degrees of mental defect from feeble-mindedness to idiocy occur, but intelligence may be preserved. Epilepsy usually begins within the first few years of life and though any form may occur, generalized convulsion is the commonest. The characteristic skin lesions are described in Section 14.

Treatment

Symptomatic treatment is needed for the epilepsy, and the patient cared for in a suitable institution.

Course and Prognosis

The course is very slowly progressive. Most patients spend their lives in institutions for mental defectives, but frequently attain a considerable age.

OTHER HEREDO-FAMILIAL DISORDERS

Down's Syndrome (*Mongolism*) is described in Section 17.

The Laurence-Moon-Biedl Syndrome is familial, more common in boys, and consists of mental defect, which is usually severe, obesity, sexual arrest, infantilism, retinitis pigmentosa and polydactyly [see Section 5].

Hereditary Optic Atrophy—Synonym: Leber's disease. This is a sex-linked hereditary disease, very rare in females. There is slow loss of central vision, usually in both eyes equally, in early adult life. This slowly progresses, with primary optic atrophy, but becomes arrested short of blindness. There is tenuous evidence that it might be due to disturbance of cyanide metabolism.

AGENESIS

CEREBRAL DIPLEGIA

Synonyms. Congenital spastic paralysis; Little's disease.

Definition

A group of clinical conditions caused by congenital damage to or imperfect development of the nerve cells of the cerebral cortex, basal ganglia or cerebellum. This may affect those cells of the pyramidal system which control the legs and the resulting clinical condition is cerebral spastic paraplegia or Little's disease, or all the cells of the pyramidal system may be affected, producing generalized spastic rigidity. Again, the higher regions of the cortex may be affected and the result is congenital idiocy. Similar affections of the cells of the basal ganglia result in congenital bilateral athetosis, and congenital chorea. When the cerebellum is involved, congenital cerebellar ataxy results. There may be any combination of these conditions.

Aetiology

A cause of congenital diplegia (Little's disease) is birth injury caused by mechanical disturbance at the vertex, and that of diffuse spasticity with intellectual defect and possibly athetosis is asphyxia neonatorum. Agenesis of the pyramidal cortex, of the frontal lobes generally or of the cortex and basal ganglia on both sides causes similar clinical pictures. The disorder may be apparent at the time of birth, but more often the signs of deficient or perverse movement, or of mental deficiency, appear during the first year of life. *Abnormalities of birth* are frequent. Premature, or precipitate birth, prolonged labour from uterine inertia rather than from dystocia, and asphyxia neonatorum are all common. The child is often the first-born.

A well-defined variety of cerebral diplegia associated with congenital deafness occurs as a result of the mother having rubella in the early months of pregnancy.

Pathology

The essential histology of the affected regions is that of non-development, paucity in numbers and degeneration of the nerve cells, with corresponding absence, poor development or degeneration of the corresponding tracts. The pyramidal tract, for example, may be found absent throughout, or it may reach to the medulla, or to the cervical region only, and so show at what period development was arrested. The changes in the nerve cells are followed by secondary gliosis. The final result is termed atrophic sclerosis. More often certain regions are profoundly affected, while others escape relatively or completely; but the distribution is always symmetrical upon the two hemispheres. The convolutions are unduly hard to the touch, and their surfaces often present a worm-eaten and faceted appearance. This irregular form of the convolutions, with wide, separating sulci, gives the brain a characteristic appearance, like that of a walnut kernel.

Symptoms

The clinical picture of the several forms of cerebral diplegia, traumatic, asphyxial or agenetic, presents a combination in varying degrees of certain characteristic symptoms, always bilaterally distributed, though sometimes more severe on one side than on the other. These symptoms are: muscular rigidity, paresis, perverse movements, contractures and increased deep reflexes. Mental deficiency, optic atrophy and ataxia are other important symptoms. The signs of the disease become obvious during the first year of life or soon after. In severe cases, soon after birth, the nurse, in washing the child, is the first to notice the stiffness of the limbs, or the regular assumption of a curious bodily attitude. Otherwise, the abnormalities may not be obtrusive until the child should sit up or learn to get about, when weakness, rigidity, involuntary movements and pes cavus may attract attention, or backwardness in learning to walk and to talk, and mental deficiency may first suggest that there is something wrong. The following are the common types of the disease, but it must be remembered that any combination of, or transition between, the types may be met with.

1. *Generalized spasticity; general congenital spastic paralysis.* There is extensive defect of the pyramidal system. The spasticity and weakness affect the whole of the musculature.

2. *Spastic diplegia; congenital spastic paraplegia; Little's disease.* The pyramidal deficiency is largely confined to that supplying the lower part of the trunk and lower limbs.

3. *Congenital bilateral athetosis and congenital chorea.* The agenesis affects the cells of the basal ganglia, with the appearance of irregularity of movement, and of spontaneous involuntary movements, which may be of an athetotic, choreic or irregular type. These movements are not present at birth but advance with maturity of the brain. A certain variable degree of general spasticity is present in these cases.

4. *Congenital cerebellar ataxia.* The agenesis affects the cerebellum with the appearance of cerebellar ataxy. In this type, the limbs are flaccid, and in mixed cerebral and cerebellar types there is a tendency to hypotonicity of the muscles, instead of rigidity.

5. *Congenital idiocy; restless idiocy.* The agenesis affects those parts of the brain concerned with the higher functions. These children are emotionless, restless and unteachable. The skull often shows frontal or occipital microcephaly.

6. *Microcephalic idiocy*—where the agenesis is of the whole brain and the skull remains very small.

Paresis and Spasticity. Except in severe cases, in which the weakness amounts to complete paralysis, there is more spasticity than weakness, and it is often astonishing that there should be so much power with so much spasticity. The legs are generally the most affected, the arms to a less degree, and the facial region still less. In severe cases movement is slow and clumsy, and spontaneous involuntary movements are often present in the limbs. Contractures accompany the spasticity, and if walking is possible the gait is digitigrade from contraction of the calf muscles, the knees are flexed, the thighs rotated inwards and the knees pressed together, causing 'scissor gait'. The rigidity and contractures, when severe, may cause peculiar attitudes A mask-like expression, with wide palpebral fissures and large open mouth, is seen. The head may be rigidly retracted, but more commonly the chin is pressed down upon the chest. The spinal column generally shows some deformity in the way of kyphosis, lordosis or scoliosis, and pes cavus or equinovarus is the rule.

Involuntary Movements. These are the constant maladroitness of voluntary movement, the facial over-action and grimacing in speech and in mimetic expression, choreic movements, athetotic movements and intention tremor. Common sensation and the muscular sense are unimpaired. The sphincters are unaffected. The deep reflexes are increased but are often difficult to obtain when rigidity is very marked. The abdominal reflexes may be present, the plantar reflexes are sometimes flexor. There may be microcephaly, asymmetry and flattening in the region of the central convolutions, or a furrow corresponding with the interhemispheric fissure, or frontal or occipital smallness and flattening. Every degree of mental reduction may be met from slight mental dullness to complete amentia, but this by no means corresponds with the severity of the bodily symptoms, for the mental defect is often most severe when the bodily symptoms are slight, and conversely. In some cases high intelligence persists, when there is utter uselessness of the limbs, and when speech is hardly intelligible. Primary optic atrophy occurs in a small number of cases. Inequality of the pupils and slowness of light reaction are not uncommon. Nystagmus is often seen. Convergent strabismus occurs in about one-third. Convulsions are common, and in about a tenth epilepsy becomes established.

Treatment

In those patients with marked backwardness, and in those which show a course of progressive degeneration, no treatment is of avail. In slighter cases of generalized spasticity, treatment is to be directed to the prevention of contractures, to regaining of voluntary control, and the improvement of mental acuity. There is, perhaps, no disease which demands greater patience and persistence in carrying out suitable treatment, and there are few in which more brilliant results may be produced from apparently hopeless cases by pertinacity. It is in the early years, when treatment is often neglected, that good results are more quickly and readily obtained. From the first, regular massage and passive movements should be employed. Voluntary movement should be encouraged, as far as possible, and as power and movement increase, gymnastic exercises of every kind should be employed. Rigid apparatus for prevention of deformity and to reduce contracture is harmful, for it increases the weight of the limb, and interferes with movement, which is the remedy with which paralysis is to be combated. Tenotomy is of great service in the relief of deformity and contracture, and should be soon followed by passive movements. It should never be performed unless a fair degree of voluntary power is present, for surgical intervention is apt to add another to the patients' many handicaps.

Prognosis

In many patients with generalized spasticity there is a tendency to slow amelioration, an increase of voluntary power and control of the muscles in the course of time, especially under the influence of careful training. If mental acuity is not impaired, laborious treatment may result in an almost normal condition of the limbs by the age of puberty. On the other hand, some children become progressively worse, and die very young. Bilateral athetosis and choreic diplegia, as a rule, follow a slowly progressive course, without tendency to a fatal result. A great many patients with all forms of diplegia die before the sixth year, and in those who survive this age, life is short, few living more than 30 years.

INFANTILE HEMIPLEGIA

CEREBRAL THROMBOPHLEBITIS

While in childhood hemiplegia of slow onset is due to the same causes as in adults, cerebral tumour being the common cause, the majority of the cases of infantile hemiplegia of rapid onset are examples of diseases peculiar to children, to which no comparable disease occurs in adults, and to such cases the term 'infantile hemiplegia' is restricted. These conditions are due to gross organic lesions of the brain, and for this reason must be strictly separated from the cerebral diplegias which are the result of cell lesions, and not of gross structural lesions.

Aetiology

In two-thirds of all the cases, the onset occurs within the first 3 years of life, becoming increasingly rare as childhood advances. A few of the cases are of prenatal origin and a few due to obstetrical events during birth, by which the cerebrum is injured. Acute infective diseases cause about one-third of all cases and by far the most important of these are measles and scarlet fever, but hemiplegia may occur in the course of pertussis, smallpox, rubella, diphtheria, dysentery, pneumonia, mumps, malaria, chorea and endocarditis. While there can be no doubt that primary vascular lesions are responsible for many of the cases in which this condition complicates the specific fevers (whooping cough, for example, may cause cerebral haemorrhage, and febrile illnesses, thrombosis of cortical veins, whilst endocarditis may cause embolism), yet in some cases an inflammatory lesion of the brain or encephalitis is present.

Pathology

The following lesions are seen: (1) atrophic sclerosis; (2) cyst formation; (3) shrunken patches resembling wet wash-leather, with some degree of atrophic sclerosis in their vicinity; and (4) porencephaly. The general appearance of these lesions, which appear to be varying degrees of the same process, suggests the end result of a vascular disturbance, but it is difficult to tell if the cause was arterial or venous. Though arterial occlusion is sometimes responsible, cerebral thrombophlebitis complicating infections is probably the most common cause.

Symptoms

The onset is rapid, and in two-thirds the first sign of trouble is a convulsion, which may be unilateral, but more often general. Multiple fits end in coma from which the child gradually emerges in the course of a few days, to show the signs of some cerebral defect, usually hemiplegia, sometimes hemianopia, or aphasia, or any other sign of local cerebral or cerebellar lesion. Pyrexia often accompanies the convulsion, and vomiting is common. The onset may be without convulsions or loss of consciousness.

The relation of the onset of the paralysis to the convulsion varies. It may reach its height immediately after the initial convulsion, or slight hemiparesis may occur which deepens after each subsequent convulsion. Sometimes the early convulsions leave no paralysis, but this appears towards the end of the first week, either suddenly with fresh convulsion, or gradually, as the patient recovers from the comatose state. The paralysis at its onset is flaccid, and involves the whole of one side of the body to a greater or smaller extent. An initial monoplegia is rare. The paralysis may not reach the greatest intensity until the end of the second week. Subsequently it lessens, in some cases disappearing completely in from a few weeks to 3 months; in others, it may show no sign of improvement. The limbs, at first flaccid, subsequently become spastic and develop contractures. In the course of years there may be great arrest of growth on the affected side, and this is not necessarily proportional to the degree of paralysis, but apparently depends upon the degree of destruction which has occurred in the parietal lobule. Post-hemiplegic spontaneous movements of an athetoid, choreic or irregular kind are common, and are attributable to lesions in the corpus striatum and subthalamic grey matter, for which regions encephalitis shows an especial predilection. Epileptic fits recur at varying intervals in about half of all cases of infantile hemiplegia. These always commence upon the affected side and are sometimes confined to it. Mental deficiency is found, in relation to the position and extent of the cerebral cortex which is involved in the lesion.

Diagnosis

The nature of the illness, with convulsions, may

possibly be suggested by prodromal pyrexia, by the severity and long duration of the convulsions, and by the prolonged subconscious state that often follows. Angiography may show occlusion of the middle cerebral artery, but more often it contributes little to knowledge of the case. Convulsions occurring several days after the onset of specific fevers should strongly suggest the diagnosis. When the signs of hemiplegia or of other local cerebral lesions appear, the diagnosis presents no difficulty.

Treatment

Too often the damage to the brain has happened as soon as a diagnosis is possible so that it is too late to consider the use of anticoagulants. When the paralysis has developed, treatment is to be directed to the prevention of rigidity and contractures by regular passive movements, to regaining voluntary control by encouragement and patient exercises, and to the improvement of mental acuity. Where there is much contracture and deformity, tenotomies are of great service, provided there be some voluntary power in the muscles. Recurring convulsions should be treated.

Severe cases of this disorder as they reach childhood and adolescence present a characteristic picture. The infantile hemiplegia is associated with some degree of failure of growth in the affected limbs and with involuntary movements. In addition, epilepsy, mental retardation and violent temper-tantrums are characteristic.

Such cases have, of recent years, been increasingly treated by complete surgical removal of the damaged hemisphere. This hemispherectomy is usually followed not only by cessation or improvement in the fits but by a marked improvement in the mental enfeeblement and the temper-tantrums. Even more surprisingly, the severity of the hemiplegia instead of being increased is diminished.

Course and Prognosis

In a few the patient does not survive the initial manifestations and dies in convulsions; apart from this, infantile hemiplegia has little tendency to destroy life. The initial flaccid hemiplegia tends to improve and gives way to a slowly resolving spastic hemiplegia, which, with the return of some power, shows perversity of movement, stiffness and slowness, ataxia, athetosis and choreic movements or tremors according to the position of the lesion. The spontaneous movements appear within a year of the onset. Slow improvement may go on for years, but cases with much mental reduction or in which recurring epilepsy is frequent, do not improve.

REFERENCES

AUSTIN, J. H. (1960) Metachromatic form of diffuse sclerosis, *Neurology (Minneap.)*, **10**, 470.

BACHER, A. B. (1934) Friedreich's ataxia, *Amer. J. Path.*, **10**, 113.

BELL, J. (1939) Hereditary ataxia and spastic paraplegia, in *Treasury of Human Inheritance*, Vol. iv, Part 3, London.

BIRD, A. (1948) The lipidoses and the central nervous system, *Brain*, **71**, 434.

CROCKER, A. C., and FARBER, S. (1958) Niemann-Pick disease: a review of eighteen patients, *Medicine (Baltimore)*, **37**, 1.

CUMINGS, J. N., ed. (1957) *Cerebral Lipidoses—A Symposium*, Oxford.

CUMINGS, J. N. (1957) Some metabolic disturbances affecting the cerebrum, in *Modern Trends in Neurology*, 2nd Series, ed. WILLIAMS, D., London.

FITZGERALD, G. M., GREENFIELD, J. G., and KOUNINE, B. (1939) Neurological sequelae of kernicterus, *Brain*, **62**, 292.

FORD, F. R. (1963) *Diseases of the Nervous System in Infancy, Childhood and Adolescence*, 4th ed., Oxford.

GREENFIELD, J. G. (1954) *The Spino-cerebellar Degenerations*, Oxford.

HASSIN, G. B. (1930) Niemann-Pick's disease, *Arch. Neurol. Psychiat. (Chic.)*, **16**, 708.

JERVIS, G. A. (1960) Infantile metachromatic leucodystrophy, *J. Neuropath. exp. Neurol.*, **19**, 323.

NORMAN, R. M. (1962) Lipid disease of the brain, in *Modern Trends in Neurology*, 3rd Series, ed. WILLIAMS, D., London.

NORMAN, R. M., URICH, H., and FINGLY, A. H. (1960) Metachromatic leuco-encephalopathy—a form of lipidosis, *Brain*, **83**, 369.

SACHS, B. (1929) Amaurotic family idiocy and general lipid degeneration, *Arch. Neurol. Psychiat. (Chic.)*, **12**, 247.

SCHEIG, R. L., and BORNSTEIN, P. (1961) Tuberous sclerosis in the adult, *Arch. intern. Med.*, **108**, 789.

THANNHAUSER, S. V. (1953) Diseases of the nervous system associated with disturbances of lipid metabolism, *Ass. Res. nerv. Dis. Proc.*, **32**, 238.

TYRER, J. H., and SUTHERLAND, J. M. (1961) The primary spino-cerebellar atrophies and their associated defects with a study of foot deformity, *Brain*, **84**, 289.

WALSHE, J. M., and CUMINGS, J. N., eds (1961) *Wilson's Disease: Some Current Concepts*, Oxford.

WILSON, J. (1963) Leber's hereditary optic atrophy, *Brain*, **86**, 347.

WOODWORTH, J. A., BECHETT, R. S., and NETSKY, M. G. (1959) A composite of hereditary ataxias, *Arch. intern. Med.*, **104**, 594.

ZUELZER, W. W. (1960) Neonatal jaundice, *Arch. Neurol. (Chic.)*, **3**, 127.

PAROXYSMAL DISORDERS

EPILEPSY

Epilepsy, in one form or another, is very common and it is estimated that about one in two hundred of the population suffer from it at some time. It is to be regarded as a symptom and not as a disease.

Definition

Epilepsy is a word that has come down to us from ancient Greece, and in general it refers to the persistent occurrence of attacks. If the attacks happen because there is disease elsewhere, such as uraemia, cardiac failure or hypoglycaemia, we do not say that the patient has epilepsy, but rather 'uraemic fits' or 'syncope' or 'hypoglycaemic convulsions'. Though there can be no sharp dividing line, where the word epilepsy is used, there is the implication of primary disorder of the brain.

The manifestations of epilepsy are many, and theoretically in so far as attacks arise within the brain, they are capable of mimicking any activity of which the brain is capable, in movement, in bodily sensations and in sight. Some of them include elaborate experiences and highly co-ordinated movements. Epilepsy then is present when there are recurring discrete disturbances of movement, of sensation or of consciousness which are primarily cerebral in origin. This definition, it will be seen, excludes attacks of any sort which are due to disease elsewhere in the body.

Classification

Epilepsy may be classified in many ways, for instance according to cause, to kind of attack, to age of patient, to severity or to electroencephalographic accompaniments. No classification is all-inclusive. Each is unsatisfactory. There are however only two sorts of epilepsy—general and focal. There are two sorts of general epilepsy—major and minor (grand mal and petit mal). Any attack, however elaborate in its manifestations, which the observer is satisfied is epileptic, other than grand mal or petit mal, is a focal epileptic attack. There is, therefore, no need to talk of epileptic equivalents or epileptoid states. Focal attacks may range from local muscle twitching to co-ordinated acts, from a feeling of pins and needles in a finger to the experience of an elaborately organized hallucination.

Another division is between constitutional (idiopathic) and symptomatic epilepsy. More and more, attacks are now recognized as due to a cause, often benign and small, and the constitutional factor in epilepsy is being reduced in importance. Heredity in epilepsy is not a major factor, but in many patients the coexistence of an unusual tendency to convulse in the presence of a recognized cerebral cause, can be seen.

SYMPTOMATIC EPILEPSY

The known causes of symptomatic epilepsy are many. The diagnosis is often based on assumption because some item in the history of the case provides a basis for supposing that organic cerebral disease or injury has occurred, and it requires much knowledge and good judgement to assess whether such an assumption is well founded. Injury of the brain, whether from violence from without or from disease within, may cause epilepsy. There are as many causes of epilepsy as there are diseases which damage the brain—cerebral tumours, agenesis, encephalitis, meningitis, abscess, vascular lesions, cysticercosis, and so on. Birth injury and birth asphyxia are the most common causes, injury in later life the next, and then incidental illness involving the brain: the younger the subject, the more likely is epilepsy to develop.

IDIOPATHIC EPILEPSY

Definition

Epilepsy is said to be idiopathic when the attacks recur over long periods of time without any discoverable organic disease of the brain or other known cause of fits.

The fit is a disturbance of function, due to a sudden excessive discharge of nervous activity attributable to a disorder of the metabolism of the cells in which the abnormal discharge originates. Of the nature of this metabolic perversion we are still ignorant and as far as we know it is not associated with any recognizable change in the histological appearances of the cells concerned. The metabolism of nerve cells in activity is accompanied by changes of electric potential which can be recorded by the electroencephalogram or electrocorticogram.

Aetiology

We must be clear in our minds what we mean by the cause of epilepsy. In symptomatic epilepsy organic disease of the brain is usually present, but in idiopathic epilepsy there is no organic disease with which the liability to fits can be associated: moreover, the same organic disease, e.g. a glioma of one frontal lobe, may be associated with fits in one case and not in others. Thus the organic disease is not the immediate cause of the liability to abnormal discharges, but it is a more remote cause. Of the more immediate cause (or causes) of the liability to attacks little is known, beyond the indications of metabolic disturbance in nerve cells that have already been referred to. Of remote causes of the liability in addition to organic disease of the brain, constitution plays a part. While this factor is regarded much less seriously now than formerly, in some cases a history of epilepsy in a near relative is obtained. Moreover, electroencephalographic observations show that in the parents of epileptic subjects changes of a constitutional kind are often present. It may be that while epilepsy is not inherited, there is some heritable instability of cortical cell function which, in combination with other factors, leads to the appearance of epilepsy in certain circumstances.

There are then remote causes and immediate—predisposing and precipitating. The remote causes include an inborn liability which is sometimes overtly hereditary, disturbances in development, injuries and anoxia at birth, and subsequent injuries and diseases. The immediate causes include normal and abnormal factors. Among the normal ones are the age of the subject, his general bodily state, his state of alertness, his degree of concentration and bodily activity at the time, the time of day, degree of hunger, and his affective condition. The abnormal factors include intercurrent illness, especially fevers, exhaustion, worry, frustration and any major psychological disorder, whether immediate or prolonged.

In the vast majority of cases of idiopathic epilepsy the tendency to fits first reveals itself in childhood or adolescence. In 70 per cent. of cases attacks have begun by the age of 20, and in 85 per cent. by the age of 25. In a small number of cases idiopathic epilepsy first appears in the fourth or fifth decade, but fits coming on after the age of 25 are more often symptomatic of organic cerebral disease. Often children starting to have fits in adolescence have had convulsions in infancy.

The frequency of fits in the same patient varies greatly, so that the liability to abnormal discharge evidently fluctuates. When it is sufficiently great, there must also be a final exciting cause which starts the attack—especially the major fit. Of the cause(s) of fluctuations in the liability to attacks and of the exciting causes of fits we are, again, quite ignorant. The most that can be said is that something is known from empirical observation of the conditions in which fits often occur. These are subject to great variability from patient to patient, but often show great uniformity for the same individual.

More than half of all convulsive attacks occur during sleep. Many patients only have attacks in sleep, nocturnal epilepsy, but the liability attaches to sleep, whether nocturnal or diurnal, including the Sunday afternoon 'nap' in front of the fire. Of the nocturnal fits, many occur soon after the patient has fallen asleep, but still more shortly before or just after waking. In general the liability to fits during sleep is greater than during the waking state. The next greatest frequency of attacks is in the first hour after waking. Many patients have attacks when washing or dressing in the morning or about breakfast time only. During the rest of the day the liability to attacks is much less, though they may occur at any time and under the most unpredictable circumstances. In general the patient is less liable to attacks while intent on the day's activities than when inactive, relaxed or lounging or dozing. In the evening, especially in the last hour before bedtime, the average liability to fits is again increased, but the evening liability is not nearly as great as that of the first morning hour.

Here the lie may be given to the idea that watching television causes epilepsy. Photic fits may be induced by the repeated bright flashing of a maladjusted set, if the face is close to the tube, but people with epilepsy spend as much time as their contemporaries before the television set, half asleep, or apathetic, or bored for hours in the evening—just the circumstances in which fits happen in the predisposed.

In women there is a pronounced increase of liability to fits in association with the menstrual period, beginning about 5 days before the onset of menstruation and lasting till the end of 48 hours after its termination, with its maximum in the 2 days preceding the menses. In many women with mild epilepsy the attacks may only occur then.

Physical disturbances such as vertigo, nausea, or vomiting increase the liability to fits, as also does physical injury. General anaesthetics often precipitate fits in epileptic subjects. The retention of water in the body, brought about by the intake of a large amount of beer or fluid and the injection of pituitrin subcutaneously, lead to the occurrence of fits. Granted that a patient is liable to epilepsy psychological factors are much more potent than physical ones as immediate precipitants. Everyone has seen instances of an attack being precipitated by the worry of an examination, the excitement of starting a holiday, the frustrations of travel, the grief of a bereavement or anticipation of bad news. It requires understanding of the patient and knowledge of his life and his attitude to his disability to realize how often epileptic attacks are aggravated and indeed maintained by affective disorders. Depression, anxiety, doubt and frustration are *invariably* associated with increase in the incidence of attacks. This is particularly so in those stoical patients of rigid and rather obsessional temperament who maintain the patterns and the poise of their life in spite of these feelings. Granted that they are more liable to epileptic attacks than the average person, in them the attacks may continue as stress symptoms. Epilepsy, a disturbance of the brain, is much affected by disorders of the mind.

Symptoms

Prodromata. The circumstances which immediately precede the occurrence of an attack are of importance. As has been mentioned, it is uncommon, speaking generally, for an attack to occur when the attention is fixed, or when some act is being performed, and from this it follows that the epileptic is relatively or absolutely free from attacks when at work, and only in rare cases comes to harm or injury from accident. Some patients are able, by effort of will in fixing attention, or by the performance of some vigorous action, to arrest attacks which threaten or have even begun.

Sometimes a change in the general condition of the patient may make him aware that an attack is pending, and such signs of altered health may last for many hours. Headache, irritability, restlessness, euphoria, depression, lethargy, somnolence, unusual appetite and a peculiar vacant look are all seen in this connexion.

Sometimes the attack is preceded by paroxysmal manifestations which are in reality minute attacks, such as partial lapses in consciousness, a sense of strangeness, a 'dreamy state', myoclonus, or giddiness.

Description of the Attacks. The varieties of the epileptic attack are legion, and more than one type may occur in the same subject—indeed, it is unusual for fits to remain always the same in one subject. They tend to vary both in degree and nature.

The division of epilepsy already given is into:

Major fits—grand mal
Minor fits—petit mal
Focal fits

This is a clinical division, based upon the events in the fit, not upon the electroencephalogram. Consequently to the clinician *petit mal* may include any small attack. This popular usage has however been modified by increasing knowledge, and now petit mal is limited to the brief frequent stereotyped *absences* of childhood, associated with the characteristic 3-a-second spike and wave discharge in the electroencephalogram. Myoclonic epilepsy, which will be described later, is a variant of this.

All other forms—of any kind—are focal attacks. It is generally held that some major fits begin generally, and some focally but it is the author's view that focal attacks may induce a major fit in the same way as may an electrical discharge or a chemical disorder, the focal disturbance does not spread to become general but it fires off the major fit.

Major Convulsions (*grand mal*). There is tonic spasm of all the muscles of the body, of sudden onset. The blood pressure falls, the face is for a moment pallid, the eyes widely open, the pupils dilated, the corneae insensitive. The tonic spasm causes head retraction and opisthotonos; the arms are stiff in flexion and adduction, the legs in extension. If standing, the patient falls, usually backwards. The respiratory muscles and larynx, going into spasm, produce the epileptic 'cry', and the respiratory movements being no longer possible the face darkens with the asphyxia. After the tonic spasm has lasted some seconds and perhaps has produced such a degree of asphyxia as seems hardly compatible with survival, it begins to break into a series of sudden shock-like, jerky movements—the clonic spasm—which continue for some seconds, becoming less regular and occurring at longer intervals until, with a final jerk, the muscles become perfectly limp. At this stage there may be incontinence. The clonic spasm is in reality interruption of the tonus, and it may be that that causes biting of the tongue. Meanwhile the relaxation of the respiratory and laryngeal spasm has allowed the respiratory movements to return and to churn up the saliva, often bloodstained, which escapes at the nose and mouth in the form of froth. At the end of the attack there is complete loss of consciousness, the pupils are dilated and insensitive to light, the corneal reflexes absent, the knee-jerks absent and the plantar reflexes extensor in type. In a short time the knee-jerks return, the plantar reflexes become flexor and consciousness is regained. Usually the patient is dazed, feels ill, has marked headache and if left to himself soon sleeps heavily for some hours. It must be noted that the general convulsive attack almost always leaves the patient face downwards, so that he has been known to drown in a puddle and has been asphyxiated by his own pillow—the commonest way in which an epilepitc meets his death from accident in a fit.

The epileptic cry. There are two quite different sounds that may occur at the commencement of an epileptic attack. The one is a natural, conscious cry at the advent. It is curious how rarely any memory of such cries or utterances remains with the patient. The other is the epileptic cry proper—a weird, hollow sound, produced by inspiratory spasm drawing air over the nearly closed vocal cords. This cry occurs in a minority even of severe cases, for the obvious reason that it is determined by a particular march of the spasm. If the inspiratory spasm occurs before the larynx has gone into spasm or after it is in spasm, there can be no laryngeal noise, but only the commonly witnessed pharyngeal and buccal grunting and gurgling. The spasm must be so timed that the inspiratory spasm must occur as the larynx is closing, and this only obtains in a minority of the cases.

Tongue-biting. Some patients always bite the tongue, others never, and some now and again. The tongue is always bitten at the side some way from the tip, because it is deviated to one side in the spasm and its thicker part brought between the molar teeth. The same side is usually bitten. The tongue cannot be bitten unless protrusor spasm occurs either before the jaw has gone into tonic spasm or after it has broken into clonic spasm. If any other march of spasm occurs, the tongue escapes. It is remarkable how little scarring occurs even from severe and repeated tongue-biting unless a piece is bitten clean out.

Incontinence. Though common, incontinence is by no means invariable even in severe attacks. More often it is the urine alone that is evacuated, much more seldom the bowel alone, still more rarely both. A rare phenomenon during an epileptic fit is seminal emission.

Secondary events. The degree of asphyxia during the attack may be severe, and blood vessels may give way under the stress, with the production of surface ecchymoses or deep haemorrhages, including cerebral haemorrhage. The spasm is powerful and may give rise to much subsequent aching, as if the patient had been beaten all over. It may rarely dislocate joints, rupture muscles and even break bones. A dislocation once produced in a fit is very liable to recur with subsequent fits.

Duration of epileptic attacks. Two minutes may be given as an outside time-limit for the duration of a major fit, from its commencement to the end of the active phenomena, and in convulsive attacks to the end of the spasm. Usually the time is much shorter than this, and often is a few seconds only. Sometimes attacks are described as of much longer duration. When analysed, such attacks will be found to be a series of attacks with very short intervals, or slight attacks with postepileptic functional spasm, or hysterical attacks.

Other varieties of convulsive disorder are commonly encountered either as heralds of a *grand mal* attack or as the sole expression of the epileptic disturbance.

Major fits are accompanied in the electroencephalogram by a ubiquitous discharge of high voltage very fast spikes which precede the clinical evidences of the attack. A focal onset may be evident; the postictal phase is associated with very slow waves.

Minor Epilepsy (*petit mal*). The disturbances to which this term is given show considerable variation in degree, but share in common the fact that there is a sudden impairment or loss of consciousness. Attacks of this sort usually occur in children with constitutional epilepsy and spontaneously improve after maturation is complete at about 14 years of age.

Simple loss of consciousness. In this, the commonest of all minor phenomena, there is a simple break in the continuity of consciousness. The train of thought and action is suddenly arrested for a few seconds, and there is a sudden stillness of posture and facial expression which attracts the attention of a witness. The face may show sudden pallor, a vacant expression and curious fixity of the eyes, with large pupils. The patient does not fall, or move or drop anything that he is holding. In a few seconds the attack is over, leaving the patient unable to describe what has happened, perhaps a little confused for some seconds, sometimes emotional and even hysterical. More often he continues what he was about as if nothing had happened. Such attacks sometimes occur very frequently, even hundreds in a day. These brief attacks of lowered consciousness aptly called by the French *absences* are invariably associated with a ubiquitous 3-a-second spike and wave discharge in the electroencephalogram.

Simple loss of consciousness with falling. The patient suddenly falls, without warning, in the extended position, and almost always prone, so that his head reaches the ground first, and his forehead receives the bruise. He regains consciousness immediately, and picks himself up as if nothing had happened. In another form of this type the head, or the head and trunk, alone are affected; the patient does not fall, but simply drops the head forward.

Myoclonic Jerking. Simple twitchings of individual muscles or groups of muscles may occur. They are conspicuous in the convulsions of childhood, where they often constitute the chief clinical feature.

Myoclonic jerks happen especially in constitutional epilepsy and in association with degenerative cerebral disease of infancy, for instance lipid disease [p. 1237]. In constitutional epilepsy the jerks involve the arms more than the legs, and they are often bilateral. Myoclonic epilepsy is the only form in which, whilst bilateral jerking occurs, the patient is conscious. They happen particularly when the muscle is being stretched, and are worst first thing in the morning and when tired in the evening. They are invariably associated with 3-a-second spike and wave discharges in the electroencephalogram.

FOCAL FITS

In local convulsive attacks the common foci of onset are the angle of the mouth, the thumb and index finger, and the great toe, but the spasm may occasionally begin elsewhere. It rarely produces conjugate deviation of the eyes as a primary movement, but usually in association with, and secondary to, deviation of the head. The convulsive movements may remain confined to their place of onset throughout the fit, or may spread widely so as to involve a whole limb, one half of the body, or the entire musculature. In fits involving the musculature of the right half of the face and tongue, speech is usually lost during the attack and returns shortly after its cessation. In some cases the convulsion leaves varying degrees of weakness in the affected muscles—Todd's paralysis or post-epileptic paralysis—with transient signs of loss of function of the pyramidal system, such as loss of trunk reflexes, increase of jerks and extensor plantar reflexes.

Epileptic spasm usually puts the hand in the position of extension at the interphalangeal joints, and flexion at the metacarpophalangeal joints, with flexion at wrist and elbow, and adduction at the shoulder. The feet are dropped and inturned, with extension at the knee and hip.

The sequence of tonic spasm, followed by clonic spasm, though usual in epilepsy, is not invariable. Purely tonic fits may occur with no clonic spasm, the tonic spasm remitting suddenly. Such fits are usually of slight severity and duration. On the other hand, the spasm may be clonic only. The simple jactitation already described may be taken as a simple clonic fit. Local fits, especially of the face and of the hand, may be purely clonic.

Jacksonian attacks are focal fits which march in a stereotyped manner determined by the functional pattern of the involved cortex. Hughlings Jackson described the march of the clonic movements of a hand and arm in a patient who subsequently was found to have a small meningioma of the motor cortex. He used the occurrence of these advancing focal attacks to study the functional integration of the cerebral cortex. It is most interesting and was also sad that that great medical philosopher's own wife had Jacksonian epilepsy in her fatal illness.

Loss of consciousness in focal fits. This seems to depend upon the extent of the cortex involved. With narrowly confined fits there may be no evident impairment at all, as in local convulsion of the face or hand, or as in a patient who vividly described a slow visual fit as it was occurring. When the fit spreads, consciousness is usually impaired, and when lost, it is lost late in the fit. For example, it is usual for a convulsion which spreads to one-half of the body to cause some impairment, and if it involves both sides generally, consciousness is always lost.

Focal Paralytic Fits (*akinetic attacks*). These are the rarest of all forms of the epileptic attack. They consist in a sudden inability, relative or complete, to use a limb or one side of the body or the whole voluntary musculature, with no preceding convulsion. There are the usual signs of cerebral paralysis—at first flaccidity with a tendency for the jerks to fail; a few moments later increased jerks, with absent trunk reflexes and extensor plantar reflexes, all of which signs soon disappear. The attack may occur as an isolated phenomenon. More often a slight 'minor' attack or a local sensory attack accompanies the onset of the paralysis. Sometimes such an attack may result from local disease of the brain. When it involves the right face or right side of the body it may cause aphasia, or the aphasia may occur alone as the attack of simple paralysis.

Sensory Epileptic Disturbances. Numerous sudden sensory disturbances may happen in epilepsy. They may be related to the organs of special sense, to those of common sensibility or to those of visceral sensibility. They may occur as isolated events and so constitute the whole epileptic attack. Often, however, the disturbance of the cortex spreads widely, involving general convulsion and loss of consciousness; but the initial phenomena are remembered by the patient as the 'warning' of the attack and have from ancient times been termed 'auras', when preceding general convulsion. In reality, they constitute an essential part of the attack as showing the region of the brain in which the disturbance starts, and in every patient who has such 'warnings' preceding his severe attacks, the warnings occur at times by themselves without any such sequel.

Visual fits. These may take the form of negative phenomena, such as dimness of vision, complete darkness or hemianopia, or of positive effects, such as flashes of light, scintillating stars or balls of fire, or of both together in the form of blindness with flashes of light. In the last case they may closely resemble the visual phenomena of migraine, and are not infrequently caused by a local lesion of the occipital region. Complex visual hallucinations may occur.

Auditory fits. The hallucinations of sound may be of any nature—hissing, booming and elaborate musical sensations, as of bells, being common. There is usually a sense of coincident deafness of 'far away' hearing, which passes off with or soon after the sound.

Olfactory and gustatory fits. These hallucinations are

described as of 'flavour', usually unpleasant. Very often, movements of the lips, tongue and jaw, or swallowing movements are present, and the 'dreamy state' referred to below may be associated. From the location of the functions of smell and taste in the cortex of the uncinate gyri, and from the common occurrence of fits of this character in lesions of these convolutions, this type of fit is often referred to as the 'uncinate fit'.

Sensory fits. These hallucinations may start in any part of the body. They may remain local, but more commonly they spread from the point of origin in terms of the local representations of the body in the cerebral cortex, and usually from the periphery towards the trunk and head, but a sensory fit may spread to the extreme periphery first. For example, commencing in the fingers, it may spread up the arm to the head, or on reaching the shoulder it may invade trunk and leg before ascending to the head. It may be bilateral, and may be confined to the anterior or posterior aspect of the body.

The sensation may be described as 'numbness', 'tingling', 'pins and needles', 'vibration', 'rushing', 'as if the limb were withering', much more rarely actual pain. Sometimes the sensation is indescribable. The sensory attacks have their origin in a local disturbance of the parietal region of the cortex, and may indicate the presence of an organic lesion in that region. They may be accompanied or followed by temporary loss of sensibility, in the form of astereognosis, loss of sense of position or anaesthesia.

Another group of sensory fits which arise in the anterior temporal and orbital frontal cortex is that of the so-called visceral auras, which are mainly referred to the distribution of the vagus nerve. Such are the commonly occurring 'epigastric' sensation, and feelings of choking, dyspnoea, nausea and cardiac discomfort. These are in fact actual local attacks, the idea that the visceral sensation is merely a warning being mistaken. The motor and sensory cortex serving the upper alimentary and respiratory tracts is in the anterior and posterior parts of the insula.

Disturbances of vestibular function are common indications of epilepsy. Sudden giddiness may be the sole indication of epilepsy, and is a common initial event in major attacks. It may be indicative of the sudden fall of blood pressure, or the feeling of rotation may be consequent upon early spasm causing conjugate deviation of the eyes. In patients with focal epilepsy the electroencephalogram recorded between the fits will usually show local disturbances corresponding with the site of onset of the trouble. There may be focal spikes or slow waves. The spikes may be potentiated by injection of leptazol and are used as a guide to surgical intervention.

Temporal Lobe Attacks (*psychomotor fits*). These may take the form of peculiar mental states, of instantaneous onset, remembered afterwards sometimes in exquisite detail, sometimes only in vague character. Emotional conditions of fear or horror, which may cause the patient to attempt with violence to escape from his surroundings—'cursive' epilepsy—may occur. Or, the attacks may take the form of a sudden feeling of misery, or an intense sense of personal wrongdoing, a sense of intense familiarity in surroundings which are unfamiliar, a sudden sense of strangeness, as in a patient whose fit was 'suddenly seeming to be somewhere else', a sense of euphoria or of intense mental energy, a 'dreamy state', often associated with smacking of the lips and champing or swallowing movements, which often has a pleasurable emotional tone. Again, the psychic fit may take the form of a highly complex and detailed hallucination. Other psychomotor attacks may express themselves as outburts of uncontrollable rage, and in rare instances the patients make attacks of great ferocity on unoffending individuals and have no recollection of these incidents afterwards. The electroencephalogram in patients with temporal lobe epilepsy may show discharges in one or both sides. These may be focal and may consist of well localized spike discharges, or episodes of monophasic 4–7-a-second rhythms.

Condition After Attacks. The epileptic fit may leave no after-effects whatever, even though it is severe, though this is unusual. On the other hand, even the slightest attacks may cause conspicuous sequels. Sleep and headache are very common, especially following convulsive attacks, and they may be alternative effects, in that if sleep occur there is no headache, but if it is prevented headache is severe. The postepileptic paralysis of Todd has already been described, and also the aphasia which may follow right-sided attacks. The mental state is usually affected by the attack, and returns to the normal sometimes quickly, sometimes slowly. Commonly the patient is dull and dazed, speaking at random, unreceptive, irritable and is unable to fully recognize his surroundings. During this state of impaired consciousness the patient may show automatism, in which acts are performed in a conscious manner but of which no recollection is afterwards retained. This fact has an important bearing as regards the criminal responsibility of the epileptic. These postepileptic conditions occur commonly after minor attacks, but they may also follow major fits; they seldom occur when convulsion has been severe.

Vomiting may follow any type of epileptic fit, but it happens often after a convulsion. As it occurs during the period of unconsciousness, there is some danger of the vomited material being drawn into the larynx.

Dementia and the 'Epileptic Temperament'. There is little evidence that occasional fits lead to dementia, though some patients with frequent fits do show dementia. As a generalization, dementia is due to the cause of the fits and not to the fits themselves, so that a patient with a cerebral tumour, with cortical atrophy or who is an alcoholic with fits may show dementia and change in personality. The confusion of the results of the lesion with the results of the fits has done great disservice to the large population of otherwise normal epileptic patients.

There is as wide a range of temperament in people with epilepsy as in the ordinary population, but otherwise normal epileptics have, through the distortions which the occurrence of the attacks themselves impose upon their life-patterns, great difficulties to contend with. This frustrating situation readily produces an intransigent neurosis, as might readily be expected.

SPECIAL VARIETIES OF EPILEPSY

Epilepsy from Local Disease of the Brain. Almost any lesion of the cerebral hemispheres may produce symptomatic epilepsy. But yet not more than 5 per cent. of them do so. The convulsions which may occur in cerebral thrombosis, encephalitis and meningitis are examples of epilepsy incident with the onset of an acute lesion. Lesions of the brain in childhood more commonly cause epilepsy than those in adult life. Agenetic states of the brain of pre-natal origin (cerebral diplegias) are associated with epilepsy in 30 per cent. of cases, and infantile hemiplegia is followed by epilepsy in about the same proportion. In adults the commonest causes of symptomatic epilepsy are birth injuries, head injury and tumours. Increased intracranial pressure by itself may produce fits, and they are usual with cerebral abscess.

The fits caused by local lesions may be in every respect identical with the usual type of epileptic manifestation, from the slightest momentary minor fit, all through the local sensory and motor fits, to the severe general convulsion of instantaneous onset and immediate loss of consciousness. There are the same auras and the same sequels.

Minor attacks with loss of consciousness are the least common of those occurring as the result of a local lesion; the general convulsion by far the most common; while the local fit holds an intermediate position, and its nature is often indicative of the position of the lesion. The sort of juvenile petit mal accompanied by 3-a-second spike and wave discharge in the electroencephalogram is never the result of an acquired local lesion.

Traumatic Epilepsy. The underlying pathological change in traumatic epilepsy is a cortical cicatrix although the occurrence of epilepsy will be largely determined by the particular brain affected.

The incidence of traumatic epilepsy is variously estimated by different writers, but is much higher in penetrating than in closed injuries of the brain. In the case of closed injuries of all severity the estimates range from 4 per cent. to 8 per cent., the liability increasing with the severity of the injury as judged by the duration of unconsciousness. In penetrating wounds of the brain estimates vary from 10 per cent. to 25 per cent. The development of epilepsy always follows a latent interval which varies from two months to many years, and averages 2–3 years.

Any form of epileptic disturbance may follow injury but the generalized convulsion is the most common, and it is often associated with focal attacks.

Myoclonus Epilepsy. In this group are included any brief attacks in which there are solitary muscle twitches. The most common is that of 'idiopathic' epilepsy, where, in addition to major fits, there are, first thing in the morning and when tired in the evening, isolated jerks of muscles which are being used. These are much more common in the arms than the legs, more often on one side or the other indiscriminately than bilateral. There is no disturbance of consciousness, or other event at all. There is always a 3-a-second spike and wave discharge in the electroencephalogram recorded at the time. They are the motor homologues of the disorder of the sensorium causing the *absences* of *petit mal*. Where there is identical spike and wave discharge this form of epilepsy has always been present from childhood, and is never symptomatic of acquired disease.

Other forms of myoclonus epilepsy are seen with degenerative diseases such as the lipodystrophies, subacute inclusion encephalitis, the leucodystrophies and Unverricht's disease. In all of these there is mental impairment too [see p. 1253].

Reflex Epilepsy. There are many cases in which fits can be produced with great regularity by certain specific stimuli. To these the term reflex epilepsy has been applied. The most frequent of such exciting causes is some tactile stimulus to a particular part of the body, especially when unexpected. In another form the stimulus may be a sudden noise or music, and recently reflex epilepsy in response to repeated light flashes (photic) has been the subject of much physiological research. Other cases are precipitated by emotion.

Epilepsia Partialis Continua (*focal status epilepticus*). Under this name have been described cases of focal epilepsy, usually consisting of clonic spasm, which remain confined to the part of the body in which they originate but which persist with little or no intermission for hours or days at a stretch.

This form of epileptic discharge is most often seen in the face and is probably always associated with local organic disease of the corresponding area of the cerebral cortex.

Status Epilepticus. In this condition severe convulsion succeeds severe convulsion at short intervals without return of consciousness. It is as if a convulsion recurred as soon as the body recovered sufficiently from the exhaustion produced by the last. Meanwhile the temperature rises, and may reach a hyperpyrexia. The difficulty in feeding and providing fluids, the severe muscular exertion and the pyrexia add their dangers to those of exhaustion and the patient may die. Status epilepticus must not be confused with frequently recurring fits in which there is some return to consciousness during the intervals, though it often develops from such a condition, for this is not accompanied by a rising temperature, the fits are more easily controlled and are not nearly so serious. If the convulsions of status epilepticus cannot be stopped by treatment, the patient usually dies from sudden collapse. Status epilepticus may occur with acute lesions of the brain but it sometimes heralds idiopathic epilepsy. It may follow sudden withdrawal of anticonvulsants.

Vasovagal Attacks. Under this misleading title, Gowers described a recurrent paroxysmal symptom-complex with some or all of the following components; a sensation of fullness in the epigastrium; precordial pain or discomfort; difficulty in breathing; a sense of impending death; a slowness of mental operations but without disturbance of consciousness; a sense of physical fatigue and coldness of face and extremities. These symptoms wax and then wane gradually, and may be present for as long as 4 hours from onset to disappearance.

Gowers stated that he used the term 'vasovagal' as a purely descriptive one, but without implying any theory of causation. Unfortunately, those who have adopted his terminology have overlooked its lack of foundation.

The term has no precise meaning, no sound basis of observation and no proper place in neurological terminology.

Differential Diagnosis

The recognition of epilepsy needs a working acquaintance with the nature of its many manifestations and especially of the slight forms, little exteriorized, which may be easily overlooked or misinterpreted. The sudden unexpected onset, without cause, the transience, the recurrence and the circumstances of the moment, are useful aids. If all these clinical features are taken into account a confident diagnosis can almost invariably be made. Epilepsy is the only condition which causes repeated attacks in sleep, with the exception of the nightmare, and this seldom causes difficulty in diagnosis. Again, if an attack occurs soon after waking, there is a very strong presumption that it is epileptic. There is, however, a syndrome which is altogether mistaken for epilepsy, the so-called functional midbrain syndrome. In this, the patient undergoes strange experiences as going from wakefulness to sleep, or from sleep to awakening. On the motor side these include jerks or compulsive movement and paralysis ('sleep paralysis') and on the sensory, disturbances of body shape or size, sounds, voices, or visions ('waking dreams'). It is associated with disorder of sleep and with cataplexy. If the patient only has the disturbances at the moment between being awake and asleep, then they are not epileptic. The electroencephalogram is seldom helpful in the primary diagnosis but may give useful information about the focal discharge in some cases of symptomatic epilepsy.

There is no corner of medicine in which it is so important to listen carefully to the patient, to believe what he says however bizarre, and to question him carefully about details which may seem unimportant to him. If there were more good doctors taking good histories from patients with epilepsy we could close some of our overworked departments of electroencephalography.

Syncopal attacks can often be distingusihed from epilepsy by their slow onset, the gradually increasing pallor of greyness, the distancing of sound, the nausea and flatulence, the presence of an obvious cause, and by their duration. Nevertheless syncope may end in a convulsion, the result of cerebral ischaemia, but then the diagnosis is that of the first cause—syncope.

The hysterical attack has to be distinguished from the convulsion of epilepsy. Hysterical convulsions which are rare today have not the manner nor the march of epileptic spasm. It never begins with conjugate deviation of head and eyes to one side, there is not the orderly spread of convulsion, and there is never anything but a poor imitation of the sequence of tonic followed by clonic spasms. The movements in the hysterical fit are purposive, spectacular, violent and are liable to be increased by restraint and are rapidly abolished by complete inattention. The hysterical fit never occurs during sleep, the tongue is never bitten, though other parts of the body and other people may be. There is no transient abolition of the tendon-jerks, nor transient appearance of the Babinski plantar response. The sphincters are never relaxed. Intense converging spasm of the eyes is a common feature of the hysterical attack, but this sign is not met with in epilepsy. When elaborate disorders of behaviour follow slight and rapidly transient epileptic attacks, the distinction between these and purely hysterical attacks is often difficult and sometimes impossible, except after long observation, for the initial epileptic attack may be practically unnoticeable, and the subsequent events may be typical of hysteria and are usually amenable to the same line of treatment. Often some point in the circumstances under which the attack occurs will settle the diagnosis. Any attack having occurred during sleep, any in which the patient has fallen in circumstances of serious danger, as among the traffic of a London street, or any occurring when the patient cannot attract the attention of others, establishes the diagnosis of epilepsy. The best plan is to regard all fits as possibly epileptic, and every fit of doubtful type as probably epileptic, until time and circumstance bring definite conviction.

Migraine may possibly simulate epilepsy when paralysis, or sensory auras, or visual hallucinations occur without headache. But while the sensory phenomena of migraine may last for 5–30 minutes, those of epilepsy have a duration of seconds only.

Diagnosis of the Cause. A careful history and detailed examinations are essential in every new case of epilepsy seen. Papilloedema, headache and vomiting may reveal increased intracranial pressure; while local paralysis, sensory loss, visual or other defect may indicate a local lesion of the brain, past or present, and this may also be suggested by the nature of a local fit. The presence of infantilism, undue adiposity, or disorder of bone may indicate the presence of metabolic or endocrine disorder. The blood pressure should always be recorded for even in infancy fits may be hypertensive. Where syphilis is likely, the reactions in the blood and cerebrospinal fluid should be examined. Lastly, any evidence of chronic intoxication by drugs or alcohol should be sought. Cysticercosis epilepsy should be thought of when the patient has lived abroad [Section 2].

These are examples only, for as stated earlier there are so many causes of fits, and fits are always just symptoms. When nothing has been found as a prime cause for the fits, investigation should include radiology of skull and chest, electroencephalography, and routine blood studies. If, however, the fits are not focal, clinical examination is negative, and the electroencephalograph does not show the signs of a local lesion. Further 'neurosurgical' investigations need not be undertaken at the time. Although late epilepsy and focal epilepsy both suggest a local gross cerebral cause for the fits, it is much less common to find a remediable cause than not, in either circumstance. A previous history of fits, such as of infantile convulsions, makes a newly acquired cause most unlikely.

Treatment

General Treatment. The general principles for the maintenance of good health should be adopted. Whenever possible, no change should be made from the regime of life of a normal person. In childhood, education, discipline and pleasures and school life should be continued upon strictly normal lines, and the adult should continue with work and occupation. The life of the epileptic should be as regular as possible and physical and emotional strains, changes in occupation and diet should be reduced to a minimum. Continuity of treatment is of great importance and any course adopted should be given a thorough trial before being modified. Frequent changes of drugs or doctors should be avoided. No advantage has accrued from the adoption of special diets, such as the prohibition of meat, the exclusion of salt or the use of purine-free foods. Alcohol in moderation is generally harmless.

The forbidding of such pastimes as may be fraught with danger should a fit occur, such as swimming, boating or cycling should be exercised with the greatest restraint, to prevent the patient feeling frustrated and different from his fellows. Unless the fits are prohibitively frequent, parents should be taught to accept the minor risk of swimming, climbing or boating, provided the child in his turn is taught to accept his share of responsibility. A child who can swim under observation or who can cycle on side roads has a much greater chance of ceasing fits than the one who stays at home under his mother's anxious care. This problem of maternal anxiety and overt surveillance is so conducive to the maintenance of fits that as an aphorism I have advised the family doctor to give the phenobarbitone to the anxious mother, not to the epileptic child.

Car Driving. This is prohibited in people with active epilepsy or with any other 'disabling attacks of giddiness or faintness'. The responsibility not to drive is therefore clearly upon the patient's shoulders and is not primarily medical. Any recurring attacks are a bar to driving; this should be pointed out to the patient who is naturally anxious to find some medical justification for his illegal intentions. When attacks of any kind have ceased, driving may be recommenced, but how soon depends upon all the circumstances of the attacks, their cause and nature, and also the circumstances in which the patient is to drive. It is only on this question of 'how soon' after cure that the doctor must shoulder responsibility. As a guide, application for a licence may be made if previously established epilepsy has ceased for 3 years, with or without treatment.

Marriage and Pregnancy. The subject of epilepsy sometimes seeks—but rarely heeds—advice on marriage, both in its effects upon himself (or herself) and on heredity. Marriage has no necessary effect upon the course of epilepsy, and, as we have seen, direct transmission of the disease is rare. Therefore the sweeping medical prohibitions once so frequent in these circumstances are not in fact warranted. It is common, though not constant, for fits to cease in pregnancy; fits at this time constitute no special danger and are not an indication for termination. On the other hand, the confirmed and serious epileptic person is clearly unlikely to be able to discharge adequately the responsibilities of parenthood.

Institutional Treatment. Where there is low mentality, dementia or insanity, and frequent fits, where no adequate care and occupation can be provided at home, there is every advantage in a colony or other institution for people with epilepsy. In them regular work, discipline, interest and contentment may bring about remarkable improvement.

Otherwise the place for the person with epilepsy is in the community at large, whether at school, at home, in the workshop or the university.

Surgical Treatment. In the present state of our knowledge surgery has no part to play in the treatment of idiopathic epilepsy. Neurosurgical procedures, such as encephalography and ventriculography, are of great value in establishing or excluding the presence of a space-occupying lesion in doubtful cases and in revealing the presence of cortical atrophy, porencephaly or ventricular dilatation. Such epileptogenic processes as cerebral tumours or abscesses may be amenable to surgical removal and the epilepsy may be relieved thereby. The place of surgery in traumatic epilepsy is more debatable. Penfield and others have demonstrated the value of the excision of scarred areas of the cortex in selected cases of traumatic epilepsy but demand as criteria for operation that ventriculography should reveal a definite ventricular distortion in that area of the brain indicated as the starting-point of the discharge by the nature of the fits, and that it should be possible to reproduce an accurate replica of the fit by electrical stimulation of the abnormal area of cortex at the time of operation. In general, the removal of brain with the apparent site of origin of the epilepsy by the best surgeons in the best centres, with most careful selection of cases, stops attacks for 5 years in about half the cases. The procedure is therefore reserved for intractable epilepsy where the nidus is in a part of the brain which can be removed without harm.

Stereotactic surgery for the relief of epilepsy is in its infancy, but is based upon acceptable physiological principles.

Medical Treatment. There are now several groups of drugs which arrest or mitigate the attacks in epilepsy. They seem to have much the same effect, and may conveniently be combined or alternated in the treatment of any given case. Sometimes one group is found to suit an individual patient better than the other. Moderate doses, which cause no deterioration in bodily or mental health even if taken regularly and for years, give the best results. All successful anticonvulsants, whatever their chemical parentage, have in common their ability to disturb carbohydrate metabolism by interfering with fractions of the vitamin B complex; in particular their anticonvulsant effect is associated with lowering of blood folate, and restoration of its level by giving folic acid modifies their therapeutic effect.

The most widely used after 50 years is still phenobarbitone. It is conveniently prescribed in doses of 30 mg., with a maximum dose of 100 mg. three times in the day to an adult. In larger doses it is an hypnotic, and in patients who have idiosyncrasy it may produce toxic symptoms. It occasionally makes the patient peculiarly quarrelsome; this is especially the case in children. People vary enormously in their tolerance for it—believe what they say.

Primidone (*Mysoline*) is as useful an anticonvulsant as phenobarbitone; from 1 to 6 tablets of 0·25 G. may be taken in the day. The toxicity of primidone is low and by itself it is not usually hypnotic, but if taken in association with phenobarbitone it may cause excessive drowsiness. Phenytoin sodium (*Dilantin*, *Epanutin*) is dispensed in capsules or tablets of 50 and 100 mg. For adults, the usual dose is up to 300 or 400 mg. daily, smaller doses for children in proportion to size. It is a slowly cumulative poison, giving an irreversible ataxia, dysarthria and diplopia in excess. Prolonged continuation may rarely lead to permanent effects. It also causes hypertrophy of the gums, and rashes.

A useful regime for major fits is to commence with phenobarbitone, 30 mg., up to 3 a day, then to add phenytoin, 100 mg. up to 3 a day, and then to substitute primidone, 250 mg. up to 6 a day, for the phenobarbitone. Succinimides are being used with success in a wide variety of forms and are well worth adding, but it is wise not to administer at any one time more than two anticonvulsants. Sulthiame (*Ospolot*), 200 mg. up to 3 a day, is a valuable adjuvant, especially for focal temporal epilepsy.

The treatment of focal fits is similar, but primidone is less reliable in its effects upon them.

The treatment of petit mal is quite different. Phenobarbitone occasionally helps, but the diones, ethosuximide (*Zarontin*) and stimulants such as amphetamine and caffeine are used. Probably the most useful regime is first to use *Zarontin*, up to one tablet 4 times a day, to try the effect of troxidone (*Tridione*) and then to add a stimulant in a dose appropriate to the age. Phenobarbitone is unlikely to help and phenacemide (*Phenurone*), though very effective, may be exceedingly toxic.

The medical treatment of petit mal is unsatisfactory; this must be accepted and the child must not be afflicted by therapy as well as by the little attacks. This view is fortified by the frequent occurrence of minor toxic effects with the substances mentioned.

In women with premenstrual epilepsy temporary dehydration with a diuretic helps, and in patients whose fits are increased by a psychological tension state, tranquillizers can act indirectly as anticonvulsants. Do not forget, though, that chlorpromazine is a mild convulsant. Whatever regime is chosen it is wise to anticipate the occurrence of the fit by the administration of the drug. Thus, if fits are nocturnal only, the treatment is given in a single large dose at night, or if diurnal only, in a single dose in the early morning. If the fits are more frequent before menstruation, they should be anticipated by increased dosage before it.

Status Epilepticus. The treatment is one of great urgency and constitutes one of the important neurological emergencies.

First stop the convulsions by inducing light anaesthesia. For this purpose paraldehyde in large doses is perhaps the safest and most effective drug. If it can be administered by mouth, 15–30 ml. should be used in the case of an average adult, or alternatively 30–60 ml. may be given per rectum. Subsequently smaller doses should be given every 2–3 hours in order to maintain a state of light narcosis, the amounts being judged by the depth of unconsciousness and the occurrence of fits. Phenobarbitone, 200 mg. in the soluble form may be given intramusculary and, if necessary, repeated in 12 hours. If an anaesthetic such as thiopentone sodium (*Pentothal*) is used intravenously, full anaesthetic facilities should be available, because of possible respiratory arrest. They may be necessary to save life but in an emergency paraldehyde, 10 ml. intramuscularly, is safer. In children, the present vogue is to use up to 40 mg. of diazepam (*Valium*) given slowly in an intravenous drip, until the fits cease. When consciousness returns, the routine treatment of epilepsy should be resumed. Status eiplepticus carries a considerable mortality, and death commonly occurs from bronchopneumonia or from cardiac failure. Status epilepticus may be the terminal event in cases of chronic epilepsy.

Prognosis

The outlook in epilepsy is so variable that only the broadest principles in prognosis can be given. In an otherwise normal subject, at school or in employment, living a natural unrestricted life, the outlook with well planned medical treatment is generally good. Almost half the patients will cease their attacks and the other half will in some degree be improved. On the other hand, patients with gross brain lesions, even if these are stationary, are liable to continue to have attacks. Intercurrent but unrelated disease makes the attacks worse and psychological illness, with depression or anxiety, with maladjustment or with major personality problems, will maintain attacks in spite of the most rigorous medical treatment.

The danger to life from the epileptic attack itself, either directly or indirectly, is not great. However severe the fit, it is rare for death to occur, and when this happens it is from turning over and smothering with the wetted pillow or by choking from the aspiration of vomited material. Injury, burning and drowning may cause death, yet the number of epileptics who meet their deaths in this way is so small as almost to remove the danger of accident from practical perspective. In status epilepticus, however, the danger to life may be great. Spontaneous cessation of the attacks occurs in some cases.

The chance of recovery is much greater when the continuance of education or of regular employment allows a fully occupied and satisfying life, and much less when education is stopped, pleasures and sports forbidden and the patient condemned to social ostracism, and a gloomy life of frustration because he has a few fits. It is perhaps smallest when severe attacks occur daily or at short intervals and when both major and minor attacks occur in the same subject.

MYOCLONUS

Synonyms. Paramyoclonus multiplex (Friedreich); Myoclonus epilepsy (Unverricht).

Definition

There are sudden shock-like contractions of the muscles, which may vary in intensity from simple fibrillary twitching to contraction causing violent movement of a limb. The movements are often symmetrical, and affect particularly the proximal limb muscles. The disease is pathophysiolgically a form of epilepsy due to diffuse brain disease, of one of a number of rare familial or sporadic kinds.

Aetiology

The disorder appears in children usually between the ages of 5 and 15 years or less often in young adults. Both sexes are liable. Many instances in which several children of the same parents have been affected, have been recorded, and in a few it has been transmitted through several generations. The condition may be associated with diffuse cerebral lipidosis, the various forms of cerebromacular degeneration, subacute inclusion body encephalitus, while in other cases the peculiar bodies described by Lafora are found in the cells of the brain and also in the liver, heart and possibly other organs.

This form of myoclonus should be distinguished from that seen in idiopathic epilepsy, which is unassociated with evident brain disease or dementia.

Symptoms

The movements of myoclonus are simple and sudden resembling those resulting from a single faradic stimulus. Each movement commonly involves a single muscle only, and it may concern no more than a few fibres, resembling then the fibrillary twitching common in progressive muscular atrophy. In other cases, many muscles may be implicated in the shock-like spasms, which may be so violent as to throw the patient to the ground. The distribution of the contraction is never determined by that of the nerve supply, nor do the muscles contract according to their synergic association. Myoclonic movements are irregular as regards rhythm and range of successive movements. The arms are more affected than the legs and the proximal parts more than the distal, while the periphery, the hand and foot, often escape. Voluntary muscular effort usually checks the myoclonic movements, but in rare instances it excites or augments the spasm. Routine examination is negative. Speech may be disturbed when the muscles of jaw, palate and larynx are implicated, and spontaneous laryngeal and pharyngeal noises may occur. The ocular muscles are never involved. Convulsions are present in the typical cases. Depending upon the nature of the primary disease of the brain there may be a varying degree of dementia and personality disorder, together with disturbances of pyramidal functions.

There are characteristic electroencephalographic changes, discharges coinciding with the movements, consisting of wide-spread spikes of high voltage with 1- and 2-a-second wave complexes.

Diagnosis

This is not difficult since the simple shock-like movements in symmetrical muscles, without any resemblance to volitional movements and entirely destitute of rhythm, occur in this disease alone.

Treatment

Drugs used for petit mal should be tried, but are not very effective.

Course, Duration and Prognosis

The movements are often phasic in their occurrence, but progress with the prime disease. Myoclonus is a symptom of a number of degenerative diseases of the brain, and its cause depends upon the cause of the prime disease. They are mainly progressive and over months or years advance to a fatal termination.

A note upon the use of the electroencephalogram appears on page 1202.

INFANTILE SPASMS

A form of epilepsy similar to myoclonic epilepsy occurs in infants, and is associated with dementia. It is due to metabolic brain disease which is rare, and temporarily responds to corticosteroids. The attacks are very frequent indeed, and have many forms—brief petit mal, local or general myoclonus and flaccid attacks in which the child falls forward (salaam attacks). The electroencephalogram shows widespread severe abnormality consisting of every variety and frequency of scan waves, to which the name of hypsarrhythmia was given by Gibbs—a name which has erroneously been used for the clinical state. Even when there is response to steroids the childs stays demented, and needs special education later.

NARCOLEPSY—CATAPLEXY—SLEEP PARALYSIS

In this remarkable syndrome there are a number of disturbances of the physiology of sleep.

Symptoms

There is the onset of apparently normal sleep, which comes on especially at time of inattention or when the desire to sleep might normally be expected to occur, as, for example, after meals, in public vehicles or during the performance of tedious duties. The sleep is preceded by a sensation of extreme drowsiness. The sleeper is easily roused and is then perfectly normal, but if left undisturbed may remain asleep for many minutes or even an hour or two. Attempts to ward off the attack by voluntary effort lead to an increase in intensity of the craving for sleep until it is satisfied. This is *hypersomnia*.

There is also the recurrence of momentary overwhelming compulsive sleep, which only lasts for a moment, to be followed by wakefulness and a sensation of great relief, as of a compulsion. This is *narcolepsy*.

When awake there is sudden onset of weakness and tonelessness in the voluntary muscles, which is *cataplexy*. These cataplectic attacks are almost invariably precipitated by sudden emotion, such as anger, pleasure, surprise or anticipation, and most often of all by events provoking laughter. In a severe attack, when the emotion reaches a certain intensity, the muscles suddenly become limp, the head falls forward, the jaw drops, the eyelids close and the face becomes expressionless, the arms fall to the sides and the legs crumple so that the patient sinks to the ground, an inert mass, speechless, and incapable of the slightest movement, but without any impairment of consciousness. In a second or two the attack passes and the muscles immediately regain their normal condition. Milder attacks may involve any part of the musculature or may consist merely of a momentary feeling of weakness of the knees. Patients can often judge with great accuracy the intensity and nature of the emotion necessary to bring on an attack.

Narcolepsy and cataplexy are associated with other disturbances in relation to sleep. In the twilight state before sleep there may be repeated jerks of the limbs, auditory or sometimes visual hallucinations. On waking there may be weakness of the body, analogous to cataplexy, which is called sleep paralysis. These disorders may be associated with disturbances of proprioception, the patient feeling himself levitated or too heavy. Functional disorders of this kind, though undoubtedly physiogenic, are much aggravated by disorders of affect. They are *hypnogogic experiences*.

Although most commonly the sleep attacks and cataplectic attacks occur under the characteristic circumstances in the same patients, each may occur in isolation. Often the patient complaining of one form of attack will admit to the other upon questioning, though it may have been of rare occurrence and have caused little inconvenience.

Epilepsy may also occur with this strange syndrome —also called the *functional midbrain syndrome*. In sleep the state of consciousness and the state of muscle control change compared with wakefulness. The sleeping person is unresponsive to expected harmless sounds but immediately alert to potentially harmful, however small; he has the flaccidity of sleep and the movements of sleep. In this syndrome the sleep mechanism is disturbed. Sleep comes too easily, lasts too long, and the transitions to and from sleep are inefficient in their sensory and motor aspects, alone or together, as if the two-pronged switch of sleep were faulty. This is where cataplexy fits in; when awake the sudden startle, preserved in sleep, produces the flaccidity of sleep.

Affective disorders disturb the pattern of sleep, they also make this sleep disturbance much worse.

The *Kleine-Levin syndrome* is the name used for a state of intermittent somnolence with withdrawal and retardation which happens in young men. The phases lasts a few days, with normality between. There is hyperphagia on recovery. The disturbance has many of the features of recurrent depression.

Course

In the majority of patients suffering from narcolepsy, examination reveals no evidence of organic disease in the nervous system or elsewhere, and pathological investigation is equally negative. In such cases the term idiopathic narcolepsy can properly be applied. Men are much more affected than women, and though the attacks may begin at any age a large proportion have their onset between the ages of 10 and 30 and may continue throughout life.

In rare cases the narcoleptic syndrome may occur as a symptom of organic disease of the nervous system, notably of encephalitis lethargica or tumours of the third ventricle. This association suggests that the site of the disturbance is in the autonomic centres of the hypothalamus and the floor of the third ventricle.

Treatment

The sleep attacks of narcolepsy are in many cases greatly improved by the regular use of amphetamine sulphate. An initial dose of 10 mg. after breakfast and lunch is often enough, but this may be increased if necessary to 20 or even 30 mg. twice daily. Patients with this symptom are most tolerant of the amphetamines, and they may respond in a most specific way to one of the three of them.

MIGRAINE

Synonyms. Hemicrania; Sick headaches.

Definition

A common disorder with recurring intense headaches, which often develop on waking in the morning, and which, while often unilateral, may be bifrontal, occipital or general. The attacks often date from childhood; they are often associated with nausea and vomiting, 'sick headaches', and also with disturbances of vision and with giddiness. Less common are sensory changes, attacks of hemiplegia or monoplegia, of aphasia, and of ophthalmoplegia. Some of these may accompany the headaches, but others occur apart, and may cause difficulty in diagnosis.

Aetiology

Migraine may start in early childhood, but commonly appears around puberty, and tends to persist, with fluctuations in the severity and frequency of attacks, throughout adult and middle life. The sexes are equally affected. Subjects of migraine are often energetic, intelligent and have a meticulous standard of thoroughness and precision almost amounting to obsessionality. These personality characteristics are very important in the causation of the disorder.

The immediate cause of the attack is a paroxysmal variation in the calibre of the cranial blood vessels, either spasm or dilatation, or the one followed by the other. The dilatation, which causes the headache, is associated with oedematous swelling of the vessel wall, which is why vasconstrictors which may be effective in stopping the pain when given early in the attack may not be if given late. The vasomotor changes may happen in either carotid or basilar arterial systems in any combination or separately, so that the resulting symptoms may be difficult to interpret. The headache may, for instance, be on the same side as hemiplegic symptoms. When the spasm is in the territory of the internal carotid system, hemiplegia, monoplegia, hemianopia, sensory changes and aphasia may happen. The spasm of the basilar artery cause many of the characteristic disturbances of nausea, vomiting, vertigo and visceral changes, as well as the majority of the visual experiences. When there is dilatation of the branches of the external carotid artery temporal and frontal headache occurs, sometimes with intense pain in the eye or face (neuralgic migraine).

Precipitating factors are numerous and may be specific. On the psychological level fatigue, anxiety and frustration play an important part. On the physical plane over-exertion and fatigue, indiscretions or irregularities of food, exposure to excessive light or noise, prolonged eye strain, especially in the presence of an uncorrected error of refraction, commonly figure in the history of migrainous subjects. Women may have attacks in association with the menstrual periods and often remain entirely free during pregnancy.

Symptoms

The subjects of migraine are otherwise healthy, and often robust. Premonitory signs of the attacks are present in some and these may take the form of an unusual feeling of well-being and intellectual acuity, or, on the other hand, of lassitude and depression.

The attack commences commonly on waking in the morning, when on raising his head from the pillow the patient experiences a sense of giddiness, ocular confusion and nausea, such as is commonly felt at the onset of sea-sickness. It is at this stage of the attack and within a few minutes of its commencement, that the visual phenomena occur if these are present. Often the patient vomits at once, but sometimes vomiting is delayed for hours but may continue throughout the attack with great prostration, sweating and coldness of the extremities. The visual disturbances last but a short time (from 10 to 30 minutes) but leave, as a rule, some confusion of vision and discomfort throughout the attack. The headache follows shortly after these initial symptoms. It is cumulative and throbbing in character and often begins constantly in a localized spot over one eye, or in the temple as a sharp boring pain which gradually spreads, and may involve the neck and arm. The pain may be unilateral, frontal, occipital or quite general, but is usually constant from attack to attack. As the headache increases in severity the face becomes pale and grey, the patient becomes much prostrated and is incapable of mental or physical effort and unable to take food. Light, noise and movement aggravate the pain intolerably and the patient seeks the refuge of his bed in a darkened room. After remaining in this condition for some hours he falls into a deep sleep and wakes next day shaken by his illness, but otherwise well.

This description covers many attacks of migraine, but there are wide variations. The attacks do not always occur on waking; they may come on at any time of the day or at night. They may be rapidly transient, lasting for a few hours only, or they may last for days and give rise to much anxiety in the attempt to provide nourishment and sleep for the patient. They sometimes change their character gradually as the patient gets older, and in cases of long standing the patient may have a persistent, annoying headache between the attacks. In other cases the headache may be relatively inconspicuous compared with the vomiting and the various sensory disturbances.

Visual phenomena. Considering how common migraine is, visual changes in attacks are quite rare. There may be general mistiness of vision, floating spots, scotomata, bright stars and colours, hemianopia, double hemianopia with complete blindness, or psychic hallucinations of vision. In connexion with scotoma and with hemianopia, the phenomenon of teichopsia may occur as follows: upon the dark background of the scotoma or hemianopic field, a ball of light appears, which grows larger and becomes dark in the centre. This ring of light breaks at one spot, opens out and becomes a series of entering and retreating angles (castellation figure) which become gloriously coloured (fortification spectrum) and which later become fragmented and fade. These visual events usually occur at the beginning of the attack, before the headache develops, and are rapidly evanescent, but they may be isolated without headache.

Aphasic attacks may consist of confusion of speech, word-blindness, or even complete aphasia. They accompany the headaches and occur at the commencement of the attacks. They are not common.

Sensory auras. These are rare, but are pathognomonic of migraine, and may occur apart from the headaches. They begin at the periphery of a limb and travel slowly proximally, taking half an hour or more to reach from the fingers to the head, and can be alarming. They disappear rapidly without further event. They may involve the lips and the tongue in numbness and tingling.

Ophthalmoplegia. This is rare; it occurs at the height of the headache, in severe attacks. It is partial paralysis of the oculomotor nerve trunks, most commonly of the sixth nerve alone, but sometimes of the third or fourth nerves, or of a combination of these three. It is generally unilateral, but may occur simultaneously on both sides. Severe diplopia results. It passes off in from a few days to a few weeks. When once it has occurred, it is apt to recur with subsequent attacks. Attacks of this kind are called ophthalmoplegic migraine, and are due to involvement of the basilar system.

Neuralgic migraine, or migrainous neuralgia, is a distinct variant. The attack of migrainous headache is accompanied by intense pain of a stabbing, crushing or gougeing quality in and around the eye and cheek, with occasionally swelling of the face, redness of the sclera and engorgement of the nose on that side. It commonly appears early in the sixth decade, particularly in those of obessional temperament, and may commence at precisely the same time of the day in any one patient, most commonly awakening him in the early hours of the night.

Diagnosis

In typical cases the diagnosis of migraine is seldom in doubt. The long history, the familial incidence and the common association of headache with vomiting and various sensory disturbances all contribute to a characteristic clinical picture.

It is important to remember that tumours of the occipital lobes and intracranial aneurysms may be associated with attacks exactly resembling migraine, and every case should be carefully examined for signs of organic nervous disease, particularly papilloedema or persistent defects in the fields of vision.

Hypertension may cause headaches like migraine. The headaches of neurosis may closely simulate migraine, particularly when, as is not infrequently the case, they are superimposed upon it. It is not common for migraine to recur more often than once in 2 or 3 weeks, or to last more than 2 days.

Those who are not familiar with the full range of sensory symptoms that may precede the onset of the headache, and do not realize the severity of the speech disturbances which in some cases accompany them, are apt to take an unduly grave view of the history. Thus, a diagnosis of epilepsy or of cerebral tumour may sometimes be made, especially in the first attack. It should, therefore, be remembered that the disturbances of sensation which occur in epileptic attacks are momentary in duration and never persist, as do the migrainous symptoms in question, for many minutes. Again, consciousness is rarely blunted or lost in migraine.

Attacks of migraine consisting wholly of vomiting and sometimes associated with diarrhoea and abdominal discomfort are readily mistaken for abdominal disorders.

Treatment

Few non-fatal disorders are more stubbornly resistant to treatment than migraine. Many victims suffer from recurring attacks throughout the most valuable years of their lives, to the serious detriment of their work and happiness. In many cases help can be given by attention to general health and physical and mental well-being, for a lowering of these in a migrainous subject often increases the number and severity of attacks. In others it may be possible to eliminate precipitating factors, whether physical or psychological in nature, but only too often when these are discoverable they are found to be amongst the unalterable features of the patient's environment. Inquiry will usually uncover a persisting frustrating life situation with which the patient must live in enforced and stoical harmony. There is, too, a marked affective disorder with much fatigue.

Drugs administered consistently over a long period may be of value in some cases, and of these phenobarbitone, 25 mg. twice daily, or 50 mg. at night, or amylobarbitone, 50 mg., chlordiazepoxide (*Librium*), 5 or 10 mg., or trifluoperazine (*Stelazine*), 2 mg. in the morning, may be tried. Methysergide, 1 mg. two or three times daily, has proved an effective prophylactic in about 50 per cent. of patients, but prolonged administration may lead to retroperitoneal fibrosis [see Section 12]. This is avoided if after each three months the drug is withdrawn for a month. More recently clonidine hydrochloride, 0·025–0·075 mg. twice daily, has been found to be valuable.

The individual attacks are equally difficult to relieve. Some people get much benefit from minor analgesics such as aspirin or paracetamol (*Panadol*) even though the headache is severe. Ergotamine tartrate (*Femergin*) in doses of ½–1 mg. by mouth or injection will sometimes cut short an attack, but it is by no means the specific that has been claimed. It is combined with caffeine with benefit and if vomiting is severe may be given in suppositories, of which suppositories of *Cafergot*—which contain 2 mg. of ergotamine tartrate—is a useful example. This substance may also be chewed and absorbed through the buccal mucosa, or ergotamine may be administered in a nasal spray. When attacks are frequent one or two tablets of ergotamine tartrate daily may be used as a prophylactic. There are many proprietary preparations containing ergotamine tartrate.

Apart from these it remains to keep the patient as comfortable as possible and to induce sleep by the use of ordinary hypnotics and to secure that he takes adequate fluids and nourishment during a prolonged attack. Neuralgic migraine usually responds well to the ergotamine preparations. Migraine occurring in the premenstrual phase may be helped by diuretics such as acetazolamide (*Diamox*), hydrochlorothiazide or by ethisterone.

REFERENCES

ALEXANDER, G. L., and NORMAN, R. M. (1960) *The Sturge-Weber Syndrome*, Bristol.

BATES, J. A. V. (1962) The surgery of epilepsy, in *Modern Trends in Neurology*, 3rd Series, ed. WILLIAMS, D., London.

BICKERSTAFF, E. R. (1961) Basilar artery migraine, *Lancet*, i, 15.

BOWER, B. D., and JEAVONS, P. M. (1959) Infantile spasm and hypsarrhythmia, *Lancet*, i, 605.

BRIDGE, E. M. (1949) *Epilepsy and Convulsive Disorders in Children*, London.

ESZENYI-HALASY, M. (1949) Histamine headache, *Brit. med. J.*, **1**, 1121.

FALCONER, M. A. (1953) Discussion of the surgery of temporal lobe epilepsy, *Proc. roy. Soc. Med.*, **46**, 971.

FALCONER, M. A., and CAVANAGH, J. B. (1959) Clinico-pathological considerations of temporal lobe epilepsy due to small focal lesions, *Brain*, **82**, 483.

FARQUHAR, H. G. (1956) Abdominal migraine in children, *Brit. med. J.*, **1**, 1082.

GIBBS, F. A., GIBBS, F. L., and LENNOX, W. G. (1937) Epilepsy: a paroxysmal cerebral dysrhythmia, *Brain*, **60**, 377.

GOWERS, W. R. (1881) *Epilepsy and Other Chronic Convulsive Disorders*, London.

GOWERS, W. R. (1907) *The Borderland of Epilepsy*, London.

HARRIS, S. (1959) Migraine and cluster headaches, *J. Amer. med. Ass.*, **171**, 1224.

HILL, D., and PARR, G., eds (1963) *Electro-encephalography*, 2nd ed., London.

Lancet (1964) Treatment of migraine, i, 541.

LENNOX, W. G. (1945) The petit mal epilepsies, *J. Amer. med. Ass.*, **129**, 1069.

LENNOX, W. G. (1960) *Epilepsy and Related Disorders*, London.

LEVIN, M. (1936) Periodic somnolence and morbid hunger. A new syndrome, *Brain*, **59**, 494.

MERRITT, H. H. (1959) Medical treatment in epilepsy, *Brit. med. J.*, **1**, 666.

PENFIELD, W., and JASPER, H. H. (1954) *Epilepsy and the Functional Anatomy of the Brain*, Boston.

SYMONDS, C. (1956) A particular variety of headache, *Brain*, **79**, 217.

SYMONDS, C. (1959) Excitation and inhibition in epilepsy, *Brain*, **82**, 133.

SYMONDS, C. P. (1962) Concussion and its sequelae, *Lancet*, i, 1.

TOWER, D. B. (1957) The status of the medical treatment of epilepsy, in *Modern Trends in Neurology*, 2nd Series, ed. WILLIAMS, D., London.

WHITTY, C. W. M. (1962) The neurological basis of memory, in *Modern Trends in Neurology*, 3rd Series, ed. WILLIAMS, D., London.

WILLIAMS, D. (1941) The significance of the abnormal electro-encephalogram, *J. Neurol. Psychiat.*, **4**, 257.

WILLIAMS, D. (1950) New orientations in epilepsy, *Brit. med. J.*, **1**, 685.

WILLIAMS, D. (1957) The temporal lobe and epilepsy, in *Modern Trends in Neurology*, 2nd Series, ed. WILLIAMS, D., London.

WILLIAMS, D. (1958) Modern views on the classification of epilepsy, *Brit. med. J.*, **1**, 661.

WILSON, S. A. K. (1928) The narcolepsies, *Brain*, **51**, 63.

WOLFF, H. G. (1950) *Headache and Other Head Pain*, New York.

DISORDERS CHARACTERIZED BY INVOLUNTARY MOVEMENTS

WILSON'S DISEASE [see p. 1239]

PARALYSIS AGITANS

Synonyms. Parkinson's disease; Parkinsonism; The shaking palsy.

Definition

A progressive disease of insidious onset and slow course, usually occurring in the second half of life, and characterized by loss of the normal associated movements and by a peculiar stiffness of the muscles, which causes a distinctive facial expression, bodily attitude and gait. The stiffness is accompanied by weakness, and often by rhythmic tremors, which caused James Parkinson, a Hoxton practitioner, to give it the name of the shaking palsy in his famous eighteenth-century monograph.

Aetiology

Little is known of the cause. It is essentially a disease of the decline of life from the fiftieth to the seventieth year. Men suffer twice as often as women. It is associated with arteriosclerosis and may well prove to be due to reduction in the rate of cerebral blood flow for most subjects of it have constitutional arterial hypotension for their ages. It is similar to the postencephalitic syndrome described in Section 2.

Pathology

The most definite pathological findings are degenerative changes in the cells and fibres of the corpus striatum and its efferent systems. These are most marked in the globus pallidus of the lenticular nucleus but occur also in the putamen, the caudate nucleus, the corpus Luysii and the substantia nigra. There is a constant loss of cells, preceded by degenerative changes in those that remain. An associated glial proliferation takes place in the affected regions, together with fibrosis in the smallest arterioles and capillaries. The relationship of these changes to the symptomatology of the disorder is not clear; in the postencephalitic cases the principal changes are found in the substantia nigra.

Symptoms

The onset is always insidious, and the paucity of movement and the muscular rigidity are almost always the first signs to appear. This *rigidity* affects the face, neck and trunk to a greater extent than the limbs, and when the limbs are affected then the proximal muscles present a greater degree of rigidity than do those of the periphery. The oncoming rigidity of the facial muscles does away with the usual play of the emotional movements in facial expression, and the face assumes a fixed, anxious and mask-like expression, with absence of the usual involuntary nictitation. The voice loses its inflexions, and becomes monotonous, from rigidity of the muscles of larynx, tongue and lips; but there is no other defect of articulation. The effect of the rigidity of the muscles of the neck is striking, for the patient carries his head and neck in one piece with his trunk as if he were a statue, never inclining or raising it in the customary expressive manner, and if he turns round to look at anything he tends to move the whole trunk round with the head. In looking sharply to one side, the eyes move before the head, whereas, in normal circumstances, the coarse adjustment of this movement is done first by the neck muscles, and the fine adjustment subsequently by the eye muscles. The stiffness of the trunk muscles gives a stooping attitude with the head inclined forwards, while that of the upper extremities causes the shoulders to be rounded, and the arms carried with the elbow semiflexed, and pressed into the sides. The gait is characteristic, for through the rigidity of muscles, it is deprived of spring and suppleness. The patient, in the characteristic attitude described, takes small gliding steps, displacing his centre of gravity as little as possible. If, by any circumstances, such as catching the feet against an unevenness of the ground, or a push, the centre of gravity is much displaced, the patient often has difficulty in regaining it, and in moving to recover his centre of gravity is unable quite to catch it up, and so continues the movement of necessity until he falls or comes in contact with some object by which he can arrest himself and restore his balance. This phenomenon is more often seen in advanced cases, and is known as 'propulsion', 'retropulsion', and 'lateripulsion', depending upon whether the centre of gravity is displaced forwards, backwards or sideways. *Festination* is the term used for the quickening of the pace sometimes seen in this attempt to overtake the displaced centre of gravity. In the hand the rigidity is greater in the interosseous muscles, and the hand therefore tends to assume the 'interosseal position' with the fingers pressed together and the thumb abducted, the metacarpophalangeal joints being flexed, and the interphalangeal joints extended. The writing becomes small as well as tremulous, and the patient finds it difficult to write in a straight line. Muscular weakness always accompanies the rigidity and the tremors. It is slight until the late stages of the disease, when it may increase rapidly and render all useful movement impossible. Because of the rigidity and consequent slowness of movement, the patient experiences a sense of weakness which is much greater than that shown by the dynamometer. *Tremor* is present in most cases. It usually begins in the hand and forearm and is worst here, but it may be seen in the face, tongue, jaw, neck and feet, while, in rare cases, it may be universal. The nature of the tremor is peculiar, and is highly characteristic. It is a regular rhythmical contraction of the muscles, alternating in the opposing groups with a frequency of from four to six oscillations per second with a range of from an eighth to three-quarters of an inch. Its rhythmic nature, its slowness and its range distinguish it from other varieties of tremor. In the hand the characteristic movement of the tremor is the rolling together of the opposed thumb and fingers, cigarette-rolling, bread-crumbling or drum-tapping movement. There is nearly always in addition a peculiar pronator-supinator tremor. The tremor is increased by excitement and by self-consciousness, and ceases during sleep. It is temporarily arrested by voluntary movements but varies greatly, and in occasional patients the tremor is more evident in movement. There seems to be an antagonism between the tremor and the rigidity, for in cases where the rigidity is conspicuous the tremor is little marked or is absent, and conversely, when tremor is universal or is of early onset, rigidity is a less noticeable feature.

Other common symptoms are difficulty in turning over in bed, the result of the rigidity of the trunk muscles, flexion of the toes into the sole of the foot, pain of a dull aching character in the trunk and limbs, produced by the rigid muscles, abnormal sensations of heat and cold and hypersensitiveness to changes of temperature—the patient cannot bear to be near the fire nor yet in a cold room. Mental symptoms are absent, except in the last stages, when profound asthenia overtakes both mind and body. The constant bodily discomfort, restlessness, sensations of fatigue, which the rigidity and the tremors bring, and the consciousness of a chronic disability often result in lasting depression. Objective sensibility is unimpaired. The special senses and the cranial nerves are not affected. The sphincters and the reflexes are normal except that some patients get frequency of micturition. Trophic changes in the periphery of the limbs, thinning and glossiness of the skin, with fluted nails and vasomotor disturbance, are common.

Diagnosis

Three diagnostic points are: (1) the general appearance of the patient, with fixed expression, and stooping attitude, round shoulders, elbows pressed into the sides and hands carried across the abdomen in the interosseal position, the immobility of the head and neck, and the curious gliding gait; (2) the rhythmic rolling tremor which is quite unlike any other, and which is worst during rest; and (3) the absence of any of the signs of disease of the pyramidal system. Difficulty may perhaps be experienced in mild cases where the tremor is limited to one part, such as the face, tongue or neck; but, if the possibility of tremor in any situation being that of paralysis agitans be borne in mind, its rhythmic rolling nature will give the diagnosis.

When paralysis agitans is confined to one side of the body, the appearance of the patient may superficially resemble that of hemiplegia; but in these cases the peculiar aspect of paralysis agitans is marked, and the organic signs of hemiplegia, such as the extensor response in the plantar reflex, the increase in the deep reflexes and the absence of the abdominal reflex upon the paretic side are not present. In senile tremor the rhythmic rolling quality is absent, movement aggravates the tremor, and the aspect is not that of paralysis agitans. In post-hemiplegic tremor the organic signs of hemiplegia are present. Toxic tremor is irregular and never rhythmical, and is (mercurial tremor excepted) a fine tremor. The intention tremor of disseminated sclerosis, cerebellar disease and lesions of the red nucleus are so peculiar and so widely different from the tremor of paralysis agitans, as to render confusion impossible.

Benign familial tremor is often and unwarrantably mistaken for Parkinsonism. There is no other disability than tremor, which appears in young adult life and takes decades to advance; the tremor affects the arms first, the major side, the neck and rarely affects the legs. It is profoundly affected by social embarrassment, and is relieved by alcohol. Characteristically the patient has great trouble in getting his glass to his mouth at a cocktail party, but he is all right after that, as might have been his father before him.

The one clinical condition which may resemble paralysis agitans so closely as to be indistinguishable is the form of Parkinsonism which may appear as a sequel of encephalitis lethargica. In this condition there are similarly placed changes in the basal ganglia. Such postencephalitic cases commonly originate much earlier in life than paralysis agitans, and there may be a history of the initial disease. The onset is often more rapid and the condition may become arrested, whereas paralysis agitans is invariably relentlessly progressive. Postencephalitic cases often manifest other sequelae of the disease, notably oculogyric crises, postencephalitic tics, alteration in the pupils or external ocular muscles and changes in temperament. There is also increased sweating, the skin being greasy, and excessive salivation. These are absent in paralysis agitans.

Treatment

Medical. Where there is much rigidity gentle exercise, passive movements and massage are useful.

Levodopa has superseded all the 'spasmolytics' as the substance of choice in treating Parkinsonism. Its introduction has initiated a new phase in research into the nature of the disorder, for it is allied to a naturally-occurring neural transmitter within the extrapyramidal system which decays in Parkinsonism. The substance has many disturbing side-effects, of which the most common early in its administration are nausea and the symptoms of hypotension; later there is fluctuation in its therapeutic action in some cases and involuntary movements in others. Fortunately these last cease if the dose is reduced sufficiently. It is best to give levodopa with meals and to start treatment with a small dose, 250 mg. three times a day, increasing as the patient tolerates it to 3–6 G. daily according to need.

Amantadine hydrochloride, a drug first introduced as an antiviral agent, has proved to have a similar, although much less marked, action on Parkinsonism as that of levodopa. It is, moreover, without untoward side-effects and can be used in doses of 200 mg. daily when levodopa is not tolerated.

There is still a place for the spasmolytic drugs in the early stage of the disease. Benzhexol (*Artane*) in 2 or 5 mg. tablets, and orphenadrine (*Disipal*), 50 mg. three to eight times daily, are the most useful.

The progress of the disease is slow and the patient should be encouraged to maintain his activities as long as possible; nothing is to be gained by rest. When the patient is bedridden, great care must be taken with the skin.

Pains may be troublesome. The immobility of the limbs may cause 'frozen shoulder', and this should be guarded against by passive movements, and when it occurs treated by the usual appropriate measures.

Surgical. The development of stereotactic neurosurgery with the discovery of Cooper that lesions of the globus pallidus would ameliorate many of the effects of Parkinsonism has given much help. Patients already leading totally dependent helpless lives are walking and even working. Techniques are still being improved, and at present thermal or chemical coagulation of tissue about 8 mm. in diameter is achieved with accuracy in the posterolateral part of the optic thalamus (lateral thalamotomy). The patient, who is given a local anaesthetic and an amnesic sedative, co-operates in the procedure during control testing of sensation and movement. He is usually in hospital for 10 days, and in established centres complications or untoward sequelae are now unusual. The operation is now undertaken at any age, but contra-indications are arterial disease, and failing memory and dementia. Thalamotomy will abolish tremor and rigidity to restore voluntary movements to normal, but it does not so greatly improve the akinesis or the speech disturbance.

In favourable cases, where an excellent result has been achieved by thalamotomy, the relief obtained may be permanent, but the advent of levodopa has greatly reduced the need for surgery.

Course and Prognosis

Paralysis agitans often begins in one limb, usually the upper, and spreads to the opposite limb, or to the other limb of the same side. In the latter case it has approximately a hemiplegic distribution, and it may remain for years much more evident upon one side of the body. The course is slowly progressive with variable rate. In some cases the illness may remain stationary for years, and this is more often seen in middle-aged subjects, before the disease has reached an incapacitating stage. Such arrest may be seen in young subjects, with postencephalitic Parkinsonism. The average duration without thalamotomy is from 10 to 15 years, and since the major incidence of the disease is in the sixth decade of life it will be seen that many of the patients are of average longevity. When operation is impracticable death may occur from intercurrent respiratory infection; but more commonly, after the lapse of many years, the patient becomes bedridden from increasing weakness and rigidity.

CHOREA

Synonyms. St. Vitus' dance; Sydenham's chorea; Rheumatic chorea.

Definition

In chorea there are involuntary movements, irregular in time, in extent and in place of occurrence, and also muscular weakness, with variable degree of psychic disturbance. It is now rare, but a quarter of a century ago was a common disease of childhood.

Aetiology

The important causal factor of the ordinary variety of chorea is acute or subacute rheumatism. Chorea was much more common among poor people and its frequency has steadily declined so that now it is an uncommon condition in England, and when seen is usually mild. Its incidence is upon tense subjects rather than upon the phlegmatic. Chorea is practically unknown during the first 3 years of life, and is rare before the fifth year has passed. Common between the ages of 5 and 10 years, it reaches its maximum incidence between 10 and 15 years. After the age of 20 it is rare, except in pregnancy. Females are affected twice as frequently as are males. Often the patient has suffered with acute or subacute rheumatism, 'growing pains', rheumatic erythema, purpura, rheumatic nodules or recurrent sore throat before the appearance of the chorea, and may be found to be already the subject of rheumatic heart disease. Many of those patients who have never shown any sign of rheumatic fever before or during the attack of chorea subsequently suffer from it. A survey showed that rheumatism preceded the chorea in 26 per cent. of the cases, and that in 46 per cent. of the remainder rheumatic signs accompanied the chorea, or appeared subsequently.

Psychical disturbances. Any emotional disturbance, such as fright, anxiety, depression, or overpressure in school or disturbed home surroundings may act as an immediate determining factor, but more often these events simply aggravate symptoms which are already present in slight degree.

Pregnancy. The relationship of pregnancy to chorea is very definite. It was seen in first pregnancies, and before the age of 25 years, and in most cases the pregnancy appeared to be the only immediate cause for the chorea, but a history of rheumatism would often be obtained in a careful history. The onset of the chorea was usually between the first and third months of pregnancy. It was liable to recur with subsequent pregnancies.

Pathology

The essential lesion has proved difficult of detection by microscopical investigation, but it consists in a diffuse meningo-encephalitis affecting mainly the basal ganglia, the cerebral cortex and the pia arachnoid.

Symptoms

The onset is usually gradual, but it may be abrupt if emotional disturbance has been the determining cause.

The appearance of choreic movements is often preceded by alterations in the mental and physical condition of the child. She becomes nervous and more emotional, increasingly inattentive, clumsy in her movements, and lets fall objects which she is holding.

The involuntary movements are always irregular in time and in the form of the movement. Similar movements are never repeated successively in the same part. Each movement begins rapidly, and ends suddenly, and one frequently sees the involuntary movement complicated by the addition of a voluntary movement to cover the fault. Most of the movements are complicated, involving several muscles and often more than one joint. In the face, the more simple movements take the form of asymmetrical twitches in the lips, and about the angles of the mouth and orbits. The symptoms of a well-marked case of chorea are: (1) involuntary movements; (2) weakness of voluntary movements; (3) ataxia or loss of precision of voluntary movement; (4) emotional instability and other psychological disturbances.

The pupils are often dilated and may be unequal and eccentric, and hippus may be present. Sensation is not impaired. The sphincters are not affected. The skin reflexes are normal. The deep reflexes are also normal in most cases, but often the knee-jerk shows an alteration which is peculiar to chorea. On tapping the patellar tendon, the resulting contraction of the quadriceps is unduly sustained, and the leg remains in a position of extension at the top of its excursion for several tenths of a second; in other cases a pendular knee-jerk is present. In severe cases, the deep reflexes may be diminished and rarely may be absent for months.

Limp chorea (*chorea mollis*). This is a more severe degree of choreic paralysis which may affect the whole musculature but is more often of hemiplegic distribution. It may be preceded by the usual symptoms of chorea. More often the paralysis is the first noticeable symptom, and this develops rapidly in from 24 to 48 hours. The paralysis is characterized by complete flaccidity of the limbs. Paretic chorea and chorea mollis run a benign course, and recovery is said to be almost invariable.

Psychological disturbances are common, with emotional instability, failure of attention and depression. The patient's behaviour changes; she may laugh or weep without sufficient reason; she may become capricious, irritable and obstinate; attention and memory are usually impaired, and less interest is taken in the surroundings. These symptoms usually disappear with the chorea, and in all cases the prognosis as regards permanent mental recovery is good.

Rheumatic manifestations. Cardiovascular changes are common in chorea. Endocarditis used to be present in 90 per cent. of the fatal cases and at least one-half of all cases present cardiac murmurs. Cutaneous affections which occur in rheumatism are met with also in chorea, namely, erythema, purpura and subcutaneous nodules. Acute articular rheumatism is comparatively rare, and when it occurs it is usually accompanied by a cessation of the choreic movements. When rheumatic phenomena are present and in the acute mania of chorea, pyrexia is usually present, but uncomplicated chorea is an apyrexial disease.

Recurrence. One-third of the subjects of chorea have more than one attack. Females are more prone to a recurrence than males in about the same proportion as they are more liable to original attacks.

Diagnosis

The diagnosis is usually easy, but occasionally a case of multiple tics in a child does present difficulties, for the movements are not—as is so commonly stated—invariably repetitive. In chorea the involuntary movements may lead to the dropping of objects from the hands. This does not happen in the case of tics. Again, when the choreic subject gives the observer a firm and sustained handclasp, the irregular waxing and waning of the muscular contraction may be felt throughout by the observer. In a case of tics, the contraction is steadily maintained as in the normal subject. In myoclonus, the movements are short and shock-like, while in athetosis they are slow and writhing. In chorea mollis or hemiplegic chorea the paresis is in itself highly characteristic. It is a flaccid paralysis which is never absolute and usually affects the arm most. There is no pain and no wasting, and while spasticity is absent the deep reflexes are usually preserved.

Treatment

It is well to begin treatment in every case with a few days' absolute rest in bed, though the ordinary periods of rest should be prolonged.

The salicylates are of value and of these aspirin is the most useful and should be continued well into convalescence. As a sedative, amylobarbitone, 25–50 mg., or diazepam (*Valium*), 2 mg., may be used. In addition to the symptomatic treatment of chorea the management is that of rheumatic fever [see Section 2].

Severe cases of chorea call for skilled nursing. The sides of the cot or bed should be well protected by pillows and the patient's hands and elbows covered with pads of cotton wool. An unbreakable feeding-cup is needed.

Course and Prognosis

The disease ends spontaneously after a few weeks to 6 months. The average duration of cases treated in hospital used to be 10 weeks. The disease may, however, last for more than a year, and slight cases with remissions may last several years—relapsing chorea.

HUNTINGTON'S CHOREA

Synonym. Hereditary chorea of adults.

This is an uncommon heredofamilial disease, in which symptoms almost identical with those of rheumatic chorea, namely, involuntary spontaneous movements, ataxia, paresis and slow and slurring articulation, gradually appear in adult life, usually about the age of 40 years, and are accompanied by progressive mental failure, and personality changes with disturbed social behaviour. The choreic movements may be severe, and the inco-ordination marked. The disease progresses slowly to death in from 5 to 30 years. General health is not affected but the patients are always thin because of the high total metabolic rate caused by the involuntary movements. It is familial, the transmission is dominant and direct from parent to child, but if a generation escapes, it does not seem to reappear. Sporadic cases, in which no heredity can be traced, do occur. The sexes are equally affected. No causal factors are known. The morbid anatomy consists in a slow progressive degeneration of the nerve cells of the basal ganglia and of the cerebral cortex, with consecutive atrophy of the convolutions, neuroglial overgrowth and meningeal thickening. There is no effective treatment other than sedatives.

APOPLECTIFORM CHOREA

This title has been given to rare cases of chorea of sudden onset in elderly subjects. The involuntary movements are usually unilateral, and are often of great severity and large amplitude (hemiballismus). They are always due to small vascular lesions.

Thrombotic softening or haemorrhage has been found in the subthalamic region, particularly in the corpus Luysii. The mechanism by which small lesions in this situation cause such violent movements is not understood, but their occurrence is obviously of great theoretical importance, in view of the research into the basis of stereotactic surgery.

SENILE CHOREA

An illness in which typical choreic movements constitute the chief feature is seen in elderly people, and is possibly due to a progressive neuronal degeneration in those regions affected in the other forms of chorea. It differs from Huntington's chorea in the late onset, the absence of heredity and in the absence of mental changes.

SPASMODIC TORTICOLLIS

Definition

Tonic movements of the superficial and deep muscles of the neck, causing the head to assume either a position in which it is turned to one side and upwards, or one of marked retraction (retrocollic spasm). It is a disturbance of movements rather than muscles, and perhaps, physiologically considered, it may be thought of as a disorder in the carriage of the head. This carriage is a more complex and highly co-ordinated function in the erect posture than in the quadrupedal posture; it is a function peculiar to man, and in this sense is of recent evolutionary development.

Aetiology

No morbid anatomical changes have been found. The disorder is most often seen in the middle-aged or elderly. It is twice as common in women. The causation is obscure. A striking feature in the aetiology of the disorder is the association in the same patient or the occurrence in a group of patients of psychogenic or physiogenic factors. The movements may occur in patients with other involuntary movements which suggest disease of the basal ganglia, and the arm may be involved in the disorder. On the other hand the subjects will show during a personality interview that they are more conscientious, more careful or meticulous, habit forming and rigid in their temperaments than the average. A fuller psychiatric interview will often expose prolonged stress of a frustrating kind without any concomittant affective disorder. Undoubtedly, though we cannot say why this disorder occurs in some subjects and not in others, it afflicts predisposed individuals. In a few cases it has developed from an occupational neurosis; it developed, for instance, in a tailor who in drawing each stitch had the habit of making a short jerking movement of the head to one side. It occasionally occurs as a symptom of hysteria; but such cases should be carefully separated from those in which there is no hysterical manifestation, as being more susceptible to treatment and having less tendency to recur when once cured. A torticollic movement may occur as a variety of tic. Typical torticollis may occur as the end result of lethargic encephalitis.

Symptoms

The onset of spasmodic torticollis is usually insidious, but in rare cases may be quite sudden, as in the case of a man aged 40 years, who, when walking along a London street suddenly turned his head at the sound of an accident which shocked him severely; he was unable to turn his head back without using his hands to do so, and he subsequently developed the most severe torticollis. The initial symptom is always spasm, either tonic or clonic; frequently both are combined in the same case. In the tonic form, the head is retracted and the face turned to one side, usually the left, and owing to the retraction of the head the face is turned upwards. The shoulder on the side to which the head is inclined is usually raised. In severe cases all the muscles of the arm, the scaleni and the face muscles, may become involved. The spasm, except in the earliest stages, always involves muscles of both sides of the neck. Where the bilateral involvement is general and equal, the rotation of the head does not recur, but it becomes strongly retracted, and the condition is then known as retrocollic spasm. This is always accompanied by marked over-action of the frontales, the skin of the forehead being thrown into transverse wrinkles. The eyes do not follow the movements of the head. The muscle primarily involved is the sternomastoid, the action of which is to incline the head forwards and towards the shoulder of the same side, and rotate the face to the opposite side. The next muscle involved is the splenius of the opposite side, which inclines the head backwards and rotates the face towards its own side, its rotary action thus coinciding with that of the opposite sternomastoid. When the splenii of both sides act together, the head is strongly retracted. Next to be affected are the upper parts of the trapezii and the deep neck muscles, and with further spread of the spasm, any neighbouring muscles of the shoulder and upper extremity may be affected. Sleep causes cessation of the spasm which is always increased by fatigue and excitement. There is no wasting of the muscles involved, but, on the other hand, they may even become hypertrophied. The amount of pain associated with the spasm varies greatly. There may be a slight feeling of cramp only, but usually there is a great deal of aching pain, which may radiate down the arm and into the side of the head, and make life unbearable to the patient. More rarely, sharp neuralgic pains are present. The patient may control the movement, partially at least by the adoption of a particular fixed posture of the head, or by placing a finger against the advancing chin. The pressure he applies is not enough to control the movement physically, yet the movement stops for a while.

The course of the disease, which has no tendency to shorten life, is chronic, exacerbations and remissions under treatment and recurrence, after temporary cure, being common.

Diagnosis

This is usually quite simple. Fixed positions of the head associated with spasm occur in disease of the cervical spine, especially in spinal caries, and are also associated with enlarged lymphatic glands in the neck. The local signs of these conditions, however, are characteristic.

Treatment

Spasmodic torticollis is a most intractable condition, and in most cases temporary alleviation is all that can be secured. It is usually best to begin treatment by rest in bed, the patient lying supine with the head low and between sandbags or pillows. No form of surgical intervention has done any good, whether to the brain, the nerves or the muscles. Mechanical restriction of the movements of any sort is as cruel as it is useless. Rest in bed with the head comfortably supported while the patient has a light narcosis will in the earlier stages give temporary relief. Supportive psychotherapy helps of course, but claims made upon the basis of individual cases by the adherents to various psychotherapeutic schools have not been substantiated by others.

There is a *congenital form of torticollis* which is of a very different nature. The disease is prenatal and analogous to congenital talipes, the sternomastoid alone is affected, and nearly always that of the right side. Such a muscle is frequently ruptured during birth, and this has given rise to the opinion that the birth injury and subsequent haematoma of the muscle were responsible for the torticollis. In many of these cases there is marked facial asymmetry, the face being smaller on the side of the affected sternomastoid. This association points strongly to some defect in the nerve centres of the medulla. Treatment consists in tenotomy of the contracted muscle.

THE TICS OR HABIT SPASMS

Definition

Tics are characterized by the occurrence of: (1) sudden, rapid, twitch-like, involuntary co-ordinated movements, always of the same nature and in the same region; or of (2) sudden psychological events, imperative ideas and explosive utterances; or (3) of a train of deliberate highly co-ordinated actions produced by an imperative idea. Any combination of these phenomena may occur.

The tics are both aetiologically and clinically related to spasmodic torticollis, into which some of the motor tics gradate. A torticollic movement may occur as a tic, and it may in rare cases pass over into an established torticollis. The patients show the same personality characteristics.

The tics may be conveniently divided for clinical purposes into the following groups, between which any combinations may occur:

(1) The clinical picture is of sudden twitch-like co-ordinated movements, which resemble reflex or defence movements. The movement is always of the same nature and occurs in the same region, though several different tics may occur in the same patient. The usual region affected is the face, with the pharynx and larynx, the neck and upper extremity. This form occurs chiefly in children, and usually runs a favourable course—simple tic.

2. The spasms are more severe and complicated than in simple tic, and imperative ideas and explosive utterances are common and important symptoms. The condition is seen soon after puberty, and more commonly in males—convulsive tic.

3. There is no spasm or other motor manifestation, but the tic is expressed by uncontrollable imperative ideas, explosive utterances, arithmomania, or obscene words—psychical tic.

While the more simple forms of motor tic from their pattern suggest strongly that they were originally associated with some peripheral irritation, from the conjunctiva in the case of a blinking tic, from the nose in a case of snuffling tic, and from the larynx in a case of laryngeal tic, and that constant irritation from these regions has set up a habit, yet it cannot be too strongly pointed out that in many cases no such peripheral irritation precedes the onset of tic, and the irritation and cause come from within the nervous system alone. The nervous symptom is that of a rigid obsessional lesion under continuing stress.

SIMPLE TIC

This is a common disorder of late childhood, most cases occurring between the fifth and tenth year in both sexes equally. The onset may be preceded by poor health, and sometimes fright and emotion bring on the tic, but often it affects perfectly healthy children without assignable cause. The children are usually 'highly strung' and intelligent. It is a rare event to see a backward child with a tic.

Symptoms

The recurring tic appears suddenly, and may reach its height in a few days. The movements are of the nature of a simple act. They occur suddenly and without warning, and are executed rapidly. Usually the movement is of one kind only; but sometimes several movements coexist. The common site of the spasm is the head, face and neck. Blinking, winking, alternate elevation and depression of the eyebrows, side to side movements of the mouth, tossing the chin in the air, sudden movements of the tongue, palate or larynx, accompanied by an unpleasant fidgeting sound, are of frequent occurrence, while any movement of the head upon the shoulders, torticollic movements, shrugging of the shoulders and any movements of the arms may be met with. Respiratory movements are often associated with those occurring in the tongue and larynx. Tic affecting the legs is much less common. The movements cease during sleep. A variable time separates the individual movements, but in severe cases these may follow one another almost unceasingly. They are increased by excitement and by observation, and can usually be controlled by the will, but only for a limited time.

Diagnosis

The movement of tic is so peculiar that it cannot be confused with any other spontaneous, involuntary movement. It is the same movement, repeated with very rapid execution, in the same place. It is short and sharp, like a twitch. In chorea the movements are slow compared with those of tic, and are irregular in nature, in time and in place.

CONVULSIVE TIC

In this form, which was first described by Gilles de la Tourette, and which bears his name, the same movements as are seen in simple tic occur, but they are more severe and more widely spread, and they involve the whole body in spasm at one time. There are also psychic tics which cause irresistible impulses, among which are explosive utterances, repetition of words, sounds and gestures, and also imperative ideas.

Symptoms

The spasmodic movements resemble at first those of simple tic in their nature and rapidity, and favour the same sites; but they are not restricted to the repetition of the same movement, but successive movements may vary widely in position and extent and sometimes involve the whole musculature of the body. The great variety of facial grimaces, head jerking, grotesque attitudes and ridiculous gestures which may occur in this affection lead commonly to the belief that the patient is shamming. The tic is not continual as in the simple form. It occurs in the form of bouts in which the same pantomime is reproduced. These are often excited by observation and emotion. They can often be controlled, but with much fatiguing effort on the part of the patient, who becomes so worn out with half-successful efforts to control them that he ceases to make the attempt. Between the attacks the patient seems quite normal. The psychological phenomena are the same as in psychical tic, about to be described, and the treatment of the two conditions is identical.

PSYCHICAL TIC

Here there is no muscular spasm; but the sudden event takes the form of explosive utterances, imperative ideas and impulsive acts. This condition often occurs as a part of convulsive tic. The exclamatory tic consists of some sound or word or group of either, which is habitually uttered, with complete irrelevancy of time, place or sense. Sometimes the words are of an obscene nature and cause the greatest distress to the patient. The utterances may be single, or may be repeated over and over in rapid succession. Echolalia, which is an uncontrollable impulse to repeat sounds heard, or to repeat words which the patient or others have just spoken, may be met. Though the patient desires above all to prevent them he cannot do so. These may also be imperative ideas and impulsive acts, and in general the symptoms of a severe obsessional state.

Diagnosis

Both in the convulsive and psychical tics the diagnosis is obvious, both by the nature of the movements and because of the peculiarity of the psychic disturbance.

Treatment

Treatment of the more severe cases should be in the hands of an experienced child psychiatrist who will be as involved in the home background and the parents' attitude as he will be in the patient himself. The difficulty is to know, early in the disorder, that expert help is needed, for most tics are transient, superficial in their causation and non-recurrent.

OCCUPATIONAL NEUROSES

Synonyms. Craft palsy; Occupational palsy; Occupational cramp.

Definition

A disorder, now uncommon, determined by the habitual use of one set of muscles for the constant repetition of an act of short range, to the exclusion of acts of wider range and acts involving a different set of muscles. The symptoms are: local pain and spasm in the muscles concerned with weakness and loss of volitional control of the range and nature of the movements. These symptoms may occur separately or together, all other movements of the affected part except the causal one being perfectly usual.

Aetiology

The disorder is apt to arise in any occupation involving rapid, repetitive movements of short range by a small portion of the body, especially the hand, as in occupations of manual writers, typists, telegraphists, musicians, seamstresses and many others. The movements concerned are always acquired, and need a high degree of precision and co-ordination, but in the course of time become so automatic that in health they are carried out without attention and almost subconsciously while the performer's thoughts are concentrated on other aspects of his work. They involve the rapid, repetitive action of small groups of muscles which may thus be supposed to be subject to especial fatigue. In many such occupations from 5 to 10 repetitive movements a second may be executed. No structural change in the cerebral cortex, nervous system or muscles has ever been demonstrated. The disability first concerns only one set of stereotyped movements and the affected parts function normally in other activities even though these involve movements of comparable rapidity and skill. Thus, the subject of writer's cramp is able to use the hand normally for shaving, eating or even for playing the piano. In severe and intractable cases, however, other similar co-ordinated movements of the hand may gradually be drawn into the ambit of the disorder, especially if they concern the patient's definitive occupation. The disorder appears when the individual is called upon to exceed a certain level of performance, or after any physical or psychological event which may lower the patient's normal level of efficiency.

Everyone who develops an occupational cramp, has, in addition to a stereotyped precise act to do in his job, a rigid punctilious temperament. He is neat, precise and conscientious to a degree; it is probably this set of attitudes that make it possible for him to perform the repetitive act in such a stereotyped way. Every subject of writer's cramp has neat, uniform writing.

Opinion has gradually moved away from the original conception that the disorder was due to structural change or uncomplicated physical fatigue towards the view that it is primarily psychogenic. That is not to say it is in the loose sense 'neurotic' or motivated, for the syndrome is stereotyped and it only occurs in subjects who by their vocation must, and by their temperament can, perform accurately repeated minute movements almost indefinitely. This creates a situation in which, presumably, an equally minute and immutable part of the physical substrate of behaviour becomes exhausted in the task. Causative factors are no doubt numerous and often multiple, and both physical and psychological in nature, but in their summation they result in the breakdown of the smooth execution of a stereotyped movement, and ultimately lead to the setting up of a faulty habit closely akin to a stammer or a tic.

Symptoms

These are of two orders, namely: subjective, consisting of discomfort, pain and the sense of fatigue; and objective, comprising muscular spasm and the abnormalities of movement arising from it and from the effort to avoid both pain and spasm. In some subjects pain, in others spasm predominates.

The onset is gradual. In the case of writer's cramp the movements of the pen become inexplicably difficult and tend to be irregular, the strokes extending too high or too low. The subject then finds himself grasping the pen with excessive force, and the correct adjustment of the finger ends becomes hard and apt to fail, the index slipping off the penholder. This he tries to correct by a still firmer grasp. The hand then begins to ache, and feels heavy and tired. With the passage of time all these symptoms increase, and the writing becomes more irregular and the nib is driven more firmly into the paper which it penetrates, the ink spluttering over the sheet. Some tremor may develop in the limb. As the condition grows worse, the cramp appears more and more readily when writing is started, so that even taking the pen in the hand may evoke cramp. At the same time, other fine and repetitive movements of the hand may be performed with normal ease and facility. The pain which in varying degree accompanies the cramp tends as the affection grows worse to spread from the small hand muscles up the limb until the whole arm and shoulder ache. With variations dependent upon the details of the movements involved, comparable disturbances are seen in the other varieties of the disorder.

Diagnosis

From what has been said of the character of the symptoms in these forms of cramp, of the mode of their production by a particular movement-complex, and of their occurrence in the absence of signs of organic nervous disease, errors of diagnosis should not occur.

Nevertheless, errors are not infrequent and consist in the diagnosing of writer's or of telegraphist's cramp when in fact some organic affection is present. Paralysis agitans, with little or no tremor, and postencephalitic Parkinsonism provide fruitful sources of error. In the clinical picture thus presented, the initial symptoms may involve the right arm and hand, and at first consist in a difficulty in the normally rapid and free performance of fine movements. Not unnaturally the handwriting may be affected early. It becomes slow in performance, spidery and progressively smaller, and the effort to continue writing may be irksome and even painful. The total clinical picture in such a case is made up of such small deviations from the normal that the inexperienced or careless observer may miss them and may note no more than the patient himself has noted; namely, that it has become difficult and uncomfortable to write.

Treatment

Occupational cramps are now rare through more enlightened conditions of work and through improved industrial design. Writer's cramp is seen from time to time and occasionally musician's cramp. Good teaching of unconstrained methods of manipulation and encouragement of ambidexterity in all the occupations concerned are important prophylactic measures. Long hours and the speeding-up of work should be avoided. After long absence from work, the work should be gradually resumed and not recommenced at full pressure. When the malady appears, rest and change of work afterwards are absolutely essential.

General treatment consists of the removal, when possible, of adverse factors in the patient's environment, such as uncomfortable working conditions, poor light, excessive noise and sources of personal friction. Full attention should be given to all aspects of the subject's physical well-being.

Psychological treatment may play a valuable part in relieving the underlying anxiety and tension, and in enabling the individual to make a better adaptation to his surroundings, and whenever necessary in giving guidance as to a change in occupation. Careful selection of personnel in occupations liable to the disorder would be of value in eliminating those with special predisposition to this form of breakdown.

When attention has been given to these factors re-education of the movements themselves can profitably be attempted, particularly in the variety of the disorder most often encountered in general practice—namely, writer's cramp. A specially large pen or pencil should be used, and held loosely and comfortably in the natural writing posture. At first the patient should practise drawing straight lines from left to right with easy movements of the forearms. Next, while the same basic movements are maintained, the lines should be made wavy by simultaneous movements of the wrist. Then the waves should be regularly interrupted so that they become series of pot-hooks, m's and n's. From this by gradual stages the smooth execution of other letters may be achieved.

Course and Prognosis

This is simply stated. The patient must stop what he is doing and take another job. Any other course is foolish.

REFERENCES

ALCOCK, N. S. (1936) A note on the pathology of senile chorea (non-hereditary), *Brain*, **59**, 376.

BELL, J. (1934) Huntington's chorea, in *Treasury of Human Inheritance*, Vol. iv, Part 1, London.

BRADSHAW, J. P. P. (1954) A study of myoclonus, *Brain*, **77**, 138.

CALNE, D. B. (1970) L-dopa in the treatment of Parkinsonism, *Clin. Pharmacol. Ther.*, **11**, 789.

CAMPBELL, A. M. G., CORNER, B., NORMAN, R. M., and URICH, H. (1961) The rigid form of Huntington's disease, *J. Neurol. Neurosurg. Psychiat.*, **24**, 71.

COTZIAS, G. C., PAPAVASILIOU, P. S., and GELLENE, R. (1969) The modification of Parkinsonism—Chronic treatment with L-dopa, *New Engl. J. Med.*, **280**, 337.

CUMINGS, J. N. (1959) *Heavy Metals and the Brain*, Oxford.

DENNY-BROWN, D. (1960) Diseases of the basal ganglia and their relation to disorder of movement, *Lancet*, ii, 1099, 1155.

FIELDS, W. S., ed. (1958) *The Pathology and Treatment of Parkinsonism*, Springfield, Ill.

GILLINGHAM, F. J., WATSON, W. S., DONALDSON, A. A., and NAUGHTON, J. A. L. (1960) The surgical treatment of Parkinsonism, *Brit. med. J.*, **2**, 1395.

HENDERSON, J. H., ed. (1961) *Cerebral Palsy in Childhood and Adolescence*, London.

INGRAM, T. T. S. (1964) *Paediatric Aspects of Cerebral Palsy*, London.

LIVERSEGE, L. A. (1961) Writer's cramp and the conditioned reflex, in *Scientific Aspects of Neurology*, ed. COPLAND, H., Edinburgh.

LIVERSEGE, L. A. (1962) Involuntary movements—a clinical review, in *Modern Trends in Neurology*, 3rd Series, ed. WILLIAMS, D., London.

LIVERSEGE, L. A., and SYLVESTER, J. D. (1955) Conditioning techniques in the treatment of writer's cramp, *Lancet*, i, 1147.

MARTIN, J. P. (1960) Further remarks on the function of the basal ganglia, *Lancet*, i, 1362.

NORMAN, R. M., URICH, H., and MCMENEMY, W. H. (1957) Vascular mechanisms of birth injury, *Brain*, **80**, 49.

PATERSON, M. (1945) Spasmodic torticollis: results of psychotherapy in 21 cases, *Lancet*, ii, 556.

RUSHWORTH, G. (1962) Muscle tone and the muscle spindle in clinical neurology, in *Modern Trends in Neurology*, 3rd Series, ed. WILLIAMS, D., London.

SCHWAB, R. S., ENGLAND, A. C. JR, POSKANZER, D. C., and YOUNG, R. R. (1969) Amantadine in the treatment of Parkinson's disease, *J. Amer. med. Ass.*, **208**, 1168.

STEWART, R. M. (1942) Observations on the pathology of cerebral diplegia, *Proc. roy. Soc. Med.*, **36**, 25.

USHER, S. J., and JASPER, H. (1941) Sydenham's chorea, *Canad. med. Ass. J.*, **44**, 365.

LOCAL LESIONS OF THE SPINAL CORD

INTRODUCTION

For the lesions of the spinal cord the general rule applies that examination enables us to find the nervous structures which are affected and also the site of a lesion, but to find the nature of the lesion we depend on the history, the general examination of the patient, and special tests.

There are many conditions in which the spinal cord is damaged only in a short portion of its extent, and it may be of the greatest importance to discover the exact site of the lesion.

The functions of the motor and sensory tracts are usually disturbed by the lesion and by examining these we can determine the level below which muscular weakness, spasticity and reflex disturbances exist and sensation is impaired. Thus the approximate level of the lesion can be deduced. Secondly the motor, sensory and reflex functions of the individual segments of the cord are known and from this we can find more exactly in which segments the functions of the cord are abolished or impaired and thus the precise level of the lesion. Myelography may confirm its site and in many cases provide additional information.

MOTOR TRACT DISTURBANCES—SPASTIC PARAPLEGIA

Motor symptoms. Interruption of the pyramidal tracts produces spastic weakness in parts below the lesion, which, when fully developed, constitutes the picture of spastic paraplegia. The clinical features are: (1) diminution of voluntary power; (2) alterations in the amount and distribution of muscle tone, and in the attitude of the limbs; (3) changes in the tendon and skin reflexes; and (4) the occurrence of certain involuntary and reflex movements.

Remember that the muscles of the leg are divided into two groups, the flexors and the extensors, and that those which dorsiflex the foot and toes are physiologically flexors, while the plantar flexors are extensors. In all that follows these muscles will be grouped accordingly. In spastic paraplegia:

1. Loss of voluntary power varies from slight weakness of one group of muscles to complete paralysis of both limbs, and depends on the degree of damage to the pyramidal tracts. It usually begins in the distal segments of the limb, and is greater in the flexors than in the extensors. Dorsiflexion is the earliest and remains the most severely impaired movement.

2. The tone in all the muscles increases early, and is greatest in the extensors. Hence an early symptom is generally stiffness of the limbs, especially a difficulty in flexing them. If the limbs are handled passively, the resistance to flexion is found to be greater than to extension. It is greatest at the beginning of a passive movement and decreases suddenly in a way that has given rise to the expression 'clasp-knife rigidity'. As power diminishes spasticity increases, until at length the limbs are held constantly in an attitude of complete extension. This combination of weakness and spasticity with extended lower limbs is known as 'paraplegia in extension'.

As the damage to the cord increases, and when certain extrapyramidal motor tracts are affected, the extensor muscles gradually lose their excessive tone for which connexions with the brain stem through these extrapyramidal tracts are essential, while the tone in the flexor muscles, which depends on a reflex arc which is purely spinal, is retained. The result is that the knee- and ankle-jerks, which indicate tone in extensor muscles, are lost while the reflexes from flexor muscles (hamstring-jerks) persist. At the same time, in some cases, the limbs are gradually drawn up by the unopposed action of the flexors. This combination of weakness and spasticity with flexed lower limbs is known as 'paraplegia in flexion'. At first, the flexed position is occasional—flexor spasms; later, it becomes constant, but is still due entirely to excess of tone in the flexors; and ultimately, contractures occur in the muscles, and the deformity becomes permanent.

3. Exaggeration of the tendon reflexes is a constant early sign of spastic paraplegia. The abdominal reflexes below the level of the lesion and the cremasteric reflexes are lost early. The normal plantar reflex is also lost, and is replaced by a different kind of reflex—Babinski's sign, the 'extensor' plantar response.

4. While the limbs are still rigid in extension, the commonest involuntary movement is a spontaneous clonus of the extensor muscles, in which the whole limb trembles, as it does when ankle clonus is elicited in a case with marked spasticity. In the later stages, when the extensor muscles are beginning to lose their tone, a new kind of movement appears, in which the limbs are drawn up suddenly from time to time by an involuntary contraction of the flexor muscles—flexor spasms. Further, by appropriate stimulation many reflex movements can be produced in the paralysed limbs. The most important of these is the 'flexion reflex of the lower limb'. This is elicited most easily by stimulating the outer border of the sole by firm pressure or a pin-prick, and in its complete form consists in flexion of the hip and knee, dorsiflexion of the foot, and an upward movement—so-called extension but physiological flexion—of the great toe. When the damage to the motor tracts is slight, when the limbs are rigid in extension and the movement of flexion is prevented by the hypertonus of the extensors, or when almost all reflex activity has disappeared, the reflex appears in its minimal form. A part of this minimal response is an 'extension' of the great toe. The normal 'flexor' plantar response is obtained from the sole alone. The pathological reflex, of which the 'extensor' reponse is a part, may be obtained not only from the sole, but when well developed by stimulating the skin and deeper structures on any part of the lower limb. In the light of this the nature of many reflexes which have been described as isolated signs of pyramidal tract disease, e.g. the 'extensor' plantar reponses, Oppenheim's and Gordon's signs, and many others, become clear. In all of them a stimulus is applied to some part of the lower limb, and the reponse is a flexion reflex, whose most obvious component is 'extension' of the great toe. It is unfortunate that the term 'extensor response' is commonly used to describe a movement which is physiologically one of flexion.

SENSORY TRACT DISTURBANCES

The level of the lesion may be determined approximately by finding where sensation is impaired, but in general, for reasons which will be given, the exact site of the lesion is usually several segments higher than the level determined by this method. When the two sides of the cord are affected unequally the anaesthesia is confined to one side or extends higher on one side than on the other. In many instances reliance has to be placed on the disturbances of pain and temperature sensation and it must be borne in mind that the spinothalamic tract in the anterolateral column of the cord is concerned with pain and temperature sensation on the opposite half of the body, and that the fibres crossing the cord to join it do so with different degrees of obliquity at different parts of the cord. In the lumbosacral enlargement the pain and temperature fibres cross slowly and in fact clinical experience suggests that they have not taken up their new position until they reach the twelfth dorsal segment. In the mid-dorsal region the decussation of pain and temperature fibres is complete one segment above the point of entry of the root by which they reach the cord. At higher levels crossing occurs more slowly, until in the upper cervical region impulses which enter together in one root ascend through five or six segments before all of them reach the opposite side. At all levels pain crosses most quickly, then cold, then heat, and touch slowest of all.

When the posterior columns of the cord are involved in the lesion, loss of sense of position occurs in the feet and legs with resulting ataxia. Disturbances of posterior column sensation cannot be used for localization in the dorsal portion of the cord, but in the cervical portion the disturbances of postural sense in the different fingers may be of localizing value.

BROWN-SÉQUARD SYNDROME

When a lesion affects one half of a segment of the spinal cord it interrupts the pyramidal tract conveying motor impulses for the lower limb of the same side, the spinothalamic tract conveying pain and temperature impulses from the opposite side of the body below the level of the lesion, and the posterior column conveying sense of position impulses from the lower limb on the same side as the lesion. Consequently a local lesion affecting one half of the cord produces a syndrome, described by Brown-Séquard, consisting of loss of power (with spasticity) on one side, and loss of pain and temperature appreciation on the other side, below the level of the lesion; and, if the posterior column is involved (and it often is not), loss of sense of position on the same side as the weakness.

The Brown-Séquard syndrome most commonly results from lesions in the thoracic portion of the cord. Occasionally it occurs with lesions in the cervical portion, and then the upper limbs as well as the lower may be involved. It does not occur with lesions in the lumbar or sacral cord, because, as has already been mentioned, the pain and temperature fibres have not crossed in these portions, and, consequently, with lumbar and sacral unilateral lesions all the sensory loss is on the same side as the weakness.

SEGMENTAL DIAGNOSIS

Motor Localization. Each segment of the cord contains groups of anterior horn cells for several muscles, and most muscles receive nerve fibres from more than one root; but as each muscle seems to have one main root of supply, the weakness, wasting and loss of tone vary in distribution with the segment affected. The muscles which suffer most when the corresponding segment is damaged are named hereunder:

> C.4, supraspinatus, infraspinatus; C.5, biceps, deltoid, brachialis, supinator longus; C.6, pronators of forearm; C.7, triceps, extensors of wrist and fingers; C.8, flexors of wrist and fingers; D.1, small muscles of the hand; D.2–10, intercostal muscles; D.7–12, muscles of the abdominal wall; L.2–3, adductors of thigh; L.4–S.1, abductors of thigh; L.2–4, extensors of knee; L.4–5, anterior tibial muscles; L.5–S.1, peronei; S.1, small muscles of foot, calf muscles; L.5–S.2, hamstrings; L.4–S.2, glutei.

Wasting of the muscles in an intercostal space is a valuable guide, as the muscles of each space are innervated from one segment alone. If the lesion is at the level of the ninth dorsal segment the rectus abdominis is weakened below a point about an inch above the umbilicus. In such a case, when an attempt is made to raise the head against the resistance of a hand placed on the forehead when the patient is in the supine position, the upper part contracts and the umbilicus is drawn upwards (excursion of the umbilicus). If the lesion is at the twelfth dorsal segment the entire rectus contracts, but the iliac regions bulge, owing to weakness of the lower part of the oblique muscles.

Localization by Changes in the Reflexes. Above the lesion, the reflexes are normal; at its level, they are diminished or lost; below it, the skin reflexes are diminished or lost, and the tendon reflexes are exaggerated. The segments on which important reflexes depend are:

> C.5, biceps- and supinator-jerks; C.6, pronator-jerks; C.7, triceps-jerks; D.7–12, abdominal reflexes; L.2, cremaster reflexes; L.3–4, knee-jerks; S.1, ankle-jerks; S.1, plantar reflexes.

In lesions involving the fifth cervical segment of the cord, such as may be found in syringomyelia and in injuries associated with dislocation of the cervical spine, Babinski has recorded that the supinator jerk may be abolished and replaced by finger flexion when the lower end of the radius is tapped. This is known as 'inversion of the radial reflex', and is a useful localizing sign of lesions of the segment in question.

Sensory Localization. The sensory areas supplied by each segment of the cord are shown in FIGURE 69. 'Root pains' in the distribution of one or more of these areas form a fairly sure guide to the affected segment. There may also be sensory loss or impairment over the same areas, and this may be continuous below with the sensory loss which is the result of interference with the sensory tracts, or there may be an interval corresponding to the distribution of one or several segments between the 'root loss' at the affected site and the upper limit of the 'tract loss'. In many other cases there is a state of hyperalgesia in the segmental areas corresponding to the segment just above the lesion or to the affected segment itself if the lesion be a relatively slight one.

DISTURBANCES OF THE BLADDER AND RECTUM

Emptying of the bladder is essentially a reflex function, but in the normal state the reflex is voluntarily controlled, being inhibited or initiated at will. The detrusor muscles of the bladder wall are innervated by parasympathetic fibres from the second and third sacral segments of the spinal cord through the vesical plexus. The sphincter muscles are also innervated by the sacral nerves as well as by sympathetic fibres coming from a higher level, from the first and second lumbar segments, with contributions from the third and fourth. The emptying reflex is excited by an appropriate degree of pressure within the bladder and it evokes a co-ordinated activity combining contraction of the detrusor with relaxation of the sphincter. Voluntary control over this reflex is exerted through the upper motor neurones, and as long as one pyramidal tract is functioning perfectly, control of the bladder remains normal. When the function of both pyramidal tracts is impaired by a spinal lesion above the lumbar region, voluntary inhibition and voluntary initiation of the bladder-emptying reflex becomes imperfect. If spinal reflex activity below the level of the lesion is greatly exaggerated, as, for instance, in many cases of disseminated sclerosis, the bladder-emptying reflex is hyperactive and with the impaired control the patient is unable to inhibit it and precipitancy of micturition results. In other instances the patient is unable to initiate the reflex when he wishes and may be able to pass urine only after long delay. While one or other form of disturbance usually predominates, they are not mutually exclusive and both may occur on different occasions in the same patient. Delay in micturition may go on to retention as a progressive spinal lesion becomes more complete.

With sudden or rapidly occurring tract lesions above the lumbar region, associated as they are with depression of spinal reflex activity, retention of urine is the rule. As soon as the bladder becomes distended retention is followed by overflow incontinence, and it should be an invariable rule in all cases of incontinence to feel for a distended bladder in the abdomen. At a later stage in many such cases spinal reflex activity increases and reflex emptying of the bladder may then occur at intervals. The bladder may act spontaneously or the reflex may be initiated by pressure on the lower abdomen or by other means. Such reflex micturition is a useful aid in the management of a case of complete paraplegia, but it should be realized that emptying of the bladder by this means is always incomplete and leaves a considerable amount of residual urine.

SWEATING

With severe lesions of the spinal cord, sweating is excessive on the paralysed parts of the body. If not evident it may be excited by cutaneous stimuli or by the injection of a small dose of pilocarpine, 10 mg., and the level of a spinal lesion may be determined by this means by an observer who is familiar with the cutaneous segmental distribution. Profuse sweating of a phasic nature sometimes happens in patients with cervical paraplegia.

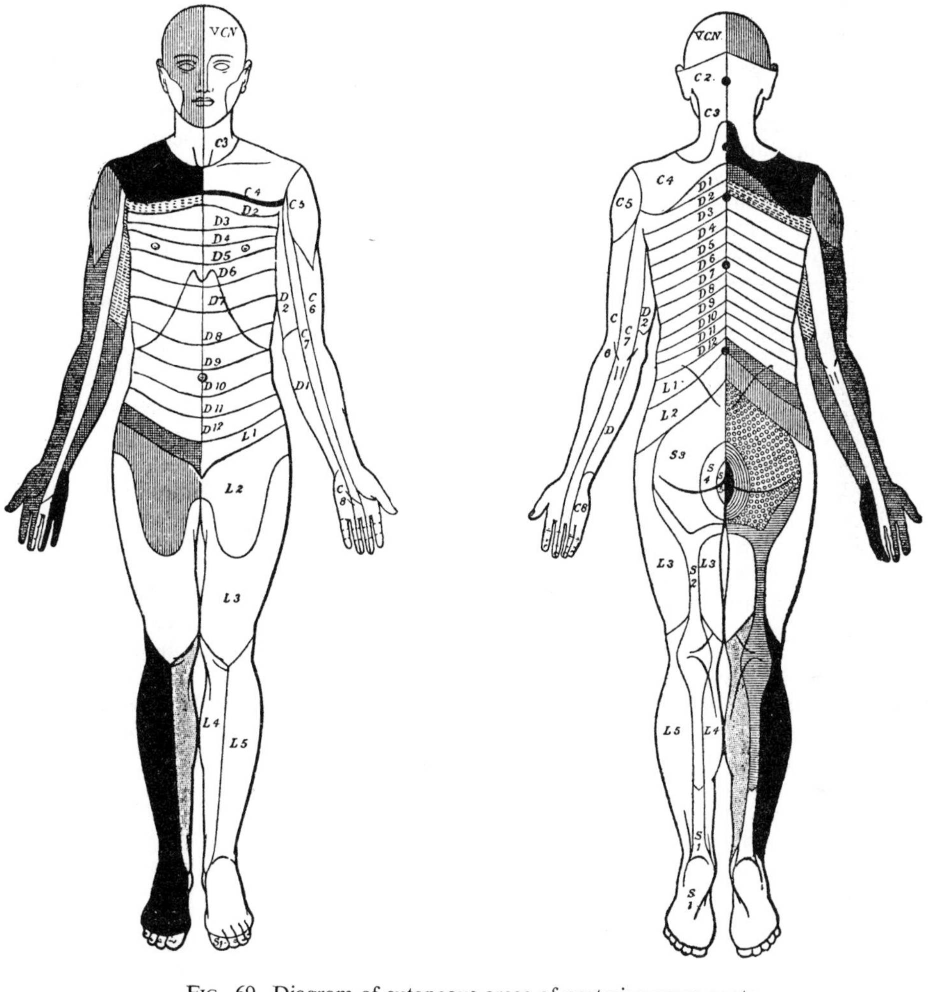

FIG. 69. Diagram of cutaneous areas of posterior nerve roots.

With lesions in the upper lumbar region of the cord, the vesical sphincter is paralysed and dribbling incontinence results. Lesions in the second and third sacral segments or in the corresponding spinal roots interrupt the arc of the emptying reflex and so cause retention, with a flaccid condition of the bladder wall. Lesions in the conus medullaris, where there is a reflex controlling centre, produce the same effect.

Control of the rectum is in nearly every respect similar to that of the bladder. Incontinence of faeces usually occurs only after aperients have been taken: retention expresses itself as constipation and may be relieved by regular enemata.

SURFACE ANATOMY

If the cord is to be exposed at the level of the affected segments their relation to the spinous processes of the vertebrae must be known. The segmental localization of a lesion having been obtained, the desired segment can be found as follows: in the cervical region of the cord, deduct one from the number of the segment—the sixth cervical segment is at the level of the fifth cervical spine; in the upper half of the thoracic cord, deduct two—the fifth thoracic segment is at the level of the third thoracic spine; and down to the first lumbar segment, deduct three—the first lumbar segment is at the level of the tenth thoracic spine. The remaining segments of the cord are shorter and so are farther separated from their corresponding vertebrae. The third lumbar segment is approximately at the level of the eleventh dorsal spine, and the first sacral segment at the level of the twelfth. The cord terminates just above the level of the first lumbar spine.

Myelography should be requested in every case where there is suspicion of a spinal lesion which might need surgical exploration.

GENERAL MANAGEMENT OF PARAPLEGIA

In all cases of severe paraplegia from a spinal cord lesion in which sensory and sphincter functions are also impaired or lost, whatever the cause, there are certain general principles of treatment. The patient should be nursed on a special bed, with a ripple mattress. This mattress distends alternate segments with air to prevent constant pressure on any point. The back should be attended to 4-hourly, first washed with soap and water, then carefully dried, rubbed with surgical spirit and powdered. These measures harden the skin and make it less likely to break down under the constant pressure of the body weight. The patient's position should be changed two-hourly. When there is incontinence of urine, care should be taken to prevent the skin from becoming wet with condom drainage in the male and large absorbent pads in the female. Retention is managed by the immediate use of an indwelling Foley catheter, tidal flow being instituted as soon as possible. An oral antibiotic controls bladder infection. Enemata will be needed. The toilet of the anus after defaecation should be careful and thorough. There are various techniques for the sacral or trochanteric bed-sore if it develops. Separation may be hastened by wet dressings of eusol. Painting with mercurochrome or acriflavine after cleaning with an antiseptic detergent such as *Savlon* will suffice for the smaller infected areas, but with larger sores dressing with tulle gras, or penicillin preparations combined with general antibiotic therapy and a high protein diet including *Complan* may be necessary. The heels should also be carefully watched for the appearance of the haemorrhagic blisters which herald the development of a sore. Rings for the heels may avert them, and air rings for the sacrum may also be needed.

Rehabilitation of the paraplegic. Experience gained during the Second World War has gone far to improve the lot of paraplegics suffering from irreparable but local damage to the spinal cord, particularly of young subjects with traumatic lesions.

Bed-sores, even of large dimensions, will heal by active treatment. Suprapubic cystotomy and tidal drainage of the bladder may gradually be replaced by the development of satisfactory automatic emptying which permits the use of a urinal. Contractures and deformities can be prevented, or where necessary corrected. Physiotherapy and training directed to the healthy muscles may enable the patient to replace to a great extent the functions of the paralysed parts, as well as overcoming the gravitational effects in the circulation, which are a conspicuous feature of thoracic cord lesions.

Finally, occupational therapy, both pre-vocational and vocational, in specialized spinal centres and mental readjustment can enable these patients to a remarkable degree to resume their places as active members of the community.

TUMOURS AND COMPRESSION OF THE SPINAL CORD

INTRAMEDULLARY TUMOURS

Aetiology and Pathology

Tumours of the spinal cord while uncommon are encountered at all ages. The ependymoma, a tumour arising from the cells of the ependyma of the central canal, is the commonest, forming about half of the total. Tumours of this variety are demarcated from the nervous tissue of the cord, and although centrally placed can be renewed. They arise most frequently in the cervicothoracic region and the filum terminale. Various types of gliomata form the remainder of the total, the astrocytoma, Grade IV, being the most common; all the tumours of this group are of an invasive character, devoid of any definite demarcation, and therefore incapable of being removed without gross damage being done to the cord. In addition to the tumours arising from the tissues of the cord medulloblastomata and oligodendrogliomata may be found on the surface of the cord as seedling metatases from cerebral and especially cerebellar tumours. Various types of haemangioma are also found.

Symptoms

In the case of any patient presenting the signs of a local lesion of the spinal cord of gradual onset the possibility of an intra- or extramedullary tumour should be remembered, and every patient should be dealt with as a neurological emergency, for delay in operation may make the difference between full recovery and survival with some degree of spastic paraplegia or bladder dysfunction.

The symptoms of an intramedullary spinal tumour often start unilaterally, with weakness and stiffness of one leg, and at a slightly later stage a partial Brown-Séquard syndrome is not uncommon. At all stages dissociated sensory disturbances are common because of different degrees of involvement of sensory tracts. Root pains are unusual, but local muscular wasting, corresponding to one or several consecutive segments, is often present. Sphincter disturbances occur at a relatively early stage.

The cerebrospinal fluid contains a moderate excess of protein, and some excess of globulin. Queckenstedt's test does not indicate any blockage in the spinal theca until the tumour has reached such a size that it occupies most of the width of the theca. Unless the tumour is at an advanced stage, there may be no obstruction to the passage of *Myodil*, and even at a late stage the obstruction may be only partial. The expanding mass within the spinal theca may cause thinning of the pedicles of several consecutive vertebrae, which may be apparent in the radiograph by an increase in the interpeduncular distance.

Diagnosis

This has to be made from other forms of spinal cord disease which produce paraplegia of gradual onset, and compression of the cord from without. Of the former, disseminated sclerosis is usually the most difficult to exclude, and is the disease to which the symptoms of spinal tumour are most often wrongly attributed. The diagnosis of disseminated sclerosis is rarely justified unless there is evidence of several lesions in the central nervous system, and if after careful examination of the whole nervous system all the signs and symptoms can be attributed to a single spinal lesion, the probability of tumour is greatly increased. Secondly, with tumour, the exacerbations and remissions of disseminated sclerosis do not occur. Finally, in a case of tumour the cerebrospinal fluid may show a considerable increase of protein; a moderate increase, however (·06 per cent. or less), does not help in the differentiation. The spinal fluid in an active case of disseminated sclerosis occasionally gives a 'paretic' type of curve with Lange's colloidal gold test, which does not occur in the case of tumour. Cases of supposed disseminated sclerosis beginning after the age of 45 should be regarded with the greatest suspicion. The diagnosis may be particularly difficult in cases of haemangioma of the cord, because in many of these there is evidence of two spinal lesions.

Disease of the vertebra and the intervertebral disc will always be considered, and as a cause for advancing paraplegia cannot be differentiated from spinal tumour without special investigations.

The diagnosis between intramedullary tumour and compression of the cord from without (e.g. by a meningeal tumour, or a neurofibroma) cannot be made with confidence on clinical grounds alone. Search should first be made for evidence of those conditions which are known to cause compression. Queckenstedt's test may, of course, indicate obstruction in the theca, but in many cases at the stage at which diagnosis is called for it gives an indefinite result, and myelography is then required. If this reveals no obstruction, or if the picture obtained indicates a fusiform expansion of the cord with a little of the oil passing down at the sides of it, the diagnosis of intramedullary tumour may be accepted. In many cases the final diagnosis is made only by exploratory operation.

Treatment

Many ependymomas have been successfully removed, the cord having been incised between the posterior columns. If operation reveals a glioma or evidence of haemangioma, surgery can do no more to benefit the patient, and the treatment thereafter is that of paraplegia in general. Radiotherapy is variable in its efficiency, but should be used after palliative decompression.

COMPRESSION OF THE SPINAL CORD

In compression, the lumen of the spinal canal is reduced in a small part of its length and the cord is injured at this point, either directly by pressure or indirectly by interference with its blood supply. Nearly all the extramedullary lesions of the cord come under this heading. Except in cases of collapse of a vertebral body such as may occur in malignant disease, compression is in general a slow process, although in a number of cases the symptoms come on abruptly. A sudden event, such as fracture-dislocation of the spine, causes laceration rather than compression of the cord.

Clinically, compression gives two sets of phenomena, local or root symptoms in the regions supplied by the roots arising from the cord at the level of the lesion; and remote or cord symptoms due to interruption of the conducting paths in the white matter. Obstruction of the spinal theca may be inferred if Queckenstedt's test [see p. 1192] is positive. In addition, complete or partial obstruction is associated with an increase of protein in the fluid below the obstruction, and Froin's syndrome [see p. 1192] may be present. In most cases the fluid shows a slight degree of xanthochromia. Myelography confirms or reveals the site of the obstruction, and the outline of the filling defect may give a valuable clue to its nature.

Compression of the spinal cord may be the result of conditions arising within the theca, the most important of these being meningeal tumours, neurofibromata and arachnoiditis; and lesions compressing the theca and subsequently the cord. Of the latter, the most important are vertebral diseases, especially secondary carcinoma and protruding intervertebral disc; and rarer causes are tuberculous disease of the spine, extrathecal abscess, myelomatosis, Hodgkin's disease, Paget's and other forms of bone disease.

INTRATHECAL COMPRESSION

MENINGEAL TUMOURS

Though fibroma and sarcoma are occasionally found, for practical purposes the 'meningioma' is the only common tumour arising from the spinal meninges.

Aetiology and Pathology

The meningioma is a firm, oval, pinkish tumour of smooth or nodular outline. When impregnated with calcareous deposits the term 'psammoma' was applied to it, and it may become so calcified as to be discernible on a radiograph of the vertebral column. The incidence of these tumours is mainly between 30 and 60 years of age, and they affect women much more often than men. Their common site is in the thoracic region and they usually lie posterior to the spinal cord.

Symptoms

Pain of root distribution and of variable severity is usually the first symptom. It is aggravated, typically, by coughing, sneezing or straining. This is followed after some time by spastic paralysis of slow onset and steady uninterrupted progress, affecting first one leg and then the other, the combination and especially the course of these symptoms being almost pathognomonic. Sensory signs of similar slow course accompany the motor signs, or follow them after a brief interval. The sense of position may be the first to be disturbed, and give rise to unsteadiness in walking and standing. By the time the patient comes under observation the cerebrospinal fluid shows considerable increase in its protein content and in the globulin fraction, and Queckenstedt's test is positive. If the tumour is in the cervical region, as is unusual, all the foregoing changes are less intense.

Diagnosis

With such manifestations the diagnosis of meningioma is most probable, but the diagnosis from other forms of intrathecal obstruction is not certain until the tumour is seen at operation. The diagnosis from extrathecal compression is usually easier. With spinal caries root pains are not so severe, signs of bone disease are rarely absent, and the paralysis is usually bilateral from the beginning and is severe by the time sensory loss develops. The distinction from vertebral new-growth is generally made or confirmed by radiographic examination, but may for a time be impossible when bone symptoms and radiographic signs are absent.

Radiographic examination may show the outline of the tumour at the level determined clinically, or, more often, it shows some change in the shape of the pedicles of the vertebral arches, or an increase of the interpeduncular distance. *Myodil* introduced into the theca is held up, and its border in contact with the obstruction displays the outlines of the surface of the tumour.

Treatment

This is obviously surgical. During recovery the treatment after the operation wound has healed is that of spastic paraplegia in general [p. 1270] including careful management of the bladder and re-education in walking.

Course and Prognosis

The tumour grows very slowly. Root symptoms may precede paralysis by months or even years, and the weakness may increase gradually for several months before walking becomes impossible. In the absence of operation it progresses eventually to complete motor, sensory and sphincter paralysis, possibly with paraplegia in flexion. Most patients with simple tumours come to operation a few weeks or months after the onset of the first symptom. The prognosis after removal depends in part on the duration of the weakness in the legs and on whether sphincter control has been lost. Recovery from severe paralysis takes many months. When the paralysis is of longer duration, recovery, though gratifying, is rarely complete. Nevertheless, full return of power has been seen after 3 years of severe paralysis. The sooner the removal the better the outlook.

NEUROFIBROMATA

Aetiology and Pathology

Neurofibromata within the spinal theca affect both sexes and occur mostly in early middle life. They arise on the spinal nerve roots, and may be solitary or multiple. In cases of neurofibromatosis the occurrence of small neurofibromata on many of the lower spinal roots is the rule, although they may not give rise to severe symptoms. A neurofibroma may be situated partly within and partly outside the vertebral canal, the constriction at the intervertebral foramen giving the tumour a dumb-bell shape. Histologically the intrathecal neurofibroma has a structure similar to that of the acoustic neuroma [see p. 1197].

Symptoms

A neurofibroma compressing the spinal cord is apt to give rise to unilateral symptoms, and to the Brown-Séquard syndrome. Root pains are often very severe, and in some cases there are spasms of intense pain on the opposite side of the body below the level of the tumour resulting from irritation of the spinothalamic tract by the growth.

Diagnosis

The unilateral nature of the spinal signs may suggest the nature of the tumour. Also, neurofibromata cause a great increase of protein in the cerebrospinal fluid; findings above 1 per cent. are common in the lumbar fluid, and even in the fluid above the tumour the protein content is raised. The fluid withdrawn at lumbar puncture may be yellow. Queckenstedt's test and myelography disclose complete or partial obstruction of the theca. Radiographic examination of the spine shows in many cases enlargement of the intervertebral foramen through which the affected nerve root emerges, and the *Myodil* picture may show the lateral situation of the obstructing mass.

Prognosis and Treatment

For the solitary neurofibroma these are similar to those of a spinal meningioma. When multiple neurofibromata are present the prognosis is less favourable, although the removal of a single tumour may completely relieve the spinal compression.

ARACHNOIDITIS

Aetiology

The condition is a rare one in Britain. As a result of a low-grade inflammation of the arachnoid membrane, adhesions occur within it and give rise to cystic formations containing cerebrospinal fluid, or the membrane, thickened and fibrous, may become bound down on to the spinal cord. Such arachnoiditis may follow injury (perhaps as a reaction to haemorrhage), infectious diseases, or meningitis, but is usually unexplained. It was encountered after spinal anaesthesia with percaine. It is much commoner in the tropics where there is evidence that it is caused by chronic tuberculous infection.

Symptoms

In the course of a year or several years, cystic adhesive material causes slowly increasing pressure on the cord. Root pains are seldom pronounced, but muscular wasting occurs corresponding to the site of the maximal local incidence of the arachnoiditis. The tract signs are usually limited to gradually increasing spasticity of the lower limbs, but sensory changes, with a definite level, may develop. Pressure measurements at the time of lumbar puncture may reveal complete or partial obstruction of the theca, and the myelogram shows a characteristic appearance of guttering, the opaque fluid being broken into droplets among the arachnoid adhesions.

Prognosis and Treatment

Even with surgical decompression, the prognosis is bad, because the disease is usually progressive and also because of the poor reparative qualities of the fibre tracts in the spinal cord.

EXTRATHECAL COMPRESSION

With extrathecal compression, the pressure on the spinal cord is apt to be more uniform, and the manifestations have in consequence a greater tendency to be equal on the two sides, especially in the lower limbs. This is, however, no more than a rule of thumb and there are many exceptions to it. As long as the compression is relatively slight, motor tracts are more affected than sensory, so that with the more slowly progressive conditions, weakness and spasticity of the lower limbs may precede sensory disturbances by a long period. The onset of paraplegia is usually rapid and, as prognosis after operation depends on the duration of compression, every case of advancing hemiplegia should be considered urgent.

TUBERCULOUS DISEASE OF THE SPINE

Synonyms. Spinal caries; Pott's disease.

Aetiology

This used to be the most common cause of slow compression, but is now rare in the British Isles. It occurs more often in children. Signs of injury to the cord are usually preceded by obvious deformity of the spine but may appear before disease of the bone is suspected. Rarely paralysis comes on for the first time in an adult who has had a curvature since childhood.

The cord may be damaged by direct pressure of displaced bone, but more commonly by an abscess beneath the periosteum of the diseased vertebrae. In almost all cases the injury is indirect, and results from oedema of the cord, arising from interference with its blood supply by tuberculous granulation tissue, which forms on the outer surface of the dura mater and fills the epidural space (pachymeningitis externa). The functions of the cord may be temporarily deranged for long periods by this oedema, without permanent damage to the nervous tissues; hence, when the disease is cured, the oedema subsides and the cord recovers. In cases of greater severity necrosis of the nervous structures follows thrombosis of the vessels, or prolonged pressure causes atrophy of nerve roots, and complete recovery is impossible.

Diagnosis

When spastic paraplegia develops in a patient who is known to suffer from tuberculosis of the spine, the cause is obvious; but today, when tuberculosis of bone is so rare, the diagnosis is difficult. In all cases of compression the spine should be examined repeatedly for deformity, tenderness and limitation of movement. If tenderness is found constantly in the same place, and the nervous symptoms are compatible with disease of the underlying segments, disease of the bones is almost certain. Severe root pains are rare in spinal caries but are the rule in vertebral new-growth. A radiograph will usually demonstrate the presence and nature of the bone disease.

Treatment

This is to be directed towards curing the bone disease in the hope that cure of the paralysis will follow, and it usually does so. Complete rest on the back and fixation of the spine for many months is the routine treatment and recovery commonly takes about 2 years. The tuberculous infection is treated in the customary way [see Section 2]. Great care is to be taken to prevent bed-sores, cystitis and deformities of the limbs. Laminectomy is not usually needed.

Course and Prognosis

The course of the bone disease does not always run parallel with the paralysis, and either may alter in severity independently, but if the caries undergoes cure the paralysis usually diminishes. Considering the severity of the paralysis, the prognosis is favourable and astonishing recoveries occur. The outlook is best in young people with disease in the dorsal region. Many recover completely, but more often, especially in adults, recovery, though considerable, is imperfect. So long as the lower limbs remain spastic in the extended position together with exaggerated tendon reflexes the prognosis for complete recovery of power is better; but if the limbs become flexed, if they become flaccid, if the knee- and ankle-jerks are lost, if sensory loss is severe, or if there is wasting in the limbs following damage to lower motor neurones, the outlook is bad. Some patients live for years with severe paralysis, but life is constantly endangered by sepsis from bed-sores, ascending infections of the urinary tract, chest complications and tuberculous disease in other parts.

TUMOURS OF THE VERTEBRAL COLUMN

Vertebral tumours are about twice as common as all the other forms of extramedullary tumours together, and almost all of them are malignant. Metastatic carcinoma from a primary tumour of the breast, lung or prostate is particularly common. Evidence of compression may appear before the existence of the primary growth is suspected, but, on the other hand, it may occur several years after its complete removal and be the first evidence of a recurrence. Tumours arising primarily in vertebrae are uncommon; the least rare is myelomatosis. Sarcoma may occur, but more often, like Hodgkin's disease, spreads from the mediastinum or retroperitoneal lymph nodes by direct extension through intervertebral foramina.

The growth of vertebral tumours is usually rapid, and extensive portions of the spinal column may be completely destroyed. The cord is compressed by the growth itself, by displaced bone, or by a process of the growth which invades the spinal canal through an intervertebral foramen. As a rule, the dura mater sets bounds to its inward extension. Benign tumours of the spine are rare. They usually grow forwards, but occasionally an osteoma, or an exostosis, produces signs of compression.

Symptoms

In most cases these are typical of spinal compression. Root pains are usually severe, but occasionally they are absent. Often the onset of paraplegia is rapid, paralysis developing in the course of 24 to 48 hours. No deformity of the spine is ordinarily apparent, but local tenderness is usual, and radiographic examination reveals bony disease at a level corresponding to it. Lumbar puncture and myelography shows thecal obstruction.

Diagnosis

When root pains occur in a patient with malignant disease, secondary growth in the vertebral column is most probable, even though radiographic examination fails to show any deposits in the vertebral bones. When pains are the first symptom, mistakes are easily made because their root origin is not recognized. Diminished sensibility in the painful area indicates the nature of the pain, and this directs attention to the spine, where tenderness or deformity is discovered. As most vertebral tumours are secondary, the next step is to examine the parts where carcinoma is common, remembering that a small primary growth, e.g. in the breast, lung, thyroid or prostate, may give rise to widespread metastases in the bones. In the absence of a history or signs of new-growth in other parts, the diagnosis is founded on the combination of local tenderness or deformity and rigidity of the spine with root or cord symptoms. The severity of the root pains, and their great aggravation by movement, are characteristic.

Treatment

When paraplegia results from malignant deposits management is directed first to the relief of local compression by laminectomy and appropriate neurosurgical intervention, simultaneously to management of the paraplegia itself, and finally to the treatment of the tumour as such. Endocrine therapy of carcinoma of breast or prostate, or radiotherapy of the primary and secondary deposits and of lymphadenoma may prolong life usefully and happily for several years in favourable cases. Even if the primary tumour is not amenable to treatment the question of relief of the paraplegia should be given careful thought, for the horrors of a short paraplegic life are well worth avoiding even though treatment is palliative.

Course and Prognosis

When sarcoma or carcinoma spreads to the vertebrae from surrounding parts, the duration of the disease is measured by the response of the primary condition to treatment. In primary sarcoma, and in some cases of carcinoma of the vertebrae, life may be prolonged for a year or two, and death is due rather to complications of the cord disease—bed-sores, cystitis, etc.

PROTRUDING INTERVERTEBRAL DISC (CERVICAL AND DORSAL)

Pathology

In this section we are only considering protrusion of a disc or secondary osteophytosis as a cause of spinal cord damage. The complex pathology of the joints and blood vessels is not discussed, neither are the orthopaedic changes, or the effects upon motor or sensory roots. The protrusion of an intervertebral disc in the cervical or dorsal region is rarer than in the lower lumbar region. The common site is between C.5 and 6. The mechanisms by which it occurs are similar at all levels; as a result of trauma the cartilaginous annular portion of the disc is ruptured, and the semi-solid nucleus pulposus is then gradually extruded. In most cases the mass is protruded backwards into the vertebral canal, and causes compression of the theca. Degenerative changes in the joint cause severe osteophytosis with consequent deformity of the canal and disorganization of the blood supply to the cord. When the joint is deranged, its innervation is also disturbed so that it becomes a neuropathic joint and the process of change is hastened. In the cervical region the degree of compression of the cord which ensues is seldom severe.

Symptoms

The clinical history of the case is that of spastic paraplegia coming on very gradually. Progress of the paraplegia is usually very slow, and after a time one arm or both arms may become spastic and may show a little muscular wasting and a diminished tendon-jerk. At this stage the condition in most instances becomes stationary. Sensory impairment is seldom demonstrable, but there is usually a zone of hyperalgesia corresponding to the segment just above the level of the lesion. Mild root pains across the shoulders are likely to be attributed to rheumatism. In some cases, however, root pains are the principal manifestation and may be ascribed to brachial neuritis.

Diagnosis

Unless there is a close association with a definite accident the diagnosis is always a matter of great difficulty and only occasionally can it be made with confidence. In the cervical region the degree of obstruction is not sufficient to give a positive result with Queckenstedt's test. After injection of *Myodil* the hold-up is at most partial. While symptoms are progressing the differentiation from an intramedullary tumour of the cervical enlargement may be impossible, but the history of an accident, and the persistent absence of objective sensory loss, should suggest a disc lesion, and the eventual arrest of the progress excludes a tumour. From disseminated sclerosis the diagnosis may be equally difficult, but as all the trouble is due to a single lesion it is unjustifiable to postulate disseminated lesions, and moreover many of the patients concerned are too old for it. A syndrome of intermittent disorder of cord function with dysaesthesiae in the legs which has been called *claudication of the cord* may develop from prolapse of a dorsal intervertebral disc.

Treatment

Although one would expect a decompressive laminectomy to relieve the paraplegia the most to be expected is relief of progression. This is because permanent damage has been done to the cord and also because the blood supply is diminished by the disc lesion, which is bony hard. In most cases a light plastic collar is used for months to immobilize the neck and to avoid operation. If there is no relief then either the bony and cartilagenous obstruction is removed by an anterolateral approach and the two vertebrae (usually C.5–6) are fused, or by laminectomy the unopened theca is allowed room to ride over the protrusion or part of it.

INJURIES OF THE SPINAL CORD

Aetiology

The spinal cord is a delicate structure with poor power of repair. Injuries of it occur in the first place in association with fractures and dislocations of the spinal column. The cord is usually lacerated, its fibres torn and its circulation interfered with so that compression plays little part in causing the persisting symptoms and its relief brings about no amelioration. Transverse lesions of the cord also result from gunshot wounds. Secondly, disruption of fibres, and minute haemorrhages occur within a localized extent of the cervical cord as a result of acute flexion of the neck. The damage is probably the result of the sudden traction exerted on the cord, as flexion of the neck causes the cord to be pulled upwards. When the muscles of the neck are relaxed, a moderate degree of violence may cause the head to fall forward, producing sudden flexion of the neck and damage to the cord. With greater violence there may be accompanying dislocation or fracture of the cervical vertebrae, but in the typical case the spinal cord is not compressed. Sudden extension of the neck, as in diving accidents, also may cause severe injury of the cord, with or without vertebral dislocation or fracture. As there can be no repair of severed fibres in the cord there is an immense difference between minor contusion and severe damage of the cord, not only at the time, but especially later; the first may leave no disability, the last a hopeless permanent paraplegia.

Fracture-dislocation of the vertebral column is most common in the region of the fifth and sixth cervical vertebrae and in the lower dorsal region. Crush fractures of vertebral bodies due to force transmitted longitudinally, as when a patient falls from a height and lands on his feet, usually affect the first lumbar or one of the adjacent vertebrae, and the corresponding lumbar spinal roots or the roots of the cauda equina may be damaged. The roots, being peripheral nerves, are generally believed to have greater power of recovery than the structures within the cord itself.

Symptoms

A sudden transverse lesion of the spinal cord causes first a condition of 'spinal shock', in which most of the automatic functions of that part of the cord below the level of the lesion are temporarily abolished. If this occurs at a high level, death is usually immediate, but if not, flaccid paralysis of all four limbs results. If the lesion is in the dorsal region the immediate result is a state of acute flaccid paraplegia, with retention of urine due to flaccid paralysis of the bladder wall (detrusor urinae); in severe cases, all the tendon reflexes and the plantar and abdominal reflexes are at first absent, and there is complete loss of sensory appreciation below the level of the lesion. In some cases the degree of spinal shock is less and the abolition of spinal function is partial.

With the traction injuries of the cervical cord there is seldom the same degree of spinal shock, but temporary paralysis may be considerable; sensory loss is usually partial, and some or all of the reflexes are preserved. Retention of urine is in most instances a matter of a few hours. Paralysis of the hands, with relative sparing of the upper arms, is common in these cases. As the fifth cervical segment is often involved in the lesion, the supinator-jerk, which depends on this segment, is often abolished, but the flexion reflexes remain, and tapping of the supinator tendon produces reflex flexion of the fingers. This is called 'inversion of the supinator reflex'. The fibres of the cervical sym. pathetic (as they descend in the cord to emerge with the first dorsal root) are often involved in the lesion, and in consequence there may be contraction of the pupil and a slight degree of ptosis of the upper eyelid on one or both sides. At a later stage, when the legs have largely recovered, wasting becomes apparent in the hands and forearms, and the case presents a superficial resemblance to one of amyotrophic lateral sclerosis, but the history of accident, the presence of sensory disturbances and such features as the absence of the supinator jerks and signs of disturbance of the sympathetic nervous system should help to make the distinction [see p. 1282].

Treatment

Cervical dislocation should be reduced under general anaesthesia, and subsequently a plaster 'Minerva' collar should be applied to the neck to prevent undue mobility until the damaged ligaments have healed. In cases of cervical fracture, a collar should also be applied, because further displacement may occur during sleep or under other conditions of muscular relaxation so that prolonged immobilization in bed, with light traction upon the neck through ice-tong calipers, is necessary, a weight of up to 4 lbs. being used.

In cases of fracture of the spinal column with injury of the cord, open operation is usually contra-indicated. Fracture of the vertebral arches, on the other hand, may call for operation and the removal of bony fragments from the spinal canal. Pressure on spinal roots is usually relieved by the Watson-Jones method of treating spinal fractures.

The further treatment of injuries of the spinal cord is that of acute paraplegia [see p. 1270], and in no condition is the most careful nursing and skilled medical supervision more urgently called for.

Course and Prognosis

In incomplete and mild cases, as spinal shock passes off, the reflexes begin to return. Retention of urine persists for a variable time, and if not prevented by catheterization, overflow incontinence ensues. The Babinski reflex appears, and is coupled after a time with withdrawal reflexes of the legs. Later, the tendon reflexes return and a variable degree of sensory and motor recovery may take place.

In severe cases this does not happen, and the condition remains one of complete physiological interruption of the cord at the site of the lesion. After an interval there are frequent flexor spasms of the legs, and a state of paraplegia-in-flexion may follow. Any stimulus below the level of the lesion may then cause violent flexion spasms in the legs, contraction of the abdominal wall and extrusion of urine from the bladder—the 'mass reflex'. In most of those cases in which the cord is completely divided, the paralysed muscles remain entirely inert and the only evidence of reflex activity is the development of automatic function of the bladder.

In severe cases, the outlook is always extremely grave. With high cervical lesions, death, if not immediate, may occur within a few hours if the patient is not in an intensive care unit. There are several paraplegic units in the country where after-care and rehabilitation makes a paraplegic life acceptable, even with cervical lesions and a paraplegia involving the arms.

REFERENCES

BROCK, S. (1960) *Injuries to the Brain and Spinal Cord and their Coverings*, 4th ed., London.

COMAR, A. E. (1959) The practical urological management of the patient with spinal cord injury, *Brit. J. Urol.*, **31**, 1.

CRUICKSHANK, E. (1962) Neurological diseases in the tropics, in *Modern Trends in Neurology*, 3rd Series, ed. WILLIAMS, D., London.

DAVIS, R. A., and WASHBURN, P. L. (1970) Spinal cord meningiomas, *Surg. Gynec. Obstet.*, **131**, 15.

DENNY-BROWN, D., and ROBERTSON, E. G. (1933) The state of the bladder and its sphincters in complete transverse lesions of the spinal cord and cauda equina, *Brain*, **56**, 397.

DRAKE, C. G. (1962) Cervical spinal cord injury, *J. Neurosurg.*, **19**, 487.

GAUTIER-SMITH, P. C. (1967) Clinical aspects of spinal neurofibromas, *Brain*, **90**, 359.

GUTTMAN, L. (1946) Rehabilitation after injuries to the spinal cord and cauda equina, *Brit. J. phys. Med.*, **9**, 162.

HARDY, A. G. (1956) The care of the bladder in traumatic paraplegia, *Postgrad. med. J.*, **32**, 328.

KERNOHAN, J. W., WOLTMAN, H. W., and ADSON, A. W. (1931) Intramedullary tumours of the spinal cord, *Arch. Neurol. Psychiat.* (*Chic.*), **25**, 679.

MONRO, D. (1961) Treatment of fractures and dislocations of the cervical spine, complicated by cervical cord and root injury, *New Engl. J. Med.*, **264**, 573.

ODOM, G. L., FINNEY, W., and WOODALL, B. (1958) Cervical disc lesions, *J. Amer. med. Ass.*, **166**, 23.

PLUM, F. (1962) Bladder dysfunction, in *Modern Trends in Neurology*, 3rd Series, ed. WILLIAMS, D., London.

REWCASTLE, N. B., and BERRY, K. (1964) Neoplasms of the lower spinal canal, *Neurology* (*Minneap.*), **14**, 608.

SHINNERS, B. M., and HORNBY, W. B. (1949) Protruded lumbar intervertebral discs, *J. Neurosurg.*, **6**, 450.

SPILLANE, J. D. (1957) Developmental anomalies in the region of the foramen magnum, in *Modern Trends in Neurology*, 2nd Series, ed. WILLIAMS, D., London.

SPILLANE, J. D., PALLIS, C., and JONES, A. M. (1957) Developmental anomalies in the region of the foramen magnum, *Brain*, **80**, 11.

SYMONDS, C. P., and MEADOWS, S. P. (1937) Compression of the spinal cord in the neighbourhood of the foramen magnum, *Brain*, **60**, 52.

WALTZ, T. A. (1967) Physical factors in the myelopathy of cervical spondylosis, *Brain*, **90**, 395.

OTHER DISEASES OF THE SPINAL CORD

ACUTE TRANSVERSE MYELITIS

Aetiology

The condition is rare during childhood, and mostly occurs during the first half of adult life. The sexes are affected equally. In most cases the cause cannot be determined. Some cases are of viral origin, some due to acute demyelination; syphilis has long ceased to be the most frequent cause.

Pathology

The cord appears healthy except in a short portion of its length comprising one or two segments. The lesion is most frequently situated in the lower half of the dorsal region, and at its site the cord shows intense signs of disease and may be wholly or partly diffluent. In some microscopic sections of the affected segments no normal spinal tissue may be found, and in others, though elements are spared in an irregular fashion, nearly every portion exhibits some pathological change. The adjoining segments are affected in lesser degree, and elsewhere the cord is healthy. Unless all the elements are necrotic there is evidence of inflammatory reaction in the diseased portions. Intense congestion of vessels and minute points of haemorrhage may be present.

Symptoms

There may be malaise and a slightly raised temperature and sometimes pain of 'root' type at the level of the lesion for a few days before the onset of paralysis. These symptoms are followed by weakness of one or both legs, and paralysis may be complete from the waist down within 24 or 48 hours; in other cases, it is complete in an hour or two; in others, though remaining incomplete, it may reach its full intensity in that time; while in still other cases, the onset is 'apoplectic', i.e. the patient feeling some weakness, sits down, and within a few minutes is completely paraplegic.

If the patient is seen soon after the onset he usually shows complete motor and sensory paralysis from the waist down, with flaccidity of the muscles and loss of reflexes; retention of urine is present and may have gone on to overflow incontinence. If some power of voluntary movement or some sensation is preserved, some of the reflexes usually persist too. There may be from the first a zone of hyperaesthesia at the upper limit of the paralysis, and later a 'girdle sensation' may develop at this site. While the limbs are flaccid and sensation is absent, bed-sores may develop with great rapidity, and in the paralysed bladder intense cystitis may occur. The patient may die in the acute stage as the result of these complications. More often sensation and the reflexes return after a few weeks, and in course of time spasticity develops in the limbs, with a variable amount of voluntary power. There may be a partial Brown-Séquard syndrome. Remarkable recovery may occur in the course of many months, but even then considerable disability usually persists. In other cases there is no return of power, and the bedridden patient succumbs in a few months to intercurrent disease.

Diagnosis

Queckenstedt's test should be done at the time of lumbar puncture, in order to exclude conditions of thecal block and full examination of the cerebrospinal fluid, including the Wassermann reaction, chromatography and if possible micro-estimations of protein fractions. Poliomyelitis is excluded by the presence of severe sensory loss. It may not be possible to make the differential diagnosis from haemorrhage into the substance of the cord, but the latter is usually associated with more pain and, after the first acute stage is over, with a syringomyelic type of sensory loss. Angioma of the cord usually causes less acute paralysis coming on with less constitutional disturbance.

Treatment

The treatment is that of the paraplegia [see p. 1270].

LOCAL VASCULAR LESIONS OF THE SPINAL CORD

Arterial and Venous Angiomas

Haemorrhage into the spinal cord is uncommon apart from pre-existing vascular abnormalities. When it occurs it produces signs of an acute segmental lesion, followed, as a rule, by those of more general haematomyelia.

Venous thrombosis in the cord may cause local lesions with paraplegia, and that following local extrathecal infective conditions has been attributed to this cause. Vascular abnormalities resulting from congenital malformation of blood vessels occur in the spinal cord. The most usual type is a racemose venous angioma, partly within the cord and partly on its posterior surface. These lesions are almost always in the lower half of the cord. Pain of root type affecting the lower limbs and recurring in acute episodes is a salient clinical feature. It may be followed, or even preceded, by wasting and weakness of one or both legs, and sphincter disturbance is usually present during the acute episodes. The reflex findings are often anomalous. The diagnosis is made upon the characteristic changes seen on myelography. The abnormal vessels show as tortuous clear channels in the contrast medium.

The superficial vessels should not be touched. There has been unresolved debate upon the use of anticoagulants if there is steadily advancing paraplegia in such a case.

SPINA BIFIDA

The most common developmental abnormality of the spinal cord results from a failure of the neural tube to close perfectly and to separate completely from the surface ectoderm. Because of the failure of separation the mesodermal tissues in which the vertebral arches develop cannot close over the posterior surface of the developing cord at the affected site, and spina bifida ensues. Spina bifida is thus usually associated with some abnormality in the cord itself, and its significance as a clinical finding is that it is a pointer to a local fault of development in the cord.

Spina bifida is common; in 90 per cent. of cases it affects the lumbosacral region and in about 5 per cent. the lower cervical. There may be some abnormality of the skin over the affected vertebral arches, or there may be a frank meningocele. Hydrocephalus may be associated.

Incomplete fusion of the lower lumbar and sacral vertebral arches is so common as to be a normal variant, and is usually unassociated with any disability. Severe degrees of malformation of the spinal cord are incompatible with life. Of the two forms, complete and occult, we are only concerned with the second, for complete spina bifida is not compatible with survival. Spina bifida occulta may be associated with deformity in the sacral region, in its minor form simply a hairy dimple.

Symptoms

Weakness of the legs may be present from birth or an early age, and may increase, or it may be noticed about puberty, when the vertebral column elongates and the spinal cord, which in these cases is often adherent at its lower end, becomes pulled upon. The ankle-jerks and possibly also the knee-jerks may be absent, the muscles of the legs poorly developed and the feet hollow. Congenital talipes may be present. Control of the sphincters of bladder and anus is often imperfect, especially the former. Trophic changes may occur on the feet, and there may be areas of anaesthesia on the feet and on the buttocks. Sometimes the sensory loss is of a dissociated type.

Diagnosis

If symptoms have been present since childhood, the diagnosis is easy and is confirmed by radiographic examination. When they appear at puberty or later, and there is no external abnormality, spina bifida may not be considered, but if tumour is suspected radiographic investigation is likely to be undertaken and the bony abnormality is seen.

Treatment

In most cases, because of the malformation of the cord, no improvement can be expected from operation.

Prognosis

In the less severe cases the symptoms become stationary, and are consistent with a normal duration of life, but the very severe die young.

SYRINGOMYELIA

Synonym. Status dysraphicus.

Definition

A chronic disease due to the formation in the spinal cord and brain stem of long cavities with surrounding gliosis. To the disease in the brain stem the term syringobulbia is often applied. The conditions are uncommon.

Aetiology

In most cases the disease causes symptoms in the period of growth, and it is rare for them to be delayed beyond 30. Both sexes may be affected, males more than females. The disease depends upon a congenital abnormality, and other somatic abnormalities may be present in the same patient. Cavitation in the spinal cord may also occur in association with intramedullary tumours, with spinal vascular disease, with pachymeningitis cervicalis and with haemangiomata of the spinal cord.

The view at present is that a congenital defect of the angle of the brain stem makes the central canal of the spinal cord subject to the direct thrust of the pulsating pressure of the spinal fluid; this distends the canal and causes distinctive pressure upon the surrounding tissues. Gardiner has advocated plugging the upper end of the canal with a small piece of muscle. In support of this view, syringomyelia sometimes occurs in association with deformity of the neuraxis—the Arnold-Chiari deformity.

Pathology

At necropsy the cord is enlarged, and cross-section shows a cavity filled with clear or yellowish fluid. Its extent is often considerable and the lower cervical and upper dorsal segments are the most frequently and the most severely affected. The cavitation is most marked in the posterior half of the cord and appears to arise at the base of one of the posterior horns, or in the middle line behind the central canal. The cavity does not represent a dilated central canal, for this can often be found separate from it, though the two usually communicate. More than one cavity may be present. It is surrounded by glial tissue which is relatively acellular and often peculiarly translucent. The blood vessels frequently show degenerative changes, and the fluid within the cavity may give evidence of old or recent haemorrhage. The cavity is so placed that it interrupts the crossing neurones which convey pain and temperature sensations. As it enlarges, the anterior horns of grey matter become involved in its surrounding gliosis and the cells degenerate. Ascending and descending tracts are affected either by pressure as a result of distension of the cavity with fluid, or by the glial process. The posterior columns always survive longest.

In the medulla the disease affects particularly the floor of the fourth ventricle in the region of the hypoglossal nucleus and tends to extend as a slit anterolaterally to a position just anterior to the descending nucleus of the trigeminal nerve. In its course it may destroy the motor nucleus of the vagus and glossopharyngeal nerves or emerging fibres of these nerves. It interrupts the internal arcuate fibres passing from the cuneate and gracile nuclei to the mesial fillet, and the fibres from the descending nucleus of the vestibular nerve to the posterior longitudinal bundle. The development of this lesion thus leads to complete sensory loss which was previously of the typical dissociated type, and causes or increases nystagmus. If it reaches far enough it also interrupts some or all of the fibres passing from the descending trigeminal nucleus to the fillet of the opposite side, and so causes dissociated sensory loss on the face on the side of the lesion. The disease may extend up into the pons and, in rare instances, higher.

Symptoms

Disturbances of Sensation. By far the most constant and characteristic feature of syringomyelia is a sensory loss of a peculiar kind, named by Charcot 'dissociated'. This is a loss of sensation to painful impressions and to thermal stimuli, while sensibility to touch, to vibration, to position, to passive movement and to the appreciation of location upon the skin, remain relatively or entirely intact. In other words, those forms of sensation which travel by a path crossing in the commissures of the spinal cord are lost, because the lesion of syringomyelia destroys especially the region of the commissures, while these forms of sensibility which travel by paths which are uncrossed in the spinal cord are not affected.

The destruction of the commissures in the lower cervical and upper dorsal regions produces the dissociated sensory loss symmetrically over the thorax and upper extremities, the distribution varying with the extent of the lesion. The symmetrical sensory loss is seldom found below the thorax because the spinal lesion does not often extend below the mid-dorsal region. Occasionally the sensory loss varies in depth, extent and symmetry of distribution according to the completeness, extent and symmetry of the lesion. Thus, in early and slight cases, the sensory disturbance may not amount to more than a relative loss of pain and temperature confined to the hands and ulnar borders of the forearms, while in an advanced case there is usually complete inability to appreciate painful and thermal stimuli over an area which would be covered by a sleeved jacket. The area often extends later over the neck and the face. Combinations of the 'sleeved jacket' sensory loss with hemianalgesia and hemithermanaesthesia often occur in cases where both the spinal lesion and the medullary lesion are present. The dissociated sensory loss comes on insidiously, and is often unnoticed by the patient and discovered for the first time on medical examination. Sometimes the patient finds that he appreciates heat and cold upon some parts of the skin and not on others. Often he injures himself or burns himself without noticing it at the time.

Subjective sensation is not often affected, and for the most part syringomyelia may be described as a painless disease; but there are notable exceptions. Sensations of heat and cold, dull fixed pains, lasting neuralgic pains, and lightning pains resembling those of tabes, may occur. These pains are confined to the regions which are the seat of the other symptoms.

Muscular Atrophy. This is found in considerably more than half the cases. Though usually bilateral, it is often asymmetrical, and may be entirely confined to one side. The intrinsic muscles of the hands, and the muscles of the ulnar side of the forearms are first and most affected in the ordinary run of cases. The atrophy is often here confined, but it may extend up the arm, though it is unusual for the whole upper limb to be affected. Sometimes the shoulder muscles are first affected, and again the scapulothoracic and humero-thoracic muscles may be early involved. The upper intercostals and that section of the muscles which supports the spine supplied from the upper six dorsal segments suffer, but the scalenes seem generally to escape. The muscular atrophy is strictly limited and is apt to become complete in the muscles affected. Fibrillation is not unusual. The lesions of the medulla may involve the motor nuclei of the cranial nerves. Wasting of the tongue occurs and its discovery in a young subject should always arouse suspicions of the presence of syringomyelia. Unilateral paralysis of the palate, pharynx and all the muscles of the larynx upon the affected side may occur from involvement of the nucleus ambiguus. Similarly, but in much rarer cases, atrophic paralysis of the face, of the trigeminal muscles, of the sternomastoid and trapezius may occur from unilateral involvement of the corresponding motor nuclei. Nystagmus is almost a constant feature.

Contractures resulting from the muscular atrophy are commonly seen in the hands, and the deformity tends to the 'claw-hand' type, but hardly reaches the degree seen in ulnar nerve paralysis, and is often much modified by trophic and vasomotor changes, and by the results of injuries and whitlows.

Other Motor Symptoms. The legs almost invariably escape so far as atrophy of muscles is concerned but usually present a slight spasticity, with the signs of involvement of the crossed pyramidal tracts. This does not often produce much disability. In cases, however, where the lesions involve the lateral region of the cord, either by direct extension or by the pressure of distended cavities, severe spastic paraplegia may result. Rarely this may lead to avascularization and a complete transverse lesion of the spinal cord with the appearance of flaccid paraplegia with incontinence, total sensory loss and absent deep reflexes.

Sphincter trouble is usually absent, or slight and occasional; but in cases in which paraplegia is severe any degree may occur.

The skin reflexes of the trunk are diminished or absent and the plantar reflexes are of the extensor type, according to the degree of pyramidal involvement. Pes cavus is often present. The knee-jerks and ankle-jerks are increased, while the arm-jerks, even in the absence of muscular wasting, are characteristically absent.

Spinal curvature is present in many cases. It consists of a kyphosis or kyphoscoliosis of the upper dorsal region, with a compensating lordosis and lateral curve in the lumbar region. The upper convexity is to the left, because of the major use of the right hand. It depends upon paralysis of the trunk muscles, from involvement of the anterior horns in the upper dorsal region, and, in addition, dystrophic changes in the bones may be factors in its production. It is more marked the earlier it begins during growth, and in cases in which heavy manual occupation has been followed.

Trophic and Vasomotor Disturbances. Thickening of the bones or a condition of osteoporosis and brittleness may be seen. More often Charcot's arthropathy occurs. It differs in no way from the similar condition in tabes dorsalis, but being confined to the joints of the analgesic region it affects those of the upper extremity. The most characteristic of the trophic changes consists in thickening of the subcutaneous tissue and of the skin itself, which is seen in the hands. The fingers become thick and swollen, and lose their natural outline, the tips become blunted and the knuckle-folds thick and coarse, and vasomotor disturbance renders them unduly red, or even blue. They have been termed 'sausage-like' fingers, and often stand out in contrast to the wasting of the intrinsic muscles of the hand. A similar condition affecting the whole hand is common, and was termed by Charcot 'la main succulente'. The analgesic condition of the hands and the thermanaes-thesia present expose them unduly to injuries and, since the injuries are likely to be unnoticed or dis-regarded, septic infection arises easily, and the results of injuries, burns and whitlows are frequently seen, giving rise to further deformity from scars, or loss of the terminal phalanges.

Considering that the efferent neurones of the cervical sympathetic system have their origin in the brain stem, and their exit from the spinal cord in the upper dorsal segments, thus traversing the whole of the region usually affected by the lesion of syringomyelia, the frequency with which *paralysis of the cervical sympathetic* occurs is easily understood. It may be complete or incomplete, unilateral or bilateral, and is recognized by smallness of the pupil, narrowing of the palpebral aperture (sympathetic ptosis) and a peculiar flatness of expression on the side of the face affected, with decrease or loss of sweating. These signs are much more obvious when unilateral than when bilateral, for, in the absence of the contrast which a normal side of the face gives, they are often overlooked when bilateral.

Morvan's Disease. This is a condition of great rarity, in which a chronic peripheral neuritis is combined with syringomyelia, with severe effects upon the extremities. There is absolute loss of all forms of sensibility in the hands and in some cases also in the feet, together with atrophy of the intrinsic muscles. The cause of this complication of syringomyelia is unknown.

Diagnosis

Syringomyelia has to be differentiated, in its early stages, from those diseases which cause slowly progressive muscular atrophy in the upper extremities, and, in its later stages, from other lesions of the central region of the spinal cord. Those cases in which the lesions are chiefly in the pontomedullary region must be distinguished from other slowly advancing lesions of the brain stem.

The age of onset, during the later years of childhood and the earlier years of adult life, is important, and during this period slowly developing paralysis with sensory loss, and with or without muscular atrophy should always suggest the possibility of syringomyelia.

Other causes, which may produce this symptom group, and which may be confused with syringomyelia, are local lesions of the brachial plexus, and, especially, the lesion produced by the presence of cervical ribs, root lesions, lesions of the central grey matter of the spinal cord, especially central tumours of the spinal cord, and haematomyelia. That the peculiar sensory changes of syringomyelia are usually the first signs of that disease is important; but this rule has many exceptions, both as to the nature of the sensory changes and their time of appearance. When sensory changes are not an early sign the diagnosis has to be made from such diseases as progressive muscular atrophy, peroneal atrophy and myotonia atrophica.

Local lesions of the peripheral nerves produce signs which are confined to the distribution of the nerve involved; the sensory loss is to all forms, and the condition is ordinarily unilateral. While these features are enough to distinguish them from syringomyelia in nearly all cases, rarely the sensory loss and the muscular atrophy may be so narrowly confined to the distribution of the ulnar nerve to resemble it. Any sensory loss over the trunk, or signs outside the distribution of the peripheral nerve, will, if present, clearly divide the two conditions.

Cervical ribs may produce slowly progressive atrophy of muscles, pain and sensory loss, difficult to distinguish from those resulting from syringomyelia. The diagnosis in these cases is beset with peculiar difficulties, for so frequently do cervical ribs produce no nervous symptoms at all that their presence, when demonstrated, does not argue that they are the cause of the symptoms. Again, cervical ribs are among the commonest of the developmental peculiarities which are so frequently seen in the subjects of syringomyelia. Slow muscular atrophy and slowly oncoming sensory loss and perhaps pain characterize both syringomyelia and cervical rib paralysis, and the distribution may be unilateral or bilateral in either condition; but it is only when the effects are confined to the arms and neck that difficulty arises. The slightest physical sign outside of this region at once turns the diagnosis in favour of syringomyelia, and of these signs cervical sympathetic paralysis, sensory loss on the trunk and alteration of the abdominal and plantar reflexes are the most important. A careful search must be made for any such signs, and the patient observed over a considerable time before a certain diagnosis is made.

Lesions of the central grey matter of the spinal cord may produce a symptom-complex closely resembling that of syringomyelia. Central tumours of the spinal cord, are hardly distinguishable, except by their rate of growth, the majority being of more rapid development, and speedily causing severe paraplegia.

Progressive muscular atrophy in its early stages may give difficulty in diagnosis, since the muscular atrophy in syringomyelia may precede the appearance of any sensory loss or may be well marked when the sensory loss is slight. In this connexion, widely distributed fasciculation indicates progressive muscular atrophy, particularly if it be seen in muscles not conspicuously wasted. In peroneal atrophy the atrophy of the intrinsic hand muscles is always preceded by a more extensive atrophy of the muscles below the knee, which are rarely atrophied in syringomyelia.

Syringobulbia may be distinguished from other lesions of this region by its insidious onset and the special tendency to the involvement of the lateral region of the medulla, causing a unilateral paralysis of palate, pharynx and larynx with hemianalgesia and hemithermanaesthesia on part of the face and even on the opposite half of the body. Often some signs of cervical syringomyelia coexist.

Treatment

With the good results reported for Gardner's operation of plugging the spinal canal, early diagnosis is important. Without it life is prolonged but disabled; with its successful completion it seems that the condition may be arrested.

Course and Duration

The disability begins insidiously, and without operation progresses slowly, often ceasing to advance for periods which may amount to many years.

HAEMATOMYELIA

Aetiology and Pathology

Haematomyelia, or haemorrhage into the spinal cord sufficient to cause symptoms is rare. It arises when there is some abnormality of the spinal vessels, and in particular some variety of angioma and in haemorrhagic diseases. Often the cause is undiscovered. Haemorrhage may occur into a syringomyelic cavity. The haemorrhage is nearly always centrally situated, spreads longitudinally and may extend over many segments.

Men are affected far more than women and mainly in the first half of adult life.

Symptoms

Prodromal symptoms may occur in the form of local weakness or transitory sensory disturbances. In most cases the actual onset is sudden, but the symptoms increase for an hour or two. They vary according to the site and the extent of the extravasation. At first there is paraplegia, with more or less complete motor and sensory paralysis up to the level of the lesion, with intense pain at the upper limit of disturbance. As the haemorrhage extends longitudinally these manifestations are quickly followed by a syringomyelic type of sensory loss.

Sometimes, but not usually, blood is found in the cerebrospinal fluid.

Diagnosis

The diagnosis of primary haematomyelia rests upon the sudden onset, the rapid development of symptoms, which soon come to a standstill, and the physical signs of a central lesion of the spinal cord. The distinction has to be made from acute myelitis. Acute myelitis, though rapid in onset, rarely shows the dramatic symptoms of haematomyelia, and the sensory loss which accompanies it is not of the syringomyelic type.

Treatment

Treatment is that of the paraplegic, laminectomy being of diagnostic value only.

SUBACUTE COMBINED DEGENERATION OF THE SPINAL CORD

Definition

A progressive disease due to deficiency of vitamin B_{12} (cyanocobalamin) and associated with pernicious anaemia, in which the white matter of the spinal cord degenerates, the effects being particularly in the posterior and lateral columns. There is an associated peripheral neuropathy. It is much less common than a few years ago, perhaps because of the ubiquitous use of the vitamin B complex.

Aetiology

The causes of deficiency of vitamin B_{12} are considered in Section 13 under Megaloblastic Anaemia for it is also essential for normal blood formation and deficiency leads to megaloblastic anaemia. Thus Addisonian pernicious anaemia is usually associated with subacute combined degeneration. The severity of the anaemia and the extent of the neural damage show no constant relationship. One may be trivial and the other profound. Indeed, anaemia may be absent when subacute combined degeneration is first recognized and the diagnosis of pernicious anaemia nowadays is never delayed until the appearance of nervous symptoms.

The cases now seen are often mild and atypical and may occur in patients with Addisonian anaemia in whom the treatment has been inadequate. The sexes are equally affected.

Pathology

The essential lesion is degeneration of the myelin sheaths and axis cylinders in the posterior and lateral columns. Similar changes occur in the peripheral nerves and hemispheres. The myelin swells and later disintegrates. This change is first seen in the centre of both posterior columns in the lower dorsal regions, and soon afterwards in the centre of either lateral column, as snall areas of a darker and more translucent appearance than the normal white matter.

From its origin in the lower dorsal region the degeneration spreads upwards and downwards in the white columns of the spinal cord, starting as small isolated spots of degeneration in the posterior, lateral and anterolateral columns, which increase in size and coalesce. The degeneration extends upwards, and in severe cases has been found as high as the internal capsule.

When degeneration in the peripheral nerves is severe the muscles are wasted in the later stages, and the muscle fibres show diminution in size and poor striation.

The Blood. Sometimes the blood is normal but usually some change can be found, although it may be no more than trivial macrocytosis. Commonly, however, the blood and the bone marrow show the typical features of a megaloblastic anaemia [see Section 13].

The serum B_{12} should be estimated; the level is greatly reduced in all untreated cases of subacute combined degeneration even in the absence of anaemia.

The cerebrospinal fluid is normal.

Symptoms

In most cases the symptoms appear insidiously and without any recognized exciting cause. Sometimes the onset is more rapid and may be preceded by gastrointestinal symptoms, or the patient may go to bed for a few days with an attack of 'influenza' and on getting up again may be grossly unsteady.

The first nervous symptom is usually numbness or tingling in the feet, and if the patient is asked he will usually admit that he has a slight sensation of the same kind in the fingers. Less often the sensation in the feet is one of swelling, or coldness, or as if walking on cotton wool; and in a few cases unsteadiness in walking is at first the only complaint. Soon weakness in the legs is felt, the numbness spreads, and the patient feels unsteady in walking.

Examination at this time shows weakness of the toes or in dorsiflexion of the feet, diminution or absence of the ankle-jerk, probably an extensor plantar reflex, and a variable degree of sensory loss; this is usually more marked for vibration and for sense of position than for light touch. There may be tenderness of the feet or calves. Romberg's sign is positive. The superficial sensory loss is at first only over the feet, then it spreads up to cover a 'sock' area, and later has a 'stocking' distribution, pain and temperature impairment meanwhile being added to it. Loss of deep sensation is marked, with consequent unsteadiness. At that stage the arms may be normal. The dysaesthesiae in the legs are generally very distressing.

If the condition is allowed to progress, either the signs of peripheral nerve disease or those of spinal cord disease may predominate. In the former case the knee-jerks become diminished and the ankle-jerks lost, the muscles below the knees become paralysed and flaccid and eventually waste, deep sensory loss is severe, and there is loss of all forms of superficial sensation over a 'stocking' area. The paralysed muscles become very tender, flexion spasms may set in and every movement is agonizing. In the upper limbs a variable degree of sensory loss may develop with astereognosis in the hands and loss of superficial sensation over a 'glove' area. The supinator-jerks may be abolished, but rarely the biceps- and triceps-jerks. If the signs of spinal cord disease predominate, the legs tend to become spastic, the knee-jerks are increased but the ankle-jerks are usually weak and the plantar reflexes are strongly extensor. Sensory loss is less marked as a rule than when the signs of peripheral disease predominate, but deep sensation is always greatly impaired, and as time goes on there is considerable loss of pain and temperature appreciation, extending over the lower limbs and to a gradually higher level on the trunk. In the arms the tendon jerks may be increased. Except in advanced cases sphincter disturbances are slight.

The cranial nerves are usually unaffected, but optic atrophy is a complication in a few cases, and the visual disturbances due to it may rarely be the first symptom. Slight nystagmus is common.

Mental changes occur in some when the anaemia is not sufficient to account for them. Apathy, mild dementia and confusional psychosis with impaired memory and disorientation are the commonest types of disturbance.

Pernicious anaemia, being also due to deficiency of vitamin B_{12}, is usually associated with subacute combined degeneration. In some patients nervous symptoms dominate the clinical picture and anaemia is trivial or absent; in others anaemia is the main problem and nervous symptoms may be lacking; in some the severity of the anaemia and of the neural damage run parallel. The patient with subacute combined degeneration may therefore show any or all of the features described as characteristic of pernicious anaemia [see Section 13].

Diagnosis

In the early stages of the disease, when peripheral paraesthesiae dominate the picture, the condition has to be distinguished from peripheral neuritis and occasionally from peripheral arterial disease. In the well-developed stages of the disease, its recognition presents no great difficulty. Attention is quickly attracted by the conspicuous anaemia and biscuit-coloured skin. Following a period of slight paraplegia, the steadily increasing paralysis of the lower extremities, producing complete and lasting helplessness, the characteristic distribution of the sensory loss, the irregular pyrexia, the anaemia and the relatively late onset of sphincter trouble serve to separate this disease from other forms of paraplegia. The change from the spastic to the flaccid type of paraplegia with loss of the deep reflexes and persistence of the extensor response, which occurs in some of the cases in the late stages, is highly characteristic.

In the earliest stages and before the appearance of any definite evidence of organic spinal disease, there may be such disability as to suggest hysterical paraplegia or ataxia, and only the examination of the blood may expose the real disease. When there is evidence of organic spinal disease, it is especially from disseminated sclerosis, spinal tumour, tabes dorsalis and polyneuritis that the diagnosis has to be made. The preponderance of peripheral subjective sensations and the anaemic appearance should always suggest a diagnosis of subacute combined degeneration. Slight spastic ataxia is the common clinical picture of subacute combined degeneration, of disseminated sclerosis and of spinal tumour. The presence of objective peripheral sensory loss is in favour of subacute combined degeneration, whereas diplopia, nystagmus, transient amblyopia and intention tremor are strongly in favour of disseminated sclerosis. Spinal tumour is especially distinguished by a sharp line of sensory loss, transverse to the axis of the body, which does not spread up from below in slow fashion.

When subacute combined degeneration starts with flaccid ataxia and loss of deep reflexes, the distinction must be made from tabes dorsalis. The extensor plantar reflex, which is almost always present in the former disease and which is rare in early tabes, the different distribution of the sensory loss in the two diseases, the loss of power and associated anaemia in subacute combined degeneration, and the results of the examination of the blood and cerebrospinal fluid for syphilitic reactions and of the latter fluid for lymphocytosis, are important aids in the differential diagnosis.

It is also necessary to bear in mind the close resemblance of the disease to polyneuritis. The differentiation may in the early stages depend chiefly, if not wholly, upon the examination of the blood and estimation of the serum vitamin B_{12} level. But, sooner or later, the appearance of an extensor response will indicate the presence of a cord lesion. On the other hand, in the spastic type, the presence of muscular tenderness in the legs is a strong indication in favour of subacute combined degeneration.

Treatment

Whatever the degree of anaemia present, intensive replacement treatment is essential. Cyanocobalamin (vitamin B_{12}) should be given for the first month in doses of 100 microgrammes on alternate days. Thereafter the dosage may be very gradually reduced provided that the blood picture is satisfactory, and the ultimate maintenance dose may be as little as 250 microgrammes monthly. Hydroxycobalamin can be given less often as a holding dose, 500 microgrammes every 2 months being adequate.

The blood count should be restored to normal as quickly as possible. The more advanced the stage of the disease the more prolonged will need to be the period of intensive treatment and the more severe the residual disability is likely to be.

Course and Prognosis

Cases of the flaccid type, in which peripheral neuritis predominates, respond better to vitamin B_{12} than do the more spastic, the disease in the latter being chiefly in the spinal cord. In cases of the latter type the extensor plantar reflex, usually the most persistent sign of spasticity, may disappear. Advanced cases of both types may fail to show much response to treatment. But no case, however advanced when first recognized, should be deprived of full treatment, and the most surprising recoveries are sometimes seen. If treatment is stopped relapse occurs sooner or later, and with renewed treatment recovery again ensues, but it is doubtful whether this process can be frequently repeated, on account of the probability of gliosis in the spinal cord.

MOTOR NEURONE DISEASE

Synonyms. Progressive muscular atrophy; Amyotrophic lateral sclerosis.

Definition

There is a large group of cases in which progressive wasting of the muscles and a moderate degree of spasticity are secondary to widespread degenerative changes in the central nervous system, the chief incidence of which is on the lower and upper motor neurones. Clinically there is great variety, according to the sites of the initial wasting and the degree of spasticity, but there are three clinical types. In the first and most common type, the wasting begins in the arms, and the legs become spastic but do not waste. This variety was called by Charcot *amyotrophic lateral sclerosis*. In the second type, the wasting commences in the muscles innervated from the medulla and pons, and the names *progressive bulbar paralysis* and *labioglossopharyngeal paralysis* are applied to it. In the third type, the wasting begins in or quickly spreads to the legs and no spasticity develops: this is called the *purely atrophic type*. Transitions between these types are common, and the first two are frequently combined.

Aetiology

The disease is rare before 25, but occurs at all ages thereafter, attaining its maximum incidence between 30 and 50. Men are affected much more often than women. No causal factors have been discovered but the disease will probably prove to be due to an intracellular biochemical disorder of the affected motor neurones, in the same sense that subacute combined degeneration and pellagra are the results of such deficiencies. There is no convincing evidence that the disease is ever due to injury, though, of course, patients may notice the first symptoms after they have hurt themselves, but we know of no pathological process whereby a peripheral injury can set up a diffuse degenerative process within the central nervous system. Injury of the cervical portion of the spinal cord may produce a syndrome embracing wasting in the arms and spasticity in the legs [see p. 1275], thus superficially resembling amyotrophic lateral sclerosis, but there is not sufficient evidence that trauma can cause the progressive and ultimately fatal malady of which true amyotrophic lateral sclerosis is the most common clinical variety [see Diagnosis, p. 1286].

In rare instances progressive muscular atrophy has been described in the subjects of old acute anterior poliomyelitis. The familial motor neurone disease which was recognized in Guam during the Second World War, and which is associated with dementia, has excited much interest, but has not really advanced knowledge of the cause.

Pathology

The essential lesion is a primary degeneration of the anterior horn cells and of their homologues in the motor nuclei of the brain stem which shrink, lose their dendrites and become oval or spherical. Similar, but always less intense changes are seen in the Betz cells and the upper motor neurones.

In the later stages of the disease all the structures of the cord are affected except the posterior columns and the fine fibres passing forward in the grey matter which have their cell bodies outside the central nervous system. It is probably their preservation which explains the strikingly brisk tendon reflexes characteristic of the wasting muscles of amyotrophic lateral sclerosis.

The changes in the muscles are those which constantly follow denervation.

The pathological picture, therefore, of progressive muscular atrophy is a widely scattered degeneration, not confined to the motor systems, though these are predominantly affected.

The condition mentioned above is pathologically the same as motor neurone disease and is the commonest cause of death amongst the native Chamorro population of Guam, but is an hereditary disorder.

It is quite extraordinary that there are still no clues at all as to the prime cause of this most distressing disorder. Nothing is similar to it in the endogenous degeneration of motor neurones.

Symptoms

The onset is gradual, but can be quite rapid, and severe incapacity may result in a few months. In rarer cases a severe disability may develop in the course of a few weeks, and then it is not uncommon to see the most remarkable temporary improvement. The nature of the onset, as a rule, indicates the course of the illness. A very slow onset is followed by a slowly advancing disease, often interrupted by long stationary periods, whereas the more rapid the onset, the quicker will be the advance. At the onset, and during the early stages of the disease, are certain sensory symptoms which, from the confusion in diagnosis they may cause deserve emphasis. These are confined to the regions where the wasting first appears, and are a subjective feeling of stiffness and uselessness, much increased when the limb or the body is cold. Or there may be dull aching pains, intermittent neuralgic pains which may be severe, or a sensation of coldness or numbness which may be intense. Painful cramp in the muscles which are about to be affected is comparatively common. The patient may first notice the atrophy, and this is more common when the onset is in the hands. More often the disability due to the weakness is noticed first; this is always the case where the commencement is in the bulbar muscles, and usually also where the muscles of the legs, proximal muscles of the arms and trunk muscles are first involved. Lastly, the fasciculation may be so marked as to attract notice first.

The *muscular wasting*, which is the most characteristic feature of the disease, may begin in any muscle group. It may be first seen in such rare situations as the facial muscles, intercostal muscles or muscles of the back and abdomen. The commonest is in the muscles of the arm, where the distal (intrinsic muscles of the hand) or the proximal muscles (deltoids and spinati) are first affected in about an equal number of cases. In the hand, the muscles of the thenar eminence are the first to waste, and this is followed by atrophy of the hypothenars, of the lumbricals and of the interossei with the usual flattening of the palm, exposure of the flexor tendons in the palm from loss of the bulk of the lumbricals, hollowing of the interosseal spaces and a tendency to the 'claw' attitude of the hand. This *main en griffe* is never so marked in this disease as in paralysis of the ulnar nerve or syringomyelia, because the wasting soon affects the long flexors of the fingers, and, moreover, contractures of the affected muscles are not marked in progressive muscular atrophy. When the upper arm is affected the wasting is usually first seen in the deltoids, whence it spreads upwards, involving the spinati and the muscles attaching arm to scapula, and arm and scapula to trunk. Among these muscles some tend to escape the atrophy, or to be affected much later than others, and these are the triceps, the latissimus dorsi, the lower half of the pectoralis major, the levator anguli scapulae and especially the upper half of the trapezius. In the limbs the wasting always begins in one, but soon spreads to the corresponding limb of the opposite side and tends ultimately to become symmetrical.

The type of muscular wasting in amyotrophic lateral sclerosis and in other forms of progressive muscular atrophy is what Gowers called *tonic atrophy*. It might be expected that when degeneration began in a group of anterior horn cells, the corresponding muscles would gradually lose their tendon reflexes and become inexcitable. But in amyotrophic lateral sclerosis, while the muscles waste, their tendon-jerks become and remain exaggerated, and the wasting muscles, though they hang flabbily on the limbs, become hyperexcitable to percussion and show spontaneous contractions of groups of fibres, known as fasciculation.

In other forms of progressive muscular atrophy, the wasting muscles are more liable to lose their tendon-jerks, they may be inexcitable to percussion of the muscle bellies, and they show less, if any, fasciculation.

Accompanying the muscular wasting there is usually wasting of the subcutaneous tissues and the skin becomes loose, and the reduced and separated muscles stand out when they are voluntarily contracted. In some cases the subcutaneous tissue is not affected and then the muscular wasting may be masked for a long time, even till paralysis becomes complete. There may be an appearance of vasomotor paralysis—redness, blueness and some swelling of the periphery—but this seems to occur much more as the result of the continual pendant position of the hands and of the absence of muscular activity which normally aids the circulation than of any definite vasomotor palsy.

While, in the usual type of case, muscular wasting is going on in the arms, signs of spasticity gradually develop in the legs. The knee-jerks and ankle-jerks become exaggerated, and after a time the plantar reflexes become 'extensor'. There is seldom a severe spasticity and it may not be palpable, although the reflex signs of pyramidal disease are present. The parts which become spastic do not, in general, develop any wasting.

Spasticity from the upper motor neurone disease may develop in the legs before there are any signs elsewhere of atrophic paralysis due to the lower motor neurone lesion, and such cases present the physical signs of a primary lateral sclerosis. It must, therefore, be borne in mind that such a case may eventually prove to be one of amyotrophic lateral sclerosis.

In some cases of progressive muscular atrophy no abnormal clinical signs are found in the legs, but, *post mortem*, degeneration of the pyramidal tracts is evident.

Next in order of frequency to initial wasting in the arms comes the incidence of the disease upon the muscles concerned in facial expression, articulation, mastication and deglutition, and in lesser degree upon the muscles of phonation. The disease may be confined to these muscles throughout the whole of its course—*progressive bulbar paralysis*, or *labioglossopharyngeal paralysis*. The wasting begins in the intrinsic muscles of the tongue and spreads to the orbicularis oris, the extrinsic muscles of the tongue, pharynx and larynx, the muscles of mastication and, eventually, but in less degree, to the facial muscles generally; but only in rare cases are the oculomotor muscles affected.

The intrinsic muscles of the palate, the constrictors of the pharynx, the intrinsic muscles of the larynx and the muscle of the oesophagus are little affected. This seems at first anomalous, considering how great and important are the troubles with deglutition in bulbar paralysis. But the anomaly disappears at once when one considers that the muscles which are concerned with buccal deglutition are the muscles of the tongue, those forming the floor of the mouth, including the mylohyoid and the diagastric, the muscles which raise and lower the jaw, and those of the lip. Further, the muscles which are most important in pharyngeal deglutition are those which raise and lower the hyoid bone and larynx as a whole, and these are the stylohyoid and stylopharyngeus, the palatoglossus and palatopharyngeus, the geniohyoid, thyrohyoid, sternohyoid, sternothyroid and omohyoid. All these muscles are early and severely affected in bulbar paralysis; and when they fail, the intrinsic muscles of the palate are unable to shut off the nasopharynx, the constrictors of the pharynx are entirely unable to perform the act of deglutition, and the intrinsic muscles of the larynx—though phonation is never lost—are unable, since the larynx is unfixed by the extrinsic muscles, to modulate the tone of the voice. The active pharyngeal reflex and the difficulty in using the laryngoscope on account of spasm of the pharynx in the subjects of this disease, are good clinical evidence that the pharyngeal constrictors are not affected.

The earliest physical sign of bulbar paralysis is the loss of the finer movements which are essential for correct articulation, and consequently a slurring dysarthria develops, and the consonants become less distinct until they are inaudible. The failure of the palate to close upon the posterior pharyngeal wall gives a nasal voice. Later, the patient becomes unable to interrupt his blast at any of the stop positions, and speech becomes a long, moaning, monotonous, inarticulate sound. His phonation remains, but he cannot alter its pitch nor divide it into parts of speech, except by taking a fresh breath. The orbicularis oris is early affected, and the lips lose their firmness and become thin, and as they weaken, the unopposed retractors of the angles produce a wide, straight mouth, both at rest and in emotional action. Whistling and pursing up the lips become impossible, and ultimately there is much dribbling of saliva for this can neither be retained by the lips nor swallowed. The tongue shows fine fasciculation, and as it wastes it loses its point, becomes rounded, and is protruded with difficulty. Its surface becomes dimpled and faceted; in the end it consists solely of the covering mucous membrane, the glands and the fibrous tissue, and lies motionless in the floor of the mouth, resembling a crinkled mushroom. The muscles of mastication all become affected. The bite becomes feeble and the mouth cannot be opened against resistance. In the late stages the jaw drops and the mouth is constantly open. The combined weakness of tongue and buccinators makes it difficult for the patient to keep his food between his teeth in mastication, and often he aids his disability by digital pressure upon the cheeks. Nasal regurgitation is not uncommon. The difficulty in swallowing is greatest with fluids, for these require quick action, and is next greatest with lumpy solids, for these necessitate powerful action. It is least with food of a porridge-like consistency, and this should be carefully borne in mind in feeding.

The other muscles of the face are affected later and to a much less severe degree than is the orbicularis oris. It is as if there were a physiological selection on the part of the disease for the nervous mechanism serving mastication and deglutition. Still, in the majority of cases there is bilateral general facial weakness and wasting which, with the peculiar mouth and dropping jaw, produce a characteristic facies. The upper facial muscles are invariably weak. Only rarely does the atrophy extend to the oculomotor muscles. As in the paralysis of the limbs, so also in bulbar paralysis, concomitant signs of both upper motor neurone and of lower motor neurone lesion may exist. When such tonic atrophy of the bulbar muscles is present, the symptomatology and clinical appearance are the same as have been described for the simple atrophic form, with the exception that the jaw-jerk and the other muscle-jerks of the bulbar region, which are absent in the latter condition, are brisk in the tonic-atrophic form.

In less common cases of progressive bulbar paralysis the upper motor neurone lesion alone is in evidence, and the bulbar paralysis is purely spastic. Here the symptomatology is the same, and the facial aspect identical with that of the simple atrophic and tonic-atrophic forms. The tendon-jerks are brisk. The appearance of the tongue, however, is quite different; it is smooth, narrow, stiff and drawn into a narrow compass by the spasm of the muscles composing it. It is too small for the mouth. There is no fasciculation, and the muscles are not wasted.

The muscles of the back of the neck are commonly the first to be affected with the wasting of progressive muscular atrophy. There is increasing difficulty in extending the head, which drops forward, with overaction of the frontales which raise the brows to clear the line of vision when the head is so placed. The lower cervical and upper dorsal spines stand out to give an appearance like that of an angular curvature.

Primary affection of the legs is much less common than that of the arms, bulbar region or neck muscles. The anterior tibial and peroneal muscles are usually attacked first, and less commonly the quadriceps. The clinical type is that of flaccid atrophy in most cases. Tonic atrophy, which is so common in the arms and in the bulbar region, is rare in the legs.

Wherever the site of onset of progressive muscular atrophy, it invariably spreads, sometimes slowly and with periods of arrest which may last for years, sometimes with remarkable rapidity. The manner of spread is usually in terms of the contiguity of the affected elements in the nervous system; but it is sometimes in terms of the physiological association of the muscles, as is commonly seen in the bulbar forms. The appearance of fasciculation, in any muscles otherwise unaffected, is a sure sign that atrophy will shortly begin.

According to the method of advance shown by the disease, cases of progressive muscular atrophy fall into two groups. In the first, the atrophy spreads locally and slowly and remains confined to one region of the body during most of the course. These cases are always of the simple atrophic type and they usually live a long time. Such cases, however, tend to become general just before death. In contrast with the local type is the group in which the signs spread to many parts of the body. The spread may be rapid, and the end may occur in a few months, or it may be slower; but it is unusual for any of the cases forming this group to survive for more than 2 years. This group comprises the generalized cases of simple flaccid atrophy; all the cases of amyotrophic lateral sclerosis and most of the bulbar cases.

Fasciculation is a most important symptom of the disease, and is an associate of the muscular atrophy. It precedes the wasting of the fibres, and is a sure herald of wasting. It ceases when the muscle is completely wasted, and is not seen when the atrophy is not progressing. The importance of fasciculation as a diagnostic sign of progressive muscular atrophy makes it desirable to consider other conditions in which it is met. It occurs in syringomyelia and in peroneal atrophy, but only when the muscular atrophy is progressing, and, therefore, it is only an occasional symptom in either disease. It occurs in a conspicuous form in certain conditions of gastro-enteritis, and is presumably due to an intoxication, and to this form the term 'myokimia' has been applied. It is not seen in polyneuritis, poliomyelitis, myopathy, nor in the common gross lesions of nerve trunks, nerve roots or spinal cord.

Electromyography, with convincing evidence of denervation of muscles in the reduction of spontaneous motor unit activity, and in the presence of fibrillary activity and the large action potentials of fasciculation will confirm the diagnosis.

Contractures are conspicuous by their absence in this disease, which is thus strongly contrasted with peroneal atrophy and some other muscular atrophies. If the atrophy becomes complete the result is a flail limb.

Mental changes are often present in the cases in which the bulbar region is affected. Emotional instability and hyperexcitability are the usual change. The patient is easily excited to tears or to laughter by trivial causes, and cannot control his expression of emotion. He himself feels little joy or grief during the paroxysms of laughing or crying. Dementia sometimes occurs.

Sphincters. In most cases these are not affected.

Reflexes. The reflexes are altered in this disease, by spasticity and by the muscular atrophy which may prevent response in the affected muscles. The pharyngeal reflex in bulbar cases is usually brisk; but the response is not normal, involving all the muscles concerned in deglutition, for these are atrophied and paralysed; it is confined to the constrictors of the pharynx and the muscles of the palate, with the feeble co-operation of such of the somatic bulbar muscles as are still able to act. The plantar reflexes are usually 'extensor' when the legs are spastic. Similarly, the abdominal reflexes do not disappear so constantly or so early as is the case in disseminated sclerosis, for example, and they may persist when the legs are markedly spastic and extensor plantar responses have appeared. In cases of tonic atrophy the tendon reflexes are everywhere increased, even in regions where the atrophy is severe, and in this type they never disappear. The same increase of the muscle-jerks occurs in the purly spastic cases. In simple atrophic cases the tendon-jerks disappear with the wasting of the muscles.

Cerebrospinal fluid. The cerebrospinal fluid is always normal.

Diagnosis

The disease has to be distinguished from the many conditions in which progressive weakness and wasting of the muscles occur, from those in which muscular wasting and spasticity are conspicuous clinical features, and lastly from other diseases in which bulbar symptoms are early evidenced. Injury of the cervical enlargement of the spinal cord causes a limited degree of wasting in the upper limbs, and spasticity of greater or less intensity in the lower limbs [see p. 1275]. The wasting in the arms becomes apparent some weeks after the injury and affects the muscles corresponding to the injured segments of the cord, which are commonly those of the forearms and hands. But weakness of these muscles and the spastic weakness of the legs are maximal immediately after the injury, and power usually shows an improvement during the succeeding weeks or months, whereas in progressive muscular atrophy the weakness, wasting and spasticity come on insidiously and progress steadily. Although bony injury is commonly present, injury of the cervical cord may occur without any fracture or dislocation of the cervical spine. Furthermore, a moderate degree of weakness of the limbs may escape observation while the patient is in bed after an accident, or it may be ascribed to other causes, and so the signs resembling amyotrophic lateral sclerosis may not be discovered until several weeks after the occurrence of the lesion responsible for them. Inversion of the supinator-jerk [see p. 1275] is a common sign in cases of injury of the cervical enlargement, but rarely, if ever, occurs in progressive muscular atrophy. Syphilitic amyotrophy, now exceedingly rare [p. 1210], may be indistinguishable from progressive muscular atrophy except for abnormalities in the pupils and the results of the Wassermann reaction. Peroneal muscular atrophy very closely resembles progressive muscular atrophy, it is usually familial, and commences in childhood. The atrophy is well marked in the periphery of all four limbs and cannot be confused with progressive muscular atrophy, which never has this distribution.

The diagnosis of progressive muscular atrophy from the primary muscular dystrophies seldom causes serious difficulty. These occur earlier and several members of a family may be affected; the wasting is almost invariably proximal, the weakness is out of proportion to the apparent wasting, fasciculation is absent, and the progress is very much slower. Dystrophia myotonica is at once separated from progressive muscular atrophy by the myotonus. When myotonus is absent, the characteristic wasting of the sternomastoids and of the muscles of the thighs, the age of the subject, and sometimes the presence of cataract should suggest the diagnosis. In the dystrophies the electromyographic changes are quite different. Arthritic muscular atrophy occurs in the regions of joints which show easily recognizable disease. Fasciculation does not occur, nor are there electromyographic changes.

Lesions of peripheral nerves or roots may be diagnosed by the history of a local cause, by the discovery of a palpable local lesion upon the course of the nerve, and by the confinement of the atrophy to the distribution of one particular nerve, while pain and sensory loss often occur in that same distribution.

Diagnosis is most difficult in those cases where spasticity in the limbs is the first sign of progressive muscular atrophy, and where such spasticity precedes the appearance of any muscular atrophy by a long time. If it is remembered that spastic paralysis may be the earliest and for a time the only sign of progressive muscular atrophy, and that among the many diseases of the nervous system which begin with the same clinical picture of spastic paralysis a certain diagnosis cannot be made until further distinguishing signs appear, error will be avoided. Special investigations including examination of the cerebrospinal fluid in doubtful cases are essential.

Treatment

This disease is entirely uninfluenced by any treatment. It remains, therefore, to secure favourable conditions of life for the patient, and to maintain the general health in as perfect a state as possible. Massage and passive movements are useful as giving bodily comfort to the patient, and satisfying him that something is being done for him. In bulbar cases, the dysphagia must be aided by avoiding liquids and solids, and by serving all the articles of diet in pultaceous form. Salivation, which is so troublesome in this condition, may be helped by hyoscine, belladonna, or benzhexol hydrochloride (*Artane*), 2 mg.

Course and Prognosis

Motor neurone disease always progresses to death. The course may be rapid, and the end may be reached in a few months, or it may be slow, and extend over several years. The local types of progressive muscular atrophy of slow onset are the most gradual, and these may have periods of arrest in the progress. The generalized simple atrophic type of the disease is the most rapid, especially when it begins with severe initial flaccid paralysis without atrophy.

In the bulbar types of the disease, and in the common type of amyotrophic lateral sclerosis, the course is, for the most, steadily progressive. Every type will show, however, upon occasion, exacerbations and remissions, and the exacerbations are the most important, and in the bulbar types may cause death in a few hours. Of particular interest are rapid extensions of a flaccid paralysis, which may occur in a few hours, and which resemble the onset of the disease with initial flaccid paralysis without atrophy, which has been already described. Whatever type of the disease is present, it tends in the end to spread and to become general.

In amyotrophic lateral sclerosis the average duration of life is seldom more than 3 years from the onset. When bulbar symptoms are present the average duration is under 2 years. In the generalized cases the average duration is under 1 year. Widely spread fasciculation in muscles, which are neither weak nor wasted, is the constant herald of generalization, and renders the immediate prognosis serious. Rapid extension of the weakness, the advent of bulbar symptoms, involvement of all the respiratory muscles, and especially general asthenia and drowsiness are the signs which usher in the fatal result.

PERONEAL MUSCULAR ATROPHY

Synonym. Charcot-Marie-Tooth type of muscular atrophy.

Definition

This is a distinct form of neurogenic muscular atrophy, often heredo-familial. It usually begins in mid-childhood, and after 20 years or so becomes arrested. The atrophy always starts in the intrinsic muscles of the feet, and is throughout strictly distal in distribution. The muscles of the face and trunk and the proximal muscles of the limbs are never affected. The atrophy leaves a peculiar elastic fibrosis in the affected muscles, so that the incapacity caused by this disease is much less than in any other form of muscular atrophy of like degree. Sensation is often slightly affected, and there may be deep sensory loss.

Aetiology

The onset is usually between the fifth and tenth years, but it may appear as late as the fourth decade. Boys and girls are both affected. Heredity plays an important part, although isolated sporadic cases occur. It may show every type of inheritance. It has been traced through five generations; it may skip a generation and then reappear.

Pathology

The anterior horn cells of the affected regions show a slowly progressive atrophy and disappearance, with corresponding atrophy of fibres in the peripheral nerves. The cells of Clarke's column degenerate, as do also some of the fibres of the posterior columns of the spinal cord, and especially those of the posterolateral column. Slight degeneration in some of the fibres of the pyramidal tracts is usually found. The affected muscles are atrophied. There is a simple shrinking of the fibres, which stain progressively and more and more deeply with haematoxylin, lose their striation, and finally disappear. Secondary fibrotic changes accompany the atrophy, together with sclerosis of the arteries of the muscle.

Symptoms

Muscular atrophy dominates the clinical picture. It is strictly distal in distribution, and this distinguishes peroneal atrophy from any other form of muscular wasting. This is to say it does not affect one particular muscle, but the distal ends of all the muscles below a certain level on the limb, leaving the proximal ends of the muscles normal, and it advances upwards, the separation of the wasted from the normal portion being transverse to its length. The muscle fibres waste in terms of the length of the spiral axons which supply them. The wasting always begins in the intrinsic muscles of the feet, and hollowness of the instep and thinness of the feet, together with retraction of the toes and the difficulty which the pes cavus so produced causes in fitting shoes, first draw attention to the disease. As the process advances, the lower segments of the anterior tibial, peroneal and calf muscles become affected, and the limb is subsequently involved until the lower third of the thigh is reached, at which stage the disease is invariably arrested. This slow spread of the atrophy from the distal towards the proximal portion of the limb causes the characteristic feature in the appearance of the legs. As an example, the complete atrophy of all the muscles below the middle and a well-developed musculature in the upper half of the leg, give rise to the inverted 'fat bottle' calf. When the atrophy has involved the lower third of the thigh, the lower end of the femur, bare of muscle and covered only by skin and tendons, contrasts strongly with the well-developed muscles of the upper thigh, and causes the thigh to resemble an inverted champagne bottle.

Some years after the atrophy has become marked in the legs, and in the usual run of cases just before puberty, the intrinsic muscles of the hands, and first those of the thenar and hypothenar groups, begin to waste, and this wasting may extend as high as the middle of the forearm. The disease may become arrested at any time, and arms often escape altogether. With the exception of the lower part of the thighs, the proximal segments of the limbs do not become involved, and the muscles of the head, neck and trunk remain unaffected.

The affected regions of the muscles waste absolutely, and leave an elastic fibrous tissue. Fasciculation occurs; it is seen only when the disease is progressing, and in the muscles which are obviously wasting. It is never general, as in some cases of progressive muscular atrophy, and since peroneal atrophy is at times advancing and at other times stationary, it may be in one case conspicuous and in another never seen. It disappears entirely when the progress becomes arrested, and is, therefore, useful as a clinical indication of active advance of the disease. Contractures always occur, and from the nature of the distribution of the atrophy are necessarily confined to the feet and the hands. In the feet, pes cavus with retracted toes is the rule; but sometimes, and in some stages of the disease, the feet and toes may be dropped and the feet inverted. The sphincters are unaffected. The ankle-jerks are diminished or lost in proportion to the wasting of the calf muscles. In the final arrested stage they are usually lost. The knee-jerk is always retained and is usually brisk. The plantar reflexes are usually lost early. Pain, tenderness and cramp are absent. Conspicuous loss of sensation is uncommon, but slight loss of deep sensibility, and of vibration sense can be detected; in rare cases all forms of sensibility may be affected, then perforating ulcers may be seen upon the soles of the feet, due to the association of sensory loss with thinness and deformity.

The most striking of all the clinical features of peroneal atrophy is the comparatively slight disability caused by the wasting of the muscles and consequent paralysis, and even the sensory loss, when it is present.

Motor nerve conduction time is increased and there is reduction in normal motor unit activity, with fibrillation of the affected muscles, and sometimes fasciculation potentials in the electromyogram.

Diagnosis

Peroneal atrophy in the early stages may be confused with progressive muscular atrophy, in that wasting of muscles and fibrillation are the conspicuous features. The onset usually in childhood and the fact that the feet are affected first, the peculiar distal distribution and the presence of any familial incidence, are important. But the only distinction which is absolute is the distribution, for progressive muscular atrophy may not appear until adult life, and a familial history may be absent. In the course of time the diagnosis always becomes clear, for progressive muscular atrophy never keeps to the classic distribution of peroneal atrophy, nor is it followed by the peculiar fibrosis which characterizes the latter.

Dystrophia myotonica when beginning in the peroneal muscles may for a time closely simulate peroneal atrophy. The presence of the least sign of myotonia, the involvement of the face and the atrophy of the sternomastoids, will establish the diagnosis.

The usual forms of myopathy are at once separated from peroneal atrophy by the distribution of the muscular weakness and wasting, which in the muscular dystrophies is conspicuously upon the face, trunk and proximal muscles of the limbs. Peripheral neuritis is more rapid in its onset, and is apt to be associated with marked sensory disturbances, both objective and subjective, and the paralysis is in terms of individual muscles, which is not the case in peroneal atrophy.

Treatment

The general health should be carefully maintained, and with a normal well-regulated life care must be taken to avoid over-fatigue of the affected muscles, but to ensure exercise compatible with their capacity. Bicycling, for example, since it employs chiefly the thigh muscles, is a better form of exercise for these patients than is walking. In no circumstances should tenotomies be performed for the deformity of the feet, for such measures tend to destroy the effect of the conservative fibrosis, so essential to the production of a useful limb. The use of heavy mechanical supports is to be avoided above all things. Light, well-fitting boots, so as to interfere as little as possible with the exercise of the damaged muscles, are essential and foot-drop is counteracted by light toe springs.

Course

The course is irregularly progressive for a number of years only, and the advance of the disease slows down in later life. Exacerbations of the weakness are likely to be followed in every case by considerable improvement, owing to the secondary fibrosis in the muscles.

PROGRESSIVE SPINAL MUSCULAR ATROPHY OF CHILDREN

Synonyms. Amyotonia congenita: 1. Infantile form—the Werdnig-Hoffmann disease. 2. Juvenile form—Oppenheim's disease.

THE WERDNIG-HOFFMANN DISEASE

Definition

The Werdnig-Hoffmann disease appears in the first year, may affect several siblings, and gives a gradual development of progressive muscular weakness and atrophy, which affects the proximal muscles first and most, increases to a complete paralysis of trunk and limbs, and finally affects the bulbar muscles. The disease is invariably fatal in from a few weeks to several months.

Aetiology

In some of the cases the paralysis is noticeable at the time of birth, and the disease is obviously of pre-natal development. In others the children are quite healthy at birth, and the disease develops some time during the first year of life, most frequently within 8 weeks of birth. Though sporadic cases may be found, usually several children of the same mother are affected. Both pre-natal and postnatal cases may be found among the children of the same mother. The sexes are equally affected. No maternal ill health during pregnancy has been noticed, and nothing is known about any other aetiological factor.

Pathology

The most extensive changes are in the ventral horn cells throughout the spinal cord and brain stem, and at many levels no normal cells whatever are to be seen. Tigrolysis, swelling and glassiness of the cells, extrusion of the nuclei, disappearance of the dendrites, shrinking of the cells and final disappearance is the sequence of the changes. Degeneration of the anterior roots and of the peripheral motor nerve fibres consequently occurs. These changes are not confined to the lower motor neurones, for in some cases examination by the Marchi method shows extensive degeneration throughout the posterior columns of the cord, indicating that lower sensory neurones were also considerably affected.

The muscles show intense degeneration with hypertrophy of some fibres and atrophy of most, waving, moniliform shape, hypernucleation of the spindles, general nuclear increase and fibrosis.

Symptoms

In the cases which are pre-natal, the disease is noticed at the time of birth because of the tonelessness, flaccidity and the poorness of movement in the trunk and proximal muscles of the limbs. In the postnatal cases there is a gradual onset of similar weakness and flaccidity in the trunk first, and in the limbs afterwards, which usually begins within 6 weeks of birth, but which may not appear until towards the end of the first year of life. The weakness seems always to be least marked in the periphery of the limbs, where curious, slow, involuntary movements of the fingers and toes have been noted in many of the cases. The paralysis is followed by a rapid and extensive wasting of the muscles, accompanied by occasional fibrillary twitchings. Since these children are not only well nourished, but often put on much fat during the illness, wasting of the muscles may not be apparent on inspection or palpation. It can, however, immediately be detected by radiography, which distinguishes sharply between fat and muscle.

As the weakness progresses the trunk muscles become completely paralysed, the intercostal muscles always before the diaphragm. The limbs become progressively weaker, and, lastly, bulbar paralysis supervenes in those cases where death has not already occurred from respiratory paralysis. Sensation may be unimpaired but pain sensation may be diminished over the limbs and trunk. The sphincters are unimpaired until the last stages of the disease. The superficial and deep reflexes are lost. The ocular muscles are not affected, and intelligence is preserved throughout. Electromyography shows the characteristic change of severe denervation.

Diagnosis

The peculiar and striking features of the disease make the diagnosis easy. Amyotonia congenita presents the same helplessness and flaccidity of trunk and limbs as does the Werdnig-Hoffmann disease, and further resembles it in being sometimes congenital, and sometimes having an onset very early in life. In amyotonia congenita, however, the paralysis is not complete, and it tends to improvement and not to progressive increase. Contractures also occur, which are not found in the Werdnig-Hoffmann disease, and, lastly, the definite spinal cord changes of the latter malady are not found in the former. Greenfield, however, considered that amyotonia congenita and Werdnig-Hoffmann paralysis are different aspects of a single disease.

Treatment

No treatment influences the course.

Course and Prognosis

The course is invariably progressive, and is more rapid the earlier in life the disease begins, and it is most rapid of all in the pre-natal cases, which are usually fatal within a few weeks. With an onset some weeks after birth, life is usually continued for several months, and a few cases have been reported with an onset towards the end of the first year, in which death has been delayed until the third or fourth year.

OPPENHEIM'S DISEASE

Definition

Oppenheim's disease occurs in early childhood and is sometimes familial. There is extreme flaccidity, smallness and weakness of the muscles, which are not actually paralysed by loss of the tendon-jerks and by contractures in the region affected. The juvenile form of progressive spinal muscular atrophy has the same pathology as the infantile form.

Symptoms

The flaccidity of the affected muscles may be noticed from the time of birth. They are small and weak, and though there is no muscular wasting and no absolute paralysis, yet in many cases the limbs cannot be raised against the action of gravity, nor can the head be held up. The great relaxation of the muscles and ligaments allows of the most fantastic attitudes being assumed without pain. When the child gets older, he is unable to sit up, but when placed in the sitting position the spine bunches up from absence of any muscular support, and he is unable to support his weight upon the weak legs. The amyotonia is symmetrical, and affects the legs always, the trunk often, the arms not infrequently, but never the face. Notwithstanding the flaccidity, some degree of flexor contracture is usually present. Sensation and the sphincters are not affected. The superficial reflexes are normal, but the deep reflexes are invariably absent in the affected regions. The children are usually intelligent, with good bodily development and growth proceeds normally.

The juvenile form is much more benign than the infantile, progresses more slowly, is not fatal and usually becomes arrested in late childhood.

REFERENCES

ALTROCCHI, P. H. (1963) Acute transverse myelopathy, *Arch. Neuroi. (Chic.)*, **9**, 11.

BRAIN, S., NETSKY, M. G., and ZIMMERMAN, H. M. (1952) Vascular malformation of the spinal cord, *Arch. Neurol. Psychiat. (Chic.)*, **68**, 339.

BYERS, R. K., and BANKER, B. Q. (1961) Infantile muscular atrophy, *Arch. Neurol. (Chic.)*, **5**, 140.

DAVISON, C. (1942) Amyotrophic lateral sclerosis, *Arch. Neurol. Psychiat. (Chic.)*, **46**, 1039.

GARDNER, W. J. (1965) Hydrodynamic mechanism of syringomyelia: its relation to myelocele, *J. Neurol. Neurosurg. Psychiat.*, **28**, 247.

GREENFIELD, J. G., and TURNER, J. W. A. (1939) Acute and sub-acute necrotic myelitis, *Brain*, **62**, 227.

HAASE, G. R., and SHY, M. (1960) Pathological changes in muscle biopsies from patients with peroneal muscular atrophy, *Brain*, **83**, 631.

HENSON, R. A., and PARSONS, M. (1967) Ischaemic lesions of the spinal cord: An illustrated review. *Quart. J. Med.*, **36**, 205.

INGRAHAM, F. D., and HAMLIN, H. (1943) Spina bifida and cranium bifidum, *New Engl. J. Med.*, **228**, 631.

Lancet (1963) Acute transverse myelopathy, ii, 1045.

LAWYER, T. Jr., and NETSKY, N. G. (1953) Amyotrophic lateral sclerosis, *Arch. Neurol. Psychiat. (Chic.)*, **69**, 171.

NETSKY, N. G. (1953) Syringomyelia. A clinico-pathological study, *Arch. Neurol. Psychiat. (Chic.)*, **70**, 741.

PANT, S., ASTBURY, A. K., and RICHARDSON, E. P. JR (1968) The myopathy of pernicious anaemia—a neurological reappraisal, *Acta neurol. Scand.*, Suppl. **35**, 44.

RICHMOND, J., and DAVIDSON, S. (1958) Sub-acute degeneration of the spinal cord in non-Addisonian anaemia, *Quart. J. Med.*, **27**, 517.

STEEGRMANN, A. T. (1952) Syndrome of the anterior spinal artery, *Neurology*, **2**, 15.

TURNER, J. W. A. (1949) On amyotonia congenita, *Brain*, **72**, 25.

UNGLEY, C. C. (1949) Sub-acute degeneration of the spinal cord, *Brain*, **72**, 382.

DISORDERS OF THE PERIPHERAL NERVES

LESIONS OF INDIVIDUAL NERVE ROOTS AND TRUNKS; MONONEURITIS

Individual peripheral nerves may be damaged by many agencies which may affect them in a variety of ways. Direct wounding may sever the nerve completely or partially. Injury by a blow or transmitted concussion in surrounding tissues, as occurs with the passage of a projectile near the nerve, may destroy the axons without interrupting the continuity of the more resistant medullary sheaths and perineurium. Recovery entails the growth of new axons down the surviving medullary sheaths. Milder injuries interrupt function for hours or days. Nerves may also be injured by pressure such as 'Saturday night paralysis', crutch palsy, palsies from pressure of plaster and other splints and chronic over-stretching as in the case of the ulnar nerve. Peripheral nerve lesions may follow a variety of general infections. Nerves may be involved in specific inflammatory processes such as leprosy. Finally they may be involved in new growths. The most important example of this is infiltration with carcinoma from a neighbouring focus, but nerves may be the site of isolated neurofibromata or multiple lesions in cases of Von Recklinghausen's neurofibromatosis.

The investigation of individual nerve injuries has been greatly helped by nerve conduction studies. A measured length of nerve is subjected to electrical stimulation through a pair of surface electrodes, and the time the resulting impulse takes to reach the end of the part under examination is evident on an oscilloscope. The stimulating electrodes are distal in sensory nerves, of course, and the muscle action potential gives the end response in motor nerves. The delay in conduction is proportional to the degree of damage.

When there is injury to motor nerves the electromyogram [p. 1314] gives information of the state of the denervated muscle. By both techniques recovery of nerve can be followed objectively.

The Sweating Test. Based upon loss of the sudomotor fibres in the territory of the sensory cutaneous distribution of a nerve, the test consists of applying a powder of starch and iodine to the skin and producing generalized sweating by warming the body; there is no change in colour in the denervated area.

A sign of nerve recovery not used enough is *Tinel's sign.* Very light digitial percussion over a sensory nerve will cause tingling when the site of injury is reached, in the same way as a hard percussion over any normal sensory nerve will. This is very useful, for instance, in determining the site of injury to the ulnar nerve at the elbow. As the damaged fibres grow after nerve injury the sign will follow the course of recovery down the nerve.

When more than one peripheral nerve is involved in disease—as in periarteritis nodosa, diabetes, or serum reactions—the term 'mononeuritis multiplex' is used, to save confusion with polyneuritis, where peripheral nerves are differently affected, distally and symmetrically, depending mainly upon their length.

THE PHRENIC NERVE (C. 2, 3, 4)

This nerve supplies the diaphragm. Paralysis results most often from disease of the spinal cord, but the roots may be implicated in disease of the spine, and the trunk may be injured, in its course through the neck and thorax, by wounds or tumours. Bilateral paralysis occurs in lesions of the cord and spine, and in acute infective polyneuritis. Other causes usually affect one side only. When the diaphragm is completely paralysed, the normal inspiratory protrusion of the upper part of the abdomen disappears, or is replaced by retraction of this part with each inspiration. During rest, so long as the lungs are healthy, the respiratory rate does not increase, but if bronchitis or pneumonia arises as a complication, or if the patient exerts himself, the diminished reserve of respiratory power is seriously felt. When one nerve only is affected the diaphragm does not move on that side, but becomes permanently raised as a result of collapse of the base of the corresponding lung. This is rarely detected by observation of the abdominal movements, but is easily seen on the radiograph screen. It produces no discomfort.

THE LONG THORACIC NERVE (C. 5, 6, 7)

This nerve supplies the serratus anterior muscle. When all the fibres of this muscle contract, the scapula moves upwards, forwards and outwards. It contracts with the pectoralis major in the action of pushing the point of the shoulder forward and in the rapier-thrust movement. It also helps the deltoid to raise the arm. When it is paralysed alone, the position of the scapula at rest is unaltered, but if the trapezius and the rhomboids are paralysed as well, the scapula drops, and its lower angle is displaced inwards. Paralysis of the serratus anterior is best demonstrated by asking the patient to hold the arms outstretched before him. The arm is not raised so high on the affected as on the normal side, because the scapula is not fixed and the deltoid works at a disadvantage. Viewed from behind the deformity is characteristic. The vertebral border of the scapula stands out prominently and the hand can be pushed between this bone and thorax—'winged scapula'. On raising the arm from the side, there is difficulty in attaining the horizontal position, but the winging of the scapula is less apparent.

The nerve may be damaged by carrying heavy weights on the shoulder, by falls or blows on the shoulder, and by continued muscular effort with the raised arm. The nerve may be injured alone in gunshot wounds, but as a rule it is associated with lesions of the brachial plexus. In addition, a serratus anterior palsy may develop suddenly in an otherwise healthy person apparently spontaneously, or as part of a rare reaction to the administration of serum or antitoxin. In such neuritic cases and in the cases caused by compression, severe neuralgic pains in the neck precede the onset of paralysis. Recovery is always very slow and the defect may be permanent.

THE BRACHIAL PLEXUS

The brachial plexus may be injured by wounding, by dislocation of the shoulder or fracture of the clavicle, or by pressure of a tumour, aneurysm or cervical rib. Further, the nerves may be torn by forcible dragging on the arm in accidents or during delivery. In most cases the lesion is partial and the symptoms conform in the main to one of the following types:

Upper Plexus Paralysis (Erb's Palsy) (C. 4, 5, 6). This results from an injury to the fifth and sixth cervical roots. The muscles paralysed are: biceps, deltoid, brachialis, brachioradialis (supinator longus), supraspinatus, rhomboideus, subscapularis, clavicular portion of pectoralis major, serratus anterior, latissimus dorsi, teres major. The arm cannot be flexed at the elbow (flexors of forearm), nor raised and abducted (deltoid). The movements of the wrist and fingers are not impaired. Adduction of the arm is weak (pectoralis major), and rotation is feeble or absent (spinati). On attempting to oppose the shoulders, the scapula on the affected side passes farther from the middle line (rhomboid). The hand of the affected side cannot be placed on the buttock of the sound side (latissimus dorsi).

The reaction of degeneration is often complete in the deltoid and flexors of the forearm and nearly so in the spinati. It is usually incomplete in the other muscles. Sensation is diminished or lost along the outer border of the whole arm immediately after the injury, but improvement is as rapid. For some time the patient experiences pins and needles and burning sensations in the affected area, which last longest in the thumb and index finger. The biceps reflex is lost.

Lower Plexus Paralysis (Klumpke's Palsy). This results from a lesion of the eighth cervical and first dorsal roots, or of the common trunk of the median and ulnar nerves. The intrinsic muscles of the hand and the flexors of the wrist and fingers are paralysed, and the inner border of the forearm and hand is anaesthetic. When the roots are damaged sympathetic fibres may be implicated with the production of myosis, narrowing of the palpebral aperture, enophthalmos and alterations in sweating on the face, neck, arm and upper part of the chest on the affected side.

Middle Plexus Paralysis (C. 6, 7, 8). This form of paralysis is a common result of gunshot injuries of the plexus. It affects the muscles supplied by the radial and axillary nerves—posterior cord. As the nerve to the latissimus dorsi arises from the same cord, this muscle is often paralysed as well. In addition to these simple types, more complicated paralyses occur, in which various parts of the plexus are injured together.

Paralysis of the Medial Cord of the Plexus (C. 8, T. 1). Atrophy is confined to the intrinsic hand muscles, and the sensory loss is to the hand.

Incomplete lesions of the brachial plexus show a remarkable tendency to spontaneous recovery. In many cases recovery is complete in 6 months to 2 years, in others it is partial, and some muscles remain paralysed.

THE RADIAL NERVE (C. 6, 7, 8)

Owing to its long course, its position in relation to the humerus, and its peculiar vulnerability to compression, paralysis of the radial nerve is one of the commonest peripheral nerve palsies; although it is a mixed nerve, containing sensory, motor and vasomotor fibres, the symptoms of an injury are almost entirely motor. In the upper arm the nerve supplies the triceps and the anconeus, in the forearm the supinators, the extensors of the wrist and fingers, and the extensors and long abductor of the thumb.

Injury to the nerve is followed by dropping of the wrist and fingers. The wrist and the first phalanges are flexed. The flexion is limp and easily reducible.

When the lesion is in the axilla the whole of the *triceps* is paralysed, and extension at the elbow is lost. Occasionally in wounds of the posterior aspect of the arm the nerves to the triceps are injured, whilst the main trunk escapes. The patient is then able to extend the arm powerfully by means of the anconeus, but if he is made to raise the elbow as high as possible with his fingers on the point of the shoulder, extension of the bent forearm is impossible.

In most cases the nerve is injured in the middle third of the arm and the triceps escapes, but the brachioradialis and *all* the extensor muscles in the forearm are paralysed. Partial paralyses, such as are seen in lesions of the median and ulnar nerves, are very rare. The brachioradialis is not a supinator. Its action is to flex the forearm, whilst the hand is in a position intermediate between pronation and supination. Paralysis of this muscle is detected by the absence of contraction when the pronated forearm is flexed against resistance. Owing to paralysis of the *supinator*, supination is abolished. During the movement of flexion of the forearm the biceps acts as a supinator, and during extension the external rotators of the shoulder correspond, though feebly.

Paralysis of the *extensors of the carpus* abolishes both extension and lateral movement at the wrist. The flexors of the carpus play no part in lateral movements. The *extensors of the fingers* extend the first phalanges *only*. Extension at the distal joints is carried out by the lumbricals and interossei. Paralysis of the *extensors and long abductor of the thumb* renders abduction of the thumb and extension of the phalanges impossible. On trying to abduct the thumb, it passes no farther than the radial border of the hand. In some cases, the second phalanx of the thumb can be feebly extended by the muscles of the thenar eminence.

Many muscles not supplied by the radial nerve work at a disadvantage when the extensors are paralysed. These defects must not be mistaken for signs of injury to other nerves. Owing to the flexed position of the hand the grasp is feeble, but if the wrist is extended passively the grasp is improved. The patient cannot make a fist properly, as the thumb does not oppose the index finger and the fingers cannot be flexed into the palm, until the thumb has been moved aside by the sound hand. The movements of the interossei in abducting and adducting the fingers are also feeble while the wrist is flexed, but are much stronger when the hand is resting flat on a table with the wrist and fingers extended. Atrophy becomes obvious in a month or two. Its extent and severity give important evidence for prognosis.

Sensory disturbances. Subjective symptoms are rare. In a few cases, paraesthesiae are felt on the posterior aspect of the forearm and on the dorsal aspect of the thumb. They are of brief duration, and are commoner with partial than with complete lesions. Sensibility to light touch, superficial pain and temperature is impaired over a small area on the radial border of the hand, including the proximal joints of the thumbs and the first two fingers. The defect is often very slight, and is only discovered on very careful examination. Deep sensation is rarely affected. Considering the extensive distribution of the superficial branch of the radial nerve, it is rather surprising that the sensory disturbances are so slight when the nerve is injured above the origin of this branch. This is due to the overlap by its neighbours.

As a rule, the brachioradialis recovers first, then the extensors of the wrist, then the extensors of the middle, ring, little and index fingers in this order, and the extensors and abductors of the thumb last of all. On palpation of the muscles during attempted extension, contractions can be felt before any movement is produced. Other signs of impending recovery are the disappearance of automatic pronation and of the flail-like drop of the hand, also diminution of automatic flexion of the fingers after passive extension. Recovery of movement is complete when the patient is able to extend the wrist and all the fingers simultaneously or separately. After this becomes possible, restoration of power is rapid.

THE MEDIAN NERVE (C. 7, 8, T. 1)

Whilst the clinical individuality of the radial nerve is shown in the preponderance of motor symptoms and in the uniform completeness of the paralysis that follows an injury, that of the median is seen in the frequency of partial and especially of painful lesions. Isolated palsy of this nerve is infrequent except as a result of direct injury.

Total Paralysis. The muscles paralysed are the pronators, the radial flexor of the wrist, the flexors of the fingers except the ulnar half of the deep flexor, most of the muscles of the thenar eminence (opponens, abductor brevis and outer head of the flexor brevis pollicis) and the two radial lumbricals. Stated briefly the symptoms are: inability to flex the phalanges of the index finger and the second phalanx of the thumb; difficulty in flexing the phalanges of the middle finger; defective opposition of the thumb. The appearance of the hand in total lesions is fairly constant. The hand inclines to the ulnar side, the index and middle fingers are more extended than is normal, and the thumb lies on a level with the fingers—the ape-hand.

Pronation is incomplete and defective. The patient tries to overcome the defect by rotating the whole limb at the shoulder. Paralysis of the *flexors of the wrist* is seen when an attempt is made to flex against resistance. The tendon of the ulnar flexor alone stands out, and the hand is drawn towards the ulnar side. Even at rest, the flexor tendons are more prominent on the sound than on the affected side.

Flexion of the fingers is good in the two ulnar fingers, though weaker than normal. The index cannot be flexed at all, and the third finger only incompletely. Flexion at the proximal joint is usually good in all fingers including the index, and flexion at this joint with extension at the last two joints is usually well done by the interossei and lumbricals. If the proximal phalanx of the thumb is immobilized, it will be seen that flexion of the terminal phalanx is abolished, owing to paralysis of the *flexor longus pollicis*.

Paralysis of the *thenar muscles* renders opposition and abduction of the thumb defective. By means of the adductor the thumb can be drawn into the palm, but as the radial fingers cannot be flexed nor the thumb opposed, it is impossible to place the tip of the thumb on the tips of the fingers. Atrophy of the muscles becomes obvious in a few weeks. The outer part of the thenar eminence is flattened, and the bulk of the muscles arising from the internal condyle is greatly diminished.

Sensory disturbances. In almost every case there is complete anaesthesia to all forms of sensation in the two terminal phalanges of the index and middle fingers. The skin outside this area may be unaffected even in complete lesions, but in most cases sensibility is diminished in the terminal phalanx of the thumb, and to a less extent over the remainder of the radial half of the palm, including the radial side of the ring finger. Stereognostic sense is lost in the outer fingers. This defect, together with the loss of power, renders the thumb and index finger useless, and makes paralysis of the median the most serious single nerve lesion of the upper limb.

Vasomotor and trophic changes. In many cases the skin in the distribution of the median nerve is red, dry and chapped, and the nails white or purple, and atrophy occurs in the pulp of the affected fingers.

Recovery is slow and is rarely complete. Sensation begins to return before power, but the stereognostic sense is often defective, long after movement in the fingers has returned. The pronator and the flexors of the wrist recover first, then the flexors of the thumb and middle finger. Flexion of the index finger and opposition of the thumb, if it is regained at all, remains defective for several years. In searching for signs of recovery, care must be taken lest some 'trick-movement' due to contractions of healthy muscles is misconstrued. For example, when told to flex the terminal phalanx of the thumb, the patient first over-extends and abducts, and then relaxes suddenly. The terminal phalanx then makes a slight passive movement of flexion, which may be mistaken for true active flexion. Recovery is complete when the patient is able to make a good fist with the fingers flexed well into the palm, and the thumb pressed firmly upon the dorsal aspect of the second phalanx of the middle finger.

Partial Lesions. Partial paralysis of the median nerve is much commoner than the complete form.

Motor symptoms. Flexion of the index finger and

opposition of the thumb are most impaired. The flexors of the middle finger and of the terminal phalanx of the thumb may suffer also, but to a less degree, whilst the pronators and the flexors of the wrist often escape entirely.

Sensory symptoms. Apart from the painful lesions to be mentioned later, sensory troubles are usually slight in partial lesions. Anaesthesia is rare, but sensibility to all forms may be diminished in the areas mentioned under complete lesions.

Vasomotor symptoms. The skin is often cyanosed in the distribution of the injured nerve, and it may perspire more freely than in healthy parts. These changes are more distinct when the paralysis is complicated by a vascular lesion.

Recovery is naturally more rapid than in complete lesions. The order in which the muscles recover and the tests for complete return of function have been mentioned above.

Painful Lesions of the Median Nerve. *Causalgia.* In many cases the most prominent symptom of injury causing an incomplete lesion of the median nerve is *pain.* It comes on about a month after the injury, at first as tingling or pricking in the finger-tips and palm, later as a constant severe smarting, dragging or *burning* pain—hence the name causalgia. Added to the constant pain, which never ceases day or night, paroxysms occur, in which the pain increases suddenly in intensity. The application of cold water gives temporary relief, and patients often wear bandages or gloves which they keep constantly moistened. The pain is greatly aggravated by emotional influences.

Vasomotor changes are a feature of this type. In many cases perspiration is diminished over the radial half of the palm, and the skin becomes dry and scaly. In others, perspiration is increased over the median area.

Motor disturbances are always present, but are usually slight, the weakness affecting mainly the flexors of the index finger and the thenar muscles.

In severe cases the limb is held flexed at the elbow and wrist, with the hand constantly raised and the fingers extended or hyperextended. The whole hand atrophies, and irreducible ankylosis occurs with the limb in this position. The skin of the hand is thin and dry. The fingers taper, and the nails are long, brittle, blackened and striated longitudinally. The pain reaches its acme 4 or 5 months after the injury, and then slowly declines, but the limb remains useless. Even in slighter cases, without much deformity, recovery of function is extremely slow, and is rarely complete. The condition is often much improved by early operation and neurolysis of the nerve, or relief may be gained by sympathectomy.

The Carpal Tunnel Syndrome. The median nerve is often compressed at the wrist as it passes through its tunnel in the transverse carpal ligament. The condition is common in middle life in women who have gained weight by fat or water retention, engaged in housework, laundrywork and other manual labour, and also at an earlier age in women who have young children. It is commoner and more severe in the active right hand, but it is seen first on the left in women who scrub on their knees and support their weight on the extended left hand. Uncommon, in men it happens in the right hand especially when there is a special occupational cause such as painting. There should always be careful questioning for these causes, in men and women, for their avoidance will bring recovery, especially when there has been unwonted activity such as house decorating in the holidays. An acute bilateral form complicates and may herald myxoedema, acromegaly, primary amyloidosis, rheumatoid arthritis or other deformities of the wrist. The chief complaint is of pain or numbness in the middle three fingers but frequently pain is felt in the forearm, and this occurs particularly at night. Pressure at the carpal tunnel causes acroparaaesthesia. In this condition tingling may be present at all times, but it occurs above all during the night and wakens the patient from sleep; some complain of the inability to sleep as much as of the discomfort. The tingling is in some way due to the use of the limbs during the day, and if the patient rests throughout the day he or she is, as a rule, soon relieved of his nocturnal symptoms. Many of the patients are middle-aged women who have been compelled to do vigorous housework to which they have not been accustomed from youth. In general, warmth aggravates the tingling and the patient who is awakened in the night puts the affected limbs outside the bedclothes. In the less severe cases the symptoms are worst during the early part of the night and after a number of hours of broken sleep the patient is able to sleep without interruption for the rest of the night. In other cases the symptoms continue throughout the night and are still present in the morning; then the hands may appear, or may feel, swollen, and the patients complain of awkwardness of the fingers, but impairment of postural or other sensation can rarely be demonstrated. In some, wasting of the upper part of the thenar eminence may be observed and in severe cases sensory impairment may be found over the affected fingers. This condition may fluctuate and recur and can be very disabling through pain, loss of sleep or insensitivity of the pads of the first two digits. The muscular branches are usually spared because the nerve passes over the ligaments to reach the adductor pollicis brevis.

It is a feature of the disorder that in all but the more severe instances no signs of nerve damage will be found though the patient complains bitterly of tingling, especially in the small hours of the morning. In these people the syndrome may be reproduced by inflating a sphygmomanometer cuff on the forearm to above venous pressure, and Tinel's sign may be elicited by lightly tapping the nerve at the carpus. There is often tenderness above it on pressure, swelling and flattening of the contour of the wrist.

An important aspect of this common syndrome, is that it has taken attention away from the thoracic outlet, and offered one rational explanation for a bewildering range of recurring syndromes in the arm.

Treatment is by avoidance of the cause, by rest to the wrist and hand and by light splinting in the mid position with an extensor splint at night. Loss of weight and dehydration help, and injection of hydrocortisone, 0·5 ml., into the carpus may give relief for months and help natural recovery. If all fails, tenotomy of the anterior carpal ligament is needed. At operation the median nerve is found compressed in its tunnel and swollen for a short distance proximal to its entry into the carpal ligament. Opening up the tunnel relieves the symptoms. In occasional cases some weakness of the fingers results in consequence of the failure of the weakened carpal ligament to retain the flexor tendons in their normal position.

THE ULNAR NERVE (C. 7, 8)

This nerve supplies the ulnar flexor of the wrist, the ulnar half of the deep flexor of the fingers, the muscles of the hypothenar eminence, the interossei, the two inner lumbricals and the adductor and inner head of the short flexor of the thumb. Its sensory area is the ulnar border of the hand, the little finger and the inner half of the ring finger.

Total Paralysis. Paralysis of the *flexor carpi ulnaris* may be detected by palpating the tendons when the wrists are flexed against resistance. The limpness on the affected side contrasts strongly with the firmness on the sound side. Lateral movements of the hand are unaffected, as these are carried out by the extensors.

Paralysis of the ulnar portion of the *flexor profundus digitorum*. In making a fist, flexion of the index finger is perfect and that of the middle finger good, whilst in the ring and little finger it is absent or very feeble. This weakness is best seen when flexion is attempted with the index and middle fingers extended. Even when the fingers can be flexed by the action of the flexor sublimis, the power of resisting passive extension is completely lost in the terminal phalanx of the two ulnar fingers. Paralysis of the *hypothenar* muscles abolishes lateral movements of the little finger, and diminishes the power of flexion at the proximal joint. Paralysis of the interossei and of the inner two lumbricals leads to the production of the 'claw-hand'.

The action of these muscles is to flex the fingers at the proximal joints with the distal joints extended. In the 'claw-hand' the posture of the fingers is just the opposite of this, namely, extension at the proximal joint with flexion of the distal joints. Although all the interossei are paralysed, the defect is seen only in the ulnar fingers, as the radial lumbricals supplied by the median are still healthy. It is produced by the action of the long extensors, which being now unopposed, over-extend the proximal joints, and by the flexor sublimis which flexes the second joint and draws the distal joint down with it. The clawing of the fingers is greatly accentuated when the nerve is paralysed below the point of origin of the fibres to the long flexors of the fingers. Other features of the 'ulnar hand' are atrophy of the interossei and of the hypothenar eminence, and persistent abduction of the little and ring fingers. The movements of abduction and adduction are lost in the inner two fingers, and often in the middle finger. Further, these fingers cannot be flexed at the distal joint, whilst the proximal joints are extended.

Paralysis of the *adductor pollicis* and of the inner head of the *flexor brevis pollicis* produces peculiar disturbances in prehensile movements. If the patient is asked to grasp a folded paper between his thumb and index finger, and to resist efforts to remove it by pulling, it will be found that this movement, which is normally very powerful, is grossly defective. He cannot grasp the object beneath the thumb with the second phalanx extended; but presses the tip of the flexed thumb against the outer margin of the index finger.

Sensory disturbances. In complete lesions, all forms of sensation are abolished in the little finger, and along the ulnar border of the hand. Beyond this there is usually diminished sensibility on the ulnar side of the ring finger, and over a narrow area towards the centre of the hand on both aspects. Spontaneous pains are rare, and vasomotor changes are usually slight.

Partial Paralysis. In partial lesions the same symptoms are found in a less degree. The small muscles of the hand suffer most. Clawing may be slight or absent. Neuralgic pains may be felt in the distribution of the ulnar nerve; but causalgia is never seen in lesions of this nerve alone.

Recovery of sensation is usually complete before movement is regained. The flexor carpi ulnaris recovers first, then the long flexors of the fingers and last the small muscles of the hand. In these recovery is extremely slow. When recovery of movement is complete the patient can abduct and adduct the middle finger with the palm flat on a table, and he can also scratch the table with the nail of the little finger without moving his wrist.

The Ulnar Groove Syndrome. The commonest site of injury is in the ulnar groove of the elbow where pressure causes a local lesion. Easily detected by eliciting Tinel's sign by lightly tapping at the site of damage which causes tingling in the ulnar two digits. In this syndrome a 'low' ulnar palsy, with sparing of the alar slips of flexor digitorum profundus results. Treatment is by avoiding the cause, by surgical transposition of the nerve to the front of the forearm, and by easing pressure on it by the fibrous retinaculum.

The nerve is involved on both sides simultaneously in leprosy.

THE MUSCULOCUTANEOUS NERVE (C. 5, 6)

This is rarely affected alone, but is often implicated with the brachial plexus. It supplies the biceps, coracobrachialis and brachialis. Flexion of the forearm can still be carried out by the brachioradialis; but the power of flexion is greatly diminished. Sensation may be diminished or lost along the radial border of the forearm.

THE AXILLARY NERVE (C. 5, 6)

This nerve supplies the deltoid and teres minor, and the skin over the deltoid. It may be injured alone in injuries of the shoulder and by pressure of a crutch. The chief symptom is paralysis of the deltoid with almost complete inability to raise the arm.

THE LUMBOSACRAL PLEXUS

In war injuries lesions of the nerves of the lower limb are frequent; but in peacetime, apart from sciatica and foot-drop, local lesions of these nerves are uncommon.

The *lumbar plexus* may be damaged by abdominal tumours, and its roots by new-growth or other disease of the vertebrae. In a certain number of cases signs of inflammation of the lumbar plexus are found in association with sciatica or neuritis of the *sacral plexus*.

The *sacral plexus* may be damaged by growths or inflammation in the pelvis, by compression during parturition, and by penetrating missiles. It is also often the seat of spontaneous neuritis.

THE FEMORAL NERVE (L. 2, 3, 4)

This is the largest branch of the lumbar plexus. It supplies the iliacus, pectineus, sartorius and quadriceps femoris. It may be injured alone by fractures of the pelvis or of the femur, by dislocations of the hip, or by implication in wounds, psoas abscesses or new-growths.

The most prominent symptoms are loss of power to extend the knee, loss of the knee-jerk, wasting of the quadriceps and sensory disturbances over the anterior surface of the thigh and inner surface of the leg. The psoas always escapes, unless the plexus itself is also damaged; but flexion at the hip may be imperfect through paralysis of the iliacus. Owing to the rapid dispersion of the branches in the thigh, wounds in this part often cause partial lesions. In these the *nerve to the quadriceps* is most often injured. The resulting paralysis causes serious disability in walking as the knee gives way at every step, especially in going down stairs, and lameness lasts for a long time after return of voluntary movement.

THE OBTURATOR NERVE (L. 2, 3, 4)

This nerve is rarely damaged alone. It supplies the three adductor muscles, the obturator externus and the gracilis. The symptoms are weakness of adduction and internal rotation at the hip.

THE LATERAL FEMORAL CUTANEOUS NERVE (L. 2, 3)

This nerve supplies an area of skin on the antero-lateral aspect of the thigh. As a result of injury, but more often without obvious cause, the skin in the territory of this nerve may show peculiar sensory disturbances, which have been described under the name of *meralgia paraesthetica*. Most cases occur in men, especially when obese and out of condition. It occurs in younger men after excessive walking. In women it is usually associated with pregnancy, pelvic tumours and other pelvic infections. The nerve is tender on pressure at the point where it passes from under Poupart's ligament, and neuralgic pain or numbness and tingling is felt in the skin, which may be slightly insensitive on objective examination or extremely hyperaesthetic, so that the slightest touch causes pain. The symptoms, which are usually unilateral, are made worse by walking, and may cause serious incapacity by their persistence and severity. In severe cases the nerve should be excised.

THE SCIATIC NERVE (L. 4, 5, S. 1, 2, 3)

This supplies the flexors of the leg and all the muscles below the knee. It may be involved in pelvic new-growths, or injured by fractures of the pelvis or femur. Next to the radial and ulnar it suffers in gunshot wounds more often than any other nerve.

Total Paralysis. The foot drops, and the toes point downwards. Walking is possible, but the patient cannot stand on the heel or toes of the paralysed foot. The knee is raised high, but the steppage is not so marked in total lesions as when the common peroneal alone is paralysed. All movement below the knee is abolished. When the wound is in the buttocks, flexion of the knee is very weak. The foot becomes oedematous if allowed to hang down. Sweating is often absent on the sole and dorsum of the foot, but is normal on the inner side of the foot, which is supplied by the femoral. The skin is dry and thin, and may be scaly. Hyperkeratosis of the sole is common. Subjective sensibility is rarely affected. The skin is completely anaesthetic over the entire foot, except the inner border of the sole and around the internal malleolus so that pressure sores may develop. The anaesthesia extends upwards on the postero-external aspect of the calf in its lower two-thirds, embracing the tendo Achillis and external malleolus. Beyond this area of complete anaesthesia there is a wide zone in which sensibility is diminished. The sense of position and passive movement is abolished in the foot and toes. The knee-jerk is present. The ankle-jerk is always lost.

Partial Paralysis. In wounds of the sciatic nerve it often happens that the fibres of the common peroneal alone are wounded, since the sciatic trunk often divides into the tibial and common peroneal branches as high as the great sciatic notch. The symptoms are described below under paralysis of these nerves. In other cases, the fibres of the tibial nerve are damaged either alone, or with some of the fibres of the common peroneal. In this case the outstanding clinical features are paralysis of the muscles of the calf and foot, anaesthesia of the sole and, with incomplete lesions, pain similar to that described in partial lesions of the median nerve.

THE COMMON PERONEAL NERVE (L. 4, 5, S. 1)

This nerve may be injured as it winds round the fibula by wounds or fractures or by compression of a tight bandage. The paralysis is usually severe, all the muscles being equally affected. The foot is dropped and inverted, and the toes are slightly flexed. Dorsiflexion of the foot, extension of the proximal phalanges of the toes and abduction of the foot are impossible. The patient can walk, and he can stand on tiptoe, but he cannot run, and walking is made difficult by the foot-drop. Subjective sensory disturbances are usually absent. The skin is anaesthetic over a narrow band which extends from the outer surface of the leg in its middle third, downwards beside the outer border of the tibia, and along the middle of the dorsal aspect of the foot as far as the base of the toes. For an inch or so, on both sides of this band, the sensibility of the skin is diminished. The knee-jerk and ankle-jerk are present. The plantar response is always flexor. Vasomotor changes are slight, and trophic changes are absent.

THE TIBIAL NERVE (L. 5, S. 1)

This nerve is rarely injured alone. It supplies the popliteus, the calf muscles, the flexors of the toes and the intrinsic muscles of the foot. When it is paralysed, the patient is unable to stand on tiptoe, or to extend or invert the ankle, or to flex his toes. Paralysis of the interossei leads to a claw-like deformity of the foot, associated with lowering of the heel and raising of the metatarsus—talipes calcaneovalgus. The calf muscles are flabby and the ankle-jerk is abolished. Sensation is lost on the sole, except along its inner border, on the outer border of the foot and on the plantar surface of the toes. Causalgia, similar to that in paralysis of the median is very often present.

The distal portion of the tibial nerve may be injured by a penetrating missile or a deep wound in the calf. Movements of the ankle are unaffected and anaesthesia is confined to the sole of the foot and heel, or merely to its inner half. The paralysis of the intrinsic muscles of the foot may escape detection, and the lesion may easily be overlooked, especially when the nerve is injured below the origin of the branches supplying the flexor longus hallucis and the flexor longus digitorum. The symptoms then are pain in the sole of the foot, anaesthesia on the sole and paralysis of the plantar muscles.

TREATMENT OF LOCAL NERVE LESIONS

Treatment must depend on the cause and degree of the lesion. During the long period which elapses between the onset of paralysis and the first signs of recovery, even in cases of simple physiological interruption of the nerves, every effort must be made to prevent degeneration of the muscles, to keep the circulation of the limb active, and to prevent the occurrence of contractures and deformities. Massage, movements, electrotherapy and suitable appliances all have their uses. With regard to operative treatment, it must be remembered that more than half the cases of nerve injuries undergo spontaneous cure. It is advisable, therefore, to wait many months before an operation is undertaken. If, then after repeated examinations, no sign of recovery has been detected, no harm can be done by exposing the nerve. If it is found to be divided completely, the ends should be 'freshened' and sutured end to end. If the nerve is notched laterally, the edges of the notch should be pared and sutured, care being taken to preserve the bridge of uninjured tissue. Sometimes the nerve at the site of the lesion appears as a fibrous, flattened band between two swellings on the nerve. In most of such cases the nerve is completely divided, and the condition calls for resection of this fibrous tissue and end-to-end suture. Another common finding, when the nerve is exposed, is a nodule or cicatricial swelling in the course of a nerve which has maintained its continuity. In these cases the continuity of the nerve should not be interrupted. It should be freed from adhesions, and incised in the long axis of the swelling. Operations which involve grafting of nerves have met with little success. For an account of the advances in the technique of the surgical treatment of nerve injuries which have been made as a result of experience gained in the First and Second World Wars, special works must be consulted.

The treatment of painful forms of nerve lesions is extremely difficult. In severe cases external applications and internal medication entirely fail. Simple freeing of the nerve sometimes gives relief. Where this fails, it may be advisable to practise complete division followed by immediate suture. In other instances sympathectomy, by excision of the stellate ganglion in the case of the upper limb and of two or more of the lumbar sympathetic ganglia in the case of the lower limb, may give lasting relief.

'INTERSTITIAL' NEURITIS

Definition

A painful disorder of plexus or nerve trunks but which may affect any peripheral nerve, once regarded as due to inflammation of the interstitial connective tissues which surround and bind together the nerve fibres into the nerve trunks. This hypothetical view of its pathology is no longer seriously entertained.

BRACHIAL NEURITIS

NEURALGIC AMYOTROPHY (SHOULDER-GIRDLE NEURITIS)

Neuralgic amyotrophy was not recognized as an entity until the Second World War but it has been common in England during recent years, and occurred in the armies abroad. The cause is unknown, but the course of the illness resembles that of an infective disease, and in many cases the onset of the neuritis has occurred while the patients were in hospital suffering from an infectious illness of the respiratory or alimentary system.

Symptoms

Severe pain in the shoulder or side of the neck, radiating down the arm is usually the first symptom, but in a few cases no significant pain occurs. In the more severe cases general malaise accompanies the onset. After a few days paralysis is noticed, affecting, as a rule, some of the more proximal muscles innervated from the brachial plexus. Paralysis of the serratus anterior, with consequent winging of the scapula, is especially common, and if the patient is in bed because of other symptoms, this disability may escape notice until he is up and about again, and begins to use the arm of the affected side. If the paralysis affects the muscles of the upper arm, wasting is soon evident. All the tendon-jerks of the affected arm or of both arms may be abolished. Tenderness is present over the brachial plexus and may persist for several weeks. Sensory loss is, as a rule, slight or absent. The cerebrospinal fluid is usually normal.

Differential Diagnosis

This disorder only needs to be known to be recognized, but in soldiers abroad the diagnosis has to be made from poliomyelitis. In poliomyelitis the onset is more abrupt and in adults is accompanied by a greater degree of malaise and fever, stiffness of the neck is usual and Kernig's sign may be present; the cerebrospinal fluid contains a considerable excess of lymphocytes, followed by a gradual rise of protein during the weeks succeeding the onset of the paralysis. The paralysis tends to have a segmental distribution, whereas in the case of brachial neuritis it has much more tendency to be limited to the muscles supplied by one or two individual nerves.

Treatment

The cause of the disease being unknown, treatment can only be on general principles. Analgesics are given for the relief of pain, and the affected limb is supported in such a position as to relax the paralysed muscles. The shoulder should be passively exercised to prevent the very painful and frequently occurring 'frozen' shoulder or pericapsulitis. Though corticosteroids have been used, they are not efficacious.

Course and Prognosis

In this variety of brachial neuritis the pain usually goes off within a few days, and sensory loss, if any, does not last for long, but the outlook for recovery of the paralysis is always doubtful, and if such occurs, it takes many months.

BRACHIAL PAIN DUE TO A PROTRUDING INTERVERTEBRAL DISC

Brachial pain, loosely called 'brachial neuritis' is often due to irritation of one or more cervical nerve roots by a displaced intervertebral disc. In these cases the onset of pain is usually sudden, and often follows forceful movement of the neck or prolonged strain on the cervical muscles with the head partially rotated, as may occur in supporting a heavy weight.

The pain is usually described as being intense in severity, and is felt across the base of the neck and between the shoulder blades, and is usually worse on one side. It is aggravated by movement or jarring of the neck or by straining. After a few days the cervical pain usually improves but pain goes down the arm to the fingers supplied by the damaged root.

When examined, the patient is found to have limitation of movement of the neck, and may show severe signs of a radicular lesion in the arm in the form of muscular wasting or weakness, sensory impairment and diminished reflexes. The root most commonly affected is the sixth cervical and the patient's chief complaint is of pain in the arm and pain, tingling and numbness in the index finger and to a less degree in the thumb; on examination some sensory impairment is found over the index finger and the triceps-jerk is diminished or lost, and, after a time, some diminution of the muscles of the forearm is apparent on comparison with the normal limb.

Such cases usually recover gradually with symptomatic treatment but some stiffness of the neck may remain. Recovery can sometimes be hastened by manipulation of the neck combined with axial traction, which should only be carried out by an expert in manipulative methods.

Absolute rest in bed may be needed, with head traction, and exceptionally a plastic collar must be worn for weeks afterwards, because of liability to recurrence. It is only in the most recalcitrant cases that operation upon the offending joint is required, for most attacks resolve spontaneously and almost all the others improve with rest and traction. Even so, the practice in the United States has been to advise immediate radicular decompression. This certainly relieves the pain but usually no more quickly than rest, immobilization and medical treatment.

THE THORACIC INLET SYNDROME

Aetiology

The development of the ribs at the thoracic inlet depends on the mode of formation of the brachial plexus, for the nerves are large structures in the embryo at a time when the ribs are soft and pliable. When the plexus is 'normal', a well-formed first rib springs from the first dorsal vertebra. If, however, the plexus is 'post-fixed', that is, when the contribution to the plexus from the fourth and fifth cervical segments is small and the fibres from the first and second dorsal segments form a powerful cord, this cord in rising over the first dorsal rib may compress and deform it to such an extent that it presents the characters of a rudimentary rib. On the other hand, and this is more frequent, when the plexus is pre-fixed, that is, when the contribution from the upper cervical segments is relatively large and that from the dorsal segments is small, a supernumerary rib is allowed to develop from the seventh cervical vertebra. When this pre-fixation is pronounced, the seventh cervical rib is often very large and is easily felt in the neck, and in these cases symptoms are usually absent. When the abnormality is intermediate in degree, symptoms are caused by compression of the lower cord of the plexus as it passes over the supernumerary rib, or over the deformed first rib. This compression may be exerted by the bony portion of the extra rib, but more often the nerves are damaged by a fibrous prolongation which connects it with the first rib.

These abnormalities in the ribs only cause symptoms in some 10 per cent. of the cases in which they are present. Further, the symptoms are often unilateral with bilateral supernumerary ribs, and the symptoms are often more prominent on the side of the smaller extra rib. Again, the onset of symptoms is usually delayed until adult life is reached. It is clear, therefore, that some contributory cause must come into play. This is found in the dropping of the shoulder girdle, which is normal in adolescents, and is often excessive in persons whose muscular tone is low. In a child the clavicle rises boldly as it passes outwards. In a normal adult male the clavicle is almost horizontal, in women it droops slightly, and in those who develop symptoms of pressure on the nerves, the outer is usually distinctly lower than the inner end. In them, the lowest cord of the plexus is submitted to constant rubbing against the extra rib which rises and falls during respiration, and it is compressed by any movement of the arm which depresses the shoulder girdle. Relief is obtained by raising the shoulders, and patients soon learn to support the limb and to assume attitudes in which pressure on the nerves is relieved.

The condition is uncommon, many instances of damage to the median nerve in the carpal tunnel having been misdiagnosed in the past because of the pain which extends up the arm in that condition. Exactly similar symptoms will be caused by involvement of the roots (C. 8 and T. 1) in carcinoma and other gross lesions in this area. An identical syndrome is caused by pressure of the branches of the lower cord within the scalenus anticus muscle (the scalenus anticus syndrome).

Symptoms

These may be sensory, motor or vasomotor, either singly or in combination. Subjective sensory disturbances are most frequent. They take the form of numbness and tingling or neuralgic pains. Paraesthesiae are most often unilateral, and are often confined to the ulnar side. Pain, when present, is usually felt below the elbow. It is often neuralgic, darting down the arm and again confining itself to one border of the limb. It hardly ever radiates from the neck. Sensory changes, if present, are in the territory of the first thoracic root.

Muscular wasting is not so common as sensory disturbance. Wasting appears first in the small muscles of the hand innervated by the ulnar nerve. In some cases all the muscles of the hand and, to a less degree, the flexors in the forearm show considerable wasting. The atrophy may be bilateral and symmetrical.

Vasomotor disturbances are very common. The hands feel hot or cold, they may be oedematous or discoloured and the changes may suggest Raynaud's disease. Pressure on the subclavian artery sometimes causes inequality of the pulse, and the pulse on the affected side may be obliterated by depression of the shoulder. The inequality disappears when the arm is raised.

Diagnosis

Motor and sensory disturbances in the territory of the first thoracic root should suggest the diagnosis, and pain in the clavicular region, with vasomotor changes make it almost certain. Dysaesthesiae in the hand on the median rather than the ulnar side, with pain up the arm, and nocturnal 'acroparaesthesiae' suggest the much more common carpal tunnel syndrome. The thoracic inlet syndrome follows—with much pain, secondary extension from carcinoma of the breast, or aneurysm of the axillary artery.

Treatment

This is that of the cause, deep X-ray therapy being used for carcinoma involving the plexus. When the cause is a mechanical one, confirmed by radiology, operative removal of the compressing bone may be needed or section of the scalenus anticus muscle. Pain may be relieved by rest with the arms suitably supported. Atrophy calls for operation to rectify the cause. Pain is always relieved by operation, either immediately or after an interval of some months. The progress of atrophy is always retarded, and complete recovery may occur if an operation is undertaken early.

SCIATICA

The term 'sciatica' is an old one applied when pain is experienced along the course and in the distribution of the sciatic nerve—that is to say, in the buttock, back of the thigh, outer side and back of the leg and the outer border of the foot. It is important at the outset to notice the limitations of this distribution and, in particular, to notice that the sciatic nerve does not supply any structures on the front of the thigh, and so pain in that region or in the groin is not included in sciatica.

Cases of sciatica as thus defined are common, and many of them have a prolonged course and other well-described features. Until 30 years ago they were all confidently attributed to interstitial neuritis (sciatic neuritis) but it is now thought that this is not an entity. Most are the result of irritation of one of the roots of the great sciatic nerve by displaced tissue; commonly a prolapsed intervertebral disc, other changes in the disc and the surrounding bone, osteophytosis or secondary fibrosis and neuroma formations. Some are due to primary and secondary tumours, but some to injury. It is probable that the prime cause in all instances is mechanical.

SCIATICA DUE TO DISEASE OF THE INTERVERTEBRAL DISC

Sciatica is the most common syndrome caused by herniation of the nucleus pulposus of a lumbar intervertebral disc.

Aetiology

Many patients give a history of injury at, or shortly before, the onset of symptoms. The injury is commonly of the variety known as a strain of the back, due to sudden bending, the lifting of heavy weights or sudden movements of the back, as when striving to avoid a fall. Men are more commonly affected. In women, childbirth, especially with instrumental delivery, is an additional cause.

Pathology

Formerly the condition under discussion was one recognized on laminectomy, and spoken of as endochondroma of the disc. Actually, the disc ruptures and its nucleus pulposus subsequently herniates into the vertebral canal. The complicated mechanical pathology at the site is discussed in orthopaedic manuals.

The commonest site of such a lesion is in the lumbar spine, below the termination of the spinal cord, and the extruded mass causes irritation and compression of one or more of the roots of the cauda equina. The disc most often ruptured is that between the fifth lumbar vertebra and the sacrum (fifth lumbar disc), and the spinal root affected is the fifth lumbar. The fourth lumbar disc is also commonly ruptured and the third lumbar occasionally so. The rupture of higher lumbar intervertebral discs is uncommon. In each case the spinal root most affected is that emerging just below the site of the lesion. Multiple ruptures are not uncommon.

Symptoms

The outstanding feature is pain. It begins in the small of the back either at the time of the injury or after an interval of some hours, days or weeks. It may remain limited to the back, but in most cases it extends, after a variable interval, down the back of one thigh, and then down the leg and possibly into the foot, so that the clinical condition becomes one of 'sciatica'. The exact distribution of the pain in the leg depends on which spinal root is affected. The pain is severe and lancinating, aggravated by stooping, by coughing and sneezing, and by turning in bed, and relieved by lying still. Flexion of the extended leg at the hip is always painful (Lasègue's sign), and the patient adopts an attitude of partial flexion of the affected limb at the knee and hip, which avoids tension on the sciatic nerve and its roots.

The objective physical signs fall into two groups: those referable to the spine, and those to impairment of function in the affected nerve root or roots. The lumbar spine is flattened and is tilted at the site of the lesion; the tilt is usually away from the side of the sciatic pain but may be towards it and in some cases the tilt alternates. Radiographic examination shows the flattening of the lumbar curve and the tilting more clearly, and it may show a suggestive reduction of one intervertebral space but this is not usual. The signs are in general those of impairment of function of a single spinal root, most commonly the first sacral, and the ankle-jerk is abolished; the muscles of the calf and the peronei become slightly wasted, and the change in outline is apparent when the two legs are compared with the patient standing up or lying prone. The power of flexion of the small toes is diminished. The glutei on the affected side are flattened. Sensation is impaired along the outer border of the foot and on the outer half of the sole, and the patient has a sensation of numbness or tingling in this area. This may be impairment of pain appreciation, and loss of tickle on the affected area of the sole, or a loss of light touch appreciation, or a loss of sense of position of the small toe, or all of these combined. When the fourth lumbar disc is ruptured and the fifth lumbar root is the most affected, the site of the worst pain is on the outer side of the leg and perhaps on the dorsum of the foot, wasting of the calf is less pronounced, and the ankle-jerk is more often diminished than abolished; an area of sensory loss for light touch or impairment of pin-prick appreciation may be found on the outer side of the calf. In severe cases some disturbances may be found in the functions of the first sacral root as well as in those of the fifth lumbar. With lesions of the higher lumbar discs the pain is maximal in the fourth or higher root distributions, and the knee-jerk may be diminished or lost.

In some cases the nervous symptoms are entirely irritative, and there are no signs of impaired root function. Spinal signs are usually present, and ultimately some wasting appears, but in a number of such cases it may still be impossible to make the differential diagnosis from sciatic pain due to other causes.

Diagnosis

When the diagnosis is in doubt myelography shows a filling defect, corresponding to the knuckle of cartilage indenting the theca or the bony overgrowth.

In almost every case the problem is to distinguish the symptoms of a ruptured intervertebral disc from 'sciatica' due to other causes. Most cases of sciatica in people under 40 years of age are due to disease of the intervertebral discs. If there is some history of injury or strain, if both the spinal and nervous groups of signs are present, and if the latter are limited to the distribution of a single root, there is little doubt about the diagnosis. In cases of referred sciatic pain, reflex changes, muscular wasting and objective sensory loss are absent. Very prolonged and, especially, recurrent sciaticas are mostly due to ruptured intervertebral discs.

Osteoarthritis of the spine, carcinoma, and benign tumours must be excluded. We are apt to forget that pelvic tumours, benign as well as malignant may, especially in women, cause sciatica and back pain. Therefore rectal and pelvic examination should be made whenever there is not a perfectly obvious story of disc protrusion.

Treatment

It is not known how the structures within the vertebral canal adapt themselves but in most instances the pain subsides without operative removal of the protruding mass. It is presumed that the affected nerve root suffers the minimum of physical irritation when the patient takes up the posture which is for him least painful. In general, the patient should remain at rest in his most comfortable position and be given such pain-relievers as aspirin, Compound Codeine Tablets, B.P., and paracetamol together with sedatives. Heavy sedation with diazepam (*Valium*), 10 mg. three times daily, may help the more severely affected who are confined to bed, possibly on weight extension. Physiotherapy may be comforting after the acute phase has passed, but it has no effect. When the patient has been free from pain for a week, while still in bed, he may be allowed to sit up and very gradually begin to move about, but he should avoid doing anything which causes pain and he should rest when pain begins. If pain is recurrent when the patient has begun to move about, support of the lumbar spine by a plaster jacket may be necessary, followed by use of a Goldthwaite or similar belt.

Operation for the removal of the protruding portion of disc is advisable: (1) if after 6 weeks or so of well organized conservative treatment with *absolute* bedrest the pain is not definitely diminished; (2) if the sciatica is recurrent; (3) if the patient's employment involves heavy work and much movement of the back. Careful selection of patients upon the basis of their general health and their attitude to their disability will influence the operative results which in general are excellent, though in some cases some pain persists or returns.

Course and Prognosis

In the absence of operative treatment, the symptoms usually subside gradually in the course of from 6 weeks to 6 months. In a very few cases they clear up more quickly, and in a small proportion they persist in some degree for years, sometimes better and sometimes worse. The muscular wasting, though obvious, never becomes severe and there is never total paralysis of the affected nerve root.

REFERRED SCIATIC PAIN

In some cases of sciatic pain there are no manifestations of disease of the sciatic nerve itself, either in the way of impaired function or of tenderness, and the pain is believed to be a referred pain excited by disease of other structures within the nerve distribution of the spinal segments from which the sciatic nerve arises. The pain is abolished by the cure of the primary disease or anaesthetization of the structure which it affects. Conditions which may cause referred sciatic pain are arthritis in the hip joint, arthritis in the sacro-iliac joint, disease of the lower lumbar vertebrae or of the sacrum, trauma of the gluteal muscles and lesions of the vertebral ligaments. It should be noted that malignant disease of the lower vertebral bones may cause severe referred sciatica at a time when no bony change is revealed by radiography, and the occurrence of sciatic pain in a patient who has suffered from carcinoma is to be interpreted in the light of this knowledge.

Referred sciatic pain is usually moderate. Its distribution is in the calf on the outer side of the leg, or on the outer side of the ankle. The calf muscles are slightly tender and uncomfortable, which causes the patient to move them often. The absence of neurological signs is the most important diagnostic feature.

In all cases of referred pain the treatment is that of the exciting condition. Injection of a local anaesthetic into the disordered structure abolishes the pain temporarily, and occasionally the relief is permanent, especially if the anaesthetic is used in oily solution, the effect of which is more lasting than that of an aqueous solution.

OBSTETRICAL PARALYSIS

It is useful to group together under this heading all those conditions of paralysis occurring, either in mother or child, which are the result of the processes of labour in the passage of the foetal head through the pelvis. Autopsies upon the still-born, and upon children who have survived birth for a few days only, have shown that haemorrhage into the meninges is of common occurrence, and it has been argued that such meningeal haemorrhages are the cause of many of the conditions of cerebral paralysis which are present immediately after birth, or which appear during the first year of life, and especially the cause of cerebral diplegia [see p. 1241]. The pathological conditions found in the brain in cases of cerebral diplegia, however, make it impossible that they could be caused by meningeal haemorrhage, for no sign of old haemorrhage is ever found, nor could haemorrhage cause a general cell atrophy of the brain without signs of any local lesion. It seems clear, then, that though meningeal haemorrhage may be common during birth, and may be the cause of stillbirth, there is no clinical or pathological evidence to show that it causes any lasting cerebral defect.

The following conditions may occur: (1) In the child: facial paralysis; hemiplegia from laceration of the brain substance; fracture-dislocation of the spine with transverse lesion of the spinal cord; injury to the brachial plexus from the separation of head and shoulder in traction; and injury to peripheral nerve trunks at the elbow, axilla or groin, in using traction with the finger.

(2) In the mother: paralysis of the lumbosacral cord and obturator nerve from prolonged pressure of the head against the sacrum and pelvis.

Facial paralysis. This is usually caused by the pressure of the forceps upon the facial nerve as it crosses the ramus of the jaw, but it has been known to occur where instruments have not been used. When unilateral, as is the common event, it gives rise to little or no difficulty with sucking, and is evidenced by the unsightly deformity of the face, which is drawn over to the sound side. When bilateral, it is one of the causes of complete inability to suck, and because of the flaccid symmetry of the face it may be missed. It necessitates spoon feeding for a time. Obstetrical facial paralysis invariably recovers within weeks. Gentle stretching and massage of the face with the finger is the only 'treatment'.

Hemiplegia from laceration of the brain may occur during delivery in contracted pelvis from the pressure upon the sacral promontory, and has been caused by the use of forceps. It is exceedingly rare, and is generally rapidly fatal from the associated haemorrhage. It may occasionally be survived, with an irreparable hemiplegic condition.

Fracture-dislocation of the spine is produced by traction upon the aftercoming head by pulling upon the trunk, and it may be associated with injury to the brachial plexus. It occurs most often in the lower cervical region, and the transverse lesion of the spinal cord is usually complete.

Injury to the brachial plexus may occur in traction either upon the head, or upon the trunk, if the head is aftercoming, and is caused by an undue separation of head and shoulder on one side rupturing or straining the brachial plexus. The paralysis is usually of the upper arm or Erb type, the fifth and sixth roots being most affected, and the deltoid, biceps and supinator longus muscles being paralysed, but the whole plexus may be involved and even torn completely across [see p. 1291]. Traction upon a prolapsed arm has caused lower arm or Klumpke type of paralysis, in which the first dorsal and eighth cervical roots are most affected, and the intrinsic hand muscles and the flexors of the forearm are paralysed [see p. 1291]. The obstetrical lesions of the brachial plexus are serious, many of the cases making no motor recovery at all, though sensation usually does.

Injury to the peripheral nerves from pressure or traction upon the flexures is seldom severe enough to prevent a rapid and complete recovery.

Paralysis of the lumbosacral cord and of the obturator nerves in the mother occurs immediately after parturition. The lumbosacral plexus is in an exposed position as regards the foetal head engaging the pelvis, especially the lumbosacral cord, and this may be subjected to such severe pressure as to cause paralysis, and in the second place, the obturator nerve actually crosses the brim of the pelvis and must be pressed upon by any large foetal head which passes the pelvic brim. The lumbosacral cord paralysis is shown by dropped foot and paralysis of the anterior tibial and peroneal muscles and if it is severe, by loss of sensation over the distribution of the fourth and fifth lumbar routes. Sometimes the third lumbar root area is affected. The obturator nerve involvement is shown by weakness or paralysis of the muscles supplied by the obturator nerve, namely, all the adductor muscles of the thigh. The paralysis may be noticed directly after parturition, or when the patient begins to get about. The lumbosacral paralysis is usually unilateral, and is nearly always upon the right side. The obturator paralysis is sometimes bilateral, and both forms of the paralysis may coexist. There may be numbness, but no pain. This condition nearly always occurs with a first delivery, and often the child's head has been unduly large. It may recur with subsequent deliveries, but this is not a common event.

The prognosis is absolutely favourable, every case making a complete recovery in from a few weeks to a few months. The treatment is rest in the first place, with gentle massage and passive movements, and when power begins to return the patient may start to get about.

POLYNEURITIS

Synonym. Multiple peripheral neuritis; Peripheral neuropathy.

Introduction

The clinicopathological condition is a striking and uniform reaction of the nervous system. In it there is degeneration from the periphery, the longest fibres being affected first and most, of sensory or motor fibres, or more commonly, both. The disorder is always symmetrical in distribution and degree. The diagnosis is simple, the cause generally obscure.

Aetiology

At first sight the factors that cause polyneuritis fall into three groups: (1) certain chemical poisons; (2) the toxins of certain bacteria; and (3) certain disorders of metabolism. Widely differing as these three causative factors may seem to be, it may be that a common underlying factor which is immediately responsible for polyneuritis may determine them all. It is probable that in the case of groups (1) and (2) the pathogenic substance gives rise to a disorder of metabolism in the course of which a toxic metabolite is produced in the body, this acting directly upon the nervous system. In the metabolic group (3) the same process is in action. Thus, in beriberi, for example, the illness ensues upon the ingestion of a diet deficient in vitamin B_1 without which carbohydrate metabolism is disordered. Beriberi is not, as the biochemists formerly insisted, a simple starvation-degeneration of the nervous system, but an intoxication strictly comparable with that obtaining in other varieties, aetiologically considered, of polyneuritis. The final and complete proof of this unity of causation of polyneuritis, in whatever circumstances it is seen, is not yet available, but there is an increasing body of evidence in favour of it.

Returning to the ordinary aetiological classifications of polyneuritis, we see that in alcoholic or arsenical polyneuritis the poison is taken by the mouth, and presumably the final common toxic substance reaches the nervous system by the blood stream. In diphtheritic paralysis, on the other hand, the exotoxins are produced locally at the site of the diphtheritic ulceration, whether on the fauces, or, as in extrafaucial diphtheria, at some other local site on the body surface. This unique channel of entry in diphtheritic paralysis causes a group of symptoms not found in other aetiological varieties of polyneuritis. This group includes palatal and accommodation paralyses, which precede the appearance of polyneuritis. It is noteworthy that in the case of extrafaucial diphtheria this initial paralysis is not palatal, but is anatomically related to the site of the diphtheritic lesion. Yet the paralysis of accommodation may occur whatever be the site of the diphtheritic lesion. It is believed, therefore, that the exotoxins gain access to the nervous system by conduction from the seat of the lesion via the axons of the nerves which innervate this region. They pass upwards in the axis cylinders to the central nervous system and produce their toxic action directly there, this action being reflected peripherally again as a motor and sensory paralysis of the muscles and skin or mucosa in the region of the lesion. Thus a diphtheritic ulcer on a finger may be followed by a local paralysis of that part before polyneuritis develops. The subsequently developing polyneuritis is then probably produced in the manner described above, while the accommodation paralysis may indicate a specific action of the toxin upon the nervous mechanism concerned. We thus have a local, a specific and a general group of symptoms. The analogy of the local, specific and general phases of tetanus will occur to the reader.

Acute and subacute polyneuritis occur as complications of metabolic and neoplastic diseases which have been described in other sections of the book: acute porphyria, lupus erythematosus, sarcoidosis, bronchogenic carcinoma and primary amyloidosis. It is evident that in all these disorders a biochemical change is responsible for the polyneuritis, but in each investigation and treatment is that of the primary disorder, and in all the polyneuritis has similar features modified by the rate of progression. Ingested causes, in addition to alcohol, are methyl alcohol, triorthocresylphosphate (Jake paralysis), thalidomide (*Distaval*) and nitrofurantoin (*Furadantin*).

Acute 'febrile' polyneuritis has no known causal factors. It appears in apparently healthy persons, adequately nourished and free from all discoverable signs of infection, and it is extremely difficult in the present state of knowledge to account for on any hypothesis of avitaminosis, or to suggest any possible mode of intoxication. In at least a half of all cases of acute polyneuritis no cause can be found however exhaustive the investigations.

Many of the intoxications of the nervous system commonly included under the heading of polyneuritis are associated with lesions and clinical manifestations which are not those of polyneuritis. Such substances, to name but a few, are lead, mercury, copper, carbon disulphide and carbon monoxide, and it would be erroneous to regard these as causes of polyneuritis.

Pathology

The changes in the nerves are those of parenchymatous neuritis, and longitudinal sections stained by the Marchi or Weigert-Pal methods show severe degeneration of the fibres. The alterations are most intense in the small branches supplying the skin and muscles, and they diminish in severity as the larger branches are approached. They are best seen in the terminal branches of the musculospiral and anterior tibial nerves. The wasted muscles often show a reduction in the size of their fibres, and an increase of connective tissue—fibrous myositis. The spinal cord may be healthy, but in almost all cases examination by modern methods shows changes in the nerve cells and degeneration in the tract fibres derived from the posterior roots.

Recent research shows that there are two main forms of degeneration of the peripheral nerves, loss of myelin which may be in patches along the length of the nerve, and primary degeneration of the axis cylinder. In some sorts the axis cylinder dies back from the periphery, primarily, and in others the prime disorder is in the neurone itself, the fibre dying back in consequence.

Symptoms

As might be expected from the composition of the peripheral nerves, the symptoms of polyneuritis may consist of disorders of movement, sensation and autonomic function, and these disorders are symmetrical and typically begin in the peripheral portions of the limbs and spread proximally. The relative severity of these disturbances varies from one variety of polyneuritis to another, and the detailed symptomatology of each variety is more fully considered below. The motor disorder is in all instances a lower motor neurone paralysis, with the characteristic weakness, reflex loss and muscle wasting with a marked propensity to contracture. Bilateral foot-drop is in a large number of cases the first objective motor manifestation. The sensory disorders are similarly peripheral and symmetrical and may involve both superficial and deep sensation and may be both positive (pains and paraesthesiae) and negative (anaesthesiae). The first complaint is usually of numbness in the feet and then in the hands; this extends proximally, and is soon accompanied by objective sensory loss, which has a 'glove and stocking' distribution. In some varieties autonomic defects are seen in alterations in sweat secretion and trophic changes in the skin, nails and other tissues.

The cerebrospinal fluid may show an increase of protein, the globulin fraction also showing an increase; the other elements of the fluid are normal.

Diagnosis

The diagnosis of polyneuritis is easy. It is made from the combination of symmetrical flaccid paralysis with sensory loss of the 'glove and stocking' distribution, and tenderness of the muscles and nerves, confined to, or most intense in, the distal part of the limbs. A variable degree of polyneuritis is an associated feature of subacute combined degeneration of the spinal cord, and this disease may be confused with polyneuritis. The differential clinical features are given on page 1282 and, as pointed out there, the distinction at an early stage may in most cases be made with confidence by the associated pyramidal signs. The development of extensor plantar reflexes is an absolute point against polyneuritis, while an excess of protein in the cerebrospinal fluid is equally against subacute combined degeneration. When sensory disturbances and diminished tendon reflexes are prominent symptoms and muscular weakness is slight, tabes dorsalis may be suggested, and the resemblance is still greater when ataxia is present. The lighting pains of tabes cannot be mistaken by anyone who is familiar with their peculiar characters. Anaesthesia of the extremities is common to both diseases, but diminished sensibility around the nose and across the chest is peculiar to tabes and is present in almost every case.

Treatment

The first essential is to try to find the cause and remove it. This is easier said than done, except perhaps with alcoholic neuritis, for usually no cause can be found.

Treatment is symptomatic, for the dyaesthesia and the affected muscles, but this has already been described for these symptoms in other neurological disorders.

Failing any cause, vitamin B preparations are used in abundance with little justification, except the theoretical basis that the carbohydrate metabolism of neurones depends upon the vitamin B group. The only circumstance in which there really is a basis for this is when there is *known* to be deficiency of the vitamin B group in alcoholic polyneuritis, beriberi, and the polyneuritis which sometimes accompanies Addisonian anaemia without spinal cord involvement. However, its use especially if injected, makes everyone feel a little better.

The debate about the use of steroids continues. There is a form of relapsing polyneuritis which can be temporarily reversed by the use of ACTH especially, but the therapeutic cynics refer to these cases as 'steroid dependent' and they may well be right.

Course and Prognosis

In a few instances myocardial failure or respiratory paralysis brings about a fatal issue at the height of the illness. Otherwise in many cases the course is a stage of invasion followed by a stage of recession, leading to complete recovery. The duration of these varies greatly. In rare cases recovery fails to occur.

Disability after recovery from the neuritis may result from muscular contractures, wasting or neuritic pains.

ALCOHOLIC NEURITIS

In former years alcoholism was perhaps the commonest cause of severe peripheral neuritis, but at present alcoholic polyneuritis is a rare disease in the British Isles. It occurs most often in women and in them it has often been the first indication of secret drinking. There is much evidence that the disorder results as much from the deficient diet and the chronic gastritis commonly found in alcoholic subjects as from the direct toxic effect of the alcohol taken.

The onset is insidious, and in most cases premonitory symptoms, such as numbness and tingling in the extremities or cramps in the muscles of the lower limbs, are present for several months before actual weakness occurs. Subjective sensory troubles are a marked feature, even in the early stages. Besides numbness and tingling the patients have feelings of excessive heat or of coldness in the limbs, or of severe aching or cutting pains in the legs. Painful cramp in the calf muscles is a common symptom. It is often worst at night, and may interfere seriously with sleep. Objective examination usually reveals sensory loss, in which the various elements of sensation are affected in a manner which is almost pathognomonic.

Stated briefly, there is anaesthesia of the skin with hyperaesthesia of the deeper structures. Light touches are not appreciated at all or many are missed, the temperature sense is defective, and the prick of a pin causes no pain, whereas even moderate compression of the muscles may cause the patient to cry out. The sensory loss is greatest in the feet and hands and diminishes towards the knees and elbows. Muscular tenderness is usually greatest in the calves. The soles of the feet are also unduly tender. Hyperalgesia is often well marked before anaesthesia of the skin appears. To the disability caused by pains and spasms, weakness of the muscles is added in all but the slightest cases. The arms may suffer first, but in most cases the extensors of the toes, the dorsiflexors of the ankle, and the extensors of the fingers and wrists are attacked in progression, and double foot-drop and wrist-drop result. To overcome the foot-drop, the knees are raised high in walking. This gives to the gait the 'steppage' character which is common to all forms of peripheral neuritis. In most cases the distal flexor muscles are also affected, but to a slighter degree. In severe cases, weakness extends to the proximal muscles and even to the muscles of the trunk. The affected muscles become soft and diminish rapidly in bulk. Unless precautions are taken, contractures occur in the flexor muscles and produce deformities of the limbs, which add greatly to the difficulties of treatment.

At the onset the knee-jerks are exaggerated, but in most cases by the time the patient comes under observation all the tendon reflexes are absent. The cutaneous reflexes may be unaltered, diminished or absent. Sphincter control is retained. Slight bilateral weakness of the face is often present but severe paralysis is rare. Ptosis, nystagmus and weakness of the external ocular muscles have been observed.

Trophic and vasomotor disturbances in the extremities are common. The hands and feet often perspire freely at first and then become unnaturally dry, and they may be white and cold or red and hot. In some cases oedema of the hands or legs is present. In chronic cases the skin of the hands and fingers is thin, smooth and shiny, and the nails are ridged and brittle.

SPECIAL TYPES OF POLYNEURITIS

Sometimes with alcoholic neuritis there is some mental change. One form—Korsakoff's psychosis—is characteristic of and almost peculiar to this disease. The most prominent feature is failure of memory for recent events and loss of appreciation of time and place. In most cases the mental defects are not gross. There is merely a failure of memory with personality change.

Alcohol must be withdrawn in hospital, with the help of sedatives, and large doses of vitamin B given intramuscularly. In view of the dietary deficiency which accompanies alcoholic polyneuropathy crude vitamin B preparations have precedence. Attention must be paid to the mental state, the accompanying gastritis, and the heart. Active bed exercises and re-education in movement and later in walking are essential. The prognosis, with abstinence from alcohol is good.

ARSENICAL NEURITIS

Peripheral neuritis may be caused by a single large dose of arsenic and it was formerly seen after prolonged therapeutic use of salts of the metal. It is now rare.

It is like alcoholic neuritis but hyperaesthesia of the skin and tenderness of the muscles are more constant and more severe, and paralysis and atrophy of the muscles are often more widespread and more rapid in their progress. Hyperkeratosis of the soles and pigmentation of the skin are characteristic of arsenical poisoning. In a suspected case, the diagnosis can be confirmed by the discovery of abnormal quantities of arsenic in the urine or in the hair and skin.

The mental changes described in connexion with alcoholic neuritis under the heading of Korsakoff's psychosis may be present, especially when repeated poisonous doses of arsenic have been taken.

MERCURIAL NEURITIS

Mercury poisoning results from ingesting organic mercury compounds, as in the outbreak in Japan caused by eating shellfish which lived in the effluent from a factory.

TRIORTHOCRESYLPHOSPHATE NEURITIS

The polyneuritis caused by this poisoning is acute, severe and often fatal. It is caused by the unintentional (as opposed to accidental) ingestion of this poison as in Jake palsy from the use of Jamaican ginger in alcoholic drinks in the United States, or the disastrous outbreak in Algeria where cooking oil was contaminated with aviation oil for nefarious gain. In that outbreak about 10,000 people were affected and a quarter died.

DIPHTHERITIC PARALYSIS

This is now almost unknown in the British Isles. The exotoxin is highly selective for nervous tissues, and some form of paralysis occurs in a very high proportion of the cases. The intensity of the paralysis bears no constant relation to the severity of the local infection, for cases in which the original disease has passed unnoticed may be followed by serious damage to the nervous system. The nervous manifestations of diphtheria fall into three distinct groups, the local. the specific and the generalized paralyses.

Local paralysis occurs in parts related anatomically by nervous connexions to the site of the diphtheritic lesion. In faucial diphtheria, the local palsy appears in the palate. In extrafaucial diphtheria, e.g. infected sores on the limbs, the local palsy appears in the muscles supplied by the segments of the cord to which afferent nerves from the infected focus pass.

The *specific* manifestation of diphtheria is paralysis of accommodation. Like trismus in tetanus, it is not due to a local lesion, but occurs in many cases, whatever the site of origin of the toxins, and is the local effect of exotoxin accepted from the general blood stream.

The third or *generalized* form of diphtheritic paralysis is multiple neuritis. It follows extrafaucial as well as faucial diphtheria, and is also a result of the action of exotoxin circulating in the blood.

As faucial diphtheria was the commonest form, the most frequent nervous symptom is *paralysis of the soft palate*. It is shown by the nasal quality of the voice and by the regurgitation of fluids through the nose. As a rule, the weakness is bilateral and equal, but in some cases it is greater on the side on which the local lesion is more severe. It appears about the end of the second week, but may come on as early as the fourth day, or as late as the sixth week. Recovery usually occurs in a few weeks. In rare instances the muscles of the pharynx and the vocal cords are paralysed. Together with palatal palsy, it is common to find marked weakness and tenderness of the sternomastoid muscles and masseters. These are also local effects.

Paralysis of accommodation appears about the same time as the palatal palsy, perhaps a few days sooner. The reaction of the pupils to accommodation as well as to light, can almost always be obtained. The trouble is subjective, and is shown by defects of near vision—for example, by inability to read small print. Hypermetropes suffer great inconvenience. In myopes it may pass unnoticed. Paralysis of any of the extrinsic ocular muscles with strabismus and diplopia may occur, and this may be either nuclear or peripheral in type.

Polyneuritis usually comes on 3–6 weeks after recovery from the throat infection when patients are convalescent. It is a severe and rapidly advancing form of polyneuritis, described in Section 2.

Cardiac failure used to be a grave but uncommon complication. It is of myocardial origin. Vasomotor paralysis and disturbances in the nutrition of the skin, which occur so often in other forms of peripheral neuritis, are never seen in diphtheria. In those that survive the attack, complete recovery from the nervous troubles always occurs.

ACUTE INFECTIVE POLYNEURITIS

Synonyms. Acute febrile polyneuritis; Landry's paralysis; the Guillain-Barré syndrome.

Pathology

This disorder is a polyradiculitis, the inflamed roots contributing protein to the cerebrospinal fluid. It is because it is radicular that the muscles are uniformly affected, proximally as well as distally.

At various times small epidemics of a form of polyneuritis with a febrile onset and by the involvement of the facial nerves have been described.

It is probably a tissue reaction, and is associated sometimes with central nervous system changes (the Guillain-Barré syndrome). It responds satisfactorily to corticosteroids.

Symptoms

The onset is with slight fever, headache and malaise, pains in back and limbs, and such general symptoms as a coryza or gastro-intestinal irritation. The fever persists for 2 or 3 days only. A few days then elapse before the signs and symptoms of polyneuritis develop. It is said that the proximal limb muscles are more severely involved than the distal muscles, a point of distinction from other forms of polyneuritis, but this relative incidence of weakness is not invariable and has probably been over-stressed. The trunk muscles do not escape, and the face is often bilaterally paralysed. As in other forms the paralysis is of the lower motor neurone type, flaccid, atrophic and with loss of tendon-jerks. Sensory loss is very slight, and there is relatively slight muscular tenderness. Sometimes the spinal cord is affected to cause paraplegic symptoms and signs. The cerebrospinal fluid shows a very high rise in the protein content, but is otherwise normal.

The clinical course is variable, and sometimes fluctuates. Death may ensue from paralysis of the respiratory muscles, but recovery in the majority of cases is fairly rapid. There is the usual tachycardia of polyneuritis. If the patient survives the acute phase, complete recovery ensues.

Treatment

Management of the condition is of great importance because of the good prognosis for ultimate recovery. The patient should always have access to a well equipped respiratory unit, so that should weakness involve the respiratory muscles life can be sustained in a respirator. It is now usual to perform tracheostomy and use a positive pressure respirator of the Beaver type for this purpose. There must be diligent attention to humidity, acid-base balance and intercurrent infection. Hope must never be lost, for once the patient is 'round the corner' remarkable recovery will ensue.

Response to the use of ACTH, 40 I.U. daily until improvement is occurring, and then slow reduction, is usually dramatic. It should be given immediately the diagnosis is made, and with its use prognosis is excellent so long as such complications as respiratory paralysis are overcome.

DIABETIC NEURITIS

In many patients with glycosuria, symptoms are present which point to changes in the peripheral nerves. In some cases the only symptom is neuralgic pain in the distribution of one or more nerves. This is commonest in the legs where it simulates sciatica, and sugar is found in the urine in the absence of any other sign of diabetes. In other cases, a single large nerve trunk suddenly becomes paralysed.

In severe diabetes mellitus the knee-jerks and ankle-jerks are diminished or lost in more than half the cases. This may accompany subjective sensory troubles in the lower limbs, or it may appear as an isolated symptom. The muscles are often tender and the vibration sense of the feet is frequently absent. To objective examination, the sensibility of the skin is usually intact. Perforating ulcers of the feet have been observed. Only in very rare instances does the neuritis proceed to the stage of generalized peripheral paralysis of motor and sensory structures.

In mild cases of diabetes, however, polyneuritis develops, and sometimes the disturbed carbohydrate metabolism is only discovered by investigation of the polyneuritis. This form is mainly sensory and causes intense dysaesthesia. It is more 'patchy' or less uniform than other forms because it has in its aetiology arteriolar degeneration of the vasa nervorum caused by the diabetes. In consequence of this its effects do not subside when the diabetes is brought under control.

POLYNEURITIS CAUSED BY COMMERCIAL AND MEDICAL TOXINS

As more than half the cases of polyneuritis—which is not an uncommon condition—have no discoverable cause, any chemical with which the patient has had contact tends to be incriminated—often unjustifiably. This has been the case for instance with agricultural and horticultural sprays used for killing plants, insects, moulds or bacteria Reports of single cases are most misleading, and indeed it would be more scientific to report the widespread use of so many new preparations by so many people who do not develop polyneuritis, with minimal precautions having been taken. The author saw a young woman with polyneuritis of unknown origin, whose occupation was that of spraying crops. She returned to her work before the neuritis had recovered, but it continued to do so. Extensive study failed to relate the spray used to her body chemistry, and none of the hundreds of other agricultural workers similarly employed had come to harm. The polyneuritis *may* have been due to the spray but it *may* have been coincidental.

PROGRESSIVE HYPERTROPHIC POLYNEURITIS

Dejerine and Sottas described an extremely rare progressive form of polyneuritis, sometimes developing in infancy, showing an heredofamilial incidence, and characterized by thickening of the nerve trunks due to hypertrophy of the sheaths of Schwann. In recent years other cases of hypertrophic polyneuritis have been described which have no hereditary or familial character. There is evidence that some, at least, of the cases described under this heading were examples of primary amyloidosis of the peripheral nervous system.

Pathology

The thickening of the nerves may be palpable during life, but is not invariably so. Miscroscopically this thickening is found to be due to masses of non-nucleated tissue arising from the sheath of Schwann.

Symptoms

The illness develops and progresses very slowly with peripheral weakness, muscular wasting, sensory loss and loss of tendon-jerks. In addition, there may be noted kyphoscoliosis, nystagmus and ataxia of movement. It was formerly thought that the Argyll Robertson pupil was an integral part of the symptom-complex, but this is not the case.

Treatment

There is no known treatment which is effective.

Prognosis

Death ultimately ensues from intercurrent disease.

REFSUM'S SYNDROME

This is an hereditary form of polyneuritis due to a disorder of lipid metabolism with storage in the body of phytanic acid. The advancing polyneuritis is of mixed form and is accompanied by deafness, retinitis pigmentosa, skeletal abnormalities, myocardial degeneration and ichthyosis. There is an increase in serum lipids and in cerebrospinal fluid protein. It is extremely rare.

SHY-DRAGER SYNDROME

This is caused by progressive degeneration of the autonomic system in its sympathetic and parasympathetic components. It occurs in adult life and its cause is unknown. Its main consequence is extreme hypotension and vasomotor paralysis, which makes it impossible for the patient to stand without fainting. There is anhidrosis, impotence and constipation, and in the fully developed disease there is also cerebellar and extrapyramidal degeneration, to cause tremor, rigidity, and ataxia.

The *Steel-Richardson syndrome* is similar. There is autonomic and basal ganglion degeneration with rigidity and tremor, associated with gross vasomotor inadequacy.

LEAD PALSY

The nervous effects of lead poisoning are confined almost entirely to motor neurones. Subjective sensory disturbances are often slight or absent, and in most instances there is no objective sensory loss.

Pathology

There is local concentration of lead in those muscles which are about to be paralysed and the paralysis is a muscular event primarily. Secondarily, the lead ascends along the motor axons and may finally cause the death of the ventral horn cell. The degenerative changes in the nerves are confined almost entirely to the motor fibres, and are most intense in the intramuscular twigs supplying muscles of the extensor groups. Normal and degenerated fibres are found side by side, the former becoming more numerous as the nerve is traced upwards. Degenerative changes due to the action of lead are also found in the affected muscles.

Symptoms

In most cases of the common *antebrachial* or *wrist-drop type*, paralysis is limited to the extensor muscles of the fingers and wrists—that is, to the muscles supplied by the musculospiral nerve. But the brachioradialis and the abductor longus pollicis, also supplied by this nerve, usually escape. Inability to extend the first phalanges of the two middle fingers, owing to weakness of the common extensor, is usually the first difficulty. The special extensors of the index and little fingers, the long extensors of the thumb and the extensors of the wrist are next attacked, and the characteristic wrist-drop appears. As a rule the paralysis becomes severe about a week after it is first noticed. By this time it is usually bilateral and symmetrical, but for several days, or even for several weeks, it may be confined to one side. The affected muscles waste rapidly and the back of the forearm becomes flattened, thus rendering the intact brachioradialis more prominent. In this form, loss of power always precedes atrophy, and some muscles may show weakness without any wasting. Recovery is almost complete. Simple weakness without atrophy usually passes off in a few weeks. If the wasting is moderate and the muscles still react to faradism, recovery may be expected in a few months. When the atrophy is severe, a year or more may elapse before recovery is complete.

REFERENCES

BOWDEN, R. F. M. (1958) *Peripheral Nerve Injury*, London.

BRAIN, W. R., and HENSON, R. A. (1958) Neurological syndromes associated with carcinoma; the carcinomatous neuropathies, *Lancet*, ii, 971.

BROWN, M. R. (1941) Alcoholic polyneuritis, *J. Amer. med. Ass.*, **116**, 1615.

BROWNE, R. C. (1955) Metallic poisons and the nervous system, *Lancet*, i, 775.

CAMPBELL, A. M. G. (1952) Neurological complications associated with insecticides and fungicides, *Brit. med. J.*, **2**, 415.

CAMPBELL, A. M. G. (1957) The aetiology of polyneuritis, *Proc. roy. Soc. Med.*, **51**, 157.

CHAMBERS, R. A., MEDD, W. E., and SPENCER, H. (1958) Primary amyloidosis, *Quart. J. Med.*, **27**, 207.

COLOVER, J. (1948) Sarcoidosis with involvement of the nervous system, *Brain*, **71**, 451.

DAVIS, D. R. (1949) Some factors affecting the results of treatment of peripheral nerve injuries, *Lancet*, i, 877.

ELLIOT, F. A., and KREMER, M. (1945) Brachial pain from lamination of cervical intervertebral disc, *Lancet*, i, 4.

FALCONER, M. A., MCGEORGE, M., and BEGG, A. C. (1948) Cause and mechanism of symptom-production in sciatica and low back pain, *J. Neurol. Neurosurg. Psychiat.*, **11**, 13.

FISHER, C. M., and ADAMS, R. D. (1956) Diphtheritic polyneuritis: a pathological study, *J. Neuropath. exp. Neurol.*, **15**, 243.

GARLAND, H. (1955) Diabetic amyotrophy, *Brit. med. J.*, **2**, 1287.

GARLAND, H., BRADSHAW, J. P. P., and CLARK, J. M. P. (1957) Compression of the median nerve in carpal tunnel and its relation to acroparaesthesia, *Brit. med. J.*, **1**, 730.

GILLIATT, R. W. (1957) Clinical electromyography, in *Modern Trends in Neurology*, 2nd Series, ed. WILLIAMS, D., London.

GUTTMANN, L. (1940) Topographical studies of disturbances of sweat secretion after complete lesions of peripheral nerves, *J. Neurol. Psychiat.*, **3**, 197.

HAYMAKER, W., and WOODHALL, B. (1953) *Peripheral Nerve Injuries*, 2nd ed., Philadelphia.

HEYMAN, A., PFEIFFER, J. B. Jr., WILLETT, R. W., and TAYLOR, H. M. (1956) Peripheral neuropathy caused by arsenical intoxication, *New Engl. J. Med.*, **254**, 401.

H.M.S.O. (1969) *Guide to Peripheral Nerve Injuries*, Reprint 7/6.

JEFFERSON, M. (1957) Sarcoidosis of the nervous system, *Brain*, **80**, 540.

KAHLKE, W., and RICHTERICH, R. (1965) Refsum's disease, *Amer. J. Med.*, **39**, 237.

Lancet (1963) Cervical ribs, ii, 1263.

LISHMAN, W. A., and RUSSELL, W. R. (1961) The brachial neuropathies, *Lancet*, ii, 941.

MARTIN, M. M. (1953) Diabetic neuropathy, *Brain*, **76**, 594.

PARSONAGE, M. J., and TURNER, J. W. A. (1948) Neuralgic amyotrophy, the shoulder girdle syndrome, *Lancet*, i, 973.

RUSSELL, W. R., and GARLAND, H. G. (1930) Progressive hypertrophic polyneuritis, with case reports, *Brain*, **53**, 376.

SCHLESINGER, A. S., DAGGINS, V. A., and MASUCCI, E. F. (1962) Peripheral neuropathy in familial primary amyloidosis, *Brain*, **85**, 357.

SEDDON, H. J. (1954) Peripheral nerve injuries, *Spec. Rep. Ser. med. Res. Coun.* (*Lond.*), No. 282.

SIMPSON, J. A. (1962) The neuropathies, in *Modern Trends in Neurology*, 3rd Series, ed. WILLIAMS, D., London.

SIMPSON, J. A. (1964) Biology and disease of the peripheral nerves, *Brit. med. J.*, **2**, 709.

SPILLANE, J. D. (1943) Localized neuritis of the shoulder girdle, *Lancet*, ii, 532.

STEVENS, H. (1957) Meralgia paraesthetica, *Arch. Neurol. Psychiat.* (*Chic.*), **77**, 557.

SULLIVAN, J. F. (1958) The neuropathies of diabetes, *Neurology*, **8**, 243.

THOMAS, P. K. (1961) Recent advances in the clinical electrophysiology of muscle and nerve, *Postgrad. med. J.*, **37**, 377.

WALSHE, F. M. R. (1942) The anatomy and physiology of cutaneous sensibility: a critical review, *Brain*, **65**, 48.

WEDGWOOD, J. (1957) Diabetes mellitus with acute polyneuritis, *Brit. med. J.*, **1**, 1346.

WILLIAMS, D. (1964) The problem of sciatica, *Practitioner*, **193**, 299.

DENIS WILLIAMS

FAMILIAL DYSAUTONOMIA

Synonym. Riley-Day syndrome.

Definition

In 1949 Riley and co-workers described a condition with disturbances of the nervous system, many of which might be due to autonomic malfunction. It was inherited as an autosomal recessive and was found mainly in families of Jewish extraction. Insensitivity to pain, excessive sweating, abnormal temperature control and postural hypotension may all result from impaired autonomic control. It has been suggested that this could be explained by a lesion in the reticular formation in the brain stem.

Clinical Features

Widespread abnormalities of function are to be anticipated and these may vary with the extent to which sympathetic and parasympathetic pathways are involved.

Abnormalities commonly present include:

Absent tear production.

Cold hands and feet, often with increased sweating.

Transient patches of cutaneous vasodilatation sometimes associated with excitement or eating.

Relative indifference to pain.

Difficulty in swallowing due to impaired muscular co-ordination and abnormal oesophageal mobility.
Absent deep tendon reflexes.
Dysarthria and excessive salivation causing difficulty in learning to speak.
Emotional lability together with psychomotor retardation.
Slow physical growth and late puberty.

Other less constant features include unexplained episodes of hyperpyrexia, breath-holding attacks and bouts of intractable vomiting. Many patients develop a scoliosis which adds to their motor difficulties. Taste and smell are often impaired and the lack of circumvallate papillae is a helpful diagnostic finding.

Diagnosis

It is thought that the condition could result from inability to synthesize a substance necessary for normal neurohumoral transmission. Examination of catecholamines in the urine would support this view since there is evidence of a block in the production of adrenaline and noradrenaline from dopamine.

Three tests are useful in making the diagnosis. If 2·5 per cent. methacholine is instilled into the conjunctival sac prompt miosis occurs whereas it is without effect in normal persons. An exaggerated response to an infusion of noradrenaline causes a marked rise of blood pressure. Again, an intradermal injection of histamine, 0·02 ml. of a 1 in 10,000 solution, produces a weal but no characteristic surrounding red flare. The flare is dependent on an axon reflex along sensory fibres and is absent in denervated limbs and in dysautonomia.

Prognosis

About 75 per cent. of these children survive to adult life. Gradual improvement occurs as the life-threatening incidents of fever and respiratory obstruction become less frequent in the pre-school era. There is a varying degree of motor and intellectual retardation, although many children learn to cope well with their limitations. Drugs such as pilocarpine have been used but probably their dangers outweigh their therapeutic value.

Occasionally the deltoid, biceps, brachialis and brachioradialis muscles are affected, either alone or in company with the forearm muscles—*upper arm* or *brachial type*. Less often paralysis occurs in the legs, the muscles supplied by the peroneal nerve, namely, the long extensors of the toes and the peronei, being chiefly involved—*peroneal type*. Like the brachioradialis in the arm, the tibialis anterior, although supplied by the peroneal nerve, usually escapes. This type is usually associated with paralysis of the forearm muscles, and runs the same course.

In this form of paralysis the features are similar to those of a traumatic lesion to a nerve. Loss of power precedes, and may be more extensive than wasting, and recovery is usually complete, it is therefore called the degenerative form. In the second form, the paralysis has the characters of progressive muscular atrophy. Weakness and wasting come on together, and the **paralysis is often permanent. Motor nerve conduction disappears and the electromyogram shows evidence of severe denervation. This is known as the primary atrophic form. It occurs especially in the small muscles of the hand—*Aran-Duchenne type*—but is sometimes irregular in its distribution and affects many muscles in all four limbs. It is often associated with the first form, but may occur alone. Wasting comes on slowly, and accompanies the loss of power, instead of succeeding it. It is much more intractable than the degenerative form, and often persists after muscles showing the first form of paralysis have recovered. [See also Lead Encephalopathy, Section 3.]**

Treatment

The first essential is to remove the source of intoxication at the same time as excretion of the heavy metal is accelerated by BAL or penicillamine, as in the treatment of Wilson's disease [see p. 1239]. The management of the case is that of all acute peripheral neuritis.

REFERENCES

Riley, C. M. (1957) Familial dysautonomia, *Advanc. Pediat.*, **9**, 157.

Shinebourne, E., Sneddon, J. M., and Turner, P. (1967) Evidence for autonomic denervation in familial dysautonomia, *Brit. med. J.*, **4**, 91.

Dennis Cottom

SECTION 16

DISEASES OF VOLUNTARY MUSCLE

DISEASES OF VOLUNTARY MUSCLE

THE ANATOMY AND PHYSIOLOGY OF MUSCLE

A voluntary muscle is composed of muscle fibres, each of which is a multinucleate cell containing myofibrils, sarcoplasm and discrete intracellular organelles including mitochondria, ribosomes and the sarcotubular system. Each fibre is enclosed within a sarcolemmal sheath beneath which the muscle nuclei are situated and each has a motor end-plate in which the nerve fibre terminates. Under normal conditions, muscle fibres never contract singly, but the functional unit of muscle activity is the motor unit, namely that group of muscle fibres supplied by a single anterior horn cell and its axon. Discharge of such an anterior horn cell causes simultaneous contraction of all of its muscle fibres. While on occasion all of the fibres of a motor unit may be localized within a single bundle or fasciculus, recent evidence suggests that the several fasciculi, and even the individual muscle fibres which make up the motor unit, may be widely separated anatomically within the muscle. The electrical activity which accompanies contraction of a motor unit and which can be recorded electromyographically, depends upon physical factors including the characteristics of the recording electrode and special features of the muscle examined. In the biceps brachii of a healthy young adult, a single motor unit action potential usually appears as a di- or triphasic wave with a duration of 5–10 msec. and an amplitude of less than 250 mV., but there is considerable normal variation in form, amplitude and duration.

In 1934 Dale first demonstrated that acetylcholine was the humoral element responsible for transmission of the nerve impulse at the myoneural junction. It seems that synaptic vesicles in the motor nerve terminal are packets of acetylcholine and that these are continually being released spontaneously to give small depolarizations (miniature end-plate potentials) which can be recorded with a micro-electrode inserted in the region of the end-plate. When a nerve impulse arrives, this causes the synchronous release of many packets of acetylcholine, giving localized depolarization of the muscle fibre membrane, the so-called end-plate potential. When the latter reaches a critical size, an action potential is induced which travels from the end-plate along the surface membrane of the fibre. At rest, the inside of the fibre membrane is some 80 mV. negative with respect to the outside, but as the action potential passes, the polarization of the membrane reverses so that the inside of the fibre becomes transiently positive. This reversal of electrical polarity is caused by increased sodium permeability of the membrane. It seems that the wave of excitation spreads into the substance of the fibre along the transverse system of tubules (T-system) and that the resulting release of calcium ions in the sarcoplasmic reticulum initiates contraction of the fibrils.

The unit of structure of the individual myofibril is the sarcomere, extending from one Z-line (situated in the midst of the I-band) to the next [Fig. 70]. Attached to each Z-line are a series of thin filaments of actin which interdigitate with thicker myosin filaments, the latter corresponding to the dark (birefringent) A-bands of the myofibrils [Fig. 71]. In cross-section, each filament of myosin is surrounded by a hexagonal array of actin filaments and the actin and myosin filaments are joined by molecular cross-bridges. It now appears that during contraction these cross-bridges repeatedly disengage and re-engage at successive sites on the actin filaments and that as a result the actin and myosin filaments slide upon one another and the myofibril shortens. The biochemical changes which accompany this process are very complex, but it seems that creatine phosphate is broken down in the presence of calcium to creatine and

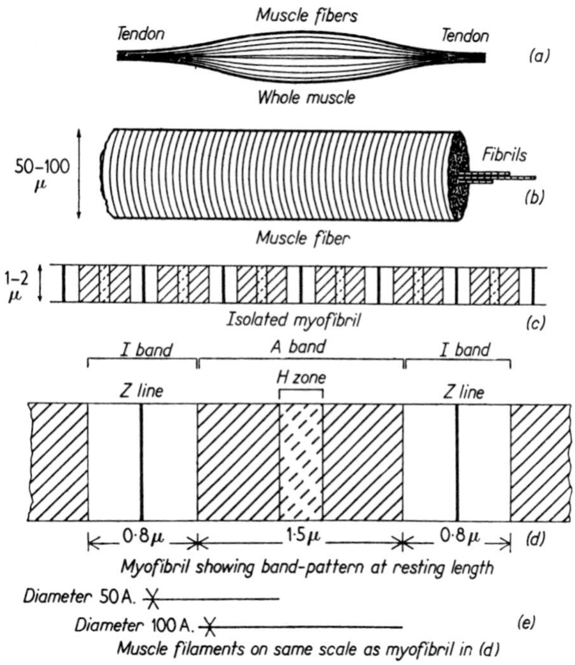

Fig. 70. Diagram illustrating the dimensions and arrangement of the contractile components in a muscle. The whole muscle (a) is made up of fibres (b) which contain cross-striated myofibrils (c, d). These are constructed of two types of protein filaments (e), put together as shown in Fig. 71. [From Huxley, H. E., and Hanson, J. (1960) in *The Structure and Function of Muscle*, ed. Bourne, G. H., Vol. 1, Academic Press Inc., New York.]

phosphate, and adenosine triphosphate (ATP) is broken down to adenosine diphosphate (ADP). This release of high-energy phosphate bonds provides much of the necessary energy.

It has recently been shown that skeletal muscles are not homogeneous and contain at least two main types of muscle fibre which are morphologically and histochemically distinct. The so-called Type I fibre is smaller than the second type, contains myofibrils which are generally somewhat slender, and a large number of mitochondria. Histochemical staining shows that these fibres contain a high concentration of oxidative enzymes and a higher concentration of fat than do the second type. In the larger Type II fibre, which generally has coarser and broader and more widely-dispersed myofibrils, there are fewer mitochondria, less fat is present, but there is a higher concentration of glycogen and a greater amount of enzymes such as phosphorylase which are concerned with anaerobic metabolism. In man, all skeletal muscles contain an admixture of Type I and Type II fibres, so that in sections stained histochemically a typical checkerboard pattern is seen. Physiologically, it is now apparent that the Type I fibres are concerned largely with the maintenance of posture and upon stimulation are found to contract and relax relatively slowly. Type II fibres, by contrast, are more rapidly-contracting (fast-twitch muscles). It now appears that the motor nerve controls not only the physiological behaviour, but also the histochemical structure of the muscle fibres in that transposition of the motor nerve supply from a group of 'fast' fibres to a group of 'slow' ones in animals may reverse the physiological and histochemical characteristics of the fibres.

Finally, certain drugs which act at the neuromuscular junction may be mentioned. Acetylcholine is normally broken down by cholinesterase which is present in the subneural apparatus of the end-plate and can be demonstrated histochemically. Curare acts on the post-junctional membrane and reduces or prevents the depolarizing effect of the acetylcholine released by the nerve impulse. Drugs such as neostigmine destroy cholinesterase and allow acetylcholine to accumulate. Initially this accumulation produces muscular contraction as a result of depolarization of the fibre membrane, but if this substance accumulates in excess, the depolarization persists and may then block the muscle action potential (depolarization block). Whereas drugs such as curare and gallamine compete with acetylcholine for the end-plate chemical receptors and are thus known as competitive inhibitors, drugs such as decamethonium and suxamethonium produce muscle paralysis as a result of depolarization block.

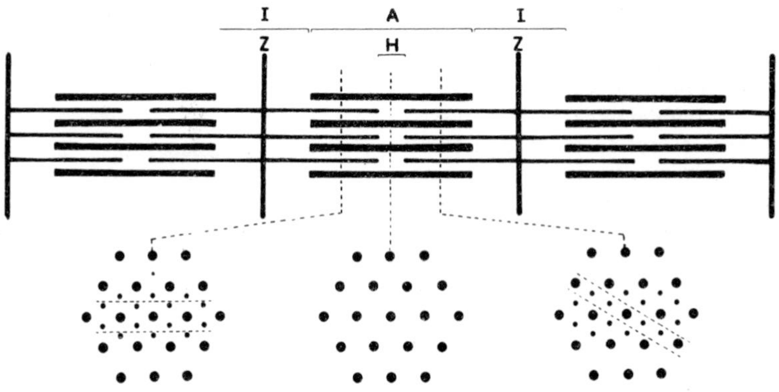

FIG. 71. Diagram illustrating the arrangement of the two kinds of protein filaments (thick filaments—myosin, thin filaments—actin) in a myofibril. At the top are three sarcomeres drawn as they would appear in longitudinal section. Below are transverse sections taken through the H zone and through the other parts of the A band where the thick and thin filaments interdigitate. The plane of section determines whether, in electron micrographs, there seem to be one or two thin (actin) filaments between two thick (myosin) ones. [From Huxley, H. E., and Hanson, J. (1960) in *The Structure and Function of Muscle*, ed. Bourne, G. H., Vol. 1, Academic Press Inc., New York.]

GENERAL COMMENTS ON MUSCLE DISORDERS

Since conditions which affect muscle through disease of the spinal cord, anterior horn cells and peripheral nerves have been dealt with in the preceding pages, this commentary will deal only with those disorders which primarily affect voluntary muscle and the myoneural junction. The term 'myopathy' may reasonably be used to define any disease or syndrome in which the patient's symptoms and/or physical signs can be attributed to pathological, biochemical or electrophysiological changes which are occurring in the muscle fibres or in the muscular interstitial tissues and in which there is no evidence that the symptoms are secondary to disordered function of the central or peripheral nervous system. This group of diseases includes many disorders which are genetically determined, as well as others of a primary biochemical character, and yet others in which the disease process appears to be inflammatory.

Clinical Nosology

Pain, muscular weakness and fatigability are the most important symptoms of muscle disease. Muscle *cramps* occurring in the elderly, particularly in bed at night, are common and may be relieved by a nocturnal dose of quinine or hydantoinates; in younger individuals cramp may follow unaccustomed exertion but can on occasion be a manifestation of metabolic muscle disease. Spontaneous muscle *pain* at rest usually occurs in inflammatory disorders of muscle, but pain experienced on exertion generally implies either muscle ischaemia or a metabolic disorder such as hypothyroidism or phosphorylase deficiency. Muscle *weakness* is the predominant symptom of most varieties of myopathy. It is important to judge its distribution and tempo of development. Thus proximal muscle weakness in the upper limbs gives difficulty in lifting the arms above the head, and in the lower limbs difficulty in climbing stairs and in rising from a low chair. In most of the genetically-determined disorders of muscle, weakness develops gradually over a period of many months or years; a more rapid onset of muscular weakness suggests that the patient is more probably suffering from an inflammatory or metabolic myopathy. Periodic attacks of weakness with complete recovery in between the episodes strongly suggest that the patient may be suffering from one of the group of periodic paralyses. *Fatigability* is characteristic of myasthenia gravis and myasthenic syndromes. The term implies that muscle weakness increases with continuing exercise; many patients mention that the more they exert themselves the weaker they become, and many notice that weakness increases towards the end of the day. The *family history* is also of great importance in that if other members of the family are affected, a genetically-determined disorder of muscle is probable.

On *physical examination*, the importance of a general physical examination must be stressed as there may be changes in the eyes, skin, lymph nodes or viscera indicating that the muscular weakness of which the patient complains is but one manifestation of a systemic multisystem disease. On examining the muscular system itself, the presence of *atrophy*, *hypertrophy* or *fasciculation* of muscle may be of diagnostic value, and so too may the presence of muscular *contractures* with consequent skeletal deformity. Fibrillation (the spontaneous contraction of single muscle fibres) is an electrical phenomenon which can be recorded electromyographically from denervated muscle, but cannot be seen through the intact skin. Fasciculation (the spontaneous contraction of individual muscle fasciculi) is a phenomenon observed most frequently in patients with disease of the anterior horn cells; it is rare in primary muscle disease but may occasionally be seen in polymyositis or thyrotoxic myopathy. Coarse fasciculation, occurring particularly in the lower eye-lid or in the calf muscles, is a benign phenomenon which may be seen in normal individuals, and when such coarse benign fasciculation is widespread and is accompanied by hyperhidrosis, this syndrome is often given the name of *myokymia*. Delayed muscular relaxation after voluntary contraction or following percussion of a muscle is the most prominent feature of *myotonia*, a diagnosis which can be confirmed electromyographically [p. 1314], but in hypothyroidism both muscular contraction and relaxation are greatly slowed and the time-course for the tendon reflexes is characteristically slower than normal. *Myoidema* is a name which has been given to the formation of a localized ridge, lasting for a few seconds after local percussion of a muscle; this type of ridge is electrically silent and the phenomenon tends to occur particularly in patients suffering from malnutrition or cachexia due to malignant disease, though it may also be seen in hypothyroidism. Physiological *contracture*, which differs from the pathological contracture resulting from permanent shortening of muscles and tendons due to fibrosis in chronic muscle disease, in that it is a reversible shortening of muscle lasting for some minutes after exercise, may be seen particularly in muscle phosphorylase deficiency (McArdle's disease). Direct *myotatic irritability* is the name which has been given to the reflex contraction which occurs in the belly of a muscle when it is percussed or stimulated directly by mechanical means. As with the tendon reflexes, this direct reflex response may be accentuated by anxiety but is particularly striking in patients suffering from tetany and hypocalcaemia.

The response of muscle to stretch, i.e. *muscle tone*, is also of diagnostic importance. Increased tone (*spasticity* or *rigidity*) implies disease in the central nervous system, but there are many primary disorders of muscle which give rise to diminished tone (limpness or *hypotonia*); the differential diagnosis of these various disorders may be particularly difficult in infancy. *Palpation* of muscles can also be of diagnostic importance. Tenderness may imply inflammation, an abnormally firm consistency, infiltration with fat, connective tissue, calcium or even the presence of a primary neoplasm, but muscle tumours are rare and localized swellings usually imply either haematoma formation, rupture of a tendon or herniation of muscle tissue through its covering fascia.

The examination of *muscle power* is sufficiently important almost to warrant a chapter to itself. It is sufficient to say that careful testing of the power of individual muscles, combined with an attempt at quantitative assessment, is one of the most important facets of the clinical examination. Different diseases show different *patterns of muscular involvement* and selective atrophy and weakness of certain muscles with sparing of others may be one of the most important clues to the nature of the patient's illness. The *tendon reflexes* in muscle disease are usually diminished or lost when the muscles subserving the particular reflex being examined are involved in the disease process. In general, however, it may be said that in muscular dystrophy the tendon reflexes tend to disappear early, in myasthenia gravis and in polymyositis they remain unexpectedly brisk even in the presence of substantial weakness, and in the myopathy which may accompany metabolic bone disease the reflexes are often exaggerated, even in markedly weakened muscles.

Diagnostic Methods

When involvement of the voluntary muscles is but one part of a systemic, inflammatory or metabolic affliction, a considerable number of investigations, including differential white cell counts, erythrocyte sedimentation rate, serum electrophoresis, estimations of the serum electrolytes and of calcium and phosphorus, may be of relevance and, where considered

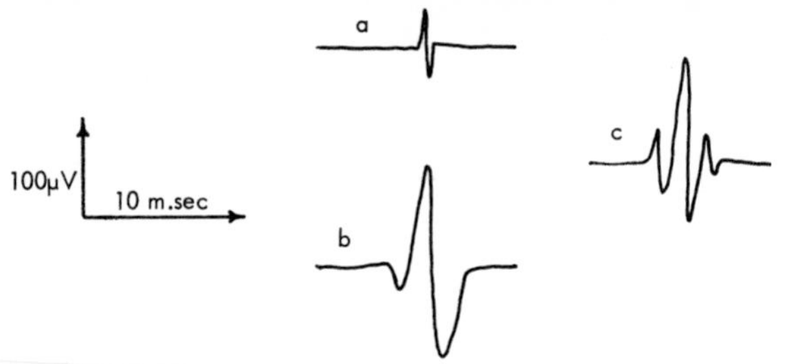

FIG. 72. Diagrammatic representation of muscle action potentials recorded in the electromyogram; a = fibrillation (single fibre) potential; b = triphasic motor unit action potential; c = polyphasic motor unit potential.

individually to be important, will be mentioned in relation to specific disease entities. In any patient suffering from muscular weakness, it is first necessary to determine whether the weakness is secondary to disease primarily involving other tissues or organs, and if such a process can be excluded, the next step is to determine whether the pathological process responsible for the syndrome lies in the lower motor neurone, at the myoneural junction or in the muscle itself. The techniques which are most valuable in providing this information, in distinguishing between neuropathic and myopathic disorders on the one hand and between specific myopathic conditions on the other, are respectively electromyography, biochemical techniques, of which serum enzyme studies are by far the most important, and finally muscle biopsy.

Electromyography. In neuropathic disorders, spontaneous fibrillation potentials may be recorded from a relaxed and resting muscle which is undergoing an active process of denervation; these fibrillation potentials are usually diphasic or triphasic spikes of about 1 msec. duration and 100 mV. in amplitude [FIG. 72] and are generally easy to distinguish from motor unit action potentials [FIG. 72]. The pattern of motor unit activity on volition is reduced [FIG. 72], but the surviving motor unit potentials are either normal or increased in size. In the myopathies, spontaneous fibrillation is uncommon though it may be seen in polymyositis and less often in muscular dystrophy. Myotonia is accompanied by a characteristic discharge of high-frequency activity evoked by movement of the exploring electrode and waxing and waning repeatedly to give a characteristic appearance on the cathode ray oscilloscope and a typical sound in the loudspeaker, the so-called 'dive-bomber' note. Volitional activity in all of the myopathies, including fatigued muscle in patients with myasthenia, demon-

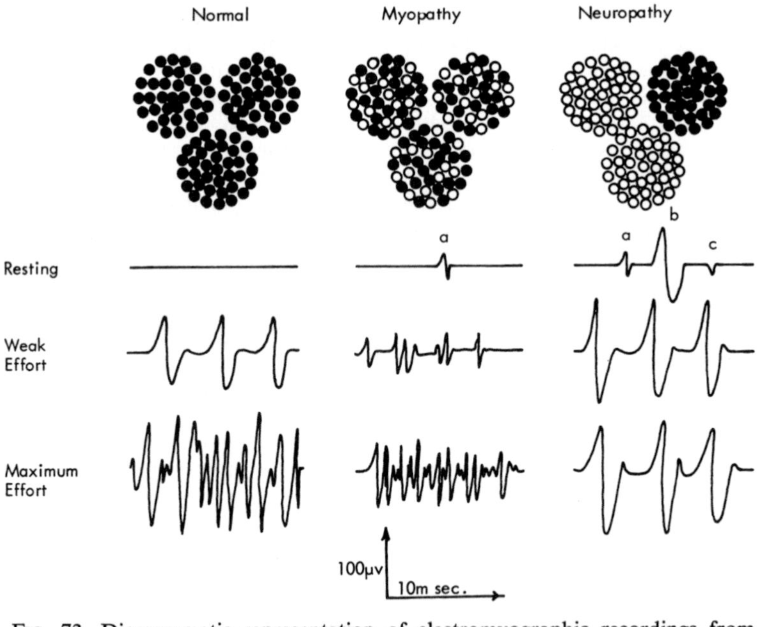

FIG. 73. Diagrammatic representation of electromyographic recordings from normal muscle, from myopathic muscle and from partially denervated muscle (redrawn from an illustration from R. J. Johns). a = spontaneous fibrillation; b = fasiculation potential; c = positive sharp wave ('saw-tooth potential').

Normal muscle is silent at rest, shows discrete motor unit action potentials during weak effort and a full 'interference pattern' of motor unit action potentials during maximum effort. In myopathy, spontaneous fibrillation is occasionally recorded, while during volition the motor unit action potentials are of short duration and of low amplitude, or else polyphasic; the interference pattern is full but of low amplitude and 'spiky' or complex. In partially denervated muscle, spontaneous fibrillation, fasciculation and positive sharp waves may be recorded, while on weak effort the surviving motor units are either normal or larger than normal in size, and on maximum effort the interference pattern is reduced and made up sometimes of discrete motor unit action potentials.

strates a breakdown of the motor unit action potentials with a consequent increase in the proportion of short-duration and polyphasic potentials [FIG. 73]. Measurement of these volitional potentials shows that the mean action potential duration is increased and that the motor unit territory is diminished.

Nerve conduction velocity measurements are normal in all of the primary myopathies. In myasthenia gravis, supramaximal stimulation of the motor nerve supply to a myasthenic muscle at a rate of 3–5 per sec. may give a progressive diminution in the amplitude of the evoked action potential [FIG. 74] (the myasthenic response). This is only seen in muscles clinically affected by the disease. At tetanic rates of stimulation (50 per sec.) the amplitude of the evoked action potential may actually increase markedly in cases of the myasthenic-myopathic syndrome which may complicate lung cancer [FIG. 74].

Biochemical Diagnosis. In the various endocrine myopathies to be described below, many tests related to the diagnosis of individual endocrine disorders may be required. In the periodic paralysis syndromes, in addition to serial estimations of serum potassium level and measures designed to precipitate attacks for diagnostic purposes, there are cases in which the sodium and potassium output in the urine, and even sodium and potassium balance, may need to be measured. In patients with generalized muscle pain and weakness, myoglobin must be sought in the urine, while in individuals suffering muscle pain after effort, it may be necessary to exclude certain forms of glycogen storage disease by measuring the lactate and pyruvate in venous blood distal to a tourniquet following a period of ischaemic work. In such cases estimations of phosphorylase and of other glycolytic enzymes in muscle biopsy samples may also be required.

In cases of muscle disease in general, there may be an excessive urinary output of creatine and diminished creatinuria, but these findings are non-specific, as is the amino-aciduria which may occur in a proportion of cases. The serum aldolase and the serum transaminases (aminotransferases) may be substantially raised in various forms of myopathy including the more rapidly progressive varieties of muscular dystrophy and polymyositis, but the most useful enzyme in the diagnosis of muscle disease is unquestionably now creatine kinase (normal <60 I.U./litre). In early cases of muscular dystrophy of the Duchenne type, a 300-fold increase in the serum activity of this enzyme may be found and changes of similar magnitude are observed in certain cases of acute and subacute polymyositis. Less striking rises in activity may be observed in patients suffering from other more indolent forms of myopathy and from the more benign varieties of muscular dystrophy. In some of the endocrine and metabolic myopathies and in the benign congenital myopathies, the activity of this enzyme is not infrequently normal, as is generally the case in patients suffering from muscular weakness secondary to disease of the anterior horn cell or motor nerve. The sole exception to the latter rule is that in some patients with benign spinal muscular atrophy (the Kugelberg-Welander syndrome) moderate increases in serum creatine kinase have been observed.

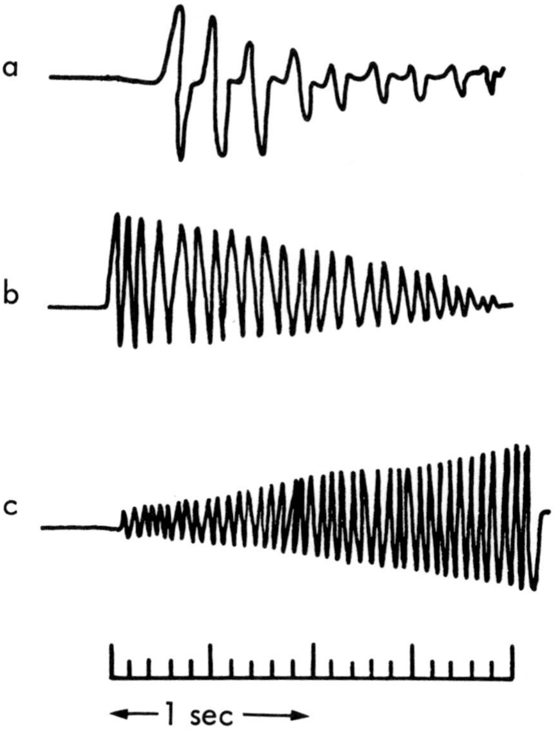

FIG. 74. Recording of evoked muscle action potentials from one hypothenar eminence during supramaximal stimulation of the ulnar nerve. a. Myasthenia gravis; stimulation at 5/sec., demonstrating a progressive decrement in the amplitude of the evoked potential. b. Myasthenia gravis; a similar decrement is observed at tetanic (30/sec.) rates of stimulation. c. Myasthenic-myopathic syndrome; during stimulation at 50/sec. there is an increment in the amplitude of the evoked potential.

Muscle Biopsy. While it is generally possible on the basis of the findings observed in sections of muscle obtained by biopsy to distinguish with reasonable confidence between muscular atrophy secondary to denervation on the one hand and that resulting from primary myopathic processes on the other, differential diagnosis between the various forms of myopathy is much less exact. Modern techniques, including intravital staining of the motor end-plate, histochemistry, tissue culture and electron microscopy, have yielded information of considerable value from the point of view of research, but have as yet added relatively little precision to histological diagnosis, except that 'fibre type grouping' (large groups of fibres of uniform histochemical type) is usually diagnostic of chronic denervation atrophy. The histological features observed in cases of muscular dystrophy are similar in all varieties of the disease, though varying considerably in severity. The most common changes are marked variations in fibre size, fibre-splitting, the central migration of sarcolemmal nuclei, patchy atrophy of individual muscle fibres, the formation of nuclear chains, the presence of segmental areas of necrosis within muscle fibres with phagocytosis of necrotic sarcoplasm, and basophilia of sarcoplasm with an enlargement of sarcolemmal nuclei showing prominent nucleoli (changes construed as being regenerative in character); there is also a progressive infiltration by fat cells and connective tissue. In subacute or chronic polymyositis, the changes may be very similar, but in this condition signs of muscle fibre destruction and repair (necrosis, phagocytosis and regeneration) are usually more striking and widespread; in addition, in this disease there may be interstitial or perivascular infiltrations of inflammatory cells such as lymphocytes or plasma cells; the absence of these does not, however, exclude the diagnosis of polymyositis. There are cases in which distinction between muscular dystrophy on the one hand and polymyositis on the other is impossible on histological grounds alone. In some cases of myasthenia gravis and in thyrotoxic and other endocrine myopathies, focal collections of lymphocytes (lymphorrhages) may be seen, either around blood vessels or between fibres, but in many patients with thyrotoxic and other endocrine myopathies, and in the myasthenic-myopathic syndrome complicating bronchial carcinoma, histological changes are frequently mild and non-specific. Striated annulets or so-called *ringbinden*, in which striated myofibrils encircle muscle fibres cut in transverse section, are often seen in biopsies from patients with myotonic dystrophy but can also be observed in other forms of muscle disease; in myotonic dystrophy, chains of nuclei within the muscle fibres are particularly prominent and there may also be peripheral masses of palely-staining homogeneous sarcoplasm (sarcoplasmic masses) but these, too, are non-specific and have been noted in some patients with muscular involvement in myxoedema.

Vacuolar change within muscle fibres, if striking and widespread, may imply the storage of abnormal metabolites within the cells and this pattern is particularly seen in cases of glycogen storage disease. Widespread but less striking vacuolar change may often be seen in muscle biopsies taken from patients with periodic paralysis during the attacks and rarely in patients with systemic lupus erythematosus and in others suffering from a myopathy resulting from long-continued chloroquine administration. In some of the rare benign congenital and non-progressive myopathies described in recent years, special stains of muscle biopsy sections may be required in order to demonstrate the specific morphological abnormalities of the muscle fibre which have been described in these various disorders and which will be mentioned in the appropriate sections.

THE MUSCULAR DYSTROPHIES

While muscular dystrophy can reasonably be defined as genetically determined primary degenerative myopathy, it must be noted that there are a number of other rare myopathies which will be referred to later which are also genetically determined but which are not normally regarded as being muscular dystrophies in the accepted sense of the term.

Classification

Classification of a case of muscular dystrophy is the only safe guide to prognosis and genetic counselling and the most satisfactory clinicogenetic classification based upon current knowledge is as follows:

The 'pure' muscular dystrophies:

1. X-linked muscular dystrophy.
   Severe (Duchenne type)
   Benign (Becker type)
2. Autosomal recessive muscular dystrophy:
   Limb-girdle type
   Childhood muscular dystrophy (except Duchenne)
   Congenital muscular dystrophies
3. Facioscapulohumeral muscular dystrophy (autosomal dominant)
4. Distal muscular dystrophy
5. Ocular muscular dystrophy
6. Oculopharyngeal muscular dystrophy

Although this classification would seem to be the most satisfactory at the present time, there are still some cases which are difficult to fit into any of the groups described.

Aetiology

Though all forms of muscular dystrophy are genetically determined, the exact nature of the process which causes the muscles to waste is as yet unknown. Some recent evidence has raised the possibility that a defect of neuronal trophic substance, rather than an abnormality of the muscle fibre itself, may be an important factor. The condition is comparatively rare, but appears to be world-wide, affecting all races; the Duchenne type is the commonest, but it has been estimated that there are probably 10,000 cases of muscular dystrophy of all kinds in the United Kingdom at any one time.

Pathology

Although the nature of the pathological process which causes the muscular weakness and wasting in these cases is similar in character though different in tempo in the various clinical and genetic types, there are certain other features, including differences in the pattern of muscular involvement and in the degree to which enzymes such as creatine kinase leak into the serum in the different forms of the disease, which strongly suggest that they may eventually prove to be different diseases from the aetiological standpoint. While fibre necrosis and phagocytosis and abortive regenerative activity are commonly seen in muscle biopsy samples obtained in the early stages of the disease, and particularly in the more rapidly-progressive clinical forms, in the later stages infiltration with fat and connective tissue, marked variation in fibre size and central nucleation of many muscle fibres are the predominant findings.

Electromyography

Electromyography reveals volitional activity characteristic of any form of myopathy, and spontaneous activity is usually absent on recording from relaxed, resting muscle.

Symptoms and Signs

These depend upon the muscles which are first involved by the disease process and upon its rate of progress. Weakness of pelvic girdle muscles gives rise to slowness in walking, inability to run, frequent falling, difficulty in climbing stairs or in rising from the floor, and eventually the patients develop accentuation of the lumbar lordosis and a characteristic waddling gait. Climbing up the legs on rising from the floor (Gowers' sign) is a characteristic feature but is not specific for muscular dystrophy as it occurs in any disorder in which pelvic girdle muscles are weakened. Involvement of the shoulder girdles gives a sloping appearance of the shoulders with a tendency for the scapulae to rise prominently when the patient attempts to abduct the arms. Many patients use trick movements by placing one hand beneath the other elbow in order to lift the hand to the face or head. Facial weakness, as seen in facioscapulohumeral dystrophy, causes inability to whistle and difficulty in pouting the lips or in closing the eyes, while distal weakness in the extremities (as seen in the distal variety) causes weakness of the grip and of fine finger movement, and footdrop. Contractures are a common feature of all forms of muscular dystrophy in the later stages, but are seen particularly in the severe Duchenne type. They may be due to weakness developing in muscles whose antagonists remain powerful (this accounts for the equinovarus deformity of the feet which occurs in advancing cases of the Duchenne type and which causes the children to walk on their toes; it is due to weakness of anterior tibial muscles while those of the calf remain powerful). Contractures are also accentuated by postural changes developing in patients confined to a wheelchair when biceps and hamstrings usually shorten. The most important clinical characteristic of all forms of muscular dystrophy is that muscles are picked out by the disease in a selective manner. Though there are certain differences in the pattern of weakness and wasting seen in the various subvarieties, it is common in the upper limbs to find that the serrati and pectoral muscles are weakened and atrophic, as are biceps and brachioradialis, while deltoid and triceps remain relatively unaffected. In the lower limbs, quadriceps and anterior tibials are usually involved first, and the calf muscles are spared, but in limb-girdle muscular dystrophy the hamstrings and quadriceps are often affected equally.

THE SEVERE X-LINKED DUCHENNE TYPE

Though there is ample evidence to indicate that this condition is due to a sex-linked recessive gene, over half of the affected boys appear to be isolated cases and in these individuals the disease is presumed to have resulted from genetic mutation occurring in the ovarian cells of the mother or maternal grandmother.

The condition usually becomes apparent clinically towards the end of the third year of life with slowness in walking, frequent falling and difficulty in climbing stairs. Enlargement of the calf muscles and sometimes of quadriceps and deltoids occurs in about 90 per cent. of cases at some stage, but later disappears. There is evidence to suggest that this phenomenon, often referred to in the past as pseudohypertrophy, is more often due to true compensatory hypertrophy of unaffected muscle fibres. Most patients deteriorate steadily and become unable to walk by about the age of 10 years, but apparent improvement may occur between the ages of 5 and 8 years when the rate of deterioration is outstripped by the processes of normal development. When the child is confined to a wheelchair, progressive deformity and skeletal distortion and atrophy occur and death usually results from inanition, respiratory infection or cardiac failure towards the end of the second decade. Some affected boys waste progressively, but others become obese; macroglossia and absence of certain incisor teeth are occasionally seen. The intelligence quotient in these cases is 10 per cent. or more lower than in a group of control children of comparable age and sex. Skeletal atrophy may so affect the shafts of long bones that they fracture on minimal trauma. Involvement of cardiac muscle is invariable, though not clinically detectable in the early stages; the electrocardiogram typically shows tall R waves in the right precordial leads and deep Q waves in the limb and left precordial leads.

THE BENIGN X-LINKED (BECKER) TYPE

This disorder differs from the severe Duchenne variety in that the onset of the disease is usually between the fifth and twenty-fifth years, the disorder may be transmitted by affected males through carrier daughters to their grandsons, there is often an initial phase of generalized muscular hypertrophy before weakness becomes apparent, and there is gradually progressive weakness and wasting of pelvic and later of shoulder-girdle muscles, so that most patients become unable to walk 25 years or more after the onset. Cardiac involvement is usually absent, contractures and skeletal deformity occur late, and many patients, though severely disabled, survive to a normal age.

Carrier Detection

The sisters of males suffering from the two X-linked forms of muscular dystrophy described above have on genetic grounds a 50-50 chance of being carriers and of passing on the disease to their sons; half of the sons of a female carrier are likely to be affected and half of her daughters will themselves be carriers. An important recent advance has been the discovery that female carriers of the gene responsible for the severe X-linked Duchenne type of the disease can usually be detected by means of serum creatine kinase estimation, quantitative electromyography and possibly by muscle biopsy. To date, a smaller proportion of carriers of the benign Becker type are detectable by these methods. This is, however, an important practical advance since if carriers can be detected and do not reproduce, the incidence of the disease will diminish in the future, though cases will continue to arise as a result of mutation.

LIMB-GIRDLE MUSCULAR DYSTROPHY

This form of the disease occurs equally in the two sexes and usually begins in the second or third decade of life, but occasionally first appears in middle life. Though usually inherited by an autosomal recessive mechanism, many cases appear to be sporadic and some may be due to manifestation in the heterozygote. In about half the cases muscle weakness begins in the shoulder-girdle muscles and may not spread to involve the pelvic girdle for many years, but in the remaining half the pelvic-girdle muscles are first involved and weakness affects the shoulders within about 10 years. Enlargement of the calf muscles is not uncommon. Sometimes muscular weakness and wasting are asymmetrical initially and occasionally the disease process arrests temporarily, but most patients are severely disabled within 20 years after the onset. The course of the disease is generally more benign in those in whom the upper limb muscles are first involved. Contractures and skeletal deformity occur late in the course of the disease but progress more rapidly when the patient is confined to a wheelchair. Most sufferers are severely disabled in middle life and many die before the normal age. Many patients regarded in the past as suffering from this condition have been found to be cases of benign spinal muscular atrophy (the Kugelberg-Welander syndrome).

CHILDHOOD MUSCULAR DYSTROPHY WITH AUTOSOMAL RECESSIVE INHERITANCE

The existence of this uncommon form of the disease has been demonstrated by the very occasional occurrence of muscular dystrophy resembling the Duchenne type in young girls and occurring in a few families in which parental consanguinity has made autosomal recessive inheritance seem likely. This form of the disease is clinically similar to the Duchenne type, but more benign. The onset may be in the second year or as late as the fourteenth, but is most often in the second half of the first decade. Progression is comparatively slow and patients usually become unable to walk in their early twenties, but sometimes as early as 15 years or as late as 40 years. The pattern of weakness is very similar to that observed in the typical severe X-linked Duchenne type and most patients die in middle life.

CONGENITAL MUSCULAR DYSTROPHY

This rare disorder presents with severe and generalized muscular hypotonia which is noted from birth and which is followed by the subsequent development of progressive muscular wasting and weakness. In many affected children there are widespread muscular contractures suggesting arthrogryposis multiplex congenita. Occasionally the muscular weakness increases rapidly after birth and the disease terminates fatally within the first year of life, but there are other cases in which the condition appears to be relatively non-progressive. Few affected patients are ever capable, however, of sitting or standing unsupported and the prognosis is uniformly unfavourable. Diagnosis from spinal muscular atrophy of infancy can only be made with confidence by means of electromyography, serum enzyme studies and muscle biopsy. The occasional involvement of sibs supports the suggestion that this rare disorder may be due to an autosomal recessive gene. It may be distinguished from the various benign congenital myopathies to be discussed later in this chapter, first by its severity and secondly by the fact that in this condition the histological changes in muscle biopsy specimens are similar to those observed in other forms of muscular dystrophy.

FACIOSCAPULOHUMERAL MUSCULAR DYSTROPHY

This variety, which is inherited by an autosomal dominant mechanism, occurs equally in the two sexes, can begin at any age from childhood until adult life but is usually first recognized in adolescence. Facial involvement, with a typical pouting appearance of the lips and difficulty in closing the eyes, is apparent early and is accompanied by weakness of the shoulder-girdle muscles with bilateral winging of the scapulae and wasting of the pectorals. Muscular enlargement is uncommon in this form of the disease; in the lower extremities the anterior tibial muscles are often the first to be involved, causing bilateral foot-drop. In most patients the disease is benign and runs a prolonged course with periods of apparent arrest, so that muscular contractures and skeletal deformity are late in developing. There are some patients in whom the condition progresses more rapidly and severe accentuation of the lumbar lordosis is seen at an early stage; by contrast, in others the disease process is abortive and after certain muscles have been affected, the spread of weakness appears to cease. Most affected individuals survive and remain active until a normal age. The heart muscle is not involved and the range of intelligence is normal.

DISTAL MUSCULAR DYSTROPHY

This variety is rare in Britain and in the United States, but is not uncommon in Sweden. It is generally inherited as an autosomal dominant character, beginning usually between the ages of 40 and 60 years and involving both sexes. Weakness begins in the small muscles of the hands and in the anterior tibial muscles and calves, but eventually spreads to proximal muscles, unlike the pattern observed in peroneal muscular atrophy with which the disorder is most often confused. In Sweden the condition is comparatively benign, but sporadic cases observed in other countries tend to be more severe and rapidly progressive.

OCULAR MYOPATHY

This disorder usually begins with progressive bilateral ptosis and goes on to give progressive bilateral external ophthalmoplegia. In the past the condition was referred to in the literature as 'progressive nuclear ophthalmoplegia', but pathological studies have shown that the muscular weakness in such cases is almost invariably myopathic. Most patients also have some weakness of the upper facial muscles (particularly orbicularis oculi) and often the neck and shoulder-girdle muscles are slender and slightly weak. Most cases are sporadic, but the condition is sometimes inherited by an autosomal dominant mechanism.

OCULOPHARYNGEAL MUSCULAR DYSTROPHY

Whereas ocular myopathy, as described above, commonly begins in early adult life, this condition usually develops first in middle life but otherwise differs only from ocular myopathy in that dysphagia is an invariable symptom due to pharyngeal muscular involvement. The condition is slow to progress, the prognosis in general is good as disability usually remains slight for many years. Many reported cases have been of French-Canadian ancestry.

DIAGNOSIS

In the typical case of muscular dystrophy showing the usual slowly progressive pattern of increasing muscular weakness and selective atrophy of the proximal limb muscles, diagnosis is rarely in doubt. If the pattern of weakness and wasting is obscured by subcutaneous fat, or when involvement is predominantly distal, it may not always be easy to distinguish muscular dystrophy from neuropathic disorders; here, electromyography may be of particular value. This is particularly true in making the distinction between limb-girdle muscular dystrophy on the one hand and benign spinal muscular atrophy (the Kugelberg-Welander syndrome) on the other, as these two conditions may be readily confused. Polymyositis may also resemble muscular dystrophy of the limb-girdle type; in polymyositis, however, the onset is often more rapid, muscular weakness and wasting are less selective, neck muscles are frequently involved and dysphagia is common, while the family history is negative; associated phenomena such as skin changes and the Raynaud syndrome occurring in such cases may be conclusive.

Estimation of the serum creatine kinase is of particular value in diagnosing muscular dystrophy of the Duchenne type, since in early cases of this type it may be increased almost 300-fold (up to 20,000 I.U./litre). Less striking increases up to 10 or 20 times the normal upper limit may be observed in the other more benign varieties of muscular dystrophy, and surprisingly in congenital muscular dystrophy the activity of this enzyme is often little increased.

The value of muscle biopsy has already been commented upon.

TREATMENT

Unfortunately no drug has any influence upon the course of the disease, though complications such as respiratory and urinary infections may demand antibiotics. Physical exercise appears to delay the march of the weakness and the onset of contractures, and a regular programme of such activities may be started under the supervision of a skilled physiotherapist and subsequently continued at home by the patients and their relatives. Passive stretching of those tendons which show a tendency to shorten should also be carried out regularly. In some cases, light spinal supports may help to delay the development of skeletal deformity and in occasional cases, too, calipers are valuable; surgical lengthening of shortened tendons is only to be advised if this can be followed by immediate mobilization of the patient in walking plasters or calipers. Immobilization or prolonged periods of bed-rest are to be avoided as these inevitably cause rapid deterioration. Psychological management may demand considerable reserves of patience and understanding on the part of parents, doctors, nurses and social workers. Optimism and encouragement, however unjustifiable in the face of continuing deterioration, are of great importance.

COURSE AND PROGNOSIS

This has been mentioned in relation to the individual subvarieties of the disease.

MYOTONIC DISORDERS

Myotonia is the continued act of contraction of a muscle which persists after the cessation of voluntary effort or stimulation; an electrical after-discharge can be seen to accompany the phenomenon in the electromyogram. Clinically it is best demonstrated as a slowness in relaxation of the grip or by a persistent dimpling after a sharp blow on a muscle belly, e.g. in the thenar eminence or tongue. It seems to be due to an abnormality of the muscle fibre, as it persists after section or blocking of the motor nerve and after curarization. It occurs in three hereditary syndromes, all of autosomal dominant inheritance, namely myotonia congenita, dystrophia myotonica and paramyotonia. While it has been suggested that these three disorders may be variants of a single disease process, in most families the three conditions breed true and they are best regarded as different diseases. While dystrophic changes occur in certain muscles in one of these conditions, namely dystrophia myotonica, these disorders are more closely related to each other than they are to the muscular dystrophies. There appears to be a definite relationship between paramyotonia on the one hand and the periodic paralyses on the other.

In a rare syndrome, variously called 'one form of myokymia', 'pseudomyotonia', 'neuromyotonia', 'the myotonia-myokymia-hyperhidrosis syndrome' and 'a syndrome of continuous muscle fibre activity and spasm', a phenomenon similar clinically but electrically different from myotonia is associated with myokymia (benign coarse fasciculation), cramps, hyperhidrosis and sometimes muscle wasting. Its nature is little understood, but the impaired relaxation in these cases, like that of myotonia, seems to be relieved by hydantoin preparations.

MYOTONIA CONGENITA

Synonym. Thomsen's disease.

This condition is usually present from birth, but symptoms may not appear until the end of the first decade. Myotonia is generalized, accentuated by rest and by cold and gradually relieved by exercise. In infancy, these children are often difficult to feed and have a peculiarly strangled cry. Later, myotonia of the tongue may give rise to difficulty in speaking. Diffuse hypertrophy of muscles usually persists throughout life, though the myotonia tends to improve with increasing age; rarely, it increases during exertion (myotonia paradoxa) but must then be distinguished from the cramping stiffness of McArdle's disease. Hypertrophia musculorum vera may well be a variant of this condition.

DYSTROPHIA MYOTONICA

Dystrophia myotonica (myotonia atrophica) is a diffuse systemic disorder in which myotonia and distal muscular atrophy are accompanied by cataracts, frontal baldness in the male, gonadal atrophy, cardiomyopathy, impaired pulmonary ventilation, mild endocrine anomalies, bone changes, mental defect or dementia, and abnormalities of the serum immunoglobulins. The affected families show progressive social decline in successive generations, diminished fertility and an increased infantile mortality rate. The condition is about as common as muscular dystrophy of the Duchenne type.

The presenting symptom is usually weakness of the hands and difficulty in walking, and myotonia is rarely obtrusive. Poor vision, weight-loss, impotence, ptosis and increased sweating are common. The condition may present in infancy and childhood with severe muscular weakness and hypotonia or delay in walking, and these children may be erroneously regarded as examples of benign congenital myopathy or hypotonia unless the existence of myotonic dystrophy in other members of the family is recognized. More commonly the condition begins between the ages of 20 and 50 years.

The facial appearance is characteristically long and haggard; ptosis is usual and occasionally there is external ophthalmoplegia. Wasting of the masseters, temporal muscles and sternomastoids is invariable and in the extremities weakness and wasting involves particularly forearm muscles, the anterior tibial group and the calves and peronei. Slit-lamp examination reveals cataracts in most cases. Cardiac involvement is common and the pulmonary vital capacity and maximum expiratory pressure are often impaired, so that many patients tolerate barbiturate anaesthesia poorly. Dysphagia can be shown to be due to disordered oesophageal contraction. The testes are usually small and histologically the changes are like those of Klinefelter's syndrome. Females often show irregular menstruation, infertility and prolonged parturition. Pituitary function is usually normal, but there may be a selective failure of adrenal androgenic function and occasionally thyroid activity and glucose utilization are impaired. Hyperostosis of the skull vault and a small sella turcica are frequently observed radiologically, while both mental defect and progressive dementia occur. There is a high incidence of abnormal electroencephalograms in such cases, and air encephalography may show progressive cerebral ventricular enlargement. Excessive catabolism of immunoglobulin-G has been demonstrated in some cases.

PARAMYOTONIA

This condition is characterized by myotonia which appears only on exposure to cold. In addition, patients experience attacks of generalized muscular weakness like those of familial periodic paralysis, but in these attacks, as in adynamia episodica hereditaria (*vide infra*), the serum potassium usually rises. Myotonia in the upper lids on looking upwards may be particularly prominent in these cases.

DIAGNOSIS

Myotonia must be distinguished from the slowness of muscular contraction and relaxation which may occur in hypothyroidism and from the similar clinical phenomenon of delayed relaxation with prolonged dimpling on percussion of muscle which may occasionally be seen in patients with polymyositis, polyneuropathy and spinal muscular atrophy. The pain and contracture which may follow exertion in patients with myophosphorylase deficiency (McArdle's disease) may also give rise to diagnostic difficulty, but these various disorders may be distinguished with confidence electromyographically. The distal muscular wasting and areflexia seen in dystrophia myotonica, and the diffuse muscular hypotonia occurring in affected infants, may readily be confused with the similar phenomena which may occur in other diseases of the neuromuscular apparatus unless the presence of myotonia is recognized either clinically or electromyographically in the patient or in his relatives. In dystrophia myotonica, the electromyogram demonstrates not only myotonic discharges evoked by movement of the exploring electrode, but myopathic potentials are recorded from the weakened and wasted muscles during volition. The serum creatine kinase activity is normal in myotonia congenita and paramyotonia, but may be raised to between 2 and 10 times the normal upper limit in myotonic dystrophy. In muscle biopsy samples, cases of myotonia congenita and paramyotonia may show nothing more than hypertrophy of muscle fibres, but in myotonic dystrophy changes similar to those of muscular dystrophy may be seen in addition to frequent long chains of nuclei in the centre of muscle fibres, combined with numerous ringed annulets and peripheral sarcoplasmic masses.

TREATMENT

In dystrophia myotonica, no treatment influences the progressive muscular wasting and weakness which eventually develops. In paramyotonia, treatment depends upon whether the paralysis is shown to be hypo- or hyperkalaemic in type (*vide infra*). Myotonia itself can, however, be relieved by drugs and this is particularly helpful in myotonia congenita and in some patients with myotonic dystrophy in whom myotonia is severe. Quinine and prednisone help in some cases, but procainamide in a dosage of 250–500 mg. three or four times daily is superior, and sodium hydantoinate in a dosage of 100 mg. three or four times daily is probably the most effective remedy of all.

Course and Prognosis

Myotonia congenita is essentially a benign disorder which does not shorten life, and the same is true of paramyotonia. Most patients with dystrophia myotonica, however, show progressive deterioration and become severely disabled and unable to walk within 15–20 years of the onset. Death from respiratory infection or cardiac failure usually occurs well before the normal age.

INFLAMMATORY DISEASES OF MUSCLE

SPECIFIC INFECTIONS

Muscle may be involved secondarily by suppuration

arising in skin, bone or connective tissue and extensive necrosis may follow trauma as a result of infection with the anaerobic organism of gas gangrene. Acute myositis can result from infection with viruses of the Coxsackie group; in Bornholm disease, pain in the trunk muscles and particularly in the chest wall related to deep breathing and coughing occurs, but the disorder usually recovers spontaneously within a few days. In trichiniasis due to the ingestion of infested pork, fleeting muscle pain and tenderness may be accompanied by periorbital oedema and the *Trichinella spiralis* is sometimes detectable on muscle biopsy.

MUSCULAR INVOLVEMENT IN COLLAGEN OR CONNECTIVE TISSUE DISEASES

In rheumatoid arthritis, muscle biopsy sections may demonstrate foci of inflammatory cell infiltration, but this focal nodular myositis is not usually accompanied by specific muscular wasting and weakness, save for that resulting secondarily from joint disease. In sarcoidosis, however, muscle involvement may cause a subacute weakness and wasting of proximal muscles and typical sarcoid granulomas may be observed on muscle biopsy. Localized muscle pain, subcutaneous oedema and tenderness can occur as a result of muscle infarction in polyarteritis nodosa. In systemic lupus erythematosus, muscular involvement is sometimes severe and diffuse and is then indistinguishable from polymyositis although in occasional such cases muscle biopsies demonstrate a vacuolar myopathy.

POLYMYOSITIS

This term is generally used to identify a group of cases in which muscular weakness and wasting may be associated with muscle pain and tenderness or with evidence of some form of connective tissue or collagen disease. The term is commonly used to include cases with florid skin change which are more properly called dermatomyositis; it is usually taken to indicate the so-called idiopathic syndrome and excludes disorders such as polymyalgia rheumatica [see Section 4] and also acute myositis resulting from infections with micro-organisms and viruses. With the exception of the specific myasthenic-myopathic syndrome [p. 1324] which has been observed in patients with lung cancer, it seems that most cases of so-called carcinomatous myopathy probably belong to the syndrome of polymyositis.

Aetiology

Recent work demonstrating that polymyositis may be produced in animals by the injection of muscle homogenates with Freund's adjuvant supports the view that this syndrome in the human may well be the result of hypersensitivity or of autoimmune processes. It may therefore be suggested that polymyositis in which clinical evidence suggests that the disease process is limited to muscle, may be regarded as an organ-specific autoimmune disease, while in cases showing involvement of skin or joints, it can be accepted as being the muscular manifestation of non-organ-specific autoimmune disease. The commonly demonstrated relationship between polymyositis and dermatomyositis on the one hand and malignant disease on the other suggests that the condition may also on occasion be the result of a conditioned auto-immune response in patients suffering from cancer. Attempts to demonstrate specific antimuscle antibodies in the serum of patients with polymyositis have to date been unsuccessful, but the close relationship of the condition to other disorders of the connective tissue group is underlined by the occurrence of certain cases which may successively present manifestations of polymyositis, systemic lupus erythematosus and/or scleroderma or systemic sclerosis.

Polymyositis is world-wide, occurs in many races and appears to be commoner in men. It is more common in adult life than muscular dystrophy, but is less common than the latter in childhood. About 15 per cent. of cases occur under the age of 15 years, another 15 per cent. between the ages of 16 and 30, about a quarter between 31 and 45, and a third between the ages of 45 and 60. It usually develops spontaneously but can follow febrile illness or the administration of various drugs including sulphonamides.

Classification

The following four clinical categories of polymyositis have been arbitrarily defined:

Group I:

- Polymyositis
  - Acute, with myoglobinuria
  - Subacute or chronic
    - in childhood
    - in early adult life
    - in middle or late life

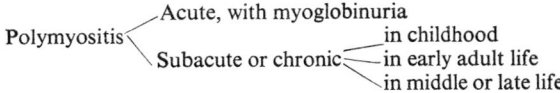

Group II: Polymyositis with dominant muscular weakness but with some evidence of an associated collagen disease or dermatomyositis with severe muscular disability and with minimal or transient skin changes.
Group III: Polymyositis complicating severe collagen disease, e.g. rheumatoid arthritis, or dermatomyositis with florid skin changes and minor muscle weakness.
Group IV: Polymyositis complicating malignant disease (including 'carcinomatous myopathy' and dermatomyositis occurring in patients with malignant disease).

Symptoms and Signs

Apart from occasional acute cases in which widespread muscle pain, fever, constitutional upset and rapidly progressive paralysis, often with respiratory weakness, may develop, the condition usually runs a subacute or chronic course. Muscle pain and tenderness occur in approximately 50 per cent. of cases, as does dysphagia. Cutaneous manifestations are seen in about two-thirds of all patients and may take the form of widespread erythema with desquamation seen particularly on the face and on other exposed areas of the trunk, but occasionally involving the whole body. Heliotrope erythema around the eyes and periorbital oedema are particularly characteristic and so, too, is congestion of the nail beds. Sometimes the skin changes are slight in the form of a faint butterfly-type rash on the face, while in others, particularly in childhood, there may be ulceration over bony prominences with subcutaneous calcification. Raynaud's syndrome is a common association and many younger patients develop loss of elasticity of the skin over the fingers, face and anterior chest wall, indistinguishable from the appearances of scleroderma or acrosclerosis.

In about a quarter of the patients joint pain and stiffness occur at some stage. Proximal limb muscles are almost invariably involved and the neck muscles are characteristically affected in about two-thirds of all cases so that patients may have difficulty in holding up the head. Involvement of distal limb muscles is less common, but weakness may be generalized in about a third of all cases, and when the condition runs a subacute or chronic course contractures sometimes develop (chronic fibrosing myositis). Facial weakness and involvement of the external ocular muscles are rare. Occasionally fatigability resembling that of myasthenia is striking and is partially responsive to edrophonium or neostigmine, but treatment with these and related drugs usually produces only temporary improvement. The deep tendon reflexes may be depressed in the affected muscles but are often surprisingly brisk despite the severity of the weakness.

Diagnosis

In many cases the clinical picture is entirely characteristic, but when involvement of the skin and joints is unobtrusive and the course of the illness is subacute, it may be mistaken for muscular dystrophy or for various forms of metabolic myopathy. The rise in basal metabolic rate which occasionally occurs in polymyositis may cause confusion with thyrotoxic myopathy, but the radioactive iodine uptake is normal. The pattern of muscular involvement does not show the selectivity characteristic of muscular dystrophy, the serum potassium, calcium and phosphorus are normal, and signs of associated endocrine disease are absent. The serum creatine kinase activity is often greatly raised in acute or subacute cases; the erythrocyte sedimentation rate is often, though not invariably, increased, and there may be a rise in the serum gamma-globulin. Electromyography demonstrates a myopathic pattern of volitional activity, but in addition there may be spontaneous fibrillation, positive sharp waves and occasional pseudomyotonic discharges recorded from the resting muscle. Muscle biopsy specimens generally demonstrate widespread necrosis and phagocytosis of muscle fibres and interstitial and perivascular infiltrations of inflammatory cells, mainly lymphocytes and plasma cells; the absence of such infiltrates in a single muscle biopsy section does not, however, exclude the diagnosis of polymyositis. In occasional cases where the clinical picture suggests this diagnosis but the exact diagnosis remains in doubt after full investigation, a therapeutic trial of steroid drugs is indicated.

Treatment

The condition should usually be treated with 60 mg. of prednisone daily, given for 4 or 5 days, thereafter reducing the dose to 40 mg. daily when clinical improvement appears, and subsequently regulating the maintenance dose according to the level of serum creatine kinase activity and the clinical response. Occasionally even higher doses of prednisone may be required for short periods, and in resistant cases ACTH, 80 Units daily, is worth trying as an alternative and has the advantage in childhood of having less effect in the suppression of growth. Maintenance therapy may have to be continued for several years before the drug can eventually be withdrawn. Respiratory and urinary infections should be treated with appropriate antibiotics and in occasional acute cases, intermittent positive-pressure respiration is necessary. Recent evidence suggests that in cases resisting treatment with steroids, there may be some value in giving immunosuppressive drugs such as methotrexate or cyclophosphamide. Following the acute stage, active and passive movements carried out under the supervision of a skilled physiotherapist help to speed recovery.

Course and Prognosis

Even without treatment, the course of the illness is variable. Sometimes it runs a fluctuating course with spontaneous exacerbations and remissions. Progressive deterioration with a fatal termination within a few weeks or months of the onset is seen particularly in acute dermatomyositis, but spontaneous arrest occasionally occurs. Slow insidious progression is seen particularly in middle-age, but spontaneous recovery may occur in childhood; nevertheless, before the introduction of steroid drugs, the over-all mortality of the disease was about 50 per cent.

The high incidence of malignant disease in such cases indicates that all patients developing this syndrome in adult life should be investigated with the possibility of occult neoplasia in mind. In general, the prognosis is best in children and in young adults; after the age of 30, some patients go on to develop evidence of diffuse connective tissue disease (lupus erythematosus or systemic sclerosis) unresponsive to treatment, while after the age of 50 the presence of malignant disease is the single factor most likely adversely to affect the prognosis.

MYASTHENIA GRAVIS

Definition

A disease with a tendency to remit and to relapse, characterized by abnormal muscular fatigability sometimes confined to, or predominant in, an isolated group of muscles and later associated in many cases with permanent weakness of some muscles. There is a disorder of conduction at the myoneural junction which can be temporarily relieved by neostigmine and similar drugs and some patients are benefited by removal of the thymus gland.

Aetiology and Incidence

Myasthenia occurs in all races and affects both sexes, but occurs in women twice as often as in men. Only rarely does it affect more than one member of the same family. While usually beginning in early adult life, it sometimes develops in childhood and occasionally as late as the ninth decade. Most remissions occur within the first 5 years of the disease process and most deaths also occur within this period. Neonatal myasthenia is seen in about one in seven of the children born to myasthenic mothers, but usually recovers within a few weeks. Myasthenia is closely related to thyrotoxicosis and the two diseases occur in the same individual more often than can be accounted for by chance. In occasional cases there is an association with diabetes mellitus, rheumatoid arthritis, systemic lupus erythematosus and sarcoidosis. This clinical observation suggested to Simpson (1950) that myasthenia might be an auto-immune disorder, and a number of workers have demonstrated a muscle-binding globulin in myasthenic serum, while it has been shown that bacterial antigen injected into the guinea-pig thymus may produce a histological reaction similar to that seen in myasthenia. Current evidence suggests that some as yet undefined autoimmune response may prevent the proper release or formation of acetylcholine at the motor end-plate. Although it has been suggested that the disease may be due to a circulating toxin ('thymin') released by the thymus, no such substance has yet been demonstrated with certainty.

Classification

The symptom of muscular fatigability or myasthenia is not peculiar to one disease as similar weakness, increasing after exercise, may be seen in muscles of patients suffering from polymyositis, systemic lupus, dermatomyositis and in one specific form of carcinomatous myopathy. However, a therapeutic response to anticholinesterase drugs is necessary for the definition of true myasthenia gravis and although some response may be found in the symptomatic myasthenias, this is rarely dramatic and often fails within a few weeks. In myasthenia gravis, by contrast, the response to treatment is usually dramatic and sustained and the disease has an individual natural history and pathology.

Pathology

Muscle sections obtained by biopsy may in early cases show no significant abnormality, but in some patients areas of focal necrosis and phagocytosis of muscle fibres are seen and sometimes collections of lymphocytes (lymphorrhages) may be found around blood vessels or between the fibres. These changes are, however, non-specific and the same appears to be true of changes which have been described in the terminal intramuscular motor nerves.

Thymic enlargement is often observed, particularly in younger patients, and histological examination of the thymus demonstrates prominent germinal centres and Hassall's corpuscles. Thymic enlargement in some patients may be shown to be due to a thymoma and some thymomas are malignant.

Symptoms and Signs

The muscles most often affected are the external ocular, bulbar, neck and shoulder-girdle muscles in this descending order, but not infrequently those of respiration and the proximal muscles of the lower extremities are also involved early. Ptosis of one or both upper lids, developing gradually, is often the first symptom and is soon associated with diplopia due to paralysis of one or more of the external ocular muscles. These symptoms typically appear in the evening when the patient is tired and disappear after a night's rest. When the bulbar muscles are first involved, difficulty in swallowing and/or in chewing is described, developing during the course of a meal, and speech may become indistinct.

On examination, there may be unilateral or bilateral ptosis accentuated by upward gaze. External ocular muscle weakness is usually asymmetrical, though it may progress to complete external ophthalmoplegia. The pupillary reflexes are usually normal. The facial muscles are almost always affected with weakness of the orbicularis oculi and of the retractors of the angles of the mouth, giving a characteristic 'myasthenic snarl'. Weakness of the jaw muscles leads to difficulty in chewing and weakness of the muscles of the soft palate, pharynx, tongue and larynx to difficulty in swallowing and in articulation. If the patient is asked to count aloud, speech becomes progressively less distinct and more nasal, and fluids may regurgitate through the nose when the patient attempts to swallow. Neck muscle weakness may cause the head to fall forwards, a sign seen most often in myasthenia but sometimes in polymyositis. In severe cases, weakness in the upper limbs is such that the hands cannot be lifted to the mouth and it is typical that muscle power may initially be satisfactory but after testing a movement several times, the strength rapidly declines. Breathlessness is always a sinister symptom as respiratory weakness may develop rapidly and may even cause sudden death.

Muscular wasting is unusual in the early stages, but in long-standing cases there may be permanent myopathic change, irreversible by drugs, in the external ocular muscles and in certain limb muscles, particularly triceps brachii. In some cases the disease remains limited to the external ocular muscles, but in the majority those of the head and neck, trunk and limbs are eventually involved. The tendon reflexes are almost always brisk even in the presence of severe weakness.

Diagnosis

Diagnosis depends not only upon the typical clinical picture and upon fatigability, which may be demonstrated electrically by means of repetitive supramaximal stimulation of a peripheral nerve while recording the evoked muscle potential from a suitable group of muscles, but also upon the clinical response to an injection of neostigmine or edrophonium chloride. The quick-acting edrophonium (*Tensilon*) is given initially in a dosage of 2 mg. intravenously, followed immediately by a further 8 mg. if there is no severe reaction. The effect lasts for only a few minutes but is usually diagnostic. Provocative tests designed to bring out myasthenic symptoms and utilizing such drugs as curare and quinine are dangerous and are rarely required.

Treatment

The standard treatment for myasthenia gravis is still neostigmine or the closely-related drug pyridostigmine. The usual initial dose of neostigmine is a 15 mg. tablet three or four times a day, and it is often necessary to give in addition atropine, 0·6 mg. twice daily, to overcome muscarinic side-effects. Recent evidence suggests that pyridostigmine is probably preferable as the standard medication and the initial dosage is 60 mg. three or four times a day, again with atropine or propantheline. The dosage is steadily increased until maximum benefit is obtained. Some patients require to take the drugs every 2, 3 or 4 hours, but this is an individual matter. Another drug of value in some cases is ambenonium hydrochloride (*Mytelase*) in which the usual dosage is 10–25 mg. three or four times daily. ACTH, immunosuppressive drugs, aldosterone inhibitors and potassium chloride all have their advocates, but none seems superior to the standard medication, though ephedrine sulphate is often helpful when given as an adjuvant in a dosage of 25 mg. three times daily.

The differential diagnosis between myasthenic and cholinergic crises can be a matter of considerable difficulty and is important as respiratory weakness in such crises may threaten life. The most useful test is to give intravenous edrophonium. If this increases muscle power, then it is likely that the weakness is myasthenic and requires more treatment, while if weakness increases it is probably cholinergic and treatment must be reduced. Any hint of impending respiratory insufficiency may indicate that all drugs should be withdrawn and that assisted respiration with positive-pressure apparatus and tracheostomy should be used. Unfortunately some patients show a differential sensitivity of different muscles to various drugs, so that a dose of pyridostigmine which improves power in the limb muscles may be sufficient to cause cholinergic paralysis of the diaphragm.

The place of thymectomy is still in doubt. The operation may benefit both sexes, but improvement is greatest in women who would otherwise have a worse prognosis than men. The results are best in young women with a short history of severe myasthenia, but any patient who is deteriorating despite optimum medication has nothing to lose in the hands of an experienced surgeon. If a thymoma is present, radiotherapy is generally recommended to the thymus before operation.

Course and Prognosis

Despite all forms of treatment, there are some patients in whom death occurs within the first 2–3 years. Spontaneous remission may occur and may sometimes be complete and long-lasting, but is more often temporary and followed by relapse after an interval of months or years. After 5–10 years the disease in many patients appears to enter a static phase with only a moderate response to treatment and a varying degree of residual disability. Even after thymectomy, two out of three patients with thymomas die within 5 years, but the survivors may benefit to the same extent as those who do not have a tumour.

THE MYASTHENIC-MYOPATHIC SYNDROME

This syndrome is generally associated with oat-cell carcinoma of the bronchus, though it has been occasionally seen in patients with carcinoma elsewhere. Muscular weakness, wasting and fatigability usually affect the proximal part of the limbs and trunk and the patient often complains of increased enfeeblement after exertion, but in many such cases muscle power may in fact be increased by brief exercise, a so-called reversed myasthenic effect. In contrast to the findings in true myasthenia, the tendon reflexes in this condition are almost always depressed or absent; muscle power is only slightly improved by treatment with neostigmine, even though definite improvement may follow an injection of edrophonium. Weakness and fatigability may be greatly improved in such cases by the oral administration of guanidine hydrochloride in a dosage of 20–50 mg./kg. body weight daily.

ENDOCRINE MYOPATHIES

DISORDERS OF THE THYROID GLAND

[see Section 5]

THYROTOXIC MYOPATHY

In severe cases of thyrotoxicosis, weakness and wasting of proximal limb muscles may occur particularly in the upper extremities, and may resolve when the thyroid disease is effectively treated. Recent quantitative electromyographic studies have shown that in thyrotoxicosis there is almost always a reversible abnormality of muscle function which may be readily overlooked, but that recovery is almost always complete following adequate treatment of the thyrotoxicosis.

EXOPHTHALMIC OPHTHALMOPLEGIA

The principal effect of this disorder is upon the external ocular muscles which are greatly increased in bulk, as are the entire orbital contents. The main symptoms are exophthalmos, pain in the eyes and diplopia. Papilloedema and even corneal ulceration may occur in the presence of severe exophthalmos and, if not relieved, the patient may go on to develop optic atrophy and blindness. Surgical decompression of the orbit is occasionally required, even as an emergency measure. Medical and hormonal treatment have been in general disappointing.

THYROTOXICOSIS AND MYASTHENIA GRAVIS

About 5 per cent. of myasthenic patients have thyrotoxicosis and the myasthenia may become worse when hyperthyroidism increases. Both conditions must be treated in the standard way, but the risks of thyroidectomy are greatly increased in patients with myasthenia.

THYROTOXIC PERIODIC PARALYSIS

An association between thyrotoxicosis and periodic paralysis has been observed particularly in the Japanese and Chinese. Adequate treatment of the hyperthyroidism results in disappearance of the periodic attacks of weakness or in a marked decrease of their number and severity; the attacks of paralysis are usually hypokalaemic.

MYOPATHY IN HYPOTHYROIDISM

Muscular hypertrophy with weakness and slowness of muscular contraction and relaxation has been described in children suffering from sporadic cretinism (the Debré-Semelaigne syndrome). A similar condition in adults, causing pain and aching in the muscles after exertion, is known as Hoffmann's syndrome and may superficially resemble myotonia, though electromyographically no myotonic discharges are found in this condition. It has recently been suggested that myxoedema may be associated with a true girdle myopathy causing mild proximal weakness and wasting which responds to treatment with thyroxin.

DISORDERS OF THE PITUITARY AND ADRENAL GLANDS

In acromegaly and pituitary gigantism, and conversely in hypopituitarism, widespread muscular weakness with some degree of atrophy has been observed but is non-specific clinically, electromyographically and pathologically. General weakness may also be seen in Addison's disease and probably results from changes in plasma and muscle water and electrolytes.

MYOPATHY IN CUSHING'S SYNDROME

Weakness of the muscles of the pelvic girdle and thighs, sometimes with pain in the quadriceps, is now well recognized as an occasional complication of Cushing's syndrome. Both electromyography and muscle biopsy may demonstrate relatively non-specific myopathic changes in such cases. Similar changes have been extensively reported to occur in patients under treatment with steroid drugs and particularly with those which have a fluorine atom in the 9α position. The myopathy of Cushing's disease improves after treatment of the condition, and steroid myopathy generally recovers completely when steroid drugs are withdrawn; the latter condition is less common in patients receiving prednisone than it is in those treated with other related drugs.

ACTH MYOPATHY

It has recently been noted that proximal muscle weakness, fatigability and minor degrees of muscle wasting may occur in pigmented patients who had previously undergone adrenalectomy for Cushing's disease. Electromyography confirms that this weakness is myopathic and muscle biopsy sections show an accumulation of fat within the muscle fibres; this disorder appears to be due to an increased quantity of circulating ACTH.

METABOLIC MYOPATHIES

MYOPATHY IN METABOLIC BONE DISEASE

Non-selective wasting and weakness of proximal limb muscles with pain and discomfort on movement, hypotonia and brisk tendon reflexes are the main features of this myopathy which may be seen in patients with hyperparathyroidism, but is more often observed in those suffering from osteomalacia. The condition may be due to interference with the excitation-contraction coupling involving the entry of calcium into the muscle fibre and may be related to abnormalities of vitamin D metabolism.

GLYCOGEN STORAGE DISEASE OF MUSCLE

McARDLE'S DISEASE

In 1951 McArdle described the case of a man of 30 who had developed generalized muscular pain and stiffness which increased during exertion. He showed that the blood lactate and pyruvate levels failed to rise after exercise and suggested that the disorder was due to a defect of glucose utilization. Subsequently it was shown that this condition is a disorder of glycogen storage due to absence or deficiency of myophosphorylase in muscle fibres; myoglobinuria is observed after exertion in some cases, and after repeated contraction the muscles may go into a state of contracture. The condition runs a benign course, though some degree of permanent muscular weakness and wasting develops in some cases. No treatment has any influence upon the symptoms.

OTHER FORMS OF GLYCOGEN STORAGE DISEASE

Recently a myopathic disorder resembling McArdle's disease clinically has been shown to be due to phosphofructokinase deficiency. Pompe's disease, due to a deficiency of amylo-1, 4-glucosidase (acid maltase), usually gives rise to glycogen storage in the heart, skeletal muscles and central nervous system and has been generally believed to be incompatible with survival beyond the first few weeks of life. Recently, however, it has become apparent that certain patients with acid maltase deficiency may present with an apparently progressive myopathy of girdle muscles in late childhood or adult life. This diagnosis must now be considered in all cases of suspected limb-girdle muscular dystrophy arising in middle life and muscle biopsy may be diagnostic as striking vacuolation of muscle fibres is usually demonstrated easily and the vacuoles contain large quantities of glycogen. Unfortunately this condition too, does not appear to be amenable to treatment.

PERIODIC PARALYSIS SYNDROMES

HYPOKALAEMIC PERIODIC PARALYSIS

This condition gives rise to attacks of flaccid weakness of the voluntary muscles, but those of speech, swallowing and respiration are usually spared. Attacks usually begin in the second decade and are commonest in early adult life. Often they start on waking, after a period of rest following exertion or after a heavy carbohydrate meal, and usually they last for several hours. During attacks the plasma potassium level is found to be low (usually less than 3 mEq. per litre); there is positive balance of potassium and some or all of the retained potassium seems to pass into the muscle cell. Muscle biopsy specimens taken during an attack usually show that many muscle fibres are vacuolated as a result of dilatation of the sarcoplasmic reticulum.

The suggestion that this form of periodic paralysis may be due to intermittent aldosteronism has not been substantiated; aldosteronism can be distinguished from periodic paralysis by the associated hypertension, alkalosis and hypernatraemia and by the persistence of hypokalaemia between the attacks. Administration of potassium chloride 4–6 G. daily, is the treatment of choice for attacks of the hypokalaemic type. Spironolactone, 25 mg. four times a day, and other similar aldosterone antagonists have been found to reduce greatly the frequency and severity of the attacks. Rarely in such cases muscle weakness is localized to one or more muscle groups and sometimes permanent atrophy of muscles develops after frequent episodes of weakness, but most patients improve spontaneously with age.

HYPERKALAEMIC PERIODIC PARALYSIS (ADYNAMIA EPISODICA HEREDITARIA)

In this condition, which, like the hypokalaemic variety, is inherited by an autosomal dominant gene, the attacks are usually much shorter in duration, lasting on an average 30–40 minutes and they may be precipitated immediately by exercise. In the attacks the serum potassium usually rises, though some patients have severe weakness when the level is no higher than 4 mEq. per litre. Some patients show definite myotonia, but in others this phenomenon seems curiously limited to the muscles around the eyes. The attacks may be cut short by the intravenous administration of calcium gluconate, while acetazolamide (250 mg. two or three times daily), hydrochlorothiazide (25 mg. two or three times daily) and dichlorphenamide have all been used successfully for prophylactic treatment.

SODIUM-RESPONSIVE NORMOKALAEMIC PERIODIC PARALYSIS

This is probably a variant of the hyperkalaemic type, except that the attacks may occasionally last for days or weeks and often develop at night. The paralysis is always increased by the administration of potassium and is improved by large doses of sodium chloride. Acetazolamide combined with 9-α-fluorohydrocortisone, 0·1 mg. daily, has been shown to prevent the attacks.

Plainly careful investigation of every case of periodic paralysis is necessary to establish the nature of the patient's illness. Attempts to demonstrate a specific disorder of carbohydrate metabolism in such cases have been unsuccessful, but treatment given either prophylactically or in order to shorten the attacks has proved to be successful in most cases once the character of the attacks has been carefully defined by investigation.

MYOGLOBINURIA

Myoglobin may appear in the urine as a result of widespread crush injury to muscle, in acute polymyositis and in localized ischaemic muscular necrosis. In a specific syndrome of paroxysmal myoglobinuria of unknown aetiology, patients suffer acute attacks of severe cramp-like muscle pain and tenderness associated with weakness or paralysis and accompanied by profuse myoglobinuria. In some cases occurring predominantly in adolescent or young adult males, pain and myoglobinuria follow exercise and recurrent attacks may lead to permanent muscular weakness and wasting. In a second type which is commonest in childhood, the attacks are severe, often follow acute infection, are accompanied by fever and leucocytosis, but occur at progressively longer intervals and usually clear up with the passage of time. The cause of this syndrome is unknown and no treatment has any influence upon it.

THE FLOPPY INFANT SYNDROME

Generalized muscular hypotonia in infancy may be due to a variety of causes, including cerebral palsy, mental retardation, cerebral degenerative disease and a number of disorders of the neuromuscular apparatus. Spinal muscular atrophy (Werdnig-Hoffmann disease) is an important cause and in such cases the hypotonia is usually profound and widespread, there is generalized areflexia, respiratory muscle weakness and often fasciculation of the tongue. The diagnosis can be confirmed by electromyography and muscle biopsy; this condition, of grave prognosis, may be mimicked by congenital muscular dystrophy which has already been described.

BENIGN CONGENITAL HYPOTONIA

This term is widely utilized to identify those floppy infants in whom hypotonia is not demonstrated to be the result of any specific metabolic disorder, nor is it shown to be secondary to mental defect, or disease in the central nervous system, and in such cases full investigation, including electromyography and muscle biopsy, may fail to demonstrate any specific abnormality of the muscle fibres other than, in some cases, an overall decrease in their diameter. The aetiology of this condition is unknown but it improves progressively with increasing age. Probably this syndrome will prove to be one of multiple aetiology. In some patients demonstrating similar diffuse hypotonia in early infancy, improvement occurs but yet the muscles remain weak, slender and hypotonic throughout life, and these cases are often identified as examples of 'benign congenital myopathy' even though electromyographic and muscle biopsy findings in such individuals are usually non-specific. In recent years, however, it has been demonstrated that some such patients are suffering from apparently specific though benign disorders of muscle.

CENTRAL CORE DISEASE

In 1956 Shy and Magee described a family in which affected children did not walk until the age of 4 years. There was widespread muscular hypotonia and muscle biopsy revealed large muscle fibres, most of which showed one or sometimes two central cores which had different staining properties from the other fibrils. The central core was shown to be devoid of oxidative enzymes and of phosphorylase activity and seemed to be non-functioning. The condition is probably due to an autosomal recessive gene and runs a benign course, but its pathogenesis is obscure.

NEMALINE MYOPATHY

This is another congenital and relatively nonprogressive myopathy in which collections of rod-shaped bodies may be found within the muscle fibres, lying usually beneath the sarcolemma. These patients show evidence of diffuse myopathy, but also facial weakness, a high arched palate, prognathism of the lower jaw and skeletal changes resembling those of arachnodactyly, though none of the other stigmata of Marfan's syndrome are present. Examination of muscle from such cases with the electron microscope has shown that the subsarcolemmal rods appear to be due to a selective swelling and degeneration of Z-bands with consequent destruction of myofilaments in the adjacent part of the muscle fibre.

MEGACONIAL MYOPATHY

In 1964 Shy and Gonatas described an 8-year-old white female suffering from a slowly progressive muscular weakness beginning at about the age of 3 and involving shoulder and pelvic-girdle muscles. Routine examination of muscle biopsy specimens revealed no abnormality, but under the electron microscope it was found that the fibres contained enormously enlarged mitochondria, many of which contained unusual rectangular crystalline-like inclusions of high density. Similarly abnormal mitochondria have been described recently in many different forms of muscle disease and the existence of this condition as an independent diagnostic entity remains somewhat in doubt. The same may well prove to be the case with so-called *pleoconial myopathy*, a disorder in which large numbers of rounded mitochondria were seen within muscle fibres. There is now evidence to suggest that abnormal numbers of mitochondria within skeletal muscle may occur in many different forms of metabolic myopathy.

MYOTUBULAR OR CENTRONUCLEAR MYOPATHY

In 1966 Spiro, Shy and Gonatas reported the case of a 9-year-old child suffering from a form of Möbius syndrome characterized by facial diplegia, external ocular palsies, a decrease in muscle mass, moderate symmetrical muscle weakness and poor development of all limb muscles. Most of the muscle fibres contained central nuclei, often lying in chains, and the appearances in the muscle were similar to those of so-called myotubes seen in normal foetal muscle in the early months of intra-uterine life. Recent work suggests that these fibres are in several respects different from foetal myotubes, but nevertheless the condition appears to represent an example of cellular developmental arrest. The condition appears to run a benign course, but so few cases have been reported to date that the prognosis is far from clear.

While it cannot be concluded that all of the syndromes mentioned represent specific disease entities within the difficult field of benign congenital myopathy, advances are occurring with great rapidity and many new and apparently specific histological abnormalities of the muscle fibre are being demonstrated by modern techniques.

SOME MISCELLANEOUS MUSCULAR DISORDERS

RESTLESS LEGS

The aetiology of this syndrome (Ekbom's syndrome) is unknown; it gives rise to unpleasant aching in the muscles of the lower limbs when the patient rests in a chair or on lying in bed. This aching, accompanied by a sense of intolerable restlessness, may be accompanied by muscular cramps which interfere with sleep. There are no abnormal physical signs on examination and electromyography, nerve conduction velocity measurements and muscle biopsy all give normal findings. Some patients are greatly helped by treatment with chlorpromazine and/or by diazepam and hydantoinates.

TIBIALIS ANTERIOR SYNDROME

Severe boring pain in the tibialis anterior muscle may occur on one or both sides after unaccustomed exercise; the condition is due to ischaemic swelling of the muscle within its tight fascial compartment. Rarely the pain is intense and widespread necrosis of the muscles occurs. In mild chronic cases recurrent pain occurs after any exertion and relief can only then be obtained by surgical decompression of the anterior crural compartment.

PROGRESSIVE MYOSITIS OSSIFICANS

Localized ossification in voluntary muscle may occur as a result of its repeated involvement in the trauma of certain exercises or occupations (as in horse-riders) and is occasionally seen in muscles around the hip joint following spastic paraparesis. Progressive myositis ossificans is, however, a genetically-determined disorder in which there is widespread ossification of the muscles which seems to be preceded by sclerosis of the intramuscular connective tissue. Most cases present in childhood and affected individuals often have associated anomalies of their great toes or other digits. The condition is probably due to a dominant gene showing incomplete penetrance; it begins usually with swelling or swellings in the neck mimicking congenital torticollis and eventually the muscles of the back, shoulder and pelvic girdles, particularly, become ossified. The overlying skin may ulcerate and terminal aspiration pneumonia is common, but the condition may run a benign course over many decades.

THE STIFF-MAN SYNDROME

This syndrome of so-called progressive fluctuating muscular rigidity and spasm predominantly affects male adults who, after a prodromal phase of aching and tightness of the axial muscles, go on to develop a symmetrical continuous stiffness of the skeletal muscles upon which painful muscular spasms are superimposed and may be precipitated by movement. The aetiology of the condition is unknown but it may be a disorder of interneurones in the spinal cord; it is usually successfully controlled by treatment with diazepam.

REFERENCES

Adams, R. D., Denny-Brown, D., and Pearson, C. M. (1962) *Diseases of Muscle: A Study in Pathology*, 2nd ed., New York.

Adamson, D. G., Salter, R. H., and Pearce, G. W. (1967) McArdle's syndrome (myophosphorylase deficiency), *Quart. J. Med.*, **36**, 565.

Astrom, K. E., Kugelberg, E., and Müller, R. (1961) Hypothyroid myopathy, *Arch. Neurol. (Chic.)*, **5**, 472.

BUCHTHAL, F. (1957) *An Introduction to Electromyography*, Copenhagen.

CAMPBELL, M. J., REBEIZ, J. J., and WALTON, J. N. (1969) Myotubular, centronuclear or pericentronuclear myopathy?, *J. neurol. Sci.*, **8,** 425.

CAUGHEY, J. E., and MYRIANTHOPOULOS, N. C. (1963) *Dystrophia Myotonica and Related Disorders*, Springfield, Ill.

COOMES, E. N. (1965) Corticosteroid myopathy, *Ann. rheum. Dis.*, **24,** 465.

DALE, H. (1934) Chemical transmission of the effects of nerve impulses, *Brit. med. J.*, **2,** 835.

DUBOWITZ, V. (1968) *Developing and Diseased Muscle*, London.

EKBOM, K. A. (1960) Restless legs syndrome, *Neurology (Minneap.)*, **10,** 868.

EMERY, A. E. H., and WALTON, J. N. (1967) The genetics of muscular dystrophy, in *Progress in Medical Genetics*, ed. Steinberg, A. G., and Bearn, A. G., Vol. V, New York.

ENGEL, A. G. (1961) Thyroid function and myasthenia gravis, *Arch. Neurol. (Chic.)*, **4,** 663.

GARDNER-MEDWIN, D., HUDGSON, P., and WALTON, J. N. (1967) Benign spinal muscular atrophy arising in childhood and adolescence, *J. Neurol. Sci.*, **5,** 121.

HOWARD, F. M. (1963) A new and effective drug in the treatment of stiff-man syndrome, *Proc. Mayo Clin.*, **38,** 203.

HUDGSON, P., GARDNER-MEDWIN, D., FULTHORPE, J. J., and WALTON, J. N. (1967) Nemaline myopathy, *Neurology (Minneap.)*, **17,** 1125.

HUDGSON, P., GARDNER-MEDWIN, D., WORSFOLD, M., PENNINGTON, R. J. T., and WALTON, J. N. (1968) Adult myopathy from glycogen storage disease due to acid maltase deficiency, *Brain*, **91,** 435.

HUXLEY, H. E., and HANSON, J. (1960) The molecular basis of contraction, in *Structure and Function of Muscle*, ed. Bourne, G. H., Vol. 1, New York.

KILOH, L. G., and NEVIN, S. (1951) Progressive dystrophy of external ocular muscles (ocular myopathy), *Brain*, **74,** 115.

KOREIN, J., CODDON, D. R., and MOWREY, F. H. (1959) The clinical syndrome of paroxysmal paralytic myoglobinuria, *Neurology (Minneap.)*, **9,** 767.

MCKUSICK, V. (1956) *Heritable Disorders of Connective Tissue*, p. 184, St. Louis.

MCQUILLEN, M. P., and JOHNS, R. J. (1966) The nature of the defect in the Eaton-Lambert syndrome, *Neurology (Minneap.)*, **17,** 527.

MOERSCH, F. P., and WOLTMAN, H. W. (1956) Progressive fluctuating muscular rigidity and spasm (stiff-man syndrome), *Proc. Mayo Clin.*, **31,** 421.

MÜLLER, R., and KUGELBERG, E. (1959) Myopathy in Cushing's syndrome, *J. Neurol. Neurosurg. Psychiat.*, **22,** 314.

OSSERMAN, K. E. (1958) *Myasthenia Gravis*, New York.

PAINE, R. S. (1963) The future of the 'floppy infant', *Develop. Med. Child Neurol.*, **5,** 115.

PEACHEY, L. D. (1968) Muscle, *Ann. Rev. Physiol.*, **30,** 401.

PEARSON, C. M., and ROSE, A. S. (1960) Myositis, the inflammatory disorders of muscle, *Res. Publ. Ass. nerv. ment. Dis.*, **38,** 422.

POSKANZER, D. C., and KERR, D. N. S. (1961) A third type of periodic paralysis with normokalaemia and favourable response to sodium chloride, *Amer. J. Med.*, **31,** 328.

PRATT, R. T. C. (1967) *The Genetic sof Neurological Disorders*, London.

PRINEAS, J. W., HALL, R., BARWICK, D. D., and WATSON A. J. (1968) Myopathy associated with pigmentation following adrenalectomy for Cushing's syndrome, *Quart. J. Med.*, **37,** 63.

PRUZANSKI, W. (1966) Variants of myotonic dystrophy in pre-adolescent life (the syndrome of myotonic dysembryoplasia), *Brain*, **89,** 563.

ROSE, A. L., and WALTON, J. N. (1966) Polymyositis: a survey of 89 cases with particular reference to treatment and prognosis, *Brain*, **89,** 747.

SHY, G. M., ENGEL, W. K., SOMERS, J. E., and WANKO, T. (1963) Nemaline myopathy, a new congenital myopathy, *Brain*, **86,** 793.

SHY, G. M., and GONATAS, N. K. (1964) Human myopathy with giant abnormal mitochondria, *Science*, **145,** 493.

SHY, G. M., and MAGEE, K. R. (1956) A new congenital non-progressive myopathy, *Brain*, **79,** 610.

SIMPSON, J. A. (1960) Myasthenia gravis: a new hypothesis, *Scot. med. J.*, **5,** 419.

SMITH, R., and STERN, G. M. (1967) Myopathy, osteomalacia and hyperparathyroidism, *Brain*, **90,** 593.

SPIRO, A. J., SHY, G. M., and GONATAS, N. K. (1966) Myotubular myopathy, *Arch. Neurol. (Chic.)*, **14,** 1.

TODD, J. W. (1961) Polymyalgia rheumatica, *Lancet*, ii, 1111.

VAN'T HOFF, W. (1962) Familial myotonic periodic paralysis, *Quart. J. Med.*, **31,** 385.

WALTON, J. N. (1966) Diseases of muscle, *Abstr. Wld Med.*, **40,** 1, 81.

WALTON, J. N. (1969) *Disorders of Voluntary Muscle*, 2nd ed., London.

WALTON, J. N., and ADAMS, R. D. (1958) *Polymyositis*, Edinburgh.

WALTON, J. N., and NATTRASS, F. J. (1954) On the classification, natural history and treatment of the myopathies, *Brain*, **77,** 169.

ZELLWEGER, H., AFIFI, A., MCCORMICK, W. F., and MERGNER, W. (1967) Severe congenital muscular dystrophy, *Amer. J. Dis. Child.*, **114,** 591.

JOHN N. WALTON

SECTION 17

PSYCHOLOGICAL MEDICINE

PSYCHOLOGICAL MEDICINE

INTRODUCTION

Psychiatry is concerned with forms of illness as widespread and diverse as those of somatic medicine. Despite the introduction of many new treatments there are still almost as many hospital beds occupied by psychiatric patients as by patients suffering from all other diseases, and there is an undoubtedly large part of the population who have mental disorder not needing in-patient hospital care. The diversity of this widespread group of illnesses depends on their being disorders of mind—disorders, that is, of the human function which comprehends and sums up all other functions of the organism, serves to relate a human being to his complex environment, and is the chief token that he is an individual, and not a type. Mental disorders are therefore varied, as are the people who suffer from them. It is only by ignoring most of what is individual in these illnesses that a few common types or categories can be recognized, comparable to the 'diseases' of somatic medicine. Such a procedure is necessary for practical ends. Material must be classified and, moreover, a biological foundation may be assumed for the psychiatric syndromes which stand for the main ways in which a human being can become mentally unhealthy. There are only a few such ways, and they are determined by the structural and functional patterns inherent in the organism. Diversity arises through their becoming manifest under the influence of each individual's special environment and in combination with his other inherited tendencies. Diversity, therefore, can be due to a combination of hereditary causes and to the effect of each individual's environment throughout his life upon his development and behaviour. There is always interplay between inheritance and environment. Part of the psychiatrist's business is to discover how this interplay can lead to illness. To do this he must, even more than the general physician, study illness in two ways: first, as showing some typical pattern of morbid behaviour with characteristic pathological changes, and tending to run along predictable lines; and secondly, as a patch of personal biography, something to be understood, rather than classified in terms of psychology and physiology. The two methods are complementary, though in a brief textbook presentation the former must be the more prominent.

There is no dividing line between somatic medicine and psychiatry. Psychiatry, although it has to work in part with social and psychological conceptions of which general medicine has hitherto felt less need, suffers greatly when it limits itself to this way of regarding mental phenomena. It cannot safely ignore the relationship between bodily happenings and the patient's state of mind. There is no mental disorder, mild or severe, in the causation of which bodily disease may not play an important part. Moreover, it is not only in crude instances of structural or chemical disease that the relationship between bodily and mental illness may be recognized. A human being does not exist as a rarefied mind united with a solid body; he is an organism all of whose subsidiary functions contribute to this highest function—his mind—which brings him not only consciousness, but also an integrated behaviour in relation to his surroundings. Disturbances, transient or permanent, of these part-functions (e.g. in the sensory apparatus or the circulatory system) will have some effect on his state of mind. Changes in the central nervous system are the most obvious instance of this, but the endocrine glands, the autonomic nervous system and the metabolic processes are often of notable significance in the various maladjustments summed up as mental disorder.

A human being is constantly responding to, and influencing, his surroundings, but his doing so is conditioned by the various parts of his body and the way they are working. It is likewise, and equally, necessary to weigh psychological influences and effects when deciding the pathogenesis or the treatment of predominantly physical illness. It is now clear that emotion may play an important part in the chain of events that cause or aggravate many physical diseases, and the interplay between psychological and physical happenings may influence the outcome of many a surgical or other illness. Much of the current interest in 'psychosomatic' medicine turns on a belated recognition of these clinical facts. It is plain that psychiatric issues must be the concern of all doctors, not merely the psychiatrist's preserve; and that psychological happenings differ from physiological in their deceptive accessibility to familiar methods of observation, in their almost Gordian complexity, and in the concepts found most useful for describing and explaining them, rather than in any essential quality which would keep them permanently distinct.

Before the categories and clinical features of mental illness are described, the principles of general psychopathology call for brief consideration, since without them psychological medicine can be little more than a tedious catalogue of details.

GENERAL PSYCHOPATHOLOGY

The term 'psychopathology' is often erroneously taken to refer exclusively to a set of meaningful connexions, couched in psychological terms, which purport to account for a psychiatric symptom or condition. This usage is unduly restrictive and too readily confounds psychological speculation with scientific inquiry. It is preferable to revert to the broader, more traditional view of general psychopathology as being concerned with the identification of those factors bearing on the causal associations and natural history of mental diseases, and with the mechanisms and interactions of such factors. As such, the subject may extend from the details of a neurochemical reaction to the abstractions of the mind-body problem. For this reason it is of central importance to pay scrupulous regard to method and to define the limits of the many techniques and concepts which are relevant to the study of psychiatric morbidity.

CAUSES

The aetiology of every mental illness is multifactorial, representing a sequence of related phenomena within and outside the patient's body. In the absence of a firm understanding of many of these factors there is a tendency to polarize them into simplified but artificial groupings: intrinsic or extrinsic, endogenous or exogenous, organic or psychological, physical or mental. It is, of course, possible in many cases to discover some indispensable or prepotent link in this chain of factors—a brain injury, for example, or a bereavement—but the more detailed the analysis of a patient's endowment and life-history, the more entangled do these factors seem to be.

With these qualifications it is permissible to distinguish between dominantly *intrinsic* and dominantly *extrinsic* causal factors. The intrinsic causes of mental disorder include those which depend on heredity and on epochal phases of psychological development. The extrinsic factors derive from the environment and may be either some form of physical damage or some variety of mental experience. In this context it may be emphasized that 'experience', denoting as it does the impact of the outer world on the human organism, also implies the organism's response, which in turn depends on previous experiences—psychosocial and physical—as well as on current state [see below].

Heredity, Personality and Constituton

The hereditary factor is not a general neuropathic taint; there are specific predispositions to one or other anomaly. These predispositions are transmitted in accordance with familiar genetic principles, summed up in the modern gene theory of inheritance. Studies of families and of twins have proved the importance of the hereditary factor in the major non-organic psychoses, though they have not yet sufficed to reveal with certainty the number and location of genes concerned in the transmission of the hereditary types of morbid reaction.

Among the main reasons for this incompleteness in our knowledge is the impossibility of concluding that an inherited trait is not present, merely because it is not manifest in some recognizable form. Some inherited predispositions, e.g. Huntington's chorea, are almost exempt from this proviso, but such are exceptional. Other inherited factors and, most of all, the environment, will in many cases determine whether an individual predisposition is to become evident or not. Thus a man may have an inherited tendency to melancholia which remains latent until a financial reverse or disease of the cerebral arteries provides the conditions necessary for its manifestation.

More than one type of proneness to mental disorder can be inherited by the same person. He may, for example, be prone not only to periodic insanity, but also to schizophrenia. Mingled proclivities of this kind account for anomalous clinical pictures, often met with and difficult to classify as either one syndrome or another. The 'either-or' kind of diagnosis is often out of place or misleading in psychiatry because of the frequency with which more than one constitutionally rooted type of illness may be found in the same patient. Syndromes are frequently combined; to grasp their clinical meaning one may have to investigate the patient's family not only as to mental disorder, but as to normal characteristics of temperament also.

The signs of a transmissible tendency to some mental disorder may not be actual illness, but only a special kind of personality. The frequency of association and similarity of form between the personality and the illness points to the constitutional background of mental illness. It also shows how hereditary tendencies can express themselves in more or less normal ways in personality before the catastrophe of an obvious illness has directed attention to them.

In studying personality, the psychiatrist can have recourse to several techniques, besides direct observation and the descriptive method based on the reports of those familiar with the individual studied. The most ambitious are projective methods, of which the Rorschach ink-blot and the thematic apperception test are examples; in these the patient's fantasy is evoked by more or less standardized stimuli, and inferences drawn from what he says and does in these circumstances. More widely employed and more direct are questionnaires which apply statistical discipline to the replies people give when asked about their social attributes, their feelings and attitudes. Expert and cautious interpretation is indispensable for the whole of the growing array of psychological methods of assessing personality.

It is not only in the personality that inherent proclivities may be revealed; certain types of bodily structure, too, occur much more frequently in those with a particular mental constitution or mental illness than in the rest of the population. The most striking instance of this is the frequency with which a 'pyknic' bodily habit and a 'syntonic' personality are found among those who have periodic attacks of mania or melancholia. It is not common to find pure examples of mental or physical types in the population, and recent work has aimed at making it possible to designate the mixture of components in any individual by a taxonomic formula rather than by ascribing them all to one or other type; but whatever method of description be employed, the association of osseous and muscular structure with a particular personality structure and perhaps with a predominant form of autonomic response seems frequent enough in healthy as well as in mentally ill persons to warrant classing physique, physiological behaviour and personality together, however tentatively. Such constitutional features, whether mental or physical, indicate that inherited tendencies can body themselves forth in normal physical and psychological structure before morbid exaggerations of them make an appearance. The relationship, however, is not a simple one. There are very many people with these types of personality who never fall mentally ill.

Although personality and constitution have been spoken of as though they were static, innate attributes of the human organism, neither of these epithets is appropriate, not even in respect of bodily constitution. Responsiveness and plasticity are essential to human development of every kind; there is a constant interplay of personality with the outer world. The main pattern of development is doubtless determined by innate, inherited factors but general directions and main patterns mean little unless they are given substance and content by individual experience. Nutrition, for example, can deflect the body from its ordained pattern or enable its fulfilment, and all sorts of physical interference can maim or improve it. The same is true of the mental side of human growth and maturity; this feeds on psychological and social stimuli which may be advantageous or deleterious. Consequently, each patient's personality is not to be assessed as conforming to a frozen artificial type, but as a complex of dynamic functions, changing in outward form, sometimes in unstable equilibrium, and none the less powerful for being subterranean.

Highlights of this process are provided by the changes that occur at certain phases of development, such as puberty, pregnancy or the climacteric. Endocrine and other physical changes at these epochs may be accompanied by psychological disturbances, the severity and form of which bring them under the notice of the psychiatrist. They are dramatic episodes in a lifelong process of growth, maturity and involution or decay, which is marked by plasticity and development of varied functions in the first stage; stability and differentiated adaptation in the second; emotional lability and suspicion, intellectual narrowing, rigidity, failing grasp and memory, in the last. The mental disturbances which may occur at different ages are much influenced by these intrinsic factors and tendencies.

Physical Damage

Some external happenings influence the mental state chiefly by way of the body: infection, physical trauma, intoxication and metabolic and endocrine disturbances due, wholly or in part, to environmental influences may result in mental disorder. In many of these instances the mental change is mediated by way of some cerebral damage, and the clinical picture is of the organic neurogenic kind, e.g. dementia. It would be wrong to attribute the whole of such mental disorder to the cerebral damage; but to it is referable the core of the psychosis. Some diseases have an incidence on special functions and parts of the central nervous system, which determines characteristic features in the mental picture. In the main, however, it is not yet possible to correlate mental symptoms with special areas or kinds of cerebral damage—partly because the brain is not the only structure concerned, but mainly because the presumptive changes in it are too evanescent and delicate to be accessible to our crude methods of examination. Even the electroencephalogram, which seemed to promise so much, has contributed little to the understanding of cerebral happenings in mental disorders other than those associated with epilepsy, though it is valuable in suggesting the presence or indicating the site of a lesion, e.g. in the temporal region.

To limit one's self to the brain in studying the somatic correlates or basis of mental phenomena would be an error. In the physical accompaniments of emotion, the whole body participates through the mediation of the vegetative nervous system and the endocrine glands. This is significant, because emotional upset is one of the most important phenomena of mental disorder. The sequence of psychophysical happenings of which an emotional upset is the climax and the outward sign, may be started not only by some mental happening, but also by physical experiences—intoxication with a drug, or a circulatory disturbance, or a metabolic upheaval such as acute hypoglycaemia. Whether the physical event—hypoglycaemia, for example—comes from outside, as an injection of insulin, or arises from within the body as a 'spontaneous' deficiency, is of little consequence in its bearing on the mental disturbance engendered. The chief emphasis lies on the physical apparatus through which so widespread an affection of the whole organism can be evoked, just as in other circumstances the emphasis would lie on the psychological apparatus which serves the same end.

Mental Experiences

There are general needs in mental life, instinctual drives or inherited functions, which provide experience by bringing us into relation with our immediate surroundings; they lead us to feed ourselves, maintain our lives, reproduce, and aim at other ends which have been variously formulated by philosophers, saints and psychologists. These biological forces, however denominated or classified, are not peculiar to human beings, but in respect of human beings are so much more accessible to minute inquiry along verbal lines, that complex conceptual systems have been built up to describe them. Comparative and experimental psychology have partly corrected unreal refinements and highly metaphorical interpretations. Contributions from physiology and ethology can also help counterbalance some of the unduly speculative subtleties which are ill-suited to medical needs.

Mental growth is dependent on daily experience for its material but human beings deal selectively, and not passively, with experience. In reacting to the multifarious world about him, a human being is constantly obliged to select what he will perceive, and in what form he will perceive it. Pure 'objective' perception never occurs; to perceive things at all, he must give them meaning by relating them to himself and to his previous experience. Unless he can do this, not necessarily consciously, he is at the mercy of his environment, as a new-born baby is. Perception is therefore an active process; it has instinctual and emotional, as well as cognitive aspects. It depends partly upon memory for being able to give meaning to what it perceives. Memory is not merely an intellectual function by which we store and later recall a happening into consciousness, but a device, or function, by which past happenings are able to influence subsequent behaviour; the ways in which they do so, and the form in which the earlier experience is reproduced into consciousness, will be greatly influenced by its original emotional, as well as more purely perceptual, aspects, and by other physical and mental experiences—a distressing repetition of the experience, for example, or a physical happening like concussion or cortical atrophy.

It follows from the foregoing that memory need not be conscious. Consciousness is only an attribute of psychological happenings, not their essence or their criterion; mental life goes on with varying degrees of consciousness attaching to it. There is no sharp division between conscious and unconscious mental life; no region called 'the unconscious' with its own rules and contents. Many of the psychological happenings most significant for psychiatry go on without clear consciousness of them, but in appropriate conditions they may be accompanied by much more, or by full, consciousness. Biologically and psychologically regarded, consciousness is an attribute, like movement or the ability to learn, immensely important for us human beings, but not a 'present-or-absent' factor decisive for our mode of mental conduct.

It is imperative to take account of these complex mechanisms if the significance of any adverse psychological or social event for the individual human being is to be evaluated. For this purpose the notion of 'stress' cannot be defined in impersonal, physiological terms alone. Whether the events be on a large scale, e.g. war, natural disaster, or on a small scale, e.g, bereavement, divorce, their role as causes or precipitants of mental illness can only be established in the setting of a psychobiological life-history. Beginners in psychiatry and adherents to holistic systems of psychogenesis both tend to seek the explanation of many forms of mental disorder in terms of an understandable sequence of psychosocial events. In reality such events often play a pathoplastic rather than an aetiological role in the genesis of the disorder.

SYMPTOMATOLOGY: THE PHENOMENA OF MENTAL ILLNESS

All too often in psychiatry the examination of a patient reveals no physical signs and laboratory investigations are negative. The clinician must then rely on no more than an account of subjective experiences and/or disordered behaviour in the setting of the patient's history and background [see below]. In essence this procedure does not differ from that which is followed by all physicians when confronted by many disorders of function, e.g. migraine. The difference lies in the ambiguity of most psychiatric symptoms and in the relative complexity of the functional disturbance.

The inadequacy of dualistic logic is clearly exposed by the genesis of psychiatric symptoms. Where a symptom is, on the face of it, definitely physical or definitely mental, its causation may not be inferred to be exclusively of the same order. The chief cause of, say, an anorexia may be a series of mental experiences or an attack of migraine or uraemia or a hypothalamic lesion; study of the anorexia alone cannot serve to discriminate them; not even study of the psychological state alone, or of the physical state alone may suffice. Very often the physical and psychological factors in causation are mingled inextricably; they represent, of course, different facets of the same series of phenomena.

The patient's present symptoms must be examined in the light of his earlier experience. Thus one elucidates in detail the content of his illness and some of the causes of its occurrence. Which experiences play a role in determining the form of mental symptoms depends much on the emotional disturbance they originally provoke and this, in turn, on the instinctual drives which they touch on and disturb. If these drives conflict the emotion accompanying the conflict may prove so disturbing that it cannot be borne in its naked form; 'repression' serves the end of making this more or less tolerable, through disguising or distributing it. So emotion may be shifted from one object to another, and paradoxical or unexpected emotions be thus aroused by objects on to which the affect has been displaced. Alternatively, energy mainly directed to plain ends, e.g. sexual love, may be diverted into less obvious channels, and when thus 'sublimated' and mingled with features derived from other instinctual sources, its origins may be hard to recognize. Sexual needs so often conflict with others that many of the most powerful motives for the production of mental symptoms come from the struggle. To describe emotional experience, however, wholly or largely in terms of sex and aggression, as has sometimes been done, is only possible if one strains the meaning of these words out of all knowledge. It is as unwise to make sexual factors paramount in psychogenesis as to burke them.

A related error is to push back all one's inquiries to a supposedly crucial stage of early childhood. The experiences of the first 2 or 3 years of life are, like all subsequent experience, contributory to mental development, and they show certain sequences of phenomena characteristic of such development. Moreover, their relative simplicity makes it possible to recognize in these early reactions the instinctual drives which become manifest when the environment supplies the necessary material. On the other hand, the functions recognizable in the relatively simple reactions of early childhood are not the same as those which may be seen in later years when the organism is more fully grown, any more than an infant's physical structure and functions are identical with those of the more differentiated adult. The obvious continuity of the actual happenings in a human being's lifetime does not justify one in trying to analyse and reduce all adult mental phenomena into terms of child psychology, nor does clinical practice require it.

Since perception is an active process which makes use of past experience, it may not only select its material and invest it with meaning, but in doing so may distort it, and give it a special 'false' meaning. Unwelcome emotions may be thus projected on to external objects or happenings, which are then regarded as hostile or contemptuous, or in some other way significantly related to one's self. This may be compared with the process in visual perception whereby one projects the image on one's retina into the external world, and is convinced of its reality there; the further process of clothing it with emotional significance depends on one's inherent tendencies and one's previous experiences. Paranoid symptoms, ideas of reference, grandiose and self-reproachful delusions exemplify this mechanism. Hallucinations and kindred phenomena are a special instance of the interplay between material substrate, e.g. in cocaine poisoning, inherent tendencies, e.g. visual fantasies of children, and past experience, e.g. hallucinations of homosexual abuse or divine commands. Similarly, by fantasy and imagination the outer world can be manipulated or denied according to the heart's desire, just as by body-images of proposed movement the way is prepared for purposive muscular action. In giving meaning to present things, personal connexions between them and earlier experiences are established; whether normal or morbid, this ascription of 'symbolic' meaning to everyday objects is indispensable to thought, and is most striking in our use of spoken or written language, where sounds and shapes are conventional symbols for the most diverse experiences. Some of our words are personal to ourselves, and are used in an individual way; in morbidly heightened form, this process may issue in schizophrenic neologisms, or oddities of expression. Similarly, an obsessional patient may feel towards some word or object a superficially incomprehensible mixture of attraction and repulsion, which is due to this word or object being the symbol of some earlier experiences that have been of great moment in his life. To see how it has come to be such a symbol calls for minute study of his earlier experiences. Physical happenings in one's own body may symbolize present emotions or earlier experience of a momentous and emotionally painful kind. A gesture of disgust may normally be evoked unconsciously by a banal happening which has somehow become emotionally coloured by past experience. A headache or nausea may embody our dissatisfaction with a present situation. So hysterical 'conversion' symptoms may reflect and symbolize an inner emotional struggle, as may also some obsessional movement, schizophrenic stereotypy or hypochondriacal fear. The body, with all its functions, is the background of psychic life, and resonates to it.

The phenomena of mental disease must also be considered in relation to social and cultural forces. A belief in witchcraft, for example, cannot be deemed morbid without regard to such factors as nationality, upbringing, religious faith, social class and educational level. Too partial a regard for subsidiary or part functions, whether physiological or psychological, leads the investigator away from a view of the human being as an integrated organism towards the study of disparate mental and physical systems. This trend can only be counterbalanced by an awareness of the social matrix in which the individual develops and lives. It is for this reason that information and concepts derived from the social sciences carry so much meaning for the study of psychiatric illness.

CLASSIFICATION AND DIAGNOSIS

An ideal system of classification in psychiatry would be securely based on aetiology; it would incorporate clinical disturbances of function, both physical and psychological, and carry prognostic implications. The present stage of knowledge renders this ideal remote. In practice the best that can be achieved is a provisional mixture of aetiological, functional and clinical categories. The problems posed by this inevitable compromise are clearly illustrated by reference to the best-known schema, the International Statistical Classification; the main categories of the 8th revision (1965) are set out below, the fourth digit sub-categories being omitted.

Psychoses:
- Senile and presenile dementia
- Alcoholic psychosis
- Psychosis associated with intracranial infection
- Psychosis associated with other cerebral condition
- Psychosis associated with other physical condition
- Schizophrenia
- Affective psychoses
- Paranoid states
- Other psychoses
- Unspecified psychosis

Neuroses, Personality Disorders and Other Non-psychotic Mental Disorders:
- Neuroses
- Personality disorders
- Sexual deviation
- Alcoholism
- Drug dependence
- Physical disorders of presumably psychogenic origin
- Special symptoms not elsewhere classified
- Transient situational disturbances
- Behaviour disorders of childhood
- Mental disorders not specified as psychotic associated with physical conditions

Mental Retardation:
- Borderline mental retardation
- Mild mental retardation
- Moderate mental retardation
- Severe mental retardation
- Profound mental retardation
- Unspecified mental retardation

A simpler, less elaborate classification will be employed in this section, as befits a brief textbook presentation. All the categories can nonetheless be readily assimilated to those of the *International Classification of Diseases.*

The first ten categories of the I.C.D. are subsumed under the traditional heading of 'psychoses' which are distinguished from a group of 'non-psychotic' disorders and from the various forms of mental retardation. Commonly the psychoses are still equated with insanity and the neuroses with the other psychiatric anomalies which are outwardly less alien to the normal mind. The distinction between neuroses and psychoses is at times convenient, but without substance. To argue whether a dubious case is neurotic or psychotic is like arguing whether a man of medium size is thin or fat: he is both and neither. A genuine decision as to aetiology, prognosis or treatment turns not on whether a case is regaded as neurotic or psychotic, but on more solid findings. Since such words die hard, the best use of them is to term a patient with mental disorder 'neurotic' if he has fair insight into his illness, is co-operative and unlikely to need care in an institution, and to term him 'psychotic' if the contrary is the case.

Within the large group of psychoses the chief division is between those mental changes accompanying distinctive somatic disorder and those for which no such physical relationship has been demonstrated. The former are called 'symptomatic' or 'organic'; the latter 'constitutional' or 'functional'. Whereas everything found in the latter may be seen also in the former, the reverse of this is not true: there are some symptoms—due to the loss or damage of essential tissues, especially in the central nervous system—which can only occur when the material substrate is grossly damaged. Yet although the 'functional' group is made up of those conditions for which no distinctive somatic disorder can be found responsible, it by no means follows that their causes or basis are therefore purely psychological. Theoretically, such a belief is untenable since, as has been observed, physiological and psychological reactions are only different aspects of the same phenomena. Further, as a matter of observation certain physical disturbances so regularly accompany these disorders, and a physical configuration may be so linked with them, as to render it probable in time that the somatic disturbances of function will be well enough worked out for the terms 'organic' and 'functional' to lapse. Only the crudity or transience of the physiological changes would then remain to distinguish 'functional' from 'organic'.

The organic psychoses are subdivided into diseases located in the nervous system and those affecting it indirectly, as uraemia or lead poisoning may. Some are toxic, e.g. delirium tremens; some degenerative, e.g. senile psychoses; some inflammatory, e.g. encephalitis lethargica; some plainly hereditary, e.g. Huntington's chorea or 'primary' mental defect; and some privative, e.g. pellagra or myxoedema. The 'functional' psychotic conditions are often arranged according to whether emotional disturbance is evident and predominant (affective disorder); whether there is profound derangement of thought, feeling and contact with the real world (schizophrenia); or whether morbid false beliefs have become fixed without intellectual or emotional deterioration (paranoia).

The large collection of 'Neuroses, Personality Disorders and Other Non-psychotic Mental Disorders' which constitute the second ten categories of the International Statistical Classification illustrate still more clearly the heterogeneous nature of the clinical groupings which command acceptance at the present time. At the one extreme are those disorders for which an aetiological factor is specified or implied, namely 'physical disorders of presumably psychogenic origin', 'mental disorders not specified as psychotic associated with physical conditions' and 'transient situational disturbances'. At the other extreme, individual symptoms have had to be recognized as dominating certain diagnostic categories. This is explicitly so in the case of 'special symptoms not elsewhere classified' which includes such clinically important phenomena as enuresis, tics and stammering. Further, particular symptoms are employed in the sub-classification of the neuroses and the personality disorders, e.g. obsessive compulsive neurosis and hysterical personality, and disorders of behaviour dominate the categories of 'sexual deviation', 'alcoholism', 'drug dependence' and 'behaviour disorders of childhood'.

Intermediate between the broad clinical groupings or types of morbid reaction and the individual symptoms there are a number of important psychiatric symptom-complexes or syndromes. These make up the weft that runs across the psychiatric pattern and are not limited to any one of the major groupings: the most important are depersonalization, hypochondriasis, twilight states, stupor and other disorders of motility, and anorexia nervosa.

The personality of the patient may also be a criterion of these groupings, with the proviso mentioned earlier that illness does not only occur in those with the appropriate psychopathic anomaly of personality, nor does the latter by any means regularly issue in definite symptoms. Unless, however, psychiatry takes account of the psychopathic personality, even when not accompanied by symptoms of illness, it cannot study delinquency, disorders of behaviour in children, sexual perversions and other anomalies which touch very closely on psychiatric problems in the stricter sense. Personality disorders are also encountered frequently in association with other psychiatric conditions and must be incorporated in any multifactorial diagnosis.

Tradition and convenience argue in favour of retaining the third large grouping of mental deficiency or subnormality which might logically be distributed among the other categories. Again, it is custom rather than reason which decrees that mental subnormality be classified primarily by degree of intellectual retardation rather than by aetiology. However, the International Statistical Classification employs the fourth digit to indicate the many causal factors which are associated with mental subnormality [see p. 1385].

COURSE AND PROGNOSIS

In the absence of any clear-cut physiopathology the classification of many functional psychiatric disorders has in the past been linked with the notion of outcome. Residual traces of this approach can still be detected in modern nosological schemata, e.g. the '*episodic* excessive drinking' or the '*transient* situational disturbances' of the International Classification, but whereas the making of a correct diagnosis may in psychiatry indicate the general drift of an illness—towards recovery, chronicity, progression or relapse—it is of even less use than in the rest of medicine for showing how far this will apply to a particular patient. Clinical observation and statistics have furnished a wealth of empirical knowledge leading to several well-established generalizations. Thus an abrupt onset is favourable, other things being equal; a gradual, especially an insidious, onset may indicate a rooted abnormality that will be hard to shift. The longer an illness has gone on, the more will it have become autonomous, i.e. independent of the immediate causes of its occurrence. A study of the ups and downs in the course of an illness may show favourable influences that can with profit be deliberately brought to bear on it, as well as harmful ones that must be avoided. The more reconciled the patient has become to his illness the less likely his recovery. The patient's age also matters. In a young man there is more chance of his being adaptable, so that the removal of various stresses may help him, and his energies be diverted in less morbid channels; as he grows older, he may gain in stability, but gradually become more disposed to fear and suspicion, bodily preoccupations and fixed attitudes of mind.

Similarly, there are prognostic conclusions to be drawn from the form of many psychiatric disorders. A predominantly affective attack will very likely clear up, but may recur; a schizophrenic syndrome is ominous in the long run; hypochondriasis and depersonalization, especially in young people, tend to last a long time, even years; sexual perversities can seldom be got rid of altogether; hysterical symptoms can easily be changed, but hysterical reactions are persistent; obsessional illnesses are either periodic or very chronic; melancholia is often a fatal disease, through suicide; delirium tremens commonly ends by crisis or lysis after about 7 days; untreated general paralysis of the insane goes downhill towards dementia and death, with partial remissions on the way.

Nonetheless, useful as these general guide-lines may be, a careful study of each life-history and illness is indispensable if a prognosis is to be assessed in the individual case. From what has been already been said about causation it follows that the complex interplay of factors is sufficiently varied in the course of each patient's life to render prognosis a matter of individual study, rather than of summary inference from a diagnostic label. Where a known external cause has been at work, its point of attack, its severity and persistence will affect the issue. This applies equally to such 'organic causes' as poisons and cerebral diseases and to 'mental causes', like economic misery or frustrated love. The physician must consider how long the environmental cause has been acting; what changes it is known to produce—cell degeneration or gloom, fibrosis or fantasy; whether it is likely to persist; and whether the patient's previous history has shown evidence of sensitivity to such a trauma. He must also ask a number of questions about intrinsic causes. How has the patient previously reacted to this sort of interference or to any disturbing circumstances? Has he fallen more and more into unsatisfactory habits in meeting his daily life and its difficulties? How has his whole character developed? Is there good evidence of his being able to cope with partial deviations from mental health? Has he inherited tendencies to benign or to progressive illness? What seem to be the most useful reparative or stabilizing features in his personality? How far are his struggles with the world an outcome of his intrinsic endowment, evident in various guises since his childhood, and how far have they been forced upon him by an adverse milieu? In addition, the physician will pay regard to the possibilities of active intervention. Is treatment likely to be efficacious, feasible and acceptable? Can the patient's living conditions and personal relationships be improved? An attempt must be made to answer such questions in formulating a prognosis for every case.

PREVENTION

Primary prevention can be achieved in only a small segment of the wide area of mental illness. By and large it is the organic disorders which are more accessible to effective preventive methods, principally because an indispensable link in the causal chain can sometimes be identified and controlled by public health measures. The reduced incidence of the psychoses associated with pellagra and alcohol in the first half of this century illustrate what can be achieved in these circumstances. While the 'functional' disorders are probably due in part to such social factors as adverse moral and cultural values or noxious upbringing, the precise role of these factors is much harder to assess and the evaluation of prophylactic measures is correspondingly more difficult. Many of the most effective programmes of community mental hygiene are still largely negative: they are concerned with what to avoid rather than with what to do.

Prophylaxis in the individual case is often uncertain in respect of both intrinsic and extrinsic causes. Eugenic precautions, such as birth-control or voluntary sterilization may under skilled guidance prevent some mentally unstable persons from being born to parents who, having had mental illness themselves, do not wish to propagate it. If physical factors, e.g. syphilis, are prominent in causation, it may be possible to prevent the mental illness, or at any rate to scotch it in its early beginnings, by dealing with the somatic disorder. Thus, there are fewer cases of syphilitic psychoses now that syphilis is less often contracted and earlier treated. The psychological reactions to a physical disease or blemish may be favourably modified or averted, when foreseen. It is for obvious reasons impossible to counteract mental disorder by regularly protecting the patient from physical or psychic trauma; in any case, a life guarded against risks and painful experiences would be almost certain to issue in mental ill health, out of its very emptiness. By altering a patient's environment and way of living one may, however, be able to avert an impending illness: only study of the individual patient can show how this end is to be achieved. Making the patient's environment easier for him may be difficult in some instances because doing so would conflict with his obligations toward other people; and even if, on balance, a change of this sort seems essential, the patient may thereafter be troubled by guilt and shame. This is particularly evident in unsettled times.

The work people do and the conditions under which they do it influence their mental health. By ensuring that good vocational advice and training is available to those about to enter the field of employment and to those whose maladjustment is connected with their occupation, useful preventive work can be done.

How far the treatment of behaviour disorders and neurotic traits in childhood can be trusted to avert outbreaks of definite mental illness in later life is a disputable matter, but it is fairly certain that by taking advantage of his plasticity and responsiveness, and modifying his human environment, help and advice can often be given to the maladjusted child, which will result in his being socially better adapted and better able to deal with his problems. In the field of sexual attitudes, for example, needless fears and harmful education are rife, as with regard to the masturbation of adolescence—a common and comparatively harmless phase of sexual development.

TREATMENT

Whether it be considered in terms of physical, psychological or social measures the treatment of mental illness represents a special instance of the environment acting on the patient: as such its power and limitations cannot be assessed without regard to the effects of other experiences in his life. Rational and effective therapy based on a full understanding of aetiology is still relatively rare in psychiatry, being available chiefly for those disorders which are closely related to some identifiable cause, e.g. the psychoses associated with myxoedema or neurosyphilis. By contrast, the great majority of remedies are empirical, though none the less efficacious in a few cases: artificial fever for general paresis, electroconvulsive therapy for some types of depression, hypnotherapy for selected hysterical symptoms have all proved their worth in the absence of established knowledge about their mode of action. The place of most of the many empirical forms of psychiatric treatment, however, depends more often on the uncertain foundations of clinical opinion than on scientific fact. Clinical opinions about therapy are notoriously unreliable when conditions of unknown aetiology and uncertain course are treated in this way, and it is still unusual for a psychiatric diagnosis to connote a method cf treatment. Further, such non-specific factors as suggestion, the so-called placebo-effect and socio-environmental influences all exercise a potent influence on mental disorders so that controlled clinical trials are indispensable for the evaluation of new, and even old, treatments in psychological medicine. In psychiatry, more than most branches of medicine, therapeutic optimism can lead to self-deception, just as therapeutic pessimism can lead to indifference.

These reservations render the management of the individual patient a matter of balanced clinical judgement. Sometimes a patient's condition demands energetic intervention; sometimes it demands restrained symptomatic treatment; sometimes social or psychotherapeutic measures are called for; sometimes drugs are required. Rarely can treatment be limited safely to one approach, though the emphasis will vary from case to case. Never can it be assumed that a heavily tainted family history or other evidence of a strong constitutional factor indicates that therapeutic endeavour must be regarded as no more than a superfluous struggle against fate.

Social and Occupational Treatments

The first task in social treatment is to decide where the patient is to be looked after. Is he fit to be at home, should he be in a hospital, attending a day hospital, or in some other environment? Although many of the social treatments of mental illness were developed to help hospital in-patients it has become increasingly necessary to apply and extend such measures in an extramural setting. Whereas a spell in hospital may be an essential component of a therapeutic programme there are disadvantages and even dangers in too protracted an institutional residence. The duration of stay in psychiatric hospitals is now much shorter than formerly; the size of resident population in these hospitals is decreasing and legal powers are employed much less frequently to admit and detain patients. This has been achieved partly through the development of new methods of treatment and partly as the result of a social policy which places greater emphasis on the management of the mentally sick in the community. Without the provision of a whole range of extramural services—hostels, day-centres, enlarged out-patient facilities, domiciliary care, and the like—the therapeutic gains of social psychiatry could not have been achieved.

The decision as to the need of psychiatric in-patient care rests in the first instance on the danger the patient presents to others, or the chance of his committing suicide. These two problems of behaviour were at one time almost the only grounds of admission to a mental hospital. Nowadays the question turns on the positive benefits the hospital setting affords. The hospital milieu can exert a powerful effect for good or ill. Much effort has been put into developing in all those who inhabit a psychiatric hospital—staff and patients alike—a feeling of tolerant understanding of oneself and others which will weld the people involved into a community striving towards mental health and coping helpfully with inevitable upsets.

If the patient's immediate environment contains many disturbing influences, it will be desirable for him to be away from them, temporarily at least, so long as this does not entail worse troubles. Summary decisions are here impossible. It may, for example, be useless to get a woman who is paranoid about her neighbours to move to another district to escape them, unless it is the actual conduct of the neighbours and not the patient's morbid attitude that is provoking her suspicion of them. It requires a close knowledge of the facts as well as wisdom and psychiatric experience to give help on matters that may wholly alter the course of a patient's life—advice, say, about separating from his wife, giving up his job or emigrating. Many instances of this might be offered. Weary, depressed patients are often harmfully urged to go to dances and lively resorts where they must try to look happy. Hysterical patients do not benefit by being put among people who are hostile and contemptuous, any more than in an atmosphere of mawkish sympathy and compliance. Neurotic patients are often advised to get married, especially if loneliness and sexual needs trouble them, as though marriage were a panacea; such advice by rule of thumb too often makes their condition worse, ruins the life of the person they marry and results in offspring that have to be treated at a child guidance clinic.

In the social treatment of patients indispensable help can be given by trained psychiatric social workers. Their assistance is not restricted to the patient's economic problems: they provide expert information and advice on all the social aspects of his illness, and carry out social measures of treatment. Similarly, a non-medical psychologist must be available for help in dealing with educational and vocational problems and the administration of specialized tests. He can also give valuable help and stimulus in the planning of therapeutic measures based on the theory of learning and conditioning.

Occupational treatment is important for all kinds of mental disorder. Where there is acute overt emotional disturbances, rest is at first desirable, as it is also for confusional and delirious states. In these conditions opportunity for occupation must be gradually offered to the patient as his disorder subsides; steady, simple work is preferable to the restless, unsatisfying, fickle activity in which he would often engage if left to himself. The less acute any mental disturbance, the more necessary is it that occupation should be urged upon the patient, and that it should be disciplined and congenial. A planned occupational regime is a central feature of any programme designed to reduce chronic disability associated with psychiatric illness. This applies equally to gross psychoses and minor affections of the neurotic sort. Allowance must be made for the patient's bent, his symptoms and personality, and especially his more or less conscious reasons for working and not working; hence there will be much diversity in the conditions of his occupation, whether it be therapeutically contrived in a hospital, offered at a Rehabilitation Unit or sought out as remunerative work in the open market. These may be stages in his progress towards normal health and life in the general community. For most people, mental health cannot be permanently retained unless one does some satisfying work; often it cannot be recovered unless one does.

Physical Treatments

'Mechanical restraint' and violence are now foreign to the treatment of insanity; the patient may be unrestrained and violent, but his treatment may not. It is still necessary, however, to restrain a patient who is bent on harming himself or others. Physical force may be the only way of doing so, but it must always be a last resort and chemical substitutes for it are now plentiful. Drugs have their place in the treatment of all kinds of mental disorder, though their use easily turns to abuse.

Since the early 1950s the introduction of a host of new pharmacological compounds has led to a revival of interest in the rapidly growing field of *psychopharmacology*, a general term which is now widely accepted as designating the study of drug action in relation to the higher functions of the central nervous system, normal and abnormal. The new compounds, often known collectively as psychotropic drugs, are a heterogeneous group: most of them have a sedative action, some relieve depression. They are credited with a favourable effect on the symptoms and course of various forms of mental disorder, and the enthusiasm generated by them has been so great that their arrival has been said to mark a psychiatric revolution. There have, however, been too few controlled trials, and some of the drugs acclaimed and popular a few years ago are now no longer used. There are grounds for regretting that well-tried and effective sedative drugs, such as the barbiturates, have often been put aside, to give way to newer, and often more toxic but not more efficacious drugs.

In 1935 treatment by induced convulsions was introduced. At first drugs, and then electrical stimulation of the brain, were used for this purpose: the electrical method, commonly referred to by the abbreviation E.C.T., is now almost always preferred to the pharmacological. Originally put forward as a way of treating schizophrenia, it has limited success there except in the acute stuporose forms and those associated with an affective syndrome. Its efficacy in involutional and some other affective disorders is, however, striking. It terminates obstinate melancholias and abbreviates attacks of depression which would otherwise take many months to clear up. Modifications, such as electronarcosis, have been tried, but the standard method is the most satisfactory.

Another physical procedure, first reported in 1936, was surgical incision of both frontal lobes—leucotomy—to sever the connexion of the anterior portions with the thalamus. Its benefits are uncertain, and its risks considerable. It should be a last resort, when other forms of treatment have failed and the condition is seriously distressing, accompanied by tension, and occurring in a person who has not had long-standing disorder of personality. The conditions for which it may be beneficial are chronic agitated depression, chronic schizophrenia punctuated by violent outbursts, and intractable obsessional disorder. The risks are death from the operation (between 2 and 3 per cent. in a large collection of cases), blunting of spontaneity and self-control, impairment of judgement and foresight, and epilepsy or urinary incontinence. Although modifications in the size and extent of the cut have been made, which are claimed to reduce the risks without reducing the benefits, the operation has become less and less favoured, especially since the advent of the psychotropic drugs. More recently, claims have been made for a stereotaxic technique of tractotomy involving the implantation of radioactive seeds into the substantia innominata.

The insulin coma treatment of schizophrenia is now fast becoming a matter of historical interest only. It has been in rapid decline during the last few years, though it was for a time highly valued by many psychiatrists who believed that it shortened the duration of schizophrenic illness and increased the number of recoveries; others, however, maintained that it scored its successes in patients who would have got well as quickly, or more quickly, with other forms of treatment if administered with equal zeal. That such diverse views could be held by responsible observers was due not only to their prejudice and temperament, but to the difficulties of judging therapeutic success in an illness which is sometimes difficult to diagnose with certainty in its early stages and has anything but a uniform prognosis; moreover, it was believed to be hopeless by many psychiatrists in pre-insulin days, so that they did not try to treat it by methods then available which would have yielded full permanent recovery in a quarter of the cases, if selected on the same basis as became customary for insulin treatment. Insulin and convulsant treatment have demonstrated that in the present state of psychiatry the value of a new therapeutic procedure should be assessed not by the reports of enthusiasts, valuable though their efforts and observations are, but by the outcome of a planned therapeutic trial in which uniform standards have been employed in the selection of cases, the method of administering the treatment and the assessment of outcome; also due regard must be paid to the choice of those 'control' cases with which the beneficiaries of the new method are to be compared.

The details of a hospital regime may include such measures as exercise, massage and hydrotherapy, beneficial as much for their psychological as for their physiological results; the latter, however, are not negligible, as may be seen in the effect on an excited or an anxious patient of a continuous bath at body temperature. On the other hand, patients with a visceral neurosis, e.g. 'effort syndrome', a hypochondriacal preoccupation, an hysterical anomaly, or a somatic delusion can be harmed by the prolonged physical investigation and treatment they receive: it confirms the symptom, localizes it all the more and may bring fresh ones in its train. Sometimes one has no choice; a progressive hysterical contracture, a dermatitis artefacta, a sore infected by constant picking, a tooth loosened by obsessional knocking at it demand treatment.

The chief importance of diet lies in the frequent refusal of food by patients who are depressive, hysterical, stuporose, paranoid, hypochondriacal or overactive. Feeding by the nasal tube may in rare instances be a necessity, after every other method has failed. A special diet may be called for, as in the symptomatic psychoses of diabetes, pernicious anaemia or pellagra, for anorexia nervosa and also for some temporary disabilities of the alimentary tract. As a rule, however, such dietetic regime, and indeed all physical treatment of localized psychogenic disturbances of function in a bodily system, is an expedient rather than a settled and adequate mode of treatment.

Psychological Treatments

There is no form of treatment which has not a psychological aspect and result. In the literal and larger sense of the term psychological treatment is needed for every variety or stage of mental and physical illness, and every degree of co-operativeness or intelligence. It is a wide notion, including all that may ease or reassure the patient, bring him to a better relationship with those around him and with himself, and protect him from being distressed by the ignorance, lack of tact, or thoughtlessness of others. It implies both positive and negative measures. The physician and the rest of those who are in contact with the patient must do certain positive things: make due allowance for his disorder influencing his conduct, use their understanding of the psychological happenings without saying so, take advantage of every opportunity created by other methods of treatment. When occupation, narcosis, a surgical operation, massage ,a physical illness or other happenings bring him more closely into contact with nurses and physicians there are chances of unobtrusive psychological treatment in the wide sense. On the negative side, one must avoid arguing with the patient, telling him lies 'for his own good' or to avoid unpleasant scenes, cajoling him, making promises that will not be kept, threatening or punishing him, jesting at his expense, losing one's patience with him, assuming he is indifferent to what goes on because he looks indifferent, provoking him by petty supervision or frequent rebukes; one should not assume that he is quite irresponsible or quite responsible, nor talk theory to him, nor get on a false footing through ready assent to his delusions and his point of view.

The term 'psychotherapy' is conventionally limited to those forms of treatment which depend upon direct and personal relationship between the patient and the physician. They have been given separate names, and divided into schools and techniques. Stress may be laid upon the prestige of the physician, as in suggestion; the patient's attachment to him, in all its complicated phases ('transference'); the trained understanding and thoroughness with which he clears up the patient's problems—persuasion, re-education, distributive analysis; or on his qualities of personality—enthusiasm, energy, warmth, candour, wisdom. In so far as psychological treatment is necessarily based on a personal relationship it cannot be made a routine except in its non-essentials: whatever rules the psychiatrist follows or whatever the training he has undergone, he himself is more important than his method in benefiting the patient. To that great extent psychotherapy is not a scientific procedure. While method and training are of some consequence they are never more than devices whereby the influence of one human being upon another's mind and conduct can be turned to the best medical ends and the dangers inherent in such a relationship minimized.

It has not proved possible to describe in general terms what the psychotherapist does, otherwise than by metaphor or analogy: he promotes the ventilation and desensitization of emotional disturbances; he elucidates latent or obvious muddles, disentangles conflicting tendencies, giving them new incentives and a different direction; and so guides the patient through the maze of his life's experience, as recalled in memory, that he is then better fitted for dealing with current experience, knows himself better and has somewhat purged himself of past harms. All 'analytic' methods review the patient's life as he recalls it under special conditions, e.g. of free association, hypnosis, biographical scheme, etc. They stop at different points, some aiming at emotional clearance by abreaction, some at a redirection and liberation of the instinctual bases of character, while others remain content with an educational achievement.

The more specialized, intricate or esoteric the method of psychotherapy, the less suitable is it to be used by any but the expert. It is inappropriate here to detail the many kinds of technique that have been employed but the following general principles apply to every method: (1) The psychological causes of the patient's illness should be sought only to the extent that the patient's well-being demands; this is often far short of what one's own interest and psychological curiosity would demand. (2) The therapist should be satisfied with the patient's recovery, and not aim at a state of ideal mental health and self-understanding. It is better that treatment should be quick and effective than drawn out to meet theoretical standards. (3) The removal of symptoms should be deemed a good thing, but the maintenance of normal social adaptation far better. It is bad to get rid of one symptom only to see it replaced by another, but much worse to get rid of all symptoms only to see the patient at the end of treatment a dependent and introspective hypochondriac of the mind, a social invalid. (4) Though the influence of psychotherapy may be profound it is not necessarily beneficial. It is always important to consider carefully whether any shock to the patient, any aggravation one produces in his illness even temporarily, may be a sign of bad treatment.

Whether psychotherapy, in the formal sense, can or should be applied will depend on the following factors: the patient should be willing to co-operate in the treatment; free from such hindering disabilities as, say, deafness; able to give the necessary time; of at any rate average intelligence; still capable of modification, as he would not be, for example, in old age, or with very long-standing and indurated habits of faulty reaction, or with organic cerebral disease; and, finally, endowed with a considerable residue of normal mental functions with which one may work. The more profound his aberrations, as in schizophrenia, or the more extreme his emotional disturbance, as in agitated melancholia, the less is he fit for psychological treatment of this individual and specialized kind.

Of late much effort has been put into the psychotherapy of patients, not as individuals, but as members of a group. Though less economical of time and labour than had been hoped, this has the advantage of utilizing for therapeutic purposes the influence that patients have on one another through candid self-revelation, disclosure of significant experiences, and search for interpretations that will make their morbid reactions understandable to them and to others. Emotions are aroused, and verbally expressed; the therapist has to regulate them. Many devices of group treatment have been employed, from social club meetings to 'psycho-drama' —plays that originate with the patients and touch on their conflicts, and are followed by a group discussion. Group procedures have not made individual treatment superfluous.

Besides these personal forms of psychotherapy, relatively impersonal methods drawn from modern learning theory and experiment are also being applied to the treatment of neurotic symptoms. The symptoms are regarded as unadaptive conditioned responses; the treatment consists in extinguishing these and replacing them by desirable or adaptive conditioned reactions. The term 'behaviour therapy' has come into fashion as a description of a group of techniques employed to this end. These techniques comprise desensitization, aversion and positive conditioning. Desensitization, often called reciprocal inhibition, is designed to reduce morbid anxiety by means of muscle relaxation combined with the graded experience of anxiety-provoking situations, either in reality or in imagination: encouraging results have been reported in the treatment of some types of phobias. In aversion therapy the objective is to remove the symptom by associating it with an unpleasant stimulus which is repeatedly administered; the stimulus in question may be pharmacological or electrical and variants of the treatment have been widely applied to alcoholism and sexual deviation. Positive conditioning techniques are best exemplified by the treatment of nocturnal enuresis with the bell and pad method, whereby a wet bed induces an electrical contact to ring a bell which wakes the patient to empty his bladder: bladder distension becomes associated with arousal and the patient learns to control vesical function. Behaviour therapy is often accompanied by strong emotional reactions on the part of the patient towards the therapist and its complete independence from the holistic forms of psychotherapy is more apparent in theory than in practice.

PSYCHIATRIC DISORDERS ASSOCIATED WITH ORGANIC DISEASES

THE ORGANIC PSYCHIATRIC SYNDROMES

The varieties of form and course of the organic psychiatric disorders—sometimes called symptomatic psychoses or exogenous reactions—are essentially few. The causes, by contrast, are numerous and cannot be inferred by study of the mental picture alone; for that the methods of somatic medicine are needed. Many different poisons and lesions may produce the same effect on the mental state. The differences depend on the degree and duration of the physical damage and its site, which may determine neurological and other symptoms of a typical kind.

Though the organic reactions are the least constitutional of all mental affections, yet even in them constitutional factors are far from negligible. It is due to such factors that one man will show a psychosis with physical illness that in another would lead to no such mental upset, and that one patient responds with a manic extravagance to the cerebral disease which makes another patient depressed. Moreover, genetic factors can be of great importance in these organic affections. The content of the disorder is often understandable in relation to the patient's previous personality and life-history.

The syndromes commonly met with must be described before seeing how particular diseases colour them and determine their course and treatment. In all organic syndromes a diminution in mental capacity is the central finding. To some extent these syndromes may occur also in patients in whom no structural damage can be found, as might be expected since the available patterns of structure and function are in all cases much the same.

NEURASTHENIA

This term has been over-used and ill-used, but it need not therefore be discarded now. It denotes a form of irritable, hypersensitive weakness and depression that is not uncommon after infections, exhausting experiences, e.g. hunger, lactation, insomnia, worry, haemorrhage, cranial injuries and chronic poisoning, e.g. with alcohol or coffee. A clinical picture indistinguishable from it frequently arises where physical causes are unlikely and emotional causes are obvious. This clinical finding carries the same significance as the fact that the anxiety of exophthalmic goitre resembles psychogenic anxiety; just as the anxiety of exophthalmic goitre or constant fear can pass into delirium, so can physiogenic neurasthenia be aggravated until it becomes plain dementia.

The symptoms are partly somatic—active deep reflexes, increased sensory irritability, feelings of pressure on the head and pains in the muscles and elsewhere, giddiness, vasomotor lability, delayed peristalsis and feelings of fullness in the abdomen, diminished libido, slight clumsiness, and tremor of the muscles of the face, tongue and hands. On the psychological side, there are feelings of languor, and incapacity to concentrate on any mental work, doubts as to the accuracy of memory, loss of interest, slight depersonalization, irritability and tenseness, lessened control of emotion, and perhaps slight paranoid, obsessional or hypochondriacal trends. This general condition is, when physiogenic, less influenced by a change in mood than would be the case with psychogenic neurasthenia, and the patient is better able to control his motor unrest than his features, which are expressive of his agitation. The chief reliance, however, must be put on the history and physical findings for telling whether the neurasthenia is physiogenic or not; psychological causes which seem adequate to explain the illness may be deceptive.

The course of neurasthenia is towards recovery unless the noxa continues to act; where the noxa persists, extreme chronicity can result. Sometimes an original physical noxa ceases to act, but meanwhile other emotional ones have entered the field, e.g. unemployment, domestic fears and frustrations, and so the illness drags on. Treatment depends on assessment of the causes and the possibility of removing them: drugs alone are insufficient.

SUBDELIRIOUS STATES

Closely akin to delirium, and indeed shading into it, is the state of *clouded consciousness* (or confusion) in which thought is very incoherent, but the patient is more eager to get in touch with his environment than in typical delirium. If consciousness is not too grossly clouded, the patient is perplexed and troubled by the disordered perceptions through which alone he can learn what is going on about him. The picture may be indistinguishable from that seen in some forms of manic excitement and in some catatonic states. Differentiation rests, not on the immediate psychiatric symptoms, but on the history and discoverable causes of the illness. The same is true of *acute hallucinosis* in which orientation and grasp are very little impaired, but auditory hallucinations—especially threatening sounds and voices—abound, and there is a tendency to the formation of delusions on the basis of these and other perceptual disturbances.

The name *twilight state* is applied to another syndrome in which consciousness is changed chiefly because of some powerful affective influence; anger or fear may so overwhelm psychic life that the patient cannot grasp his surroundings, his thinking is interrupted and slow (except where it falls in tune with the affective disturbance), and his motor behaviour is in keeping with his mood. It is as often of psychogenic as of organic origin: one can hardly, for example, by direct observation tell an epileptic twilight state from an hysterical one. Like delirium and the other conditions just mentioned, it is prone to subside and to be followed by amnesia for what happened during it: where there is some recollection, it may be associated with a conviction that the hallucinations and other morbid phenomena were real external happenings.

DELIRIUM

Delirium, most familiar in fevers, can also be produced by drugs and other causes of acute cerebral disturbance: moreover, severe affective disturbance may be accompanied by delirium. Its characteristics are general malaise, restlessness, irritability and sensitiveness to external stimuli, headache, anxiety and troubled sleep or insomnia. Mild forms are met with in so transient an affection as cold in the head. Severe forms are marked by illusions and hallucinations of all the special senses, especially vision. Anxiety often becomes extreme, and the patient is terrified of his fantastic visions. Thought becomes as chaotic and fleeting as in dreams, activity is incessant and past experiences of daily life are revived, as in the occupational delirium of alcoholics. Attention is weakened, and orientation in time and space much impaired. There are striking variations in the severity of the condition in the same patient: it becomes worse in the evening or when the patient has hardly any external stimuli to keep him in touch, cf. delirium at night and after a cataract operation. The extent to which consciousness is clouded usually corresponds to the amount of perceptual and affective disturbance. Auditory hallucinations occur with clearer consciousness, visual ones very profusely with a clouded mind. The auditory hallucinations are commonly of an elementary, undifferentiated kind rather than of voices. Vestibular hallucinations may occur, e.g. of floating in the air. Distressing and incoherent ideas pursue each other—ideas of being torn to pieces, burnt, poisoned, buried alive and so on. Ideas of grandeur can also be held and occasionally residual belief in the content of a delirious experience is maintained.

THE AMNESTIC SYNDROME

In the *amnestic syndrome*, often associated with the name of Korsakoff, the memory disturbance is in the forefront. There is reduced capacity to register, retain, recall and recognize impressions. Gaps in memory may be filled in by active fantasy (confabulation). The patients may be very ready to adopt suggestions, so that one can lead them to tell absurd tales about their recent movements. They do not show an intellectual damage or incapacity to deal with ideas that is at all comparable in degree to their memory disorder, but they are always out in their appreciation of time-relationships, especially where the present is concerned. At first blush they often seem to be behaving like mentally healthy people, but one presently discovers that their memory is much impaired, their orientation as to space, time and personal identity correspondingly poor, and their interest and general mood duller than is normal. Though the amnestic syndrome is closely connected with dementia, the disorder of memory is never, as in dementia, a general weakness reaching back even to childhood.

The Korsakoff syndrome is most often seen in alcoholics, in whom it was first described associated with polyneuritis, but it also occurs in a great variety of organic disorders, e.g. intoxication with lead, carbon monoxide and other poisons, uraemia, vitamin B_1 deficiency, cranial trauma, cerebral syphilis and arteriosclerosis. Apoplexy may precede it and the amnestic syndrome be thus complicated by asphasia. That it should sometimes follow on delirium is not surprising, since in delirium the same memory disturbance is present, but covered up by the concomitant excitement, disturbance of consciousness and hallucinations. Whether a Korsakoff syndrome will clear up depends on the cerebral damage which produces it; the alcoholic form occasionally does so eventually in uncomplicated and treated cases [see p. 1347].

DEMENTIA

Of all gross encephalopathic syndromes this is the gravest and most typical. It corresponds to a diffuse cerebral disease, and is made up of intellectual impairment and lessened control of emotion. Its form depends so much on the stage of the patient's development at which it occurs, that it is customary to consider as dementia only those cases in which the cerebral damage has occurred in later childhood, adolescence or adult life, and to regard earlier cases, e.g. cretins, as showing mental deficiency or arrest of development. Nonetheless, mental subnormality in some of its forms is a special instance of cerebral impairment though it is considered, for the sake of convenience and tradition, in a separate section [see p. 1385]. The distinction is rather artificial at whatever age it be made but only the adult form will be described here.

The order in which functions are impaired corresponds to Hughlings Jackson's principle of dissolution: thus, recently acquired memories are soonest lost, though there are exceptions. There is intellectual weakness—the patient cannot reason, grasp and remember as he could, his attention is less concentrated and sharp, his ideas are fewer, he cannot take in anything complicated or be sure about time and place, he loses himself. His emotions are likewise affected—he weeps over trifles in spite of efforts to control himself, his feelings are shallow and transient, he may be foolishly euphoric, or may burst into anger whenever he cannot get his own way. There are wide variations in the severity of the condition, and its symptoms may be much influenced by the local incidence of the pathological changes in the brain. The extent to which various cerebral functions are impaired may differ widely in the same patient: a man who seems hopelessly demented may be able to play a good game of chess; while another in whom it is hard to demonstrate any intellectual inpairment may micturate into his shoes or do something equally stupid and inappropriate; unexpected sexual misdemeanours are not uncommon in demented persons before they show gross intellectual damage.

Psychological tests have been increasingly used in dementia. Although they are untrustworthy for diagnostic purposes, they can be of value in measuring the degree and progress of the impairment.

PSYCHIATRIC DISORDERS ASSOCIATED WITH INFECTIOUS TOXAEMIAS

Delirium and a Korsakoff syndrome are the more acute, and neurasthenia the milder, signs of mental disorder due to an infectious fever. In many of the cases in which mental disorder is attributed to infection, however, either the mental changes are unconnected with the infectious process or there has been no infectious process, as is often found when one inquires into an alleged attack of 'influenza' and finds it was nothing of the kind. There are three possibilities: either the mental changes, especially of the delirious variety, are mainly due to the infection; or they are independent of the infection, as when some non-organic syndrome is put down to sepsis; or they are partly due to the infection and partly to other, usually constitutional causes, e.g. a post-infectious depression.

No mental symptoms specific to any one infection can be demonstrated. Wherever a delirium or other mental disturbance of one infection differs from that of another, e.g. the delirium of typhoid from that of pneumonia, the difference lies in the severity and duration of the physical effects of the intoxication and in the peculiarities of the affected person. Among these individual characteristics must be included a constitutional predisposition or readiness to respond with symptomatic psychoses to mainly physical ills.

There are a few infections that rarely cause mental disturbance, e.g. tetanus and diphtheria; others do so by their local cerebral incidence, e.g. malaria and encephalitis. Tuberculosis, by virtue of its chronicity and its occasional incidence on the central nervous system occupies a special position. Its treatment, moreover, may necessitate an abnormal, unsatisfying life for a time, and this with the toxaemia seems to be responsible for a euphoric or anxious restlessness in which erotic tendencies and irritability are often prominent. Spes phthisica is partly attributable to toxic euphoria; in part it is a form of over-compensation for fear.

PSYCHIATRIC DISORDERS ASSOCIATED WITH METABOLIC AND ENDOCRINE DISEASES

Various metabolic disorders can affect mental health in a non-specific way. In the metabolic disorders to be mentioned here the physical phenomena are relatively coarse and obvious. It is in some cases proven and in others highly probable that less obvious metabolic disturbances are among the primary symptoms of 'functional' mental illness, or are its pathological basis. The electrolytes of the blood, the metabolism of carbohydrate, fat and protein, and the chemical regulation of the vegetative activities are all, in such forms of mental illness as schizophrenia and mania, subject to changes which have not as yet been used in the pathology or treatment of these conditions, because the findings are not sufficiently constant and specific. Similarly, endocrine disorders play a more prominent role in the investigations than in the clinical practice of psychiatry. Many endocrine preparations have been administered to schizophrenic, sexually perverted and melancholic patients, either empirically or in accordance with a premature theory, but their therapeutic value remains controversial.

Diabetes mellitus is especially frequent in families with a predisposition to affective psychosis and may be accompanied by transient phases of depression, anxiety or excitement which correspond to changes in the blood-sugar level, or a ketosis may be ushered in by mild delirium. A diabetic pseudoparesis, with peripheral neuropathy, may cause difficulty in diagnosis. In children, mild hypoglycaemia may be responsible for anxiety, naughtiness and other disturbances of behaviour. Anomalous psychic states, often mistaken for hysteria or an anxiety state, may be induced by the hypoglycaemia associated with the rare condition of hyperinsulinism; this may be functional or due to an islet-cell tumour of the pancreas.

Gout may occur in people predisposed to affective disorder; often a depressive phase precedes an attack. Alkalosis and anoxaemia may each be the cause of mental disturbance of the organic type.

Deficiency diseases, especially of the vitamin B complex [see Section 4], are not infrequently associated with psychiatric symptoms. The nutritional deficiencies are usually multiple, though the clinical picture may be dominated by one or other syndrome. *Pellagra*, resulting principally from a lack of nicotinic acid, is most commonly productive of mental disorder. The clinical picture is sometimes very like that of hysteria; or the usual organic syndromes may be produced, especially florid confusion with perhaps hallucinations of fire. It must be remembered that a long-standing anorexia, of psychogenic origin or occurring in the course of a chronic melancholia, may itself lead to a pellagroid condition, so that the symptoms of mental disorder will then be those of the original illness plus those due to the deficiency.

The *Wernicke syndrome*—ophthalmoplegia, ataxia, clouding of consciousness and memory disturbances—results from a thiamine deficiency which may or may not also be associated with *beriberi*. It is seen most often in chronic alcoholics and in such emaciating conditions as advanced carcinoma, hyperemesis gravidarum or starvation.

In *pernicious anaemia* there may be mental symptoms, e.g. an acute confusional state, referable to the structural changes in the central nervous system, but more often depression occurs without 'organic' features; mania can also occur, and in some cases a chronic paranoid condition. Indeed, mental symptoms may be the only signs of vitamin B_{12} deficiency. The more 'organic' the picture, the poorer the prognosis for a return to mental health. The megaloblastic anaemia with disturbances in the metabolism of vitamin B_{12} and folic acid is associated with anticonvulsant medication and is sometimes accompanied by mental symptoms.

Uraemia may disturb consciousness greatly in the form of any of the organic syndromes, from a twilight state to a euphoric dementia; a Korsakoff condition can occur, but is infrequent.

Hepatic disease may lead to an encephalopathy with delirium and coma when liver failure develops. Jaundice may be accompanied by severe depression.

Exophthalmic goitre is more prone to occur in anxious nervous people, especially after some sudden shock. The usual concomitants—restlessness, tension, irritability, difficulty of concentration and liability to sudden changes of mood—may be complicated by a definite mania or depression. If the disease be severe or advanced, delirium and confusion may supervene. Though such organic syndromes mean, as a rule, a bad prognosis, they sometimes clear up dramatically after operation. The interaction of constitutional and psychogenic factors with the intoxication makes treatment by psychological as well as other methods desirable in many cases of exophthalmic goitre, either as a preliminary or supplement to partial thyroidectomy.

In adult *myxoedema* the slowing of mental activity may sometimes be accompanied by a chronic paranoid psychosis, or there may be a phase of excitement with hallucinations; the variety of syndromes that can occur is referable to pre-existing constitutional tendencies and to the varying severity and rapidity of development of the thyroid deficiency. An apparently 'functional' syndrome may precede the overt myxoedema. Juvenile and congenital myxoedema are described elsewhere [see Section 5].

Disorders of *calcium metabolism* may be accompanied by mental symptoms. The clinical features of tetany can follow the removal of the parathyroid glands if hypocalcaemia results. It may be signalized by epileptiform seizures, or there may be a proneness to psychogenic fits; thus the patient may spontaneously overbreathe until a convulsion is induced. Hysterics sometimes use hyperventilation in this way. In severe tetany a resistive lethargy or an excited, incoherent confusion may occur. Manic, depressive and other psychotic conditions may develop in hyperparathyroidism.

Pituitary diseases are more often accompanied by mental symptoms that are a comprehensible reaction to the physical symptoms than by organic syndromes; the latter, when they occur, may be due to increased intracranial tension. In acromegaly depression, reserve, touchiness and irritability are not surprising, though some acromegalics remain cheerful as long as their disabilities are moderate, and sometimes there is a blindness to the disease, a lack of insight, even when it is advanced. In dystrophia adiposogenitalis a rather childish placidity may be met. In adiposis dolorosa depression may be severe, or hysterical symptoms may develop. Sheehan's syndrome may be accompanied by depression, reaction to the psychosexual disturbance, and, in the later phases, by organic syndromes due to the cachexia. In Cushing's basophil syndrome depression and other mental disturbances can occur.

Among the disorders of the *adrenal glands* Addison's disease is accompanied by a neurasthenia of which for a time the physical basis may be quite overlooked (as may also occur in myasthenia gravis, so often misdiagnosed as hysteria); in the later stages delirium has been known to occur. Acute anxiety attacks may occur from a phaeochromocytoma. The adrenogenital syndrome, whether due to adrenal hyperplasia or to a neoplasm, can be accompanied by serious mental symptoms. During the course of treatment with cortisone or corticotrophin some people develop an acute psychosis which clears up if the drug is withdrawn.

PSYCHIATRIC DISORDERS ASSOCIATED WITH SEXUAL EPOCHS

In women sexual epochs may be associated with mental disorder of the organic type, e.g. some psychoses of pregnancy and the puerperium. *Menstruation* is apt to be associated with depression, irritability and languor in many women, especially during the few days before the period begins; there are no true menstrual psychoses but the liability to suicide and to psychopathic reactions is somewhat higher at this time.

Puberty and the *climacteric* are periods of stress during which schizophrenic and affective disorders may occur.

During *pregnancy* psychosis is rare, but depression and anxiety are fairly common, especially if the mother is reluctant to have another baby; a psychotic illness may, however, break out during the later months of pregnancy. The organic mental syndromes may develop along with polyneuritis, eclampsia or chorea gravidarum. Termination of the pregnancy is called for on account of the mental condition when there are symptoms of organic psychosis which are likely to get worse, a history of suicidal attempts or infanticide in connexion with previous pregnancies and a depression again in this one; or if on other grounds there is a clear risk of suicide or other untoward result of the mental illness, should pregnancy continue. The decision is often a very difficult one, requiring an expert knowledge of psychiatry for the careful appraisal of aetiology and prognosis essential in every case. The question must turn mainly on the therapeutic value of terminating the pregnancy so far as the mother's mental state is concerned, as well as upon the stage of pregnancy reached. Termination for purely psychiatric reasons is, on the whole, seldom necessary.

In the *puerperium* 'functional' psychoses often develop in predisposed women; if there be septicaemia as well, a confusional state or a delirium, followed by a period of neurasthenia, may occur. In many cases the delirious puerperal psychosis clears up in a week or two; the more endogenous varieties have sometimes a less satisfactory outcome than their form and onset suggest. Infanticide may occur in a puerperal psychosis, especially if the mother has, while pregnant, felt resentful at having a baby or been troubled by murderous preoccupations, e.g. obsessions. Psychoses of lactation are rare, and seldom of the organic type.

There is no satisfactory evidence that the affective disorders of later middle life ('involutional melancholia') in women are caused by the endocrine changes of the menopause; they are not benefited by oestrogen therapy. The effects of *castration* are dependent on the age at which the gonads are removed: intellectual development is unaffected, but the emotional and conative activities of those castrated in adult life may be impaired. Neurasthenic symptoms are frequent, and in women anxiety symptoms may appear.

PSYCHIATRIC DISORDERS ASSOCIATED WITH OTHER NON-CEREBRAL PHYSICAL CONDITIONS

Cardiac disorders predispose to an anxiety, which at night may take the form of mild delirium, with restlessness, terror, disorientation, auditory and sometimes visual hallucinations. With improvement in the circulation, the mental symptoms disappear, or remain only as a moody unrest. Reference is made elsewhere to arterial hypertension [see Section 8].

The connexion between many *alimentary* disorders and neurasthenic states is well attested, and is striking in children.

Exhaustion, especially if conjoined with distressing experiences, e.g. an earthquake or bombardment, can induce a delirium or a twilight state. 'Light-headedness' is a common complaint among patients who have suffered a severe haemorrhage or who have become cachectic as a result of physical disease.

The most common *post-operative* psychiatric disorder is a confusional state but 'functional' syndromes are also encountered, often after a short interval of a few days. These reactions can occur after any type of operation but they occur most frequently after surgery on the eye, uterus and heart. Several factors play a part in the development of mental symptoms in such cases—biochemical disturbances, anaesthetic effects, anxiety and fear about the procedure.

Porphyria [see Section 4] is a rare and often misdiagnosed cause of psychiatric disorder. Mental symptoms occur most frequently in association with the acute intermittent form of the disease and may be protean, ranging from an organic psychosis to seemingly hysterical conduct.

Patients with *systemic lupus erythematosus* [see Section 4] may exhibit prominent psychiatric symptoms, most often of the organic variety. These reactions are related to the occurrence of the characteristic lesions in the cerebral hemispheres.

It should be emphasized that in addition to the foregoing list there are many other physical disorders, e.g. *bronchial carcinoma*, *hepatolenticular degeneration*, in which mental symptoms can be dominant or presenting. Also some of the genetically-determined conditions which are often associated with mental subnormality can occur in patients of normal intelligence with psychiatric disorders [see Section 4].

'PSYCHOSOMATIC' DISORDERS

Many psychiatric disorders associated with physical illness have been designated 'psychosomatic'. Ill-defined as it is, this term has been loosely applied to a number of conditions characterized by tissue damage or physiopathological disorder in which emotional factors have been claimed to play a significant aetiological role. The problems raised by such claims are intricate, and the nature of the interplay between the psychological and the physiological aspects of the disease processes has still to be disclosed in the major conditions studied, e.g. peptic ulcer, coronary thrombosis, ulcerative colitis, bronchial asthma, and rheumatoid arthritis. Until the evidence is more secure advocates of the 'psychosomatic' hypothesis could profitably adopt the terminology of the I.C.D. where such conditions appear as 'physical disorders of presumably psychogenic origin'.

Many of the difficulties posed by illness in this category are well illustrated by *anorexia nervosa* in which self-induced starvation and its sequelae dominate a clinical picture which is characteristically seen in young women. The disinclination to eat may be associated with various psychiatric features, e.g. hysterical, depressive, obsessional, but it is difficult to account for the anorexia wholly in terms of psychogenesis. The often intractable amenorrhoea which accompanies, and may precede, the phase of anorexia points to an endocrine disturbance, and it is probably also relevant that in experimental animals lesions of the hypothalamic region cause severe reduction in food intake.

DRUG INTOXICATIONS AND DRUG DEPENDENCE

Many centrally-acting drugs can induce psychiatric syndromes of the organic type. These untoward effects may arise as a result of accident or intention: exposure to industrial toxins, therapeutic mismanagement, self-poisoning and drug dependence all contribute to the large, and probably increasing, number of patients with these disorders. In recent years particular attention has been drawn to the concept of 'drug dependence' which has come to replace the older, less satisfactory terms 'drug addiction' and 'drug habituation'. Drug dependence has been defined as '. . . a state of psychic or physical dependence, or both, on a drug, arising in a person following administration of that drug on a periodic or continuous basis. The characteristics of such a state will vary with the agent involved, and these characteristics must always be made clear by designating the particular type of drug dependence in each specific case.' The withdrawal of a drug from a physically dependent subject leads to a state of intense and distressing somatic disturbances, the phenomena varying with different drugs, which make up the abstinence or withdrawal syndromes. Psychological dependence on a drug represents an interaction between the pharmacodynamic action of the drug and the personality of the subject. Many drug-dependent patients also exhibit drug *tolerance*, an adaptive state in which either a larger dose of drug is needed to induce the same pharmacodynamic action or the same dose induces a diminished action. The causes of drug dependence are manifold and account must always be taken of personal and sociocultural factors as well as of the physical properties of individual drugs. Many people become dependent on more than one of the common habit-forming drugs.

ALCOHOL

The physical effects of intoxication with alcohol resemble those which are associated with barbiturates so closely as to have evoked the term 'dependence of barbiturate-alcohol type'. There are, however, important differences in the social and psychological settings of usage between the two drugs. Alcohol is consumed so widely in so many countries that dependence on it cannot be characterized without reference to culturally accepted patterns of drinking as well as to impairment of health and social relationships. Psychological dependence occurs in different degrees, and physical dependence is marked by an abstinence syndrome with clinical features including nausea, sweating, tachycardia, hyperpyrexia, tremors, convulsions and delirium. Some measure of tolerance to alcohol occurs and there is incomplete cross-tolerance between alcohol and the barbiturates.

Alcohol is so permissible and trusted a poison, so easy of access for those who wish to escape from their troubles, that it is resorted to in excess by maladjusted persons; consequently its effects may complicate or be complicated by the psychopathic anomaly which favoured the taking of the drug, e.g. episodic excitement or depression, anxiety, cerebral arterial disease, paranoid states, hysteria. The acute effects of a single dose of alcohol are either the well-known phenomena of intoxication, or an excitement (*mania à potu*) sometimes with clouding of consciousness. The excitement is commoner in people with cerebral trauma, arteriosclerosis, epilepsy or unstable hysterical personality, and in them may lead to acts of violence; rarely it may occur in normal persons who have taken alcohol when they were exhausted or upset.

In chronic drunkards, a dementing *demoralization* can occur. Their narrowing of interest, superficiality of thought, weakness of memory and moral decrepitude are reminiscent of what may happen in epileptics and some early general paralytics. The crudeness and even brutality of their conduct is in ill accord with their maudlin prating about virtues and their pot-house jollity. The mood of these men can be as labile as their abandonment to it is constant: they pass from rage to weeping, and laugh soon after, with no shame for themselves and no thought for the miseries they put on their families. Such degradation is, of course, far from being the rule: some chronic alcoholics become only cheap editions of themselves, with their former qualities underlined or smudged rather than defaced; they are perhaps weak and irritable, untrustworthy or lying, but not given to savage fury, nor grossly damaged in judgement and social feeling. Some of them develop delusions, especially of infidelity; they collect, as paranoid people of other kinds do, scraps of alleged evidence which they piece together to prove their jealous suspicions right; complicated delusions of persecution, however, are rarely developed. Sometimes the delusions of infidelity fade as the patient gets more and more facile, but more often they persist as a form of chronic insanity and are of the greatest danger to the suspected wife; murder is not unknown in such cases. The nature of the delusions is to be attributed in part to the lessened sexual potency of chronic drunkards and to the domestic wretchedness and aversion they often create, as well as to the same causes as in 'functional' paranoid states, where such delusions are also common, especially in middle life.

The symptoms of *delirium tremens* would appear to differ in nothing but severity from the essential symptoms of any delirium [see p. 1342]. Some observers, however, deny this. In some cases the syndrome is precipitated by the abrupt withdrawal of alcohol. The anxiety amounts to terror, mixed oddly enough with euphoria; optic and cutaneous hallucinations are vivid and restlessness can be extreme. There is almost complete sleeplessness, and much disorientation as to time and place, but not as to personal identity. The patient's attention wavers between his hallucinated and his actual surroundings, but can usually be caught and held for a few moments. He is very suggestible, as most chronic drunkards are; pressing on his eyeballs, for example, will very likely make him see whatever one tells him he sees, and he will read aloud from a blank sheet if one wants him to. Among the visual hallucinations may be miniature ones (micropsia), and many illusional perceptions. The content of the hallucinations changes rapidly, and a false perception in one field, e.g. a vestibular one, tends to evoke others, e.g. of sight, touch or hearing. Insight is commonly lacking; afterwards there is patchy amnesia for what has happened in the delirium. The death rate, with adequate treatment, has been about 1 in 7; and of those who die most of the men are under 40, and most of the women under 45.

In *acute alcoholic hallucinosis* auditory hallucinations of a persecutory kind are prominent and consciousness is not notably clouded. It is rarer than delirium tremens, and is more prone to follow a bout or orgy of drunkenness. The patient is frightened, but not obviously out of his mind; he is correctly orientated and may be able to go about his business for days. Auditory hallucinations are vivid and insistent, after a premonitory phase in which there are sensitiveness to sounds, and roaring, singing, hissing, etc. in the ears. Tormenting voices, sharply localized but seldom fastened upon bystanders, abuse, threaten or discuss the patient: they may say his wife plays him false, order him to kill himself, describe his every movement, especially at private moments in the bath or lavatory, cast up his more shameful secrets at him, shout his thoughts aloud. There may be many voices of men, women and children, all talking together and perhaps rising and falling in the same rhythm as his pulse. They are so real that the patient answers them; he may be in doubt about the presence of his tormentors and may shout back insults to see if a blow will follow from the owners of these evasive pursuing voices. Hallucinations of sight and other senses are far less prominent than those of hearing; cutaneous ones, e.g. of being sprayed with a cold liquid, are not uncommon. Delusions are usually inconspicuous: they are, as a rule, attempts to account for the hallucinations, and they commonly fade out of the picture or pass into a chronic persecutory disorder. Flight or acts of violence may result from the patient's fear or anger. Usually it is a matter of only 2 or 3 weeks before the hallucinosis clears up, if no further alcohol be drunk; sometimes, however, a delusional state, more rarely a Korsakoff picture, supervenes in predisposed persons. After recovery, there is little or no amnesia for the events of the hallucinosis. Relapse is to be expected if the drinking goes on.

The *Korsakoff* syndrome is not invariably associated with polyneuritis. Nor, as stated on page 1343, is it limited to alcoholism; it can follow other severe chemical and mechanical injuries to the brain. In alcoholics it is commoner in middle life, developing either insidiously in the course of chronic alcoholic demoralization, or after delirium tremens; women are especially prone to develop this syndrome after the delirium. The symptoms have already been described [p. 1342]. The disorientation, superficial appearance of clarity, incapacity for initial perception and subsequent recall (extending often to most of the material of memory) yet with retention of some capacity for learning by repetition, along with confabulation, dullness of emotion and initiative, and grossly impaired judgement make a striking picture. Complete recovery is on the whole uncommon, occurring in less than a quarter of all cases. The mortality rate is higher in women and older people, in those with acute onset and with a red-cell count below 3,000,000, or with a rise in the protein content of the cerebrospinal fluid. It does not correlate with the severity of the peripheral neuritis.

Chronic delusional states have been referred to above; they are sometimes called alcoholic paranoia, but inappropriately so; jealousy is the commonest and most dangerous feature. Alcoholic epilepsy has been described. It is a symptomatic epilepsy, often atypical; sometimes in unstable hysterical patients it may be brought about through overbreathing when intoxicated.

Diagnosis

The diagnosis of alcoholism and the alcoholic psychoses must depend much more on a history of drunkenness in any patient than on his clinical psychiatric features, none of which is limited to alcoholic disorder. Since, however, alcohol is far the commonest cause of most of the toxic abnormalities described, it can be safely presumed in some cases in which the certain history of addiction is unobtainable.

Differential diagnosis of the alcoholic psychoses, so far as aetiology is concerned, will turn on somatic findings, including the results of chemical tests. If the form of the disorder is in question, the chief diagnostic difficulty arises with acute hallucinosis and the chronic delusional varieties. A hallucinosis of similar type can occur in schizophrenia and in affective disorders, but in the latter is recognizable by the ideas of self-reproach expressed; the differentiation from schizophrenia is difficult, since in many of the cases the progress of the disorder is towards a chronic schizophrenic psychosis, and one may suppose that in these patients the intoxication has activated the same mechanisms as those involved in schizophrenia, or had complicated a schizophrenic illness. This applies also to the chronic psychosis with delusions of infidelity. There is limited value in differentiating carefully the clinical varieties of alcoholic psychoses, since they overlap so often.

Treatment

Social prophylaxis is the main thing. The incidence of alcoholic psychoses in England is less than it was 40 years ago, and this may be attributed almost entirely to social influences. Individual prophylaxis is scarcely to be considered, save as a by-product of psychiatric treatment, since a great proportion of unstable persons are potential drunkards, and in any case we cannot yet tell which alcoholics will become mentally ill through their drinking. Social prophylaxis is so immeasurably better in forestalling alcoholism and the psychoses and degradation that sometimes spring from alcoholism, that the value of deliberate individual prevention is here negligible.

When alcoholism is itself to be treated, independently of its ill-effects upon mental health, the problem is that of any drug addiction. Withdrawal of the drug is essential in the first place. This may be effected for a time by getting the patient into a hospital or home where he cannot obtain the alcohol he desires, but to ensure that the patient who has had years of excess shall henceforward be able to put aside alcohol while it is within his reach a great emotional upheaval, e.g. bereavement, religious conversion, fear of death, and considerable changes in his human environment are required. These are provided, for instance, by a semi-religious organization of former drunkards, called Alcoholics Anonymous, which had its rise in America and which has had notable success in the last decade. For the most part, treatment of alcoholism without restrictions upon access to the drug is a failure; the restrictions must at first be imposed from without, not left to the patient's self-control and judgement. Psychotherapy is a necessary feature of the treatment in the many cases in which inner struggles and neurotic disabilities have been the basis for the addiction; it must, however, be conjoined with vigorous social measures [see p. 1338].

Methods which aim at 'conditioning' the patient to have a distaste for alcohol are sometimes successful. The unconditioned reflex of nausea and vomiting (evoked by apomorphine or emetine) is linked up with the sight, smell and taste of alcohol. Thoroughly carried out, the method has yielded fairly good results; half of those treated are reported as still abstinent 4 years afterwards. It is impossible, however, to benefit the addict who does not seriously want to stop drinking. In a small proportion of chronic alcoholics amphetamine sulphate is said to diminish the craving.

Drugs which may help the patient's efforts to remain abstinent are disulfiram (*Antabuse*) and citrated calcium carbimide (*Abstem*); taken daily by the mouth this ensures that a drastic reaction will ensue if the patient drinks any alcohol, since acetaldehyde is then liberated within the circulatory system. Knowledge of this very disagreeable consequence deters the former addict from drinking, but he can evade the risk, if he wants to, by ceasing to take the drug. It is therefore pointless to administer it unless the patient sincerely wishes to be abstinent. The risks of the method and its dependence upon the patient's co-operation make it desirable that it should be initiated in hospital and undertaken only as part of a general plan of treatment and rehabilitation.

The grosser mental disorders due to alcohol need hospital treatment. Delirium tremens should be treated as far as possible without hypnotics, which have little effect upon the excitement and sleeplessness unless employed in dangerous doses; chlorpromazine may allay excitement. A useful drug is chlormethiazole, 1–2 G. initially by mouth followed by 1–2 G. every five hours until the desired sedation is achieved. Not more than 8 G. should be given in 24 hours. Circulatory failure and accidental self-injury are most to be guarded against. The continuous bath at body temperature is sometimes beneficial; otherwise the patient should be in bed with a minimum of necessary restraint, under the care of an experienced nurse and ensurance of adequate diet—mainly fluids and glucose and large amounts of thiamine or the whole vitamin-B complex. No alcohol should be given. Insulin in small doses and chlorpromazine have been found beneficial, but the evidence is not impressive.

Especial care must be taken against the early discharge from hospital of alcoholics with delusions of infidelity. If they have been brought to hospital against their will, they may add a deep resentment on this score to their other grounds of jealous hatred, and there is grave danger that they may, if they resume drinking, attack their wives murderously.

BARBITURATES

The barbiturates are among the most widely prescribed drugs in medical practice. They may be taken alone or in combination with other substances. Their therapeutic uses include the relief of insomnia and anxiety, the treatment of epilepsy and the induction of anaesthesia, continuous narcosis and abreaction. Acute intoxication is most often the outcome of a suicidal attempt: the signs include drowsiness, agitation (especially in the elderly), intellectual impairment, emotional instability, slurred speech, incoordination, a staggering gait and, eventually, coma. Conservative treatment is best for the majority of these patients. Serious intoxication can call for diuretic therapy with alkalinization and haemodialysis or peritoneal dialysis may be needed.

The principal symptoms of chronic intoxication are confusion, defective judgement and loss of emotional control with an accentuation of any pre-existing morbid personality traits. The neurological findings—dysarthria, ataxia, hypotonia, tremor and a transient extensor reflex—may suggest a diagnosis of cerebellar disease, disseminated sclerosis, alcoholism, or general paresis. Treatment is essentially the same as in other forms of drug dependence.

Both psychological and physical dependence are induced by the barbiturates. The occurrence and severity of the withdrawal syndrome is closely related to the dose of barbiturate being ingested. It can be alarming and occasionally fatal. The first few hours following abstinence are marked by a phase of well-being, followed by anxiety, headaches, twitching, insomnia and sometimes vomiting. After some 24 hours the disturbance becomes more severe and is characterized by nausea, abdominal cramps, a high pulse rate, convulsions and often a delirious state with systematized delusions. Small doses of barbiturate are useful in the general management of this state. Tolerance is less well developed than with morphine.

THE AMPHETAMINES

The amphetamines have been used to treat depression, narcolepsy, obesity, enuresis and over-active children, to counteract fatigue and to facilitate psychotherapeutic interviews. A moderate dose can induce euphoria, wakefulness, increased initiative and a heightened sense of confidence.

These effects, which can be enhanced by amphetamine-barbiturate mixtures, easily lead to chronic administration, especially among adolescents and susceptible subjects receiving the drugs for obesity or the alleviation of minor conditions. Tolerance is readily induced but the dependence which develops is psychological rather than physical. Unwanted effects include anxiety, tremulousness, insomnia, irritability, tachycardia, headache, impotence, anorexia and dryness of mouth. Some patients also develop psychotic reactions. These are occasionally organic in form but are most often paranoid states with hallucinosis in clear consciousness; as such they can be clinically indistinguishable from paranoid schizophrenia, but a clear history and the detection of amphetamine degradation products in the urine usually clinch the diagnosis.

The active principle of the khat plant is closely related to the amphetamines chemically and pharmacologically. In some parts of the world khat is chewed to induce similar subjective reactions, but tolerance is not a feature of this practice.

THE OPIATES

Dependence on the opiates, of which morphine may be taken as the characteristic example, can be initiated by small doses of the drug, often within the therapeutic range. The dependence is both physical and psychological, and tolerance is also rapidly induced. Further, the intensity of the physical dependence and tolerance increase in relation to an increase in dosage.

Weak, unstable, unhappy people, e.g. many homosexuals, are most likely to become addicts; it is rare to meet an addict who has not shown pronounced psychopathic traits before his addiction began; and few of those who profess to have been seduced into the habit by more or less injudicious administration of morphine for some pain they had, are in that telling the whole truth. Yet it is a wise caution that withholds morphine from all chronic disease that is not hopelessly progressive, and hesitates to prescribe it at all for those whose personality or opportunities make the risk of addiction greater.

Symptoms

These are not at first noteworthy, unless the patient be seen during the next 2 or 3 hours after he has taken his drug. The symptoms of withdrawal, sometimes severe, are more likely to occur in those whose tolerance has been raised by the habit; they consist of yawning, sneezing, overflow of tears and saliva, fullness in the head, then restless movements, malaise, twitching in the face, tremors, palpitation, indigestion, vomiting, diarrhoea, strangury, sleeplessness and circulatory upset which may go on to collapse.

It is difficult to judge how far the drug itself is responsible for the demoralization that is met with in chronic morphine addicts; probably as important in causing it are the psychopathic personality of the addict, and the underhand life he must lead. Laziness and lying are frequent, and the patient may resort to subterfuges, or even crimes, to get his drug. Dementia does not occur; delirium is rare. The physical effects of chronic morphinism are dryness of the skin, hair and nails, constipation and anorexia, partial impotence and poor resistance to infection.

Treatment

This is best carried out in an appropriate institution; general hospitals seldom have the necessary facilities. Treatment at home is bound to be a failure. It should be impossible for the patient, however skilled in stratagems, to get hold of morphine. He should, if possible, contract to stay for at least 2 months. The mode of withdrawal of the drug is a controversial matter. Some advocate that it should be abrupt and total; others, expressing the more widely held opinion, reduce it gradually, over about a fortnight, or substitute for the morphine gradually lessening doses of methadone for 8 or 9 days, while alleviating withdrawal symptoms by chlorpromazine or barbiturates for a few days. When an end has been put to the taking of morphine, the rigours of the first 4 or 5 days (after which the worst is over) can be alleviated by sedatives in fairly large doses, copious fluids, warm baths and massage. Insulin in subcoma doses has also been used to ease the period of withdrawal. After this phase is past, sleeplessness may still be intractable: sedatives or hypnotics should be used sparingly with frequent changes and complete refusal to let the patient know what he is having. Psychological treatment is of importance, but there is no specific technique applicable to this addiction. To be successful, the psychological treatment requires the co-operation of the patient's family as well as of the patient himself, who will be well advised to keep in touch with his physician for years. The difficulty of getting the drug in this country, because of the vigilance of the Home Office, is an immensely favourable factor after active medical treatment has ceased. It is wise for the patients to eschew alcohol and, of course, hypnotic drugs.

Prognosis

This is poor as regards recovery from the addiction, especially if the patient's profession makes access to the drug easy. The more normal the patient's personality, the better the outlook. After apparent cure, however, relapse is frequent, and the outlook is then correspondingly worse unless the patient can be stopped from getting the drug. Many morphine addicts also take alcohol, cocaine and such other drugs as they can get. Suicide with morphine is not uncommon, for obvious reasons. Death is sometimes the result of cutaneous infections, especially when the patient is grossly undernourished.

CANNABIS

The reported rise in the incidence of cannabis taking in recent years has led to considerable interest in the psychiatric implications of this practice. The physical effects of cannabis intoxication include a raised blood pressure and pulse rate, injected ciliary vessels, a tremor of tongue and mouth and an oropharyngitis. There is much individual variation in the psychological effects, the more important being euphoria, a distortion of the senses of space and time, increased suggestibility, an impairment of memory and judgement and emotional upheaval. Repeated administration is also associated with a lowering of the sensory threshold for visual and auditory stimuli, illusions and hallucinations, anxiety, aggressiveness and sleep disturbances.

Though cannabis is often taken by mentally unstable people and may be associated with a psychotic reaction in predisposed individuals there is no unequivocal evidence that it is a major or sufficient cause of psychosis.

Neither tolerance nor physical dependence has been established but there can be a strong psychological dependence because of the drug's subjective effects. The abuse of cannabis is often associated with the social conditions and mores of sub-groups within the general population, in which asocial or antisocial elements may be found. Many of the harmful effects attributed to cannabis arise indirectly from the economic and psychosocial consequences of a way of life rather than from any pharmacodynamic action of the drug.

THE HALLUCINOGENS

Among the better known substances of this type are lysergic acid diethylamide (LSD), mescaline and psilocybin. There is much individual variation in the responses to these drugs, but autonomic and perceptual reactions are prominent: they include somatic and psychological manifestations of anxiety, mood changes, anomalies of space-perception, body schema and the passage of time, distortion of visual perspective and the awareness of an intense luminosity of colour. In some individuals such direct effects are elaborated to constitute more complex, dramatic experiences but these depend on the setting in which the drug is taken, the expectations of the subject and his personality and background. Abnormal mental states, akin to psychotic reactions, can occur. The use of LSD for therapeutic purposes should be undertaken only with great circumspection, if at all.

Tolerance is readily induced by hallucinogenic drugs and cross-tolerance has been demonstrated between mescaline, LSD and psilocybin. Physical dependence does not occur, but a minority of individuals become psychologically dependent on these substances.

COCAINE

Cocaine is a drug which induces neither physical dependence nor tolerance. Its stimulant effects, however, readily lead to psychological dependence. Most commonly it is self-administered by the practice of chewing coca-leaves from which relatively small quantities of the active substance are released. In higher doses, especially when derived from intravenous administration, cocaine induces a pronounced euphoria, often with paranoid delusional experiences and hallucinosis; microptic and cutaneous sensations, e.g. of bugs under the skin, are prominent. Physical effects include anorexia, nausea, insomnia, emaciation and convulsions. The prognosis of cocaine addiction is bad and moral deterioration may be extreme.

OTHER SUBSTANCES

The introduction of many new psychotropic agents has been attended by a variety of adverse effects which have assumed some clinical significance in view of the increasing frequency with which these drugs are being prescribed. The various *phenothiazine* derivatives do not induce dependence but common unwanted effects include drowsiness, hypotension, dryness of the mouth, gain in weight, menstrual disturbances, skin rashes and extrapyramidal phenomena; the latter may present as a typically Parkinsonian state, as akathisia or as a dystonic reaction and may require the administration of an anti-Parkinsonian drug, e.g. benzhexol or orphenadrine. Other well-recognized complications of treatment with the phenothiazines are cholestatic jaundice, blood dyscrasias, an increased deposition of melanin in exposed skin with corneal and lenticular opacities, and sudden, unexpected death.

The administration of *reserpine* can also lead to extrapyramidal, autonomic and epileptiform adverse effects but the most serious complication is a depressive reaction which can constitute a suicidal risk.

Of the two principal groups of drugs employed in the treatment of depression the *monoamine oxidase inhibitors* are associated with a variety of unwanted reactions. These include headaches, ankle oedema, autonomic effects, skin reactions, leucopenia, hepatocellular jaundice, states of excitement and toxic psychoses. The monoamine oxidase inhibitors also interact with many other drugs. They potentiate, often to a dangerous degree, the effects of pethidine, morphine, ether, alcohol, sympathomimetic agents, barbiturates and the tricyclic antidepressants. The so-called 'cheese reaction' exemplifies an important effect which consists in a hypertensive crisis with a severe headache, and sometimes a subarachnoid haemorrhage which can be fatal. The mechanism of this reaction depends on the ingestion of pressor amines like tyramine which are normally metabolized by the enzyme monoamine oxidase; the blocking of this process by a monoamine inhibitor, especially tranylcypromine, results in the entry of the amine into the circulation where it induces a pressor reaction. As many foodstuffs contain amines capable of inducing this reaction dietary precautions are advisable for patients receiving monoamine oxidase inhibitors. The main dangers are cheese, especially cheddar cheese, game, yeast extract, sliced broad bean pods and some wines, particularly Chianti.

The *tricyclic antidepressants*, of which imipramine is the best-known representative, have anticholinergic properties which make for adverse clinical effects, especially dryness of the mouth. Tremor, tiredness, dizziness, Parkinsonism, allergic reactions, excitement and confusional states have all been reported.

Many of the newer drugs which have been introduced for the relief of anxiety and mental strain can produce some degree of psychological dependence and physical dependence in higher doses. In this respect compounds like *glutethimide*, *chlordiazepoxide* and *meprobamate* resemble the barbiturates and must be prescribed with caution.

Of the older drugs *ether*, *chloral* and *paraldehyde* occasionally lead to dependence. *Bromide intoxication*, now rare, often passes unrecognized. A delirium and a paranoid confusional state or lacrimose amnesic syndrome are the usual forms. Diagnosis rests on the history and the mount of bromide found in the blood, more than 50 mg. per 100 ml. being indicative of a considerable intake or retention of bromide. Treatment consists in complete withdrawal of the drug, and promotion of its excretion by giving sodium chloride and fluids in large quantities.

Mercury and *lead* poisoning may lead to mental disorder [see Section 3]; *manganese* to a Parkinsonian syndrome with compulsive symptoms (reminiscent of encephalitis lethargica) and a mild paranoid or euphoric dementia; and *benzene* or *carbon disulphide* may cause delirium.

Acute carbon monoxide poisoning in rare instances leaves behind severe mental disorder of the amnesic-aphasic kind, which may not become apparent until several weeks after the recovery of consciousness. More commonly, it results in a clinical picture almost indistinguishable from hysteria; this may take months to clear up, and is in no wise benefited by psychotherapy. Chronic poisoning by small quantities of carbon monoxide causes neurasthenia.

PSYCHIATRIC DISORDERS ASSOCIATED WITH CEREBRAL DISEASES

CEREBRAL TRAUMA

Concussion is commonly followed by retrograde amnesia, and later there may be also amnesia for events following the injury; the extent of this depends on the severity of the damage. Delirium may ensue; it has little that is characteristic, and is more frequent in alcoholic and elderly people. A Korsakoff syndrome may develop. Twilight states are rather more common; during them acts of violence may be committed, as in epilepsy, and afterwards quite forgotten. Traumatic epilepsy may follow. Though the later changes in personality are commonly those that may be found lingering after any toxic or other structural impairment of the brain, sometimes the disturbance of consciousness is more persistent, the intellectual damage greater, the deterioration progressive. In such cases there is usually cerebral arterial disease, an unrecognized alcoholism, cerebral tumour, general paralysis of the insane, or some other complicating factor. In predisposed persons the cranial injury may be responsible for a melancholic attack, schizophrenia or other 'functional' syndrome; the prognosis is usually good even if the illness lasts many months.

Minor symptoms which may be hysterical occur frequently after cerebral trauma. This is partly because of the site of the injury, which favours vague physiogenic symptoms that respond readily to emotional and other psychological influences. Many of these symptoms are, however, due to psychological rather than physical causes. Mental attitudes rather than injured cells are at the bottom of the tremblings, faintings, weakness, paraesthesiae and other troubles so often the sequel of a trauma in itself little likely to have such effects. They are not responses to the actual injury, but to the situation created by the injury. It is as unwise to dub all such vague post-traumatic phenomena hysterical as to attribute them entirely to the direct injury. If there is slight amnesia of the typical kind, with difficulty in concentration and headache, it is probable that these are physiogenic residues; if there has been an interval between the actual concussion and the appearance of the indeterminate symptoms, a history of psychopathic predisposition and an adequate psychogenesis, e.g. economic fears and insecurity, or claims for compensation with repeated medical examinations and patent uncertainty among the experts, the condition is likely to be neurotic. Much will, of course, depend on the neurological and other findings, including the demonstration of localized lesions; thus, damage to the frontal lobes may change the personality, and in other sites be responsible for an apraxia, say, or a visual defect. Too rigid and doctrinaire an insistence on discriminating neurogenic from psychogenic residues of the injury can be harmful; the main objective is to prevent neurotic attitudes and symptoms from developing, or if already there, from continuing.

The degree of intellectual impairment can sometimes be measured, and the departure from normality demonstrated, by psychometric methods [see p. 1388]. Among the tests employed those which require a capacity to deal with abstract concepts, e.g. sorting objects according to qualities they have in common, are particularly informative.

CEREBRAL INFECTION

MENINGITIS

There may be delirium, preceded during the prodromal stage by irritable apathy, and followed by months of moody neurasthenia.

CEREBRAL ABSCESS

The mental symptoms are those of tumour with or without others due to meningitis.

SYDENHAM'S CHOREA

The usual mental changes here are lability of affect and irritability; these are seen in children as naughtiness, outbursts of anger or crying, resentment at sudden noise or light. In other patients there is lessened spontaneity, often masked by the choreic movements. In more severe cases, especially in older children, these changes are accentuated; in the fleeting phases of anger or terror there may be slight delusional trends. Still more severe forms, with delirium, hallucinations, delusions of persecution and much excitement, are seen in adults, e.g. in chorea gravidarum.

The tics and compulsive utterances (Gilles de la Tourette's syndrome) which may follow chorea are evidence of the interplay between hereditary, psychological and structural factors. Chorea is more prone to occur in those whose families show nervous disorders, especially schizophrenia. The motor after-effects, especially tics, appear and disappear under emotional influences; they are also conditioned by the original choreic disturbance of neuromuscular function. They illustrate well how psychological influences work through available bodily structures and functions, whether morbid or healthy. The obsessional element in this affection is comparable to that in encephalitis lethargica.

ENCEPHALITIS

Though now sporadic and rare, lethargic encephalitis has thrown much light on the neurological substrate of some psychiatric symptoms. Non-lethal and chronic forms of inclusion body encephalitis may produce similar clinical pictures to those that were common after epidemic encephalitis.

The mental disturbance of the acute attack may merge into a hyperkinetic excitement, with choreiform and athetoid movements, insomnia, generalized pains, mild delirium and, occasionally, catatonic symptoms: this seldom lasts more than a few weeks. There may be subsequently a neurasthenic fatigue and irritability with headaches and poor sleep. The distinction between what is neurological and what is psychiatric in the symptoms could scarcely be more difficult than in this disease. The motor disturbances, such as oculogyric crises, are not merely responsive to emotional and other psychogenic influences; they are inseparable from concomitant mental happenings, e.g. the surging up of anxiety or obsession, and whole patterns of complicated behaviour, e.g. breathing, may be involved. The motor rigidity of the patient's Parkinsonian state may be paralleled by a lack of the normal drive and fluidity of thought or behaviour. Memory and grasp, however, are unaffected. The obsessional symptoms sometimes occur quite apart from oculogyric crises, and may greatly distress the patient. Depressive phases may result in suicide, which can be fostered by the keen appreciation which many patients have of their ruined careers and their almost imbecile appearance, so different from what they were and, indeed, from what they still know themselves to be. Paranoid, and especially schizophrenic, symptoms may develop in the later stages.

The younger the patient the more likely is it that he will develop disagreeable anomalies of personality, and have attacks of restlessness or even be permanently restless. Many children and adolescents after their acute attack become social problems: they play stupid or cruel tricks, they set every one they can by the ears, they may steal, behave sexually in an outrageous way or accuse others of sexual offences against them. Their activity is not always purposive, not always antisocial; they make the same impression as a monkey might who is sometimes mischievous but always on the move. There may be no Parkinsonism in these cases. The prognosis is not good, and they almost always do better when subjected to the regime of an appropriate institution; they do badly at home or in places where what may be termed normal delinquents and 'social problems' are cared for.

Many less common neurotropic viruses induce neurological disorders with psychiatric sequelae. These tend to be most pronounced in children.

NEUROSYPHILIS

Only the mental symptoms will be described here. Hypochondriacal and depressive reactions sometimes follow infection, or the risk of infection: such psychogenic illnesses do not belong under this rubric; occasionally, however, a patient's anxiety lest he be developing neurosyphilis turns out to be justified. A syphilitic neurasthenia can occur in the early stages of the disease, due to a mild meningitis. The more severe meningo-encephalitis—*cerebral lues*—may be accompanied by disturbance of consciousness, even to the point of delirium or mild dementia: loss of initiative, euphoria or moroseness, poor judgement and impaired memory may persist and the patient be aware of them in greater measure than he is in general paralysis. These conditions are often complicated by the signs of premature arterial degeneration in the brain. The psychoses that accompany tabes are due to syphilitic changes in the brain, often complicated by alcohol, trauma, heart and kidney disease, and other exogenous factors; there are also depressive hypochondriacal reactions to the pains and other disabilities which the patient suffers.

GENERAL PARALYSIS OF THE INSANE

Dementia is the constant sign of this mental picture; the old descriptions of a 'classical' course with an expansive onset are fallacious, but general dementia is almost certain to occur in every case that is not treated. All the other symptoms are either neurological and focal, or due to the patient's constitutional predisposition and previous experiences.

The dementia may at first be quite undetectable as such, because it appears under the deceptive guise of a neurasthenia, melancholia or mania; only gradually does the intellectual impairment become manifest. In the beginning of general paralysis, which is seldom abrupt (though it may need a careful inquiry to verify the prodromal symptoms), 'functional' syndromes can be so 'typical' and organic changes so slight that the most expert psychiatrist is misled; only by physical and serological examinations can he avoid a blunder. A faint degradation of personality, a lapse in social refinements may be the first indication of what is wrong. Then memory for the events of yesterday and last week becomes less trustworthy, what seemed at first a trivial absence of mind becomes serious incapacity, and yet the patient remains serene and outwardly indifferent to his lapses. As in senile and arteriosclerotic dementia, he may be all right so long as he is in an accustomed rut, but a holiday or a change reveals his infirmity. His mood and interests as the illness goes on become dull or labile, his rages are fleeting, his activities fussy; if, however, he is in a manic excitement, with little dementia as yet, the affective changes can be violent, and indeed dangerous, just as in a depressive phase the patient may kill himself. Sleepy and slow, careless about social usages, inattentive and ignorant of what he once knew well, the more demented patient cannot escape recognition as having an organic cerebral affection. Elementary problems in arithmetic and questions of general information are more than he can cope with. He gives easy assurances that he can do them, or puts his questioner off with airy explanations, e.g. that he has not had his spectacles by him lately, when pressed, he makes bad mistakes or becomes angry. The extent of his failure will, of course, depend not only on his dementia, but on his previous intelligence and habits, e.g. a bank manager retains the capacity to do mental arithmetic when much else has gone. Inability to receive new impressions and to relate them to earlier memories co-operates with impaired judgement to give a gross but patchy and fluctuating amnesia. Because of these disturbances, and especially the bad judgement, patients may commit offences, ruin themselves by grotesque extravagance and brush aside facts that stare them in the face. They will put up with restrictions on their freedom, forgetting their protests soon after making them; silly reasons are sufficient for their compliance, and a tactfully offered cigarette or joke may divert their thought and feeling from some serious matter that angers them. Their delusions may be due to the same disorders of memory and judgement, coloured by their general personality; sometimes they are confabulations, rationalizations for their having forgotten or spoilt something. If the patient had in health tendencies to euphoria and expansive behaviour, grandiose delusions and boasting will be to the fore. It is, however, not uncommon to find a fatuous euphoria, though there had not previously been affective swings and hypomania; in such patients one finds abundant proof of gross impairment of judgement, especially shown as defective insight. The most advanced dementia appears as a helpless, vegetative, bedridden state, sometimes accompanied by gross focal symptoms, such as aphasia and agnosia. The physical symptoms [see Section 15] are much intermingled with the mental ones, as in the patient's clumsy movements and disturbed speech and handwriting: thus, in his writing he leaves out letters, syllables and words, repeats and transposes them, messes the paper with blots and sputters, writes across the lines, puts in meaningless strokes and leaves his mistakes uncorrected; the tremulous script shows interruptions in the usual smooth alternation and tempo of movement, the letters are of very uneven size and ill spaced. Articulatory and aphasic disturbances may affect the sense, intonation, timbre, rhythm and precision of utterance; they must not be evaluated in diagnosis, any more than the writing disorder may, without regard to the patient's previous normal script and speech and the circumstances under which he was writing or talking, since people, habitually untidy in their enunciation or handwriting, can exhibit many of these symptoms when tired or in a hurry.

A simple progressive dementia is by far the commonest clinical picture; depressive, confusional and hyperkinetic states are almost as frequent as the expansive. Atypical mental pictures may be seen either ordinarily or as the outcome of treatment. Paranoid states, hallucinosis, a Korsakoff syndrome, epileptiform excitement, hysterical disorders and catatonic symptoms of every kind (except flexibilitas cerea) may occur. Hallucinations are uncommon, except during fever or after malarial treatment; in the latter case they are often of paranoid colouring. In the 'Lissauer' form the slowness of the dementia is remarkable in comparison with the conspicuous focal symptoms, such as the seizures without convulsions or loss of consciousness.

In the '*juvenile*' form there may be premonitory symptoms of excitability, grizzling, timidity and backwardness at school. Gradually the symptoms of dementia become plain, and if the onset be early enough, symptoms usually found in severe mental deficiency naturally appear, such as rhythmic or iterative movements, grimaces, repetitive chewing and sucking of an automatic kind, great restlessness and screaming attacks. Simple dementia is the usual form; grandiose ideas are exceptional. If the illness begins before the age of 10 or 11 years, speech and writing may be completely lost, or reduced to a senseless smattering.

The effects of treatment upon the mental state are of great social moment. In many patients who do well the personality has the edge taken off it, and there may be less initiative and force in mental activity, emotion may be less controlled, especially in the proneness to anger or to frivolous levity, yet the patient is able to return to his former work, even though it is responsible and complex; he could scarcely, however, except in the most favourable cases, learn a new job or adapt to new and exacting situations.

For prognosis and treatment, see Section 15.

DEGENERATIVE CEREBRAL DISEASES OF THE SENIUM AND PRE-SENIUM

SENILE DEMENTIA

Aetiology

Constitutional factors are obviously the most important. A tendency to become dotards may be evident in successive generations of a family; heredity is held responsible for the wide differences in mental health among elderly people. The symptoms of senile psychosis may not be revealed until the patient is exposed to some sudden stress—the death of his wife, the need to move house, the loss of his occupation, some new set of circumstances. Social factors are of great importance. Senile psychoses are more common in people with lifelong nervous symptoms or psychopathic personality.

Pathology

The tissues show the general signs of age, i.e. a diffuse atrophy, which makes the convolutions narrower and the weight of the brain less. The nerve cells and fibres are fewer, while the mesodermal and neuroglial tissues are increased; fatty pigment accumulates. In senile dementia there are also striking histological features in the grey matter, especially of the cortex, namely, thickening of the neurofibrils, which are characteristically twisted and aggregated; there are also remarkable plaques, seldom seen except in this condition. The main change is probably in the brain colloids so that condensation and coagulation take place; the plaques and thickened neurofibrils are secondary to this change. This is no close correspondence between the kind or extent of the tissue changes and the mental state. Plaques and neurofibrils can occur also in the brains of mentally healthy old people. Many senile brains also show arterial degeneration.

Symptoms

The symptoms need not be obvious. Often the illness has developed so slowly that no one can say when it first passed beyond what is normal in old age. An apparent change of character—a kindly man becoming selfish, a respectable churchwarden assaulting little girls sexually—may usher it in; this is not so much a change in character as a release of primitive trends, hitherto controlled. The previous tendencies of the patients may greatly colour the symptoms. The psychosis may take various forms—depressive, manic and paranoid. In the *depressive* variety there is seldom retardation, the affect is rather empty, the patient is irritable and hysterical symptoms may be commingled with hypochondriacal ones. Obscure somatic preoccupations and disturbances in time appreciation lead often to fantastic delusions about eternity and what is happening in the body. Ideas of poverty, wickedness and disease are often grotesque in their exaggeration—the patient's urine drowns the whole world, his body is an undying shell of corruption, he is as tiny as a baby—and are monotonously reiterated. The *manic* variety is rarer: pointless activity and a diarrhoea of words, with silly boasting, may be accompanied by a disturbance of memory, giving a total picture of the Korsakoff type: it is sometimes called 'presbyophrenia'. Many of these patients have always been of hypomanic temperament; their illness may be only slightly progressive and not so severe as to call for hospital care. The *paranoid* variety is especially likely to occur in people who have always been of a suspicious turn of mind. They hide things because they feel surrounded by thieves, and then forget where they have hidden them; their failing senses, especially of hearing, feed their distrust and they project their awareness of sexual impotence or waning intellect. Hallucinations and delusions are mingled—gases are pumped into their room, their food is poisoned, people throw bombs at the house by night, greedy heirs are doing them out of their possessions. Some of these patients barricade themselves against their enemies or call in the police. Whereas the depressive and manic forms are commoner in people with corresponding heredity, this paranoid form is genetically often connected with schizophrenia, though the distinction between the three varieties is not a sharp or important one. The name 'involutional paranoia' has been given to the chronic delusional condition of this type that may develop in single women between the ages of 40 and the early fifties.

Memory is poor for recent events; the extent of the damage may increase until only the recollections of childhood and early adult life remain. People and places are falsely identified with those once familiar, and transient pseudomemories are invented. Events with a strong affective tone, especially if unpleasant, are remembered better. The memory of the remote past is not entirely spared; even matters of personal identity may at last be forgotten. Grasp and judgement, the capacity to follow a train of thought and to eliminate the irrevelant are faulty. Obstinacy and perseveration go with a rigid adherence to old habits. Prolix and garrulous, the patient does not recognize how little interest there is for others in his repetitive and ill-arranged talk. He may partly cover its emptiness with long and resounding sentences; on the other hand, some patients become monosyllabic, because of their failure to find words to express themselves, and others again will use a word loosely associated with the one they are vainly seeking, or will quite seriously give a punning meaning to a word, and even act accordingly, e.g. whistling because 'You said I could whistle for my money'.

There is a narrow range of interests, in which food, possessions and bodily well-being are prominent. Grotesque hypochondriacal delusions are common. Patients hoard rubbish and are angry if interfered with in this. On the whole, however, their affective responses are greatly reduced; they meet calamities with composure, partly due to their failure to grasp what has happened. Now and then they show depression and resentment at a slight, and may bear a grudge long after. Their activities are sometimes considerable, on the lines of determined rummaging and collecting; others show no more than a dull inactivity. They become dirty and unable to look after themselves; this applies as much to those who are excited and active as to the inert. The former may fight against being fed and washed, and it is not possible to get them to understand what is being done. Delirium and confusional states are prone to occur at night, accompanied by fear and bewilderment. Sleep is bad, and often the patients busy themselves about the place all night long.

Legal difficulties arise through the heightened readiness to accept some suggestions (as in the matter of making a will, or giving away property), the poorer judgement and the lessened capacity to control sexual desire which is sometimes seen in the early stages. Hoarding may lead to petty thieving. Occasionally the patient sets fire to the house during his nocturnal prowlings.

Bodily symptoms are those of old age, especially in the central nervous system, where it leads to a slow, careful gait, with short steps and legs wide apart, apraxia and poor co-ordination, tremulous rather whining utterance, small sluggish pupils and occasionally epileptic seizures. The disorder of movement is conspicuous in the handwriting—pointed, small or erratic in size, and sometimes jerky and tremulous.

Senile dementia of the depressive variety must be differentiated from depression coming on in an elderly person. A history of previous attacks and freedom from any signs of intellectual impairment or deterioration are significant indications.

PICK'S DISEASE AND ALZHEIMER'S DISEASE

The conditions known by the names of Pick and Alzheimer can be regarded as atypical varieties of senile or presenile psychosis. Clinically it is often difficult to distinguish between Pick's disease and Alzheimer's disease: mixed forms occur. A progressive dementia, often with aphasia and apraxia, coming on at a comparatively early age and progressing rapidly, points to one or other of these closely linked conditions. They form about 5 to 10 per cent. of all such psychoses.

Pick's disease consists pathologically of a circumscribed cerebral atrophy, mostly in the frontal or the temporal lobe, or in both; the motor area, however, is seldom affected, nor are Wernicke's zone and the transverse temporal convolutions; other areas of the brain, especially the parietal, may be involved. Histologically, the ganglion cells are swollen and contain argentophil globules. There is an hereditary determinant: it is almost twice as frequent in women as in men —the opposite of what has been found to hold for cerebral arteriosclerosis. The onset, which is gradual, can be at any age from 40 onwards, but is usually between 50 and 60. Symptoms depend on the localization of the atrophy. Memory and affect are not impaired till late; they are preserved at a stage in which the patient behaves stupidly—stealing, lying or otherwise making a fool of himself. Spontaneous attention is poor; at first moody, the patient becomes dull and unresponsive; judgement deteriorates and initiative fails. Stereotypies, echolalia and repetition of empty phrases, monotonous talking and laughing or singing, and outbursts of bellowing or whining appear in the later stages. There may be aphasia. Diagnosis can be difficult during life; it may be assisted by an encephalogram showing the shrinkage of cerebral tissue from atrophy, or by biopsy. The condition may last from 2 to 12 years.

In *Alzheimer's disease* the senile plaques and neurofibril changes are very numerous. The onset may be between 40 and 60. Women predominate. Indefinite premonitory symptoms (headache, irritability, forgetfulness) are quickly followed by progressive dementia; aphasia and apraxia are prominent, though less coarse and sudden than in cerebral arteriosclerosis. In the earlier stages the patients are in fair contact with their environment, and look as though they grasp much more than they actually can. Their deficiencies are shown up in writing and talking. They may be restless and depressed. As the disease advances they are less open to affective influences: they sink into themselves and say little. Stereotyped words or syllables and movements take the place of embarrassed remarks and gestures. In the aphasia there is a rather characteristic stringing together of syllables like each other in sound, but meaningless. Disturbances of gait and increased muscular tone are common. Muscular rigidity may lead to contractures. Convulsions are not uncommon. The progress of this disease to severe dementia is faster than in typical senile deterioration and the onset is rather earlier.

Treatment

Since the breakdown of old people is often brought about by their inability to cope with the demands and stresses of a society that is organized for younger people, social measures can do much to delay the time when senile mental changes will make special care necessary. The more satisfying their mode of life, the less will maladjustment and gross failure be the effect of their senility. When senile dementia is clearly evident, treatment will partly consist in providing as easy, familiar and considerate an environment as possible; none the less, it would be harmful to leave senile patients idle because they seem listless, or let them be lonely because they are fretful. Whether institutional treatment is necessary depends not only on the mental impairment but also on the patient's social level and the willingness of his relatives to look after him well enough. Patients often fit surprisingly well into hospital life and routine when this makes due allowance for their infirmities, and provision for their social and psychological as well as their physical needs. Sedative drugs may be needed but the risk of inducing confusion or nocturnal delirium must be watched.

Prognosis

This depends partly on environmental factors and partly on the previous rate of development of the condition, the general physical health of the patient and any special pathological basis, e.g. Pick's atrophy, that may be recognized. Delirious and confusional phases may give a deceptively bad impression for sometimes, after they clear up, the patient can resume his old routine tolerably well.

CEREBRAL VASCULAR DISEASE

CEREBRAL ARTERIOSCLEROSIS

The characteristic features here are the focal symptoms. All else is indistinguishable clinically from senile and other cerebral conditions. The early or mild symptoms of cerebral arteriosclerosis are the same as those of 'essential' hypertension; and very like those of many benign melancholias of late middle age. Cerebrovascular disorders with psychiatric symptoms can complicate many general diseases with an inflammatory or an allergic pathology.

Pathology

Atheroma of the cerebral arteries is accompanied by nutritional changes—softening—in the brain tissue, falling into three stages, viz. necrosis, degeneration (with masses of granular phagocytes, containing fats and haemosiderin) and sclerosis in which cavities and scars of glial, astrocyte and mesodermal tissue take the place of the necrotic cells) [see also Section 15]. The cortex on the convexity of the brain may show microscopic areas of perivascular gliosis, but no softening. These findings often go with the pathological changes of old age. It is not yet possible to correlate the mental and the cerebral changes in these psychoses, except for the focal lesions.

Symptoms

Since 'essential' hypertension often precedes definite vascular disease and itself produces mental symptoms, a description of these symptoms serves also to describe the earlier stage of cerebral arterial degeneration. Along with headache, giddiness, tinnitus, faintness and insomnia, there may be disturbance of speech and writing—the former becoming slow and at times indistinct—and transient pareses and apraxia. Certain traits of personality may be intensified: the patient becomes irritable, egotistic, moody and easily tired; his conversation lumbers along where once it moved easily; he is depressed or paranoid; but there may be wide variation in the intensity of these changes, which are by no means always found. Brief phases of disturbed consciousness, lasting up to 3 weeks, may suddenly occur either in a form very like the 'absences' of the epileptic, or as twilight states with hallucinations, ecstasy, incoherence, disturbed motility and agitation.

After this stage of neurasthenia and episodic disturbances, the patient with cerebral vascular disease may begin to have trouble in finding words: he perseverates a little, and is at a loss when anything unusual is required of him. His depression and hypochondriacal worries increase; he is distressed by his own slowness and failures, and may attempt to kill himself. Emotional control falls off so that he weeps and storms when he would rather be calm. Nihilistic ideas may abound—his bowels have not been opened for 6 months, his trunk is a hollow cavity. Nocturnal delirium is frequent. Aphasia and apraxia are commonest after a focal complication. The most important feature is the way the patient continues to look normal and sensible when already mildly demented. Sometimes transfer to the strange surroundings of hospital is too much for the hitherto well-preserved outward normality, and the patient goes to pieces, as he also may if he has to give up his usual work or move house.

Diagnosis

Because a patient has generalized arterial disease, it does not follow that any psychiatric symptoms he may show are due to the cerebral vessels being thus affected. Unless there are definite focal symptoms, or evidence of dementia, it is unsafe to hold the cerebral arteries responsible and to give a prognosis based on this. If there has not been any history of depressive tendencies until an attack at the age of 60 or over, the probability that it is an organic vascular disease is much higher. The distinction is all the more difficult because so many unstable persons develop arterial disease in later life, especially those prone to anxiety and other affective disorders. Neurological findings [see Section 15] may be decisive in a doubtful case. The condition of the retinal arteries is not a guide.

It is not always easy to be sure about mild dementia; it can be counterfeited by passing emotional disturbances.

Treatment

Besides the general medical care of such patients, not a little can be achieved by psychiatric methods. In the early stages, where there is much anxiety and depression, too energetic physical investigation and treatment may do harm: reassurance and sedation can do much good. The less said to the patients about their blood pressure and their arteries the better. They should keep at work and in their accustomed surroundings as long as they can, unless an acute phase of the illness or depression intervene. Emotional upsets more often aggravate their condition than physical ones, so they should be cushioned against such jolts. Their depression may necessitate hospital care, especially because of the risk of suicide, or because they are too irritable and neglectful to be at home any longer. If there be dementia, even of mild degree, the patient will probably remain in a mental hospital once he has gone there.

Course and Prognosis

In definite cases of cerebral arterial disease with mental disorder the prognosis is necessarily bad, though the mental symptoms may only progress slowly, and the patient live another 10 or 20 years. Much will depend on such sudden accidents as thrombosis or haemorrhage. An episodic confusional state, perhaps even one produced by drugs, may suggest a needlessly gloomy prognosis. In cases of 'essential' hypertension, the course of the mental illness is dependent on the general disturbance, and is often quite favourable. Symptoms that are apparently hysterical, occurring for the first time in middle life, are of bad omen.

MIGRAINE

Occasionally sharp changes of mood, behaviour and personality may take the place of the ordinary attack with headache. It has often been observed that emotional stress may precipitate an attack, and psychological guidance which improves emotional stability has been found to lessen the frequency and severity of attacks in many patients.

CEREBRAL TUMOUR

The many neurological phenomena associated with cerebral neoplasms are described in Section 15, but it is important to appreciate that psychiatric symptoms may be prominent and not infrequently constitute the presenting features of the disorder. Apart from any aphasia and apraxia, the mental state here is more closely related to general intracranial tension than to any local disturbance. The size and rate of growth of the tumour are therefore important in this regard. If rapidly growing, there is more disturbance of consciousness, with impaired memory, disorientation, incoherence and, sometimes, hallucinations and confabulation; this clouding of the mind fluctuates a good deal. In more slowly growing tumours, lucidity is preserved and change of disposition is the prominent feature. The patient's earlier tendencies get freer play, unsuspected ones appear, and a series of foolish investments, for example, or homosexual escapades may for years divert attention from the organic disease. The moria, or fatuous wit and cheerfulness, often attributed to frontal tumours but also found in other cerebral diseases, may give the impression of being a hysterical pseudodementia; other apparently psychogenic symptoms may prove misleading. A straightforward depressive attack can occur, or indeed any 'functional' syndrome.

Hallucinations may depend on a focal lesion, as in the cases in which they are limited to the hemianopic field, or are solely of taste and smell.

EPILEPSY

Although the motor seizure is the chief symptom of epilespy and the decisive one in diagnosis, there are minor or equivalent symptoms, as well as delirium, twilight states and dementia, to be included among the mental disorders of this illness. The association of these with lesions of the temporal lobe is well established. Hallucinations, which may be olfactory, gustatory or visual; disturbed recognition and sense of reality; and automatic behaviour with clouding of consciousness are features of the temporal lobe syndrome. Fifty per cent. of temporal lobe epileptics have disorders of personality; twenty-five per cent. have psychotic episodes. Psychomotor epilepsy, however, does not invariably originate in the temporal lobe.

Instead of a major fit the patient may become unconscious; or he may pass into a twilight state in which for a few minutes or longer he wanders about in a dazed way and does inappropriate things, having afterwards complete amnesia for all this; or there may be a sudden interruption of action and speech, during which the patient remains immobile or makes some automatic or aimless movements. Epileptic furor is a delirious state in which acts of violence may be committed: it lasts often for several days, is accompanied by disorientation and hallucinosis, and is much rarer than is popularly or forensically supposed. Twilight states may precede the motor attack, follow it, or be accompanied by a few violent clonic movements.

Apart from their seizures, epileptics are prone to swings of mood—towards anger, shallow sentimentalism or depression—which may pass over into a fugue, during which the patient wanders a long way from home. Chronic paranoid hallucinatory states which resemble schizophrenia may develop.

The likelihood of dementia later cannot be inferred from the symptoms of the epilepsy, except that it is greater if attacks occur very often. Apparent dementia may be the result of intoxication with anticonvulsant drugs, or of the idleness and sterile life in an institution. When there is genuine dementia, it often begins as a faint loss of interest and concentration, with increased sensitiveness to supposed slights; then memory falls off somewhat, the trivial and the important are muddled together, and the patient talks with much circumlocution; he is fond of needless system, assumes and parades virtues he has not, e.g. an intellectual bias or a devout spirit, and is childishly pleased when anyone praises him. Later, a profound dementia may supervene, but this is not common. It is unlikely that the changes of character just described are part of a dementing process; many epileptics who exhibit some of the most disagreeable features of this sort never become plainly demented, and many severe epileptics are free not only from dementia but also from these traits. They are much less evident, or not evident at all, in those who in spite of their epilepsy live comparatively normal lives.

The treatment of epilepsy is described elsewhere [p. 15]. Here it need be emphasized only that anticonvulsant medication can induce a megaloblastic anaemia which is occasionally accompanied by mental symptoms.

OTHER CEREBRAL DISEASES

DISSEMINATED SCLEROSIS

Slight deviations from mental health are frequent, but obvious ones rare in this disease. Affective lability may be conjoined with a slight disorder of judgement, so that a baseless euphoria develops, but this is not universal, and many of the patients are depressed. Acute outbursts of excitement, hallucinosis or delirium occur in a few cases, and dementia in the advanced stages. An important mental disorder is that which appears as hysteria. A hysterical personality has not been present in these patients before the disease began, and the symptoms are in that respect only dubiously hysterical: they do, however, in other respects conform, in that they can be evoked psychologically and removed psychologically; they may centre on, and elaborate, actual anomalies, e.g. of movement or sensation, and may still yield to hypnosis or other psychological measures. They can greatly confuse the diagnosis.

SCHILDER'S DISEASE

In this disease profound dementia gradually develops along with the blindness, deafness, aphasia and agnosia and other focal symptoms. In the juvenile cases there may be at first disturbances of behaviour like those of juvenile encephalitis lethargica.

PARALYSIS AGITANS

This may be accompanied by hypochondriacal depression. Sometimes this is an expression of the cerebral disease which also causes the Parkinsonism, and in that case the prognosis is bad; sometimes it is a recurrence of depressive attacks which have occurred at times of stress earlier in the patient's life, and then the outlook is fairly favourable. Senile dementia is, of course, not infrequent in these elderly patients.

HUNTINGTON'S CHOREA [see Section 15]

FUNCTIONAL PSYCHOSES

SCHIZOPHRENIA

Definition

The forms of illness under this name are so diverse that many efforts have been made to distribute them, so far in vain. What is common to them all is a detachment from the world without, and a breaking up of normal psychological connexions within. The personality is not integrated as in normal people; thinking, emotion and conduct are discrepant and morbid, yet there is no impairment of formal intelligence such as is found, for example, in organic dementia. The obsolescent name 'dementia praecox' is not a synonym for schizophrenia, but a reminder of its recent history. At the end of the last century a large number of patients in mental hospitals were found to have begun their illness before they were 30, and to have passed ultimately into a deteriorated state that looked like dementia; their illness was closely studied, delimited and called 'dementia praecox'. When the same clinical picture, however, came to be found in cases that had not such an outcome or onset, the latter criteria were waived in favour of a descriptive analysis of the actual symptoms, and along with this larger conception came the new word 'schizophrenia', which betokened a more psychological approach, and a more elastic and generous notion of what might be included. Theories of causation, psychopathology and clinical boundaries are implicit in any view of 'schizophrenia' or, more properly, the schizophrenias; consequently, it is still possible for two experts to disagree about what should properly be included under this name, yet over the diagnosis and prognosis of any particular patient they will attain a measure of agreement and certainly surprising to those who know the condition only from reading or limited experience.

Aetiology

The role of *genetics* is undoubtedly important, but recent observations suggest that although genetic factors may be necessary they are not always sufficient for the occurrence of a schizophrenic illness; environmental influences can also play their part in the causal chain. Studies of the incidence in twins and in the members of a family demonstrate an hereditary factor in a majority of cases. The results of a number of studies have shown that if one of a monozygotic pair of twins be schizophrenic, the concordance rate is at least 60 per cent., whereas the corresponding percentage among dizygotic twins is in the region of only 10 per cent. The nature of the mode of transmission is still in doubt. Spontaneous mutations probably occur frequently. Variations in the manifestation of the disorder may be in part dependent on a non-specific character controlled by a multifactorial genetic mechanism.

The *constitutional* features that betoken an innate predisposition to this illness are more of the psychological than the physical kind. The bodily attributes have been said to be an 'asthenic' or 'ectomorph' (weedy and lank), 'athletic' or 'dysplastic' build; but, since these are found in much the same proportion among healthy people as among schizophrenics, and the correlations between habitus and diagnosis are not convincing, there is little to be said for them here. It is, however, certain that 'pyknic' build [see p. 1366] is uncommon among schizophrenics. The commonly termed 'schizoid' features of personality, are to be found in a large number of cases, though not by any means in all. A single 'typical' schizoid personality is a myth. It is, moreover, to be stressed that a 'frozen' description of the schizoid varieties of personality does not do justice to the true state of affairs: characteristic deviations from the conventional norm of behaviour can always be understood better if the patient's way of dealing with his circumstances is viewed historically as a biography of individual tendencies and experiences, rather than described as a bundle of traits. By paying heed to the development of faulty as well as healthy habits of response, the psychiatrist can often see the march of events that led up to the patient's illness, and escape too artificial a sundering of inherent tendencies from the external happenings by which these tendencies have been evoked and given shape and substance.

With regard to *physical precipitants* a schizophrenic illness sometimes breaks out after childbirth or an acute infection. None of the efforts made to inculpate some specific infection have succeeded, nor has intoxication in general been found to play any considerable part in the causation of schizophrenia. The same is true of cerebral trauma. There are, however, many instances of a chronic schizophrenia supervening on an intoxication, and of schizophrenic symptoms, especially of the catatonic sort, appearing in the course of an organic disorder, such as encephalitis lethargica. In these, the same structural and functional systems must be supposed to have suffered impairment as in the 'endogenous' forms of schizophrenia, and it has been urged that the chronic paranoid conditions which may follow an acute alcoholic psychosis are no different from schizophrenic reactions that happen to be associated with alcoholism, if not partly activated or released by it. It is further to be remembered that certain intoxications, e.g. with mescaline or lysergic acid, produce a mental disturbance that is in some respects similar to schizophrenia, and that any chronic hallucinosis comes in time to look very like a long-established schizophrenia, probably because the possibilities for abnormality of any human mind are few, the deprivation symptoms almost uniform, and our methods of clinical examination imperfect. Endocrine disorders, especially of the gonads, have been held responsible, but are more probably manifestations of emotional disturbance; findings are not consistent and the relation between endocrine and psychological events still obscure.

Recent *mental stress* may sometimes be the starting

point of an attack, but in a considerable proportion of these cases the reported overwork, disappointment in love or other painful experience, is found to have been a product of the already existing illness, or the last of a long series of disturbing events. No recent or remote experience is ever sufficient to account for the illness without regard to intrinsic causes. No matter how searchingly the patient's life be resurrected and analysed, it is scarcely ever possible to discover that anything happened to him which would have led to his adopting a schizophrenic way of shunning daily life unless he had been somehow disposed to it from the beginning; although, of course, much may have happened to him that has strengthened and fostered the disposition.

Among contributory factors, age and sex are noteworthy. An onset after the age of 40 is uncommon. In three-quarters of the cases that later exhibit the characteristic chronic syndrome, the illness begins between 15 and 25. The condition may become overt before puberty and some autistic children develop states which are clinically indistinguishable from schizophrenia. Men are probably more often affected than women.

Pathophysiology

Histological changes in the brain are not characteristic; it is doubtful if they are even frequent. A cellular loss in the third and fifth layers of the cortex, with lipoid accumulation, has been found, but it occurs in many other conditions. Swelling of the oligodendroglia has been described in brain tissue obtained at biopsy.

Many claims about cerebral pathology, and the chemical and physiological changes in schizophrenia have now been discredited, so that all findings in this difficult field have come to be matters of suspicion. Variations in the same individual may be wide. Investigations have purported to show: changes in general and intermediate carbohydrate metabolism (including a factor in schizophrenic plasma which decreases the amount of glucose oxidized by the brain); a toxic component in schizophrenic urine (dimethoxyphenylethylamine) which disturbs a number of biological test systems; lowered levels of neuraminic acid in the cerebrospinal fluid of schizophrenics; and sensitiveness to L-methionine. These findings represent apparent disorders of metabolism and regulation which may be a concomitant of the characteristic mental disorder. It is, however, salutary to remember that abnormal indoles found in the urine of schizophrenics were due to absorption from the gut of bacterial degradation products of tryptophan.

Some inferences have been drawn from the similarity of catatonia to the extrapyramidal syndrome that can be produced in animals by bulbocapnine and from the similarity of schizophrenic hallucinosis with clear consciousness to the perceptual and other disturbances produced by mescaline or lysergic acid. The argument from analogy cannot be pushed further than to say that certain functional systems are available in the brain, disorders of which are sometimes evident in schizophrenia, as they also may be in poisoning or in encephalitis and other diseases.

Very significant are the well-attested metabolic findings in the rare cases of cyclical catatonia. In these the nitrogen balance varies periodically, with alternating phases of retention and over-excretion, corresponding to the mental change from excitement to stupor or vice versa. By means of thyroxine a thorough emptying of the patient's nitrogen store can be brought about and subsequent nitrogen retention prevented, thus leading to clinical improvement.

Psychopathology

The large and inconclusive literature on the psychopathology of schizophrenia derives from several sources:

1. Minute description of the phenomena observed, and abstraction from them of general principles of disordered function.
2. Experimental study, using projective, sorting, reasoning and other tests, as far as possible under controlled conditions.
3. Studies of artificial hallucinoses (e.g. mescaline intoxication) and parallel experiences.
4. Comparative study of animals, children, poets, primitive people, etc.
5. Intuitive or speculative interpretation.

It will be obvious that these methods overlap and that they differ widely in acceptability and usefulness. The findings of almost all can sound plausible, when stated in general terms; discrepant and abstruse, when stated in detail. Their exposition touches on the most intricate problems of normal and morbid psychology, and therefore is highly technical and unsuitable here. Experimental studies have shown anomalies of concept-formation, psychomotor reactions, internal inhibition, and the use of verbal symbols: but none of these is pathognomonic. A working clinical hypothesis is that in schizophrenia there are inherent faulty dispositions, whose manifestation depends, in severity and persistence, on upbringing and other external circumstances. It is characterized by, among other things, a perversion and failure of synthesis, so that there is an inco-ordination, an 'intrapsychic ataxia', as it has been called, a dissociation and splitting up of the mental life, which justifies the name 'schizophrenia'. The whole psychic life of the patient, cognitive, emotional and conative, may be changed in a way that is alien to normal understanding. We can observe the change but to enter into it or describe it adequately in terms of our own experience is far more difficult than if we try to do this for depression, manic excitement, hysteria or obsessions. It shows itself also as a turning away from the contacts and realities of daily life, a preference for what the mind can supply from its own stores, however morbidly, rather than for the current experience that the outer world affords.

Recent epidemiological studies strongly suggest that the well-recognized association between schizophrenia and poor socio-economic conditions is due to the drift of patients into lower social class life than to any causal nexus.

Symptoms

Schizophrenia may be regarded for clinical purposes as a form of maladaptation in which there are characteristic defects of inner harmony and consistency in behaviour, thought and emotion. These are not common in childhood, but from puberty onwards they may appear in varied combinations, often in persons who for years have been introspective and unsociable. There is discrepancy between mood and utterance, disturbance of conduct (briefly summed up as catatonic or hebephrenic), self-absorption and incapacity for sustained thinking along normal lines. A guarded or artificial demeanour may conceal these essential features, whereas they may be conspicuous in a florid or 'deteriorated' case. Hallucinations and delusions may fill out the picture; affective or other morbid types of reaction may complicate it.

The onset is not always abrupt. There is often a long history of preliminary symptoms in which it is arbitrary to decide where personality has merged into illness. Complaints of headache, weakness, anxiety attacks, loss of appetite and dysmenorrhoea may have accompanied slight oddities of behaviour, such as rudeness or apparent absence of mind, and indecision. The patient may have felt an alarming change in himself, in his capacity to think and feel normally; he may have been notably depressed and anxious. Ideas of persecution or of exaltation may occasionally escape him, or he may have become stilted in his talk and shown other affectations and mannerisms. The more gradual the onset—and in many cases it has spread over many years—the more unlikely is it that it will have been recognized as morbid.

The commonest or *basic symptoms* are: *disorder of thinking; emotional incongruity; characteristic hallucinations; disturbed impulses or conduct.* From these can be derived most of the other symptoms, such as delusions, feelings of influence, autism, catatonic phenomena, anomalies of speech, negativism and the rest.

There are three main clinical tasks set by any schizophrenic symptom: (1) to search out its psychological origins and its meaning for the patient in his actual situation; (2) to link it with other presenting functional disorders; and (3) to consider its background of physical structure and function. It is not always practicable to attempt all three, nor is it as yet possible to do them well, but none can be ignored without detriment to a full analysis.

The *disorder of thinking* is a characteristic and central feature. The patient cannot command the whole range of an act of consecutive thought; he misses the point, fastens on details and brings in irrelevant associations which are correct in themselves, but which divert him from the main end of his original process of thought; consequently his thinking is incoherent, rambling and jumbled. He brings together the most far-fetched topics, so that the connexions are sometimes so superficial as to be empty of meaning, and at another time profoundly influenced by symbolism and highly individual values. The usual logical sequences are ignored: cause and effect are interchanged; temporal, spatial, verbal and accidental relationships are unduly turned from abstract to concrete, treated as grounds of identity, played with or flouted. Things linked only by analogy and chance association are taken to be the same. The condensation of several concepts in one, or transference of a set of attributes to some inappropriate object, may become a matter of course, so that only the closest knowledge of the patient and his surroundings will enable the psychiatrist to follow his meaning. It is not necessary, however, that such extreme incoherence be evident in the patient's talk; he may not show any at all when speaking, or may suddenly obtrude a startling lapse from normal ways of thought which he then ignores, justifies or explains away. Inconsistent thoughts can be present together in a way impossible for normal people; and the same object or notion can appear to him in several interchangeable guises, each of which would normally exclude the others. The patient himself is often aware of his disordered thinking, and may describe it: he feels his thoughts are suddenly taken out of his mind; other thoughts, foreign to him, are put into his head; his mind is not his own; his thinking is suddenly interrupted; some external power controls it.

The thought-disorder is illustrated by the following characteristic remarks of patients: 'There were bats and bees coming through the window; of course that was because my brother-in-law kept teasing me. He said I had bees in my bonnet.' 'If I should return during my absence, keep me here until I come back.' 'I have a lot of forced thoughts. My thoughts are all drawn-out words, they ought to be pin-pricks. There is an unnatural stoppage in my thoughts, too . . . I have heard voices say, "He is conscious of his life" . . . To get my feeling back to normal I feel like changing motor-cars into battleships, to be superior to them.'

This disorder may only be demonstrable when the patient speaks on the topic of his delusions; in other matters he may seem quite sensible. In many respects it resembles what normal people experience during states of altered consciousness, e.g. in dreams, or when falling asleep; the schizophrenic, however, has it with clear consciousness, so that a listener often feels that the patient is making fun of him in giving such transparently absurd answers with an air of knowing exactly what he is about. A chronic well-preserved schizophrenic has been known to make his living as a comedian, the audience much enjoying the allusive, half-comprehended nonsense, with its background of innuendo and symbolism. Autism, i.e. immersion in his own fantasies and preoccupations, may account for much of the oddity and detachment the patient shows; it accounts also in part for his 'negativism', in that he resents any stimulus that interferes with his daydreams.

Delusions arise mainly out of the thought-disorder. They are often bizarre; they may occur to the patient with a suddenness of conviction that puts them beyond all argument; and they are egocentric in that they commonly bring indifferent happenings or people into a special relationship with the patient—e.g. he suddenly knows that when his cousin yesterday said he had been reading about Napoleon's divorce of Josephine, it was a subtle way of telling the patient that his wife was committing adultery with this cousin, whose name is Joseph. The delusional ideas may not be firm convictions, but fleeting notions, readily given up, and based upon some casual instance of the thought-disorder; sometimes they are schizophrenic ways of saying something commonplace—e.g. the patient declares his wife has poisoned him, but when he is further questioned says airily that he means she gives him ill-cooked food which is bad for his digestion.

Fixed delusions are, however, common, and are usually of a paranoid complexion; they may develop out of more or less ephemeral ideas of reference. They are often intermixed with hallucinations. The patient gets into a state of mind in which he feels there is meaning in everything, something is going on behind the scenes, he is perplexed by all this, and mystified, it has to do with him in some uncanny way. Presently, he begins to 'see through it all', sometimes he gives it some religious or cosmic significance, especially if he has much anxiety as well—the Last Judgement is at hand, he is to be responsible for the regeneration of the whole world. The delusions are not always enacted on so grand a stage; there may be homely fancies about neighbours who whisper and sneer, or about some bogy like the Jesuits or the Jews. Often, the patient complains that people work on his mind, hypnotize him, influence him for his own good, set about to drive him mad or ruin him. Delusions of grandeur may be linked up with these paranoid ones, e.g. he is being persecuted because he is the Messiah, and may be likewise pedestrian or lofty, according to the patient's previous education and interests, the severity of his disorder, the copiousness of his fancy and the amount of normal mental function still in evidence. Here, as elsewhere in psychiatry, the symptoms are a mixed outcome of impaired or perverted function on the one hand, and of normal function on the other, the latter either reacting to and modifying the disorder, or obtaining freer play through it. If, for example, a patient feels his thoughts are being controlled by some external influence and he has queer tinglings in his body, his conviction that he is being hypnotized, and that someone is playing an electrical instrument on to him, must be regarded as a normal attempt to find the cause of an almost inexplicable happening. The delusions are sometimes about past events, which are falsified retrospectively, e.g. the patient relates details of his having been a changeling or a predestined hero. Delusions about bodily transformation or disease are frequent, and may be complicated and bizarre.

Patients often do not act in accordance with their delusional beliefs, especially when these are fleeting or chronic; they may, for example, be friendly towards a nurse whom they believe to be persecuting them cruelly. On the whole, however, this is unusual in the early or acute stages of the illness: a patient will then act on his beliefs violently or in terror; he may go to the police or be driven to suicide.

Constantly the matter of a patient's delusions will be found to be intimately dependent on his experiences, his emotional attachments and sufferings, his struggles and frustrations; it is impossible, none the less, by any such analysis and derivation of his delusions to account for the fact of their occurrence, i.e. for the patient's choice of this way of dealing with the experiences in question. The same is true of the general thought-disorder: e.g. interruption or 'blocking' of the train of thought may take place only when some emotionally weighted topic, some complex, is touched on. This accounts for the place where 'blocking' occurs, but not for the 'blocking' itself; that, like the other fundamental disturbances of function in schizophrenia, eludes a wholly psychological explanation.

Intellectual defect does not occur, though the patient may find it difficult to form concepts necessary for abstract thinking. There is usually no clouding of consciousness. Intellectual laziness or evasion is often conspicuous; the patient may repeat questions in a musing way, or profess ignorance. Orientation and memory are not, as a rule, diffusely impaired, though hallucinations, delusions and lack of interest may interfere with them, and consciousness may be disturbed in stupor or excitement. Many a patient who has long borne the appearance of gross dementia will suddenly show that his intelligence is still a sharp instrument: drugs, e.g. amylobarbitone sodium or insulin, and intercurrent disease or shock can thus dramatically reveal how little ground there is for calling this illness a dementia. Schizophrenics often do the unexpected. Amnesias and deliria, when they occur in schizophrenia, may be hysterical; obsessional and hysterical symptoms, like anxiety and depression, are compatible with schizophrenia, and are often an intimate component of the illness.

The speech and writing of the schizophrenic betray the extent of his thought-disorder. Stiffness, pedantry, fantastic euphuisms, words of his own coining, queer symbols and grammar, stereotyped repetition and infantile twists like speaking of himself always in the third person may be conspicuous features of the patient's use of language. There may, on the other hand, be little or nothing outwardly amiss in his conversation and writings. In florid or chronic cases the patient may talk in an unnatural voice, or without any modulation. Writing may be set forth as though it was painting, and the converse: in subject and matter the patient's insanity may be patent, but his treatment of his matter, however odd, is seldom odder than some forms of art, and it cannot be called typical of the illness. These anomalies of symbolical representation are as open to psychological as explanation are the delusions mentioned above; the neologisms, for example, can be analysed up to a point; and these phenomena have enriched our knowledge of the psychopathology of schizophrenia.

The *emotional incongruity* is the chief, but not the only, sign of disturbed affect. Often the patient himself notices in the beginning of his illness that he is less moved by habitual affection, or even feels hatred towards a parent he has loved. The strongest and rarest of human passions are not infrequent in this illness: ecstasy, mystic communion, despair, horror, agony of death, limitless abandon, apotheosis, salvation, are approximate names for these exceptional states that are probably indescribable in the current language of normal people. Apart from these, and much the commonest of the affective changes, is apparent emotional shallowness: the patient receives moving news without any sign of being touched by it, or his response is perfunctory; he smiles or looks bored when talking of a recent tragedy in his own family. This shallowness and incongruity of affect is, however, not to be taken at face value. What the patient says, and what he means with his words, may be very different; so may what we say be very different from the meaning the patient attaches to it. It is unsafe to assume that the patient's words have reference to what is mainly going on in his mind at the moment, or that his outward expression is a trustworthy index of his emotional state. Violent emotional outbursts—of anxiety, rage, love, misery—can certainly occur in a patient who has lately seemed empty of all affect. The schizophrenic patient is undoubtedly different from normal people in his emotions, but not in so negative a way as his seeming apathy and lack of affective rapport would suggest. His attitude towards the same person may change quickly, in accordance with conflicting or opposite tendencies in himself; this ambivalence is often understandable in the light of his earlier history. Sometimes the illness leads to a blunting of ordinary reserve, a lack of reticence, or a levelling down of the gravest matters, so that frivolous or cynical indifference and imperturbability are signs of the patient's morbid condition.

Hallucinations are not so frequent as superficial examination of patients might suggest; many of the patient's assertions about queer sights and sounds are not the expression of vivid perceptions but of passing fantasies, imagined more plastically than is normal; this is particularly true of many of the so-called visual hallucinations, or of cases where the unreal perceptions occur in several senses together. Hallucinations are nevertheless extremely common and persistent in schizophrenia: auditory ones occur most often, diffuse somatic ones not infrequently, those of smell, taste and sight more rarely.

The 'voices' are sometimes so closely linked with the thought-disorder that it is difficult to tell whether the patient is relating what he has heard or what he has thought. He may show the intermediate stages between the two, declaring that people repeat his thoughts or that everything which passes through his mind is spoken aloud inside his head; his actions are described publicly, he cannot go to the lavatory without shameless comments. What the voices say may be abuse or encouragement, trivial repetition or threats and commands; this content can usually be accounted for by the psychiatrist when he knows the patient and his history well. The voices may come from strange places, e.g. from inside the patient's own chest or abdomen, and are then often accompanied by curious somatic hallucinations, indicative of morbid attitudes, both physiogenic and psychogenic, towards parts of the body. The latter often occur independently. Queer sexual feelings, or distortions and impossible growth of various organs, may be reported. They are usually bound up, as any schizophrenic symptom is likely to be, with delusional and emotional components, which are partly derived from the patient's experiences and psychological development. The visual disturbance, like the gustatory, is more often illusional than hallucinatory, e.g. people's faces look fiendish or artificial or transfigured.

The *actions and bearing* of the patient are often characteristic. Abruptness or lack of grace in movement may be seen early; it can be indistinguishable from the fidgety self-conscious hobbledehoy stage of adolescence. The patient may pull faces at himself in the mirror, or may be unaware of his grimaces. Asymmetrical movements of expression, twitchings, mannerisms, queer rituals and tic-like gestures are to be met with. The meaning of the patient's movements can usually be worked out, but after they have been present for long their sharpness is rubbed off, as it were, and the empty stereotyped movement may at last give little clue to what was once a significant emblem of experience and feeling. The movements often seem to become automatic, like the 'verbigeration' of empty phrases in the patient's speech. Negativism, talking and acting beside the point, and bizarre escapades may be seen at any stage of the illness.

There may be a suspension of movement, or the reverse: akinesis or hyperkinesis. Both may occur in the same patient, who may lie for weeks or months in a catatonic stupor, from which he suddenly emerges into swift action. He may carry out some impulsive action and then promptly return to bed and stupor; or he may become wildly excited and imperil his life by his blind and raving activity. During catatonic stupor, patients may adopt strange postures, e.g. holding their head off the pillow all day, pursing their lips. They may be indifferent to cleanliness about faeces and urine, or actively dirty in this regard. Waxy flexibility is rare, but many patients are automatically obedient so that they keep up an imposed posture.

The variety of schizophrenic anomalies of conduct is too great to be described here. They must not be assessed absolutely, but always in relation to the setting in which they occur. Then they have meaning in the individual case, and are not merely so many examples of 'ambivalence', or 'mutism' or 'negativism'. It is, however, true in this matter also that understanding the content of an anomaly does not render its occurrence explicable. Much of the schizophrenic's conduct is so close to that seen in organic disease of the central nervous system and its connexions, that somatic, especially subcortical, mechanisms may be assumed to play a part in this condition.

Often the most significant yet intangible effect of the illness is upon the patient's *personality*. After florid symptoms have died away, or when there are no definite symptoms at all, a change in the patient's ways is remarked by his intimates. Not only is he outwardly different—more 'peculiar', less understandable and predictable, rather shut-in upon himself, remote, with queer values and impulses—but in many cases he is also aware of this change, and may complain of an inner perversion of himself, a loss of that unity which we take for granted when we say 'I', or 'me'. Insight in schizophrenia, in this respect and more generally too, may be penetrating and just, as many self-descriptions attest. There may also be varying degrees of impairment up to gross lack of insight.

None of the *bodily symptoms* are characteristic of this illness, though many occur. Besides the somatic complaints and preoccupations already mentioned, patients, especially if young, show vegetative anomalies. Thus, vasomotor disturbance may take the form of cold bluish extremities, exanthems or oedema. Plethysmographic studies show gross anomalies.

Seborrhoea is common. Abnormal growth of hair occasionally occurs in women. Loss of weight in the acute stages, and fatness in the chronic condition, interruption or irregularity of menstruation, and fluctuations of temperature may also be observed, especially in catatonic cases; of the schizophrenic states, stupor is the richest in demonstrable bodily changes. Fleeting neurological signs, e.g. pupillary anomalies, may be found. In states of acute excitement attacks of unconsciousness may occur, but epileptic seizures are rare.

Clinical Varieties

There are three main forms—*catatonic* (with acute outbursts); *hebephrenic* and simple (early onset, chronic course); *paranoid* (fairly late onset, delusional). They are not exclusive categories, and it is usually profitless to try and apportion a doubtful case to one or the other. They do not correlate closely enough with outcome or effective form of treatment to be of much use clinically.

In *hebephrenia*, the least common variety, delusions and hallucinations are inconsiderable, but abnormal conduct is to the fore: the patient may be silly and mischievous, abruptly eccentric or inert and without initiative. The illness may progress without acute episodes ('dementia simplex'), or be interrupted by phases of excitement or obvious insanity, which subside, leaving the patient worse than before. In *catatonia*, the most favourable variety, the symptoms are plain even to the layman: akinetic or hyperkinetic states may appear and subside quickly, sometimes for good or for several years. There are usually, also, characteristic disorders of thought and emotion, which may clear up with the abatement of stupor or excitement.

In the *paranoid* form, generally rather late and insidious in its development, but less damaging to the personality than the hebephrenic, partial systematization of the delusions is common in the earlier stages, but may be later swallowed up in the general thought disorder and deterioration ('dementia paranoides'). The more bizarre the delusions, the more likely is affective emptiness to replace gradually the initial resentment and distress, but sometimes the patient passes into a chronic paranoid state, obviously schizophrenic to the psychiatrist, but compatible with ordinary life outside a hospital. Hallucinations and luxuriant delusions may, however, be conspicuous in the paranoid form (paraphrenia and 'dementia phantastica').

Diagnosis

The chronic and advanced cases—'typical dementia praecox'—that used to abound in mental hospitals, are easy to diagnose: early or inconspicuous cases can often be extremely difficult. The chief positive points to look for are: characteristic thought-disorder, a qualitative change of affect, and other evidence of 'intrapsychic ataxia', as well as feelings of being under external influence. Catatonic symptoms are of limited diagnostic value, because of their frequency in organic and symptomatic psychoses. More important than any single feature is the impression of the cases as a whole, the development away from normal interest and response to the real world, and the establishment, instead, of 'autistic' self-satisfactions so that the patient's personality is twisted awry, as it were, and withdrawn from easy contacts.

It is unsafe to lay much weight on the diagnostic help afforded by projective and other psychological tests. The intuitive element in the interpretation of Rorschach and other findings of this kind is greater than is consistent with a reliable diagnostic procedure. The psychological data may suggest schizophrenia but should not be the decisive factor.

From *organic syndromes*—syphilis of the central nervous system, alcoholic psychoses, disease of the cerebral vessels, etc.—the differentiation turns on the physical findings, more than on the mental state: a schizophrenic syndrome may appear in an organic condition, because the brain, as Kraepelin said, is like an organ whose stops give out the same sound, whoever works them. Often it is not a matter of deciding whether the syndrome is organic or schizophrenic, but whether, being schizophrenic, it has a discoverable somatic basis or not. Alcoholic delusional states are an instance of the complicated relationship that may be found [see p. 1347]: if, after consciousness has become clear again, the other phenomena of toxic confusional psychosis persist, then schizophrenia is the more probable diagnosis.

Diagnosis of schizophrenia from an *affective syndrome* is difficult, because both are often combined in the same patient. Some of the significant points are discussed on page 1371. Catatonic excitement differs from mania in that the speech and acts of the latter are intelligible as expressing a general affect and are conformable to the situation in some measure; the onset and cessation are not so abrupt as in catatonic excitement; and there are usually characteristic features which make the distinction easy. Melancholia becomes suspect when delusions are repeated without the appropriate affect, and there is a readiness to project responsibility for the illness, to complain of external influence. The inertia of the depressive is not so complete as that of catatonic stupor, or so likely to be abruptly broken through. States of severe agitation are not always easy to distinguish from schizophrenic excitement, but a more frequent problem is that of deciding whether some bodily fear or conviction of disease is schizophrenic or not. Whether in regard to a preoccupation or a delusion, the chief point to consider is the appropriateness of the affect to the alleged hypochondriacal notion; the more bizarre the bodily change described, the more likely to be schizophrenic. Depersonalization is sometimes at the bottom of these somatic complaints; what is significant is not the depersonalization, but the way it is elaborated and regarded by the patient.

Hysteria can offer great difficulties, largely because hysterical mechanisms are so often operative in schizophrenia. Plain motor or sensory disturbances commonly give less trouble than hysterical dissociation, stupor and pseudodementia. The previous history, the relationship of the outburst to a particular set of happenings, the behaviour in the intervals, the demands upon the attention or response of bystanders must all be taken into account. The mistakes and oddities of the hysterical pseudodement may be theatrical, in accordance with his ignorant notion of what insanity is like; the deliriously dissociated hysteric does not identify correctly the people around him, as the schizophrenic usually does, even when in a dream-like state; the hysteric who is acting some imagined scene does so without discrepancies or gross interpolations, whereas the schizophrenic is seldom so consecutive and persistent. The degree to which the patient is being influenced by his immediate surroundings is, however, the chief guide, apart from definite schizophrenic features.

Obsessional states offer difficulty when the patient is in doubt as to whether his alien thought or impulse comes from within his own mind or is imposed upon him. If he shows indifference as to the occurrence and content of the compulsive ideas, it is suggestive of schizophrenia; but careful examination of the development of the symptom, and the patient's attitude towards it, permits a clear diagnosis in most cases. Complicated rituals, odd obsessions and chronicity make an obsessional illness look very like schizophrenia; so does intoxication of an obsessional patient by bromides. Obsessions may rarely develop into schizophrenic symptoms [see p. 1380].

Treatment

Prophylactic measures, whether eugenic or individual, are limited and uncertain. Even if effective, they can reach only a minority at present, and their effectiveness is a matter of faith. Mental hygiene in childhood may do good in averting potential schizophrenia, but no one can be sure of this. Such treatment aims at diverting the child into social activities and keeping him out of situations in which he will be mortified or otherwise troubled emotionally. However wordily or abstrusely the prophylactic treatment be described, it is essentially a matter of trying to make an unusual child into an average one, or changing his surroundings to suit him.

Treatment in a psychiatric clinic or mental hospital is usually necessary at some stage of the disorder, and must be decided chiefly by the severity and social risks at the time. Painstaking attempts at readjustment of the patient's outlook and behaviour by means of suitable psychotherapy, occupation and direction of interests, are then the most systematic way of making a change for the better. The co-operation of the patient is here necessary; it is also desirable to enlist the help of a social worker who may do much to modify and arrange the patient's circumstances in the interests of his mental health, e.g. getting him suitable occupation and schooling his relatives in a sensible attitude towards him. Such treatment may not be practicable for those acutely ill, but for the mild, the convalescent or the imperfectly recovered case it is of great value. By means of it most patients can be discharged from hospital before they have settled into apathy, or become unresponsive to the claims of the external world; it is better not to keep a schizophrenic patient in hospital waiting for complete recovery, but to get him back into ordinary life as soon as possible, provided conditions there are not too adverse for him, or he too abnormal to cope with them.

For those who become in need of long-term institutional care, much of the deterioration which was formerly customary may now be averted by the energetic use of occupational therapy and recreation which make the patient's life less sterile and bring him into responsive, friendly, active relation with other people. Many schizophrenics are prone to withdraw into a private world of autistic fantasy. Isolated from external stimuli and correctives, they will deteriorate in surroundings which leave them much to their own devices and take little account of their emotional needs, wishes and fears. If nurses and others who come into frequent contact with these patients treat them always as potentially responsive individuals, troubled and uncertain, but desirous of affection and achievement, they can help avert 'institutionalization' and promote a return to ordinary life in the general community. The term 'total push' has been applied to a programme having this object, and attaining its social end in proportion to its vigour in using all available means of stimulating and encouraging the individual patient. Planned occupation is indispensable for this purpose: it is best carried out in conditions approximating closely to those of normal remunerated work, in workshops like those designed for the rehabilitation of physically handicapped people. The more his supervision here rests in the hands of one person whom the patient knows and trusts, the better.

There are few conceivable ways of altering a human being's mind that have not been tried in schizophrenia but no one treatment of schizophrenia has manifest superiority over any other. Many forms of treatment have been those believed to be efficacious in other illnesses; some have been intended to shock the patient somehow. Of the former may be mentioned thyroid and other endocrine preparations (in large doses), transplantation of gonads, removal of supposed septic foci, induction of fever by malaria, injection of human serum, manganese salts, production of aseptic meningitis, hypothermia and continuous narcosis. Of the latter, i.e. shock methods, many of the procedures of a bygone time are examples: the whirling chair, precipitation from a height, immersion in ice-cold water and so forth. More recent methods which entail a profound disturbance are those which use insulin or a convulsant [see p. 1339]. The convulsant method has been of value in some acute stupors and conditions in which, along with the schizophrenia, there is a considerable affective admixture.

The phenothiazines and the butyrophenones are often beneficial during the earlier stages of an acute schizophrenic attack, especially where there is over-activity or recently developed paranoid symptoms. The drugs are often continued after the apparent disappearance of symptoms. Chlorpromazine is still the drug of choice, though for patients who have become inactive and deluded trifluoperazine and other phenothiazine derivatives, e.g. prochlorperazine, may be more effective. Long-acting preparations of the drugs can be administered by injection and have a place in the management of some patients. The usefulness of these drugs in the management of schizophrenia is now generally accepted but they do not by themselves bring about recovery. Further, the reduction in the number of schizophrenic patients in mental hospitals cannot be attributed to the introduction of these drugs without regard to the more energetic, personal and confident approach to the treatment of schizophrenic patients by doctors and nurses working in both the hospital and the community.

The psychotherapy of schizophrenics varies according to the personality and training of the psychiatrist. Good listeners get better results than active therapists who steadily put forward interpretations of the patient's behaviour and motives. Intensive psychotherapy carries the risk of aggravating the patient's condition, and is safe only in experienced hands. Regular discussion of current difficulties in the patient's daily life, in and out of hospital, and in his relations with members of his family can, however, be of much benefit to him. Although group psychotherapy has been found valuable by some psychiatrists, individual treatment is in most cases much to be preferred.

Prognosis

Schizophrenia is always a serious condition. Though some patients recover, the tendency of this morbid change is to do permanent damage to mental function. In the individual case, however, pessimism is not justified. It is certainly never possible in the early stages of the illness to be certain that recovery is out of the question.

Heredity is a poor guide to the prognosis, except in the rare cases in which an identical twin of the patient has for some years had a schizophrenic illness, or in which one parent is schizophrenic, and the other has schizophrenic relatives; even then it is difficult to prognosticate with assurance regarding the present attack. If one parent has had an affective illness the prospects of recovery are brighter, but this can better be assessed from the patient's own bodily and mental constitution. If he is of pyknic build, the outlook is much better. Similarly, the patient who has for years tended more and more to withdraw from his surroundings, to be careless of social requirements, to lie late and live alone, given up to daydreaming and eccentricity—such a one, should he become overtly schizophrenic, has a poorer chance of doing well than the active, suspicious and impulsive man, or the self-conscious, introspective worrier who similarly falls ill. A narrow and rigid previous personality makes deterioration more likely than if there had been wide interests and possibilities of adaptation.

The more abrupt and stormy the onset, the better the outlook. This is one of the most reliable guides. When the onset has followed upon a recent painful experience, and the content of the patient's talk and his behaviour refer to this, or when a physical damage appears to have provoked the symptoms (e.g. influenza or head injury), the outlook is rather better than when the provoking factors are obscure; but this is by no means always the case. If the attack occurs during puberty or adolescence, prognosis must be cautious, because of the difficulty of distinguishing between the transient upsets of this period of adjustment, and the progressive schizophrenia that may then show itself plainly. The earlier history is of great help.

The nature of the symptoms is not a safe guide. Very severe departures from normality may clear up, yet an outwardly mild condition be of grave omen. Symptoms such as stereotypies of movement and speech, which indicate that the illness has been going on for a long time and that there is a general narrowing and fixity, are grave; as are also hebephrenia, and a long-drawn-out stupor. with negativism, impulsive violence and vasomotor changes. The more manic or depressive features, the better the outlook. Previous attacks, with an interval of normality between them, are prognostically favourable. If the patient first falls ill after 30, he will rarely go downhill in the tragic way young people sometimes do. He may develop fixed delusions, which are often rigid and encapsulated, so to speak, and therefore he may be able to return to ordinary life, with reservations; or it may be that his morbid beliefs will absorb all his mental powers, and compel institutional life. The more the psychiatrist can discover healthy modes of response in the illness itself, as well as in the previous personality, the happier the outlook. Some patients, after an attack, do not return to work, but have narrower interests and less spontaneity than before; they are more easily tired, and may be hypochondriacal, or show other symptoms thought to be 'neurotic'. Such patients have sometimes made a poorer recovery than others who return to work and can meet most social demands, though careful inquiry reveals definitely schizophrenic sequelae in their thinking and emotions.

The simplest rule is that an abrupt onset of the illness, an adequate cause for its occurrence and a well-adapted non-schizoid personality are the criteria of good prognosis. Sensible early treatment may avert disaster. A constricting, empty, institutional life of routine will conduce to the development of gross disturbances of conduct, and many of the most extreme instances of 'schizophrenic deterioration' are to a large extent artefacts produced in the schizophrenic by the conjunction of his autistic and other morbid tendencies with the sterile life formerly imposed upon him in some hospitals.

PARANOID STATES

The words 'paranoia' and 'paranoid' are used loosely by many. Kraepelin gave paranoia its modern meaning, describing it as the endogenous, insidious development of a permanent and unshakable delusional system, with complete preservation of clarity and order in thought, will and action. If the illness cleared up, if it showed symptoms of an organic, affective or schizophrenic syndrome, or if it was provoked by external happenings, it could not be paranoia. Thus delimited, the condition is exceptionally rare; so rare, indeed, that there is hardly any use in having such a category. Moreover, cases that Kraepelin himself called paranoia have since become obviously schizophrenic. The same is true of paraphrenia. There is now no profit in thinking of paranoid states as syndromes in their own right and of the same order as schizophrenia or affective disorders. They are on the same subsidiary level as stupor, hypochondriasis, anxiety and depersonalization. When met with, they must be distributed according to the accompanying symptoms and the general trend of the illness; and their prognosis and treatment must be assessed accordingly.

Besides the paranoid beliefs and attitudes referred to in previous sections, there are a number of instances of this unhealthy relationship between the patient and his surroundings, which may be mild in their outward form, easily understandable in the light of the patient's history and fairly responsive to treatment. Some *deaf* people become distrustful, misinterpreting what they cannot hear plainly, and construing it into a jeer or an insult. *Sensitive* and shy people are often troubled by doubts and shame as to their physical or moral worth; and, by projection, attribute to others the dislike or contempt they do not acknowledge in themselves. This occurs in youths who masturbate, and suppose others to remark it, and in old maids who believe men to be pursuing them. There are many variations on the theme of *sexual jealousy* which come into this category. In addition, other varieties of shame and desire may lead to such ideas of reference or persecution. The development of paranoid reactions of this sort is usually plain. So is that of the *querulous*, resentful type of reaction, e.g. in the man who believes himself done out of his rights and who becomes a persistent litigant or writer of memorials. Before judging such a man psychopathic, the extent of the injustice he has suffered must be compared with the degree of his resentment and his relevant conduct. Commonly the injustice is found to be fanciful or trifling and the man's sense of grievance immoderate, so that he comes to believe there is a veritable conspiracy to wrong him, and devotes most of his time to useless appeals or threats. He may persuade his wife or his children of the justice of his complaints, inducing delusional ideas in them, i.e. *folie à deux*, etc. Many such patients, however, never become deluded: they are contentious about their wrongs, and waste years, perhaps, in proclaiming them or seeking redress, but they are well aware how other people regard them, and what has actually happened. Many claimants of compensation, 'grousers', 'old soldiers' and unstable adherents of more or less cranky movements, are to be placed here. There is no sharp dividing line between these psychopathic people, and the more or less normal, often socially precious, leaven who detest injustice and are willing to do much to defeat it.

AFFECTIVE DISORDERS

The range of affective phenomena is wider than a brief textbook account can convey, but for descriptive purposes the clinical features may be subdivided into three main types, each with a major and a minor form. These are: (1) manic excitement and hypomania; (2) melancholia and mild or neurasthenic depression; and (3) agitated depression and anxiety state.

Each of these types is related to a more or less characteristic personality, and for each the cause of occurrence may be chiefly environmental or chiefly hereditary. Combinations are frequent (mixed forms), or there may be successive appearance of the different types, often with an interval between the attacks. A benign outcome or periodic course is the rule for the major forms, but not for the minor, which often tend to become chronic. This is partly because the environment can have more influence, whether for good or bad, on the course of the minor than of the major, more explosive and sweeping forms.

It would be very convenient if endogenous cases could be sharply differentiated from psychogenic ones, as in the Kraepelinian scheme, but this cannot be done. Recent work suggests that depressive illnesses may be best regarded as one or more continua, extending between the classical psychotic and neurotic archetypes. On this basis there is little purpose, apart from administrative convenience, in trying to diagnose affective disorder from psychogenic depression, cyclothymia, anxiety neurosis, neurasthenia or involutional melancholia: these are only subdivisions of it, in which the age of onset, reactivity, severity or chronicity of the condition is being stressed. Periodic recurrence is sometimes made the hallmark of affective psychosis; this historically interesting point of view is hard to apply because so many patients have only one definite attack in their lifetime, and because periodicity can be striking in other conditions, such as obsessional disorder and schizophrenia.

Aetiology

Heredity is the most constant single cause. Research has been mainly into the major manic-depressive cases, where the genetic factor is weakly dominant. It may be that more than one gene is concerned, but this is hard to tell, because the predisposition to an affective disorder may be latent in persons who have not been subjected to the stresses that would make it manifest, and consequently the usual Mendelian figures are not to be expected. The present state of knowledge is illustrated by studies on manic-depressive twins, among whom more than two-thirds of the monozygotic subjects were alike affected with the disorder, while the corresponding figure was less than one quarter for the dizygotic pairs. In the monozygotic twin pairs who were not alike in respect of mental illness, the difference must have lain in the environment, thus showing the relative importance of external factors in causing the inherited tendency to become manifest. Although not manifest as illness, the inherited tendency may express itself in bodily and mental constitution.

The *bodily habit* that is found in a majority (not the overwhelming majority) of those with affective psychoses is called pyknic or eurymorph. It is best seen in men after the age of 30. It is characterized by large visceral cavities (head, thorax, belly), a tendency to fat on the trunk, slender shoulder girdle and extremities, stocky build, a broad face on a short massive neck, thick receding hair and, later, baldness, venules on the cheeks, and a disposition to arthritis, gout, diabetes and especially arteriosclerosis. As this John Bull build is so common in mentally healthy people, it cannot be regarded as a precursor of mental illness, but only as an indication that some of the constitutional and genetic causes, or biological requirements, for affective psychoses are present.

The same is true of the mental constitution or *personality*. Here there are several groups, shading off on the one side, by way of cyclothymia and other intermediate forms of mild disorder, into definite affective psychosis, and on the other into normal and stable personality. There are those with a pervading gloominess, pessimism and feeling of insufficiency that spoil their lives; others who are for ever anxious, keyed-up, wondering whether something has gone wrong or will go wrong, and whether it is their fault—careworn worrying creatures; while a third group is made up of the lively, enterprising, confident, sociable people, whose euphoria is patent. Irritability may be found in any of these groups, especially the second and the last. Contrasted or different features are often found mixed in the same patient. The most striking characteristic of the personality of manic-depressive patients is their ready responsiveness and lability of mood; they fluctuate with their surroundings, and in many instances pass suddenly and with small occasion from one mood into another far removed from it.

There is little to choose between the curves of *age* incidence for morbid depression and morbid anxiety of whatever degree; for mania the frequency is highest before the age of 30, as also for affective illnesses with a strong confusional flavour. The influence of *sex* as a whole is obscure. Women have this illness more than men, though the manic form is relatively more frequent in men. The reactivity is often greater and the syndrome less clear-cut in women. The signs of affective illness may appear in childhood, though major outbreaks of mania, depression or agitation are rare before puberty. When these occur, the phases are usually brief and the environmental influences strong. Milder forms are often regarded as normal, since night-terrors and other fears, mischievous gaiety and sulky gloom are all familiar enough in children; it is the degree, occasion and persistence of the affect which must decide whether it is morbid.

The psychological crises of puberty are only occasionally affective—chiefly self-reproachful depression or agitation—but during adolescence the illness becomes more frequent; it seldom, however, calls for mental hospital care. Each *menstrual period* may be accompanied by depression or restlessness, usually coming on about 2 days before the period. *Pregnancy* is frequently accompanied by depression and agitation; psychological factors are mainly responsible. After childbirth, though there be no septicaemia, affective illness can occur, running a typical and often lengthy course.

In the third decade of life the number of cases steadily rises, and there is another peak in frequency between the ages of 45 and 55. The latter, 'involutional', cases show the influence of age strikingly, so much so that they are often considered as separate disorders. The female *climacteric* is a time when anxiety usually mounts, and is accepted as an ineluctable effect of 'the change'. It may become a definite illness, persisting even for 2 or 3 years. It is doubtful whether there is a specific connexion between the endocrine causes of the menopause and so-called climacteric insanity; the melancholia then coming on is like the melancholia of 5 or 10 years later, or the melancholia of middle-aged and elderly men in whom the endocrine changes are not the same.

There are geographical differences, sometimes thought to be racial, in the incidence, but the little that is known points to environmental rather than intrinsic causes for this. It has been suggested that affective psychoses are commonly linked with high intellectual gifts; another says they have affinity with mental defect. The former statement has better support than the latter, but both probably are fallacies depending on the material selected for study.

Physical precipitants such as toxaemia and acute infections, especially influenza and pneumonia, can play a part in the illness. Various drugs help to heighten the anxiety to a morbid degree, e.g. alcohol in certain circumstances. Cerebral trauma may provoke an attack. The list of physical factors could be expanded, but it must be borne in mind that wherever a distinctive, rather than incidental, physical cause can be found, the condition passes over into the category of organic psychoses. The most difficult cases in practice are those in which there is a question of cerebral arteriosclerosis or exophthalmic goitre; the affective disorders indisputably due to these two diseases may be quite indistinguishable from others for which there is no such organic basis. The problem here is clinical rather than fundamental; since vascular, cerebral, endocrine and autonomic functions are particularly concerned in the mechanism of emotional change, certain disturbances of the physical apparatus will necessarily be accompanied by many of the psychological phenomena of these emotional changes. The depression of paralysis agitans and the anxiety of coronary disease are of the same order. The notion that coitus interruptus and other sexual practices produce anxiety is unfounded, but they may contribute to it by psychological means.

Psychological precipitants may include any recent misfortune, commonplace or tragic. However trivial it seems to outsiders, the event that has precipitated an affective attack has been felt as a catastrophe by the patient; there are no records of great and sudden happiness causing an affective psychosis. The nearest approach to a specific connexion between the precipitating event and the type of affective illness is seen in the anxiety disorders which follow a terrifying experience such as exposure to shell fire and bombardment from the air; morbid depression following bereavement, financial setbacks or degradation is an understandable response, but to ascribe the type of response always directly to the nature of the experience is specious, since on another occasion the reaction may be one of hilarious mania.

No clear-cut evidence has been adduced to support the contention that early childhood environment is aetiologically related to the affective disorders. It is more important to emphasize that the experiences of a lifetime will have determined what calamities are most felt; they need not be calamities in other people's eyes at all and, indeed the effects of experience in bringing about this illness cannot be explained in terms of a logical and coherent system, unless one accepts the premises of that system and infers what cannot be observed. Consequently, as there are several such psychological systems, there are several explanations. They state the conjectured ways in which instinctual energy or libido may become misdirected because of environmental conditioning, frustration and loss.

Life experiences, spread over years, are the common extrinsic cause of the more chronic neurotic forms of affective illness; this applies least to chronic hypomania. In these chronic conditions the patient's own behaviour has so much to do with what happens to him, as it were, from outside that to separate extrinsic from intrinsic is very hard.

Pathophysiology

The *physiological* changes are characteristic only of emotional disturbance, not of morbid emotional disturbance; and therefore they are not of diagnostic value. They consist in lability of blood pressure and pulse rate, abnormal motility of plain muscle, especially in the alimentary tract, carbohydrate disturbances, variations in either direction of the rates of salivary and other secretions and decreased psychogalvanic activity. The changes are variable from patient to patient and are not always discoverable. More significant are changes in basal metabolism, weight, sleep and menstruation; loss of weight is the rule during the illness. Irregularity of menses often occurs. Rise in the blood iodine content, changes in the potassium/calcium ratio, diminished cellular respiration, hypercholesterolaemia and signs of adrenocortical hyperactivity have been alleged but not conclusively demonstrated. There is a higher level of total exchangeable sodium during severe depressive illness than after recovery: the level of exchangeable potassium remains constant. A dose of radioactive sodium brings about a slower rise in the level of radioactivity in the cerebrospinal fluid of depressed patients during an attack than in normal subjects or depressed persons after they have recovered. It has been suggested that changes in the cerebral concentration of biogenic amines may be implicated in affective disorders, but the evidence from human studies is still inadequate.

Symptoms

The *psychological* changes, in spite of great external differences, have the following general features in common: the morbid phenomena are in accordance with the prevailing mood, though not wholly derivable from it; thought is less purposively directed to impersonal ends than it would normally be, but more purposively to personal ones; there is a small number of topics of preoccupation in each patient, but his ways of arranging and embellishing them can be many; the whole body (or parts of it) often receives much of the patient's attention, because of more or, it may be, less feeling in it (hypochondria, depersonalization); misconstructions abound, with consequent ideas of self-reference and persecution as well as misidentification; and there is a feeling of inner tension, unrest and excitement, however apathetic or carefree the patient's demeanour.

Patients with affective disorder are more irritable and excitable than is normal. Time appreciation may be grossly disturbed: personal time seems to pass very differently from clock time; time may seem to stand still; no future is conceivable. Perplexity may be conspicuous, and explanations of this in terms of Gestalt psychology, conditioned reflexes and toxaemia have been proffered.

Symptoms of Excitement (Mania). There is excitability of mood and movement. The *mood* is mostly one of jollity, rather infectious, but likely to become boring or overbearing; occasionally it turns to anger and resentment. It is labile; tears will flow readily on some trivial occasion, to pass into laughter in a twinkling.

The seemingly greater quickness and capacity of manic patients has not been confirmed by psychomotor, intellectual and association tests; hypomanic patients sometimes, however, do better than in their normal state. This can be compared to the effects of increasing doses of alcohol.

Thinking is apparently rapid. There is flight of ideas, with successive words and phrases loosely connected only by similarities of sound or chance associations. Consequently, the patient wanders from the point; whether he can come back to it depends on the severity of his condition. Jokes, self-praise, flighty comment on his surroundings and facile optimism make up the tenor of his exuberant conversation. Nevertheless, the number of topics he touches on in the course of the day is often more limited than if he were in normal health: he reverts to a few matters over and over again. He may criticize himself, with cynical bitterness or humour, as he criticizes others; he may talk a lot about bodily disturbances, e.g. his varicose veins or his sore throat. His mood and expression are consonant with what he says. He is distractable, herein seeming at the mercy of his sensations and of every small detail, whether it be inside himself, or, as is more common, connected with things about him. Judgement is impaired.

Delusions are less common than *distortions* and misstatements. People are wilfully called out of their names, events misrepresented, bodily sensations exaggerated, and accusations of ill-treatment or persecution irresponsibly preferred and sometimes long persisted in. The more confused and excited the patient, the more likely to be deluded and even hallucinated. Most of the seeming hallucinations are *façons de parler* or illusions; sometimes the patient is, as it were, pretending or acting the part of a hallucinated person.

Activity is exaggerated, and in severe cases incessant. Its object may change from moment to moment, but sometimes the main end is kept pertinaciously in view. The patient, if tactlessly thwarted, gets angry, sulky or violent. He feels very strong, and seems untiring. He has many schemes, of an optimistic cast, and, in the course of putting them into action, may be extravagant, inconsiderate or interfering. Sexual excesses or drunkenness may occur and bring much harm, especially when the patient is a young woman. Troubles with the police arise through silly pranks or self-confident exploits.

Sleep is brief but deep. In the early and mild stages the patient looks exceptionally well, but after weeks or months of over-activity and little sleep he looks exhausted, with sordes on his lips, hoarse voice, drawn skin and perhaps less total activity but many unfinished little movements. Food is welcomed in the mild stages; when the activity is great, the patient does not give himself time to eat, but plays with his food or is continually diverted to something else. Sexual desire is at first heightened but potency is diminished.

The symptoms vary widely in degree. Mild hypomania may be an enviable time of well-directed expansive energy, unencumbered by some habitual restraints; gross mania may be a delirious, hallucinatory condition, with incoherent talk and little free activity.

Symptoms of Depression. In the early stages or milder forms of depression, the patient finds concentration and recollection difficult, he has less interest and pleasure in life, he feels that this world is unreal and himself changed, he dreads effort or responsibility.

The *mood* is one of grief and misery, the patient looking in every direction for material to feed on. The past supplies peccadilloes or graver lapses; what is wretched in the present is dwelt on inordinately; the future is foreseen as hopeless ruin. Anxiety is mixed with it, often in extreme degree. Weeping is less common in the extreme forms. The patient's expression usually conforms to his affect.

Thinking is more difficult. This 'retardation' in thinking shows itself as incapacity to deal quickly and purposively with impersonal topics, while brooding on personal matters goes on, with a press of inner activity, a ceaseless roundabout of painful thought. The making of decisions is dodged. Conversation may become meagre, even monosyllabic, though some patients are ever ready to tell their troubles. The content of their thought is sombre—the product of ruthlessly unfair examination of their frailties and misfortunes. Some criticize themselves remorsefully or with cynical detachment; some bewail their losses; others abandon themselves to resigned and world-shunning despair. There are many varieties of misery, and melancholia knows them all—as many varieties as can be made from the experiences, character and imagination of a human being. Consequently they reflect the moral, economic or hygienic standards of what is good and bad that are imposed on us by modern society and our particular education.

Delusions occur in proportion to the depth of affect; they are the extreme form of the doubts or preoccupations just mentioned. Patients often fluctuate between uncertainty and conviction about their troubles even during the same day or the same conversation. Insight may be good and judgement sound, when the affect is not overwhelming. The delusions are the product of the depression, which is primary; they are not its occasion, though often adduced as that. Most of them concern the future as well as the past; anxiety is prominent. Wickedness to be visited with damnation; secular crime to be punished in this world; loss of property that will mean starvation and beggary for one's family; mortal or corrupting diseases—these are the common substance of delusions and are often commingled. For example, some patients blame themselves for having caught venereal disease which will expose them to the loss of their job and of their hope of salvation, exclude them from decent society and do loathsome damage to their bodies; no evidence, no argument shakes the erroneous belief. The delusions may be grandiose in that the patient affirms himself the chief of sinners, no one has ever been as wretched or wicked as he, he alone has done the unpardonable sin; or they may be of a minimizing sort—nobody cares about him, he is of no account, let him go into a corner to hide, people despise him. This last belief is often understandably associated with ideas of reference or persecution—people make contemptuous gestures or remarks as he passes, they set detectives to watch him, they tell each other how bad he is. He accepts this almost always as his desert, though occasionally there may be overt resentment. Apart from this resentment, his beliefs derive understandably from his affective state. There are, however, features that betoken undercurrents at variance with the professed attitude or delusions. Thus many depressed patients, professing humility, are importunate in their demands on those around them.

Such *hallucinations* as occur are in keeping with the patient's affect and are of much the same nature as the delusions, though expressed more in perceptual terms. People are making derisive remarks, his body gives off foul smells, food has a different and disagreeable taste —it is often the mode of expression rather than of subjective experience that decides whether these are hallucinations or delusions. This is notably the case with bodily preoccupations, when, for example, patients report their food to be stagnating in their belly, their skin dull or foetid, their eyes impaired, their head empty. Much of this depends on *depersonalization*, in which the body as a whole feels bereft of life and feeling, and emotional deprivation or emptiness is translated into bodily experience. In mild forms of depression there is no question of delusion or hallucination, and often no recognizable content to the gloom; the patient cannot say why he is sad. In the more chronic forms a settled and partly justified conviction about ill health, present troubles, and the dark future prevails; the ideas may be obsessional and partly divorced from the prevailing affect.

Activity is limited, thus contributing to the 'retardation'. The more severe the depression the less does the patient do, unless the concomitant anxiety makes him restless. It is possible, however, for a patient to be depressed without 'retardation'. In typical cases facial expression is rather fixed and movements delayed, as though done against resistance; more or less complex activities, e.g. dressing or writing a letter, take unduly long. The most extreme form is stupor or lack of all spontaneous activity; it is seldom absolute. Patients rarely become wholly indifferent to cleanliness in defaecation and micturition.

Suicide is the greatest danger in depression. It is most often encountered among older people who have suffered a recent bereavement or physical illness. Whereas manic patients thoughtlessly do themselves harm or get into a fight but do not try to get hurt, depressive patients are often bent upon doing away with themselves. The risk is not proportionate to the degree of depression; many very retarded and melancholy patients make no attempt, while in depersonalized mild cases a fatal outcome is not uncommonly brought about in this way. There is consequently much risk during the phase of improvement—often more risk then than during the preceding severe 'retardation'. Deliberate self-mutilation is rare.

Sleep is bad—hard to come by, light and unrefreshing. The *appetite* is bad too: food may be constantly refused for this reason. Commonly also the patient eats too little because of feelings of fullness and other discomfort in the abdomen, or because of delusions about his bowels or his food. Mild constipation is common, but is often given much exaggerated importance by the patient. The *weight* diminishes, chiefly, but not wholly, because of insufficient intake of food. Daily fluctuation in the general condition, with improvement towards evening, is common. The skin may be dry and sallow, and in some severe cases pigmented, as it is in pellagra. Menstruation may lessen or cease; sexual desire is much diminished. There may be autonomic disturbance, generalized or limited to a single system.

Here, too, there are wide variations, between the mild 'neurasthenic' and the grossly deluded melancholic who craves death. There is every gradation between the two extremes, and a single patient may exhibit them all during the course of an illness.

Symptoms of Anxiety. The *mood* ranges from uneasiness to panic-stricken terror. It may be an abiding or a recurrent state. Though chiefly turned to the future, as fear must always be, it rests on past experience, often painful and largely repressed, and it reverts to the past to account for the troubles in store. Herein, as with rationalization and some other psychological devices, there is evident a strong desire to make things understandable in a causal nexus—a tendency to be found not only in patients but also in those who observe them. The patient's expression varies with the strength of his fear.

Thinking is troubled, the disorder showing itself in speech somewhere between frightened dumbness and the voluble talk that seems designed to cover up embarrassment and disquiet. The patient can seldom follow a train of thought for long without a limited number of preoccupations forcing themselves in. How far this interferes with daily life or set tasks depends on the amount of anxiety, as does also the impairment of judgement and insight. The content of thoughts is as manifold as in depression; every normal matter of human concern enters into it. Fears centring strictly on a few special topics, e.g. the fear of being run over in the street, may be to the fore; the fear of insanity is particularly common. Phobic states, whether monosymptomatic or diffuse, occur frequently in association with states of anxiety or depression [see p. 1380].

Delusions are frequent in the grosser forms of agitation, which are most strikingly, though not exclusively, seen in patients of late middle life. They may say that their bowels are stopped up and their bodies about to rot; their enemies are waiting to tear them to pieces; their families will be tortured; their names abhorred for ever. Hell, they are certain, awaits their souls though their bodies cannot die; time stands still and no redemption is possible. There are many delusions less extreme than these mainly hypochondriacal and nihilistic ones, e.g. beliefs that employment will be unobtainable, or that the patient will be victimized for having had such an illness. Hallucinations can occur: at the height of fear every sound and sight and smell may be misinterpreted as meaning some pain to come; but most of this is illusional colouring of actual percepts. Depersonalization is common with all degrees of anxiety.

Activity is much disturbed. There may be sudden attacks of panic in which the patient rushes blindly out into the open, or aimless wandering, ceaseless agitation, with movements especially at the small joints—wringing of the hands, rubbing the face, picking at sores, pulling out hair. Starting many tasks and finishing none is as characteristic of anxiety as of mania. Anxious people are distractable: their eyes follow a trivial movement—a fly walking on the window-pane—though they only comment on it when some interpretation that chimes with their mood can be fitted; their ears are sharp for hints of alarm. During an attack of anxiety with strong somatic repercussions activity may be completely interrupted—so-called collapse—while the patient, terror-stricken, expects his death; alternatively he may run for air or help. Very agitated patients may lie or sit in semi-stupor, with staring eyes and parted lips, incapable of speech unless under some strong stimulus.

Suicide is uncommon in those with episodic, highly somatic attacks of fear, and in those with chronic mild hypochondriacal anxiety, but not infrequent in the grosser forms and in those mingled with depression.

Sleep is bad: in the mild forms the patient may be afraid to fall asleep because of his horrifying dreams and the terror into which he suddenly awakes.

Sudden highly *somatic episodes of anxiety* are common: the patient feels his heart palpitating, his bowels turning over within him, he sweats, his limbs tremble, his mouth is dry, he feels he will fall or collapse or die; he turns pale, his pulse rate changes, usually becoming more rapid, his blood pressure rises, he may want to open his bowels or pass his urine. When anxiety is long-standing and severe, such attacks are rare. It is possible for parts of this general affective disturbance to be isolated, and to occur with little conscious anxiety, as in effort syndrome, aerophagy, neurotic indigestion, enuresis, impotence, ejaculatio praecox, psychogenic asthma and hyperidrosis. The factors determining such special emphasis on one or other system are partly physical (some organic defect or innate functional anomaly) and partly psychological. In anxiety thyroid enlargement can occur; weight falls off; menstruation is irregular or ceases; the deep reflexes are very active. [See also *anxiety states*, p. 1374.]

Diagnosis

Typical cases are easy to recognize. The common errors of diagnosis lie in: (1) Missing organic disease (e.g. general paralysis, cerebral arteriosclerosis); or the converse (e.g. mistaking the expansive manic patient for a general paralytic). (2) Forgetting how mixed the symptoms of mania, melancholia and anxiety may be, so giving rise to atypical pictures that may be mistaken for schizophrenia, if too superficial an examination or too static and rigid a diagnostic criterion be used. (3) Forgetting the influences of age, general personality, cultural background and milieu on the content of a patient's mind, e.g. his having lived among spiritualists may lead to deceptively fantastic statements. (4) Expecting to be able to diagnose solely on presenting symptoms, without regard to previous history and constitution; the reverse is also to be avoided. (5) Expecting diagnosis always to lie between distinct entities which could not possibly be mixed together in the same person, as though hysteria were incompatible with affective psychosis, or either of these with schizophrenia; in fact, they often are mingled.

It may be possible from the mental state of a patient with affective disorder to exclude an organic basis such as general paralysis or cerebral arteriosclerosis. This decision must turn on the physical findings. The problem becomes simpler when signs of dementia supervene [see p. 1343]. The clinical picture may resemble that of *Parkinsonism* in some cases.

From *schizophrenia*, diagnosis depends on a picture of the whole illness, on the presence of characteristic thought-disorder, incongruity of affect and bizarreness of behaviour, as well as on the previous personality and constitution, rather than on any positive features of affective psychosis; the remoteness and unconvincing manner of the schizophrenic, so hard to describe but almost conclusive when recognized, may help. Later, when complaints have become empty and repetitive to the point of stereotypy, and catatonic symptoms mix with the anxiety, diagnosis is easier. As between schizophrenic and manic excitement, the setting in which the excitement occurs is almost more important than the *prima facie* symptoms. In young people schizophrenic features may often be found without their being of much significance; in the elderly what seem to be catatonic features may rest on an organic cerebral basis. The more easily one can get in touch with the patient, enter into his mood and understand what he says and does, the more is it likely to be an affective, not a schizophrenic, disorder.

From *obsessional disorder* the diagnosis may be difficult when there is localized anxiety or depression with sharp content and good insight; so closely alike are the conditions, that some authorities have proposed to include obsessional disorder also in the manic-depressive group, thus disposing of the diagnostic problem. It is best, however, to keep them distinct, and to discover in a particular case whether the characteristic subjective rejection of the obsession occurred at its first appearance; often the anxious or depressive patient at the beginning has accepted the thought which accords with his affect, though later he struggles against it and may disclaim it. Genuine obsessions, however, are common in affective psychoses.

The numerous somatic symptoms associated with morbid anxiety and depression can raise the possibility of many forms of *physical disorder*.

Treatment

Genetic *prophylaxis* is occasionally possible, as when two persons with affective disorders marry each other and are advised not to have any children. Rules of thumb do not apply in this matter; it is wrong to tell a patient he should marry or not marry, procreate or not, unless one has been able to weigh the dubieties of our genetic knowledge, the pedigree of the patient and all his transmissible qualities with an informed and cautious judgement.

Individual prophylaxis is not usually practicable until after symptoms have appeared which bring the patient to the doctor; social prophylaxis and child guidance may, however, have value in staving off or mitigating affective illness, especially in those who are temperamentally very responsive to adverse circumstances, e.g. in their domestic life, their upbringing or their employment. No satisfactory evidence is forthcoming that such measures can forestall the grosser affective disturbances, necessitating mental hospital care, which occur in highly predisposed persons. In so far as one finds that environmental factors, e.g. heavy responsibility, unemployment, or sexual frustrations, have been important in provoking an attack, advice on these matters may be helpful; it may be practicable by psychological and social treatment during the healthy interval to do much good in this way. But some cases, in which intrinsic factors seem all powerful, are proof against such measures, and in any case it is not easy to persuade the patient when he is well again to put himself for a long time in the doctor's hands.

In considering the treatment of established illness it is convenient to consider separately the acute major forms, and the minor more chronic cases.

For the major forms of affective disorder, the treatment other than by convulsions and drugs is directed to safeguarding life, relieving distress and providing the best conditions for the emotional disturbance to subside. Exhortations to 'pull yourself together' are as out of place as advice to take a voyage or an argument about the delusions. If the attack is sufficiently severe to render the patient unfit for ordinary duties, treatment at home is probably inadvisable. Although in such attacks argument is futile and active psychotherapy harmful, yet the loss of relation between current experience and emotion is never absolute; there is virtue in separating the patient from real trouble and distressing associations, reassuring him, giving him firm, kind management. The essential combination of these, and especially the last, is rarely obtainable at home. The patients, however boisterous or suicidal, usually recognize their need of treatment and are willing to enter hospital. They should not transact any business if it can be helped; their judgement may be too much disturbed, they lay up trouble for themselves. Continuous narcosis sometimes curtails an attack; it demands experience and care.

Convulsant treatment is valuable; most of all for involutional conditions, least for mania. Among involutional patients those with baseless suspicion and resentment respond less well than the self-reproachful and agitated. It is still uncertain how much benefit can be obtained in younger patients with acute affective disorder; many of the figures purporting to show that in manic-depressives (thus distinguished from involutional melancholics) the recovery rate after convulsant treatment is also high, have been compiled from a series of patients the majority of whom had reached later middle life and might therefore have been properly classified as involutional. It is, moreover, difficult to evaluate recovery rates for this purpose in a condition in which recovery is often obtained by other therapeutic methods, such as would probably have been employed along with the convulsant treatment. Whereas in the depressive conditions of late middle life there can be little doubt about the general superiority of convulsant treatment to any other available method, in the affective disorders of earlier life it is only by the effect on the duration of the attack, and the subsequent frequency and severity of attacks, that the efficacy of convulsions can be judged; the restricted information available does not give any conclusive general answer, though it is evident that, on the one hand, many young patients have their attacks of depression promptly cut short by this method of treatment, whereas previous attacks not treated thus had lasted for many months, and on the other hand some of them soon relapse. For manic patients it is on the whole disappointing.

Convulsant treatment by the electrical method has superseded chemically induced convulsions. It is important that the psychiatrist should not use subconvulsant doses if he can help it. The number of fits required varies from patient to patient but it is unwise to give a total of more than twenty fits. In order to lessen the chance of spinal or other fracture, a relaxant is administered, usually in conjunction with barbiturate intravenously. Claims for the superiority of the unilateral administration of electroconvulsant treatment have still to be substantiated.

For the depressions of middle life convulsant treatment has enough success to justify regarding it as the method of choice. By the electrical method, fits lasting less than a minute are induced three times a week; not more than ten fits are usually required. A relapse may necessitate repetition of the treatment. Fragile bones or vertebral deformity may preclude use of the method, unless special precautions are taken and the dangers made known to the patient or his responsible relative. Patients with circulatory or pulmonary disease should have convulsions only after the risks have been fully weighed. The treatment causes temporary cerebral damage though the forgetfulness or disturbance of consciousness which may follow the fits usually clears up after a few hours. In spite of the simplicity of the actual procedure—hardly more complicated than turning on the wireless—the tiro can do harm with it by selecting patients who are unsuitable on either mental or physical grounds or by giving too many or too few fits.

Patients with severe and chronic agitated depression sometimes are improved by *leucotomy* [see p. 1339].

Drugs play a large part in treatment. The introduction of 'tranquillizers' and 'anti-depressant' drugs has greatly reduced the use of electroconvulsant therapy for depression; and these drugs have superseded morphine, hyoscine, paraldehyde and other narcotics in allaying excitement.

Chlorpromazine has a considerable effect in calming excited patients. The dose varies between 25 and 30 mg. three times daily, by mouth, and 0·6 G. per day, or more: there is little agreement about dosage but the large doses which may be required to quieten a manic patient carry a risk of severe toxic symptoms, e.g. liver damage, or gross extrapyramidal disorder of motility. Alternative phenothiazine derivatives are said to be less toxic, but their effect on excitement is less dependable. Barbiturates are valuable adjuncts to chlorpromazine, but it has to be remembered that potentiation may occur. Haloperidol is another drug which allays excitement and lithium carbonate is also used for this purpose.

For depression there is now a large array of drugs alleged to relieve the condition. Undoubtedly in some patients the improvement which follows their administration is attributable to them, and cannot be accounted for as a 'placebo' effect or a misleading change for the better in the natural course of the illness. At the same time controlled studies of their efficacy are few, and the interpretation of results is complicated and seldom unequivocal. If a patient fails to respond to one of them, he may be benefited by another. Of the drugs currently available, imipramine and its congeners enjoy most esteem. It is given in increasing doses, working up in five days from 100 mg. a day to 0·25 G. daily, and then gradually adjusted to maintain whatever improvement has taken place. The group of mono-amine oxidase inhibitors may also benefit depression, though their use is attended by serious risks [see p. 1350]. If any of these drugs has failed to improve a depressed patient in three weeks, it is usually unlikely to do so on further administration.

For morbid anxiety it is doubtful whether any other drug is to be preferred to a barbiturate. So far from their familiarity being a demerit, it enables one to prescribe them with a very good knowledge of what they can be expected to do and confidence that troublesome and unpredictable toxic effects are not lurking in the wings. Of the newer drugs the benzodiazepines have been widely used for reducing agitation and tension.

Food must be given in adequate quantity and kind. The induction of mild hypoglycaemia by insulin each morning may be helpful in inducing a willingness to take more food. Artificial feeding, preferably by nasal tube, may rarely and for a short time be necessary because otherwise the patient would die of starvation. The presence of acetone in the urine and a falling weight curve are strong indications that nutrition must be attended to promptly. A good nurse may, by unusual patience and sense, get over an obstinate refusal to take enough food and drink. Attention to the bowels and other measures of general hygiene are desirable, but care must be taken that aperients are not needlessly given to patients with nihilistic delusions who declare that their bowels are never opened.

Suicide is of the first importance. Prevention of it can be better ensured by close knowledge of the patient and his day-to-day condition than by mechanical precautions, but if he is bent upon it, these may be unavoidable. It is possible to make them unobtrusive without nullifying them, for bolts and bars can defeat their own ends and excessive supervision aggravates a patient's misery, his fears or his resentment. Two good rules are: (1) to discredit the maxim that those who talk of suicide never commit it, and (2) to remember that many suicides are surprises. Convalescence from melancholia is a risky time.

Occupational therapy is good, as soon as the patient can be got to co-operate; though it is not rational treatment to pester a melancholic, to encourage the fretful restlessness of the agitated, or to give the manic patient more things to muddle himself with and destroy. None the less, it is often surprising to find how soon, under tactful guidance, these patients will enter into ordered activity of a more or less simple sort, and how helpful it can be to them. During the stage of improvement the same is true of recreations and social activities. Patients should not leave hospital till recovery is assured, unless it is obvious that the hospital surroundings and the absence from home and work are an actual cause of their persistent anxiety or dejection.

To revert to the *milder* forms, which tend more to become chronic: here manipulation of the conditions in which the patient lives at home and at work may be conjoined with psychological treatment (individually or in a group), depending on an appraisal of the causes of his illness. There is nothing distinctive (though much that takes account of the individual patient's needs) in the psychotherapy and social treatment called for [see p. 1338]; danger signals must be recognized as they occur. Zeal must give way to the real needs and resources of the patient, which are often not appropriate to a drastic or very lengthy treatment. Simple measures of inquiry, explanation and reassurance, together with small environmental changes, may have much effect. A fixed regime imposed in detail by the doctor is helpful; this becomes more and more necessary as the affect dwindles in long-standing cases. Hypomania does not usually respond to causal treatment of any kind; it seems to run a largely autonomous course. Anxiety may yield very satisfactorily to patient psychotherapy and environmental adjustment. Some patients are helped symptomatically by medication but the possibility of drug-dependence must be borne in mind when treating chronic affective disorders.

Course and Prognosis

The varieties of outcome and sequence are many. They depend on the balance between particular intrinsic and extrinsic causal factors in each case, and on the extrinsic factors which are brought to bear on it in the form of treatment. The more typical the illness, the surer the recovery in favourable circumstances.

A history of definite affective psychosis in a parent or grandparent points to recovery from the attack, but it is unsafe to infer the course of the illness from hereditary data alone. A well-adapted personality and a pyknic build, a history of similar illness followed by complete recovery, a fairly sharp and fairly recent onset, and precipitation by external troubles which will not be likely to continue are all of them points to the good. Advancing years make the prognosis poorer, but a first attack of melancholia in late middle life, if there be no vascular disease, eventually clears up in two-thirds of the cases; convulsant treatment has further improved the prognosis for this group. Bodily changes are often the best indication of coming recovery. Improved appetite and regularity of the bowels, cessation of anxiety symptoms, clearing of the complexion, increase of weight and return of menstruation may be noted even before any increase of activity and long before any admission of feeling better can be obtained from the patient.

A first attack of excitement or anxiety will seldom be the only one; of depression it may. Periodic depression and anxiety is less likely to cease in middle life than periodic excitement. The occurrence of hallucinations or delusions is in itself of little consequence prognostically. A transition from anxiety to depression or mania, and from mania to depression, or vice versa, is commonly gradual. Only in predominantly reactive attacks can one surmise how long the illness will last, or when another attack is to be feared. After recovery complete insight into what happened during the illness may not be attained, especially by resentful manic patients, melancholics who are sensitive and suspicious, and agitated patients who fear personal harm.

Generalized somatic disturbances, e.g. loss of weight, especially if acute and brief, are of good prognostic import, other things being equal. The more the somatic preoccupations or symptoms are diffused over a period of time and localized to one system, the poorer the prognosis; this, however, does not apply so much to children as to adults. Hypochondriasis and depersonalization suggest a long illness, as do nihilistic delusions (e.g. denying that one's bowels are opened at all), and, to a far less extent, an admixture of hysterical or schizophrenic features. The more the psychogenic causes have been obviously operative for a long period, the greater the tendency to chronicity. In the more chronic forms, or after a series of attacks, there may be impaired initiative and judgement, irresoluteness, dullness and social deterioration—none of them conspicuous. Puerperal and pregnancy psychoses have a good outlook. The milder forms of anxiety and depression, if not already chronic, respond well to treatment, especially to psychotherapy.

Death may occur from suicide, insufficient food and intercurrent disease, especially pneumonia.

NEUROSES AND PERSONALITY DISORDERS

Reference has already been made to the concepts of neurosis [see p. 1336] and personality disorder [see p. 1336]. It is evident from what has been said that some mental states may be clinically indistinguishable from conditions in one or other of these categories and yet be closely related to either organic brain disease, e.g. a post-traumatic reaction [see p. 1353] or to a functional psychosis, e.g. schizoid personality [see p. 1358]. In most cases, however, patients with neurotic and personality disorders are more usefully regarded as exhibiting morbid deviations from normally distributed traits and behaviour patterns. These characteristics are, of course, founded on a somatic or constitutional basis but while psychophysiological anomalies are not uncommon they are overshadowed by psychological, behavioural and social phenomena. In evaluating the significance of these phenomena the physician must pay particular regard to the role of interpersonal and environmental factors in relation to the life-history of the patient as well as to such innate factors as heredity, age and sex.

The principal clinical groupings are summarized below but it must be emphasized that considerable overlap may occur in practice.

ANXIETY STATES

As already stated, the so-called anxiety state is best regarded as part of the group of affective disorders, in which depression and manic excitement are also included. For a description of the clinical features, aetiology, diagnosis, treatment and prognosis see Affective Disorder [p. 1366]. It would be indefensible to put into a special category all the forms of mental illness in which anxiety is conspicuous, for it can be severe in the most diverse conditions, ranging from delirium tremens to schizophrenia. The outwardly mild form, tending to chronicity and often largely psychogenic, is most often commingled with frankly depressive symptoms. As it responds well to treatment in the less advanced stages it is therefore important that its recognition should not be delayed because of a doubt as to physical disease. Yet often the correct diagnosis is overlooked while the patient is being investigated or treated for some local disorder. This arises partly because of the quasi-physical signs of fear which he may show—dizziness, tremor, nausea and vomiting, indigestion, diarrhoea, palpitation, a sense of oppression in the chest, rapid pulse, flushing, sweating, frequent passage of urine, etc. It is still more due to the patient's anxiety turning on his health, especially his physical health, and leading him to ask for more and more medical opinions, radiographs, laboratory investigations, etc., the favourable results of which, however, may not allay his worry. Over-cautious advice as to regime, based on a possibility that there may be some early physical disease, can be harmful to the patient's mental health in that it restricts his normal life, and may constantly recall and reinforce his anxiety. The converse error of mistaking some early symptoms of physical illness for hypochondriacal anxiety is equally to be avoided. Physical investigation of doubtful cases is, in short, indispensable, and should be prompt as well as thorough. When it fails to confirm the presence of a physical disorder the patient should not be treated as though he will still be in danger of the physical illness unless he takes special precautions in diet, exercise, etc. This is well illustrated by such a condition as *effort syndrome*, where care taken to avoid any damage to the heart intensifies the illness. The patient should be fully investigated on the psychological side and treated accordingly; this does not mean that he should be treated only by psychotherapy. The discovery of a possible psychological cause for the symptoms does not prove that there is not also a physical cause for them, but it makes it less likely. The converse is also true.

HYSTERIA

In hysteria, symptoms of illness are represented by the patient for the sake of some advantage, without his being fully conscious of this motive. The form of representation will vary widely according to the circumstances that have provoked the illness, the patient's experience of what the symptoms are that he is trying to represent, and his somatic resources. These factors, presently to be discussed, bear on the hysterical symptoms that simulate physical disease. But it is impossible to restrict hysteria to this physical form. The illness that is represented by the hysteric may be a mental one; moreover, it is not possible to consider hysteria without regard to the mechanisms of its occurrence which manifest themselves in the personality and are mainly psychological. Hysteria is the most psychogenic of all illnesses. Its recognition is therefore a double problem: (1) exclusion of what may be called 'genuine' illness, i.e. of a recognized morbid pattern; and (2) discovery of an adequate motivation. To ignore either of these requirements is to court error, since hysteria may occur along with physical or mental disorder, elaborating upon it and mimicking it; and, on the other hand, some physical diseases give rise to symptoms indistinguishable in their form and apparent psychological mechanism from those of hysteria.

Aetiology

A hereditary factor can be inferred in many cases though it has not proved possible to tell the mode of transmission or the nature of what is transmitted. At the same time the occurrence of hysterical mechanisms in children, and their frequency in healthy adults, especially after calamities or in unendurable conditions, such as may occur in war, suggest that hysteria is potentially present in most people and that environment is more important here than heredity. The combination of heredity and environment may result, long before actual illness occurs, in a *hysterical personality*. This is not found in all patients who show hysterical symptoms, but nearly all people of hysterical personality show hysterical symptoms at some time. Many of the features of this personality are socially obnoxious, but other features are not, and it is wrong to use 'hysterical' as a depreciatory epithet for a set of qualities that one dislikes. These people are unduly responsive to the situation they are in, especially if by their excessive response they can fulfil wishes of which they are hardly aware, or evade what is painful in the situation, instead of meeting it and disposing of it adequately. Unsatisfied with their own capacities, they seek to cut a better figure than their endowment warrants, and are constantly posing and pretending. This, like all their behaviour and aims here described, is not done with full consciousness, but with a more or less sincere ignorance or ambiguity of purpose; it is not a question of deliberate deceit, of studied histrionics or malingering. In thus responding to situations and turning the response to some inadequate end, the hysterical person is characterized by a lack of inner stability and of constant standards of behaviour, and also by a lability of affect and an exuberant fancy. The fantasies normal in childhood are here seen in physically mature adults, who, like children, can temporarily live their fantasies, absorbed in this unreal compound of past experiences and longings, yet not so wholly divorced from their real surroundings as might appear. In an attentuated form, this is evident when they almost unwittingly manufacture some situation, according to their needs —literally 'making a scene'—and enter into it emotionally with a rapidity and fervour impossible for more stable people. Egotism and untruthfulness (pseudologia phantastica) may be pushed to the point of delinquency. There may be a longing for prestige, sympathy, love or some other emotional relationship, which leads the hysteric to behave in a way strikingly out of keeping with his demeanour on other occasions; the inappropriateness of his behaviour even at the time may be obvious to a detached onlooker, but is not always so. Many of these people can use illness or well-acted fantasies of illness to satisfy their hardly conscious needs; they may also gain their ends by forgetting what it would be painful to remember. Here again the onlooker may find it hard to tell how genuine or complete is this forgetfulness, but the question is of little moment compared with discovery of the motive for the hypomnesia. Hysterics are often regarded as unduly suggestible because they respond so readily or violently to situations and to people with whom they develop an emotional relationship, often unrecognized by themselves as such. The emotional attitude of a hysteric towards others is often influenced by sexual factors. Hysterical personality is believed to be commoner in women than in men, and may be associated with psychosexual immaturity. Coquetry and frigidity are not uncommonly allied in hysterics; there may be much flirting and sexual excitation, stopping short of coitus. It is, however, juster to say that the sexual lives of hysterics show instability and inadequacy than to specify any particular aberration.

The precipitating factor for the onset of hysterical symptoms is usually a situation, emotionally charged, out of which the patient's symptoms will bring him more or less overt, but unacknowledged, gain. This gain need not be material and obvious, and may run directly counter to such accepted values as health and ability to work. One of the plainest instances of a partial unsubstantial gain is that created by an injury, and the resulting insecurity and claim for compensation or pension; hysterical symptoms flourish in such a soil, and are usually influenced for the worse by repeated medical examinations. Hysteria occurs among soldiers under active service conditions, and can readily be fostered in them by injudicious measures.

Psychopathology

This is almost wholly a matter of psychological disorder. It is true that disseminated sclerosis and many other organic diseases of the brain may be accompanied by hysterical symptoms, but the association is not a constant one. The psychological changes can usually be traced further back than the happening that provoked the illness; often they are the continuation of normal tendencies of childhood that have been fostered and extended by ill-judged upbringing. The hysterical symptoms that appear as motor or sensory phenomena show the patient's readiness for the translation of experience into bodily symbols; this is a special instance of the universal tendency for somatic representation of experience, converting it into action. It is the facility and exaggeration, not the existence, of this 'conversion' mechanism that is characteristic of hysteria. What is thus translated or 'converted' into physical terms has been something painful and unacceptable; the partial exclusion of it from consciousness, 'repression' of it, is therefore understandable; in its physical, symbolic form it is tolerable and may even be prized. Identification with other people is responsible for the frequent imitation of symptoms and for the epidemics of hysteria. Clearly the mechanism need not be limited to the production of physical symptoms, though bodily structure and local weaknesses may conduce to this. There can be hysterical phenomena, such as the dissociation seen in fugues and so-called splitting of personality, which are instances of the exclusion of recent and remote painful experience from clear consciousness. The wishes and fears that deviously attain outward expression as hysterical symptoms do not derive solely from the recent past, though much of their strength may come from it. It must be admitted that there are some hysterics in whom this psychopathology cannot be demonstrated, and that such cases are among the most intractable.

Symptoms

These may be divided into: (1) sensory; (2) motor, including fits; and (3) quasi-psychotic.

The symptoms can be like those of any conceivable affection of which the patient has a notion. The cruder his notion, the less will his symptoms be like those of the simulated condition, but after he has been demonstrated to a class or repeatedly examined he may better his notion, and consequently his symptoms come closer to those of organic disease. Or, if he has had opportunity of seeing insanity, his pseudo-insanity may smack less of the stage than it otherwise usually does. The range of hysterical symptoms is so great that to describe them all in detail would take inordinate space, and there is no need to do so. The crude physical manifestations have become rather uncommon.

Sensory. The sensory or, more properly, the *perceptual* symptoms include *clavus* and *globus hystericus*, *blindness*, *deafness* and *anaesthesia*. The two former are so common in all sorts of mental disorder, especially those accompanied by anxiety, that they are of little specific importance in hysteria; inquiry as to their presence will often in these rather hypochondriacal patients lead to their occurrence. The difficulty in swallowing reported by hysterical women may be associated with a disinclination to eat—anorexia nervosa [p. 1346]. Any cutaneous disturbance of sensation that the patient has a notion of can be presented, e.g. anaesthesia, either uni- or bilateral, or of stocking and glove distribution, and analgesia of any part. The anaesthesia seldom corresponds to any nerve trunk, nerve root, or spinal segment, unless the patient has had special opportunities of knowing the relevant anatomical areas. With an anaesthetic hand objects may be identified, and any test which the patient does not recognize as referring to this disability he will perform satisfactorily. Such tests are not a means of 'catching the patient out' as though he were a malingerer, but of ascertaining whether the symptoms express only his notion of some illness. The tests for a malingerer, it is true, amount to the same thing, though one assumes the malingerer to be clearly conscious of his purpose; consequently any distinction between hysteria and malingering must depend on the observer's impression as to the patient's honesty and self-knowledge; certainly it cannot be decided by tests. The tests for blindness (e.g. using a stereoscope with a supposedly blind eye), deafness (e.g. effect on pulse, respiration and psychogalvanic reflex of exciting remarks addressed to the patient), and for other forms of perceptual defect all depend on the physician's greater knowledge of what should or should not accompany the symptoms of which the patient complains; they are not intended to discover hysterical 'stigmata' or characteristic anomalies. The ovarian and other hyperaesthetic spots, the pharyngeal anaesthesia and the concentric limitation of the field of vision formerly used diagnostically, were all products of suggestion or, as in the last instance, phenomena that may occur in normal fatigue, in hypochondria and in certain cerebral lesions.

Motor. The motor symptoms are *paralyses*, *pareses*, *spasms*, *contractures* and *tremors*. Hysterical paralysis or paresis never affects individual muscles, but always movements. By various devices it can be shown that the patient can still use the affected muscles, as long as he does not know that the movement in question requires their use. The paralyses affect chiefly the left side of the body, are common in the legs (preventing proper walking or standing), and often occur in limbs or other structures that have earlier been the seat of an organic disability, e.g. trauma or paresis. If the paralysis be flaccid, no loss of tone or of reflex response is found, and the patient, through his ill-informed notions of what should happen, behaves otherwise than a patient with organic paralysis would—e.g. if asked to rise from the supine to the sitting posture, without using his hands, he keeps his paralysed leg flat on the bed. If the paretic part be kept stiff, the antagonists will be found to come into action first when the patient is asked to perform the movement he says he cannot; and if the movement has to be made against resistance, sudden removal of the resistance reveals how much of the apparently tremendous effort was going into associated irrelevant or antagonistic movements. Passive movement to overcome the spasticity or subsequent contractures cause the patient to be more upset than could be accounted for by any pain he may complain of. The varieties of abnormal gait are numerous; many of them fantastically elaborate and, from the look of them, exhausting. Not only the musculature of the limbs may be affected but of the trunk (leading to curvatures and odd postures) and indeed any voluntary muscles, e.g. of the tongue, larynx, pharynx or eye. In hysterical aphonia the voice may sink to a whisper, or there may, more rarely, be complete mutism; the voice can, however, be used normally for coughing and similar purposes. The aphonia often comes on after some local inflammation that has caused hoarseness, or after a fright. Stammering, usually of the exaggerated kind, may also occur. Spasm of the external ocular muscles, leading to a convergent squint, may accompany a spasm of accommodation. Ptosis and blepharospasm sometimes occur. Many of the tics and spasms that used to be thought hysterical are now recognized to be often physiogenic, e.g. residual symptoms of encephalitis lethargica and chorea; spasmodic torticollis, for instance, is far less often psychogenic than used to be supposed. When a spasm or paresis has long been maintained, trophic disturbance may follow: blueness and oedema, shiny skin, fibrosis of periarticular structures and similar effects of rigidity and disuse. Tremor may occur and is often gross, as in many of the war cases. It is variable in degree and rhythm, and often disappears when the patient's attention is turned from it; this, however, is not a safe criterion.

Hysterical *fits* commonly occur in patients with obviously hysterical personality. They may be little more than a fainting attack or an outburst of temper, significantly like the tantrums of an ill-behaved child. Often, however, they are more differentiated than this, and diagnosis from an epileptic fit may be difficult. Sometimes the fit grows out of a tremor induced by fright or anxiety, or it may express some emotional state, such as great pain, anger or erotic excitement. Occasionally the patient shows plainly by her expression and movements that the fit is erotic; it may be a typical orgasm. The 'classical' four-phase fits which Charcot described were artefacts of the clinic.

Sometimes the patient's fit becomes very like an epileptic one after he has spent some time at a neurological clinic, or he may be an epileptic who also has hysterical fits. Some hysterics, by overbreathing, induce an epileptiform convulsion, which can be abruptly terminated if an injection of calcium chloride or gluconate be given. They may pass from one such fit into another, so that the condition suggests a status epilepticus. The unconsciousness that often appears to accompany a hysterical fit is seldom as complete as it looks; neither is the subsequent amnesia. There may, however, be a delirium, corresponding to the emotional upheaval. Patients very rarely hurt themselves seriously in the fit, however violent, or have a fit when alone or asleep. The length of the attack and its degree often depend on the audience; the more the bystanders try to restrain the movements, the wilder do the kicking, struggling, biting, shouting, panting, spitting, etc., become and the longer they go on. There is neither the pallor nor the cyanosis, the regular sequence nor the subsequent headache and sleepiness of epilepsy; urine is not passed, nor the bowels opened; reflexes, including the corneal response, are unaffected, and the end of the fit may be abrupt.

Quasi-psychotic. The commonest quasi-psychotic symptoms are *stupor*, *twilight state*, *fugue* and *pseudodementia*.

In the *stupor*, seen typically in harassed weary soldiers under bombardment, the patient lies motionless, taking food like a 12-months' baby, non-resistive, sometimes incontinent of urine or faeces, and without any predominant emotional tone. It is of brief duration if the exciting circumstances cease to prevail. In less acute forms there may be a sullen resistive akinesia, or a condition lasting even for years, with an occasional break; this is a rare form. Only with great caution and reserve should such stuporose or semi-stuporose conditions be regarded as hysterical; physical factors often play a large part in causing them, or they may be schizophrenic.

The *confusional* or *delirious* states may accompany a fit or represent an important emotional experience, e.g. some sexual episode. They are often histrionic, and represent wishes of a religious or grandiose sort; or the patient may behave as though he were an animal or a child. Sometimes they occur during the night, and in a somnambulist state the patient repeats some past happening, or may do complicated work. This is closely akin to the hysterical fugue, in which there is not so much a clouding as a narrowing of consciousness, a 'dissociation'. In the *fugue* the patient may live out some fantasy or—as more commonly happens—simply says that he does not know who he is or where he lives. The patient says he has forgotten some or all of his life before a certain date, and later he may profess to remember nothing of what has happened during the fugue. There is, in short, a double set of memories, which may alternate, and since the patient's own identity is commonly included in the repressed and temporarily forgotten material, he may be said to have two personalities, and sometimes three or four. Actually there are no cases in which it is strictly correct to speak thus of multiple personalities; it is only a matter of different aspects or fragments of the one personality.

Nearly always a hysterical fugue with gross amnesia turns out to have been a means of evading some predicament, and it is well to keep in mind in such cases that the patient may have broken the law or otherwise exposed himself to disgrace and punishment. The amnesia is seldom as complete as the patient states. Fugues may occur as a hysterical mechanism in an organic psychosis: for example, in a man with arrested general paralysis who had been prominently and in detail reported as a case of multiple personality which responded to psychotherapy. Psychogenic fugues are not invariably hysterical; they may be symptoms of a reactive depression in which despair and perplexity are conspicuous.

'*Pseudodementia*' covers the large group who behave as though insane. It may occur, as in the so-called Ganser syndrome, in prisoners awaiting trial. Whatever the circumstances, its motive is escape from a disagreeable situation. It is likely, however, that it is mainly those with a predisposition towards severe mental illness, especially schizophrenia and high-grade defectives who have recourse to this kind of hysterical behaviour. It sometimes comes on after brain injury. The patients' behaviour corresponds necessarily to their notion of insanity, which is usually far enough removed from anything the psychiatrist knows as such. Occasionally, however, it is very near the buffoon-like conduct of some schizophrenics. The patients say that they do not know their own age, affect not to understand simple remarks, give absurd answers which nevertheless indicate that they know the right answer, e.g. by inverting the correct order of the figures in a sum. When asked about some simple matter, they look as though they were making strenuous efforts to remember, herein behaving differently from the schizophrenic. The most characteristic feature is the disparity between the patient's alleged deficiencies and his general alertness: he says he does not know anything about his own past, he cannot read or spell or do the simplest arithmetic, and yet he may be behaving quite naturally and adapting himself to the situation in a way which would be inconceivable if he had actually so advanced a dementia.

Some hysterics go to great lengths in their representation of ideas of illness. They will allow themselves to be put among grossly insane people, or submit to repeated operations, such as amputation. Self-inflicted injuries, e.g. keeping wounds and sores open, are sometimes met with, cf. dermatitis artefacta. In some such cases masochistic tendencies can be recognized, but by no means in all. Suicidal attempts are not infrequent. They often have as their purpose revenge, the satisfaction of some spite, and the patient may leave behind a lying, fantasy-coloured letter, indicting someone. Frequently the suicidal attempt is in the nature of a theatrical demonstration, or an appeal for sympathy and help, carried out in such circumstances as make it unlikely to be fatal; and if the patient kills herself, it is more through bad management than intention.

Diagnosis

It will be plain from what has been said that diagnosis must be both negative and positive—negative, by excluding any organic cause for the symptoms; positive, by finding motives and relating the symptoms to them. Neither method is alone sufficient, because of the occasional concurrence of structural disease with psychogenic symptoms. As to the former, i.e. the negative method, it is unnecessary to enter here into all the differentiating points. Many of them have been mentioned in the foregoing description of symptoms, and all turn on the disparity between what experience tells us would occur if these symptoms were of organic origin, and what the patient knows about such matters. Consequently a doctor who has hysterical symptoms is extraordinarily, difficult to diagnose, in this negative sense. The method of arriving at a diagnosis by suddenly taking the patient unawares, and seeing if the symptoms persist, is to be deprecated; it antagonizes her. Similarly undesirable is the procedure of seeing whether one can suggest new symptoms to the patient, e.g. an anaesthesia; it can be both misleading and harmful. Neither is the hysterical nature of a symptom to be judged solely by whether it can be removed by suggestion; for some organic symptoms are temporarily got rid of thereby, and many hysterical symptoms are not. An intimate knowledge of the range of symptoms of physical disease is much more useful to the physician than an equipment with special tests and lists of differences between 'functional' and 'organic'. It is not only a problem of neurology but of the whole of medicine, since the hypochondriacal tendencies of many hysterics lead them to complain of visceral symptoms; usually, in doubtful cases, the symptoms are those which might well occur in the earlier stages of some physical disease. It is, however, in neurology that the most difficult cases of all arise, e.g. in disseminated sclerosis, carbon monoxide poisoning, cerebral vascular disease or encephalitis lethargica; here there is more likelihood of the organic disease being overlooked than of its being wrongly diagnosed. The patient's previous personality, any provocative situation or emotional disturbance, the previous occurrence of organic signs, e.g. transient diplopia, and the age of the patient must be considered. Hysterical symptoms appearing for the first time in middle or later life in someone whose personality has been stable, are probably not solely psychogenic. If the symptoms diminish when little or no attention is paid to them, they are more likely to be hysterical.

Treatment

Too much treatment is worse than too little. Injudicious physical or psychological treatment of hysterics often makes their symptoms worse and their illness intractable. Recondite methods should be eschewed by all but experts. Common sense is as important as psychological understanding; and social usefulness more to be aimed at than eradication of symptoms or attainment of self-knowledge. In short, it is often not so much the hysterical illness or the mechanism of repression and conversion that calls for remedy, as the patient's inadequate way of dealing with difficult situations. Consequently, the whole treatment must aim at the patient's return to ordinary conditions of life as soon as possible, and at a re-education of his ways of meeting difficulties. To this end it is profitable to go over with the patient the situations, emotional disturbances and motives that led up to the illness, and to do this without implying moral judgement or social indifference—certainly without teaching the patient one's psychological theories. It is a matter of general psychotherapy [see p. 1340]; and it may entail a far-reaching analysis of the patient's past life, her emotional development and her instinctual tendencies. It is questionable, however, whether anyone without special psychiatric experience is wise to enter lightly upon this way of benefiting the patient. For, on the one hand, he may be misled into a wilderness of fantasy masquerading as once-repressed, now-recalled psychological trauma; and, on the other, he may be at a loss how to deal with the attachment and dependence upon him which the patient will come to show, and which may in fact be the chief influence in bringing about her precarious recovery. A great deal may be achieved—perhaps as much as by more thoroughgoing methods—if the physician, himself mature and with impartial insight into the psychological motivation of the symptoms, leaves aside in his dealings with the patient any very detailed inquiry into the more remote causes of the illness and the purposes it served; and, instead, directs her towards a better social adaptation, by advising her to avoid when possible the situations that, as he sees, favour the production of symptoms, getting her into a disciplined way of living, and stepping in with explanation, support and advice whenever fresh difficulties arise. His success in getting rid of individual symptoms at the beginning may be an important factor in establishing the necessary relationship with the patient. Such a line of treatment is not heroic or dramatic, and it demands a great deal of the physician; but it avoids some of the commonest blunders and may be strikingly successful. For this, or indeed any treatment, admission to hospital is not obligatory; but it will help when there are adverse factors in the patient's situation and, of course, will be essential if there be such symptoms as self-injury, suicidal attempts, pseudodementia or gross paralysis. The danger of the patient's picking up new symptoms in hospital should also be weighed. Isolation is usually inadvisable.

Many of the symptoms of hysteria will not wait upon general treatment, but demand energetic intervention. Anorexia, for instance, cannot be allowed to go on to an avoidable inanition, nor a paralysis to the stage of contracture; a mute patient, or one who is deaf or blind or ignorant of his own identity, offers such practical obstacles to almost any kind of treatment that the symptoms must be tackled and disposed of early. For this purpose suggestive measures are valuable and appropriate physical treatment may be called for, e.g. supervision during feeding in anorexia to ensure adequate intake, physiotherapy for paralysis, voice exercises. Suggestive measures need not take the form of hypnosis; suggestion in the normal waking state has many advantages over hypnosis, though those expert in the latter are sometimes very successful in their treatment. Suggestion, like almost every form of treatment of hysteria, has pitfalls; its triumphs, like those of every other method, sometimes prove vain, but in the hands of a physician who is at once confident and cautious, this method may result in a satisfactory recovery. In using suggestion, such physical devices as faradization should be avoided. As a means of demonstrating that the illness is not due to local disease, however, such methods sometimes take their place in a detailed plan of treatment. Motor and sensory symptoms can usually be removed if the physician is patient, determined and confident in the use of persuasion and suggestion. Intravenous injection of a barbiturate, such as amylobarbitone sodium, may facilitate such treatment, and may help the patient to disclose motives and happenings she had been reluctant or unable to talk about; disclosures of this kind, however, must be received and utilized with caution, and lasting benefit is not to be expected from such catharsis alone.

The choice of occupation, the settlement of any social cause of illness (e.g. claims for compensation), and the obtaining of a healthy attitude—neither complaisant, much-enduring nor harsh—on the part of the patient's relatives and friends, are all important factors in treatment. The hysterical reactions to injury call for special mention because of their frequency. Though often of transparent motivation, they are not by any means to be regarded as outright malingering; for the patient's feeling of illness may be sincere, his symptoms distressing, his anxiety typical and his irritability and insomnia symptoms that he would gladly lose. They are none the less psychogenic. It is often assumed that so far as an illness is psychogenic, it must be treated only by psychotherapy. This is false theory. There are few mental disorders in which psychotherapy alone produces such small benefit as in hysterical conditions due to the compensation or pension situation that may follow an injury. Putting an end to the situation early and the resumption of ordinary activity as soon as any physical injury has been repaired are the most potent measures in the earlier stages. Even if the symptoms have been present a long time, the ending of disputes about claims and the return to ordered routine and regular occupation achieve more than do frequent medical interviews. Psychotherapy is then an adjunct, not an essential feature, of the treatment.

Marriage should never be recommended as treatment for hysteria; the superstition about this has resulted in lamentable troubles, especially for the person the hysteric marries. This is not to say that every hysteric is to be dissuaded from marrying; there are more things than treatment to be considered then. Married hysterics, however, should not be recommended to have—or to adopt—a child. Contrary to popular notions, pregnancy and puerperium more often aggravate than benefit hysteria. Moreover, hysterical women are not usually satisfactory parents, and may induce psychological disorders in their children.

Course and Prognosis

This depends mainly on the patient's personality and social setting, and on the treatment employed. A long history of hysterical traits prior to the illness, a continuance of circumstances favourable to the symptoms, and inadequate or excessive treatment are all unfavourable. This is, however, an illness that sometimes confounds prediction, patients recovering when many adverse factors have been operative and the symptoms have been present for years. In children the prognosis is fairly good if treatment can be undertaken promptly; it is best if the hysteria is monosymptomatic and has come on after a fright. In all cases in which the situation which provoked the illness persists, the outlook is bad; for example, in compensation cases for which no medical treatment is of any avail—for obvious reasons—until the litigation is settled once and for all. Similarly, during war, psychotherapeutic successes are often dazzling while the hysterical soldier is under treatment in hospital, but the symptoms return when he must go back to duty. There are many varieties of outcome, chronic invalidism being the commonest. A few patients later become schizophrenic, and a few become involutional melancholics. The prognosis in respect of the patient's hysterical personality is more important than that of his hysterical illness; it is, however, no more to be assessed by rules than the general future of any human being's life and personality. Patients do not necessarily tend to become antisocial; delinquency is certainly a likelihood in some hysterical people, but bravery and self-devotion may be conspicuous in others.

OBSESSIONAL DISORDER

Definition

In this condition the characteristic feature is that, along with some mental happening, there is an experience of subjective compulsion and of resistance to it. Commonly the mental happening—which may be a fear, an impulse or a preoccupation—is recognized, on quiet reflection, as senseless; nevertheless it persists.

Aetiology

The *hereditary* factor is strong. A third of the parents of obsessional patients, and a fifth of their brothers and sisters, have themselves shown pronounced obsessional traits; the proportion is in each case higher if all forms of mental abnormality be included, since both schizophrenia and affective illnesses occur with more than average frequency in families of obsessionals. The abnormal personality of the parents is probably also potent as an environmental cause. Very many obsessional patients have for years before they became ill shown a rather characteristic mental constitution: they are excessively cleanly, orderly and conscientious, sticklers for precision; they have inconclusive ways of thinking and acting; they are given to needless repetition. Those who have shown such traits since childhood are often morose, obstinate, irritable people; others are vacillating, uncertain of themselves and submissive. 'Obsessional' traits occur, however, in many people who never become mentally ill, and in many who become mentally ill otherwise than with an obsessional disorder. Consequently these traits cannot be rigidly held to be the forerunners or non-morbid counterparts of obsessional illness.

Environmental factors must always be considered. The influence of strict, morose, cruel, over-conscientious or obsessional parents is difficult to evaluate; certainly in some cases it plays no part. There is nothing specific in the situations which supply the content of an obsession: they might equally well have preceded hysterical symptoms, for example, in a person so predisposed. Nevertheless, the fright or pain which once accompanied a particular experience, or a long series of experiences, must not be overlooked in working out the multiple causes of some obsession psychologically related to this experience.

Encephalitis lethargica and a few other cerebral diseases may produce typical obsessional symptoms in persons previously free from demonstrable tendencies in this direction.

Psychopathology

Apart from the difficult instances in which lesions of the brain are accompanied by obsessions, this is at present wholly a matter of abnormal psychology. Some elements of an obsession are universal human attributes: all little children tend to ritualize and repeat; all human beings are at times uncertain of the rightness or sense of what they have done; they try to avert trouble by symbolical acts and other magical devices, whose effectiveness they may question, e.g. superstition; many normal people, moreover, have mild obsessions that do not bother them, e.g. scruples. The manifest struggle going on in the obsessional patient may be restated in terms of hypothetical instinctual tendencies. His symptoms can be recognized as a symbolic representation of emotionally significant earlier experiences; by means of protective mechanisms he tries to ward off the painful and overwhelming obsession, with the result that he develops complicated rituals and similar devices which may be mistaken for the essential symptom. The transition from obsessional to schizophrenic is easy to understand psychopathologically, since in both some contents of consciousness are separated from the main stream.

Symptoms

Obsessions are conveniently classified as: (1) *ideas* or *images*; (2) *impulses*; (3) *phobias*; and (4) *rumination*. These overlap constantly.

Among obsessional *ideas and images* are tunes, phrases, mental pictures of a disagreeable sort, e.g. of a mutilated corpse, and obscene associations, e.g. every cranny reminds the patient of a vulva. Obsessional *impulses* are often of a suicidal or aggressive character: the patient may feel an urge to kick people in the street, to push his friend over a cliff, or to throw himself under a passing train. In many other cases, however, they are less alarming; e.g. impulses to swear loudly in church, or to laugh at a funeral; or more of an intellectual sort, such as an impulse to count and manipulate numbers senselessly or to avoid typing any word with a given number of letters or beginning with a particular consonant.

Phobias are closely bound up with the other varieties of obsession: thus, the patient who has an impulse to plunge a knife into his friend's or his own neck has an understandable phobia of knives; the patient who is troubled by obscene thoughts whenever he looks at a naked statue develops a phobia of museums. Not all phobias can be so accounted for; they may rest on some forgotten alarm, and take a queer form, such as a phobia of lavatories or of one-legged men. It is loose usage to give the name 'phobia' to every case in which an individual develops fear that is excessive or inexplicable; the essential features of an obsession, already mentioned, should also be present. The term 'claustrophobia', for example, is often loosely applied to a fear or dislike of being in an enclosed place, which is not obsessional. Fears of dirt or infection are very common phobias: they are symbols of moral, usually sexual, taint, and they lead to much washing, etc.; thus, a patient who has blamed himself for masturbation may be constantly washing his hands, or following a complicated ritual of touching nothing with his bare hands for fear of contamination. Often the rituals and defensive precautions seem grotesque when compared with their ostensible purpose, as in the case of a patient who is perpetually putting himself to the greatest trouble in order to ensure that he never steps on a worm inadvertently. Ludicrous as his behaviour may seem, it is often tragic in the distress, and indeed ruin, it may cause him. Another phobia is that which has fear as its object, i.e. the patient is afraid of any situation in which he may feel fear; some such patients do not leave their homes for years, because they fear they may have 'agoraphobia' once they get outside.

Obsessional *rumination* usually takes the form of endless questioning or search. The patient has to ask himself 'Why' with pointless insistence about all manner of problems beyond his or anybody's grasp; or he has to keep casting round in his mind after some forgotten name or word which he could easily do without. Religious scruples sometimes fall into this category, as when a penitent is continually running to his confessor with some venial trifle he has come upon in his interminable self-questioning and doubt.

Obsessional patients are in many cases *depressed*; their illness is a depressing one. Besides this secondary depression, however, there is frequently an association of a more intimate kind, in which depression—or mania—is the essential or the main part of the illness, and the concurrent obsessions seem to be symptoms of this affective disorder. In such cases the obsessional illness is very often cyclical in its course. *Anxiety* is a common accompaniment of obsessions; in phobias it is most conspicuous. The anxiety is inseparable from the patient's struggle against the subjective compulsion which is so alarming to his feeling of integrity in self and mind, such a shock to his belief that he is a free agent. *Depersonalization* may occur in the course of an obsessional illness.

Diagnosis

If the essential features, i.e. feeling of subjective compulsion and immediate resistance to this, be kept in view, it is seldom difficult to distinguish between obsessions, on the one hand, and delusions, hallucinations, ideas of reference or self-reproach, feelings of being influenced and schizophrenic stereotypies, etc., on the other. Schizophrenic symptoms may be in the offing, or actually present, when the obsessional ideas are of the magical kind, e.g. the patient feeling that the effect of his obscene thoughts upon others may be averted by some gesture, or when his rituals are carried to bizarre lengths, e.g. having to save the last drops of his urine because of some recurring doubt. In differential diagnosis it must be remembered that obsessions may occur in the course of almost any mental illness in a person of obsessional tendencies, and that the psychological mechanism for the production of obsessions, like that for hysterical symptoms, is present in almost everybody in varying degree. Anorexia nervosa, for example, frequently has obsessional characteristics: the patient is well aware of the senselessness of her abstention from food and she struggles, though vainly, to overcome the compulsion—in this case a denial and an avoidance—by efforts of will or by some ritual. Consequently, an illness is not to be regarded as obsessional unless obsessions are the chief symptoms. The only difference between obsessions and many schizophrenic phenomena towards which the patient retains insight and which he regards as alien to him, lies in the nature of the compulsion he experiences: in obsessions it is subjective—he feels that it comes from within his own mind, whereas in the schizophrenic phenomena he feels that it comes from without, it is imposed upon him. It is a difference, however, that may be obliterated, i.e. what was once obsessional may become schizophrenic, but this is an uncommon outcome when the obsessional disorder is definite and well-established.

Treatment

Patients should be encouraged to continue at their occupation and not to test themselves, or to try to overcome their obsession, by repeatedly putting themselves in a situation in which it will occur. So long as their impulses are not likely to get them into trouble, they should be dissuaded from 'fighting' them; external restrictions are more helpful than reliance on 'will-power'. The physician should aim at getting a patient well by putting an end to his anxiety and struggle; if that is not wholly attainable, the patient must be educated to deal with his obsessional tendencies by acknowledging their existence, their psychological origins, and, often, their harmlessness in those very respects in which he thought them most harmful, e.g. obscenity. Frank recognition of obsessional tendencies, which everyone has in some degree, is an important step in learning to control them. In some patients the obsessional attack is so cyclical and almost self-limited that a brief rest and general care are all that are needed. In others, whose affection is chronic, recovery is out of the question, but advice about the management of their lives, varying according to their individual circumstances, helps them greatly. In some such patients frontal leucotomy lessens or removes the distress that formerly accompanied their obsession. Obsessional patients, so prone to rumination and endless questioning, often clamour to be psychoanalysed. There is no evidence that psychoanalysis, however prolonged, benefits them more than methods that are not so exigent of time and money.

Various forms of behaviour therapy based on the application of learning theory [p. 1341] have been employed with some success in the treatment of patients suffering from phobias which are evoked in more or less specific situations. Large claims for the effectiveness of this type of treatment in the management of various forms of obsessional behaviour are currently under examination.

Course and Prognosis

The outlook for recovery is worse if obsessional symptoms have been present since childhood, if they now fill up most of the patient's time, and if he is weakly resigned to his illness. The best outlook is when the obsessional illness comes on suddenly in a person who has not had conspicuous obsessional traits or who has had previous benign attacks. A cyclical course is not uncommon. The situation is ominous when the ritual gets more and more systematized and remote from what previously occasioned it. The development along schizophrenic lines, already mentioned, is more to be feared in such cases and in those with bizarre obsessional thoughts; the great majority of gross obsessionals, however, do not become schizophrenic or anything else than obsessional. About half the patients recover from an attack, which may, however, last for a year or even more. Many people are subject to brief attacks, lasting only a few days, and largely due to fatigue or physical illness reducing their mental health. Intercurrent happenings influence the course of the illness, e.g. some men were free from symptoms during their period of war-service, with its routine and lack of responsibility or need for decision. The content of the obsessions is of little use prognostically. Old age is not in itself an adverse factor, but attacks in childhood suggest a strong constitutional bias and are therefore unfavourable on the whole. Few obsessionals give way to antisocial impulses, e.g. to suicide, homicide, delinquency. It is true that obsessionals who are also depressed may kill themselves, and that obsessionals who are irritable and angry may injure others; but obsessionals rarely yield directly to an impulse they have resisted, or need to have 'irresistible impulse' urged in extenuation of a crime. Sexual offences and perversions are rarely obsessional.

PSYCHOPATHIC PERSONALITY

All abnormality of personality that does not amount to manifest illness may properly be called 'psychopathic personality'. There are many people who do not regard themselves as ill, nor do others think them so, yet their behaviour is abnormal enough to upset or puzzle other people, and sometimes themselves. In this it is like mental illness, and calls similarly for psychiatric understanding and treatment. But since they are not deemed to be ill, their behaviour must be attributed to abnormal personality, much as an aberration like alkaptonuria must be attributed to abnormal physical constitution.

In some cases anomalies of cerebral structure may contribute to the condition. In childhood and even in maturity damage to the brain, by infection, poisoning, malnutrition or trauma, can lead to changes in personality, such as occur after encephalitis, carbon monoxide intoxication, pellagra, operations and accidental violence to the brain. They do not conform to a single pattern, and may be complicated by intellectual impairment. They depend to some extent on the part of the brain affected; in perhaps the most striking group—encephalopaths whose emotional control is much reduced so that they easily become violent when they cannot get their own way—the hypothalamus and other structures in the rhinencephalon are suspect. Electroencephalographic data have recently been added to the clinical, psychological and experimental evidence for this. Some writers believe that most of those with psychopathic personality characterized by violent outbursts have an innate or acquired cerebral abnormality, and even, though on inconclusive grounds, that there is a kinship between the aggressive psychopath and the epileptic. It has also been demonstrated that sex-chromosome anomalies can be associated with antisocial conduct: in particular, the so-called XYY male can be unusually tall, aggressive and sometimes of subnormal intelligence. It would, however, be a mistake to attribute psychopathic personality, even when marked by excitability and impulsive acts of violence, necessarily to anomalies of cerebral constitution; emotional deprivation or insecurity during childhood, parental mismanagement, and in adult life severe frustration and adversity constitute psychological causes which are often in evidence.

Such questions arise in only a small group of instances. The large majority of individuals with psychopathic personalities exhibit no evidence of cerebral or other physical disorder. As a clinical concept 'psychopathic personality' is an essentially descriptive term. It does not connote an evaluation of character, according to how useful such a person is to society; nor is it a prediction about the likelihood of subsequent illness of a particular type. None the less, people of abnormal personality will often come into conflict with organized society and with individuals more normally constituted; they will be on the whole more vulnerable to stresses; their peculiarities, intensified into symptoms of illness or proofs of delinquency, will earn them pity, contempt, dislike, punishment or compulsory treatment. It is therefore common for 'psychopathic personality' to be used as a pejorative term, limited to those who will afflict society in some way—the 'antisocial psychopath', the 'psychopathic tenth', are significant phrases, akin to 'psychopathic inferiority' and the still earlier 'moral insanity'; it is, however, wrong to apply to the concept 'psychopathic personality' so shifting and subjective a criterion as social disapproval. The term is also used to denote those who stand in danger of insanity—the 'schizoid psychopath', for instance—but mental illness cannot be assumed to be a certain outcome in even pronounced aberrations of personality. Among mystics and poets, men of action, scholars and scientists are some who have properly been classified as of 'psychopathic personality', their abnormality consisting nevertheless in unusually high, rare and valuable if peculiar qualities, rather than in a blemish or handicap. St. Teresa, Joan of Arc, T. E. Lawrence, Cavendish, Cellini, Tolstoy, Mozart, Michelangelo—or any of the lists of famous people that have been cited as examples of psychopathic personality—testify to this.

Apart from any judgement about the good or harm they do to society, people are therefore said to have psychopathic personalities if they fall outside the wide range agreed upon as normal—not quite the same thing as healthy—yet are not ill. Society being ordered as it is, the majority of such abnormal people will at some time come into conflict with it or fail to meet its demands and their conduct will often rightly be called antisocial. The antisocial group of persons with psychopathic personality is large; its size will very according to the culture in which they live and the allowances or opportunities it makes for them. This is obviously true if their adjustment as adults to the demands of the community is the measure of their 'antisocial' trends; it is true also of their development and the way in which social influences may be such as to foster their smooth participation in a very diverse pattern of human relationships, or may mar them, giving neither free play nor direction to their peculiarities. Success in preventing many of these abnormal people from becoming a nuisance or a danger is, therefore, a test of the educational methods, the pliancy and the psychiatric hygiene of a community. This is not to ignore the hereditary and narrowly individual factors which determine psychic constitution, but to stress the social causes of later social failure, should it occur; such failure, however, need not be regarded as inevitable in people of psychopathic personality. It is unfortunate that in the Mental Health Act, 1959, the term 'psychopathic disorder' is restricted, by definition, to those whose persistent disorder or disability of mind results in abnormally aggressive or seriously irresponsible conduct, and 'requires or is susceptible to medical treatment'. The obscure final clause runs ahead of present knowledge; it has not yet been determined which forms of psychopathic disorder require medical treatment or will respond to it.

Classification of psychopathic personality can be (1) arbitrary, (2) psychological or (3) psychiatric. The first picks out what seem serviceable characteristics that occur often and conspicuously; thus, one well-sponsored list is made up of the excitable, the unstable, the impulsive, the eccentric and perverse, the quarrelsome, the antisocial, and the liars and swindlers, and makes further reference to aesthetes, scatterbrains, enthusiasts and fanatics. The second, which is the ideal method, is based on the varieties of normal personality. Unfortunately, the types, trait-clusters and other classificatory groups so far proposed do too little justice to the complexity and range of human personality to be satisfactory or lasting.

The third, or psychiatric, classification, is likewise provisional but it has the advantage of grouping these non-morbid abnormalities in the same categories as the severe, morbid ones (with which there is reason to believe them genetically connected). To do this begs some fundamental questions, but it is for the present useful to recognize several clinical varieties of psychopathic personality: these include the schizoid [p. 1358], the affective [p. 1366], the paranoid [p. 1365], the obsessional [p. 1379] and the hysterical [p. 1374]. This list is open to the objections that must be made to any attempt at stating types of personality, and it is wrong to suppose that any of the varieties mentioned must always precede, or indicate proneness to, the illness from which its epithet is derived. Nevertheless, they give the psychiatrist afamiliar frame of reference and they leave room for manifold combinations of traits and attitudes within each class, so that the individual drug-addict, the sexual pervert, the hypochondriac and the fanatic can be included. If this psychiatric classification were to be judged by as rigorous a standard as the psychological, it could not stand; it will no doubt eventually give way before a surer psychology of personality and a surer psychopathology. For the time being, it is convenient to use these derivative terms, such as schizoid, and to give them no more weight than the bare labelling of personality deserves. Understanding a psychopathic person's motives and conduct, of course, requires full consideration of his development, circumstances and traits and goes beyond their classification for clinical purposes.

Any adequate description of forms of psychopathic personality must be lengthy, as must also any consideration of current views about their psychopathology and treatment. Crime, juvenile misbehaviour, habitual or sporadic drug-taking, incapacity for certain occupations and public duties (e.g. school teaching, military service), the temperamental concomitants of inferior intelligence and, at the other extreme, some of the characteristics of genius; these are intimately linked with the problem of psychopathic personality, and their exposition would demand a fuller treatment than space allows. Separate mention, however, should be made of the various forms of *sexual deviation*, unrelated to other forms of mental illness, which are often referred to psychiatrists. Some of these, like fetishism, may be private anomalies of sexual behaviour; others, like paedophilia and exhibitionism, involve public conduct with forensic implictions. Two of these anomalies, homosexuality and trans-sexualism, have been regarded as expressions of psychological intersexuality: there is no evidence to suggest that the chromosomal, gonadal or apparent sex in these individuals is abnormal. The expectations of any treatment of well-established sexual deviation, whether by physical or psychological means, should always be guarded.

CHILD PSYCHIATRY

The psychiatry of childhood has come to occupy an increasingly important place in the field of psychological medicine. Like the psychiatry of old age it raises clinical questions which are peculiar to an extreme life-epoch, but there are additional features which distinguish it from adult psychiatry. In the first place, the study of child psychiatry must take into account the many factors affecting the several phases of child development, both physical and psychological: the changes which occur in the human organism between infancy and adolescence are much greater than those which are exhibited over the whole remaining life-span. Secondly, since the child is much more dependent on his personal and social environment than is the adult, an understanding of the influence exercised by the family and, later, the school is indispensable to the clinician: for this reason the child psychiatrist usually works closely with the social worker and the clinical psychologist. Thirdly, the relative inability of children to describe their thoughts and feelings clearly renders their behaviour—or, all too often, their reported behaviour—a central feature of child psychiatry. The accurate interpretation of this behaviour demands skill and experience which take account of both biological and environmental factors: thumb-sucking, for example, cannot be evaluated without reference to the child's age, while an assessment of reading difficulties will demand some knowledge of the child's intellectual endowment and scholastic milieu.

The classification of psychiatric disorders in children reflects the uncertainties implicit in these considerations. While the same broad categories as those employed in adult psychiatry—psychosis, neurosis, personality disorder and organic reaction—are applicable to childhood, the large majority of psychological disturbances in the early years of life manifest themselves as anomalies of conduct which cannot easily be fitted into such categories. In consequence the I.C.D. includes not only a separate category of 'behaviour disorders of childhood' but also 'transient situational disturbances', in which some of the short-lived reactions of adolescence may be placed, and 'special symptoms not elsewhere classified' which include such phenomena as feeding disturbances, enuresis, stammering and specific learning disturbances. In addition, antisocial behaviour which may or may not include delinquency should, in the opinion of some authorities, be given a separate rubric. Finally, the various forms of mental subnormality are traditionally allocated to a category of their own [see p. 1385].

With so much of his clinical activity dependent on the evaluation of patterns of behaviour the task of the child psychiatrist would clearly be facilitated by the availability of standardized, quantitative information with which deviations from the norm could be assessed at different phases of development and in different environmental situations. The most serviceable measures which have yet been constructed to meet this situation relate to the sphere of intelligence, the assessment of which consists in the administration of tests which have been standardized on average samples of the population. What is average or normal at a given age is therefore known, and the child's performance can be compared with this. The most widely used tests are modifications of those put forward by Binet and Simon in 1908. As these may give a rating that depends unduly on the child's educational opportunities and facility in language, and may not indicate special abilities, e.g. in mechanical matters, many other tests have been worked out which supplement or, in certain cases, replace the Binet scale. Any satisfactory intelligence test must be both reliable, i.e. measuring the subject's ability accurately and consistently, and valid, i.e. correlating effectively with other measures of the ability being tested. The validation of intelligence tests is sometimes carried out by comparing test scores with ratings of intelligence by teachers and other judges or with subsequent educational achievement, and sometimes by the statistical procedure of factorial analysis in which all the test items are compared with each other to determine internal consistency.

Despite the care which has been taken in their construction it must none the less be emphasized that measures of intelligence cannot be regarded as objectively as, say, measures of height and weight. They depend on the tests employed, they have varying reliability, and they cannot be translated into the language and recommendations of practical life unless the interpreter has a clear knowledge of the theoretical and technical limitations implicit in their method. Intelligence tests are intended mainly to measure native ability and not acquired experience but they do not wholly succed in this. Since test scores have no absolute significance any test which has not been standardized on an appropriate population cannot be safely employed, and the choice of such a population may be a complex matter. Further, in all tests the emotional state of the subject is a factor that may influence his performance.

The foregoing account indicates the range of data about intelligence necessary for the child psychiatrist to make a rational assessment in this sphere of performance. Very little comparable information is available on the many other forms of widely distributed behaviour about which a clinical decision may have to be taken. Without such information the limits of normal variation can only be defined in an arbitrary fashion so that, as a leading authority has pointed out: 'There is no absolute criterion for the normalcy of any of the common forms of behaviour problems of children. Their evaluation is bound up tightly with the general outlook of the evaluating agent.' The same proviso applies to other diagnostic categories where behaviour is a central feature, e.g. personality disorder or neurosis, but none the less a great deal of clinical description exists and can be found in specialized textbooks. Here only a brief survey is justified, with special reference to particular phenomena or syndromes.

The *behaviour disorders* of childhood embrace a large, heterogeneous, ill-defined collection of phenomena. Some of these are problems of individual conduct, either real or perceived as such by responsible adults, e.g. thumb-sucking, nail-biting, masturbation. Others are problems of interpersonal conduct, e.g. anger, jealousy, fear. Still others are problems of social or antisocial conduct, e.g. stealing, truancy. Regardless of its nature, however, the behaviour or reported behaviour does not constitute a diagnosis in its own right. In every case it must be examined both in its own right and in the light of knowledge about the child's physical state as well as the personality, background and social adjustment: many physical disorders in childhood can manifest themselves as disorders of behaviour.

The 'special symptoms' of the I.C.D. include a number of well-recognized patterns of clinical behaviour. *Enuresis nocturna*, defined as involuntary urination during sleep in children more than 3 years old, is a common, widespread and troublesome disturbance of function. A number of factors have been suggested as being causally important—physical conditions, constitution, depth of sleep, psychological factors. *Encopresis*, involuntary defaecation unassociated with physical disorder, is a much rarer phenomenon than enuresis and usually betokens a more serious degree of psychological disturbance. *Stuttering*, essentially a disorder of speech rhythm, is the commonest speech disorder in childhood. Heredity, brain dysfunction (lack of dominance by one cerebral hemisphere over the other) and emotional upsets have all been postulated as causes. Of the specific learning disturbances *dyslexia* is probably the most important. While many children experience reading difficulties as a result of such diverse factors as low intelligence, defects of vision or hearing, emotional difficulties and school problems, dyslectic subjects exhibit a specific verbal disability with a tendency to reverse letters and words in both reading and writing; their intellectual performance is otherwise unimpaired and they are sometimes, though not always, left-handed. Of the *psychomotor disorders* the most important numerically are the various forms of *tics* or habit spasms, some of them sequelae to an encephalitic illness, others apparently determined by psychological factors. Though an extremely rare condition, *Gilles de la Tourette's syndrome*—tics, compulsive utterances which usually become coprolalic, and echo-phenomena—is of particular interest because of the unique clinical picture. While the obscene ejaculations of this syndrome are dependent on much the same articulatory and respiratory hyperkinesias as are the breathing spasms of encephalitis lethargica, they are also related to psychological tendencies and experiences: in many cases it has not proved possible to find evidence of cerebral disease. The term *hyperkinetic syndrome* is applied to children who display extreme over-activity, distractibility, aggression, impulsiveness, fluctuations of mood and a short attention-span, often but not always with evidence of organic brain dysfunction. In milder forms hyperkinesis may be a component of other reactions, especially morbid anxiety. A wide variety of disorders of *sleep* and *feeding* are encountered in children.

The relationship between *physical illnesses* and the psychological disorders of childhood is of clinical importance. Any chronic or disabling disease poses a threat to intellectual and emotional development, particularly if it necessitates long periods of time in medical institutions away from familial security. While such dangers can be minimized by appropriate measures, the effects of *organic brain damage* can be associated more specifically with psychiatric problems. Cerebral damage may lead to manifest neurological sequelae which depend on such factors as the pathology of the disease, the area of brain affected, the provocation or otherwise of abnormal cerebral function, and the child's age at the time of the insult; it may also result in more subtle forms of disorder in which there are delays in or limitations to the development of normal function, e.g. severe motor clumsiness, retarded speech. Psychiatric disorder in brain-damaged children is related to the site and area of the pathology. In most cases, however, the clinical picture is not distinctive, suggesting that there is not so much a direct effect on behaviour as an increased vulnerability to the external influences which may affect development in an adverse manner. Psychiatric syndromes specific to brain damage are uncommon: they include acute and chronic organic reactions, though sometimes a dementing process with regressive behaviour in early childhood (Heller's disease) is unaccompanied by clear evidence of brain damage; episodic disturbances of behaviour associated with ictal phenomena; the hyperkinetic syndrome; and some instances of infantile psychosis or autism.

Other forms of *psychosis* are also relatively unusual in the earlier years of childhood, though in adolescence the functional psychoses are encountered more frequently. Adolescents may react to personal difficulties with symptomatic disturbances which are difficult to distinguish from the manifestations of a functional psychosis: such reactive psychoses, however, tend to have a better prognosis than their counterparts in later years. A frank manic-depressive illness is rare before adolescence and much less common between the ages of fifteen and twenty than is schizophrenia. While the phenomena of schizophrenia after puberty do not differ essentially from those in later life the occurrence and form of this condition in earlier childhood remain controversial. The so-called infantile psychosis— characterized by autism, language and perceptual defects, ritualistic and stereotyped behaviour and non-distractibility—can be associated with cerebral damage or severe mental subnormality, and its relationship to childhood schizophrenia has still to be clarified.

All the well-established neurotic reactions and morbid personality traits can be identified in childhood, though the clinician must find his evidence in terms of the child's world. The features of *hysteria* [p. 1374] can be recognized before puberty. In younger children, however, they must be extreme to attract attention because of the frequency of such mechanisms in otherwise normal children, e.g. counterfeiting illness, somnambulism, behaving as though fantasies were real. Some of the grossest instances of hysterical behaviour have been recorded in girls not yet adolescent, e.g. the children who created havoc in the New England town of Salem at the end of the seventeenth century. The *schizoid* 'model child' demonstrates slight peculiarities from his earliest years, often being reported as quiet, shy and solitary, given more to daydreaming or abstract speculation than to ordinary interests and activities; sometimes he has been unduly submissive and sentimentally affectionate, or touchy, suspicious, obstinate, and resentful of advice and control. Overt *depression*, interestingly enough, is comparatively rare in children and a depressed mood is more often expressed as a behaviour disorder, hypochondriacal complaints or a manifestation of anxiety [see p. 1374]. *Obsessional* children may be beset with fears of contamination and religious scruples.

Treatment

The management of a psychiatric disorder in childhood can rarely be confined to the child. An assessment of the mental status, including cognitive abilities, and the physical condition are invariably to be supplemented by information about the immediate environment, e.g. family, school, and often by further specialized investigations. Only then can logical decisions be reached about the basis for intervention. This may entail a number of measures—social work, speech therapy, advice to parents, institutional placement, coaching with school work, prescription of drugs, psychological treatments, play therapy—alone or in combination, according to the nature of the problem.

MENTAL SUBNORMALITY

As already stated [p. 1336], there is nothing in principle to separate the various forms of subnormality from other forms of mental anomaly save that they occur at an earlier stage of life. Like mental disorder, they shade into normality; no man can say where stupidity ends and feeble-mindedness begins. Again, as with mental disorder, the same clinical picture may be due to a variety of causes ranging from heredity to trauma. They are, moreover, delimited to a large extent by social criteria, and they are not definitely associated with any constant pathological findings, except in the numerically limited group of special clinical types. The effects of encephalitis, parenchymatous syphilis and thyroid deficiency upon the mental state and development at different ages, or the varying results of amaurotic familial idiocy in the infantile and the delayed juvenile forms, illustrate how important is the stage of growth or maturity at which damage is done. In that mental retardation is capable of only limited improvement when well established, and that the intellectual functions are more obviously damaged than any others, its similarity to cerebral impairment in adult life is easily seen.

Mental subnormality is not by any means a matter of purely intellectual defect. It represents, it is true, one extreme on the scale which has people of great intellectual ability at its other end; but it also comprises of a general impairment of mind, affecting the emotional and conative functions, and often associated with a more general impairment of the whole organism, which may be seen in the physical structure. Since the milder forms are indistinguishable (except on an arbitrary reckoning) from what may be termed normal stupidity, it is difficult to use rigorously the statutory definition of mental subnormality, as a 'state of arrested or incomplete development of mind which indicates subnormality of intelligence and is of a nature or degree which requires or is susceptible to medical treatment or other special care or training of the patient'. In the severe form, the patient cannot live an independent life or guard himself against serious exploitation. It should be recognized that, just as 'psychosis' differs from 'neurosis' only in a rough social sense, turning on the need for special care, and 'neurosis' from 'normality' only in respect of the limitations the former imposes on one's daily life as a social organism, so does the distinction between normality and feeble-mindedness, and between gross or certifiable deficiency and the lesser forms, turn on the social adaptation of the person in question.

Aetiology

Heredity plays a large part. In those defectives in whom a characteristic metabolic anomaly has been identified, the condition is usually a recessive character, attributed to a single gene; the affected person is homozygous for it. The mode of transmission of amaurotic familial idiocy is similarly recessive. Chromosome anomalies have been established in a number of conditions, of which Down's syndrome is numerically the most important. These conditions are all rare, and individuals affected by them make up less than 5 per cent. of all defectives. There is a further, much larger percentage—the 'subcultural' group representing the lower extreme of normal variation—in whom the hereditary factors are due to the interaction of many genes.

Environmental causes include cerebral damage, e.g. from kernicterus due to Rhesus incompatibility, meningitis, encephalitis, maternal rubella, birth injury and anoxia, cerebral syphilis; malformation; and deprivation of sensory and social stimuli, as in a neglected deaf-mute. Another sort of deprivation leads to cretinism. Of prenatal influences, those operating during the first trimester of pregnancy are most likely to impair normal development.

Pathology

In the large 'subcultural group with mild retardation' there are no significant somatic findings.

In the small genetically determined groups there are some highly specific *biochemical anomalies*, showing a defective synthesis of an enzyme necessary for normal metabolism. The best studied metabolic error of this sort is *phenylketonuria*, in which there is a block in intermediary metabolism at the point where phenylalanine is hydroxylated to form tyrosine. Excessive concentration of phenylalanine in the blood and other body fluids is associated with a disturbance of the normal metabolic processes in the brain during the first few months of life which causes lasting impairment. *Other amino-acid disturbances* appear in 'maple syrup disease, histidinaemia, homocystinuria, cystathioninuria, argininosuccinic aciduria and Hartnup disease. Disorders of carbohydrate metabolism associated with mental defect include galactosaemia.

Among the various *chromosome abnormalities* the autosomal anomalies, of which Down's syndrome (mongolism) is the best known, are in general associated with more severe somatic stigmata, a greater degree of intellectual retardation and a shorter expectation of life than sex-chromosome imbalance. *Down's syndrome* is characterized by an anomaly in the number of chromosomes; the patients usually have 47 instead of the usual 46 with trisomy for No. 21. The extra chromosome, which matches one of the smallest pairs of autosomes, is probably the result of non-disjunction during gametogenesis. The discovery of this anomaly explained the widespread bodily changes of the disease, and the fact that monozygotic twins are concordant in respect of mongolism. In rare cases an extra chromosome is not detectable but a compound chromosome is seen to have been formed through translocation. The chromosomal anomaly has not provided an answer to questions about the causation of most cases of Down's syndrome. The condition is prone to occur in children born to relatively elderly mothers; but the reason for this is obscure. In about 20 per cent. of cases, however, the age of the mother does not seem to have been a factor in determining abnormal maturation of the ovum; in these (who include the patients with translocation of a chromosome) there is evidence of hereditary influence, through the mother.

Anomalies of the sex chromosomes have been found in some mentally subnormal patients with ovarian dysgenesis, and in Klinefelter's syndrome, which may be associated with high-grade defect. These are rare conditions.

Structural and chemical abnormalities may be found in the brain. General hypoplasia and microgyria may be mingled with evidences of a past lesion, as in porencephaly or hemiatrophy, or with signs of a disease actually present, as in amaurotic idiocy and tuberose sclerosis. Localized lipid deposits (cerebrosides) are found in amaurotic idiocy.

Symptoms

The traditional classification is into *idiots* (who are too defective to be able to guard themselves against common physical dangers like falling into the fire), and *imbeciles* and *feeble-minded* persons (who need to be looked after because of their incapacity to manage their affairs or to profit by instruction). A preferable classification is based on psychometric assessment: the customary tests for mental age (usually the Stanford-Binet or the Wechsler) are applied and the subject's intelligence quotient $\left(\frac{\text{mental age}}{\text{actual age}} \times 100\right)$ measured. At the same time it must be recognized that while mental defect is mainly, though not solely, a matter of intellectual capacity, no intelligence test, however valuable and trustworthy, can give a complete indication of the degree of mental defect. Even the intellectual defect may be uneven, showing much more in some tasks than in others, and it would be a gross error to suppose that a mentally defective person with a mental age of, say, 9½ years is mentally in the same state as a normal child aged 9½ years.

The *physical* symptoms are chiefly due to lesions of the central nervous system: birth trauma may have led to paralysis, spasticity, athetosis; or there may be evidence of an inflammatory condition of the brain and its membranes, as from syphilis. The whole clinical picture may be greatly coloured by the motor disturbance, e.g. continual rocking and twisting movements, grimaces and abnormal posture. The special senses may be affected, as the result of an independent anomaly, e.g. coloboma, misshapen ears; or from a common cause, e.g. interstitial keratitis, the retinal changes of amaurotic idiocy. It is very dubious whether the 'stigmata of degeneration', such as a 'Gothic' palate or a Darwinian tubercle, occur any more frequently among defectives than in the rest of the population: at all events, there is none that can be used diagnostically, except in the case of Down's syndrome. There are, however, some correlations between somatic anomalies and mental defect. Thus, there are more physical defects among these people than in the average population, and this becomes more evident as one looks lower in the scale of mental defect, in which skeletal and cardiovascular anomalies may fairly often be found, sometimes, but not always, due to thyroid or pituitary disorders.

The *mental* symptoms are lack of intelligence and of the normal exercise and control of primitive tendencies. This may be extreme, as in those who cannot be taught to feed themselves and keep clean or who can only just recognize their companions and make their elementary needs known—they are, indeed, much less intelligent than an animal. Imbeciles are usually incapable of learning and remembering any but very simple matters. They may, however, be able to do automatically what they cannot understand or put to independent purpose: thus, 'idiots savants' are especially clever at doing mental arithmetic, recalling dates and other such operations. What they manage to learn they cannot utilize in any but the most familiar circumstances. Abstract concepts are too hard for them, and their judgement is as poor as their grasp or awareness of what is relevant in any situation. Though in many ways suggestible and accessible to flattery, they may be obstinate and egotistical, and readily fall into antisocial courses, e.g. prostitution, vagrancy, crime. Crude sexual offences or murder may be committed as lightly as some minor deception.

The personality of imbeciles varies widely: some are docile and kindly, others rough or deceitful and vindictive. This depends much on their upbringing. It has been found that in satisfactory conditions only about 8 per cent. of defectives show antisocial or troublesome behaviour, but though the deviations of personality may not lead to delinquency it is common to find in mentally deficient persons defects of temperament and character, as well as of intelligence, which are reflected in social inefficiency. This is most important in the feebleminded, who have intelligence enough to learn an occupation; whether they can earn their living by it will depend on their character and the way they have been brought up. Many persons who are high-grade defectives, when measured by formal tests, are not taken to be such because of their social adaptability, their fluency and capacity for keeping their heads above water as long as economic and other stresses are light. There are instances of people classed as mentally subnormal during childhood, because of their backwardness in school and their low score in tests, who later in life amass money by their own efforts, or even hold responsible positions. Many high-grade defectives, however, live dependent and often troublesome lives; at most they do simple repetitive work. Hysterical trends may show themselves in crude phenomena, e.g. convulsions, counterfeit insanity or fantastic lying; and religious and artistic pretensions may take in gullible followers and even lead to the founding of ephemeral movements.

Defectives are prone to disturbances of mood, sometimes arising out of awareness of their inferiority and its social consequences. Sudden outbursts of excitement may show similarity to manic or catatonic hyperkinetic states; they may be accompanied by a paranoid hallucinosis, mainly auditory, which clears up with startling rapidity in a day or two. In respect of these psychotic episodes, defectives are like epileptics and juvenile encephalitics, in whom a cerebral impairment has likewise occurred before the attainment of maturity. Some of the morbid phenomena, especially in idiots, are very similar to the disorders of motility seen in schizophrenics, because, it may be assumed, the same bodily mechanisms are implicated.

Of the special forms *Down's syndrome* is characterized by striking physical changes, widespread through the body. The condition is usually present from birth; physical growth is slow, and has stopped by the time the child is 15. Defective growth of the skull, leading especially to abnormalities of the base and the orbit, is responsible for the peculiarities of cranial shape. The appearance of these usually happy idiots and imbeciles is rather suggestive of a Mongol or of a foetus. The skull is small and round, and the junction of occiput and back of neck flat; an epicanthic fold across each inner canthus, narrow tilted eye-slits and lids without lashes, red cheeks, fissured and often protruding tongue, stubby depressed nose with nostrils looking forward, irregular late-appearing teeth, coarse hair on the scalp, small facial bones and occasional neurological anomalies, such as nystagmus, make the head of every patient a disagreeable but ready index to his disorder. That the disorder is a general one the rest of his body testifies; his limbs are lax and over-mobile at the joints; he has broad, clumsy feet and hands (with short fingers, a special pattern between the base of the third and fourth fingers, and a crease across the palm), protuberant belly and low stature; and perhaps a congenital cardiac lesion. The similarity in a few respects to juvenile myxoedema, and the occasional concurrence of the two conditions sometimes make differential diagnosis difficult; not all of the signs here mentioned need be present in any one case. On the mental side, there is a liveliness and amiability not often seen with so much intellectual defect: the patients like music and little jokes of a primitive sort; they will imitate gestures, but seldom learn to speak properly with their rough harsh voices.

The forms of deficiency due to *thyroid insufficiency* and *cerebromacular degeneration* are referred to elsewhere [Sections 5 and 15]. *Epiloia* is the name given to the rare condition in which tuberose sclerosis of the brain, adenoma sebaceum and tumours of the kidney and heart may be associated; epilepsy is common, and there are gross mental disturbances [see Section 4]. *Gargoylism* is a rare chondrodystrophy, with hepatosplenomegaly and mental deficiency [see Section 4]. In *phenylketonuria* there is increased urinary excretion of phenylpyruvic acid, phenyllactic acid and phenylalanine; high concentrations of phenylalanine occur in the blood plasma and the cerebrospinal fluid. In *galactosaemia*, another biochemical 'error', there is evidence of a specific failure in the formation of a transferase concerned in the conversion of galactose into glucose-1-phosphate [see Section 4]. The other rare metabolic anomalies associated with subnormality likewise have a specific enzyme deficiency; in the case of *Hartnup disease* the characteristic pellagrous rash and neuropsychiatric signs and symptoms may be present without mental subnormality [see Section 4].

Diagnosis

Recognition of gross mental deficiency calls for no skill. The degree and kind of impairment, however, and the somatic variety or cause have to be worked out in every case. The latter problem—a minor one, except in the case of juvenile myxoedema and syphilis—is to be settled by careful physical examination and inquiry into the history. The former is a matter of assessing intelligence and social aptitude.

A child under the age of 5 cannot be satisfactorily dealt with by the Binet tests, which moreover have only limited value for measuring the intelligence of adults. It is difficult to agree about what in a normal child must be regarded as the limiting age at which he becomes of adult intelligence; it is generally taken as 14 or 16 years. The emotional reactions to being tested must always be assessed, along with responses to more familiar situations, e.g. at home or at school, as evidence of the soundness or instability of the child's personality; by such criteria must be judged the social development of the patient, his fitness for living in the community or being put under lasting surveillance and control.

Mental age and intelligence quotient are familiar devices for stating the results of the Binet test and its derivatives. In spite of their convenience, they are open to so many objections that they might well be dropped now in favour of a percentile scale or one in which test scores are converted into standard scores, the statistical properties of which are known. The percentile method, which requires less familiarity with statistics, indicates whereabouts on the curve of distribution a given score comes when a large representative sample of the population is tested. Thus, whatever the test, the score obtained on it can with such a scale permit the conclusion that the person tested falls within, say, the upper 5 per cent. of the population in this respect or within the bottom 1 per cent. The alternative is to use levels of measured intelligence, expressed in terms of standard deviation units which describe the distribution of scores that can be expected for a particular test if the abilities it measures are normally distributed in the general population. Valuable for children, such a method of assessing intelligence (and other qualities) is particularly needed for adults, in whom the mental age method is inapplicable. Since it has become very plain that it is useful to test the intelligence of adults, the inadequacy for this purpose of the Binet scale has led to its being superseded by several tests, of which the Wechsler-Bellevue and the Progressive Matrices are probably the best known and most serviceable. The Bellevue-Adult scale has been standardized on a large adult population; it consists of verbal tests (of comprehension, information, digit span forwards and backwards, recognition of similarities, arithmetical reasoning) and performance tests (picture completion, picture arrangement, object assembly, block design, digit symbol).

Tests of intelligence are by no means chiefly employed for detecting and measuring defect; they have their main field of application in indicating a child's educability and potential attainment, and an adult's capacity to undertake certain activities. They are used for judging fitness rather than unfitness, selecting rather than rejecting. At all times they must be applied judiciously. To take a 'self-administering' test or a group test of intelligence and to draw merely from the score obtained on it by a child or adult the conclusion that he is mentally subnormal, would be as inept and gross an error as to diagnose active syphilis merely because an unknown laboratory on one occasion reported a positive Wassermann reaction in the patient's blood.

There are general observations about mental tests which it is particularly necessary for occasional or inexpert testers to bear in mind. The scores must be accurately and as far as possible objectively arrived at; therefore the personal opinion of the tester should not enter into them, though his skill in administration may have influenced the result and his comments will be informative. Test scores must always be compared with 'norms', and it is imperative that these norms shall have been collected on a suitable group since it would be misleading, for example, to judge an English child to be less intelligent than an American one because he could not do a test the reliability and validity of which had been established in a setting of American habits and ideas.

Intelligence tests are different from educational tests. While educational attainment like intelligence depends largely on innate qualities, the more an intelligence test relies on tasks which demand some acquirement not equally available to all those tested, the more misleading may be its results. The application of this to verbal tests is obvious; a subject who has poor command of English or who has aphasia cannot do himself justice on a test that is satisfactory for the bulk of literate people. Performance tests, which do not use words, are not entirely free from similar defects, and in spite of certain merits, e.g. greater attractiveness for children, tendency to evoke informative temperamental reactions, they have disadvantages: they are seldom cheap or handy, are sometimes unreliable, and have poor validity; on some of them the subject's performance is much influenced by any emotional or neurotic disturbance he may have. Consequently, whereas a single predominantly verbal test like the Stanford-Binet may suffice to indicate the child's or adult's intelligence (provided there is no special verbal difficulty), it would be unsafe to rely on one, or even two or three, performance tests; a median or average score based on half a dozen performance tests is preferable.

Group tests have become increasingly popular because they save so much time. They are not suitable for testing young children (under the age of 7 or 8), and are not so objective and standardized in application as they seem; further, they are by no means foolproof, depending as they do to some degree on the subject's attitude and situation at the time, about which the group-tester will know little or nothing, and they cannot be trusted when a low score has been obtained. In all instances where a decision must be taken that depends partly on the results of the test, any puzzling or unduly low score on a group test should be reinforced by an individual test, such as the Binet or Bellevue. It must, however, be admitted that the inexpert administration of individual tests can yield as rich a crop of wrong conclusions as can the uncritically accepted group test. The truth is that 'no one ought to use tests who is not willing to familiarize himself with the underlying principles which must be understood if tests are to be applied and interpreted properly, and with the literature which bears on the particular tests that he employs. In skilled hands, testing provides a far surer and more accurate tool for the assessment of abilities than do subjective impressions or the ordinary examination paper. But human nature is far too complex to be measured in the simple and direct ways in which physical quantities can be measured, and the over-enthusiastic but unskilled tester is only too likely to make serious mistakes.'

The distinction between mental subnormality and juvenile autism, i.e. a mute withdrawal akin to that of schizophrenia, may be hard to make in an individual case: it may require a prolonged period of close observation.

Treatment

Defect may be prevented or lessened by specific medical treatment when it is due to certain physical abnormalities. Cretinism was for long the outstanding example of this, but there is now evidence that phenylketonuric children can be benefited if given a phenylalanine-free diet from an early age. It is not certain how much improvement in the mental level can be thus brought about, because insufficient data have so far been collected to judge the long-term outcome of treatment persevered with for years. It is, however, indisputable that this rational treatment, and that of galactosaemia by a galactose-free diet, will effect remarkable physical improvement, and there are grounds for inferring that corresponding improvement in mental development can be achieved.

These methods of treatment are at present applicable only to a tiny minority of mentally subnormal children. The majority have either a physical disease for which there is no effective treatment that will promote normal cerebral functioning, or their retardation calls for general educational treatment, training and rehabilitation rather than for anything specific.

Educational and social. Much improvement may be attained by the training of defectives: it is work for experts. Many high-grade defectives who would otherwise spend their lives in an institution can be prepared by suitable graduated work under sheltered conditions for an independent life in the general community. Where there are special disabilities, e.g. of the senses, or of such capacities as reading and writing, attention to these may lift the child out of the class of mental defectives altogether; so may education designed to promote emotional stability and self-confidence. Whether a child lives at home or in an institution will depend not only on the degree of his intellectual and social deficiency, but also on the adequacy of his home circumstances. Much improvement in verbal ability and verbal intelligence can be effected by upbringing in a nursery unit where the children are cared for on family group lines. There are many kinds of provision for the care of defectives in England and Wales, ranging from special schools to mental hospitals. Well-run centres providing adequate psychological and occupational as well as psychotherapeutic and other clinical services succeed in socializing many defectives hitherto vicious or violent, who can then go out and live usefully in the community or in hostels. Some, however, prove intractable, especially those who have epileptic fits.

REFERENCES

ACKERKNECHT, E. (1969) *A Short History of Psychiatry*, 2nd ed., trans. WOLFF, S., New York.

ASTRUP, C., FOSSUM, A., and HOLMBOE, R. (1959) A follow-up study of 270 patients with acute affective psychoses, *Acta psychiat. scand.*, **135**, Suppl.

BLEULER, E. (1950) *Dementia Praecox or the Group of Schizophrenias*, trans. ZINKIN, J., New York.

BROWN, G. W., BONE, M., DALISON, B., and WING, J. K. (1966) *Schizophrenia and Social Care*, Maudsley Monograph No. 17, London.

CROME, L., and STERN, J. (1967) *The Pathology of Mental Retardation*, London.

DEPARTMENT OF HEALTH AND SOCIAL SECURITY (1970) Report on Public Health and Medical Subjects, No. 24. *Amphetamines, Barbiturates, LSD and Cannabis: their Use and Misuse*, London.

DURKHEIM, E. (1951) *Suicide*, trans. SPAULDING, J. A., and SIMPSON, G., Springfield, Ill.

EDDY, N. B., HALBACH, H., ISBELL, H., and SEEVERS, M. H. (1965) Drug dependence: its significance and characteristics, *Bull. Wld Hlth Org.*, **32**, 721.

FRANK, J. D. (1961) *Persuasion and Healing, a Comparative Study of Psychotherapy*, Baltimore.

FREUD, S. (1943) *Introductory Lectures on Psycho-analysis*, trans. RIVIÈRE, J., London.

GENERAL REGISTER OFFICE (1968) *A Glossary of Mental Disorders*, Studies on Medical Population Subjects, No. 22, London, H.M.S.O.

HILL, D., and PARR, G., eds (1963) *Electroencephalography*, 2nd ed. London.

HIMWICH, H. ed. (1971) *Biochemistry, Schizophrenias and Affective Illnesses*, Baltimore.

HOENIG, J., ANDERSON, E. W., KENNA, J. C., and BLUNDEN, R. (1962) Clinical and psychological aspects of the mnestic syndrome, *J. ment. Sci.*, **108**, 541.

ISBELL, H., FRASER, H. F., WIKLER, A., and BELLEVILLE, R. E

(1955) An experimental study of the aetiology of 'rum fits 'and delirium tremens, *Quart. J. Stud. Alcohol*, **16**, 1.

JANET, P. (1920) *The Major Symptoms of Hysteria*, 2nd ed., New York.

JANET, P. (1925) *Psychological Healing*, trans. PAUL, E. and C., London.

JASPERS, K. (1963) *General Psychopathology*, trans. HOENIG, J., and HAMILTON, M. W., Manchester.

JELLINEK, E. M. (1960) *The Disease Concept of Alcoholism*, New Haven.

KANNER, L. (1962) *Child Psychiatry*, 3rd ed., Springfield, Ill.

KENDELL, R. E. (1968) *The Classification of Depressive Illnesses*, Maudsley Monograph No. 18, London.

KRAEPELIN, E. (1921) *Manic-Depressive Insanity and Paranoia*, trans. BARCLAY, E. M., ed. ROBERTSON, G. M., Edinburgh.

KRAUPL TAYLOR, F. (1966) *Psychopathology: Its Causes and Symptoms*, London.

LEWIS, A. (1967) *Inquiries in Psychiatry*, London.

LEWIS, A. (1967) *The State of Psychiatry*, London.

LEWIS, A. (1970) Paranoia and paranoid: a historical perspective, *Psychol. Med.*, **1**, 2.

LJUNBERG, L. (1957) Hysteria, a clinical, prognostic and genetic study, *Acta psychiat. scand.*, **112,** Suppl.

MARKS, I. M. (1969) *Fears and Phobias*, London.

MILBANK MEMORIAL FUND (1961) *Causes of Mental Disorders, a Review of Epidemiological Knowledge*, 1959, New York.

O'CONNOR, N. (1968) Psychology and intelligence, in *Studies in Psychiatry*, ed. Shepherd, M., and Davies, D. L., London.

PENROSE, L. S. (1966) *The Biology of Mental Defect*, 2nd rev. ed., London.

PENROSE, L. S., and SMITH, G. F. (1966) *Down's Anomaly*, London.

POLANI, P. E. (1967) Chromosome anomalies and the brain, *Guy's Hosp. Rep.*, **116**, 365.

PORTER, R., ed. (1968) *The Role of Learning in Psychotherapy*, London.

POST, F. (1962) *The Significance of Affective Symptoms in Old Age*, Maudsley Monograph No. 10, London.

ROSENTHAL, R., and KETY, S., eds (1968) *The Transmission of Schizophrenia*, Oxford.

RUSSELL, G. F. M., and BEARDWOOD, C. J. (1968) The feeding disorders, with particular reference to anorexia nervosa and its associated gonadotrophin changes, in *Endocrinology and Human Behaviour*, ed. MICHAEL, R. P., London.

RUTTER, M., TIZARD, J., and WHITMORE, K., eds (1970) *Education, Health and Behaviour*, London.

SAINSBURY, P. (1955) *Suicide in London*, Maudsley Monograph No. 1, London.

SCHNEIDER, K. (1958) *Psychopathic Personalities*, trans. HAMILTON, M. W., London.

SHEPHERD, M. (1961) Morbid jealousy: some clinical and social aspects of a psychiatric symptom, *J. ment. Sci.*, **107,** 687.

SHEPHERD, M., and COOPER, B. (1964) Epidemiology and mental disorder: a review, *J. Neurol. Neurosurg. Psychiat.*, **27,** 277.

SHEPHERD, M., LADER, M., and RODNIGHT, R. (1968) *Clinical Psychopharmacology*, London.

SHEPHERD, M., OPPENHEIM, B., and MITCHELL, S. (1971) *Childhood Behaviour and Mental Health*, London.

SKOOG, J. (1959) The anancastic syndrome and its relation to personality attitudes, *Acta psychiat. scand.*, **134,** Suppl.

SLATER, E., and COWIE, V. (1971) *The Genetics of Mental Disorders*, London.

STEINBERG, H., ed. (1969) *Scientific Basis of Drug Dependence*, London.

TIZARD, J., and GRAD, J. C. (1961) *The Mentally Handicapped and their Families*, Maudsley Monograph No. 7, London.

WOLSTENHOLME, G. E. W., and O'CONNOR, M. eds (1970) *Alzheimer's Disease and Related Conditions*, London.

MICHAEL SHEPHERD

INDEX